PATHOLOGY

IMPLICATIONS *for the* PHYSICAL THERAPIST

FOURTH EDITION

PATHOLOGY
IMPLICATIONS *for the* PHYSICAL THERAPIST

CATHERINE CAVALLARO GOODMAN, MBA, PT, CBP
MEDICAL MULTIMEDIA GROUP
PRIVATE PRACTICE
MISSOULA, MONTANA

KENDA S. FULLER, PT
ABPTS BOARD CERTIFIED SPECIALIST IN NEUROLOGIC PHYSICAL THERAPY
CO-OWNER SOUTH VALLEY PHYSICAL THERAPY, PC
DENVER, COLORADO
INVITED LECTURER, PHYSICAL THERAPY PROGRAM
UNIVERSITY OF COLORADO HEALTH SCIENCES CENTER
DENVER, COLORADO

MEDICAL DIRECTOR: CELESTE PETERSON, MD

SECTION EDITOR: PATHOLOGY OF THE MUSCULOSKELETAL SYSTEM: KEVIN HELGESON, DHSc, PT
PROFESSOR
ROCKY MOUNTAIN UNIVERSITY OF HEALTH PROFESSIONS
PROVO, UTAH

SECTION EDITOR: WOMEN'S HEALTH: BETH SHELLY, PT, DPT, WCS, BCB PMD*
DOCTOR OF PHYSICAL THERAPY
BOARD CERTIFIED SPECIALIST IN WOMEN'S HEALTH
SPECIALIZING IN PELVIC HEALTH AND LYMPHEDEMA
1634 AVENUE OF THE CITIES
MOLINE, ILLINOIS

**THIS TEXT HAS BEEN REVIEWED BY BETH SHELLY, PT, DPT, WCS, BCB, PMD, AND IS IN COMPLIANCE WITH SUGGESTED
SECTION ON WOMEN'S HEALTH GUIDELINES FOR FIRST PROFESSIONAL CONTENT IN WOMEN'S HEALTH.*

PHARMACOLOGIC CONSULTANTS: TANNER HIGGINBOTHAM, PharmD
DRUG INFORMATION SPECIALIST
UNIVERSITY OF MONTANA SKAGGS SCHOOL OF PHARMACY
DEPARTMENT OF PHARMACY PRACTICE
MISSOULA, MONTANA

GENINE THORMAHLEN, PharmD, AE-C
UNIVERSITY OF MONTANA SKAGGS COLLEGE OF HEALTH PROFESSIONS AND BIOMEDICAL SCIENCES
SCHOOL OF PHARMACY DRUG INFORMATION SERVICE
MISSOULA, MONTANA

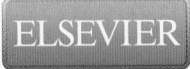

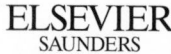

ELSEVIER
SAUNDERS

3251 Riverport Lane
St Louis, Missouri 63043

Executive Content Strategist: Kathy Falk
Content Development Manager: Jolynn Gower
Publishing Services Manager: Julie Eddy
Senior Project Manager: Celeste Clingan
Design Direction: Ashley Miner

Printed in China

Last digit is the print number: 9   8   7   6   5   4   3   2

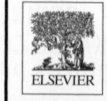

Kathleen L. Allen, PT, DPT
Center for Health and Fitness
Swedish Medical Center
Cherry Hill Campus
Seattle, Washington

Annie Burke-Doe, PT, MPT, PhD
Associate Professor
University of St. Augustine for Health Science
San Marcos, California

Tamara L. Burlis, PT, DPT, CCS
Assistant Director, Professional Curriculum
Associate Director of Clinical Education
Assistant Professor Program in Physical Therapy
    and Internal Medicine
Washington University Program in Physical Therapy
St. Louis, Missouri

Mary Calys, DPT, PT
Coordinator, Cancer Rehabilitation
    and Fatigue Management
Kansas City, Missouri

Heather Campbell, PT, DPT, MA
Physical Therapist
South Valley Physical Therapy
Denver, Colorado

Michael S. Castillo, PT, MHS, MPA, GCS, NCS
Senior Physical Therapist
Physical Therapy Department – Inpatient
Kaiser Permanente
Walnut Creek Medical Center
Walnut Creek, California

Joy C. Cohn, PT, CLT-LANA Lymphedema Team Leader
Penn Therapy and Fitness
Good Shepherd Penn Partners
Abramson Cancer Center
Philadelphia, Pennsylvania

Erica DeMarche, MSPT
Physical Therapist
South Valley Physical Therapy and Parkinson's
    Association of the Rockies
Denver, Colorado

Susan S. Deusinger, PT, PhD, FAPTA
Director, Program in Physical Therapy
Professor, Physical Therapy and Neurology
Washington University School of Medicine
St. Louis, Missouri

Janice T. Dinglasan, MPT
Physical Therapy Department – Inpatient
Kaiser Permanente
Walnut Creek Medical Center
Walnut Creek, California

Jan Dommerholt, PT, DPT, MPS
Myopain Seminars LLC
Bethesda Physiocard, Inc.
Bethesda, Maryland

Kimberly Dunleavy, PT, PhD, OCS
Associate Professor of Physical Therapy
University of Florida
Gainesville, Florida

Lara A. Firrone, PT, NCS
Methodist Healthcard University Hospital
Memphis, Tennessee

Beth Anne Fisher, PT, DPT, CSCS, CBP
Clinical Instructor
University of Colorado
Anschutz Medical Campus
Physical Therapy Program
Denver, Colorado

Joseph A. Fraietta, PhD
Laboratory of Carl H. June, MD
Abramson Family Cancer Research Instituter
University of Pennsylvania School of Medicine
Philadelphia, Pennsylvania

Courtney Frankel, PT, MS, CCS
Duke University
Durham, North Carolina

Denise Gaffigan-Bender, PT, GCS, MEd, JD
Associate Professor-Program Director for
    DPT Program
Department of Rehabilitation Science
College of Allied Health
University of Oklahoma Health Sciences Center
Oklahoma City, Oklahoma

Paula Richley Geigle, PT, PhD
Assistant Professor, Dept. of Physical Therapy
University of Delaware
Newark, Delaware

Allan M. Glanzman, PT, DPT, PCS, ATP
Co-Chair, Scientific Review Committee
Physical Therapy Department
The Children's Hospital of Philadelphia
Philadelphia, Pennsylvania

Robyn Gisbert, PT, DPT
Assistant Professor
School of Medicine
University of Colorado
Aurora, Colorado

Eva Gold, PT
University of Minnesota Medical Center
Minneapolis, Minnesota

Stephen A. Gudas, PT, PhD
Associate Professor of Anatomy and Neurobiology
Medical College of Virginia
Virginia Commonwealth University
Richmond, Virginia

Kevin Helgeson, DHSC, PT
Professor
Rocky Mountain University of Health Professions
Provo, Utah

Tanner Higginbotham, PharmD
Drug Information Specialist
Department of Pharmacy Practice
Skaggs School of Pharmacy
University of Montana
Missoula, Montana

Glenn L. Irion, PhD, PT, CWS
Associate Professor of Physical Therapy
University of South Alabama
Mobile, Alabama

David M. Kietrys, PT, PhD, OCS
Associate Professor
Doctor of Physical Therapy Program
Graduate School at Camden
Rutgers University
Stratford, New Jersey

Patricia (Trish) M. King, PT, PhD, OCS, MTC
Professor and Chair
Department of Physical Therapy
East Tennessee State University
Johnson City, Tennessee

Bonnie Lasinski, MA, PT, CSCI, CLT-LANA
Lymphedema Therapy
Woodbury, New York

Rolando T. Lazaro, PT, PhD, DPT, GCS
Associate Professor and Chair
Department of Physical Therapy
Samuel Merritt University
Oakland, California

Alan W. Chong Lee, PT, PhD, DPT, CWS, OCS
Associate Professor
Doctor of Physical Therapy Program
Mount St. Mary's College
Los Angeles, California

Kim Levenhagen, PT, DPT, WCC
Assistant Professor
Program in Physical Therapy
Saint Louis University
St. Louis, Missouri

Harriet B. Loehne, PT, DPT, CSW, FACCWS
President, Wound & Integumentary Specialty Education
Thomasville, Georgia

Lisa A. Massa, DT, WCS, CLT
Director Women's Health
Physical Therapist Residency
Adjunct Assistant Professor
Duke University Health System
Durham, North Carolina

Karen L. McCulloch, PT, PhD, NCS
Professor
Division of Physical Therapy
Allied Health Department
School of Medicine
University of North Carolina
Chapel Hill, North Carolina

Charles L. McGarvey, PT, MS, DPT, FAPTA
President, CLM Consulting Services
Rockville, Maryland

G. Stephen Morris, PT, PhD, FACSM
Associate Professor
Wingate University
Department of Physical Therapy
Wingate, North Carolina

Charlotte O. Norton, PT, DPT, ATC, CSCS
Building Bridges
Sacramento, California

Lora Packel, PhD, MSPT, CCS
Assistant Professor
Department of Physical Therapy
University of Sciences
Philadephia, Pennsylvania

Kathleen J. Pantano, PT, PhD
Doctor of Physical Therapy Program
Cleveland State University
Cleveland, Ohio

Gina Pariser, PT, PhD
Associate Professor
Doctor of Physical Therapy Program
Bellarmine University
Louisville, Kentucky

Celeste Peterson, MD
Medical Consultant
Missoula, Montana

Karen Rushby, PT, MScHA
Olympic Medical Center
Port Angeles, Washington
Olympic Medical Cancer Center
Sequim, Washington

Darina Sargeant, PT, PhD
Associate Professor
Department of Physical Therapy and Athletic Training
Doisy College of Health Science
Saint Louis University
St. Louis, Missouri

Lynzie Schulte, PT, DPT
Middleburg Heights, Ohio

Beth Shelly, PT, DPT, WCS, BCB, PMB
Doctor of Physical Therapy
Board Certified Specialist in Women's Health
Specializing in Pelvic Health and Lymphedema
Moline, Illinois

Irina V. Smirnova, PhD, MS (Hon)
Assistant Professor
University of Kansas Medical Center
Kansas City, Kansas

Susan Ann Talley, PT, DPT, C/NDT
Director, Physical Therapy Program
Eugene Applebaum College of Pharmacy and Health Sciences
Department of Health Care Sciences
Wayne State University
Detroit, Michigan

Holly Tanner, PT, MA, OCS, WCS, LMP, BCB-PMB, CCI
Board Certified, Orthopedics and Women's Health
Faculty, Pelvic Rehabilitation Institute
Duluth, Minnesota

Candy Tefertiller, PT, DPT, NCS
Director of Physical Therapy
Craig Hospital
Englewood, Colorado

Lisa VanHoose, PhD, PT, CLT-LANA, WCC
Assistant Professor and Director of Survivorship Optimization Lab and Clinic
Physical Therapy and Rehabilitation Science
University of Kansas Medical Center
Kansas City, Missouri

Karen von Berg, PT
Johns Hopkins Hospital
Baltimore, Maryland

Meredith A. Wampler, PT, DPTSc
Adjunct Faculty Member
Harrison Medical Center
University of Puget Sound
Bremerton, Washington

Valerie Wang, PT
St. Luke's Rehabilitation Institute
Spokane, Washington

Laura S. Wehrli, PT, DPT, ATP
Physical Therapy Supervisor, SCI
Craig Hospital
Englewood, Colorado

Chris L. Wells, PT, PhD, CCS, ATC
Clinical Associate Professor
Department of Physical Therapy and Rehabilitation Services
University of Maryland School of Medicine
Baltimore, Maryland

Patricia A. Winkler, PT, DSc, NCS (retired)
Assistant Professor
Regis University
Denver, Colorado

Bonnie Yost, PT, LCCE
Pathway to Full Freedom, LLC
Be Your Best Consulting
Elizabeth, Colorado

CHAPTER AND SECTION REVIEWERS

Karen Abraham, PT, PhD
Associate Professor and Director
Division of Physical Therapy
Shenandoah University
Winchester, Virginia

Susan Barth, PT
Legacy Good Samaritan Hospital Cancer Institute
Portland, Oregon

Renata Beaman, PT, MS, MA, OCS, CLT-UE
Breast Cancer Rehabilitation Specialist
Spooner Physical Therapy – Ahwatukee Office
Phoenix, Arizona

Andrea R. Branas, MSE, MPT, CLT
Lead Therapist
Abramson Cancer Center
Philadelphia, Pennsylvania

Michelle H. Cameron, MD, PT, OCS
Oregon Health and Sciences University
Portland, Oregon

Nancy D. Ciesla, PT, DPT, MS
Outcomes After Critical Illness and Surgery
Group Division of Pulmonary and Critical
    Care Medicine
Johns Hopkins University
Baltimore, Maryland

Cydney Dashkoff, PT, CSLT
Legacy Good Samaritan Hospital Cancer Institute
Portland, Oregon

James W. Farris, PT, PhD
Associate Professor, Physical Therapy
A.T. Still University
Mesa, Arizona

Meryl R. Gersh, PT, PhD
Professor and Chair
Doctor of Physical Therapy Program
Eastern Washington University
Spokane, Washington

Barbara Gladson, PT, PhD
Director, UMDNJ Biopharma Educational Initiative
MS in Clinical Trial Sciences, SHRP
Associate Professor of Physiology & Pharmacology
Professor of Physical Therapy
University of Medicine and Dentistry of New Jersey
Newark, New Jersey

John Heick, PT, DPT
Assistant Professor, Physical Therapy
Arizona School of Health Science
A.T. Still University
Mesa, Arizona

Patricia Rayellen Hoover, PT
Hoover Physical Therapy
Camp Hill, Pennsylvania

Catherine Johnston, MAppSc, BAppSc
Lecturer
Clinical Education Coordinator
Faculty of Health
Displicine of Physiotherapy
School of Health Sciences
The University of Newcastle
New South Wales, Australia

Loraine Lovejoy-Evans, MPT, DPT, CLT-Földi
Independence Through Physical Therapy
Sequim, Washington

Jennifer Mackney, MClinEd, BAppSc
Faculty of Health
Displicine of Physiotherapy
School of Health Sciences
The University of Newcastle
New South Wales, Australia

Daniel Malone, PT, PhD, CCS
Assistant Professor
Physical Therapy Program
School of Medicine
University of Colorado
Aurora, Colorado

Christine Mamawag, PT
Physical Therapist
Cedars-Sinai Medical Center
Los Angeles, California

Kerry Ann McGinn, MSN
Author and Nurse Practitioner

Willis H. Navarro, MD
Medical Director
Transplant Medical Services
National Marrow Donor Program
Minneapolis, Minnesota

Joni C. Nichols, MD
Medical Oncologist and Hematologist
Co-Medical Director of Hospice of Spokane
Spokane, Washington

Christiane Perme, PT, CCS
Senior Physical Therapist
The Methodist Hospital
Houston, Texas

Margaret E. Rhinehart-Ayers, PT, PhD
Associate Professor of Physical Therapy
Director of Clinical Education
College of Health Professions
Thomas Jefferson University
Philadelphia, Pennsylvania

Susan E. Roush, PT, PhD
Professor, Physical Therapy Department
University of Rhode Island
Kingston, Rhode Island

Anne K. Swisher, PT, PhD, CCS
Graduate & Distance Education Coordinator
WVU Division of Physical Therapy
Morgantown, West Virginia

Linda Tripp, DPT
Adult Inpatient Physical Therapy
Rehabilitation Services
University of Minnesota Medical Center
Minneapolis, Minnesota

Karen E. Wilk, PT, DPT
Administrative Director of Rehabilitation Medicine
Englewood Hospital and Medical Center
Englewood, New Jersey

Each edition of this text gives an opportunity to thank all the members of the Elsevier team, but especially one individual in the background who richly deserves applause. This one honors David Stein, Senior Project Manager, an amazing man who knows no equal in all respects: work ethic, attention to detail, the "eagle eye," speedy turnaround time, not to forget mentioning being fun, smart, and witty.

CCG

To my many patients who rise above the effects of neurological dysfunction. You have been my inspiration to learn, and you have taught me so much about how to live my life.

KSF

Being a physical therapist has two special joys. One is seeing the progress that our patients make each day in our care. Another is the satisfaction found in knowing and growing with our colleagues. This text epitomizes both of these joys for me.

Pathology: Implications for the Physical Therapist represents an important contribution to the quality of care that we provide to our patients. Knowledge of the pathology of disease has always stood as one of the fundamental prerequisites to safe and effective health care practice. By understanding principles of pathology, we can put names to the problems we find in our patients. These names, or diagnoses, allow us to then classify our patients to lead to effective interventions with maximum outcome.

With the development and application of the disablement model, physical therapists, along with others, have been able to place pathology in its appropriate context. Rather than seeing pathology as the primary, and perhaps single, basis for understanding and naming illness, the disablement model places pathology as the initiation of a cascade of affects that can lead to impairments, functional limitations, disability, and handicap. Physical therapists recognize that we also name these impairments and functional limitations in diagnosing and classifying our patients.

Catherine Goodman and Kenda Fuller set their presentation of pathology in this context. This text not only provides the basis for our conversations with other health care practitioners about our patients but also frames that conversation in the clinical decisions that we, as physical therapists, make about and with our patients. We must understand pathology and the changes it induces in our patients, and then we must use this knowledge to help us make accurate diagnoses that lead to accurate prognoses about the ability of our patients to benefit from our interventions. The format of this text, with its grounding in the disablement model, its presentation of pathology, the addition of the medical and surgical management of patients with specific pathology, and, finally, special implications for physical therapists, provides students and clinicians alike with the basis for our clinical decisions. In addition, the authors provide extensive text and journal references so that readers can seek the evidence that supports the authors' contentions.

The authors' concern about the quality of our care is imbued throughout the text. Because of this concern, the authors' attention to detail, and the application of the disablement model, the text offers us an important and useful tool to improve our patient care. It can be used successfully by students, faculty, and clinicians as a reference for patient care, helping them to experience the true joy of providing the best possible physical therapy care to their patients.

This text has also given me the opportunity to experience the second joy to be found in our field. Physical therapy continues to grow and expand, but it remains a closely-knit group, offering many opportunities for development of a true community, with all of the interrelationships found in a community of colleagues.

I have had the great pleasure to meet and interact with almost all of the authors and reviewers of this text. They continually impress me with their professional expertise and their dedication to improving physical therapy. But I take special pride in my professional relationship with Catherine Cavallaro Goodman. I first met Cat many years ago when she was a student and I was a teacher and her advisor in the physical therapy program at the University of Pennsylvania. In the intervening years, we have each taken a different path. How wonderful it is to have these paths occasionally intertwine, to be able to point with pride and joy to her many contributions to our field, and to see the excitement, enthusiasm, and expertise she brings to her writing and teaching.

Physical therapy is truly a source of joy and excitement for those of us blessed to be part of this profession. *Pathology: Implications for the Physical Therapist* offers us one more opportunity to strengthen the quality of the care we provide our patients. I am confident that readers will agree with me that this is indeed cause for celebration. May they all enjoy the contribution of this text to our profession!

Laurita M. Hack, PT, MBA, PhD, FAPTA

PREFACE

The community of physical and occupational therapists has responded to this text in an overwhelmingly positive way. That is good because health professionals more frequently encounter illnesses, diseases, and conditions that limit mobility and function among people of all ages, but especially the aging population.

Physical therapy should be provided when pathology limits mobility and function and let's face it: there is often some amount of lingering disability after many health problems. The older we get, the longer it seems to take to recover to our former level of function, if indeed we do get back to what we consider "normal."

Improving functional abilities that contribute to independent living, returning home following hospitalization, less reliance on medical and support services, and reduced health care costs are major contributions made by the physical therapy community.[3] We are able to achieve these goals through a unique appreciation of pathology as it fits within the continuum of care for each patient.[2] Understanding the relationship among the problems, the intervention, and goals for physical therapy often requires knowledge of pathology, including risk factors, etiology, and prognosis.[4]

The information in this text is designed to provide therapists with a place of reference and clinical direction. As often as possible, the most up-to-date information and references are provided. Critical thinking based on evidence is intended to yield better outcomes. Communicating with and informing others (e.g., our patients/clients, their family members, and other members of the health care team), our plan of care and rationale, will aid in placing value on what we do.

Prevention and wellness have become more mainstream now. Therapists play an important role in disease prevention and health promotion across the life span so, whenever possible, risk-factor reduction and prevention strategies are a part of the discussion surrounding each disease. By communicating our consideration of these variables and our ability to meet the comprehensive needs of individuals both in staying well and in recovering from illness, disease, or injury, we demonstrate our unique contribution to health care and the field of rehabilitation.[3,4]

Although therapists do not usually devise intervention strategies for primary systemic conditions, we must be aware of the impact that such diseases may have on the rehabilitation process. Gaining a level of understanding of the pathogenesis and medical treatment beyond just the basics enables us to communicate more effectively with other health care personnel across the continuum of health care delivery settings.

In addition to integrating information from the APTA's Guide and updating scientific and medical information, this fourth edition continues to offer details about the clinical impact of diseases and "dis-eased" body systems on clinical interventions. Toward that end, whenever possible, a special section on the role of exercise and each condition or pathology is included to reflect the current understanding of the importance of exercise as a primary intervention for many diseases.

The key strength of this text continues to be the *Special Implications for the Therapist*, whether the therapist is a student with that first client or a seasoned clinician of many years. This edition boasts the collaborative effort of over 57 contributors who have banded together to provide you with the clinical expertise of seasoned practitioners.

This edition offers a new feature entitled "A Therapist's Thoughts" in the *Special Implications* sections. Here you can find comments, suggestions, and reflections based on observation, experience, and expertise. As always, we encourage you to search for high-quality, evidence-based studies to support all that you do in the clinic. But listen to the voice of experience and let a modicum of common sense prevail when making clinical decisions and applying the results of research.

We remind ourselves and our readers that this text is meant to help students and clinicians in all settings to appreciate the role of pathology in our patients'/clients' clinical presentation and participation in their various life roles.

We deliver cost-effective care that is affected by underlying pathology(ies) and impacts not only the immediate, but also the long-term health of each patient/client. Our differential diagnostic skills, education of diverse caregivers and patients/clients, and dynamically evolving status of the patient/client demands a dynamic bridge between physical therapists and physicians, and attention to post-acute continuity of care for optimal outcomes.[1]

Whenever possible, we have used language from the International Classification of Functioning, Disability, and Health (ICF) recognizing that the material in this text is really "in the front of the ICF" . . . meaning knowledge of each patient's pathology comes before incorporation of the ICF format. The information on pathologic conditions, diseases, and illnesses offered within this text follows a traditional medical model in order to assist us in communicating with physicians and other health care professionals who use this framework for evaluation and treatment while we ourselves treat movement impairments rather than medical pathology.

Catherine Cavallaro Goodman

[2] German SI: Nationwide acute care physical therapy practice analysis identifies knowledge, skills, and behaviors that reflect acute care practice, *Phys Ther* 90(10):1453-1467, 2010.

[3] Smith J: President's message, *J Acute Care Phys Ther* 2(3):86-87, 2011.

[4] Sullivan KJ: A vision for society: Physical therapy as partners in the national health agenda, *PTJ* 91(11):1664-1672, 2011.

[1] Bose S: Quote from Acute Care List Serve. February 25, 2012.

ACKNOWLEDGMENTS

We wrote the first edition of this text without the benefit of e-mail and only Internet access to the National Library of Medicine. We were naïve in the undertaking! Now that we know better and are armed with the benefits of electronic communication, there are many people who deserve our thanks and praise.

First, to the reviewers and contributors who gave their time and expertise (often without financial reward) ... your names are in lights on the Reviewers/Contributors pages! Each one of these individuals took the time and effort to carefully review, revise, or update specific chapters or sections within a chapter to make sure everything was up to date and/or to offer insight from their own years of clinical practice in specialty areas. Special thanks to the physical therapy community across the United States and those closer to home in our own communities for their ongoing support of this project.

Likewise, to the daring and courageous clinical therapists who offered their case examples for instructors to use with students to engage them in dialog, discourse, and discussion, we thank you and praise you: Susan Barth, Kathy Bell, Mary Calys, Nancy Ciesla, Lara Firrone, Pat Hoover, Alan Lee, and Karen Rushby.

To the many, many people who have helped in previous editions...reviewers, contributors, brain stormers, and hand holders. We started writing them down and it was too many to print. So we are limiting the list to former contributors. If you do not find your name on this list (and you expected to see it there), please know you are in our minds and hearts with thanksgiving: Dana Austin, William Boissonnault, John R. Corboy, Sharon Funk, Ira Gorman, Steve Gudas, Kathleen Harris, Julie Hobbs, Elizabeth Ikeda, Milagros Jorge, Zoher F. Kapasi, Sharon Konecne, Michael Koopmeiners, D. Michael McKeough, G. Stephen Morris, Charlotte Norton, Sue Queen, Nancy Rich, Susan A. Scherer, Marcia Smith, Teresa E. Snyder, Steve Tepper, Margaret (Peg) Waltner, Patricia A. Winkler, and Bonnie Yost.

We offer thanks to those people and organizations who shared their PowerPoint slides, handouts, notes, abstracts, poster presentations, and other resources with us... and to all who contributed to the formation of the *Guide to the Physical Therapist Practice.*

A special thanks to Celeste K. Peterson, MD, our medical consultant who had a direct hand in reviewing and editing much of the medical information in Section II and to all the unnamed but not forgotten physicians who answered questions, reviewed materials, responded to countless phone calls and e-mail requests for information.

Thanks go to the staff of St. Patrick Hospital and Health Sciences Center, Center for Health Information, Missoula, Montana, especially the medical library staff, Dana Kopp and Lisa Autio, for seeing us through four editions of this text now.

The many professional partners of all kinds at Elsevier Science from editors to indexers, marketing, production, design specialists ... many whose names we don't know, but to those we do know, we thank you: Kathy Falk, Jolynn Gower, Christie Hart, David Stein, and Celeste Clingan.

And to each of you who contributed an important piece to this project...maybe you don't remember doing that, but WE do! William G. Boissonnault for getting the first edition started, Sujoy Bose, Kevin Carroll [Hanger Prosthetics and Orthotics], Nancy Ciesla, Amy Nordon-Craft, Carol M. Davis, Jackie Drouin, Kim Ericsson, Lara A. Firrone, Eva Marie Gold, Brant Goode, Steve Gudas, Laurita Hack, Ellen Hillegass, Sharon Konecne, Bonnie Lasinski, Alan Chong W. Lee, Daniel Malone, Charles L. McGarvey, G. Steven Morris, Christiane Perme, Jaque Pokorney, Alessander D. Santos, and Shirley Sahrmann.

Tamara Kittelson-Aldred, MS, OTR/L, ATP, Assistive Technology Practitioner (RESNA), Access Therapy Services, for the wonderful photos of individuals using a variety of adaptive equipment and assistive technology.

To those who offered advice, counsel, and/or direction: Rose Bjorklund, Jessa Brown, Elizabeth Cole, Rebecca Craik, Jackie Drouin, Barbara Gladson, Laurita Hack, Fatima Hakeem, Daniel J. Malone, Janet B. Hulme, Reed Humphrey, Elizabeth Ikeda, Bonnie Lasinski, Andréa Leiserowitz, Ruth Mulvany, G. Stephen Morris, Barbara J. Norton, Michael J. Parisi, Cindy Pfalzer, Kathryn Ryans, Angelo Rizzo, Beth Shelly, Barbara A. Tschoepe, and Jennifer Tucker.

Folks who provided special photographs: Jane Kepics, MS, PT, CLT-LANA, Phoenixville Hospital, Phoenixville, Pennsylvania, for the photos and documentation of axillary web syndrome; Rosalie Bush, RN, MSN, CNS Billings Clinic (Cystic Fibrosis classification); and to Bonnie Lasinski; Karen Rushby, Jarvik (heart transplant); Darlene Haven, Senior Manager. Medical Marketing, National Marrow Donor Program; and Chris Wells.

Colleagues who made useful comments on the Acute Care and Oncology Section list serves including: Nancy Abodeely, Kathy Bell, Mary Calys, Alisa Curry, Daniel Drummer, Loraine Lovejoy-Evans, Lara Firrone, Nancy Gessner, Colleen Lettvin, Daniel J. Malone, Nancy Roberge, Marisa Perdomo, Jennifer Ryan, and Katesel Strimbeck. It is likely someone was missed—our apologies!

Contributing/supportive friends: Rick Beck, Royal Beck, Cheryl Hanson, Kerry Resch, Jill Hansen-Twardoski, Sean O'Brien, Valerie B. Wang, and Matt Zdanek.

And always, to our families for standing by our sides, sometimes day and night, putting aside their time schedules, and contributing intangible love and support. In particular, for Catherine: Cliff Goodman, Ben and Ellen Goodman, and Guy Goodman.

To these people and to the many others who remain unnamed but not forgotten, we say thank you. Your support and encouragement have made this text possible.

Catherine Cavallaro Goodman

Kenda S. Fuller

CONTENTS

SECTION 3
PATHOLOGY OF THE MUSCULOSKELETAL SYSTEM

CHAPTER 1

Introduction to Concepts of Pathology

CATHERINE CAVALLARO GOODMAN

PATHOGENESIS OF DISEASE

Pathology is defined as the branch of medicine that investigates the essential nature of disease, especially changes in body tissues and organs that cause or are caused by disease.[45] *Clinical pathology* in medicine refers to pathology applied to the solution of clinical problems, especially the use of laboratory methods in clinical diagnosis. *Pathogenesis* is the development of unhealthy conditions or disease, or more specifically, the cellular events and reactions and other pathologic mechanisms that occur in the development of disease.

This text examines the pathogenesis of each disease or condition—that is, the progression of each pathologic condition on both its cellular level and clinical presentation whenever signs and symptoms are manifested. Advances in medicine have resulted in a population with greater longevity but also with a more complex pathologic picture. Orthopedic and neurologic conditions are no longer present as singular phenomena; they often occur in a person with other medical pathology. We must be knowledgeable of the impact other conditions and diseases have on the individual's neuromusculoskeletal system and the necessary steps that must be taken to provide safe, effective treatment.

For the physical therapist, clinical pathology has a different meaning regarding the effects of pathologic processes (i.e., disease) on the individual's functional abilities and limitations. The relationship between impairment and functional limitation is the key focus in therapy. In addition, how the person with the pathologic condition is able to participate in his or her family and community is paramount. Current clinical practice should include an emphasis on the person's activity level, participation, level of supports, and environment. Thus, despite the disease process and related loss of function, the whole person must be considered.

Pathology and the Guide to Physical Therapist Practice

The American Physical Therapy Association (APTA) *Guide to Physical Therapist Practice*[3] was developed for clinical use by physical therapists as an expert consensus document. Panels of clinicians were involved in the first step of formulating the *Guide,* and then more than 1000 therapists across the country participated in reviewing the document.

Three conceptual models are integrated throughout the *Guide:* the (Nagi) Disablement Model, the Integration of Prevention and Wellness Strategies, and the Patient/Client Management Model. The *Guide* uses an expanded version of the disablement model to provide therapists with a common language to understand and communicate about our clients. The *Guide* is currently in its second (revised) edition and being revised for a third edition that will reflect how the profession has moved toward using the World Health Organization (WHO) International Classification of Functioning, Disability, and Health (ICF) to describe the impact of a pathology on a person's lifestyle and plan of care. This model expands on the previous disablement model by also a considering the individual's participation and environmental constraints or supports.

The *Guide* includes a section of specific diagnostic groups referred to as *Preferred Practice Patterns* that represent the major body systems and are designed to facilitate a systems approach to patient/client management. The Practice Patterns are described in four sections: musculoskeletal, neuromuscular, cardiopulmonary, and integumentary. The therapist will encounter multiple medical comorbidities that extend beyond the four categories of the Preferred Practice Patterns outlined in the *Guide.*

However, the physical therapist will not be devising intervention strategies for systemic or visceral diseases, but must be aware of the impact that such diseases may have on the human movement system and rehabilitation process. In previous editions of this text, the most likely practice patterns associated with each disease or disorder discussed were presented in the *Special Implications for the Therapist* boxes, but in this edition they are now available on the Evolve site in a feature called "Preferred Practice Patterns." These patterns may vary with each episode of care, depending on clinical presentation.

CONCEPTS OF HEALTH, ILLNESS, AND DISABILITY

Health

Many people and organizations have attempted to define the concept of health, but no universally accepted definition has been adopted. A dictionary definition describes health in terms of an individual's ability to function normally in society. Some definitions characterize health as a disease-free state or condition. The WHO[66] has defined *health* as a state of complete physical, mental, and social well-being and not merely as the absence of disease or infirmity. All of these definitions present health as an either/or circumstance, meaning an individual is either healthy or ill.

Health is more accurately viewed as a continuum on which wellness on one end is the optimal level of function and illness on the other may be so unfavorable as to result in death. Health is a dynamic process that varies with changes in interactions between an individual and the internal and external environments. This type of definition recognizes health as an individual's level of wellness.

Health reflects a person's biologic, psychologic, spiritual, and sociologic state. The *biologic* or physical state refers to the overall structure of the individual's body tissues and organs and to the biochemical interactions and functions within the body. The *psychologic* state includes the individual's mood, emotions, and personality.

The *spiritual* aspect of health addresses the individual's religious/soul needs, which may be affected by illness or injury. The spiritual dimension in health care focuses on the integration of mind, body, and spirit, with the goal of promoting whole-person healing. The *sociologic* or social state refers to the interaction between the individual and the social environment. A high level of wellness or holistic health is achieved when the biopsychosocial-spiritual needs of a person are met.

Illness

Definition

Illness is often defined as sickness or deviation from a healthy state, and the term has a broader meaning than disease. *Disease* refers to a biologic or psychologic alteration that results in a malfunction of a body organ or system. *Disease* is usually a term used to describe a biomedical condition that is substantiated by objective data such as elevated temperature or presence of infection (as demonstrated by positive blood cultures).

Illness is the perception and response of the person to not being well. Illness includes disturbances in normal human biologic function and personal, interpersonal, and cultural reactions to disease. Disease can occur in an individual without that person being aware of illness and without others perceiving illness. However, a person can feel very ill even though no obvious pathologic processes can be identified.

Incidence and Prevalence

When discussing various diseases, disorders, and conditions, incidence and prevalence may be reported. Incidence is the number of new cases of a condition in a specific period of time (e.g., 6 months or 1 year) in relation to the total number of people in the population who are "at risk" at the beginning of the period. Prevalence measures all cases of a condition (new and old) among those at risk for developing the condition. Measures of prevalence are made at one point in time (e.g., on a specific day).

Natural History

The natural history of a condition, disorder, or disease describes how it progresses over time. The natural history of some conditions, such as cancer, can be judged based on the stage of the tumor at the diagnosis and response to treatment. Scientists are actively engaged in identifying predictive factors that help tell what the patient/client's prognosis and outcome might be. In medicine, predictive factors (both negative and positive) are the closest thing we have to a crystal ball.

Even with known predictive factors, the natural history is not always clear; predicting what is going to happen and when it is going to happen can have wide or narrow margins, depending on the condition. For example, individuals with some forms of muscular dystrophy have a more predictive natural history, whereas individuals with cerebral palsy may not be so easy to gauge, especially during the early years of growth and development.

The therapist must develop a plan of care keeping in mind the natural history of the condition and where the individual is in the life span or life stage. Some thought should be given to dovetailing our view of impairments, dysfunctions, and disabilities with the natural history of the disease, condition, and illness. This is particularly important when working with individuals who have long-term, degenerative or progressive neurologic, or chronic conditions.

Improvements in treatment for neurologic and other conditions previously considered fatal (e.g., cancer, cystic fibrosis) are now extending the life expectancy for many individuals. Improved interventions bring new areas of focus such as quality of life issues. With some conditions (e.g., muscular dystrophy, cerebral palsy, cystic fibrosis, fetal alcohol syndrome), the artificial dichotomy of pediatric versus adult care is gradually being replaced by a lifestyle approach that takes into consideration what is known about the natural history of the condition.

Many individuals with childhood-onset diseases now live well into adulthood. For them, their original pathology or disease process has given way to secondary impairments. These secondary impairments create further limitation and issues as the person ages. For instance, a 30-year-old with cerebral palsy may experience chronic pain, changes or limitations in ambulation and endurance, and increased fatigue. These symptoms result from the atypical movement patterns and musculoskeletal strains caused by chronic increase in tone and muscle imbalances that were originally caused by the condition. In this case, the therapy would not be focused on decreasing the primary signs and symptoms of cerebral palsy, but rather on the issues that have developed as a result of the cerebral palsy.[27]

Acute Illness

Acute illness usually refers to an illness or disease that has a relatively rapid onset and short duration; it is not synonymous with "severe." The condition often responds to a specific treatment and is usually self-limiting, although exceptions to this definition are numerous.

If no complications occur, most acute illnesses end in a full recovery and the individual returns to the previous level of functioning.

Subacute refers to how long a disease has been present, but there is no set time that divides subacute from the other time descriptions (i.e., acute and chronic). Subacute describes a time course that is between acute and chronic. A symptom that is subacute has been present for longer than a few days but less than several months. Chronic conditions sometimes flare up and may be referred to as subacute.

Acute illnesses usually follow a specific sequence, or stages of illness, from onset through recovery. The first stage involves the experience of physical symptoms (e.g., pain, shortness of breath, fever), cognitive awareness (i.e., the symptoms are interpreted to have meaning), and an emotional response, usually one of denial, fear, or anxiety.

Subsequent stages of an acute illness may include assumption of a sick role as the person recognizes the problem as being sufficient to require contact with a health care professional. If the illness is confirmed, the individual continues in the sick role; if it is not confirmed, a return to normalcy may occur or the person may continue to seek health care to identify the illness.

A stage of dependency occurs when the person receives and accepts a diagnosis and treatment plan. This type of dependency in the psychologically and emotionally balanced person represents awareness, acceptance, reliance on diagnosis, and care beyond self-help. This definition of dependency differs from dependency associated with dependent personality disorder, in which the affected person lacks self-confidence or the ability to function independently, and allows others to assume responsibility for his or her care. Depending on the severity of the illness, the individual may give up independence and control and assume a more dependent sick role. During this stage, sick people often become more passive and concerned about themselves.

Most people move from acute or subacute to the final stage of recovery or rehabilitation. During this stage, the individual gives up the sick role and resumes more normal activities and responsibilities. Individuals with long-term or chronic illnesses may require a longer period to adjust to new lifestyles.

Chronic Illness

Chronic illness describes illnesses that include one or more of the following characteristics: permanent impairment or disability, residual physical or cognitive disability, or the need for special rehabilitation and/or long-term medical management. Chronic illnesses and conditions may fluctuate in intensity as acute exacerbations occur that cause physiologic instability and necessitate additional medical management (e.g., diabetes mellitus, fibromyalgia, rheumatoid arthritis, multiple sclerosis). A person who has exacerbations of chronic illness may progress through the stages of illness described in the previous section.

Psychologic Aspects

One of the most important factors influencing psychologic reactions to illness is the premorbid (before illness) psychologic profile of the affected person. For example, a person with a dependent-type personality may become very dependent, perhaps seeking unusually large amounts of advice or reassurance from the health care specialist or expecting attention beyond that required for the degree of illness present. A narcissistic (self-centered) person may be particularly concerned about the need to take medication or the loss of the ability to work. The stoic person (indifferent to or unaffected by pain) may have difficulty admitting to being sick at all.

Other factors that affect a person's psychologic reaction include the extent of the illness and the particular symptoms that develop. Extremely mild disease may have little effect, whereas completely unexpected and debilitating illness may be very distressing. A common reaction to any illness is fear or anxiety related to the loss of control over one's own body. Denial is an unconscious defense mechanism that allows a person to avoid painful reality as long as possible. Denial can be a natural part of the process of dealing with illness, which culminates in acceptance.

Noncompliance with treatment may have a psychologic basis (e.g., denial: "There is nothing wrong with me, so I do not need medical treatment."), but it may also occur as a result of previous experience. For example, noncompliance with prescribed corticosteroid therapy may be based on aversion to side effects experienced during use of this drug in a previous disease flare. With chronic autoimmune diseases (e.g., connective tissue diseases), denial may continue for years as a coping mechanism for the individual who continues to decline in physical functional capacity.

It is important to recognize that psychologic or psychiatric symptoms, such as impairment of memory, personality changes (e.g., paranoia), loss of impulse control, or mood disorders (e.g., persistent depression or elation), can have a functional or organic basis. Functional symptoms occur without significant physical dysfunction of brain cells, whereas organic symptoms can be caused by abnormal physiologic changes in brain tissue. An example of a functional symptom is depression that is considered to be the psychologic consequence of a general medical condition (e.g., myocardial infarction).

Organic symptoms occur as a direct physiologic consequence of a medication or medical condition. For example, onset of corticosteroid-induced psychologic symptoms is often dose-related, and symptoms subside as the corticosteroids are tapered. Another example of an organic basis for symptomatology is the person with systemic lupus erythematosus who experiences symptoms of organic mental disorders secondary to systemic lupus erythematosus–mediated vasculitis, called lupus cerebritis, or the person with end-stage liver disease who develops hepatic encephalopathy when toxic substances in the blood, such as ammonia, reach the brain.

Disability

Disability is a large public health problem in the United States affecting more than 50 million Americans, who report disabling conditions. This figure illustrates that nearly 20% of the U.S. population currently lives with a disability. Prevalence of disability is higher among women than men and is reported highest among people 65 years of age and older. One of the national health goals for 2010 is to eliminate health disparities among different segments of the population, including among people with disabilities.

National estimates of disability range from 15% to 20% for adults over the age of 18 years.[16] Although these figures were determined in 1999, the Centers for Disease Control and Prevention reports that the number of adults reporting a disability has not changed since that time. However, the number of baby boomers (persons aged 45–64 years) reporting disabilities is expected to rise over the next decade as increasing numbers enter the 65 years of age and older group, which has a much higher risk for disability. When this happens, the absolute number of persons affected is expected to increase substantially. The added number of persons reporting disabilities will likely place more demands on the health care and public health systems. This trend will impact physical therapists directly as there will be an increased need for additional health care providers trained in musculoskeletal conditions.[16]

Disability is often viewed by physical therapists from a biopsychosocial model (see description and discussion in Chapter 3), which incorporates and integrates the traditional medical model with the less stringent and more flexible social model of disability. The medical model confines disability as a descriptor of the affected individual. In this context, disability requires intervention by others (usually health care providers) to correct the problem. The social model of disability is more likely to see an unaccommodating environment and lack of social response to individuals with disabilities as the problem requiring a social or political response.[35]

Disablement and Classification Models

There are many contemporary models proposed today to describe disability classifications and give us a framework for identifying the consequences of diseases, disorders, and injuries. Some are strictly medical models that emphasize the cause of disability as a medical condition or disorder. Others are economic models that examine the likelihood of employment or reemployment. Sociopolitical models present disability as a human (civil) rights issue that must be addressed in order to provide full access to (and participation in) society for the affected individual.[31]

Individually, none of these models focus on what or how the person with a disability experiences his or her problems. The APTA's adoption of the WHO's International Classification of Functioning, Disability, and Health (ICF) helps physical therapists avoid some of the pitfalls associated with other models of disability. The ICF can be used to more accurately identify and address the multiple factors that affect and contribute to an individual's recovery.[65] The model briefly summarized here has been incorporated into this text whenever possible.

> **Note to Reader:** There are numerous articles written for the physical therapist further discussing the use of the IC that may aid you in applying the ICF to specific problems related to the human movement system.[4,5,21,26,35,55,56,57] Readers are encouraged to take a look at these publications; additional information can be found on the APTA website at http://www.apta.org/ICF/.

International Classification of Functioning, Disability, and Health. The WHO's framework to classify and code information about health and provide standardized language is the *International Classification of Functioning, Disability, and Health*, established in 2001. The ICF is presented as the international standard to describe and measure health, function, and ability (rather than disability) from a biopsychosocial perspective by all health care professionals. The ICF Health and Disability Model is a good framework for research from a global perspective—this one instrument can provide an international health information system. It will allow for research and clinical study describing function that can be combined and compared for better statistical significance and understanding.

While traditional health indicators are based on the mortality (i.e., death) rates of populations, the ICF shifts focus to "life" (i.e., how people live with their health conditions and how these can be improved to achieve a productive, fulfilling life). The ICF model is an interactive, integrative, and universal model that focuses on human functioning, not disability. Most notable in the current structure is the inclusion of "host factors" that impact the behavior of the individual such as demographic background, physical and social environments, and psychologic status. The full description of this model can be found at www.who.int/classification/icf.

The ICF Health and Disability Model includes the following five components (Fig. 1-1); each component has subsets or "qualifiers" to help define the level of functioning and health for the problem being described or evaluated:

- Body functions
- Body structures
- Activities and participation
- Environmental factors
- Personal factors

The ICF describes how people live with their health condition. The ICF uses these health-related domains to describe body functions and structures and activities and participation from body, individual, and societal perspectives. Because an individual's functioning and disability occur in a context, the ICF also includes a list of environmental factors.[68]

The ICF changes our understanding of disability, no longer presenting disability as a problem of a minority group, or just of people with a visible impairment or in a wheelchair. For example, a person living with HIV/AIDS could be disabled in terms of his or her ability to participate actively in a profession. In that case, the ICF provides different perspectives as to how measures can be targeted to optimize that person's ability to remain in the workforce and live a full life in the community.[69]

Bu using this model, physical therapists can describe the changes that occur in the body, the whole person, the person's ability to perform tasks, his or her social roles, and the environment that forms the context of that person's life. Using this model makes it possible to more accurately portray the function and disability state of an individual by describing (rather than classifying) individuals according to their functioning.

ICF—Language. The ICF introduces new "enablement" language to replace older disablement terminology that

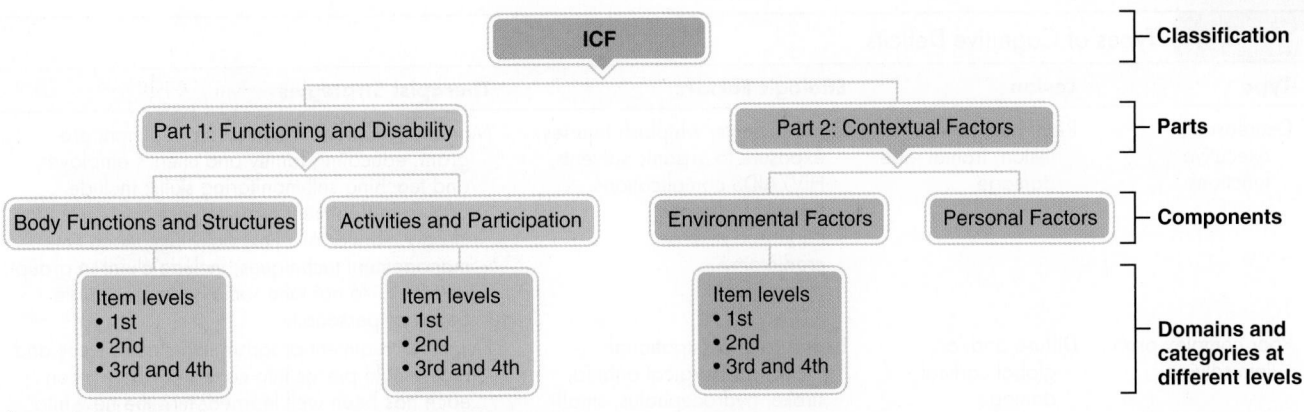

Figure 1-1

Structure of the International Classification of Functioning, Disability, and Health (ICF). (From World Health Organization [WHO]: *Principles and process for including classifications in the Family of International Classifications*, Geneva, Revised 2004, WHO.)

implied distinctions between individuals who are healthy and those who have disabilities. The new language defines *body functions and structures* as physiologic or psychologic functions of body systems or anatomic parts (e.g., organs, limbs). *Impairments* are defined as problems in body function or structure.

Activity is defined as the execution of specific tasks or actions by an individual. *Activity limitations* are the difficulties that an individual might have in executing activities, and *participation* is the individual's involvement in life situations. *Participation restrictions* are problems the individual might have in real-life situations.[34,68]

Secondary conditions or impairments of body structures can result from limitation of activity and participation. Joint contractures, disuse atrophy, and heart disease are examples of changes from inactivity. If not prevented, these changes can lead to further limitation of activity but are not part of the underlying health condition. It is important to remember that the same impairments may not result in the same extent of activity limitation or that activity limitation may not limit the participation in a life role in the same way in two different individuals.

An example of this continuum could be described this way: a person has survived a stroke in the left side of the brain and has the impairments of hemiparesis and aphasia. This person may not be able to walk or talk but can participate in work with the assistance of a walker and communication board. On the other hand, a person who survived a stroke on the right side of the brain may be able to walk but not be able to participate in work because of loss of executive function and poor judgment.

If the first individual does not have access to a walker and communication board because of lack of funding, he or she may not be able to return to work. In many cultures, it is tradition that if a person is injured or has a medical condition, it is the responsibility of the family to provide passive or palliative care; that person may never have the opportunity to rehabilitate to full potential.

The ICF framework takes a broad biopsychosocial view that looks beyond mortality and disease to focus on how people live with their conditions.[34,35] The ICF framework promotes international exchange using a common and consistent framework and universal language to discuss disability and related phenomena.[35] The APTA has joined the WHO, the World Confederation for Physical Therapy, the American Therapeutic Recreation Association, and other organizations in endorsing the ICF model.

Cognitive Disability[64]

Disabilities are not just limited to the physical body. Problems such as mental illnesses like depression, alcoholism, schizophrenia, and cognitive impairments, although responsible for only about 1% of deaths, are seriously underestimated sources of disabilities that account for 11% of the world's disease burden.[67] These conditions are often undiagnosed, and although therapists cannot diagnose these impairments, recognizing the deficits is important. Only cognitive disability is discussed in this section; common mental illnesses are discussed in Chapter 3. Five types of cognitive deficit most commonly encountered by the physical therapist are presented here. Each one is associated with a specific area of brain damage and linked to possible causes that may be barriers to successful treatment (Table 1-1).

Executive functions may be described as cortical functions involved in formulating goals and in planning, initiating, monitoring, and maintaining behavior.[38] Behavior is defined here in its broadest terms to include not only overt motor behavior but also affective and social behavior. A person with executive function deficits typically appears inert or apathetic. Clinically, these clients typically have a right hemisphere lesion and apraxia, unilateral neglect, or both. When frontal lobe damage occurs, the effects of impaired executive functions may be attributed to depression. Although the two may occur simultaneously, depression is usually characterized by a lack of energy, whereas impaired executive functions are demonstrated by a lack of involvement.

Complex problem solving may be described as the effective handling of new information. Impaired problem solving results in concrete thinking, inability to distinguish the relevant from the irrelevant, erroneous application of rules, and difficulty generalizing from one situation to another. For example, when a client learns how to accomplish wheelchair transfers and then generalizes that information to various settings (bed to chair, chair to toilet, chair to car, in hospital, at home), he or she is using new information in complex problem solving.

Table 1-1	Types of Cognitive Deficits		
Type	**Lesion**	**Etiologic Factors**	**Therapist Strategies**
Decreased executive functions	Right hemisphere lesion, frontal lobe damage	Car accidents, whiplash injuries, exposure to organic solvents, HIV/AIDS complications, Korsakoff disease, Parkinson disease, craniotomy	More active role in maintaining treatment program, educating family and client's employer, and teaching self-monitoring skills; include pacing in treatment regimen; use home trainers; closely monitor all clinic activities; teach time management techniques; include client in group activities; do not take socially inappropriate behavior personally
Poor complex problem solving	Diffuse and/or global cortical damage	Exposure to occupational toxins, postsurgical anoxia, stroke, hydrocephalus, small-vessel disease associated with hypertension	Fragment treatment program into small pieces and reassemble pieces into coherent whole when each has been well learned; turn the new into the familiar through repetition; reduce complexity of treatment components; avoid abstract visual aids and abstract verbal explanations
Slowed information processing	Diffuse cortical or subcortical system damage, reticular activating system of the brainstem	Alcohol abuse, drug abuse, exposure to toxins, developmental delays, traumatic brain injury	Slow the rate of presentation; remove environmental distractors; do not speak loudly as though client were hearing impaired; simply present one type of information at a time, making sure the client understands you before you move on
Memory deficits	Temporal lobe damage	Alcohol abuse, temporal lobe injuries, seizures, traumatic brain injury, exposure to toxins, age-related deterioration	Make certain that no learning or emotional disorder is involved; use external aids and multichannel approaches to improve retention of information; determine which aid or approach works best for each individual
Learning disabilities	Unclear	Unknown; possibly traumatic birth or genetic predisposition, early acquired brain damage, metabolic abnormalities	Avoid written material unless it is appropriate to the person's reading level; use nonverbal modes of communication

Modified from Woltersdorf MA: Beyond the sensorimotor strip. *Clin Manage* 12:63–69, 1992.

Information processing involves the speed with which information travels from one part of the brain to another and the amount of information assimilated at that speed.[38] Whereas complex problem solving has to do with the orchestration of information, information processing involves the efficient transfer of information.

As a result of genetic, environmental, and educational factors, some people are more proficient processors than others. As a result of trauma, some people may lose processing ability and speed. Noise levels, external sensory stimulation (e.g., presence of other people and other activities), and presentation of more than one kind of information at a time (e.g., providing a written home program then discussing the time of the next appointment) are examples of distractions to people with reduced information-processing abilities.

Memory deficits result from a failure to store or retrieve information. Before it can be determined that the person is experiencing a memory lapse, it must be established that the material was learned in the first place. Memory problems typically are acquired rather than developmental. Depression may masquerade as memory loss, but the depressed person is usually less attentive or interactive with the environment and therefore registers (or learns) less. For example, a client may appear to be suffering from a memory dysfunction when, in fact, the decreased attention span is a result of depression that has reduced learning.

Learning disability occurs in a person with normal or near-normal intelligence as difficulty acquiring information in specific domains such as spelling, arithmetic, reading, and visual–spatial relationships. Therapists most commonly encounter learning disabilities manifested as noncompliance with written treatment programs, repeated tardiness or absence for treatment sessions, and an overly anxious approach to the physical symptoms that have brought the client to the therapist in the first place.

SPECIAL IMPLICATIONS FOR THE THERAPIST   **1-1**

Disability Classifications

Both the medical model and the ICF Health and Disability Model are reflected in this text. Diagnosis and treatment of disease are presented after the medical model, along with the ICF Model's assessment of the impact of acute and chronic conditions on the functioning of specific body systems (impairments) and basic human performance (functional limitations).

The ICF Model extends the scope of the medical model of disease with its primary emphasis on diagnosis and treatment of disease by placing the focus on the functional consequences of disease. Thus the reader will see terminology reflecting these two models such as *etiology, pathogenesis, diagnosis,* and *prognosis* from the traditional medical model and *impairments, interventions, desired outcomes,* and *functional limitations* from the Disablement Model.

Using these tools and the definition of clinical pathology, we ask the following: How does this particular disease or condition affect this person's functional abilities and functional outcome? What precautions should be taken when someone with this condition is exercising? Should vital signs be monitored during therapy for this disease? How will that information affect the plan of care or intervention?

Physical Disability

Each individual client must be evaluated on the basis of the clinical presentation in conjunction with the underlying pathology. For example, the person with osteoporosis may require joint mobilization, but this technique must be modified for the presence of osteoporosis. The individual with cardiac valvular disease may need a different exercise program than that prescribed for a healthy athlete. The adult with musculoskeletal symptoms of thoracic spine pain, muscle spasm, and loss of thoracic motion who has a primary medical diagnosis (e.g., posterior penetrating ulcer) will be unaffected by therapy techniques aimed at the human movement system.

Cognitive Disability

Although therapists cannot diagnose cognitive deficits, the therapist's evaluation and clinical observations may help identify cognitive deficits that might interfere with treatment. Appropriate referral is always recommended when problems beyond our expertise are suspected.

There is a new prevalence of executive function impairments as a result of new information regarding the impact of multiple concussions on cognitive performance.[8,61] Soldiers serving in combat zones or training to serve have a large incidence of blast injuries and concussions. In addition, athletes are being monitored for the effects of single concussion versus multiple concussions.[14,36] These topics will be discussed in more depth in subsequent chapters related to neurologic pathologies.

Overall, a person with cognitive impairments requires adapted intervention and follow-up strategies. The treatment area may have to be modified to reduce noise, reduce lighting, and reduce the amount of activity so that the person can concentrate and improve. Hope programs may need to be in an altered format and not exclusively written. Multisensory formatting such as audio recording, video recording, or many repetitions may need to be implemented to assist the client in succeeding with the home program.[27]

THEORIES OF HEALTH AND ILLNESS

Germ Theory

Many theories exist as to the cause of illnesses. In the latter part of the 19th century, Louis Pasteur took medicine out of the Dark Ages. It was not "bad air" or "bad blood" that caused diseases like malaria and yellow fever but pathogens transmitted by mosquitoes.

Pasteur's germ theory promoted our understanding of infectious disease and helped reduce deaths from infection. Pasteur proposed that a specific microorganism was capable of causing an infectious disease. Infections, such as poliomyelitis, tuberculosis, HIV associated with AIDS, or legionellosis (legionnaires' disease), are caused by a known agent. Once the causative agent is identified, specific treatment methods can be determined.

Pasteur's germ theory has been labeled Germ Theory, Part I, and has been expounded on by today's biologists in what is referred to as Germ Theory, Part II. Taken from Darwin's description of how an organism and its environment fit together, it is now restated that the success of an organism is relative to competing organisms. According to this theory, genetic traits that may be unfavorable to an organism's survival or reproduction do not persist in the gene pool for very long. Natural selection, by its very definition, weeds them out in short order. By this logic, any inherited disease or trait that has a serious impact on fitness must fade over time because the genes responsible for the disease or trait will be passed on to fewer and fewer individuals in future generations. Common illnesses that cannot be linked to genetics or to some hostile environmental element (including lifestyle) must have some other explanation.

The current germ theory suggests that diseases present in human populations for many generations that still have a substantial negative impact may have an infectious origin. Chronic diseases of the late 20th century that have been considered hereditary, environmental, or multifactorial may in fact be caused by an infectious pathogen. For example, herpesviruses have been linked to multiple sclerosis, Kaposi sarcoma, B-cell lymphomas, Burkitt lymphoma, and several other forms of cancer.

Heart disease is now being linked to infections such as herpes simplex virus, enterovirus, and *Chlamydia pneumoniae*, a bacterium that causes pneumonia and bronchitis. Several studies have now shown that people who have had a heart attack have high levels of antibodies to one or more of these infections from previous exposure, often during childhood.[1,33,35,49] But the germ theory does not account for all illness and disease as seen by the fact that chronic inflammation is also a large part of the underlying pathology of heart disease (as well as depression, diabetes, and cancer).[9,24,25,59,63]

Biomedical Model

The biomedical model explains disease as a result of malfunctioning organs or cells. Within this model, conditions can be classified as diseases if they have a recognized cause, if a change occurs in the structure or function of an organ, and if a consistently identifiable group of signs and symptoms is apparent. The biomedical model focuses on cause-and-effect relationships but does not take into account psychosocial components of disease, such as varying reactions to a disease because of age, lifestyle, personality, and compliance with therapy.

Neither the germ theory nor the biomedical model can explain the widespread increase in noninfectious chronic diseases that affect modern civilizations. In the past, the high death rate from epidemics of infectious diseases meant that many people did not live long enough for chronic illnesses to develop, especially those that occur

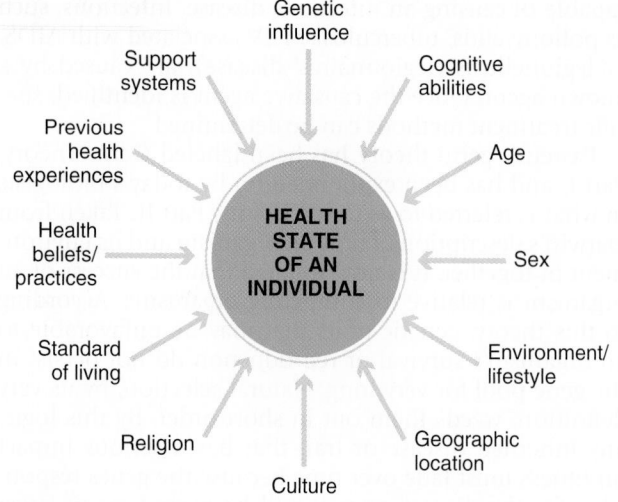

Figure 1-2

Multiple variables influence the health and illness of an individual. (From Ignatavicius DD, Workman ML: *Medical-surgical nursing: patient centered collaborative care*, ed 7, Philadelphia, 2010, WB Saunders.)

with aging. With the development of penicillin in 1928 and the subsequent development of other antibiotics, people in the 20th century have had reduced mortality from infectious disease.

Multicausal Theory

It is now recognized that lifestyle, diet, and stress response contribute to the development of diseases, and treatment interventions are focusing more on the relationship of the individual with his or her external and internal environment. Multicausal theories have been proposed to take into account the many additional factors associated with health and the development of illness (Fig. 1-2). Many of these variables are discussed further in Chapter 2.

Homeostasis Theory

Homeostasis theories developed in the 19th century continue to be expanded on through the 21st century. Homeostasis is the body's ability to maintain its internal environment in a constant state of equilibrium despite external influences that promote imbalance. Homeostasis begins at the cellular level in that the cell receives nutrients, oxygen, water, and essential minerals from the environment. It uses these resources to generate energy, maintain its own integrity, and contribute to the body's internal stability. The body's ability to maintain temperature, blood pressure, and levels of fluid and electrolytes, serum glucose, blood oxygen, and carbon dioxide within a given range are examples of dynamic homeostasis that begins at the cellular level. External stimuli can alter the body's equilibrium or homeostasis. External demands may exceed the capacity of the cell to adapt, resulting in a permanent disequilibrium and injury or illness.

Injury occurs when the cells or tissues have been required to adapt beyond their limitations. Like a muscle that has exceeded its ability to stretch, has ruptured, and is no longer able to contract, cells can be irreparably

damaged and unable to return to the original steady state. Illness is the result of an imbalance in the body's (cell's) ability to regulate the internal environment. The concept of "fight, flight, or freeze" to explain the body's reactions to emergencies was added to the homeostasis theory and continues to be used today to explain homeostasis as a dynamic equilibrium designed to maintain a steady state.

General Adaptation Syndrome

The general adaptation syndrome continued to build on the homeostasis theory and the concept of fight, flight, or freeze by describing a response to stress that, regardless of diagnosis, has common symptoms such as appetite loss, weight loss, myalgias, and fatigue. The entire body responds to stress in an attempt to maintain or adapt through the autonomic and central nervous systems. If the demand or stress continues, the adaptive capacity of the body can be exceeded, and disease may result.

This theory suggests that stress causes disease by placing excessive demands on the body, which in turn produces high levels of adaptive hormones, such as glucocorticoids, which reduce inflammation, and mineralocorticoid hormones, which regulate electrolyte and water metabolism. These hormones lower the body's resistance to disease and cause organ damage. When stress is continuous, the adaptive capacity of the body may be exceeded, and disease (or even death) may result.

Psychosocial Theory

Psychosocial theories of disease attempt to integrate physiologic, psychologic, and social factors to explain disease. An individual's degree of resistance to microbes depends largely on how well he or she is coping with internal and external stresses. Resistance to infectious disease, allergies, and possibly cancer depends on a well-functioning immune system. People who cope poorly with stress have significantly impaired immune responses, as manifested by a diminished activity level in natural killer cells. These are a special type of leukocyte that destroy viruses and cancer cells without having previously encountered them. Biopsychosocial-spiritual concepts as they relate to health are discussed more fully in Chapter 3.

Psychoneuroimmunology Theory

As new research added important information, the psychosocial theory has been modified to become the psychoneuroimmunology (PNI) model, first described in the 1980s. PNI is the study of the interactions among behavior and neural, endocrine, enteric, and immune system functions.

Those who founded the research in this area point out that PNI is a misnomer because it reveals only part of the process and redundantly includes the brain as psycho and neuro, leaving out the powerful impact of the endocrine system.[39] The literature refers to this theory by a variety of names, such as neuroendocrine immunology, neurogastroimmunology, or psychoimmunology, and is seemingly dependent on the system under investigation.

Illness was once thought of as the result of a breakdown within the immune system alone, but immune function is now recognized as the integrative defense mechanism of multiple systems. This theory has outlined the influence of the nervous system on immune and inflammatory responses and how the immune system communicates with the neuroendocrine systems. This information is very relevant in understanding host defenses and injury/repair processes.

Further, the integration of the hypothalamic–pituitary–adrenal axis and the neuro–endocrine–enteric axis has a biologic basis first discovered in the late 1990s. Physiologically adaptive processes occur as a result of these biochemically based mind–body connections. We now know that each thought and emotion is a message to the rest of the body, mediated by an intricate array of nerve signals, hormones, and various other substances.[19]

Candace Pert,[39,51] formerly a molecular biologist at the National Institutes of Health, made a groundbreaking discovery when she identified the biologic basis for emotions (neuropeptides and their receptors). This new understanding of the interconnections between the mind and body goes far beyond our former understanding of psychosomatic or psychosocial theories of health and illness.

It is now known that these chemical messengers (sometimes referred to as peptides, neuropeptides, ligands, neurotransmitters, or information molecules) move through the bloodstream to every cell of the body. When these chemicals find body cells with receptors that attract them like magnets, they attach and make significant changes in that cell structure and organ system. These information molecules are the messengers the body uses to communicate between all the major body systems. For example, both the digestive (enteric) system and the neurologic system communicate with the immune system via these peptides. These three systems can exchange information and influence one another's actions.

Knowledge of PNI sheds new light on many of the previously postulated theories of health and illness, whereas understanding dysfunctions in the PNI system may highlight a wide variety of system disorders and diseases. For example, explaining how the body maintains homeostasis through autonomic temperature regulation (homeostasis theory) will now have an added dimension when considering the role of these information molecules or understanding that the sympathetic nervous system controls cardiovascular and immune functions, hormones control energy balance, and neurohormones control salt and fluid balance (general adaptation syndrome) via the interactions of the PNI.

Continued research in this area has brought new information to light about the effects of variables, such as stress and coping, personality, mental status, socioeconomic status, and work and family life, and their role in the outcome of surgery or the development and progression of disease, morbidity, and mortality (e.g., Multicausal Theory, Psychosocial Theory).[7,22,42]

Energy Medicine

Many well-known scientists (e.g., Candace Pert, James Oschman, Larry Dossey) with extensive training and research in the areas of biophysics and biology have attempted to bring together evidence from a range of disciplines to provide an acceptable explanation for the energetic exchanges that take place in all therapies.[18,50] Studies in biophysics have shown that physical instabilities result in fluctuations, the quantum properties of which can be applied to regulatory control mechanisms in living organisms with promising results. The discovery of the existence of macroscopic quantum coherence in living systems has led to a new field of mind–body medicine and a new understanding of the role of natural "energy forces" within the body in maintaining normal health and well-being.[31]

At the same time, behavioral scientists have been exploring the concept that consciousness in the form of beliefs, expectations, and intention plays a central role in healing. Studies of prayer and the spiritual aspects of medicine have moved many health care professionals away from a biomedical model of health care to a model of whole-person caring.[36] This in turn has led to interest in how these energies or forces may be used to assist in healing and the restoration of normal health. The concept of energy medicine has resulted in a new discipline called complementary and alternative medicine or complementary and integrative medicine.

HEALTH PROMOTION AND DISEASE PREVENTION

The topic of health promotion and disease prevention has taken front and center stage in many arenas within the health care industry. There has been a change in health care focus from intervention for cure and healing to healing, health, wellness, and prevention. Traditional health promotion has not been to take care of the sick and disabled but rather to prevent disease and disability in the healthy.[23] Today's concepts of health place all health on a continuum. The focus is on practicing healthy behaviors, even in the presence of disease and disability. Although disability can increase a person's risk of or susceptibility to secondary health conditions, the primary disability does not mean that individual is "unhealthy."

Research has proved without a shadow of a doubt that many of today's illnesses, disorders, and conditions can be prevented altogether. Diseases of longevity, lifestyle, and health behaviors are prevalent, and more people are living longer with chronic diseases, all of which drive up the cost of health care. The health care industry as a whole and especially third-party payers have been slow to respond with ways to change our approach to this information.

The first set of national health targets was published in 1979 in Healthy People: The Surgeon General's Report on Health Promotion and Disease Prevention. Healthy People 2000 was released in 1990 as a management tool with goals to reduce mortality, increase independence among older adults, reduce disparities in health among different population groups, and achieve access to preventive health services.

This program has become an ongoing comprehensive program of public health planning now called *Healthy People 2020* that is a tremendously valuable asset to all who work to improve health. *Healthy People 2020* (available at http://health.gov/healthypeople/) has a series of objectives to bring better health to all people in this country and to eliminate disparities among different segments of the population. These include differences that occur by gender, race or ethnicity, education or income, disability, residence in rural localities, and sexual orientation. This program has a built-in means to measure progress toward achieving 10-year targets across a broad range of health behaviors and outcomes.

Health Promotion

Health promotion as a concept and as an active process is built on the principles of self-responsibility, nutritional awareness, stress reduction and management, and physical fitness. Health promotion is not limited to any particular age or level of ability but rather extends throughout the life span from before birth (e.g., prenatal care) through old age, including anyone with a disability of any kind.

Health promotion programs that encompass the entire life span are applicable to people of both genders and all socioeconomic and cultural backgrounds, to those who have no health problems, and to those with chronic illnesses and disabilities. Many types of health promotion programs are in existence such as health screening, wellness, safety, stress management, or support groups for specific diseases.

Disease Prevention

Even since the last edition of this text, disease prevention has gained momentum and today is at the forefront of the health care industry. It is now recognized and addressed by greater numbers of health care professionals that preventing disease is more cost-effective than treating disease. Many new areas of study have developed as a result of this paradigm shift in focus from treatment to prevention. Scientists are revolutionizing the way we fight infection, manage chronic illness, and stay well. For example, one group has coined the term immunotics to describe this new approach to preventing and treating disease.[17]

Immunotics is to the 21st century what antibiotics were to the 20th century—but perhaps even better. Whereas antibiotics are used to treat illness after it occurs, immunotics is designed to prevent illness in the first place. Unlike antibiotics, which can have serious side effects, immunotics has no side effects; at the very least it adopts the Hippocratic philosophy of do no harm.[17]

In another area, cancer prevention strategies to reduce the incidence of cancer occurrence and recurrence have commanded the attention of oncology researchers. Chemoprevention, the use of agents to inhibit and reverse cancer, has focused on diet-derived agents. Another term, preventive oncology, is a relatively new branch of medicine that includes both primary and secondary prevention.

Preventive medicine as a branch of medicine is categorized as primary, secondary, or tertiary. Primary prevention is geared toward removing or reducing disease risk factors, for example, by maintaining adequate levels of calcium intake and regular exercise as a means of preventing osteoporosis and subsequent bone fractures or by giving up or not starting smoking to reduce multiple causes of morbidity. Use of seat belts, use of helmets by motorcyclists and bicyclists, and immunizations are other examples of primary prevention strategies.

Secondary prevention techniques are designed to promote early detection of disease and to employ preventive measures to avoid further complications. Examples of secondary prevention include skin tests for tuberculosis or screening procedures such as mammography, colonoscopy, or routine cervical Papanicolaou smear.

Tertiary prevention measures are aimed at limiting the impact of established disease (e.g., radiation or chemotherapy to control localized cancer). Tertiary prevention involves rehabilitation and may end when no further healing is expected. The goal of tertiary prevention is to return the person to the highest possible level of functioning and to prevent severe disabilities.

Specific therapy interventions are not the focus of this text but, whenever possible, risk factor reduction strategies are offered because risk factors are a part of the discussion surrounding each disease and therapists play an important role in disease prevention and health promotion.

SPECIAL IMPLICATIONS FOR THE THERAPIST **1-2**

Health Promotion and Disease Prevention

The practice of physical and occupational therapies is becoming increasingly complex. Rapid changes in the health care system are placing increased pressure on therapists for effective and efficient management of clients amid fast client turnover and high productivity quotas. Additionally, many individuals seeking physical and occupational therapy services have extensive medical histories requiring careful evaluation. Yet diagnosis, prediction of prognosis, intervention, and client-family education must be done quickly and accurately. The integration of examination, evaluation, diagnosis, prognosis, and intervention (including health promotion and prevention education) is an important part of routine client management.[33]

In many hospitals, decreased acute care length of stay means that physical and occupational therapists are being consulted or called on to treat clients earlier in the course of the hospitalization to help prevent secondary complications of immobility. For example, in the acute care setting, decreasing mortality from critical illness has led to an increasing number of ICU survivors. A new approach for managing critically ill patients includes reducing deep sedation and increasing rehabilitation therapy and mobilization soon after admission to the ICU. Survivors of severe critical illness commonly have significant and prolonged neuromuscular complications that impair their physical function and quality of life after hospital discharge (see "Discussion" in Chapter 5).

Understanding the diseases, surgeries, and medications frequently encountered in practice is necessary for safe and appropriate interventions and establishing a reasonable prognosis. The APTA Guide to Physical Therapist

Practice[3] *describes the components that make up the history portion of an examination. These components include the investigation of a client's coexisting health problems, such as illnesses, surgeries, and medications that have implications for health promotion, disease prevention, and direct treatment interventions.*[10]

Role in Secondary and Tertiary Care[3]

Physical and occupational therapists play major roles in secondary and tertiary care. Clients with musculoskeletal, neuromuscular, cardiopulmonary, or integumentary conditions are often treated initially by another health care practitioner and then referred to the therapist for secondary care. Therapists provide secondary care in a wide range of settings from hospitals to preschools.

Tertiary care is provided by therapists in highly specialized, complex, and technologically based settings (e.g., transplant services, burn units, emergency departments) or when supplying specialized services (e.g., to clients with spinal cord lesions or closed-head trauma) in response to requests for consultation made by other health care practitioners.

Role in Prevention and Wellness[3]

Physical and occupational therapists are involved in prevention and wellness activities, screening programs, and the promotion of positive health behavior. These initiatives decrease costs by helping clients achieve and restore optimal functional capacity; minimize impairments, functional limitations, and disabilities related to congenital and acquired conditions; maintain health and thereby prevent further deterioration or future illness; and create appropriate environmental adaptations to enhance independent function.

Prevention is not confined to a single form of presentation but rather takes one of three forms: primary, secondary, or tertiary. All individuals are included—even those who already have one or more primary disabilities.

Primary prevention involves preventing disease in a susceptible or potentially susceptible population through general health promotion. Secondary prevention comprises decreasing duration of illness, severity of disease, and sequelae through early diagnosis and prompt intervention. Tertiary prevention includes limiting the degree of disability and promoting rehabilitation and restoration of function in clients with chronic and irreversible diseases.

As mentioned, acute care therapists are especially involved in secondary and tertiary prevention regarding complications of mechanical ventilation and immobility in the ICU. Early mobility is decreasing length of stay with greater likelihood of discharge to home and rehab versus extended care facilities.

The beneficial role of prescriptive exercise for health and disease has been documented many times and in many ways. When prescribed appropriately, exercise, including cardiovascular training, endurance training, and strength training, is effective for developing fitness and health, for increasing life expectancy, for the prevention of injury and disease, and for the rehabilitation of impairments and disabilities (see Box 2-2).

Prescriptive exercise programs to develop and maintain a significant amount of muscle mass, endurance, and strength contribute to overall fitness and health. Exercise plays a significant role in reducing risk factors associated with disease states (e.g., osteoporosis, diabetes mellitus, heart disease), the risk of falls and associated injuries, and the morbidity associated with chronic disease.[22]

Although not as abundant, the evidence also suggests that involvement in regular exercise can provide a number of psychologic benefits related to preserved cognitive function, alleviation of depression symptoms and behavior, and an improved concept of personal control and self-direction. It is important to note that although participation in physical activity may not always elicit increases in the traditional markers of physiologic performance and fitness in older adults (e.g., maximum oxygen consumption [VO_2max], body composition, blood pressure changes), it does improve health as measured by a reduction in disease risk factors and improved functional capacity and quality of life in the aging population.[2]

As always, when planning treatment interventions, including client education, the therapist must take into consideration the comorbidities and pathologic processes present. This requires identification of lifestyle factors (e.g., amount of exercise, stress, weight) that lead to increased risk for serious health problems, identification of risk factors for disease or injury, and performance of screening examinations (e.g., osteoporosis, skin cancer).

As a final reminder, the study and understanding of basic mechanisms of disease physiology and pathokinesiology along with the identification of lifestyle or risk factors are necessary but insufficient guides for clinical practice. Many variables affect the relationships among pathology, impairments, and disability. Attention must be paid to the psychosocial, spiritual, educational, and environmental variables that can modify client outcomes.[19]

GENETIC ASPECTS OF HEALTH AND DISEASE

Advances in immunology and molecular genetics have accelerated our understanding of the genetic and cellular basis of many diseases. Remarkable progress has been made in recombinant deoxyribonucleic acid (DNA) technology, making it possible to offer molecular and cellular treatments for infectious diseases, inherited disorders, and cancer. Development of the monoclonal antibody technique is finding ever-increasing uses in the treatment of diseases such as rheumatoid arthritis, cancer, and AIDS.[46]

At the same time, innovations in gene therapy have advanced the field of vaccine development, especially recombinant vaccine technology. Although the field of vaccination has historically focused on the prevention of infectious diseases, this technology provides a broader base for immune modulation of pathologic responses underlying other conditions.[46]

The completion of the Human Genome Project just 50 years after the discovery of the structure of DNA, combined with advances in technology, has enabled researchers to begin identifying the actual genes that encode particular disorders.[48] It may be possible in the near future to treat altered gene structure (gene therapy) in an attempt to cure or control previously incurable diseases. The laboratory studies and advances in the collection of immune cells made it possible to begin clinical trials of gene therapy in the early

1990s. The recent explosion in biotechnology has advanced the field of genetic testing, which is a necessary component in the genetic treatment of diseases and disorders.

The development of epigenetics, the study of the molecular mechanisms by which the environment controls gene activity, is one of the most active areas of scientific research today. The genetic code that we call the "blueprint of life," our DNA, changes with the environment. Environment includes not just the toxins in our air and water and electromagnetic noise from cell phone towers, power lines, and transformer stations but our beliefs, emotions, and thoughts as well. Epigenetics is beginning to show us that we are not just "victims" of heredity or other environmental factors that are out of our control.[11]

The role of the environment in regulating gene activity has taken a more front and center priority in research investigating control above genetics. Environmental influences, including nutrition, stress, thoughts, and emotions can influence the behavior of cells without changing the genetic code but can also modify genes and be passed on to future generations. It is starting to look like epigenetic mechanisms have a much larger role to play in diseases such as cancer, cardiovascular impairments, and diabetes than even heredity.[41]

The Human Genome Project

The Human Genome Project, an international project led in the United States by the National Human Genome Research Institute and the Department of Energy, was completed in April 2003 and provides a reference DNA sequence of the human genome. Researchers identified 25,000 genes existing in 23 pairs of chromosomes and deciphered the genetic code by sequencing the 3.1 billion base pairs of human DNA and mapping their location in the chromosomes.

Genes are the chemical messengers of heredity. Two hundred thousand (200,000) human genes composed of DNA molecules along a double helix and carrying instructions for synthesizing every protein that the body needs to function properly (Fig. 1-3) have been identified. Their order determines the function of the gene. Genes determine everything from appearance to the regulation of everyday life processes (e.g., how efficiently we process foods, how effectively we fight infection).

DNA is composed of different combinations of molecules called *nucleic acids.* The sequence of nucleic acids provides instructions for assembling amino acids, which are the basic structural units of proteins (Fig. 1-4). A change in the normal DNA pattern of a particular gene is called a *mutation.* Some illnesses are caused by a tiny change in the DNA of just one gene, whereas others are caused by major changes in the DNA of multiple genes.

Most illnesses, including many cases of cancer, are caused by acquired mutations. Acquired mutations arise during normal daily life, usually during the process of cell division. Each day the body replaces thousands of worn-out cells. Some genetic errors are inevitable as old cells replicate and pass DNA flaws along to replacement (daughter) cells. When all goes well, daughter cells recognize these mutations and repair them, but the repair mechanism can fail or be disabled by environmental toxins and diet. Although acquired mutations can be passed on to daughter cells, they cannot be inherited.

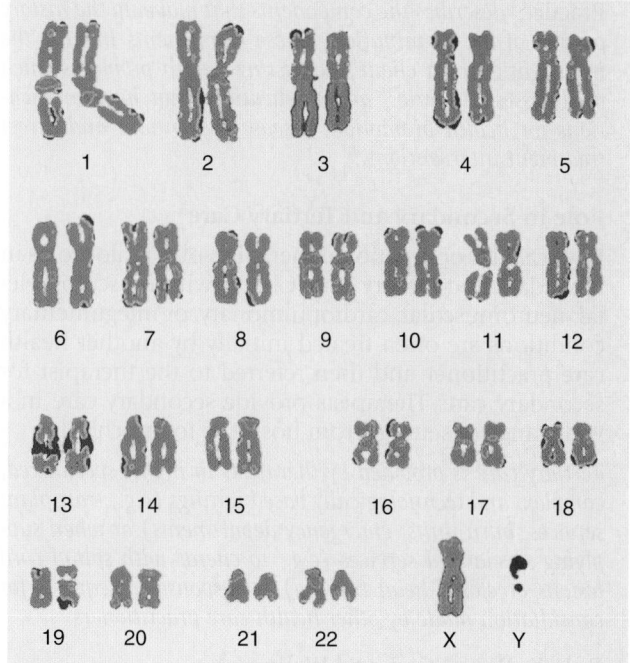

Figure 1-3

Example of genetic basis for cancer found in early cervical carcinoma. The gain of chromosome 3q (tumor DNA seen as *green*) that occurs with human papillomavirus 16 infection defines the transition from severe dysplasia/carcinoma in situ to invasive carcinoma of the uterine cervix. Genetic testing can help identify chromosomal aberrations such as this that occur during carcinogenesis. (From Heselmeyer K, Schrock E, du Manoir S, et al: Gain of chromosome 3q defines the transition from severe dysplasia to invasive carcinoma of the uterine cervix. *Proc Natl Acad Sci U S A* 93:479–484, 1996.)

The goals of the Genome project have been to identify all human genes, map the genes' locations on chromosomes, and ultimately provide detailed information from the genetic coding about how the genes function. Because virtually every human illness and even many lifestyle-related conditions have a hereditary component, the Human Genome Project may hold the key to the prevention or cure of many, if not all, diseases and disorders.[38]

The Human Genome Project dispelled the idea that race- or ethnicity-based biologic differences existed when they discovered that 99.99% of the genome is the same across the human population, regardless of race or ethnic origin. Individual variations can increase the risk of disease as some people can become more vulnerable to bacteria, viruses, toxins, and chemicals, but the Human Genome Project disproved many previously held beliefs about biologically based racial differences.

Knowing the order in which these chemical units are arranged on each strand of DNA does not tell where the genes are located within the genome, the specific function of each gene in the sequence, or which genes make which proteins. The study of genomes has been labeled *genomics,* which includes the investigation of an organism's entire hereditary information encoded in the DNA. The term comes from the words *gene* and *chromosome.*

The genome of any organism (including humans) is a complete DNA sequence of one set of chromosomes.

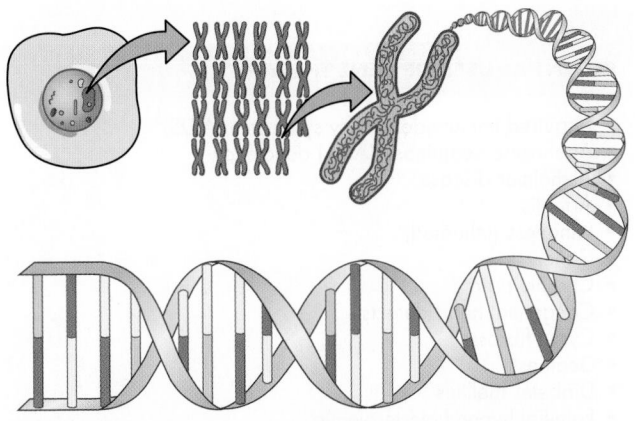

Figure 1-4

Schematic diagram of deoxyribonucleic acid (DNA). Inside the nucleus of nearly every cell in the body, a complex set of genetic instructions, known as the *human genome*, is contained on 23 pairs of chromosomes. Chromosomes are made of long chains of a chemical called *DNA*, packaged into short segments called *genes*. Every cell of every human body contains a copy of the same DNA. Genes contain instructions to direct all body functions written in a molecular language. This molecular language is made up of four letters; each letter represents a molecule on the DNA: adenine, cytosine, guanine, thymine. The As, Cs, Gs, and Ts form in triplets, constituting a code; each triplet of letters instructs the cell to attach to a particular amino acid (e.g., TGG attaches to amino acid tryptophan). Amino acids combined together form proteins. If the DNA language becomes garbled or a word is misspelled, the cell may make the wrong protein or too much or too little of the right one—mistakes that often result in disease.

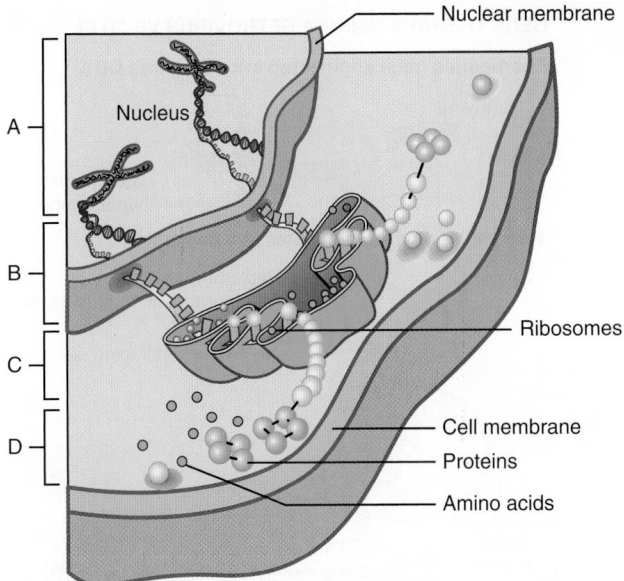

Figure 1-5

The chain of events from DNA; this is how the DNA directs the cell. A, Ribonucleic acid (RNA) receives instructions from the DNA code in the chromosomes. **B,** The RNA travels from the nucleus to link up with ribosomes (protein-making units). **C,** Instructions from the code contained within the DNA are used by the RNA–ribosome complex to assemble amino acids. **D,** Cellular function is now directed by proteins containing the amino acids.

Genomics is different from genetics, which is generally the study of single genes or groups of genes. Genomics with its unfolding of the complete DNA sequences will provide a basis for the study of susceptibility to disease, the pathogenesis of disease, and the development of new preventive and therapeutic approaches.

Additionally, the completion of the Human Genome Project has enhanced the widespread use of prenatal diagnosis and DNA chip technology and will make it possible to analyze a sample of DNA collected from saliva. Drugs designed and prescribed to accommodate individual differences in metabolism may be possible from the data derived from this project. All of these areas of interest will be the substance of future studies.

Information about the genes is made available immediately on the Internet to scientists, clinicians, librarians, educators, and the general public. The cataloging and filing of this information are under the auspices of the Cancer Genome Anatomy Project. The Human Cancer Genome Project is another program that is attempting to develop a comprehensive description of the genetic basis of human cancer and specifically the complete identification and characterization of genetic alterations present in a large number of major types of cancer (Fig. 1-5).

Gene Therapy

Gene therapy is the science of replacing genes or other defective cells; it is a means of treating diseases by genetic manipulation.[58] Gene therapy may be able to help heal injuries or replace worn out tissue that lead to pain and disability from degenerative processes.

More specifically, gene therapy (also known as human genetic engineering) is the process in which specific malfunctioning cells are targeted and repaired or replaced with corrected genes (Fig. 1-6). A gene can be delivered to a cell using a carrier known as a "vector." The most common types of vectors used in gene therapy are genetically altered viruses, but nonviral vectors are being developed as potential gene delivery vehicles as well. Essentially, DNA is used like a drug, allowing it to replace or repair defective genes. It is hoped that the altered cells will yield daughter cells with healthy genes; these offspring cells will help eliminate the diseased cells. Alternatively, cells can be genetically altered to contain a toxin-producing suicide gene to treat some cancers.[40]

Uses for Gene Therapy

Research is ongoing into such cures for a wide variety of hereditary disorders and diseases caused by aging (Box 1-1); some diseases, such as hemophilia, are being studied as a good model for gene therapy. At present, there are three main gene therapy strategies for treatment of cancer: oncolytic viruses, suicide gene therapy, and gene-based immunotherapy. Gendicine, the first approved anticancer drug based on the gene therapy principle, makes use of oncolytic viruses.[58] Gene therapy for the treatment of diseases in children before birth is being actively pursued at many medical centers using animal models. In utero gene therapy could be beneficial for those with genetic diseases if gene therapy is performed before symptoms are manifested.[47,64,49]

Gene therapy is being investigated as a means of helping injuries heal, replacing worn-out tissue, reducing scar

GENE THERAPY USING A RETROVIRUS VECTOR

Therapeutic gene engineered into retrovirus DNA

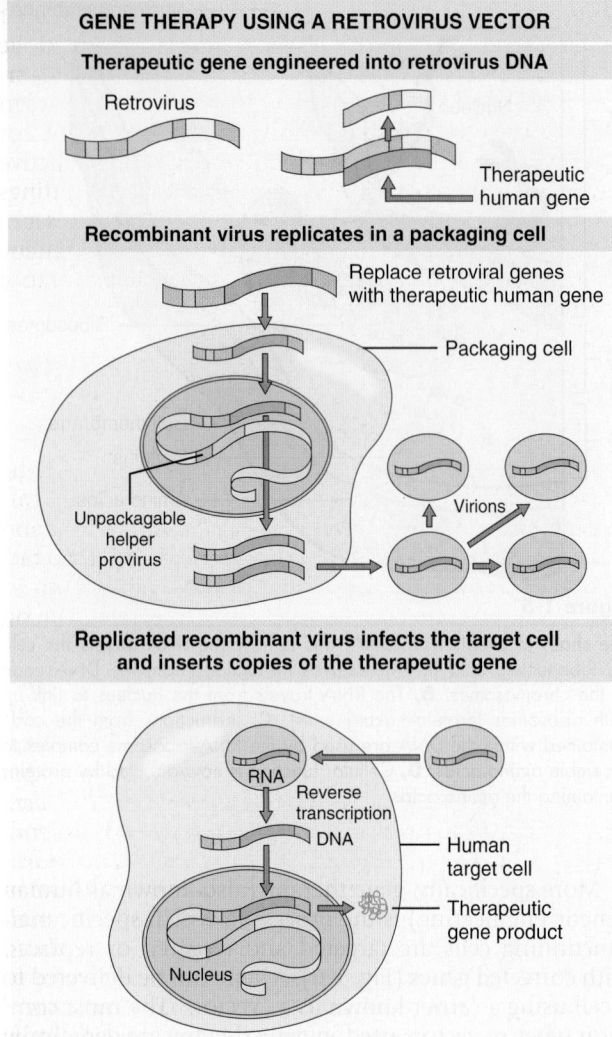

Recombinant virus replicates in a packaging cell

Replicated recombinant virus infects the target cell and inserts copies of the therapeutic gene

Figure 1-6

Gene therapy. A therapeutic gene is engineered genetically into the retrovirus DNA and replaces most of the viral DNA sequences. The recombinant virus that carries the therapeutic gene is allowed to replicate in a special "packaging cell," which also contains normal virus that carries the genes required for viral replication. The replicated recombinant virus is allowed to infect the human diseased tissue, or "target cell." The recombinant virus may invade the diseased tissue but cannot replicate or destroy the cell. The recombinant virus inserts copies of the normal therapeutic gene into the host genome and produces the normal protein product. (From Yanoff M, Duker JS: *Ophthalmology*, ed 3, St. Louis, MO, 2008, Mosby.)

tissue, or fusing spinal segments together. The gene for bone growth has been injected into the disk space and shown to signal enough bone growth to bridge the bone on either side of the space. Investigational studies using animals may find an injectable method to fuse bone to replace the costly and complicated spinal fusion surgery.[53]

Gene insertion has been used to successfully treat humans with inoperable coronary artery disease. Researchers injected a gene that makes a protein called vascular endothelial growth factor into the hearts of candidates with severe chest pain caused by ischemia that could not be corrected with bypass surgery or angioplasty. Tests suggest that once installed, the gene produces blood vessel–promoting proteins for 2 or 3 weeks (enough

POTENTIAL USES OF GENE THERAPY*

- Acquired immunodeficiency syndrome (AIDS)
- Adenosine deaminase (ADA) deficiency
- Alzheimer disease
- Arthritis
- Blindness (inherited)
- Cancer
- Chronic pain
- Congenital heart defects
- Cystic fibrosis
- Deafness
- Diabetes mellitus
- Familial hypercholesterolemia
- Heart disease
- Hemophilia
- Hepatitis
- Huntington disease
- Hypertension
- Immunodeficiency syndrome (HIV/AIDS)
- Liver failure
- Marfan syndrome
- Mesothelioma
- Muscular dystrophy (Duchenne)
- Neurofibromatosis
- Parkinson disease
- Peripheral vascular disease
- Schizophrenia
- Severe combined immunodeficiency (SCID)
- Sickle cell disease

* This is only a partial list of diseases or disorders being studied and compiled from research reported but should give the reader an idea of the broad and varied applications of genetic manipulation intended to treat, cure, or prevent disease.

to grow a permanent new blood supply) before ceasing to work. The heart actually sprouts tiny new blood vessels (therapeutic angiogenesis) too small to be seen but with improved blood flow to the heart readily demonstrated.[30,54] Investigations continue to examine gene therapy strategies to deliver genes coding for the angiogens.

Approaches to Gene Therapy

Gene therapy may take a number of different approaches. The original design was to inject one or more genes into the person to replace those that are absent or not functioning properly. A second approach called small-molecule therapy injects a small molecule (i.e., a drug) to modify the function of one or more genes in the body that is making a normal product but just too much or too little of it.

Other approaches include transferring a gene into cancer cells to sensitize them to drugs[20] or restoring immune function in HIV[32] by transferring a therapeutic gene into target cells, rendering them resistant to HIV replication. Infusion of protected cells may limit virus spread and delay AIDS disease progression. Efforts are underway to deliver antiviral genes to hematopoietic stem cells to ensure a renewable supply of HIV-protected cells for the life of the individual.[13,15,39]

Germ-line gene therapy is an approach that delivers genes to sperm or egg (or to the cells that produce them). It might prevent defective genes from being transmitted to subsequent generations by repairing the original genetic defect in germ cells. Gene modification at an early stage of embryonic development might also be a way of correcting gene defects in both the germ-line and body cells. This therapy is highly controversial because it carries an unknown level of risk (interference with another gene, specificity of the insertion). As a consequence, germ-line gene therapy is not being considered for application to humans at this time. In the future, if scientists determine ways to make sure that a transferred gene goes into the cell's genome at the same position as the already mutated gene, then the safety of germ-line gene therapy procedures might be dramatically increased.

Obstacles to Gene Therapy

Some obstacles to gene therapy must be overcome before this procedure can be considered a viable treatment option. Examples include finding appropriate harmless viral vectors to carry the normal gene to the target cells that do not provoke an immune response against them as foreign invaders or cause toxic side effects, engineering the transplanted genes to be efficient and effective, and finding ways to modify retrovirus vectors so they can carry the genes into nondividing cells (presently, genes can only be delivered to actively dividing cells when delivered by retrovirus vectors).

Ethical concerns have also been raised about the use of human genetic engineering for purposes other than therapy (e.g., eugenics).[43] These include the use of genes to improve ourselves cosmetically, improve memory, increase intelligence,[37] accomplish ethnic cleansing ("designer babies" genetically engineered before birth),[44] or cause permanent changes in the gene pool. Some researchers are advocating the use of human genetic engineering for the treatment of serious diseases only.[6]

Gene Doping. Gene therapy in sports athletes, called *gene doping*, involves transferring genes directly into human cells to blend with an athlete's own DNA, enhancing muscle growth and increasing strength or endurance. Gene doping is banned in sports, and although there has been no direct evidence yet to prove it, there is some concern that gene doping has already begun.[28,62]

Concerns have been raised about long-term effects such as leukemia, other forms of cancer, and unknown effects, including the potential harm in passing changes on to the athlete's children. Although not currently in use, the potential for gene doping to enhance performance has been discussed in the literature.[29,60]

Gene Testing. The rapidly expanding field of genetic testing holds great promise for detecting many devastating illnesses long before their symptoms become apparent. Such testing identifies people who have inherited a faulty gene that may (or may not) lead to a particular disorder. In the last 15 years, such predictive tests have been developed for more than 200 of the 4000 diseases thought to be caused by inherited gene mutations. The result has been earlier monitoring, preventive treatments, and in some cases, planning for long-term care.

However, gene testing is not without its difficulties. For example, the presence of a particular mutation does not mean that illness is inevitable, making the interpretation of test results a highly complex task. The psychologic implications of predictive testing must be considered. Identifying who is a candidate for testing remains to be determined. Inheritance accounts for a limited number of diseases, suggesting that genetic testing should be reserved for people with a strong family history of a particular disease. Safeguards and protocols are not always in place before testing finds its way into general practice. For these reasons, it has been recommended that predictive testing should be confined to research or clinical settings where skilled counseling is available. Other ethical issues and privacy concerns, such as the potential use of genetic testing to screen job applicants or to qualify for insurance coverage, must also be settled.

SPECIAL IMPLICATIONS FOR THE THERAPIST   1-3

Genetic Aspects of Disease

As scientists strive to unravel the complex etiologic factors of diseases, such as obesity, diabetes, and cardiovascular disease, through the use of molecular and genetic tools now available, understanding the interaction and influence of environmental factors, such as exercise, on gene expression and function has taken on increasing importance.

The Human Genome Project emphasizes the importance of other factors in disease susceptibility when genetic differences are eliminated. For example, regular exercise has been shown to improve glucose tolerance, control of lipid abnormalities, diabetes mellitus, hypertension, bone density, immune function, psychologic function, sleep patterns, and obesity, with the greatest benefits realized by sedentary individuals who begin to exercise for the first time or after an extended period of inactivity. Responses to exercise interventions are often highly variable among individuals, and research has indicated that response to exercise may be mediated or influenced in large part by variation in genes.[12]

The study of acute and chronic effects of exercise on the structure and function of organ systems is now a field of research referred to as exercise science. During the last 30 years, exercise-related research has rapidly transitioned from focus on an organ to a subcellular/molecular focus. It is expected that genetic research will focus on translating fundamental knowledge into solving the complexities of a number of degenerative diseases influenced heavily by activity/inactivity factors such as cardiopulmonary disease, diabetes mellitus, obesity, and the debilitating disorders associated with aging.[6]

Individual genotypes and other genetic information may eventually help therapists assess a client's risk for conditions, enable us to understand why some people respond to the same intervention faster or better than others who have the same diagnosis, and develop and execute an appropriate plan of care. Gene therapy and the elimination of some diseases and conditions may contribute to the continued trend to focus on health and fitness for physical therapists of the future.[52]

REFERENCES

To enhance this text and add value for the reader, all references are included on the companion Evolve site that accompanies this textbook. The reader can view the reference source and access it online whenever possible.

CHAPTER 2

Behavioral, Social, and Environmental Factors Contributing to Disease and Dysfunction

TAMARA L. BURLIS • SUSAN S. DEUSINGER • DENISE GAFFIGAN-BENDER

OVERVIEW

Using the concepts of health and disease presented in Chapter 1, we recognize that the consequences of disease include effects on tissues (pathology), on organs or organ systems (impairments), and on the person's ability to function in daily life (disability, activity limitations) and in society (handicap, participation restrictions). As rehabilitation specialists, physical therapists reduce (mitigate) the impact of the effects of disease by focusing on improving physical function and/or performance of daily activities.

Aside from the pathology itself, many behavioral, social, and environmental factors influence health and may mitigate (or alternately, enhance) the effects of disease. The impact of these factors on the disease process or the consequences of disease will be a major focus of this chapter. The influence of selected behavioral, social support, and environmental factors on health will be reviewed separately with models or theories described that integrate these components in defining and characterizing health.

During the last two decades of the 20th century, health care professionals developed a better understanding of the importance of behavioral and social issues and how unhealthy behaviors are linked to many conditions and diseases. This shift in emphasis encourages the development of new treatments or interventions that can impact an individual's health.

The Centers for Disease Control and Prevention (CDC) has responded to a growing awareness of these changes by establishing three new internal units to deal with them directly: (1) the National Center for Chronic Disease Prevention and Health Promotion; (2) The National Center for Injury Prevention and Control; and (3) the National Center for HIV, STD, and TB Prevention. The task of these groups is to focus on conditions, diseases, and injuries that have clear behavioral risks.[152]

Other areas of behavioral and social research have focused on social forces affecting the environment that could impact health and the influence of class, family structure, and ethnicity on health and illness.[154] In keeping with these changes in the direction of behavioral and social sciences in public health, the intent of this chapter is to increase the physical therapists' understanding of behavioral, social, and environmental issues in addition to the pathology that can affect health and physical function.

Role of the Physical Therapist in the Current Health Care Environment

Physical therapists have received recognition as essential health care professionals within the current health care delivery system. The American Physical Therapy Association (APTA) has provided a vision for physical therapists in society as partners in the national health agenda.[291] The physical therapist will be the recognized specialist in the human movement system. In this role, physical therapists provide primary care (including rehabilitation), primary and secondary prevention, and health promotion while also reducing the effects of disease to protect the physical health and mobility of the human movement system.[291]

Our practice as physical therapists takes us from birth to death through all health care settings (e.g., emergency departments, schools, home health, inpatient, outpatient, transitional unit, assisted living, long-term care, hospice, and so on). We must not be constrained to the medical model with its emphasis on the diagnosis and treatment of disease or injury in an environment of episodic care, but rather address the effects of disease or injury on the human movement system across the life span[291] or life stages.

In accordance with *Healthy People 2020*,[306] physical therapists are involved in guiding others to practice safe physical activity across the many life stages (infancy and childhood, preadolescence, adolescence, young adult, middle-aged adult, older adult, and senior and frail adult).[291,67] This includes preventing disease or injury at the community level, risk reduction at all life stages, preventing early disability, promoting the health and well-being of people with disabilities, and assisting children and adults who have comorbid health conditions.

CLINICAL MODELS OF HEALTH

The theories of health and illness presented in Chapter 1 are the basis for many different models of health; most can be narrowed down to the following main approaches:

- Biomedical model focuses on the disease process.
- Biopsychosocial model describes the role of biological, psychological, and social factors on a person's health.
- Biopsychosocial-spiritual model develops the biopsychosocial model one step further so that the physical, mental, social, *and* spiritual aspects of a person's life are viewed as an integrated whole.
- Social-ecologic model describes multiple levels of interaction that influence health.

Biomedical Model

The biomedical model of health care has governed the thinking of most health practitioners for the past three centuries holding to the premise that all illness can be explained based on disorder and disease of bodily anatomy and physiologic processes. This model assumes that psychologic, social, and spiritual influences are independent of the disease process. Chemical or mechanical treatments are aimed at the underlying pathophysiology and pathoanatomy in order to treat the underlying disease process and improve health, if not provide a cure.[321]

Traditionally, physical therapists have approached rehabilitation from a medical model mediated through the mechanism of physiologic impairments. The medical model generally considers the underlying assumptions that pathology should be treated or cured and that pathology leads directly to consequences, including impairment, limitations in physical function, and diminished quality of life. The medical model is then logically focused on eliminating pathology or the resulting impairments, which would then lead to improved function.

Although this model is important for understanding medical care, it does not address the other factors that influence a person's physical or mental health. The medical model focuses on factors internal to the individual that directly affect an individual's health status; however, considerable information now indicates that factors external to an individual also play a significant role in a person's health status.

Biopsychosocial Model

By contrast, the biopsychosocial model of health and illness supports the idea that biologic, psychologic, and social variables are key factors in health and illness. The mind and body cannot be separated because they both influence the state of health. The biopsychosocial model emphasizes health and illness, rather than considering illness as a deviation of the healthy state.

In this model, a person's psychologic system, including aspects of cognition, emotion, and motivation, interacts with biologic and environmental factors to produce various states of health. Likewise, how an individual interacts with family, community, and society also influences health outcomes.[321] The World Health Organization's (WHO's) *International Classification of Functioning, Disability, and Health* (ICF) adopted by the APTA is a biopsychosocial model of health.

Compared to the biomedical model, the biopsychosocial approach has several benefits. First, it includes factors other than physical condition that influence health. For example, this approach helps explain differences in outcomes for individuals with persistent pain as a result of living in difficult social conditions. And it encourages health care professional and clients to work together to find solutions to problems in order to enhance the healing process.[87] The downside of this approach is to place blame on the individual for his or her health status, while neglecting the influence of social or environmental factors on the individual.

Biopsychosocial-Spiritual Model

During the 1980s, the medical model was influenced by a movement toward what was then called *holistic health*, the notion that the physical, mental, social, and spiritual aspects of a person's life must be viewed as an integrated whole. During the 1990s, basic scientists and clinicians continued to recognize the healing potential of faith, spirituality, and religious beliefs and started to consider the complex biopsychosocial-spiritual phenomena associated with disease, illness, and injury.

Since that time, it has become well established that social and spiritual support play important roles in promoting health, decreasing susceptibility to disease, and facilitating recovery from illness or injury. Multidisciplinary team and managed care approaches to such conditions address the needs of the client in terms of the emotional and psychologic impact, social and spiritual needs, and comprehensive biologic picture that goes beyond medication and surgical intervention as the primary forms of medical treatment. Physical therapists can use this information to guide clinical decision making to enhance the physical therapist–patient/client relationship, potentially improve compliance with the physical therapist's plan of care, and improve the quality of care.[117]

Social-Ecologic Model

From the field of social community health and health promotion, the social-ecologic model was developed on a broader view of health issues. Social ecology is viewed as an overarching framework or a set of theoretic principles for understanding the interrelations among diverse personal and environmental factors in human health and illness.[335] Social-ecologic theory, an extension of the biologic concept of ecology, creates a framework in which to place and discuss health at a level beyond the individual.

Four primary assumptions regarding social-ecologic theory have been outlined.[287,288] First, intrapersonal, social, and physical environments work jointly to influence health behavior. Second, environmental influences on health are the result not only of physical and social components but also the perception of these variables by the individual. Recognition of various collective levels of human interaction with the environment (e.g., individual-environment, community-environment, or population-environment) comprises the third assumption.

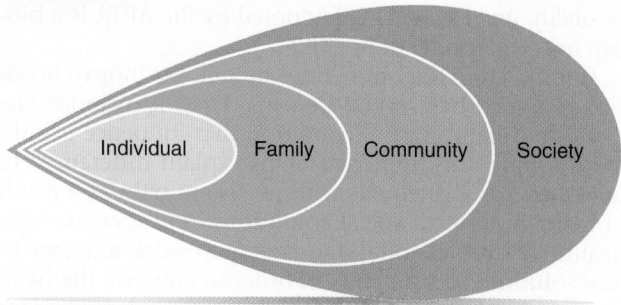

Figure 2-1

Social structures influencing the individual. Aside from the pathology itself, many behavioral, social, and environmental factors influence health and may mitigate or enhance the effects of disease. The individual is influenced in various ways by family, community, and society. Each of these nested social structures influences the individual and can shape behavior, including the ability to make health decisions, compliance with regimens, or even with initial health choices. (Courtesy Ira Gorman, PT, MSPH, Regis University, Department of Physical Therapy, Denver, CO.)

The fourth and critical assumption of social-ecologic theory is the relationship between environmental levels and collections of individuals. In short, altering behaviors among individuals will influence environmental level characteristics, which will in turn further influence groups of individuals within a community or population.

Various models of social ecology have been described and applied in intervention programs. The most common construction of social ecology, provided by Sallis and Owen,[271] proposes that behaviors are influenced by *intrapersonal, sociocultural, policy,* and *physical-environmental* factors.

In another social ecology model, Bronfenbrenner's[48] model describes three levels of environmental-individual interaction, the *microsystem* (i.e., interpersonal interactions), the *mesosystem* (i.e., interactions among various settings such as work, family, and social networks), and the *exosystem* (i.e., cultural, political, and economic forces).

The model proposed by McLeroy et al in 1988[202] is composed of five classes of factors: *intrapersonal factors, interpersonal processes* and *primary groups, institutional factors, community factors,* and *public policy.* Behavior is the outcome of interest and is determined by the five classes, with four of the five pertaining to the person's environment and clearly beyond the intrapersonal. Moos's[210] ecologic model is geared toward health behavior and constructed of *physical settings, organizational factors, human aggregates,* and *social climate.*

The important point in recognizing the diversity of the models used to describe social-ecologic theory is to observe the common threads that run among them. Each reflects the interrelationship between individual-level characteristics and large-scale social forces (Fig. 2-1). Increasingly larger social structures influence the individual and can shape behavior, including the ability to make health decisions such as adherence with regimens or even initial health choices.

This model attempts to identify the various levels of influence that have an impact on health, from the individual to the environment. This view greatly broadens the types of interventions that can improve health and helps us understand the role pathologic processes have at the cellular level as they interact with the environment to cause disease, impairment, functional limitations, and disability.

VARIATIONS IN CLIENT POPULATIONS

Healthy People 2020[307] recognizes the need for all Americans to benefit from advancements in quality of life and health, regardless of race, ethnicity, gender, geographic location, disability status, income, sexual or spiritual orientation, or educational level. Recognizing variations in client populations is important in helping all health care professionals to provide health-promoting and preventive programs.

Sociodemographics

Sociodemographic information and the results of the 2010 Census have provided us with a composite picture of America never before so broad based or so complete. Americans are more diverse ethnically, with an estimated ethnic racial mix of 72% white alone, 12% black or African American alone, 12% Hispanic, and 4% Asian and Pacific Islander. Statistics collected for the Census now also include a Two or More Races population. It is estimated that in the next decade, the number of people of Asian descent will double from 10 million to 20 million, and by 2050, whites will comprise only 53% of the U.S. population.

Rapid population shifts to the mountain states and resurgent growth in suburbs have changed the urban–rural configurations. More than 70% of all rural counties gained population in the last decade. Finally, the percentage of Americans who are married continues to drop—with unmarried partner households and multigenerational households being relatively new categories.[300]

Health Status

The health status of the United States is a description of the health of the total population using information that is representative of most people living in this country. However, it must be noted that our current epidemiologic system does not keep data on people who do not obtain treatment; no universal or uniform registry is available in the United States.

Health status of a nation can be measured by birth and death rates, life expectancy, quality of life, morbidity from specific diseases, risk factors, the use of ambulatory care and inpatient care, accessibility of health personnel and facilities, financing of health care, health insurance coverage, and many other factors.

The leading causes of death are often used to describe the health status of a nation. For example, in the United States, obesity, alcoholism, sedentary lifestyle, and tobacco use have contributed significantly to the most common causes of morbidity and mortality in 2010. This is in contrast to the year 1900, when infectious diseases ran rampant in the United States and worldwide and topped the leading causes of death. In the year 2010, 65% of all deaths were caused by cardiovascular disease, cancer, and diabetes.[68]

Deaths, permanent disability, and unnecessary suffering from medical errors (e.g., medication errors, health care–acquired infections, falls, handoff errors, diagnostic

Table 2-1 Leading Causes of Death in the United States*

Cause of Death in 1900	Cause of Death in 2010	Etiology of Death in 2010 (Lifestyle/behaviors: modifiable)
Pneumonia, influenza	Heart disease	Tobacco use
Tuberculosis	Cancer	Poor diet and physical inactivity
Heart disease	Stroke	Alcohol consumption
Diarrhea, enteritis	Chronic lower respiratory disease	Toxic agents (e.g., environmental pollutants)
Stroke	Stroke	Microbial agents (e.g., influenza)
	Accidental injuries	Motor vehicles
	Alzheimer disease	Firearms
		Sexual behavior
		Illicit drug use

*Listed in descending order of incidence; five leading causes of death accounted for 63% of all deaths in the United States. Causes may vary when evaluated by age (e.g., unintentional injuries and suicide account for more deaths in younger individuals, whereas chronic conditions are attributed more to deaths among older adults).
Data from National Center for Health Statistics. Death in the United States, 2010. Available online at http://www.cdc.gov/nchs/data/databriefs/db99.htm.

errors, and surgical errors) are an escalating problem that remains largely unreported. It is estimated that medical errors account for almost 100,000 death each year in the United States.[252] Studies show that nursing home residents may be at higher risk for experiencing adverse medical events that lead to serious safety and quality of care concerns. These risks may be attributable to lack of effective communication among caregivers who help transition patients across acute care settings.[270] Statistics are not available for similar errors in other health-related settings such as same-day surgery centers, outpatient clinics, retail pharmacies, nursing homes, and in-home care. Deaths from medication errors that occur both in and out of hospitals (more than 7000 annually) exceed those caused by injuries in the workplace.

Chronic Diseases

Over the last century, a shift from infectious to noncommunicable chronic diseases such as heart disease, cancer, and diabetes has occurred. As a result of the control of many infectious agents, eradication of childhood diseases, and the current increasing age of the population, chronic diseases now top the list as causes of morbidity and mortality in the United States (Table 2-1). Many of these illnesses are modifiable through changes in behavior and lifestyle. This trend has led to a new focus in rehabilitation: chronic disease management. In some places, chronic disease management is a new term for rehabilitation.

Cost of health care delivery has increased exponentially with the rise in aging, risky lifestyle behaviors, and associated medical conditions. Chronic conditions, such as heart disease, hypertension, diabetes, and mental disorders reportedly affect more than 130 million Americans (nearly half the population) at a cost into the billions of dollars.[136] Up to half of Medicare patients aged 65 and older have at least three chronic medical conditions, and one-fifth has five or more.[297]

Medical spending has increased as more people have chronic disorders with multiple complex comorbidities. In addition, some conditions have become more expensive to treat, and the number of people diagnosed with these conditions has increased.[297]

With modifiable behavioral risk factors as leading causes of mortality in the United States, identifying trends and gearing prevention strategies and opportunities toward these specific behaviors may help offset escalating health care costs.[207] The new Patient Protection and Affordable Care Act of 2010 created the Prevention and Public Health Fund to invest in public health and disease prevention. The intent is to reorient U.S. health care toward wellness while restraining cost and expenses created by the high prevalence of chronic disease.[153]

Americans with Disabilities

Over 50 million Americans (one in five people) are living with at least one disability and it is predicted that most Americans will experience a disability some time in their lives.[60] Traumatic brain injury (TBI) is a leading cause of death and disability in the United States.[82] Older adults have the highest rates of TBI hospitalizations and deaths among all age groups. TBI is the leading cause of injury-related death in children and young adults in the United States and other industrialized countries. Overall rates of disability (including TBI) are higher among older adults who also have higher rates of chronic diseases.[82]

Almost half of all seniors (over age 65) have a physical, sensory, mental, or learning disability of some kind. One difficulty in identifying how many people have a disability is the wide range of definitions for disability used in social research situations. In some cases, disability is any difficulty with activities of daily living (ADLs) or limitations associated with over 30 associated health conditions.[203] Other definitions include those receiving federal benefits on the basis of an inability to work or those with any limitation in the ability to work at a job or business, yet over half (56%) of working-age individuals with a disability are employed.[301]

According to the U.S. Census, there are 21.5 million military veterans in the United States in 2011. For a breakdown of number based on demographics (e.g., race, gender, income, when they served, and where they are located) go to http://www.census.gov/newsroom/releases/pdf/cb12ff-21_veteran.pdf. An estimated 3.5 million have a service-connected disability rating, with the most typical injuries being TBI, amputations, and post-traumatic stress disorder.[303] Physical therapists are seeing many combat-related disabilities among men and women in the military, as well as in the civilian sector once they are discharged.

With increasing life expectancy and the aging of America, health issues related to disability are likely to increase in prevalence and importance over the next few decades. Living longer means increasing percentages of individuals with disabilities.[203]

Geographic Variations

The concept of "community" as it relates to where individuals live geographically and the characteristics of that place has a definite impact on the status of people's health. Although somewhat controversial and highly debated, some of the most stressful U.S. cities and jobs have been identified. Some published lists base their findings on cost of living, crime index, education, divorce, population density, unemployment, and average commuting time. Likewise, suggestions have been made as to the least stressful locations and occupations.[15,44,76]

Other factors, such as urban pockets of minority groups (usually associated with increased levels of poverty), access to fresh fruits and vegetables (or lack thereof), and even local smoking ordinances, contribute to the geographic variations people experience that can impact their health.[239]

The geographic and political climates of countries also play a role in determining how people live and the health problems that commonly develop. A half-century ago, a few physicians cultivated an interest in diseases that seemed to have strict geographic boundaries. As a result, a discipline called *geographic pathology* developed. Geographic pathology was concerned with diseases endemic (present in a community at all times) to certain areas of the world, most often parasitic and infectious diseases that seemed unique to individual geographic regions. A component called *occupational disease* was added with the discovery that chemical agents are mediators of a variety of tissue changes and the recognition that many of these causative agents are environmental contaminants. Disease caused by contaminants was included to constitute the field of *environmental pathology*. For further discussion, see Chapter 4.

One other issue related to geographic variations is the fact that treatment for a single medical condition can vary significantly from one geographic location to another. Rates and types of surgical procedures differ from one geographic location to another, depending on the prevailing health care system, physician and hospital preferences (notably not client preferences or needs), and where the physician was trained.[39,201,230]

Race and Ethnicity

The use of the terms "race" and "ethnicity" are seldom well defined and are generally thought to have less scientific and biologic significance than sociologic and cultural importance. The CDC defines race as "an arbitrary classification based on physical characteristics; a group of persons related by common descent or heredity." The CDC defines ethnicity as "an arbitrary classification based on cultural, religious, or linguistic traditions; ethnic traits, background, allegiance, or association."[217]

Identification of race and ethnicity is widely used when collecting vital statistics and demographic data for documenting health patterns among population groups living in the United States and globally. The National Health and Nutrition Examination Survey (NHANES) I, II, and III (developed in 1959, the 1970s, and the 1980s, respectively) used race and ethnicity data when evaluating the health and nutrition status of the civilian, noninstitutionalized population of the United States. This survey is updated annually.[220]

The Hispanic HANES (HHANES) was conducted to obtain sufficient numbers to produce estimates of the health and nutritional status of Hispanics in general, as well as specific data for Puerto Ricans, Mexican Americans, and Cuban Americans. Included in the survey were Mexican Americans from Texas, Colorado, New Mexico, Arizona, and California; Cuban Americans from Dade County, Florida; and Puerto Ricans from the New York area, including parts of New Jersey and Connecticut.[66,309]

In the past, it was believed that race or ethnic background predisposed people to certain diseases and chronic conditions. However, during the last 50 years, "race" has been scientifically disproved—that is, race is not a real, natural phenomenon. Data on human variation come from studies of genetic variation, which are clearly quantifiable and replicable. Genetic data show that no matter how racial groups are defined, two people from the same racial group are as different as two people from any two different racial groups.

Current information about biologic and genetic characteristics of various groups (e.g., blacks, Hispanics, Native Americans, Alaskan Natives, Native Hawaiians, or Pacific Islanders) does not explain the health disparities experienced by these groups. These differences are thought to be the result of the complex interaction among genetic variations, environmental factors, and specific sociocultural and health behaviors.

Data indicate that some conditions are more prevalent in certain groups; for example, nonwhite people (black, Native Americans, and Asians) are three times more likely to die of hypertension than whites of the same age group. In the past, causes of death were identified that together accounted for more than 80% of mortality in nonwhite people, including cancer; cardiovascular disease and stroke; chemical dependency; cirrhoses; diabetes; homicides, suicides, and accidents; and infant mortality.[233]

Other conditions that are peculiar to ethnic or racial groups include Tay-Sachs disease (Jewish people of northeastern European origin are most susceptible); cystic fibrosis (incidence is highest in whites and rare in Asians); and sickle cell anemia, which affects blacks, especially Africans.

Health Disparities and Inequities

Health disparities have been defined as the differences in individual or regional community health due to lack of access, high cost, or other factors that create barriers to health services.[291] Although over the last 100 years health care has dramatically improved the life span and the quality of life for many through advances in public health, medical discoveries, and technology, not every segment of the population has benefited equally from the advances in health care.

Social factors, such as socioeconomic status, access to health care, language differences, place of birth, residential segregation, and access to nutrition, have all been variables that help explain the disparities in health care that result in higher morbidity and mortality rates among groups of Americans.[2] For example, statistics show a broad gap between the death rates for blacks and whites, but blacks differ more from each other than they do from whites.[106] Whites living in higher socioeconomic areas have lower mortality rates than whites living in predominantly black areas for all age groups, and elderly blacks living in black areas (despite their less favorable socioeconomic status) have lower mortality rates for all causes than those living in white areas.[107]

Education and health care resources often are not accessible to minorities and rural residents with limited financial means. Routine programs, such as antismoking campaigns and cancer screenings (e.g., breast, prostate, or colon), tend to be focused on affluent Americans who are better educated and can afford regular medical care.[95]

The general understanding regarding health care was that those who could afford health care had access to health care and those who could not afford health care did not have access to health care. Thus, there was disparity in health care related to access based on socioeconomic factors. As previously mentioned, the new Patient Protection and Affordable Care Act of 2010 has been passed in an effort to address these kinds of disparities but remains under considerable debate and controversy.[153]

Factors Contributing to Health Disparities and Inequities

The impact of social and economic determinants of health status and the existence of racial and ethnic health care access disparities have been well documented.[268] The Institute of Medicine (IOM) is one agency in the forefront that continues to examine, investigate, research, and report on health disparities. A brief presentation is provided here but more information is available on their website at www.iom.edu including free access to a document updating progress made in this area over the past decade.[13]

The IOM has also identified several factors that contribute to health disparities and inequities. First, health systems have financial expectations that influence health care practice. For example, increased productivity demands utilize scheduling practices that often limit health practitioner contact with clients and require health care practitioners to engage in multiple duties at the same time. Health systems also provide financial incentives to physicians for limiting services including diagnostic procedures and interventions.

Second, there is disparity in the quality of health care in different populations. For example, the IOM report indicates that minority populations are more likely to be diagnosed with late-stage cancer than whites.[3] Minority individuals typically have less access to preventive care, causing later diagnosis and more severe disease.[168,272] Health status is consistently higher among individuals with more social advantage—people of low income and little education have worse health indicators.[47]

Third, clients are not always followed by the same health care provider, and inconsistencies exist when one health practitioner orders certain tests and procedures for a medical workup while another practitioner does not. There is evidence of this type of fragmentation of health care along socioeconomic lines. Clients in lower socioeconomic groups are less likely to receive a complete array of medical tests routinely ordered for individuals with a higher socioeconomic status. Other factors contributing to racial and ethnic health disparities include cultural and linguistic barriers, discrimination, bias, stereotyping, and uncertainty and a lack of cultural competence on the part of the health practitioner.[38,58]

Another model has been proposed by well-known researchers in this content area[58]—one that provides a practical framework for understanding and working with modifiable barriers to health care access. The Health Care Access Barriers Model (HCAB) describes three categories of modifiable health care access barriers: financial, structural, and cognitive. The three types of barriers reinforce one another and affect health care access individually or in concert together. These barriers are associated with screening, late presentation to care, and lack of treatment. Each of these factors contributes to poor health outcomes and health disparities. By targeting those barriers that are measurable and modifiable, the model facilitates root-cause analysis and intervention design.[58]

Despite best intentions to avoid such practices, health practitioners engage in stereotyping and bias that may be conscious or unconscious. The health care provider may experience uncertainty in the clinical encounter and rely on a previous experience as the basis for the clinical decision making. The bias, stereotyping, and uncertainty may be the result of cultural differences and linguistic issues and affect the clinical management and ultimate health outcomes.[264]

Strategies to Eliminate Disparities

The health of individuals within the society directly influences the health of the nation in the collective. Citizens contribute to the culture and the society to create the fabric of national life. The health of the citizens of the nation is of paramount importance; every effort must be made to eliminate racial and ethnic disparities in health care. The IOM has recommended the following strategies to that end; other proposed local solutions to reduce inequities in health are available[78] on their website (e.g., www.iom.edu and http://www.iom.edu/~/media/Files/Activity%20Files/SelectPops/HealthDisparities/Commissioned_local_disp.pdf).

- Education to address discrimination, bias, stereotyping, and uncertainty that contribute to health disparity; engage health practitioners in reflective practice that can alter conscious and unconscious behavior.
- Cross-cultural education provided to current and future health care practitioners to develop attitudes, knowledge, and skills in working with diverse populations.
- Standardize data collection to include race and ethnicity data for both the client and the provider, primary language data, socioeconomic data, and monitoring of performance outcomes.
- Policy and regulatory strategies that address:
  - Reduction in fragmentation of health plans along socioeconomic lines
  - Use of clinical guidelines and best practice recommendations
  - Increases in the number of racial and ethnic minorities in health professions
  - Use of interpreter services for health care

See Evolve Box 2-1, Strategies to Eliminate Health Disparities, on the Evolve website for more information on this topic.

Beyond Cultural Competence: Transnational Competence

Understanding of cultural diversity and cultural competence has become a familiar topic in the physical therapist's education. Likewise, some consideration of these topics has become a part of all U.S. medical schools. Cultural competence has been linked with quality assurance and cost-containment programs to help reduce disparities in health care.[175] A new goal is to prepare students for multiple (international) practice sites.[175]

Given rapidly changing global demographics and the continued health disparities, social scientists propose a need to move beyond cultural competence to embrace *transnational competence* (TC). TC teaches the health care professional how to address issues of physical and mental health along with experiences related to geographic dislocation and adaptation to unfamiliar settings.[175]

Consistent with global trends, demographic patterns are changing rapidly in the United States. Disparities in health and health care are increasing. More than 35 million foreign-born persons are living in the United States—more than 12% of the total population. Currently, 6 of every 10 babies born in New York City have at least one foreign-born parent.[37]

It is not enough to consider lists of ethnocultural characteristics and single-factor explanations such as health-belief systems. Relevant links between health and postmigration stressors may include employment status and experiences, discrimination, insecurity of immigration status, or family fragmentation.[174] TC requires a multidimensional approach that takes into account the current era of globalization and migration and their impact on health beliefs, disparities, and diversity within ethnic groups.

Age and Aging

Age and gender play important roles in the development of most diseases. Age often represents the accumulated effects of genetic and environmental factors over time. Intrinsic cellular mechanisms play a role in aging, though these can be modulated by extracellular factors such as hormones. Discriminating between causes and effects of aging is often impossible. Separating aging from pathology remains a major challenge in our understanding of these two concepts.

There are many theories to explain what changes occur that lead to aging, but no universal theory of aging or consensus over what causes aging or determines the rate of aging exists. Theories of aging that have gathered more experimental support than others are presented here.

Theories of Aging

Senescence, the process or condition of growing old, may be the result of continuous cellular metabolism, cellular damage, and inefficient repair systems throughout the entire life span. Some researchers in gerontology (specifically biogerontologists) regard aging itself as a "disease" that may be curable. Understanding aging from this framework is referred to as a *damage-based theory*. Examples of damage-based explanations of aging include *error theory*, the *wear and tear theory*, the *free radical theory*, the *neuroendocrine theory*, and the *waste accumulation theory*. To those who accept the damage-based view, aging is an accumulation of damage to macromolecules, cells, tissues and organs.

Examples of environmentally induced damage range from alterations to deoxyribonucleic acid (DNA), formation of free radicals from oxidative processes causing damage to tissues and cells, and increased cross-linking of tendon, bone, and muscle tissue reducing tissue elasticity and obstructing the passage of nutrients and waste between cells. These concepts are discussed in greater detail in Chapter 6.

An alternate explanation for the aging process is *programmed-based*, which presumes that aging is a genetically driven process and not primarily the result of ongoing and accumulated cellular or environmental processes. In other words, aging is regulated by a biologic clock. Changes in gene expression are either preprogrammed or derived from DNA structural changes and affect the systems responsible for maintenance, repair, and defenses.[54] Examples of the programmed-based explanation of aging include the *gene mutation theory*, the *genetic control theory*, and the *planned obsolescence theory*. Both damage-based and programmed-based theories acknowledge that aging is influenced to some degree by intrinsic and extrinsic factors. It is also possible that elements of both theoretic models apply.

A newer theory in the field of antiaging medicine is the *telomerase theory* of aging. The basis of this theory is the shortening of telomeres in the process of DNA replication during cell division. Telomeres are sequences of nucleic acids extending from the ends of chromosomes. Telomeres do not encode genes; rather they act to maintain the integrity of our chromosomes by ensuring that the sequence lost during replication is a nonessential, noncoding sequence. However, every time our cells divide, telomeres are shortened. Once the safety margin provided by a telomere is consumed, gene coding regions of the chromosome are no longer protected during replication leading to replicative senescence, progressive damage to the chromosome, and eventual cellular damage and cellular death associated with aging.[170]

Researchers also found that the enzyme *telomerase* is a key factor in rebuilding the disappearing telomeres. Telomerase is found only in germ cells and cancer cells. Telomerase may be manipulating the biologic clock that controls the life span of dividing cells. Future development of telomerase inhibitor may be able to stop cancer cells from dividing. The hope is to convert them back into normal cells.

Life Expectancy

Life expectancy at birth for persons born in the United States is now about 78.7 years for white women and 75 years for white men, compared with 48 years at the turn of the last century.[219,302] These estimates have continued increasing for both genders[216] but some researchers predict a decline in U.S. life expectancy based on the dramatic rise in obesity, especially among young people and minorities.[236] Whites and blacks have similar life expectancies at age 65, but a higher death rate exists among younger blacks. Once adults reach age 65, men can expect to live an additional 15.8 years, and women can expect an additional 17.6 years. Individuals 75 years of age can be expected to live an average of 11 more years for a total of 86 years.[300]

The majority of cancers occur in adults over the age of 65, with about 70% of all cancer deaths in this population. Mortality rate from cancer remains higher for blacks who are not diagnosed and treated early. For many cancers, a person's advanced chronologic age is considered a major adverse prognostic factor. Many older adults tolerate cancer treatment, but they experience delayed recovery and are at increased risk of serious infectious and bleeding complications.[339]

Centenarians and Supercentenarians

A dramatic extension of longevity has occurred in the last 100 years. In 1900, people over age 65 constituted 4% of the U.S. population. By 1988, that proportion was up to 12.4%, and it is predicted that by 2025, one-third of all Americans will be age 65 or older, and 30% of the over-65 population will be nonwhite by 2050, representing an even greater cultural diversity among the aging.[18]

The most rapid population increase in the past decade has been among those over age 85 and the "oldest old" over 100 years of age (centenarians: those who live to the age of 109; supercentenarians: those who live to the age of 110 or more).[205] More than half (62.5%) of the 53,364 centenarians alive at the 2010 census were age 100 or 101: 82.5% were white alone and 12.2% were black or African American alone; 5.8% were Hispanic, and the Asian alone share was 2.5%. Women outnumbered men in all ages and ethnic groups; there were 330 total reported supercentenarians.[205]

This aging trend of the U.S. population is reflected in the kinds of clients and problems therapists will treat in the coming decades. Confusion; fractures and other injuries related to falls; strokes; infections; and effects of polypharmacy, inappropriate medications, and decline in drug clearance are just a few of the more common characteristic problems this group of older adults faces.

Finally, the older adult can be assessed for modifiable risk factors that contribute to functional decline. Slow gait, short-acting benzodiazepine use, depression, low exercise level, and obesity with its associated comorbidities are significant modifiable predictors of functional decline in both vigorous and basic activities. Weak grip predicts functional decline in vigorous activities, whereas long-acting benzodiazepine use and poor visual acuity predict decline in basic activities. Known nonmodifiable predictors of functional decline include age, education, medical comorbidity, cognitive function, smoking history, and presence of previous spine fracture.[276]

Children and Adolescents

Research has produced dramatic advancements in children's health that have an impact on adulthood. The long-term benefits of childhood intervention to prevent adult disease are documented. For example, preventing osteoporosis in the aging adult begins by providing necessary dietary calcium intake during bone development and calcification in childhood.

Tobacco use remains the leading cause of preventable morbidity and mortality in the U.S. The health consequences of tobacco use include heart disease, multiple types of cancer, pulmonary disease, adverse reproductive effects, and the exacerbation of chronic health condition.[69] There has been a slowing in the decline of smokers among younger adults but smoking remains widespread among all age groups suggesting that tobacco use will remain an important public health issue for the foreseeable future unless effective tobacco control strategies are fully implemented and sustained.[69]

Preventing tobacco-related cancer and lung diseases begins with educating children about the risks of initiating smoking. *Healthy People 2020* leads the country in trying to develop effective and economic self-management strategies and interventions for children and families to prevent disease and improve health.

As the young and the aging continue to garner attention, teenagers are falling between the cracks of medical care. Prenatal and well child prevention programs have boosted the care given to the under-12 age group, but most physicians do not categorize teenagers as adults and may not be adequately addressing the needs of this group.

Adolescents as a group are the primary users of illicit drugs, tobacco, and alcohol and comprise the largest group with unwanted pregnancies, abortions, and sexually transmitted diseases. Preventive health care and intervention among this age group are the next targets for the *Healthy People 2020* campaign.

Gender or Sex?

Although the terms *gender* and *sex* are often used interchangeably, technically, these terms are not the same. According to the Society for Women's Health Research (SWHR),[285] *sex* refers to our biology, or genetics (XX for women, XY for men); *gender* refers to social roles, behaviors, and environmental influences. Sex and gender affect health independently as well as interactively.

After almost two decades of research, we now know that these differences between the sexes and implications are significant even in terms of promotion of wellness, as well as prevention (or cure) of diseases.[187] A move toward more personalized medical care in regards to the integration of sex and gender competency is now part of the IOM's 2010 recommendations.[157]

Gender/Sex Bias and Gender/Sex Equity

Gender bias on the part of health care providers (whether conscious or unconscious) can affect health outcomes.[273] Fortunately, the importance of gender equity in health is receiving more attention, with increasing focus on gender roles linked with health-related problems. Until the late 20th century, evidence for gender bias, usually against women, was seen in three areas: (1) the historical use of public monies to fund research predominantly in men, (2) the perpetuation of the view in medicine that the 70-kg man is the norm for representing all humans in medicine, and (3) the use of federal funds through Medicare to provide better reimbursement for conditions more prevalent in men compared with those more prevalent in women.[57]

The National Institutes of Health (NIH) issued guidelines in 1990 requiring the inclusion of women and minorities in all NIH-sponsored clinical research and revised these guidelines in 1994 to require analysis of clinical trial outcomes by gender. Although most clinical studies since that time have included women as study subjects, only a small percentage of research findings are analyzed by gender.[315]

Gender-Based Biology and Physiology

> **Note to Reader:** Having made the distinction between gender and sex, you will still see ways in which the terms are used in the literature and at large that do not follow the definition provided above. The subtitle here, "Gender-Based Biology and Physiology," is a good example; by the SWHR definition, these topics would not be labeled "gender"-based biology and physiology, but rather, sex-based biology and physiology.

Increasingly, research efforts are finding that the differences between men and women go far beyond the reproductive organs to affect every physiologic function and organ in the body, including the aging process. Physiologic or biologic differences between males and females are clearer now than ever before and form the basis for a new area of medicine referred to as *gender-specific medicine* (sometimes referred to as just *gender medicine*).

Gender-based biology has demonstrated major gender differences in such things as risk factors, response to medications, response to surgical procedures, and response to treatment. Striking physiologic differences exist between men and women.[261] For example, women's hearts beat faster, which is now recognized as a result of the configuration and activity of the cardiac cell membrane as they function differently between the genders. Men's brains are larger than women's, but women have more brain cells. Diagnostic scanning shows that different areas of the brain light up in response to an identical task between men and women.[187] Age-related changes that differ in men and women are just now coming to the forefront of science.

Gender-Based Patterns of Disease

It is clear now that men and women experience different patterns of disease. Some gender differences may represent either environmental or genetic factors. Diseases with rates of occurrence that differ between men and women may reflect lifestyle or environmental differences or anatomic and hormonal differences.

Women are twice as likely as men to contract a sexually transmitted disease (STD) and 10 times more likely to contract HIV, in particular during unprotected sex with an infected partner. Women smokers are more likely to develop lung cancer than men who smoke. Women are more likely to have a second heart attack within a year of the first, and nearly one-half of men but only one-third of women survive 1 year after a heart attack.

Women constitute 80% of those who have bone loss (osteoporosis) severe enough to increase fracture risk significantly; women have higher blood alcohol levels than men after both consume the same amount; and women tend to regain consciousness after anesthesia more quickly than men.[96] Additionally, the incidence of health risks to women, such as depression, anxiety, alcoholism, and eating disorders, is increasing.[90,155]

Men, however, face some unique health challenges. Deaths from malignant melanoma are 50% higher in men than in women, despite a 50% lower incidence of the disease in men. In general, men die an average of 5 years earlier than women, develop heart disease a decade earlier, and are more likely to participate in dangerous jobs and recreational activities. Men are two times more likely than women to die from unintentional injuries and four times more likely to die from firearm-related injuries.

Additionally, researchers are now examining whether people are more vulnerable to environmental and biologic challenges during periods of critical biochemical change than in times of relative quiescence. For example, are social, biologic, or psychologic changes that affect health influenced by hormonal fluctuations associated with puberty, premenstrual cycles, pregnancy, and menopause, compared with other periods in a woman's life cycle?

LIFESTYLE FACTORS THAT INFLUENCE HEALTH

Overview

According to the World Health Organization (WHO), the highest number of deaths are attributed to the risk factors of tobacco use, high blood pressure, high body mass index (BMI), high cholesterol, low fruit and vegetable intake, alcohol consumption, and lack of physical activity, in that order.[240] More than half of deaths from the leading causes in the United States (see Table 2-1) are associated with behavioral and lifestyle factors such as diet, exercise, smoking, and substance abuse. These factors not only contribute to the number of deaths but also contribute significantly to disability and the burden of disease.

More than any other intervention, changing behavior and lifestyle could help prevent death, enhance the quality of life, and reduce the escalating costs of treating chronic illnesses. For example, although heart disease remains the number one cause of death in the U.S. adult population, the cardiac death rate has been reduced by 52% over the last 2 decades as a result of changes in diet and lifestyle.

Other risk factors in lifestyle affecting health status and health care are considered individually modifiable and include personal habits such as rest and sleep; diet, including calcium, fat, and fiber intake; level of activity and exercise (fitness); stress and coping ability; substance abuse; travel; environmental or occupational status; and high-risk sexual activity.

The gay and lesbian population comprises a diverse community with disparate health concerns. Major health issues for gay men are HIV/AIDS and other STDs, substance abuse, depression, and suicide. Gay male adolescents are two to three times more likely than their peers to attempt suicide. Some evidence suggests lesbians have higher rates of smoking, obesity, alcohol abuse, and stress than heterosexual women. The issues surrounding personal, family, and social acceptance of sexual orientation can place a significant burden on mental health and personal safety.[92]

This section examines selected lifestyle and behaviors that affect health and directly influence physical therapy practice. Psychologic and behavioral risk factors that influence health outcomes presented include physical activity, nutrition, tobacco use, alcohol and other drug use, stress and coping, and domestic violence. Some current theories about health behavior change that can influence effectiveness of physical therapy interventions will also be discussed.

Cultural Influences

Variations in lifestyle influencing clients' perceptions of health care may occur as a result of cultural, religious, socioeconomic, or even age factors. Although clinical manifestations of a disease or condition are essentially the same across cultures, how a person (or family member) responds or interprets the experience can vary.

This phenomenon of response based on cultural influence is called *cultural relativity*—that is, behavior must be judged first in relation to the context of the culture in which it occurs. For example, some groups consider health as a function of luck (good or bad), whereas others see health problems as a punishment for bad behavior and good health as a reward for good behavior.

Cultural factors may also prevent illness. For example, people belonging to religious faiths that forbid drinking or smoking have lower cancer rates than the general population. Religious beliefs related to health must be recognized and respected. Research to study the effects of religiosity as a predictor of outcome in a variety of disorders is beginning to draw definitive conclusions about the efficacy of prayer, religious practices and activities, and philosophic orientation toward health.[16,176,282] Research suggests that one of the principal reasons people are attracted to alternative medicine is that they find many of these therapies in keeping with their personal beliefs.[17]

Demographics by Generation

Generational differences are seen among groups such as the Matures, also known as postwar/depression-era (born from 1900 to 1946); the baby boomers (born from 1946 to 1964); the Generation X-ers (born from 1965 to 1979); the Millennials, also referred to as Generation Y (born from 1980 to 1999), Generation Z or the Digital Natives (the first generation to grow up using technology as a way to communicate, study/educate, record personal/societal history, and understand and make global connections[257]), and now Homelanders, the name suggested for the youngest generation (other names suggested for this group include iGen or Generation Net since they were born into the world with the Internet).

Many people born before 1946 tend to assume a passive role in their own health and in receipt of health care by accepting whatever happens to them and whatever treatment is outlined. However, baby boomers have grown up questioning authority, and their offspring are even more likely to consider themselves consumers asking for treatment rationales, seeking second opinions, and combining allopathic treatment with alternative/integrative approaches (e.g., naturopathy, aroma therapy, acupuncture, massage therapy, Reiki, BodyTalk, yoga, tai chi, qi gong).

Socioeconomic Status

The most adverse influence on health is socioeconomic status, with a higher percentage of low-socioeconomic-class members experiencing health-related problems than any other group. Adults with higher incomes tend to experience better health and can expect to live more than 3 years longer than those in the lowest income bracket.

The percentage of people in the lowest-income families reporting limitation in activity caused by chronic disease is three times that of people in the highest-income families.[307] Lack of health insurance coverage and/or access to quality health care may result in delayed or postponed diagnosis and treatment of health problems.

Differences in attitudes toward health have been found to be greater between social classes than between races or ethnic groups. Ninety percent of all health care dollars is spent on extraordinary care in the last 2 to 3 years of life. This style of death-based medicine assigns the greatest financial and professional resources to treating the diseases of aging.[125]

The homeless have become one of the fastest growing populations in need of health care in the United States. Traditionally, the homeless consisted primarily of older, single men, often alcoholics, but now this group includes families and children who are runaways or adolescent throwaways.

Declining public assistance, a shortage of affordable rental housing, and an increase in poverty are contributing factors to the rise in homelessness. Although estimates of homeless people vary, the National Coalition for the Homeless[221] reports that on any given night, 700,000 Americans are homeless and up to 2 million homeless people are reported in a year's time. This number includes an estimated 100,000 children in the United States who are homeless; more than half are under age 5.

Adverse Childhood Experiences

Adverse experiences in childhood are linked to the development of problems later in life, including alcohol and other drug use, drug and/or tobacco addiction or addictions, obesity, fibromyalgia, or other autoimmune disorders. Children who have been exposed to four or more adverse experiences in childhood are more likely to have attempted suicide and to have had multiple sex partners, increasing their risk of STDs. Dangerous or apparently counterproductive behaviors can serve a purpose (e.g., coping mechanism, barrier against social contact).

The strong relationship between exposure to abuse or household dysfunction during childhood and multiple risk factors for several of the leading causes of death in adults is beginning to be recognized in the health care setting.[12,109] *Healthy People 2020* has set goals of primary prevention of adverse childhood experiences and improved treatment of exposed children to reduce self-destructive behaviors, such as smoking, among adolescents and adults. For a more complete understanding of the impact of adverse experiences in general, see Chapter 3.

Variations in Lifestyle: Adapting Treatment Intervention to the Individual

In the final decades leading to the 21st century, the demographics of the United States changed rapidly, bringing with it a better understanding of the biopsychosocial-spiritual variables that affect the episode of care seen in a physical therapist's practice, especially health care issues centered around minorities and economic variables. The physical therapist's role in education and prevention has never been more important as we come to understand the effect individual modifying (risk) factors have on pathology and recovery. A biopsychosocial-spiritual model is essential because risk factors correlate with results, especially in chronic disease/disorders.

Cultural Awareness

Race/ethnicity, culture, and religion are important factors in an individual's response to pain, disability, and disease. It is essential to remember that people of any culture may deal with pain, impairment, movement dysfunctions, and disability differently than expected.

The culturally sensitive health professional must screen for cultural practices, such as fasting or the use of alternative remedies; document these practices; and communicate appropriate information to other members of the team providing care for that individual. This is especially important for the client who may have a medical condition (e.g., diabetes mellitus, hypertension) that could be compromised by these practices.

The APTA is committed to ensuring equality in physical therapy services through education of physical therapy professionals. This education focuses on increasing knowledge about the inequalities that currently exist in health care and in the education of culturally competent and transnational professionals who engage in evidence-based physical therapy that eliminates racial, ethnic, geographic, and socioeconomic health disparities.[10]

In any setting, it is important for therapists to be aware of their own attitudes and values regarding lifestyle choices; responses to pain, illness, and disability; and health practices. It may be beneficial to adapt the individual intervention program to ethnic practices and beliefs. Health care education may be most effective if provided without trying to change the individual's or family's longstanding beliefs. Knowing what is needed to effectively rehabilitate an individual does not assure success unless provided within a cultural and socioeconomic framework acceptable to the individual or family.

Some cultures have a very conservative view of physical contact, requiring a modified approach to the hands-on or manual therapist. In all situations where control may be an issue, the rationale and specifics for direct intervention must be clearly communicated and acceptable to the client.

Illness, especially life-threatening illness, often results in feelings of loss of control. Control, modes of control (e.g., passive acceptance, positive yielding or acceptance, or assertive control), and the desire for control are considered important variables that may influence physiologic function and health outcomes. Balancing active and yielding control styles and matching control strategies to client control styles and preferences may lead to optimal psychosocial adjustment and quality of life in the face of life-threatening illnesses.[29,42]

Language barriers make health care literature unavailable to many individuals who do not speak English and who require an interpreter (often unavailable) or for whom English is a second language, especially if English is spoken but not read. Keeping an open mind, asking questions, and respecting cultural differences are other ways to improve health care quality and delivery among minority groups.

Disabilities

The Americans with Disabilities Act of 1990 was designed to eliminate discrimination against people with disabilities, including discrimination in health care services. Although the Americans with Disabilities Act has improved access, barriers still exist for many people in receiving full age-appropriate primary care services. Disabled individuals, especially disabled women age 65 and older, often do not receive appropriate primary care. The more severe the disability, the less likely a person is to receive adequate care and undergo health screening.[49]

The physical therapist can be instrumental in assessing the disabled person's access to important screening and prevention services, advocate for the care of the disabled, encourage these people to become their own advocates for health care, and conduct research on people with disabilities.

Homelessness

Physical therapists are increasingly faced with addressing the needs of the homeless, who often experience frostbite, poor nutrition and hygiene, fatigue, mental illness, and a host of other minor medical problems. Many have additional secondary diagnoses (e.g., diabetes mellitus, hypertension, peripheral vascular disease, HIV, previous or present untreated orthopedic injuries) that complicate rehabilitation services. A third of the homeless clients have histories of past (and current) alcohol addiction and substance abuse.[52]

Physical Activity

The benefits of physical activity have been recognized since the time of Hippocrates, as evidenced by this quote attributed to Hippocrates (460–377 BC): "All parts of the body which have a function, if used in moderation and exercised in labours in which each is accustomed, become thereby healthy, well-developed and age more slowly; but if unused and left idle they become liable to disease, defective in growth, and age quickly." The importance of physical activity is as relevant today as it was then.

Physical activity is defined as any bodily movement produced by skeletal muscles that results in an expenditure of energy.[308] Physical activity is different from other lifestyle behaviors, in that all individuals have to move, although some move more and some move less. Physical activity contributes both directly and indirectly to health status and outcomes. Physical activity levels appear to contribute directly to disease mortality and morbidity, as well as indirectly by the influence of physical activity on conditions such as obesity, diabetes, and osteoporosis.

Physical fitness may be defined as "a set of attributes a person has in regards to a person's ability to perform physical activities that require aerobic fitness, endurance, strength, or flexibility and is determined by a combination of regular activity and genetically inherited ability."[308] Physical fitness and physical activity are related since increased physical activity is required to improve physical fitness, although one can perform a modest amount of physical activity without seeing improvements in fitness.

Effects of Physical Activity on Morbidity and Mortality

Much has been learned in the last decade about the adaptability of various biologic systems and the ways that regular physical activity and exercise can influence them. Participation in regular physical activity (both aerobic and strength training) is an effective intervention modality to reduce and/or prevent a number of functional declines associated with aging and to elicit a number of favorable responses that contribute to healthy aging[42] (Box 2-1).

The effect of training intensity, psychosocial variables influencing exercise, and the breadth of emotional benefit from physical activity has not been fully determined, although studies in this area are ongoing. The risks and benefits of exercise among people with disabilities are not fully known; more research is needed in this area. As people with disabilities live longer, the need for addressing long-term health issues, assessing the risk for secondary disability, and prescribing exercise from the perspective of disease prevention while reducing the risk for injury is needed.[80]

Other research to determine the potential links between oxidative stress and physical activity/exercise in the aging adult is ongoing. Exercise, especially when performed strenuously, is associated with increased free radical formation (see Fig. 6-2) that damages key cellular components.[186] In the older adult, the benefit of exercise is influenced by sedentary lifestyle, nutritional deficiencies, and comorbidities that can all deplete the individual's antioxidant reservoir.

Aging adults face additional problems of deconditioning or loss of balance and stability as a result of disease or illness. The most successful exercise programs take into consideration the person's functional capacity, medical status, and personal interests. Some helpful strategies for facilitating an exercise program (whether for a specific body part or as an overall fitness program) are listed in Box 2-2.

Morbidity. Physical inactivity contributes to the incidence of some chronic diseases. According to the WHO, there is convincing evidence that physical inactivity increases the risk of obesity and type 2 diabetes. In other words, regular physical activity decreases the risk of

---

Box 2-1

BENEFITS OF REGULAR PHYSICAL ACTIVITY AND EXERCISE

Note to Reader: You can access the ACSM's position stands on exercise for specific population groups (e.g., female athlete triad; individuals with coronary artery disease, hypertension, diabetes; healthy adults, older adults, wrestlers, etc.) at http://www.acsm.org/access-public-information/position-stands.

- Reduces/prevents functional declines associated with aging
- Maintains/improves cardiovascular function; enhances submaximal exercise performance; reduces risk for high blood pressure; decreases myocardial oxygen demand
- Aids in weight loss and weight control
- Improves the functioning of hormonal, metabolic, neurologic, respiratory, and hemodynamic systems
- Alters carbohydrate/lipid metabolism, resulting in favorable increase in high-density lipoproteins
- Strength training helps to maintain muscle mass and strength, especially in the aging group
- Reduces age-related bone loss; reduction is risk for osteoporosis
- Improves flexibility, postural stability, and balance; reduces risk of failing and associated injuries
- Psychologic benefits (e.g., lowers risk of cognitive decline and dementia, prevents and alleviates symptoms/behavior of depression and anxiety, improves self-awareness, promotes sense of well-being)
- Reduces disease risk factors for stroke, type 2 diabetes, coronary heart disease, and some forms of cancer (colon, breast)
- Improves functional capacity
- Improves immune function (excessive exercise can inhibit immune function)
- Reduces age-related insulin resistance
- Contributes to social integration
- Improves sleep pattern

Data from American College of Sports Medicine (ASCM) Position Stand: Exercise and physical activity for older adults. *Med Sci Sports Ex* 41:1510–1530, 2008. Available online at http://www.acsm.org/access-public-information/position-stands/position-stands. See also Garber CE. Quantity and quality of exercise for developing and maintaining cardiorespiratory, musculoskeletal, and neuromotor fitness in apparently healthy adults: guidance for prescribing exercise. *Med Sci Sports Ex* 43(7):1334–1359, 2011. Available online at http://journals.lww.com/acsm-msse/Fulltext/2011/07000/Quantity_and_Quality_of_Exercise_for_Developing.26.aspx.

---

cardiovascular disease, type 2 diabetes, obesity, and osteoporosis and decreases the risk of some types of cancers (e.g., colorectal).[319]

Regular physical activity appears to modify or reverse cardiovascular disease severity in individuals with known cardiovascular disease.[294] These effects include decreased risk of death from cardiovascular causes,[295] decreased atherosclerotic plaque formation,[93] and improved health status.[238]

Aerobic and resistive exercise appear to be associated with a decreased risk for type 2 diabetes, even among people at high risk for the disease.[144] In one large study, the risk of type 2 diabetes decreased 6% for every increase in

STRATEGIES TO FACILITATE SUCCESSFUL EXERCISE PROGRAMS

- Ask the client if he or she is currently exercising regularly (or was before illness or injury). Provide a brief description of benefits that the person could achieve from such a program.
- Stress exercise benefits of improving health rather than achieving weight loss.
- Allow the person to respond to the recommendation for an exercise program. Encourage the person to verbalize any thoughts or reactions to your suggestions.
- Determine whether the person believes that an exercise program will benefit him or her personally. Help the individual to set personal goals for exercise.
- Establish a patient/client self-charge contract and plan to monitor one's own success
- Be aware of any cultural or philosophical beliefs the person may have regarding exercise
- If resistance to the idea of an exercise program is encountered, give the person an opportunity to list potential barriers to exercise. Ask the person to suggest ways to overcome potential barriers.
- Whenever possible, provide a written (preferably just pictures because of the potential of undisclosed illiteracy) of the proposed exercise program. Review progress and reward attempts, successes, and progression of the exercise program.
- Make it fun to foster a lifestyle approach characterized by long-term adherence.

energy expenditure of 500 kilocalories (kcal)/week.[143] In addition, moderate physical activity was shown to be as effective as one type of diabetes medication (metformin) in reducing risk of diabetes.[173]

Osteoporosis is associated with increased disability and frequency of some types of fractures. The greatest benefits to bone mineral density and the incidence of osteoporosis appear to come from resistance training.[318] Exercise training programs have been found to prevent the 1% of bone loss per year observed in the lumbar spine in premenopausal and postmenopausal women.[330]

In regard to cancer, physical activity has an effect on some kinds of cancers.[184] Physical activity decreased the risk of colon cancer for men and women by 30% to 40% and also demonstrated a risk reduction of 20% to 30% for breast cancer in physically active women.[184]

Since there is an association of improved health with increased physical activity, it is important to define how much physical activity is beneficial. There is debate over the optimal amount of exercise needed for health benefits, although the general agreement is that more is better. Current discussion centers on whether the volume or intensity of exercise is most important for health.[103] Given that moderate exercise appears to provide significant health benefits and that vigorous exercise is difficult for individuals to achieve, public health policy has emphasized regular moderate exercise as an achievable goal for the greatest number of individuals.

The current recommendation of the U.S. Surgeon General indicates that adults gain substantial benefits from 2½ hours a week of moderate-intensity aerobic physical activity, or 1 hour 15 minutes of vigorous-intensity aerobic physical activity; each person is encouraged to accumulate 30 minutes of moderate exercise on most days of the week. Minimum increments of 10 minutes are advised. Additional wording indicates that people who are already active may benefit from more intense levels of physical activity.[308] For details of key guidelines by age, see the U.S. Department of Health and Human Services Physical Activity Guidelines, available online at http://www.health.gov/paguidelines/guidelines/default.aspx.

Mortality. Physical activity patterns appear to have a direct effect on deaths. In the 1990s, activity patterns and nutrition contributed to 14% of all deaths in the United States.[200] In addition, 23% of deaths from major chronic diseases were also linked to lack of physical activity.[137] Increased levels of physical activity appear to reduce the relative risk of death in both men and women by 20% to 35%.[197,198] In addition, increased physical activity by 1000 kcal/week or 1 metabolic equivalent (MET) of fitness is associated with a 20% decrease in mortality, at least among women.[158,185]

Physical fitness appears to confer a greater benefit than physical activity alone. A clear relationship between fitness and all-cause mortality and deaths from cardiovascular disease has been established.[96] These studies demonstrate that death rates are highest in the lowest quartile of fitness. The greatest improvement in mortality occurs between the lowest and next lowest category of fitness, suggesting there is a graded effect of improved fitness on mortality. This is consistent with other research that demonstrates that small improvements in fitness are associated with significant reduction in risk of cardiovascular events and death.[319]

Occupational Versus Leisure-Time Physical Activity

Early investigation of the role of physical activity in mortality compared people in sedentary versus physically active occupations.[212] Much of the literature, including the Surgeon General's report, has investigated leisure-time physical activity.[308] Taking the evidence together, it appears that the overall volume and intensity of physical activity are most important, whether at work or during leisure time. However, there may be additional effects of strenuous work on health status or musculoskeletal pathology. For example, self-reported health was lower in people with active and strenuous jobs.[242]

In a study of industrial workers over a 28-year period of time, vigorous leisure-time activity was associated with low risk of poor physical function, but strenuous work activity increased the risk of poor physical function.[186] In addition, low levels of physical activity were associated with higher rates of low back pain.[146] Future investigations may clarify the various effects of leisure versus occupational physical activity.

Aerobic Capacity Versus Musculoskeletal Fitness

Physical activity, regardless of aerobic capacity level, appears to provide health benefits. Musculoskeletal performance is increasingly linked to improved physical function and prevents or modifies disability.[211] Many ADLs require more musculoskeletal performance and rely less on aerobic capacity.[319] Furthermore, a decline in physical performance, defined by activities such as rising from a chair and climbing stairs, is associated with dependence in ADLs and assisted living placement.[135]

Prevalence of Physical Activity Behaviors

Two behavioral strategies for reducing the risk for chronic disease have been identified: (1) consuming fruits and vegetables five or more times per day and (2) engaging in regular physical activity. Despite the importance of physical activity, only a minority of Americans are meeting physical activity guidelines.

Data for the prevalence of physical activity behaviors are available from a variety of population surveys. One common source of information is the Behavioral Risk Factor Surveillance System,[62] a population-based, random digit–dialed telephone survey of the U.S. population older than age 18 years conducted by the CDC.[208] Information regarding health risk behaviors, clinical preventive health practices, and health care access, primarily related to chronic disease and injury, is obtained from a representative sample of adults in each state.[208] Respondents are asked to recall the overall frequency and time spent in a variety of leisure time activities, as well as in moderate and vigorous physical activity.

The current Behavioral Risk Factor Surveillance System indicates that less than half (48%) of U.S. adults meet the physical activity guidelines; less than 30% of high school students get at least 60 minutes of daily physical activity. Rates of activity and inactivity vary across states and regions: for example, individuals living in the South are less physically active than any other region. Adults with higher education and socioeconomic status are more likely to remain physically active.[63]

There are differences in physical activity and nutrition reported by ethnicity. Among men, engaging in regular physical activity was significantly less common for non-Hispanic blacks, Hispanics, and Asian/Pacific Islanders than for non-Hispanic whites. Among women, regular physical activity was significantly lower among non-Hispanic blacks and Hispanics than among non-Hispanic whites.[63]

Compared with non-Hispanic white men, the combined prevalence for eating fruits and vegetables five or more times per day and engaging in regular physical activity was significantly higher for men of multiple/other races. Among women, the combined prevalence of eating fruits and vegetables five or more times per day and engaging in regular physical activity was significantly lower for non-Hispanic blacks and Hispanics than for non-Hispanic whites.[133]

There is also great concern about children's activity levels. Based on the study Youth Risk Behavior Surveillance System conducted in 2010, most children and youth are not meeting current physical activity guidelines. About 15% of children reported no recent physical activity of any intensity during leisure time. Inactivity is higher in girls than in boys and in black girls than in white girls.

Approximately 25% of youth reported no vigorous physical activity; however, 25% also reported walking or biking nearly every day (equivalent to light or moderate activity). Participation in physical activity decreases significantly as age or grade in school increases. Additionally,

the Youth Risk Behavior Surveillance System reports that one-third of all students in grades 9 to 12 did not meet national guidelines for physical activity in 2010; only 31% attended physical education class daily.[71]

Regular physical activity is beneficial in improving both physical and mental health outcomes. There is evidence that physical activity decreases blood pressure, improves lipid profile by decreasing triglycerides and total cholesterol while increasing high-density lipoprotein, improves insulin sensitivity, and enhances endothelial function, all of which contribute to decreasing cardiovascular risk.[228] Regular physical activity helps build and maintain healthy bones and muscles. In addition, regular physical activity is associated with an increased sense of well-being, can modify the symptoms of depression, and increase self-efficacy (the ability or confidence of a person to implement an effective behavior).[71]

Interventions for Increasing Physical Activity

Given the benefits of physical activity, it is helpful to know what type of interventions are successful in changing health behaviors, including increasing physical activity. There are a variety of strategies used to encourage physical activity, including self-directed behavior, exercise referral schemes,[247] supervised programs, online interventions,[102] specific reminders (including electronically generated), or combined approaches. However, it is difficult to compare the success of interventions since they are so varied.[245,246]

A review of physical activity interventions examined randomized controlled trials for different interventions for community-living adults with a 6-month follow-up and no more than 20% participant loss over the time period.[149] In this study, all types of interventions were successful at increasing physical activity levels, including individual and positive encouragement and group or individual exercise programs.[149] This implies that all medical practitioners, including physical therapists, should encourage individuals to exercise. Cardiopulmonary fitness also improved in people who exercised, as compared to controls. However, few studies were able to demonstrate success for individuals in achieving a predetermined amount of physical activity.[194]

The interventions that appear to improve physical activity the most include physician advice; counseling from a health educator on action planning and follow-up phone calls, emails, monitoring cards; and a pedometer.[149] Adding weekly classes on skills for increasing physical activity and educational materials appears to help women achieve higher fitness goals, although these additions do not significantly influence men.[337] Success appears to increase with ongoing support in which there are four or more contacts among exercise participants and staff.[149]

SPECIAL IMPLICATIONS FOR THE THERAPIST 2-2

Physical Activity

Promoting Physical Activity

Healthful exercise and eating behaviors have been shown unequivocally to reduce the risk for health compromise and chronic disease. Physical therapists are in an ideal position to promote healthy behaviors and reduce the risk of chronic disease in all individuals by including each of the following steps.

- *Assess physical activity along with other health indicators and risk factors such as smoking, heart disease, and hypertension*
- *Work with other public health groups to address the importance of increasing physical activity*
- *Recommend physical activity as part of a physical therapy plan of care*

Physical Activity Recommendations[305]

> **Note to Reader:** For full details of Physical Activity Guidelines for Americans by age group (life stage) with a review of the strength of the scientific evidence, go to http://www.health.gov/paguidelines/guidelines/default.aspx. These are general guidelines and provide a starting point to help people of all ages engage in more physical activity. The complete publication can be accessed at http://journals.lww.com/acsm-msse/Fulltext/2011/07000/Quantity_and_Quality_of_Exercise_for_Developing.26.aspx
>
> There are additional health benefits from increasing activity levels beyond these initial guidelines. The physical therapist's understanding of pathophysiology and ability to consider patient/client goals and individual factors (age, general health, lifestyle, comorbidities) positions us as the health professional best suited to prescribe exercise programs for all ages and all groups (e.g., pregnant or postpartum women, individuals with disabilities, athletes, centenarians, individuals with chronic conditions, and so on).

- *Accumulating 30 minutes of daily physical activity for adults and 60 minutes daily for children and adolescents (ages 6–17) has been shown to have health benefits; however, the minimum amount of time to be spent in physical activity is 10 minutes. Most of this time should be either moderate- or vigorous-intensity aerobic activity.*
- *Adults are advised to complete a total of 2½ hours of moderate-intensity physical activity each week or 75 minutes (1 hour 15 minutes)/week of vigorous-intensity aerobic physical activity.*
- *Moderate exercise is defined as reaching a certain threshold of energy expenditure. Energy expenditure estimated in METs gives a guideline for energy expenditure. By definition, 1 MET is equivalent to the amount of oxygen consumed at rest, averaged at 3.5 mL/kg^{-1}/min^{-1}. Moderate activity ranges from 3 to 6 METs, or 10.5 to 21.0 mL of oxygen consumed for each kilogram of body weight per minute. This leads to approximately 100 calories burned for 30 minutes of exercise in an individual who weighs 150 lb.*
- *Muscle- and bone-strengthening exercises should be performed at least 3 days a week for children and teens and a minimum of twice a week (more often is preferable) for adults of all ages.*
- *Older adults should do exercises that maintain or improve balance.*
- *How can physical therapists estimate energy expenditure?*

Table 2-2 provides some estimates of energy expenditure for the average person that can be used in physical therapy settings.

Table 2-2	Estimates of Energy Expenditure			
METs	**Oxygen consumption**	**Kcal/ min**	**Kcal for 30-min exercise**	**Walk speed**
3	10.5 mL/ kg^{-1}/min^{-1}	3.5	100	2.6 mph
4	14 mL/kg^{-1}/ min^{-1}	4.5	135	3.9
5	17.5 mL/ kg^{-1}/min^{-1}	5.75	175	3.0 mph 4.2% grade
6	21 mL/kg^{-1}/ min^{-1}	7	210	3.0 mph 9.2% grade

METs, Metabolic equivalents; Kcal/min, kilocalories per minute; mph, miles per hour.

Nutrition

Nutrition is a modifiable risk factor for chronic disease; there is increased evidence that diet has significant effects (positive or negative) on health. Studies by the WHO indicate that diet has an important role in preventing and controlling both morbidity and mortality.[332] The chronic diseases most influenced by diet and creating the greatest cost in deaths or disability include obesity, diabetes, cardio- and/or cerebrovascular disease, cancer, and osteoporosis.

The National Cholesterol Education Program and the American Cancer Society both emphasize lifestyle modifications that include diet and physical activity to reduce disease risk. Diets high in fruits and vegetables combined with participation in regular physical activity are associated with a lower risk for all individuals, especially those whose health is at risk from lifestyle factors and individuals with chronic diseases and conditions.[32,228] These are also two of the strategies implemented by states participating in the CDC Nutrition and Physical Activity Program to Prevent Obesity and Other Chronic Diseases.[178]

Significant changes have occurred in the world food economy with profound effects on diets and lifestyles. These shifting dietary patterns include increased consumption of energy-dense foods high in saturated fat and low in unprocessed carbohydrates at the same time there has been a decline in energy expenditure associated with a sedentary lifestyle and ageing population.[333] Nutritional patterns indicate that in industrialized countries, energy intake averages 3380 kcal per capita per day, with a large increase (26%) from 1969 to 1999 in energy supplied by animal fat. North America remains above the recommended average of fat-to-energy ratio defined as the percentage of energy derived from fat in the total number of calories supplied, as well as above the recommended amount of saturated fat per total calories (10%).[334]

Obesity

Definition and Measurement

Obesity is defined as an excessive accumulation of fat in the body that contributes to numerous chronic diseases as well as early mortality and morbidity. *Bariatrics* is the branch of medicine concerned with the management of obesity.[286]

Prior to the development of the *Clinical Guidelines on the Identification, Evaluation and Treatment of Overweight and Obesity in Adults: The Evidence Report*,[224] measures used to determine weight status varied (e.g., weight–height tables, skinfold measurements, 20% higher than normal weight).

Currently, most studies use one of three commonly accepted measures to define obesity in adults: BMI, waist circumference, and waist-to-hip ratio. All of these measures are clinically feasible to administer and have been shown to relate to health risk. Ranges of BMI, calculated as a ratio of height to weight, are used to categorize body weight status and health risk (Table 2-3).

The National Institutes of Health[223] clinical guidelines and the WHO[336] define overweight as a BMI equal to or greater than 25 kg/m^2. Obesity, defined as a BMI equal to or greater than 30 kg/m^2, is further divided into three classes. A BMI greater than or equal to 25 kg/m^2 is associated with increased risk for premature death and disability. As one progresses to a higher class of obesity, health risk and morbidity increase.[120] The term *morbid obesity* has been used by some authors to refer to a BMI greater than 40 kg/m^2.[159] BMI varies with age and sex in children and adolescents, necessitating the CDC to develop BMI guidelines that uniquely account for growth using weight and height. BMIs greater than or equal to the 85th and less than or equal to the 95th percentile signify a risk for being overweight; BMI greater than or equal to the 95th percentile signifies risk for being obese. Regardless of the person's age, gender, or socioeconomic status, all medical practitioners should track weight and height regularly and address any concerns or weight-related risks with their patients/clients.

Waist circumference is used to determine an individual's measure of abdominal fat and to further elucidate disease risk. The presence of excess fat in the abdomen is a predictor of cardiovascular risk factors and disease.[311] Waist circumference provides an independent prediction of risk beyond what BMI alone can provide. However, once waist circumference is beyond the level predictive of high risk, the values lose their predictive power. Waist-to-hip ratio is also used as an indicator or measure of obesity and the risk of developing serious health conditions. Waist-to-hip ratio shows a graded and highly significant association with myocardial infarction risk worldwide (85% or higher ratio for women and 90% or higher for men increases the risk).[88,192] Redefinition of obesity based on waist-to-hip ratio instead of BMI has been suggested. The waist-to-hip method increases the estimate of myocardial infarction attributable to obesity in most ethnic groups.[341] Of the three measures, only the waist-to-hip ratio takes into account the differences in body conformation and distribution of adiposity in the trunk and extremities ("apple vs. pear" shape).

Table 2-3	Body Mass Index to Determine Obesity Classification	
NHLBI Terminology	**Body Mass Index (BMI) Range (kg/m^2)**	**WHO Classification**
Underweight*	<18.5	Underweight
Normal	18.5–24.9	Normal
Overweight	25.0–29.9	Preobese
Obesity Class 1	30.0–34.9	Obese Class 1
Obesity Class 2	35.0–39.9	Obese Class 2
Obesity Class 3	≥40.0	Obese Class 3

NHLBI, National Heart, Lung, and Blood Institute.
*BMI less than 17.5 is classified as anorexic.

New strategies for measurement are being considered as researchers and practitioners seek the best measures for describing the extent of the obese condition and its relationship to health risk. For example, the Body Adiposity Index (BAI), a relationship between hip circumference and height, has been proposed as a clinically feasible strategy for measuring percentage body fat. Thus far, however, the BAI measure is still being studied for its accuracy and ability to predict health risk.[33] Although BMI may not accurately reflect individual variations in fat-free mass, this measure is currently the most common measure of obesity and is an internationally accepted and understood definition of the condition. Regardless of the measure used, obesity is a condition that is inherently risky for health and longevity, especially if the distribution of such fat is in and around the abdomen (see Fig. 11-8).[341]

See further discussion of the diagnostic relevance of measures of obesity under "Diagnosis" later in this topic.

Incidence and Prevalence

Obesity is now regarded as a pandemic (affecting all people globally),[266] with implications for 300 million people across the world.[10,175] Obesity has begun to replace other known causes of mortality (e.g., undernutrition and infectious diseases) as the most significant contributor to ill health. It is second only to cigarette smoking as a leading cause of preventable death in the United States and contributes to 500,000 deaths annually; out of these deaths, the CDC reports that 30,000 are premature deaths. In the United States, it is estimated that 65% of adults can be categorized as overweight or obese.[171]

The prevalence of obesity among adults continues to increase[43,64] From 1980 to 2002, obesity doubled in adults and overweight prevalence tripled in children and adolescents.[64] Rates of obesity have been expected to increase more quickly than overweight, resulting in a predicted prevalence in the United States by 2015 of 40% for men and 45% for women.[314]

Other countries' estimates of future obesity prevalence and health-related concerns are similarly troublesome. For example, in Australia, estimates of weight gain project the prevalence of adult obesity to rise by 65% if the rate of change occurring between 2000 and 2005 continues. Further, the impact on longevity of both men and women who are obese will be a loss of life expectancy of 43.3 years and 42.2 years, respectively, in comparison to normal-weight individuals.[317] Thus, obesity is a worldwide concern with a significant impact on life and health.

This growth in the percentage of people who are now overweight or obese is occurring across all age groups and is of significant concern in both pediatric and geriatric populations. The disease burden created by obesity is not felt equally across all populations; disparity exists across race, gender, age, socioeconomic status, and education level.[114,328] Also of concern is the medical cost associated with obesity in the United States, estimated to be at least $147 billion and 37% more than for adults who are not obese.[111]

The U.S. Department of Health and Human Services (DHHS) reports that nearly one out of every five children 6 to 11 years old is obese, with prevalence rates being slightly lower for children 2 to 5 years (10.4%) and for adolescents 12 to 29 years of age (18.1%).[234] Of great concern is the 147% increase in obesity rates that occurred from 1971 to 1994 among children ages 6 to 11[42] because of the socioeconomic disparities associated with these rates.[235] The increase in numbers of people who are obese is paralleled by a considerable reduction in daily energy expenditure and physical activity that leads to a decrease in aerobic capacity and deficiencies in the ability to perform physical activities.[65,200,225,299]

Existing evidence indicates that physical inactivity is strongly associated with body weight gain and that participation in purposeful and regular exercise and maintenance of a physically active lifestyle can be effective in maintaining a healthy body weight.[48,74,80,121,233,327] Although sedentary lifestyles have not been shown to be the cause of obesity, sedentary behavior (i.e., muscular inactivity) has been linked to metabolic risks,[94] and the risk of becoming sedentary increases with BMI.[214] Research has confirmed the importance of physical activity to maintain weight loss, especially if exercise commitment reached or exceeded 200 minutes per week.[160,164] Prescribing regimens to meet this criterion is definitely in the scope of practice for physical therapists.

Etiologic and Risk Factors

The development of obesity depends on an imbalance between energy intake and energy expenditure, with more energy consumed than is expended. Inactivity and an energy-dense diet (i.e., highly processed and refined foods without fiber) are known contributors for weight gain. Environmental factors (including lack of access to full-service grocery stores, increasing costs of healthy foods and the lower cost of unhealthy foods, and lack of access to safe places to play and exercise) all contribute to the increase in obesity rates by inhibiting or preventing healthy eating and active living behaviors.[171]

Absolute reasons why energy imbalance leads to obesity remain to be determined. However, several factors associated with the development of the energy imbalance and that may lead to excessive fat deposition and obesity are listed in Box 2-3. In addition, the failure of aging people to adjust food intake in response to lowered metabolism and diminished activity, and weight cycling with fluctuations of body weight produced by repeated

---

Box 2-3

RISK FACTORS FOR OBESITY

- Sedentary lifestyle
- High glycemic diet*
- Underlying illness (e.g., hypothyroidism, polycystic ovary syndrome)
- Genetic disorder (Prader-Willi syndrome)
- Genetic, familial, or biologic factors
- Medications (e.g., increased appetite or food cravings associated with prescription medications)
  Corticosteroids (see Box 5-5)
  Antidepressants
  Antihypertensives
  Anticonvulsants
  Diabetes medications (short acting insulin)
- Environmental or psychosocial/behavioral factors (e.g., history of sexual abuse, socioeconomic status, eating disorders, lack of sleep, stressful lifestyle, smoking cessation)

* High glycemic diet refers to foods that are high in sugar, salt, and fats with little or no nutritional value because of the absence of vitamin, mineral or fiber content.

---

cycles of weight loss and gain appear to contribute to the inability to lose weight on a long-term basis.

Medication-induced weight gain also may occur as a result of increased appetite, episodes of hypoglycemia, or water retention. Other drugs, such as corticosteroids, make the body less able to absorb blood glucose, leading to increased fat deposits in the trunk. Antihypertensive medications, such as beta-blockers, may produce fatigue or shortness of breath, leading to reduced activity levels and increased weight gain.

A growing body of evidence suggests that some forms of obesity may result from biochemical defects rather than just consumption of excess calories.[167,326] After a 40-year search, scientists originally found three genes linked to obesity (ob, neuropeptide Y [Npy], and the Beacon gene). Npy and the Beacon gene produce a protein that stimulates the appetite, whereas the ob gene produces a protein (leptin) that switches off the appetite. In some obese people, the body does not respond to leptin; in others, the Beacon gene is working in overdrive, producing too much appetite-stimulating protein.[79]

Despite the new discoveries of single-gene mutations resulting in obesity, most cases of obesity are more likely the result of subtle interactions of several related genes with environmental factors that favor the net deposition of calories as fat resulting in obesity. The increasing rates of obesity cannot be exclusively explained by changes in the gene pool, although genetic variants that were previously silent may now be triggered by the high availability of energy- and fat-dense foods and by the increasingly sedentary lifestyle of modern societies.[199]

Pathogenesis

The mechanisms proposed to explain the development or effects of obesity on the human body target neurologic, metabolic, and energy regulation systems.

Accumulating evidence indicates that obesity is a central nervous system–mediated *neuroendocrine dysfunction*. Because the central nervous system plays a key role in the regulation of food intake and energy balance, one explanation may be that either spontaneous genetic mutations or targeted gene deletions that impair central nervous system signaling cause disrupted food intake and body-weight control.[31] Researchers are studying the highly complex process of signaling molecules involved in the regulation of food intake and how inherited or acquired defects in the function of these hormonal and neuropeptide signaling pathways contribute to obesity.[279,331]

Another explanation involves the neuroendocrine system and suggests that *hormonal dysfunction* affecting the hypothalamic–pituitary–adrenal (HPA) axis results in a complex series of events. Stress stimulates daily, periodic elevations of cortisol secretion and results in impaired cortisol secretion, prolonged stimulation of the sympathetic nervous system, and subsequent hypothalamic arousal. The net effects of this neuroendocrine–endocrine cascade are poorly regulated cortisol secretion, insulin resistance, elevated blood pressure, and visceral accumulation of body fat (central obesity).[40] The result can be a collection of metabolic risk factors, referred to as the *metabolic syndrome*, which includes abdominal obesity, atherogenic dyslipidemia, elevated blood pressure, insulin resistance, and prothrombotic and proinflammatory state of the blood (see "Metabolic Syndrome" in Chapter 11).

Energy regulation also has been a target for explaining the mechanism(s) of obesity. In this case, the sodium (Na^+)/potassium (K^+)/adenosine triphosphatase (ATPase) pump is thought to play a major role in the development of obesity. This enzyme pump transports sodium out of the cell and potassium into the cell at the expense of cellular energy in the form of adenosine triphosphate (ATP). Obese people are thought to have fewer ATPase pumps than the non-obese; the obese person uses less energy and expends fewer calories, keeping a state of equilibrium within the body.

The *adipose cell* theory postulates that some people inherently have an excessive number of fat cells (adipocytes), and the size of the fat cells is increased. Similarly, the *lipoprotein lipase* theory suggests that the enzyme lipoprotein lipase, which helps fat to be deposited in adipocytes, is elevated in obese persons, and weight reduction stimulates even more production of the enzyme, causing fat cells to return to their hypertrophic size.

More recently, researchers have proposed the theory that for some people, obesity is the result of intestinal microorganisms. The *microbial* theory of obesity suggests a biologic cause of weight gain from an altered level of bacterial intestinal microbes called *gut microflora*.[19,188] Gut microbes contribute to body weight regulation through an effect on the metabolic and immune system of each individual resulting in an improved ability to extract and store energy from ingested food.[189,274]

In recent years, *viral infections* have been recognized as a possible cause of obesity, along with the traditionally recognized causes. A human virus *adenovirus-36* (Ad-36) has been recognized as a potential cause of obesity (referred to as infectoobesity). This virus is known to increase the replication, differentiation, lipid accumulation, and insulin sensitivity in fat cells and reduce those cells' leptin secretion and expression (gene that switches off appetite).[312]

Box 2-4

COMPLICATIONS ASSOCIATED WITH OBESITY

- Metabolic syndrome
- Type 2 diabetes mellitus
- Liver diseases
- Osteoarthritis
- Sleep apnea
- Atherosclerosis; hypertension; cardiovascular diseases
- Stroke
- Asthma
- Cancer
- Menstrual disorders and infertility
- Lymphedema
- Impaired mobility
- Gallbladder disease
- Psychologic disturbances such as irritability, loneliness, depression, binge eating, and tension
- Premature death

Data from Deusinger SS et al: The obesity epidemic: health consequences and implications for physical therapy. *PT Magazine* 12(6):82–104, June 2004.

Linked to the regulation of leptin, there is some evidence that people who sleep less, weigh more. Chronic sleep deprivation defined as sleeping only 4–5 hours/24-hour cycle alters levels of the appetite-regulating hormones leptin and ghrelin, leading to increased appetite. Weight gain may occur as a result of increased wake time, altered appetite, and the resultant fatigue, which makes exercise more difficult.[244]

Clinical Manifestations

Regardless of the mechanisms of the condition, the outward signs and symptoms of obesity are readily observable (excess body fat). However, the effects and complications of obesity are less easily identified at onset.

Obesity is associated with significant increases in both morbidity and mortality from many conditions (Box 2-4) and is associated with three leading causes of death: cardiovascular disease, cancer, and diabetes mellitus. The roles of obesity in inflammation, fat (adipose tissue) as an endocrine gland, and the relationship of obesity and fat accumulation to cancer are discussed in Chapters 9 and 11.

Diabetes Mellitus. Type 2 diabetes mellitus is often associated with obesity. Excessive food intake, with or without physical inactivity, stimulates hyperinsulinemia. Through a negative-feedback mechanism, excessive insulin levels decrease the number of insulin receptor sites on adipose cells. The decrease in insulin receptor sites decreases the amount of glucose that can enter the cells. This promotes high blood levels of glucose. The excess glucose is stored as glycogen in the liver or as triglycerides in adipose cells, thereby enhancing hypertrophy and hyperplasia of fat cells in the already obese person. Weight reduction can reverse this process.

Asthma. Rising asthma rates and poor management of the disease are increasingly linked to obesity.[45,55] The mechanism for the causality is thought to be related to an inability of the person to take deep breaths, which leads to more reactive airways and, if severe enough, asthma.

Research is mixed as to whether the link between obesity and asthma is the same for women and men. One study concluded that independent of age, women with a BMI greater than or equal to 30 kg/m² were about twice as likely to develop asthma as women of a normal weight.[73]

Functional Impairments. Obesity also is associated with significant functional deficits or problems that lead to functional impairments. Shortness of breath; fatigue; ADL limitations[274]; increased risk for falls[81]; and an increased incidence of hip, knee, and back pain in those who are obese[14] are potential problems. Given a strong association between obesity and osteoarthritis (OA) of the knee, the risk for dysfunction in functional activities, such as walking and stair climbing, has been investigated.[77,206] Weight loss has been shown both to reduce the risk of OA and to improve function in the face of this condition.[206]

Both perceptions and observed measures of functional limitations have been tested and found to be associated with difficulty of accomplishing daily tasks related to housework and self-care.[181,182] Thus the clinical manifestations of obesity have broad implications for numerous body systems and health dimensions.

Lower Extremity Lymphedema. Obesity may be a cause of lower extremity lymphedema. Individuals with a BMI greater than 59 have been documented with lymphedema. It has been hypothesized that this may be the threshold above which lymphatic flow becomes impaired.[134] The mechanism for this relationship between BMI and lymphedema has not been established. Lymphatic vessels may be compressed or inflamed, resulting in impaired lymph flow, or alternately, elevated production of lymph from the enlarged limb may overwhelm the lymph system's capacity to move/remove fluid.[134]

Complications with Pregnancy. Obesity in pregnancy is of concern and affects maternal–fetal outcomes. Women who are obese face high risk of developing health problems during their prenatal and postnatal periods, increased risk of spontaneous abortions and still births,[86] gestational diabetes mellitus,[124] pregnancy induced hypertension,[1,124] development of deep venous thrombosis,[86] and prolonged pregnancy and labor.[338] Risks to the fetus include birth defects,[162] macrosomia (birthweight more than 4000 g [9 lb]),[86] and shoulder dystocia[142] during birth; in addition, there is a higher risk of developing childhood obesity and glucose intolerance in adulthood.[142]

Other Complications. Other complications may include nephrotic syndrome and renal vein thrombosis; other thromboembolic disorders; digestive tract diseases, such as gallstones and reflux esophagitis; asthma; obstructive sleep apnea; carpal tunnel syndrome; subfertility- and pregnancy-related issues in women; and subsequent pulmonary compromise with decreased gas exchange, vital capacity, and expiratory volume. As discussed, dietary patterns, portion control, and energy-dense choices in combination with physical inactivity contribute to obesity and metabolic consequences.

MEDICAL MANAGEMENT

PREVENTION. Preventing obesity from occurring or worsening is an important part of achieving a healthier population. Prevention includes maintenance of healthy weight, maintenance of weight loss, and prevention of weight gain. Identifying risk factors that can lead to obesity or cause related health problems and learning strategies toward achieving a healthy weight are the keys to successful prevention.[9] The CDC has recommended 24 strategies and appropriate measurements to help communities create environments that promote good nutrition and physical activity (available at http://www.cdc.gov/mmwr/preview/mmwrhtml/rr5807a1.htm?s_cid=rr5807a1_e). These strategies confirm the importance of a multidimensional approach to the causes and solutions for the obesity epidemic.

Physical therapists' scope of practice includes an imperative for involvement in all levels of prevention (primary, secondary, tertiary) of this important health risk. Physical therapists have been traditionally comfortable with tertiary prevention, which aims to limit the sequelae of chronic health conditions, and actively involved with secondary prevention, which focuses on reducing the severity or duration of existing conditions. Providing primary prevention services is a contemporary expectation that involves vigilance about health risk and promotion of lifestyle strategies that reduce risk and impart health. With regard to obesity, primary prevention would be aimed at achieving appropriate energy balance to avoid weight gain in the first place—especially during biological or personal stages of life (e.g., puberty) shown to be related to potentially unhealthy weight gain.

Diagnosis. Physical examination should be directed at determining the presence and distribution of body fat by measuring height, weight, body circumference (extremity and waist), and nutritional status. In addition, the presence of associated causes of obesity should be investigated.

Abdominal (visceral) fat is metabolically active. Measurement of abdominal circumference is needed to identify the distribution of body fat and to determine the risks associated with increased waist circumference. Waist circumferences that are higher than 40 inches for men and 35 inches for women increase the risk for premature death and disability as a consequence of overweight or obesity. Waist circumference is the best predictor of visceral (intraabdominal) fat and total fat. The most clinically telling physical sign of serious underlying disease is increased waist circumference, which is linked to insulin resistance, hypertension, dyslipidemia, type 2 diabetes, coronary heart disease, sleep apnea, and gallbladder disease.[139]

Although BMI and waist circumference measurements are the most clinically feasible methods to identify clients who are overweight or obese, additional methods may be used to measure subcutaneous fat or body composition.[97] Methods that are known for accuracy but often only used in research settings include hydrostatic weighing and dual-energy x-ray absorptiometry.[51,177]

Additional methods that require less expensive equipment include the use of skinfold measurement calipers and the measurement of bioelectrical impedance. Skinfold measurements using calipers (the pinch test) are performed in several locations on the body (e.g., midbiceps, midtriceps, and subscapular areas). Measurements greater than 1 inch are thought to indicate excessive body fat. Interobserver variability may be high with skinfold measurement, thus raising questions about the accuracy of this method of assessing obesity.[193] Any use of skinfold measures should include consideration of adiposity distribution and height.

Another way to measure obesity is through bioelectrical impedance analysis (BIA). BIA measures the impedance or resistance to an electrical signal that is circulated through the body. A person who has more fat mass will have larger impedance because there will be more resistance to the electrical signal traveling through the body since fat mass contains less water. BIA measures have been shown to be reliable and valid; however, variability among individuals can be high, and inaccuracy can occur in situations of altered hydration status and extreme obesity in those being measured.[30,151] BIA has not been shown to be superior to BMI as a predictor of overall adiposity in a general population.[324] Although inexpensive BIA machines are in common use, they typically lack reliability. It is anticipated that the measurement of body composition will become more reliable and accurate as technology improves.

All of these measures can provide a baseline measurement for relative fat mass and can be used to monitor progress of body composition as people advance through a weight loss program. BIA is commonly used in community health clubs and health fairs.

Treatment. Both physical activity and nutrition are important in addressing obesity. Physical activity and nutrition are modifiable factors that respond similarly to the same interventions. To maintain a healthy weight, it is important to keep energy expenditure at or above energy intake. This can be accomplished by decreasing caloric intake, increasing exercise energy expenditure, or both.

Weight Loss. Weight loss is regarded as a major aspect of treatment for the person who is obese. Although the amount of weight loss necessary may be individual, 10% loss in body weight is regarded as a standard that improves health. The National Weight Control Registry (www.nwcr.ws/) reports that weight loss and maintenance of the weight loss are best accomplished if individuals participate in regular intensive exercise, attend support groups, restrict the amount and kinds of food eaten, and weigh themselves often.

A multidisciplinary approach with emphasis on weight loss and maintenance of that loss is appropriate for anyone with a BMI of 30 and above and for those people with a BMI in the 25 to 29 range who have associated health problems. Such a treatment program includes moderate calorie intake, behavior modification, exercise, and social support. The same recommendations are appropriate for individuals who have not yet become overweight but are at risk for the condition because of genetics, personal habits, or environment.

Medications. Medications for obesity are widely available over the counter and by prescription. The use of pharmacologic agents to calm cravings, inhibit appetite, reduce fat absorption, and increase metabolic rate is highly controversial and provides at best only a short-term benefit. Drug therapy is thought to work best when it is part of an overall program aimed at lifestyle change involving dietary changes, exercise, and behavior modification.[317,322] To be effective, drug treatment for obesity should be continued indefinitely, much like treatment for any chronic condition.[8,105,322] Researchers continue to look for drugs that can prevent or alter the physiology of obesity.

Surgery. Surgical treatment, referred to as *bariatric surgery,* may be considered for some obese people if serious attempts to lose weight have failed, if BMI is greater than 40 kg/m^2 with or without comorbidities, or if there is a BMI of 35 kg/m^2 with significant health-related comorbidities[8,105,227,290,322] and complications of obesity that are life-threatening. Surgical approaches rely on reconfiguring or redirecting the gastrointestinal system through bariatric weight loss surgery (e.g., Roux-en-Y gastric bypass, laparoscopic adjustable gastric banding, vertical banded gastroplasty). Bariatric surgery has been shown to provide the greatest degree of sustained weight loss in people with morbid obesity.[190] Other benefits and complications of bariatric surgery are listed in Table 2-4.

Laparoscopic Roux-en-Y gastric bypass has been referred to as the "gold standard" operation for surgical control of obesity. It is effective in achieving weight loss, improving comorbidities and quality of life, and reducing recovery time and perioperative complications.[277] This procedure is safe and effective and decreases overall costs.[227]

Evidence supports this shift in surgical approach for individuals having laparoscopic surgery based on studies demonstrating improved SF-36 scores,[2,127,226,290]

Table 2-4	Potential Benefits and Complications of Bariatric Surgery	
Potential Benefits	**Potential Complications**
Weight loss	Nephrolithiasis
Improved serum lipids	Hepatic failure
Remission of type 2 diabetes*	Cholelithiasis
Decreased blood pressure	Malnutrition; vitamin and
Improved or resolved	mineral deficiencies
comorbidities:	Reflux
• Diabetes mellitus	Small bowel obstruction (SBO)
• Improved or resolved	Hemorrhage
sleep apnea	Iron-deficiency anemia
• Reduced hypertension	Gastric prolapse
Reduced venous stasis	Postoperative bleeding
Decreased joint pain	Atelectasis; pneumonia
Improved quality of life	Death
Overall improved function	
Improved quality of life	

American Society for Metabolic and Bariatric Surgery: Benefits and complications of bariatric surgery. Available online at http://asmbs.org/.
*After gastric bypass, more than 80% of diabetics cease to be diabetic; essentially 100% of prediabetics are spared from developing the disease in the first place. Individuals with type 2 diabetes treated with gastric bypass are reportedly more successful at keeping diabetes in remission. (Mingrone G: Bariatric surgery versus conventional medical therapy for type 2 diabetes. *N Engl J Med* March 26, 2012. Epub ahead of print; Schauer PR: Bariatric surgery versus intensive medical therapy in obese patients with diabetes. *N Engl J Med* 366(17):1567–1576, 2012.)
Courtesy Tamara L. Burlis, PT, DPT, CCS, Washington University Program in Physical Therapy, St. Louis, MO. Used with permission, 2012. Data compiled from a variety of published studies.

decreased recovery times,[2,226] earlier return to work,[226] less postoperative pain,[226,277] and comparable amounts of weight loss.[89,226]

Behavioral and Lifestyle Changes. The relationship(s) between biologic and behavioral factors influencing obesity is not yet completely understood. However, regardless of the medical and surgical treatments available to treat obesity, behavioral change in the frequency and type of eating and exercise habits remains the foundation of both prevention and intervention.[316]

Behavior in both prevention and treatment is influenced by what options are available (e.g., vending machines, safe parks in which to walk), how and to whom health information is portrayed (e.g., media vs. health practitioner), and what type of support is given to individuals who seek and/or need to make a change.[165]

Practitioners require knowledge of what motivates change, how behavioral change occurs, what resources are needed to make change, and strategies useful for promoting change. Across the theoretic foundations guiding this knowledge, the combined merits of providing accurate information, understanding barriers preventing change, anticipating personal readiness for change, and providing structure and support over extended periods to enable sustained new behaviors have been recognized as helpful.[24]

Although lifestyle programs have been shown to be the most successful in creating durable change, regulation of body weight (to either prevent gain or maintain loss) is still affected by a myriad of intrapersonal and environmental factors that interact to make obesity control difficult. Tailoring all interventions to the "personal environment" of each individual is critical in overcoming the intrinsic and extrinsic pressures in the American culture that affect the current epidemic of obesity.[195]

Prognosis. The management of obesity continues to be challenging, particularly because its effect on the whole person is so broad and the causes/influences are so numerous that prognosis relies on significant and sustained lifestyle changes that must last a lifetime. When therapy is confined to dietary measures alone, treatment of obesity is less likely to be successful. Because the risk of mortality and morbidity from obesity rises in proportion to the degree of obesity and the presence of complications, treatment is essential. For example, among the cardiovascular problems associated with obesity, hypertension in combination with obesity increases the risk for development of cerebrovascular disease, specifically cerebral thrombosis.

Weight loss alters conditions associated with obesity, and even moderate weight loss in an obese person (i.e., 10–20 lb) provides substantial changes in risk factors. Following weight loss in individuals who are obese, a decrease in blood pressure usually occurs with a regression of left ventricular hypertrophy, total and high-density lipoprotein cholesterol are favorably changed, and glucose tolerance improves in those people with type 2 diabetes mellitus.

The addition of exercise to a comprehensive program of caloric reduction and behavior modification can improve results. Regular exercise can maximize body composition change and increase the probability of maintaining weight loss.

Patterns of fat distribution are important in determining the risks associated with obesity. Visceral fat within the abdominal cavity is more hazardous to health than subcutaneous fat around the abdomen. Upper body obesity around the waist and flank is a greater health hazard than lower body obesity marked by fat in the thighs and buttocks.

People who are obese with high waist-to-hip ratios (greater than 1.0 in men and 0.8 in women) have a significantly greater risk of diabetes mellitus, stroke, coronary heart disease, and early death than equally obese people with lower ratios. Waist circumference alone has also been designated as an independent predictor of health risks and may replace the waist-to-hip measurement as a predictor of increased risk. For women, weight-related health risks increase when the waist measurement is 35 inches or more; for men, this figure is 40 inches or more.

Although the connection between obesity (BMI greater than 30) and coronary heart disease is well established, it remains unknown whether a similar link exists for those who are mildly overweight. Research has shown that people whose BMI at midlife (30–55 years of age) was between 23 and 24.9 had a 50% higher risk of heart attack compared with those whose BMI was under 20. Women whose BMI was greater than 29 had a 3.6 times greater risk of heart attack compared with the leanest group.[325] Moderately higher adiposity at younger ages (18 years) is associated with increased premature death in younger and middle-aged women.[310]

SPECIAL IMPLICATIONS FOR THE THERAPIST   2-3

Obesity

Obesity has negative effects on overall health; emerging evidence indicates that obesity has effects beyond those associated with chronic disease. For example, obesity has negative effects on overall physical function and mobility, although the contributions of obesity to overall musculoskeletal function are not well understood. For example, for every day someone lies in bed or remains immobile, it takes even more time to regain the strength from that day of bedrest. Also, presumably the person was not losing weight at the same rate he or she was losing strength. Because sedentary habits have increased the disparity between body mass and strength over the last 5 years, those conditions create an even greater challenge when treating someone who is obese and who is chair or bed bound.

Problems associated with obesity commonly seen in a therapy program include back pain; arthritis; biomechanical dysfunction affecting the hips, knees, and ankle/foot; skin breakdown; and cardiopulmonary compromise. Obesity is a known risk factor in the development of type 2 diabetes mellitus often accompanied by diabetic neuropathy, foot ulcerations, and neuropathic fractures (see "Diabetes Mellitus" in Chapter 11).

For the physical therapist, working with the individual who is obese poses a definite risk to personal safety and health. Using proper body mechanics, careful planning for transfers, and obtaining adequate help are essential during any lifting, transfers, and hands-on therapy. A screening tool, developed by Michael Dionne (Dionne's Egress Test, or DET) can be used to predict the safety of bariatric patient transfers. It provides a three-step process to evaluate a person's mobility to go from sit-to-stand, march in place, and step forward and back. The DET takes into account neurologic deficits that may be linked to balance, not muscle weakness, and may assist health care clinicians to determine whether someone with extreme obesity can safely mobilize out of bed or whether mechanical conveyance is indicated. The DET has been shown to be moderately reliable in a pilot study; validity has not been established.[284]

Obesity and Body Composition

Body composition (i.e., the relationship of fat mass to lean body mass) is an important variable in judging health risk and one that many people may seek to understand. The public has become aware that BMI is not a sufficient measure of body composition and is flawed when used (for example) in reference to professional athletes who have a high ratio of lean body mass, or the elderly who have less lean body mass.[104,313] Standard expectations for percent body fat are 10% to 22% for men and 20% to 32% for women.[5] Clearly, it is important to provide education about health risk from adiposity, not from accumulation of muscle from resistance training or other exercise strategies.

Obesity and Back Pain

A relationship between obesity and low back pain has not been definitively established. Studies show mixed results, with only severe obesity (BMI greater than 40) being consistently linked with back pain.[126,243] The link between obesity and the incidence of symptomatic lumbar disease manifested by low back pain is a weak one at best. Whereas some studies demonstrate a high incidence, others report no correlation between the conditions.[204,243]

Obesity and Joint Pain

Obesity contributes to increases in musculoskeletal pain, demonstrated by increased odds ratios of 1.7 to 9.9 of work-restricting pain in obese subjects as compared to the general population.[250] There is an association between obesity and knee OA but not hip OA or general OA.[289]

There is also some relationship between BMI and the frequency of hip and knee replacement surgery[323] and poorer outcomes after total knee arthroplasty,[116] but no association is demonstrated between BMI and the need for total hip or knee revision surgery.

Obese individuals should have greater joint loading forces; however, at least one study demonstrated that obese individuals could have gait loading forces in the knee that are less than normal-weight individuals, if they adjust their gait by adopting a slower self-preferred speed.[91]

Obesity and Mobility/Balance

Individuals with moderate and severe obesity have been found to report that their mobility is less than very good or excellent. They also demonstrate low levels of mobility on performance-based measures. Higher BMI categories are not associated with statistical differences in self-reported or physical measures of balance; however, a trend was observed, with a greater percentage of subjects with higher BMIs being unable to complete tests of unilateral stance.[145]

Obesity and Physical Activity

Obesity might have a negative effect on performance of activities that require muscular strength or power, because the muscle would have to apply a greater force to move a larger mass. This was demonstrated in one study of children where obesity limited the ability to perform lower extremity activities such as vertical jump and standing long jump.[148]

In addition, walking requires a training level of moderate to high intensity in most obese women, 56% VO_2max in obese women versus 35% in normal-weight women.[200] Therefore, long and brisk walks should not be regarded as low intensity and fat-burning for obese women. Because walking in obese adults also has been shown to require more energy than in nonobese counterparts, pursuing greater participation in physical activity may not be motivating.[50]

Compliance may be improved with exercise and activity programs that require a lower VO_2max level, for example, bicycling, water activity, and simple calisthenics and weight resistance training. Another ADL that requires significant lower extremity strength is rising from a chair. One study demonstrated that in 8- and 9-year-old obese children, 69% needed assistance in rising from a chair.[148] This difficulty may accelerate the cycle of obesity and encourage sedentary behavior as a result of the difficulty in getting up to perform physical activity.

Obesity and Operative Complications

There are technical challenges in preparing and operating on an obese individual. Imaging equipment may not be large enough to accommodate the very obese individual and the quality of the image may be poor. Motion studies using flexion and extension radiographs may not assess range of motion adequately. Additional considerations include maintaining an open airway and accessing venous or arterial blood vessels because of adipose tissue getting in the way.[243]

There is no strong correlation between obesity and perioperative complications,[166,215] but there are many reports of operative complications in obese individuals after many different kinds of procedures (e.g., gynecologic, orthopedic, cardiovascular, transplantation, urologic). There are reports of positional neuropathies after surgery in morbidly obese individuals (BMI greater than 40). Positional palsies are attributed to increased weight causing traction or compression on peripheral neurovascular bundles, especially when the individual is placed in the prone position without adequate support and padding.[243]

Increased body mass also increases blood volume, placing added strain on the cardiovascular and respiratory systems. Over time, this can lead to decreased lung compliance and hypoxia. Preventing respiratory complications must be a team priority.[85] Early mobility to help prevent both respiratory complications and venous thromboembolism is advised. The American Society for Metabolic and Bariatric Surgery recommends early postoperative ambulation, perioperative use of lower extremity sequential compression devices, and chemoprophylaxis (anticoagulation regimen) unless contraindicated.[11]

Bariatric Weight Loss Surgery

After bariatric surgery, vitamin and mineral deficiencies can occur; the physical therapist should watch for signs and symptoms such as brittle nails, poor wound healing, easy bruising, paresthesias of the hand and feet, and bone pain. Dumping syndrome, a problem associated with Roux-en-Y gastric bypass procedure is characterized by nausea, weakness, perspiration, and diarrhea.

Changes in physical function and mobility following gastric bypass surgery (e.g., increased distance during the 6-minute walk test), and quality of life have been reported.[298] Additional research is needed to examine individual-specific interventions that can further enhance improvements in functional mobility and further define the role of the physical therapist with this patient population.

Postoperative complications can include chronic inflammation of the lower extremities; increased pendulous tissue in the abdomen, trunk, and extremities; and lymphedema of the head, neck, trunk, genitals, and extremities. Individuals with diabetes and/or vascular problems may have lower extremity lymphedema complicated by slow- or non-healing wounds.

Techniques of lymphatic massage and compression strategies may be needed. Care must be taken to address postural and breathing issues (e.g., forward head, rounded shoulders, deep breathing in the upright position). The plan of care should also emphasize cardiopulmonary endurance, muscle strengthening, and adaptive techniques for hygiene and self-care.

Prevention

Prevention and screening programs for adults and children were advocated by *Healthy People 2010* and again reinforced in *Healthy People 2020* toward the goal of promoting health and reducing chronic disease associated with diet and weight because no state achieved the intended reduction in prevalence of adult obesity to 15%.[70] The physical therapist's role in prevention and wellness, including screening programs and health promotion, is discussed in Chapter 1 and presented in detail in the APTA *Guide to Physical Therapist Practice*.

In the face of a true epidemic of obesity, our roles will undoubtedly be focused on secondary prevention (e.g., adapting exercise regimens to avoid high-impact activity for people carrying excess weight) or tertiary prevention (e.g., prescribing support stockings to potentially prevent vascular insufficiency). However, primary prevention of weight gain is a must for individuals still at low risk for obesity and could include prescription of multiple exercise strategies that sustain long-term participation and referral to literature or professionals dealing with proper (not fad) nutrition

habits. See also previous discussions of physical activity and nutrition in this chapter.

Physical therapists must be involved in screening for obesity and its comorbidities as suggested by the Surgeon General to reinforce how important regular exercise is in enhancing physical and mental well-being and prevention of the comorbidities associated with obesity. Since obesity is often associated with an increased prevalence of cardiovascular risk factors, graded exercise testing may be indicated before prescribing an exercise program. Even morbidly obese people can be evaluated on the treadmill with some modification in the testing protocol such as beginning with slow walking without treadmill elevation, followed by gradual increases in speed to achieve maximal exertion. Submaximal exercise testing overcomes many of the limitations of maximal exercise testing and may be applicable to this population.[6,95]

Exercise

The effects of overconsumption in adults can be addressed with just 3 minutes more walking per day. This means that closing the gap between energy intake (i.e., eating) and energy expenditure (e.g., moving) may require minimal additional energy expenditure.[314] Physical therapists recognize the challenges of encouraging lifestyle change in their patients/clients and must seek creative and individualized ways to promote healthy approaches to balancing the energy equation associated with the epidemic of obesity.

Hill and colleagues,[147] using National Health and Nutrition Examination Survey[147,218] data over an 8-year period, have determined that the median energy accumulation is 15 kcal/day and that 90% of the population accumulates an excess of less than 50 kcal/day. On the basis of this information, much of the weight gain seen in the population could be eliminated by some combination of increasing energy expenditure and reducing energy intake, thus closing the energy gap.[90] For example, this can be accomplished for many people simply by walking an extra mile per day or for 15 to 20 minutes, or by reducing intake with smaller portions of food.

Prescribing exercise for obese people follows the principles used with healthy people (see Box 2-2), including modifications for mechanical limitations, awareness of potential hazards during exercise (Box 2-5), and awareness of the greater heat intolerance of the obese. Some equipment modifications may be necessary if the client is too large to use a stationary bicycle or exceeds the manufacturer's recommended weight capacity. For example, the client can pedal some stationary bikes while seated in a chair behind the bike.

A higher incidence of exercise-related injury exists among the obese that requires extra caution in the first few weeks of exercise participation. Recommendations include adequate warm-up and stretching and progressive increases in intensity, frequency, and duration. Severe obesity contributes to back pain and back injury and affects foot mechanics, which can lead to foot and ankle problems. Selection of appropriate footwear with possible orthotic devices that provide heel support or compensatory foot pronation is recommended to make exercise safer and more comfortable.

The American College of Sports Medicine[6,7] presents the benefits of low-intensity, short-duration regular exercise. Exercise regimens, paired with appropriate nutritional change have healthful effects and may produce significant weight loss. Long-term continuation of this dual lifestyle change is required for both weight loss and maintenance. Accumulation of 60 minutes of formal exercise and daily physical activity is recommended. Performance at an appropriate frequency and intensity are the early goals toward achieving a habit of regular exercise rather than weight loss.

Developing an exercise program the person likes and can complete over time is the initial focus. Finding the right match may take some time and several unsuccessful attempts. Moreover, studies indicate that improved fitness through regular physical activity reduces cardiovascular morbidity and mortality for overweight individuals even if they remain overweight. The ultimate goal for the exercising obese person is to make a lifelong commitment to achieving reasonable energy expenditure through routine physical activity.[281]

The influence of body weight on exertion and lower-extremity trauma may support an initial program of stationary cycling. Aquatic exercise programs can be an important part of reducing strain on joints by providing non–weight-bearing exercise for the obese person. Resistive exercises and weightlifting can be structured to produce aerobic gains by using a circuit style with low resistance, multiple repetitions, and short rests between sets. For most individuals, caloric expenditure with traditional strength-training techniques is not as great as with circuit lifting or aerobic conditioning, but strength training does use calories and can increase lean body mass.

Behavior modification focusing on routine daily activities that require no special equipment and involve only simple lifestyle changes may be the only type of physical activity that is continued for any length of time. For example, less reliance on vehicular transportation, parking a distance from the destination, avoiding elevators and using stairs, delivering messages within the work structure rather than telephoning, and walking 10 minutes during lunch are useful and easily accommodated suggestions for increasing energy expenditure.

Smoking and Tobacco Use (See Discussion, Chapter 3)

Smoking and the use of tobacco products are associated with a number of chronic diseases, including chronic pulmonary diseases and cardiovascular conditions, as well as many types of cancers. Besides the obvious health risks associated with tobacco use as a lifestyle choice, it can become a psychologic problem because of the addictive qualities of this substance. For this reason, we have chosen to include tobacco use as part of a discussion of substance abuse in Chapter 3.

Box 2-5

POTENTIAL COMPLICATIONS OF OBESITY DURING EXERCISE

- Precipitation of angina pectoris or myocardial infarction
- Excessive rise in blood pressure
- Aggravation of degenerative arthritis and other joint problems
- Ligamentous injuries
- Injury from falling
- Excessive sweating
- Skin disorders, chafing
- Hypohydration and reduced circulating blood volume
- Heat stroke or heat exhaustion

From Skinner JS: *Exercise testing and exercise prescription for special cases: theoretical basis and clinical application*, ed 3, Philadelphia, 2005, Lea & Febiger.

Alcohol and Other Drugs (See Discussion, Chapter 3)

Addiction specialists and drug educators want to make it clear that alcohol is a drug. The commonly used phrase today when discussing substance use and abuse is "alcohol and other drugs." Whether to consider substance use/abuse a behavioral condition or a psychologic problem remains uncertain. Many psychologists and addiction counselors say it is a condition, illness, or problem with multiple factors, including physical, psychologic, social, economic, and spiritual. Others place it on a continuum from behavior to disorder, depending on the individual's relationship to the substance(s) and how that individual's friends, family, colleagues, or coworkers are affected. Substance use is considered by some a "choice," whereas addictions may be diagnosed as a disorder and then categorized as a pathologic psychologic disorder.

Culturally and socially, we live in a world that advertises and encourages the use of alcohol and other drugs as part of the American lifestyle. Addictions may be considered unique disorders that have their start in personal or lifestyle behaviors and choices but later become addictions with diagnosable pathology. Someone who drinks or uses drugs recreationally may not be an alcoholic or addicted, but when the use of substances has consequences in other areas of their life, then a problem is identified. There can be a fine line between lifestyle choices and behaviors and addictions and psychologic disorders. For now, we have chosen to place alcohol and other drug use in Chapter 3 but mention it here as a possible lifestyle, behavior, or choice that can affect the health of the individual and/or family members.

Domestic Violence

Domestic violence (DV) can be classified under categories of child abuse, intimate partner violence (IPV), and elder abuse. Because of the wide variety of practice settings in which they work, physical therapists are likely to encounter individuals of all ages who have been victims or survivors of DV.

DV includes the physical, emotional/psychological, or sexual abuse; financial exploitation; neglect; or stalking of an individual by a person with whom they have a marital, familial, social, or dependency relationship. DV occurs in all socioeconomic and racial/ethnic groups as well as across genders. Despite cultural stereotypes to the contrary, a large number of males experience domestic violence. A combination of male underreporting, societal beliefs, and the failure of officials to classify reported injuries as the result of a domestic violence may account for the widely held belief that it is a crime committed solely against females.[278]

Even with abuse that crosses gender lines, certain subgroups of women are more vulnerable than the rest of the population. Women with disabilities have indicated that their primary health concern is abuse.[140] In all forms of DV, the incidence of abuse, especially from partners or caregivers, of individuals with disabilities is much greater than occurs in the nondisabled population.[26,255,292,304,340] Abuse resulting from domestic violence can take many forms:

- *Physical abuse* involves nonaccidental physical injury, which can range from superficial bruises and welts to broken bones, burns, serious internal injuries, and death.
- *Emotional and psychologic abuse* can result from acts or omissions that cause or could cause serious behavioral, cognitive, emotional, or mental disorders as a result of actions such as confinement or the constant use of verbally abusive language and criticism.
- *Sexual abuse* ranges from nontouching offenses, such as exhibitionism, to the contact offenses that include fondling, rape, molestation, or the forced use of a child or an adult in the production of pornographic materials.
- *Neglect* can involve the withholding of or failure to provide adequate food, shelter, clothing, hygiene, emotional support, medical care, and/or supervision needed for optimal health and well-being. Neglect also includes refusal or delay in seeking health care, abandonment, inadequate supervision, and expulsion from home.
- *Stalking*, another form of DV, is defined by the National Criminal Justice Association as "a course of conduct directed at a specific person that involves repeated visual or physical proximity, nonconsensual communication, or verbal, written or implied threats, or a combination thereof, that would cause a reasonable person fear."[222]

Child Abuse

Child abuse involves the physical or emotional abuse or neglect or sexual abuse of a child under the age of 18 years, unless a state's protection law specifies a different age limit. Estimates suggest that 12 out of every 1000 children in the United States are victims of physical or sexual abuse or neglect and that many other cases are never reported.[304] Almost 1500 children die each year as the result of abuse; the majority of these children are younger than 3 years of age.[304]

Because children are prone to accidents, it is important for pediatric clinicians to carefully distinguish between accidental or inflicted injuries and to determine if there is a reasonable suspicion of abuse or neglect. Generally,

accidental bruising, fractures, and burns are rarely found in infants who are not yet crawling or walking. Even in older children, accidental injuries, such as those occurring from falls, usually result in contusions over bony prominences rather than soft tissue areas. Bruises on the buttocks or other areas of the body are suspicious for abuse. Contusions around the mouth of infants and young children often are the result of force-feeding. Other potential indicators of abuse include marks resembling finger imprints, which may occur when a child is forcibly held, shaken, or slapped, and injuries that resemble imprints of straps, cords, human bites, or utensils.

Shaken baby syndrome (SBS) usually occurs in a child under the age of three. The syndrome results after a caregiver rapidly shakes the unsupported neck and head in an attempt to prevent an infant or child from crying or performing other unwanted behaviors.

Because of the weakness of an infant's neck muscles and the size of the head, shaking results in multiple forces of the fragile brain against the skull. This impact can result in direct trauma to the brain, swelling, subdural hematoma, and subarachnoid hemorrhaging. This in turn can lead to TBI, seizures, cerebral palsy, brain damage, and death.

Other sequelae of SBS include retinal hemorrhage, blindness, spinal paralysis, intellectual disability, and learning disabilities. Symptoms of SBS include irritability, seizures, vomiting, diminished eating, decreased responsiveness, and changes in breathing. Fractures of the ribs and long bones often accompany SBS and cannot be attributed to accidental falls. These symptoms of SBS warrant emergency attention. SBS is the most common cause of mortality in infants,[260] and one of four shaken infants dies as the result of these injuries.[254] In many cases, the caregiver is not aware that shaking can result in serious, sometimes fatal, injury or disability.

Burn and scald injuries account for 10% of child abuse cases.[249] These injuries typically occur in children under 10 years of age, with the majority of inflicted burns occurring in children less than 2 years old.[249] *Accidental* burns are not always easy to distinguish from *intentional* burns. Accidental burns tend to be superficial because of the tendency to pull away when something hot is encountered. For example, brushing against a hot object causes a burn pattern that is shallow and irregular.

Contact burns can result from accidental and deliberate injuries. Accidental contact burns often occur when young children pull pots of hot liquid off a stove. In this case, the first point of contact occurs on the face, chin, neck, and axilla (because they look up as they reach for the handle) and the flow pattern lessens as it moves down along the torso. Other accidental contact burns occur when a child touches or falls against an unshielded heated surface.

Intentional burns will result in a more defined or deeper pattern, such as *immersion* burns that can be identified by sharply delineated water lines. These marks often present with a glove or stocking distribution pattern that result from holding the child's hands or feet in very hot water. A doughnut pattern may result if a child is forcibly seated in a tub of scalding water. This pattern occurs when the buttocks are spared from burns because they make contact with the bottom of the tub instead of the hot water that burns the legs and lower trunk. "Sparing" may also occur in the creases of the body and palms of the hands when, as a defensive mechanism, a child flexes the body or hands away from the hot water. Deliberate contact burns can occur when hot liquids are thrown at a child or when a heated object is used to intentionally burn a child. These burns often display a symmetrical and deep pattern. These burns are often found inside the palm of the hand or on the back or buttocks. Sometimes the shape of the object used in the abuse is outlined on the burned tissue.

The physical therapist must judge whether the caregiver's explanation of the injury is reasonable and accounts for the child's age, height, and motor abilities. Health care professionals should be alert to indicators of abuse suggested by atypical parent–child interaction Examples include parents who do not respond to a child's distress or who believe that a child does things, such as soiling themselves, to annoy the parents. A less common but perhaps underreported condition, Munchausen syndrome by proxy, is suspected when the caregivers meet their own psychological needs by creating, falsifying, or exaggerating the child's medical signs and symptoms.[125] Identification and management of any abuse issues are dependent on the careful observation and documentation by any health providers who are involved in providing clinical services.

The medical history of children should be carefully reviewed since many medical disorders can mimic signs of child abuse. Osteogenesis imperfecta is a collagen defect in which fractures can occur with minimal or even no apparent force.[241] Hemophilia, a clotting factor disorder, often causes persistent bleeding with little or no injury. Illness and medical treatment involving platelet irregularities can also result in excessive bleeding/bruising. Allergies can result in "allergic shiners" that resemble the contusions associated with a "black eye."

Mongolian spots, a condition also known as congenital dermal melanocytosis, are darkly pigmented areas caused by entrapment of melanocytes; they are often found on the sacrum or lower back of many African-American and Hispanic infants (Fig. 2-2). Although these spots resemble bruises, they do not change in size and fade over a period of years. Another cultural consideration is that contusions may be difficult to perceive in darkly pigmented children.

On autopsy, significant bleeding related to severe trauma may be discovered although the records show that health providers did not observe any external bruising. If reasonable suspicions exist, then health providers should report findings to the appropriate child abuse agencies. The clinical manifestations often associated with abuse are listed in Table 2-5.

Intimate Partner Violence

Although often used synonymously with DV, IPV occurs between current or former partners in both heterosexual and homosexual relationships. Unfortunately, the limited amount of research published on this topic that exists in allied health literature, as well as variations in the definition used to explain the term, may contribute to the lack of awareness of therapists in practice.[253]

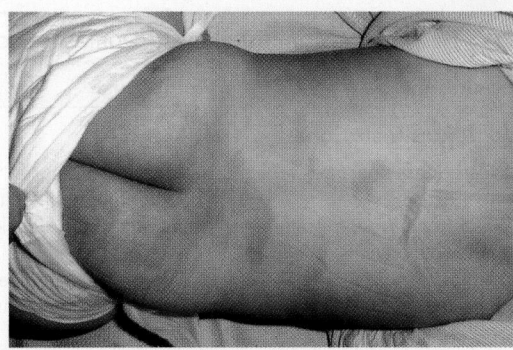

Figure 2-2

Mongolian spots (congenital dermal melanocytosis). The physical therapist must be aware of Mongolian spots, which can be mistaken for bruising from child abuse in certain population groups (e.g., Asian, East Indian, Native American, Inuit, African, and Latino or Hispanic heritage). They are also present in about 1 in 10 fair-skinned infants. Mongolian spots are bluish gray to deep brown to black skin markings that often appear on the base of the spine, on the buttocks and back, and even sometimes on the shoulders, ankles, or wrists. Mongolian spots may cover a large area of the back. When the melanocytes are close to the surface, they look deep brown. The deeper they are in the skin, the more bluish they look, often mistaken for signs of child abuse. These spots "fade" with age as the child grows and usually disappear by age 5. (From Goodman CC, Snyder TE: *Differential diagnosis for the physical therapist: screening for referral*, ed 5, Philadelphia, 2013, WB Saunders. Courtesy Dr. Dubin Pavel.)

IPV is usually a recurrent pattern of abuse that often worsens with time. It is responsible for a wide range of injuries and accounts for approximately 33% of homicides of women in the United States.[262] The U.S. Department of Justice estimates that each year there are more than 8.5 million physical assault and rape victimizations by intimate partners. They also estimate that victims of physical assault and rape account for more than 2.3 million visits to physical therapy annually.[276] Although approximately 92%–95% of IPV victims are women, men are also victims of abuse.[72] The potential for IVP exists regardless of whether the individuals involved are cohabiting or involved in sexual activity.

Physical injury may occur to any area of the body, although there are frequently occurring patterns associated with IPV. Head, neck, and facial injuries are commonly seen, and this pattern is suggestive of battering. Perciaccante[251] found that women involved in IPV were 7.5 times more likely to have sustained head, neck, and facial injuries than women with other forms of trauma.

Injuries resulting from IPV often occur in a central pattern, involving the breasts/chest, abdomen, and genital areas. Bruises, cuts, and/or fractures to the hands or arms, consistent with raising them to protect the head and face, suggest a pattern of injuries related to attempts at self-defense. Medical problems resulting from IPV include chronic neck, back, and pelvic pain; headaches; temporomandibular joint dysfunction; bone fractures; and musculoskeletal pain.

IPV survivors also have a higher rate of central nervous system symptoms, suggesting that individuals with TBI, mild TBI, and postconcussive syndrome should be screened for IPV. The pattern, frequency, and severity of injuries

Table 2-5	Clinical Manifestations of Domestic Violence		
All Populations	**Child Abuse**	**Intimate Partner Violence**	**Elder Abuse**
Physical Manifestations			
Cuts, lacerations, puncture wounds, fractures Bruise, welt, and wound patterns that resemble utensils, bite marks, cords, etc. Any injury incompatible with history Untreated injuries; delay in obtaining medical care Burns from cigarettes, acids, friction from ropes or chains Defensive pattern of injuries when the hands and arms are used to protect the face, head Injuries in various stages of healing Injuries to genitals and inner thighs from sexual abuse	Explanation of injuries incompatible with child's age, size, and developmental skills History of frequent illness affecting the ears, throat, lungs, chest, and GI tract Shaken baby syndrome—retinal hemorrhage, signs of TBI Subdural hematoma; skull fracture in infants Upper lip and frenulum injuries from forced feedings	Head, neck, and facial injuries; temporomandibular joint pain Injuries in a central pattern that involves the breasts/chest, abdomen, and genital areas TBI; mild TBI; postconcussive syndrome Back, neck, and chest pain; abdominal and pelvic pain Vague symptoms of pain; chronic pain Posttraumatic distress symptoms Frequent headaches; migraine headaches Pregnancy complications	Soiled clothing or bed; fecal or urine smell; health or safety hazards in living environment Absence of hair and/or hemorrhaging below scalp Dehydration and/or malnourishment/weight loss without illness-related cause Poor skin condition, poor skin hygiene, rashes, pressure ulcers Marks around mouth indicating that the person has been gagged Rope burns or abrasions on the wrists, ankles, torso, and neck from restraints Inadequate clothing, heat, food
Behavioral Manifestations			
Mood and appetite disturbances; eating disorders Depression/suicidal tendencies Sleep disturbances Use of emergency departments for health care Frequently missed/cancelled therapy/medical appointments	Neglect may result in head banging and rocking Failure to thrive; developmental delays Speech delays Aversion to touch	Increased use of alcohol and drugs Partner answers all questions; partner always present Fatigue	Increased use of alcohol and drugs Caregiver answers all questions; caregiver always present

Courtesy Claudia B. Fenderson, PT, EdD, PCS, Mercy College, Dobbs Ferry, New York.

resulting from IPV are identified through careful screening to distinguish between those injuries more typically associated with household and sports-related accidents.

Pregnancy and the postpartum period represent a time of significantly higher risk for IPV. The reported incidence of abuse of pregnant women varies from 0.9% to 24%.[128,130,163] They face twice the likelihood of experiencing an episode of domestic violence within 12 months of a pregnancy.[263] These rates indicate that violence during pregnancy is more common and just as potentially dangerous as pregnancy-related conditions such as placenta previa, preeclampsia, or gestational diabetes.[128] Ferris[110] reported that previous abuse is the strongest indicator that abuse will occur during pregnancy. Additionally, if abuse occurs during the first trimester, it will most likely continue in the postpartum period. Often the abuse and injuries worsen throughout the course of the pregnancy.

Elder Abuse

The term *elder abuse* refers to any intentional or negligent act by a caregiver or other person that causes harm, or a serious risk of harm, to an older person. Legislation regarding elder abuse, including reporting requirements, varies widely from state to state.

Although elder abuse is usually defined as occurring in anyone over 60 or 65 years of age, it is estimated that more than 1.8 million seniors in the United States are victims of abuse.[248] The true incidence is difficult to ascertain because many cases of abuse are never reported. The objective findings associated with elder abuse are similar to those seen with IPV and are categorized as neglect, as well as physical, psychological, sexual, or financial abuse.[118] *Neglect*, which can involve passive or active actions, is the withholding of adequate and appropriate food, clothing, health-related services, or housing with the potential for deleterious effects on the person's health.[83]

- *Physical abuse* is more likely to involve the use of physical restraints and overmedication.
- *Emotional/psychologic abuse* can involve isolating the elderly from acquaintances and threatening abandonment or unwanted placement in a long-term care facility as a means to control the actions of the older adult.
- *Financial exploitation*, the illegal or improper use of funds or assets, is more common in this age group compared with other age groups. Self-neglect occurs when an older person fails to provide for his or her own welfare and medical care. Passive neglect is the

nonwillful failure to provide care and often occurs when an elderly person is unable to take care of his or her spouse.

- *Sexual abuse* is usually committed by a person in a position of power or authority against one who is vulnerable to their control. It includes physical acts as well as forced observation of acts or participation in creation of pornography.[83]

Indicators of elder abuse include being fearful, withdrawn, or hesitant to talk and/or demonstrating signs of depression and extreme changes in mood. Issues in detecting abuse are hampered by the victim's shame, reluctance to report abuse because of reliance on the perpetrator for financial support, fear that the abuse will worsen, and concern about victimization of other family members or pets. Detection of abuse of older adults is also difficult because so many live in isolation and see few outsiders. Perpetrators of elder abuse may attribute an older person's complaints of abuse to dementia or other cognitive changes.

In the aging adult, additional signs of abuse may include dehydration or malnourishment in the absence of illness, poor skin condition and hygiene, and the presence of sores and pressure ulcers. These signs and symptoms may indicate abuse but are also associated with the physical and cognitive changes that accompany aging. A health provider who fails to evaluate findings in the light of potential abuse could easily attribute these changes to other causes.[269]

If abuse is suspected or cannot be ethically ruled out as a possibility, the physical therapist must act to protect the client. All states have hotlines and established systems for reporting abuse. This is generally done through Adult Protective Service agencies that receive and investigate reports of suspected elder abuse.

SPECIAL IMPLICATIONS FOR THE THERAPIST 2-4

Domestic Violence and Intimate Partner Abuse

The APTA, along with many other health care organizations, advocates screening of all clients for domestic violence. Physical therapists are well situated to recognize abusive situations. During the course of an examination, therapists often view body areas that are usually covered by clothing and accordingly may observe hidden contusions, welts, burns, and other injuries. They generally see clients over the course of multiple visits, which provides an opportunity to develop trusting relationships in which they can broach a discussion concerning clinical observations.

In pediatric settings, therapists already work closely with families and caregivers on abuse prevention strategies such as modeling appropriate interactions with children, teaching about age-appropriate behaviors such as an infant's constant need for attention, and emphasizing the importance of using positive reinforcement to manage challenging behavior. Pediatric therapists have the opportunity to observe the child and caregiver's relationship over time and identify potentially abusive behaviors.

Screening, Observation, and Assessment

Although many therapists may not directly receive referrals or provide intervention related to sexual or emotional abuse, the trauma associated with these events may manifest in ways that affect our relationship and interactions with the client. Unlike physical abuse, emotional and sexual abuse does not always result in visually observable signs and symptoms. Instead, these existing or previous episodes of abuse may be the unspoken but underlying reason that could fully explain the back pain, headaches, fatigue or other symptoms that have caused the client to seek physical therapy services.[53] Details of effects of sexual abuse on patients/clients and guidelines for the physical therapist from Schachter 1999 are available on the Evolve site in Evolve Box 2-2.

A therapist who encounters a client who seems to respond in an atypical manner to routine interactions or procedures should consider whether the possibility of abuse has been adequately explored before continuing with the proposed plan of care.[93] Across all client populations, therapists should view inconsistent explanations for injuries, atypical physical findings, and unexplained delays in seeking prompt medical attention, as possible red flags that require further investigation.

Despite the prevalence of every type of abuse, therapists often fail to routinely address it during patient/client interactions. Reasons vary, but include a lack of knowledge, feelings of helplessness about the situation, fear of offending others, limited time to spend with the client, and holding the false belief that the victims can readily remove themselves from the situation.[259]

Sometimes, personal biases of health care professionals prevent them from recognizing that both perpetrators and victims of abuse come from all racial/ethnic, socioeconomic, gender, sexual orientation, educational, religious, and occupational groups. Suspicion of abuse should not be based on a belief that a person is too nice or too respectable to be either abused or an abuser.

The APTA recommends that all physical therapists routinely ask their clients about the existence of abuse. Literature suggests that asking direct, nonjudgmental questions about abuse can open the door, allowing clients an opportunity to disclose abuse and possibly seek help. To avoid offending clients, the physical therapist should explain that it is routine to ask all clients about domestic violence because it is so common. By doing so, the physical therapist communicates reassurance that abuse can happen to anyone and that the therapist is knowledgeable about how to address the situation.

Evidence supports that most women in abusive relationships are in favor of being asked about abuse[46] and might feel empowered to discuss the abuse if health care workers raise the issue in a sensitive physical manner.[36] Suggestions to increase sensitivity include broaching the subject while the client is still fully dressed, sitting at eye level during the discussion, and allowing enough time for the individual to fully respond.[141]

Documentation

Over the course of several visits, the original injuries may change in size, color, and level of discomfort. Long before any legal action is concluded, any evidence of injuries may have resolved. Physical damage may have occurred at different times, thus causing variation in their stages of healing. Documentation is a critical part of managing the care of the person with suspected abuse. Whenever possible, therapists should interview clients in private to allow them an opportunity to request assistance.

Recorded descriptions should include the size, shape, color, and anatomic location of injuries, as well as the type of wound. If written permission can be obtained, photographs should be taken of bruises and injuries, with care to include the person's face in some of the pictures in case they are needed for evidence at criminal trials. Documentation created during several treatment sessions, especially if all observed information is objectively recorded on a body map, allows the physical therapist to create an ongoing record of injuries.

Documentation should also include any agencies that are contacted. It is essential, however, that physical therapists obtain permission from the individual before contacting anyone. Reporting suspected abuse or providing DV written materials may put the person at increased risk if the abuser finds out. The most dangerous time for someone in an abusive relationship is when they attempt to leave that relationship. Reports of abuse should include the client's own description of how the injuries occurred. If a person fears for his or her immediate safety, local law enforcement should be contacted and the physical therapist should stay with the victim until they arrive. One of the most important services therapists can provide to victims of DV is appropriate referral for medical care and counseling. Most states have free materials on child abuse, IPV, and elder abuse, and these resources should be readily available in a private area and in a format that can be shared easily with clients.

Reporting Issues

Reporting requirements differ according to the state and the age or perceived vulnerability of the client. All states have legislation regarding the reporting of child abuse. It is essential that therapists are knowledgeable about the reporting regulations of states in which they work. Health care professionals do not have to have evidence of abuse but instead are legally obligated to report even "suspected" child abuse, since this will facilitate an investigation of the matter.

In addition to the ethical reasons for reporting abuse, there are legal implications for health care professionals who do not report child abuse. Therapists, and their employers, may be subject to criminal penalties. Therapists also risk suspension or revocation of their license to practice and can be sued in civil court for monetary damages for any injuries that occur that are attributed to the failure to report the abuse. All states have a 24-hour child abuse hotline. The National Child Abuse Hotline (1-800-4-A-CHILD/800-422-4453) provides information and services for parents and professionals in 140 languages.

When elder abuse is identified, reporting requirements may vary across the country but most states have established Adult Protective Agencies. Information about state agencies can be obtained through Eldercare Locator, a public service of the U.S. Administration on Aging at 1-800-677-1116. If the safety and welfare of an elderly person are at risk, 911 should be called.

Reporting suspected IPV can be problematic, since it may put the victim in more danger, especially if they are not willing to press charges. Additionally, victims of IPV often have multiple issues that may prevent them from leaving an abusive situation, including lack of housing options and financial resources and children and their educational needs, as well as religious and cultural beliefs. If an issue of safety exists, therapists should call 911. Resources should be provided for clients and should include the National Domestic Violence Hotline at 1-800-799-SAFE (7233).

Regardless of legal implications, therapists have an ethical responsibility to inquire and offer assistance if abuse is suspected. It is recommended that all settings in which therapists work have established protocols and policies regarding DV. These should include ongoing training about the recognition of abuse (including abuse or violence in the workplace), state reporting laws, and referrals to local and state agencies, as well as routine screening for DV. Appropriate handling of DV situations for all populations is the moral and ethical responsibility of all therapists because timely intervention can protect clients and save lives.

BEHAVIORAL INFLUENCES ON HEALTH

Individual behaviors as they relate to lifestyle significantly influence health, including morbidity/disability and mortality. Specific individual behaviors that are important in health and disease include coping with stressful situations. Because of the importance of lifestyle choices in health and wellness, it is also important to understand the process by which individuals are effective at changing behaviors. These models, broadly described as health behavior models, assist health professionals in developing effective strategies to improve lifestyle choices and thus to improve health. In the following section, we will be discussing how stress, coping, and self-efficacy affect health and then describe models of behavior change.

Stress, Coping, and Self-Efficacy

People react to a stressful event using coping mechanisms, also called *relief behaviors*. Behavioral or cognitive coping mechanisms are used to resolve, reduce, or replace the level of stress, depression, and anxiety. When the stress is resolved, accepted, or changed, adaptation occurs, implying that a sense of equilibrium is restored to the person disordered by stress.

The body also has physiologic coping mechanisms, referred to as the *generalized adaptation response*, to stressors with multiple physiologic events (see Fig. 2-4). The human stress response has been characterized, both physiologically and behaviorally, as the "fight, flight, or freeze" response. The autonomic nervous system activates the body's involuntary responses such as hormone secretions, metabolism, and fluid regulation.

Once the body recognizes a continued threat, physiologic forces are mobilized to maintain an increased resistance to stressors and return to a state of homeostasis. Chronic resistance eventually causes damage to the involved systems as the body enters a stage of exhaustion, possibly resulting in diseases of adaptation or stress-related responses or conditions.

A landmark University of California–Los Angeles study[296] suggests that women may physiologically respond to stress with a cascade of chemicals that causes them to seek social support by making and maintaining friendships with other women. This response is referred to as "tend-and-befriend." When the hormone oxytocin is released as part of the stress response in a woman, it buffers the fight-or-flight response.

A link between the oxytocin receptor and psychologic resources such as optimism and self-esteem has been suggested.[275] Seeking emotional support in times of distress is more likely in individuals who have the oxytocin receptor genotype.[172] When the woman engages in tending or befriending, more oxytocin is released along with endogenous opioids, which further counters stress and produces a calming effect. The fact that women respond differently to stress than men has significant implications for their health. It may take time for new studies to reveal all the ways oxytocin helps women manage stress physiologically.[296]

Stress

Definition and Overview. Alterations in an individual's personal health or social situation can create significant stress for that individual. The term *stress* can be used to describe many social (e.g., change in job, residence, or marital status), psychologic (e.g., anxiety, fear of the unknown), and physiologic (e.g., blood loss, anesthesia, pain, immobility, infection) factors that cause neurochemical changes within the body.

Stress and other emotional responses are components of complex interactions of genetic, physiologic, behavioral, and environmental factors that affect the body's ability to remain or become healthy or to resist or overcome disease. Regulated by nervous, endocrine, and immune systems, stress exerts a powerful influence on other bodily systems with important implications for the initiation or progression of cancer, cardiovascular disease, HIV, autoimmune diseases, and other illnesses.[3]

Holmes and Rahe[130] first developed the notion that personal or work-related life changes as a source of stress can eventually lead to disease. Their findings rank-ordered major life change events, giving each event an assigned number to represent units of stress that could be totaled and scored.

At that time, it was thought that a direct link could be established between stress events and illness or between

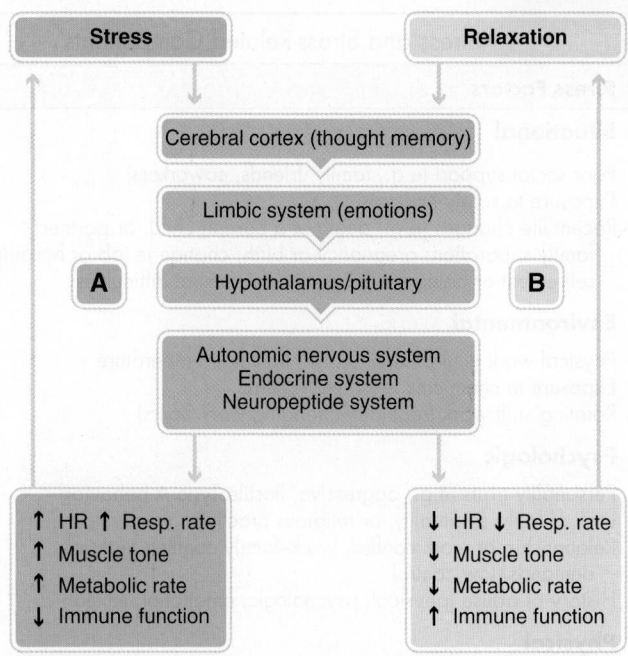

Figure 2-3

A simplified model of the cyclic mind–body and body–mind influences of stress (A) and relaxation (B) on health. As our body experiences the physical responses to stress or relaxation, the central nervous system remembers each event, causing a continuation of the cycle and resulting in long-term positive or negative physiologic responses and consequences. (Modified from Rakel D: *Integrative medicine*, ed 3, Philadelphia, 2012, WB Saunders.)

personality type and illness. It was not uncommon to hear professionals speak of a colitis-, ulcer-, or stroke-personality. Research supports a strong correlation between chronic stress response and the manifestation of various disorders, but a direct link has not been established; only personality (angry, hostile type A behavior) has been directly linked with heart disease.

Type A beliefs may predispose individuals to health problems through impaired interactions with their interpersonal environment, as will mechanisms that increase cardiovascular and neuroendocrine responses.[320] Type A behavior pattern is characterized by excessive competitiveness and aggression and a fast-paced lifestyle. Persons exhibiting type A behavior are constantly struggling to accomplish ill-defined or broadly encompassing goals in the shortest time possible. This type of behavior has been shown to be as significant as other risk factors in the development of coronary artery disease and myocardial infarction when accompanied by hostility associated with anger.[119] The opposite type of behavior, exhibited by people who are relaxed, unhurried, and less aggressive, is sometimes referred to as the type B personality.

The body's response to any stress, whether caused by events perceived as positive or negative, is to mobilize its defenses to maintain homeostasis (Fig. 2-3 and Table 2-6). The success of the stress response in maintaining homeostatic balance is determined by biobehavioral factors such as a person's age, gender, physical condition, coping mechanisms, health enhancing or

Table 2-6	Stress and Stress-Related Components		
Stress Factors		**Stress Response**	**Symptoms of Stress**
Situational		Increased heart rate and blood pressure	Hypertension
		Changes in respiratory system	Chest pain
Poor social support (e.g., family, friends, coworkers)		Release of glucose, adrenaline	Headache
Exposure to safety hazards		Redirection of blood supply (brain, muscles)	Myalgia, arthralgia, fibromyalgia
Recent life changes (e.g., death of a parent, child, or partner; family separation; pregnancy or birth; change in job or housing; retirement or being fired; heavy debt; sexual difficulties)		Decrease in blood clotting time	Allergic responses
		Dilation of pupils	Gastrointestinal symptoms
Environmental		Contraction of the spleen	Depression, anxiety, panic attacks
		Increased sweat production	Discouragement, boredom
Physical work environment; noise, lighting, temperature		Decreased peristalsis and gut function	Eating disorder
Exposure to chemicals, dust, pathogens		Decreased immune response (chronic stress)	Prolonged fatigue (chronic fatigue syndrome)
Rotating shift work (regularly changing work hours)			Poor work or school performance; errors in judgment
Psychologic			Sleep disturbance
Personality traits (e.g., aggressive, hostile Type A behavior)			
Lack of faith, spirituality, or religious practices			
Relationship or work conflict, work–family conflict, high job demands/low control			
History of abuse (physical, psychologic, emotional, sexual)			
Physical			
Sleep disturbances and/or sleep deprivation			
Chemical or biologic triggers (e.g., foods, poor nutrition, caffeine)			
Medical events, change in personal health, injury			
No exercise or excessive exercise			

impairing behaviors (e.g., diet, exercise, tobacco use, exposure to sunlight), and the duration of the stress.[239]

Research suggests a possible role of early life factors (e.g., adverse or traumatic life events) in altering the stress response. Stressful experiences that occur very early in life can alter the responsiveness of the nervous and immune systems.[131] Individuals may become more vulnerable to future adverse events after early stressors have affected cortisol secretion, diurnal rhythm, and HPA axis function.[283] Combined together, psychologic stress and aging can impact the immune system and the effects are interactive. Psychologic stress can mimic and exacerbate the effects of aging. Older adults often show greater immunologic impairment to stress than younger adults.[131]

Risk Factors. A growing consensus among stress researchers is to understand the relationship between stress and illness outcomes, so the factors that modify or mediate the relationship must be identified. There is evidence suggesting that immunosenescence (decline associated with aging) can be accelerated by external factors such as chronic stress leading to premature aging.[27]

A stressor may produce an extreme reaction in one person but no reaction in another, or the same stressor may produce variable reactions in the same individual at different times. This suggests that factors exist that alter the responses to stressors.

Stress and Aging. The idea that stress is a risk factor for multiple diseases of aging, premature aging, and death is not new.[232] For example, chronic depression has been linked with heart disease and immune system dysfunction and anxiety disorders elevate inflammation, a common risk factor for diseases of aging.[231] Heightened

levels of stress hormones (i.e., glucocorticoids) and the increased activity of the sympathetic nervous system as exaggerated neurobiologic responses to threat also increase the rate of oxidative damage, formation of free radicals, and shortening of telomeres.[232] The end result of cumulative psychosocial stress and real or perceived threat is acceleration in the aging of leukocytes.[99,101] In fact, there is accumulating evidence to support the idea that leukocyte telomere length is a biologic marker of cellular aging.[256]

There is some evidence that maternal psychologic stress during pregnancy can exert an effect on the developing telomere system in the fetus that is measurable in the newborn.[99,100] It is possible that life stressors do not necessarily cause shortened chromosomes. Some research suggests it could be the other way around: people with intact telomeres are better able to resist psychologic and emotional stress right from birth.[197] Researchers are now focused on individual genetic differences in the vulnerability of telomeres to stress.[41]

The process of coping with chronic pain, trauma, or illness is ongoing. Each change in the downward course of the illness requires new and painful acceptance of the disease and its limitations. Behavioral or cognitive coping may be adaptive (e.g., talking or reading about the problem, prayer, or seeking God) or maladaptive (e.g., denial and distancing or the use of alcohol or other drugs). When a person is unable to mobilize the necessary resources to manage stress, death from disease may result or suicide may be the final step to conflict resolution.

Other Factors. Another factor that can alter a stress response is the environment, such as social support, which tends to buffer individuals from the potentially

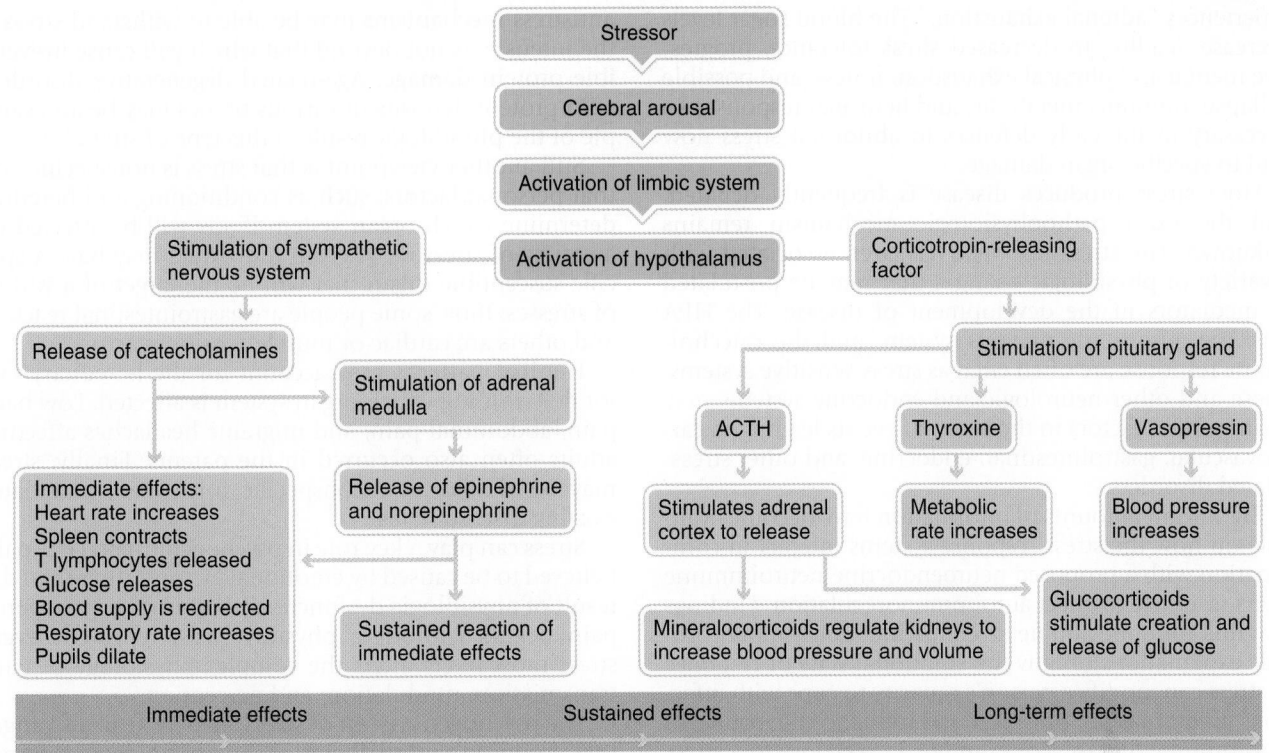

Figure 2-4

The general adaption syndrome. See text discussion. (From Ignatavicius DD, Workman M, Mishler MA: *Medical-surgical nursing*, ed 2, Philadelphia, 1995, WB Saunders.)

negative effects of stressors. Those people with strong social supports live longer and have a lower incidence of physical illness.

Several large studies have established that women feel stress more than men do at comparable life stages and in similar circumstances. Women's catecholamines and blood pressures tend to remain elevated long after the end of the workday or after a stressful situation, whereas men's blood pressures start to decline as soon as they leave work or end a stressful conversation.[118,138] Other potential factors are listed in Table 2-6.

In addition to early stressful life events, negative life events in adults, especially work-related, are associated with adverse physiologic responses. Depressed mood and mental strain have been reported as a result of chronic stress. Depressed mood and mental strain are also directly linked with increased tobacco consumption in labor workers and increased alcohol consumption in professional workers.[265] Although many factors causing stress have been studied, the ability to predict a stress response in any given individual remains poor.

Even transient physical and psychologic stressors can cause immune dysregulation and delay healing. For example, acute pain, academic examinations, and other anxiety and perceived stress have been reported as risk factors for health problems.[131]

Pathogenesis. Over the past century, many theories to describe the biologic response of the body to acute and chronic stress have been proposed. Today there is evidence that stress is a neurophysiologic, hormonal, and behavioral event. The body's response to stress is a complex combination of biologic and behavioral mechanisms that are regulated by the neurohormonal axis. According to Selye, who introduced the theory of the *general adaptation syndrome* (Fig. 2-4), the three phases that occur in response to prolonged stress are alarm, resistance, and exhaustion.

In the alarm phase, the body releases adrenaline and a variety of other chemicals to combat the stress and to stay in control. This is called the *fight, flight, or freeze* response. The muscles tense, the heart beats faster, breathing and perspiration increase, and the eyes dilate. All of these autonomic nervous system responses are protective in nature and critical to survival. Once the cause of the stress is removed, the body will return to a state of homeostasis.

If the stressor is not removed, the general adaptation syndrome goes to its second stage called *resistance* or *adaptation*. The body is responding now to the need for long-term protection. It secretes further hormones that increase blood sugar levels to sustain energy and raise blood pressure. The adrenal cortex produces corticosteroids for this resistance reaction.

Overuse by the body's defense mechanism in this phase can lead to disease. If this adaptation phase continues for a prolonged period of time without relaxation or rest to counterbalance the stress response, sufferers become prone to fatigue, concentration lapses, irritability, and lethargy as the effort to sustain arousal slides into negative stress.

The third stage of the general adaptation syndrome is called *exhaustion*. In this stage, the body has run out of its reserves of body energy and immunity. Mental, physical, and emotional resources are depleted. The body experiences "adrenal exhaustion." The blood sugar levels decrease, leading to decreased stress tolerance, progressive mental and physical exhaustion, illness, and possible collapse. Immune, metabolic, and neuronal responses so necessary in the early defenses to abnormal stress now lead to specific organ damage.

How stress produces disease is frequently debated, and the exact pathophysiologic mechanism remains unknown. The stress response has been associated with a variety of physiologic changes that may be postulated as mediators in the development of disease. The HPA axis, the autonomic nervous system, and the catecholamine response are often cited as stress-sensitive systems. These and other neurologic and endocrine systems may be important factors in the chain of events leading to cardiovascular, gastrointestinal, endocrine, and other stress-related disorders.

Significant amounts of information have become available on how the stress response systems interact in combination with a proposed neuroendocrine-neuroimmune stress response to effect autoimmunoregulation. Findings that link immune and neuroendocrine function may provide explanations of how the emotional state or response to stress can modify a person's capacity to cope with infection, inflammation, or cancer and influence the course of autoimmune disease. For example, in response to a stress impulse, the amygdala in the brain signals the hypothalamus to release adrenocorticotropic hormone (ACTH)–releasing factor. This stimulating hormone causes ACTH (corticotropin) to be released from the pituitary gland.

ACTH is the major hormone regulator of the body's adaptive response to stress and the physiologic stimulus for the release of stress hormones (e.g., adrenaline, noradrenaline, cortisol) from the adrenal glands (target organ). These powerful hormones and glucocorticoids (cortisol) create within the body the fight, flight, or freeze response. This cascade of events can lead to hypercortisolism and inappropriately elevated catecholamines, resulting in immunosuppression (i.e., decreased numbers of lymphocytes [white blood cells]) and antibodies and thus increasing vulnerability to infectious diseases, including viral-induced cancers and other diseases.

Studies of the HPA axis as a potential psychobiologic mediator of these effects are underway.[28] Understanding the biochemical mechanisms underlying stress may permit the development of more effective strategies to treat chronic stress and possibly prevent the development of stress-related disorders.

In 1995, researchers identified a peptide known as *pre-pro-TRH178-199* that had been shown to reduce the secretion of corticotropin, or ACTH, by 50%. Administration of this corticotropin release–inhibiting factor in animal studies before exposure to stress revealed significantly reduced levels of ACTH and other hormones elevated in response to stress. This peptide also decreased fear and anxiety-related behaviors.[98] Ongoing studies continue to look for ways to use this peptide for therapeutic purposes.

Another theory holds that certain kinds of stress are consistently likely to produce given physiologic responses and, consequently, specific pathologic states. The impact of stress on cells directly or indirectly causes protein denaturation and elicits a stress response. A cell with normal antistress mechanisms may be able to withstand stress if the intensity is not beyond that which will cause irreversible protein damage. Age-related degenerative disorders with protein deposits in various tissues may be an example of the physiologic result of this type of stress.[196]

Still another viewpoint is that stress is nonspecific and that personal factors, such as conditioning and heredity, determine which organ system if any will be affected by a variety of stressors. A given individual may have a specific susceptible organ that will be the target of a variety of stresses; thus, some people are gastrointestinal reactors and others are cardiac or muscle-tension reactors.

Familial patterns may account for the hereditary factor determining which organ system is affected. Low back pain, abdominal pain, and migraine headaches affecting adults often also occurred in the parents. Finally, stress may be viewed as a nonspecific force that exacerbates existing disease states.

Stress can play a key role in psychogenic pain (i.e., pain believed to be caused by emotional factors rather than the result of physiologic dysfunction). Although psychogenic pain begins without a physical basis, repeated severe stress most likely alters the complex physiology of pain transmission, modulation, and perception.

The psychogenic effect of stress, anxiety, fear, and anger that produces painful alterations in physiology is referred to as *psychophysiologic* pain. For example, stress can produce chronic excessive muscle contraction with resultant ischemia and pain with eventual functional impairment.

Clinical Manifestations. Therapists often treat people with neuromusculoskeletal dysfunction, especially head, neck, and back pain, without an identified point of injury or cause. Stress, reaction to stress, and posttraumatic stress disorder are common causes of physical manifestations treated by the physical therapist. Muscle tension and pain, restlessness, irritability, fatigue, increased startle reaction, breath holding, hyperventilation, tachycardia, palpitations, and sleep disturbances are some of the more common symptoms reported to the physical therapist (see Table 2-6). Clients often self-medicate using chemical (alcohol, nicotine, drugs) or food substances; the alert therapist may help assist the client by facilitating treatment intervention for this aspect of the person's stress response.

There is clear and convincing evidence that chronic psychosocial stress contributes significantly to the pathogenesis and exacerbation of coronary artery atherosclerosis, whereas acute stress induces ovarian dysfunction, hypercortisolism, and accelerated atherosclerosis. Acute stress triggers myocardial ischemia, stimulates platelet function, increases blood viscosity, and causes coronary vasoconstriction in the presence of underlying atherosclerosis (coronary heart disease).[267]

Some individuals also experience exaggerated heart rate and blood pressure responses to psychologic stress. Emotionally responsive individuals report less satisfaction with social support and higher levels of perceived daily stress, anxiety, and depressive symptoms. Psychosocial traits that have been linked to cardiovascular disease may be associated with more marked cardiovascular activation occurring in response to negative emotions experienced throughout the day.[56]

Researchers hypothesize the exaggerated systemic vascular resistance responses during stress may be caused by endothelial dysfunction. This association may help explain the growing evidence of a relationship between stress hemodynamics and cardiovascular disease risk. It is postulated that the interplay between the sympathetic nervous system and the endothelium accounts for the regulation or dysfunction of vascular tone.[280]

Coping and Self-Efficacy

Coping strategies refer to the tools individuals use to manage, tolerate, or control stressful events. Whether an individual has effective or maladaptive coping strategies can significantly influence both physical health and the level of disability associated with a particular medical condition. It is important for physical therapists to support effective coping strategies. Generally, there are two main ways of coping: an active problem-solving strategy and an emotion-based strategy.[191] Active coping strategies appear to be more effective in dealing with stressful events.[150] For example, cognitive restructuring guides the client to focus on active coping behaviors and improving function instead of focusing on physical symptoms and pain. Reinforcing positive active behaviors and ignoring pain-related behaviors is called *operant conditioning* (see Box 3-20).

Measuring Coping. Several tools are frequently used to measure coping strategies. The Ways of Coping tool developed by Folkman and Lazarus[115] identifies specific strategies such as seeking social support, planned problem solving, self-control, distancing, or escape/avoidance. The COPE measure asks participants to identify specific traits that typify their response to stressful events. These trait scales include topics that are similar to the ways of coping, such as active coping, planning, seeking social support, religion, or acceptance.[59]

Using the Ways of Coping and COPE measures, it appears that active coping strategies have a positive influence on physical health. Active coping was better than avoidance for improving immune status of HIV-positive men.[129] Active coping was associated with fewer recurrences of melanoma.[108] Physical therapists may want to familiarize themselves with these coping tools or work with team psychologists to support active coping strategies for their clients.

Although coping is a mechanism used by individuals to manage stressful events, greater improvements in health can be observed if certain lifestyle behaviors are changed. Changing individual behaviors is a complex and dynamic process affected by many factors. Several models of health behavior have been examined to assist health professionals in understanding the process of behavior change and developing effective strategies to improve lifestyle choices and thus to improve health.

Changing Health Behaviors. Helping people change behavior has become more important in the plan of care for all individuals in the health care setting. Addressing lifestyle modification for disease prevention, long-term disease management, addictions, chronic pain, and many other areas of health care is increasing in importance and a necessary component of whole-person care.[342] Understanding readiness to make changes, recognizing barriers to change, and helping clients anticipate relapse can improve patient/client satisfaction, and lower frustration on the part of the provider during the change process.

Much has been written about the success and failure in helping people change behaviors. People clearly understand the need to change and often make efforts to make lifestyle modifications, but consistent, lifelong behavior changes are difficult and relapse is common. Repeated suggestions, record-keeping, a "just do it" attitude, and other behavior modification approaches do not always work. Individuals are often labeled as "noncompliant" or "unmotivated" when behavior change does not take place.[342]

The behavioral change approach to disease prevention and health promotion focuses on the modification of individual health-related behaviors. Research into smoking cessation and alcohol abuse has advanced our understanding of the change process, including what works and what is not effective. Clearly, there is not a "one-size-fits-all" approach.[342] Four models and theories often cited in the literature using a health behavior change approach are presented here.

Models of Health Behavior Change. The Health Belief Model (HBM) was initially developed in the 1950s by the U.S. Public Health Service in order to help explain why there was limited success of early screening programs such as free mobile x-ray screening for tuberculosis.[161] Its foundation was based on the social psychology literature of the time, which included the confluence of two learning theories: Stimulus Response Theory and Cognitive Theory.

The HBM is a value-expectancy model in which the desire to avoid illness or get well is considered the value and the belief that a certain action will prevent or limit illness is the expectation. This model embraces the cognitive theorists' and behaviorists' understanding of learning versus the traditional stimulus response or operant conditioning theories popular at the time. The HBM proposes that in order for persons to change their behaviors they must first believe they are susceptible to a particular condition and that the severity of that condition is serious.[161] Changes in behavior are based on six key components: perceived susceptibility, perceived severity, perceived benefits, perceived barriers, cues to action, and self-efficacy.

The HBM model assumes individuals act on the basis of their rational appraisal of a given situation. The model is not designed to account for social pressures that might persuade the individual to partake in the unhealthy behavior.[75,123] This is a limiting factor when one considers that a problem like obesity often has stigma and social pressure attached to it; therefore the intervention must acknowledge this.

Rating the severity, susceptibility, benefits, barriers, and self-efficacy associated with a health behavior is just the first of many steps to understanding why (or why not) individuals adopt a specific health behavior. Prospective studies performed on the HBM in the early 1980s provided support of earlier research, demonstrating that perceived barriers were the most powerful predictor of the HBM concepts.[161] Any attempt to change behavior, such as eating habits or physical activity, must address the perceived barriers, which are often at the family or community level rather than the individual level.

The *Theory of Reasoned Action* (TRA) and the *Theory of Planned Behavior* (TPB) are also based on a value-expectancy theory similar to the HBM,[209] which was originally designed in order to understand the relationship between attitudes and behavior.[112] A key aspect is the difference between the attitudes toward the object of health (in this case breast cancer) versus the attitude toward the behavior of health with respect to that object (specifically a mammogram).[113]

The TRA assumes that the most important determinant of behavior is the individual's intent to change behavior. The person's attitude toward the behavior is determined by his or her belief about the outcomes of performing the behavior. If a positive outcome is the expected result, then there will be a positive attitude toward that behavior. These intentions are measured on a bipolar scale, such as agree/disagree or likely/unlikely, although the behavior itself is not usually measured. One limitation to the TRA is that individuals usually have only incomplete volitional control of behavioral choices.

The TPB builds on the TRA to help predict behaviors over which people have incomplete volitional control.[4] The TPB includes some understanding of environmental factors that may prevent the individual with high motivation from performing that behavior. This has been the case in fighting obesity since the individual may not have access to facilities to perform physical activity or the availability to obtain healthy food choices.

Perceived behavioral control indirectly measured by control beliefs and perceived power were components added to the TPB. By including normative belief and norms, which impact intentions, this model shows that the individual can be affected by external influences that can mix with the social environment.

The *Transtheoretical Model*, also known as the *Stages of Change Model*, utilizes a stage construct to represent change over time. The stages of change were used to attempt to systematically integrate various theories of intervention, hence the Transtheoretical Model.[258] Six stages are used to demonstrate that behavior change is a process rather than a finite event or single activity. The stages include precontemplation (uninterested, unaware, or unwilling to change), contemplation (considering a change), preparation (getting ready to change), action (taking actual steps to effect change), maintenance, and termination.

This model looks beyond the intention aspect of a decision and includes an observable action of behavior change. It takes into account the fact that most people will relapse or even fail, but they can reengage with the stages and may even do so several times before a change becomes genuinely established.[342] This is essential with physical activity in that the individual must demonstrate the behavior and then even continue into the maintenance stage with less temptation to relapse into the previous behavior pattern. As self-efficacy improves in this model, an individual is able to move into maintenance and eventually into termination, although very few people (<20%) attain this final stage.[258]

Changing an overt behavior for more than 6 months constitutes the maintenance stage. Success using the Transtheoretical Model involves the delivery of "tailored" interventions versus targeted or one-size-fits-all programs. This would seem to match the clinical model in which an individually tailored program can be designed, providing the provider is willing and capable of recognizing the stage the person is in and then developing a tailored intervention. These stage-matched interventions take additional time and effort, and more research is needed using modern tools of communication, such as the Internet, that would improve the efficiency and ability to reach more diverse populations.[258]

Social Cognitive Theory (SCT) is a health behavior model that is more dynamic in nature than the HBM. Bandura initially felt that children can learn through observational learning and therefore the behavior is modeled and the reward is gained through vicarious reinforcement versus direct reward.[25] These became two important constructs of the SCT.

The SCT is similar to ecologic models in the sense that it shares the perspective that environmental factors can be influential in shaping health-promoting behaviors.[22] SCT not only incorporates factors associated with the environment but also personal and behavior-specific factors. These three components are constantly influencing each other and became the concept known as *reciprocal determinism*.[25]

Behavior under SCT is not focused independently on factors external to the individual or the environment. The situation is the person's perception of that environment. The combination of these two constructs provides an ecologic framework for the understanding of the behavior.

This model also includes a significant acknowledgment of the sociologic concept of agency and that personal efficacy constitutes a key factor of human agency. Human agency operates within the structure of these three determinants and acts reciprocally at various strengths, times, and circumstances.[21,23]

Finally, outcome expectations are also constructs within the overall theory. Self-efficacy (the ability or confidence of a person to implement an effective behavior) is considered the most important construct and necessary prerequisite for behavior change.[22] Self-efficacy is based on the combination of the attitudes, cognition, and expectations of an individual and can be improved through successful attainment of tasks, skills, or behaviors. Self-efficacy has been used in previous studies of healthy eating behaviors and food choices among third and fourth grade students. It was the primary predictor of the intention to engage in these healthy food choices.

Although SCT encompasses the environment more so than other behavioral models or theories, there is still limited ability to measure long-term sustainability and in some cases even action beyond the person's stated intention. Other limitations of SCT include the criticism that the theory is too comprehensive with too many constructs that allow researchers to explain almost any phenomena observed.[25]

Winters and colleagues[329] used the SCT to explain the variance in predictor variables for moderate and vigorous exercise in high school students. They determined that although educational methods can be effective, the specific psychosocial variables relating to self-regulation, self-efficacy perception, and outcome expectation within the SCT should be the focus.

These theories have been utilized in other large studies and programs, such as the Multiple Risk Factor Intervention Trials and the Minnesota Heart Health Program, in an attempt to reduce cardiovascular disease, although the modest impact of these interventions demonstrates a limitation in focusing on the individual behavior change models for health promotion.[335]

SPECIAL IMPLICATIONS FOR THE THERAPIST 2-5

Stress, Coping, and Self-Efficacy

Health Behavior Change

It is not easy for people to make necessary changes (or they would have done so long ago), and denial often obscures the picture. The physical therapist has a key role in bringing multiple dimensions of wellness into the plan of care. A higher level of wellness includes more than just the physical. It embraces the emotional, social, intellectual, and spiritual dimensions of health and well-being.[156] Toward this end, the physical therapist can do the following:

- *Assess readiness to change before prescribing lifestyle changes, including exercise.*
- *Provide opportunities for improving self-efficacy. For example, observe and monitor the client performing the recommended intensity of exercise (on the treadmill) and provide feedback.*
- *Allow opportunities for self-regulation, self-efficacy perception, and outcome expectations described by the participant.*
- *Promote wellness and select strategies appropriate for ability to change and perception of self-efficacy.*

The physical therapist may need to develop his or her own personal coping mechanisms when working with clients who have chronic illnesses, major stress, or psychologic disturbances. Preexisting character issues or the presence of psychologic problems in a client or for the provider (e.g., anxiety, panic disorder, depression) can create obstacles to rehabilitation or prevent progress.

True behavior change rarely has a starting and ending point but exists on a continuum of time and effort. The client moves from being uninterested, unaware, or unwilling to make a change, to thinking about making a change, to deciding to do so, and getting on with it. It is easy to encourage and support someone in the change process until discouragement and relapse occur.

Understanding the processes required to make behavior change will enable the physical therapist to recognize which stage the patient/client may be in and identify the next step of action needed to help the individual move to the next state. Patience is needed if the individual is still in the precontemplation or contemplation stage. The client may seem in denial or argumentative. The physical therapist's efforts to convince him or her usually results in increased client resistance.

The physical therapist may need to shift back to find ways of engaging the client in contemplating change by asking thought-provoking questions and personalize risk factors while maintaining a positive, nonjudgmental attitude. For example, to help the individual think about change, the physical therapist can ask, *"What would have to happen for you to know that this is a problem?"* To help the individual examine barriers to change, ask, *"What is keeping you from changing?"* or *"What has helped you change in the past?"* or *"What are your reasons for not changing?"* Additional tools and techniques to help facilitate behavior change are available.[342]

Stress

The physical therapist may be called on to assist the client in reducing the physical impact of stress on the body as well as providing a means of physical or emotional control. *Progressive muscle relaxation*, breathing exercises, physical activity and exercise, and biofeedback are the primary tools used in therapy to teach the client effective stress-reducing techniques.

Since stress commonly causes muscle tension, producing somatic symptoms such as headaches and neck and back pain, control of muscle tension appears to help reduce the physical effects of such tension as well. Progressive muscle relaxation involves the alternate tensing and relaxing of all major muscle groups, usually in sequential steps. It is easy to teach and inexpensive.

Breathing exercises can be helpful in restoring normal respiration by providing moments of deep breathing because the person in a stressful situation tends to breathe shallowly or even unconsciously hold his or her breath. Teaching diaphragmatic breathing skills and suggesting ways clients can remember to check their breathing (e.g., whenever the telephone rings, setting their watches to beep on the hour, at every stop sign when in an automobile) can aid in reducing the chest and upper body muscle tension and diaphragmatic tension and dysfunction that accompany altered breathing patterns.

Biofeedback can be an effective means of training people to reverse the subtle changes in blood pressure, muscle tension, and heart rate that accompany a stress-induced somatic response. Biofeedback involves using electronic instrumentation to signal selected somatic changes. Surface electrodes are sensitive to small changes in the electrical activity of the muscles, signaling to the client by way of sound or sight the need to practice physiologic quieting techniques (e.g., visualization, imagery, deep breathing).

Physical Activity, Exercise, and Stress

Physical activity and exercise is only one of the behavioral and psychologic therapies recommended for the treatment of stress. Moderate exercise can aid in balancing cortisol/dehydroepiandrosterone (DHEA), lower serum proinflammatory cytokines, and lower counts of senescent T cells, thereby potentially altering immunosenescence.[27]

Exercise training, along with behavior modification, psychologic counseling, smoking cessation, and dietary modification, are all considered important in the overall holistic treatment approach to many people. For example, aerobic exercise has been found to consistently attenuate (weaken, blunt, or reduce) the cardiovascular and adrenal responses to stress, particularly in type A personalities.

Although physical exercise may be considered a stressor itself, significant differences are apparent in the way the body responds to exercise versus the way the body responds to a mental stressor. A key difference is between the diastolic and systolic blood pressure responses. Exercise results in a rise in the systolic pressure and possibly a small increase in diastolic pressure, whereas mental stress produces a significant increase in both diastolic and systolic blood pressures. Blood vessels dilate during physical exercise to increase the blood supply to the muscles.

During this vasodilation, the diastolic blood pressure tends to stabilize or increase mildly, whereas during mental stress the muscles may isometrically contract (muscle tension), but no substantial movement of the body by the muscles and no metabolic reason for vasodilation occur. Decreased vagal activity may contribute to the exaggerated diastolic blood pressure reactivity to mental stress.

Social Support, Networks, and Roles That Influence the Effects of Illness

There are several key terms that describe the role of social relationships and the effect it has on health. *Social epidemiology* is the branch of epidemiology that studies the social distribution and social determinants of health. Social epidemiology provides a systematic and comprehensive study of health, well-being, social conditions or problems, and diseases and their causes. Public health activists rely on social epidemiology to develop interventions, programs, policies, and institutions that may reduce the extent, adverse impact, or incidence of a health or social problem and promote health.[84,229]

Social network refers to the web of social relationships that encompass an individual.[142] They are the linkages between people. Network analysis focuses on the characteristic patterns of social ties between individuals. Previous work has demonstrated that the strength of weak ties (acquaintances) between people are as important if not more as the strength of strong ties (close friends).[132] Unfortunately, these weak ties have been measured indirectly, such as membership in religious or voluntary civic organizations. Social networks are not always positive influences. For instance, cigarette smoking by peers is among the best predictors of smoking for adolescents.[180] Social support is the functional content of relationships, the aid and assistance exchanged through interpersonal relationships. Social support is always intended to be helpful and is consciously provided by the sender.[142]

There is a two-way directional pathway between social networks and social support and health outcomes or disease (social epidemiology). A person's health status is affected by social support, whereas the ability to maintain a social network is in turn affected by the person's health status.

Data collected over the last 20 years connect social support and social networks to physical and mental health, including studies that looked at all-cause mortality[36]; cardiovascular disease[179,237]; stroke[34,169]; infectious disease,[213] including the common cold; and HIV/AIDS.[183]

Berkman and Glass[35] describe the impact on health by social networks as being along a continuum of factors (e.g., cultural, socioeconomic, political, religious, geographic, psychologic). More specifically, poverty, discrimination, and conflict are social-structural conditions that can exert a negative influence on health, whereas factors such as access to resources and material goods, close family ties, and help-seeking behaviors provide positive social support. The future success of our health care system may depend on reducing social inequities and lack of support that keep people from experiencing optimal health and well-being.

SPECIAL IMPLICATIONS FOR THE THERAPIST   2-6

Social Support

Whereas the medical model focuses on factors internal to the individual that directly affect an individual's health status, a considerable body of knowledge indicates that factors external to an individual also play a significant role in a person's health status. Not only does pathology impact the level of disability, but personal characteristics, social networks, and the environment also affect an individual's daily function.

This shift in emphasis encourages the development of new treatments or interventions that impact an individual's health. Physical therapists need information not only about the impact of pathology on individual health, but also on the role of social and environmental factors that can lead to improved outcomes in our clients.

- *Assess social support in the initial intake.*
- *Ask about social support components, including family, partners, peers, organizations such as church or synagogue, work, and culture.*
- *Social support may have an impact on the prognosis of individuals suffering from acute or chronic conditions and may differ between conditions.*

ENVIRONMENTAL BARRIERS TO HEALTH CARE

Although there are environmental exposures that lead to disease, the nature of the physical environment has an impact on health and disease outcomes. The environmental influences on eating, physical activity, and subsequent obesity have been reviewed in detail.[122]

Eating behavior is affected by food supply trends, nutritional content of foods, larger portion sizes, and eating away from home regularly. Individuals are subjected to television advertising and media campaigns, and are affected by pricing. Grocery store chains in high-income markets offer fewer energy-dense foods than in low-income markets, which further affects the income disparity in obesity.[122]

Present trends in the reduction of physical activity because of increased screen time, increased automobile use, change in types of occupational activities, the increase in availability of labor-saving devices, and the reduction of accessibility to parks and recreational space have caused the obesity epidemic to spread in all populations and demonstrate the need to intervene at the environmental level.

Simple environmental interventions, such as placing music and artwork in stairwells, have led to a 39% increase in stair use.[122] Further architectural changes such as designing buildings with stairwells that are easier to access than elevators can make differences that would surpass the 100 kcal/day recommendation for daily activity.[147]

In an effort to combat reluctance to prepare healthy meals at home because of lack of time, cooking utensils, ingredients, and expertise, companies around the country are opening and marketing state-of-the art kitchens that will allow individuals or groups to come in and prepare 10 to 14 healthy meals. Such meals can be eaten at home without further preparation time.

At the same time, grocery stores offer a wide variety of high-sodium, high-fat microwaveable meals that appeal to busy people on the go. Teenagers who do not want to take the time and older adults who can no longer prepare meals are likely targets for this type of low-nutrition food.

Pilot projects at some universities have been instigated to increase walking on campus. Signs and campus-wide competition encouraging increased walking, as well as structural environmental changes, such as changing the locations of various parking lots, are strategies employed in this effort. These activities and programs are all consistent with the recommendations of the 2002 Task Force on Community Preventive Services.[293]

SPECIAL IMPLICATIONS FOR THE THERAPIST 2-7

Environmental Barriers

As mentioned earlier in this chapter, more than 50 million Americans (18% of the total U.S. population) have a disability.[60] Data suggest that substantial disparities in health behaviors and overall health status exist between persons with and without disabilities.[61] The WHO's *International Classification of Functioning, Disability, and Health (ICF)* stresses the importance of environment, including physical environment, attitudes of others, or policies enforced as barrier or facilitator in the daily activities of persons with disabilities.[334] The extent to which environment affects the lives of people with disabilities may depend on the person's demographic characteristics (e.g., level of income, level of education, urban versus rural setting) and severity of disability.[20]

Disabilities can be physical, sensory, mental, emotional, or learning. Environmental barriers related to disability can include restricted social activity, not knowing where or how to obtain disability resource information, needing home modifications but having no way to obtain them, having difficulty accessing a health care provider's office because of physical layout or location, and being treated unfairly at a health care provider's office.[20]

There remains a need for environmental improvements to reduce social isolation and facilitate ADLs among persons with disabilities. Physical therapists can take an active and proactive role in educating the public and removing barriers. Therapists can help community leaders ensure that public places, such as restaurants, stores, and movie theaters, comply with the Americans with Disabilities Act.[20]

Within our own clinical practice, we can modify our actions to meet the needs of the disabled. For example, physical therapists should sit down when speaking with a person in a wheelchair and speak directly to the client rather than to the person with them. If needed, schedule extra time for people who have trouble undressing or difficulty getting on and off the table.

When talking with someone who is hearing impaired, say their name first and get their attention before speaking. This can help avoid repeating everything you say. You may or may not have to speak louder, but clearly enunciate your words when speaking to a person with a hearing loss.

REFERENCES

To enhance this text and add value for the reader, all references are included on the companion Evolve site that accompanies this textbook. The reader can view the reference source and access it online whenever possible.

CHAPTER 3

The Psychosocial-Spiritual Impact on Health Care

SUSAN ANN TALLEY • BETHA ANNE FISHER • KATHLEEN J. PANTANO • DARINA SARGEANT • KIMBERLY DUNLEAVY • BONNIE YOST

If we consider our profession to be one of "helping," it is inconsistent that we should extensively attend to physical pain, dysfunction, and symptoms without recognizing and attending to the nonphysical contributors to those physical maladies.

— BONNIE YOST

Increasing focus and attention are being brought to the concepts of whole systems healing and integrative care along with offering prevention and wellness in providing health care for the total person. As a result of this shift in thinking, a concept referred to as *whole systems healing* is making its way into the health care arena.[508]

Whole systems healing is a way of enhancing the health and well-being not only of individuals, but also communities and the environment in which we live. Change is needed in the way we deliver and practice health care. Understanding complex human and environmental systems and finding ways to improve well-being and outcomes associated with health care will become the focus of care in the future. Toward that end, therapists must understand the value of their own wellbeing while attending to the health and care of others. An effective approach to health care is one that supports and maximizes each person's potential physically, emotionally, socially, and spiritually. This chapter does not cover every aspect of these dimensions but does, hopefully, draw the reader's personal as well as professional attention to the importance of these concepts.

PSYCHOLOGIC CONSIDERATIONS IN HEALTH CARE

Trauma and psychologic contributors to pain and dysfunction can cause extensive comorbidity for people seen by rehabilitation providers. Trauma can be defined as an *overwhelming or life-threatening event—experienced or witnessed—resulting in intense fear, helplessness, and horror* (Box 3-1). The physiologic responses to trauma—the "fight-or-flight" responses of the sympathetic nervous system—are immediate and automatic, appropriate responses to avoid danger or imminent harm. The emotional responses to trauma are more complex and individual, with different coping responses that may be influenced by family history, genetic influences, and emotional development.

Medical diagnostics and treatment are often directed toward physical causes without consideration of emotional and psychologic symptoms and reactions as primary diagnoses, secondary responses, or comorbid conditions. Psychologic diagnoses are also extremely important to consider for overall prognosis.[162,163,281,368] If medical and rehabilitation professionals ignore the psychologic elements of a person's diagnosis or the causative factors, outcomes are often adversely impacted.[368] Contemporary practice must attend to the personal and environmental factors including psychosocial elements following the World Health Organization's International Classification of Functioning, Disability and Health endorsed by the American Physical Therapy Association (APTA) in 2008.[12]

The cognitive, physical, emotional, and spiritual systems of human beings are intricately intertwined and interdependent and vague symptoms can be the result of complex psychologic contributions or multifaceted problems. The amount of time spent with patients/clients provides opportunities for physical therapists to recognize physical and nonphysical contributions to pathology and, in concert with other health care professionals, to attend to the rehabilitation of the whole person.[342] There is the possibility that individuals who have a history of psychologic trauma may have psychologic symptoms reactivated during health care encounters, even if their physical impairments are being addressed.[113,128,342,343,427]

It is important to remember that physical pain and symptoms that have nonphysical roots will not resolve unless the underlying causes of the problems are addressed. It is vital, as health care professionals, that we are sensitive to the effects of our care on the *whole* person. Attention to psychologic resources, personal beliefs, support systems, resiliency, self-efficacy and spiritual reserves are critical to healing and enhanced outcomes.[389]

Incidence of Trauma

(See also "Domestic Violence" in Chapter 2.)

TRAUMA-RELATED TERMINOLOGY

Trauma

Definitions of *trauma* include:
- An event that threatens serious bodily injury or survival of self or others—experienced or witnessed—resulting in intense fear, helplessness and horror
- The meaning of the event may be as important as the physical trauma
- In psychology—emotional shock: an extremely distressing experience that causes severe emotional shock and may have long-lasting psychologic effects
- In medicine—bodily injury: a physical injury or wound to the body

Torture

Definitions of *torture* include:
- The deliberate, systematic or wanton infliction of physical or mental suffering by one or more persons acting alone of on the orders of any authority, to force another person to yield information, to make confession or for any other reason
- To inflict pain on someone; to inflict extreme pain or physical punishment on people; cause somebody anguish: to cause somebody mental or physical anguish; distort something: to twist or distort something into an unnatural form

Ritual Abuse

Definitions of *ritual abuse* include:
- Ritual abuse is a brutal form of abuse of children, adolescents and adults, consisting of physical, sexual, and psychologic abuse involving the use of rituals. Ritual abuse rarely consists of a single episode. It usually involves repeated abuse over an extended period of time.
- Alleged systematic child abuse: the alleged physical abuse of children by adults taking part in supposed satanic rituals

Dissociation

Definitions of *dissociation* include:
- An unconscious process by which a group of mental processes is separated from the rest of the thinking processes, resulting in an independent functioning of these processes and a loss of the usual relationships; for example, a separation of affect from cognition.
- In psychiatry: separation of emotions: the separation of a group of normally connected mental processes, for example, emotion and understanding, from the rest of the mind as a defense mechanism

Data compiled by Bonnie Yost; sources available upon request.

Table 3-1 Incidence of Interpersonal Trauma

Type of Trauma	Reported Incidence
Child Abuse	• A global meta-analysis concluded that 12.7% of the population reported that they had been victims of childhood sexual abuse: 18% females, 7.6% males[469] • In the United States, more than 740,000 children are treated in hospital departments as a result of violence each year • Youth violence resulted in more 656,000 emergency room treatments in 2008 with nearly 6,000 homicides in 2007
Adult/Elder Abuse	• 1-2 million adults older than age 65 yr are estimated to suffer abuse or neglect annually • Violence accounts for approximately 51,000 deaths in the United States annually
Rape	• In a national survey of 9,684 adults, 10.6% female and 2.1% male respondents reported being raped at some stage in their lives, with 60%-70% of these individuals being raped before age 18,[49] while another survey reported as many as 17.6% of women and 3% of men reporting forcible rape[494]

Modified from Centers for Disease Control and Prevention (CDC). *Injury center: violence prevention.* Available online at http://www.cdc.gov /ViolencePrevention/; Stoltenborgh M: The neglect of child neglect: a meta-analytic review of the prevalence of neglect. *Soc Psychiatry Psychiatr Epidemiol* 48(3):345–355, 2013.

Whether it is apparent, health care professionals in all specialties work with individuals who have a history of trauma (physical, sexual, or emotional). The incidence of psychologic trauma is high and researchers and clinicians suggest that these statistics are low because unreported incidents[193] and ritual abuse (intentional and repeated torture) statistics are difficult to monitor (Table 3-1).

Although family and interpersonal violence is more common, torture and war provide intense, repeated and extremely damaging stressors for those directly involved, for their families, and sometimes even for medical personnel who are called upon to assist with individuals who are being tortured.[99] Large numbers of refugees who now reside in the United States have experienced or witnessed torture to varying degrees.[180] They have also been exposed to death on a large scale with high prevalence of major depressive disorders, post-traumatic stress disorder (PTSD), anxiety and panic attacks, as well as physical and psychologic pain.[180,250]

Combat

The trauma of war can affect not only the warriors, but also their partners and children. Trauma associated with war can cause problems with self-esteem, communication, sexuality, and parenting. A condition of hyperawareness or hyperarousal is common long after the euphoria of returning home has worn off. Adrenaline rushes from constantly being on alert in war zones do not just get "turned off" once the soldier is home or in a safe environment.

Combat trauma can lead to depression, PTSD, and other forms of emotional pain. The most common problems confronting families of combat veterans include emotional numbing, sexual difficulties, anger, family violence, and guilt. Healing the wounds of war is becoming the focus of new research and clinical attention.[297] For further discussion, see "Posttraumatic Stress Disorder" below.

World Events and Cultural Trends

Currently, our world is threatened by terrorist activity. Along with our society's saturation of fear-based marketing strategies and victim mentality, the general public in the United States is a prime target for psychogenic illness. The resulting sequelae directly impact medical care and the clinician's perspective.

The Department of Homeland Security believes that our country and the world need to prepare for outbreaks of mass psychogenic illness.[509] World and U.S. events point to the effects of fear and terrorist attacks on the general public and specifically on people in the real or perceived exposure areas. The number of individuals suffering psychogenic illness could far exceed the number of actual casualties in a chemical, biologic, or radiologic or other life-threatening event.

Support for this perception based on real events has been published.[336] Distress experienced in populations and various social groups well outside the involved communities include feelings of distrust for authority figures and organizations, anxiety over potential future threats, feelings of grief and loss, a sense of loss of control, and doubting local wisdom that persists for at least 18 months. The study punctuated the importance of open and consistent communication, personal involvement with those perceiving or recovering from trauma, and community support in trauma healing.[336]

The 21st century cultural guidelines in the United States have become more ambiguous and obscure, especially in comparison to the more tangible social constructs of the 20th century.[310] Fear-based living leads to victim mentality and can result in an unrealistic perception of life with associated loss of personal awareness and stress-management potential.

Medical remedies for common concerns serve as backups and safety nets when personal management skills are unsuccessful or nonexistent. Loss of confidence in innate coping ability propels us into seeking an external cause and source of remedy (including substances, food, and other addictive behaviors). Evidence of this trend is seen in medicine and in everyday life.

Psychologic Responses to Stress and Trauma

Trauma including physical, sexual or emotional abuse, violent physical injury such as motor vehicle accidents (MVAs), injuries sustained during combat, assault, even an unexpected event perceived as a threat (e.g., dog bite) can result in acute psychologic stress symptoms such as anxiety, dissociation (detachment of the mind from the emotional state and/or even the body), intense fear, helplessness or horror, reexperiencing the event and increased arousal.[18] Observation of physical trauma such as torture, disasters, or violent personal assaults[462] can result in the development of *Acute Stress Disorder*, which is the appropriate diagnosis if the characteristic anxiety, dissociative and other symptoms occur within 1 month of the trauma.[26] If these symptoms are still present beyond 4 weeks, the diagnosis changes to *Posttraumatic Stress Disorder*.

Physiologic Responses to Stress

Stress Reactions

Worry, fear of the unknown, and other anxieties are normal occurrences, which usually resolve. Empathetic support from caring people who listen, offer reassurance, and point out options for dealing with the event may help alleviate fear or anxiety.[448] In the presence of danger, fear is helpful for the purpose of initiating an appropriate short-term survival response referred to as the sympathetic fight, flight, or freeze response already mentioned. Anxiety or fear of potential threat in the absence of real danger or for extensive time periods can cause damaging psychologic and physiologic patterns.

Animal studies confirm that in repeated experiences of overwhelming trauma, freezing becomes the default coping mechanism, even when other options for escape or defense are available. *Dissociation* (lapses in consciousness, decreased awareness of the surroundings, loss of memory or occasionally loss of identity) is an extreme manifestation of the freeze response that occurs as a response to severe trauma.[340,433,436,513] The concept of dissociation is defined as *a detachment of the mind from the emotional state or body*. This condition can be as mild and fleeting as daydreaming, or it can be so severe that the personality is shattered into adaptive "parts" such as in Dissociative Personality Disorder.

Living in the shadow of unresolved trauma and depending constantly on coping systems designed as temporary, short-term defenses for survival have implications for physical, emotional, mental, and spiritual health. Individuals whose dysregulated responses to unresolved trauma (including dissociation) are often unaware of their fractured state until the coping mechanisms begin to break down and functioning becomes increasingly difficult.

There is also a negative impact on the brain and sympathetic nervous system as a result of the long-term effects of living in a constant state of anxiety and survival mode. Persistent fear and a sense of being unsafe (perceived or real) has devastating effects on every aspect of health. The normal acute stress responses include activation of the hypothalamic-pituitary-adrenal system with release of cortisol, epinephrine and norepinephrine resulting in the fight-or-flight responses described here.[175] The release of cortisol reduces metabolic activity, elevates blood glucose. After prolonged stress responses, the body responds by activating a negative control on the hypothalamic-pituitary-adrenal system to stop the acute responses when high levels of cortisol are present.[175,533] Persistent, long-term stress without resolution therefore results in a downregulated system with low cortisol levels and the possibility of decreased immune function. The physical effects of low cortisol are closely related to inadequate immune responses to microtrauma,[175] infection, or neoplasms.[181]

Impairments in the regulatory cycle of the hypothalamic-pituitary-adrenal system may correspond with physical pain, excessive fatigue, and tension with negative effects on the anatomy and function of the brain. Young children who experience abuse or neglect show abnormal cortisol levels, indicative of a dysregulated stress response. These changes often remain after the child has been removed to a safe, caring environment and are persistent in individuals who show clinical or subclinical symptoms of PTSD.[182,468]

Individuals with PTSD have also been shown to exhibit high levels of inflammatory cytokines partly attributed to low cortisol levels.[175,181] However, the opposite relationship has also been proposed whereby chronic inflammation results in changes in dopamine activity in the hippocampus and amygdala, contributing to fear responses and memory retrieval of trauma with similar symptoms to individuals with major depression.[175,181] Research continues to explore these relationships, as well as pharmacologic management, including serotonin uptake inhibitors and responses to hydrocortisone.

Pain Perception: The Link Between Psychologic and Physical Connections?

Pain has been defined as an unpleasant sensory and emotional experience associated with actual or potential tissue damage.[325] The extent of pain experiences are shaped by psychologic factors such as the attention or importance of the pain, interpretation of the pain (based on previous experience, beliefs, attitudes and expectations), coping strategies and resultant behaviors.[282] Psychologic variables, such as pain catastrophizing (exaggerated negative attitude in response to a minimal physical event),[474] fear-avoidance behaviors,[273,277] and pain-related anxiety,[429,521] can impact postsurgical and rehabilitation outcomes.[155]

These and other psychologic risk factors (such as unhelpful beliefs about pain, expectations of poor treatment outcome, clinical depression and/or personality disorder) are identified and considered "yellow flags."[368] When the physical therapist observes or identifies yellow flags, it may be possible to address or accommodate the comorbidities during treatment; otherwise, an appropriate referral may be needed.[282,368] By addressing yellow flags, it may be possible to limit long-term disability and fear behaviors,[520] or to explain poor outcomes.[368,538]

Acute pain serves as a warning system and carries the expectation of resolution. Chronic pain is less well-defined, provides no biologic benefit, and does not resolve. The neurophysiologic changes that occur in the presence of chronic pain are complex with prolonged neurochemical changes, increased sensitization of peripheral and central nociceptive pathways and receptors and changes in areas of sensory appreciation in the cortex. Noxious stimuli to dorsal horn neurons cause substance P and glutamate to produce cellular changes, which can enhance pain transmission to the brain.

Prolonged central sensitization or decreased threshold of neural excitability eventually requires lower or no external stimuli to be self-perpetuating. In addition to sustaining cellular changes in the spinal cord, individuals with chronic pain have a more complex brain response to additional pain experiences than people without chronic pain histories. Chronic pain can impair sleep, cognitive function, mood, cardiovascular health, sexual function and influence every facet of an individual's social interactions.[148]

Psychologic Considerations in Health Care

Physical therapists are ideally placed to bridge the gap between the physical and psychologic realms and broaden the scope of caring for the whole person. Repeat visits over time set the stage for developing trust and sharing at deeper levels.[115] Knowledge of neurophysiology and biopsychosocial trends, along with careful listening and reflection, helps the clinician address subconscious needs of the client, thereby allowing the therapist to evaluate more carefully (and the individual to participate more fully) in treatment choices.

As health care professionals, we frequently encounter people suffering from childhood and adult trauma in our clinical practices. Health care professionals must be sensitive to the most wounded and complicated client so as to maximize the potential for whole-person healing. Today's political and social events are precipitating real and perceived trauma. Domestic, sexual, ritual, and other abuses permeate all social strata. It is impossible to identify a perpetrator or survivor of abuse by outward appearances. Perpetrators are skilled at cover-up, and survivors cope through dissociation to look "normal" because of conditioned fear.

Many individuals with unresolved, unseen emotional and psychologic wounds do not know the reasons for their comorbid diagnoses; failed treatments; reactive, destructive lifestyles; and bankrupt relationships. They have survived by hiding their pain, disability, and terror from themselves and from others. Triggers, flashbacks, and nightmares often do not intrude into daily life until well into adulthood, when the survivor is unable to continue the exhausting "cover-up," fear-based façade, and denial stemming from overwhelming shame and trauma. Signs of unresolved trauma can be found in Table 3-3.

Common health care practices often significantly hinder the recovery of abuse and trauma survivors. Medical practitioners are trained to take control and move through treatment within limited time allowances. Medical offices are filled with sights, sounds, smells, and items that can make even a person without a traumatic background feel uneasy or unsafe. The clinician may use hands-on techniques, such as pushing, pulling, stretching, compressing, touching, rubbing, and other sensory or sudden changes, that can impact a client with a history of abuse in a negative way. Persistence in cajoling, cheerleading, or demanding compliance meant as encouragement may further victimize the individual.[245]

Problems of this type in practice can be remedied and significant improvements can be seen in patient/client satisfaction and response when involved professionals understand the specific needs of the individual and the dynamics of the deeper, heart-mind-body pathology.

EFFECTS OF TRAUMA ON BRAIN DEVELOPMENT

A-Type (Neglect) Trauma and B-Type (Abuse) Trauma

The terms *type A* and *type B* psychologic trauma have been used to describe *neglect* (type A) and *abuse* (type B).Type A trauma results from the absence of positive support for psychologic health and well-being, such as nurturing by and healthy bonding with parents. Physiologically, lack of early childhood support results in changes in the limbic and related areas of the brain where strong emotions are processed and stored. Type A traumas will present as painful feelings emerging when the wounded person realizes the impact of lack of nurturing in his or her own development.

Type B traumas are negative events that take place during childhood or adulthood. Dissociative coping mechanisms and barriers or distortions to memory are more likely to result from negative events. The harbored reactions, feelings, and beliefs related to the psychologic trauma stimulate flight or fight fear reactions and sympathetic system activation and influence the ability to receive or express joy. Dissociative amnesia is the brain's coping mechanism for overwhelming, life-threatening trauma and can occur any time after infancy.[18,434]

Both type A and type B traumas increase the individual's conscious and unconscious need for self-protection, activating the sympathetic system and escalating adrenal activity. Self-perpetuation of mixed messages (the inability of the brain's two hemispheres to make sense of and resolve the cognitive message and sensory input) results in a persistent sense of helplessness. The conflicting and stressful input causes elevated, sustained cortisol levels, expressed physically as somatic pain and psychologically as emotional representations of the ongoing internal, mental conflict.

If the trauma is severe, the sense of self can be shattered confounding identity and destroying the concept of personal boundaries. Childhood trauma disrupts the course of normal development and perpetuates brain dysregulation. Consistent character traits and functional difficulties can be traced from deficits in early development. Major deficits in any of the normal developmental steps can lead to the unhealthy tendencies and traits listed in Table 3-2.

Identification and Disclosure of History of Trauma

Mild-to-extreme incidents of sexual trauma and domestic violence are frequently well hidden. Often individuals do not disclose their history of abuse because of feelings of shame and guilt, and fear of retribution.[193] The fear of not being believed, as well as implications for further violence or loss of support, also may result in not disclosing the trauma. The effects of trauma in early development on brain cognition and memory can destroy victim credibility and promote denial in the victim. Physicians and therapists who serve as entry points into the health care system need to be able to recognize signs of psychologic trauma presenting as primary diagnoses, secondary comorbidities, or somatic symptoms in order to be able to refer to mental health professionals, as well as to adapt evaluation and treatment strategies.[128,203,282,435,436]

Table 3-2	Developmental Impact of Trauma	
Age	**Normal Developmental Steps**	**Potential Tendencies and Traits**
Birth to 3 years	• Caregivers meet needs in healthy ways (temperature, caring/protective touch) • Caregiver relationships, faces and voice tones confirm personal value/belonging • Child experiences safety; healthy conflict resolution and management of emotions is modeled by caregivers	• Fear and insecurity in relationships • Manipulative, self-centered, isolated or discontented personality • Difficulty regulating emotions; emotional outbursts, worry, depression • Narrow scope of emotional tolerance
4 to 12 years	• Child learns to identify needs, ask and receive appropriately • Child discovers and owns up to the consequences of own choices/behaviors • Child sees benefit in doing tasks the child does not feel like doing • Child experiences success exercising own talents and initiative	• Passive-aggressive; persistent frustration/disappointment when needs and expectations are not met • Addictive; searching for satisfaction • History of repeated failure; "stuck," undependable, focuses on comfort, daydream fantasies • Unproductive goals and activities
13 years to birth of first child	• Young adult cares for self and others • Young adult able to tolerate and successfully manage difficult situations • Young adult recognizes and owns effects of personal actions on self and others; able to contain self; avoids harm to others • Young adult is able to maintain healthy relationships over time and distance	• Self-centered; difficult to be around • Conforms to negative/destructive group activities • Insensitive to others; defensive, controlling, harmful, victim mentality, • Shows excessive self-importance, loner

Note: Failure to receive healthy nurture and instructions listed as part of Normal Developmental Steps can lead to unhealthy tendencies and traits listed. Data from Wilder EJ: *The life model*, Pasadena, CA, 2004, Shepherd's House.

There is a high incidence of concurrent mental health problems, substance abuse (see "Substance Use and Addictive Disorders" in this chapter), and physical disorders observed in the general population. Women who have a history of violence have been found to have a high rate of chronic illness,[269] often complain of multiple nonspecific physical problems,[315] and have a high rate of disability claims.[418] There is also an association between the severity of childhood abuse or domestic violence with poor health behavior, disabling health conditions, and severity of somatic symptoms.[534] The ability to provide trauma-cognizant and patient-sensitive effective care for those with or without an identified history of physical and/or psychologic trauma may depend on recognizing the symptoms of abuse without an explicit disclosure.[128]

Many physical, mental, and emotional pain and behavioral problems are common to abuse, trauma, and torture survivors. Although psychologic sequelae are frequently the outcome of traumatic experiences, survivors often experience their problems as primarily somatic.[513] Because of dissociation, amnesia, and survival reactions at the time of trauma, the person may not have any conscious awareness of the abuse and trauma history until much later, especially if the trauma occurred during childhood.[512]

People suffering from unresolved trauma often work to cover their severe distrust of people and unfamiliar environments. Safety, real or perceived, is foreign and unidentifiable because of their past history. The effects of past trauma can be expressed physically or emotionally and are set off by normal daily events, especially medical treatment. Sensory information through sound, smell, taste, sight, touch, and position or movement similar to the original trauma can elicit physical or emotional reactions, apparently unrelated to the current treatment focus or context.[433,435,436]

Medical offices may be associated with care following the trauma and can make even a person without a traumatic background feel uneasy or unsafe. The clinician may use hands-on techniques, such as pushing, pulling, stretching, compressing, touching, rubbing, and other sensory or sudden changes, that can impact a client with a history of abuse in a negative way. Persistence in cajoling, cheerleading, or demanding compliance meant as encouragement may further victimize the individual. In addition, default coping strategies surface repeatedly and reinforce the physical, emotional, and mental survival reactions as if past trauma was occurring in the present. This often presents as "freeze" reactions accompanied by shallow breathing or breath holding.

These "triggers" might be difficult for the physical therapist or the patient/client to identify without careful observation of body language, consistency of verbal responses with body language, or through questioning.[128,435,436] The astute provider can look beyond the superficial and obvious symptoms to consider the contributions from all systems and underlying pathology. Dissociative changes are very subtle, allowing the survivor to conceal tremendous turmoil internally. Table 3-3 lists the most common signs and symptoms of unseen wounds and unresolved trauma; this list is not exhaustive as there may be other symptoms experienced by some people.

Sensitive observation, attentive listening, and appropriate questions help the clinician to grasp subtle changes that indicate client status.

SPECIAL IMPLICATIONS FOR THE THERAPIST 3-2

Effects of Trauma

Identification of Psychologic Contributions to Physical Diagnoses

Physical therapists are ideally situated to screen for and respond to family violence and all forms of trauma and abuse. As a client is treated over a period of time, and with repeated visits, a relationship is formed that is conducive to growing trust and openness. As the client verbally discloses this information to the physical therapist, observations of function, affect, reactivity, receptiveness, and appropriateness can be gathered. Receiving and comparing information from the client's musculoskeletal, neurologic, verbal, and nonverbal communication provides a wealth of confirming or contradictory evidence.

Observe the client for:
- *Excessive tension, rapid breathing, and freeze patterns observed during positioning and hands-on activities*
- *Inappropriate responses to questions or evaluation techniques*
- *Excessive fear responses (body language, facial expressions, declining treatment)*
- *Sudden fear, muscle guarding, sweating or the need to move from a specific location*
- *Darting eye movements, sweating or lack of conscious attention*
- *Treatment or touch results in excessive reports of pain, or muscle spasm that are inconsistent with the area or the extent of pressure.*

Evaluation tools that may assist in identifying psychologic contributions:
- *Questions on the intake evaluation related to abuse or emotional trauma*[436]
- *Sensitive open-ended questions to allow disclosure*[436]
- *Tampa Kinesophobia Scale (>39 elevated score)*[2,258,537,538]
- *Pain catastrophizing scale (>20 elevated score)*[2,537,538]
- *Beck Depression Inventory (>13 elevated score)*[68,195,538]
- *PTSD Scale*[152]
- *Evaluation of inconsistencies between subjective reported pain or influence on function and observed functional capabilities*

Evaluation of progress and identification of:
- *Failure to progress*
- *Difficulty complying with his or her independent self-care program*
- *Belief that there is an answer to physical discomfort that will take away all the pain such as another health care provider opinion, explanations derived from MRI or other sophisticated testing, surgery or pharmaceutical management*

Strategies to enable disclosure or identify if referral to a psychologist is needed or modifications to physical therapy treatment are required[436]:
- *Establish an environment of personal safety and trust*

Table 3-3	Signs of Unresolved Trauma		
Physical	**Emotional**	**Behavioral**	**Mental**

• Hypervigilance
• Cannot differentiate between healthy and unhealthy pain
• Joint and muscle pain
• Headaches, shoulder and neck pain, and tension-related problems
• Balance, vestibular problems, and dizziness
• Visual disturbances or loss
• Hearing loss and tinnitus
• Recurrent high blood pressure
• Gait abnormalities
• Paresis
• Disconnection from body
• Syndromes and diseases, such as:
  • Chronic fatigue syndrome
  • Fibromyalgia
  • Irritable bowel syndrome
  • Reactive bladder
  • Restless legs syndrome
  • Meniere disease
  • Lupus erythematosus
  • Multiple sclerosis
  • Autoimmune diseases
• Teeth clenching and bruxing (grinding)
• Digestive and intestinal problems
• Blood pressure problems, heart arrhythmias, chest pain
• Nervous tics, tremors
• Rashes, itching
• Exhaustion
• Allergies
• Insomnia
• Short of breath
• Diagnoses unresolved by medical tests and treatment; comorbidity
	• Egocentric, self-blame ("I am the cause of everything that happens")
	• Inability to tolerate feelings or conflicts
	• Intense self-blame and feeling unworthy
	• Staying stuck in victim or perpetrator roles
	• Disconnection from feelings, emotions
	• Feeling very isolated, alone, vulnerable
	• Anxious, fearful, panic attacks—fear of the unknown, consistently anticipating the worst
	• Depression, doubt, discouragement
	• Paranoia, distrust
	• Secrecy, guilt, shame
	• Insecurity/poor self-worth
	• Feeling out-of-control, overwhelmed, at the end of one's rope
	• Sudden, exaggerated emotional reactions
	• Flaring anger, rage, hatred; abusive talk/actions
	• Quarreling, fighting, complaining, judging
	• Nightmares, sleep disorders; flashbacks, "triggers"
	• Bitterness, resentment, shame
		• Cannot recognize, define, or emulate healthy behaviors, relationships
		• Does not know what is "normal"
		• Does not know how to model or live "normal"
		• Child-like, unrefined, or harsh social skills
		• Difficulty with relationships; unhealthy boundaries
		• Self-injury, self-persecution/blame; destructive lifestyle
		• Inappropriate threat/defense reactions
		• Failure to own responsibility; victim mentality
		• Greed, materialism
		• Cheating; lying; stealing; apathy; laziness; procrastination
		• Obsessive impulse, driven
		• Disorganization, procrastination
		• Difficulty keeping promises, appointments
		• Reactive, inconsistent personality traits
		• Reckless driving, accident prone
		• Impatience, irritability, inappropriate social reactions
		• Disorders in eating, sleeping, sexual desire
		• Addictions—alcohol, drugs, sexual, smoking, food
		• Inability to speak needs or feelings
		• Withdrawn, isolated, loner
		• Disorganized attachment patterns—clinging or avoidance behaviors
		• Out-of-control, self-injurious and/or suicidal behaviors and patterns
			• Difficulty with problem solving and intentional focus
			• Confusion, forgetfulness
			• Difficulty saying "No" and/or making decisions
			• Intrusive, negative, or destructive thoughts, images, feelings
			• Failure to recognize and act on available options
			• Identity confusion and deception; overriding focus on self

Data compiled by Bonnie Yost; sources available upon request.

- *At the appropriate time, explain that sharing apparently unrelated reactions is important to successful intervention because thoughts, feelings, and sensations reveal factors contributing to the symptoms and may interfere with positive outcomes*
- *Identify triggers that increase stress reactions through careful observation, discussion with the patient/client and ongoing monitoring of both physiologic and psychologic responses*
  Referral for psychologic management:
- *Identification of clients who might benefit from referral for psychologic services is an important element of*

evaluation with possible elements such as identification of "yellow flags," client reported history of abuse or emotional trauma, identifying inconsistencies or exaggerated responses to physical diagnoses, fear-avoidance behaviors or lack of progress[332]
- *It is important to inform the client of options in obtaining those services and the benefits of receiving such services. Have a prepared referral list with contact information for carefully screened interdisciplinary professionals. A list to consider can help smooth the client's transition in thinking about taking advantage of adjunct services[436]*

RIGHT BRAIN HEMISPHERE FUNCTION

The right hemisphere of the brain is *dominant* for:

- Receiving, expressing, interpreting and communicating emotional states (right hemisphere to right hemisphere)
- Sending and receiving subconscious, nonverbal communication
- Retaining the most deeply ingrained message (the nonverbal, which overrides the verbal message)
- Registering emotional messages from the subconscious facial expression and tone of voice of the sender then generating a somatosensory bodily representation of how the sender feels about self (receiver) and about the emotional status of the sender
- Primary-process cognition
- Adapting to complex, internally contradictory information
- Processing of "image thinking:" simultaneous, multilevel incorporation of varied image messages and components
- Processing of stress and negative emotions, utilizing negative environmental stimulus for error compensation
- Storing emotions that are then expressed physically and nonverbally, mostly subconsciously, by the right hemisphere

SUPPORTING PSYCHOLOGIC HEALING

The time constraints under present financial and insurance restrictions result in health care practitioners having less and less time to listen and make a personal connection with the individual. As physical therapists may have more consistent interactions with clients than other professionals on the health care team, clients might reach out to physical therapists for support or choose to disclose their psychologic problems. The physical therapist should therefore be able to refer to appropriate mental health professionals, be familiar with methods of psychologic management in order to support interdisciplinary care, and be able to apply some behavioral and learning techniques to facilitate improvement in physical function. Conversely, physical therapists will also need to be aware of how to manage dysfunctional patterns and avoid client dependency or transference. These skills take time and additional exploration and training to develop; therapists are encouraged to seek opportunities for such training throughout their careers.[441]

Psychologic Healing Potential

The areas of the brain involved in receptive and expressive communication are distributed across both hemispheres. The left hemisphere controls linguistic communication and analytical interpretation, whereas the right hemisphere is responsible for nonverbal receptive and expressive communications (Box 3-2). Both brain hemispheres work together to seek and verify consistency and accuracy of information and stimulus. Traumatic experiences interrupt brain function and precipitate conflicting interpretation of sensory and cognitive input.

Maturation of the right brain in infancy is equated with the early development of self (brain-mind-body). The right hemisphere of the brain, more than the left, develops vast connections with the emotion-processing limbic areas of the brain, which have a powerful influence on behavior. Nonverbal communication (facial and body language, tone of voice) relays the dominant message when receiving, expressing, and communicating emotional states.[438,440] These messages are operate at a subconscious level and are derived from past experiences, deep emotions, and base perceptions of both the sender and receiver. The receiver's brain generates a somatosensory, physical representation of how the sender is perceived to be feeling during the interaction and the related "message" or meaning to the receiver.[439]

Emotional interpretations, such as impressions of joy, frustration, contentment, insecurity, confidence, fear, and peace, are often the first, strongest, and most lasting messages, no matter what words or ideas are verbalized. The right hemisphere of the brain is also responsible for processing stress and emotions and for learning how to compensate for negative or stressful experiences (even positive events and experiences can be perceived as "stressful" although not in a negative way).[441,442]

The Development of Joy

From birth and throughout life, connection with other people or lack thereof impacts every aspect of our health, perspective, and function. Just as neglect and abuse interfere with normal development, nurture and relational joy promote healthy growth and development and a secure, resilient identity. Joy has been identified as a necessity for human development.

Humans will mirror nonverbal interpersonal communication paths. A child will mirror what the child receives nonverbally from interaction with older children and adults, and behavior is mimicked from exposure to the more mature models.[438-440] The attitude and emotions of the sender, conveyed nonverbally, carry the deepest and most lasting message to the receiver. The more healthy and mature a person is, the better able that person is to accurately understand left and right hemisphere communications and resolve conflicting verbal and nonverbal messages while retaining a solid and consistent self-perception and response stability.[438,439] Tone of voice and facial expression result in much faster messages than verbal communication. Subconscious messages from facial expressions occur as fast as 40 milliseconds or the time it takes for one brain cell to fire. The complete cycle of sent and received nonverbal messages occurs at six times per second.[438-440]

The Right Orbital Prefrontal Cortex[428]

The importance of right brain function in the development of joy and the ability to resolve emotional, personal, and psychologic conflicts can be understood better by reviewing a description of the role of the right orbital prefrontal cortex (ROPC). ROPC of the human brain develops between birth and 18 months of age. How much and how fast this area grows depends directly on the nature and quality of stimulation this area receives through interaction with a caregiver. Growth in a person's ROPC occurs when the child receives nonverbal messages that they are valued and cared for through eye contact, voice tone, and touch, which becomes a positive motivator for the child younger than 12 months old.[440,442]

There are normal growth spurts of the ROPC between birth and 18 months of age, with peaks at 3 months and 9 months of age; between 3 and 5 years of age with the peak at 4 years of age; between 7 and 10 years of age; at 15 years of age; and at the birth of the first child.[438] Biochemical changes during pregnancy prepare the mother's brain for ROPC growth. The last identified growth spurt of the ROPC occurs at the birth of the first grandchild.[438-440] Throughout life, the ROPC retains its ability to grow, and thus its ability to heal, to the same extent as from infancy. ROPC deficits can be restored in persons suffering previous developmental or trauma losses.[439,440]

Brain scans confirm that the ROPC grows in response to joy, targeting the left eye.[438-440,539,540] For clarity, "joy" is differentiated from "happiness" in that joy is relational and results in positive growth and health beyond circumstances. Happiness can be manipulated and governed by circumstances and by the person's will. Although some growth of the ROPC will occur with even minimal joy experiences, the most favorable growth and healing of the ROPC occurs during frequent and consistent experiences of joy such as genuine smiles. ROPC function is enhanced when the right hemisphere messages are in agreement with the verbal left hemisphere content and when there is synchrony of communication. In the absence of "joy" stimulation, the ROPC will atrophy and the full growth and potential will not be achieved.

Phases of Healing

> **Note to Reader:** This section is written from the perspective of a psychologic health care provider but is intended to provide the physical therapist with an understanding of the concepts as they are currently understood and employed by that professional discipline because we often share clients and integrate services. Recognizing where our patients/clients may be in the healing phases can aid and assist us in providing compassionate and effective care. The physical therapist must be in touch with, able to successfully process, and model healthy responses to physical therapist's own pain in order to remain clear of the client's painful experiences and pain reactions.
>
> The physical therapist can impact physical and nonphysical healing in all phases in a powerful way. From the initial establishment of safety, choice, and trust to equipping the individual with knowledge, problem-solving skills, and personal awareness for self-care, the physical therapist can comprehensively serve the client. The physical therapist can support and enhance the client's work with a counselor, providing insights, and promoting mind, emotion, and body connection.

Most stress- and trauma-related pathologies can be managed as the brain has great potential for healing. Psychologic healing occurs when consistent messages are received and confirmed by both the cognitive (more logical) left hemisphere and the more emotional right hemisphere. The reconciliation between the two aspects of communication, learning, and emotional development may be unfamiliar and initially uncomfortable to the person who has lived with mixed messages and emotional, mental, and spiritual wounds for prolonged periods.

Healing often requires the assistance of a mental health provider who understands that the ability to tolerate disruption and uncertainty is fundamental to life, health, and growth and who is able to assist and mentor the individual in exploring that truth during treatment. Physical therapists may not have the full repertoire of psychologic treatment tools to enable psychologic healing, and referral to appropriate providers is an important step, especially as the client/patient may not seek help on their own. However, reinforcement of psychologic strategies, consistent support and caring, and avoidance of further stress may assist with alleviation or adaptation to physical diagnoses.

The phases of healing move from recognizing the need for healing (Phase I), to recognizing options for improvement (Phase II), to weighing the costs/benefits (Phase III), to facing healing challenges (Phase IV), to celebrating healing victories (Phase V), to reconciliation with health and wellness (Phase VI), to, finally, full reconciliation (Phase VII). Each of these phases provides unique challenges for the patient/client and for the physical therapist working with those individuals who are addressing their personal psychologic trauma or condition. The resolution and healing process is not necessarily linear and reactivation of stress can also occur.[128,436] Psychologic management during healing may consist of individual or group techniques[57,443] and at times is accompanied by pharmacologic management using antianxiety or antidepressive medications.[207]

Phase 1: Recognizing the Need for Healing

(See Fig. 3-1, *A* and *B*.)

The initial phase of healing from psychologic trauma is the recognition that there are options to manage the symptoms and developing a desire for improvement. The goal for health care providers during this phase is to help the individual learn to feel safe and develop a sense of trust, which is often difficult for survivors of sexual, emotional, and physical trauma.[436] In this phase, the person begins to reflect on his or her life patterns and to identify destructive thoughts, negative messages, and unnecessary limitations. The individual will begin to recognize and reveal established survival coping mechanisms and habits and how the old reactions influence relationships and daily function. The internal conflicts become clearer to the individual, which can produce fear of the unknown, of what may be revealed to others, and of people. Acknowledging hidden or "secret" trauma can generate feelings of panic, shame, guilt, and hopelessness and may interfere with keeping appointments and treatment strategies.

Sensitive care will help create a sense of safety while the dissociative, internally shattered person breaks down the barriers between emotions and perceptions (right hemisphere function) and cognitive function and thoughts (left hemisphere) and gains verbal descriptions and comprehension. The rehabilitation provider will need to understand that this can be a very frightening and confusing time for the individual. The client may become antagonistic and the connection can be difficult for both the clinician and

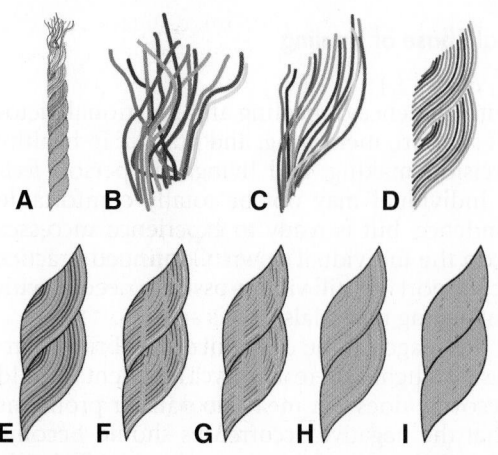

Figure 3-1

Phases of healing. Rope analogy to demonstrate how dissociation, function, and healing can be described and quantified. **A,** Rope shown as a progression from fractured, dissociative, and surviving *(top)* to functional health—whole, integrated, and thriving *(bottom)*. **B,** Frayed rope depicts the fractured, wounded condition of the individual existing in "parts" or "alters" used as a coping mechanism before healing. Colored threads represent hidden parts or alters that emerge as needed. In the initial phase, survival coping mechanisms break down and the person recognizes growing physical, emotional, and relational problems, motivating them to seek healing. **C,** Recognizing options for improvement. As the individual recognizes options for improvement, the individual begins to feel some hope and empowerment. **D,** Weighing the costs/benefits. Although the healing is challenging and healthy habits are new, the person experiences improved function and order as negative reactions are replaced with positive responses. **E,** Healing challenges. Difficult healing challenges provide vital opportunities to model and practice problem-solving and stress management skills. **F,** Healing victories. As the individual experiences the efficiency and success of system healing and integration, difficulties are outweighed by victories. **G,** System integration. This is a time of personal exploration and rejecting "surviving" habits to practice "thriving" skills. **H,** Early final phase. The client prepares for independence from the mentor/provider with a new, more tangible sense of identity, discovering how to take ownership of his or her life, choices, and actions. **I,** Final phase. The client moves into independence with healthy relationships and connection to others—not dependent and not isolated but able to appropriately give and receive (i.e., autonomous). (Courtesy Bonnie Yost. Used with permission.)

client, as the client tests acceptance and trustworthiness in this new relationship. In pushing away those who can and want to help, the affected individual is also testing their prolonged defense mechanisms and perceptions such as, "No one cares. You are not worth caring about. You are hopeless. There is no way out of this way of life and you cannot improve." With persistence and the guidance of a mental health professional, the client can eliminate these beliefs and open the way to healing. Unwavering, effective nonverbal communication and quiet acceptance of the person by the physical therapist through all challenges and emotions are crucial during this phase of healing, along with healthy, caring, well-established boundaries—vital for both clients and clinicians.

Phase 2: Recognizing Options for Improvement

(See Fig. 3-1, *C.*)

In this phase of healing, the client recognizes that there is help and healing available and should be able to report back what the client is working on with their psychologist

if the client chooses to share information about what works or does not work for them. The client experiences some personal control, safety, and respect from others. The client begins to understand how to state needs, ask for help, and see that it is possible to receive without resorting to high-energy survival coping strategies.

The individual's scope of self-awareness and assertiveness is growing through questioning his or her past beliefs and behaviors. Testing of reality and safety continues in this phase as the person explores healthy, sincere interaction. As the reality of safety grows, the individual risks replacing the escape-focused dissociative tendencies with staying in the present. This step of trust carries the risk of feeling, which can be very frightening for the individual. Additional effects, such as nightmares and hypervigilance, may become more evident as memories resurface or issues become apparent.

Previously unknown coping mechanisms come to light and more conditioned reactions or different triggers are revealed and the individual begins to grow in internal and external awareness. The conflicting messages may heighten before it begins to decrease. Learning to trust and receive without fear of repercussion takes time and practice. Physical therapists need to realize that new triggers can surface progressively and that there may be differences in the extent of communication at different times and with different clients.

Phase 3: Weighing the Cost/Benefits

(See Fig. 3-1, *D.*)

The client starts to appreciate how difficult healing is and can be overwhelmed. Questions such as, "How long will this take?" and "Must I relive my past abuse or pain?" are common. The clinician's truthful, open answers are most valuable along with facilitating support from other clinicians, family, and friends. "Your healing will take as long as it needs to take, depending on the severity of your condition and how able you are to move through each step of healing" is an accurate answer that helps break an overwhelming process down into manageable steps. During this phase, the client will have enough experiences that are different from past trauma that the potential of healing is appealing. Probably the greatest challenge to this healing phase is commitment. Fear of the unknown, of what may be revealed, of abandonment by caregivers, or other anxieties will cause some people to resist or give up this worthwhile effort.

Phase 4: Healing Challenges

(See Fig. 3-1, *E.*)

During this phase of healing, the client works through progressive steps and deeper psychologic support with the assistance of psychology professionals. Repetitive care, such as provided by the physical therapist, allows the clinician to develop a deeper understanding and safe relationship with the individual.

Difficulties in this phase can include testing the therapeutic relationship; the fear of losing parts of self by healing; and feeling insecurity, shame, and guilt when receiving joy. Familiar behaviors that appeared to rescue the client and take care of necessary functions might seem to be disappearing as the new behaviors are coordinated and integrated. The concept of personal identity, while retaining and improving the strengths and function of all parts, starts to become more comfortable. The client needs to know that healing is worth the effort and that it will take time and practice to adjust. The experiences of joy, improved function, and support persuade the affected individual to continue the healing journey while still experiencing residual thought, image, and emotional intrusions from the past. Lifestyle options and changes can be discussed and introduced during this phase. The client begins to experience how unity of body, mind, and feelings becomes much less exhausting, much more fulfilling, and more efficient.

Phase 5: Healing Victories

(See Fig. 3-1, *F.*)

This phase of healing is very rewarding and joy is experienced more frequently as the person works through issues that previously blocked ROPC healing and growth. Physical problems stemming from stress reactions, faulty perceptions, and reacting to previous triggers or memories improve or resolve.

Safe relationships and healthy boundaries are recognized, practiced, and appreciated. The internal hunger begins to abate, as joy is no longer feared but welcomed without striving, as a flow, not a flood. Through testing honest, open relationships in treatment and in personal circles, the client learns that physical and relational discomfort, healthy confrontation, and feelings can be acknowledged and faced. Healthy proactive problem-solving and choices are used to identify options rather than being driven by circumstances. Taking initiative becomes more comfortable and a proactive way of life. Through continued practice, the client learns that challenges can be addressed effectively and successfully, with less energy, time, and stress.

Phase 6: Moving Deeper into Health and System Integration

(See Fig. 3-1, *G.*)

This phase of healing consists of practicing and refining new insights and skills. Realistic, objective assessment of life and situations becomes more routine and efficient, although relationship discernment may still be challenging. Hypervigilance continues to diminish, but sensory hypersensitivity may increase temporarily at times. After prolonged periods of avoiding feelings and practicing emotional and sensory numbness, individuals in this phase go through a period of sensory activation and accommodation, even describing more acute hearing, vision, taste, smell, and tactile sensation.

Evidence of healing in mind, body, and spirit is confirmed by being able to manage triggers or avoiding dissociation or exaggerated emotional responses, less-frequent urges to react impulsively and return to unhealthy, unsafe thoughts, habits, places, and people. Fear and avoidance behaviors slowly decrease and the client is able to slowly start feeling safe with people, as well as in crowds, have the capacity to focus and complete tasks efficiently, and recognize his or her options to exercise choice and control. The desire to participate in self-punishment, mutilation, or other negative health behaviors diminishes or abates.

Phase 7: Final Phase of Healing

(See Fig. 3-1, *H* and *I.*)

Finally, with evidence of healing and functional victories and with support, mentoring, and practice in healthy thinking, decision making, and living, the person *feels* healed. The individual may not be totally comfortable with independence, but is ready to experience successes and failures on the individual's own. Continued practice and periodic support are still vital to assist as needed with facing and managing new trials.

People at this stage can be destabilized by brief recurrences of past thoughts or reactions. The client should know that recovery does not mean no pain or problems but rather that the negative occurrences should become less frequent, less intense, and easier and more efficiently addressed with practice. Issues and areas left unattended may come to light at some point, offering an opportunity for further healing and growth.

Sensory hypersensitivity and habitual hypervigilance decrease and often resolve. The person is able to recognize negative thoughts quickly and choose alternative options. Self-control improves while self-centered immaturity transforms into more mature altruism. Appropriate responding and proactivity replace past reactivity.

SPECIAL IMPLICATIONS FOR THE THERAPIST   3-3

Supporting Phases of Healing

- *Physical therapists are primarily involved in the treatment and rehabilitation of physical manifestations and comorbidities but might need to support healing of unresolved trauma (see Table 3-3) at any of the different phases.*
- *The sensitive clinician will recognize that unfamiliar positive or safe experiences can be quite scary for some clients. The insightful clinician is able to stay within the client's fragile tolerance while building trust through quietly communicating caring, consistency, confidence, and assurance through vocal tone and facial expression.*
- *Both therapist and client need to understand that stress can build up, as well as break down, a person, and that some uncertainty and discomfort is foundational to a healthy growth and healing process.*[438]
- *Avoid second-guessing your client and reacting out of your fears about what the client might feel or think, which will foster distrust.*
- *Often psychologic healing does not follow a linear course and both physical therapists and clients will need to be aware that some improvement may not always result in progressive resolution.*[128,436]

Nonverbal and Verbal Communication

- *Communicate consistent messages by ensuring that your body language matches verbal and cognitive educational, treatment, and self-care information.*
- *Psychologic healing can be supported by the health care professional's ability to empathize with the person's distress, and model appropriate management of stress. This requires the therapist to synchronize with the client visually, by vocal tone, and through the use of body language and space.*

- *Reinforce verbal communication with written instructions. Ask the client to review what was conveyed and exercise healthy boundaries.*
- *Listen without bias, encourage without coercion, offer options and step back, allowing the individual to make the choice—good or bad.*
- *Monitor nonverbal body language.*
- *Listen attentively to the client and reflect feelings and circumstances.*
- *Responding sensitively both verbally and most importantly, nonverbally.*

Maintaining Healthy Boundaries

- *To distinguish between personal feelings and reactions and to separate them from the client's emotional circumstances, the physical therapist must be attuned to his or her own emotional state and psychologic vulnerabilities and strengths. It is extremely easy to be influenced by a client's transference and neediness, and clinicians need emotional strength to prevent reacting or jumping to resolve the client's distress.*
- *Burnout or "compassion fatigue" can occur rapidly when the care provider is invested in or desires the client's healing more than the client desires it himself or herself.*
- *Healthy clinicians take the time to scrutinize themselves to determine positive and negative effects in caring for needy people. It is a valuable exercise for the protection of yourself and your clients to assess how difficult or complex individuals generate internal fears, insecurities, anger, or other emotions in you. Personal examination and healing allow you to know yourself, develop and practice healthy boundaries, and remain consistent in your thinking and interactions.*
- *Personal boundaries are critical to a person's identity and function. Boundaries can be flexible or rigid, open like fences or solid like walls, or versatile like a gate. Whereas positive life experiences promote exploration and testing of boundaries, negative or painful life experiences cultivate avoidance behaviors, especially every real or perceived trauma-related boundary.*
- *People with harbored hurts tend to keep the darker emotions (e.g., anger, shame, fear) hidden and avoid positive events (e.g., safe connection and trust, joy, helpful support) out of their lives. With healing, the function of boundaries reverses to allow and keep the positive, healthy and keep out negative, harmful elements. As health improves, personal boundaries help strengthen and magnify coping ability.*
- *Healthy boundaries maintain an adult-to-adult equality in the relationship, prevent the provider from taking on unrealistic responsibility for outcomes, and keep the focus on the needs of the client. Practicing healthy, personal boundaries is critical for the client, as a model of safety, respect, and health, and for the clinician to be above reproach, upholding ethical integrity and moral excellence. Establishing healthy boundaries allows others to know who you are and what to expect, facilitating a safe and trusting relationship.*
- *Initially, the clinician is encouraged to clearly define the clinical relationship with the client, including goals, expectations, roles, policies, and options. The therapist is advised to follow established policies; do not pacify the client by changing the rules. If concessions are made within established policies and healthy boundaries, let the client know what concessions are available and clearly identify the sustaining or limiting parameters.*
- *Appeasing the client may give relief for the moment, but changing the policies can cause confusion and insecurity in the future. Recognize and reflect on what your client is feeling and expressing and then clarify your desire to do the best you can for the individual. Clearly explain the policy and what is expected of both sides and document the interaction well.*
- *Participate in regular consultation with peers for healthy accountability, support, and perspective. Practice clear statements and interactions that convey empathy, clarity, confidence, and decisiveness. Be objective, not defensive or emotion-laden.*
- *Do not be in a hurry to respond to highly charged, emotional messages or phone calls. Seek counsel from peers and other providers, write out your response, offer options that are "win-win." Document thoroughly in an objective, nonjudgmental way as if the client, the client's family, lawyers, and other professionals will read your notes.[294]*

Patient-Sensitive and Trauma-Cognizant Approaches

- *The late Jules Rothstein, PhD, PT, FAPTA, and former editor of the professional journal, Physical Therapy, stated that, "Cynics might dismiss the concept of sensitive practice, but reality tells us that only by listening to our clients can we know about them and their condition. The knowledgeable listener who can act on what the patient/client says needs to couple that skill with keen observations of unspoken messages. All the while, the physical therapist must be wary about receiving messages never meant to be sent, messages that come from within the practitioner, born out of bias and personal agendas."[422]*
- *A primary goal for a physical therapist working with anyone with a history of psychologic trauma is to encourage patient/client control and responsibility in his or her own care.[128,436,536]*
- *Schachter et al[128] have suggested nine principles of sensitive practice for individuals with a history of sexual abuse: respect, taking time, developing rapport, sharing information, sharing control, respecting boundaries, fostering mutual learning, understanding nonlinear healing, and demonstrating awareness of interpersonal violence. They provide more detail on specific suggestions to promote these principles gleaned from interviews with survivors of childhood sexual abuse.*
- *Monitor the patient/client for stress responses through attentive listening and observation.[128]*
- *Sensitive inquiry about discomfort is usually appreciated by everyone.[436]*
- *Work with the individual to identify and avoid triggers and hyperarousal, such as allowing the person to discontinue or change positions, treatment, and equipment.[128,436]*
- *Encourage clients to identify and exercise options and choices and to report what they are thinking and feeling.[128]*

- If stress reactions are observed direct questioning or redirecting attention may diffuse somatic responses.[128]
- Provide a safe environment by adjusting surrounding space, proximity to other clients (especially if opposite gender or specific characteristics trigger stress).[128,436]
- Offer a choice of gender of therapist, especially if the client has a history of abuse.[436]
- Provide positive feedback for achievement of psychologic and physical goals.
- Support the individual's coping strategies (developed with a psychology professional); for example, this may include cognitive reframing, conscious attention to the present circumstances, breathing techniques.[128]
- Simple spirituality screening questions give the physical therapist information that can enhance client coping, trust and hope and inform the physical therapist's plan of care.

Goal Versus Task Orientation Challenges to Patient-Sensitive and Trauma-Cognizant Approaches

- Goal- or task-oriented training and treatment are necessary for immediate medical management, such as emergency medicine or surgery, when the person is incapacitated. However, goal orientation may induce feelings of loss of control, particularly when memories of the initial trauma are connected to health care management or health care settings. Goal orientation and lack of time with the patient/client can impose the physical therapist's agenda onto the client initiating further stress rather than assisting with disclosure or blocking the desire to address previous trauma.[128,436]
- The provider-client relationship can easily become stressed if the provider desires improvement more than the client, preventing the client from taking ownership of the process and the outcomes as the client's own.[438] Although task-oriented treatment can build independence through appropriate instruction and client compliance, this approach can also build dependence or discourage addressing the psychologic comorbidities.
- Client-focused, process-oriented care fosters healing and melds physical and psychologic needs, significantly increasing client satisfaction and positive outcomes. This approach not only emphasizes nonverbal communication, but also meets the individual where the individual is and actively involves the person in his or her own healing and future care. By maintaining a safe physical and nonphysical environment, the client can begin to feel, explore, mimic, and learn appropriate self-regulation.[438]

Psychologic and Physical Strategies During Rehabilitation

There are a variety of psychologic techniques that may be of benefit at different times during healing or with different types of coping strategies. Addressing physical pain and impairments can influence the psychologic wellbeing.

- Behavioral techniques such as lack of support for unrealistic expectations or clear explanations of the negative effect of avoidance behaviors or catastrophizing can be used to manage pain or movement avoidance.[282]

Positive reinforcement and support for addressing issues are important throughout to promote progress through phases of healing (both physical and psychologic).

- Cognitive restructuring involves clear explanations and learning about physical impairments as well as mechanisms to avoid exacerbation of pain or disability. If the patient/client is able to control his or her own goals (process-oriented care), the fear related to loss of control or the unknown can also be addressed.[282]
- Exercise has been used to address anxiety and PTSD. Studies of children with PTSD have provided support for reduction of PTSD symptoms, depression, and anxiety through aerobic exercise.[365a] For further discussion see "Anxiety and Exercise" in this chapter.

SPIRITUAL DEVELOPMENT IN THE HEALTH CARE PROFESSION

Spirituality can be viewed as one's search for purpose, meaning, and relationship with the transcendent or others. Spirituality is recognized as a factor that contributes to health in many persons.[252,420] The concept of spirituality is found in all cultures and societies. It is expressed in an individual's search for ultimate meaning through participation in, among other things, religion or belief in God, family, work, naturalism, rationalism, and humanism.[399] For some people, religion is viewed as beliefs, rituals, or rules, whereas for others this definition is too restrictive.[248]

In the last 20 years, the impact of human spirituality and beliefs has come under closer scrutiny in research, secular publications, and clinical education. In that same time period, there has been an increase in the number of required courses in spirituality and medicine in U.S. medical schools. In February 2009, a national consensus conference developed spiritual care guidelines for interprofessional clinical spiritual care. These guidelines, as well as the educational advances, research, and ethical principles, have supported the developing field of spirituality and health.[400] Professional development now offers more ways to develop spirituality, especially as it relates to the health care professional's sense of calling to their profession, the basis of relationship-centered care, and the provision of compassionate care.[401]

Studies show an association between religion or spirituality and health outcomes such as hypertension, lower fasting glucose levels, recovery from surgery, coping with illness, and the will to live.[208,252] Many studies demonstrate the importance of religion, specifically prayer, in the coping process of individuals with cancer, pain control and other chronic conditions has been shown to decrease the medical costs associated with end-of-life care.[42,45,119,253]

Individuals whose spiritual needs are not met are less satisfied with their care.[38] Most people polled want a more holistic approach to health care and do not mind (actually prefer) conversation with their health care provider about spirituality, their faith, their spiritual needs.[44] Some organizations, such as the National Cancer Institute, have published materials to help health care professionals learn how to talk about spiritual beliefs, values, and practices and their effect on health, illness, disease, and stress.[345]

According to a Gallup poll, 92% of Americans believe in God or a Higher Power; 50% polled said that religion was very important to them.[165] Prayer is a common practice in the United States. According to a national survey, more than one-third of Americans pray for good health. Many people who are ill may turn to prayer as a means of coping with their illness. Yet only about 1 in 10 people who pray for health reasons mention it to their health care provider.[307]

The health care provider's openness and ability to address a client's spiritual issues as the client reveals such concerns or beliefs are essential to the health and healing of the whole person. Jensen and Mostrom conclude that a physical therapist's level of comfort in addressing the spiritual domain with others is related to the physical therapist's own level of comfort with the spiritual domain.[227] Spiritual care is not in any one provider's domain. It is the responsibility of everyone on the health care team to listen to what is important to the individual, respect the individual's spiritual beliefs, and be able to communicate appropriately with the person as those issues and beliefs are shared. Health care providers can ask patients/clients in a nonbiased, nonjudgmental way about their spirituality for a more holistic approach to health and healing.[307]

A study surveying more than 200 hospital inpatients found that 77% said physicians should consider patients' spiritual needs. Furthermore, 37% wanted their physician to discuss spiritual beliefs with them more frequently, and 48% wanted their physicians to pray with them.[246] Another study involving primarily white women (92%) with a mean age of 62 years revealed that only 8% of those with religious or spiritual tendencies desired spiritual interaction with their physicians.[137] However, spiritual support from others, such as chaplains, pastoral care professionals, or family members and friends, as well as personal spiritual beliefs was highly important. Various reasons were postulated by the researchers regarding why respondents did not desire a spiritual interaction with their physicians, including good internal and external support; lack of a close relationship with the physician; focus on the illness itself; patient perception of the severity of the illness; and physician attitude.[137]

Spiritual Perceptions and Health

How an individual perceives his or her condition determines how the person will respond to a disease, illness, or other physical or mental health condition. Spiritual experience, beliefs, and perspectives can have a powerful impact on an individual's understanding of his or her illness.[209] For example, in numerous studies, African American women identified the tremendous support spirituality provided in coping with breast cancer.[483] Religious convictions can affect an individual's scope of options and decision-making process. Spiritual convictions may constitute a foundational need in health care or may cause a person to refuse procedures or treatment altogether.

A person who has experienced spiritual abuse might actively avoid anything with a religious or spiritual connotation. Knowing the pertinent history will allow the caregiver to gather information about words, expressions, and other triggers that might cause a negative reaction in the client. Spiritual health fosters coping beyond normally accepted parameters by giving the following[252,399]:

- *Sense of control:* Faith and trust are choices. Making the choice to trust beyond understanding eradicates helplessness, actively engages the person in self-awareness and assessment, and expands coping potential through the experience of empowerment.
- *Hope for restoration, for healing, for attaining goals, for a peaceful death:* People can find the ability to accept and deal with current conditions through belief in a Higher Power.
- *Acceptance:* Inconceivable stresses and demands can be tolerated when trust in a Higher Power gives meaning and purpose to life and suffering beyond understanding.
- *Strength and endurance:* A personal faith imparts peace beyond understanding or explanation, strength beyond self, and the ability to focus outwardly instead of being overwhelmed by internal suffering.

Human history is replete with accounts of people going through extreme, incomprehensible, life-threatening experiences or severe loss and finding the resolve to survive and the strength to endure through their faith and trust in God. Healing, beyond medical understanding or imagination, termed *miracles* or *spontaneous healing* by both clients and health care providers, is attributed to prayer and supernatural intervention. Although the tangible, consistent differences between those who spontaneously heal and those who do not are still being sought, the impact of spirituality is being considered and studied.

Consistently living in trust beyond circumstances and purpose beyond what we can see and understand relieves stress for many people. Instead of being reactive and allowing external pressures and demands to take control and dictate the results, problem-solving and life choices become responsive in nature. Challenges are addressed responsively, through weighing the options, making reasonable choices, and taking action on those choices.

Unfamiliar situations and apparently threatening events are entrusted to the Higher Power, who is believed to know the big picture beyond the individual's scope of comprehension and is powerful enough to direct, protect, and provide through any event in life. For people who do not identify with a Higher Power, belief in personal strength, mindfulness or connectedness with others can provide similar positive outcomes.[45,373] This type of belief brings the individual an ability to cope and hope and a joy that is above difficult circumstances. The health benefits of preventing damaging effects of persistent stress through abated fears, coming to terms with death and eternity, and knowing place and purpose in life through faith are experienced by many individuals.[132,208]

Distant Healing

Distant healing, the concept that human beings can intentionally cause healing effects in others, is an ancient concept, but one that has gained much attention in the last decade. Researchers in the field of distant healing cite formal laboratory and clinical studies with reported significant effects.[8,36,37,110,232]

Broadly defined, distant healing is a conscious, dedicated act of another person who is physically and emotionally at a distance.[59,121,122] Although this concept has come under fire and remains heavily debated, the use of intercessory prayer for patients in a coronary care unit has been established as a landmark study in the areas of both medicine and religion. Limitations of the study have been discussed as well.[78,79,130] The relationship between religious activities and lowered blood pressure, improved mental health, and decreased depression in older adults also has been reported.[254,255,334]

Other researchers have evaluated whether receiving intercessory prayer or knowing intercessory prayer was being offered has any effect on recovery after cardiac surgery. It seems that individuals who know they are being prayed for may have a higher incidence of complications.[60]

The topic of intentional healing from a distance is not standard conversation among rehabilitation providers. This is a complex and highly emotional subject for many people. The Holistic Nursing Association has brought this topic forward for the nursing profession with a commitment to the well-being of others, integrating intentionality in healing, caring, and communication.[412] Research conducted jointly by medical researchers, philosophers, and theologians may bring greater clarity to the topic in future years.

Practicing Sensitive Care

Sensitive care for the spiritual elements of each individual includes the following[29a,42,147,299,394,399]:

- Providing a safe environment by giving attention to the physical environment and to nonverbal messages.
- Listening attentively to the client and reflecting feelings and responding appropriately, both verbally and most importantly, nonverbally.
- Accepting the individual as a person whether you agree or approve, verbally and nonverbally respecting and valuing the person as you partner in discovering truth and evaluating options.
- Obtaining a spiritual history or identifying the person's need for avoidance of discussion of spiritual topics.
- Honoring spiritual practices, as appropriate; each clinician would benefit from discussing this issue and defining the professional, ethical, and personal boundaries involved.
- Recognizing pastors, chaplains, pastoral care professionals, rabbis, and other spiritual leaders as part of the interdisciplinary team and making appropriate referral for spiritual care

SPECIAL IMPLICATIONS FOR THE THERAPIST   **3-4**

Spiritual Development

The health care provider's spiritual condition, as well as the client's spirituality, impacts the caring relationship and each individual's perspective of illness, healing, and wholeness.[399] Therapists are encouraged to grow in understanding of the seen and unseen conditions of patients/clients; to explore and attend to their own emotional, mental, physical, and spiritual condition; and to

incorporate sensitive practice skills into client care as part of offering comprehensive care in the health care setting.

Spirituality and Stress

Stress in the form of anxiety (fear in the absence of actual danger), unresolved burdens, and strain and tension can create negative stress or distress. Stress that is chosen, such as a desire to serve above and beyond, triumph over a challenge, or master new situations, can foster eustress (good, pleasant, or curative stress). Eustress is not defined by the type of stressor but rather by how the individual person perceives that stress (e.g., negative or threatening versus positive or challenging).[447,466,480] Therapists and clients can benefit by an understanding of this concept.

Spiritual emptiness allows for no resource outside of self and understandably leads to self-limited, humanly limited coping, strength, and potential. If we believe there are no resources outside of ourselves, we tend to struggle under unrealistic expectations and pressures on self and others. Shouldering responsibility for managing life and circumstances can deplete and stress every system. Dependence on human fallibility, frailty, and limitation alone can result in exhaustion and pervasive feelings of burnout, depression, loneliness, hopelessness, and helplessness for some people.

Subsequently, physical therapists should be familiar with levels of spiritual distress. O'Brien identified seven levels of spiritual distress: spiritual pain, spiritual alienation, spiritual anxiety, spiritual guilt, spiritual anger, spiritual loss, and spiritual despair.[371] *Spiritual pain* may be expressed during routine conversation when patients/clients disclose that normal spiritual support is not available because of decreased mobility or other pathology.

Spiritual alienation is related to concerns about material resources, such as finances or care of a spouse or child. *Spiritual anxiety* reflects the individual's fear of judgment from members of her normal spiritual support group. *Spiritual guilt* is the fear that the situation is caused a result of sin or poor choices. When people blame God for the situation they are demonstrating *spiritual anger*. When a person expresses that life no longer has meaning or they no longer feel supported by others, *spiritual loss* is present. Finally, the most severe form of spiritual distress is *spiritual despair* or loss of hope. Physical therapists who recognize that spiritual distress is present can assist their patients/clients in the healing process through referral to pastoral care professionals.

Studies of both positive and negative coping have found that religious or spiritual experience and practices extend the individual's coping resources and are associated with improvement in health care outcomes. People who perceive their suffering as punishment from God or a Higher Power, who have excessive guilt or anger about failed expectations, or who feel betrayed by God, experience more depression, a poorer QOL, and greater callousness toward others. People who depend on God for strength, guidance, and help show less psychologic distress. In asking for forgiveness or by forgiving others, their spiritual beliefs provided strength and comfort beyond themselves.[383,399,480] Research examining the physiologic benefits of forgiveness among various groups (e.g., Christian women, individuals with PTSD, different faith traditions) report early findings of association between forgiveness and cardiovascular health, stress levels, and improved overall health.[231,266,268,404] Future studies in this area are anticipated.

A spiritual community can provide individuals with tangible support and value through a larger support system. Spiritual relationships, finding meaning, trust, and dependence on a Higher Power can fulfill deep needs; provide extraordinary hope, strength, endurance, and resiliency; and promote overall well-being.

SPECIAL ROLE OF THE PHYSICAL THERAPIST

It is virtually impossible to discern or identify *all* of the contributing factors in a person's pathology. Given this, however, it is to the clinician's and the client's benefit to consider the whole person during the physical therapist's assessment and intervention so as to avoid limiting perspective. Utilization of the World Health Organization's International Classification of Functioning, Disability, and Health can assist the physical therapist in determining environmental and personal factors that influence health outcomes. Simple spirituality screening questions give the physical therapist information that can enhance client coping, trust, and hope, and inform the physical therapist's plan of care.

Pathology is never purely physical, mental, emotional, or spiritual. Those systems are intimately connected and interdependent; to believe that comprehensive care can come from treating a single cause or system, while ignoring other components, is naïve and negligent. For example, in the physical realm physical therapists are ideally situated to screen for and respond to family violence and all forms of trauma and abuse that have mental, emotional, and spiritual effects. As a client is treated over a period of time, and with repeated visits, a relationship is formed that is conducive to growing trust and openness. Even though physical therapists are less comfortable with screening solely for what appear to be the client or patient's spiritual needs, it remains our responsibility develop our skills in the spiritual care of our patients/clients and their families keeping in mind the interrelationship between body, mind, spirit, and emotions.

The task before us is not easy, but all of our skills and knowledge will matter little unless we bring to our practice the sensitivity that is the right of all of our clients.[435] Exercising sensitive, compassionate, and insightful care, the physical therapist is able to identify and attend to situations of abuse, neglect, and domestic violence.[115] See Chapter 2 for further discussion of domestic violence.

Other elements that strengthen the position of the physical therapist in identifying and treating underlying contributors to physical pathology include the fact that we monitor a variety of information sources. As the client verbally informs the physical therapist, observations of function, affect, reactivity, receptiveness, and appropriateness can be gathered. Receiving and comparing information from the person's musculoskeletal, neurologic, verbal, and nonverbal communication provides a wealth of confirming or contradictory evidence.

Physical therapists are primarily involved in the treatment and rehabilitation of most of the signs of unresolved trauma (see Table 3-3) arising from a combination of contributors over time. The importance of listening, observing, and responding carefully to understand the person's reports of pain, thinking, and living patterns beyond the presenting organic components cannot be overemphasized and reinforces the tenets of the World Health Organization's International Classification of Functioning, Disability, and Health. Balance of the mind-body-spirit is essential in the provision of care based on the biopsychosocial model of health.[70]

The late Jules Rothstein, PhD, PT, FAPTA and former editor of the professional journal, *Physical Therapy*, stated that, "Cynics might dismiss the concept of sensitive practice, but reality tells us that only by listening to our clients can we know about them and their condition. The knowledgeable listener who can act on what the patient says needs to couple that skill with keen observations of unspoken messages. All the while, the physical therapist must be wary about receiving messages never meant to be sent, messages that come from within the practitioner, born out of bias and personal agendas."[422]

This chapter on nonphysical contributors to physical pain and pathology serves as a practical introduction to the potential we have as physical therapists to integrate neuromusculoskeletal health and function with cognitive, emotional, and spiritual health and function. As we step out in bridging the gap between medical and psychologic training and treatment, we need to seek insightful resources and competent ancillary professional teammates to partner with us in the rehabilitation of the whole person—heart, mind, spirit, and body.

Boundary Basics for the Provider[553]

Personal boundaries are critical to a person's identity and function. Boundaries can be flexible or rigid, open like fences or solid like walls, or versatile like a gate. Whereas positive life experiences promote exploration and testing of boundaries, negative or painful life experiences cultivate avoidance behaviors, especially every real or perceived trauma-related boundary.

People with harbored hurts tend to keep the darker emotions (e.g., anger, shame, fear) in and positive events (e.g., safe connection and trust, joy, helpful support) out of their lives. With healing, the function of boundaries reverses to allow in and keep in good and healthy elements and keep out negative, harmful elements. As health improves, personal boundaries help to monitor internal and external status, which strengthens and magnifies coping ability.

Healthy boundaries maintain an adult-to-adult equality in the caring relationship, prevent the provider from taking on unrealistic responsibility for outcomes, and keep the focus on the needs of the client. Practicing healthy, personal boundaries is critical for the client, as a model of safety, respect, and health, and for the clinician to be above reproach, upholding ethical integrity and moral excellence. Establishing healthy boundaries allows others to know who you are and what to expect, facilitating a safe and trusting relationship.

Guidelines for the Health Care Professional

Initially, the clinician is encouraged to clearly define the clinical relationship with the client, including goals, expectations, roles, policies, and options. The therapist is advised to follow established policies; do not pacify the client by changing the rules. If concessions are made within established policies and healthy boundaries, let the client know what concessions are available and clearly identify the sustaining or limiting parameters.

Appeasing the client may give relief for the moment, but changing the policies can cause confusion and insecurity in the future. Recognize and reflect on what your client is feeling and expressing and then clarify your desire to do the best you can for the individual. Clearly explain the policy and what is expected of both sides and document the interaction well.

Participate in regular supervision and consultation with peers for healthy accountability, support, and perspective. Practice potentially difficult sessions with peers before the session(s). Practice clear statements and interactions that convey empathy, clarity, confidence, and decisiveness. Be objective, not defensive or emotion-laden.

Do not be in a hurry to respond to highly charged, emotional messages or phone calls. Seek counsel from peers and other providers, write out your response, offer options that are "win-win." Document thoroughly in an objective, nonjudgmental way as if the client, the client's family, lawyers, and other professionals will read your notes.[294]

Start and stop each session on time, allowing time for "cool down," settling, and refreshment, with about 5 minutes dedicated to reviewing victories, independent preparation, and rescheduling.

Avoid rescuing and becoming the "savior." Know your roles and personal boundaries and make an appropriate referral when necessary. The therapist should have signed permission from the client (in accordance with Health Insurance Portability and Accountability Act of 1996 [HIPAA] standards) to contact members of the extended team if there is a crisis or suicide threat.

Useful Tools

Tools streamline the therapist's practice and help maintain consistency in treatment. Clinical tools, such as a comprehensive patient/client entry questionnaire, can save time and provide crucial, possibly elusive, pertinent hints as to the individual's needs, thinking, and status. Have a prepared referral list with contact information for carefully screened interdisciplinary professionals. A list to consider can help smooth the client's transition in thinking about taking advantage of adjunct services.

SPECIFIC PSYCHOLOGIC CONDITIONS

Physical therapists are likely to encounter individuals with mental health disorders in two distinct practice settings: (1) mental health units in an inpatient setting and (2) any other setting a physical therapist may practice. Although physical therapists do not generally provide intervention directly for a mental health disorder, it is likely that the therapist will encounter clients who have a psychiatric comorbidity sometime in their practice. This section is a brief review of the most common mental health disorders but is not complete in the information offered. The information in this section is designed to help the therapist recognize the need for referral and to better understand clients who have mental health disorders that can bring many unique challenges to the rehabilitation process. Additional resource materials are suggested and available on the Evolve site in Evolve Box 3-1.

The disorders in this chapter can be found in the American Psychiatric Association's taxonomy, the *Diagnostic and Statistical Manual of Mental Disorders, Fifth Edition* (DSM-5), which was published in 2013.[18] The DSM-5 replaces the *Diagnostic and Statistical Manual Disorders, Fourth Edition–Text Revisions (DSM-IV-TR),*[6] the primary handbook used in diagnosing mental disorders in the United States

The *International Statistical Classification of Diseases and Related Health Problems* (*ICD*) is used more frequently internationally to categorize mental health disorders. The most recent version (*ICD-10*) was revised at the same time the *DSM-IV* was being revised.[547] Both taxonomies utilize a medical paradigm and identify categorical disorders that can be diagnosed by set lists of criteria.

Mental health disorders are widespread in the U.S. adult population. The National Institute of Mental Health (NIMH) reports that the number of persons with a mental disorder that impacts activity and participation in a given year is 26.2%.[399] It is estimated that 1 in 17 persons experience a significant negative impact in their ability to participate fully in life roles because of a serious mental disorder. Men and women are equally likely to experience a mental health disorder; non-Hispanic blacks are 30% less likely than non-Hispanic whites to have a mental health disorder in their lifetime.[358] The Agency for Health Care Research states that more than $57.5 billion dollars was spent on mental health care in 2006 ($8.9 billion on children ages 0-18 years) in addition to $193 billion in lost income.[356,358]

The *International Classification for Functioning, Disability, and Health*[548] addresses mental health disorders through coding the impact on body function, body structure, activities and participation. In addition, the *International Classification for Functioning, Disability, and Health* emphasizes the impact of personal characteristics, such as motivation, attention, and drive as well as environmental factors on both activities and participation in life roles. Mental health disorders can widen the gap between a person's capacity to do an activity (i.e., his/her best performance in a controlled setting) and their performance (i.e., what the person actually does in the person's own environment).

Physical therapists must understand the impact psychopathology has on a client, on interaction with the client and on implementing a plan of care in order to most effectively maximize the individual's performance of activities and minimize participation restrictions.[467] It is important to remember that professional, clinical care can either exacerbate psychopathology or enhance healing. In addition to the benefits of sensitive, insightful therapeutic care, referral to counseling or medical services intervention may be required.

The number of diagnostic categories included in the *DSM* has increased dramatically from just over 100 in the first edition[15] to more than 200 in the proposed DSM-5. The proposed DSM-5 has been reorganized, abandoning the five-axes approach, instead proposing organizing mental disorders into chapters (Box 3-3). A second major paradigm change is the consideration of the dimensionality of mental health disorders. Previous versions of the *DSM* have taken a dichotomous approach to diagnosis, that is, "yes" or "no." The DSM-5 is attempting to recognize degrees of severity and other dimensions of the disorder. One example is the inclusion of Asperger syndrome within the *Autism Spectrum Disorder* classification rather than as a separate diagnosis. Many of these changes have sparked considerable political, social, and professional debate.

Therapists may choose to have a physical copy of the DSM-5 available in the clinic. Alternatively, there are numerous reliable and user-friendly online resources, for example, through the American Psychiatric Association,[19,20] the NIMH,[352] and the Mayo Clinic,[301] among others. The DSM-5 can be a useful tool for physical therapists during all phases of patient/client management, particularly examination, evaluation, and the development/implementation of a plan of care.

Physical therapists should be alert to symptoms (physical, behavioral, cognitive and/or language) that may by symptomatic of a mental health disorder (Table 3-4) and be prepared to make a referral to a mental health professional as indicated. Physical therapists may need to modify client interactions and the provision of interventions to maximize effectiveness and improve the client's quality of life (QOL) in the presence of mental illness. While all DSM-5 diagnostic categories are important, physical and occupational therapists are most concerned with how the mental health condition impacts the individual's ability to perform activities and participate in life roles, and to develop a plan of care that helps to manage or adapt to the individual's particular mental health disorder(s). Conditions most likely encountered in the provision of physical therapy services are included in this chapter.

Neurodevelopmental Disorders

Intellectual Developmental Disorders

Overview and Incidence. This diagnostic category represents a name change from "mental retardation" used in previous *DSM* editions. "Mental retardation" is no longer an accepted term internationally and in many contexts nationally. An intellectual developmental disorder (IDD) is diagnosed when three criteria are met: (1) impairment in general mental abilities, (2) impairment in adaptive functioning that leads to significant activity limitations and participation restrictions in life roles (e.g., communication, activities of daily living, social skills), and (3) occurs prior to age 18 years of age. IQ is often used as a measure of impairment: profound (less than 20), severe (20-34), moderate (35-49), mild (50-69), and borderline (70-84).[16,547] Controversy exists in the use of IQ scores as there are cross-cultural effects on IQ scores[454]; however, it is clear that individuals with this diagnosis function significantly below their age level. The prevalence of IDD is 1% to 3%; the majority is classified as mild.

Etiology and Pathogenesis. The etiology of IDD is known in 50% to 70% of individuals. Genetic causes include Down syndrome (trisomy 21), fragile X syndrome,[276] Williams syndrome, and phenylketonuria. Primary in utero causes include fetal alcohol syndrome, maternal malnutrition, microcephaly, and an infection such as rubella. Environmental factors after birth include lead exposure, inadequate nutrition, low birth weight, meningitis, insufficient stimulation, and educational deprivation.[114]

Clinical Manifestations. Severity of IDD based on IQ testing is correlated with the individual's function.

Box 3-3

COMMON MENTAL DISORDERS

Neurodevelopmental Disorders

- Intellectual Developmental Disorders
- Communication Disorders
- Autism Spectrum Disorder (poor social interaction/communication skills with repetitive, stereotypic behaviors)
- Attention Deficit/Hyperactivity Disorder (distractible, impulsive, lack of focus)
- Motor Disorders
  - Developmental Coordination Disorder (significantly delayed gross/fine motor development not secondary to a medical condition)
  - Stereotypic Movement Disorder (repetitive, non-purposeful movement)
  - Tourette Disorder (multiple motor tics and at least 1 vocal tic)

Schizophrenia Spectrum and Other Psychotic Disorders (least to most severe)

- Schizotypal Personality Disorder (odd, eccentric, lack empathy, intimacy, withdrawn)

- Delusional Disorder (include Erotomania, Grandiose, Jealous, Persecutory)
- Brief Psychotic Disorder (may include delusions, hallucinations, disorganized speech and behavior, 1 month or less duration)
- Schizophreniform Disorder (similar to schizophrenia; less severe impact on participation)
- Schizoaffective Disorder (combination of schizophrenia and major mood disorder)
- Schizophrenia (delusions, hallucinations, disorganized speech, bizarre movement patterns)

Bipolar and Related Disorders

- Bipolar I Disorder (at least 1 Manic episode)
- Bipolar II Disorder (at least one Major Depressive episode and Hypomanic episode)
- Cyclothymic Disorder (numerous brief episodes of hypomania and minor depression)

Depressive Disorders

- Disruptive Mood Dysregulation Disorder
- Major Depressive Disorder, Single Episode

Continued

Box 3-3

COMMON MENTAL DISORDERS—cont'd

- Major Depressive Disorder, Recurrent
- Dysthymic Disorder
- Premenstrual Dysphoric Disorder

Anxiety Disorders

- Separation Anxiety Disorder
- Panic Disorder
- Agoraphobia (anxiety experienced in open spaces, transportation, outside of home, etc.)
- Specific Phobia (anxiety specific to a stimulus, e.g., heights, spiders, physicians)
- Social Anxiety Disorder (anxiety in situations in which person fears being judged)
- Generalized Anxiety Disorder (anxiety related to preoccupying worries)

Obsessive-Compulsive and Related Disorders

- Obsessive-Compulsive Disorder
- Body Dysmorphic Disorder (excessive focus on perceived flaws in physical appearance)

Trauma and Stressor Related Disorders

- Reactive Attachment Disorder of Infancy/Early Childhood (lack of attachment behavior)
- Disinhibited Social Engagement Disorder (lack of fear approaching unknown adults)
- Acute Stress Disorder
- Posttraumatic Stress Disorder (PTSD)
- Adjustment Disorders (behavioral or emotional response deemed excessive to stressor)

Dissociative Disorders

- Depersonalization Disorder
- Dissociative Amnesia
- Dissociative Identity Disorder

Somatic Symptom Disorders

- Somatic Symptom Disorder
- Illness Anxiety Disorder
- Conversion Disorder (Functional Neurological Symptom Disorder)
- Factitious Disorder

Eating Disorders

- Pica
- Avoidant/Restrictive Food Intake Disorder
- Anorexia Nervosa
- Bulimia Nervosa
- Binge Eating Disorder

Elimination Disorders
Sleep-Wake Disorders
Sexual Dysfunctions

- Gender Dysphoria (strong conflict between assigned and desired gender identity)

Disruptive, Impulse Control, and Conduct Disorders

- Oppositional Defiant Disorder
- Intermittent Explosive Disorder
- Conduct Disorder
- Antisocial Personality Disorder (APD) (impulsive, aggressive, manipulative)

Substance Use and Addictive Disorders

- Substance-Induced Mental Disorder
- Alcohol Related Disorders
- Caffeine-Related Disorders
- Cannabis Related Disorders (marijuana, grass, pot, weed, reefer, hashish, bhang, ganja)
- Hallucinogen Related Disorders (psychedelics, LSD, mescaline, peyote, psilocybin, DMT)
- Inhalant Dependence (sniffing: glue, gasoline, toluene, solvents)
- Opioid Related Disorders (heroin, methadone, morphine, Demerol, Percodan, opium, codeine, Darvon)
- Sedative Related Disorders (sleeping pills, barbiturates, seconal, valium, Librium, Ativan, Xanax, Quaaludes)
- Stimulant Related Disorders (amphetamines, speed, uppers, diet pills)
- Tobacco-Related Disorders
- Gambling Disorder

Neurocognitive Disorders

- Delirium
- Mild Neurocognitive Disorder
- Major Neurocognitive Disorder
- Subtypes, e.g., Alzheimer Disease, Vascular Neurocognitive Disorder, Lewy Body Dementia, Huntington Chorea

Personality Disorders

- BPD (impulsive, self-destructive, unstable)
- OCPD (perfectionist, rigid, controlling)
- Avoidant Personality Disorder (shy, timid, "inferiority complex")
- Schizotypal Personality Disorder
- APD (Antisocial Personality Disorder)
- NPD (boastful, egotistical, "superiority complex")

Other Disorders

- Non-Suicidal Self Injury
- Suicidal Behavior Disorder

Data from *Diagnostic and Statistical Manual of Mental Disorders-5* (DSM-5), American Psychiatric Association, 2013 (www.dsm5.org).

Table 3-4   Signs of Potential Mental Health Disorders

Physical	Behavioral	Cognitive/Thinking	Language
• Psychomotor agitation or retardation • Increased or decreased activity levels • Difficulty falling asleep or staying asleep	• Agitation • Cutting or other self-injury • Impulsive • Outbursts • Withdrawal	• Lack of focus • Difficulty concentrating • Hallucinations • Delusions • Suicidal ideation	• Rapid or slow speech • Unusual phrasing • Tangential speech • Flight of thought

Environmental barriers and supports and personal characteristics are able to influence the performance of activities of a person with IDD, as well as that person's ability to participate in social/occupational roles. Consequently, functional performance can exceed predicted expectations when positive supports are available. Individuals in the most-severe categories will present with pervasive functional deficits, including limited or no capacity to speak, have independent mobility or limited activities of daily living.

MEDICAL MANAGEMENT

DIAGNOSIS. IDD is diagnosed using both standardized developmental psychologic testing as well as clinical assessment of the child's capacity and performance of skills in multiple domains including conceptual, social and practical. The criteria in the DSM-5 are used to diagnosis IDD.[20]

TREATMENT AND PROGNOSIS. Life expectancy has increased for many individuals and long-term community living environments have been developed to meet the need.[363] There is no treatment specifically for IDD. However, improvement may occur if the underlying cause is treated and potentially reversed. For example, early detection and treatment of meningitis will minimize the severity of IDD or prevent it entirely. Psychotropic medications are used to treat comorbid conditions such as depression or aggression. Ensuring environmental facilitators, such as maintaining good health, providing a stimulating and interactive environment, and providing training and behavioral interventions will help maximize performance of activities and participation within the limits of the severity of the disorder. Andriolo et al[32] and others found evidence that aerobic exercise improves health, both physical and mental, in persons with developmental delay, including IDD.

Autism Spectrum Disorder

Overview and Incidence. Autism spectrum disorder (ASD) is a new diagnostic category in the DSM-5[22] that combines four disorders from the DSM-IV-TR (autism, Asperger, childhood disintegrative disorder, and pervasive developmental order not otherwise specified).[16] The formation of ASD as a new category is an example of the DSM-5 approach to dimensional qualities of previously isolated disorders, reflecting the broad range of impairments, activity limitations, and participation restrictions that individuals with ASD can have. This dimensional approach to ASD has met resistance. ASD is diagnosed in childhood; however, an increasing number of adults are diagnosed with ASD.

Children diagnosed with ASD have impairments in two primary domains: (1) social communication and interaction and (2) restricted, repetitive patterns of behavior, interests, or activities.[22] Social communication and interaction is characterized by activity limitations in three specific contexts as defined by the DSM-5:

- Social-emotional reciprocity.
- Use of nonverbal communication in social interactions.
- Developing and maintaining relationships.

Repetitive patterns of behaviors can be manifested by activities such as stereotypic movements or nonpurposeful patterns of speech, fixations, perseverations, ritualistic patterns of behavior, and abnormal sensory processing. Children functioning at the most severe end of the spectrum experience significant activity limitations and have little or no ability to participate in social/occupational roles. Children who have mild ASD (Asperger, high-functioning autism in the DSM-IV-TR)[17,378] may be perceived as socially awkward but experience few activity limitations or participation restrictions (e.g., higher IQ, absence of language impairments).

The prevalence of ASD has increased from 6.6 to 11.3 per 1000 children between 2002 and 2008.[39] The Centers for Disease Control and Prevention (CDC) estimates the prevalence of ASD in 2012 was 1 in 88 eight-year-old children, a 78% increase from the CDC's first report in 2007. The increase can be partially explained by better methods for identification and diagnosis as well as an increased public awareness of ASD, perhaps counting for as much as 25% of the increase.[247] The CDC is actively looking for causative and correlated factors to account for the unexplained increase.

Etiology and Pathogenesis. The cause of ASD is unclear but it is likely that it is caused by a variety of factors, including biologic/genetic and environmental factors. Two factors, inadequate parenting (particularly "mothering")[532] and the measles-mumps-rubella vaccine,[133] have largely been discounted as causative. There is a definitive, although small, familial link (identical twins have ASD 90% of the time); siblings have a 35-times increased risk of having ASD,[33] which suggests a genetic link.[107] However, the majority of people with ASD do not have a familial link. Specific genetic markers have not yet been identified and it is likely that multiple genes are involved. Changes in brain structure (cerebellum, limbic system, and the cortex), changes in neurotransmitters, and decreased lateralization of the brain have been identified as related to spatial attention deficits in some children with ASD.[499] A number of recent studies link increasing paternal age with random genetic mutations and an increased risk of having a child with autism.[83] Researchers are also searching for environmental factors that cause or predispose a child for ASD.

Clinical Manifestations. Children with severe ASD often lack speech or have nonpurposeful speech patterns or demonstrate echolalia (the automatic repetition of vocalizations made by another person), do not initiate social interaction (may seem oblivious, showing no interest in interaction), fail to respond to their name, avoid eye contact, may be tactilely defensive or indifferent to sensory stimulation, may perform repetitive self-stimulatory behaviors (hand clapping, hair twirling, jumping, spinning), and may be fixated on routines and rituals—becoming very disturbed at even the slightest change. Individuals with mild ASD may demonstrate awkwardness in social interactions, missing nonverbal cues, flat facial expressions, and diminished capability to be empathetic or see another point of view, and may move with less coordination than their peers.[18,301,378]

MEDICAL MANAGEMENT

DIAGNOSIS. The diagnosis of the more-severe forms of ASD is often made by the age of 3 years. Diagnosis of ASD is difficult because of the variation in symptoms. The examination often utilizes a team approach and assesses developmental milestones, social behavior, and interactions. During the diagnostic process the criteria established by the American Psychiatric Association related to impairments of social communication and interaction as well as criteria regarding restricted, repetitive behaviors published in the DSM-5 must be met.[18,352] The symptoms are apparent in early childhood and they impact participation in social/occupational roles including play and interaction. TREATMENT. Interventions are not well grounded in evidence because the disorder is not yet well understood and because of the wide range of symptoms and severity. The plan of care is best if it is multidisciplinary as the impairments are pervasive. Intervention focused on behavior and communication is common with the intent to improve social communication and interaction and to decrease nonpurposeful movements, vocalizations, and rituals. Education and training programs can be successful, but there are no psychotropic medications that are effective. Drugs may be prescribed for concurrent behavioral problems or anxiety. Sensory integration therapy may be used to enhance sensory processing.[88]

Interventions for children on the high end of the spectrum are similar for those with severe symptoms: training to improve social communication and interactions, modify and interpret nonverbal behaviors, and cognitive behavior therapy to manage behaviors that interfere with relationships. Psychotropic drugs may be prescribed for concurrent problems, including hyperactivity (e.g., guanfacine [Intuniv]), depression (selective serotonin reuptake inhibitors [SSRIs]), agitation (risperidone [Risperdal]), or repetitive behaviors (e.g., olanzapine [Zyprexa]). PROGNOSIS. Prognosis for persons with severe symptoms of ASD is poor, with significant impact activity limitations which markedly or completely preclude participation in social/occupational roles. The prognosis is proportionately better as the symptoms become less severe, having little, if any, impact on activities and participation in social/occupational roles.

Schizophrenia Spectrum and Other Psychotic Disorders

Overview and Incidence

These severely disabling psychotic disorders are listed in Box 3-3 in order of increasing severity. Considered the least severe, a person with *Schizotypal personality disorder* has difficulty with interpersonal relationships (e.g., lack of empathy). In addition, that person exhibits odd personality characteristics that interfere with relationships (e.g., odd beliefs, behaviors, thought processes, aversion to social contacts). *Schizophrenia*, the most severe form, is characterized by impairments that severely impact the ability to perform activities, participate in social/occupational roles and QOL. Performance is markedly below the person's capacity to function prior to onset. Individuals with schizophrenia usually experience at least two of the following: hallucinations (visual or auditory are most common), disorganized speech, delusions, extreme motor behaviors, or flat affect.[17,20] Schizophrenia is often characterized by periodic exacerbations of symptoms, referred to as an active phase. This is preceded by a prodromal phase in which behavior declines and the person begins to withdraw from reality. The active phase is followed by a residual phase, with behaviors not unlike the prodromal phase.[346] In a 12-month period, the prevalence of schizophrenia

in adults is 1.1% in the United States.[359] The age of onset often is in the late teens or early 20s; women are generally diagnosed less frequently and at an older age then men.[481]

Etiology and Pathogenesis

Although the cause of schizophrenia is unknown, a variety of possible contributing factors include biologic, psychologic, and socioeconomic. There is evidence of a genetic predisposition for schizophrenia. First-degree relatives have a 10-times higher risk; a child who has two parents diagnosed with schizophrenia has a 40% risk of developing the disease.[241] However, it is thought that psychosocial stressors may be required in addition to the genetic predisposition to trigger active symptoms, as well as exacerbate symptoms. Current investigations are seeking a model that can explain the complex patterns of disease transmission within families and explain the expression and function of risk genes during brain development.[105,214,215] Research implicates the neurotransmitter dopamine, particularly in the prefrontal cortex, as a contributing factor.[337] Imaging studies have identified changes in brain structure including changes in connectivity and decreased gray matter volume in the superior and middle temporal gyri and anterior cingulated among other areas.[502]

Clinical Manifestations

Schizophrenia is sometimes characterized by periods when the symptoms are less severe, but people with schizophrenia rarely recover completely. Symptoms include apathy, emotional unresponsiveness, social withdrawal, limited or odd patterns of speech, and confused thinking with periodic outbreaks of psychotic symptoms such as hallucinations and delusions. Hallucinations are most commonly auditory or visual and delusions may vary in type. Symptoms will be persistent in approximately 50% of individuals.

MEDICAL MANAGEMENT

DIAGNOSIS. Specific criteria established by the DSM-IV-TR[16] must be met including at least two of the following: delusions, hallucinations, disorganized speech, grossly disorganized behavior, negative symptoms. The DSM-5[18] requires that one of the symptoms be one of the first three in the list. TREATMENT. A multimodal approach is used in the treatment of an individual with schizophrenia. Psychotropic drugs are the primary intervention. Traditional drugs (e.g., chlorpromazine, Haldol) seem to be more effective than newer drugs, but tardive dyskinesia is a serious side effect of these drugs. Psychosocial, behavioral, and training interventions are also used. PROGNOSIS. The long-term outcome is much more variable than commonly believed, with 33% to 50% of individuals having good outcomes.[139,228,405] Environmental barriers and facilitators, as well as personal factors, including family support, age, gender, education, and financial status impact long-term outcomes. In addition, there are multiple subtypes of schizophrenia. After a first schizophrenic episode, only 14% to 20% of individuals will recover completely. A study in Europe indicated that QOL was poor in persons with chronic symptoms: 79% were chronically unemployed, 65% were unmarried, and many had unmet needs.[492] Differences in QOL are different for men and women, with

SIDE EFFECTS OF ANTIPSYCHOTIC MEDICATIONS

Dopaminergic Side Effects

- Pseudoparkinsonism
  - Cogwheel rigidity
  - Shuffling gait
  - Parkinsonian tremor
  - Masked facies
- Acute dystonias, such as opisthotonus, torticollis, and laryngospasm, which may cause acute airway obstruction
- Increased prolactin secretion that may lead to galactorrhea
- Akathisia—subjective or observable restlessness ("Thorazine shuffle")
- Tardive dyskinesia, tardive dystonia
- Neuroleptic malignant syndrome (NMS)

Anticholinergic Side Effects

- Dry mouth
- Blurred vision
- Constipation that may lead to adynamic ileus
- Urinary hesitancy or obstruction
- Memory and concentration difficulties, up to frank delirium

α-Adrenergic Blockade

- Hypotension; orthostatic hypotension

Antihistaminergic Side Effects

- Sedation, drowsiness
- Weight gain

Others

- Agranulocytosis
- Electrocardiogram (ECG) changes (prolonged QT interval)
- Elevated liver function tests
- Elevated creatine phosphokinase
- Fetal toxicity
- Photosensitivity
- Pigmentary retinopathy
- Seizures (decreased seizure threshold)
- Sexual dysfunction (erectile problems, impotency, delayed, absent, or retrograde ejaculation, priapism)
- Skin rashes

Data from Jacobson JL: *Psychiatric secrets*, ed 2, St. Louis, Hanley and Belfus, 2001.

men experiencing more unmet needs.[493] The prevalence of cardiovascular disease in persons with schizophrenia is above average.[444] Antipsychotic medications have significant side-effects that can result in serious activity limitations and participations in addition to the condition (Box 3-4).

Bipolar and Related Disorders

Overview and Incidence

Bipolar I, Bipolar II and *Cyclothymic Disorders* are characterized by cyclical mood swings between depressed episodes and manic or hypomanic episodes (previously referred to as manic-depressive illness). A *Manic Episode* manifests as a rapid elevation of mood, which severely disrupts the ability to perform activities and restricts participation in social/occupational roles. A *Hypomanic Episode* is a less-severe elevation in mood with less disruption in

CLINICAL MANIFESTATIONS OF MANIC EPISODE

Mood Changes

- Excessive high or euphoric feelings
- Irritable, agitated, uncomfortable

Behavior Changes

- Increased energy, activity, restlessness, racing thoughts, and rapid talking
- Decreased need for sleep
- Unrealistic beliefs in one's abilities and powers
- Distractibility and restlessness
- Uncharacteristically poor judgment
- Impulsivity
- Increased high risk or pleasurable activities: sex, shopping, drug abuse
- Denial that anything is wrong

From National Institute of Mental Health (NIMH): What are the symptoms of bipolar disorder?, 2013. Available at http://www.nimh.nih.gov/health/publications/bipolar-disorder/what-are-the-symptoms-of-bipolar-disorder.shtml.

function. *Depressed Episodes* also vary in severity and can include a major depressive disorder (MDD). Bipolar I is the most severe form, with mood shifting between manic and MDD. Bipolar II is less disruptive with mood swings between hypomania and MDD. Cyclothymic disorder is the least-severe form with mood swings that are not extreme. Epidemiologic studies indicate that it is more prevalent than previously thought.[204] Prevalence of the bipolar disorders is estimated at 1.0% (bipolar I), 1.1% (bipolar II), and 2.4% (cyclothymic), or 3.5% of the adult population.[75,322] Onset of bipolar disorders is usually in the 20s.

Etiology and Pathogenesis

Genetic-based pathogenesis is suspected for bipolar disorder based on a clear familial pattern and chromosomal linkage studies. Evidence exists that the key gene involved in the transmission of bipolar disease is X-linked. Linkage studies implicate chromosome 18 or 21, but this has not yet been proved.[151,168] Late-onset of a bipolar disorder is often associated with another medical condition, for example, hyperthyroidism.[344] Mania is linked to excessive levels of norepinephrine and dopamine.

Clinical Manifestations

Clinical manifestations of Bipolar and Related Disorders are listed in Boxes 3-5 and 3-6. Mania is characterized by abnormal and persistent euphoria and/or irritability, grandiose thoughts, decreased need for sleep, increased energy and activity, racing thoughts, rapid speech, and increased risk taking. Mania severely limits activities and participation in social/occupational roles.[361] Bipolar I is characterized by mood swings between manic and depressive episodes. Bipolar II is characterized by distinct periods of depression and hypomania, and periods of depression tend to last longer than the hypomania.

The bipolar disorders are characterized by cyclical mood swings that may last from days to months,

Box 3-6

CLINICAL MANIFESTATIONS OF MAJOR DEPRESSIVE EPISODE

Mood Changes

- Depressed mood (sad, empty, lack of hope, pessimism)
- Loss of interest or pleasure in almost all ordinary activities, including sex (anhedonia)

Behavior Changes

- Decreased energy, feeling fatigued, or being slowed down
- Feelings of guilt, worthlessness, or helplessness
- Difficulty concentrating, remembering, making decisions, initiating activities
- Irritability
- Sleep disturbances (insomnia or hypersomnia)
- Change in appetite and weight (unintentional loss or gain)
- Change in activity level (lethargic or restlessness)
- Chronic pain or other persistent bodily symptoms that are not caused by physical disease
- Thoughts of death or suicide; suicide attempts

From National Institute of Mental Health (NIMH): What are the symptoms of bipolar disorder?, 2013. Available at http://www.nimh.nih.gov-/health/publications/bipolar-disorder/what-are-the-symptoms-of-bipolar-disorder.shtml.

switching back and forth quickly or with normal periods in between. Heightened creativity and creative talent are sometimes associated with all phases of bipolar disorder.

MEDICAL MANAGEMENT

DIAGNOSIS. A physical exam is often performed to rule out predisposing medical conditions. The criteria in the DSM-5 are used to diagnosis the various Bipolar and Related Disorders. Bipolar I requires at least one manic episode with a severe impact on function. Bipolar II requires a MDD, one or more episodes of hypomania, and no history of a manic episode. Cyclothymic disorder requires symptoms of at least 2 years' duration, with symptoms less severe than those of a hypomanic episode and no history of a MDD or manic or hypomanic episode.

TREATMENT. A multimodal approach is often used to manage bipolar disorders. Mood-stabilizing drugs (lithium, Depakote,) are often the first drug of choice. Antipsychotics (e.g., risperidone [Risperdal], olanzapine [Zyprexa], aripiprazole [Abilify]); and antidepressants (Prozac, Paxil, Lexapro, Zoloft) are often used in conjunction with a mood stabilizer.[361] Some people prefer to experience the extremes of this disorder so as to avoid losing the creative edge that can occur when the medication balances mood swings. Group, family, and individual psychotherapy, educational approaches and behavior modification are common interventions. Some programs advocate a predetermined plan of action to put in place if and when warning signs of mania develop.

PROGNOSIS. Bipolar and Related Disorders are chronic with recurring episodes, often separated by symptom free periods of time. Insight can be impaired with 55% of individuals diagnosed with bipolar denying any psychiatric problems.[388] Bipolar disorder is frequently accompanied by alcoholism and/or other drug abuse. It is not clear if alcohol is a trigger for bipolar episodes or if the individual is using alcohol to self-medicate. Comorbidity of alcohol abuse with bipolar disorder often delays early diagnosis, especially when alcohol abuse has been the primary focus of intervention. Other comorbidities may also exist (e.g., migraine headaches, asthma, anxiety and panic attacks, allergies, eating disorders).[82,134]

SPECIAL IMPLICATIONS FOR THE THERAPIST 3-5

Schizophrenia Spectrum and Other Psychotic Disorders; Bipolar and Related Disorders

The role of the physical therapist in providing multidisciplinary care for people with schizophrenia spectrum and other psychotic disorders is not clearly differentiated, but efforts have been made to identify the value added by physical therapy.[511] The role of exercise (aerobic and strength training), yoga, and breathing techniques and progressive muscle relaxation in providing reduced psychiatric symptoms and distress, and improving short-term memory and health-related QOL has been identified but not fully quantified.[511] No adverse effects of this approach have been found. More study is needed to investigate the efficacy of physical therapy for people with these disorders and possibly create specific targeted or tailored interventions for this patient population.

Adverse Effects of Medications

Antipsychotic medications are used in a number of conditions to treat psychotic symptoms, including hallucinations, delusions, paranoia, combativeness, agitation and hostility, insomnia, catatonia, hyperactivity, bizarre psychomotor behaviors, and poor grooming and self-care.[223] Antipsychotics are often used in long-term care settings to help normalize disturbances of thought. They do not cure psychosis associated with acute mania and schizophrenia but help manage signs and symptoms. Some are able to control fluency of ideas and language and alleviate the diminished ability to concentrate, express emotions, pursue goal-directed activity, and experience pleasure.[65]

The therapist must be aware of anyone taking these medications because of the potential adverse side effects (see Box 3-4). Increased levels of serotonin may have an effect on the regulation and release of antidiuretic hormone requiring close monitoring for dehydration; watch for headache, confusion (or increased confusion), loss of appetite, and muscle cramps.

There may be extrapyramidal effects or movement disorders commonly observed with their use. Dystonias, sustained abnormal postures, and disruption of movement caused by muscle tone alterations can develop within 5 days of administration. Other common extrapyramidal effects may include restlessness, anxiety, or pacing (akathisia) and Parkinson-like symptoms. Long-term use of antipsychotics can result in permanent involuntary choreoathetoid muscle movements of the face, jaw, tongue, and extremities.

Depressive Disorders

Overview and Incidence

Depressive disorders were categorized in the DSM-IV-TR under mood disorders. The DSM-5 chapter currently has seven diagnostic disorders, but several are under review. Therapists are most likely to encounter individuals with MDDs (possibly with a seasonal pattern) and Depressive Disorder Associated with Another Medical Condition.

Major Depressive Disorder, Single Episode, and Major Depressive Disorder, Recurrent. MDD occurs when an individual experiences one or more Major Depressive Episodes a severely depressed mood characterized by symptoms such as those listed in Box 3-6. MDD interferes with the individual's ability to perform activities and may prevent participation in social/occupational roles. Depression is the most commonly seen mood disorder within a therapy practice. According to a National Health Interview of adults ages 18 years and older, during 2010–2011, women were more likely than men to often feel depressed (10.7% compared with 7.7%) overall and among those ages 18 to 44, 45 to 64, and 65 to 74 years. For both men (9.9%) and women (13.0%), the prevalence of depression was highest among those ages 45 to 64 years.[349,403] Data are from a subset of the adults randomly selected for the Sample Adult Component of the National Health Interview Survey questionnaire. Prenatal and postpartum depression occurs in approximately 20% of all pregnancies. As the DSM-5 is being developed, debate continues whether depression experienced after bereavement can be diagnosed as MDD, with the prevailing opinion that it should not be excluded.

Major Depressive Disorder with Seasonal Pattern. *MDD with Seasonal Pattern* is a variation of MDD commonly referred to as *Seasonal Affective Disorder (SAD)*. SAD has a consistent pattern of depressive symptoms that occur with the advent of colder weather and fewer hours of daylight and dissipate as daylight hours increase in the spring. SAD is most prevalent in geographic areas north of 40-degrees latitude. Interestingly, Native Alaskans are less likely to have SAD than people who move there from some other geographical location. Women are affected by SAD three times more often than men.

Etiology and Pathogenesis

Predisposing factors for the development of depression may be genetic, familial, biologic, psychosocial, and medical or surgical conditions. MDD is considered a risk factor for cardiac morbidity and mortality. Vascular depression accounts for 30% to 40% of all depression in people older than age 65 years. Treating depression to reduce cardiac disease is under investigation.[86] Depression may occur as a result of medications (Box 3-7), especially sedatives, hypnotics, cardiac drugs, antihypertensives, and steroids; as well as alcohol or drug abuse, especially cocaine dependence; or exposure to heavy metals or toxins (e.g., gasoline, paint, organophosphate insecticides, nerve gas, carbon monoxide, carbon dioxide).[30]

There appears to be a genetic predisposition for depression. Psychosocial stressors may be required in addition to the genetic predisposition to trigger active symptoms, as well as exacerbate symptoms. Psychosocial factors include psychologic trauma (e.g., childhood

sexual abuse), significant life events (e.g., death of a loved one, divorce, childbirth),[55] or chronic stress. Psychosocial stressors may play a more significant role in the precipitation of the first or second episodes of MDD, but less of a role in subsequent episodes.

Psychoneuroimmunology studies study possible links among neural activity, the endocrine system, and altered immune responses in people with depressive disorders. Although the literature indicates some type of relationship exists between these systems, the exact mechanisms remain unknown.[220,239] Neuroendocrine abnormalities, such as in the limbic hypothalamic-pituitary-adrenal axis, are implicated in the cause of depression. This abnormality is common in survivors of repeated abuse and the sequelae related to chronic sympathetic system stimulation.

Box 3-7

DRUGS COMMONLY ASSOCIATED WITH DEPRESSION

Psychoactive Agents

- Amphetamines
- Cocaine
- Benzodiazepines
- Barbiturates
- Neuroleptics

Antihypertensive Drugs

- β-Blockers, especially propranolol (Inderal)
- α_2-Adrenergic antagonists
- Methyldopa (Aldomet)
- Hydralazine (Apresoline)

Analgesics

- Salicylates
- Propoxyphene (Darvon, Darvocet-N)
- Pentazocine (Talwin)
- Morphine
- Meperidine (Demerol)

Cardiovascular Drugs

- Digoxin (Lanoxin)
- Procainamide (Pronestyl)
- Disopyramide (Norpace)

Anticonvulsants

- Phenytoin (Dilantin)
- Phenobarbital

Hormonal Agents

- Corticosteroids
- Oral contraceptives
- Anabolic steroids

Miscellaneous

- Alcohol, illicit drugs
- Histamine H_2 receptor antagonists, especially cimetidine (Tagamet)
- Metoclopramide (Reglan)
- Levodopa
- Nonsteroidal antiinflammatory drugs
- Antineoplastic agents
- Disulfiram (Antabuse)
- Cytokines (interferons)

Box 3-8

MEDICAL AND SURGICAL CONDITIONS COMMONLY ASSOCIATED WITH DEPRESSION

Cardiovascular

- Atherosclerosis
- Hypertension
- Myocardial infarction
- Angioplasty or bypass surgery

Central Nervous System

- Parkinson disease
- Huntington disease
- Cerebral arteriosclerosis
- Cerebrovascular accident/stroke
- Alzheimer disease
- Temporal lobe epilepsy
- Postconcussion injury
- Multiple sclerosis
- Miscellaneous focal lesions

Endocrine, Metabolic

- Hyperthyroidism
- Hypothyroidism
- Addison disease
- Cushing disease
- Hypoglycemia
- Hyperglycemia
- Hyperparathyroidism
- Hyponatremia
- Diabetes mellitus
- Pregnancy (postpartum)

Viral

- Acquired immunodeficiency syndrome
- Hepatitis
- Pneumonia
- Influenza

Nutritional

- Folic acid deficiency
- Vitamin B_6 deficiency
- Vitamin B_{12} deficiency
- Anemia

Immune

- Fibromyalgia
- Chronic fatigue syndrome
- Systemic lupus erythematosus
- Sjögren syndrome
- Rheumatoid arthritis
- Immunosuppression

Cancer

- Pancreatic
- Bronchogenic
- Renal
- Ovarian

Miscellaneous

- Pancreatitis
- Sarcoidosis
- Syphilis
- Porphyria

Box 3-9

SOMATIC SYMPTOMS ASSOCIATED WITH MAJOR DEPRESSIVE DISORDERS*

- Fatigue
- Sleep disturbance
- Weakness
- Headaches
- Back pain
- Joint pain (arthralgia)
- Muscle pain (myalgia)
- Chest pain
- Dizziness
- Palpitations
- Excess perspiration
- Rapid breathing
- Dry mouth or excessive salivation
- Dry skin
- Blurred vision
- Tinnitus
- Flushing
- Slurred speech
- Confusion
- Sexual dysfunction
- Amenorrhea, polymenorrhea
- Difficulty with urination
- Digestive problems, constipation

* Refers to nonmedicated persons.
Data from Tykeem A, Gandhi P: The importance of somatic symptoms in depression in primary care. *Prim Care Companion J Clin Psychiatry* 7(4):167–176, 2005.

The role of neurotransmitters, particularly norepinephrine, dopamine, and serotonin, has been studied, but the evidence is not clear. The theory is that these neurotransmitters are either produced in inadequate amounts or the receptor sites are not functioning properly. Brain abnormalities have been identified in persons with depression including abnormal electroencephalograms and MRIs.[264] MRI studies indicate that lesions of the striatopallidothalamocortical pathways and other areas are evident in older adults diagnosed with vascular depression, which is correlated with vascular disease.[6,46,415] It appears to be a biologic alteration rather than a chemical one with black holes (lacunes) observed in the basal ganglia representing cerebral ischemia or silent strokes.[260]

Major Depressive Disorder with Seasonal Pattern. With shorter days and less exposure to sunlight the body produces more melatonin, a hormone secreted by the pineal gland that is made almost exclusively at night to help us sleep and may help to synchronize other circadian rhythms.[531] It is possible that some people with SAD do not produce more melatonin but are hypersensitive to the hormone.

Depressive Disorder Associated with Another Medical Condition. This diagnostic category is biologically based and associated with other physical illnesses (Box 3-8). Chronic general medical conditions are a risk factor for more persistent depressive episodes. Structural changes in the brain associated with disease (e.g., multiple sclerosis) or brain trauma (e.g., left-sided cerebrovascular accident, traumatic brain injury [TBI]) can cause depressive reactions, either on a short-term or recurring basis.

Clinical Manifestations

MDD can occur as a single, isolated episode lasting weeks to months, or intermittently throughout a person's life. Severely depressed mood and loss of interest in usually pleasurable activities are the hallmarks of MDD (see Box 3-6). More than 95% of depressed people report having decreased energy, even for minor daily tasks; 90% report having problems with concentration and memory. The inability to accomplish new or challenging activities often restricts participation in social/occupational roles.[111]

People with MDD may present with somatic complaints, most commonly headache, gastrointestinal disturbances, or unexplained pain (Box 3-9). Depression is also associated with elevated heart rate and reduced heart rate variability, which are known risk factors for cardiac disease.[86,465] Family members who live with individuals with depressive illness report additional behavior symptoms previously unknown and unreported in the literature.[180a] Depression is strongly correlated with increased severity of chronic musculoskeletal pain, decreased health related QOL and participation restrictions in social/occupational roles.[43] Individuals who have both medical conditions and depression tend to have more severe physical and mental impairments, leading to greater activity limitations and participation restrictions as well as increased health care cost.[89]

Almost 80% of depressed people report problems with sleep, including early morning and frequent nocturnal awakenings Sleep abnormalities associated with depression[264] include decreased rapid eye movement (REM) latency (the time between falling asleep and the first REM period), longer first REM period, less continuous sleep, and early morning awakenings. Whether these sleep

CLINICAL MANIFESTATIONS OF MAJOR DEPRESSIVE DISORDER IN CHILDREN AND ADOLESCENTS*

- Reluctance to go to school
- Decreased performance in school
- Negative behaviors (e.g., acting out, aggression, sullenness)
- Withdrawal

*May be concurrent with symptoms in Box 3-6.
Data from National Institute of Mental Health: Bipolar disorder, 2013. Available at http://www.nimh.nih.gov/health/publications/ bipolar-disorder/what-are-the-symptoms-of-bipolar-disorder.shtml; and American Psychiatric Association–Diagnostic and Statistical Manual of Mental Disorders (DSM-5) 2013. http://www.psych.org/practice/ dsm/dsm5 and http://www.dsm5.org/Pages/Default.aspx

abnormalities represent causes or effects of depression remains unknown.

Other mental disorders often cooccur with MDD such as substance-related disorders, panic disorder, obsessive-compulsive disorder, generalized anxiety disorder, PTSD, anorexia nervosa, bulimia nervosa, and borderline personality disorder.

Depression in children and adolescents is of significant concern, both in the present and the lifelong impact of the disorder.[328] The lifetime prevalence of depressive disorders in 13- to 18-year-olds is 11.2%.[323] Children and adolescents with depression often present differently than adults (Box 3-10) and may have difficulty expressing their feelings.

Hallmarks of adolescent depression may include helplessness, anger, aggressiveness, withdrawal, avoiding friends and classmates, apathy, low self-esteem, and resistance to authority, in addition to signs and symptoms typically experienced by adults. These activity limitations may lead to decreased performance at school and risky behaviors, including sex and drugs.

Depressive orders are difficult to identify in older adults because they typically present as medically complex. Occasions for bereavement are more frequent with aging; depression may be misidentified as normal grieving. Depression in older adults may manifest itself in difficulty concentrating and marked forgetfulness, which may be mistaken as symptoms of dementia. Depression in older adults is often a cause of sleep disturbances. Older adults with depression are often reluctant to talk about how they feel.

MEDICAL MANAGEMENT

DIAGNOSIS. Although depressive disorders are one of the most common mental health disorders, accurate diagnosis is inconsistent. Mitchell[331] found that 15% of patients in primary care received a false-positive diagnosis of depression, while the diagnosis of depressive disorder was missed 10% of the time. One intent of the DSM-5[18] revisions is to increase the sensitivity and specificity in the diagnosis of MDD.

The criteria in the DSM-5 are used to diagnosis MDD. The diagnosis of MDD requires the individual to have five or more of the criteria of a major depressive episode (see Box 3-6) within a 2-week period, which significantly restricts participation in social/occupational roles. There can be no history of a manic or hypomanic episode.

The physician will use the history, laboratory findings, and physical examination to determine whether the MDD is independent of or is associated with a medical or surgical condition (e.g., as in Box 3-8) or the side effect of a drug or other substance.

TREATMENT. There are three primary interventions for the treatment of depressive disorders: (1) psychotropic medications, (2) psychologic/psychosocial interventions, and (3) electroconvulsive therapy (ECT). These may be used individually or in combination. In addition to traditional therapies, there are a number of complementary therapies that may provide symptom relief.

Psychotropic Medications. There are six primary categories of antidepressant medications.[303,354] Mechanisms of action vary between classes, as do the type, number, and severity of side effects (Table 3-5). Many of these drugs take 4–6 weeks to reach therapeutic levels. Trial and error is often involved in finding the right pharmacologic regimen for a specific individual. A serious concern with antidepressants is the potential increased risk of suicide, particularly in children, adolescents, and young adults; this may also be a concern in older adults.[113]

- *Selective serotonin reuptake inhibitors* (SSRIs) are newer medications, generally have fewer and less severe side-effects compared to older classes of drugs. Consequently, they are prescribed more frequently than other antidepressants. SSRIs inhibit the reabsorption of the neurotransmitter serotonin, making serotonin more available for postsynaptic receptors with a resultant elevation of mood (e.g., citalopram [Celexa], paroxetine [Paxil], fluoxetine [Prozac], sertraline [Zoloft], escitalopram [Lexapro]).
- *Serotonin and norepinephrine reuptake inhibitors* (SNRIs) work similar to the SSRIs except that they effectively increase the availability of both neurotransmitters simultaneously (e.g., duloxetine [Cymbalta], venlafaxine [Effexor], desvenlafaxine [Pristiq]).
- *Norepinephrine and dopamine reuptake inhibitors* effectively increase the availability of the two neurotransmitters without impacting the availability of serotonin. Norepinephrine and dopamine reuptake inhibitors are one of the few classes of antidepressants that do not have sexual side-effects.
- *Atypical.* Because these antidepressant drugs have various mechanisms of action, they do not fit into other classes.
- *Tricyclic antidepressants* (TCAs) is an older class of drugs but the outcomes on depression are generally as effective as the newer classes. However, the side effects are often much less tolerable. TCAs block absorption of serotonin and norepinephrine, but are less focused as they also have an effect on other neurotransmitters. TCAs sometimes work when the newer drugs are not effective (e.g., amitriptyline [Elavil], demexiptiline [Deparon]).
- *Monoamine oxidase inhibitors* (MAOIs). MAOIs are used reluctantly and as a last resort because of the seriousness of side effects (potentially lethal) especially from food or drug interactions. The mechanisms of action of MAOIs prevents removal of serotonin, dopamine and norepinephrine from the brain. However, MAOIs also act on other neurotransmitters in the brain and digestive system (e.g., phenelzine [Nardil], tranylcypromine [Parnate], selegiline [Emsam]).

Table 3-5 Side Effects of Antidepressants

Drug Class	Tricyclic Antidepressants (TCA)	Selective Serotonin Reuptake Inhibitors (SSRIs)	Monoamine Oxidase (MAO) Inhibitors
Examples:	• Amitriptyline (Elavil/Endep) • Amoxapine (Asendin) • Desipramine (Norpramin, Pertofrane) • Doxepin (Adapin, Sinequan) • Imipramine (Janimine, Tofranil)	• Citalopram (Celexa) • Fluoxetine (Prozac) • Fluvoxamine (Luvox) • Paroxetine (Paxil) • Sertraline (Zoloft)	• Phenelzine (Nardil) • Tranylcypromine (Parnate) • Selegiline (Deprenyl)
Function:	Increase norepinephrine and serotonin levels	Block reuptake of serotonin resulting in higher circulating levels of active serotonin	Inactivate MAO, the enzyme responsible for degradation of norepinephrine and serotonin

Effects:	• Anticholinergic effects
	  • Dry mouth
	  • Blurred vision
	  • Nausea, vomiting
	  • Abdominal bloating
	  • Constipation
	  • Confusion (older adults)
	• Heart arrhythmia
	• Tachycardia
	• Orthostatic hypotension
	  • Low blood pressure or sudden drop
	  • Dizziness
	  • Weakness
	• Sedation/drowsiness
	• Sleep disturbance/nightmares
	• Sexual dysfunction
	• Weight gain
	• Fine tremor (older adults)
	• Skin rash/photosensitivity
		• Nervousness/jitteriness
		• Gastrointestinal distress
		  • Appetite loss
		  • Nausea
		  • Diarrhea
		• Headache
		• Insomnia/sleep disturbance
		• Sexual dysfunction
			• Hypertensive crisis
			• Postural hypotension
			• Insomnia
			• Headache
			• Anemia
			• Hyperreflexia
			• Muscle weakness, tremors
			• Syndrome of inappropriate antidiuretic hormone (SIADH)-like syndrome
			• Sexual dysfunction
			• Gastrointestinal disturbance

Psychosocial Interventions. Psychosocial interventions for depressive disorders include various types of psychologic therapies. Cognitive-behavioral therapy (CBT) changes the focus of thought patterns, or "cognitive chatter," to more positive thoughts. As thought patterns become more positive, the individual begins to perceive their environment and those they interact with more positively. Problem solving and concentration may also improve. CBT may be sufficient for those with mild to moderate depression. Interpersonal therapy focuses on examining relationships that may be the foundation of the individual's depression or making the symptoms worse. Interpersonal therapy focuses on enabling the person to develop better communication and interpersonal skills.[352]

Electroconvulsive Therapy. ECT, formerly known as electroshock therapy, is an intervention whereby electrical currents are passed through the brain. Theories on how ECT works are speculative, but relief is usually immediate, including in severe cases of depressive disorders.[380] Side effects include memory loss and confusion, usually short-lived. It is a painless and safe procedure used for depressed people with dementia who do not improve with antidepressant therapy[406] or who are severely suicidal, self-mutilating, catatonic, or unable to eat or function. Repetitive transmagnetic cranial stimulation seems to have effects similar to ECT.[116,143]

Vagal nerve stimulation, originally used to control epilepsy, has been used with severe depression that is intervention-resistant in 30% to 44% of cases. Vagal nerve stimulation changes the concentration of neurotransmitters in the cerebrospinal fluid or their metabolites (e.g., γ-aminobutyric acid [GABA]).[425] The device, implanted under the clavicle with direct attachment to the vagus nerve, sends electrical pulses to the brain and improves mood.

Interventions for SAD include phototherapy, psychologic therapy, and/or psychopharmacology (e.g., serotonin).[189] Negative air ionization, which acts by liberating charged particles on the sleep environment, has also become effective in treatment of SAD.[189] Light therapy is often the first line of treatment for SAD.[262,486] The light system uses white fluorescent light (10,000 lux) with a diffusing screen that filters out ultraviolet rays that can cause eye damage and skin cancer. Light therapy begins in the fall and is done in the early morning for 30 minutes. The light must reach the retina or it will not produce any results. A *dawn simulator* uses a bedside timer to gradually increase the bedroom light in the morning to create an artificial early dawn.[13,262,486]

Complementary therapies have gained popularity as people seek out alternative strategies to cope with depression. A program of self-care, including exercise, stress reduction, social contact, and positive self-talk, is advocated. Outdoor activities are encouraged. Exercise of any kind that increases the heart rate even mildly is advised by most experts in this field.[242] Cardiovascular (aerobic) exercise five to six times a week for at least 30 minutes may be optimal. Research is limited, but some evidence exists to support the beneficial effects of process-oriented treatment and right brain communication in medical care, trauma-sensitive body work[553]; exercise; herbal therapy (*Hypericum perforatum* [St. John's wort], S-adenosyl-L-methionine [SAM-e]); and, to a lesser extent, acupuncture and relaxation therapies.[142,242]

Prognosis. Recurrent MDD is a chronic relapsing disorder associated with high morbidity and mortality; the severity of the initial depressive episode appears to predict persistence.[460] Adolescent-onset depressive disorder may carry an increased risk for poor outcome.[535] Researchers are investigating whether treating depression will improve medical prognosis in people who have a depressive disorder and a history of coronary artery disease or who have suffered an acute myocardial infarction.[87]

Up to 15% of people diagnosed with MDD die by suicide. Epidemiologic evidence also suggests a fourfold increase in death rates in people with MDD who are older than age 55 years. In fact, adults older than age 65 years, particularly those with major depression, are at a higher risk for suicide than any other age group.[426] And depression affects an estimated 15% to 19% of Americans ages 65 years and older living in a variety of settings, yet the illness often goes unrecognized and untreated.[81] People with depression admitted to nursing homes may have a markedly increased likelihood of death in the first year.[1,423,424,457]

SPECIAL IMPLICATIONS FOR THE THERAPIST　3-6

Depressive Disorders
Depression

In addition to MDDs, depression is associated with many medical conditions (see Box 3-8). Consequently many patients/clients in physical therapy may present with depressive disorders. If the therapist suspects the possibility of depression, baseline information can be obtained and provided to the physician when referring that client. Screening tests, such as the Beck Depression Index (BDI),[54] the McGill Pain Questionnaire,[320] the Multidimensional Pain Inventory (MDI),[31] and the Geriatric Depression Scale,[552] are noninvasive, easy to administer, and do not require interpretation outside the scope of a therapist's practice. It is recommended that routine screening for depression and anxiety be included in the examination for all clients. Asking for permission to discuss symptoms of depression with the referring practitioner or other appropriate health care professional is recommended; in the case of a minor, parental consent may be needed.

The acronym **PLISSIT** may help provide the therapist with some direction early on in the intervention. Although this model was originally developed and used for sexuality assessment, it works quite well with depression, too.

- Permission: *Acknowledge the presence of the depression and give the person permission to feel depressed.*
- Limited Information: *"Of course you are feeling down. You broke your hip, it hurts, and you cannot get around." This acknowledges and validates the person's experience.*
- Specific Suggestions: *For example, knowing that depression often causes the person to avoid social contact and seek isolation, which then contributes to the depression, encourage the person to make telephone contact*

with at least one person every day, or listen to upbeat music every morning and evening, or make arrangements to exercise with someone else (even if only for 10 minutes once a week).

- Intensive Therapy: *The client is referred to appropriate specific therapy from other trained professionals.*

When depression is noted, it should be included as a problem in the care plan; the team can then develop strategies to help the person. A client who is not progressing in rehabilitation and who is moderately or severely depressed but not receiving intervention for the depression may need to delay rehabilitation until the depression is under control. Under these circumstances, the therapist should not hesitate to refer a client for evaluation and treatment.

Box 3-6 lists the signs and symptoms of depression. Because of the rapport developed early in the client–therapist relationship, the therapist may identify early signs of depression separate to or in conjunction with a response to a medical condition. Lack of motivation, lack of interest in participation, and/or nonadherence during therapy with minimal or no adherence in following a home program may be indicative of depression. The depressed client may cry easily, and often for no apparent reason. Such a situation can be handled by offering reassurance and redirecting the person's attention toward the instructions, activity, or other more positive topics.

Depression may also lead to anger, which is observed as outbursts of hostility, attempts to sabotage treatment efforts, or blaming the worksite, employer, significant other, or the therapist for the injury. Active listening without communicating judgment when the client expresses despair, anger, or negative feelings is appropriate.

Depressive disorders occur in more than 50% of people with Parkinson disease and stroke. People with depression commonly have global memory loss, whereas dementia results in loss of recent memory but retention of detail. Depression is a risk factor for osteoporosis; it increases the risk for fracture in older people.[326] Increases in the stress hormone cortisol could account for some of the loss. An alternative mechanism is that demineralization is a side effect of medication use. The physical therapist's intervention for people who are experiencing major depression should include fracture prevention. Depression and anxiety have also been associated with slowed wound healing also potentially attributed to elevated cortisol levels.[104,518]

Exercise and Depression

A recent systematic review on the effect of exercise on the symptoms and management of depression suggests exercise reduces mild-to-moderate depressive symptoms, especially in those individuals with a chronic illness.[200] More recent research supports the link between exercise and improvement of depressive symptoms in persons with MDD.[141] The authors hypothesize that exercise increases of the number of serotonin neurotransmitter receptors in the hippocampus via stimulation of neurogenesis. The release of endorphins during aerobic exercise and the reduction cortisol levels in the bloodstream elevate mood, reduce pain, and mediate stress reactions.

Increased aerobic exercise or strength training has been shown to reduce mild-to-moderate depressive symptoms significantly in people younger than 60 years of age, although habitual physical activity has not been shown to prevent the onset of depression. Studies of older adults and adolescents with depression have been limited, but physical activity and exercise appear beneficial in these populations as well.[351] In some cases, exercise can alleviate depression immediately, independent of achieving fitness, although some evidence exists that exercise must be continued to remain effective.[40] Ströhle reports that further study on how type of exercise and dosage (intensity, frequency, duration) impact depression (and anxiety) is needed.[471]

Antidepressant Medications

For the client taking TCAs, heart rate during peak exercise should be monitored (see Appendix B) because the anticholinergic effect of these medications significantly increases heart rate. Drugs used to treat depressive disorders may cause a number of other side effects as a result of increased norepinephrine levels such as dry mouth, blurred vision, urinary retention, constipation, and palpitations (see Table 3-5).

Orthostatic hypotension can be the source of dizziness and fainting, increasing the risk of falls and accidents, especially in older adults. Older adults taking TCAs are at greater risk for heat stroke as a consequence of decreased ability to adjust easily to ambient air temperatures, which may affect their exercise program or pool therapy. The therapist should always encourage the client to report any breakthrough symptoms and/or side effects to the prescribing physician.

Withdrawal from antidepressants must be monitored by the physician as tapering of the dosage is required to prevent withdrawal symptoms. If the physical therapist is aware that the client has decided to discontinue use of these medications without physician approval, appropriate counsel should be offered. Abrupt cessation of SSRIs (e.g., in preparation for surgery or at the time of admission) is the most frequent complication in patients in the hospital, resulting in the SSRI discontinuation syndrome within 24 to 72 hours. It can be very uncomfortable for the patient and signs and symptoms (neurologic, gastrointestinal, psychologic, and somatic) can last 1 to 2 weeks if untreated.[217] The therapist may be the first to recognize withdrawal signs and symptoms such as nausea, vomiting, dizziness, poor balance, tremors, twitching, paresthesias, fatigue, lethargy as a complication of SSRI withdrawal. The therapist should communicate the findings with the physician or other appropriate provider.

Anxiety Disorders

Overview and Incidence

Anxiety is defined as a generalized excessive emotional state of fear and apprehension usually associated with a heightened state of physiologic arousal. The experience of anxiety is the common thread among the specific anxiety

---

Box 3-11

DIAGNOSTIC SYMPTOMS OF PANIC ATTACK*

- Palpitations
- Pounding heart
- Tachycardia
- Sweating
- Trembling or shaking
- Perceived shortness of breath or choking
- Feeling heat or chills
- Cold, clammy feeling
- Chest tightness, pain or discomfort
- Dizziness
- Light headedness
- Unsteadiness
- Numbness or tingling
- Feeling detached, disconnected
- Nausea
- Diarrhea
- Fear of losing control, going crazy
- Fear of dying

* Multiple symptoms are experienced at one time.
Data from American Psychiatric Association. DSM-5 *Development: Panic Attack.* Retrieved from http://www.psych.org/practice/dsm and Mayo Clinic Staff: Panic attacks and panic disorder, 2013. Available at http://www.mayoclinic.com/health/panic-attacks/DS00338/DSECTION=symptoms.

---

disorders[17,21] (see Box 3-3). *Generalized Anxiety Disorder* is characterized by excessive and persistent worry and concern about everyday things (e.g., money, health, family) sometimes just worrying how to get through the day or night. Obsessive-compulsive disorder and posttraumatic stress disorders are classified separately from the anxiety disorders. Approximately 18.1% of the adults in the United States have an anxiety disorder in any given 12-month period (prevalence) and 28.8% of adults will experience an anxiety disorder at least once during their life.[244] The most common anxiety disorders encountered in the therapy practice include general anxiety disorder, panic disorder, and specific phobia and possibly agoraphobia in the home care setting. The 12-month prevalences in the adult population of these anxiety disorders are 3.1% (general anxiety disorder), 2.7% (panic disorder), 8.7% (specific phobia), and 0.8% (agoraphobia).[244]

A *panic attack* is an acute onset of intense or excessive anxiety, fear, and/or discomfort that includes four or more of the symptoms in Box 3-11. Panic attacks typically occur without warning and can occur at any time, even during sleep. A panic attack is not an anxiety disorder but may be a component of any of the anxiety disorders or may occur in the absence of an underlying anxiety disorder. A panic attack (or anxiety) may occur comorbidly with medical conditions (e.g., asthma,[178] hyperthyroidism, hypoglycemia). Initial panic attacks may develop during a period of extreme stress or after surgery, a serious accident, illness, or childbirth. The premenstrual period is one of heightened vulnerability for women. Panic attacks occur at least once in approximately 3% of the population.[459] It is not uncommon for an individual experiencing a panic attack to believe that he or she is having a heart attack and, consequently, go to a hospital emergency department.[4,395]

Panic disorder is an anxiety disorder in which the person experiences recurring panic attacks with no known precipitating event. Having experienced panic attacks, the person with panic disorder begins to become preoccupied with worry, fear and/or dread about having another. The person may even begin to avoid situations in which a panic attack has occurred, hoping that the avoidance will prevent future attacks.

Specific phobias are manifested as persistent significant, irrational (or disproportionate) fear toward an object or specific situations that cause marked distress for the person. Common phobias involve heights, flying, storms, animals (mice, spiders, cats), enclosed spaces, and medically related situations (injections, blood, "white coats"). *Agoraphobia* occurs when anxiety prevents a person from participating in social/leisure/occupational roles because of fear of panicking in the situation. The "lived-world" of the person becomes smaller and smaller.

Etiology and Pathogenesis

The cause of panic attacks and anxiety disorders is not clear. Proposed factors that contribute to anxiety disorders include genetics; biologics, including neurocircuitry, neurotransmitters, and neuronal hormones; and environmental factors (e.g., family relationships, stress, abuse).[69,202,464] Inducing GABA synthesis in the dorsomedial-perifornical hypothalamus increases the likelihood of panic attacks in rats by activating orexin neurons. Persons who have panic anxiety have increased levels of orexin in their cerebrospinal fluid. Development of an orexin antagonist may be useful in the treatment of panic and/or anxiety.[230]

Neurocircuits potentially involved in regulating anxiety and panic have been studied with positron emission tomography scans. The number of 5-HT$_{1A}$ serotonin receptors in the anterior cingulate, posterior cingulate, and the raphe nuclei, central structures in the brain, were reduced by almost one-third in persons with panic disorder.[365] Efferent neurons from the raphe nuclei secrete serotonin throughout most of the brain as well as in the spinal cord. This may help explain why SSRIs are effective in treating anxiety disorders. Other imaging studies have linked the prefrontal cortex and the amygdala with anxiety disorders.[298]

Increased pain perception (intensity, related activity limitations and participation restrictions and health-related QOL) in persons with anxiety.[43] The hippocampus and associated areas have long been implicated in the modulation of pain.[321] Increased activity in the entorhinal cortex of the hippocampus found during functional MRI studies is associated with induced anxiety resulting in decreased modulation of pain.[392] Changes in autonomic nervous system function have been implicated in panic disorder, indicating decreased sympathetic nervous system activity and poor heart rate variability.[308]

Clinical Manifestations

Box 3-11 and Table 3-6 list symptoms associated with panic attack and anxiety disorders, respectively. These represent the most common symptoms, but other manifestations of anxiety include irritability, difficulty with memory or concentration, uncertainty, hypervigilance to somatic symptoms, muscle tension, and headache. Symptoms range in severity: Mild anxiety may cause

Table 3-6	Symptoms of Anxiety	
Physical	**Behavioral**	**Cognitive**
• Increased sighing respiration • Increased blood pressure • Tachycardia • Shortness of breath • Dizziness • Lump in throat • Muscle tension • Headaches • Dry mouth • Diarrhea • Nausea • Clammy hands • Sweating or chills • Pacing • Chest pain*	• Hyperalertness • Irritability • Uncertainty • Apprehensiveness • Difficulty with memory or concentration • Sleep disturbance	• Fear of losing one's mind • Fear of losing control • Sense of terror • Fear of dying

*Chest pain associated with anxiety accounts for more than half of all emergency room admissions for chest pain. The pain is substernal, a dull ache that does not radiate, and is not aggravated by respiratory movements, but is associated with hyperventilation and claustrophobia.

minor activity limitations or participation restrictions, while severe anxiety can completely prohibit the ability to participate in social/occupational and leisure roles, as in agoraphobia.

Panic disorder is characterized by periods of sudden, unprovoked, intense anxiety with associated physical symptoms lasting a few minutes up to 2 hours. Residual sore muscles and fatigue are a consistent finding after the panic attack. Recurrent panic attacks during sleep occur in approximately 30% of panic disorders. The person with sleep panic attacks awakens feeling fatigued, stiff, and sore. Persons with generalized anxiety disorder experience restlessness and muscle tension that can lead to body aches, headaches, procrastination, and delayed decision making in response to their worries.

Persons with anxiety disorders often feel frustrated and embarrassed that they cannot control their symptoms on their own. Anxiety can become self-generating because the symptoms reinforce the reaction, causing a spiral effect. Stimulants, such as caffeine, cocaine, or other stimulant drugs; medications containing caffeine; or stimulants used in treating asthma can trigger anxiety disorders.

Anxiety is associated with a heightened perception of pain, particularly musculoskeletal pain.[43] Persons with both anxiety and depression report increased pain intensity, as well as increased impact of pain on activities, health-related QOL and participation in occupational/social/leisure roles. Persons with musculoskeletal pain reported 32.2 days of disability over a 3-month period compared to only 18.1 days in those with pain and no anxiety[43] and 42.6 days among those with pain with both anxiety and depression.

MEDICAL MANAGEMENT

DIAGNOSIS. A physical exam is often performed to rule out predisposing medical conditions. The criteria established by the American Psychiatric Association in the DSM-5 are used to diagnose the various anxiety disorders. The required duration varies with disorder; for example, symptoms must be present for at least 1 month for a diagnosis of panic disorder whereas the excessive worry associated with generalized anxiety disorder must be present for at least 3 months.

TREATMENT. A combination of pharmacologic and psychotherapy interventions are most effective for the various anxiety disorders.[192,306,355,449,525] The goal of therapeutic intervention is to manage or relieve levels of anxiety and preventing panic attacks or minimizing the impact and duration of a panic attack. CBT is a particularly effective psychotherapeutic intervention. CBT focuses on the way the person thinks, reducing "cognitive chatter," and how the person responds to the person's own thoughts.

Two types of psychoactive medications are typically used, in various combinations, depending on the type and severity of the anxiety disorder: (1) antidepressants (SSRIs, SNRIs [see "Depressive Disorders" above]), which primarily increase the availability of serotonin and (2) antianxiety medications such as buspirone (BuSpar) and benzodiazepines (e.g., lorazepam [Ativan], diazepam ([Valium], alprazolam [Xanax], clonazepam [Klonopin]). Benzodiazepines help control the symptoms of a panic attack and have various pharmacokinetic characteristics. For example, Xanax acts more quickly than Klonopin but has a shorter half-life so blood levels of the drug decrease more quickly as well. Benzodiazepines can be addictive and should be used with care. More severe anxiety disorders (e.g., agoraphobia) may require TCAs or MAOIs, but they cause more significant side effects.

A number of complementary/integrative therapies may be useful, such as exercise (including tai chi, qi gong, yoga), prayer/meditation, the HeartMath approach,[100,218,309] acupuncture, hypnosis, Reiki, BodyTalk, and other relaxation techniques. Herbal supplements are sometimes used (kava, valerian, vitamin B). The evidence is strongest for meditation, exercise, and relaxation. Kava is associated with liver dysfunction.

PROGNOSIS. The prognosis is quite good for most individuals with anxiety disorders as CBT and psychopharmacologic interventions are very effective alone or in combination.[192,449,525] Persons with poorly controlled panic disorder may develop avoidance behaviors in an attempt to avoid situations that become perceived as possible triggers (e.g., driving, going to a movie theater). Generalized anxiety disorder can lead to significant sleep disorders, gastrointestinal conditions, persistent headaches, and bruxism (teeth grinding). Specific phobias can lead to activity limitations and participation restrictions, for example, avoiding medical care, social situations, driving out of the way to avoid a bridge. Agoraphobia may become so severe that the individual can no longer leave the house or, in the worst case, a specific room in the home. Depression, suicidal thoughts, and substance use disorders are serious potential complications of poorly managed anxiety disorders.

SPECIAL IMPLICATIONS FOR THE THERAPIST 3-7

Anxiety Disorders

A client explained how panic disorder impacts her ability to participate in therapy: "First, what if I have a panic attack while I am at therapy? The therapist will think I am crazy, or stupid—that I should be able to control this. This fear frequently makes me want to cancel my appointment. Then I worry about doing my exercises. When I have a panic attack my heart beats fast and pounds in my chest. What if exercising increases my heart rate and that triggers a panic attack? I can't let that happen. What if I can't tell the difference between a panic attack and a heart attack, or a stroke? I've been to the emergency room several times already. One of these times it really might be a heart attack….How will I know? How will I know when to say something?"

Recognizing that our clients may experience anxiety or panic during our intervention is critical. The therapist must differentiate between a hypoglycemic episode, a panic attack, and a true cardiac event. A hypoglycemic episode will resolve quickly in response to ingestion of orange juice or similar source of sugar. During a panic attack, symptoms decrease if the person walks around and talks it out. If it is a true cardiac event, symptoms will increase with increased activity. If a client experiences an initial panic attack during a therapy session referral to a physician or mental health professional is appropriate.

Hyperventilation may be an accompanying symptom requiring intervention. Breath awareness and breath retraining can be helpful.[135] Clients may be hypervigilant of their vital and other somatic signs and symptoms during therapy. Redirection of the client's focus may lessen anxiety. Some individuals, including children, may have "white coat" phobias. Not wearing a lab coat and making the therapeutic environment welcoming and less clinical may help with this specific phobia.

Client preparation, reviewing options, and equipping the client to control symptoms through treatment participation and direction are very beneficial. This is especially important for clients whose perception of pain (intensity, impact on activities and participation) is magnified by anxiety or depression (or a combination) as preparatory information decreases pain perception by suppressing hippocampal activity.[43,392]

Anxiety and Exercise

Regular aerobic exercise and/or resistance training is a direct intervention for anxiety disorders, especially generalized anxiety disorder, and among sedentary adults with a chronic illness.[35,200,224,430] The exact mechanism whereby exercise reduces symptoms of anxiety has not been determined but differing psychologic and physiologic mechanisms have been proposed.

Combining physical therapy with behavioral therapy and/or appropriate medications can often accelerate both the physical and psychologic rehabilitation process.[224] New approaches to anxiety disorders developed by the HeartMath Institute focus on interrupting the brain patterns and changing the individual's biochemistry and neural patterning.[100,218] Physical therapists may have a role in helping affected individuals establish new neural connections.

When working with an individual with an anxiety disorder, physical therapists must remain alert to the possibility of suicide or alcohol abuse sometimes combined with dependence on sedatives. Screening for suicide potential is consists of asking a few questions (see Box 3-18). Suspicion of either suicide or alcohol abuse should be reported to the case manager, counselor, or physician (see "Suicidal Behavior Disorder" discussed previously). The Generalized Anxiety Disorder-7 is also a useful screening tool for anxiety that can be used by therapists.[463] A high score on the Generalized Anxiety Disorder-7 should be reported to the case manager, counselor, or physician.

Obsessive Compulsive and Related Disorders

Obsessive-Compulsive Disorder

Overview and Incidence. Obsessive-compulsive disorder (OCD) is characterized by obsessions (constantly recurring thoughts, such as fear of exposure to germs) and compulsions (repetitive actions, such as washing the hands hundreds of times a day, repeated checking such as repeatedly checking door locks, and nervous rituals, such as opening and closing a door a certain number of times before entering or leaving a room).[12,381] The client has no control over the thoughts and their uncontrolled presence results in anxiety. The compulsive behaviors are an attempt to manage the anxiety related to the obsessions. A person is not considered to have a disorder unless the obsessive and compulsive behaviors are extreme enough to interfere with daily activities. Major depression is present in two-thirds of cases of OCD, making it a notable comorbidity. The 12-month prevalence of OCD is 1.0%; 19 years is the mean age of onset.[279,244]

Etiology and Pathogenesis. Although the cause is not well understood, OCD is linked to genetic, biologic, and environmental factors. Family history and significant stressful events may trigger OCD. Serotonin is not well regulated and evidence of increased blood flow to the orbital-frontal lobes and the basal ganglia are indicative of structural brain changes. There is some thought that OCD may be a learned component. Researchers are narrowing in on an area near the gene BTBD3 on the human genome as an area of interest. OCD is likely to have multiple genetic links.[382]

Clinical Manifestations. Obsessions tend to be centered on one or more themes (e.g., fear of exposure to germs, order, or symmetry). The first may be manifested by repetitious hand washing, refusing to touch certain objects or shake hands, refusal to eat at a pot luck meal, and so on. Order and symmetry might manifest by continually lining up objects, performing tasks in a specific order, or repeatedly checking a door to see if it is locked. Most clients do not mention the symptoms or the disorder (if diagnosed) and must be asked about their presence and effect on the person's life and rehabilitation. People

with OCD should not be confused with a much larger group of individuals who are sometimes considered compulsive because they hold themselves to a high standard of performance in their work and even in their recreational (or rehabilitation) activities.

OCD is a dimensional disorder with a wide range of symptom manifestation. Impact on activities and participation in occupational/social/leisure roles can be minimally impaired or severely restricted.

MEDICAL MANAGEMENT

DIAGNOSIS. Diagnosis is made according to the criteria established in the DSM-5 based on observation, history, and interview.[24] A physical examination is also completed to rule out or identify comorbid medical conditions.

TREATMENT. The interventional approach for persons with OCD is multimodal: pharmacologic and psychotherapy. CBT is the usual psychologic approach. Antidepressants (SSRIs and SNRIs) and antianxiety medications are the drugs of choice (see "Depressive Disorders" and "Anxiety Disorders" above). It may take up to 3 months for the medications to have a therapeutic effect.

PROGNOSIS. OCD is a chronic condition but symptoms may ebb and flow over time. OCD is one of the most common causes of severe participation restriction as a consequence of a mental health condition. MDD may be linked to OCD through the prefrontal cortex and is present in approximately two-thirds of people with OCD.

SPECIAL IMPLICATIONS FOR THE THERAPIST 3-8

Obsessive-Compulsive and Related Disorders

Clients with obsessive-compulsive tendencies must be given specific guidelines for any home program prescribed. Specific limits for numbers of repetitions must be provided, including the strict admonishment to avoid checking or forcing through their pain or loss of motion to see if any improvement has occurred. Changes in therapy schedules, sequence of interventions or individuals providing therapeutic interventions may induce significant stress in clients with OCD. Similarly, people with OCD may be reluctant to touch equipment, sit or lay on mats, and so on. Using linens on large surfaces and having a container of antiseptic wipes and easy access to a sink with soap and water may facilitate the flow of the therapy session.

Trauma- and Stressor-Related Disorders

Posttraumatic Stress Disorder

Overview. PTSD is a traumatic stress disorder that can occur at any age, including childhood. The disorder was fully described as a psychiatric diagnosis in 1980.[550] War, military combat, natural disasters, acts of terrorism (local and global), sexual and criminal assaults, and domestic violence have contributed to a rise in recognition of the prevalence of this condition. PTSD may occur as a result overwhelming personal experience of an actual or threatened death or serious injury; threat to one's physical integrity; or witnessing of an event that involves death, injury, or threat to someone else.

Other traumatic events may include violent personal assault (sexual assault, physical attack, robbery, mugging); being kidnapped or taken hostage; torture; incarceration as a prisoner of war or in a concentration camp; natural or manmade disasters; experiencing a significant medical event (e.g., cardiac arrest and resuscitation); or being diagnosed with a life-threatening illness (e.g., cancer) or being treated in an intensive care unit for critical illness.[198,233]

PTSD can result from emotional, mental, spiritual, physical, or sexual trauma. The traumatic event does not have to be experienced directly. Health care workers dealing with the aftermath of violence or natural disasters have developed PTSD.[173] Individuals who did not witness the World Trade Center or Pentagon attacks of September 11, 2001 were later diagnosed with delayed-onset PTSD attributed to the terrorist attacks.[432]

The acute stress responses to a major stressor can consist of: (1) reminders of the event, including flashbacks, intrusive thoughts and images, and nightmares, (2) sensory hyperactivation (hyperarousal, sleep disturbances, agitation, irritability, anger, impulsiveness), and (3) hypoactivation (numbing, withdrawal, avoidance, confusion, depression, dissociation).[17,450] If symptoms in each of the above categories are present for more than 1 month, the diagnosis of PTSD is applicable.

Risk Factors. Despite the large number of individuals exposed to significant traumatic events, only a minority develop PTSD. There is still controversy about the exact risk factors for development of chronic or delayed-onset PTSD. Some of the risk factors more commonly described are the magnitude of the stress,[339] previous history of traumatization,[164] and presence of both physical and psychologic trauma.[450] There is also research that suggests genetic predisposition may increase the vulnerability of individuals exposed to physical or psychologic trauma who develop PTSD.[432,550,551] A high percentage of individuals with a history of childhood sexual abuse develop PTSD symptoms. Sexual assault is the most common precipitating cause reported by women with PTSD; combat deployments are the most commonly identified etiology in men. Sleep disturbances of other factors that can diminish resiliency have also been linked with an increased risk for PTSD.[376,446]

Clinical Manifestations. The diagnosis of PTSD is made if symptoms from each of the five DSM-5 categories of symptoms are experienced: category A: history of significant physical or emotional trauma; category B: reexperiencing; category C: avoidance numbing; category D: negative alterations in thoughts and mood; and category E: hyperarousal.[26] The presence of both numbing and hyperarousal symptoms are relatively unique to PTSD.[128,513]

The person with PTSD experiences persistent symptoms of anxiety, unwanted and distressing thoughts and nightmares, increased arousal, or hypervigilance not present before the trauma. Symptoms also may include difficulty falling or staying asleep, exaggerated startle response, or difficulty concentrating on or completing tasks. Children may also exhibit various physical symptoms such as headaches and stomach aches. Emotional numbing symptoms leave affected individuals unresponsive and unattached emotionally to other people.[129]

Symptoms of PTSD can be divided into three types: intrusion, avoidance, or arousal. *Intrusion* refers to reexperiencing the trauma in nightmares; daytime flashbacks; or unwanted memories, thoughts, images, or sensations. Certain cues (*triggers*) associated with the traumatic event trigger these thoughts or memories, which then reproduce excessive autonomic responses. In all age groups (from young children to adults), distressing dreams of the traumatic event may evolve into generalized nightmares of monsters, of rescuing others, or of threats to self or others.

Avoidance symptoms are represented by social withdrawal and becoming numb to feelings of any kind (positive or negative emotions). The affected individual avoids any stimuli that might trigger memories or experiences similar to the trauma. People who suffer from PTSD frequently say they cannot feel emotions, especially toward those to whom they are closest. As the avoidance continues, the person seems to be bored, cold, or preoccupied. Family members often feel rebuffed by the person because he or she lacks affection and acts mechanically.

Other individuals with avoidance symptoms (e.g., combat or military veterans) avoid accepting responsibility for others at the time of the PTSD because they think they failed in the past to ensure the safety of people who did not survive the trauma. Some people also feel guilty because they survived a disaster while others (particularly friends or family) did not. In combat veterans or survivors of civilian disasters, this guilt may be worse if they witnessed or participated in behavior that was necessary to survival but unacceptable to society.[515] Such guilt can deepen depression as the person begins to look on himself or herself as unworthy, a failure, or a person who violated his or her predisaster values.

Arousal symptoms are the final type of PTSD symptom. These symptoms, sometimes referred to as hyperarousal, put the person on guard and may lead to panic attacks. The persistence of a biologic alarm reaction is expressed in exaggerated startle reactions. They may feel sweaty, have trouble breathing, and may notice their heart rate increasing. They may feel dizzy or nauseated. Difficulty with relationships, insomnia, irritability, difficulty concentrating, and being easily startled are hallmark symptoms of PTSD. War veterans may revert to their war behavior, diving for cover when they hear a car backfire or firecrackers exploding.

Other symptoms include inappropriate responses triggered by sensory aspects associated with the initial trauma including more passive, fearful responses, and inappropriate cognitive or behavioral responses to perceived threats. Individuals with PTSD also have problems with sustained attention and working memory with contributions from the intrusive memories, persistent hypervigilance disturbing present concentration and sleep disturbances.[128,513]

There may also be increased pain responses or lower thresholds to pain,[170] which may be part of the inability to distinguish between relevant and irrelevant sensory stimuli or to association with pain experienced during the initial stressor.[513] There are also some occasions when the psychologic stress is misinterpreted as somatic complaints or somatization.[513] Many traumatized children and adults may have physical symptoms, such as stomachaches and headaches, in addition to symptoms of increased arousal.[517]

There is a high rate of comorbid psychologic conditions such as anxiety disorders.[311] Other associated conditions can exist in those with PTSD, such as agoraphobia, OCD, social phobia, specific phobia, MDD, somatization disorder, and substance abuse disorders. Recent studies show a link between combat-related PTSD and heart attack in military veterans even when accounting for known cardiac risk factors.[263] Physical therapists should keep this diagnosis in mind when working with clients who have a history of military combat, history of major trauma including MVAs, domestic violence (including child abuse, sexual abuse, or violence against other family members), or any other major stressor.[206,263]

After a traumatic event, people often report using substances to relieve their symptoms of anxiety, irritability, and depression. Alcohol may relieve these symptoms temporarily because drinking compensates for deficiencies in endorphin activity after a traumatic experience. Long-term success is unlikely unless the underlying PTSD along with the alcohol and substance abuse.[370]

Pathogenesis. Modern imaging technology has provided insight into brain function in individuals with PTSD.[211,452] There is less activity in the prefrontal cortex visible with functional magnetic imaging in individuals with PTSD. Disturbances in self-referential processing are increasingly recognized in PTSD.[66] In healthy adults, self-referential processing tasks engage the medial prefrontal cortex and posterior cingulate cortex brain regions that have shown altered function in PTSD.[66] The prefrontal cortex is the area of the brain responsible for inhibition of emotions and repression of memories, as well as allowing verbal relay of the history (see section on ROPC and responses to trauma earlier in this chapter).[211]

The excessive and continuous fight-or-flight responses result in abnormal hypothalamic-pituitary-thyroid activity and maladaptive stress responses.[450] Adrenaline and norepinephrine in the brain stimulate the amygdala, which is the seat of emotional memories associated with threat.[387] In PTSD, the amygdala becomes overactive, causing the individual to be on high alert with disproportionate fear responses to ordinary circumstances that interfere with normal fear–memory function. Abnormalities in amygdala pathways can affect both the acquisition and expression of fear conditioning.[166]

After endorphin levels gradually decrease, a period of endorphin withdrawal lasting from hours to days occurs, producing emotional distress and contributing to the symptoms of PTSD. Areas of the brain that normally balance the amygdala, such as the hippocampus, anterior cingulate cortex, prefrontal cortex, insula, and superior temporal and inferior frontal cortex, are smaller in size and do not function as well in people with PTSD.[73,408]

MEDICAL MANAGEMENT

DIAGNOSIS. Diagnosis is based on clinical presentation and psychologic evaluation (see APA DSM-5, 2013). The recognition of symptoms of PTSD requires referral to an appropriate mental health and/or primary care professional. Although it can be normal to feel anxious or distressed after a significant event, nightmares and persistent thoughts about the event can signal PTSD. Avoiding situations, thoughts, or feelings that remind the person of the stress or trauma is another indication of a potential problem. Being easily startled, feelings of detachment, or any of the other clinical manifestations listed, signal the need for medical evaluation.

TREATMENT. Pharmacologic interventions may include antidepressants, antianxiety medications, mood-stabilizing drugs, and antipsychotics when appropriate.[219] The long-term effects on the neural bases of memory with the use of β-adrenergic antagonists to prevent or erase pathologic emotional memories in the amygdala remain unknown at this time.[176]

Psychologic options for treatment include trauma-focused CBT[64] (neural patterning techniques[100]) progressive desensitization, stress management techniques, hypnosis, supportive therapies such as relaxation techniques, and psychodynamic therapy offered in individual or group environments.[64] Of particular importance for rehabilitation professionals is the use of exercise. Lifestyle and psychologic changes, such as decreased anger levels, increased mental awareness, and increased energy levels, have been reported after an exercise program for individuals with PTSD.[262,377]

Eye movement desensitization and reprocessing, a variation on behavioral treatment for PTSD and panic disorder, is becoming a recognized form of psychotherapy for PTSD.[226,272] Once the client learns to relax and feel safe in a behavioral counseling setting, the person is exposed to distressing memories and images. At the same time, specific hand motions that elicit REMs are used to stimulate information-processing areas of the brain. The neurologic basis and benefit of this kinesthetic stimulation remains under investigation.[379]

Adjustment Disorders

The *adjustment disorder* is usually a temporary phenomenon in response to a stressor such as a traumatic injury (e.g., spinal cord injury, cerebrovascular accident, total-body burns); change in family system because of debilitation of the wage earner; or a known organic condition such as a pulmonary embolus with a life-threatening status. During the adjustment phase, the person gathers resources to maintain self-worth, acceptance, and ability to cope. For some people, the adjustment stage becomes more of a maladjustment stage, in which case the person remains unable to come to terms with fear, disbelief, anger, guilt, or depression, and remains hampered by the disease's real or perceived impairment. When viewed by the client as an unpredictable, variable, and disabling condition, chronic illnesses, such as chronic obstructive pulmonary disease or multiple sclerosis, are often associated with such an adjustment disorder.

Somatic Symptom Disorders

Overview and Incidence

The DSM-IV-TR[17] had a chapter on somatoform disorders. However, because of poor reliability and validity of the various disorders included in this chapter, a major revision has been recommended by the DSM-5 Somatic Symptom Disorders Work Group.[27] Several disorders have been combined and disorders such as somatoform or hypochondriasis are no longer considered diagnostic categories. Five disorders are included in this chapter: *Somatic Symptom Disorder, Illness Anxiety Disorder, Conversion Disorder (Functional Neurological Symptom Disorder), Psychological Factors Affecting Medical Conditions,* and *Factitious Disorder.* Approximately 75% of disorders previously identified as hypochondriasis are now included in Somatic Symptom Disorder, while 25% are included in Illness Anxiety Disorder. All of the disorders included in this group involve physical symptoms and/or excessive focus on medical illness. Table 3-7 identifies the primary presentation of each of these disorders.

Etiology and Pathogenesis

Symptoms of somatic symptom disorders (SSDs) are consistent with unresolved trauma, conflict, or stress, and can coexist with a concurrent physical illness, emphasizing the need for ongoing evaluation. There is evidence of a biologic component related to either an inflammatory or an immune process or some combination of both.

Clinical Manifestations

The essential markers for the SSDs are the absence or inadequacy of physical findings, insatiable complaints, excessive social and occupational consequences, preoccupation with problems, and lack of obvious secondary or material gain. This is not to say that adopting the sick role (although sometimes enjoyable) has no gain associated with it—just not material or monetary gain. In short, the person with a somatoform disorder often presents with vague pain complaints that ultimately cannot be cured or successfully managed. In the case of conversion disorder, the person demonstrates a deficit in voluntary sensory or motor function that cannot be explained by a known organic etiology. The most common symptoms are neurologic with paralysis, blindness, loss of sensation, or loss of voice, hearing, or smell. Symptoms are unconscious, meaning the individual is unaware that the problem has a psychologic, emotional, or stress-induced etiology.[120]

MEDICAL MANAGEMENT

DIAGNOSIS. SSDs can account for 80% of all physician visits and make up a large portion of clients in a therapy setting. Diagnosis is made following a thorough physical examination in order to rule out any possible medical condition. If a medical condition is ruled out, the physician will diagnose a SSD depending on the cluster of presenting symptoms (see Table 3-7). It is important that an accurate diagnosis is made in order to provide optimal care for this diverse group of people.

TREATMENT AND PROGNOSIS. SSD clients can have a bewildering array of symptoms, all of which can be highly resistant to improvement through therapy or other medical or psychologic treatment. Psychotherapeutic intervention includes the identification and alleviation of factors that amplify and perpetuate the person's symptoms and cause functional impairment. CBT used in conjunction with antidepressants seems to be the most effective.[150,261,476,546] Antidepressants alone have not been as successful alone.[390] Persons with SSDs often seek treatment from several physicians concurrently, which may lead to complicated and sometimes hazardous combinations of treatment (polypharmacy). Frequent use of medications may lead to side effects and substance-related disorders.

Conversion disorder is often of short duration, and hospitalized individuals have remission within 2 weeks in most cases. A good prognosis for conversion is associated with acute onset; presence of clearly identifiable stress at the time of onset; a short interval between onset and the initiation of treatment; above-average intelligence; and symptoms of paralysis, aphonia, and blindness. Poor prognostic indicators include symptoms of tremors and seizures. The course of factitious disorder may be limited to one or more brief episodes, but it is more often of a chronic nature with a lifelong pattern of hospitalization.

Table 3-7	Somatic Symptom Disorders
Disorder	**Presentation**
Somatic Symptom Disorder	• One or more distressing somatic symptoms* • Preoccupation with symptoms: thoughts, feelings, behaviors • Associated with increased anxiety related to the physical symptoms • Chronic
Illness Anxiety Disorder	• Somatic symptoms only mild or nonexistent • Preoccupation with the fear of having or the idea that one has, a serious disease • Constantly scanning or checking for symptoms • Chronic
Conversion Disorder	• Unexplained symptoms affecting voluntary motor or sensory functions • Symptoms are not indicative of known neurologic or medical condition • Significant activity limitations and decrease participation in social/occupational roles
Psychological Factors Affecting Medical Conditions	• Diagnosed with a medical condition • Psychologic/behavioral factors: (1) correlate with onset, exacerbation, or prolongation of condition, (2) interfere with treatment, (3) contribute to additional health risks, (4) impact the pathophysiology, worsening the condition
Factitious Disorder	• Intentionally fake physical or psychologic signs/symptoms; inflict injury • Tell others that they have impairments, activity limitations, disability • No apparent reward for initiating or continuing the behavior • Can be related to self or to another by proxy

*Digestive; pain in back, extremities, head, chest; dizziness, fatigue, sleep disturbances.

Data from American Psychiatric Association (APA), DSM-5 Development, Somatic Symptom Disorders, http://www.psych.org/practice/dsm.

Somatic Symptom Disorders

A therapist may encounter individuals with SSDs or malingering. The health care professional who can communicate a willingness to consider both physiologic and psychologic aspects of illness can foster a trusting relationship with the client that is foundational to healing. Such an attitude promotes client self-disclosure and a reliance on confidentiality. The presence of these diagnoses frequently requires behavioral and treatment modifications. As with all psychologically based illnesses, the therapist is encouraged to practice in cooperation with the other team members, especially when behavioral or psychologic approaches are the basis of medical treatment. Working solo with these individuals can result in frustration as each approach or intervention provided by the physical therapist has an unsuccessful outcome.

Physical therapists do not usually provide direct intervention for persons with SSDs as the activity limitations and participation restrictions are attributable to biopsychosocial factors that are generally beyond the physical therapy scope of practice. A physical therapist may be integral to the examination and evaluation process as differential diagnosis of an SSD often requires a team approach. Physical therapist evaluation will shed light onto the likelihood that symptoms are physical or psychologic in nature. Persons with conversion disorder are not intentionally faking their impairments (usually severe with significant activity limitations and participation restrictions) but the physical therapist will determine that the pattern does not fit any known cluster of signs and symptoms.

It is often challenging for a physical therapist to work with persons with SSDs, as it can be frustrating to not be able to identify a cause or make sense of the presenting symptoms. The provider should accept and treat highly involved clients in the same way as any other client while establishing healthy boundaries, letting time and confirming evidence, or lack thereof, provide client feedback and treatment direction.

After the client–provider relationship is established, a discussion of the confirming or contradictory evidence, along with the client's needs and perspectives, can occur. Such a discussion can help give clients an explanatory model that focuses on processes and functioning rather than on structural or biomedical abnormalities. It is better to stay supportive, conservative, and treat only what is objectively found and not what is subjectively reported.[544] A list of Table 3-8 lists possible clinical strategies for physical therapists.

The therapist is encouraged to maintain close communication with the physician(s) if the client appears to have multiple medications prescribed from multiple physicians or if evidence of substance use, intoxication, or withdrawal exists.

Factitious disorder involves a client who falsifies signs or symptoms through self-injury, ingestion of substances that will create symptoms, etc. There often is no apparent direct gain for this behavior. When a person has factitious disorder by proxy, the parent fosters a close relationship with the medical team and pushes for findings not supported by the physical examination or laboratory tests of the child. The perpetrator may even convince the therapy staff of the need for support in obtaining invasive diagnostic procedures.

The health care professional should be observant of the following red flags: (1) a parent with little formal education or training who has extensive knowledge of the child's medical condition, (2) a history of repeated hospitalizations or trips to the emergency department accompanied by an apparent lack of concern on the part of the parent, (3) inconsistent medical history, (4) clinical presentation does not fit the history and/or does not match any neuromuscular or musculoskeletal pattern of symptoms, and (5) the child's condition develops only when left alone with the parent in question.

Because these are also red flags for child abuse or ritual abuse, any of these findings requires a consultation with the physician and a competent counselor. The child will rarely verbally report or confirm experiences of abuse out of fear, but careful observation of body language, facial expression, physical condition, and discerning palpation will allow the body to speak. If time and red flags lead the clinician to suspect abuse, it is wise to confer with the attending physician and a knowledgeable counselor to report your findings and concerns, as local laws vary.

Table 3-8	Clinical Strategies for Persons with Somatic Symptom Disorders
Do…	**Don't…**
• Assess regularly • Keep accurate records of all physical findings • Assess and focus on physical needs of the client • Remain professional • Document objectively and unemotionally • Demand regular improvement and set criteria early in treatment for what improvement looks like • Focus on a client's strengths • Focus on what you can change (e.g., stiffness) and avoid what you cannot (e.g., nausea) • Mention progress often • Praise strengths • Remember pain cannot be measured directly, focus on the indirect effects of pain • Utilize a multidisciplinary approach • Stay upbeat • Downplay any undue attention to the actual area of disfigurement • Gently confront inconsistencies • Refer appropriately	• Tell the client that it is in his or her "head," even if you are right • Confront the obvious contradictions • Become more than a physical therapist • Get angry with your client • Have the client talk about his/her feelings about the body part in question • Tell the client that he/she is being unreasonable • Say, "I know how you feel" • Try to be a friend • Take the client's responses or behaviors personally • Allow emotions to creep into your documentation

Modified from Woltersdorf MA: Hidden disorders: psychologic barriers to treatment success, *PT Mag* 3(12):58–66, 1995.

Malingering

Malingering is the intentional exaggeration of physical or mental conditions for some type of gain—typically financial as in workers compensation or following a MVA. However, psychosocial gain may be a factor, such as missing work or school, being taken care of, gaining sympathy, etc.

A health care provider cannot rely on any single test to determine malingering, and symptoms of unresolved trauma can easily be confused with malingering tendencies, especially early on. It is important to document completely, and to compare and triangulate data collected at different times and settings with other members of the health care team. The physical therapist may see that pain patterns and activity limitations observed during treatment either change or disappear outside of the clinical setting as the client arrives or leaves the clinic or is seen outside of the professional relationship. Observations regarding effort, motivation, and inconsistent behavior offer valuable feedback.

If the physician has ruled out the possibility of an underlying systemic disorder accounting for the client's clinical manifestations, then the best approach is to discuss the therapist's concerns with the client over the lack of effort and/or inconsistent findings that have no apparent clinical meaning and consider referral to a competent counselor. The therapist should avoid confrontation or directly labeling the person as a malingerer but remain focused on objective data and function. The therapist may need to make the difficult decision to terminate the episode of care after carefully considering all evidence.

It is not wise to conclude too quickly that the person is malingering as systemic disorders, complex medical conditions and unresolved trauma can masquerade as neuromusculoskeletal pathology and can present with apparent mismatching of disproportionate symptoms for the injury or pathology.

Feeding and Eating Disorders

Overview

Eating disorder is the general term used to describe an obsession with food and weight in adolescence or adulthood, including anorexia nervosa, bulimia nervosa, and binge-eating disorder (BED). According to the National Eating Disorders Association, the prevalence of eating disorders in the United States is 10 million.[347]

The cause of eating disorders is unknown, although it is likely that a variety of factors (e.g., biologic, psychologic, genetic, sociocultural) affect whether an individual may develop an eating disorder. Typically, an underlying dissatisfaction with body image exists that is based on the faulty belief that weight, shape, or thinness is the primary source of self-worth and value.

Whereas an eating disorder is considered an illness, *disordered eating* is a reaction to life situations or a habit that can be changed through attending to the underlying need, education, self-help, or nutritional or other counseling. Disordered eating does not include persistent thinking and altered behaviors centered around body, food,

and eating, and does not lead to health, social, school, or work problems as is common with eating disorders. Disordered eating may lead to transient weight changes or nutritional problems, but rarely causes major medical complications. For further discussion see "Disordered Eating and the Female Athlete Triad" below.

A form of body image disturbance in male bodybuilders and weightlifters has been described as *muscle dysmorphia*. Previously referred to as "reverse anorexia," this disorder is characterized by an intense and excessive preoccupation or dissatisfaction with a perceived defect in appearance, even though men with this disorder are usually large and muscular. The goal in disordered eating for this group of men is to increase body weight and size. The use of performance-enhancing drugs and dietary supplements is common in this group of athletes.[50]

Risk Factors

Researchers are advocating moving away from female gender as a primary risk factor associated with eating disorders. An estimated 25% of eating disorder cases now occur in boys and men.[213] Other more relevant risk factors for both sexes include personality traits or disorders (e.g., perfectionist, rigid, risk-avoiding)[191]; dieting and family history of eating disorders; and social pressure such as military personnel required to meet certain weight requirements, elite athletic performance, or activities valuing thinness (e.g., dancing, gymnastics, modeling, acting).

Several groups of athletes are at greater risk for eating disorders. This includes women who participate in sports that emphasize the importance of low body weight, such as distance running or cheer squad involving lifts overhead and pyramid formations; sports in which judging is based on aesthetic criteria, such as gymnastics and figure skating; and sports where being lean improves performance such as gymnastics or diving. Critical comments about eating from teacher/coach/siblings and a history of depression have also been reported as potent risk factors.[222]

Men at risk are those who participate in sports that use weight classes such as wrestling and rowing. Horseracing jockeys of both genders also exhibit eating disorder behaviors.[470] Gay men tend to be more dissatisfied with their body image and may be at greater risk for symptoms of eating disorders compared to heterosexual men.[236]

A personal or family history of obesity, drug and/or alcohol abuse, depression, or sexual abuse or other forms of trauma are additional risk factors for this type of problem.[101,153] Having a past history of eating disorders is also a significant risk factor for recurrent episodes or the development of other types of eating disorders. Family issues, such as separation, divorce, parental/guardian overinvolvement, or abandonment, are also reported risk factors for development of an eating disorder.[256]

Up to 20% of women with type 1 diabetes mellitus have some kind of eating disorder; this, in turn, predisposes them to further complications with glucose control. The treatment of diabetes mellitus greatly emphasizes weight control, dietary habits, and food. This focus, combined with stress, poor self-esteem, and altered body image that can result from any chronic illness, contributes to the risk of eating disorders in this population. In addition, these individuals may discover that they can lose weight through excessive urination, noting that by skipping insulin injections, hyperglycemia can be induced.[318] This practice in addition to other consequences leads to a higher mortality rate for individuals who have anorexia nervosa coupled with type 1 diabetes mellitus.[369]

MEDICAL MANAGEMENT

PREVENTION. More needs to be done in the areas of prevention, early detection, and early treatment of eating disorders. Education efforts should be focused on girls in early middle school or junior high because of the rapid bone formation during puberty that will be necessary for the rest of their lives. Again, physical therapists are uniquely and ideally placed to identify the client's presenting symptoms, attend to their underlying needs, and refer appropriately to other professionals. Targeting preventive interventions at females with high weight and shape concerns, a history of critical comments about eating weight and shape, and a history of depression may reduce the risk for eating disorders.[222]

Several national organizations provide valuable educational and prevention information: Eating Disorders Awareness and Prevention (EDAP): http://www.edap.org; National Association of Anorexia Nervosa and Associated Disorders (ANAD): http://www.anad.org. Women identified as meeting the criteria for the female athlete triad (see "Clinical Manifestations" below) should not be disqualified from athletic participation but rather provided with appropriate education and treatment intervention.

The prevention of eating disorders in at-risk college-age women has been demonstrated using an 8-week Internet-based cognitive-behavioral psychosocial intervention. Women with high weight and shape concerns participated with follow-up for 3 years with appropriate weight reduction and decreased risk for eating disorders.[222,484] Other online family-based programs for adolescents have provided easily accessible, brief programs when therapist support is minimal or unavailable.[234]

DIAGNOSIS. Diagnostic criteria may be taken from the American Psychiatric Association's DSM-5 (Table 3-9). The gold standard for eating disorder assessment is the investigator-based interview: Eating Disorder Examination.[144] Other self-report eating disorder questionnaires are also available based on population (males vs. females, adolescents vs. adults, acute vs. chronic condition). The Clinical Impairment Assessment is another tool under investigation but appears to provide valid and reliable results when used with individuals who are at high risk for eating disorders.[514] Various laboratory tests may be performed to evaluate hormone levels in men and women, and imaging studies may include a dual-energy x-ray absorptiometry scan to evaluate bone density.

It is important to note that eating disorders are often accompanied by associated psychiatric disorders. Additional psychiatric disorders tend to be connected with anorexia nervosa and to bulimia nervosa.[279] Concomitant psychiatric disorders may include mood disorders such as major depression or bipolar disorder, anxiety disorders, obsessive compulsive disorders, alcohol/drug abuse, and personality disorders.[318]

TREATMENT. Eating disorders can be treated successfully, but recovery is often a long process with a high risk of relapse (recidivism). Overall, degrees of response range along a continuum. With good treatment, 70% of people with eating disorders can be cured. However, it may take years, and the chance of relapse on the road to recovery is as high as 30%.[201] Family-based approaches are possibly the most effective; one newer technique (the Maudsley method, a family-based approach) boasts an 80% recovery rate with no further treatment required after only 20 sessions over a 6-month period of time.[67,274,413,500]

The role of pharmacology has also increased in the treatment of eating disorders with the availability of antidepressants such as SSRIs and SNRIs. It is thought that these medications help control depression, anxiety, and compulsive behaviors (especially around food and exercise) so that behavioral, cognitive, and family therapy can be more effective.

Anorexia Nervosa

Definition. Anorexia nervosa is a refusal to eat. It is characterized by severe weight loss in the absence of obvious physical cause and is attributed to emotions such as anxiety, irritation, anger, and fear. This condition is characterized by distorted thinking, including a fear of becoming obese despite progressive weight loss, accompanied by

Table 3-9	Diagnostic Criteria for Eating Disorders	
Anorexia Nervosa	**Bulimia Nervosa**	**Binge-eating Disorder**

• Body weight 15% below expected weight for age and height; less than minimally normal
• Intense fear of weight gain; refusal to maintain or gain weight
• Inaccurate perception of own body size, weight, or shape
	• Recurrent binge eating (at least once/week for at least 3 months)
	• Recurrent purging, excessive exercise, or fasting (at least twice/week for 3 months)
	• Excessive concern about body weight or shape
	• Absence of anorexia nervosa
		• Recurrent binge eating (at least once/week for 3 months)
		• At least 3 of these behavioral symptoms:
		  • Eating rapidly
		  • Eating alone or in secret
		  • Eating until bloated or full
		  • Eating when not hungry
		  • Feeling shame, guilt, or disgusted after binging
		• Absence of anorexia nervosa

Bingeing is defined as eating large amounts of food at one time or over a short period of time.
Data from Hoffman L: *Eating disorders*, Bethesda, MD, 1993, National Institutes of Health, NIH Publication No. 93-3477, and the American Psychiatric Association: *Diagnostic and Statistical Manual of Mental Disorders*, ed 5 (DSM-5), Washington, DC, 2013, American Psychiatric Association, Available at http://www.psych.org/practice/dsm.

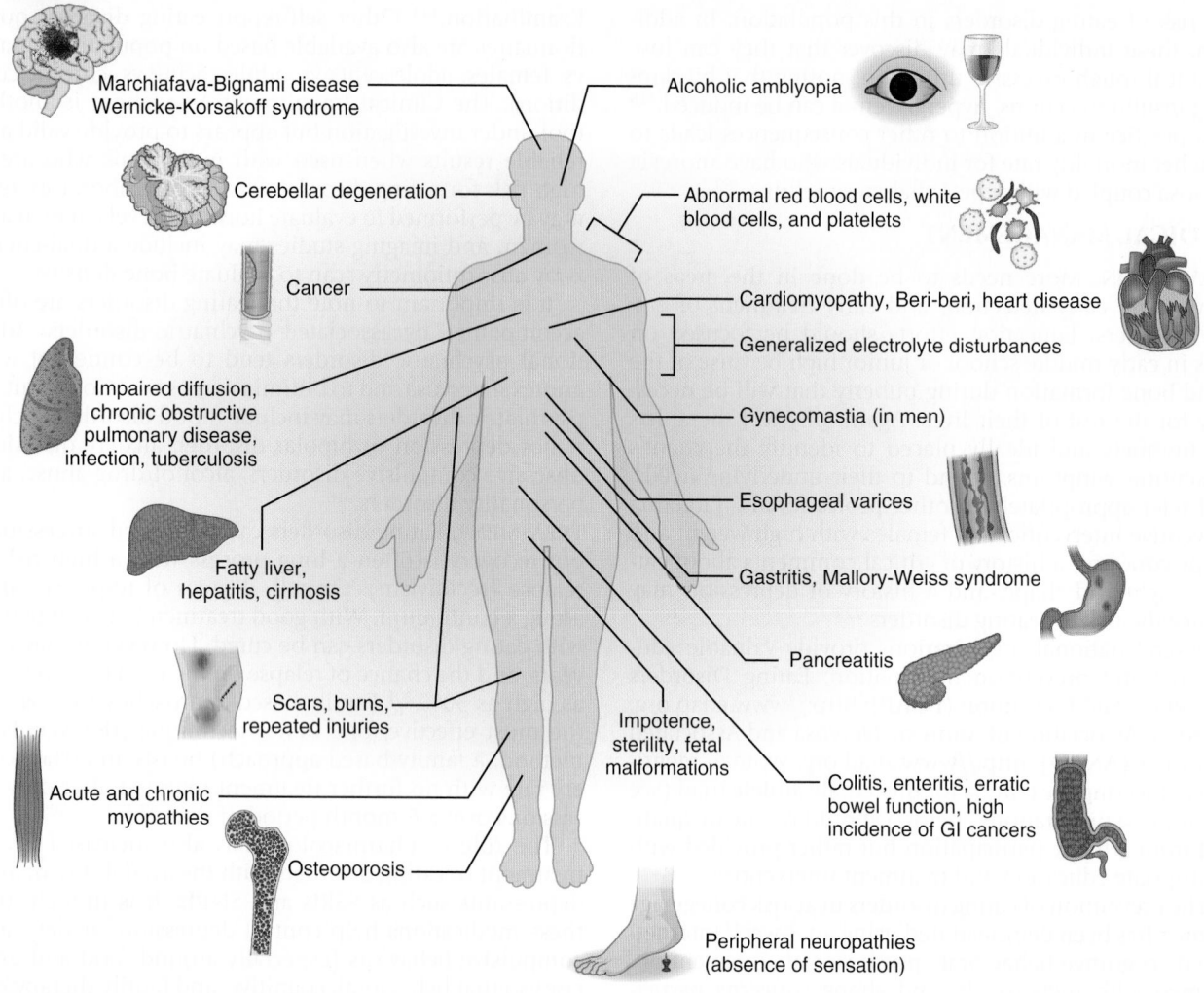

Figure 3-2

Biopsychosocial model for anorexia nervosa. See text discussion. (From Lucas AR: Toward an understanding of anorexia nervosa as a disease, *Mayo Clin Proc* 56:254, 1981.)

body dysmorphia, or the perception that the body is fat when it is underweight.

Although some individuals only restrict kilocalorie intake by eating small, insufficient portions of food, others may use laxatives, diuretics, fasting, exercise, and self-induced vomiting to achieve additional weight loss. The effects of starvation have psychologic, emotional, and physical sequelae, and medical complications that may lead to death.

Anorexia nervosa has been characteristically observed in adolescent and young adult females from middle- and upper-class families, often at or near the onset of menstruation (menarche), but this has spread to include younger girls, older women (midlife and beyond),[555] boys, and all economic classes. Experts are exploring the genes that control hormone production as a potential underlying factor in the development of anorexia.

Etiology and Risk Factors. An increased incidence of anorexia occurs among sports participants, especially sports that emphasize leanness, such as gymnastics, wrestling, diving, figure skating, and distance running, and in ballet dancers. Approximately 5% to 10% of anorexia

cases occur in men; it is suspected that this figure is a low estimate, as it is likely that more males experience anorexia but do not inform their health providers.

Although attributed to psychologic and emotional factors (e.g., the need for control is a common variable; fear of growing up; fear of sexuality; rejection of self), the cause of anorexia remains unknown. During the past several decades, single-factor causal theories have been replaced by the view that anorexia nervosa is a multifactorial biopsychosocial disorder (Fig. 3-2).

Specific early experiences and family influences may create intrapsychic conflicts that determine the psychologic predisposition. The challenges and conflicts of pubertal endocrine changes (biologic factors) may initiate the disorder. Social factors, such as the American cultural obsession with thinness, reinforce the pursuit of thinness.

The cumulative effects lead to dieting (a known risk factor for eating disorders) and other means of weight loss. This, in turn, results in malnutrition and starvation neurosis. The vicious circle of psychologic dysfunction fostering further dieting and psychologic denial becomes established and may lead to death.

More recently, pilot studies have found higher levels of homocysteine in women with anorexia compared to women with bulimia or healthy controls. Because homocysteine can induce neuronal cell death leading to brain atrophy and is linked with depressive disorders, this finding has potential significance and remains the topic of further investigation.[160,161]

Anorexia may have a genetic component and possibly inherited biologic basis. Genetically transmitted variation in gene expression may play a role in vulnerability to anorexia.[41,76] Although rare in the general population (2 in 1000), a person with a family history of anorexia has a 1 in 30 chance of developing it; a biologic twin has a 50% increased risk of anorexia when the twin sibling has this condition.[456]

The biologic basis for anorexia suggests that individuals who lose too much weight may trigger adaptive mechanisms designed for survival when in starvation conditions. Denial of starvation, hyperactivity, and food restriction may be characteristic of ancestral nomadic foragers leaving depleted environments. Genetically susceptible individuals may trigger these adaptations when they lose too much weight.[108,187]

Clinical Manifestations. Besides the obvious lack of appetite and refusal to eat accompanied by weight loss, other signs and symptoms may occur as a result of starvation, vomiting, and chronic laxative or diuretic abuse (Box 3-12). These practices also lead to alternating periods of dehydration and "rebound" excessive water retention observed as swelling or reported as "puffiness" in the abdomen, fingers, ankles, and/or face. Edema is usually noticed most immediately after vomiting and laxative abuse have been stopped. Normalization of food intake and discontinuation of the purging practices will gradually reduce the wide swings in water balance, but the individual often becomes so alarmed at the sudden weight gain or swelling that they repeat the cycle by returning to vomiting or laxatives.[168,501] Box 3-13 provides a comprehensive list of behavioral symptoms associated with these disorders.

It is important to distinguish the edema associated with the cessation of purging practices from that related to the refeeding process itself. Individuals who have lost more than 30% of their ideal body weight are at high risk for a process known as "refeeding syndrome" within the initial weeks of reintroducing appropriate proportions of nutrients and fluids.[318] While the complexity of this process is still being studied, the physical therapist should be aware that these individuals will be at high risk for cardiac failure.

Typically individuals with this level of malnutrition should initiate the weight restoration process in an inpatient, medically monitored setting. The physical therapist should be persistent in checking vital signs throughout activity episodes and communicating with the multidisciplinary team consistently to determine appropriate activity levels in this stage.[151]

Starvation seriously affects growth and compromises cardiac functioning. Altered cardiac function, which generally includes bradycardia and hypotension, when combined with electrolyte disturbances may result in life-threatening arrhythmias. Mitral valve prolapse may occur

---

Box 3-12

PHYSICAL COMPLICATIONS OF EATING DISORDERS

- Electrolyte disturbances
- Edema and dehydration
- Cardiac abnormalities:
  - Bradycardia
  - Tachycardia
  - Hypotension
  - Ventricular arrhythmias
  - Mitral valve prolapse (Mitral valve prolapse)
  - Cardiomyopathy (ipecac use)
  - Cardiac failure
- Kidney dysfunction
- Hematologic disorders:
  - Leukopenia (low white blood cell count)
  - Anemia (low iron count)
  - Thrombocytopenia (less common, low platelet count)
- Neurologic abnormalities:
  - Cerebral atrophy (apathy, poor concentration, poor recall or memory)
  - Seizures
  - Muscular spasms (tetany)
  - Peripheral paresthesia
- Endocrine dysfunction:
  - Cold intolerance, hypothermia
  - Hair loss, growth of lanugo (fine hair)
  - Dry, yellow skin
  - Brittle nails
  - Constipation
  - Fatigue
  - Diabetes insipidus
  - Menstrual dysfunction (amenorrhea)
  - Reproductive dysfunction (delayed sexual development, infertility, prenatal complications)
  - Osteopenia, osteoporosis
  - Sleep disturbance
- Musculoskeletal Impairments:
- Proximal muscle weakness (ipecac use):
  - Abnormal muscle biopsy
  - Abnormal electromyography
  - Gait disturbance
- Bone fractures (associated with osteopenia/osteoporosis)
- Gastrointestinal disturbances:
  - Hypertrophy of salivary glands/facial swelling
  - Atrophy of small and large intestine musculature (causes delayed emptying and bloating, reflux)
  - Esophagitis
  - Abdominal pain/bloating
  - Diarrhea/constipation
  - Rectal bleeding
- Dental deterioration/discoloration
- Finger clubbing
- Anemia
- Emotional/psychologic disturbance:
  - Depression
  - Anxiety
  - Irritability
  - Mood swings
  - Personality changes

COMMON BEHAVIORAL SYMPTOMS OF EATING DISORDERS*

- Excessive weight loss in relatively short period of time
- Continuation of dieting although bone-thin
- Dissatisfaction with appearance; belief that body is fat, even though severely underweight
- Unusual interest in food and development of strange eating rituals
- Eating in secret
- Obsession with exercise
- Serious depression
- Bingeing (consumption of large amounts of food)
- Vomiting or use of drugs to stimulate vomiting, bowel movements, and urination
- Bingeing but no noticeable weight gain
- Disappearance into bathroom for long periods of time to induce vomiting
- Abuse of alcohol or other drugs
- Self-esteem based on weight and shape

* Some individuals experience anorexia and bulimia and have symptoms of both disorders.

From National Institutes of Mental Health (NIMH), *Eating disorders,* 2013. Available online at http://www.nimh.nih.gov./index.shtml.

secondary to starvation-induced decrease in left ventricular volume (see "Special Implications for the Therapist: Mitral Valve Prolapse" in Chapter 12).

Brain scans are abnormal in more than half of all anorexia cases and in some cases of bulimia nervosa. In both eating disorders, this condition appears to reverse itself with renourishment.[497] Loss of body fat results in cessation of menstrual cycle (amenorrhea), hypothermia (cold intolerance), and the subsequent development of lanugo (the fine hair sometimes seen on the body of the newborn infant).

There are other serious sequelae associated with anorexia and bulimia. Skeletal myopathy can be seen in these disorders. The typical presentation is proximal muscle weakness from extreme weight loss; this may have a metabolic basis. Fortunately, this type of metabolic myopathy resolves with improved nutrition.[313] Bone density is also decreased in women with anorexia and bulimia, possibly resulting from estrogen deficiency, low intake of nutrients, low body weight, early onset and long duration of amenorrhea, low calcium intake, reduced physical activity, and hypercortisolism. This type of reduced bone density is associated with a significantly increased risk of fracture even at a young age.[184]

Bone density is decreased in anorexic and bulimic women, possibly resulting from estrogen deficiency, low intake of nutrients, low body weight, early onset and long duration of amenorrhea, low calcium intake, reduced physical activity, and hypercortisolism. This type of reduced bone density is associated with a significantly increased risk of fracture even at a young age.[184]

MEDICAL MANAGEMENT

DIAGNOSIS. As mentioned earlier, diagnostic criteria may be taken from the DSM (see Table 3-9). Eating disorder assessments are valuable tools. Various laboratory and imaging studies may be performed to identify the effects of anorexia nervosa and plan a management program appropriately.

TREATMENT. No universally accepted treatment for anorexia nervosa exists. A multidisciplinary approach is needed to normalize eating patterns and increase weight gain. Treatment can be difficult and lengthy if the eating disorder becomes entrenched or if medical complications exist. Treatment may include behavior therapy, demand feeding, behavioral contracts, psychotherapy, family therapy, nutritional counseling, and correction of nutritional status, which may require hospitalization.

Hospitalization is indicated if the body weight or body mass index (BMI) drops below a certain minimum (e.g., less than 16 BMI for adults), treatment-resistant bingeing occurs, or vomiting and/or laxative abuse persist.[30] As mentioned, starvation-induced cardiac failure and death are possible. The use of estrogen hormone replacement for low bone density as a consequence of nutritional and hormonal alterations associated with eating disorders, although beneficial in treating bone loss in menopause has demonstrated mixed results and remains controversial.[62,317,330] It is agreed that early diagnosis and treatment of anorexia nervosa are essential to prevent initial weight loss and subsequent loss of bone.[317]

PROGNOSIS. Unfortunately, the prognosis for individuals diagnosed with anorexia nervosa is very poor. This illness carries a significant risk of suicide.[256] Although 84% of affected individuals achieve a partial recovery at some point in the course of the illness, the rate of sustained full recovery is approximately 33%.[201] A poorer prognosis for recovery exists for those who have been repeatedly hospitalized for eating disorder treatment, have a later age of onset for the disorder, or have had a longer duration of illness.[151]

Bulimia Nervosa

Definition. Bulimia nervosa is characterized by episodic binge eating (consuming large amounts of food at one time) followed by purging behavior such as self-induced vomiting, fasting, laxative and diuretic abuse, and excessive exercising. Before the 1970s, this disorder was relatively uncommon, but since that time its incidence has increased to exceed that of anorexia.

Etiology and Risk Factors. The exact cause of bulimia nervosa is unknown, although low tryptophan levels (precursor to serotonin) have been implicated. Several theories include a primary neurologic dysfunction, an electrical disorder similar to epilepsy, disturbance in the appetite and satiety center of the hypothalamus, and a learned behavior for dealing with stress and unpleasant feelings. A vicious cycle of depression, overeating to feel better, vomiting and purging or fasting and exercising to maintain normal weight, and subsequent depression perpetuates this disorder.

Risk factors are the same as for anorexia nervosa, and the bulimic person has a preoccupying pathologic fear of becoming overweight despite the fact that she or he is usually within normal weight standards. The individual is usually aware that the eating pattern is abnormal, and self-recrimination is frequent.

Clinical Manifestations. Unlike individuals with anorexia nervosa who restricts food as a means of gaining control over problems, people with bulimia react to distress by the binge-purge cycle.[453] For many people with bulimia, the binge-purge cycle is initiated by a period of starving or extreme dieting and excessive exercising to lose weight. Periods of normal eating may occur, but the pattern of fasting or bingeing with compensatory behaviors (e.g., vomiting; fasting; use of diuretics, laxatives, or enemas) will resume at some point in time.

Whereas individuals with anorexia nervosa are severely undernourished, the person with bulimia nervosa may appear to be of normal weight or even overweight. The effects of bulimia nervosa are similar to self-induced vomiting in anorexia nervosa: erosion of the tooth enamel and subsequent dental decay, irritation of the throat and esophagus, fluid and electrolyte imbalances, and rectal bleeding associated with laxative abuse. Comorbid psychiatric conditions may include depression, anxiety disorders, substance abuse, and personality disorders.[256]

MEDICAL MANAGEMENT

DIAGNOSIS AND TREATMENT. In making the diagnosis of bulimia nervosa, the physician relies on physical findings, laboratory testing (e.g., electrolyte abnormalities, increased serum amylase levels), and diagnostic criteria from the DSM-5 (see Table 3-9). Controlled trials have established CBT as the psychosocial treatment of choice for people with bulimia nervosa.[29] Other treatment interventions may include interpersonal therapy, group therapy, antidepressants, and nutritional counseling.

PROGNOSIS. The prognosis for bulimia nervosa is much better than for individuals with anorexia. Full recovery is possible for those individuals who seek treatment.[201]

Binge-Eating Disorder

Definition. Bingeing, sometimes referred to as *compulsive overeating*, has been defined as eating an unusual amount of food in a discrete period (e.g., within any 2-hour period) while feeling out of control (i.e., being unable to stop eating or control what or how much is eaten). It occurs as a normal consequence of restrictive eating or dieting.

Usually, the binge eater is waiting too long between meals and snacks, avoiding certain types of food (usually considered high in calories and/or fat), or is not obtaining the necessary caloric or nutrient needs. A fear of weight gain underlies this eating disorder; purging by the use of laxatives or induced vomiting is not typical.

Binge eating is considered a core feature of bulimia but differs in that the person binge eating does not engage in compensatory behaviors (e.g., vomiting, diuretics, laxatives, fasting). Binge eating is also frequently observed in obesity. It differs from overeating by normal individuals in that during binge eating, the food is eaten more rapidly than normal, the person eats until uncomfortably full, eats large amounts when not feeling physically hungry, and experiences feelings of embarrassment by how much is being eaten or disgust with oneself. Guilt and depression are often part of the behavioral characteristics.[402]

Etiology and Risk Factors. BED, a syndrome often seen in obese individuals, may be a familial disorder caused in part by factors distinct from other familial factors for obesity. BED-specific familial factors may independently increase the risk of obesity, especially severe obesity. In other words, BED may be a distinct behavioral pattern with a familial etiology.[213] This emerging disorder is designated in the DSM-5 as a condition requiring further study.

Clinical Manifestations. Binge eating results in abdominal distention and discomfort or pain until relieved by fasting, vomiting, or laxative use. Obesity is more commonly associated with BED than with purging or nonpurging bulimia nervosa.[402] Persons with BED do not routinely engage in the compensatory behaviors found in bulimia nervosa (purging, exercise, fasting) and represent a substantial number of people in weight-loss programs.[117,118] Nighttime eating often accompanies BED but is still considered by many experts as a separate eating disorder. Nighttime eating disorder may be an eating, sleep, and mood disorder with distinctive behavioral characteristics.[472]

Other symptoms may include mood changes, secretiveness, impulsive behaviors, sleep difficulties, and obsession with food and exercise (see Boxes 3-12 and 3-13). An increasing number of reports of seasonal mood fluctuations (e.g., SAD, discussed later in this chapter; see "Major Depressive Disorder with Seasonal Pattern") are associated with bulimia nervosa. This connection is likely a result of a common neurobiologic abnormality in the serotonergic dysfunction common to both disorders.[171]

MEDICAL MANAGEMENT

DIAGNOSIS AND TREATMENT. The DSM-5 provides diagnostic criteria for this condition. Surveys for eating disorders, such as The Eating Disorder Inventory,[167] Binge Eating Scale,[179] or Eating Disorder Examination[144] may be used to confirm the diagnosis. Treatment is also similar to the intervention recommended for anorexia, including psychotherapy, family therapy, and self-help groups. Pharmacotherapy may include SSRIs such as Prozac, Zoloft, Luvox, Celexa, and Paxil. Treating bulimia with antidepressant drugs to increase serotonin levels may decrease the number of binge episodes and ease the depression associated with bulimia.

PROGNOSIS. BED is possible to overcome with CBT in a self-help format. This method of treatment has been shown to be the most effective for this disorder, including individuals who are obese in addition to having BED.[541] Goals of treatment include cessation of binge eating and improvement of eating-related psychopathology (e.g., concerns about weight and shape), weight loss or prevention of further weight gain, and improvement of physical health.[118] Remission rates are as high as 50% in the treatment of BED, but the overall prognosis is better than for individuals with bulimia nervosa.[118]

SPECIAL IMPLICATIONS FOR THE THERAPIST   3-10

Eating Disorders

Individuals with eating disorders may be relatively open about severely restrictive dieting, but they are usually less likely to spontaneously offer information about purging or the use of exercise to compensate for eating. Denial of the illness is quite common among individuals with eating disorders, and interview techniques to obtain information are often unsuccessful. The therapist should be aware there are other less-common eating issues that have not been discussed in this chapter, including selective eating, restrictive food refusal, appetite loss secondary to depression, and pervasive refusal syndrome.

Establishing a strong therapeutic relationship characterized by genuineness, acceptance, honesty, and warmth is a prerequisite to eliciting accurate information. The therapist should be aware that people with eating disorders may be very resistant or ambivalent about seeking counseling, nutritional guidance, or direct intervention of any kind.

Therapists who work with athletes or anyone with an altered sense of body image can help promote acceptance of a healthy body image. The National Eating Disorders Association (NEDA) provides helpful tips for health care professionals discussing body image.[348,451] For example, the therapist can help affected individuals do the following:

- *Remember that treatment requires a receptive client, as well as a competent provider. Meeting the individual where the individual is, listening carefully and skillfully, appropriately interviewing while attending to both verbal and nonverbal cues, and seeking to identify the underlying needs of the client are the first priorities.*
- *Using worksheets and self-awareness techniques that allow the client to realize and accept healthy truth is most helpful for lasting improvement. We can tell the client what the realities are, but until that individual is able to receive our suggestions and make the concepts their own, professional advice is useless and sometimes increases guilt or shame.*
- *Recognize that bodies come in all different sizes and shapes. Everyone is unique; accept your own individuality. There is no one "right" body size.*
- *Look critically at messages from the media and our culture that emphasize a certain body type as ideal. Do not set obtaining a perfect body as a goal.*
- *Remember that body size, shape, or weight does not determine value, intelligence, or identity. Identify other unique qualities to develop or enhance such as sensitivity, cooperation, caring, patience, having feelings, or being artistic or musical.*
- *Be aware of negative self-talk and substitute positive inner dialogue. For example, if you start giving yourself a message like, "I look gross," substitute a positive affirmation, "I accept myself the way I am," or "I'm a worthwhile person, no matter what I look like."*
- *Learn how to express yourself by developing meaningful relationships, learning how to solve problems, establishing goals, and contributing to life. View exercise and balanced eating as aspects of your overall approach to a life that emphasizes self-care.*

Routine screening for eating disorder risk factors will increase early detection. Appropriate evaluation and intervention can help decrease the consequences of eating disorders. Female athletes should be monitored for female athlete triad (disordered eating, amenorrhea, osteopenia; see section on "Disordered Eating and the Female Athlete Triad," earlier in this chapter) with special attention to preventing stress fractures now and the development of osteoporosis later in life.[523]

Anorexia Nervosa

It is important for the therapist to be aware of the physical side effects of previously diagnosed anorexia. Rehabilitation may be required for the person with anorexia to regain muscle mass lost as a result of low-calorie diets, malnutrition, bingeing, and purging. Key strategies for physical therapist intervention may include vigilant medical monitoring in the early stages of weight restoration, creating interventions with an awareness of the potential for exercise misuse, and consistent communication as part of a multidisciplinary team.[151]

The physical therapist should never treat an individual with an eating disorder without regular consultation with the individual's dietitian and/or primary care physician to ensure the individual is restoring weight appropriately during the physical therapy episode of care. Regaining lost bone density without weight gain and supplementation is impossible and even with weight gain improving bone density is a challenge.

Vital sign instability can be severe, including orthostatic hypotension, irregular and decreased pulse, and bradycardia and hypothermia, which can result in cardiac arrest. This should be monitored especially in the older adult who has had an eating disorder for years (often unrecognized or undiagnosed). Heart rate must be monitored and maintained within safe limits during exercise for all individuals affected by this disorder. Profound heart abnormalities have been observed during exercise and can be associated with sudden death.

Electrolyte imbalance and dehydration, fatigue, muscle weakness, and muscle cramping are physical complications associated with starvation, self-induced vomiting, and purgative abuse. Poor nutritional status and dehydration also contribute to easy bruising and poor wound healing. The client should also be monitored for lower extremity edema and cardiac abnormalities due to refeeding syndrome as earlier discussed, as these complications may require further attention if severe.

Posture is often poor because of the loss of upper body muscle mass. Exercise tolerance may be low and endurance reduced significantly as a result of malnutrition. Clients may resist exercise or may engage in excessive exercise to vent or work off their feelings and to burn up caloric intake.

Individuals with anorexia nervosa demonstrate decreased bone mass when compared with healthy controls in 90% of cases. Therefore weight-bearing exercises provided at the proper time, with the proper intensity may be indicated. It is important to note that timing is key, as it has been found that exercises that excessively load the client's body while still recovering may adversely affect bone mass[529]

The therapist can be instrumental in screening for undiagnosed eating disorders, especially among preadolescents, adolescents, and young adults. Physical therapists may use tools such as the SCOFF questionnaire to screen clients suspected to demonstrate signs consistent with an eating disorder.[335] The therapist may notice the presence of a painless swelling of the salivary glands and accompanying facial swelling during a head and neck examination. Although this finding may require further examination by a physician for other causes, it can be associated with bulimia nervosa, as the parotid glands tend to swell 2 to 3 days after an episode of vomiting activity is discontinued.[318]

A musculoskeletal problem can be an indication of an eating disorder. Overuse injuries, such as shin splints, tendinitis, stress fractures, or hip or back pain, can occur from excessive exercise; the individual may continue to exercise despite fatigue, weakness, and pain. The therapist can assess exercise habits of clients with the following list of questions[364]:

- *Do you force yourself to exercise, even if you don't feel well?*
- *Do you prefer to exercise rather than being with friends?*
- *Do you become very upset if you miss a workout?*
- *Do you base the amount you exercise on how much you eat?*
- *Do you have trouble sitting still because you think you're not burning calories?*
- *Do you worry that you'll gain weight if you skip exercising for a day?*

In addition to observation of clinical manifestations, the therapist can identify the presence of risk factors and ask screening questions presented elsewhere.[177] Early detection and prompt referral to an appropriate center with expertise in treating this illness are essential. Consulting with other members of the health care team, such as psychologists and psychiatrists, can help in providing a behavioral approach to physical therapy and especially to an exercise program (Box 3-14).

Bulimia Nervosa

Bulimia contributes to problems associated with fluid depletion and temperature regulation. For people who use vomiting to purge and abuse laxatives or diuretics, significant dehydration and potassium loss are quite frequent. The immediate outcome of such behavior is usually muscle cramping, including irregular heartbeat as the heart muscle cramps; fatigue; and low blood pressure on standing.

In such situations, the physical therapist should delay intervention until electrolyte levels are within normal limits and encourage fluid intake and reduced activity level. In the more extreme condition, motor incoordination, confusion, and disorientation may be observed requiring medical attention.

Most deadly among the forms of purging is the abuse of ipecac, an emetic (syrup that induces vomiting) used to treat poison victims. Many people who try it once find it so unpleasant that they avoid further use, but repeated use of ipecac can cause toxic levels in the body, producing myopathy with arm or leg weakness or affecting the heart and causing sudden death.

Exercise and Eating Disorders

A medical provider must assess when an individual is safe to exercise no matter what the weight or BMI.[199] Guidelines are usually individualized and vary from program to program (e.g., some treatment teams use the 10th percentile for child and adolescents and a BMI of 18 kg/m^2 for adults; others use BMI of 19 or return of menses as a guideline for "permission" to participate in exercise). When considering the plan of care, it is vital to be aware of the tendency for individuals with eating disorders to use exercise as a means of controlling calorie consumption. This may typically be done through aerobic activities, but also may be achieved through repetitive completion of strengthening activities as well, such as abdominal crunches. It is not unusual to hear reports of the individual performing hundreds of abdominal crunches each day.

Physical therapists are uniquely positioned to provide client education in the proper boundaries for these activities, and to help clients understand the calorie requirements for activity. Clients must learn to balance calorie intake and output to achieve a healthy balance to prevent weight loss. Clients should also be monitored for over-exercising behaviors in the course of a physical therapy episode of care. The physical therapist may communicate with the client's psychotherapist to integrate concepts from psychotherapeutic treatment into the physical therapy plan.

After entering a recovery program or during hospitalization, a graduated exercise program may be introduced when clinically safe. Any exercise program must be adjusted for bone density and cardiac status, and laboratory values must be monitored for signs of dehydration, low white blood cell count, or anemia (see Chapter 40).

Exercise is not recommended if the body weight is below a BMI of 18, although clients with BMIs lower than 18 may require the expertise of a physical therapist because of a lack of functional independence or the presence of postural stability impairments caused by severe weakness associated with the advanced starvation process. In these cases, physical therapy intervention should be initiated slowly with close monitoring of vital signs and a "deemphasis" on typical exercise perceptions.[151] Strenuous exercise programs such as aerobics are not introduced until the person is in a maintenance weight range and then only if the client is medically stable. If the individual loses weight or cannot control the amount of exercise, then the exercise program is reduced or stopped temporarily.

The therapist can guide the client in avoiding excessive exercise, which is defined as exercise that is accompanied by intense guilt when it is postponed or exercise solely to burn calories and influence weight or shape. Addressing dysfunctional exercise behavior is both part of prevention and intervention for eating disorders.[333] More research is needed to define more clearly the role of exercise in the treatment of people with eating disorders. The investigation of prescribed exercise training for eating disorders is limited but has been growing in recent years.[419,495] Several resources are available, including Pauline Powers and Ron Thompson's book *The Exercise Balance*[396] and a chapter on "Normalizing Exercise" in Herrin and Matsumoto's *The Parent's Guide to Eating Disorders*.[199] See the helpful website, http://www.marciaherrin.com, for more information on eating disorders.

A THERAPIST'S THOUGHTS*
Working with Individuals who have Eating Disorders

Working with an individual who has an eating disorder in any practice setting can be a unique experience. The physical therapist should be aware of a few key items to ensure success in implementing the plan of care, in addition to keeping the individual safe. Regardless of the reason for the physical therapist's consultation, communication with the client's medical team is essential. Throughout the episode of care, the physical therapist should communicate with the physician managing the client's eating disorder and the client's dietitian, if such a practitioner is also involved.

It is not necessary to know the client's weight with every session; however, it is important to confirm that the client is consistently meeting prescribed calorie intake requirements. This may best be accomplished through monitoring vital signs with every session and communicating with the individual's care team. Strategies such as using a food log done directly with the client may overemphasize food intake too much. If at any time during the episode of care, the physical therapist determines the person demonstrates inadequate food intake, if the client's appearance changes in an unhealthy manner, or new complaints from the client surface regarding pain or symptoms such as dizziness, lightheadedness, near falls, or generalized numbness and tingling, the session should be terminated and the individual's physician should be contacted in a timely manner. The physical therapy episode of care should not resume until the client has followed up with his or her medical team, and the physician has given clearance for the client to resume physical therapy treatment.

Finally, the physical therapist should never assume that a client with an eating disorder has already received all of the necessary education to successfully prevent injury when comorbidities are present, such as osteopenia or osteoporosis, muscular atrophy of starvation origin, or central neurologic changes associated with starvation. Helping the client to objectively understand particular sequelae of the starvation process is critical as it may affect the client's neuromuscular and/or skeletal systems, and empower the client with self-care knowledge. For example, clients often do not understand the potential harm done to the spine by repetitive trunk flexion in the setting of osteoporosis for abdominal strengthening. Providing education to clients regarding such precautions will help to create a safe and successful physical therapy treatment plan, not only during the physical therapy episode of care, but for the client's long-term self-management strategies.

*Beth Anne Fisher, PT, DPT, CSCS

Box 3-14
BEHAVIORAL GOALS AND GUIDELINES FOR EATING DISORDERS

- Obtain an accurate exercise history.
- Determine the person's target heart rate and teach how and why it is important to monitor heart rate during exercise.
- Develop a well-rounded program of exercise, including stretching exercises, breathing techniques, light weights for upper-extremity toning, aerobic exercise, and cool down.
- Convey to the person that the treatment or exercise plan is to help and protect the person's overall health status and is not meant to control the person.
- Instruct each person on how to determine the appropriate frequency, intensity, and duration of each component of exercise. Monitor daily and weekly amounts of exercise using a chart or written record and use this tool to help the person develop a consistent and appropriate level of exercise.
- Make clear upper limits on number of repetitions and/or sets, since a tendency to over exercise exists.
- Encourage the client whenever possible to make decisions about the treatment plan; this will help provide a sense of control and increase self-confidence.
- Discern the person's attitude toward exercise and consistently encourage recognition of exercise as part of the overall health plan, not just as a means of losing weight.
- Exercise is only one tool for stress relief; encourage each individual to develop alternative ways of expressing feelings.
- Modifying thought patterns and changing behavior is a slow process. Encouragement and support are essential. Reinforce even small steps and successes.
- Watch for signs of dissociation (e.g., glazed look or far-away expression) and assist the person to remain aware of the effect of exercise on the physical body; paying attention to the physical discomfort helps prevent working through fatigue, striving for the runner's high, over exercising, and overuse injuries.
- Avoid making value judgments about the client's body or physical condition. When the client makes comments such as "I lost/gained a pound this week" or "I cannot believe how fat my arms are," do not react or judge by saying, "You are not supposed to be weighing yourself" or "You are not fat at all!" Seek professional guidance to handle such situations.

eating, amenorrhea, and osteopenia or osteoporosis, a situation that often goes unrecognized and untreated.[5,103]

Disordered eating is more discreet and difficult to recognize than *eating disorders* because they encompass a wide-spectrum of eating patterns that may not necessarily be perceived as abnormal behaviors and may not be regularly or consistently practiced on a daily basis. Examples of disordered eating include the restriction or elimination of certain food's from one's diet, for example, eliminating fats or carbohydrates.

Other disordered eating behaviors may include general caloric restriction, compulsive dieting or fasting, poor food selections, and the use of laxatives, diuretics, or diet pills for the purpose of losing weight or increasing lean body mass.[437,478] Individuals who adopt vegetarian (and vegan diets) for the sole purpose of losing weight or becoming lean may also practice behaviors that fall under the classification of disordered eating. Often the rationale for adopting the behavior, rather than the behavior itself,

Disordered Eating and the Female Athlete Triad

Kathleen J. Pantano, PT, PhD

Definition and Overview. Whereas *Eating Disorders* (Anorexia Nervosa, Bulimia Nervosa, Binge-Eating Disorder) fall under the American Psychiatric Association's DSM-5 diagnostic criteria[367] as separate illnesses, the term *Disordered Eating* refers to a spectrum of subclinical abnormal or atypical eating patterns that are often episodic in nature (engaged in before or during stressful events, or during major athletic competitions).[437,478] The term *female athlete triad* is being used to describe the interrelationship of energy availability, menstrual function, and bone density.[488] It is a combination of disordered

Box 3-15

DISORDERED EATING AND FEMALE ATHLETE TRIAD

Risk Factors for Female Athlete Triad

- Poor body image
- Intensive exercise training schedule
- Perceptions of competition, performance, and success
- Eating disorder with negative energy balance
- Loss of menstrual cycle or delay of starting
- Family dysfunction such as depression, alcoholism, abuse
- Personal traumatic life event

Clinical Manifestations

- Osteoporosis/osteopenia
- Amenorrhea/suppressed luteal phase
- Anorexia/eating disorders/negative energy balance
- Common components
  - Negative energy balance—calorie intake less than calorie output
  - External and internal pressure lead to disordered eating
  - Often resulting in lean body fat below 12%
  - Decreased estrogen occurs
  - Leading to amenorrhea and eventually osteoporosis
- Further resulting in:
  - Increased illness—calcium imbalance with cardiac effect
  - Increased injury
  - Longer recovery times
  - Decreased performance

Data from Papanek PE. The female athlete triad: an emerging role for physical therapists. *J Orthop Sports Phys Ther* 33:594–614, 2003. Compiled by and courtesy of Beth Shelly, PT, DPT, WCS, BCB-PMD.

may be the delineating factor between normal behavior and a pathological response.

Disordered eating is often considered benign to the health of an individual because it may not inevitably affect one's long-term health or ability to function in society. In children, adolescents, and some genetically susceptible individuals, however, disordered eating may be a risk factor for the development of a clinical eating disorder.

Without early recognition and the use of effective strategies for intervention, disordered eating that is severe and persistent enough can cause deleterious effects on reproductive function and long-term bone health. In certain young, active female populations disordered eating can lead to an unbalanced state in which available energy in the form of kilocalories becomes compromised. When this deficit reaches a certain threshold, it can cause menstrual irregularities or the cessation of menstrual function, thereby limiting hormonal release, such as estrogen. Low estrogen states can cause an increase in bone resorption, therefore, poor nutrition can eventually impair bone formation and the development of peak bone mass in growing adolescents and young adults. The link between disordered eating, menstrual dysfunction, and compromised bone health (low bone density) has been referred to as the *female athlete triad* (Box 3-15).

Prevalence. The exact prevalence of disordered eating is not known. Most of the available data has focused on disordered eating, eating disorders,[53,80,372,411,458,479] or menstrual dysfunction[13,52,284,285,410] in female athletes,

and the results of these studies vary. The prevalence of disordered eating in gymnasts, for example, was found to be as high as 62%[417] compared to 5.5% to 9% in matched nonathletic control groups.[52,410] Other studies report no differences between female collegiate athletes and nonathletes with regard to the prevalence of disordered eating, and abnormal menstrual cycles.[6,44] Athletes participating in lean-type sports (distance running, gymnastics, dance), however, are more likely to display greater disordered eating symptoms than athletes involved in nonlean sports and college students who are not athletes.[479]

Few studies have measured the simultaneous existence of disordered eating (low energy availability), menstrual dysfunction, and low bone density as they occur with the female athlete triad.[51,367,496] The prevalence of having all of the components of the triad has been reported in various studies as 1.2% (2/170) in high school athletes involved in eight different sports,[367] 2.7% (3/112) in collegiate athletes representing seven sports,[51] and 4.3% (8/186) in elite Norwegian athletes, compared to 3.4% (5/145) in matched controls.[496] Eighteen percent of the high school athletes and nearly 27% of the elite athletes in the Torstveit and Sundgot-Borgen (2005) study met the criteria for disordered eating behaviors.

Disordered eating has been reported to be more prevalent in athletes who were told that they were overweight by their coach and were unsupervised when dieting to lose weight.[437] More recently, female high school athletes who reported disordered eating were found to be more than twice as likely to suffer a musculoskeletal injury compared to those reporting normal eating behaviors; those who already had a history of prior injury were five times as likely to sustain an injury during the season in which they practiced their sport.[409,489]

Etiology and Risk Factors. The causes and risk factors for disordered eating are multifactorial (see Box 3-15). A person may be motivated to practice disordered eating to reduce body weight (particularly if they partake in a weight-class sport), to remain lean or thin to achieve a desired physical appearance, or because of a belief that leanness may enhance physical performance. Young women participating in endurance-type sports (cross-country, track), weight-class sports (crew), and activities or sports that accentuate aesthetic value and physical appearance (gymnastics, figure skating, ballet, cheerleading, dancing) may be more susceptible to disordered eating behaviors.

A poor body image, frequent weight cycling (weight gain and loss), the early start of sports-specific training, injuries, sudden increases in training volume, and traumatic life events (change of a coach, family illness, personal relationship problems) have also been reported as significant predictors of disordered eating, particularly in female college athletes.[63,437]

In athletes, high levels of competition anxiety are also associated with disordered eating, which may be influenced by the level of sport in which an athlete plays (Olympic vs. collegiate), the importance of the competition, how the athlete perceives success in sports may affect other factors (coaches, peers, or parents expectations; future scholarships, public recognition), and how winning or losing impacts their self-esteem.[479]

Although disordered eating is associated with the female athlete triad, it can occur in male and female individuals alike. Any factor that causes a person to restrict dietary intake, or exercise for prolonged periods of time, could be considered a risk factor for disordered eating and low energy availability, whether the behavior is intentional or not. Gender differences in body composition and societal influences and expectations regarding body image may explain why women may be more susceptible to disordered eating than men. Risk factors for disordered eating may go unrecognized as these practices are often considered to be acceptable and harmless.

Pathogenesis and Clinical Manifestations. The physical effects of disordered eating are most likely related to the degree that *energy availability* is affected in the body. Energy availability is defined as dietary energy intake minus exercise energy expenditure, and represents the amount of energy or calories that remain after exercise training that are available for essential metabolic bodily functions. In women, low energy availability as a result of disordered eating can affect normal menstrual cycle function because it inhibits hormonal release in the hypothalamus, pituitary gland, and ovaries.[287]

Initially, gonadotropin-releasing hormone (GnRH) from the hypothalamus gets suppressed,[286a,437,528] which normally triggers the release of luteinizing hormone (LH) and follicle-stimulating hormone from the pituitary gland.[77,437,528] When GnRH release is inhibited, normal pulses of LH and follicle-stimulating hormone may be disrupted or reduced, causing amenorrhea or irregular menstrual cycles.[286a] Leptin, a hormone secreted by adipocytes, is speculated to play a role in the process because it regulates basal metabolic rate and critical thresholds of leptin (1.85 mg) are required to maintain normal menstrual cycles. Hypothalamic dysfunction results in the reduction of normal LH pulses, causing inadequate release of estrogen and progesterone by the ovaries (hypoestrogenemia), which can lead to menstrual cycles that occur at intervals longer than 35 days (oligomenorrhea) or a loss of menstruation (hypothalamic amenorrhea).[284,410] Increasing evidence suggests that low estrogen levels may also cause impaired endothelial cell function and impaired arterial dilation, precursors to cardiovascular disease.[267]

The degree of disruption of reproductive function and the effect on bone health as a result of low energy availability depends on the severity of GnRH and estrogen deficiencies.[77] It has been determined that the amount of energy that needs to be available to maintain energy balance in young adults is about 45 kcal/kg of fat-free body mass per day (kcal/kgFFM/day).[286] In women, this is the amount of dietary energy that must remain, after exercise expenditure has been accounted for, to allow normal menstrual function to occur. Low energy availability as a result of disordered eating can impede skeletal growth and maturation when it occurs during adolescence and young adulthood. The development of peak bone mass can be compromised and may increase risk for stress fractures[186,339] and low bone mineral density, which, if left untreated, can contribute to a greater risk of osteoporotic fracture in adulthood.[375]

Athletes at greatest risk for stress fractures include those with dietary insufficiency (including low calcium and vitamin D intake), menstrual disturbances, late menarche, low bone mineral density, a previous stress fracture, and genetic predisposition,[58,286,329,338] as well as other modifiable factors that the physical therapist can directly impact. Women who become amenorrheic as a result of disordered eating and who have not been treated within the first year the condition manifests (when bone loss is most rapid), and those who do not reach normal age levels of bone mineral density when menses resume, may be most susceptible to developing osteoporosis in the future.[124,125,240]

MEDICAL MANAGEMENT

Medical management of disorder eating depends on the degree in which the condition is adversely affecting one's health and is likely to be influenced by the severity of the condition and the length of time in which adverse eating behaviors have been practiced. Nutritional counseling by a dietitian is the priority for treatment because disordered eating can potentially lead to more detrimental long-term effects, such as unhealthy weight loss, low energy (caloric) availability, loss of menstruation (amenorrhea) or menstrual irregularity (oligomenorrhea) in women, compromised bone health, and the development of an eating disorder.

SCREENING AND PREVENTION. Medical management is often focused on preventing the cascade of events that can result from disordered eating through adequate screening and early intervention using a multidisciplinary team-approach.[527] Screening begins with a thorough physical examination that includes age, sex, height, weight, vital signs (pulse, blood pressure), BMI, a history of physical activity and nutrition diary, a history of musculoskeletal injury (particularly stress fractures), and in women, a detailed menstrual history. Screening exams can be performed during annual health checkups for children and adolescents involved in team sports, or it can conveniently be administered during pre-participation (sport) physical examinations.[9]

When disordered eating is associated with sport performance and a desire to achieve or maintain physical leanness certified athletic trainers and coaches can work together in recognizing athletes who display unhealthy behaviors and attitudes toward training and require modifications in their exercise routines or should refer that person to a dietitian to assist them in increasing their dietary intake.

Physical therapists and certified athletic trainers are well-equipped to examine, correct, and modify training errors and recovery from exercise that may lead to overuse injury. When a history of musculoskeletal injury is present, physical therapists are an important part of the team in treating musculoskeletal and biomechanical faults responsible for injury, as well as providing tools for preventing future injury.

Each team member involved in the care of the individual with disordered eating should be responsible for knowing when to treat and when to refer the individual to another team member or health professional when intervention is out of the scope of their knowledge base. Referring an individual to an appropriate health care professional requires having knowledge and awareness of the condition, as well as good communication skills, so they can best serve the individual with disordered eating.

NUTRITIONAL EDUCATION. An individual's general health and any medical complications that exist from disordered eating are typically monitored by a physician. A registered dietitian, preferably one who specializes in sport nutrition, can address individual nutritional needs by reviewing a nutritional diary and exercise and training habits to identify those with *disordered eating* who may be at risk for low energy availability. Food logs can provide a record of nutritional inadequacies, triggers leading to *disordered eating*, and can help monitor positive changes and progress that occur with healthy eating behaviors.

The role of a registered dietitian is to ensure that daily refueling (energy intake from calories and nutrients) is appropriately matched with daily energy expenditure (calories burned during exercise).[126] Currently there is no test that definitively identifies low energy availability as it exists in an individual. However, the method described above can indirectly identify a person who is at risk for a state of negative energy balance and may be used as a starting point for effective treatment of disordered eating.[496]

The amount of energy that needs to be available to maintain energy balance in young adults is about 45 kcal/kgFFM/day.[286a] Research indicates that, in women, energy availability that falls below 30 kcal/kgFFM/day is associated with menstrual dysfunction and therefore could be defined as a state of low energy availability.[286a]

It must be noted that while it is possible for energy balance to be restored in 1 day, changes in menstrual function may not become apparent for at least a month or more, therefore, apparent markers of success with restoration of menstrual function require time and persistence. If disordered eating results in menstrual dysfunction, medical management may also include an assessment of bone health as menstrual dysfunction has an adverse effect on bone density and could lead to irreversible bone loss.[158]

Under the guidance of a physician, dual-energy X-ray absorptiometry can differentially diagnose for stress fractures, or other bone fractures, as well as for the presence of osteopenia and osteoporosis. In adolescent girls and young women who experience menstrual dysfunction as a result of disordered eating, resumption of menses is a clear indication that a minimal healthy weight has been met.

Standards on minimal healthy weights established by the Centers for Disease Control and Prevention indicate that in adults (older than 20 years) a BMI less than 18.5 is classified as being underweight.[9,92] For children and teens up to age 20 years age-specific BMI values are used; values that are less than the fifth percentile of the normal BMI range for that age are considered underweight.[9,92] Caution should be exercised when using body composition measurements to establish weight management goals for this population because body composition changes during normal pubertal growth and maturation can be significant and can considerably affect BMI values.[50,462] General treatment goals when disordered eating results in low energy availability or an underweight condition are to increase energy intake (or decrease energy expenditure), optimize nutritional status, and normalize eating behaviors.[127]

PSYCHOLOGIC COUNSELING. Even though nutritional education is first and foremost in addressing the physical affects that can result from disordered eating, modifying and treating the emotional thought processes, fears, and concerns that trigger the behaviors may require concurrent psychologic counseling by a licensed mental health expert. The goals of such an intervention would be to identify the psychologic barriers that preclude healthy eating patterns and to provide support to increase the likelihood that permanent attitudinal and behavioral change are made.

PROGNOSIS WITH TREATMENT. As previously stated, the first line of intervention in the individual with disordered eating is nutritional: restoring healthy eating patterns and achieving energy balance by increasing energy intake, reducing energy expenditure, or a using combination of both.[372] Although it has been suggested that nutritional recovery should be based on having the necessary reserve of kilocalories per day to prevent the continuum of health concerns related to menstrual dysfunction and low bone density (the second and third components of the female athlete triad), little research has been conducted proving the efficacy of this type of intervention. Even so, convincing evidence based on case studies is emerging.[127,257,527]

It is important to note that strategies for treating a person with disordered eating be individualized so that the most important concerns for that individual are addressed and maximal use of the multidisciplinary team involved in the intervention are identified. Although a limited amount of evidence exists, preliminary research[127,257,527] indicates that the prognosis for disordered eating is good when early intervention is implemented and the more harmful long-term effects of the condition have been avoided or prevented.

SPECIAL IMPLICATIONS FOR THE THERAPIST   3-11

Disordered Eating and the Female Athlete Triad

Physical therapists play an important part of the multidisciplinary team that not only screens and treats clients with disordered eating but, most importantly, can act to prevent complications that exist as a result of the condition. Although physical therapists do not directly treat disordered eating, they can be indirectly involved in recognizing warning signs that indicate disordered eating and make the appropriate referral so that early intervention can begin. Physical therapists should be aware of the secondary complications that can result if disordered eating results in low energy availability and is not treated.

As previously stated, in young athletic populations, preparticipation physical examinations provide an excellent opportunity for assessing current and previous activity levels, menstrual history, identifying and treating musculoskeletal and biomechanical faults, and modifying activities to prevent injury.[9,270] In the clinic, when treating physically active children and young adults, physical therapists should routinely assess daily activity patterns (both during formal training and on the athlete's own time). Any signs that indicate nutritional needs are not being met (excessive fatigue, preoccupation with weight or food, history of stress fractures) should raise a red flag.

Table 3-10 includes some guidelines of what questions to ask when assessing disordered eating and the potential consequences that can occur as a result of this condition.[270] Because disordered eating behaviors are not easily admitted to, especially if there is a belief that negative consequences may result if the behaviors are exposed, menstrual history at least provides an indication for young women that disordered eating or an eating disorder may exist. Menstrual dysfunction can be caused by other factors besides disordered eating, so it is important that other causes for the dysfunction are first ruled out by a qualified endocrinologist. Girls not menstruating after age 16 years should be referred for medical evaluation, including baseline screening for osteoporosis.

During stages of rehabilitation of an injury, a physical therapist's expertise can be used to determine whether the selection of exercise is appropriate to the stage of tissue healing, particularly when stress fractures are present. An exercise program should be carefully modified to minimize risk rather than having the individual limit or stop activity, which often leads to frustration, depression, and noncompliance, and may actually provoke disordered eating behaviors. Young female athletes with unexplained pain should be screened for osteoporosis and/or fracture(s).

When determining the appropriateness of an exercise, the desired effect on bone should be considered. For example, choosing strength (weight) training versus impact (weight-bearing) exercise or alternating modes of exercise should be determined by the goals set for that individual at that particular stage of rehabilitation. Educating and helping an individual understand that incorporating days of recovery from exercise and complying with dietary recommendations enhances (rather than hinders) mental and physical performance are important concepts in promoting trust and successful behavioral changes. When suspicious of disordered eating in athletes, education should extend to coaches, parents, and teammates[212] so that normal and realistic body images and healthy habits become a part of everyone's knowledge and awareness.

Sleep–Wake Disorders

Overview

There are at 12 sleep disorders identified in the DSM-5, including insomnia, sleep apnea, and restless legs syndrome. Lack of adequate sleep appears to be increasing in the general population. Sleep deprivation can lead to learning and memory problems, decreased eye–hand coordination, decreased metabolism and weight gain, depression, decreased immune system function, hypertension, irregular heart rhythm, increased medical errors, and heightened perception of pain. There is evidence that a sleep-deprived driver may be more impaired by alcohol than when adequately rested.[196]

Etiology and Pathogenesis

Sleep abnormalities are consistently associated with depression, including decreased REM latency (the time between falling asleep and the first REM period), longer first REM period, less continuous sleep, and early morning awakenings. Animal studies show that many antidepressants can reset the internal clock. Whether these sleep abnormalities represent causes or effects of depression remains unknown.

Table 3-10	Questions a Physical Therapist May Ask Clients to Screen for Disordered Eating and Complications Related to Disordered Eating*

Disordered Eating

1. What is your present weight?
2. Are you happy with your weight?
3. How much would you like to weigh?
4. Are you trying to lose weight?
5. In the last year, what was your highest weight? Lowest weight?
6. Has anyone recommended you change your weight or eating habits?
7. Do you lose weight regularly to meet weight requirements for your sport?
8. At what weight do you intend to compete?
9. Do you limit or carefully control what you eat?
10. Have you ever tried diet pills, sitting in a sauna, diuretics, laxatives, vomiting, or similar techniques to lose weight?
11. Have you ever been diagnosed with anorexia, bulimia, or another type of eating disorder?

Menstrual Disorders

1. Have you ever had a menstrual period?
2. How old were you when you had your first period?
3. How many periods have you had in the last 12 months?
4. How much time do you usually have from the start of 1 period to the start of another?
5. What was the longest time between periods in the last year?
6. Do you take birth control pills or any form of estrogen replacement?

Osteoporosis

1. Have you had any broken or fractured bones?
2. Have you ever had a stress fracture? If so, how many, when, and where in your body?
3. Have you ever had a bone density test?
4. Is there a history of osteoporosis in your family?
5. Do you take calcium, vitamin D, or other supplements for bone health?

From Sundgot-Borgen J: Disordered eating In Ireland ML, Nattiv A, eds: The Female Athlete, Philadelphia, Saunders, 2002:242–243.

Substance Use and Addictive Disorders

Overview and Incidence

Substance abuse is defined as the excessive use of mood-affecting chemicals that are a potential or real threat to either physical or mental health. Substance abuse has become increasingly prevalent in American society among people of every age, social, economic, professional, and educational status. Addiction may lead to a lifestyle (e.g., prostitution, theft, violent crime) that puts the person at considerable risk for illness, disease, and injury.

Substance Use and Addictive Disorders[28] are disorders that were included in the DSM-IV-TR *Substance-Related Disorders* category.[17] Non–substance addictive disorders (e.g., gambling disorder) are also included. The DSM-IV-TR addressed four primary diagnoses—dependence, intoxication, abuse, and withdrawal—and the various substances were addressed under each. The disorders are now organized into nine specific substance-related categories, each with three possible specific diagnoses (Use, Intoxication, Withdrawal) (Table 3-11). Substance-induced mental health disorders (e.g., substance-induced bipolar disorder disorders) are also included.

Substance Use Disorders indicate that the person chronically (for 12 or more months) uses the substance to the extent that it impairs function, limits activities, and interferes with participation in social/occupational/leisure roles and/or interactions in those roles. The severity of impaired function varies from mild to severe. Use disorders may include overuse (versus intended use), preoccupation with obtaining or using the substance, craving, continued use despite adverse physical and/or psychologic consequences, etc. *Substance Intoxication* refers to the single use of substantial quantities of the substance resulting in significant impairment of psychologic status and/or behavior that restricts participation in social/occupational/leisure roles combined with additional specific signs and symptoms (see Table 3-11).

Substance Withdrawal is the pattern of physical responses severe enough to create restrictions in participation when regular drug use is discontinued. The onset of withdrawal signs and symptoms may occur within minutes or after a few days when a physically dependent person abruptly stops consumption. Withdrawal can cause emotional, psychologic and/or physical distress, and with certain substances, can be so severe that it results in death (see Table 3-11).

Alcoholism is the most common drug abuse problem in the United States, affecting more than 15 million Americans, including the adolescent and aging populations. The frequency of binge drinking (defined as five or more drinks at a time for men or four or more drinks for women on an occasion during the past 30 days)[95] among college students has increased dramatically in the last decade with an increase in the number of alcohol-related injuries, property damage, and disruption.[95,210] Evolve Table 3-1 lists the incidence of substance use.

Tobacco-related deaths number more than 440,000 per year among U.S. adults and direct medical costs attributable to smoking total at least $75 billion per year and an estimated $82 billion in lost productivity.[90] American Indian adults (18 years or older) have a much higher rate (32.7%) reported by the CDC.[48] Epidemiologic data suggest that smoking among high school students peaked in the late 1990s and is now declining. Previously reported rates of 36% in 1997 dropped to 28.5% in 2001, went down to 20.9% in 2005,[93] and then down to 18.1% in 2012. Smoking appears to be correlated with low income, persons with a GED or formal education of less than 12 years, military personnel, and specific groups such as Native Americans and Alaskan Natives. Men have only somewhat higher rates of smoking than women within the total U.S. population.[300]

Etiology and Pathogenesis

Dopamine, a neurotransmitter, plays a pivotal role in substance dependence by activating mesolimbic pathways (nucleus accumbens, amygdala, hippocampus, prefrontal cortex) in the brain that register feelings of arousal, reward, and satisfaction the so-called reward pathway.[102] For people who become drug dependent, the pathway becomes more deeply ingrained with each use and becomes linked with cues evoking drug use, such as smells, location, paraphernalia, or certain companions. When a person who is substance dependent encounters a use-associated cue, a spontaneous and overwhelming desire for the substance occurs, triggered by a dopamine release in the brain. Stimulation of the mesolimbic dopamine reward pathway way may induce neuroplastic changes in the prefrontal-striatal networks, impairing impulse control, further augmenting the addictive behavior and increasing the likelihood of relapse (recidivism).[98]

Two neurotransmitters, GABA (inhibitory) and glutamate (excitatory) are implicated in addictive behavior. Various substances impact the availability of these neurotransmitters, explaining the psychotropic effects of certain classes of drugs. Alcohol increases GABA activity and decreases glutamate activity, resulting in sedative effects on the brain, leading to feelings of pleasure, calmness, or sleepiness. Sedatives increase GABA availability (sedative effects) while caffeine inhibits GABA and increases glutamate (stimulating effects) and phencyclidine (PCP) and other stimulants increase glutamate availability (stimulating effects).

Alcohol-Related Disorders. Alcohol use/abuse was initially thought to be a sign of poor morals. Currently, problems of alcohol use and intoxication are recognized as a medical and/or a mental health disorder. Research provides evidence of a genetic predisposition in alcohol and other substance-related disorders.[398] Twin and adoption studies show that approximately 50% of individual variation in susceptibility to addiction is hereditary. Although the etiology is not well understood, it is thought that psychosocial or environmental stressors may be required in addition to a genetic predisposition to trigger active addiction.[247] Stress, depression, peer pressure, anxiety, and mental illness, such as schizophrenia, PTSD, antisocial personality disorder, and borderline personality disorder, increase the risk of addiction.

Familial-related alcohol abuse tends to manifest differently. Early-age-onset substance use disorder involves multiple phenotypes (biochemical, physiologic, and psychologic) interacting with the environment beginning at conception. Alterations in biobehavioral phenotypes have been linked with substance use, first as difficult or abnormal temperament in infancy, progressing to conduct disorder in childhood and culminating in early adolescence substance abuse, becoming severe by young adulthood.[482,526] Protein kinase C-epsilon (PKC-ε) has been implicated in both nicotine and alcohol addictions. Studies involving mice show that in the absence of PKC-ε, alcohol makes the GABA receptor system even more sensitive. Alternatively, PKC-ε may impact the reward system

Table 3-11   Specific Effects of Substance Use, Intoxication, and Withdrawal

Substance	Behavioral or Psychological Impairments that Impact Activities and Participation in Social, Leisure or Occupational Roles	Intoxication/Adverse Effects	Signs and Symptoms of Withdrawal
Alcohol (wine, beer, liquor)	• Inappropriate sexual behavior • Mood lability • Impaired judgment	• Slurred speech • In-coordination • Unsteady gait • Nystagmus • Impaired attention • Impaired memory • Stupor or coma	• Hyperactive SNS* • Tachycardia • Sweating • Hand tremor • Insomnia • Nausea/vomiting • Hallucinations • Psychomotor agitation • Anxiety • Generalized tonic-clonic seizures
Caffeine (some soda pops, energy drinks, coffee, black tea, chocolate, some over-the-counter medications)		• Restlessness • Irritability • Nervousness • Excitement • Headache • Insomnia • Flushed • Diuresis • GI disturbance • Muscle twitching, tension • Rambling flow of thought/speech • Tachycardia/arrhythmia • Periods of inexhaustibility, sleep disturbances • Psychomotor agitation • Enhances pain perception	• Headache • Marked fatigue or drowsiness • Dysphoric mood, depressed mood, irritability • Difficulty concentrating • Flu-like symptoms, nausea, vomiting, muscle pain/stiffness
Cannabis marijuana (pot, weed), THC, hashish	• Impaired motor coordination • Euphoria • Anxiety • Sensation of slowed time • Relaxed inhibitions • Impaired judgment • Paranoia, social withdrawal	• Red sclera • Increased appetite • Dry mouth • Tachycardia	• Irritability, anger or aggression • Nervousness or anxiety • Sleep difficulty • Decreased appetite or weight loss • Restlessness • Depressed mood • Sweating • Chills • Headache
Hallucinogens LSD, PCP, peyote, psilocybin (mushrooms, "schrooms," "rooms")	• Marked anxiety or depression • Ideas of reference • Paranoid ideation • Impaired judgment	• Pupillary dilation • Tachycardia • Sweating • Blurring of vision • Tremors • Incoordination	• Persisting perception disorder • Continued signs/symptoms of intoxication
Inhalants (gasoline, nitrous oxide, nitrite gases, aerosols)	• Belligerent • Assaultiveness • Apathy • Impaired judgment	• Dizziness • Nystagmus • Incoordination • Slurred speech • Unsteady gait • Lethargy • Depressed reflexes • Psychomotor retardation • Tremor • Generalized muscle weakness • Blurred vision or diplopia • Stupor or coma • Euphoria	

Table 3-11   Specific Effects of Substance Use, Intoxication, and Withdrawal—cont'd

Substance	Behavioral or Psychological Impairments that Impact Activities and Participation in Social, Leisure or Occupational Roles	Intoxication/Adverse Effects	Signs and Symptoms of Withdrawal
Opioids (morphine, Demerol, Dilaudid, Vicodin, codeine)	• Euphoria • Psychomotor agitation/ retardation • Impaired judgment	Pupil constriction plus 1 or more: • Drowsiness or coma • Slurred speech • Impairment in attention or memory	• Dysphoric mood • Nausea/vomiting • Muscle aches • Lacrimation or rhinorrhea • Pupil dilation, piloerection, sweating • Diarrhea • Yawning • Fever • Insomnia
Sedatives/ Hypnotics Benzodiazepines (Xanax, Valium), barbiturates (Seconal), heroin	• Inappropriate sexual behavior • Mood lability • Impaired judgment	• Slurred speech • Incoordination • Unsteady gait • Nystagmus • Impairment in cognition (e.g., attention, memory) • Stupor or coma • Death (overdose)	• Autonomic hyperactivity (sweating, HR > 100) • Hand tremor • Insomnia • Nausea or vomiting • Hallucinations (visual, tactile, auditory) • Psychomotor agitation • Anxiety • Grand mal seizures
Stimulants amphetamines ("speed"), cocaine (crack), metham- phetamine, ecstasy	• Euphoria or affective blunting • Hypervigilance • Anxiety • Tension • Interpersonal sensitivity	• Tachycardia or bradycardia • Pupillary dilation • Elevated or lowered blood pressure • Increased pulse rate • Perspiration or chills • Nausea or vomiting • Weight loss • Psychomotor agitation/ hallucinations • Muscle weakness, • Respiratory depression • Chest pain • Arrhythmias • Confusion • Seizures • Dyskinesias • Dystonias • Coma • Death (overdose)	• Dysphoric • Fatigue • Vivid, unpleasant dreams • Insomnia or hypersomnia • Increased appetite • Psychomotor retardation or agitation
Tobacco (cigarettes, cigars, chewing or spit tobacco, pipe tobacco)		• Increased risk of heart disease, respiratory disease, and many types of cancer • Poor wound healing • Back pain, spinal disk disease • Osteoporosis	• Irritability, frustration or anger • Anxiety • Difficulty concentrating • Increased appetite or weight gain • Restlessness • Depressed mood • Insomnia

by signaling α(6)-containing nicotine receptors, reducing dopamine release in the nucleus accumbens (part of the brain's pleasure center).[271] Inhibiting this enzyme may remove the rewarding effects of alcohol.[205]

Women feel the effects of alcohol sooner and more intensely than do men. Women produce substantially less of the gastric enzyme alcohol dehydrogenase, which breaks down ethanol in the stomach. As a result, women absorb 75% more alcohol into the bloodstream. Women (and older adults of either gender) have less water in their tissues than men of comparable height and build. Because alcohol is soluble in water, it tends to dissolve more slowly resulting in longer lasting intoxication after fewer drinks.

Caffeine-Related Disorders. Adenosine, among other functions is an inhibitory neurotransmitter. Caffeine acts as an adenosine receptor antagonist, binding with receptors on cell walls that normally respond to adenosine affecting sleep patterns, cognition, learning and memory.[414] These effects are being examined relative to diseases such as Alzheimer and Parkinson diseases, among others. Functional MRI studies indicate that caffeine increases responses in the bilateral medial frontopolar cortex (BA 10) and the right anterior cingulate cortex (BA 32), brain structures associated with executive function and attention during working memory.[176] Caffeine inhibits GABA and increases glutamate resulting in a stimulatory effect. Caffeine also decreases cerebral blood flow.

Cannabis-Related Disorders. Marijuana and other cannabis drugs are often considered a gateway drug. Cannabis use is often initiated experimentally in social situations and is perceived by many to be relatively harmless. The psychoactive compound in cannabis-related substances is Δ9-THC (Δ9-tetrahydrocannabinol). Although the mechanism of action of Δ9-THC is not fully understood, it does act as a cannabinoid (CB1) receptor agonist, impacting motor activity, pain, affective state, and appetite among other functions.[385] Δ9-THC is stimulates the dopamine reward system via the CB1 receptors. Evidence indicates that the interaction of Δ9-THC with A_{2A} adenosine receptors contributes to physical dependence, tolerance, and motivation in mice.[461] The effects of cannabis derivatives usually last a few hours. As a result of a long half-life and the development of tolerance, less of the drug is needed to produce the same effects. The agent persists in the body as an active metabolite for as long as 8 days after use.

Hallucinogenic-Related Disorders. Users usually begin by experimenting with these drugs. The pathogenesis of hallucinogenic drugs is not well understood. There is preliminary evidence that the neurotransmitter, serotonin and/or postsynaptic serotonergic receptors are the site of action.[366]

Inhalant-Related Disorders. The number of possible inhalants makes it impossible to pinpoint a pathogenic action. Inhalants can alter brain chemistry and may induce lifelong damage to the nervous system. Some inhaled gases can replace oxygen in the lungs and result in *Sudden Sniffing Death.*

Opioid-Related Disorders. Opioids bind to specific opioid receptors in the central and peripheral nervous systems as well as to receptors in the gastrointestinal system. Opioid receptors are found in the substantia gelatinosa, periaqueductal gray, reticular formation, hypothalamus, thalamus, and the cortex. Binding with the opioid receptors principally blocks pain but results in multiple side effects, including a profound sense of euphoria. Opioids increase the amount of dopamine in the dopamine reward system (mesolimbic system).

Sedative-Related Disorders. The pathogenesis of sedatives is similar to alcohol. Sedatives increase the availability of the neurotransmitter, GABA, resulting in a generalized sedative effect on the brain.

Stimulant-Related Disorders. Stimulants increase the availability of the neurotransmitter, glutamate, in the brain resulting in excitation and increased activity. Many stimulants act similar to monoamine neurotransmitters (e.g., dopamine, norepinephrine), enhancing the influence of dopamine on the dopamine-reward system. Methamphetamine has toxic effects on dopamine axon terminals.

Tobacco-Related Disorders. Tobacco is one of the most addictive agents, with even greater development of dependence than cocaine and heroin. The active substance in tobacco products is nicotine, a mild stimulant. Brain imaging studies of addicted smokers suggest that nicotine leads to a rapid increase in dopamine levels, promoting further nicotine use.[6] Persons who smoke have an increased risk of lung cancer, chronic obstructive pulmonary disease (emphysema), and bronchial conditions as the result of the tar in cigarette smoke. Carbon monoxide in the smoke increases the risk of cardiovascular disease. The presence of certain genes involved may predispose individuals to both alcohol dependence and habitual tobacco use.[185]

Clinical Manifestations

The clinical manifestations of substance use and addictive disorders can be found in Table 3-11. Additional substance-specific details are described below

Alcohol-Related Disorders. Individuals with alcohol-use disorder are likely to drink in one of three patterns: (1) regular binge drinking (e.g., college students on "Thursday Bar Night" or the weekend drinker), (2) consistent heavy drinking, or (3) occasional heavy binge drinking interspersed with periods of no drinking. Drowsiness, perceptual changes, and motor impairments (e.g., decreased balance, coordination, reaction and movement time) result in restricting participation in social/occupational/leisure roles. These impairments also lead to an increased incidence of MVAs (40% of all MVAs) and a large percentage of accidents that occur on the job.[237] Drug seeking behaviors can further restrict participation and social behavior may revolve around either drinking or avoidance of drinking.

Alcoholism is extremely prevalent yet underdiagnosed among adults with symptomatic terminal cancer.[28] Binge drinking (more than six drinks at a time for men or four drinks for women) has also been identified as a risk factor for all strokes.[477] Alcohol withdrawal usually begins 3–36 hours after the last drink and may be accompanied by behavioral manifestations or physiologic complications such as electrolyte disorders, dehydration, polyneuropathy, or myopathy.[145]

Individuals with more advanced physiologic effects of chronic alcohol abuse may be impaired cognitively from Wernicke-Korsakoff syndrome. Wernicke-Korsakoff syndrome is a well-described syndrome of neurologic and cognitive problems that comprises both Wernicke encephalopathy and Korsakoff syndrome. When Wernicke encephalopathy is undiagnosed or inadequately treated, it can progress to Korsakoff syndrome (also known as Korsakoff dementia).[491]

Wernicke encephalopathy is an acute neuropsychiatric disorder caused by thiamine deficiency to the brain. Korsakoff syndrome is a consequence of chronic thiamine deficiency from malnutrition that often accompanies chronic alcohol abuse. Signs and symptoms of the neurotoxicity associated with Wernicke encephalopathy include impairment in memory formation and "confabulation" (making up information), gait ataxia (loss of coordination), ophthalmoplegia (eye paralysis), and confusion. The symptoms of Korsakoff alcohol neurotoxicity present as amnesia, blackouts, apathy (low or flat affect), and poor executive brain function (decision making, organization of thought, logic).[221,288]

Caffeine-Related Disorders. Caffeine is the most common behaviorally active drug that can result in physical dependence. The most common source of dietary caffeine is coffee, with average consumption around 200 mg/day; soda pop and energy drinks are a common and growing source. High daily doses of caffeine in excess of the equivalent of 5 cups of coffee may increase the chance of miscarriage or fetal growth retardation, although it is possible that some of this risk is a result of confounders such as cigarette smoking and alcohol use.[251]

Cannabis-Related Disorders. The intensity of these effects tends to be perceived as less pervasive than other classes of substances, for example, opioids and stimulants. Consequently, the impact of cannabis use on activities of daily living and on participation in social/occupational/ leisure activities is of less consequence. Significant impact on function is correlated with long-term, frequent use and may lead to lethargy and lack of motivation.[524] Marijuana has been used medically to treat nausea associated with chemotherapy and for persons with intractable pain. The use and regulation of marijuana for medicinal purposes is controversial.

Hallucinogenic-Related Disorders. These drugs result in an experience of an altered perception of the environment. Hallucinogens may be experienced positively but negative experiences ("a bad trip") are not uncommon. Individuals often experiment with these drugs and then either quit or progress to other drugs.

Inhalant-Related Disorders. The variety of substances that may be inhaled is large—paint, gasoline, glue, nail polish, hair spray, lighter fluid, and more. Inhalants are more likely to be used by children and teens than any other groups.

Opioid-Related Disorders. This is a particularly addictive class of drugs. The person's experience of opioids tends to be calming, relaxing, and antidepressive, resulting in a feeling of euphoria but also followed quickly by lethargy. Continued and increased use of opioids is often an attempt to avoid the signs and symptoms of withdrawal. Use of opioids often severely impacts activities and participation in occupational/leisure/social roles. Costs (social and financial) to maintain use of opioids is high. Consequently, the individual is more likely to turn to criminal activity to support the habit.

Sedative-Related Disorders. Similar to alcohol, drowsiness, perceptual changes and motor impairments (e.g., decreased balance, coordination, reaction and movement time) result in restricting participation in social/ occupational/leisure roles. These impairments also lead to an increased incidence of MVAs. Drug seeking behaviors can further restrict participation and social behavior focuses on drug use.

Stimulant-Related Disorders. There are two patterns of use: (1) frequent, habitual use and (2) binge use. The half-life of these substances tends to be short, leading to frequent cravings to regain the heightened psychologic state. Irritability can be pronounced and interfere with interpersonal relationships. Use disorders may include prescription drugs that were initially legitimately prescribed or purely illicit

drugs such as cocaine. Methamphetamine is also known as "speed" or "crystal" when it is swallowed or sniffed, "crank" when it is injected, and "ice" or "glass" when it is smoked. Addiction is often immediate with the first methamphetamine use—as opposed to a longer period of use required to become addicted to some of the other illicit drugs. Hyperthermia and convulsions can result in death.

Tobacco-Related Disorders. Nicotine addiction requires daily use of tobacco products to maintain nicotine levels in the brain, primarily to avoid withdrawal but also to modulate mood. Regular tobacco users exhibit altered levels of stress, arousal, and impulsivity.[61] Nicotine dependence is the single most common psychiatric diagnosis in the United States. Substance abuse, major depression, and anxiety disorders are the most prevalent psychiatric comorbid conditions associated with nicotine dependence.

Smokeless (chew) tobacco can lead to nicotine addiction and long-term use can lead to health problems including periodontal disease. Chronic use of any tobacco products can lead to cancer and cerebrovascular and cardiovascular disease as long-term consequences. There is a known link between active smoking and cervical cancer; a similar association likely exists between passive smoke exposure and cervical carcinogenesis.[503] The Surgeon General's report on the consequences of involuntary exposure to tobacco smoke reports the following major conclusions[84]:

- Secondhand smoke causes premature death in children and adults who do not smoke.
- Children exposed to secondhand smoke are at an increased risk for sudden infant death syndrome, acute respiratory infections, ear problems, anxiety and depression,[47] and more-severe asthma;
- Exposure of adults to secondhand smoke has immediate adverse effects on the cardiovascular system and causes coronary heart disease and lung cancer.

Driving and Substance Use/Intoxication. In addition to alcohol, marijuana and benzodiazepines impair driving performance. New users of opioid analgesics likely have impaired driving skills. Alcohol is the most common drug associated with fatally injured drivers, followed by marijuana, cocaine, benzodiazepines, and amphetamines.[237] Combining alcohol with other drugs and the use of multiple drugs increase the overall risk for crashes.[237]

MEDICAL MANAGEMENT

DIAGNOSIS. Diagnosis of Substance Use and Addictive Disorders is made primarily through examination, particularly a thorough history, identification of the various signs and symptoms of substance use, intoxication, and withdrawal (see Table 3-11), and appropriate questionnaires. The DSM-5[18] delineates the criteria that must be met to diagnose the individual disorders. A thorough physical examination is also required to rule out medical conditions that may mimic substance use, to measure levels of substances in the body, and to identify comorbid medical conditions. In older adults, slowed response, hypersomnia, and increasing confusion are sometimes thought to relate to aging when actually they are symptoms of toxic drug levels. Signs and symptoms of withdrawal may not be readily diagnosed in older adults.

Prevention is the key to any successful substance abuse program. The American Medical Association has released guidelines recommending that all people older than age 60 years be screened and treated for substance abuse problems.

TREATMENT. Substance abuse can be characterized as a psychologic condition, a medical condition, or a combination of both. From a substance recovery perspective, a biopsychosocial approach is most common and effective. Interventions include education, counseling, CBT, behavior modification, and for many substances, pharmacologic help. Success depends on the individual's desire to correct the problem and adherence with treatment regimens.

A mindfulness-based intervention called *urge surging* has been developed for calming, curbing, or extinguishing cravings. This behavioral approach relies on the idea that urges for addictive substances or activities rarely last very long and can be used to deal with the internal struggle that feeds cravings. This approach may not initially reduce urges but may change the response to such thoughts.[71] More specific information about this technique is available online at: http://www.mindfulness.org.au/urge-surfing-relapse-prevention/.

Detoxification is required in many cases of substance use resulting in withdrawal symptoms. This may need to be an inpatient, medically controlled process to protect the individual.

Alcohol-Related Disorders. Treatment may occur in outpatient, intensive outpatient or inpatient settings. Treatment may be one-to-one or in a group setting. Twelve-step programs (e.g., AA, Celebrate Recovery), which combine a social and spiritual approach, seem to be effective for many.[146] Other psychosocial approaches include cognitive behavior and motivational enhancement therapies. Pharmacologic interventions include SSRIs (e.g., sertraline),[389a] naltrexone and nalmefene, which block opioid receptors thus diminishing the pleasurable effects, in turn decreasing cravings,[333a,421] and disulfiram (Antabuse), which causes nausea when alcohol is consumed.[302] Detoxification may take 2 to 7 days depending on severity of use. Prevention of relapse is a key component of intervention.[542]

Cannabis-Related Disorders. There is a lack of evidence for the success of specific treatment regimens. As in other substance-related disorders a biopsychosocial approach may be most effective. Many users of cannabis quit of their own accord after a period of experimentation.

Hallucinogenic-Related Disorders. Most individuals use hallucinogenic drugs as a temporary experiment, often stopping after having a negative experience.

Opioid-Related Disorders. Tolerance to opioids develops quickly and withdrawal symptoms are difficult and can be fatal. Discontinuation of severe opioid use may take multiple days and often is done "cold-turkey" (all at once) in a medically supervised inpatient facility. Intensive outpatient therapy, including CBT, 12-step programs, and other psychosocial approaches, may be helpful. Pharmacologic interventions (e.g., naloxone, buprenorphine) are sometimes used in conjunction with psychologic and behavioral approaches.

Sedative-Related Disorders. Withdrawal from sedatives can be complicated by the *kindling* phenomenon. This is a neurologic condition in which withdrawal symptoms magnify with each subsequent withdrawal attempt and become very severe, including seizures.

Stimulant-Related Disorders. The pleasurable aspects of the "high" (euphoric feelings) make it difficult to be motivated to discontinue use. A multimodal approach is likely necessary, combining behavioral, psychologic, and pharmacologic interventions. Treatment is further complicated by the social nature of stimulant drugs.[542]

Tobacco-Related Disorders. Of the estimated 48 million adult smokers in the United States, approximately 16 million attempt to stop smoking cigarettes for at least 24 hours annually; another 2-3 million attempt to stop but cannot abstain for 24 hours. CBT and pharmacologic interventions for any tobacco addiction, including smokeless tobacco, increase the success rates.[131] However, 1.2 million people stop smoking each year, often without the behavioral and pharmacologic aids. Pharmacologically assisted quit attempts per year jumped from 1–2 million to approximately 7 million, corresponding with the availability of nicotine gum and the nicotine patch as nonprescription products. Nonnicotine medications include antidepressants and drugs that interfere with nicotine receptors. Pharmacologic interventions double the success rates. All health care workers are encouraged to recommend smoking cessation to all clients while providing appropriate treatment referral and support.[91,94,391] See further discussion of the role of physical therapists in smoking cessation in *Special Implications* following this section.

PROGNOSIS. Substance abuse is associated with child and spousal abuse; sexually transmitted diseases, including HIV infection; teen pregnancy; school failure; motor vehicle crashes; mental health conditions; escalation of health care costs; low worker productivity; and homelessness. Individual characteristics, length and severity of use, and support networks all impact the prognosis.

Alcohol-Related Disorders. Treatment for alcohol abuse is a life-long process, either as an active alcoholic (currently drinking) or a recovering alcoholic (currently not drinking). The prognosis is good for those whom a biopsychosocial approach aligns with their values and personality. Chronic alcohol use/intoxication is correlated with increased incidence of liver damage, cognitive impairments, peripheral neuropathy, chronic pancreatitis, cardiomyopathy, and certain cancers (e.g., upper respiratory, gastrointestinal, breast, pancreatic).[265,487,556] Excessive alcohol consumption kills approximately 75,000 people each year in the United States.[498] Alcohol-related deaths outnumber deaths related to other drugs 4 to 1, and alcohol is a factor in more than half of all domestic violence and sexual assault cases.[350]

Pregnant women are advised to avoid alcohol because no safe level has been identified. Even as little as 1 drink per day has been shown to cause teratogenic effects (i.e., consequences of consuming harmful substances) in offspring. Drinking early in pregnancy and binge drinking are associated with the greatest risk. The most severe consequence associated with alcohol use during pregnancy is fetal alcohol syndrome. Research suggests that the destruction of millions of neurons in the developing human brain could explain the reduced brain mass and associated dysfunction.[216]

Cannabis-Related Disorders. Long-term use has been correlated with cognitive changes and decreased motivation. For some individuals, this is a gateway drug (i.e., first drug used that leads to the experimentation and use of other, often more potent, substances).

Hallucinogenic-Related Disorder. Long-term abuse of hallucinogenic drugs is not common. PCP, often manufactured in home laboratories, can result in brain impairments, even with minimal use. Persons high on PCPs can also experience rage, psychotic episodes and/or suicidal ideation.

Inhalant-Related Disorders. Use is often temporary; death can occur the first time an inhalant is used.

Opioid-Related Disorders. It is difficult to discontinue opioid use and craving for the effects of the drug is strong. Comorbid personality, adjustment or psychotic conditions, as in cocaine use, complicate an individual's ability to successfully recover from opioid use.[278] Overdose and death from heroin intoxication is of particular concern. The prognosis for recovery from opioid use is more positive for those who use the drugs recreationally, that is, less consistently.

Stimulant-Related Disorders. Successful treatment is difficult to achieve because of the highly addictive nature of these drugs and frequent cravings.[3] There is a high rate of relapse/recidivism. Recovery is more difficult for individuals who have been diagnosed with a MDD or with alcohol and drug dependency. These individuals who are dual diagnosed are using stimulants to self-medicate, making successful treatment more difficult.[278]

Tobacco-Related Disorders. The use of tobacco products continues to be the single most preventable cause of disease and death in the United States. Smoking results in more deaths each year in the United States than AIDS, alcohol, cocaine, heroin, homicide, suicide, motor vehicle crashes, and fires combined.

Smoking harms nearly every organ of the body, damaging the smoker's overall health even when it does not cause a specific illness.[85] Smoking has been linked conclusively to acute myeloid leukemia and cancers of the cervix, kidney, pancreas, and stomach. Smoking is known to cause elevated blood pressure, pneumonia, abdominal aortic aneurysm, cataracts, and periodontitis. Smokers are at an increased risk of developing diabetes, heart disease,[156] major depression,[249] and suicide.[74] Smokers may be at increased risk of low back pain[7] as nicotine has been linked with accelerated disk degeneration.

Smoking impairs the normal processes of fibroblasts. In the lung, smoking slows fibroblast proliferation and makes fibroblasts less mobile, leading to slower repair of injured lung tissue.[341] Smoking also has a well-known negative effect on wound healing, bone graft incorporation, and pain reduction.[197] These last three effects are particularly important to some aspects of physical therapy practice. Smoking impairs the normal processes of fibroblasts. In the lung, smoking slows fibroblast proliferation and makes fibroblasts less mobile, leading to slower repair of injured lung tissue.[341]

SPECIAL IMPLICATIONS FOR THE THERAPIST 3-12

Substance Use and Addictive Disorders

Primary intervention or care for the chemically dependent person is essential. However, the realistic picture is more often one of a person who has a pattern of substance abuse and either denies the problem or admits failure in the past. For example, people who smoke or chew tobacco and have repeatedly tried to quit most commonly admit failure. Failure to stop or correct unhealthy habits when the person desires to do so often indicates that (1) the underlying need associated with the destructive behavior has not been addressed or (2) the person may need more equipping or support to attain and maintain the desired correction.

Many people who seek medical attention for seemingly unrelated conditions fail to disclose their use of alcohol or other drugs. Behavioral research shows that most excessive drinkers (79%) are insured and even have contact with health care professionals. Low screening rates among excessive drinkers may be more a matter of missed screening opportunities (i.e., failure of the health care professional to conduct a comprehensive screening examination).

As part of the assessment process, therapists using a systems approach can screen for the presence of chemical substances by asking about the use of prescribed drugs, nonprescription drugs, and self-prescribed drugs such as nicotine, caffeine, and alcohol or other drugs. Therapists must be alert to alcohol and other drug use and abuse. Recognition of the problem is crucial to successful patient/client management. Because physical therapists generally spend more time with patients/clients than many other health professionals, they may be the ones best able to recognize substance abuse that would be hidden from those who spend less time with the client or who do not have the skills to recognize impairments of the cognitive or motor systems.

It may be helpful to assess the behavioral impact of substance abuse by asking one or more of the following questions:

- *When is it that you feel you need these substances?*
- *How do these activities help you?*
- *Are you concerned about your dependence?*
- *Do you have a pattern of cutting back or stopping the use of alcohol, cigarettes/tobacco, sleeping aids, or other substance but then restarting it?*
- *Have you been concerned or has anyone around you raised concern about your use of these substances?*

An appropriate final question may be "Because it is important to the results of your treatment, do you take (use) any drugs or substances that you have not told me about yet?"

The National Council on Alcoholism and Drug Dependence (http://www.ncadd.org or (800) NCA-CALL) has a self-test available for assessing the signs of alcoholism. If the client reports the use of substances, the therapist may want to ask whether the person has discussed this with his or her physician or other health care personnel. Encourage the client to seek medical attention, or inform the individual that this will be addressed as a medical problem in your communication with the physician.

The physical therapist can take the approach that this situation is no different from a case of undiagnosed or untreated angina, high blood pressure, cataracts, or other health problem that can be treated. The client's health is impaired by the use and abuse of substances, and therapy will not be effective as long as the person is under the influence of chemicals.

In the acute care setting, it is estimated that one in five patients suffers from an alcohol use disorder (abuse or dependence)[384] and may be at risk for the adverse effects of alcohol withdrawal, a potentially life-threatening condition. Signs and symptoms of alcohol withdrawal syndrome, such as hand tremors, headaches, palpitations, diaphoresis, anxiety, insomnia, motor hyperactivity, nausea or vomiting, and transient hallucinations or illusions, can be easy to miss or attribute to adverse effects of medications.[109,136,519]

With all inpatients, especially including the spinal cord injury and TBI population, the therapist must be alert to any suspicious signs or symptoms of substance abuse (see Table 3-11). More than half of all people with spinal cord injury or TBI incurred their disabilities while under the influence of drugs or alcohol; some studies report as much as 80%. It is estimated that two-thirds of people with disabilities who abuse drugs and/or alcohol did so before their injury, and many turn to substance use afterward to cope with life changes caused by the disability. Medical professionals should also be observant for excessive sleeping and unusual symptoms, such as muscular inflammation and myopathies, which can occur with the use of street drugs.

The Clinical Institute Withdrawal of Alcohol Scale (CIWA)[473] is an assessment tool used to monitor alcohol withdrawal symptoms. Although it is used primarily to determine the need for medication, it can provide the therapist with an indication of stability level when determining patient safety before initiating physical therapy. The assessment requires about 5 minutes to administer and is available online with no copyright restrictions. A CIWA score greater than zero suggests the individual is still detoxing, and therefore will still need some time. If the score equals zero, then physical therapy intervention may be appropriate to address any residual impairments.

Substance abuse can impair or slow the rehabilitation process, especially delaying wound healing. The client using any substances discussed in this section should be encouraged to reduce (eliminate if possible) intake of these chemicals during the rehabilitation process. Not only will the healing process accelerate but levels of perceived pain can also be reduced when these substances are eliminated. Of course, as with any addiction, this type of approach has a limited appeal and limited success. And individuals with more advanced physiologic effects of chronic alcohol abuse impaired cognitively from Wernicke encephalopathy and/or Korsakoff syndrome are often unable to shift their thinking from apathy to motivation.

Interaction of Alcohol with Prescription and Nonprescription Drugs

The therapist should be aware of potential hazards of treating anyone who appears to have been consuming alcohol before coming to the treatment session. Physical therapists must know about all drugs clients are taking on a regular basis.

If the physical therapist suspects the client may be consuming alcohol in excessive amounts, remember that certain medications, both prescribed and nonprescription have the potential for adverse reactions when taken with alcohol. Many of these adverse interactions can have a serious, negative impact on the physical therapy plan of care. Many medications, both prescription and nonprescription, contain significant percentages of alcohol. Some of the medications physical therapy clients may be taking (and their interaction with alcohol) are listed in Box 3-16.[510]

Tobacco

Tobacco use can be associated with several negative outcomes. For example, smoking may exacerbate circulatory problems leading to foot amputation in people with diabetes. This population generally has a lower oxygen supply to the lower extremities because they are subject to advanced atherosclerosis. Because good oxygen supply is required for wound healing in soft tissue, it is imperative that people with a history of diabetes and smoking, now presenting with pressure ulcers or other foot complications, receive adequate arterial blood supply to the lower extremities (see Chapters 10 and 11).

The detrimental effects of cigarette smoking on wound healing, ability to cope with pain, and peripheral circulation are well documented. Heavy smoking is commonly associated with chronic alcohol abuse, and both addictions have a negative influence on bone formation, probably the result of defective osteoblastosis. Women who smoke are at significantly higher risk of developing osteoporosis late in life and subsequent bone fractures compared with nonsmokers (see "Special Implications for the Therapist: Osteoporosis" in Chapter 24).

The relationship between smoking and pain has also been documented, including an association with the incidence and prevalence of back pain in all ages. A link between smoking and back pain in occupations requiring physical exertion was also established possibly as a result of smoking-related reduced-oxygen perfusion and malnutrition of tissues in or around the spine, causing these tissues to respond inefficiently to mechanical stresses.[140] Study findings may have implications for targeting at-risk groups for back care education or intervention programs.

The effects of tobacco use (see Table 3-11) have a direct impact on the client's ability to exercise and must be considered when starting a treatment intervention or exercise program. Smokers are more likely than nonsmokers to suffer fractures, sprains, and other physical injuries even at an early age; these detrimental effects of smoking on injuries appear to persist at least several weeks after cessation of smoking.

Box 3-16

INTERACTION OF ALCOHOL WITH PRESCRIPTION AND NONPRESCRIPTION DRUGS

Many medications, both prescription and nonprescription, have the potential for adverse reactions when taken with alcohol. Age is an additional risk factor as older adults are more likely to mix alcohol and other drugs.

Some of the more common medications physical therapy clients may be taking (and their interaction with alcohol) are presented here. With many new drugs developed each year, it is difficult to make sure such a list of this type is always current. Individuals can and should always consult with their physician or pharmacist for any specific medications prescribed.

Analgesics (e.g., aspirin [Percodan], acetaminophen [Darvocet, Datril, Tylenol] propoxyphene [Darvon]):
- May result in increased alcohol intoxication, excessive sedation, stomach and intestinal bleeding, also increased susceptibility to liver damage from acetaminophen. Affected individuals may fall asleep during treatment or have balance problems as a result of the apparent increased intoxication.
- Aspirin may increase the bioavailability of alcohol, increasing the effects of the alcohol. Chronic alcoholic ingestion activates enzymes that transform acetaminophen into liver-damaging chemicals. Even small amounts of acetaminophen with varying amounts of alcohol can have this harmful effect.

Antianxiety (e.g., benzodiazepines):
- Benzodiazepines are often used to treat anxiety and insomnia. The sedative effect of these medications is enhanced by alcohol ingestion. Severe drowsiness can result in household and MVAs. Older adults often have an increased response to these drugs and can experience impaired driving ability, breathing difficulties, and depressed cardiac function.

Antibiotics (e.g., furazolidone [Furoxone], griseofulvin [Grisactin], metronidazole [Flagyl], quinacrine [Atabrine]):
- The client may experience nausea, headache, possible convulsions, or respiratory paralysis. Some of these medications are rendered less effective by chronic alcohol use.
- The availability of antitubercular drugs such as isoniazid and rifampin used together to treat tuberculosis is decreased with alcohol consumption. The effectiveness of the medication is reduced. Older adults and homeless alcoholics are especially at risk for both tuberculosis and chronic use of alcohol.

Anticoagulants (e.g., warfarin [Coumadin], heparin):
- Acute alcohol consumption enhances anticoagulation, increasing the person's risk for life-threatening hemorrhages. The therapist must be alert to the effects of increased anticoagulation, such easy bruising, bleeding from any opening, and joint bleeds. Physical therapy interventions, such as soft-tissue mobilization, can result in more hemorrhage or bruising, and excessive bleeding may occur with sharp debridement.

Antidepressants (e.g., amitriptyline, doxepin, sertraline [Zoloft], paroxetine [Paxil], mirtazapine [Remeron], citalopram [Celexa], bupropion [Wellbutrin]):
- There are many commonly used psychiatric drugs affected by the ingestion of alcohol. Metabolism of these drugs is generally (but not always) delayed by alcohol. Alcohol increases the sedative effects of tricyclic antidepressants.
- Tyramine, a chemical found in some beers and wine interacts with some antidepressants (e.g., monoamine oxidase inhibitors) to cause dangerously elevated blood pressure.
- The combination of alcohol and amitriptyline results in a marked increase in body sway. The interaction between alcohol and antidepressants also is noted for adverse effects on psychomotor skills. The combination of alcohol and psychiatric drugs is often reported as a cause of death in accidental or nonaccidental (suicide) deaths.

Antidiabetics (e.g., metformin [Glucophage], tolbutamide [Orinase]):
- When oral hypoglycemic drugs used to help lower blood sugar levels are taken concurrent with alcohol consumption, increased antidiabetic effect or excessive low blood sugars may occur. Acute alcohol consumption prolongs, and chronic alcohol use decreases, the availability of Orinase. Alcohol also interacts with some oral hypoglycemics causing nausea and headache.
- The individual whose plan of care includes more vigorous physical activity may experience problems related to low blood sugar.

Antihistamines (e.g., all nonprescription asthma, hay fever, and cold remedies and nasal decongestants; acetaminophen [Actifed, Benadryl], carbinoxamine [Dimetane], dimenhydrinate [Dramamine], orphenadrine [Norflex], hydroxyzine [Vistaril]):
- When taken concurrent with alcohol consumption, the individual may experience increased interference with the central nervous system, increased sedation, reduced alertness, dizziness, or increased danger when operating machinery or autos, thus resulting in potential difficulties during an intervention session requiring alertness or fine motor skill.

Antihypertensives (e.g., methyldopa [Aldomet], chlorothiazide [Diuril], propranolol [Inderal], furosemide [Lasix], reserpine [Serpasil]):
- When taken concurrently with alcohol, increased blood pressure, orthostatic hypotension, or lowered effectiveness of some of these medications may occur. The client whose plan of care includes more vigorous physical activity may readily experience problems normally associated with uncontrolled hypertension, or lose consciousness while standing.

Antipsychotics (e.g., chlorpromazine [Thorazine]):
- Drugs used to diminish psychotic symptoms such as delusions and hallucinations can cause breathing problems, impaired, coordination, and liver damage when combined with alcohol.

Antispasmodics/Muscle Relaxants (e.g., cyclobenzaprine [Flexeril], diazepam [Valium], methocarbamol [Robaxin]):
- When taken concurrently with alcohol, muscle relaxants can cause increased drowsiness, blurred vision, rapid pulse, excessive sedation, or mental confusion. Physical therapy interventions that require alertness and cooperation on the part of the patient or client may be compromised.

Cardiovascular (e.g., nitroglycerin for angina and many antihypertension medications):
- Alcohol consumption with many of the medications prescribed to treat cardiac and vascular problems can cause orthostatic hypotension accompanied by dizziness and fainting. Chronic alcohol use decreased the availability of some drugs (e.g., propranolol [Inderal]) used to treat high blood pressure. Monitoring vital signs is important.

Narcotic Pain Relievers (e.g., meperidine [Demerol], propoxyphene [Darvon], morphine and morphine derivatives, codeine, oxycodone [OxyContin]):
- When taken concurrent with alcohol consumption, dangerous depression of autonomic nervous system, increased intoxication, or excessive sedation may occur. Use of thermal agents may be contraindicated because of the potential for enhanced anesthetic effects of alcohol and excessive sedation.
- Coingestion of alcohol and long-acting opioids for chronic pain relief can accelerate release of the extended release capsules. This effect is called *dose dumping* and has resulted in removal of some drugs from the market. Serious side effects, such as respiratory depression, coma, and even death, have been reported and remain potential problems when alcohol is combined with other slow-release morphine-based opioids.

Sources: DiPiro JT, Talbert RL, Yee GC, et al, editors: *Pharmacotherapy. A pathophysiologic approach*, ed 8, New York, 2011, McGraw Hill; Brunton LL, Chabner BA, Knollmann BC, editors: *Goodman & Gilman's the pharmacological basis of therapeutics*, ed 12, New York, 2011, McGraw Hill; Micromedex Healthcare Series [Internet database]. Greenwood Village, CO, Thomson Reuters (Healthcare), updated periodically. From Drug Facts and Comparisons. *Facts & comparisons eAnswers* [online], 2012. Available from Wolters Kluwer Health, Inc.

All of the adverse effects of tobacco need to be considered and discussed with women who are pregnant. Many lifestyle improvements occur when a woman and her family are expecting a child. Taking the time to educate your prenatal clients about the negative effects of smoking on fetal development, pain tolerance in labor/delivery, healing postpartum, and potential harm to her own body and family can have a significant positive impact.[553]

In addition to the overall effects of nicotine, inhaled nicotine has additional pulmonary effects. The combination of smoking and coffee ingestion raises the blood pressure of hypertensive clients about 15/33 mm Hg for as long as 2 hours,[159] requiring careful monitoring of vital signs during exercise.

Smoking Cessation

The tobacco industry is actively promoting product substitution (cigars, pipe smoking) and use as an alternative to complete cessation. The fact remains that cardiopulmonary function is compromised by these alternate sources of tobacco and life-years lost have been estimated at 5 years compared with cigarette smokers 7 years.[416] A clear need to increase the frequency of smoking cessation advice and counseling on the part of all health care providers for all tobacco users is evident.

Health care providers should offer culturally appropriate or tailored interventions for racial/ethnic populations as it has been reported that receiving advice to quit for racial/ethnic groups may be influenced by social or cultural factors. For example, among older Hispanic and Asian-American adults, language barriers may affect the lower rates of receiving advice to quit or in understanding the advice. To aid in counseling all individuals regarding smoking cessation, the APTA endorsed the Agency for Healthcare Policy and Research's *Clinical Practice Smoking Cessation Guideline.* This has been superseded by an updated Tobacco Cessation Guideline released by the Public Health Service and available at http://www.surgeongeneral.gov/tobacco/treating_tobacco_use08.pdf. The guidelines recommend that every client who smokes or uses tobacco products should be advised on the known dangers of tobacco use and increased success of smoking cessation programs.

The therapist is often in a unique position as the health care professional that the client feels most comfortable with and able to trust for supportive education. Unequivocally, quitting smoking reduces the risk of cancer, cardiovascular disease, and pulmonary disease caused by continued smoking.[123,391] Brief advice (as little as 5 minutes) has been shown to have a positive impact on attempts to quit and actual cessation.[554] Explaining some of the immediate and long-term benefits of smoking cessation may be helpful (Table 3-12), as well as discussing the effects of tobacco on the integumentary, musculoskeletal, and neuromuscular systems as outlined by Pigmataro.[391] Younger people benefit the most, but even those who are age 65 years or older can add years to their life by quitting.[485] *A Youth Tobacco Cessation Guideline*[96] and *Role of the Physical Therapist in*

Table 3-12	Benefits of Smoking Cessation
Time Since Last Cigarette	**Benefit**
20 min	Vital signs return to person's baseline normal level (blood pressure, pulse, temperature)
8 h	Oxygen levels increase; carbon monoxide levels decrease
1 day	Risk of myocardial infarction (heart attack) decreases
2 days	Increased ability to smell and taste; nerve endings begin repair
2 wk to 3 mo	Improve circulation and lung function; reduces shortness of breath, improved exercise capacity
1-9 mo	Cilia in lungs regenerate improving movement of secretions; reduced coughing and sinus congestion; decreased fatigue and increased energy levels
1 y	Risk of coronary heart disease reduced to one-half that of a smoker
5 y	Risk of lung cancer reduced by 50%; reduced risk of cerebrovascular accident (stroke); risk of oropharyngeal cancer (mouth, throat) reduced to one-half that of a smoker
10 y	Lung cancer death rate corresponds to nonsmoker's rate; risk of other tobacco-related cancers reduced
15 y	Risk of coronary heart disease equals that of a nonsmoker

Data from American Cancer Society, 2013 (http://www.cancer.org/).

Smoking Cessation[391] have also been published to help guide physical therapists in this type of counseling.

Whenever possible, clients who smoke should be encouraged to stop smoking or at least reduce tobacco use before surgery and when recovering from wounds, pressure ulcers, or injuries resulting from trauma (including surgery) or disease. The National Cancer Institute (800-4-CANCER) provides educational materials for health professionals that contain practical steps toward stopping smoking.

Smokers trying to quit may benefit from a medication approved by the Food and Drug Administration (FDA), either nicotine replacement therapy (gum, inhaler, nasal spray, or patch) or a nonnicotine pharmacologic aid (e.g., bupropion). The goal is to wean off of tobacco products and then to decrease and cease the use of pharmacologic aids. The American Cancer Society Quit For Life program can be reached by calling 866-784-8454.

Injection Drug Use

Injection drug use is associated with a high rate of skin and soft-tissue infections from the use of unsterile intravenous and subcutaneous injection (skin popping). This factor, combined with the presence of pathogenic microorganisms on the skin, results in a wide range of clinical problems from simple cellulitis and abscess to life-threatening necrotizing fasciitis and septic thrombophlebitis.

The clinical appearance of the skin is often atypical and subtle because of longstanding damage to the skin and to venous and lymphatic systems, resulting in underlying lymphedema, hyperpigmentation, scarring, and regional lymphadenopathy. The therapist may observe redness, warmth, and tenderness of inguinal or axillary lymph nodes. Skin ulcers resulting from skin popping consisting of low-grade foreign-body granulomatous inflammation and necrosis are common and easily become superinfected (coinfected with more than one virus at a time), requiring local wound care, occasionally requiring skin grafting.

Impaired Professionals

Substance (especially alcohol) abuse can be a real problem among our own profession at all levels including students, clinicians, researchers, educators, and administrators. Physical therapists should be able to recognize and deal with their colleagues who are abusing alcohol and other drugs. The following APTA position statement is directed toward the impaired professional[14]:

> The American Physical Therapy Association (APTA) recognizes the responsibility of the profession to meet the physical therapy needs of society; to promote the well-being of physical therapists, physical therapist assistants, and students; to uphold the ethical and legal responsibilities of the profession; and to follow the guidelines put forth in the APTA Board of Directors' document Peer Assistance/Impaired Provider Program. Physical therapists, physical therapist assistants, and students shall address the problems associated with alcohol and substance abuse within the profession.

APTA recognizes that alcoholism and other chemical dependencies are treatable diseases. Therefore, it is the duty of the physical therapist, the physical therapist assistant, and students to help themselves and their colleagues acknowledge that health and professional roles are adversely affected by these impairments.

Additionally, APTA believes that appropriate treatment should continue to be available for impaired physical therapy practitioners and their family members to facilitate re-entry of practitioners into the profession as accountable and reliable professionals. Reentry should occur when the well-being of the physical therapy practitioner and the patient/client are assured.

The practitioner's entry into the recovery process should be confidential and should be instituted in a nonpunitive manner. APTA seeks to create a supportive environment for impaired physical therapy practitioners in their recovery and thereby enhance the well-being of its members and the profession. APTA encourages chapters to advocate for the establishment of non-punitive programs for impaired practitioners.

A THERAPIST'S THOUGHTS*

Alcohol Withdrawal and Detoxification

Alcohol abuse is encountered in the acute care setting overtly and in more subtle ways. It is likely we will see more in combination with addiction to pills as the Baby Boom generation ages. Although physical therapy intervention is not advocated as a direct treatment when alcohol abuse is the primary problem, associated comorbidities, such as fractures, head trauma from falls, and chronic neurologic impairments, may need to be addressed. Often, these individuals are impulsive, unsteady, and unsafe when hospitalized and physical therapy receives a consult.

We have an in-patient detoxification unit and a very-well-established community rehabilitation program for alcoholics and addicts. The elderly alcoholics I see often suffer from alcoholic neuropathy or severe memory impairments secondary to Wernicke-Korsakoff syndrome (previously described in "Clinical Manifestations"). These individuals and their family members may benefit from education on how to accommodate to those impairments and may need an assistive device.

Some individuals have severe neurologic impairments from chronic addiction, so I may need to work on a safe plan for discharge. The plan may be for discharge to a shelter, which may not be the best option for them at the time.

Most of our inpatient rehabilitation programs won't take them because they don't have a "rehab" diagnosis, the programs don't want to deal with the addiction part of the person's rehab needs, or the programs are not equipped to do so. Sometimes I lobby for a day or two of "two hots and a cot," some good nutrition and rest. Then we work in physical therapy on some safety strategies and education, get them an assistive device, and off they go—hopefully detoxed and steadier.

I suggest that physical therapists meet addictions head on and explain to our patients/clients what neurologic problems can develop as a result of chronic addiction. They may nod and smile, and they may have heard it all before, but we do it with smokers, so why not these folk? Sometimes they need to be confronted with how they are being affected physically.

Safe is a tough word these days. Everyone in the hospital wants me to say a patient is "safe for discharge," but unsafe is not a reason in itself to stay in the hospital, which seems ironic to me. Often after detox, they are good to go, steady, and on their feet again. We really aren't needed to see them at that point if the impairments have cleared up. I have seen some very interesting neurologic impairments in individuals who abuse alcohol chronically and 2 days later—boom—all cleared up without physical therapy intervention.

The health care professional is cautioned against actively or passively encouraging the use of substances out of an attempt to normalize socialization or out of a sense of compassion or pity. This concept is termed *entitlement* and may take the form of endorsement, subtle agreement with the use of substances, or even active participation with the client (e.g., going out for a few drinks together, providing marijuana and getting "stoned" together).

The concept of moderation is acceptable for some people but for anyone with a past history or current use of substances, the best advice health care professionals can offer is to avoid all substances at all times. The risk of dangerous interactions with medications or further injury from the effects of these chemicals is too great to offer anything but abstinence as an acceptable treatment goal. Considering the predisposing conditions and needs of the client, it is the position of the health care professional to offer, train, and support the individual toward integration of healthy options.[553]

*Katesel Strimbeck, PT, MS.

Neurocognitive Disorders

Delirium

Overview. Delirium is a cluster of signs and symptoms rather than a specific disorder or disease. Delirium is an acute change in attention and in orientation to the environment that occurs suddenly, usually within hours to a few days.[18] Symptoms fluctuate throughout the day and tend to worsen late in the day (nocturnal delirium) or "sundowner's syndrome." Delirium can elicit fear and distressed emotions (e.g., fear, anxiety) in the client as well as the client's caregivers.[304] Older adults are at greater risk for delirium; 30% to 70% experienced delirium during a single hospital stay [157,314] Delirium associated with mechanical ventilation results in longer hospital stays and is correlated with significantly increased health care costs.[327]

Etiology and Pathogenesis. Delirium is a secondary complication of a wide variety of conditions, including serious medical illness, surgery, high fever, head trauma, medications (alone or interaction effects), organ failure (e.g., lung or liver), drug/substance withdrawal, mechanical ventilation, and treatment in a critical care unit, among others.[97,157,289] Exact mechanisms leading to delirium are not known but it is recognized as a global cerebral impairment without primary structural brain disease.[97] The impairment may be a global decrease in brain metabolism with impacts levels of neurotransmitters. Another theory is that high levels cortisol may impair brain function.

Delirium is a frequent complication of mechanical ventilation and admission to a critical unit. Contributing factors include a serious medical condition, immobilization, often complicated with restraints, bladder catheters, sleep deprivation, and loss of the circadian rhythm because of continuous light, noise and activity, and sensory overload characteristic of a critical care unit.[312,327]

Clinical Manifestations. Individuals experiencing delirium appear extremely confused and have poor attention as well as poor orientation to their environment. Attention impairments include inability to maintain or shift focus, distractibility, and poor short-term memory. Other impairments include difficulty with language (receptive speech, rambling or nonpurposeful speech, reading, writing and word-finding difficulties), disorientation (place, time and person), or hallucinations (visual are the most frequent).

MEDICAL MANAGEMENT

DIAGNOSIS. Diagnosis of delirium is made per the criteria listed in the DSM-5.[23] Examination and evaluation of a client with delirium focuses on identifying the underlying cause and ruling out life-threatening and other psychotic conditions. Comorbid conditions include cancer, malnutrition, dementia, major surgery, and polypharmacology.[157] Delirium in the intensive care or critical unit is considered a serious, yet underdiagnosed condition.[138]
TREATMENT. Treatment of the underlying condition(s) and modification of contributing factor is the primary intervention for delirium. Factors to be addressed include adequate nutrition and hydration, pain management, minimize use of restraint, maintain the day–night cycle,

and avoid overstimulation.[157] Sedatives (e.g., diazepam [Valium] or lorazepam [Ativan]) or antipsychotics, (e.g., haloperidol [Haldol], olanzapine [Zyprexa], risperidone [Risperdal]) may be required if the client is at risk of injuring him-/herself or others.[397]

There is growing evidence that using a holistic intervention that includes periodic interruption of sedation combined with early mobilization by physical therapists for mechanically ventilated clients results in fewer impairments and activity limitations, and better participation in social/occupational roles postdischarge, in addition to decreasing the cost of care.[72,259,327,445]
PROGNOSIS. Delirium is a temporary disorder that usually dissipates when the underlying conditions and factors are resolved. While the client has delirium, the symptoms may ebb and flow during the day, gradually becoming less prominent. Delirium may prolong critical care unit and overall hospital stay and cost; subacute or home care may be required to enable the transition to home.[157,327] Delirium, especially when it is persistent, results in poorer medical outcomes and increased morbidity.

Personality Disorders

Overview and Incidence

A personality disorder is a fixed and maladaptive interpersonal style that causes significant restriction of social and/ or occupational roles. Personality disorders include both a disordered personality (self and interpersonal) and pathologic personality traits. Personality disorders are distinct and separate from personality types. Some personality types may not blend well together and therefore create conflicts, but personality disorders do not blend with anything.

Individuals with personality disorders are unable to respond to various people and situations according to the demands of the moment but rather tend to respond in the same way, lacking the social, interpersonal, and life problem-solving tools that allow optimal flexibility in hectic or changing situations.

The proposed DSM-5[25] may reduce the number of personality disorders to likely to include: Borderline Personality Disorder (BPD), Obsessive-Compulsive Personality Disorder (OCPD), Avoidant Personality Disorder, Schizotypal Personality Disorder, Antisocial Personality Disorder (APD), and Narcissistic Personality Disorder (NPD).

Clinical Manifestations

Persons with BPD are known for a pervasive instability of identity, interpersonal relationships, and mood. They can be supportive and inviting one minute and vicious and attacking the next. They tend to be impulsive and reckless. Symptoms of BPD are varied and usually manifest in adolescence or early adulthood interfering with most (if not all) skills necessary for functional relationships.

Persons with OCPD identify their sense of worth through their work, are often perfectionists, and are rigid in their view of how things should be done. Persons with *avoidant personality disorder* have low self-esteem, are uncomfortable in social situations, overly sensitive to perceived criticism, and avoid interpersonal relationship for fear of rejection. A person with *schizotypal personality disorder* has difficulty with interpersonal relationships (e.g., lack of empathy) as well as exhibiting odd personality characteristics that interfere with relationships (e.g., odd beliefs, behaviors, thought processes, aversion to social contacts). APD (antisocial personality disorder) is characterized by a focus on self and personal gratification, lack of empathy, behaviors that include those that are hostile, deceitful, impulsive, and aggressive, and an absence of remorse for these behaviors. A person with NPD has grandiose behavior, being critical in the evaluation of others, and a lack of empathy. This person may have an exaggerated sense of self-importance, demanding special treatment with a sense of entitlement.

The 12-month prevalence of any personality disorder is 9.1% of the population. BPD occurs in 1.6% of the adult population, APD in 5.2%, and antisocial in 1.0% of the adult population.[183,275] BPD and OCPD are more common in women, whereas NPD and APD are more common in men.

Etiology and Pathogenesis

The etiology of the personality disorders is not well understood. Many of the personality disorders are thought to be learned behaviors in response to dysfunctional family relationships and/or childhood trauma, including sexual and physical abuse, particularly in BPD,[431] NPD, and avoidant personality disorder. BPD is the result of type A and type B traumas (discussed earlier in this chapter, "Effects of Trauma on Brain Development"), especially when occurring in childhood; 80% of physically and sexually abused victims demonstrate borderline personality symptoms.

A new model of BPD[316] presents this disorder as a result of dissociation and a lack of sense of self involving developmental, neurobiological, and behavioral factors. The Meares model emphasizes failure of synthesis among the elements of psychic life and points to the need for both personal and social development, integration of unconscious traumatic memory, affect regulation, and restoration of the self.[316]

There is some evidence that NPD may be found more often in older individuals, men, and in individualistic societies.[154] Genetics may be a factor in BPD[283] and APD.[516] Biologic factors have also been implicated in various personality disorders. Persons with BPD often have cognitive-perceptual impairments suggesting a central nervous system component. OCPD may have similar central nervous system involvement as OCD, and some consider it to be a mild form of OCD—perhaps part of a continuum, rather than a distinct disorder.[149] Structural brain changes have been recorded in persons with APD, including decreased gray matter in the prefrontal cortex and the right superior temporal gyrus and decreased size of the amygdale and hippocampus.[530,549]

MEDICAL MANAGEMENT

DIAGNOSIS. Psychiatrists, other physicians, psychologists, or trained counselors/licensed social workers can make the diagnosis. They rely on history and clinical presentation, particularly focusing on disordered personality traits involving the self and/or interactions and specific pathologic personality traits. Observed traits and behaviors are evaluated by the criteria established by the American Psychiatric Association.

TREATMENT[305]. Medical management of personality disorders requires a collaborative alliance between the health care provider and the client that makes restoration of function (rather than elimination of symptoms) the goal of treatment. Accordingly, the treatment approach may vary depending on the clinical presentation and client profile, and may require periodic inpatient treatment. Psychotherapeutic approaches are the primary interventions for individuals with personality disorders. CBT is commonly used. Training, education and structuring the environment may be helpful. Psychoactive medications may be used to treat comorbid conditions.

Dialectic behavior therapy is another psychotherapeutic approach. The aim of dialectic behavior therapy is to help individuals with BPD replace maladaptive behaviors with skillful behavior. This type of therapy helps the individual learn to regulate emotions, tolerate distress, self-manage, and be more effective with other people. Increasing skills use can be a mechanism of change for suicidal behavior, depression, and anger control.[362] Meares offers a three-stage neurobiologic treatment model that may be of interest to those working with individuals with this disorder.[316]

The following are examples of treatment techniques used to help reduce symptoms such as impulsive behavior and unstable relationships:

- Behavior therapy that helps the person feel cared about and understood.
- Short-term, structured time in the hospital for self-inflicting injuries, such as self-cutting, self-burning (self-mutilating activities), or suicide attempts.
- Learning healthy ways to cope when under stress (e.g., what to do besides self-mutilation).
- Day treatment programs, including structured activities and group therapy every day.
- Medication, especially for symptoms of anxiety, panic, depression, or mood swings.
- Treatment for any alcohol or drug abuse problems.

PROGNOSIS. The natural course of personality disorders varies, but each tends to be stable across time and context. Impact on activities and participation in social/leisure and occupational roles varies with the severity and type of personality disorder. BPD and antisocial behavior disorder are particularly difficult to treat. Depression is associated with several personality disorders and persons with BPD are more likely to attempt suicide.[256]

SPECIAL IMPLICATIONS FOR THE THERAPIST   3-13

Personality Disorders

Personality disorders cannot be "fixed" but rather should be approached by the therapist with an eye toward the therapist's own personal health, while providing sensitive care and accepting the client without bias or resistance. This can be accomplished through self-awareness and understanding of the disorder involved. The healthy, sensitive, and insightful therapist who offers consistent professional help in the therapist's area of expertise will fare well. Progressively, the client learns from the clinician's ability to appropriately respond to emotional changes while upholding healthy boundaries. The therapist should be familiar with specific strategies for dealing with personality disorders.[543]

People with BPD have stormy and unpredictable ways of relating to other people. This behavior covers up poor self-esteem and feelings of anger and of not deserving anything good. BPD impacts the person's ways of thinking, feeling, and behaving, which causes many problems, socially and medically. BPD can impact medical care in the following ways:

- *Passive-aggressive behaviors (the clinician is great/awful)*
- *Playing one caregiver against another and manipulating to prevent accountability*
- *Poor compliance in self-care and appointment times*
- *As people reconnect with feelings, expect to see an increased urgency to regress in cognitive, emotional, and behavioral areas*
- *Misunderstanding of instructions, relationships, boundaries*
- *Prolonged treatment time required because of nonphysical triggering and the development of extensive, subtle physical symptoms*
- *Self-persecution and egocentric perspective ("I caused it, it's my fault")*
- *Insurance challenges as a result of complexity of diagnoses/failed care*

Healing is accomplished as the healthy clinician works with the individual diagnosed with BPD in the same way as with any other person suffering from brain injury. As the caregiver practices sensitive care, within individual client tolerances, and remains true to self through whatever the client presents, the individual with BPD benefits from consistent right and left hemisphere messages from the healthy provider.[438,539,540]

Other Disorders

Suicidal Behavior Disorder

Overview and Incidence. This is a new diagnostic category for inclusion in the DSM-5. Suicide is by far the most devastating outcome of depression; however, people who are not clinically depressed also commit suicide. In addition, there are many people with significant major depressive and other disorders who do not end their lives.

In 2012, suicide was the 10th leading cause of death in people age 10 years and older; more than 38,000 deaths are attributed to suicide each year.[11,92a] The suicide rates vary by race/ethnicity, age, and gender. Non-Hispanic whites and American Indians/Alaskan Natives had the highest suicide rates (15.99 and 17.4/100,000, respectively). Until 2006 persons age 65 years and older had the highest suicide rate; from 2006 to 2009 persons between 25 and 65 years of age had the highest rate. In 2007, suicide was the third leading cause of death for those individuals between the ages of 15 and 24 years.[360] Males consistently have a higher suicide rate than females, white

(non-Hispanic) males older than the age of 85 years had a suicide rate of 47/100,000, the highest rate in the United States (mean of 11.3 for the general population). The overall suicide rate has been rising since 2000.[92a,360]

Most people (approximately 90%) who kill themselves have a treatable mental disorder but do not seek medical care[11] because of social stigma or financial limitations. Many who do see a physician are misdiagnosed. New research in the area of the biologic basis for depression and suicide may result in better care and fewer deaths in the future.

Etiology, Pathogenesis, and Risk Factors. Great progress has been made in identifying the clinical, genetic, social, and biochemical factors that contribute to suicidal behavior. Positron emission tomography is now being used to pinpoint biologic markers commonly found in people who are at greatest risk of attempting or completing suicide.[291,292] These imaging studies show impaired metabolic activity in the prefrontal cortex of the brains of people who have attempted suicide, compared with depressed individuals who have not attempted suicide. The prefrontal cortex is the area of the brain involved in mood regulation. An important factor in setting an individual's threshold for acting on suicidal impulses is brain serotonergic function; serotonin is the neurotransmitter that keeps impulsive and aggressive behaviors in balance. Although the signaling and functional roles of serotonin have been implicated in the psychopathology of suicide, the exact physiologic phenomenon remains unknown. Fewer serotonin transporter sites with local reduction of serotonin binding may be associated with the predisposition to act on suicidal thoughts.[290,291]

People who are both impulsive or aggressive and depressed have a much higher likelihood of attempting suicide. Studies continue to examine the relationship of these (and other) variables. Box 3-17 lists the risk factors for suicide. Many have a depressive illness that their

---

Box 3-17

RISK FACTORS FOR SUICIDE

- Past history of attempted suicide
- Suicidal ideation, talking about suicide, determining a suicide method
- Mood disorders or mental illness:
  - Clinical depression, especially manic depressive illness
  - Schizophrenia
  - Personality disorders, especially borderline and antisocial
- Chronic alcohol and other drug abuse
- Comorbidities (chronic pain and nonpsychiatric conditions)
- Circumstantial risk factors: stressful life events
- Exposure to suicide or suicidal behavior, especially in adolescents and young adults
- Genetic predisposition/family history of suicidal behaviors
- Decreased levels of serotonin
- Availability of firearms (most common method of completed suicide)
- Gender (males are 5 times more likely to commit suicide)
- Age (younger than age 40 years or older than age 65 years; risk increases 5x in white males older than age 80 years)

Data from the American Foundation for Suicide Prevention, New York, 2013 (http://www.afsp.org; [888] 333-AFSP).

doctors are not aware of, even though many of these suicide victims visit their doctors within 1 month of their deaths.[56,360] Half of all successful suicide victims were described by family or friends as being depressed or suffering some other mental health problem just before their death.[386] Suicidal mass murders currently on the rise in the United States are theorized to be part of a suicide wish on the part of the perpetrator.[280]

Substance use is implicated in half of all cases tested.[238] Psychoactive drugs, specifically antidepressants, may increase the risk of suicide, particularly in adolescents and young adults.[188] Males are five times more likely to take their own lives, and suicide rates are highest for people younger than age 25 years and for white men older than age 80 years. Chronic medical illness in older adults has been linked with increased rates of suicide. The risk is greatly increased in individuals with multiple illnesses.[235]

Older adults do not necessarily attempt suicide more often than younger people. Instead they are more likely to succeed when they make an attempt. They are more likely to use a lethal method (e.g., gun) and less likely to tell anyone their intentions, compared to younger people. Older adults living alone are less likely to be found in time to be saved.

Although some risk factors are the same as for adults, additional risk factors for children include the loss or death of a family member or close friend, traumatic experiences such as physical or sexual abuse, and being bullied.[304]

Warning Signs of Suicide. Warning signs of suicide, such as mood changes (e.g., irritability, sadness, difficulty getting along with others); loss of interest in family, work, or social activities; and significant changes in sleep pattern or appetite are common signs of depression serious enough to lead to suicide (see Box 3-6). Suicide threats or previous suicide attempts, and even statements revealing a desire to die, are other warning signs of suicide. Making final arrangements, giving away prized possessions, saying goodbye to friends and family, and purchasing a gun or collecting prescription drugs are red flag signs of suicide. There may be subtle or overt signs of acute distress, expressions of hopelessness about the future, or a desire to "end it all."

MEDICAL MANAGEMENT

PREVENTION. Focus on suicide prevention has increased in the last 10 years. The National Institute of Mental Health[353] and the American Foundation for Suicide Prevention[10] have a major focus on education, research, and health information related to depression and suicide. Other organizations with a focus on suicide prevention target specific groups.[225]

Age-appropriate tools to screen for depression are available. For example, the Center for the Advancement of Children's Mental Health at Columbia University has developed a Youth Depression Screening test.[106] The Geriatric Depression Scale can be used with older adults. It should be noted that for now the accuracy of methods to screen for high risk of suicide is unknown. Likewise, few studies have shown that screening reduces suicide attempts or mortality rates from suicide. More research is needed in this area.[510]

DIAGNOSIS AND TREATMENT. A physician will complete an physical examination, interview, and psychologic examination to identify or rule out potential causes of suicidal ideation. New diagnostic neuroimaging now offers an opportunity to visualize serotonin function in a more direct way than has previously been available. Although this technology may provide the possibility of timely therapeutic intervention in people at high risk for suicide, it is not available everywhere.

Major depression can be treated via counseling and trauma/stress resolution and/or pharmacologically, although it is often undertreated, even in the presence of a history of suicide attempt. Some suicide attempts may be preventable if depression is diagnosed early and treated adequately. The need for psychoeducation for health professionals and the public is evident.[544]

PROGNOSIS. Treatment with SSRIs brings complete resolution of depressive symptoms for up to half of the people taking these agents. In addition, there is a lower risk of fatal overdose or serious heart arrhythmia reported with SSRIs compared with other antidepressants. Despite earlier concerns, there is no convincing evidence that SSRIs are linked with higher rates of suicide; however, TCAs are the leading cause of death by overdose after illicit drugs.[172,229]

SPECIAL IMPLICATIONS FOR THE THERAPIST	3-14

Suicide

Treatment of depression does not change or alleviate symptoms immediately; most drugs used to treat depression require 4–6 weeks before a true mood-elevating effect is perceived. The physical symptoms of sleep and appetite disturbances, fatigue, and agitation are the first to improve with medication. Cognitive and emotional symptoms, such as low self-esteem, guilt, uncertainty, pessimism, and suicidal thoughts, resolve more slowly but benefit significantly from modifying the health care approach to process-orientation rather than goal-orientation.[438,553]

Side effects of antidepressant medications are common and may affect multiple systems (see Table 3-5). The therapist should be alert to any mention of these and encourage the affected person to continue taking the prescribed medications and to contact his or her physician before discontinuing or tapering dosage. Unpleasant side effects combined with the delay in attaining therapeutic effects of medication contribute to discontinuation of the drug prematurely. The therapist can offer some practical suggestions, such as an nonprescription artificial saliva spray for dry mouth; an education and prevention and management program for orthostatic hypotension (see "Postural Hypotension" in Chapter 12); or reduced caffeine intake for people experiencing tremor.

Although some severely depressed people lack the energy necessary to complete an impulsive act such as suicide, close observation is required during the early weeks of pharmacologic treatment. As energy is restored but before a stable elevation of mood is achieved, the individual is at increased risk for suicide.

All suicidal thoughts and acts must be taken seriously and responded to appropriately. Three-fourths of all suicide victims give some warning of their intentions to a friend or family member. Many older adults who commit suicide have contact with a health care professional (usually their primary care physician) in the month before killing themselves; 40% are in contact with their physicians sometime in the week before taking their own lives.[510]

Observe for changes in client mood such as calmness or tranquility in a formerly hostile, angry, or depressed client. Such a behavior change may be a prelude to a suicidal event. Comments such as, "I won't be seeing you again," or "My family would be better off without me" may be a form of suicidal communication. Developing a contract with the client and identifying when and who should be contacted, as well as the consequences of breaching the contract, may be helpful to the caring relationship and to treatment success.

Use the QPR for Suicide Prevention model to potentially save a life (Box 3-18). Do not hesitate to ask whether a person is considering suicide or even if the person has a plan or particular method in mind. Do not attempt to argue someone out of suicide; instead, let that person know that you care and understand and that depression can be treated. Avoid the temptation to offer reasons for living such as "You have so much to live for," "You have come so far to throw your life away," or "Your suicide will hurt your family; think about them."

People who are suicidal may also be manipulative; therefore all health care providers need to be aware of and manage their own feelings while empathizing with the client's point of view. When in doubt, report concerns to the appropriate resource (e.g., physician or counselor when one is involved).

The physical therapist should chart accurately anything the client says or does that might suggest a suicide threat. It is better to meet the required standard of care and err on the side of caution through documentation and the referral process.

In an acute crisis, do not leave the person alone. In addition, remove all potential objects that could be used for suicide. Get the person to the nearest emergency department—call 911 if necessary. A national suicide resource is available by calling 800-SUICIDE (800-784-2433) or 800-273-TALK (800-273-8255) while waiting for transportation or to talk to a counselor.

Chronic Pain Disorders

Overview

Chronic pain has been recognized as pain that persists past the normal time of tissue healing assumed to be more than 3 months.[324] Chronic pain can occur with a wide variety of musculoskeletal, neurologic, endocrine, and oncology diagnoses.[148] The progression of acute to chronic pain can result in more complex and devastating physical, psychologic, and socioeconomic sequelae than the original disease entity.[148] Box 3-19 lists the most common chronic pain conditions encountered by the physical therapist.

Chronic pain is associated with increased rates of depressive disorders[374] and suicidal tendencies.[407] The

---

> **Box 3-18**
>
> ### QPR FOR SUICIDE PREVENTION
>
> **Q**—Question the person about suicide. Do you have thoughts of suicide? *If yes*, do you have a suicide plan in mind? Tell me about your plan?
>
> Indirect questions:
> - Are you unhappy enough to wish you were dead?
> - Do you wish you could go to sleep and never wake up?
> - Have you ever wanted to stop living?
> - Do you feel your life is no longer worth living?
>
> **P**—Persuade the person to get help. Listen carefully. Offer to help by making a referral or accompany the person to get help.
>
> **R**—Refer for help. Contact the individual's physician, minister, rabbi, counselor, tribal leader, or call 1-800-SUICIDE (1-800-784-2433) for assistance in finding local agencies or services in your area.
>
> PLEASE NOTE: QPR is not intended as a form of counseling or prevention. It is a screening and prevention tool to help assess warning signs of suicide and potentially prevent a successful suicide. Asking questions about suicide does NOT increase the risk of suicide attempts or success.

> **Box 3-19**
>
> ### COMMON CHRONIC PAIN CONDITIONS
>
> - Arthritis
> - Persistent neck/back pain
> - Neuralgias
> - Peripheral neuropathies
> - Peripheral vascular disease
> - Causalgia
> - Chronic regional pain syndrome (formerly reflex sympathetic dystrophy)
> - Hyperesthesia
> - Myofascial pain syndrome
> - Fibromyalgia syndrome
> - Phantom limb pain
> - Cancer
> - Postoperative pain
> - Spinal stenosis

---

associated mental disorders may precede the pain disorder (and possibly predispose the individual to it), cooccur with the pain, or result from the pain.[17]

The International Association for the Study of Pain has proposed an updated system for categorizing chronic pain. This etiologic classification describes pain according to (1) anatomic region, (2) organ system, (3) temporal characteristics of pain and pattern of occurrence, (4) person's statement of intensity and time since onset of pain, and (5) etiologic factors. This five-axis system focuses primarily on the physical manifestations of pain but provides for comments on the psychologic factors on both the second axis where the involvement of a mental disorder can be coded and on the fifth axis where possible etiologic factors include psychophysiologic and psychologic components.[324]

Chronic pain disorders can occur at any age and are extremely common with some estimating that approximately one third of adults in the United States are influenced by chronic pain.[393] Thus far, the role of gender in chronic pain has been found to be less important than psychologic and behavioral responses to chronic pain condition such as coping mechanisms and strategies.[506]

Etiology

Chronic pain disorders can be psychologically based (SSD), the result of a general medical condition, or a mixture of both. Chronic pain may also be linked to psychologic trauma through memories of physical trauma, transference of psychologic distress, or by decreased immune responses and healing.[181]

An increasing number of studies now support the concept that spinal pain is commonly triggered by biopsychosocial factors that may influence prognosis,[368,475] transitioning from acute to chronic pain[281] and development of disability.[210,273,319,475] Among the most common general medical conditions associated with chronic pain are musculoskeletal conditions (e.g., disk herniation, osteoporosis, osteoarthritis or rheumatoid arthritis, myofascial syndromes), neuropathies (e.g., diabetic neuropathies, postherpetic neuralgia), and malignancies (e.g., metastatic lesions in bone, tumor infiltration of nerves).[17]

Chronic postoperative pain occurs after some procedures, such as tumor resection and subsequent regrowth anywhere in the body, tumor invasion of the chest wall, mastectomy with pain from interruption of the intercostobrachial nerve (branches from the brachial plexus to the thoracic region), surgical amputation followed by phantom limb pain, and chemotherapy when associated with neuropathies producing painful dysesthesias (abnormal sensations) of the feet and hands.

Physiologic, Psychologic, and Behavioral Responses to Chronic Pain

Behavioral, cognitive, and affective factors have direct effects on the report of pain, adaptation to pain, and response to treatment, as well as indirect effects by influencing sympathetic nervous system and neurochemical factors associated with nociception.[504,505] Physiologic responses to chronic pain depend in part on the amount of time pain is experienced (e.g., low back pain, migraine headache). Intermittent pain produces a physiologic response similar to that of acute pain, whereas persistent pain allows for physiologic adaptation (e.g., normal heart rate, blood pressure, and respiratory rate) but can result in detrimental chronic cortisol release.[433]

The extent of pain is not directly associated with the extent of physical pathology. People report pain in the absence of physical pathology and individuals demonstrate objective physical pathology without symptoms. Individuals with chronic pain are less able to discriminate muscle tension and sensory stimulus levels compared with control subjects without pain symptoms. Biologic factors may initiate and maintain physical symptoms, whereas psychosocial factors influence pain perception.[174] The reproduction of pain is also complex and direct association between impairments and disability is not always consistent.

Chronic anxiety and depression (see sections on anxiety and depression) may produce heightened irritability, overreaction to stimuli, and a heightened awareness of symptoms. The person may become preoccupied with the details of anatomic function and how each movement or external event affects the symptoms. This self-focus should be redirected toward improving function. The focus on chronic pain differs from the overdramatization of the discomfort that is sometimes common in certain cultures.

The presence of chronic pain can be associated with significant behavioral and psychologic changes that are accompanied by neural changes similar to those found in PTSD. Women with chronic pelvic pain related to endometriosis have been found to demonstrate decreased gray matter volume in the areas of the brain associated with pain perception.[34]

The extent of pain symptoms is important to evaluate to distinguish if painful symptoms are disproportionate to the injury or are inconsistent with the objective findings which may indicate systemic disease or a psychogenic pain disorder. Chronic pain syndrome is characterized by multiple complaints, excessive preoccupation with pain or physical symptoms, and, often, excessive pain medication or substance abuse, but underlying physical causes of pain always need to be ruled out. There are cases in which chronic pain occurs and a diagnosis is elusive (e.g., spinal stenosis or thyroiditis). In those cases, treatment is specific to the identified underlying cause and not simply a program of pain management.

People with chronic pain often are depressed, have sleep disturbances, and may become preoccupied with the pain. The person exhibiting symptoms of a chronic pain syndrome may isolate himself or herself socially from other people and be fatigued, tense, fearful, and depressed. A constellation of life changes that produce altered behavior and persists even after the cause of the pain has been eradicated are characteristics of chronic pain syndrome. They may attempt to maintain their former lifestyle to appear as normal as possible, even engaging in activities that exacerbate their painful symptoms. They may not report the full extent of their pain, for fear of being labeled a complainer, mentally ill, or a hypochondriac. The need to hide the pain may conflict with the need to have someone understand the pain. The result is emotional and all conflicts.

Fear-Avoidance Behavior

Fear-avoidance behaviors can also be a part of disability from chronic pain. The Fear-Avoidance Model of Exaggerated Pain Perception was first introduced in the early 1980s.[277,455] The concept is based on studies that show a person's fear of pain (not physical impairments) is the most important factor in how he or she responds to low back pain.

Fear of pain commonly leads to avoiding physical or social activities. Screening for fear-avoidance behaviors can be done using the Fear-Avoidance Beliefs Questionnaire (FABQ).[522] Elevated fear-avoidance beliefs are indicative of someone who has a poor prognosis for rehabilitation. They indicate psychosocial involvement, provide insight into the prognosis, and indicate the need to modify intervention with consideration for referral to a psychologist or behavioral counselor.

When the client shows signs of fear-avoidance beliefs, then the therapist's management approach should include education that addresses the client's fear and avoidance behavior, while considering a graded approach to therapeutic exercise.[169] The therapist can teach clients about the difference between pain and tissue injury. Chronic ongoing pain does not mean continued tissue injury is taking place. This common misconception can result in movement avoidance behaviors.

Symptom Magnification Syndrome

Symptom magnification syndrome is defined as a self-destructive, socially reinforced behavioral response pattern. Individuals who magnify symptoms allow symptoms to negatively influence their QOL. This disorder is not listed in the DSM-5, although it is possibly a variant of SSD. Conscious symptom magnification is referred to as malingering, whereas unconscious symptom magnification is labeled illness behavior or somatoform disorder.[295]

The following signs indicate symptom magnification: (1) Reported symptoms are excessive while activities are still possible. (2) The client acts as if the future cannot be controlled because of the presence of symptoms and limitations are blamed on symptoms: "My (back) pain won't let me...." (3) The client may exaggerate limitations beyond those that are reasonable in relation to the injury; they apply minimal effort on maximum performance tasks and overreact to loading during objective examination.[295]

Identification of symptom magnification has focused on screening for less than full effort performance during a functional capacity evaluation. Most methods of identification are not significant predictors of the syndrome and even the best methods frequently lead to misclassification.[296] Again, these symptoms can easily be associated with unresolved trauma and the related psychologic needs.

MEDICAL MANAGEMENT

Considering recent research discussing the impact of perception on pain and psychosocial impact on medical care, it may seem overwhelming to ferret out and attend to all of your client's physical and psychologic contributing factors. Remember that medical management and healing is a process wherein the client and provider(s) need to take one small step at a time—together. Addressing the client's basic developmental needs through sensitive care while treating the presenting physical complaints is a very effective and consistent way of caring for the whole person.[508,553]

DIAGNOSIS. The clinical evaluation of pain currently involves identification or diagnosis of the primary disease/etiologic factors considered responsible for producing/initiating the pain; placing the individual within a broad pain category, typically nociceptive, inflammatory, or neuropathic pain; and then identifying the anatomic distribution, quality, and intensity of pain. Although identifying the disease is essential, especially when disease-modifying treatment is possible (e.g., acute herpes zoster, diabetes, tumor), the vast majority of people with persistent or chronic pain have irreversible disease or pathology (e.g., peripheral/segmental nerve lesions, brachial avulsion, spinal cord injury, poststroke central pain).[545]

There is still some discussion about how to label normal but less helpful psychologic reactions to injury compared to psychopathology such as depression and PTSD. Nicholas et al[368] suggest that yellow flags are those psychologic reactions that are amenable to change by trained health care providers, such as the belief that pain implies damage, while the more-severe symptoms are labeled as orange flags, which require referral to a mental health specialist.[368] Valid criteria for assessing malingering and symptom embellishment do not exist, thereby requiring careful clinical judgment on the part of the physician and all other health care professionals.[490]

PROGNOSIS. A wide range of variability exists in the course of chronic pain. The identification of "yellow flags" or psychologic prognostic factors is possible and have been suggested to lead to better results than not addressing the identified issues[368]; however, questions related to appropriate interventions, timing, and skills required for treatment have yet to be answered.

One of the strongest prognostic factors for persistent symptoms in individuals with low back pain is depression.[112] In a large study of 20 psychosocial prognostic factors, self-efficacy, perception of personal control, catastrophizing, and illness identity were independently predictive of long-term disability.[155] Although most research has focused on establishing if psychosocial factors are predictive of prognosis, fewer studies have established if these factors can be targeted for treatment intentions or as mediators of outcomes.[203]

Prognostic factors predict outcome based on initial levels, while mediators can change to influence outcome.[203] In an intervention study using CBT for individuals with chronic temporomandibular pain, improvements in activity interference, pain, and limitations with jaw use explained the most changes in the patients' perceptions of their ability to control their pain (mediator); self-efficacy also contributed to positive outcomes.[507] The Fear-Avoidance Model of Exaggerated Pain Perception was first introduced in the early 1980s.[277,455] Individuals who exhibit an excessive fear of pain that leads to avoidance of movement or activity have been shown to have poor outcomes postinjury, postsurgery, or with rehabilitation. Fear of pain commonly leads to avoiding physical or social activities.

SPECIAL IMPLICATIONS FOR THE THERAPIST   3-15

Chronic Pain Disorders

- *It is counterproductive to speculate on whether the client's pain is real. Pain is real to the person, and working with the client to develop mutually acceptable goals and improving functional outcomes should be the focus of treatment rather than on reducing the pain alone.*
- *The cornerstone of a unified approach to chronic pain syndrome is a comprehensive behavioral program. Whenever possible, the physical therapist should reinforce the behavioral approaches used by the other members of the team. Box 3-20 outlines some general guidelines.*
- *A more extensive social history can be used to assess the client's recent life stressors and history of depression,*

drug, or alcohol abuse. Pain may lead to inactivity and social isolation, which in turn can lead to additional psychologic problems (e.g., depression) and a reduction in physical endurance results in fatigue and additional pain.

- *The FABQ[177,522] can be useful to indicate clients who have high fear avoidance and indicate the need to modify intervention choices and consider referral to a psychologist or behavioral counselor. The work subscale of the FABQ is the strongest predictor of work status. There is a greater likelihood of return-to-work for scores less than 30 and less likelihood of return-to-work or increased risk of prolonged work restrictions for scores greater than 34.[163]*

- *Screening for depression in patients with chronic pain related to musculoskeletal diagnoses can be conducted using a brief 2 question screening tool using yes or no responses from the Primary Care Evaluation of Mental Disorders Procedure: (1) "During the past month, have you often been bothered by feeling down, depressed or hopeless?" (2) "During the past month, have you often been bothered by little interest or pleasure in doing things?"[190]*

- *Management approaches could include education that addresses the client's fear and avoidance behavior, and a graded approach to therapeutic exercise.[169] The exact relationship of fear-avoidance behavior as a predictor or how to progressively increase movement is still to be determined.[203] However, cognitive-behavioral interventions designed to decrease the influence of pain on function, such as understanding the extent of their injury and that chronic pain does not mean continued tissue injury is taking place, has been found to be useful for improving understanding, addressing pain-related anxiety, and catastrophizing.[5,293,368] This common misconception can result in movement avoidance behaviors.*

- *Treatment progress feedback is useful for clients and may prompt joint problem solving and education that will influence exploring pain behavior or other factors influencing the patient's/client's perceptions, including self-control and self-efficacy.[194,507]*

Box 3-20

BEHAVIORAL GOALS AND GUIDELINES FOR CHRONIC PAIN

- Identify and eliminate pain reinforcers.
- Decrease drug use.
- Use positive reinforcers that shift the focus from pain.
- Concentrate on abilities, not disabilities.
- Avoid the concept of cure; concentrate on control of pain and improved function.
- Avoid discussion of pain except as arranged by the team (e.g., only during monthly reevaluation, only with a designated team member).
- Use a home program to focus on function and functional outcome (e.g., self-help tasks within capabilities).
- The client should keep a log of accomplishments so that progress can be measured and remembered.
- Measure success by what the individual client can accomplish, not based on others' success or expectations.
- Take one day at a time. Direct energy toward solving today's problems rather than focusing on the future.
- Avoid negative reinforcers such as sympathy and attention to symptoms, especially pain.
- Encourage tolerance to increasing activity levels.
- Gradual progress is better than quick results with increased symptoms.
- Teach the client how and when to ask for and accept help when necessary. Do not offer help or yield to the demands of someone who does not need help.

REFERENCES

To enhance this text and add value for the reader, all references are included on the companion Evolve site that accompanies this textbook. The reader can view the reference source and access it online whenever possible.

CHAPTER 4

Environmental and Occupational Medicine

LYNZIE SCHULTE

INTRODUCTION

Environmental medicine is a broad term that encompasses industrial and occupational medicine and environmentally induced illnesses and conditions. It is used throughout this chapter to refer to all three branches of study. Environmental medicine and a separate branch of medicine called *clinical ecology* both study the results of interaction between humans and the environment. *Occupational medicine* is a specialty involving the health of workers and workplaces and can be considered a special form of environmental medicine.

Clinical ecology encompasses little-understood health disorders and chronically fluctuating illnesses mainly attributed by clinical medicine to psychosomatic complaints. Considerable polarization occurs over the issues of environment-related illnesses. People affected by environment-related illnesses consider themselves victims of medical ignorance, and the medical community is skeptical of the physiologic basis for the often numerous and vague symptoms described.

The *environment* is defined as all agents outside the body, including infectious organisms, toxins, and food. Intrinsic factors include the genetic makeup of the host and the individual's underlying state of health and history of past illnesses. Cell injury and resultant disease result from interplay of the environment and these intrinsic factors when the host defenses are overcome. Whether at home, in the workplace, or in the community at large, chemical, physical, biologic, psychosocial-spiritual, and traumatic hazards exist.

Usually the focus of environmental medicine is on chemical and physical hazards in the environment. Many diseases, disorders, and defects (contact dermatitis, obstructive lung disease, nephropathy, neuropathy, autoimmune disorders, various cancers, and birth defects are a few examples) occur when the body is exposed to some agent or stressor in the environment.

Industrial, occupational, and environmental illnesses, injuries, and diseases widely affect the population. Hazardous waste sites, nuclear energy leaks, contaminated drinking water, low-level exposures to untested chemical compounds, and repeated exposure to electromagnetic waves and secondhand smoke are examples of problems the American public continues to face. However, it should be noted that in comparison to all the possible hazards listed, morbidity and mortality from the voluntary intake of tobacco smoke, alcohol, and illicit psychoactive drugs far exceed effects from all other environmental hazards combined.

Molecular Epidemiology

Another area of research called *molecular epidemiology* is specifically aimed at measuring biologic effects and the influence of individual susceptibility to carcinogens and mutagens. Completed in 2003, the Human Genome Project (a 13-year project) has increased genetic and population-based association studies focused on identifying underlying susceptibility genes and contributions from gene–environment interaction to common complex diseases.

Exposure to environmental contaminants can now be measured using biomarkers such as metabolites in urine, chromosomal aberrations, mutations in specific genes, or deoxyribonucleic acid (DNA) measure of exposure to hydrocarbons or tobacco smoke. Biomonitoring involves looking for "pollution in people" by testing bodily substances, usually blood and urine, for the presence of harmful substances such as dioxins, polychlorinated biphenyls, and DDT.

Epidemiologic studies support the use of chromosomal breakage as a relevant biomarker of neurodegenerative disorders, cancer, diabetes, cardiovascular and inflammatory diseases as well as aging.[179] For example, particulate air pollution can cause damage to DNA and eating fruits and vegetables or ingesting antioxidants may be able to reduce the breakage and initiate repair.[127]

Regulation of Environmental Health Care

Multiple agencies exist for the investigation and regulation of environmental health care. The National Institute for Occupational Safety and Health is the federal research agency that conducts studies to develop safety and health standards. It does not have legal authority to adopt or enforce regulations.

The Occupational Safety and Health Administration (OSHA) is the primary regulatory agency that determines which of the standards proposed by the National Institute for Occupational Safety and Health are adopted and

122

enforced. Its standards are law throughout the United States, and its compliance officers can inspect the workplace at any time to determine the status of health and safety.

Risk assessment used by the Environmental Protection Agency (EPA) in regulating new chemicals determines how much harm is acceptable to human health, animals, or the environment. For example, risk assessment can determine how much hormone or pesticide residue is allowed in food, how much of a toxic substance can be discharged into a river, and how much pollutant can be released as automobile exhaust. Based on evaluation by a risk assessor, it is determined what type of current or future consequence there will be from human or ecological exposure. Some scientists are advocating an alternative to this type of risk assessment by asking whether this toxin is necessary instead of how much is safe.[100]

Applying a precautionary principle and questioning whether a new substance is needed requires the industry to find alternatives when there is evidence of damage to the environment. For example, the industry did find an alternative to chlorofluorocarbons when damage to the ozone was identified. Many countries around the world have already established this approach by offering financial incentives for organic farming, resisting importation of beef treated with growth hormones, and seeking alternatives to new chemicals.

ENVIRONMENTAL MEDICINE

Definition and Overview

Environmental medicine takes into account risk factors in the environment and human health and how they interact with one another. The environment exposes individuals to numerous physical, biological, and chemical agents and can create concern for a person's health and well-being.

In 2010, there was close to 3.1 million nonfatal workplace injuries and illnesses reported in the private sector, making the incidence rate 350 cases per 10,000 full-time workers. The number of nonfatal occupational illness cases accounted for 5.1% of those 3.1 million injuries and illnesses with an incidence rate of 18.1 per 10,000 full-time workers.[225] It has also been estimated that there are as many as 100,000 deaths from occupational diseases each year.

It is likely that because of the difficulty of diagnosis and the likelihood that occupational illness claims will be disputed by employers, these figures are most likely gross underestimates of the true incidence of environmentally induced illnesses. An estimated 23% of preventable illnesses worldwide and 16% of preventable illnesses in the United States can be attributed to poor environmental quality.[89] Air pollution alone is estimated to cost $40 to $50 billion in health-related costs annually (preterm birth, infant mortality, diabetes, or lung disorders, including asthma).

The Clean Air Act of 1970, which was last amended in 1990, requires the EPA to set National Ambient Air Quality Standards for pollutants considered harmful to public health and the environment. This Act established two types of national air quality standards. *Primary standards* set limits to protect public health, including the health of sensitive subgroups such as children, older adults, and anyone with conditions such as asthma or chronic obstructive pulmonary disease. *Secondary standards* set limits to protect public welfare, crops, vegetation, and buildings.[232] These standards are reviewed and revised every 5 years and include a very thorough review of scientific information.

The federal government continues to propose stricter standards for particulates with the latest standards set in 2013. Particulates are pollutants that are a mixture of solid particles and liquid droplets that are found in the air. Some can be seen by the naked eye, whereas others require microscopes to see. Primary particles are emitted from a direct source including construction sites, unpaved roads, fields, smokestacks, and fires while secondary particles come from reactions of chemicals in the atmosphere.[232]

Effects of Environmental Contaminants on Children

Children especially are more likely to be adversely affected by environmental contaminants. Children are born with immature nervous, respiratory, reproductive, and immune systems. They absorb a greater proportion of substances through their intestinal tract and lungs and detoxify and excrete toxins differently than adults. Children are outdoors more often, engage in hand-to-mouth activity, and often play in the dirt or on the floor or carpet, which places them closer to the source of many pollutants. Studies are looking at exposure of children from disadvantaged, low-income neighborhoods and have found that these children are at the high end of exposure to environmental contaminants compared to national averages. These include pesticides, metals, tobacco smoke, and other chemicals.[197]

The EPA has established an Office of Child Care Protection to increase its studies on the welfare of children in its environment. Researchers are investigating the possible causal relationship between environmental exposure and the increased incidence of childhood onset of asthma, lead exposure, childhood cancers, and developmental disabilities including mental retardation, autism, and attention deficit disorders.

Polybrominated diphenyl ethers (PBDEs) are flame retardants that have been added to a multitude of products to reduce flammability. In America, 97% of the population has detectable levels in their blood. There are more than 200 different formulas of PBDEs with the pentaBDE, octaBDE, and decaBDE formulas being banned for use in several U.S. states, including California. PBDEs have been found in breast milk samples from around the world, including both the northern and southern hemispheres, indicating this chemical has become a worldwide pollutant. Studies are looking at the effect of PBDEs on fertility in women and have found initial evidence of decreased fecundability (the probability that conception will occur in a given population of couples during a specific time period); with those women who have increased levels of PBDEs requiring increased time to conceive.[77,98,110,198,219,260]

Bisphenol A (BPA) is a chemical that is widely used in the production of polycarbonate plastics and epoxy resins. They have been used in food and drink packaging including baby bottles, water bottles, safety equipment and medical devices as well as food cans, bottle tops, and water supply pipes. BPA is poorly soluble in water and can leach out of materials readily, especially if put through repeated wear and tear and heating. In their 2003–2004 National Health and Nutrition Examination Survey, the Centers for Disease Control and Prevention (CDC) found that out of 2517 urine samples gathered, 93% of them had detectable levels of BPA.[151] The Environmental Working Group collected and analyzed the blood of 10 umbilical cords from minority infants born between the years 2007 and 2008. They were able to identify up to 232 industrial compounds and pollutants and BPA was detected in nine out of ten of the cords.[76] In 2005, the EWG looked at 10 umbilical cord samples from babies born in U.S. hospitals and found 287 industrial chemicals and pollutants. The blood harbored pesticides, chemicals from nonstick cooking pans and plastic wrap, long-banned polychlorinated biphenyls, and wastes from burning coal, gasoline, and garbage. These studies confirm that the placenta does not shield cord blood and the baby from chemicals and pollutants.[106] As a result of this study, there has been a call for more publicly funded studies of the impact of chemical exposure to children and biomonitoring of exposure to environmental contaminants throughout the life span. The National Children's Study established in 2000 is examining the effects of environmental influences on the health and development of more than 100,000 children across the United States, following them from before birth until age 21. The goal of the study is to improve the health and well-being of children.[18,149] Results of the study are available online at www.nationalchildrensstudy.gov.

Etiologic Factors

Chemical (organic and inorganic), physical, and biologic agents that can be considered environmental hazards are numerous (Box 4-1). Despite the many restrictions on industries placed by the EPA, according to the Toxic Release Inventory (TRI), the increased number of polluters in the United States (and worldwide) and underreporting practices have resulted in the release of more toxic chemicals into the environment each year. The TRI is a publicly available EPA database that contains information on more than 650 toxic chemical releases and other waste management activities reported annually by some industry groups, as well as federal facilities.[239]

These agents, combined with psychosocial factors, can lower the body's resistance, making a person more susceptible to infectious diseases. Only chemical and physical agents are discussed here; biologic agents are discussed in Chapter 7; behavioral, social, and lifestyle factors are presented in Chapter 2; and psychosocial-spiritual factors are discussed in Chapter 3.

Chemical Agents

Chemical agents can be classified by use (e.g., agricultural chemicals, automotive products, pharmaceutical agents, cleaning agents, paints, dyes, or explosives); mechanism of action (e.g., enzyme disruption, metabolic poison,

---

Box 4-1

ENVIRONMENTAL HAZARDOUS AGENTS

Chemical Agents

- Pollution or occupational exposure
  - Air (carbon monoxide, smog, radon, acid rain, tobacco smoke, household cleaning products, sick building syndrome; see text for others)
  - Water (industrial chemicals, pesticides, disease)
  - Food (pesticide residues, hormone residues, irradiation, genetic modification, food additives, preservatives)
  - Soil contamination
- Asbestos
- Manmade minerals
- Aging polyvinyl chloride (PVC) (e.g., dolls, toys)
- Fire and pyrolysis products
- Heavy metals
- Waste
  - Solid waste
  - Hazardous waste
  - Incinerator waste
  - Medical/infectious waste

Physical Agents

- Electromagnetic fields
- Vibration
- Heat stress
- High-altitude and aerospace medicine
- Mechanical factors
  - Cumulative or repetitive trauma
  - Accidents/injury
- Noise

Biologic Agents

- Bacteria
- Viruses
- Allergens
- Fungi (molds)
- Parasites

Psychosocial-Spiritual Factors (see Chapters 2 and 3)

---

irritants, or free radical formation); and target organ(s) (e.g., neurotoxins, hepatotoxins, or cardiotoxins). Although many toxic effects can occur, they can be broken down into three main categories: local acute effects, systemic effects, and idiosyncratic (unpredictable) effects.

Air Pollution. Many investigations of home and workplace environments have clearly documented the role of air pollutants in causing health complaints and disease. Although exposure to air pollution is classified separately as indoor and outdoor, the concept of total personal exposure whether exposure occurs in the home, office, outdoors, in a car, in a movie theater, and so on is relevant to every individual. Anecdotal evidence and statistical studies have made a correlation between pollution and a variety of diseases, particularly asthma, heart disease, respiratory disorders, and cancer and can cause damage to the brain, nervous system, liver and kidneys. Short term effects of air pollution can cause eye, nose and throat irritation, upper respiratory infections, headaches, nausea and allergic reactions.

People considered especially susceptible to air pollution include the elderly, the very young, pregnant

Table 4-1	New Air Quality Index	
Air Quality Index Levels of Health Concern	**Numerical Value**	**Meaning**
Good	0–50	Air quality is considered satisfactory, and air pollution poses little or no risk.
Moderate	51–100	Air quality is acceptable; however, for some pollutants, there may be a moderate health concern for a very small number of people who are unusually sensitive to air pollution.
Unhealthy for sensitive groups	101–150	Members of sensitive groups may experience health effects. The general public is not likely to be affected.
Unhealthy	151–200	Everyone may begin to experience health effects; members of sensitive groups may experience more serious health effects.
Very unhealthy	201–300	Health alert; everyone may experience more serious health effects.
Hazardous	>300	Health warnings of emergency conditions. The entire population is more likely to be affected.

The air quality index shows how clean or polluted the air is in a specific geographical area. The higher the index number, the greater the level of air pollution and the greater the health concern. The index number is based on the number of harmful particles in the air on any specific day (or time). You can access this information at www.airnow.gov.

From AirNow: Today's AQI forecast. Available at www.airnow.gov.

women, cigarette smokers (or those exposed to secondhand smoke), people with heart disease, asthma, or lung disease including chronic obstructive pulmonary disease, emphysema, or chronic bronchitis.

Increased rates of heart attacks and other cardiovascular events are reported with increased exposure to air pollution for individuals with known heart and blood vessel disease. Fine particulate matter that travels directly into the bloodstream, constricting arteries, is considered to be the mechanism for this effect.[35,36] It has been found that there is an increase in hospital admissions for cardiovascular diagnoses on the days there is an increase in elemental carbon in the air and an increase in admissions for respiratory diagnoses on the days there is an increase in organic carbon matter in the air. This increase in air pollution containing elemental carbon and organic carbon matter comes primarily from vehicle emissions, diesel, and wood burning.[164] The prevalence of diabetes has also been shown to increase with long-term exposure to fine particulate matter. In other words, air pollution may be an emerging risk factor for diabetes.[12,163]

Indoor Air Pollution. Other sources of indoor air pollution include tobacco smoke; fireplaces; space heaters; stoves; pilot lights; gas ranges; mothballs; cleaning fluids; glues; photocopiers; formaldehyde in foam, glues, plywood, particleboard, carpet backing, and fabrics; and infectious and allergic agents such as dust mites, cockroaches, bacteria, fungi, viruses, and pollen. Toxic chemicals found in every home, from drain cleaners to furniture polish, are three times more likely to cause respiratory distress than airborne pollutants.

The National Pollution Control Center estimates that the average home has approximately 62 different chemicals and that more than 2 million poisonings involving children age 6 and younger occur every year in the United States. Another 2 million poisonings are for those older than 6, which results in the poison centers answering a phone call every 8 seconds.

Construction and architectural modifications introduced in the 1970s as a result of the worldwide energy crisis have resulted in better insulated and tighter buildings with reduced ventilation. Illnesses that develop from indoor air pollution in tight, energy-efficient homes and buildings with poor ventilation and reduced air-exchange rates are known as *sick building syndrome* or *building-related illness*. The EPA has created an Indoor AirPLUS program to help home builders distinguish themselves as being able to offer a home with improved air quality.

Radon, a product of the breakdown of radium, poses an environmental risk because of its carcinogenic (especially lung cancer) properties. It is estimated to cause around 21,000 lung cancer deaths each year.[234] Radon comes from the natural breakdown of uranium in soil, rock, and water and can be found all over the United States. Exposure is predominantly naturally occurring rather than generated by human polluters and is present in poorly ventilated homes in the form of an odorless gas. Other sources include radioactive waste and underground mines; exposure to tobacco smoke multiplies the risk of concurrent exposure to radon.[56,124]

Outdoor Air Pollution. The Air Quality Index (AQI) reports daily air quality and says how clean or polluted the air is and the health effects that may be of concern based on breathing in that AQI level (Table 4-1). The EPA calculates the AQI based on five major air pollutants including ground-level ozone, particulate matter, carbon monoxide, sulfur dioxide, and nitrogen dioxide. The AQI runs from 0 to 500, the higher the number, the more pollutants that are present in the air and the more risk of health problems arising.

As part of the Clean Air Act of 1990, the EPA set air quality standards to protect sensitive population groups from outdoor air pollutants. The Clean Air Act regulates oxide emissions, making these particles less available to react with volatile organic compounds that form ozone. *Healthy People 2020* sets goals to improve the health of Americans by establishing science-based objectives that were last updated in 2010. These are 10-year objectives meant to increase length of life and quality of life and promoting good health. Included in these objectives are to reduce the number of days the AQI exceeds 100 (in 2008, 11 days exceed 100 and the goal for 2020 is 10 days) and to reduce the air toxic emissions from mobile sources such as cars (from 1.8 million tons reported in 2005 to 1.0 million tons in 2020).[100]

Preliminary research on pollutants indicates that biofiltration technology used to clean up airborne waste stream removes 94% of the total hazardous air pollutants. Studies are showing that biofilters and biotrickling filters are effective in treating waste air and have the potential to reduce the amount of overall toxicity and carcinogens in waste air.[85,111]

Carbon monoxide (CO), an odorless, tasteless, and colorless gas, is a common environmental pollutant from automobile exhaust emissions; the use of liquefied petroleum gas (LPG)–powered forklifts in inadequately ventilated warehouses and production facilities; fires; and home heating systems. CO is responsible for around 15,000 emergency department visits and roughly 500 deaths annually in the United States. CO exposures typically occur between November and February and those most often affected live in the Midwest or the Northeast. Inexpensive CO-monitoring devices have helped identify many previously undetected cases of high levels of CO in private homes.

CO is commonly recognized for its toxicologic characteristics, especially central nervous system (CNS) and cardiovascular effects. CO combines 240 times more quickly with hemoglobin (or myoglobin affecting muscles) than oxygen, so when carbon dioxide is bound to hemoglobin, its oxygen-carrying capacity is decreased. In the presence of CO, oxygen is not released normally by the blood, resulting in tissue hypoxia.

Tissue hypoxia has serious functional consequences for organ systems that require a continuous supply of oxygen such as the brain and the heart. Exposure to CO also causes impaired visual acuity, headache, nausea, vomiting, fatigue, seizures, behavioral change, and ataxia. In addition, when tissue partial pressure of oxygen is low, CO binds to intracellular hemoproteins, such as myoglobin, inhibiting their function and thereby affecting muscle function.

More severe CO poisoning can produce metabolic acidosis, pulmonary edema, coma, and death. The classic clinical findings of cherry-red lips and nail bed cyanosis caused by the bright-red color of carboxyhemoglobin may occur if its concentration is above 40%, but this is rarely observed.

Other air pollutants include *smog*, a combination of smoke and fog that develops when vehicle emissions and exhaust fumes containing nitrous oxides and hydrocarbons are photochemically oxidized. Ozone and nitrogen, the components of smog, result from the action of sunlight on the products of vehicular internal combustion engines. Both of these by-products are toxic to the respiratory tract, damaging ciliated endothelial cells lining bronchioles and impairing the mucociliary clearance mechanism.

New technology is aimed at reducing smog, including roof tiles that are "smog-eating." The EPA found that over 1 year, a 2000-square-foot roof with these tiles would destroy as much nitrogen oxide as that produced by a car driven 10,800 miles.

Growing evidence from around the world shows that the harmful effects of smog extend even to the unborn in utero. More than a dozen peer-reviewed studies in the United States, Brazil, Europe, Mexico, South Korea, and Taiwan have linked smog to low birth weight, premature births, stillbirths, and infant deaths. In the United States, research has documented ill effects on infants even in cities with modern pollution controls. Although this research shows a correlation between air quality and infant illnesses, it does not establish a conclusive cause–effect connection.[174]

Acid rain is an air pollutant that is caused by the interaction of sulfur dioxide and nitrogen oxides in the atmosphere that forms fine sulfate and nitrate particles. These materials come from sources such as volcanoes and decaying vegetation as well as man-made sources like emissions from fossil fuel combustion. The sulfur dioxide and nitrogen dioxide interaction is then transported by wind currents over long distances through the air. It is damaging to lakes, streams, and forests as well as all of the plants and animals that live there. Outdoor sulfate and nitrate particles can penetrate indoors and can be inhaled deep into the lungs. No known correlation exists between elevated levels of these fine particles and bronchoconstrictive disorders such as asthma, emphysema, and bronchitis.

A study that looked at the trends and effects of acid rain between 1984 and 2009 found that sulfite emissions dropped more than 50% and nitrate emissions dropped more than 30% over that time frame. Researchers believe this is due in part by the Clean Air Act of 1990 amendments that regulated emissions of these gases, which, when mixed with rain water, becomes sulfuric and nitric acid.[222] Although these numbers have continued to decline, acid rain is still an issue and tends to affect the Northeastern United States the greatest.

Outdoor air pollution has long been associated with clinically significant adverse health effects. The very young, very old, heavy smokers or those with preexisting lung disease are at increased risk in the presence of these toxins. Pollution from coal power plants in the United States results in 13,000 premature deaths, 20,000 heart attacks, and hundreds of thousands of asthma attacks annually. The cost of these health impacts exceeds $100 billion each year.[60] Although it is unclear whether outdoor air pollution contributes to the development of asthma, it does trigger asthma episodes.[1]

Water Pollution. Water pollution in the form of contamination of drinking water by toxic chemicals has become widely recognized as a public health issue since the late 1970s. Increased monitoring since then has shown that many pesticides and industrial chemicals can be detected in drinking water. The EPA, in conjunction with public health officials and the drinking water industry (e.g., Partnership for Safe Water), has worked diligently to survey and reduce waterborne-disease outbreaks, chemical contamination from leached industrial waste chemicals, and toxins released into recreational and drinking water.[20] From 1998 to 2005, there was a 4-billion-pound decrease in certain toxic chemicals in industrial waste, reducing the amount of waste materials by 16%.[240]

In 1996, the Safe Drinking Water Act was amended to require all community water systems to deliver an annual water quality report to their customers, including levels of any detected contaminants. The EPA has placed limits on the amount of certain contaminants in water provided by public water systems. Anyone with a private source of water (e.g., cistern or well water) does not come under this type of protection. The EPA has a list of possible water contaminants with their maximum contaminant level (MCL) based on primary drinking water regulations. These contaminants include microbial contaminants, such as viruses and bacteria, that come from sewage treatment plants, septic systems, agricultural livestock operations, and wildlife as well as inorganic contaminants, such as salts and metals, which may be present from urban storm water runoff, industrial or domestic wastewater discharges, oil and gas production, mining, or farming.

Pesticides and herbicides from a variety of sources (e.g., agriculture, urban storm water runoff, or residential uses) and organic chemical contaminants from by-products of industrial processes and petroleum production (including from gas stations) are additional source-water contaminants.

Some subgroups of people may be more vulnerable to contaminants in drinking water than the general population. Immunocompromised individuals, such as those with cancer who are undergoing treatment; organ transplant recipients; people with human immunodeficiency virus/acquired immunodeficiency syndrome (HIV/AIDS) or other immune system disorders; some older adults; and infants are at increased risk from infections.

Disinfection with chlorine is the most common method to ensure drinking water safety in the United States. A dramatic decline in waterborne diseases, such as cholera and typhoid fever, occurs when water systems are disinfected this way. One potential downside of this disinfectant treatment is the increased genotoxicity that occurs with water treatment. Ways to evaluate the toxicity and genotoxicity of disinfected drinking water are under investigation. A study looking at detection of a cholesterol lowering drug in U.S. wastewater found that water chlorination may increase the toxicity of pharmaceutically active compounds in surface water.[39]

A different form of water pollution has also raised concerns. Billions of gallons of treated sewage are released offshore into deep waters via long undersea pipelines called *outfalls*. Wastewater is filtered and processed, but many contaminants including estrogenic compounds and human pharmaceutical drugs remain and settle into ocean sediment, where they are consumed by bottom-feeding organisms that become food for other ocean life. Evidence of abnormalities in animals and fish exposed to sewage and industrial contaminants has been reported, but the effect on overall health and abundance of fish populations and the rest of the marine ecosystem remains unknown.[129,220]

In other areas of the United States, past abuses from mining thousands of tons of arsenic, copper, manganese, and other metals harmful to humans and aquatic life polluted the soil and groundwater, leaving areas barren and unable to support vegetation. Acid-generating deposits called *slickens* scattered throughout the floodplain continue to send toxic metals directly into rivers through runoff. Not all areas have undergone cleanup and restoration.

The effect on health and potential for higher incidences of cancer and other diseases remains underdetermined at this time.

Food. Food as a pollutant is one of the major environmental agents to which people are exposed. In many documented cases, reversible and irreversible human and ecologic damage has occurred as a result of pollution-induced food contamination. As scientific and epidemiologic information accumulates, society is questioning to what degree these technologies and by-products contribute to the steadily rising incidence of certain cancers, autoimmune and other chronic diseases, birth defects, autism, learning disorders, and other health problems for which the cause is not well understood.

Pesticides, Insecticides, and Herbicides. Pesticide, insecticide, and herbicide residues in food; hormone residues; food irradiation (a method of preservation and protection from microbial contamination); genetically modified foods; and food additives and preservatives are major consumer concerns. The EPA sets limits on how much of a pesticide may be used on food while growing and processing it as well as how much may remain on food purchased by consumers. In 1992, the EPA revised the Workers Protection Standard for agricultural pesticides that protects workers from exposure to pesticides on the job. There are over 1055 active ingredients registered as pesticides, which can create thousands of pesticide products. In 2009, 57.4% of food samples contained detectable pesticide residue which is an increase from 46.1% in 2003.[241] Pesticide and herbicide exposure can cause many different health effects, from acute problems, such as dermatitis, asthma exacerbations, and gastroenteritis to chronic problems, such as chronic obstructive pulmonary disease and cancer.[185] There is also evidence to suggest that increased pesticide exposure can cause birth defects, fetal death, and neurodevelopmental disorder.[114,184] Acute pesticide poisoning has been reported among food handlers (e.g., clerks, baggers, stockers, or shipping/receiving handlers) and janitors in retail establishments that sell food products, especially fruits and vegetables.[45]

Among the people most in danger from pesticide exposure are farmers and agricultural workers. Many studies of these groups have shown an increase in soft tissue sarcomas, presumably from herbicide exposure.[87] Children, especially very young children, are also at greater risk from exposures to pesticides and other environmental toxins compared to adults because, pound for pound of body weight, children drink more water, eat more food, and breathe more air than adults.

Childhood leukemia, non-Hodgkin lymphoma, and Hodgkin lymphoma have also been linked with the use of home and pet insecticides, garden fungicides, and to a lesser degree herbicides during pregnancy and early childhood.[181] The treatment of pediculosis (lice) with an insecticidal shampoo also may be associated with an increased risk of childhood leukemia.[138] School-aged children are also at increased risk for acute illnesses from repellants and pesticides applied within school grounds, pesticide drift exposure from farmland, and pesticide use at parks.[7]

In the United States, environmental exposure to chlorophenoxy herbicides used in wheat production has been linked to musculoskeletal and respiratory-circulatory birth defects, cancer, type 2 diabetes, and heart disease.[190,191] Counties in which wheat is produced have a high rate of defects among infant boys conceived during April or June when herbicide application takes place. Boys conceived during other times of the year and born in counties with low wheat production have far fewer birth defects.[189]

Pesticides that are not registered or are restricted for use in the United States can be imported in fruits, vegetables, and seafood produced abroad. Environmental quality is a global concern as increasing numbers of people and products cross national borders, transferring health risks such as infectious diseases and chemical hazards.

Contaminated Soil. Contaminated soil is often the main source of chemical exposure for humans, and an active interchange of chemicals occurs between soil and water, air, and food. Direct contact and ingestion of soil are important exposure pathways, and inhalation of volatile compounds or dust must also be considered. The movement of contaminants through soil is very complex, some moving rapidly and others slowly, eventually reaching and contaminating surface or ground water on which people rely for drinking and other purposes.

Asbestos. Asbestos continues to be a significant occupational hazard. It was not until the late 1960s and early 1970s that the public was made aware that asbestos used in products ranging from automotive brake linings to building insulation caused chronic respiratory illnesses, cancer, and other illnesses. Since then, commercial use of asbestos has decreased dramatically.

Abatement workers employed to remove asbestos in buildings wear protective clothing to decrease exposure but still are considered at risk. Long latency (exposure occurring 30 or more years ago continues to affect former workers) and long-term, low-level exposure to the presence of indoor asbestos remain risk factors. It is not just asbestos but other long, thin mineral fibers in the workplace or in the environment that can have similar effects. See Chapter 15 for a discussion of asbestosis.

Manmade vitreous fibers containing mineral wool, glass wool or fiber, and ceramic fiber have replaced asbestos in the workplace. The nonoccupational exposure to manmade minerals does not put consumers at substantial risk; health issues related to these materials mainly occur among workers with long duration of exposure. Clinical consequences are similar to those of asbestos, including pulmonary fibrosis, bronchogenic carcinoma, mesothelioma, and possibly other types of cancers.

Other Chemical Compounds. Polyvinyl chloride (PVC), a type of plastic made flexible through the addition of a chemical, is used in a variety of medical products, including saline bags that store medical solutions as well as blister packs, medical shrink wrap, and IV lines. Vinyl chloride production has doubled in the last 20 years, with current production of 27 million tons per year worldwide. Concern exists over the possibility of chemical plasticizers leaching into the solutions used long-term by certain populations, including people on dialysis, individuals with hemophilia, or neonates exposed at critical points in development.

Additionally, measured changes in the acidity of IV solutions in PVC packaging have been reported.[212] Dioxin,

a by-product of PVC plastics manufacturing, was declared a carcinogen by the EPA in June 2000. Dioxin accumulates in fatty tissues of mammals and fish. The observed toxicities of these chemicals have been linked to cancers, birth defects, and immune system disorders, resulting in the request for PVC-free medical devices and reduction of environmental contamination with these compounds to the lowest level possible.[121,217] High levels of dioxin exposure are associated with chloracne, a distinctive form of acne (Fig. 4-1), and with porphyria cutanea tarda (Fig. 4-2).

In 2005, Catholic Healthcare West, one of the largest hospital networks in the United States, signed a contract for vinyl-free IV bags and tubing and in 2012 Kaiser Permanente, another major U.S. health care provider, announced that it will no longer buy IV medical equipment made with PVC and di-(2-ethylhexyl) phthalate–type plasticizers.[41,205]

In early 2012, the EPA finalized stronger air emissions standards for PVC production facilities in order to improve air quality and health in the surrounding communities. The new standards would reduce annual emissions from major production sources by 238 tons of total air toxics.[235]

Most adult blood tests show the chemical perfluorooctanoic acid (PFOA), a chemical compound widely used in Teflon-coated cookware, water- and stain-resistant

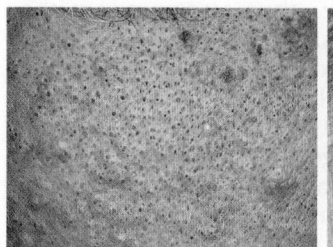 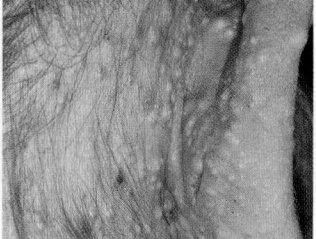

Figure 4-1

Chloracne. (From Bolognia JL, Jorizzo JL, Rapini RP: *Dermatology*, St. Louis, 2003, Mosby.)

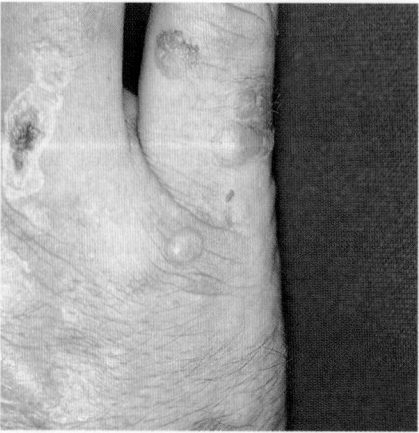

Figure 4-2

Porphyria cutanea tarda. Erosion, crusting, and vesicles on the dorsum of the hand in an individual with porphyria cutanea tarda. (From Goldman L: *Cecil textbook of medicine*, ed 22, Philadelphia, 2004, WB Saunders.)

clothing, cosmetics, and many other products. There has been growing concern about the effects of this compound. Research has found that PFOA causes a modest increase in cholesterol and uric acid, and further research is looking into the effects on thyroid function, cancers, diabetes, sexual reproduction, and fetal development.[211] PFOA has been linked to testicular, liver, and pancreatic cancer in animals.[44,118,160] In 2005, the EPA scientific advisory board concluded that PFOA was likely to be a carcinogenic in humans and is considered an animal carcinogen.

PFOA never breaks down in the environment so will always be around. In 2006, the EPA began the PFOA Stewardship Program with eight major fluoropolymer and telomere manufacturers with goals to reduce PFOA emissions and products by 95% no later than 2010 and to work on eliminating these chemicals from emissions and products by 2015.[231]

Fire and Pyrolysis. Fire and pyrolysis directly affect 2 million people annually who are treated for burns, including civilians and firefighters. Pyrolysis, or incomplete combustion, of wood releases many highly toxic compounds that can react with other organic substances to produce new toxic and irritant chemicals. Incomplete combustion and fire-fighting water also produce highly acidic aerosols. Smoldering or partially controlled fires release many toxic products.

The most common type of injuries is in the category of smoke inhalation and respiratory problems followed by lacerations, contusions, and falls. Death can occur as a result of smoke inhalation and myocardial infarction. In fact, the number one cause of on-the-job deaths for firefighters is sudden cardiac death.[207] See "Occupational Burns" in this chapter.

Pyrolysis can also be used to reprocess scrap tires into activated carbon, carbon black, Boudouard carbon, and fuel gas.[256] In 2007, the United States had 262 million waste tires. More than 89% of these waste tires were recycled or reused, with 54% of them being converted into fuel and was consumed by power plants, industrial boilers, and cement kilns.[180] Research continues to be done to determine whether recycling tires in this manner is profitable. This could decrease the amount of tire waste tremendously and utilize tires to our benefit.

Waste. Waste from solid, hazardous, and incinerator by-products is not likely to be encountered directly in a therapy practice. However, the effects of exposure to medical/infectious waste may be more problematic. Standard precautions for handling all medical/infectious waste are available (see Chapter 8 and Appendix A).

Heavy Metals

Heavy metals, such as lead, arsenic, and mercury, actually fall under the chemical agents category but are mentioned separately because of their former prevalence and uniqueness as classic occupational and environmental hazards. In the early 1990s, environmental concerns shifted attention away from lead, mercury, arsenic, and asbestos exposure despite continued high production volume chemical development, toxicology testing, and issues centered around environmental justice.[125]

However, new findings from the TRI have resulted in a resurgence of interest and research in this area. The TRI is a publicly available EPA database that contains information on toxic chemical releases and other waste management activities reported annually by some industry groups, as well as federal facilities. The 2010 TRI findings report 3.93 billion pounds of combined on-site and off-site disposal or other releases of toxic chemicals. Total disposal or other releases of mercury and mercury compounds amounted to 4.8 million pounds in 2004.

Lead Poisoning. A normal blood lead level is 0. An elevated blood lead level in adults is defined as concentrations greater than 10 µg/dL. This level was reduced in 2010 from an original level of 25 µg/dL. Apparent toxicity is not usually demonstrated until the blood serum lead levels exceed 10 µg/dL in adults. Lower levels (5 µg/dL) have been identified as toxic for pregnant women. A significant association has been found between low-level lead exposures and elevations in maternal blood pressure during labor and delivery, which was seen with umbilical blood lead levels <2.5 µg/dL.[254] Infant blood lead amounts at birth is about 85%–90% as high as the mother's blood lead level. There is more recent evidence that low-dose lead exposure from chronic dose exposures <30 µg/dL can result in adverse effects in multiple organ systems, including effects in neurologic, cardiovascular, reproductive, and renal function. Any levels above these marks require intervention. OSHA prohibits workers with levels greater than 50 µg/dL or higher for construction workers and 60 µg/dL or higher for general industry workers from returning to the workplace where lead is present. Workers are permitted to return to work when their blood lead level is <40 µg/dL.[8]

Lead poisoning is on the decline in the United States as a result of federal initiatives to end the use of lead in gasoline, lead solder in the seams of food cans (beware of foods in cans manufactured outside the United States), lead-based paints, and plumbing in homes. There has been a reduction in blood lead levels between 1994 and 2009. Data collected by the CDC in 40 states that have the Adult Blood Lead Epidemiology and Surveillance program showed that in 1994 there were 14 per 100,000 employed adults who have ≥25 µg/dL, whereas in 2009 it dropped to 6.3 per 100,000.[49] In 2010, when the National Institute for Occupational Safety and Health changed the elevated blood lead levels to 10 µg/dL, there were 26.4 adults per 100,000 with an elevated lead level. The CDC continues to work with the Adult Blood Lead Epidemiology and Surveillance program to ensure these numbers decline with the new definition for an elevated blood lead level of >10 µg/dL.[51]

Adults are more likely to be exposed to lead in the manufacture of brass, storage batteries, bullets, solder, or glass; furniture refinishing; home renovations; stained-glass or pottery making; mining of lead and zinc ores, and painting and paper hanging. The most common nonoccupational exposures are shooting firearms, retained bullets (gunshot wounds), and prolonged exposure to the burning of metallic wick candles (e.g., home use, restaurant, religious, or ceremonial).[8]

Consumers should also be aware that the porcelain glaze of old bathtubs and the glaze on imported dishware (ceramics, china, or porcelain) often contain lead and are a potential source of lead exposure. Internet purchases of dishware and ceramics online present a particular threat.

Lead can leach out of dishware when the glaze is improperly fired or when the glaze has broken down because of wear from daily usage, especially after repeated use in a microwave or dishwasher. Chips and cracks in ceramic ware also allow leaching of lead. Children's risk for such exposures is increased with frequent consumption of acidic juices that promote lead leaching from ceramics.[50]

Children. Lead is particularly toxic to infants and children for several reasons, including (1) the blood-brain barrier is immature before the age of 3, allowing lead to enter the brain more readily; (2) ingested lead has a 40% bioavailability in children, compared with 10% in adults; and (3) the behavioral hand-to-mouth habits. Apparent toxicity in children is not usually demonstrated until the blood serum lead levels exceed 10 μg/dL. In the United States there are approximately 250,000 children between the ages of 1 and 5 years who have blood lead levels >10 μg/dL.[53] Ingestion of lead paints found in older residential neighborhoods and exposure to lead dust particles during home renovation projects remain continuing problems among the pediatric population. Likewise, dust and soil containing lead particles too small to see expose children, who are more likely to be on the ground or outside and who engage in more hand-to-mouth activities.

After lead is absorbed it enters the blood stream and attaches to proteins in the blood which carry it to various organs and tissues throughout the body. In adults more than 95% of the total body stores of lead are found in bone and in children around 70% is found in bone.[19] Lead can also adversely affect many organ systems, including the CNS and the gastrointestinal, hemopoietic, reproductive, and renal systems. The body is able to rid itself of lead through the urinary and gastrointestinal tract but most people are unable to get rid of as much lead as they take in.

Health effects in infants born to women with moderately elevated blood lead levels include preterm birth, decreased gestational maturity, lower birth weight, reduced postnatal growth, increased incidence of minor congenital anomalies, and early neurologic or neurobehavioral deficits. It remains unclear how long these neurologic effects persist, but some evidence suggests a link between prenatal elevated lead levels and decreased intelligence in children up to age 7 years.[46]

Serum levels once thought to be safe have been shown to be associated with intelligence quotient (IQ) deficits, behavioral disorders, slowed growth, decreased competency in verbal performance and auditory processing, and impaired hearing. The impairment of cognitive function begins to occur at levels greater than 10 μg/100 mL, even though clinical symptoms may not be apparent; serum levels are required for diagnosis. Other studies show cognitive and delayed puberty at levels below 10 μg.[48,176,196]

Arsenic. Arsenic is a naturally occurring metal-like element found in the earth's crust. It was used extensively in pesticides and herbicides until the late 1960s, with most agricultural uses being banned. Until 2004, arsenic was utilized in the preservatives for pressure-treated lumber. It can be found in most foods in very low levels and some fish and shellfish build up the organic form in their tissues, which is not toxic.[154] Arsenic binds to tissue proteins and is concentrated in the liver, skin, kidney, nervous system, and bone, with bone being affected to a lesser extent than with lead. The symptoms of acute inorganic arsenic poisoning may include severe burning of the mouth and throat, abdominal pain, nausea, vomiting, diarrhea, hypotension, and muscle spasms.

Typically the arsenic is excreted in the urine within 1 week of exposure, with any remaining arsenic mostly found in the hair, nails, and skin. With chronic arsenic poisoning, the first sign is small dark spots appearing on the trunk, neck, face, arms, and legs. Then the palms of the hands and soles of the feet develop corn-like growths. Increased exposure would produce neurologic symptoms, including numbness, tingling or burning sensations; fluid accumulation; and anemia, with eventual liver, kidney, and CNS damage.[226] In severe cases, cardiomyopathy, jaundice, renal impairment, red cell hemolysis, ventricular arrhythmias, coma, seizures, and intestinal hemorrhage are seen. Painful dysesthesia in the hands and feet, bone marrow depression, transverse white striae of the nails, altered mentation, and occasionally garlicky perspiration odor may occur.

Epidemiologic studies have demonstrated a correlation between environmental or occupational arsenic exposure and a risk of vascular diseases related to atherosclerosis. It appears that arsenic induces endothelial dysfunction as a result of impaired nitric oxide balance, and inflammatory and coagulating activity. Arsenic may accelerate atherosclerosis, but the mechanism for this event remains under investigation.[201]

Cancers of the skin, kidney, bladder, and lungs have been associated with arsenic poisoning, but the mechanisms responsible for arsenic carcinogenesis have not been established. Increasing evidence indicates that arsenic acts at the level of tumor promotion by modulating the signaling pathways responsible for cell growth.[202,247] The risk of arsenic-induced cancer is associated with 20 or 30 years of drinking polluted water, not from a brief or occupational exposure. The current standard in the United States is 10 parts per billion. Any water supply that has much higher arsenic levels is not considered safe for human consumption.

Arsenic trioxide, which is an inorganic oxide of arsenic, has been utilized for cancer treatment over the last 15–20 years. It is used specifically for relapsed acute promyelocytic leukemia (APL) and has demonstrated good results with these patients. Current research being done shows that combining arsenic trioxide with standard treatment for APL improves survival outcomes and may reduce the amount of cytotoxic chemotherapy exposure to this patient population. Arsenic trioxide has also shown efficacy in treating other malignancies including multiple myeloma and myelodysplastic syndrome.[75]

Mercury. Mercury is a naturally occurring element found in air, water, and soil. It can be dangerous when ingested, inhaled, or absorbed through the skin. Most people have some amount of mercury in their bodies, but random testing of individuals has revealed higher than the acceptable, safe limit of 1 part per million set jointly by the EPA and the Food and Drug Administration (FDA). Mercury is usually released in elemental form and then converted into methylmercury by bacteria. Methylmercury is more toxic to humans because it is more easily absorbed into the body. Current research has found no safe level of methylmercury in the blood.[238]

Sources of Mercury. Mercury is found in the earth's crust and can be found in many rocks, including coal. In the United States, more than 50% of mercury emissions in the air are from coal-burning power plants. Common products created with mercury include thermometers, switches, and some light bulbs. Phasing out these mercury-containing products has already become a national trend.

Inorganic mercury compounds take the form of mercury salts, which are generally white powders or crystals. Both inorganic and organic mercury compounds have been commonly used as fungicides, antiseptics, or disinfectants and in some medicines including some nasal sprays and ophthalmic solutions.

Harmful mercury vapors can be transferred to water and soil where they can be introduced into the food chain, causing renal and neurologic disorders. Although eating contaminated fish is the leading cause of mercury accumulation in humans, elevated levels of emissions from coal-burning power plants and petroleum refineries, mining-related wastes, and the improper disposal of mercury products have resulted in increased mercury in the environment, with the trickle-down effects on fish, with the larger fish having higher concentrations of mercury. In 2004, the EPA and FDA issued consumer advice about mercury in fish and shellfish intended for women who might become pregnant, women who are pregnant, nursing mothers, and young children. The recommendations are to eat those fish and shellfish that are lower in mercury content, including shrimp, canned light tuna, salmon, pollock, and catfish and avoid those that are higher in mercury content including shark, swordfish, tilefish, and king mackerel.[236]

Exposures to women of childbearing age, pregnant and nursing women, and children younger than age 15 are of great concern because of the susceptibility of these groups and resultant adverse effects. According to analysis of data gathered by the National Health and Nutrition Examination Survey, between 200,000 and 400,000 children born in the United States each year have been exposed to mercury levels in their mothers' wombs high enough to impair neurologic development.[150]

Hospitals generate a daily average of 26 pounds of waste per staffed bed. There is increasing concern about mercury release from medical waste incinerators. In 2012, the Healthier Hospitals Initiative began which is a national campaign to implement a new approach to improve environmental health and sustainability in the health care sector. Healthier Hospitals Initiative will be gathering data from participating hospitals over their first 3 years to demonstrate the impact their initiatives are having on the health and safety of patients, workers, and communities as well as a reduction in health care expenditures. Hospitals and health systems produce 11,700 tons of waste each day with some of the medical supplies containing mercury. Hospitals and health systems are beginning to eliminate mercury-containing thermometers, sphygmomanometers, and clinical devices and replacing them with nonmercury items.[99]

There is considerable controversy as to whether dental amalgams ("silver fillings") may cause significant health effects in humans. They are made up of about 40%–50% mercury, 25% silver, and 25%–35% mixture of copper, zinc, and tin. There is some evidence that a sustained release of mercury and other metals occurs from the amalgam into the body. Researchers have measured a daily release of mercury on the order of 10 µg from the amalgam into the body. In response to a need for a greater concentration of research in this area, a group of concerned dentists formed the International Academy of Oral Medicine and Toxicology in 1984. One of their objectives was to scientifically explore the safety of amalgam restorations. A study looking at neurologic findings in children with dental amalgams found that even children with 7–10 amalgam surfaces had no change in neurologic status after 7 years. This may show that neurologic factors from amalgam mercury exposure in children are insignificant.[122] Consequently, there are a growing number of scientific studies that document pathophysiologic effects associated with amalgam mercury. In the interest of protecting their citizens' health, Sweden, Norway, Germany, Denmark, Austria, Finland, and Canada have recently taken steps to limit and phase out the use of amalgam restorations. About one-third of the dentists in the United States no longer use mercury-containing products. Resin composite fillings, which match the tooth color, are used instead.

Despite consumer concerns about mercury exposure from dental fillings, clients and dental personnel are at greatest risk when amalgams are removed. The aerolization during removal creates greater mercury exposure than the hardened and intact filling in the mouth. It is advised by some that amalgams should only be removed when the filling (or tooth) is no longer intact, rather than to eliminate mercury exposure. Dental personnel are at greatest risk for this type of repeated exposure.

Clinical Manifestations (Mercury Exposure). The EPA reports that 3% of women of child-bearing age had at least 5.8 parts per billion of mercury in their blood in 2005–2008. About 42% of the women of child-bearing age in the United States have at least 1 part per billion of mercury in 2005–2008. They also noted that children born to women with blood concentrations of mercury above 5.8 parts per billion are at some risk of adverse health effects, especially decreased IQ and problems with motor skills.

The National Academy of Sciences and EPA determined that pregnant women with between 32 and 58 parts per billion of mercury in the blood corresponds to an approximate doubling in the risk of poor performance on neurodevelopmental tests including those measuring attention, fine motor function, language skills, visual spatial abilities, and verbal memory.[237] Exposure to hazardous levels of mercury can cause permanent neurologic heart and kidney impairment. Neurologic or neurodegenerative diseases, mental retardation, cerebral palsy, seizures, memory loss, learning disabilities, developmental delays, autoimmune disorders, mental health disorders, and birth defects are among the many conditions blamed on mercury exposure.[255]

Vaccines commonly given to children before 2001 contained a preservative (Thimerosal) that contained mercury. There were concerns raised over the total number of vaccinations given to children during the first 6 months of life that could lead to toxic levels of mercury. There was some suspicion that increased rates of autism could be the result of mercury poisoning from vaccines, but this has not been proved conclusively. A 2011 study comparing urinary mercury between children with autism and control children showed no statistical differences in levels of urinary mercury levels even when controlled for age, gender, and amalgam fillings.[258]

Acute exposure to high levels of elemental mercury results in CNS effects such as tremors, mood changes, and slowed sensory and motor nerve function. Chronic exposure can also cause CNS effects such as increased excitability, irritability, tremors, and a chronic personality disorder called the Mad Hatter syndrome, characterized by unusual shyness, labile affect, and decline in intellect. Acute exposure to inorganic mercury orally may result in nausea, vomiting, and severe abdominal pain. Kidney damage is a major effect from chronic exposure to inorganic mercury. Acute exposures to very high levels of methylmercury can result in CNS effects such as blindness, deafness, and impaired consciousness levels. Chronic exposure may lead to paresthesia, blurred vision, malaise, speech difficulties, and constriction of the visual field.[6]

Mercury Regulation. In 2005, the EPA took its first step toward reducing mercury pollution from coal-fired power plants with the Clear Air Mercury Rule, designed to reduce mercury emissions by 70% over the next 20 years. In December of 2011, the EPA announced the Mercury and Air Toxics Standards, which is the first national standards to protect families from power plant emissions. The plants will have up to 4 years to comply with these new standards. The EPA has estimated that in 2016, the health benefits of these changes would be between $37 billion and $90 billion and would avoid 4200 to 11,000 premature deaths, 2800 cases of chronic bronchitis, 4700 heart attacks, 130,000 cases of aggravated asthma, 5700 hospital and emergency department visits, 6300 cases of acute bronchitis, 140,000 cases of respiratory symptoms, 540,000 days of missed work, and 3.2 million days when people restrict their activities.

Xenoestrogens/Xenobiotics

Xenoestrogens are also part of chemical environmental exposure but are discussed separately because of their unique place as a hazardous agent. In the early 1970s, scientists from around the world met together to discuss the cumulative efforts of researchers investigating various endangered species. Together they identified that exposure to petrochemicals (previously called *xenoestrogens* but now referred to as *xenobiotics*, meaning "foreign to life") is the underlying cause of dwindling births in these species.

Petrochemicals, such as pesticides and insecticides, are the primary xenobiotics and constitute substances totally foreign to nature—that is, they are not found in the natural world but rather are synthesized chemicals. Other petrochemicals are present in commonly used items or products such as emollients in lotions and creams, spreaders in salad dressing, carpet glues, paints, solvents, automobile gasoline, plastics, and a multitude of other

common household objects. Researchers concluded that the effect of these residues is selective to the reproductive systems of the developing fetuses so that exposure in the developing fetuses resulted in infertility or sterility. Since that time, it has been recognized that these chemicals can affect other systems, including the thyroid, immune function, and nervous system.

The effect of these chemicals has been to create what is referred to as an *estrogen-dominant environment* because the chemicals have estrogenic activity. Estrogen dominance on humans (both men and women, although women are more susceptible) is the subject of intense scrutiny by scientists and researchers.

This biologic phenomenon may be linked to autoimmune dysfunction, thyroid disruption, increased body fat, metabolic regulation, decreased sex drive and sperm production (infertility), altered blood clotting, early menarche, zinc deficiency associated with prostate dysfunction, endometriosis, and headaches associated with fluid retention.

The official opinion of the Endocrine Society is that there is sufficient evidence for adverse reproductive outcomes including genital birth defects, cancers, and infertility to be concerned. For complete research data and references from peer-reviewed scientific journals, see the Endocrine Society website (www.endo-society.org).

Physical Agents

Electromagnetic Radiation. The long-term effects of exposure to electromagnetic radiation or electromagnetic fields (EMF), including radiofrequency and microwave, ultraviolet light, x-ray, and gamma rays, remain under intense scrutiny (Fig. 4-3). Ionizing radiation is the result of electromagnetic waves entering the body and acting on neutral atoms or molecules with sufficient force to remove electrons, creating an ion. The most common sources of ionizing radiation exposure in humans are accidental environmental exposure and medical, therapeutic, or diagnostic irradiation.

All living material is vulnerable to ionization by high-energy radiation because the disruption of atoms joined into molecules producing ions and free radicals (see Chapter 6 and Fig. 6-2) can result in further biochemical damage, including somatic effects, such as cell death, and genetic effects, including reproductive effects and cancer. Radiation-induced changes can cause genetic mutations and structural rearrangements in chromosomes that can be transmitted from generation to generation.[25,221]

A wide range of other adverse health effects have been attributed to ionizing radiation, including visual, thermal, behavioral, CNS, and auditory effects; effects on the blood–brain barrier; and immunologic, endocrinologic (including effects on biorhythm), hematologic, developmental, and cardiovascular effects.

Exposure to nonionizing radiation (i.e., the electromagnetic wave does not have enough energy to strip an atom of its electron) occurs most commonly as a result of the use of a wide variety of industrial and electronic devices (e.g., microwave ovens, scanning lasers in stores, high-intensity lamps, video display terminals, scanning radars, or electronic antitheft surveillance).

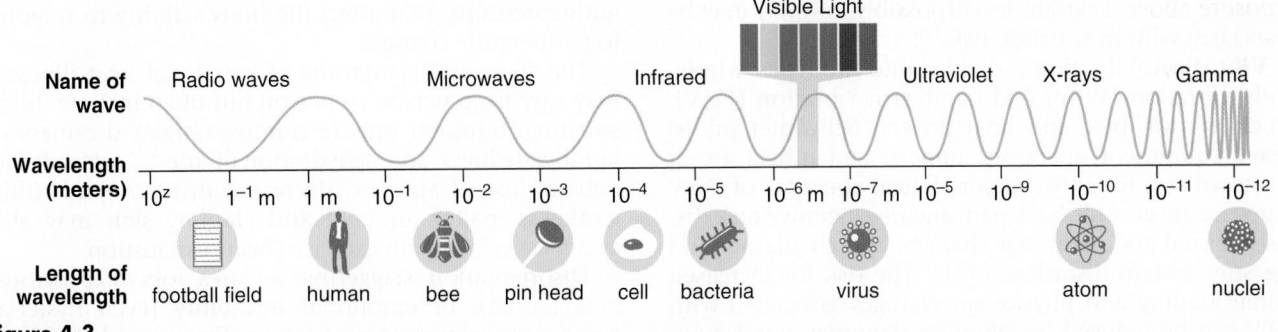

Figure 4-3

Electromagnetic (EM) spectrum. Different types of electromagnetic radiation have different frequency or wavelengths. Radio waves, television waves, and microwaves are all types of electromagnetic waves. The electromagnetic spectrum includes, from longest wavelength to shortest: radio waves, microwaves, infrared, optical, ultraviolet, x-rays, and gamma rays. Waves in the electromagnetic spectrum vary in size from very long radio waves the size of buildings, to very short gamma rays smaller than the size of the nucleus of an atom. The frequency is the rate at which the electromagnetic field goes through one complete oscillation (cycle) and is usually given in Hertz (Hz), where 1 Hz is one cycle per second. As the frequency rises, the wavelength gets shorter.

Chemical compounds from plastic wrap surrounding food or covering dishes used in a microwave can leach into the foods and affect the body. Packaging and plastic wraps that contain polyethylene are preferred for use in the microwave, because these do not have plasticizers (materials that make the wrap more pliable). Containers meant for cold foods, such as margarine or whipped topping, should also be avoided for microwave use, because these containers can melt, dispersing some of their components into the food.

Considerable speculation has gone on around the world that long-term exposure to EMFs is correlated with the development of breast cancer, leukemia, miscarriage, and neurodegenerative diseases such as Alzheimer disease, Parkinson disease, and amyotrophic lateral sclerosis (ALS).[95]

The unexplained high incidence of breast cancer in industrialized nations is suspected as being linked to electric power generation and consumption. The proposed biologic mechanism is the inhibition of melatonin caused by the products of electric power generation, EMFs, and light at night, but this has not been proved and further investigation is warranted.[71,137,158]

Most exposures to electromagnetic interference are transient and pose no threat to people with pacemakers and implantable cardioverter defibrillators; however, magnetic resonance imaging (MRI) and prolonged exposure to EMFs are contraindicated in anyone who is pacemaker-dependent.[166]

Concerns that cellular telephone radiation is linked to tumors of the head and neck (including brain and salivary gland tumors) or causes a variety of serious problems (e.g., genetic damage, pacemaker or implantable cardioverter defibrillator disruption, interference with heart/lung monitors, or compromise to the blood–brain barrier) have not been substantiated.[220] Long-term studies of longer induction periods, especially for slow-growing tumors with neuronal features, conclude that the data do not support the hypothesis that mobile phone use is related to an increased risk of brain tumors.[128,178,193]

In 2011, the WHO and International Agency for Research on Cancer (IARC) classified radiofrequency electromagnetic fields as *possibly carcinogenic to humans* (2B Classification) based on an increased risk for glioma associated with wireless phone use. The evidence was shown to be limited among users of wireless phones for glioma and acoustic neuroma and was shown to be inadequate to draw conclusions for other cancers.

The lack of ionizing radiation and the low-level electromagnetic energy emitted from mobile phones and absorbed by human tissues is not strong enough to change the structure of atoms, making it unlikely that these devices cause DNA changes that can lead to cancer. But these devices do emit enough energy to heat tissue, and the effects of prolonged exposure have not been determined. The only health hazard of mobile phones that has been confirmed is the increased risk of having an accident while driving and using a mobile phone.[62] In 2009, there were 5474 people killed and around 448,000 injured in motor vehicle crashes involving distracted driving. Of those killed, 995 (18%) involved reports of mobile phone use, whereas 24,000 (5%) of those injured reported mobile phone use.[227] There has been some indication that there is an increased risk for glioma in those who report the highest 10% of mobile phone usage; however, the results were not consistent.[257] Until conclusive evidence is available, consumers may want to purchase phones with the lowest emissions (for more information, see Environmental Working Group at http://www.ewg.org/cellphone-radiation).

The American Society for Reproductive Medicine found that the more men used their mobile phones, the lower their sperm count was, the poorer the quality of the sperm was, and the lower the sperm mobility was. Using a mobile phone for more than 4 hours per day caused a 25% decrease in the sperm produced, with only 20% of them looking normal. Research on the ovaries of mice is looking at the effects of radiofrequency exposure and is limited at this time. Research on the effects of radiofrequency exposure during pregnancy is also limited.[4,5,252]

Likewise, a previous concern that living in close proximity to power lines was correlated to cancer has not been proved[31,204] nor have reports linking video display terminals to miscarriages been substantiated.[80] A study looking at exposure to magnetic fields during pregnancy found strong evidence that prenatal maximum magnetic field exposure above a certain level (possibly 16 mG) may be associated with miscarriage risk.[126]

Vibration. Vibration is divided into two types: whole-body vibration (WBV) and hand–arm vibration (HAV). Truck, tractor, bus, and boat drivers; helicopter pilots; heavy equipment operators; miners; and others are at increased risk for WBV. Major clinical concerns of WBV exposure are chronic back pain and degenerative disk diseases, visual and vestibular changes, and circulatory and digestive system disorders.[27,94,141] The risk for increased spinal loading and physiologic changes associated with WBV can be reduced by vibration damping, good ergonomic design, reducing exposure, and reducing other risks such as lifting.[167]

Vibration-induced white finger disease is the most common example of an occupational injury caused by vibration of the hands. This condition occurs secondary to the use of hand tools, such as power saws, grinders, sanders, pneumatic drills, and jackhammers, and other equipment used in construction, foundry work, machining, and mining.

WBV is used as a neuromuscular training method for a range of individuals from athletes to geriatrics. WBV has been found to increase the mechanical power output of muscles and improve neuromuscular efficiency in athletes and can increase walking speed, step length, and single-leg stand time in the geriatric population. WBV therapy as a treatment for osteoporosis has been researched over the last several years and there has been very little information on potential harms of WBV. However, there are safety concerns including possible long-term harm. Further research is needed for whether this would be an advantageous treatment choice in this population.[33,78,116,139,161,173,259]

Heat Stress. Heat stress exceeding human tolerance can result in heat-related disorders (e.g., exertional heat stroke, exhaustion, cramps, dehydration, or prickly heat) and heat illnesses (e.g., chronic heat exhaustion, reduced heat tolerance, anhidrotic heat exhaustion, or exertional hyponatremia), some of which are fatal. Heat illness is more likely in hot, humid weather but can occur in the absence of hot and humid conditions.

Between 1999 and 2003, there was a total of 3,442 deaths resulting from exposure to extreme heat, with 2,239 of them having hyperthermia as the cause of death and 1,203 with hyperthermia as a contributing factor. This means on average there are more than 650 heat-related mortalities in the United States.[52] In a therapy setting, the groups of people most likely to experience heat stress include older adults during temperature extremes, industrial workers, construction workers, firefighters, outdoor sports participants, agricultural workers, pregnant women, and people taking mood-altering drugs (i.e., they lose touch with their environment).

Those at higher risk of heat stress include the elderly, young children, and those with chronic medical conditions. This population is also at an increased risk for heat-related mortality. Individuals receiving medications that interfere with salt and water balance are at increased risk for heat-related illness and death. Watch for diuretics, anticholinergic agents, and tranquilizers that impair sweating, as well as antidepressants, such as tricyclic antidepressants, that affect the body's ability to respond to temperature changes.

The signs and symptoms of exertional heat illnesses may vary from person to person but often include thirst, sweating, transient muscle cramps, fatigue, dizziness or lightheadedness, and dehydration (Table 4-2). Headache, nausea, loss of appetite, decreased urine output, chills, weakness, pallor, or cool and clammy skin may also occur, especially with exercise (heat) exhaustion.

Disorientation, staggering, seizures, loss of consciousness (coma), or emotional instability (even hysteria) occur with exertional heat stroke. Exertional hyponatremia is characterized by increased body-core temperature, low blood-sodium level, progressive headache, confusion, lethargy, significant mental compromise, seizures, swelling of the hands and feet, and even coma.[28]

High Altitude. High-altitude environment (8000-14,000 feet) is characterized by atmosphere with decreasing partial pressure of oxygen and decreasing temperature. Hypoxia (reduced availability of oxygen to the body) appears to be the underlying cause of most of the physiologic changes of elevated altitude.

Acute altitude sickness includes *acute mountain sickness, high-altitude pulmonary edema,* and *high-altitude cerebral edema.* These three probably represent a continuum of disease, but each has different symptom complexes, pathogenesis, and slightly different treatment interventions. With high-altitude pulmonary edema, fluid accumulates in the lungs when the arteries become constricted because of a lack of oxygen and the decrease in air pressure. Symptoms include fatigue; breathlessness at rest; fast, shallow breathing; cough that produces pink, frothy sputum; blue or gray lips or fingernails (cyanosis); chest tightness; and drowsiness.

High-altitude cerebral edema is brain swelling severe enough to interfere with brain function. The affected individual may experience confusion, inability to think or concentrate, confusion, and loss of physical coordination. Vision can become blurred if bleeding occurs from blood vessels at the back of the eye.

Not everyone gets sick at higher altitudes, but health risks increase the higher and faster one climbs, especially if early warning signs are ignored (e.g., headache, fatigue, dizziness or lightheadedness, nausea, or vomiting). People with cardiopulmonary and other diseases (e.g., sickle cell disease) are at increased risk for worsening of the medical disorder and possibly at increased risk for acute altitude illnesses with ascent to high altitudes. Aviation and aerospace illnesses are rarely encountered by the therapist and are beyond the scope of this book.

Risk Factors

Environmental pathogenesis requires an understanding of latency, the concept that a hazardous or toxic agent may initiate a series of internal reactions that do not manifest as overt disease for many years or even decades as the body strives to maintain a state of optimal health or homeostasis. Exposures to any of the agents discussed in the previous section on etiology are in fact risk factors. Many additional factors, such as route of exposure (e.g., inhalation, ingestion, or absorption through the skin); magnitude or

Table 4-2	Clinical Manifestations of Exertional Heat Illnesses		
Heat Illness	**Risk Event**	**Signs and Symptoms**	**Intervention**
Dehydration	Fluids are not maintained or replenished	Dry mouth, thirst, irritability, headache, dizziness, cramps, fatigue, decreased athletic performance	Move to a cool environment, rehydration
Heat cramps	Intense exercise; fluid deficiencies; electrolyte imbalance	Intense muscle pain; prolonged muscle contraction	Rehydration, replace sodium if needed, light activity (stretching, slow walking), massage, relaxation
Heat syncope	Exposure to high environmental temperatures; first 5 days of acclimatization; prolonged standing	Orthostatic dizziness; dizziness or fainting, tunnel vision, pallor, sweaty skin, decreased pulse rate	Move to cool (shaded) area, adequate hydration, modified activity levels until acclimatized, elevate legs above level of heart, instruct person to increase venous return before standing (e.g., ankle pumps, arms over head, change positions slowly)
Heat exhaustion	Hot, humid conditions (e.g., indoor pool, sauna or hot tub, outdoor weather)	Unable to continue exercise or activity; unable to sustain cardiac output; loss of coordination; dizziness or fainting; profuse sweating; headache; nausea and vomiting; diarrhea; muscle cramps	Move to cooler environment; remove excess clothing; recline and elevate legs above heart; cool with fans, ice towels, or ice bags; rehydration if possible (no nausea or vomiting)
Exertional heat stroke	Temperature regulation system is overwhelmed by excessive heat production or inhibited heat loss in challenging environmental conditions	Elevated core body temperature (more than 40° C/104° F); tachycardia; hypotension; vomiting; sweating or dry skin; altered mental status, seizures, coma, death	Whole body cooling (e.g., immersion), monitor body temperature recovery every 5–10 minutes, avoid overcooling, medical referral if physician is not on-site

Data from Centers for Disease Control and Prevention (CDC): Extreme heat: a prevention guide to promote your personal health and safety. Available at www.bt.cdc.gov/disasters/extremeheat/heat_guide.asp. Accessed August 30, 2012.

concentration (dose) of exposure; duration (e.g., minutes, hours, days, lifetime); and frequency (e.g., seasonal, daily, weekly, or monthly), play into the development of progressive and overt disease.

Likewise, personal factors that vary from one person to another may affect pathogenesis and must be considered. These include age, gender, ethnicity, nutritional status, personal habits and lifestyle, genetic makeup and host susceptibility, and the strength of individual defense mechanisms. The host–agent–environment interactions are immensely complex and poorly understood at this time.

Pathogenesis

Once a hazardous substance is released into the environment, it may be transported and transformed in a variety of complex ways. For example, a chemical may be modified by the environment before entering the body; transformed by chemical or biochemical processes; or undergo vaporization, diffusion, dilution, or concentration by physical or biologic processes. Plants and animals may accumulate small doses of a chemical agent and bioconcentrate them to the degree that they become hazardous when consumed by humans.

All cells respond to a variety of different adverse environmental stimuli with a cellular defense response now commonly referred to as the *stress response*. Molecules released by the cells in response to stress (e.g., hyperthermic shock, radiation, toxins, or viral infections) are called *heat shock* or *stress proteins*. Increased levels of these proteins after a cellular injury from any of the environmental hazardous agents seem to act as molecular chaperones that facilitate the synthesis and assembly of new reparative proteins.

Cells that produce high levels of stress proteins seem better able to survive ischemic damage; stress proteins may be influential in certain immunologic responses and may also be a requirement for cells to recover from a metabolic insult.[79] Research looking at the role of stress proteins is being done and has found that heat shock proteins increase the level of maturation and expression of cells and they could regulate cell differentiation and proliferation both physiologically and pathologically.[3]

Once some people are sensitized to chemicals, they develop increasingly severe reactions to more and more chemicals at smaller and smaller concentrations. The allergic response that occurs does not appear to be a typical response, perhaps suggesting altered immune system modulation. Immunologists have also discovered a possible connection between stress proteins and autoimmune disease, which may lead to preparations of specific protective vaccines.[59,253] Research is also being done on the role of stress proteins on chronic inflammatory diseases like multiple sclerosis, with the results being controversial.[130,144]

Chronic exposure to air particulate matter leads to inflammation and oxidative stress, precursors to pulmonary and cardiovascular diseases and cancer.[172] Exposure to environmental pollutants has been linked with oxidative DNA damage in humans.[107,203] Exposures are genotoxic and interfere with DNA repair and inhibit the cellular apoptosis needed to prevent cancer. Biomonitoring studies show that DNA damage is influenced by a variety of lifestyle and environmental exposures, including exercise, air pollution, sunlight, diet, and the chemical and physical agents discussed in this chapter.[26,142,213]

Clinical Manifestations

An environmental illness may manifest in a variety of ways. The illness may present as a newly developed clinical syndrome or an aggravation or change in a preexisting condition. The EPA identifies the following seven categories of human health effects from hazardous exposures[233]:

- *Carcinogenicity:* can cause cancer.
- *Heritable genetic and chromosomal mutations:* can cause mutations in genes and chromosomes that will be passed on to the next generation, such as caused by ionizing radiation.
- *Developmental toxicity:* can cause birth defects or miscarriages.
- *Reproductive toxicity:* can damage the ability of men and women to reproduce.
- *Acute toxicity:* can cause death from even short-term exposure to the lungs, through the mouth, or the skin.
- *Chronic toxicity:* can cause long-term damage other than cancer, such as liver, kidney, or lung damage.
- *Neurotoxicity:* can harm the nervous system by affecting the brain, spinal cord, or nerves.

Local toxicities from exposure to environmental agents, such as ocular damage, mucous membrane complaints (eye, nose, and throat irritation), chemical burns to skin, noise-induced hearing loss, and vestibular disorders, can occur. Systemic toxicities can involve any organ system (Table 4-3). The clinical syndrome may mimic a wide range of psychiatric, metabolic, nutritional, inflammatory, and degenerative diseases.

Over the last 15 years, a new syndrome of environmental symptoms associated with chemicals, called *multiple chemical sensitivity* (MCS), has been observed both in the United States and in European countries. MCS is characterized by a chronic condition with symptoms that recur reproducibly in response to low levels of exposure to a wide variety of chemicals found in everyday substances. Those chemicals rated as causing the most symptoms include pesticides, formaldehyde, fresh paint, new carpet, diesel exhaust, perfume, and air fresheners.[88]

Symptoms occur in multiple organ systems and improve or resolve when irritants are removed.[66] Two to four times as many cases of MCS exist among Gulf War veterans compared with undeployed controls[169,214] (see "Gulf War Syndrome" in this chapter). Objective physical findings and consistent laboratory abnormalities or biomarkers associated with MCS are typically nonexistent, leading some in the medical community to call this condition *idiopathic environmental intolerance*, a psychosomatic or neuropsychiatric disorder. Reported symptoms range from runny nose to difficulty breathing and heart palpitations but also include fatigue, headaches, weakness, malaise, decreased attention/concentration, memory loss, disorientation, confusion, and mood changes—with the most often seen symptoms being tiredness/lethargy,

Table 4-3	Systemic Manifestations of Toxicity
Systems	**Clinical Manifestations**
Optic	Optic nephropathy, optic neuritis, optic atrophy
Integument	Atopic dermatitis
	Urticaria
	Pain, itching, erythema
	Pustules, papules
	Chemical burns
Cardiovascular	Cardiac arrhythmia
	Coronary artery disease
	Hypertension
	Myocardial injury
	Nonatheromatous ischemic heart disease
	Peripheral arterial occlusive disease
Respiratory system	Airway inflammation and hyperreactivity
	Bronchitis
	Asthma
	Hypersensitivity pneumonitis
	Pneumoconiosis
	Interstitial fibrosis
	Asbestosis
	Silicosis
	Granuloma formation
	Diffuse alveolar damage
Gastrointestinal (GI) tract	Cancer
Liver	Acute or subacute hepatocellular injury
	Cirrhosis
	Angiosarcoma
	Carcinoma
	Hepatitis
Kidney and urinary tract	Acute renal disease
	Chronic renal failure
	Tubulointerstitial nephritis
	Nephrotic syndrome
	Rapidly progressive glomerulonephritis
Central nervous system	Sensorimotor polyneuropathies (mild system to severe weakness)
	Muscular fasciculations and weakness
	Reduced or absent reflexes
	Cranial neuropathy
	Prominent autonomic dysfunction
	Encephalopathy
	Cerebellar ataxia
Hematopoietic system	Aplastic anemia
	Hemolytic anemia
	Myelodysplastic syndromes
	Multiple myeloma
	Toxic thrombocytopenia
	Porphyria
Immune system	Allergic disease
	Allergic rhinitis
	Bronchial asthma
	GI allergy (food)
	Anaphylaxis
	Autoimmune diseases
	Neoplasia
Reproductive system	Menstrual disorders
	Altered fertility or infertility
	Spontaneous abortion or stillbirth
	Birth defects, low birth weight
	Cancer
	Reduced libido or impotence
	Altered or reduced sperm production
	Premature menopause

difficulty concentrating, muscle aches, memory difficulties, and long-term fatigue.[88]

Studies looking into treatment strategies for those affected by MCS have found that there can be learned behaviors and symptoms in response to specific toxins. This can cause an overreactive response as well as anxiety.[140] The mechanism of response to toxins is still not understood; therefore, an effective treatment strategy does not exist at this time.

The treatment focus of this philosophy is to overcome the affected individual's belief in a toxicogenic explanation for the symptoms,[210] whereas other health care professionals are calling for accurate diagnostic assessment, agreement on the use of specific questionnaires, clinical and technical diagnostic procedures, and prospective clinical studies of people with MCS, comparative groups, and experimental approaches.[10] All in all, the concept of MCS has ignited considerable controversy in the fields of medicine, toxicology, immunology, allergy, psychology, and neuropsychology.[120]

Neurotoxicity

Of particular interest to the therapist may be the effects of hazardous or toxic agents on the nervous system. Neurologic symptoms are common presenting symptoms in people seen by occupational and environmental health professionals. Confusion and other cognitive difficulties, headaches, fatigue, dizziness, limb paresthesias, and abnormal gait patterns are often experienced, but these are nonspecific and seldom point to a single disease or cause.

Many toxins manifest as a nonspecific syndrome of distal sensorimotor impairment that is indistinguishable from the neuropathy caused by common systemic diseases (e.g., diabetes mellitus, vitamin B_6 deficiency, alcoholism, or uremia). Toxins, such as lead, have a striking predilection for motor fibers and usually produce minimal sensory symptoms.

Neurologic symptoms that appear immediately after acute exposure are usually a result of the physiologic effects of the specific (usually chemical) agent. These symptoms subside with cessation of exposure and elimination of the compound from the body. By contrast, delayed neurologic disorders are generally a result of pathologic alterations of the nervous system.

Symptoms appear in a subacute manner over days or weeks after short-term exposure. In the case of long-term exposure, symptoms may appear insidiously and progress over many weeks or months. Recovery can be expected after cessation of exposure, but recovery is slow and depends on the extent of neuronal damage, the half-life of the chemical (i.e., continued exposure until the drug is out of the system), and the adverse effects of chelates used in the chemotherapy of metal poisoning.

Neurotoxicants do not cause focal (asymmetric) neurologic syndrome. Neurotoxins reach the nervous system by the systemic route and cause neurologic symptoms and deficits in a diffuse and symmetric manner, resulting in polyneuropathy. Any significant asymmetry in the presentation, such as weakness or numbness affecting one limb or one side of the body, is not likely to be attributed to neurotoxicity. Multiple neurologic syndromes are possible from a single toxin. Although the effects of neurotoxins are symmetric, neurons from different parts of the nervous system react differently to the agent.

Toxic polyneuropathy affects the distal limbs first, reflecting the greater vulnerability of the longest nerve axons. Sensory disturbances are usually reported as a tingling or burning sensation distributed in a stocking-and-glove pattern (see Fig. 39-5). The toes and the feet are affected first; hand symptoms are seldom present during the early stage. Involvement of the motor nerve fibers, if present, manifests first as atrophy and weakness of the intrinsic foot and hand muscles, bilaterally. More severe cases may present with footdrop or wristdrop, reflecting degeneration of motor axons to the lower leg and forearm muscles.

Neuropathic pain is commonly encountered in people with peripheral neuropathies regardless of the cause. In other words, pain patterns associated with chemically induced peripheral neuropathies do not differ significantly from the clinical picture of pain associated with neuropathy of other causes. Often this pain bears little relationship to the severity of neuropathy and may intensify during a period of recovery, or it may remit paradoxically as the neuropathy progresses, often with further loss of sensation. Pain is not a reliable indicator of neurologic progression or recovery.

MEDICAL MANAGEMENT

Clinical assessment may include assessing the details of exposure and correlating them with the medical condition. Various testing procedures may be developed on the basis of the historical information provided by the client. The clinical presentation, environmental history, and results of laboratory tests assist the physician in demonstrating a correlation between exposure and the clinical manifestations. Nerve conduction velocity (NCV) studies and electromyography are the primary tools for the laboratory evaluation of neuromuscular disorders. A toxic polyneuropathy is characterized by a diffuse and relatively symmetric pattern of nerve conduction velocity abnormalities.

Removal from exposure and decontamination of the exposed victim are essential in the treatment of exposure-linked toxicity. Specific intervention protocols depend on the agent involved (e.g., pesticide poisoning requires symptom-specific therapy such as IV anticonvulsants to halt a seizure; antihistamines are used for allergic reactions), the particular organ system involved, and the presenting pathologic condition.

SPECIAL IMPLICATIONS FOR THE THERAPIST 4-1

Environmental Medicine

Environmental Hazards

Given the context of industrial, occupational, and environmental medicine and the single overriding factor of latency, health care professionals must view each client's health status holistically, as a composite of the individual's total life experience. Whenever symptoms present in the absence of a clearly identifiable history or cause, the client's past medical history must be carefully reviewed.

An environmental and occupational history includes dates of employment, a list of current and longest-held jobs, average hours worked per week, exposure to potential hazards in the workplace, common illnesses in coworkers, and personal protective equipment worn (or not worn) on the job.

Many health care providers use the mnemonic CH²OPD² (Community, Home, Hobbies, Occupation, Personal habits, Diet and Drugs) as a tool to identify an individual's history of exposures to potentially toxic environmental contaminants.[134] Specific questions for the therapist to ask are available.[92,134] Any information elicited by the therapist but unknown to the physician must be documented and reported.

Each geographic area has its own specific environmental/occupational concerns. The therapist must find out about specific local exposures and community concerns. Overall, the chronic exposure to chemically based products and pesticides has escalated the incidence of environmental allergies and cases of multiple chemical sensitivity. Frequently, these conditions present in a physical therapy setting with nonspecific neurologic and/or musculoskeletal manifestations.

The therapist must be aware that chemically induced illnesses may present as generalized muscle rigidity, peripheral neuropathy, or neurocognitive impairment as a result of neurotoxicity. Any unexplained muscle weakness and atrophy, sensory loss, depressed or absent deep tendon reflexes, memory loss, delirium, ataxia, or global change in muscle tone should raise a red flag for possible chemical etiology.[162]

Air Pollution

Vigorous exercise outdoors, which increases the dose of pollution delivered to the respiratory tract, should be avoided during periods of ambient air pollution.[84,183] Health care providers can reasonably advise all clients, especially anyone with respiratory disorders, as well as athletes in training,[170] to stay indoors during pollution episodes.

Respiratory protective equipment has been developed for use in the workplace to minimize exposure to toxic gases and airborne particles. Many of these devices, particularly those likely to be most effective, add to the work of breathing and are not well tolerated by some people, especially those with respiratory disease. The major limitation of respiratory protective equipment is that the anticipated protection is only achieved if the equipment fits properly. Much remains unknown about the efficacy of respiratory protective equipment, and concerns have been raised about the risk of dangerous carbon dioxide accumulation within the device, proper fit and inward leakage, resistance to airflow as the filter load increases, and individual breathing rates and filter replacement schedules. Research to answer these questions is necessary before specific recommendations can be made for the general population, as well as for individuals with known respiratory disease.

Studies have shown that high efficiency–filter air cleaners improve airway hyperresponsiveness and decrease peak flow amplitude in people with allergic asthma (studies to date have centered on children) who are sensitized and exposed to pets.[243] Future studies are needed to develop biologic markers to identify more accurately people who have a clinical improvement after allergen reduction.

Carbon Monoxide

Anyone with lung injury or reduced lung capacity may have a reduced ability to diffuse carbon monoxide when it is encountered. Individuals with low lung volumes for any reason (e.g., restrictive lung disease, sickle cell anemia, or lobectomy) who try to exercise may be at risk for CO poisoning under conditions a healthy individual would be able to tolerate.[108]

The main symptoms of CO poisoning are dizziness, headache, nausea, weakness, and tachypnea, followed at higher amounts by loss of consciousness, coma, convulsions, and death. As CO binds to hemoglobin to form carboxyhemoglobin, the reduced capacity of the blood to deliver oxygen to the tissues results in increased frequency of congestive heart disease and arrhythmias and stresses the immune system.[67,91,118,200]

Acute myonecrosis (death of individual muscle fibers) has been associated with CO poisoning. Clinical studies of people with heart disease have been carried out to evaluate the effects of CO exposure on exercise capacity. During exercise, persons with coronary artery disease experience a decreased time to occurrence of myocardial ischemia when exposed to CO compared to healthy subjects.[2,9] Neurologic recovery in people with mild to moderate CO poisoning is good. The prognosis after severe poisoning is variable and correlates with the extent and duration of the insult. Short-term memory impairment, depression, and syndromes related to lesions of the basal ganglia are well known. A syndrome of delayed neurologic deterioration occurs in about 10% of victims of serious CO intoxication. Risk factors for the delayed syndrome include age older than 40 years, prolonged exposure, and abnormalities of the brain on computed tomography (CT).[165]

In a small study of 16 healthy ice hockey players exposed to CO from a faulty ice resurfacer, chronic cough and dyspnea persisted 6 months after the exposure. Conventional pulmonary function tests did not reveal airway abnormalities but impulse oscillometry showed evidence of increased airway resistance and small-airway disease, which correlated with players' symptoms and reduced the players' ability to play effectively under exertion.[115]

Initial treatment following CO poisoning includes removing the person from the source of CO, initiating cardiac pulmonary resuscitation if they are not breathing and have no pulse, and initiating 100% inspired oxygen via a tight-fitting mask. Hospitalization normally is needed when carboxyhemoglobin levels in normal healthy individuals are greater than 25%, greater than 15% in those with heart or lung disease, and greater than 10% in pregnant women. Hyperbaric oxygen has been thought to provide even better treatment; however, these are limited among health care facilities. Current research does not support hyperbaric oxygen treatment to reduce the incidence of adverse neurologic outcomes. Additional research is needed to better define the role of hyperbaric oxygen.[38]

Lead

The brain is the target of lead toxicity in children, but adults usually present with manifestations of peripheral neuropathy. Typically, the radial and peroneal nerves are affected, resulting in wristdrop and footdrop, respectively. Anyone presenting with vague or nonspecific symptoms of myalgias, paresthesias, arthralgias accompanied by fatigue, irritability, lethargy, abdominal discomfort, poor concentration, headaches, tremors, and known risk factors may be suffering from lead poisoning.

Pica (compulsive chewing on nonnutritive objects such as dirt, paint, plaster, or clay) observed in children may be associated with lead toxicity and must be evaluated. Lead anemia and lead nephropathy may also occur (see "Neurotoxicity" in this chapter). For more information, contact the National Lead Information Center Clearinghouse at (800) 424-5323.

Vibration

Equipment and tools can be modified to reduce some of the dangerous levels of vibration. Seat upgrades have been found to help reduce vibration by up to 60% on large equipment that workers drive.[65] Utilizing antivibration gloves, taping handles with vibration-dampening tape, maintaining and balancing hand tools regularly, and using lower-vibration tools can also help decrease vibration. When vibration increases, muscles tend to tighten, and the tighter the grip on the equipment the more vibration gets transmitted to hands and arms.

Heat Stress

Even with a heat-illness prevention plan that includes medical screening, acclimatization, conditioning, environmental monitoring, and suitable practice adjustments for the athlete, heat illness can and does occur. Monitoring vital signs in anyone at risk will help identify early signs of heat exhaustion (e.g., weak, rapid pulse; elevated body temperature; shallow and fast breathing; or changes in blood pressure).

Observe for or ask about heat rash, a red cluster of pimples or small blisters on the neck and upper chest, in the groin, under the breasts, and/or in the elbow creases. The therapist must be prepared to respond quickly to alleviate symptoms and minimize morbidity and mortality.[28]

Exercise-associated muscle (heat) cramps represent a condition that presents during or after intense exercise sessions as an acute, painful, involuntary muscle contraction. Muscle cramps and distal extremity edema, dehydration, and electrolyte imbalance are the most commonly observed phenomena associated with heat stress in a therapy practice. The implications surrounding these adverse effects are discussed fully in Chapter 5.

For athletes with spinal cord injuries, regulating heart rate, circulating blood volume, production of sweat, and transferring heat to the surface varies with the level and severity of the spinal cord lesion. The therapist must monitor these athletes closely for heat-related problems and be prepared to provide more fluids, lighter clothing, or cooling of the trunk, legs, and head.[28]

Individuals who experience heat stroke may have compromised heat tolerance for up to a year or more. For an athlete, this can affect training and competition. Gradual return to sports is advised with close monitoring during exercise. The National Athletic Trainers' Association has guidelines for heat acclimatization for athletes that have recommendations for returning athletes affected by heat stress back to their sport located at www.nata.org/health-issues/heat-acclimatization. Older athletes have a decreased ability to maintain an adequate plasma volume during exercise, which may put them at risk for dehydration. Regular fluid intake is essential to avoid hyperthermia. The older athlete may need cardiovascular stress testing before participating in sports or strenuous activities in hot environments.[28]

The National Athletic Trainers' Association has published a position statement on exertional heat illnesses with helpful guidelines and recommendations for anyone working with athletes.[28] Representatives from 18 leading medical, nutritional, and sports medicine–related organizations have formed the Inter-Association Task Force on Exertional Heat Illnesses with additional helpful information.[148]

High Altitude

Many issues are related to altitude change (e.g., effects on fetal size and development, ultraviolet intensity with increases in altitude, sympathetic nervous system changes during acclimatization, air pollution at higher elevations, or physiologic changes and pathologic conditions occurring in military and aerospace personnel) that are being researched and reported in the literature. These are beyond the scope of this text. Implications here are confined to the more common issues in a therapy practice related to exercise capacity.

Chronic exposure to high altitude is known to result in changes in the mechanisms regulating oxygen delivery to the contracting muscles, but the underlying cause of changes in exercise capacity associated with high altitude is not completely understood.[93]

The primary effect of altitude on exercise capacity is through effects on the cardiovascular system, with a decrease in maximum oxygen consumption (VO_2max), a decrease in maximum heart rate, and pulmonary vascular resistance. Studies of oxygen saturation during submaximal exercise in natives of high-altitude areas compared with individuals born at sea level and acclimated to high altitudes suggest that oxygen saturation during exercise may be influenced by adaptation during growth and development and larger lung volume and pulmonary diffusion capacity for oxygen in the native high-altitude population.[37] Research continues to look at the effects of high altitude on the cardiovascular system, including effects of medications at high altitudes.

With continued exposure to increased altitude, exercise capacity does seem to improve, but never reaches that which is attained by the native population at sea level.[188] People with congestive heart failure or coronary artery disease are more likely to be symptomatic at high altitudes. Those with either of these conditions are likely to experience reduced exercise capacity.[109,143] With chronic carbohydrate loading at high altitudes, it has been found that athletes have a reduced rate of perceived exertion and improved physical performance. This was found to be especially true during prolonged and high-intensity exercise tasks.[159]

Mild sensory neuropathy may also occur at high altitudes, both as part of the burning feet/burning hands syndrome (distal limb burning and tingling paresthesias) associated with chronic mountain sickness and as a separate entity among control groups studied. This condition resolves with low-altitude sojourn (even for high-altitude natives), suggesting that a mechanism of altered axonal transport may be involved. Additionally, reduced thickness of microvessels observed implies that adaptive structural changes to hypobaric hypoxia may also occur in peripheral nerves and are similar to those reported in other tissues of high-altitude natives.[215]

Neurotoxicity

Neurologic recovery is facilitated by the plasticity of the nervous system. Peripheral sensory and motor nerve fibers have a remarkable capacity to regenerate after removal of the neurotoxin. Although the neurons in the CNS lack the ability to multiply, the surviving neurons may eventually take over the function of degenerated neurons and partially restore neurologic function. Physical and occupational therapy is beneficial during the recovery time to facilitate this process. When given sufficient time (18 to 24 months), partial clinical improvement is demonstrable in the majority of cases.

Coasting is the phenomenon of continuing clinical progression of neurologic deficits after removal of the offending toxin. Weakness or sensory deficits of these neuropathies often worsen for as long as 4 to 5 months after cessation of exposure, reflecting the delayed neuronal death or degeneration induced by the toxin.

Litigation and other potential sources of secondary gains often complicate environmental or occupational exposures that result in neurologic disorders. Psychologic factors may have profound effects on the client's perception of neurologic symptoms, even in those people with genuine organic disease. Emotional issues must be recognized and addressed throughout the rehabilitation process.

OCCUPATIONAL INJURIES AND DISEASES

Overview

Each year, millions of the estimated 140 million U.S. workers are injured on the job or become ill from exposure to hazards at work. These work-related injuries and illnesses result in substantial human and economic costs for workers, employers, and society; estimated direct and indirect costs of work-related injuries and illnesses are approximately $170 billion each year.[216]

Data collected through a National Electronic Injury Surveillance System report an estimated 3.4 million nonfatal injuries and illnesses among workers of all ages. More than three-fourths of all nonfatal workplace injuries/illnesses were attributed to contact with objects or equipment (e.g., being struck by a falling tool or caught in machinery), sprain or strain, and falls. Male workers under the age of 25 have the highest rate of workplace injuries.[73]

In 2010, there was a total of 4690 U.S. workers who died from occupational injuries, which is the second lowest number that has been recorded by the Bureau of Labor Statistics. There were around 3.4 million workers treated in the emergency room and about 94,000 workers who were hospitalized in 2007 because of work-related injuries and illnesses.[58] The most common fatal work injury continues to be highway incidents, with 1044 in 2010.[223]

The most common three events/exposures in 2010 included contact with objects and equipment, with 284,140 incidents; overexertion, with >100,000 incidents; and fall on same level, with >100,000 incidents. These accounted for 62% of total injuries and illnesses requiring days away from work.

The most common occupational injuries are referred to as *musculoskeletal disorders* (MSDs) and can involve cumulative trauma disorders caused by prolonged static positioning while using force (e.g., exerting constant force with the thumb pressed in while holding a computer mouse or constant gripping of tools or handles) and forceful repetition of work (repetitive strain injury) while using incorrect muscle groups or posture (e.g., keyboarding, meat cutting, or repetitive lifting and turning).

The lifetime cost of all injuries (including occupational and others) occurring in a single year in the United States totals an estimated $406 billion in medical expenses and productivity losses, including wages, fringe benefits, and the ability to perform normal household duties. The actual cost of these injuries is likely much higher when other related costs not included in the analysis are considered (e.g., police services, caregiver time, pain and suffering, decreased quality of life, or nonmedical expenditures such as wheelchair ramps or hand controls for vehicles).[81]

Computers and other time-saving devices have resulted in less physically demanding jobs, but new physical challenges and risk of impairments occur from incorrect ergonomics and prolonged (static) postures and positions, as well as repetitive motions. The prevalence of computers in modern society's workplace and leisure activities has also contributed to the increase in the "weekend warrior syndrome," or injuries to sedentary workers who go out on a weekend (or on an occasional basis during free time) and participate in sports or other strenuous physical activities. Overuse injuries and muscle strains are common, especially in the middle-aged and older adult. Activities such as gardening, hiking, or household repairs can be more strenuous than they seem in these age groups.[112]

Faster travel for business or pleasure in smaller spaces for long periods of time may also be contributing to an increase in injuries, deep vein thrombosis (DVT), or neck and back strain. Some individuals are at increased risk for these problems. For example, people are more prone to DVT if they have had a previous history of DVT, stroke, heart disease, or cancer. Anyone who has a neurologic disorder, lower extremity impairment, or mobility impairments may be at risk for DVT under these circumstances.[112]

Risk Factors for Occupational Injury

Risk factors for musculoskeletal occupational injury have been identified by OSHA. If workers are exposed to two or more of these factors (Box 4-2) during their shift, they are at increased risk and require preventive intervention. Additionally, in April 2000, Congress adopted the Senior Citizens' Freedom to Work Act that allows retired seniors to continue working without losing their Social Security benefits. The growing silver collar workforce (adults of the baby boomer generation working past the age of 65) may represent a unique risk factor, because aging is associated with a progressive decrement in various components of physical work capacity, including aerobic power and capacity, muscular strength and endurance, flexibility and coordination, and the tolerance of thermal stress.[199] Aging may thus contribute to additional workplace injuries and accidents.

Other risk factors in the general population may include psychosocial stress, gender, and personality. For example, psychosocial stress increases the physical demands of lifting for people with certain personality traits, making those people more susceptible to spine-loading increases and suspected low-back disorder risk.[133]

Those who work in nursing homes, including nurses, aides, and therapists, will come across frequent heavy lifting and repositioning of residents that may exceed their capacity. In 2003, there were 211,000 occupational injuries with caregivers, and this has likely increased because of the expanding aging population and increased workforce. Not only do proper body mechanics need to be learned by those working with the patients, but they need to have proper equipment to protect them. This can

---

Box 4-2

RISK FACTORS FOR OCCUPATIONAL INJURY

Worker Characteristics

- Age
- Psychosocial stress
- Gender
- Personality
- Physical fitness, including aerobic capacity, endurance, strength, flexibility, range of motion
- Health status, including lifestyle and presence of pregnancy or disease(s) such as chronic fatigue, fibromyalgia, Raynaud, diabetes, arthritis, coronary artery disease
- Individual anatomy and physiology (e.g., body capacity vs. job requirements, tissue resilience, functional reach)
- Work experience and training

Occupational Risk Groups

- Manufacturing (e.g., assembly line work, meat packing, automobile plants)
- Health care workers, especially in hospitals, nursing and personal care facilities
- Lumber and building material retailing
- Trucking (over the road) and ground courier (e.g., United Parcel Service, Federal Express)
- Sawmills, planing mills, millwork
- Construction
- Computer operators (keyboarding)
- Crude petroleum and natural gas extraction
- Retail store clerks and cashiers, especially grocery stores
- Musicians
- Agriculture production
- Beauty salons

Work Site Factors

- Lighting, temperature, noise
- Poor workstation ergonomics
- Poor ergonomic practices; inadequate injury prevention training

- Vibration
- Overtime, irregular shifts, length of workday; recovery time between shifts
- Infrequent or no breaks during work shift
- Continuing to work when injured or hurt (voluntarily or involuntarily)

Task-Specific Factors

- Performance of the same motions or motion pattern every few seconds for more than 2 hours at a time (repetition)
- Fixed or awkward work postures for more than a total of 2 hours (e.g., overhead work, twisted or bent back, bent wrist, kneeling, stooping, or squatting)
- Use of vibrating or impact tools or equipment for more than a total of 2 hours
- Unassisted manual lifting, lowering, or carrying of anything weighing more than 25 lb more than once during the work shift
- Piece rate or machine-paced work for more than 4 hours at a time
- Using hands/arms instead of available tool(s)
- Improper positioning or use of tools
- Static or awkward postures
- Contact stress (placing the body against a hard or sharp edge)
- Computer keyboard usage more than 15 hours/week

For the Health Care Worker*

- Performing manual orthopedic techniques
- Assisting clients during transfers and gait training activities
- Working with confused or agitated clients
- Unanticipated sudden movements or falls by client
- Treating a large number of clients in one day
- Rehabilitation, acute care, long-term care facilities
- Working with TBI, SCI, stroke individuals (high physical demands)

TBI, traumatic brain injured; *SCI*, spinal cord injured.

*From Cromie JE, Robertson VJ, Best MO: Work-related musculoskeletal disorders in physical therapists: prevalence, severity, risks, and responses. *Phys Ther* 80(4):336–351, 2000.

include mechanical lifts, stand lifts, transfer boards, slide boards, various types of beds and chairs and gait belts as well as making sure adaptive equipment is safe, not broken, and that they are using equipment appropriate for each individual.[64] This can also apply to therapists treating patients in the acute rehabilitation setting, the acute care setting, the skilled nursing setting, and the home health care setting.[55]

The National Institute for Occupational Safety and Health has a revised lifting equation which is a tool to evaluate two-handed lifting tasks. It was created to assist with a solution in reducing physical stress for workers who perform manual lifting. Studies are looking at whether this equation is able to accurately predict low back pain risk. It has been found that as the lifting index (which is an estimate of the physical stress associated with a particular manual lifting task) increases, the risk of low back pain increases as well.[249,250]

Research continues to be done on lifting techniques. Studies have looked at the recommended weight limits for lifting and holding limbs in the orthopedic setting as well as safe patient handling in the orthopedic setting. Research is also looking at various lifting devices and the amount of force required for operating them as well as the effectiveness of curriculum in schools that target safe patient handling and movement. This needs to be a continued area of focus in order to provide quality patient care in each setting with decreased risk for injury.[153,171,195,251]

Obesity may also be a co–risk factor for the development of occupational asthma and cardiovascular disease that may modify the worker's response to occupational stress, immune response to chemical exposures, and risk of disease from occupational neurotoxins. The interrelationship of work, obesity, and occupational safety and health is under further investigation.[192]

Ergonomics

Derived from the Greek terms *ergon*, meaning work, and *nomos*, meaning law, *ergonomics* is the study of work and of the relationship between humans and their working and physical environment. Over the last two decades, ergonomics has become a branch of industrial engineering that seeks to maximize productivity by minimizing worker discomfort and fatigue. Ergonomics is the science of fitting the task or the job to the worker.

Ergonomics is an interdisciplinary field of study that integrates engineering, medicine, and physical and behavioral management sciences and addresses issues arising from the interaction of humans in an increasingly technologic society. As a field of study, ergonomics deals with job design, work performance, health and safety, stress, posture, body mechanics, biomechanics, anthropometry (measurement of body size, weight, and proportions in relation to the task requirements), manual material handling, equipment design, quality control, environment, workers' education and training, and employment testing.

The goal is to provide an environment that allows the individual to adequately absorb and dissipate forces placed on the body. Fitting the work to the worker makes it possible to enhance productivity while controlling errors and reducing musculoskeletal strain and fatigue.

Ergonomics reduces risk factors known to contribute to occupational ergonomic-related injuries.

Humans have limitations arising from factors such as gender differences; differences in size, weight, and body proportions; aging; physical fitness and lifestyle choices; diet; stress; and pain and injury. Our abilities (and limitations), combined with the necessary acquired skills, determine how well we perform our daily tasks. Ergonomics helps people recognize their abilities and limitations for safe and effective performance within the environment. Work environments are often designed without adequate consideration for the people who will use them. Inadequate workplace design can contribute to stress, injury, pain, job-related impairments, disabilities, and subsequently, lost productivity. If products are designed without considering the human factor, health and safety hazards can occur.

A substantial body of validated scientific research and other evidence (epidemiologic, biomechanical, pathophysiologic studies) support the positive outcomes of ergonomic programs.[147,152] The evidence strongly supports two basic conclusions: (1) a consistent relationship exists between musculoskeletal disorders and certain workplace factors, especially at higher exposure levels; and (2) specific ergonomic interventions (e.g., proper equipment, postural education, and use of correct body mechanics) can reduce these injuries and illnesses.

Participatory ergonomics is the involvement of people in planning and controlling their work activities with knowledge and power to influence the process and outcome in order to achieve their goals. Most workplaces have an ergonomics team to work on participatory ergonomics interventions. The team can include employees, managers, ergonomists, health and safety personnel, and research experts. Combined with outside experts, they create a unique ergonomic intervention for the specific workplace and personnel. Participatory ergonomics interventions have shown some positive effects on health outcomes, including reducing musculoskeletal symptoms, injuries, worker's compensation claims, and the number of lost days from work due to sickness or injury.[63] Further research is needed on participatory ergonomic intervention to determine the benefit and costs.

A new branch of ergonomists, *rehabilitation ergonomists*, are health care professionals who, in addition to functioning as an ergonomist practitioner, also use knowledge of the relationship between pathology and work to match the demands of the job to the capacity of the worker. The practitioners are therapists and other specialists who have a background of anatomy, physiology, kinesiology, pathology, and ergonomics. They analyze the person performing the work as well as analyze the setting in which they work in order to make positive ergonomic changes. Rehabilitation ergonomists will work with people who do not fit the normal standards and assist in creating modifications to safely and productively perform their job or task. Concentrating on improved safety focuses on physiologic improvement, which in turn increases productivity.

The CDC has several ergonomic programs and interventions for various occupations, including construction workers, manual material handling, children and adolescents working in agriculture, workers who use non-powered hand tools, and many more. These are located at www.cdc.gov/niosh/topics/ergonomics.

Ergonomic Certification

Certification as an ergonomist practitioner is available through two national boards: the Board of Certified Professional Ergonomists and the Oxford Research Institute. These two are nonprofit board certification programs that are nationally and internationally recognized. Competency is demonstrated through experience, work samples, and a passing grade on a board examination. Previously, board certification in professional ergonomics accredited engineering ergonomists through a certification examination. Today, psychologists, therapists, and others have joined engineers in the pursuit of ergonomics as a career.

A wide range of private certification programs are available to the health care professional seeking training and certification as an ergonomist. The Occupational Injury Prevention and Rehabilitation Society supports the accreditation of therapists through the Board of Certified Professional Ergonomists and the Oxford Research Institute but recognizes other programs that meet the minimum criteria for certification as an ergonomist. These criteria and a listing of ergonomic certification options for therapists are available.[21,101] The orthopedic section of the American Physical Therapy Association (APTA) also has an occupational health special-interest group.

Musculoskeletal Disorders

MSDs are often referred to as *ergonomic injuries* and encompass cumulative trauma disorders, work-related musculoskeletal disorders (WMSDs), and repetitive strain injuries. WMSDs are defined as an injury or disorder of the muscles, tendons, ligaments, cartilage, or spinal disks as diagnosed by a health care professional, resulting in a positive physical finding sufficient to require medical intervention and/or days away from work or assignment (i.e., an "OSHA-recordable" injury).[157]

MSDs do not include injuries resulting from slips, trips, falls, or accidents. The disorder must be directly related to the employee's job and specifically connected to activities that form the core or a significant part of the job (e.g., a poultry processor might report tendinitis, but a back injury while occasionally changing the water bottle on a water cooler would not be covered).[157]

There were a total 346,400 WMSDs in 2010, with the back being injured in nearly half of the cases. In 2010, sprains, strains, and tears accounted for 40% of total injury and illness cases requiring days away from work, with soreness and pain accounting for 11% of total cases. The sprains, strains, and tears were a result of overexertion 43% of the time. The back was injured in 36% of the sprain, strain, and tear cases, with 12% involving the shoulder and 26% involving the lower extremities. Although the cases involving the back occur most frequently, they are also decreasing in frequency faster than all of the other body parts and required a median of 7 days to recover. For those cases involving the shoulder, they required a median of 21 days to recover, which is more than any other sprain, strain, or tear cases.[224]

WMSDs account for more than one-third of all occupational injuries that are serious enough to result in days away from work. Back injuries and carpal tunnel syndrome (CTS) are the most prevalent, most expensive, and most preventable MSDs. Men tend to have more severe injuries compared to women, with men requiring a median of 9 days to recover compared to women, who require 7 days to recover. Each year more than 100,000 women experience work-related back injuries that cause them to miss work. It is estimated that 300,000 injuries and $9 billion in worker's compensation can be saved with improved industry safety and ergonomic practices.

Seventy percent of the repeated trauma cases are in manufacturing industries.[40] The shift in the U.S. economy to service industries, such as nursing homes and other long-term care facilities, in which staff members are required to perform heavy lifting, has contributed significantly to the number of back injuries.[123] Other commonly sustained workplace injuries include eye injuries, hearing impairment, fractures, amputations, and lacerations severe enough to require medical intervention.

Etiology and Risk Factors

Risk factors for MSDs are divided into four major categories: genetic, morphologic, biomechanical, and psychosocial. Among the various biomechanical risk factors, exposure to repetitive, static, and vibratory activities is known to result in MSDs.[119] Differences in physical, occupational, and physiologic factors may contribute to MSDs. For example, CTS is associated with pregnancy as well as rheumatoid arthritis, which is a condition that affects women more often than men. Women comprise 70% of the CTS cases and 62% of tendinitis cases that are serious enough to warrant time off work.[156]

CTS accounts for more days away from work than any other workplace injury, requiring a median of 27 days to recover in 2010.[224] In addition to workers who spend hours at the computer, CTS has been reported in meat packers, assembly line workers, retail clerks scanning labels, jackhammer operators, athletes, physical and occupational therapists, and homemakers. In both genders, CTS can be associated with other medical conditions, such as thyroid problems, liver disease, multiple myeloma, and diabetes, as well as with other musculoskeletal disorders that may or may not be work-related (see Box 39-1). For all work-related CTS, poor worksite design, poor posture and body mechanics, and industrial equipment and computers that take out the automatic pauses of work must be evaluated as possible contributors. An in-depth discussion of CTS is included in Chapter 39.

Pathogenesis

The exact pathomechanisms of MSDs remain obscured because of the difficulty of analyzing tissues of individuals in the early stages of work-related MSDs. Tissue injury caused by repeated motion may involve an inflammatory response, but why one worker develops symptoms while others doing the same task do not remains unknown and a topic of discussion and study. The relationship between repetition rate, forcefulness of tasks, cellular responses to these activities, number of strains, and inflammatory response is under investigation. The role of genetics and psychosocial factors is also being considered.[15-17,209]

A systematic review of the literature looking at work-related MSDs in 2009 found the following risk factors with reasonable evidence of a causal relationship for the development of MSDs: heavy physical work, smoking, high body mass index, high psychosocial work demands, and the presence of comorbidities. The most common biomechanical risk factors with reasonable evidence of a causal relationship for the development of work-related MSDs include excessive repetition, awkward postures, and heavy lifting.[69]

It is likely that the development of MSDs is multifactorial, with variations in individual tissue tolerances. Each individual may have his or her own threshold below which tissue integrity is preserved and above which injury results. It is possible that the combined and/or accumulative effects of risk factors for MSD can exceed tissue tolerance capacity and cause injury. When continued task performance is superimposed on injured and inflamed tissues, a cycle of injury, inflammation, and motor dysfunction occurs.[16,17]

MSDs in the lumbar spine may have a different mechanism. Static lumbar loading applied to ligaments results in creep (e.g., stretch of viscoelastic tissue over time that is not fully restored immediately after load removal). In theory, ligaments that remain stretched beyond their resting length may result in increased laxity of intervertebral joints and risk of instability and injury. In the spine, ligaments have a secondary role in maintaining intervertebral stability.[206]

Static lumbar flexion under constant load results in long-lasting viscoelastic creep that does not fully recover after 7 hours of rest. The creep developed gives rise to a neuromuscular disorder with reduced reflexive muscle activity, muscle spasms during flexion, and hyperexcitability of muscle activity during rest that may last 24 hours or more. The viscoelastic creep and associated neuromuscular disorder can occur even with low loads, which may help explain how cumulative low back problems develop.[206]

Clinical Manifestations

Workers suffering from MSDs, especially upper extremity MSDs, may experience decreased grip strength and range of motion, impaired muscle function, and inability to complete activities of daily living. Symptoms are persistent (although intermittent, they return and progress over time) and most commonly include pain (e.g., headache, neck, back, shoulder, wrist, hip, or knee); burning sensation, numbness, and/or tingling (hands or feet); Raynaud phenomenon; and myalgias and arthralgias with spasm, stiffness, swelling, or inflammation.

Neural tissues at the cervical spine, carpal tunnel, cubital tunnel, or thoracic outlet can be compressed as a result of the swelling associated with the biomechanical microtrauma. The individual may perceive weakness and drop objects or have difficulty with handwriting. Common MSDs and upper extremity MSDs are listed in Box 4-3.

A predictable sequence of events leads up to MSDs of a repetitive nature or those caused by static postures (e.g., some tasks such as prolonged writing or typing at a

---

Box 4-3

COMMON WORK-RELATED MUSCULOSKELETAL DISORDERS

- Carpal tunnel syndrome
- Carpet layers' knee
- Cubital tunnel syndrome
- de Quervain's disease
- Epicondylitis (medial or lateral tennis elbow)
- Focal hand dystonia
- Hand-arm vibration syndrome
- Herniated spinal disc
- Pronator syndrome
- Radial tunnel syndrome
- Raynaud phenomenon
- Rotator cuff syndrome
- Sciatica
- Tendinitis (shoulder, elbow, wrist)
- Tenosynovitis (finger flexors or extensors; trigger finger)
- Tension neck syndrome, thoracic outlet syndrome, cervical radiculopathy
- Thoracic outlet syndrome
- Ulnar nerve syndrome

---

keyboard require cocontraction of the agonists and antagonists). Fatigue and the inability to recover from fatigue brought on by additional hours and pressured deadlines, combined with emotional stress and improper posture, improper use of tools, or an ergonomically inadequate workstation, result in muscle soreness.

Over time and without intervention or a change in the contributing factors, the body strains to keep up and pain develops, followed by injury or trauma. In the case of tendinitis or focal hand dystonia, it is possible that a sensory problem rather than just a motor problem occurs and is caused by a dysfunction in cortical sensory processing.[43] Evidence suggests that aggressive sensory discriminative training complemented by traditional exercises to facilitate musculoskeletal health can improve sensory processing and motor control.[42]

SPECIAL IMPLICATIONS FOR THE THERAPIST   4-2

Occupational Injuries and Diseases

In 2008, there were 28% of workers who stated they were in "excellent health" compared to 34% of workers in 2002. The variables of an effective workplace where workers are more likely to report excellent health include having learning opportunities and challenges, good work and personal life balance, autonomous practice, a supervisor who promotes success and supports economic security, and a place where there is respect and trust.[61]

In 2003, OSHA put into place a comprehensive plan designed to reduce ergonomic injuries through the development of guidelines, enforcement measures, workplace outreach, and research. OSHA targeted approximately 2500 nursing or personal care facilities that reported high injury and illness rates, and it inspected approximately 1000 of those facilities, focusing on specific hazards that account for the majority of nursing home staff injuries and illnesses. Those hazards include ergonomics (primarily back injuries from patient handling); bloodborne pathogens/tuberculosis; and slips, trips, and falls. OSHA's recommendations include minimizing and eliminating manual lifting of residents and having employers implement an effective ergonomics process that includes management support, involvement of employees, identification of problems, implementation of solutions, addresses reports of injuries, provides training, and evaluates ergonomic efforts.[225]

Therapists can have an important role in the development of health and safety programs that will accurately assess hazards in the workplace and reduce the risk of musculoskeletal injuries, amputations, and illnesses. For all clients with MSDs, questions related to occupation and exposure to toxins, such as chemicals or gases, are included because well-defined physical (e.g., cumulative trauma disorder) and health problems occur in people engaging in specific occupations.[155] For example, pesticide exposure is common among agricultural workers, who may also experience musculoskeletal problems from repetitive loading. Asthma and sick building syndrome are reported among office workers.

Ergonomics

The therapist can have a significant role in the prevention (e.g., worksite analysis and workstation redesign) and rehabilitation of occupational injuries. The role of ergonomics in injury management includes a prompt and safe return to work, cost savings, and prevention of injuries or reduction of injury progression or recurrence. There is evidence that workstation exercises can reduce musculoskeletal discomfort for workers sitting in front of a computer or other video display terminal. The therapist can devise easy-to-do, appropriate workstation exercises for individuals at risk for postural immobility and the resultant musculoskeletal discomfort.[80,131]

With the increased and prolonged use of computers at home, school, and work, upper extremity MSDs are becoming more prevalent. It is estimated that some individuals may use up to 100,000 keystrokes in an average day. Computer keyboard usage greater than 15 hours per week can contribute to MSDs affecting the upper extremity, shoulder, neck, and low back. The therapist can offer guidance to workers regarding keyboard workstation designs and features.[132]

When conducting a job analysis, the therapist evaluates job duties and environmental factors that put physical stress on the worker; stressors most typically include force (any weight that is lifted, pushed, or carried), repetition, and posture. The therapist will assess the amount of force needed to produce the necessary work, the number of repetitions, and the postural tolerances required by the job.

These variables are evaluated for both newly developing programs or job tasks and in industrial rehabilitation programs for cases of work conditioning and work hardening. The APTA defines work conditioning as "an intensive, work-related, goal-oriented program designed specifically to restore systemic neuromusculoskeletal functions, motor function, range of motion, and cardiovascular/pulmonary functions. It is meant to restore physical capacity and function to enable the worker to return to work." The APTA defines work hardening as "a highly structured, goal-oriented, individualized intervention program designed to return a worker to work. They are multidisciplinary, use real/simulated work activities designed to restore physical, behavioral, and vocational functions. Work hardening addresses the issues of productivity, safety, physical tolerance and worker behaviors." The main goal of these programs are to return injured or disabled workers to work or to improve the work status of the worker The focus is on simulating the worker's job tasks in a safe and supervised location. Throughout the program, there is focus on psychological, physical, and emotional tolerance as well as improving endurance.[136,187] The APTA has guidelines for occupational health physical therapy, including work conditioning and work hardening programs.[11]

Quantifying the requirements for each job is essential in both prevention and return-to-work situations. Therapists can provide analysis and management of injury-related job hazards, injury prevention training, examination/evaluation management of MSDs, development of job/task alterations, and return-to-work program planning.[14]

Silver Collar Workers

Therapists also need to modify traditional intervention strategies for prevention and treatment of injuries in the silver collar workforce previously mentioned. Although older workers may have lower injury rates compared with younger workers, their injuries are likely to be more severe with a longer recovery time. The fatality rate for older workers was found to be 3 times that of younger workers in 2003.[177]

Therapists can assist industries and job sites to adapt job duties to accommodate for age-related conditions such as reduced muscle strength and motion. Providing ergonomically correct worksites and work areas, implementing diagnostic and training programs to prevent specific conditions (e.g., CTS, tendinitis, or back injuries), and instituting wellness programs to include home- or gym-based exercise programs and organized stretch/walk breaks will help keep all employees, particularly seniors, in good health and injury free.[22]

There is a need for the development of distinct fall prevention programs specific to the older population in the workforce. Efforts should be made to minimize fall hazards in all occupational sectors. More attention must be paid to the sensory impairments of the older worker, especially in vision and hearing, with job modifications as needed. Motor learning theory suggests that older adults may need different types of safety training. Emphasizing task analysis and repeated practice may be needed in this population.[90]

Physical Therapists with Work-Related Symptoms

Interventions employed by therapists can lead to WMSDs among themselves although little is known about this segment of the population. A summary of prevalence, severity, risks, and responses associated with MSDs in physical therapists suggests that therapists at greatest risk are the more inexperienced therapists who may not know their limits (more than 50% have their first episode as a student or in their first 5 years of practice), those in neurology and rehabilitation, and those performing manual orthopedic techniques.[37] Other studies have found that older and younger therapists have similar WMSDs but that the older therapists had more severe pain and were more likely to change jobs because of their injury.[117] It has been reported that one in six physical therapists change their work setting or leave the profession because of a WMSD and around 57% of physical therapists will have a work-related musculoskeletal complaint.[47]

One study found that the most frequently injured body part of a physical therapist is the low back, followed by hand and wrist, neck and shoulder. It also found that the settings with the highest number of WMSDs were the school system, "other," and private practice.[47]

Researchers have demonstrated that knowledge of ergonomics, injury, and intervention strategies is not associated with a reduced risk of injury among therapists.[68,104] For example, maintaining good body mechanics is not always protective when a client is starting to fall and pulls the therapist down. Lifting with sudden maximal effort, bending and twisting, repetitive movement, awkward postures maintained for a prolonged period of time, and using high levels of force are correlated with work-related injuries among therapists.[32,104]

Activities in specific practice areas have been associated with increased therapist injuries. These areas include performing functional activities with patients in acute care, preventing patient falls in skilled nursing facilities, and working on motor vehicle activities with patients in home care.[70] Therapists working in rehabilitation units with individuals who have brain injuries, stroke, and spinal cord injuries with high physical demands are at increased risk of work-related injuries. Clients who are less mobile in long-term care facilities, skilled nursing facilities, or acute care often put the greatest demands on therapists.[245]

Other risk factors include heavy client loads, working with combative clients, increased number of hours performing manual therapy, and injuries that occur outside the workplace that are not treated or healed before returning to work. Manual therapy and transfers/lifts has been associated with 54% of all physical and occupational therapy injuries.[70] The cultural context in which therapists work might contribute to WMSDs. For example, the need to demonstrate hard work and care for patients/clients along with the need to appear knowledgeable and skilled by remaining injury-free may increase risk for therapists. The therapist may put the needs of the patient/client first, subsequently suffering an injury. They fail to report the injury to avoid being perceived as incompetent. There is also a tendency to try and manage their own condition, which can lead to delays in recovery.[67]

Therapists are encouraged to maintain good body mechanics, change position often, ask for help, and report injuries when they occur. Using gait belts for patient transfers, using appropriate adaptive equipment such as a walkers for ambulation, having a wheel chair behind for anyone who is unsteady, using parallel bars for gait training, and using mechanical aids such as Hoyer lifts or stand-lifts is advised when appropriate for patient and therapist safety and injury prevention. The therapist should seek care and modify work or take time off when necessary. It is not a good idea to try to work through the injury.[245]

Understanding risk factors, identifying what causes injury, and changing behaviors are the keys to preventing injuries to therapists in the workplace setting. Therapists frequently believe their knowledge of physical therapy and skills will prevent WMSDs from occurring. Further research is needed to identify aspects of therapy practice that place the therapist at greatest risk and ways to reduce that risk.[245]

Occupational Burns

Of the more than 1 million firefighters employed in the United States, over 300,000 are career firefighters, with the rest being volunteer firefighters. The rate of injury and death occurring on the fire ground (49% of all injuries in 2011) or while responding to or returning from an incident (6% of all injuries in 2011) has declined since the late 1980s with the mandatory use of gloves, self-contained breathing apparatus, and full personal protective clothing. National trends for firefighter injuries are sprain/strain- and stress-related injuries. Overexertion and strain account for 25% of all fire-related firefighter injuries and is the leading cause of injury. In 2011, 38% of all fire-related injuries resulted in missed work time. Studies support the longstanding assertion that the number of firefighters responding to a fire is a factor that affects injuries.[242,244]

Aside from the acute injurious effects of fire, clinicians must be alert to the pathophysiologic changes associated with exposure to heat and smoke and to the chronic sequelae, both physical and psychologic (Table 4-4). In addition to the management of burns and trauma, it is necessary to evaluate clients for all acute systemic effects of exposure to smoke, heat, or toxic substances; recognize toxic effects that may be obscured by more serious traumatic effects; be alert for delayed consequences; and recognize acute and chronic exposure and health effects as a result of toxic chemicals in smoke, especially among firefighters.

Occupational Pulmonary Diseases

Materials inhaled in the workplace can lead to all the major chronic lung diseases, except those as a result of vascular disease. Exposure in office buildings and hospitals is now included as a known workplace-related cause of disease. As new industries are developed, new problems are

Table 4-4	Types of Fire-and-Rescue–Related Acute and Chronic Injury

Acute	Chronic
Lacerations, contusions	Chronic cardiovascular disease
Falls (including on site and from moving apparatus)	Chronic respiratory disease
Burns (superficial, deep, internal)	Noise-induced hearing loss
Dermal reactions to toxicants	Posttraumatic stress disorder
Eye irritation, injuries, and burns	Physical disability
Smoke inhalation	Hepatitis C
Sore throat, hoarseness, cough	
Exacerbated asthma	
Dyspnea, tachypnea, wheezing	
Headaches	
Cyanosis	
Cardiovascular strain	
Musculoskeletal trauma	
Heat stress and fatigue	
Neuropsychiatric effects	
Renal damage	
Death (motor vehicle accidents, falls, asphyxiation, burns)	

Modified from National Institute for Occupational Safety and Health (NIOSH) and Centers for Disease Control and Prevention: Fire fighter investigation and prevention program. Available at http://www.cdc.gov/niosh/fire/. Accessed August 30, 2012.

Box 4-4

ASTHMA-TRIGGERING SUBSTANCES IN THE HEALTH CARE SETTING*

- Latex (primarily latex gloves)
- Glutaraldehyde (sensitizing agent used in cold sterilization)
- Ammonia and chlorine (cleaning and disinfecting solutions)
- Antimicrobial pesticides (sterilizers, disinfectants, sanitizers)
- Dust and irritating particles in the air (construction and remodeling projects)
- Mold and fungus (carpeting, ceiling tiles exposed to water)
- Perfumes, scented personal care products worn by clients/patients, coworkers, visitors
- Isocyanate (a class of extremely hazardous substances found in orthopedic casting materials)
- Pharmaceutical drugs (e.g., psyllium, rifampin, penicillin, tetracycline)
- Formaldehyde used in specimen preparation
- Diacetyl (ingredient in artificial butter and other flavoring)

*Includes hospitals, medical and dental clinics, nursing and personal-care facilities, dialysis centers, specialty outpatient facilities, and medical laboratories.

From Bain EI: Perils in the air: Avoiding occupational asthma triggers in the workplace. *Am J Nurs* 100(6):88, 2000; and Mehler L: Acute antimicrobial pesticide-related illnesses among workers in health care facilities. *MMWR* 59(18):551–556, 2010.

reported. For example, obstructive lung disease has been reported in workers in the microwave popcorn and flavor manufacturing business who have not been adequately protected from chemical exposures.[135]

Identifying the source of illness is important because it can lead to cure and prevention for others.[23] Disorders caused by chemical agents are classified as (1) pneumoconioses, (2) hypersensitivity pneumonitis, (3) obstructive airway disorders, (4) toxic lung injury, (5) lung cancer, and (6) pleural diseases. These conditions are discussed more fully in Chapter 15.

Asbestos and other silicates, such as kaolin, mica, and vermiculite, can cause *pneumoconiosis*. Asbestos-induced diseases cause lung inflammation and fibrosis as a result of activation of alveolar macrophages. Coal worker's pneumoconiosis is another parenchymal lung disease caused by inhalation of coal dust.

Hypersensitivity pneumonitis has many other names, such as extrinsic allergic alveolitis, farmer's lung, mushroom picker's disease, humidifier or air conditioner lung, bird breeder's or bird fancier's lung, and detergent worker's lung, and is characterized by a granulomatous inflammatory reaction in the pulmonary alveolar and interstitial spaces. Silicosis is a parenchymal toxic lung disease caused by inhalation of crystalline silica, a component of rock and sand. Workers at risk include miners, tunnelers, quarry workers, stonecutters, sandblasters, foundry workers, glass blowers, and ceramic workers.

The pathogenesis of these occupational lung diseases varies among different pneumoconioses, but the bottom line is that cilia and mucus-secreting cells are absent in the small bronchioles and alveoli. The body depends on macrophages to remove any of the tiny particles that lodge in these areas. The macrophages then carry them to the mucociliary elevator or dump them into the lymphatics. The process is often sabotaged because substances, such as silica dust, can destroy the macrophages. In the process, substances are released that trigger inflammation and pulmonary fibrosis. See Chapter 15 for more details about these diseases.

Exposure to allergens and irritants has resulted in the recognition of a new disease called *work-related (or occupational) upper airway disease* or *united airway disease*, which although not life-threatening, has been reported to cause sufferers to experience reduced quality of life. Occupational allergens identified are many and varied, including plants (e.g., tobacco leaf dust, grapes, asparagus, or flowers), insects (e.g., bees or locusts), powder paints, and others. Reports of upper airway disease in various occupational groups involved in rescue, recovery, and cleanup at the World Trade Center identified a new work hazard from irritants. This was due to a large amount of dust, smoke, and combustion products in the air of New York City, causing tens of thousands of workers and volunteers to inhale this air pollution.[72,246]

Health problems caused by these irritants range from runny nose to full-blown allergic rhinitis. Up to 40% of individuals in the workplace with allergic rhinitis also have asthma and 92% of workers with occupational asthma report symptoms of occupational rhinitis. The link between rhinitis and asthma is the presence of inflammation of the nasal and bronchial mucosae. The incidence of having both occupational asthma and rhinitis is highest for farmers and woodworkers.[145,246]

Occupational asthma is asthma that is attributable to or is made worse by environmental exposures (e.g., inhaled gases, dusts, fumes, or vapors) in the workplace. The air in health care institutions may contain irritating and sensitizing chemicals and particles that can aggravate asthma (Box 4-4).

Occupational asthma has become the most prevalent occupational lung disease in developed countries, is more common than is generally recognized, and can be severe and disabling. The reactions can be immediate or delayed, sometimes hours after leaving the workplace. Identification of workplace exposures causing and/or aggravating the asthma and appropriate control or cessation of these exposures can often lead to reduction or even complete elimination of symptoms and disability.[86]

OSHA requires employers to provide a safe and healthy work environment free from recognized hazards. In addition, the Americans with Disabilities Act of 1990 requires employers to accommodate workers with asthma. Suspected episodes of occupational asthma should be documented, including symptoms, suspected exposures, visits to health services, and similar symptoms reported by other employees. Many effective and appropriate substitutions and controls are available that can be incorporated to eliminate or prevent airborne and topical exposures.[13]

Occupational Cancer

Each year it is estimated that there are 20,000 cancer deaths and 40,000 new cases of cancer in the United States that are attributed to occupation (Table 4-5). It is also estimated that less than 2% of chemicals used in workplaces have been tested for carcinogens.[54] Despite increased knowledge of occupational risk for cancer, it is estimated that 30% to 40% of the population in the industrialized world will develop malignant disease during their lifetime. Changes in wood processing and decreased duration of occupational exposure because of more frequent job changes may have altered the picture somewhat.

Studies continue to provide evidence that cancer in humans has environmental causes (e.g., exposure to arsenic is associated with increased risk of skin, urinary bladder, and respiratory tract cancers; chronic exposure to ultraviolet light is associated with skin cancer; vinyl chloride is associated with liver cancer; dry cleaning solvents are associated with kidney and liver cancer and non-Hodgkin lymphoma). Research is ongoing to assess combined genetic and environmental contributions to risk.[74,102,186]

Alteration or mutation in the genetic material (deoxyribonucleic acid [DNA]) may occur as a result of exposure to carcinogenic chemicals or radiation. Both experimental animal models of cancer and the study of human cancers with known causes have revealed the existence of a significant interval between first exposure to the responsible agent and the first manifestation of a tumor. This period is referred to as the *induction period, latency period,* or *induction-latency period.*

For humans, the length of the induction-latency period varies from a minimum of 4 to 6 years for radiation-induced leukemias to 40 or more years for some cases of asbestos-induced mesotheliomas. For most tumors, the interval ranges from 12 to 25 years; such a long period may easily obscure the relationship between a remote exposure and a newly discovered tumor.

In the future, individuals with a high environmental risk of developing cancer may benefit from immune

Table 4-5	Cancers Related to Occupational Processes
Cancer	**Examples of Substance/Process**
Lung	Arsenic, asbestos, beryllium, cadmium, coke oven fumes, chromium compounds, coal products, nickel refining, foundry substances, radon, soot, tars, silica, vinyl chloride, diesel exhaust, radioactive ores like uranium
Bladder	Paint/dyeing products, printing processes, benzidine, beta-naphthylamine, arsenic, chemicals used in rubber, leather, and textile industries
Nasal cavity and sinuses	Formaldehyde, textile industry, mustard gas, nickel refining, chromium dust, leather dust, wood dust, baking, flour milling, radium
Larynx	Asbestos, wood dust, paint fumes, chemicals used in metal working, petroleum, plastics and textile industries
Mesothelioma	Asbestos
Lymphatic and hematopoietic	Benzene, herbicides, insecticides, radiation
Skin	Arsenic, coal tars, paraffin, certain oils, sunlight
Soft-tissue sarcoma	Radiation
Liver	Arsenic, vinyl chloride
Lip	Sunlight

From American Cancer Society: Occupation and Cancer. 2007. No. 300214-Rev. 02/12. Available at http://www.cancer.org/acs/groups/content/@nho/documents/document/occupationandcancerpdf.pdf. Accessed August 1, 2012.

stimulation as a means of cancer prevention by inducing specific immunity through the use of vaccines.[83] Oncoantigens continue to be researched as preventative vaccines as well as to cure more advanced stages of cancer lesions.[30] Research continues to be completed on both animal and human models for various types of cancer vaccines and has had some positive results.[24] Individual cancers and their treatment are discussed in organ-specific chapters in this text; see also Chapter 9.

Occupational Infections

Occupational infections are diseases caused by work-associated exposure to microbial agents, including bacteria, viruses, fungi, and protozoa. Occupational infections are distinguished by the fact that some aspect of the work involves contact with a biologically active organism. Occupational infection can occur after contact with infected people, as in the case of health care workers; infected animal or human tissue, secretions, or excretions, as in laboratory workers; asymptomatic or unknown contagious humans, as happens during business travel; or infected animals, as in agriculture (e.g., brucellosis).

Physical therapists should be aware of all types of occupational infections in order to treat anyone who may have signs/symptoms of an occupational infection. Therapists also need to be aware of the occupational infections they may come across during a day of work. Common occupational infections therapists may encounter include hepatitis, HIV/AIDS, herpes simplex and herpes zoster (shingles), methicillin-resistant *Staphylococcus aureus*, *Clostridium difficile*, and tuberculosis. Another occupational infection therapists should also be aware of is outbreaks of the flu, including H1N1 (swine flu).

Occupational Skin Disorders

There are roughly 13 million U.S. workers who are exposed to chemicals that absorb through the skin. Occupational skin diseases are the second most common type of occupational disease, accounting for 20% of all cases of occupational disease in the United States, with 61,000 new cases reported each year. It is likely that many cases of work-related skin disorders are underreported, because it is often not a life-threatening condition and never diagnosed or treated. The health care industry reports 4000 cases of skin illness each year, but the highest rates are in agriculture and manufacturing. Other industries commonly affected included food service, cosmetology, cleaning, painting, mechanics, printing/lithography, and construction.

The most common forms of occupational skin diseases include irritant contact dermatitis, allergic contact dermatitis, skin cancers, skin infections, skin injuries, and miscellaneous skin diseases. Dermatoses are more prevalent in some states such as California and Florida; contact dermatitis from plants, particularly in combination with sunlight, and chemicals, such as pesticides or fertilizers, is common among agricultural workers especially since the use of fertilizers has increased by 300% over the last 46 years.[240] Contact dermatitis (acute, chronic, or allergic) is the most common of occupational skin disorders, with an estimated annual cost to treat that exceeds $1 billion, but other types include contact urticaria, psoriasis, scleroderma, vitiligo (areas of depigmentation), chloracne (see Fig. 4-1), actinic skin damage known as farmer's skin or sailor's skin, cutaneous malignancy, and cutaneous infections.

There can be four different causes of occupational skin diseases, which includes chemical agents, mechanical trauma, physical agents, and biological agents. Chemical agents are the most common cause and can be divided into primary irritants, which act directly on the skin, and sensitizers, which react with repeated exposure. Physical agents include extreme temperature and radiation; mechanical trauma includes friction, pressure, abrasions, lacerations, and contusions; and biological agents include parasites, microorganisms, plants, and other animal materials.

Skin cancer is an important occupational illness and is most often the result of excessive exposure to ultraviolet light; farmers, fishermen, roofers, and road workers who continuously work in the sun are at greatest risk. For further discussion of specific skin disorders, see Chapter 10.[57]

Rubber Latex Allergy

During the recent past, the incidence of natural rubber latex allergy (LA) has dramatically increased not only among the general population but also among health care workers, the latter because of repeated contact as a result of standard precautions and subsequent increased occupational exposure.

LA occurs predominantly in certain high-risk groups (Box 4-5); the estimated prevalence in health care workers varies widely (2.8%–18%), and studies do not always distinguish between those who are positive in an assay for latex-specific immunoglobulin E (IgE) and those with clinical allergy.[168] The prevalence of LA in the general population ranges from 0.1% to 1.0%, compared with as high as 60% for those with spina bifida or other chronic medical conditions associated with repeated exposure to latex.[146]

This occupational sensitivity to natural rubber latex (NRL; i.e., latex proteins and in some cases the associated cornstarch glove powder serves as a carrier for the allergenic proteins from the NRL) has resulted in the following three types of reactions:
- Immediate hypersensitivity (type I hypersensitivity; IgE-mediated) with urticaria (hives), watery eyes, rhinitis, respiratory distress, and asthma or skin rash, which can spread from the hands, up the arms, and to the face (it can also cause swelling of the lips, eyes, ears, and larynx [laryngeal edema can prevent the person from speaking]).
- Irritation or irritant contact dermatitis manifested as dry, crusty, hard bumps; sores; and horizontal cracks on the skin (Fig. 4-4)
- Mild-to-severe allergic contact dermatitis (delayed type IV hypersensitivity; cell-mediated) (Fig. 4-5)

The first two reactions are related to mechanical and chemical exposure, whereas LA is caused by sensitization to the proteins in NRL. These responses occur when items containing latex touch the skin, mucous membranes (eyes, mouth, nose, genitals, bladder, or rectum), or open areas.

Latex exposure has become one of the leading causes of occupational asthma. Once sensitized, some health care

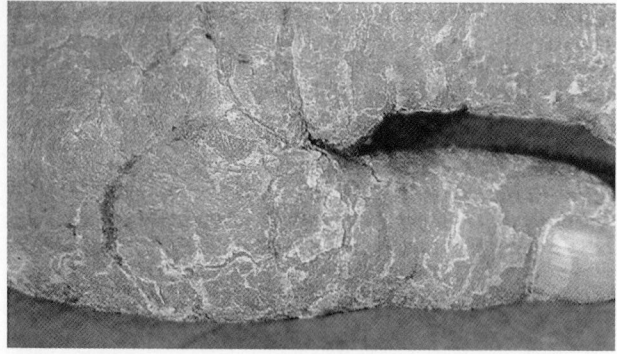

Figure 4-4

Rubber glove dermatitis. (From Baxter PJ et al: *Hunter's diseases of occupations*, ed 9, CRC Press, 2000.)

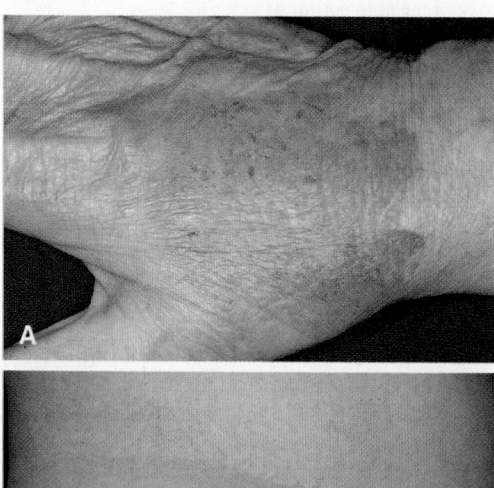

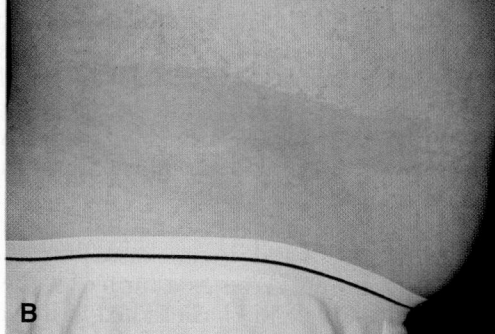

Figure 4-5

Latex allergy dermatitis. A, Latex glove allergy should be suspected in health care workers who present with eczema, blistering, or skin peeling anywhere on the hands. **B,** Allergy to the rubber band of underwear. Washing clothes with bleach may make the rubber allergenic. Similar skin reactions can be seen in women across the midback under the bra strap (not shown). (From Habif TP: *Clinical dermatology*, ed 4, St Louis, 2004, Mosby.)

workers are at risk for severe systemic allergic reactions, which can be fatal in some cases. In susceptible individuals, airways react to low levels of a variety of sensitizers and irritants in the environment. The two major routes of exposure include dermal exposure and inhalation exposure. The elimination of wearing latex gloves has been successful in reducing the rate of latex sensitization 16-fold. Complete elimination has not occurred because latex allergens are airborne and can be carried in dust through air ducts.[248] Exposure by the respiratory route occurs when

the NRL protein becomes airborne, especially because glove powder becomes airborne, acting as a carrier for the NRL protein when gloves are donned or doffed.

Latex-induced rhinitis and occupational asthma are new forms of occupational illness secondary to airborne latex allergens in operating rooms, intensive care units, and dental suites. Anyone with latex allergies should be treated as the first case of the day, whether in the operating room or in a therapy department, to avoid latex in the air and to avoid introducing any latex from clothes or materials from previous contacts.

SPECIAL IMPLICATIONS FOR THE THERAPIST   4-3

Rubber Latex Allergy

In the hospital setting or therapy clinic, latex is not only in the disposable gloves, it can be found in stethoscopes, blood pressure cuffs, syringes, electrode pads, exercise bands, mats, and rubber balls. Other products that often have latex include spatulas, balloons, swimming goggles, condoms, mouse pads, erasers, and expandable fabrics.

All clients should be screened for known LA or risk factors on admission. It is not enough to ask if someone is allergic to latex; risk factors and medical history must be assessed. This is especially important because anaphylaxis could be the first sign of LA.

If anyone in the rehabilitation or therapy department develops symptoms in association with the use of latex gloves, emergency medical care may be required. The presence of hives, perioral itching, respiratory distress, watery eyes, and facial swelling may indicate a type I hypersensitivity response and requires immediate medical attention. In a hospital setting, a physician can be paged immediately; other locations may require an emergency medical team (calling 911 or an emergency medical service). Check with the facility for incident report requirements.

For the health care worker with a known sensitivity, a medical-alert bracelet should be worn, and the individual should have autoinjectable epinephrine (EpiPen) for use if another reaction occurs. Anyone experiencing the first reaction should not ignore the symptoms; further episodes must be avoided by developing a latex-safe environment and using nonlatex products.

All clients with myelomeningocele are to be treated as if latex allergic. The therapist, family members, and caregivers must avoid using toys, feeding utensils, pacifiers, nipples, or other items made of latex that the infant or child might put in the mouth. Clothes and shoes with elastic anywhere must be avoided. Parents must be advised to read all labels and avoid all items containing latex. If no indication of latex content is evident, the manufacturer should be contacted for verification before purchase or use of the item. More information on this topic is available at the American Latex Allergy Association website (www.latexallergyresources.org).

A latex-safe environment may be required for complete recovery for people with LA and is essential for all pediatric cases and anyone with known LA. A latex-safe environment, including the operating room, is described as one in which no latex gloves are used by any personnel, no direct client contact with latex devices (e.g., catheters, condoms, diaphragms, adhesives, tourniquets, rubber backing on bath mats or other materials, hot water bottles, or anesthetic equipment) occurs; and all medical and patient/client care items have been assessed for latex and labeled.

Handwashing before donning and after removing gloves must be carried out at all times, with special care given to using a pH-balanced soap and rinsing well to remove all residue. All medical products containing NRL that could come in contact with clients must be labeled. Keep in mind that many latex-free supplies have packaging that contains latex (glue), and those workers in the production or packaging of these products may have worn latex gloves.

No latex balloons or toys containing latex should be allowed in health care facilities; crash carts should be latex free. Personnel in the therapy department must be aware of the many items in the department that contain latex and replace these with latex-free products or a latex-free barrier (Table 4-6). Almost all equipment, supplies, and personal protective equipment is

Table 4-6	Potential Sources of Latex in a Rehab Department*	
Item	**Replacement Item**
Personal Protective Equipment	
Gloves (sterile and nonsterile)	Nitrile, neoprene, or thermoplastic elastomer examination gloves
Goggles	
Hair covers	
Respirators	
Rubber aprons	
Shoe covers	
Surgical masks	
Equipment/Supplies	
Bandages	
Casting material	
Compression sleeves/garments	
Crash cart	
Crutch and walker handgrips	Cover with stockinette
Crutch axillary pads	Cover with stockinette
Dressings	
Elastic netting	Band Net Latex Free (Western Medical, Ltd.)
	Stretch Net: Latex Safe (DeRoyal)
	The Net Works (Wells Lamont Medical)
Electrode pads, especially disposable TENS	
Exercise balls	Cover ball with a towel
Exercise bands	Use the following latex-free brand:
	REP Band (Magister Corporation)
	Theraband Latex Free
	Latex-free CANDO exercise band (SPRI)
	Use free weights that are not covered with materials containing latex
Exercise mats	
Foam rubber lining splints, braces, mattresses and inside pillows	Cover with sheet or blanket
Mini trampoline	Line with cloth, felt
Positioning supports and pads of foam rubber without complete coverings	Cover with stockinette
Reflex hammer	Cover with latex-free plastic bag
Rubber bands	String, paper clips
Shoe orthotics	
Stethoscope tubing	Cover with gauze or premade cover
Sphygmomanometer	Cover cuff or extremity with gauze
Tape (all kinds)	Cover skin first with gauze; tape over gauze
Toys; toys made from latex gloves	Toys made without latex
Vascular stockings	
Wheelchair cushions	Cover with cloth
Wheelchair tires	Propel with leather or cloth gloves

*Many manufacturers now make latex-free items. Any medical supply with latex must be so marked.
Courtesy Harriett B. Loehne, PT, DPT, CWS, FCCWS.

available in latex-free form, although not by all manufacturers. Complete guidelines for prevention and protection are available through the American Nurses Association at (800) 274-4ANA.

Several potential sources of powder-free, natural hypoallergenic latex gloves may be tolerated by latex-sensitive individuals, but no single replacement glove has been found for all people affected. Cotton liners or barrier creams can be effective interventions. Vinyl gloves are generally less protective than latex and more prone to tearing. Some of the new synthetic materials such as nitrile, neoprene, and thermoplastic elastomer offer equal or superior barrier protection and durability and are a reasonable alternative to latex or vinyl, offer better protection than latex types when handling lipid-soluble substances and chemicals, and are reasonably priced.[182]

However, like latex, synthetic glove products can cause allergic reactions because they may contain chemical additives similar to those found in latex and both are manufactured using the same process, called *vulcanization*. Additionally, synthetic gloves also provide a poorer fit than their latex counterpart and come with environmental concerns (e.g., the production and disposal of vinyl gloves releases toxic substances, such as dioxins, into the environment). Watch out for reactions to neoprene and spandex as some people who are allergic to latex are also sensitive to these materials. Therapists working with individuals to control lymphedema must be aware of all materials in compressive garments and monitor for sensitivities and reaction.

Ideas for controlling latex allergies in the therapy clinic include the following: stop wearing powdered gloves, frequently clean work areas that are contaminated with latex dust, don't ignore symptoms of latex allergies, know the high-risk groups to protect everyone in the clinic, and encourage the clinic manager to eliminate or replace as many latex products as possible.

Military-Related Diseases

Military personnel are exposed to a wide range of chemical, physical, and environmental hazards during their military service. Agent Orange is an herbicide used during the Vietnam War, and the Gulf War has had the Gulf War Syndrome pop up in its veterans. Radiation exposure can be found in those that participated in radiation-risk activity such as Hiroshima and Nagasaki, Japan, and personnel can be subject to contact with uranium in military tank armor and bullets, chromium in contaminated sodium dichromate dust, polychlorinated biphenyls used in coolant and insulating fluid, burn pits for waste disposal at military sites, and a sulfur fire that released large amounts of sulfur dioxide into the air in Iraq.

Seven diseases (asthma, laryngitis, chronic bronchitis, emphysema, and three eye ailments) have been identified by the Department of Veterans Affairs for compensation as a result of exposure to toxic chemicals during World War II. The Department of Veterans Affairs has added Parkinson, ischemic heart disease, and B-cell leukemias to the disorders it automatically considers to be service connected. For a full list of the diseases that may qualify a Vietnam veteran (or that veteran's spouse or widow) for disability compensation and Department of Veterans Affairs (VA) health care, go to www.publichealth.va.gov/exposures and http://www.publichealth.va.gov/exposures/agentorange/diseases.asp.

Posttraumatic stress disorder (PTSD) is a type of anxiety disorder found among those who have seen or experienced a traumatic event that involved the threat of injury or death. Military personnel are at higher risk than the general population for this disorder because of the nature of their work. Veterans groups have introduced the idea that this condition is more accurately called *posttraumatic stress* (without the *disorder* because the stress responses to conditions soldiers are exposed to are normal, not disordered).

Agent Orange

The VA recognizes some cancers and other health problems possible diseases associated with exposure to Agent Orange or other herbicides during military service. Survivors of the Vietnam War who served between January 1962 and May 1975 are presumed to have been exposed to dioxin (2,3,7,8-tetrachlorodibenzo-*p*-dioxin [TCDD]) contained in the herbicide mixture Agent Orange (sprayed from the air, by boat, and on the ground in Vietnam to defoliate jungles where the enemies were hiding). These Veterans are known to be at risk for numerous diseases, including diabetes, AL amyloidosis, chronic B-cell leukemias, chloracne, Hodgkin disease, ischemic heart disease, multiple myeloma, non-Hodgkin lymphoma, Parkinson disease, peripheral neuropathy, porphyria cutanea tarda, prostate cancer, respiratory cancers, and soft tissue sarcomas. The risk for other types of cancer has never been conclusively proven, but as Vietnam veterans continue to age, additional research will yield more information about cancer risk.[87,230]

There has been concern about the reproductive effects of Agent Orange such as birth defects in the children of exposed veterans. Neural tube defects, neurotoxicity, neuropsychiatric dysfunction, deficits in motor function, and peripheral neuropathy may be linked to Agent Orange exposure but considerable uncertainty exists about these associations.[87] The VA has recognized spina bifida as being associated with Veterans' exposure to Agent Orange or other herbicide during those specific dates during the Vietnam War.

Gulf War Syndrome

Overview. Once a hotly debated topic, Gulf War Syndrome (GWS) has more scientific research indicating that it is real and a result of neurotoxic exposures during Gulf War deployment. According to the CDC, Americans who served in the Persian Gulf War are significantly more likely than others to experience more than a dozen disorders known generically as *GWS* or otherwise known as Gulf War Illness. However, the Department of Defense does not support the existence of this illness, reporting only that the results of medical examinations of 10,000 veterans and family members affected revealed multiple illnesses with overlapping symptoms.[113]

Gulf War Veterans have also been linked to increased incidences of ALS or Lou Gherig disease. It has been found, looking back at medical record reviews, that there is a significant elevated risk of ALS that occurred among deployed personnel, deployed active duty military, deployed Air Force, and deployed Army personnel. Elevated but nonsignificant risks were seen in deployed Reserves and National Guard, deployed Navy, and deployed Marine Corps personnel. Overall, the risk found that was associated with deployment was 18%.[105] Other research studies have looked at incidences of ALS in veterans outside of the Gulf War and whether military service itself is associated with increased risk of ALS. There are increased death rates from ALS in men who served in the military compared with those who did not serve and there may be a link between ALS and specific branches of the military.[208]

VA does not like to use the term "Gulf War Syndrome" because it is a cluster of unexplained symptoms reported by Gulf War Veterans and the symptoms vary so widely that it does not meet the definition of a syndrome. They prefer to use "medically unexplained chronic multisymptom illnesses" and "undiagnosed illnesses" to describe these individuals. The VA does presume that certain chronic, unexplained symptoms existing for 6 months or more are related to their Gulf War service without regard to its cause. The symptoms must have appeared during active duty in the Southwest Asia theater of military operation or by December 31, 2016, and be at least 10% disabling. The illnesses included are chronic fatigue syndrome, fibromyalgia, functional gastrointestinal disorders, and undiagnosed illnesses, and they can receive VA disability compensation.[228]

Incidence and Clinical Manifestations. The Gulf War Research Panel has found that one in four of the 697,000 U.S. veterans of the 1991 Gulf War suffer from Gulf War illness.[34] As of January 2007, more than 100,000 veterans have filed with the federal registry reports of symptoms that include (in order of frequency) fatigue, skin rash, headache, muscle and joint pain, memory loss, shortness of breath, sleep disturbances, diarrhea and other gastrointestinal symptoms, and depression. CDC data show that GWS affects 27% of veterans, compared with 2% of nonveterans. Fatigue has been reported to affect 54% of Gulf War veterans compared with 16% of non–Gulf War veterans.

Etiologic Factors. No single cause has been identified, but possible factors include chemical or biologic weapons used on allied forces, insecticides, oil well fires in Kuwait, nerve agents from the demolition of Iraqi chemical weapons, parasites, pills protecting against nerve gas, and inoculations against petrochemical exposure administered by the military that had unexpected side effects or reacted with one another to create adverse symptoms.

Pathogenesis. The pathogenesis for GWS remains unknown but researchers are investigating the similarities between the underlying mechanisms of chronic fatigue syndrome, fibromyalgia, migraine headaches, and GWS. MRI studies of veterans with different GWS have biochemical evidence of neuronal damage in different distributions in the basal ganglia and brain stem, supporting the theory of neurologic toxicity related to chemically induced injury to dopaminergic neurons in the basal ganglia.[96,97,218]

MEDICAL MANAGEMENT

No specific intervention beyond management and symptomatic measures exists. Focusing on triggering events rarely helps define treatment for people with syndromes such as GWS. Understanding the entire spectrum of illnesses from chronic fatigue syndrome to fibromyalgia to ALS to GWS in light of treatment must be the means to developing multidisciplinary treatment programs for affected people that includes allopathic, naturopathic, and alternative treatment.

Post-Traumatic Stress (Disorder)

Overview. PTSD is a type of anxiety disorder that can occur after seeing or experiencing a traumatic event that involves the threat of injury or death. It can occur at any age and can occur after a natural disaster, or from events such as assault, domestic abuse, prison stay, rape, terrorism, or from war.

Incidence. PTSD occurs in our military veterans as they have seen and experienced traumatic events in war. The most recent veterans, those from Operations Enduring Freedom and Iraqi Freedom (OEF/OIF) have endured high combat stress and are at risk for PTSD and psychosocial problems.[194] According to the Department of Defense Report in 2008, the Military Health System had recorded 39,365 military personnel that were diagnosed with PTSD. This resulted in an estimated $63.8 million on direct and purchased care for these individuals and $13.1 million spent on prescriptions filled after the diagnosis of PTSD.[82] Going forward 4 years into 2012, the numbers (which includes veterans of Operations Enduring Freedom, Iraqi Freedom and New Dawn) totaled 228,361 who were coded with PTSD. This number will likely continue to climb as we have troops returning home to the United States.[229]

Clinical Manifestations. There are three categories of symptoms with PTSD. The first category is reliving the event, which can disturb day-to-day activity. It is filled with flashbacks, repeated upsetting memories, repeated nightmares, and strong uncomfortable reactions to situations that are a reminder of the event. The second category is avoidance. This includes numbing of emotions; feeling detached; being unable to remember important aspects of the traumatic incident; lack of interest in normal activity; decreased affect; avoiding places, people, or thoughts that are a reminder of the event; and having the feeling that you have no future. The third category is arousal, which causes difficulty in concentrating, being startled easily, having exaggerated responses to being startled, feeling more aware, feeling irritable, and having trouble falling or staying asleep.

Pathogenesis. The cause is unknown. It is a combination of psychological, genetic, physical, and social factors and it changes the body's response to stress. It is also unknown why some people affected by traumatic events have PTSD and others do not.

MEDICAL MANAGEMENT

There are no tests for diagnosis of PTSD, it is based on symptoms. For PTSD the symptoms are present for at least 30 days. If the time period is shorter, they may be diagnosed with Acute Stress Disorder. Mental health exams, physical exams, and blood tests will be done to rule out other illnesses that can look like PTSD.

It is advised for those with PTSD to have a good social support system. Treatment of individuals with PTSD include desensitization, which helps reduce symptoms by encouraging the person to remember the traumatic event and express their feelings about it with the idea that over time these memories of the event should become less fearful. Support groups with those who share similar experiences can also be helpful. It is important to watch for other problems developing in this population

including alcohol or substance abuse, depression, suicidal thoughts or plans, and other medical conditions related to these problems. A combination of pharmacotherapy and psychological therapies may help people recover from PTSD more effectively than just one or the other.[29,103,175]

REFERENCES

To enhance this text and add value for the reader, all references are included on the companion Evolve site that accompanies this textbook. The reader can view the reference source and access it online whenever possible.

CHAPTER 5

Problems Affecting Multiple Systems

CELESTE PETERSON • MEREDITH A. WAMPLER • JOY C. COHN • LARA A. FIRRONE

Many conditions and diseases seen in the rehabilitation setting can affect multiple organs or systems (Box 5-1). With the kinds of multiple comorbidities and system impairments encountered in the health care arena, the therapist must go beyond a systems approach and use a biopsychosocial-spiritual approach to client management. Chronic diseases and multiple system impairments require such an approach because risk factors correlate with health outcome; early intervention and intervention results are correlated with improved outcome.

Individual modifying (risk) factors, such as lifestyle variables and environment, affect pathology and modify how a person responds to health, illness, and disease. For example, adverse drug events are correlated with increasing age and obesity, whereas fitness level has a profound impact on recovery from injury, anesthesia, and illness.

Additionally, a single injury, disease, or pathologic condition can predispose a person to associated secondary illnesses. For example, the victim of a motor vehicle accident (see "Special Implications for the Therapist: Cell Injury" in Chapter 6) suffered a traumatic brain injury and concomitant pelvic fracture then developed pneumonia and pulmonary compromise, subsequently experiencing a myocardial infarction.

This type of clinical scenario involving multiple organs and comorbidities is not uncommon. Also consider the medically complex person who needs a splint. The therapist must first review laboratory values (see Chapter 40) to determine albumin levels (nutritional status) and platelet levels (potential for bleeding), perform a skin assessment (see Chapter 10), and consult with both nursing staff and the nutritionist before providing an external device that could create skin breakdown and add to an already complex case.

Although medical conditions encountered in the clinic or home health care setting are discussed individually in the appropriate chapter, the health care provider must understand the systemic and local effects of such disorders. This chapter provides a brief listing of the systemic effects of commonly encountered pathologic conditions and a basic presentation of acid–base and fluid and electrolyte imbalances. The scope of this text does not allow for an in-depth discussion of each condition or disease and its related multiple systemic effects.

SYSTEMIC EFFECTS OF PATHOLOGY

Systemic Effects of Acute Inflammation

Acute inflammation can be described as the initial response of tissue to injury, particularly bacterial infections and necrosis, involving vascular and cellular responses. Local signs of inflammation (e.g., redness, warmth, swelling, pain, and loss of function) are commonly observed in the therapy setting. Local inflammation can lead to abscesses when excessive suppuration (formation of pus) occurs.

Systemic effects of acute inflammation include fever, tachycardia, and a hypermetabolic state. These effects produce characteristic changes in the blood, such as elevated serum protein levels (C-reactive protein, serum amyloid A, complement, and coagulation factors) and an elevated white blood count (leukocytosis).[152] For a complete discussion of inflammation and its effects, see Chapter 6.

Systemic Effects of Chronic Inflammation

Chronic inflammation is the result of persistent injury, repeated episodes of acute inflammation, infection, cell-mediated immune responses, and foreign body reactions. The tissue response to injury is characterized by accumulation of lymphocytes, plasma cells, and macrophages (mononuclear inflammatory cells) and production of fibrous connective tissue (fibrosis). Fibroblasts and small blood vessels, along with collagen fibers synthesized by fibroblasts, constitute fibrosis. Grossly, fibrotic tissue is light gray and has a dense, firm texture that causes contraction of the normal tissue.

The associated fibrosis may cause progressive tissue damage and loss of function. Systemic effects of chronic inflammation may include low-grade fever, malaise, weight loss, anemia, fatigue, leukocytosis, and lymphocytosis (caused by viral infection).[69] Inflammation is reflected by an increased erythrocyte sedimentation rate. In general, as the disease improves, the erythrocyte sedimentation rate decreases.

Systemic Factors Influencing Healing

In addition to local factors that affect healing (e.g., infection, blood supply, extent of necrosis, presence of

Box 5-1

CONDITIONS THAT AFFECT MULTIPLE SYSTEMS

- Autoimmune disorders
- Burns
- Cancer
- Cystic fibrosis
- Congestive heart failure (CHF)
- Connective tissue diseases:
  - Rheumatoid arthritis
  - Progressive systemic sclerosis (scleroderma)
  - Polymyositis
  - Sjögren syndrome
  - Systemic lupus erythematosus
  - Polyarteritis nodosa
- Endocrine disorders (e.g., diabetes, thyroid disorders)
- Environmental and occupational diseases
- Genetic diseases
- Infections (e.g., tuberculosis, human immunodeficiency virus [HIV])
- Malnutrition or other nutritional imbalance
- Metabolic disorders
- Multiple organ dysfunction syndrome (MODS)
- Renal failure (chronic)
- Sarcoidosis
- Shock
- Trauma
- Vasculitis

foreign bodies, protection from further trauma or movement), a variety of systemic factors influence healing as well (see Box 6-3). Systemic factors may include general nutritional status, especially protein and vitamin C; psychologic well-being; presence of cardiovascular disease, cancer, hematologic disorders (e.g., neutropenia), systemic infections, and diabetes mellitus; and whether the person is undergoing corticosteroid or immunosuppressive therapy.[207]

Healing in specific organs varies according to the underlying cause and site of the injury. For example, myocardial infarctions heal by scarring, and the heart may be weakened. A cerebrovascular accident, or stroke, may cause permanent disability, and healing occurs by the formation of glial tissue (e.g., astrocytes, oligodendrocytes, and microglia) rather than by collagenous scar formation; this process is called *gliosis*.

In other organs, effective tissue regeneration depends primarily on the site of injury. Necrosis of only parenchymal (functional visceral) cells with retention of the existing stroma (framework or structural tissue) may permit regeneration and restoration of normal anatomy, whereas necrosis that involves the mesenchymal framework (connective tissue, including blood and blood vessels) usually results in scar formation (e.g., as in hepatic cirrhosis). For further discussion, see Chapter 6.

Consequences of Immunodeficiency

Immunodeficiency diseases are caused by congenital (primary) or acquired (secondary) failure of one or more functions of the immune system, predisposing the affected individual to infections that a noncompromised immune system could resist. The therapist is more likely to encounter individuals with acquired (rather than congenital) immunodeficiency from nonspecific causes, such as those that occur with viral and other infections; malnutrition; alcoholism; aging; autoimmune diseases; diabetes mellitus; cancer, particularly myeloma, lymphoma, and leukemia; chronic diseases; steroid therapy; cancer chemotherapy; and radiation therapy.[117]

Predisposition to opportunistic infections, resulting in clinical manifestations of those infections, is the primary consequence of immunodeficiency. Selective B-cell deficiencies predispose an individual to bacterial infections. T-cell deficiencies predispose to viral and fungal infections. Combined deficiencies, including AIDS, are particularly severe because they predispose to many kinds of viral, bacterial, and fungal infections.

Systemic Effects of Neoplasm

Malignant tumors, by their destructive nature of uncontrolled cell proliferation and spread, produce many local and systemic effects. Locally, the rapid growth of the tumor encroaches on healthy tissue, causing destruction, necrosis, ulceration, compression, obstruction, and hemorrhage.

Pain may or may not occur, depending on how close tumor cells, swelling, or hemorrhage occur to the nerve cells. This process also occurs locally at metastatic sites. Pain may occur as a late symptom as a result of infiltration, compression, or destruction of nerve tissue. Secondary infections often occur as a result of the host's decreased immunity and can lead to death.[392]

The person with a malignant neoplasm often presents with systemic symptoms such as gradual or rapid weight loss, muscular weakness, anorexia, anemia, and coagulation disorders (granulocyte and platelet abnormalities). Continued spread of the cancer may lead to bone erosion or liver, gastrointestinal (GI), pulmonary, or vascular obstruction. Other vital organs may be affected; increased intracranial pressure in the brain by tumor cells can cause partial paralysis and eventual coma. Hemorrhage caused by direct invasion or necrosis in any body part leads to further anemia or even death if the necrosis is severe.

Advanced cancers produce cachexia (wasting) as a result of tissue destruction and the body's nutrients being used by the malignant cells for further growth. Multiple mechanisms may be involved in this process, including release of cytokines such as tumor necrosis factor (also called *cachectin*).

Paraneoplastic syndromes (see Chapter 9) are produced by hormonal mechanisms rather than by direct tumor invasion. For example, hypercalcemia can be caused in cases of lung cancer by the secretion of a peptide with parathyroid hormone, and polycythemia can be caused by the secretion of erythropoietin by renal cell carcinoma. Neuromuscular disorders, such as Eaton-Lambert syndrome, polymyositis/dermatomyositis, and hypertrophic pulmonary osteoarthropathy, are other examples of paraneoplastic syndromes that can occur as a systemic effect of neoplasm (see Tables 9-4 and 9-5).

Systemic Effects of Pathology[80,81]

Medical advances, the aging of America, the increasing number of people with multisystem problems, and the expanding scope of the therapist's practice require that the therapist anticipate, assess, and manage the manifestations of disease and pathology. Physical and occupational therapists are primary health care professionals who focus on maximizing functional capacity and physical independence by optimizing healthy active lifestyles and community-based living.

Interventions to maximize oxygen transport (e.g., mobilization, positioning, breathing control, and exercise) should be an important focus even in people who are acutely and critically ill. Enhancing oxygen transport centrally and peripherally improves the body's ability to respond to stress. At the same time, many therapy interventions elicit an exercise stimulus that stresses an already strained oxygen transport system. Exercise is now recognized as a prescriptive intervention in pathology that has indications, contraindications, and side effects. These factors necessitate careful and close monitoring of cardiopulmonary status, especially in the person with multisystem involvement.

Hematologic abnormalities require that the results of the client's blood analysis and clotting factors be monitored so that therapy intervention can be modified to minimize risks. Individualized treatment programs are developed for each person addressing the special needs of that client and the family, responding to physical, psychologic, emotional, and spiritual needs. The reader is encouraged to review an excellent article[80] for an additional in-depth discussion of specific implications for physical therapy management in systemic disease.

ADVERSE DRUG EVENTS

Drugs were once developed through a hit-or-miss process in which researchers would identify a compound and test it in cells and animals to determine its effect on disease. When a compound appeared to be successful, it was often tested in humans with little knowledge of how it worked or what side effects it might have. Today, biochemists know much more about disease processes and work at the molecular level designing drugs to interact with specific molecules. Disease-modifying antirheumatic drugs, selective estrogen receptor modulators (SERMs), and monoclonal antibodies are examples of such "designer drugs."

Drugs in the future will have greater molecular specificity, possibly with the ability to accommodate for gender, age, and genetic differences between individuals. Despite these advances, reactions still remain a significant problem in the health care industry today.

Definition and Overview

Adverse drug events (ADEs) are defined as unwanted and potentially harmful effect(s) produced by medications or prescription drugs. The term usually excludes nontherapeutic overdosage such as accidental exposure or attempted suicide. Most ADEs are medication reactions or side effects. A *drug–drug* interaction occurs when medications interact unfavorably, possibly adding to the pharmacologic effects. A *drug–disease* interaction occurs when a medication causes an existing disease to worsen. *Side effects* are usually defined as predictable pharmacologic effects that occur within therapeutic dose ranges and are undesirable in the given therapeutic situation. Overdosage toxicity is the predictable toxic effect that occurs with dosages in excess of the therapeutic range for a particular person.[114]

ADEs may be dose-related (predictable drug injury) or non–dose-related (unpredictable or idiosyncratic drug injury). Dose-related effects may include drug toxicity from overdose, variations in pharmaceutical preparations, preexisting liver disease, presence of comorbidities such as renal or heart failure, or drug interactions. Non–dose-related effects may occur as a result of hypersensitivity, resulting in acute anaphylaxis or delayed hypersensitivity or other nonimmunologic idiosyncratic reactions, according to individual susceptibility.

ADEs are classified as *mild* (no antidote, therapy, or prolongation of hospitalization necessary), *moderate* (change in drug therapy required, although not necessarily a cessation of therapy; may prolong hospitalization or require special treatment), *severe* (potentially life-threatening, requires discontinuation of the drug and specific treatment of the adverse reaction), and *lethal* (directly or indirectly leads to the death of the person).

Incidence

ADEs have been declared a national public health problem with more than 700,000 emergency department visits and 120,000 hospitalizations required for further treatment after the emergency visit.[52] The annual incidence of death caused by ADEs is estimated to be between 0.08/100,000 and 0.12/100,000 people.[323] According to one study of primary care outpatients, ADEs were common (25%) and often preventable.[136]

Adults older than age 65 years are twice as likely to go to an emergency department because of an ADE and are almost seven times more likely to experience an ADE requiring hospitalization than a younger person.[43,44] Older adults often take multiple medications, increasing the possibility of a detrimental interaction.[332] Death rates secondary to an ADE are also highest in people older than age 55 years, with the greatest risk in those older than 75 years.[323] The Centers for Disease Control and Prevention report inappropriate medications are prescribed to older adults in about 1 of every 12 visits (8%).[149]

Inappropriate use of pain medications has led to significant increases of both emergency department visits and death. In 2009, there were 475,000 visits to the emergency department.[340] In 2008, there were 14,800 deaths from unintentional overdose of opioid analgesics (methadone, oxycodone, and hydrocodone)—greater than the number of people who died secondary to illicit drug use of cocaine and heroin.[53,373] Care should always be taken to prescribe only the needed dose and type of medication to match pain relief goals. Many states have prescription drug monitoring programs to aid in this effort.

Specific studies have been conducted to determine the rate of ADE-related medication-dispensing errors in hospital pharmacies[60] and outpatient chemotherapy clinics,[135] and the rate of ADEs associated with immunizations.[178] Medication changes are also common during transfer between hospital and nursing home and are a cause of ADEs. Most changes are discontinuations, dose changes, and class substitutions.[38]

Etiologic and Risk Factors

Definite risk factors for experiencing a serious ADE can include age (older than age 75 years, younger for some pharmaceuticals), gender, polypharmacy, ethnicity, concomitant alcohol consumption, new drugs, number of drugs, dosages, concomitant use of herbal compounds,[77] duration of treatment, noncompliance (e.g., unintentional repeated dosage), small stature, and presence of underlying conditions (e.g., hepatic or renal insufficiency).[58,65,279]

Of all the risk factors, age has the most prevalent effect in the aging American population. Factors that contribute to ADEs in older people include age-related physiologic changes, a greater degree of frailty, an increased number of underlying diseases, and the presence of polypharmacy.[109,221] Age-related physiological changes affect the distribution of drugs. A decrease in lean body mass and an increase in the proportion of body fat result in a decrease in body water. As a result, water-soluble drugs (e.g., morphine) have a lower volume of distribution that speeds up onset of action and raises peak concentration. High peak concentrations are associated with increased toxicity.

On the other hand, lipid-soluble drugs are distributed more widely, have a delayed onset of action, and accumulate with repeated dosing. Aging adults are also at risk for drug accumulation because of changes in both metabolism and elimination. With advanced age, functional liver tissue diminishes and hepatic blood flow decreases. Consequently, the capacity of the liver to break down and convert drugs and their metabolites declines. This may be exacerbated by other changes such as age-related reduction in renal mass and blood flow, the accompanying decline in glomerular filtration and tubular reabsorption rates, and other conditions such as dehydration, cancer, heart failure, and cirrhosis.

There are also changes in the sensitivity of the cardiovascular system with age. For example, with the addition of β-adrenergic agonists and antagonists, there is less responsiveness of the cardiovascular system and orthostatic events increase.[109]

Additionally, drugs commonly prescribed for older clients, such as the calcium-channel blockers verapamil and diltiazem and the antigout drug allopurinol, further slow drug metabolism, potentially contributing to toxicity and adverse drug reactions.

In the older adult population, emergency department visits as a result of medications classified as always potentially inappropriate were only implicated in 3.6% of visits.[45] The medications most commonly causing emergency department visits included warfarin, insulin, and digoxin (33.3% of visits). Warfarin, insulin, oral

---

Box 5-2

DRUGS THAT ARE COMMONLY ASSOCIATED WITH ADVERSE DRUG REACTIONS IN THE AGING

- Anticholinergics
- Antidiarrheals
- Antihistamines (first-generation)
- Antiplatelets
- Benzodiazepines (anxiolytics)
- β-Blockers
- Calcium channel blockers
- Corticosteroids (systemic)
- Digoxin
- Diuretics
- Hypoglycemics (e.g., sulfonylureas, insulin)
- Muscle relaxants
- Neuroleptics
- Nonsteroidal antiinflammatory drugs (NSAIDs)
- Opioids
- Tricyclic antidepressants
- Vasodilators (e.g., nitrates)
- Warfarin

Based on data from Fick DM, Cooper JW, Wade WE, et al: Updating the Beers criteria for potentially inappropriate medication use in older adults: results of a US consensus panel of experts. *Arch Intern Med* 163(22):2716–2724, 2003; Thomsen LA, Winterstein AG, Søndergaard B, et al: Systematic review of the incidence and characteristics of preventable adverse drug events in ambulatory care. *Ann Pharmacother* 41(9):1411–1426, 2007; Gallagher P, O'Mahony D. STOPP (Screening Tool of Older Persons' potentially inappropriate Prescriptions): application to acutely ill elderly patients and comparison with Beers' criteria. *Age Ageing* 37(6):673–679, 2008; Budnitz DS, Lovegrove MC, Shehab N, Richards CL: Emergency hospitalizations for adverse drug events in older Americans. *N Engl J Med* 365:2002–2012, 2011; Budnitz DS, Shehab N, Kegler SR, Richards CL: Medication use leading to emergency department visits for adverse drug events in older adults. *Ann Intern Med* 147:755–765, 2007.

---

antiplatelet agents, and oral hypoglycemic agents were the medications most often implicated in emergency hospitalizations as a consequence of ADEs (67%).[45] Box 5-2 lists the drugs most commonly associated with ADEs in the aging.

Cardiac or pulmonary toxicity may occur as a result of irradiation and immunosuppressive drugs given to prepare recipients for organ transplantation or for treatment of cancer. Box 5-3 lists some of the more common specific target organs and effects.

Clinical Manifestations

Rashes, fever, and jaundice are common signs of drug toxicity. Adverse skin (cutaneous) reactions include erythema, discoloration, itching, burning, urticaria, eczema, acne, alopecia, blisters, or purpura (Fig. 5-1). Onset may be within minutes to hours to days. Signs and symptoms suggestive of a mild reaction include anxiety, dizziness, headache, nasal congestion, shakiness, and brief vomiting. Persons with a moderate drug reaction may present with abdominal cramps, dyspnea, hypertension or hypotension, palpitations, tachycardia, and persistent vomiting. Severe reactions can include arrhythmia, seizures, laryngeal edema, profound hypotension, pulmonary

Box 5-3

TARGET ORGANS AND EFFECTS OF ADVERSE DRUG EVENTS

Heart

- Arrhythmia
  - Adenosine
  - Flecainide
  - Propafenone
  - Digoxin
  - Procainamide
- Cardiomyopathy
  - Adriamycin
  - Antipsychotics
  - Anthracyclines (i.e., doxorubicin, daunorubicin, epirubicin)
  - Trastuzumab
- Myocardial infarction/acute coronary syndrome
  - Oral contraceptives
  - Selective cox-2 inhibitors (NSAIDs)
  - Abacavir
  - Didanosine
- Orthostatic hypotension
  - Atypical antipsychotics
  - Antihypertensives
    - Calcium-channel blockers
    - Centrally acting α-adrenergic agonists
    - Peripheral α-blockers
    - β-Adrenergic blockers
    - Peripherally acting vasodilators
    - Diuretics

Lung

- Interstitial lung disease/pulmonary fibrosis
  - Methotrexate
  - Cyclophosphamide
  - Amiodarone
  - Tamoxifen
  - Bleomycin
- Asthma/bronchospasms
  - Aspirin
  - NSAIDs
  - Sulfites
  - Acetaminophen

Gastrointestinal Tract

- Gastritis and peptic ulcer
  - Aspirin
  - NSAIDs
  - Bisphosphonates
  - Potassium chloride
- Gingival hyperplasia
  - Phenytoin
  - Cyclosporine
  - Nifedipine
  - Verapamil
- Pseudomembranous colitis
  - Broad-spectrum antibiotics
- Hepatic and cholestatic disease
  - Tacrine
  - Nucleoside reverse transcriptase inhibitors
  - Isoniazid
  - Protease inhibitors
  - Amiodarone

- Quinidine
- Rifampin
- Dapsone
- Leflunomide

Fetal Injury

- Phocomelia
  - Thalidomide
- Vaginal carcinoma
  - Diethylstilbestrol
- Discoloration of teeth
  - Tetracyclines
  - Minocycline
  - Ciprofloxacin
- Multiple congenital anomalies
  - Disulfiram
  - Estrogens
  - Progestins
  - Human chorionic gonadotropin
  - Antineoplastic agents
  - Phenytoin
  - Warfarin
  - Isotretinoin

Kidneys

- Acute interstitial nephritis
  - Rifampin
  - Lithium
  - NSAIDs
  - β-Lactam antibiotics
- Acute tubular necrosis
  - Aminoglycosides
  - Amphotericin B
  - Radiocontrast media
  - Cisplatin
- Nephrolithiasis
  - Indinavir
  - Topiramate
  - Sulfonamides
- Glomerulonephritis
  - Allopurinol
  - Lithium
  - NSAIDs

Endocrine System

- Adrenocortical atrophy
  - Corticosteroids
- Hypothyroidism
  - Amiodarone
  - Interferon-α and -β
  - Lithium
  - Thalidomide
- Hyperthyroidism
  - Amiodarone
  - Interferon-β

Skeletal System

- Osteoporosis/osteomalacia
- Corticosteroids
- Antineoplastic agents
- Aromatase inhibitors
- Methotrexate
- Heparin

Nervous System

- Seizures
  - Tramadol
  - Propofol
  - Bupropion
  - Tricyclic antidepressants
  - Cyclosporine
- Movement disorders
  - Droperidol
  - Metoclopramide
  - Prochlorperazine
  - First-generation antipsychotics
  - Atypical antipsychotics
- Peripheral neuropathy
  - Leflunomide
  - Didanosine
  - Stavudine
  - Carboplatin
  - Cisplatin
  - Vincristine
- Delirium
  - Opioids
  - Clozapine
  - Valproic acid
  - Lithium
  - Digoxin
- Depression
  - Phenobarbital
  - Primidone
  - Interferon-α and -β
  - Gonadotropin-releasing hormone agonists
  - Triptans
  - Corticosteroids
- Anxiety
  - Amphetamines
  - Antipsychotics
  - Bupropion
  - Caffeine
  - Dopamine agonists and antagonists
  - Theophylline

Blood and Bone Marrow

- Anemias
  - Penicillins
  - Cephalosporins
  - Methyldopa
  - Antimalarial drugs
  - Sulfonamides
  - Nitrofurantoin
  - Methotrexate
  - Phenytoin
  - Antineoplastic agents
- Thrombocytopenia
  - Abciximab
  - Heparin
  - Valproate
  - NSAIDs
- Deep vein thrombosis
  - Heparin
  - Erythropoietin
  - Estrogen-containing hormones
  - Raloxifene

Continued

TARGET ORGANS AND EFFECTS OF ADVERSE DRUG EVENTS—cont'd

- Tamoxifen
- Anastrozole
- Megestrol
- Contrast agents

Skin

- Allergies, pseudoallergies
  - Radiocontrast media
  - Angiotensin-converting enzyme inhibitors
  - Heparin
  - Penicillins
  - Omalizumab
  - Cephalosporins
- Photosensitivity
  - Voriconazole
  - Methotrexate

- Diclofenac
- Ibuprofen
- Amiodarone
- Alopecia
  - Anticonvulsants
  - Chemotherapy agents
  - Immunosuppressants
  - Interferons
  - Retinoids
- Hirsutism
  - Cyclosporin
  - Danazol
  - Testosterone

Ears, Nose, and Throat

- Ototoxicity
  - Carboplatin

- Cisplatin
- Doxycycline
- Gentamicin
- Interferon
- Minocycline
- Neomycin
- Tobramycin

Eyes

- Severe visual disturbances
  - Amiodarone
  - Clomiphene
  - Digitalis
  - Isotretinoin

NSAIDs, nonsteroidal antiinflammatory drugs.
Data from Tisdale JE, Miller DA, editors: *Drug-induced diseases*, ed 2, Bethesda, MD, 2010, American Society of Health-System Pharmacists.

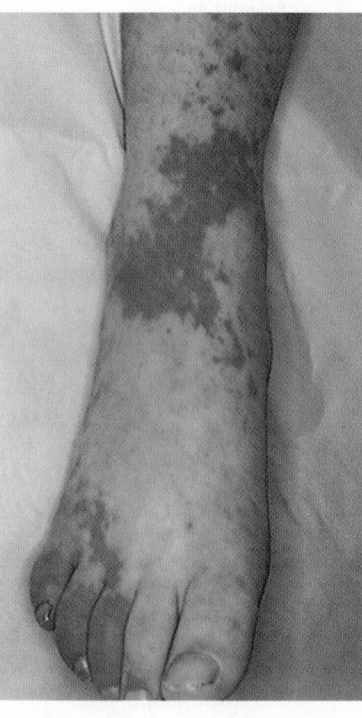

Figure 5-1

Purpura. Hemorrhaging into the tissues, particularly beneath the skin or mucous membranes, producing raised or flat ecchymoses or petechiae. Seen most often in a physical therapy practice as a result of thrombocytopenia (e.g., drug-reaction or medication-induced, especially nonsteroidal antiinflammatory drugs, methotrexate, Coumadin or warfarin; radiation- or chemotherapy-induced); also occurs in older adults as blood leaks from capillaries in response to minor trauma. (From Hurwitz S: *Clinical pediatric dermatology: a textbook of skin disorders of childhood and adolescence*, ed 2, Philadelphia, 1993, Saunders.)

COMMON SIGNS AND SYMPTOMS OF ADVERSE DRUG REACTIONS IN THE AGING

- Dry mouth
- Dyspepsia
- Restlessness
- Orthostatic hypotension (dizziness, weakness, decreased blood pressure, falls)
- Depression
- Dehydration
- Confusion, delirium
- Impaired memory or concentration
- Nausea
- Loss of appetite
- Constipation
- Incontinence
- Extrapyramidal syndromes (e.g., parkinsonism, tardive dyskinesia)
- Fatigue, weakness
- Sedation

edema, and cardiopulmonary arrest. Arthralgias and myalgias can be part of the mild or moderate reactions.

Older adults may develop ADEs that are clearly different from those seen in younger persons, with mental status changes as one of the more common symptoms (Box 5-4).[294] The therapist should be aware of increased bruising indicative of warfarin toxicity or nausea/vomiting with/without cardiac manifestations suggestive of digitalis toxicity. Elevated levels of both medications can be life threatening (see Table 12-5). Early symptoms of salicylate intoxication include tinnitus, disequilibrium, drowsiness, and a moderate delirium.[279]

The therapist may observe motor tics called *tardive dyskinesia*, which is a neurologic syndrome caused by the long-term use of neuroleptic drugs. Neuroleptic drugs are usually prescribed for psychiatric disorders but may be used for some GI and neurologic disorders. Tardive dyskinesia is characterized by repetitive, involuntary, purposeless movements. The client may demonstrate repetitive grimacing, tongue protrusion, lip smacking, puckering and pursing, and rapid eye blinking. Rapid movements of the arms, legs, and trunk may also occur. Involuntary movements of the fingers may give the person the appearance of playing an invisible guitar or piano.

MEDICAL MANAGEMENT

Differentiating an ADE from underlying disease requires a thorough history, especially when a symptom appears 1 to 2 months after a medication regimen has been started. Monitoring blood cell counts, liver enzymes, electrolytes, blood urea nitrogen (BUN), and creatinine is indicated for certain drugs. Cardiotropic drugs can cause arrhythmias that require electrocardiogram monitoring. With dose-related ADEs, dose modification is usually all that is required, whereas with non–dose-related ADEs, the drug therapy is usually stopped and reexposure avoided.

The federal initiative Partnership for Patients has a goal to reduce the number of preventable rehospitalizations by 20% and the reduction of ADEs is a key focus of the partnership.[159,193] Hospitals, clinics, nursing facilities, pharmacies, etc., are expected to evaluate their prescribing, testing, and follow-up methods in order to reduce ADEs.

SPECIAL IMPLICATIONS FOR THE THERAPIST   5-2

Adverse Drug Events

Many people treated by physical therapists today have a pharmacologic profile. It is not unusual to find out during the client interview that the person is taking many different prescription or nonprescription medications. Often there is an equally long list of nutritional aids, supplements, herbs, or vitamins, sometimes referred to as nutraceuticals. Adults age 65 years or older commonly have complicated medication regimens that may result in ADEs. Age-related physiologic changes result in altered pharmacokinetic and pharmacodynamic response to medications that contribute to adverse responses.[127]

Knowing when a person is having an ADE to medication or supplements versus experiencing symptoms of disease or illness is not always easily distinguished. Knowing about potential drug effects and using a drug guide to look up potential side effects is a good place to start.

Client/patient education is important. The therapist can remind his or her clients to take their medication as prescribed and to report any unusual signs and symptoms to their doctor, physician's assistant, or nurse practitioner. Encourage your clients to keep follow-up appointments with the health care professional who prescribed the drug and to make sure that person knows all drugs and supplements currently being taken.

If the therapist suspects drug- or nutraceutical-related signs or symptoms, several observations can be made and reported to the physician, such as correlation between the time medication is taken and length of time before signs and symptoms appear (or increase). Additionally, family members can be asked to observe whether the signs or symptoms increase after each dosage. Documentation of observed or reported behavior or signs and symptoms and the date first observed is important. Make note of the client's clinical condition and your interventions. Follow your facility's policies for notification of suspected ADE.

Interpretation of drug-related or disease-induced signs and symptoms is beyond the scope of a therapist's practice, but the therapist can identify when these clinical manifestations are interfering with rehabilitation and make the necessary referral for evaluation. Any time a client has reached a plateau or has demonstrated poor potential for improvement, the therapist should consider that these responses may be a result of an ADE.

Any signs of tardive dyskinesia should be reported to the physician. There is no standard treatment for tardive dyskinesia. The first step is generally to stop or minimize the use of the neuroleptic drug. This may not be possible for anyone with a severe underlying condition. Replacing the neuroleptic drug with substitute drugs may help some people. Other drugs, such as benzodiazepines, adrenergic antagonists, and dopamine agonists, may also be beneficial.

Symptoms of tardive dyskinesia may continue even after the person has stopped taking the drugs (usually neuroleptics). Some symptoms may improve and/or disappear over time with proper medical management.

Exercise and Drugs

Exercise can produce dramatic changes in the way drugs are absorbed, distributed, localized, metabolized, and excreted in the body (pharmacokinetics). The magnitude of these changes is dependent on the characteristics of each drug (e.g., route of administration, chemical properties) and exercise-related factors (e.g., exercise intensity, mode, and duration).

A single exercise session can cause sudden changes in pharmacokinetics that may have an immediate impact on people who exercise during therapy. Exercise training can also produce changes in pharmacokinetics, but these tend to occur over a longer period and cause a slower and fairly predictable change in a person's response to certain medications.

Drugs that are administered locally by transdermal techniques or by subcutaneous or intramuscular injection may have altered or increased absorption in the presence of exercise, local heat, or massage of the administration site. Diuretics, herbal products, nonsteroidal antiinflammatory drugs, statins, and insulin medications are some of the more common medications that can affect physiologic function during exercise causing a wide range of potential adverse effects.

In addition, allergic and potentially fatal anaphylactic drug reactions are mediated by exercise. The therapist should always consider the possibility that anyone in therapy taking drugs may have an altered response to those drugs as a result of interventions used in therapy.[320] The possibility of drug-exercise interactions requires careful and consistent monitoring of vital signs.

Table 5-1	Nonsteroidal Antiinflammatory Drugs*
Generic	**Common Brand Names**
Nonprescription	
Aspirin	Ascriptin,* Bayer,* Bufferin,* Ecotrin*
Ibuprofen	Advil, Midol, Motrin
Naproxen	Aleve, Midol Extended Relief
Prescription Traditional COX-inhibitors	
Diclofenac	Cataflam, Flector, Voltaren
Diflunisal	Dolobid
Etodolac	Lodine
Fenoprofen	Nalfon
Flurbiprofen	Ansaid
Ibuprofen	IBU-Tab
Indomethacin	Indocin
Ketoprofen	Orudis
Ketorolac	Toradol
Meclofenamate	Meclomen
Mefenamic acid	Ponstel
Meloxicam	Mobic
Nabumetone	Relafen
Naproxen	Anaprox, Naprelan, Naprosyn
Oxaprozin	Daypro
Piroxicam	Feldene
Sulindac	Clinoril
Tolmetin	Tolectin
Prescription COX-2 Selective Inhibitors	
Celecoxib	Celebrex

*These all have additives to minimize GI side effects but are known as aspirin products. Many nonselective (standard) NSAIDs are available nonprescription at a lower dosage (e.g., 200 mg) and by prescription at a higher dosage (e.g., 500 mg).

Courtesy Tanner Higginbotham, PharmD. Drug Information Specialist, University of Montana Skaggs School of Pharmacy, Department of Pharmacy Practice, Missoula, Montana.

SPECIFIC DRUG CATEGORIES

Nonsteroidal Antiinflammatory Drugs

Nonsteroidal antiinflammatory drugs (NSAIDs) are a heterogeneous group of drugs that reduce inflammation, provide pain relief, and reduce fever. NSAIDs are commonly used postoperatively for discomfort; for painful musculoskeletal conditions, especially among the older adult population; and in the treatment of inflammatory rheumatic diseases.

These medications may consist of nonprescription preparations, such as acetylsalicylic acid or aspirin; other salicylates; ibuprofen (e.g., Advil, Motrin, Nuprin, Medipren, Rufen), naproxen (Aleve); or prescription drugs (Table 5-1). Because of their extensive clinical uses, NSAIDs are taken by more than 30 million Americans.[327]

Mechanism of Action

The mechanism of action of NSAIDs involves inhibiting the production of prostaglandins from arachidonic acid by reversibly or irreversibly binding to cyclooxygenase

(COX). There are two principal forms of COX: COX-1 and COX-2. COX-1 is necessary for cells to function normally and is found in most cells. It is responsible for hemostasis, platelet aggregation, and the production of prostacyclin. COX-2 is an inducible enzyme and produced when cytokines and other proinflammatory factors are present because of fever, inflammation, or pain. NSAIDs affect both the peripheral and central nervous systems.[48]

NSAIDs are reversible platelet inhibitors resulting in antiplatelet activity. Aspirin is the most powerful agent because it irreversibly binds to platelets. A single dose of aspirin impairs clot formation for 5 to 7 days, and two aspirin can double bleeding time. These characteristics of acetylsalicylic acid also make it an important drug in the treatment of coronary artery disease, myocardial infarctions, and stroke.

Adverse Effects

Although the incidence of serious side effects from using NSAIDs is rather low, the widespread use of readily available nonprescription NSAIDs results in a substantial number of people being adversely affected.[266] The use of NSAIDs is associated with a wide spectrum of potential clinical toxicities (Table 5-2), but serious side effects are most often seen with the GI tract, kidneys, and cardiovascular system.

Gastrointestinal System. Many NSAIDs are nonselective and inhibit both COX-1 and COX-2. However, because COX-1 is involved with prostacyclin formation, which normally protects the stomach, NSAIDs have been designed to selectively inhibit COX-2 in attempts to reduce unwanted GI side effects. NSAIDs can cause GI symptoms ranging from mild dyspepsia to more serious complications, such as GI bleeding, ulceration, and perforation. These serious side effects may occur without previous symptoms (e.g., dyspepsia) and are particularly more likely to occur in persons taking higher doses, in older adults, and with chronic use.

GI toxicity from NSAIDs is a serious problem in the United States, with more than 70,000 people hospitalized because of serious complications and more than 7000 deaths each year. Medications should be used prophylactically for clients requiring NSAID treatment (e.g., osteoarthritis or rheumatoid arthritis [RA]), such as proton pump inhibitors and misoprostol, which have been shown to reduce the development of symptomatic ulcers.[198] Misoprostol may also reduce the risk for other serious GI complications.[169] COX-2 inhibitors have shown a reduction in GI-related toxicities, but their connection to cardiovascular events has led to their careful use.[346]

Although the stomach has received most of the attention for GI-related NSAID toxicities, new technology has revealed that the small intestine can sustain damage as well. Approximately 55% to 75% of asymptomatic NSAID users have evidence of injury to the small bowel.[131,215] Erosions, ulcers, and strictures[402] from chronic NSAID use have been documented. Studies are evaluating medications that may reduce the incidence of small bowel injury caused by NSAIDs.

Renal System. In the kidney, COX-dependent prostaglandins are also involved with renin release, sodium

Table 5-2	Possible Systemic Effects of Nonsteroidal Antiinflammatory Drugs
Site	**Sign/Symptom**
Gastrointestinal	Abdominal pain
	Anorexia
	Gastroesophageal reflux
	Gastric ulcers
	GI hemorrhage and perforation
	GI obstruction
	Nausea
	Diarrhea
Hepatic	Jaundice
	Transaminase elevation
Renal	Sodium and water retention
	Hypertension (particularly in clients with hypertension)
	Hyperkalemia
	Renal insufficiency
	• Papillary necrosis
	• Nephrotic syndrome
	• Interstitial nephritis
	Renal dysgenesis (infants of mothers given NSAIDs during third trimester)
	Decreased urate excretion (especially with ASA)
Hematologic	Thrombocytopenia
	Anemia
	Prolonged bleeding time
	Increased risk of hemorrhage
Cardiovascular	Blunt action of cardiovascular drugs (e.g., diuretics, ACE inhibitors, β-blockers)
	Hyper- or hypotension
	Congestive heart failure (for those on diuretics or otherwise volume depleted)
	Edema (exacerbation of CHF)
	Premature closure of ductus arteriosus
	Myocardial infarction
	Stroke
	Thrombosis
Cutaneous	Rashes
	Pruritus
	Flushing
	Urticaria (hives), angioedema
	Sweating
Respiratory	Bronchospasm—ASA sensitive asthma
	Rhinitis
Central nervous system	Headache
	Vertigo
	Dizziness, lightheadedness
	Drowsiness
	Aseptic meningitis—rarely seen with ibuprofen therapy
	Tinnitus
	Hyperventilation (salicylates)
	Confusion (elderly treated with ASA, indomethacin, ibuprofen)
Ophthalmologic	Blurred vision, decreased acuity
	Scotomata
Other	Anaphylaxis
	Shock
	Prolongation of gestation
	Labor inhibition

ACE, Angiotensin-converting enzyme; ASA, aspirin; CHF, congestive heart failure; NSAIDs, nonsteroidal antiinflammatory drugs.
From Grosser T, Smyth E, FitzGerald GA. Anti-inflammatory, antipyretic, and analgesic agents; pharmacotherapy of gout. In: Brunton LL, Chabner BA, Knollmann BC, eds: *Goodman & Gilman's the pharmacological basis of therapeutics*, ed 12, New York, 2011, McGraw Hill, pp. 959–1004.

excretion, and maintenance of renal blood flow, especially during times of volume contraction. To varying degrees, all NSAIDs can cause sodium retention and edema in susceptible people. Inhibition of COX enzymes leads to hyperkalemia, a result of the suppression of the renin-aldosterone system; sodium retention, with resulting

edema; and decreased glomerular filtration rate (GFR), resulting in edema, hypertension, and rarely acute renal insufficiency.[54,45,369]

Cardiovascular System. Recent studies confirm the toxicity of NSAIDs to the heart, noting both poor clinical outcomes and changes in gene expression of cardiac cells in the laboratory.[271] NSAIDs are documented to interfere with platelet aggregation, lipid oxidation, endothelial function, apoptosis, cardiac fibrosis, acute myocardial infarction, arrhythmias, blood pressure, antihypertensive therapy, sodium and water retention, and aggravation of congestive heart failure.[129,137] These changes persist with continued use.[314]

NSAIDs are also known to interact with hypertension medications, particularly angiotensin-converting enzyme inhibitors, angiotensin receptor blockers, and β-blockers, thereby modestly increasing blood pressure in persons with hypertension.[288,374] Papillary necrosis, nephritic syndrome, and interstitial nephritis infrequently occur as a result of NSAID treatment. Nephrotoxicity occurs, especially in older clients with volume depletion, congestive heart failure (CHF), or underlying renal disorders.[22] Careful monitoring is required of older adults taking NSAIDs in both the short and long term.[272]

Although COX-2 inhibitors were designed to reduce GI bleeding, an unexpected finding was an increase in myocardial infarctions and stroke.[37,42] Several COX-2 inhibitors were removed from the market, and the remaining drug, celecoxib (Celebrex), carries a black-box warning. Questions continue as to whether this increase in cardiovascular events is a class-wide problem.[332,388] COX-2 inhibitors may effectively reduce inflammation, yet they do not inhibit thromboxane, a prothrombotic enzyme, leading to continued platelet aggregation and serious cardiovascular complications.

Risk Factors

When prescribing NSAIDs, consideration of side effects must be taken into account, individualizing treatment according to risk factors the client may have.[2,125,312,355] Risk factors associated with increased toxicities include advanced age, higher doses, volume depletion, concurrent use of corticosteroids or anticoagulants, previous history of GI bleed or ulcer, or serious comorbidities.[55,312,389] Risk factors for NSAID-induced cardiovascular events include established cardiovascular disease or an estimated 10-year cardiovascular risk greater than 20%.[312]

SPECIAL IMPLICATIONS FOR THE THERAPIST 5-3

Nonsteroidal Antiinflammatory Drugs

The therapist is advised to observe for any side effects or adverse reactions to NSAIDs, especially among older adults; those taking high doses of NSAIDs for long periods (e.g., for RA); those with peptic ulcers, renal or hepatic disease, CHF, or hypertension; and those treated with anticoagulants. NSAIDs have antiplatelet effects that can be synergistic with the anticoagulant effects of drugs such as warfarin (Coumadin). Easy bruising and bleeding under the skin may be early signs of hemorrhage.

Ulcer presentation without pain occurs more often in older adults and in those taking NSAIDs. Often, people who take prescription NSAIDs also take Advil or aspirin. Combining these medications or combining these medications with drinking alcohol increases the risk for development of peptic ulcer disease.[279] Any

client with GI symptoms should report these to their physician.

Musculoskeletal symptoms may recur after discontinuing NSAIDs because of the pain-relieving effects of antiinflammatory agents and the fact that they do not prevent tissue injury or affect the underlying disease process.[230]

Depending on the therapy intervention planned, the therapist may schedule the client according to the timing of the medication dosage. For example, with a chronic condition such as adhesive capsulitis, the goal may be to increase joint accessory motion, which requires more vigorous joint mobilization techniques. Relieving local painful symptoms may help the client remain relaxed during mobilization procedures.

When pain can be predicted (i.e., pain is brought on by treatment intervention), the drug's peak effect should be timed to coincide with the painful event. For nonopioids, such as NSAIDs, the peak effect occurs approximately 2 hours after oral administration. However, in a condition such as shoulder impingement syndrome, teaching the client proper positioning and functional movement to avoid painful impingement may require treatment without the maximal benefit of medication. The therapy session could be scheduled for a time just before the next scheduled dosage.

NSAIDs produce modest increases in blood pressure, averaging 5 mm Hg, and should be avoided in people with borderline blood pressures or who are hypertensive.[288] All NSAIDs are renal vasoconstrictors with the potential of increasing blood pressure, resulting in increased fluid retention, especially lower-extremity edema. NSAIDs also reduce the antihypertensive effects of β-blockers and angiotensin-converting enzyme inhibitors and should generally be avoided in people receiving these cardiac medications. Interaction between most NSAIDs and loop and thiazide diuretics reduces the effects of the diuretic and may lead to a worsening of CHF in a person predisposed to this condition.

It is important to check blood pressure the first few weeks of therapy and to periodically check thereafter to identify any adverse blood pressure response to the combination of NSAIDs, antihypertensive agents, and activity. In addition, NSAIDs may increase serum potassium and lithium levels. Indomethacin may increase the plasma concentration of digoxin, requiring close monitoring of digoxin levels.

Immunosuppressive Agents

Immunosuppressive agents are used traditionally and most frequently in organ and bone marrow transplantation. These medications have also been found to be helpful in treating other diseases, but because of their significant toxicities are only indicated for serious, debilitating, and nonresponding disease.

Immunosuppressive agents for transplantation are used to initially induce immunosuppression (induction therapy), maintain immunosuppression (maintenance therapy), or treat acute rejection. Induction therapy refers to a baseline immunosuppressive agent accompanied by the addition of a prophylactic antibody. Maintenance therapy involves the use of a corticosteroid, a calcineurin inhibitor, and an antiproliferative agent. Acute rejection is treated by increasing maintenance drugs and adding an antibody.

Drug Classes and Mechanisms of Action

Immunosuppressive drugs fall into five classes and have various mechanisms of action. The five main types of immunosuppressives are: (1) corticosteroids, (2) calcineurin inhibitors, (3) antiproliferative agents, (4) monoclonal antibodies,[216,300] and (5) polyclonal antibodies.

Corticosteroids are used in maintenance therapy and are first-line agents in treating acute graft rejection. They principally block T-cell activation and the production of interleukin (IL)-1, IL-2, and IL-6 (cytokines that communicate with other immune cells). Because of the global suppression of the immune system and possibility for severe side effects, most transplant recipients are weaned off corticosteroids a few months following transplantation.[391]

Maintenance of immunosuppression is most frequently accomplished with *calcineurin* drugs. Well-known examples of this class of medication are cyclosporine and tacrolimus. T cells play a key role in graft rejection, so one method of reducing rejection is to block T-cell activation. The calcineurin agents act in a way that ultimately inhibits calcineurin, a protein phosphatase, and the production of IL-2. IL-2 is required for the activation and differentiation of B and T cells. Careful drug monitoring is required for cyclosporine and tacrolimus, because toxicities are often dosage dependent. Nephrotoxicity is the most common prominent toxicity.

Antiproliferative medications, such as sirolimus (Rapamune), azathioprine (Imuran), and mycophenolate mofetil (CellCept),[192] are used for both maintenance therapy and for treatment of acute rejection. These agents inhibit DNA synthesis and block T cells from proliferating. Complete blood counts are needed with azathioprine therapy, and lipid monitoring is required for the drug sirolimus. After several months, most clients can be safely weaned from antiproliferative medications without an increased incidence of graft rejection.

Monoclonal antibodies are designed to target a specific antigen that is required for graft rejection. Muromonab-CD3, one of the first monoclonal antibodies approved, had significant side effects and marketing was discontinued in 2010 because of the availability of other effective, but less toxic, drugs. The IL-2 receptor antagonist,[220] basiliximab, is available for use in early rejection prophylaxis and treatment of acute rejection. Monoclonal antibodies block T-cell activation by binding to T-cells, which are then removed from the circulatory system by phagocytic cells, thereby depleting T cells from the circulation. Numerous monoclonal antibodies are currently approved for many types of disease,[300] such as RA, Crohn disease, hematologic cancers, and dermatologic diseases.

The last class of immunosuppressants is *polyclonal antibodies*, which treat acute rejection and are given as a prophylaxis for early rejection. Unlike monoclonal antibody medications, which are targeted against a specific antigen involved in rejection, polyclonal antibody agents are directed against multiple antigens. These medications are similar to monoclonal antibody agents and lead to a depletion of T cells in the circulation. Examples of this class of agents are antithymocyte globulin-equine (Atgam) and antithymocyte globulin-rabbit (thymoglobulin), with thymoglobulin shown to be more effective.[156]

Adverse Effects

All immunosuppressants have adverse side effects; some of the most serious being an elevated risk of infection[76,122] and transplant-related malignancies.[376] Adverse effects related to immunosuppression are often the most serious consequences of transplantation. Most immunosuppressive agents render transplant recipients prone to infection, particularly cytomegalovirus. There is also an increased risk of developing fungal (especially *Candida* species) and bacterial infections. Viruses, such as herpes simplex virus and varicella zoster, may disseminate or reactivate.

An increase in certain kinds of malignancy occurs with long-term use of immunosuppressants, including lymphoma and other lymphoproliferative malignancies and nonmelanoma skin cancers.[282] Host and graft survival are improving, making infection and cancer more relevant complications. Newer protocols are being developed to reduce the risk for infection and cancer.[154]

The goal of therapy is to provide an adequate balance of immunosuppression so that transplant clients do not experience rejection, while endeavoring to minimize side effects. Drugs are administered at the lowest possible doses while still maintaining adequate immunosuppression. Individual medical factors often determine the choice of immunosuppressive agent. For example, clients who have hypertension or hyperlipidemia may be given tacrolimus instead of cyclosporine. Usually, intensive immunosuppression is required only during the first few weeks after organ transplantation or during rejection crises. Subsequently, the immune system accommodates the graft and can be maintained with relatively small doses of immunosuppressive drugs with fewer adverse effects. Table 5-3 provides a summary of drug-related adverse effects of immunosuppressive agents.

SPECIAL IMPLICATIONS FOR THE THERAPIST 5-4

Immunosuppressants

Careful handwashing is essential before contact with any client who is immunosuppressed. If the therapist has a known infectious or contagious condition, the therapist should *not* work with the immunosuppressed client (see Table 8-5). Both client and therapist can wear a mask in the presence of an upper respiratory infection.

Peripheral neuropathies and subsequent functional impairment can be addressed by the therapist while the client waits for resolution of these side effects. Upper-extremity splinting (e.g., cockup splint for the hand) may be appropriate, or an ankle-foot orthosis to prevent falls and assist in continued and safe ambulation may be provided.[47] Delayed response in the fingers and toes to temperature may require education to prevent injuries.

Table 5-3   Major Immunosuppressive Agents and Adverse Effects*

Agent	FDA-labeled Indications for Use	Adverse Effects
Antithymocyte globulin (rabbit [thymoglobulin] and equine [Atgam])	Renal transplant	Fever, hypertension, peripheral edema, tachycardia, hyperkalemia, shivering, leukopenia, thrombocytopenia, anaphylaxis, cytokine release syndrome
Azathioprine (Imuran)	Renal transplant Rheumatoid arthritis	Opportunistic infections, leukopenia, thrombocytopenia, anemia, nausea, vomiting, pancreatitis, interstitial pneumonitis, rashes
Basiliximab (Simulect; always used with cyclosporine [or equivalent] and corticosteroids)	Renal transplant	Vomiting, asthenia, insomnia, edema, hypertension, anemia, dysuria, candidiasis, cough, cytomegalovirus infection, fever
Corticosteroids (see Box 5-3)	Various inflammatory conditions Neoplasms Autoimmune diseases	Hypertension, atrophy of skin, fluid retention, decreased body growth, hypernatremia, opportunistic infections, osteoporosis, depression, Cushing syndrome, hyperglycemia, adrenocortical insufficiency, cataract, glaucoma, pulmonary tuberculosis
Cyclosporine (Sandimmune, Neoral)	Renal, cardiac, hepatic transplant	Opportunistic infections, renal disease, hypertension, malignant neoplasms, hirsutism, gingival hyperplasia, hyperuricemia, electrolyte abnormalities
Cyclophosphamide (Cytoxan)	Leukemias Lymphomas Hodgkin disease	Opportunistic infections, malignant neoplasms, leukopenia, thrombocytopenia, anemia, hemorrhagic cystitis, bladder cancer, nausea, vomiting, diarrhea, pulmonary fibrosis
Intravenous immune globulin (IVIG)	Immunodeficiency Immune thrombocytopenia purpura Inflammatory diseases	Hypotension, injection site reaction, diarrhea, pharyngolaryngitis, fatigue, fever, tachycardia, erythema multiforme, Stevens-Johnson syndrome, hemolysis, thrombosis, hepatitis, backache, rigor
Leflunomide (Arava)	Rheumatoid arthritis	Alopecia, respiratory tract infection, Stevens-Johnson syndrome, toxic epidermal necrolysis, agranulocytosis, pancytopenia, thrombocytopenia, opportunistic infection, pneumocystis pneumonia, sepsis, interstitial lung disease
Muromonab-CD3 (Orthoclone OKT3)	Renal transplant Cardiac and hepatic transplant (in steroid resistant acute rejection)	Cytokine-release syndrome (can be life threatening), pulmonary edema, cardiac arrest, seizures, cerebral edema (and other central nervous system events), acute renal failure
Mycophenolate mofetil (CellCept) Mycophenolate sodium (Myfortic)	Renal, cardiac, and hepatic transplant	Opportunistic infections, leukopenia, diarrhea, nausea, dyspepsia, elevated transaminases
Sirolimus (Rapamune)	Renal transplant	Opportunistic infection, renal disease, hypertension, malignant neoplasms, hyperlipidemia, pneumonitis, interstitial lung disease
Tacrolimus (Prograf)	Hepatic, cardiac, and renal transplant Atopic dermatitis	Opportunistic infections, renal disease, hypertension, malignant neoplasms, diabetes mellitus, neurotoxicity (tremor, headaches, sensory changes), hirsutism, gingival hyperplasia, myocardial hypertrophy

*All immunosuppressive agents (except basiliximab) increase the incidence of infection and may increase the potential for malignancies (posttransplantation lymphoproliferative disease, skin malignancies).

Data from Cannon GW. Immunosuppressing drugs including corticosteroids. In Goldman L, Shafer AI, Arend WP, et al, eds. *Goldman's Cecil medicine,* ed 24. New York, 2012, Elsevier, pp. 159–165; and DRUGDEX System [Internet database], Greenwood Village, CO, Thomson Reuters, updated periodically.

Corticosteroids

Corticosteroids are naturally occurring hormones produced by the adrenal cortex and gonadal tissue. These hormones are steroid-based with similar chemical structures but quite different physiologic effects. Generally, they are divided into *glucocorticoids* (cortisol), which mainly affect carbohydrate and protein metabolism; *mineralocorticoids* (aldosterone), which regulate electrolyte and water metabolism; and *androgens* (testosterone), which cause masculinization. Many steroid hormones can be synthesized for clinical use. Box 5-5 contains a list of commonly prescribed synthetic corticosteroids.

Glucocorticoids are used to decrease inflammation in a broad range of local or systemic conditions (Box 5-6), for immunosuppression (see "Immunosuppressive Agents" above), and as an essential replacement steroid for adrenal insufficiency.

Therapists most often see people who have received prolonged, systemic glucocorticoid therapy in the treatment of cancer, transplantation, autoimmune disorders, and respiratory diseases (e.g., asthma). Mineralocorticoids are given for adrenal insufficiency or type IV renal tubular acidosis (RTA), whereas androgens are given for deficiency states.

Box 5-5

COMMONLY PRESCRIBED CORTICOSTEROIDS

- Betamethasone (Celestone; Diprolene)
- Beclomethasone (Qvar [inhaler])
- Budesonide (Symbicort [combination product inhaler])
- Cortisone (Cortone)
- Desoximetasone (Topicort)
- Dexamethasone (Decadron; Dexameth; Dexone;)
- Fludrocortisone (Florinef)
- Fluticasone (Flonase [nasal spray]; Advair [inhaler])
- Hydrocortisone (Solu-Cortef; Cortef; Hydrocortone)
- Methylprednisolone (Medrol; Solu-Medrol; Depo-Medrol; A-Methapred)
- Prednisolone (Pediapred; Delta-Cortef; Prelone)
- Prednisone (Deltasone; Liquid Pred)
- Triamcinolone (Aristocort; Kenacort; Kenalog; Nasacort AQ [nasal spray])

Generally, glucocorticoids cause fluid imbalances, and mineralocorticoids cause electrolyte imbalances. However, mineralocorticoids are used less frequently (e.g., for adrenal insufficiency or adrenogenital syndrome). Most adverse effects seen by the clinical therapist will be related to glucocorticosteroids. Adverse effects of anabolic steroids primarily occur in an athletic or sports-training setting.

Adverse Effects of Glucocorticoids

Glucocorticoids have multiple actions; they exert both antiinflammatory and immunosuppressive properties. However, long-term use of glucocorticoids to sustain disease benefits is accompanied by an increased risk of side effects and adrenal suppression.[384] Fortunately, glucocorticoids for treatment of most illnesses are used for a limited time along with disease-modifying medications, whereas long-term use is only necessary for adrenal insufficiency and a few other diseases (e.g., RA and inhaled steroids for asthma).

Glucocorticoids affect many functions of the body, especially in persons taking long-term steroids. Therapists should be familiar with common adverse effects such as change in sleep and mood, GI irritation, hyperglycemia, bone loss, and fluid retention (Table 5-4); side effects are related to dose and duration of treatment.[98] The most serious side effect of steroid use is increased susceptibility to infection and the masking of inflammatory symptoms from infection or intraabdominal complications.

Mood. Most clients taking glucocorticoids notice a change in mood, behavior, or sleep. Individuals often describe a nervous or "jittery" feeling. Symptoms may range from mild anxiety to confusion or psychosis. Changes are typically noted 5 to 14 days after glucocorticoid therapy begins; improvement is seen with withdrawal of the medication.

Effects on Skin and Connective Tissue. Effects on the skin and connective tissue include thinning of the subcutaneous tissue accompanied by splitting of elastic fibers with resultant red or purple striae (stretch marks). Ecchymoses (bruising) and petechiae are caused by decreased vascular strength.[33]

Glucocorticoids alter the response of connective tissue to injury by inhibiting collagen synthesis,[59] which is why these agents are used to suppress manifestations of collagen diseases. Clients who are taking steroids experience delayed wound healing with decreased wound strength, inhibited tissue contraction for wound closure, and impeded epithelization.

Steroid-Induced Myopathy. In high doses, glucocorticoids can cause muscle weakness and atrophy called *steroid-induced myopathy.* Glucocorticoids reduce protein synthesis (mediated by a reduction of growth factors), while increasing muscle catabolism (by increasing the expression of genes involved with atrophy).[298] This results in muscle wasting and atrophy severe enough to interfere with daily function and activities.[280]

Steroid-induced myopathy can begin abruptly and painfully, but is more often insidious, appearing as painless weakness weeks to months after the initiation of treatment.[17] There is no special or definitive test to make the diagnosis of myopathy. Electromyograms and muscle enzymes are often normal, and muscle biopsies are nonspecific.

Clients present with bilateral atrophy and weakness of proximal muscles; the pelvis, hips, and thighs are typically affected first.[195] Upper limb muscles can be affected; occasionally distal limb muscles are involved. The diaphragm may also be involved, which results in difficulty breathing, especially in people with underlying pulmonary disease. Physical therapy intervention may be helpful in counteracting this glucocorticoid-induced muscle dysfunction.[106]

Recovery from chronic myopathy (with cessation of drug) is possible with reduction or discontinuation of the drug but may take from 1 to 4 months up to 1 to 2 years.[280] Prognosis depends on the underlying diagnosis before treatment with corticosteroids (e.g., organ transplantation requiring long-term administration of glucocorticoids). Four functional classifications of muscle weakness can occur in people with steroid-induced myopathy (Table 5-5).

Effect on Growth and Bone. Long-term use of glucocorticoids in children causes apoptosis of the chondrocytes at the epiphyseal plate, leading to growth retardation.[101] Although there is an increase in bone synthesis once the drug is discontinued, full height may not be achieved.[361] In adults, prolonged use of glucocorticoids inhibits bone mineralization, induces apoptosis of osteoblasts, and encourages osteoclastic activity.[41] There is also decreased GI calcium absorption and increased calcium excretion by the kidneys. These combined changes result in osteoporosis.[59,205] Strategies should be in place before extended therapy of glucocorticoids (greater than 3 months) to avoid bone loss.[281,303]

Long-term exposure to corticosteroids increases the risk of avascular necrosis, which often requires orthopedic intervention (e.g., total hip replacement). Glucocorticosteroids are also associated with an increase in the prevalence of vertebral fracture compared with individuals who are not treated with corticosteroids.[145,307,310]

Hyperglycemia. Elevated blood glucose due to corticosteroids is a frequently encountered problem. Total dose and duration of therapy are predictors for the

Box 5-6

THERAPEUTIC USES OF GLUCOCORTICOIDS

Allergy/Immunology

- Allergy
- Immunosuppression

Dermatologic

- Discoid lupus
- Eczema
- Lichen simplex chronicus
- Lichen planus
- Pemphigus
- Bullous dermatitis herpetiformis
- Stevens-Johnson syndrome
- Mycosis fungoides
- Severe psoriasis
- Angioedema
- Dermatitis (exfoliative, seborrheic, atopic)

Endocrine

- Adrenal cortical insufficiency
- Congenital adrenal hyperplasia
- Nonsuppurative thyroiditis
- Hypercalcemia associated with cancer

Gastrointestinal

- Alcoholic hepatitis
- Intractable sprue
- Crohn disease
- Ulcerative colitis

Hematologic

- Idiopathic thrombocytopenic purpura
- Secondary thrombocytopenia
- Acquired hemolytic anemia
- Erythroblastopenia
- Congenital hypoplastic anemia

Nephrology

- Nephrotic syndrome

Oncologic

- Autoimmune anemia/thrombocytopenia in chronic lymphocytic leukemia

- Bowel obstruction (in nonsurgical situations)
- Chemotherapy-induced nausea/vomiting
- Hemolytic anemia
- Immune thrombocytopenic purpura
- Metastatic multiple myeloma
- Spinal cord compression
- Reduce intracranial pressure from brain metastasis
- Palliative care of leukemias and lymphomas

Ophthalmic

- Acute respiratory distress syndrome
- Allergic conjunctivitis
- Keratitis
- Allergic corneal ulcers
- Optic neuritis

Pulmonary

- Acute respiratory distress syndrome
- Aspiration pneumonitis
- Asthma
- Chronic obstructive pulmonary disease (exacerbation or severe disease)
- Interstitial lung disease
- Sarcoidosis
- Seasonal or perennial allergic rhinitis

Rheumatologic

- Ankylosing spondylitis
- Giant cell arteritis
- Henoch-Schönlein purpura
- Osteoarthritis
- Psoriatic arthritis
- Rheumatoid arthritis
- Crystal-induced arthritis

Inflammatory Myopathies

- Polymyalgia rheumatica
- Steroid-induced myopathy
- Systemic lupus erythematosus
- Systemic dermatomyositis

From Glucocorticoids. Drug Facts and Comparisons. Facts & Comparison eAnswers [online], 2012. Available from Wolters Kluwer Health, Inc. Accessed March 22, 2012.

development of hyperglycemia.[63] Glucocorticoids produce hyperglycemia through insulin resistance/tolerance and reduced insulin production (reduced islet cell function). Because of the insulin resistance, the liver is not as sensitive to the presence of insulin and continues gluconeogenesis despite elevated blood glucose levels. Fat and muscle cells also exhibit insulin resistance and do not readily take up glucose.[197] Individuals already requiring oral diabetic agents or insulin frequently need an increase in their dosage. Persons at risk for diabetes (e.g., glucose intolerance) may require a diabetic agent. Glucose monitoring is essential. New therapies may be available to prevent the development of steroid-induced hyperglycemia.[363]

Other Side Effects. For clients with asthma, long-term treatment with inhaled glucocorticoids is common.

Glucocorticoids decrease inflammation and aid in counteracting the vasodilation caused by β_2 agonists. Researchers initially hoped that the inhaled delivery of the glucocorticoids would eliminate or significantly reduce the side effects of the glucocorticoids; but bone loss and other adverse effects remain problematic in people with asthma or chronic obstructive pulmonary disease (COPD) using inhaled steroids.[74,179,189]

The GI effects of steroids are fewer than with NSAIDs, yet they are known to cause gastritis, esophageal irritation, GI bleeding, and, less commonly, peptic ulcers. Many clients take both glucocorticoids and NSAIDs, increasing their risk for adverse GI events (e.g., ulcer with perforation). For these individuals, a GI protective agent (e.g., proton pump inhibitor or misoprostol) may be beneficial.

Table 5-4	Possible Adverse Effects of Prolonged Systemic Corticosteroids

System	Symptom
Metabolic	Increases glucose/protein metabolism
	Stimulates appetite
	Weight gain with truncal obesity
	Hypokalemia
	Suppresses hypothalamic–pituitary–adrenal axis
Endocrine	Delays puberty
	Reduces estrogen and testosterone production
	Menstrual irregularities and amenorrhea
	Hyperglycemia
	Insulin resistance
	Diabetes
	Cushing syndrome (hypercortisolism)
Cardiovascular	Dyslipidemia
	Increases blood pressure
	Fluid retention/edema
	Capillary fragility
	Heart failure
	Ischemic heart disease
Immune	Increases risk of opportunistic infections
	Activates latent viruses
	Masks infection
Musculoskeletal	Increases muscle catabolism (degenerative myopathy, muscle wasting)
	Retards bone growth
	Tendon rupture
	Osteoporosis
	Osteonecrosis, avascular necrosis of femoral head
	Bone fractures
Gastrointestinal	Peptic ulcer disease
	Gastrointestinal bleeding
	Gastritis
	Pancreatitis
	Nausea
Nervous	*Central*: Changes behavior (insomnia, euphoria, nervousness)
	Psychosis, depression
	Changes cognition, mood, and memory
	Cerebral atrophy
	Pseudotumor cerebri
	Autonomic: Autonomic nervous system dysfunction
	Peripheral: Peripheral neuropathy
Ophthalmologic	Cataracts
	Glaucoma
Integumentary	Acne
	Striae (stretch marks)
	Bruising, petechiae
	Dermal thinning
	Delays wound healing
	Hirsutism
	Facial erythema
	Increases sweating

Based on data from Moghadam-Kia S, Werth VP: Prevention and treatment of systemic glucocorticoid side effects, *Int J Dermatol* 49(3):239–248, 2010; Stanbury RM, Graham EM: Systemic corticosteroid therapy—side effects and their management, *Br J Ophthalmol* 82(6):704–708, 1998; Barnes PJ: Pulmonary pharmacology. In Brunton LL, Chabner BA, Knollmann BC, editors: *Goodman & Gilman's the pharmacological basis of therapeutics*, ed 12, New York, 2011, McGraw Hill, pp. 1031–1066; Cannon GW: Immunosuppressing drugs including corticosteroids. In Goldman L, Shafer AI, Arend WP, et al, editors: *Goldman's Cecil medicine*, ed 24, New York, 2012, Elsevier, pp. 159–165.

Glucocorticoids are also known to cause cataracts, both cortical and posterior subcapsular. Cataract formation is dependent on dose and duration of use. They typically develop bilaterally but slowly. Development of glaucoma is also related to glucocorticoid use. Clients with a history of glaucoma and taking glucocorticoids long term may have an increase in pressure while taking glucocorticoids, making pressure checks advisable.

Because glucocorticoids cause adrenal suppression, withdrawal must be slow and tapered to allow for endogenous hormones to be produced by the adrenal cortex. Severe adrenal insufficiency may follow sudden

Table 5-5	Functional Classifications of Corticosteroid-Induced Myopathy
Level	**Function**
Advanced	Person has difficulty climbing stairs
High	Person cannot rise from a chair
Intermediate	Person cannot walk without assistance
Low	Person cannot elevate extremities or move in bed

Modified from Askari A, Vignos PJ, Moskoweitz RW: Steroid myopathy in connective tissue disease, *Am J Med* 61:485–492, 1976.

withdrawal of the medication, particularly in the presence of infection or other stress. The person may experience vomiting, orthostatic hypotension, hypoglycemia, restlessness, arthralgia, anorexia, malaise, and fatigue. These symptoms should be reported to the physician.

Designer Glucocorticoids

The hypothesis that most of the beneficial antiinflammatory effects of glucocorticoids are a result of "repressing" inflammatory genes, whereas most of the adverse side effects are mediated by activating genes, has led to the attempted development of "designer" glucocorticoids that could uncouple the benefits from the side effects. More recent research, however, demonstrates that there is more complexity to the interaction of the glucocorticoid/glucocorticoid receptor with genes and other proteins, resulting in both benefits and adverse effects.[62] No current glucocorticoid demonstrates a complete separation of benefits and adverse effects.[23] These newer glucocorticoids are referred to as selective glucocorticoid receptor agonists or selective glucocorticoid receptor modulators.[33,83,311] Studies[299] and further trials will ultimately verify if there is a beneficial use of these new agents.

Anabolic–Androgenic Steroids

Anabolic–androgenic steroids (AASs), anabolic steroids, or "roids," are synthetic derivatives of the hormone testosterone. They are most commonly used in a nonmedical setting to develop secondary male characteristics (androgenic function) and to build muscle tissue (anabolic function).[30-32] The use of anabolic steroids to enhance physical performance by athletes has been declared illegal by all national and international athletic committees. Even so, an estimated 3 million individuals in the United States alone are current or past nonmedical users of AASs.[92] Administration of these compounds can be orally, intramuscularly, or by injection.

In 2006, 500 AAS users who frequented AAS Internet sites were questioned about their habits. Ninety-nine percent stated they most frequently injected the steroids and 13% used unsafe needle practices.[276] One survey reports the average age at first-time use is 14 years with a significant number of children (15%) taking an AAS before the age of 10.[335]

Users. Studies indicate that adolescent AAS[194] users are significantly more likely to be males and to use other illicit drugs, alcohol, and tobacco.[14] Previously, more athletes were found to use AASs than nonathletes to enhance

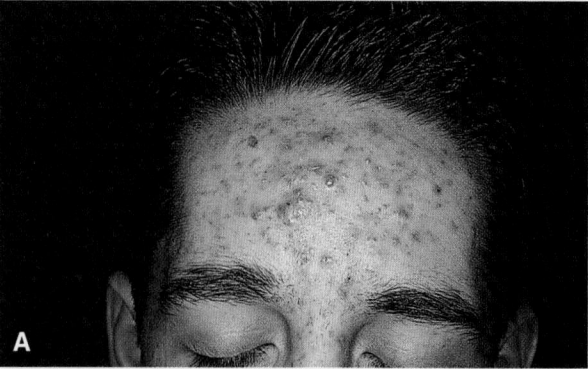
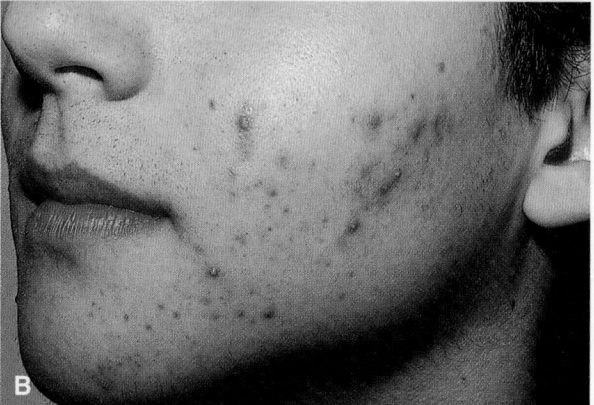

Figure 5-2

Acne vulgaris on the forehead and lower face associated with the use of anabolic steroids. It is considered an abnormal response to normal levels of the male hormone testosterone. The face, chest, back, shoulders, and upper arms are especially affected. There are many other causes of this form of acne; its presence does not necessarily mean the individual is using anabolic steroids. (From Callen JP: *Color atlas of dermatology,* ed 2, Philadelphia, 2000, WB Saunders.)

their sport.[18] However, now a broader spectrum of users are found among professionals working in emergency services—casual fitness enthusiasts and women.[11] Questions are being raised as to the percentage of people who now use AASs for cosmetic reasons alone.[276] The goal is to advance to a more mature body build and enhance the masculine appearance.

The use of this type of steroid is illegal and potentially unsafe, unless given under the direction of a licensed physician; most of these drugs cannot even be prescribed legally but are still obtained from other athletes, physicians, and coaches.[335]

Athletes tend to take doses that are 10, 100, or even 1000 times larger than the doses prescribed for medical purposes. They cycle the drugs before competition, a technique known as *stacking,* alternately tapering the dosage upward and downward before a competitive event. Human growth hormone has been used alone and in combination with anabolic steroids to further enhance athletic performance.

Adverse Effects. Nearly all users of AASs report side effects. The most common include an increase in sexual drive, acne vulgaris (Fig. 5-2), increased body hair, and an increase in aggressive behavior.[259] Individuals may also exhibit an increase in low-density lipoproteins and a decrease in high-density lipoproteins, complicating atherosclerosis and coronary artery disease.[11,158,222] The development of thrombosis (i.e., venous thromboembolism, stroke, retinal vein occlusion) is also seen in persons taking AAS.[208]

Misuse of supraphysiologic doses of AASs for nonmedical reasons has been linked with serious side effects such as hypertension, left ventricular hypertrophy, myocardial ischemia, peliosis hepatis (liver tissue is replaced by hemorrhagic cysts), hepatocellular carcinoma, and sudden and premature death.[3,96,157,201,232,341]

Users of anabolic steroids may experience an increased susceptibility to tendon strains and injuries, especially biceps and patellar tendons, because muscle size and strength increase at a rate far greater than tendon and connective tissue strength. Adolescent steroid use may lead to accelerated maturation and premature epiphyseal closure.[339]

Homicides, suicides, poisonings, and other accidental deaths associated with AAS use have been attributed to impulsive, disinhibited behavior characterized by violent rages, mood swings, and/or uncontrolled drug intake.[284,348] Shared use of multidose vials, dividing drugs using syringes, and increased sexual risk-taking behavior are risk factors associated with AAS use and are potential routes for HIV and hepatitis infection.[224]

Therapeutic Use. There are, however, legitimate medical uses for anabolic steroids that have come about as a result of physiologic evidence that anabolic steroids prevent loss of lean body mass. Oxandrolone, a synthetically derived testosterone, is approved as an adjuvant therapy to promote weight gain after weight loss secondary to chronic infections (HIV wasting), severe trauma (severe burns),[291] Turner syndrome,[128] and extensive surgery and to relieve bone pain associated with osteoporosis.[96-98,130] Other areas of testosterone use include premenopausal women with a loss of libido and aging men to prevent loss in muscle mass and strength.[32,116,144,211,344]

Another anabolic steroid with a practical use is Anadrol. It is indicated for the adjuvant treatment of anemia secondary to a lack of red blood cell production such as occurs in acquired and congenital aplastic anemia and myelofibrosis. Because of the side effects and drug interactions, these agents should be used with caution.

SPECIAL IMPLICATIONS FOR THE THERAPIST 5-5

Corticosteroids
Inflammation and Infection

In the rehabilitation setting, large doses of steroids are administered early in the treatment of traumatic brain injury and in some spinal cord–injured clients to control cerebral or spinal cord edema. Suppression of the inflammatory reaction in people who are given large doses of steroids may be so complete as to mask the clinical signs and symptoms of major diseases, intraabdominal complications, or spread of infection (blocking of inflammatory mediators). In the orthopedic population, local symptoms of pain or discomfort are also masked, so the therapist must exercise caution during evaluation or treatment to avoid exacerbating the underlying inflammatory process.

Increased susceptibility to the infections associated with impaired cellular immunity and the decreased rate of recovery from infection associated with corticosteroid use requires careful infection control. Special care should be taken to avoid exposing immunosuppressed clients to infection, and everyone in contact with that person should follow strict handwashing policies (see "Special Implications for the Therapist: Control of Transmission" in Chapter 8).

Some facilities recommend that people with a white blood cell count of less than 1000 mm³ or a neutrophil count of less than 500 mm³ wear a protective mask. Therapists should ensure that anyone who is immunosuppressed is provided with equipment that has been disinfected according to standard precautions (see Appendix A).

If back pain occurs in a person who is receiving corticosteroids, diagnostic measures should be undertaken to rule out osteoporosis or compression fracture.

Intensive Care Setting

Although clients in the intensive care unit (ICU) are often treated with steroids for various serious illnesses, the use of these medications may increase the risk for complications, such as infection, impaired wound healing, ICU-acquired paresis (ICUAP) or muscle weakness,[85] or death. Individuals who develop ICUAP have been found to require mechanical ventilation for a longer period of time compared to those without ICUAP, supporting clinical observations that clients treated with glucocorticoids often experience difficulty weaning from the ventilator or clearing lung secretions.

Glucocorticoids (methylprednisolone) do not improve persistent acute respiratory distress syndrome, and if begun 2 weeks after the initial episode, may increase the risk for death.[107] Glucocorticoids, however, may be of benefit to clients with COPD requiring mechanical ventilation.[257] Studies are ongoing to determine the most efficacious use of glucocorticoids in this fragile population.

Intraarticular Injections

Occasionally, intraarticular injections of corticosteroids are necessary to control acute pain in a joint that is not responding to oral analgesics, particularly if an effusion is present. Such injections can provide short-term relief and improve the client's mobility and function.[186] The rationale for use in the joint is to suppress the synovitis because no evidence currently indicates that intraarticular injections retard the progression of erosive disease. Intraarticular injections must be carefully selected, and no single joint should have more than three or four injections before other procedures are pursued.[252]

Most steroid injections are accompanied by an anesthetizing agent, such as lidocaine or bupivacaine, which usually provides immediate pain relief, although the antiinflammatory effect may require 2 to 3 days. During this time, the client should be advised to continue using proper supportive positioning and avoid movements that would otherwise aggravate the previous symptoms.

Some controversy remains as to whether the person can bear weight on the joint for several days after the injection; a less conservative approach permits nonstrenuous activity. Vigorous exercise may speed resorption of the steroid from the joint and reduce the intended effect. Intraarticular injection of corticosteroids may also result in pigment changes that are most noticeable among dark-skinned people.

Exercise and Steroids

The harmful side effects of glucocorticoids can be delayed or reduced in their severity by physical activity, regular exercise (aerobic or fitness), strength training, and proper nutrition. Unfortunately, these clients are often too sick to engage in exercise at all, much less at a level of intensity that would reverse myopathy. When possible, the therapist can help emphasize the importance of exercise, especially activities that produce significant stress on the weight-bearing joints (e.g., walking; jogging is not usually recommended), to decrease the calcium loss from long bones that is attributable to prolonged steroid use. It is essential to consult with the client's physician before initiating aerobic exercise.

Glucocorticoid-induced changes in body composition in heart transplant recipients occur early after transplantation. However, 6 months of specific exercise training restores fat-free mass to levels greater than before transplantation and dramatically increases skeletal muscle strength. Resistance exercise, as a part of a strategy to prevent steroid-induced myopathy, should be initiated early after transplantation (see Chapter 21).[40]

Strength training or stair exercise is one way to maintain the large muscle groups of the legs, which are most affected by the muscle-wasting properties of corticosteroids. The treatment plan should also include closed-chained exercises to prevent shearing forces across joint lines and to allow for normal joint loading, prevention of vertebral compression fractures, and education about proper body mechanics during functional activities.[342]

Client education on the importance of proper footwear and choice of exercise surfaces is important for the individual receiving long-term corticosteroid therapy. For the person who is at risk for avascular necrosis of the femoral head, exercising the surrounding joint musculature in a non–weight-bearing position may be required.

Monitoring Vital Signs

Long-term use of corticosteroids may result in electrolyte imbalances (e.g., hypokalemia, hypocalcemia, metabolic alkalosis, sodium and fluid retention, edema, and hypertension), which necessitates monitoring of vital signs during aerobic activity because of the demand placed on the cardiovascular system in conjunction with these adverse effects. (See "Guidelines for Activity and Exercise" in Appendix B.)

Many glucocorticoids have mineralocorticoid activity as well. This causes sodium and fluid retention and enhanced angiotensin II activity, leading to hypertension. Careful monitoring of blood pressure should be performed in clients with previously existing high blood pressure, as glucocorticoid administration may require an increase in the dosage of antihypertensives.

Increased fluid retention may also lead to an exacerbation of CHF in susceptible people; monitoring for signs and symptoms of heart failure is important. Clients may develop hypokalemia secondary to potassium loss from the kidneys; individuals with a history of hypokalemia or taking diuretics benefit from monitoring of blood chemistries.

Steroids, Nutrition, and Stress

People taking steroids may be advised to increase their dietary intake of calcium and vitamin D to counteract the loss of calcium in the urine.[278] Clients may also require a medication to decrease the loss of bone such as a bisphosphonate.[298] Protein intake is recommended for muscle growth to offset steroid-induced catabolism. Individuals may also require potassium supplementation because of increased potassium loss in the urine.

Corticosteroids stimulate gluconeogenesis and interfere with the action of insulin in peripheral cells, which may result in glucose intolerance or diabetes mellitus or may aggravate existing conditions in diabetes. Regular blood glucose monitoring is recommended to detect steroid-induced diabetes mellitus.

Some facilities establish exercise protocols based on blood glucose levels. Exercise is not recommended for people with blood glucose levels greater than 300 mg/dL without ketosis or greater than 250 mg/dL with ketosis.[9]

Clients taking glucocorticoids long-term for Addison disease or RA may need to increase the required dosage during medically stressful situations, particularly with infections or surgery. Temporary mineralocorticoid dosage increases may also be indicated if the client receiving replacement mineralocorticoid experiences profuse diaphoresis for any reason (strenuous physical exertion, heat spells, or fever).[123] Either of these situations requires physician evaluation.

Psychologic Considerations

Corticosteroid use can result in a range of mood changes from irritability, euphoria, and nervousness to more serious depression and psychosis. Insomnia is often also a reported problem during corticosteroid therapy. The intensity of changes in mood may depend on the dosage administered, the sensitivity of the individual, and the underlying personality. When intense changes are observed, the physician should be notified so that an adjustment in dosage can be made.

Chronic corticosteroid use may alter a person's body image because of changes in adipose tissue distribution, thinning of skin, and development of stretch marks. The classic characteristics of a cushingoid appearance may develop, including a moon-shaped face; enlargement of the supraclavicular and cervicodorsal fat pads (buffalo hump); and truncal obesity (see Figs. 11-6 to 11-8).

Some people may be extremely self-conscious about these cosmetic changes, and others may be emotionally devastated by them; caution is required in discussing assessment findings with the client. These cosmetic changes do reverse when the drug is discontinued slowly.

The therapist needs to be aware of the affected individual's coping abilities. Treatment intervention can include educating the individual about traditional stress-management techniques. Therapists can facilitate psychosocial support by contacting social work and clinical nurse specialists to integrate programs such as survivorship support groups and image consultants.

Anabolic Steroids[190]

Therapists working with athletes, especially adolescent athletes, may observe signs and symptoms of (nonmedical, illegal) anabolic steroid use, including rapid weight gain (10-15 lb in 3 weeks); elevated blood pressure and associated peripheral edema; acne on the face, upper back, and chest; alterations in body composition with marked muscular hypertrophy; and disproportionate development of the upper torso along with stretch marks around the back and chest. After prolonged anabolic steroid use, jaundice may develop.

Therapists working with adolescents may see cases of recurrent tendon or muscle strain. Soft tissues working under the strain of added muscle bulk and body mass take longer than expected for physiologic healing to occur. Reinjury is not uncommon under these conditions.

Other signs of steroid use include needle marks in the large muscle groups, development of male pattern baldness, and gynecomastia (breast enlargement). Abscesses from injection use may also develop. Among females, secondary male characteristics may develop, such as a deeper voice, breast atrophy, and abnormal facial and body hair. Irreversible sterility can occur (females being affected more than males), and menstrual irregularities may develop in women.

Changes in personality may occur; the user may become more aggressive or experience mood swings and psychologic delusions (e.g., believe he or she is indestructible). "Roid rages," sometimes referred to as *steroid psychosis* and characterized by sudden outbursts of uncontrolled emotion, may be observed. Severe depression is one of the signs of withdrawal from steroids. Withdrawal from AASs is a risk factor for suicide.

Despite the side effects of AAS use, steroid users are not readily apparent. The therapist who suspects an athlete may be using anabolic steroids should report findings to the physician and consider approaching that person to discuss the situation. The U.S. Olympic Committee provides a toll-free hotline ([800] 233-0393) for questions on steroids, medications, and prohibited substances. The U.S. Antidoping Agency also offers an online drug reference at http://www.usantidoping.org.

Testing for elevated blood pressure may provide an opportunity for evaluation of anabolic steroid use. Information as to the long-term adverse effects of anabolic steroids should be provided as part of the education process for all athletes. The therapist or trainer can provide healthy and safe strength training, stressing the importance of nutrition and proper weight-training techniques.

RADIATION INJURIES

Joy C. Cohn, PT, CLT-LANA

Definition and Overview

Radiation therapy, or radiotherapy, is the treatment of disease (usually cancer) by delivery of radiation to a particular area of the body. Radiation therapy is one of the major treatment modalities for cancer and is used in approximately 60% of all cases of cancer (see Chapter 9 for further discussion). Radiotherapy is used in the local control phase of treatment but has both direct and indirect toxicities associated with its use. Radiation reactions and injuries are the harmful effects (acute, delayed, or chronic) to body tissues of exposure to ionizing radiation.

Today, a pencil-thin beam of radiation can be targeted to deliver extremely high doses of radiation to within a millimeter of a cancer site. Advanced computer technology creates a three-dimensional model of the tumor to allow target mapping. Careful preplanning and delivery of targeted, modulated radiation doses have contributed to a reduced number of radiation side effects.

Etiologic and Risk Factors

Risk factors for developing radiation toxicities arising from therapeutic radiation are often multifactorial, depending on the organ radiated, individual variations and tolerance, tumor type, volume radiated, and fraction size (Table 5-6).

People may also be exposed to radiation found in the environment, such as radon in their homes, or when rare nuclear events release large amounts of radioactivity, exposing people to total-body irradiation. Bone marrow transplant clients may receive total-body irradiation as a preparative regimen.

According to the seventh report on the Biological Effects of Ionizing Radiation issued by the National Academy of Science, exposure to even low-dose imaging radiology (including CT scans) can result in the development of malignancy. Exposure to medical x-rays is linked with leukemia, thyroid cancer, and breast cancer. There is a 1 in 1000 chance of developing cancer from a single CT scan of the chest, abdomen, or pelvis. The latency period for leukemias is 2 to 5 years and 10 to 30 years for solid tumors.[242]

Pathogenesis

Radiation therapy uses high-energy ionizing radiation to kill cancer cells. Irradiation is an effective treatment for cancer because it directly destroys hydrogen bonds between DNA strands within cancer cells. This prevents ongoing cellular replication. Although cells in all phases of the cell cycle can be damaged by radiation, cells in G_2 and M phases (see Fig. 9-3) have the greatest sensitivity to radiation, making rapidly dividing cells most likely to be damaged.

Ionizing radiation interacts with nuclear DNA directly or indirectly to inhibit replicating capacity, resulting in apoptosis (programmed cellular death) or cellular necrosis. The radiation causes the breakage of one or both strands of the DNA molecule inside the cells, thereby preventing their ability to grow and divide.

Table 5-6	Factors Contributing to Radiation Toxicity				
		ENTEROCOLITIS			
Neurotoxicity	**Dermatitis**	**Acute**	**Chronic**		**Pulmonary**
• High total dose • High fractionation dose • Large field size • Increased Edema • Age less than 12 years and greater than 60 years • Concurrent chemotherapy • Presence of underlying diseases which affect the vasculature (diabetes, hypertension) • Stereotactic surgery and interstitial brachytherapy	• Total dose/volume irradiated • Fractionation dose • Surface area exposed	• Large volume irradiated • High total dose • High fractionation dose • Receiving concurrent chemotherapy	• Older age • Received postoperative radiation • Presence of collagen vascular disease • Received concurrent chemotherapy • Poor radiation technique		• Older age • Lower performance status • Lower baseline pulmonary function • Large volume treated

Based on data from Cross NE, Glantz MJ: Neurologic complications of radiation therapy. *Neurol Clin* 21(1):249–277, 2003; Hymes SR, Strom EA, Fife C: Radiation dermatitis: clinical presentation, pathophysiology, and treatment 2006. *J Am Acad Dermatol* 54(1):28–46, 2006; Nguyen NP, Antoine JE. Radiation enteritis. In Feldman M, Friedman LA, Sleisenger MH: *Sleisenger & Fordtran's gastrointestinal and liver disease: pathophysiology, diagnosis, management*, ed 7, Philadelphia, 2002, Saunders; Machtay M: Pulmonary complications of anticancer treatment. In Abeloff MD, Armitage JO, Niederhuber JE, Kastan MB, McKenna WG, editors, *Clinical oncology*, ed 3, New York, 2004, Churchill-Livingstone.

Ionizing radiation also causes the production of free radicals (see discussion of free radicals Chapter 6), which leads to membrane damage and breakdown of structural and enzymatic proteins, resulting in cell death. Often arterioles supplying oxygenated blood are damaged, resulting in inadequate nutritional supply, leading to ischemia and death of the irradiated tissues. The damage to nucleic acids may result in gene mutations, possibly leading to neoplasia years later (see "Mechanisms of Cell Injury" in Chapter 6).

Clinical Manifestations and Medical Management

The clinical manifestations of radiation, similar to risk factors associated with radiation therapy, depend on individual variations, location and type of tumor, radiation volume and fraction dose, and organ system involved. Although newer techniques allow for organ shielding and lower volumes and fraction doses, radiation therapy continues to cause symptoms and injuries.

Each organ has its own tolerance to radiation, therefore injuries vary between organ systems. Yet there are some general principles that encompass radiation therapy injuries. Most organ systems exhibit both acute injuries that occur within 30 days of irradiation and delayed injuries that occur more than 30 days later (Table 5-7). Acute injuries are frequently self-limiting, whereas delayed effects are often irreversible and difficult to treat. Acute symptoms may delay further radiation treatments because of damage to GI mucosa, bone marrow, and other vital tissues.

Management of acute injuries is often treated symptomatically with red blood cells and platelet transfusions, antibiotics, fluid and electrolyte maintenance, and other supportive medical measures as needed. With prognosis poor in many cases of delayed radiation complications, more effort is being placed on prevention. Clinicians

have been attempting to optimize total dose, fractionation size, and total volume being radiated.[108,210]

Modifications are made when chemotherapy is used in conjunction with radiation and prophylactic medications are under investigation to prevent damage or complications.[172,298,352,396] Researchers are also developing more targeted therapy, which would increase tumor sensitivity while reducing damage to adjacent, normal tissue.[251,377]

Because there are unique or specific injuries to different organ systems, the following section specifies clinical manifestations, treatment, and research pertaining to different organ systems.

Radiation Esophagitis and Enterocolitis

The esophagus is a centrally located organ in the mediastinum and is often involved in the radiation fields under treatment for lung cancer. An acute reaction may occur within 2 to 3 weeks after the initiation of radiation therapy manifested by abnormal peristalsis activity, odynophagia (pain with swallowing), and dysphagia (difficulty swallowing).

Although uncommon with radiation alone (1.3% for lung cancer), clients are more likely to develop severe esophagitis after the use of a chemosensitizer (14%-49%),[379] requiring hospitalization for tube feeding, pain control, and hydration. The medication amifostine, presumed to be a free radical scavenger, may be helpful in reducing the frequency and/or severity of esophagitis.[380] Resolution of symptoms typically occurs 1 to 3 weeks after completion of radiotherapy. Late esophagitis is a result of inflammation and fibrosis of tissue, causing stricture and fistula formation. Dilation and surgical repair may be necessary.[381]

As in other organs receiving radiation, the intestines exhibit both acute and chronic symptoms of radiation treatment. Acutely, the rapidly dividing stem cells located in the crypts of Lieberkühn are induced into apoptosis, or programmed cellular death. This increased rate of stem cell loss contributes to acute radiation enteritis, reducing

Table 5-7	Immediate and Delayed Effects of Ionizing Radiation*	
System Affected	**Immediate**	**Delayed Effect**
Musculoskeletal		Soft-tissue (collagen) fibrosis, contracture, atrophy Orthopedic deformity
Neuromuscular	Fatigue Decreased appetite Subtle changes in behavior and cognition Short-term memory loss Ataxia (subacute)	Myelopathy (spinal cord dysfunction) Cerebral injury, neurocognitive deficits Radionecrosis (headache, changes in personality, seizures) Plexopathy (brachial, lumbosacral, or pelvic plexus) Gait abnormalities
Cardiovascular/ pulmonary	Fatigue, decreased endurance Radiation pneumonitis	Radiation fibrosis (lung) Cardiotoxicity Coronary artery disease Myocardial ischemia/infarction Pericarditis Lymphedema
Integumentary	Erythema Edema Dryness, itching Epilation or hair loss (alopecia) Destruction of nails Epidermolysis (loose skin) Delayed wound healing	Skin scarring, delayed wound healing, contracture Telangiectasia (vascular lesion) Malignancy (basal cell, squamous cell, melanoma)
Other	Gastrointestinal: anorexia, nausea, dysphagia; vomiting, diarrhea, xerostomia (dry mouth); stomatitis (inflammation of mouth mucosa); esophagitis; intestinal stenosis	Bone marrow suppression (anemia, infection, bleeding) Cataracts Endocrine dysfunction (cranial radiation) including amenorrhea, menopause, infertility, decreased libido Hepatitis Nephritis, renal insufficiency Malignancy
	Renal/urologic: urinary dysfunction	Skin cancer Leukemia Lung cancer Thyroid cancer Breast cancer

*Some of the delayed effects of radiation (e.g., cerebral injury, pericarditis, pulmonary fibrosis, hepatitis, nephritis, GI disturbances) may be signs of recurring cancer. The physician should be notified of any new symptoms, change in symptoms, or increase in symptoms.

the surface area required for nutrient absorption and leading to dehydration and malnutrition.

Intestinal motility also changes, causing diarrhea, abdominal cramping, and nausea. If the terminal ileum is included in the radiation field, there may be a reduction in the absorption of B_{12} and bile acids leading to B_{12} deficiency and steatorrhea, respectively.[249] Abnormal intestinal motility can occur after the first treatment, but symptoms become most pronounced around the third week of treatment.

Dehydration may require hospitalization and a break in the radiation schedule, but is usually not life-threatening. Concurrent chemotherapy causes an increase in cellular damage when compared to radiation alone, with resulting neutropenia leading to serious infections and sepsis.

The incidence of chronic radiation enteritis is unknown and probably underreported but may occur in up to 15% of cases involving the intestines. Symptoms are insidious, occurring 6 months to 25 years after treatment.[249] Unlike acute radiation symptoms, chronic symptoms often require treatment or surgery with more serious outcomes.

Radiation frequently causes fibrosis of tissues that may lead to strictures in the intestines, bowel obstruction, fistulas with abscess formation, ulceration with bleeding, and malabsorption. Intracavitary implants can also cause rectal damage.

Preventive strategies under investigation include free radical scavengers, antioxidants, and use of cytoprotective agents.

Radiation Heart Disease

Radiation to the chest can cause pericarditis, coronary heart disease, and myocardial disease. Early cardiovascular disease is the leading noncancer cause of death in the population of cancer survivors. This risk is related to chemotherapy as well, and is thought to be the result of damage to the endothelium of the blood vasculature.[239] People at greatest risk for radiation-induced heart disease include those who received mediastinal radiotherapy for breast cancer, testicular cancer, or Hodgkin disease before associated risks were known and radiation regimens were changed. Radiation-induced aortic valve disease has been reported in people who had radiation of the mediastinum for Hodgkin disease 20 to 30 years ago.[160,176] Studies from survivors of atomic bombings suggest that the risk of mortality from radiation-induced heart disease is greatest when the dose is between 0 and 4 Gy and usually occurs at least a decade after irradiation.[347,359] The risk of stroke/transient ischemic attacks is doubled in patients after irradiation for head and neck cancer.[68] Radiation of the left breast has also been linked with coronary artery stenosis (four times the risk compared with right-sided breast radiation).[254]

Radiation Lung Disease

The lung is a radiosensitive organ that can be affected by external beam radiation therapy. Pulmonary toxicity is fairly uncommon and determined by the volume of lung radiated, the dose and fraction rate of therapy, concurrent chemotherapy, older age, lower baseline pulmonary function, and lower performance status.[213]

The two syndromes of pulmonary response to radiation are an acute phase (radiation pneumonitis) and a chronic phase (radiation fibrosis). *Radiation pneumonitis* is caused by significant interstitial inflammation creating a reduction of gas exchange. The hallmark of this toxicity is symptoms disproportionate to other findings, including appearance on radiographs. It usually occurs 2 to 3 months (range: 1 to 6 months) after completion of radiotherapy and typically resolves within 6 to 12 months.

Symptoms range from a dry cough with dyspnea on exertion to severe cough and dyspnea at rest.[213] Rarely, clients may develop acute respiratory distress requiring intubation and ventilation. The National Cancer Institute has developed a grading system called Common Terminology Criteria for Adverse Events (CTCAE), version 3 (Grades 0–5), which does not recognize acute versus chronic symptoms, but rather grades events, such as aspiration or dyspnea. (This grading system is available online at http://ctep.cancer.gov/forms/CTCAEv3.pdf.)

Diagnosis of radiation pneumonitis can prove difficult if underlying disease, such as COPD, is present. Clients with grade 1 or 2 radiation pneumonitis respond well to corticosteroids, although their use can increase the risk for serious infection. Grades 3 and 4 radiation pneumonitis typically have a poor outcome.

Pulmonary radiation fibrosis may occur months after radiation therapy. Radiation fibrosis is progressive and symptoms may develop slowly. Only supportive therapy is available, such as oxygen supplementation, bronchodilators, and treating infection. Corticosteroids have no value, but studies are ongoing to find preventive measures.[12,229,304]

Other radiation-induced pulmonary problems include formation of bronchopleural fistulas, pneumothorax, hemoptysis, and bronchial stenosis.

Radiation Dermatitis

Damage to the skin is one of the more common side effects of radiation as it is involved in most therapies, despite tumor location. Although most injury to the skin is reversible, severe reactions can cause delay in therapy or a change in dosing. The cutaneous effects of radiation can be separated into acute, consequential-late, and chronic.

The National Cancer Institute has provided guidelines for grading acute cutaneous damage to the skin after radiation including erythema, dry desquamation, moist desquamation, and necrosis. Grade 1 reactions resemble sunburn and are accompanied by hair loss, dry

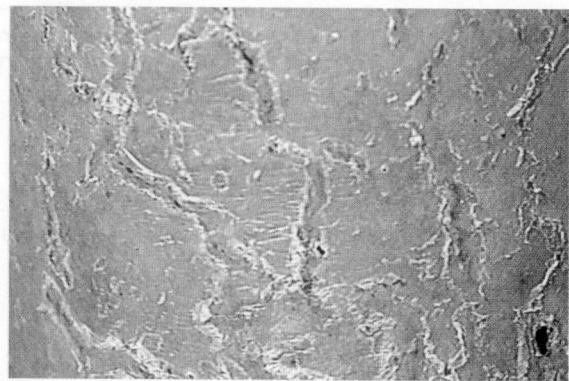

Figure 5-3

Dry desquamation with scaling associated with radiation. (From Habif TP: *Clinical dermatology,* ed 4, Edinburgh, 2004, Mosby.)

desquamation, pruritus, dyspigmentation, and scaling (Fig. 5-3). These changes are secondary to damage of the hair follicles and sebaceous glands. The term *desquamation* is preferred to "radiation burn"; the latter term is unacceptable and no longer used in clinical practice.

Grade 2 reactions produce persistent erythema or patchy moist desquamation in the folds and creases of the skin, often associated with pain and edema. Bullae may form, rupture, and become superinfected. These changes present 4 to 5 weeks into therapy and peak 1 to 2 weeks after treatment completion. Complete healing requires 1 to 3 months.[177]

Confluent, moist desquamation of the skin with pitting edema characterizes grade 3 reactions. Compared to grade 2 reactions, the edematous erythema of grade 3 is not confined to the skin folds. Grade 4 reactions (rare) are severe with skin necrosis or ulceration of full-dermis thickness associated with bleeding. Infrequently, grade 4 reactions do not heal and progress into consequential late effects, eliciting fibrosis with breakdown of necrotic tissue, ulceration, and exposure of underlying structures such as bone.[102] These injuries are difficult to heal, as much of the tissue is avascular secondary to radiation.

Although consequential late effects are persistent acute changes, chronic radiation-induced effects develop months to years after treatment. These late effects in skin and soft tissue are caused by decreased vascular perfusion as a result of late damage to the endothelial cells of the blood vessel walls and deposition of collagen. This leads to fibrosis of small vessels and narrowing of larger vessels.[68] Repeated doses of radiation without sufficient time between doses to repair can lead to significant cutaneous injury. This injury is often manifested by atrophic skin, telangiectasia, hyperpigmentation, and hypopigmentation.

Sebaceous glands, hair follicles, and nails may be permanently affected. Fibrosis of the dermis accompanied by absorption of collagen creates contracted, atrophic skin, which is susceptible to tearing and ulceration (Fig. 5-4). An abnormal proliferation of arteriole cells may occur, causing thrombosis of the vessels, which combined with fibrosis, inhibits healing and predisposes ulcers to infection. These complex ulcers are painful and difficult to heal.

Treatment of acute cutaneous injury is typically symptomatic. For grades 1 and 2 reactions, washing with water

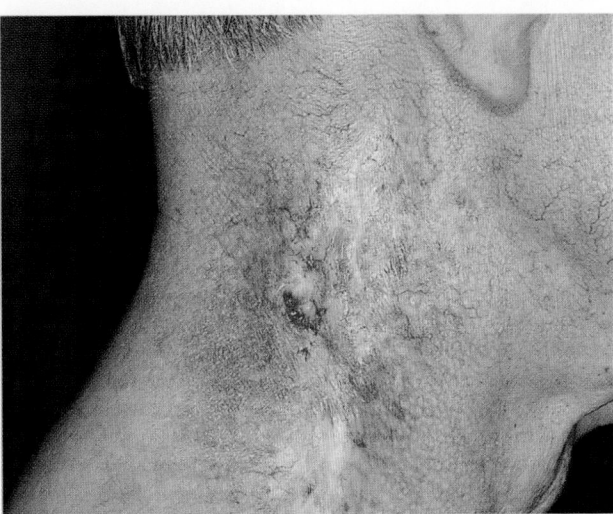

Figure 5-4

Radiation dermatitis. Acute or chronic inflammation of the skin caused by exposure to ionizing radiation (radiation therapy for cancer). Symptoms may include redness, blistering, and sloughing of the skin. The condition can progress to scarring, fibrosis, and atrophy as shown here. (From Callen JP: *Color atlas of dermatology*, ed 2, Philadelphia, 2000, WB Saunders.)

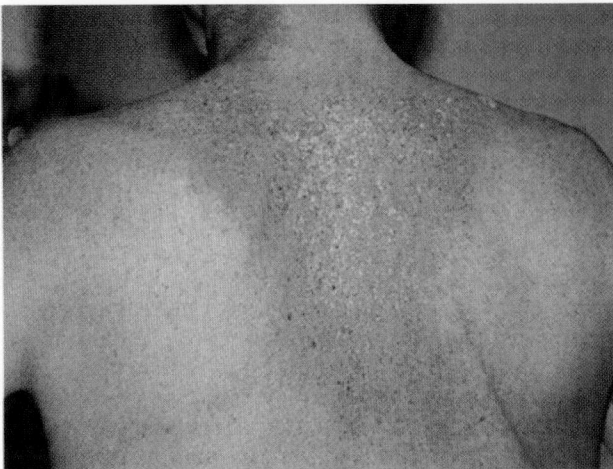

Figure 5-5

Radiation recall. This person had small cell cancer of the lung treated with radiation. Cytoxan treatment some months later elicited erythema and desquamation within the portal of radiation. This lesion is in the healing phase. (From Abeloff MD: *Clinical oncology*, ed 3, Philadelphia, 2004, Churchill Livingstone.)

or a gentle, low pH agent is sufficient to keep the skin clean and reduce bacterial load. Antiperspirants and talcum powders should be avoided in the radiation field. Ointments and creams can often benefit irritated and dry skin after radiotherapy.

Treatment of ulcers and erosions from radiation does not require specific therapy, but the same general principles of wound care apply (such as providing a moist environment, pain control, removing necrotic tissue, and protection against infection).[177] Various dressings may be utilized, depending on the wound type (e.g., burn pads or foam dressings can be used for exudative wounds).

Other modalities that have been used include biosynthetic, artificial, and bioengineered skin; lasers[313]; and recombinant platelet-derived growth factor.[390] Diligence is required to keep fibrotic tissue intact. Active and passive range-of-motion exercises are important to retain mobility and reduce contractures.

The drug pentoxifylline[86] and hyperbaric oxygen therapy (HBOT)[113] have been used to enhance healing, and studies exploring prophylactic uses are ongoing. HBOT administers 100% oxygen under higher-than-atmospheric pressure, helping the body recognize damaged tissue and restoring up to 80% of the preinjury vascular density. High levels of oxygen in the tissues support healing by facilitating angiogenesis.

Another type of radiation-induced reaction is *radiation recall*. Radiation recall reactions (Fig. 5-5) are inflammatory reactions that occur in a previously irradiated site after the administration of certain chemotherapeutic drugs (e.g., dactinomycin, doxorubicin, bleomycin, methotrexate, gemcitabine, and paclitaxel) or antibiotics.[167,187] The reaction is characterized by a "recalling" of inflammation in the entire skin region previously exposed to radiation therapy. Treatment consists of topical agents and discontinuation of the drug regime.

Exposure to ultraviolet rays (e.g., tanning booths or outdoor exposure) is also a risk factor for radiation recall. Anyone undergoing radiation therapy is advised to use sunscreen and avoid exposure to ultraviolet A or B rays (which enhance the effect of radiation therapy) to prevent radiation recall.

Recall may occur in the skin, mucous membranes, lungs, central nervous system (CNS), esophagus, and GI tract, although the skin is most frequently involved.[306] Months, and even years, may pass from the time of the initial radiation therapy to the onset of this reaction. A more immediate reaction (within 2-3 days) often occurs after the initiation of chemotherapy and is usually characterized by a mild, sunburned appearance. The skin may itch or burn; the reaction can last hours to days.

More significant reactions exhibit moist desquamation with blister formation and may even progress to full dermis necrosis and ulceration. Radiation recall involving other organs can be problematic but may respond to supportive measures, corticosteroids, or antiinflammatory medications.[182]

Effects of Radiation on Connective Tissue

Radiation therapy, especially teletherapy, is well known to cause significant long-term or chronic effects on the connective tissue. Acute irradiation toxicity is less likely because connective tissue has a slower turnover or reproductive rate and striated muscle tolerates relatively high doses of radiation.

Late changes, such as fibrosis, atrophy, and contraction of tissue, can occur to any area irradiated but especially to collagen tissue. In growing bones and limbs, irradiation can cause profound and irreversible changes resulting in limb-length discrepancies and scoliosis requiring orthopedic surgical correction.

Weakness of the bone may lead to pathologic fractures because of osteoradionecrosis characterized by hypovascularity, hypoxia, and hypocellularity because of relative sensitivity of the osteoblasts to injury as compared to osteoclasts.[367] Osteoradionecrosis of the jaw either from radiation alone or in conjunction with oral surgery after jaw irradiation was reported in one study assessing HBOT in chronic radiation injuries.[155]

Fibrosis of connective tissue can result in edema, decreased range of motion, and functional impairment. Radiation of the pelvic cavity often causes dense pelvic adhesions that may cause painful motion restrictions and more rarely, plexopathy. Subsequently, these effects lead to soft-tissue fibrosis, resulting in decreased range of motion, pain, and, in some cases, lymphedema.

The fibrotic effect of radiation on the circulatory and lymphatic system is typically seen in a loss of elasticity and contractility of the irradiated vessels that are required to transport the blood, lymph, and waste products from the area of the body being exposed.[16]

Although lymphatic vessels maintain their structural integrity after being irradiated, fibrosis occurs in the surrounding tissue. This effect can inhibit normal growth of lymphatic vessels into healing tissues and delay lymphatic proliferation in response to inflammation.[222] These types of effects can be minimized by sparing lymphatics from the radiation portal, but presently, up to 30% of breast cancer survivors in the United States develop lymphedema sometime in their lifetime.

Partial breast irradiation appears to cause a lower risk of breast lymphedema as compared to whole-breast irradiation and whole-breast irradiation provided by intensity-modulated radiation therapy (IMRT–a radiation technique using computer driven controls to more closely "conform" the radiation delivered to the tissues at highest risk) also reduced the incidence of breast edema as compared to standard whole breast irradiation.[203]

It is important to remember that lymphedema may not be a side effect of radiation but rather a sign of advanced progressive metastases associated with cancer recurrence. Lymphedema can develop when lymphatic overload contributes to systemic congestion; a medical differential diagnosis is required.

Currently, physical therapy and supportive measures are the mainstay of therapy, although newer modalities and medications are under investigation.[265]

Effects of Radiation on the Nervous System

As radiation therapy is used more frequently and aggressively in treating malignancies, toxicities to the nervous system increase. The incidence of nervous system toxicity related to radiation increases as the volume of nervous tissue being irradiated increases and the total dose and fraction size increase.[72]

Despite knowing risk factors for nervous system damage, toxicities continue to occur because individual reactions vary, safe thresholds are not known in all cases, and excessive doses may be used in an attempt to cure a malignancy. Studies determining the incidence of long-term effects of radiation are lacking but high total dose, high fractionation dose, and concomitant chemotherapy probably increase the risk.

Clinical manifestations of nervous system radiation toxicity can be separated into three categories: acute, subacute, and delayed. Neurologic symptoms relating to acute

and subacute complications are most often self-limiting, requiring only supportive measures. The chronic or delayed complications are more often severe and progressive. Therapies for these complications are often palliative at best, although hyperbaric oxygen and anticoagulation have demonstrated questionable improvement.[143,209,295,397]

Acute Symptoms. Acute symptoms generally occur during the period of treatment. The most common symptom is progressive and sometimes debilitating fatigue. Other clinical manifestations of cranial irradiation may include lethargy, short-term memory difficulties, and subtle changes in behavior and cognition. General symptoms that may occur during brain irradiation include decreased appetite, dry skin, hearing loss, hair loss, and decreased salivation.

Cranial radiation can often cause changes in short-term memory, cognition, and personality, ultimately leading to radiation-related encephalopathy or frank dementia.[73] Clients infrequently demonstrate hydrocephalus accompanied by ataxia and incontinence.[82,349]

Acute radiation encephalopathy, probably related to edema, is an uncommon reaction secondary to brain irradiation, causing headache, nausea and vomiting, lethargy, seizures, new focal deficits, and mental status changes. Because of careful planning and use of the drug dexamethasone, the incidence has significantly decreased, although it can be life-threatening in clients that do develop this complication.

Subacute Symptoms. Subacute symptoms (early delayed), noted 1 to 4 months after the completion of therapy, are fairly uncommon. If treatment included the cervical spine (and to a lesser degree the thoracic), clients may experience subacute myelopathy, a tingling, shock-like sensation passing down the arm or trunk when the neck is flexed (Lhermitte sign). This sign occurs in up to 15% of clients receiving mantle radiation therapy for Hodgkin disease. Newer methods of irradiation (IMRT) have reduced exposure of the cervical spinal cord and have reduced the incidence of Lhermitte sign to 3.9% in a population of patients with radiotherapy for head and neck cancer; symptoms resolved in a median duration of 6 months (range: 1-30 months).[238]

Symptoms are usually self-limiting and peak 4 to 6 months after treatment. Irradiation of the brainstem may cause ataxia, nystagmus, and dysarthria. Occasionally, a transient brachial plexopathy occurs, causing paresthesias and muscle weakness, which improves over time.

"Pseudoprogression" is a phenomenon described particularly in individuals with glioblastomas treated with temozolomide and external beam irradiation to the brain. Brain imaging suggests tumor progression and the person demonstrates symptoms of headache, nausea, vomiting, impaired cognition or weakness (also suggestive of tumor reoccurrence). The symptoms are thought to be caused by edema and loss of myelin. They occur in up to one-third of patients and are reversible by steroid usage.[308]

Delayed Complications. Even though many of the acute and subacute complications of radiation are self-limiting or mild, late or delayed complications (late delayed) can be more serious and do not appear for months to years after therapy. For example, when exposed to radiation, cerebral vasculature, as well as other arteries, such as the carotid and coronary arteries, may be damaged, leading to coronary artery disease, transient ischemic attacks, stroke, or myocardial infarction.[175] Other late effects are described as follows and in Table 5-7.

Radionecrosis. One of the best-described complications of whole-brain radiotherapy is delayed cerebral radionecrosis. Symptoms occur in approximately 5% of persons who receive more than 5000 cGy of cranial radiation and include headache, changes in cognition and personality, focal neurologic deficits, and seizures. Another serious long-term complication of radiotherapy of the brain is the development of tumors, including meningiomas, gliomas, lymphomas, fibrosarcomas, and malignant schwannomas. These tumors are often aggressive and difficult to cure.

Radiation of the brain may affect the hypothalamic system. Abnormalities in growth hormone, gonadotropins, thyrotropin, and corticotropin may be seen. Hyperprolactinemia commonly occurs and can resolve spontaneously.[72] Hyperprolactinemia is a condition of elevated serum prolactin, which is an amino acid protein produced in the anterior pituitary gland. Its primary function is to enhance breast development during pregnancy and to induce lactation. Women present with changes in menstruation and infertility; men present with visual disturbances or headache.

Myelopathy. Radiotherapy of the spinal cord may cause a radiation-induced myelopathy. This can present as the Brown-Séquard syndrome or as a motor neuron syndrome. The Brown-Séquard syndrome displays muscle weakness that ultimately leads to paraparesis or quadriparesis. Motor neuron syndrome is uncommonly seen after pelvic radiation (testicular cancer). Clients develop muscle weakness with atrophy of muscles, fasciculations, and areflexia. Sensory examination remains unchanged. This syndrome can progress over years before reaching a plateau.

Plexopathy. The brachial and lumbar plexuses may also be damaged after treatment. Clinical manifestations of radiation-induced brachial plexopathy include paresthesias with progressive motor deficits, lymphedema, and pain. Many clients lose hand function or develop arm paralysis with associated loss of sensation.[20,112]

The incidence of brachial plexopathy after radiation therapy has been reduced significantly with improved treatment, but women who were given large daily fractions of postoperative telecobalt therapy to the axillary, supraclavicular, and parasternal lymph node regions years ago have shown a progression of both prevalence and severity of the late effects many years later, including arm paralysis.[183] Irradiation for apical lung tumors also carries a risk of brachial plexopathy and limits the dosage of radiation possible in tumors that are unresectable. IMRT treatment protocols are being studied that would allow effective treatment of this region of the lung with reduced exposure of the brachial plexus.[10]

Today, with improved irradiation techniques (e.g., matching fields, maintaining the client's position between fields, and avoiding overlapping fields that can cause hot spots), the overall incidence is approximately 0.5% of all cases of irradiated breast cancer. Plexopathies can be caused by cancer recurrence or new cancer onset rather than the effects of irradiation and must be differentially diagnosed by a physician.

Factors seen most often in association with radiation-induced brachial plexopathy include upper trunk plexus involvement, no pain (in some people), lymphedema, and radiation changes in the skin. This is thought to be a result of more exposure in the radiation field of the upper plexus with less overlying soft-tissue protection.[146] Lumbar plexopathy is also possible when the pelvic area is irradiated. Clinical manifestations of radiation-induced plexopathy appear to be a result of fibrosis around the nerve trunks and include paresthesias, hypesthesia, progressive weakness, decreased reflexes, and pain.

Currently, no curative treatment is available for either brachial or lumbar plexopathies, although therapeutic interventions can achieve significant pain control and improve strength and function in the affected limb.[151] Neurolysis surgeries to release fibrotic entrapment of the plexus provides only short-term improvement.[147] Comprehensive strategies may be required in cases of lymphedema (see Chapter 13).

Loss of neural mobility from radiation fibrosis can be addressed using neural mobility assessment and treatment techniques. Treating all tissues of the radiated field (skin, muscle, joint mobility) along with neural mobilization addresses the big picture rather than just focusing on the loss of nerve gliding. Caution should be used to avoid stretching the nerve tissue in the acute phase until the individual demonstrates symptom stability and nonirritation of the nerve(s) in question. The therapist can begin with restoration of the glide component without reaching end ranges and without using overpressure until the individual responses can be monitored and treatment advanced accordingly.

Pregnancy

The fetus is very sensitive to radiation. Pregnant women or those who suspect they may be pregnant must avoid all possible exposure to sources of radiation. Congenital anomalies that develop after intrauterine exposure, especially if it occurs during early pregnancy or 2 to 12 weeks after conception during organ development, may include microcephaly, growth and intellectual developmental disorder, hydrocephalus, spina bifida, blindness, cleft palate, and clubfoot. Later development of cancer, especially leukemia and thyroid cancer, is most often reported when the fetus is exposed to a source of radiation.[365]

| SPECIAL IMPLICATIONS FOR THE THERAPIST | 5-6 |

Radiation
Radiation Hazard for Health Care Professionals

People who receive external radiation do not give off radiation to those who come in contact with them. Likewise, patients coming to physical therapy after a nuclear medicine scan pose no hazard to the therapist. Internal implants can present some hazards to others as long as the implant is in place. Pregnant staff members should avoid all contact with the internally radiated client. Radiation from internal implants (brachytherapy) is usually exhausted after 12 months.

When administering direct care, staff members should plan interventions so that each task can be accomplished as quickly as possible. Because distance provides some protection, it is advisable to use positions that place the staff person as far away from the radioactive implant as possible. For example, if the implant is in the pelvis, the caregiver might stand at the head or foot, not the side, of the bed.

The use of protective lead aprons or portable shields may be recommended according to the hospital protocol. Each staff member is encouraged to know and follow the recommended policies and procedures for the given institution. A film badge or ring badge worn on the outside of any protective devices or clothing of the caregiver records the cumulative dose of radiation received and is used to monitor exposure over a period. When removed, this badge should be stored in a location where no additional radiation exists.

Some sources of radiation (e.g., iodine-131, phosphorus-32) are excreted in body fluids (e.g., urine, sweat, tears, or saliva) for several days after administration to the client. Detectable radioactivity is emitted for up to 3 days after a bone or thyroid scan; up to 51 days for cardiac scans; and up to 95 days after iodine therapy. These clients are placed in strict radioactive isolation during hospitalization and treatment. All articles used by the client, such as urinals, toothpicks, tissues, and bed linens, are considered as a possible radiation hazard. Disposal of all such items should follow hospital protocol. Good quality examination gloves made of latex or a strong synthetic material (not vinyl) are adequate for general care, although the use of 2 sets of gloves is recommended when in direct contact with body fluids deemed radioactive.[393]

Careful removal and disposal of any personal protective equipment worn by the therapist must be done according to radiation safety instructions posted. Thorough handwashing after glove removal is essential.[393]

Postradiation Therapy

For the client who is in the process of receiving external radiation therapy, handwashing before treating the client is essential to protect him or her from infection. Skin care precautions include the following:

- *Avoid topical use of alcohol or other drying agents, lotions, gels, oils, or salves; creams and gels on the skin can potentiate the received skin dosage and lead to increased adverse effects; do not wash away markings for the target area.*
- *Avoid positions in which the client is lying on the target area.*
- *Avoid exposure to direct sunlight, heat lamps, or other sources of heat, including thermal modalities.*
- *Avoid friction to the tissue in the radiation field (i.e., by direct manipulation of the tissue or application of compression in or near affected skin until acute effects of radiation have resolved).*
- *Delayed wound healing associated with radiotherapy requires assessment early on of other factors that impair*

wound healing such as smoking or tobacco use, poor nutrition, weight loss before the start of treatment, and infection.[290]

Radiation to the low back may cause nausea, vomiting, or diarrhea because the lower digestive tract is exposed to the radiation.[243] Radiation of the pelvic cavity often causes dense pelvic adhesions that can cause painful motion restrictions. The therapist's role in the postradiation treatment of these clients is to increase range of motion and provide stretching exercises. Early intervention by the therapist is essential to prevent or minimize restrictive scarring through instruction in effective, focused and efficient flexibility exercises for long term use.

Some effects of radiation on the nervous system can develop years after treatment. Radiation plexopathy can develop many years after exposure to the radiation doses used 20 or 30 years ago. Pain relief has been achieved with surgical release of the nerves from surrounding soft tissue, but improvement in sensation or motor function may not be seen in chronic cases or in situations of delayed diagnosis.[183] With early diagnosis of radiation-induced neuropathies new disease-modifying treatments may improve outcomes in the future.[293]

The therapist should be aware of anyone at risk for seizures, observe for any signs of seizure activity, and take appropriate actions to ensure client safety. Anyone with neurologic signs or symptoms of unknown cause must be questioned about past medical history (cancer, heart disease) and the possibility of prior radiation treatment, keeping in mind that progressive disease or a vascular event can also cause an acute or subacute neurologic event. The physician must rule out cancer recurrence in anyone with a previous history of cancer and evaluate for the presence of some other cause of new onset neurologic signs and symptoms.

Postradiation Infection

Signs and symptoms of infection are often absent because the immunosuppressed person cannot mount an adequate inflammatory response. Fever may be the first and only sign of infection. Swelling, redness, and pus may be absent in infected tissue. The therapist must observe very carefully for any sign of infection, anemia, or bleeding and other signs of thrombocytopenia (see Chapter 14) and refer the individual immediately for physician assessment/treatment the same day.

Radiation Therapy and Exercise

Radiation and chemotherapy can cause permanent scar formation in the lungs and heart tissues, whereas drug-induced cardiomyopathies can contribute to limitations in cardiovascular function (see "Chemotherapy and Exercise" in this chapter, "Cancer and Exercise" in Chapter 9, and Tables 40-8 and 40-9).

Both of these variables require monitoring of vital signs when working with people who are recovering or in remission from cancer treatments. Clients should be taught to monitor their own vital signs including pulse rate, respiratory rate, perceived exertion rate, which is not to exceed 15 to 17 for moderate-intensity training or submaximal testing, and observe for early signs of cardiopulmonary complications of cancer treatments, such as dyspnea, pallor, excessive perspiration, or fatigue during exercise.

Low- to moderate-intensity aerobic exercise (e.g., self-paced walking) during the weeks of radiation treatment can help manage treatment-related symptoms by improving physical function and lowering reported levels of fatigue, anxiety, depression, and sleep disturbance.[228,317] Patients must be educated that avoidance of exercise due to fatigue can increase their fatigue and deconditioning and adoption of a daily "dose" of activity as prescribed can be beneficial in both the short and long term. An American College of Sports Medicine roundtable publication stated: "The advice to 'avoid inactivity,' even in cancer patients with existing disease or undergoing difficult treatments, is likely helpful."[315] Excellent guidelines for many cancer diagnoses and safe prescription of exercise are included.

A successful aerobic training protocol for a client with cancer should include client education, an exercise evaluation, and an individualized exercise prescription. Ideally, these components of cancer treatment should begin when the person receives the diagnosis. Current guidelines recommend that clients should be advised not to exercise within 2 hours of chemotherapy or radiation therapy because increases in circulation may increase the effects of the treatments.[138] Guidelines for choosing an exercise test and prescribing an exercise prescription are available.[8,104]

Radiation and Soft Tissue

Direct treatment of the radiated tissue is not advised during the acute inflammatory phase other than to teach gentle global flexibility for the general area and discuss simple skin care (which the radiation oncology nurses have usually covered well). Postirradiated tissue can tear when stretching. Therapist and client must directly observe for blanching of the skin during exercise and avoid stretching beyond that point.

Soft-tissue mobilization can be performed carefully and judiciously *around* the immobile area. Direct tissue work over the irradiated area must be postponed until after the subacute phase of healing (usually after four months). Active range of motion for generalized tissue mobility is the therapist's first-line approach with maximum respect for irradiated tissue. Remember to teach diaphragmatic breathing during all activities. This is particularly true for the individual who has had surgery/irradiation to the chest wall as ipsilateral rib excursion is often reduced because of scarring and soft-tissue fibrosis. Active motion to the end range as a means of stretching the soft tissues must be continued for at least 18 to 24 months postirradiation as the fibrotic process continues for that amount of time or longer (up to 5 years).[68]

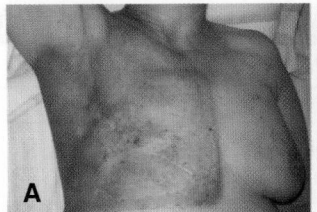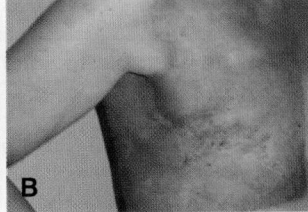

Figure 5-6

Overview of skin changes from radiation therapy. Note the scar/incision site and boundaries or borders between radiated and nonradiated tissue. **A,** Individual nearing the end of her radiation treatment postmastectomy for breast cancer. There is mild-to-moderate erythema with some dry desquamations (skin toxicity also known as *radiation dermatitis*) for which the individual has received topical skin care products for self-application. Areas of redness shows "hot" or radiated tissue; areas of brown skin show healing following damage from radiation. Note that the more red the tissue (just like a sunburn on steroids) the more fragile and damaged the skin and underlying tissue. No visible wet desquamations, which would usually cause the radiation oncologist to put a temporary hold on treatment. These side effects usually appear after about 4 to 5 weeks of radiation. Although there is no visible sign of chest lymphedema, it is important to know that there is a risk of lymphedema for the entire quadrant (not just the upper extremity). With irradiated tissue, assessment should include the borders of the irradiated field (in these photos very obvious because of the erythema, but often must be found by exploration for the reference tattoos), the temperature of the tissue to touch, the mobility of the tissue (adherent to underlying structures versus mobile), the presence of telangiectasia (dilated capillary beds at surface of skin reflecting damage to the autonomic innervation causing permanent vasodilation in that region), and blanching of the tissue to light touch (a sign of acute inflammation still resolving). **B,** Close-up view of same individual postmastectomy during radiation treatment. (A and B, Courtesy Catherine C. Goodman. Used with permission.)

With irradiated tissue, assessment should include the borders of the irradiated field (seen clearly in Fig. 5-6, **A** and **B** as a result of the erythema) but often must be found by exploration for the reference tattoos), the temperature of the tissue to touch, the mobility of the tissue (adherent to underlying structures versus mobile), the presence of telangiectasia (dilated capillary beds at surface of skin reflecting damage to the autonomic innervation causing permanent vasodilation in that region), and blanching of the tissue to light touch (a sign of acute inflammation still resolving).

Once the area no longer blanches with light palpation, then the therapist can begin to apply gentle compression with frequent checks for irritation due to almost certain decreased sensation in the field. Generalized flexibility exercises can be progressed at this time. There is reduced vascularity and sensation so the tissue is at increased risk for injury and reduced capacity to heal; for these reasons, the application of deep tissue techniques to free soft tissue if fixed to underlying structures is not advised at any time. Additionally, increased erythema created by deep techniques may be the inciting event for a lymphedema in this "at risk" tissue (see Chapter 13, Lymphatic System).

Adjuvant Therapies: Radiation

Note to Reader: It is difficult to discuss separate effects of adjuvant therapies (radiation therapy vs. chemotherapy) when so many individuals receive both. Comments here are directed toward radiation therapy although many of the concepts apply to all people who have been treated for cancer with adjuvant therapy; see also discussion of Adjuvant Therapies: Chemotherapy in the next section below in this chapter.

There were an estimated 13.7 million cancer survivors in the United States in 2012 and that number was expected to rise dramatically in the coming years as mortality from a cancer diagnosis continues to trend downward.[7] This means that there is a high likelihood that an individual seeking physical therapy evaluation and treatment may have a history of cancer with adjuvant treatment such as radiation or chemotherapy. In particular, the therapist's understanding of the tissue and sensory changes associated with previous cancer treatment is critical for patients seeking physical therapy for pain or other musculoskeletal problems.

Evaluation

Eliciting a complete past medical history is essential as people often fail to mention previous cancer diagnoses! Careful inspection of scars on the abdomen and trunk will often lead to additions to the history obtained on an intake form. Many people understandably avoid the emotions/reminder associated with a previous cancer diagnosis.

General sensory testing for protective sensation, balance, and proprioception are indicated with a history of radiation (and chemotherapy). Careful examination of the individual who has received radiation treatment is necessary to find boundaries of a previous field of radiation; look for tattoos, skin mobility, surgical scars, sensory changes, temperature and color. Specific signs associated with radiation changes may include:

- Telangiectasia—seen usually in areas of thinner skin such as the axilla and trunk.
- Collateral veins—seen in unusual areas such as the chest wall; these can represent collateralization of the venous circulation caused by obstruction from deep radiation fibrosis, tumor, or previous deep venous thrombosis (DVT) and always require a physician clearance prior to treatment.
- Lymphedema—assess for lymphedema but keep in mind that a significant swelling of rapid onset or progression (days to weeks) in the proximal aspect of a limb associated with complaints of neurogenic pain is almost *never* a benign presentation and requires a physician's assessment. This clinical presentation is often a sign of recurrence of a cancer—even if the person has been previously treated for lymphedema of this same region (see Chapter 13, The Lymphatic System). Cancer patients are at increased risk for DVT, which also suggests that physician evaluation is needed when this type of change develops.

Treatment Planning

The use of modalities is a standard treatment option in treating many musculoskeletal conditions; however, the use of modalities in the region of previous tumor growth/irradiation/surgery requires very careful consideration (see "Physical Agents" in Chapter 9). It is important to keep in mind that impaired sensation and circulation, acute inflammation, loss of skin integrity, and acute DVT are common occurrences in this population with exposure to adjuvant therapies. Additionally, there are several risks associated with use of these interventions including possible stimulation of tumor growth/metastasis, increased blood flow allowing potentiation of active chemotherapy or radiation, and increased tissue injury.

Tissue fibrosis is often a significant factor in limitations of active range of motion seen in this population long term. Deep tissue mobilizations in regions of tissues adherent to the underlying structures is not recommended because of the risk of tissue damage in avascular structures including underlying bone (ribs in particular). However, careful consideration of the layers of musculoskeletal tissue in an irradiated region can lead to the development of focused flexibility exercises to address rib cage, spinal, scapular, and extremity mobility. Instruction in self-mobilization with visual monitoring of the tissue via use of a mirror or direct visualization can assist a patient in maintaining mobility in tissue less amenable to exercise (e.g., the breast).

The emphasis in this population must be on the development of a long-term home exercise program, which is focused in effect and time needed for execution. This is critical given the extended timeframe for tissue remodeling in irradiated tissue and the prolonged nature of the effects of radiation and chemotherapy with regards to cancer fatigue. Flexibility exercises that incorporate multiplanar and multijoint motions are preferable. Practical suggestions as to how to incorporate the needed exercise into daily activities (e.g., while showering) can be very effective in encouraging long-term adherence.

Discomfort and reduced tissue flexibility in a region treated with radiation often leads a patient to consider applying superficial heat to the affected region. Patients must be educated as to the risk of application of superficial heat to tissues that have been exposed to radiation even in the distant past. The tissue is relatively avascular/insensate leading to a greater risk of thermal injury with increased scarring and extended time to heal. Additionally, local heating of the tissues may trigger lymphedema in a region at risk.

*Joy C. Cohn, PT, CLT-LANA

CHEMOTHERAPY[233]

Joy C. Cohn, PT, CLT-LANA

Systemic chemotherapy plays a major role in the management of the 60% of malignancies that are not curable by regional modalities. As with radiation therapy, chemotherapy acts by interfering with cellular function and division. Chemotherapy may be used to cure cancer, to palliate or stabilize disease as preliminary therapy before bone marrow transplantation, or as adjuvant therapy.

In contrast to most cells in the body, tumor cells undergo frequent cell division, leading to an accumulation of cells that are cytologically and histologically defective. Cellular processes needed to support this increased cell division, such as DNA synthesis, DNA repair, DNA replication, and RNA transcription, are themselves accelerated. The principal goal of chemotherapy is to destroy malignant cells with the least harm to normal cells or the host. However, most chemotherapeutic agents are nonspecific and therefore affect both malignant and normal cells.[302]

Researchers first used these unique characteristics of tumor cells as targets for antitumor drugs in the mid-1940s. Goodman and Gillman successfully reduced tumor size in adults with non-Hodgkin lymphoma with mustine, a drug that disrupts the normal structure of DNA.[185] This discovery led to the development of many new drugs, commonly referred to as *chemotherapeutic drugs*, which specifically target those processes needed to support mitotic activity and cell division. Although such drugs have been successful in treating a wide variety of cancers, they are unable to distinguish cancerous from noncancerous cells (i.e., they lack specificity) often attacking normal, as well as cancerous, cells.

Characteristics and Categories of Chemotherapeutic Drugs

Chemotherapeutic drugs are *systemic drugs*, meaning that they travel throughout the body rather than remain confined to a specific area. They are able to reach cells in the primary tumor and cancerous cells that may have escaped from the primary tumor. Many chemotherapeutic agents are systemic and nonspecific, which means they can reach and exert their toxic effects on noncancerous cells as well.

Normal cells most at risk for damage by chemotherapeutic agents are those that normally have high mitotic rates such as hepatic cells, cells that make up epithelial layers, bone marrow cells, and hair cells. However, virtually every organ in the body can be affected by these drugs; for this reason, chemotherapy is often accompanied by multisystem problems and disease.

Four broad categories of systemic chemotherapeutic agents are generally recognized, each of which interferes in some manner with compounds or processes that contribute to cell growth (Table 5-8). Specifically, *alkylating agents* insert themselves into DNA strands, disrupting the normal structure of the strand, preventing the successful replication of an exact copy of that DNA strand, creating a break in the DNA strand. These compounds are mutagenic and potentially carcinogenic.

Table 5-8	Major Toxicities Commonly Associated with Cancer Chemotherapeutic Agents
Chemotherapy Agents	**Major Toxicities**
Alkylating Agents	
Busulfan	Myelosuppression,* nausea/vomiting
Lomustine	Myelosuppression, nephrotoxicity
Carmustine	Myelosuppression, nephrotoxicity
Chlorambucil	Myelosuppression
Cyclophosphamide	Hemorrhagic cystitis, myelosuppression, nausea/vomiting
Ifosfamide	Neurotoxicity, myelosuppression, nephrotoxicity, hemorrhagic cystitis
Bendamustine	Myelosuppression, mucositis
Temozolomide	Myelosuppression, liver toxicity, nausea/vomiting
Dacarbazine	Myelosuppression, liver toxicity, nausea/vomiting
Heavy Metal Compounds	
Cisplatin	Neurotoxicity, peripheral neuropathy, nephrotoxicity, ototoxicity, nausea/vomiting
Carboplatin	Myelosuppression
Oxaliplatin	Peripheral neuropathy, nausea and vomiting
Antimetabolites	
Pemetrexed	Mucositis, myelosuppression, nausea/vomiting
Methotrexate	Mucositis, hepatotoxicity, myelosuppression, neurotoxicity, nephrotoxicity
Thioguanine	Myelosuppression, hepatotoxicity
Mercaptopurine (6-MP)	Myelosuppression, hepatotoxicity
Capecitabine	Myelosuppression, hand-foot syndrome, diarrhea
5-Fluorouracil (5-FU)	Mucositis, diarrhea, myelosuppression
Cytarabine	Myelosuppression, hepatotoxicity, neurotoxicity, nausea/vomiting
Gemcitabine	Myelosuppression, hepatotoxicity, neurotoxicity, nausea/vomiting
Decitabine	Myelosuppression
Azacytidine	Myelosuppression
Fludarabine	Myelosuppression, immunosuppression
Cladribine	Immunosuppression
Pentostatin	Immunosuppression
Topoisomerase Inhibitors	
Teniposide	Myelosuppression
Etoposide	Myelosuppression
Doxorubicin	Cardiotoxicity, alopecia

Continued

Table 5-8	Major Toxicities Commonly Associated with Cancer Chemotherapeutic Agents—cont'd

Chemotherapy Agents	Major Toxicities
Daunorubicin	Myelosuppression, cardiotoxicity
Idarubicin	Myelosuppression, cardiotoxicity
Epirubicin	Myelosuppression, cardiotoxicity
Mitoxantrone	Myelosuppression, cardiotoxicity, mucositis
Topotecan	Myelosuppression, diarrhea
Irinotecan	Diarrhea, myelosuppression
Agents with Diverse Mechanisms of Action	
Mitomycin	Myelosuppression, reversible and nonreversible pulmonary fibrosis, nausea/vomiting
Bleomycin	Dermal toxicities, reversible and nonreversible pulmonary fibrosis, nausea/vomiting
Hydroxyurea	Myelosuppression, interstitial pneumonitis
L-Asparaginase	Hypersensitivity reactions, protein synthesis inhibition
Arsenic Trioxide	QT prolongation, reversible hyperglycemia, fatigue, dysesthesias, and hepatic enzyme elevations
Vorinostat	Fatigue, nausea, diarrhea, thrombocytopenia, QT prolongation
Microtubule-Targeting Agents	
Vinblastine	Myelosuppression, neurotoxicity
Vincristine	Neurotoxicity
Vinorelbine	Myelosuppression
Paclitaxel	Myelosuppression, neurotoxicity
Docetaxel	Myelosuppression, edema
Estramustine	Myelosuppression, estrogenic side effects
Ixabepilone	Myelosuppression, neurotoxicity
Cell Surface Glycoprotein-Targeting Agents	
Rituximab	Infusion-related toxicity, B-cell depletion, neutropenia
Ibritumomab tiuxetan	Hematologic toxicity, myelodysplasia
Tositumomab	Hematologic toxicity, myelodysplasia
Alemtuzumab	Infusion-related toxicity, T-cell depletion, myelosuppression
Growth Factor Receptor- and Ligand-Targeting Agents	
Cetuximab	Infusion-related toxicity, skin rash
Panitumumab	Infusion-related toxicity, skin rash
Trastuzumab	Cardiomyopathy, infusion-related reactions, myelosuppression
Erlotinib	Rash, diarrhea, interstitial lung disease
Lapatinib	Diarrhea, hepatotoxicity, rash, QT prolongation
Bevacizumab	Hypertension, bleeding, thrombotic events
Sunitinib	Diarrhea, fatigue, rash, congestive heart failure
Sorafenib	Diarrhea, fatigue, rash, hand-foot syndrome
Other Biologic and Targeted Agents	
Imatinib	Diarrhea, nausea/vomiting, edema, hepatotoxicity, myelosuppression
Dasatinib	Diarrhea, nausea/vomiting, edema, hepatotoxicity, myelosuppression, pleural effusions
Nilotinib	Diarrhea, nausea/vomiting, edema, hepatotoxicity, myelosuppression, QT prolongation
Bortezomib	Myelosuppression, fatigue, peripheral neuropathy
Temsirolimus	Rash, mucositis, myelosuppression, fatigue, pulmonary infiltrates
Everolimus	Rash, mucositis, myelosuppression, fatigue, pulmonary infiltrates
Thalidomide	Sedation, constipation, peripheral neuropathy, thromboembolic events
Lenalidomide	Myelosuppression, hepatotoxicity, renal dysfunction, thromboembolic events
Retinoids	Dry skin, cheilitis, retinoic acid syndrome
Interferons	Flu-like symptoms, depression, anxiety, myelosuppression
Interleukin-2	Capillary leak syndrome, arrhythmia, rash
Denileukin Diftitox	Hypersensitivity reaction, capillary leak syndrome

*Myelosuppression: bone marrow suppression resulting in anemia, leucopenia, and/or thrombocytopenia.

Data from DiPiro JT, Talbert RL, Yee GC, et al, editors. *Pharmacotherapy. A pathophysiologic approach*, ed 8, New York, 2011, McGraw Hill; and Brunton LL, Chabner BA, Knollmann BC, editors. *Goodman & Gilman's the pharmacological basis of therapeutics*, ed 12, New York, 2011, McGraw Hill.

Drugs known as *antimetabolites* are structurally similar to the purine and pyrimidine bases that form the backbone of each DNA strand. These drugs act either by being incorporated into the DNA strand, leading to the synthesis of a defective DNA strand, or by inhibiting enzymes necessary for DNA and RNA replication, as well as protein synthesis.

Several chemotherapeutic agents are *antibiotics*. These compounds are incorporated into the DNA strand, preventing the synthesis of DNA and RNA. These compounds also lead to the formation of free radicals (see discussion of free radicals in Chapter 6), which can damage DNA and cell membranes. Finally, a variety of *plant alkaloids* are effective in treating cancers, because they interfere with the formation of the mitotic spindle, subcellular structures that transfer genetic material from the mother cell to the two daughter cells.

Although systemic chemotherapy drugs remain the mainstay of chemotherapy, drugs targeting critical biochemical pathways unique to tumor cells have become available. These so-called *targeted therapies* include imatinib mesylate (Gleevec) and trastuzumab (Herceptin). Gleevec specifically attacks the Philadelphia chromosome, which is a chromosome translocation found in chronic myelogenous leukemia.

The anti-HER2 antibody trastuzumab (Herceptin) is used to treat some women with breast cancer. Approximately 30% of individuals with breast cancer have increased expression of the human epidermal growth factor receptor (HER2), resulting in aggressive tumors and poor prognosis. Herceptin specifically targets these receptors and in doing so, increases the likelihood of tumor regression in select individuals. These targeted therapies do not randomly attack rapidly dividing cells, so they generally cause fewer and less severe side effects than do chemotherapy drugs.[150]

Chemoprevention

Chemoprevention drugs have been developed to reduce the risk of reoccurrence of a cancer after primary treatment by surgery/radiation/chemotherapy. The best known of these drugs are the ones developed to reduce the reoccurrence of breast cancer in women who had tumors responsive to estrogen (or estrogen receptor positive tumors). Tamoxifen and Raloxifene are SERMs. SERMs block the ability of estrogen to stimulate tumor growth in estrogen positive tumors and are therefore indicated for use in premenopausal and postmenopausal women after primary treatment ends. These drugs are usually prescribed for 5 years of use after completion of primary treatment.

The side effects of these medications include hot flashes; vaginal bleeding, atrophy, and dryness; endometrial cancer; blood clots; depression; fatigue; and vaginal atrophy. A study called the STAR trial compared tamoxifen to raloxifene in thousands of women after breast cancer and found an equivalent effect in reducing the reoccurrence of invasive breast cancer.[368] Women taking Raloxifene were found to have a reduced risk of endometrial cancer and blood clots. Raloxifene also increases bone density (the purpose for its original development).

An additional class of drugs have been developed called *aromatase inhibitors*. Aromatase inhibitors block an enzyme called aromatase, which changes androgens produced by the adrenal gland in postmenopausal women into estrogen.[1]

Women taking these medications also have a lower risk of blood clots and endometrial cancer as compared to individuals on Tamoxifen, but aromatase inhibitor drugs are associated with a significant percentage of women reporting symptoms of arthralgia or myalgia. The arthralgias involve multiple joints and are reported most often as morning stiffness/pain that diminishes as the day progresses with increased activity. Approximately 25% of women taking Arimidex in one trial reported joint symptoms. A significant number of women with joint symptoms (46%) have reported that a preexisting joint problem was made worse, but in the rest the arthralgia/myalgia symptoms were of new onset.[351]

Symptoms occurred usually within the first 2 years of taking the drugs and were reported to have resolved in 50% of affected individuals within 6 months and in 75% within 18 months. However, there is a high rate of nonadherence with reported rates of 31% to 73% of women having discontinued treatment before completing 5 years of therapy,[240] so the full impact of these medications and their associated side effects (such as arthralgias and myalgias) may be underestimated. General recommendations for symptom management include exercise, weight management and nonsteroidal medications.[386] Other interventions noted for symptoms include switching to a different aromatase inhibitor, acupuncture, and vitamin D. In one study, yoga was seen to have a positive impact on aromatase inhibitor side effects.[132]

Adverse Effects of Chemotherapy

Many chemotherapy agents have unique, dose-limiting toxicities. Chemotherapy drugs are used in combination for their specific actions on cells and care is taken not to use agents with significant overlapping toxicities. Table 5-8 outlines the short- and long-term toxicities of commonly used chemotherapy drugs (see also Table 9-8).

Most chemotherapeutic agents have the propensity to cause nausea and vomiting with the administration of the drug, and mucositis, diarrhea, myelosuppression, and alopecia often occur after treatment. Many cause sterility and are toxic to a fetus.[283]

Cognitive deficits referred to as chemotherapy-related cognitive dysfunction can have a dramatic effect on a person's quality of life. These deficits can be subtle or dramatic, transient or permanent, or stable or progressive.[134]

Alopecia

Alopecia (hair loss) is the most noticeable cutaneous side effect of chemotherapy and often the most distressing because it has a profound social and psychologic impact on the individual. Actively growing hair or anagen hair is the most rapidly proliferating cell population in the human body and therefore very susceptible to the effects of systemic chemotherapeutic agents.

Depending upon which drugs and doses are used, clients may experience varying amounts of hair loss, ranging from thinning of hair to complete loss of hair, including eyelashes, eyebrows, and body hair.

Hair loss typically occurs within 1 to 3 weeks after the initiation of chemotherapy. Hair loss is temporary, with regrowth of hair 2 to 3 months after termination of treatment. Full hair restoration may require 1 to 2 years and may be accompanied by changes in hair color, texture, and type.[165] Clients should be encouraged to prepare for hair loss and given treatment options.[399] Standard advice includes use of a gentle shampoo, wearing scarves, shaving the head, or purchasing a wig.

The scalp may be tender and require special care such as routine application of sunscreen and keeping warm. The application of 2% minoxidil is one treatment option some people choose. Although minoxidil does not reduce hair loss, it can be helpful in speeding hair regrowth.[399]

Although no treatment has been found to be completely effective at reducing hair loss, scalp cryotherapy (scalp hypothermia) has been shown to provide significant benefit.[356,360] This treatment consists of placing ice packs or similar cooling devices on the scalp during chemotherapy infusion. Side effects include feeling uncomfortably cold and headaches. Because the scalp does not receive the same dose of chemotherapy as the remainder of the body, there is a slight risk of cancer recurrence to the scalp for specific types of tumors.

Gastrointestinal Toxicity

Chemotherapy drugs cause the most damage to cells that are rapidly growing. Although this is the means by which eradication of tumor cells occurs, these cytotoxins also affect cells that normally divide quickly, such as cells of the oral cavity and GI tract. This damage leads to mucositis, which is defined as ulcerations or damage of the mucous cells lining the GI tract because of cytotoxic cancer chemotherapy and/or radiation.[343] Clinical symptoms include abdominal pain, bloating, nausea/vomiting, diarrhea, and constipation. These side effects are the most common reasons to reduce doses of chemotherapy drugs, delay treatment, or stop treatment.[13,227] Cytotoxic agents and radiation each have their own potential for causing mucositis and in varying degrees. Mucositis occurs in approximately 40% of persons receiving chemotherapy and in nearly all those receiving high-dose chemotherapy and stem-cell transplantation.[188] Current treatment for mucositis is determined by symptoms and the portion of the GI tract that is affected.

Chemotherapy drugs have a varying ability to cause nausea/vomiting, known as emetogenic potential. High-dose platinum-based agents are among the most strongly emetogenic drugs. Chemotherapy-induced nausea and vomiting (CINV) can be acute or delayed. Acute CINV typically occurs 1 to 2 hours after the administration of the agent, with the effects peaking at 4 to 10 hours after administration and lasting approximately 12 to 24 hours.

Risk factors for CINV include sex (women affected more frequently than men), age (younger clients), and a previous history of nausea/vomiting (motion sickness, chemotherapy, pregnancy), among others. Potential medical complications of chemotherapy-induced emesis include dehydration, electrolyte and acid–base disturbances, and anorexia with accompanying weight loss.[21] Prophylaxis is the best treatment strategy and a variety of antiemetic drugs are currently available to be given prior to treatment and after a treatment.[124]

Other agents, such as platinum-based agents (i.e., oxaliplatin, cisplatin), are known to cause delayed nausea and vomiting, with symptoms occurring 1 to 5 days after drug administration. Some people suffer nausea and vomiting before drug administration apparently in anticipation of becoming sick. Acute nausea and vomiting is usually the most severe, whereas the course of delayed nausea and vomiting can be prolonged, leading to dehydration and poor nutrition.

The mechanisms responsible for acute and delayed CINV are varied and not completely understood, and different drugs may cause nausea by utilizing different pathways. Acute nausea and vomiting are often related to serotonin release in the small intestine which triggers the vomiting reflex via afferent vagal fibers, making serotonin receptor antagonists the agents of choice. Delayed emesis appears to involve other neurotransmitters such as substance P and is best treated with neurokinin-1 receptor antagonists, which block substance P. New antiemetics are being developed that are able to block specific neurotransmitters in order to treat CINV.

Constipation and diarrhea are common side effects of chemotherapy/radiation that significantly impact the physical and emotional well-being of clients receiving cancer treatment. Constipation is most frequently a consequence of pain medication and inadequate fluid intake. Fecal impactions can be uncomfortable and even life-threatening, particularly in the elderly, and clients should be educated and frequently questioned regarding bowel habits in order to avoid complications. Fecal incontinence may be an undisclosed problem. Clients with severe diarrhea can develop life-threatening conditions such as sepsis or severe acid–base disturbances. One rare but life-threatening side effect of intensive chemotherapy is neutropenic enterocolitis,[140] reportedly caused by Gram-negative bacteria. Clinical signs/symptoms include diarrhea, fever, neutropenia, and abdominal pain. Early diagnosis and intervention are keys to successful treatment.

Myelosuppression

Myelosuppression, defined as the inhibition of bone marrow cells resulting in fewer red cells, white cells, and platelets, is a frequent side effect of many cancer treatments. Myelosuppression often results in anemia, infections, and bleeding, as a result of a reduced number of cells. A reduction of white cells, referred to as leukopenia, or more specifically neutropenia (reduced number of neutrophils), is a major dose-limiting toxicity of cancer treatment and often delays further treatment, possibly compromising outcomes. It is also one of the most serious adverse effects of chemotherapy resulting in significant morbidity, mortality and cost.[213] Prolonged neutropenia can result in severe, life-threatening infections requiring prolonged hospital stays and aggressive antibiotic therapy.

Fever is common once an individual is neutropenic, termed febrile neutropenia. This typically occurs during the first cycle of chemotherapy because the person is usually receiving a full dose.[91] Because of the lack of white blood cells, the cause of fever may be bacterial, fungal, or viral. With prolonged neutropenia fungal infections become more likely (particularly persons who have undergone myeloablative therapy). For individuals with a solid tumor who experience febrile neutropenia, the mortality is approximately 5%.[91] For those with hematologic tumors, the mortality can be as high as 11%.[91] Gram-positive bacteremia is the most common cause of febrile neutropenia, whereas the incidence of antibiotic resistant infections continues to rise.

Individuals who develop neutropenic infections (infections that occur while a client is neutropenic) are treated with antibiotics/antifungals and various colony-stimulating factors (CSFs) to stimulate the proliferation and differentiation of hematopoietic progenitor cells. CSFs aimed at increasing white blood cell count include granulocyte colony-stimulating factor (G-CSF) and granulocyte-macrophage colony–stimulating factor (GM-CSF). The use of CSFs is often limited by cost and indicated for persons with a high likelihood of developing complications from neutropenia.[213] G-CSF is currently indicated for clients undergoing myelosuppressive chemotherapy to prevent chemotherapy-induced neutropenia. GM-CSF is indicated for use in clients with acute myeloid leukemia following induction chemotherapy and in the setting of stem cell transplantation.[245]

Although erythropoietin analogues increase red blood cell synthesis and reduce anemia, questions have arisen over adverse outcomes in certain cancer patient populations[20] and administration has become more targeted.[269] Interleukin-11 can be used to reduce thrombocytopenia[34,394] for clients with chemotherapy-induced thrombocytopenia. Administration of blood products, such as blood and platelet transfusions, can also help alleviate adverse effects and symptoms.[110]

Fatigue

It has been estimated that between 70% and 100% of all individuals with cancer will experience cancer-related fatigue.[126] Symptoms of cancer-related fatigue may include persistent sense of tiredness that is not relieved by rest, shortness of breath, decreased ability to focus or concentrate, and decreased ability to perform daily tasks.[270] Although most people will experience fatigue during treatment (chemotherapy, postsurgery, or postradiation), upwards of 35% still experience fatigue 24 months after completing therapy.[244]

Fatigue often peaks within a few days after receiving cyclic chemotherapy then declines until the next treatment cycle. Fatigue significantly reduces quality of life. It is generally agreed that fatigue has multiple cancer-related or treatment-induced causes that can be described as being either physiologic or psychologic. Physiologic causes of fatigue include underlying cancer; cancer treatment; anemia; infection; accompanying pulmonary, hepatic, cardiac, and renal disorders; sleep disorders; poorly controlled pain; lack of exercise, hormonal changes, and malnutrition. Psychologic causes of fatigue include anxiety disorders, depressive disorders, and cognitive losses that include decreased attention span and concentration.[292]

Because cancer-related fatigue is multifactorial, multidimensional interventions involving both physical and psychologic components are required to successfully treat it.[378] Such an approach has proved to be successful.[364]

Cardiotoxicity

Over the last 20 years, therapies for cancer have improved and more people are surviving cancer. However, the aggressive therapies have led to more toxicities with resulting long-term effects, including toxicities of the heart.[225] Cytotoxic agents and targeted therapies used to treat cancer, including classic chemotherapeutic agents, monoclonal antibodies, antiangiogenic drugs, and chemoprevention agents (such as COX-2 inhibitors) all affect the cardiovascular system.[5] Combining chemotherapy and other agents with cardiotoxic effects or with radiation often amplifies cardiovascular injury.

Cardiotoxicity can be categorized as either class I, which is permanent damage to the myocardium, or class II, which is usually reversible and less serious than class I. Each agent used in treating cancer varies in its capacity to cause cardiac damage. Cardiotoxicity may occur acutely (during or immediately after exposure), subacutely (days to weeks after treatment), or chronically (exhibiting injury weeks to months following administration).[328] Cardiotoxicity may be revealed as a cardiomyopathy with a reduced left ventricular ejection fraction, symptomatic heart failure, arrhythmias, myocarditis, myocardial infarction, and pericarditis.[5,318]

The mechanisms of cardiovascular injury are complex and most drugs have more than one means of causing injury. The following is a brief summary of some of the more common cardiotoxic drugs; for more details see Table 5-8 for a list of chemotherapy toxicities.

The most common chemotherapy drug to cause significant cardiotoxicity is doxorubicin (an anthracycline, topoisomerase inhibitor), which can lead to cardiomyopathy with heart failure. The toxicity is cumulative and dose-dependent.[324] Clients receiving this drug can experience cardiac complications up to 10 years posttreatment.[261] Mitoxantrone, another type of chemotherapy, is known to cause arrhythmias during infusion and an acute myocarditis.

Antimetabolite therapies (such as cytarabine) can induce cardiac ischemia and pericarditis. Cardiac ischemia with resultant myocardial infarction can be seen with the use of fluoropyrimidines, such as 5-fluorouracil.[5] Antimicrotubular agents, particularly the vinca alkaloids and paclitaxel, can cause arrhythmias and cardiac ischemia.[400]

Newer treatments, such as monoclonal antibodies, epidermal growth factor receptor targeting agents, tyrosine kinase inhibitors,[268] antiangiogenic (vascular disrupting agents),[168] interleukins, and interferon-α can lead to arrhythmias, CHF, hypertension, and hypotension.[400] The drugs sorafenib and sunitinib, antiangiogenic and tyrosine kinase inhibitors,[78] are known to induce hypertension and other cardiotoxicities. Antiangiogenic agents have hypertension, reduction in left ventricular ejection fraction, and thrombosis as possible side effects. Trastuzumab, a tyrosine kinase inhibitor, is associated with the risk of developing cardiac dysfunction, which increases substantially when this drug is used in combination with anthracyclines or cyclophosphamide (Cytoxan).[139,318] Imatinib mesylate (Gleevec) and nilotinib (Tasigna), indicated for leukemia, can cause CHF and fatal arrhythmias (QT prolongation), respectively.

High-dose regimens and the total dose per course increase the likelihood of developing cardiac disease.

Cessation of the drug will often decrease symptoms.[400] Complicating risk factors for the development of cardiovascular injury caused by drugs include dose, infusion rate, younger and advanced age, exposure to mediastinal radiation, previous heart disease, and hypertension.

Clients with risk factors or who are to receive agents known to cause cardiotoxicities are monitored carefully. They may receive cardioprotective medications, serial echocardiograms[267] or multiple gated acquisition scans to evaluate heart function, or blood tests evaluating troponin levels,[50] looking for myocardial damage.[287] More accurate biomarkers are needed in order to find cardiovascular injury earlier.

Preventive medications that have been shown to slow or reduce the effects of cardiotoxic drugs include angiotensin-converting enzyme inhibitors and β-blockers.[321] Carvedilol, antioxidants (such as salidroside),[403] and others have displayed potential benefits as well. Dexrazoxane has been used effectively and recently metformin has shown promise to reduce the cardiotoxicity related to anthracycline agents.[15,333] As more cardioprotective therapies are developed, each agent, because of unique mechanisms of action, may require several different therapies.

Pulmonary Toxicity

Pulmonary toxicity as a result of cancer treatments is relatively uncommon, but for those clients who do develop lung disease, the consequences can be life-threatening. Many classes of chemotherapy agents are known to have pulmonary toxicities that range from bronchospasm to pneumonitis to acute lung injury. The most common classical chemotherapy drugs to induce pulmonary toxicities are bleomycin, and mitomycin. Newer agents have also been rarely connected with pulmonary toxicities, such as erlotinib, an epidermal growth factor receptor tyrosine kinase inhibitor.[236] Unfortunately, it is often difficult to determine if disease complications or drugs are causing pulmonary disorders.[358] Clients with a history of underlying pulmonary disease are monitored to minimize any further pulmonary decline.

Risk of pulmonary toxicity is increased with advancing age, tobacco use, concomitant irradiation, and size of accumulated dose. For those clients with previous unrelated pulmonary disease, the development of pulmonary pneumonitis or fibrosis may be life-threatening. Symptoms of lung toxicity can occur up to 2 years after completion of treatment.[356]

Renal Toxicity (Nephrotoxicity)

Many chemotherapy agents, antibiotics, and other drugs used in cancer treatment are metabolized and excreted by the kidneys, making the renal system prone to injury or exacerbating underlying disease. Renal abnormalities are one of the most commonly encountered problems associated with cancer therapy, which may alter dosing or require a change in therapy. Renal impairment can be manifested as a range of abnormalities spanning from an asymptomatic increase in BUN and creatinine on laboratory tests, to more serious disorders such as acute renal failure.

As with other systems affected by chemotherapy, clients with underlying kidney disease require special care and monitoring to maintain kidney function. Special biomarkers are currently being studied in order to identify early renal impairment.[93] The classical chemotherapy agents that are most often related to renal injury include cisplatin, methotrexate, and the alkylating class of drugs. Cyclophosphamide and ifosfamide are particularly known to cause hemorrhagic cystitis. The metabolite created from these agents (acrolein) irritates the bladder, causing bleeding, pain, and irritation. Mesna (2-mercaptoethanesulfonate) can be administered with the drug in order to reduce the risk of hemorrhagic cystitis by binding acrolein and forming an inactive compound that is excreted.

A serious complication of chemotherapy that has serious adverse effects on the kidneys is tumor lysis syndrome. Tumor lysis syndrome occurs when cytotoxic drugs destroy malignant cells, releasing large amounts of intracellular ions and metabolic byproducts into the bloodstream (e.g., potassium, phosphate, and uric acid). The kidneys are unable to tolerate the sudden load, leading to hyperkalemia, hyperuricemia, and hyperphosphatemia. Hypocalcemia subsequently develops because of hyperphosphatemia. This can be life-threatening, leading to cardiac dysrhythmias and renal failure.

Clients who have renal insufficiency before treatment, large tumors, or rapidly dividing tumors that are sensitive to chemotherapy, such as acute leukemias and some lymphomas, are at highest risk for this syndrome. Treatment consists of early recognition, hydration, and treatment of metabolic abnormalities. The medications allopurinol and, most recently, rasburicase have been used successfully to treat hyperuricemia associated with tumor lysis syndrome.[105] The most common adverse effects of rasburicase are vomiting and fever; others include nausea, headache, abdominal pain, constipation, diarrhea, respiratory distress, sepsis, neutropenia, mucositis, and rash.

Hepatic Toxicity

Because many cancer treatments use agents that are metabolized by the liver, acute as well as chronic liver injury is possible. Classic chemotherapy drugs that are known to cause hepatotoxicity include methotrexate, L-asparaginase, carmustine, mercaptopurine, dacarbazine, etoposide, gemcitabine, fluorouracil (5-FU), irinotecan, cisplatin, oxaliplatin, and capecitabine[296] (see Table 5-8). Imatinib is a tyrosine kinase inhibitor that is rarely associated with hepatotoxicity.

Risk factors for drug-induced liver disease include age, gender, genetic or familial predisposition, interaction with currently used drugs, past history of drugs that caused liver injury, alcohol (abuse), poor nutritional status, and the presence of underlying liver disease (such as viral hepatitis).[188]

Steatosis, chemotherapy-induced steatohepatitis, and sinusoidal injury are a few of the common or significant hepatic side effects that result from chemotherapy. Approximately 85% of people receiving chemotherapy develop steatosis, which is the synthesis of fatty acids and retention of lipids in hepatocytes.[296] This can be problematic in that hepatocytes with a high lipid content may be more prone to injury from subsequent treatment.[57] Steatohepatitis, inflammation and injury of hepatocytes, although less common, is more serious than steatosis because it can progress to fibrosis and cirrhosis. Sinusoidal injury may range from sinusoid dilation to obstruction.

Sinusoidal obstruction syndrome or venoocclusive disease of the liver is typically seen in clients receiving high-dose chemotherapy in preparation for bone marrow transplant.[27] Damage to endothelial cells of the central veins by toxic agents activates clotting pathways. This leads to occlusion of central and sublobular veins, and, in some cases, liver veins.[296] The incidence of sinusoidal obstruction syndrome has significantly decreased in recent years as a result of therapies that are less hepatotoxic, better hydration, and early use of prophylactic ursodiol (a bile acid).[184] Clients who may receive therapy utilizing a drug known to cause liver injury should also avoid hepatotoxic agents such as alcohol and acetaminophen.

Chemotherapy is also frequently given prior to surgery for metastatic colorectal cancer to the liver, in order to shrink the size of tumor(s). The damage caused by chemotherapy often leaves the liver with little reserve to tolerate surgery,[305] and postsurgical outcomes are accompanied by complications.

Neuropathies

Meredith A. Wampler, PT, DPTSc

Many chemotherapeutic agents adversely affect the nervous system either peripherally or centrally, depending on the pharmacologic properties of the class of chemotherapy drug. Chemotherapy-induced peripheral neuropathy (CIPN), a toxicity-related injury of peripheral neurons, is commonly observed in several classes of chemotherapy agents—microtubule targeting agents (i.e., taxanes and vinca-alkaloids), heavy metal compounds (i.e., platinum compounds), and some biologic agents (i.e., bortezomib, thalidomide) (see Table 5-8 for a specific list).

Although the mechanism of injury is not fully understood, these drugs tend to be found in higher concentration in the dorsal root ganglion, where sensory nerve cell bodies are found, compared to ventral horn cell bodies of motor neurons.[286,354,395] In addition, it has been documented that clients with CIPN have a dying back of sensory neurons[46,202] more than motor neurons. These observations are consistent with the predominately sensory symptoms experienced by clients. However, some clients also experience motor and autonomic symptoms.

CIPN symptoms can develop within hours after an infusion or may not appear for several days to weeks after treatment has stopped. Although most symptoms will improve or resolve, some clients report their symptoms persist for years after completing treatment.[297] Clients will often describe numbness, tingling (paresthesias/dysesthesias), or burning of their hands or feet, that will progress in a distal to proximal pattern as the neuropathy becomes more severe.

Other common impairments include diminished or absent deep tendon reflexes, increased vibration and touch thresholds, hyperalgesia, allodynia, and reduced sural and peroneal nerve conduction amplitudes. In cases where motor neuropathy occurs, clients will present with weakness and/or cramping of distal muscles in the hands and feet; and in the rare case of autonomic neuropathy, orthostatic hypotension, constipation, and dysfunction of sexual organs and urinary bladder may be reported.

The severity of neuropathy is related to several factors, including cumulative dose, coexisting peripheral neuropathy, and combination therapy of several neurotoxic chemotherapy agents.[385] As a result of impairment to peripheral nerve function, clients may experience deficits in the activity and participation realm such as decreased balance, gait instability, and decreased fine motor coordination.[103,354,387]

Oncology physicians and nurses monitor their patients for the development and severity of CIPN. Physical therapists can also assess CIPN severity, but often are more concerned with the functional implications of the neuropathy as it progresses (see tools used by the physical therapist in the "Special Implications: Chemotherapy/Neuropathy" section of this chapter). The most commonly used method by physicians is the CTCAE version 4.0.[357] There are two scales, one for sensory symptoms and one for motor symptoms. In grade 1 neuropathy, clients are asymptomatic for motor symptoms, and/or present with loss of deep tendon reflexes or paresthesias. In grade 2, clients experience moderate symptoms that limit instrumental activities of daily living. In grade 3, symptoms are severe and limit self-care activities of daily living. And in grade 4, symptoms are life-threatening. Many physicians will not change drug dose or drug type unless the client experiences a severe, grade 3 or 4, neuropathy. However, it is becoming recognized by the medical community that a prospective surveillance model for CIPN that includes early intervention for symptoms and mobility-related limitations, such as a referral for physical therapy, will help minimize acute and long-term morbidity associated with CIPN.[338]

Central nervous system toxicity may present as an acute or delayed complication from some chemotherapy drugs. Impairments can manifest as a range of problems, including neurovascular complications, headaches, focal neurologic deficits, generalized neurologic decline with cognitive impairment, seizure activity, spinal cord damage with myelopathy, cortical atrophy, and white matter abnormalities. The mode of administration (intrathecal vs. intravenous) and cumulative dose impacts the severity of toxicity.

Alkylating agents, such as cisplatin or ifosfamide, are known to be neurotoxic. Like many other chemotherapy-related impairments, symptoms may be transient or chronic in nature.[95,248] Antimetabolites, such as methotrexate, cytarabine, and gemcitabine also cause neurotoxicity. Methotrexate, in particular, may cause acute (within hours of administration) symptoms, including headache, neck pain, nausea/vomiting, fever, and photophobia as the result of an aseptic meningitis. Subacutely (within 2 weeks of a dose),[51] recipients may develop acute stroke-like symptoms with focal weakness/seizures or myelopathy-like symptoms with bladder dysfunction, back pain, or local limb weakness.

Chemotherapy-related cognitive impairment, sometimes referred to as "chemobrain," continues to be a controversial topic in oncology care. The subjective and objective measures vary making it difficult to have a clear definition of this phenomenon. Regardless, many clients will report changes to their attention, memory, or other cognitive function (e.g., learning and speed of processing information) during or after chemotherapy treatment. Individuals treated with high-dose protocols or increased number of cycles of chemotherapy are more likely to complain of impairment.[225] There are several measurement tools available to the therapist to document these changes.[142] A case study series has shown that complementary therapies, such as yoga, may be beneficial for this problem.[133] Referral for speech or occupational therapy for cognitive retraining may also be helpful.

Adverse Effects of Hematopoietic Cell Transplantation

See Chapter 21 for full discussion of the adverse effects of hematopoietic cell transplantation.

SPECIAL IMPLICATIONS FOR THE THERAPIST   5-7

Chemotherapy
Chemotherapy Hazard for Health Care Professionals

Questions are often raised by therapists working directly with clients during chemotherapy or during the period shortly after infusion. Are contact precautions required? Is there any evidence to support this practice? The general consensus of clinical oncology specialists is that although chemotherapy is excreted through the person's body fluids (urine, feces, saliva, vomit, blood), very few agents are secreted through sweat glands and/or skin, and only in high doses, such as in transplant settings. Two drugs known to exit the body via sweat are thiotepa (Thioplex) and cyclophosphamide (Cytoxan).[214,329] Gloves for skin-to-skin contact during and within 24 hours of infusion of these medications may be advised. Otherwise contact precautions are not required in most facilities while working with patients on chemotherapy. Until there is evidence to support this policy, some health care professionals are choosing to wear gloves as a contact precautionary measure.

Note to Reader: When we asked our PharmD consultant to research this topic for us, here's what he reported: "This has been a frustrating search for me. Unfortunately, I cannot find any good references that support using gloves when in contact with a chemotherapy patient's sweat. I've found some general recommendations that suggest using gloves for 48 hours after chemotherapy when in contact with a chemotherapy patient's body fluids. But again, no good supporting evidence. I think the recommendations in this section are accurate and safe. The following are links to some information describing this same precaution:"

- American Cancer Society (ACS). Understanding chemotherapy: a guide for patients and families. Available online at http://www.cancer.org/treatment/treatmentsandsideeffects/treatmenttypes/chemotherapy/understandingchemotherapyaguideforpatientsandfamilies/understanding-chemotherapy-chemo-safety-for-those-around-me
- St. Jude Children's Research Hospital. Patient medications: cyclophosphamide. Available online at: http://www.stjude.org/SJFile/cyclophosphamide.pdf
- St. Jude Children's Research Hospital. Patient medications: thiotepa. Available online at: http://www.stjude.org/SJFile/thiotepa.pdf

---

Chemotherapy-Related Considerations for the Client

The period during chemotherapy administration is critical for each client who may be susceptible to spontaneous hemorrhage and infection. Anyone receiving chemotherapeutic drugs is at increased risk of acquiring an infection because these drugs often reduce white blood cell numbers; almost one-third of all chemotherapy patients are impacted by febrile or severe neutropenia most commonly in the first cycle.[71,212] Because neutropenia can occur with a normal white blood cell count, the number of absolute neutrophil count is often used as a measure of neutropenia. An absolute neutrophil count of less than 1500 cells/mm^3 defines neutropenia.

The usual precautions for infection control must be strictly adhered to, including proper hand hygiene and the usual precautions for thrombocytopenia (see Chapter 14). The importance of strict handwashing technique with an antiseptic solution cannot be overemphasized.

The therapist should be alert to any sign of infection and report any potential site of infection such as mucosal ulceration or skin abrasion or tear. Check skin for petechiae, ecchymoses, cellulitis, and secondary infection.

Myelosuppression or bone marrow suppression is the most frequent side effect of many chemotherapeutic drugs. These drugs can cause the circulating numbers of one or more of the mature red blood cells to fall to dangerous levels. Significantly decreased hemoglobin, hematocrit, and red blood cell numbers can compromise an individual's ability to engage in physical activity.

Drug-induced mood changes ranging from feelings of well-being and euphoria to depression and irritability may occur; depression and irritability may also be associated with the cancer. Knowing these and other potential side effects of medications used in the treatment of cancer can help the therapist better understand client reactions during rehabilitation or therapy intervention. Collectively, the therapist should do the following:

- *Be aware of the possibility of myelosuppression in the person on chemotherapy drugs.*
- *Monitor the hematology values in these individuals.*
- *Be aware of the signs and symptoms of the major side effects of myelosuppression (e.g., anemia, infection, and bleeding).*
- *Treat clients appropriately within the context of the limitations and risks represented by myelosuppression.*

As part of the cancer care team, the therapist should keep abreast of reliable up-to-date information about treatment. The American Cancer Society publishes educational materials such as *Understanding Chemotherapy: A Guide for Patients and Families.* These types of introductory materials may help the therapist come to a better understanding of the patient's own early experiences and questions. Educational materials are usually provided free. Contact the local American Cancer Society office; if there is no local or district office, contact the national organization (www.cancer.org or (800) ACS-2345).

Late Effects of Chemotherapy

It is important for the therapist to realize that the adverse effects of many chemotherapeutic agents may not appear for many years after treatment has been completed. For example, bleomycin can cause significant pulmonary fibrosis resulting in decreased pulmonary function; Adriamycin can cause significant cardiac damage 5 to 20 years after treatment; and growth hormone deficiency is the most common endocrinopathy after cranial radiation for brain tumor.

Survivors face an increased risk of morbidity, mortality, and diminished quality of life associated with cancer treatment. Risk is further modified by the survivor's genetics, lifestyle habits, and comorbid health conditions. The Childhood Cancer Survivor Study provides much information on survivorship, occupational outcomes, health-related quality of life issues, long-term complications, and the underutilization of physical therapy among cancer survivors.[191,231,262]

Because a therapist is less likely to see individuals receiving these drugs acutely, the greater concern is for the cardiac and other organ damage, which manifests itself months to years after the cancer treatment has ended. Survivors of childhood and adolescent cancer are one of the higher risk populations seen. The curative therapy administered for the cancer also affects growing and developing tissues.[262]

Careful history taking is important in gaining this information. The therapist must be aware of this because it may explain the symptoms the therapist is evaluating or create comorbid conditions that impact the plan of care. See Chapter 12 for more information regarding the cardiotoxicity of chemotherapeutic agents.

Neuropathy*

CIPN is a toxic neuropathy that may cause sensory, motor or autonomic nervous system impairments (see Table 5-8 for a list of neurotoxic drugs). Sensory symptoms often predominate and include numbness, tingling, and burning of the hands and feet and may progress in a proximal pattern. Motor symptoms include weakness and/or cramping of distal muscles. Autonomic symptoms of orthostatic hypotension, constipation and dysfunction of sexual organs and urinary bladder may also be observed.

There are many methods to measure the severity of CIPN, including symptom based-questionnaires like the chemotherapy-induced peripheral neuropathy assessment scale,[353] touch thresholds using Semmes Weinstein monofilaments, or quantitative vibration thresholds. Many feel that it is best to use a polymodal test, such as a modified or reduced total neuropathy scale, to capture sensory, motor, large and small fiber impairments in one test. These reduced scales have shown high reliability to the gold standard Total Neuropathy Scale, but because they exclude nerve conduction testing, they are more clinically feasible.[141,142,330,371]

The severity of CIPN and which types of nerves have been impaired, will impact the therapist's treatment plan. If the client has impaired protective sensation, then education in proper foot wear and how to protect him- or herself from cuts or burns is warranted. In the case of hypersensitivity to cold (seen acutely after oxaliplatin therapy) or touch, therapists can use sensory reeducation and desensitization techniques to minimize pain. Weakness of ankle or hand muscles would necessitate a strengthening program. If the weakness is severe, an ankle–foot orthotic for foot drop or adaptive equipment to assist weak hand muscles in activity of daily living tasks may be helpful.

The therapist will want to assess balance in all individuals taking neurotoxic chemotherapy, because even low scores on the modified total neuropathy scale, indicating a mild neuropathy, have been associated with significant balance impairments.[372] Breast cancer survivors, even up to 2 years out from completing their chemotherapy, have been documented to report falls and balance problems.[166,387] When developing a balance intervention, the therapist should consider strengthening exercises as well as static and dynamic skill practice with various sensory challenges (i.e., eyes open, eyes closed, on foam, with head shakes).[370] The therapist may also recommend an assistive device in cases of severe balance problems.

Finally, if the therapist recommends aerobic exercise for other impairments, such as cancer-related fatigue, then several CIPN impairments may need to be considered. If the client is unsteady with walking, then it may be better to recommend biking or swimming. The therapist will need to monitor for abnormal heart rate and blood pressure responses in clients with autonomic peripheral neuropathy.

Chemotherapy and Exercise

For a discussion of chemotherapy and exercise, see "Cancer, Physical Activity, and Exercise Training" in Chapter 9.

*Meredith A. Wampler, PT, DPTSc

SPECIFIC DISORDERS AFFECTING MULTIPLE SYSTEMS

Vasculitic Syndromes

Vasculitis is a term that applies to a diverse group of diseases characterized by inflammation in blood vessel walls that causes narrowing, blockage, aneurysm formation, or rupture. Vasculitis is classified according to the size of the vessel affected (i.e., large-vessel, medium-vessel, and small-vessel vasculitis). The primary forms of vasculitis encountered in a therapy practice include: giant cell (temporal) arteritis, polymyalgia rheumatica, and Takayasu arteritis (all large-vessel disease); polyarteritis nodosa and Kawasaki disease (medium-vessel disease); and Wegener granulomatosis and Henoch-Schönlein purpura (small-vessel disease). These are discussed in greater detail in Chapter 12.

Large-vessel disease often produces headache, aching in the shoulders/neck/hip, limb claudication, hypertension, aortic dilation, and bruits. Vasculitis of the medium vessels causes cutaneous nodules (Fig. 5-7), edema or erythema of the digits, coronary aneurysms, mononeuritis multiplex, and abdominal pain. Sinusitis, palpable purpura, glomerulonephritis (renal disease), and alveolar hemorrhage (pulmonary disease) can be seen in disease affecting small vessels.

Most clients with vasculitis will exhibit constitutional symptoms such as fever, arthralgias, arthritis, weight loss, and malaise.[336] Vasculitis may occur as a primary disease (as described above) or as a secondary manifestation of other illnesses such as autoimmune diseases (RA or systemic lupus erythematosus), infection (hepatitis B), malignancy (hairy cell leukemia), or as a drug-induced illness (hydralazine).

Rheumatoid Arthritis

See the complete discussion of RA in Chapter 27.

RA is best known as a progressive, autoimmune disease affecting the synovial tissue and joints. Yet RA has many extraarticular manifestations involving bone, muscle, eyes, lung, heart, and the skin.[66] The presence and severity of extraarticular manifestations generally depends on the duration and severity of the RA. The most frequent skin manifestation is the rheumatoid nodule. These are most commonly found subcutaneously on extensor surfaces, such as the forearm, or pressure points, such as the sacrum in immobile clients, but have been noted on the heart, lung, larynx, and leptomeninges.

Other extraarticular conditions that can occur with RA include vasculitis, anemia/thrombocytopenia, and osteopenia/osteoporosis. *Rheumatoid vasculitis* has become

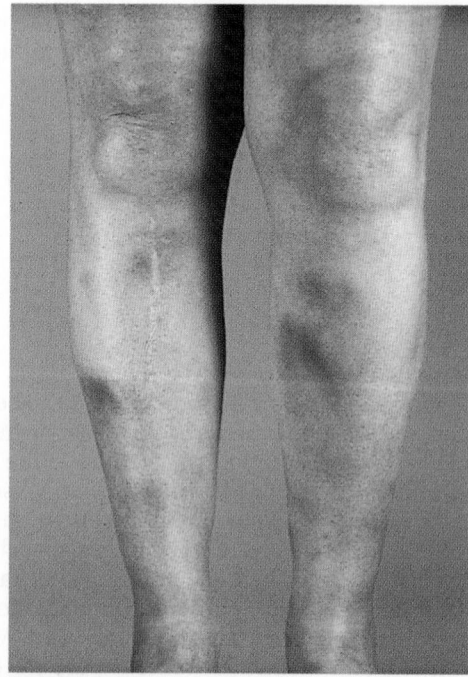

Figure 5-7

Nodular vasculitis caused by inflammation of the medium blood vessels.
(From du Vivier A: *Atlas of clinical dermatology*, ed 2, London, 2002, Gower.)

much less frequent over the last decade, probably because of disease-modifying agents, yet it remains the most feared complication of RA, with considerable morbidity and mortality. Vasculitis is more common in men and usually develops in persons with the most significant active disease (deforming arthritis and high rheumatoid factor titers).

Clinical features of systemic rheumatoid vasculitis are diverse because the disease affects both medium and small vessels throughout the body. The most common findings are cutaneous lesions such as nail-edge infarctions (e.g., splinter hemorrhages; see Fig. 27-14), purpura (see Fig. 5-1), and skin ulcers (e.g., pyoderma gangrenosum). Skin ulcers usually develop suddenly as deep, punched-out lesions at sites that are unusual for venous ulceration, such as the dorsum of the foot or the upper calf.

Neurologic manifestations of RA vasculitis present most commonly as either a mild distal sensory neuropathy (paresthesia or numbness) or as a severe sensorimotor neuropathy such as wrist or foot drop (mononeuritis multiplex). These may be the only extraarticular manifestations of RA.

Vasculitis of the heart is one of the leading causes of death in people with RA. Affected individuals may already have traditional risk factors for heart disease, which are then superimposed with chronic inflammation from RA.[258] Aggressive treatment of RA has been shown to decrease the development of heart disease.[223] Lung involvement may be manifested as pulmonary effusions or interstitial lung disease. Infarction of the intestine may occur, requiring bowel resection.

Systemic manifestations of rheumatoid vasculitis may include unexplained weight loss, anorexia, and malaise. Malaise may be related to the release of cytokines (substances released by lymphocytes with various immunologic functions) and may be accompanied by fatigue, low-grade fever, and night sweats. Individuals with severe RA who experience any of these symptoms should be referred to the physician for further evaluation. Clients with multiple manifestations of vasculitis have a poor prognosis and require aggressive treatment.

Anemia secondary to RA is usually mild with normocytic/normochromic features and is proportional to the disease severity. More than three-fourths of people with RA and anemia have anemia of chronic disease; one-quarter will respond to iron supplementation. In addition, either group may have superimposed B_{12} or folate deficiency.[277] If an individual with RA is noted to have iron deficiency, sources of bleeding must be explored, such as GI bleeding from therapy with NSAIDs. Anemia with a hemoglobin value less than 10 is rarely associated with RA and should be investigated aggressively for another cause. The therapist should follow special precautions related to anemia until the disease is under control (see "Special Implications for the Therapist: Anemia" in Chapter 14).

Thrombocytosis is frequently seen in clients with RA, particularly in people who have extraarticular manifestations and severe disease. Felty syndrome is an uncommon but serious manifestation of severe RA. Clients exhibit splenomegaly, thrombocytosis, and neutropenia and are at risk for infection, skin ulcerations, and other complications.

Osteopenia and osteoporosis may result from post-menopausal bone loss, treatment with glucocorticoids, or general immobility, but it may also be an inherent part of RA. Because most clients with RA may have all these risk factors for bone loss, they should be aggressively treated to reduce bone loss. With longstanding disease, osteoporosis may become generalized and can lead to fractures after minimal stress, particularly the fibula.

Systemic Lupus Erythematosus

Lupus erythematosus is an autoimmune disease that appears in two forms: discoid lupus erythematosus, which affects only the skin, and systemic lupus erythematosus (SLE), which affects both the skin and multiple organ systems. SLE most commonly causes rashes of the skin, polyarthritis, alopecia, and myalgias. The most serious complications affect the heart (pericarditis, endocarditis, myocarditis), kidneys (nephritis and glomerulonephritis), and CNS (vasculitis associated transverse myelitis, aseptic meningitis, stroke, seizure, encephalitis). Like RA, SLE is characterized by recurring remissions and exacerbations. Morbidity and mortality are increasing related to side effects from medications (infection, malignancy) and long-term organ damage from severe disease (chronic kidney disease or neurologic complications). SLE is also an independent risk factor for cardiovascular disease. (For further discussion, see Chapters 7 and 10).

Systemic Sclerosis

Systemic sclerosis (SSc), or scleroderma, is a generalized connective tissue disorder of unknown etiology characterized by immune dysregulation (autoantibody production), microangiopathy (vasculitis and obstruction of small vessels), and fibrosis of skin and internal organs. It may affect the heart, lungs, GI tract, and kidneys.

Although there are many subgroups termed *scleroderma*, it is often categorized into three main subgroups to help clinically prognosticate: limited and diffuse cutaneous scleroderma and systemic sclerosis sine scleroderma (ssSSc). Limited cutaneous scleroderma (lcSSc) is characterized by skin thickening that does not progress proximal to the elbows and knees. A subset of clients with lcSSc demonstrates a syndrome known as the CREST syndrome (*C*alcinosis, *R*aynaud phenomenon, *E*sophageal dysmotility, *S*clerodactyly, and *T*elangiectasia).

Diffuse cutaneous scleroderma (dcSSc) extends proximally to the elbows and knees. Both limited and diffuse disease can involve the head and neck. Clients with lcSSc are more likely to develop pulmonary hypertension, whereas those with dcSSc are more likely to develop interstitial lung disease and/or renal disease. ssSSc is characterized by fibrosis of internal organs without the presence of skin manifestations.

There is significant variability of symptoms and organ involvement between clients. It affects women more than men, especially between ages 35 and 50 years. Although SSc has no current significant disease-modifying treatments, there has been a significant improvement in survival. This is most likely a result of better management of specific organ disease, such as renal crisis and pulmonary hypertension. One survey found that for clients with dcSSc, 5-year survival increased from 69% between 1990 and 1993 to 84% during 2000–2003.[253] (See Chapter 10 for discussion of this condition.)

Tuberculosis

Tuberculosis (TB) is an acute or chronic infection caused by *Mycobacterium tuberculosis*, an acid-fast staining bacillus. Although the primary infection site is the lung, mycobacteria commonly exist in other parts of the body; this is referred to as *extrapulmonary TB*. Extrapulmonary TB is often present without symptomatic lung disease or abnormalities on chest radiographs. The extrapulmonary sites may include the renal system, skeletal system (osteomyelitis; vertebral TB is known as *Pott disease*), GI tract, meninges (tuberculous meningitis), and genitals. Extrapulmonary TB occurs with increased frequency in people with HIV infection. New assays are available to aid in diagnosing extrapulmonary TB[204] (see Chapter 15 for more on pulmonary TB; see Chapter 25 for more on tuberculous spondylitis [Pott disease]).

Sarcoidosis

Sarcoidosis is a multisystem disorder characterized by the formation of noncaseating granulomas, defined as a core of monocyte-derived epithelioid cells and multinucleated giant cells interspersed with or surrounded by lymphocytes. These granulomas may develop in any organ but often are noted in multiple organs at once, including the lungs (90% of clients with sarcoidosis will have lung involvement), heart, lymph nodes, liver, bones, or eyes (see Box 15-10) and may be accompanied by skin lesions (see Fig. 15-21).

Presenting symptoms of sarcoidosis can often be confused with other inflammatory or infectious processes which form granulomas, making the diagnosis difficult and unsure.[25,345] In the United States, sarcoidosis occurs predominantly among blacks (3 times higher than whites) and affects women more often than men.[382]

There is significant morbidity and mortality associated with this multisystem disease. Treatment is focused on cutaneous disease or symptomatic systemic disease, as the disease process is not completely understood.[25] Most deaths are related to disease involvement of the heart or lung (see Chapter 15 for a complete discussion of this condition).

Sepsis

Overview

Sepsis is a systemic syndrome that affects all ages, is found in communities, hospitals, and extended-care facilities, and involves all medical specialties. It encompasses a range of signs and symptoms from the mild to the severe. International conferences have been held to better define sepsis and risk factors. The 2001 International Sepsis Definitions Conference formulated definitions that would be helpful for both researchers and clinicians.[206] *Sepsis* is defined as involving both the invasion of microorganisms and the response of the host resulting in hyperinflammation and tissue injury. Unlike sepsis, *bacteremia* is defined only as the presence of bacteria in the blood.

Other terminology has been developed to further describe the continuum of sepsis and characterize the severity. For example, *systemic inflammatory response syndrome* (SIRS) is a generalized hyperinflammatory response to various insults (trauma, burns, infection, etc.). There are four clinical signs that define SIRS: (1) temperature greater than 38°C (100.4°F) or less than 36°C (96.8°F), (2) heart rate greater than 90 beats/min, (3) respiratory rate greater than 20 breaths/min, (4) white blood cell count greater than 12,000 or less than 4000. Sepsis can be further defined as SIRS (2 criteria) because of infection. *Severe sepsis* is sepsis with tissue hypoperfusion and organ dysfunction,[326] whereas septic shock is severe sepsis accompanied by hypotension that is resistant to aggressive and adequate volume resuscitation. Severe sepsis may result in multiple organ dysfunction syndrome (MODS; see next section), which carries a high mortality.

Incidence and Risk Factors

Sepsis is relatively common with more than 700,000 cases of severe sepsis reported in 2007. The estimated annual mortality is 30–50/100,000 people,[100] making sepsis one of the top 10 causes of death. Severe sepsis is also more common in the elderly,[218] who account for the majority of sepsis cases. Another risk factor, other than age, includes the presence of comorbidities such as COPD, CHF, diabetes mellitus, and cancer.[75,217] Not all people with sepsis have bacteremia but certain conditions that are associated with bacteria can lead to sepsis and include total parenteral nutrition, liver dysfunction, and an indwelling catheter.[24]

In the elderly, the respiratory and genitourinary tracts are the source of sepsis in more than 65% of cases, whereas younger people develop infections from GI and skin, bone, and soft-tissue sources. African American men may also have a greater risk for sepsis compared to white men,[217] possibly from a lack of presepsis care of underlying conditions.[99] The elderly also have a higher incidence of resistant organisms, often as a result of recent hospitalization, recent antibiotic use, and indwelling urinary catheters.[301] Gram-negative organisms are more likely to be responsible for sepsis in the elderly compared to younger clients, principally because of the increase in the involvement of the urinary tract (urosepsis). For people who develop bacteremia with sepsis, the most common organism seen in the elderly (community-acquired) is *Escherichia coli*, whereas *Staphylococcus aureus* is more common in the young adult population.[94] There also has been an increase in fungi as a source for sepsis, observed most often in persons who are immunocompromised, have recently undergone surgery or been hospitalized, or received antibiotics or parenteral nutrition.[153,331,366]

Pathogenesis

Infectious organisms are composed of foreign molecules termed *pathogen-associated molecular patterns*, which are recognized by the immune system as foreign, triggering both immunologic and inflammatory pathways. *Damage-associated molecular patterns* are the noninfectious molecules that are released after cellular injury of the host (i.e., trauma) and can also induce the immune response. Pathogen-associated molecular patterns are recognized by proteins called *pattern-recognition proteins* that can be found in cell membranes (transmembrane) or cytosol, or can be secreted.

Once pattern-recognition proteins are activated, various pathways are triggered leading to the release of interleukins and tumor-necrosis factor. Some bacteria produce toxins, or exotoxins, which act as "superantigens" by interacting with T cells in a way that activates a much higher percentage of T cells than other toxins. This results in the release of multiple cytokines and tumor-necrosis factor, the primary mediators of inflammation. Fungi, viruses, and parasites also activate pattern-recognition proteins, but the process isn't as well characterized as it is for bacteria.

Primary mediators then induce the release of secondary mediators that amplify the inflammation process. Endothelial cells become damaged from the presence of leukocyte adhesion molecules on the surface that recruit neutrophils and other immune cells to the site of the infection.[61] This further drives the inflammatory response. The coagulation system is also altered with an increase in proinflammatory and procoagulant tissue factors and an inhibition of natural anticoagulants, such as protein C. Low levels of activated protein C, are thought to contribute to thrombosis and severe sepsis.[28] The complement pathway is also stimulated and induces macrophages to produce proinflammatory mediators.

Normally the immune response is balanced and remains in the area of the infection. However, under certain conditions, the inflammatory response becomes systemic, known as SIRS, where the response is uncontrolled, unregulated, and self-sustaining. Alterations in multiple systems lead to sepsis, including changes in cellular metabolism, oxygen utilization, apoptosis, coagulation, and inflammatory and immune pathways (see Chapter 6).

Clinical Manifestations

Signs and symptoms related to sepsis frequently depend upon the location of the infection, which are seen in conjunction with the generalized signs associated with SIRS (fever, tachycardia, and tachypnea). If the infection begins in the lungs, shortness of breath, productive cough, and chest pain accompanied with an elevated white blood count, hypoxia, and low oxygen saturations may be present. A GI infection may exhibit nausea/vomiting, diarrhea, ileus and/or abdominal pain. Other enzymes could also be elevated including liver enzymes (shock liver).

Severe sepsis is often signaled by markers for tissue injury and hypoperfusion such as an elevated serum lactate level or blood pH that demonstrates acidosis, increased BUN/creatinine, and decreased urine output. In addition to an elevated white blood cell count, septic shock may reveal a prolonged bleeding time, prothrombin time (PT), or partial thromboplastin time, and elevated D-dimer levels. Mental status may be altered, particularly in the elderly. Cultures should be obtained from blood, urine, lung, or other possible source of infection (i.e., skin abscess).

MEDICAL MANAGEMENT

DIAGNOSIS, TREATMENT, AND PROGNOSIS. Mild cases of sepsis can often be managed outside the ICU and are treated with fluids, supplemental oxygen, and antibiotics according to the source of infection. Severe sepsis requires emergent recognition and treatment. Central IV access should be obtained followed by aggressive fluid resuscitation with crystalloid. A central venous catheter can aid in providing adequate resuscitation. Vasopressors may be required if hypotension persists despite adequate fluid.

People with severe sepsis often require intubation as a result of generalized vascular permeability and pulmonary edema. Broad-spectrum antibiotics are given until cultures are available. Questions still persist as to treatment of elevated glucose levels. In studies related to clients who have undergone heart surgery, there is an improved outcome when a low-dose insulin infusion is used to keep glucose levels less than 150. Current studies have not supported using low-dose infusion insulin to keep glucose levels less than 150[118,383] in critically ill clients with severe sepsis.

Prognosis depends upon age, underlying conditions, presence of immunocompromise, delay in diagnosis, and the type of organism responsible for the infection. Overall mortality rate is around 40% but may be as low as 5% for healthy persons or 80% for people with significant health problems.[150]

The Medically Complex Patient: Critical Illness

Lara A. Firrone, PT, NCS

> **Note to Reader:** The December 2012 issue of the *Journal of the American Physical Therapy Association* (Vol. 92, No. 12) features a special series on rehabilitation for people with critical illness. The publication is an excellent compilation of information about this condition for the physical therapist.

Overview

To a certain extent people admitted to the hospital are there because they are sick and it is assumed that those in the ICU must be the sickest. One factor to consider is that the ICU contributes to that sickness. Some patients in the ICU can develop severe ICU-related complications.[398] It seems to be more so with those who have required prolonged mechanical ventilation (depending on the setting that could be as few as 3 days or many more).[36,199,404] It can also be those who develop sepsis or multiple system organ dysfunction. There is a debate about individuals who have been on high doses of corticosteroids and neuromuscular blocking agents and their frequency of developing lasting complications.[84,275] The short-term issues range from difficulty or failure to wean from the ventilator to severe muscle weakness and loss of muscle function; many face chronic disability.

Of the individuals in the ICU who require advanced life support, there are those who handle it well; 75% are weaned from the ventilator on the first try. Once off ventilation, that patient can make a recovery that leads to discharge from the hospital. Unfortunately, others struggle and develop complications when they fail to wean, which can impact all systems in the body, from cardiovascular and respiratory to neuromuscular, as well the more difficult to identify (e.g., psychologic and social).[163,256]

As the medically complex patient who has been sedated becomes more stable, the medical staff (e.g., physicians, nurses, and occasionally the respiratory therapists) may begin to realize that the patient is functionally impaired or that the medical issues present on admission are much worse now. This group of symptoms or conditions can go by many names. Terms like ICU-acquired weakness (ICU-AW), critical illness polyneuropathy (CIP or CIPN), critical illness myopathy or neuromyopathy (CIM), ICU-acquired paresis, and others are used interchangeably.

These are all ways of saying that there has been an impact on nerves and/or muscles to the point that movement and function reach critical levels of impairment. In other words, the impact reaches a level that becomes clinically demonstrable and lasting and is out of proportion to the patient's pre-admission baseline considering the primary medical problem. There is also being added into this mix the use of "postintensive care syndrome" to cover those patients who leave the ICU and hospital with lasting deficits.[111]

Incidence

Incidence of critical illness is compounded by how the disorder is defined, what diagnostic tools and tests are used, and when those diagnostic measures are initiated and repeated. Studies report incidence in a range from 25% to 58%.[85,246,334] Some studies that had more restricted criteria for their cohorts and the reported incidence rate for neurologic and muscular deficits rise even higher, from 50% up to 100%.[255,319]

Etiology and Risk Factors

The cause or etiology of these deficits in strength and sensation is still under debate and research. Part of the problem is related to the fact that there may be more than one type of illness being grouped together. For example, in one study patients were excluded if they were older than 75 years or younger than 18 years, if they had diabetes or renal problems, a stroke or spinal cord injury or prior neuropathy, cancer, or certain infections. This same study started with 490 survivors of the ICU and 102 were excluded because of the criteria described. So essentially, 20% had some kind of weakness, but they were not going to call it ICU-AW because it may have had another cause. Other studies have tried to link the weakness to the use of certain drugs (e.g., corticosteroids, insulin)[85,161,174,241,334] or the diagnosis of sepsis or hyperglycemia,[162,334] the use of sedative or paralytics, and orders for strict bedrest, but nothing conclusive has been shown.[27,70,95,126]

With the debate about the cause, there is also some question as to risk factors. From a practical standpoint, the more systems involved and the more medical support the person needs (especially if it is invasive, like intubation or dialysis) the greater the risk that the patient will develop measurable weakness with a drop in functional performance compared to the prehospitalization baseline. Sepsis, SIRS, and multiorgan failure are risk factors for CIP and CIM.[199]

As noted above, the more problems the individual develops, the less likely a formal diagnosis of ICU-AW (or CIP, or CIM, etc.) will be made. If the individual happened to have had a stroke in the past then some might call it a decompensation due to the stress of the current illness. Or perhaps there was a previous history of polio so the diagnosis becomes postpolio; for multiple sclerosis it might be presumed to be an exacerbation.

Pathogenesis

CIP and CIM are not isolated events; they are an integral part of the process leading to multiorgan dysfunction and failure. Peripheral nerves and muscle (excitable tissues) are key targets, and are probably damaged by a combination of ischemic and toxic means.[120,325] Therefore, shared microcirculatory, cellular, and metabolic pathophysiologic mechanisms are likely.

When considering a body that is affected by illness like multiple organ involvement and sepsis, there should be an awareness of the changes the body undergoes on the physical and chemical level and the system level (see further discussion in Chapter 5). The nerves can be damaged by the impaired delivery of oxygen and nutrition on a cellular level. But this alteration is also directly linked to the person's whole-body medical status. Impaired glucose metabolism (hyperglycemia) can affect microcirculation to peripheral nerves and cytokines can be toxic to the tissues. Prolonged disuse of muscle with muscle wasting (prominent features of sepsis) can be linked to increased muscle protein breakdown that may contribute to the myopathic symptoms seen in these individuals.[49]

During critical illness, microcirculation is impaired throughout the body (ischemic hypoxia). Mitochondrial function is impaired with reduced adenosine triphosphate biosynthesis, energy generation, and use (cytopathic hypoxia), which is thought to be a cause of cellular and organ dysfunction in critical illness. For more details of the proposed pathophysiologic mechanisms, as well as electrophysiologic and histologic features of CIP and CIM, the reader is referred to any of the recent studies referenced in this section, especially Latronico and Bolton[199] and Nordon-Craft et al.[255]

Diaphragmatic weakness, injury, and atrophy develop rapidly during mechanical ventilation (especially when combined with sedation),[260] and the scale of damage is significantly correlated with the duration of this medical treatment.[181] Subsequent weakness of the diaphragm makes breathing harder thus contributing even more to the affected individual's immobility.

The therapist must always keep in mind that skeletal muscle immobility can contribute substantially to muscle wasting even in the absence of systemic inflammatory changes.[260] Muscle atrophy begins within hours of bed rest or deep sedation, and even healthy people can have large loss of muscle mass and strength within 10 days of bed rest, particularly from the lower limbs.[196] Bower[39] does an excellent job detailing how the body declines and changes as a result of extended inactivity.

Clinical Manifestations

Muscle weakness is the hallmark finding of this condition; onset of clinical signs can be rapid. This is first generally observed when the individual fails to wean from the ventilator. Then when the sedation is lifted other areas of motor weakness become apparent; sensation can also be impaired. Although a patient may demonstrate elements of delirium or impaired consciousness, these are usually related to effects of medication or coma or a separate pathology (e.g., stroke, septic encephalopathy).

Most affected individuals will demonstrate both sensory and motor impairments. Weakness and sensory loss is symmetric, somewhat more distal than proximal for CIP affecting limb and respiratory muscles. Facial muscles are not usually affected.[199]

For primary myopathy associated with CIM, muscle weakness and atrophy are usually symmetric and more proximal, but without sensory impairments. There can be flaccid limbs and deep tendon reflexes may be reduced. Some individuals have difficulty coughing and clearing and may speak in a hoarse voice.[67,199]

Differentiating CIP from CIM can be difficult in the ICU setting; if the individual makes a favorable recovery it is likely because that individual had CIM alone versus CIP alone.[319] Practically speaking, the average therapist is going to see patients with combined damage.

MEDICAL MANAGEMENT

DIAGNOSIS. Difficulty weaning an individual who has been critically ill from mechanical ventilation and that is unexplained by increased respiratory or cardiac load, metabolic disturbances, nutritional deficiencies, delirium, or other medical condition points to the possible diagnosis of CIM and/or CIP.[35] CIP/CIM is suspected when there is weakness and/or flaccid limbs or what little limb movement the patient initially shows does not improve over time. Diagnosis relies on clinical presentation and physical examination findings, testing that can include radiologic, electrophysiologic, or laboratory services, and potentially tissue studies.[67]

Muscle strength can be tested using the Medical Research Council (MRC) scale. The MRC can be found at www.medicalcriteria.com as well as on the official MRC website (www.mrc.ac.uk). Instructions as well as reliability and validity information are provided. For an excellent summary of the MRC, see Confer et al.[67] The MRC composite score examines the results from three muscle groups from each limb.

Nerve function can also be examined, but the type of testing depends on the resources available. Some patients in some facilities may be tested with monofilaments or the more complete nerve conduction and electromyography tests. Simple light touch may be all that is done because of concerns for infection and overall infection control issues. Swelling and skin integrity issues may limit the validity of any of the tests used. Noninvasive testing of reflexes like deep tendon reflexes may be performed.

Respiratory muscle strength can be tested by measurement of the maximal inspiratory and expiratory pressures and vital capacity. Low scores on these measures are correlated with limb muscle weakness[199,200] associated with delayed extubation, prolonged ventilation, and unplanned readmission to the ICU.

Imaging studies may include a CT or MRI of the head and spine to rule out other conditions. The same guidelines are used when determining the need for a lumbar puncture. Unfortunately there is no simple blood test that is definitive for this condition. The medical differential diagnosis is more a process of elimination and a bit of presuming it is present with treatment accordingly.

Prevention. Ideally the health care team works to prevent this condition from developing in the first place. The medical team can adjust some of the drugs on board and can attempt strict control of the blood glucose to reduce the hyperglycemic effects, as well as stabilizing the individual's electrolytes and ensuring there is adequate nutrition provided. The attempt should be made to wean the patient from the use of ventilator support as quickly as possible. The primary cause or initial presenting diagnosis should be addressed as quickly as possible; however, as previously noted, the various types of critical illness weakness can be difficult to diagnose and differentiate from other diseases. Thus a person with multiorgan failure may have so many issues that weakness is the least of the team's concerns as they work to keep the individual alive. There may come a time when everyone gets the preventative care regardless.

Treatment. Medical treatment is very limited and more of a management approach than a medical cure. There is no one drug or combination of drugs that will reverse the weakness and/or sensation losses. Once the condition is recognized, the health care team continues to provide the same care used for prevention. Gaining adequate glycemic control, getting the patient off the ventilator as quickly as possible, and reducing the use of medications that may be toxic are the best ways to prevent this condition from progressing.

Prognosis. When looking at survival with CIM, CIP, and ICU-AW, the more severe the case, the more it can be anticipated that there will be a poor prognosis for full recovery; muscle weakness has been linked with increased mortality.[6]

Studies show that up to two-thirds of the people in the ICU will develop one of the disorders, and of those, 23% die in the hospital and another 33% die within 6 months after hospital discharge.[322] Many who have this disorder do not make it home. If discharged from the hospital with an opportunity to stay at home, they can exceed the care the family can provide and end up in community placement, either skilled or intermediate. Unfortunately, many families may see this occur in a relatively short period of time.

Investigations show there is a favorable chance for a return to functional independence in the long term, but only in those affected individuals who are young (the average reported age was 56 years) and for those who have no concomitant diseases.[260,319] Survivors of critical illness conditions may demonstrate significant residual disability.[180] Muscle weakness can persist months and even years with serious exercise limitations.[163]

There is growing evidence of additional changes in the quality of life for a survivor. Cognitive impairments, delirium, and inability to return to work or be active at a community level have been observed and reported.[170] According to Nordon-Craft et al,[255] these physical and psychologic and social limitations are now being quantified by tools like the 6-Minute Walk Test, 36-Item Short Form Health Survey, and RAND 36-Item Health Survey.

Cox et al[70] reported at 1 year posthospitalization that only 9% of the patients were alive and functionally independent (out of the 56% that survived the hospitalization), whereas 61% of the survivors needed daily assistance. The societal impact was significant with 84% of caregivers having to alter or quit their job to accommodate the care the affected family member needed. There was also a very poor prognosis for emotional recovery for the person who survived as well as for the caregivers regardless of the patient's survival.

SPECIAL IMPLICATIONS FOR THE THERAPIST   5-8

The Medically Complex Patient: Critical Illness

The role of the therapist is both in prevention and treatment of the deconditioning and respiratory conditions that can occur in critically ill individuals. Reductions in functional performance, exercise or respiratory capacity, and quality of life are indicators that rehabilitation following a stay in the ICU should be recommended.[164]

Recent evidence suggests that early rehabilitation can be safely and effectively implemented in the ICU to maintain patients' physical function, provided that patients are given an appropriate amount of sedation.[199] The therapist's focus is most often directed toward the functional limitations, reduced respiratory capacity, decreased cardiac reserve, and other limitations imposed by the physiologic deficiencies. The therapist also has an important role in providing emotional support and facilitating communication with patient, family, and staff.

More information and details of treatment protocols specific to the physical therapist are being investigated and researched and will be available in the literature at the time of this publication.[263] This adds to the studies that are already published including targeted activity and exercise with the appropriate mode and at the recommended intensity.[111,148,273,309] Considerations for when to move a critically ill individual versus the risk of immobility, safety concerns, and approaches to acutely ill, cooperative but also sometimes uncooperative patients are discussed.[148] Some protocols might be difficult to reproduce depending on constraints based on a particular facility's staffing, funding, and philosophy.

Review of Systems

The principal of "Keep It Simple" seems impossible when there are so many factors to consider. However, approaching any patient requires that the therapist look at all the systems, make appropriate assessments, and devise a plan of care that addresses those deficits. There are always more factors to consider when working with patients in a critical care unit.

The therapist must step back and look at the big picture: Is there just a single organ involvement or multiple organ systems impaired? For example, did the patient have a car accident with some broken limbs or did he or she have a heart attack and were otherwise healthy prior to admission? Or, as the case seems to be more and more, were there multiple comorbidities and then an acute event that sent them over the edge? For instance, there may be the patient with diabetes who came in for an amputation, got into some kidney trouble, ending up on dialysis, and then had a stroke and respiratory failure that required mechanical ventilation.

Once the number of systems or organs that are involved are known, then the therapist can start looking at the clinical manifestations and see if any signs and symptoms present are related to the known issues or if there might be another medical condition playing a part. Sometimes a therapist can identify an underlying or new problem and alert the team and participate in active management before permanent issues arise.

The Role of Early Mobilization

The benefit of early mobilization has been well-documented.[19,39,70,234,235,247,273,285,309,316,322] More and more studies are being done that support getting the patient up and moving as quickly as possible. Early mobilization can decrease the length of stay in an ICU as well as aid the person who is difficult to wean. PTs have an active role in the initiation of an early mobilization program. Starting strengthening and mobilization as early as clinically indicated and feasible may be the most valuable thing for anyone at risk for these disorders. There is a flip side to this as noted by Berney and Haines,[29] regarding the benefit from continuing the care started in the ICU to the outpatient setting, but they also note that maintaining compliance over the long term can be difficult.

A THERAPIST'S THOUGHTS*
Early Mobilization

Physical therapists may not know that they have had experience with this condition. Some medical records do not include it in the problem (diagnosis) list, despite the fact that they might have 20 or more diseases and as many medications. It might be that a therapist treated patients when on a rotation in the ICU of an acute care setting. However, as the studies showed, there are survivors of the various ICU-related disorders, and they frequently do not go home but end up in inpatient rehab, extended acute care, or long-term care facilities.

When seen in the ICU, the environment can be challenging, especially as these individuals tend to be more complex and more fragile. The patient's diagnosis or multiple diseases the patient is facing can be strongly impacted by the environment, the critical care that the patient requires, and by real-world problems like staffing and equipment. Clinical manifestations of ICU-AW will necessitate longer term physical therapy intervention; this can be very challenging when in alternative care settings (i.e., outside the ICU).

And as the saying goes "the times, they are 'a changing'"—in health care that seems particularly true. Clinicians are seeing overall larger, more obese, and sicker patients than ever before. When I started work as a therapist almost 20 years ago, a 300-pound patient was considered large. Today, individuals this size are more the average; I regularly see people in the very severely obese category (Obese Class 3 body mass index: over 40; largest man I ever walked was more than 800 lb and the largest patient I ever treated approached 1200 lb).

Diseases once thought to be the hallmark of old age are striking much younger people. Patients with stroke are now regularly in their 20s and 30s and the patients who are older than 70 years are seeing more devastating effects. Staff on the various medical and rehab teams are also seeing newer complications that their predecessors never had to deal with such as superbug infections, multiple organ failure, and newer disorders that are just now being recognized. It is also the case for comorbidities, that is, patient diagnoses now routinely include 20 to 30 medical diagnoses instead of the 2 to 5 when I started. Coronary artery disease CHF, diabetes mellitus, hypertension, hypercholesterolemia, peripheral vascular disease, gastroesophageal reflux disease, cardiovascular accident, and

COPD are almost standard in my ICU patients, except the occasional frank trauma who was otherwise fit. This doesn't even include their past and current list of surgical and invasive procedures, which can number in the dozens (or more).

Some facilities are not staffed to permit the type of evidence-based best care described in the literature. A hospital may not be able to have a therapist be in the ICU throughout the day. Having adequate staffing allows the timing of interventions for the most opportune moment. Knowing when a patient is going to get a "sedation vacation" allows the therapist to see the patient in a more active state and better assess their actual deficits. It would also allow active movement, which is key to regaining muscular function. Another consideration might be seen as the opposite line of thought by having the therapist provide range of motion and stretching at a time when the patient is sedated; this schedule permits the sedation vacation to be used for active weaning from the ventilator. The question becomes how to most effectively use the patient's available energy, apply it first to strengthen the limbs or to the lungs?

Other barriers to consider when mobilizing patients include the actual equipment and hospital policy. Some facilities do not permit mobilizing with an endotracheal tube in place or only if certain staff members are present (e.g., a respiratory therapist must be present in the event of accidental extubation). Practical matters can be additional speed bumps, like the fact that the patient is being taken to tests or having bedside procedures. This may mean that having daily and lengthy physical therapy sessions is more difficult to reproduce consistently. But that does not necessarily mean it should not be tried.

In an ideal world, ICUs would be staffed with a therapist similarly to the way nursing is staffed, with one therapist covering a small number of patients. The rehab staff would have access to appropriate and necessary equipment. For example, the availability of tilt tables with a sliding mechanism that permits gradual body weight tasks such as a modified squat at a 45-degree angle would be very helpful. As the patient improves, the angle can be increased to increase the patient's work load until the point that they are ready to step off the end. Some ICUs have a modified walker with the ability to support the patient and a portable vent along with all the IV pumps and

Continued

equipment that attached to the patient. This set up would leave the therapist's hands free to assist the patient. Other useful tools include weights and resistance bands that meet infection control policies and interactive games like the Wii for individuals who are restricted to the bed for other reasons.

For those who are in less-well-funded facilities, it means being more creative. If the tilt table is too big to put next to the patient's bed to permit transfers and there are no power outlets that can power it in the hall where there might be more space, then the therapist can direct intervention toward gradually increasing the head of the bed. This approach will improve patient tolerance to a more upright position. Pulmonary hygiene will be part of the plan-of-care until the patient can tolerate a functional supine-to-sit transition on the side of the bed. Marching in place at the side of the bed is suggested when there are not additional staff members to permit walking in the hallway, for instance when nursing and respiratory staff are on transport with another patient. Manual resistance can replace bands and weights when the patient is in isolation.

An area that rehab staff can also impact with very little cost but show a big payoff is in communicating with the patient and the family. Therapists are at the bedside longer than most of the other professionals. RNs come to give a med and then leave. RT might apply a treatment to the vent and the return to draw an arterial blood gas. These take a few minutes. Doing exercises and giving appropriate

rest breaks and mobilizing out-of-bed takes time. The return on that time can be increased considerably by using those extra minutes to answer questions and give additional information and later alert staff to any deficits that other team members may need to address.

Rehab staff can provide honest assessments of functional tasks that a patient and family member can relate to more than numbers from lab values. When a patient becomes visibly fatigued with 5 minutes of static sitting, the physical therapist can point out that it might take 10 minutes to eat a small meal, which is a vital dynamic task. In this way, the therapist can demonstrate more clearly how far the patient has to improve to accomplish this basic task. Or when the family says the patient must be able to be left alone for 4 hours while a caregiver works a part-time job, the therapist can use this guideline to create appropriate goals and outcome measures.

In conclusion, patients can be very sick; some are more complicated than others. Sometimes the therapy staff is working with a known diagnosis and other times we are dealing with the unknown. As long as the therapist looks at the whole patient and an attempt is made to address all of that patient's needs, then an appropriate plan of care can be developed. The focus is on returning the individual to his or her highest level of function and, hopefully, preparing the individual for the day when discharge from the ICU is possible (and eventually return to home or transition to another facility from the hospital).

*Lara A Firrone, PT, NCS

Multiple Organ Dysfunction Syndrome

Overview

Care of critically ill people has progressed significantly during the last 50 years. Substantial advances have been made in the care of shock, acute renal failure, acute brain injury, and acute respiratory failure, with more people surviving these conditions.

However, despite these advances, progressive deterioration of organ function may occur in people who are critically ill or injured. People often die of complications of disease, rather than from the disease itself. MODS is often the final complication of a critical illness; it is one of the most common causes of death in the ICU.[119]

Definition and Etiologic and Risk Factors

MODS, also called *multiple organ failure syndrome*, is the progressive failure (over more than 24 hours) of two or more organ systems after a severe illness or injury. Although sepsis and septic shock from infection are the most common causes,[401] infection is not required for its development. MODS also can be triggered by acute respiratory distress syndrome, severe inflammatory processes (e.g., pancreatitis), other types of shock, and traumatic injury (e.g., burns or surgery). MODS carries a high mortality rate that increases with each organ that fails.

Several scoring systems have been developed, such as the Sequential Organ Failure Assessment or the Multiorgan Dysfunction Score, which correlate with mortality.[226] MODS may result in persons who develop SIRS that progresses to septic shock. Systemic inflammatory response,

sepsis, septic shock, and MODS are a result of excessive activation of inflammatory pathways.

After an initial insult or injury, other factors can increase the risk of developing MODS/SIRS, including inadequate or delayed resuscitation, age older than 65 years, alcoholism, diabetes, surgical complications (e.g., infection, hematoma formation), bowel infarction, or the previous existence of organ dysfunction (e.g., renal insufficiency).

Pathogenesis

Although MODS may be a final common pathway in critical illnesses, actual causes and cellular changes leading to MODS are not completely understood. Most likely multiple mechanisms and factors are responsible or contribute to the development of MODS. In response to illness or traumatic injury, the neuroendocrine system activates stress hormones (e.g., cortisol, epinephrine, norepinephrine, or endorphins) to be released into the circulation, whereas the sympathetic nervous system is stimulated to compensate for complications such as fluid loss and hypotension.

Because of the initial insult, proinflammatory cytokines (e.g., interferons and tumor necrosis factor) and enzymes are released with the overall effect of massive uncontrolled systemic immune and inflammatory responses. Coagulation factors, such as protein C and antithrombin III, are phagocytized (consumed), resulting in systemic hypercoagulation and later bleeding. This uncontrolled hyperinflammation and hypercoagulation leads to the development of edema, cardiovascular instability, endothelial damage, and clotting abnormalities.

Dysregulated cytokine-induced apoptosis and immune system paralysis are also evident.[173]

At the same time, initial oxygen consumption demand increases because the oxygen requirements at the cellular level increase. Blood flow and oxygen consumption are mismatched because of a decrease in oxygen delivery to the cells caused by maldistribution of blood flow, myocardial depression, and a hypermetabolic state. The end result is abnormal cellular respiration and function (tissue hypoxia with cellular acidosis and death), resulting in the multiple organ dysfunction characteristic of MODS.[274]

CLINICAL MANIFESTATIONS

A clinical pattern in the development of MODS has been well established. After the precipitating event, low-grade fever, tachycardia, dyspnea, SIRS, and altered mental status develop. The lung is the first organ to fail, resulting in acute respiratory distress syndrome (see Chapter 15).

Between 7 and 10 days, the hypermetabolic state intensifies, GI bacteremia is common, and signs of liver and kidney failure develop. During days 14–21, renal and liver failures progress to a severe status and the GI and immune systems fail, with eventual cardiovascular collapse. Ischemia and inflammation are responsible for the CNS manifestations. Protein metabolism is also affected, and amino acids derived from skeletal muscle, connective tissue, and intestinal viscera become an important energy source. The result is a significant loss of lean body mass.

MEDICAL MANAGEMENT

Prevention and early detection and supportive therapy are essential for MODS, as no specific medical treatment exists for this condition. A way to halt the process, once it has begun, has not yet been discovered. Pharmacologic treatment may include antibiotics to treat infection, inotropic agents (e.g., dopamine or dobutamine) to counteract myocardial depression, and supplemental oxygen and ventilation to keep oxygen saturation levels at or above 90%. Fluid replacement and nutritional support are also provided.

Attempts to develop inflammatory modulators have yet to prove helpful. Current investigations are centered on balancing proinflammatory and counterinflammatory mechanisms.[130] Research into biomarkers that could identify people at risk for MODS is also in development.[362]

MODS is the major cause of death (usually occurring between days 21 and 28) after septic, traumatic, and burn injuries. If the affected individual's condition has not improved by the end of the third week, survival is unlikely. The mortality rate of MODS is 60% to 90% and approaches 100% if three or more organs are involved, sepsis is present, and the individual is older than 65 years.

SPECIAL IMPLICATIONS FOR THE THERAPIST 5-9

Multiple Organ Dysfunction Syndrome
Only the critical care or burn unit therapist will encounter the client with MODS/SIRS. The hypermetabolism associated with this condition is accompanied by protein catabolism, primarily of skeletal muscle and

---

visceral organs. Lean body mass can be significantly depleted in 7 to 10 days, necessitating skin precautions and skin care.

FLUID AND ELECTROLYTE IMBALANCES

Observing clinical manifestations of fluid or electrolyte imbalances may be an important aspect of client care, especially in the acute care and home health care settings. Identifying clients at risk for such imbalances is the first step toward early detection.

The causes of fluid and electrolyte imbalance are many and varied and include disease processes, injury, medications, medical treatment, dietary restrictions, and imbalance of fluid intake with fluid output.[350] The most common causes of fluid and electrolyte imbalances in a therapy practice include burns, surgery, diabetes mellitus, malignancy, alcoholism, and the various factors affecting the aging adult population (Box 5-7).

This is a brief presentation of the normal homeostatic processes of fluid and electrolyte balance. The interactions of these systems and how they maintain fluid and electrolyte balance and acid–base regulation are beyond the scope of this text. For a more in-depth study of these concepts, the reader is referred to the latest edition of Guyton AC, Hall JE: *Textbook of medical physiology*, ed 12, Philadelphia, 2011, WB Saunders.

Aging and Fluid and Electrolyte Balance

The volume and distribution of body fluids composed of water, electrolytes, and nonelectrolytes vary with age,

---

Box 5-7

FACTORS AFFECTING FLUID AND ELECTROLYTE BALANCE IN THE AGING

- Acute illness (fever, diarrhea, vomiting)
- Bowel cleansing for GI diagnostic testing
- Change in mental status
- Constipation
- Decreased thirst mechanism
- Difficulty swallowing
- Excessive sodium intake:
  - Diet
  - Sodium bicarbonate antacids (e.g., Alka-Seltzer)
  - Water supply or water softener
  - Decreased taste sensation (increased salt intake)
- Excessive calcium intake:
  - Alkaline antacids
- Immobility
- Laxatives (habitual use for constipation)
- Medications:
  - Antiparkinsonian drugs
  - Diuretics
  - Propranolol
  - Tamoxifen (breast cancer therapy)
- Sodium-restricted diet
- Urinary incontinence (voluntary fluid restriction)

gender, body weight, and amount of adipose tissue. Throughout life, a slow decline occurs in lean body or fat-free mass with a corresponding decline in the volume of body fluids. Only 45% to 50% of the body weight of aging adults is water compared with 55% to 60% in younger adults. This decrease represents a net loss of muscle mass and a reduced ratio of lean body weight to total body weight and places older people at greater risk for water-deficit states.

There are also changes in the kidney that further potentiate the risk for fluid and electrolyte disturbances. With increasing age, there is a decrease in renal mass and GFR. This, in turn, may lead to the inability of the aging kidney to excrete free water in the face of fluid excess, causing hyponatremia.

Yet hypernatremia can also be problematic in the aging adult secondary to a defect in the ability of the kidney to concentrate urine combined with a decreased thirst despite dehydration, often seen with age. Although these changes are seen in normal aging, factors that depress the sensorium in the frail and sick elderly (stroke and medications) further complicate hypernatremia by suppressing the natural compensatory mechanism for fluid intake.

Infection, dementia, neurologic disorders, and other systemic illnesses can decrease the release of arginine vasopressin, further placing older adults at high risk for dehydration.[56] Renin and aldosterone decrease with age, accompanied by a blunted response to aldosterone. These changes can lead to hyperkalemia, particularly if other factors are present, such as the use of potassium-sparing diuretics.

Fluid Imbalances

Overview

Approximately 45% to 60% of the adult human body is composed of water, which contains the electrolytes that are essential to human life (see "Electrolyte Imbalances" below). This life-sustaining fluid is found within various body compartments, including the intracellular (within cells), interstitial (space between cells), intravascular (within blood vessels), and transcellular compartments.

Fluid in the transcellular compartment is present in the body but is separated from body tissues by a layer of epithelial cells. This fluid includes digestive fluids, water, and solutes in the renal tubules and bladder, intraocular fluid, joint-space fluid, and cerebrospinal fluid. The fluid in the interstitial and intravascular compartments comprises approximately one-third the total body fluid, called the *extracellular fluid* (ECF). Fluid found inside the cells, called the *intracellular fluid* (ICF), accounts for the remaining two-thirds of total body fluid.

The cell membrane is water permeable with equal concentrations of dissolved particles on each side of the membrane maintaining equal volumes of ECF and ICF and preventing passive shifts of water. Passive shifts occur only if an inequality occurs on either side of the membrane in the concentration of solutes that cannot permeate the membrane. For example, water will move from one compartment to another if there is a change in sodium ion concentration.

The following five types of fluid imbalances may occur:
1. ECF volume deficit
2. ECF volume excess
3. ECF volume shift
4. ICF volume excess
5. ICF volume deficit

A simpler approach to this subject is to view fluid shifts in terms of intravascular or extravascular movement. Movement from the vascular space to the extravascular areas and vice versa takes place easily and is the first mechanism of extracellular movement.

The material in this section is presented on the bases of three broad categories: fluid deficit, fluid excess, and fluid shift (see Chapter 13).

Etiologic Factors and Pathogenesis

Maintaining constant internal conditions (homeostasis) requires the proper balance between the volume and distribution of ECF and ICF to provide nutrition to the cells, allow excretion of waste products, and promote production of energy and other cell functions. Maintenance of this balance depends on the differences in the concentrations of ICF and ECF fluids, the permeability of the membranes, and the effect of the electrolytes in the fluids.

A fluid imbalance occurs when either the ICF or ECF gains or loses body fluids or electrolytes, causing a fluid deficit or a fluid excess. Sodium is the major ion that influences water retention and water loss. A deficit of total-body fluid occurs with either an excessive loss of body water/fluids or an inadequate compensatory intake. The result is an insufficient fluid volume to meet the needs of the cells. It is manifested by dehydration (Box 5-8), hypovolemia, such as blood or plasma loss, or both. Severe fluid volume deficit can cause vascular collapse and shock.

An *excess* of water occurs when an overabundance of water is in the interstitial fluid spaces or body cavities

---

Box 5-8

CLINICAL MANIFESTATIONS OF DEHYDRATION

- Absent perspiration, tearing, and salivation
- Body temperature (subnormal or elevated)
- Confusion
- Disorientation; comatose; seizures
- Dizziness when standing
- Dry, brittle hair
- Dry mucous membranes, furrowed tongue
- Headache
- Incoordination
- Irritability
- Lethargy
- Postural hypotension
- Rapid pulse
- Rapid respirations
- Skin changes:
  - Color: gray
  - Temperature: cold
  - Turgor: poor
  - Feel: warm, dry if mild; cool, clammy if severe
- Sunken eye
- Sunken fontanel (children)

(edema) or within the blood vessels (hypervolemia). This may occur as a consequence of an inability to excrete excess fluid, as with renal disease, or an inability of the heart to move fluid/blood from the venous system to the arterial system, as with CHF. A *fluid shift* occurs when vascular fluid moves to interstitial or intracellular spaces or interstitial or ICF moves to vascular fluid space.

Fluid that shifts into the interstitial space (i.e., fluid not in the vascular compartment) and remains there is referred to as *third-space fluid*. Third-space fluid is commonly seen in a therapy practice as a result of altered capillary permeability secondary to tissue injury or inflammation, but the most common cause is liver disease. Decreased serum protein (albumin) associated with liver disease and/or states of malnutrition results in third-space fluid accumulation in the abdomen because there is a higher concentration of protein outside the vascular system than inside the vascular system and fluid shifts to a space with a higher protein concentration.

Other areas, called *potential spaces* (normally not fluid-filled), can fill with fluid in the presence of inflammation or fluid imbalances. Examples of potential spaces include the peritoneal cavity fluid (e.g., ascites) and the pleural cavity (e.g., pleural effusion).

Clinical Manifestations

Fluid volume deficit (FVD) is most often accompanied by symptoms of decreased vascular volume, such as decreased blood pressure, increased pulse, oliguria, and orthostatic hypotension. FVD can occur from loss of blood (whether obvious hemorrhage or occult GI bleeding), loss of plasma (burns or peritonitis), or loss of body fluids (diarrhea, vomiting, diaphoresis, or lack of fluid intake), resulting in dehydration. The affected individual experiences symptoms of thirst, weakness, dizziness, decreased urine output, weight loss, and altered levels of consciousness (i.e., confusion). Significant decreases in systolic blood pressure (less than 70 mm Hg) result in symptoms of shock and require immediate medical treatment and possibly life-sustaining emergency management.

Fluid volume excess is primarily characterized by weight gain and edema of the extremities. With intravascular fluid volume excess, other clinical manifestations include dyspnea, engorged neck veins, and a bounding pulse. In the early stages, if the fluid is in the third space (interstitial fluid between cells), the person may not exhibit any of these symptoms.

Fluid shift from the vascular to the extravascular (interstitial) spaces (e.g., burns or peritonitis) is manifested by signs and symptoms similar to FVD and shock, including skin pallor, cool extremities, weak and rapid pulse, hypotension, oliguria, and decreased levels of consciousness. When the fluid returns to the blood vessels, the clinical manifestations are similar to those of fluid overload such as bounding pulse and engorgement of peripheral and jugular veins.

MEDICAL MANAGEMENT

The ECF is the only fluid compartment that can be readily monitored; clinically, the status of ICF is inferred from analysis of plasma and the condition of the person. A fluid balance record is kept on any individual who is susceptible or already experiencing a disturbance in the balance of body fluids. In addition, medical evaluation of clinical signs and laboratory tests are helpful in the assessment of a person's hydration status. Laboratory tests may include serum osmolality, sodium, hematocrit, and BUN measurements (see "Laboratory Values" in Chapter 40).

Serum osmolality measures the concentration of particles in the plasma portion of the blood. Osmolality increases with dehydration and decreases with overhydration. Serum sodium is an index of water deficit or excess; an elevated level of sodium in the blood (hypernatremia) would indicate that the loss of water from the body has exceeded the loss of sodium such as occurs in the administration of osmotic diuretics, uncontrolled diabetes insipidus, and extensive burns. Hematocrit increases with dehydration and decreases with excess fluid. BUN serves as an index of kidney excretory function; BUN increases with dehydration and decreases with overhydration (see Table 40-2).

Treatment is directed to the underlying cause; in the case of FVD, the aim is to improve hydration status. This may be accomplished through replacement of fluids and/or electrolytes by oral, nasogastric, or IV means.

SPECIAL IMPLICATIONS FOR THE THERAPIST   5-10

Fluid Imbalances
Monitoring Fluid Balance

Fluid balance is so critical to physical well-being and cardiopulmonary sufficiency that fluid input and output records are often maintained at bedside. The therapist may be involved in maintaining these records, which also include fluid volume lost in wound drainage, GI output, and fluids aspirated from any body cavity. Body weight may increase by several pounds before edema is apparent. The dependent areas manifest the first signs of fluid excess. Individuals on bed rest show sacral swelling; people who can sit on the edge of the bed or in a chair for prolonged periods tend to show swelling of the feet and hands.[79]

Water and fluids should be offered often to older adults and clients with debilitating diseases to prevent body fluid loss and hypernatremia. However, increasing fluid intake in clients with CHF or severe renal disease is usually contraindicated.

Caffeinated fluids and alcohol can increase water loss, thereby increasing the serum sodium level; these beverages should be avoided to prevent fluid loss as a consequence of this diuretic effect. Water is the preferred fluid for hydration except in athletic or marathon race situations, which require replacement of electrolytes.[121]

Thirst is not always a reliable signal for fluid intake or even dehydration. A person may not feel "thirsty" until the body reaches a dangerous point of fluid loss. Therapists and clients should both be encouraged to keep water and clear fluids on hand and drink on a schedule rather than wait until they feel thirsty. Many people confuse thirst for hunger and eat instead of drinking when the thirst mechanism does kick in.

Urine is good gauge of adequate hydration. A low volume of dark or highly concentrated urine is a yellow flag. When accompanied by other signs of dehydration (e.g., dry mouth, irritability, constipation, fatigue, or muscle weakness), it becomes a red flag.

Dehydration

Healthy older adults can become at risk for dehydration for many physiologic and psychosocial reasons. Older individuals have an impaired thirst response to dehydration; abnormal circadian rhythm of AVP leads to nocturia and increased fluid loss. Other contributing medical factors include diabetes, urinary tract infections, renal failure, and medications such as diuretics.[237]

Psychosocial factors also play a key role in the development of dehydration in the older age group. Isolation, depression, and confusion are associated with reduced oral intake and impaired fluid status and can make dehydration worse.[237]

Dehydration (water deficit) degrades endurance exercise performance, and physical work capacity is diminished even at marginal levels of dehydration (defined clinically as a 1% loss of body weight through fluid loss). Alterations in VO_2max (aerobic capacity) occur with a 2% or more deficit in body water loss. Greater body water deficits are associated with progressively larger reductions in physical work capacity.

Dehydration results in larger reductions in physical work capacity in a hot environment (e.g., aquatic or outdoor setting) for individuals in any age group, as compared with a thermally neutral environment. Prolonged exercise that places large demands on aerobic metabolism is more likely to be adversely affected by dehydration than is short-term exercise.[26]

Core body temperature increases predictably as the percentage of dehydration increases. The heart rate increases about 6 beats/min for each 1% increase in dehydration. This is not true for older adults, who may have limited rate changes with increased activity.

Older individuals are especially at risk for negative sequelae associated with dehydration. Hospitalization for dehydration is common and mortality is high. Almost 50% of Medicare patients who are hospitalized with dehydration die within a year of admission.[237,374,375]

Anyone with hypovolemia cannot compensate as easily with an increased heart rate like younger people can, so shock is more difficult to treat. In addition, aging individuals are often being treated with cardiac medications, such as β-blockers or digoxin that block or inhibit a rapid heart rate and limit rate changes with increased activity. Heart transplant recipients also have a unique situation because the heart has been denervated (see "Special Implications for the Therapist: Heart Transplantation" in Chapter 21).

Individuals exercising in the heat, including aquatic exercise, should be encouraged to drink water in excess of normally desired amounts. When exercise is expected to cause an increase of more than 2% in dehydration, target heart rate modifications are necessary.[219]

Severe losses of water and solutes can lead to hypovolemic shock. It is important for the therapist to be aware of possible fluid losses or water shifts in any client who is already compromised by advanced age or by the presence of an ileostomy or tracheostomy resulting in a continuous loss of fluid.

Dehydration may contribute to underlying disabilities caused by orthostatic hypotension and dizziness. It may result in symptoms, such as confusion and weakness that can interfere with rehabilitation outcomes, especially after orthopedic surgery.[237]

Because the response to fluid loss is highly individual, it is important to recognize the early clinical symptoms of fluid loss (see Box 5-6) and to carefully monitor clients who are at risk (e.g., observe for symptoms and monitor vital signs). People at risk for profound and potentially fatal FVD, as in severe and extensive burns, should be assessed frequently and regularly for mental acuity and orientation to person, place, and time.

Skin Care

Careful handling of edematous tissue is essential to maintaining the integrity of the skin, which is stretched beyond its normal limits and has a limited blood supply. Turning and repositioning the client must be done gently to avoid friction. A break in or abrasion of edematous skin can readily develop into a pressure ulcer.

Client education may be necessary in the proper application and use of antiembolism stockings or other appropriate compression garments, lower-extremity elevation, and the need for regular exercise. Clients should be cautioned to avoid crossing the legs, putting pillows under the knees, or otherwise creating pressure against the blood vessels.[97,250]

Electrolyte Imbalances

Overview

Electrolytes are chemical substances that separate into electrically charged particles, called *ions*, in solution. The electrolytes that consist of positively charged ions, or *cations*, are sodium (Na^+), potassium (K^+), calcium (Ca^{2+}), and magnesium (Mg^{2+}). Those that consist of negatively charged ions, or *anions*, are chloride (Cl^+); bicarbonate (HCO_3^-); and phosphate (PO_4^{3-}).

Concentration gradients of sodium and potassium across the cell membrane produce the membrane potential and provide the means by which electrochemical impulses are transmitted in nerve and muscle fibers. *Sodium* affects the osmolality of blood and therefore influences blood volume and pressure and the retention or loss of interstitial fluid. Sodium imbalance affects the osmolality of the ECF and is often associated with fluid volume imbalances.

Adequate *potassium* is necessary to maintain function of sodium–potassium membrane pumps, which are essential for the normal muscle contraction–relaxation sequence. Imbalances in potassium affect muscular activities, notably those of the heart, intestines, and respiratory tract, and neural stimulation of the skeletal muscles.

Calcium influences the permeability of cell membranes and thereby regulates neuromuscular activity. Calcium plays a role in the electrical excitation of cardiac cells and in the mechanical contraction of the myocardial and vascular smooth muscle cells. An imbalance in calcium concentrations affects skeletal muscle, bones, kidneys, and the GI tract. Conditions that can cause movement of calcium from the bones into the ECF (e.g., bone tumors, multiple fractures, or osteoporosis) can cause

hypercalcemia. (Table 5-9 lists other causes of hypocalcemia or hypercalcemia.)

Magnesium, an important intracellular activator for more than 300 enzymatic processes, exerts physiologic effects on the nervous system that resemble the effects of calcium. Two-thirds of the body's magnesium is found in the bones; most of the rest is located in the ECF, including the vascular compartment and interstitial spaces. As a result, the normal serum magnesium concentration is relatively low (1.5% to 2.5 mg/dL).

Magnesium plays a role in maintaining the correct level of electrical excitability in the nerves and muscle

Table 5-9	Causes of Electrolyte Imbalances
	Risk Factors for Imbalance
Potassium	
Hypokalemia	Dietary deficiency (rare)
	Intestinal or urinary losses as a result of diarrhea or vomiting (anorexia, dehydration), drainage from fistulas, overuse of gastric suction
	Trauma (injury, burns, surgery): damaged cells release potassium, are excreted in urine
	Medications such as potassium-wasting diuretics, steroids, insulin, penicillin derivatives, amphotericin B
	Metabolic alkalosis
	Cushing syndrome, severe magnesium deficiency
	Hyperaldosteronism
	Integumentary loss (sweating)
	Type 2 renal tubular acidosis
	Diabetic ketoacidosis
Hyperkalemia	Conditions that alter kidney function or decrease its ability to excrete potassium (chronic renal disease or renal failure)
	Intestinal obstruction that prevents elimination of potassium in the feces
	Addison disease
	Chronic heparin therapy, lead poisoning, insulin deficit, NSAIDs, ACE inhibitors, cyclosporine
	Trauma: crush injuries, burns
	Metabolic acidosis
	Rhabdomyolysis
	Tumor lysis syndrome
	Hyperglycemia
	Digitalis toxicity
	Hypoaldosteronism
Sodium	
Hyponatremia	Inadequate sodium intake (low-sodium diets)
	Excessive intake or retention of water (kidney failure and heart failure)
	Excessive water loss and electrolytes (vomiting, excessive perspiration, tap-water enemas, suctioning, use of diuretics, diarrhea)
	Loss of bile (high in sodium) as a result of fistulas, drainage, GI surgery, and suction
	Trauma (loss of sodium through burn wounds, wound drainage from surgery)
	IV fluids that do not contain electrolytes
	Adrenal gland insufficiency (Addison disease) or hypoaldosteronism
	Cirrhosis of the liver with ascites
	SIADH: brain tumor, cerebrovascular accident, pulmonary disease, neoplasm with ADH production, medications, pain, nausea
	Hypothyroidism
	Nephrotic syndrome
Hypernatremia	Decreased water intake (comatose, mentally confused, or debilitated client)
	Water loss (excessive sweating, osmotic diarrhea), fever, heat exposure, burns
	Hyperglycemia
	Excess adrenocortical hormones (Cushing syndrome)
	IV administration of high-protein, hyperosmotic tube feedings and diuretics
	Diabetes insipidus
	Central: loss of neurohypophysis from trauma, surgery, neoplasm, CVA, infection
	Nephrogenic: renal resistance to ADH drugs (lithium), hypercalcemia papillary necrosis, pregnancy

Table 5-9	Causes of Electrolyte Imbalances—cont'd
	Risk Factors for Imbalance

Calcium

Hypocalcemia	Inadequate dietary intake of calcium and inadequate exposure to sunlight (Vitamin D) necessary for calcium use (especially older adults)
	Impaired absorption of calcium and Vitamin D from intestinal tract (severe diarrhea, overuse of laxatives, and enemas containing phosphates; phosphorous tends to be more readily absorbed from the intestinal tract than calcium and suppresses calcium retention in the body)
	Hypoparathyroidism (injury, disease, surgery)
	Severe infections or burns
	Overcorrection of acidosis
	Pancreatic insufficiency
	Renal failure
	Hypomagnesemia (especially with alcoholism)
	Medications—anticonvulsive medications
Hypercalcemia	Hyperparathyroidism, hyperthyroidism, adrenal insufficiency
	Multiple fractures
	Excess intake of calcium (excessive antacids), excess intake of vitamin D, milk alkali syndrome
	Osteoporosis, immobility, multiple myeloma
	Thiazide diuretics
	Sarcoidosis
	Tumors which secrete PTH (bone, lung, stomach, and kidney)
	Multiple endocrine neoplasia tumors (types I and II)

Magnesium

Hypomagnesemia	Decreased magnesium intake or absorption (chronic malnutrition, chronic diarrhea, bowel resection with ileostomy or colostomy, chronic alcoholism, prolonged gastric suction, acute pancreatitis, biliary or intestinal fistula)
	Excessive loss of magnesium (diabetic ketoacidosis, severe dehydration, hyperaldosteronism and hypoparathyroidism)
	Vitamin D deficiency
	Impaired renal absorption
	Parenteral nutrition/enteral feeding with inadequate magnesium replacement
	Acute tubular necrosis
	Medications: diuretics, cisplatin, foscarnet, cyclosporine, amphotericin B, some proton pump inhibitors
	Hyperthyroidism
	Metabolic acidosis
	SIADH
	Pregnancy
Hypermagnesemia	Chronic renal failure or renal insufficiency*
	Overuse of antacids and laxatives containing magnesium
	Severe dehydration (resulting oliguria can cause magnesium retention)
	Overcorrection of hypomagnesemia
	Diabetic ketoacidosis
	Tumor lysis syndrome
	Near-drowning (aspiration of sea water)
	Intestinal obstruction
	Trauma, burns
	Hypothyroidism
	Addison disease (adrenal insufficiency)
	Shock, sepsis

ACE, angiotensin-converting enzyme; ADH, antidiuretic hormone; CVA, cardiovascular accident; GI, gastrointestinal; IV, intravenous; NSAIDs, nonsteroidal antiinflammatory drugs; SIADH, syndrome of inappropriate antidiuretic hormone.
*Hypermagnesemia is much less common than hypomagnesemia because normally functioning kidneys easily excrete magnesium.
Data from Porth CM. *Essentials of pathophysiology*, ed 3, Philadelphia, 2011, Lippincott Williams & Wilkins.

cells by acting directly on the myoneural junction. Magnesium depresses acetylcholine release at synaptic junctions. Magnesium influences cardiovascular function because of its vasodilatory effect.[289]

Neuromuscular irritability results from hypomagnesemia (e.g., malnutrition from poor diet, chronic alcohol abuse, diuretic use [renal loss of magnesium], or prolonged diarrhea with impaired intestinal absorption of magnesium), and magnesium excess (rare but occurs with renal failure or the overuse of magnesium-containing antacids) causes neuromuscular depression affecting the musculoskeletal and cardiac systems.[4]

Etiologic and Risk Factors

An electrolyte imbalance exists when the serum concentration of an electrolyte is either too high or too low.

Stability of the electrolyte balance depends not only on adequate intake, distribution, and excretion of the electrolyte, but is often tightly connected to and dependent on fluid balance, particularly sodium. Many conditions can interfere with these processes and result in an imbalance (see Table 5-9). For example, cell death (from ischemia, chemotherapy, trauma) results in the release of electrolytes such as potassium, calcium, phosphate, and magnesium. Medications (i.e., diuretics) lead to an excessive excretion of electrolytes, and diseases (i.e., renal failure) interfere with the excretion of electrolytes. Often, as with sodium, the laboratory value may appear too high or too low, yet the total amount of sodium is normal; it is frequently an imbalance in fluid that alters the concentration of sodium.

Clinical Manifestations

In a therapy practice, paresthesias, muscle weakness, muscle wasting, muscle tetany, and bone pain are the most likely symptoms first observed with electrolyte imbalances (Table 5-10) (see "Clinical Manifestations" under "Common Causes of Fluid and Electrolyte Imbalances" below).

MEDICAL MANAGEMENT

Potassium, calcium, sodium, and chloride can be measured in plasma. Intracellular levels of electrolytes cannot be measured; consequently, all values for electrolytes are expressed as serum values. Serum values for electrolytes are given as milliequivalents per liter (mEq/L) or milligrams per deciliter (mg/dL) (see Table 40-2). As with fluid imbalances, the underlying cause of electrolyte imbalances must be determined and corrected. Electrolyte supplementation, when needed, can be given orally or intravenously.

SPECIAL IMPLICATIONS FOR THE THERAPIST　　5-11

Electrolyte Imbalances

With appropriate medical therapy, cardiac, muscular, and neurologic manifestations associated with electrolyte imbalances can be corrected. Delayed medical treatment may result in irreversible damage or death. That is why continual assessment for signs and symptoms of electrolyte imbalance must be ongoing, and changes need to be reported immediately. Observing for accompanying signs and symptoms of fluid and electrolyte imbalances will help promote safe and effective exercise for anyone with the potential for these disorders.

Encourage adherence to a sodium-restricted diet when prescribed. The use of nonprescription medications for people on a sodium-restricted diet should be approved by the physician. Encourage activity and alternate with rest periods. Monitor for worsening of the underlying cause of fluid or electrolyte imbalance and report significant findings to the nurse or physician.

If dyspnea and orthopnea are present, teach the client to use a semi-Fowler position (head elevated 18 to 20 inches from horizontal with knees flexed) to promote lung expansion. Frequent position changes are important in the presence of edema; edematous tissue is more prone to skin breakdown than normal tissue.

Hypokalemia

Older adults have frequent problems with hypokalemia most often associated with the use of diuretics. Decreased potassium levels can result in fatigue, muscle cramping, and cardiac dysrhythmias, usually manifested by an irregular pulse rate or complaints of dizziness and/or palpitations. Fatigue and muscle cramping increase the chance of musculoskeletal injury.

Hypomagnesemia

Monitor carefully any individual being medically treated for hypomagnesemia because administration of magnesium for hypomagnesemia can result in hypermagnesemia and signs and symptoms associated with magnesium toxicity (e.g., loss of deep tendon reflexes).

Hypermagnesemia

For hospitalized patients with severe hypermagnesemia (usually secondary to renal failure), monitor vital signs carefully and initiate safety precautions as appropriate. Watch for hypotension, bradycardia, and respiratory depression. Assess neuromuscular function and level of consciousness regularly. Frequently, individuals with hypermagnesemia are restricted from mobility activities (sitting up, ambulating) without supervision.

Postoperative Electrolyte Imbalances

Electrolyte imbalances associated with complex spinal surgeries have been reported in more than 40% of all cases.[337] It is believed that this figure has previously been underreported and thanks to a spinal specific tool used to report and classify severity of complications, this information has come to light. Therapists in the acute care setting and early outpatient rehab for these individuals should keep this in mind and monitor closely for electrolyte disturbances. Again, early recognition and intervention may reduce morbidity and mortality.[337]

Common Causes of Fluid and Electrolyte Imbalances

Overview

The exact mechanisms of fluid and electrolyte imbalances are outside the scope of this text. A brief description of the common causes and overall clinical picture encountered in a therapy practice is included here. Burns, surgery, and trauma may result in a fluid volume shift from the vascular spaces to the interstitial spaces. Tissue injury causes the release of histamine and bradykinin, which increases capillary permeability, allowing fluid, protein, and other solutes to shift into the interstitial spaces.

Table 5-10	Clinical Features of Various Electrolyte Imbalances

	SYSTEM DYSFUNCTION	
Potassium Imbalance		
	Hypokalemia	**Hyperkalemia**
Cardiovascular	Dizziness, hypotension, arrhythmias, electrocardiogram (ECG) changes, cardiac arrest (with serum potassium levels 2.5 mEq/L)	Tachycardia and later bradycardia, ECG changes, cardiac arrest (with levels >7.0 mEq/L)
Gastrointestinal (GI)	Nausea and vomiting, anorexia, constipation, abdominal distention, paralytic ileus or decreased peristalsis	Nausea, diarrhea, abdominal cramps
Musculoskeletal	Muscle weakness and fatigue, leg cramps	Muscle weakness, flaccid paralysis
Genitourinary	Polyuria	Oliguria, anuria
Central nervous system (CNS)	Malaise, irritability, confusion, mental depression, speech changes, decreased reflexes, pulmonary hyperventilation	Areflexia progressing to weakness, numbness, tingling, and flaccid paralysis
Acid–base balance	Metabolic alkalosis	Metabolic acidosis
Calcium Imbalance		
	Hypocalcemia	**Hypercalcemia**
CNS	Anxiety, irritability, twitching around mouth, laryngospasm, seizures, Chvostek sign, apathy, irritability, confusion	Drowsiness, lethargy, headaches, depression, or Trousseau sign
Musculoskeletal	Paresthesia (tingling and numbness of the fingers), tetany or painful tonic muscle spasms, facial spasms, abdominal cramps, muscle cramps, spasmodic contractions	Weakness, muscle flaccidity, bone pain, pathologic fractures
Cardiovascular	Arrhythmias, hypotension	Signs of heart block, cardiac arrest in systole, hypertension
GI	Increased GI motility, diarrhea from dehydration	Anorexia, nausea, vomiting, constipation, dehydration, polyuria, prerenal azotemia
Sodium Imbalance		
	Hyponatremia	**Hypernatremia**
CNS	Anxiety, headaches, muscle twitching and weakness, confusion, seizures	Agitation, restlessness, seizures, ataxia, confusion
Cardiovascular	Hypotension; tachycardia; with severe deficit, vasomotor collapse, thready pulse	Hypertension, tachycardia, pitting edema, excessive weight gain
GI	Nausea, vomiting, abdominal cramps	Rough, dry tongue; intense thirst; severe hypotension
Genitourinary	Oliguria or anuria	Oliguria
Respiratory	Cyanosis with severe deficiency	Dyspnea, respiratory arrest, and death (from dramatic rise in osmatic pressure)
Cutaneous	Cold clammy skin, decreased skin turgor	Flushed skin; dry, sticky mucous membranes
Magnesium Imbalance		
	Hypomagnesemia	**Hypermagnesemia**
Neuromuscular	Muscle tremors and weakness; athetoid movements Hyperirritability, tetany, leg and foot cramps, Chvostek sign (facial muscle spasms induced by tapping the branches of the facial nerve)	Diminished reflexes, muscle weakness, flaccid paralysis, respiratory muscle paralysis that may cause respiratory impairment and even respiratory arrest
CNS	Confusion, apathy, depression, delusions, hallucinations, psychosis, seizures	Drowsiness, flushing, lethargy, confusion, diminished sensorium
Cardiovascular	Arrhythmias (ventricular tachycardia, ventricular fibrillation), vasomotor changes (vasodilation and hypotension), occasionally hypertension	Bradycardia, weak pulse, hypotension, heart block, cardiac arrest

In the case of burns, the fluid shifts out of the vessels into the injured tissue spaces, as well as into the normal (unburned) tissue. This causes severe swelling of these tissues and a significant loss of fluid volume from the vascular space, which results in hypovolemia. Severe hypovolemia can result in shock, vascular collapse, and death. In the case of major tissue damage, potassium is also released from the damaged tissue cells and can enter the vascular fluids, causing hyperkalemia.

In an attempt to treat shock, large quantities of fluid are administered intravenously to maintain blood pressure, cardiac output, and renal function. After 24–72 hours, capillary permeability is usually restored and fluid begins to leave the tissue spaces and shift back into the vascular space. If renal function is not adequate, the accumulation of fluid used for treatment and fluid returning from the tissue spaces into the vascular space can cause fluid volume overload. Fluid overload can then lead to CHF or pulmonary edema.

Diabetes mellitus (type 1) may result in a condition called *diabetic ketoacidosis*, which is caused by a lack of insulin. This leads to hyperglycemia, polyuria, and an overproduction of ketones that results in metabolic acidosis (see Chapter 11). Hyperglycemia draws ICF into the extracellular compartment (fluid shift) causing an intracellular dehydration; it also leads to an osmotic diuresis with not only loss of fluid, but also loss of electrolytes (potassium, sodium, and phosphate). Although many clients present with a laboratory value consistent with hyperkalemia (a result of metabolic acidosis), once adequate fluid has been restored, it is evident that there is actually hypokalemia, which, unless treated immediately, can cause life-threatening cardiac dysrhythmias.

Hyponatremia is one of the most common electrolyte imbalances affecting hospitalized patients. Hyponatremia is typically caused by an increase in water with normal sodium stores (increased extracellular volume) and is most frequently seen as a result of CHF, renal failure (nephrotic syndrome), or liver disease (ascites). Treatment is to manage the underlying condition along with fluid restriction.

Hyponatremia may also be seen when extracellular volumes are normal, but sodium is elevated. This is typically secondary to the syndrome of inappropriate antidiuretic hormone, but may also be a result of severe hypothyroidism or water intoxication (psychogenic polydipsia). *Tumors* and pulmonary and CNS disorders often inappropriately produce antidiuretic hormone (ADH), which is not regulated by normal suppression feedback loops; consequently, the ectopic hormone continues to be released by the tumor, often causing serious electrolyte imbalances. One example of this phenomenon is the ectopic production of ADH by lung carcinomas, resulting in hyponatremia.

A more local effect of malignancy occurs when metastases to the skeletal system produce hypercalcemia from the osteolysis of bone. The treatment of malignancies also can create fluid and electrolyte imbalances such as occurs with hormonal treatment for breast cancer (e.g., tamoxifen can cause hypercalcemia). Hyponatremia and hypokalemia may also result from nausea and vomiting caused by chemotherapy. Certain chemotherapeutic drugs (e.g., vincristine and cyclophosphamide) are associated with syndrome of inappropriate antidiuretic hormone, causing hyponatremia.

Alcohol withdrawal and *eating disorders* are also associated with physiologic changes that can include electrolyte imbalances. See discussion of each individual condition in Chapter 3.

Hypernatremia may be seen with severe systemic disease (i.e., sepsis, surgery), volume loss without adequate water replacement (i.e., diarrhea or osmotic diuresis), or impaired sensorium or physical disability that prevents access to water. Diabetes insipidus also leads to hypernatremia because of a lack of ADH or resistance to ADH.

Hyperkalemia can be life-threatening. Mild hyperkalemia may be a consequence of improper potassium supplementation; moderate to severe hyperkalemia can be seen with renal failure, acidosis (i.e., diabetic ketoacidosis), digitalis toxicity, rhabdomyolysis, and insulin deficiency.

Hypokalemia may result from diarrhea, vomiting, acute leukemia, magnesium deficiency, diabetic ketoacidosis, and diuretics.

Clinical Manifestations

The effects of a fluid or electrolyte imbalance are not isolated to a particular organ or system (Box 5-9). Symptoms most commonly observed by the therapist may include skin changes, neuromuscular irritability (muscle fatigue, twitching, cramping, or tetany), CNS involvement, edema, and changes in vital signs, especially tachycardia and postural (orthostatic) hypotension (see Box 12-11).

Skin changes include changes in skin turgor and alterations in skin temperature. In a healthy individual, pinched skin will immediately fall back to its normal position when released, a measure of skin turgor. In a person with FVD, such as dehydration, the skin flattens more slowly after the pinch is released and may even remain elevated for several seconds, referred to as *tenting* of tissue (Fig. 5-8). Tissue turgor can vary with age, nutritional state, race, and complexion, and must be accompanied by other signs of FVD to be considered meaningful.

Skin turgor may be more difficult to assess in older adults because of reduced skin elasticity compared with that of younger clients. Skin temperature may become

---

Box 5-9

CLINICAL MANIFESTATIONS OF FLUID/ELECTROLYTE IMBALANCE*

Skin Changes
- Poor skin turgor
- Changes in skin temperature

Neuromuscular Irritability
- Muscle fatigue
- Muscle twitching
- Muscle cramping
- Tetany

CNS Involvement
- Changes in deep tendon reflexes
- Seizures
- Depression
- Memory impairment
- Delusions
- Hallucinations

Edema
- Changes in vital signs:
- Tachycardia
- Postural hypotension
- Altered respirations

* Only signs and symptoms most likely to be seen in a therapy practice are included here.

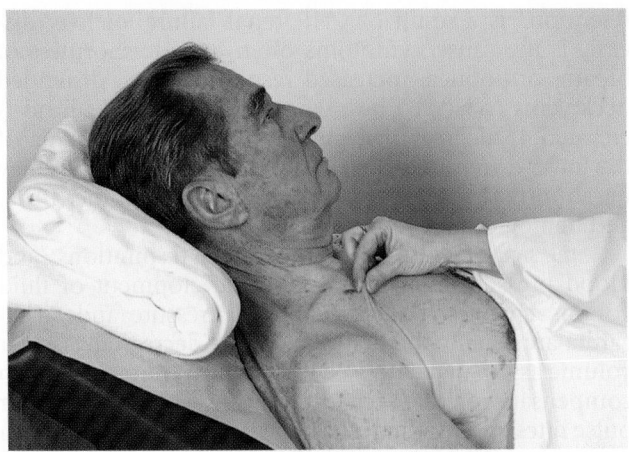

Figure 5-8

Testing skin turgor (normal resiliency of a pinched fold of skin). Turgor is measured by the time it takes for the skin and underlying tissue to return to its original contour after being pinched up. If the skin remains elevated (i.e., tented) for more than 3 seconds, turgor is decreased. Normal turgor is indicated by a return to baseline contour within 3 seconds when the skin is mobile and elastic. Turgor decreases with age as the skin loses elasticity; testing turgor of some older persons on the forearm (the standard site for testing) is less valid because of decreased skin elasticity in this area. (From Jarvis C: *Physical examination and health assessment,* ed 4, Philadelphia, 2004, WB Saunders.)

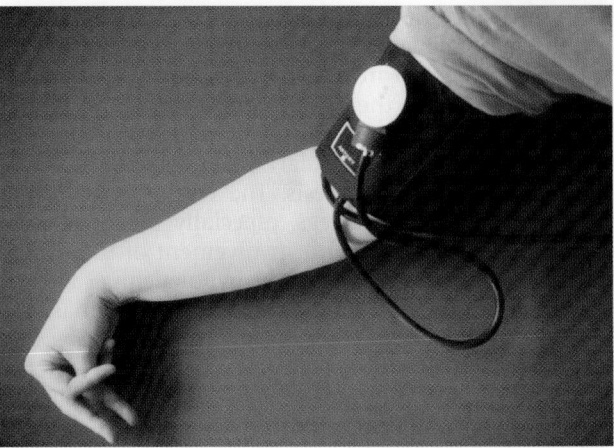

Figure 5-9

Carpopedal attitude of the hand, a form of latent tetany associated with hypocalcemia, is called the *Trousseau sign.* This can be tested for by inflating a blood pressure cuff on the upper arm to a level between diastolic and systolic blood pressure and maintaining this inflation for 3 minutes. A positive test results in the carpal spasm shown here. (From Ignatavicius DD, Workman ML: *Medical-surgical nursing: critical thinking for collaborative care,* ed 5, Philadelphia, 2006, WB Saunders.)

warm and flushed as a result of vasodilation (e.g., in metabolic acidosis) or pale and cool because of peripheral vasoconstriction compensating for hypovolemia.

Neuromuscular irritability can occur as a result of imbalances in calcium, magnesium, potassium, and sodium. (See Chapter 24 for discussion of osteoporosis associated with calcium loss.) Specific signs of neuromuscular involvement associated with these imbalances occur because of increased neural excitability, specifically increased acetylcholine action at the nerve ending, resulting in lowering of the threshold of the muscle membrane.

Tetany (continuous muscle spasm) is the most characteristic manifestation of hypocalcemia. The affected person may report a sensation of tingling around the mouth (circumoral paresthesia) and in the hands and feet, and spasms of the muscles of the extremities and face. Less-overt signs (latent tetany) can be elicited through the Trousseau sign (Fig. 5-9), the Chvostek sign (Fig. 5-10), and changes in deep tendon reflexes (DTRs) (Table 5-11). Many other factors can produce abnormalities in DTRs, requiring the therapist to evaluate altered DTRs in light of other clinical signs and client history.

Nervous system involvement may occur in the peripheral system (hyperkalemia) or the CNS (hypocalcemia, hypercalcemia, hyponatremia, and hypernatremia). CNS manifestations of hypocalcemia may include seizures, irritability, depression, memory impairment, delusions, and hallucinations. In chronic hypocalcemia, the skin may be dry and scaling, the nails become brittle, and the hair is dry and falls out easily.

Signs and symptoms of hyponatremia occur when a drop in the serum sodium level pulls water into cells. When this happens, the client may experience headaches, confusion, lethargy, muscle weakness, and nausea. These

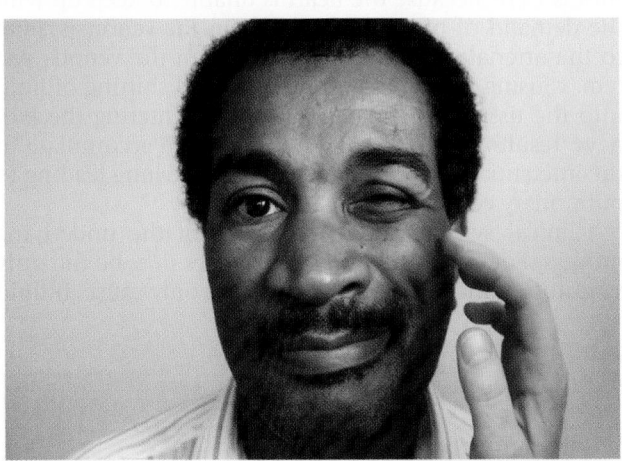

Figure 5-10

To check for the *Chvostek sign,* **tap the facial nerve above the mandibular angle, adjacent to the ear lobe.** A facial muscle spasm that causes the person's eye and upper lip to twitch, as shown, confirms tetany. (From Ignatavicius DD, Workman ML: *Medical-surgical nursing: critical thinking for collaborative care,* ed 5, Philadelphia, 2006, WB Saunders.)

Table 5-11	Changes in Deep Tendon Reflexes Associated with Fluid–Electrolyte Imbalance

Increased (Hyperactive)	**Decreased (Hypoactive)**
Hypocalcemia	Hypercalcemia
Hypomagnesemia	Hypermagnesemia
Hypernatremia	Hyponatremia
Hyperkalemia*	Hyperkalemia
Alkalosis	Acidosis

*Generally hyperkalemia is accompanied by decreased or absent deep tendon reflexes (DTRs); some sources do report hyperactive DTRs with hyperkalemia. In the clinical situation, DTRs are never used to determine a potassium imbalance. They are a warning sign for the therapist to assess the client further and report all pertinent findings.

symptoms are easily mistaken for complications from anesthesia or analgesia.

Hypokalemia seen in a therapy practice can be associated with diuretic therapy; excessive sweating, vomiting, or diarrhea; diabetic acidosis; trauma; or burns. It is accompanied by muscular weakness that can progress to flaccid quadriparesis. The weakness is initially most prominent in the legs, especially the quadriceps; it extends to the arms, with involvement of the respiratory muscles soon after.[264] Severe hypokalemia can cause paralysis, respiratory failure, cardiac arrhythmias, and hypotension. Finally, a condition called *rhabdomyolysis* (disintegration of striated muscle fibers with excretion of myoglobin in the urine) can occur with potassium or phosphorus depletion.

Edema is defined as an excessive accumulation of interstitial fluid. Many disease processes result in edema in various locations of the body. Because of gravity, the most common location is the lower extremities. Fluid may accumulate in the ankles and legs secondary to incompetent veins or from a lack of protein in the blood (low albumen), leading to a shift of fluid into the tissues.

Another common cause of edema in the lower extremities is CHF. Because the heart is unable to keep up with the demand of pumping blood from the venous system to the arterial system, fluid backs up in the venous system, causing an increase in pressure and shifting of fluid into the tissue. There is also less fluid entering the kidneys, resulting in oliguria. Fluid may also accumulate in the interstitial tissues and airspaces of the lung leading to pulmonary edema.

Clinical symptoms are indicative of the underlying process. Edema of the lower extremities may be the only symptom if incompetent veins are the only cause. If fluid

retention, as a result of CHF, renal failure, or liver disease, is the cause, symptoms often include shortness of breath, orthopnea, increased respiratory rate, distended neck veins (observed best when the individual's head is elevated 45 degrees), weight gain, and pitting edema of the lower extremities (Fig. 5-11). Laboratory findings may be abnormal (e.g., electrolytes, serum creatinine, BUN, and hemoglobin).

Vital sign changes, including pulse, respirations, and blood pressure, may signal early development of fluid volume changes. Decreased blood pressure and tachycardia are usually the first signs of the decreased vascular volume associated with FVD, as the heart pumps faster to compensate for the decreased plasma volume. Irregular pulse rates and dysrhythmias may also be associated with magnesium, potassium, or calcium imbalances.

Orthostatic hypotension is another sign of volume depletion (hypovolemia). Moving from a supine to standing position causes an abrupt drop in venous return, which is normally compensated for by sympathetically mediated cardiovascular adjustments. For example, in the healthy individual, increased peripheral resistance and increased heart rate maintain cardiac output. Blood pressure is unaffected or characterized by a small decrease in systolic pressure, and the diastolic pressure may actually rise a few millimeters of mercury (mm Hg).

In contrast, for the person with FVD, systolic pressure may fall 20 mm Hg or more, accompanied by an increase in the pulse rate greater than 15 beats/min.[171] The decreased volume results in compensatory increases in pulse rate as the heart attempts to increase output in the face of decreased stroke volume.

As fluid volume depletion worsens, blood pressure becomes low in all positions from loss of compensatory mechanisms and autonomic insufficiency. Conditions such as diabetes, associated with autonomic neuropathy, can also produce orthostatic blood pressure and pulse changes (see "Orthostatic Hypotension" in Chapter 12).

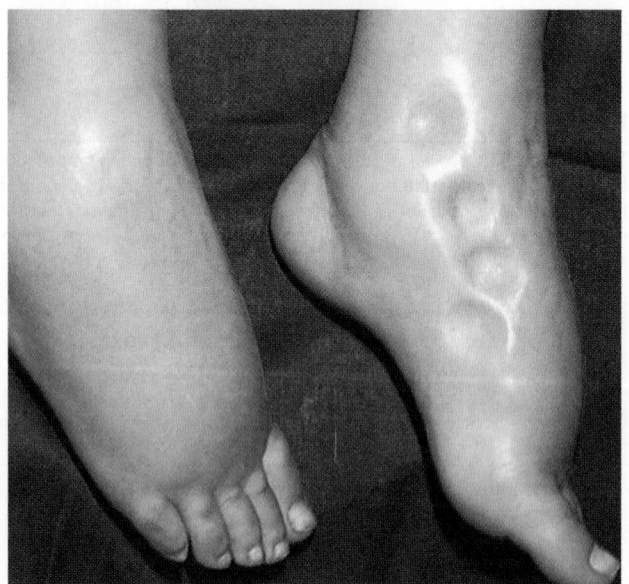

Figure 5-11

Severe, dependent, pitting edema occurs with some systemic diseases, such as congestive heart failure and hepatic cirrhosis. Note the finger-shaped depressions that do not refill after pressure has been exerted by the examiner. (From Thibodeau GA, Patton KT: *The human body in health and disease*, ed 4, St. Louis, 2005, Mosby.)

| SPECIAL IMPLICATIONS FOR THE THERAPIST | 5-12 |

Assessment of Fluid and Electrolyte Imbalance

Assessment of fluid and electrolyte balance is based on both subjective and objective findings (Table 5-12). At the bedside or in the home health care setting, the therapist must be alert to complaints of headache, thirst, and nausea and changes in dyspnea, skin turgor, and muscle strength. More objective assessment of fluid and electrolyte balance is based on fluid intake, output, and body weight. (See "Special Implications for the Therapist: Fluid Imbalances and Electrolyte Imbalances" above.)

ACID–BASE IMBALANCES

Overview

Normal function of body cells to maintain homeostasis depends on regulation of hydrogen ion concentration

(H+) so that H+ levels remain within very narrow limits. Acid–base imbalances occur when these limits are exceeded and are recognized clinically as abnormalities of serum pH (i.e., the measure of acidity or alkalinity of blood). Normal serum pH is 7.35 to 7.45. Cell function is seriously impaired when pH falls to 7.2 or lower or rises to 7.55 or higher (see "Laboratory Values" in Chapter 40).

Three physiologic systems act interdependently to maintain normal serum pH: immediate buffering of excess acid or base by the *blood buffer systems*, excretion of acid by the *lungs* (occurs within minutes to hours), and excretion of acid or reclamation of base by the *kidneys* (occurs within 24–48 hours). The four general classes of acid–base imbalance are respiratory acidosis, respiratory alkalosis, metabolic acidosis, and metabolic alkalosis. Table 5-13 summarizes these four imbalances (see also Table 40-3).

Acidosis (metabolic or respiratory) refers to any pathologic process causing a relative excess of acid in the body (pH less than 7.35). This can occur as a result of accumulation of acid or depletion of the alkaline reserve (bicarbonate content, HCO_3^-) in the blood and body tissues.

Acidemia refers to excess acid in the blood and does not necessarily confirm an underlying pathologic process. The same distinction may be made between the terms *alkalosis* and *alkalemia*; alkalosis indicates a primary condition resulting in excess base in the body. Although efforts have been made to standardize acid–base terminology, these terms are often used interchangeably.

Incidence

The incidence of acid–base imbalances in hospital settings is high. Acid–base imbalances are often related to respiratory and/or metabolic problems typical of the critically ill or injured individual. Some people have more than one acid–base imbalance at the same time.

Clinical Manifestations

Table 5-13 is a guide to the clinical presentation of acid–base imbalances. Besides the major distinguishing

Table 5-12	Assessment of Fluid and Electrolyte Imbalance	
Area	**Fluid Excess/Electrolyte Imbalance**	**Fluid Loss/Electrolyte Imbalance**
Head and neck	Distended neck veins, facial edema	Thirst, dry mucous membranes
Extremities	Dependent pitting, edema, discomfort from weight of bed covers	Muscle weakness, tingling, tetany
Skin	Warm, moist; taut, cool feeling when edematous	Dry, decreased turgor
Respiration	Dyspnea, orthopnea, productive cough, moist breath	Changes in rate and depth of breathing sounds
Circulation	Hypertension, distended neck veins, atrial arrhythmias	Pulse rate irregularities, arrhythmia, postural hypotension, tachycardia
Abdomen	Increased girth, fluid wave	Abdominal cramps

Modified from Briggs J, Drabek C: Fluid and electrolyte imbalance. In Phipps WJ, Sands J, Marek J, editors: *Medical-surgical nursing: concepts and clinical practice*, ed 6, St Louis, 1999, Mosby.

Table 5-13	Overview of Acid–Base Imbalances		
Mechanism	**Etiologic Factors**	**Clinical Manifestations**	**Treatment**
Respiratory Acidosis			
Hypoventilation	Acute respiratory failure COPD Neuromuscular disease • Guillain-Barré • Myasthenia gravis Respiratory center depression Drugs • Barbiturates • Sedatives • Narcotics • Anesthetic CNS lesions Tumor Stroke Inadequate mechanical ventilation	Hypercapnia, restlessness, disorientation, confusion, sleepiness, visual disturbances, headache, flushing, dyspnea, cyanosis, decreased deep tendon reflexes, hyperkalemia, palpitation, pH <7.35, $PaCO_2$ >45 mm Hg	Treatment underlying cause; support ventilation; correct electrolyte imbalance
Excess carbon dioxide production	Hypermetabolism Sepsis Burns		

Continued

Table 5-13 Overview of Acid–Base Imbalances—cont'd

Mechanism	Etiologic Factors	Clinical Manifestations	Treatment
Respiratory Alkalosis			

Hyperventilation	Hypoxemia
	  Pulmonary embolus
	  High altitude
	Impaired lung expansion
	  Pulmonary fibrosis
	  Ascites
	  Scoliosis
	  Pregnancy*
	Congestive heart failure
	Stimulation of respiratory center
	  Anxiety hyperventilation
	  Encephalitis/meningitis (hepatic failure)
	  Salicylates (aspirin overdose)
	  Theophylline
	  CNS trauma
	  CNS tumor
	  Excessive exercise
	  Extreme stress
	  Severe pain
	Mechanical overventilation
		Tachypnea, hypocapnia, dizziness, difficulty concentrating, numbness and tingling, blurred vision, diaphoresis, dry mouth, muscle cramps, carpopedal spasm, muscle twitching and weakness, hyperreflexia, arrhythmias pH >7.45, $PaCO_2$ <35 mm Hg, hypokalemia, hypocalcemia (see Table 5-10)	Treat underlying cause; increase carbon dioxide retention (rebreathing, sedation)

Metabolic Acidosis			

Acid excess	Renal failure (acid retention)
	Diabetic or alcoholic ketoacidosis
	Lactic acidosis (see text)
	Starvation and fasting
	Ingested toxins
	  • Aspirin
	  • Antifreeze
	  • Cyanide
	  • Iron
		Hyperventilation (compensatory), muscular twitching, weakness, malaise, nausea, vomiting, diarrhea, headache, hyperkalemia (cardiac arrhythmias), pH <7.35, HCO_3^-, <22 mm mEq/L, $PaCO_2$ normal (35-45 mm Hg) or slightly decreased, coma (death)	Treat underlying cause, correct electrolyte imbalance; $NaCO_3$ for severe acidosis (pH <7.2)

Base deficit	Severe diarrhea (HCO_3^- loss) Renal failure (inability to reabsorb HCO_3^-)		
Metabolic Alkalosis			

Fixed acid loss (with base excess)	Hypokalemia
	  Diuretic therapy
	  Steroids
	Vomiting
	Nasogastric suctioning
		Hypoventilation (compensatory): dysrhythmias, nausea, prolonged vomiting, diarrhea, confusion, irritability, agitation, restlessness, muscle twitching, cramping, hypotonia, weakness, Trousseau sign, paresthesias, seizures, coma, hypokalemia, pH >7.45, $PaCO_2$ normal (35-45 mm Hg) or slightly increased	Treat underlying cause; administer potassium chloride

Excessive HCO_3^- intake	Peptic ulcer
	  • Milk-alkali syndrome
	  • Excessive intake of antacidsOvercorrection of acidosis
	Massive blood transfusion
		Hypochloremia	

Excessive HCO_3^- resorption	Hyperaldosteronism Cushing disease		

COPD, chronic obstructive pulmonary disease; HCO_3^-, bicarbonate ion; $NaCO_3$, sodium bicarbonate; $PaCO_2$, partial pressure of carbon dioxide.
*In the third trimester of pregnancy, the hormone progesterone also stimulates respiration.

characteristics of acid–base imbalance described in this chapter, potassium excess (hyperkalemia) is associated with both respiratory and metabolic acidosis, and neuromuscular hyperexcitability is associated with both respiratory and metabolic alkalosis.[79]

MEDICAL MANAGEMENT

DIAGNOSIS. Pulse oximetry is used most often to measure oxygen saturation, yet it does not provide needed information regarding the effectiveness of ventilation or the pH of the blood. A more comprehensive procedure is the arterial blood gas test (see Table 40-18).

This measurement is important in the diagnosis and treatment of ventilation, oxygen transport, and acid–base problems. The test measures the amount of dissolved oxygen and carbon dioxide in arterial blood and indicates acid–bases status by measurement of the arterial blood pH. The pH is inversely proportional to the hydrogen ion concentration (H^+) in the blood. Therefore, as the hydrogen ion concentration (H^+) increases (acidosis), the pH decreases; as the hydrogen ion concentration (H^+) decreases (alkalosis), the pH increases.

The PCO_2 is a measure of the *partial pressure of carbon dioxide* in the blood. PCO_2 is termed the *respiratory component* in acid–base measurement because the carbon dioxide level is primarily controlled by the lungs. As the carbon dioxide level increases, the pH decreases (respiratory acidosis); as the carbon dioxide level decreases, the pH increases (respiratory alkalosis).

Treatment. Treatment in acid–base imbalances is directed toward the underlying cause and correction of any coexisting electrolyte imbalance. For example, respiratory infections contributing to ventilatory failure (respiratory acidosis) are managed with appropriate antibiotic therapy, pulmonary hygiene, oxygen support, and possibly, continuous mechanical ventilation. Use of pharmaceutical agents that depress the respiratory control center is minimized. Dialysis may be indicated in renal failure (metabolic acidosis) or overdose of toxins.

Respiratory Acidosis

Respiratory acidosis is nearly always a result of hypoventilation and subsequent retention of carbon dioxide (CO_2). In a therapy setting, respiratory acidosis is most commonly observed in the population with COPD or asthma, depressed CNS (drugs, infection, or brain injury), or whenever the diaphragm is impaired (e.g., Guillain-Barré syndrome, myasthenia gravis, or chest wall deformities); secondary to burns; and as a result of lesions of the CNS (e.g., tumor, stroke, or muscular dystrophy).

The respiratory system has an important role in maintaining acid–base equilibrium. In response to an increase in the hydrogen ion concentration in body fluids, the respiratory rate increases, causing more CO_2 to be released from the lung.

Anything that impairs this CO_2 exhalation causes the CO_2 to accumulate in the blood, where it unites with water to form carbonic acid (H_2CO_3), decreasing the blood pH. In addition, the kidneys begin to excrete more acid and retain more bicarbonate to further correct the acid imbalance.

Respiratory acidosis can be acute because of a sudden failure in ventilation, or chronic, as with long-term pulmonary disease (e.g., COPD). In the *acute* episode, the blood buffer systems cannot compensate to restore the acid–base balance because normal blood circulation and tissue perfusion are impaired. The lungs may not be functioning properly and the kidneys require more time to compensate than the acute condition permits.

Chronic respiratory acidosis results from gradual and irreversible loss of ventilatory function. Although there is increased retention of CO_2, the kidneys have time to compensate by retaining bicarbonate and thereby maintaining a pH within tolerable limits. However, if even a minor respiratory infection develops, the person is subjected to a rapidly developing state of acute acidosis because the lungs remove only a limited amount of carbon dioxide.

Clinical Manifestations

Acute respiratory acidosis produces CNS disturbances. Effects range from restlessness, confusion, and apprehension to somnolence (sleepiness), with a fine or flapping tremor (see "Asterixis" in Chapter 17) or coma. The person may report headaches and shortness of breath with retraction and use of accessory muscles. On examination, DTRs may be depressed. This disorder may also cause cardiovascular abnormalities such as tachycardia, hypertension, atrial and ventricular arrhythmias, and in severe acidosis, hypotension with vasodilation.

Respiratory Alkalosis

Respiratory alkalosis, the opposite of respiratory acidosis, occurs as a result of a loss of acid without compensation and most commonly when the lungs excrete excessive amounts of carbon dioxide (hyperventilation).

Conditions associated with respiratory alkalosis fall into the following two categories:

1. *Pulmonary*, caused by hypoxemia in early stage pulmonary problems (e.g., pulmonary edema, pulmonary embolism, pneumonia, and acute asthma) and by overuse of a mechanical ventilator
2. *Nonpulmonary*, which includes anxiety, pain, fever, high environmental temperature, pregnancy, drug toxicities (salicylates, theophylline), CNS disease (brainstem tumors, infection), high altitude, and hyperthyroidism (see Table 5-13).

Hyperventilation and the subsequent respiratory alkalosis is a common finding in ICU patients.

Clinical Manifestations

The cardinal sign of respiratory alkalosis is deep, rapid breathing, possibly exceeding 40 breaths/min (much like the Kussmaul respirations that characterize diabetic acidosis) (see Table 5-13). Such hyperventilation usually leads to CNS and neuromuscular disturbances such as dizziness or light-headedness (caused by below-normal CO_2 levels that decrease cerebral blood flow); inability to concentrate; tingling and numbness of the extremities and around the mouth; blurred vision; diaphoresis; dry mouth; muscle cramps; carpopedal (wrist and foot) spasms; twitching (possibly progressing to tetany); and muscle weakness. Severe respiratory alkalosis may cause cardiac arrhythmias, seizures, and syncope.

Metabolic Acidosis

Metabolic acidosis is an accumulation of acids or a deficit of bases in the blood. This type of acidosis can occur with an acid gain (e.g., ketones with diabetic ketoacidosis, lactic acid with hypoxia, toxins such as ethylene glycol, and renal failure) or bicarbonate loss (e.g., diarrhea).

Metabolic acidosis can be divided into two categories: (1) metabolic acidosis with an anion gap and (2) metabolic acidosis with a normal anion gap. An anion gap is based on the principle of electrical neutrality in the body (i.e., cations should equal anions). The anion gap can be estimated from the equation: anion gap = sodium – (chloride + bicarbonate). A normal anion gap is positive (sodium constitutes over 90% of cations), usually 12±4 (some labs may use 7±4).

However, if the anion gap is elevated, there are unmeasured (and unaccountable) anionic molecules present in the blood. The osmolal gap can also be calculated (expected osmolality – calculated osmolality), which demonstrates the presence of low-molecular weight substances seen in toxic overdoses. Table 5-13 lists specific etiologic factors. Metabolic acidosis with an elevated anion gap can be caused by toxic ingestions (methanol, ethylene glycol, isoniazid, iron, ethanol, salicylates, paraldehyde, solvents, and inhalants), uremia, diabetic ketoacidosis, lactic acidosis, and starvation.

Ketoacidosis, a major cause of metabolic acidosis, occurs when insufficient insulin for the proper use of glucose results in increased breakdown of fat (lipolysis). This accelerated fat breakdown produces ketones and other acids. Although the body attempts to neutralize these increased acids, the plasma bicarbonate (HCO_3^-) is depleted.

In the case of uremia associated with *renal failure*, the failing kidney cannot produce the necessary bicarbonate to buffer the acid load that accumulates in the body. *Lactic acidosis* occurs as excess lactic acid is produced during strenuous exercise or when oxygen is insufficient (hypoxemia). Other risk factors for developing lactic acidosis include cardiopulmonary failure, shock, acute pulmonary edema, carbon monoxide poisoning, smoke inhalation, sepsis, trauma, grand mal seizure, adverse reactions to medications or toxins, alcohol abuse, liver disease, cancer, and AIDS.

Alcoholic ketoacidosis occurs when a person abruptly stops drinking alcohol and has prolonged vomiting associated with a background of fasting or starvation. This most often occurs in adults with alcoholism, although it can be seen in younger, inexperienced binge drinkers. Because of a low nutritional state, insulin production is reduced while other counterregulatory hormones are increased. Lipolysis is upregulated with release of fatty acids, which are then oxidized to ketone bodies. Many other processes such as dehydration and the metabolism of alcohol contribute to further ketone production.

Metabolic acidosis with a normal anion gap is caused by a loss of bicarbonate (e.g., loss from GI sources),[264] but can also be seen with the addition of hydrochloric acid (e.g., parenteral hyperalimentation) or decreased ammonia production (e.g., moderate renal failure). Another important cause is RTA.

RTA is further categorized as an RTA associated with hypokalemia or hyperkalemia. RTA with hypokalemia is the result of a defect in the kidney that results in decreased bicarbonate reabsorption (proximal type II) or a defect in hydrogen ion secretion (distal type 1). Hyperkalemic RTA can be either mineralocorticoid-sensitive or mineralocorticoid-resistant (rare). Mineralocorticoid-sensitive is secondary to adrenal insufficiency (primary hypoaldosteronism, Addison disease) or hyporeninemic hypoaldosteronism (diabetes mellitus, chronic renal disease).

Clinical Manifestations

The symptoms of metabolic acidosis can include muscular twitching, weakness, malaise, nausea, vomiting, diarrhea, and headache (see Table 5-13). If the acidosis is severe, myocardial depression and hypotension can occur. Compensatory hyperventilation may occur as a result of stimulation of the hypothalamus as the body attempts to rid itself of excess CO_2. As the acid level goes up, these symptoms progress to stupor, unconsciousness, coma, and death.

Some causes of metabolic acidosis have symptoms that may be present and point to the diagnosis. Diabetics with ketoacidosis may have breath with a fruity odor in the presence of ketone production. Methanol ingestion produces visual changes, whereas salicylate overdose leads to tinnitus and vertigo.

Metabolic Alkalosis

Metabolic alkalosis occurs when either an abnormal loss of acid or excess accumulation of bicarbonate occurs. The most common cause is chloride and volume depletion from either a GI source or hydrogen chloride loss through the kidneys (diuretics). Postoperative loss of acids through vomiting or gastric suctioning may also result in metabolic alkalosis. In the outpatient setting, diarrhea, excessive use of laxatives, diuretics, antacids, and milk (milk alkali syndrome) may also lead to metabolic alkalosis. Bulimia with vomiting and diuretic abuse associated with an eating disorder are notable causes, particularly in the young (see discussion of eating disorders, chapter 3). Table 5-13 lists other causes.

Clinical Manifestations

Signs and symptoms occur as the body attempts to correct the acid–base imbalance, primarily through hypoventilation. Respirations are shallow and slow as the lungs attempt to compensate by building up carbonic acid stores. Clinical manifestations may be mild at first, with muscle weakness, irritability, confusion, and muscle twitching (see Table 5-13). If untreated, the condition progresses and the person may become comatose, with possible seizures, cardiac arrhythmias, and respiratory paralysis.

Aging and Acid–Base Regulation

Acid–base disturbances are common in the elderly and frequently determine outcome and prognosis.[347] The normal aging process results in changes in the lung such as decreased ventilatory capacity and loss of alveolar surface area for gas exchange; thus older adults are prone to respiratory acidosis caused by hypoventilation and to respiratory alkalosis caused by hypoxemia and subsequent hyperventilation. Older adults are often taking multiple medications for hypertension (diuretics) or cardiovascular disease that may contribute to hypokalemia and metabolic alkalosis. Respiratory compensation in these conditions can be compromised because of the structural and functional changes mentioned. Respiratory alkalosis may be the result of hyperventilation caused by anxiety, CNS infection/infarction, pulmonary embolism, or pulmonary edema.

Several alterations in the kidney of the elderly lead to an inability to compensate for acid–base changes in order to maintain homeostasis. There is a decline in the GFR and capacity to excrete an acid load, resulting in a chronic, low-level metabolic acidosis. Complications may be nephrolithiasis, bone demineralization, and muscle wasting. Aldosterone is less effective in older adults, as is ammonia buffering. These changes limit renal compensation for respiratory imbalances and place the individual at higher risk for metabolic imbalance.[294,350]

SPECIAL IMPLICATIONS FOR THE THERAPIST 5-13

Acid–Base Imbalances

The therapist must observe clients at risk for acid–base imbalance for any early symptoms. This is especially true for people with known pulmonary, cardiovascular, or renal disease; clients in a hypermetabolic state, such as occurs in fever, sepsis, or burns; clients receiving total parenteral nutrition or enteral tube feedings that are high in carbohydrates; mechanically ventilated clients; clients with insulin-dependent diabetes; older clients whose age-related decreases in respiratory and renal function may limit their ability to compensate for acid–base disturbances; and clients with vomiting, diarrhea, or enteric drainage.[294] Specific reference values in acid–base disorders are listed in Tables 5-13 and 40-3.

Client and family education in the prevention of acute episodes of metabolic acidosis, particularly diabetic ketoacidosis, is essential. A fruity breath odor from rising acid levels (acetone) may be detected by the therapist treating someone who has uncontrolled diabetes.

The therapist should not hesitate to ask the client about this breath odor, as immediate medical intervention is required for diabetic ketoacidosis. Dehydration occurs rapidly as a result of severe hyperglycemia. A rising pulse rate and a drop in blood pressure are critical (and often late) indicators of a fluid volume deficit caused by dehydration.

Safety measures to avoid injury during involuntary muscular contractions are the same as for convulsions or epileptic seizures. Vigorous restraint can cause orthopedic injuries as the muscles contract strongly against resistance. Placing padding to protect the person is a key to prevention of injury.

Measures that facilitate breathing are essential to client care during respiratory acidosis. Frequent turning, coughing, and deep breathing exercises to encourage oxygen–carbon dioxide exchange are beneficial. Postural drainage, unless contraindicated by the client's condition, may be effective in promoting adequate ventilation.

In the case of respiratory hyperventilation, rebreathing CO_2 in a paper sack is helpful, as well as encouraging the individual to hold the breath. Oxygen may be given to reduce respiratory effort and the resultant blowing off of CO_2 by the person who has anoxia caused by pulmonary infection or CHF. Individuals with COPD may retain CO_2; the use of oxygen is contraindicated in these clients because it can further depress the respiratory drive, causing death.

Any client receiving diuretic therapy must be monitored for signs of potassium depletion (e.g., postural hypotension, muscle weakness, and fatigue; see Table 5-10) and alkalosis (see Table 5-13). Decreased respiratory rate may be an indication of compensation by the lungs, but the physician must make this assessment. Signs of neural irritability, such as the Trousseau sign (see Fig. 5-8), may be seen when taking blood pressure measurements, and they are helpful in detecting early stages of tetany caused by calcium deficiency.

REFERENCES

To enhance this text and add value for the reader, all references are included on the companion Evolve site that accompanies this textbook. The reader can view the reference source and access it online whenever possible.

CHAPTER 6

Injury, Inflammation, Healing, and Repair*

ROLANDO T. LAZARO • ANNIE BURKE-DOE

OVERVIEW

Pathology is defined as the structural and functional changes in the body caused by disease or trauma. Understanding the normal structure and function of the tissues is required before the discussion of pathology.

The organization of the material presented in this chapter parallels the processes underlying pathology—that is, cell injury and the factors causing this injury, inflammation as a secondary response to cell injury, and tissue healing and repair, which are essential components to return the tissue into optimal function. Figure 6-1 illustrates the possible cellular responses to stress and injury and serves as a roadmap for our discussion in this chapter. A thorough understanding of the concepts that underpin cellular injury, inflammation, healing, and repair provides a solid foundation to facilitate comprehension of the other topics presented in this text.

CELL INJURY

Introduction

The structural and functional changes produced by pathology start with injury to the cells that make up the tissues. Mild injury produced by stressors leads to sublethal alterations of the affected cells that may be reversible, whereas moderate or severe injury leads to lethal alterations that are likely irreversible, and can lead to cell death. We start by discussing the most common causes of cellular injury.

Causes of Cell (Tissue) Injury

Cells may be damaged by a variety of factors. The most important causes are listed in Box 6-1. As mentioned earlier, cell injury may be reversible or irreversible. Whether the injury is reversible is dependent on the cell's ability to withstand the derangement of homeostatic mechanisms and its adaptability (i.e., ability to return to a state of homeostasis). Reversing the injury and achieving homeostasis are determined by a combination of factors including the mechanism of injury, length of time the injury is present without intervention, and the severity of the injury.

Ischemia

At the tissue or organ level, ischemia occurs when the blood flow is insufficient to maintain cell homeostasis and metabolic function. This can be due to a reduction in flow or an increase in metabolism of the tissue beyond the capability of the arterial vascular system. Insufficient blood flow results in a partial (hypoxia) or total (anoxia) reduction in oxygen supply; a decreased delivery of nutrients; and decreased removal of waste products from the tissue. The lack of oxygen leads to loss of aerobic metabolism. The resulting reduction in adenosine triphosphate synthesis leads to accumulation of ions and fluid intracellularly. The cells swell and their function is compromised. This concept is discussed further in the section on *Reversible Cell Injury* in this chapter.

Hypoxia or anoxia may occur under many circumstances, including obstruction of the respiratory tree (e.g., suffocation secondary to drowning), inadequate transport of oxygen across the respiratory surfaces of the lung (e.g., pneumonia), inadequate transport of oxygen in the blood (e.g., anemia), or an inability of the cell to use oxygen for cellular respiration (e.g., carbon monoxide poisoning).[117]

Ischemia is usually the result of arterial lumen obstruction and narrowing caused by atherosclerosis and/or an intravascular clot called a *thrombus*. Ischemia, resulting in myocardial infarction (MI) and stroke (lack of blood flow to the heart or brain, respectively), can cause death of tissue (necrosis) and accounts for two of the three leading causes of mortality in industrialized nations.[230]

Infectious Agents

Infectious agents, such as bacteria, viruses, mycoplasmas, fungi, rickettsiae, protozoa, prions, and helminths (see Chapter 8), may also cause cell injury or death. Bacterial and viral agents are responsible for the vast majority of infections.

Bacterial infections cause cell injury primarily by invading tissue and releasing exotoxins and endotoxins that can cause cell lysis and degradation of extracellular matrix and aid in the spread of the infection. Injury can also result from the inflammatory/immunologic reactions induced by bacteria in the host. For example, exotoxins may be released by clostridial organisms that cause gas gangrene, tetanus, and botulism.

*The authors would like to acknowledge the contributions of Steve Tepper and Michael McKeough in the second and third editions of this text.

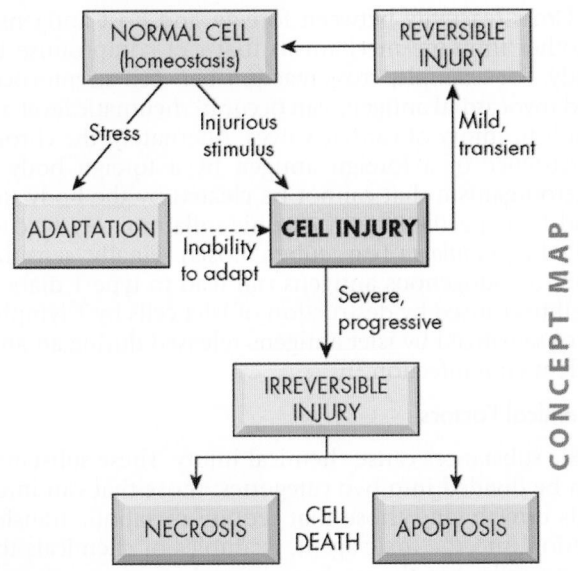

Figure 6-1

Cellular response to stress and injurious stimuli. (From Kumar V, et al: *Robbins and Cotran pathologic basis of disease,* ed 8, Philadelphia, 2010, Saunders Elsevier.)

Box 6-1

CAUSES OF CELL INJURY

- Ischemia (lack of blood supply)
- Infectious agents
- Immune reactions
- Genetic factors
- Nutritional factors
- Physical factors
- Chemical factors

Box 6-2

ACTIONS OF CYTOKINES: INTERLEUKIN-1 AND TUMOR NECROSIS FACTOR

Local

- Stimulates leukocyte adhesion to endothelium
- Modulates the coagulation cascade
- Stimulates production and/or secretion of inflammatory mediators (including IL-1 itself)
- Activates fibroblasts, chondrocytes, osteoclasts

Systemic

Metabolic

- Induces fever
- Increases body metabolism
- Decreases appetite
- Induces sleep
- Induces adrenocorticotrophic hormone release to secrete corticosteroids
- Nonspecific resistance to infection

Hemodynamic

- Causes hypotension
- Hypovolemia (sepsis)

Hematologic

- Changes blood chemistry (see text)
- Activates endothelial, macrophage, and resting T cells
- Increases neutrophils in circulation
- Decreases lymphocytes in circulation
- Stimulates synthesis of collagen and collagenases

Clostridium tetani, for example, releases an exotoxin that is preferentially absorbed by the alpha motor neurons and delivered into the central nervous system (CNS). Once inside the CNS, the exotoxin crosses the synapse of the anterior horn cell and interferes with release of inhibitory neurotransmitters. This disruption of homeostasis eventually causes the activation of motor neurons that in turn cause involuntary muscular contractions (tetanus).

When microorganisms or their toxins are present in the blood, a condition called *sepsis* can occur (see further discussion in Chapter 5). Endotoxins released from gram-negative bacteria induce the synthesis of cytokines (extracts of normal leukocytes such as tumor necrosis factor [TNF] and interleukins [ILs]) that are responsible for many of the systemic manifestations of sepsis (Box 6-2). In sepsis, endothelial cell damage, loss of plasma volume, and maldistribution of blood flow result in hypovolemia. Cardiovascular collapse may ensue and lead to a condition called *septic shock*. The detection of an infectious agent initiates an inflammatory reaction designed to contain and inactivate the pathogen, but the magnitude of this defensive response by the host may also cause cellular or tissue destruction in the infected area.

Viruses kill cells by one of two mechanisms (Fig. 6-2) and are the consequence of complete redirection of the cell's biosynthesis toward viral replication. The first is a direct cytopathic effect usually found with ribonucleic (RNA) viruses. These viruses kill from within by disturbing various cellular processes or by disrupting the integrity of the nucleus and/or plasma membrane.

The second mechanism is an indirect cytopathic effect mediated by immune mechanisms. In this process, virally encoded proteins become inserted into the plasma membrane of the host cell (forming a channel) and alter the permeability of the cell membrane to ions. The resulting loss of the ionic barrier leads to cell swelling and death. DNA type viruses also kill cells through an indirect cytopathic effect by integrating themselves into the cellular genome. These viruses encode the production of foreign proteins, which are exposed on the cell surface and recognized by the body's immune cells. Immunocompetent cells, such as the T lymphocyte, recognize these virally encoded proteins inserted into the plasma membrane of host cells and attack and destroy the infected cell. When the immune system is compromised or if the number of invading microorganisms overwhelms the immune system, disease (and the symptoms of illness) occurs (see further discussion, Chapter 7).

Immune Reactions

Although the immune system normally functions in defense against foreign antigens, sometimes the system becomes overzealous in its activity, leading to hypersensitivities ranging from a mild allergy to life-threatening anaphylactic reactions or autoimmune (attacking oneself) disorders. The mechanisms by which the immune system can lead to cell

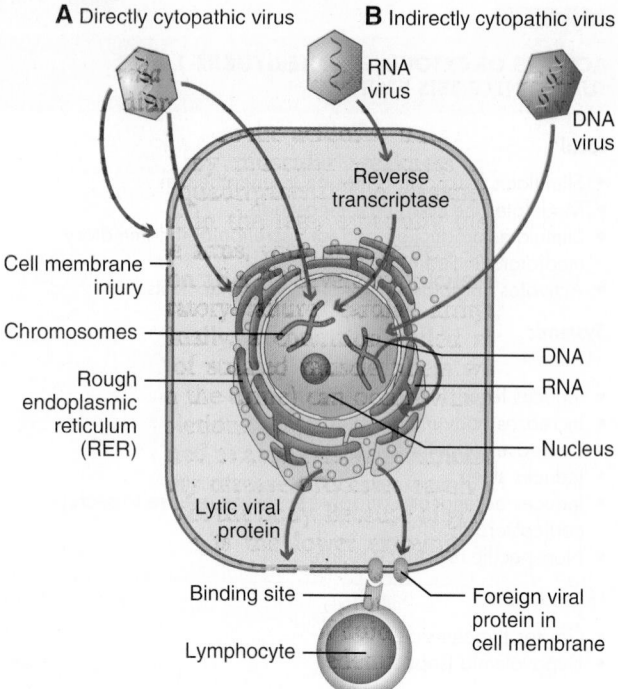

A Directly cytopathic virus   **B** Indirectly cytopathic virus

RNA virus

DNA virus

Reverse transcriptase

Cell membrane injury

Chromosomes

Rough endoplasmic reticulum (RER)

DNA

RNA

Nucleus

Lytic viral protein

Binding site

Lymphocyte

Foreign viral protein in cell membrane

Figure 6-2

Mechanisms of cell destruction by viruses. A, Direct cytopathic effect: RNA virus inserts itself in a receptor on the cell membrane and is brought into the cell. The RNA virus is altered into DNA by reverse transcriptase. The DNA within the nucleus of the cell forms various types of RNA that allows for protein synthesis in the rough endoplasmic reticulum (RER). The protein formed inserts itself into the cell membrane, forming a channel that allows ions and extracellular fluid to enter, leading to cell lysis (directly killing the cell). **B,** Indirect cytopathic effect mediated by immune mechanisms: DNA virus inserts itself in a receptor on the cell membrane and is brought into the cell. The DNA virus within the nucleus of the cell forms various types of RNA that allow for protein synthesis in the RER. This foreign viral protein inserts into the cell membrane and becomes a neoantigen. This neoantigen will be recognized by the T lymphocytes that will react to and kill (indirectly) the infected cell. (From Damjanov I: *Pathology for the health-related professions,* ed 4, St. Louis, MO, 2012, Elsevier.)

injury or death include antibody attachment, complement activation, and activation of the inflammatory cells (e.g., neutrophils, macrophages, T and B lymphocytes, mast cells, and basophils). See Chapter 7 for a complete discussion of the immune system and its function.

Cell injury and disease can be caused by the immune system in numerous ways. For example, allergies are caused by the presence of high numbers of a specific antibody-E (IgE) on the surface of specialized cells (mast cells and basophils, which release histamine), resulting in mild, moderate, or severe allergic reactions. Examples of mild reactions include the runny nose and watery eyes caused by a mild allergic response.

Moderate reactions include severe hypoxia caused by asthmatic bronchoconstriction. Severe reactions can result in a potentially life-threatening circulatory collapse seen in anaphylaxis (a whole-body allergic reaction). The presence of what would normally be considered optimal ratios of antigen to antibody in the circulation may lead to damage of filtration in the kidney because of excess deposition of antigen-antibody complexes in the glomeruli.

Cross-reactivity between foreign and host antigens is another immune mechanism that can compromise the body. For example, cross-reaction between streptococcal and myocardial antigens can occur in rheumatic fever and result in injury of cardiac valves. Alternately, the chronic persistence of a foreign antigen by a foreign body or microorganism that cannot be cleared by the body may lead to a specific type of chronic inflammatory reaction called a *granuloma* (e.g., tuberculosis). Finally, sensitization to endogenous antigens can lead to type 1 diabetes mellitus caused by destruction of islet cells by T lymphocytes sensitized by islet antigens released during an antecedent viral infection.[217]

Chemical Factors

Toxic substances cause chemical injury. These substances can be divided into two categories: those that can injure cells directly and those that require metabolic transformation into the toxic agent. Examples of chemicals that injure cells directly are heavy metals, such as mercury, that bind to and disrupt critical membrane proteins and a number of toxins and drugs, such as alkylating agents, used in chemotherapy.

Alkylating agents, such as nitrogen mustards, induce cross-linking of DNA and inactivation of other essential cellular constituents. Carbon tetrachloride and acetaminophen are examples of inert substances that must be metabolized to reactive intermediates to cause cell injury. Taken in large amounts, most medications can be toxic, and many are even lethal. Suicide by drug overdose is a common example of drug-induced chemical toxicity.

Free Radical Formation. An important mechanism of cell injury and disease is the production of reactive oxygen species (ROS) sometimes referred to as the formation of *free radicals.* Free radicals are an integral part of metabolism and are formed continuously in the body. They can exert positive effects (e.g., on the immune system) or negative effects (e.g., lipid, protein, or DNA oxidation). A variety of normal and pathologic reactions can lead to the activation of oxygen by the sequential addition or subtraction, respectively, of one electron at a time (Fig. 6-3).

For example, the body's natural process of using oxygen and food to produce energy can create free radicals as a by-product of these functions. These unpaired electrons are reactive and commonly bind to oxygen for stabilization. The oxygen then binds to hydrogen for stabilization. This series of reactions generated by normal cellular metabolism results in a phenomenon referred to as *oxygen toxicity* and yields superoxide (O_2^-), hydrogen peroxide (H_2O_2), and hydroxyl radical (OH^-). These forms of reactive oxygen are referred to as *oxygen radicals,* which are toxic to cells.

The cellular enzymes always scavenging the body to protect cells from this type of injury normally inactivate these radicals and convert the free radical back to usable oxygen. Some unstable oxygen molecules (i.e., free radicals) enable the body to fight inflammation, kill bacteria, and help regulate the autonomic nervous system.

However, if produced in excess amounts (a situation referred to as *oxidative stress*), these radicals can become the mechanism of cell injury and subsequent cell death. Free radicals have been considered central to the damaging effects that can lead to conditions such as heart disease, cerebrovascular disease, diabetes mellitus, cataracts,

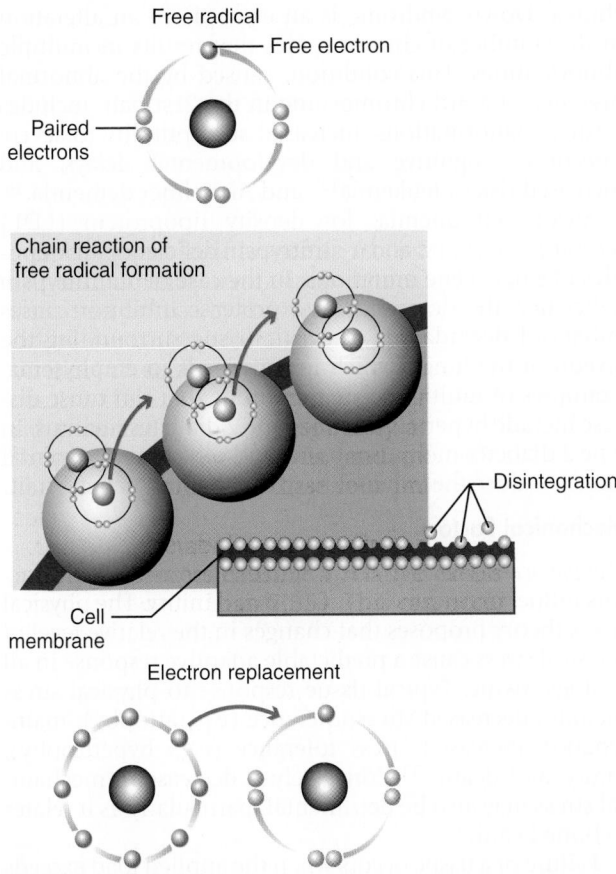

Figure 6-3

The oxidative process and formation of free radicals. Normal metabolic processes and a variety of other extrinsic factors, such as pollution, poor nutrition, and exposure to toxic chemicals, can result in the formation of free radicals when normal oxygen atoms lose one of their four paired electrons. The resulting unstable atom attempts to replace the missing electron by "stealing" an electron from a healthy cell, creating another unstable atom (free radical) and setting off a chain reaction referred to as oxidation. Oxidation as a by-product of metabolism damages cell membranes, leading to intrinsic cellular damage, a part of the normal aging process. Free radical damage (oxidation) is believed to alter the way cells encode genetic information in the DNA and may contribute to a variety of diseases and disorders. Antioxidant molecules freely give up an electron to stabilize the oxygen atom without becoming unstable and without initiating a chain reaction.

Parkinson disease, Alzheimer disease, premature aging, and cancer.[203] In fact, research has shown that oxidative stresses caused by ROS are factors in more than 90% of lifestyle-related diseases.[146]

Reactive oxygen species or free radical formation occurs as a result of many events such as prolonged exercise; exposure to high levels of oxygen, irradiation, ultraviolet or fluorescent light, pollutants, tobacco smoke, and pesticides (airborne or in food); drug overdose; heat stress; and the reperfusion injury that is induced by the restoration of normal blood flow after a period of ischemia such as occurs during organ transplantation or after MI.

Free radical toxicity may also be the underlying cause of degeneration of neurons located in the *substantia nigra* leading to the loss of dopamine necessary for the normal control[203] of movements that produces the abnormal movements seen in Parkinson disease.[187]

Antioxidants. Oxygen-like atoms are the most likely source of free radicals in the human body; the utilization of oxygen as a life-supporting mechanism means oxidative stress is an inescapable part of the human biologic system. The simultaneous presence of antioxidants is an adaptive response to help the body ward off the potentially harmful effects of oxygen and its derivatives, including free radicals.[232]

Antioxidants neutralize the extra free radicals and keep them from taking electrons from other molecules that would otherwise result in cellular and DNA damage. A variety of enzymatic and nonenzymatic defense mechanisms are present within cells to perform the function of antioxidants detoxifying ROS and protecting the cells from this type of injury. These are called *endogenous antioxidants*. Researchers are finding a variety of uses for natural antioxidants in combating the effects of aging and disease.

There are also *exogenous antioxidants* that can be taken from outside the body through our diet. Vitamin C, E, and beta-carotene are three important exogenous antioxidants. Over 200 antioxidants have been identified through food or plant substances. For example, the Age-Related Eye Disease Study (AREDS) study concluded that high doses of antioxidants such as vitamin C and E; beta-carotene and copper significantly slow the progression of age-related macular degeneration. Researchers postulated that the antioxidants bind with the free radicals that are produced following the absorption of light in the retina.[3]

In the case of the prostate, lycopene, the compound that makes tomatoes red, is a potent antioxidant that may be potentially effective in promoting prostate health.[83,121]

Multiple trials are ongoing to investigate oxidation and its effect on cellular injury, aging, and disease (e.g., cancer, heart disease, and cataracts) and the use of antioxidants found naturally in food and plants to combat oxidative stress, thereby preventing or possibly modifying diseases at the cellular level. Animal and human studies have confirmed that regular, moderate physical activity and exercise strengthen the antioxidant defense system, whereas intense or prolonged, strenuous exercise (especially in a person who has a sedentary lifestyle) lead to oxidative stress and may be potentially harmful.[61,66,86,90,169]

Nitric Oxide. The nitric oxide (NO) molecule is composed of one nitrogen atom and one oxygen atom. It is present in all mammals including humans and is one of the few gaseous signaling molecules known. NO should not be confused with nitrous oxide (N_2O), a general anesthetic, or with nitrogen dioxide (NO_2), which is a poisonous air pollutant.

The nitric oxide molecule is a free radical, which is relevant to understanding its high reactivity. NO is recognized as an important modulator of an enormous number of physiologic responses. Reduced NO bioavailability that is a result of oxidative stress seems to be the common molecular disorder causing many pathologic effects within the body. For example, decreased NO bioavailability is associated with risk factors for cardiovascular disease.[77]

NO assists in long-term memory. It also influences neuronal transmission by increasing the permeability of nerve endings, making acetylcholine transfer across the synapses easier. NO alters the ability of the gastrointestinal mucosa to resist injury induced by toxins, thereby influencing the immune system. NO inhibits virally induced cytokine and chemokine production, possibly combating the common cold.[170] It also stimulates collagen synthesis for wound healing, modulates fracture healing, and is useful in the treatment of tendinopathy.[160,161,174]

NO is an antilipid that provides a nonstick coating to the lining of blood vessels, much like *polytetrafluoroethylene*, more commonly known as Teflon® (DuPont Corporation, Wilmington, DE). This helps explain how NO might prevent heart attacks and strokes and why nitroglycerin works—nitroglycerin is converted to NO inside vascular tissue, where it relaxes smooth muscle in arteries and causes blood vessels to dilate. It also controls platelet function by preventing platelets from clumping together, thus preventing the formation of blood clots.

Exercise and Free Radicals. Physical activity and exercise can have positive or negative effects on oxidative stress depending on training load, training specificity, and basal level of training. Oxidative stress seems to be involved in muscular fatigue and overtraining.[73] Excessive exercise has been shown to induce DNA damage in peripheral leukocytes. Exhaustion of the leukocyte ROS may reduce the body's ability to combat microbial invasions (i.e., infections) before the system has been restored.[157] On the other hand, moderate stress in the form of regular exercise training may have protective effects against exercise-induced DNA damage.[181]

Current evidence supports improved NO bioavailability with exercise training. Up-regulation of endogenous antioxidant defense systems and complex regulation of repair systems are seen in response to training and exercise.[36] Up-regulation of antioxidants and modulation of the repair response may be mechanisms by which exercise can influence our health in a positive way.[71] Regular, long-term aerobic exercise has been shown to reduce migraine pain severity, frequency, and duration, possibly a result of increased NO production.[154]

Researchers are studying the effect of NO on free radicals that cannot be stabilized or removed. Studies show that NO appears to play a role in exercise-induced dilation of blood vessels supplying cardiac and skeletal muscle. Exercise training enhances NO-mediated vasodilation. The exact mechanism is not clear yet, but a growing number of studies suggest that exercise training, perhaps via increased capacity for NO formation, retards atherosclerosis.[136] There is also accumulating evidence that NO is involved in skeletal muscle glucose uptake during exercise.[137,156]

Genetic Factors

Genetic alterations lead to cellular injury or death by three primary means: (1) alterations in the structure or number of chromosomes that induce multiple abnormalities, (2) single mutations of genes that cause changes in the amount or functions of proteins, and (3) multiple gene mutations that interact with environmental factors to cause multifactorial disorders. These genetic alterations can be severe enough to cause fetal death in utero, resulting in spontaneous abortion. Some may cause congenital malformations, whereas others do not manifest pathologic alterations until midlife such as Huntington chorea. Down syndrome is an example of an alteration in the number of chromosomes that results in multiple abnormalities. This condition, caused by the abnormal presence of a 3rd chromosome in the 21st pair, includes cardiac malformations, increased susceptibility to severe infections, cognitive and developmental delays, and increased risk of leukemia[135] and Alzheimer dementia.[46]

Sickle cell anemia, low-density lipoprotein (LDL) receptor deficiency, and α-antitrypsin deficiency are examples of single gene mutations. In the case of α-antitrypsin deficiency, the deficiency in a protease inhibitor causes enhanced degradation of elastic tissue surrounding the alveoli of the lungs, which in turn leads to emphysema. Examples of multiple gene mutations that can cause disease include hypertension and type 2 diabetes mellitus. In type 2 diabetes mellitus, obesity and other environmental factors induce the expression of the diabetic genetic trait.

Mechanical Factors

The *physical stress theory* may help explain mechanical factors influencing tissue adaptation and injury. The physical stress theory proposes that changes in the relative level of physical stress cause a predictable adaptive response in all biologic tissue. Typical tissue response to physical stress includes decreased stress tolerance (e.g., atrophy), maintenance, increased stress tolerance (e.g., hypertrophy), injury, and death.[152] Conversely, a decrease in mechanical stress may also be detrimental, particularly as it relates to bone health.[6]

Failure of a tissue occurs when the applied load exceeds the failure tolerance of the tissue. Soft tissues are influenced by the history of recent physical stresses, so that the accumulation of individual stresses can cause injury. Characteristics of the load, such as rate, compression, and forces (e.g., torsion, shear), along with the properties of the affected tissue determine the type and extent of tissue damage. The time elapsed since injury and the extent of tissue damage determine the inflammatory response.[17]

With repetitive and/or forceful tasks, the initiating stimuli for inflammatory responses include repeated overstretch, compression, friction, and anoxia. These insults lead to mechanical injury of cellular membranes and intracellular structures and a localized release of proteins such as collagen, fibronectin, and cytokines.[17]

A single high load or stress from a traumatic fall, car accident, or other traumatic event can cause significant injury. Bones can fracture and ligaments can rupture from one episode of high-magnitude force. These tissues could also fail from repeated bouts of moderate magnitude loads. Stress fractures or stress reactions in the bones could result from repeated episodes of moderate-magnitude force,[102] whereas slow degradation of tissue tolerance can occur in workers lifting heavy boxes repeatedly. Decreasing tissue tolerance may explain why there are no active acute inflammatory indicators in tendons associated with chronic tendinopathy.[78] Instead, antiinflammatory mediators and fibrotic proliferation are observed, suggesting the acute inflammatory phase has resolved. Conditions such as tennis elbow and/or golfer's elbow are recognized in many cases as a noninflammatory condition after an inflammatory episode.[10,17,69,70] In fact, research is ongoing to find ways to reinitiate the inflammatory cascade and promote healing in an otherwise degenerative process.[60] Low loads sustained over a long period of time, such as workers who remain in a fixed, flexed posture for prolonged periods of time, can also result in tissue injury because of decreased tissue tolerance.[152]

Altering mechanical stress (either increasing or decreasing forces) can be used to benefit individuals under varying circumstances. For example, reducing mechanical stress by offloading or pressure reduction is a concept used for healing ulcers and preventing their recurrence.

Controlled increase in physical stress is the underlying principle of progressive resistive exercise used to cause muscle fibers to hypertrophy and thereby able to withstand and generate greater force. Moreover, higher than normal levels of physical stress can promote remodeling in bone. Musculoskeletal tissues subjected to higher than normal levels of stress become more tolerant to subsequent physical stresses and are more resistant to injury.[152]

Nutritional Factors

Imbalances in essential nutrients can lead to cell injury or cell death. For example, deficiencies of essential amino acids interfere with protein synthesis. Synthesis of proteins is required to replace cell proteins lost through normal catabolism, through growth, and in preparation for cell replication. Cell replication is essential for the healing processes after cell injury and the replacement of cells lost through normal turnover.

The consequence of protein malnutrition is a condition called *kwashiorkor*; marasmus, another form of malnutrition, is a consequence of generalized dietary deficiency. These two diseases are still leading causes of death in impoverished countries. In many industrialized countries, excessive nutrient intake leads to obesity and its many complications.

Nutritional imbalance can also occur as a result of abnormal levels of either vitamins or minerals. These nutrients function as cofactors for biosynthetic reactions or are essential components of proteins or membranes; their deficiency usually affects selected cells or tissues. For example, a deficiency of iron leads to anemia, and the presence of excessive amounts of iron in the tissues can cause damage by the formation of free radicals.

Physical Factors

Trauma and physical agents can lead to cell injury and/or death. Blunt trauma caused by motor vehicle accidents is a leading killer in the United States.[132] Massive brain contusions, injury to internal organs and soft tissues, and blood loss may lead to immediate mortality. Survivors may succumb to infections and multiple organ failure. Repair of injuries to soft tissue, skeletal and muscular systems, and internal organs often requires prolonged periods of physical rehabilitation. Penetrating trauma inflicted by a variety of weapons can result in multiple complications.

Cells may be damaged by extremes of physical agents, such as temperature, radiation, and electricity. Generalized increases in body temperature (hyperthermia) or reduction in body temperature (hypothermia) can lead to cell injury; high or low tissue temperatures can cause

tissue injury or death. With increased temperature, the resulting morbidity and mortality are dependent on the severity of the burn and the total surface area that was burned. Markedly reduced temperatures may induce the freezing of tissue (frostbite). Ice crystals in cellular tissue rupture the cell membrane, which leads to cell death.

Irradiation for the treatment of cancer can cause injury of susceptible normal cells. Ionizing radiation causes radiolysis of water and the production of hydroxyl radicals ($\overline{O}H$). These radicals will lead to membrane damage and breakdown of structural and enzymatic proteins that result in cell death. Often, arterioles that supply oxygenated blood are damaged by ionizing radiation, resulting in inadequate nutritional supply leading to ischemia and death of the irradiated tissues. Irradiation also causes damage to nucleic acids and may result in gene mutations, possibly leading to neoplasia years later.

Psychosocial Factors

Psychosocial factors can have an impact on tissue adaptation, especially as related to tissue injury.[138] Psychosocial factors (e.g., fear, tension, or anxiety) may influence individual threshold values for tissue adaptation and injury. Many studies have investigated the role of mechanical and psychosocial factors in the onset of musculoskeletal (and other regional) acute and chronic pain. For example, people who are only occasionally or never satisfied in their work settings or who describe their work as "monotonous" have a higher risk of injury than those who are satisfied or completely satisfied with support from supervisors and colleagues.[24,92,93,153]

CELLULAR AGING

Aging and age-related changes can significantly influence homeostasis and the recovery process. The ability of a cell to resist microorganisms or to recover from injury or inflammation is dependent in part on the underlying state or health of the cells. Age-related changes at the cellular level are present but remain difficult to measure or quantify; researchers are working toward finding satisfactory biomarkers of aging at the cellular level. Age-associated deterioration in cells leads to tissue or organ deficiencies and ultimately to the expression of aging or disease.

Various components of cells (e.g., mitochondria, ribosomes, or cell membrane) are subject to changes associated with aging. Mitochondrial deoxyribonucleic acid (DNA) is considered a prime target for age-related changes. DNA has to replicate and maintain itself to preserve the primary genetic message. This takes place through division, which can result in alterations of the genetic code by anything that can damage DNA (e.g., physical, chemical, or biologic factors; spontaneous mutations of genes; exposure to radiation). Anything that can alter the information content of the cell can cause changes in function and affect the ability of the cell to maintain homeostasis.

The presence of a component called *lipofuscin* is the most well described age-associated change in the subcellular structure (lysosomes) of postmitotic cells. Lipofuscin is an aging-pigment granule that is found in high concentrations in old cells. The explanation for the increase of lipofuscin with age and the effects of these intracellular deposits on function remains under investigation. It is suspected that pressure from this pigmented lipid on the cell nucleus may interfere with cellular function.[176,184]

Theories of Cellular Aging

With aging, the cells demonstrate deceased capacity to respond to stress, resulting in a progressive decline in homeostatic balance and may lead to pathology.[223] More than 300 theories exist to explain the aging phenomenon from a cellular level. Many of these theories originate from the study of changes that accumulate with time. In organs composed of cells that cannot regenerate, such as those of the heart and brain, the *wear-and-tear theory* may account for the decline in function of these organs. Other factors may also play a role, such as the influence of genetics suggested by the genetic hypothesis that aging is a genetically predetermined process.

The *free radical theory* of aging is the most popular and widely tested and is based on the chemical nature and wide presence of free radicals causing DNA damage and cellular oxidative stress as it relates to the aging process (see "Chemical Factors" under "Mechanisms of Cell Injury" earlier in this chapter).

The discovery of the telomeres, the structure at the end of chromosomes, has added the *telomere aging clock theory* for the molecular mechanisms that lead to senescence. This theory suggests that the telomere acts as a molecular clock signaling the onset of cell senescence. Normal human cells will not divide forever but eventually enter a viable non-dividing state (senescence). The progressive accumulation of senescent cells contributes to but does not exclusively cause the aging process. Cell senescence acts as an anticancer mechanism to control the potential for cellular proliferation (see further discussion in Chapter 9).[2,105,216] Because of the close association between telomere dysfunction and malignancy, both pathologists and clinicians expect this molecule to be a useful malignancy marker.

Pathologic changes associated with aging vary from individual to individual but usually consist of reduced functional reserve caused by atrophy of tissues or organs. Resistance to infection declines with age, and pathologic processes such as atherosclerosis result in increased cardiovascular and cerebrovascular injuries or death.

Of particular value to physical therapists is the ability of our interventions to influence some of the processes that may lead to cellular aging. For example, studies have shown that considerable potential exists for improving aerobic capacity by training. This observation has cellular implications, as mitochondria of cardiac and skeletal muscle cells improve function under appropriate training conditions.[30] Moreover, changes in diet and exercise or treatment with hormones or compounds, such as antioxidants (see Fig. 6-3), are able to modify damage by ROS, which may allow the body to reestablish cellular norms.

TYPES OF CELL INJURY

Alteration in a cell's functional environment, either acute or chronic, produces a stress to the cell's ability to attain or maintain homeostasis. The extent to which the cell is able to alter mechanisms and regain homeostasis in the altered environment is considered an adaptation by the cells or tissues. When the cell is unable to adapt, injury can occur. A *reversible cell injury* occurs if the stress is sufficiently small in magnitude or short enough in duration that the cell is able to recover homeostasis after removal of the stress. If the injurious or stressful stimulus is of sufficient magnitude or duration or if the cell is unable to adapt, *irreversible cell injury* occurs (see Fig. 6-1).

Reversible Cell Injury

Cells react to injurious stimuli by changing their steady state to continue to function in a hazardous environment. Reversible (sublethal) injury caused by any of the mechanisms of cell injury listed in Box 6-1 is a transient impairment in the cell's normal structure or function. Normal cell structure and function can return after removal of the stressor or injurious stimulus (Fig. 6-4).

Acute reversible injury causes an impairment of ion homeostasis within the cell and leads to increased intracellular levels of sodium and calcium. An influx of interstitial fluid into the cell accompanies these ionic shifts and causes increased cell volume (swelling). Swelling occurs within the cytosol (liquid medium of the cytoplasm) and within organelles such as mitochondria and the endoplasmic reticulum. Swollen mitochondria generate less energy. Thus, instead of oxidative adenosine triphosphate production, the cell reverts to less efficient anaerobic glycolysis, which results in excessive production of lactic acid. The pH of the cell becomes acidic, which slows down the cell metabolism, resulting in further cellular damage. The injured cell forms plasma membrane *blebs* that can seal off and detach from the cell surface. In severely injured cells, ribosomes detach from the rough endoplasmic reticulum, and a decrease in the number of polysomes occurs. These changes lead to reduced protein synthesis by the affected cells and the cycle of damage can continue.

However, if the cell nucleus remains undamaged and the energy source is restored or the toxic injury is neutralized, the cell is able to recover and pump the ions and excess fluid back out. The swelling disappears, and the cell is returned to the original steady state, constituting a reversible cell injury.

Cellular Adaptations in Chronic Cell Injury

When a sublethal stress remains present over a period of time, stable alterations (adaptations) take place within the affected cells, tissues, and organs. Adaptation enables the cells to function in an altered environment and thereby avoid injury. Characteristics of cell adaptation, such as change in size, number, or function, increase the cell's ability to survive; these changes are also potentially reversible. In many but not all cases, these changes benefit the function of the parent organ or structure within which the cell resides. Common cellular adaptations include atrophy, hypertrophy, hyperplasia, metaplasia, and dysplasia (Fig. 6-5).

Atrophy is a reduction in cell and organ size. Atrophy can occur with vascular insufficiency, reduction in hormone levels, malnutrition, immobilization, and pain

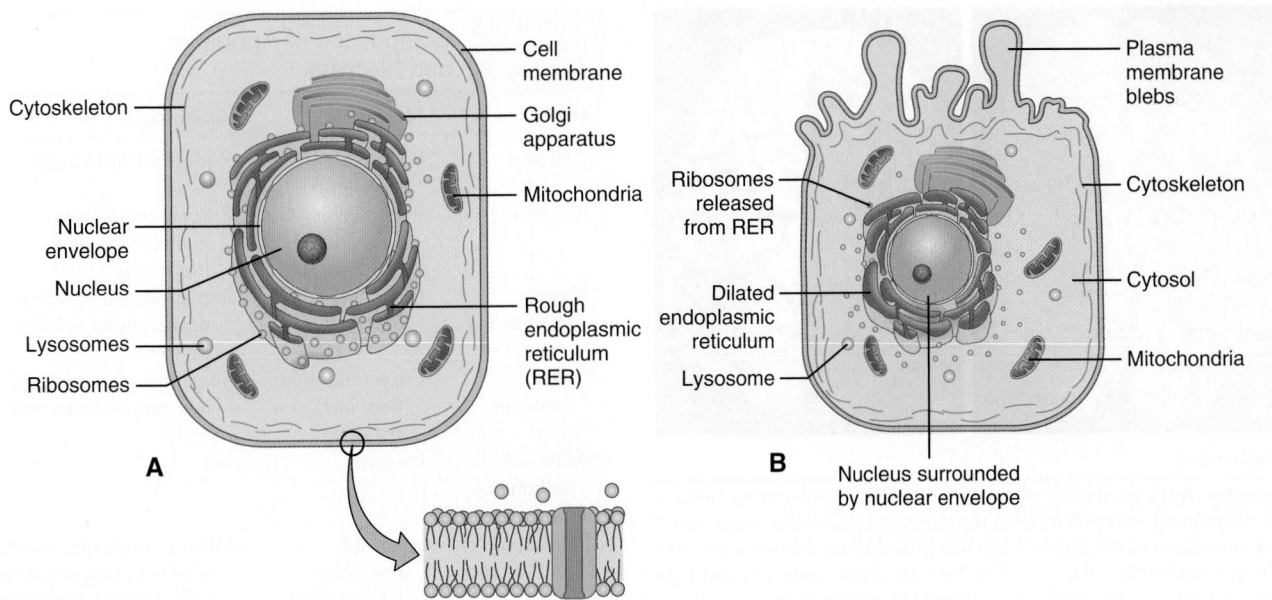

Figure 6-4

A, A normal cell with its organelles. **B,** Reversible cell injury with cellular swelling, accumulation of fluid in endoplasmic reticulum, and the release of ribosomes and formation of membrane blebs. (Courtesy SH Tepper, PhD, PT.)

that limits movement and function, and chronic inflammation. Bone loss, muscle wasting, and brain cell loss (Fig. 6-6) are examples of either tissue or organ atrophy associated with aging. Pathologic atrophy occurs as a consequence of cell injury due to ischemia, inadequate nutrition, or physical factors previously mentioned (see previous section on causes of cell injury). For example, ischemia of the viscera results in atrophied organs; cancer or malnutrition can result in cachexia, a general wasting of the body; and spinal cord injury results in atrophy of the affected muscles.

Hypertrophy is an increase in the size of the cell and organ. Hypertrophy can occur when increased functional demands are placed on the cells, tissue, or organs and with increased hormonal input (e.g., exercise stress can induce skeletal muscle hypertrophy). Pure hypertrophy only occurs in the heart and striated muscles because these organs consist of cells that cannot divide. Hypertrophy of the heart is a common pathologic finding that occurs as an adaptation of heart muscle to an increased workload. Specifically, hypertrophy of the left ventricle is a typical complication of hypertension. Increased blood pressure requires that the heart produce more force to eject the blood. The additional force is produced by hypertrophy of muscle fibers in the left ventricle.

Hyperplasia is an increase in the number of cells leading to increased organ size. In tissues consisting of cells that are capable of dividing, the presence of excessive functional demands can cause a consequent increase in cell number. Pure hyperplasia typically occurs because of hormonal stimulation (e.g., prolonged estrogen exposure causes the endometrium of the uterus to become thick) or chronic stimulation (e.g., persistent pressure on the skin induces hyperplasia and the formation of a callus). Some hyperplasia has no discernible cause and may represent early neoplasia. Hypertrophy and hyperplasia often occur together such as in the case of prostate enlargement and

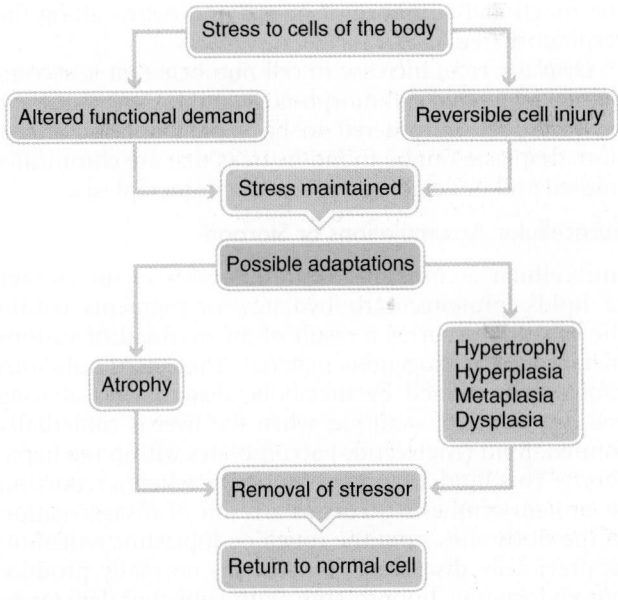

Figure 6-5

Cellular adaptations and reversible cell injury in response to stress. When the body is under persistent stress leading to either reversible cell injury or altered functional demand, the tissues adapt. Adaptations could include atrophy, hypertrophy, hyperplasia, metaplasia, or dysplasia. All of these changes are reversible with removal of the stressor. (Courtesy SH Tepper, PhD, PT.)

obstruction of the urethra and bladder. The result is an increase in size and number of smooth muscle cells in the wall of the urinary bladder.

Metaplasia is a change in cell morphology and function resulting from the conversion of one adult cell type into another. For example, in smokers, portions of the respiratory tract change from ciliated pseudostratified columnar epithelium into stratified squamous epithelium, leading

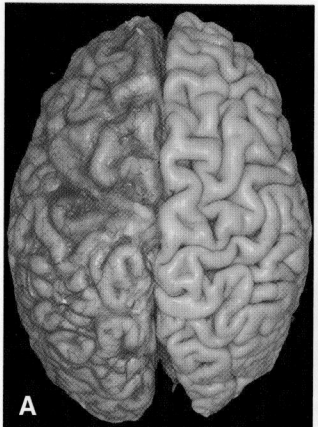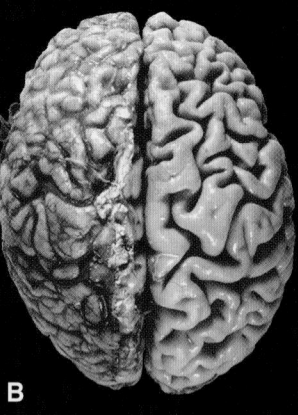

Figure 6-6

Atrophy. A, Normal brain of a young adult. **B,** Atrophy of the brain in an 82-year-old man with atherosclerotic cerebrovascular disease, resulting in reduced blood supply. Note that loss of brain substance narrows the gyri and widens the sulci. The meninges have been stripped from the right half of each specimen to reveal the surface of the brain. (From Kumar V, et al: *Robbins and Cotran pathologic basis of disease,* ed 8, Philadelphia, 2010, Saunders Elsevier.)

Table 6-1	Comparison of Apoptosis and Necrosis	
Feature	**Necrosis**	**Apoptosis**
Cell size	Enlarged (swelling)	Reduced (shrinkage)
Nucleus	Pyknosis → karyorrhexis → karyolysis	Fragmentation into nucleosome-size fragments
Plasma membrane	Disrupted	Intact; altered structure, especially orientation of lipids
Cellular contents	Enzymatic digestion; may leak out of cell	Intact; may be released into apoptotic bodies
Adjacent inflammation	Frequent	No
Physiologic or pathologic role	Invariably pathologic (culmination of irreversible cell injury)	Often physiologic, means of eliminating unwanted cells; may be pathologic after some forms of cell injury, especially DNA damage

From Kumar V, et al: *Robbins and Cotran Pathological Basis of Disease,* ed 8, Philadelphia, 2010, Saunders Elsevier.

to a thickening of the respiratory epithelium and loss of the functional clearance of mucus and debris along the respiratory tree.

Dysplasia is an increase in cell numbers that is accompanied by altered cell morphology and loss of histologic organization. Considered to be a preneoplastic alteration, dysplasia can be found in areas that are chronically injured and undergoing hyperplasia or metaplasia.

Intracellular Accumulations or Storage

Intracellular accumulations are increases in the storage of lipids, proteins, carbohydrates, or pigments within the cell that occur as a result of an overload of various metabolites or exogenous material. These accumulations can also be caused by metabolic disturbances altering cell function. For example, when the liver is sublethally injured, lipid (triglyceride) accumulates within the hepatocyte. This lipid accumulation occurs when a reduction in protein synthesis occurs as a result of disaggregation of the ribosomes from the rough endoplasmic reticulum as previously discussed. Hepatocytes normally produce our endogenous lipoproteins. With sublethal damage to hepatocytes (e.g., due to alcohol abuse), a lack of protein shell formation occurs so that lipoproteins cannot be packaged and transported to the plasma. As a result, lipids remain within the hepatocyte, causing the characteristic "fatty liver" found in alcoholics.

Irreversible Cell Injury

Irreversible cell injury is synonymous with cell death. Cell death occurs due to *apoptosis* or *necrosis*.[112] Table 6-1 summarizes the features of apoptosis and necrosis, whereas Figure 6-7 illustrates the changes in the cellular structure during these two processes.

Apoptosis, or programmed cell death, is a genetically mediated and managed process that causes cells to die. This type of cell death is generally physiologic, but could also be pathologic. Apoptosis begins with either an activation of a trigger or stimulus, or the suppression of a specific agent that then allows the process of cell death to occur. It is typically not associated with an inflammatory response.

The active process of degradation of dead cells is called *necrosis*. Necrosis is the end point of a pathologic process that results in lethal, irreversible cell injury. Hallmarks of lethally injured cells include alterations in the cell nucleus, mitochondria, and lysosomes and the rupture of the cell membrane (see Fig. 6-7).

Damage to the cell nucleus can present in three forms: pyknosis, karyorrhexis, and karyolysis. Nuclei undergo clumping or pyknosis, which is a degeneration of the cell as the nucleus shrinks in size and the chromatin condenses to a solid mass. The pyknotic nuclei can fragment, a process termed *karyorrhexis*, or it can undergo dissolution (karyolysis).

Mitochondria lose their membrane potential and become unable to synthesize adenosine triphosphate, leaving the cell without the necessary energy production for cell function. Morphologically, irreversibly injured mitochondria appear swollen, contain large lipid-protein aggregates called *flocculent densities*, and may also contain dense crystalline deposits of calcium (Fig. 6-8).

After cell death, lysosomes release their digestive enzymes within the cytoplasm of the cell, initiating enzymatic degradation of all cellular constituents, a process that may be aided by enzymes released from inflammatory cells. Enzymes help dissolve the dead tissue, making it easier for phagocytic cells to remove the dead tissue in preparation for healing by repair (laying down of a collagenous tissue scar) or regeneration (regrowth of parenchymal tissue). Dead cells release their contents into the extracellular fluid, eventually making their way into the circulation, where they can be measured as clinically

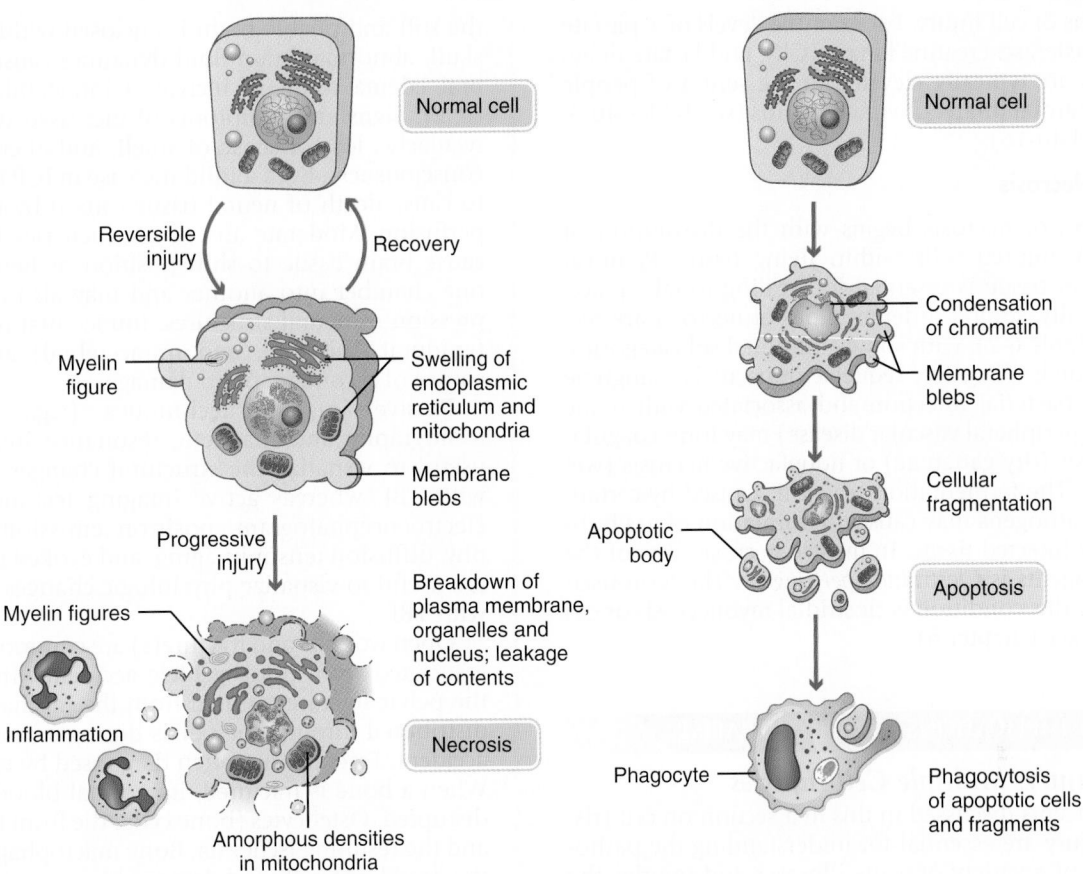

Figure 6-7

Schematic illustration of the morphologic changes in cell injury culminating in necrosis or apoptosis. (From Kumar V, et al: *Robbins and Cotran pathologic basis of disease*, ed 8, Philadelphia, 2010, Saunders Elsevier.)

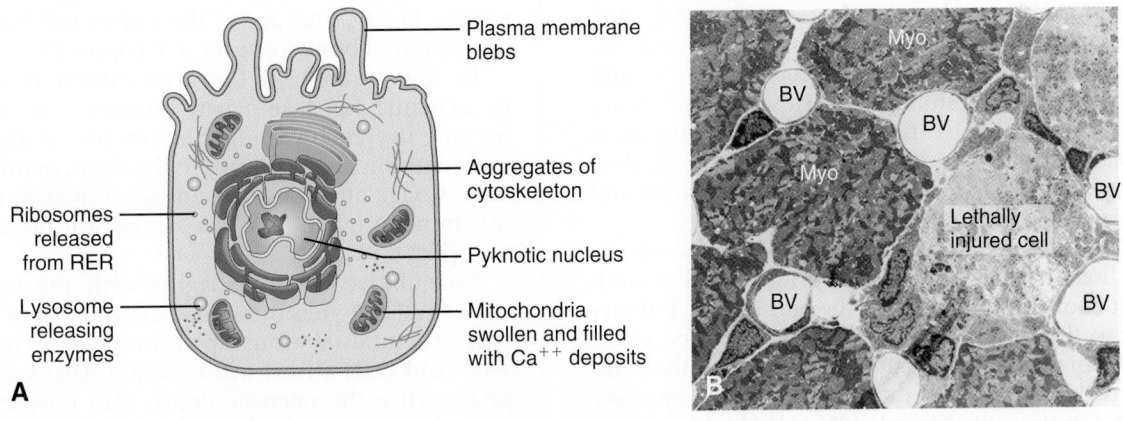

Figure 6-8

Irreversible cell injury: ultrastructural alterations in an irreversibly killed cell. A, Mitochondria are nonfunctional and filled with flocculent densities (particles suspended together in a cluster). Lysosomes are releasing their digestive enzymes. The nucleus is condensing upon itself (pyknosis). Membrane breakdown allows intracellular enzymes to be released into the interstitial area. **B,** Electron micrograph of lethally injured cardiomyocytes next to healthy viable cardiomyocytes (*Myo*). Note lethally injured cells to the right of the Myo are swollen, mitochondria are filled with flocculent densities, there is a loss of myofilaments, and mononuclear phagocytic cells are beginning to remove these dead cells. *BV*, Blood vessel. Original magnification ×1500. (A, Courtesy SH Tepper, PhD, PT; B, From Tepper SH, Anderson PA, Mergner WJ: Recovery of the heart following focal injury induced by dietary restriction of potassium. *Path Res Prac* 186:265–285, 1990.)

useful signs of cell injury. For example, levels of aspartate aminotransferase, creatine kinase (CK), and lactate dehydrogenase are typically elevated in the serum of people with myocardial infarct or viral hepatitis (see Tables 40-5, 40-15, and 40-16).

Types of Necrosis

The process of necrosis begins with the dissolution of irreversibly injured cells within living tissue. Removal of this dead tissue is essential for healing to take place. Histologically, several different types of necrosis are recognized (Table 6-2), with some additional subcategories.

Gangrene is a negative sequelae of necrosis. Gangrene caused by bacterial infection and associated with tissue ischemia (peripheral vascular disease) may form coagulative necrosis (dry gangrene) or liquefactive necrosis (wet gangrene). The fermentation reactions caused by certain bacterial pathogens may cause the formation of gas bubbles in the infected tissue. In muscle necrosis, one of the causative agents is *Clostridium perfringens*. The term used to describe this condition is clostridial myonecrosis or gas gangrene (see Chapter 8).

SPECIAL IMPLICATIONS FOR THE THERAPIST   **6-1**

Cell Injury: Multiple Cell Injuries

The concepts discussed in this first section on cell (tissue) injury are essential for understanding the pathogenesis of a variety of acute illnesses and injuries the therapist may see in any clinical setting. Often, multiple episodes of care with complex cases involving comorbidities occur in clinical practice. For example, the victim of a motor vehicle accident experiencing a traumatic brain injury (TBI) and concomitant pelvic fracture may develop pneumonia and pulmonary compromise and subsequently experience MI. The therapy staff following this client throughout the entire continuum of care—from the intensive care unit (ICU) through rehabilitation to a home health service setting and possibly as an outpatient—can better meet the needs of such an individual during the healing process by understanding these concepts of injury and recovery.

TBI could occur during motor vehicle accidents. With direct trauma to the head, primary and secondary injury can lethally damage the brain tissue. Primary injury to the brain may occur in the following areas: (1) local brain damage occurs at the site where the brain impacts the skull (coup injury) and the site opposite impact (contrecoup injury); (2) polar brain damage occurs at the tips (poles) of the frontal, temporal, and occipital lobes and the undersurface of the frontal and temporal lobes when the brain moves inside the skull; or (3) diffuse axonal injury occurs throughout the subcortical white matter (and brain stem if the magnitude of force is great enough) with sufficient shear force to injure axons. The extent of primary damage to the brain depends on the nature, direction, and magnitude of the forces applied to the skull.

Secondary injury is usually the result of hypoxic-ischemic injury caused by cerebral edema. Because the soft and pliable brain is enclosed within the rigid skull, abnormal brain fluid dynamics caused by cerebral edema result in increased intracranial pressure (ICP). Signs and symptoms of increased ICP include headache, loss of sense of smell, and altered level of consciousness. Even a mild increase in ICP is sufficient to cause death of neural tissue caused by inadequate perfusion. Moderate and severe increases in ICP can cause brain tissue to shift position or herniate from one chamber into another and may also cause compression of neural structures. Intracranial hematomas (epidural, subdural, and intracerebral) are another source of secondary brain damage.

Passive imaging techniques (e.g., computed tomography and magnetic resonance imaging) are useful to visualize the structural changes that occur with TBI, whereas active imaging techniques (e.g., electroencephalogram, positron emission tomography, diffusion tensor imaging, and evoked potentials) are useful to visualize physiologic changes that occur with TBI.

Open wounds and fracture(s) are common sequelae associated with motor vehicle accidents. In this case, the pelvic fracture resulted from the mechanical force distributed through the pelvis during a motor vehicle accident. Fractures are often diagnosed by radiograph. When a bone is fractured, its normal blood supply is disrupted. Osteocytes (bone cells) die from the trauma and the resulting ischemia. Bone macrophages remove the dead bone cells and damaged bone.

A precursor fibrocartilaginous growth of tissue occurs before the laying down of primary bone, eventually followed by the laying down and remodeling on normal adult bone. This process from fracture to full restoration of the bone will take weeks to months depending on the type of fracture, location, vascular supply, health, and age of the individual. See further discussion of bone fractures in Chapter 27.

In this example, if the myocardium is subjected to ischemia for a sufficient duration, the myocytes become irreversibly injured. A cascade of physiologic and anatomic changes leads to the death of myocardial cells. Coagulative necrosis ensues, followed by acute inflammation, and finally repair by scar tissue formation (Fig. 6-9).

Coagulative necrosis begins with the release of lysosomal enzymes that cause dissolution of the normal structural relationships found within myocytes. The dead cells attract acute inflammatory cells that phagocytize the necrotic debris and release growth factors. The growth factors initiate the proliferation of blood vessels (angiogenesis) and fibroblasts, resulting in the eventual production of a collagenous scar.

Signs and symptoms correlate with the different stages of lethal cell injury and differ according to the organ or structure(s) involved. During acute MI, the individual often experiences angina, shortness of breath, sweating, and nausea. These symptoms of physiologic stress are caused by the release of histamines, bradykinins, and prostaglandins such as substance P from the lethally injured myocytes.

An electrocardiogram reveals ST-segment elevation and Q waves over the affected area. The person is also at an increased risk for life-threatening dysrhythmias due to the loss of electrical conductivity of lethally injured myocytes and disrupted conductivity (irritability) of the adjacent cells. If a significant percentage of the myocardium is infarcted, cardiogenic shock or congestive heart failure may ensue.

Cytoplasmic enzymes or proteins (e.g., myocardial isoenzyme of creatine kinase [CK-MB]) are released from the dead cells. Normally, the plasmalemma is impermeable to these large molecules and contains them within the confines of the cytoplasm. After lethal injury, the plasmalemma is broken down by the actions of phospholipases, and these molecules are released from inside the cell. A number of cytoplasmic proteins are released into the interstitial area and are taken up by adjacent lymphatic vessels and finally enter the bloodstream. Lactate dehydrogenase, CK-MB, and troponin (see Tables 40-15 and 40-16) are clinically relevant for diagnosis and assessment of the severity of a MI.

The therapist must understand the process of injury and repair to the brain, pelvic bones, and myocardium (or other involved organs and/or structures) as appropriate client care is determined by the different stages of this process. For example, recovery from TBI tends to follow the progression outlined by the Rancho Los Amigos Levels of Cognitive Function (LOCF) (see Table 33-2).

In general, intervention is directed by the person's current LOCF level. During LOCF levels I to III, primary goals involve increasing tolerance of activities, including intervention, tolerating upright posture, and increasing interaction with the environment. During levels IV to VI, the emphasis shifts to increasing physical and cognitive endurance. During levels VII and VIII, intervention focuses on the skills necessary to reenter the community.

After fracture of bone, a period of immobilization usually occurs to remove longitudinal stress. This period allows for the phagocytic removal of necrotic bone tissue and the initial deposition of the fibrocartilaginous callus. As the fracture heals as revealed by radiograph, gradual progression of stress is applied. Mobilization of this individual will occur depending on the type of fixation used on the pelvis. For example, if an external fixation is applied for fracture stabilization, mobilization can occur almost immediately within tolerance of the person's symptoms.

The highest risk of death during the first hours after MI stems from dysrhythmias. Rupture of the myocardium is possible during days 3 through 10 after a transmural MI (from outside epicardium to inside endocardium). The risk of these events dictates that exercise during this time must not subject damaged cells to excessive stress. Proper mobilization of the individual soon after infarction may decrease the likelihood of succumbing to the negative effects of bedrest but may be complicated by variables such as pelvic fracture, pneumonia, and the TBI in this case.

INFLAMMATION

Overview and Definition

After cell injury, the body reacts by initiating the process of inflammation. The amount, type, and severity of the inflammatory reaction are dependent on the amount, type, and severity of the injury. As part of the healing process, the inflammatory process is responsible for the removal of the injurious agent, removal of cellular debris, and the initiation of the healing process. The healing process occurs to allow restoration of structure and function whenever possible.

Inflammation serves a vital role in host defense against pathogens and in response to cell injury. The inflammatory process provides us with the capability to both get rid of the initial cause of cell injury (trauma, bacteria, and toxins) and the consequences of such an injury (damaged cells and tissue). It proceeds as a complex set of overlapping reactions of vascular and cellular responses. Each reaction serves a specific purpose and is necessary as the body responds to tissue injury or damage.

There are several mechanisms by which injury can cause inflammation and the vascular and cellular reactions it triggers. If microbes are introduced, they can stimulate potent inflammatory cells,[180] particularly innate immune cells such as neutrophils (white blood cells [WBCs]) and macrophages (phagocytes).[42] Traumatic stimulation of mast cells and nerves can also lead to the release of proinflammatory mediators (histamine, serotonin, prostaglandins, and leukotrienes).[8,200] If trauma causes bleeding, then hemostatic mechanisms (platelets and clotting) that are triggered can also generate inflammatory mediators.[114,120] Additionally, cell death is a universal and potent stimulator of sterile inflammation (inflammation in the absence of microorganisms).[42,180] These soluble factors produced by cells and plasma proteins can initiate and amplify the response, as well as determine the pattern, severity, and clinical and pathologic manifestations.[123]

The termination of inflammation occurs when the injurious agent is removed. The reaction resolves quickly, because cytokines are broken down and dissipated and leukocytes have short life spans in the tissues. Additionally, antiinflammatory mechanisms are activated that serve to control the response and prevent it from causing excessive damage to the host.[123]

The inflammatory process is closely intertwined with the process of repair and stimulates the necessary response to try and heal the damaged tissue. Repair begins during inflammation but reaches completion usually after the injurious influence has been neutralized. The process of healing occurs either by regeneration (regrowth of original tissue) or by repair (formation of a connective tissue scar) or, most commonly, by a combination of these two processes.

Normally, inflammation has a protective role and is generally beneficial to the body. However, inflammation, whether in the acute or chronic stage (and with all of its components), can be detrimental and has the potential of causing damage (and even death) to adjacent healthy tissue.

The degree and persistence of the inflammatory response is a major factor in the outcome of the repair

Table 6-2 Types of Necrosis

Type	Cause	Effects	Area of Involvement	Example
Coagulative	Ischemia (lack of blood supply	Cell membrane is preserved; nucleus undergoes pyknosis and karolysis (dissolution), organelles dissolve	Solid internal organs (e.g., heart, liver, kidneys)	Wedge-shaped kidney infarct
Caseous ("cheesy")	*Mycobacterium tuberculosis* (TB); seen with other fungal infections	Cell membrane is destroyed; debris appears cheese-like and does not disappear by lysis but persists indefinitely; damaged area is walled off in a fibrous calcified area forming a granuloma	Lungs, bronchopulmonary lymph nodes, skeletal bone (extrapulmonary TB)	Tuberculosis of the lung, with yellow-white and cheesy debris.
Liquefactive	Pyogenic bacteria (e.g., *Staphylococcus aureus*)	Death of neurons releases lysosomes that liquefy the area, leaving pockets of liquid and cellular debris (abscess of fluid-filled cavity), shapeless, amorphous debris remains	Brain tissue (e.g., brain infarct); skin, wound, joint infections	Infarct of the brain, showing dissolution of the tissue
Fatty necrosis	Acute pancreatitis, abdominal trauma	Formation of calcium soaps by the release of pancreatic lipases	Abdominal area	White chalky deposits indicating fatty necrosis in the mesentery
Fibrinoid	Trauma in blood vessel wall	Plasma proteins accumulate; cellular debris and serum proteins form pink deposits	Blood vessels (tunica media, smooth muscle cells)	Fibrinoid necrosis in an artery

Photographs from Kumar V, et al: *Robbins and Cotran pathologic basis of disease*, ed 8, Philadelphia, 2010, Saunders Elsevier.

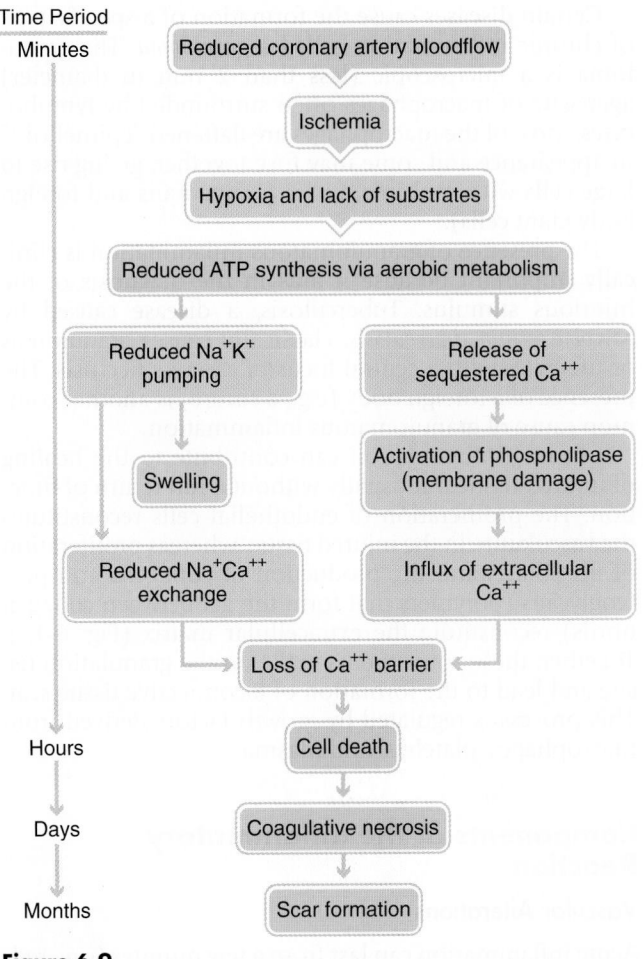

Time Period

Minutes

Figure 6-9

Pathogenesis of myocardial infarction (MI). With reduction in coronary artery blood flow (CABF) caused by a thrombus formation, ischemia results in a reduction of aerobic metabolism. Irreversible cell injury occurs, followed by necrosis of the heart tissue. Release of intracellular enzymes (myocardial isoenzyme of creatine kinase [CK-MB], troponin) from the dead heart tissue serve as biochemical markers in the early diagnosis of MI (see Tables 40-15 and 40-16). In the following weeks, healing occurs by repair, the formation of a connective tissue scar. (Courtesy SH Tepper, PhD, PT.)

Table 6-3	Four Cardinal Signs/Symptoms of Inflammation

Sign	Precipitating Events
Erythema	Vasodilation and increased blood flow
Heat	Vasodilation and increased blood flow
Edema	Fluid and cells leaking from local blood vessels into the extravascular spaces
Pain	Direct trauma; chemical mediation by bradykinins, histamines, serotonin; internal pressure secondary to edema; swelling of the nerve endings

chronic inflammation and is associated with the presence of lymphocytes and macrophages, the proliferation of blood vessels and fibrosis, and tissue destruction.[123]

In the *acute inflammation* stage, the inflammatory stimulus acts on blood cells and plasma constituents in order to deliver leukocytes and plasma proteins to sites of infection and tissue injury. Acute inflammatory reactions can be triggered by many stimuli such as infections, tissue necrosis, foreign bodies, and immune reactions. All inflammatory reactions share the same basic features, although different stimuli may induce reactions with some distinctive characteristics.[123] The clinical manifestations of inflammatory reaction are redness, swelling, increased temperature, pain, and decreased function of the affected site (Table 6-3). Arteriolar vasodilation gives rise to the redness and heat. The exudation and leukocyte infiltration give rise to the swelling. Pain and loss of function occur as a result of the increased pressure from the edema on the peripheral nerves[17] (Fig. 6-10).

Once the injurious agent is removed, acute inflammation subsides. If little necrosis is present and replacement of lost parenchymal cells is possible, restitution of normal structure and function of the tissue occurs.

Chronic inflammation may occur in the presence of extensive necrosis or if regeneration of parenchymal cells is not possible (e.g., heart, CNS, or peripheral nervous system cells). The inflammatory reaction may also become chronic if the underlying cause is not addressed and the injurious agent persists for a prolonged period. Repeated episodes of acute inflammation in the same tissue over time or low-grade, persistent immune reactions can also result in a chronic inflammatory response (Fig. 6-11).

The hallmark of chronic inflammation in a tissue is the accumulation of macrophages, lymphocytes, and plasma cells (Fig. 6-12). The macrophage accumulation is the result of chemotaxis (locomotion or movement) of monocytes (precursors to macrophages) to the area of injury. Macrophages modulate lymphocyte functions and promote growth of endothelial cells and fibroblasts by the release of growth factors. Eosinophils may also be present, particularly if allergic reactions or parasite invasions are involved.

Granulation tissue made up of proliferating endothelial cells and fibroblasts is also seen in areas of chronic inflammation. Granulation tissue can be seen in well-healing, open wounds. Inspection of the wound site reveals red "beefy" tissue with pinpoint red dots (new capillaries) and a granular surface composed of newly formed collagen.

process. Complete regeneration and repair without scar can be expected if the inflammation is minimal and there are no complicating factors. However, if the inflammation is chronic and persistent, and comorbidities, risk factors, and complications are present, resulting chronic wounds could be expected.

Inflammation has been linked with many other conditions in the absence of infection[42] (e.g., Alzheimer disease, atherosclerosis, cancer, diabetes, insulin resistance syndrome, and obesity). The focus of this chapter is inflammation in relation to the musculoskeletal system.

Acute Versus Chronic Inflammation

Inflammation of sudden onset and short duration is referred to as *acute inflammation*; its main characteristics are exudation of fluid and plasma proteins (edema) and the migration of leukocytes, predominately neutrophils (called polymorphonuclear leucocytes).[123] Inflammation that does not resolve but persists over time is called

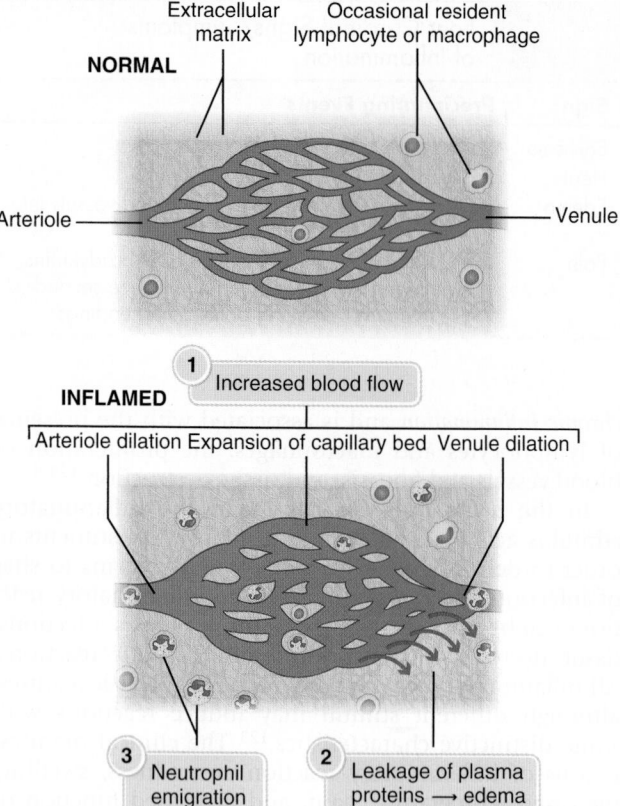

NORMAL

Extracellular matrix

Occasional resident lymphocyte or macrophage

Arteriole

Venule

INFLAMED

1 Increased blood flow

Arteriole dilation Expansion of capillary bed Venule dilation

3 Neutrophil emigration

2 Leakage of plasma proteins → edema

Figure 6-10

The major local manifestations of acute inflammation, compared to normal. (1) Vascular dilation and increased blood flow (causing erythema and warmth); **(2)** extravasation and extravascular deposition of plasma fluid and proteins (edema); **(3)** leukocyte emigration and accumulation in the site of injury. (From Kumar V, et al: *Robbins and Cotran pathologic basis of disease*, ed 8, Philadelphia, 2010, Saunders Elsevier.)

Certain diseases cause the formation of a specific type of chronic inflammation called a *granuloma*. The granuloma is a microscopic (less than 2 mm in diameter) aggregate of macrophages often surrounded by lymphocytes. Most of the macrophages are flattened "epithelioid" in appearance and some may fuse together, giving rise to large cells with multiple nuclei (Langerhans and foreign body giant cells).

The presence of granulomatous inflammation is clinically important because it aids in the diagnosis of the injurious stimulus. Tuberculosis, a disease caused by *Mycobacterium tuberculosis*, classically causes granulomas or tubercles with a central focus of caseous necrosis. The presence of a foreign body (e.g., a suture) is another common cause of granulomatous inflammation.

Chronic inflammation can contribute to the healing of injured tissue but usually without a full return of function. The proliferation of endothelial cells reconstitutes the vasculature in the injured tissue, whereas proliferation of fibroblasts and the production of collagens and proteoglycans (polymers that form the gel between collagen fibrils) reconstitute the extracellular matrix (Fig. 6-13). Together, these constituents make up the granulation tissue and lead to the formation of a connective tissue scar. This process is regulated by growth factors derived from macrophages, platelets, and plasma.

Components of the Inflammatory Reaction

Vascular Alterations

Acute inflammation can last from a few minutes (e.g., redness and swelling from scratching your skin) to a few days (e.g., after an open cut on the finger), during which time a series of vascular events occurs. The goal of the series of vascular changes is to increase the movement of plasma proteins and circulating cells out of the intravascular

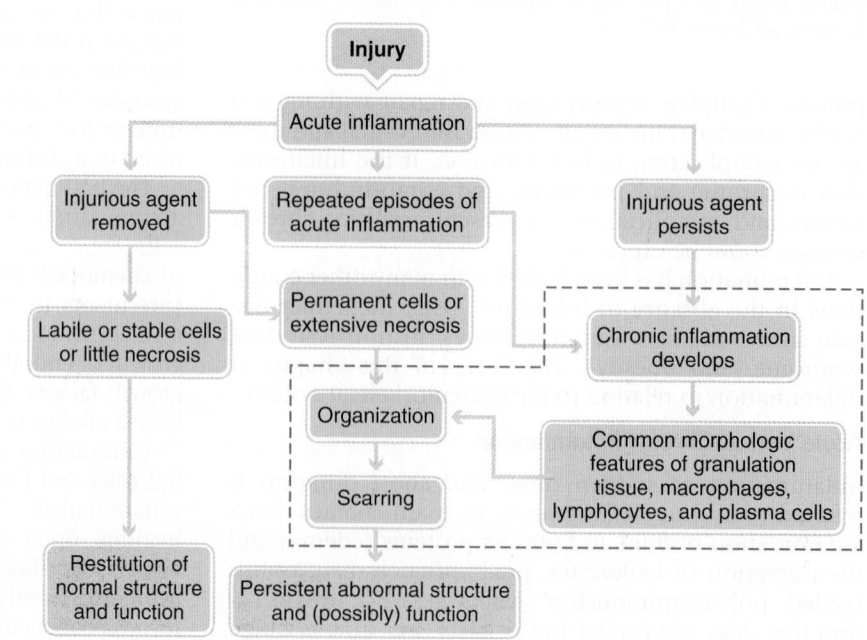

Injury

Acute inflammation

Injurious agent removed

Repeated episodes of acute inflammation

Injurious agent persists

Labile or stable cells or little necrosis

Permanent cells or extensive necrosis

Chronic inflammation develops

Organization

Common morphologic features of granulation tissue, macrophages, lymphocytes, and plasma cells

Scarring

Restitution of normal structure and function

Persistent abnormal structure and (possibly) function

Figure 6-11

Overview after tissue injury: acute inflammation, chronic inflammation, and the likely healing process. (Courtesy SH Tepper, PhD, PT.)

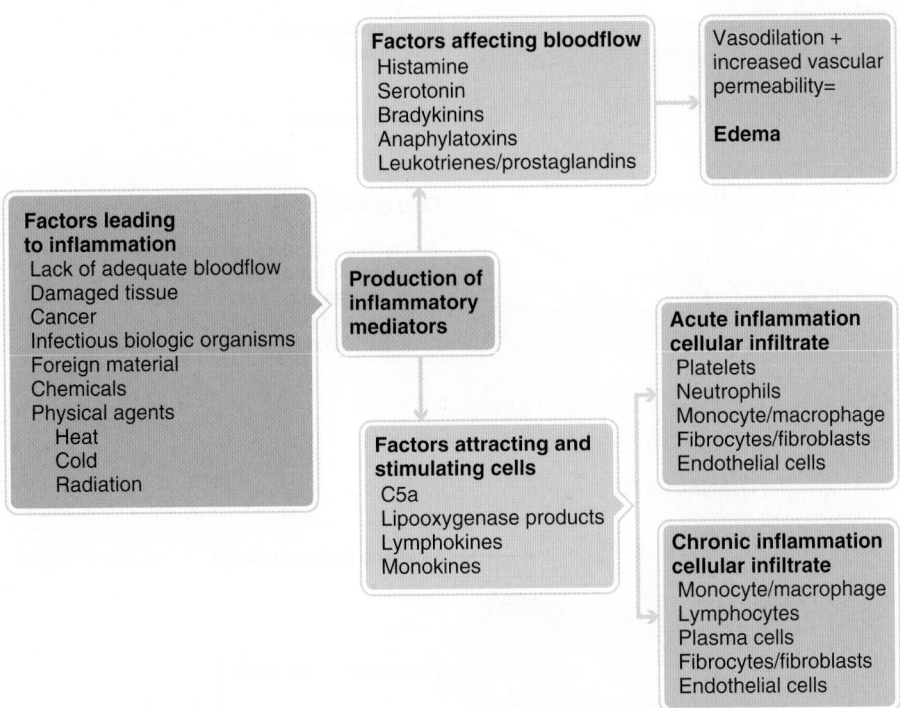

Figure 6-12

Contributing factors and components of inflammation. Note the vascular alterations associated with factors affecting blood flow (vasoactive mediators) leading to edema and the factors attracting and stimulating cellular alterations (chemotactic factors) resulting in acute (and sometimes) chronic inflammation. (Courtesy SH Tepper, PhD, PT.)

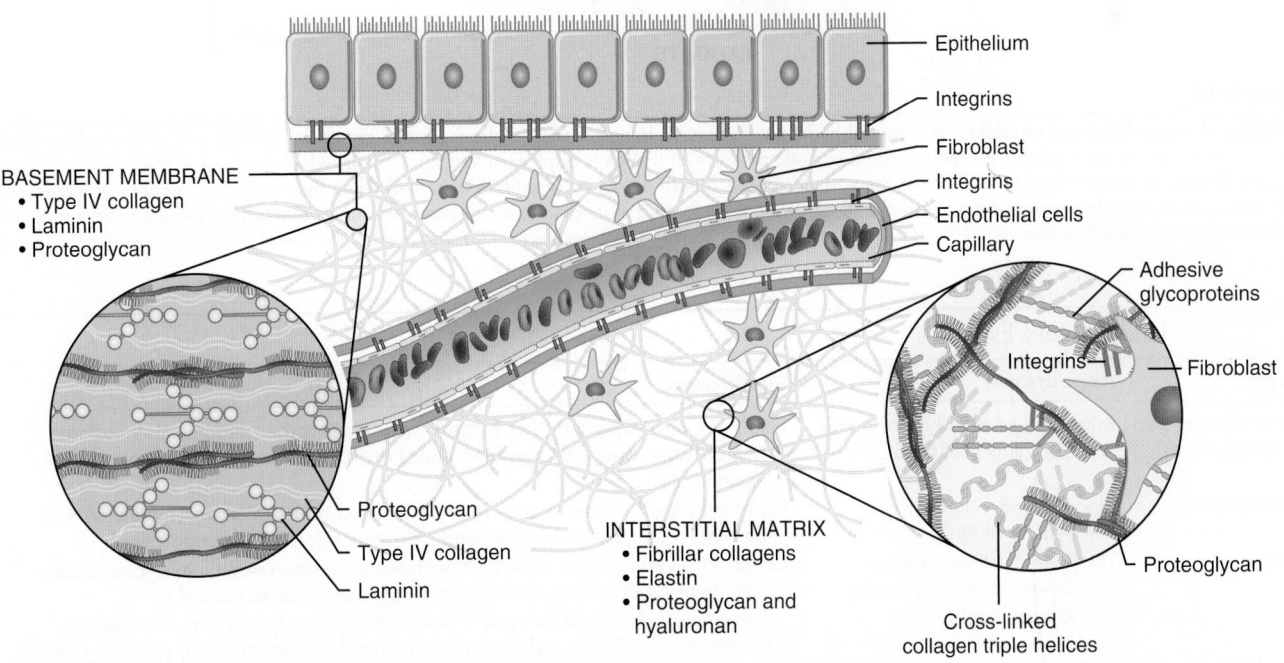

Figure 6-13

Main components of the extracellular matrix (ECM), including collagens, proteoglycans, and adhesive glycoproteins. Both epithelial and mesenchymal cells (e.g., fibroblasts) interact with ECM via integrins. Basement membranes and interstitial ECM have different architecture and general composition, although there is some overlap in their constituents. For the sake of simplification, many ECM components (e.g., elastin, fibrillin, hyaluronan, and syndecan) are not included. (From Kumar V, et al: *Robbins and Cotran pathologic basis of disease*, ed 8, Philadelphia, 2010, Saunders Elsevier.)

space and into the site of injury. The escape of fluid, protein, and blood from the vasculature system into tissue or body cavities is known as *exudation*.[41] Exudate is an extravascular fluid that contains a high protein concentration, cellular debris (phagocytic cells), and has a high specific gravity.[123] Exudation occurs when an increase in capillary permeability allows proteinaceous fluid and/or cells

to leak out primarily through openings created between adjacent endothelial cells in the capillaries or venules (Fig. 6-14).[41,123] Various types of exudate are evident in the tissue, depending on the stage of inflammation and its cause (Table 6-4). In contrast, a *transudate* is a fluid with low protein content, little or no cellular material, and low specific gravity. It is essentially an ultrafiltrate of

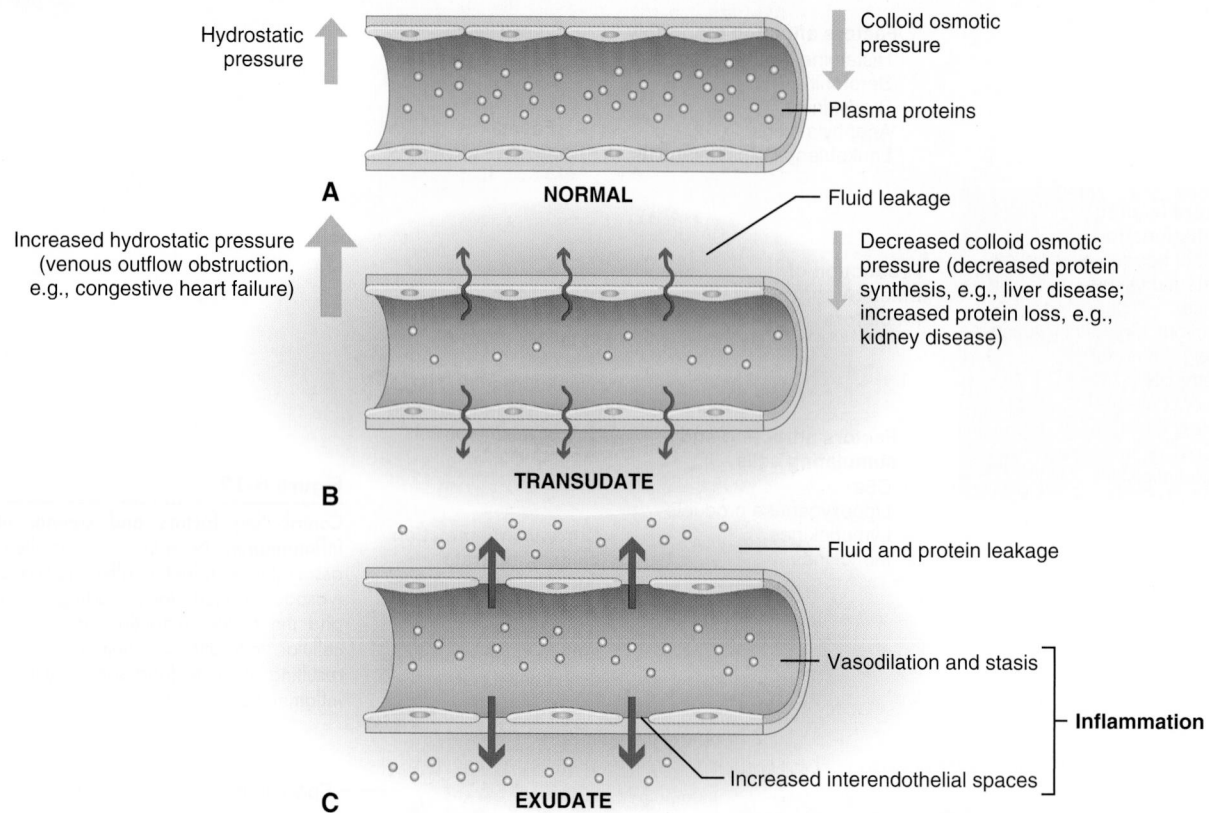

Figure 6-14

Formation of transudates and exudates. A, Normal hydrostatic pressure (*blue arrows*) is about 32 mm Hg at the arterial end of a capillary bed and 12 mm Hg at the venous end; the mean colloid osmotic pressure of tissues is approximately 25 mm Hg, which is equal to the mean capillary pressure. Therefore, the net flow of fluid across the vascular bed is almost nil. **B,** A transudate is formed when fluid leaks out because of increased hydrostatic pressure or decreased osmotic pressure. **C,** An exudate is formed in inflammation, because vascular permeability increases as a result of increased interendothelial spaces. (From Kumar V, et al: *Robbins and Cotran pathologic basis of disease,* ed 8, Philadelphia, 2010, Saunders Elsevier.)

Table 6-4	Inflammatory Exudates	
Type	**Appearance**	**Significance**
Hemorrhagic; sanguineous	Bright red or bloody; presence of red blood cells (RBCs)	Small amounts expected after surgery or trauma. Large amounts may indicate hemorrhage. Sudden large amounts of dark, red blood may indicate a draining hematoma.
Serosanguineous	Blood-tinged yellow or pink; presence of RBCs	Expected for 48-72 hours after injury or trauma to the microvasculature. A sudden increase may precede wound dehiscence (rupture or separation).
Serous	Thin, clear yellow, or straw-colored; contains albumin and immunoglobulins	Occurs in the early stages of most inflammations; common with blisters, joint effusion with rheumatoid arthritis, viral infections (e.g., skin vesicles caused by herpesvirus); expected for up to 1 week after trauma or surgery. A sudden increase may indicate a draining seroma (pocket of serum within tissue or organ).
Purulent	Viscous, cloudy, pus; cellular debris from necrotic cells and dying neutrophils (PMNs)	Usually caused by pus-forming bacteria (streptococci, staphylococci) and indicates infection. May drain suddenly from an abscess (boil).
Catarrhal	Thin, clear mucus	Seen with inflammatory process within mucous membranes (e.g., upper respiratory infection).

Modified from Black J: Wound healing. In Black JM, Matassarin-Jacobs E, editors: *Luckmann and Sorensen's medical-surgical nursing,* ed 8, Philadelphia, 2009.

blood plasma that results from osmotic or hydrostatic imbalance in a vessel without an increase of vascular permeability (e.g., left ventricular failure, cirrhosis, and nephrosis).[14] When fluid transudates or leaks from blood vessels and accumulates inside an anatomic space, such as the pleural, pericardial, or peritoneal cavities or the joint space, these accumulations are called effusions. *Effusion* is a more general term referring to the escape of a fluid and can either be a transudate or an exudate.

Removal of the fluid for analysis is required when differentiating between transudates and exudates and helps establish a specific diagnosis. Sometimes exudates are described by visual appearance (e.g., serosanguineous exudate, a fluid containing erythrocytes, or red blood cells [RBCs]).

Although nerve reflexes at the site of injury can cause immediate vasoconstriction,[59a] the rapid response of chemical mediators result in the characteristics of acute inflammation, listed as follows: (1) vasodilation, one of the earliest manifestations, causing increased blood flow with resultant heat and redness (erythema); (2) increased capillary permeability, which permits the passage of plasma proteins and leukocytes into the extravascular space, causing edema; (3) the loss of fluid due to increased vessel permeability that leads to slower blood flow, a higher concentration of red blood cells in small vessel, and increased viscosity of the blood; (4) clotting of the fluid in the interstitial spaces because of increased fibrinogen and other proteins to wall off the invader; and (5) migration of leukocytes from the microcirculation, their accumulation in the focus of injury, and their activation to eliminate the offending agent, resulting in swelling of the tissues.

Leukocyte Accumulations

An important consequence of the exudation of protein and fluid from the vasculature is the engorgement of vessels with blood cells. This causes a slowing or cessation of blood flow in the affected vessels, a phenomenon called *stasis.*[123] During stasis, the leukocytes (WBCs) accumulate and adhere to the endothelial cells of blood vessel walls at the site of injury in a process called *margination.* Inflammatory mediators cause an increased expression of specific glycoproteins called *adhesion molecules* on the surface membrane of leukocytes and endothelial cells. These adhesion glycoproteins, by adhering to each other, function as receptors and counterreceptors. The adhesion glycoproteins are the glue that binds the leukocytes to each other and to the endothelium of venules and capillaries.

The binding of leukocytes to receptors on endothelial cells of venules is the first step in the migration of leukocytes from the vasculature to the interstitial tissues. This process initiates the circulation of leukocytes through the extravascular space in normal conditions and the infiltration of leukocytes into the site of inflammation.

In the next stage, the leukocytes actively migrate out of the vessels, passing through the vascular walls without damaging the blood vessels and entering the interstitial space in a process called *diapedesis,* or oozing (see Fig. 6-15). The continued migration of leukocytes in interstitial space is directed by a chemical trail created by a concentration gradient of one of many possible attractants. The attractants are called *chemotactic agents,* and the process of locomotion is called *chemotaxis.* In other words, leukocytes are attracted to and accumulate at the site of an inflammatory reaction in response to a chemical stimulus.

The presence of leukocyte accumulations in tissue or fluid specimens is diagnostic of an inflammatory process. The predominant cell type found in a specimen identifies the type of inflammation and/or its duration and original stimulus (see Table 40-11). Typically, during acute inflammation, neutrophils predominate (neutrophilia). Neutrophils inhibit bacterial growth by releasing lactoferrin, a protein that binds with iron, thus preventing

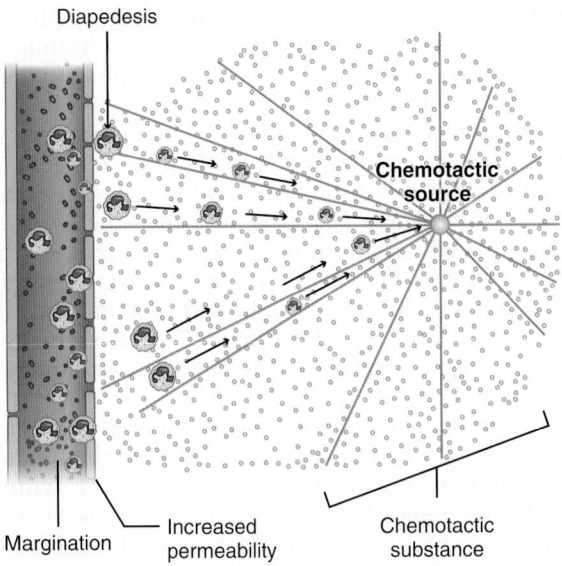

Figure 6-15

Many different chemical substances in the tissues cause both neutrophils and macrophages to move through the capillary pores in a process called *diapedesis* and toward the area of tissue damage by chemotaxis. Chemotaxis depends on the concentration gradient of the chemotactic substance. The concentration is greatest near the source, which directs the unidirectional movement of the WBCs. Chemotaxis is effective up to 100 µm away from an inflamed tissue. Because almost no tissue area is more than 50 µm away from a capillary, the chemotactic signal can easily move vast numbers of WBCs from the capillaries into the inflamed area. (From Hall JE, Guyton AC: *Textbook of medical physiology,* ed 12, Philadelphia, 2011, WB Saunders.)

microorganisms from using iron for growth and development. Neutrophils also demonstrate direct cytotoxic activity toward viruses, fungi, and bacteria by releasing defensin, which are peptides with natural antibiotic activity.

If the inflammatory stimulus subsides, the neutrophils rapidly die out because their life span (after extrusion from the circulation) is approximately 24 hours; they are replaced by monocytic/macrophage cells responsible for cleaning up the cellular debris left after neutrophils have done their job. Certain inflammatory stimuli can induce a sustained neutrophil response (e.g., first defense against pyogenic bacteria), a predominantly lymphocytic response (e.g., fight tumor cells or respond to viruses), or an eosinophilic response (e.g., plays a role in asthma and allergies or attacks parasites).

In addition to the types of WBCs present, the total and differential counts of the leukocytes in the circulating blood are also very important diagnostic tools (see Table 40-11). An increased number of circulating leukocytes (leukocytosis) is often an indication of an active inflammatory reaction (typically to an infection or tissue injury). A decreased WBC count (leukopenia) can, for example, be seen in certain types of infections and is an indicator of grave prognosis in severe systemic infections (sepsis).

The main function of the leukocytes recruited to the affected tissue is to remove or eliminate the injurious stimulus. Leukocytes achieve this function by releasing enzymes and toxic substances that kill, inactivate, and degrade microbial agents, foreign antigens, or necrotic tissue. Leukocytes also take up these materials by phagocytosis and release growth factors necessary for healing or regeneration (please refer to the section on phagocytosis later in this chapter).

In addition to the role played by blood vessels in inflammation, a contribution is made from a system of thin-walled channels formed by endothelial cells with loose junctions. These channels are called the *lymphatics* and ultimately drain into the subclavian vein via the thoracic duct (see Fig. 13-8). These channels in physiologic conditions help drain fluid and protein from the interstitium, thereby reducing edema. They also serve as a conduit for the removal of certain leukocytes and inflammatory stimuli.[173]

The movement of the phagocytic cells into the lymphatic vessels allows presentation of the engulfed material to immunocompetent cells located in the lymph nodes. Hyperplasia of immunocompetent cells (T and B lymphocytes) in the lymph nodes leads to an enlargement of the nodes called lymphadenopathy. During the process of removing infectious agents, lymphatics and their lymph nodes may become actively inflamed. Clinically, the inflamed lymphatics may appear as red streaks under the epidermis and may be painful to palpation; this condition is called *lymphangitis* (see Chapter 13).

Chemical Mediators of Inflammation. A large number of chemical mediators are responsible for the vascular and leukocyte responses generated by the cells involved in an acute inflammatory response. These mediators are either released from inflammatory cells (cell-derived) or are generated by the action of plasma protease (plasma-derived). Mediators of inflammation are multifunctional and have numerous effects on blood vessels, inflammatory cells, and other cells in the body. Some of their primary effects in the inflammatory response include vasodilation or vasoconstriction, modulation of vascular permeability, activation of inflammatory cells, chemotaxis, cytotoxicity, degradation of tissue, pain, and fever. These mediators include histamine, serotonin, bradykinin, the complement system, platelet-activating factors, arachidonic acid derivatives (e.g., prostaglandins, leukotrienes), and cytokines (Table 6-5).

Histamine. Histamine is synthesized and stored in granules (for quick availability and release) of mast cells, basophils, and platelets. Histamine causes endothelial contraction leading to the formation of gaps, which increase blood vessel permeability and allow fluids and blood cells to exit into the interstitial spaces (vascular leak). Histamine's effect occurs quickly but is short-lived because it is inactivated in less than 30 minutes. Histamine is also a potent vasodilator and bronchoconstrictor. Serotonin is another mediator released from platelets. It induces vasoconstriction, but its effect is usually overridden by the vasodilator action of histamine.

Platelet-Activating Factor. Leukocytes and other cells on stimulation also synthesize three classes of inflammatory mediators that are derived from phospholipids (the major lipids present in cell membranes). The first of these mediators is an acetylated lysophospholipid named *platelet-activating factor* (PAF). The other two classes of mediators are derived from a fatty acid (arachidonic acid) of membrane phospholipids and are called *prostaglandins*

Table 6-5	Mediators of Inflammation
Cell-Derived Sources	**Plasma Cell–Derived Sources**
Circulating platelets (platelet-activating factor, histamine, serotonin)	Blood coagulation cascade
	Fibrinolytic system
Tissue mast cells (histamine)	Kinin enzymatic system:
Basophils (histamine)	• Bradykinin
Polymorphonuclear leukocytes (neutrophils)	• Hageman factor
Endothelial cells	Complement system: C3a, C3b, C5a, C5b
Monocytes/macrophages	Membrane attack complex
Injured tissue itself	
Arachidonic acid derivatives (prostaglandins, leukotrienes)	
Cytokines (TNF, IL-1)	

TNF, tumor necrosis factor; *IL-1*, interleukin-1

and *leukotrienes*. All three of these lipid mediators have potent and wide-ranging inflammatory activities. In addition, these mediators have hormone-like functions that modulate physiologic responses and induce pathology in a variety of organ systems.

PAF was so named because it was first found to induce platelet activation and secretion. PAF is now known to be a potent activator of cells, such as smooth muscle cells, endothelial cells, and leukocytes, by receptor binding and intracellular signaling mechanisms. As a consequence, PAF can induce the aggregation of leukocytes and leukocyte infiltration in tissues and can profoundly affect vasomotor tone and permeability.[195] PAF can potentiate (increase or strengthen) the activity of other inflammatory mediators.

Arachidonic Acid Derivatives. The synthesis of prostaglandins and leukotrienes begins with the cleavage (splitting) of arachidonic acid from membrane phospholipids by the action of the phospholipase (Fig. 6-16). Once this step is completed, either a cyclooxygenase enzyme or a lipoxygenase enzyme further metabolizes the arachidonic acid. The cyclooxygenase pathway leads to the production of several types of prostaglandins that modulate vasomotor tone and platelet aggregation (e.g., thromboxane is a strong platelet aggregator and vasoconstrictor, whereas prostacyclin [PGI$_2$] is a strong platelet inhibitor and vasodilator). Clinically, prostaglandins are also important because they are mediators of the fever and pain responses associated with inflammation.[155]

The lipoxygenase pathway leads to the production of leukotrienes. Leukotrienes occur naturally in leukocytes and produce allergic and inflammatory reactions similar to those of histamine. They are extremely potent mediators of immediate hypersensitivity reactions and inflammation, producing smooth muscle contraction, especially bronchoconstriction; increased vascular permeability; and migration of leukocytes to areas of inflammation. They are thought to play a role in the development of allergic and autoimmune disease such as asthma and rheumatoid arthritis. Certain leukotrienes (C4, D4, and E4) are collectively known as a slow-reacting substance of

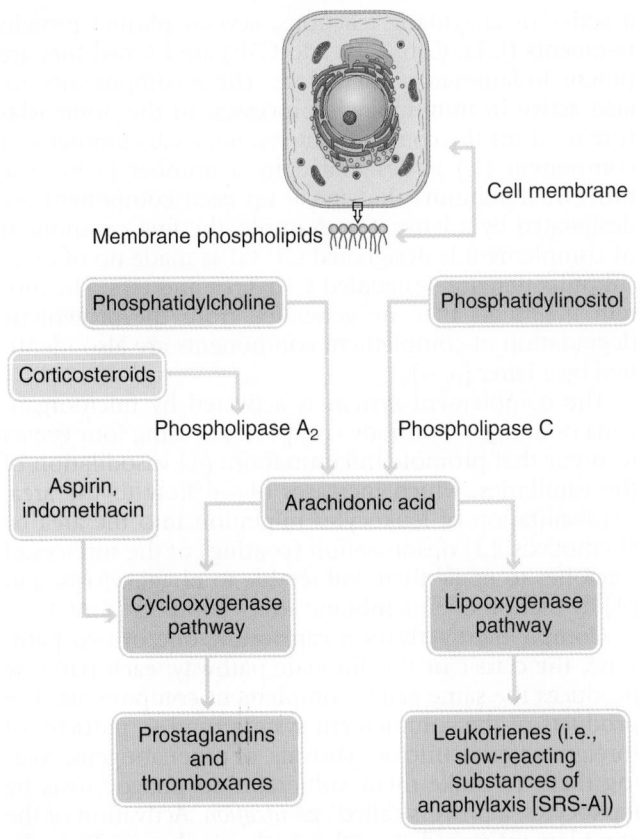

Figure 6-16

Production of prostaglandins and leukotrienes from damaged cell membranes. Note sites for pharmacologic (aspirin and prednisone) interventions. (Courtesy SH Tepper, PhD, PT.)

anaphylaxis (SRS-A), which is the name given when their potent bronchoconstrictor activity was discovered; they also cause leakage of fluid and proteins from the microvasculature.

The importance of the arachidonic acid metabolites in the inflammatory process is made evident by the excellent clinical response to treatment of acute and chronic inflammatory conditions with drugs that block the production of arachidonic acid (corticosteroids) or inhibit the enzyme and block the production of prostaglandins and cyclooxygenase (nonsteroidal antiinflammatory drugs [NSAIDs] such as aspirin or the newer cyclooxygenase-2 inhibitors). These antiinflammatory medications are commonly used for people with somatic pain or inflammatory conditions, especially rheumatoid arthritis.

Cytokines. Leukocytes also produce polypeptide substances called *cytokines* (see Chapter 7) that have a wide range of inflammatory actions affecting either the cytokine-producing cells themselves (autocrine effects) or adjacent cells (paracrine effects). Cytokines also have a number of systemic "hormonal" inflammatory effects.

Two important cytokines with overlapping functions are IL-1 and TNF. As many as 15 ILs are now identified. Most ILs direct other cells to divide and differentiate, each interleukin acting on a particular group of cells that have receptors specific for that interleukin. TNF is thought to be capable of inducing most of the actions of IL-1 with the exception of activation of lymphocytes.

IL-1 has a number of local actions that promote the inflammatory reaction and a number of systemic actions that induce metabolic, hemodynamic, and hematologic alterations (see Box 6-2). These alterations are discussed in some detail because of their importance in the clinical and laboratory diagnosis of inflammation. IL-1 causes fever by raising the production of prostaglandins in the hypothalamus and thereby resetting the threshold of temperature-sensitive neurons.

Fever in turn raises the systemic metabolism and increases the systemic consumption of oxygen by approximately 10% for each degree Celsius of body temperature elevation. As a result, a decrease in systemic vascular resistance occurs, thereby producing hypotension and an increase in cardiac output to increase the flow of blood and the delivery of oxygen to various organs. These hemodynamic changes are characteristic of severe systemic infections and a febrile condition.

IL-1 also causes characteristic changes in blood chemistry. Albumin and transferrin levels are decreased, while levels of coagulation factors complement components, C-reactive protein, and serum amyloid A increase. These changes occur because IL-1 alters the rate of synthesis of these proteins by the liver. IL-1 also increases the number of neutrophils and decreases the number of lymphocytes in the circulation.

The Blood Coagulation, Fibrinolytic, and Complement Systems. Plasma proteins produce chemical inflammatory mediators by the enzymatic activity of proteases on plasma proteins. Plasma proteases are enzymes that act as a catalyst in the breakdown of proteins. These plasma protein systems are the blood coagulation and fibrinolytic, kinin enzymatic, and complement systems.

All of these systems can become activated by contact with by-products of cell injury or foreign materials. Examples include contact with components of denuded vascular endothelial cells revealing their underlying basement membrane, which occurs with trauma to the vessel wall and contact with bacterial endotoxins. The key plasma protein in the activation sequence of these systems is clotting factor XII, also known as *Hageman factor*.

The blood coagulation system (Fig. 6-17) is formed in part by plasma proteins. The design is to bandage injuries with clots (coagulation), then disassemble (lyse) the clots when the job is done. The system protects against both hemorrhage and catastrophic clotting. To maintain homeostasis, these two processes must remain in balance.

Platelets circulating throughout the bloodstream are always ready to seal any damage to blood vessels with a hemostatic plug. When there is no need for the platelets, the smooth vascular walls prevent platelets from adhering and aggregating. At the same time, endothelial cells in the walls of the blood vessels make tissue plasminogen activator to prevent fibrin deposits from forming and for breaking down existing clots.

More specifically, when injury or bleeding occurs, a series of enzymes are activated sequentially to generate the enzyme thrombin, which converts the plasma protein fibrinogen to fibrin, the essential component of a blood clot. Fibrin forms a meshwork at bleeding sites to stop the bleeding and trap exudate, microorganisms, and foreign materials and keep this content contained in an area

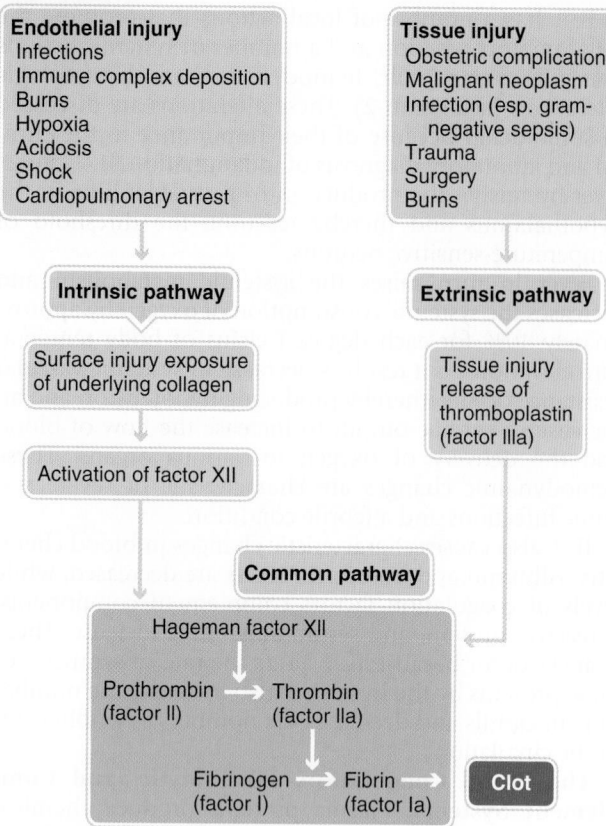

Figure 6-17

Clinical causes of the activation of a clotting cascade, intrinsic and extrinsic pathways of activation, and the mechanism by which both pathways lead to the formation of fibrin threads, or clot. In the chain reaction, inactive proenzymes (represented by Roman numerals) are converted into active enzymes (represented by Roman numerals followed by the letter "a"). The clotting cascade can follow two pathways: intrinsic and extrinsic. The intrinsic pathway is activated within the vascular compartment. The extrinsic pathway is activated outside the vascular compartment, when blood comes in contact with any tissue other than blood vessels. In the case of internal bleeding, both pathways are activated. (Courtesy SH Tepper, PhD, PT.)

where eventually the greatest number of phagocytes will be found. This localizing effect prevents the spread of infection to other sites and begins the process of healing and tissue repair.

The fibrinolytic system (designed to dissolve these clots) is activated by the conversion of plasminogen to the enzyme plasmin (also known as *fibrinolysin*, which means "to loosen"). Plasmin splits or divides fibrin and lyses the blood clots. Both the coagulation and the fibrinolytic systems are activated in inflammation and function together in a system of checks and balances to preserve vascular function.

The products of fibrin degradation are chemotactic for leukocytes and increase vascular permeability. The kinin enzymatic system is also activated by Hageman factor and functions to produce bradykinin. Bradykinin is a mediator that causes dilation and leakage of blood vessels and induces pain.

The complement system is composed of a group of plasma proteins that normally lie dormant in the blood, interstitial fluid, and mucosal surfaces. Then, through a series of enzymatic reactions, several plasma protein fragments (C3a, C3b, C5a, and C5b) are formed that are potent inflammatory mediators. These components are also active in immunologic processes. In the nomenclature used for the complement system, each complement component (C) is designated by a number (1-9). The individual subunits that make up each component are designated by a letter. For example, the first component of complement is designated C1. C1 is made up of three subunits that are designated C1q, C1r, and C1s. The protein fragments that are generated from the proteolytic degradation of complement components are also identified by a letter (a, b).

The complement system is activated by microorganisms or antigen–antibody complexes causing four events to occur that promote inflammation: (1) vasodilation of the capillaries, which increases blood flow to the area, (2) facilitation of leukocytes migration into the area by chemotaxis, (3) opsonization (coating) of the surfaces of microbes to make them vulnerable to phagocytosis, and (4) formation of a membrane attack complex (MAC).

Complement activation can follow one of two pathways, the classic or the alternate pathway; each pathway produces the same active complement components. The products of the complement system bind to particles of foreign material, microorganisms, or other antigens, coating them to make them vulnerable to phagocytosis by leukocytes, a process called *opsonization*. Activation of the complement cascade by either pathway also results in the formation of the MAC. The MAC is inserted in cell membranes of the microorganism where it creates an opening (pore or channel) in the cell membrane, leading to influx of sodium and extracellular fluid, eventually leading to its lysis (Fig. 6-18). For example, in hemolytic anemia, MAC bores holes in the cell membrane of RBCs, causing their destruction.

The plasma protease systems (blood coagulation, fibrinolytic, kinin enzymatic, and complement systems) are interconnected at several steps. This arrangement serves to amplify the stimulus for the inflammatory reaction as a balance mechanism. For example, the activation of the plasma protein Hageman factor can initiate both the coagulation (blood clotting) and the kinin systems (produces bradykinin causing dilation and vascular leakage).

The kinin system can in turn activate the fibrinolytic system by producing plasmin (splits or divides fibrin and lyses blood clots). Plasmin then can activate the complement system and further amplify these protease loops by activating Hageman factor, once again starting the cycle (Fig. 6-19).

Phagocytosis. One of the most important functions of the inflammatory reaction is to inactivate and remove the inflammatory stimulus and to begin the process of healing. The process of ingestion (phagocytosis) of microorganisms, other foreign substances, necrotic cells, and connective tissue constituents by specialized cells (phagocytes) is important in achieving this goal. As mentioned earlier, the chemical mediators attract the phagocytic cells to the area for removal of the dead tissue or microorganisms. After ingestion by phagocytic cells, microorganisms are killed or inactivated, and necrotic debris is removed to allow tissue healing to proceed.

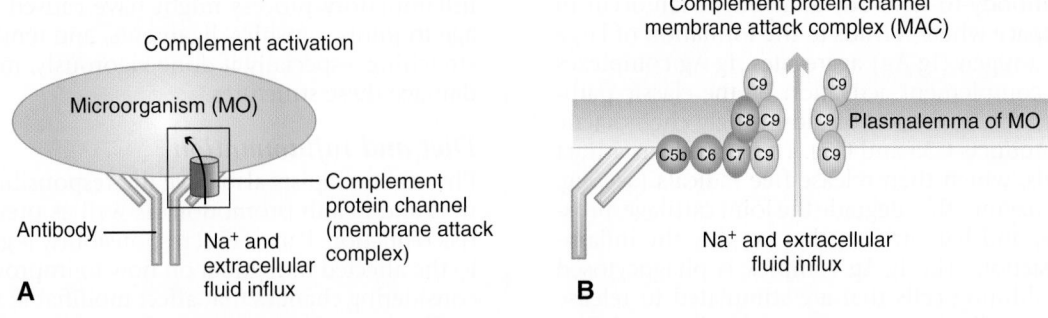

Figure 6-18

A, When an antibody attaches to an antigen (foreign protein) on a microorganism (MO), the antibody–antigen stimulates plasma-derived complement proteins to attach and form the membrane attack complex (MAC). **B,** This MAC forms a channel through the membrane of the invading cell and allows ions and extracellular fluid to enter, causing cytolysis (death of the microorganism). (Courtesy SH Tepper, PhD, PT.)

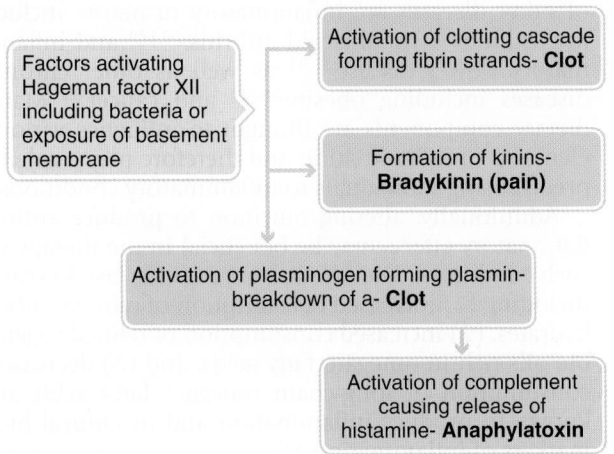

Figure 6-19

Clot formation. Revealed in this figure are the mechanisms for activating both the intrinsic and the extrinsic pathways for clot formation. Either of the above pathways leads to activation of the Hageman factor XII that results in the formation of a fibrin clot. (Courtesy SH Tepper, PhD, PT.)

The most important phagocytes involved in the inflammatory and healing reactions are neutrophils, monocytes, or when found in tissues of the body, macrophages. Macrophages have different names depending on their location (e.g., histiocytes in the skin, osteoclasts in bone, and microglial cells in the CNS).

The mechanism of phagocytosis is well understood. Phagocytosis is facilitated by the coating (opsonization) of particles to be ingested by immunoglobulin G (IgG) antibody or by the C3b component of complement. These opsonins bind to specific receptor sites located on the cell surface of neutrophils and macrophages. This receptor binding initiates a process of transmembrane signaling, allowing calcium influx that activates cytoskeletal proteins within the cell. These cytoskeletal structures allow the movement of cell membranes that is necessary for phagocytosis.

The internalization of the opsonized particle begins by the enfolding of the cell surface membrane (Figs. 6-20 and 6-21). The membrane folds surround the particle to be ingested and seal it within a pouch that separates it from the cell surface and becomes an intracellular vacuole called the *phagosome*. The phagosomes fuse with

lysosomes (containing digestive materials and bactericidal components) and acquire enzymes and other substances that allow the killing and degradation of microorganisms and other ingested materials. Many neutrophils (e.g., polymorphonuclear neutrophils [PMNs]) die in their battle with bacteria. Dead and dying leukocytes, mixed with tissue debris and lytic enzymes, form a viscous yellow fluid known as *pus*. Inflammations identified by their pus formations are called *purulent* or *suppurative* (see Table 6-4).

SPECIAL IMPLICATIONS FOR THE THERAPIST   6-2

Inflammation

Clinical Example: Rheumatoid Arthritis
Inflammation, which involves all of the processes described in this section, is a normal, healthy response to tissue injury, but it can also damage adjacent healthy tissue. Chronic activation of inflammatory cells can cause tissue injury such as occurs with rheumatoid arthritis. The role of the therapist is important in supporting the healing process and, when appropriate, to limit inflammation and its consequences. The therapist must remember that finding and correcting the cause of inflammation is the goal, not just addressing the inflammatory process. Poor lifestyle choices including poor nutrition, improper posture and body mechanics, and poor breathing habits can contribute to the chronicity of this condition.

Rheumatoid arthritis illustrates how the inflammatory mediators discussed are activated and how this process leads to clinical manifestations observed in a therapy practice. Inflammatory activity can be detected by the erythrocyte sedimentation rate. The therapist can review laboratory values (see Table 40-7) to assess systemic factors; in general, as the inflammation improves, the erythrocyte sedimentation rate decreases. Systemic effects of acute and chronic inflammation are discussed in Chapter 5.

The majority of people with rheumatoid arthritis produce rheumatoid factor, an antibody that is made against the person's own antibodies of the IgG class. In this case, the IgG antibody actually functions as an antigen (Ag) capable of inducing an immune response.

This antibody-to-antibody attachment can occur in the joint space where it leads to the formation of large antibody–antigen (Ig-Ag) aggregates. Ig-Ag complexes stimulate complement activation by the classic pathway and to the formation of the strongly chemotactic cleavage products C3a and C5a. These products attract neutrophils, which then release free radicals (see Fig. 6-3) and enzymes that degrade the joint cartilage, prostaglandins, and leukotrienes that amplify the inflammatory reaction. The Ig-Ag complex is phagocytosed by synovial-lining cells that are stimulated to release collagen-degrading enzymes, prostaglandins, and IL-1.

Lymphocytes contribute to the acute reaction by the production of rheumatoid factor and are responsible for the evolution of a chronic inflammatory reaction by producing cytokines that attract and activate macrophages. The macrophages produce cytokines, such as IL-1, that further amplify the inflammatory reaction by attracting more neutrophils and lymphocytes and by stimulating the synthesis and release from fibroblasts, chondrocytes, and osteoclasts of enzymes that degrade cartilage and bone.

Clinically, the joints affected by the inflammatory process appear red and swollen and are painful; a low-grade fever may also be present. A prominent symptom is joint stiffness that is relieved by activity. With disease progression, damage to the joints occurs; with loss of cartilage, narrowing of the joint space occurs, and resorption of bone is evident on radiograph. These changes are associated with a decrease in the range of motion of the affected joints. In later stages, obvious joint deformities develop that are accompanied by muscle wasting. Antiinflammatory agents, such as aspirin and corticosteroids and disease-modifying antirheumatic drugs, are effective in providing symptomatic relief and in slowing the progression of the disease.

The inflammatory process associated with rheumatoid arthritis may also affect other organ systems (see Box 27-9). Foci of chronic inflammation can develop in muscles, tendons, blood vessels, nerves, and various organs of the body (e.g., heart and lungs). In the skin, these foci cause the deposition of connective tissue called *subcutaneous nodules*.

In the inflammatory phase of the condition, physical therapy may be of benefit for pain control, preservation of available motion, and protection of joint retardation or atrophy. The therapist should avoid exercises that will cause compression and irritation of the joints, potentially prolonging the inflammatory process. At this stage, limitation of joint motion is primarily due to joint swelling; therefore, stretching exercises may overstretch the tissues and cause joint hypermobility when the swelling subsides. Furthermore, because osteoporosis and ligamentous laxity are potential side effects of steroid medication, the bones and joints must be protected from excessive loads.[119]

During the remission phase of the condition, there is strong evidence that exercise of various modes and intensities is effective in improving the functional performance of people with rheumatoid arthritis.[142] The therapist must still exercise extreme care when performing stretching exercises as the previous active inflammatory process might have caused some damage to joints, capsules, ligaments, and tendons,[119] and stretching, especially if done vigorously, might further damage these structures.

Diet and Inflammation

Physical therapists also have the responsibility in wellness and health promotion, as well as prevention and risk reduction. Part of that responsibility is giving advice to the affected individual on how to improve health by considering changes that affect modifiable risk factors.

There has been an abundance of recent evidence about inflammatory markers and their relationship to various diseases, especially coronary artery disease and diabetes mellitus, both among the top 10 causes of mortality in the United States.[147] A number of other diseases are inflammatory in nature including asthma,[207] rheumatoid arthritis,[20,129] and inflammatory bowel disease,[51,95] as well as other chronic diseases including obesity[20,229] and cancer.[85] Many dietary components are thought to influence various elements of inflammation and therefore play a role in predisposing individuals to inflammatory conditions.

Additionally, altering nutrition to produce antiinflammatory effects may be beneficial in the therapy of such conditions. Dietary changes over the last 30 years, including (1) increased consumption of refined carbohydrates, (2) increased consumption of refined vegetable oils rich in omega-6 fatty acids, and (3) decreased consumption of long-chain omega-3 fatty acids are known to produce inflammation and its clinical biomarkers of inflammation.[186]

Clinical biomarkers of inflammation are used to study the effect of dietary components on development of inflammatory conditions, treatment, and prevention. C-reactive protein, which is an acute phase reactant protein, is a common clinical biomarker of cardiac related inflammation[104,175] and also a general marker of inflammation. Other common clinical indicators of inflammation include high erythrocyte sedimentation rate, high WBC count, and a low albumin level.[129] However, these tests are nonspecific, meaning an abnormal result might result from a condition unrelated to inflammation. Various cytokines and adhesion molecules are not commonly used clinically because they do not identify the source of inflammation.[23,115,185]

Diseases or conditions with a well-recognized inflammatory component are often treated with general or specific antiinflammatory pharmaceuticals.[35] Antiinflammatory nutrition is the understanding how individual nutrients affect the same molecular targets affected by pharmacologic drugs.[186] Identification of dietary changes that may decrease inflammation may improve function and reduce need for medications in some cases.[134]

Exercise and Inflammation

Animal and human studies have found that various forms of physical activity decrease both acute and chronic inflammation, as measured by reductions in CRP and certain proinflammatory cytokines.[68,229] Additionally, regular physical activity is important in reducing one's risk for obesity and chronic diseases associated with inflammation.[31] However, excessive exercise can increase systemic inflammation and suppress immune function. For example, overtraining syndrome in athletes is associated with systemic inflammation and suppressed immune function.[7] The mechanisms of exercise-associated muscle damage and the initiation of the inflammatory cytokine cascade are further discussed in Chapter 7 (see "Exercise and the Immune System").

TISSUE HEALING

The process of tissue healing begins soon after tissue injury or death and occurs either by regeneration (regrowth of original tissue) or by repair (formation of a connective tissue scar). The inflammatory cells that are recruited from the blood circulation begin the healing process by breaking down and removing the necrotic tissue. This is accomplished primarily by phagocytes that secrete degradative enzymes and also phagocytose the cellular debris, connective tissue fragments, and plasma proteins present in the dead tissue (Fig. 6-22).

The healing process is complex and influenced by many components such as fibronectin, proteoglycans and elastin, collagen, and parenchymal and endothelial cells. In addition, there is a wide range of factors that affect tissue healing and must be taken into account during recovery and rehabilitation. Both the components and the factors that affect tissue healing are presented in this section, followed by a discussion of the multiphasic process of tissue healing and recovery.

Components of Tissue Healing

Fibronectin

Fibronectin has numerous functions in wound healing, the most important of which are the formation of scaffold, the provision of tensile strength, and the ability to "glue" other substances and cells together. It is one of the earliest proteins to provide the structural support that stabilizes the healing tissue. Plasma proteins that leak from inflamed vessels are the first source of fibronectin for the healing tissue. Plasma-derived fibronectin binds to and stabilizes fibrin, a protein that makes up the blood clots that are present in the injured tissue.

Fibronectin binds together several types of proteins present in the extracellular matrix and can also bind to debris, such as DNA material derived from necrotic cells, thereby acting as an opsonin (molecule that acts as a binding enhancer to facilitate phagocytosis) during the breakdown of necrotic tissue. Fibronectin is also responsible for attracting fibroblasts and macrophages by chemotaxis to the healing tissue. The stimulated fibroblasts, in turn, secrete more fibronectin. Fibronectin binds to proteoglycans and collagens, and this binding further stabilizes the healing tissue.

The importance of fibronectin can be seen as researchers seek to explain the lack of a functional healing

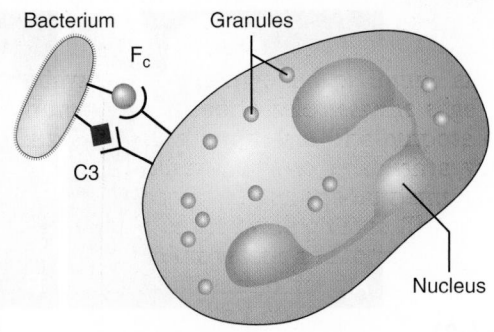

A

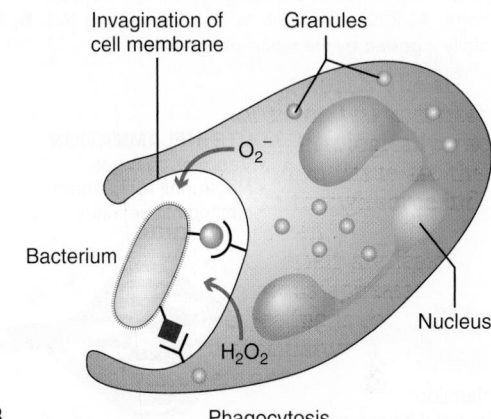

B   Phagocytosis

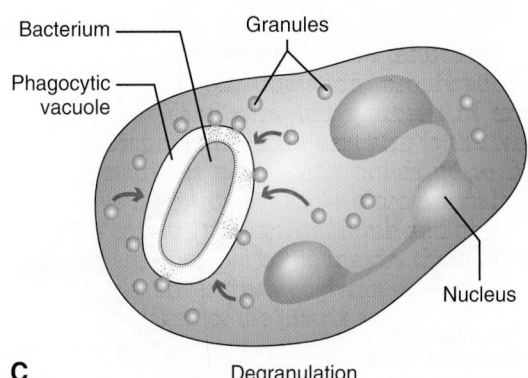

C   Degranulation

Figure 6-20

Phagocytosis of bacteria. A, The bacterium that was opsonized (coated with IgG and complement [C3]) binds to the Fc and complement receptors on the surface of the leukocytes. **B,** Engulfment of the bacterium into an invagination of surface membrane is associated with an oxygen burst and formation of oxygen radicals that are bactericidal and thus kill the bacterium. **C,** Inclusion of the bacterium into a phagocytic vacuole is associated with the fusion of the vacuole with lysosomes and specific granules of the leukocyte. The contents of the lysosomes and specific granules are bactericidal and contribute to final inactivation and degradation of the bacterium. The cytoplasm of the leukocyte becomes devoid of granules in a process referred to as degranulation of leukocytes. (From Damjanov I: *Pathology for the health-related professions,* ed 4, St. Louis, MO, 2012, Elsevier.)

response in the anterior cruciate ligament (ACL) after injury.[131] Studies focusing on the signaling pathways and on binding to fibronectin for specific tissues, such as the ACL, may yield improved prevention and intervention strategies in the future.[140,212]

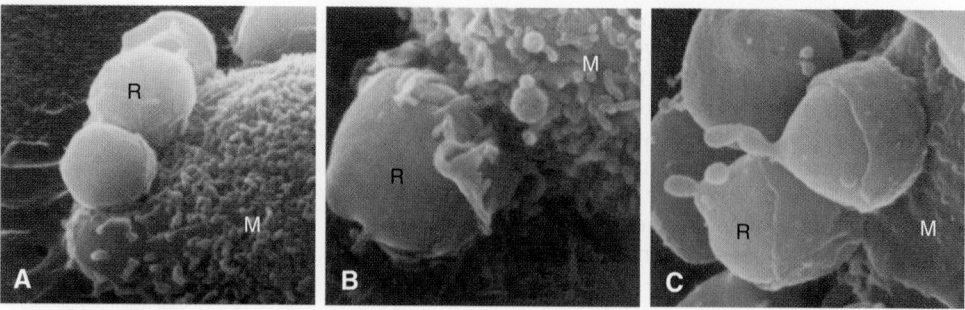

Figure 6-21

Phagocytosis. This series of scanning electron micrographs shows the progressive steps in phagocytosis of damaged red blood cells (RBCs) by a macrophage. **A,** RBCs (*R*) attach to the macrophage (*M*). **B,** Plasma membrane of the macrophage begins to enclose the RBC. **C,** The RBCs are almost totally ingested by the macrophage. (From Patton KT, Thibodeau GA: *The human body in health and disease*, ed 6, St. Louis, MO, 2014, Mosby. Courtesy Emma Shelton.)

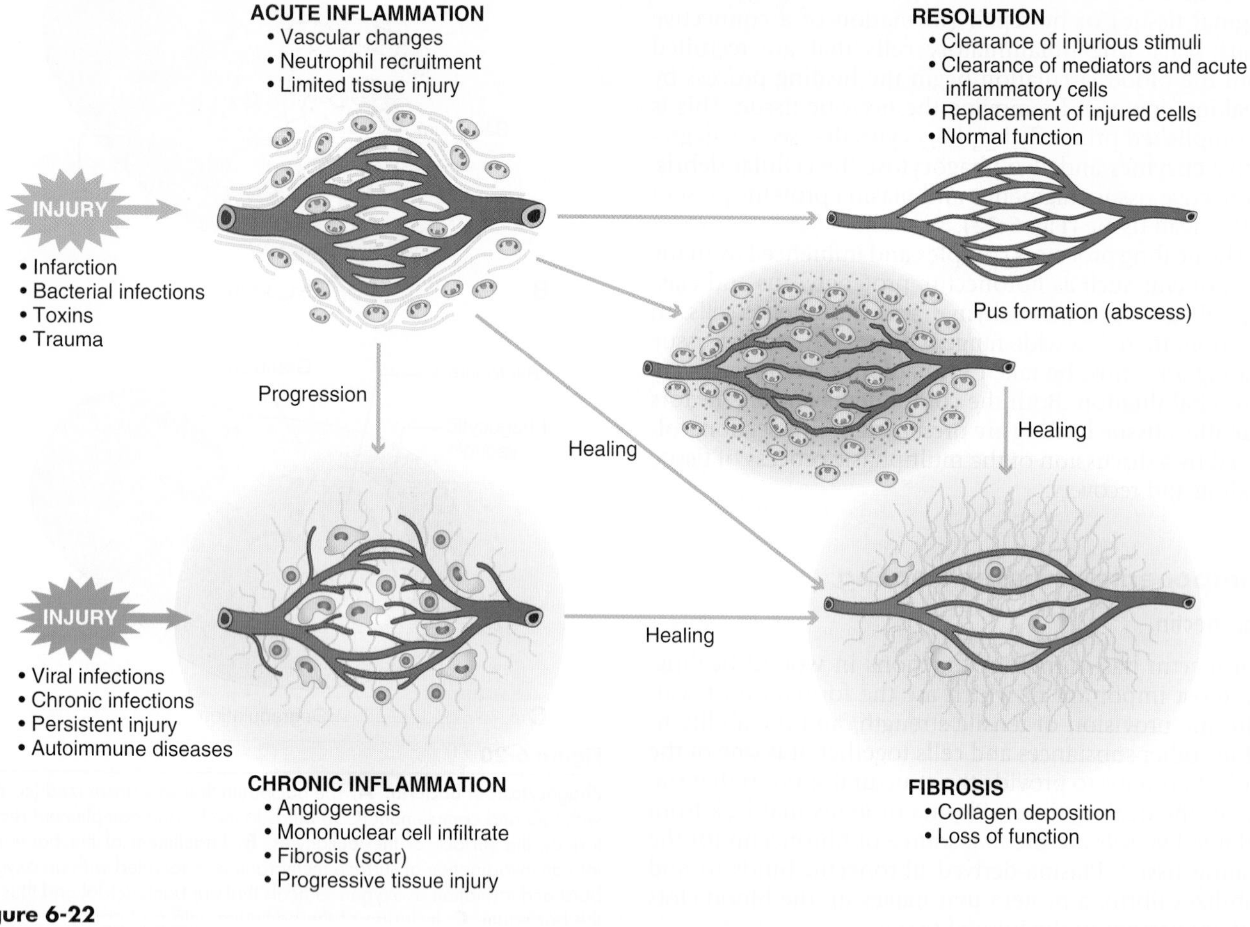

ACUTE INFLAMMATION
- Vascular changes
- Neutrophil recruitment
- Limited tissue injury

RESOLUTION
- Clearance of injurious stimuli
- Clearance of mediators and acute inflammatory cells
- Replacement of injured cells
- Normal function

INJURY
- Infarction
- Bacterial infections
- Toxins
- Trauma

Progression

Pus formation (abscess)

Healing

Healing

Healing

INJURY
- Viral infections
- Chronic infections
- Persistent injury
- Autoimmune diseases

CHRONIC INFLAMMATION
- Angiogenesis
- Mononuclear cell infiltrate
- Fibrosis (scar)
- Progressive tissue injury

FIBROSIS
- Collagen deposition
- Loss of function

Figure 6-22

Outcomes of acute inflammation: resolution, healing by fibrosis, or chronic inflammation. The components of the various reactions and their functional outcomes are listed. (From Kumar V, et al: *Robbins and Cotran pathologic basis of disease*, ed 8, Philadelphia, 2010, Saunders Elsevier.)

Proteoglycans and Elastin

Proteoglycans, proteins containing carbohydrate chains and sugars, are secreted in abundance by fibroblasts early during the tissue repair reaction. Proteoglycans bind to fibronectin and to collagen and help stabilize the tissue that is undergoing repair. Proteoglycans also retain water and aid in the hydration of the tissue being repaired. Once the tissue is healed, proteoglycans contribute to the organization and stability of collagen and create an electrical charge that gives basement membranes the property of functioning like molecular sieves. Fibroblasts also synthesize and secrete elastin, a protein that becomes cross-linked to form fibrils or long sheets that provide tissues with elasticity.

Collagen

Collagen is the most important protein to provide structural support and tensile strength for almost all tissues

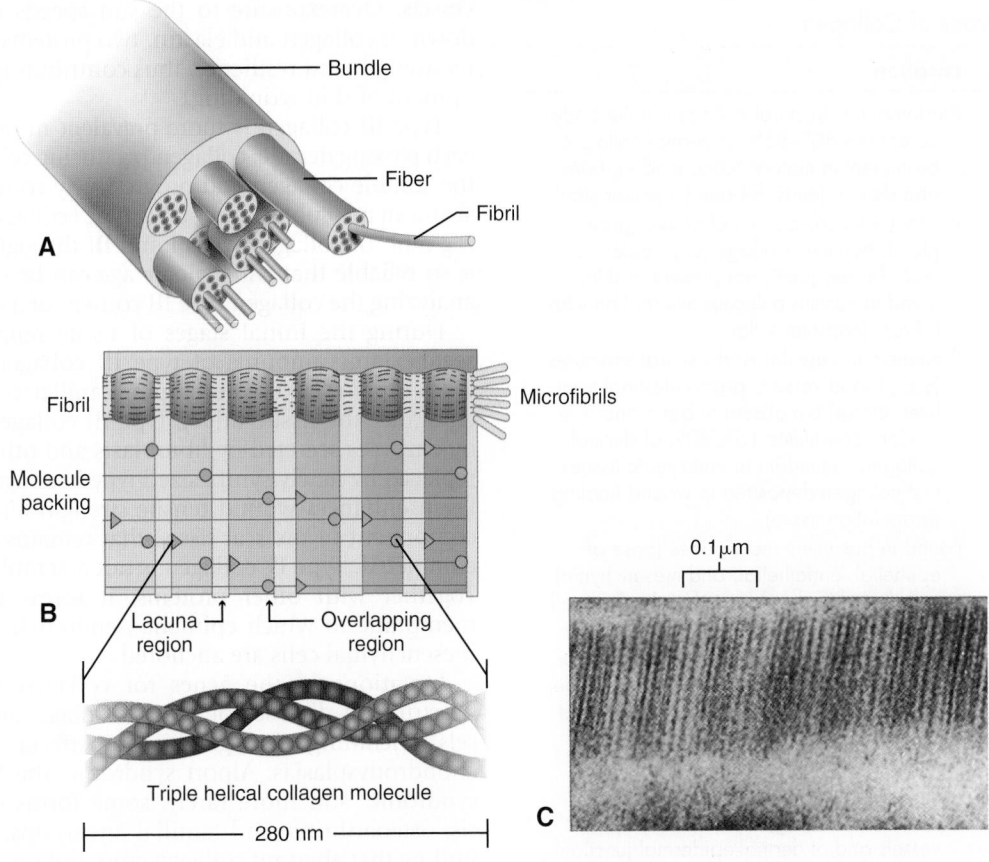

Figure 6-23

Structure of collagen. A, The collagen fiber is composed of fibrils, each of which is composed of microfibrils. **B,** The molecule itself consists of three polypeptide chains called alpha chains that wrap around each other in a triple helix. The helix is made possible because each third amino acid in the polypeptide chain is glycine. The molecules are quarter-staggered one to another, which ensures that no weak points occur across the fibril to prevent overload and slippage. **C,** Visualized by transmission electron microscopy, the individual collagen fibrils are seen to have two orders of banding. The larger bands result from the gaps between the individual molecules of collagen, which then overlap the adjacent molecules to form a strong bond. (From Bullough PG: *Bullough and Vigorita's orthopaedic pathology,* ed 3, St. Louis, MO, 1997, Mosby.)

and organs of the body. The different types of collagen give stability to healing tissue; the word *collagen* is derived from Greek and means "glue producer." Collagen is a fibrous protein molecule consisting of three chains of amino acid coiled around each other in a triple helix (Fig. 6-23). Improved technology has made it possible to identify collagen types and measure protein turnover. It is the most abundant protein in the body; at least 28 collagen types have been identified.[88]

We know that exercise is a potent stimulus for protein synthesis in skeletal muscle. Collagen in the extracellular matrix of muscle and tendon is also sensitive to mechanical stimuli. Collagen does not appear to be nutritionally sensitive, which may contribute to the loss of muscle during aging. It is possible that the tissue is unable to respond adequately to increased availability of nutrients.[219]

Organization of Collagen. Each collagen type has a specialized function (Table 6-6). The amino acid makeup of the collagen molecule and the manner in which the molecules are assembled together vary for each one of the collagen types. The differences in organization and composition account for the structural properties of each collagen type. For example, collagen organized in unidirectional or parallel bundles contributes to the strength of tendons. Collagen is the principal extracellular component of normal tendon.

Collagen in random arrangement provides flexibility of the skin and rigidity of bone. When organized at right angles, collagen allows transmission of light in the cornea and vitreous. Collagen laid down in a tubular fashion contributes to the elasticity of the blood vessels.

Some collagen molecules are assembled into progressively thicker and stronger filamentous structures, allowing the molecules to become cross-linked. These cross-links impart tensile strength to collagen fibers and prevent slippage of molecules past one another when under tension. The structural stability of the extracellular matrix is primarily a consequence of collagen and the extent of cross-linking.[44]

Types of Collagen. Type I collagen, the most common form, is assembled as a thick bundle that is structurally very strong and can be found in all body tissues, where it forms bundles together with other collagen types. Type I collagen is the main component of mature scars and is also predominant in strong tissues such as tendons and bones.

Table 6-6	Types of Collagen

Type	Location
Type I	Predominant structural collagen of the body; constitutes 80%-85% of dermal collagen; prominent in mature scars, tendon, bone, and dentin; joints; labrum (capsular side)
Type II	Predominant component of physis (growth plate), hyaline cartilage (e.g., outer ear, end of nose, joint); not present in skin; found in nucleus pulposus external annulus; labrum (capsular side)
Type III	Prominent in vascular and visceral structures (e.g., blood vessels, gastrointestinal tract, liver, uterus) but absent in bone and tendon; constitutes 15%-20% of dermal collagen; abundant in embryonic tissues; first collagen deposited in wound healing (granulation tissue)
Type IV	Found in basement membranes (base of epithelial, endothelial, and mesenchymal cells found in developing fetus), glomeruli of kidney nephron
Type V	Present in most tissues but never as a major component; prominent in fetal membrane, cornea, heart valve; minor component of skin; synovial membranes
Type VI	Prevalent in most connective tissues
Type VII	May be involved in matrix and bone disorders, anchoring filaments of lymphatic vessels and at dermal-epidermal junctions
Type VIII	Secreted by rapidly proliferating cells; found in basement membranes; may provide a molecular bridge between different types of matrix molecules
Type IX	Minor component in hyaline cartilage; vitreous humor (fluid of the eye); also found in the physis (growth plate)
Type X	Only formed in the epiphyseal growth plate cartilage; may have a role in angiogenesis; may be involved in matrix and bone disorders
Type XI	Hyaline cartilage; physis
Type XII	Embryonic skin and tendon, periodontal ligament
Type XIII	Endothelial cells
Type XIV	Fetal skin and tendons; similar to type I
Types XV-XXVII	Identified but not clearly understood

Type II collagen is assembled into thin supporting filaments and is the predominant collagen type found in cartilaginous tissue and the physis (growth plate).[15] Type II fibers of the external annulus have a half-life of about 3 months. This allows maintenance of the nutritive exchanges between degenerative external annulus and any healthy remaining tissue, possibly delaying or avoiding further degeneration.[220]

Type III collagen is assembled into thin filaments that make tissues strong but supple and elastic.[202] It contains interchain disulfide bonds or bridges not found in type I or II and is the collagen type first deposited in wound healing (i.e., fresh scars). This type of highly soluble collagen accounts in part for the plasticity of skin and blood vessels. Overexposure to the sun speeds up the breakdown of collagen and elastin, two proteins that give skin its strength and resilience, thus contributing to the development of skin wrinkling.

Type III collagen is more prevalent in newborns; with each passing decade, collagen-producing cells make less of the soluble collagen and progressively convert to synthesizing an insoluble, more stable type I collagen. The changing ratio of collagen types I and III throughout the body is so reliable that chronologic age can be determined by analyzing the collagen type III content of a skin sample.[14]

During the initial stages of tissue repair, fibroblasts secrete large amounts of type III collagen, which provides support for the developing capillaries. Within a few days after the tissue injury, type III collagen is degraded by enzymes secreted by fibroblasts and other cells and is replaced by newly synthesized type I collagen. Type I collagen enhances wound tensile strength and is the main component of the scar tissue that remains after repair is completed. Type IV collagen is not assembled into fibers. Together with other proteins, it forms the basement membrane to which epithelial, endothelial, and certain mesenchymal cells are anchored.

Mutations in the genes for collagen cause a wide spectrum of diseases of bone, cartilage, and blood vessels, including osteogenesis imperfecta, a variety of chondrodysplasias, Alport syndrome, the Ehlers-Danlos syndrome, and more rarely, some forms of osteoporosis, osteoarthritis, and familial aneurysms. Scientists are finding that aberrant collagen cross-linking and increased collagen synthesis are present in some malignancies,[21,25] whereas the presence of free radical scavengers inhibits the rate of collagen formation.[143]

When either collagen or elastin becomes resorbed, elements are released into blood and concentrate in urine. Determining the presence of these components in tissues and body fluids provides important markers in the clinical investigation of various diseases.[193] Methods to quantify the number of collagen cross-links in tissue are also being further developed at this time.[165,192,218]

SPECIAL IMPLICATIONS FOR THE THERAPIST   6-3

Tissue Healing (Part 1)

Collagen

Much debate has been directed toward the role of the therapist in using myofascial and soft tissue mobilization techniques (including deep/cross-friction massage) to change collagen structures and improve mobility, increase joint range of motion, or alter scar tissue. Whether these techniques can break the collagen cross-links and allow slippage to lengthen or realign the collagen fibers continues under investigation at this time.[16,182,183,214] The use of instrument-assisted cross-friction massage on animal ligaments has been shown to increase strength and stiffness while improving the ability of the soft tissue to absorb energy compared with untreated (acute) ligament injuries. Electron microscopy images demonstrated improved collagen fiber bundle formation and orientation with the scar region in injured ligaments treated with cross-fiber massage.[130] Human studies evaluating the effectiveness of friction massage (whether instrument assisted or not) in improving physical impairments and function have generated mixed results. Most studies have investigated the effectiveness of friction massage in combination with other interventions; therefore, its therapeutic value as an individual treatment remains to be confirmed.[22,27,111] It has been found that regular mobility of affected tissues helps maintain lubrication and critical fiber distance.[4] Immobilization is associated with excessive deposition of connective tissue in associated areas. This is accompanied by a loss of water and subsequent dehydration. The result is an increase in intermolecular cross-linking, which further restricts normal connective tissue flexibility and extensibility.[47]

Another topic that has elicited considerable attention is the use of manual or movement techniques to elicit a corresponding change to the myofascial structures. It is possible that some of divergent points of view can be attributed to varying definitions of fascia[124] and therefore conflicting expert opinions about its function and relevance. More studies are needed to conclusively determine the efficacy of these techniques in decreasing pain, improving muscular and connective tissue extensibility, and facilitating performance of activity.

Related to this topic is the increasing attention to the concept of *tensegrity* as a framework to understand how the human body is structured and organized, and how physical movement, whether self-generated or provided by an external force (as in manual therapy or soft tissue mobilization techniques), affect biochemistry of the cells and physiology of the tissues.[103] This framework posits that the human body is in itself a transegrity structure, with compression structures (primarily the skeletal system) providing strength and stability while a network of fascia, tendons, and muscles provide the tension force that is transmitted through the body, thereby resulting in movement. Transegrity also highlights the interconnectedness of the components of the system, such that a dysfunction in one component affects the entire structure. Examples of therapeutic approaches such as myofascial release, rolfing, and other bodywork techniques are based on the concept of biotransegrity. Research, both at the basic and clinical science levels, is ongoing and will deepen our understanding of the importance of this emerging viewpoint in facilitating movement and function.

Therapeutic Ultrasound in Tissue Healing

The use of ultrasound to increase collagen tissue extensibility, increase enzymatic activity at the site of wound healing, absorb joint adhesions, and reduce fibrous tissue volume and density in scar tissue has been widely accepted, although some of these effects have to be definitively proven. Ultrasound has been shown to facilitate the development of stronger and better-aligned scar tissue[37]; studies have been published that examined the ability of ultrasound to heat human tendon and muscle.[38,58] Ultrasound as a therapeutic intervention in the treatment of human tendinopathy remains under investigation.[59,82,174,179,221,224]

In the physiologic response of injury or wound healing, the key to growth or replacement tissue at sites of injury is stimulation of protein synthesis in fibroblasts. Exposure of injured tissue to ultrasound at clinically practical doses seems to provide this stimulation.[228] The pulsed mode of ultrasound is used to achieve its nonthermal effects. It is thought that these nonthermal effects include cellular diffusion, membrane permeability, and fibroblastic activities such as protein synthesis, which speeds up tissue regeneration during the proliferative phase.[38,110] Pulsed ultrasound at the lower ranges of intensity may be used during the acute phase to stimulate the release of vasodilator amine histamine from mast cells.[74]

Continuous ultrasound during the first week of wound healing may hinder repair because the consequent heating of the tissues will exacerbate the inflammatory response. After 3 weeks, collagen synthesis continues to occur for remodeling during the subacute stage of healing, and ultrasound can be used as an adjunct to other interventions to promote this collagen synthesis[171] and to minimize adhesions. Reducing adhesions occurs by raising the tissue temperature to increase viscoelastic properties during the proliferation to remodeling stage.[58,63] It has been reported that ultrasound, laser, or a combination of ultrasound and laser are all equally as effective in facilitating tendon healing.[54]

Ultrasound aids in reabsorption of joint adhesions by depolymerization of mucopolysaccharides, mucoproteins, or glycoproteins and may reduce the viscosity of hyaluronic acid in joints, thereby reducing joint adhesions. In terms of mature scar tissue, the mechanical effects of ultrasound disrupt the glucoside bonds forming scar tissue, which could assist in the remodeling process.[159] Tight capsular tissue and tendon can also obtain increased extensibility when ultrasound is properly applied and followed immediately by slow, static stretching. Proper dosing of the ultrasound treatment is critically important to achieve the necessary tissue temperature rise to alter the viscoelastic properties of the connective tissue.[58] This must be immediately followed by a slow, controlled stretching and then active motion through the full available range of motion to assist in restoring mobility in tissue and between the tissue interfaces.[38,96] The stretch must be held until the collagen reaches a deformation phase. Without these follow-up techniques, the bond will re-form in its original position.[194]

The therapist is advised to make careful assessment of the phase of injury and clinical results in the use of ultrasound and discontinue its use if there are increases in pain or edema or decreases in range of motion or function. When using ultrasound, it is very important to select the appropriate treatment parameters including the mode (pulsed or continuous), intensity, and duration based on the stage of tissue healing and treatment goals.

Factors That Affect Tissue Healing

Many variables regulate or affect the healing process and either facilitate, inhibit, or delay wound healing (Box 6-3). Because local blood supply is vital to the delivery of the materials necessary for wound healing, factors that impede local circulation or depletion of the necessary materials could delay rehabilitation. Certain tissues (e.g., tendons, ligaments, cartilage, disk) have a decreased blood supply; thus, the healing process may require additional time.

Growth Factors

The cells involved in the tissue repair response produce proteins called *growth factors* that regulate a number of cellular reactions involved in healing. Growth factors regulate cell proliferation, differentiation, and migration; biosynthesis and degradation of proteins; and angiogenesis. Through all of these varying functions, growth factors integrate the inflammatory events with the reparative processes. When these complex mechanisms are disturbed, the result can be delayed healing and an inferior scar (hypotrophic) or elevated levels of growth factor, resulting in hypertrophic scarring such as occurs after a burn injury or in the formation of keloids.[213]

Growth factors act by binding to receptors on the plasma membranes of specific cells and have a stimulatory or inhibitory effect on these cells. This binding initiates a process of transmembrane signaling that results in the phosphorylation of proteins (the process of attaching a phosphate group to the protein). These steps lead to the activation of gene expression and DNA synthesis in the cell.

The signals that turn on proliferation of normal cells and cause tissue healing are also responsible for turning on proliferation of cancer cells. With continued growth of neoplastic cells, a neoplasm or tumor may occur.

The significant difference between the healing process and cancer is that the growth of the cancer cells goes on unchecked. These analogies have led to the designation of cancers as wounds that do not heal.

Platelets, endothelial cells, fibroblasts, macrophages, and cytokines are important sources of growth factors. Two important growth factors are platelet-derived growth factor, which activates fibroblasts and macrophages, and fibroblast growth factor, which stimulates endothelial cells to form new blood vessels. An example of a growth factor that inhibits cell growth and inactivates macrophages is transforming growth factor–β.

Recombinant human (Rh) platelet-derived growth factor–BB (becaplermin) is an FDA-approved growth factor that has been proven to be effective in facilitating the healing of lower extremity ulcers of persons with diabetes.[198] This is available in a gel form and applied to wounds usually once daily, with the wound being dressed after application.[43,53] Another growth factor, granulocyte colony–stimulating factor, has been shown to reduce the need for amputation and decrease length of hospitalization stay in people with diabetic foot ulcer, when used as an adjunct to usual wound care. Granulocyte colony–stimulating factor acts by facilitating the release of neutrophil endothelial progenitor cells, resulting in improved neutrophil function.[48]

Researchers continue to explore the most appropriate medium to effectively deliver these growth factors to the wound bed. Currently several of these wound dressings are already FDA approved, while others are still being investigated.[53] Platelet-rich plasma is also being used successfully for the treatment of tendon, ligament, muscle, cartilage injuries, and early osteoarthritis. The presence of critical growth factors and signaling molecules (e.g., cytokines, fibrinogen) in platelets that govern and regulate the tissue-healing process speeds up the healing process through the inflammatory, reparative, and remodeling phases.[45]

Finally, it should be mentioned that cytokines, such as IL-1, IL-2, IL-15, and TNF, can also regulate some aspects of the healing response. Some ILs have been identified as T-cell growth factors with proinflammatory properties or the transforming growth factor associated with hypertrophic scarring. Further studies are necessary to clarify the mechanism of cytokine release in normal postoperative wounds before therapeutic use can be developed.[99]

Nutrition

Nutrition is an important factor influencing healing. Adequate nutritional intake is necessary to support the active metabolism of cells involved in repair. Trauma, including surgery, infections, or large draining wounds, often increases the systemic rate of protein catabolism (loss), which further limits the body's ability to synthesize proteins required for healing. Inadequate intake of specific nutritional factors can specifically affect collagen production and remodeling, and increase risk for infection.[197]

Zinc is essential for the activity of enzymes that degrade collagen and of enzymes that are responsible ultimately for the induction of protein synthesis. Zinc deficiency therefore impairs healing. People with cancer often manifest delayed healing because of poor nutritional

---

Box 6-3

FACTORS INFLUENCING HEALING

- Physiologic variables (e.g., age, growth factors, vascular sufficiency)
- General health of the individual; immunocompetency; psychologic/emotional/spiritual well-being
- Presence of comorbidities (examples):
  - Diabetes mellitus
  - Decreased oxygen perfusion (e.g., COPD, CHF, CAD, pneumonia)
  - Hematologic disorders (e.g., neutropenia)
  - Cancer (local and systemic effects)
  - Incontinence
  - Alzheimer disease
  - Neurologic impairment
  - Immobility
- Tobacco, alcohol, caffeine, other substance use/abuse
- Nutrition
- Local or systemic infection; presence of foreign bodies
- Type of tissue
- Medical treatment (e.g., prednisone, chemotherapy, radiation therapy)

COPD, chronic obstructive pulmonary disease; *CHF,* chronic heart failure; *CAD,* coronary artery disease.

status associated with the cancer process or the medical treatment (e.g., chemotherapy); particularly notable is the poor healing in tissues that have been subjected to radiation therapy. For an excellent source of information related to nutrition and healing in the therapist's practice, see *Nutrition Applied to Injury Rehabilitation and Sports Medicine*.[32]

Other Factors

Other factors that influence healing include vascular supply, presence of infection, immune reaction, client's age, and the presence of other medical conditions referred to as *comorbidities*. Healing is often adversely affected in people who smoke, who are immunosuppressed, or who have other compromising medical conditions. For example, incontinence, peripheral vascular disease, confusion associated with dementia or Alzheimer disease, or other neurologic impairment can contribute to delayed wound healing.

Diseases associated with decreased oxygen (tissue) perfusion (e.g., anemia, congestive heart failure, chronic obstructive pulmonary disease, or diabetes mellitus) can also delay healing. Diabetes mellitus is associated with poor healing; one of the causes appears to be impaired function of phagocytic cells and another is a defect in granulation tissue formation.[67,125]

Medications can directly affect healing, especially the prolonged use of corticosteroids, or undergoing chemotherapy or radiation treatment. Anyone taking prednisone or other corticosteroids may be at risk, as steroids are well known to impair the healing process by inhibiting the inflammatory response necessary for tissue regeneration or repair.

An adequate vascular supply is critical to provide oxygen and nutrients to support healing. Vascular insufficiency, particularly in the lower limbs, is an important cause of slow-healing or nonhealing wounds. When blood return is not normal, a buildup of fluid can occur, reducing the body's ability to supply nutrients and oxygen to the wound site.

Infection interferes with healing by inciting a severe and prolonged inflammatory reaction that can increase tissue damage. Certain microorganisms can also release toxins that directly cause tissue necrosis and lysis. Foreign bodies may retard healing by inducing a chronic inflammatory reaction, by interfering with closure of a tissue defect, and by providing a site protected from leukocytes and antibiotics where bacteria can multiply.

It may be necessary to offload weight-bearing surfaces to relieve pressure on the wound and surrounding area. Immobility, lack of desire to exercise or follow a plan of care, and refusal to change dietary or other lifestyle behaviors contributing to poor wound healing must also be considered.

Healing may be delayed or inhibited for individuals who are in a constant state of survival or sympathetic nervous system stimulation. When the sympathetic nervous system is locked in a hyperactive mode, exaggerated responses to relatively minor stimuli cause the body to work against itself for healing and recovery. Concepts discussed in Chapter 3 can be applied with these individuals to "reset" the system and facilitate forward movement in the healing process.

Tissue Healing (Part 2)

Healing in Relation to Chronic Tissue Injury

The therapist is often involved with individuals who have chronic tissue injury, often caused by stresses of moderate magnitude that are repeated many times a day. Injuries from this mechanism range from cervical and back pain to patellofemoral dysfunction, tendinopathies, impingement syndromes, stress fractures, and carpal tunnel syndrome.[152] The therapist must identify and modify all factors that may contribute to excessive stress on injured tissues. This includes movement and alignment (e.g., motor control, posture, and muscle length), extrinsic factors (e.g., footwear, gravity, and ergonomic environment), psychosocial factors, medications, age, obesity, or other comorbidities.[152]

After sources of excessive stress have been addressed, injured tissues are still less tolerant of stress than before the injury. Once pain and inflammation have subsided, previously injured tissue must be exposed gradually to higher levels of physical stress. This progression will help restore the tissues' ability to tolerate greater levels of stress. Once healing occurs and tissue integrity is restored, activity tolerance can be increased.[152]

Mueller and Maluf offer a good example of how to think about our clients in this way. An older adult has asked the therapist to help her stand independently from a sitting position. The examining therapist identifies the primary modifiable factors limiting this activity as being lower extremity muscle atrophy resulting in poor force production, decreased ankle dorsiflexion, poor motor control (movement and alignment factors), and a low seat surface (extrinsic factor).[152]

A plan of care that considers her age as an important physiologic factor includes a progressive resistive exercise program for lower extremity extensor muscles with at least 70% of maximum effort, 2 to 3 times a week, to increase muscle force production. At the same time, the client is instructed in stretching exercises to increase ankle range of motion and appropriate movement strategies with good alignment to practice going from a seated to a standing position. Finally, the client is advised to use a higher chair to lower muscle force needed to meet his or her goal of independently standing from a seated position.[152]

Delayed Wound Healing

Understanding the interaction of the wound, wound microorganisms, and the immune response is central to developing successful therapeutic interventions for wound care and management. This chapter has carefully explained how wounding of normal tissue initiates an inflammatory response that ordinarily contributes to the healing process orchestrated by specific and nonspecific immune responses. Inflammatory cells provide growth factors and stimulate the deposition of matrix proteins and phagocytose debris. However, the maturation and resolution of a wound may be complicated by the presence of microorganisms. The effects of microorganisms on oxygen consumption and pH or toxin production may interrupt the natural course of wound healing.

Numerous other factors may delay or inhibit wound healing (see Box 6-3). Because local blood supply is vital to the delivery of the materials necessary for wound healing, factors that impede local circulation or a depletion of the necessary materials could delay rehabilitation. The healing process may even be longer for certain tissues that have a decreased blood supply, such as tendons, cartilage, and disks.

It is also important for therapists to thoroughly screen a client's medical history for the presence of conditions, such as diabetes, chemical dependency (alcoholism), cigarette smoking, because these factors could delay healing and recovery.

Finally, local infection delays healing. If an abscess is present, the expected fever, chills, and sweats associated with infection may not be present in someone who is taking steroid medications. A sudden worsening of symptoms; the presence of a hot, acutely inflamed joint; or the onset of fever should warn the therapist that something more serious may exist. In general, the more compromised the host, the greater the chance of a slow or incomplete recovery.

The wound may not progress from the acute phase but may become a nonhealing chronic or recalcitrant wound as long as the antigens from microorganisms or underlying pathology remain, leading to wound infection. Even so, most chronic wounds progress toward healing, depending on the wound care strategy employed.[208] For example, a venous leg ulcer will heal once the proper compression and support have been provided to counteract the underlying venous hypertension and appropriate wound care has been provided. Similarly, diabetic neuropathic foot ulcers do not heal until the disordered glucose metabolism is controlled, adequacy of the vascular supply is ensured, and causative pressure on the foot is offloaded.

Successful healing of chronic wounds involves intervention to address the underlying causes and clinical wound management that provides an environment to tip the balance in favor of healing.[52] The therapist is more likely to select appropriate intervention measures if the evaluation and assessment process takes into consideration the physiology of tissue repair along with the many factors that can affect wound healing. Investigating the status of these other factors (e.g., nutritional status; mobility status; turning schedule for the immobile; continence status; use of substances such as tobacco, alcohol, or caffeine; and medication schedule) requires collaboration with other health care specialists and with the family.[204]

Laboratory values, such as prealbumin levels, indicating nutritional status 48 hours before may be helpful (see Table 40-5). Glucose levels, hemoglobin, and hematocrit (see Table 40-8) provide the therapist with necessary information to monitor wound healing when setting up and carrying out an appropriate intervention plan.

Specific techniques for wound management are beyond the scope of this text. The reader is referred to other texts for this information.

PHASES OF HEALING

Acute wounds caused by trauma or surgery usually heal according to a well-defined process that has the following four phases that overlap each other and can take months to years to complete[12,225]:
- Hemostasis and degeneration
- Inflammation
- Proliferation and migration
- Remodeling and maturation

Hemostasis and Degeneration

When tissue injury occurs, hemostasis is the first step. Hemostasis occurs immediately after an acute injury as the body tries to stop the bleeding by initiating coagulation. Blood fills the gap, and the coagulation cascade commences immediately, clumping platelets together to form a loose clot. Platelets release bioactive proteins that act as chemical messengers, including growth factors that summon inflammatory cells to the wounded tissue. Growth factors stimulate proliferation and migration of epithelial cells, fibroblasts, and vascular endothelial cells. Growth factors also regulate the differentiation of cells such as expression of extracellular matrix proteins.[12]

The inflammatory process described in detail in the next section begins right away, bringing fluid to the area to dilute harmful substances and support infection-fighting and scavenger cells (neutrophils and macrophages). Some sources describe this first phase as degeneration and inflammation.

The degeneration phase is characterized by the formation of a hematoma, necrosis of dead cells, and as mentioned, the start of the inflammatory cell response. After the removal of the dead tissue, the healing process undertakes the repair of the tissue defect that remains. Tissue repair begins within 24 hours of the injury with the migration of fibroblasts from the margins of the viable tissue into the defect caused by the injury. The fibroblasts proliferate and synthesize and secrete proteins such as fibronectin, various proteoglycans and elastin, and several types of collagen. The function of these proteins is to reconstitute the extracellular matrix and provide a scaffolding-like framework for the developing endothelial and parenchymal cells.

It is at this point that proliferation and migration occur as epidermal skin cells in the top layer move down the sides of the wound to help fill in the gap. Fibroblasts move in from the dermis, and new blood vessels form to create granulation tissue, which later becomes scar tissue. The next phase of remodeling eventually progresses into the final maturation phase as the regenerated tissue reorganizes into healthy scar tissue.

But we have just jumped ahead to tell you the "rest of the story" by discussing proliferation and migration before describing the inflammatory process. Because the phases of tissue healing overlap, it is difficult to describe the process from start to finish without interrupting the discussion.

Inflammation

This phase of healing has been discussed in great detail in the previous section of this chapter. As a review, please remember that inflammation serves a vital role in the healing process. Inflammation has both protective and curative features. Every step serves a specific purpose and is necessary as the body responds to tissue injury or damage. The ultimate goal of the inflammatory process is to replace injured tissue with healthy regenerated tissue, a fibrous scar, or both.[17]

The inflammatory phase begins once the blood clot forms. Vasodilation and increased capillary permeability activate the movement of various cells, such as polymorphonuclear leukocytes and macrophages, to the wound site. These cells destroy bacteria; release proteases, such as elastase and collagenase; and secrete additional growth factors.

Growth factors, cytokines, and chemokines are the key molecular bioregulators of the inflammatory phase of tissue healing. The functions of these three bioregulators overlap considerably. About 5 days after injury, fibroblasts, epithelial cells, and vascular endothelial cells move into the wound to form granulation tissue. This newly developing tissue is not strong, so there is a higher risk of wound dehiscence during this time.[12]

In contrast to cell injury, which occurs at the level of single cells, inflammation is the coordinated reaction of body tissues to cell injury and cell death that involves vascular, humoral, neurologic, and cellular responses. Regardless of the type of cell injury or death, the inflammatory response follows a basically similar pattern. As a result of all of these factors, inflammation occurs only in living organisms.

The functions of the inflammatory reaction are to inactivate the injurious agent, to break down and remove the dead cells, and to initiate the healing of tissue. The key components of the inflammatory reaction are as follows:

- Blood vessels
- Circulating blood cells
- Connective or interstitial tissue cells (fibroblasts, mast cells, and resident macrophages)
- Chemical mediators derived from inflammatory cells or plasma cells
- Specific extracellular matrix constituents, primarily collagen and basement membranes

Basement membranes are thin, sheetlike structures deposited by endothelial (cells that line the heart, blood vessels, lymph vessels, and serous body cavities) and epithelial cells (cells that cover the body and viscera) but are also found surrounding nerve and muscle cells. They provide mechanical support for resident cells and function as a scaffold for accurate regeneration of preexisting structures of tissue. Basement membrane tissue also serves as a semipermeable filtration barrier for macromolecules in organs, such as the kidney and the placenta, and acts as regulators of cell attachment, migration, and differentiation. The major constituents are collagen type IV and proteoglycans.

Proliferation and Migration Phase

Within 2 days after a skin wound or injury, endothelial cells from viable blood vessels near the edge of the necrotic tissue begin to proliferate. The purpose of the endothelial cell proliferation is to establish a vascular network that can transport oxygen and nutrients and support the metabolism of the healing tissue. The endothelial cells bud out from the vessels and form new capillary channels that merge with each other as they develop and grow toward the tissue defect caused by the injury. This process of formation of new blood vessels is called *neovascularization* or *angiogenesis*.

The rich network of developing blood vessels with its connective tissue matrix can be seen with the naked eye in healing wounds. As described previously, the appearance of a reddish granular layer of tissue was therefore given the name "granulation tissue." Histologically, the main cellular components of granulation tissue are the endothelial cells and the fibroblasts, although some inflammatory cells are also commonly present.

Initially, the newly formed vessels are leaky, and this leak contributes to the edematous appearance of tissue undergoing repair. As tissue healing is completed, blood flow to the newly formed vasculature shuts down, and the nonfunctional vessels are degraded, leaving few blood vessels in mature scar tissue.

Tissue gaps are replaced during the proliferation phase when the number of inflammatory cells decreases and fibroblasts, endothelial cells, and keratinocytes take over synthesis of growth factors. The result is the continued promotion of cell migration, proliferation, and formation of new capillaries and synthesis of extracellular matrix components.[12] The next step is the removal of damaged matrix as new matrix builds up to fill the wound. The wound initially fills with provisional wound matrix, which consists primarily of fibrin and fibronectin. As fibroblasts are drawn into the matrix, they synthesize new collagen, elastin, and proteoglycan molecules, which cross-link the collagen of the matrix and produce the initial scar.[12]

Damaged proteins in the matrix have to be removed before the newly synthesized matrix components can be properly integrated. This process is facilitated by proteases secreted by neutrophils, macrophages, fibroblasts, epithelial cells, and endothelial cells. Epithelial cells are at the front of the wound edge, traveling across the highly vascularized extracellular matrix, forming granulation tissue to re-form the epidermal layer. This process can take several weeks.[12]

Remodeling and Maturation Phase

In the maturation phase of healing, the scar tissue is reduced and remodeled, leaving tissue smoother, stronger, less dense, and less red in color (in fair-skinned individuals) as the concentration of blood vessels in the area decreases. In all skin colors, the scar tissue becomes more like the natural skin tones of the person. The density of fibroblasts and capillaries needed in the early phase of healing but no longer needed now declines, primarily through apoptosis or programmed cell death. The remodeling phase can take years as the skin first produces collagen fibers, which are broken down and rearranged to withstand stress. Over time, scar tissue grows stronger, relaxes, and then lightens.

Tissue Contraction and Contracture

As the healing process proceeds, the newly formed extracellular matrix draws together, causing shrinkage (contraction) of the healing tissue. In this manner, the size of the tissue defect caused by the injury is diminished. Some fibroblasts within the healing tissue differentiate and acquire some of the morphologic and functional characteristics of smooth muscle cells (myocytes). These specialized fibroblasts are called *myofibroblasts*. Myofibroblasts contain abundant contractile proteins and apparently contract and contribute to the shrinkage of the healing tissue.

Tissue contraction is a normal process that contributes to tissue repair by approximating the margins of the healing tissue and speeding up the closure of wounds. In some cases, excessive shrinkage of the healing tissue occurs, in addition to the pulling of the deeper tissue to approximate the healing site.[64] This condition is called *contracture*. Contracture is an undesirable outcome of healing because it can limit mobility and organ function, and can be disfiguring. For example, people with severe burns often develop skin contractures because of the process of "hypertrophic scarring" that can result in significant movement impairments and subsequent disability.

Contracted tissue with excessive arthrofibrosis can occur in the joints (most often the shoulder and knee) after either injury or surgery. Postoperative or posttraumatic arthrofibrosis is characterized by local or global periarticular scarring that can restrict, and in some cases a thickened, fibrotic capsule inhibits motion. Arthrofibrosis can be caused by a variety of factors including prolonged immobilization, infection, or graft malposition after ligament reconstruction (e.g., ACL reconstruction).[144]

There is anecdotal evidence suggesting that immature scar tissue can be successfully treated conservatively (e.g., analgesia and antiinflammatory medications, early motion, bracing, strengthening, electrical stimulation, or manual therapy techniques). However, a recent systematic review reported weak evidence regarding the use of soft tissue mobilization in scar management.[190]

Exactly when scar tissue becomes mature is variable and remains a topic of debate. Some estimate an open window of 3 to 4 months after which time interventions such as surgical manipulation (open or arthroscopic) or manipulation under anesthesia may be performed. In a systematic review, these three methods resulted in increases in knee range of motion in individuals with arthrofibrosis following total knee replacement.[81] It should be noted however that forceful manipulation of the stiff joint can create excessive joint compression leading to articular cartilage damage and even fracture.[145]

Tissue Regeneration

Within a few hours after lethal injury to skin, epithelial cells, the viable cells that surround the necrotic tissue, detach from their extracellular matrix anchorage sites and separate from the other epithelial cells. The remaining epithelial cells flatten out to cover the area left bare by the necrotic cells. These epithelial cells also divide and migrate into the tissue using the extracellular matrix support provided by the proteins secreted by the fibroblasts. This process of replacement of dead parenchymal cells by new cells is called *regeneration*. Regeneration is a very desirable healing process because it restores normal tissue structure and function. In most cases, healing of tissue is achieved by both cell regeneration and replacement by connective tissue (scarring) called *repair*. In the case of skin, for example, this type of healing occurs after wounds that involve both the epidermis and dermis. In some instances, tissue healing occurs almost exclusively by the progress of regeneration (regrowth of original tissue).

Regeneration can only occur if the parenchymal cells can undergo mitosis. Cells are classified as *permanent*, *stable*, and *labile* based on their ability to divide. Regeneration does not occur in permanent tissues that cannot divide (e.g., cardiac myocytes or central or peripheral neurons); they are long-lived and irreplaceable. Regeneration can also only occur in labile or stable tissues and only if the inflammatory reaction that follows injury is short-lived and does not disrupt the basement membranes, other extracellular components, and vascular structures of labile or stable parenchymal cells. Labile cells, such as epithelial cells of the skin and gastrointestinal (GI) system, and bone marrow divide continuously. Hematopoietic (blood cell–forming) stem cells continuously divide, giving rise to specialized cells, such as erythrocytes and neutrophils, with finite life spans (see Fig. 21-6).

Under these conditions the regenerating parenchymal cells can use the existing connective tissue scaffolding to reconstitute the normal structure and function of the organ. This type of tissue healing can be seen after superficial mechanical injury to epithelia. An example is a superficial abrasion of the skin that causes only necrosis of the epidermis. In this case, regeneration occurs with little or no scarring.

Stable cells, such as hepatocytes, skeletal muscle fibers, and kidney cells, normally do not divide but can be induced to undergo mitosis by an appropriate stimulus. For example, if a portion of the liver is removed by surgery or if liver cells are killed by a viral infection (hepatitis), the remaining hepatocytes divide and sometimes can fully replace the missing liver tissue.

Studies have revealed some capability of neurons to regenerate (neurogenesis) but only in certain areas of the brain (e.g., hippocampus, olfactory bulb, and subventricular zone).[49] The reasons for the restriction of neurogenesis to a few regions of the brain in mammals compared to a more widespread neurogenesis in other vertebrates remain unknown.[158] It may be that neuronal stem cells persist in these areas throughout the life span but why they do not persist in all areas is still a mystery.[8] What we do know is that neural stem cells residing in specific niches are able to proliferate and differentiate, giving rise to migrating neuroblasts, which in turn mature into functional neurons. These new neurons integrate into the existing circuits and contribute to the structural plasticity of certain brain areas.[163]

Scientific evidence suggests that the process could become more general under pathologic conditions. For example, adult neurogenesis increases under acute and chronic brain diseases. Neuronal precursors are directed to the lesions where they contribute to tissue repair. Investigations are underway to find ways to manipulate and direct the neurogenic process toward the amelioration of neurodegenerative diseases.[1,87,164,209]

Tissue Repair (Formation of Scar Tissue)

Skin has the remarkable ability to heal, often without scarring. Growth factors, blood components, and epithelial (skin) cells mobilize to seal off wounds and protect the body. Scarring does not occur unless the cut, incision, damage, or trauma extends beneath the surface layer (epidermis).

Tissue repair, including the formation of a connective tissue scar, requires removal of the connective tissue matrix. Without this matrix, labile cells do not regenerate or else they regenerate in an incomplete fashion. Therefore, the structural integrity of the parenchymal tissue depends on the formation of this connective tissue scar (dense, irregular laying down of collagen). In many cases, however, healing of tissue is achieved by both cell regeneration and replacement by connective tissue (which is what constitutes scarring). In the case of skin, for example, both types of healing occur in wounds that involve both the epidermis and dermis.

Minimizing tissue scarring is important not only for cosmetic reasons, as is the case in skin, but also because excessive scarring can interfere with organ function. Very large tissue defects may require the use of grafts or flaps of tissue to achieve optimal healing. It is possible to minimize scarring by surgical obliteration of the tissue defect caused by injury and cell necrosis. For example, treatment of skin wounds begins with careful cleansing of the wound to remove foreign materials and bacterial contamination, which interfere with healing. This is followed by debridement to remove nonviable tissue that normally would be broken down by the inflammatory reaction.

Careful attention to hemostasis minimizes the deposition of blood into the wound. During closure, the wound margins are closely apposed under the right amount of tension by surgical sutures. A clean, closed wound is free of infectious and other foreign material, fibrin, and necrotic debris. As a result, the duration and intensity of the inflammatory reaction are minimized. Little granulation tissue forms, and the epithelial cell surface is readily reconstituted.

The healing that occurs in the type of wound described is called *primary union* or *healing by first intention* and results in a small scar (Fig. 6-24). In the presence of large tissue defects or infections, and in other conditions where surgical closure is not possible or desirable, healing occurs by secondary union. In this situation, the time required for healing is longer and the amount of scarring is greater. There is a distinction between closure and healing; the wound or skin may close but healing takes much longer, as much as 2 years in some situations.

Even after wound closure is complete, degradation and resynthesis of collagen continue. This is a response at least in part to shifts in the stress forces to which the tissue is subjected. Cross-linking of collagen fibers continues for a period of several weeks, providing progressive

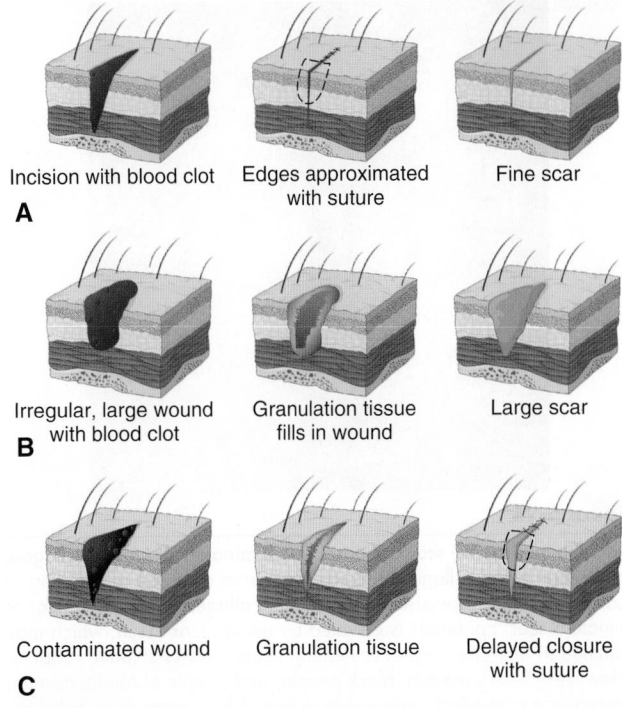

Figure 6-24

A, Healing by primary intention is the initial union of the edges of a wound, progressing to complete healing without granulation. **B,** Healing by secondary intention is wound closure in which the edges are separated, granulation tissue develops to fill the gap, and epithelium grows in over the granulations, producing a scar. **C,** Healing by tertiary intention is wound closure in which granulation tissue fills the gap between the edges of the wound, with epithelium growing over the granulation at a slower rate and producing a larger scar than results from healing from second intention. Suppuration is also usually found in tertiary wound closure. (From Lewis SL, Heitkemper MM, Dirksen SR: *Medical surgical nursing: assessment and management of surgical problems,* ed 8, St. Louis, 2011, Mosby.)

strengthening of scar tissue. However, even under optimal conditions, the repaired tissue never fully regains its original stability. In the case of skin, a fully mature fibrous scar requires 12 to 18 months and is about 20% to 30% weaker than normal skin.

In some people, especially people of African or Asian descent, there is an inherited tendency to produce excessive amounts of collagen during the healing process, causing large amounts of collagen arranged in thick bundles to accumulate in the tissue. These collagenous masses are called *keloids* and can be seen protruding from the skin surface (Fig. 6-25). Keloids are more than just raised, hypertrophic scar tissue. Both keloid and hypertrophic scar tissue result from excess collagen formation, but hypertrophic scars generally calm down in 12 to 24 months, whereas keloids tend to grow larger and appear worse, often invading surrounding tissue.

Several methods are used to treat keloids, although none of them are 100% successful. Surgical keloid excision, form pressure garments, radiation therapy, laser therapy, and pharmacologic interventions have some reported success.[226] Necrosis of heart tissue (myocardial infarct) results in a fibrous scar because cardiac myocytes do not replicate to any great extent. Outcomes that can result from tissue

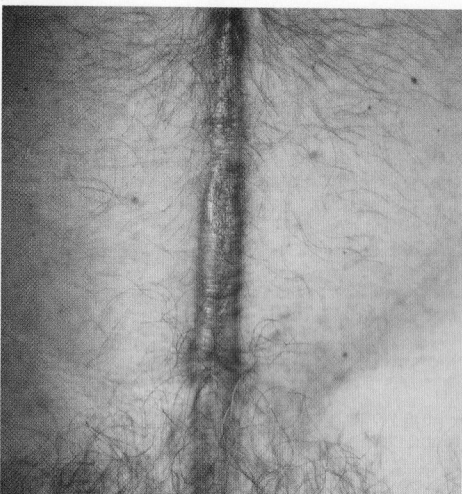

Figure 6-25

Keloid (hypertrophic) scar composed predominantly of type III collagen, rather than type I collagen. Keloids result from defective remodeling of scar tissue and the persistence of type III collagen, which is typical of immature scar. Epidermis is elevated by excess scar tissue, which may continue to increase long after healing occurs. Looks smooth, rubbery, "clawlike." Young women, black people, and people of Mediterranean descent are particularly susceptible to keloid formation. (From Rakel RE: *Textbook of family medicine*, ed 7, Philadelphia, 2007, Saunders.)

repair in various tissue and conditions are summarized in Fig. 6-11. The CNS differs in its healing process because neurons are permanent cells and do not replicate.

After tissue necrosis, neither regeneration nor tissue scarring occurs. No fibroblasts are present in the brain parenchyma, and no collagen is produced. After a brain infarct (stroke), the inflammatory cells arrive from the blood circulation and clear away the necrotic tissue, leaving behind an empty cavity (cyst). Specialized CNS cells called *astrocytes (glial cells)* proliferate, forming dense aggregates around the necrotic area called *glial scars* or *gliosis.*

Special Mention: Chronic Wounds

When a wound fails to heal normally, reepithelialization and closure do not occur. Chronic wounds can occur when the wrong biochemicals are present in the wrong amounts at the wrong times and fail to function effectively. There may be a deficiency in endogenous growth factors, which have the primary role of stimulating cell migration, proliferation, and extracellular matrix deposition. Chronic wounds remain in the inflammatory and proliferative phases.[62] Understanding the normal repair process and factors that affect tissue healing can help guide the therapist in removing barriers to healing. Preparing the wound bed appropriately changes the wound's biochemical environment back to an acute wound, thus reinitiating the healing cascade.

SPECIAL IMPLICATIONS FOR THE THERAPIST   **6-5**

Tissue Healing (Part 3)
Healing of Scar Tissue

The clinical implications of tissue repair can be seen in the example presented earlier in this chapter (see

"Special Implications for the Therapist: Collagen and Cell Injury," in this chapter). In this example, after a transmural MI, a symptom-limited stress test will usually be given after phase II of cardiac rehabilitation, around 8 to 12 weeks after MI. With understanding of the material presented in this chapter, one can see the logical explanation.

As mentioned previously, the damaged human heart muscle is not capable of regeneration.[65] Healing of the myocardium occurs primarily through the process of tissue repair, and requires 8 to 12 weeks to form a dense connective tissue scar. This dense scar allows for structural integrity and force transduction of the viable myocardium, leading to a complete heart contraction. Because the connective tissue scar is not contractile, this area of the heart will never return to full function. Of great importance is the fact that after MI, a person's aerobic fitness can improve (or exceed) to the level before his or her premorbid state with proper exercise. Studies have shown that regular exercise that includes aerobic conditioning improves quality of life, tolerance to activities, and results in the improvement of modifiable risk factors in individuals who have had a previous myocardial infarction.[80]

TISSUE REPAIR

Introduction

The intent of the repair process is to attempt to restore the injured healing tissue to its optimal function. Healing and repair are intricately connected. Throughout this chapter, examples of cell types and healing processes within various organs and systems of the body have been discussed. Some organs are composed of cells that cannot regenerate (e.g., heart, CNS, or peripheral nervous system cells), whereas other organs such as the liver and epithelial cells of the integumentary and GI systems can replace missing tissue through cell division (mitosis). Some cells, such as skeletal muscle cells and renal cells, do not divide but can be induced to undergo mitosis. The extent to which cells can regenerate depends on the type of cell (e.g., permanent, stable, labile), the cell's ability to divide, the type of damage incurred (e.g., lethal, sublethal), and other factors discussed (e.g., nutrition, age, immunocompetency, vascular supply, or presence of microorganisms leading to infection).

Also, it is important to note that advances in the fields of biotechnology and biomaterials are providing new techniques for regeneration or repair of tissue lost to injury, disease, or aging. Bioengineered tissues, including skin, bone, articular cartilage, ligaments, and tendons, are under investigation for clinical use (see "Tissue Engineering" in Chapter 21).[13,106]

Using an example of a person with TBI who also experiences MI, healing of brain and myocardial tissue was discussed earlier in this chapter (see "Special Implications for the Therapist 6-1: Cell Injury"). In this final section, only those tissues not specifically included in the main body of this chapter are presented further.

Lung

After lethal injury to alveolar cells (type I and II pneumocytes), regeneration can occur only when the basement membrane remains intact. After the phagocytic removal of the necrotic cells, adjacent living epithelial cells migrate onto the remaining basement membrane and differentiate into type II pneumocytes (cells that primarily produce surfactant). Eventually, some of these cells differentiate into type I pneumocytes (cells that permit gas exchange) and full lung function is restored. If the damage to the lung disrupts the basement membrane, healing must be achieved by repair, which is characterized by fibrosis and scar formation—epithelial cells that may be dysfunctional.[18] Also, certain injurious agents such as inhalation of asbestos can trigger the formation of scar tissue, leading to restrictive lung disease.

Digestive Tract

The healthy gut is lined with multiple rows of villi structures. These fingerlike projections are responsible for nutrient absorption and the production of digestive enzymes. Gut cells grow single file from the base of the villi up toward the top. They slough off into the intestinal tract and pass out of the body every five days or so. Damaged or injured cells are constantly leaving, whereas healthy cells renew the GI environment. It takes about 3 to 4 weeks for a complete turnover of all gut cells throughout the digestive tract.

Because two-thirds of all immune system function and 90% of serotonin function take place in the gut, healing the gut can assist in bringing both of these functions back into balance. Serotonin is needed to produce melatonin, which is an essential component for good, restful sleep; the proper amount of circulating and functioning serotonin is also needed to stabilize mood.[50]

Peripheral Nerves

When a nerve is cut, the peripheral portion rapidly undergoes myelin degeneration and axonal fragmentation. The lipid debris is removed by macrophages mobilized from the surrounding tissues in a process referred to as *Wallerian degeneration*. Within 24 hours of section, new axonal sprouts from the central stump are observed with proliferation of Schwann cells from both the central and peripheral stumps.

Careful microsurgical approximation of the nerve may result in reinnervation, especially those with gaps less than 3 mm.[55] The most important factor in achieving successful nerve regeneration after repair is the maintenance of the neurotubules (basement membrane and connective tissue endoneurium), along which the new axonal sprouts can pass.[33]

Skeletal Muscle

Skeletal muscle is composed of contractile and connective tissue elements. Actin and myosin myofilaments make up the sarcomere units of muscle fibers. Each individual myofiber is surrounded by a delicate sheath called the *endomysium* (basement membrane) and then arranged in bundles. Satellite cells surround the muscle fibers and are important for tissue regeneration following injury. The greater the degree of muscle injury, the larger the amount of connective tissue that is disrupted.[28]

Contrary to widespread belief, muscle tissue can regenerate, but the restoration of normal structure and function is strongly dependent on the type of injury sustained. In *severe infections*, the muscle fibers may be extensively destroyed. However, the sarcolemmal sheaths (basement membrane and connective tissue endomysium) usually remain intact, and rapid regeneration of muscle cells within the sheaths occurs so that the function of the muscle may be completely restored.

After *transection of a muscle*, muscle fibers may regenerate either by growth from undamaged stumps or by growth of new, independent fibers.[33] Once again, this type of regeneration after lethal cell injury to skeletal muscle fibers is possible when the basement membrane remains intact through mitotic division of "satellite cells." Satellite cells play an integral role in normal development of skeletal muscle and are essential to the repair of injured muscle by serving as a source of myoblasts for fiber regeneration. These proliferating satellite cells support the process of regeneration by either combining with other myogenic cells causing the development of new fibers, or by fusing with remaining muscle fibers.[211]

A muscle that is contused or strained has the capability to repair itself but the period of recovery is markedly prolonged, and results in strength losses. At the conclusion of the healing process, the repaired site shows a high rate of reinjury.[39,101] Recovery is largely dependent on the severity of the injury but follows the same phases of degeneration, inflammation, regeneration, and fibrosis described in this chapter.

As with all healing, muscle fiber injury is regenerated or repaired through a consistent sequence of events that go into motion as soon as an injury occurs. Hemostasis with hematoma formation and inflammation overlap in the first phase, starting in the first 24 to 48 hours after injury. This phase is followed by phagocytosis with the removal of detritus, activation of satellite cells, and subsequent myofiber regeneration. This second phase can last 6 to 8 weeks after injury. The final phase involves tissue remodeling. This phase is characterized by complete reorganization and maturation of the regenerated muscle.[40,101,127]

With death of the muscle cell and ensuing necrosis, chemotactic agents attract macrophages within the basement membrane confines to engulf the remnants of the dead cell. Macrophages release growth factors, stimulating the division of the satellite cells. These cells migrate to the central region and begin to differentiate into expressing the usual characteristics of a skeletal muscle fiber. This healing process can occur after lethal cell injury (e.g., muscular dystrophy) when the connective tissue matrix (primarily basement membrane) is disrupted and regeneration is attempted. But disruption of basement membrane leaves the satellite cells no place to set up and multiply.

The end result is that the muscle tissue heals by forming a connective tissue scar (i.e., repair). This at least maintains the structural integrity of the tissue but not the complete functional capability. This type of healing of muscle (repair vs. regeneration) could occur after the trauma of a motor vehicle accident or a knife wound.

The complete recovery of injured skeletal muscle appears to be further hindered by fibrosis, which begins during the second week after muscle injury. The formed scar tissue that replaces the damaged muscle fibers is disorganized and therefore has decreased ability to withstand tensile forces. The result is that these repaired muscles have a higher risk of injury.[128]

Bone

Bone is composed of two types of tissue: cortical and cancellous (trabecular). Cortical bone accounts for approximately 80% of skeletal tissue. It is the tough outer layer of bone, densely packed, and surrounds trabecular or cancellous bone. The remaining 20% is cancellous bone, which consists of spongy, intermeshing thin plates (trabeculae) that are in contact with the bone marrow. Bone has two surfaces, referred to as *periosteal* (external) and *endosteal* (internal).

Loss of bone occurs when there is an imbalance between destruction and production of bone cells or when there is a defective mineralization of bone matrix. An increase in osteoclasts or failure of osteoblasts to assemble can result in bone resorption faster than bone is being built up.

A variety of conditions can affect bone and require a reparative process, including fracture, infection, inflammation (e.g., tuberculosis or sarcoidosis), metabolic disturbances (e.g., Paget disease, osteoporosis, or osteogenesis imperfecta), tumors, response to implanted prostheses, bone infarction, and any other systemic diseases that have skeletal manifestations (e.g., sickle cell disease, amyloidosis, or hemochromatosis). For a discussion of these specific conditions and their impact on bone, the reader is referred to each individual chapter that includes those diseases. Only the bone response to injury and the reparative process (specifically fracture) will be discussed in this chapter.

Fracture Healing and Repair

See also "Bone Fractures," Chapter 27. Fracture repair is a healing process by regeneration and remodeling (i.e., without a scar) and with the potential for a return of optimal function in many cases. After an uncomplicated fracture, bone heals in similar overlapping phases previously discussed in this chapter (Fig. 6-26). At the moment bone injury occurs, secondary to fracture, tiny blood vessels through the haversian systems are torn at the fracture site. A brief period of local internal bleeding occurs, resulting in a hematoma around the fracture site called a fracture hematoma. Bleeding from the fracture site delivers fibroblasts, platelets, and osteoprogenitor cells, which secrete numerous growth factors and cytokines. They stimulate transformation of the initial hematoma into a more organized granulation tissue, eventually promoting callus formation.

The *inflammatory phase* occurs as inflammatory cells arrive at the injured site accompanied by the vascular response and cellular proliferation. Clinical evidence of this phase includes pain, swelling, and heat.

Clotting factors from the blood initiate the formation of a fibrin meshwork. This meshwork is the scaffolding for the ingrowth of fibroblasts and capillary buds around and between the bony ends. By the end of the first week, phagocytic cells have removed a majority of the hematoma, and neovascularization and initial fibrosis are occurring.

The *reparative phase* begins during the next few weeks and includes the formation of the soft callus seen on radiographs around 2 weeks after the injury, which is eventually replaced by a hard callus. During this phase,

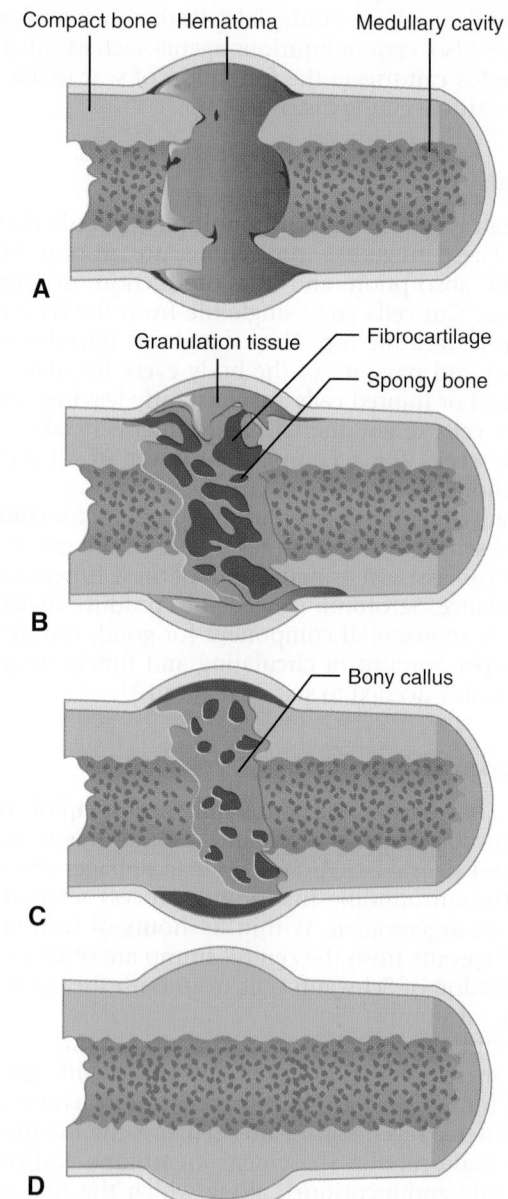

Figure 6-26

Fracture healing occurs in overlapping stages or phases. A, Immediate vascular response with hematoma formation and inflammatory response. **B,** Granulation tissue and fibrocartilage formation during early reparative phase. **C,** Fibrocartilaginous union (soft callus) is replaced by a fibroosseous union (bony callus). **D,** Remodeling phase with complete restoration of the medullary canal. (From Damjanov I: *Pathology for the health-related professions,* ed 4, St. Louis, 2012, Elsevier.)

osteoclasts (bone macrophages) clear away the necrotic bone while the periosteum and endosteum regenerate and begin to differentiate into formation of hyaline cartilage (soft callus) and primary bony spicules (hard callus). Bone growth factors, including bone morphogenetic proteins, fibroblast growth factor, insulin-like growth factors, platelet-derived growth factor, transforming growth factor–β, and vascular endothelial growth factor, are major components of the fracture healing (reparative) phase.[56]

Once the callus is sufficient to immobilize the fracture site, repair occurs between the fractured cortical and medullary bones when the fibrocartilaginous union (soft callus) is replaced by a fibroosseous union (hard callus). The process is called enchondral ossification. Delayed union and nonunion fractures result from errors in this phase of bone healing. The completion of the reparative phase (usually occurring between 6 and 12 weeks) is indicated by fracture stability. Radiographically, the fracture line begins to disappear.[100]

The *remodeling phase* begins with clinical and roentgenographic union (no movement occurs at the fracture site) and persists until the bone is returned to normal, including restoration of the medullary canal. During this phase, which may take months to years, the immature, disorganized woven bone is replaced with a mature organized lamellar bone that adds further stability to the fracture site. The excessive bony callus is resorbed, and the bone remodels in response to the mechanical stresses placed on it.

In the normal adult skeleton, approximately 10% to 30% of the bone is replaced or remodeled to replace microfractures from stress and maintain mineral balance. Bone remodeling is carried out by bone cells, including osteoblasts, osteoclasts, and osteocytes. Osteoblasts produce the bone matrix and initial bone mineralization while osteoclasts resorb bone. Osteocytes detect local mechanical loading and send signals to the surface osteoblasts to initiate bone remodeling.[5]

The time for overall bone healing varies depending on the bone involved, the fracture site and type, treatment required (e.g., immobilization vs. surgical repair, the need for bone grafting or use of bone graft substitutes), degree of soft tissue injury, treatment complications, and other factors mentioned previously (e.g., age, vascular supply, nutritional status, or immunocompetency). New biotechnologies have resulted in new approaches to facilitate repair in cases of insufficient bone regeneration.[57] The physical therapist should be aware of how these new approaches affect implicate rehabilitation management. Specific types of fractures, their treatment, and special implications for the therapist are discussed in greater detail in Chapter 27.

Tendons and Ligaments

Tendons and ligaments are dense bands of fibrous connective tissue composed of 78% water, 20% collagen, and 2% glycosaminoglycans. This composition allows them to sustain high unidirectional tensile loads, transfer forces, provide strong flexible support, and help the tissue respond to normal loads while resisting excessive mechanical or shearing forces and deformation. The viscoelastic characteristics of these tissues make them capable of undergoing deformation under tensile or compressive force, yet still capable of returning to their original state after removal of the force. Both are made up of parallel fibers of type I collagen produced by fibroblasts/fibrocytes, glycosaminoglycans/proteoglycans, a small vascular supply, and sensory innervation. The mechanical properties of tendons and ligaments are dependent not only on the architecture and properties of the collagen fibers but also on the proportion of elastin that these structures contain (e.g., minimal elastin in tendons and ligaments of the extremities, substantial elastin in the ligamentum flavum). Also, thicker tendons with higher collagen content have more tensile strength.

Tendon Injury and Healing

It has been reported that when forces are applied rapidly and obliquely, tendons have the highest risk for rupture. Another significant risk for tendon rupture is the presence of degenerative changes in the tendon itself because tensile strength is decreased under degenerative conditions.[189]

In the case of acute injury and tendon rupture, tendons may heal either as a result of proliferation of the tenoblasts from the cut ends of the tendon or more likely as a result of vascular ingrowth and proliferation of fibroblasts derived from the surrounding tissues that were injured at the time of the tendon injury. Because the surrounding tissues contribute so much to the healing of a tendon, adhesions are very common. With rupture of the Achilles tendon, rotator cuff tendons, or cruciate ligament(s), functional restoration requires surgical repair to appose and suture the cut ends.[33]

The healing and reparative process progress through the same three overlapping phases as other tissues: hemostasis and inflammation, cellular proliferation and matrix deposition, and long-term remodeling. Hemostasis begins immediately followed by the inflammatory process, which begins during the first 72 hours (3-5 days) after injury and/or surgical intervention.

Hemostasis occurs as platelets from blood plasma enter the tear to initiate clot formation. Fibrin and fibronectin form cross-links with collagen fibers to form a fragile bond, which helps reduce hemorrhage. The activity of phagocytic cells clears away the debris in the area from damaged and devitalized tissue. Chemotactic mediators attract inflammatory WBCs to the area, including polymorphonuclear leukocytes and monocytes.

The *inflammatory phase* overlaps and transforms into the *proliferative phase*, which usually occurs 2 to 3 weeks after tendon injury or repair but can begin as early as 48 hours after injury.[34] Granulation tissue is formed by the migration and proliferation of fibroblasts and vascular buds from the surrounding connective tissue. Capillary sprouts grow out of blood vessels around the edges of the wound-forming loops by joining with each other or with capillaries already carrying blood. The new blood vessels enhance delivery of nutrients to the healing tissue. While this is occurring, the fibroblasts are secreting soluble type III collagen molecules, which form fibrils. A new extracellular matrix is formed. In this step, the original fibrin clot and scaffolding are replaced with more permanent repair tissue.

Approximately 2 weeks into the healing process, the collagen fibrils are oriented and rearranged into thick bundles, providing the tissue with greater strength. During this period, the affected area remains immobilized to relieve stress from the healing tissue and prevent rupture recurrence. The lack of stress causes the newly forming collagen to be deposited in random alignment without the formation of cross-links. The immature collagen is randomly oriented and has limited strength.

Now the transition from the proliferative phase to the *maturation phase* takes place. The maturation and remodeling phase begins around week 3 after the initial injury. The immature type III collagen is replaced by mature type I collagen; the latter aligns along tensile forces. The collagen is continually remodeled until permanent repair tissue is formed that is oriented along the lines of stress and organized to provide increasing resistance to stretch and tearing.[212] On the basis of animal models, we know that tendon healing takes at least 12 to 16 weeks to reach a level at which the tendon can be stressed.[145]

When the healing tissue has achieved adequate integrity, motion is permitted once again. The remodeling collagen then aligns to the lines of stress produced by the motion, thereby permitting the healed tendons and ligaments to provide support in line with the stress. Realignment of collagen to its usual parallel arrangement also permits the restoration of full, normal range of motion after repair. The tensile strength of lacerated and repaired tendons was only 40% to 60% of healthy intact tendon.[91] Human tendons and ligaments regain normal strength in 40 to 50 weeks postoperatively; this means that even as long as a year after injury, the tendon or ligament may not have achieved premorbid tensile strength.

Although the process of healing is by repair (formation of a connective tissue scar), this constitutes regeneration because tendons and ligaments are originally composed of connective tissue. However, the scar tissue is weaker and larger and has compromised biomechanical integrity with an increased amount of minor collagens (types III, V, and VI), decreased collagen cross-links, and an increased amount of glycosaminoglycans.[97] These changes lead to impaired function, increased risk of reinjury, and increased risk of osteoarthritis.

Healing of intrasynovial tendon injuries is complicated by the formation of adhesions between the tendon and surrounding synovial sheath. It has been postulated that adhesions result from the infiltration of tenocytes from the surrounding tissue to the site of the injured tendon, thereby attaching to the site.[189] In hand injuries, range of motion can be limited because adhesions disrupt normal tendon gliding. Adhesions account for about a fourth of fair to poor functional outcomes following tendon repairs.[227]

Tendinopathy, a term used to denote clinical conditions with pain and pathologic changes, includes both tendinitis (implying an inflammatory process) and tendinosis, a degenerative process with little or no inflammation but histopathologic changes in the collagen matrix. Overuse and chronic overload with repetitive microtrauma are the most common etiologic risk factors.[189]

Chronic tendon disorders are usually caused by overuse. There are many theories to explain the exact mechanism by which tendons are injured under conditions of overuse (e.g., mechanical or overload theory, neural theory, vascular insufficiency theory, and exercise-induced hyperthermia theory).[174] Clearly, load applied has a major effect on location of tendon injuries. Older age, gender (female) with hormone fluctuations, and decreased joint motion and tendon/muscular flexibility seem to contribute to the problem.[174] Achilles tendon ruptures have been reported with the use of a particular family of antibiotics (the quinolones) and with prolonged use of steroids. Running or training on concrete surfaces will also increase the risk of tendon problems, especially of the patellar (knee) tendon.

Ligament Injury and Healing

Sprains and tears of the tendinous or ligamentous structures around a joint can be caused by abnormal or excessive joint motion. These injuries can be classified as first, second, or third degree, depending on the changes in structural or biomechanical integrity (ranging from injury of a few fibers without loss of integrity to a complete tear).

Common sites for this type of injury include the ankle, knee, and fingers with clinical manifestations of local pain, edema, increased local tissue temperature, ecchymosis, hypermobility or instability, and loss of motion and/or function. If, after injury, the therapist notes quick onset of joint effusion, and the joint feels hot to the touch with extremely painful and limited movement, the joint needs to be examined by a physician to rule out hemarthrosis.

In many extraarticular ligaments (e.g., medial collateral ligament), healing occurs by the same basic phases described in the previous section (i.e., hemorrhage, inflammation, repair, and remodeling). However, there is variation in the manner in which ligaments heal; some intraarticular ligaments (e.g., anterior cruciate ligament) have a poor healing response. After the ligament ruptures, the thin synovial sheath is disrupted and blood dissipates, preventing clot and hematoma formation. Healing cannot take place without a foundation for repair or localization of chemotactic cytokines and growth factors.[166]

Studies have revealed that after injuries, ligament tissues such as the ACL release large amounts of matrix metalloproteinases. These enzymes have a devastating effect on the healing process of the injured ligaments. Matrix metalloproteinases are critically involved in the extracellular matrix turnover, which may help explain one of the reasons why the injured ACL repairs minimally. In addition, matrix metalloproteinase activity is less in the medial collateral ligament (MCL), which may account for the difference in healing capacities between the MCL and the ACL.[206]

The remodeling phase of ligament healing consists of a continuous cycle of collagen synthesis and degradation with the intent of generating a ligament that is as close to normal as possible. This process can take months to years, and evidence exists that the replacement tissue is similar to scar tissue and does not have the histologic and biomechanical properties of a normal ligament.[94]

Moreover, the quality of the repaired tissue has been found to also be dependent on the load and stresses subjected to the ligament during the healing process. For example, returning to aggressive high-impact sports activities too soon in the healing process will subject the ligament to excessive amounts of load and stress, thereby risking ligament failure. On the other hand, too little load and stress brought about by prolonged immobilization will result in a very inferior ligament and delayed healing process. Immobilization during the healing phase leads to significant decreases in failure load at 6 to 14 weeks after ligament injury. Joint laxity is a clinical problem brought about by an inferior ligament healing process and increases the risk of reinjury to the structure. These findings reinforce the clinical importance of early mobilization in ligament injuries.[149,210]

Another potential hindrance to healing is the use of NSAIDs. Animal studies have demonstrated decreases in load-to-failure in healing ligaments when NSAIDs were used in the first 2 weeks following injury.[222] As mentioned earlier, an important component of the healing is the initiation of the inflammation process mediated by prostaglandins. Therefore, as NSAID use blocks the production of prostaglandins, the healing process is impaired. It is therefore recommended that individuals use NSAIDs judiciously during the healing process.[94]

Cartilage Injury and Healing

Several forms of cartilage are recognized, including articular cartilage found at the ends of the bones; fibrocartilage found in the menisci of the knee, at the annulus fibrosus, at the insertions of the ligaments and tendons into the bone, and on the inner side of tendons as they angle around pulleys (e.g., at the malleoli); and elastic cartilage found in the ligamentum flavum, external ear, and epiglottis (Table 6-7).

Articular cartilage has many individual zones that make up the whole (Fig. 6-27). It is composed of hyaline cartilage made up of water (75%), chondrocytes, type II collagen (20%), and glycosaminoglycans/proteoglycans (5%). It is aneural, avascular, and alymphatic and does not appear to regenerate well after adolescence, most likely because of its avascularity and low cell-to-matrix ratio. Proteoglycan, produced by the chondrocytes and secreted into the matrix, is responsible for the compressive strength of cartilage. It binds growth factors and traps and holds water used to regulate matrix hydration.

Ideal conditions for healing of articular cartilage require a source of cells, provision of matrix, removal of stress concentration, and intact subchondral bone plate with some mechanical stimulation. Following cartilage injury, the normal inflammatory process that involves the migration of repair cells to the site is impeded because the articular cartilage lacks the vascularization to bring these cells to the area.[148] Therefore, in adults without intervention, the healing of articular cartilage occurs by fibrous scar tissue or fails to heal at all. This replacement tissue does not function as well as the original, and the adjacent joint surface can be affected.

Table 6-7	Types of Cartilage
Types of Cartilage	**Location**
Articular (Hyaline)	Joint surfaces, bone apophyses, epiphyseal plates, costal cartilage (ribs), fetal skeleton
Fibrocartilage	Tendon and ligament insertion, meniscus, disk
Elastic	Trachea (epiglottis), earlobe, ligamentum flavum
Fibroelastic	Meniscus

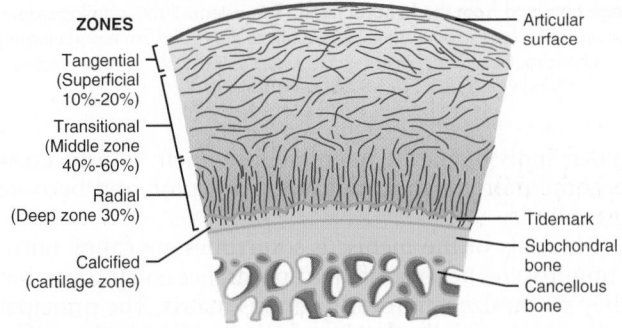

ZONES

Tangential (Superficial 10%-20%)
Transitional (Middle zone 40%-60%)
Radial (Deep zone 30%)
Calcified (cartilage zone)

Articular surface
Tidemark
Subchondral bone
Cancellous bone

Figure 6-27

Zones of cellular distribution in adult articular cartilage. **A,** Superficial tangential zone: type II collagen fibers are oriented tangentially to the surface providing the greatest ability to resist shear stresses. **B,** Transitional (middle) zone: composed primarily of proteoglycans but collagen fibers present are arranged obliquely to provide a transition between the shearing forces of the surface layer and the compression forces in the cartilage layer. **C,** Radial (deep) zone: collagen fibers are attached vertically (radial) into the tidemark; distributes loads and resists compression. **D,** Tidemark layer is located in the calcified zone; the Tidemark is the line that straddles the boundary between calcified and uncalcified cartilage; it separates hyaline cartilage from subchondral bone. **E,** Calcified zone: layer just above subchondral bone containing type X collagen. **F,** Subchondral bone. **G,** Cancellous bone.

Fibrous scarring of the articular cartilage leads to local degenerative arthritis (Fig. 6-28). This is the reason why several treatment approaches designed to repair cartilage healing induce the formation of precursor cells to the injured area to assist healing. For example, microfracture techniques to enhance chondral resurfacing have made it possible to stimulate the formation of a durable repair cartilage cap over the lesion, thereby facilitating cartilage healing and repair.[172,196,201]

Menisci (Knee)

The menisci are fibrocartilaginous structures consisting of cartilage bundles composed mainly of collagen, although proteins such as elastin and proteoglycan are also present. The amount of proteoglycan increases dramatically in the injured, degenerate meniscus. Water accounts for 70% of meniscal composition, contributing to the meniscal function of joint lubrication. Water in the menisci also provides resistance to compressive loads. Collagen makes up to 70% of the dry weight; 90% of it is type I collagen fibers, with types II, III, V, and VI present in much smaller amounts.[89] In the young individual, the menisci are usually white, translucent, and supple on palpation. In the

Normal   Osteoarthritis

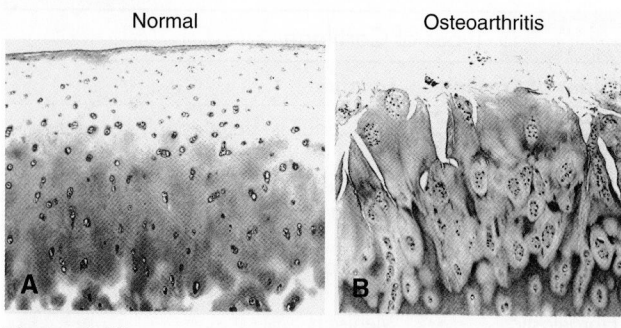

Figure 6-28

**Histologic sections of normal (A) and osteoarthritic (B) articular carti-
lage obtained from the femoral head.** The osteoarthritic cartilage demonstrates surface irregularities, with clefts to the radial zone and cloning
of chondrocytes. (From Harris ED: *Kelley's textbook of rheumatology,*
ed 7, Philadelphia, 2005, WB Saunders.)

older individual, the menisci lose their translucency,
become more opaque and yellow in color, and become
less supple.

The cells of the meniscus sometimes are called fibro-
chondrocytes because of their appearance and the fact that
they synthesize a fibrocartilaginous matrix. The principal
orientation of collagen fibers in the menisci is circumferential, designed to disperse compressive load, resist shear,
aid in shock absorption, and withstand the circumferential tension within the meniscus during normal loading
(Fig. 6-29). A few small, radially oriented fibers present
on the tibial surface probably act as ties to resist lateral
splitting of the menisci from undue compression.

At birth, the entire meniscus is vascular; by age
9 months, the inner one-third has become avascular.
By adulthood, only the outer 10% to 30% of vascularity
remains, with blood supplied via the perimeniscal capillary
plexus off the superior and inferior medial and lateral
genicular arteries.[188] Blood supply to the meniscus flows
from the peripheral to the central meniscus principally
through diffusion or mechanical pumping (movement).[9]

Meniscal tears heal by migration of cells from the synovial membrane adjacent to the meniscus. The remodeling
events of the healing process remain unknown. Healing
of meniscal tears may be inhibited based on the location
of the tear; less vascular locations have less vigorous healing capability.

Similarly, nerve fibers originating in the perimeniscal
tissues radiate into the outer one-third of the menisci.
Nerves in the densely populated anterior and posterior
horns play a proprioceptive role in protecting the joint
through reflexive neuromuscular control of joint motion
and loading.[84,89]

Injury and degeneration leading to laceration are the
two most common causes of symptoms that require
surgical intervention.[33] The presence of clinical symptoms of pain, swelling, locking and catching, and loss
of motion often require surgical intervention. Proper
management depends on the type of tear and its location (Fig. 6-30).[89] Meniscectomies cause alterations in
the biomechanical functioning of the menisci, causing
alterations in the normal loading mechanism of the
joint, and ultimately increasing the risk for development
of osteoarthritis.

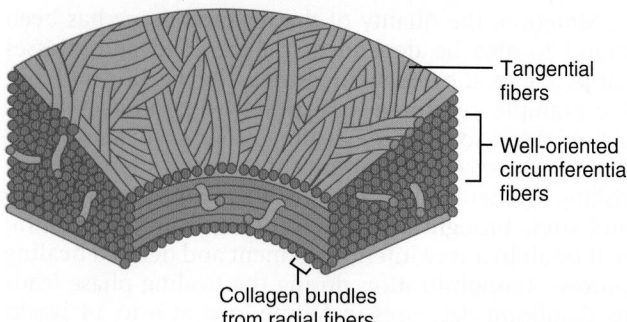

Figure 6-29

**Diagrammatic representation of the distribution of collagen fibers in the
meniscus of a knee.** Collagen is oriented throughout the connective tissues in such a way as to maximally resist the forces placed upon these
tissues. The majority of the type I collagen fibers in the meniscus are
circumferentially arranged, with a few fibers on or near the tibial surface placed in a radial pattern. This structural arrangement enables the
meniscus to resist the lateral spread that occurs during high compressive
loads generated during weight bearing. Longitudinally arranged collagen fibers facilitate shock absorption and sustain the tension generated between the anterior and posterior attachments. (From Bullough
PG: *Bullough and Vigorita's orthopaedic pathology,* ed 3, St. Louis, MO,
1997, Mosby.)

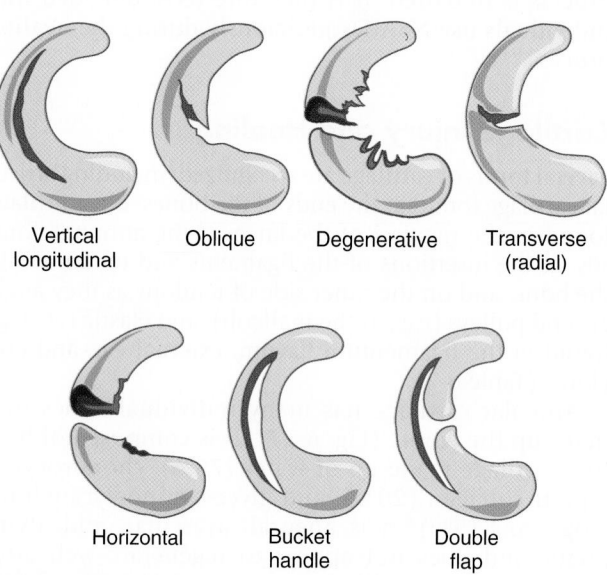

Figure 6-30

Classification of most common meniscal tears.

Synovial Membrane

The synovial membrane lines the inner surface of the joint
capsule and all other intraarticular structures (e.g., subcutaneous and subtendinous bursae sacs, tendon sheaths),
with the exception of articular cartilage and the meniscus. Synovial membrane consists of two components: the
intimal (cellular layer or synoviocytes) layer next to the
joint space and the subintimal or supportive layer made
of fibrous and adipose tissue.

The synovial membrane has three principal functions:
secretion of synovial fluid hyaluronate, phagocytosis of
waste material, and regulation of the movement of solutes, electrolytes, and proteins from the capillaries into

the synovial fluid. This latter function provides a regulatory mechanism for maintenance of the matrix through various chemical mediators such as ILs.

Injury to any of the joint structures affects the synovium and results in hemorrhage, hypertrophy, and hyperplasia of the synovial lining cells and mild chronic inflammation.[33] In the case of prolonged, chronic synovitis, such as occurs in hemophilia, abnormal synovial fluid, joint immobilization, and fibrous adhesions, a progressive destructive condition in the joint can result.

Any type of immobilization leads to contraction of the capsule. Loss of glycosaminoglycans with the associated water loss further increases capsule stiffness and results in decreased joint motion. The synovial membrane lining the inside of the capsule hypertrophies and forms adhesions between itself and the adjacent articular cartilage.[150]

Disk and Disk Degeneration

The intervertebral disk sits between each pair of vertebrae and is made of connective tissue (collagen fibers) that helps the disk withstand tension and pressure (Fig. 6-31). The disk is made of three zones: (1) the outer annulus fibrosus, a lamellated ring of alternately obliquely oriented, densely packed type I collagen fibers that insert onto the vertebral bodies; (2) the fibrocartilaginous inner annulus fibrosus, consisting of a type II collagen fibrous matrix; and (3) the viscoelastic central nucleus pulposus with type II collagen fibers along with various mucopolysaccharides and a high concentration of proteoglycans.[11] This composition supports the high water content of the nucleus, which behaves biomechanically as a fluid cushion that transmits loading forces to the outer annulus fibrosus, as well as to the vertebral endplate.[168]

The nucleus is held in place by the *annulus*, a series of strong ligament rings surrounding it. The annulus is primarily composed of type I collagen arranged in multiple concentric layers. This fiber arrangement allows the annulus to resist tensile, radial, and torsional forces. With acute trauma or degenerative changes and microtrauma over time, the fibers of the annulus may be disrupted.[168] The normal disk's blood supply is restricted to the peripheral outer annulus. The vertebral body's blood vessels lie directly against the endplates but do not enter the disk itself. The nutrition of the more centrally located disk cells is derived from diffusional and convection transport of nutrients and wastes through the porous solid matrix.[11] The metabolism of the avascular disk is so slow that the turnover of proteoglycans takes 20 years.[205]

Although the nucleus has no nerve supply, the outer third of the annulus is innervated, receiving supply from both the sinuvertebral nerve, which innervates the posterior and posterolateral regions, and the gray ramus, which is distributed primarily anteriorly and laterally. More recent studies have confirmed that the annulus is a source of pain in people with chronic low back pain.[199]

Aging and Disc Degeneration

Our intervertebral disks change with age and demonstrate degenerative changes relatively early in life, because of their large size and poor vascular supply. Cell senescence in the disk has been linked with degenerative disease,

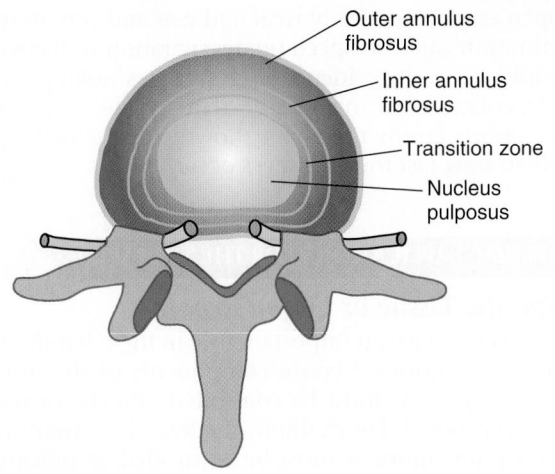

Figure 6-31

Zones of the adult human lumbar intervertebral disk.

with more senescence of cells in the nucleus pulposus compared to the annulus fibrosus in individuals with herniated disks.[178]

Disk degeneration follows a predictable pattern. First, the nucleus in the center of the disk begins to lose its ability to absorb water. This occurs as a result of a decrease in cell density in the disk that is accompanied by a reduction in synthesis of cartilage-specific extracellular matrix components such as type II collagen.[79]

As the proteoglycan content of the disk decreases, a loss of water-binding capacity by the disk matrix occurs and the disk becomes dehydrated. Then the nucleus becomes thick and fibrous, so that it looks much the same as the annulus. As a result, the nucleus is not able to absorb shock as well. Routine stress and strain begin to take a toll on the structures of the spine. Tears called *fissures* form around the annulus. In addition to these, continued compressive forces to the spine due to inactivity, weight gain, poor posture, and poor tone of the muscles supporting the spine further slow the ability of the disk to heal.[199] As the disk weakens, it starts to collapse, and the bones of the spine compress.

Along with the pathology of degeneration, changes in the extracellular matrix content affecting collagen fibers can reduce the disk's load-bearing capacity. Calcification of the vertebral endplates is another factor thought to contribute to disk degeneration. Alterations in permeability adversely affect chondrocyte metabolism. The passage of nutrients and waste products across the endplate depends on fluid flowing into the disk during the night while resting and flowing out during the day when we move about.[79]

Injury to the disk (herniation) is more likely in the morning soon after waking, when the nucleus pulposus is maximally hydrated after a prolonged period of rest. Vigorous early morning activities increase the vertical load beyond the strength of the collagen in the annulus. Other proposed risk factors for lumbar disk herniation include lifting heavy loads, torsional stress, strenuous physical activity, and occupational driving of motor vehicles.[11]

Conditions, such as a major back injury or fracture, can affect how the spine works, making the changes happen even faster. Daily wear and tear and certain types of vibration can also speed up degeneration in the spine. In addition, strong evidence suggests that smoking speeds up degeneration of the spine. Scientists have also found links among family members, showing that genetics play a role in how fast these changes occur.

SPECIAL IMPLICATIONS FOR THE THERAPIST   6-6

Specific Tissue or Organ Repair

Therapists have an important role in the rehabilitation of acute injuries. Certain components of the inflammatory process must be controlled quickly for recovery to proceed. For example, if edema is a component of a joint injury, it must be controlled as quickly as possible. Studies have demonstrated that joint edema can inhibit or hinder local muscle activity, which could result in altered joint mechanics and further irritation.[75] The anticipated goals are to facilitate healing of the injured structure and maintain the normal function of noninjured tissue and body regions. The overall goal of the rehabilitation program is to return the person to normal activity as soon as possible, yet not so fast that irritation and further inflammation of the injured area occur. A fine line exists between maximizing activity and overdoing the activity to the point of injury aggravation.

Client education is essential regarding the injured individual's role in facilitating tissue healing. Adherence to weight-bearing guidelines, avoiding aggravating movements, applying ice appropriately, and performing the prescribed exercises are key to the recovery process.

Recent studies have further clarified the role of exercises prescribed by physical therapists in the promotion of tissue repair from a cellular standpoint.[116,122,126] The mechanical loading brought about by appropriate exercise prescription produces a consequent cellular response that promotes changes in the tissue structure. This process, called *mechanotransduction*, has been shown in many studies to promote healing of tendon, muscle, articular cartilage, and bone. For example, physical loads brought about by shear or compressive forces during exercise perturb the cells. This physical perturbation results in a variety of intra- and intercellular chemical signals. In muscles and tendons, these chemical signals could result in the upregulation of growth factors that facilitate healing and repair. Loading of mechanosensitive cells in the articular cartilage (chondrocytes) and bone (osteocytes) has also been postulated to promote tissue growth via the same processes.[116] The concept of transegrity and mechanotransduction (transegrity is discussed earlier in the text) could also explain the positive effects of other physical therapy interventions such as soft tissue mobilization.[103,191]

Lastly, advances in the fields of biotechnology and biomaterials are providing new techniques for regeneration or repair of tissue lost to injury, disease, or aging. Bioengineered tissues, including skin, bone, articular cartilage, ligaments, and tendons, are under investigation for clinical use (see "Tissue Engineering" in Chapter 21).[106,107]

Prevention

Appropriate rehabilitation is necessary for soft tissue injuries, especially severe muscle strains and frank rupture of any tendon or muscle. Return to full activity, especially high-impact sports, can (and often does) result in recurrence of injury. Injury prevention should include addressing issues such as muscle fatigue, weakness, and lack of flexibility. Stronger muscles are better able to absorb energy and thereby limit the magnitude of tissue stretch. In other words, muscle strengthening is an important way to avoid muscle strain. The value of stretching prior to activity continues to be a topic of controversy. Although some studies have shown that a warm-up program that includes stretching may reduce strain injuries, more studies are needed to confirm this relationship.[139]

Rehabilitation of Repaired Soft Tissues

Careful monitoring of the timeline for tissue recovery, observing presenting signs and symptoms, and monitoring response to specific activities, movements, and treatments could guide the therapist in deciding when and how to progress intervention and activity level. The type of tissue involved also makes a difference because tendon tear/repair requires a period of rest to avoid disrupting the healing process and subsequent reinjury, whereas prolonged rest and immobilization after muscle strain can result in unwanted consequences such as stiffness. This monitoring can also be taught so the client understands the limits of his or her condition.

The process is somewhat more difficult with acute back or neck injuries than with peripheral injuries. Owing to the depth of the tissues of the spine, increased temperature and erythema are not always present or palpable if present. It is important for the therapist to pay close attention to the degree of pain, changes in movement limitation, and possible presence of protective muscle tone in deciding when the program can be progressed.

If the repair process involves sutures, the therapist must remember that as a general guideline for tissue healing, during the inflammatory phase after injury or surgery (first 3 to 5 days), the soft tissue's (e.g., tendon, ligament, or muscle) ability to hold sutures is at an all-time low. Protected rest is imperative during this stage. Gradually increasing tensile force on the healing tissue comes next. An incremental approach that is slow enough to allow and promote the stages of proliferation, maturation, and fiber realignment while at the same time being mindful of the deleterious effects of inactivity (such as the development of adhesions, stiffness, or muscle atrophy) is important to optimize the healing process and return the individual to optimal function at the soonest possible time.

Tendon or Muscle Rupture

During the proliferative phase (usually 5-28 days after tendon injury/repair), controlled passive movement is allowed. The repaired tissue is kept protected to avoid excessive force. Passive range of motion is continued as healing progresses and until the tissue moves into the remodeling phase of healing (around 4-8 weeks after injury/repair). Aggressive early motion that stresses the repair and exceeds the mechanical strength of the repair should be avoided. During the early weeks of the remodeling phase, the force required to rupture a lacerated and repaired tendon can be less than the force generated by a maximum muscle contraction. These findings suggest that maximum muscle contraction forces should be avoided for at least 8 weeks after tendon repair; the therapist can expect to see significant tendon weakness for a considerable period afterward.[34]

Active range of motion is then initiated with controlled movements (e.g., gravity-eliminated positions). The idea is to prevent excessive resistance from the weight of the limb while still working on gradually increasing the force of the muscle contraction. As the repair strengthens, the therapist can allow increased muscle force through increased antigravity movements.[34]

Resistance with weights, rubber tubing, elastic bands, and so on is not started until at least 8 weeks after the repair. Once again, resistance is increased progressively (between 8 and 12 weeks). At the end of 12 weeks, if there have been no complications (e.g., infection, wound dehiscence) and there are no comorbidities to delay healing (e.g., tobacco use, diabetes, peripheral vascular disease), then full force muscle contraction can be tolerated.

In terms of the muscle, surgical repair of a complete muscle tear has its own protocol. Clinicians must be aware that muscle repair is difficult as the muscle fibers do not hold sutures well.[28] More importantly, guidelines for nonsurgical and postoperative rehabilitation for ligament, tendon, and muscle tear/repair vary based on geographical regions and physician preferences and protocols and are reported widely in the literature. The plan of care should always be based on an understanding of the healing stages of injured tissue. As mentioned previously, the goal is to restore motion and strength without subjecting the healing tissue to excessive forces that may hinder healing or rupture the repair.

Health promotion, injury prevention, and risk reduction are important roles of the physical therapist. Clinicians have the responsibility of educating patients on risk factors that predispose an individual to soft tissue injuries to prevent the onset of injuries or recurrence of the condition if an injury is sustained.

Muscle Injury

Muscle injuries, including contusion, strain, or laceration, are common injuries, occurring particularly in sports; about 90% of all muscle injuries are either contusions or strains. A muscle *contusion* occurs when the muscle is subject to a sudden, heavy compressive force such as a direct blow to the muscle. Muscle *strains* occur when excessive tensile force leads to overstraining of the myofibers.[109] This is more likely to occur during eccentric contraction when the muscle is lengthening because tension is greater than the muscle's resistance

to stretch; the resultant forces are large. Muscles that cross two joints (e.g., hamstrings or gastrocnemius) are especially vulnerable to stretch injury because they are simultaneously affected by angular positions and velocities of the adjacent joints.[28]

The most common site of strain injury is the myotendinous junction, a region of highly folded basement membranes between the end of the muscle fiber and the tendon. These involutions maximize surface area for force transmission. The transition from compliant muscle fibers to relatively noncompliant tendon may account for the vulnerability of the myotendinous junction. If the force of stretch on a muscle is too great to be resisted by the contractile unit, resistance shifts from the contractile unit to the connective tissues. Pathogenic stretch (passive or active) that is beyond the threshold length of the entire musculotendinous unit can result in disruption at the myotendinous junction. Complete tears do occur but less often than muscle strain.[28]

Recovery from severe muscle strain may begin with a short period of immobilization and application of appropriate electrotherapeutic and physical agents to provide pain relief and protect the tissue during the initial phase of healing. Immobilization followed by mobilization of muscle may help muscle fiber regeneration and fiber orientation with reduced scar formation.[108,113] As soon as pain and swelling subside, a program can be initiated to recover range of motion, strength, and endurance. Return to sports is considered safe when there is 80% return of strength compared to the noninvolved side.[118]

Modalities

Physical therapy modalities, such as thermotherapy (application of heat and cold), and electrical modalities such as transcutaneous electrical nerve stimulation, iontophoresis, and ultrasound, may be used to manage pain and limited motion, but their impact on the underlying tear and healing tissue is not fully known.

In his text, Belanger[19] clearly articulates the evidence behind the use of these modalities according to the phases of tissue healing. The reader is advised to consult this text for an in-depth discussion of the evidence. As an example, although there is evidence supporting the use of cryotherapy in minimizing wound bleeding, it must be applied immediately after the injury for it to be effective.[19] Also, cryotherapy, when applied within the first 24 to 48 hours of the injury, is effective in reducing the consequent tissue damage following the inflammatory process.[19] Several modalities may be used to promote the development of new blood vessels and repair cells in the proliferative stage, and finally to enhance remodeling with the intent of optimizing functional gains in the maturation phase. Examples of these modalities have been included in the respective sections that discuss the healing process for each type of tissue.

Motor Control and Muscle Inhibition

As mentioned previously, injury to the muscle and the consequent repair and healing process causes alterations in movement patters. Chronic pain could be a complication of the healing process and may also be a factor in abnormal movement. Neurophysiologic adaptation to chronic pain appears to result in changes in motor control and muscle recruitment strategies. Recent research has also documented the role of cortical reorganization in abnormal movement patterns related to chronic pain following a musculoskeletal injury.[151] Physical therapy interventions that are aimed at altering these abnormal cortical representations may be of benefit for individuals with chronic pain and abnormal motor control. New information regarding muscle injury and repair, pain, and movement mirrors this complex relationship and highlights the interaction of multiple body systems in the production of movement.[98]

Medications

A significant percentage of those coming to outpatient therapy clinics are taking salicylates or NSAIDs.[26] These medications can play a key role in recovery from an acute injury, facilitating the therapist's role and clinical decision making. The common clinical practice to administer NSAIDs should be limited to early symptom control during the early phases of tissue healing. Prolonged NSAID use may be counterproductive for the biologic healing process, because complete tissue recovery involves delicate and finely coordinated elements of cellular and metabolic inflammatory reactions, which can be interrupted by NSAIDs.[141,162] Moreover, because NSAIDs also help control pain, patients may put more strain on the injured tissue (because of lack of pain), thereby exacerbating the injury and delaying the healing process.[222]

Considering the widespread use of salicylates and NSAIDs, therapists must also be aware of potential side effects that would warrant communication with a physician (see Chapter 5). Irritation of the GI system is the most common potential side effect. The risk of developing peptic ulcer disease increases significantly if someone is taking more than one of these types of drugs. This pattern of drug use exists in the therapy population, in which significant numbers of subjects are taking one or more over-the-counter antiinflammatory agents along with a prescribed NSAID.[26] Please see "Special Implications for the Therapist 5-3: Nonsteroidal Antiinflammatory Drugs" in Chapter 5 for more information on side effects of NSAIDs, and Chapter 16 for a description of peptic ulcer disease.

Tissue Response to Immobilization or Decline in Joint Mobility

In addition to having an important role in the rehabilitation of acute injuries, therapists often deal with clinical problems secondary to the effects of immobilization. Although not traumatic in the classic sense, immobilization of a limb or joint can result in significant impairment and activity limitations.

Immobilization takes a variety of forms, including bed rest, casting or splinting of a body part, or non–weight-bearing status of a lower extremity. On a tissue level, significant changes can occur with immobilization (Table 6-8). Besides the inert joint structures, changes

Table 6-8	Effects of Prolonged Immobilization
Tissue	**Results of Immobilization**
Muscle	Atrophy, decreased strength, contracture, reduced capillary to muscle fiber ratio, reduced mitochondrial density, reduced endurance
Bone	Generalized osteopenia of cancellous and cortical bone
Tendons and ligaments	Disorganization of parallel arrays of fibrils and cells; increased deformation with a standard load or compressive force
Ligament insertion site	Destruction of ligament fibers attaching to bone, reduced load to failure
Cartilage	Adherence of fibrofatty connective tissue to cartilage surfaces; loss of cartilage thickness; pressure necrosis at points of contact where compression has been applied
Synovium	Proliferation of fibrofatty connective tissue into joint space
Menisci	Adhesions of synovium villi; decreased synovial intima length; decreased synovial fluid hyaluronan concentrations; decreased synovial intima macrophages
Joint	*0 to 12 weeks:* Impaired range of motion; increased intraarticular pressure during movements; decreased filling volume of joint cavity
	After 12 weeks: Force required for the first flexion-extension cycle is increased more than 12-fold
Heart	Reduced strength of contraction (SV), reduced maximal cardiac output, reduced endurance, increased work of the heart for a submaximal load
Lung	Reduced airway clearance of mucous, increased likelihood of pneumonia, reduced maximal ventilatory volume
Blood	Reduced hematocrit and plasma volume, reduced endurance and temperature regulation

also occur in muscle, particularly a loss of strength. Such changes can occur without injury, which magnifies the importance of maintaining function in noninjured tissue and body areas. A rehabilitation program should be designed to address the needs of each of the tissues.

As previously mentioned, prolonged immobilization negatively impacts tendon and ligament healing. During immobilization, the lack of strain and loading on these tissues will cause corresponding decreases in the cross-sectional area and strength of these tissues, resulting in joint hypermobility and laxity. With restoration of loading and movement, these deleterious effects are reversed.[231] The therapist must therefore commence mobilization activities as soon as safely possible to counter these negative effects.

The use of orthotic devices such as a brace has been a common intervention to prevent reinjury of individuals who have either deficient or reconstructed ligaments. Although results of studies on the use of knee bracing to prevent ligament injuries have been mixed, there is some evidence that knee bracing provides 20% to 30% greater ligament protection,[177] increased strain relief for the medial collateral ligament, increased knee stiffness, and perception of the ability of the brace to protect and/or affect performance.[29]

Stiffness

Muscle stiffness is a common problem with advancing age. As humans get older, the elasticity of muscle decreases, due to connective tissue changes involving the musculotendinous unit. Small amounts of fibrinogen (produced in the liver and normally converted to fibrin to serve as a clotting factor) leak from the vasculature into the intracellular spaces, adhering to cellular structures. The resulting microfibrinous adhesions among the cells of muscle and fascia cause increased muscular stiffness. Activity and movement normally break these adhesions; however, with the aging process, production of fewer and less efficient macrophages combined with immobility for any reason result in reduced lysis of these adhesions.[167]

Other possible causes of aggravated stiffness include increased collagen fibers from reduced collagen turnover, increased cross-links of aged collagen fibers, changes in the mechanical properties of connective tissues, and structural and functional changes in the collagen protein. Stiffness related to impairments in tissue extensibility may respond well to a regimen of application of heat[76] followed by low-load, long-duration stretching.[72] Age-related muscular stiffness could be improved by increased physical activity and movement. A general conditioning program for the older adult will not only result in improved mobility and decrease muscular pain but also improve cardiovascular performance and overall health.

Deep Venous Thrombosis

While initiating rehabilitation after immobilization, the therapist must remain vigilant for the possible presence of deep vein thrombosis (DVT). A potential complication of DVT is pulmonary embolus, which represents one of the leading causes of morbidity and mortality, and is reported to account for 10% of hospital deaths.[133] Although a large percentage of clients with DVT are asymptomatic, severe local pain and edema, fever, chills, and malaise are all possible manifestations. The types of immobilization that carry the risk of DVT include bed rest, a limb being placed in a cast or splint, and non–weight-bearing status following a lower extremity injury, a surgical procedure, or a long car or plane ride. In terms of interventions for DVT, studies have shown that early mobilization does not increase the risk of developing pulmonary embolism[215] in people with DVT. (See Chapter 12 for more information about DVT.)

Special Note on Regenerative Rehabilitation

There has been an increased focus on the implications of advances in regenerative medicine in physical therapy. Regenerative medicine is an emerging medical practice area that seeks to identify approaches that could potentially replace, repair, or regenerate organs and tissues. These new treatments further deepen our understanding of alternative repair and healing mechanisms in human tissues and organs. Within the PT profession, the FiRST Initiative (Frontiers in Rehabilitation Science and Technology) seeks to clarify the role of regenerative rehabilitation in optimizing movement and function in individuals. See also "Tissue Engineering and Regenerative Medicine" in Chapter 21 of this text. For further information, please refer to the article by Wolf (FiRST and foremost: Advances in Science and Technology impacting neurologic physical therapy, J Neurol Phys Ther 37[4]:147-8, 2013); and the proceedings of the FiRST Initiative lecture series during the American Physical Therapy Association (APTA) 2014 NEXT Conference. The APTA website also provides an overview of genetics in physical therapy (http://www.apta.org/genetics/). This web page contains additional links pertaining to regenerative rehabilitation.

REFERENCES

To enhance this text and add value for the reader, all references are included on the companion Evolve site that accompanies this textbook. The reader can view the reference source and access it online whenever possible.

CHAPTER 7

The Immune System

JOSEPH A. FRAIETTA • DAVID M. KIETRYS

INTRODUCTION

Joseph A. Fraietta, PhD

Immunology is the study of the physiologic mechanisms that allow the body to differentiate between self and nonself and how it reacts when a nonself component is encountered. The immune system is highly adaptable and capable of generating enormous diversity that provides protection against a multitude of threats. Effective immunity (resistance) requires the orchestration of intricate networks of molecules, cells and tissues that function through various mechanisms to protect self. This resistance can be acquired by infection with microorganisms, as well as deliberate immunization with microbes or their subunits in the form of vaccines. Immune responses are crucial for the survival of the host and are usually beneficial. The goal of eliciting an immune response is to prevent infection entirely or limit the dissemination of a pathogen without causing long-term harm to the body.

Following recognition of an invader, the immune system triggers an effector response that neutralizes or eliminates the threat. One of the remarkable complexities of the immune system is the way that it translates the initial recognition event into various effector responses, each tailored specifically for a particular type of pathogen. Certain infections result in a memory response that is characterized by a more rapid immune reaction of greater magnitude upon subsequent exposure to the same disease-causing microorganism. This phenomenon, known as *immunologic memory*, is a way of "educating" the immune system and preventing disease, should the invader return.

In an attempt to eliminate a threat, damage is occasionally done to host tissues. Although this injury is typically transient, the immune system can sometimes malfunction and give rise to hyperresponses (hypersensitivities) and autoimmunity that may have mildly debilitating to life-threatening consequences. These excessive or inappropriate responses include common conditions such as allergies to plant or animal products, foods, medications, and less-well-known autoimmune diseases in which the immune system attacks "self" tissues of the host. In addition, not all immune responses are helpful, as in the case of introducing a nonself component for the purpose of medical intervention (e.g., organ transplants and prosthetic devices).

When the immune system is functioning properly, it protects the host against infection and disease; when it is not, the failure of the immune system can result in localized or systemic infection or disease. In fact, the significance of a healthy immune system is apparent in states or diseases characterized by immunodeficiency, such as those that occur in human immunodeficiency virus (HIV) infection and in individuals who are taking immunosuppressive drugs.

Without an effective immune system, an individual is at risk for the development of overwhelming infection, malignant disease (abnormal self-components), or both.

For a complete understanding of the immune system as it relates to injury, inflammation, healing, and repair the reader is encouraged to read this chapter along with Chapter 6.

TYPES OF IMMUNITY

The body uses two major immune responses to combat a potential threat: innate (natural or nonspecific immunity) and adaptive immunity (acquired or specific immunity) (Fig. 7-1). Innate immunity consists of molecular and cellular defense mechanisms that are present prior to exposure to a threat that can function as a first line of defense. If the innate immune response fails to control and eliminate the pathogen, the adaptive immune response is activated and begins a few days following the initial infection.

In general, acquired immunity adapts to recognize, eliminate, and establish long-term memory against a threat, which provides protection against future attacks by the same or a closely related invader. Because of these different roles, both innate and adaptive arms of the immune system possess a series of unique properties that are critical for host defense. It is important to recognize that innate and adaptive branches of the immune system do not function independently, but instead collaborate in a coordinated manner to increase immune responsiveness.

Innate Immunity

Innate immunity acts as the body's first line of defense to prevent the entry of pathogens and is actually capable of resolving most threats. The innate immune system is comprised of early host defense mechanisms that are able to limit the spread of infection and, in some cases, eliminate the invading pathogen, mediate the initiation and development of adaptive immunity that is pathogen-specific,

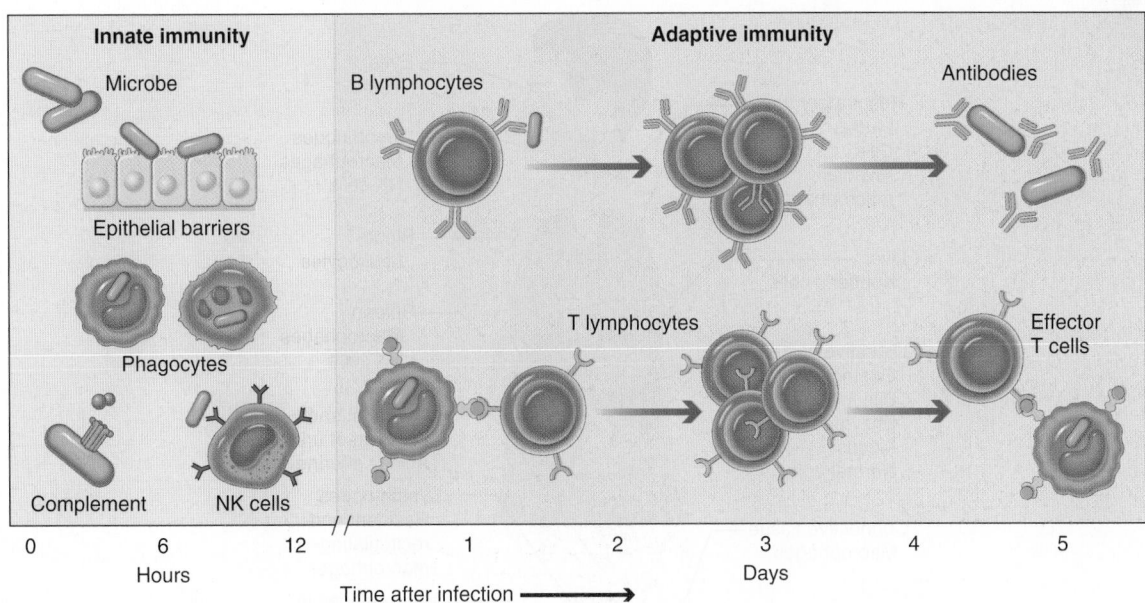

Figure 7-1

The principal mechanisms of innate and adaptive immunity and their development over time. Physical mechanisms (e.g., epithelial barriers) prevent initial microbial colonization. If the invading microbe breaches this first line of defense, non-specific innate immune mechanisms (e.g., phagocytes, NK cells, and the complement system) function to eliminate the pathogen. When innate immunity fails to prevent the spread of infection, adaptive immunity serves as a specific and comprehensive third line of defense. The adaptive immune response takes time to develop and is mediated by lymphocytes and their products. The kinetics of these responses may differ, depending on the type of infection. (Reprinted from Kumar V: *Robbins and Cotran: pathologic basis of disease*, ed 8, Philadelphia, 2009, WB Saunders.)

and work in concert with adaptive immune responses to effectively clear a microbial threat.

Certain innate immune defenses are broadly effective against a diverse array of insults, whereas other components are most effective against certain classes of pathogens (e.g., viruses, bacteria, fungi, or parasites). Innate immune system components include external defenses that are present at the site infection (e.g., physical, mechanical, chemical and biochemical barriers) and internal defenses (cellular and soluble components). A diverse array of threats that an individual may encounter in his or her lifetime is dealt with by the innate arm of the immune system through recognition molecules that identify patterns common to many different types of pathogens. Therefore, although the innate immune system responds to common features of multiple threats, it has a limited number of specificities. Furthermore, it does not remember the interaction with a specific invader for help during potential future encounters (Fig. 7-2).

Adaptive Immunity

Adaptive immunity is characterized by specificity and memory. The goal of this comprehensive line of defense is to specifically recognize the threat, promote an effective immune response, destroy/remove the invading pathogen, and establish long-term memory.

Adaptive immunity results when a pathogen gains entry into the body and a specific response is elicited against the invader. This type of immunity requires pre-activation (days to weeks for a full effect). The adaptive immune system is activated if a threat is present at a high enough level for a prolonged period of time (activation threshold). Adaptive immunity continually

"develops" throughout life following exposure to a particular threat and has memory so that when the same disease-causing microorganism is encountered again, the body can respond even more rapidly and with a heightened immune response. The two components of adaptive immunity, humoral immunity and cell-mediated immunity (see Table 7-2 and Fig. 7-8), are discussed in greater detail later in this section.

Adaptive immune responses can occur as a result of active or passive immunity. Active immunity includes natural immunity and artificial immunity, which is intended or deliberate (Table 7-1). *Active immunity* refers to protection acquired by introduction (either naturally from environmental exposure or artificially by vaccination) of an antigen (any molecule that binds specifically to an antibody or T-cell receptor) into a responsive host.

The concept of vaccination is based on the fact that deliberate exposure to a harmless version or component of a pathogen generates immunologic memory but not disease induced by the infectious agent itself. In this way, the immune system is primed to mount a secondary immune response with strong and immediate protection should the pathogenic version of the microorganism be encountered in the future.[73]

Some of the most promising prophylactic and therapeutic vaccine strategies are currently being investigated for malaria, cancer, HIV, asthma, influenza, diabetes, hepatitis C, and many other diseases.

Passive acquired immunity occurs when immune products such as antibodies or sensitized lymphocytes produced by an immune person are transferred to a nonimmune individual (see Table 7-1). For example, the transplacental transfer of antibodies from mother to fetus, the transfer of antibodies

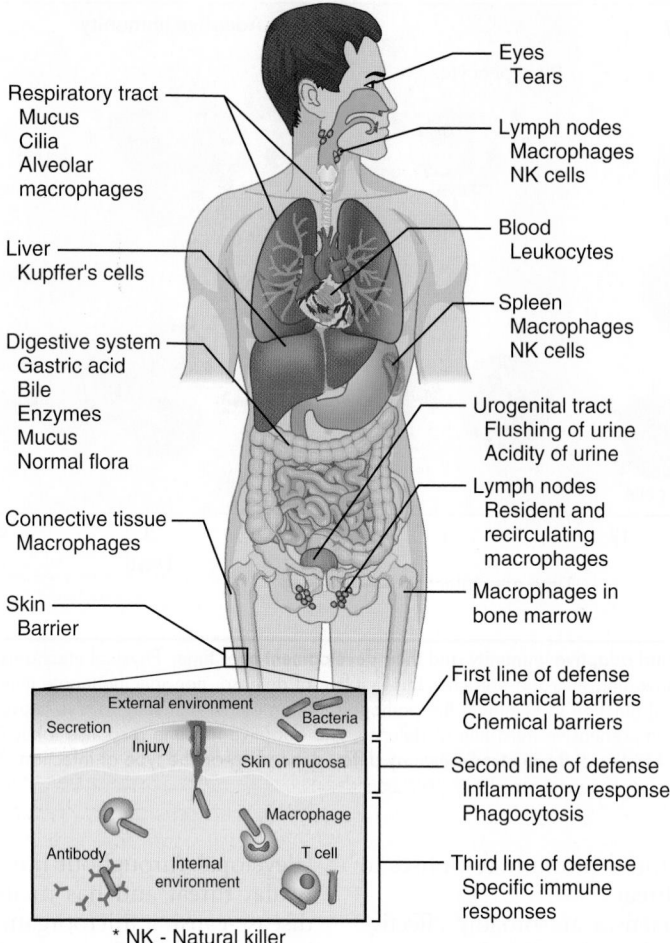

Figure 7-2

Natural protective mechanisms of the human body. The structural integrity of epithelial and mucosal surfaces is critical to the formation and maintenance of an effective barrier against initial invasion or penetration by pathogenic microorganisms. Clearance of an invading pathogen may involve complex interactions between innate and adaptive immune responses. (Reprinted from Damjanov I: *Pathology for the health professions*, ed 3, Philadelphia, 2006, WB Saunders.)

Table 7-1	Types of Acquired Immunity	
Type of Acquired Immunity*	**Method Acquired**	**Length of Resistance**
Active		
Natural	Natural contact and infection with the antigen (environmental exposure)	Usually permanent but may be temporary
Artificial	Inoculation of antigen (vaccination)	Usually permanent but may be temporary (occasional exceptions)
Passive		
Natural	Natural contact with antibody transplacentally (mother to fetus) or through colostrum and breast milk	Temporary
Artificial	Inoculation of antibody or antitoxin; immune serum globulin	Temporary

*Active immunity occurs when a person produces his or her own antibodies to the infecting organism; passive immunity occurs when the antibody is formed in another host and transferred to an individual.

to an infant through breast milk, or the administration of immune serum globulin (γ-globulin) provides immediate protection, but does not result in the formation of memory cells and therefore provides only temporary immunity.

MECHANISMS OF DEFENSE AND IMMUNE RESPONSES

See Table 7-2.

External Defenses

Anatomical barriers are the most obvious innate immune defense mechanisms that are in place to provide early protection against microbial invasion. For most pathogens to establish localized infection and proliferate at that initial site, they must first attach to and penetrate host tissues.

Physical/mechanical barriers aid in defense by inhibiting the attachment and invasion of infectious agents. These include skin, mucus, cilia lining of mucosa (mucociliary escalator), coughing, sneezing, and peristalsis. As a covering for the entire body with the exception of any openings, the skin offers a physical line of protection (see Fig. 7-2), and its importance is clearly demonstrated

Table 7-2	The Immune System and Its Response		
		ADAPTIVE IMMUNITY	
Innate Immunity		**Humoral**	**Cell-Mediated**
Nonspecific interaction with different antigens; lacks immunologic memory		Specific interaction with different antigens	Specific interaction with different antigens
Exterior defenses: Skin, mucosa, secretions, nasal hair, ear wax		Mediated by antibody, present as serum globulins	Mediated by T lymphocytes
Phagocytes (leukocytes): Neutrophils (polymorphonuclear neutrophils) Monocytes/macrophages		Antibodies are produced by plasma cells (differentiated form of B lymphocytes)	Secretion of cytokines
Eosinophils Basophils Mast cells and platelets (inflammation)			Production of helper T cells (CD4+), cytotoxic T cells (CD8+) and regulatory/suppressor T cells (CD4+CD25+)
Soluble mediators: Complement and interferons; see Table 6-5 Natural killer cells or large granular lymphocytes		Primary and secondary (memory) antibody response	Primary and secondary (memory) T-cell response

in cases of significant burns when infection becomes a major problem for the host.

The body also possesses unique defenses in the form of chemical and biochemical barriers, such as lysozyme (found in tears, saliva and nasal secretions) that can break down bacterial cell walls, wax in the ear canal to prevent bacteria from advancing inside, nasal hair, stomach acid and a rapid pH change at the gastroduodenal junction for the destruction of ingested organisms, protective low pH vaginal secretions, acidic urine, lactoferrin and transferrin (iron chelators) present in a variety of secretory fluids, and antimicrobial peptides (e.g., defensins) in the lung and gastrointestinal tract that form pores in the membranes of microbes. In addition, the normal flora that colonizes the skin, urogenital tract, upper respiratory tract and lower gastrointestinal tract competes with pathogens for nutrients, as well as attachment to epithelial and mucosal surfaces.

Internal Defenses

The innate immune system is comprised of many different internal defenses that can be classified as soluble factors (e.g., complement system, cytokines, chemokines, acute phase proteins) and cellular components (neutrophils, monocytes/macrophages, natural killer cells). Cell-membrane bound receptors can also be utilized as effectors (remember: able to neutralize or eliminate the threat). Unlike the finely tuned specificity of adaptive immunity, innate immune system components recognize repeating patterns of molecular structure that are common to certain classes of pathogens. These pathogen-associated molecular patterns (PAMPs) are of limited variability and usually part of structures that are essential to the invading pathogen (e.g., double- and single-stranded viral RNA, endotoxin of Gram-negative bacteria, peptidoglycan in bacterial cell wall, terminal mannose residues of bacterial and viral surface components).[24,286]

The interaction of innate pattern recognition receptors (e.g., Toll-like receptors) with their cognate PAMPs may result in phagocytosis and killing of the pathogen and/or recruitment of immune cells to the site of infection. Upon detection of PAMPs by soluble or membrane-bound pattern recognition receptors, certain immunologic response modifiers are produced that act locally, whereas others travel through the bloodstream and function at distant target sites. These effector molecules may serve to restrict proliferation of the pathogen, recruit and activate additional immune cells to the site of infection, and/or facilitate the development of an adaptive immune response.

Examples of these immune mediators include *cytokines* (soluble proteins or glycoproteins synthesized by a variety of cells that can modify cellular behavior) and *chemokines* (small cytokines that can induce chemotactic migration of leukocytes and enhance inflammation). Local actions of cytokines and chemokines include increased vascular permeability, activation of vascular epithelial tissue, changes in blood flow and white blood cell (leukocyte) migration patterns, and the generation of a chemotactic gradient of leukocytes to the site of inflammation.

Type I interferons (IFNα and IFNβ) are cytokines produced by cells infected with viruses early in infection (usually a few hours) and these cytokines limit the spread of the infection by protecting surrounding (uninfected) cells. Interferons also inhibit tumor growth. Most cells in the body express receptors for type I interferons that upon ligation by IFNα/β, signal the host cell to activate or increase the synthesis of large sets of proteins. Although responses may differ depending on the cell type, the result is resistance to viral replication in all cells and the initiation of effector responses to destroy virally infected cells.

Acute-Phase Response

An acute-phase response occurs when high levels of proinflammatory cytokines (e.g., interleukin [IL]-1, IL-6, tumor necrosis factor [TNF]α) are produced. Systemic effects of proinflammatory cytokines include fever, occlusion of blood vessels, leukocytosis, mobilization of energy from muscle and fat stores, and increased production of acute phase proteins, such as fibrinogen (factor I). Mannose-binding protein and C-reactive protein are other acute-phase proteins that participate in activation of the lectin-associated complement pathway.

The Complement System

The complement system consists of more than 30 proteins that are key components of the acute inflammatory response. When activated, these proteins interact in a cascade-like process and aggregate to damage the membranes of microbial cells, resulting in their death by lysis. The complement system also possesses serum glycoproteins that upon activation, aid in phagocytosis of the target (opsonization; see further discussion in Chapter 6). Another role of complement in the inflammatory response is to promote the clearance of immune complexes that are formed by the specific binding of an antibody to a soluble antigen.

It is important to appreciate that the complement system is involved in both innate immune responses (alternative complement pathway activated by PAMPs; lectin-associated complement pathway activated by binding of acute phase proteins), as well as adaptive immunity (classical complement pathway activated by antibodies bound to specific antigens of a particular threat). (See "The Complement System" in Chapter 6; see also Table 6-5.)

Natural Killer Cells

Natural killer (NK) cells are large granular lymphocytes that are distinct from T cells and B cells. Mature populations of NK cells found in the blood and spleen are localized to infected tissues in response to inflammatory cytokines. The function of NK cells is to kill cells infected with viruses and other intracellular pathogens, as well as tumor cells. Unlike T cells and B cells, NK cells do not express antigen-specific receptors. Instead, NK cells express activating and inhibitory receptors on their surfaces that interact with ligands on the target cell. The signals that are transmitted by these receptors are integrated to determine whether the NK cell will detach and move on or stay and respond. Effector functions associated with NK cells include cytotoxicity and cytokine production (Fig. 7-3).[166]

When activated, proteins contained within cytoplasmic granules of NK cells are released onto the surface of a cellular target. These granules create pores in the plasma membrane of the infected cell and this allows for other proteins to enter and activate a programmed death cascade. NK cells also collaborate with the adaptive immune system in the process of antibody-dependent cellular cytotoxicity.

When antibody-dependent cellular cytotoxicity occurs, specific antibodies bound to a pathogen trigger a receptor on an NK cell to release its cytotoxic contents. In addition to direct cytotoxic effects, NK cells secrete cytokines such as IFNγ (type II interferon) and TNFα. These two cytokines can induce the maturation of dendritic cells, which are the critical coordinators of innate and adaptive immunity that are discussed later in this chapter.

IFNγ produced by NK cells is also important for the recruitment and activation of macrophages that are able to phagocytose and kill pathogenic microbes, as well as secrete additional cytokines, chemokines, and antimicrobial effector molecules. The cytokine milieu produced early during infection is extremely important for the initiation of adaptive immunity and greatly influences the nature of these responses.

Mononuclear Phagocytes and Granulocytic Cells

Phagocytes participate in innate immunity by readily ingesting pathogens, such as bacteria or fungi, and killing them in order to protect the body against infection. The two principal families of professional phagocytes are *neutrophils*

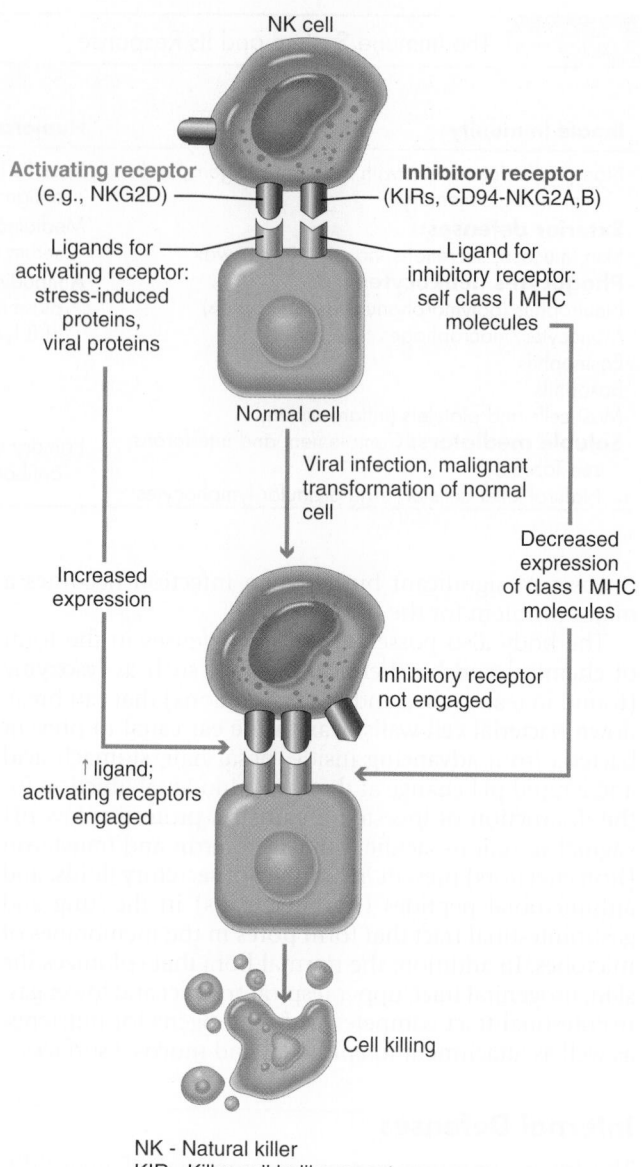

NK - Natural killer
KIR - Killer cell Ig-like receptors
MHC - Major histocompatibility complex

Figure 7-3

Schematic of NK cell receptors and cell killing. NK cells express activating and inhibitory receptors; some examples of each are indicated. Normal cells are not killed because inhibitory signals from normal major histocompatibility complex class I molecules override activating signals. In tumor cells or virus-infected cells, there is increased expression of ligands for activating receptors and reduced expression or alteration of major histocompatibility complex molecules, which interrupts the inhibitory signals, allowing activation of NK cells and lysis of target cells. (Reprinted from Kumar V: *Robbins and Cotran: pathologic basis of disease,* ed 8, Philadelphia, 2009, WB Saunders.)

and *monocytes.* These cells are classified as *leukocytes.* The five major types of leukocytes are neutrophils, eosinophils, basophils, monocytes, and lymphocytes. Because of their granular appearance, neutrophils, eosinophils, and basophils are collectively referred to as *granulocytes.* Granulocytes are short-lived (2-3 days) compared with monocytes and macrophages, which may persist for months or years.

Phagocytes emigrate from the blood into tissues in which an infection has developed, and each of these cell types has a specific effector function in the immune system (see "Disorders of Leukocytes" in Chapter 14).

Neutrophils, eosinophils, basophils, and monocytes are classified as phagocytic leukocytes that function in innate immunity. A large decrease in the absolute numbers of these cells in the blood is the principal cause of susceptibility to infection in people treated with intensive radiotherapy or chemotherapy. These treatments suppress the bone marrow, resulting in deficiencies of these phagocytic cells.

Neutrophils

Neutrophils, also referred to as polymorphonuclear cells (PMNs), are small short-lived cells with a multilobed nucleus that are produced in bone marrow. Neutrophils are the predominant leukocytes of the peripheral blood and increase dramatically in number in response to infection and inflammation. During phagocytosis, bacteria or debris is engulfed and then digested by certain molecules contained within the neutrophils (see Fig. 6-18; see also discussion of phagocytosis in Chapter 6 and Fig. 6-17).

Primary granules of neutrophils possess myeloperoxidase and cationic proteins, whereas their secondary granules contain lysozyme and lactoferrin. Although these factors allow neutrophils to effectively kill invading threats, damage is sometimes done to host tissues in the process. Neutrophils die after phagocytosis; the accumulation of dead neutrophils and phagocytosed bacteria contributes to the formation of pus. Importantly, neutrophils are the first cells to arrive at sites of inflammation and constitute a major line of defense against pus-forming bacteria such as *Neisseria, Staphylococcus,* and *Streptococcus.*

Monocytes

Monocytes are large, long-lived cells with a bilobed (dimpled) nucleus that originate in bone marrow. Monocytes circulate in the blood and when they migrate into tissues in response to infection and inflammation, they mature into residing *macrophages,* which means "large eaters."

After neutrophils kill the invading organism and the process of phagocytosis has begun, macrophages appear to "filter" the debris produced by the neutrophils and to kill any damaged, but not dead, bacteria or bacteria that are too large for neutrophils to eliminate. Phagocytosis of bacteria by neutrophils and macrophages depends on cell-surface receptors, including scavenger receptors, mannose receptors on macrophages, and receptors for complement components.

Eosinophils, Basophils, and Mast Cells

Eosinophils are the next group of leukocytes that participate in innate immunity. Eosinophils are derived from bone marrow and are involved in both allergic responses and parasitic infections. When invading organisms are too large for neutrophils and macrophages to eliminate, eosinophils localize within close proximity to the pathogen and release the contents of their granules to induce membrane damage and the subsequent death of the threat.

Basophils are granulocytes that circulate in peripheral blood and function by releasing active substances from their cytoplasmic granules that play a major role in certain allergic responses. Basophils and mast cells are located close to blood vessels throughout the body and have similar functional characteristics; *mast cells* possess granules containing histamine and other molecules that dilate blood vessels when released. Antihistamines function by neutralizing the histamines and reducing this type of excessive immune (allergic) response.

Mast cells are derived from stem cells and are released into the blood in an undifferentiated form. These cells do not differentiate until they enter tissues. Mast cells are usually found in small numbers in the connective tissue of organs. In addition to playing a major role in allergy and anaphylaxis, they participate in wound healing and are important for defense against invading pathogens. Basophils and mast cells cause an increase in blood supply in the area where a pathogen is located. This increase in circulation also helps to recruit more phagocytes to the site of infection. Increased circulation is typically accompanied by the feeling of congestion during an allergic reaction; antihistamines function by neutralizing the histamines and reducing this type of excessive immune (allergic) response.

Erythrocytes and Platelets

The role of erythrocytes and platelets in immune responses is sometimes overlooked, but because they have complement receptors, they play an important role in the clearance of immune complexes consisting of antigen, antibody, and components of the complement system.[73]

Antigens and Antibodies

The adaptive immune response involves recognition components with a higher degree of specificity than the detection mechanisms of innate immunity that distinguish features common to groups of foreign molecules. The antibody and T-cell receptor are the unique molecules of adaptive immune system that recognize specific antigenic determinants or *epitopes*. An epitope is an immunologically active site on an antigen that binds to a T-cell receptor or to an antibody (Fig. 7-4).

Antigens

Bacteria, viruses, parasites, foreign tissues, and large proteins possess constituents that are defined as antigenic because they can interact specifically with antigen receptors (i.e., T-cell receptors and/or antibodies). Although molecules may be antigenic, some may not necessarily induce a specific immune response. In other words, they do not possess immunogenicity.

Conversely, an *immunogen* is a foreign substance that induces an immune response when bound to an antigen receptor. Immunogenicity and antigenicity are two terms that are used almost interchangeably in discussions of immune responses; however, they have different meanings. For example, haptens are antigenic molecules that by themselves are too small to function as immunogenic epitopes. However, when many molecules of a single hapten are covalently conjugated to a nonimmunogenic carrier, the hapten-carrier complex becomes immunogenic when introduced into the host, as evidenced by the generation of antihapten antibodies. Haptens can be used as immunologic tools that allow researchers to determine how subtle changes in particular determinants affect the specificity of antibody–antigen interactions.

Factors that may influence the immunogenicity of a particular antigen include its degree of foreignness, structural and chemical complexity, molecular size, the genetic makeup of the host, mode of administration (route, dose and timing), as well as any substance that enhances specific responses elicited by an immunogen.[110] For example, an adjuvant is an immunostimulatory substance that is frequently included in vaccine preparations and serves to increase the response to a vaccine.

Antibodies

Antibodies are produced by B cells and consist of two identical heavy (H) chains and two identical light (L) chains (Fig. 7-5). The heavy chain possesses four or five

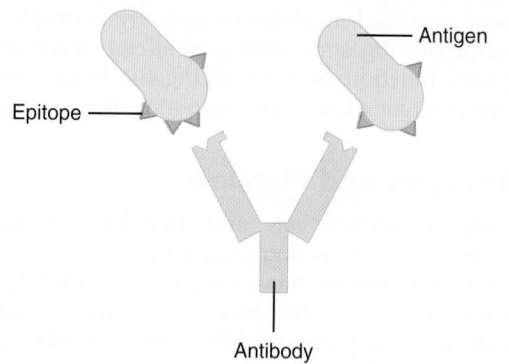

Figure 7-4

Antibodies bond to epitopes. Epitopes protrude from the surface of an antigen and combine with the appropriate binding site of an antibody. For small antigens, the binding site on the antibody may be a pocket or cleft, but in most cases it more closely resembles an undulating surface.[225] (Reprinted from Black JM, Hawks JH, Keene AM: *Medical-surgical nursing: clinical management for positive outcomes*, ed 7, Philadelphia, 2005, WB Saunders.)

immunoglobulin domains. Each light chain is bound to a heavy chain and these polypeptides are held together by intra-/interchain disulfide bonds, as well as hydrophobic and electrostatic interactions to form heterodimers.

In simplest form, an antibody resembles a Y-shaped molecule with two antigen-binding sites. The fragment antigen-binding (Fab fragment) is the portion of an antibody that binds to antigens. Aminoterminal ends of the light or heavy chain possess a high degree of variation among antibodies with different antigen specificities and are thus designated as variable (V) regions (V_H for the heavy chain and V_L for the light chain). Sequence variation in V_H and V_L confers the antigen specificity of an antibody. Hypervariable regions within V_H and V_L known as complementarity-determining regions constitute the antigen binding site of the molecule. Differences in specificity between antibodies are usually found in these areas.

In contrast, other regions of an antibody that do not contain antigen binding sites and are relatively invariant within an immunoglobulin (Ig) class are known as constant regions (designated C_L for the light chain and C_H1, C_H2, C_H3, C_H4 for the heavy chain). The region between the C_H1 and C_H2 regions is known as the *hinge region* and allows for flexibility between the two Fab arms of the *antibody* molecule. The heavy chain determines the type (isotype/class) of the antibody (IgM, IgG, IgE, IgA, or IgD). Each constant region of the immunoglobulin heavy chain is encoded by a gene segment that corresponds to a lower case Greek letter: μ (mu) encodes IgM, γ (gamma) encodes IgG, ε (epsilon) encodes IgE, α (alpha) encodes IgA, and δ (delta) encodes IgD.

The gene segments within the heavy chain are exchanged by isotype switching, which allows the antibody to change

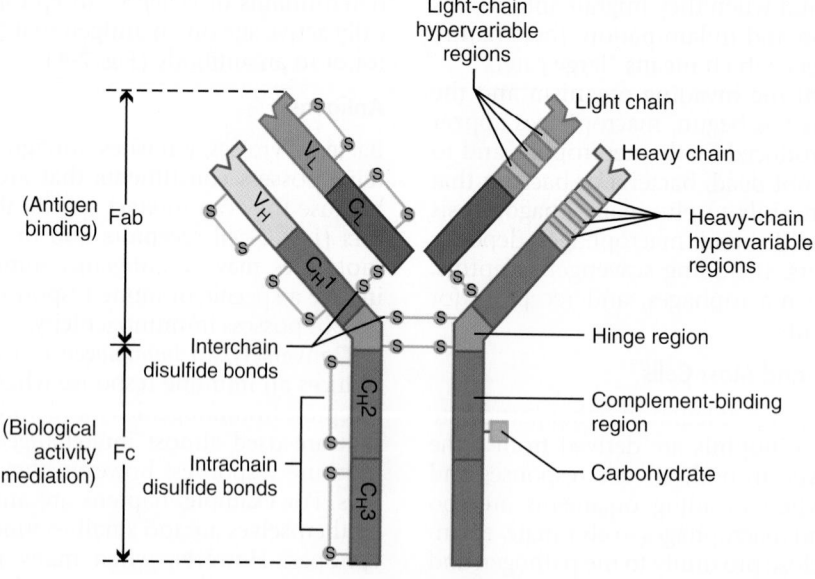

V_L and V_H: Variable regions
C_L and C_H: Constant regions

Figure 7-5

Chain and domain structure of an immunoglobulin (Ig) molecule with hypervariable regions within variable regions of both H and L chains. Fab and Fc refer to fragments of the IgG molecule formed by protein cleavage. The former contains the VH and CH1 H chain regions and intact L chain; the latter consists of the CH2 and CH3 regions of two H chains linked to one another by disulfide bonds. *(From Wasserman RL, Capra JD: Immunoglobulin. In Horowitz MI, Pigman W [eds]: The Glycoconjugates. New York, Academic Press, 1977, pp 323–348, with permission.)*

its effector characteristics and distribution. The heavy chain also contains the Fc ("fragment, crystallizable") portion of the antibody that possesses binding sites for the C1q complement protein and Fc receptors expressed on macrophages, lymphocytes, and other accessory cells. There are two light-chain types, kappa (κ) and lambda (λ) and a B cell expresses either κ or λ, but never both. These peptides are encoded by one of two genes at different chromosomal loci and can be associated with any heavy chain isotype.[96]

Immunoglobulins. Each immunoglobulin isotype possesses unique biochemical properties. Box 7-1 lists the major functions of immunoglobulins. *IgM* is an antibody produced by and expressed on the surface of a B cell. It is the first secreted antibody and is predominate in a primary or initial immune response. As a monomer, it can function as a B-cell receptor (BCR) on B cells that have not encountered antigen (naïve B cells). Pentameric forms of IgM are found in the blood; because of its large size, it is almost exclusively localized in the intravascular compartment. IgM is most efficient at activation of the classical complement pathway and its other effector functions include agglutination and neutralization of foreign invaders.

IgG is the major antibacterial and antiviral antibody in the blood and is carried by plasma into tissues. It is the major immunoglobulin synthesized during a secondary immune response (after IgM initially responds to foreign pathogens), conferring long-term immunity. IgG can activate complement via the classical pathway, promote phagocytosis (opsonization) of pathogens, and neutralize them. IgG can also cross the placenta and provide passive protection against infections in newborns during the first months of life.

IgA is found in serum and secretions. Secretory IgA defends external body surfaces, is the predominant immunoglobulin on mucous membrane surfaces, and is found in secretions such as saliva; breast milk (colostrum); urine; seminal fluid; tears; nasal fluids; and respiratory, gastrointestinal (GI), and urogenital secretions. IgA binds to pathogens and prevents their adherence to mucosal surfaces and colonization at the site of entry.

IgE is present at very low levels in the blood and is predominantly found bound to high-affinity receptors on mast cells and basophils. This immunoglobulin serves as a primary factor in the elimination of helminthic parasites, such as roundworms. *IgE* also functions during

allergic reactions by triggering the degranulation of mast cells and basophils, resulting in histamine release in association with allergies, anaphylaxis, extrinsic asthma, and urticaria (hives). This response of *IgE* is a normal reaction but becomes excessive in people with allergies.

IgD is found at low levels in the blood. Its primary function is to serve as an antigen receptor on mature naïve B cells.

Antigen Sequestration, Presentation, and Recognition in Adaptive Immunity

The elicitation of antigen-specific adaptive immune responses poses a very interesting challenge for the immune system: that is, tailoring individual responses against the limitless multitude of threats. Because interactions between antigens and their receptors are highly specific, millions of receptors are required for effective immune surveillance. The solution to this dilemma was revealed when it was discovered that virtually every characterized antibody molecule had a unique molecular signature in its variable region.

Through gene rearrangement processes, the genes that encode the BCR undergo permanent changes in DNA sequence during B-cell development to create millions of unique antigen receptors. Thus, the generation of immunoglobulin diversity occurs through the process of gene rearrangement. In addition, different forms of antibodies are created by RNA processing.[187] The result is the generation of 10^9 to 10^{11} different immunoglobulins. Accordingly, the DNA in a mature B cell is unique from every other cell, including B cells, unless the daughter cell was derived from the same original clone.

The generation of a diverse T-cell repertoire also depends upon rearrangement of genes that comprise the variable region of the T-cell receptor (TCR) (10^7-10^{10} unique TCRs are generated). More information about organization and rearrangement of BCR and TCR genes is available.[40,69] It should be noted that the genes encoding TCRs and immunoglobulins are different and are present on different chromosomes. Furthermore, variable regions of certain immunoglobulin genes only rearrange in B cells, whereas TCR gene arrangement only occurs in T cells.

B cells and T cells detect different types of antigens.[241] In addition to existing in a secreted form, antibodies may serve as membrane-bound antigen receptors on the surface of a B cell. TCRs exist only as membrane-bound antigen receptors of T cells. The BCR recognizes three-dimensional epitopes of macromolecules including nucleic acids, proteins, carbohydrates, lipids, and small chemical groups. Soluble or membrane-bound antigens in a native or denatured form can directly bind/crosslink the BCR.[241] For the antigens to be recognized, they must be accessible to the BCR. By contrast, the TCR recognizes constituents of protein antigens (peptides) that are presented (bound) by a major histocompatibility complex (MHC) on host cells. The TCR cannot detect free antigens (e.g., virus particles) that are not processed and presented in the context of an MHC. Thus, T-cell recognition depends on detection of both self-MHC and peptide antigen (MHC-restricted antigen recognition).

Antigen receptors are composed of unique recognition domains that will differ between lymphocytes, as well as

---

Box 7-1

MAJOR FUNCTIONS OF IMMUNOGLOBULINS*

- Immunoglobulins directly attack antigens, destroying or neutralizing them through the processes of agglutination, precipitating the toxins out of solution, neutralizing antigenic substances, and lysing the organism's cell wall.
- Immunoglobulins activate the complement system.
- Immunoglobulins activate anaphylaxis by releasing histamine in tissue and blood.
- Immunoglobulins stimulate antibody-mediated hypersensitivity.

*Globulins with antibody activity are referred to as *immunoglobulins*. From Firestein GS: *Kelley's textbook of rheumatology*, ed 9, Philadelphia, 2012, WB Saunders.

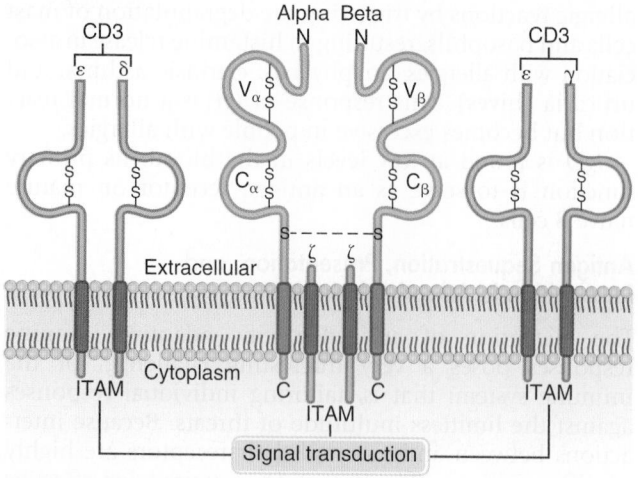

Figure 7-6

Schematic diagram of the T-cell receptor (TCR). The receptor is a complex of two main glycoprotein alpha and beta chains (defining an αβ TCR) noncovalently linked to the CD3 proteins (γ, δ, ε) and the ζ chain. As in other Ig superfamily products disulfide bonds form domains, and the carboxyl terminus of each chain is inserted into the plasma membrane. The amino terminus extracellular domains are variable in amino acid sequence and form the site of recognition of MHC-peptide complexes. The CD3 and ζ chains have intracytoplasmic ends (O) with signaling functions termed immunoreceptor tyrosine based activation motifs (ITAMs). The phosphorylation of the tyrosines in ITAMs represent the initial intracellular signaling events induced by TCR interaction with antigen.

nonvariable regions that are necessary for structural maintenance and effector function. These invariant domains are relatively conserved among all antigen-specific immune cell clones. For example, the chains of the TCR possess one variable (V) region and one constant (C) region. The variable regions of certain TCR subunits contact the MHC and antigen complex.[9] Similar to antibodies, areas of hypervariability or complementarity-determining regions within the V region vary greatly between different TCRs. Although the TCR and BCR can recognize antigens, the receptors themselves cannot transmit signals within the cell. For this reason, antigen receptors are linked to conserved molecules that function to transmit intracellular activation signals. Therefore, the recognition of a specific antigen and the resulting targeted response involves specific molecules (the receptors), and conserved sets of molecules that maintain the structure of the complex or facilitate signal transduction (Fig. 7-6).

Importantly, the signaling that is mediated by antigen receptors requires the aggregation or crosslinking of two or more receptors through association with adjacent antigenic molecules. When this receptor triggering takes place, enzymes localize to signaling portions of the receptor complexes within the cell cytoplasm and initiate the phosphorylation of downstream proteins. These phosphorylation events activate a number of complex signaling pathways that ultimately result in the synthesis of molecules responsible for mediating immune responses. More information about the processes of T and B lymphocyte signaling and activation is available.[1]

The Major Histocompatibility Complex. MHC molecules are membrane proteins that function to present antigenic peptides for recognition by T cells. MHC molecules were first identified as transplantation antigens because immunologic reactions against antiserum or skin grafts were traced to MHC differences between donors and recipients. In cases of graft rejection, the T cells of the recipient recognize the donor's MHC/peptide complexes as foreign antigens. Conversely, graft-versus-host disease occurs when the T cells from donor tissue mount immune responses against the host MHC/peptide. Although it is clear that nonself MHC molecules are a major determinant of graft rejection, this is not a natural immunological phenomenon, and therefore, MHC genes and the proteins that they encode could not have evolved for the sole purpose of mediating the rejection of foreign tissues. It is now known that the principal function of MHC molecules is to present peptides derived from protein antigens to T cells possessing distinct specificity for a particular epitope.

The MHC locus is a collection of genes that are present in all mammals. MHC proteins found in humans are known as human leukocyte antigens (HLAs), because of the discovery that these molecules could be identified with specific antibodies. The linked genes of the HLA locus are located on the short arm of chromosome 6. Because of their close proximity, these genes are typically inherited as a group or block known as a *haplotype*. MHC genes are highly polymorphic, meaning that are alternative forms of genes or *alleles* that exist among different individuals in a particular population. As a result of this high degree of polymorphism, all individuals that comprise a typical outbred population will have different sets of MHC genes and molecules.[185] However, regardless of extreme MHC polymorphism, no individual will express more than two alleles of each gene. In most cases, a person will express one allele from each parent at each MHC locus. HLA alleles inherited from both parents are expressed equally or codominantly and therefore, MHC molecules encoded by maternal and paternal alleles are present on the surface of each cell.

The three polymorphic MHC class I genes in humans, designated HLA-A, HLA-B, and HLA-C, encode antigen presentation complexes that are expressed on almost all nucleated cells. Because each individual inherits one set of paternal genes and another set of maternal genes, each cell can express six different MHC class I molecules. There are also three sets of polymorphic MHC class II genes, known as HLA-DR, HLA-DP, and HLA-DQ. The antigen presentation complexes encoded by these genes are expressed on professional antigen-presenting cells such as dendritic cells, activated macrophages and mature B lymphocytes. Many different MHC class II molecules can be expressed on the cell surface because of "mixing" of the alleles encoding certain domains of the presentation complex. Unlike MHC class I and class II genes, MHC class III genes do not encode antigen presentation complexes, but, rather, secreted proteins associated with immune processes, including, complement system proteins, soluble serum proteins, and tumor necrosis factors. MHC genes are regulated by cytokines such as IFNα/β and IFNγ, which can increase the expression of classes I and II, respectively. In addition, corticosteroids can decrease the expression levels of MHC class II genes, whereas MHC class I gene expression can be downregulated by certain viruses.[224]

Certain MHC alleles have been associated with a statistically significant increase in the incidence of autoimmune diseases (see Table 40-21 for examples). Such diseases encompass many conditions that affect the joints, endocrine glands, and skin, including rheumatoid arthritis, Graves disease, psoriasis, and a number of others listed in Table 40-21. Although these diseases occur more frequently among persons who express a particular MHC/HLA, no HLA allele is associated with disease in 100% of the cases. Therefore, MHC/HLA is likely to be only one of the contributing factors involved in disease development.

Class I and class II MHC molecules are very similar in terms of molecular structure. Both MHC class I and class II molecules possess four immunoglobulin domains, and a peptide binding groove that is large enough to accommodate small antigenic peptides (Fig. 7-7). Each class I MHC molecule (HLA-A, HLA-B, and HLA-C) is noncovalently linked to a nonpolymorphic protein, β_2-microglobulin, and has a conserved region for binding a TCR coreceptor, CD8. Class II MHC molecules (HLA-DR, HLA-DP, HLA-DQ) are composed of both an α-chain and a β-chain. These molecules are held together by noncovalent interactions. CD4 (also a TCR coreceptor) is able to bind a conserved region of the MHC class II molecule.

The binding of CD4 or CD8 to their respective MHC molecules promotes interactions between antigen-presenting cells and T cells. The peptide-binding groove of MHC class I and class II facilitates the attachment of short (8-18) amino acid chains derived from the antigen. Most MHC diversity exists in the peptide-binding groove. Despite the presence of hundreds of MHC class I and class II alleles in humans, an individual possesses only one allele from each parent for each class I gene (HLA-A, HLA-B, and HLA-C) and class II gene (HLA-DR, HLA-DP, and HLA-DQ). Therefore, only a limited repertoire of molecules encoded by these genes exists to present a multitude of antigens to T cells. Unlike the very specific antigen recognition systems of the BCR and TCR, "promiscuous binding" allows for each MHC molecule to present multiple peptides.[201]

There are two major antigen-processing pathways: the endogenous (cytosolic) pathway and the exogenous (endocytic) pathway. The endogenous pathway generally presents antigens from cytosolic sources, whereas the exogenous pathway presents antigens from the extracellular environment (Fig. 7-8). The separation of antigens by source allows for different classes of T cells to recognize antigens from different compartments. In this way, different classes of T cells can respond to both extracellular and intracellular invaders, resulting in a more effectively targeted cellular immune response.

MHC class I molecules are capable of binding constituents of proteins that have been synthesized in the cellular cytoplasm. In theory, any protein (self, viral, bacterial, tumor, etc.) that was generated in cytoplasm of a cell could be expressed on an MHC class I molecule. In this pathway, endogenous antigen (e.g., protein synthesized by a virus replicating within a cell) is broken down in the cytoplasm by a degradation "machine" known as the proteasome. The digested cytosolic protein constituents are then transported into the rough endoplasmic reticulum by the *transporter associated with antigen processing (TAP)*. The class I MHC α-chain is appropriately folded and complexed with β_2-microglobulin through interactions mediated by chaperone proteins. The MHC class I presentation complex is then loaded with peptide and moves from the rough endoplasmic reticulum through the Golgi apparatus to the plasma membrane. If the protein fragment is distinguished as nonself, the peptide/MHC complex present on the surface of the cell is recognized by cytotoxic CD8+ T cells. Once activated through their TCR, CTLs will destroy the cell presenting foreign antigen.[158]

MHC class II molecules can bind fragments of proteins that have been phagocytized, pinocytosed or endocytosed from the extracellular environment (i.e., extracellular antigens). Hypothetically, any protein that was synthesized elsewhere in the body and was taken up by professional antigen-presenting cells could be expressed on an MHC class II complex. Following internalization into the cell, foreign proteins move into intracellular vesicles known as endosomes or phagosomes, which may fuse with lysosomes. The proteins are then broken down by proteolytic enzymes to produce peptide fragments. Antigen-presenting cells synthesize MHC class II

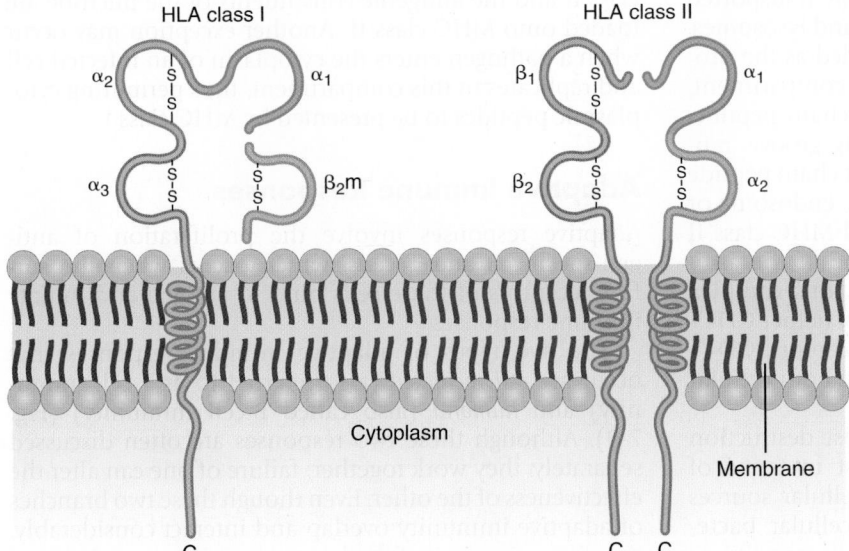

Figure 7-7

Schematic comparison of the highly homologous heterodimeric structures of HLA class I and class II molecules. The peptide-binding cleft of each molecule is formed by the α_1 and α_2 domains in the case of class I, whereas the α_1 and β_1 domains form this structure in class II molecules. S = disulfide bonds. (Reprinted from Goldman: *Goldman's Cecil Medicine*, ed 24, 2011.

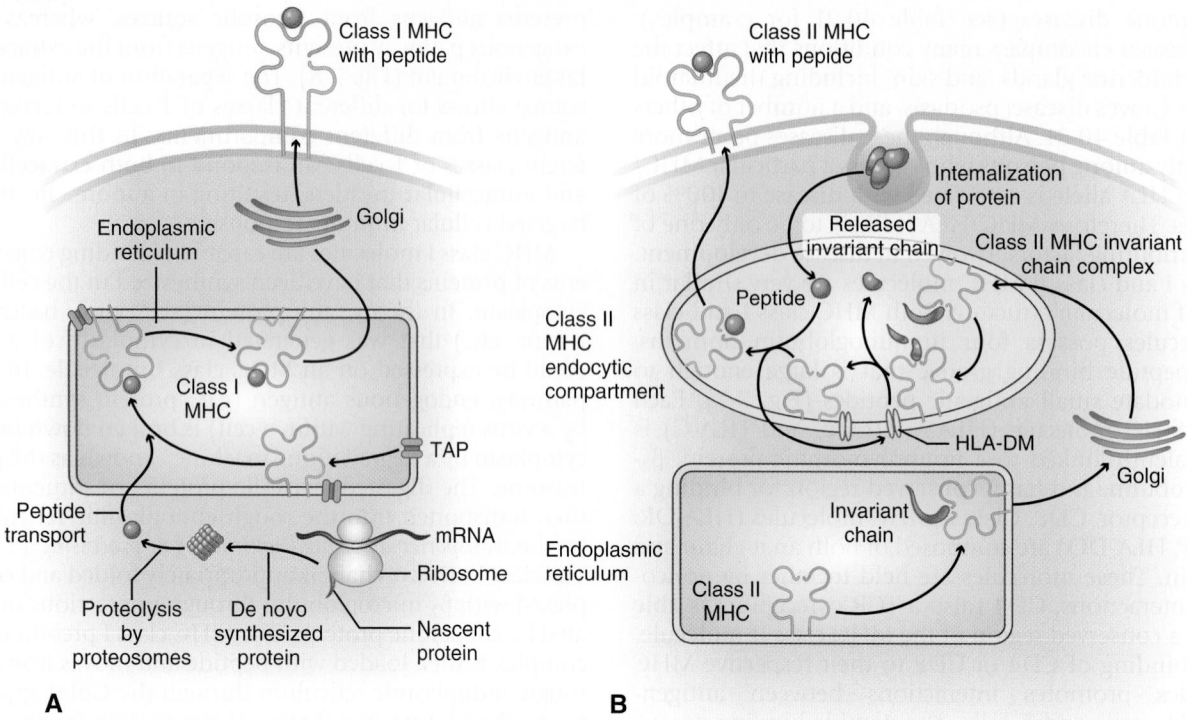

Figure 7-8

Intracellular pathways of antigen presentation. A, Foreign peptides that bind to major histocompatibility complex (MHC) class I are predominantly derived from cytoplasmic proteins synthesized de novo within the cell. Viral proteins entering cells after fusion of an enveloped virus with the cell membrane may also enter this pathway. Dendritic cells are particularly efficient at taking up proteins for the MHC class I pathway by micropinocytosis or macropinocytosis. These cells can also transfer proteins taken up as part of necrotic or apoptotic debris into the MHC class I pathway, a process known as cross-presentation. Cytoplasmic proteins are degraded by proteasomes into peptides, which enter into the endoplasmic reticulum via the transporter associated with antigen processing (TAP) system. Peptide binding by de novo synthesized MHC class I occurs within the endoplasmic reticulum. **B,** Foreign peptides that bind to MHC class II are mainly derived from internalization of proteins found in the extracellular space or that are components of cell membrane. The invariant chain binds to recently synthesized MHC class II and prevents peptide binding until a specialized cellular compartment for MHC class II peptide loading is reached. In this compartment, the invariant chain is proteolytically cleaved and released, and peptides derived from internalized proteins may now bind to MHC class II. The HLA-DM molecule facilitates the loading of peptide within this compartment. In dendritic cells, proteins that enter into the MHC class II antigen presentation pathway can be transferred to the MHC class I pathway by cross-presentation. (From Remington: Infectious Diseases of the Fetus and Newborn, 7th ed.)

molecules in the endoplasmic reticulum. Each newly generated class II molecule carries an attached protein called the invariant chain. The complexes are transported through the Golgi complex to endosomes and lysosomes. The invariant chain is progressively degraded as the proteolytic activity increases in each successive compartment, ultimately leaving only class II invariant chain peptide, which binds tightly to the peptide-binding groove, rendering it inaccessible. After class II invariant chain peptide is removed, an exogenous peptide from the endosome or lysosome is added and the peptide-loaded MHC class II molecule moves to the plasma membrane. If the antigenic peptide is distinguished as nonself, this complex on the cellular surface can be recognized by helper CD4+ T cells. Once activated through antigen receptors, CD4+ T cells will produce cytokines that regulate both cellular and humoral immunity.[158]

Certain pathogens have evolved to resist destruction by phagocytes. Therefore, exceptions exist in terms of the separation of extracellular and intracellular sources of antigen. For example, forms of intracellular bacteria can survive and reproduce in the acidic conditions generated in the intracellular phagocytic vesicles (e.g.,

phagolysosome). In this case, pathogens are present in a compartment that is used as the source of antigen for MHC class II and the antigenic constituents of the microbe are loaded onto MHC class II. Another exception may occur when a pathogen enters the cytoplasm of an infected cell and replicates in this compartment, thus permitting cytoplasmic peptides to be presented by MHC class I.

Adaptive Immune Responses

Adaptive responses involve the proliferation of antigen-specific B and T cells, which occurs when the surface receptors of these cells bind to antigen and initiate immune responses.

The two types of adaptive immune responses that occur are *cell mediated* (also referred to as T-cell immunity) and *humoral* (also called B-cell immunity) (Fig. 7-9). Although these two responses are often discussed separately, they work together; failure of one can alter the effectiveness of the other. Even though these two branches of adaptive immunity overlap and interact considerably, the distinction is useful when attempting to understand how the immune system is activated (see Fig 7-8).

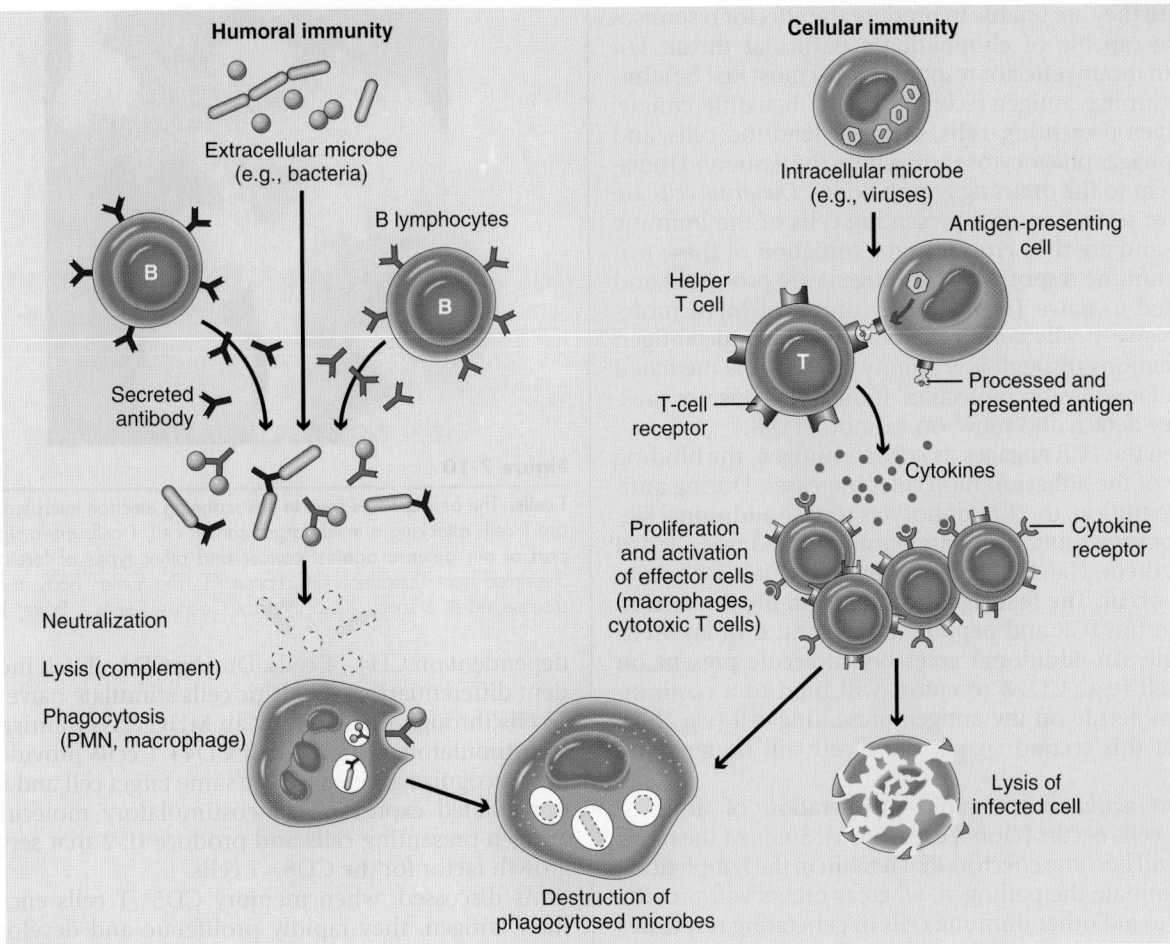

Figure 7-9

Humoral and cell-mediated immunity. Different types of lymphocytes detect distinct types of antigens. B cells recognize soluble or cell-surface antigens and differentiate into antibody-producing cells. Effector functions of B lymphocytes include neutralization of the microbe, complement activation, and phagocytosis. T cells recognize processed antigens that are displayed in the context of MHC molecules on the surfaces of antigen-presenting cells. Helper T cells secrete cytokines that elicit various mechanisms of immunity and inflammation. Cytotoxic T cells kill infected cells expressing processed microbial antigen. (Reprinted from Kumar V: *Robbins and Cotran: pathologic basis of disease*, ed 8, Philadelphia, 2009, WB Saunders.)

Cell-Mediated Immunity

Cell-mediated immunity is the arm of the adaptive immune response that protects the host against infection by intracellular pathogens. The destruction of microbes that are able to survive in the cytoplasm or phagocytic vesicles of infected cells is the principal function of T cells. Cell-mediated immune responses can sometimes be harmful to the host, as they are responsible for the rejection of transplanted tissue and certain autoimmune diseases.

T-cell development begins when a progenitor cell from the bone marrow migrates to the thymus gland which is a primary lymphoid organ. Immature T cells enter the cortex of the thymus and mature as they travel toward the medulla via a "web" created by the thymic stroma. While in the thymus, T cells encounter both soluble and membrane-bound components that direct their development. Rearrangement of TCR genes occurs in the thymus, and this determines the antigen specificity of the cells.

After the TCR is expressed, both CD4 and CD8 will be coexpressed to produce double- positive cells. During this stage, positive selection occurs to ensure that the T cell can identify peptides restricted by the MHC of the host.

Negative selection also takes place to delete cells that recognize "self" peptides of the host.

This selection process is a form of *immunological tolerance* in which the immune system is rendered nonreactive to self. Failure of negative selection will lead to autoimmune disease in which T cells recognize and react against "self" antigens presented by "self" MHC. It should be noted that mechanisms of peripheral tolerance also exist to suppress autoreactive lymphocytes that have escaped selection in the central lymphoid organs. Peripheral tolerance may involve regulatory T cells (T_{regs}) (also known as suppressor T cells), which are discussed later in this section.

As thymocytes become more mature, they express or lose different cell surface markers. The double-positive cells that survive selection downregulate the CD4 or CD8 coreceptor and become single-positive cells expressing either CD4 or CD8. Mature naïve T cells exit the thymus and migrate through the peripheral blood to secondary lymphoid organs, such as the lymph nodes and spleen, where they encounter antigens and exert appropriate effector functions.[318]

T cells recirculate through the peripheral lymphoid organs on a constant basis in search of nonself antigens. Although naïve T cells are capable of recognizing foreign antigens, they are unable to produce the effector responses that are capable of eliminating a particular threat. For T cells to mount effector responses, they must first be stimulated through antigen recognition and then differentiate.

Antigen-presenting cells such as dendritic cells and macrophages phagocytose antigens in the tissue and transport them to the draining lymph nodes. *Dendritic cells* are the most potent antigen-presenting cells of the immune system and are thus crucial in the initiation of these primary immune responses. The antigens are processed and presented to naïve T cells in the context of MHC molecules. Naïve T cells sample various MHC/peptide antigen combinations through low affinity interactions mediated by cellular adhesion molecules. If the antigen is not present, they detach and move on to another cell.

When the TCR engages its cognate antigen, the binding affinity of the adhesion molecules increases. During antigen recognition, the T lymphocytes receive additional signals from microbes or innate immune responses elicited against them. Naïve T cells require two signals for activation to occur. The first signal comes from the interaction between the TCR and peptide in the context of an MHC molecule. An additional accessory molecule present on the T cell (e.g., CD28 receptor) will bind to a costimulatory molecule on the antigen-presenting cell (e.g., B7). Without this second signal, the T cell will be rendered anergic.

Upon activation, a rapid proliferation of antigen-specific cells occurs (clonal expansion). Some of the naïve T cells will become effectors that remain in the lymph node and eliminate the pathogen, whereas others will provide signals to aid other immune cells in generating responses against the pathogen (e.g., production of antibodies by B cells). Other effector cells will exit the lymph nodes and migrate to the site of infection to eradicate the threat. Furthermore, some of the T cells that have proliferated in response to antigenic stimulation will become long-lived memory T cells that can persist for months or even years.

When the host is reexposed to an antigen, a secondary immune response is generated in which memory T cells rapidly differentiate into effectors that can respond more rapidly and with heightened immune responses, resulting in pathogen clearance. This phenomenon, known as *immunologic memory*, is the basis for vaccination. Following removal of a pathogen by effector T cells, the antigenic stimulus is eliminated and the immune system returns to its basal state.[1]

Cytotoxic T lymphocytes (CTLs) are effector cells that can kill other cells (Fig. 7-10). These lymphocytes are critical players in immune responses against intracellular threats such as viruses, abnormal/cancer cells, and intracellular bacteria. CTLs recognize and destroy infected cells or "nonself" cells (e.g., rejection of transplanted tissue). CTLs are primarily CD8+ T lymphocytes and thus MHC class I restricted. CTLs play a critical role in controlling viral infections by directly killing virally infected cells and producing cytokines such as IFNγ that inhibit viral replication.

CTLs kill their target cells by inducing programmed cell death (apoptosis). Naïve CD8+ T cells (CTL precursors) differentiate into effector cytotoxic CD8+ T cells by a number of mechanisms that can be either independent or

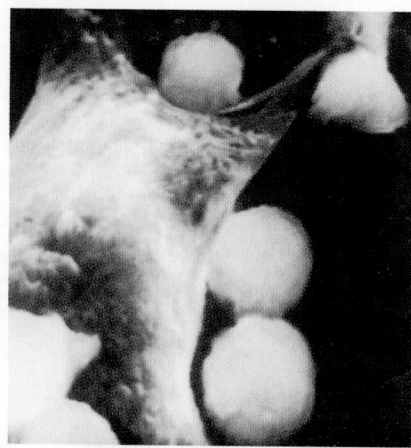

Figure 7-10

T cells. The *blue spheres* seen in this scanning electron microscope view are T cells attacking a much larger cancer cell. T cells are a significant part of our defense against cancer and other types of foreign cells. (Reprinted from Thibodeau GA, Patton KT: *The human body in health & disease*, ed 4, St Louis, 2005, Mosby. Courtesy James T. Barrett.)

dependent on CD4+ T cells. During CD4+ T-cell independent differentiation, dendritic cells stimulate naïve CD8+ T cells through their TCR by an MHC class I/antigen and a costimulatory signal. When CD4+ T cells provide help, they recognize antigen on the same target cell and induce upregulated expression of costimulatory molecules on antigen-presenting cells and produce IL-2 that serve as a growth factor for the CD8+ T cells.

As discussed, when memory CD8+ T cells encounter their antigen, they rapidly proliferate and develop into effector cytotoxic cells. Memory T cells produce their own IL-2 and do not require costimulation (i.e., "signal 2") to proliferate and become effectors. When the TCR is triggered on a CTL, granules containing perforin (forms pores in the membrane of the target cell) and granzyme (proteolytic enzyme that activates the apoptotic program) are released onto the target cell, resulting in its destruction.[250]

CD4+ T lymphocytes are helper T cells that promote immunity against both intracellular and extracellular pathogens. It is important to appreciate that most threats are extracellular at some point (e.g., viruses). CD4+ T cells produce different cytokines that modulate the immune system and help it to mount effective responses against foreign invaders. Some of these functions include (1) helping B cells augment the production of antibodies, (2) activating macrophages and helping them to destroy bacterial pathogens, (3) helping CTLs to proliferate and destroy virally infected cells, (4) helping NK cells kill infected cells, (5) neutrophil recruitment, and (6) downregulation of the adaptive immune response. As discussed later in this chapter, HIV infection results in the gradual decline of CD4+ T cells, rendering the host susceptible to a multitude of infectious agents.[245]

The adaptive immune system also consists of T_{regs} that prevent inappropriate responses against "self" antigens of the host or commensal microorganisms. T_{regs} accomplish this through the generation of inhibitory cytokines such as IL-10 and transforming growth factor (TGF)-β. T_{regs} are characterized as expressing both CD4 and high levels of CD25 (the α-subunit of the IL-2 receptor) and by the

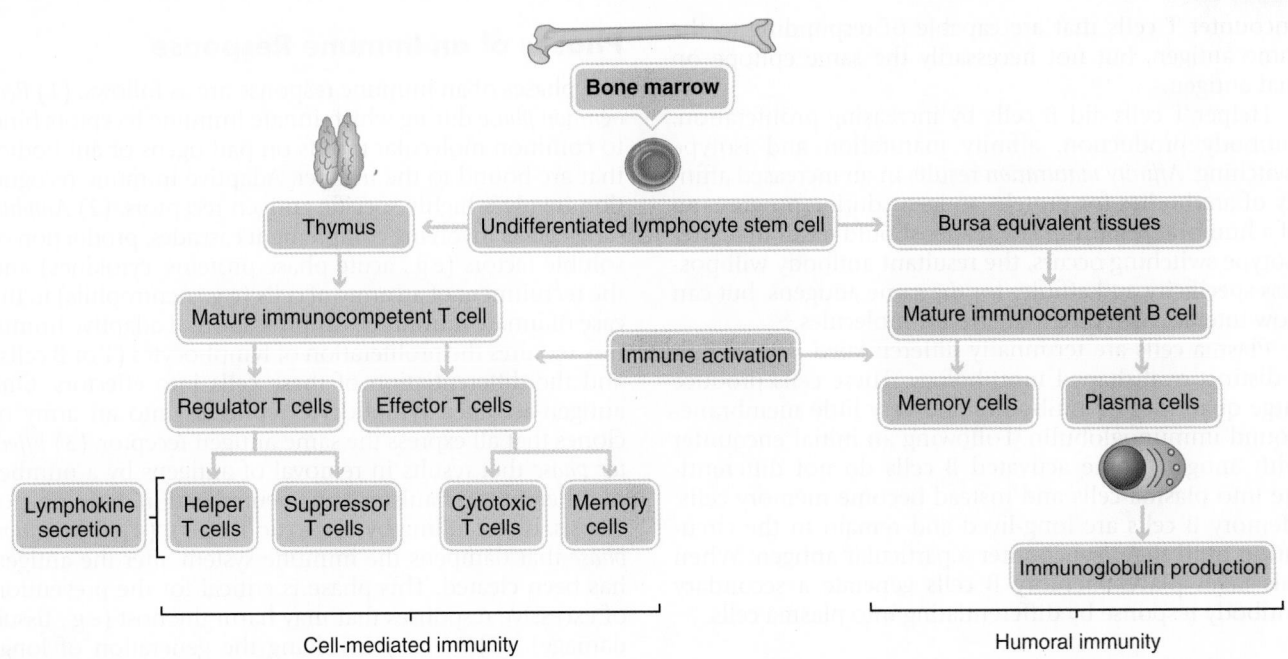

Figure 7-11

The pathway of lymphocyte maturation. Undifferentiated lymphocyte stem cells are derived from the bone marrow. B cells reach maturity within the bone marrow, but T cells must travel to the thymus to complete their development. Activation of either T or B cells by antigens leads to proliferation of immune cells that mediate either cell-mediated immunity or humoral immunity, respectively. (Reprinted from Black JM, Matassarin-Jacobs E, editors: *Medical-surgical nursing: clinical management for continuity of care*, ed 5, Philadelphia, 1997, WB Saunders, p. 597.)

production of IL-10 and TGFβ. T_{regs} are generated when naïve CD4+ T cells are stimulated by dendritic cells that are producing high levels of TGFβ, but none of the other cytokines involved in helper T cell differentiation.[296]

Humoral Immunity

The humoral immune response is mediated by antibodies present in different body fluids or secretions, such as saliva, blood, or vaginal secretions. Antibodies produced by B lymphocytes are very effective against organisms that are free floating in the body that can be easily accessed and neutralized. B cells develop in the bone marrow and migrate to secondary lymphoid organs such as the spleen and lymph nodes. Membrane-bound antibodies on the surface of a B cell bind to immunogens present at these sites and this signals the cell to become activated. The B cell then proliferates and differentiates into plasma cells, which produce soluble antibodies, and memory B cells. All of the daughter cells and antibodies that are generated by plasma cells have the same antigenic specificity as the surface receptor of the parent B cell. The secreted antibody or immunoglobulin binds to antigens and triggers one or more effector functions in order to eliminate a particular threat.

B lymphocytes originate from pluripotent stem cells in the bone marrow (Fig. 7-11). The development of a B cell is independent of antigen and occurs as the result of interactions with bone marrow stromal cells, which produce a microenvironment that is conducive to early growth and differentiation. Once committed to the B lineage, cells progress through a series of developmental stages that are defined by the status of immunoglobulin heavy and light chain genes. If gene rearrangement is successful, an immature B cell that possesses an antigen receptor in the form of a cell membrane-bound IgM that interacts with its environment.[119]

For a B-cell response to be effective, it must establish and maintain a diverse array of B-cell clones that can react to foreign antigens, but not "self" antigens. Immature B cells exit the bone marrow and recirculate throughout circulatory and lymphatic systems in order to sample antigens. Upon migration into secondary lymphoid organs such as the spleen, lymph nodes, bone marrow, and mucosal-associated lymphoid tissues, they receive critical survival signals. At this stage, immature B cells express IgD on the cell surface and become mature B cells. Naïve B cells express BCRs of the IgM and IgD isotypes. The IgM and IgD molecules expressed on the same cell have the same V region and therefore the same antigenic specificity. These cells are now prepared to be activated by antigen.[2]

B cells encounter antigens that crosslink the BCR and activate them. Like naïve T cells, B cells also require a second signal for proliferation. This signal can come from helper T cells or from innate immune components such as complement proteins. In an antigen-dependent fashion, activated B cells divide, differentiate, and begin producing antibodies in secreted rather than membrane-bound form. IgM is the first isotype that is made. Activated B cells migrate toward a compartment where helper T cells are localized. In the spleen, T and B cells can encounter one another near the blood vessels (central arteriole) that are centered in the white pulp. Activated B and T lymphocytes form germinal centers in these areas.

The interaction between B cells and T cells can also occur in other secondary lymphoid tissues, such as the lymph nodes. B cells enter a lymph node either from the lymphatic vessels or from the bloodstream by high endothelial venules. While in the lymph node, B cells encounter T cells that are capable of responding to the same antigen, but not necessarily the same epitope on that antigen.

Helper T cells aid B cells by increasing proliferation, antibody production, affinity maturation and isotype switching. *Affinity maturation* results in an increased affinity of antibodies for protein antigens during progression of a humoral response. The reader should recall that after isotype switching occurs, the resultant antibody will possess specificity and affinity for the same antigens, but can now interact with different effector molecules.[32]

Plasma cells are terminally differentiated B cells with a distinct oval-shaped morphology. These cells produce large quantities of antibodies and very little membrane-bound immunoglobulin. Following an initial encounter with antigen, some activated B cells do not differentiate into plasma cells and instead become memory cells. Memory B cells are long-lived and remain in the circulation until they reencounter a particular antigen. When this takes place, memory B cells generate a secondary antibody response by differentiating into plasma cells.

SUMMARY OF THE IMMUNE SYSTEM

The immune system has evolved to protect multicellular organisms from a vast array of threats. Immunology is the study of how the immune system works and the consequences of its dysfunction. Through past and present research on various immune response mechanisms, ways in which the immune system can be manipulated to benefit the host are being discovered. The principal function of the immune system is to eliminate infectious agents and abnormal "self" components (e.g., cancer cells) without attacking the body's own tissues. The immune system must maintain a state of balance such that when an external or internal threat is encountered, an appropriate response is generated to control the invader, and then the system returns to equilibrium. This encounter with a particular insult educates the immune system to produce memory so that upon reencountering a foreign invader, it reacts more rapidly and with a stronger response.

Most pathogens are encountered after they are inhaled or ingested. Antigens entering the body through mucosal surfaces activate cells in the mucosa-associated lymphoid tissues, including the tonsils, adenoids, and Peyer patches.[74]

Keeping in mind that innate immunity and adaptive immunity function in concert (see Fig 7-1), and that within the adaptive immune system humoral immunity and cellular immunity are also working simultaneously, a variety of immune responses can occur when a pathogen attempts to invade the body. The first line of defense consists of exterior barriers that prevent microbial colonization and host invasion. If the pathogen manages to cross these barriers, the innate immune system is equipped to detect it through a limited repertoire of molecules that recognize motifs which are common to many different pathogens. If innate immunity fails to eliminate the pathogen, the adaptive immune response provides a comprehensive third line of defense to clear the threat and prevent reinvention or recurrence of illness.

Phases of an Immune Response

The phases of an immune response are as follows: (1) *Recognition phase* during which innate immune receptors bind to common molecular motifs on pathogens or antibodies that are bound to the invader. Adaptive immune recognition involves highly specific antigen receptors. (2) *Amplification phase* involving complement cascades, production of soluble factors (e.g., acute phase proteins, cytokines) and the recruitment of an army of cells (e.g., neutrophils) in the case of innate immunity. Amplification of adaptive immunity requires the proliferation of lymphocytes (T or B cells) and the differentiation of these cells into effectors. One antigen-activated lymphocyte replicates into an army of clones that all express the same antigen receptor. (3) *Effector phase* that results in removal of antigens by a number of different mechanisms (e.g., neutralization, lysis, phagocytosis, direct killing by cytotoxic T cells). (4) *Termination phase* that dampens the immune system after the antigen has been cleared. This phase is critical for the prevention of excessive responses that may harm the host (e.g., tissue damage). (5) *Memory* involving the generation of long-lived T and B lymphocytes. These types of cells have a lower threshold for activation and will react more quickly and in an amplified fashion. It should be appreciated that although memory is maintained by adaptive immunity, it functionally involves both innate and adaptive responses.

Dysfunction of the immune system can contribute to a variety of diseases. For example, two general types of genetic alterations could lead to immunologic abnormalities: mutations that inactivate the receptors or signaling molecules involved in innate immune recognition and mutations that render them active all of the time. The first type of mutation would be expected to result in various types of immunodeficiencies. The second type of mutation would trigger aberrant immune responses and contribute to a variety of conditions with inflammatory components (e.g., asthma, allergy, arthritis, autoimmune diseases).[191]

FACTORS AFFECTING IMMUNITY

In addition to the effects of aging, other factors can affect the immune system. These factors may include nutrition; environmental pollution and exposure to chemicals that influence the host defense; prior or ongoing trauma or illnesses; medications; splenectomy (removal of the spleen); influences of the enteric, endocrine, and neurochemical systems; stress; and psychosocial-spiritual well-being and socioeconomic status.

Box 7-2 lists these factors, as well as clinical conditions that contribute to an immunocompromised state. Sleep deprivation also has important effects, similar to stress, on the immune system by reducing cellular immunity.[18,239] Some factors, such as the iatrogenically introduced interventions listed and sexual practices, do not alter the immune system directly but increase a person's exposure to pathogens.

New information is being discovered about the sensory functions of the intestine and how neural, hormonal, and immune signals interact. Representatives of all the major categories of immune cells are found in the gut or can be rapidly recruited from the circulation in response to

FACTORS AFFECTING IMMUNITY

Factors That Alter the Immune System

- Aging
- Sex and hormonal influences
- Nutrition/malnutrition
- Environmental pollution
- Exposure to toxic chemicals
- Trauma
- Burns
- Sleep disturbance
- Presence of concurrent illnesses and diseases:
  - Malignancy
  - Diabetes mellitus
  - Chronic renal failure
  - HIV infection
- Medications, immunosuppressive drugs
- Hospitalization, surgery, general anesthesia
- Splenectomy
- Stress, psychospiritual well-being, socioeconomic status

Factors That Increase Exposure to Pathogens

- Iatrogenic
  - Urinary catheters
  - Nasogastric tubes
  - Endotracheal tubes
  - Chest tubes
  - Peripherally inserted central catheter (PICC line)
  - Intracranial pressure monitor
  - External fixation devices
  - Implanted prostheses
- Sexual practices

an inflammatory stimulus. The gut immune system has 70% to 80% of the body's immune cells, and the protective blocking action of the secretory response in the gut is crucial to the integrity of the GI tract immune function and host defense.[21]

Nutritional status can have a profound effect on immune function. Nutrients have fundamental and regulatory influences on the immune response of the GI tract and, therefore, on host defense. Reduction of normal bacteria in the gut after antibiotic treatment or in the presence of infection may interfere with the nutrients available for immune function in the GI tract.

Severe deficits in calories, protein intake, or vitamins such as vitamin A or vitamin E can lead to deficiencies in T-cell function and numbers. Deficient zinc intake can profoundly depress both T- and B-cell function. Zinc is required as a cofactor for at least 70 different enzymes, some of which are found in lymphocytes and are necessary for their function.

Secondary zinc deficiencies may be associated with malabsorption syndrome, chronic renal disease, chronic diarrhea, or burns or severe psoriasis (loss of zinc through the skin). Dietary changes may alter aspects of immunity, although research in this area is ongoing. Additionally, morbid obesity may alter the immune system by creating a vulnerability to certain diseases, including cancer.

Some *medications* (e.g., cancer chemotherapeutic agents) profoundly suppress blood cell formation in the bone marrow. Other drugs (e.g., analgesics, antithyroid

medications, antiseizure, antihistamines, antimicrobial agents, and tranquilizers) induce immunologic responses that destroy mature granulocytes.

Many drugs also affect B- and T-cell function, especially against antigens that require the interaction of helper T cells and B cells for antibody production. These complications have been observed since the advent of potent immunosuppressive (e.g., corticosteroids) and chemotherapeutic drugs as treatment of people with autoimmune diseases, transplants, or cancer. Depression of B- and T-cell formation is manifested as a progressive increase in infections with opportunistic microorganisms (e.g., *Pneumocystis carinii*, cytomegalovirus (CMV), *Candida albicans*, and other fungi).

Surgery and *anesthesia* can also suppress both T- and B-cell function for up to 1 month postoperatively.[183] Because of the invasive nature of any surgical procedure and because defects in immunity have been described in most major illnesses, it is logical to assume that the majority of hospitalized surgical clients are immunocompromised to some degree.

Surgery to remove the spleen results in a depressed humoral response against encapsulated bacteria, especially *Streptococcus pneumoniae*, *Haemophilus influenzae*, *Staphylococcus aureus*, the group A streptococci, and *Neisseria meningitidis* (see Chapter 8).

Burns cause increased susceptibility to severe bacterial infections as a result of decreased external defenses (intact skin), neutrophil function, decreased complement levels, decreased cell-mediated immunity, and decreased primary humoral responses. Blood serum from clients with burns also contains nonspecific immunosuppressive factors that suppress all immune responses, regardless of the antigen involved.

The relationship between *stress, psychosocial-spiritual well-being*, and *socioeconomic status* and susceptibility to disease through depressed immune function has become an area of intense research interest. In the past, there were anecdotal reports of increased incidence of infection, diseases, and malignancy associated with periods of both intense and relatively minor stress (see Table 2-6).

EXERCISE IMMUNOLOGY

The effect of physical activity and exercise (aerobic, endurance, and resistance) on the immune and neuroimmune systems has been a growing area of research interest.[298] A brief summary of the results is presented here, but a more detailed accounting of exercise and the immune system and future direction for studies is available.[208,215,298]

Depending on the intensity, activity or exercise can enhance or suppress immune function. In essence, the immune system is enhanced during moderate exercise. Moreover, regular, moderate physical activity can prevent the neuroendocrine and detrimental immunologic effects of stress.[93]

In contrast to the beneficial effects of moderate exercise on the immune system, strenuous or intense exercise or long-duration exercise such as marathon running is followed by impairment of the immune system. Intense exercise can suppress the concentration of lymphocytes, suppress NK cell activity, and leave the host open to microbial agents, especially viruses that can invade during this open window of opportunity, and may lead to infections.

Extreme and long-duration strenuous exercise appears to lead to deleterious oxidation of cellular macromolecules. The oxidation of DNA is important because the oxidative modifications of DNA bases are mutagenic and have been implicated in a variety of diseases, including aging and cancer.[226]

Effect on Neutrophils and Macrophages

Exercise triggers a rise in blood levels of PMNs and stimulates phagocytic activity of neutrophils and macrophages. The exercise-evoked increase in the PMN count is greater if the exercise has an eccentric component, such as downhill running. If the exercise goes beyond 30 minutes, a second, or delayed, rise in PMNs occurs over the next 2 to 4 hours while the exerciser is at rest.

This delayed rise in PMNs is probably the result of cortisol, which spurs release of PMNs from the bone marrow and hinders the exit of PMNs from the bloodstream.[189] After brief, gentle exercise, the PMN count soon returns to baseline, but after prolonged, strenuous exercise, this return to normal may take 24 hours or longer.[86]

In many instances, exercise enhances macrophage function and can increase antitumor activity in mice, but many questions still remain regarding the mechanism(s) by which short- or long-term exercise affects macrophage function.[312]

Effect on Natural Killer Cells

Most researchers agree that the number of NK cells and the function or activity of these cells in the blood increase during and immediately after exercise of various types, duration, and intensity.[215,236,268] Promoting the natural cytotoxicity of NK cells, referred to as *NK enhancement*, is temporary and seems to be the result of a surge in epinephrine levels and from cytokines released during exercise.[299] NK enhancement by exercise occurs in everyone regardless of sex, age, or level of fitness training; however, once a person is accustomed to a given exercise level, the NK enhancement falls off, suggesting it is a response not to exercise per se, but to physiologic stress.

After intense exercise of long duration the concentration of NK cells and NK cytolytic activity declines below preexercise values. Maximal reduction in NK cell concentrations and lower NK cell activity occurs 2 to 4 hours after exercise.[215] Although this depression in NK cell count seems too brief to have major practical importance for health, there may be a cumulative adverse effect in athletes who induce these changes several times per week.[265]

Effect on Inflammatory Response

Regular moderate exercise as well as resistance training and long-lasting endurance exercise is known to induce proinflammatory cytokines.[11,97,283,298] Brisk exercise (even brief, heavy exertion such as maximal bicycle ergometry for 30 or 60 seconds) increases the white blood cell count in proportion to the effort.[116,206] This exercise-induced increase in white blood cells (including lymphocytes and NK cells) is largely the result of the mechanical effects of an increased cardiac output and the physiologic effects of a surge in serum epinephrine concentration. Lymphocytes may be recruited to the circulation from other tissue pools during exercise (e.g., the spleen, lymph nodes, or GI tract). The number of cells that enter the circulation is determined by the intensity of the stimulus.[215]

The number of lymphocytes in circulation increases during exercise but decreases below the normal levels for several hours after intense exercise. Decreased numbers of lymphocytes are associated with decreased lymphocyte responsiveness and antibody response to several antigens after intense exercise.[142]

Strenuous or high-intensity exercise, defined as exercising at a minimum of 80% of maximal oxygen consumption (VO_2max), can suppress immune function and damage enough tissue to evoke the *acute-phase response* in human beings.[214,317] This complex cascade of reactions can modulate immune defense by activating complement and spurring the release of TNF, INFs, ILs, and other cytokines.

Plasma IL-6 increases in an exponential fashion with exercise (without muscle damage) and is related to exercise intensity, duration, the mass of muscle recruited, and endurance capacity. The antiinflammatory effects of IL-6 are demonstrated by the fact that IL-6 stimulates the production of antiinflammatory cytokines IL-1ra and IL-10.[219] The possibility exists that, with regular exercise, antiinflammatory effects of an acute bout of exercise will protect against chronic systemic low-grade inflammation. This long-term effect of exercise may be ascribed to the antiinflammatory response elicited by a short-term bout of exercise, which is partly mediated by muscle-derived IL-6.[219]

Exercise, Aging, and Apoptosis

Aging is associated with a decline in the normal functioning of the immune system that is described by the term *immunosenescence*. Habitual exercise is capable of regulating the immune system and delaying the onset of immunosenescence.[263] Regular exercise is associated with enhanced responses to vaccinations, lower numbers of exhausted/senescent T cells, increased T-cell proliferative capacity, lower circulatory levels of inflammatory cytokines, increased neutrophil phagocytic activity, lowered inflammatory response to bacterial challenge, greater NK cell cytotoxic activity, and longer leukocyte telomere lengths in aging humans.[27,84,151,270]

The role of apoptosis, or programmed cell death, in exercise is the focus of much research in the area of exercise science. Some exercise conditions have been shown to delay apoptosis.[196] Accelerated apoptosis has been documented to occur in a variety of disease states, such as AIDS and Alzheimer disease, and in the aging heart. In striking contrast, failure to activate this genetically regulated cell death may result in cancer and certain viral infections. It is surmised that exercise may delay apoptosis and separately, exercise-induced apoptosis is a normal regulatory process that removes certain damaged cells without a pronounced inflammatory response, thereby ensuring optimal body function.[196,203,217,222]

Exercise Immunology

Physical therapists use exercise in the treatment of people of all ages with a variety of clinical problems, thereby influencing immune function. Exercise as a means of preventing illness and attaining a healthy lifestyle and as an intervention tool in immunodeficiency states is becoming a larger part of preventive services. Research in the area of exercise immunology is growing. Keeping abreast of research results is the first step to examining the clinical implications in this area.[298]

Aged adults constitute a growing and important consumer group of therapy services. Because immune function declines with advancing age, it is important that we understand the effects of exercise on immune function. Very few absolute guidelines have been developed; it seems intense or strenuous exercise may be detrimental to the immune system, whereas a lifetime of moderate exercise and physical activity enhances immune function. Further research is needed to clarify or modify this guideline.

It takes 6 to 24 hours for the immune system to recover from the acute effects of severe exercise. Each individual client must be evaluated after exercise to determine the perceived intensity of the exercise or intervention session. For example, in the deconditioned older adult with compromised cardiopulmonary function, reduced oxygen transport, and impaired mobility, ambulating from the bed to the bathroom may be perceived by their body as strenuous exercise.

Although intense exercise causes suppression of immune parameters in young subjects, data from aged animals[142,143] and human beings[144] show that intense exercise has no detrimental effect on immune function or rate of infections in older adults. Thus relatively intense exercise programs may be prescribed that could maximize cardiopulmonary and musculoskeletal function without impairing immune function in frail elderly people.[298]

Nevertheless, intense exercise during an infectious episode should be avoided. For anyone, especially competitive athletes, who wonders whether to exercise in the presence of an acute viral or bacterial infection (e.g., when manifesting constitutional symptoms), a "neck check" should be conducted. If the symptoms are located above the neck, such as a stuffy or runny nose, sneezing, or a scratchy throat, exercise should be performed cautiously through the scheduled workout at half speed. If after 10 minutes the symptoms are alleviated, the workout can be finished with the usual amount of frequency, intensity, and duration.

If instead the symptoms are worse and the head is pounding or throbbing with every footstep, the exercise program should be stopped and the person should rest. If a fever or symptoms below the neck are evident, such as aching muscles, a hacking cough, diarrhea, or vomiting, exercise should not be initiated.[86] (See the specific exercise guidelines for the person with HIV in Special Implications 7-3 this chapter.)

IMMUNODEFICIENCY DISEASES

In immunodeficiency, the immune response is absent or depressed as a result of a primary or secondary disorder. Primary immunodeficiency reflects a defect involving T cells, B cells, or lymphoid tissues. Secondary immunodeficiency results from an underlying disease or factor that depresses or blocks the immune response.

Primary Immunodeficiency

The recognition of impaired immunity in children 50 years ago has resulted in a tremendous increase in knowledge of the functions of the immune system. More than 95 inherited immunodeficiency disorders have now been identified. Genetically determined immunodeficiency can cause increased susceptibility to infection, autoimmunity, and increased risk of cancer (Fig. 7-12).

The defects may affect one or more components of the immune system, including T cells, B cells, NK cells, phagocytic cells, and complement proteins. No further discussion of these conditions is included in this book because the therapist rarely encounters these congenital conditions. A review of the pathophysiology of primary immunodeficiency is available.[35]

Secondary Immunodeficiency

Secondary immunodeficiency disorders such as leukemia and Hodgkin disease follow and result from an earlier disease or event. Multiple, diverse, and nonspecific defects in the immune defenses occur in viral and other infections and also in malnutrition, alcoholism, aging, autoimmune disease, diabetes mellitus, cancer, chronic disease, steroid therapy, cancer chemotherapy, and radiation. More specific causes such as HIV disease also contribute to secondary immunodeficiency.

Iatrogenic Immunodeficiency

Immunodeficiency induced by immunosuppressive drugs, radiation therapy, or splenectomy is referred to as *iatrogenic immunodeficiency*. Immunosuppressive drugs fall into several categories, including cytotoxic drugs, corticosteroids, cyclosporine, and antilymphocyte serum or antithymocyte globulin.

Cytotoxic drugs kill immunocompetent cells while they are replicating, but because most cytotoxic drugs are not selective, all rapidly dividing cells are affected. Not only are lymphocytes and phagocytes eliminated, but these drugs also interfere with lymphocyte synthesis and release of immunoglobulins and cytokines.

Other effects of this nonselectivity of cytotoxic drugs are discussed in Chapter 5 and may include bone marrow suppression with neutropenia, anemia, and cytopenia; gonadal suppression with sterility; alopecia; hemorrhagic cystitis; and vomiting, nausea, and stomatitis. The risk of lymphoproliferative malignancy is also increased.

Corticosteroids are used to treat immune-mediated disorders because of their potent antiinflammatory and immunosuppressive effects. Corticosteroids stabilize the vascular membrane, blocking tissue infiltration by

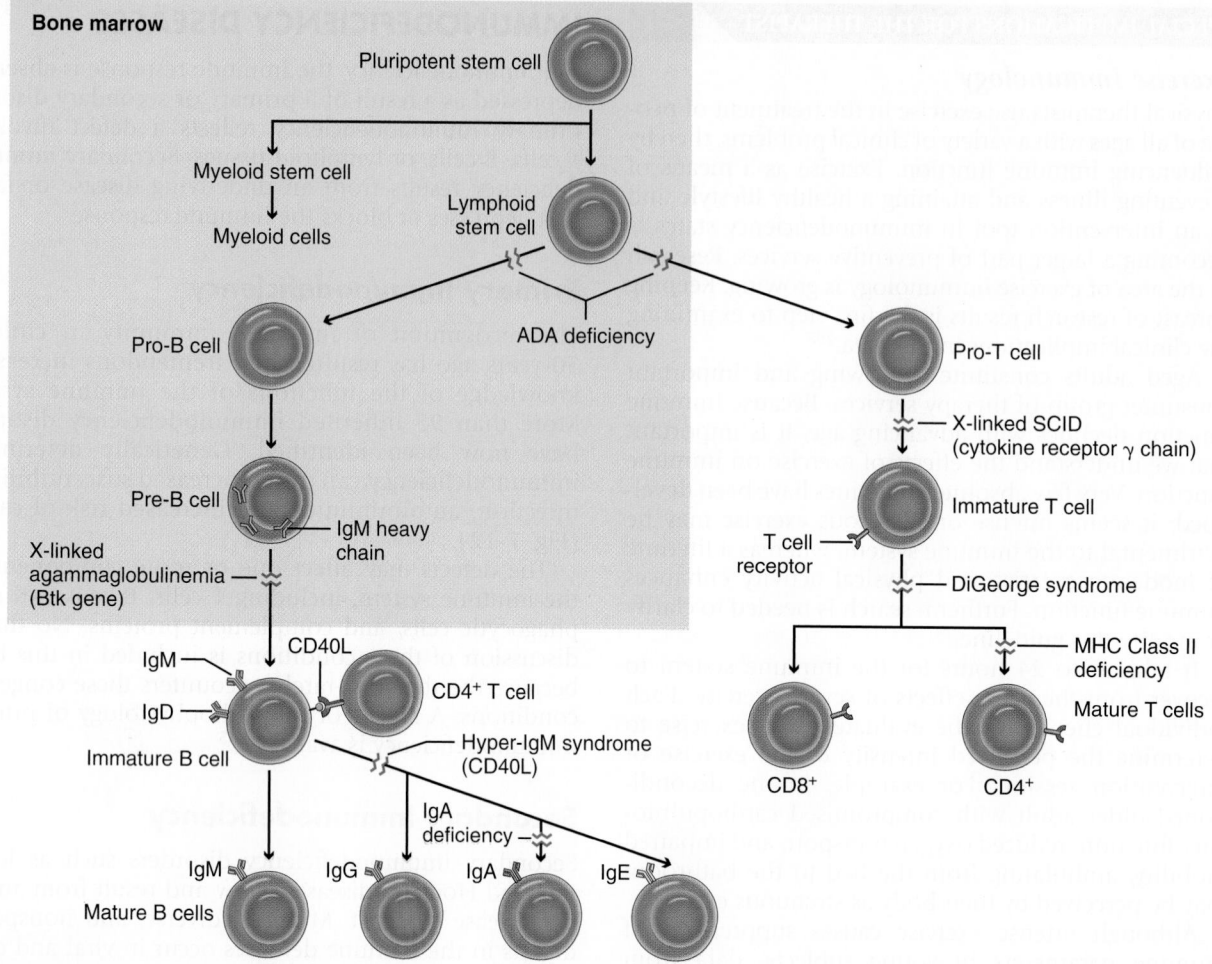

Figure 7-12

Scheme of lymphocyte development and sites of block in primary immunodeficiency diseases. The affected genes are indicated in parentheses for some of the disorders. ADA, adenosine deaminase; CD40L, CD40 ligand; SCID, severe combined immunodeficiency. (Reprinted from Kumar V: *Robbins and Cotran: pathologic basis of disease*, ed 8, Philadelphia, 2009, WB Saunders.)

neutrophils and monocytes, thus inhibiting inflammation. They also kidnap T cells in the bone marrow, causing lymphopenia. Corticosteroids also appear to inhibit immunoglobulin synthesis and interfere with the binding of the immunoglobulin to antigen.

Cyclosporine (immunosuppressive drug) selectively suppresses the proliferation and development of helper T cells, resulting in depressed cell-mediated immunity. This drug is used primarily to prevent rejection of organ transplants but is also being investigated for use in several other disorders. *Antilymphocyte serum* or *antithymocyte globulin* is an anti–T-cell antibody that reduces T-cell number and function, thereby suppressing cell-mediated immunity. It has been used effectively to prevent cell-mediated rejection of tissue grafts and transplants (see "Immunosuppressants Under Adverse Drug Reactions" in Chapter 5).

Radiation therapy is cytotoxic to most lymphocytes, inducing profound lymphopenia, which results in immunosuppression. Irradiation of all major lymph node areas, a procedure known as *total nodal irradiation,* is used to treat disorders such as Hodgkin lymphoma. It is being investigated for its effectiveness in severe rheumatoid arthritis and lupus nephritis and the prevention of kidney transplant rejection.

Splenectomy increases a person's susceptibility to infection, especially with pyogenic bacteria such as *S. pneumoniae.* This risk of infection is even greater when the person is very young or has an underlying reticuloendothelial disorder. These people should be observed carefully for any signs of infection (see Box 8-1).

Consequences of Immunodeficiency

People who are immunocompromised from any of the immunodeficiency disorders are at increased risk of developing infection because their impaired immune system does not provide adequate protection against invading microorganisms. Normal mechanical defense mechanisms may be affected (respiratory, GI systems). Body flora that are normally harmless, such as *Candida,* may become pathogenic and a source of infection.

Additional risk factors for people who are already immunocompromised include poor physiologic and psychologic health status, old age, coexistence of other diseases or conditions, invasive procedures (e.g., surgery, invasive lines), and treatments (e.g., chemotherapy, radiation therapy, bone marrow transplantation).

The weakened immune system can cause the person to become susceptible to common everyday infectious agents, such as influenza viruses and *S. aureus*, as well as the more exotic organisms such as *Histoplasma capsulatum* and *Toxoplasma gondii*.

SPECIAL IMPLICATIONS FOR THE THERAPIST   7-2

Infection Control in Immunodeficiency Disorders

Although infection control strategies, such as handwashing, standard precautions, and disinfection, are important for all people treated in the health care system, they are especially critical for individuals whose immune systems are altered by primary immunodeficiency disorders, secondary immunodeficiency disorders, and HIV infection.

It is important that health care providers are aware of altered defense mechanisms, infectious agents, reservoirs, and modes of transmission, and employ infection control strategies to prevent infection in this population (Fig. 7-13).

Pulmonary complications are common among the immunocompromised, accompanied by poor cough reflexes, an inability to cough effectively, and susceptibility to pulmonary and other opportunistic infections. Additionally, these individuals are often debilitated and easily fatigued. Frequent mobilization and body positioning enhance gas exchange and promote comfort while maintaining strength.[70]

Human Immunodeficiency Virus Disease

David M. Kietrys, PT, PhD

Overview

HIV disease is an infection of the immune system. If untreated, it results in progressive and ultimately profound immune suppression. Advanced HIV disease is also known as acquired immune deficiency syndrome (AIDS). AIDS was first recognized in homosexual men in 1981 (the earliest sample of HIV-infected blood dates back to 1959,[129] but computer analysis suggests an emergence date of 1930[177]).

A viral cause of AIDS was identified in 1983. Shortly thereafter, it was labeled HTLV-III, and later renamed HIV. HIV has been since classified into two types: HIV-1 and HIV-2. HIV-1 is the cause of most of the AIDS cases in the United States, whereas HIV-2 is largely confined to west African countries.[17]

AIDS is characterized by progressive destruction of cell-mediated immunity via destruction of T4 lymphocytes (also known as CD4 cells) and changes in humoral immunity. Elements of autoimmunity are also involved because of the central role of the CD4 cell in immune reactions (see "Monocytes" earlier for a discussion of CD4+ cells).

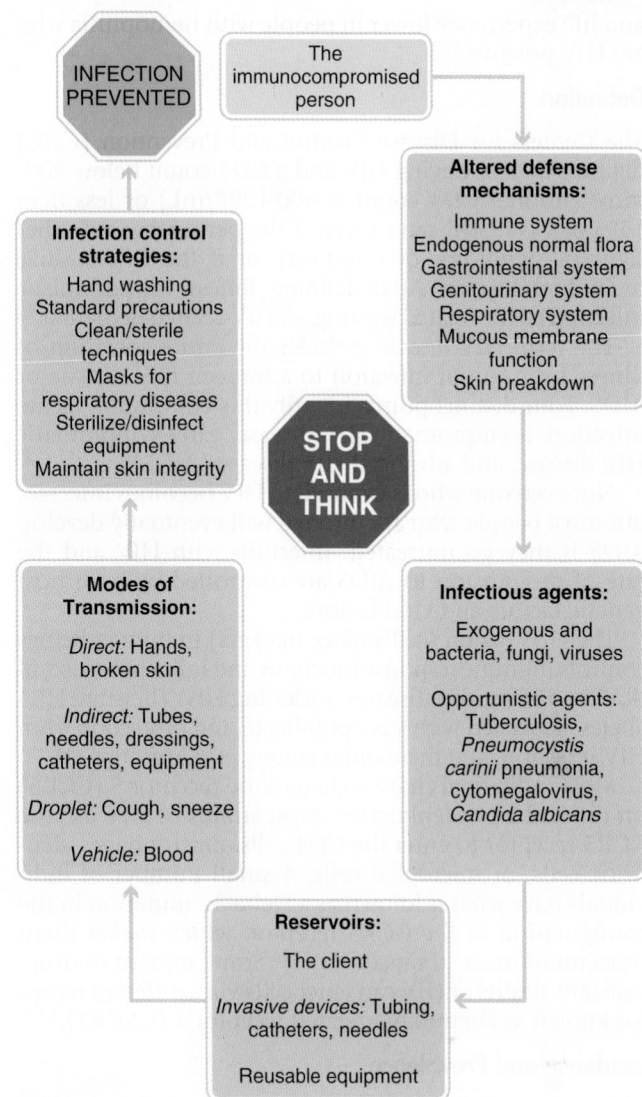

Figure 7-13

Factors affecting the immunocompromised person, leading to the selection of the correct infection control strategies to prevent infectious complications. (Reprinted from Schaffer SD, Garzon LS, Heroux DL, et al: *Pocket guide to infection prevention and safe practice*, St Louis, 1996, Mosby, p. 222.)

The resultant immunodeficiency leaves the affected person susceptible to opportunistic infections, including unusual cancers, tuberculosis, and other abnormalities that characterize this disease. Opportunistic infections are defined as infections that occur or are more severe because of immunosuppression. For example, HIV-positive individuals are nearly 2.5 times more likely than HIV-negative persons to have a recurrence of tuberculosis[275] and 8 to 10 times more likely to develop Hodgkin disease when compared with the general population.[174]

Additionally, approximately 25% of Americans with HIV are thought to be coinfected with the hepatitis C virus (HCV), and an estimated 10% of individuals infected with HIV are coinfected with hepatitis B virus.[49,266] The incidence of coinfection is higher in injection-drug users and in those with hemophilia as a result of blood products used to treat the hemophilia.[14] Mortality rates are higher and life expectancy lower in people with hemophilia who are HIV positive.[225]

Definition

The Centers for Disease Control and Prevention (CDC) defines AIDS as having HIV and a CD4 count below 200/mm[3] (normal CD4 count is 600-1200/mL) or less than 15% of CD4:CD8 ratio (even if the person has no other signs or symptoms of infection), or if the HIV-positive individual has an AIDS-defining illness (opportunistic infection), HIV-related wasting, or HIV-related dementia.[42]

The term *HIV disease* includes the entire spectrum of illness from initial infection to advanced HIV disease or AIDS. Four distinct points identify this continuum: acute infection, asymptomatic HIV disease, early symptomatic HIV disease, and advanced HIV disease (AIDS).

Not everyone who is exposed to HIV becomes infected, but most people who are infected will eventually develop AIDS if they go untreated. Infection with HIV and the rate of progression to AIDS are controlled by both host genetic factors and viral factors.

The HLA region (cell surface markers) in human beings controls immune response functions and influences susceptibility to infectious diseases, including HIV. There are HLA alleles associated with susceptibility to and protection from HIV infection, and these differ among ethnic groups.[244]

Most individuals have a chemokine receptor 5 (CCR5) on the surface of leukocytes. Most strains of HIV use the CCR5 receptor to enter the CD4 cells, macrophages, dendritic cells, or microglial cells. A small number of individuals have what is known as a Delta 32 mutation in the configuration of the CCR5 receptor, which makes them resistant to most strains of HIV.[254] Some mutant or drug-resistant strains of HIV can enter cells via a different receptor known as chemokine-related receptor 4 (CXCR4).[197]

Incidence and Prevalence

Although global new infection rates and global AIDS related deaths are on the decline, AIDS remains an epidemic of vast proportions in many parts of the world, especially sub-Saharan Africa. In 2010, approximately 68% of people with HIV disease, an estimated 5.6 million, resided in sub-Saharan Africa. In Africa, the number of deaths from AIDS has exceeded the estimated 25 million caused by the Black Death in the 14th century.[109,280]

However, AIDS is a global pandemic. Other regions that have been especially hard hit include south and southeast Asia, eastern Europe, central Asia, and North America.[294] Twenty percent (6.6 million) of people with HIV disease are in Asia and the Pacific.[109] In some parts of the world, such as eastern Europe and central Asia, new infections and AIDS-related deaths have been accelerating since 2008.[294]

Of the 33.2 million people worldwide living with HIV/AIDS, 30.7 million are adults (half of whom are women)[50] and 2.5 million are children younger than 15 years. In 2010, there were 2.7 million newly infected individuals worldwide, including 390,000 among children.[294]

In 2010, the CDC estimated that 1.2 million people in the United States were living with HIV infection, and approximately 1 in 5 were unaware of his or her HIV status.[53] The first AIDS cases were reported in the United States in 1981. The number of cases and AIDS-related deaths increased rapidly during the 1980s and early 1990s. As a result of advances in antiretroviral therapy and prevention efforts there have been substantial declines in new cases and AIDS-related deaths since the late 1990s.[50]

In the United States, the greatest impact of the epidemic is among men who have sex with men (MSM) and injection-drug users (IDUs).[109,267,292] In 2010, adult and adolescent transmission of HIV in the United States was attributed to MSM in 61% of cases, IDU in 8% of cases, MSM+IDU in 3% of cases, and heterosexual sex in 28% of cases. Infection rates are higher in racial/ethnic minority groups such as blacks and Hispanics.[41,154] Increases have been observed in the number of cases attributed to heterosexual transmission among minority women and women older than 50 years.[47]

In the United States in 2010, women accounted for 21% of all new HIV/AIDS diagnoses. Women of color are disproportionately affected; 80% of new infections were in women were in blacks or Hispanic/Latinas in 2010.[53] Women are infected most often through the use of shared injection-drug needles and sex with infected men (Fig. 7-14).[292]

Most people diagnosed with AIDS in the United States are 20 to 49 years of age; however, the number of adolescents and young adults (age 13-19 years) with HIV in the United States has been on the rise in recent years.[54] Teens account for 25% of the cases of new sexually transmitted diseases (STDs) reported each year, and AIDS in older adults accounts for 11% of all AIDS cases.[48]

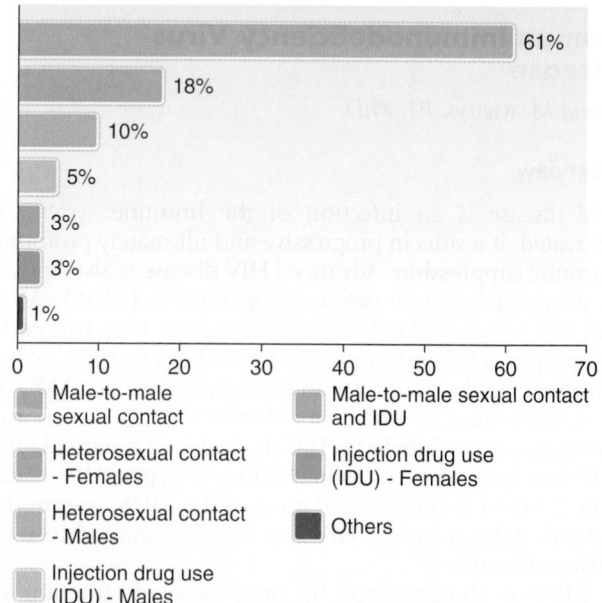

Diagnoses of HIV infection among adults and adolescents, by transmission category, 2010—46 States and 5 U.S. dependent areas, N = 48,079

61%
18%
10%
5%
3%
3%
1%

0   10   20   30   40   50   60   70

■ Male-to-male sexual contact

■ Male-to-male sexual contact and IDU

■ Heterosexual contact - Females

■ Injection drug use (IDU) - Females

■ Heterosexual contact - Males

■ Others

■ Injection drug use (IDU) - Males

Figure 7-14

Proportion of AIDS cases and population by race/ethnicity, reported in 2010 (50 states and Washington, DC). (Reprinted from Centers for Disease Control and Prevention: HIV/AIDS surveillance by race/ethnicity (through 2010). http://www.cdc.gov/hiv/topics/surveillance/resources/slides/race-ethnicity/.

Etiologic Factors, Transmission, and Risk Factors

The cause of AIDS is infection with the HIV retrovirus, most commonly type 1. Transmission of HIV occurs by exchange of body fluids (notably blood and semen) and is associated with high-risk behaviors.[55]

High-risk behaviors include unprotected anal, vaginal, and oral sex, including having six or more sexual partners in the past year, sexual activity with someone known to carry HIV, or IV drug use. HIV is not transmitted by fomites (e.g., coffee cups, drinking fountains, or telephone receivers) or casual household or social contact. Cases of HIV transmission from bone or tendon allograft are extremely rare and are generally preventable via donor screening and testing of allograft material.[200]

As mentioned, IDU also continues to play a key role in the HIV epidemic. In some drug-using communities, HIV seroincidence and seroprevalence among IDUs have declined in recent years.[77] This decline has been attributed to several factors, including needle exchange programs, shifts from injection to noninjection methods of using drugs, and cessation of drug use.[7] However, IDU among young adult heroin users has increased substantially in some areas, an indication that, as with sexual behaviors, changes to less-risky behaviors may be difficult to sustain.[134,292]

Transmission of HIV varies by gender. In 2010, 77% of male HIV infections were related to MSM, 7% were related to IDU, and 12% of the infections resulted from heterosexual sex. In the same year in females, 86% of HIV infections were related to heterosexual sex and 14% resulted from IDU.[55]

A woman is twice as likely as a man to contract HIV infection during vaginal intercourse, and the presence of some STDs greatly increases the likelihood of acquiring or transmitting HIV infection. The rates of gonorrhea and syphilis are higher among women of color, especially between the ages of 15 and 24 years.[46]

In the United States, MSM has been the most common mode of HIV transmission, followed by IDU and heterosexual contact. To avoid social isolation, discrimination, or verbal or physical abuse, many MSM, especially young and minority MSM, do not disclose their sexual orientation.

Young MSM who do not disclose their sexual orientation (nondisclosers) are thought to be at particularly high risk for HIV infection because of low self-esteem, depression, or lack of peer support and prevention services that are available to MSM who are more open about their sexuality (disclosers). Homophobia and stigmatization create additional barriers to effective prevention and treatment, especially in minority communities.

Additionally, one in three nondisclosers reports having recent female sex partners, suggesting that nondisclosing MSM may have an important role in HIV and STD transmission to women.[255] This is especially relevant in black nondisclosing MSM. New HIV diagnoses in black MSM increased by 93% from 2001 to 2006, with an estimated HIV prevalence of 28% in black MSM in 2008.[51,55]

The chief determinant of whether HIV is transmitted during intercourse is the viral load in the infected partner's bloodstream or semen. Viral load refers to the number of viral RNA particles present in the blood and correlates strongly with the stage of disease. To use a train crash analogy, CD4 values represent the distance to the crash, whereas viral load counts represent the speed of the train, that is, how fast the person is declining.[253]

Viral load tests measure the amount of HIV-specific RNA in the bloodstream, which is highest during the period of acute infection or in untreated late stage disease. However, a viral load also exists in untreated individuals and may exist in treated individuals, and thus contagion is a concern across all stages of disease. Viral load is a useful measurement for determining the effectiveness of drug treatment and also directly correlates with the risk of perinatal transmission in pregnant women with HIV.

Transmission is less likely to occur when serum HIV-1 RNA levels are less than 1500 copies/mL (i.e., low viral load).[234] However, in some cases, viral load in semen is higher than in blood, and thus an undetectable viral load in blood is no guarantee that transmission will not occur through contact with semen.[163] Uncircumcised men have a greater risk of contracting HIV through sexual contact than do circumcised men. The thinner epithelial lining of the glans penis may be susceptible to increased trauma during sexual activity, increasing the likelihood of viral transmission.[167] Nearly all transmissions of HIV through transfusion of blood or blood products occurred before testing of the blood supply for HIV antibody and self-referral programs were initiated in 1985. People with hemophilia were especially vulnerable and susceptible to transmission. In 1991, approximately 70% of people with hemophilia had seroconverted to being positive for HIV; however, since 1986 no further HIV transmission has occurred by that mechanism.

Ethnicity is not directly related to increased AIDS risk, but it is associated with other determinants of health status such as poverty, illegal drug use, access to health care, and living in communities with a higher prevalence of HIV infection. Adolescents are one of the groups at greatest risk for HIV infection, particularly minority inner-city youth. Runaway and homeless youth are especially likely to engage in high-risk sexual activity. The use of amphetamines, ecstasy, and amyl nitrate is associated with increased frequency of unprotected anal sex, especially among homosexual and bisexual individuals younger than 23 years.[80]

The prevalence of HIV infection is nearly five times higher in incarcerated populations than for the general population. HIV transmission among inmates in correctional and detention facilities is associated with MSM and potentially tattooing. Sex among inmates occurs, and laws or policies prohibiting sexual contact between inmates are difficult to implement and enforce. Condom distribution is unavailable in most correctional facilities.

Although no case of HIV transmission by tattooing has been documented, the procedure carries a theoretical risk for transmission if nonsterile equipment is used. In some instances, receipt of a tattoo has been associated with HIV seroconversion.[287] Although rare, transmission through living-donor organ transplantation has been confirmed. To reduce the risk for transmission of HIV through living-donor organ transplantation, transplant centers are advised to screen living donors for HIV as close to the time of organ recovery and transplantation as possible.[22]

Pathogenesis

The rapid convergence of information from diverse areas of AIDS research conveys the importance of obtaining the most up-to-date information. Scientists continue to report new discoveries about the pathogenesis of HIV disease.

Untreated HIV infection eventually leads to profound pathology through destruction of CD4+ cells, other immune cells, or neuroglial cells, or indirectly through the secondary effects of immunosuppression. The natural history of HIV disease begins with infection by the HIV retrovirus detectable only by laboratory tests. This retrovirus predominantly infects human T4 (helper) lymphocytes (also known as CD4 cells). CD4 cells are major regulators of the immune response, and HIV destroys or inactivates them. Macrophages, B cells, dendritic cells, and microglial cells are also infected (Fig. 7-15).

HIV is classified as a lentivirus, a subclass of retroviruses that contain RNA. When the RNA virus initiates replication in the living host cell, it must convert its RNA genetic information into a DNA template to replicate. HIV is unique in that despite the body's immune responses after initial infection, some HIV invariably escapes. Large amounts of HIV have been discovered hiding in the immune cells lining the surface of adenoids.[93] Thus, the virus's growth continues slowly in the period between acute infection and the onset of symptoms.

Once HIV enters the body, cells with CCR5 or CXCR4 receptors, such as CD4 cells and macrophages, serve as receptors for the HIV retrovirus, allowing direct passage of the infection into other target cells in the GI tract, uterus/cervix, and neuroglia. After attaching to and fusing with a cell, the HIV *virion* injects the core proteins and the two strands of viral RNA into the cell.

HIV virions contain enzymes including reverse transcriptase, integrase, and protease. All are required for successful reproduction. Before viral replication can occur in the host cell, reverse transcriptase enables the copying all the genetic information from the HIV RNA strand to make viral DNA. Once the viral genome is transcribed, integrase enables it to be is integrated into the host's DNA and duplicated many times. Final assembly of new HIV virion particles is enabled by protease (Fig. 7-16).

Replication of the virus can cause cell death, although the person remains asymptomatic for a period of time. Seroconversion refers to the emergence of HIV antibodies in the bloodstream (i.e., the person becomes positive for HIV antibodies) and usually takes place 3 to 6 weeks after infection; however, it can take up to 6 months for seroconversion to occur. Thus, an antibody test used for screening will yield a negative result for a period of time after exposure. During this preseroconversion period, contagion is possible because of the viral loads being high immediately after acute infection. After seroconversion, less virus is found in the blood; but HIV antibodies can be detected.

During asymptomatic HIV disease, the virus migrates from the serum into the tissues to infect CD4 cells in lymph tissue. The virus continues to kill the CD4 cells in

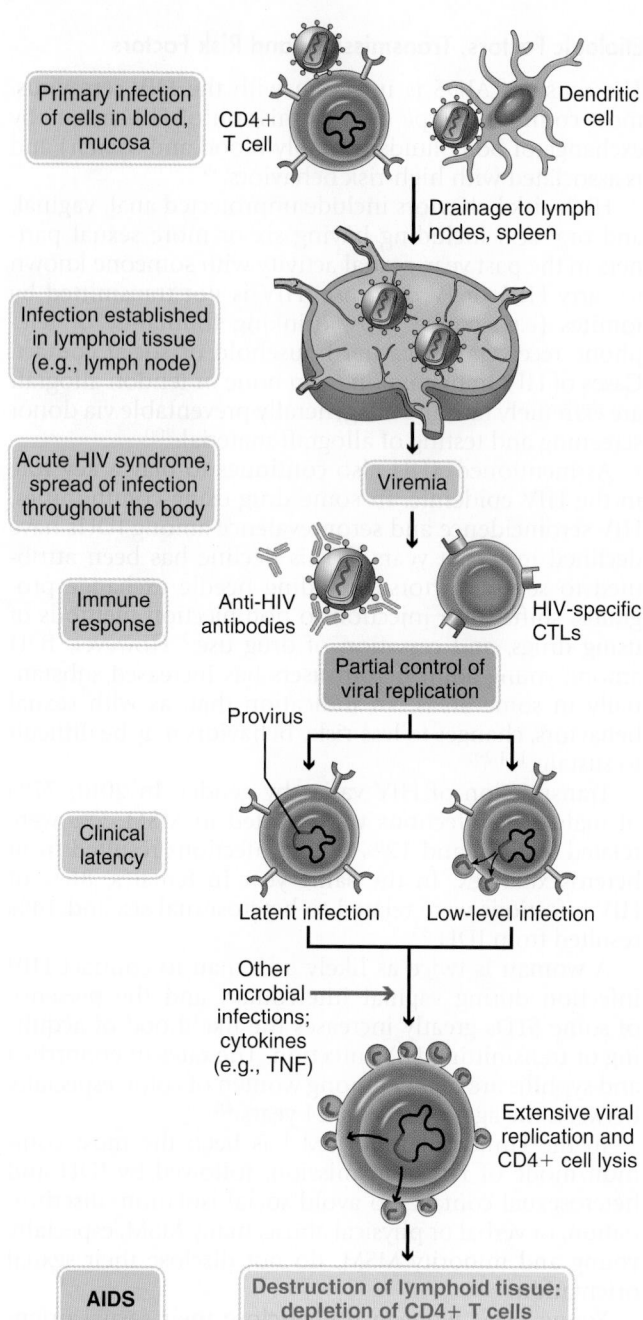

Figure 7-15

Pathogenesis of HIV-1 infection. Initially, HIV-1 infects T cells and macrophages directly or is carried to these cells by Langerhans cells. Viral replication in the regional lymph nodes leads to viremia and widespread seeding of lymphoid tissue. The viremia is controlled by the host immune response (not shown), and the patient then enters a phase of clinical latency. During this phase, viral replication in both T cells and macrophages continues unabated, but there is some immune containment of virus (not illustrated). A gradual erosion of CD4+cells by productive infection (or other mechanisms, not shown) continues. Ultimately, CD4+cell numbers decline, and the patient develops clinical symptoms of full-blown AIDS. Macrophages are also parasitized by the virus early; they are not lysed by HIV-1, and they may transport the virus to tissues, particularly the brain. (Reprinted from Kumar V: *Robbins and Cotran: pathologic basis of disease*, ed 8, Philadelphia, 2009, WB Saunders.)

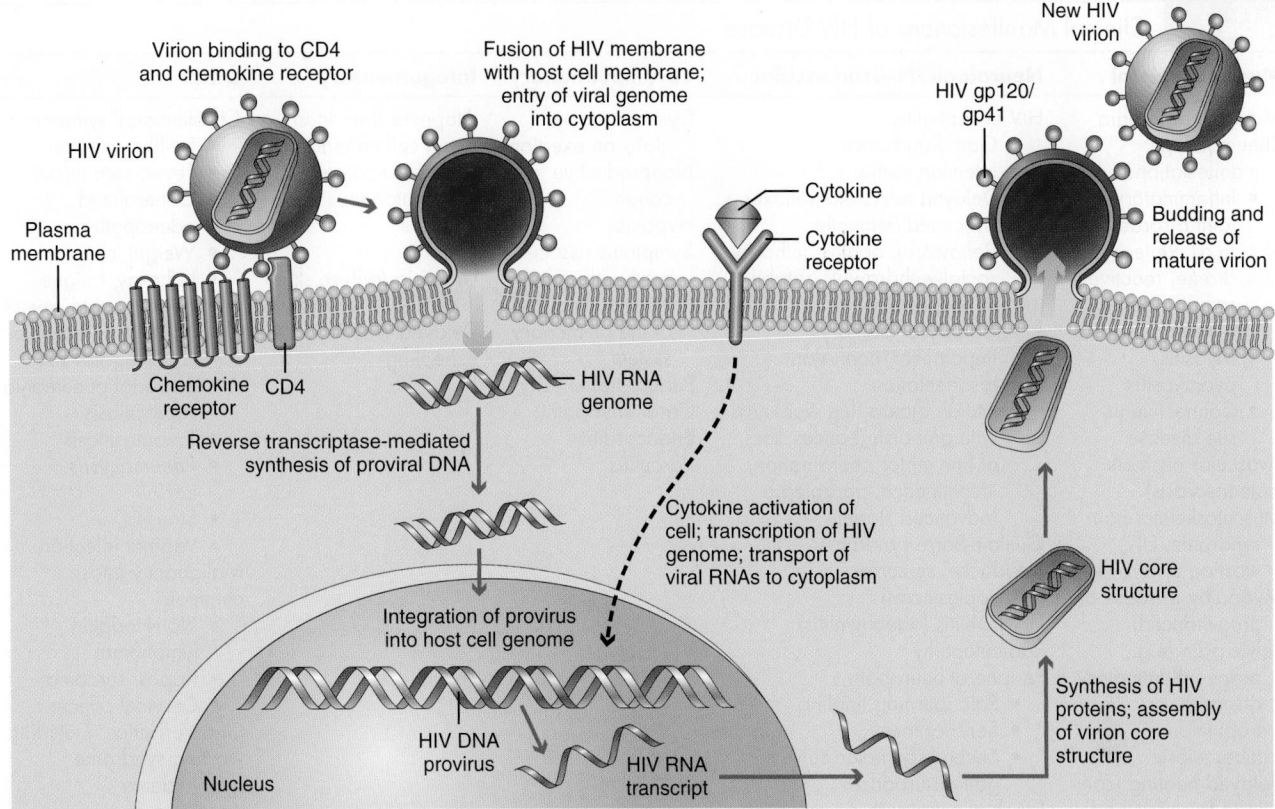

Figure 7-16

The life cycle of HIV. The steps from viral entry to production of infectious virions are illustrated. (Reprinted from Kumar V: *Robbins and Cotran: pathologic basis of disease*, ed 8, Philadelphia, 2009, WB Saunders.)

the lymph nodes, although the CD4 count remains above 500 cells/mm³.

As CD4 cells in lymph nodes are depleted, the virus once again enters the blood to infect any remaining lymphocytes and clinically apparent disease, known as symptomatic HIV disease, emerges. By the time this happens, the immune system has been compromised and is ineffective and unable to mount a specific immune response to these virions. The immune system dysfunction places the individual at risk for opportunistic diseases.

The decline in CD4 cells results in progressive loss of immune system function and the development of a wide variety of clinical signs and symptoms (see Table 7-3). In this symptomatic phase CD4 count ranges between 200 and 500 cells/mm³.

When the CD4 count declines less than 200 cells/mm³ and/or when an AIDS defining illness (opportunistic infection), wasting, or dementia occurs, the person is classified as having advanced HIV disease, or AIDS. Immunocompromise and elevated viral load occur during the advanced stage and are associated with the development of opportunistic infections (Fig. 7-17).

This infectious process and subsequent immunosuppression may result in one or more of the following: immunodeficiency with opportunistic infections and unusual malignancies; autoimmune conditions such as rheumatoid arthritis, lymphoid interstitial pneumonitis, hypergammaglobulinemia, and production of autoimmune antibodies; or neurologic dysfunction, including HIV-associated dementia, HIV encephalopathy, and peripheral neuropathies.

HIV has an extremely high mutation rate even within a single individual, producing competing strains of the same virus that fight for survival against the weapons produced by the immune system, and contribute to the development of resistance to antiretroviral medications.

Clinical Manifestations

HIV infection manifests itself in many different ways (Table 7-3) and differs between adult and pediatric populations. Great variation exists among individuals as to the amount of time that passes between acute HIV infection, the appearance of symptoms, the diagnosis of AIDS, and death.

Acute Infection. One to 6 weeks after an exposure and acute infection with HIV, the person may experience a transient period of flu-like symptoms and lymphadenopathy. Viral loads are typically high after an acute infection; however, antibody tests used the screen for HIV disease will remain negative until the point of seroconversion.

Asymptomatic HIV Disease (CD4 Count of 500 cells/mm³ or more). During the asymptomatic stage, the person demonstrates a positive antibody test for HIV but remains asymptomatic, for a period that can range between 1 and 20 years.

During the asymptomatic period, the infected person is clinically healthy and capable of normal daily activities, normal work habits, and unrestricted level and duration

Table 7-3   Clinical Manifestations of HIV Disease

Musculoskeletal	Neurologic/Neuromuscular	Cardiopulmonary	Integumentary	Other
Myalgia/arthralgia Rheumatologic manifestations: • Inflammatory joint disorders (e.g., Reiter syndrome, reactive arthritis, psoriatic arthritis) • Myositis/pyomyositis • Connective tissue disease Avascular necrosis (osteonecrosis) Musculoskeletal pain syndrome/HIV wasting syndrome Myopathy (disease or drug-induced) Pelvic pain (e.g., pelvic inflammatory disease) Extrapulmonary tuberculosis Delayed healing (can lead to sepsis and death) Myositis ossificans	HIV encephalitis: • Gait disturbance • Intention tremor • Delayed release of reflexes HIV-associated dementia: • *Behavioral:* apathy, lethargy, social withdrawal, irritability, depression • *Cognitive:* memory impairment, confusion, disorientation • *Motor:* ataxia, leg weakness with gait disturbances, loss of fine motor coordination, incontinence, paraplegia (advanced stage) Guillain-Barré syndrome Headache, seizures (toxoplasmosis) HIV myelitis (osteomyelitis) Radiculopathy Peripheral neuropathy: • Pain (burning tingling) • Sensory loss • Secondary motor deficits, gait disturbances Brachial neuropathy Vacuolar spinal myelopathy	Dyspnea, especially on exertion Nonproductive cough Hypoxia Symptoms associated with opportunistic infections of the pulmonary system Pericardial effusion Cardiomyopathy Endocarditis Vasculitis	Alopecia (hair loss) Basal cell carcinoma Kaposi sarcoma Mucocutaneous ulcers Rash Urticaria (diffuse skin reaction, wheals) Delayed wound healing	Constitutional symptoms: • Flu-like symptoms • Fever, sore throat • Generalized adenopathy • Weight loss • Lethargy, fatigue • Night sweats, fevers Opportunistic infections: • Cytomegalovirus • Bacterial pneumonia • Tuberculosis • Toxoplasmosis • *Pneumocystis carinii* • Sinusitis • Vaginal infection Malignancy (most common • Non-Hodgkin lymphoma • Kaposi sarcoma • Cervical cancer GI disturbance, including wasting syndrome Lymphedema Lipodystrophy Renal (kidney) failure Hepatic (liver) failure Oral thrush Gingivitis Visual disturbance HIV-related psychiatric disorders

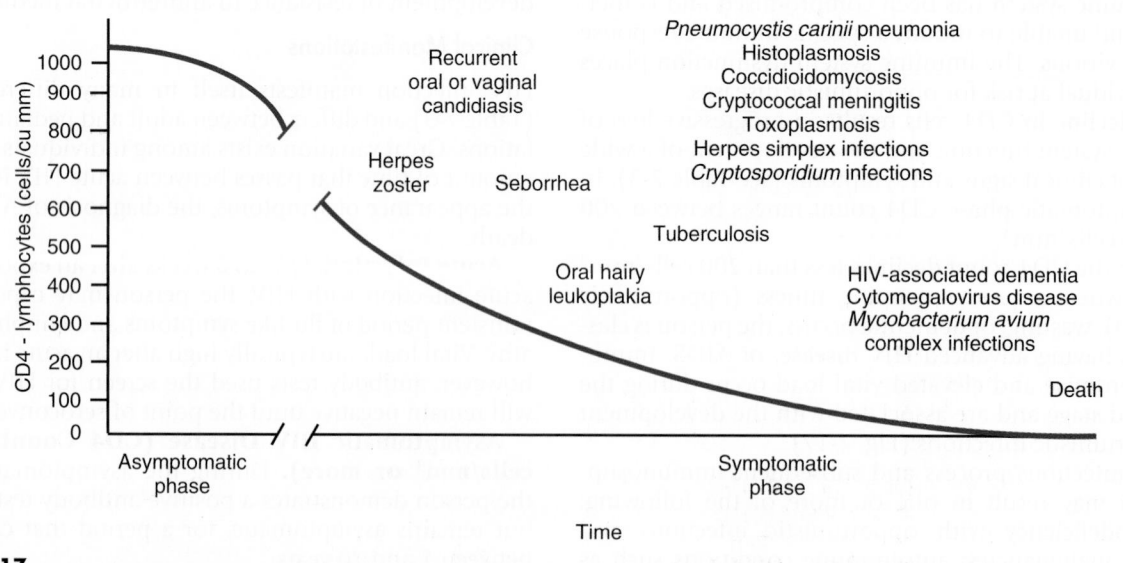

Figure 7-17

Complications of HIV disease as related to lymphocyte count.

of exercise. Fatigue and generalized lymphadenopathy with swollen and firm lymph glands may be reported during this stage.

Symptomatic HIV Disease (CD4 Count Between 200 and 500 cells/mm³). As the infection progresses and the immune system becomes increasingly more compromised, a variety of symptoms may develop, including persistent generalized adenopathy, nonspecific symptoms (such as diarrhea, weight loss, fatigue, night sweats, and fever), or neurologic symptoms resulting from HIV encephalopathy. The length of this phase is variable. If untreated, the person will eventually progress to advanced HIV disease.

Advanced HIV Disease (AIDS) (CD4 Count of 200 cells/mm³ or Less, and/or Occurrence of an AIDS-defining Illness [Opportunistic Infection], Wasting, or Dementia). The neurologic manifestations of advanced HIV disease are numerous and can involve the central, peripheral, and autonomic nervous systems. In addition to the symptoms that may occur from opportunistic diseases, treatment with multiple medications can cause adverse side effects, sometimes creating a confusing clinical picture. The immune system dysfunction, as evidenced by a precariously low CD4 counts, places the person at risk for an opportunistic infection (such as *P. carinii* pneumonia, CMV, toxoplasmosis) or malignancy.

CMV can cause peripheral neuropathy and HIV retinitis (with possible blindness). *P. carinii* pneumonia is a fungal infection of the lungs that causes symptoms such as dyspnea on exertion, chest discomfort, nonproductive cough, and weight loss. Toxoplasmosis is a parasitic disease that affects the central nervous system (CNS).

More than half the adults with HIV in this stage report fatigue that limits physical and recreational activities. Half the adults who report fatigue are unable to attend school or work.[260] HIV or AIDS encephalopathy, also referred to as HIV-associated dementia is thought to be caused by a primary infection of the brain by HIV. Symptoms can vary and are listed in Table 7-3. In some cases of advanced HIV disease, severe dementia, mutism, incontinence, and paraplegia may occur. A detailed summary of nervous system disorders associated with HIV, including treatment, is available.[103,256,295]

Dermatologic conditions are common in individuals with advanced HIV disease and can be extensive, including malignancies, bacterial, viral, or fungal infections (Fig. 7-18), and reactions to drug treatment. Cutaneous manifestations of HIV can present as dry flaking skin, telangiectasias, and thinning of the skin (and hair).

Other dermatologic conditions such as seborrheic dermatitis, psoriasis, Reiter syndrome, acquired ichthyosis, or Kaposi sarcoma may occur. Kaposi sarcoma (purple nodular skin lesions) predominantly affects homosexual men (Figs. 7-19 and 7-20). HIV-associated nutritional disorders may also contribute to nail and hair changes. HIV-associated wounds may occur as a result of Kaposi sarcoma, herpes simplex virus, syphilis, IDU ("tracks"), candidiasis and other fungal infections, postoperative infections, and herpes zoster (see Fig. 8-7).[126]

Pain Syndromes in Individuals with HIV Disease. Pain syndromes seen in HIV-infected individuals are divided into three groups: pain associated with HIV

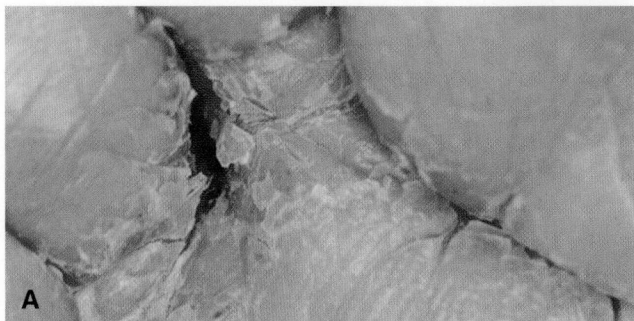

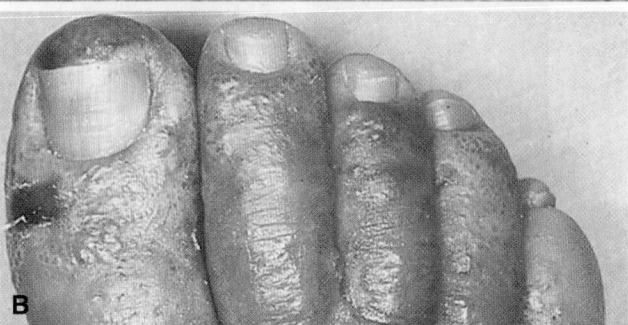

Figure 7-18

Tinea pedis. A, Fungal infections, such as tinea pedis (also known as athlete's foot), often begin between the toes and extend to the surface of the toes and foot. Red, itching skin may begin to peel or cause foot odor. **B,** The condition can progress, as shown here. Skin changes can become even more severe, with complete destruction of the nail beds (not shown). (A, Reprinted from Seidel H: *Mosby's guide to physical examination*, ed 5, St Louis, 2003, Mosby. B, Reprinted from Cohen J, Powderly WG: *Infectious diseases*, ed 2, St Louis, 2004, Mosby.)

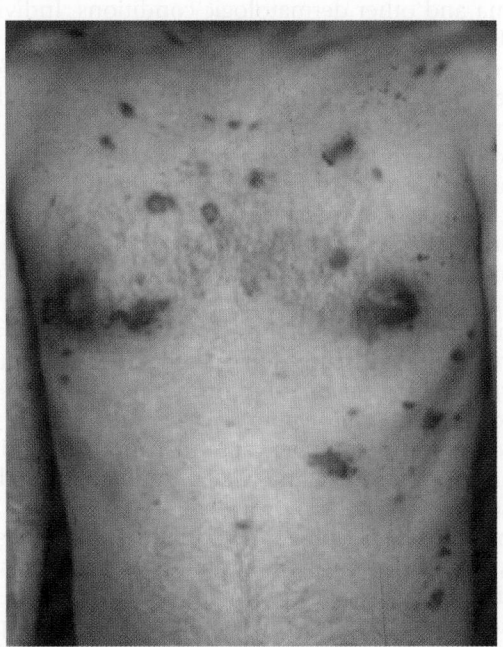

Figure 7-19

Kaposi sarcoma. There is a reduced incidence of Kaposi sarcoma in the HIV population because of better treatment, so fewer people progress this far in the disease. With better treatment have come fewer complications. Kaposi sarcoma appears primarily in the upper body, sometimes starting as a bulbous lesion on the end of the nose but also involving the face, chest, and lymph nodes. (Courtesy Julie Hobbs, Kingwood Medical Center, Kingwood, TX.)

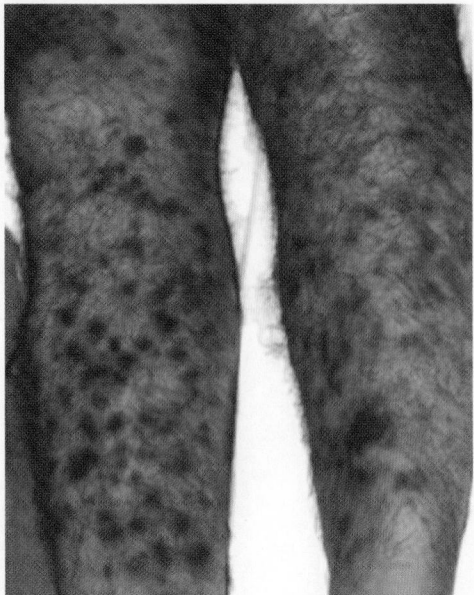

Figure 7-20

Kaposi sarcoma is not limited to the upper body; it can also appear in the lower quadrant. (Courtesy Julie Hobbs, Kingwood Medical Center, Kingwood, TX.)

infection, immunosuppression, opportunistic infections or comorbidities; pain caused by HIV diagnostic procedures and treatment; and pain unrelated to HIV disease or its treatment (e.g., diabetic neuropathy, discogenic pain).

For example, pain is associated with extensive Kaposi sarcoma and other dermatologic conditions. Individuals with HIV disease may experience headache, abdominal pain, chest pain, and arthralgias and myalgias. Women infected with HIV experience pain more often and with greater intensity than men; women also have unique gynecologic syndromes related to opportunistic infections and cancers of the pelvis and genitourinary tract.[285] Lower genital tract infections and HIV are major causes of morbidity and mortality among women.[284] As the HIV epidemic affects more women, increasing cases of pelvic inflammatory disease are being reported.[132,133] Pain is a common symptom in all these conditions. Pelvic inflammatory disease is discussed in greater detail in Chapter 20.

Peripheral Neuropathies. A form of peripheral neuropathy known as *distal sensory polyneuropathy* (DSP) is the most common neurologic cause of pain in HIV disease, affecting between 30% and 62% of individuals with HIV disease.[81,271]

Symptoms of peripheral neuropathies, as well as pain and symptoms of musculoskeletal disorders, occur most often in advanced stages of HIV disease but can occur earlier and may be the presenting manifestation. Neuropathic conditions in the HIV disease population may develop as a result of neurotoxic antiretroviral medications, chronic HIV infection, vitamin deficiencies resulting from poor nutrition, metabolic abnormalities, and opportunistic infections such as CMV.[104]

Peripheral neuropathies affect a large portion of people with AIDS. Although DSP is the most common form, other peripheral neuropathies may occur and other parts of the body may be affected such as the face or trunk. DSP symptoms present in a stocking-glove distribution, with the feet and legs more commonly affected than the hands and arms. Involvement of the upper extremities is less common and often occurs much later in the disease process.

Symptoms of DSP include sensory disturbances (paresthesias, numbness), impaired sensation (vibration, pain, light touch, temperature), burning pain, allodynia, hyperalgesia, leg cramping, weakness in intrinsic foot muscles (in advanced cases), sleep disturbances, difficulty with activities of daily living, and impaired balance.

DSP can be caused by neurotoxic effects of certain antiretroviral drugs. In this case, changes in the antiretroviral regimen can alleviate symptoms. More commonly, however, DSP occurs as a consequence of the prolonged effects of living with HIV infection and is linked to exposure to HIV proteins,[89] indirect damage from products of immune activation after HIV infection,[258] or prolonged exposure to inflammatory cytokines that can injure mitochondria in muscle and nerve.[198] In the individual with HIV and newly acquired neuropathy with a strong major motor component, vasculitis may be the underlying cause (see "Vasculitis" in Chapter 12).[199]

Neuromusculoskeletal Diseases. AIDS is associated with *neuromusculoskeletal diseases* such as osteomyelitis, bacterial myositis, and infectious (reactive) arthritis. Osteonecrosis, osteopenia, and osteoporosis are increasingly observed in clients who have been living with HIV disease for long periods. Avascular necrosis (osteonecrosis) of the femoral head(s) has been reported with the use of antiretroviral therapy containing protease inhibitors.[95]

The increased incidence of osteonecrosis in HIV/AIDS may be a result of the use of protease inhibitors or possibly as a result of an increased frequency of risk factors previously associated with osteonecrosis, such as hyperlipidemia, corticosteroid use, alcohol abuse, and hypercoagulability.[259] It is possible that HIV disease itself may have an independent effect on bone loss regardless of antiretroviral therapy.[190,213] Others suggest a link between lipodystrophy and bone loss.[233]

Some *musculoskeletal pain syndromes* seen in individuals with HIV disease may be associated with *HIV wasting syndrome.* HIV wasting is characterized by a disproportionate loss of metabolically active tissue, specifically body cell mass (i.e., tissue involved with glucose oxidation, protein synthesis, and immune system function).

These conditions occur secondary to low food intake, altered metabolism, and poor nutrient absorption with manifestations such as extreme weight loss, chronic diarrhea, unexplained weakness, fever, and malnutrition (e.g., mineral and vitamin deficiencies).

Studies show a clear relationship between vitamin B_{12} deficiency and dysfunction of the CNS and peripheral nervous system. Some of the clinical abnormalities of the nervous system seen in people with HIV are similar to the nervous system abnormalities described in those with vitamin B_{12} deficiency.

HIV-associated myopathy presents with a progressive weakness in the proximal limb and trunk muscles. The weakness is symmetrical and often involves the muscles of the face and neck. This type of myopathy may occur in individuals with HIV at every stage of illness. Muscle biopsies have shown necrosis of muscle fibers with and without inflammatory infiltrates. No evidence has been found of direct HIV infection of the muscle, and the underlying cause has not been determined. The fact that these clients improve on corticosteroids or plasmapheresis may point to an underlying autoimmune defect. Inflammatory myopathy is associated with serial escalation of creatine phosphokinase levels. In acute myopathy, exercise is contraindicated.

Rheumatologic Diseases and IRIS. Rheumatologic manifestations may be transient, subtle, or severe, and appear more often as HIV disease progresses. HIV-related arthritis does not necessarily respond to conventional medications. Arthritis may precede or accompany seroconversion. Polymyositis involves bilaterally symmetrical proximal muscle weakness.

There has been a decline in reactive arthritis, psoriatic arthritis, and various forms of connective tissue disease for adults, but *immune reconstitution inflammatory syndrome* (IRIS) following initiation of highly active antiviral therapy (HAART) may cause musculoskeletal symptoms in some individuals.

IRIS describes a group of clinical syndromes that occur as a complication of antiretroviral drugs used to boost immune function. IRIS presents as a flare-up of signs and symptoms when the recovering immune system begins to respond to an existing infection such as tuberculosis or CMV, *P. carinii* pneumonia, toxoplasmosis, HBV and HCV, or varicella-zoster virus infection.[145]

IRIS manifestations are diverse and have not been defined precisely; they are usually characterized by fever and worsening of the clinical manifestations of the underlying opportunistic infection. These clinical manifestations might be at the site of previously recognized opportunistic disease or might "unmask" disease at new sites previously unknown to be infected by the pathogen. They also might represent a response to a previously unrecognized additional pathogen. The majority of individuals who manifest IRIS do so within the first 4 to 8 weeks after starting antiretroviral therapy, and have had high viral loads and low CD4+ T-lymphocyte (CD4+) counts. However, IRIS has occurred weeks after antiretroviral therapy was started and in sequestered sites such as bone.

Lipodystrophy or Lipodystrophic Syndrome. Lipodystrophic syndrome, a syndrome of defective fat metabolism, dyslipidemia, and insulin resistance, manifests as central fat accumulation (Fig. 7-21) with visceral fat deposition documented by computed tomographic scans. It is a common problem that may occur soon after starting HAART. Loss of fat occurs in the arms, leg, or face with concomitant fat deposits in the abdomen, breasts (men and women), and back of the neck ("buffalo hump"; see Fig. 11-7).

AIDS-Related Lymphomas. AIDS-related lymphomas, including Burkitt lymphoma, non-Hodgkin lymphoma, Hodgkin lymphoma, and other more uncommon types (e.g., primary effusion lymphoma), are more likely to occur in HIV-infected people when compared with the general population. AIDS-related lymphomas are now the

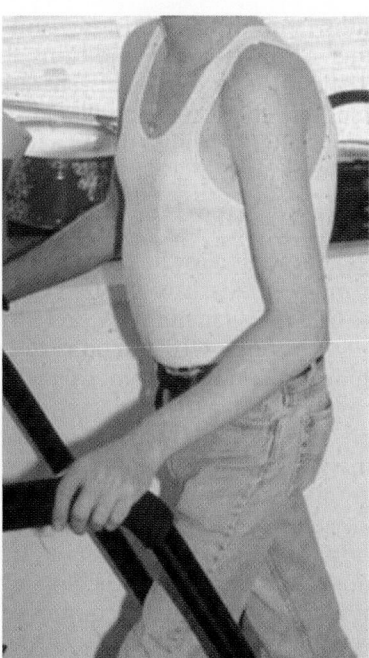

Figure 7-21

Lipodystrophic syndrome (LDS) in clients with HIV/AIDS has become more prevalent as a result of HAART treatment. LDS with cardiac complications from hyperlipidemia affects men and women, with fat deposits in the upper body and breasts contributing to body image problems, emotional trauma, and cardiac involvement. Additional fat deposits in the upper thoracic area and abdomen with loss in the extremities are seen in this client with AIDS. (Courtesy Julie Hobbs, Kingwood Medical Center, Kingwood, TX.)

second most common cancer associated with HIV after Kaposi sarcoma and increase with time after infection. The incidence of non-Hodgkin lymphoma appears to be declining with the use of HAART, whereas the incidence of Hodgkin lymphoma may actually have increased in the HIV-infected population.[174]

AIDS-related lymphoma can occur at any CD4+ level, but the risk is increased with declining CD4+ lymphocyte counts.[6,117] The course of disease is often aggressive, with extranodal metastases involving unusual sites such as the jaw, heart, body cavities, gallbladder, skin, and soft tissues.[1]

Cardiopulmonary Diseases. Cardiopulmonary diseases continue to be an important cause of illness and death in people with HIV disease. Bacterial pneumonia, bronchitis, tuberculosis (pulmonary and extrapulmonary), and CMV are common opportunistic diseases in the HIV/AIDS population. Emphysema, asthma, and pulmonary hypertension are also observed in this population. Cardiac involvement (heart and blood vessels) occurs as a result of a combination of the HIV infection, medical management, and secondary opportunistic infections. Both HIV infection and HAART can cause changes in lipid and glucose metabolism as well as elevation of blood pressure, promoting the development of atherosclerosis.

Cardiovascular diseases have become a major cause of mortality among HIV-infected people who respond well to antiretroviral therapy. Myocardial infarction, cardiomyopathy, pericardial effusion, and pericarditis are some other cardiovascular conditions that occur as a result of HIV and/or its treatment. There is increasing evidence to suggest that cardiovascular disease appears earlier and more often among HIV-infected adults than in the general public.[131,145,191]

MEDICAL MANAGEMENT

PREVENTION. Education regarding sexual activity and IDU has been the main emphasis of public health prevention programs. The CDC's overarching HIV prevention goal is to reduce the number of new HIV infections and to eliminate racial and ethnic disparities by promoting HIV counseling, testing, and referral and by encouraging HIV prevention among persons living with HIV and those at high risk for contracting the virus.[293] Socioeconomic factors (e.g., high rates of poverty and unemployment, lack of access to health care) are associated with high rates of HIV risk behaviors among minority MSM and are barriers to accessing HIV testing, diagnosis, and treatment. Reaching minority MSM who may not identify themselves as homosexual or bisexual with prevention messages remains a challenge.

The CDC now recommends routine HIV testing for all individuals between the ages of 13 and 64 years, with annual testing for those in high-risk groups. The CDC also recommends routine HIV testing of all pregnant women and routine screening of any infant whose mother was not screened.[30,136] Routine screening, along with partner notification and availability of sustained treatment for infected individuals contributes to prevention of transmission. Increased availability and use of simple, rapid HIV tests and at-home HIV tests may help overcome some of the traditional barriers to early diagnosis and treatment of infected persons.

Two simple but effective interventions limit the horizontal spread of HIV: condoms and counseling. Prophylactic use of the antiretroviral drugs, known as PrEP has been shown to reduce infection rates in MSM and heterosexual serodiscordant couples, when used in conjunction with condoms and education.[49,115]

However, education on safe sex and reducing or eliminating risky drug-abuse behavior has not been enough to stop the spread of AIDS. Unfortunately "prevention fatigue" has made prevention of HIV transmission less attainable as time goes by. An increase has been reported in HIV-associated behaviors such as sharing syringes or injection equipment among HIV-infected injection-drug users, unprotected vaginal sex, or unprotected sex with more than one sexual partner.[2]

Behavior intervention, the primary prevention tool, includes school-based programs, peer-to-peer interventions, strategies that limit needle sharing, parent-to-child communication, client-centered counseling, and personalized risk-reduction strategies (Box 7-3). The introduction of routine counseling, voluntary testing for women with HIV, and providing zidovudine (commonly known as *AZT*) antiretroviral drugs to infected pregnant women and their infants have dramatically reduced mother-to-child transmission rates.[48,293]

Effective behavior change programs need to address possible behavioral disinhibition (i.e., continuing or returning to high-risk behaviors when one feels protected) among persons who receive preventative interventions.

Box 7-3

RISK REDUCTION BEHAVIORS FOR THE PREVENTION OF HIV TRANSMISSION

Obtain testing for HIV* if any of the following is true:
- You received blood or blood products before 1985.
- You have (or have had) sex, especially if with multiple partners.
- You inject drugs and share needles.
- You have sexual intercourse (vaginal, anal, or oral) with someone else who injects drugs and shares needles.
- You have sex without a condom ("rubber") with someone who has HIV.
- You share used needles for tattooing or body piercing.

Protect yourself during sexual activities as follows:
- Abstinence or a monogamous relationship (sex with only one partner; both partners must be HIV free) is the only known prevention for the transmission of HIV.
- Use latex glove when inserting finger(s) into vagina or rectum.
- Use a new condom each time you have oral, anal, or vaginal sex.
- Latex or polyurethane is best because HIV can pass through lambskin or natural condoms.
- Do not use outdated condoms (check expiration date).
- Use the new condom with each sexual act from beginning to end (i.e., put on the condom before genital contact with partner and when the penis is erect; hold the condom firmly against base of penis during withdrawal; withdraw penis while still erect).
- Use water-based lubricants (e.g., KY jelly), *not* oils, lotions, or Vaseline that can cause a condom to tear or break.
- Ensure that no air is trapped in tip of condom.

Protect yourself as follows if you use drugs:
- Never share drug needles or "works."
- Participate in clinic needle exchange programs or clean drug needles with 100% bleach, leave 30 seconds, repeat three times and then rinse three times with water between uses.
- Mixing sex, drugs, and alcohol increases your risk. If you are drunk or high, it is harder to make good decisions about sexual practices.

Protect yourself as follows if you are pregnant:
- You can pass on HIV to your unborn child during pregnancy, birth, or breastfeeding. If you are pregnant and you have engaged in HIV risk behaviors, obtain HIV testing and appropriate treatment if you test positive for HIV.
- Medications taken during pregnancy can reduce your risk of HIV transmission to the fetus during pregnancy.

---

*A simple blood test (some centers offer a saliva test) can determine HIV infection 6 months after exposure. This test can be obtained anonymously (without giving out your name) and is free or low cost in most states. Contact your local Health Department.

Data from Centers for Disease Control and Prevention (CDC) (http://www.cdc.gov/hiv/prevention/programs/pwp/risk.html), Accessed 7/6/2014.

Prevention counseling that addresses safe sex, reducing the number of sex partners, and using condoms correctly and consistently, and other reproductive health needs (e.g., STD treatment and family planning) must be incorporated alongside any other potential prevention interventions such as preexposure prophylaxis.[293]

Restricting sex to partners of the same serostatus does not protect against transmission of other STDs or the possibility of HIV coinfection or superinfection (resistance to two or more classes of antiretroviral drugs) unless condoms are used correctly and consistently.[134] Controlling the AIDS epidemic requires sustained prevention programs in all affected communities, particularly programs targeting MSM, sexually active individuals with multiple partners, IDUs, and minorities.

Even though potent antiviral treatment can eradicate HIV from the blood, these drugs cannot completely eliminate the virus from the body, especially in semen. Although antiretroviral therapy reduces shedding of HIV in semen, thereby reducing HIV transmissibility, a substantial portion of people with HIV may still be infectious and may have drug-resistant strains of the virus.[16] Safe sex practices should continue to be reinforced in all people with HIV.

Researchers are working to find a topical inhibition strategy that would prevent sexual HIV-1 transmission by using a microbicide that can target a diversity of HIV-1 strains without causing mucosal inflammation in the lining of the vagina and have a minimum of adverse side effects, all while maintaining effectiveness for prolonged periods.[232] For individuals with HIV disease, prevention of other infections is important. For example, *P. carinii* pneumonia prophylaxis can be achieved with drugs such as Bactrim. *Mycobacterium tuberculosis* has a higher prevalence in the HIV population. It is communicable, preventable, and treatable. One in three adults with HIV disease is coinfected with *M. tuberculosis*. Tuberculin skin testing should be available and routinely offered to individuals at HIV testing sites. Guidelines for the prevention of other opportunistic infections in people with HIV are also now available.[52,145]

DIAGNOSIS. Early diagnosis is important so that effective treatment can be initiated in a timely manner. Sex partners should be notified of their risk of HIV and the subsequent need for HIV testing. Tests that determine the presence of antibodies to HIV are used for screening. Antibody tests indicate HIV infection indirectly by revealing HIV antibodies (indicating exposure to the virus). Rapid tests use an oral fluid from a swab of the gums, or a small amount of blood from a finger stick. The OraQuick Rapid HIV-1 Antibody test can be completed in as little as 10 minutes and has up to 99.6% accuracy. Rapid testing means that individuals who are HIV-positive can receive immediate counseling, early treatment to preserve their health, and prompt education on preventing disease transmission.[171]

HIV-1 antibody enzyme immunoassay tests use a small vial of blood obtained from a vein and lab results typically take several days. The CDC estimates that one-third of all individuals tested in this way do not return for their test results. If a rapid test or an enzyme immunoassay test is positive, results are confirmed with a follow-up test such as a Western blot.

For a variable period of time after acute infection, antibody testing will not be positive because the body takes a variable amount of time to produce a detectable level of antibodies. Consequently, a person with HIV could test negative for HIV antibodies until the point of seroconversion, which could be as long as 6 months after the initial exposure. Although a negative antibody test may assure some individuals they are negative for HIV, this does not necessarily translate into reduced risk without continued education regarding effective prevention.

Additional laboratory confirmation of HIV infection is required; HIV RNA viral load testing (as measured by the plasma HIV RNA assay), CD4+ (T4 lymphocyte) count,

and CD4:CD8 ratios are used to determine the clinical status. CD4 counts normally range from 500 to 1200 cells/mm^3, and values lower than the normal range suggest immunocompromise. However, because of normal fluctuations in CD4 counts, the CD4:CD8 ratio is considered a more stable indicator of the health of the immune system. The normal ratio if CD4:CD8 is between 32% and 68%.

TREATMENT. No cure has been found for AIDS, but advances in treatment have successfully transformed AIDS into a manageable chronic condition for most individuals who have access to treatment. The national HIV Vaccine Trials Network has been established to develop and test possible vaccine compounds, but an effective vaccine is not imminent. Ongoing research is investigating the use of gene therapy and immune reconstitution or restoration in the context of HIV disease. Until a vaccine is available, the goals of intervention are to stop HIV from replicating, increase the number of CD4 cells, and prevent or delay HIV disease progression.

Pharmacologic Treatment

Medical management centers on use of HAART and its effects on CD4 cell count and viral load. When CD4 cell counts drop below 500 cells/mm^3, HAART is initiated. In some cases, HAART is initiated even earlier. HAART involves a combination of antiretrovirals drugs from different drug classes. Typical HAART combinations consist of a nonnucleoside reverse transcriptase inhibitor plus two nucleoside reverse transcriptase inhibitors, or a boosted protease inhibitor plus two nucleoside reverse transcriptase inhibitors, or a integrase inhibitor plus two nucleoside reverse transcriptase inhibitors. These drugs act by preventing the function of enzymes that are involved in the replication process.

Another class of antiretroviral drug known as *entry inhibitors* is sometimes used to prevent entry of the HIV virion through the CD4 cell membrane via inhibiting the CCR5 receptor or preventing fusion between the virion and the cell membrane. The goal of HAART is to achieve sustained suppression of HIV replication, reducing the amount of virus in the blood to undetectable levels. These drugs do not completely eradicate the virus; despite undetectable levels in blood, the virus can hide in sanctuary sites that include latent CD4 cells, macrophage, and follicular dendritic cells, the CNS, lymph tissue, and semen. Lifelong HAART therapy is required to maintain viral suppression and health of the immune system.

Factors in HAART include: (1) simplifying the drug regimens to improve adherence (in most cases, once-daily dosing is now possible), (2) developing alternatives for those in whom the current medications have failed (known as "salvage regimens"), (3) preventing viral rebound (return of high levels of the virus when drugs are discontinued), and (4) managing the wide range of pharmacologic side effects.

Development of drug resistance is the inevitable consequence of incomplete suppression of virus plasma levels in individuals with HIV treated with HAART. Noncompliance with the drug regimen can lead to mutation of the virus and resistance to the treatment. Drug resistance is one of the most significant threats to effective therapy.

Genotypic and phenotypic testing of an individual's HIV strains may be used to direct the initial choice of antiretroviral drugs, and is also carried out when the individual is not responding to drug therapy, as indicated by an increase in the viral load and a decrease in the CD4+ cell count. Genotyping detects viral mutation, whereas phenotyping detects a decrease in the sensitivity of the virus to the drugs.[138]

Concurrent medical management of comorbidities and side effects is needed when they are present. Palliative treatment for individuals with osteonecrosis may include nonsteroidal antiinflammatory drugs and pain medications. Surgical procedures to improve blood flow to the affected area or joint replacement to improve function may be considered. When present, hyperlipidemia may be associated with accelerated atherosclerosis and insulin resistance, contributing to increased cardiovascular morbidity and mortality rates in the population with HIV.[108,159]

Medical interventions also may be needed to manage opportunistic infections or malignancies in individuals with advanced HIV disease. Treatments used to address various clinical manifestations of HIV disease include antibiotics, corticosteroids, interferon therapy, or chemotherapy, depending on the nature of the problem.

Adverse Effects of Treatment. A listed of commonly seen side effects of drugs used in HAART can be found at AIDS Education and Training Centers National Resource Center (www.aids-etc.org). Potential toxicities and side effects from drug treatment include peripheral neuropathy, metabolic disorders such as lipodystrophy, avascular necrosis of the femoral head(s), osteonecrosis, renal toxicity, and lactic acidosis. Lactic acidosis may occur as a result of injured cell mitochondria giving off lactic acid in response to the effects of nucleoside reverse transcriptase inhibitors. AZT myopathy, a toxic mitochondrial myopathy, is much less often seen today and is limited to people taking high doses of AZT. Comorbidities directly linked to AZT can often be managed with a change in antiretroviral drugs.[262]

Nonpharmacologic Treatment. Nonpharmacologic interventions include nutritional therapy, exercise, and mental health support. Nutrition counseling can help with AIDS-associated weight loss, nutritional deficiencies, loss of muscle mass (wasting syndrome). Over the counter nutritional supplements should be reviewed by the individual's infection disease physician, as some can interact or interfere with certain medications used in HAART.

The use of complementary and alternative medicine interventions, such as yoga, tai chi, or acupuncture, is common in HIV-positive individuals. Josephs et al reported that 60% of HIV-positive individuals claim use of complementary and alternative therapies.[139] Effectiveness of complementary and alternative medicine therapies to help manage some of the symptoms or comorbidities associated with HIV disease is an area of ongoing study. There is no evidence that complementary and alternative medicine therapies can cure or successfully treat HIV disease itself.[139]

Prognosis. Since the early 1980s, HIV disease has evolved from a devastating disease with a high mortality rate into a manageable chronic illness for those who have access to treatment and adhere to treatment. Use of HAART is extending the lives of individuals with HIV disease to life expectancy in many cases. For those not diagnosed until they have advanced disease, HAART can help restore health, extend survival, and restore function.

HAART has reduced mortality rates from AIDS by more than 80%. Current research efforts to provide a "functional cure" would allow affected individuals to be treated with medications that lower levels of HIV such that the person's own immune system would keep the virus in check once the drugs are discontinued. People who get effective treatment can live healthy, normal lives. Although HAART improves survival, it often comes at the price of a variety of metabolic (and other) side effects.

Patterns of morbidity and mortality are changing; a leading cause of death is now kidney or liver failure as a result of medical treatment (e.g., protease inhibitors are metabolized by the liver) or HCV.[39]

The widespread use of HAART has helped reduce deaths caused by opportunistic illnesses. However, opportunistic illnesses still continue to cause considerable morbidity and mortality in individuals unaware of their HIV infection or in those who delay initiation of treatment for HIV.[52,145]

Prognosis is worse for those who has both HIV and HCV or those who manifest wasting syndrome. For individuals who are coinfected with HCV, concurrent treatment of HCV makes HIV treatment more complex because of the hepatotoxicity of antiretroviral medications and the important role the liver has in maintaining health. IDUs have a higher burden of comorbidities of HIV disease, possibly contributing to poor response to HAART. Active drug use is most commonly associated with nonadherence to the required antiretroviral treatment regimen and prophylaxis for opportunistic infections.[195]

A considerable body of evidence suggests that psychosocial factors influence the progression of HIV infection, its morbidity, and its mortality. Psychosocial influences relating to faster disease progression include life-event stress, sustained depression, denial or avoidance coping, concealment of gay identity, and negative outlook. Conversely, protective psychosocial factors include active coping, collaborative relationship with health care professionals, and effective stress management.

Biologic factors such as genetics, age, viral strain and virulence, and immune response are also major determinants of disease progression and also have an impact on outcome. Scientists are continuing to investigate psychoneuroimmunologic pathways by which immune and neuroendocrine mechanisms might link psychosocial factors with health and survival.

Pediatric Population. Clinical presentation in the pediatric population is often more devastating due to the immaturity of the immune system. Children become sicker faster, with death within 2 years in many untreated cases. The immature CNS is very vulnerable to direct infection by HIV. Developmental delays are often the first sign of HIV and contribute to morbidity in this group.

SPECIAL IMPLICATIONS FOR THE THERAPIST   **7-3**

Human Immunodeficiency Virus Disease

With advances in treatment, improved care, and longer survival, therapists can expect to see increasing numbers of people in their practices who may have HIV. Maximal effectiveness from physical therapy requires a therapist who is knowledgeable about HIV disease and the rehabilitation issues surrounding individuals with HIV disease.[251]

It is possible for HIV-positive individuals to come to a therapy practice undiagnosed or unwilling to disclose their HIV status. Remember, the CDC estimates that 1 in 5 HIV-positive individuals in the United States are unaware of their HIV status. Women who have been raped have an increased risk of HIV transmission and may not report this information.

Consideration of HIV status should be integrated into history and/or medical screening. For example, anyone presenting with musculoskeletal or neuromuscular symptoms of unknown origin, with or without constitutional symptoms, should be interviewed more specifically about medical history, including whether they have had a HIV test (especially if the person is in a high-risk group). This may potentially lead to medical referral, diagnosis, and appropriate therapy.

Health care providers who routinely assess the sexually transmitted disease risks of their clients can encourage at-risk individuals to test annually for HIV, syphilis, gonorrhea, and chlamydia, and to seek vaccination against hepatitides A and B.[313] Providing a discreet and nonjudgmental environment with assurance of confidentiality while emphasizing the importance of disclosing accurate risk information may help facilitate risk disclosure.

Clients at any stage of HIV disease may need psychosocial support to deal with depression, anxiety, or emotional problems that may develop. Thus, screening for depression and anxiety is essential; referral for further treatment may be indicated.[148]

Therapists also may have a role in osteoporosis education, prevention, and screening. Risk factor assessment is advised for anyone with HIV infection. Anyone at high risk for osteopenia or osteoporosis should be referred for dual x-ray absorptiometry measurement of bone mineral density. Clients should be encouraged to minimize risk for developing osteoporosis with dietary calcium and vitamin D intake, maintaining a normal body mass index, avoiding tobacco and alcohol abuse, and maintaining a long-term weight-bearing exercise program.[233]

Prevention of Transmission in the Health Care and Athletic Settings

The risk of transmission of the virus from client to health care worker is exceedingly small. Sources of HIV that may pose a risk of transmission through these routes include blood, visibly bloody fluids, tissues, and other body fluids, including semen; vaginal secretions; and cerebrospinal, synovial, pleural, peritoneal, pericardial, and amniotic fluids. In addition, any direct cutaneous or mucosal contact, without barrier protection to concentrated HIV in a research laboratory or production facility is considered to be an exposure.[184] In the absence of visible blood in the saliva, exposure to saliva from a person with HIV is not thought to pose a risk for HIV transmission. Exposure to tears, sweat, or nonbloody urine or feces from individuals with the virus does not constitute exposure to HIV. Occupational exposure to breast milk does not constitute an exposure unless ingested directly.[184]

The CDC estimates that percutaneous exposure (needlestick) to HIV-infected blood is 0.3%, whereas mucous membrane exposure to HIV-infected blood is 0.09%. Non–intact skin exposure to HIV-infected blood is estimated to be lower than risk for mucous membrane. The risk of transmission via exposure to fluids or tissues other than HIV-infected blood have not been quantified, but is probably lower than risk from blood exposures.

Factors affecting HIV transmission risk include the quantity of blood and the viral load in the blood. Prolonged contact (i.e., several minutes or more) of intact skin with infected blood has not been associated with HIV transmission but is considered a potential exposure, in part because the skin may have unrecognized areas of disruption that could serve as portals of entry.[184]

Because of the nature of their work, physical therapists are at negligible risk unless they work in a setting that involves contact with blood or body fluids containing blood, such as wound care or debridement. The health care worker is at far greater risk for the transmission of HBV and should consider prophylactic vaccination for HBV or become familiar with postexposure prophylaxis for HBV (see Chapter 17).[212]

In all health care settings, standard precautions (e.g., using barriers for working with any liquid that comes from another person, excluding sweat [see Appendix A]) should be observed to prevent the transmission of any blood borne pathogens. Box 7-4 includes specific recommendations for health care professionals working with HIV-positive clients. Individuals with advanced HIV disease are likely to be immunodeficient, and every precaution must be taken to prevent infection for that person.

There are no documented cases of HIV being transmitted during participation in sports. The very low risk of transmission during sports participation would involve exposure to infected blood, typically through open wounds or mucosal membranes. There is no risk

---

Box 7-4

STANDARD HIV PRECAUTIONS FOR HEALTH CARE WORKERS

- Use protective barriers (gloves, eye shields, gowns) when handling blood, body fluids, and infectious fluids.
- Wash hands, skin, and mucous membranes immediately and thoroughly if contaminated by blood or other body fluids.
- Prevent needle or scalpel sticks.
- Ventilation devices are available for resuscitation.
- Any health care worker with open wounds or skin lesions should not treat clients or handle equipment until the lesion(s) heals.
- Pregnant health care workers should take extra precautions. See Appendix A for additional information.
- Occupational exposure to HIV should be followed immediately by evaluation of exposure source and postexposure prophylaxis.

From Centers for Disease Control and Prevention (CDC): *Occupational HIV transmission and prevention among health care workers*, 2011. Available online at: http://www.cdc.gov/hiv/resources/factsheets/hcwprev.htm.

of HIV transmission through sports activities in which bleeding does not occur. Athletes in contact and collision sports are at greater risk of HBV transmission and should be vaccinated against this virus.[156] The NCAA Handbook is an excellent resources for guidelines regarding bloodborne pathogens and working with athletes. In general, standard precautions apply.[202]

Postexposure Prophylaxis

Postexposure prophylaxis (PEP) is used to prevent HIV infection after occupational exposure, unsafe sex with an infected partner, sexual assault, or high-risk IDU.[192,212] Occupational exposure should be considered an urgent medical concern requiring timely postexposure management.[45] Health care providers with occupational exposure to HIV should receive follow-up counseling, postexposure testing, and medical evaluation regardless of whether they receive PEP treatment.

PEP consists of a 28-day course of HAART and must be initiated as quickly as possible (within hours) after exposure. The antiretroviral medications may help to diminish or end viral replication, thereby reducing the viral inoculum to a more potentially manageable target for the host's defenses. Determining level of risk and appropriateness of drug selection should be conducted as soon as possible after an exposure has occurred. Information should be provided about potential drug interactions and drugs that should not be taken with PEP, side effects of prescribed drugs, measures to minimize side effects, and methods of clinical monitoring for toxicity during the follow-up period. Symptoms of rash, fever, back or abdominal pain, pain on urination or blood in the urine, or symptoms of hyperglycemia (e.g., increased thirst or frequent urination) should be reported to the physician immediately.

Exposed health care providers are advised to use precautions to prevent secondary transmission, especially during the first 6 to 12 weeks postexposure (e.g., avoid blood or tissue donations, breastfeeding, or pregnancy). Other guidelines for HIV PEP are available.[45,192,212]

Guidelines for Health Care Workers with HIV

Guidelines for HIV-positive health care workers are available from The Center for HIV Law and Policy. A chart summarizing guidelines and policies currently in place regarding HIV-positive health care workers for all 50 states is available online on the Center's website at http://hivlawandpolicy.org/resources/guidelines-hiv-positive-health-care-workers-center-hiv-law-policy.

In general, all health care workers should use standard precautions in all health care and athletic settings. For the therapist, internal pelvic floor examination and wound care, including debridement and dressing changes might be excluded. According to guidelines drafted by the CDC, at a minimum the potential client must be informed of the worker's HIV, HBV, or HCV status if the therapist is to engage in high-risk activity such as vaginal examination of the pelvic floor muscles, debridement, or other wound care (see response and comments above).[44]

As stated on the Center for HIV Law & Policy website, given the limited ways in which HIV is a genuine risk and the absence of such risk to health care patients, guidelines, statutes, and regulations adopted by the CDC in the early 1990s should be reevaluated and rewritten. According to Gostin,[112] the national policy restricting the practices of HIV-positive health care workers is not necessary.

According to the Center for HIV Law & Policy:

> States differ slightly in their guidelines on restrictions on an HIV-positive HCW's [health care worker's] practice and on patient notification. Regarding restrictions on an HCW's practice, all states agree that infection alone is not a basis for imposing restrictions and each employ some form of committee or expert review panel to make the decision regarding use of restrictions. Some states require that HIV-positive HCWs cease performing invasive procedures until they have sought the advice of the panel. Other states, however, make the decision to seek the advice of the panel more voluntary. Most states provide for continued review and/or supervision following the imposition of any restrictions. Regarding patient notification, many states leave that decision to the review committee to make on a case-by-case basis, while others require the consent of the patient before the HCW can participate in an invasive procedure.[290]

HIV and Rehabilitative Therapy

Over the past 30 years, the rehabilitation of the person with HIV or AIDS has changed significantly. In the middle of the 1980s, the person with AIDS often developed opportunistic infections that led to death. During that period, the physical therapist's role was primarily that of pain control, energy conservation, and instruction in the use of adaptive equipment to maximize functional ability.

Today, chronic conditions such as cardiovascular disease related to lipodystrophic syndrome and rheumatologic and musculoskeletal conditions are much more common in those living with HIV. Therefore, physical therapists are generally focused on assisting the individual with the management of specific impairments and functional limitations related to chronic HIV infection and/or its comorbidities and/or opportunistic infections when they arise.

The individual with HIV disease may demonstrate clinical manifestations of overlapping pathologic processes and disabilities that need appropriate rehabilitation intervention.

For example, the CNS can be the site of more than one opportunistic disease process simultaneously,[103] or the individual may sustain a stroke in addition to having an already existing peripheral neuropathy or other neuromusculoskeletal manifestations. The therapist may be involved in wound intervention when integumentary impairment is caused by HIV opportunistic infections while also providing intervention to relieve problems associated with rheumatologic dysfunctions.[251]

Physical therapists need to consider physical fitness, quality-of-life issues, work, activities of daily living, including community management skills such as access to transportation, socialization opportunities, shopping, banking, ability to negotiate health care and insurance systems[103]; and participation in church, synagogue, or other spiritual network. Home programs must be simple and easily incorporated into the patient's lifestyle.

Often individuals with AIDS are overwhelmed by the disease process, the complicated treatment, the multiple health care appointments, and scheduling to manage all of these tasks. Adding an exercise program may result in frustration and noncompliance unless the person can see a clear benefit and way to manage yet another aspect of the treatment program.

For individuals with CNS involvement, rehabilitation therapy may help the client optimize functional ability. These clients may respond to an eclectic blend of rehabilitation strategies such as those for other individuals who have CNS involvement as a result of stroke or head injury.[147]

Distal sensory peripheral neuropathy is one of the most common causes of pain in people with chronic HIV disease. It may be related to certain drugs used to treat HIV or related to effects of the chronicity of the infection.[105] The use of conventional transcutaneous electrical nerve stimulation may be helpful in addressing peripheral pain in HIV-related peripheral neuropathies; there is no known evidence that this modality is contraindicated but studies are needed to verify its true benefit. Joint and soft tissue mobilization, stretching, gait and balance training, and desensitization techniques can also be very effective. The alternate use of microcurrent electroacupuncture has been reported to reduce pain, improve functional status, and increase perceived strength. Discussion of the possible mechanisms for these effects is available.[105]

The presence of peripheral neuropathies may also signal nutritional deficiencies requiring nutritional counseling. This is especially true for the client who has the wasting syndrome that often accompanies advanced HIV disease. In addition, without proper nutrition, therapy involving balance training, extremity strengthening and stretching, and motor skills may be limited in benefit.

Diminished sensory information associated with peripheral neuropathies of the lower extremities makes balance and gait control more difficult. Clients with HIV disease may have balance deficits at lower movement speeds compared to healthy adults. Motor slowness is associated with both neuropathy and myopathy.[178] Formulating a rehabilitation approach must be based on the underlying neurophysiologic deficit(s) present.[104] Other guidelines for management of the lower extremity complications, balance, and postural derangements associated with distal symmetrical polyneuropathy are available.[106,261]

For individuals with acute inflammatory myopathy, exercise is generally contraindicated until the inflammatory condition is managed medically. For many other musculoskeletal conditions, progressive resistance training with weights or elastic bands or tubing to strengthen specific muscles may be beneficial.

Improper body mechanics, poor postural alignment and postural instability, balance and gait problems, and other biomechanical changes may occur in the person who has developed muscle weakness and fatigue from progression of the disease process, malnutrition, or the wasting syndrome. Postural awareness, stretching and strengthening of specific muscles, and attention to nutrition may be part of the treatment plan.

Cardiopulmonary complications (see Table 7-3) in advanced stages of HIV disease contribute to morbidity and mortality. Oxygen transport mechanisms can be adversely affected. Muscle and joint mobilization techniques and breathing exercises are essential for the person who has been immobilized for any length of time as a result of respiratory or other disease involvement. Cardiac rehabilitation principles should be applied as needed for individuals with specific cardiopulmonary conditions such as myocardial infarction, pericardial effusion, or myocarditis.

For the client with malignancy, guidelines for management and interventions are discussed in Chapter 9 (see also the section on Kaposi sarcoma in Chapter 10).

Exercise and HIV Disease

As discussed in "Exercise Immunology" in this chapter, exercise has clinically significant effects on immune responsiveness and thus potentially can alter the natural history of HIV infection in a beneficial manner. A growing number of studies are now addressing the issue of the relationship between exercise and HIV infection.[85,150]

Exercise in any stages of HIV disease may provide pain relief; improve appetite, reduction of muscle atrophy, and regular bowel activity; and improve function; it can also enhance immune function by increasing CD4 cells and the inducer subset, which activate suppressor/cytotoxic (CD8) cells. Exercise can improve overall cardiovascular and pulmonary function to improve endurance and cardiac function and help prevent pneumonia and other respiratory infections.

Moderate exercise often reduces anxiety and improves mood, which may be the mechanism by which it enhances or stabilizes the immune system. Exercise can benefit psychoneuroimmunology interactions by reducing stress and improving mood, potentially improving quality of life, which, in turn, can influence disease progression.

Results of group aerobic exercise and tai chi on functional outcomes and quality of life for persons living with HIV disease showed improved physiologic and physical changes along with improved functional outcomes and quality of life. Group intervention provides a socialization context for the management of HIV disease with enhanced psychologic coping and improved social interactions.[107]

Exercise training at 70% to 80% of maximal heart rate is recommended to achieve the benefits listed. Higher intensities increase strength and aerobic fitness but have not been shown to change total lymphocyte cell counts or ratios.[243] A rate of perceived exertion no greater than 14 is recommended[170] (see Table 12-13); other recommendations established by the American College of Sports Medicine are available for all three stages of HIV disease.

Monitoring vital signs (see Appendix B) and laboratory values (see Chapter 40) is an important part of determining exercise intensities, especially in the presence of comorbidities such as anemia, vitamin deficiency, wasting syndrome, or opportunistic infections. Proper caloric intake is also important in setting the standard for each type of exercise to meet energy expenditure required for the activity. Seeking the advice of a nutritionist is recommended.[103]

The effects of exercise demands on a high-level athlete with HIV in competition on levels of psychologic stress and immune function remain unclear. Potential adverse effects of the stresses of competition include increased upper respiratory infections in marathon runners.[207] Exercise recommendations for athletes with HIV are summarized in Box 7-5.

Exercise programs to increase strength and body mass are particularly relevant to HIV because lean body mass wasting is one of the most devastating aspects of this infection.

Exercise training, including strength training, may have the potential to arrest (possibly only temporarily) and/or reverse the wasting effects. Improved muscle function and increased body dimensions and mass can occur following progressive resistive exercises three times per week for 6 weeks.[88,276] Fillipas et al reported improved self-efficacy, cardiovascular fitness, and quality of life in HIV-positive men after a 6-month program of combined resistive and aerobic exercise.[91] A systematic review reported that progressive resistance exercise or a combination of progressive resistance exercise and aerobic exercise may lead to statistically significant increases in body weight and arm and thigh girth, appears to be safe, and may be beneficial for medically-stable adults living with HIV.[211]

Early Asymptomatic Stage of HIV Disease

Exercise is considered safe for people with HIV and an important way to increase the CD4 cells at earlier stages of the disease, possibly delaying symptoms while increasing muscle strength and size. During asymptomatic stages of HIV disease, metabolic parameters are within normal limits, with no limitations placed on the individual. Individuals with asymptomatic HIV disease should be encouraged to exercise regularly, including both aerobic and resistance exercise components.[150]

The effect of HIV and its treatment with protease inhibitors on exercise and activity tolerance has been reported. Physical activity intolerance resulting in functional limitations may be caused by diminished aerobic capacity (decreased peak VO_2) far below that occurring as a result of physiologic deconditioning alone. Individuals who receive HAART may have a reduced ability to extract and use oxygen from the muscle during exercise, limiting their ability to increase the intensity of activity.[37]

Symptomatic and Advanced Stages of HIV Disease

During symptomatic and advanced stages of HIV disease, functional capacity is reduced, requiring more individualized exercise prescription and lower intensities.[170] Neurologic dysfunction and deconditioning are common. Regular physical activity and exercise are just as important in this group but are more difficult and symptom limited. Among people with HIV disease who have known cardiovascular disease, pulmonary limitations, or muscle dysfunction, exercise prescription should address impairments and limitations. Collaboration with the physician to determine any contraindications for exercise is advised.

Strenuous or exhaustive exercise training is not recommended; aerobic exercise at moderate levels of intensity is suggested with medical clearance.[282] Constant or interval aerobic exercise for at least 20 minutes, at least three times per week for 4 weeks, may lead to improved cardiopulmonary fitness and improved psychologic status, with an accompanying maintenance of immunologic function.[209] Supervised aerobic exercise training safely decreases fatigue, weight, body mass index, fat, and central fat in HIV-1–infected individuals. It may not affect dyspnea.[272]

Clients with advanced disease may be at greater risk for exercise-related injuries due to chronic myopathic and neuropathic tissue changes. Recovery periods after exercise may be prolonged. Response to exercise should be carefully monitored.[150]

Individuals with acute inflammatory myopathy or myositis should not perform strenuous or resisted exercises until creatine phosphokinase levels normalize. Bouts of acute inflammatory arthralgia may require periods of joint protection and relative rest as well as medical management.[150]

Exercise has beneficial effects for those with the AIDS-related wasting syndrome. Progressive resistance exercise can increase lean body mass significantly.[246,247]

The role of exercise in the treatment of lipodystrophic syndrome is important[26] and has been shown to have potential in normalizing insulin resistance, to be effective in managing metabolic abnormalities without causing further side effects,[67] and to reduce trunk fat mass.[248] Short-term intervention of aerobic exercise combined with a low-lipid diet can increase functional capacity but may not change plasma lipid levels.[289]

A THERAPIST'S THOUGHTS*

Working with the Individual Who Has HIV Disease

Almost all individuals with HIV disease have experienced some form of prejudice, social ostracism, or bigotry as a result of being HIV-positive. Some patients have even had such unfortunate experiences in their interactions with health care workers. Individuals with HIV disease do not need sympathy or any special treatment from health care workers. However, we must be mindful that they do need our compassion and empathy, as well as the best possible evidence-based therapy. Providers need to be nonjudgmental, understanding, and ethical with all patients, including those who are HIV-positive. With approximately 1.2 million HIV-positive individuals in the United States (about 1 in every 250 people), it is a certainty that all health care providers will at some point work with HIV-positive individuals.

*David M. Kietrys, PT, PhD, OCS

Chronic Fatigue and Immune Dysfunction Syndrome

Overview

Chronic fatigue and immune dysfunction syndrome, chronic fatigue syndrome (CFS), chronic Epstein-Barr virus, myalgic encephalomyelitis, neuromyasthenia, all denote a highly publicized but not new illness. The name *chronic fatigue syndrome* indicates that this illness is not a single disease but the result of a combination of factors and is actually a subset of *chronic fatigue*, a broader category defined as unexplained fatigue of greater than or equal to 6 months' duration. This distinction is made to facilitate epidemiologic studies of populations with prolonged fatigue and chronic fatigue.

Incidence and Risk Factors

Two U.S. community-based CFS studies found prevalences among adults of 0.23% and 0.42%; the rates were higher in women, members of minority groups, and people with lower educational attainment and occupational status.[137,242]

People of every age, gender, ethnicity, and socioeconomic group can have CFS. Demographic data show that in most studies 75% or more of people with CFS are female. The mean age at onset of CFS is between 29 and 35 years. The mean illness duration ranges from 3 to 9 years.[38] Although CFS is much less common in children than in adults, children can develop the illness, particularly during the teen years.

Etiologic Factors and Pathogenesis

Many studies have investigated the etiology and pathogenesis of CFS.[164] More than half of the CFS studies between 1980 and 1995 concentrated on the physical etiology of CFS, with a slight shift toward psychologic and psychiatric research in the next few years.[64]

Many somatic and psychosocial hypotheses on the etiology of CFS have been explored. Explanations for CFS were sought in viral infections, immune dysfunction, neuroendocrine responses, dysfunction of the CNS, muscle structure, exercise capacity, sleep patterns, genetic constitution, personality, and (neuro)psychologic processes.

Although several studies found abnormalities, only a few were diagnosed in large groups of people with CFS and were independently confirmed in well-controlled studies, an exception being the subtle changes in the hypothalamopituitary–adrenal axis.

Neuroendocrine challenge tests have found a lower-than-normal cortisol response to increased corticotrophin concentrations and upregulation of the serotonergic system. Studies of neuroendocrine function in individuals with CFS have found no evidence for uniform dysfunction of the hypothalamopituitary–adrenal axis or stress hormones.[65] Increasing evidence points to acquired neuroendocrine dysregulations in people with CFS.[102]

However, abnormalities of the neuroendocrine system and CNS alone are not sufficient to explain the symptoms of CFS. More complex interactions between regulating systems are assumed to be at work and seem to involve the CNS, the immune system, and the hormonal regulation system. The etiology and pathogenesis are generally thought to be multifactorial.[58,66]

Personality and lifestyle are presumed to influence vulnerability to CFS. Personality characteristics of neuroticism and introversion have been reported as risk factors for the disorder.[231]

Inactivity in childhood and inactivity after infectious mononucleosis have been found to increase the risk of CFS in adults.[296,303] Also, acute physical or psychologic stress might trigger the onset of CFS.

Three quarters of the individuals with this disorder have reported an infection, such as a cold, flu-like illness, or infectious mononucleosis, as the trigger,[72,252] and high rates of chronic fatigue after Q fever and Lyme disease have been found.[176] Finally, serious life events, such as the loss of a loved one or a job, and other stressful situations have been found to precipitate the disorder.[121,291]

Clinical Manifestations

At illness onset, the most commonly reported CFS symptoms are sore throat, fever, muscle pain, and muscle weakness. As the illness progresses, muscle pain and forgetfulness increase along with prolonged (lasting more than 6 months), often overwhelming fatigue that is exacerbated by minimal physical activity.

Neurally mediated hypotension, caused by disturbances in the autonomic regulation of blood pressure and pulse, is common in people with CFS. This condition is characterized by lowered blood pressure and heart rate accompanied by lightheadedness, visual dimming, or slow response to verbal stimuli. Many people with neurally mediated hypotension experience lightheadedness or worsening fatigue as they stand for prolonged periods or when in warm places (e.g., hot shower, sauna, indoor pool environment).

The severity of CFS varies from person to person, with some people able to maintain fairly active lives. By definition, however, CFS significantly limits work, school, and family activities.

Although symptoms vary from person to person in number, type, and severity, all individuals with CFS are functionally impaired to some degree. CDC studies show that CFS can be as disabling as multiple sclerosis (MS), lupus, rheumatoid arthritis, heart disease, end-stage renal disease, chronic obstructive pulmonary disease, and similar chronic conditions.

CFS often follows a cyclical course, alternating between periods of illness and relative well-being. Some people experience partial or complete remission of symptoms during the course of the illness, but symptoms often reoccur.

This pattern of remission and relapse makes CFS especially hard for clients and their health care professionals to manage. People who are in remission may be tempted to overdo activities when they are feeling better, which can exacerbate symptoms and fatigue and cause a relapse. In fact, postexertional malaise is a hallmark of the illness.[43]

MEDICAL MANAGEMENT

DIAGNOSIS. There are no physical signs or diagnostic laboratory tests that help identify CFS. People who suffer the symptoms of CFS must be carefully evaluated by a physician because many treatable medical and psychiatric conditions are hard to distinguish from CFS.

Common conditions that should be ruled out through a careful medical history and appropriate testing include mononucleosis, Lyme disease, thyroid conditions, diabetes, MS, various cancers, depression, and bipolar disorder.

To aid the identification of this disease, the CDC has developed a working case definition with three criteria to distinguish CFS from other forms of fatigue (Box 7-6). The symptoms must have persisted or recurred during 6 or more consecutive months of illness and must not have predated the fatigue. Research conducted by the CDC indicates that less than 20% of the people with CFS in this country have been diagnosed.[43]

TREATMENT. Because there is no known cure for CFS, treatment is aimed at symptom relief and improved function. A combination of drug and nondrug therapies is usually recommended.

No single therapy exists that helps all individuals with CFS.

Lifestyle changes, including prevention of overexertion, reduced stress, dietary restrictions, gentle stretching, and nutritional supplementation, are frequently recommended in addition to drug therapies used to treat sleep disturbances, pain, and other specific symptoms.

Carefully supervised physical therapy may also be part of treatment for CFS. However, symptoms can be exacerbated by overly ambitious physical activity. A very moderate approach to exercise and activity management is recommended to avoid overactivity and to prevent deconditioning.[43] Systematic reviews have investigated the effectiveness of several CFS treatments, and cognitive behavior therapy and graded exercise therapy are the only interventions found to be beneficial.[230,240,304]

PROGNOSIS. CFS affects each individual differently. Some people with CFS remain homebound and others improve to the point that they can resume work and other activities, even though they continue to experience symptoms.

Box 7-6

CDC DEFINITION OF CHRONIC FATIGUE SYNDROME

Chronic fatigue syndrome (CFS) is a debilitating and complex disorder characterized by intense fatigue that is not improved by bed rest and that may be worsened by physical activity or mental exertion. People with CFS often function at a substantially lower level of activity than they were capable of before they became ill. The cause or causes of CFS have not been identified, and no specific diagnostic tests are available. Therefore, a CFS diagnosis requires three criteria:

1. The individual has had severe chronic fatigue for 6 or more consecutive months that is not due to ongoing exertion or other medical conditions associated with fatigue (these other conditions need to be ruled out by a doctor after diagnostic tests have been conducted)
2. The fatigue significantly interferes with daily activities and work
3. The individual concurrently has 4 or more of the following 8 symptoms:
   - postexertion malaise lasting more than 24 hours
   - nonrestorative sleep
   - significant impairment of short-term memory or concentration
   - muscle pain
   - pain in the joints without swelling or redness
   - headaches of a new type, pattern, or severity
   - tender lymph nodes in the neck or armpit
   - a sore throat that is frequent or recurring

These symptoms must have persisted or recurred during 6 or more consecutive months of illness and must not have predated the fatigue.

Reprinted from Centers for Disease Control and Prevention (CDC): *Chronic fatigue syndrome case definition, 2012.* Available at http://www.cdc.gov/cfs/case-definition/index.html. Accessed February 4, 2013.

The CDC's research shows that those who have CFS for 2 years or less are more likely to improve. It remains unknown if early intervention is responsible for this more favorable outcome; however, the longer a person is ill before diagnosis, the more complicated the course of the illness appears to be.

Recovery rates for CFS are unclear. Improvement rates varied from 8% to 63%, with a median of 40% of clients improving during follow-up. However, full recovery from CFS may be rare, with an average of only 5% to 10% sustaining total remission.[43]

SPECIAL IMPLICATIONS FOR THE THERAPIST   7-4

Chronic Fatigue Syndrome

The client with CFS is treated following guidelines and protocols for autoimmune disorders such as fibromyalgia (see "Fibromyalgia" in this chapter). Pacing, energy conservation (see Box 9-8), stress management, and balancing life activities are extremely helpful in preventing worsening of fatigue and maintaining an even flow of energy from day to day. Support groups may be beneficial in providing emotional and psychologic support and in helping the individual keep up with the latest research results and progress in medical intervention.

Exercise and Chronic Fatigue Syndrome

Carefully controlled and graded exercise is the center of effective intervention for CFS.[99,100,216,227] Many affected individuals fear a relapse and avoid physical activity and exercise, but deconditioning and muscle atrophy increase fatigue and make other symptoms even worse.

The physical therapist can be very instrumental in providing a prescriptive program of regular, moderate exercise to avoid deconditioning while advising against overexertion during periods of remission. During the acute onset or during flare-ups, people with CFS are unable to sustain physical activity or exercise. Beginning with low-level, intermittent physical activity throughout the day to accumulate 30 minutes of exercise has been shown to be effective without exacerbating symptoms.[61]

People with CFS may also have a significantly reduced exercise capacity. Always assess for conditioning before initiating even a simple exercise program with anyone who has had CFS longer than 6 months. Athletes and sports participants may require special help to develop a progressive exercise regimen. Impairments of peak aerobic power and muscle strength may occur with self-imposed or physician-imposed inactivity.[264]

Although abnormal lung function or low concentration of oxygen with accompanying dyspnea or shortness of breath is not a clinical feature of this disease, anyone who is severely deconditioned and then tries to do even light exercise may experience dyspnea. Reaching age-predicted target heart rates may be limited by autonomic disturbances.[71] It may be better to begin a strengthening program before challenging the cardiovascular system.

The therapist must evaluate for altered breathing patterns, components of poor posture, and inefficient or biomechanically faulty movement patterns contributing to pain. Addressing these areas is an important part of the rehabilitation process.

Stretching, strengthening, and cardiovascular training are essential aspects of therapy. Like people with fibromyalgia, those diagnosed with CFS must progress slowly and avoid overexertion since they often do not have the internal mechanism to alert them to stop an activity.

Soft tissue and joint mobilization combined with stretching are important components of intervention, especially in the presence of postural components or faulty mechanics. Prolonged inactivity, rest in poorly supported positions for long periods, and assuming postures dictated by pain can contribute to muscle shortening (see "Modalities and Fibromyalgia" in this chapter).

Over time, some individuals can be progressed to graded aerobic exercise therapy (some can begin at this level depending on the individual clinical presentation). Continuous exercise must be started at a short duration appropriate to the client's baseline ability. A more specific description of how to deliver a graded exercise therapy program to people with CFS is available.[98] This is significantly more effective than just stretching and relaxation exercises.[99,301]

Monitoring Vital Signs

Assessment of vital signs in adults with CFS may demonstrate very large fluctuations in pulse rate and blood pressure, which are not consistent with the person's position or movement. Whereas the blood pressure and pulse rate normally show a slight increase as a physiologic response to a change in position from sitting to standing, orthostatic hypotension is marked in the CFS population. Vital signs may stay the same or even decrease, resulting in dizziness, lightheadedness, or loss of balance. The symptoms may result in decreased self-confidence in the ability to pursue activities.

During the initiation of an exercise program, it is advised to monitor blood pressure, rate of perceived exertion (see Table 12-13), heart rate, and respiratory rate for any signs of physiologic distress. Although the rate of perceived exertion may not change during the exercise session, the individual may perceive fatigue as worse after initiating exercise. However, if this increase in fatigue does not exceed 1 unit on a scale of 1 to 5 from the baseline level established before exercise, symptom exacerbation following exercise can potentially be avoided.[61]

HYPERSENSITIVITY DISORDERS

An exaggerated or inappropriate immune response may lead to various hypersensitivity disorders. Such disorders are classified as type I, II, III, or IV, although some overlap exists (Table 7-4).

Overreaction to a substance, or hypersensitivity, is often referred to as an *allergic response*, and although the term *allergy* is widely used, the term *hypersensitivity* is more appropriate. Hypersensitivity designates an increased

Table 7-4 Clinical Manifestations of Hypersensitivity Disorders

Type I	Type II	Type III	Type IV
Varies according to the allergies present Classic symptoms: • Wheezing • Hypotension • Swelling • Urticaria • Rhinorrhea Anaphylaxis	*General:* malaise, weakness *Dermal:* hives, erythema *Respiratory:* sneezing, rhinorrhea, dyspnea *Upper airway:* hoarseness, stridor; tongue and pharyngeal edema *Lower airway:* dyspnea, bronchospasm, asthma (air trapping), chest tightness, wheezing *Gastrointestinal:* increased peristalsis, vomiting, dysphagia, nausea, abdominal cramps, diarrhea *Cardiovascular:* tachycardia, palpitations, hypotension, cardiac arrest *Central nervous system:* anxiety, seizures	Headache Back (flank) pain Chest pain similar to angina Nausea and vomiting Tachycardia Hypotension Hematuria Urticaria	Fever Arthralgias Lymphadenopathy Urticaria Anemia

immune response to the presence of an antigen (referred to as an *allergen*) that results in tissue destruction. The damage and suffering come predominantly from the immune response itself rather than from the substances that provoke it.

The several types of hypersensitivity reactions include immediate, late phase, and delayed, based on the rapidity of the immune response. *Immediate hypersensitivity reactions* usually occur within minutes of exposure to an allergen. If the skin is affected, blood vessels dilate and fluid accumulates, causing redness and swelling. In the eyes and nose, increased fluid and mucous secretions cause tearing and a runny nose.

Late-phase inflammation and symptoms persist for hours to days after the allergens are removed and can cause cumulative damage (e.g., progressive lung disease) if they persist. *Delayed hypersensitivity reaction* occurs after sensitization to certain drugs or chemicals (e.g., penicillin, poison ivy). These reactions often take several days to cause symptoms.

Type I Hypersensitivity (Immediate Hypersensitivity, Allergic Disorders, Anaphylaxis)

Type I hypersensitivity reactions include hay fever, allergic rhinitis, urticaria, extrinsic asthma, and anaphylactic shock. In this type of immediate hypersensitivity response, IgE, instead of IgG, is produced in response to a pathogen (allergen).

The term *atopy* is often used to describe IgE-mediated diseases. People with atopy have a hereditary predisposition to produce IgE antibodies against common environmental allergens and have one or more atopic diseases.

Allergens are a special class of antigens that cause an allergic response. These normally harmless substances are inhaled (e.g., mold spores, animal dander, dust mites, grasses, weeds), eaten (e.g., nuts, fruits, shellfish, eggs), or injected (e.g., venom from fire ants, wasps, bees, hornets), or they come in contact with the skin or mucous membranes (e.g., plants, cosmetics, metals, drugs, dyes, latex).

IgE resides on mast cells in connective tissue, especially the upper respiratory tract, GI tract, and dermis. When IgE meets the pathogen again, an immediate response occurs with histamine release, along with other inflammatory mediators (e.g., chemotactic factors, prostaglandins, and leukotrienes) that enhance and prolong the response initiated by histamine (Fig. 7-22).

If this response becomes systemic, widespread release of histamine (rather than just local tissue response) results in systemic vasodilation, bronchospasm, increased mucus secretion, and edema, referred to as *anaphylaxis*.

Classic associated signs and symptoms are wheezing, hypotension, swelling, urticaria, and rhinorrhea (clear, runny nose often accompanied by sneezing) (Fig. 7-23). Anaphylaxis is a life-threatening emergency and requires immediate intervention with injected epinephrine to restore blood pressure, strengthen the heartbeat, and open the airways. Bee stings remain the number one cause of anaphylaxis; other triggers include penicillin, foods, animal dander, children, semen, and latex.

A marked increase in the prevalence of atopic disease has occurred in the United States during the last 2 decades, indicating the importance of environmental influences. The mechanisms for this action are outlined in greater detail elsewhere.[146]

Type II Hypersensitivity (Cytotoxic Reactions to Self-Antigens)

When the body's own tissue is recognized as foreign or nonself, activation of complement occurs with subsequent agglutination (clumping together) and phagocytosis of the identified pathogens. This means the cellular membrane of normal tissues (e.g., red blood cells, leukocytes, and platelets) is disrupted and ultimately destroyed. Self-antigen disorders include blood transfusion reactions, hemolytic disease of the newborn, autoimmune hemolytic anemia, and myasthenia gravis (Fig. 7-24).

A second type of hypersensitivity response occurs when there is a cross-reaction between exogenous pathogens and endogenous body tissues, such as in rheumatic fever. For example, group A hemolytic streptococci (the exogenous pathogen) are attacked by the immune system, but the body also misinterprets the mitral valve (endogenous body tissue) as a foreign microorganism (i.e., as streptococci) and attacks normal, healthy tissue in the same way it attempts to destroy the true pathogenic microorganisms. Another example of this type of cross-reaction is an exogenous virus causing the immune system to attack the peripheral nervous system as nonself, such as in acute Guillain-Barré syndrome.

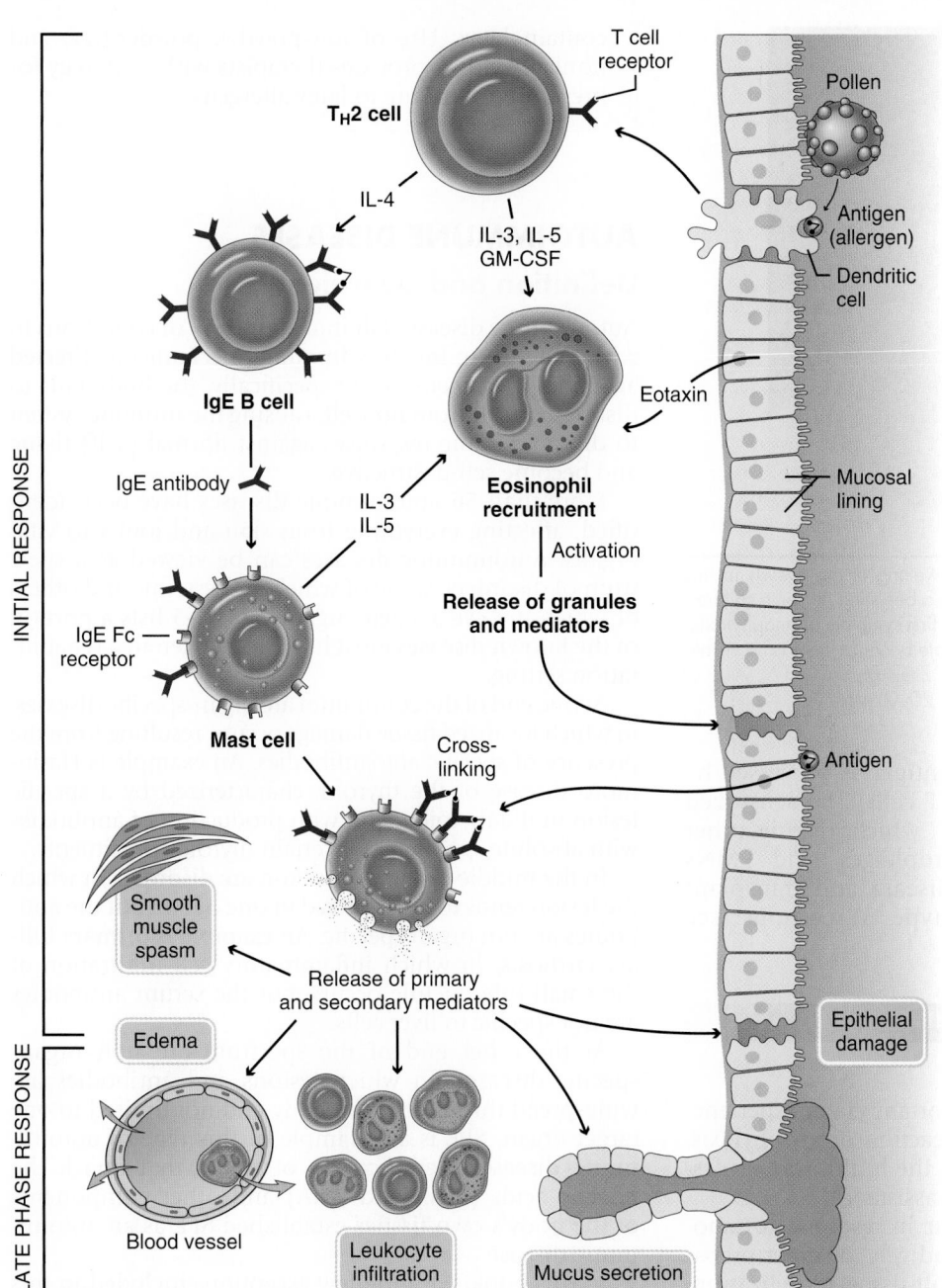

Figure 7-22

Pathogenesis of immediate (type I) hypersensitivity reaction. The late-phase reaction is dominated by leukocyte infiltration and tissue injury. TH2, T-helper type 2 CD4 cells. (Reprinted from Kumar V: *Robbins and Cotran: pathologic basis of disease,* ed 8, Philadelphia, 2009, WB Saunders.)

Type III Hypersensitivity (Immune Complex Disease)

Normally, excessive circulating antigen–antibody complexes called *immune complexes* are effectively cleared by the reticuloendothelial system. When circulating immune complexes (antigen–antibody complexes) successfully deposit in tissues around small blood vessels, they activate the complement cascade and cause acute inflammation and local tissue injury (Fig. 7-25).

The subsequent vasculitis most commonly affects the skin, causing urticaria (wheals); joints, causing synovitis, such as in rheumatoid arthritis; kidneys, causing nephritis; pleura, causing pleuritis; and pericardium, causing pericarditis.

Systemic lupus erythematosus (SLE) is the classic picture of vasculitis, occurring in various organ systems. The antigen is the individual's own nucleus of cells; antinuclear antibodies (ANAs) are made, which, in turn, form a complex with the antigen and are deposited in the skin, joints, and kidneys, causing acute immune injury. Other examples of this hypersensitivity reaction occur in association with infections such as hepatitis B virus and bacterial endocarditis, malignancies, or after drug or serum therapy.

Type IV Hypersensitivity (Cell-Mediated Immunity)

Type IV is a delayed hypersensitivity response such as the reaction that occurs in contact dermatitis after sensitization to an allergen (commonly a cosmetic, adhesive, topical medication, or plant toxin such as poison ivy), latex sensitivity, or the response to a tuberculin skin test present 48 to 72 hours after the test.

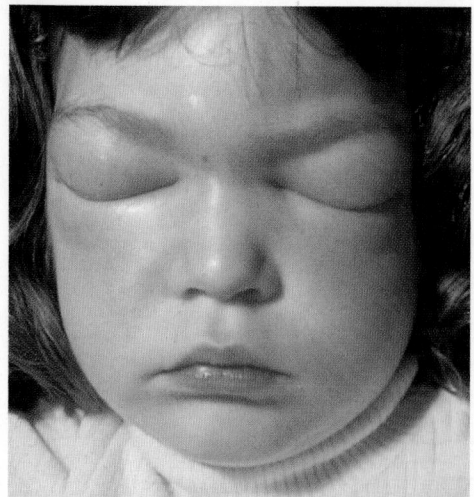

Figure 7-23

Type I hypersensitivity reaction. Severe swelling of the eyelids in this child is the result of an allergic response to a bee sting. In some children and adults, difficulty breathing may be the first symptom of anaphylaxis. Intervention can be delayed until it is too late because there is no visible sign of narrowed airways. (Reprinted from Zitelli BJ, Davis HW: *Atlas of pediatric physical diagnosis*, ed 4, St Louis, 2002, Mosby.)

In this type of reaction, the antigen is processed by macrophages and presented to T cells. The sensitized T cells then release cytokines, which recruit other lymphocytes, monocytes, macrophages, and PMNs (Fig. 7-26). Graft-versus-host disease and transplant rejection are also examples of type IV reactions (see Chapter 21).

SPECIAL IMPLICATIONS FOR THE THERAPIST	7-5

Hypersensitivity Disorders

Immediate action is required for any client experiencing a type I hypersensitivity reaction or anaphylaxis. When a severe reaction occurs, the health care professional must call for emergency assistance.

Type IV reactions may occur in response to lanolin added to lotions, ultrasound gels, or other preparations used in massage or soft-tissue mobilization, requiring careful observation of all people for delayed skin reactions to any of these substances.

With the first exposure, no reaction necessarily occurs but antigens are formed, and on subsequent exposures, hypersensitivity reactions are triggered. Anyone with known hypersensitivity should have a small area of skin tested before use of large amounts of topical agents in the therapy setting. Careful observation throughout treatment is recommended.

Beginning in the 1980s, the use of latex gloves to protect health care workers against exposure to blood and body fluids increased. Since then, the number of reported cases of latex sensitivity also has increased. Reactions to latex range from contact dermatitis (type IV hypersensitivity) to anaphylactic shock (type I hypersensitivity).

Therapists who are allergic to latex should avoid contact with latex gloves and other products that contain latex. Use of low-powder, powder-free, and nonlatex gloves provides therapists with a strategy for preventing exposure to latex allergens.[177]

AUTOIMMUNE DISEASES

Definition and Overview

Autoimmune diseases fall into a category of conditions in which the cause involves immune mechanisms directed against self-antigens. More specifically, the body fails to distinguish self from nonself, causing the immune system to direct immune responses against normal (self) tissue and become self-destructive.

More than 56 autoimmune diseases have been identified, affecting everything from skin and joints to vital organs. Autoimmune diseases can be viewed as a spectrum of disorders, some of which are systemic and others of which involve a single organ. Table 7-5 lists a portion of the known diseases most likely to be seen in a rehabilitation setting.

At one end of the continuum are organ-specific diseases, in which localized tissue damage occurs, resulting from the presence of specific autoantibodies. An example is Hashimoto disease of the thyroid, characterized by a specific lesion in the thyroid gland with production of antibodies with absolute specificity for certain thyroid constituents.

In the middle of the continuum are disorders in which the lesion tends to be localized in one organ, but the antibodies are not organ specific. An example is primary biliary cirrhosis, in which inflammatory cell infiltration of the small bile ductule occurs, but the serum antibodies are not specific to liver cells.

At the other end of the spectrum are non–organ-specific diseases, in which lesions and antibodies are widespread throughout the body and not limited to one target organ. SLE is an example of this type of autoimmune disease. Identification of ANAs that attack the nucleic acids (DNA and RNA) and other components of the body's own tissues established SLE as an autoimmune disease.

In this book, with the few exceptions included in this chapter (e.g., fibromyalgia, CFS, SLE), autoimmune disorders are discussed individually in the most appropriate chapter. For example, Reiter syndrome, rheumatoid arthritis, and Sjögren syndrome are discussed in Chapter 27. Polymyositis, dermatomyositis, and progressive systemic sclerosis are discussed in Chapter 10. Giant cell arteritis is discussed in Chapter 12, sarcoidosis in Chapter 15, and so on. More information is available on autoimmune-related diseases.[12]

Etiologic and Risk Factors

Although the autoimmune disorders are regarded as acquired diseases, their causes often cannot be determined. Autoimmunity is thought to result from a combination of factors, including genetic, hormonal (women are affected more often than men by autoimmune diseases), and environmental influences (e.g., exposure to

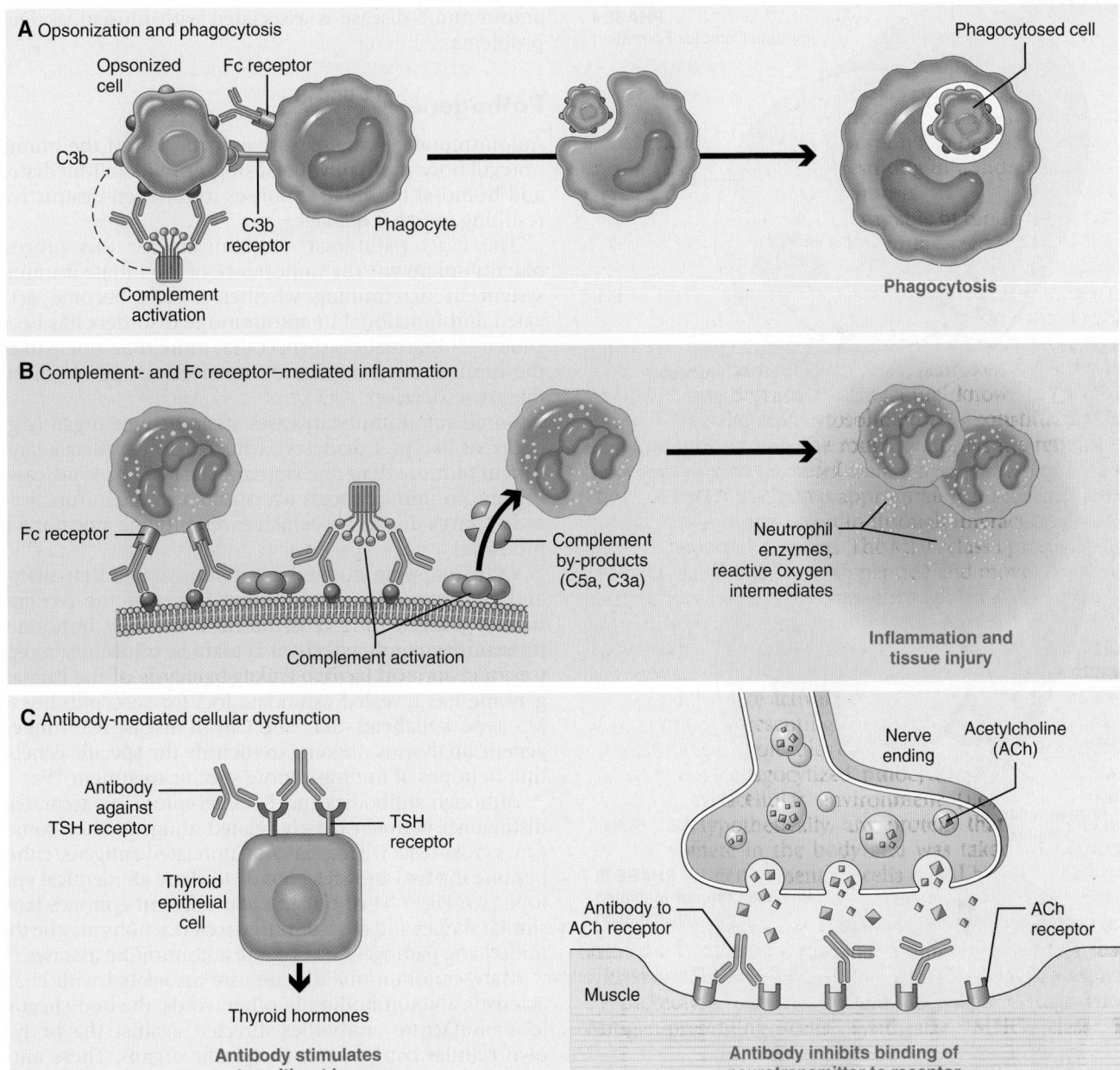

Figure 7-24

Schematic illustration of the three major mechanisms of antibody-mediated injury in type II hypersensitivity reactions. **A,** Opsonization of cells by antibodies and complement components and ingestion by phagocytes. **B,** Inflammation induced by antibody binding to Fc receptors of leukocytes and by complement breakdown products. **C,** Antireceptor antibodies disturb the normal function of receptors. In these examples, antibodies against the thyroid-stimulating hormone (TSH) receptor activate thyroid cells in Graves disease, and acetylcholine (ACh) receptor antibodies impair neuromuscular transmission in myasthenia gravis. (Reprinted from Kumar V: *Robbins and Cotran: pathologic basis of disease,* ed 8, Philadelphia, 2009, WB Saunders.)

chemicals, other toxins, or sunlight and drugs that may destroy suppressor T cells).

Although no single gene has been identified as responsible for autoimmune diseases, clusters of genes seem to increase susceptibility. In most autoimmune disorders, a known or suspected genetic susceptibility is evident, and certain HLA types show increased risk, such as ankylosing spondylitis with HLA-B27 (see Table 40-21).

The influence of hormonal factors is confusing as some autoimmune diseases occur among women in their 20s and 30s, when estrogen is high, and others develop after menopause or before puberty, when estrogen levels are low. During pregnancy, many women with rheumatoid arthritis or MS experience complete remission, whereas pregnant women with SLE often experience exacerbations.

Other factors implicated in the development of immunologic abnormalities resulting in autoimmune disorders include viruses, stress, cross-reactive antibodies, and various autoimmune diseases occurring in women who have had silicone gel breast implants. This organ-specific

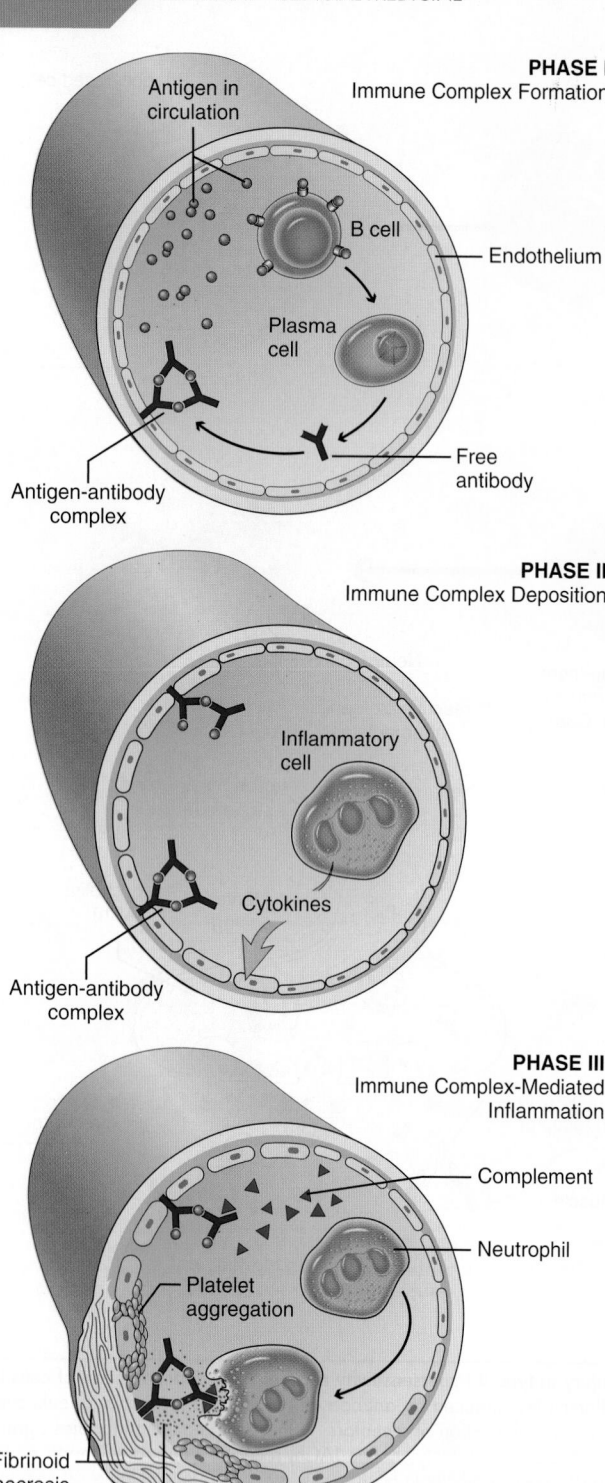

PHASE I
Immune Complex Formation

PHASE II
Immune Complex Deposition

PHASE III
Immune Complex-Mediated Inflammation

Figure 7-25

Schematic of the three sequential phases in the induction of systemic immune complex–mediated disease (type III hypersensitivity). (Reprinted from Kumar V: *Robbins and Cotran: pathologic basis of disease*, ed 8, Philadelphia, 2009, WB Saunders.)

autoimmune disease is associated with musculoskeletal problems.

Pathogenesis

Autoimmune disorders involve disruption of the immunoregulatory mechanism, causing normal cell-mediated and humoral immune responses to turn self-destructive, resulting in tissue damage.

The exact pathologic mechanisms for this process remain unknown. The importance of the innate immune system in determining whether T cells become activated and functional in autoimmune disorders has been shown.[191] Researchers suspect that more than one part of the immune system must be involved for autoimmune disease to develop.

Some autoimmune diseases affect a single organ (e.g., pancreas in type 1 diabetes), whereas others affect a large system or more than one system (e.g., MS). In some cases the autoimmune process overstimulates organ function, as in Graves disease, in which excess thyroid hormone is produced.

Gene-mapping studies have demonstrated that allergy and autoimmunity must involve not only the recognition of antigen by T cells, but also the very important immunoregulatory effects of cytokines, inhibitory receptors, and survival factors. Linkage analysis of the human genome has revealed candidate loci for susceptibility to MS, type 1 diabetes, SLE, and Crohn disease. Continued genetic analysis is ongoing to identify the specific genetic link in hopes of finding a more specific treatment.[141]

Although antibodies and T-cell receptors can accurately distinguish between closely related antigens, they sometimes cross-react with apparently unrelated antigens, either because the two antigens happen to share an identical epitope (see Fig. 7-4) or because two different epitopes have similar shapes and charges. Such cross-reactions may be the underlying pathogenesis of some autoimmune diseases.[74]

Many autoimmune diseases are associated with characteristic autoantibodies. In other words, the body begins to manufacture antibodies directed against the body's own cellular components or specific organs. These antibodies are known as *autoantibodies*, in this case, producing autoimmune diseases.

For example, SLE is associated with anti-DNA and anti-spliceosomal (Sm) antigen, Sjögren syndrome is associated with antiribonucleoproteins (SS-A and SS-B), progressive systemic sclerosis is associated with anticentromere and anti–Scl-70 (DNA topoisomerase), psoriasis and psoriatic arthritis are associated with HLA-B13, and mixed connective tissue disease is associated with antiribonucleoprotein without anti-DNA.

Antibodies specific to hormone receptors on the surface of cells have been found and determined to be partially responsible for some conditions. Examples include myasthenia gravis, in which anti–acetylcholine receptor antibodies are involved; Graves disease, in which antibodies against components of thyroid cell membranes, including the receptors for thyroid-stimulating hormone, are responsible; and certain cases of insulin-resistant diabetes mellitus, in which the antibodies affect insulin receptors on cells.

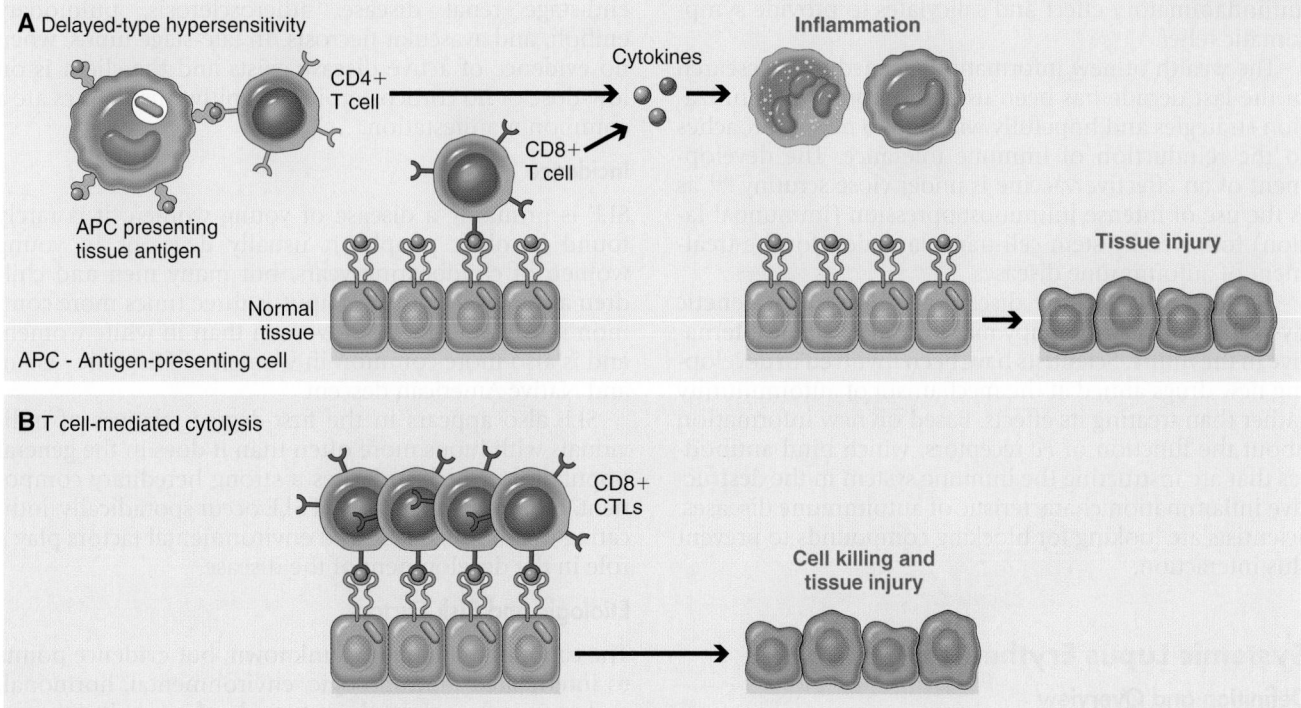

Figure 7-26

Mechanisms of T cell–mediated (type IV) hypersensitivity reactions. A, In delayed-type hypersensitivity reactions, CD4+ T cells (and sometimes CD8+ cells) respond to tissue antigens by secreting cytokines that stimulate inflammation and activate phagocytes, leading to tissue injury. **B,** In some diseases, CD8+ cytolytic T lymphocytes (CTLs) directly kill tissue cells. (Reprinted from Kumar V: *Robbins and Cotran: pathologic basis of disease,* ed 8, Philadelphia, 2009, WB Saunders.)

Table 7-5	Autoimmune Disorders	
Organ-Specific	**Systemic**	
Addison disease	Amyloidosis	
Crohn disease	Ankylosing spondylitis	
Chronic active hepatitis	Mixed connective tissue	
Diabetes mellitus	disease	
Giant cell arteritis	Multiple sclerosis	
Hemolytic anemia	Myasthenia gravis	
Idiopathic thrombocytopenic	Polymyalgia rheumatic	
purpura	Progressive systemic sclerosis	
Polymyositis/dermatomyositis	(scleroderma)	
Postviral encephalomyelitis	Psoriasis (psoriatic arthritis)	
Primary biliary cirrhosis	Reiter syndrome	
Thyroiditis	Rheumatoid arthritis	
Graves disease	Sarcoidosis	
Hashimoto disease	Sjögren syndrome	
Ulcerative colitis	Systemic lupus erythematosus	

Other diseases involving autoimmune mechanisms include rheumatic fever, rheumatoid arthritis, autoimmune hemolytic anemia, idiopathic thrombocytopenic purpura, and postviral encephalomyelitis.

Clinical Manifestations

Autoimmune disorders share certain clinical features, and differentiation among them is often difficult because of this. Common findings include synovitis, pleuritis, myocarditis, endocarditis, pericarditis, peritonitis, vasculitis, myositis, skin rash, alterations of connective tissues, and nephritis. Constitutional symptoms such as fatigue, malaise, myalgias, and arthralgias are also common.

MEDICAL MANAGEMENT

DIAGNOSIS. Diagnosis can be difficult because autoimmune diseases are poorly understood, mimic one another, and often consist of vague symptoms such as lethargy or migratory joint pain. Laboratory tests may reveal thrombocytopenia, leukopenia, immunoglobulin excesses or deficiencies, ANAs, rheumatoid factor, cryoglobulins, false-positive serologic tests, elevated muscle enzymes, and alterations in serum complement. The Coombs test is positive when hemolytic anemia is present.

Some of the laboratory alterations that occur in autoimmune diseases (e.g., false-positive serologic tests, rheumatoid factor) occur in asymptomatic people. These changes may also be demonstrated in certain asymptomatic relatives of people with connective tissue diseases, in older individuals, those taking certain medications, and people with chronic infectious diseases.

TREATMENT. Treatment of autoimmune diseases varies with the specific disease. Treatment must maintain a delicate balance between adequate suppression of the autoimmune reaction to avoid continued damage to the body tissues and maintenance of sufficient functioning of the immune mechanism to protect the person against foreign invaders. In general, autoimmune diseases are treated by the administration of corticosteroids to produce an antiinflammatory effect and salicylates to provide symptomatic relief.

The wealth of new information gleaned from research in the last decade has been used to improve immunization strategies and hopefully will lead to new approaches to the reinduction of immune tolerance. The development of an effective vaccine is under close scrutiny,[141] as is the use of intense immunosuppression (immunoablation) followed by stem cell transplantation for the treatment of autoimmune diseases.

Because autoimmune disease is the result of genetic dysregulation, gene therapy may become a viable alternative in the future. Scientists have been involved in developing new drugs aimed at the mechanism of autoimmunity rather than treating its effects. Based on new information about the function of *Fc* receptors, which bind antibodies that are instructing the immune system in the destructive inflammation characteristic of autoimmune diseases, scientists are looking for blocking compounds to prevent this interaction.

Systemic Lupus Erythematosus

Definition and Overview

Lupus erythematosus, sometimes referred to as *lupus*, is a chronic inflammatory autoimmune disorder that appears in several forms, including *discoid lupus erythematosus* (*DLE*), which affects only the skin (usually face, neck, scalp) (see Chapter 10), and *SLE*, which can affect any organ or system of the body.

The clinical picture of SLE presents on a continuum with different combinations of organ system involvement. The most common of these presentations are latent lupus, drug-induced lupus, antiphospholipid antibody syndrome, and late-stage lupus. *Latent lupus* describes a constellation of features suggestive of SLE but does not qualify as classic SLE. Many people with latent lupus persist with their clinical presentation of signs and symptoms over many years without ever developing classic SLE.

Drug-induced lupus may be diagnosed in people without prior history suggestive of SLE in whom the clinical and serologic manifestations of SLE develop while the person is taking a drug (most often hydralazine used to treat hypertension or procainamide used to treat arrhythmia). The symptoms cease when the drug is stopped, with gradual resolution of serologic abnormalities.

Antiphospholipid antibody syndrome describes the association between arterial and venous thrombosis, recurrent fetal loss, and immune thrombocytopenia with a variety of antibodies directed against cellular phospholipid (lipids in cell membranes containing phosphorus) components. This syndrome may be part of the clinical manifestations seen in SLE, or it may occur as a primary form without other clinical features of lupus.

Late-state lupus is defined as chronic disease duration of greater than 5 years. In such cases, morbidity and mortality are affected by long-term complications of SLE that result either from the disease itself or as a consequence of its therapy. These late complications may include end-stage renal disease, atherosclerosis, pulmonary emboli, and avascular necrosis. In late-stage lupus, when no evidence of active disease exists and the client is on low-dose or no corticosteroids, cognitive disabilities are a common manifestation.

Incidence

SLE is primarily a disease of young women; it is rarely found in older people. It usually develops in young women of childbearing years, but many men and children also develop lupus. Lupus is three times more common in African American women than in white women, and is also more common in women of Hispanic, Asian, and Native American descent.

SLE also appears in the first-degree relatives of individuals with lupus more often than it does in the general population, which indicates a strong hereditary component. However, most cases of SLE occur sporadically, indicating that both genetic and environmental factors play a role in the development of the disease.

Etiologic and Risk Factors

The cause of SLE remains unknown, but evidence points to interrelated immunologic, environmental, hormonal, and genetic factors. With its periods of intermittent exacerbations and flare ups, the theory of a latent virus infection (e.g., Epstein-Barr virus), which occasionally switches to lytic cycle, also makes sense.[82]

But whether SLE represents a single pathologic entity with variable expression or a group of related conditions remains unknown. Immune dysregulation in the form of autoimmunity is thought to be the prime causative mechanism. SLE shows a strong familial link, with a much higher frequency among first-degree relatives. Evidence for genetic susceptibility is present, and linkage studies in conjunction with genome scans may delineate this more specifically in the future.[314]

Genetically determined immune abnormalities may be triggered by both exogenous and endogenous factors. Although the predisposition to disease is hereditary, it is likely to involve different sets of genes in different individuals. As the human genome becomes more extensively mapped, a susceptibility gene may be found, although it remains possible that the differences in disease course among ethnic groups relate solely to their environment and other social factors.

Other factors predisposing to SLE may include physical or mental stress, which can provoke neuroendocrine changes affecting immune cell function; streptococcal or viral infections; exposure to sunlight or ultraviolet light, which can cause inflammation and tissue damage; immunization; pregnancy; and abnormal estrogen metabolism.

Whether pregnancy induces lupus flare-ups has not been established; existing data suggest both that it does and does not. More studies are needed to further determine the effects of pregnancy on this condition.

A higher incidence of SLE exacerbation occurs among women taking even low-dose estrogen contraceptives. Because an increased risk of thrombosis is possible in young women with SLE, estrogen-containing contraceptives are avoided or used at the lowest effective dose.

No evidence exists that postmenopausal estrogen replacement therapy is associated with SLE flare-ups, and because women in this age range are at increased risk for coronary artery disease and osteoporosis, estrogen replacement therapy can be taken. For all women with SLE who have been treated with cyclophosphamide, an increased risk of gynecologic malignancy is evident.[220]

The role of the Epstein-Barr virus as a possible risk factor for SLE remains under investigation.[82,135,179,249] SLE may also be triggered or aggravated by treatment with certain drugs (e.g., quinidine, hydralazine, anticonvulsants, penicillins, sulfa drugs, and oral contraceptives), which could modify both cellular responsiveness and immunogenicity of self-antigens.

Pathogenesis

Three main mechanisms are implicated in the development of lupus: autoantibodies, vascular abnormalities, and inflammatory mediators. The central immunologic disturbance in SLE is autoantibody production (e.g., antineuronal, antiribosomal P, antiphospholipid). The body produces antibodies against its own cells and antigens. Deposition of the combined antigen-antibody complexes at various tissue sites can suppress the body's normal immunity and damage tissues.

In fact, one significant feature of SLE is the ability to produce antibodies against many different tissue components such as red blood cells, neutrophils, platelets, lymphocytes, or almost any organ or tissue in the body. This wide range of antigenic targets has resulted in SLE being classified as a disease of generalized autoimmunity. Given the clinical diversity of SLE, the disease may be mediated by more than one autoantibody system and several immunopathogenic mechanisms.

Specific pathologic findings are organ dependent; for example, repeat biopsies of the kidney show inflammation; cellular proliferation; basement membrane abnormalities; and immune complex deposition comprised of IgM, IgG, and IgA.

Skin lesions demonstrate inflammation and degeneration at the dermal-epidermal junction, with the basal layer being the primary site of injury. Other organ systems affected by SLE are usually studied only at autopsy. Although these tissues may show nonspecific inflammation or vessel abnormalities, pathologic findings are sometimes minimal, suggesting a mechanism other than inflammation as the cause of organ damage or dysfunction.

Clinical Manifestations

Generally, SLE is more severe than discoid lupus, and no two people with SLE will have identical symptoms. For some people, only the skin and joints will be involved. For others, joints, lungs, kidneys, blood, or other organs and/or tissues may be affected.

Musculoskeletal. Arthralgias and arthritis constitute the most common presenting manifestations of SLE, but the onset of SLE may be acute or insidious and may produce no characteristic clinical pattern. Other early symptoms may include fever, weight loss, malaise, and fatigue.

Acute arthritis can involve any joint but typically affects the small joints of the hands, wrists, and knees. It may be migratory or chronic; most cases are symmetrical, but asymmetrical polyarthritis is not uncommon.

Unlike rheumatoid arthritis, the arthritis of SLE is not usually erosive or destructive of bone, and symptoms are not usually severe enough to cause joint deformities, but pain can cause temporary functional impairment. When deformities do occur, ulnar deviation, swan-neck deformity, or fixed subluxations of the fingers often occur as well. Tenosynovitis and tendon ruptures may occur.

Cutaneous and Membranous Lesions. The skin rash occurs most commonly in areas exposed to sunlight (ultraviolet rays) and may be exacerbated by the use of cosmetic products containing alpha hydroxy acids. The classic butterfly rash over the nose and cheeks is common (Fig. 7-27).

Discoid lesions associated with discoid lupus erythematosus are raised, red, scaling plaques with follicular plugging and central atrophy (see Fig. 10-20). This raised edging and sunken center gives them a coinlike appearance (see further discussion in Chapter 10).

Vasculitis (inflammation of cutaneous blood vessels) involving small- and medium-size vessels may cause other skin lesions, including infarctive lesions of the digits (Fig. 7-28) splinter hemorrhages, necrotic leg ulcers, or digital gangrene. Raynaud phenomenon occurs in approximately 20% of people.

Diffuse or patchy alopecia (hair loss) may be temporary, with hair regrowth once the disease is under control. However, permanent hair loss can occur from the extensive scarring of discoid lesions. Painless ulcers of the mucous membranes are common involving the mouth, vagina, and nasal septum.

Cardiopulmonary System. Signs of cardiopulmonary abnormalities may develop as immune complexes are deposited in the pericardial and pleural spaces, (e.g., pleuritis, pericarditis, and dyspnea). Myocarditis, endocarditis, tachycardia, and pneumonitis (acute or chronic) may also occur. Pulmonary hypertension and congestive heart failure are less common and usually secondary to a combination

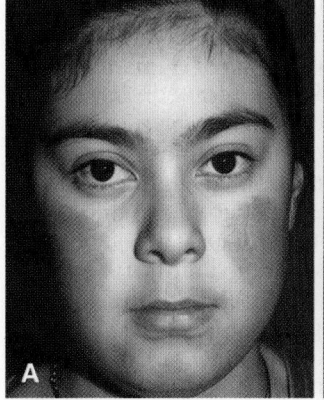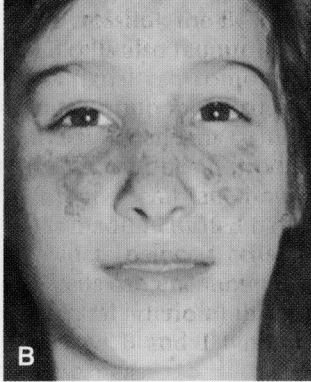

Figure 7-27

The butterfly rash of SLE. The rash can vary from an erythematous blush **(A)** to thickened epidermis to scaly patches **(B).** (Reprinted from Kliegman R, et al: *Nelson textbook of pediatrics,* ed 19, Philadelphia, 2011, WB Saunders.)

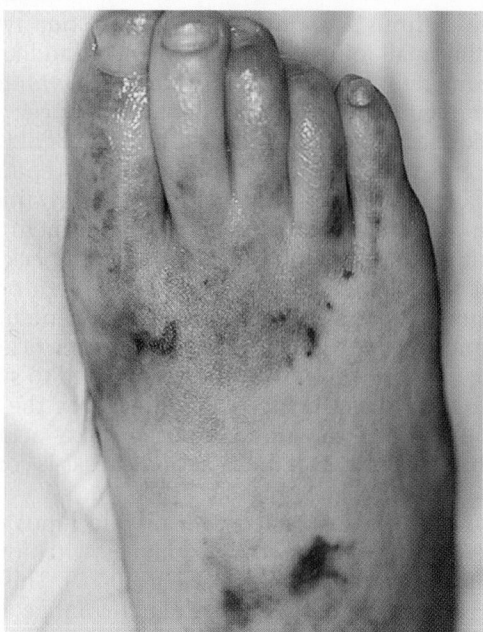

Figure 7-28

A 12-year-old girl with SLE and antiphospholipid antibodies with painful cutaneous vasculitis of the right foot. Arterial thrombosis documented by angiography resulted in cyanosis of the large toe. Symptoms resolved with treatment with heparin and corticosteroids. (Reprinted from Kliegman R, et al: *Nelson textbook of pediatrics*, ed 19, Philadelphia, 2011, WB Saunders.)

of factors. Anyone with SLE with the antiphospholipid antibody syndrome is at a high risk of thrombosis (see "Collagen–Vascular Disease" in Chapter 12).

Central Nervous System. A significant number of people with SLE will have CNS involvement at some point in their illness, sometimes referred to as *neuropsychiatric manifestations*. Clinical manifestations may be related to specific autoantibodies that react with nervous system antigens and/or cytokine-mediated brain inflammation and include headaches, irritability, and depression (most commonly).

Emotional instability, psychosis, seizures, cerebrovascular accidents, cranial neuropathy, peripheral neuropathy, and organic brain syndrome can also occur. Return to the previous level of intellectual function may follow remission of the neuropsychiatric flare, or permanent cognitive impairment may occur.

The pattern of cognitive dysfunction is diverse; intensity can vary within the same person and can be affected by mood.[204] The person may have difficulties with verbal memory, attention, language skills (verbal fluency, productivity), and psychomotor speed. Progressive cognitive impairment, sometimes subtle and sometimes obvious, may develop even in the absence of clinically diagnosed episodes of neuropsychiatric disease.[76] People with SLE may or may not have other signs of lupus when they experience neurologic symptoms.

Renal System. Approximately 50% of individuals with SLE have renal disease (e.g., glomerulonephritis), usually from deposition of immune complexes and resultant inflammation and tissue damage.

Other Systems. Anemia from decreased erythrocytes is a common finding, with associated amenorrhea

(cessation of menstrual flow) among women. Sometimes the spleen and cervical, axillary, and inguinal nodes are enlarged; hepatitis may also develop. Nausea, vomiting, diarrhea, and abdominal pain may occur with GI involvement. All symptoms mentioned in this section can occur at the onset or at any time during the course of lupus. Nearly all people with SLE experience fluctuations in disease activity with exacerbations and remissions.

MEDICAL MANAGEMENT

PREVENTION. There is no known way to prevent SLE, but preventive measures can reduce the risk of flare-ups. For photosensitive people, avoidance of (excessive) sun exposure and/or the regular application of sunscreen usually prevents rashes. Regular exercise helps prevent muscle weakness and fatigue. Immunization protects against specific infections.

Support groups, counseling, and reliance on family members, friends, and health care professionals can help alleviate the effects of stress. Lifestyle choices and personal behavior, such as smoking, excessive consumption of alcohol, too much or too little of prescribed medication, or postponing regular medical checkups, are very important for people with SLE.[162]

DIAGNOSIS. Diagnosis of SLE is difficult because it often mimics other diseases and the symptoms are often vague, varying greatly from individual to individual. The diagnosis and subclassification of SLE is based on a combination of clinical findings and laboratory evidence including pattern of organ involvement.

The Systemic Lupus International Collaborating Clinics (SLICC) group revised and validated the American College of Rheumatology (ACR) SLE classification criteria in 2012. The proposed SLICC classification criteria are based on new knowledge regarding the immunology of SLE.[221] According to this new rule, the diagnosis of SLE depends on the person having at least one clinical or one immunologic criterion *or* biopsy-proven lupus nephritis in the presence of ANAs or anti–double-stranded DNA antibodies.

Clinical criteria include acute or chronic cutaneous lupus, oral ulcers, nonscarring alopecia, synovitis involving two or more joints or tenderness in two or more joints and at least 30 minutes of morning stiffness, serositis (pleurisy, pericardial pain), renal involvement, neurologic manifestations, hemolytic anemia, leucopenia, and thrombocytopenia. *Immunologic criteria* are evaluated through lab studies, including levels of ANA, anti–double-stranded DNA antibody, anti-Sm, antiphospholipid antibody, and low complement. For details of the SLICC classification validation and comparison to previous American Rheumatism Association Diagnostic Criteria for SLE, see Petri et al.[221]

Magnetic resonance imaging scans of the head are usually ordered for all people experiencing new episodes of focal neurologic deficits, seizures, altered consciousness, or psychosis. Neuropsychologic assessment may be helpful for identifying subtle, clinically latent sequelae of CNS events, such as stroke, and in monitoring the response to drug treatment.[75]

TREATMENT. The objectives of medical intervention are to control disease activity, prevent damage from disease, and prevent flare ups that can cause further damage. At the present time, pharmacologic interventions are the primary means of accomplishing these goals and must be customized for each individual to accomplish the treatment goals and spare the person adverse effects of the medications.[101]

Mild symptoms can be managed with nonsteroidal antiinflammatory drugs to relieve muscle and joint pain while reducing tissue inflammation. Corticosteroid-sparing agents (e.g., methotrexate) used earlier preserve bone and offer protection from premature cardiovascular disease. Anticoagulants for individuals who have antiphospholipid antibody syndrome and coagulopathies ensure a more favorable outcome.

Antimalarial agents (e.g., chloroquine [Aralen], hydroxychloroquine [Plaquenil]) are useful against the dermatologic, arthritic, and renal symptoms of this disease. Immunomodulating drugs (e.g., azathioprine [Imuran], cyclophosphamide [Cytoxan]) are immunosuppressive drugs used to suppress inflammation and subsequently the immune system. These are used only with active disease, especially with severe kidney involvement. Corticosteroids and cytotoxic drugs are given in more severe disease that has not responded to these other types of drug therapy.

Biologic immune-targeted treatments such as B-cell–targeted therapy, cytokine blockade, and peptide-based treatments are being developed based on current understanding of the dysregulated immunologic pathways involved in SLE pathogenesis.[25] Stem cell transplantation for severe SLE remains under investigation; early results have not been favorable.[186]

PROGNOSIS. The prognosis improves with early detection and intervention that prevents organ damage and improves life expectancy. The overall reduction in the use of large doses of corticosteroids over the past 2 decades has significantly reduced morbidity and mortality rates.

People with SLE have an increased prevalence of valvular and atherosclerotic heart disease, apparently because of factors related to the disease itself and to drug therapy necessary in severe cases. Symptomatic large-vessel occlusive disease in SLE, occurring several years after the diagnosis of the disease, is associated with a relatively poor short-term outcome. There is an increased risk of certain cancers in SLE; the risk appears to be most heightened for lymphoma.[22]

Prognosis is less favorable for those who develop cardiovascular, renal, or neurologic complications or severe bacterial infections. High stress, poor social support, and psychologic distress are modifiable factors associated with health outcomes for people with SLE.[78,299]

SPECIAL IMPLICATIONS FOR THE THERAPIST   **7-6**

Systemic Lupus Erythematosus

Physical and occupational therapy intervention can be important components of the overall treatment plan for lupus. Recurrence of disease can be managed with carefully controlled and sometimes restricted activities. After an exacerbation, gradual resumption of activities must be balanced by maximum rest periods, usually

8 to 10 hours of sleep a night and several rest periods during the day.

Most of the principles and reference materials outlined in the following section on fibromyalgia also apply to SLE. Management of joint involvement follows protocols for rheumatoid arthritis (see "Special Implications for the Therapist: Rheumatoid Arthritis" in Chapter 27). Clients with skin lesions should be examined thoroughly at each visit. The therapist can be instrumental in teaching and assisting with skin care and prevention of skin breakdown.

Functional limitations among people with SLE vary according to the type and degree of the disease. Generalized fatigue, defined as "the inclination to rest, even though pain and weakness are not limiting factors," is a common problem and can be very debilitating, especially for those individuals with both SLE and fibromyalgia.[8]

The therapist can be very instrumental in teaching clients how to avoid lupus flares by spacing activities and conserving energy (see Box 9-8), following a prescriptive exercise plan, avoiding excessive bed rest, and protecting joints. Excessive bed rest can worsen fatigue, promote muscle disuse and atrophy, and promote osteoporosis. Prescriptive exercise should strengthen the muscles and improve endurance while avoiding undue stress on inflamed joints. Patient education should include identifying triggers (e.g., too much work, not enough rest, emotional stress, poor diet, ultraviolet light exposure) and self-monitoring for the earliest signs of a flare-up. The person with SLE must limit exposure to direct sunlight (and take sun exposure precautions), fluorescent light, halogen lamps, overhead lights, computer screens, and photocopiers both at home, in public, and at work.

Attention to socioeconomic factors is important because women of color are disproportionately affected by this autoimmune disease and may not receive the full care needed to manage a chronic condition of this type. Working with other members of the health care community, especially social workers can be very helpful in meeting the goals and needs of these individuals.[125]

Septic arthritis or osteonecrosis may develop as a complication of SLE or its treatment (e.g., steroid medications). Septic arthritis is uncommon in SLE, but it should be suspected when one joint is inflamed out of proportion to the others. People with SLE may develop a drug-related myopathy secondary to corticosteroids or as a complication of antimalarials (see "Corticosteroid Myopathy" in Chapter 5).

Anyone taking corticosteroids or immunosuppressants must be monitored carefully for signs of infection, especially people at heightened risk of infection such as those with renal failure, cardiac valvular abnormalities, or ulcerative skin lesions. (See specific side effects and "Special Implications for the Therapist 5-5: Corticosteroids" in Chapter 5). The client should contact the physician if a fever or any other new symptoms develop. The therapist can provide osteoporosis prevention and intervention management.

High-dose oral corticosteroid treatment remains the major predisposing cause of avascular necrosis in SLE and other autoimmune disorders. The most common site is the femoral head of the hip; less commonly, the femoral condyle of the knee is affected. Although the condition may be bilateral, it most often presents with an insidious onset of unilateral hip or knee pain that is worse with ambulating but often present at rest. Symptoms are progressive over weeks to months.

Observe carefully for any sign of renal involvement such as weight gain, edema, or hypertension. Take seizure precautions if there are signs of neurologic involvement. The therapist may recognize signs of cognitive dysfunction or decline, either directly observed in the client or by family report. These manifestations should be reported to the physician for consideration in evaluating medications. If Raynaud phenomenon is present, teach the client to warm and protect the hands and feet (see "Special Implications for the Therapist: Peripheral Vascular Disease/Raynaud Phenomenon" in Chapter 12).

A discussion of pregnancy and SLE is beyond the scope of this text but may be of importance to the therapist involved in women's health issues. More detailed information is available elsewhere.[193,237,238,281]

Fibromyalgia

Definition and Overview

Fibromyalgia or fibromyalgia syndrome (FMS), formerly mislabeled or misdiagnosed as fibrocytis, fibromyositis, myofascial pain, CFS, or SLE, is a chronic muscle pain syndrome. Fibromyalgia is defined as chronic widespread pain with allodynia or hyperalgesia to pressure pain, and is classified as one of the largest groups of soft-tissue pain syndromes (not a disease).[3] Simply stated, it is a disorder of pain processing (i.e., abnormal pain modulation with hypersensitivity to painful stimuli and reduced pain inhibition).[277]

Sometimes FMS occurs as a result of some other medical condition. For example, individuals with inflammatory conditions (e.g., rheumatoid arthritis, polymyalgia rheumatic, SLE), metabolic dysfunction (e.g., thyroid problems), or cancer often develop a type of FMS referred to as *reactive* fibromyalgia. It is important to identify whether or not the FMS is *primary* (the main problem) or *secondary/reactive* (caused by other problems).

Fibromyalgia has been differentiated from myofascial pain (see "Myofascial Pain Syndrome" in Chapter 27) in that fibromyalgia is considered a systemic problem involving biochemical, neuroendocrine, and physiologic abnormalities, with widespread multiple tender points as one of the key symptoms.

Myofascial pain is a localized condition specific to a muscle and may involve as few as one or as many as several areas with characteristic trigger points that are painful and refer pain to other areas when pressure is applied. The person with FMS may have both tender points and trigger points requiring specific treatment interventions for each.

The person with myofascial pain syndrome does not exhibit other associated constitutional or systemic signs or symptoms unless palpation elicits a painful enough response to elicit an autonomic nervous system response

with nausea and/or vomiting, increased blood pressure, and increased pulse.

It has been proposed that fibromyalgia and CFS are two names for the same syndrome, with CFS being an early form of FMS, but at present CFS is thought to differ by the greater degree of fatigue. People with fibromyalgia tend to experience more pain. In contrast to CFS, fibromyalgia is associated with a variety of initiating or perpetuating factors such as psychologically distressing events, primary sleep disorders, inflammatory rheumatic arthritis, and acute febrile illness.

Fibromyalgia and CFS have similar disordered sleep physiology, and evidence suggests a reciprocal relationship of the immune and sleep–wake systems. Interference with either system has effects on the other and will be accompanied by the symptoms of CFS.[194] A significant number of people with FMS meet the criteria for CFS and vice versa.

Incidence

Fibromyalgia occurs in more than 6 million Americans. It has now surpassed rheumatoid arthritis as the most common musculoskeletal disorder in the United States.[168] Women are affected more often than men (90% are women), with symptoms appearing between the ages of 20 and 55 years, although it has been diagnosed in children as young as 6 years and adults as old as 85 years.

Risk Factors

Risk factors or triggering events for the onset of fibromyalgia may include prolonged anxiety and emotional stress, trauma (e.g., motor vehicle accident, work injury, surgery), rapid steroid withdrawal, hypothyroidism, and viral and nonviral infections. Exposure to tobacco products has been suggested as a possible risk factor for the development of fibromyalgia but this has not been investigated fully or proven.[302]

Fibromyalgia may also develop with no obvious precipitating events or illnesses. It is more prevalent in minimally to moderately physically fit persons and is not usually found in highly trained athletes. Anxiety, depression, and posttraumatic stress disorder (perhaps associated with physical and/or sexual abuse in childhood and adulthood)[122,274] also seem to be linked with FMS.[29] Having a bipolar illness increases the risk of developing FMS dramatically.[297]

Claims that fibromyalgia is linked with cosmetic breast implants are not supported by the scientific literature.[175] However, it has been reported that women with extracapsular silicone (silicone gel outside of the fibrous scar that forms around breast implants) as a result of rupture are more likely to report having fibromyalgia.[33,34] At the time of this text revision, no new data had been reported to support or refute this finding.

Etiologic Factors

Research is now ongoing to determine the cause of fibromyalgia; most likely the initiation of this condition is multifactorial (Fig. 7-29). Possible etiologic theories include diet; viral origin; sleep disorder; occupational, seasonal, or environmental influences; and adverse childhood experiences, including sexual abuse[92,225] Psychologic and

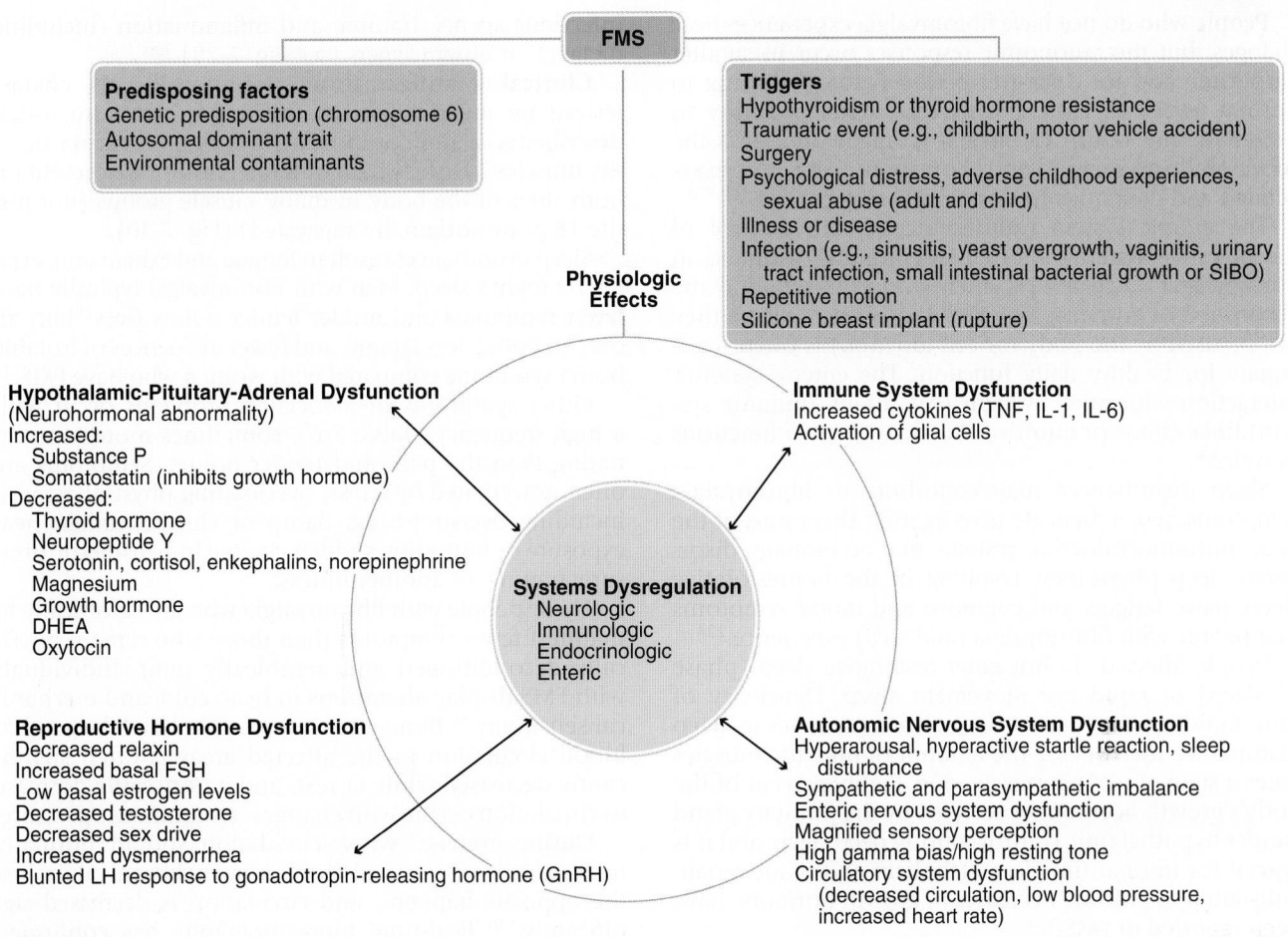

FMS

Predisposing factors
Genetic predisposition (chromosome 6)
Autosomal dominant trait
Environmental contaminants

Triggers
Hypothyroidism or thyroid hormone resistance
Traumatic event (e.g., childbirth, motor vehicle accident)
Surgery
Psychological distress, adverse childhood experiences,
    sexual abuse (adult and child)
Illness or disease
Infection (e.g., sinusitis, yeast overgrowth, vaginitis, urinary
    tract infection, small intestinal bacterial growth or SIBO)
Repetitive motion
Silicone breast implant (rupture)

Physiologic Effects

Hypothalamic-Pituitary-Adrenal Dysfunction
(Neurohormonal abnormality)
Increased:
    Substance P
    Somatostatin (inhibits growth hormone)
Decreased:
    Thyroid hormone
    Neuropeptide Y
    Serotonin, cortisol, enkephalins, norepinephrine
    Magnesium
    Growth hormone
    DHEA
    Oxytocin

Immune System Dysfunction
Increased cytokines (TNF, IL-1, IL-6)
Activation of glial cells

Systems Dysregulation
Neurologic
Immunologic
Endocrinologic
Enteric

Reproductive Hormone Dysfunction
Decreased relaxin
Increased basal FSH
Low basal estrogen levels
Decreased testosterone
Decreased sex drive
Increased dysmenorrhea
Blunted LH response to gonadotropin-releasing hormone (GnRH)

Autonomic Nervous System Dysfunction
Hyperarousal, hyperactive startle reaction, sleep
    disturbance
Sympathetic and parasympathetic imbalance
Enteric nervous system dysfunction
Magnified sensory perception
High gamma bias/high resting tone
Circulatory system dysfunction
    (decreased circulation, low blood pressure,
    increased heart rate)

Figure 7-29

Multifactorial causes of FMS. There are many hypotheses and models of how multiple factors contribute to the development of FMS. This model represents data thus far to support FMS as a biologic (organic) disorder caused by neurohormonal dysfunction of the autonomic nervous system. The physiologic effects of four primary systems dysfunction are listed.

cognitive/behavioral factors seem to cooccur with FMS including psychiatric disorders such as major depression, anxiety disorders, personality disorders, altered pain perception and catastrophizing.[305]

Familial aggregation of fibromyalgia and a reduced pain threshold in first-degree female relatives of affected individuals (even in family members without obvious clinical symptoms) provides evidence of fibromyalgia as a heritable disorder. Clear genetic markers have not been identified; candidate genes linked to fibromyalgia support a genetic (biologic) basis for this condition in some people.[169] How much is genetic influence and how much can be attributed to shared environment remains unknown at this time.[5,23]

Pathogenesis

Its pathogenesis is not entirely understood, although it is currently thought to be the result of a CNS malfunction that increases pain transmission and perception[3] accompanied by ineffective pain inhibition.[277] Fibromyalgia syndrome is currently perceived by rheumatologists and pain physicians alike as representing the classic condition of central sensitization.[4] Accumulating evidence suggests the underlying cause of fibromyalgia pain results from abnormal pain processing particularly in the CNS rather than from dysfunction in peripheral tissues where pain is perceived.[218]

Previous theories that abnormalities of the hypothalamic–pituitary–adrenal axis were the cause of FMS have been set aside as only a small subset of individuals demonstrate these abnormalities as a precipitating factor. There is no doubt the hypothalamic–pituitary–adrenal axis is involved, but it looks more like the onset of fibromyalgia may bring about disturbances in the regulatory systems of the body, not the other way around.[305]

Autonomic Nervous System. Many researchers have shown that people with fibromyalgia have an autonomic nervous system with a hyperactive sympathetic branch (fight-flight-fright-freeze mode) and an underactive parasympathetic (rest and digest) branch. The activity of the skeletal muscles, heart, stomach, intestines, blood vessels, and sweat glands during daily stress tends to be excessive in fibromyalgia. These organs overactivate, resulting in the heart beating faster, the stomach secreting excessive digestive juices and contracting erratically, the smooth muscles of the intestines and bowel contracting abnormally, breathing becoming rapid and shallow, and blood vessels constricting, which decreases blood flow to body parts. These and other autonomic nervous system responses may occur in response to a relatively mild life stressor and linger even after cognitive memory of the event is gone.[79]

People who do not have fibromyalgia experience these changes, but the autonomic responses occur in smaller amplitude and for a shorter period before returning to normal levels. In FMS, the nervous system's ability to modulate and return to normal is fragile and lacks the subtle ability to respond quickly; responses are more exaggerated and the return to normal takes more time.[130,315]

The enteric system (autonomic nervous control of the digestive system) is often significantly disrupted in fibromyalgia. Digestion is often compromised, and the absorption of nutrients into the bloodstream (where they can be used by the body for cell function) is often inadequate for healthy daily function. The enteric system's interaction with other systems (e.g., brain, immune system) links effects of nutritional deficits to other functions as well.[130]

Sleep disturbances may contribute to fibromyalgia symptoms; researchers are investigating alterations of the neuroimmunoendocrine systems that accompany disordered sleep physiology, resulting in the nonrestorative sleep, pain, fatigue, and cognitive and mood symptoms that people with fibromyalgia (and CFS) experience.[228]

People affected do not enter restorative sleep (phase IV sleep) or rapid eye movement sleep. Deficiency of non–rapid eye movement sleep also contributes to sleep disturbance by reducing the amount of time the muscles enter a state of resting muscle tone. Eighty percent of the body's growth hormone is secreted by the pituitary gland (under hypothalamic control) during deep sleep, and it is crucial for normal muscle metabolism and tissue repair. Substantial nighttime decreases in growth hormone have been reported in FMS.[164]

These types of sleep disturbances are not unique to fibromyalgia but have been observed in many people with rheumatoid arthritis, osteoarthritis, and other painful rheumatic diseases.

Immune System. Finally, a model for pathologic pain syndromes such as FMS and CFS has been formulated based on pain facilitory effects produced by the immune system. Immune cells, activated in response to infection, inflammation, or trauma, release proinflammatory cytokines that signal the CNS to release glia within the brain and spinal cord. Pain has been classically viewed as being mediated solely by neurons, but the discovery that spinal cord glia (microglial and astrocytes) amplify pain has changed this view.

When glial cells become activated by sensory signals arriving from the periphery, they can release a variety of substances known to be involved in chronic pain (e.g., nerve growth factor, excitatory amino acids, nitric oxide), and they can also control the release of neurotransmitters (e.g., substance P).

Once activated, such as when viruses and bacteria enter the CNS, glial cells cause prolonged release of proinflammatory cytokines (e.g., TNF, IL-1, IL-6), creating an exaggerated pain state. Glia may be the key driving force for the pain created by tissue inflammation and nerve injury because they can increase the release of pain transmitters and cytokines from the neurons in the surrounding area, and they are connected to large networks that allow activation of glia at distant sites.

This pain model emphasizes again the need for anyone with FMS to minimize pain-generating aggravants such as

infectious agents, trauma, and inflammation (including dietary), or other triggers (see Fig. 7-29).[300]

Clinical Manifestations. Fibromyalgia is characterized by muscle pain as the major symptom, often described as aching or burning, a "migraine headache of the muscles." Diffuse pain or tender points are present on both sides of the body in many muscle groups (not just the 18 points originally suggested) (Fig. 7-30).

Sleep disturbances result in fatigue and exhaustion, even after a night's sleep. Men with fibromyalgia typically have fewer symptoms and milder tender points (less "hurt all over" reports), less fatigue, and fewer incidences of irritable bowel syndrome compared with women who have FMS.[3]

Other symptoms or associated problems occur with a high frequency (Table 7-6), sometimes more incapacitating than the pain and tender points. Symptoms are often exacerbated by stress; overloading physical activity, including overstretching; damp or chilly weather; heat exposure or humidity; sudden change in barometric pressure; trauma; or another illness.

Those people with fibromyalgia who are aerobically fit manifest fewer symptoms than those who remain physically deconditioned and aerobically unfit. Individuals with FMS display alterations in heat, cold, and mechanical sensitivity.[31] Biofeedback specialists have shown that blood circulation to the affected areas is often significantly decreased while at rest, and a noticeable decrease in circulation occurs with changes in barometric pressure.

During exercise, when circulation should normally increase to muscles and the brain, in fibromyalgia just the opposite happens, and circulation is decreased significantly.[130] Real-time ultrasonography has confirmed the lower magnitude of muscle vascularity following dynamic and during static exercise. The immediate flow response to muscular activity was lower in magnitude and of a shorter duration in people with fibromyalgia compared to healthy controls.[87]

The diaphragm is significantly affected in fibromyalgia to the point that it ceases to function as the major breathing muscle, and accessory muscles of the neck and upper chest take over. This overwork results in tender points or tightness of the neck and chest muscles.

In general, the level of muscular activity in fibromyalgia is high, even when the body is sitting or reclining. During daily activities such as cleaning, cooking, typing, and even socializing, the muscles used for these activities are at a higher level of activity than the muscles of a normal person doing the same tasks.

When the activity is over and the person with fibromyalgia is resting, those same muscles continue to repeat the activity over and over at a lower intensity so that no outward movement is apparent. At the same time, increased pain sensation after repeated exposure to a stimulus creates central sensitization. This phenomenon called the "wind-up response," combined with increased central pain processing, may lower tender point thresholds and result in prolonged after-sensations.[305]

MEDICAL MANAGEMENT

DIAGNOSIS. No definitive test is currently available to determine the presence of fibromyalgia, and usually the organs involved are not the cause but merely the

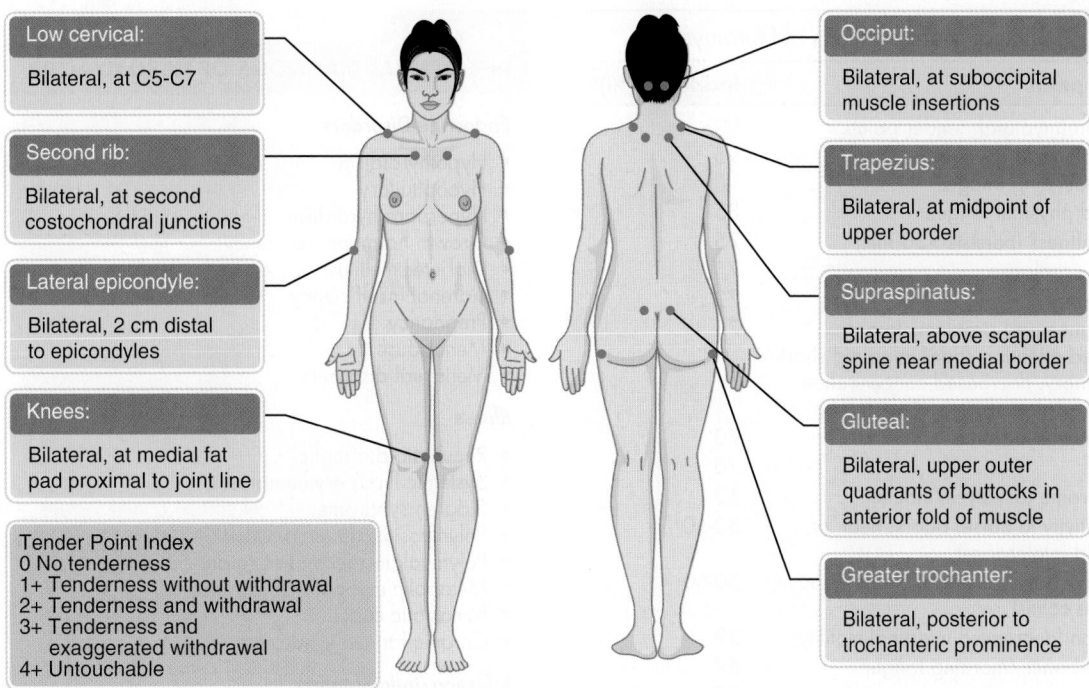

Low cervical:
Bilateral, at C5-C7

Second rib:
Bilateral, at second costochondral junctions

Lateral epicondyle:
Bilateral, 2 cm distal to epicondyles

Knees:
Bilateral, at medial fat pad proximal to joint line

Tender Point Index
0 No tenderness
1+ Tenderness without withdrawal
2+ Tenderness and withdrawal
3+ Tenderness and exaggerated withdrawal
4+ Untouchable

Occiput:
Bilateral, at suboccipital muscle insertions

Trapezius:
Bilateral, at midpoint of upper border

Supraspinatus:
Bilateral, above scapular spine near medial border

Gluteal:
Bilateral, upper outer quadrants of buttocks in anterior fold of muscle

Greater trochanter:
Bilateral, posterior to trochanteric prominence

Figure 7-30

Anatomic locations of tender points associated with fibromyalgia. According to the literature, digital palpation should be performed with an approximate force of 4 kg (enough pressure to indent a tennis ball), but clinical practice suggests much less pressure is required to elicit a painful response. For a tender point to be considered positive, the subject must state that the palpation was "painful." A reply of "tender" is not considered a positive response. Counting the number of points as part of the clinical diagnosis of FMS has been discounted[215]; however, the presence of multiple tender points is still a key feature of FMS. (Reprinted from Goodman CC, Snyder T: *Differential diagnosis for physical therapists: screening for referral*, ed 5, Philadelphia, 2013, WB Saunders.)

messenger of a problem originating elsewhere in the body. Research underway to find biomarkers for CFS and fibromyalgia has discovered increases in the expression of sensory, adrenergic, and immune genes not found in normal subjects. These changes were only observed after sustained moderate exercise.[173]

The ACR has used two criteria for a medical diagnosis of FMS: (1) widespread (four-quadrant) pain both above and below the waist present for at least 3 months and (2) subjective report of pain when pressure is applied to 11 of the 18 common FMS tender points on the body (see Fig. 7-30).

Subjective assessment of tender points can be elicited by the use of an instrument called a *dolorimeter*, which distributes pressure equally over a discrete point. With a dolorimeter, the pressure required to produce pain in a given area can be recorded.

Controversy also exists regarding current use of the ACR's criteria for tender point count in clinical diagnosis of FMS. In fact, the original author of the ACR criteria has suggested that counting the tender points was "perhaps a mistake" and has advised against using it in clinical practice as the only means of diagnosis.[308,310]

A Symptom Intensity Scale was subsequently developed and validated by Wolfe to help differentiate FMS from other rheumatologic conditions (e.g., SLE or polymyalgia rheumatica) with similar widespread pain.[307,311]

Since that time, Wolfe and associates have proposed new diagnostic criteria, which the ACR has adopted.[309,310] The new tool focuses on measuring symptom severity rather than relying on the tender point examination. The new criteria use a clinician-queried checklist of painful sites and a symptom severity scale that focuses on fatigue, cognitive dysfunction, and sleep disturbance. Tender point assessment still has value; people with fewer than 11 of the 18 tender points included in the ACR classification criteria may still be diagnosed with fibromyalgia if they have other clinical features consistent with fibromyalgia.[23,149]

Often, the diagnosis is determined as a process of elimination by ruling out other conditions based on clinical presentation and past medical history (Box 7-7). In addition to the presence of tender points, skin fold tenderness, increased reactive skin hyperemia, and low tissue compliance (in the trapezius and paraspinal regions) provide further diagnostic information.

No special laboratory or radiologic testing is necessary for making a diagnosis of FMS; routine testing for rheumatoid factor or ANAs is not recommended. Although routine inexpensive tests, including complete blood count, basic chemistry (blood urea nitrogen, creatinine, hepatic enzymes, serum calcium), and thyroid function, should be undertaken (if not done in the past year), any other test to rule out other conditions, unless clinically indicated (by both symptoms and physical examination), is a waste of time and resources.

A routine complete blood count test may demonstrate anemia caused by medications or another disease, which may contribute to fatigue, and cytopenia; a baseline chemistry test is useful in monitoring various medication side effects. Because spinal pain in FMS and pain caused by pathologic changes in the spine (e.g., osteoarthritis

Table 7-6   Clinical Manifestations of Fibromyalgia

Sign/Symptom	Incidence (%)*
Muscle pain (myalgia), tender points	99
Visual problems (e.g., blurring, double vision, bouncing images)	95
Mental and physical fatigue	85
Morning stiffness (persists >30 min)	75
Mitral valve prolapse	75
Global anxiety	72
Cognitive (memory) problems (e.g., decreased attention span, impaired short-term memory, decreased concentration, increased distractibility)	71
Irritable bowel syndrome	70
Headaches	70
Sicca syndrome (dry eyes/mouth)	63
Hypersensitivity to noise, odors, heat, or cold (cold intolerance)	50-60
Inflammatory bowel disease (Crohn disease, ulcerative colitis)	50-60
Constipation (decreased intestinal motility)	59
Sleep disturbance/morning fatigue	57
Dizzy or faint going from sit-to-stand	57
Paresthesias	50
Swollen feeling (joint or soft tissues)	50
Muscle spasms or nodules	50
Reactive hypoglycemia (e.g., weakness, irritability, disorientation)	45-50
Pelvic pain	43
Irritable bladder syndrome, female urethral syndrome	40
Hypotension (low blood pressure, elevated heart rate); neurally mediated hypotension or vasopressor syncope	40
Raynaud phenomenon	38
Respiratory dysfunction (e.g., dyspnea, erratic breathing patterns during exertion)	33
Lack of libido	33
Restless leg syndrome, nocturnal myoclonus, periodic leg movement disorder	30-60
Diaphoresis (unexplained sweating)	30
Auditory problems	30
Temporomandibular dysfunction	25
Depression	20
Allergies	Unknown
Skin discoloration	Unknown
Sciatica	Unknown

*These figures were compiled from a variety of sources but represent a fairly accurate clinical perspective.

Data from Solano C: Autonomic dysfunction in fibromyalgia assessed by the Composite Autonomic Symptoms Scale (COMPASS), *J Clin Rheumatol* 15(4):172–176, 2009.

and osteopenia with vertebral compression fracture) cannot always be distinguished clinically, a spinal x-ray may be necessary for a middle-aged or older adult, especially considering other risk factors for these conditions. It is important not to miss these diagnoses, because the management approach is likely to be different from FMS alone. A sleep study should be considered only when history suggests a primary sleep disorder.[316]

Box 7-7

DIFFERENTIAL DIAGNOSIS OF FIBROMYALGIA

Endocrine Disorders

- Hypothyroidism
- Hypopituitary
- Hyperparathyroidism
- Growth hormone deficiency
- Diabetes mellitus
- Adrenal insufficiency
- Pregnancy
- Menopause
- Menstrual disorders

Illness

- Rheumatoid arthritis
- Systemic lupus erythematosus
- Sjögren syndrome
- Polymyositis/dermatomyositis
- Polymyalgia rheumatica/giant cell arteritis
- Metabolic myopathy (e.g., alcohol)
- Metastatic cancer
- Chronic fatigue syndrome

Infection/Inflammation

- Subacute bacterial endocarditis
- Lyme disease
- Hepatitis C
- AIDS
- Chronic syphilis
- Tuberculosis

Other

- Temporomandibular joint dysfunction
- Disk disease
- Myofascial pain syndrome
- Silicone breast implant
- Neurosis (depression/anxiety)
- Substance abuse
- Malnutrition
- Allergies (including food intolerances)

Data from Cleveland Clinic: *Current clinical medicine*, ed 2, Philadelphia, 2010, WB Saunders.

TREATMENT. Effective treatment of the widespread pain of FMS attributed mainly to an increase in the processing and handling of pain by the CNS must be directed toward function of the CNS.[4] Current clinical practice guidelines of several American and European medical societies recommend a multimodal, holistic, and multidisciplinary[13,120,257] approach, including education and support, stress management, nutrition and lifestyle training (e.g., coping strategies, applying work simplification and ergonomic principles, and cognitive-behavioral therapy), medications (e.g., antidepressants,[123] muscle relaxants, analgesics, and anticonvulsants), local modalities and techniques for muscle pain (e.g., relaxation techniques, biofeedback, Physiologic Quieting, or soft-tissue techniques, electrotherapy), and conditioning and aerobic exercise.

Cognitive behavioral therapy, especially combined with exercise, is strongly recommended.[120,155] This approach is aimed at altering sensory, affective, cognitive, and behavioral aspects of chronic pain (e.g., pain severity, emotional distress, depression, anxiety, pain behavior) and is effective over a long period, even when the disease process cannot be controlled and symptoms worsen. Based on current evidence, a stepwise program emphasizing education, certain medications, exercise, cognitive therapy, or all four should be recommended.[305]

Complementary intervention and integrative medicine (e.g., acupuncture, herbal or vitamin supplements, chiropractic, hypnotherapy, and meditative movement therapy such as qi gong, tai chi, yoga) often provides palliative relief from symptoms and depression severity for varying periods of time.[83,165] Like most interventions (allopathic or integrative medicine), no single intervention is effective all the time, and the person with FMS may cycle through various treatment approaches over time.

PROGNOSIS. Many people with mild symptoms are managed without a specialist and have an expected good long-term outcome, but most people experience persistent symptoms of fibromyalgia for many years or a lifetime. Good therapy must be instituted early in the client's course if there is to be any chance of achieving substantial improvement or a remission.

SPECIAL IMPLICATIONS FOR THE THERAPIST 7-7

Fibromyalgia

Therapists are often the first to recognize the history and clinical manifestations suggestive of fibromyalgia and then request medical diagnosis and intervention. The Composite Autonomic Symptoms Scale (COMPASS) can be used to document symptoms produced by abnormal function of the autonomic nervous system.[273]

Efforts to assess the accuracy of thumb nail-bed blanching as a means of determining the presence of tender points suggest that the therapist can quickly learn to use the 4 kg/cm^2 of force required to administer a tender point examination (manual tender point survey).[3] Nail-bed blanching refers to the definition of tender point being one that is painful when 4 kg of pressure are applied (the amount of pressure needed to blanch the examiner's thumbnail when palpating the palm of the examiner's own hand).

Accurate assessment allows the therapist to establish a baseline sensitivity to aid in determining progress and direct intervention.[59] Specific procedures for identifying and palpating each site are available.[160,279] A complete compendium of blank assessment forms and information on how to obtain assessment instruments for FMS are also available.[130,181]

Rehabilitative therapy is an important component in managing fibromyalgia. Many people with FMS have undergone unnecessary exploratory or corrective surgery and have residual functional limitations. Chronic musculoskeletal conditions that are sources of noxious neural input to the CNS often involve the shoulder(s) and spine.

Therapy is helpful first in directing individuals to reach goals of lessening pain and fatigue and eliminating sleep disturbance. Outcomes can be measured in a variety of ways, not only by reduction in tender points but also by global scores of pain, fatigue, sleep, reduction of other distressing symptoms, improved quality of life, reduced visits to the physician, reduction or elimination of medications, increased sexual activity, improved work performance, and so on.

Therapists should listen for reports of adverse effects from pharmaceuticals used to treat FMS. The tricyclic antidepressants (such as amitriptyline) and the serotonin noradrenaline (norepinephrine) reuptake inhibitors (e.g., duloxetine and milnacipran) are first-line options for the treatment of individuals diagnosed with FMS. There is evidence that a small number of people experience substantial symptom relief with no or minor adverse effects from these medications. At the same time, a large number of people stop taking them because of intolerable adverse effects or they only get a small amount of relief from symptoms, which do not outweigh the adverse effects.[123]

Many people with FMS have been told they must "learn to live with it." A more positive approach is to suggest working together to learn how to move forward with FMS, respecting limitations but not being controlled by them. The therapist can be very instrumental in guiding that person to understand how to manage this condition. Prevention programs for osteoporosis and falls related to low blood pressure are additional services the therapist can provide.

Strategies for work modification and applying ergonomic techniques to increase efficiency and decrease pain are important interventions. A chronic pain program may be appropriate. The reader is referred to more specific literature for treatment regimens, self-stabilizing techniques, and therapy protocols for this condition.[2,57,130,235]

Monitoring Vital Signs

Monitoring tests provide an indication of the present physiologic status but cannot predict future status, so regular monitoring is necessary. Depending on the current status, the individual may have to self-monitor every 2 hours, whereas others are able to maintain a balance by monitoring twice daily or less often. For most people with FMS, the sensory system and the autonomic nervous system (ANS) are overactive. Monitoring tests are a helpful tool in developing techniques to quiet these hypersensitivities and achieve a state of physiologic quiet.[130]

Blood pressure and heart rate are indicators of cardiac and circulatory system function and should be monitored. Most people with FMS have low blood pressure and usually an elevated pulse rate even at rest (some individuals have a slow pulse). Hypotension in people with FMS is now referred to as *neurogenic hypotension*. It has been suggested that thyroid hormone regulation will normalize the heart rate and contractility and often normalizes the blood pressure.[182]

For some individuals with a hypoglycemic component, blood glucose assessment may be necessary. Hand temperature is one indicator of ANS function and can be easily assessed using a handheld biofeedback device (e.g., PhysioQ[223]) designed to measure hand temperature. This tool along with a program of physiologic quieting provides a mean of modulating the ANS, improving circulation, and reducing pain levels. The therapist can monitor medical and physical therapy intervention outcomes by assessing vital signs and documenting results.

Modalities and Fibromyalgia

Very little research is available to determine the outcomes of modality use (e.g., physical therapy intervention with thermal or mechanical properties such as physical agents, cryotherapy, moist heat, massage, manual therapy, soft-tissue treatment) with FMS.

The use of noninvasive cranial electrotherapy stimulation (sending minicurrents of electricity through the brain) for the treatment of refractory pain associated with FMS is under investigation.[210] Limited study shows that this treatment intervention can provide a significant improvement in tender point scores and in self-rated scores of general pain level, along with dramatic gains in six stress-related psychologic test measures.[153,172]

Ultrasound can be an effective therapeutic modality for the treatment of pain in people with FMS when combined with connective tissue manipulation and high-voltage pulsed galvanic stimulation.[60] Also, pulsed ultrasound has been shown to be effective in treatment of pain in FMS as combined therapy with interferential current.[10]

There are some reports on the use of ultrasound as an effective therapeutic modality for its thermal effects and for the treatment of myofascial trigger points often present in people with FMS. Continuous ultrasound is preferable to pulsed ultrasound and should be combined with a complete trigger point protocol.[288] The intensity must be reduced from standard settings to accommodate hypersensitivity in most people with FMS. Specific positions, tissue effects, intervention techniques, and treatment parameters are available.[127,128]

Again, additional steps must be taught to sustain pain relief, for example, using biofeedback or Physiologic Quieting[130] to avoid contracting the involved muscle; gentle stretching combined with moist heat several times each day; appropriate changes in work style, patterns of movement, or postures; and nonprescription analgesics such as ibuprofen or naproxen (when approved by the physician).[128]

Soft-tissue techniques may correct the neurocirculatory abnormality and thereby reduce or eliminate the nociceptive signal transmission from the muscle. The result should be to relieve pain and improve tender point index scores or other FMS pain scores assessed.

Given the proposed mechanism of muscle pain (hyperresponsive myofascial mechanoreceptors/impaired CNS pain-inhibiting system), soft-tissue techniques must be applied gently and slowly to increase circulation while avoiding an increase in nociceptive signal transmission. With the typical FMS client, post-treatment discomfort can be avoided by keeping the discomfort level during treatment between 1 and 5 on a self-assessment scale of 1 to 10. Cross-friction massage is not advised.[182]

Exercise and Fibromyalgia

The primary nonpharmacologic modality in the management of FMS is prescriptive exercise. Low-to-moderate intensity aerobic exercise and strength training are strongly recommended.[36,306] Improvement in both subjective pain and objective measurement has been demonstrated with cardiovascular fitness training or simple flexibility training.[132,305] Increases in β-endorphin, adrenocorticotropic hormone, and cortisol levels in response to exercise at aerobic levels (i.e., 60% of maximal oxygen consumption) also have been shown in this population.[205]

Aerobic exercise also contributes by increasing the metabolic rate of the lean tissues for those individuals with a thyroid component.[267] Resistance exercise contributes to the increase in metabolism by increasing lean tissue mass, which has a higher metabolic rate than fat tissue.[229] Resistance exercise can reduce acute pain perception in women with fibromyalgia if they are able to exercise at a workload level high enough to reach the threshold necessary to trigger this response.[152] Well-managed prescriptive exercise regimens improve sleep and result in a decrease in pain and fatigue.[63]

Only general concepts are included in this text; other texts are available for specific exercise regimens.[19,111,130] Comprehensive reviews of evidence for effectiveness of exercise programs for individuals with fibromyalgia have recently published.[113,114,157] The therapist should reinforce the fact that although medications may reduce the individual's symptoms, they are often more effective if taken in conjunction with exercise, stretching, and stress management.[23]

Combining self-care and management strategies with an exercise program helps the individual reach the goals of optimal function and fitness while maintaining decreased pain and fatigue and increasing endurance for daily activities. A number of excellent self-care books are available for consumers.[56,68,94,278] Gentle stretching exercises performed routinely throughout the day may reduce fatigue. The Fibromyalgia Impact Questionnaire can be used to measure changes in pain, fatigue, stiffness, and other measures of functional performance.[90] A cardiopulmonary fitness component should be included at whatever level the individual presents with at the time of assessment.

Sometimes the person's condition is so acute that exercise is not tolerated immediately. This is often the reason for using modalities in the early stage of therapy. Exercising too soon and committing to too much can set the person back considerably, but at the same time the therapist must keep in mind the long-term goal to increase strength and improve aerobic fitness.

Aquatic therapy is an ideal way to begin conditioning, especially for those individuals with FMS who have injuries, are overweight, or are sensitive to axial load. Aquatic therapy provides low-load progressive exercises, gradually increasing strength and endurance while improving overall cardiovascular fitness.[15,118] Ideal pool temperature is between 28.9° C (84° F) and

32.2° C (90° F) (compared with 27.8° C [82° F] to 28.9° C [84° F] for the general population and 32.2° C [90° F] to 34.4° C [94° F] for people with arthritic conditions).[161]

As with all exercise programs with this population (whether aquatic or other therapy), people with fibromyalgia fatigue quickly and may have a low tolerance for exertion. The key is to avoid activating the peripheral sensory mechanisms in order to avoid increasing pain postexercise.

The person with FMS will respond to stimuli that would not ordinarily be perceived as painful (referred to as *allodynia*). This requires short exercise sessions, according to individual tolerance using the rate of perceived exertion (see Chapter 12), that are possibly even only 3 to 5 minutes at first.

The client is encouraged to increase exercise duration in small daily increments, sometimes only by seconds or minutes. Reaching a goal of 30 minutes of daily exercise may take weeks to months; some individuals are only able to tolerate one to three daily exercise cycles, each lasting only 5 to 10 minutes, but this will produce beneficial effects.

The individual with FMS must be taught to set aside the philosophy of "no pain, no gain" and to avoid "pushing through the pain." In the normal individual, growth hormone is increased with exercise, but this does not happen in the person with FMS.

Rather, as a result of ANS dysfunction, reduced microcirculation (capillary flow and other small vessels that supply muscles) causes microtrauma in muscles with vigorous, strenuous, or excessive exercise. The resulting postexertional muscle pain or discomfort aggravates the abnormal pain filter experienced by this population. All causes of increased pain should be minimized, reduced, or eliminated.[20]

Poor compliance is common when the use of muscle relaxants, sedatives, or other medications reduce desire or drive to exercise. Symptoms of pain and fatigue increase during exercise, resulting in limited compliance and limited long-term benefits. The therapist can explain that pain may result in part from muscle spasm and reduced blood flow to muscles, both of which can be aided by persistence in managing exercise.

Using training intensity as a measure of improvement may be helpful. Before performing the physical activity or exercise, compute the maximum heart rate (MHR = 220 − Age). During the activity/exercise, take the pulse and record this for later calculations.

Once the activity/exercise is completed, compute the intensity of work (I_W): I_W = Pulse/MHR. Multiply I_W by the number of minutes exercised to determine the training index (TI): TI = I_W × number of minutes. Keep track of the TI for each activity/exercise session and total them up for 1 week. Track this value over time to assess improved outcomes.[62]

People with fibromyalgia are also more vulnerable to overuse syndromes than are people with normal muscle histology, requiring a slower, longer rehabilitation process. This may not be activity induced as once thought, but rather may occur as a result of sarcolemmal abnormality.[140] At present, until more is known and understood about this phenomenon, whenever possible an aerobic exercise routine should become a part of the client's life before individual muscle group strengthening is started.

Additionally, trigger points, a separate entity from tender points, must be detected and eliminated before initiating exercise using those muscles. Specific assessment and intervention for trigger point therapy is available,[57,124,269] but it should be noted that trigger points are treatment resistant in some individuals with inadequate thyroid hormone at the cellular level. For these individuals, treatment of the underlying hypothyroidism and/or thyroid resistance is essential first.[180]

Other resources include the *Fibromyalgia Network Newsletter* (www.fmnetnews.com) and the American Fibromyalgia Syndrome Association (www.afsafund.org).

ISOIMMUNE DISEASE

Organ and Tissue Transplantation

With recent advances in technology and immunology, organ and tissue transplantation is becoming commonplace. In fact, transplantation of almost any tissue is feasible, but the clinical use of transplantation to remedy disease is still limited for many organ systems because of the rejection reaction. Transplant rejection, an isoimmune phenomenon, occurs in response to transplantation because the body usually recognizes the donor tissue as nonself and attempts to destroy the tissue shortly after transplantation.

In all cases of graft rejection, the cause is incompatibility of cell surface antigens. The rejection of foreign or transplanted tissue occurs because the recipient's immune system recognizes that the surface HLA proteins of the donor's tissue are different from the recipient's.

For this reason, HLA matching of donor and recipient greatly enhances the probability of graft acceptance. Certain antigens are more important than others for a successful transplant, including ABO and Rh antigens present on red blood cells and histocompatibility antigens, and most importantly, the HLA. As expected, a better chance of graft acceptance is evident with syngeneic or autologous transplants because the cell surface antigens are identical.

For a complete discussion of histocompatibility, graft rejection (acute vs. chronic), graft-versus-host disease, and immunosuppression, see Chapter 21.

REFERENCES

To enhance this text and add value for the reader, all references are included on the companion Evolve site that accompanies this textbook. The reader can view the reference source and access it online whenever possible.

CHAPTER 8

Infectious Disease

KIM LEVENHAGEN • CELESTE PETERSON

Although human beings are continually exposed to a vast array of microorganisms in the environment, only a small proportion of those microbes are capable of interacting with the human host in such a way that infection and disease result. With the steady advances being made in medicine, people are living longer, but infection is still a frequent cause of hospital admission and remains an important cause of death, especially in the aging population.

From 1950 until 1980 the management of communicable infectious diseases was well under control; morbidity and mortality from infectious diseases such as yellow fever, cholera, typhus, malaria, typhoid fever, and plague were no longer serious threats in the United States.

The widespread availability and use of antibiotics successfully treated tuberculosis, syphilis, gonorrhea, bacterial meningitis, scarlet fever, and rheumatic fever. Organized efforts to immunize all children lowered the incidence of vaccine-preventable diseases such as measles, mumps, rubella, diphtheria, tetanus, and poliomyelitis; more recently children have also been vaccinated against chickenpox (varicella), human papilloma virus (HPV), and hepatitis A and B.

Unfortunately, this period of reduced morbidity and mortality secondary to infectious disease did not last, and in the 1970s and 1980s new infectious agents appeared. *Legionella*, human immunodeficiency virus (HIV), antibiotic-resistant organisms, avian flu, and a resurgence of tuberculosis are examples of infectious processes that have returned focus to the prevention and treatment of infectious diseases. Infectious diseases have the ability to spread more rapidly throughout the world than in the past, facilitated by a combination of environmental disruption and increasing human mobility.

At the same time, infectious agents are suspected in disorders such as cancer (liver and cervical), gastric and duodenal ulcers, heart disease, neurologic diseases, and autoimmune diseases.[67,154,177] In addition, an area of major public health concern is the continued emergence of antibiotic-resistant microorganisms that appear in hospitals and communities.

Infectious pathogens (a pathogen is any microorganism that has the capacity to cause disease) almost invariably mutate, leading to eventual resistance to antibiotics/antivirals and other treatments. This is compounded by the misuse and overuse of antibiotics in treatment of infections or potential infections.[59]

Other variables include large numbers of children in daycare facilities; a sicker population base when hospitalized (therefore more susceptible to infection); crowding of prisons, military facilities, or multifamily dwellings; and modern agriculture's reliance on antibiotics to boost growth and limit disease among animals. Poor immunologic resistance (e.g., premature infants, aging adults, and those with debilitating disease, burns, or wounds) are contributing factors in the rapid and progressive spread of human bacterial infections.

The resistant organisms spread quickly and easily when inadequate precautions are taken to prevent transmission (e.g., poor use of handwashing and contact precautions). The presence of these multidrug-resistant organisms in health care facilities limits the number of effective antimicrobials available for treatment.

The most common of these resistant bacteria are methicillin-resistant *Staphylococcus aureus* (MRSA); vancomycin-resistant enterococci, and multidrug-resistant *Mycobacterium tuberculosis*. Additionally, certain *S. aureus* strains demonstrate various levels of resistance to vancomycin (vancomycin-intermediate/resistant *S. aureus*), which makes treatment of this organism difficult.[37]

Multidrug resistance in *Pseudomonas aeruginosa* is increasing, and carbapenem-resistant *Klebsiella* strains are emerging. Recent increases in the frequency and severity of *Clostridium difficile*–associated illness are associated with the emergence of a hypervirulent *C. difficile* strain with increased resistance to the fluoroquinolones.[192]

Although a number of new infectious diseases have appeared in recent years, a worldwide resurgence of long-standing diseases once thought to be well controlled has occurred. Among infectious diseases in the world, *M. tuberculosis* is one of the world's leading causes of death in adults, killing 1.5 million people a year.[227] Organisms travel on the shoes of tourists, in the ballast of cargo ships, within the confines of jetliners, and in the blood of human beings.

When natural systems are weakened or altered by ecologic stresses (e.g., pollution, habitat destruction, weather disasters, climate change, famine), they become more vulnerable to damage or destruction by invading organisms, which can result in the spread of infection. Opportunistic organisms take advantage of the weakened defenses.

All health care professionals must maintain a vigilant attitude to preventing infectious disease. This requires an understanding of the infectious process, the chain of transmission, and selected aspects of control. In this chapter, a basic understanding of these concepts is provided along with a discussion of a few infectious diseases. Other pertinent infectious diseases are presented in appropriate chapters according to the primary clinical pathology (such as pneumonia in Chapter 15 and bacterial meningitis in Chapter 29).

SIGNS AND SYMPTOMS OF INFECTIOUS DISEASES

Clinical manifestations of infectious disease are many and varied depending on the etiologic agent (e.g., viruses, bacteria) (see "Types of Organisms" below) and the system affected (e.g., respiratory, central nervous system [CNS], gastrointestinal [GI], genitourinary).

Systemic symptoms of infectious disease can include fever and chills, sweating, malaise, and nausea and vomiting. Changes in blood composition may occur, such as an increased number of leukocytes or a change in the types of leukocytes. Older adults may experience a change in mentation (e.g., confusion, memory loss, difficulty concentrating). When observing any person for early signs of infection, the therapist will most likely see one or only a few symptoms (Box 8-1).

A change in body temperature is a characteristic systemic symptom of infectious disease, but fever may accompany noninfectious causes such as inflammatory, neoplastic, and immunologically mediated diseases (Box 8-2). *Fever*, a sustained temperature above normal, can be caused by abnormalities of the hypothalamus, brain tumors, dehydration, or toxic substances affecting the temperature-regulating center of the hypothalamus. Certain protein substances and toxins can cause the set point of the hypothalamic thermostat to rise. This results in activation of the hypothalamus to conserve heat and increase heat production. Substances that cause these effects are called *pyrogens*.

In infectious disease, the endotoxins of some bacteria and the extracts of normal leukocytes (cytokines) are pyrogenic. They act to raise the thermostat in the hypothalamus, thus raising the body temperature. Fever patterns may differ depending on the specific infectious disease present and occur clinically on a continuum from fever associated with an acute illness lasting 7–10 days, to sepsis and ongoing infection lasting longer than 10 days, to fever of unknown origin associated with a possible infectious origin lasting at least 3 weeks.

Fever patterns can include *intermittent fever* (temperature returns to normal at least once every 24 hours), which is usually associated with sepsis, abscesses, and infective endocarditis; *remittent fever* (temperature fluctuates but doesn't return to normal), associated with viral upper respiratory infection, *Legionella*, and *Mycoplasma* infections; *sustained* or *continuous fever* (temperature remains above normal with minimal variations); and *recurrent* or *relapsing fever* (episodic fevers lasting 1 to 3 days with 1 or more days of normal temperatures between episodes).

Other causes of fever include neoplasm (lymphoma and leukemia are the most common); autoimmune disorders (systemic lupus erythematosus and polyarteritis nodosa) and miscellaneous diseases, including temporal

---

Box 8-1

SIGNS AND SYMPTOMS OF INFECTIOUS DISEASE

- Fever, chills, malaise (most common early symptoms)
- Enlarged lymph nodes

Integument

- Purulent drainage from abscess, open wound, or skin lesion
- Skin rash, red streaks
- Bleeding from gums or into joints; joint effusion or erythema

Cardiovascular

- Petechial lesions
- Tachycardia (see "Aneurysm" and "Thrombophlebitis" in Chapter 12)
- Hypotension
- Change in pulse rate (may increase or decrease depending on the type of infection)

Central Nervous System

- Altered level of consciousness, confusion, seizures
- Headache
- Photophobia
- Memory loss
- Stiff neck, myalgia

Gastrointestinal

- Nausea
- Vomiting
- Diarrhea

Genitourinary

- Dysuria or flank pain
- Hematuria
- Oliguria
- Urgency, frequency

Upper Respiratory

- Tachypnea
- Cough
- Dyspnea
- Hoarseness
- Sore throat
- Nasal drainage
- Sputum production
- Oxygen desaturation
- Decreased exercise tolerance
- Prolonged ventilatory support

In the Older Adult

Signs and symptoms may be subtle and atypical:
- Change in mental status
- Subnormal body temperature
- Bradycardia or tachycardia
- Fatigue (or increased fatigue)
- Lethargy
- Decreased appetite

arteritis, thromboembolic disease, alcoholic hepatitis, and drug-induced fever, among others.

A general guideline, the 39° C (102° F) rule divides conditions into two groups: those that do not cause temperature elevations exceeding 39° C (102° F) and those that regularly exceed 39° C (102° F). Table 8-1 reflects hospital data; the outpatient population is more likely to experience fever accompanied by generalized arthralgias and myalgias associated with a self-limiting illness or fever with localized symptom(s), such as a sore throat, cough, or right lower quadrant pain, as occurs with bacterial infection. Temperature elevation to 40° C (104° F)

Box 8-2

COMMON* INFECTIOUS AND NONINFECTIOUS CAUSES OF FEVER IN THE HOSPITALIZED PERSON

Infectious

- Urinary tract infection
- Respiratory tract infections
- Catheter-related infection
- Surgical wound infection
- Infected pressure ulcers
- Other (less common): colitis, peritonitis, meningitis

Noninfectious (Injured or Abnormal Cells Incite Production of Pyrogens)

- Drug reaction
- Pulmonary emboli
- Neoplasm
- Tissue necrosis (e.g., stroke, myocardial infarction)
- Autoimmune diseases

*The most common infectious causes are urinary tract infections, bacteremia, and pneumonia. Medical charting often lists "primary bloodstream infection," which includes catheter line–associated bloodstream infections (instead of recording the condition as bacteremia, septicemia, or catheter line–associated infection).

Data from Bor DH: Fever in hospitalized medical patients: characteristics and significance, *J Gen Intern Med* 3(2):119–125, 1988.

---

may cause delirium and seizures, particularly in children. An extremely high fever may damage cells irreversibly.

It is important to note that some people with serious infection do not initially develop fever but instead become *tachypneic* (rapid breathing), *confused*, or develop *hypotension*. Most often this situation occurs in older adults, individuals with a health care–associated infection (HAI), or in immunocompromised persons.

Inflammation and its exudates may remain localized, permeate the tissue, or spread throughout the body via the blood or lymph. For example an *abscess* begins as a localized infection with inflammation and purulent exudate. Leukocytes form a wall around the organisms. The abscess deepens as more leukocytes are drawn into the area, more organisms are killed, and more necrotic tissue is dissolved. The exudate may eventually be autolyzed and resorbed by the body, in which case the inflammation and infection are resolved. Rupture of the abscess and drainage into other tissues can spread the infection to other areas of the body.

For example, infectious abdominal disorders (e.g., diverticulitis, appendicitis), tuberculosis of the spine, pelvic inflammatory disease, vertebral osteomyelitis, septic arthritis of the sacroiliac joint, and tumor of the thigh can result in abscess formation in the space between the posterior peritoneum and the psoas and iliac fascia.[60,122] A psoas abscess is usually confined within the psoas fascia, but occasionally, because of anatomic relations, infection extends to the buttock, hip, or upper thigh (see further discussion in Chapter 16).

Such an abscess causes true musculoskeletal symptoms of back pain, or pain referred to the hip or knee, and limited range of hip motion from an underlying systemic cause. Flexion contracture of the hip (positive Thomas test) may develop from reflex spasm, and extension of the thigh is very painful; hip abduction and adduction evoke minimal discomfort. An unexplained limp may be the initial symptom, an important clinical clue when taking a history (see Figs. 16-14 and 16-15). Only days to weeks

---

Table 8-1 | Most Common Causes of Prolonged Fever*

Conditions in Which Fever Generally Does Not Exceed 39° C (102° F)	Conditions in Which Fever Regularly Exceeds 39° C (102° F)
Catheter-associated bacteriuria	Malignant hyperthermia (secondary to anesthesia)
Atelectasis	Transfusion reactions
Phlebitis	Urosepsis
Pulmonary emboli	Intravenous (IV) line sepsis
Dehydration	Prosthetic valve endocarditis
Pancreatitis	Intraabdominal or pelvic peritonitis or abscess
Myocardial infarction	*Clostridium difficile* colitis
Uncomplicated wound infections	Procedure-related bacteremia
Any malignancy	Health-care associated pneumonia
Cytomegalovirus	Drug fever
Hepatitis	HIV infection
Infectious mononucleosis (Epstein-Barr virus)	Heat stroke
Subacute bacterial endocarditis	Acute bacterial endocarditis
Tuberculosis	Tuberculosis (usually disseminated or extrapulmonary)
	Lymphoma
	Metastasizing carcinoma to liver or central nervous system

*The evaluation of fever magnitude with the 39° C (102° F) rule is most often done in the acute care setting. This is a general guideline that must be taken into consideration with other presenting factors.

later does lower abdominal pain develop and the person become acutely ill with a high fever.

Rash with fever can result from an infectious process caused by any microbe that has successfully penetrated the stratum corneum (see Fig. 10-1) and multiplied locally. Skin rashes may also occur with infection elsewhere in the body unrelated to local skin disease (e.g., scarlet fever caused by streptococci, also called *scarlatina*).

The most common types of skin lesions associated with infectious disease are maculopapular eruptions (e.g., classic childhood viral illnesses such as measles, rubella, roseola, fifth disease), nodular lesions (e.g., *Streptococcus, Pseudomonas*), diffuse erythema (e.g., scarlet fever, toxic shock syndrome), vesiculobullous eruptions (e.g., varicella, herpes zoster), and petechial purpuric eruptions (e.g., Epstein-Barr virus [EBV] and cytomegalovirus [CMV]). Specific types of skin lesions are discussed in Chapter 10.

Red streaks may develop from an infection site in the direction of regional lymph nodes, known as acute lymphangitis. Lymphangitis usually occurs as a result of group A streptococci entering the lymphatic channels from an abrasion or local trauma, wound, or infection. The red streak may be obvious, or it may be faint and easily overlooked, especially in dark-skinned people. As bacteria travel to the lymph nodes, septicemia, or bacteria in the bloodstream, may result, leading to a rapid systemic deterioration. Involved nodes are usually tender and enlarged (greater than 3 cm).

Inflamed lymph nodes can be associated with other infectious diseases and may be palpated by the therapist, especially in cervical, axillary, or inguinal areas when presenting musculoskeletal symptoms are evident in those areas. For example, intraoral infection may cause an inflamed cervical node leading to spasm of the sternocleidomastoid muscle, causing neck pain. Palpation may appear to aggravate a primary spasm as if originating in the muscle, when in fact a lymph node under the muscle is the source of the symptom.

In acute infections, nodes are tender, asymmetrical and enlarged. The overlying skin may be erythematous (red) and warm. Unilaterally warm, tender, enlarged, and fluctuant lymph nodes sometimes associated with elevated body temperature may be caused by pyogenic infections and require medical referral.

Supraclavicular and inguinal nodes are also common metastatic sites for cancer. Nodes involved with metastatic cancer are usually hard and fixed to the underlying tissue. Any suspicious lymph node (e.g., changes in size greater than 1 cm; changes in shape, such as matted together; or changes in consistency, such as rubbery) or the presence of painless, enlarged lymph nodes must be evaluated by a physician. (See the section on lymph nodes in "Special Implications for the Therapist: Anatomy of the Lymphatic System" in Chapter 13.)

Joint effusion, usually of one joint (monarticular), associated with infectious arthritis can occur as a result of bacterial, mycobacterial, fungal, or viral etiologic agents. Streptococcal bacteremia from any cause can result in suppurative arthritis (inflammation with pus formation). Bone and joint infections are discussed more completely in Chapter 25.

AGING AND INFECTIOUS DISEASES

As a group, older adults (those older than 65 years of age) are more susceptible to infectious diseases and experience increased morbidity and mortality compared with younger people; this is especially noted in the frail and debilitated older adult. This increased susceptibility is most likely multifactorial, encompassing changes in immune function,[48] called immunosenescence, as well as comorbidities, such as decreased circulation, reduced gag reflex, and poor wound healing.[79]

The immune system is complex and requires well-orchestrated adaptability and responsiveness.[81] With aging, there are modest changes in cell-mediated or T-cell function with a decrease in the number of naïve T cells but an increase in the number of memory T cells. These memory cells, however, are slower to respond and require a stronger stimulus.

Diminished cell-mediated immunity results in the reactivation of dormant infections, such as herpes zoster and tuberculosis, as well as a decreased response to vaccines.[81] Although studies are lacking, it appears most older adults retain antigen-presenting cell function. The elderly also appear to have the presence of chronic low-grade inflammation (termed inflamm-aging). This changes the balance of inflammatory mediators toward the proinflammatory cytokines and oxidative stress,[70] which then alters the function of the immune cells.[21] The health of the immune system appears to be associated with longevity and biologic age.[52]

Extrinsic factors apart from the immune system can lead to increased susceptibility to infection in the older adult. Atrophic skin is more easily damaged, decreased cough and gag reflexes make it more difficult to control secretions, and decreased bronchiolar elasticity and mucociliary activity contribute to the development of pneumonia.

In many aging people, physical decline or psychologic impairment may result in indifference to personal hygiene and loss of manual dexterity, body mobility, or vision. This may lead to an increased risk for falls, with accompanying injuries and fractures resulting in hospitalizations or surgery, therefore increasing their risk of developing an infection.

Denture-associated infections may occur in up to 60% of older adult denture-wearing clients. Predisposing factors include flaccid, sagging cheeks; deepened labial angles constantly moistened by saliva; and ill-fitting dentures, often worn for a considerable time without replacement or repair. These age-related changes compromise the individual's first line of defenses leaving them at increased risk for infection.

Many types of infections are seen in the aging adult, but early recognition of infection in the older adult is difficult because people underreport symptoms, the presentation is often vague, blunted or atypical, and symptoms are difficult to assess.[148] The older adult may be unable to describe the present illness or past history or list the medications being taken. A complete physical examination may be difficult because of the person's uncooperativeness, cognitive impairment, neurologic deficits, or physical impairments. Pain may be poorly localized or absent, or it may be confused with preexisting conditions, such as in septic arthritis in a client with degenerative joint disease.

Another important reason recognition of infection in older adults can be difficult is the presence of implanted devices. The elderly are more likely to have an implanted device such as joint prostheses, pacemakers, defibrillators, peripherally inserted central catheter lines, stents, and grafts. Implanted devices can develop a biofilm, which consists of organisms surrounded by a self-produced protective layer of polysaccharides, proteins, nucleic acids and lipids, which adhere to the synthetic device.[65] Frequently there is no overt initial response and the infection subtly grows.

The aging person also can have more serious infections with little or no fever because of an impaired thermoregulatory system or the masking effects of drugs such as aspirin, other antiinflammatory drugs, and corticosteroids.

Fever in older people may not be high enough to cause concern because the basal body temperature is low. A lower threshold for infection should be used (e.g., oral temperature of 37.2° C [99° F] or 37.8° C [100° F]), especially if the person is taking a medication that masks fever. Watch for (or ask family about) any recent episodes of confusion, memory loss, or other change in mental status; these may be the first symptoms of infection.[61]

If the febrile response is absent in an older adult with a serious infection, it is a grave sign. Acute infections in the older adult may cause delirium or a sudden change in mental status. Chronic infections of the lungs, bone, skin, kidneys, and CNS may cause mental status changes perceived as dementia.

Many frail elderly are in acute or extended-care settings and are therefore more likely to be exposed to healthcare associated pathogens such as gram-negative bacilli, *S. aureus*, and vancomycin-resistant enterococci.

INFECTIOUS DISEASES

Definition and Overview

Infection is a process in which an organism establishes a parasitic relationship with its host. This invasion and multiplication of microorganisms produces an immune response and subsequent signs and symptoms. Such reproduction injures the host by causing cellular damage from microorganism-producing toxins or intracellular multiplication or by competing with the host's metabolism.

The host's immune response may compound the tissue damage; such damage may be localized (e.g., as in infected pressure ulcers) or systemic. However, in some instances, microorganisms may be present in the tissues of the host and yet not cause symptomatic disease. This process is called *colonization of organisms*. The person with colonization may be a carrier and transmit the organisms to others but does not have detectable symptoms of infection unless or until the immune system is weakened or compromised.

The development of an infection begins with transmission of an infectious organism (agent, pathogen) and depends on a complex interaction of the pathogen, an environment conducive to transmission of the organism,

and the susceptibility of the human host. Even after successful transmission of a pathogen, the host may experience more than one possible outcome.

The pathogen may merely contaminate the body surface and be destroyed by first-line defenses such as intact skin or mucous membranes that prevent further invasion, or a subclinical infection may occur in which no apparent symptoms are evident other than an identifiable immune response of the host. A rise in the titer of antibody directed against the infecting agent is often the only detectable response. Antibiotic treatment is not necessary, although infection control procedures remain in force to prevent spreading the bacteria to others.

A third possible outcome is the development of a clinically apparent infection in which the host-parasite interaction causes obvious injury and is accompanied by one or more clinical symptoms. This outcome is called *infectious disease* and ranges in severity from mild to fatal depending on the organism and the response and underlying health of the host.[93]

The period between the pathogen entering the host and the appearance of clinical symptoms is called the *incubation period*. This period may last from a few days to several months, depending on the causative organism and type of disease. Disease symptoms herald the end of the incubation period. A *latent* infection occurs after a microorganism has replicated but remains dormant or inactive in the host, sometimes for years (e.g., tuberculosis, herpes zoster). The host may harbor a pathogen in sufficient quantities to be shed at any time after latency and toward the end of the incubation period. This time period when an organism can be shed is called the *period of communicability*.

From this concept of communicability, communicable diseases can be defined as any disease whereby the causative agent may pass or be carried from one person to another directly or indirectly. It usually precedes symptoms and continues through part or all of clinical disease, sometimes extending to convalescence; but it is important to note that an asymptomatic host can still transmit a pathogen. The communicable period, like the incubation period and mode of transmission, varies with different pathogens and different diseases.[188]

Types of Organisms

A great variety of microorganisms are responsible for infectious diseases, including viruses, mycoplasmas, bacteria, rickettsiae, chlamydiae, protozoa, fungi (yeasts and molds), helminths (e.g., tapeworms), mycobacteria, and prions. All microorganisms can be distinguished by certain intrinsic properties such as shape, size, structure, chemical composition, antigenic makeup, growth requirements, ability to produce toxins, and ability to remain alive (viability) under adverse conditions such as drying, sunlight, or heat.

These properties provide the basis for identification and classification of the organisms. Knowledge of the properties permits diagnosis of a specific pathogen in specimens of body fluids, secretions, or exudates. All these properties are important to consider when looking for ways to interfere with the mechanisms of transmission.

Viruses are subcellular organisms made up only of a ribonucleic acid (RNA) or a deoxyribonucleic acid (DNA) nucleus covered with proteins. They are the smallest known organisms, visible only through an electron microscope. Viruses are completely dependent on host cells and cannot replicate unless they invade a host cell and stimulate it to participate in the formation of additional virus particles.

The estimated 400 viruses that infect human beings are classified according to their size, shape (spherical, rod shaped, or cubic), or means of transmission (respiratory, fecal–oral, or sexual). Viruses are not susceptible to antibiotics. However, antiviral medications can mitigate (moderate) the course of the viral illness. For example, acyclovir, an antiviral medication used for herpesvirus, interferes with DNA synthesis, causing decreased viral replication and decreasing the time of lesional healing.

Mycoplasmas are unusual, self-replicating bacteria that have no cell wall components and very small genomes. For this reason, antibiotics that are active against bacterial cell walls have no effect on mycoplasmas. At present, mycoplasmas remain sensitive to some antibiotics. They require a strict dependence on the host for nutrition and sustenance and are able to pass through many bacteria-retaining filters or barriers because they are very small.

Bacteria are single-celled microorganisms with well-defined cell walls that can grow independently on artificial media without the need for other cells. Bacteria can be classified according to shape. Spherical bacterial cells are called *cocci*, rod-shaped bacteria are called *bacilli*, and spiral-shaped bacteria are called *spirilla* or *spirochetes*.

Bacteria can also be classified according to their response to staining (gram-positive, gram-negative, or acid-fast), motility (motile or nonmotile), tendency toward capsulation (encapsulated or nonencapsulated), and capacity to form spores (sporulating or nonsporulating) (Fig. 8-1).

Bacteria can also be classified according to whether oxygen is needed to replicate and develop (aerobic) or whether they can sustain life in an oxygen-poor (anaerobic) environment. Normal human flora is primarily anaerobic, and disease can be produced when these normal organisms are displaced from their usual tissue sites (e.g., mouth, skin, large bowel, female genital tract) into other tissues or closed body spaces. Other common anaerobic organisms include the spore-forming bacilli such as *Clostridium botulinum* or *Clostridium tetani* that thrive in a strictly anaerobic environment.

Rickettsiae are primarily animal pathogens that typically produce disease in human beings through the bite of an insect vector such as a tick, flea, louse, or mite. They are small, gram-negative obligate intracellular organisms that often cause life-threatening infections. Like viruses, these microorganisms require a host for replication. Three categories of the family Rickettsiaceae are *Rickettsia*, *Coxiella*, and *Bartonella*.

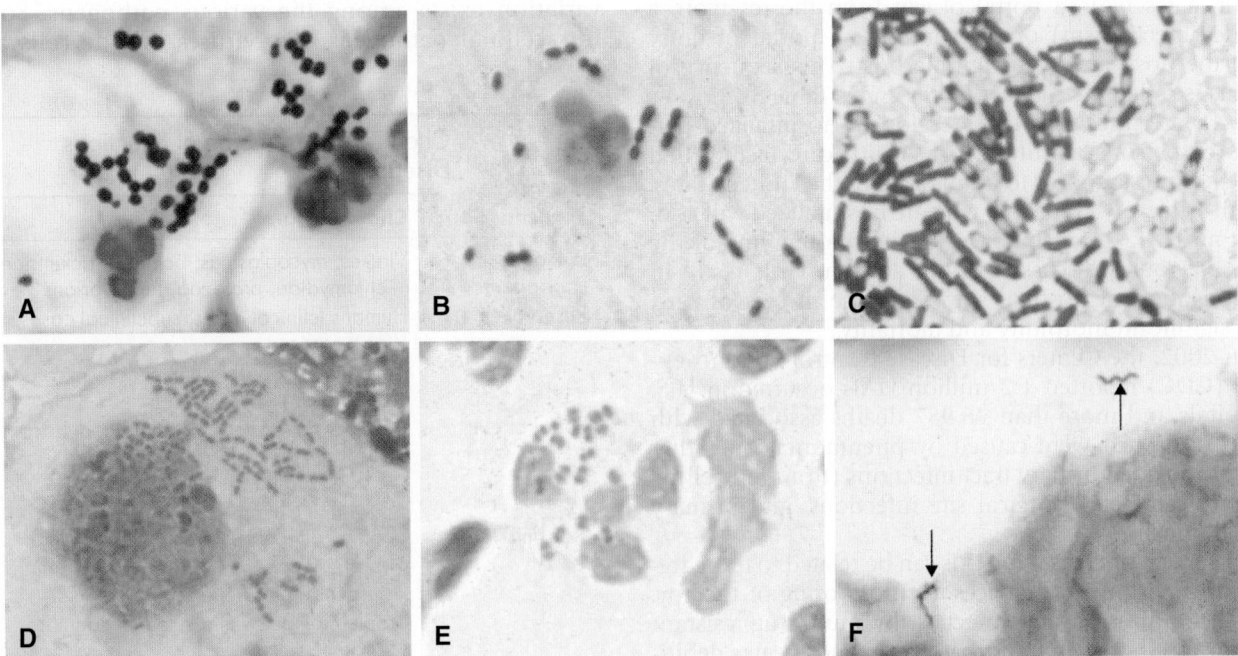

Figure 8-1

A variety of bacterial morphology. A, Gram stain of sputum from person with pneumonia. There are gram-positive cocci in clusters *(Staphylococcus aureus)* with degenerating neutrophils. **B,** Gram stain of sputum from an individual with pneumonia. gram-positive elongated cocci in pairs and short chains *(Streptococcus pneumoniae)* and a neutrophil are seen. **C,** Gram stain of *Clostridium sordellii* grown in culture. A mixture of Gram-positive and gram-negative rods, many of which have subterminal spores (clear areas), are present. *Clostridia* species often stain as both Gram positive and negative, although they are true gram-positive bacteria. **D,** Gram stain of a bronchoalveolar lavage specimen showing gram-negative intracellular rods typical of Enterobacteriaceae such as *Klebsiella pneumoniae* and *Escherichia coli.* **E,** Gram stain of urethral discharge from someone with gonorrhea. Many gram-negative diplococci *(Neisseria gonorrhoeae)* are present within a neutrophil. **F,** Silver stain of brain tissue from a person with Lyme disease meningoencephalitis. Two helical spirochetes *(Borrelia burgdorferi)* are indicated by *arrows.* The panels are at different magnifications. (A to C, Reprinted from Kumar V, Abbas AK, Fausto N: *Robbins and Cotran: pathologic basis of disease,* ed 7, Philadelphia, 2005, WB Saunders, courtesy Dr. Kenneth Van Horn. D, Courtesy Karen Krisher, Clinical Microbiology Institute, Wilsonville, OR.)

Chlamydiae are smaller than rickettsiae and bacteria but larger than viruses. They, too, depend on host cells for replication, but unlike viruses they always contain both DNA and RNA and are susceptible to antibiotics.

Protozoa have a single-cell unit or a group of nondifferentiated cells loosely held together and not forming tissues. They have cell membranes rather than cell walls, and their nuclei are surrounded by nuclear membranes. Larger parasites include roundworms and flatworms. *Fungi* are unicellular to filamentous organisms possessing hyphae (filamentous outgrowths) surrounded by cell walls and containing nuclei (eukaryocyte). Fungi show relatively little cellular specialization and occur as yeasts (single-cell, oval-shaped organisms) or molds (organisms with branching filaments). Depending on the environment, some fungi may occur in both forms. Fungal diseases in human beings are called *mycoses*.

Prions are proteinaceous, infectious particles consisting of proteins but without nucleic acids. These particles are transmitted from animals to human beings and are characterized by a long latent interval in the host. When reactivated, they cause a rapidly progressive deteriorating state in the host (e.g., Creutzfeldt-Jakob disease, bovine spongiform encephalopathy, or "mad cow disease").[164]

The Chain of Transmission

Infection begins with transmission of a pathogen to the host. Successful transmission depends on a pathogenic agent, a reservoir, a portal of exit from the reservoir, a mode (mechanism) of transmission, a portal of entry into the host, and a susceptible host. This sequence of events is called the *chain of transmission* (Table 8-2).

HAIs are infections that develop in hospitalized persons or persons admitted to a health care facility that were not present prior to admission. In the United States, about 1 in every 20 people who are hospitalized will contract an HAI.[28] Transmission can be through any of the possible routes discussed in this section. HAIs result in prolongation of hospital stays, increase in cost of care, and significant morbidity and mortality.

In 2002, the Centers for Disease Control and Prevention (CDC) reported 1.7 million HAIs occurred in U.S. hospitals and more than 98,987 deaths associated with an HAI.[26] Most were caused by pneumonia, but other causes included urinary tract infections (from indwelling urinary catheters), surgical site infections, and primary blood infections.

In general, increases in HAIs can be related to more frequent use of invasive devices for monitoring or therapy, more colonization and infection by multidrug-resistant organisms (both viral and bacterial), and greater debilitation and severity of illness of hospitalized clients who acquire these infections.

The increased use of invasive and surgical procedures, immunosuppressants, antibiotics, and the lack of handwashing predispose people to such infections and superinfections. At the same time, the growing number of personnel who come into contact with the client makes the risk of exposure greater.

Prevention is of critical importance in controlling HAIs. The concept of standard precautions emphasizes that all clients must be treated as though each one has a potential bloodborne, transmissible disease; thus all body secretions are handled with care to prevent disease. Handwashing has been cited as the easiest and most effective means of preventing HAIs and must be done routinely, even when gloves are used. See further discussion under "Control of Transmission" below.

Pathogens

Humans coexist with many microorganisms in complex, mutually beneficial relationships. Even so, many organisms are parasitic, maintaining themselves at the expense of their host. Some parasites arouse a pathologic response in the host and are called *pathogens* or *pathogenic agents*. A *pathogen* as defined at the beginning of this chapter is any microorganism that has the capacity to cause disease.[169] As such, pathogens are ineffective parasites because they stimulate a disease response, which may harm the host and eventually kill the pathogen.

The ability of a pathogen to stimulate an immune response in the host (antigenicity) varies greatly among organisms, depending on the site of invasion, the number of pathogenic organisms, and the dissemination of organisms in the body. The immune status of a person plays the largest role in determining the risk for infection and the ability of the host to combat organisms that have gained entry.

The mode of action of a pathogen refers to how the organism produces a pathologic process. Great variation exists among the various pathogens. Some intracellular pathogens, like viruses, invade cells and

Table 8-2	Chain of Transmission of Infectious Disease	
Transmission	**Chain Factors**
Pathogen or agent	Viruses, mycoplasmas, bacteria, rickettsiae, chlamydiae, protozoa, fungi, prions
Reservoir	Humans (clinical cases, subclinical cases, and carriers)
	Animal, arthropod, plant, soil, food, organic substance
Portal of exit	Genitourinary tract, gastrointestinal tract, respiratory tract, oral cavity, open lesion, blood, vaginal secretions, semen, tears, excretions (urine, feces)
Transmission	Contact (direct or indirect)
	Airborne (float on air currents and remain suspended for hours; small particles)
	Droplet (fall out within 3 feet of source; large particles)
	Vehicle (through a common source such as water or food)
	Vectorborne (carried by insects or animals)
Modes of entry	Ingestion, inhalation, percutaneous injection, transplacental entry, mucous membranes
Susceptible host	Specific immune reactions
	Nonspecific body defenses
	Host characteristics: age, sex, ethnic group, heredity, behaviors
	Environmental and general health status

interfere with cellular metabolism, growth, and replication, whereas others invade and cause hyperplasia and cell death. Yet other organisms, such as the influenza virus, have the potential to alter their antigenic characteristics. This virus is capable of extensive gene rearrangements, resulting in significant changes in surface antigen structure. This ability allows new strains to evade host antibody responses directed at earlier strains.

Some viruses (e.g., all members of the herpesvirus group) cause a persistent latent infection that can be reactivated in certain circumstances. HIV causes immunosuppression by destroying helper T lymphocytes. Some pathogens, such as the tetanus bacillus, produce a toxin that interferes with intercellular responses. Some bacteria, such as diphtheria and tetanus, secrete water-soluble antigenic exotoxins that are quickly disseminated in the blood, causing potentially severe systemic and neurologic manifestations. Larger parasites, such as roundworms, cause anemia and interfere with the function of the GI system.

The characteristics of the organism and the susceptibility of the host influence the likelihood of a pathogen producing infectious disease and the type of disease produced. Not all pathogens have an equal probability of inducing disease in the same host population. *Principal* pathogens regularly cause disease in people with apparently intact defense systems.

Opportunistic pathogens do not cause disease in people with intact host defense systems but can clearly cause devastating disease in many hospitalized and immunocompromised clients. Organisms that may be harmless members of normal flora in healthy people may act as virulent invaders in people with severe defects in host defense mechanisms.

Pathogenicity, the ability of the organism to induce disease, depends on the organism's speed of reproduction in the host, the extent of damage it causes to tissues, and the strength of any toxin released by the pathogen. *Virulence* refers to the potency of the pathogen in producing severe disease and is measured by the case fatality rate (i.e., the number of people who die of the disease divided by the number of people who have the disease). Virulence provides a quantitative measure of pathogenicity. The amount and destructive potential of released toxin are closely related to virulence.

Reservoir

A reservoir is an environment in which an organism can live and multiply, such as an animal, plant, soil, food, or other organic substance or combination of substances. The reservoir provides the essentials for survival of the organism at specific stages in its life cycle. Some parasites have more than one reservoir, such as the yellow fever virus, which can maintain life in human beings and other animals. Some parasites require more than one reservoir at different growth stages and still others, such as most sexually transmitted organisms, require only a human reservoir.

Human and animal reservoirs can be symptomatic or asymptomatic carriers of the pathogen. A carrier maintains an environment that promotes growth, multiplication, and shedding of the parasite without exhibiting signs of disease. Hepatitis is a common example of this carrier state in human beings.

Portal of Exit

The portal of exit is the place from which the parasite leaves the reservoir. In general, this is the site of growth of the organism and corresponds to the system of entry into the next host. For example, the portal of exit for GI parasites is usually the feces, and the portal of entry into a new host is the mouth. Exceptions to the case include hookworm eggs, which are shed in the feces but enter through the skin of a person walking barefoot in soil containing hatched eggs.

Common portals of exit include secretions and fluids (e.g., respiratory secretions, blood, vaginal secretions, semen, tears), excretions such as urine and feces, open lesions, and exudates such as pus from an open wound or ulcer. Some organisms, such as HIV, have more than one portal of exit. Knowledge of the portal of exit is essential for preventing transmission of a pathogen.

Mode of Transmission

For infection to be transmitted, the invading organism must be transported from the infected source to a susceptible host. Microorganisms are transmitted by several possible routes, and the same microorganism can travel by more than one route. The five main routes of transmission are contact, airborne, droplet, vehicle, and vector borne.

Contact transmission occurs directly or indirectly. Direct contact is the direct transfer of microorganisms that come into physical contact either by skin-to-skin contact or mucous membrane–to–mucous membrane contact (e.g., sexual contact, biting, touching, kissing).

Indirect contact involves transfer of microorganisms from a source to a host by passive transfer from an inanimate, intermediate object, called a *fomite*. Inanimate objects can include items such as the telephone, sphygmomanometer, bedside rails, tray tables, countertops, and other items that come into direct contact with the infected person, thus emphasizing the need for thorough handwashing at all times.

An example of indirect transmission is transfer of human immunodeficiency virus from a contaminated source to a host through a needlestick. Another example of indirect contact includes fecal–oral transmission by the ingestion of enteric pathogens from a food prepared by a person who does not wash his or her hands.[93]

Airborne transmission occurs when disease-causing organisms are so small (less than 5 microns) that they are capable of floating on air currents within a room and remain suspended in the air for several hours. They are often propelled from the respiratory tract through coughing or sneezing. A host then inhales the particles directly into the respiratory tract (e.g., tuberculosis, chickenpox, rubeola measles).

Droplet transmission is different from airborne transmission because droplets are larger particles (greater than 5 microns) than airborne particles and they do not remain suspended in air but fall out within 3 feet of the source. They are produced when a person coughs or sneezes and then travel only a short distance. A common example of droplet-spread infection is influenza. Those people who are in closest proximity to the infected source have the highest risk for infection.

Vehicle transmission occurs when infectious organisms (e.g., salmonellosis) are transmitted through a common source (e.g., contaminated food, water, and IV fluid) to many potential susceptible hosts. *Vectorborne* transmission of infectious organisms involves insects and/or animals that act as intermediaries between two or more hosts. Lyme disease and Rocky Mountain spotted fever are examples of vectorborne diseases.

Portal of Entry

A pathogen may enter a new host by ingestion (GI tract), inhalation (respiratory tract), or bites or injury of the skin. Microbes commonly enter through contact with mucous membranes and less frequently transplacentally. Infectious diseases vary as to the number of organisms and the duration of exposure required to start the infectious process in a new host.

Host Susceptibility

Each person has his or her own susceptibility to infectious disease, and this susceptibility can vary throughout time. A susceptible host has personal characteristics and behaviors that increase the probability of an infectious disease developing.

Biologic and personal characteristics such as age, sex, ethnicity, and heredity influence this probability. General health and nutritional status, hormonal balance, and the presence of concurrent disease also play a role. Likewise, living conditions and personal behaviors such as drug use, diet, hygiene, and sexual practices influence the risk of exposure to pathogens and resistance once exposed.

Older adults in hospitals and long-term care facilities are already susceptible hosts, especially if poorly nourished. Immunosuppressive agents and corticosteroids decrease the body's ability to resist infection. Inadequate or absent handwashing or other breaches of aseptic technique result in spread of microorganisms from health care workers (HCWs) to clients and between individuals receiving health care.

Surfaces of equipment can become contaminated and then transmit microorganisms that cause infection. Incorrect isolation procedures such as leaving doors open to rooms in which airborne precautions are in effect or not using masks increase the risk of transmitting organisms that cause health care–associated infections.

The presence of underlying medical disorders (e.g., malignancy, diabetes, renal failure, acquired immune deficiency syndrome [AIDS], and cirrhosis) decreases T-cell– and B-cell–mediated immune function. Breaches of body integrity, such as nasogastric and chest tubes, intubation, urinary catheters, and IV devices, impair the body's defense mechanisms, decreasing the ability of the integumentary, GI, genitourinary, and respiratory systems to resist invasion by microorganisms.

Lines of Defense. Susceptibility is also influenced by the presence of anatomic and physiologic defenses, sometimes called *lines of defense*. The *first-line defenses* are external, such as intact skin and mucous membranes; oil and perspiration on skin; cilia in respiratory passages; gag and coughing reflexes; peristalsis in the GI tract; and the flushing action of tears, saliva, and mucus.

These first-line defenses act to inhibit invasion of pathogens and remove them before they have an opportunity to multiply. The chemical composition of body secretions such as tears and sweat, together with the pH of saliva, vaginal secretions, urine, and digestive juices, further prevents or inhibits growth of organisms. Compromise in any of these natural defenses increases host susceptibility to pathogen invasion.

Another important first-line defense is the normal flora of microorganisms that inhabit the skin and mucous membranes in the oral cavity, GI tract, and vagina. These organisms occur naturally and usually coexist with their host in a mutually beneficial relationship. Through a mechanism called *microbial antagonism* they control the replication of potential pathogens.

The importance of this mechanism is evident when it is disturbed, as happens when extensive antibiotic therapy destroys normal flora in the oral or vaginal cavity, resulting in *Candida albicans*, an overgrowth of yeast. Some normal flora can become pathogenic under specific conditions such as immunosuppression or displacement of the pathogen to another area of the body. Displacement of normal flora is a common cause of HAIs. This can occur when *Escherichia coli*, ordinarily normal flora in the GI tract, invade the urinary tract. Invasive procedures increase the risk of displacing these organisms.

The *second-line defense*, the inflammatory process, and the *third-line defense*, the immune response, share several physiologic components. These include the lymphatic system, leukocytes, and a multitude of chemicals, proteins, and enzymes that facilitate the internal defenses.

Once a microorganism penetrates the first line of defense, the inflammatory response is initiated. Inflammation is a local reaction to cell injury of any type whether from physical, chemical, or thermal damage, or microbial invasion. As a response to microbial injury, inflammation is aimed at preventing further invasion by walling off, destroying, or neutralizing the invading organism.

The early inflammatory response is protective, but it can continue for sustained periods in some infections, leading to granuloma formation. The production of new leukocytes may be stimulated for weeks or months and is reflected in an elevated white blood cell count. However, sustained inflammation can become chronic and result in destruction of healthy tissues. Extensive necrosis from persistent inflammation can increase tissue susceptibility to the infectious agent or provide an ideal setting for invasion by other pathogens.

The first- and second-line defenses are nonspecific; that is, they operate against all infectious agents in the same way. In contrast, the immune system responds in a specific manner to individual pathogens as long as the organism has antigenic characteristics. In general, antigens are proteins, large polysaccharides, or large lipoprotein complexes that stimulate an immune response.

Not all microorganisms are antigenic, but some are bound by complement or other host-produced substances to form an antigen that elicits an immune response. An immune response is triggered after foreign materials have been cleared from an area of inflammation. For specific details regarding cell-mediated versus humoral immune responses, see Chapter 7.

Control of Transmission

Much can be done to prevent transmission of infectious diseases, including the use of barriers and isolation; comprehensive immunizations, including the required immunization of travelers to or emigrants from endemic areas; drug prophylaxis; improved nutrition, living conditions, and sanitation; avoiding risk-taking behaviors, and correction of environmental factors.

Breaking the transmission chain at any of these links can help control transmission of infectious diseases. The link most amenable to control varies with the characteristics of the organism, its reservoirs, the type of pathologic response it produces, and the available technology for control. The general goal is to break the chain at the most cost-effective point or points—that is, the point at which the greatest number of people can be protected with available technology and the least amount of resources.

Isolation and barriers can be used to prevent the transmission of microorganisms from infected or colonized people to other unaffected people. In hospital or institutional settings, the purpose of isolating individuals or residents is to prevent the transmission of colonized or infectious microorganisms among clients, visitors, and HCWs.

New isolation guidelines for health care settings were published in 2007 by the CDC and the Hospital Infection Control Practices Advisory Committee (CDC 2007). The guidelines outline a two-tiered approach with specific recommendations categorized as Standard Precautions or Transmission-Based Precautions. A brief summary is offered here in context of the material in this chapter, but the reader is directed to Appendix A for a complete discussion of these precautions.

Standard Precautions assume any person may be contagious. These precautions continue to be the foundation for preventing the transmission of infectious organisms and include hand hygiene, wearing personal protective gear, and, new for these guidelines, respiratory hygiene/cough etiquette. Box 8-3 presents a list of what is considered infectious and safe waste. Boxes 8-4 and 8-5 present hand hygiene indications and technique. Appendix Table A-1 presents a summary of the Standard Precautions.

Standard Precautions apply to all clients, whereas Transmission-Based Precautions apply to anyone with documented or suspected infection or colonization with highly transmissible or epidemiologically important organisms that require additional precautions (i.e., in addition to Standard Precautions) to prevent transmission.

Transmission-Based Precautions are defined according to the major modes of transmission of infectious agents (contact, airborne, and droplet) in the health care setting (Table 8-3). Specific recommendations have been published according to the type of infection and condition and can be found at http://www.cdc.gov/hicpac/

Box 8-3

INFECTIOUS AND SAFE MEDICAL WASTE

Infectious Waste	Safe Waste
Blood and components	Cotton balls, Band-Aids
All disposable sharps (used or unused)	Gloves (latex and latex-free), masks, or other personal protective devices
Urine, stool, or emesis if visibly contaminated with blood	Nasal secretions
Vaginal secretions	Sputum
Semen	Feces
Cerebrospinal fluid	Urine
Synovial fluid	Vomitus
Pericardial fluid (mediastinal tubes)	Tears
Amniotic fluid	Sweat

Regulation of medical waste disposal is primarily regulated at the state level. To determine the laws that apply in your state, go to U.S. Environmental Protection Agency: http://www.epa.gov/osw/nonhaz/industrial/medical/programs.htm. Click on your state for information about your state medical waste regulations and programs.

2007IP/2007ip_appendA.html. Guidelines are also given for colonization or infections with multidrug-resistant organisms at http://www.cdc.gov/hicpac/mdro/mdro_toc.html. These precautions are in addition to Standard Precautions.

Immunizations have become a mainstay for curtailing if not eliminating infectious diseases. The World Health Organization has estimated that more than 2.5 million lives are saved by the use of about 120 vaccines, and 2 million more lives could be saved by the expanded use of vaccines.[125] Immunizations, by decreasing host susceptibility, can now control many diseases, including diphtheria, tetanus, pertussis, measles, mumps, rubella, some forms of meningitis, poliomyelitis, hepatitides A and B, pneumococcal pneumonia, influenza (certain strains), and rabies.

Each year the CDC issues updated information on the vaccine and antiviral agents available for controlling influenza during the current influenza season. Vaccines contain either live but attenuated (altered) microbes or killed microbes; these actively induce immunity to diseases by stimulating white cells to produce antibodies. When a virus or bacteria invades the body, antibodies are produced and attach to specific proteins on the virus or bacteria. Other immune defenses are then stimulated to destroy it.

Another mode of providing immunity to certain organisms is to manufacture specific immune globulins, rather than stimulate the production of antibodies. Immune globulins are previously formed antibodies from hyperimmunized donors or pooled plasma and provide temporary passive immunity (they bind to the virus or bacterium, which then stimulate destruction). Passive immunization is generally used when active immunization is life threatening or when complete protection requires both active and passive immunization (e.g., immunoglobulins used for hepatitis B or for tetanus) (see Table 7-1).

INDICATIONS FOR HAND HYGIENE AND HAND ANTISEPSIS*

Handwashing with soap (microbial or non-antimicrobial) and water:

- When hands are visibly soiled with blood or body fluid
- Before eating
- After using the restroom
- If proven or suspected exposure to *Bacillus anthracis* or *C. difficile*
  Decontaminate hands with alcohol-based rub:
- After exposure to body fluids or excretions but hands not visibly soiled
- After having direct contact with a client
- Before and after putting on gloves for client care
- Before and after putting on gloves for a nonsurgical procedure
- After contact with intact client skin
- After attending to a contaminated-body site and before moving to a clean-body site on the same client
- After contact with objects in client area

Data from Boyce JM, Pittet D; Healthcare Infection Control Practices Advisory Committee; HICPAC/SHEA/APIC/IDSA Hand Hygiene Task Force: Guideline for hand hygiene in health-care settings. Recommendations of the Healthcare Infection Control Practices Advisory Committee and the HICPAC/SHEA/APIC/IDSA Hand Hygiene Task Force. Society for Healthcare Epidemiology of America/Association for Professionals in Infection Control/Infectious Diseases Society of America, *MMWR Recomm Rep* 51(RR-16):1-45, 2002. Available online at http://www.cdc.gov/mmwr/PDF/rr/rr5116.pdf.

*For visual orientation to handwashing, see the World Health Organization's poster: How to Handwash. Available online at http://www.who.int/gpsc/5may/How_To_HandWash_Poster.pdf. Video presentations are also available at http://www.who.int/gpsc/5may/.

PROPER HAND-HYGIENE TECHNIQUE

Alcohol-Based Rubs

Using alcohol-based hand rubs may reduce contamination better than soap and water. Apply product in the palm of the hand and rub hands together, remembering to cover all areas of the hands, including the back or the hands and webs of the fingers, until dry.

Washing Hands with Soap and Water

Wet hands prior to beginning then add soap. Rub hands together vigorously for at least 15 to 20 seconds, covering all areas of the hands and fingers. Rinse soap from hands and dry completely with a disposable towel. Turn the water off using the towel. Avoid hot water since this may increase the risk for dermatitis.

Special Considerations

- Jewelry may sequester gram-negative organisms, but more studies are needed to determine if this translates to increased transmission of the organisms.
- Artificial nails or extenders can harbor high concentrations of coagulase-negative staphylococci and gram-negative rods. Although more studies are needed to determine if artificial nails increase the likelihood of transmitting organisms, the CDC recommends that artificial nails or extenders not be worn when in contact with clients at high risk for infection (http://www.cdc.gov/mmwr/PDF/rr/rr5116.pdf).
- Wear gloves if potentially coming into contact with blood, body fluids, mucous membranes, nonintact skin, or environmental surfaces.
- For therapists in outpatient settings, the source reference for this box listed below is a valuable tool when reviewing infection control. This is especially helpful when your facility does not have an infectious disease department.

For more information on hand hygiene and infection control, visit the web sites for the Centers for Disease Control and Prevention (CDC) (http://www.cdc.gov) and the Association for Professionals in Infection Control and Epidemiology (http://www.apic.org).

Data from Boyce JM, Pittet D; Healthcare Infection Control Practices Advisory Committee; HICPAC/SHEA/APIC/IDSA Hand Hygiene Task Force: Guideline for hand hygiene in health-care settings. Recommendations of the Healthcare Infection Control Practices Advisory Committee and the HICPAC/SHEA/APIC/IDSA Hand Hygiene Task Force. Society for Healthcare Epidemiology of America/Association for Professionals in Infection Control/Infectious Diseases Society of America, *MMWR Recomm Rep* 51(RR-16):1-45, 2002. Available online at http://www.cdc.gov/mmwr/PDF/rr/rr5116.pdf.

Side effects to immunization can occur, but the incidence of significant adverse effects of immunization among human beings remains very small. The potential increase in susceptibility to influenza and death from respiratory illness in high-risk people (e.g., those with rheumatoid arthritis, the aging adult, and chronically ill or immunosuppressed individuals) suggests that the influenza and pneumococcal vaccines should include these groups in standard immunization programs.

Prophylactic antibiotic therapy may prevent certain infections and is usually reserved for people at high risk of exposure to dangerous infections or adverse outcomes (e.g., *Pneumocystis carinii* pneumonia in clients with HIV/AIDS, postexposure of HCWs to percutaneous contamination from individuals with HIV, preoperatively before joint replacement surgery).[72] Prophylactic antibiotics are also beneficial following the removal of a urinary catheter after abdominal surgery to avoid urinary tract infections.

Improved nutrition, living conditions, and *sanitation* through the use of disinfection, sterilization, and antiinfective drugs can inactivate multidrug resistant organisms such as *S. aureus*.

Two distinct strains of MRSA have become common causes of hospital and community-acquired infections (HA-MRSA and CA-MRSA). More cases of CA-MRSA linked with skin, soft-tissue infections, and pneumonia are being reported than ever before. MRSA usually develops when multiple antibiotics are used in the treatment of infection, and in older adults who are debilitated, having surgery or multiple invasive procedures, or being treated in critical care units. Depending on whether it is HA-MRSA or CA-MRSA, other risk factors include incarceration, homelessness, living in close quarters (e.g., barracks, dormitories, hospitals, extended care facilities), and comorbidities such as diabetes mellitus and infection with HIV. CA-MRSA is associated with contact sports and shared athletic equipment.[30,84]

Table 8-3	Type of Transmission-Based Precautions and Prevention Guidelines	

Type of Precaution	**Type of Microorganism**	**Measures Taken**
Standard Precautions	Bloodborne pathogens; applies to all clients	See Appendix A
Airborne Precautions	Microorganism transmitted by small particle residue; can suspend in the air and be dispersed by air currents (i.e., coughing, sneezing, talking) *Examples:* • Measles (rubeola) • *Mycobacterium tuberculosis* (MDRT) • Varicella (chickenpox) • Zoster (disseminated shingles)	• Private room with monitored negative airflow (airborne infection isolation room) • ROOM DOOR CLOSED and client in room • Respiratory protection when entering room (specialized, approved filter masks [e.g., N95 mask] in suspected or known tuberculosis) • Restrict entry of certain susceptible people (immunosuppressed, pregnant women) when rubella or varicella is suspected or known • Limited transport of client from room (only when essential); place surgical mask on restricted individual transported
Droplet precautions	Microorganisms transmitted by large particle droplets about 3 feet from the source; generated by sneezing, coughing, talking or during procedures *Examples:* • Invasive *Haemophilus influenzae* type B including meningitis, pneumonia, epiglottis, sepsis • Invasive *Neisseria meningitidis* • Diphtheria, pertussis • *Mycoplasma pneumoniae* • Pneumonia plaque • Streptococcal pharyngitis, pneumonia, or scarlet fever in infants and young children • Adenovirus • Influenza, RSV • Mumps, rubella • Parvovirus B19	• Private room or house with others with same infection • Door may remain open • Wear mask when working within 5 feet of affected person • Limit client transport to only when necessary; place surgical mask on person when transported
Contact precautions	Microorganisms that can be transmitted by direct contact with the client (hand/skin to skin contact); or indirect contact (touching environmental surfaces or client/care items) *Examples:* • Gastrointestinal, respiratory; skin or wound infections • Multidrug-resistant bacteria (MRSA, VRE) • Enteric infections (low infectious dose or prolonged environmental survival) (*Clostridium difficile*) • Diapered or incontinent clients (enterohemorrhagic *Escherichia coli*; *Shigella*; hepatitis A; rotavirus) *In infants and young children* • RSV • Parainfluenza virus • Enteroviral infections • Highly contagious skin infections or those that may occur on dry skin • Diphtheria; herpes simplex virus; impetigo; noncontained abscesses, cellulitis or decubiti; pediculosis; scabies; herpes zoster (disseminated) • Viral/hemorrhagic conjunctivitis • Viral hemorrhagic infections (e.g., Ebola)	• Private room • Glove when entering room • Changes gloves after having contact with infective material that may contain high concentrations of microorganism (e.g., fecal material; wound drainage) • Remove gloves before leaving the client environment and wash hands immediately with antimicrobial soap or waterless antiseptic • After removing gloves and washing hands, DO NOT TOUCH potentially contaminated surfaces or materials • Wear a clean gown when entering the room if you anticipate substantial contact with the contaminated materials or surfaces (particularly if the person is incontinent, has diarrhea, ileostomy, colostomy, or noncontained draining wound) • Remove gown before leaving; do not touch contaminated areas • Limit transport of person from room • Dedicate use of noncritical client care items to only this person (e.g., stethoscope) • Disinfect equipment with approved disinfectant if to be used with other people

MDRT, multidrug-resistant tuberculosis; MRSA, methicillin-resistant *Staphylococcus aureus*; RSV, respiratory syncytial virus; VRE; vancomycin-resistant enterococci.

Modified from Siegel JD, Rhinehart E, Jackson M, Chiarello L, and the Healthcare Infection Control Practices Advisory Committee: 2007 Guideline for isolation precautions: preventing transmission of infectious agents in healthcare settings. Available online at http://www.cdc.gov/hicpac/2007IP/2007isolationPrecautions.html (Alternate URL: http://www.cdc.gov/hicpac/pdf/isolation/Isolation2007.pdf). See page 35 in this document for reference to risk in ambulatory care centers. The delineation of the different facilities in this document confirms the need to keep in mind the importance of appropriate environmental cleaning and hand hygiene in all settings. Refer to pages 77–90 for that information.

Correction of environmental factors, particularly water treatment, food and milk safety programs, and control of animals, vectors, rodents, sewage, and solid wastes, can best eradicate nonhuman environments (reservoirs) and thus control pathogens.

Other prevention methods in this category include proper handling and disposal of secretions, excretions, and exudates; isolation of infected clients (doors must remain closed, especially in negative-pressure rooms); and quarantine of contacts.

The CDC has recommended specific transmission precautions based on knowledge of the transmission chain for individual infections. The precautions were designed to prevent transmission of pathogens among hospitalized people, HCWs, and visitors (see Table 8-3). Specific recommendations have been made for individual diseases.

SPECIAL IMPLICATIONS FOR THE THERAPIST   **8-1**

Control of Transmission

The impact of infections cannot be underestimated in a physical therapy practice or rehabilitation setting. Infections, and especially HAIs, decrease patients' endurance and delay recovery and progression toward discharge or transfer to a more independent setting. We must do everything we can to halt the spread of organisms that can cause or contribute to infections leading to morbidity and mortality at all levels of care.

The CDC has set up guidelines for the care of all clients regarding precautions against the transmission of infectious disease (see Appendix A). These should be used with all clients regardless of their disease status. All blood and body fluids are potentially infectious and should be handled as such (see Box 8-3).

All clients receiving therapy (and thus in contact with HCWs) may be asymptomatic hosts during the period of communicability. The careful use of precautionary measures severely limits the transmission of any disease. Keep in mind risk factors that make people more susceptible to infections (any opening in the skin from wounds, pressure ulcers, surgical incisions; diabetes mellitus or even elevated blood glucose levels; bowel or bladder incontinence following spinal surgery) and include appropriate preventive measures in the plan of care.[152]

In addition, each hospital has transmission-based precautions organized according to categories of transmission routes to prevent the spread of infectious disease to others. Every HCW must be familiar with these procedures and follow them carefully. Transmission prevention guidelines and accompanying basic isolation procedures are provided in Table 8-3 and in greater detail in Appendix A.

Note to Reader: Although we have elected to move the majority of information on infection control to Appendix A, we want to make it clear that this is for ease of reference and not an indication that the material is not important. We think this information is *extremely* important and encourage everyone to read through Appendix A carefully and review this information periodically.

HCWs should be concerned about improving their own resistance and decreasing their susceptibility to infectious diseases. Maintaining an adequate immunization status is one approach. Every HCW should be adequately immunized against hepatitis B, measles, mumps, rubella, polio, tetanus, diphtheria, and varicella. Table 8-4 lists the most recent CDC recommendations for immunization of HCWs. A complete schedule of recommended adult immunizations is available.[23,34]

Health Care–Associated Infections

Therapists can help prevent transmission of HAIs from themselves to others, from client to client, and from client to self by following standard precautions and guidelines presented in Box 8-6, Table 8-5, and Appendix A.

A THERAPIST'S THOUGHTS*
Health Care–Associated Infections

In the past, the term "nosocomial" infection was used to refer to hospital- or nursing home–based infections, but this is considered an older term now. There is mention of this in Appendix A in the section on historical perspective. In fact, it is important to note that another term, "hospital infection control," is also outdated. The new nomenclature is "health care–associated infection." You will still see the term "nosocomial" in use, but most of the literature is using "heath care associated" because patients are receiving their care in a variety of places, including outpatient surgery centers, laboratory centers, dialysis centers, nursing homes, and hospitals. The true definition would include all of these places but they are not all hospitals or nursing homes. The CDC revised its guidelines in 2003 and removed the word "nosocomial" and replaced it with "health care associated." It's important that we all realize that this problem is not just isolated to hospitals and nursing homes. For up-to-date details, see Centers for Disease Control and Prevention: *Healthcare-Associated Infections*, which is available online at: http://www.cdc.gov/hai/.

*Kim Levenhagen, PT, DPT, WCC

Central Line–Associated Bloodstream Infections

The use of central venous catheters is an integral part of modern health care, allowing for the administration of intravenous fluids, blood products, medications, and parenteral nutrition, as well as providing access for hemodialysis and hemodynamic monitoring. The use of central venous catheters is associated with the risk of bloodstream infection caused by microorganisms that colonize the external surface of the device or the fluid pathway when the device is inserted or manipulated after insertion. These serious HAIs, termed *central line–associated bloodstream infections* (CLABSIs), are associated with increased morbidity, mortality, and health care costs.[130] It is now recognized that CLABSIs are largely preventable when evidence based guidelines are followed for the insertion and maintenance of central venous catheters.[204]

As part of an effort to address preventable infections, the Joint Commission has released a document with the most current, evidence-based guidance for the prevention of CLASBIs. Mortality for CLABSIs is as high as 25% in the United States.[204]

Although this is more of a nursing-directed prevention program, therapists must be aware of the potential for central or peripheral line infections and remain vigilant in assessing dressing integrity anywhere near these lines and assist in maintaining entry points that are waterproof and shielded from the external environment. It is truly a team effort to keep patients safe and infection free.[75] Hand hygiene remains an integral part of team effort to prevent all infections, including CLABSIs.

Hydrotherapy and Therapeutic Pool Protocol

See discussion in Appendix A.

Home Health Care

See discussion in Appendix A.

SPECIFIC INFECTIOUS DISEASES

Most infections are confined to specific organ systems. In this book, many of the important infectious disease entities are discussed in the specific chapter dealing with the affected anatomic area. Only the most commonly encountered infectious problems not covered elsewhere are included in this chapter.

Bacterial Infections

Enterobacteriaceae

Enterobacteriaceae is a family of gram-negative bacteria including *Klebsiella*, *E. coli*, *Proteus*, *Serratia*, and *Yersinia*, many of which cause significant disease. This group is typically found in the GI tract of humans, although the oropharynx can also be colonized. These species are also the most commonly isolated gram-negative bacteria in the hospital setting.

Similar to other bacteria such as *S. aureus*, this family continues to develop resistance to multiple classes of antimicrobials. Initially *Enterobacteriaceae* developed resistance to cephalosporins, including third- and fourth-generation cephalosporins, aztreonam, and extended-spectrum penicillins (termed extended-spectrum β-lactamases).

Because this resistance is conferred by plasmid, resistance to aminoglycosides, trimethoprim-sulfamethoxazole and fluoroquinolone drugs are frequently included. Organisms exhibiting this extended-spectrum of resistance were often treated with carbapenems. However, bacteria termed carbapenem-resistant *Enterobacteriaceae* (CRE) or carbapenemase-producing *Enterobacteriaceae* (see Fig. 8-1) now exhibit resistance to carbapenems and are causing increasing cases of infections in acute care settings.

Table 8-4	CDC Recommendations for Immunization of Health Care Personnel (HCP)
Vaccine	**Schedule**
Hepatitis B	Give recombinant vaccine (IM) in a three-dose series; obtain anti-HBs serologic testing 1-2 months after last dose
Influenza	Annual influenza vaccination is recommended for all persons aged 6 months and older who have no medical contraindications; therefore, vaccination of all HCP who have no contraindications is recommended
Measles, mumps, rubella (MMR)	For anyone born in 1957 or later without serologic evidence of immunity or prior vaccination (adults born before 1957 generally are considered immune); contraindicated in pregnancy
Varicella zoster (chickenpox)	HCP who have no serologic proof of immunity, prior vaccination, or history of chickenpox; contraindicated in pregnancy
Tetanus and diphtheria (Td)	Recommended for all adults with booster every 10 years; tetanus prophylaxis advised for HCP in wound management; advised after needle-stick injury. New ACIP recommendations for Tdap (combined tetanus, diphtheria, and pertussis vaccine) in adults and HCP were released in 2011.*
Meningococcal	Not recommended routinely for all HCP; recommended for HCP in direct contact with respiratory secretions from infected persons without proper use of precautions; microbiologists who are routinely exposed to *Neisseria meningitidis*; postexposure prophylaxis advised
Bacille Calmette Guérin (BCG)	Not used in the United States as prophylaxis; foreign-born HCP who have received this vaccine outside the United States must be aware that it does *not* provide lifelong immunity.

HCWs should consult with their physicians for individual recommendations based on medical and other indications.

*Updated recommendations for use of tetanus toxoid, reduced diphtheria toxoid, and acellular pertussis (Tdap) vaccine from the advisory committee on immunization practices, 2010. *MMWR Morb Mortal Wkly Rep* 60(1):13–15, 2011.

For more complete information visit the CDC Vaccines and Immunizations website (http://www.cdc.gov/vaccines), Immunization Action Coalition (IAC) website (http://www.immunize.org/acip), and check with the CDC for updates (http://www.cdc.gov/vaccines/hcp/acip-recs/vacc-specific/index.html).

Data from Centers for Disease Control and Prevention (CDC): Immunization of health-care personnel: recommendations of the advisory committee on immunization practices (ACIP) *MMWR* 60(RR07); 1-45, 2011. Available online at: http://www.cdc.gov/mmwr/preview/mmwrhtml/rr6007a1.htm. Accessed June 23, 2014.

Currently carbapenem-resistant *Klebsiella pneumoniae* (CRKP) is the species of CRE most commonly encountered in the United States. CRKP is resistant to almost all available antimicrobial agents. Infections with CRKP are associated with high rates of morbidity and mortality, particularly in intensive care units and in persons who have undergone an organ transplant.[105,143]

Individuals who have been in the hospital for prolonged periods and those who are critically ill and exposed to invasive devices (e.g., ventilators, central venous catheters) are at increased risk for complications associated with CRKP.[116]

Carbapenem resistance has been on the radar since the late 1990s when imipenem was frequently used in infections associated with hematologic cancers/treatment. Imipenem is an intravenous β-lactam antibiotic developed in 1985. It belongs to the subgroup of carbapenems with an extremely broad spectrum of antimicrobial activity against aerobic and anaerobic gram-positive as well as gram-negative bacteria. It is particularly important for its activity against *P. aeruginosa* and the *Enterococcus* species. Imipenem and other drugs in the carbapenem class are now restricted in use, in order to avoid widespread bacterial resistance.

A new form of carbapenemase ("superbug") that is highly resistant to antibiotics and easily transmitted has been identified: New Delhi metallobeta-lactamase–1 (NDM-1). These bacteria cause a wide range of infections including wound, respiratory, bloodstream, and urinary tract infections. There is concern that increasing human air travel and migration will allow strains of this bacteria to disseminate world-wide. Only two current antibiotic drugs can combat NDM-1.[147,217]

All individuals with CRE are managed by using (and reinforcing the use of) meticulous hand hygiene and contact precautions, including environmental cleaning and disinfecting with appropriate cleaners. Aggressive detection and control strategies are employed to prevent the spread of CRKP and other types of CRE as a public health threat regarding antimicrobial resistance among Gram-negative bacteria.[111,116,132]

Clostridium difficile Infections

Overview. *C. difficile* has become an important public health issue as the most common cause of health care–associated diarrhea worldwide. Once thought to be only associated with antibiotic use in medical settings, it is now also detected in healthy persons in the community without a history of antibiotic exposure. It is an anaerobic, spore-forming bacillus that can cause symptoms ranging from mild diarrhea to severe colonic inflammation leading to death. It is the only anaerobe that poses a health care–associated risk. *C. difficile* infections (CDIs) are most often recognized among residents of long-term care facilities or persons in acute care or short-stay hospitals because of the high rates of antibiotic use.

Box 8-6

TIPS FOR PREVENTING INFECTION

Chest Tube

- Prevent chest tube from kinking by carefully coiling the tubing on top of the bed and securing it to the bed linen (usually according to nursing protocol), leaving room for the person to turn.

Tracheostomy

- Maintain the head of bed at 30 degrees; this helps minimize the risk of HA pneumonia
- Contact with secretions occurs with a tracheostomy; follow standard precautions. When direct contact is made and potential splash secondary to expelled secretions occurs, gown, mask, protective face wear, and gloves are needed.

Urinary Catheter

- Follow standard precautions for hand hygiene.
- Do not allow the drainage bag spigot to come in contact with a contaminated surface.
- When the drainage tubing becomes disconnected, do not touch the ends of the tubing or catheter. Contact the nursing staff for reconnecting.
- Before turning, moving, or transferring a catheterized person, locate the proximal end of the tubing and either clamp it to the person's gown or hold it to allow necessary slack during movement. This will help prevent the catheter from accidentally and traumatically being pulled out.
- Whenever possible, avoid raising the drainage bag above the level of the person's bladder.
- If it becomes necessary to raise the bag during transfers, clamp the tubing but avoid prolonged clamping or kinking of the tubing (except during bladder conditioning).

- Avoid allowing large loops of tubing to dangle from the bedside, wheelchair, or walker.
- Drain all urine from tubing into the bag before the person exercises or ambulates.

Intravenous Devices

- If you have exudative lesions or weeping dermatitis, refrain from all direct contact with intravenous (IV) or invasive equipment until the condition resolves.
- Notify the nursing staff of any suspicious observations such as if the IV device is not dripping at a steady rate (either none at all or flowing very fast); if the IV bag is empty; or if blood is flowing from insertion of the IV catheter tip into the person's body out into the IV line.

Nasogastric and Feeding Tubes

- Care must be taken to avoid excessive movement or pulling and tugging of these tubes.
- Wash your hands before and after touching the entry point of the tube into the body.

Hydrotherapy

- Hydrotherapy for wound care (pulsatile lavage with suction) should be performed in a private treatment room with all walls and doors closed.
- Proper personal protective equipment must be worn when treating the client and/or cleaning hydrotherapy equipment.
- Whirlpool equipment should be cleaned before and after treatment.

Table 8-5 Summary of Important Recommendations and Work Restrictions for Personnel with Infectious Diseases

Disease/Problem	Work Restriction	Duration
Conjunctivitis	Restrict from client contact with the client's environment	Until discharge ceases
Cytomegalovirus infections	No restriction	
Diarrheal diseases		
Acute stage (diarrhea with other symptoms)	Restrict from client contact, contact with the client's environment, or food handling	Until symptoms resolve
Convalescent stage, *Salmonella*	Restrict from care of high-risk clients	Until symptoms resolve; consult with local and state health authorities regarding need for negative stool cultures
Diphtheria	Exclude from duty	Until antimicrobial therapy completed and 2 cultures obtained ≥24 hours apart are negative
Enteroviral infections	Restrict from care of infants, neonates, and immunocompromised persons and their environment	Until symptoms resolve
Hepatitis A	Restrict from client contact, contact with client's environment, and food handling; use proper handwashing	Until 7 days of onset of jaundice
Hepatitis B		
Personnel with acute or chronic hepatitis B surface antigenemia who do not perform exposure-prone procedures	No restriction*, refer to state regulations; standard precautions should always be observed	
Personnel with acute or chronic hepatitis B e antigenemia who perform exposure-prone procedures	Do not perform exposure-prone invasive procedures until counsel from an expert review panel has been sought; panel should review and recommend procedures the worker can perform, taking into account specific procedure and skill and technique of worker; refer to state regulations	Until hepatitis B e antigen (a marker of a high titer of virus) is negative
Hepatitis C	No recommendation	
Herpes simplex		
Genital	No restriction	
Hands (herpetic whitlow)	Restrict from client contact and contact with client's environment	Until lesions heal
Orofacial	Evaluate for need to restrict from care of high risk clients	
HIV	Do not perform exposure-prone invasive procedures until counsel from an expert review panel has been sought; panel should review and recommend procedures the worker can perform, taking into account specific procedure and skill and technique of the worker; standard precautions should always be observed; refer to state regulations	
Measles		
Active	Exclude from duty	Until 7 days after rash appears
Postexposure (susceptible)	Exclude from duty	From 5th day after first exposure through 21st day after last exposure and/or 4 days after rash appears
Meningococcal Infections	Exclude from duty	Until 24 hours after start of effective therapy
Mumps		
Active	Exclude from duty	Until 9 days after onset of parotitis
Postexposure (susceptible personnel)	Exclude from duty	From 12th day after first exposure through 26th day after last exposure or until 9 days after onset of parotitis
Pediculosis	Restrict from duty	Until treated and observed to be free of adult and immature lice

Continued

Table 8-5	Summary of Important Recommendations and Work Restrictions for Personnel with Infectious Diseases—cont'd	

Disease/Problem	Work Restriction	Duration
Pertussis		
Active	Exclude from duty	From beginning of catarrhal stage through 3rd week after onset of paroxysms or until 5 days after start of effective antimicrobial therapy
Postexposure (asymptomatic personnel)	No restriction, prophylaxis recommended	
Postexposure (symptomatic Personnel)	Exclude from duty	Until 5 days after start of effective antimicrobial therapy
Rubella		
Active	Exclude from duty	Until 5 days after rash appears
Postexposure (susceptible personnel)	Exclude from duty	From 7th day after first exposure through 21st day after last exposure
Scabies	Restrict from client contact	Until cleared by medical evaluation
Staphylococcus aureus infection		
Active, draining skin lesions	Restrict from contact with client and client's environment or food handling	Until lesions have resolved
Carrier state	No restriction, unless personnel are epidemiologically linked to transmission of the organism	
Streptococcal infection, group A	Restrict from client care, contact with client's environment or food handling	Until 24 hours after adequate treatment started
Tuberculosis		
Active disease	Exclude from duty	Until proved noninfectious
PPD converter	No restriction if not an active case and if cleared medically	
Varicella		
Active	Exclude from duty	Until all lesions dry and crust
Postexposure (susceptible personnel)	Exclude from duty	From 10th day after first exposure through 21st day (28th day if VZIG given) after last exposure
Viral respiratory infections, acute febrile	Consider excluding from the care of high-risk clients[†] or contact with their environment during community outbreak of RSV influenza	Until acute symptoms resolve
Zoster		
Localized in healthy person	Cover lesions; restrict from care if high-risk clients[‡]	Until lesions dry and crust
Generalized or localized immuno-suppressed person	Restricted from client contact	Until lesions dry and crust
Postexposure (susceptible personnel)	Restrict from client contact	From 10th day after first exposure through 21st day (28th day if VZIG given) after last exposure or, if varicella occurs, until all lesions dry and crust

PPD, purified protein derivative; RSV, respiratory syncytial virus; VZIG, varicella zoster immunoglobulin.
*Unless epidemiologically linked to transmission of infection.
[†]High-risk patients defined by the Advisory Committee of Immunization Practices for complications of influenza.
[‡]Those susceptible to varicella and who are at increased risk of complications of varicella, such as neonates and immunocompromised persons of any age.
Modified from Centers for Disease Control and Preventions: Guidelines for infection control in health care personnel, *Am J Infect Control* 26(3):289–343, 1998. Changes have been made since publication in 1998. wonder.cdc.gov/wonder/prevguid/p0000446/p0000446.asp. Accessed June 26, 2014.

Incidence. CDI rates continue to increase sharply in the United States and Canada and show no sign of decline. The U.S. hospital discharges for which *C. difficile* was listed as a diagnosis more than doubled from 82,000 in 1996 to 178,000 in 2003, with the highest rate reported in adults age 65 years or older. Between the years 1996 and 2009, the incidence of CDI rates in persons older than age 65 years increased 200%. The reason for rising rates of CDIs has been ascribed to the appearance of hypervirulent strains, misuses of antibiotics, and an increase in the number of susceptible people (immune deficiency, advanced age, etc.).[117] The severity of disease has also increased with higher rates of morbidity and mortality.

Etiology, Transmission, and Risk Factors. *C. difficile* is a bacterium that is commonly present in our everyday environment in natural water sources, soil, and animal and human feces. Because *C. difficile* exists in a hardy spore form, it is able to survive for weeks or months. Disease is thought to develop once these spores are picked up and inadvertently ingested (fecal–oral route).

Typically, healthy people do not develop symptoms because of the high numbers of normal bacteria in the intestine. Susceptible persons often have decreased levels of normal flora as a consequence of antibiotic treatment, which allows *C. difficile* to spread quickly. Contamination of the patient care environment also plays an important role. Spores have been found on cart handles, bedrails, bedside tables, toilets, sinks, stethoscopes, thermometers, telephones, and remote controls.

Risk factors include age (65 years and older), use of antibiotics (even many months prior to symptoms), recent hospitalization, residence in a long-term care facility, serious underlying illness or weakened immune system, or a previous diagnosis with *C. difficile* infection. Almost all classes of antibiotics are associated with CDIs; however, the most common antibiotics include fluoroquinolones, cephalosporins, clindamycin, and penicillins.

Factors that disrupt the intestinal mucosa also increase the likelihood of developing a CDI such as chemotherapy, GI surgery, prolonged nasogastric tube placement, and decreased gastric acidity from the use of proton pump inhibitors and H_2 blockers.

Pathogenesis. Disease itself is secondary to the release of toxins (A and B) produced by *C. difficile*. These toxins then induce an inflammatory response which damages the intestinal cells. More virulent strains overproduce toxins leading to severe inflammation and therefore more severe illness.

Clinical Manifestations. CDI is typically recognized by persistent diarrhea associated with antibiotic use in conjunction with abdominal cramping and tenderness. Although loose stools are frequently associated with antibiotic use without infection, *C. difficile* infection is noted by watery diarrhea at least three times a day for 2 or more days. Fever and an elevated white blood count are often not present in mild to moderate infections. Severe disease can be manifested by fever, abdominal pain, ileus, sepsis, toxic megacolon, perforation, and/or sepsis.

MEDICAL MANAGEMENT

DIAGNOSIS AND TREATMENT. The gold standard of diagnosis is by stool culture followed by the identification of toxigenic isolate. However, because of time constraints, faster methods of diagnosis include a two-step procedure that identifies specific toxins in the stool. CT of the abdomen demonstrating thickened bowel or colonoscopy identifying pseudomembranous lesions (present in severe disease) may help identify difficult-to-diagnose cases.

Although no treatment has been shown to be significantly more efficacious than another,[55] standard treatment consists of prompt discontinuation of the antibiotic agent with administration of oral metronidazole (Flagyl) or oral or rectal vancomycin. Relapse is common, occurring in approximately 20% to 30% of patients. Of these, approximately 45% have only a single recurrence, whereas the remaining 55% have two or more relapses. This is often caused by abnormalities in the colonic flora rather than drug resistance. Retreatment of the relapse is again based on severity, although second relapses are often treated with vancomycin because of metronidazole's cumulative neurotoxicity.

Other therapies under investigation include vaccines,[157] monoclonal antibody treatment,[92] and intestinal transplanting of donor fecal specimens, referred to as fecal bacteriotherapy.[8,17,82,108] For more information on fecal bacteriotherapy, go to http://www.medscape.com/viewarticle/765243?src=mp&spon=38.[100]

PREVENTION. Prevention of this HAI is imperative to reduce patient morbidity and mortality and reduce health care costs associated with infection control, medication, and excess hospital days.

CDI is, by and large, a HAI disease and, therefore, most prevention and control efforts take place in the health care setting. Proven strategies include hand hygiene, environmental disinfection, barrier precautions, and antimicrobial stewardship.[191]

Proper handwashing is the most effective prevention, requiring 1 to 2 minutes of washing followed by proper hand drying to remove spores. Only chlorine-based disinfectants and high-concentration vaporized hydrogen peroxide are able to kill spores. Of note, alcohol-based hand products are not sporicidal and are ineffective in removing spores from the hands. Sporicidal wipes that may reduce the transmission of *C. difficile* are now available.[22]

Contact precautions are recommended to prevent the transmission of *C. difficile* in the health care setting consisting of using private rooms or rooms shared by CDI patients, using gloves and gowns for all contact, and using disposable equipment or cleaning equipment between use with each patient.[71] Bundles (grouping together practices rather than performing each separately) can also control infection rates in hospitals.[135]

Preventing oral ingestion of the *C. difficile* organism is important whenever suction devices are used in the oral cavity. A strong correlation has been noted between ventilator-associated pneumonia rates and CDI rates in the critical care population, emphasizing again the importance of cleanliness of anything introduced into an individual's mouth and stomach. A significant means of reducing risk is through the careful use of antimicrobial drugs, as risk may be associated with cumulative antibiotic exposure.[201]

SPECIAL IMPLICATIONS FOR THE THERAPIST | **8-2**

Clostridium difficile

With *C. difficile* illness rates increasing along with the strain's pathogenicity, therapists have an important role in taking measures to reduce transmission, thus potentially preventing the severity of the disease among those at increased risk (e.g., older adults, those who are immunocompromised).

Keep in mind that anyone who has had a history of *C. difficile* is also at increased risk for relapse or recurrence. Half of all individuals experiencing a relapse of *C. difficile* within 2 months of the primary infection are likely infected with a new strain. In these cases, disease-control practices are key to preventing recurrence.

Appropriate measures include adequate hand hygiene with soap and water before and after contact.

Spores are resistant to alcohol so alcohol-based hand rubs are not considered adequate when the disease is in a spore state; most *C. difficile* organisms released during disease outbreaks are in the vegetative form and can be killed by alcohol.[202] Without knowing the exact state of the condition, it is difficult to know when alcohol-based products will be effective.

One other important step the therapist can take to help prevent reinfection is to ensure the environment around the affected individual is clean.[42] Only a few disinfectants (e.g., bleach) are capable of killing the spore-forming organism that causes *C. difficile,* but sanitizers potent enough to kill these organisms can also can damage equipment and surfaces. As discussed in detail in Appendix A (see section on "Environmental Surfaces, Medical and Other Equipment"). CDC guidelines for preferred cleaning, disinfection, and sterilization methods are available online at http://www.cdc.gov/hicpac/pubs.html. See also *Guide to Elimination of Clostridium Difficile in Healthcare Settings,* Washington, DC, Association for Professionals in Infection Control and Epidemiology (APIC), 2008 (http://www.apic.org/Resource_/EliminationGuideForm/5de5d1c1-316a-4b5e-b9b4-c3fbeac1b53e/File/APIC-Cdiff-Elimination-Guide.pdf).

Staphylococcal Infections

Overview and Incidence. Staphylococci bacteria are among the most common bacterial pathogens normally residing on the skin. Although there are more than 30 species of staphylococci, only a few are clinically relevant. They are hardy and able to survive on inanimate objects for an extended period.

S. aureus has become a significant health problem both in the hospital and the community. *S. aureus* isolates can be divided into various categories, based on their molecular and clinical characteristics. MRSA signifies that the isolate is resistant to β-lactam antibiotics including cephalosporins and penicillins. MRSA isolates can be further distinguished as CA-MRSA and HA-MRSA.

CA-MRSA typically refers to cases where the client has not been in a hospital or medical facility within a year of diagnosis; these strains are molecularly unique from HA-MRSA with clinically distinguishable symptoms. HA-MRSA is defined as cases acquired within a year of hospitalization or admission to a medical facility. However, with more cases of CA-MRSA introduced to hospitals, the line of distinction is beginning to blur with CA-MRSA endemic in some hospitals.[53]

Between the years 1992 and 2003, the rates of MRSA infections in ICUs doubled while the proportion of HAIs caused by MRSA tripled.[151] The number of persons colonized with MRSA has significantly increased, particularly with CA-MRSA.[77,167] *S. aureus* and *Staphylococcus epidermidis* continue to be the leading causes of orthopedic implant infections.[131]

Risk Factors. *S. aureus* spreads by direct contact with colonized surfaces or people (typically skin-to-skin). People at risk for CA-MRSA are those living in close quarters, such as households, military personnel, jail detainees, children in daycare and daycare workers, and athletes.[30,54,84,107,186] Other groups include Native Americans, Pacific Islanders, and men who have sex with men. Risk factors for HA-MRSA include recent hospitalization or admission to a medical facility, recent surgery, dialysis, or having an indwelling device, such as a urinary catheter.

The most common location of human colonization of *S. aureus* is the nares (nasal passages), although the skin, axilla, groin, intestines, perineum, vagina, and oropharynx can also be colonized. Infections occur more frequently in individuals who are colonized than those who are not (typically with their own colonized strain). Colonization, therefore, is a significant risk factor for developing a *S. aureus* infection.[145,175] Transient contamination of HCWs' hands can also transmit the bacteria to clients and is an important cause of spreading bacteria in health care settings.[47]

Individuals more likely to develop a *Staphylococcus* infection include surgical and burn patients (from damaged skin); individuals with diabetes (from needlesticks, decreased leukocyte function)[161]; anyone who is neutropenic (polymorphonuclear neutrophils dangerously low); and anyone with prosthetics, chronic skin disease, rheumatoid arthritis, catheters, or on corticosteroid therapy (unable to control local infections sufficiently).

Predisposing factors are multiple and varied depending on disease location (Table 8-6).

Pathogenesis. *S. aureus* cannot invade through intact skin or mucous membranes; infection usually begins with inoculation of the organism though damaged skin. Once inside the body, the organism is a virulent pathogen, secreting membrane-damaging enzymes and toxins that and cause harm to host tissues.

Staphylococci stimulate a significant host immune response, forming a suppurative or pustular local response. If the bacteria are then able to evade local host defenses, they can spread via the bloodstream to almost any location in the body. The bones, joints, kidney, lung, and heart valves are the most common sites of *S. aureus* infections. *Staphylococcus* species are frequently involved in sustaining chronic infections (particularly bones and prosthetic devices) because of their ability to create a biofilm. A biofilm is composed of pockets of surface-attached cells surrounded by an extracellular matrix, which is resistant to antimicrobials and host defense systems.[109]

Clinical Manifestations. CA-MRSA has a predilection for causing pneumonia, and skin and soft-tissue infections, characteristically inducing a suppurative response with abscess formation. The abscesses range in size from microscopic to lesions several centimeters in diameter filled with pus and bacteria (Fig. 8-2). HA-MRSA is often associated with bacteremia, septicemia, endocarditis, osteomyelitis, and surgical incision infections.

Infective syndromes include osteomyelitis, infections of burns or surgical wounds, pneumonia (particularly in newborns and intubated or ICU patients), bacterial arthritis, septicemia, bacterial endocarditis, and toxic shock syndrome. Consumption of toxins produced by staphylococcal species in contaminated food is a common cause of food poisoning. Fever, chills, and symptoms associated with the affected area may accompany staphylococcal infection of any body part.

Staphylococcus-associated *skin infections* include cellulitis (see "Cellulitis" in Chapter 10), furuncles and carbuncles

Table 8-6	Staphylococcal Infections
Type	**Predisposing Factors**
Bacteremia	Infected surgical wounds
	Abscesses
	Infected intravenous or intraarterial catheter sites; catheter tips
	Infected vascular grafts or prostheses
	Infected pressure ulcers
	Osteomyelitis (see further details below in this table)
	Injection-drug abuse
	Source unknown (primary bacteremia)
	Cellulitis
	Burns
	Immunosuppression
	Debilitating diseases (e.g., diabetes, renal failure)
	Infective endocarditis
	Cancer (leukemia) or neutropenia after chemotherapy or radiation
Pneumonia	Immunodeficiency (especially older adults and children [2 yr])
	Chronic lung disease and cystic fibrosis
	Malignancy
	Antibiotics that kill normal respiratory flora but spare *Staphylococcus aureus*
	Viral respiratory infections, especially influenza
	Bloodborne bacteria spread to the lungs from primary sites of infections (e.g., heart valves, abscesses, pulmonary emboli)
	Recent bronchial or endotracheal suctioning or intubation
Enterocolitis	Broad-spectrum antibiotics as prophylaxis for bowel surgery or treatment of hepatic coma
	Elderly; newborn infants (associated with staphylococcal skin lesions)
Osteomyelitis	Hematogenous organisms (bloodborne)
	Skin trauma
	Infection spreading from adjacent joint or other infected tissues
	S. aureus bacteremia
	Orthopedic surgery or trauma
	Cardiothoracic surgery
	Usually occurs in growing bones, especially femur and tibia of children <12 yr
	Male sex
Food poisoning	Contaminated food
Skin infections	Decreased immunity
	Burns or pressure ulcers
	Decreased blood flow
	Skin contamination from nasal discharge
	Foreign bodies
	Underlying skin diseases, such as eczema and acne
	Common in persons with poor hygiene living in crowded quarters

(boil-like lesions), and small macules that may develop into pus-filled vesicles. Associated symptoms may include mild or spiking fever and malaise. Scalded skin syndrome is typically seen in infants with exfoliation of skin secondary to staphylococcal-produced toxins.

Coagulase-negative staphylococci are most often associated with prosthetic device infections: prosthetic cardiac valves and joints, vascular grafts, intravascular devices, and CNS shunts. Coagulase-negative staphylococci do not typically produce fulminant symptoms.[153] Individuals may present with mild fever, pain, and slightly elevated leukocytosis with a subtle course of illness.

MEDICAL MANAGEMENT

DIAGNOSIS, TREATMENT, AND PROGNOSIS. Gram stain and culture of the organism from the infected site, blood, or other fluid is usually diagnostic; antibiotic sensitivity testing is important. A 2-hour blood assay can now detect both MRSA and *S. aureus* rapidly, making it possible to start treating MRSA infections within hours rather than within days.

Gram stain is a laboratory staining technique used to distinguish between two groups of bacteria by identifying differences in the structure of their cell walls. The Gram stain was named after Danish bacteriologist Christian Gram, who developed this technique. Gram stain has become an important laboratory tool, distinguishing between so-called gram-positive bacteria, which remain colored after the staining procedure, and gram-negative bacteria, which do not retain dye.

Polymerase chain reaction (PCR)–based assays are becoming more available for rapid diagnosis of *S. aureus*,

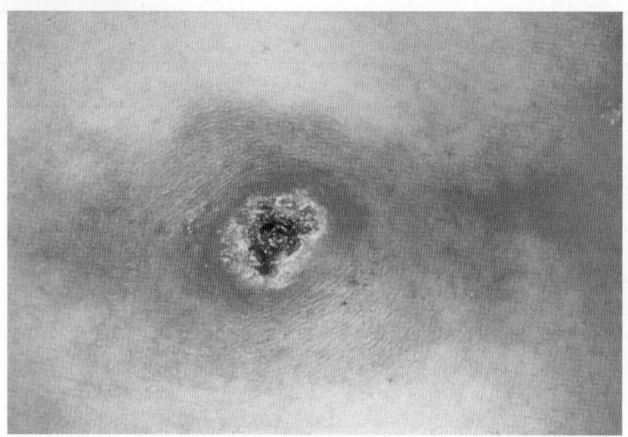

Figure 8-2

Staphylococcus **skin abscess.** (Reprinted from Braverman IM: *Skin signs of systemic disease*, ed 3, Philadelphia, 1998, WB Saunders.)

especially in areas where resistance is high. Because coagulase-negative staphylococci are ubiquitously found on the skin and are a common contaminant, the isolation of coagulase-negative staphylococci does not always indicate infection.

Isolation of *S. aureus* in blood cultures usually confirms bacteremia, and several positive blood cultures can be diagnostic of endocarditis in the presence of a new murmur or echocardiogram demonstrating valvular vegetations.

CA-MRSA retains susceptibility to some oral medications, such as trimethoprim-sulfamethoxazole and tetracyclines, which may be used for minor soft-tissue and skin infections. Not all purulent soft-tissue infections require antibiotics. For small abscesses (less than 5 cm) without associated systemic symptoms (i.e., fever, tachycardia, or blood pressure instability), incision and drainage may suffice. For moderate to severe infections with systemic symptoms, hospitalization with intravenous antibiotic treatment (typically vancomycin) is warranted with appropriate incision/drainage.[50] Treatment of HA-MRSA often requires IV treatment with vancomycin.

Prevention still remains key to reducing the number of HA-MRSA cases. The Veterans Administration was able to implement a bundling system to significantly decrease HA-MRSA infections by 62%. This consisted of universal admission surveillance, contact precautions, hand hygiene, and a change in institutional culture.[97] They found an admission colonization rate of 13.6%. Debate continues concerning universal screening surveillance when clients are admitted to a medical facility and studies are needed to determine cost-effectiveness of this approach.

Reports of reduced susceptibility to vancomycin among strains of *S. aureus* are on the rise. Strains may be determined to be vancomycin-intermediate and -resistant *S. aureus*. Novel antibiotics are being developed to deal with such strains. There are vancomycin alternatives and other compounds in early development.[155]

Studies are underway to develop an effective vaccine to prevent *S. aureus*. Although it may be several years before vaccines against *S. aureus* are available for human beings,

immunization may represent an important step toward solving the problem of antimicrobial resistance.[163]

Prognosis is good with treatment, although antibiotic-resistant strains are increasingly associated with increased morbidity and mortality. Infective endocarditis with *S. aureus* remains a serious life-threatening illness, with 20% to 40% mortality. Visceral abscesses, osteomyelitis, and staphylococcal sepsis are illnesses that are potentially lethal.

SPECIAL IMPLICATIONS FOR THE THERAPIST 8-3

Staphylococcal Infections

Some organisms, such as *S. aureus* (and streptococci), are considered resident organisms because they are not easily removed by scrubbing and often can be cultured from the HCW's skin. Many HCWs carry *S. aureus* without sequelae and are able to shed organisms into nonintact skin areas of susceptible hosts, causing infections.

For the most part, good handwashing with soap or an alcohol-based rub is adequate in the therapy or home setting, but therapists need to consistently educate family members and caregivers about infection control through proper hand hygiene and environmental management.

Antimicrobial soaps that contain chemicals to kill transient and some resident organisms may be recommended, although debate continues over questions of long-term resistance. The choice of using an antimicrobial soap or plain soap is usually based on the need to reduce and maintain minimal counts of resident organisms and to mechanically remove transient organisms such as *Pseudomonas*, *E. coli*, *Salmonella*, or *Shigella*.

When working with people who are infected with drug-resistant, gram-positive cocci such as MRSA[127] or vancomycin-resistant enterococci, antimicrobial soap may be recommended because some studies show that these organisms persist on hands until an antimicrobial product is used.[76]

Some questions have been raised regarding isolation procedures for methicillin- or vancomycin-resistant clients who have been discharged from an isolation setting as an inpatient but are now returning to therapy as an outpatient. Is a separate area required? Are special precautions necessary?

Anyone with an active, resistant infection should not be discharged from an inpatient setting. However, if such a case is encountered, the therapist must remember that these organisms are spread by contact. Symptoms may improve but the patient is still colonized for days to months later still placing the caregiver and others at risk. Therefore the same germicidal cleaning measures used in a hospital or institutional setting are required.

All equipment that comes in direct contact with a draining area needs to be cleaned with an approved germicidal before and after use. Isolation (e.g., private room or separate area of the gym or clinic) is not required. The American Physical Therapy Association infection control guidelines for hydrotherapy and physical therapy aquatic programs recommend that clients with MRSA may attend therapy programs provided the area of colonization can be contained. If it is in a wound, the drainage must be contained within the dressing without evidence of breakthrough.

Streptococcal Infections

Group A Streptococci. *Streptococcus pyogenes*, the prototype of group A streptococci (GAS), is one of the most common bacterial pathogens of humans of any age. It causes many diseases of diverse organ systems, ranging from skin infections to acute self-limited pharyngitis to postinfectious syndromes of rheumatic fever and poststreptococcal glomerulonephritis (Box 8-7).

GAS is typically transmitted via contact with respiratory droplets, although other, less-common mechanisms have been identified, such as foodborne. In health care settings, personnel may spread GAS after contact with clients who have infected secretions or may become infected themselves. The infected personnel subsequently acquire a variety of GAS-related illnesses (e.g., toxic shock–like syndrome, cellulitis, and pharyngitis).

HCWs who are GAS carriers have infrequently been linked to sporadic outbreaks of surgical site, postpartum, or burn wound infection and to foodborne transmission of GAS causing pharyngitis. Adherence to standard precautions or other transmission-based precautions can prevent health care–associated transmission of GAS to personnel. Restriction from client care activities and food handling is indicated for personnel *with* GAS (see Table 8-5).

Box 8-7

STREPTOCOCCAL INFECTIONS

***Streptococcus pyogenes* (Group A Streptococci)**

Suppurative

- Streptococcal pharyngitis
- Scarlet fever (scarlatina)
- Impetigo (streptococcal pyoderma)
- Streptococcal gangrene (necrotizing fasciitis)
- Streptococcal cellulitis
- Streptococcal myositis
- Puerperal sepsis (following vaginal delivery or abortion)
- Toxic shock syndrome (TSS)
- Pneumonia (rare)

Nonsuppurative

- Rheumatic fever
- Acute poststreptococcal glomerulonephritis

***Streptococcus agalactiae* (Group B Streptococci)**

- Neonatal streptococcal infections
- Adult group B streptococcal infection

Streptococcus pneumoniae

- Pneumococcal pneumonia
- Otitis media
- Meningitis
- Endocarditis

Signs, symptoms, and complications of GAS depend upon the location of the infection.

Streptococcal Pharyngitis. Streptococcal pharyngitis, commonly known as *strep throat*, occurs most commonly in children and accounts for 15% to 36% of all sore throats in children and only 10% of adults.[13,112] It is also the only pharyngitis requiring antibiotic treatment.

The infection occurs most commonly from October to April in children ages 5 to 10 years, but a recent increase has occurred among adults ages 30 to 50 years. This organism often colonizes in throats of people with no symptoms; up to 20% of schoolchildren may be carriers.[14]

The incubation stage is 2 to 4 days. Clinical manifestations vary but may include a fever, sore throat with pain on swallowing (may be severe), beefy red pharynx, edematous tonsils with exudate, swollen lymph nodes along the jaw line, generalized malaise and weakness, anorexia, and occasional abdominal discomfort (particularly in children). Affected children may have symptoms too mild for diagnosis.

Complications have significantly been reduced with the advent of antibiotics but may include otitis media, sinusitis, peritonsillar or retropharyngeal abscess, bacteremia, endocarditis, meningitis, pneumonia, and osteomyelitis. Poststreptococcal sequelae include acute rheumatic fever or acute glomerulonephritis. Diagnosis is usually by rapid diagnostic kits, but if negative a throat culture (the gold standard) should be performed. Treatment is with antibiotics to avoid poststreptococcal syndromes. A positive test for *Streptococcus* should be obtained prior to treatment in order to avoid overuse of antibiotics.

Scarlet Fever. Scarlet fever usually follows untreated streptococcal pharyngitis but may also occur after wound infections. It is caused by a streptococcal strain that releases pyogenic exotoxins and is most common in children ages 2 to 10 years.

The streptococcus is acquired by inhalation or direct contact with oral secretions and presents with a sore throat, fever, strawberry tongue (white-coated tongue with prominent red papillae), and a fine erythematous rash that blanches on pressure and has been described as feeling like sandpaper. The white coat on the tongue disappears, leaving a red, "beefy" tongue. The rash first appears on the upper chest and then spreads to the extremities, sparing the soles and palms. The rash fades over a week and after 6 to 9 days there is a general desquamation of the skin, which can last for weeks.[14] Because of the availability of antibiotics, severe disease and complications are rarely seen. Complications and disease may include high fever, hypotension, arthritis, and jaundice. Rare poststreptococcal complications are acute rheumatic fever and acute poststreptococcal glomerulonephritis.

Impetigo. Impetigo is included here so the reader may appreciate that it is principally caused by GAS, although other streptococcal or staphylococcal species may be involved. See Chapter 10 for complete discussion of this condition. Colonization with GAS most often precedes the skin lesions, so good hygiene is essential.

Streptococcal Cellulitis. Streptococcal cellulitis, an acute spreading inflammation of the skin and subcutaneous tissues, usually results from infection of burns, wounds, or other breaks in the skin, although in some cases no entry site is noted.[14] Recurrent episodes of cellulitis may occur in extremities in which lymphatic drainage has been impaired (e.g., postaxillary node dissection, site of saphenous vein harvest) or chronic fungal infections serve as a reservoir.[183]

The skin is painful and swollen with accompanying erythema. Systemic symptoms such as fever and chills are often associated with the skin infection. Cellulitis can rapidly spread or involve bacteremia or lymphangitis. Lymphangitis is readily recognized by the presence of red, tender, linear streaks directed toward enlarged, tender regional lymph nodes. It is accompanied by systemic symptoms such as chills, fever, malaise, and headache (see "Cellulitis" in Chapter 10 and "Lymphangitis" in Chapter 13).

Erysipelas. This skin infection is a type of cellulitis typically caused by GAS and involves the upper dermis and superficial lymphatics. The skin is painful, very red, shiny, and swollen in appearance (Fig. 8-3) (elevated above the surrounding normal skin). This type of cellulitis develops

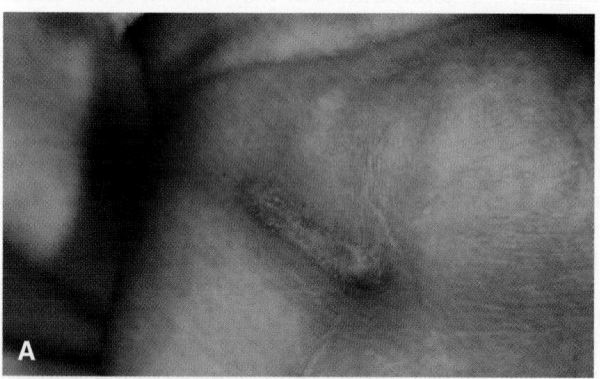

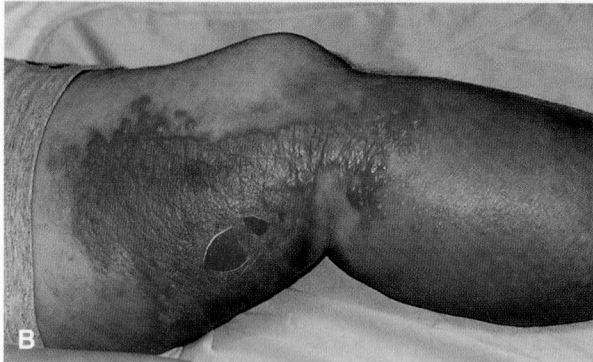

Figure 8-3

Cellulitis and lymphangitis. A, Infection in a wound is usually caused by streptococcal bacteria, but often in combination with *Staphylococcus.* Infection can be local without streaking (cellulitis), local infection with streaking toward the heart (lymphangitis or blood poisoning), or pus forming (boil or abscess). This boy stuck a needle into a burn blister on his palm the previous day. Note the redness and the streaking. **B,** Erysipelas, a type of cellulitis, is more of a clinical diagnosis describing an infectious skin condition characterized by sharp, elevated, demarcated borders; redness; swelling; vesicles; bullae; fever; pain; and lymphadenopathy. Erysipelas affects the face and legs most often. It is almost always caused by GAS but can be caused by *Staphylococcus.* (A, Courtesy Bruce Argyle, Utah Mountain Biking, http://www.utahmount ainbiking.com/firstaid/infect.htm. B, Reprinted from Black JM, Hawks JH: *Medical-surgical nursing: clinical management for positive outcomes,* ed 7, Philadelphia, 2006, WB Saunders.)

over a few hours; vesicles and bullae may form in the affected areas after 2 to 3 days. The margins between normal and infected skin are well demarcated. Systemic symptoms such as fever and chills are common.

The most common area affected is the legs followed by the face, although erysipelas can occur anywhere.[83] The disease is more common in women and may be especially severe in anyone with a debilitating condition. Antibiotics that cover GAS are the treatment of choice, but may need to be broadened to include staphylococcal species.

Streptococcal Toxic Shock Syndrome. Streptococcal toxic shock syndrome (STSS) is any streptococcal infection that leads to shock and organ failure. Streptococcal species involved in STSS typically carry virulence factors, allowing for aggressive, penetrating behavior.[43] Most cases are sporadic, although reports of transmission from one infected person to another have been published. It may occur in persons of any age and in previously healthy individuals.

STSS is a component of many subtypes of streptococcal infections, such as streptococcal necrotizing fasciitis, postpartum infection, and joint infection.[14] *Streptococcus* enters the body via the vagina, pharynx, mucosa and skin (trauma) or during a surgical procedure. Viruses such as varicella and influenza provide a means for *Streptococcus* to enter the skin. *Streptococcus* pharyngitis rarely leads to STSS.

Once the microbe has entered the body, it may be able to penetrate into deeper tissue and the bloodstream secondary to an existing injury or wound, or invade intact tissue.[14] Pyrogenic exotoxins are produced, leading to shock and organ failure.

Initial symptoms (24-48 hours) are influenza-like, including fever, chills, nausea, and vomiting. For those individuals who subsequently develop necrotizing fasciitis, pain is typically their first symptom. Systemic symptoms including tachycardia, persistent fever, and tachypnea then appear, followed by sudden shock exhibited by hypotension, delirium, and evidence of organ failure (i.e., renal and liver impairment, coagulopathy, respiratory distress syndrome). Treatment consists of locating the source of the infection, surgical debridement, supportive measures, and intravenous antibiotics.[14]

Streptococcal Necrotizing Fasciitis. Necrotizing fasciitis (NF; also called necrotizing soft-tissue infections) is a rare but serious infection. The CDC estimates there are approximately 500 to 1500 cases per year,[4] but the National Necrotizing Fasciitis Foundation suggests a higher figure based on cases reported to them.[141] NF progresses rapidly along fascial planes, usually in the legs, causing severe tissue damage as it spreads and consumes whatever soft tissue is in its path (fat, muscle, nerves, connective tissue).

Although many bacteria can be involved in causing NF, *Streptococcal* species are often implicated. One classification system separates NF into type I and type II. Type I is a polymicrobial infection (often including *Enterobacteriaceae* and anaerobes) that typically occurs following surgery when protective mucosa of the GI or genitourinary tract is damaged or when seeding occurs from an occult abscess. Gas formation may also form. *S. pyogenes* accounts for more than 60% of type II NF and often originates from a distal break in the skin or transient bacteremia.

Something as simple as a rug burn, punch on the arm, paper cut, blood draw, or toothpick injury can precede this condition. NF is a rare but serious complication of chickenpox lesions and should be suspected in children with progressive pain, fever, and lethargy.[223]

NF may be difficult to diagnose initially. Pain (usually disproportionate to the appearance) and fever are present but the overlying skin often is without abnormalities. In approximately 20% of all NF cases, a precipitating lesion is not found; this is more common in NF caused by *Streptococcus* species than other bacteria.[4]

The infection spreads rapidly, causing edema and tenderness. Changes later occur in the skin as thrombosis of blood vessels occurs. The skin turns a dark red color with accompanying induration. Bullae form and fill with dark fluid. Later the skin becomes friable and turns a maroon or black color consistent with ischemia.

The bacteria produce several pyogenic endotoxins, causing severe breakdown of tissue in multiple organs. Affected individuals commonly experience toxic shock syndrome with hypotension, nausea, vomiting, and delirium. There is often renal and hepatic compromise as well as pulmonary infiltrates, leading to respiratory distress. Mortality rate is high, with 1 in 4 persons dying from the infection.[151]

Immediate surgery with aggressive debridement of all necrotic tissue along with appropriate intensive IV antibiotics is essential to save muscles and limbs. Gram stain and culture of the site is essential to identify the organism(s) and antimicrobial susceptibility. Multiple procedures and serial debridement may be necessary with secondary closure as the demarcation line of infection is difficult to identify.

Streptococcal Myositis. Streptococcal myositis is a rare but potentially life-threatening entity characterized by severe pain and inflammation in the affected muscle with few abnormalities of overlying skin. Typically blunt, nonpenetrating trauma or hematologic seeding of bacteria to the muscle leads to the infection. Streptococcal myositis is fulminant with systemic symptoms, high fever, bacteremia, and a high mortality rate (80%).[14]

This condition can also be caused by other bacteria (usually *S. aureus*), mycobacteria, fungi, viruses, and protozoan forms. Clinical features of myositis and NF often overlap and are distinguished at surgery and by biopsy.[1] Therapy includes aggressive surgical debridement and IV antibiotics (see "Myositis" in Chapter 25 and "Streptococcal Necrotizing Fasciitis" in this chapter).

Puerperal Sepsis. Puerperal sepsis follows abortion or normal delivery when streptococci colonizing the woman or transmitted from medical personnel invade the endometrium and surrounding structures, lymphatics, and bloodstream.[193] The resulting endometritis and septicemia may be complicated by pelvic cellulitis, septic pelvic thrombophlebitis, peritonitis, or pelvic abscess. Before the antibiotic era and the benefits of handwashing between clients were known, this disease was more common and associated with a high mortality rate.

SPECIAL IMPLICATIONS FOR THE THERAPIST   **8-4**

Streptococcal Infections

Health care personnel can transmit and acquire streptococcal infections. Guidelines for preventing transmission must be followed at all times (see Boxes 8-4 and 8-5, Table 8-4, and Appendix A).

Group B Streptococci. Group B streptococcal infection (*Streptococcus agalactiae*) is the leading cause of neonatal pneumonia, meningitis, and sepsis. More than 1000 neonatal infections with group B streptococci occur in the United States each year, and approximately 5% of the infants with the infection die.[30,181] Among preterm infants born with the disease, the mortality rate is high, around 22%.[25] The frequency of infections in adults has increased two- to fourfold over the last 2 decades, particularly in older adults and persons with underlying disease.[58]

Group B streptococci are part of the normal vaginal flora and are found in more than 20% of women.[57] Most newborns born to colonized women acquire the organism as they pass through the birth canal. Approximately 50% become colonized,[57] but only 1% of these infants develop group B streptococcal infections. With the implementation of maternal antibiotic prophylaxis guidelines, the rate of early-onset group B streptococcal infections has significantly decreased.

Neonates who develop early infections (birth to 1 week) may present with hypotension, pneumonia (and respiratory distress), bacteremia, or meningitis. Late disease (1 week to 3 months) is acquired either at birth or from contact with the infected mother or other personnel. These babies demonstrate fever, bacteremia, meningitis, and pneumonia.

Rapid administration of IV antibiotics is essential. The CDC recommends that pregnant women be screened for carriage of group B streptococci and appropriate antibiotics be given to prevent transmission to the baby.[38] A vaccine is under development that would reduce the number of women and babies exposed to antibiotics.[88]

Group B streptococci can cause peripartum infections in women, such as endometritis or chorioamnionitis. Resulting bacteremia can lead to endocarditis or meningitis. Appropriate antibiotics are required for treatment.

Adults (men and nonpregnant women) now comprise the majority of cases (approximately 65%) of group B streptococcal infections.[57,181] Most affected individuals are elderly, in a nursing home, or have a chronic disease or are immunocompromised.[158]

The most common infections in adults are skin and soft tissue infections (approximately 33% of cases),[182] primary bacteremia, and pneumonia. Other infections include arthritis, osteomyelitis, and endocarditis. Adults are more likely to die from group B streptococcal infections than neonates, with a mortality rate between 5% and 25%, depending on the location of the infection.[58,181] Mortality increases with age and presence of underlying disease.

Streptococcus pneumoniae

Etiologic and Risk Factors. Pneumonia and other infections, such as sepsis, otitis media, and meningitis, can be caused by *Streptococcus pneumoniae* (pneumococcal pneumonia or pneumococcus) (see Box 8-7). This organism is thought to be responsible for more than 700,000 deaths worldwide in children younger than age 5 years.[228] In the United States, during 2009 there were more than 43,500 cases with 5000 deaths.[38] *S. pneumoniae* colonizes the oropharynx and nasopharynx and can be found in 5% to 10% of healthy adults and 20% to 40% of children.[73,90] Once colonized, the host can develop illness related to *S. pneumoniae* by spreading to the sinuses or eustachian tubes or inhaling the bacteria into the lungs. Hematogenous spread occurs, creating disease in other organs (i.e., endocarditis).

Transmission from person to person is by direct contact or inhalation of droplets of respiratory secretions. *S. pneumoniae* causes disease particularly in the very young and the old. It is the most common cause of community-acquired pneumonia. Pneumococcal pneumonia often follows influenza or viral respiratory infections and is often seen in clients with chronic diseases or immunosuppression and in alcohol abusers. Box 8-8 lists other risk factors.

S. pneumoniae is the most common cause of meningitis in adults, infants, and toddlers. Head trauma, cerebrospinal fluid leaks, otitis media, and sinusitis may precede pneumococcal meningitis, creating an extension of disease or opportunity for direct infection. Pneumonia may lead to bacteremia with subsequent seeding of the meninges.

Clinical Manifestations. Clinical manifestations of pneumonia include acute onset of fever, chills, pleuritis with pleuritic chest pain, and dyspnea with productive cough or purulent sputum that may be blood tinged. Because pneumococcal disease occurs most commonly in the very young and the very old, the presenting features will vary. Older adults may have only a slight cough or delirium but lack a fever. An elevated respiratory rate is frequently present. Increased morbidity and mortality is associated with a lack of fever and hypothermia.[134] Complications from pneumococcal pneumonia may include empyema (approximately 2% of cases), bacteremia, sepsis, or meningitis.

Infection of the meninges (meningitis) stimulates a robust inflammation, leading to increased intracranial pressure and brain edema with headache and nausea/vomiting, mental status changes, stiff neck, and fever. The disease progresses rapidly over 24 to 48 hours and mortality rate is high without treatment.

Rare complications of *S. pneumoniae* include pericarditis, endocarditis, peritonitis, and septic arthritis. Septic arthritis can occur in a natural or prosthetic joint or in damaged joints from rheumatoid arthritis; underlying chronic joint disease may delay diagnosis.

MEDICAL MANAGEMENT

DIAGNOSIS, TREATMENT, AND PREVENTION. Diagnosis of pneumococcal disease is by laboratory examination of sputum (pneumonia), cerebrospinal fluid (meningitis), or blood (bacteremia) with Gram stain and culture of the organism. Treatment is with antibiotics that are effective against local pneumococcal strains and take into consideration resistance patterns in the community. In the year 2010, a 13-valent pneumococcal polysaccharide conjugate vaccine became available for young children and infants.[150]

Currently, the 23-valent pneumococcal polysaccharide vaccine is available for adults.[38] Immunization for pneumococcal disease is available and is recommended in specific circumstances as defined by the CDC. Adults age 65 years and older should receive 1 dose of the vaccine. Individuals ages 19 to 64 years with defined conditions, such as immunocompromise, HIV, asplenia, chronic liver or renal dysfunction, pulmonary disorders (chronic obstructive pulmonary disease), and diabetes mellitus, should be vaccinated.

Persons with asthma or who smoke should also be vaccinated. With the introduction and implementation of vaccine programs, rates for hospitalization and clinic visits for infections relating to *S. pneumoniae* have significantly decreased.[150] Efficacy has not been proven in the very old and the immunocompromised.[38]

Overall, the rate of antibiotic-resistant invasive pneumococcal infections has decreased for all ages,[99] with the expanded valence vaccines (more serotypes are covered). As a bonus, the use of vaccines against pneumococcal bacteria in children has also reduced the rate of pneumococcal disease in adults because fewer bacteria are passed from children to adults. Prudent use of antibiotics will aid in decreasing the presence of drug resistant species.

Gas Gangrene (Clostridial Myonecrosis)

Definition and Overview. *Gangrene* is the death of body tissue, usually associated with loss of vascular (nutritive, arterial circulation) supply and followed by bacterial invasion and putrefaction. The three major types of gangrene are dry, moist, and gas gangrene.

Dry and moist gangrene results from loss of blood circulation from various causes. Gas gangrene occurs in wounds infected by anaerobic bacteria (in this case, *Clostridium*), leading to the production of exotoxins that

---

Box 8-8
RISK FACTORS FOR PNEUMOCOCCAL DISEASE

Age
- Children age younger than age 2 years
- Adults age 65 years or older

Recent episode of influenza or viral respiratory infection

Chronic illness
- Diabetes mellitus
- Heart disease
- Pulmonary disease
- Renal disease
- Liver disease

Immunosuppression/unable to make antibodies
- HIV
- Multiple myeloma
- Leukemia
- Lymphoma
- Hodgkin disease
- Transplant recipients
- Chronic use of corticosteroids

Neurologic impairment (cerebrospinal fluid leak)

History of alcoholism

Asplenia (absent, removed, or nonfunctioning spleen)

Crowding or close contact with infected persons (shelters, nursing homes, prisons, military camps, daycare centers)

break down cells, leaving necrotic tissue. Gas production is a by-product.

This is a rare but severe and painful condition that usually follows trauma or surgery (70% of cases).[2] Of this type of gas gangrene, approximately 80% are caused by *Clostridium perfringens*. Another category of clostridial myonecrosis occurs without a known injury termed spontaneous or nontraumatic gangrene (seen in persons with malignancy or intestinal tract abnormalities).[200] The disease spreads rapidly to adjacent tissues and can be fatal within hours of onset.

Pathogenesis. Fortunately, the anaerobic conditions necessary to foster clostridial growth are uncommon in human tissues and are produced only in an environment low in oxygen. Contributing factors include the presence of devitalized tissue, such as occurs with trauma, wartime injuries, and septic abortions; hypoxia from obstructed microvasculature (clotting of small vessels secondary to toxin production), injured vessels, pressure dressings, local injection of vasoconstrictors; and foreign bodies.

Gas gangrene is most often found in deep wounds, especially those in which tissue necrosis further reduces oxygen supply.

Clinical Manifestations. The incubation period for *Clostridium* ranges from 24 hours to 3 days. Sudden, severe pain occurring at the site of the wound, which is tender and edematous, is an early sign and symptom of gas gangrene. The skin darkens because of hemorrhage and cutaneous necrosis. The lesion develops a thick discharge with a foul odor and may contain gas bubbles. Crepitation may be felt on palpation of the skin from the gas bubbles in muscles and subcutaneous tissue.

True gas gangrene produces myositis and anaerobic cellulitis, affecting only soft tissue. The skin over the wound may rupture, revealing dark-red or black necrotic muscle tissue accompanied by a foul-smelling watery or frothy discharge. Associated symptoms may include sweating, low-grade fever, and disproportionate tachycardia followed by hemolytic anemia, septic shock (e.g., decrease in blood pressure), liver necrosis, and renal failure. Details on any of these conditions can be found in individual chapters (see index).

MEDICAL MANAGEMENT

DIAGNOSIS, TREATMENT, AND PROGNOSIS. Radiographs may demonstrate evidence of gas formation, although gas may not be seen in early stages, whereas CT or MRI may show infection along fascial planes. Diagnosis can be established by frozen section of muscle. Gram stain and culture also verify the diagnosis but not as rapidly.

Early, immediate intervention is necessary (diagnostic tests should not delay surgery) with surgical debridement and excision of necrotic tissue. Delay of more than 12 hours is associated with an increase in mortality.[2] Antibiotics are administered, but if significant gangrene develops then amputation may be necessary. Hyperbaric oxygen therapy following surgery is controversial.[103,113] Mortality can be very high, often depending upon the location of the

infection; of the 50% of people who develop shock, 40% will die.[199]

Gas Gangrene
Careful observation may result in early diagnosis. With any postoperative or posttraumatic injury, look for signs of ischemia such as cool skin; pallor or cyanosis; sudden, severe pain; sudden edema; and loss of pulses in the involved limb. Record carefully and immediately report these findings to the medical staff. Throughout this illness, adequate fluid replacement is essential; assess pulmonary and cardiac functions often.

Special care to prevent skin breakdown is important, and meticulous wound care following surgery is imperative. To prevent gas gangrene, routinely take precautions to render all wound sites unsuitable for growth of *Clostridia* by attempting to keep granulation tissue viable; adequate debridement is imperative to reduce anaerobic growth conditions. Notify the physician immediately of any devitalized tissue. Position the client to facilitate drainage.

Psychologic support is critical, as these clients can remain alert until death, knowing that death is imminent and unavoidable. The therapist must be prepared for the foul odor from the wound and prepare the client emotionally for the large wound after surgical excision. Wound care may require sterile procedures to prevent spread of bacteria; dispose of drainage material and dressings in double plastic bags for incineration. No special cleaning measures are required after the client is discharged.

Pseudomonas
Overview. *P. aeruginosa* is a major opportunistic pathogen and one of the most common hospital- (particularly ICU) and nursing home–acquired pathogens. *Pseudomonas* is uncommon in community-acquired infections and healthy individuals.[69] The organism is ubiquitous in nature and infrequently colonizes humans (upper respiratory tract), but it can cause disease, particularly in the hospital environment, where it is associated with pneumonia, wound infections,[187] urinary tract disease, and sepsis in debilitated people.

Burns, urinary catheterization, cystic fibrosis, chronic lung diseases, neutropenia associated with chemotherapy, and diabetes all predispose to infections with *P. aeruginosa*. It thrives on moist environmental surfaces, making swimming pools, whirlpool tubs, respiratory therapy equipment, flowers, endoscopes, bronchoscopes and cleaning solutions prime targets for growth.

This organism produces several virulence factors and is inherently antibiotic resistant. Spread of the organism in a health care setting is by contact, typically from a reservoir as described above. HCWs have been known to pass the organism on their hands or under fingernails.[16]

Pathogenesis. *P. aeruginosa* is a versatile bacterium that relies on complex signaling pathways in order to produce acute or chronic disease or simply colonize a tissue.[40] *P. aeruginosa* produces an array of proteins, which allow it to attach to, invade, and destroy host tissues while avoiding host inflammatory and immune defenses. Injury to epithelial cells uncovers surface molecules that serve as binding sites for *P. aeruginosa*.

Many strains of this pathogen produce a proteoglycan that surrounds the bacteria (i.e., a biofilm),[124] protecting them from mucociliary action, complement, and phagocytes. The organism releases extracellular enzymes, which facilitate tissue invasion and are partially responsible for the necrotizing lesions associated with *Pseudomonas* infections. This pathogen can also invade blood vessel walls and produce systemic pathologic effects through endotoxin and several systemically active exotoxins.

Clinical Manifestations. Signs and symptoms of *Pseudomonas* infection vary with the site of infection and the state of host defenses. If the host has the capacity to respond to the invading bacteria with neutrophils, an acute inflammatory response results.

The *Pseudomonas* organism often invades small arteries and veins, producing vascular thrombosis and hemorrhagic necrosis, particularly in the lungs and skin. Blood vessel invasion predisposes to bacteremia, dissemination, and sepsis. This bacterium causes infections of the respiratory tract (pneumonia), bloodstream, CNS, skin (see Fig. 8-4) and soft tissues, bone and joints, and other parts of the body.

Respiratory Tract Infections. Pneumonia caused by *P. aeruginosa* is one of the most common causes of healthcare acquired pneumonia.[69] Of all sites which may become infected with *P. aeruginosa*, lung infections carry the highest mortality.[69] Lung infections occur as three principle syndromes: (1) in persons with chronic lung disease, such as chronic obstructive pulmonary disease; (2) hospital-acquired, typically in the intensive care unit; and (3) secondary to a bacteremia which spread to the lungs, often seen in neutropenic individuals.[69] With the advent of highly active antiretroviral therapy (HAART) for the treatment of AIDS, pneumonia caused by *P. aeruginosa* in people with HIV has significantly decreased.

The signs and symptoms of pneumonia caused by *Pseudomonas* are typical of pneumonias seen with other organisms, such as dyspnea, fever, productive cough, low oxygenation, elevated white cell count, and delirium. In the lungs, infection with *P. aeruginosa* causes necrosis of tissue and hemorrhaging. Diagnosis may be challenging as most blood cultures (excepting clients with bacteremia) are negative. Endotracheal tubes can also be colonized without a true infection, adding to the diagnosis difficulty. Bronchoalveolar lavage is most sensitive for the diagnosis.[209]

Chronic infections with *Pseudomonas* are noted in children or young adults with cystic fibrosis.[215] Over time there is chronic progression of symptoms with acute exacerbations of disease. Clients typically experience mucous plugging and airway inflammation, which predispose to *P. aeruginosa* infection. The bacteria then contribute to further mucous plugging and cause a chronic inflammatory reaction leading to lung damage and fibrosis.

Bacteremia

Pseudomonas bacteremia typically occurs in persons with significant underlying diseases (approximately 90%) such as cancer, diabetes, renal failure, congestive heart failure, immune system deficiencies, or posttransplant.[203] It is an important cause of serious, life-threatening bloodstream infections in clients with neutropenia. *P. aeruginosa* bacteremia is usually acquired in the hospital and may be primary (no identifiable source) or secondary to a focal infected site (e.g., skin, lungs, intravascular source, indwelling catheters, GI or urinary tracts).

As with other *Pseudomonas* infections, bacteremia is rapidly progressive without treatment, with high morbidity and mortality rates. Clients experience fever, tachypnea, tachycardia, hypotension, and delirium, which can lead to renal failure, acute respiratory distress syndrome, and death. Rarely characteristic lesions of *Pseudomonas* bacteremia, *ecthyma gangrenosum*, develop on the skin. These vesicles are initially hemorrhagic with progressive necrosis and ulceration. They occur as single lesions or in small groups.

Central Nervous System Infections. *Pseudomonas* infections of the CNS result from extension from a contiguous structure such as the ear, mastoid, or paranasal sinus; direct inoculation into the subarachnoid space or brain by means of head trauma, surgery, or invasive diagnostic procedures (e.g., lumbar punctures, spinal anesthesia, intraventricular shunts); and bacteremic spread from a distant site of infection such as the urinary tract, lung, or endocardium.

The clinical manifestations of *Pseudomonas* meningitis are like those of other forms of bacterial meningitis (see Chapter 29) and include fever, headache, stiff neck, nausea, and confusion. The onset of disease may be acute and occur suddenly or may be more gradual and insidious.

Skin and Soft-Tissue Infections. *Pseudomonas* disease of the skin and mucous membranes can result from primary or metastatic foci of infections. Common predisposing factors for primary skin and soft-tissue infections are a breakdown in the integument, especially resulting from surgery, burns, trauma, and pressure ulcers; whirlpool use; and chemotherapy-induced neutropenia.

The wound is hemorrhagic and necrotic and rarely may have a characteristic fruity odor (sweet, grape-like odor) with a blue-green exudate that forms a crust on wounds (Fig. 8-4). *Pseudomonas* bacteremia may produce distinctive skin lesions known as *ecthyma gangrenosum*, as described in "Bacteremia" above.

Pseudomonas burn wound sepsis is a dreaded complication of extensive third-degree burns and is characterized by multifocal black or dark-brown discoloration of the burn eschar; degeneration of the underlying granulation tissue with rapid eschar separation and hemorrhage into subcutaneous tissue; edema, hemorrhage, and necrosis of adjacent healthy tissue; and erythematous nodular lesions on unburned skin.

Systemic manifestations may include fever, hypothermia, disorientation, hypotension, oliguria (low output of urine), ileus, or leukopenia. The diagnosis is based on clinical signs and symptoms; biopsy of the burn site,

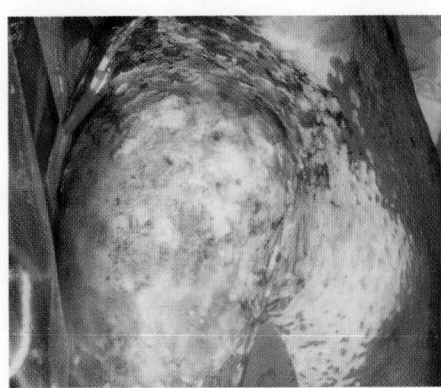

Figure 8-4

Pseudomonas. Blue-green color in a burn wound indicates infection by *P. aeruginosa.* (Reprinted from Gould BE: *Pathophysiology for the health professions,* ed 3, Philadelphia, 2006, WB Saunders, courtesy Judy Knighton, Ross Tilley Burn Center, Sunnybrook and Women's College Health Center, Toronto, Ontario, Canada.)

which demonstrates evidence of invading bacteria; and culture positive for *Pseudomonas.*

Bone and Joint Infections. Pseudomonas infections of the bones and joints result from hematogenous spread from other sites or extension from contiguous sites of infection. Contiguous infections are usually related to penetrating trauma, surgery, or overlying soft-tissue infections. Injection-drug users may contaminate drugs or water with *Pseudomonas,* which often seeds the sternoclavicular or other joints.[173]

P. aeruginosa is the most common cause of osteochondritis of the foot following a puncture wound.[98] Infection involves the cartilage of the small joints and the bones of the foot. Typically, the person experiences early improvement in pain and swelling following a puncture wound only to have the symptoms recur or worsen several days later.

The average duration of symptoms before diagnosis is several weeks; fever and other systemic signs are usually absent. An area of superficial cellulitis is evident on the plantar surface of the foot, or there may merely be tenderness to deep palpation.

Bloodborne *Pseudomonas,* from injection drug use or pelvic surgery, appears to have a predilection for fibrocartilaginous joints such as the symphysis pubis.[172] Vertebral osteomyelitis caused by *P. aeruginosa* is occasionally associated with complicated urinary tract infections and genitourinary surgery or instrumentation. This disease occurs most often in older adults and involves the lumbosacral spine. Physical signs include local tenderness and decreased range of motion in the spine; fever and other systemic symptoms are relatively uncommon. Mild neurologic deficits may be present (see further discussion in Chapter 27).

Other Pseudomonas Infections. Pseudomonas is noted to cause disease of the external ear, which may be benign ("swimmer's ear") or malignant (invasion of bone, soft tissue, and cartilage). *P. aeruginosa* infection of the cornea causes bacterial keratitis or corneal ulcers.

Corneal ulcers can progress rapidly with complications such as corneal perforation, anterior chamber

involvement, and endophthalmitis. Native heart valves or prosthetic valves can become infected with *P. aeruginosa,* causing endocarditis. *P. aeruginosa* is the most common cause of health-care associated urinary tract infections often arising from urinary catheters, instrumentation, or surgery. The prostate or kidney stones may harbor the bacteria, resulting in recurrent infections.

MEDICAL MANAGEMENT

DIAGNOSIS, TREATMENT, AND PROGNOSIS. Diagnosis requires isolation of the *Pseudomonas* organism in blood, spinal fluid, urine, or exudate culture. Antibiotic therapy should be initiated immediately because of the virulent nature of the bacteria. Typically, *Pseudomonas* is treated with two antipseudomonal drugs (different classes); although with increasing drug resistance (including to imipenem),[234] there are suggestions of using monotherapy except for neutropenic persons with bacteremia.[101] More studies are needed to determine the best therapy practices.

P. aeruginosa infections are among the most aggressive human bacterial infections, often progressing rapidly to sepsis, especially in people with poor immunologic resistance (e.g., premature infants; aging adults; and those with debilitating disease, burns, or wounds).

In local *Pseudomonas* infections, treatment is usually successful and complications are rare. Immediate medical intervention is necessary; septicemic *Pseudomonas* infections are associated with a high mortality rate. Medical management is directed according to the site of infection and may include antibiotics, surgery, pulmonary therapy, respiratory assistance if necessary, and other supportive measures dictated by the presence of septic shock and other complications.

Local *Pseudomonas* infections or septicemia secondary to wound infection requires debridement or drainage of the infected wound. For older children with cystic fibrosis and chronic *Pseudomonas* lung infection, long-term inhaled antibiotic treatments are recommended and have been used with some success at reducing hospitalizations and reducing exacerbations. Novel methods are under development including new anti-pseudomonal drugs and devices.[78]

SPECIAL IMPLICATIONS FOR THE THERAPIST 8-6

Pseudomonas Infections

Reservoirs for *P. aeruginosa* are most often medical equipment or moist areas in the health care setting, such as sinks. However, the source of some outbreaks has been traced to HCWs' hands or nails.[66,220] *P. aeruginosa* can be removed from the skin by following proper hand hygiene guidelines, which prevents further spread of the organism.[16,178] Proper cleaning of any equipment in contact with mucous membranes or a moist environment is absolutely critical.[138]

Anyone who is immunocompromised should be protected from exposure to this infection. Wound care requires strict sterile technique.

Viral Infections

Bloodborne Viral Pathogens

The bloodborne viruses that most endanger HCWs are the bloodborne pathogens hepatitis B virus (HBV), hepatitis C virus (HCV), and HIV. In 1991, the U.S. Congress passed the Bloodborne Pathogens Standard, prepared by the Occupational Safety and Health Administration and written to help eliminate or minimize occupational exposure to HBV, HCV, HIV, and other bloodborne pathogens.[212]

The guidelines are based on the use of standard precautions, including appropriate hand hygiene and barrier precautions, to reduce contact with body fluids potentially contaminated by these viruses. The use of safety devices and techniques to reduce the handling of sharp instruments can help in the reduction of significant contact with body fluids, particularly blood or blood-containing fluids.[222]

SPECIAL IMPLICATIONS FOR THE THERAPIST   8-7

Bloodborne Viral Pathogens

Mention of bloodborne viral pathogens is made here to help the reader appreciate the big picture of patient problems. Taking a moment to recognize that hepatitis and HIV are transmitted through blood and blood products renews our understanding of why standard precautions is so very important in preventing the transmission of these pathogens. An in-depth discussion of hepatitis can be found in Chapter 17; discussion of HIV is located in Chapter 7.

Herpesviruses

Overview and Definition. The term *herpes* is derived from the Greek word *herpein*, which means "to creep." The word refers to the tendency for this type of viral infection to become chronic, latent, and recurrent. The known human herpesviruses (HHVs) are divided by genomic and biologic behavior into eight types (Box 8-9).

All herpesviruses are morphologically similar, but the biologic and epidemiologic features of each are distinct. Subclinical primary infection with the herpesviruses is more common than clinically symptomatic illness, and each type then persists in a latent state for the rest of the life of the host.

With the herpes simplex virus (HSV) and varicella-zoster virus (VZV), the virus remains latent in sensory ganglia and, upon reactivation, lesions appear in the distal sensory nerve distribution. Virus reactivation in immunocompromised hosts may lead to widespread lesions in affected organs such as the viscera or the CNS.

Severe or fatal illness may occur in infants and the immunocompromised. Association with malignancies includes EBV with Burkett lymphoma and nasopharyngeal carcinoma and HHV-8 with Kaposi sarcoma and body cavity lymphoma.[44,180]

Box 8-9

TYPES OF HERPESVIRUSES

Herpes simplex virus (HSV)	Type 1
Herpes simplex virus (HSV)	Type 2
Varicella-zoster virus (VZV)	Type 3
Epstein-Barr infectious mononucleosis virus (EBV)	Type 4
Cytomegalovirus (CMV)	Type 5
Roseola (exanthema subitum) human (HHV)	Type 6 human herpesvirus
Herpesvirus serologically associated with roseola (HHV)	Type 7 human herpesvirus
Human herpesvirus associated with Kaposi sarcoma (HHV)	Type 8 sarcoma

---

Herpes Simplex Viruses Types 1 and 2. See Table 8-7.

Incidence, Etiologic Factors, and Risk Factors. Approximately 70% of Americans older than 12 years harbor HSV-1, which is usually responsible for cold sores.[179] Herpes type 2 is one of the most common sexually transmitted diseases in the world, and the principal cause of genital ulcers and genital herpes. It is estimated by the CDC that more than 50 million people live with HSV-2.[232] Since 1999, the seropositivity of the population for HSV-2 has decreased from 21% to 16.2% in 2008, but the majority of initial cases go unrecognized (81%).[231]

Both strains can infect any visceral organ or mucocutaneous site, and HSV-1 can be transmitted to the genital area during oral sex. HSV creates a significant health risk as infection with HSV-2 can increase the risk of acquiring HIV infection by at least twofold.[68] Seroprevalence for both viruses increases with age and with sexual activity for HSV-2.

Intermittent, asymptomatic shedding is common and is the typical time of transmission, usually during the period immediately preceding appearance of sores. Sexual contact during asymptomatic periods is less likely to result in transmission of the virus than when sores are present. However, because people with genital herpes are more likely to engage in sexual contact when they are free of sores, the rate of asymptomatic transmission is still significant.

Infants born to women with genital herpes can be infected with HSV when they pass through an infected birth canal. The virus can also be passed to other regions of the body by hand contact, particularly in people who are immunosuppressed (e.g., older adults, transplant recipients, people with cancer undergoing chemotherapy, and anyone with HIV or other conditions that weaken the immune system).

Pathogenesis. Even though HSV-1 and -2 are the two most closely related herpesviruses and share antigenic cross-reactivity, these two agents are genetically and serologically distinct and produce different clinical

Table 8-7 Most Common Sexually Transmitted Infections*

Infection	Incidence	Transmission	Clinical Manifestations	Treatment†
Human papilloma virus (HPV) (genital warts)	6 million new cases/year	Unprotected sexual contact (including oral sex; condoms do not provide 100% protection as the virus can be spread by contact with an infected part of the genitals not covered by a condom); vertical transmission from mother to newborn with vaginal delivery (rare)	Often asymptomatic; warts on the vulva, anal region, vagina, cervix, mouth, penis, scrotum, or groin: 1-6 months after sexual contact with infected person; can also cause oropharyngeal cancer; *in women*: abnormal Pap smear; HPV can cause cervical cancer	Usually is cleared by the immune system (90% within 2 years). When it is not, no treatment exists for the virus but symptoms can be treated. Warts can be removed using topically applied chemicals, cryotherapy, or surgical therapies. Recurrence is not uncommon
Chlamydia	>1 million new cases/year	Unprotected vaginal or anal intercourse, oral sex; infection transmitted from infected mother to infant during delivery	*In men*: none or urethritis with discharge or burning with urination *In women*: commonly none or vaginal discharge or pain with urination; can cause pelvic inflammatory disease (PID) with fever, abdominal pain, and pain with intercourse; infertility if untreated; eye infections and respiratory tract infections in newborn	Can be cured with antibiotics. Partner must be treated as well. PID may require additional treatment
Herpes simplex virus 2 (genital herpes)	1 million new cases/year 50 million carriers	Oral, genital, or anal sex; kissing or touching an infected area where there is a break in the skin; can be spread by asymptomatic person; transmission from mother to child during vaginal birth	None or vesicular (blister-like) lesions on the genitals, vagina, cervix, anal region, mouth, or throat; can cause serious complications if untreated	Cannot be cured but healing can be accelerated and recurrence of outbreaks can be reduced with antivirals; partner must be informed
Gonorrhea (the "clap")	300,000 new cases/year	Unprotected oral, vaginal, or anal sex; transmission to baby during delivery	*In men*: urethritis with discharge, frequent urge to urinate and pain during urination; may be asymptomatic *In women*: none or slight vaginal discharge or difficulty or pain during urination; pelvic pain; vaginal bleeding between periods; PID *Both*: arthritis (if untreated)	Most cases can be cured with antibiotics (third-generation cephalosporins) although strains are resistant to fluoroquinolones and are becoming resistant to available cephalosporins
Hepatitis B	43,000 new cases/year (significant decrease since vaccination of children began)	Infected blood; sexual contact; occupational needle sticks; sharing needles; baby infected during delivery	May be asymptomatic; jaundice, arthralgias, dark urine, anorexia, nausea, abdominal pain, cirrhosis, liver failure, liver cancer, clay-colored stools, fever	Can be prevented with hepatitis B vaccine In unvaccinated people, hepatitis B immune globulin and hepatitis B vaccine given as postexposure prophylaxis; antiviral agents are used but relapse on cessation of treatment is common
Syphilis primary	13,700 new cases/year (primary and secondary combined); overall incidence increased between 2000 and 2009, with a slight decrease in 2010	Unprotected sexual contact (vaginal, oral, anal); sexual contact with exudates of skin and mucous membranes of infected person; transplacental infection of fetus if mother is infected; can be transmitted through blood transfusions‡	Painless papule or chancre at site of infection (genitals, mouth) occurring 3-8 weeks after infection; lymphadenopathy	Can be cured with antibiotics in primary, secondary, and latent stages. Late-stage disease may cause irreversible damage to the brain, nerves, heart, blood vessels, eyes, liver, bones, joints

Continued

Table 8-7 Most Common Sexually Transmitted Infections*—cont'd

Infection	Incidence	Transmission	Clinical Manifestations	Treatment†
Syphilis (secondary)	See Syphilis primary above	Progression of untreated primary-stage syphilis (spirochetes spread throughout body)	Can be asymptomatic Flu-like symptoms, lymphadenopathy, mucocutaneous lesions (chancres) and rash (maculopapular) occurring 6-12 weeks to 1-2 years after infection (but has a wide range of clinical symptoms; e.g., fatigue, fever, headache, myalgia, sore throat, weight loss); can cause fetus to abort in untreated pregnant women	
Syphilis (latent)		Can still transmit disease to others	Test positive but no symptoms of clinically active disease	
Syphilis (late; can occur up to 20 years after second stage)		Progression of untreated primary, then secondary syphilis	Cardiovascular and central nervous system damage (e.g., ataxia, paresis, paresthesias, dementia, visual loss)	
HIV/AIDS	50,000 new cases/year; majority of transmissions caused by sexual contact (men who have sex with men)	Exposure to blood/blood products; exposure to body fluids (blood, semen, vaginal secretions, breast milk); sexual contact; shared needles in injection-drug users; transmission from mother to child during vaginal delivery or breast feeding	Widespread illness because of immune system decline; may not develop symptoms for 10 years or more after infection	Cannot be cured, but combined antiviral therapy can prolong life for many people

*Listed in descending order by incidence.

†All sexually transmitted diseases can be prevented by sexual abstinence and mutually monogamous sex between two uninfected partners. The Centers for Disease Control and Prevention has come under criticism by the medical community for not stressing this point in their prevention programs for young people.

‡Centers for Disease Control and Prevention (CDC): *Control of communicable diseases manual*, ed 19, Atlanta, 2008, U.S. Department of Health and Human Services.

From Centers for Disease Control and Prevention (CDC): *2010 Sexually transmitted disease surveillance*, Atlanta, 2011, U.S. Department of Health and Human Services. Available at http://www.cdc.gov/std/stats10/chlamydia.htm. Accessed on Feb 4, 2011.

symptoms. HSV-1 and -2 primarily affect the oral mucocutaneous (cold sores and mouth sores) and genital areas (genital herpes), respectively. Primary infection occurs through a break in the mucous membranes of the mouth, throat, eye, or genitals or via minor abrasions in the skin. Initial infection can be asymptomatic, although minor localized vesicular lesions may be evident.

Local multiplication occurs, followed by viremia and systemic infection with a subsequent lifelong latent infection and periodic reactivation of the virus. During primary infection, the virus enters peripheral sensory nerves and migrates along axons to sensory nerve ganglia in the CNS, allowing the virus to escape immune detection and response.

During latent infection of nerve cells, viral DNA is maintained and not integrated into surrounding cellular structures, thus maintaining true latency. Various disturbances such as physical or psychologic stress can disrupt the delicate balance of latency, and reactivation of the latent virus occurs. The virus travels back down sensory nerves to the surface of the body and replicates, forming new lesions. Although painful, most recurrent infections resolve spontaneously, recurring at a later time.

Clinical Manifestations. Primary HSV-1 (first episode) typically affects the mouth and oral cavity, causing vesicles in the mouth, throat, and around the lips. Vesicles typically open to form moist ulcers after several days. Systemic symptoms can accompany the lesions such as fever, myalgias, and malaise. Symptoms and lesions resolve within 3 to 14 days.

Primary infection is often asymptomatic. Recurrences are usually milder, involve fewer lesions, are of shorter duration, and in immunocompetent hosts are usually confined to the lips (herpes labialis). Recurrent genital

HSV-1 is milder and less frequent than HSV-2. Recurrences are most commonly induced by stress, fever, sunlight, infection, or other factors.

HSV-2 is most often acquired through sexual contact. Primary HSV-2 causes vesicles to form on the mucosal and cutaneous surfaces of the genital area. Lesions are usually painful, small, grouped, and vesicular, with possible burning and itching. The blister-like lesions break and weep after a few days, leaving ulcer-like sores that usually crust over and heal in 1 to 3 weeks.

Genital ulcers may occur on the genital area, cervix, buttocks, rectum, urethra, or bladder, causing vaginal and urethral discharge, dysuria, cervicitis, proctitis, and tender inguinal adenopathy. Systemic symptoms occasionally noted include headache, malaise, myalgias, and fever. Primary infection is often asymptomatic. Genital HSV-2 reactivation may be associated with a prodrome such as tingling or pain.

First symptomatic episodes may not be the initial infection. Known as nonprimary infections, individuals may have been previously exposed to HSV-1 and produced antibodies but not developed symptoms until exposed to HSV-2 or vice versa. In these cases, the initial symptomatic nonprimary infection has fewer symptoms and complications as compared to a first episode without previous exposure.

HSV can be responsible for other infections. Viral meningitis from HSV is caused by inflammation of the meninges surrounding the brain. This occurs more commonly from HSV-2 than HSV-1. Aseptic meningitis may develop 3 to 12 days following the appearance of lesions, but may also occur without skin lesions. Typical symptoms are headache, nausea, stiff neck, and fever. Meningitis may develop concomitant with the primary infection or recurrent episodes. Because of the latent nature of HSV-2, episodes of recurrent meningitis also occur.[11] The prognosis is good for immunocompetent hosts.

Herpes encephalitis (an infection of the brain tissue), although rare, is a more serious infection and carries a 70% mortality without treatment.[211] Typically caused by HSV-1, HSV-2 can also be implicated.[174] In children and young adults, primary infection is the main cause. Adults may have reactivation as the principal source.

Presenting symptoms include fever, headache, behavioral and speech disturbances, and seizures. Abnormalities caused by HSV can be seen on MRI. Encephalitis carries high morbidity and mortality rates, and permanent neurologic sequelae often result despite treatment.[211] Neonatal herpes simplex encephalitis is a devastating infection of the fetus, typically from primary HSV-2 (30% of cases are HSV-1). The majority (70%) of babies born with this rare infection were born to mothers who did not manifest symptoms of the infection.[11]

The risk of the fetus of acquiring HSV from a primary maternal infection is approximately 50%.[11] The most severe complications of neonatal HSV infection are dissemination and CNS involvement. Neonatal herpes may also occur from unknown shedding in the mother's genital tract at the time of delivery. If untreated, babies can develop visceral dissemination or infection of the CNS, with an 80% mortality rate. Cesarean section reduces the risk of neonatal herpes in mothers known to be shedding the virus.[18,219]

Herpetic keratitis (ulceration of the cornea from infection) is one of the most common causes for corneal blindness in the United States. Onset is acute, accompanied by blurred vision, conjunctivitis, and pain. Despite treatment, recurrences are common and cause scarring, making this a chronic disease. Severe scarring is an indication for corneal grafting.

Herpetic whitlows (herpetic infection of the fingers) can result from inoculation of the finger from a herpes lesion (Fig. 8-5). Prior to implementation of standard glove precautions, herpetic whitlow was most often seen in HCWs. In children, herpetic whitlow is typically caused by HSV-1, whereas HSV-2 is implicated in cases involving adults.[230]

HSV can also disseminate to visceral organs, causing severe consequences such as hepatitis, thrombocytopenia, arthritis, and pneumonitis. Disseminated infection typically occurs in pregnant women (primary genital HSV) or immunocompromised persons (primary or recurrent HSV). HSV esophagitis is seen in immunocompromised hosts, but rarely noted in immunocompetent persons.

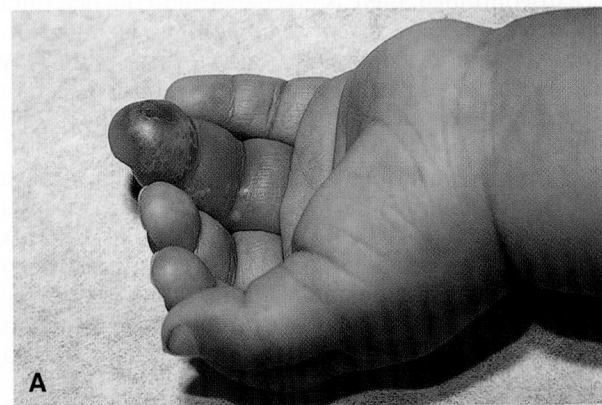

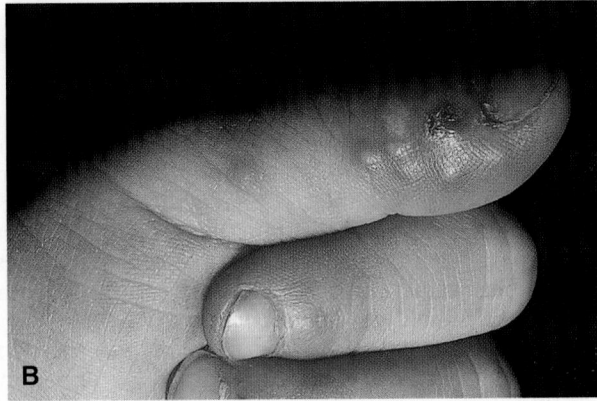

Figure 8-5

Herpetic whitlow. Herpetic whitlow is an intense, painful infection of the hand involving one or more fingers and typically affecting the terminal phalanx. HSV-1 is the cause in approximately 60% of cases of herpetic whitlow, and HSV-2 is the cause in the remaining 40%. **A,** Herpes simplex infection of the finger in a child. **B,** Herpetic whitlow of the thumb in an adult. (Reprinted from Callen JP: *Color atlas of dermatology,* ed 2, Philadelphia, 2000, WB Saunders.)

MEDICAL MANAGEMENT

DIAGNOSIS, TREATMENT, AND PREVENTION. Clinical diagnosis of herpes is often insensitive. Up to 30% of first-episode genital herpes are caused by HSV-1, which has a low recurrence rate compared to HSV-2, making distinction between the two types important.

Viral cultures of vesicular fluid are the standard laboratory test. The sample must be collected during the first few days the lesion is present in order for the results to be accurate. PCR tests are also available and are the test of choice for detection of HSV in spinal fluid.

Although elusive, research continues in order to develop an HSV vaccine.[39] Although no immunization against HSV infection is available, antiviral drugs can be used to treat initial cases, reduce the frequency and degree of viral shedding, and suppress recurrences.

The CDC has released recommendations and guidelines for the treatment of HSV-2. Acyclovir, famciclovir, and valacyclovir are approved for the treatment and suppression of HSV-2. Famciclovir can be used to treat recurrent mucocutaneous HSV in individuals infected with HIV. Acyclovir is used for neurologic complications of HSV and Penciclovir is approved for the treatment of cold sores.

These medications do not eradicate the virus and, once discontinued, there is no change in frequency, duration, or severity of recurrences. In recent years, mutations have led to the development of acyclovir-resistant HSV. This should be suspected when the diagnosis is certain but there is no clinical response. Foscarnet is the drug of choice in this situation.

Counseling regarding transmission and education on how to recognize symptoms and defer sex are essential in preventing new cases. Daily suppressive use of valacyclovir along with safe sex can reduce transmission of HSV-2.[45] Proper use of condoms can also reduce the risk of acquiring HSV-2.[216] This is particularly helpful for couples in which one is seropositive and the other seronegative for HSV.

SPECIAL IMPLICATIONS FOR THE THERAPIST 8-8

Herpes Simplex Virus

Recurrent disease is best treated with acyclovir, and recurrent genital disease requires barrier precautions during sexual activity in addition to medication. Although herpes simplex is contagious, health care–associated transmission is rare. However, it has been reported in some high-risk areas, such as nurseries, ICUs, burn units, and other areas where immunocompromised individuals might be placed.

Transmission of HSV occurs primarily through contact with lesions or with virus-containing secretions such as saliva, vaginal secretions, or amniotic fluid. Exposed areas of skin, particularly when minor cuts, abrasions, or other skin lesions are present, are the most likely sites of viral entry. The incubation period of HSV is 2 to 14 days.

HCWs may acquire a herpetic infection of the fingers (herpetic whitlow or paronychia) from exposure to contaminated oral secretions. Such exposures are a distinct risk for HCWs who have direct contact with either oral or respiratory secretions from clients.

HCWs can protect themselves from acquiring HSV by adhering to standard precautions and hand hygiene before and after all client contact and by the use of appropriate barriers such as a mask, gloves, or gauze dressing to prevent hand contact with the lesion. Some work restrictions may be appropriate for affected HCWs when active lesions are present (e.g., herpetic whitlow) (see Table 8-5). No reports are evident that HCWs with genital HSV infections have transmitted HSV to clients, so no work restriction for people with HSV-2 is indicated.[212]

During the prodromal stage of herpes simplex, the levator scapulae becomes vulnerable to activation of its trigger points by mechanical stresses that are usually well within its tolerance. However, a stiff neck syndrome can develop a day or two before the fully developed symptoms of herpes simplex.[190]

Careful questioning regarding previous history of herpes, presence of prodromal symptoms, and observation for the development of a new outbreak of sores during the episode of care will help the therapist in making an accurate assessment of the client's presentation.

Varicella-Zoster Virus (Herpesvirus Type 3)

Incidence. VZV is known to cause *chickenpox* and *shingles* (see "Viral Infections: Herpes Zoster" in this chapter). Prior to the availability of the varicella vaccine, primary or first-infection VZV accounted for about 3 to 4 million cases of chickenpox per year in the United States. Postvaccination data show a significant decline in hospitalizations and death from varicella.[123]

One in 3 people will develop the secondary, or reactivation, form of VZV in their lifetime, resulting in herpes zoster, or shingles. Approximately 1 million cases of shingles occur in the United States every year and cause significant pain and disability.[87] The risk of developing shingles starts to rise around age 50 years. Anyone who is immunocompromised (e.g., HIV infection, receiving chemotherapy, corticosteroid therapy, or has cancer) is also at increased risk. Young adults such as college students living in dormitories are at increased risk for VZV as either chickenpox (first time) or shingles (recurrence).

Pathogenesis. Like other herpesviruses, VZV has the capacity to persist in the body (dorsal root ganglia next to the spinal cord) following an initial infection of chickenpox. VZV is acquired from contact with infected airborne droplets (from coughing or sneezing) into the respiratory tract or by direct contact with vesicular fluid to mucous membranes or eye.

The virus is thought to initially multiply at the site of entry, with subsequent viremia (spreading to the blood) occurring 4 to 6 days after infection. The virus then disseminates to other organs such as the liver, spleen, and sensory ganglia and further replicates in the viscera, followed by a secondary viremia with viral infection of the skin and mucosa (mouth, respiratory tract, or eye).

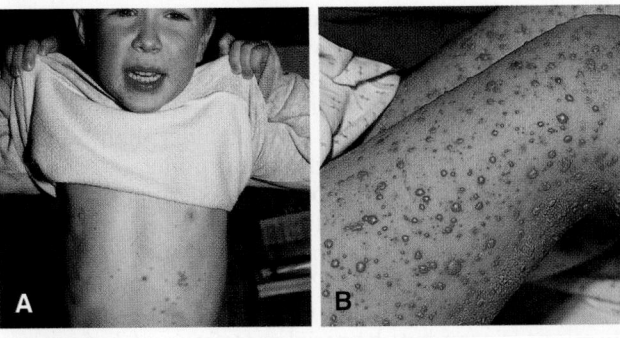

Figure 8-6

A, Early onset of varicella (chickenpox) in a young child. Painful itching can cause severe distress. Note the lesions on face and trunk. **B,** Varicella (chickenpox) with the more characteristic rash classically described as a "dewdrop on a rose petal," with a vesicle on an erythematous base. (A, Courtesy Catherine Goodman. B, Reprinted from Callen JP: *Color atlas of dermatology,* ed 2, Philadelphia, 2000, WB Saunders.)

Viral infection of the skin and mucosa produces vesicles filled with high titers of infectious virus, which, when broken, then shed more viruses. The incubation period is 14 to 16 days from exposure with a range of 10 to 21 days. This may be prolonged in immunocompromised persons. VZV is present in white blood cells up to 5 days before the rash is present, and individuals can be contagious a day or two prior to the appearance of the rash. Individuals remain contagious until the lesions have crusted.

The exact mechanism for reactivation of VZV remains unknown, although it is most likely multifactorial and involves cell-mediated immunity. Shingles occur more often in immunocompromised adults such as older adults, those with hematologic malignancies, especially leukemia and lymphoma, and people with HIV. Other factors associated with recurrent disease include intra-uterine exposure to VZV and varicella at a young age (less than 18 months).[6]

Clinical Manifestations. Disease manifestations are either chickenpox (varicella) or shingles (herpes zoster). Primary VZV is virtually always symptomatic. Second episodes of chickenpox are uncommon unless the child is younger than 1 year at the time of the first episode. A mild prodrome consisting of headache, photophobia, and malaise may precede the onset of the rash in adults, whereas in children the rash is often the first sign of disease.

The rash is classically described as a "dewdrop on a rose petal," with a vesicle on an erythematous base. The lesions begin as macules that quickly progress to papules, vesicles, and then pustules before crusting. VZV usually appears first on the scalp and moves to the trunk and then the extremities. Successive crops appear over several days, with lesions present in several stages of evolution at any one time.

The generalized pattern of eruption without specific dermatome distribution distinguishes varicella from herpes zoster (Fig. 8-6). Shingles in the adult present as blister-like lesions that erupt unilaterally along a specific dermatome supplied by a dorsal root ganglia. The highest concentration of lesions on the trunk corresponds with dermatomes from T3 to L3 (Fig. 8-7). Pain and itching are common symptoms during the eruption of the vesicles.

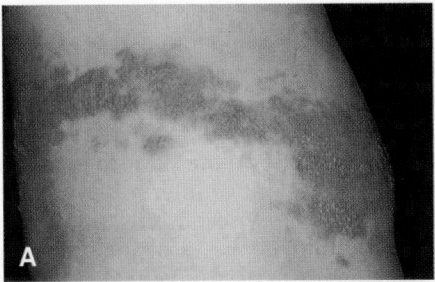

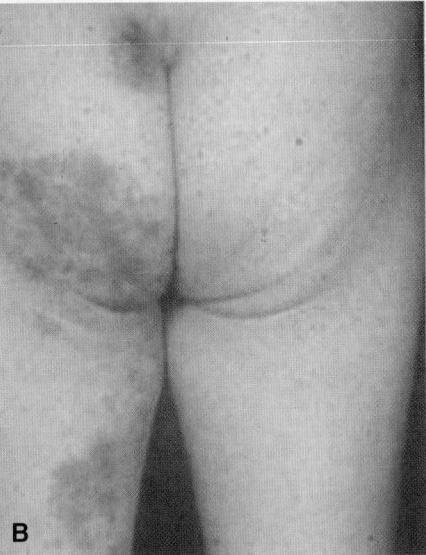

Figure 8-7

Herpes zoster (shingles). Small grouped vesicles occur along the cutaneous sensory nerve, forming pustules that crust over. Reactivation of VZV, the dormant chickenpox virus, is the underlying cause of this condition. **A,** Commonly seen on the trunk, these outbreaks can occur anywhere along the dermatome of the affected nerve. **B,** Lesions appear unilaterally and do not cross the midline. Usually external, these lesions can occur internally as well. Pain is often severe and can become chronic, a condition called *postherpetic neuralgia.* (A, Reprinted from Hurwitz S: *Clinical pediatric dermatology: a textbook of skin disorders of childhood and adolescence,* ed 2, Philadelphia, 1993, WB Saunders. B, Courtesy Mary Lou Galantino, Richard Stockton College of New Jersey, Pomona, NJ.)

Complications of varicella occur more often in adults, infants, and the immunocompromised. Adults are more likely to develop pneumonitis and CNS involvement (cerebellar ataxia and encephalitis) than are healthy children. The immunocompromised, especially those with leukemia or lymphoma who are receiving continuous chemotherapy, can develop disseminated disease with severe visceral involvement, including pneumonitis and encephalitis. The most common complication among persons affected with VZV is secondary bacterial skin infections.

When contracted during the first or second trimesters of pregnancy, varicella carries a low risk of congenital malformations. Yet if a mother develops varicella within 5 days before delivery to 2 days after delivery, the newborn is at risk of serious disseminated disease.

Shingles also can lead to chronic, often debilitating nerve pain called *postherpetic neuralgia* (PHN), lasting months to years and often resulting in significant morbidity and reduction in quality of life. The risk of developing PHN with each episode of zoster is 10% to 18%.[87]

Pain, hyperalgesia, and allodynia are typical of PHN. Examples of allodynia include pain from the touch of clothing (touch allodynia) or pain that occurs from a draft of warm or cold air on the skin (thermal allodynia). The pain may be constant or intermittent and vary from light burning to a deep visceral sensation. The cause of PHN is not fully understood. Scarring and degenerative changes involving the nerve trunks, ganglia, and skin may be important factors. The incidence of scarring and hyperpigmentation is much higher in older adults.

For those who develop shingles, factors that predict the severity and occurrence of PHN include the severity of pain both before and after onset of the rash, the extent of the rash, occurrence in the face and eye distribution, and the occurrence of viremia.[87]

Occasionally herpes zoster involves the cranial nerves, especially the trigeminal and geniculate ganglia or the oculomotor nerve. Geniculate zoster may cause vesicle formation in the external auditory canal, ipsilateral facial palsy, hearing loss, dizziness, and loss of taste. Trigeminal ganglion involvement causes eye pain and possibly corneal and scleral damage with loss of vision. Herpes zoster ophthalmicus is considered a medical emergency. All persons with VZV near the eye should be evaluated by an ophthalmologist.

In rare cases, herpes zoster leads to generalized CNS infection, muscle atrophy, motor paralysis (usually transient), acute transverse myelitis, and ascending myelitis. More often, generalized infection causes acute retention of urine and unilateral paralysis of the diaphragm.

MEDICAL MANAGEMENT

DIAGNOSIS AND TREATMENT. Diagnosis is usually made based on clinical symptoms; however, with the advent of the varicella vaccine, the number of atypical cases has increased, making laboratory diagnosis more relevant. Fluid from a vesicle may be stained and viewed under a microscope in order to identify multinucleated giant cells. Direct fluorescent antibody staining is the fastest and most sensitive.[87]

Treatment is supportive (not curative) in order to relieve symptoms and should begin within 24 hours of the appearance of the rash (preferably when the pain begins). Bed rest is recommended until the fever has gone down, and the skin should be kept clean to avoid secondary bacterial contamination. Itching can be relieved with oral antihistamines, topical calamine lotion, and other skin-soothing lotions and baths.

All contaminated items should not be reused. Nondisposable items should be washed in boiling water or disinfected before reuse. Infected persons may need to be isolated (especially in hospitals or other medical facilities or long-term care facilities) in order to prevent transmission.

Antiviral medications can be used to treat individuals at high risk for complications but are not recommended for children with uncomplicated disease. Valacyclovir and famciclovir are only approved for treatment of adults with varicella. Oral acyclovir is recommended by some experts for pregnant women in their second or third trimesters,

whereas children who are immunocompromised should receive IV acyclovir. Persons with chronic lung or skin disease should also be considered for treatment.

For the treatment of zoster (shingles), the CDC recommends antiviral therapy for persons older than 50 years who have moderate or severe pain, moderate or severe rash, or involvement of nontruncal dermatomes (particularly near the eye).[86] Antivirals may reduce the number of days new lesions appear, the severity of systemic symptoms, and the risk for PHN, but they have not been shown to reduce transmission risk or reduce other complications. Secondary bacterial infections of lesions are treated with antibacterial ointment or oral antibiotics if severe. Recovery from varicella infection usually results in lifetime immunity.

Treatment for PHN can be complex, with various trials of medications needed in order to find the treatment that provides the best relief. Nonopioid analgesics, tricyclic antidepressants, anticonvulsants, capsaicin cream, or topical local anesthetics based on the type of pain experienced (e.g., antidepressants for diffuse pain, paroxysmal and local pain treated by anticonvulsants and local anesthetics).

Corticosteroids are reported to diminish acute zoster pain and decrease the time to cutaneous healing, reduction of analgesic therapy, and return of uninterrupted sleep and normal daily activities. However, no evidence indicates that use of corticosteroids prevents development of PHN.[87,221,225]

For individuals who are exposed but are without immunity to varicella, the varicella vaccine can be used up to 3 days postexposure (particularly in outbreaks) to aid in modifying symptoms or preventing the infection. For those individuals at high risk for severe complications and for whom the vaccine is contraindicated (such as immunocompromised persons, pregnant women, or in neonatal situations), postexposure prophylaxis can include VariZIG (a varicella zoster immune globulin).[27]

PREVENTION. The varicella vaccine (Varivax) is recommended for all persons age 12 months or older as a routine vaccination and for those who do not have evidence of immunity (children, adolescents, adults),[87] especially in those persons who have close contact with individuals at high risk for severe disease and complications.

For those individuals who are uncertain whether they had childhood varicella, a variety of serologic tests for the varicella antibody are available. Adults who are at high risk for exposure and transmission should also receive the vaccine (such as teachers of young children, child care employees, and residents and staff at medical facilities). The varicella vaccine is also available with the measles, mumps, and rubella (MMR) vaccine (ProQuad).

It is also recommended that all children who have not developed immunity by the age of 13 years should be vaccinated. Because the vaccine is a live attenuated vaccine, it is contraindicated in pregnant women and in those who may become pregnant within 4 weeks of receiving the vaccine; guidelines are available for individuals with HIV.[123]

The vaccine provides long-lasting (but not lifelong) immunity, with a 70% to 90% efficacy.[123] Vaccine breakthrough cases are common but mild. Persons present with fewer lesions (usually less than 50) and lack systemic symptoms (such as fever).[123]

The shingles vaccine (Zostavax; live attenuated virus) reduces the incidence of shingles by 51% and the incidence of PHN by 67% in adults age 60 years and older.[87] Among people who develop shingles despite being vaccinated, the vaccine can reduce the disease's severity. The FDA has approved the use of Zostavax among adults ages 50 to 59 years, although at this time, the CDC continues to recommend its use for adults 60 years and older because of lack of data and supply limitations.[86]

PROGNOSIS. Overall prognosis is good unless the infection spreads to the brain (rare). Most people recover completely, with the possible exception of scarring and, with corneal damage, visual impairment. One of the most significant complications associated with VZV is PHN. Occasionally, intractable pain associated with PHN may persist for months or years. PHN pain can be very difficult to treat, but many options are available. Signs of the disorder in immunocompetent persons resolve within a month, but the area that was affected may be partly insensitive or show postinfectious skin changes. Studies are lacking on recurrent zoster, although it is thought that one episode of zoster is not protective against a second.[233]

SPECIAL IMPLICATIONS FOR THE THERAPIST   8-9

Varicella Zoster Virus

Varicella is highly contagious. The period of communicability extends from 1 to 2 days before the onset of the rash through the first 4 to 5 days or until all lesions have formed crusts. Immunocompromised individuals with progressive varicella are probably contagious during the entire period new lesions continue to appear.

Any patient or client suspected of having herpes zoster (shingles) requires immediate medical attention. Reports of prodromal pain, symptoms, or onset of rash are red flags to warrant immediate diagnosis and early treatment. Early intervention can reduce morbidity.

Because airborne transmission of VZV occurs, affected individuals in a hospital setting should be isolated in negative pressure rooms until crusts have dried.

HCWs who do take care of VZV clients should use contact precautions, including careful use of barriers such as gloves, gowns, and masks whenever in contact with active lesions. If serologic immunity of the HCW cannot be verified, varicella vaccine is recommended (see Table 8-4).

Health care–associated transmission of VZV is well known. Sources for exposure include clients or residents, HCWs, and visitors, including children or HCWs, with either varicella or zoster.

The CDC has set up guidelines for the care of all clients regarding precautions for the transmission of infectious skin diseases (see Table 10-3; see also Table 8-5). These Standard Precautions (see Appendix A) should be used with all clients regardless of their disease status.

All skin lesions are considered potentially infectious and should be handled as such. The careful use of these precautionary measures severely limits the transmission of any disease. In addition, each hospital has isolation precautions organized according to categories of disease to prevent the spread of infectious disease to others. Every health care professional must be familiar with these procedures and follow them carefully. See also the section on Isolation Procedures in Appendix A and Table 8-3.

Neither heat nor ultrasound should be used on a person with shingles because these modalities can increase the severity of the person's symptoms. For the person with severe herpetic pain, relaxation techniques may be useful. In the case of unresolved PHN, the individual may benefit from a program of chronic pain management.

For the Therapist

Adults with shingles are infectious to persons who have not had chickenpox, and the person with shingles can develop shingles more than one time. To develop shingles, it is necessary to have been exposed to chickenpox and harbor the virus in your nervous system.[140] For this reason, therapists who have never had chickenpox should receive the vaccination; complications and morbidity associated with adult onset of varicella warrant this precaution. It is generally advisable to allow only HCWs who are immune to varicella to take care of clients with VZV.

Any female therapist who is pregnant or planning a pregnancy should be tested for immune status if unsure about her previous history of varicella. This is especially important because transmissibility of the virus occurs 2 to 3 days before symptoms develop; immunocompromised clients with shingles are probably contagious during the entire period new lesions are appearing until all lesions are crusted over.

This means that anyone receiving intervention by a therapist may be an asymptomatic host during the period of communicability; exposure to self and further transmission to others can occur without the therapist's awareness.

Susceptible health care workers with significant exposure to varicella should be relieved from direct client contact from day 10 to day 21 after exposure. If workers develop chickenpox, varicella lesions must be crusted before they return to direct client contact.

Because of the possibility of transmission to and development of severe illness in high-risk clients, HCWs with localized zoster should not take care of such clients until all lesions are dry and crusted. However, they may take care of others if they cover their lesions.

When vaccinated HCWs are exposed to varicella, serologic testing for antibodies may be done, and exclusion from duty can occur if they are seronegative or develop varicella symptoms. Varicella-zoster immunoglobulin and acyclovir are not routinely recommended postexposure for healthy HCWs (exceptions may be made for pregnant or immunocompromised HCWs).[5]

Infectious Mononucleosis (Herpesvirus Type 4)

Overview. Infectious mononucleosis is a clinical syndrome most commonly associated with EBV, a member of the herpesvirus family. Although it may be seen at any age, it primarily affects young adults and children. In children, it is usually so mild that the symptoms are attributed to nonspecific illnesses.

Once thought to have an association with chronic fatigue syndrome (CFS), it now seems clear that no one infectious agent causes CFS. The CDC conducted a four-city surveillance to determine if an infectious etiology for CFS existed, and found no one organism was responsible. It may be that CFS has multiple causes with the same end point[24] (see "Chronic Fatigue and Immune Dysfunction Syndrome" in Chapter 7).

Incidence, Etiologic Factors, and Risk Factors. Infection with EBV is common in the United States, with 95% of people between the ages of 35 and 40 years having been infected.[119] When an adolescent or young adult becomes infected with EBV, 30% to 50% of the time they will develop the symptoms of infectious mononucleosis. Both genders are affected equally. Incidence varies seasonally among college students but not among the general population. The reservoir of EBV is limited to human beings, and transmission is through contact with oral secretions, blood or transplanted organs infected with the virus.[210] Because people shed EBV in the saliva during the acute infection and for an indefinite period afterward, it is sometimes called the "kissing disease."[208]

Pathogenesis and Clinical Manifestations. EBV causes lymphoid proliferation in the blood, lymph nodes, and spleen. Characteristically, the virus produces fever, sore throat, and tender cervical lymphadenopathy; headache, malaise, and abdominal pain (from splenic enlargement or hepatitis) may also be present. The incubation period is about 4 to 6 weeks.

Temperature fluctuations occur throughout the day, peaking in the evening. There is often an increase in the white blood cell count, with an elevation in atypical lymphocytes. Hepatomegaly (accompanied by elevated liver enzymes), palatal petechiae, and splenomegaly are clinically detectable in 15% to 65% of cases, although most affected persons have splenomegaly on ultrasound. The spleen may enlarge to two to three times its normal size, causing left upper quadrant pain with possible referral to the left shoulder and left upper trapezius region. Although uncommon, affected individuals are at risk for splenic rupture (occurring in approximately 1% of cases), and care should be taken to avoid trauma.

Both the peripheral nervous system and CNS can be involved (1%-5% of cases) producing neurologic abnormalities including Guillain-Barré syndrome, encephalitis, aseptic meningitis, peripheral neuritis, and optic neuritis. Although typically mild, the most common complications are hematologic (25%-50%) and include hemolytic anemia, aplastic anemia, thrombocytopenia, and thrombotic thrombocytopenic purpura.[119] Symptoms subside about 6 to 10 days after onset of the disease but may persist for weeks. Symptoms from EBV-related infectious mononucleosis rarely last longer than 4 months.

MEDICAL MANAGEMENT

DIAGNOSIS, TREATMENT, AND PROGNOSIS. Diagnosis is based on clinical examination, laboratory tests, and a positive heterophil (monospot) test. In clients with acute EBV, there are generally 10% atypical lymphocytes on the peripheral blood smear. Heterophil antibodies (a group of immunoglobulin [Ig] M antibodies, which cause agglutination of sheep red blood cells) are negative in 25% of people during the first week of acute infection and in 5% to 10% in the second week. In children younger than 12 years, the heterophil test is positive in only 25% to 50% of cases. Once antibodies are present, they may persist for up to a year.[119] If a definitive diagnosis is required, tests specific for EBV (IgM and IgG antibodies for portions of the virus) are available.[41]

EBV may have a pathogenic role in causation of cancers such as Burkitt lymphoma, nasopharyngeal carcinoma, Hodgkin disease,[91,205] and lymphoproliferative disorders in immunosuppressed and posttransplant clients.[126,171] Oral hairy leukoplakia, Hodgkin, and non-Hodgkin lymphoma are diseases that are linked with EBV in HIV-positive individuals.[96,142]

Studies support an association between infectious mononucleosis and the subsequent development of multiple sclerosis for both adults and children.[118,189] Young people who have had a strong immune response to the EBV are twice as likely to develop multiple sclerosis in adulthood. Studies are underway to determine the cause and develop a therapy.[176]

The prognosis is excellent with rest and supportive care. Clinical symptoms typically improve within a month, although the fatigue and lymphadenopathy may persist longer. Most people are back to normal activities within 2 to 3 months.[9] Questions still remain as to the most appropriate time for athletes to resume contact sports. Because the majority of splenic ruptures have occurred within 3 weeks of symptoms, it is generally recommended that clients wait at least 3 weeks after initial symptoms.[166]

No other specific interventions appear to alter or shorten the disease process, although studies have evaluated antiviral medications and corticosteroids.[20] Larger trials are needed to determine if either of these treatments is beneficial, particularly in clients with immunodeficiencies or severe complications. If given ampicillin, clients often develop a maculopapular rash. Because the virus can live indefinitely in B lymphocytes and the oropharynx, reactivation of the virus frequently occurs. The virus is commonly found in the saliva, although most often without symptoms.

SPECIAL IMPLICATIONS FOR THE THERAPIST 8-10

Infectious Mononucleosis

Infectious mononucleosis is probably contagious before symptoms develop until the fever subsides and the oral and pharyngeal lesions disappear. Although infectious mononucleosis appears to be only mildly contagious, adherence to standard precautions, especially good hand hygiene and avoidance of shared dishware or food items with other people, is essential in preventing the HCW from contracting this condition.

The person with infectious mononucleosis should be cautioned against engaging in excessive activity, especially contact sports, which could result in splenic rupture or lowered resistance to infection. Usually this guideline is appropriate for a period of at least 1 month.

Any sign of splenic rupture (e.g., abdominal or upper quadrant pain, the Kehr sign, sudden left shoulder pain, or shock) requires immediate medical evaluation. Any soft-tissue mobilization or myofascial techniques necessary in the left upper quadrant, especially up and under the rib cage, must take into consideration the enlarged liver and/or spleen; indirect techniques away from the spleen are indicated.

In rare cases, mononucleosis impairs the CNS. Any change in neurologic status must be evaluated and reported to the physician. Changes in respiration or signs and symptoms of airway obstruction may require emergency intervention.

Cytomegalovirus (Herpesvirus Type 5)

Overview and Incidence. CMV (herpesvirus type 5) is a commonly occurring DNA herpesvirus. It increases in frequency with age. One percent of newborns have it, and two-thirds of adults older than 35 years have CMV (usually contracted during childhood or early adulthood) and are seropositive.

For the majority of people who are infected with the virus after birth, there are few symptoms or complications. However, for unborn babies or the immunocompromised (posttransplant or with HIV disease), the consequences can be severe or life-threatening. In the literature, a distinction is made between CMV infection and CMV disease. Infection signifies a positive laboratory result, whereas disease refers to an infection with associated symptoms.

Etiologic and Risk Factors. CMV is transmitted by human contact with infected secretions, such as urine, saliva, breast milk, feces, blood, semen, and vaginal and cervical secretions. It may also be transmitted through the placenta. The virus can be acquired from transplanted organs and rarely via blood transfusions. As with other herpesviruses, CMV can remain dormant to evade detection and persists in multiple organs. There is frequent intermittent reactivation with asymptomatic shedding of virus.

Pathogenesis and Clinical Manifestations. CMV probably spreads through the body via lymphocytes or mononuclear cells to the lungs (CMV pneumonitis), liver (CMV hepatitis), GI tract (CMV gastroenteritis), eyes (CMV retinitis), and CNS, where it produces inflammatory reactions. Complications include diffuse interstitial pneumonitis, leading to respiratory distress syndrome, hepatitis, GI ulcerations and bleeding, vision loss, and loss of transplanted organs.

In normal adolescents or adults, the infection is usually asymptomatic or presents as an infectious mononucleosis-like illness with a self-limiting course of fever and mild hepatitis. Unlike infectious mononucleosis from EBV, CMV rarely causes pharyngitis or adenopathy.

In approximately 1% to 4% of women who have their first or primary infection during pregnancy, 30% to 40% of the babies become infected.[234] The course of the illness for the fetus ranges from mild splenomegaly or hepatitis to disseminated disease. Approximately 10% to 20% of those infected are born with acute symptoms. Of these babies, up to 20% die while the remainder have moderate to severe complications.[56] The most common complications include hearing loss, vision impairment, and varying degrees of intellectual developmental disorder. Approximately 5% to 15% of congenitally infected babies born without initial symptoms, will go on to develop later sequelae.[234] Approximately 80% of babies born with CMV do not have symptoms or further problems.

In immunosuppressed people, particularly transplant recipients and those with HIV, various manifestations of disease develop with CMV infection. Transplant clients who are at greatest risk for severe disease are those who are negative for CMV, but receive a donor-positive organ/tissue. Fever, splenomegaly, hepatitis, pneumonitis, esophagitis, gastritis, colitis, encephalitis, or retinitis may occur in individuals who are immunocompromised.

CMV is also associated with an increase in risk of infection by other viruses and bacteria.[63,89] The specific transplanted organ is particularly susceptible to disease (e.g., hepatitis in liver transplants). Transplant recipients are most at risk the first 100 days following transplantation (see Chapter 21). With improved treatment of HIV using HAART, CMV retinitis has significantly decreased but remains an important cause of blindness in advanced HIV disease.

MEDICAL MANAGEMENT

DIAGNOSIS, TREATMENT, AND PROGNOSIS. Diagnosis of an acute infection is made either by culture (blood, sputum [from bronchoalveolar lavage], urine, throat swabs, or tissue samples) antigen-detection assays, or PCR. Traditional viral culture requires time; however, expedited results can be obtained for immunocompromised clients through PCR or antigen-detection assays.

Enzyme-linked immunosorbent assay (ELISA) is the most common serologic test available and is able to distinguish between previous or active infection when samples are drawn at least 2 weeks apart to demonstrate increasing titers of antibodies and an active infection. Newer techniques of measuring antibody maturity also provide for a clearer method of determining acuity of infection, although these tests are not widely available.

Because most people infected with CMV are asymptomatic or display nonspecific and self-limiting symptoms, treatment is not required. In immunocompromised clients, pharmacologic treatment has proven effective.

The prognosis for people with transplanted organs or who are immunocompromised can be associated with poor outcome, as they may have fatal disseminated infections with multiple organ involvement. Clients undergoing transplant receive prophylaxis medications, which help reduce subsequent CMV infection and disease.[63,224] Those with HIV and reactivated CMV disease benefit from

HAART which may aid the immune system in recovering enough to suppress the virus, making anti-CMV treatment unnecessary.[95]

Infants who are born with severe symptoms related to CMV infection may be treated with ganciclovir, although there is little data to guide treatment and is not currently licensed for newborns. Some evidence suggests that CMV hyperimmune globulin given to a pregnant woman with a primary infection can reduce the risk of congenital infection.[234] Babies with congenital CMV should have their hearing and vision checked regularly.

Vaccines are currently in development.[12]

SPECIAL IMPLICATIONS FOR THE THERAPIST   8-11

Cytomegalovirus

Other practice patterns depend on organ systems involved and clinical presentation. The two principal reservoirs of CMV in health care institutions are (1) infants and young children and (2) immunocompromised individuals. However, HCWs who provide care to these high-risk populations have a rate of primary CMV that is no higher than among personnel without such client contact.

CMV transmission appears to occur directly, either through close, intimate contact with contaminated secretions or through excretions, especially saliva or urine.[46] Transmission by the hands of HCWs or individuals with the virus has also been suggested. The incubation period for person-to-person transmission is not known, and although CMV can survive on environmental surfaces or objects for a very short time, no evidence of fomite transmission exists.[212] There is some evidence to suggest there is an occupational risk of transmission (to daycare employees) via environmental surfaces at daycare facilities.[102]

Pregnant women and immunosuppressed people should avoid exposure to confirmed or suspected CMV infection. Pregnant women or women of childbearing age need to be counseled regarding the risks and prevention of transmission of CMV, but no data show that HCWs can be protected from infection by transfer to areas with less contact with individuals who have been diagnosed with CMV. Work restrictions for HCWs who contract CMV are not necessary as the risk of transmission of CMV can be reduced by careful adherence to hand hygiene and standard precautions.[212]

Clients with CMV infection should be encouraged to wash their hands thoroughly and frequently to prevent spreading it. It is especially important to impress this on young children. As difficult as it may be, the child should not be allowed to kiss others, and parents and others should also avoid kissing the affected child.

HERPESVIRUSES TYPES 6, 7, AND 8. HHV-6 is a B-cell lymphotropic virus that is the principal cause of exanthema subitum (roseola infantum, or sixth disease). Primary HHV-6 is common in children, with 90% infected by the age of 2 years. Although classically described as 3 to 5 days of high fever followed by a macular rash on the neck and trunk (roseola), children more commonly develop a fever, runny nose, and fussiness. Its occurrence in adults is more complicated and associated with immunocompromised states such as HIV, transplant recipients, and lymphoma. It is associated with graft rejection[115] and bone marrow suppression in transplant recipients. Both HHV-6 and HHV-7 reactivation have been implicated in the exacerbation multiple sclerosis.[146]

HHV-7 is a T-cell lymphotropic virus that is biologically similar to HHV-6. HHV-7 does not appear to be as clinically significant as other herpes viruses, although may at times explain a "recurrent" case of roseola. HHV-8 is associated with Kaposi sarcoma in AIDS and other immune-related diseases (e.g., primary effusion lymphoma).[115] (See "Kaposi Sarcoma" in Chapter 10.)

Viral Respiratory Infections

Viral respiratory infections (influenza, respiratory syncytial virus [RSV]) are common problems in health care settings. Many viral pathogens can cause respiratory infections, but influenza and RSV are associated with significant morbidity and mortality rates.

Influenza. Each year in the United States influenza viruses cause serious illness and even death, especially in young children; persons with chronic diseases; immunocompromised adults; and the frail elderly. Between the years 1990 and 1999 there were approximately 36,000 deaths attributable to influenza epidemics.[207] Influenza is caused by influenza viruses A or B and occurs in epidemics between late fall and early spring.

In recent years, two influenza A viruses emerged that have caused significant morbidity and mortality worldwide. In 2005, an avian influenza A virus made the news for its ability to cause severe symptoms with fatal outcomes in humans. The subtype is H5N1 and was originally identified in Asia. In 2009, the subtype H1N1 (previously seen in swine) led to a pandemic outbreak of influenza. The complication rate reported in the normally healthy age range of 19 to 64 years was greater than typically seen.

The mode of transmission is from person to person by inhalation of aerosolized virus (sneezing, coughing into the air) or by direct contact. Health care–associated transmission of influenza has been reported in acute and long-term health care facilities and has occurred from clients to HCWs, from HCWs to clients, and among HCWs. The incubation period is usually 1 to 4 days (average of 2 days).

Influenzas A and B resemble other respiratory illnesses such as parainfluenza, RSV, rhinovirus, *Mycoplasma pneumoniae*, and adenovirus. The onset of symptoms is usually abrupt, with high fever, chills, malaise, muscular aching (myalgia), headache, sore throat, nasal congestion, and nonproductive cough. The fever lasts about 1 to 7 days (usually 3-5). Children often manifest nausea, vomiting, and otitis media. The infection can progress rapidly in the first few days, causing pneumonia and respiratory failure, predominantly in high-risk groups. Secondary bacterial pneumonia may also develop, usually 5 to 10 days after the onset of viral symptoms, particularly in the older adult.

MEDICAL MANAGEMENT

PREVENTION. In 2010, the Advisory Committee on Immunization Practices recommended that all persons 6 months of age and older should be vaccinated.[38] This policy changed because under the old guidelines, many people at risk for complications from influenza were being missed. The new plan recognizes that mass immunization programs based on age have been more successful than those targeting people with chronic diseases.

Vaccination of HCWs has shown a total reduction in mortality in clients in long-term care facilities,[162] whereas vaccinations given during an epidemic reduce the risks for pneumonia, hospitalization, and death in elderly persons.[80]

Two types of vaccines are available. One is the trivalent inactivated influenza vaccine, which can be used in any person 6 months old or older, including those with high-risk conditions. It is typically given intramuscularly, although a new intradermal formulation is now available for adults age 18 through 64 years (Fluzone Intradermal). The live attenuated influenza vaccine may be used for healthy nonpregnant persons ages 2 to 49 years (FluMist, given intranasally). Either vaccine may be used in healthy, nonpregnant persons between the ages of 2 and 49 years.[33] Because the safety and effectiveness of live attenuated influenza vaccine in persons with underlying medical conditions has not been established, it is recommended that these people continue to be vaccinated with only trivalent inactivated influenza vaccine.[32]

DIAGNOSIS. The virus may be isolated from nasopharyngeal or nasal swab, and nasal wash or aspirate. These can be sent for a rapid detection of antigen (ELISA or immunofluorescent assay [IFA]) and culture. With the advent of improved antiinfluenza medications requiring initiation within 48 hours, the antigen detection method is a mainstay in many laboratories. Culture requires 3 to 10 days but should be performed if the rapid detection test is negative and the likelihood high that the person has influenza (i.e., false negatives are more common than false positives). Like other antigen detection methods, culture provides information regarding the subtype of influenza virus, yet provides a definitive diagnosis.

Genetic mutations in the influenza virus create hundreds of variations within the two main types; being immune to one variant does not ensure immunity to another. Trivalent influenza virus vaccine provides partial immunity (approximately 85% efficacy) for a few months to 1 year. The CDC updates the vaccine annually to include the most current influenzas A and B virus strains.

TREATMENT. There are currently several licensed medications available for the treatment of influenza. Many influenza A virus strains have become resistant to some of these drugs. Early antiviral treatment should be administered for persons with severe symptoms or at high risk for severe complications (either suspected influenza or confirmed).

Approved antiviral medications should be used when influenza A (H1N1) from 2009, influenza A (H3N2), or influenza B viruses are suspected or confirmed. Children younger than 1 year should be treated with antiviral medication in order to reduce the risk of severe complications.[62] Influenza antiviral agents can be given in conjunction with vaccine during institutional outbreaks of influenza.

Antiviral agents used to treat influenza help decrease the duration and severity of signs and symptoms. Treatment must be initiated within the first 2 days of the illness and benefits those at high risk for complications. Resistance to these antivirals does occur, and the CDC monitors and recommends specific, effective treatment for each season.

Many people with influenza prefer to rest in bed; analgesics and a cough medicine mixture are often used. Droplet precautions (see Table 8-3) are imperative for all diagnosed and suspected cases of influenza. Antibacterial antibiotics are used only for treatment of bacterial complications.

PROGNOSIS. The duration of the uncomplicated illness is 3 to 7 days, and the prognosis is usually very good in previously healthy people. Reye syndrome is a rare (almost eradicated) and severe complication of influenza and other viral diseases, especially in young children (to avoid Reye syndrome, acetaminophen should be used for fever instead of aspirin in children).

Most fatalities related to influenza are caused by bacterial and viral pneumonia. People at greatest risk for influenza-related complications are (1) individuals older than 65 years, (2) children younger than 2 years of age, and (3) persons of any age who have medical conditions that place them at increased risk for complications from influenza.[206] Epidemiology studies from the 2009 pandemic also showed that Native Americans and persons who were morbidly obese were at a higher risk for complications from the influenza A (H1N1) virus.[62]

RESPIRATORY SYNCYTIAL VIRUS. RSV is the leading cause of lower respiratory tract infections in children worldwide.[139] In the United States, between 75,000 and 125,000 hospitalizations related to RSV occur among children younger than 1 year old, and 1.5 million outpatient visits occur in children younger than age 5 years.[35]

In adults and older children, reinfection is common and manifests itself as mild upper respiratory tract infection and tracheobronchitis. Serious pulmonary RSV infections have been described in older and immunocompromised individuals, and there is a high mortality rate in bone marrow and solid organ transplant recipients. In addition, infants with congenital heart disease, individuals in intensive care units, those with cystic fibrosis, and older adults are at high risk for serious and complicated RSV. Clients with HIV tend to have a less-severe course of the illness than transplant clients and although hospitalization for RSV is high, it rarely causes death.

Annual epidemics occur in fall, winter, and spring, although there is geographic variation. The incubation period is between 3 and 8 days. Inoculation occurs through the eyes or nose but rarely the mouth.

Health care–associated transmission of RSV occurs among clients, visitors, and HCWs. RSV is present in large numbers in the respiratory secretions of children with symptomatic RSV infections. It can be transmitted through large droplets (although not aerosolized) during close contact with such individuals or indirectly by hands or fomites that are contaminated with RSV. Hands can become contaminated through touching or handling of fomites or respiratory secretions and can transmit RSV by touching the nose or eyes.

Usually people shed the virus for 3 to 8 days, but young infants may shed the virus for as long as 3 to 4 weeks. Symptoms of RSV can be similar to those of other common respiratory pathogens, such as influenza, including low-grade fever, tachypnea, and wheezing. Hyperinflated lungs, decreased gas exchange, and increased work of breathing are also often present, and otitis media is a common complication.

Rapid diagnosis of RSV may be made by viral antigen identification of nasal washings, using an ELISA or IFA, or shell vial culture technique. Culture of nasopharyngeal secretions is the standard for definitive diagnosis but requires 4 to 15 days. Real-time PCR assays for RNA of the virus are becoming more available but are used most frequently in large medical centers.

Treatment consists of hydration, humidification of inspired air, and ventilatory support as needed. Aerosolized ribavirin (an antiviral agent used in chronic HCV therapy) is FDA approved for the treatment of RSV in children, but close monitoring must be provided. Pregnant women should avoid ribavirin exposure as it is associated with fetal malformation or fetal death.

Evidence also supports the use of aerosolized ribavirin for the treatment of RSV in immunocompromised adults with or without palivizumab (a humanized monoclonal antibody [IgG]) or intravenous immunoglobulin.[185] Palivizumab has been approved for prevention of serious lower respiratory tract illness in infants and young children who are at high risk of serious RSV,[94] but it is expensive and must be administered intramuscularly on a monthly basis during the RSV season.

Avoidance of exposure to tobacco smoke, cold air, and air pollutants is also beneficial to long-term recovery from RSV bronchiolitis. A number of vaccines to prevent this infection are currently being studied, but because the immune response is neither durable nor complete it has been a difficult task.

SPECIAL IMPLICATIONS FOR THE THERAPIST   **8-12**

Viral Respiratory Infections
Influenza

HCWs must follow the guidelines in Tables 8-3 and 8-5 regarding prevention of transmission of influenza, both for themselves and their clients. Recommendations for immunization must be reviewed and acted on individually. Because the immunization for influenza does not provide immunity for the entire year or for all strains of influenza, common sense must prevail in the case of a HCW who suspects he or she has early signs and symptoms of influenza.

An early diagnosis can result in the use of antivirals to minimize intensity and duration of symptoms, especially in those at high risk for complications.

HCWs must be aware of their responsibility to avoid transmission of infectious diseases such as influenza and either use personal protective equipment or practice self-isolation by staying home. This is especially important for the therapist in a setting with aged, immunocompromised, or chronically ill individuals.

Influenza can cause substantial morbidity and mortality among persons age 65 years and older and among adults age 50 years and older who have chronic illnesses. Anyone in these two groups is vulnerable to the serious complications of influenza. Routine influenza vaccination is associated with reductions in influenza-associated and all-cause mortality during influenza season.[144] Despite the benefits from vaccination, utilization remains below target rates. Physical therapists can be instrumental in reducing morbidity and mortality rates by encouraging clients in these two groups to get a flu shot each year and by getting one themselves.

Miscellaneous Infectious Diseases

Prostheses and Implant Infections

Any device implanted into the body of any synthetic material (e.g., titanium, cobalt, silicone) can give rise to serious life-threatening infections. Bioprostheses, implanted in large numbers in the 1970s and early 1980s, have now gone into the second decade of life since implantation, a time when biodegradation becomes more common. Multiple reoperations carry a higher risk of infection.

Likewise, as the population ages, an increasing number of primary and revision arthroplasties are being done. Early detection of infection or other problems can reduce complications and morbidity associated with these devices. Anyone with implants of any kind with onset of increasing musculoskeletal symptoms (especially in the area of the surgery) must be screened for the possibility of infection.

Normal radiographs and negative needle aspirates can delay medical diagnosis of infection. Knowing the risk factors for developing an antibiotic-resistant infection (e.g., multiple surgical procedures, previous *S. aureus* infection, multiple antibiotics) and recognizing red flag symptoms of infection can help the therapist recognize the need for persistence in obtaining follow-up medical care.

See Chapter 25 for a complete discussion of this topic.

Lyme Disease

Definition and Overview. Lyme disease is an infectious multisystemic disorder caused by three closely related tickborne spirochete species, collectively referred to as *Borrelia burgdorferi senso lato*. In the United States, most cases of Lyme disease are caused by *B. burgdorferi senso stricto*. In Europe and Asia, it is most often caused by *Borrelia afzelii* and *Borrelia garinii*.

Lyme disease was first recognized in 1976 when a group of children in Lyme, CT, developed an unusual type of arthritis and a bull's-eye rash.[196] Some of these children also had a history of tick bites. Not until 1982 was the organism recovered from affected individuals and tick vectors established the relationship between the spirochete and the infection.[19]

In the United States, the disease is only transmitted to human beings by certain ticks of the *Ixodes* species: *Ixodes scapularis* (formerly called *Ixodes dammini*), known as the deer or black-legged tick in the Northeast (from Massachusetts to Maryland) and North Central United States (Wisconsin and Minnesota), and *Ixodes pacificus*, the Western black-legged tick found on the western coast of northern California and Oregon. The ticks are extremely small, measuring approximately 1 to 2 mm.

Incidence. Lyme disease has become the most prevalent vectorborne infectious disease in the United States.[133] In 1982, when the CDC began national surveillance, only 229 cases were reported, whereas in 2006 a total of 19,931 cases were brought to medical attention.[7] This increased frequency is most likely multifactorial, a result of a heightened awareness of the illness in endemic areas as well as an increase in overdiagnosis.[168]

Most cases (more than 90%) have been reported from the Mid-Atlantic, Northeastern, and North Central regions of the country. In 2008, the CDC stated that more than 248,074 cases had been reported between the years 1992 and 2006 from all 50 states and the District of Columbia. Children, typically between the ages of 5 and 14 years, were the most often affected.[7] In the United States, Lyme disease is often seen in the late spring and summer months when the tick nymphs are most active and human outdoor activities are greatest.

Pathogenesis. *I. scapularis* exists in larval, nymphal, and adult stages. Larvae contract *B. burgdorferi* by feeding on infected rodents (white-footed mouse or other small rodents). The bacteria are then passed to nymphs and then to adults. The host of the adult is the white-tailed deer, which is required for survival of the ticks.

Human beings generally acquire the infection from nymphs when they attach to the skin to feed. The tick becomes engorged with blood and turns a grayish color. The ticks require at least 36 hours or more (up to 72 hours) of feeding before the bacteria move from the midgut to the salivary glands and then injected into the host.[150] Most commonly, however, the tick falls off or is removed before the bacteria are injected into the host's bloodstream.

After incubating for 3 to 32 days, the spirochetes cause an inflammatory response, resulting in characteristic skin lesions at the site of the tick bite (see "Clinical Manifestations" below). The bacteria then disseminate to other organs via the bloodstream or lymphatic system if not treated.

The human host activates an immune response, producing cytokines and antibodies against the bacteria. Despite the host's response and if untreated, *B. burgdorferi* can survive for years in certain areas of the body by genetically adapting and inhibiting host immune responses.[160,194]

Human vertical transmission—that is, infected mother to child in utero—can occur and is more likely when the mother is infected in the first trimester. The incidence of transmission is believed to be quite low. Perinatal transmission of *B. burgdorferi* can result in a multisystemic

illness that can prove fatal, although there is no evidence for the converse situation, that is, asymptomatic infection for a prolonged period.[149]

Clinical Manifestations. Like syphilis, Lyme disease can be described as an imitator because its signs and symptoms mimic those of many other diseases. Symptoms vary widely and may not develop for as long as 1 month after a bite; in some cases, symptoms do not develop at all. Clinical manifestations of the infection occur in three stages.

Stage 1, the early, localized stage, usually occurs within 5 to 14 days following a tick bite. Approximately 80% to 90% of affected individuals will have a red, slowly expanding rash called *erythema migrans* (Fig. 8-8).[137] Not all people with the disease develop the telltale rash, and because early symptoms are often mild, some people may remain undiagnosed and untreated. Erythema migrans resolves spontaneously without treatment within an average of 4 weeks. Flu-like symptoms suggestive of early dissemination such as fatigue, chills, fever, headache, lethargy, myalgias, or arthralgias may also develop early in the course of the infection and may be the presenting symptoms for anyone without a rash.

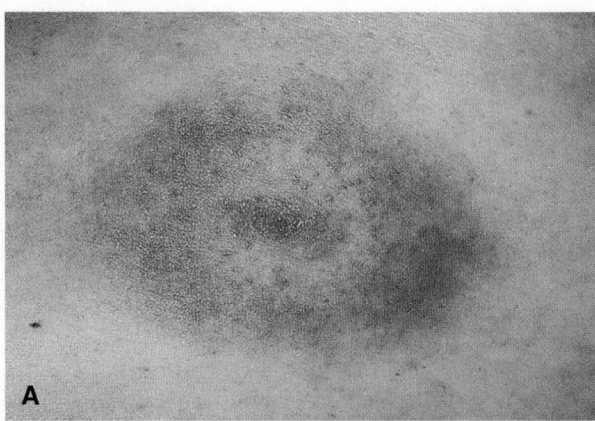
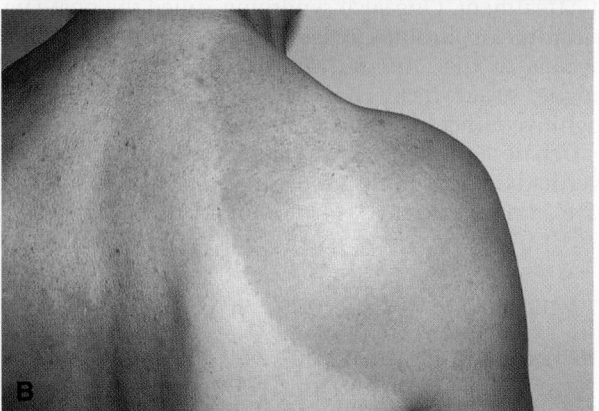

Figure 8-8

Examples of erythema migrans associated with Lyme disease. **A,** Many sources describe a characteristic bull's-eye rash with Lyme disease. **B,** However, there is a wide range of skin reactions labeled as erythema migrans possible with Lyme disease, as shown. Some skin rashes may be so minor as to be ignored or go unnoticed by the affected individual. (**A,** From Swartz MH: *Textbook of physical diagnosis: history and examination,* ed 4, Philadelphia, 2002, WB Saunders. **B,** Reprinted from Mandel GL: *Principles and practice of infectious diseases,* ed 6, Edinburgh, 2005, Churchill Livingstone.)

Stage 2, disseminated infection, occurs within weeks to months after the tick bite, particularly to the skin, nervous system, heart, and joints. Skin manifestations include multiple, smaller erythema migrans, similar to the original rash. Neurologic symptoms may be the first to arise and occur in 15% of all cases, most commonly manifested as aseptic meningitis with mild headache, stiff neck, and difficulty with mentation; cranial neuropathies, particularly Bell palsy (involvement of cranial nerve VII); and radiculopathies (Box 8-10).[85] Even if untreated, neurologic symptoms may improve or resolve.

Early treatment can prevent the development of arthritis.[87] If untreated, approximately 80% develop joint involvement.[197] Lyme disease related arthritis is typically of a relapsing/remitting pattern. Migratory musculoskeletal pain in joints, bursae, tendons, muscle, and bone may occur in one or a few locations at a time, often lasting days to weeks in a given location.

Some people (approximately 5%) experience cardiac signs and symptoms. The most common is conduction abnormalities (usually atrioventricular block) and dysrhythmias, which can result in irregular, rapid, or slowed pulses; dizziness; fainting; and shortness of breath. Symptoms typically resolve after a several days. Myocarditis is less commonly seen.[160]

Stage 3, late persistent infection, may become apparent months to years after the initial infection. In the United States approximately 60% of individuals left untreated develop stage 3 joint symptoms characterized by intermittent or chronic monarticular (one joint) or oligoarticular (affecting only a few joints) arthritis. This arthritis is associated with marked pain and swelling, especially in the large joints, such as the knees (Fig. 8-9). Rarely, affected individuals may go on to develop erosions or permanent joint abnormalities.

Postinfection Syndromes. Several syndromes have been reported describing persistent symptoms despite antibiotic treatment. One such syndrome, called the post-Lyme syndrome or chronic Lyme disease, more resembles fibromyalgia or CFS. Affected individuals describe disabling fatigue, severe headache, diffuse muscle or joint pain, cognitive difficulties, and sleep abnormalities.

Debate continues as to whether affected individuals ever had an active infection with *B. burgdorferi,* and may have another disease.[133] Most evidence demonstrates that

the diagnosis of Lyme disease is appropriate for only a minority of patients in whom it is suspected.[114]

In studies that followed persons with an accurate diagnosis of Lyme disease, few went on to demonstrate chronic syndrome complaints. Of those with documented, treated disease, it is hypothesized that the bacteria may trigger a neurohormonal or immunologic process that causes symptoms despite eradication of the spirochete.[165] Although evidence of the spirochete exists in the synovial fluid prior to treatment, posttreatment joint fluid is often negative for infection. This may be immune rather than infection related.[195]

MEDICAL MANAGEMENT

PREVENTION. Prevention is the key to avoiding Lyme disease.[133] Lyme disease is most common during the late spring and summer months in the United States when nymphal ticks are most active and human populations are frequently outdoors and most exposed. People who live or work in residential areas surrounded by woods or overgrown brush infested by ticks or favored by white-tailed deer and live in the endemic geographic areas are at risk. In addition, people who participate in outdoor recreational activities in tick habitat are also at risk for Lyme disease.

Prophylactic treatment is controversial, but a single dose of doxycycline for ticks that have been attached to the skin for between 36 and 72 hours may be helpful.[136] Box 8-11 provides specific strategies available for Lyme disease prevention.

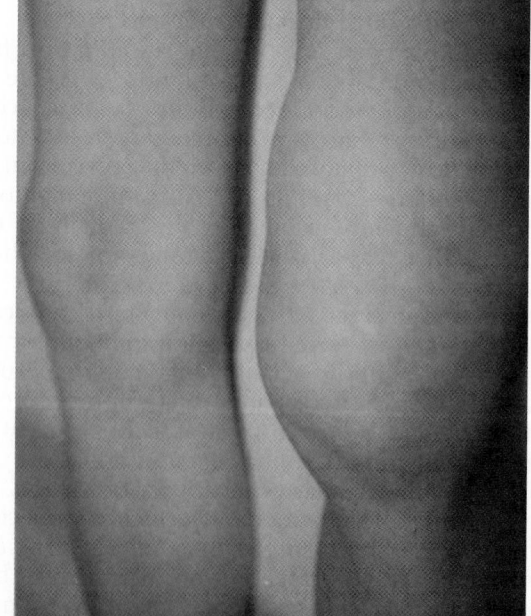

Figure 8-9

Swollen knee of a youth with Lyme arthritis. (Reprinted from National Institutes of Health: *Lyme disease: the facts, the challenge,* NIH publication no. 92-3193, Bethesda, MD, 1992, U.S. Department of Health and Human Services, p. 12.)

Box 8-10

NEUROLOGIC MANIFESTATIONS OF LYME DISEASE

Facial Nerve Palsy (Bell Palsy)
Cognitive impairment (e.g., forgetfulness, decreased concentration, personality changes)
Inflammation of the brain, spinal cord, or nerves
- Cranial neuritis
- Encephalitis
- Encephalomyelitis
- Encephalopathy
- Meningitis
- Radiculoneopathies

Box 8-11

PREVENTION OF LYME DISEASE

These precautions are provided for people living in tick-infested areas:

- Avoid tick-infested areas, especially in May, June, and July (check with local health departments or park services for the seasonal and geographic distribution in your area).
- Walk along cleared or paved surfaces rather than through tall grass or wooded areas.
- Wear long-sleeved shirts, long pants tucked into socks, and closed shoes (no part of foot exposed).
- Wear light-colored clothing to make it easy to detect ticks.
- Always check for ticks after being outdoors. If ticks are removed within 36 hours of attachment, the risk of infection decreases significantly.
- Shower as soon as possible after being outdoors. Ticks take several hours to attach themselves to the skin and can be washed away first.
- Wash clothing worn outdoors immediately and use a dryer (heat kills the ticks). If no access to laundry facilities is available, the clothing should not be stored in the bedroom, or if camping, the clothing should not be stored in the same area where people are sleeping.
- If bitten by a tick, remove the tick immediately by grasping it as close to the skin as possible with tweezers and tugging gently. Do not twist or turn the tweezers; pull straight away from the skin. Do not use petroleum jelly, fingernail polish, or a hot match to remove ticks.
- To lessen the chance of contact with the bacterium, do not crush the tick's body or handle the tick with bare hands. Clean the bite area thoroughly with soap and water, then swab the area with an antiseptic to prevent bacterial infection.
- Whenever possible, save the tick in a glass jar for identification should symptoms develop.
- If living in an area in which deer ticks are common, keep the weeds and grass around the house mowed. Consider using wood chips where lawns meet forested areas. Ticks are less able to survive in a dry environment.
- Use flea and tick collars on pets; brush and examine them carefully after they have been outdoors. People can use insecticides such as permethrin or insect repellents containing diethyltoluamide (DEET).*

*The use of such chemicals may be objectionable to some people because they may cause neurotoxicity in children. Alternative methods are available.

DIAGNOSIS. Persons with the typical erythema migrans do not require testing nor is it recommended. There are no consistently reliable tests for early disease since antibodies are not present for 1 to 2 weeks following infection.

For clients who have had symptoms longer than a few weeks, the CDC suggests a two-step process in diagnosing Lyme disease. The first step is to test the blood for antibodies to the spirochete. This is done with a sensitive enzyme immunoassay or IFA. If this test is positive or equivocal, a Western immunoblot should be performed to confirm the diagnosis.[31]

More recent reports suggest that the two-tier Lyme disease test relies on a serologic assay and can only indicate possible past exposure.[1a] No direct test can indicate whether living *Borrelia* are present in the blood. There is some concern and controversy currently over the use of this new culture method for the diagnosis of Lyme disease. The CDC has issued a direct warning against using any "unapproved" tests.[2a] Care must also be taken not to overdiagnose. Often serum antibody tests are done for "screening" purposes when clients have nonspecific symptoms. In this case, a false-positive result[184] could lead to unnecessary treatment with antibiotics[198] and an incorrect diagnosis. Antibodies can be present for years after successful treatment[104] and are not indicative of an infection causing the current symptoms.

TREATMENT. Early Lyme disease is treated with oral antibiotics, typically doxycycline, or amoxicillin for children or pregnant women. Antibiotics are given for 14 days. If third-degree heart block or meningitis develop, IV antibiotics are given for 14 to 28 days. Other neurologic symptoms are treated for 14 to 28 days, most often with oral antibiotics.[85] Lyme arthritis can be treated with oral or IV antibiotics, depending on the severity of symptoms, although oral therapy is easier and often equally effective.

For anyone with continued arthritis despite recommended treatment, PCR may be helpful in determining if further treatment may be beneficial. If symptoms persist despite the second treatment, data do not support the continued use of antibiotics.[229] Nonsteroidal medications, disease-modifying antirheumatic drugs, and arthroscopic synovectomy have been used as alternatives to treat arthritis, although studies are lacking for these approaches.[165]

PROGNOSIS. For most people, Lyme disease is curable with standard antibiotic therapy at any stage, and the effects of Lyme disease resolve completely within a few weeks or months of treatment. Nonspecific symptoms, such as fatigue, muscle and joint pain, may persist for weeks to months, but do not necessarily indicate failure of treatment. For a minority of clients who continue to have symptoms 6 months following treatment, efforts should be made to determine if they have continued infection, inflammation resulting from infection (postinfection), or another disease.[133] Unfortunately, no natural immunity develops from exposure to Lyme disease, and anyone can be reinfected. Although Lyme disease is rarely fatal, heart complications may cause life-threatening cardiac arrhythmias.

SPECIAL IMPLICATIONS FOR THE THERAPIST 8-13

Lyme Disease

Chronic arthritis is the most widely recognized result of untreated Lyme disease in the United States. Unlike other forms of rheumatoid arthritis, Lyme arthritis does not affect the joints bilaterally, although both sides may be affected alternately.

The condition has been called chronic because episodes can last months, occurring intermittently over a period of 1 to 3 years. Permanent joint damage and cartilage destruction can occur if excessive use occurs during the inflammatory period. Range-of-motion and strengthening exercises are important but must be carried out carefully and without overexertion.

Nervous system abnormalities can develop weeks, months, or even years following an untreated infection.

These symptoms often last for weeks or months and may recur. The therapist may treat such a client at any time during the course of symptomatic presentation.

For anyone with known Lyme disease, frequent assessment of the person's neurologic function and level of consciousness is important. Any signs of cardiac abnormality or increased intracranial pressure and cranial nerve involvement (e.g., ptosis, strabismus, diplopia) must be reported to the physician immediately. Both upper- and lower-extremity peripheral nerve problems can occur and are managed as any neuropathy from other causes.

It has been hypothesized that people who present with symptoms of multiple sclerosis but respond to antibiotics may have been bitten by ticks years ago. Along the same lines, the question has been raised whether Lyme disease triggers fibromyalgia since symptoms consistent with fibromyalgia and chronic fatigue syndrome develop in individuals with clear-cut Lyme disease, even after adequate treatment. To date, no biologic relationship has been proven between these conditions and Lyme disease.[128]

Sexually Transmitted Diseases

HIV/AIDS is covered in Chapter 7, but it is mentioned here to remind us that it is an infectious disease with a specific chain of transmission and control of transmission as discussed in this chapter.

Overview and Incidence. Sexually transmitted diseases (STDs) are a variety of clinical syndromes caused by pathogens that can be acquired and transmitted through sexual activity. Each year about 19 million Americans contract an STD. Accurate data are often difficult to obtain because of underreporting. Currently, only three STDs require reporting to the CDC: syphilis, gonorrhea, and chlamydia. States require reporting syphilis, gonorrhea, chlamydia, chancroid, HIV infection, and AIDS. It is likely that the incidence of STDs is underreported for several reasons.[226]

Not all STDs have symptoms and infected persons may not seek medical attention. There also continues to be significant social stigma related to STDs, which may lead individuals to postpone or avoid seeking treatment. Physicians may fail to report STD cases to local health departments despite being mandated to do so. Physicians also rely on patients to notify their sexual partners, who may or may not be tested and/or treated. A lack of free screening or reimbursement for screening may also be a contributing factor.

Syphilis was once thought to be trending toward elimination, but the incidence steadily increased from 2000 to 2009, before slightly decreasing in 2010, particularly in men who have sex with men.[226] Although the incidence of gonorrhea has reached an all-time low in the United States, chlamydia and HPV remain significant health problems. *Chlamydia* is the most common bacterial STD in the United States, with more than 1.3 million cases reported to the CDC in 2010.[36] It is estimated that the actual number of people infected (not just reported cases) is approximately 2.8 million annually.[214] Untreated chlamydia and gonorrhea can progress to pelvic inflammatory disease, infertility, ectopic pregnancy, and chronic pelvic pain.[3]

HPV, a collection of more than 40 serotypes that can infect the genital area, infects more than 6 million men and women per year. Specific serotypes of HPV (e.g., 16 and 18) can cause cervical cancer in women and are linked with oral squamous cell carcinoma. The national oral infection incidence is high at 6.9% of the population.[74] Other serotypes (e.g., 6 and 11) can cause genital warts.

Although the number of seropositive HSV-2 cases has been trending down, it is a chronic disease and most cases remain undiagnosed.[226] It is estimated that more than 50 million people carry the HSV-2 virus.[232]

STDs are spread primarily through sexual contact, but some cases may also be spread by sharing infected needles or by transmission from mother to child during vaginal childbirth. Many STDs are easily treated and cured, but others remain chronic. More than 50 different STDs have been described; only the most common ones are included here (see Table 8-7).

Risk Factors. All groups of people are potentially at risk for STDs, but women, teens, men who have sex with men, and minorities have been disproportionately affected. Although 25% of all STDs occur in people younger than 25 years, numerous surveys of healthy adults verify that older people are sexually active and less likely to practice safe sex. Direct contact with an infectious lesion is the main risk factor.

Other risk factors include multiple sex partners, persons who initiate sex early in adolescence, a partner with a known risk factor, persons residing in detention facilities, men having sex with men, obstacles in obtaining health care, a history of a blood transfusion between 1977 and 1984, failure to use a condom (or use it properly) during sexual intercourse, and sharing needles during illicit drug use. The presence of STDs is a risk factor itself for facilitating the transmission of HIV. In fact, persons with an STD are three to five times more likely than a person without an STD of sexually acquiring HIV.[64,218]

Pathogenesis and Clinical Manifestations. STDs are caused by bacteria, viruses and, occasionally, parasites and may have a considerable latency period when the infectious organism lies dormant before triggering symptomatic presentation (Fig. 8-10).

Clinical manifestations vary according to the STD present (Figs. 8-11 and 8-12; see also Table 8-7). STDs may be completely asymptomatic and therefore are less likely to be diagnosed until serious problems develop. Complications of STDs are often more severe and more frequent among women than men. Once infected, women are more susceptible to reproductive cancers, infertility, and contracting other STDs, including HIV.

MEDICAL MANAGEMENT

A brief summary of these key points is provided; for details, the reader is referred to the CDC's updated treatment guidelines published in 2010.[226]

PREVENTION. Prevention is the most important key to managing STDs. The CDC has identified five principal strategies for the prevention of STDs: (1) education and counseling

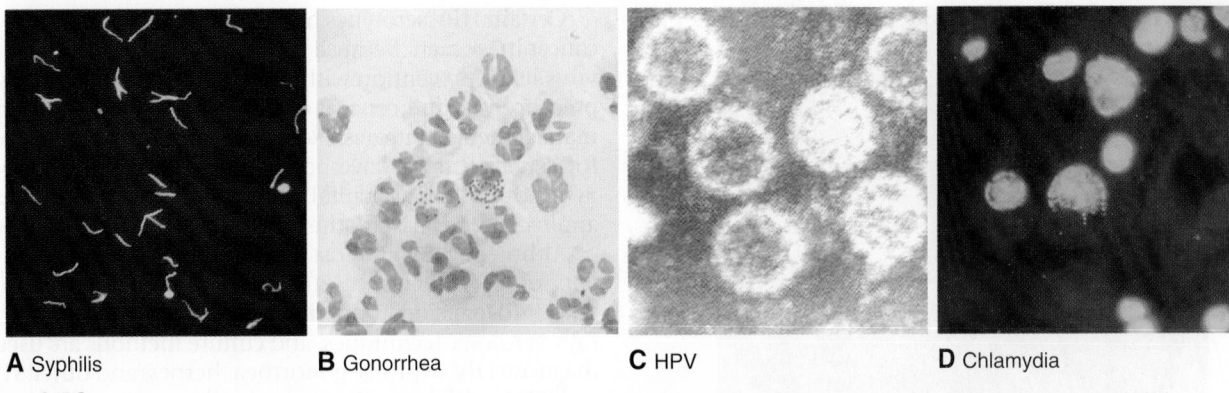

A Syphilis   **B** Gonorrhea   **C** HPV   **D** Chlamydia

Figure 8-10

Sexually transmitted infections. A, *Syphilis* mimics so many diseases it is called "the great imitator. " Dark-field microscopy showing several spiro-chetes in scrapings from the base of a syphilitic chancre. **B,** *Gonorrhea,* called the "preventer of life," can cause sterility. Gram-stained smear of urethral discharge showing intracellular gram-negative diplococci characteristic of gonorrhea. **C,** HPV is the most common cause of cervical and other reproductive cancers. **D,** *Chlamydia* is the most common STD reported in the United States. (A, Reprinted from Kumar V: *Robbins and Cotran: pathologic basis of disease,* ed 7, Philadelphia, 2005, WB Saunders, courtesy Paul Southern, Department of Pathology, University of Texas Southwestern Medical School, Dallas. B, Reprinted from Mandell GL: *Principles and practice of infectious diseases,* ed 6, Philadelphia, 2005, Churchill Livingstone. C, Reprinted from Kumar V: *Robbins and Cotran: pathologic basis of disease,* ed 7, Philadelphia, 2005, WB Saunders, courtesy Ian Frazer, Princess Alexan-dra Hospital, University of Queensland, Australia. D, Reprinted from Mandell GL: *Principles and practice of infectious diseases,* ed 6, Philadelphia, 2005, Churchill Livingstone, courtesy Robert Suchland, Seattle, WA.)

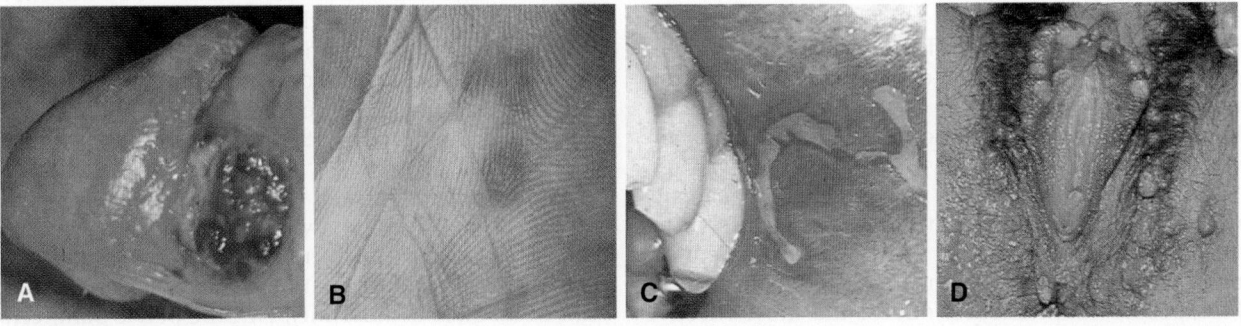

Figure 8-11

Clinical manifestations of syphilis. Many sexually transmitted infections present with lesions of the skin and/or genitals. Each one presents differ-ently based on the stage of the disease. **A,** Chancre in primary syphilis on the penis. **B,** Palmar lesions of a coppery color in secondary syphilis. **C,** Mucous patch of the mouth in secondary syphilis. **D,** Genital lesions called condylomata lata in a female (secondary syphilis). (A, C, and D, Reprinted from Forbes CD, Jackson WF: *Color atlas and text of clinical medicine,* London, 2003, Mosby. B, Reprinted from Habif TP: *Skin disease: diag-nosis and treatment,* St Louis, 2001, Mosby.)

of persons at risk on ways to avoid STDs through changes in sexual behaviors and use of recommended prevention services; (2) identification of asymptomatically infected persons and of symptomatic persons unlikely to seek diag-nostic and treatment services; (3) effective diagnosis, treat-ment, and counseling of infected persons; (4) evaluation, treatment, and counseling of sex partners of persons who are infected with an STD; and (5) preexposure vaccination of persons at risk for vaccine-preventable STDs.[226]

Primary prevention of STDs begins with changing the sexual behaviors that place persons at risk for infection. The only prevention that is 100% effective is abstinence from oral, vaginal, and anal sex, and/or to be in a mutu-ally monogamous sexual relationship (single partner) with an uninfected partner.

For those who are sexually active, condoms, consis-tently and properly used, are able to reduce the transmis-sion of STDs spread by mucosal fluid (e.g., gonorrhea, chlamydia, and HIV). However, condoms do not cover all surfaces and only protect the skin they cover, and are,

therefore, less likely to protect against diseases acquired from skin-to-skin contact, such as syphilis, HPV, and HSV. Genital warts caused by HPV are contagious; avoid touch-ing them. Spermicides with nonoxynol-9 may not be effective against gonorrhea, chlamydia, or HIV infection; the CDC does not recommend the use of nonoxynol-9 with or without condoms for STD or HIV protection.[226]

To prevent transmission of STDs to newborns, preg-nant women should have blood tests for syphilis, HBV, and HIV. Early syphilis, if untreated in pregnant women, can cause fetal death, particularly seen after 20 weeks. Even if syphilis is acquired up to 4 years before pregnancy, infection of the fetus can occur in 50% of cases. All preg-nant women should be routinely tested for hepatitis B surface antigen during the first trimester, even if they have been previously vaccinated or tested.[213]

A vaccine is available to protect anyone, especially women of childbearing age, against HBV (see Table 8-4). Pregnant women should also be routinely tested for chlamydia and those at high risk should be tested for

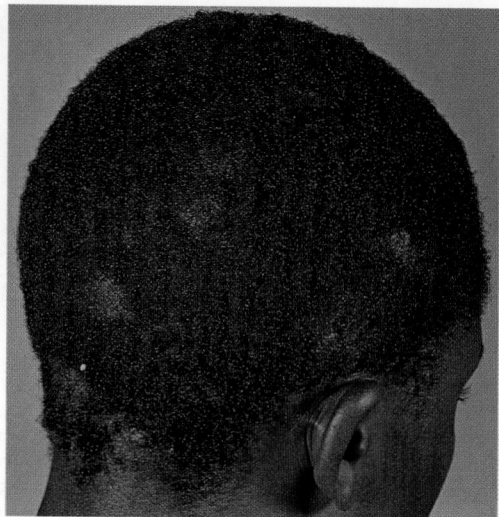

Figure 8-12

Alopecia of the scalp (balding) associated with secondary syphilis. This is a temporary, irregular presentation of alopecia sometimes referred to as "moth-eaten" alopecia. (Reprinted from Habif TP: *Clinical dermatology,* ed 4, St Louis, Mosby, courtesy Subhash K. Hira.)

gonorrhea and hepatitis C.[226] Those with recurrent genital herpes and open sores benefit from cesarean section delivery to protect the child.

Drug users, especially injection-drug users, can prevent transmission of disease best by discontinuance of drugs. However, in most cases this is not immediately realistic. Programs have been set up to help reduce needle sharing by providing needle exchange centers and street education programs aimed at teaching more sterile practices.

Preexposure vaccination is one of the most effective methods for preventing transmission of some STDs. Two HPV vaccines are available for females age 9 to 26 years to prevent cervical precancer and cancer: the quadrivalent HPV vaccine (Gardasil) and the bivalent HPV vaccine (Cervarix). Gardasil also prevents genital warts. Routine vaccination of females age 11 or 12 years is recommended with either vaccine, as is catch-up vaccination for females age 13 to 26 years. Gardasil can be administered to males age 9 to 26 years to prevent genital warts. Details regarding HPV vaccination are available at http://www.cdc.gov/hpv.

SCREENING, DIAGNOSIS, TREATMENT, AND PROGNOSIS. STDs can often be identified by the clinical manifestations, but many remain asymptomatic. Various tests are available to aid in diagnosis. The U.S. Preventive Services Task Force recommends annual screening for chlamydia of all sexually active adolescents and women younger than 25 years of age and older women with risk factors (new sex partner or multiple sex partners),[129] as well as pregnant women. With the advent of urine-based testing, more frequent screening has been accomplished, which may partly account for such high prevalence rates.

Treatment includes antibiotics and referral of all sexual contacts for testing and treatment from at least 60 days prior to symptoms or date of diagnosis. Follow-up testing is not recommended except in pregnant women.[226]

Certain HPV serotypes have been found to cause cervical cancer in women. Because there is currently no cure for the virus itself, prevention with immunizations and testing for precancerous and cervical cancer are the most appropriate management strategies. Recommendations for screening for cervical cancer have been published (see Table 20-2). Symptoms, such as genital warts, are treated with topically applied chemicals, cryotherapy, or surgical removal.

Although HPV is most often acquired in younger clients, older women continue to be at risk, so testing should take into consideration risk factors. Various immunoassays, serologic techniques, and culture methods are used to diagnose HIV, syphilis, gonorrhea, herpes, and other STDs.

HSV is a lifelong disease and only symptoms are managed. Antibiotics can cure some STDs (see Table 8-7), although some may be drug resistant. Currently, there is concern that gonorrhea, known to be resistant to fluoroquinolones, may become resistant to the only effective antibiotics, third-generation cephalosporins.[15] Limiting the number of sexual partners, practicing abstinence, and safe sex (proper use of condoms) are recommended to prevent the transmission of disease. Intercourse during an active infection dramatically increases the risk of transmitting STDs and sexually transmitted infections.

When working with clients with active disease, following contact precautions, frequent hand hygiene, and avoiding touching the affected areas are essential practices. A vaccine is now available for HBV, and HPV (HPV-2 or HPV-4 for women ages 19 through 26 years and HPV-4 for men ages 9 to 26); vaccines against HIV and herpes are under investigation.

The prognosis varies with each STD, but with treatment symptoms can be minimized and complications prevented. Without treatment, serious complications can occur such as infertility, chronic pelvic pain, ectopic pregnancy and miscarriage, cardiovascular disease, CNS impairment, blindness, cervical cancer, and even death.

SPECIAL IMPLICATIONS FOR THE THERAPIST | 8-14

Sexually Transmitted Diseases and Infections

Any therapist treating men or women with clinical presentation of pelvic, buttock, hip, or groin pain of apparent unknown cause must be prepared to ask the client about past history of STDs and sexually transmitted infections, sexual activity, changes in sexual function, and presence of urogenital signs or symptoms (e.g., discharge from penis or vagina, painful urination, difficulty initiating or continuing a stream of urine). Any suspicion that the clinical manifestations may be correlated to an STD must be further evaluated by a physician. A 2010 document from the CDC[226] provides treatment guidelines for STDs along with guidelines for gathering information for client education regarding prevention and protection that may be of interest to the therapist. See Evolve Box 8-1, "The Five Ps: Partners, Prevention of Pregnancy, Protection from STDs, Practices, and Past History of STDs," on the Evolve website for more information on this topic.

Infections in Drug Users

Drug use in the United States continues to be a significant health problem, with 9.2% of people older than the age of 12 years using illicit drugs each month.[29] Serious illnesses, such as HIV and hepatitis, are transmitted with injection-drug use.

Drug users as a whole also have a higher incidence of bacterial infections because of the various drugs used, the route and sites of administration, and preparation of the drug. Each of these factors determines risk for infection and the likelihood of specific bacterial infections.

IV use of black-tar heroin causes sclerosis of the veins and leads to "skin popping," or injecting the drug subcutaneously. Continued injection into the same site creates a necrotic environment suitable for clostridial germination and toxin production.[51] Necrotizing fasciitis with toxic shock syndrome can result from the spread of a clostridial infection.[2]

Drug users, particularly IV drug users, vary the site of administration. Local abscess formation or infections from hematogenous seeding are seen in unusual places because of the site of injection (the femoral vein, or "groin hit," and the neck, or "pocket shot"). Osteomyelitis may develop in the sternoclavicular, sacroiliac, or vertebral spine. Septic arthritis is often seen in the knees.

Environmental factors frequently contribute to infections. Some users may lick the skin or needle prior to injecting, leading to polymicrobial infections. Others crush tablets between their teeth or blow clots out of needles before reusing. Sharing of needles and paraphernalia is also common. Because of these habits, drug users are more likely to develop certain types of bacterial infections with specific organisms.

The four types of infections most often seen are of the skin or soft tissue, endovascular infections, respiratory infections, and musculoskeletal infections.[106] *S. aureus* and streptococcal species (flora from the user's skin) are the most common pathogens in drug-related infections. Drug users are more likely to be colonized with MRSA in the nares and skin than non–drug users; this most likely occurs because of tissue damage from inhaling or injecting drugs.[10]

Abscess formation is common. More serious infections such as endocarditis, septic thrombophlebitis, mycotic aneurysms, and sepsis occur from hematogenous spread of organisms. In injection-drug users, *S. aureus* is the most common organism causing endocarditis. Although polymicrobial endocarditis is rare, it is most often seen in injection drug users. Complications of endocarditis include brain, lung, and splenic abscesses.

Drug users are more likely to develop a respiratory tract infection compared with nonusers, and respiratory infections, particularly pneumonia, are the most common infection in drug users. Smoking cocaine also leads to direct damage of the lung, causing disease such as interstitial fibrosis, pulmonary hypertension, and alveolar hemorrhage.[170] Damage to cells from inhaling drugs and chronic cigarette use (many drug users also smoke) may lead to inability to clear secretions. Aspiration may occur because of decreased mental alertness. Sharing of paraphernalia also increases the risk for infectious diseases.[121]

Clients with HIV may present with atypical features and radiographs, so a good history and physical examination are important. Pulmonary tuberculosis (and drug-resistant tuberculosis) is encountered more frequently in drug users who practice "shotgunning" (inhaling cocaine and blowing smoke into the mouth of another person),[156] live in crowded spaces, delay diagnosis, or have HIV.

Musculoskeletal infections may occur in unusual places, as discussed above. Flora from the skin is the most common pathogen, although polymicrobial infections are seen, especially if saliva contaminates the skin, drugs, or needles. The infection may be subtle, with mild fever and pain.

SPECIAL IMPLICATIONS FOR THE THERAPIST 8-15

Infections in Drug Addicts

See "Special Implications for the Therapist 3-12: Substance Use and Addictive Disorders" in Chapter 3.

Being aware of the signs of substance abuse or drug addiction and the patterns of infection associated with drug addiction may assist the therapist in recognizing early signs of infection requiring medical evaluation and treatment.

Any therapist involved in wound care management, needle electromyography, or other high-risk practice techniques who has not already been immunized against HBV should be vaccinated. Because of the high risk of infection with CA-MRSA with open wounds in these individuals, environmental surfaces in the area of treatment need to be cleaned by U.S. Environmental Protection Agency–approved products.

REFERENCES

To enhance this text and add value for the reader, all references are included on the companion Evolve site that accompanies this textbook. The reader can view the reference source and access it online whenever possible.

CHAPTER 9

Oncology

CHARLES L. MCGARVEY • LISA VANHOOSE • MARY CALYS •
JOSEPH A. FRAIETTA

Cancer is a term that refers to a large group of diseases characterized by uncontrolled cell proliferation and spread of abnormal cells.[248] Other terms used interchangeably for cancer are *malignant neoplasm, tumor, malignancy,* and *carcinoma.* According to the American Cancer Society (ACS), about 5% of cancer is genetic, whereas 95% is related to other (often modifiable) factors. Only oncologic concepts are presented in this chapter; individual cancers are discussed in the chapters devoted to the affected system. Because cancer and cancer treatment can affect multiple systems, the reader is encouraged to read this chapter along with Chapter 5 for a more complete understanding of its potentially wide-ranging systemic effects.

Two case studies about cancer patients are provided in Evolve Box 9-1 on the Evolve site that accompanies this textbook. Each one includes patient data and questions to answer.

DEFINITIONS

Differentiation

Normal tissue contains cells of uniform size, shape, maturity, and nuclear structure. Differentiation is the process by which normal cells undergo physical and structural changes as they develop to form different tissues of the body. Differentiated cells specialize in different physiologic functions.

In malignant cells, differentiation is altered and may be lost completely so that the malignant cell may not be recognizable in relationship to its parent cell. When a tumor has completely lost identity with the parent tissue, it is considered to be undifferentiated (anaplastic). In this case, it may become difficult or impossible to identify the malignant cell's tissue of origin. In general, the less differentiated a tumor becomes, the faster the metastasis (spread) and the worse the prognosis.

Dysplasia

A variety of other tissue changes can occur in the body. Some of these changes are benign, whereas others denote a malignant or premalignant state. *Dysplasia* is a general term that indicates a disorganization of cells in which an adult cell varies from its normal size, shape, or organization. This is often caused by chronic irritation such as is seen with changes in cervical (uterine) epithelium as a result of long-standing irritation of the cervix. Dysplasia may reverse itself or may progress to cancer.

Metaplasia

Metaplasia is the first level of dysplasia (early dysplasia). It is a reversible and benign but abnormal change in which one adult cell changes from one type to another. For example, the most common type of epithelial metaplasia is the change of columnar epithelium of the respiratory tract to squamous epithelium.

Another example of metaplasia is Barrett esophagus (also called Barrett syndrome), in which the squamous epithelium of the esophagus is replaced by the glandular epithelium of the stomach. Although metaplasia usually gives rise to an orderly arrangement of cells, it may sometimes produce disorderly cellular patterns (i.e., cells varying in size, shape, and orientation to one another). Anaplasia (loss of cellular differentiation) is the most advanced form of metaplasia and is considered the hallmark feature of malignant disease.

Hyperplasia

Hyperplasia refers to increased number of cells in tissue, resulting in increased tissue mass. This type of change can be a normal consequence of physiologic alterations (physiologic hyperplasia) such as increased breast mass during pregnancy, wound healing, or bone callus formation. Neoplastic hyperplasia, however, is the increase in cell mass because of tumor formation and is an abnormal process. Presence of hyperplastic tissue increases the risk of later development of breast cancer, as well as other solid tumor cancers.[268]

Tumors

Tumors, or neoplasms, are defined as abnormal new growth of tissue that serve no useful purpose and may harm the host organism by competing for vital blood supply and nutrients. These new growths may be benign or malignant (see following discussion of classification) and primary or secondary.

A primary tumor arises from cells that are normally local to the given structure, whereas a secondary tumor arises from cells that have metastasized from another part of the body. For example, a primary neoplasm of bone arises from within the bone structure itself, whereas a secondary neoplasm occurs in bone as a result of metastasized cancer cells from another (primary) site.

Carcinoma in situ refers to a localized, preinvasive, and possibly premalignant tumor of epithelial tissue. At this stage of dysplasia, these tumors are contained within the host organ and have not broken through basement membrane. In situ tumors commonly occur in the cervix, bladder, skin, oral cavity, esophagus, bronchus, and breast. Carcinoma in situ that affects glandular epithelium occurs most commonly in the cervix, breast, stomach, endometrium, large bowel, and prostate gland (prostate intraepithelial neoplasia). The time period between advent of cell dysplasia and invasion beyond local tissue is variable for different cancers.

CLASSIFICATIONS OF NEOPLASM

A neoplasm (new growth) can be classified on the basis of cell type, tissue of origin, degree of differentiation, anatomic site, or whether it is benign or malignant.

A benign growth is usually considered harmless and does not spread to or invade other tissue. Certain benign growths, recognized clinically as tumors, are not truly neoplastic but rather represent overgrowth of normal tissue elements (e.g., vocal cord polyps, skin tags, hyperplastic polyps of the colon). However, benign growths can become large enough to distend, compress, or obstruct normal tissues and impair normal body functions, as in the case of benign central nervous system (CNS) tumors. These tumors can cause disability and even death.

Tumors (benign or malignant) are classified by cell type, and are named according to the tissue from which they arise (Table 9-1). The five major classifications of normal body tissue are epithelial, connective and muscle, nerve, lymphoid, and hematopoietic tissue. Not all tissue types fit into one of these five categories, thus requiring a miscellaneous category for other tissues (not included in Table 9-1), such as the tissues of the reproductive glands, placenta, and thymus.

Epithelium covers all external body surfaces and lines all internal spaces, organs, and cavities. The skin, mucous membranes, gastrointestinal tract, and lining of the bladder are examples of epithelial tissue. The functions of epithelial tissues are to protect, excrete, and absorb. Cancers originating in epithelial tissue (endodermal origin) are called carcinomas. A common example of a tumor derived from glandular tissues is called an *adenocarcinoma*. Carcinomas represent the most common solid tumors prevalent in adults.

Connective tissue consists of elastic, fibrous, and collagenous tissues such as bone, cartilage, and fat. Cancers originating in connective tissue and muscle (mesenchymal origin) are called *sarcomas*. Sarcoma are relatively rare tumors and are generally classified as either soft tissue (e.g., rhabdomyosarcoma: striated muscle) or osteo (Ewing bone) sarcomas. Further, osteosarcoma is generally diagnosed in children or adolescents while soft

Table 9-1	Classification of Neoplasms by Cell Type of Origin	
Tissue of Origin	**Benign**	**Malignant**
Epithelial Tissue		
Surface epithelium (skin) and mucous membrane	Papilloma	Squamous cell, basal cell, and transitional cell carcinoma
Epithelial lining of glands or ducts	Adenoma	Adenocarcinoma
Pigmented cells (melanocytes of basal layer)	Nevus (mole)	Malignant melanoma
Connective Tissue and Muscle		
Fibrous tissue	Fibroma	Fibrosarcoma
Adipose	Lipoma	Liposarcoma
Cartilage	Chondroma	Chondrosarcoma
Bone	Osteoma	Osteosarcoma
Blood vessels	Hemangioma	Hemangiosarcoma
Smooth muscle	Leiomyoma	Leiomyosarcoma
Striated muscle	Rhabdomyoma	Rhabdomyosarcoma
Nerve Tissue		
Nerve cells	Neuroma	
Glia		Glioma or neuroglioma
Ganglion cells	Ganglioneuroma	Neuroblastoma
Nerve sheaths	Neurilemoma	Neurilemic sarcoma
Meninges	Meningioma	Meningeal sarcoma
Retina		Retinoblastoma
Lymphoid Tissue		
Lymph nodes Spleen Intestinal lining		Lymphoma
Hematopoietic Tissue		
Bone marrow		Leukemias, myelodysplasia, and myeloproliferative syndromes
Plasma cells		Multiple myeloma

tissue sarcomas are predominantly identified in the adult population.

Nerve tissue includes the brain, spinal cord, and nerves and consists of neurons, nerve fibers, dendrites, and a supporting tissue composed of glial cells. Tumors arising in *nerve tissue* are named for the type of cell involved. For example, tumors arising from astrocytes, a type of glial cell thought to form the blood-brain barrier, are called *astrocytomas*. Tumors arising in nerve tissue are often benign, but because of their critical location they are more likely to be harmful than benign tumors in other sites.

Malignancies originating in *lymphoid tissues* are called *lymphomas*. Lymphomas can arise in many parts of the body, wherever lymphoid tissue is present. The most common sites to find lymphoid malignancies are the lymph nodes and spleen. However, lymphomas can appear in other parts of the body such as the skin, CNS, stomach, small bowel, bone, and tonsils.[72]

Hematopoietic malignancies include leukemias, multiple myeloma, myelodysplasia, and the myeloproliferative syndromes.

Eponyms are used to describe the tumors as either benign or malignant depending on the cell of origin. For example, a neoplastic lesion of adipose tissue (fat) if benign would be described as a lipoma, and a malignant lesion would be identified as a liposarcoma (see Table 9-1).

Staging and Grading

Staging is the process of describing the extent of disease at the time of diagnosis to aid treatment planning, predict clinical outcome (prognosis), and compare the results of different treatment approaches. The stage of disease at the time of diagnosis reflects the rate of growth, the extent of the neoplasm, and the prognosis. A simplified way to stage cancer is as follows:

- Stage 0: Carcinoma in situ (premalignant, preinvasive)
- Stage I: Early stage, cancer is usually localized to primary organ.
- Stage II: Increased risk of regional spread because of tumor size or grade.
- Stage III: Local cancer has spread regionally but may not be disseminated to distant regions.
- Stage IV: Cancer has spread and disseminated to distant sites.

In some cases, cancer may be staged as II or III depending on the spread of the specific type of cancer. For example, in Hodgkin disease, stage II indicates lymph nodes are affected on one side of the diaphragm. Stage III indicates affected lymph nodes above and below the diaphragm.[177,330]

Systems of Staging

Staging systems are specific for each type of cancer. The TNM (tumor, node, metastases) system is used most often for solid tumors and has been adapted for other types of tumor. In the TNM classification scheme, tumors are staged according to the following basic components (Box 9-1):

- Tumor (T) refers to the size of primary tumor and carries a number from 0 to 4.
- Regional lymph nodes (N) represents regional lymph node involvement; also ranked from 0 to 4.
- Metastasis (M) is zero (0) if no metastasis has occurred or 1 if metastases are present.

Numbers are used with each component to denote extent of involvement; for example, T0 indicates undetectable and T1, T2, T3, and T4 indicate a progressive increase in size or involvement.

Some cancers do not have a staging system (e.g., brain cancer) and some can be staged using more than one system. The International Union Against Cancer (UICC) is the universally accepted staging system, which incorporates the TNM classification of malignant tumors; the American Joint Committee on Cancer (AJCC) 7th edition released in 2010 is the current reference used by most institutions.[111] The National Cancer Institute provides more detailed information about staging.[247]

Box 9-1

TNM STAGING SYSTEM

T: Primary Tumor

T_X	Primary tumor cannot be assessed
T_0	No evidence of primary tumor
T_{IS}	Carcinoma in situ (confined to site of origin)
T_1, T_2, T_3, T_4	Progressive increase in tumor size and involvement locally

N: Regional Lymph Nodes

N_X	Nodes cannot be assessed
N_0	No metastasis to regional lymph nodes
N_1, N_2, N_3	Increasing degrees of involvement of regional lymph nodes

M: Distant Metastasis

M_X	Presence of distant metastasis cannot be assessed
M_0	No distant metastasis
M_1	Distant metastasis

Note: Extension of primary tumor directly into lymph nodes is considered metastasis to lymph nodes. Metastasis to a lymph node beyond the regional ones is considered distant metastasis.

From Abeloff MD: *Abeloff's clinical oncology*, ed 4, Philadelphia, 2008, Churchill Livingstone.

It is important to realize the TNM staging system is an anatomic staging system that describes the anatomic extent of the primary tumor, as well as the involvement of regional lymph nodes and distant metastases. In the TNM system, clinical stage is denoted by a small "c" before the stage (e.g., cT2N1M0) or by a small "p" to indicate the pathologic stage (e.g., pT2N0). Clinical staging is based on clinical examination and testing of the individual prior to definitive treatment and is the stage of disease generally presented at tumor boards. The pathologic stage is determined by direct examination of the tumor by the pathologist once it has been removed and is considered a more accurate reflection of the tumor and its spread. Not all tumors are resected or excised so pathologic staging is not always available.

Pathologic staging presented during tumor boards after resection of the tumor, may alter the original clinical stage of the disease allowing for a more accurate assessment of extent or degree of malignancy. Such information is critical to the oncologist in the determination of the best treatment intervention based on clinical practice guidelines.

Conversely, pathologic staging may underestimate the true stage for individuals who received adjuvant treatment (radiation or chemotherapy) before surgery. Errors in the preparation or examination of tissue examined may result in false positive or false negative findings resulting in mis-staging and possibly altering diagnosis and treatment.

Staging, as a process, continues to evolve with new, more precise levels of screening sensitivity and specificity. Molecular screening for the presence of markers characteristic of some diseases will enable more accurate staging, treatment planning, and the ability to monitor the effectiveness of targeted therapies.[177,330]

ANN ARBOR STAGING

Ann Arbor Staging is used for lymphomas (Hodgkin disease and non-Hodgkin lymphoma).

Stage I: Local cancer in one area such as one lymph node and the local surrounding area; usually here are no other systemic or clinical symptoms

Stage II: Cancer is located in two separate regions on one side of the diaphragm (above or below the diaphragm); two separate regions refers to an affected lymph node or organ within the lymphatic system and a second affected area

Stage III: Cancer has spread to both sides of the diaphragm (above and below); includes one organ or area near the lymph nodes or the spleen

Stage IV: Diffuse or disseminated spread to one or more extralymphatic organ or area near the lymph nodes or the spleen; liver, bone marrow, or nodular involvement of the lungs is possible

Letters such as *A*, *B*, *E*, and *X* may be used to modify or append the stage:

A = absence of constitutional symptoms.

B = presence of constitutional symptoms.

E = extranodal (not in the lymph nodes or has spread from the lymph nodes to adjacent tissue).

X = used to describe mass larger than 10 cm or mediastinum wider than one-third of the chest on a chest x-ray.

From Abeloff MD: *Abeloff's clinical oncology*, ed 4, Philadelphia, 2008, Churchill Livingstone.

Revisions to the TNM staging system are made as the understanding of the natural history of tumors at various sites improves with advancing technology. Beyond the TNM UICC systems, other staging systems are used in certain cases. For example, cervical cancer is staged using the International Federation of Gynecology and Obstetrics (FIGO) System of Staging, which is based on clinical examination, rather than surgical findings (see Box 20-3). Lymphomas are staged using the Ann Arbor staging (Box 9-2).

Immune Classification. As mentioned above, tumor staging (the AJCC/UICC-TNM classification) summarizes data on tumor burden (T), presence of cancer cells in draining and regional lymph nodes (N), and evidence for metastases (M). However, this classification provides limited prognostic information in estimating the outcome in cancer and does not predict response to therapy.

It is recognized that cancer outcomes can vary significantly among individuals within the same stage. Cancer development may be controlled by the host's immune system, which points to the importance of including immunologic biomarkers for the prediction of prognosis and response to therapy. Data collected from large cohorts of human cancers has shown that the immune-classification has a prognostic value that may be superior to the AJCC/UICC TNM-classification. Efforts are under way to begin incorporating immune scoring as a prognostic factor and to introduce this parameter as a marker to classify cancers, as part of the routine diagnostic and prognostic assessment of tumors.[127,128]

Grading

Grading of tumor tissue is done by the pathologist using different grading for different types of tumors. For example, the Bloom-Richardson (or Nottingham) scale is used in breast cancer, the Gleason score in prostate cancer, and the Fuhrman scale in grading cancers of the kidney. Each grading method may use a different numerical score or scale but generally the lower the value, the lower the grade tumor and the better differentiation of tissue within the tumor. A highly scored/scaled tumor is considered a high-grade tumor with poor cellular differentiation and a tendency to metastasize early.

Grading provides a measure of the anaplasia or differentiation of the tissue of the tumor. Additional important information is the size, shape, and rate of nuclear (mitotic division) within the specimen; these factors further define the aggressiveness of the tumor.

In general, grading is classified in three categories: low, intermediate, and high. Low-grade tumors have better predictive and prognostic clinical outcomes versus those identified as high grade. Grading of the tumor specimen when considered with anatomic staging (local, regional, and distant involvement) is critical in effective treatment planning, surveillance, and prognosis.

INCIDENCE

Estimates of worldwide incidence, mortality, and prevalence of 26 cancers are available from the International Agency for Research on Cancer (IARC). Geographic variations between 20 large areas (182 countries) of the world are studied. The most recent report published in 2011 identified a 12.7 million incidence of new cases and 7.6 million deaths. Rate of survivorship in developing countries is less than one-half of those of developed countries because of late diagnosis and lack of availability of care. Additional international variation is due to exposure to known or suspected risk factors related to lifestyle or environment. The IARC has been researching and providing a database of global cancer estimates (GLOBOCAN) for the last 30 years.[113,114,179]

The most commonly diagnosed cancers are lung, prostate, breast, and colorectal; the most prevalent cancer in the world is lung cancer and accounts for the most number of cancer deaths worldwide.[174] In the United States, the ACS publishes annual cancer statistics and estimates cancer trends (Fig. 9-1). Each year the ACS calculates estimates of the number of new cancer cases and expected cancer deaths in the United States and compiles the most recent data on cancer incidence, mortality, and survival.[10,337]

Based on statistical estimates, in the year 2014, the ACS predicts about 1.6 million new cases of invasive cancer in the United States and approximately 585,720 cancer-related deaths. This figure does not include most skin cancers, which are expected to affect 1 million people per year.[10,337]

It is estimated that at least one in three people will be diagnosed with some form of invasive cancer in their lifetime and 3 of 5 people will be cured and/or survive 5 years after cancer treatment. However, cancer is still the second

Estimated New Cases*

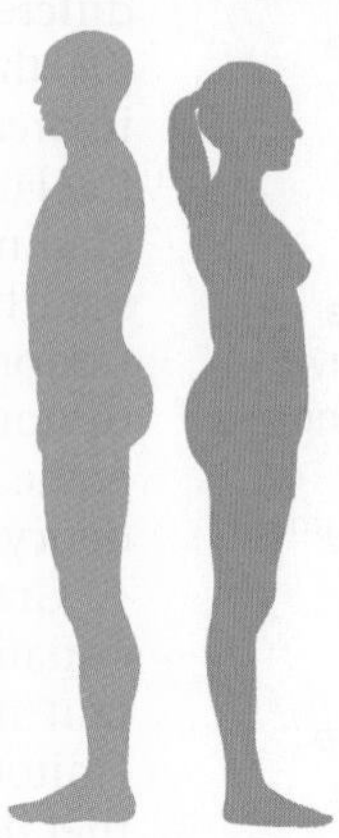

Males   Females

Prostate	233,000	27%		Breast	232,670	29%
Lung and bronchus	116,000	14%		Lung and bronchus	108,210	13%
Colon and rectum	71,830	8%		Colon and rectum	65,000	8%
Urinary bladder	56,390	7%		Uterine corpus	52,630	7%
Melanoma of the skin	43,890	5%		Thyroid	47,790	6%
Kidney and renal pelvis	39,140	5%		Non-Hodgkin lymphoma	32,530	4%
Non-Hodgkin lymphoma	38,270	4%		Melanoma of the skin	32,210	4%
Oral cavity and pharynx	30,220	4%		Kidney and renal pelvis	24,750	3%
Leukemia	30,100	4%		Leukemia	22,280	3%
Pancreas	23,530	3%		Ovary	21,980	3%
All sites	**855,220**	**100%**		**All sites**	**810,320**	**100%**

Estimated Deaths

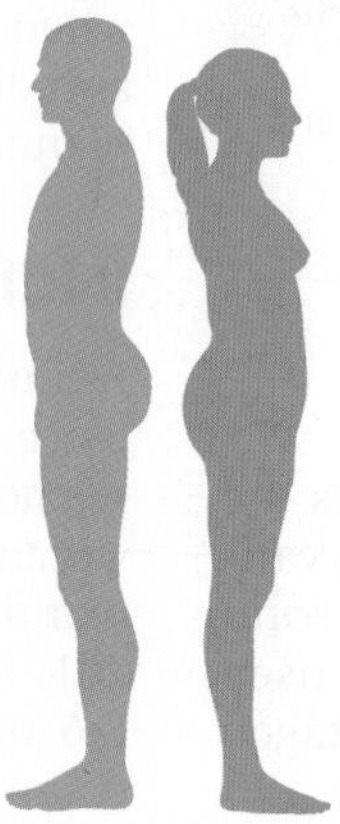

Males   Females

Lung and bronchus	86,930	28%		Lung and bronchus	72,330	26%
Prostate	29,480	10%		Breast	40,000	15%
Colon and rectum	26,270	8%		Colon and rectum	24,040	9%
Pancreas	20,170	7%		Pancreas	19,420	7%
Liver and intrahepatic bile duct	15,870	5%		Ovary	14,270	5%
Leukemia	14,040	5%		Leukemia	10,050	4%
Esophagus	12,450	4%		Uterine corpus	8,590	3%
Urinary bladder	11,170	4%		Non-Hodgkin lymphoma	8,520	3%
Non-Hodgkin lymphoma	10,470	3%		Liver and intrahepatic bile duct	7,130	3%
Kidney and renal pelvis	8,900	3%		Brain and other nervous system	6,230	2%
All sites	**310,010**	**100%**		**All sites**	**275,710**	**100%**

Figure 9-1

Estimated new cancer cases *(top)* **and cancer deaths** *(bottom)*, **2014, in the United States (percent distribution of sites by gender).** (From Siegel R, Naishadham F and Jemal A: Cancer Statistics 2014. *CA: A Cancer Journal for Clinicians* (62) (1) Jan/Feb 2014 10-29. http://www.ca-journal.org/.)

leading cause of death in the United States, exceeded only by heart disease. Poor health and nutrition habits, continued smoking, ozone destruction, and a long-term lack of exercise among many people continue to be discussed as contributors to the overall rise of this disease.[196]

The National Cancer Institute established the Surveillance, Epidemiology, and End Results (SEER) program in 1973 as a way to report population-based data of site-specific incidences and outcomes of cancer. Estimates of new cancer cases are based on data collected and analyzed from 20 population based registry sites. These sites serve as a representative sample of the general and minority-based population. The estimation of new cancer cases occurring annually is estimated using complex statistical measures.[69,402] Age-adjusted mortality rates are more accurate and are based on certificates of death as recorded by individual states. These statistics are reported on an annual basis through the National Vital Statistics Reporting Unit of the National Center for Health Statistics, part of the Centers for Disease Control and Prevention (CDC).[231]

Additional information related to the incidence of cancer of the American population is easily retrieved through the following website: http://seer.cancer.gov/faststats.

Trends in Cancer Incidence and Survival

Incidence

Overall incidence of cancer peaked in 1990 and has declined in the last decade by an average of 1.1% annually, with a 1.4% decline in cancer death rates. In 2003 and 2004, the rate doubled to 2% per year, largely attributed to smoking cessation among men, which peaked in the mid-1960s. The latest drop in cancer deaths occurred across all four major cancer types (lung, colon and rectal, prostate, and breast; lung cancer deaths in women stayed relatively constant).

Targeted cancer therapies (i.e., drugs that seek out and selectively destroy cancer cells, leaving most normal cells unharmed) promise to reduce adverse events and improve these statistics in the coming years.[330] Cancer prevention strategies (e.g., smoking cessation, regular physical activity, and maintaining a healthy weight) may reduce the incidence of cancer occurrence and recurrence.[19,35,158]

Survivorship

At the same time, survival rates for cancer are on the rise, increasing from 50% to 64% over the last 30 years. A cancer survivor has been defined by the ACS as *any person who has been diagnosed with cancer, from the time of diagnosis through the balance of life*,[335] with three distinct phases associated with cancer survival: (1) the time from diagnosis through the end of initial treatment, (2) the transition from treatment to extended survival, and (3) long-term survival.[240]

The ACS reports that there are nearly 13.7 million Americans with a history of cancer alive as of January 1, 2012.[335] Further, it is estimated that the number of survivors will climb to 18 million by 2022. Most common male cancer survivors are prostate (43%), colorectal (9%), and melanoma. For females, the most common survivors are those diagnosed with breast (41%), uterine (8%), and colorectal (8%).[12]

Currently, more focus and attention are being given to survivors and their unique needs. The Institute of Medicine (IOM) defines the essential needs of cancer survivorship care as[160]:

* Prevention and detection of new cancers and recurrent cancer
* Surveillance for cancer spread, recurrence, or second cancers
* Intervention for consequences of cancer and its treatment
* Coordination between specialists and primary care providers to ensure that all of the survivor's health needs are met

Consequences of cancer and especially cancer treatment are wide ranging but often include medical problems such as lymphedema and sexual dysfunction; symptoms, including pain and fatigue; psychological distress experienced by both cancer survivors and their caregivers; and concerns related to employment and insurance. Coordination of care for survivors should include health promotion, immunizations, screening for both cancer and noncancerous conditions, and the care of concurrent conditions).[160]

The American Cancer Society publishes an annual document dedicated to cancer survivorship titled *Cancer Treatment and Survivorship: Facts and Figures*.[12] This document provides survivorship statistics, descriptions of common adverse effects of treatment and issues related to quality of life, long-term and late effects, risk of recurrence, and healthy behaviors. This document, based on SEER statistics, provides the basis and rationale for the importance of rehabilitation in the continuum of care and medical management of survivors of cancer.

Gender-Based Incidence

Among men, the most common cancers are predicted to be cancers of the prostate, lung and bronchus, and colon/rectum. Among women, the three most commonly diagnosed cancers are expected to be cancers of the breast, lung and bronchus, and colon/rectum.

The largest decreases in deaths occurred among men (especially among black men), who bear the heaviest overall cancer burden and colorectal cancer in particular. Officials have attributed the steady downward trends to improved vigilance among Americans, who are benefiting from early screening and advances in treatment, as well as smoking less, improving their diets, and exercising more.

For the period 2004–2008, overall cancer incidence declined 0.6% per year in men and was stable in women. In the same period, death rates decreased 1.8% in men and 1.6% in women.[337] Breast cancer alone accounted for approximately 235,030 new cancer cases in women in 2014 compared with 178,400 in 2007.[337] The decline in rates of breast cancer deaths has been attributed in part to increased mammography but also to more aggressive therapy; overall decline in deaths among women may also be the result of the recent falloff in hormone replacement therapy.

Likewise, improved screening, detection, and treatment of prostate cancer have resulted in a decline in the death rate associated with this type of cancer. About a dozen cancers continue to rise in incidence or mortality, including melanoma, non-Hodgkin lymphoma, thyroid, esophageal cancer, breast (increased incidence but decreased mortality), and female lung cancer.

ETIOLOGY

The cause of cancer varies, and causative agents are generally subdivided into two categories: those of endogenous (genetic) origin and those of exogenous (environmental or external) origin. It is likely that most cancers develop as a result of multiple environmental, viral, and genetic factors working together to disrupt the immune system along with failure of an aging immune system to recognize and scavenge cells that have become less differentiated.

Certain cancers show a familial pattern, giving people a hereditary predisposition to cancer. The most common cancers showing a familial pattern include prostate, breast, ovarian, and colon cancers. One of the potential objectives of The Human Genome Project completed in 2003 was to begin investigating and cataloguing genes that might be associated with various cancers. Such information would assist in identifying high-risk individuals for screening and early detection. Examples of such genetic testing include *BRCA1* and *BRCA2* for breast cancer. These genes belong to a family of cancer suppressor genes for which mutation (if inherited), significantly increases the lifetime risk of breast and/or ovarian cancer.

The ACS estimates that 50% of all cancers are caused by one or more of nearly 500 different cancer-causing agents (e.g., tobacco use, viruses, chemical agents, physical agents, drugs, alcohol, hormones).[196] Etiologic agents capable of initiating the malignant transformation of a cell (i.e., carcinogenesis) are called *carcinogens*. The study of *viruses* as carcinogens is one of the most rapidly advancing areas in cancer research today.

Researchers now have evidence that viruses play a role in the pathogenesis of cervical carcinomas, some hepatomas, Burkitt lymphomas, nasopharyngeal carcinomas, adult T-cell leukemias, and indirectly, many Kaposi sarcomas. Viruses, such as the human immunodeficiency virus

(HIV), the causative agent of acquired immunodeficiency syndrome (AIDS), weaken cell-mediated immunity, resulting in malignancies.

Chemical agents (e.g., tar, soot, asphalt, dyes, hydrocarbons, oils, nickel, or arsenics) and *physical agents* (e.g., radiation or asbestos) may cause cancer after close and prolonged contact with these agents. Most people affected by chemical agents are industrial workers. Radiation exposure is usually from natural sources, especially ultraviolet radiation from the sun, which can cause changes in deoxyribonucleic acid (DNA) structure that lead to malignant transformation. Notable exceptions include history of radiation treatment for acne, thymus, or thyroid conditions. Basal and squamous cell carcinomas and malignant melanoma are all linked to ultraviolet exposure. See "Chemical and Physical Agents" in Chapter 4.

Some *drugs*, such as cancer chemotherapeutic agents, are in themselves carcinogenic. Cytotoxic drugs, including steroids, decrease antibody production and destroy circulating lymphocytes. Cancer clients treated with chemotherapy are at risk for future development of leukemia and other cancers.

Hormones have been linked to tumor development and growth, such as estrogen stimulating the growth of the endometrial lining, which over time becomes anaplastic. Other types of cancer occurring in target or hormone-responsive tissues include ovary and prostate cancers.

Excessive *alcohol* consumption is associated with cancer of the mouth, pharynx, larynx, esophagus, breast, and pancreas. It can also indirectly contribute to liver cancer (i.e., alcohol causes liver cirrhosis, which is associated with cancer).

The reader is directed to the following website for additional information on causation and risk factors for the development of cancer: http://www.cancer.gov/cancer topics/causes.

RISK FACTORS

Advancing age is one of the most significant risk factors for cancer. In addition to age and the carcinogens described earlier in "Etiology," predisposing factors also influence the host's susceptibility to various etiologic agents (Box 9-3), which are discussed further in the next section below.

Nine modifiable risk factors are responsible for more than one-third of cancer deaths *worldwide* (tobacco, alcohol, obesity, inactivity, diet/nutrition, unsafe sex, urban air pollution, indoor smoke from household fuels, or contaminated injections in health care settings). Of these, smoking and alcohol consumption are the most damaging. This means that even without the potential benefits of early detection and treatment, at least one-third of cancer deaths are preventable.[86,361]

Experimental and epidemiologic evidence has established an association between at least eight viruses and various cancer sites. At least 10% of cancer worldwide is caused by viruses, tobacco, and diet. Some risk factors are interactive and become exponential rather than additive (e.g., alcohol and smoking for oral pharyngeal cancers).

There is no evidence to support popular theories that some people are more likely to develop cancer because

---

Box 9-3

CANCER RISK FACTORS

Advancing age	Exposure to hormones
Previous cancer	(e.g., estrogen, testosterone)
Lifestyle or personal	Geographic location and
behaviors	environmental variables
Tobacco use	(see Chapter 4)
Diet and nutrition	Previous cancer treatment
(high fat, low fiber)	(e.g., radiotherapy)
Obesity/type 2 diabetes	Gender
Alcohol use	Ethnicity
Sexual and reproductive	Socioeconomic status
behaviors	Occupation (see Chapter 4)
Physical inactivity	Heredity (family history of
Exposure to viruses	cancer)
Human papillomavirus	Presence of precancerous
(HPV)	lesions, polyps or other
Epstein-Barr virus (EBV)	Stress
Hepatitis B virus (HBV)	Inflammatory, bowel disease
Hepatitis C virus (HCV)	(IBD)
Helicobacter pylori	
Herpesvirus 8	

---

of specific personality traits such as anger, hostility, frustration, sexual repression, or conflicted parent–child relationship. Additionally, cancer survival is not predicted by personality type, including neuroticism, extroversion, or low self-esteem.[147,245]

Heredity

Cancer is a disease of genes, which are vulnerable to mutation, especially over the course of a long human life span. However, evidence shows that only a small proportion of cancers (5%-10%) linked to a single gene are inherited. It is abundantly clear that the incidence of all the common cancers in humans is determined by various controllable external factors making it, in large part, a preventable disease.[393]

Evidence showing that patterns of cancer are altered by environmental factors rather than being genetically determined come from studies describing changes in the rates of different cancers in genetically identical populations that migrate from their native countries to other countries. Changes in the rates of the most common cancers (e.g., stomach, colorectal, breast, prostate) are significant after only one or two generations.[393]

Aging

Age over 50 years (some experts say age over 40 years) is a significant risk factor for the development of cancer, but cancer is not an inevitable consequence of aging. The association of cancer and aging is becoming more common because of the aging of the general population. According to SEER report for the period 2002–2006, the median age for all races and gender at time of primary diagnosis is approximately 66 years. The median age is expected to increase over the next several decades.[166]

The risk of multiple diseases (comorbidity) also increases with age, creating limitations in the life expectancy of individual aging adults and enhancing the likelihood of treatment complications. Older people may be more susceptible to cancer simply because they have been exposed to carcinogens longer than younger people. The effects of age on immune function and host defense are being studied to determine what the association is between cancer and age (see "Aging and the Immune System" in Chapter 7).

Factors such as accumulated nonlethal damage to DNA by free radicals, increased proinflammatory factors, and age-associated declines in DNA repair are important.[166] Studies on mutations in cancer-causing structures, such as telomeres (a region of DNA at the end of chromosomes), DNA repair aberrations, and dysregulation of important hormonal and immune modulators, are all being reported as potential reasons for the increasing incidence of cancer in older adults.[34,331]

Clues about the life span of a cell and about aging in general are emerging from research on telomeres. In normal cells, the telomere shortens each time a cell divides. Telomeres provide chromosomal stability by protecting the ends from degradation and recombination. A minimal telomere length is needed to maintain tissue homeostasis.[243]

The cell dies when the telomere becomes so short that it can no longer divide. An important enzyme, telomerase, helps keep normally dividing cells healthy by rebuilding the telomeres. Telomerase normally shuts down when cells are mature, but in cancer, the enzyme enables cancer cells to grow with unlimited cell divisions. Telomerase is active in up to 85% of all human cancers.[60,61,273] See also "Cellular Aging" in Chapter 6. This understanding has led to discoveries regarding the life span of human cells, their relationship to aging, and the development of many illnesses associated with aging such as cancer. It has been reported that normal cells do not divide indefinitely during the life span of a human because of a phenomenon called the *Hayflick limit* and a stopping process or permanent growth arrest called *cellular senescence*.

The Hayflick limit was discovered by Leonard Hayflick in 1965.[151] Hayflick observed that cells dividing in cell culture divided about 50 times before dying. As cells approach this limit, they show more signs of old age. For most differentiated cells, the limit to the number of times a cell divides has been determined in all cell types. The human limit is around 52, but there is some variation from cell type to cell type and, more significantly, from organism type to organism type (e.g., mice and humans). This limit has been linked to the shortening of telomeres and is thought to be one of the causes of aging. Telomeres may act as cellular clocks that control aging. This is called the *telomere theory of aging*. If the shortening of telomeres can be slowed or prevented, life expectancy may be extended but perhaps at a higher risk of tumorigenesis.[159]

Many in vitro and in vivo studies support the idea that telomere length is strongly correlated with life span. Longer telomeres have been associated with shorter life span (e.g., mice have very long telomeres and a short life span; the opposite is true for humans). Telomeres shorten progressively with each cell division; when a critical telomere length (Hayflick limit) is reached, the cells undergo senescence and subsequently apoptosis (programmed cell death).[159]

An alternate view is the *theory of dysfunctional senescence*. Some researchers have proposed that failure of cells or tissues to enter into cellular senescence occurs as a result of defects in genomic maintenance mechanisms after years of mutation and leads to cancer.[54,370] In other words, cellular senescence may reduce cancer mortality rather than promote it late in life, thus positively contributing to longevity in organisms with renewable tissues.[210]

Cancer cells constitute one exception to the limits on cell division. It is thought that the Hayflick limit exists principally to help prevent cancer. If a cell becomes cancerous and the Hayflick limit is approaching, the cell will only be able to divide a limited number of times before it dies. Once it reaches this limiting number of divisions, the formed tumor will no longer be able to reproduce and the cells will die off.

Cancer cells that have found ways around the Hayflick limit are referred to as "immortal." Such immortal cells may still die, but the group of immortalized cells produced from cell division of an immortal cell has no limit as to how many times cell division might take place. Telomeres in immortal cells are maintained by telomerase. Irrespective of telomere length, if telomerase is active, telomeres can be maintained at a sufficient length to ensure cell survival.[159] This presents a unique challenge in preventing and killing cancer cells. Creating telomerase inhibitors may possibly produce a means of supporting anticancer activity.

People age 65 years and older have a risk of cancer development much greater than younger persons, and some cancers in the older adult population seem to be biologically different from those in younger people. For example, the poor prognosis for older adults with acute leukemia is not just due to poor tolerance of aggressive chemotherapy but is more likely associated with cytogenetic resistance to chemotherapy.[169]

All the highest-incidence cancers affect older adults in larger numbers. In both men and women over 65 years, cancers of the colon/rectum, stomach, pancreas, and bladder accounted for two-thirds to three-fourths of the total number of these malignancies. More than 65% of lung cancers and 50% of non-Hodgkin lymphomas occur in older men and women; 77% of the cases of prostate cancer occurred in men older than age 65 years; and 48% of breast cancer and 46% of ovarian cancer occurred in women older than age 65 years.[398]

As previously mentioned, malignancies of the lung, colon/rectum, breast, and prostate account for the highest number of cancer deaths in the United States. Malignancies of the pancreas, stomach, ovary, and bladder and non-Hodgkin lymphomas are also a major cause of cancer deaths. For each of these cancers, more than one-half of the cancer deaths occur in persons older than 65 years.[398]

Lifestyle

Lifestyle or personal behaviors, such as tobacco use, diet and nutrition, alcohol use, and sexual and reproductive behavior, are cited as risk factors for the development of cancer. Lifestyle-related risk factors for cancer combined with cancer-causing substances in the environment and the presence of genes that increase the risk of cancer account for 70% of the total risk for developing cancer.

Tobacco

Both epidemiologic and experimental data support the conclusion that tobacco (including smokeless tobacco) is carcinogenic and remains the most important cause of cancer. Tobacco use accounts for approximately 30% of cancer deaths, with lung cancer now the leading cancer causing deaths in both genders.[93] Cigarette smoking is related to nearly 90% of all lung cancers, and accumulating evidence suggests that cigarette smoking increases the incidence of cancer of the bladder, pancreas, and to a lesser extent, the kidney, larynx, oral cavity, and esophagus.

Diet and Nutrition

The major role of diet and nutrition in affecting cancer risk is well established.[13,15,50,356] It is estimated that approximately one-third of cancer mortality in developing countries may result from dietary causes.[18,196,385] The reader is encouraged to read an excellent summary (by Kushi et al[196]) on the role of nutrition (including the role of specific food items, additives, contaminants, dietary supplements, sweeteners/substitutes, spices, and antioxidants) and physical activity available at http://cacancer journal.com.

Consumption of a poor diet may blunt the immune system's natural defense mechanisms against genetic damage caused by long-term exposure to an environmental carcinogen. Diet and nutrition can directly influence various hormonal factors affecting growth and differentiation in the carcinogenic process. A healthful diet is thought to act, at least in part, to detoxify carcinogens and to inhibit certain processes in carcinogenesis, particularly at the stage of growth and spread. Diet and nutrition can influence these processes (positively or negatively) by providing bioactive compounds to specific tissues via the circulatory system or by modulating hormone levels.

Differences in certain dietary patterns among populations explain a proportion of cancers. These dietary patterns in combination with physical inactivity contribute to obesity and metabolic consequences such as increased levels of growth factor, insulin, estrogen, and possibly testosterone. New evidence suggests that elevated serum insulin levels (insulin resistance) may be a risk factor for postmenopausal breast cancer. These hormones tend to promote cellular growth; high levels of circulating insulin increase the availability of insulin-like growth factors promoting cell growth and reproduction, including cells with damaged DNA that can develop into cancer.[133,183] A history of obesity and/or type 2 diabetes is a risk factor for breast, prostate, pancreatic,[208] and colorectal cancer. Excess weight also contributes to cancers of the uterus, kidney, esophagus, pancreas, gallbladder, and less commonly to leukemia, multiple myeloma, and non-Hodgkin lymphoma.[298,299] Fat (adipose tissue) as an endocrine gland and its role in cancer is discussed in Chapter 11.

Cancer survivors are often highly motivated to improve nutrition and begin an exercise program after receiving a diagnosis of cancer. The ACS continues to publish and update best clinical practices related to optimal nutrition and physical activity during and after cancer treatment.[16]

In the absence of scientific evidence that diet, nutrition, and physical activity[35] can prevent cancer recurrence, reasonable conclusions are offered.[196]

Cancer and cancer treatment can cause profound metabolic and physiologic alterations affecting the body's needs for adequate nutritional intake. Gastrointestinal side effects of treatment can lead to loss of appetite and weight loss accompanied by malnutrition. All the major treatment modalities (e.g., surgery, chemotherapy, or radiation) can adversely impact how the body digests, absorbs, and uses food. Preserving lean body mass is an important goal of nutritional care for survivors, especially during active cancer treatment.[316]

The use of nutritional supplements and antioxidants remains controversial. Until more evidence is available that suggests more benefit than harm, the Institute of Medicine suggests it is prudent for cancer survivors receiving chemotherapy or radiation therapy to avoid exceeding more than 100% of the daily value for antioxidant-type vitamins during the treatment phase.[171,172,196]

Alcohol

Alcohol consumption has been linked to increased rates of cancer of the mouth, pharynx, larynx, esophagus, liver, breast, and probably colon. In people who have been diagnosed with cancer, alcohol intake could also affect the risk for new primary cancers of these sites. Alcohol intake can increase the circulating levels of estrogens, theoretically increasing the risk for breast cancer recurrence.[306,343]

With tobacco use, alcohol interacts with smoke synergistically, increasing the risk of malignant tumors by acting as a solvent for the carcinogenic smoke products and thus increasing the absorption of carcinogens. Evidence is suggestive (but not yet convincing) in associating alcohol consumption and cancers of the colon, pancreas, breast, bladder, and head and neck.[153]

Sexual and Reproductive Behaviors

Sexual and reproductive behaviors are linked to the risk of developing various cancers. For example, the risk of developing cervical cancer is linked with early sexual intercourse and multiple partners. Pregnancy and childbearing seem to be protective against cancers of the endometrium, ovary, and breast. Prolonged lactation may also have a significant impact in the reduction of breast cancer risk by reducing the cumulative exposure of breast tissue to estrogen.[153] Other risk factors for breast cancer are discussed in Chapter 20.

Hormonal Exposure

Hormonal exposure is a factor for women. For example, prolonged exposure to estrogen (e.g., early onset of menses, menopause after age 50, nulliparity or no children, first child after age 30, never breastfed children, or use of first-generation oral contraceptives before 1975) is a risk factor for estrogen-sensitive breast cancer.

Prolonged use of estrogen hormone replacement therapy for relief of menopausal symptoms has been linked with increased rates of breast cancer. Data from the Women's Health Initiative resulted in a halt to the routine use of estrogen and progestin in combination (Prempro) in 2002 and estrogen alone (Premarin) in 2004. When compared with a placebo group, it was clear that hormone users were experiencing more breast cancer, heart disease, stroke, and blood clots. Estrogen showed some benefit, but it was not enough to outweigh the risks.[390]

Growth factors, such as insulin growth factor 1 (IGF-1), and hormones, such as estrogen and testosterone, are considered risk factors linked with cancers other than breast and prostate (e.g., lung, endometrial, and colon). A growing body of literature indicates that besides its essential role in growth and development, growth hormone may play a role in the development and progression of cancer.[26,397]

The *insulin-cancer hypothesis* postulates that complex links between excess body weight, the insulin–IGF axis, and cancer suggest molecular mechanisms are present that lead to increased availability of IGF-1, providing a cellular environment that favors tumor formation.[300] Growth factor signaling pathways appear to be upregulated in hormone-resistant tumors and interact with estrogen receptor signaling, which remains functional even after long-term endocrine deprivation. Intensive research efforts to develop antitumor agents that inhibit IGF signaling in human tumors are under way, with mixed results. A need has been identified to develop biomarkers, gain a clearer understanding of insulin receptor function, and find ways to combine treatment regimens that are safe and effective while yielding positive outcomes [26,399]

Geographic Location and Environmental Variables

The incidence of different types of cancer varies geographically. People living in rural areas are less likely to use preventive screening services or to exercise regularly. Colon cancer is more prevalent in urban than in rural areas, but in rural areas, especially among farmers, skin cancer is more common. Availability of specialty care is a possible contributing issue for this group of people.

The greater susceptibility of certain geographic areas within the United States is probably related to exposure to different carcinogens.[81] The increased incidence of cancer found in urban areas may be related to the increased pool of minorities, increased poverty represented in this group, local smoking ordinances, and diet (e.g., cost and availability of fresh fruits and vegetables).[279]

Occupational or environmental exposure to chemicals (e.g., herbicides, insecticides, dyes), fibers (e.g., asbestos), radon, and air pollution is a risk factor for lung and hematologic cancers. Researchers are investigating the possible causal relationship between environmental exposure and the increased incidence of childhood cancers. The U.S. Environmental Protection Agency (EPA) has identified the carcinogenic effects from hazardous exposures. Heritable genetic and chromosomal mutations caused by environmental or occupational exposures to agents (e.g., chemicals, radiation) can be passed on to the next generation. For further discussion, see Chapter 4.

According to the seventh report on the Biological Effects of Ionizing Radiation (BEIR VII) issued by the National Academy of Science, exposure to even low-dose imaging radiology (including computed tomographic [CT] scans) can result in the development of malignancy. Exposure to medical x-rays is linked with leukemia, thyroid cancer, and breast cancer. There is a 1 in 1000 chance of developing cancer from a single CT scan of the chest, abdomen, or pelvis. The latency period for leukemias is 2 to 5 years and 10 to 30 years for solid tumors.[246]

Ethnicity

Despite advances in cancer diagnosis, treatment, and survival, racial and ethnic minorities suffer disproportionately from cancer. Differences among ethnic groups represent a challenge to understand the reasons and an opportunity to reduce illness and death while improving survival rates. Diagnosis at more advanced stages with lower survival rates at each stage of diagnosis is evident in African Americans compared to whites.

Poverty has emerged as a significant factor influencing poor cancer outcomes for all races, especially among minorities.[283] Inequities in insurance status adversely affect low-income families, preventing individual members from obtaining screening, access to quality care, or the entire range of cancer care available.[338] Other barriers to adequate screening and treatment include cultural issues around testing and treatment, fear, and scarcity of or difficulty with transportation.[286]

African Americans

In particular, racial disparities exist between whites and other groups, especially African Americans. Overall, incidence and mortality from cancer is 10% higher in African Americans compared to whites.[49,338] Studies have shown that equal treatment yields equal outcomes among individuals with equal disease.[32,173] At present, this increased incidence is attributed to preventable risk factors such as the absence of early screening, delayed diagnosis, and smoking and diet. Although the number of African American men who smoke is decreasing and tobacco-related cancers are slowly declining, the incidence of lung cancer and other smoking-related diseases still remains high, possibly because black men tend to smoke cigarettes with a higher tar and nicotine content. The incidence rates of prostate cancer (the most commonly diagnosed cancer among African American men) are at least 50% higher than rates for this group of men compared with other ethnic groups. [11]

Lung cancer is the leading cause of cancer death among both African American men and women. The number of African American women (aged 45-54 years) who have died from lung cancer has increased 30% over the last 2 decades.[387] The number of African American women of all ages who have died from breast cancer has risen nearly 20% over the last 25 years. Breast cancer is the second leading cause of death for African American women. Colorectal cancer has increased in both African American men and women; black women are twice as likely to develop cervical cancer and nearly three times as likely to die from it as other women; African American men have a 60% higher incidence rate of prostate cancer than white men in the United States and the highest rate worldwide.[11]

Some specific forms of cancer affect other ethnic groups at rates higher than the national average (e.g., stomach and liver cancers among Asian American populations and colorectal cancer among Alaska Natives).

African Americans have a lower incidence of bladder cancer but higher mortality rates compared to whites.[364] The incidence of and mortality rates for esophageal cancer are twice as high for African Americans compared to whites.[36]

Hispanics/Latinos

Hispanic people originate from 23 different countries with a wide range of diversity. Racial variations exist in tumor growth, susceptibility, and treatment response. For example, Latino populations have different drug resistance gene expression than non-Latino whites.[260]

Hispanics have lower incidence and death rates than non-Hispanic whites for all cancers combined but the risk increases with the duration of U.S. residence. Cancer is the leading cause of death among U.S. Hispanics.[334] The association between infectious agents (e.g., hepatitis B virus, *Helicobacter pylori*) and cancer may account for higher rates of stomach, liver, uterine cervix, and gallbladder cancers but lower screening rates, differences in lifestyle and dietary patterns, and genetic factors are highly prevalent risk factors.[334] Readers interested in an update on cancer statistics for Hispanics can find this information available online at www.cancer journal.com.[76,334]

Asian Americans

Asian Americans have a unique situation in that they are the only racial/ethnic group to experience cancer as the leading cause of death with proportionately more cancer of infectious origin (e.g., human papillomavirus–induced cervical cancer, hepatitis B virus–induced liver cancer, and stomach cancer) than any other minority group. Cultural barriers to intervention exist such as overcoming resistance to physician visits, reducing tobacco use, and increasing exercise.[70]

The Office of Minority Health and Health Equity (OMHHE) of the Centers for Disease Control and Prevention has been the leading federal agency charged with identifying the national impact of disparity on cancer diagnosis and treatment among various ethnic groups in the United States. The site also describes specific research programs designed to investigate various contributing factors associated with cancer types and ethnic populations. The following website provides a summary of their findings and activities: http://www.cdc.gov/Features/CancerHealthDisparities/.

Public Law 106-525, enacted by Congress in November 2000, specifically created a federal definition, authority, and commitment to the study and investigation of survivorship among minorities and health disparity in the United States.[232] Partnerships between the federal government and other agencies and the private sector have begun to address many of these socioeconomic and accessibility issues as well.[258]

In addition, newer federal legislation, the Patient Protection and Affordable Health Care Act (PPACA) (Public Law 111-148 and 111-152), signed into law in 2010 and upheld by the Supreme Court in 2012, provided the authority for preventive screening for certain cancers (breast, cervical, and colorectal). It also provided insurance coverage for those with a preexisting chronic condition, such as cancer, traditionally denied in the past.

Elements of the law will be incorporated over the next 8 years until 2020.

Precancerous Lesions

Precancerous lesions and some benign tumors may undergo later transformation into cancerous lesions and tumors. Common precancerous lesions include pigmented moles, burn scars, senile keratosis, leukoplakia, and benign adenomas or polyps of the colon or stomach. All such lesions need to be examined periodically for signs of changes.

Stress

Support continues to grow for links between biobehavioral and psychological factors such as stress, depression, and social isolation and the progression (but not necessarily the initiation) of cancer.[238] Depression is a disorder of both immune suppression and immune activation. Markers of impaired cellular immunity (decreased natural killer cell cytotoxicity) and inflammation (elevated IL-6, tumor necrosis factor alpha [TNF-α], and C-reactive protein) have been associated with depression, suggesting the potential for a direct relationship between depression and cancer.[44] Chronic inflammation (with or without accompanying depression) may also be implicated in the progression of cancer.[44,77,81]

The interaction between stromal cells (connective tissue cells of any organ) and tumor cells is known to play a major role in cancer growth and progression. Here again, the influence of stress hormones comes into action as the crosstalk between tumor and stromal cells changes signaling pathways contributing to disease progression.

Research with animal models (animals with a disease that is similar to or the same as a disease in humans) suggests that the body's neuroendocrine response (release of hormones into the blood in response to stimulation of the nervous system) can directly alter important processes in cells that help protect against the formation of cancer, such as DNA repair and the regulation of cell growth.[25] Although substantial evidence supports a positive effect of psychosocial interventions on quality of life in cancer, the clinical evidence for efficacy of stress-modulating psychosocial interventions in slowing cancer progression remains inconclusive, and the biobehavioral mechanisms that might explain such effects are still being investigated.[216]

The possibility that psychological interventions and social support may enhance immune function and survival is under further investigation.[216] Proponents of psychooncology[266] (psychoneuroimmunology and cancer) suggest that advances in mind–body medicine research combined with healthy nutrition and lifestyle choices can have a significant impact on health, health maintenance, disease, and disease prevention, including cancer.[28] See "Psychoneuroimmunology Theory" in Chapter 1; see also "Stress" in Chapter 3.

Additional information about stress can be found on the National Institute of Mental Health's website at http://www.nimh.nih.gov on the Internet. The National Institute of Mental Health, a part of the National Institutes of Health, provides national leadership in the study of mental and behavioral disorders, including the causes and effects of psychological stress.

PATHOGENESIS

Early in the study of cancer, the concept that neoplasia originates in a single cell by acquired genetic change was proposed and remains today the view of cancer pathogenesis most supported by experimental evidence. This hypothesis, called the *somatic mutation theory*, was first substantiated when investigations of tumors confirmed that tumor cells are characterized by chromosomal abnormalities, numerical and structural.

The discovery that chromosomal aberration is one of the basic mechanisms of tumor cell proliferation laid the foundation of modern cancer cytogenetics (study of chromosomes in cancer). Chromosomal changes can include addition or deletion of entire chromosomes (numerical changes) or translocations, deletions, inversions, and insertions of parts of chromosomes (structural changes). Translocations occur when two or more chromosomes exchange material and are common in leukemias and sarcomas. Deletions or losses of chromosomal material are common in epithelial adenocarcinomas of the large bowel, lung, breast, and prostate. Chromosomal deletions may lead to neoplastic development when a tumor suppressor gene is lost. Chromosomal inversions and insertions are less common but still cause abnormal juxtaposition (side-by-side placement) of genetic material.[303]

At first the question arose: Are acquired chromosomal abnormalities the cause of the neoplastic changes in cells or merely the result of the neoplastic state? Chromosomal banding techniques developed in the 1970s have allowed precise identification of chromosomal changes. This information, along with molecular genetic techniques developed during the 1980s, has enabled researchers to investigate this question by examining tumor cells at the level of individual genes.

From these studies, two functionally different classes of cancer-relevant genes have been detected: (1) the dominant oncogenes and (2) the recessive tumor suppressor genes. Oncogenes and tumor suppressor genes are present in all cells. In their normal, nonmutated form, they contribute to the regulation of cell division and death. The activation of oncogenes along with the inactivation of tumor suppressor genes is an important driver of cancer progression.

Current Theory of Oncogenesis

The study of viruses in tumors has led researchers to discover small segments of genetic DNA called *oncogenes*. Oncogenes, also called *cancer-causing genes*, have the ability to transform normal cells into malignant cells, independently or incorporated with a virus. More than 100 oncogenes have been identified. *Protooncogenes* are the normal, nonmutated form of an oncogene that aid in regulating biologic functions, such as cell division, in normal cells. Oncogenes are thought to be the abnormal counterparts of protooncogenes.

Oncogenes may be activated by carcinogens, at which point they alter the regulation of growth in the cell. Oncogenes force a cell to grow even when its surroundings contain none of the cues that normally provoke growth. Oncogenes are hyperactivated versions of normal cellular growth-promoting genes. By releasing strong, unrelenting growth-stimulating signals into a cell, oncogenes can drive cell growth ceaselessly.

Researchers have also discovered a group of regulatory genes, called *antioncogenes* and now called *tumor suppressor genes* that have the opposite effect of oncogenes. When activated, tumor suppressor genes can regulate growth and inhibit carcinogenesis. Tumor suppressor genes (e.g., p53 or telomeres) are the "brakes" to the "stuck accelerator" of the activated oncogene. When defects in the oncogene occur simultaneously with inactivation of growth-suppressing genes, aggressive cell proliferation takes place with the creation of certain types of tumor cells.

Exactly how chromosomal changes contribute to the malignant process remains unclear. Chromosomal rearrangements may lead to oncogene activation, either by a regulatory change causing increased production of normal oncogene-encoded peptides or by creating a deranged oncogene template that codes for an abnormal protein product.

Another proposed mechanism suggests that chromosomal changes inactivate a tumor suppressor gene through chromosomal deletion. Loss of tumor suppressor genes is suspected because chromosomal regions found to be consistently missing in tumor cells have been observed in carcinomas of the lung, breast, bladder, and kidney.

The *p53* gene appears to trigger programmed cell death (apoptosis) as a way of regulating uncontrolled cellular proliferation. p53 is activated by cellular stresses that could facilitate tumor development such as hypoxia, lack of nucleotides, or DNA damage. Mutations in the *p53* tumor suppressor gene result in loss of the ability of the gene protein to bind with DNA and act as a suppressor for the division of that cell.[263] When the p53 pathway has been altered by cancer, the mutated protein product cannot protect the genome. Mutations accumulate and produce resistance to chemotherapy and radiation therapy.

Additionally, researchers have demonstrated that cancer cells develop multiple mechanisms of their own to evade apoptosis. Cancer cells can inactivate proapoptotic factors or upregulate antiapoptotic factors. Strategies to induce apoptosis specifically in tumor cells are currently under investigation. One proapoptotic protein that has been shown to induce apoptosis in a wide variety of tumor cells is a member of the TNF superfamily called *TNF–related apoptosis-inducing ligand* (TRAIL).[68,307]

Another genetic suppressor of cell growth and division also plays a part in the aging process. As cells divide and grow older, there is continuous progressive shortening of the end portions of the chromosomes or telomeres of those cells. Studies of human fibroblasts and other human tissues have shown a very close association between the development of cancer and the overproduction of the enzyme telomerase. When this enzyme is present, it prevents the telomeres from shortening, thus lengthening the life span of the cell indefinitely. Telomerase has been found to be present in more than 85% of human cancer cells but is absent in most normal human tissues.[273,309,366]

Recurrent or persistent inflammation may induce, promote, or influence susceptibility to carcinogenesis by causing DNA damage, inciting tissue reparative proliferation, and/or creating an environment (soil) rich with cytokines and growth factors. Chronic inflammation and the metabolic products of phagocytosis are often accompanied by the excessive formation of reactive oxygen and nitrogen that are potentially damaging to DNA, lipoproteins, and cell membranes.[355]

Although much remains to be learned about the cascade of genetic changes for every kind of cancer, increasing understanding may suggest a means for interrupting the genetic events leading to cancer and for diagnosing the early stages of tumorigenesis. Current research continues to focus on the following major areas of biologic study:

- Regulation of cellular proliferation and expression of oncogenes and tumor suppressor genes
- Telomere length and telomerase
- Free radical–induced DNA damage (see Fig. 6-3) and regulation of apoptosis
- Immune function and response (e.g., senescence, surveillance, enhancement)
- Cellular, metabolic, and humoral factors associated with the chronic inflammatory process[355]

Cancer Stem Cell Hypothesis

Cancer stem cells have been identified in certain types of cancers such as leukemia, giving support to the idea that not all cancer cells are the same and leading to the development of the *cancer stem-cell hypothesis.*

The cancer stem-cell hypothesis predicts that there are different functional and morphologic cancer cells within a single tumor and a hierarchical order in which the abnormal stem cells form and feed a cancer. Emerging evidence indicates that these cells are also resistant to chemotherapy and radiation therapy because their DNA repair mechanisms are more highly developed. Targeting and eliminating the tumor-initiating stem cells may be a more efficient and direct way to eradicate cancer without killing fast-growing normal cells. This information, first reported more than 10 years ago, set off a new direction in cancer research.[97,259,330]

Tumor Biochemistry and Pathogenesis

Carcinogenesis is the process by which a normal cell undergoes malignant transformation. Usually, it is a multistep process, involving progressive changes after genetic damage to or alteration of cellular DNA through the development of hyperplasia, metaplasia, dysplasia, carcinoma in situ, invasive carcinoma, and metastatic carcinoma in that order.[237] These discrete stages in tumor development suggest that a single altered gene only suffices to push a cell part of the way down the path to actual malignancy. The process is completed when multiple, successive changes occur in distinct cellular genes, including activation or overexpression of oncogenes and loss or mutation of tumor suppressor genes.

The number of genetic events required for conversion of normal cells to malignant cells is still debated, but, at least in the case of many solid tumors (e.g., colon carcinomas), this number may be as great as seven or eight. This high number of genetic events may imply that genetic instability occurs during cancer progression.[237] This requirement for multiple changes creates an important protective mechanism against cancer.

If a small number of genetic changes sufficed to transform a normal cell into a malignant one, multiple tumors would develop easily. These multiple barriers, along with the normal circuitry inside cells, ensure that only the rare cell will sustain the requisite number of changes for making a cancer cell.

On the other hand, cancer has developed multiple methods centering on genetic mutation to promote self-survival and perpetuation. The pliability of cancer cells to mutate in several different phenotypes in an attempt to find one that will survive and colonize at a metastatic site makes finding effective treatment difficult at best. The next section, "Cancer and the Immune System," will further demonstrate the complexity of carcinogenesis and give the reader an understanding of current treatment focus through translational medicine.

Cancer and the Immune System

Joseph A. Fraietta, PhD

There is a considerable amount of clinical and scientific evidence to suggest that the human body responds immunologically to tumors. Over a century ago, it was first conceived that a primary function of the immune system is to prevent an "overwhelming frequency" of carcinomas.[112] In 1957, emerging discoveries on immune control of neoplastic disease were incorporated into the formal hypothesis of cancer *immunosurveillance,* which states that the immune system is continuously searching out and destroying potentially cancerous cells before they become harmful tumors.[51] These transformed cells are thought to constantly arise during the life span of the host.

Immunosurveillance

The phenomenon of immunosurveillance is supported by the following observations: (1) a higher incidence of cancer after immunosuppression or in immunodeficiency,[130,274] (2) infiltration of tumors by lymphocytes and macrophages (i.e., positive correlation between the extent of *in situ* lymphocyte infiltration in tumors and patient survival rates),[74] (3) lymphocyte proliferation in response to tumors, (4) regression of metastases after ablation of the primary tumor, and (5) immune-mediated spontaneous regression of human tumors (especially in malignant melanoma, but also in neuroblastoma and other tumors).[313] Although the theory of cancer immunosurveillance has been challenged, a large amount of current data obtained by many independent researchers supports the basic principles of this concept that an unmanipulated immune system detects and eliminates primary tumors and this is heavily dependent on lymphocytes and the various factors they produce.[108]

Interestingly, recent experimental evidence suggests that inactivation of an oncogene with therapeutic agents (i.e., curing the oncogene addiction) leads to regression of tumors in immunocompetent hosts, but this effect is only transient in immunodeficient hosts.[296] Despite the fact that the immune system reacts against tumors, these immune responses may be associated with tumor inhibition but not elimination. Furthermore, recognition of tumor antigens by the immune system may result in tolerance rather than activation of a response. The fact that tumors arise in otherwise healthy individuals suggests that antitumor immunity is often insufficient and easily overwhelmed by a rapidly proliferating malignancy. For this reason, researchers have endeavored to identify and characterize various types of tumor antigens against which immune responses are elicited and continue to explore how immunity against cancer can be bolstered to benefit the patient. For a complete understanding of the immune system as it relates to cancer, the reader is encouraged to read this chapter along with Chapter 7.

Tumor-Specific Antigens

A key feature of cancer immunology is the interaction between the immune system of the tumor-bearing individual and a constantly changing source of foreign molecules (tumor antigens). Tumor-specific antigens (TSAs) are tumor antigens that are uniquely expressed by tumor cells and are not expressed by normal cells. TSAs are often referred to as *neoantigens* or "new antigens" that may exist in the nucleus, cytoplasm, or cell membrane and may be excreted from the cell. Altered proteins are the result of gene mutations that give rise to new peptides (mutant peptides). If a portion of these peptides can be loaded onto major histocompatibility complexes (MHCs), the immune system will recognize a TSA as foreign.

Fusion proteins are a type of TSA that can be generated by translocations in which part of one gene moves to a different chromosome and recombines with another gene (e.g., BCR/ABL). The joining part of the two genes produces a new sequence because it spans the genes and is translated into a protein that does not normally exist. In addition to translocations and recombination, fusion proteins can be generated by deletions that resulted in joining of two or more genes that originally coded for separate proteins.

TSAs can also consist of *viral proteins* that are component proteins or new enzymes that aid in the replication of the virus. Tumor viruses can induce benign or malignant proliferation of the cells that they infect. The resultant tumors express viral antigens—these are not host proteins or unique in some way; they are simply viral proteins. Viral constituents found in tumors form a major part of the evidence that establishes a causal link between viruses and human cancers (e.g., human papillomavirus E6 and E7 proteins) (Fig. 9-2).[365]

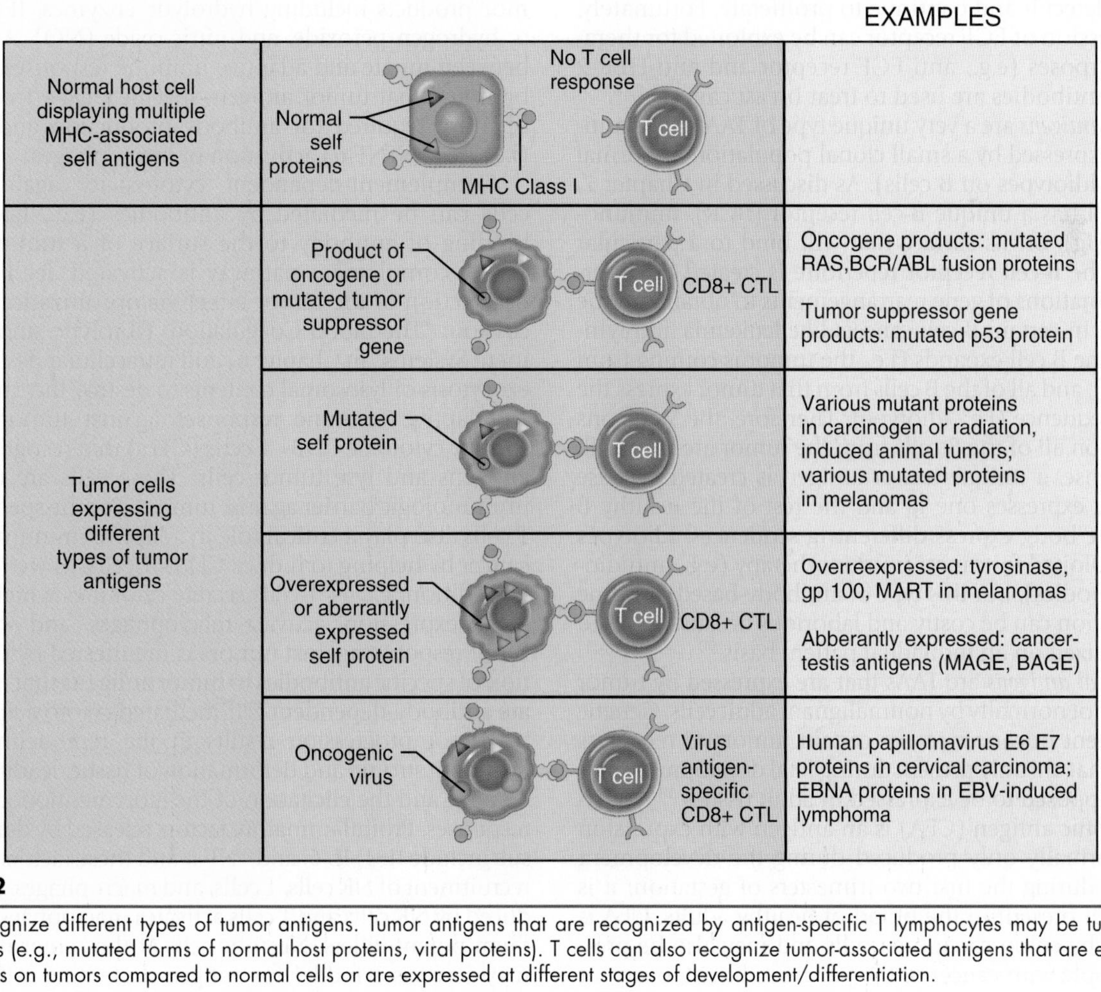

EXAMPLES

Normal host cell displaying multiple MHC-associated self antigens	Normal self proteins — No T cell response — T cell — MHC Class I	
Tumor cells expressing different types of tumor antigens	Product of oncogene or mutated tumor suppressor gene — T cell — CD8+ CTL	Oncogene products: mutated RAS, BCR/ABL fusion proteins Tumor suppressor gene products: mutated p53 protein
	Mutated self protein — T cell	Various mutant proteins in carcinogen or radiation, induced animal tumors; various mutated proteins in melanomas
	Overexpressed or aberrantly expressed self protein — T cell — CD8+ CTL	Overreexpressed: tyrosinase, gp 100, MART in melanomas Abberantly expressed: cancer-testis antigens (MAGE, BAGE)
	Oncogenic virus — T cell — Virus antigen-specific CD8+ CTL	Human papillomavirus E6 E7 proteins in cervical carcinoma; EBNA proteins in EBV-induced lymphoma

Figure 9-2

T cells recognize different types of tumor antigens. Tumor antigens that are recognized by antigen-specific T lymphocytes may be tumor-specific neoantigens (e.g., mutated forms of normal host proteins, viral proteins). T cells can also recognize tumor-associated antigens that are expressed at higher levels on tumors compared to normal cells or are expressed at different stages of development/differentiation.

Tumor-Associated Antigens

Tumor-associated antigens (TAAs) are antigens that are expressed by tumors and normal cells. These tumor antigens are expressed at higher levels on tumors relative to normal cells or are expressed at different stages of development or differentiation. *Oncospermatogonal antigens* or cancer-testis antigens are expressed in spermatocytes and cancer cells, but not normal cells of the tissue of tumor origin (non–lineage-specific expression). For example, melanoma antigen–encoding gene (MAGE-1) is a normal testicular protein that is expressed by melanoma cells.[369] *Differentiation antigens* are TAAs that are expressed on a tumor and are also expressed at some stage of differentiation of nonmalignant cells of the tumor's cell lineage (lineage-specific antigens). Melanocyte differentiation antigens (e.g., MART-1/Melan-A) are antigens that are expressed by melanomas, but also by normal melanocytes. A normal melanocyte will express the antigen during its development and differentiation, and tumor cells will reexpress the antigen.[165] Prostate differentiation antigen (PSA) is another common differentiation antigen.

In some cases, overexpression of normal protein/antigen constitutes a TAA. For example, the epidermal growth factor (EGF) receptor is typically found on epithelial cells, as well as other cell types. Certain adenocarcinomas are characterized by EGF receptor expression that is manyfold higher than levels found on normal cells. In this way, the tumor is expressing a growth factor at very high levels and can detect it and continue to proliferate. Fortunately, overexpression of EGF receptor can be exploited for therapeutic purposes (e.g., anti-EGF receptor and anti-HER-2 receptor antibodies are used to treat breast cancer).[228]

Clonal antigens are a very unique type of TAA. These antigens are expressed by a small clonal population of normal cells (i.e., idiotypes on B cells). As discussed in Chapter 7, each B cell has a unique B-cell receptor (BCR), immunoglobulin (Ig), on its surface that will bind to a particular antigen. The B-cell receptor repertoire is created by different combinations of gene rearrangements to obtain unique V regions. In certain B-cell cancers like leukemia and lymphoma, one B cell expands (i.e., the tumor is coming from one B cell), and all of the B cells from that tumor express the same Ig sequence (i.e., idiotype). Therefore, the V regions of the Igs on all of the B cells from the tumor are identical. In that sense, a unique tumor antigen is created because the tumor expresses one Ig and the rest of the healthy B cells in the body express different Ig sequences. Idiotypes can be exploited for cancer immunotherapy (e.g., antiidiotypic antibodies), but this type of antibody-based immune manipulation can be costly and laborious because it has to be customized on an individual patient basis.[90]

Oncofetal antigens are TAAs that are expressed by tumor cells, but not normally by nonmalignant adult cells. Genetic derangement in cancer causes certain tumors to reexpress antigens that are only present during fetal development and are not supposed to be expressed in adult tissues.[383] Carcinoembryonic antigen (CEA) is an antigen with expression that is normally only produced during the development of a fetus during the first two trimesters of gestation; it is usually not present in the blood of healthy adults. CEA is expressed by colon carcinoma cells and may also be present in people with cancer of the pancreas, breast, ovary, or lung. Alpha-fetoprotein is another oncofetal protein that is expressed by fetal liver as well as yolk sac cells and is also found on tumors of the liver and testis.[56,365]

Major Immune Responses Against Tumors

Major immune responses elicited against tumors that have been described in humans and animal models involve both innate and adaptive immunity. Innate immune responses against tumors may include natural killer (NK) cells that directly kill cancer cells without any previous exposure to the tumor. As discussed in Chapter 7, NK cells are activated by a balance of activating and inhibitory receptors. MHC class I is a ligand for an inhibitory receptor and without inhibitory signals, NK cells are activated against tumor cells that have decreased MHC expression. Once contact with the tumor cell has been made, the NK cell releases soluble cytotoxic factors such as perforin, proteases, nucleases, and TNF-α. NK cells also have an Fc receptor (CD16) that binds to antibody-coated tumor cells and triggers antibody-dependent cell-mediated cytotoxicity.

Macrophages can function as effectors (antibody-dependent cell-mediated cytotoxicity, cytokine release, TNF-α production) that kill tumor cells. This activity does not require tumor antigen recognition directly. Macrophages do not recognize a specific tumor antigen, but similar to NK cells, they can distinguish normal cells from cancer cells. Detection by macrophages may involve phospholipids that are expressed ectopically in the membrane of a malignant cell. These innate immune cells generate many different antitumor products including hydrolytic enzymes, IFN-α, TNF-α, hydrogen peroxide, and nitric oxide (NO). As a bridge between innate and adaptive immune responses, it should be noted that tumor antigen–specific CD4+ T cells and B cells are required for antibody production and cytokine (i.e., IFN-α; TNF-α) activation of macrophages.

Complement-dependent cytotoxicity against tumor cells can be mediated by antibodies (e.g., IgM). Upon binding of antibody to the surface of a tumor cell, the classic complement pathway is activated, leading to the destruction of the tumor target via opsonization (see discussion, "The Blood Coagulation, Fibrolytic, and Complement Systems" in Chapter 6) and intracellular destruction or exocytosis of lysosomal contents to destroy the cancer cell.

Adaptive immune responses against tumors include specific cytotoxic CD8+ T cells (CTLs) that recognize tumor antigens and lyse tumor cells. These cells are the major immunologic barrier against tumors. Tumor-specific CD4+ T cells also play a critical role in adaptive immunity against cancer by helping to induce CD8+ T cells, as well as B cells. In addition, CD4+ T cells secrete cytokines which increase MHC expression, activate macrophages, and so on. The B-cell response against tumors is manifested by the formation of specific antibodies to tumor antigens that may mediate antibody-dependent cell-mediated cytotoxicity.[62,363,374]

Tumor progression results in the remodeling of surrounding stroma and deformation of tissue, leading to local damage and the elicitation of the aforementioned immune responses. Proinflammatory factors released by damaged tissue include IL-1, IL-6, and TNF-α and these factors aid in the recruitment of NK cells, T cells, and macrophages. IFN-γ produced by NK cells and T cells activates macrophages, making them potent killers. Necrotic cells at the center of a tumor may serve as a fodder for antigen-presenting cells, such as dendritic cells (DCs). DCs phagocytose tumor debris and

EXAMPLES

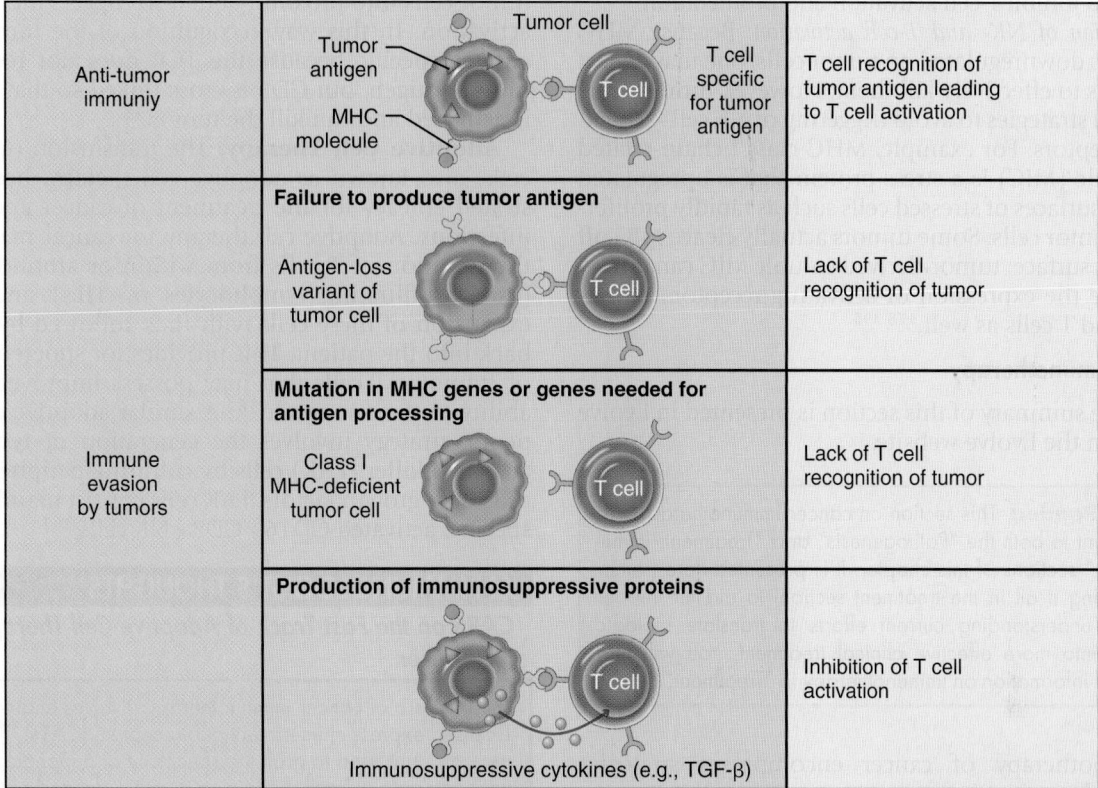

Figure 9-3

Mechanisms of immune evasion by tumors. T cell–mediated antitumor immunity develops upon recognition of a cognate tumor antigen and lymphocyte activation. Tumor cells have the capacity to evade immune responses by losing expression of antigens or MHC molecules or via the elaboration of immunosuppressive factors.

migrate to the draining lymph nodes. Antigen is presented to CD4+ T cells in the context of MHC class II and to CD8+ T cells in the context of MHC class I. Activated CD4+ T cells and CD8+ T cells migrate to the tumor and differentiate into effector cells. CD4+ T cells are differentiated by the cytokine milieu into different helper T (T_H) cell subsets that aid other immune cells in mediating tumor clearance. CD8+ T cells acquire cytotoxic function. This is enhanced by T_H1 production of IFN-γ. In addition to helping B cells to produce antibodies, T_H2 cells may induce potent antitumor immune responses through IL-4–induced activation of NK cells.[56,189]

Tumor Evasion Strategies

Despite the fact that immunity is mounted against neo-antigens or antigens that are inappropriately expressed, one may ask why these responses are often insufficient to clear tumors. In other words, why does cancer develop in an immunocompetent individual? As it turns out, the immune system faces a daunting challenge of eliminating malignancies that are proliferating at such a rapid rate that immune defenses are simply overtaken. In addition, many tumor antigens are weak immunogens, perhaps because they vary only slightly from self-antigens.

Tumors have also evolved to evade innate and adaptive immune responses.[294] This is known as *immune escape* and can occur through many different mechanisms (Fig. 9-3), including the following:

1. *Loss of immunogenicity.* In the same way that virus infection induces MHC class I downregulation, selection of

tumor cell variants with low levels of MHC class I occurs and this prevents the induction of NK cells and cytotoxic CD8+ T cells. Tumors will also mutate antigenic peptides so that they cannot be loaded onto the class I MHC and be presented to CD8+ T cells. It should be appreciated that tumors are not professional antigen-presenting cells. As discussed in Chapter 7, T cells require two signals for activation—signal I through the T-cell receptor (TCR) and signal II, which is costimulation. Even if the tumor cell presents antigen to T cells, it does not express costimulatory molecules (e.g., B7-1) that could bind to CD28 on the T cell. In this situation, the tumor cell may be providing signal I, but not signal II and that often leads to *tolerance* of T cells.[219] In addition, some tumors downregulate adhesion molecules like ICAM-1. In order for a CD8+ T cell to kill its target, it needs to bind and tumors evolve to express very low levels of adhesion molecules. As a result, the cytotoxic T cell cannot make good contact with the tumor cell and undergo the remaining steps of triggering its killing mechanism.

2. *Antigenic modulation* refers to the loss of a surface antigen. When this occurs, tumor antigens are internalized or downregulated so that antibodies cannot bind.

3. *Induction of immune suppression.* Tumors produce a variety of suppressive factors that inhibit T cells directly, and also downmodulate the function of antigen-presenting cells like DCs that infiltrate the tumor. These antigen-presenting cells pick up antigen from dying tumor cells to present to T cells. Immunosuppressive cytokines such

as TGFβ and IL-10 will keep DCs in an immature state and also inhibit T-cell activation and proliferation.

4. *Prevention of NK- and T-cell activation*: Because MHC class I is downregulated on tumor cells, one may expect NK cells to effectively kill them. However, tumors have evolved strategies to avoid triggering of NK cell–activating receptors. For example, MHC class I chain-related molecule (MIC) is a stress protein that is upregulated on the surfaces of stressed cells such as rapidly proliferating tumor cells. Some tumors actually cleave MIC off of their surface; tumor-derived soluble MIC can downregulate the expression of activating receptors on NK cells and T cells as well.[178,395]

Cancer Immunotherapy

An outline summary of this section is presented in Evolve Box 9-2 on the Evolve website.

> **Note to Reader:** This section on cancer immunotherapy is a complement to both the "Pathogenesis" and "Treatment: Immunotherapy" sections of this chapter. It is presented here (rather than placing it all in the treatment section) to aid the reader in better understanding current efforts to translate biologic research into more effective clinical treatment. You will find additional information on immunotherapy in "Treatment" below.

Immunotherapy of cancer encompasses strategies aimed at boosting immune responses against tumors through the administration of immunomodulatory factors (e.g., cytokines, adjuvants) or more specific approaches such as monoclonal antibodies directed against a particular tumor antigen. Cytokines such as IFN-α, IFN-β, IFN-γ; IL-2, IL-4, IL-6, IL-12, and TNF have been used alone or in combination to bolster immune responses against cancer.[104] Similarly, a variety of adjuvants such as attenuated strains of *Mycobacterium bovis* (bacillus Calmette-Guérin) have been used to augment antitumor immunity by activating macrophages to generate various cytokines, increase MHC class II expression, and upregulate costimulatory molecules (e.g., B7).[56]

Antibody-Based Therapy. If the tumor antigen is known, monoclonal antibodies can be administered that are "naked" or conjugated with agents that increase their efficacy. If a patient is injected with monoclonal antibodies against a tumor antigen, NK cells can bind through their Fc receptors and get triggered to kill the tumor cell.

Complement may also play a role in the destruction of tumor cells following the binding of antibodies. In addition, monoclonal antibodies can induce apoptosis of certain malignant cells (i.e., by cross-linking of surface immunoglobulin or CD20) or block/downregulate a receptor for a tumor growth factor (e.g., EGF receptor and HER-2 receptor blockade). Monoclonal antibodies are often coupled with immunotoxins (e.g., ricin) or to radionuclides in order to concentrate the substance/radiation at the tumor site, while sparing healthy tissues.[2]

A clever antitumor immunotherapy strategy involves the engineering of *bispecific antibodies* in which the binding sites of the immunoglobulin recognize different targets. For example, these antibodies have been used to simultaneously target tumor cells and CD3. Thus, this type of bispecific antibody not only brings the T cells and tumor cells into proximity but also triggers the T cells for activation. In this way, recognition of the tumor is not antigen-specific because the TCR does not recognize a tumor antigen, but CD3 is cross-linked so that the T cell is activated and can kill the tumor.[33]

Adoptive Cell Therapy. The transfusion of immune cells, also known as adoptive cell therapy, has demonstrated efficacy for the treatment of cancer and chronic infections. Adoptive cell therapy for cancer may include the isolation of T cells from within or around a tumor (tumor-infiltrating lymphocytes or TILs) and *ex vivo* expansion of these cells with IL-2, followed by infusion back into the patient. This provides for superenrichment of cytotoxic T cells that may possess improved homing ability to the tumor site.[182] A similar adoptive cell therapeutic strategy involves the generation of lymphokine activated killer (LAK) cells by culturing peripheral blood cells with growth factors. LAK cells consist mainly of non-specific, activated CD16+ CD3– NK cells.[163]

AN IMMUNOLOGIST'S THOUGHTS*

CARS on the Fast Track of Adoptive Cell Therapy for Cancer

The new era of cancer immunotherapy involves engineering T cells to express chimeric antigen receptors (CARs). These receptors are used to graft the specificity of a monoclonal antibody onto a T cell, endowing it with a defined antigen recognition capability that is independent of the natural TCR.[142] The signaling domains of the CD3/TCR complex and costimulatory receptors (e.g., 4-1BB and CD28) are incorporated into CARs to potentiate T-cell effector functions and activation of costimulatory pathways (see Chapter 7) upon binding to its target. Therefore, a patient's T cells can be directed against virtually any tumor antigen in a non–MHC-restricted fashion. Remarkable clinical success utilizing CAR T cells has recently been achieved in patients with chronic lymphocytic leukemia who had a high tumor burden and exhibited resistance to conventional forms of therapy.[184] Part of my own research involves manipulating CAR T cells to expand and persist in strongly immunosuppressive tumor microenvironments.

*Joseph A. Fraietta, PhD

Cancer Vaccines. See further discussion of cancer vaccines in "Treatment" below.

Cancer vaccines are available to either treat individuals with an existing malignancy (*therapeutic* vaccines) or to prevent the development of cancer (*prophylactic* vaccines). In the context of therapeutic vaccines, when the tumor antigen has been identified, autologous antigen-presenting cells such as dendritic cells (DCs) can be isolated from the patient, loaded with the tumor antigen and then reinfused into the subject with the hope of stimulating anticancer immunity. Viral vectors (e.g., adenovirus) can also be engineered to encode a particular tumor antigen. Because viruses strongly activate antigen-presenting cells, the immune system can be "tricked" so that there is enhanced presentation of tumor antigen, resulting in a more potent response.[198]

Although still experimental, DNA vaccines allow for tumor antigens to be encoded, along with cytokines and perhaps costimulatory molecules so that T cells can be activated to inhibit tumor growth.[371] In addition, autologous tumor cells can be isolated from the patient and manipulated to express costimulatory molecules to activate T cells in the host.[7] Tumor cells can also be engineered to express granulocyte-macrophage colony–stimulating factor (GM-CSF) and when reinfused into the patient, these cells will facilitate the activation and differentiation of antigen-presenting cells to enhance presentation of tumor antigen to T cells.

Another useful strategy that can be employed when the tumor antigen is unknown is to immunize cancer patients with autologous tumor-derived heat shock proteins. Heat shock proteins are chaperones that pick up antigenic peptides and shuttle them to MHC class I and class II. The rationale behind this strategy is that if heat shock proteins are isolated from a tumor, they should be loaded with immunogenic peptides from the cancer cells.[347]

The major challenge involved with developing prophylactic cancer vaccines is identifying a tumor antigen to immunize individuals against. This is further complicated by the tremendous amount of heterogeneity observed in human cancers. However, there are some conditions such as viral infections that tumors are known to be associated with. Therefore, if a population is immunized against certain oncogenic viruses, it will be protected against the future development of tumors induced by these viruses (e.g., human papillomavirus or hepatitis B virus). It should be noted that although these vaccines constitute very effective preventive strategies, they target viral and not tumor antigens.

INVASION AND METASTASES

Malignant tumors differ from benign tumors in their ability to metastasize or spread from the primary site to other locations in the body. Metastasis occurs when cells break away from the primary tumor, travel through the body via the blood or lymphatic system, and become trapped in the capillaries of organs. From there, they infiltrate the organ tissue and grow into new tumor deposits. Cancer can also spread to adjacent structures and penetrate body cavities by direct extension. For example, ovarian tumors frequently shed cells into the peritoneal cavity where they grow to cover the surface of abdominal organs and cause ascites.

Patterns of metastasis differ from cancer to cancer. Although there is no clear explanation of the exact mechanism of metastasis, certain cancers tend to spread to specific organs or sites in the body in a predictable manner (Table 9-2). The five most common sites of metastasis are the lymph nodes, liver, lung, bone, and brain. The spread of cancer may be influenced by a variety of host factors such as the aging or dysfunctional immune system, increasing age, hormonal environment, pregnancy, and stress. Factors that may slow the spread of metastasis include radiation, chemotherapy, anticoagulants, steroids, and other antiangiogenic agents.

Seed Versus Soil Theory of Metastasis

Some cancers favor certain sites of metastasis over others so that metastases only occur if the cancer cell (the seed) finds a favorable microenvironment at the site of the host (the soil). Certain tumor cells seem to have specific affinity for certain organs. The idea that metastasis is organ specific was first proposed in 1889 by Stephen Paget, an English surgeon who first published the seed versus soil hypothesis to explain the pattern of metastasis.[115]

Studies in the 1990s showed that there is "crosstalk" between metastatic cells and the organ microenvironment. Host cells secrete growth factors that prompt tumor cell replication and allow the tumor to take over the homeostatic mechanisms of the host. Angiogenesis, the process by which blood vessels from preexisting vessels grow into the solid tumor, is one way that tumor cells take over homeostatic mechanism for their own gain.[115]

Traditional cancer treatment targets the seed, whereas today's research is focused on approaches that target the soil, making the sites of metastasis unsuitable for the growth of cancer cells. There are many challenges in preventing metastasis because the microenvironments of metastasis sites can be very different. For example, lung cancer that spreads to the femur can behave very differently from lung cancer that spreads to the spine. Treatment that is optimal in the primary organ may not work in the metastatic sites.[267]

Animal studies show that the surgical removal of a primary tumor can result in the rapid growth of previously dormant metastatic cells. Additional challenges to preventing metastases are possible if this phenomenon occurs in humans.[53]

Incidence of Metastasis

Approximately 30% of clients with newly diagnosed cancers have clinically detectable metastases. At least 30% to 40% of the remaining clients who are clinically free of metastases harbor occult (hidden) metastases. Unfortunately, most people have multiple sites of metastatic disease, not all of which present at any one time. The formation of metastatic colonies is a continuous process, commencing early in the growth of the primary tumor and increasing with time.

Even metastases have the potential to metastasize; the presence of large, identifiable metastases in a given organ can be accompanied by a greater number of micrometastases that have been disseminated more recently from the primary tumor or the metastasis. The size variation in metastases and the dispersed anatomic location of metastases can make complete surgical removal of disease impossible, limiting the effective concentration of anticancer drugs that can only be delivered to tumor cells in metastatic colonies.

Mechanisms of Metastasis

For rapidly growing tumors, millions of tumor cells are shed into the vascular system each day. Only a very small percentage of circulating tumor cells initiate metastatic colonies because most cells that have invaded the bloodstream are quickly eliminated. Classic isotope studies have shown that 99% of circulating potentially tumorigenic cells are killed by blood vessel turbulence within 24 hours.[115,116,135] Metastases of the remaining 1% require

Table 9-2 Pathways of Cancer Metastases

Primary Cancer	Mode of Dissemination	Location of Primary Metastases
Breast	Lymphatics	Bone (shoulder, hips, sacrum, ribs, vertebrae); CNS (brain, spinal fluid, brachial plexus)
	Blood (vascular or hematogenous)	Lung, pleural cavity, liver, bone
Bone	Blood	Lungs, liver, bone, then CNS
Cervical (cervix)	Local extension and lymphatics	Retroperitoneal lymph nodes, bladder, rectum; paracervical, parametrial lymphatics
	Blood	CNS (brain), lungs, bones, liver
Chordoma	Direct extension	Neighboring soft tissues, spine
	Blood	Liver, lungs, heart, brain, spine
	Lymphatics	Lymph nodes, peritoneum
Colorectal	Direct extension	Bone (vertebrae, hip, sacrum)
	Peritoneal seeding	Peritoneum
	Blood	Liver, lung
Ewing sarcoma	Blood	Lung, bone, bone marrow
Giant cell tumor of bone	Blood	Lung
Kidney	Lymph	Pelvis, groin
	Blood	Lungs, pleural cavity, bone, liver, brain
Leukemia		Does not really "metastasize" because it is present throughout the body and therefore causes symptoms throughout body
Liver	Blood	CNS (brain)
Lung (bronchogenic sarcoma)	Blood	CNS (brain, spinal cord)
	Blood	Bone (ribs, sacrum, vertebrae)
	Direct extension, lymphatics	Mediastinum (tissue and organs between the sternum and vertebrae such as the heart, blood vessels, trachea, esophagus, thymus, lymph nodes)
Lung (apical or Pancoast's tumors)	Direct extension	8th cervical and 1st and 2nd thoracic nerves within the brachial plexus
	Blood	CNS (brain, spinal cord), bone
Lung (small cell)	Blood	CNS (brain, spinal fluid)
Lymphomas	Blood	CNS (spinal cord, spinal fluid), bone
	Lymphatics	Can occur anywhere, including skin, visceral organs, especially liver
Malignant melanoma	No typical pattern	Mets can occur anywhere; skin and subcutaneous tissue; lungs; CNS (brain, spinal fluid); liver; gastrointestinal tract; bone
Multiple myeloma	Blood	Bone (sacrum)
Nonmelanoma skin cancer	Usually remain local without metastases; local invasion	Bones underlying involved skin; brain
Osteogenic sarcoma (osteosarcoma)	Blood	Lungs, CNS (brain)
	Lymphatics	Lymph nodes, lungs, bone, kidneys
Ovarian	Direct extension into abdominal cavity	Nearby organs (bladder, colon, rectum, uterus, fallopian tubes); spread beyond abdomen is rare
	Lymphatics, peritoneal fluid through the abdomen	Liver, lungs; regional and distant
Pancreatic	Blood	Liver
Prostate	Lymphatics	Pelvic, sacrum, and vertebral bones, sacral plexus
		Bladder, rectum
		Distant organs (lung, liver, brain)
Soft tissue sarcoma	Blood; lymphatics (rare)	Lung (first) but also bone, brain, liver, soft tissue (distant)
Spinal cord	Local invasion; dissemination through the intervertebral foramina	CNS (brain, spinal cord)
Stomach, gastric	Blood	Liver, vertebrae, abdominal cavity (intraperitoneum)
	Local invasion	
Testes	Local invasion	Bone (pelvis, lumbar spine, hip)
	Blood, lymphatics	Lung
Thyroid	Direct extension	Bone; nearby tissues of neck
	Lymphatics	Regional lymph nodes (neck, upper chest, mediastinum)
	Blood	Distant (lung, bone, brain)

CNS, Central nervous system.

From Goodman CC, Snyder TE: Differential diagnosis for physical therapists: Screening for referral, ed 5, Philadelphia, 2013, Saunders.

Steps for metastasis

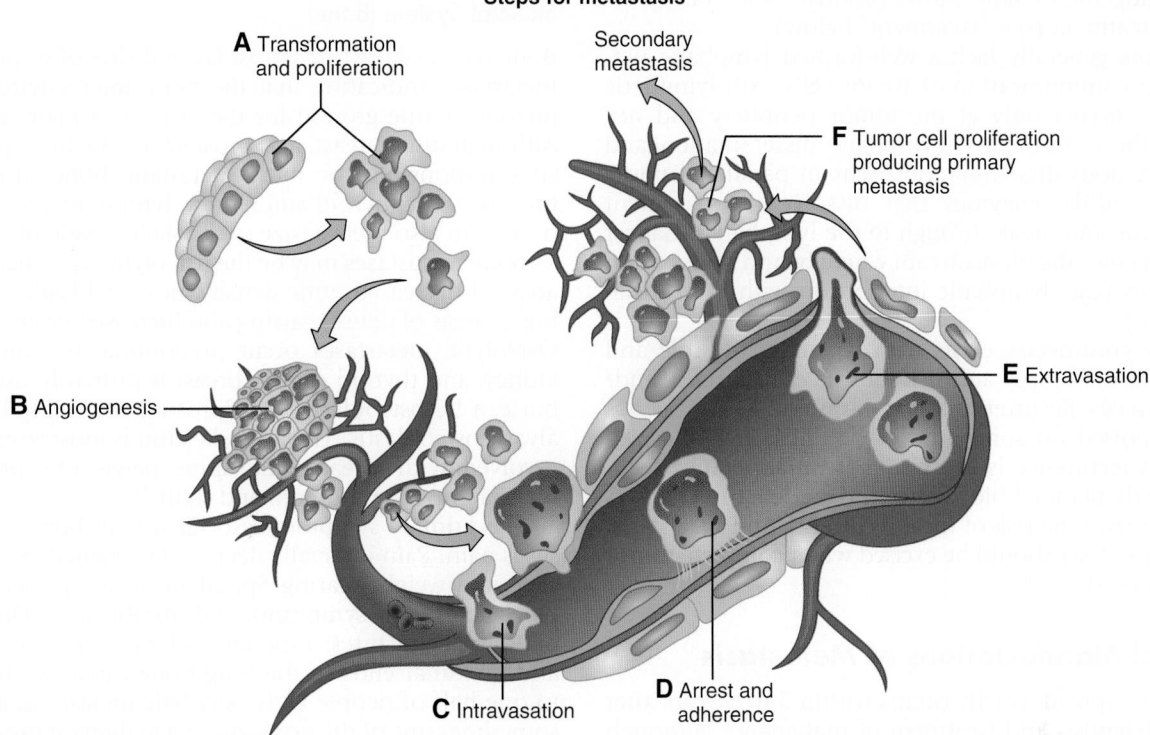

Figure 9-4

Major mechanisms of metastases. To metastasize, tumor cells must gain several unique biologic properties such as invasive growth **(A)**, induction of vascular growth **(B)**, vascular invasion **(C)**, adherence to endothelial cells or thrombosis of peripheral sinusoids **(D)**, continuation of invasive growth with extravasation **(E)**, and formation of primary and secondary metastatic foci **(F)**. Not all tumor cells develop all the abilities shown here; some cell clones may subspecialize and just create angiogenesis; others may invade and move on. (From Dorfman HD, Czerniak B: *Bone tumors,* St. Louis, 1998, Mosby.)

a good deal of coordination between the cancer cells and the body (Fig. 9-4).

The greater the number of invasive tumor cells in the bloodstream, the greater the probability that some cells will survive to form metastases. Metastasis is more likely to occur via the veins as opposed to the arteries because the cancer cannot break through the arterial wall. The major challenge in treating cancer is not eradicating the primary tumor because surgery or radiation is effective in these early cases. Eradicating metastases, often already present at the time of diagnosis, is the key factor to cancer cure.

A complicated series of tumor–host interactions resulting in a metastatic colony is called the *metastatic cascade* and is similar for all tumor cells. Once a primary tumor is initiated and starts to move by local invasion, then blood vessels from preexisting vessels grow into the solid tumor, a process called *tumor angiogenesis* (see Fig. 9-4). As a normal physiologic process, angiogenesis is crucial to tissue growth, repair, and maintenance.

The ability of a tumor to grow beyond a very small mass (1-2 mm) depends on its ability to gain access to an adequate supply of blood and in some cases (e.g., breast and prostate) the presence of hormonal factors. The supply of blood allows the tumor to obtain essential nutrients, such as oxygen, and to eliminate metabolic waste products, such as carbon dioxide and acids. The blood supply to tumors is provided by growth of new capillaries and larger vessels into the tumor mass from the blood supply of adjacent normal tissues.

The normal process of angiogenesis begins with the formation of endothelial cell sprouts followed by proliferation and migration of neighboring endothelial cells along the preformed extensions. The initiating event and mechanism of sprouting are unknown; in apoptotic cells, endothelial cell sprouting occurs via electrostatic signaling. Negatively charged membrane surfaces in apoptotic cells initiate the formation of directional endothelial cell sprouts that extend toward the dying cells.[127]

Tumor-derived proteins called *angiogenesis factors* also facilitate the use of nearby blood vessels from normal tissues and promote the growth of new blood vessels into the malignant tissue.[303] The actual factors involved in tumor angiogenesis are very complex, but two cytokines have been identified as primary stimulators of vascular proliferation.

Both vascular endothelial growth factor and fibroblast growth factor stimulate proliferation of vascular cells and even allow the newly formed blood vessels to be easily invaded by the cancer cells that are closely adjacent to them.[110] Increased tumor contact with the circulatory system provides tumors with a mechanism to enter the general circulation and colonize at distant sites. Resection without clear margins has the potential to provide remaining tumor cells with a means of metastasizing as new blood vessels form during the healing process.

Antiangiogenic therapy shows promise as a strategy for cancer treatment (see "Treatment" below).

Tumors generally lack a well-formed lymphatic network, so communication of tumor cells with lymphatic channels occurs only at the tumor periphery and not within the tumor mass. Lymphatic dissemination and hematogenous dissemination occur in parallel. Tumors excrete acidlike enzymes that dissolve the basement membrane and break through to the lymphatics. Cancer cells can enter the bloodstream where lymph nodes drain into veins (e.g., lymphatic intersection with the subclavian vein).

Some controversy exists with regard to the role and risk of needle biopsy and risk for cancer recurrence and/or metastasis. Recurrence along the surgical pathway has been reported for some tumors.[29,117] It is hypothesized that this recurrence is the result of intraoperative seeding. Poorly planned biopsies or incomplete tumor resection increases the risk of local recurrence and metastasis. The biopsy tract should be excised when complete tumor removal occurs.

Clinical Manifestations of Metastasis

Metastatic spread usually occurs within 3 to 5 years after initial diagnosis and treatment of malignancy, although some low-grade lesions can reappear as much as 15 to 20 years later. It is therefore very important to conduct a thorough past medical history as part of any client interview. As mentioned before, metastases occur most commonly to areas of the body that provide an environment rich in nutrition to the colonized tumor cells, such as the lung, brain, liver, and bone; metastases can be found in other areas as well (e.g., the lymph nodes, skin, ovaries, and adrenal glands).

Pulmonary System (Lungs)

Pulmonary metastases are the most common of all metastatic tumors because venous drainage of most areas of the body is through the superior and inferior venae cavae into the heart, making the lungs the first organ to filter malignant cells. Parenchymal metastases are asymptomatic until tumor cells have obstructed bronchi, resulting in pulmonary symptoms, or until tumor cells have expanded and reached the parietal pleura where pain fibers are stimulated.

A dry, persistent cough is often the first symptom of pulmonary metastases. Pleural pain can indicate pleural invasion, and shortness of breath (dyspnea) usually occurs in the presence of a malignant pleural effusion. If hemoptysis occurs, there is usually bronchial tissue invasion either by a primary lung malignancy or metastatic disease.[359]

Hepatic System (Liver)

Liver metastases are among the most ominous signs of advanced cancer. The liver filters blood coming in from the gastrointestinal tract, making it a primary metastatic site for tumors of the stomach, colorectum, and pancreas. Symptoms include abdominal and/or right upper quadrant pain, general malaise and fatigue, anorexia, early satiety and weight loss, and sometimes low-grade fevers.

Skeletal System (Bone)

Bone is one of the three most favored sites of solid tumor metastasis, indicating that the bone microenvironment provides fertile ground for the growth of many tumors. Although lung, breast, and prostate are the three primary sites responsible for most metastatic bone disease,[384] tumors of the thyroid and kidney, lymphoma, and melanoma can also metastasize to the skeletal system.

Bone metastases may be the osteolytic type, marked by areas of decreased bone density, or osteoblastic, appearing as areas of dense scarring and increased bone density. Osteolytic metastases occur predominately from lung, kidney, and thyroid cancer; breast is primarily osteolytic but can be osteoblastic, and prostate is usually but not always osteoblastic. The axial skeleton is most commonly involved, with spread to the spine, pelvis, ribs, proximal femora, proximal humeri, and skull.[242]

The primary symptom associated with bone metastases is pain. Pain is usually deep and worsened by activity, especially weight bearing. Spinal metastases presents with pain, neurologic symptoms, and instability.[384] Disabling pathologic fractures, especially of the vertebral bodies and proximal ends of the long bones, may occur in up to one-half of people with osteolytic metastases and are sometimes one of the first signs of a malignant process.[143] Blastic lesions often result in an elevated serum alkaline phosphatase, whereas lytic lesions may not.[222]

Hypercalcemia (abnormally high concentration of blood calcium) is a frequent complication of neoplastic disease and is associated with bony metastases, particularly osteolytic lesions as a result of increased bone resorption. The presence of tumor cells in the bone disturbs the balance between new bone formation and bone resorption, resulting in abnormal bone remodeling.

Carcinoma cells secrete a variety of factors that stimulate tumor growth, as well as osteoclast recruitment and activation. Osteoclasts are bone cells that break down bone tissue. Although more than 80% of people with hypercalcemia have bony metastasis, the severity of the hypercalcemia does not correlate with the extent of the bony disease.

Assessment of risk for fracture in individuals with known metastasis to bone is often determined using a scoring system published by Mirel in 1989. The total score is based on the location of the lesion, degree of pain, type of lesion, and percentage of cortex involved. The higher the score (maximum of 12), the higher the risk for fracture.[233]

Hydration and administration of oral or intravenous bisphosphonates (e.g., alendronate [Fosamax], risedronate [Actonel], ibandronate [Boniva], zoledronate [Zometa]) are the mainstays of current treatment and have contributed to the decrease in the frequency of hypercalcemia and to minimizing or preventing bone loss. Bisphosphonates prevent thinning of the bone by inhibiting osteoclast function, thereby inhibiting bone resorption. There is no life-prolonging benefit with bisphosphonates, but there is a substantial reduction of morbidity (e.g., decreased pain, prevention of fracture and/or deformity) associated with bone metastases and improved quality of life (QOL).[45,75,91,342]

Central Nervous System

Brain. Many primary tumors may lead to CNS metastases. Lung carcinomas account for approximately one-half of all metastatic brain lesions. Breast carcinoma and malignant melanoma also commonly metastasize to the brain. Metastatic disease in the brain is life-threatening and emotionally debilitating. Metastatic brain tumors can increase intracranial pressure, obstruct the normal flow of cerebrospinal fluid, change mentation and contribute to cognitive impairment, and reduce sensory and motor function. The management of cognitive impairments is important, and the therapist can use the same strategies known for people with traumatic brain injury (see Chapter 33).

Clinical manifestations of brain metastases depend on the location, either in the brain or outside the brain in the bony cranium exerting compression externally. The therapist can look at CT scan results, see the location of pathologic conditions, and correlate these to signs and symptoms observed clinically (see Table 30-3). Primary tumors of the CNS rarely develop metastases outside the CNS despite the highly invasive capacity of these tumors. Microscopically, some CNS (brain) tumor cells (astrocytomas) may spread widely within the CNS but rarely metastasize outside it.

Tumor cells traveling from the lung via the pulmonary veins and carotid artery can result in metastases to the CNS. Lung cancer is the most common primary tumor to metastasize to the brain. Any neurologic sign may be the presentation of a silent lung tumor.[143]

Spinal Cord. Metastatic involvement of the vertebrae may result in epidural spinal (usually anterior) cord compression. In addition, severe, destructive osteolytic lesions can lead to fracture and fragility of one or more vertebral bodies. In such cases, compression of the cord occurs as a result of the subsequent deformity.[241] Spinal cord and nerve root compression cause either insidious or rapid loss of neurologic function. This compression phenomenon occurs in approximately 5% of people with systemic cancer and is most often caused by carcinoma of the lung, breast, prostate, or kidney. Lymphoma and multiple myeloma may also result in spinal cord and nerve root compression.

The earliest neurologic symptoms include gradual onset of distal weakness and sensory changes, including numbness, paresthesias, and coldness. The incidence of permanent motor dysfunction has markedly decreased in the past 2 decades because of earlier diagnosis and treatment.[91] The client who presents with spinal cord symptoms caused by metastatic epidural disease and resultant compression may have only transient symptoms with proper medical treatment. More than 95% of people with spinal cord compression complain of progressive central or radicular back pain often aggravated by recumbency, weight bearing, sneezing, coughing, or Valsalva maneuver. Sitting often relieves it. Later symptoms may include a major change or loss of bowel or bladder function, which is considered by many as a serious condition requiring immediate assessment for possible spinal stabilization.

Lymphatic System

Previous cancer-related surgery or adverse effects involving radiation fibrosis can affect the lymph nodes and may result in dysfunction of the lymphatic system presenting as lymphedema. It has a wide range of onset from weeks to years from the initial insult to the lymphatic system. The therapist may be the first health care professional to recognize subtle abnormalities or changes in the extremities. See further discussion in Chapter 13.

Diagnosis of Metastasis

Metastases usually reproduce the cellular structure of the primary growth well enough to enable a pathologist to determine the site of the primary tumor. For example, bone metastases from a carcinoma of the thyroid not only exhibit a microscopic structure similar to the original tumor but also may produce thyroid hormone. Sometimes, symptoms of a cancer will present in the metastatic site rather than the site of origin (primary site). If the primary tumor cannot be found, the malignant tissue is called *carcinoma of unknown primary*. Special histologic stains can be done on the unknown tissue and compared to slides of a previous malignancy to determine similarity.

Cancer Recurrence

Disease-free survival describes the time between diagnosis and recurrence or relapse. Recurrences may be local, regional, disseminated, or a combination of these. The most important predictors of recurrent cancer are the stage at the time of initial therapy and histologic findings. Recurrence of cancer may be first recognized by the return of systemic symptoms associated with paraneoplastic phenomena. The metabolic or toxic effects of the syndrome (e.g., hypercalcemia or hyponatremia) may constitute a more urgent hazard to life than the underlying cancer.

CLINICAL MANIFESTATIONS
Local and Systemic Effects

In their earliest stages, most cancers are asymptomatic but treatable if found. Primary site cancers cause certain symptoms that are recognizable causes for suspicion or concern. For example, endometrial cancer causes abnormal bleeding so often that it is usually detected in its early stages. Laryngeal cancer causes hoarseness, which is also an early sign. Conversely, lung cancer is usually quite extensive before it causes enough symptoms to warrant investigation, similarly, breast cancer or tumors deep to the chest wall may also be difficult to palpate and therefore not detected. Current imaging techniques including computed tomography (CT), magnetic resonance imaging (MRI), and positron emission tomography (PET) allow for early detection and therapeutic intervention.

As cancer progresses, symptoms characteristic of the involved organ or tissue may start to develop. With advanced cancer, nausea, vomiting, and retching accompanied by anorexia and subsequent weight loss are common as a result of the malignant process and its treatment. Nausea, vomiting, and retching is especially prevalent in association with lung carcinoma, hypernephroma, and pancreatic carcinoma.

Anorexia has been attributed to tumor production of TNF, which is a polypeptide protein (a cytokine) also called *cachectin*. TNFs are thought to play an important role in mediating inflammation and cytotoxic reactions (along with interleukins). TNFs produce necrosis of tumor cells by eliminating the blood supply to these growths. Small amounts of TNF are beneficial in promoting wound healing and preventing tumors, but uncontrolled production is accompanied by symptoms of fever, weight loss, and tissue damage that can cause more problems than the benefits provided.

Cancer-related anorexia/cachexia is a complex phenomenon in which metabolic abnormalities, proinflammatory cytokines produced by the host immune system, circulating tumor-derived catabolic factors, decreased food intake, and possibly other unknown factors all contribute. Profound muscle loss is prominent in cancer-related anorexia/cachexia syndrome as a result of decreased protein synthesis and abnormal muscle proteolysis.

Later, rapid growth of the tumor encroaches on healthy tissue, causing destruction, necrosis, ulceration, and hemorrhage resulting in many local and systemic effects. Pain may occur as a late symptom caused by infiltration, compression, or destruction of nerves. With advanced or stage IV cancer, the host presents systemically with muscular weakness, anemia, and coagulation disorders such as granulocyte and platelet abnormalities. See "Disorders of Hemostasis and Thrombocytopenia" in Chapter 14.

Pyrexia or fever may be seen with cancer in the absence of infection and is produced either by white blood cells inducing a pyrogen (an agent that causes fever) or by direct tumor production of a pyrogen. Continued spread of the cancer may lead to gastrointestinal, pulmonary, or vascular obstruction. Secondary infections frequently occur as a result of the host's decreased immunity and can lead to death.

Other vital organs may be affected, such as the brain, in which increased intracranial pressure by tumor cells can cause strokelike symptoms. In addition to the local effects of tumor growth, cancer can produce systemic signs and symptoms that are not direct effects of either the tumor or its metastases (e.g., paraneoplastic syndromes or fever with renal cancer).

Cancer Pain

Overview

One of the most common symptoms of cancer is pain, affecting between 50% and 70% of clients in its early stages and 60% to 90% of clients in late stages of the disease. It is estimated that 1.1 million Americans experience cancer-related pain annually.[71] Alternately stated, pain occurs in approximately one-quarter of adults with newly diagnosed malignancies, one-third of individuals undergoing treatment, and three-quarters of all people with advanced disease.[139,352]

Depression and anxiety may increase the person's perception of pain or may be the result of the cancer pain. Symptoms often go unreported or underreported because clients are reluctant to take the pain medication prescribed. An unfounded fear of tolerance, addiction, or adverse effects from pain medication may result in underreporting of painful symptoms with subsequent inadequate cancer pain control and unnecessary pain-induced loss of function. Likewise, physicians may hesitate to provide adequate pain medications based on this misconception of client addiction.

Etiology and Pathogenesis

The cause of cancer pain is multifaceted, and the characteristics of the pain depend on the tissue structure, as well as on the mechanisms involved (Table 9-3). Some pain is caused by pressure on nerves or by the displacement of nerves. Microscopic infiltration of nerves by tumor cells can result in continuous, sharp, stabbing pain generally following the pattern of nerve distribution. Ischemic pain (throbbing) may also result from interference with blood supply or from blockage within hollow organs.

A common cause of cancer pain is metastasis of cancer to bone. Lung, breast, prostate, thyroid, and the lymphatics are the primary sites responsible for most metastatic bone disease. Bone metastasis results in increased release of prostaglandins and cytokines and subsequent bone destruction caused by breakdown and resorption. Bone pain may be mild to intense. Movement, weight bearing,

Table 9-3	Common Patterns of Pain Referral	
Pain Mechanism	**Lesion Site**	**Referral Site**
Somatic	C7, T1-5 vertebrae	Interscapular area, posterior shoulder
	Shoulder	Neck, upper back
	L1, L2 vertebrae	Sacroiliac joint and hip
	Hip joint	SI and knee
	Pharynx	Ipsilateral ear
	TMJ	Head, neck, heart
Visceral	Diaphragmatic irritation	Shoulder, lumbar spine
	Heart	Shoulder, neck, upper back, TMJ
	Urothelial tract	Back, inguinal region, anterior thigh, and genitalia
	Pancreas, liver, spleen, gallbladder	Shoulder, midthoracic, or low back
	Peritoneal or abdominal cavity (inflammatory or infectious process)	Hip pain from abscess of psoas or obturator muscle
Neuropathic	Nerve or plexus	Anywhere in distribution of a peripheral nerve
	Nerve root	Anywhere in corresponding dermatome
	Central nervous system	Anywhere in region of body innervated by damaged structure

SI, Sacroiliac; *TMJ*, temporomandibular joint; *CNS*, central nervous system.
From Goodman CC, Snyder TE: Differential diagnosis for the physical therapist: Screening for referral, ed 5, Philadelphia, 2013, Saunders.

and ambulation exacerbate painful symptoms from bone destruction. Pathologic fractures with resultant muscle spasms can develop; in the case of vertebral involvement, nerve pain may also occur.

Pain may also result from diagnostic or therapeutic procedures such as surgery, radiation therapy, or chemotherapy (e.g., mucositis, stomatitis, esophageal inflammation, localized skin burns; see Table 9-7).

Clinical Manifestations

Signs and symptoms accompanying mild-to-moderate superficial pain may include hypertension, tachycardia, and tachypnea (rapid, shallow breathing) as the result of a sympathetic nervous system response. In severe or visceral pain, a parasympathetic nervous system response is more characteristic, with hypotension, bradycardia, nausea, vomiting, tachypnea, weakness, or fainting.

Spinal cord compression from metastases may present as radicular back pain, leg weakness, and unilateral loss of bowel or bladder control. Back pain may precede the development of neurologic signs and symptoms. The presence of jaundice in association with an atypical presentation of back pain may indicate hepatobiliary obstruction and/or liver metastasis. Signs of nerve root compression may be the first indication of a cancer, in particular, lymphoma, multiple myeloma, or cancer of the lung, breast, prostate, or kidney. Other neurologic or musculoskeletal manifestations of neoplasm are discussed in Paraneoplastic Syndromes" that follows.

Immobility and inflammation can lead to pain. Inflammation with its accompanying symptoms of redness, edema, pain, heat, and loss of function may progress to infection, necrosis, and sloughing of tissue. If the inflammatory process alone is present, the pain is characterized by tenderness. Pain may be excruciating in the presence of tissue necrosis and sloughing.

Pain Control

Pain management and control may depend on its underlying etiology. For example, epidural metastases with impending spinal cord compression require treatment with steroids, radiation, chemotherapy, or neurosurgery. Abdominal pain caused by obstruction of the hollow organs requires evaluation for surgical intervention.[92]

Treatment approaches depend on whether the individual is experiencing acute or chronic pain. The hope is to begin by gaining control of the pain during the acute phase and then to sustain that pain relief while minimizing side effects.

Pain should be screened, assessed, and managed according to clinical practice guidelines. Clinical practice guidelines for the treatment of cancer-related pain in adults outlining the process of screening, evaluation, and intervention have been published by the National Comprehensive Cancer Network (NCCN).[251] A similar clinical practice guideline is available from the NCCN for pediatric cancer pain[249] and one for senior adult oncology.[250]

Before starting therapy, the physician determines the underlying pain mechanism and diagnoses the pain syndrome. Pain control measures used include narcotic and nonnarcotic analgesics; chemotherapy or radiation therapy or both; surgery; nerve blocks; or other more invasive pain control measures, such as intraspinal, rhizotomy, or cordotomy. Newer drugs, such as the bisphosphonates, have been useful in the treatment of refractory bone pain.[71]

Opioids. Appropriate opioid selection may be difficult and depends on the individual's pain intensity and any current analgesic therapy. Morphine, hydromorphone, fentanyl, and oxycodone are the opioids commonly used in the United States. A balance between analgesia and side effects might be achieved by changing to an equivalent dose of an alternative opioid. This approach, known as *opioid rotation*, is now a widely accepted technique used to address poorly responsive pain.[251]

Several methods of continuous infusion that are widely used in clinical practice include "around the clock," "as needed," and "patient-controlled analgesia" (PCA). Around the clock dosing is provided to chronic pain patients for continuous pain relief. A "rescue dose" should be provided as a subsequent treatment for individuals receiving these controlled-release medications. Rescue doses of short-acting opioids should be provided for pain that is not relieved by sustained/controlled-release opioids.

Opioids administered on an as-needed basis are for individuals who have intermittent pain with pain-free intervals. The as-needed method is also used when rapid dose escalation is required.

The PCA technique allows a person to control a device that delivers a bolus of analgesic "on demand" (according to and limited by parameters set by a physician). This system permits the person to self-administer a premeasured dose of analgesic by pressing a button that activates a pump syringe containing the analgesic. Small intermittent doses of the analgesic administered via intravenous (IV) line maintain blood levels that ensure comfort and minimize the risk of oversedation. Clinical studies report that people using PCA effectively maintain comfort without oversedation and use less drug than the amount normally given by intramuscular injection.

Nonpharmacologics. Nonpharmacologic modalities, such as massage, simple-touch,[197] acupuncture, imagery/hypnosis, reflexology, relaxation training, and other forms of complementary therapies, are recognized as part of integrative oncology used to manage procedural pain and distress and improve mood even among children, especially when fear, anxiety, and tension heighten pain perception.[15,92,197,214,312]

Whereas severe cancer pain is treated pharmaceutically, mild to moderate joint and muscle pain can be addressed by the rehabilitation professional. Pain elimination through the use of medication may not be possible without accompanying severe loss of function, which is an undesirable outcome.

Massage

Much debate exists about the safety and efficacy of massage therapy for individuals with cancer, especially anyone with lymphedema or at risk for developing lymphedema.[80] A review of data included in the Cochrane Database of Systematic Reviews suggests that conventional care for people with cancer can safely incorporate massage therapy, although individuals with cancer may be at higher risk for adverse events. There is no evidence that massage therapy can spread cancer, although direct pressure over a tumor is usually discouraged.[80]

The strongest evidence for the benefits of massage is stress and anxiety reduction. Research regarding the use of massage for pain control and management of other symptoms is promising. Massage therapists may advocate the use of massage to reduce constipation, improve immune system function, help promote postoperative wound healing, and reduce scar tissue formation, as well as to help release metabolic waste by improving circulation. Published trials for these indications have not been reported.[80]

Modifications to massage (e.g., lighten pressure or avoid deep tissue massage) may be necessary to prevent potential harm such as bleeding, fracture, or increased pain when individuals with cancer receiving massage have a coagulation disorder (low platelet count or when receiving warfarin/heparin/aspirin therapy). Similar precautions are required for anyone with cancer metastases to the bones. Massage should be avoided over open or healing wounds or radiation dermatitis.[80]

Physical Agents

Michelle H. Cameron, MD, PT, OC.S

Empirical evidence regarding the use of various modalities and physical agents with cancer patients is not available to support the indication/contraindication or efficacy of these agents at this time. Future targeted research and clinical investigations may aid in producing consensus or even clinical practice guidelines.

Various forms of electric, electromagnetic, and other biophysical energy sources have beneficial physiologic effects on tissue and therefore the potential to relieve some of the symptoms and side effects of cancer; these modalities are not meant to treat the cancer. However, because physical modalities have the capacity to break down cell membrane barriers and stimulate changes in transmembrane potentials (potentially triggering growth and development of abnormal tissue), there is the potential for providing conditions that could favor cancer growth and metastases. This topic remains confusing and controversial.[85]

The use of ultrasound and transcutaneous electrical stimulation for the treatment of pain associated with cancer and/or cancer treatment remains under investigation.[305,322] At the present time, the application of therapeutic ultrasound (especially continuous ultrasound) or electrical stimulation over tumors is contraindicated, presumably because it is thought that there is an increased risk of metastasis.[354] Studies conducted on mice have shown that a tumor given large doses of ultrasound will spread because of increasing blood supply to the area.[164,204,220,332]

Low-level laser treatment has been approved by the FDA for the treatment of breast cancer-related lymphedema. The laser-beam pulses produce photochemical reactions at the cellular level, thereby increasing shoulder motion and scar mobility while also reducing limb volume of the affected arm, extracellular fluid, and tissue hardness.[57,102,221,264] The effect of low-level laser on melanoma has been studied in mice with the conclusion that the use of this modality should be avoided over melanomas as melanoma tumor growth was significantly increased.[215]

Manufacturers of laser equipment suggest that a history of carcinoma is a contraindication for the use of Class 3 laser. Information is lacking regarding the use of Class 1 laser. When considering the method of action of the laser (increased transport across the mitochondrial barrier), prior carcinoma is a contraindication in the use of laser. Research in this area is needed and evidence provided before safe recommendations can be developed with any measure of confidence.

Additional references related to laser in the treatment of lymphedema are available.[5,38,42,43,58,102,129,187,192,200] For other expert opinions, go to http://www.cancer.org/treatment/treatmentsandsideeffects/complementaryandalternativemedicine/manualhealingandphysicaltouch/transcutaneous-electrical-nerve-stimulation and http://www.oncolink.org/experts/article.cfm?id=2241.

A THERAPIST'S THOUGHTS*
Modalities for the Oncologic Patient

Many other noninvasive physical agents, including thermotherapy, electrical stimulation, diathermy, lasers and light, and ultrasound are often considered for pain management; however, because all of these agents may increase circulation and promote cell function, growth, and replication, their use in individuals with cancer or a history of cancer is controversial. There are no studies in humans evaluating the effects of these physical agents on tumor growth or metastasis, but given the concern for such adverse effects, such studies could not be performed ethically. However, the few studies demonstrating increased rates of tumor growth and metastasis with the application of therapeutic ultrasound in animals support this concern.[332,333]

Although the mechanism of action of physical agents suggests that their use may be safe if not used over an area where cancer is present, the very nature of cancer is that it can metastasize to other areas and therefore the clinician cannot know with certainty where cancer is or is not. Many clinicians avoid the use of physical agents in patients for 5 years after the patient has had cancer. Although this approach has appeal as most cancers do not recur after 5 years, given the variability in recurrence patterns for different malignancies it is recommended that the clinician discuss the potential risks and benefits of using a physical agent in anyone with a history of cancer at any time in their life.

One exception commonly made to the contraindication for using physical agents in patients with a history of cancer is during hospice or palliative care where the priority is patient comfort over survival. In such circumstances, physical agents may provide pain relief with fewer and less severe side effects than medications and are sometimes used in place of, to supplement, or to allow lower doses of analgesic medications.

We all want to help our patients feel better. We often use physical agents to achieve this. Physical agents reduce pain and can promote tissue healing. However, in the person with cancer, or a history of cancer, I worry. I worry that despite helping the patient feel better now, I may, conceivably, be contributing to cancer growth, metastasis, or recurrence. I know the evidence is very limited but still, I worry. I wonder, is the benefit worth the risk? I don't know. None of us really knows. We don't know how great the benefit will be. We don't know the level of risk. We each get to decide, together with our patients, what makes the most sense in a specific circumstance. For me, the risk is rarely worth it. I recognize that physical agents can help but there's no going back if cancer recurs, and there's no knowing why it did.

*Michelle H. Cameron, MD, PT, OCS

Neuropathic Pain. People with cancer may also experience pain because of nerve damage. This damage can be caused directly by tumor invasion or indirectly as a side effect of cytotoxic drug therapy (e.g., taxanes or platinum agents). The treatment of neuropathic pain remains a dilemma because conventional analgesic drugs do not always provide relief.

Recommended treatment for neuropathic pain includes infrared (Anodyne), antidepressant drugs (e.g., amitriptyline); antiepileptics (e.g., carbamazepine and gabapentin); and steroids (e.g., methylprednisolone and dexamethasone). Pain relief is usually not immediate, and the drugs used must be taken continuously; thus side effects, such as sedation and bone marrow depression, can be additional problems.[71,161] Many people seek alternative therapies such as Reiki, acupuncture, BodyTalk, TouchTherapy, and craniosacral therapy for relief from neuropathies.

Management of pain in people with cancer who live in long-term care facilities remains an ongoing concern. Consistent, daily pain is prevalent among nursing home residents with cancer and is frequently untreated, particularly among older and minority clients.[41] For individuals with difficult-to-control chronic pain, complementary therapies can help even if it is only to reduce the level of analgesics required to maintain pain control.

Cancer-Related Fatigue

Much has been written about cancer-related fatigue (CRF) and its impact on clients. CRF is a distressing, persistent, and subjective sense of tiredness or exhaustion related to cancer or cancer treatment that is not proportional to recent activity and interferes with usual functioning.[252] CRF syndrome is a collection of symptoms with multiple characteristics and problems. Fatigue is a nearly universal symptom in all people receiving chemotherapy, radiotherapy, and treatment with biologic response modifiers; reduced physical performance and fatigue are universal after bone marrow transplantation.

Up to 30% of cancer survivors report a loss of energy for years after cessation of treatment. For many people with cancer, fatigue is severe and imposes limitations on normal daily activities.[60] Many people's perceptions are that fatigue is more distressing than pain or nausea and vomiting, which can be managed with medication for most clients.

Fatigue should be screened, assessed, and managed according to clinical practice guidelines, which have been published for CRF.[252] All individuals should be screened for fatigue at their initial visit, at regular intervals during and after cancer treatment, and as clinically indicated. Fatigue should be recognized, evaluated, monitored, documented, and treated promptly for all age groups, at all stages of disease, during and after treatment. Clients and their families should be informed that management of fatigue is an integral part of total health care.[252]

Using a numeric rating scale, fatigue can be rated as mild (1-3), moderate (4-6), or severe (7-10).[287,323] Children can be asked whether they are "tired" or "not tired." Fatigue that causes distress or interferes with daily activities or functioning should be treated according to its severity and the presence of other treatable factors known to contribute to fatigue (e.g., pain, emotional distress, sleep disturbance, anemia, nutritional deficits, deconditioning, and comorbidities).

Clients should be reassured that treatment-related fatigue is not necessarily an indicator of disease progression. It may be the result of anemia, deconditioning, or the presence of certain cytokines (e.g., interleukin [IL]-1, IL-6, or TNF-α). There may be contributing psychosocial factors such as anxiety, depression, and disrupted sleep pattern.

Despite the prevalence of CRF, the exact mechanisms involved in its pathophysiology are unknown. Abnormal accumulation of muscle metabolites, production of cytokines, changes in neuromuscular function, abnormalities in adenosine triphosphate (ATP) synthesis, serotonin dysregulation, and vagal afferent activation are just a few more of the proposed theories. Comorbidities, such as cardiopulmonary impairments, may put an individual at greater risk for fatigue.[252]

Likewise, the cause of fatigue in posttreatment disease-free individuals is unclear and likely multifactorial. Higher serum markers, such as interleukin-1 receptor antagonist (IL-1ra) and soluble TNF type II (sTNF-RII), and lower cortisol levels have been observed in fatigued cancer survivors compared with nonfatigued survivors. Significantly higher levels of circulating T lymphocytes have also been observed in fatigued survivors. These findings together point to a chronic inflammatory process involving T cells as a possible fatigue-inducing mechanism.[252]

Additional clinical practice recommendations published by the NCCN on adolescent, young adult and senior adult oncology care are available from the NCCN website.[249,250]

Paraneoplastic Syndromes

Overview and Definition

In addition to the local effects of tumor growth, cancer can produce systemic signs and symptoms that are not direct effects of either the tumor or its metastases. When tumors produce signs and symptoms at a site distant from the tumor or its metastasized sites, these remote effects of malignancy are collectively referred to as *paraneoplastic syndromes.*

Although malignant cells frequently lose the function, appearance, and properties associated with the normal cells of the tissue of origin, they can acquire in some cases new cellular functions uncharacteristic of the originating tissue. Many of these syndromes involve ectopic hormone production by tumor cells or the secretion of biochemically active substances that cause metabolic abnormalities. For example, tumors in nonendocrine tissues sometimes acquire the ability to produce and secrete hormones that are distributed by the circulation and act on target organs at a site other than the location of the tumor. The most common hormone-secreting tumor associated with paraneoplastic syndromes is small cell cancer of the lung, which can produce adrenocorticotropic hormone (ACTH) in amounts sufficient to cause Cushing syndrome.

Malignancy is often associated with a wide variety of musculoskeletal disorders, which may be the presenting symptoms of an occult tumor. Although musculoskeletal symptoms often result from direct invasion by the malignancy or its metastases into bone, joints, or soft tissue, they may also occur without invasion as a result of the paraneoplastic disorders, including well-recognized syndromes, as well as less well defined disorders referred to as *cancer arthritis*.[350]

Incidence

Previously, paraneoplastic syndromes occurred in 10% to 20% of all cancer clients, but this figure may be increasing because of greater physician awareness and the availability of serodiagnostic tests for some syndromes. Neurologic paraneoplastic syndromes are rare, occurring in 1% to 2% of people with malignancy, but physical therapists are often treating these individuals because of the neuromuscular and musculoskeletal manifestations.

Etiology and Pathogenesis

The causes of paraneoplastic syndromes are not well understood, but the following four groups of mechanisms and their effects have been identified:

- A variety of vasoactive tumor products (e.g., serotonin, histamine, catecholamines, prostaglandins, and vasoactive peptides), which usually occur in the small bowel and less commonly in the lung or stomach.
- The destruction of normal tissues by tumor, such as occurs when osteolytic skeletal metastases cause hypercalcemia.
- Unknown mechanisms, such as unidentified tumor products or circulating immune complexes stimulated by the tumor (e.g., osteoarthropathy as a result of bronchogenic carcinoma).
- Autoantibodies (antibodies directed against the host's tissue), for example, cancer cells, produce antibodies that impair presynaptic calcium channel activity, hindering the release of the neurotransmitter acetylcholine, resulting in muscle weakness.

There is increasing evidence that many of the neurologic paraneoplastic syndromes appear to be an immune reaction against antigens shared by the cancer and the nervous system. The immune response is triggered by and directed against the tumor, which then cross-reacts with protein expressed by the peripheral or central nervous system. Consequently, any part of the nervous system can be affected.[122,213]

Clinical Manifestations

The paraneoplastic syndromes are of considerable clinical importance because they may accompany relatively limited neoplastic growth and provide an early clue to the presence of certain types of cancer. Nonspecific symptoms, such as skin changes, neurologic changes, anorexia, malaise, diarrhea, weight loss, and fever, may be the first clinical manifestations of a paraneoplastic syndrome. Even these types of nonspecific symptoms occur as a result of the production of specific biochemical products by the tumor itself.

Paraneoplastic syndromes with musculoskeletal manifestations are listed in Table 9-4. Gradual, progressive muscle weakness may develop over a period of weeks to months. The proximal muscles (especially of the pelvic girdle) are most likely to be involved; the weakness does stabilize. Reflexes of the involved extremities are present but diminished. Proximal leg weakness seen in Lambert-Eaton myasthenic syndrome is most often associated with small cell carcinoma of the lung. Diagnosis is made by needle electromyography and has a characteristic "dive bomber" sound upon insertion of the needle into a muscle. Additional blood studies assist in further diagnosis and differentiation from myasthenia gravis, a related disorder.

Muscular, neurologic, and cutaneous disorders associated with malignancy are presented in Table 9-5. Many of these conditions can occur in association with or in the absence of underlying malignant disease. The appearance of any of these conditions requires a full medical evaluation but does not guarantee that a tumor will be found. Early tumor recognition, before metastasis occurs, may improve survival rates. Myositis may precede, follow, or arise concurrently with the malignancy and tends to occur most often in older people. Paraneoplastic dermatoses are a large group of paraneoplastic syndromes that may be associated with an internal malignancy.[358]

Carcinoma Polyarthritis. There may be rheumatologic symptoms referred to as *carcinoma polyarthritis*. This condition can be differentiated from rheumatoid arthritis by the presence of asymmetric joint involvement, involvement of primarily the lower extremity (although symmetric involvement of the hands has

Table 9-4	Paraneoplastic Syndromes: Rheumatologic Associations and Clinical Features	
Malignancy	**Rheumatologic Associations**	**Clinical Features**
Lung cancer, particularly small cell lung cancer	Lambert-Eaton myasthenic syndrome (LEMS)	Proximal leg weakness
Lymphoproliferative disease (leukemia)	Vasculitis	Necrotizing vasculitis
Plasma cell dyscrasia	Cryoglobulinemia	Vasculitis, Raynaud's disease, arthralgia, neurologic symptoms
Hodgkin disease	Immune complex disease	Nephrotic syndrome
Ovarian cancer	Complex regional pain syndrome	Palmar fasciitis and polyarthritis
Carcinoid syndrome	Scleroderma	Scleroderma-like changes: anterior tibia
Colon cancer	Pyogenic arthritis	Enteric bacteria cultured from joint
Mesenchymal tumors	Osteogenic osteomalacia	Bone pain, stress fractures
Renal cell cancer	Severe Raynaud's phenomenon	Digital necrosis (and other tumors)
Pancreatic cancer	Panniculitis	Subcutaneous nodules, especially males

been reported),[350] explosive onset, late age of onset, and the presence of malignancy and arthritis together. Neurologic paraneoplastic syndromes are of unknown cause and include subacute cerebellar degeneration, amyotrophic lateral sclerosis, sensory or sensorimotor peripheral neuropathy, Guillain-Barré syndrome, myasthenia gravis, and the Lambert-Eaton myasthenic syndrome.

Stiff-Person Syndrome. Isolated cases of paraneoplastic stiff-person syndrome have been reported in association with small cell lung cancer, thymoma (thymus), melanoma, breast adenocarcinoma, and graft versus host disease.[176,255,288] Women are affected twice as often as men, most likely because of the association with breast cancer. Paraneoplastic stiff-person syndrome is characterized by progressive symptoms of neuropathy or myelopathy with increased muscle tone and rigidity in the spine and lower extremities, especially the ankle dorsiflexors with loss of ankle motion.[154,244]

The disease may take years to manifest but in some individuals, symptoms develop over a period of weeks. The first symptom may be a persistent progressive stiffening of the back or leg that is triggered by sudden noise, touch, or fatigue or made worse by stress such as time pressure (e.g., hurrying to cross a street). Stiffness progresses to hypertonia, spasm, and then severe, painful rigidity, postural abnormalities, and musculoskeletal deformities. Walking becomes difficult, and the individual is at increased risk for unprotected falls (i.e., they fall like a tin soldier). Symptoms are greatly relieved during sleep.

Although rare, this condition has been encountered by therapists in an oncology practice.[154] Stiff-person syndrome is normally associated with a viral cause, such as meningitis or encephalitis, but in the case of cancer-induced stiff-person syndrome, it is chemically induced by the tumor, classifying it as a paraneoplastic syndrome.[176] It is seen more often in clients with a history of diabetes and other autoimmune diseases (e.g., hyperthyroidism, hypothyroidism, or anemia).[244]

Diagnosis of stiff-man syndrome is made by physical examination and immunocytochemistry methods demonstrating the presence of anti-GAD (glutamic acid decarboxylase) autoantibodies in the blood. Diagnosis may be confirmed by a positive response to medications used to treat this condition (e.g., benzodiazepines).

Physical therapy may have a role in the management of this disease,[154,293] as these patients/clients need to be taught how to properly stretch and maintain joint mobility as a lifelong commitment. Physical therapy interventions may include ultrasound, soft tissue mobilizations, manual stretching, and exercise. The therapist may need to assess for home adaptations, orthoses, and the need for durable medical equipment.[154]

MEDICAL MANAGEMENT

DIAGNOSIS, TREATMENT, AND PROGNOSIS
Serodiagnostic tests are available for some paraneoplastic syndromes, and characteristic abnormalities in MRI have been identified in association with neurologic paraneoplastic syndromes. Biochemical markers in urine provide specific monitoring of the response of bone metastases to treatment. This early diagnosis of paraneoplastic syndromes provides for prevention of tumor progression and subsequent problems such as bone pain, fracture, and hypercalcemia. In the case of cancer polyarthritis, the absence of rheumatoid nodules, absence of rheumatoid factor, and absence of family history of rheumatoid disease help in the diagnostic process.

Paraneoplastic syndromes usually parallel the course of the disease. Treatment of the tumor leads to regression of the syndrome (especially the cutaneous dermatoses). In some cases, the condition is related more to the amount of antibody present rather than the amount of tumor volume. Some of the cutaneous paraneoplastic syndromes will respond to specific measures, such as systemic corticosteroid therapy, but for the most part, successful resolution requires eradication of the underlying malignancy.

MEDICAL MANAGEMENT OF CANCER

Prevention and Survivorship

The goal of *Healthy People 2020* is to reduce the number of new cancer cases, as well as the illness, disability, and death caused by cancer.[367] There are 20 specific objectives listed under cancer in the *Healthy People* 2020 summary of objectives. Two objectives specifically target survivorship and quality of life:

- C-13 Increase the proportion of cancer survivors who are living years or longer after diagnosis
  Target: 72.8%; Baseline: 66.2% of persons with cancer were living 5 years or longer after diagnosis in 2007. Target setting method: 10% improvement.
- C-14 (Developmental) Increase mental and physical health-related quality of life of cancer survivors.

Evidence suggests that several types of cancer can be prevented and that the prospects for surviving cancer continue to improve. The ACS estimates that half of all cancer deaths in the United States could be prevented if

Table 9-5	Muscular, Neurologic, and Cutaneous Disorders Associated with Malignancy
Muscular	**Cutaneous**
Amyloidosis	Acanthosis (diffuse thickening)
Amyotrophic lateral sclerosis	Dermatomyositis
Polymyositis	Extramammary Paget's disease
Lambert-Eaton myasthenic syndrome (LEMS)	Nigricans (blackish discoloration; changes in skin pigmentation)
Myasthenia gravis	Pemphigus vulgaris (water blisters)
Metabolic myopathies	
Primary neuropathic diseases	Pruritus (itching)
Type II muscle atrophy	Pyoderma gangrenosum (eruption of skin ulcers)
	Reactive erythemas (skin redness)

Data from Gilkeson GS, Caldwell DS: Rheumatologic associations with malignancy. *J Musculoskelet Med* 7(1):70, 1990; Cohen PR: Cutaneous paraneoplastic syndromes. *Am Fam Physician* 50:1273-1282, 1994.

Americans adopted a healthier lifestyle and made better use of available screening tests.[290]

The ability to reduce cancer death rates depends in part on the existence and application of various types of resources. *First,* the means to provide culturally and linguistically appropriate information on prevention, early detection, and treatment to the public and to health care professionals are essential. *Second,* mechanisms or systems must exist for providing people with access to state-of-the-art preventive services and treatment. *Third,* a mechanism for maintaining continued research progress and for fostering new research is essential. Personalized prevention may become a tool in the future thanks to desktop oncology in the postgenome era of research.

Desktop oncology refers to the genomics data produced by high technology. Desktop oncology provides knowledge on demand to anyone regarding cancer-related biomarkers. Combining genetic screening for cancer predisposition in the general population and selecting individualized targeted chemoprevention may dramatically improve cancer rates in the future.[186]

Primary Prevention

Prevention is the first key to the *management* of cancer. Epigenetics may be the first step in the *prevention* of cancer. Primary prevention may include *screening* to identify high-risk people and subsequent reduction or elimination of modifiable risk factors (e.g., tobacco use, diet high in unsaturated fats and low in fiber, and sun or radiation exposure). Physical activity and weight control also can contribute to cancer prevention.

Epigenetics is a relatively new science that has brought to light the control we have as individuals on whether or not cancer develops in our bodies. Epigenetics is the study of long-lasting changes in gene *function* that do not necessarily involve changes in gene *structure.* Scientists are beginning to understand through the study of epigenetics how nutrients and certain drugs can change the way cells age, reproduce, and ultimately die. Epigenetics addresses ways we can block the formation and progression of cancer cells through nutrigenomics and chemoprevention.

Nutrigenomics. Nutrigenomics is a new field seeking to identify ways to prevent cancer through the impact of nutrition on gene structure and stability. Research is focusing on the impact of food, nutrition, obesity, and physical activity on the cancer process as the genetic message in the DNA code is translated into RNA and then into protein synthesis leading to metabolic processes.[212,368] Gene sequencing and function as well as changes in DNA sequence and modulation of oxidative stress in response to foods and beverages are an area of future research focus in nutrigenomics.[84,311,393]

Studying older adults who do not develop cancer may help identify the genetic changes associated with age-resistant protective mechanisms. Genetic information that can be used to improve disease prevention strategies is emerging for many cancers and may provide the foundation for improved effectiveness in clinical and preventive medicine services.

Even though we know that healthy everyday choices can reduce our chances of getting cancer, it is recognized that in the current American cultural environment, it is difficult for many people to make healthy choices. Far too often, the unhealthy choice is the choice that is more convenient, more affordable, and more socially accepted. For those who are interested in more information in this area, the *Policy and Action for Cancer Prevention* examines the factors—economic, environmental, and social—that influence what we eat and how much we move. The success of studies that have been designed to change our behaviors and thus our risk of cancer are available.[393]

Chemoprevention. Chemoprevention, the use of agents to inhibit and reverse cancer, has focused on diet-derived agents. Chemoprevention is effective in inhibiting the onset of cancer by eliminating premalignant cells and blocking the progression of normal cells into invasive tumors in experimental animal models. The transferability of similar results to humans remains under investigation.[177,229]

More than 40 promising agents and agent combinations (e.g., green and black tea phenols, lycopene, soy isoflavones, vitamins D and E, selenium, and calcium) are being evaluated clinically as chemopreventive agents for major cancer targets, including breast, prostate, colon, and lung cancer.[20,188,203] In addition, low-dose aspirin intake and nonsteroidal antiinflammatory drug (NSAID) intake have shown promising results in the prevention of gastrointestinal, endometrial, pancreatic, and other cancers.[48,66,67] Chemoprevention is intended to stop a cancer before it ever reaches a size that could alter the body's homeostasis, cause symptoms, or be detected.

Cancer Vaccine. (See previous discussion of cancer vaccines in "Pathogenesis" above.) Two types of *cancer vaccine* (prophylactic and therapeutic) are being investigated in clinical studies, although currently no known specific immunization prevents cancer in general. With therapeutic vaccines, the person's own tumor cells are obtained during surgery, irradiated to inactivate them, and then reinfused. This stimulates the immune system to react and make antibodies against these specific cells. The vaccine specifically evokes the activity of immune-surveillance cells to find the specified cancer cells and send killer T cells to directly target and destroy tumors in all vaccine recipients. Immunologic memory can be created so that if the cancer recurs, the immune system will respond before it becomes widespread.[103,321] A vaccine given on an outpatient basis would be less dangerous than surgery and less toxic than other cancer treatments such as chemotherapy and radiation therapy. Right now, efforts to develop such vaccines have been hampered by the fact that cancer cells seem to have the ability to evade immune-surveillance cells (see "Tumor Evasion Strategies" above).

Secondary Prevention

Secondary prevention aimed at preventing morbidity and mortality uses early detection[342] and prompt treatment. The ACS recommendations for early detection of cancer in average-risk, asymptomatic individuals including cancer site (breast, cervix, colorectal, endometrial, prostate), population to be screened, recommended test or procedure, and frequency of testing are readily available online at cacancerjournal.com (volume 62, number 2, page 131ff)[341] or http://onlinelibrary.wiley.com/doi/10.3322/caac.20143/full.

Some drugs, such as tamoxifen (Nolvadex), are used in both primary and secondary prevention of breast cancer. Tamoxifen has been approved by the FDA as a preventive agent in women who have a high risk for possible development of breast cancer.[386] The preliminary results of a randomized trial comparing tamoxifen to a placebo in women considered at high risk for breast cancer suggested that the risk of breast cancer in this group of high-risk women could be decreased by approximately 50% with the administration of tamoxifen.[268]

Multifactor risk reduction is an important part of secondary prevention for people diagnosed with cancer at risk for recurrence. This is especially true because the adverse effect of several risk factors is cumulative and many risk factors are interrelated.

A THERAPIST'S THOUGHTS*

Screening Recommendations

Recommendations for screening including who to screen, when to screen, and frequency of screening are published by different organizations and aren't always consistent from group to group. To name a few groups engaged in education, research, and recommendations, there is the U.S. Preventative Task Force (USPSTF), American Cancer Society (ACS), National Cancer Institute (NCI), American Urologic Association, American Society of Clinical Oncology (ASCO), National Comprehensive Cancer Network (NCCN), and International Agency for Research on Cancer (IARC). Recent reports by various consumer and professional organizations advising changes to cancer screening frequency and importance have been somewhat controversial among professional provider groups.

The U.S. Preventative Task Force, although sponsored by the federal government, serves as an independent advisory group and submits reports with recommendations based on literature and evidence reviewed. The reports and guidelines can be accessed at http://www.uspreventiveservicestaskforce.org/recommendations.htm. These recommendations are not considered official statements or positions of the U.S. Public Health Service or the U.S. Department of Health and Human Services. The Agency for Healthcare Research and Quality (AHRQ) also publishes evidence-based reports that can be found at http://www.ahrq.gov/clinic/epcquick.htm.

The American Cancer Society recently published a review of current guideline and issues in cancer screening.[342] This comprehensive chapter provides a history of past updates, recommendations for early detection by site, population test, and frequency and reviews prevalence of cancer screening in the United States by test, race health insurance, and educational level.

In past editions of this text, we tried to provide the therapist with a summary of the most current and appropriate screening guidelines. But with recent changes and controversies, it seems more prudent to provide you, the reader, with information that will allow you to stay as current as possible with each individual type of cancer. In this way, you can adopt whatever screening or intervention is appropriate for your personal and/or practice situation.

Keep in mind that political and economic influences on health care policy provided by organizations such as the U.S. Department of Human Health Services and the Centers for Medicare & Medicaid Services (CMS) affecting third party payers will influence coverage for various screenings and treatments. Ultimately, these forces may direct clinical practice rather than evidence-based findings.

*Charles L. McGarvey, PT, MS, DPT, FAPTA

Tertiary Prevention

Tertiary prevention focuses on managing symptoms, limiting complications, and preventing disability associated with cancer or its treatment.

Diagnosis

Medical history and physical examination are usually followed by more specific diagnostic procedures. Useful tests for the early detection and staging of tumors include laboratory values, radiography, endoscopy, isotope scan, CT scan, mammography, MRI, and biopsy. Advances in nuclear medicine have made it possible to examine images of organs, structures, and physiologic or pathologic processes and detect the distribution of radiopharmaceuticals according to their uptake and metabolism.

Tissue Biopsy

Biopsy of tissue samples is an important diagnostic tool in the study of tumors. Tissue for biopsy may be taken by curettage (Papanicolaou [Pap] smear), fluid aspiration (pleural effusion, lumbar puncture, or spinal tap), fine-needle aspiration (breast or thyroid), dermal punch (skin or mouth), endoscopy (rectal polyps), or open surgical excision (visceral tumors and nodes).

An incision or *open biopsy* consists of making an incision and removing a portion of the abnormal tissue. An incisional biopsy takes a slice or wedge of the lesion but does not attempt to remove the entire pathologic structure. The amount removed depends on the abnormality, but it is usually a piece of tissue about one inch in diameter.

An excisional biopsy (sometimes referred to as lumpectomy) consists of making an incision to excise all gross, abnormal tissue that is either visually apparent or identified using a needle placed to localize the lesion. Needle localization employs either ultrasound or MRI to accurately place a thin wire as a marker for the surgeon to locate and excise the specimen. The size of the specimen removed depends on the abnormality and the judgment of surgeon to ensure a negative margin as assessed under the microscope by a pathologist. If the specimen contains tumor cells within the margin, a reexcision by the surgeon is usually to obtain a negative margin before proceeding with other adjuvant therapies.

Core needle biopsy (sometimes referred to as Tru-Cut needle biopsy) uses a large diameter needle to take a core or plug of tissue. Core needle biopsies can be accomplished directly by employing a manual approach to remove a single or multiple specimens from the organ. For example, the surgeon uses ultrasound or fluoroscopy in conducting a biopsy of the prostate gland for diagnosis and staging. Multiple samples of a specimen can be also be removed indirectly by using computers and automation such as in the case of stereotactic biopsy of the breast.

Stereotactic (mammotome) biopsy of the breast uses digital x-rays of the breast taken from two angles to locate the abnormality seen on the mammogram. A computer then calculates the proper angle and depth of insertion of a core biopsy needle. This needle is inserted into the breast, using local anesthesia, and multiple (a dozen or more) core specimens are removed. Each core is about 2 mm by 15 mm long. These cores are then sent to the pathologist for diagnosis. As described previously, a second type of stereotactic procedure places a wire into the exact location of an abnormality within the breast. Ultrasound or mammography is used to find the lesion. The surgeon uses the wire to relocate the abnormality within the breast during an open biopsy. The procedure for placing the wire is the same as for taking a core biopsy, but a thin needle is used instead of a core biopsy needle. Once the needle is in place, a thin wire is inserted through the needle, and the needle is removed.

Sentinel lymph node biopsy (SLNBx) has become a standard diagnostic procedure to assess lymph node status of various tumors (e.g., breast, melanoma, endometrial, valvular, or head and neck) and to assess staging. A blue dye is injected around the cancerous tumor (or the biopsy site if the tumor has been removed). The dye flows through the ducts, and the first node or nodes it reaches is identified as the sentinel node(s). An incision is made over the nodes, and the blue-stained sentinel node or nodes (1-3) are removed and analyzed. The removal of more than three SLNs is considered to be a lower-level axillary dissection. Complications of SLN biopsy include allergic reaction to the blue dye (<1%), pneumothorax from unintended opening of the parietal pleura, sensory or motor nerve injury (small risk), lymphedema, surgical site infections (<1%), and seromas (10%).[148]

Information on the lymphatic drainage from the cancer can have a direct impact on surgery. SLN biopsy has reduced the number of unnecessary axillary dissections in breast cancer. The status of axillary nodes is the most important prognostic factor in breast cancer and in determining the medical management.

A recent randomized controlled trial study by the American College of Surgical Oncology Group concluded that "among patients with limited SLN metastatic breast cancer treated with breast conservation and systemic therapy, the use of SLND alone compared to ALND did not result in inferior survival."[134,400]

Biological Tumor Markers

Tumor markers, substances produced and secreted by tumor cells, may be found in the blood serum. The level of tumor marker seems to correlate with the extent of disease. A tumor marker is not diagnostic itself but can signal malignancies. CEA is one tumor marker that may indicate malignancy of the large bowel, stomach, pancreas, lungs, and breasts. CEA and other serum titers, such as CA-125 (ovarian), CA-27-29 (breast), and prostate-specific antigen (PSA), may be valuable during therapeutic intervention (adjuvant therapy) to evaluate the extent of response and detect tumor recurrence.

Other tumor markers found in the blood (no more specific than CEA) include alpha-fetoprotein, a fetal antigen uncommon in adults and suggestive of testicular cancer. The beta-2 (β_2) microglobin is used in the monitoring of lymphomas, and lactic dehydrogenase is particularly elevated in fast-growing malignancies. Human chorionic gonadotropin (β subunit) may indicate testicular cancer or choriocarcinoma. PSA helps evaluate prostatic cancer. Because of the lack of specificity of the

markers individually (except PSA), test panels are used more frequently rather than just individual tumor marker evaluations.[282]

Several research institutes have developed a monoclonal antibody that identifies breast cancer and other cancer cells. The monoclonal antibody is used to devise a simple blood test for use in diagnosis and monitoring treatment of breast and ovarian cancers and will be used in the future to diagnose colon cancer. Combining the breast cancer antibody with nuclear medicine scanning techniques will provide a noninvasive means of determining lymphatic spread and guide surgeons in determining the extent of surgery required.[30]

Molecular Profiling

Molecular profiling using specific cancer biomarkers provides additional information for the oncologist in determining aggressiveness of the tumor, potential response to treatment, and prediction of risk for cancer diagnosis with a family. Such tests are classified accordingly:

- Immunohistochemistry (IHC), which identifies the presence of specific proteins at the cellular level.
- Gene expression by microarray provides an illustration of the signal status of particular genes. These tests can predict fairly accurately what certain tumors may respond to certain interventions such as chemotherapy. Research has shown that tumors, like any other living tissue, contain genetic information that can be read with increasing accuracy. The goal is to analyze the genetic makeup of the tumor and then choose the specific treatment most likely to be effective given that gene profile, while avoiding exposing the person to toxic therapies that might not be helpful or necessary. Two gene-profiling tests—Oncotype Dx (21 genes) and Mammaprint (70 genes)—are currently available for breast cancer; others are being evaluated for non-Hodgkin lymphoma, head and neck cancer, prostate cancer, kidney cancer, melanoma, and ovarian cancer.
- Fluorescence in situ hybridization is a technique used by pathologists to identify genes with multiple copies or arrangements.
- DNA sequencing via polymerase chain reaction is able to identify mutation in selected genes.

Primary Antineoplastic Treatment Modalities

Changes in the health care system have shifted much of cancer care to the ambulatory and home settings. The medical management of cancer may be curative (i.e., with the intent to cure) or palliative (i.e., provides symptomatic relief but does not cure). Major therapies of curative cancer treatment at this time include surgery, radiation, chemotherapy, immunotherapy (or molecularly based therapy), antiangiogenesis therapy, and hormonal therapy.

Historically, the sequence of treatment of solid tumors would begin with surgery to remove the primary tumor burden, followed by adjuvant therapies (chemotherapy and radiation therapy) to obtain local regional or systemic control and possibly finally long-term (5 years or greater) hormonal treatment. However, studies have indicated excellent results of neoadjuvant (prior to definitive surgical intervention) treatment with chemotherapy or radiotherapy to shrink the primary tumor or provide local or systemic control. As such, the decision to initiate neoadjuvant versus adjuvant therapies is based on the size, extent of involved tissue and often the stage or grade of the tumor as assessed by multiple professionals and discussed at the cancer staging conference.

Following such analysis by the oncologists, a balanced discussion of the findings and recommendation of the group is shared with the patient/family and a mutually agreeable plan of care instituted intended to result in ablation of primary disease and the highest level control for future recurrence or metastasis. The desired outcome of such antineoplastic treatment is complete remission of disease.

Effective cancer treatment requires an understanding of the biology of metastasis and how tumor cells interact with the microenvironment of different organs to design effective therapies.[115] Each of the curative therapies described here may be used alone or in combination, depending on the type, stage, localization, and responsiveness of the tumor and on limitations imposed by the person's clinical status.

The administration of repeated or cyclical chemotherapy and/or radiation is designed to interrupt cell proliferation (the cell growth cycle; Fig. 9-5). Significant advances in altering the molecular biology and cellular signaling mechanisms that trigger or foster carcinogenesis are now being translated into treatment that will target cancer cells without affecting normal, healthy cells. With improved cancer targets, it may be possible to end the repeated doses of chemotherapeutic agents.[109,191,217,272]

Cell Proliferation

One round of cell division requires duplication of DNA during the *S* phase and proper segregation of duplicated chromosomes during mitosis (M phase; see Fig. 9-5). *G0* are the "resting cells" temporarily out of the proliferative cycle; when stimulated by growth factors and/or hormones, these cells move into the *G1* phase and begin to multiply. *G1* is a postmitotic period of growth and preparation of the chromosomes for replication. This is a checkpoint to stop the cell cycle if the DNA is damaged. In this phase, the cell can either repair the DNA or undergo apoptosis. DNA repair is aided by retinoids/vitamin A, vitamin D, folate, coenzyme Q10, and selenium. The *S* phase represents the synthesis of DNA.

G2 is the premitotic period and the last step in the mitotic cycle followed by M (mitosis) when cell division takes place. *G2* is another checkpoint when the cell cycle can be stopped if DNA is damaged or unreplicated, in which case repair or apoptosis occurs. During the *M* phase, there is a check to ensure each daughter cell gets the correct DNA. The end result of one full cycle is the formation of two identical (*G0*) daughter cells. Most organ cells that are hormonally linked take approximately 19 to 33 days to complete one full cycle. Chemotherapy eliminates up to 95% of cancerous cells in the body; this is called the "kill rate." Not all cancer cells will be eradicated; the immune system may be able to eliminate the remaining cells but not always.

Adjuvant treatment, such as chemotherapy and radiation therapy, is administered in repeated doses over time in an attempt to kill cells in the most susceptible phases. For example, chemotherapy is most effective during DNA synthesis and mitosis. Cells are most sensitive to radiation therapy in the *G2* phase. A certain percentage of cells will be unaffected because they are in the *G0* or resting phase. Cells in the *G0* phase are undifferentiated or stem (mesenchymal) cells waiting until called on by the body to serve a particular (differentiated) need. Stem cells in the *G0* phase are resistant to chemotherapy and radiation therapy and they may be the reason chemotherapy and radiation therapies are not 100% effective modalities in the ablation of microcirculation of tumor cells. The repeated or cyclical treatment is designed to catch *G0* cells later in the growth cycle.

Researchers are looking for ways to selectively target (and kill) cancer stem cells but because not all cancers (e.g., pancreatic cancer) contain stem cells, there are ongoing attempts to answer the question of whether cancer stem cells are the result of a cancer or the cause of it.[227,291]

Surgery

Surgery, once a mainstay of cancer treatment, is now used most often in combination with other therapies. Surgery may be used curatively for tumor biopsy and tumor removal or palliatively to relieve pain, correct obstruction, or alleviate pressure. Surgery can be curative in persons with localized cancer, but 70% of clients have evidence of micrometastases at the time of diagnosis, requiring

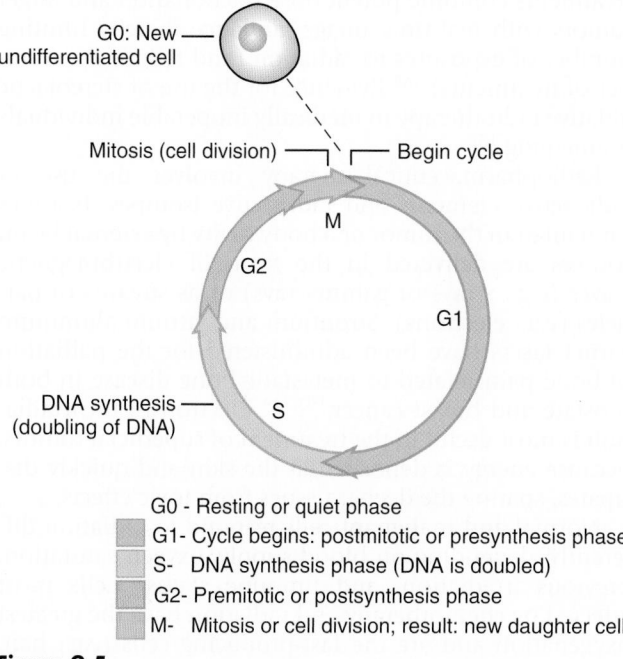

G0 - Resting or quiet phase
G1 - Cycle begins: postmitotic or presynthesis phase
S - DNA synthesis phase (DNA is doubled)
G2 - Premitotic or postsynthesis phase
M - Mitosis or cell division; result: new daughter cell

Figure 9-5

Cell cycle. *G0* represents the resting phase of cell proliferation. *G1* is the growth and preparation of the chromosomes for replication. *S* phase is the synthesis of DNA. *G2* is the preparation of the cell for division, and *M* represents mitosis (cell division). The final result of the cell cycle is the production of two identical daughter cells. [See text for complete description of the cell cycle in relation to chemotherapy and radiation therapy.] (Modified from Abeloff MD, Armitage JO, Niedruhuber JE, et al: *Clinical oncology,* ed 3, 2004, London, Churchill Livingstone.)

surgery in combination with other treatment modalities to achieve better response rates. Adjuvant therapy used after surgery eradicates any residual cells.

Surgical oncologists are beginning to employ new technologies to assist in access to tumors with minimal time and tissue disruption and impact on other normal organs. Such newer methods employ the use of robotics (da Vinci), which allow for percutaneous entry into body cavities and removal of primary tumor without open surgical procedures.

Irradiation Therapy

Irradiation therapy (RT or XRT), also known as radiotherapy, plays a vital role in the multimodal treatment of cancer. It is used to destroy the dividing cancer cells by destroying hydrogen bonds between DNA strands within the cancer cells, while damaging resting normal cells as little as possible. Advances in RT have primarily involved improvements in dose delivery and the use of Cyberknife, a relatively new technology that incorporates robotic and precision mapping and treatment of nonoperable tumors. The focus of future treatment is on combining RT with targeted therapies such as angiogenesis inhibitors.

Radiation consists of two types: ionizing radiation and particle radiation. Both types have the cellular DNA as their target; however, particle radiation produces less skin damage. The goal is to ablate as many cancer cells as possible while simultaneously sparing surrounding normal tissues. Radiation is given over a period of weeks to capture cells at each stage of the cell cycle. Radiation is particularly effective at the end of the G2 phase (see Fig. 9-5) when the cells are most susceptible to radiation.

Radiation treatment approaches include external beam radiation and intracavitary and interstitial implants. Radiation may be used preoperatively to shrink a tumor, making it operable while preventing further spread of the disease during surgery. After the surgical wound heals, postoperative doses prevent residual cancer cells from multiplying or metastasizing.

RT may be delivered externally or internally depending on the type and extent of the tumor by (1) external beam (teletherapy), (2) sealed source (brachytherapy), and (3) unsealed source (systemic therapy). When the distance between the radiation source and the target is short, the term *brachytherapy* is used. Brachytherapy allows for a rapid falloff in dose away from the target volume. When the radiation source is at a distance from the target, the term *teletherapy* is used. Teletherapy allows for a more uniform dose across the target volume.

X-rays generated by linear accelerators and gamma rays generated by radioactive isotopes (e.g., cobalt-60, radium-226, or cesium-137) are referred to as *sealed source* radiation therapies (or brachytherapy). This form of radiation is used for the treatment of visceral tumors because the rays penetrate to great depths before reaching full intensity and thereby spare the skin from toxic effects.

Modern radiology has advanced to include site-specific techniques that take into account complex tissue contours and irregular shapes, visceral movement, digestion, and the effect of respiration on the lungs when the lungs are the target organ.

A new delivery procedure known as intensity-modulated radiation therapy (IMRT) allows for very precise delivery of radiation dose with less exposure to surrounding normal tissue. Interventional radiology includes newer technologies, including brachytherapy, accelerated partial breast irradiation, radiofrequency ablation, and radiopharmaceutical therapy.

Radiofrequency ablation and stereotactic body radiotherapy (also known as stereotactic ablative radiation therapy) represent two forms of thermal ablation. IMRT allows for sculpting the radiation field and dose to match the area being irradiated. Computer optimization techniques help determine the distribution of beam intensities across a treatment volume. Improving accuracy and treatment time is also possible with RapidArc radiotherapy, an image-guided IMRT that is eight times faster than conventional or IMRT machines. The same number of treatments is required as for traditional radiotherapy but sessions are 5 to 10 minutes instead of 15 to 30 minutes, with tighter margins around a smaller targeted treatment area. The hope is for fewer side effects, less damage to surrounding healthy tissue, improved quality of life, and cost-effectiveness.[162] The equipment rotates 360 degrees around the person, delivering a precisely sculpted three-dimensional dose during one revolution of the machine.[256,380]

Radiofrequency ablation involves the insertion of a needle electrode through the skin and underlying soft tissues and into the tumor. Retractable tines are deployed and radiofrequency excitation generates a zone of heat that destroys the tumor. Stereotactic body radiotherapy treatments combine potent dose fractionation and target tumors with real-time image guidance thereby limiting number of exposures to radiation (and reduce the number of treatments).[362] Evidence for the use of stereotactic ablative radiotherapy in medically inoperable individuals is emerging.[156]

Radiopharmaceutical therapy involves the use of radioactive elements and radioactive isotopes. Isotopes implanted in the tumor or a body cavity by external beam sources are delivered in the form of electromagnetic waves (e.g., x-rays or gamma rays) or as streams of particles (e.g., electrons). Strontium and yttrium aluminum garnet lasers have been administered for the palliation of bone pain related to metastatic bone disease in both prostate and breast cancer.[193,349] Electron beam irradiation is most useful in the treatment of superficial tumors, because energy is deposited at the skin and quickly dissipates, sparing the deeper tissues from toxic effects.

Normal and malignant cells respond to radiation differently, depending on blood supply, oxygen saturation, previous irradiation, and immune status. Cells most affected by chemotherapy and radiation have the greatest oxygenation and are the fast-producing cells (e.g., hair, skin). In general, normal cells recover from radiation faster than malignant cells; damaged cancer cells cannot self-repair. Success of the treatment and damage to normal tissue also vary with the intensity of the radiation.

Standard radiation fractionation is a course of 1.8 to 2.0 Gy per day in single daily doses. Accelerated or hypofractionation refers to delivering the same total dose over a shortened treatment time (one or just a few treatment sessions). Hyperfractionation refers to the same total delivered dose over the same treatment time but in an increased number of fractions; in other words, smaller fractions are delivered more often than once a day. Although a large single dose of radiation has greater cellular effects than fractions of the same amount delivered sequentially, a protracted schedule allows time for normal tissue to recover in the intervals between individual sublethal doses.[52]

Challenges with radiation treatment still remain because of the inability to identify microscopic disease with accuracy. Immobilizing people and keeping them completely still for the duration of treatment is also difficult. Weight loss associated with treatment alters body geometry, requiring further corrections in dosimetry.

The next step in radiation oncology is to account for physiologic movements during irradiation. This may be accomplished with adaptive radiation with daily modulation of prescription and delivery using real-time imaging called four-dimensional (4-D) conformal RT (CRT).[52] See Chapter 5 for a more complete discussion of the effects of RT.

Proton Therapy. Proton therapy is also among the new and growing areas in radiation oncology. Highly targeted proton beam therapy, now available in a small number of advanced medical centers, may replace radiation therapy (if something even better does not come along first). Proton therapy is able to destroy tumor DNA so completely that the repair mechanisms are ineffective. Proton beam therapy is most useful when the tumor is close to nerves, blood vessels, the eyes, or vital organs. The beam acts like a smart weapon as it is able to locate the tumor using precise coordinates obtained from CT and/or MRI scans. Computer programs can design a course of radiation that conforms to the silhouette of the tumor.

Chemotherapy

Chemotherapy includes a wide array of chemical agents to destroy cancer cells. It is particularly useful in the treatment of widespread or metastatic disease, whereas radiation is more useful for treatment of localized lesions. Chemotherapy is used in eradicating residual disease, as well as inducing long remissions and cures, especially in children with childhood leukemia and adults with Hodgkin disease or testicular cancer. Several major chemotherapeutic agents are listed in Table 9-6. For a more complete discussion of chemotherapy and its effects, see Chapter 5.

Chemotherapy (and RT) kills most of the billion or more cells in each cubic centimeter of tumor tissue. However, cytotoxic therapies do not always eradicate every tumor cell for several reasons. Unlike normal cells, cancer cells are genetically unstable and replicate inaccurately. As the tumor grows, multiple subpopulations of cells with different biologic characteristics develop. Some of the cells will be resistant to treatment. After the treatment-sensitive cells are eliminated, the resistant cells may divide rapidly, re-creating a tumor that is now resistant to the therapy.[351]

Almost all chemotherapy agents kill cancer cells by affecting DNA synthesis or function, a process that occurs through the cell cycle. Each drug varies in the way this occurs within the cell cycle. Chemotherapy interferes with the synthesis or function of nucleic acid targeting cells in the growth phase and therefore does not kill all cells (e.g., 5% are in the quiet or quiescent phase and are unaffected by chemotherapy) (see Fig. 9-5).

Combination therapies are often used because some drugs work better during different cell cycles. For example, antimetabolites are most effective during the presynaptic (G1) phase, whereas alkylating agents target cells during the synthesis of DNA (S phase) and the postsynthesis (G2) phase. Treatment is designed to capture cell cycles at different phases for optimum cell death.[223]

Chemotherapeutic drugs can be given orally, subcutaneously, intramuscularly, intravenously, intracavitarily (into a body cavity such as the thoracic, abdominal, or pelvic cavity), intrathecally (through the sheath of a structure, such as through the sheath of the spinal cord into the subarachnoid space), and by arterial infusion, depending on the drug and its pharmacologic action and on tumor location. Administration in any form is usually intermittent to allow for bone marrow recovery between doses.

Traditional chemotherapies and newer targeted agents are known to cause neurologic symptoms that can impact quality of life.[202] Not all chemotherapy recipients develop problems with cognitive or mental function, but if it does happen, the effects can last several years. MRIs of brain structures have shown temporary shrinkage in the brain structures that are responsible for cognition and awareness. Shrinkage may be a possible physiologic explanation for chemotherapy-related cognitive difficulties.[170]

Mediating the Effects of Chemotherapy. Colony-stimulating factors (CSFs) may be used to support the person with low blood counts related to chemotherapy. CSFs function primarily as hematopoietic growth factors, guiding the division and differentiation of bone marrow stem cells. They also influence the functioning of mature lymphocytes, monocytes, macrophages, and neutrophils.

Currently, erythropoietin, human granulocyte colony–stimulating factor (G-CSF), GM-CSF, and thrombopoietin (oprelvekin) and various interleukins are being used for chemotherapy-induced pancytopenia (deficiency of all cellular components of blood). Erythropoietin is used to treat anemia by stimulating bone marrow production of red blood cells. Interleukins are a large group of cytokines sometimes called *lymphokines* when produced by the T-lymphocytes or *monokines* when produced by mononuclear phagocytes. Interleukins have a variety of effects, but most interleukins direct other cells to divide and differentiate. Both G-CSF and GM-CSF are very useful in protecting individuals from prolonged neutrophil nadirs (lowest points after neutrophil count has been depressed by chemotherapy). Thrombopoietin (oprelvekin) has been recently identified and has shown promise in promoting elevation in platelet counts.[310] In addition, GM-CSF has shown significant antitumor effects that prolong survival and disease-free survival in adults with stage III and IV melanoma who are at high risk for recurrence after surgical resection.[346]

Immunotherapy

(See also "Cancer Immunotherapy" above.)

Immunotherapy (also known as biologic therapy or biotherapy) relies on biologic response modifiers to change

Table 9-6	Major Chemotherapeutic Agents	
Class and Agent	**Mechanism of Action**	**Indications for Use**
Alkylating Agents		
Busulfan Carmustine Chlorambucil Cyclophosphamide Dacarbazine	Bind to DNA and prevent DNA replication	Acute and chronic leukemias, Hodgkin and non-Hodgkin lymphomas, brain tumors, breast cancer, and melanomas
Heavy Metal Compounds		
Cisplatin Carboplatin Oxaliplatin	Bind to DNA, distorting the DNA structure and causing cellular damage	Breast, bladder, testicular, colon, and ovarian cancers
Antimetabolites		
Cytarabine Decitabine Fluorouracil (5-FU) Methotrexate Mercaptopurine (6-MP)	Block cell growth by interfering with DNA, RNA, and nucleic acid synthesis	Acute and chronic leukemias, non-Hodgkin lymphomas, and breast, colon, rectum, pancreatic, lung, head and neck, and stomach cancers
Topoisomerase Inhibitors		
Teniposide Doxorubicin Daunorubicin Topotecan	Inhibit the actions of enzymes responsible for maintaining DNA structure (topoisomerases)	Acute leukemias, Hodgkin disease, and bone, thyroid, lung, breast, gastric, ovarian, cervical, and bladder cancers
Microtubule-Targeting Agents		
Vinblastine Vincristine Paclitaxel	Disrupt cellular mitosis by inhibiting microtubule assembly or disassembly	Acute leukemias, Hodgkin and non-Hodgkin lymphomas, and breast, ovarian, lung, and testicular cancers
Agents that Target Cell Surface Glycoproteins, Growth Factor Receptors, and Ligands		
Rituximab Ibritumomab Tiuxetan Cetuximab Trastuzumab Erlotinib Bevacizumab Sunitinib	Bind to targets on or in cancer cells and either transmit intracellular signals resulting in cell death, deliver chemotherapeutic agents to the disease site, or prevent cell growth and proliferation	Chronic leukemias, Hodgkin and non-Hodgkin lymphomas, and colorectal, gastric, breast, lung, pancreatic, renal, and head and neck cancers
Other Biologic Agents		
Interferons Interleukin-2	Increase the proliferation and activity of immune cells that destroy cancer cells without harming normal cells	Leukemias, melanomas, non-Hodgkin lymphoma, and renal cancer

Data from pharmacotherapy update: DiPiro JT, Talbert RL, Yee GC, et al: *Pharmacotherapy: A pathophysiologic approach*, ed 8, New York, 2011, McGraw Hill; Brunton LL, Chabner BA, Knollmann BC: *Goodman & Gilman's the pharmacological basis of therapeutics*, ed 12, New York, 2011, McGraw Hill.

or modify the relationship between the tumor and host by strengthening the host's biologic response to tumor cells. Much of the work related to biologic response modifiers is still experimental, so the availability of this type of treatment varies regionally within the United States.

Agents include interferons, which have a direct antitumor effect, and IL-2, one type of cytokine, a protein released by macrophages to trigger the immune response.[157] In addition to their desired immune effects, interferons cause a number of significant toxicities, including constitutional, hematologic, hepatic, and prominent effects on the nervous system, especially depression.

Hematopoietic Cell Transplantation. Hematopoietic cell transplantation including bone marrow transplantation is used for cancers that are responsive to high doses of chemotherapy or radiation. These high doses kill cancer cells but are also toxic to bone marrow; hematopoietic cell transplantation provides a method for rescuing people from bone marrow destruction while allowing higher doses of chemotherapy for a better antitumor result.

Bone marrow transplantation was a technique developed to restore the marrow to people who had lethal injury to that site because of bone marrow failure, destruction of bone marrow by disease, or intensive chemical or radiation exposure. At first, the source of the transplant was the marrow cells of a healthy donor who had the same tissue type (human leukocyte antigen; markers on the white blood cells) as the recipient (usually a sibling or close family relative). Now donor programs have

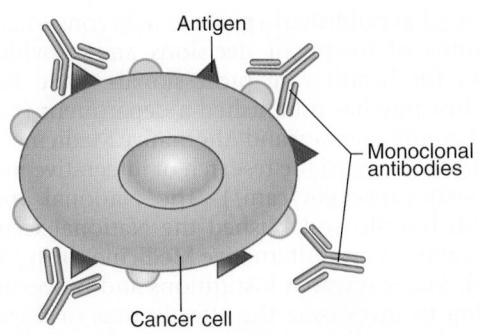

Figure 9-6

Mechanism of action of monoclonal antibodies (mAbs). mAbs are large, complex, Y-shaped molecules that bind to specific antigens on the surface of some cells. The mAb is like a key and the antigen is the lock. When they fit together, the cancer cell is destroyed. Binding of extracellular receptor results in signals that block intracellular signaling inducing cellular lysis and apoptosis (death).

been established to identify unrelated donors who have a matching human leukocyte antigen.

The transplant product is a very small fraction of the marrow cells called *stem cells*. These cells occur in the bone marrow and also circulate in the blood and can be harvested from the blood of a donor by treating the donor with an agent or agents (e.g., G-CSF) that cause a release of larger numbers of stem cells into the blood and collect them by hemapheresis. Because blood (peripheral site), as well as marrow, is a good source of cells for transplantation, the term *hematopoietic cell transplantation* has replaced the general term for these procedures (see "HCT Transplantation" in Chapter 21).

Targeted Therapy. Targeted therapy or "smart drugs" are a form of immunotherapy and include two broad groups: monoclonal antibodies (mAb) and small molecules (e.g., tyrosine kinase enzyme). By interfering with the pathway by which a normal cell becomes a cancer cell, targeted therapies are intended to spare surrounding healthy cells compared with treatment with radiation or chemotherapy (Fig. 9-6).[261,377,401]

Small molecules block enzymes and receptors involved in cancer cell growth and proliferation. Monoclonal antibody therapy uses specifically designed antibodies made by a pharmaceutical company instead of those produced by a person's own immune system. These antibodies are biologic therapies that act specifically against a particular antigen. They can also be bound with radioisotopes and injected into the body to detect cancer by attaching to tumor cells. The antibody may not actually kill target cells, but rather it marks the cells so that other components in the immune system attack it or initiate a signaling mechanism that leads to the target cell's self-destruction.[326] Monoclonal antibodies have been developed to help combat specific cancers, including colorectal cancer and some forms of non-Hodgkin lymphoma.

Research is ongoing to use these antibodies as a means of destroying specific cancer cells without disturbing healthy cells. Rituximab (Rituxan), trastuzumab (Herceptin), bevacizumab (Avastin), alemtuzumab (CamPath), and cetuximab (Erbitux) are a few of the monoclonal antibodies currently in use for cancer treatment (e.g., lymphoma, breast, colorectal, chronic leukemia, and head and neck cancer).

Bevacizumab, formerly known as anti–vascular endothelial growth factor, is an antibody used in combination with chemotherapy in the treatment of colon, lung, and breast cancer. This antibody binds to vascular endothelial growth factor made by the tumor cells and prevents it from forming new blood vessels to supply the tumor cells.

Rituximab is used primarily in the treatment of non-Hodgkin lymphoma. Rituximab binds to lymphoid cells in the thymus, spleen, lymph nodes, and peripheral blood in order to lyse and destroy specific immune target cells.

Trastuzumab is used in the treatment of metastatic breast cancer in women who have overexpression of the human epidermal growth factor receptor 2 (HER2) protein. It binds with this protein and inhibits proliferation of cells with this protein and also mediates an antibody-mediated destruction of the cancer cells that have the HER2 receptor overexpression.[125] Both agents are usually used in combination with or in addition to other chemotherapeutic agents for treatment.

Not all people respond to mAbs, presumably because of differences in the receptors being targeted. Molecular testing will have to become part of designer biologic therapy in which drugs are chosen on an individual basis after genetic profiling and immunoassay. Antibodies also function as carriers of cytotoxic substances, such as radioisotopes, drugs, and toxins, making them a key focus area of cancer research right now.[326]

Antiangiogenic Therapy

Antiangiogenic therapy shows promise as a means of blocking the formation of new blood vessels supplying cancer cells but remains limited in use and under investigation.[87,180] Research has shown that the one common area of vulnerability of all cells in any phase of growth is the nonnegotiable need for oxygen. Tumor cells cannot survive without oxygen and other nutrients transported by the blood. In fact, tumor cells cannot survive at distances greater than 150 μm from a blood vessel.[351]

Antiangiogenic therapy may be able to put a stop to pathologic angiogenesis, the process by which a malignant tumor develops new vessels and is the primary means by which cancer cells spread. Antiangiogenesis factors, their receptors, and the signaling pathways that govern angiogenesis in solid tumors have been discovered. Treatment with antiangiogenesis factors (e.g., endostatin, angiostatin, or calpastatin) approved for use in the United States focuses on blocking the general process of tumor growth by cutting off their blood supply rather than on the destruction of an already formed cancerous mass.[120] Scientists expect that combinations of angiogenesis inhibitors or broad-spectrum angiogenesis inhibitors will be needed for long-term use in cancer if tumor cells have or develop multiple molecular signaling pathways, a characteristic called *redundancy*.[121]

In the future, antiangiogenic agents may be used as maintenance therapy to control cancer much the same way that medications are used to control hypertension or hyperlipidemia. It is expected that different mutations in cancer will require individualized therapy based on current knowledge of specific tumors, their patterns of resistance, and response to angiogenesis inhibitors.[158]

The National Cancer Institute has produced a fact sheet addressing the most common questions and concerns regarding the use of antiangiogentic agents in the treatment of cancer. It is suggested that the reader consider viewing the website for additional information and references: http://www.cancer.gov/cancertopics/factsheet/Therapy/angiogenesis-inhibitors.

Hormonal Therapy

Hormonal therapy is used for certain types of cancer shown to be affected by specific hormones. For example, tamoxifen, an antiestrogen hormonal agent, is used in breast cancer to block estrogen receptors in breast tumor cells that require estrogen to thrive. See further discussion regarding hormonal therapy for breast cancer in Chapter 20.

The luteinizing hormone–releasing hormone leuprolide is now used to treat prostate cancer. With long-term use, this hormone inhibits testosterone release and tumor growth. Goserelin acetate (Zoladex) is a newer hormone used in prostate cancer that is a synthetic form of luteinizing hormone–releasing hormone. Goserelin acetate inhibits pituitary gonadotropic secretion, thus decreasing serum testosterone levels.[386]

Other cancers, such as myelodysplasia and hematologic malignancies (e.g., lymphoma, myeloma, leukemia), can be treated effectively in older adults, although advanced age does present many challenges.

The future of oncologic care may rest on the model of individualized (tailored/targeted) therapy based on a pretreatment assessment of the each individual's organ reserves, physical condition, and cognitive function. Identifying predictive factors of successful outcome will help assess who could benefit from more aggressive treatment and have the greatest chance for successful outcomes.[34,166] When curative measures are no longer possible or available, palliative treatment may include radiation, chemotherapy, physical therapy (e.g., physical agents, exercise, positioning, relaxation techniques, biofeedback, or manual therapy), medications, acupuncture, chiropractic care, alternative medicine (e.g., homeopathic and naturopathic treatment), and hospice care.

Complementary and Alternative (Integrative) Medicine

Many people are seeking help in the cure and palliation of cancer through complementary and alternative medicine (CAM) therapies, sometimes referred to as "integrative medicine," "energy medicine," or "bioenergetics" (the field of biochemistry that concerns energy flow through living systems). Some examples of these modalities include acupuncture, Reiki, BodyTalk, hypnosis, mind–body techniques, massage, music, tai chi, qi gong, yoga, meditation, and other methods to improve physical and mental well-being. Conventional treatments do not always relieve symptoms of pain, fatigue, anxiety, and mood disturbance. Some people cannot tolerate the side effects of conventional treatment. CAM has received consumer attention and concern on the part of those who provide conventional or standard medical therapy.

The ACS has published a guide to help consumers make these kinds of treatment decisions and provide some direction for health care professionals.[8] The National Cancer Institute has established a department (Office of Cancer Complementary and Alternative Medicine) specifically directed toward the research of integrative medicine (http://www.cancer.gov/cam/). The National Institutes of Health has also established the National Center for Complementary and Alternative Medicine (http://nccam.nih.gov). Major research institutions and universities are beginning to investigate the effectiveness of these types of interventions for cancer (e.g., Society for Integrative Oncology sponsored by the New York Academy of Medicine, Cochrane CAM Field—University of Maryland School of Medicine). A new movement toward integrative medicine combining the best of complementary modalities with mainstream conventional therapies has been launched. Several texts on this topic are available for physical therapists.[89,95]

Prognosis

Thirty years ago, a cancer diagnosis was often a death sentence; survivors referred to themselves as "victims." Cancer is no longer considered a death sentence, and many return to the mainstream of family life, community activities, and work. Medical treatment is often provided in outpatient settings, making it possible to work during treatment though not without some return-to-work issues (e.g., decreased physical functioning, fatigue, lack of workplace support) for many individuals.[141,224,382]

Today, there are 12 million cancer survivors in the United States; 67% of all people diagnosed with cancer have a 5-year survival rate. In general, this means that the chance of a person recently diagnosed with cancer being alive in 5 years is 67% of the chance of someone not diagnosed with cancer. Such statistics adjust for normal life expectancy (accounting for factors such as diabetes, heart disease, injuries, or dying of old age).[9]

In general, improved survival rates occur with screening and early detection/treatment, especially for cancers that have a highly effective treatment. Prognosis is influenced by the type of cancer, the stage and grade of disease at diagnosis, the availability of effective treatment, the response to treatment, and other factors related to lifestyle such as smoking, alcohol consumption, diet, nutrition, and exercise. Despite advances in early diagnosis, surgical techniques, systemic therapies, and patient care, the major cause of death from cancer is due to metastases that are resistant to therapy.[115]

The prognosis is poor for anyone with advanced, disseminated cancer. Researchers continue to search for the mechanisms responsible for cancer metastases and chemotherapeutic failure and develop new strategies to circumvent drug resistance. In general, the earlier cancers are found, the simpler treatment may be and the greater likelihood of a cure.

There are many different terms used to describe treatment outcomes, such as *disease-free survival, event-free survival, progression-free survival, complete response, stable disease, near complete response, partial response,* and *progressive disease.*[357] The term *no evidence of disease* (NED) may be used when all signs of the disease have disappeared after treatment but before the end of 5 years occurs. There are no signs of the disease using current tests. If the response is maintained for a long period, the term *durable remission* may be used. The person who is alive and without evidence of disease for at least 5 years after diagnosis is considered cured. The terms *survival* and *cure* do not always portray the functional status of a cancer survivor. Many people considered cured are left with physical limitations and movement dysfunctions that interfere with their daily lives.

Even without complete remission, cancer can be controlled to provide longer survival time and improved QOL, but these factors are not reflected in survival rates. Cancer statistics reported usually include a lag time so that rates may not reflect the most recent treatment advances. Survival rates for many cancers have increased from 1960 to the present, but not all cancers have been characterized by this increase. For example, while survival rates for Hodgkin disease and prostate, testicular, and bladder cancers have increased by at least 25%, the survival rates for cancers of the oral cavity and pharynx, liver, pancreas, esophagus, and colon have decreased or increased less than 5% during the same period.

A significantly lower survival rate in African American men for most cancer classifications has been noted. This difference may be due to a variety of factors, including limited access to health care, little or no insurance, lack of a primary health care provider, limited knowledge of the benefits of early diagnosis and treatment, and greater exposure to carcinogens. Central to these social forces is access to health care, including prevention, information, early detection, and quality treatment.[387]

In terminally ill individuals, rates of change are more important indicators of survival than absolute measures. Using a modified Barthel Index composed of 10 activities of daily living, each with five levels of dependency (maximum score more than 100 points), can provide important predictions about length of time until death. Half of those individuals with advanced cancer who lose 10 or more points per week die within 2 weeks, and three-fourths are dead at 3 weeks. In contrast, 50% of all cases without declines in score survive for 2 months or more. This may be a useful tool for planning and end-of-life issues in a hospice setting.[39]

Clinical Prediction of Outcomes

New approaches to prognostication are being used and/or developed. These techniques focus on the tumor itself or on the body's immune response to the tumor. For example, a test that focuses on the tumor to predict response to adjuvant chemotherapy is the Oncotype DX test for women with breast cancer. This test uses a core sample of the tumor to analyze gene mutations and can predict who would benefit from adjuvant chemotherapy in addition to estrogen-inhibiting drugs.

A test that looks more at the body's response to treatment is the immunoscore. The immunoscore approach provides a prediction of clinical outcome through histopathologic evaluation of tissue samples obtained during surgical resection of the tumor.[127] This technique measures cytotoxic T lymphocytes that infiltrate the tumor; the more T lymphocytes present, the stronger the immune response against the tumor. The immunoscore measures markers of tumor infiltrating T lymphocytes. Clinical trials have established that patients identified as being positive for CD3 and CD8 (showing an immune response against the tumor) have a better prognosis than patients who test negative for these markers.[123,127,146]

Two instruments are commonly used by providers to assess the functional level of newly diagnosed cases of cancer, the Karnofsky Functional Scale (see Table 30-6)[185] and the Eastern Cooperative Oncology Group (ECOG) Function Assessment Tool.[262] The Karnofsky Functional Scale is an older scale which uses a score of 100 to 0 (normal to dead) to score function, and the newer Eastern Cooperative Oncology Group tool uses a 0 to 4 scale (normal, unrestricted activity, to bedridden, fully dependent).

Selected older adults with cancer can benefit from intensive care. Age is associated with higher mortality, especially for adults older than age 60 years and when combined with multiple comorbidities.[344] A comprehensive geriatric assessment can be helpful in identifying individuals likely to benefit from cytotoxic treatment. Therapies may be adjusted based on renal and cardiac function. Cardiac toxicity and neurotoxicity are common in persons aged 65 years and older.[34]

SPECIAL IMPLICATIONS FOR THE THERAPIST 9-1

Oncology/Cancer
The Role of the Physical Therapist in Cancer Treatment

> We must expand our paradigm thinking from treating "post-op" to treating from diagnosis to survivorship.
> Leslie J. Waltke, PT[376]

The therapist should be involved in all phases of care, including prevention, restoration, support, and palliative care. Prevention lessens the impact of anticipated disability through education and training. Restorative care focuses on restoring physical function as much as possible. Supportive care assists in coping with the condition while maintaining maximal functional capacity. Palliative care provides comfort during function and activities of daily living to minimize dependence while offering emotional support.[205]

There are many individuals with cancer who would benefit from consultation with a physical therapist during the early stages of their cancer treatment. Treatment for cancer has improved over the past 20 years, but often results in functional deficits caused by fibrosis, tissue or segmental bone resection, joint, or limb amputation.

There are site-specific cancer issues (e.g., cognitive impairment with brain tumors) and postsurgical problems (e.g., limited motion, soreness, disuse, pain, fatigue, sensory loss, weakness, deep venous thrombosis and emboli, lymphedema, or sleep disturbance). There are side effects of radiotherapy, chemotherapy, and bone marrow or stem cell transplantation. Any of these problems require physical therapy intervention and education.[278,281]

The therapist is not just treating the disease but the effects of medical intervention; medical oncologists must be encouraged to refer based on treatment effects, not type of disease.[376] Treatment can result in severe disfigurement; cancer is the major cause of amputation in children. Weakness, fatigue, inflexibility, osteoporosis, risk of falls, altered or diminished breathing patterns, and lymphedema are just a few of the challenges faced by many of our cancer clients—no matter what kind of cancer they have been diagnosed with.

Therapists need to advocate as a group that appropriate oncology patients see a physical therapist—for example, targeting individuals ahead of time for immediate postoperative or post lymph node dissection consultation. Automatic referral to a physical therapist once the diagnosis of cancer has been made is preferred over waiting until radiation-induced fibrosis causes disabling contractures. More evidence is needed to identify people at risk for poor outcomes that could be improved with physical therapy and predictive factors supporting the need for physical therapy intervention.

As medical innovations help people with cancer live longer, there has been a shift in the way we approach cancer treatment. Shifting from the search for a cure to managing the disease as a chronic condition necessitates a more comprehensive and integrated management approach from diagnosis through survivorship.[304] There is greater emphasis on maximizing function and improving QOL with a more holistic approach throughout the various phases of intervention and management.

Psychosocial-spiritual issues (e.g., loss, grief, and anger) and client diversity (e.g., life span, socioeconomic class, cultural beliefs, and ethnicity) require consideration in planning an effective therapeutic approach.[281] The psychosocial-spiritual status and cultural beliefs can be a driving factor in successful outcomes. Engaging the individual in honest discussion, listening to concerns or feelings, and sharing rehabilitation needs to set mutually achievable goals will enhance outcomes.[31,194]

Benign Tumors

The therapist may be asked by clients to examine unusual skin lesions or aberrant tissue such as unusual moles, ganglion, fibromas, or lipomas. A general screening examination is required with history, age, and risk factors taken into consideration. The ABCDE (asymmetry, border, color, diameter, evolving) skin cancer screening examination can be employed with documentation of findings for any skin changes.

Benign fatty (lipoma) or fibrous tumors (fibroma) commonly located in the subcutaneous tissues can be located anywhere in the body. Lipomas are found most often in locations where fat accumulates, such as the abdomen, thighs, upper arms, back, and breast. These masses are usually round or oval in shape, soft, lumpy, and easily moveable. They may be small (pea-size) or as large as 3 to 4 inches across. Palpation reveals defined borders and a mass that is not fixed but moves readily with pressure along the edge.

These benign tumors are usually painless but can be tender when palpated. Many people who discover the lump are understandably concerned about cancer. Any suspicious integumentary or soft tissue mass must be evaluated medically, especially in the client with any additional risk factors. Only a pathologist can diagnose or rule out these types of lesions.

Side Effects of Cancer Treatment

Although it may make more sense to include a discussion of the side effects of cancer treatment in this chapter, we have opted to place that topic in Chapter 5 to help emphasize the point that the long-term effects of cancer treatment are often problems that affect multiple systems. The therapist must take this approach when planning intervention and offering patient/client education.

With improved survival rates, we expect to see more delayed reactions and long-term sequelae to today's cancer treatment modalities. With improved survival and longevity, we may also see an increased prevalence of cancer recurrence in the future. This may mean worsening of symptoms such as peripheral neuropathy or lymphedema from second and third rounds of treatment. In time, with the identification of genetic traits of cancer, treatment may become more targeted to the cancer cells and less toxic to healthy cells and tissue, eventually reducing and maybe even eliminating side effects experienced by many of today's cancer survivors.

Table 9-7 compares the potential side effects associated with the major treatment modalities discussed in this section. See Chapter 5 for discussion of the intended and adverse systemic effects of chemotherapy agents, radiation sickness, radiation recall, CNS effects of immunosuppression, and steroid-induced myopathy.

The ACS provides an online guide to drugs used in the treatment of cancer with common side effects listed.[14] The NCCN offers a number of clinical practice guidelines for cancer in general and for specific types of cancer.[252] The ACS offers suggestions for optimizing the preservation of fertility for men and women after cancer therapy.[17]

Each individual will experience and report discomfort in a slightly different way. The occurrence of symptoms is a stressor of its own, sometimes initiating a response of fear behaviors and distress. The idea of symptom distress (SD) as an additional side effect of cancer treatment is a fairly new concept.[201,235] Individual perception of symptoms includes whether the person notices a change in how he or she usually feels or behaves, intensity of the symptoms, and the impact of both the presence and intensity of symptoms on daily activities, function, and QOL. Response to SD includes physiologic, psychological, sociocultural, and behavioral components. The therapist may have a role in helping people assess their symptoms and amount of distress associated with symptoms, helping them to monitor their own level of health.[199]

The most common and often distressing side effect of cancer and cancer-related treatment is fatigue. The

| Table 9-7 | Side Effects of Cancer Treatment |

Surgery	Radiation (see Table 5-7)	Chemotherapy (see Table 5-8)	Biotherapy	Hormonal Therapy	Transplant (bone marrow, stem cell)
Fatigue	Fatigue	Fatigue	Fever	Hypertension	Severe bone
Disfigurement	Radiation sickness	Gastrointestinal	Chills	Steroid-induced	marrow
Loss of function	Immunosuppression	effects	Nausea	diabetes	suppression
Infection	Decreased platelets	Anorexia	Vomiting	Myopathy	Mucositis
Increased pain	Decreased white	Nausea	Anorexia	(steroid-induced)	Nausea and
Deformity	blood cells	Vomiting	Fatigue	Weight gain	vomiting
Bleeding,	Infection	Constipation	Fluid retention	Hot flashes	Graft versus
hemorrhage	Fatigue	Anxiety and	CNS effects	Erectile dysfunction	host
Scar tissue	Fibrosis	depression	Slowed thinking	(ED)	disease
Fibrosis	Radiation recall	Fluid/electrolyte	Memory problems	Decreased libido	(allogenic
	Mucositis	imbalance from GI	Inflammatory reactions	Vaginal dryness	graft only)
	Diarrhea	effects	at injection sites	Joint symptoms	Delayed
	Edema	Hepatotoxicity	Anemia	(arthralgia,	wound
	Hair loss	Hemorrhage	Leukopenia	arthritis)	healing
	Ulceration, delayed	Bone marrow	Altered taste sensation		Venoocclusive
	wound healing	suppression	Targeted therapies:		disease
	CNS/PNS effects	Anemia	Skin rash		Infertility
	Malignancy	Leukopenia (infection)	Paronychia		Cataract
		Neutropenia	Diarrhea		formation
		Decreased bone	Hypertension		Thyroid
		density with ovarian	Thrombus formation		dysfunction
		failure	Prolonged bleeding		Growth
		Muscle weakness	Renal toxicity		hormone
		Joint pain	Infusion reaction		deficiency
		Skin rashes	(fever, chills, short-		Osteoporosis
		Neuropathies	ness of breath, chest		Secondary
		Hair loss	pain, back pain,		malignancy
		Sterilization	flushing, changes in		
		Stomatitis, mucositis	heart rate and blood		
		(oral, rectal, vaginal)	pressure)		
		Sexual dysfunction	Mouth sores		
		Weight gain or loss			

CNS, Central nervous system; PNS, peripheral nervous system; GI, gastrointestinal.

therapist can be very instrumental in offering information and ideas about energy conservation (Box 9-4). The therapist can help the client set priorities, pace and delegate activities and responsibilities, and provide labor-saving devices and ideas. Scheduling activities at times of peak energy is important along with a structured daily routine that focuses on one activity at a time. The importance of socializing, relaxing, and finding quiet moments of pleasure cannot be emphasized enough. The therapist may also be involved in relaxation and stress management with referral for nutrition consultation, sleep therapy, and depression when indicated.[252]

Exercise to improve functional capacity, increase activity tolerance, manage stress, and improve mood is an integral part of fatigue management. See in-depth discussion "Cancer, Physical Activity, and Exercise Training" below.

Physical Therapist's Evaluation

In a physical therapy practice, anyone with a history of cancer, known cancer risk factors, and/or over the age of 40 should be screened for red flags suggestive of cancer. The therapist is a key professional in offering education for risk factor modification and cancer prevention. For the individual with a current diagnosis of cancer, an overall health assessment is important in providing the optimal exercise program. Physical examination will include observation, inspection, auscultation, percussion, palpation, and special tests. Guidelines for physical assessment, review of systems, and visceral assessment by physical therapists are available.[136] Gilchrist[132] suggests rehabilitation protocols during medical intervention with consideration for the specific cancer treatment.

The clinical behavior of the majority of musculoskeletal tumors is such that the symptoms are shared with a wide range of nontumorous orthopedic disorders. Pain, swelling, and local heat accompanying musculoskeletal tumors are also common to inflammatory conditions. In addition, the most likely sites of musculoskeletal tumors are regions frequently involved in sports injuries.[207] Occasionally the client does recall some sort of injury at the site of a previously unsuspected tumor, and this information further confuses the relationship between trauma and malignancy.[220]

Box 9-4

TIPS FOR ENERGY CONSERVATION

- Energy conservation is an organized procedure for finding ways to reduce the amount of effort and energy needed to accomplish a given task. By reducing the amount of energy needed to accomplish a task, more energy is available.
- Applying principles of energy conservation requires self-examination and assessment of habits and priorities. Making these types of changes requires patience but can result in continued activity over a longer period of time:
- Schedule the most strenuous activities during periods of highest energy.

  Before starting any activity, analyze the task and answer the following questions:

  Is the task necessary?

  Can it be eliminated or combined?

  Am I doing this out of habit?

  Can it be simplified by combining or eliminating steps?

  Can a larger job be divided into smaller tasks?

  Are there any assistive devices, small appliances, or tools that could make the task easier?

  Can this be done by someone else?

Alternate more strenuous tasks with easier ones (e.g., heavy – light-heavy-light)

Plan frequent rest periods, sit down, or take naps as needed. A slow steady rate with short rests in between is advised; working to the point of fatigue should be avoided.

Cluster activities so that it is not necessary to make frequent trips or walk long distances at home, school, or work.

Avoid or keep to a minimum the climbing of stairs.

Keep certain tasks, such as driving, shopping, and housekeeping, to a minimum. Delegate as many responsibilities and jobs as possible!

Sit down to perform activities of daily living (e.g., tooth brushing, hair combing) or household tasks, including meal preparation.

Avoid sitting on low or soft furniture that requires more energy expenditure to get up again. Store items where they are easy to reach (neither too low requiring stooping or too high to retrieve).

Encourage children to climb up on your lap or into a chair rather than lifting them up.

Minimize carrying objects; use a wheeled cart to carry things whenever possible.

Modify your living space to include grab rails in the bathroom, elevated toilet seat, chairs placed appropriately throughout to provide rest steps.

Data from Eaton LH, Tipton JM: *Putting evidence into practice: improving oncology patient outcomes.* Pittsburgh, 2009, Oncology Nursing Society; National Comprehensive Cancer Network (NCCN): *Practice Guidelines for Cancer-Related Fatigue.* Version 1.2012. Available at http://www.nccn.org/professionals/physician_gls/pdf/fatigue.pdf. Accessed June 27, 2014.

Cardiovascular and pulmonary tests and measures, including heart rate; breath sounds and respiratory rate, pattern, and quality; blood pressure; aerobic capacity test (e.g., 6-minute walk test); and pulse oximetry establish a baseline when developing an exercise program. This is especially important with the aging demographics of cancer survivors. The older people are when diagnosed with cancer, the greater the likelihood of other problems being present such as heart disease, hypertension, stroke, diabetes, osteoporosis, and so on.

Observe for and document any cluster of signs and symptoms for accompanying health conditions or comorbidities from cancer or cancer treatment such as hypoxia, decreased peripheral vascular supply, deep vein thrombosis, hypercalcemia, fluid or electrolyte imbalances, anemia, hypertension, integumentary changes, infection, and so on.

Integumentary, neuromuscular, musculoskeletal, and neurologic assessment should include but is not limited to skin characteristics and condition (including lymph node palpation); anthropometrics (e.g., limb length, limb girth, and body composition); functional strength testing; range of motion; flexibility; arousal, attention, and orientation tests; cranial and peripheral nerve integrity; motor function (e.g., dexterity, coordination, voluntary postures, and movement patterns); deep tendon and postural reflexes; and sensory testing (e.g., light touch, sharp/dull, temperature, deep pressure, proprioception, vibration, and stereognosis).[137]

The risk of falling is one of the more serious sequelae of both the local effects of cancer and the systemic consequences of cancer treatment. Weakness, pain, fatigue, orthostatic hypotension, peripheral neuropathy, decreased bone density (osteoporosis), and diminished flexibility, in various combinations, may result in falls. Some individuals will fail to inform their oncologist of debilitating peripheral neuropathies for fear of having their treatment delayed or prolonged.

The therapist can be very instrumental in patient/client education about the need to report side effects so the oncologist can evaluate dosage and treatment regimen. Anyone with neuropathies is at increased risk of falling; anyone with metastasized cancer to the spine or long bones may fracture these bones in a fall (or fall because of pathologic fractures), which can result in a serious, long-term disability.

Falls prevention and education are important aspects of the rehabilitation or exercise program. Assessment of the home environment is essential in providing a falls prevention program (see Box 27-19). In addition, the therapist must evaluate each client individually, possibly selecting an assistive device in appropriate cases. A walker with auto-stop wheels in the front may be a safer choice for some people than a standard walker that must be repeatedly lifted during ambulation. A wheelchair may be necessary for someone who experiences dizziness, weakness, fatigue, or signs of disorientation.

Higher incidences of osteoporosis and osteopenia are found in individuals with cancer, especially women taking aromatase inhibitors, exemestane for the primary prevention of breast cancer,[160] or with chemotherapy-induced ovarian failure.[325] Men with prostate cancer on androgen deprivation therapy are also more likely to develop osteoporosis.[88] Management of long-term bone health is an important aspect of comprehensive cancer care.[79,140]

Precautions

Cancer patients are immunocompromised and immunodeficient and therefore at risk for various viral, bacterial, and fungal infections but with preventive

Box 9-5

SYMPTOMATIC PRECAUTIONS DURING EXERCISE TESTING OR TRAINING

Anyone with cancer experiencing any of the following (especially brought on or exacerbated by exercise) should contact his or her physician.

- Fever
- Extreme or unusual tiredness or fatigue
- Unusual muscular weakness
- Irregular heartbeat, chest palpitations, or chest pain
- Sudden onset of dyspnea
- Leg pain or cramps
- Unusual joint pain
- Recent or new-onset back, neck, or bone pain
- Unusual bruising, nosebleeds, or bleeding from any other body opening
- Sudden onset of nausea during exercise
- Rapid weight gain or weight loss
- Severe diarrhea or vomiting
- Disorientation, confusion, dizziness, or light-headedness
- Blurred vision or other visual disturbances
- Skin pallor or unusual skin rash
- Night pain

Data from Drouin J, Pfalzer LA: Aerobic exercise guidelines for the person with cancer. *Acute Care Perspectives* 10(1&2):18–24, 2001; Drouin J, Pfalzer LA: Cancer and exercise (2012). National Center on Health, Physical Activity, and Disability (NCHPAD). Available online at http://www.ncpad.org/disability/fact_sheet.php?sheet=195&section=1465.

measures, the possibility of such complications can be reduced. The therapist must practice standard precautions carefully (especially proper handwashing and infection control principles; see chapter 8 and Appendix A) to help the individual undergoing cancer treatment avoid infection. Closely monitoring blood counts (and other laboratory values) and vital signs and observing for signs of infection, bleeding, or arrhythmias are important.

The therapist should contact the physician when the client exhibits fever or cluster of constitutional symptoms, unusual fatigue or tiredness, irregular heart beat or palpitations, chest pain, unusual bleeding, or night pain (see complete list in Box 9-5). Radiated tissue must be treated with care to avoid local trauma; extreme temperatures must be avoided; management of lymphedema may be required.

Many people undergoing cancer treatment are using complementary and alternative herbs or supplements that can have an adverse effect when combined with radiation or chemotherapy. If the client perceives disapproval, this information may not be relayed to the appropriate health care professional. By being open and nonjudgmental and inviting more discussion about the use of these techniques, the therapist may be able to bring to light potential risks involved. The client should be advised that most herbal or natural supplements and complementary interventions are designed to support, not replace, traditional medical interventions that have been proved effective.

There are many areas of question for therapists treating clients with a current or past history of cancer.

Clinical research in this area is sorely needed. In the absence of evidence-based practice, we must fall back on clinical decision making based on what evidence is available, understanding of the pathophysiology involved, and common sense in pursuing what is considered "best practice." Toward that end, any therapist working with this population group may want to take advantage of the collective ideas and suggestions made available through the American Physical Therapy Association Oncology Section's list server, an excellent resource for asking questions of therapists actively engaged in the treatment of cancer patients/clients. The oncology section also publishes an excellent peer-reviewed journal with pertinent and practical articles written by physical therapists in the field.

Oncologic Emergencies

Oncology patients/clients can present complex challenges for the physical therapist. Treatment regimens and their potential side effects top the list of important considerations during the physical therapist's intervention. Early recognition of potential emergencies, such as superior vena cava syndrome, tumor lysis syndrome, emergent spinal cord compression, severe thrombocytosis, and other conditions, is extremely important in reducing morbidity and mortality.[353]

Most of these conditions are uncommon or rare, making knowledge of them even more important so the therapist does not miss early clinical manifestations. Each one is typically associated with a particular type of cancer; knowing the patterns of potentially serious problems linked with individual cancers can help the therapist conduct surveillance with appropriate clients. For example, superior vena cava syndrome associated with small cell lung cancer and lymphoma is caused by mediastinal metastasis and central lung lesions compressing the superior vena cava. Presentation of superior vena cava syndrome is insidious with dilated neck veins and facial and arm lymphedema. Treatment may be palliative if the malignancy causing the compressive force is not curable; curative chemotherapy for lymphoma is the exception.[353]

Tumor lysis syndrome (TLS) refers to a constellation of metabolic disturbances that occur often in high-grade non-Hodgkin lymphoma after initiation of cancer treatment. TLS occurs in people with myeloproliferative disorders, such as acute leukemia and high-grade lymphoma, when chemotherapy causes lysis of a massive number of cells in a short period of time. The malignant cells die and release their contents. Acute renal failure may occur from the inability to clear the rapid deposition of potassium, phosphate, and uric acid from the cell lysis.[194,353]

Symptoms of TLS are most common 6 to 72 hours after chemotherapy begins and reflect the severity of the underlying metabolic abnormalities. TLS may only become clinically apparent in a small number of affected individuals. The therapist may hear reports of and observe muscle weakness, spasm, and cramping from TLS. Rapidly increasing uric acid levels may lead to arthralgia and renal colic. Neurologic signs and symptoms can include paresthesia and paralysis (hyperkalemia); seizures, tetany, and lethargy (hyperphosphatemia); lethargy, malaise, sleepiness, and seizures (hyperuricemia); and paresthesia, tetany, confusion, delirium, hallucinations (hypocalcemia).[194]

In addition, the therapist must monitor for cardiovascular effects such as arrhythmias, abnormal changes in blood pressure, and tachycardia during activity. Symptoms associated with volume overload may develop (e.g., dyspnea, pulmonary crackles, edema, hypertension). Accompanying gastrointestinal signs and symptoms can include anorexia, nausea, vomiting, diarrhea, hyperactive bowel sounds, and abdominal pain, bloating, or cramps. Electrolyte imbalances can trigger the clotting cascade, leading to disseminated intravascular coagulation. Any of these sequelae can be fatal. Early reporting of symptoms can prevent dangerous complications from this condition.

Spinal cord compression affects up to 30% of individuals with disseminated cancer from lung, breast, prostate, multiple myeloma, and colon. The thoracic spine is targeted most often, followed by the lumbosacral region. Back pain, muscle weakness, gait changes, or other signs and symptoms of cord compression may develop slowly or may progress rapidly; prognosis is better with slow onset.

The therapist should conduct surveillance examinations of serial muscle testing to detect decline in motor function potentially associated with spinal cord compression for individuals undergoing treatment for any of the cancers listed. A stable spine is essential before progressing to out-of-bed activities; surgical stabilization or use of an orthosis may be needed.[353]

Many individuals undergoing treatment for cancer are *thrombocytopenic* (low platelet levels). Severe thrombocytopenia (the definition of "severe" may vary from institution to institution but generally is noted as less than 10,000 cells/mm³; some institutions go as low as 5,000) increases the risk of spontaneous bleeding (e.g., intracranial, intramuscular, or joint bleeds). Precautions for thrombocytopenia are discussed further in Chapters 14 and 40. The therapist may be instrumental in preventing intracranial bleeds and falls for anyone with this complication.

Sexual Issues

Sexual dysfunction is a frequent side effect of cancer treatment, especially for those adults with cancer of the reproductive organs (e.g., breast, prostate, testicle, ovary, and uterus) and after Hodgkin disease. The most common problems include loss of desire for sexual activity, erectile dysfunction in men, interrupted childbearing and/or infertility,[55] and dyspareunia in women. Unlike many other physiologic side effects, sexual problems do not tend to resolve within the first year or two of disease-free survival but remain constant.[230,320]

Physical therapists are often in a unique position to assist people with sexual concerns because of their repeated close contact with the affected individual. Sexual function is an important aspect of QOL and requires a brief assessment. In oncology settings, it is often helpful to have a physical therapist who specializes in pelvic floor dysfunction and sexuality issues.[144,320] The therapist who is comfortable and knowledgeable in discussing sexual issues may be able to provide more focused assistance to the individual who is trying to adjust to changes in sexual style and practices as a result of the illness. Understanding the range of values and sexual history that clients bring to the clinical situation and respecting appropriate provider–client boundaries are important.[289] More specific information on this topic is readily available.[23,167,275,324]

Palliative and Hospice Care

> Palliative care is an approach that improves the quality of life of patients and their families facing the problem associated with life-threatening or serious illnesses, through the prevention and relief of suffering by means of early identification and impeccable assessment and treatment of pain and other problems, physical, psychosocial and spiritual.
> World Health Organization[394]

When curative measures have been exhausted and a cure is no longer possible or available, symptom management or palliative care may be offered regardless of how long the individual lives. The goals are to prevent symptoms; side effects caused by treatment of the disease; and psychological, social, and spiritual problems related to the disease or its treatment. When prevention is not possible, then treatment becomes the intervention.[249,300]

The CARING criteria are a practical tool to help identify those individuals who may benefit from a palliative approach with end-of-life discussions and aggressive symptom management. The criteria are simple items easily identified upon hospital admission. The criteria include the following:[118]

C: *Primary diagnosis of Cancer (especially if cancer has metastasized)*

A: *Two or more hospital Admissions for a chronic illness in the last 12 months*

R: *Resident in a nursing home*

I: *ICU admission with multiple organ failure (MOF)*

N: *Noncancer hospice (meeting two or more of the National Hospice and Palliative Care Organization's (NHPCO)*

G: *Guidelines)*

Scoring for risk of death is as follows:

Low:	<5
Medium:	5-12
High:	≥13

This set of screening criteria is highly predictive of death within 1 year in a hospitalized population. Even if the person ends up with a better result than predicted, there is no harm in instituting palliative care. The client ends up with a completed advance directive and is less likely to experience untreated pain. When death is imminent, hospice, defined as support and care given for people in the last phase of an incurable disease so they may live as fully and comfortably as possible,[254] may be provided in a free-standing hospice center, hospice hospital unit, long-term care facility, or at home. At the center of hospice and palliative care is the belief that everyone has the right to die pain-free and with dignity and that families should receive the necessary support to allow this to occur.

According to the guidelines of the World Health Organization (WHO),[402] the term *terminally ill patient* refers to an individual with cancer whose life expectancy is less than 90 days, and the index of his or her physical state (defined by the Karnofsky Performance Scale; see Table 30-6) is below 50. Individual hospice agencies may use time periods other than 90 days as their qualification standard.

Although the cost of hospice may be covered by private insurance or by the client/family out-of-pocket, Medicare has three key eligibility criteria as follows: (1) the patient's doctor and the hospice medical director use their best clinical judgment to certify that the patient is terminally ill with a life expectancy of 6 months or less, if the disease runs its normal course, (2) the patient signs a statement choosing to receive hospice care rather than curative treatments for his/her illness, and (3) the patient enrolls in a Medicare-approved hospice program.

Palliative care for the terminally ill is aimed at improving the QOL of both the individual and family members. The primary goal is to decrease the physical and psychological suffering of the individual while providing spiritual and emotional support. Every effort is made to help the individual achieve as full a life as possible, with minimal pain, discomfort, and restriction. Many medications, especially morphine, are used for pain control. Emphasis of hospice care is toward emotional and psychological support for the client and the family, focusing on death as a natural end to life.[253]

Physical therapy may enhance the QOL of individuals receiving palliative care, as well as dying individuals receiving hospice care. Disability in individuals with advanced cancer often results from bed rest, deconditioning, and neurologic and musculoskeletal complications of cancer or cancer treatment. Weakness, pain, fatigue, and dyspnea are common symptoms.

Physical therapy intervention aims to improve level of function and comfort. Physical function and independence should be maintained as long as possible to improve QOL and reduce the burden of care for the caregivers.[218] Pain management and relief, positioning to prevent pressure ulcers and aid breathing, endurance training and energy conservation, home modification, and family education are just a few of the services the physical therapist can offer hospice clients and families. The therapist is an important team member in helping clients remain functional and retain dignity and control at the end of life.[302]

At the present time, there is very little evidence that rehabilitation interventions can impact function and symptom management in individuals who are terminally ill. Clinical experience suggests that the application of rehabilitation principles is likely to improve their care.[314] Evidence-based research may help expand reimbursement under Medicare to include physical therapy as a core service.[302] Therapists working with hospice programs are encouraged to attend interdisciplinary team meetings whenever possible—even if reimbursement for the time is not possible or the therapist has not been specifically invited or included. Discussing and demonstrating ways in which the physical therapist can benefit clients, while acknowledging the costs (and cost savings), can help advance the overall work of physical therapists in hospice care.[302]

For physical therapists interested or involved in hospice care, there is an APTA Oncology Section–sponsored special interest group (SIG) available for support and information: Hospice and Palliative Care SIG (http://www.oncologypt.org/special-interest-groups/hospice-palliative-care-sig/index.cfm). The Hospice and Palliative Care SIG can help therapists who have a common interest in the treatment of life-limiting conditions meet, confer, and promote these interests.

Radiation Hazard for the Health Care Worker

Implant radiation therapy requires personal radiation protection for all staff members who come in contact with the client (this topic is discussed in "Radiation Hazard for Health Care Professionals" in Chapter 5).

CANCER, PHYSICAL ACTIVITY, AND EXERCISE TRAINING

Lisa VanHoose, PhD, PT, CLT-LANA

In the last decade, the body of knowledge focused on the relationship between exercise and cancer has exponentially increased. As with the prevention and management of heart disease, obesity, osteoporosis, and diabetes, exercise plays an important role in cancer prevention and ameliorating the side effects of cancer treatment, and promoting improved health among cancer survivors. The various modes of exercise have resulted in clinical and statistical heterogeneity in the literature. Modes of exercise include aerobic, resistive, flexibility, balance training, and conditioning or any combination of these forms. Studies using a normal, healthy adult population have indicated that each type of exercise has its own physiologic and psychological benefits, and researchers are currently investigating the effects in individuals with cancer.

Not all cancers are alike or affect the body in the same way. Exercise benefits may vary based on cancer type, stage, treatment, side effects of treatment, and other extraneous factors. Exercise appears to be safe, but long-term outcomes have not been reported. Some types of exercise, aggressive weight and aerobic training, have been shown detrimental to the immune system and this must be considered when developing a physical therapy care plan (see discussion in Chapter 7). Therapists working with the oncology population are encouraged to evaluate the literature to find the best choice of prescriptive exercise for a specific cancer. Because of the various cancer types and the breadth of literature, only a composite summary is provided in this chapter. A summary of the current evidence and suggestions for guiding individuals in this area has recently become available[226] that might be of interest to all health care providers.

Exercise as a Cancer Prevention Strategy

Physical activity is defined as body movement caused by skeletal muscle contraction that result in quantifiable energy expenditure. Exercise is distinguished from other types of physical activity by the fact that the intensity, duration, and frequency of the activity are specifically designed to improve physical fitness. Intensity of exercise is commonly stratified based on heart rate, with 40% to 54% of maximum heart rate (MHR) defined as low. Activities that are part of one's daily routine are typically of low intensity and duration. Both epidemiologic and laboratory data indicate that physical activity of at least a moderate level may affect cancer risk.[24,35,181] Moderate intensity is defined as 55% to 69% of MHR and include, but not limited to, walking, dancing, volleyball, and golfing. Fast bicycling, jogging, and like activities increase the heart rate to 70% or greater of the MHR.[64,327] However, therapists should be aware that the 220 – Age equation (MHR) does not account for differences in resting heart rate. The Karvonen Formula is a better method although slightly more complicated. The Karvonen Formula uses the MHR and heart rate reserve in calculating target heart rates or classifying the intensity of a task.[138,265]

Being sedentary is a risk factor for several of the most common types of cancer (e.g., breast and colon). A role for exercise in specifically reducing cancer risk has been shown for breast and colorectal cancer, with more equivocal evidence for others such as melanoma, lung, and prostate cancers.[329] The mode and dosage of exercise needed to prevent cancer is debatable. Therapeutic responsiveness is currently based on cancer type, stage of disease, or treatment.[168] The ACS advises moderate habitual physical activity as a potentially protective measure against certain types of neoplasms, particularly tumors of the breast, colon, kidney, lung, pancreas, prostate, and the female reproductive tract.[196] The Women's Health Initiative reported that 1.25 to 2.5 hours per week of brisk walking lowered breast cancer risk by 18% in women.[227] Moderate-intensity physical activity should be performed for 30 minutes or greater, at least 5 days a week.[284] Until results of systematic studies are available, the ACS agrees with recommendations of at least 30 to 60 minutes of moderate to vigorous physical activity at least 5 days per week to reduce the risk of cancer, cardiovascular disease, and diabetes.[196,209]

Research is elucidating the protective mechanisms of exercise. Exercise-induced changes in the activity of macrophages, natural killer cells, lymphokine-activated killer cells, neutrophils, and regulating cytokines suggests that immunomodulation may contribute to the protective value of exercise (see also "Exercise, Physical Activity, and the Immune System" in Chapter 7).[236,391]

At the present time, cytokine modulation with exercise is receiving considerable research attention. Researchers theorize that exercise can regulate production of certain hormones, which when unregulated, may spur tumor growth.[372] Also, exercise may enhance host defense against the tumor.[373] See further discussion in the "Exercise and the Immune System" in Chapter 7. Exercise also improves energy balance, which increases one's ability to maintain a healthy weight. Being overweight or obese increases the risk of various cancers,[21,37,195,271,297,298,392] possibly because of inflammation and abnormalities in immune function[339] and hormone metabolism. Exercise can normalize many of these functions with appropriate dosing.

Exercise for Cancer Survivors

The diagnosis of cancer begins the survivorship continuum from diagnosis to end of life. Exercise programs appear to have a beneficial influence throughout the continuum and especially during the early stages of the disease. However, survivors tend to decrease levels of physical activity and exercise at diagnosis, during treatment, and/or after completion of their treatment, especially if they were sedentary before their cancer diagnosis.[175] Low-intensity exercise can seem like high intensity for these individuals. In addition, some cancer therapies reduce exercise capacity because of cardiopulmonary, neurologic, and musculoskeletal impairments.

Therefore, the type, frequency, duration, and intensity of exercise should be individualized on the basis of the survivor's age, previous fitness level, type of cancer and cancer treatment, and the presence of any additional comorbidities. Some specific guidelines are available in Box 9-6. The American College of Sports Medicine (ACSM) has recommended that survivors follow the same exercise as the general population (150 minutes of moderate-level physical activity) with slow progression of resistance exercise.

Survivors should be educated to understand that any exercise has a linear benefit, with increasing health benefit with higher volume of physical activity. However, caution should be provided that extremely high levels of exercise might increase the risk for infections and exercise-related

---

Box 9-6

SPECIFIC EXERCISE PRECAUTIONS FOR CANCER SURVIVORS

- Survivors with severe anemia may need to delay exercise; medical evaluation is required
- Survivors with compromised immune function or who have had bone marrow transplantation should avoid public gyms and other public places until white blood cell counts return to safe levels; this could take up to 1 year or longer
- Severe fatigue can keep an individual from doing any exercise; daily stretching is advised and even 5-minute increments of mild activity (e.g., walking, sit-to-be-fit) should be encouraged
- Avoid exposure of irradiated skin to chlorine (e.g., swimming pools) until medically approved
- Survivors with indwelling catheters must observe additional precautions: avoid water or other microbial exposures that can lead to infection; avoid resistance training of muscles that can dislodge the catheter
- Recumbent stationary biking may be a better option than walking on a treadmill for those individuals with significant peripheral neuropathies or gait disturbances

Data from Rock CL: Nutrition and physical activity guidelines for cancer survivors, *CA Cancer J Clin* 62(4):243-74, 2012.

injuries.[257] With 12 million Americans alive today who have been through the cancer experience,[65] it is important to develop interventions to enhance immune function and prevent or minimize muscle wasting, thus counteracting the detrimental physiologic effects of cancer and chemotherapy, and maintaining quality of life (QOL) after cancer diagnosis.

Physical activity and exercise training are interventions that address a broad range of QOL issues, including physical (e.g., muscular strength, body composition, nausea, and fatigue), functional (e.g., functional capacity), psychological (e.g., coping and mood changes), spiritual, emotional, and social well-being.[36] Studies examining the therapeutic value of exercise for people with various cancers during primary cancer treatment suggest that exercise is safe and feasible, improving physical functioning and some aspects of QOL.[6,82,190,317,318]

Screening and Assessment

Medical screening should be conducted with all clients before their participation in an exercise program.[1,317] This type of screening is especially important for people with cancer who receive various levels of treatment that can affect the physiologic response to exercise. For example, fatigue is a common symptom of nearly every form of cancer treatment.

The therapist will need to take a detailed history of treatment administered to date, examine laboratory results, and distinguish between fatigue from deconditioning and fatigue from medical interventions to determine the most effective and efficient approach to rehabilitation. The medical history should also identify conditions, which may or may not be related to cancer and its treatment, such as hypertension, diabetes, coronary artery disease, and preexisting orthopedic conditions. The person's current physical condition, condition before disease onset, age, and living environment are also important variables.[389] Based on a 2012 study in the *Physical Therapy Journal*, most clinicians rely heavily on the patient/client assessment for exercise prescription and progression.[145] Therefore, a thorough assessment is crucial and multiple assessment tools are available to aid the physical therapist.

A self-reporting survey instrument called the Cancer Rehabilitation Evaluation System (formerly called the Cancer Inventory of Problem Situations) is a useful tool for evaluating rehabilitation needs and interventions.[63,157] The SF-36 has been validated in multiple cancer populations and allows the therapist to assess disease burden.[239,285,301] Another tool commonly reported in the literature is the Functional Assessment of Chronic Illness Therapy surveys. Instruments are available for several cancer types and evaluate physical, social, functional, and emotional well-being.[47,63,396]

The therapist must understand the stages of the disease and know the type and timing of the medical interventions, especially radiation and chemotherapy treatment. The body's physiologic response to these agents (e.g., fatigue, neuropathy, or chemo brain or chemo "fog") may alter the normal training response, affect tolerance for exercise, and compliance with exercise programs.

Cognitive rehabilitation techniques may be needed to improve patient/client compliance, function, and QOL.[124]

Cardiac dysfunction can result in left ventricular failure, cardiomyopathy, and/or congestive heart failure months to years after chemotherapy. These conditions may impact the client's ability to exercise. Signs and symptoms of subclinical cardiac conditions may develop with the initiation of an exercise program. Careful history taking and clinical assessment may result in early detection and intervention, potentially reducing morbidity.

Auscultation to screen for abnormal lung or heart sounds is important to identify any precautions or contraindications to exercise. The individual is not likely to be able to sustain exercise levels if there are any physiologic abnormalities present. Medical consult may be required before initiating or continuing a training program when high-risk medical conditions are identified by the physical therapists.

Older adults, especially older adults with bone disease or significant comorbidities and impairments, such as arthritis or peripheral neuropathies, will need an assessment of balance, strength, and coordination to remain safe from falls and injuries during exercise.

Monitoring Vital Signs

Monitoring physiologic responses to exercise is important in the immunosuppressed population. Baseline testing is important to determine safe guidelines and to provide a starting place against which to measure improvement and to identify the individual's functional exercise level. A hypertensive response to exercise is common among individuals with cancer and undergoing cancer treatment. Starting an aerobic training program is not advised if such a response is observed during testing.

Exercise intensity determined by training heart rate may be difficult because some people have inappropriate heart responses to exercise and large physiologic changes on a day-to-day basis from disease and treatment (e.g., changes in medications). Exercise intensity can be guided by heart rate ranges based on oxygen consumption or metabolic equivalent (MET) levels. The therapist can use test results to prescribe a program starting at approximately 60% of the individual's maximum level. The therapist is advised to use prior exercise levels, prior exercise capabilities, baseline function, and individual abilities even when using the predictive formula because each client may respond differently (unpredictably).

The therapist (or client) should always monitor oxygen saturation with pulse oximetry and evaluate heart rate (for arrhythmias), pulse rate, breathing frequency, and blood pressure before, during, and after the treatment session. Borg Scale for Rating of Perceived Exertion (RPE) (see Table 12-13) or other scales can be used to determine level of symptom distress or severity. RPE is also used when the client is taking cardiac medications that blunt heart rate response to exercise or when other conditions and comorbidities are present that may prevent the use of target heart rate formulas.

Watch closely for early signs (dyspnea, pallor, sweating, and fatigue) of cardiopulmonary complications of cancer treatment. Monitoring vital signs helps the therapist recognize early when an individual is reaching his or her tolerance level. The therapist must keep in mind the need to balance activities that push the heart rate up with energy conservation so the individual can remain functional for the rest of the day. The activity level of someone with anemia also may require adjustment. This client may have elevated pulse and respiratory rates due to hypoxia, with increased cardiac output resulting from the body's effort to maintain an adequate oxygen supply.

Prescriptive Exercise

Types, limitations, and precautions of exercise intervention in the treatment of cancer, especially cancer pain, are being studied. The programs studied vary in length from 6 weeks for individuals who were going through radiation therapy to 6 months for those in chemotherapy and the entire duration of bone marrow transplantation. Exercise interventions vary somewhat but most include progressive programs of 15- to 30-minute sessions, 3 to 5 days a week, at an intensity equal to 60% to 80% of MHR (RPE 11-14). A perceived exertion of no greater than 12 may be used as a guide when exercise testing is not possible (see Table 12-13). Although variations will occur in research and clinical protocols, the American College of Sports Medicine has recommended the FITT principles for clinical exercise prescription.[360] The acronym stands for frequency, intensity, time, and type of exercise. The goal is that exercise promotes fitness, under the FITT principle, with improvements in cardiorespiratory and muscular function, flexibility, and body composition.

The frequency and duration/time of exercise are determined by the clinical status of the person. If weight training is prescribed, high-repetition, low-weight circuit programs are recommended that do not exceed RPE of 14.[206] Other clinical tools for monitoring and more specific guidelines for exercise are available.[100,105,278]

Clinical observations and case studies have reported that individuals who exercised more than 60 minutes per day were more likely to report higher levels of fatigue, suggesting a maximum effective dose for individuals receiving adjuvant chemotherapy. However, research has suggested that the type of exercise may have a greater effect on fatigue and immunity compared to the duration of exercise.[328] Moderate levels of exercise may enhance immunity, and vigorous activity may impair the immune response and increase fatigue symptoms.[348] No serious adverse events were reported in any of the studies, although anyone in the high-risk category with serious comorbidities was excluded, and most exercise programs were flexible and symptom-limited.

The reported outcomes of these and other studies show that exercise has a powerful effect on CRF, with fatigue levels reported as 40% to 50% lower in exercising participants. Exercise reduces fatigue and emotional distress and improves QOL.[73,295,378] Without exception, all of these studies showed lower levels of fatigue and emotional distress as well as decreased sleep disturbance (if this was studied as an outcome) in people who exercised during treatment compared to controls or to baseline scores in single-group designs. A summary of the studies included is available.[252]

Not all people with cancer are able to participate in aerobic exercise. People who ambulate less than 50% of the time, those confined to bed, and those who fatigue with mild exertion may not be candidates for aerobic exercise.[388] Range-of-motion and gentle resistive work may be appropriate until tolerance for activity improves. Energy-conservation techniques and work simplification (see Box 9-4) may be necessary for the person with chronic fatigue and for those whose functional status is declining. Therapeutic exercise should be scheduled during periods when the person has the highest level of energy.

Interval exercise or a bedside exercise program may be preferred at first. Interval exercise may be the only treatment possible in this circumstance. This is performed during frequent but short sessions throughout the day with work-rest intervals beginning at the person's level of tolerance. This may be no more than 1 minute of exercise activity followed by 1 minute of rest, then 1 minute of exercise, and so on. As the person's endurance level increases, the duration of work may be increased and the interval of rest decreased. See also "Special Implications for the Therapist: Anemia" in Chapter 14.

Generalized weakness associated with cancer treatment can be more debilitating than the disease itself. Whenever possible, exercise, including strength training and cardiovascular training, is an essential component for many people with cancer. Improving strength and endurance aids in countering the effects of the disease and the effects of medical interventions. Increased physical activity may increase the homeostatic sleep drive to increase nighttime sleep and may help relieve CRF.[78]

Exercise for CRF

CRF is common and disabling for up to 100% of survivors undergoing chemotherapy and/or radiation.[96,340,375,381] Fatigue is defined as "persistent, subjective sense of tiredness related to cancer or cancer treatment that interferes with usual functioning."[234] People in cancer treatment are often advised to rest after chemotherapy, but aerobic exercise and physical activity have been shown to help improve energy level and stamina, reduce fatigue, reduce nausea, increase muscle mass, and increase daily activities without increasing fatigue.

Approximately 30% of survivors will continue to report fatigue as a barrier to function after treatment.[22,40,119] The use of exercise as an intervention for CRF has been proven as an effective strategy.[371] A 2010 Cochrane Summary indicated that exercise can attenuate fatigue throughout the cancer continuum. However, the authors stated that the type and intensity of exercise is variable and additional research is needed to determine the most effective dosage.[83] Traditional (e.g., walking or aerobics) and alternative forms of exercise (e.g., Tai chi, dance, or yoga) are being investigated.[46,59,123,126,225,308,379]

Much of the exercise-related research is focused on breast cancer,[155,276] but aerobic exercise after bone marrow transplantation[98,315] and exercise during treatment of cancers, such as multiple myeloma,[78] solid tumors, and lymphoma, have been studied.[379] Exercise combined with improved nutrition for CRF and deconditioning has also been reported successful in demonstrating significant improvements in the 6-minute walk test distance, the squat test, and fatigue level.[269]

Clients receiving chemotherapy and radiation therapy experiencing CRF who are already on an exercise program may need to exercise temporarily at a lower intensity and progress at a slower pace; the goal is to remain as active as possible. For sedentary individuals, low-intensity activities such as stretching and brief, slow walks can be implemented and slowly advanced.[52]

However, it can be difficult to convince someone who is extremely tired (and especially those who did not exercise before their cancer diagnosis) that exercise will improve his or her symptoms. The therapist may have to begin with discussions over a period of time about the importance of exercise and the pathophysiology of CRF.

The National Cancer Institute has provided and frequently updates its Fatigue PDQ, which can be used for patient education. This is especially important if the person is significantly deconditioned. The therapist can begin with an assessment of previous exercise or activity patterns. Ask the following questions:

- Can you do your normal daily activities?
- Can you participate in a formal or informal exercise program?
- What is your normal amount and frequency of exercise?
- Have you had to modify or change your exercise level or other activity patterns since the development of fatigue?

Symptoms of fatigue, headache, and lethargy begin in most people when hemoglobin falls to 12 g/dL. Mild-to-moderate graded exercise is possible for many people at this level. Symptoms become more pronounced when hemoglobin decreases to 10 g/dL, reducing exercise capacity.

Exercise is not always possible for most people when the hemoglobin level is 8 g/dL or less. Hemoglobin levels should be maintained around 12 g/dL during the administration of chemotherapy,[34] but protocols vary from institution to institution and even from one physician to another within the same facility. Bloodless medicine (see discussion in Chapter 14) has made it possible for clients to tolerate lower hemoglobin levels previously thought unacceptable without compromising oxygen delivery. See also exercise guidelines provided in Tables 40-8 and 40-9, keeping in mind that most oncology settings have their own guidelines that may be more liberal. For example, in some oncology settings, exercise is contraindicated when white blood cell count drops below 500/mm³ (compared to 5000/mm³ listed in Table 40-8) and when platelets drop below 5000/mm³ (compared to 20,000/mm³ listed in Table 40-9).

The National Center on Health, Physical Activity, and Disability guidelines on Cancer and Exercise[106] and the American College of Sports Medicine guidelines for termination of testing or training may also be consulted.[1] People with cancer are advised to contact their physician if any of the abnormal responses listed in Box 9-5 develop.

Exercise During and After Radiation Therapy or Chemotherapy

Bone marrow suppression is a common and serious side effect of many chemotherapeutic agents and can be a side effect of radiation therapy in some instances such as when radiation dosage exceeded 50 Gy in the past or currently when high levels of radiation are used to prevent death despite potential radiotherapy toxicities later. Therefore, it is extremely important to take a client history of current or past radiation therapy dosages and to monitor the hematologic values in clients receiving these treatment modalities.

The therapist must review these values before any type of vigorous exercise or activity is initiated. Current guidelines recommend that individuals undergoing chemotherapy or radiation therapy should not exercise within 2 hours of the treatment because increases in circulation may attenuate the effectiveness of the treatment[131] and increase the risk of side effects. Although this recommendation is not based on evidence-based research, it is a guideline followed by the National Institutes of Health (NIH) because of the physiologic effects of moderate to vigorous physical activity and exercise on the redistribution of cardiac output and blood flow to the working muscle. In the case of both radiation therapy and chemotherapy, there is a potential to enhance treatment toxicity with the shift in blood flow. The suggested 2-hour delay is reasonable given the half-life of most chemotherapeutic agents and the rate of decay of fractionated doses of radiation.[280] However, moderate-intensity aerobic exercise (walking for 20-45 minutes, 3-5 times per week at 50%-70% of measured MHRs during 7 weeks of radiation) has been shown to maintain erythrocyte levels during radiation treatment (of breast cancer).[107]

Exercise may increase the body's ability to recover from the effects of chemotherapy.[27] Physical activity can also improve mood and reduce anxiety and mental stress for people undergoing chemotherapy. Independence and QOL improve as functional ability improves.[3,99,101,292] A helpful guideline to indicate when aerobic exercise is contraindicated (or when reevaluation of the exercise program is indicated) in chemotherapy clients is given in Box 9-7. Keep in mind these values are primarily educated

---

Box 9-7

PRECAUTIONS TO AEROBIC EXERCISE IN CHEMOTHERAPY CLIENTS*

Platelet count	<50,000/mL
Hemoglobin	<10 g/dL
White blood cell count	<3000/mL; 10,000 with fever (no exercise)
Absolute granulocytes	<2500/mL

* Single threshold values are not usually clinically relevant but provide a *general guideline*. For example, hemoglobin levels have the most variability from client to client; protocols can vary from center to center and even from physician to physician. These general guidelines are for use as *precautions* to aerobic exercise. What constitutes aerobic can also vary from individual to individual and requires monitoring of vital signs and/or the use of rate of perceived exertion (Borg scale).

Data from:

Winningham ML, MacVicar MG, Burke CA: Exercise for cancer patients; guidelines and precautions. *Phys Sportsmed* 14:125-134, 1986.

Please keep in mind that Winningham levels often cited may be considered quite conservative in today's oncologic practice as these values were set by a research council more than 25 years ago. At that time there were more unknowns and greater concern for mortality compared with today's more evidence-based, aggressive approaches.

Stiller K: Safety issues that should be considered when mobilizing critically ill patients. *Crit Care Clin* 23(1):35-53, 2007.

estimates based on clinical consensus; there is a need for further research and stronger evidence to support these values.

Exercise and Bone Metastases

See "Special Implications for the Therapist: Metastatic Tumors" in Chapter 26.

Exercise and Lymphedema

In the past, therapists were cautioned to carefully design a program that did not cause or exacerbate cancer-related complications such as lymphedema. It was advised that repetitive or strenuous exercise would increase the production of lymph fluid, and lymphedema would be the result because lymph nodes were removed during surgery, damaged by radiation therapy, or invaded by the tumor, leaving scar tissue that prevented normal lymph drainage. In fact, it is now known that exercise activates muscle groups and joints in the affected extremity, increases lymph flow,[94] and does not induce lymphedema.[149,150] Resistance training has not been shown to adversely affect lymphedema.[6,319]

Combining a specific exercise program for each individual with the use of sufficient compression will facilitate the process of decongestion by using the natural pumping effect of the muscles to increase lymph flow while preventing limb refilling. Most clinicians experienced in lymphedema treatment agree on basic guidelines for exercise. See further discussion in Chapter 13.

Exercise and Advanced Cancer

With improved detection and treatment, more and more people are living with cancer as a controllable chronic disease or in advanced stages of cancer. Although the body of knowledge is evolving, there is insufficient research on exercise in such individuals to make specific recommendations for physical activity and exercise. In such cases, therapists are advised to prescribe exercise based on individual needs and abilities.

General training precautions for warm-up and cool down should be followed while monitoring for abnormal heart rate or blood pressure responses and observing each individual for pathologic symptomatic responses (e.g., hypertension, chest pain, onset of wheezing, claudication or leg cramps, shortness of breath, and dizziness or fainting). Clients should be encouraged to remain adequately hydrated at all times unless medically directed otherwise.

Compromised skeletal integrity, especially in the presence of muscle wasting, increases the risk of fracture and may prevent weight-bearing activities. Aerobic exercise may have to begin with non–weight-bearing exercise, such as cycling, rowing, or swimming (for those who are not immunocompromised or neutropenic), with a gradual return to weight-bearing activities whenever possible to prevent loss of bone density. People with severe muscle weakness may tolerate cycling better than walking[277] and seated exercises may be another strategy.[152] Interval exercise (periods of exercise alternated with periods of rest) may be used with a goal in mind of increasing the exercise time and decreasing the rest.[277] Exercise has been suggested to improve fatigue in advanced disease[292] and

therapists should also consider the psychosocial benefits of group exercise.[4,270]

CHILDHOOD CANCER

Incidence and Overview

Each year approximately 12,060 children (birth to 14 years) in the United States are diagnosed with cancer. According to SEER data, the death rate has decreased by more than half over the past 30 years from 4.9 per 100,000 in 1975 to 2.2 in 2008[337] With advances in treatment, 82.5% of these children will survive 5 years or more (improved from 58% for children diagnosed 30 years ago and an increase of almost 40% since the early 1960s). Currently it is estimated that there are 58,510 child survivors of cancer living in the United States.

Cancer is the second leading cause of death among children between 1 and 14 years of age.[337] Treatment-related deaths have declined as a result of advances in clinical supportive care (e.g., antibiotic therapy, indwelling venous-access lines, blood products, and enteral and parenteral nutrition) that maximize the benefits and minimize the side effects of cancer therapy.

The types of cancers that occur in children vary greatly from those seen in adults. Leukemias, particularly acute lymphocytic leukemia (ALL); lymphomas (almost half of all childhood cancers involve the blood or blood-forming organs); brain tumors; embryonal tumors; and soft tissue sarcomas are the most common pediatric malignancies, whereas adenocarcinomas (e.g., lung, breast, or colorectal) are more common in adults.

Other differences that must be taken into account when treating the child with cancer include the stage of growth and development, stage of psychosocial and cognitive development, and emotional response of the child to the illness and its treatment. The immaturity of the child's organ systems often has important treatment implications.

Types of Childhood Cancers

The most common pediatric malignancies are ALL, non-Hodgkin lymphoma, Hodgkin disease, and primary CNS tumors. Neuroblastoma, Wilms (kidney) tumor, rhabdomyosarcoma, and retinoblastomas are the types of solid tumors occurring most frequently in children.

ALL, the most common childhood malignancy, accounts for almost one-third of all pediatric cancers. White males are affected most often, and although the exact cause is unknown, radiation, chromosomal abnormalities, viruses, and congenital immunodeficiencies have all been associated with an increased incidence of leukemia. See also "The Leukemias" in Chapter 14.

Wilms tumor, a malignancy that may affect one or both kidneys, occurs in children under the age of 14 years and is slightly more prevalent in females than males. Epidemiologic research suggests an increased incidence in children of men exposed to lead or hydrocarbons. An association between Wilms tumor and chromosomal abnormalities has been established, specifically deletion of a suppressor gene located on the short arm of chromosome. This chromosomal anomaly is an autosomal dominant trait requiring evaluation of other family members.

Neuroblastoma is the most common extracranial solid tumor in children and the most commonly diagnosed neoplasm during the first year of life. Approximately 500 new cases are diagnosed annually in the United States, and the incidence is higher among whites than nonwhites. Neuroblastoma can originate anywhere along the sympathetic nervous system, but more than half the tumors occur in the retroperitoneal area and present as an abdominal mass. Other common sites include the posterior mediastinum, pelvis, and neck. If the bone marrow is involved, bone pain may occur. See "Neuroblastoma" in Chapter 30.

Rhabdomyosarcoma is the most common soft tissue sarcoma and the seventh leading cause of cancer in children. This tumor, which is more prevalent in males than females, originates from the same embryonic cells that give rise to striated muscle. The peak incidence is between the age of 2 and 5 years and a second peak occurs between 15 and 19 years, with much improved survival rates with early detection and treatment today. The most common tumor sites include the head and neck, genitourinary tract, and extremities. Rhabdomyosarcoma of the head and neck can lead to CNS involvement, including cranial nerve palsies, meningeal symptoms, and respiratory paralysis. See further discussion in Chapter 26.

Other common cancers seen in children are bone cancers, both osteogenic and Ewing sarcomas (see Chapter 26), and brain tumors (see Chapter 30).

Late Effects and Prognosis

As advances in cancer therapy improve, the prognosis of children with malignancies continues to improve. Over the past 25 years, there have been significant improvements in the 5-year survival rate for many childhood cancers, especially ALL and acute myeloid leukemia, non-Hodgkin lymphoma, and Wilms tumor. Between 1974 and 1996, 5-year survival rates among children for all cancer sites combined improved from 56 to 75%.[337] With increasing survival rates, there is a growing concern about the late effects of disease and treatment.

The term *late effects* refers to the damaging effects of surgery, radiation, and chemotherapy on nonmalignant tissues, as well as to the social, emotional, and economic consequences of survival. These effects can appear months to years after treatment and can range in severity from subclinical to clinical to life-threatening. Fortunately, not all children experience such effects, but those who do often end up in the rehabilitation setting.

Late effects have been identified in almost every organ system. Treatment involving the CNS can cause deficits in intelligence, hearing, and vision. Treatment involving the CNS, head and neck, or gonads can cause endocrine abnormalities such as short stature, hypothyroidism, or delayed secondary sexual development. Children treated with anthracyclines (e.g., doxorubicin [Adriamycin]) are at risk for development of cardiomyopathies, especially with increasing cumulative doses.[345]

Surgery and radiation involving the musculoskeletal system have been associated with defects such as kyphosis, scoliosis, and spinal shortening. Finally, the child who has received radiation or chemotherapy has a tenfold greater chance of developing a second malignancy than a child who has never had cancer.

REFERENCES
To enhance this text and add value for the reader, all references are included on the companion Evolve site that accompanies this textbook. The reader can view the reference source and access it online whenever possible.

CHAPTER 10

The Integumentary System

HARRIETT B. LOEHNE • ALAN W. CHONG LEE

The integumentary system is an essential component of physical therapist practice. The *Guide to Physical Therapist Practice* includes the integumentary system to address superficial and partial- and full-thickness skin involvement, including prevention of wounds. Practitioners must identify common skin lesions and skin conditions secondary to pathology of disease or sequelae of clinical medicine.

Skin is the largest body organ, constituting 15% to 20% of the body weight. It differs anatomically and physiologically in different areas of the body, but the overall primary function of the skin is to protect underlying structures from external injury and harmful substances. The skin is primarily an insulator but has many other different functions, including holding the organs together, sensory perception, contributing to fluid balance, controlling temperature, absorbing ultraviolet (UV) radiation, metabolizing vitamin D, and synthesizing epidermal lipids. The three primary layers of the skin are presented in Figure 10-1. The structures included in each layer are listed in Table 10-1.

SKIN LESIONS

Approximately one in every four people who consult a physician has a skin disorder. Skin lesions can occur as a result of a wide variety of etiologic factors (Box 10-1). Lesions of the skin or skin manifestations of systemic disorders can be classified as *primary* or *secondary* lesions.

The primary lesion is the first lesion to appear on the skin and has a visually recognizable structure (e.g., macule, papule, plaque, nodule, tumor, wheal, vesicle, pustule). When changes occur in the primary lesion, it becomes a secondary lesion (e.g., scale, crust, thickening, erosion, ulcer, scar, excoriation, fissure, atrophy). These changes may result from many factors, including scratching, rubbing, medication, natural disease progression, or processes of healing.

Birthmarks, commonly caused by a nevus (pl., nevi), may involve an overgrowth of one or more of any of the normal components of skin, such as pigment cells, blood vessels, and lymph vessels. Birthmarks may be classified as pigment cell (e.g., mongolian spot, café au lait spot), vascular (e.g., port-wine stain, strawberry hemangioma), epidermal (e.g., epidermal nevus, nevus sebaceus), or connective tissue (e.g., juvenile elastoma, collagenoma) birthmarks.

Most birthmarks do not require treatment. Vascular birthmarks may be removed with laser therapy for cosmetic reasons. The presence of six or more café au lait spots over 5 cm in length requires medical investigation, because these may be diagnostic of neurofibromatosis or Albright syndrome. Mongolian spots (blue-black macules) can easily be mistaken for a large bruise by uninformed individuals; therefore, complete history and physical examination of the integumentary system may be necessary (see "Child Abuse" in Chapter 2 and Figure 2-2).

SIGNS AND SYMPTOMS OF SKIN DISEASE

Pruritus (itching) is one of the most common manifestations of dermatologic disease and can be a symptom of underlying systemic disease in people with generalized itching, especially among the chronically ill and older populations. Xerosis is the most common cause of pruritus.[137] It can lead to damage if scratching injures the skin's protective barrier, possibly resulting in increased inflammation, infection, and scarring. Many systemic disorders may cause pruritus, most commonly diabetes mellitus, drug hypersensitivity, and hyperthyroidism (Box 10-2).

Urticaria, more commonly known as hives, is a vascular reaction of the skin marked by the appearance of smooth, slightly elevated patches (wheals). These are redder or paler than the surrounding skin and are often accompanied by severe itching. These eruptions are usually an allergic response to drugs or infection and rarely last longer than 2 days, but may exist in a chronic form, lasting more than 3 weeks and, rarely, months to years. There is approximately a 50% reduction in numbers of mast cells responsible for urticaria in intrinsically aged skin. This explains the relative rarity of urticaria in the older adult population.

Rash is a generalized term for an eruption on the skin, most often on the face, trunk, axilla, and groin, and is often accompanied by itching. As such, a rash can present as a continuum anywhere from erythema, to macular lesions, to a raised papular appearance. Rashes typically occur as a secondary response to some primary agent, such as exposure to the sun, allergens, irritants, or medications or in association with systemic disease.

The most common rashes are diaper rash, drug rash, heat rash, and butterfly rash (see Fig. 7-26 and "Systemic Lupus Erythematosus" in Chapter 7). Rash appearing on the breast, especially a rash on the areola or nipple with or without accompanying symptoms of itching, soreness, or burning, may be a sign of Paget disease of the nipple, a rare form of breast cancer.

Blisters (vesicle or bulla) are fluid-containing elevated lesions of the skin with clear watery or bloody contents. They can occur as a manifestation of a wide variety of diseases. Blisters may be primarily associated with diseases of a genetic or autoimmune origin or may be secondary to viral or bacterial infections of the skin (e.g., herpes simplex, impetigo), local injury to the skin (e.g., burns, ischemia, pressure, dermatitis), or drug induced (e.g., penicillamine, captopril).[27] Blisters associated with

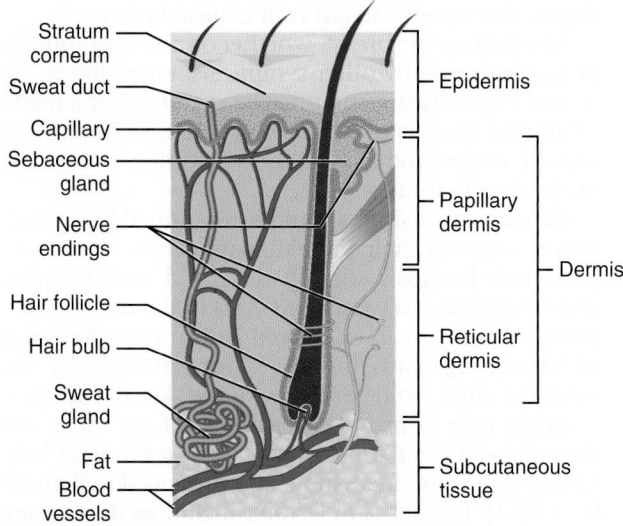

Figure 10-1

Overall skin structure.

Table 10-1	Skin Structure	
Layer	**Structure***	**Function**
Epidermis	Stratum corneum	Protection (from trauma, microbes); barrier (prevents fluid, electrolyte, and chemical loss)
	Keratinocytes (squamous cells)	Synthesis of keratin (skin protein)
	Langerhans cells	Antigen presentation; immune response
	Basal cells	Epidermal reproduction
Dermis	Collagen, reticulum, elastin	Skin proteins; skin texture
	Fibroblasts	Collagen synthesis for skin strength and wound healing
	Macrophages	Phagocytosis of foreign substances, initiates inflammation and repair
	Mast cells	Provide histamine for vasodilation and chemotactic factors for inflammatory responses
	Lymphatic glands	Removal of microbes and excess interstitial fluids; provide lymphatic drainage
	Blood vessels	Provide metabolic skin requirements; thermoregulation
	Nerve fibers	Perception of heat and cold, pain, itching
Epidermal appendages	Eccrine unit	Thermoregulation by perspiration
	Apocrine unit	Production of apocrine sweat; no known significance
	Hair follicles	Production; cavity enclosing hair
	Nails	Protection; mechanical assistance
	Sebaceous glands	Produce sebum (oil to lubricate skin)
Subcutaneous tissue	Adipose (fat)	Energy storage and balance; trauma absorption

Modified from Nicol NH: Structure and function: assessment of clients with integumentary disorders. In Black JM, Matassarin-Jacobs E, editors: *Medical-surgical nursing*, ed 5, Philadelphia, 1997, Saunders, p 2176.

*Understanding the structure of the integument is important in wound management. Knowing why a wound closes the way it does is an essential assessment tool.

underlying neoplasm, called *paraneoplastic pemphigus*, may be the first sign of underlying malignancy.

Xeroderma is a mild form of ichthyosis or excessive dryness of the skin characterized by dry, rough, discolored skin with the formation of scaly desquamation (shedding of the epithelium in small sheets). This problem is accentuated by the use of drying skin cleansers, soaps, disinfectants, and solvents, and by dry climates.

Other symptoms, such as unusual spots, moles, cysts, fibromas, nodules, swelling, or changes in nail beds, may be observed frequently, because more than half of all people have some basic skin problem at some point in their lives (Box 10-3). Any unusual spot that has appeared recently or changed since its initial appearance should be documented and brought to the physician's attention. On the legs, varicosities and stasis changes from poor venous return may be signaled by changes in skin pigmentation, skin turgor (see Fig. 5-7), and skin texture. Edema of the lower extremities can be a sign of multiple systemic illnesses, such as heart, kidney, or liver disease.

SPECIAL IMPLICATIONS FOR THE THERAPIST | **10-1**

Skin Lesions

Any time a client reports signs or symptoms of skin lesions, further evaluation is necessary, and documentation and medical referral may be required. The therapist must remain alert to any skin changes that may indicate the onset or progression of a systemic condition. It is best to use proper lighting, measurement tools, and digital photography to aid your clinical findings.

Any rash on the breast, whether or not symptomatic or accompanied by other symptoms, raises the suspicion of Paget disease and must be examined by a medical doctor. Blisters of unknown cause may be the first sign of underlying malignancy requiring immediate medical evaluation.

Certain skin lesions should be examined by a physician because of their premalignant status—for example, actinic keratosis, slightly raised, red, scaly papules; and sebaceous cysts, enclosed cysts in the dermis. Seborrheic keratosis can be moved with friction and may bleed, causing alarm, but this is not a malignancy; the therapist must avoid contact with the skin in that area.

In the case of pruritus, regardless of the cause, the therapist can offer some practical suggestions to help soothe skin, ease the itching, and prevent skin damage (Box 10-4). Bullous skin lesions, including blisters, are associated with risk of exposure to human immunodeficiency virus (HIV) at least comparable to that from

---

Box 10-3

SIGNS AND SYMPTOMS OF SKIN DISORDERS (NOT INCLUSIVE)

- Pruritus
- Urticaria
- Rash
- Blisters
- Xerosis (dry skin)
- Unusual spots, moles, nodules, cysts
- Edema
- Changes in appearance of nails
- Changes in skin pigmentation, turgor, texture

Box 10-4

SKIN CARE STRATEGIES

Reduce Pruritus

- Avoid scratching.
- Keep fingernails trimmed short to prevent damage in case of unconscious or nighttime scratching.
- Bathe with nondrying, nonfragranced, or unscented soap or other agent when indicated.
- Use soothing bath products, such as Aveeno oatmeal, mineral oil, cottonseed oil, or cornstarch (make a paste with 2 cups cornstarch and 4 cups warm water) added to warm, not hot, bath water.
- Scleroderma: Apply cooling agents, such as menthol or camphor (e.g., contained in Sarna lotion), to the affected areas.
- Psoriasis: Try skin preparations such as creams containing capsaicin,[94,149] chaparral, or aloe (some advocate the use of pure aloe). Do not apply hot-pepper creams on broken skin.
- Discuss with your physician the possible use of an alpha-hydroxyl acid (AHA) product or other prescription cream containing urea to dissolve the outer layer of skin and get rid of the dead scales.
- Second-rinse all clothing and bedding to remove residual laundry soap; avoid the use of fabric softeners.
- Wear open-weave, loose-fitting, cotton-blend fabrics to allow air to circulate and minimize perspiration, thereby reducing the risk of pruritus; avoid rough, wool, or tightly woven fabrics.

- Avoid temperature extremes that can trigger itching secondary to vasodilation and increased cutaneous blood flow. Avoid hot water (baths or hot tubs) for this same reason.
- Take antihistamines to reduce itching according to physician recommendation.
- Take a shower or bath immediately after swimming; wash with mild soap to remove any residual chlorine or chemicals from the skin.

Reduce Inflammation

- Apply topical steroids (available as lotion, solution, gel, cream, or ointment) to affected areas twice daily or as directed. Topical steroids are used to reduce skin inflammation, relieve itching, and control flare-ups of dermatitis and psoriasis. The proper preparation depends on the location and severity of the lesions and should not be applied to normal skin.
- Apply tar preparations (available as lotion, solution, gel, cream, ointment, or shampoo) to affected skin as directed. (Some tar preparations can be added to bath water.) The antiinflammatory properties of tars are not so fast-acting as topical steroids, but the effect is longer-lasting with fewer side effects.
- Tar preparations should not be used on acutely inflamed skin because this may cause burning or irritation.

Box 10-4

SKIN CARE STRATEGIES—cont'd

Maintain Skin Hydration

- Bathing has been discouraged because of its alleged drying effect, but some skin care professionals advocate the use of long soaks in a warm (not hot) bath for 15 to 20 minutes, suggesting that soaking for 15 to 20 minutes allows the stratum corneum to become saturated with water.
- Others recommend only showers or brief baths. Both groups agree that drying of the skin is the result of failure to immediately apply the appropriate occlusive moisture, thereby allowing evaporation to occur. Avoid vigorous or brisk towel drying because this removes more water from the skin and increases vasodilation; gently and quickly pat dry. Immediately (within 2 to 4 minutes of leaving the bath) apply an appropriate emollient or prescribed topical agent.

Avoid Sun (Light) Exposure

- Wear sun-protective clothing with tightly woven material covering as much of the body as possible (e.g., long sleeves, long pants, neckline with a collar, hat with broad brim, UVA/UVB-protective sunglasses).
- Avoiding sitting near a window at work or for prolonged periods of time.

- Avoid outdoor activities during peak sunlight hours (10:00 AM to 4:00 PM in most time zones but may vary geographically). Limit sun exposure during nonpeak hours.
- Avoid fluorescent lighting or reflected sunlight.
- Wear sunscreen daily and year round, even if driving inside an automobile or on cloudy days.
- Apply sunscreen 20 to 30 minutes before sun exposure to ensure maximum absorption. Sunscreen preparations must provide a minimum ultraviolet B sun protective factor (SPF) of 30 plus an ultraviolet A sunscreen for anyone with a current skin condition or who is at risk for skin cancer. A sunscreen of SPF 15 is considered adequate for anyone else who does not meet this criterion.
- Reapply every 2 hours if you are in the water, exposed to wind, or perspiring. Sunscreens are not recommended for infants under 6 months of age.
- Do not increase sun exposure because you are wearing a sunscreen. High SPF has been shown to lead to increased time spent in the sun by 25%. Sunscreen is most effective against squamous cell carcinoma.[61]

blood. Standard Precautions while treating anyone with skin lesions or burns are required.[34]

When examining and documenting the presence of a skin disorder, note the location, size, and any irregularities in skin color, temperature, moisture, ulceration, texture, thickness, mobility, edema, turgor, odor, and tenderness (Box 10-5). If more than one lesion is present, note the pattern of distribution: localized or isolated; regional; general; or universal (total), involving the entire skin, hair, and nails.

Note whether the lesions are unilateral or bilateral, note whether they are symmetric or asymmetric, and note the arrangement of the lesions (clustered or linear configuration), especially if these occur as a result of contact with clothing, jewelry, or another external object.

Blisters may be associated with a variety of skin conditions, such as frostbite, dermatitis, burns, pressure, or malignancy, or may possibly occur as a side effect of medications. Blisters over joints, limiting motion, and/or infected should be opened and debrided, except hemorrhagic frostbite blisters and stable, noninfected arterial and heel blisters, which subsequently should be monitored carefully for signs of infection or deep injury.

Although an intact blister is theoretically sterile, few blisters are substantial enough to remain intact for long. Blister fluid will "set" into a gelatinous film if debridement is delayed. In a burn, this film is the beginning of eschar and is an ideal culture medium for bacteria.

Blister fluid impairs normal function of neutrophils and lymphocytes, which reduces the effectiveness of local immunity. Blister fluid also contains arachidonic acid metabolites that increase the inflammatory response and retard the fibrolytic process. All these effects delay healing of the wound.

Special care always must be taken when working with the older adult. Avoiding shear and friction forces

Box 10-5

DOCUMENTATION OF SKIN LESIONS

Characteristics

- Size (measure all dimensions)
- Shape or configuration
- Color
- Temperature
- Tenderness, pain, or pruritus
- Texture
- Mobility; skin turgor
- Elevation or depression
- Pedunculation (stem-like connections)

Exudates

- Color
- Odor
- Amount
- Consistency

Pattern of Arrangement

- Annular (rings)
- Grouped
- Linear
- Arciform (bow-shaped)
- Diffuse

Location and Distribution

- Generalized, localized, or universal
- Region of the body; unilateral or bilateral; symmetric or asymmetric
- Patterns (dermatomal, flexor or extensor, random, related to clothing lines)
- Discrete or confluent (running together)

Modified from Hill MJ: *Skin disorders*, St Louis, 1994, Mosby, p 18.

during treatment and particularly during repositioning is essential. Extreme caution is also necessary whenever using electrical or thermal modalities (heat or cold) with older people.

Decreased circulation, reduced subcutaneous adipose tissue, and altered metabolism create a situation where initial skin resistance to electricity or poor dissipation of heat or cold can lead to tissue damage. Close supervision is necessary to prevent complications. Utilize appropriate dressings and skin moisturizers for treatment intervention, and avoid using adhesives.

Laboratory Values

Many factors affect the progression of a skin lesion to wound status and subsequent ability to heal, including use of tobacco, psychosocial status (e.g., comatose, homeless), and nutritional status. Laboratory values, such as prealbumin levels to indicate nutritional status and glucose levels, hemoglobin, and hematocrit to monitor wound healing, provide the therapist with necessary information when setting up and carrying out an appropriate intervention plan.

AGING AND THE INTEGUMENTARY SYSTEM

The skin undergoes numerous changes that can be seen and felt throughout the life span. The most obvious changes occur first during puberty and again during older adulthood. Hormone changes during puberty stimulate the maturation of hair follicles, sebaceous glands, and apocrine and eccrine units in certain body areas. Mild acne, perspiration and body odor, freckles (promoted by sun exposure), and pigmented nevi (moles) are common occurrences.

During adolescence and adulthood, the use of birth control pills or pregnancy may result in temporary changes in hair growth patterns or hyperpigmentation of the cheeks and forehead known as *melasma* or *pregnancy mask*. Other hormonal abnormalities may result in excessive facial and body hair in women (androgen-related). Hormonal and genetic changes also produce male-pattern baldness (alopecia). Smoking is an independent causative factor of facial wrinkles.[45]

The skin exhibits changes that denote the onset of senescence (the process or condition of growing old). These changes may be due to the aging process itself (intrinsic aging), to the cumulative effects of exposure to sunlight (photoaging), or to environmental factors (extrinsic aging). As aging occurs, both structural and functional changes occur in the skin (Table 10-2), resulting clinically in diminished pain perception, increased vulnerability to injury, decreased vascularity, and a weakened inflammatory response.

Visible indications of skin changes associated with aging include grey hair, balding and loss of secondary sexual hair, and increased facial hair. For women, excessive facial hair may occur along the upper lip and around the chin. Women may also experience balding after menopause. Men frequently develop increased facial hair in the nares, eyebrows, and helix of the ear.

Table 10-2	Effects of Aging on the Skin
Structural	**Functional**
Epidermis	
Flattening of the dermal–epidermal junction	Altered skin permeability
Changes in basal cells	Decreased inflammatory responsiveness
Decreased number of Langerhans cells	Decreased immunologic responsiveness; increased risk of skin cancer; increased sensitivity to allergens
Decreased number of melanocytes	Impaired wound healing; loss of photoprotection with increased risk of skin cancer
Dermis	
Decreased dermal thickness; degeneration of elastin fibers	Decreased elasticity; increased wrinkling, slow wound healing, less scar tissue (cosmetic benefit)
Decreased vascularization	Decreased vitamin D production
Appendages	
Decreased number and distorted structure of sweat glands	Decreased eccrine sweating; altered skin thermoregulation
Decreased number and distorted structure of specialized nerve endings	Impaired sensory perception; increased pain threshold
Decreased hair bulb melanocytes and decreased number of hair follicles	Change in hair color (gray, white); hair loss

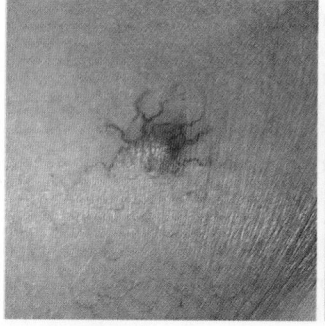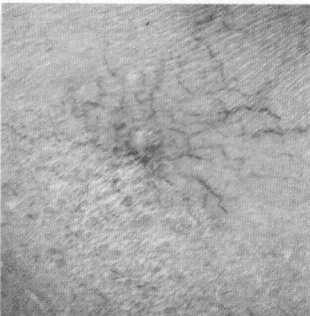

Figure 10-2

Spider angioma (arterial spider, spider telangiectasia, vascular spider) is so called because it consists of a central arteriole, radiating from which are numerous small vessels resembling a spider's legs (ranging from pinhead size to 0.5 cm in diameter). Common sites are the necklace area, face, forearms, and dorsum of the hand; may be associated with rosacea, basal cell carcinoma, scleroderma, pregnancy, liver disease, or estrogen therapy or may occur by itself. (From Habif T: *Clinical dermatology*, ed 4, St. Louis, 2004, Elsevier, Figs. 23-20, 23-21, p 830.)

Other common age-related integumentary changes include lax skin, vascular changes (e.g., decreased elasticity of blood vessel walls; angiomas) (Fig. 10-2), dermal or epidermal degenerative changes, and wrinkling. Wrinkling signifies loss of elastin fibers, weakened collagen, and decreased subcutaneous fat and is accelerated by smoking and excessive sun exposure.

Blood vessels within the reticular dermis are reduced in number, and the walls are thinned. This compromises blood flow and appears physiologically as pale skin and an impaired capacity to thermoregulate, a possible contributing factor to the increased susceptibility of older individuals to hypothermia and hyperthermia. Many other benign changes may occur, including seborrheic keratoses (brown or black, wart-like growths), lentigines (liver spots, unrelated to the liver but rather secondary to sun exposure), and skin tags (small, flesh-colored papules).

A primary factor in the loss of protective functions of the skin is the diminished barrier function of the stratum corneum (outermost layer of the epidermis; see Fig. 10-1). As this layer becomes thinner, the skin becomes translucent and paper-thin, reacting more readily to minor changes in humidity, temperature, and other irritants. There are fewer melanocytes, with decreased protection against UV radiation.

A significant decrease in the number of Langerhans cells occurs, so that by the time a person reaches 70 years of age there is only half the number of Langerhans cells compared to the number in early adulthood. A reduction in Langerhans cell counts represents a loss of immune surveillance and an increased risk of skin cancer.[136]

The epidermis is also one of the body's principal suppliers of vitamin D, which is produced when a hormone, 7-dehydrocholesterol, is exposed to sunlight. At 65 years of age, the levels of that hormone are only about 25% of what they were in youth, contributing to vitamin D deficiency and, because vitamin D plays a vital role in building bone, to osteoporosis as well.

It is generally agreed that one of the major and important contributions to skin aging, skin disorders, and skin diseases is the oxidative damage that occurs to the skin as a result of environmental exposures and endogenous (within the skin itself) factors.

The skin is rich in lipids, proteins, and deoxyribonucleic acid (DNA), all of which are extremely sensitive to the oxidation process. Scientists are developing methods of decreasing protein crosslinking and accelerating increased collagen to slow down/aide in reversing the oxidation process.[205]

SPECIAL IMPLICATIONS FOR THE THERAPIST 10-2

Aging and the Integumentary System

The therapist must remain alert to all skin changes, because age-associated blunting of vascular and immune responses may make skin findings more subtle in older adults compared to younger clients with similar disorders. Vascular changes affecting thermoregulation and wound healing require careful consideration when planning therapy intervention.

Likewise, loss of collagen increases susceptibility to shearing force trauma, increasing the risk for pressure ulcers. Wound healing is impaired in intrinsically aged as compared to young skin in that the rate of healing is appreciably slower, but paradoxically the resultant scar is usually more cosmetically acceptable.

Skin diseases and symptoms caused by skin disorders are exceedingly common among the older population. Although these disorders are not usually life threatening, they provoke anxiety and psychologic distress. Often, the client has not brought these concerns to the attention of a physician, and the therapist is the first health care professional to observe the skin lesion.

It is important to ask about physical findings in other parts of the body (e.g., the client may not mention genital lesions or may be unaware of the significance of other symptoms). All dermatologic lesions must be examined by a physician, and anyone with evidence of sun damage, particularly those with actinic keratoses (see discussion), should have a full skin examination annually.

A THERAPIST'S THOUGHTS*

Older adults may present with intrinsic, extrinsic, and iatrogenic factors that may impact wound healing. It is best to consider collaborative health care team approach to address modifiable factors in older adults. Be aware that research has shown a strong direct and indirect relationship between psychological stress and wound healing.[105] Psychological stress may impair cellular immunity. Therefore, the practitioner should mitigate stress for optimal wound healing.

*Alan Chong W. Lee, PT, PhD, DPT, CWS, GCS

COMMON SKIN DISORDERS

Atopic Dermatitis

Definition and Incidence

Atopic dermatitis (AD) is a chronic inflammatory skin disease. It is the most common type of eczema, frequently already present during the first year of life and affecting more than 10% of children.

AD is considered an early manifestation of atopy that appears before the development of allergic rhinitis or asthma. The word *atopic* (from *atopy*) refers to a group of three associated allergic disorders: asthma, allergic rhinitis (hay fever), and AD. There is usually a personal or family history of allergic disorders present, and AD is often associated with food allergies as well.

Etiologic and Risk Factors and Pathogenesis

The exact cause of AD is unknown, but it is thought to be a result of dry, irritable skin with a malfunction of the body's immune system. Genetics may play a part, but this has not been proved. Stress and emotional problems can worsen AD but do not cause it.[204]

The pathomechanisms associated with AD are also unknown but most likely include both immediate and cellular immune responses. Two possibilities include the release of inflammatory mediators by autoallergens and the release of proinflammatory cytokines by autoreactive T cells in response to autoallergens mediated by immunoglobulin E.[192]

AD is often associated with increased levels of serum immunoglobulin E and with sensitization to food allergens.[168] Some foods may be responsible for exacerbations of skin inflammation, but their pathogenic role must be clinically assessed before an avoidance diet is recommended.[78] Xerosis (abnormal dryness) associated with AD is usually worse during periods of low humidity and over the winter months in northern latitudes.

The underlying biochemical abnormality in xerosis is unknown, and the pathologic findings may be a result of the dry skin rather than the cause of the drying effects of this condition. Compared with normal skin, the dry skin of AD has a reduced water-binding capacity, a higher transepidermal water loss, and a decreased water content. Rubbing and scratching of itchy skin are responsible for many of the clinical changes seen in the skin. Hands frequently in and out of water make the condition worse.

Clinical Manifestations

AD begins in many people during infancy in the form of a red, oozing, crusting rash classified as acute dermatitis (Fig. 10-3). As the child grows, the chronic form of dermatitis results in skin that is dry, thickened, and brownish-grey in color (lichenified). The rash tends to become localized to the large folds of the extremities as the person becomes older. It is found mainly on flexor surfaces such as the elbows and knees, neck, sides of the face, eyelids, and the backs of hands and feet. Hand and foot dermatitis can become a significant problem for some people.

Xerosis and pruritus are the major symptoms of AD and cause the greatest morbidity with severely excoriated lesions, infection, and scarring. Viral, bacterial, and fungal secondary skin infections may cause further changes in the skin. *Staphylococcus aureus* is the most common bacterial infection, resulting in extensive crusting with serous weeping, folliculitis (inflammation of hair follicles), pyoderma (pus), and furunculosis (boils).

MEDICAL MANAGEMENT

DIAGNOSIS, TREATMENT, AND PROGNOSIS. Although no cure exists, AD often resolves spontaneously, and more than 90% of cases of AD can be effectively controlled through proper management. Each person is evaluated individually because of the symptomatic variability of the disease. The goal of medical therapy is to break the inflammatory cycle that causes excess drying, cracking, itching, and scratching.

Personal hygiene, moisturizing the skin, avoidance of irritants, topical pharmacology, and systemic medications (e.g., antibiotics, antihistamines, and rarely, systemic corticosteroids) are treatment techniques currently available. *S. aureus*, known to colonize the skin of people with AD, may exacerbate skin lesions and needs to be treated with antibiotics. Superinfection with disease exacerbation is also treated with antimicrobial medications.[153,154]

Adjuvant therapy includes UV irradiation preferably with UVA1 wavelength or UVB 311 nm. Dietary recommendations should be specific and given only in diagnosed individual food allergy. Allergen-specific immunotherapy to aeroallergens may be useful in selected cases. In the case of stress-induced exacerbations, behavioral counseling may be helpful.[153,154]

Advancing knowledge in understanding the immunologic basis of this disease will continue to result in effective new local and systemic treatments in the decade to come.[128,169] Updated guidelines for the treatment of this condition are available.[153,154]

SPECIAL IMPLICATIONS FOR THE THERAPIST | 10-3

Atopic Dermatitis

The therapist may be instrumental in providing client education that results in avoiding factors that precipitate or exacerbate inflammation and then teaching proper management techniques for flare-ups. Daily care (hydration and lubrication) of the skin is important, and applications (two or three times daily) of emollients that occlude the skin to prevent evaporation and retain moisture should be recommended.

Creams or ointments containing petrolatum may be used (see "Contact Dermatitis" below for sensitivity to lanolin), and those that contain urea or lactic acid improve the binding of water in the skin and prevent evaporation. In the case of skin redness, the skin lesion must be identified first because of possible fungal origin requiring an antifungal preparation.

Understanding the individual disease pattern and identifying exacerbating factors are crucial to effective management of this disorder. It is important to identify and eliminate triggers that cause the AD to flare.

Older clients should be encouraged to bathe with tepid water using a nondrying, nonfragranced, or unscented soap or other agent when indicated. Emollients must be applied to the body within 5 minutes after showering or bathing, especially in dry, winter weather, to prevent further skin drying.

Dermatitis must be considered a precaution, if not a contraindication, to some treatment modalities used by therapists. The use of water, alcohol, or any topical agents containing alcohol should be avoided. Topical agents, such as ultrasound gel and mobilization creams, must be used carefully, observing for any skin reaction. A nonreactive response does not guarantee the client will not react when such agents are subsequently applied in future interventions. Caution and careful observation are encouraged.

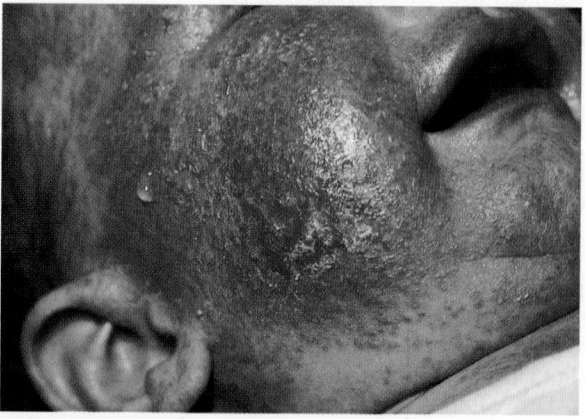

Figure 10-3

Infantile atopic dermatitis with oozing and crusting lesions. (From Paller A, Mancini A: *Hurwitz clinical pediatric dermatology: a textbook of skin disorders of childhood and adolescence,* ed 3, Philadelphia, 2006, Saunders.)

Contact Dermatitis

Etiologic Factors, Incidence, and Pathogenesis

Contact dermatitis can be an acute or chronic skin inflammation caused by exposure to a chemical, mechanical, physical, or biologic agent. It is one of the most common environmental skin diseases occurring at any age. As people age, they may develop delayed cell-mediated hypersensitivity to a variety of substances that come in contact with the skin.

Common sensitizers include nickel (found in jewelry and many common foods), chromates (used in tanning leathers), wool fats (particularly lanolin found in moisturizers and skin creams), rubber additives (see "Latex Rubber Allergy" in Chapter 4), topical antibiotics (typically neomycin and bacitracin),[31] and topical anesthetics, such as benzocaine or lidocaine.[65] Dermatitis of unknown cause is more commonly diagnosed in the older population.

A small percentage of the population is allergic to silicone. The therapist is most likely to see this reaction in a sensitized person with an amputation using a silicone type of interface in a prosthetic device (designed to reduce shear, decrease repetitive stress, and absorb shock). Silicone sheets used for scar reduction in the postburn population may also result in an episode of contact dermatitis.

Clinical Manifestations

Intense pruritus (itching), erythema (redness), and edema of the skin occur 1 to 2 days after exposure in previously sensitized persons. Clinical manifestations begin at the site of exposure but then extend to more distant sites. These conditions may progress to vesiculation, oozing (watery discharges), crusting, and scaling (Fig. 10-4). If these symptoms persist, the skin becomes thickened, with prominent skin markings and pigmentation changes.

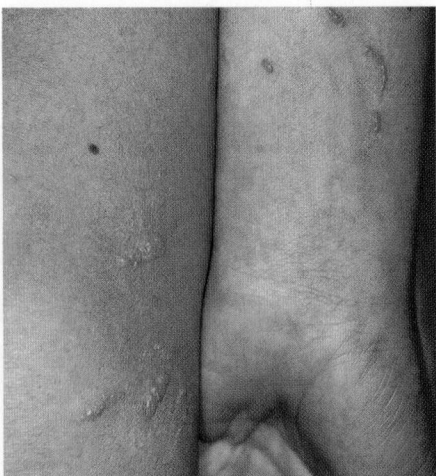

Figure 10-4

Primary contact dermatitis, a local inflammatory reaction, can occur in response to an irritant in the environment or an allergy. Characteristic location of lesions often gives a clue to the cause. Erythema occurs first, followed by swelling, wheals or urticaria, or maculopapular vesicles accompanied by intense pruritus. The example shown here is a result of contact with poison ivy. (From Paller A, Mancini A: *Hurwitz clinical pediatric dermatology: a textbook of skin disorders of childhood and adolescence*, ed 3, Philadelphia, 2006, Saunders.)

Older people have a less pronounced inflammatory response to standard irritants than do younger persons.

MEDICAL MANAGEMENT

DIAGNOSIS, TREATMENT, AND PROGNOSIS. If contact dermatitis is suspected, the client should be referred to a physician. Acute lesions usually resolve in 3 weeks; chronic lesions persist until the causative agent has been removed. A detailed history and careful examination frequently are all that are needed to make the diagnosis. It may be necessary to perform patch testing to identify the causative agent. However, with increasing age, there are more cases of hypersensitivity (positive patch test) without clinical symptoms, which among other possible causes may reflect acquisition of tolerance (hapten hyposensitization).[172]

Primary treatment is removal of the offending agent; treatment of the skin is secondary. The client should be instructed to avoid contact with strong soaps, detergents, solvents, bleaches, and other strong chemicals. The involved skin should be lubricated frequently with emollients. Topical anesthetics or steroids (topical or sometimes systemic) or both may be prescribed. For those people unable to avoid known allergens, immunosuppressant therapies (including phototherapy) can be helpful.[13]

Future research in oral hyposensitization to nickel is needed for allergic contact dermatitis.[172]

SPECIAL IMPLICATIONS FOR THE THERAPIST 10-4

Contact Dermatitis

The therapy professional should always consider the client's reactions to external substances. This is of particular importance when applying any cream, topical agent, or solution. Various modalities used within the profession may involve causative substances (e.g., whirlpool additives, ultrasound gels, self-sticking electrode pads).

Whirlpools should be used rarely, and with no additives. The client's skin always must be examined before and after intervention for the appearance of any adverse reactions. The client should be instructed to report any discomfort or unusual findings during or after treatment to the therapist.

The person with contact dermatitis associated with the use of a silicone sleeve or interface with a prosthetic device should be cautioned about the use of soaps that do not include a rinsing agent. Many antibacterial and antiperspirant soaps leave particles on the surface of the skin that act as a barrier on the skin's surface against bacterial invasion. A rash or blister may occur in patchy areas corresponding to pressure points when the friction of the interface drives the soap particles back into the skin.[23]

The therapist may suggest one of several care plans for this type of contact dermatitis. The use of alcohol-based lubricants or soaps, antifungal or antibacterial soaps without a rinsing agent, and lanolin should be avoided. Soap-free cleansing agents or a soft soap should be used for daily cleansing, and a petroleum-based ointment can be applied to the limb before putting on the liner.

Water-based ointments should be avoided when using urethane liners, because these can cause the normally tacky urethane to adhere to the skin so that when the liner is removed, bits of skin may be pulled off as well. Alcohol-based lubricants or soaps should also be avoided with urethane products because these components act as a solvent on urethane, increasing the stickiness of the urethane.[23]

Eczema and Dermatitis

Definition and Overview

Eczema and *dermatitis* are terms that are often used interchangeably to describe a group of disorders with a characteristic appearance. Eczema or dermatitis is a superficial inflammation of the skin caused by irritant exposure, allergic sensitization (delayed hypersensitivity), or genetically determined idiopathic factors.

Many types of dermatitis are represented according to these major etiologic categories (e.g., allergic dermatitis, irritant dermatitis, seborrheic dermatitis, nummular eczema, AD, stasis dermatitis).

Eczema or dermatitis has three primary stages. This condition can manifest in any one of the three stages, or the three stages may coexist. *Acute dermatitis* is characterized by extensive erosions with serous exudate or by intensely pruritic, erythematous papules and vesicles on a background of erythema.

Subacute dermatitis is characterized by erythematous, excoriated (scratched or abraded), scaling papules or plaques that are either grouped or scattered over erythematous skin. Often the scaling is so fine and diffuse the skin acquires a silvery sheen.

Chronic dermatitis is characterized by thickened skin and increased skin marking (called *lichenification*) secondary to rubbing and scratching; excoriated papules, fibrotic papules, and nodules (prurigo nodularis); and postinflammatory hyperpigmentation and hypopigmentation.

Incidence and Etiologic Factors

Dermatitis is a common skin disorder in older people. It may be caused by hypoproteinemia, venous insufficiency, allergens, irritants, or underlying malignancy, such as leukemia or lymphoma. Because older people often take multiple medications, dermatitis from drug–drug interaction can occur. The normal aging process with the flattened epidermal–dermal junction and loss of dermis results in skin fragility, which contributes to the development of skin tears and dermatitis.

Stasis Dermatitis

Stasis dermatitis is the development of areas of very dry, thin skin and sometimes shallow ulcers of the lower legs primarily as a result of venous insufficiency. The client commonly has a history of varicose veins or deep vein thrombosis (see also "Venous Diseases" in Chapter 12).

The process of stasis dermatitis begins with edema of the leg as a result of slowed venous return. As the venous insufficiency continues, the tissue becomes hypoxic from inadequate blood supply. This poorly nourished tissue begins to necrose.

The clinical manifestations include itching, a feeling of heaviness in the legs, brown-stained skin, and open shallow lesions (Fig. 10-5). The lesions are very slow to heal because of a lack of oxygenated blood. Gait training is an important part of compression, the gold standard, in the treatment of stasis dermatitis. Gradient compression wraps and stockings work well in the recumbent position, but ambulation with the muscular contract–relax cycle pushes the venous return within the compressive field. Ambulation is required for use of Unna's Boot.

Environmental Dermatoses

It is well documented that exposure to various environmental chemicals and to physical stimuli is capable of inducing adverse cutaneous responses. Common environmental skin diseases seen in a therapy practice may include irritant and allergic dermatitis, acne lesions, pigmentary changes (hyperpigmentation, hypopigmentation, absence of pigment), photosensitivity reactions, scleroderma, infectious disorders, and cutaneous malignancy. Each of these environmentally induced skin conditions is discussed separately in this chapter (see also Chapter 4).

Rosacea

Rosacea is a common chronic facial disorder of middle-aged and older people affecting approximately 10% of the general population.[9] Although it is a form of acne, it is differentiated by age, the presence of a large vascular component (erythema, telangiectasis), and usually the absence of comedones.

An acneiform rosacea can occur with inflammatory papules, pustules, telangiectasia, and oily skin. No known cause or factor has been identified to explain the pathogenesis of this disorder. It is currently considered a condition with vascular and inflammatory components in the presence of an altered innate immune response.[30,42]

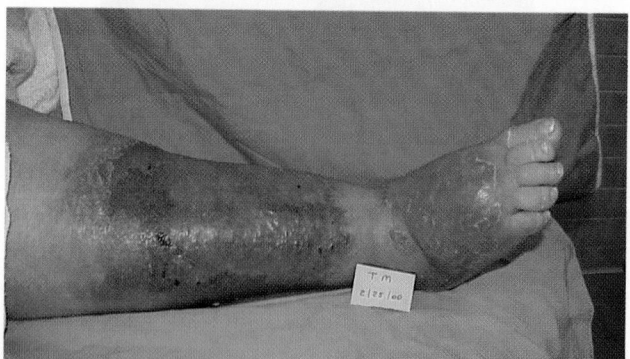

Figure 10-5

Stasis dermatitis secondary to venous insufficiency. Hemosiderin staining (dark pigmentation) indicative of venous insufficiency is evident. This staining is caused by the leakage of hemosiderin (an iron-rich pigment, the product of red cell hemolysis) as a result of blood that cannot return because of valvular incompetence. (Courtesy Harriett B. Loehne, PT, DPT, CWS, FACCWS, Archbold Center for Wound Management & Hyperbaric Medicine, Thomasville, GA. Used with permission.)

A statistically significant incidence of migraine headaches accompanying rosacea has been reported.

Rosacea has often been linked with gastrointestinal (GI) disturbances, and a causal relationship between *Helicobacter pylori* (a bacterium that causes gastritis) and rosacea was reported in the early 1990s.[189] Many studies linking rosacea to *H. pylori* infection were uncontrolled and were performed in areas where the endemic rates of both *H. pylori* infection and rosacea are high.[181] Continued investigation of this issue has suggested that *H. pylori* has a significant role in rosacea patients who have dyspeptic symptoms. *H. pylori* triggers an intense leucocyte infiltration of the gastric submucosa, an action that is mediated by proinflammatory cytokines.[189] It has been proposed that certain virulent bacterial strains increase the inflammatory response in gastric mucosa and also in cutaneous lesions.[40]

Clinically, the cheeks, nose, and chin (sometimes the entire face) may have a rosy appearance marked by reddened skin. This benign but obvious condition is most common in people with fair skin who flush easily. Sun, hot weather, and humidity can all trigger flare-ups; the condition is worse in the summer.

The affected person reports burning or stinging with episodes of flushing that come and go, but the condition may worsen over time, causing lasting redness, pimples, telangiectasias, or nasal hypertrophy (rhinophyma). Inflammatory papules are prominent, and there may be pustules. It is not uncommon to have associated ophthalmic disease, including blepharitis and keratitis.

Medical management aimed at the inflammatory papules, pustules, and surrounding erythema may include topical or systemic therapy that act as immunomodulators to restore cutaneous homeostasis.[42] Rosacea tends to be a persistent condition that can be controlled with drugs. Chronic rosacea has long been treated by pulsed dye lasers. A newer system, the Intense Pulsed Light system, allows deeper and wider area treatments.[99,158,193]

Rosacea associated with *H. pylori*–induced gastritis can be effectively treated by addressing the underlying problem. Although therapists do not treat this condition, clients with other diagnoses often present with this condition also. Clients with this condition should see a physician for adequate medical treatment.

Incontinence-Associated Dermatitis

Incontinence-associated dermatitis (IAD; formerly referred to as "diaper rash") describes skin damage resulting from urine or feces exposure. Some health care providers refer to this condition as "peri-rash" (affecting the perineum between the anus and external genitalia), but the term *IAD* is recommended because usually a larger area than the perineum is affected.[60] IAD is clinically and pathologically distinct from pressure ulcers and intertriginous dermatitis[37] (dermatitis of the skin folds).

IAD is associated with pressure ulcers; distinguishing between these two conditions in the buttocks area can be very difficult but important because prevention and treatment for each condition are different. There is a clear link between IAD and pressure ulcers, with a 37.5% increased risk of developing a pressure ulcer when IAD is present.[109]

IAD is characterized by redness with or without blistering, erosion, or loss of skin barrier function as a result of chronic or repeated exposure to urine or fecal matter.[60] Associated skin changes in individuals with dark skin tones may appear as a different color (e.g., yellow, dark red, purple, white). The affected individual may report burning, itching, or tingling. The description is very similar to the National Pressure Ulcer Advisory Panel (NPUAP) stage I pressure ulcer, with the primary difference being the underlying factors causing the condition. IAD injuries will not be confined necessarily over areas of bony prominences and will not cause full-thickness skin injury unless there is an infection.

Research supports the use of a defined skin care regimen based on principles of gentle perineal cleansing, moisturization, and application of a skin protectant. Clinical experience also supports application of an antifungal ointment or cream (powder is *not* recommended) in patients with evidence of cutaneous candidiasis, briefless policy with urinary or fecal incontinence, and highly selective use of a mild topical antiinflammatory product in selected cases.[59] Wearing disposable briefs only makes matters worse; a high-grade underpad that wicks moisture away from the skin should be used and the patient kept clean and dry; frequent monitoring to maintain this state is necessary.

SPECIAL IMPLICATIONS FOR THE THERAPIST | 10-5

Incontinence-Associated Dermatitis

Early assessment and recognition of skin changes (e.g., color, induration, tenderness) is important so that the plan of care can include appropriate interventions to minimize and prevent worsening (tissue weeping, infection, skin denudement). IAD should be categorized as a superficial wound; the NPUAP pressure ulcer staging system is not to be used for this and other skin injuries.[82] The Kennedy and Lutz skin assessment tool can be used to classify IAD.[88]

A special tool called the Incontinence-Associated Dermatitis Intervention Tool (IADIT) is available to guide nursing and physical therapy staff in providing appropriate skin care based on specific assessment to identify IAD. This tool is presented on the Evolve website as Evolve Table 10-1. As mentioned, differentiating IAD from pressure ulcers in the buttocks area is important in providing focused problem-specific care. Individuals with IAD may not need position changes or pressure redistributing devices (e.g., specialty mattress) saving time and reducing costs. It is important to remember, however, that excess moisture puts the patient at high risk for developing pressure ulcers. Accurately assessing and diagnosing these two conditions can aid in more accurate reporting statistics for related skin problems, especially the prevalence and incidence of pressure ulcers.[82]

Experts agree that evidence is lacking to provide best-practice guidelines for products and protocols in the prevention and treatment of this condition, but efforts have been made to provide health care providers with consensus statements.[37,59] More information is expected in the near future as the results of clinical experience and studies are published.

Table 10-3	Infections of the Skin
Type of Infection	**Transmission**
Bacterial	
Impetigo contagiosa	Contagious
Pyoderma	Contagious
Folliculitis (pimple, boil)	Contagious; minimal chance of spread
Cellulitis	Contagious*
Viral	
Verrucae (warts)	Contagious; autoinoculable†
Verruca plantaris (plantar wart)	Contagious; autoinoculable
Herpes simplex	
Type 1: cold sore, fever blister	Contagious
Type 2: genital lesion	Contagious
Varicella-zoster virus (herpes zoster; shingles)	Contagious; chickenpox can occur in anyone not previously exposed
Fungal	
Tinea corporis (ringworm)	Person-to-person Animal-to-person Inanimate object-to-person
Tinea capitis (affects scalp)	Person-to-person Animal-to-person
Tinea cruris (jock itch)	Person-to-person
Tinea pedis (athlete's foot)	Transmission to other people rare despite general opinion to the contrary
Candidiasis	Person-to-person; sexually transmitted during birth from colorized vagina to neonatal oropharynx
Other	
Scabies	Person-to-person; sexually transmitted during birth from colonized vaginal to neonatal oropharynx Inanimate object-to-person
Lice	Same as scabies

*Technically, cellulitis is contagious, but from a practical point of view the chances of this spreading are very low and would require a susceptible host, for example, an open cut on the therapist's hand coming in contact with blood or pus from the client's open wound.

†Capable of spreading infection from one's own body by scratching.

SKIN INFECTIONS

Many bacterial, viral, fungal, and other parasitic skin infections encountered by the therapist are not the primary focus of intervention but rather occur in clients who are hospitalized or being treated for some other condition. Many of these skin disorders are contagious (Table 10-3) and require careful handling by all health care professionals to avoid spreading the infection and becoming contaminated themselves.

Sources of infection differ depending on the disease and mode of transmission (see also Chapter 7). Predisposing factors to skin infections include decreased resistance, dehydrated skin, burns or pressure ulcers, decreased blood flow, contamination from nasal discharge, poor hygiene, and crowded living conditions. Only the most common skin infections encountered in the therapy or rehabilitation setting are discussed further in this section.

Bacterial Infections

Normally the skin harbors a variety of bacterial flora, including the major pathogenic varieties of staphylococci and streptococci. The degree of their pathogenicity depends on the invasiveness and toxigenicity of the specific organisms, the integrity of the skin, the barrier of the host, and the immune and cellular defenses of the host. Organisms usually enter the skin through abrasions or puncture wounds of the hands.

In the therapist's practice, periwound care requires cleaning away from the wound opening to avoid introducing bacteria from the surrounding skin into the wound. Clinical infection develops 3 to 7 days after inoculation. Septicemia can develop if treatment is not provided or if the person is immunocompromised.

People at risk for the development of bacterial infections include children and adults who are immunocompromised, such as occurs with acquired or inherited immunodeficiency; anyone in a debilitated physical condition; those receiving immunosuppressive therapy; and those with a generalized malignancy, such as leukemia or lymphoma.

All these factors emphasize the importance of careful handwashing and cleanliness to prevent spread of infection before and after caring for infected people and their lesions.

Some conditions (e.g., impetigo) are easily spread by self-inoculation; therefore, the affected person must be cautioned to avoid touching the involved area. Follicular lesions should not be squeezed because this will not hasten the resolution of the infection and may increase the risk of making the lesion worse or spreading the infection.

Impetigo (Bisno 2009)[17]

Definition and Overview. Impetigo is a superficial skin infection commonly caused by staphylococci or streptococci. It is most commonly found in infants, young children 2 to 5 years of age, older people, and occurs most often during hot, humid weather. Predisposing factors include close contact in schools, overcrowded living quarters, poor skin hygiene, anemia, malnutrition, and minor skin trauma. It can be spread by direct contact, environmental contamination, or an arthropod vector. Impetigo often occurs as a secondary infection in conditions characterized by a cutaneous barrier broken to microbes, such as eczema or herpes zoster excoriations.

Clinical Manifestations. Small macules (flat spots) rapidly develop into vesicles (small blisters) that become pustular (pus-filled). When the vesicle breaks, a thick yellow crust forms from the exudate, causing pain, surrounding erythema, regional adenitis (inflammation of gland), cellulitis (inflammation of tissue), and itching.

Scratching spreads infection, a process called *autoinoculation*. Lesions frequently affect the face, heal slowly, and leave depigmented areas. Neither fever nor pain is typically a component of impetigo and if present suggests another diagnosis. If the infection is extensive, then malaise, fever, and lymphadenopathy may be present. A less common presentation occurs with few isolated bullae.

MEDICAL MANAGEMENT

Single small lesions can often be managed by soaking them for 10 minutes with drying agents (Burow solution). Antibiotic treatment should cover both staphylococcal and streptococcal species. Untreated skin infections do not lead to rheumatic fever, although they can trigger poststreptococcal glomerulonephritis. A skin swab culture may be necessary to determine the contaminating organism.

Cellulitis

Cellulitis is a rapidly spreading acute inflammation with infection of the skin and subcutaneous tissue that spreads widely through tissue spaces. *Streptococcus pyogenes* or *Staphylococcus* is the usual cause of this infection in adults and *Haemophilus influenzae* type b in children, although other pathogens may be responsible.

Clients at increased risk for cellulitis include older adults and people with lowered resistance from diabetes, malnutrition, steroid therapy, and the presence of wounds or ulcers. Because cellulitis is not a reportable disease, the exact prevalence is uncertain; however, it is a relatively common infection, affecting all racial and ethnic groups.[72,116]

Other predisposing factors include the presence of edema or other cutaneous inflammation, skin irritation, or even (tiny) wounds (e.g., tinea, eczema, burns, trauma, bug bites). Venous insufficiency or stasis, thrombophlebitis, surgery, substance abuse, and immunocompromise (e.g., HIV infection, chemotherapy, autoimmune diseases, chronic use of immunosuppressants) also predispose individuals to this condition.

Recurrent episodes of cellulitis may occur in extremities in which lymphatic drainage has been impaired (e.g., postaxillary node dissection, site of saphenous vein harvest). Sometimes "repeated" episodes of cellulitis occur because the initial infection was "controlled" but not adequately resolved; recurrent episodes may really be the same infection that has progressed from a subclinical to clinically apparent status. Animal studies also suggest that simply eradicating the infection-causing bug is not enough to restore immune function. Full recovery requires the immune system to inactivate the signaling molecule that starts the invasion. Immune system suppression may persist as long as the molecule is still activated.[104]

See also "Streptococcal Cellulitis" in Chapter 8 and "Lymphangitis" in Chapter 13.

Cellulitis of the breast can occur following breast conservation therapy for breast cancer. Although only a minority of women who undergo this therapy will develop breast cellulitis, the therapist may be the first to observe signs of this disorder. A definitive pathogen has not been identified, and recurrent breast cellulitis is possible months to years after the procedure is completed. Local breast findings include the skin changes typical of cellulitis with or without fever.[7,119]

Cellulitis usually occurs in the loose tissue beneath the skin, but it may also occur in tissues beneath mucous membranes or around muscle bundles. The skin is erythematous, edematous, tender, and sometimes nodular. It can develop under the skin anywhere but affects the extremities most often.

Erysipelas, a surface cellulitis of the skin, affects the upper dermis and is characterized by patches of skin that are red and painful with sharply defined borders and that feel hot to the touch. Red streaks extending from the patch indicate that the lymph vessels have been infected. Facial cellulitis involves the face, especially the cheek or periorbital or orbital tissues; the neck may also be affected. Pelvic cellulitis involves the tissues surrounding the uterus and is called *parametritis*.

Intravenous (IV) antibiotic infusion is the primary treatment. Oral antibiotic can be effective if the infection is caught early; individuals who are susceptible to recurrent cellulitis may have a prescription for oral antibiotics on hand (or at least a prescription that can be filled at the first sign of infection). The therapist can draw around the red area and take photos to look for progression. If there are signs of progression and/or new onset of constitutional symptoms (especially fever), the person must be seen by medical personnel immediately. Good nutrition and hydration are advised to help fight infection, repair tissue, and remove bacteria and their by-products. Extensive cellulitis requires surgical debridement of the necrotic tissue. Lymphangitis may occur if cellulitis is untreated, and gangrene, metastatic abscesses, and sepsis can result.

Viral Infections

Viruses are intracellular parasites that produce their effect by using the intracellular substances of the host cells. In a viral infection the epidermal cells react with inflammation and vesiculation (as in herpes zoster) or by proliferating to form growths (warts). See Chapter 8 for details.

Herpes Zoster

See discussion in Chapter 8.

Warts (Verrucae)

Warts are common, benign viral infections of the skin and adjacent mucous membranes caused by human papillomaviruses (HPVs). Transmission is probably through direct contact, but autoinoculation is possible.

Warts may appear singly or as multiple lesions with thick white surfaces containing many pointed projections. Clinical manifestations depend on the type of wart and its location. The most common wart (verruca vulgaris) is referred to as such and appears as a rough, elevated, round surface most frequently on the extremities, especially the hands and fingers. Plantar warts are slightly elevated or flat, occurring singly or in large clusters referred to as *mosaic warts*, primarily at pressure points of the feet.

MEDICAL MANAGEMENT

DIAGNOSIS. Diagnosis is usually made on the basis of visual examination. Plantar warts can be differentiated from neuropathic ulcers, corns, and calluses by certain distinguishing features. Plantar warts obliterate natural lines of the skin, may contain red or black capillary dots that are easily discernible if the surface of the wart is shaved down with a scalpel, and are painful on application of pressure. Both plantar warts and corns have a soft, pulpy core surrounded by a thick callous ring; plantar warts and calluses are flush with the skin surface.

TREATMENT. Some warts respond to simple treatment, and some disappear spontaneously. The specific choice of treatment method is influenced by the location of the wart or warts, size and number of warts, presence of secondary infection, amount of tenderness present on palpation, age and gender of the client, history of previous treatment, and individual compliance with treatment. Over-the-counter salicylic acid preparations applied topically may be used to induce peeling of the skin. Other methods are cryotherapy and use of acids.

Electrodesiccation and *curettage* of warts are widely used for common warts and occasionally for plantar warts. High-frequency electric current destroys the wart and is followed by surgical removal of dead tissue at the base with application of an antibiotic ointment and dressing for 48 hours. Atrophic scarring may occur.

The use of mechanical (nonthermal) ultrasound has been advocated by some in the treatment of plantar warts, but this has not been widely accepted by the medical community.

Fungal Infections (Dermatophytoses)

Fungal infections such as ringworm are caused by a group of fungi that invade the stratum corneum, hair, and nails.[65] These are superficial infections by fungi that live on, not in, the skin and are confined to the dead keratin layers, unable to survive in the deeper layers. Because the keratin is being shed (desquamated) constantly, the fungus must multiply at a rate that equals the rate of keratin production to maintain itself; otherwise the organisms would be shed with the discarded skin cells.

Fungal infections will spread without treatment; antifungal creams are available over the counter, but diagnosis is required to identify the skin lesion.

Ringworm (Tinea Corporis)

Dermatophytoses, or fungal infections of the hair, skin, or nails, are designated by the Latin word *tinea*, with further designation related to the affected area of the body (see Table 10-3). Tinea corporis, or ringworm, has no association with worms but rather is marked by the formation of ring-shaped pigmented patches covered with vesicles or scales that often become itchy (Fig. 10-6). Transmission can occur directly through contact with infected lesions

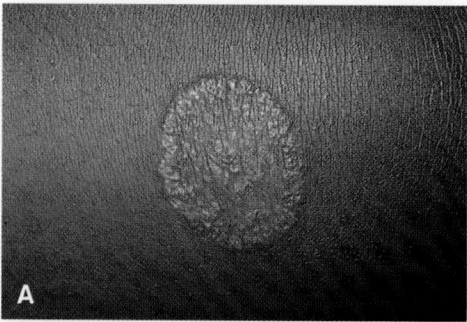
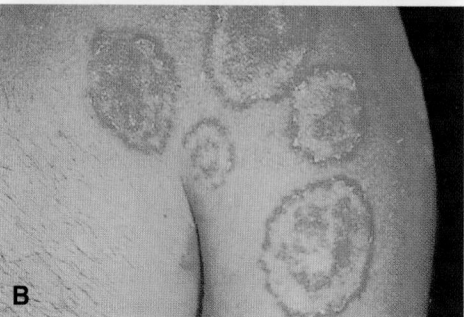

Figure 10-6

Tinea corporis (ringworm). A, Scales forming circular lesions with clear centers are characteristic of tinea corporis (ringworm). **B,** Most adults or children present with multiple lesions that are hyperpigmented in whites and depigmented in dark-skinned people. The lesions occur most often on the face, chest, abdomen, and back of arms. (**A,** From Zitelli BJ, Davis HW: *Atlas of pediatric physical diagnosis,* St Louis, 2002, Mosby. **B,** From Habif T: *Clinical dermatology,* ed 4, St Louis, 2004, Elsevier.)

or indirectly through contact with contaminated objects, such as shoes, towels, or shower stalls.

Diagnosis can be made through laboratory examination of the affected skin. Treatment for any type of ringworm requires maintaining clean, dry skin and applying antifungal powder or topical agent as prescribed.

Treatment with the drug griseofulvin may take weeks to months to complete and should be continued throughout the prescribed dosage schedule even if symptoms subside. Possible side effects of this agent include headache, GI upset, fatigue, insomnia, and photosensitivity. Prolonged use of this drug requires monitoring of liver function. Oral medication is reserved for clients with more involved cases.

Occasionally an obese client with tinea corporis is referred to therapy for wound management secondary to skin breakdown. Advanced wound dressings may be applied to areas of moist, denuded skin to optimize healing.

Athlete's Foot (Tinea Pedis)

Tinea pedis, or athlete's foot, causes erythema, skin peeling, and pruritus between the toes that may spread from the interdigital spaces to the plantar surface of the foot (see Figure 7-17). Severe infection may result in inflammation, with severe itching and pain on walking. Some individuals develop a strong foot odor as well.

Clean, dry socks and adequate footwear (well-ventilated, properly fitting) are important. After washing the feet and drying thoroughly between the toes, antifungal cream or powder (the latter to absorb perspiration and prevent excoriation) can be applied.

A history of antibiotic use, yeast infections (candidiasis, including intestinal yeast), and other risk factors for *candidiasis* may contribute to athlete's foot. If symptomatic treatment including topical preparations does not eradicate the problem, treatment of intestinal yeast may be required.

Yeast (Candidiasis)

Candidiasis also is frequently a complication of moisture-associated skin damage (MASD) due to chronic wetness from wound exudate, urine, stool, and/or perspiration. It can be found periwound, peristoma, in skin folds, and with IAD. Usually appearing as a bright red rash with tiny macules and papules, it also can appear scaly.

SPECIAL IMPLICATIONS FOR THE THERAPIST 10-6

Fungal Infections
The infectious nature of fungal infections requires specific hygienic measures common to all infectious conditions. Affected persons should not share hair care products (e.g., combs, brushes, headgear), clothes, or other articles that have been in proximity to the infected area. Affected persons must use their own towels and linens.

Because fungal infections are superficial (living on the skin), the therapist and all health care personnel are required by the Centers for Medicare and Medicaid Services (CMS) to cut body hair rather than shave it, for the application of electrodes or other adhesives and with wound management. Cutting the hair closely will avoid providing microscopic nicks that can give entrance for the transmission of surface pathogens.[47]

Ringworm
Because ringworm can be acquired by animal-to-human transmission (see Table 10-3), all household pets must be examined for the presence of ringworm as well. Other sources of infection include seats with headrests (e.g., theater seats, seats on public transportation, or other public seats that can be shared).

Athlete's Foot
Athlete's foot, often observed by the therapist (see previous description), should be discussed with the client. Although the client may consider this condition a nuisance or a minimal problem that does not require medical attention, it can be an entry point for bacterial infections, especially in older adults. Keeping athlete's foot under control is an important way to prevent cellulitis, a bacterial infection in the legs, and is especially important in the presence of diabetes.[67]

Yeast
People who take immunosuppressive medications or have immune system disorders such as diabetes or cancer are at higher risk for developing yeast infections due to MASD. Therapists involved in wound management should be aware of the difference between IAD and pressure ulcers in documentation, which is legally and financially (reimbursement) important in today's

environment. Antifungal ointments that are not prescription are available, as well as an antimicrobial silver infused fabric, InterDry® (Coloplast), for skin folds. Powder is not recommended because of clumping, and possible allergic reactions.

Other Parasitic Infections

Some parasitic infections of the skin are caused by insect and animal contacts. Contact with insects that puncture the skin for the purpose of sucking blood, injecting venom, or laying their eggs is relatively common. Substances deposited by insects are considered foreign to the host and may create an allergic sensitivity in that individual and produce pruritus, urticaria, or systemic reactions of a greater or lesser degree, depending on the individual's sensitivity.

Scabies

Definition. Scabies (mites) is a highly contagious skin eruption caused by a mite, *Sarcoptes scabiei*. It is a common public health problem with an estimated prevalence of 300 million cases worldwide. The female mite burrows into the skin and deposits eggs that hatch into larvae in a few days.

Scabies is easily transmitted by skin-to-skin contact or by contact with contaminated objects, such as linens or shared inanimate objects. Infections with human T-cell leukemia/lymphoma virus 1 (HTLV-1) and HIV are associated with scabies.[27] Mites can spread rapidly between members of the same household, nursing home, or institution, but the inflammatory response and itching do not occur until approximately 30 to 60 days after initial contact.

Clinical Manifestations. The symptoms include intense pruritus (worse at night), usually excoriated skin, and the burrow, which is a linear ridge with a vesicle at one end. The mite is usually found in the burrow, commonly in the interdigital web spaces, flexor aspects of the wrist (volar surface), axillae, waistline, nipples in females, genitalia in males, and the umbilicus. Intense scratching can lead to severe excoriation and secondary bacterial infection. Itching can become generalized secondary to sensitization.

MEDICAL MANAGEMENT

DIAGNOSIS AND TREATMENT. The mite can be excavated from one end of a burrow with a needle or a scalpel blade and examined under a microscope. In longstanding cases, a mite may not be found. At that point, treatment is based on a presumptive diagnosis.

Treatment has traditionally been with a scabicide, usually a lotion or cream containing permethrin or lindane, applied to the entire body from the neck down. Single oral-dose therapy of ivermectin (Stromectol) is an effective treatment for this infestation. Permethrin is generally the treatment of choice for head lice and scabies because of its residual effect and because toxicity and absorption are minimal. Ivermectin may be reserved for cases where permethrin fails[38]; further research is advocated regarding the safety and effectiveness of ivermectin.

SPECIAL IMPLICATIONS FOR THE THERAPIST   10-7

Scabies

If a hospitalized person has scabies, prevent transmission to self and others by practicing good handwashing technique and by wearing gloves when touching the affected person and a gown when in close contact. Observe wound and skin precautions for 24 hours after treatment of scabies. Gas-autoclave blood pressure cuffs or other equipment used with the affected person before using them on other people. All linens and toweling used must be isolated after use until the person is noninfectious. If the person is treated anywhere outside the hospital room (e.g., on a plinth or treatment mat), the area must be thoroughly disinfected after each session.

In using a scabicide, the individual must understand that NO area can be missed. After 24 hours, the affected person should bathe. All bed linens and clothes must be laundered in hot water or dry-cleaned. Other household members and those in close contact with the affected person should be treated. A second application of the cream or lotion may need to be applied 7 days later. The same procedure is followed.

Itching may persist for 1 to 2 weeks after treatment until the stratum corneum is replaced, but lesions on the forearms or legs can be occluded with Unna's boots to eliminate the scratch–itch cycle (Fig. 10-7). Widespread bacterial infections require additional treatment with systemic antibiotics.

Pediculosis (Lousiness)

Pediculosis is an infestation by *Pediculus humanus*, a very common parasite infecting the head, body, and genital area. Transmission is from one person to another, usually on shared personal items, such as combs, lockers, clothes, or furniture. Lice are not carried or transmitted by pets. School-age children are easily infected as are people who live in overcrowded surroundings and those older adults who have poor personal hygiene, depend on others for care, or live in a nursing home.

Pediculus humanus var. *capitis*, the head louse, is transmitted through personal contact or through shared hairbrushes or shared head wear. Severe itching accompanied by secondary eczematous changes develops, and small greyish or white nits (eggs) are usually seen attached to the base of the hair shafts.

Pediculus corporis, the body or clothes louse, produces intense itching, which in turn results in severe excoriations from scratching and possible secondary bacterial infections. The lice or nits are generally found in the seams of the affected individual's clothing.

Pediculus pubis (*Phthirus pubis*), the pubic or crab louse, is usually transmitted by sexual contact but can be transferred on clothing or towels. The lice and nits are usually found at the base of the pubic hairs. Sometimes dark brown particles (louse excreta) may be seen on underclothes.

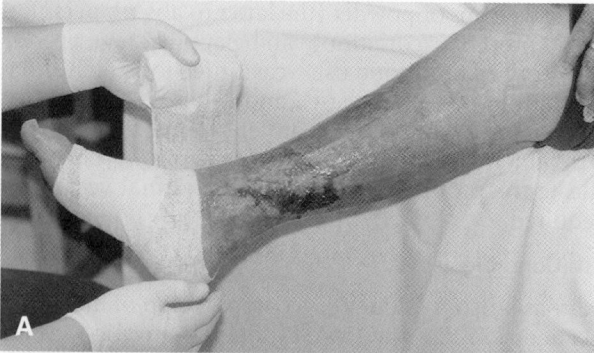
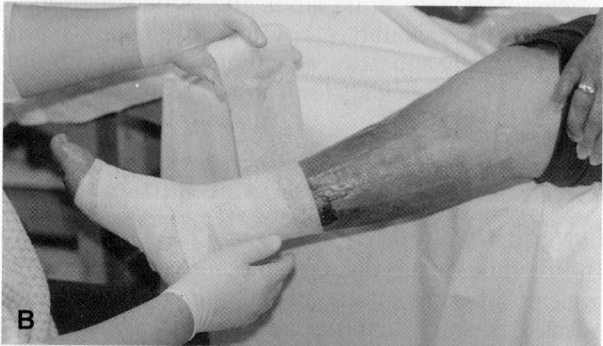
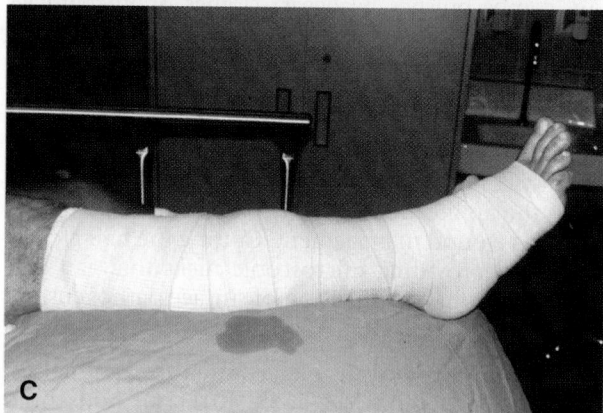

Figure 10-7

A, Unna's boots. Although most often used in cases of venous insufficiency (the client must be ambulatory to enlist the calf muscle pump), the application of Unna's boot to the forearms or legs can be used with a variety of skin lesions to eliminate the scratch–itch cycle. Unna's boot is a dressing made of gauze impregnated with gelatin, zinc oxide, calamine, and glycerin. **B,** The bandage is applied in a spiral fashion and allowed to dry, forming a semi-rigid dressing. This dressing can be allowed to stay intact for 7 days. **C,** A four-layer gradient compression wrap (Profore) provides sustained compression for up to 1 week, for both ambulatory and nonambulatory clients. (A and B, Courtesy Pam Unger, PT, Community General Hospital, Center for Wound Management, Reading, PA, 1995. C, Courtesy Harriett B. Loehne, PT, DPT, CWS, FACCWS, Archbold Center for Wound Management & Hyperbaric Medicine, Thomasville, GA. Used with permission.)

MEDICAL MANAGEMENT

Traditional treatment has been with the appropriate cleaning solution (e.g., shampoo or soap containing permethrin) specific to the type of louse present. As with scabies, single oral-dose therapy of ivermectin (Stromectol) is an effective treatment for this infestation (see previous section on Scabies).

Pediculosis

The therapist must always be conscious of the personal hygiene of all clients. Anyone can get pediculosis regardless of age, socioeconomic status, or status of personal cleanliness. Wear gloves while carefully inspecting the head of any adult or child who scratches excessively. Look for bite marks, redness, and nits or movement that indicates a louse. If exposure to lice occurs, treatment for the client as well as the therapist may be required depending on the exposure level. Use the same precautions outlined earlier in "Scabies."

All combs and brushes should be soaked in the cleaning agent, and clothing must be boiled, dry-cleaned, or washed in a machine (hot cycle). The seams of the clothing should be pressed with a hot iron. Carpets, car seats, pillows, stuffed animals, rugs, mattresses, upholstered furniture, and similar objects that come in contact with the affected person must be vacuumed or cleaned thoroughly with hot water and the cleaning agent. Any item that cannot be cleaned can be stored in a sealed plastic bag for 2 to 3 weeks until all lice have been killed.

SKIN CANCER

The American Cancer Society (ACS) estimates that skin cancers are the most prevalent form of cancer, eventually affecting nearly all white people older than 65 years of age. Skin cancer is the most rapidly increasing cancer in the United States, with more than 1 million new cases of nonmelanoma (i.e., basal and squamous cell) skin cancer diagnosed annually in the United States. There is no evidence that this epidemic has peaked.[171]

Solar radiation (exposure to midrange-wavelength ultraviolet B [UVB] radiation) causes most skin cancers, and protection from the sun during the first two decades of life significantly reduces the risk of skin cancer. The melanoma rate is rising most rapidly in persons younger than 40 years of age and is now the most common cancer in women between the ages of 25 and 29 years and second only to breast cancer in the age group from 30 to 34 years.

In this chapter, skin cancer is discussed in three broad categories: benign, premalignant, and malignant (Box 10-6). Malignant lesions of the skin are considered as either melanoma or nonmelanoma. Kaposi sarcoma, which occurs in the skin, is not included in these categories and is discussed separately in this chapter.

Benign skin lesions, such as seborrheic keratosis or nevi (moles), do not usually undergo transition to malignant melanoma and do not usually require treatment. Although most moles remain benign skin lesions, when malignant melanoma does occur, it often arises from a preexisting mole, derived from pigment cells (melanocytes) of the skin.

Keratoacanthomas do require treatment. Precancerous lesions, such as actinic keratosis or Bowen disease, may progress to malignancy and must be carefully evaluated. The most common types of (nonmelanoma) malignant

Box 10-6

TYPES OF SKIN CANCER

Benign	Premalignant	Non-melanoma	Melanoma
Seborrheic keratosis	Actinic keratosis	Basal cell carcinoma	Superficial spreading melanoma
Nevi	Bowen disease	Squamous cell carcinoma	Nodular melanoma
			Lentigo maligna melanoma
			Acral lentiginous melanoma

skin cancer are basal cell carcinoma and squamous cell carcinoma.

These carcinomas occur twice as often in white men as in white women, and the incidence increases steadily with age. A third type of malignant skin cancer (also affecting white men more than white women), malignant melanoma, is the most serious skin cancer, resulting in early metastasis and possible death.

Benign Tumors

Seborrheic Keratosis

Seborrheic keratosis is a hereditary benign proliferation of basal cells occurring most frequently after middle age and presenting as multiple lesions on the chest, back, and face. The lesions also often appear following hormonal therapy or inflammatory dermatoses. The areas are waxy, smooth, or raised lesions that vary in color from yellow to flesh tones to dark brown or black. Their size varies from barely palpable to large verrucous (wart-like) plaques. These tumors are usually left untreated unless they itch or cause pain. Otherwise, cryotherapy with liquid nitrogen is an effective treatment.

Nevi (Moles)

Nevi are pigmented or nonpigmented lesions that form from aggregations of melanocytes beginning early in life. Most moles are brown, black, or flesh-colored and may appear on any part of the skin. They vary in size and thickness, occurring in groups or singly.

Nevi seldom undergo transition to malignant melanoma, but as previously mentioned, when malignant melanoma does occur, it often arises from a preexisting mole; the chances of cancerous transformation are increased as a result of constant irritation. Any change in size, color, or texture of a mole; bleeding; or any excessive itching should be reported to a physician.

Precancerous Conditions

There are two common premalignant skin lesions: actinic keratosis and Bowen disease.

Actinic Keratosis

Actinic keratosis (also known as *solar keratosis*) is a skin disease resulting from many years of exposure to the sun's UV rays. The damage caused by overexposure to sunlight results in abnormal cell growth, causing a well-defined, crusty, or sandpaper-like patch or bump that appears on chronically sun-exposed areas of the body (e.g., face, ears, lower lip, bald scalp, dorsa of hands and forearms).

The base may be light or dark, tan, pink, red, or a combination of these, or it may be the same color as the skin. The scale or crust is horny, dry, and rough; it is often recognized by touch rather than sight. Occasionally it itches or produces a pricking or tender sensation. The skin abnormality or lesion develops slowly to reach a size that is most often 3 to 6 mm. It may disappear only to reappear later. Often there are several actinic keratoses present at one time.

Actinic keratosis affects nearly 100% of the older white population. It is most common in fair-complexioned, blue- or green-eyed, middle-aged men with a history of sun exposure (solar radiation). The number of lesions that develops is directly related to heredity and lifetime exposure to the sun.

There is a known risk of malignant degeneration and subsequent metastatic potential in neglected lesions. Almost half of the estimated 5 million current cases of skin cancer began as actinic keratosis lesions. It is important that this condition be diagnosed properly, because it is often difficult to distinguish a large or hypertrophic actinic keratosis from a squamous cell carcinoma. A biopsy may be indicated.

Not all keratoses need to be removed. The decision about treatment protocol is based on the nature of the lesion, the number of lesions, and the age and health of the affected person. Treatment may be with 5-fluorouracil (Efudex), a topical antimetabolite that inhibits cell division, or masoprocol cream; cryosurgery using liquid nitrogen; or curettage by electrodesiccation (superficial tissue destruction through the use of bursts of electrical current).

These clients should be advised to avoid sun exposure and use a high-potency (sun protection factor [SPF] 15) sunscreen 30 to 60 minutes before going outside. SPF 30 is recommended for people of fair complexion. Sunscreens are not recommended for infants under 6 months of age. Infants should be kept out of the sun or shaded from it. Fabric with a tight weave, such as cotton, is suggested.

Some conditions call for more invasive treatments, such as laser resurfacing (outer layers of the skin are vaporized) or chemical peels (outer layers are burned off via chemical solution). In June 2000, the U.S. Food and Drug Administration (FDA) approved the use of photodynamic treatment of actinic keratosis of the face and scalp using a topical application (Levulan Kerastick) followed by exposure to a nonlaser blue light source. This is a painful and involved treatment requiring application of Levulan 16 hours prior to exposure to the light source. In 2007, the FDA warned the company manufacturing Levulan to change its advertising, as it stated there were no risks, as well as made false claims.[43] This was done, and it still is being used today. A randomized controlled trial was completed in November 2012, but the results were not published. Only summary data (provided by the pharmaceutical company on their website) is available (http://www.dusapharma.com/high-clearance-rates.html). Additional information about this medication is available through Drugs.com, an independent source of information on prescription drugs (http://www.drugs.com/pro/levulan-kerastick.html).

Bowen Disease

Bowen disease can occur anywhere on the skin (exposed and unexposed areas) or mucous membranes (especially the glans penis in uncircumcised males). It presents as a persistent, brown to reddish brown, scaly plaque with well-defined margins. Often the person has a history of arsenic exposure in youth. Multiple lesions have been associated with an increased number of internal malignancies and therefore require close follow-up. Treatment is with surgical excision and topical 5-fluorouracil.

Malignant Neoplasms

Basal Cell Carcinoma

Definition and Overview. Basal cell carcinoma is a slow-growing surface epithelial skin tumor originating from undifferentiated basal cells contained in the epidermis. This type of carcinoma rarely metastasizes beyond the skin and does not invade blood or lymph vessels but can cause significant local destruction.

Incidence. Until recently, this tumor rarely appeared before age 40 years and was more prevalent in blond, fair-skinned males. In the age group under 30 years, more women than men develop skin cancer associated with the use of indoor tanning devices with concentrated doses of UV radiation.[98] It is the most common malignant tumor affecting whites, with a reported 100,000 new cases each year; African Americans and Asians are rarely affected.

Etiologic and Risk Factors. Prolonged sun exposure and intermittent sun exposure are the most common causes of basal cell carcinoma, but immunosuppression (e.g., organ transplant recipients, individuals who are HIV positive), genetic predisposition with defects in DNA replication and repair (xeroderma pigmentosum), and rarely, the site of vaccinations are other possible causes. Immunosuppressed organ transplant recipients are more likely to develop squamous cell carcinoma, whereas HIV-infected adults are far more likely to have basal cell carcinoma.

These lesions are seen most frequently in geographic regions with intense sunlight in people with outdoor occupations and on those areas most exposed, the face and neck. Dark-skinned people are rarely affected because their basal cells contain the pigment melanin, a protective factor against sun exposure. Anyone who has had one basal cell carcinoma is at increased risk of developing others. Recurrences of previously treated lesions are possible, usually within the first 2 years after initial treatment.

Pathogenesis. The pathogenesis of basal cell tumors remains uncertain, and basal cell carcinoma is considered biologically unusual. It is a stable growth characterized by monotonous structure (the same in small as well as large tumors), the absence of progression to metastasis, and a small amount of chromosomal damage (as compared with moderate chromosomal damage associated with squamous cell carcinoma).

To the dismay of investigators seeking to design experiments, basal cell carcinomas are very seldom seen in animals and not found in laboratory rodents at all. Whereas squamous cell carcinoma is often preceded by a precursor (actinic keratosis), there are no known precursors to basal cell carcinoma. This fact suggests that basal cell carcinoma tumors need only a few mutations to induce malignant transformation.[36,139]

One theory suggests that these tumors arise as a result of a defect that prevents the cells from being shed by the normal keratinization process. The process of epidermal cell maturation is called *keratinization* because the cells synthesize a fibrous protein called *keratin*. Basal cells that lack the normal keratin proteins form basal cell tumors. Another hypothesis is that undifferentiated basal cells become carcinomatous instead of differentiating into sweat glands, sebum, and hair. See also "Squamous Cell Carcinoma" (Pathogenesis) below.

Clinical Manifestations. Basal cell carcinoma (Fig. 10-8) typically has a pearly or ivory appearance, has rolled edges, and is slightly elevated above the skin surface, with small blood vessels on the surface (telangiectasia) (see Fig. 10-3).

The nodule is usually painless and slowly increases in size and may ulcerate centrally. More than 65% of basal cell carcinomas are found on the head and neck. Other locations are the trunk, especially the upper back and chest.

They also can appear similar to Bowen disease, chronic venous ulcer (Fig. 10-9), or squamous cell carcinoma in a flatter, scaling lesion, usually on the trunk or extremities.

MEDICAL MANAGEMENT

DIAGNOSIS AND TREATMENT. Diagnosis by clinical examination of appearance must be confirmed via biopsy and histologic study. Treatment depends on the size, location, and depth of the lesion and may include curettage and electrodesiccation, chemotherapy, surgical excision, and irradiation.

Mohs micrographic surgery is the gold standard treatment, in which the specimen is excised, frozen-sectioned, and examined for positive margins while the client waits, thus ensuring clean margins before complex repairs are performed. Irradiation is used if the tumor location requires it and in older or debilitated people who cannot tolerate surgery.

Radiation therapy is generally contraindicated in persons less than 50 years of age because of the risk of recurrence and the development of secondary radiation-induced tumors of the skin. Radiotherapy can be followed by chronic skin ulcers that are difficult to close, much less heal. Some radiation-induced ulcers open on and off for years, and some just develop 10 to 20 years after the radiation therapy.[162]

If the tumor is identified and treated early, local excision or even nonexcisional destruction is usually curative. Skin grafting may be required in cases where large areas of tissue have been removed. A new experimental treatment called *photodynamic therapy* is being investigated in the treatment of superficial nonmelanoma skin cancers. This technique requires the administration of a drug that induces photosensitivity, followed in 48 to 72 hours by exposure to light that helps outline the tumor. The tumor cells concentrate this drug so as to allow selective destruction of the cancer cells when exposed to a laser light of 630 nm.[84,183]

Clinical trials are under way investigating the use of chemopreventive agents, such as vitamin A analogues called *retinoids*. These topical agents may potentially complement sunscreens and result in decreased incidence, morbidity, and mortality of skin cancer.[175]

Tretinoin has proven effective in preventing UV-induced lesions and can be considered for individuals with high-risk basal or squamous cell carcinoma, as well as those with actinic keratosis, realizing that it is off-label use.[157] Topical imiquimod was approved by the FDA in 2004 for individuals who have superficial basal cell carcinoma.[54]

Cytokine therapy, including interferon and interleukin, is a type of systemic immunotherapy used to treat skin cancer. Both cytokines mentioned here have been FDA approved for metastatic melanoma.[152]

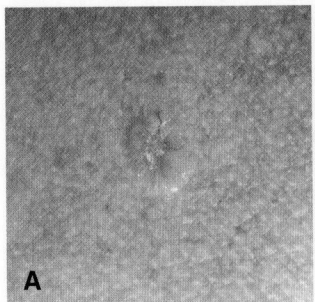
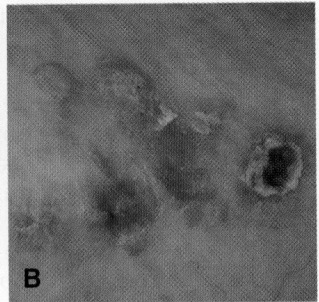

Figure 10-8

Basal cell carcinoma. A, Skin cancer in the form of basal cell carcinoma can appear as a shiny, pearly, or translucent pink, red, or white bump. There may be a rolled border with an indented center. **B,** This type of skin cancer may also present as a red patch; a crusty, open sore that will not heal; or a scar-like area. (**A,** From Lookingbill D, Marks J: *Principles of dermatology,* ed 3, Philadelphia, 2000, Saunders. **B,** From Townsend C, Beauchamp RD, Evers BM, Mattox K: *Sabiston textbook of surgery,* ed 17, Philadelphia, 2004, Saunders.)

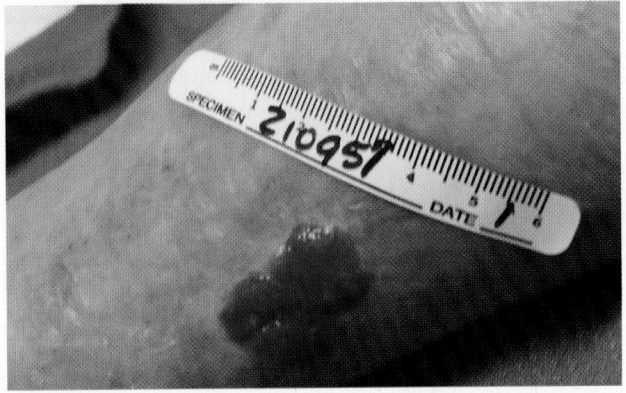

Figure 10-9

Chronic venous ulcer. Basal cell carcinoma can also mimic a chronic venous ulcer, potentially causing a delay in diagnosis. Biopsy is required to make the definitive medical diagnosis. (Courtesy Harriett B. Loehne, PT, DPT, CWS, FACCWS, Archbold Center for Wound Management & Hyperbaric Medicine, Thomasville, GA. Used with permission.)

PROGNOSIS. If left untreated, basal cell lesions slowly invade surrounding tissues over months and years, destroying local tissues such as bone and cartilage, especially around the eyes, ears, and nose.

Squamous Cell Carcinoma

Definition and Overview. Squamous cell carcinoma is the second most common skin cancer in whites/light-skinned individuals, usually arising in sun-damaged skin, such as the rim of the ear, the face, the lips and mouth, and the dorsa of the hands (Fig. 10-10). It is a tumor of the epidermal keratinocytes and rarely occurs in dark-skinned people.

Squamous cell tumors may be one of two types: in situ (confined to the site of origin) and invasive (infiltrate surrounding tissue). *In situ* squamous cell carcinoma is usually confined to the epidermis but may extend into the dermis. Common premalignant skin lesions associated with in situ carcinomas are actinic keratosis and Bowen disease (see earlier section).

Invasive squamous cell carcinoma can arise from premalignant lesions of the skin, including sun-damaged skin, actinic dermatitis, scars, whitish discolored areas (leukoplakia), radiation-induced keratosis, tar and oil keratosis, and chronic ulcers and sinuses.

Incidence. As with basal cell carcinoma, fair-skinned people have a higher incidence of squamous cell carcinoma. This particular type of tumor has a peak incidence at 60 years of age and affects men more than women.

Etiologic and Risk Factors. Predisposing factors associated with squamous cell carcinoma include cumulative overexposure to UV radiation (e.g., outdoor employment or residence in a warm, sunny climate), burns, presence of premalignant lesions such as actinic keratosis or Bowen disease, radiation therapy, ingestion of herbicides containing arsenic, chronic skin irritation and inflammation, exposure to local carcinogens (tar,

oil), and hereditary disease such as xeroderma pigmentosum and albinism.

Organ transplant recipients who are chronically immunosuppressed are at risk for the development of recurring squamous cell carcinoma. Rarely, squamous cell carcinoma may develop on the site of a small-pox vaccination, psoriasis, or chronic discoid lupus erythematosus.

Pathogenesis. UV radiation continues to be one of the most important causes of skin cancer, because the sun's UV rays damage the DNA inside the nuclei of the epidermal cells, triggering enzymes to repair the damage. UV-damaged cells are usually removed by apoptosis (programmed cell death) in a process involving the p53 protein. In non-melanoma skin cancer, the p53 tumor-suppressor gene is often damaged by UVB irradiation, so faulty cells are not removed from the skin. Both UVB and UVA rays have direct and indirect effects on the cutaneous immune system, lowering the skin's cell-mediated immunity, which is another factor in carcinogenesis. We also differ in our ability to produce repair enzymes, which may explain our differences in tanning ability as well as susceptibility to skin cancer. Not all DNA lesions are properly repaired, increasing the risk of skin cancer.

Newer studies show that when DNA damage occurs, a cell surface molecule (Fas ligand; FasL) belonging to the tumor necrosis factor family binds to its receptor Fas and attaches to the damaged cells, inducing them to die by apoptosis (i.e., programmed cell death).

These suicidal cells known as *keratinocytes* take themselves out of action, and the less damaged ones repair themselves. After many years of cumulative sun exposure, keratinocytes can become malignant. But even then, the cancers (either basal or squamous cell) grow slowly and do not spread easily.

On the other hand, melanocytes, the cells that give rise to melanomas, seem highly resistant to self-destruction. After a person gets badly sunburned, damaged melanocytes continue to replicate, increasing the chance that some will turn malignant. These studies suggest that Fas ligand is a critical defense against the accumulation of mutations caused by sunlight exposure. Its absence or inactivation may be key to the development of skin cancer.[77,134]

Clinical Manifestations. Squamous cell lesions are more difficult to characterize than basal cell tumors. The squamous cell tumor has poorly defined margins, because the edge blends into the surrounding sun-damaged skin.

This type of carcinoma can present as an ulcer, a flat red area, a cutaneous horn, an indurated plaque, or a nodule. It may be red to flesh-colored and surrounded by scaly tissue. More than 80% of squamous cell carcinomas occur in the head and neck region.

Malignant transformation of any chronic wound can occur (Fig. 10-11). *Marjolin ulcer* is the term given to aggressive epidermoid tumors that arise from areas of chronic injury and form squamous cell carcinomas. Healed burn wounds are common sites, but any chronic wound can transform into a malignancy. Dr. Jean Nicolas Marjolin first described the occurrence of ulcerating lesions within scar tissue in 1828. If these lesions are not detected and

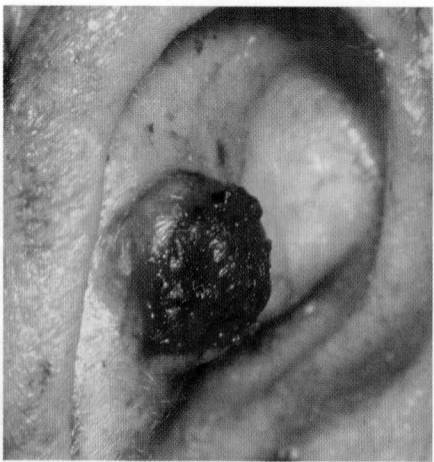

Figure 10-10

Squamous cell carcinoma can take the form of a persistent, scaly, red patch that sometimes crusts or bleeds or an open sore that does not heal. This type of skin cancer may also present as a raised or wart-like growth that may bleed. (From Goldman L: *Cecil textbook of medicine,* ed 22, Philadelphia, 2004, Saunders.)

treated early, they may invade deep tissues and ulcerate (see Prognosis section of "Diagnosis, Treatment, and Prognosis" that follows).

Usually lesions on unexposed skin tend to be more invasive and more likely to metastasize, with the exception of lesions on the lower lip and ears. These sites tend to metastasize early, beginning with the process of induration and inflammation of the lesion. Metastasis can occur to the regional lymph nodes, producing characteristic systemic symptoms of pain, malaise, fatigue, weakness, and anorexia.

A THERAPIST'S THOUGHTS*

Chronic Wounds

Therapists should consider recommending a biopsy for any chronic wound that does not progress toward healing with advanced wound management interventions.

*Harriett B. Loehne, PT, DPT, CWS, FACCWS

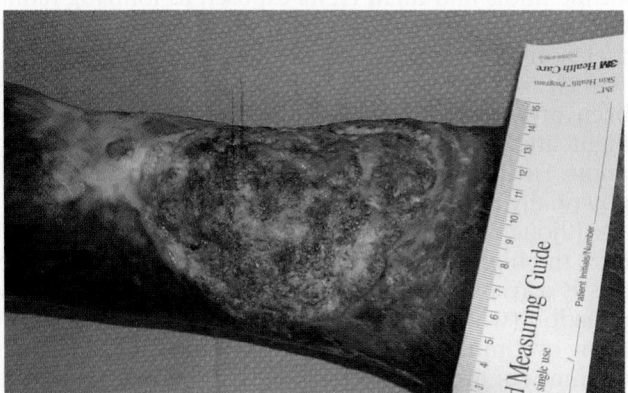

Figure 10-11

Marjolin ulcer. This large lesion constitutes a Marjolin ulcer. The client had a history of venous ulcers and had been treated for many months by home health nurses with no improvement. She was seen at the Archbold Center for Wound Management; a biopsy was done immediately with a fresh-frozen section, and a diagnosis of Marjolin was made. The cancer had metastasized to the bone, and a below-knee amputation was required. It was never clear whether the cancer began in a new ulcer or in scar tissue from a previous ulcer. (Courtesy Harriett B. Loehne, PT, DPT, CWS, FACCWS, Archbold Center for Wound Management & Hyperbaric Medicine, Thomasville, GA. Used with permission.)

MEDICAL MANAGEMENT

DIAGNOSIS, TREATMENT, AND PROGNOSIS. An excisional biopsy provides definitive diagnosis and staging of squamous cell carcinoma. Other laboratory tests may be appropriate depending on the presence of systemic symptoms. The size, shape, location, and invasiveness of a squamous cell tumor and the condition of the underlying tissue determine the treatment method selected (see "Basal Cell Carcinoma," above). A deeply invasive tumor may require a combination of techniques. As with all benign, premalignant, or malignant skin lesions, sun protection is vitally important (see Box 10-4).

All the major treatment methods have excellent rates of cure; generally, the prognosis is better with a well-differentiated lesion in an unusual location.

Malignant Melanoma

Definition and Overview

Malignant melanoma is a neoplasm of the skin originating from melanocytes or cells that synthesize the pigment melanin. The melanomas occur most frequently in the skin but can also be found in the oral cavity, esophagus, anal canal, vagina, or meninges or within the eye. The clinical varieties of cutaneous melanoma are classified into four types (Fig. 10-12)[5,20]:

1. *Superficial spreading melanoma* is the most common type of melanoma and accounts for 70% of cutaneous melanomas. It can occur on any part of the body, especially in areas of chronic irritation, the legs of females between the knees and ankles, or the trunk in both genders. It is usually diagnosed in people between 20 and 60 years of age. It usually arises in a preexisting mole and presents as a brown or black, raised patch with an irregular border and variable pigmentation (red, white, and blue; brown-black; black-blue). It is usually asymptomatic. With advanced lesions, itching and bleeding may occur.

2. *Nodular melanoma* is the most aggressive form and can be found on any part of the body with no specific site preference. Men 60 years of age and older are

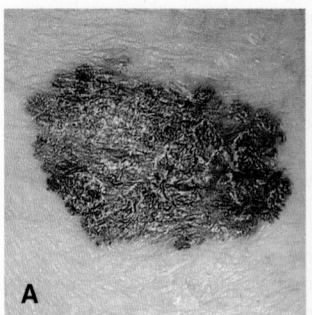
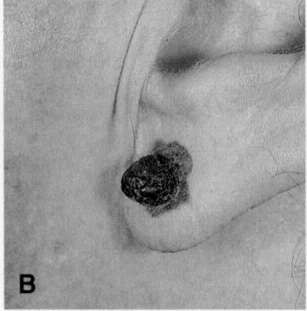
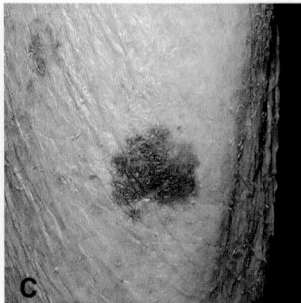
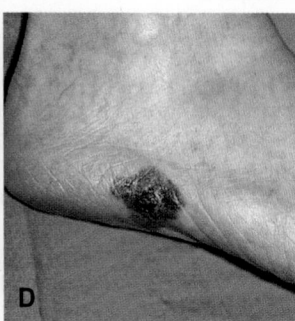

Figure 10-12

A, Superficial spreading melanoma. An irregular margin with multiple colors of black, blue, pale red, and white may be seen. **B,** Nodular lesion of melanoma. This lesion developed on top of a benign compound nevus. **C,** Lentigo maligna. If left alone, progression to lentigo maligna melanoma occurs. **D,** Acral lentiginous melanoma. This brown to black, flat lesion has irregular borders and variable pigmentation. (From Callen JP, Greer K, Paller A, Swinyer L: *Color atlas of dermatology,* ed 2, Philadelphia, 2000, Saunders. D, Courtesy Dr. Neil A. Fenske, Tampa.)

affected more often than women. It is often described as a small, suddenly appearing but quickly enlarging, uniformly and darkly pigmented papule (may be greyish) and accounts for approximately 15% of cutaneous melanomas. This type invades the dermis and metastasizes early.

3. *Lentigo maligna melanoma* is a less common type of lesion occurring predominantly on sun-exposed areas, especially the head, neck, and dorsa of hands or under the fingernails, in the 50- to 80-year-old age group, accounting for 10% of cutaneous melanomas. This lesion looks like a large (3- to 6-cm), flat freckle with an irregular border containing varied pigmentation of brown, black, blue-black, red, and white found in a single lesion. These lesions enlarge and become progressively irregularly pigmented over time. Approximately one-third develop into malignant melanoma and therefore bear careful watching.

4. *Acral lentiginous melanoma* is a relatively uncommon form of melanoma accounting for 5% of all cutaneous melanomas. It is the most common form of melanoma in dark-skinned people (e.g., Africans, Asians). These lesions usually have flat, dark brown portions with raised bumpy areas that are predominantly brown-black or blue-black. Most common areas include low-pigment sites where hair is absent, such as the palms of the hands, soles of the feet, nail beds of fingers and toes, and mucous membranes.

Incidence

Malignant melanoma accounts for up to 5% of all cancers, with a lifetime probability of developing melanoma at 1 in 36 for men and 1 in 55 for women. This has increased dramatically from a 1 in 1500 risk of developing melanoma in the 1930s.

Epidemiologists, who report that the incidence of melanoma is more than doubling every 10 to 20 years, call this a melanoma epidemic. The ACS estimates 76,250 new cases of malignant melanoma in 2012,[170] accounting for 9180 deaths, more than from any other skin disorder. The peak incidence is between 40 and 60 years. The incidence is rising in younger age groups, but the disorder remains rare in children before adolescence.

Etiologic and Risk Factors

Most people who develop melanoma have blond or red hair, fair skin, and blue eyes; are prone to sunburn; and are of Celtic or Scandinavian ancestry (Box 10-7). These risk factors are thought to be linked to variations in a gene called *MC1R* that assists in producing melanin pigment to help protect the skin against UV rays.[70,148] Not all UVB radiation (280-320 nm) but all UVA radiation (320-400 nm), the type produced by sun lamps, may promote skin cancer. For these reasons, the use of tanning devices is considered a significant risk factor for the development of skin cancer. In fact, the risk of melanoma reportedly increases 75% when the use of tanning devices starts before age 30.[39] The greater the frequency and intensity of exposure, the greater the risk. The risk is even higher for individuals using high-intensity or high-pressure devices.[98]

Melanomas appear to be more prevalent among whites of high socioeconomic status who work indoors and tend to take short vacations with intense sun exposure than in people who are at risk of chronic sun exposure. This correlation appears to be related to education, not income.[68]

Melanoma occurs more often within families and among people who have dysplastic nevus syndrome, also known as the *atypical mole syndrome*. This is a familial disorder that results in a large number of irregular moles that have an almost 50% chance of developing into melanoma during the person's lifetime. Puberty and pregnancy may enhance growth. Previous history of melanoma places the individual at greater risk of developing a second melanoma.

Other risk factors include excessive exposure to UV radiation through sunlight or tanning devices, especially intense intermittent exposure, and immune suppression from chemotherapy. There are some reports that airline pilots and flight crews exposed to ionizing radiation of cosmic origin have increased rates of malignant melanoma.[18,96,143]

Increased cancer risk among all flight personnel has been previously noted, including breast cancer among flight attendants and acute myeloid leukemia among pilots. Further studies are needed to identify specific and potentially preventable risk factors.[10,44]

Although the evidence is clear that flight personnel have the highest incidence ratio of skin cancer, whether this is a result of excessive exposure to cosmic and UV radiation (which can easily penetrate the cockpit), from flying over multiple time zones (disturbance of circadian rhythm), or from factors related to lifestyle (excessive sunbathing) rather than work conditions remains inconclusive.[66,145] Supportive research shows that an 8% to 10% increase in UVB radiation occurs for every 1000 feet

---

Box 10-7

RISK FACTORS FOR THE DEVELOPMENT OF MALIGNANT MELANOMA*

- Personal (previous) or family history of malignant melanoma
- Fair skin, light hair, blue or green eyes
- Presence of marked freckling on the upper back; dysplastic nevi (moles); congenital melanocytic nevi
- Ultraviolet light exposure
  - History of three or more blistering sunburns before age 20 years
  - History of 3 or more years of an outdoor summer job during adolescence
  - Exposure to tanning devices
- Immune suppression (e.g., medications, organ transplant recipients)
- Genetic disorder: xeroderma pigmentosum
- Age: older adults or in people younger than 30; melanoma that runs in families may occur at a younger age

*Several risk factors that alone or in combination increase the risk of developing melanoma.

Data from American Cancer Society: *Melanoma Skin Cancer*. Last revised January 11, 2012. Available online at: http://www.cancer.org/Cancer/SkinCancer-Melanoma/DetailedGuide/melanoma-skin-cancer-risk-factors.

of elevation, suggesting a higher incidence of skin cancer at higher elevations.[152]

To reduce risk for and prevent incidence of skin cancer, the U.S. Preventive Services Task Force (USPSTF) recommends counseling children, adolescents, and young adults aged 10 to 24 years who have fair skin about minimizing their exposure to UV radiation (grade B recommendation).[11]

Pathogenesis

See "Pathogenesis" under "Squamous Cell Carcinoma" above.

The majority of malignant melanomas appear to be associated with the intensity rather than the duration of sunlight exposure; that is, most people who develop melanoma work indoors and have intense but limited exposure to the sun on weekends or vacations. This accounts for the location of melanomas most commonly on skin that is covered most of the year.

Clinical Manifestations

Melanoma can appear anywhere on the body, not just on sun-exposed areas. Common sites are the head and neck in men, the legs in women, and the backs of people exposed to excessive UV radiation. Up to 70% arise from a preexisting nevus. Any change in a skin lesion or nevus (increased size or elevation; bleeding; soreness or inflammation; changes in color, pigmentation, or texture) must be examined for melanoma (Fig. 10-13).

MEDICAL MANAGEMENT

DIAGNOSIS. Early recognition of cutaneous melanomas can have a major impact on the surgical cure of this disease. The ACS suggests a monthly self-examination. A skin biopsy with histologic examination can distinguish malignant melanoma from other lesions, determine tumor thickness, and provide staging.

There are several techniques for staging skin cancer. The Breslow method measures the thickness of the melanoma; the thinner the melanoma, the better the prognosis. Generally, melanomas less than 1 mm in depth have a very small chance of spreading. A second system (Clark levels) used to determine the appropriate stage evaluates the layers of skin that are invaded by the melanoma (Fig. 10-14).

A third method of staging, TNM, combines both previously described methods. Depending on the depth of the tumor invasion and metastatic spread, other testing procedures may be used, including baseline laboratory studies, a bone scan for metastasis, or computed tomographic (CT) scan for metastasis to the chest, abdomen, central nervous system, and brain.

Diagnostic accuracy will continue to improve as digitalized images of lesions can be analyzed, enabling the physician to determine whether a biopsy is needed. Computer-aided microscopic examination of biopsy slides may lead to better diagnosis, and teledermatology will add additional assistance in melanoma diagnosis. This technology makes it possible to compress digital images of suspicious lesions and transmit them electronically anywhere in the world, making consultation easier.[151]

Scientists are continuing to seek complementary ways of predicting metastatic potential so that preventive therapies can be initiated earlier. Tests that can detect submicroscopic melanoma cells circulating in the blood vessels and lymphatics could prove invaluable, because melanoma generally metastasizes via these systems.

The reverse transcriptase polymerase chain reaction (RT-PCR) assay designed to detect genetic markers or indicators of potential metastatic melanoma in the blood has been seriously hampered by false-negative reports. A study in 2005 concluded that RT-PCR does not correlate with traditional indicators for prognosis of melanoma.[146,194]

Additional assays that make use of multiple melanoma markers are being investigated.[35,57] Adhesion markers have proved valuable[135] as well as microtubule-associated

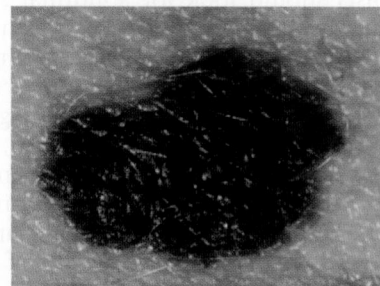

Figure 10-13

Malignant melanoma. Warning signs of malignant melanoma include asymmetry, irregular border, two or more shades of color, and diameter as outlined in Box 10-8. Any other changes in moles or skin lesions (e.g., itchiness, tenderness, swelling, redness, softening, or hardening) should be evaluated by a physician. (From Goldman L: *Cecil textbook of medicine*, ed 22, Philadelphia, 2004, Saunders.)

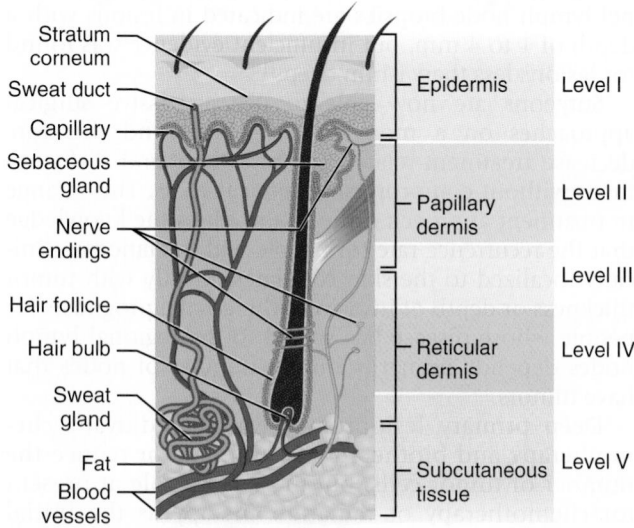

Figure 10-14

Clark levels, a system of classifying tumor progression according to skin layer penetration. Level I involves only the epidermis, level II has spread to the dermis, level III involves most of the upper dermis, level IV has spread to the lower dermis, and level V indicates that the cancer has spread to the subcutis. The higher the level, the greater the chance that metastasis has occurred.

protein 2 (MAP2), a marker of neuronal differentiation that induces mitotic defects, inhibits growth of melanoma cells, and predicts the metastatic potential of cutaneous melanoma.[50]

TREATMENT. Neither cryosurgery with liquid nitrogen nor electrodesiccation is used to treat melanoma, although they are among the acceptable procedures for squamous cell and basal cell tumors. The treatment of choice for melanoma without evidence of distant metastatic spread is surgical excision. Surgery is combined with postoperative adjuvant radiation therapy and/or chemotherapy when there is evidence of regional spread. Surgery is not usually recommended for tumors that have metastasized to distant sites.[123]

Previously, surgical excision of the primary lesion site may have been accompanied by removal of regional lymph nodes (regional lymphadenectomy), but sentinel node biopsy (see Chapter 9) has been shown to be a reliable diagnostic tool for selecting individuals to be submitted to lymph node dissection, thereby reducing the extent of surgery for those who do not need this procedure.[22,112,124]

There is considerable debate about the use of sentinel node biopsy in staging melanoma at this time. Some studies report that this type of biopsy is highly reliable in experienced hands but a low-yield procedure in most thin melanomas,[25,198] whereas others argue against its use except in clinical trials[184] and claim that there is not enough evidence to support the current combined use of sentinel node biopsy and systemic interferon (IFN) for melanoma.[133]

In 2005, a study indicated that children with high-risk melanoma could be treated with sentinel lymph node biopsy and IFN-alfa-2b with tolerable toxicity.[127] A more recent study found that seven biomarkers can be used as a prognostic tool to select appropriate therapy. Sentinel lymph node biopsies are indicated in lesions with a depth of 1 to 4 mm, but insufficient evidence was found for lesions less than 1 mm deep.[118]

Surgeons are now able to use aggressive surgical approaches on a more selective basis and therefore decrease treatment-related complications and disfigurement without compromising surgical goals. This change in treatment approach came as a result of the knowledge that the recurrence rate for people with melanoma clinically localized to the skin correlates directly with tumor thickness or depth of invasion, whereas the prognosis for people whose disease has spread to the regional lymph nodes depends primarily on the number of nodes that have tumors.[155]

Deep primary lesions may warrant adjuvant chemotherapy and biotherapy to eliminate or reduce the number of tumor cells, but there is no role at present for chemotherapy or radiation therapy as the initial treatment. Radiation therapy is used for metastatic disease to reduce tumor size and provide palliative relief from painful symptoms; it does not prolong survival time.

Ongoing research to develop immunomodulation therapy remains a large area of study. In addition to immunotherapy to stimulate the immune system, research to treat people with a vaccine made from their own cancer cells is under way.[86,108,185]

PROGNOSIS. Malignant melanoma is a more serious problem than other skin cancers because it can spread quickly and insidiously, becoming life-threatening at an earlier stage of development. However, it is essentially 100% curable if detected early.

The prognosis for all types of melanoma depends primarily on the tumor's thickness and depth of invasion, not on the histologic type. The more superficial or thin the tumor, the better the prognosis. For example, melanoma lesions less than 0.76 mm deep have an excellent prognosis (5-year survival rate is 90%), whereas deeper lesions (more than 0.76 mm) carry the risk for metastasis (5-year survival rate is 65% with local metastasis; 30%-35% when distant metastases are present). Metastases to the brain, lungs, bones, liver, and central nervous system are universally fatal, usually within 1 year.[199] Metastatic melanoma has a very poor prognosis with a median survival of less than 8 months and a 5-year survival rate of less than 5%.[186]

Prognosis is better for a tumor on an extremity that is drained by one lymphatic network than for one on the head, neck, or trunk drained by several lymphatic networks. Tumors can recur more than 5 years after primary surgery, requiring close long-term medical follow-up. Local recurrence without metastases may not represent a poor prognosis if the recurrence is simply an outgrowth of residual undetected microscopic cells from the previously excised primary tumor.[21] Education on the effects of UVB exposure can dramatically reduce the incidence and recurrence of skin cancer.

SPECIAL IMPLICATIONS FOR THE THERAPIST   10-9

Malignant Melanoma

During observation and inspection of any client, the therapist should be alert to the potential signs of skin cancer. Therapists should not become overly concerned about small pink spots on the client's skin, because other common skin conditions, such as eczema, psoriasis, and seborrheic dermatitis, are prevalent in more than half of all people at some time in their lives.

Therapists should look for abnormal spots, especially in sun-exposed areas, that are rough in texture, are persistently present, and bleed on minimal contact or with minimal friction. Keep in mind that seborrheic keratosis commonly bleeds; once diagnosed, this bleeding should not cause undue alarm.

As discussed in the text, *any* change in a wart or mole (color, size, shape, texture, ulceration, bleeding, itching) should be inspected by a physician. The Skin Cancer Foundation advocates the use of the ABCD method of early detection of melanoma and dysplastic (abnormal in size or shape) moles (Box 10-8).

Other signs and symptoms that may be important include irritation and itching; tenderness, soreness, or new moles developing around the mole in question; or a wound that does not progress toward healing within 6 weeks. For any client with a previous history

ABCDE METHOD OF EARLY MELANOMA DETECTION

A: Asymmetry: uneven edges, lopsided in shape, one half unlike the other

B: Border: irregularity, irregular edges scalloped or poorly defined edges

C: Color variability: black, shades of brown, red, white, pink, occasionally blue

D: Diameter: Larger than a pencil eraser (more than 6 mm)

E: Evolution or change; one mole looks different from all the others on an individual; mole changes, itches, or bleeds

SUNAWARE GUIDELINES FOR PREVENTION OF SKIN CANCER

Teach everyone to decrease their risk of skin cancer using the AWARE acronym:

A Avoid unprotected exposure to sunlight; avoid peak hours of sunlight (10 AM to 4 PM); seek shade; never use tanning devices

W Wear close-woven protective clothing, including long-sleeve shirts, pants, wide-brimmed hat and approved sun-protective (sun) glasses every day of the year

A Apply sunscreen of SPF 15 (if no risks and no previous problems) or 30 or greater (when there are risk factors or a previous history of skin cancer) 20 min before going outdoors to all exposed skin; reapply every two hours, especially if exposed to wind, water, or perspiration

R Routinely examine your skin and have a health care provider evaluate any skin changes

E Educate family and community children about these guidelines; protect babies from day 1 and begin education early with young children

NOTE: The AWARE acronym is based on the advice given by countless organizations, including the Skin Cancer Foundation, The World Health Organization, The American Academy of Dermatology, the Environmental Protection Agency, and The American Cancer Society.
Data from SunAWARE 2012, Nashville, Tennessee. For more information see http://www.sunaware.org/be-sunaware/avoid/.

of skin cancer, emphasize the need for continued close follow-up to detect recurrence early. Education on the effects of UV radiation and taking precautions (Box 10-9) can dramatically reduce the incidence of skin cancer.

If surgery included lymphadenectomy, the therapist may be involved in minimizing lymphedema or treating residual lymphedema (see "Lymphedema" in Chapter 13). Wound management may involve care of a skin graft and the associated donor site; the donor site may be as painful as the tumor excision site and just as much at risk for infection. Standard Precautions (see Appendix A) are essential for the postoperative as well as immunosuppressed client.

For the dying client, hospice care may include pain control and management. It is important that pain relief not be delayed until after pain occurs but rather that a schedule of analgesia to prevent pain or to prevent an increase in pain level is instituted. Wound management must include standard of care unless the client declines it.

Kaposi Sarcoma

Definition and Overview

Kaposi sarcoma (KS) is a malignancy of vascular tissue that presents as a skin disorder. In the past, this tumor was most commonly seen in older men of Mediterranean or Eastern European origin, especially men of Jewish or Italian ancestry (now referred to as *classic KS*).

The sudden emergence of this malignancy in the Western world was directly related to AIDS-associated immunodeficiency, and the incidence has risen dramatically along with the incidence of AIDS (*epidemic KS*). KS may also occur in kidney transplant recipients taking immunosuppressive drugs.[121]

Etiologic Factors and Incidence

Research in the mid-1990s confirmed that KS is caused by a herpesvirus infection. Among the people who develop AIDS, KS is seen almost exclusively among homosexual or bisexual men. If a person contracts AIDS as a result of IV drug use or from a transfusion, the chance of developing KS is less than 2%.

Rates are lower (10%) among HIV-infected women, people with hemophilia, and injection drug users. Overall incidence has been reduced among adults with AIDS associated with the use of antiretroviral therapy to control HIV replication and limit the associated immunodeficiency.[25,58]

Pathogenesis

KS is an angioproliferative tumor. It is suspected that endogenous substances produced by HIV-infected cells and/or a viral-induced tumorigenesis may promote angiogenesis and the growth of KS.[1,120,190]

Studies have demonstrated the role of vascular endothelial growth factor A (VEGF-A) and its receptors in the pathogenesis of KS.[6] VEGF-A is needed in the pathogenesis of KSHV, because of its ability to mediate angiogenesis.[3] In KS, VEGF was also increased in cells from lesions as a result of organ transplants and even more so in normal cells around the KS lesion.[173]

Clinical Manifestations

This neoplasm involves the skin and mucous membranes as well as other organs and can lead to tumor-associated edema and ulcerations. Classic KS occurs commonly on the lower extremities, and the affected areas are red, purple, or dark-blue macules (Fig. 10-15) that slowly enlarge to become nodules or ulcers. Itching and pain in the lesions that impinge on nerves or organs may occur; and as the sarcoma progresses, causing lymphatic obstruction, the legs become edematous. The lesions may spread by metastasis through the upper body to the face and oral mucosa.

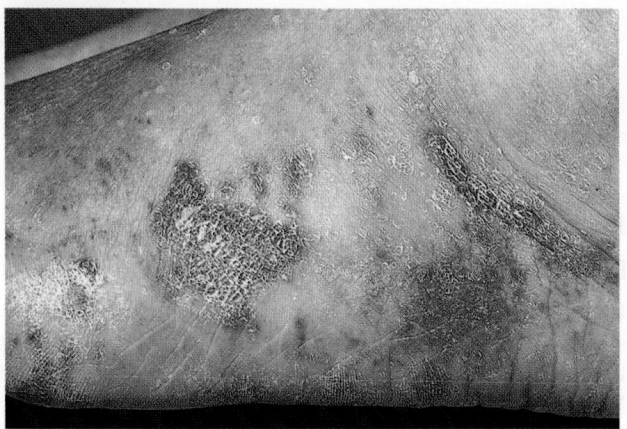

Figure 10-15

Classic Kaposi sarcoma is present as typical nodular lesions on this ankle and foot. (From Kumar V, Abbas AK, Fausto M: *Robbins and Cotran pathologic basis of disease*, ed 7, Philadelphia, 2005, Saunders.)

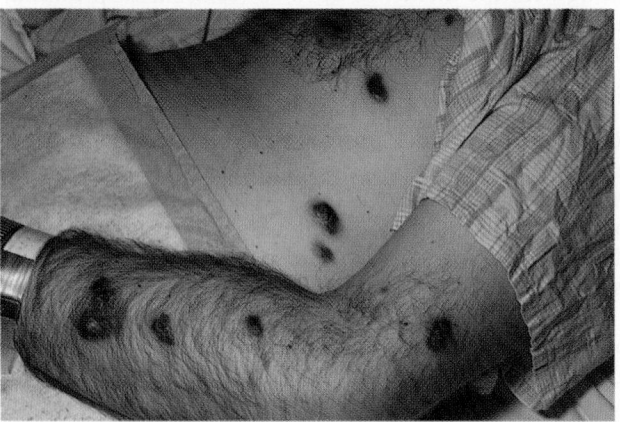

Figure 10-16

Epidemic Kaposi sarcoma in the plaque stage. Evolving lesions develop into raised papules or thickened plaques that are oval in shape and vary in color from red to brown. (From Swartz MH: *Textbook of physical diagnosis*, ed 6, Philadelphia, 2009, Saunders.)

Unlike classic forms of the disease, AIDS-associated KS is a multicentric entity that appears on the upper body (including face, chest, and neck) but can occur on the legs (Fig. 10-16; see also Fig. 7-18). Early lesions are faint pink and can easily be mistaken for bruises or nevi and be ignored.

MEDICAL MANAGEMENT

DIAGNOSIS, TREATMENT, AND PROGNOSIS. Diagnosis is by skin biopsy using a highly sensitive and specific test for this neoplasm. A CT scan may be performed to detect and evaluate possible metastasis. Dermatologic manifestations of KS can be alarming, but it is visceral involvement associated with AIDS KS that is most life-threatening.

However, new antiretroviral therapies, in particular the protease inhibitors, appear to be changing the clinical course of KS. It is now possible to see a complete resolution and control of KS with the use of these new agents. As researchers continue to unravel the pathogenesis of KS, new treatment modalities will target its pathogenic pathways.

Chemotherapy remains an integral part of treatment, and new agents are becoming available. Experimental therapies being evaluated in ongoing clinical trials include angiogenesis inhibitors, pregnancy hormone (human chorionic gonadotropin), photodynamic therapy, isotretinoin, antiviral medications ganciclovir and foscarnet, retinoic acid derivatives, and immune modulators, such as interleukin-12.[53,122,201] See discussion of AIDS in Chapter 7.

SPECIAL IMPLICATIONS FOR THE THERAPIST **10-10**

Kaposi Sarcoma

The KS skin lesions in the AIDS client are not contagious, and the health care provider need have no fear of transmission of KS or HIV through daily contact with the client. Standard Precautions must be followed whenever providing care for clients with KS to prevent the spread of infection to the client.

Prevention of skin breakdown and wound management is the usual focus of intervention. Clients receiving radiation therapy must keep the irradiated skin dry to avoid possible breakdown and subsequent infection (see the feature "Special Implications for the Therapist 5-6: Radiation" in Chapter 5).

A THERAPIST'S THOUGHTS*

One of the very few times a whirlpool is useful for wound care is the first time treating an individual with KS with multiple lesions all over the body. After that the wounds usually can be irrigated with PLWS (pulsed lavage with suction) or with Sal Jet™. Lower extremities should not be in a dependent position. Treatment in a traditional rehab setting should not include interventions that cause increased edema; the therapist must be cautious of fragile skin.

*Harriett B. Loehne, PT, DPT, CWS, FACCWS

SKIN DISORDERS ASSOCIATED WITH IMMUNE DYSFUNCTION

Psoriasis

Definition and Incidence

Psoriasis is a chronic, inherited, recurrent inflammatory but noninfectious dermatosis characterized by well-defined erythematous plaques covered with a silvery scale (Fig. 10-17). There are several types of psoriasis, including plaque, guttate, erythrodermic, and pustular psoriasis.

Psoriasis occurs equally in both genders and most commonly in young adults (mean age of onset is 27 years) but can occur at any point in a person's life and, once present, becomes a chronic condition that may go in and out of remission. Although psoriasis can occur in infancy, it is uncommon in children under the age of 6 years. It is uncommon among blacks but affects 1% to 2% of the white population; more than 6 million Americans are affected, with more than 100,000 classified as severe cases.

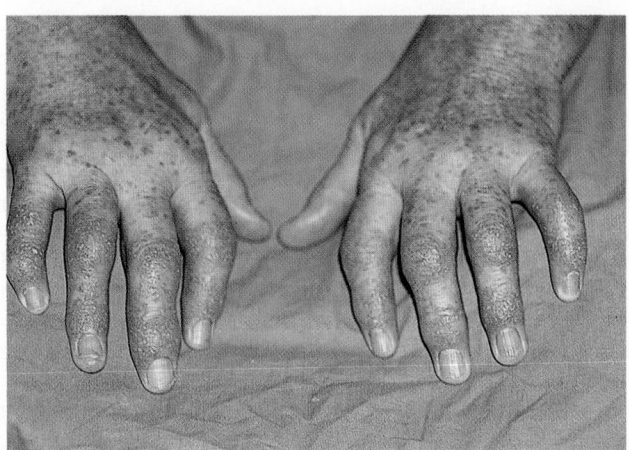

Figure 10-17

Deforming arthritis of the hands in a person with psoriasis (psoriatic arthritis). (From Callen JP, Greer K, Paller A, Swinyer L: *Color atlas of dermatology*, ed 2, Philadelphia, 2000, Saunders.)

Etiologic and Risk Factors

The cause of psoriasis is unknown, but it appears to be hereditary; that is, the tendency to develop psoriasis is genetically determined. Researchers have discovered a significantly higher than normal incidence of certain human leukocyte antigens (HLAs) in families with psoriasis, suggesting a possible immune disorder.

In the search for a psoriasis gene, researchers have discovered that, although there may be a primary "gatekeeper" gene, multiple genes seem to be involved. If one parent has psoriasis, a child has a 10% to 15% chance of developing the disease; if both parents have psoriasis, the chances increase to 50%.

Although psoriasis is thought to be genetically linked, it may be triggered by mechanical, UV, and chemical injury; various infections (especially by β-hemolytic streptococci); prescription drug use; psychologic stress; smoking; and pregnancy and other endocrine changes.[138]

Cold weather and severe anxiety or emotional stress tend to aggravate psoriasis. Flare-ups are often related to specific systemic and environmental factors but may be unpredictable. New epidemiologic studies present evidence that both smoking and drinking have an influence on psoriasis, suggesting that simple modifications in lifestyle may reduce both the prevalence and the severity of psoriasis.[76,144]

Pathogenesis

The underlying abnormality in psoriasis has not been definitively identified. It is a disorder of the keratinocytes, which form in the lower epidermis, flatten with age, and move toward the surface as new cells are generated below.

Normally, the life cycle of a skin cell is 26 to 28 days: 14 days to move from the basal layer to the stratum corneum and 14 days of normal wear and tear before the cell is sloughed off. In contrast, the turnover time of psoriatic skin is 3 to 4 days. This shortened cycle does not allow time for the cell to mature; thus cells stick and build up on the skin, resulting in a thick and flaky stratum corneum, which in turn produces the cardinal manifestations of psoriasis.

A second component in the pathogenesis of psoriasis is the immune system reaction, because T cells appear at the sites of heightened keratinocyte activity, much as they would at the site of an infection or tumor. The accelerated activity also triggers capillary growth supplying blood and nutrients to the tissue at that site.

It remains uncertain whether the accelerating keratinocyte turnover initiates the immune system reaction. One theory is that psoriasis is an autoimmune condition in which T-cell attack is provoked by a protein present in the skin, yet other animal studies suggest the pathogenesis begins in the T lymphocytes and initiates the disease process.[132]

Clinical Manifestations

Psoriasis appears as erythematous papules and plaques covered with silvery scales. The lesions in ordinary cases have a predilection for the scalp, chest, nails, elbows, knees, groin, skin folds, lower back, and buttocks. The occurrence may vary from a solitary lesion to countless patches covering large areas of the body in a symmetric pattern. Two clearly distinguishing features are the tendency for this condition to recur and to persist.

Lesions that develop at the site of a previous injury are known as the *Koebner phenomenon*. Flare-ups are more common in the winter as a result of dry skin and lack of sunlight, and, as is true for many skin ailments, the severity of psoriasis varies over time, and its exacerbations and remissions often correlate with stress levels and mental outlook.

The most common subjective complaint is itching and, occasionally, pain from dry, cracked, encrusted lesions. In approximately 30% of cases, psoriasis spreads to the fingernails, producing small indentations and yellow or brown discoloration. In severe cases, the accumulation of thick, crumbly debris under the nail causes it to separate from the nail bed (nail dystrophy).

Approximately 10% of people with psoriasis (usually moderate to severe) develop arthritic symptoms referred to as psoriatic arthritis (see Chapter 27). Psoriatic arthritis usually affects one or more joints of the fingers or toes, or sometimes the sacroiliac joints, and may progress to spondylitis. These clients report morning stiffness that lasts more than 30 minutes.

Joint symptoms show no consistent linkage to the course of the cutaneous manifestations of psoriasis but rather demonstrate remissions and exacerbations similar to those of rheumatoid arthritis. No other systemic effects of psoriasis have been reported, but hyperuricemia (gout) is fairly common in clients, precipitated by treatment with methotrexate and as a result of nucleic acid turnover caused by cellular breakdown in lesions of psoriasis.[200]

MEDICAL MANAGEMENT

DIAGNOSIS. Diagnosis depends on the previous history, clinical presentation, and, if needed, skin biopsy to identify psoriatic changes in skin or rule out other causes for the lesions.[52] Typically, the serum uric acid level is elevated because of accelerated nucleic acid degradation but without the corresponding gout usually associated with increased uric acid levels. Psoriasis must be distinguished from eczema, seborrheic dermatitis, and lichen-like papules.

TREATMENT. In the absence of a cure, the goal of treatment is to maximize remission and lessen outbreaks. Psoriasis therapy is highly individualized and often determined by trial and error because different people respond to different treatments. Psoriasis does not spread, and early treatment does not prevent the condition from progressing.

New options exist that adequately suppress the disease process and help provide better control of the psoriasis through the use of a combination of therapies. Various forms of local or systemic treatment routinely offered fall into five general categories: (1) topical preparations, (2) phototherapy, (3) antimetabolites, (4) oral retinoid therapy, and (5) immunosuppressants. Biologic systemic drugs for moderate to severe psoriasis are now available.[92]

Topical treatment of psoriasis is usually the first line of therapy, and therapeutic agents include corticosteroids; synthetic vitamin D_3; vitamin A analogues (retinoids); occlusive ointments (e.g., petroleum jelly, salicylic acid preparations, urea-containing topical ointments); oatmeal baths and emollients to relieve pruritus; and occasionally tar preparations.

Corticosteroids are the most commonly prescribed therapy for psoriasis but should be used sparingly because of the incidence of side effects, which have increased with the use of the superpotent fluorinated preparations. Only weak preparations, such as 0.5% or 1.0% hydrocortisone, should be used on the face, perineum, or other sensitive areas (e.g., the flexor surfaces of the arms, abdomen).

The major concerns with all corticosteroid preparations are dermal atrophy, skin fragility, fast relapse times, and, in rare cases, adrenal suppression resulting from systemic absorption. See also "Corticosteroids" in Chapter 5.

Crude coal tar, one of the oldest remedies for psoriasis, is assumed to work by an antimitotic effect (helps retard rapid cell production). This treatment consists of the daily application of 2% to 5% crude coal tar combined with a tar bath and UV light. The disadvantages of this treatment are the extended time commitments required by the client and the associated mess. Products (e.g., gels, creams, bath additives) with liquor carbonis detergens, an extract of crude coal, are also used to facilitate healing.

Exposure to UV light (phototherapy), such as UVB or natural sunlight, also helps retard rapid cell production. Widespread involvement may improve with whole-body irradiation with UV light. *PUVA* refers to the combination of an orally administered photosensitizing drug plus exposure to 1 to 1½ hours of UVA radiation. It is more effective for the thick plaque type of psoriasis, pustular psoriasis, and generalized erythroderma.

PUVA also has its disadvantages as a treatment option, including premature skin aging, increased risk of nonmelanoma skin and other cancers, and premature cataract formation. This type of therapy is contraindicated in pregnancy and for anyone with abnormal moles or otherwise at risk for skin cancer.

Methotrexate, originally an anticancer drug, affects DNA synthesis and inhibits reproduction in rapidly growing cells, such as the prolific keratinocytes in psoriasis. Methotrexate also has an immunosuppressant effect, tempering the inflammatory response. Cyclosporine (Neoral), an immunosuppressant most often used to prevent organ transplant rejection, has also been approved as a psoriasis treatment. These pharmaceuticals have potentially serious side effects and must be monitored closely.

A treatment strategy called *sequential therapy* involving a deliberate sequence to optimize therapeutic outcome is being explored for those who require systemic therapy without methotrexate. The rationale for this strategy in psoriasis is that it is a chronic disease requiring long-term maintenance therapy as well as quick relief of symptoms and that some medical interventions are better suited for rapid clearance whereas others are more appropriate for long-term care. In sequential therapy, an acute exacerbation of psoriasis is brought under control promptly with the use of cyclosporine followed by phototherapy and then acitretin is administered in a maintenance phase.[90,91]

To minimize side effects and maximize efficacy of rapidly clearing lesions and maintaining remission, topical sequential therapy is widely used. A class I corticosteroid and calcipotriene are applied in three different phases—the clearance, transition, and maintenance phases.[93]

PROGNOSIS. Psoriasis usually recurs at intervals and lasts for increasingly longer periods, but treatment advances bring relief during flare-ups in approximately 85% to 90% of cases. Spontaneous cure is uncommon, and the risk of infection is high because of the greater than normal amounts of staphylococci present on psoriatic plaques.

People with psoriasis who are HIV positive are at high risk of infection from self-inoculation. As many as 20% of clients who develop psoriatic arthritis may sustain early and severe joint damage with accompanying deformity and disability.

Finally, psoriasis treatment involving PUVA has been shown to contribute to an increased risk of skin cancer decades after the treatment has stopped.[174] Research shows that it may be possible to reduce the risk of skin cancer from PUVA with meditation and stress reduction techniques (e.g., biofeedback, yoga, self-help approaches) that reduced healing time to half, thus reducing UV exposure.[12]

SPECIAL IMPLICATIONS FOR THE THERAPIST   10-11

Psoriasis

Physical therapy and occupational therapy are key components in the treatment of moderate to severe psoriasis, with desired outcomes based on minimizing functional limitations. Consensus guidelines for the management of psoriasis including phototherapy protocols are available.[79,97]

Client instruction and direct intervention to provide skin care should emphasize the following: (1) steroid cream application must be in a thin film, gently rubbed into the skin until all the cream disappears; (2) all topical medications, especially those containing anthralin and tar, should be applied with a downward motion to avoid rubbing them into the hair follicles causing inflammation (folliculitis); (3) medication should be applied only to the affected lesions, avoiding contact with normal surrounding skin; and (4) gloves must be worn when applying the cream because anthralin stains and injures the skin.

After application, the client must dust himself or herself with powder to prevent anthralin from rubbing off on the clothes. Mineral oil followed by soap and water can be used to remove the anthralin; the skin should never be rubbed vigorously, but a soft brush can be used to remove the scales.

Any side effects, especially allergic reactions to anthralin, atrophy and acne from steroids, and burning, itching, and nausea, must be reported to the physician immediately. Squamous cell epithelioma may develop from PUVA. Cytotoxins from methotrexate therapy may cause hepatic or bone marrow toxicity; methotrexate may be teratogenic (harmful to fetal development) and should not be prescribed for women who are pregnant, trying to become pregnant, or breast feeding.

Other immunosuppressants, when used over a long period, have an accumulative effect and therefore the potential to cause serious side effects, such as poor wound healing, high blood pressure, kidney damage, and many other complications (see "Immunosuppressants" in Chapter 5).

Relaxation techniques and stress management are valuable tools whose use should be encouraged on a daily basis but especially during periods of exacerbation.

Psoriatic Arthritis

Clinically, psoriatic arthritis differs from rheumatoid arthritis in the more frequent involvement of the distal interphalangeal joints, asymmetric distribution of affected joints, presence of spondyloarthropathy (including the presence of both sacroiliitis and spondylitis), and characteristic extraarticular features (e.g., psoriatic skin lesions, iritis, mouth ulcers, urethritis, colitis, aortic valve disease).

Joints are less tender in psoriatic arthritis, which may lead to underestimation of the degree of inflammation. Pain and stiffness of inflamed joints are usually increased by prolonged immobility and alleviated by physical activity. Evidence of inflammation is pain on stressing the joint, tenderness at the joint line, and the presence of effusions.

The increasing use of nuclear magnetic resonance imaging (MRI) techniques, with their ability to delineate cartilage and ligamentous structures and to identify edema, is providing a radical improvement in ascertainment of musculoskeletal abnormalities associated with this disease. It is expected that in the decade to come new information about this aspect of the disease will offer greater information and improved treatment regimens.[197]

Psychologic Considerations

Psoriasis can result in psychologic problems because the skin lesions may cause the person to feel contagious and untouchable. In addition, ongoing treatment may not work, and the smell of some topical preparations and the stain may add to the psychologic reaction. Assure the client that psoriasis is not contagious. Flare-ups can be controlled with treatment, and stress control can help prevent recurrences. Relaxation techniques, group counseling, stress management, and medications to treat depression or anxiety may be suggested.

Lupus Erythematosus

Lupus erythematosus is a chronic inflammatory disorder of the connective tissues. It appears in several forms, including cutaneous lupus erythematosus primarily affecting the skin and systemic lupus erythematosus (SLE), which affects multiple organ systems (including the skin) with considerably more morbidity and associated mortality (see complete discussion in Chapter 7). *Lupus* is the Latin word for "wolf," referring to the belief in the 1800s that the skin erosion of this disease was caused by a wolf bite. The characteristic rash of lupus is red, hence the term *erythematosus*.

Cutaneous Lupus Erythematosus

Overview and Incidence. The subsets of lupus erythematosus (LE) involving the skin include chronic cutaneous LE, acute cutaneous LE, and subacute cutaneous LE. Only the skin-related components of LE are discussed in this chapter. See also "Systemic Lupus Erythematosus" in Chapter 7.

Chronic cutaneous LE, formerly known as discoid lupus, is marked by chronic skin eruptions on sun-exposed skin that can lead to scarring and permanent disfigurement if left untreated. Usually a systemic disorder does not develop, but in 5% to 10% of cases SLE does develop later; conversely, discoid lesions occur in 20% of people with SLE.[160] It is estimated that approximately 60% of persons with chronic cutaneous LE are women in their late 20s or older. The disease is rare in children.

Acute cutaneous LE occurs in 30% to 50% of clients who have SLE and includes malar erythema, widespread erythema, and bullous lesions. Association with systemic disease is highest in acute cutaneous LE, with virtually all clients meeting the American College of Rheumatology criteria for SLE (see Chapter 7).

Etiologic and Risk Factors and Pathogenesis. The exact cause of cutaneous LE is unknown, but evidence suggests an autoimmune defect. There appear to be interrelated immunologic, environmental, hormonal, and genetic factors involved. Smoking is considered a risk factor for the development of the discoid lesions associated with chronic cutaneous LE and for

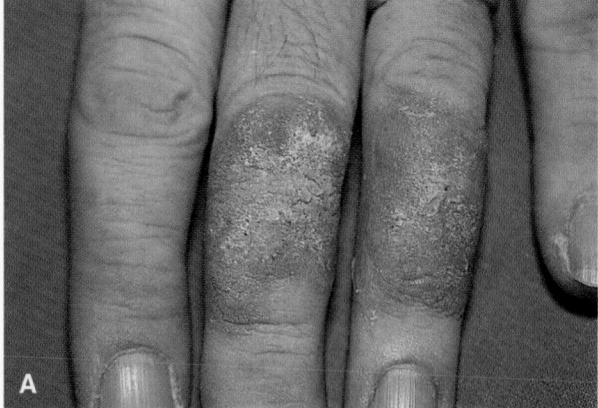

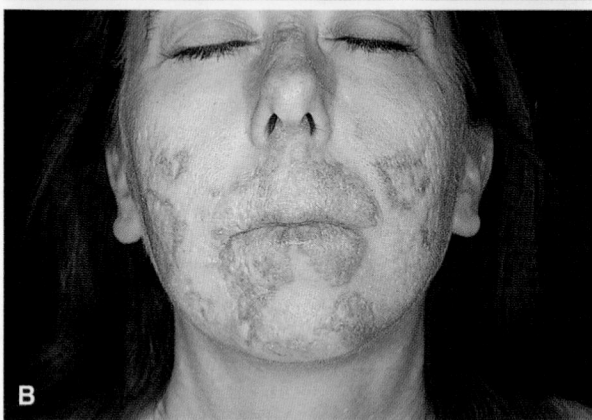

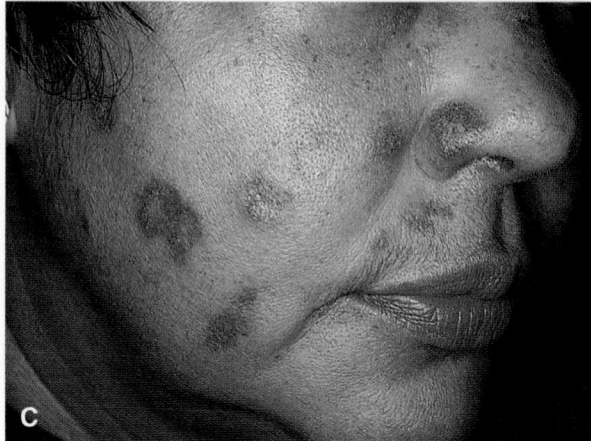

Figure 10-18

Discoid lupus erythematosus. Skin changes associated with *discoid* lupus erythematosus can present in a variety of ways. **A,** Hypertrophic discoid lupus erythematosus with prominent adherent scale. **B,** Round or oval cutaneous lesions can occur on the face or other parts of the body. **C,** Round or oval cutaneous lesions as they appear on a dark-skinned individual. (From Callen JP, Greer K, Paller A, Swinyer L: *Color atlas of dermatology,* ed 2, Philadelphia, 2000, Saunders.)

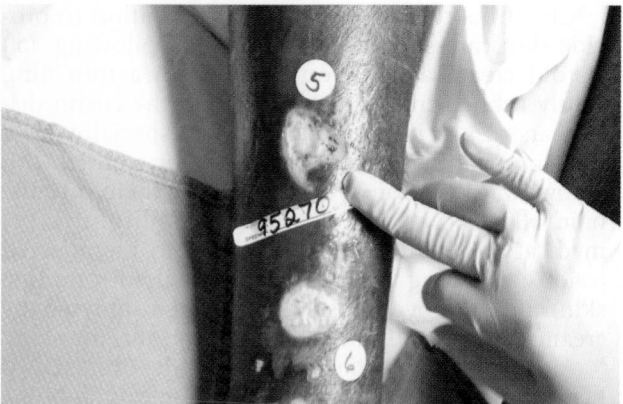

Figure 10-19

The lesions here are typical of *systemic* **lupus found on the lower extremities.** They are ulcerated, punched-out wounds with necrotic bases. *Discoid* lupus lesions (Fig. 10-20) are usually found on the face and scalp, and are raised, flat, coin-shaped wounds. (Courtesy Harriett B. Loehne, PT, DPT, CWS, FACCWS, Archbold Center for Wound Management& Hyperbaric Medicine, Thomasville, GA. Used with permission.)

thus more deposition of immune complexes in the skin at the dermal–epidermal junction. The photosensitivity is most commonly associated with LE and not other rheumatologic diseases.

Clinical Manifestations. Discoid lesions (*chronic cutaneous LE*) can develop from the rash typically seen in lupus and become raised, red, smooth plaques with follicular plugging and central atrophy. The raised edges and sunken centers give them a coin-like appearance (Fig. 10-18). Although these lesions can appear anywhere on the body, they usually erupt on the face, scalp, ears, neck, and arms or any part of the body that is exposed to sunlight. Lesions more typical of systemic lupus discussed in Chapter 7 are shown in Figure 10-19.

Hair tends to become brittle, and scalp lesions can cause localized alopecia (bald patches). Facial plaques sometimes assume the classic butterfly pattern with lesions appearing on the cheeks and the bridge of the nose. The rash may vary in severity from a sunburned appearance to discoid (plaque-like) lesions. These lesions can occur in the absence of other lupus-related symptoms and tend to leave hypopigmented and hyperpigmented scars that can become a cosmetic concern.

The most recognized skin manifestation of SLE (*acute cutaneous LE*) is the classic butterfly rash over the nose, cheeks, and forehead (see Fig. 7-25) commonly precipitated by exposure to sunlight (UV rays). This classic rash over the nose and cheeks occurs in a large percentage of affected people, but rash can occur on the scalp, neck, upper chest, shoulders, extensor surface of the arms, and dorsum of the hands. These rashes begin abruptly and last from hours to days. They may be precipitated by sun exposure and often coincide with a flare of systemic disease.[160]

Other skin manifestations may point to the presence of vasculitis (inflammation of cutaneous blood vessels)

resistance to treatment with antimalarial agents in this subgroup.[49,80]

Just how the sun causes skin rash flare-ups remains unknown. One theory is that the DNA of people with lupus, when exposed to sunlight, becomes more antigenic (able to induce a specific immune response). This antigenicity causes accelerated antigen–antibody reactions and leading to infarctive lesions in the digits (see Fig. 27-14), necrotic leg ulcers, or digital gangrene.

Acute cutaneous LE is usually accompanied by other symptoms of SLE, commonly including malaise, overwhelming fatigue, arthralgia, fever, arthritis, anemia, hair loss, Raynaud phenomenon, and urologic symptoms associated with kidney involvement.

MEDICAL MANAGEMENT

DIAGNOSIS AND TREATMENT. The client history and appearance of the rash itself are diagnostic. Skin biopsy of the discoid lesions may be performed. The client must report any changes in the lesions to the attending physician. Drug treatment consists of topical, intralesional, or systemic medication.

Potential side effects of systemic therapy (antimalarial agents) for chronic cutaneous LE include diarrhea, nausea, myopathy, cardiomyopathy, and anemia. The lesions resolve spontaneously in 20% to 40% of affected individuals or may cause hypopigmentation or hyperpigmentation, atrophy, and scarring. Discoid lesions are not life-threatening (unless accompanied by complications of SLE) but are associated with psychologic distress and altered quality of life.

Skin lesions require topical treatment, maintaining an optimal wound environment (moist enough to allow tissue healing but not swamp-like) while preventing further deterioration or infection. Most often, topical corticosteroid creams are used. The disease process can cause loss of skin integrity and subsequent loss of function.

Clients with any form of cutaneous lupus should avoid prolonged exposure to the sun, fluorescent lighting, or reflected sunlight. They are encouraged to wear protective clothing, use sun-screening agents, and avoid engaging in outdoor activities during periods of intense sunlight (see Box 10-4).

Prognosis

The survival rate has improved dramatically in recent years, although death can occur from renal failure when there is kidney involvement causing progressive changes in the glomeruli; cardiac involvement with deposition of immune complexes in the coronary vessels, myocardium, and pericardium; or cerebral infarct.

| SPECIAL IMPLICATIONS FOR THE THERAPIST | 10-12 |

Cutaneous Lupus Erythematosus

Clients with lupus erythema with skin involvement require careful assessment, supportive measures, and emotional support. Skin lesions should be checked thoroughly at each visit. The client should be urged to get plenty of rest, follow energy conservation guidelines, and practice good nutrition.

The therapist can be instrumental in teaching and assisting with skin care and prevention of skin breakdown, range-of-motion (ROM) exercises, prevention of orthopedic deformities, ergonomic and postural training, and relief of joint pain associated with SLE. Persons with LE exposed to the long-term effects of corticosteroids should be followed carefully. See specific side effects in the feature "Special Implications for the Therapist 5-5: Corticosteroids" in Chapter 5. See also the feature on SLE in Chapter 7: "Special Implications for the Therapist 7-6: Systemic Lupus Erythematosus."

Systemic Sclerosis

Definition and Overview

Systemic sclerosis (SSc, progressive systemic sclerosis, scleroderma) is a diffuse connective tissue disease that causes fibrosis of the skin, joints, blood vessels, and internal organs from deposition of excessive amounts of collagen. SSc is a chronic disease, lasting for months, years, or a lifetime, and is classified according to the degree and extent of skin thickening.

The presence of a distinctive, widespread vascular lesion characterized by endothelial abnormalities as well as by proliferative reaction of the vascular intima was a significant factor in changing terminology from *scleroderma* to *systemic sclerosis*. General clinical vernacular still refers to this condition as *scleroderma*, although that term simply refers to thickening or hardening of the skin.

There are two distinct subtypes: systemic scleroderma and localized scleroderma. *Systemic scleroderma* can take one of three forms: limited (lSSc), diffuse (dSSc), and an overlap form with either diffuse or limited skin thickening.

Limited cutaneous SSc was previously known as the *CREST syndrome* from its manifestations (*c*alcinosis, *R*aynaud phenomenon, *e*sophageal dysmotility, *s*clerodactyly, *t*elangiectasia). Persons with this form of SSc have a much lower incidence of serious internal organ involvement, although pulmonary hypertension and esophageal disease are not uncommon. Skin tightness is limited to the hands and face (excluding the trunk).

Although the diffuse form is less common than the limited form, it is by far the more debilitating because of the more frequent renal and pulmonary involvement. Some measurable degree of heart, lung, or kidney involvement, or any combination of these, can be found in the majority of people with SSc.

Diffuse scleroderma is characterized by involvement of all body parts, including the skin. In most people, this involvement tends to progress slowly, if at all, but if involvement is to become severe, it tends to do so early, within the first 5 years. The severity of the disease depends on the number of organs affected and the extent of the effect.

Localized scleroderma affects primarily the skin in one or many different areas without visceral organ involvement and is therefore a benign form of this disease. Localized scleroderma should not be confused with limited cutaneous scleroderma. The latter is a form of systemic rather than localized disease.

There is further differentiation of localized scleroderma: *morphea* is characterized by hard, oval-shaped patches on the skin, generally on the trunk. These patches are usually white with a purple ring around them. *Linear* refers to the band-like lesions that occur in the areas of the arms, legs, and forehead. The bones and muscles beneath these areas may also be affected. Ultimately, range of motion (ROM) and a child's growth are greatly affected. Linear scleroderma often occurs in childhood.

Other forms include *chemically induced localized scleroderma*, *eosinophilic myalgia syndrome* (previously associated with ingestion of L-tryptophan), toxic oil syndrome (associated with ingestion of contaminated rapeseed oil), and *graft-versus-host disease*.

Incidence

The annual incidence of SSc based on epidemiologic studies of hospital records and death certificates is 20 cases per 1 million, affecting approximately 400,000 Americans. Until the 1980s, SSc was considered a rare (1 per 2000 individuals) disease, but studies at that time reported a prevalence as much as five times greater than the highest prevalence rate previously reported. Some evidence suggests continued rising incidence rates among adults as well as children, but whether this reflects worldwide incidence or merely regional differences remains unknown.[19,41]

SSc affects women two to three times more often than men, with the female/male ratio peaking at 15 : 1 during the childbearing years. However, the rate of mortality is higher in men (and in African Americans) than in others. Preliminary studies show that fetal cells persist in maternal blood for as long as 27 years postpartum even if the pregnancy does not go to full term. This phenomenon, referred to as *fetomaternal cell trafficking*, may provide an explanation for the increased prevalence of autoimmune disorders such as SSc in adult women following childbearing.[16]

Etiologic and Risk Factors

The cause of scleroderma is reportedly unknown. However, several groups suggest that scientific evidence accumulated over the last 50 years strongly points to SSc as an acquired disease triggered by bacteria (mycoplasma).[24,100] It has also been suggested that an autoimmune mechanism is the underlying cause, because specific autoantibodies occur in the sera of these clients. Other possible triggers suggested include cytomegalovirus (CMV; increased levels of anti-CMV antibodies present in scleroderma) or immune reactions to viral or environmental factors.[83]

The potential role of placental transfer of fetal cells in the pathogenesis of autoimmune diseases has been mentioned (see Incidence). In childbearing women with scleroderma, fetal cell–derived DNA is detected more frequently in the peripheral blood than in controls. This finding of a limited number of fetal cells in maternal tissues leading to microchimerism (see explanation of chimerism in Chapter 21) has been proposed to have a role in the induction of scleroderma.[179]

The occasional onset after trauma suggests the possibility of trophoneurosis (a trophic disorder consequent to disease or injury to nerves). The onset of scleroderma immediately following a severe emotional

shock is in some cases a manifestation and result of a psychosomatic disturbance that causes vascular spasm.

Chemicals, especially from occupational exposure to silica, vinyl chloride, or various organic solvents (whether through direct contact or by inhalation), may also induce scleroderma-like changes. Exposure to organic solvents such as benzene and trichloroethane, chemicals common in paint thinners, stains, epoxy resins, and degreasers, associated with recreational hobby or occupation causes the body to produce an antibody called *Scl-70* associated with scleroderma-like illnesses.[129,130] The toxic oil syndrome and eosinophilia-myalgia syndrome are best-known examples of chemically induced localized forms of scleroderma.[32]

Pathogenesis

Widespread small-vessel vasculopathy and fibrosis set SSc apart from other connective tissue diseases. The relentless deposition of extracellular matrix (collagen) produced by activated fibroblasts and myofibroblasts in the intima of blood vessels, the pericapillary space, and the interstitium of the skin is distinctive for SSc and distinguishes it from other autoimmune disorders.

Microvascular damage provokes immune cells to produce autoantibodies, pro-inflammatory and pro-fibrotic cytokines and chemokines.[8] Endothelial injury, obliterative microvascular lesions, and increased vascular wall thickness preferentially affecting small arteries, arterioles, and capillaries are present in all involved organs. Autonomic nerve dysfunction (parasympathetic impairment and marked sympathetic overactivity) seems to be linked to the development of microvascular, cardiac, and GI alterations.[55]

The vascular pathologic condition is characterized by altered vascular function with increased vasospasm, reduced vasodilatory capacity, and increased adhesiveness of the blood vessels to platelets and lymphocytes. The connection between the vascular pathologic condition and development of tissue fibrosis remains unknown, but it is hypothesized that SSc modifies the activity of both the endothelium and the peripheral nervous system, eventually leading to the clinical manifestations of this condition.[56] The extent of injury and dysfunction is reflected by changes in the circulating levels of vascular markers.[83]

Clinical Manifestations

The three stages in the clinical development of scleroderma are the *edematous stage*, the *sclerotic stage*, and the *atrophic stage*. In the edematous stage, bilateral nonpitting edema is present in the fingers and hands and, rarely, in the feet. The edema can progress to the forearms, arms, upper chest, abdomen, back, and face. After a few weeks to several months, edema is replaced by thick, hard skin. Peripheral nervous system involvement affects nerve terminals, reducing sensory fibers in SSc skin. Neuropeptides released by sensory nerve endings are reduced, resulting in vasoconstriction in the skin.

Integument. The replacement of edema takes place in the sclerotic stage, when the skin becomes tight, smooth, and waxy or shiny and seems bound down to underlying structures. Accompanying changes include a loss of normal

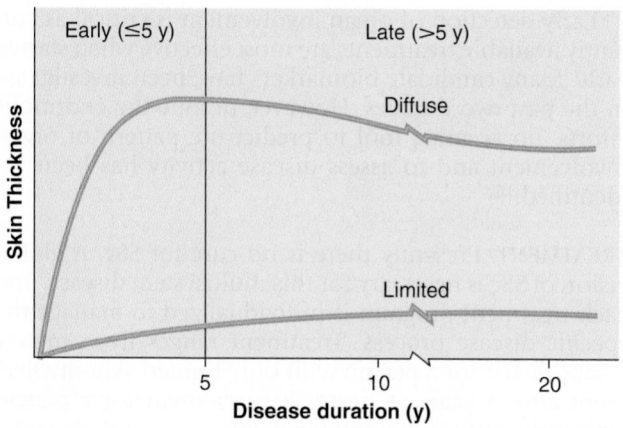

Figure 10-20

The progression of skin thickening in systemic sclerosis is greatest in the early period (first 5 years), especially in those with diffuse disease. (Modified from Clements PJ: Systemic sclerosis: natural history and management strategies. *J Musculoskelet Med* 11[11]:43-50, 1994.)

skin folds, decreased flexibility, and skin hyperpigmentation and hypopigmentation. Facial skin may also become tight and inelastic, and the face takes on a stretched and mask-like appearance, with thin lips and a pinched nose.

The skin changes may stabilize for periods (years) and may then either progress to the third stage or soften and return to normal. Actual atrophy of skin may occur, particularly over joints at sites of flexion contractures, such as the proximal interphalangeal joints and the elbows. Flexion contractures are especially severe in people with dSSc (Fig. 10-20).

Thinning of the skin contributes to the development of ulcerations at the sites of joint contractures. Softening and return to normal of the skin may occur to some extent. Improvement typically begins centrally, so that the last areas to become classically involved are the first to show regression.

Not all people pass through all the stages. Individuals with SSc who develop diffuse cutaneous thickening usually do so within 1 to 4 years after disease onset. If a person with lSSc does not develop skin thickening and progress into diffuse SSc within the first 3 to 4 years, it is not likely to happen later. The difference is important because the mortality rate is higher for individuals with diffuse SSc because of the involvement of the heart, lungs, and kidneys.[89] Subcutaneous calcification (calcinosis) is a late-developing complication that is considerably more frequent in lSSc. Sites of trauma are often affected, such as the fingers, forearms, elbows, and knees. These calcifications vary in size from tiny deposits to large masses ulcerating the overlying skin.

Raynaud Phenomenon. Scleroderma affects everyone in a different fashion. Each previously mentioned form affects the body in different ways (Box 10-10). Raynaud phenomenon is very often the first manifestation of SSc, preceding the onset of all the other signs and symptoms of the disease by months or years.[56] It appears almost universally in lSSc and in approximately 75% of cases of dSSc.

Raynaud phenomenon is characterized by sudden blanching, cyanosis, and erythema of the fingers and toes as the walls of the blood vessels that supply the hands and

---

Box 10-10

CHARACTERISTICS LIKELY TO BE SEEN IN CLIENTS WITH SYSTEMIC SCLEROSIS EARLY AND LATE IN THE DISEASE COURSE

EARLY (≤5 years)
Limited Disease

- Rapidly progressive
  - Renal crisis (5%)
  - Interstitial lung disease (severe in 10%-15%)
- Slowly progressive
  - Raynaud phenomenon
  - Cutaneous ulceration
  - Esophageal dysmotility

Diffuse Disease

- Rapidly progressive
  - Skin thickening
  - Heart involvement (severe in 10%-15%)
  - Interstitial lung disease (severe in 15%)
  - Renal crisis (15%-20%)
  - Contractures, joint pain
  - Cutaneous ulcerations
  - Esophageal dysmotility
  - Gastrointestinal complications

LATE (>5 years)
Limited Disease

- Slowly progressive
  - Raynaud phenomenon
  - Cutaneous ulcerations
  - Esophageal dysmotility
  - Gastrointestinal complications
- Very late
  - Pulmonary artery hypertension
  - Biliary cirrhosis

Diffuse Disease

- Improvement
  - Skin thickening
  - Musculoskeletal pain
- Slowly progressive
  - Heart, lung, kidney involvement
  - Raynaud phenomenon
  - Esophageal dysmotility
  - Gastrointestinal complications

Modified from Clements PJ: Systemic sclerosis: natural history and management strategies. *J Musculoskelet Med* 11(11):43-50, 1994.

---

feet become narrowed, making it difficult for the blood to pass through. Closure of the muscular digital arteries, precapillary arterioles, and arteriovenous shunts of the skin causes the hands or feet to become white and numb and then bluish in color as blood flow remains blocked.

As the spasm eases and blood flow returns (approximately 10 to 15 minutes after the triggering stimulus has ended), rewarming occurs and the fingers or toes become red and painful. This cycle is initiated in response to stress or exposure to cold. Progressive phalangeal resorption may shorten the fingers, and compromised circulation resulting from abnormal thickening of the arterial intima may cause slowly healing ulcerations on the tips of the fingers or toes that may lead to gangrene.[196]

Neuromusculoskeletal System. Most persons with dSSc have disuse atrophy of muscle because of limited joint motion secondary to skin, joint, or tendon involvement. A small percentage of people may have overlap syndromes and demonstrate marked weakness and inflammatory myopathy indistinguishable from polymyositis or dermatomyositis.

Some individuals develop myositis or erosive arthropathy that complicates the joint retraction induced by skin fibrosis. SSc also targets the peripheral nervous system with distal mononeuropathy of the median nerve as a frequent and early feature.[55] Neuropathy from carpal tunnel syndrome is also common.

Polyarthralgias and polyarthritis affect both small and large joints and are especially frequent early in dSSc associated with 30 or more minutes of morning stiffness. Tenosynovial involvement with inflammation and fibrosis of the tendon sheath or adjacent tissues is characterized by the presence of carpal tunnel syndrome and by coarse, leathery friction rubs palpated during motion over the extensor and flexor tendons of the fingers, distal forearms, knees, ankles, and other sites. These friction rubs are found almost exclusively in persons with dSSc, and their presence signifies a poorer overall clinical outcome.[196]

Viscera. GI motility dysfunction affects the esophagus and anorectal regions, causing frequent reflux, heartburn, dysphagia, and bloating after meals. Other effects include abdominal distention, diarrhea, constipation, and malodorous, floating stools. In advanced disease, cardiac and pulmonary fibrosis develops.

Cardiac involvement can be manifested as myocardial disease, pericardial disease, conduction system disease, or arrhythmias. Pulmonary involvement is characterized by pulmonary arterial hypertension and pulmonary vascular disease with a decline in forced vital capacity (FVC) and impaired diffusing capacity for carbon monoxide.[33] Kidney involvement and scleroderma renal crisis are now considered rare because of the introduction of angiotensin-converting enzyme (ACE) inhibitors.[55]

Other. Nearly 50% of adults with scleroderma report other symptoms, such as major depression, sexual dysfunction, trigeminal neuralgia, hypothyroidism, dental involvement, and corneal tears.

MEDICAL MANAGEMENT

DIAGNOSIS. Early diagnosis and accurate staging of visceral involvement are fundamental for appropriate management and therapeutic approach to this disease. However, diagnosis can be delayed because there is no single laboratory test diagnostic for SSc. A thorough physical examination and history are the first steps to a definitive diagnosis.

Laboratory tests (skin biopsy, urinalysis, blood studies, including erythrocyte sedimentation rate, presence of rheumatoid factor [results found to be positive in 30% of SSc cases], presence of antinuclear antibodies) are used to determine the extent of involvement and rule out other disease processes. Distinctive serum autoantibodies are found in more than 90% of cases.[117] Other tests may include chest films and pulmonary function studies, GI series, and electroencephalogram (EEG).

Early detection of organ involvement is critical as currently available treatments are most effective when started early. Many candidate biomarkers have been investigated in the past two decades. However, despite the enormous efforts, no accurate tool to predict the pattern of organ involvement and to assess disease activity has been yet identified.[163]

TREATMENT. Presently there is no cure for SSc. A global vision of SSc is necessary for this multisystem disease, and each treatment program is individualized to manage the specific disease process. Treatment ranges from merely symptomatic for a person with only limited skin involvement after 5 years to aggressive treatment for a person with early, diffuse skin involvement.

When organ involvement occurs, it most often develops early in the disease course, and in the acute phase it requires aggressive management. The program may include medications (e.g., immunosuppressants, penicillamine, antiinflammatory drugs), exercises, joint protection techniques, skin protection techniques, and stress management. See also "Raynaud Phenomenon" in Chapter 12.

Penicillamine, a disease-modifying drug, is a penicillin derivative immunomodulating agent that has been shown to improve the skin by interfering with crosslinking of collagen and to prolong survival in people with early, rapidly progressive SSc. Oral tetracyclines have been found to be the most effective and have the fewest side effects, with minocycline or doxycycline being the antibiotic of choice. Brand-name drugs (Minocin, Vibramycin) are preferred because some generics are ineffective.[188]

Better understanding of SSc pathogenesis has resulted in the development of drugs, such as prostanoids, endothelin-1, and phosphodiesterase inhibitors, for treatment of pulmonary arterial hypertension and digital ulcers. The use of targeted therapies and antifibrotic agents to modify disease is under investigation.[205] Stem cell transplantation seems to be promising in restarting the immune system to diminish fibrosis and restore microvasculature. Future research will be directed at genetic factors, diagnostic and prognostic markers for fibrosis and microangiopathy, and development of drugs directed to pathogenic key cells and mediators.[8]

PROGNOSIS. Short-term prognosis has improved with advances in pharmacologic intervention but the long-term prognosis in SSc is generally poor with significant morbidity and mortality, especially when there is pulmonary and renal involvement.[29,163,164] Prognosis principally depends on early diagnosis and treatment; the intensity and rapidity of involvement of the lungs, heart, gut, and kidneys; and appropriate medical management. A model to predict mortality based on a combination of three factors (proteinuria, elevated erythrocyte sedimentation rate, low carbon monoxide diffusing capacity) has been reported to have an accuracy of more than 80% in predicting mortality. The absence of these three factors is associated with 93% 1-year survival.[29,164]

Spontaneous recovery is common in children, but approximately 30% of clients with SSc die within 5 years of onset. Persons with dSSc who have lived beyond the 5-year mark with no significant visceral involvement are unlikely to experience such organ involvement. Those in whom significant visceral disease developed early can expect a slowing in its progression or at least a stabilization of its course. This 5-year mark is also a time when skin softening begins and musculoskeletal aches and pains begin to ease.

Treatment with ACE inhibitors, started early, now prevents previously fatal complications (acute hypertension, renal failure). Aggressive treatment of early interstitial lung disease may further survival.[62] Localized scleroderma may reach an end point beyond which the disease does not progress.

SPECIAL IMPLICATIONS FOR THE THERAPIST   10-13

Systemic Sclerosis

Skin (Pruritus and Ulcers)

Itching can be a major problem in this condition, and excoriation from scratching can cause open wounds susceptible to infection. The therapist can offer some simple suggestions to soothe skin, ease the itching, and prevent skin damage (see Box 10-4).

Local management of digital tip ulcers may include an advanced dressing to promote wound healing and protect against trauma and infection. Commercial dressings are particularly helpful with larger noninfected ulcers. Recent vasodilative combination therapy (Bosentan) may be effective in people with diffuse SSc and multiple digital ulcers.[95]

Infected ulcers are treated with a trial of oral antistaphylococcal antibiotics as well as topical antimicrobials and may require surgical and/or sharp debridement of necrotic tissue. Local skin care requires avoidance of excessive bathing or using moisturizing creams containing glycerin. (See also "Peripheral Vascular Disease: Special Implications for the Therapist," and "Raynaud Phenomenon" in Chapter 12).

Muscle

Myositis (muscle inflammation) is treated with corticosteroids and sometimes requires the addition of immunosuppressive drugs, whereas fibrotic myopathy (fibrotic tissue laid down within the muscle) is best managed with strengthening and ROM exercises. The efficacy of using soft tissue mobilization or similar techniques has not been investigated. Caution must be used when attempting such treatment, because the skin of these people is usually very sclerosed and sensitive to pressure. Aquatic therapy is an excellent choice for clients with this condition.

Joints and Tendons

Joint and tendon sheath involvement is common and may be treated successfully with nonsteroidal antiinflammatory drugs (NSAIDs). In early dSSc, tenosynovitis can be very painful, limiting joint movement. In addition to NSAIDs, early aggressive therapy is important in preventing or minimizing contractures.

For clients with scleroderma, regular exercise will assist with keeping the skin and joints flexible, maintaining better blood flow, and preventing contractures. Active and passive stretching exercises are necessary but difficult in the presence of extreme pain.

Analgesia is required to optimize participation in an exercise program. Protecting swollen and painful joints from stresses and strains is also an important factor. This may require teaching ways to carry out activities of daily living (ADLs) without causing strain on the joint or joints.

Lightweight splints may be necessary to provide joint protection, with regular close monitoring of integumentary integrity. Dynamic splinting has not been found effective in preventing flexion contractures. Carpal tunnel syndrome, which often occurs before the diagnosis of scleroderma, usually responds well to conservative treatment without requiring surgery.

Exercise

Practice patterns in this area will vary depending on the form of cardiovascular or pulmonary involvement manifested. When cardiopulmonary involvement occurs, intervention must take into consideration effects of this disease on the individual's activity and lifestyle. The client's primary diagnosis and primary intervention may be integument or orthopedic related, but functional limitations may be present secondary to systemic involvement (e.g., decreased aerobic capacity, endurance, and overall general physical condition secondary to cardiovascular and/or pulmonary involvement).

Psychologic Considerations

Persons with early dSSc with or without organ involvement are often anxious because their bodies are changing rapidly and in unexpected ways. They may not understand the grave nature of the disease.

Because persons with dSSc are at greatest risk for early visceral disease and early mortality, education about the disease is important, as is identifying where they are in the natural history of SSc. They should be encouraged to take their blood pressure at home at least three times per week, because this is the best method of screening for acute hypertension. The therapist may screen blood pressure as well.

Polymyositis and Dermatomyositis

Definition and Overview

Polymyositis and dermatomyositis are the two most common idiopathic inflammatory diseases of muscle (Box 10-11). Other types of inflammatory muscle disease have been distinguished, but no satisfactory classification of the idiopathic inflammatory myopathies exists; however, histologic analysis allows differentiation among the types of dermatomyositis.[21] They are diffuse, inflammatory myopathies that produce symmetric weakness of striated muscle, primarily the proximal muscles of the shoulder and pelvic girdles, neck, and pharynx. These related illnesses belong to the family of rheumatic diseases. These diseases often progress slowly, with frequent exacerbations and remissions.

Incidence

Polymyositis and dermatomyositis are not very common in the United States, affecting approximately 5 to 10 persons per 1 million; the incidence appears to be increasing. Myositis can affect people of any age, but mostly adults between 45 and 65 years and children between 5 and 15 years are affected. Twice as many women as men are affected with the exception of dermatomyositis associated with malignancy, which is most common in men over age 40 years.

Etiologic Factors

The cause of these conditions remains unknown, although there appears to be some autoimmune mechanism whereby the T cells inappropriately recognize muscle fiber antigens as foreign and attack muscle tissue. Autoantibodies are present in most cases. Polymyositis and dermatomyositis may be drug induced; possibly triggered by a virus; or associated with other disorders as listed in Box 10-11. The association of dermatomyositis with malignancy, particularly ovarian, lung, gastric, pancreatic, colorectal malignancies, and non-Hodgkin lymphoma may suggest that the neoplasm may stimulate the dermatomyositis.[21]

Pathogenesis

If these conditions are caused by an autoimmune reaction, diffuse or focal muscle fiber degeneration is followed by regeneration of new muscle cells, producing remission. Muscle biopsy reveals focal or diffuse inflammatory infiltrates consisting primarily of lymphocytes and macrophages surrounding muscle fibers and small blood vessels. Muscle cells show evidence of degeneration and regeneration, and fiber atrophy is often most severe at the periphery of the muscle bundle. Extensive interstitial fibrosis and fatty replacement are common in longstanding cases. Biopsies from individuals with chronic inflammatory disease display a low proportion of type I and a high proportion of type II muscle fibers. This has raised a suspicion that the low proportion of type I fibers might play a role in the muscle fatigue.[103]

Clinical Manifestations

Symmetric proximal muscle weakness is the dominant feature of these diseases, although it is variable in its onset, progression, and severity. In some people, symptoms appear suddenly, progress rapidly, and quickly result in a bedridden state, sometimes requiring ventilatory assistance and tube feeding.

More typically, malaise and weight loss develop insidiously over months or even years, with some people either unable to identify the onset of the disease or unaware of the gradual disability developing. Fatigue, rather than weakness, is a commonly reported symptom, but close questioning usually reveals functional losses indicating weakness as well. Pain is not a key feature of these diseases in the adult population, although aching muscles are not uncommon. Muscle wasting is observed in longstanding or severe cases.

Cardiac involvement is not uncommon and contributes significantly to mortality. Nearly half of all people with polymyositis or dermatomyositis have arrhythmias, congestive heart failure, conduction defects, ventricular hypertrophy, or pericarditis.

Pulmonary disease (progressive pulmonary fibrosis) can result from weakness of the respiratory muscles, intrinsic lung pathologic conditions, or aspiration. Swallowing difficulties, nasal regurgitation, and esophageal dysphagia and reflux are common, especially in severe cases.

Polymyositis. Polymyositis begins acutely or insidiously with muscle weakness, tenderness, and discomfort. The proximal muscles of the shoulder and pelvic girdle are affected more often than the distal muscles, usually in a symmetric pattern, but asymmetry is common.

The legs are affected more often than the arms, and the anterior thigh is more frequently involved than the posterior thigh. Initially, the muscles may be slightly swollen, but as the disease progresses muscular atrophy and induration become more noticeable, reflecting the deposition of fibrous tissue. Some persons have a mild peripheral neuropathy with loss of deep tendon reflexes.

Early signs of muscle weakness may include impaired functional status, such as difficulty climbing stairs, getting up from a chair, reaching into an overhead cupboard, combing the hair, or lifting the head from a pillow; difficulty with balance; or a tendency to fall, often resulting in a fracture.

Other muscular effects may include decreased deep tendon reflexes, contractures, arthralgias, arthritis, an inability to move against resistance (e.g., pushing open a heavy door, opening a car door), proximal dysphagia (difficulty swallowing), and dysphonia (difficulty speaking).

Dermatomyositis. When a rash is associated with polymyositis, it is referred to as *dermatomyositis*. A characteristic purplish rash appears on the eyelids (heliotrope erythema), accompanied by periorbital edema (puffy eyelids). The rash may progress to the anterior neck, upper chest and back, shoulders, and arms and may appear

---

Box 10-11

TYPES OF INFLAMMATORY MYOPATHIES*

- Primary idiopathic polymyositis
- Primary idiopathic dermatomyositis
- Dermatomyositis or polymyositis associated with malignancy (lung, breast, ovarian, gastric, colon)
- Juvenile polymyositis or dermatomyositis
- Polymyositis associated with other connective tissue diseases (overlap):
  - Sjögren syndrome
  - Mixed connective tissue disease
  - Rheumatoid arthritis
  - Systemic lupus erythematosus
  - Scleroderma

*Listed in descending order of frequency. Primary idiopathic polymyositis and dermatomyositis account for nearly three-fourths of all cases.

around the nail beds. Gottron papules (red or violet, smooth or scaly patches) may appear on the knuckles, elbows, knees, or medial malleoli (Fig. 10-21).

Although the disease usually begins with erythema and swelling of the face and eyelids, cutaneous manifestations can develop concomitantly or even afterward with proximal muscle weakness manifested as reaching overhead, difficulty getting up out of a chair, going up stairs, shortness of breath, and difficulty swallowing. Some people report muscle tenderness as well. The cutaneous lesions of dermatomyositis are nearly always present by the time proximal muscle weakness manifests itself. In some persons, muscle involvement is minimal, whereas in others it may progress to wasting and contractures associated with extreme disability.[182]

MEDICAL MANAGEMENT

DIAGNOSIS. The diagnosis of myositis is often difficult because it resembles closely several other diseases, and the pathologic manifestation can be localized, sometimes resulting in nondiagnostic biopsies. The physician must rule out internal malignancy first, requiring appropriate medical testing.

The presence of progressive, symmetric weakness is a hallmark diagnostic finding. Laboratory studies to evaluate muscle enzymes, biopsy to assess muscle fibers, and electromyography to measure the electrical activity of the muscles are all necessary to properly diagnose myositis.

Most people with these diseases have an elevated creatine kinase (CK) level at presentation. The CK represents striated muscle involvement, although in people with chronic disease CK may be of the cardiac MB isotype (see Table 40-15). MRI can reveal muscle inflammation and may help to select the site on which to do a biopsy in difficult cases.

TREATMENT. The treatment must be individualized; the components include medication, exercise, and rest. High-dose daily oral systemic corticosteroid therapy is the usual initial pharmacologic treatment for polymyositis or dermatomyositis. Steroids reduce the inflammation, shorten the time to normalization of muscle enzymes, and reduce morbidity. Persons who do not respond well to steroids or who are unable to tolerate the high dosages required may be treated with immunosuppressive drugs. Individuals with skin involvement will need to avoid sun exposure and follow the SunAWARE guidelines (see Box 10-9).

PROGNOSIS. The adult prognosis varies depending on age and progression of the disease process, but overall prognosis has improved with the introduction of systemic glucocorticoid therapy. At present, 85% of people with dermatomyositis can be expected to survive. Approximately 50% are left with residual weakness and have persistently elevated serum CK levels or experience a relapse when corticosteroids are reduced, and 20% are substantially disabled.

Generally, the prognosis is worse with visceral organ involvement, and death occurs from associated malignancy, respiratory disease, or heart failure. Side effects of therapy (corticosteroids, immunosuppressants) contribute to long-term morbidity. The prognosis for children is guarded if the disease is left untreated; it progresses rapidly to disabling contractures and muscular atrophy.

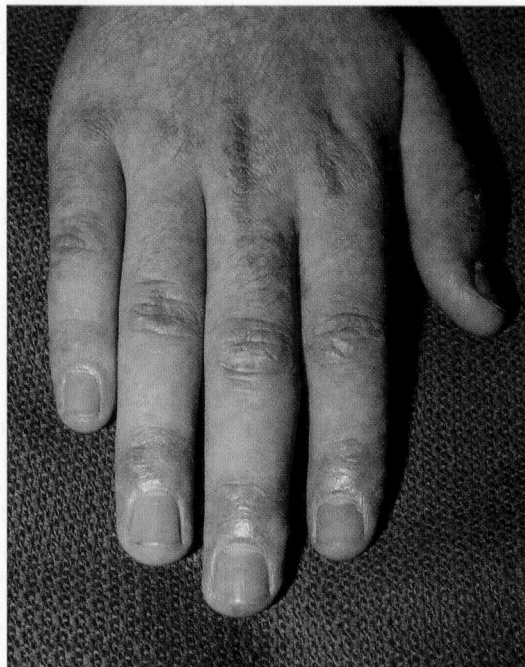

Figure 10-21

Gottron papules or Gottron sign. Typical lesions over bony prominences on the extensor surfaces of the hand. (From Bolognia JL, Jorizzo JL, Rapini RP: *Dermatology*, 2 volume set, St Louis, 2003, Mosby.)

| SPECIAL IMPLICATIONS FOR THE THERAPIST | 10-14 |

Polymyositis and Dermatomyositis

The abrupt onset of any of the cutaneous lesions associated with polymyositis or dermatomyositis could also be a sign of underlying malignancy, particularly genitourinary or GI. The differential diagnosis requires medical evaluation before proceeding with therapy intervention.

The therapist plays a pivotal role in the management of myositis. Manual muscle testing and tests of functional abilities are useful tools in following disease progression and therapeutic response over a long period. Therapists may want to look into the use of the *Myositis Damage* Index (MDI), a tool that assesses damage in adults who have idiopathic inflammatory myopathy. One study of the interrater reliability of this tool suggested it is a valuable tool with good interrater reliability for use in longitudinal studies.[177]

Exercise training is one way to prevent or delay the negative effects of the disease and the impairments seen in people with inflammatory myopathies.[64] The individualized exercise program can help improve muscle strength and function.[71] Aerobic exercise testing may be a useful functional assessment tool in some cases.[63,131,195]

It has been suggested that the medication regimen be well established before beginning exercise. In the early stages of treating myositis, the muscle fibers are fragile and could be damaged further, causing rhabdomyolysis (disintegration of muscle fibers) from exercises and other forms of therapy. Strengthening exercises should therefore be timed to begin after the acute inflammatory phase has passed.

Newer studies have shown that moderate exercise training in combination with immunosuppressive medications can improve muscle performance. In one small study,[126] resistance exercise training was shown to induce a reduction in inflammation and fibrosis in skeletal muscle. Molecular changes and changes in gene expression were demonstrated and associated with improved muscle performance.[126] Therapists treating individuals with this condition will want to stay abreast of any new developments in this area when developing a plan of care.

The therapist treating a client with myositis should keep in close contact with the physician, who will be using physical examination and laboratory tests to determine the most opportune time for initiating a graded exercise program (i.e., when muscle enzyme levels fall to acceptable levels indicating effective medical intervention). Often heat, whirlpools, and massages are very effective adjunctive treatments. Pool therapy may be initiated sooner than other forms of exercise.

Early goals are to preserve functional mobility and activities of daily living skills. If the person is confined to bed, protection from foot drop and contractures and prevention of pressure ulcers are essential. If the client has a skin rash, the therapist should caution about the possibility of infection from scratching. If antipruritic medications do not relieve severe itching, tepid sponges or compresses can be applied (see also Box 10-4). If the client is receiving corticosteroids, observe for side effects (weight gain, acne, edema, hypertension, purplish stretch marks [striae], easy bruising).

Long-term use of steroids lowers resistance to infection, may induce diabetes, causes myopathy and/or neuropathy, and is associated with loss of potassium in the urine and gastric irritation (see Table 5-4 and "Corticosteroids" in Chapter 5). If side effects are marked, advise against abruptly discontinuing corticosteroids until the client consults the physician first. A low-sodium diet will help prevent fluid retention.

Progressive pulmonary fibrosis complicates dermatomyositis and polymyositis in 10% of adults. During the acute phase of illness, clients must be closely monitored for signs of respiratory weakness that requires ventilatory assistance and for overwhelming infection that can lead to circulatory collapse.[21]

THERMAL INJURIES

Cold Injuries

Cold injuries result from overexposure to cold air or water and occur in two major forms: localized injuries (e.g., frostbite) and systemic injuries (e.g., hypothermia). Untreated or improperly treated frostbite can lead to gangrene and may necessitate amputation requiring therapy and rehabilitation. Hypothermia is a medical emergency and is not discussed in detail here.

Incidence and Etiologic and Risk Factors

Cold injuries, once almost exclusively a military problem, are becoming more prevalent among the general population, especially in athletes using localized cryotherapy or participating in outdoor sports. Frostbite results from prolonged exposure to dry temperatures far below freezing.

The risk of serious cold injuries is increased by lack of insulating body fat, old age, homelessness, drug or alcohol use, cardiac disease, psychiatric illness, motor vehicle problems, or smoking when combined with unplanned circumstances leading to cold exposure without adequate protective clothing.[176]

Research is ongoing to reduce the risk of hypothermia and frostbite through the use of nuclear, biologic, and chemical (NBC) protective clothing combined with the Extreme Cold Weather Clothing System (ECWCS) for those individuals engaging in cold weather outdoor activities. It is undetermined yet whether wearing protective clothing may increase the risk of hypothermia during periods of strenuous activity followed by subsequent periods of inactivity accompanied by sweat accumulation in clothing, which may compromise insulation.[202]

Pathogenesis and Clinical Manifestations

Cold-induced injuries can be local or systemic. Severe cold affects all organ systems and especially the central nervous and cardiovascular systems. Many biologic reactions and pathways become distorted or slowed at low body core temperatures. Low body shell temperature can interfere with athletic ability by weakening and slowing muscle contractions, by delaying nerve conduction time, and by facilitating injury.[161]

Typically, an initial vasoconstriction in the skin will protect body parts from a drop in core temperature, but when tissue temperature drops to 35.6° F (2° C), ice crystals form in the tissues and expand extracellular spaces, resulting in localized cold injuries. With compression of cells, cell membranes rupture, interrupting enzymatic and metabolic activities.

Additional injury occurs with thawing when increased capillary permeability accompanies the release of histamine, resulting in aggregation of red blood cells and microvascular occlusion. Research into the pathophysiology of cold injuries has revealed marked similarities in inflammatory processes to those seen in thermal burns and ischemia/reperfusion injury.[125]

Frostbite may be deep or superficial. Superficial frostbite affects the skin and subcutaneous tissue, especially of the face, ears, extremities, and other exposed body areas. Although it may go unnoticed at first, after return to a warm place, frostbite produces burning, tingling, numbness, swelling, and a mottled, blue-grey skin color.

When the affected area begins to rewarm, the person will feel pain and numbness followed by hypoesthesia. Deep frostbite extends beyond subcutaneous tissue and

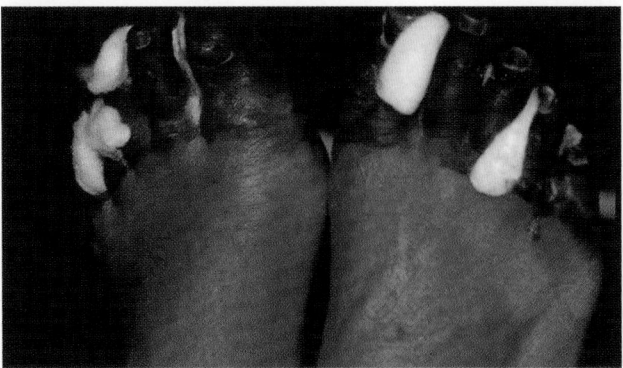

Figure 10-22

Frostbite of the feet. Blackened areas in the photo show tissue necrosis and gangrene, the result of deep frostbite that extends beyond the subcutaneous tissue. (From Auerbach PS: *Wilderness medicine: management of wilderness and environmental emergencies*, ed 4, St Louis, 2001, Mosby.)

usually affects the hands or feet. The skin becomes white until it has thawed and then turns purplish blue. Deep frostbite produces pain, blisters, tissue necrosis, and gangrene (Fig. 10-22).

MEDICAL MANAGEMENT

DIAGNOSIS AND TREATMENT. Diagnosis is usually made based on the history and presenting symptoms; measures to prevent and treat general hypothermia are taken before managing the local frostbite injuries. Evidence of the role of thromboxanes and prostaglandins in cold injuries has resulted in more active approaches in the medical treatment of frostbite wounds, including the use of vasodilators, thrombolysis, and hyperbaric oxygen.[125]

Adequate first aid, which focuses on the prevention of refreezing and mechanical injury, and rapid rewarming together with the administration of ibuprofen, are of the greatest importance for limiting eventual tissue damage. Proper positioning to avoid weight bearing (with gauze between the toes to prevent maceration) is advised. More severe and deeper injuries should not be thawed until medical treatment can be given in a hospital.

Intravenous iloprost (Ventavis) infusion and possibly (r)tPA are indicated if an affected individual presents within 24 hours after the tissue has thawed and the injury is such that severe morbidity can be expected. If the person presents after this time period, hyperbaric oxygen therapy may be considered; however, the evidence available on this type of treatment is limited.[14]

Triple-phase bone scans can be used to distinguish between tissue that is irreversibly destined for necrosis and tissue that is at risk for necrosis but potentially salvageable. These improvements in radiologic assessment have led to earlier surgical intervention to provide at-risk tissue with a new blood supply and preserve both function and length in an extremity.[176]

All frostbitten areas should be treated with topical aloe vera cream. Foam dressings may be applied to maintain a moist wound bed, absorb drainage, and provide protection. A bed cradle may be needed to keep the weight of bedcovers off the affected part or parts.

In the case of a developing compartment syndrome, a fasciotomy may be performed to increase circulation by lowering edematous tissue pressure. If gangrene occurs, amputation may be necessary. Smoking causes vasoconstriction and slows healing; the client should be advised to quit smoking, at least during the recovery period.

PROGNOSIS. The prognosis depends on the extent of localized cold injury and development of any complications, such as compartment syndrome, necrosis, or gangrene. Rapid triage and treatment of frostbite can lead to dramatic improvements in outcome and prognosis.[147] Long-term effects may include increased sensitivity to cold, burning and tingling on reexposure to cold, and increased sweating of the affected area.

Future cold injuries may be prevented through the use of wind-proof, water-resistant, many-layered clothing; moisture-wicking socks; a head covering; mittens instead of gloves; and heat-generating devices (except for those with peripheral neuropathy) in pockets or battery-operated socks.

SPECIAL IMPLICATIONS FOR THE THERAPIST 10-15

Cold Injuries

Local cold injury subsequent to prolonged exposure may not be seen in a therapy practice until complications such as necrosis and gangrene result in amputation. Whirlpool with gentle agitation directed away from the affected area may be prescribed as part of the rewarming procedure. Water temperature is based on tissue temperature and should be determined in conjunction with the medical staff.

Use of cryotherapy by the physical therapist as a modality among the general population can result in a cold injury with localized tissue damage requiring documentation (e.g., filing an accident report) and possible medical evaluation and treatment. Massage may cause further tissue damage and should not be carried out until local tissue has healed.

Burns

Definition and Overview

Injuries that result from direct contact with or exposure to any thermal, chemical, electrical, or radiation source are termed *burns*. Burn injuries occur when energy from a heat source is transferred to the tissues of the body. The depth of injury is a function of temperature or source of energy (e.g., radiation) and duration of exposure.

The severity of burn injury is assessed with respect to the risk of infection, mortality, and cosmetic or functional disability.[142] Factors that influence injury severity include burn depth, burn size (percentage of total body surface area [TBSA]), burn location, age, general health, and mechanism of injury. Burn depth can be divided into categories based on the elements of the skin that are damaged (Fig. 10-23). Most burn wounds that require

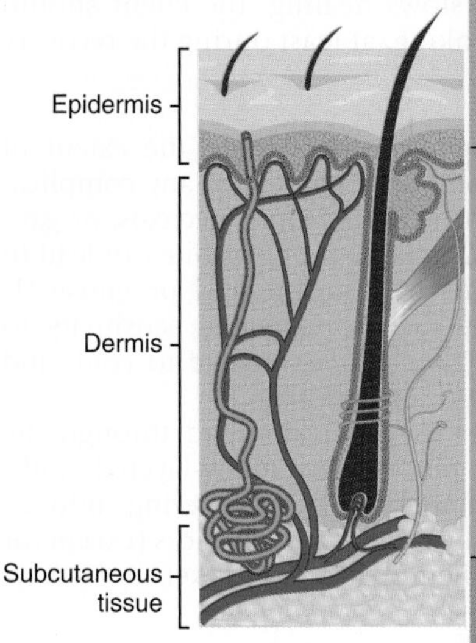

		CAUSE	APPEARANCE	SENSATION	COURSE
Epidermis	**SUPERFICIAL BURN** First-degree burn	Sunburn Ultraviolet exposure Brief exposure to flash, flame, or hot liquids	Mild to severe erythema; skin blanches with pressure; dry, no blisters; edema variable amount	Painful Hyperesthetic Tingling Pain eased by cooling	Discomfort lasts about 48 hours Desquamation in 3-7 days
Dermis	**PARTIAL-THICKNESS BURN** Second-degree burn	Superficial: Scalding liquids, semiliquids (oil, tar), or solids Deep: Immersion scald, flame	Large thick-walled blisters covering extensive area (vesiculation) Edema; mottled red base; broken epidermis; wet, shiny, weeping surface	Painful Sensitive to cold air	Superficial partial-thickness burn heals in 14-21 days Deep partial-thickness burn requires 21-28 days for healing Healing rate varies with burn depth and presence or absence of infection
Subcutaneous tissue	**FULL-THICKNESS BURN** Third-degree or fourth-degree burn	Prolonged exposure to: Chemical, electrical, flame, scalding liquids, steam	Variable (e.g., deep red, black, white, brown) Dry surface Edema Fat exposed Tissue disrupted	Little or no pain Insensate	Full-thickness dead skin suppurates and liquefies after 2-3 weeks Spontaneous healing may be impossible but small areas may be left alone to form scarring without grafting (called secondary intent) Requires removal of eschar and subsequent split- or full-thickness skin grafting Hypertrophic scarring and wound contractures likely to develop without preventive measures

Figure 10-23

Burn injury classification according to depth of injury. This information is important to review because it will help determine the practice pattern to use when making a physical therapy diagnosis. A *partial-thickness* burn involves loss of epidermis and/or a portion of the dermis. Because part of the dermis is intact and that is where the regenerating elements are, a partial-thickness wound has the ability to heal via epithelialization. A *full-thickness* burn involves total destruction of the epidermis and dermis and cannot heal independently without granulation and contraction, sometimes requiring a flap or skin graft procedure.[29]

medical intervention are a combination of partial- and full-thickness burns.

Burn size is determined by one of two techniques: the rule of nines (Fig. 10-24) and the Lund-Browder method (Figs. 10-25 and 10-26). The rule of nines is based on the division of the body into anatomic sections, each of which represents 9% or a multiple of 9% of the TBSA. This is an easy method to quickly assess the percentage of TBSA injured and is most commonly used in emergency departments where the initial evaluation takes place.

The Lund-Browder method modifies the percentages for body segments and provides a more accurate estimate of burn size according to age. For the most accurate estimate of burn size, the burn diagram should be confirmed following the initial wound debridement.[107]

Incidence

In the United States, approximately 1.4 to 2 million burn injuries occur each year; 70,000 people are hospitalized with severe injuries; and 7500 are fatalities. Extensive autografts are required in over 1500 third-degree burns every year and 40,000 second-degree burns.

Burn injuries are the third leading cause of accidental death in all age groups. Males tend to be injured more frequently than females, except for the older population (older than 70 years).[141] The incidence of burn injuries is expected to increase as an aging society characterized by a striving for independence becomes more apparent.[113]

Etiologic Factors

Burn injuries are categorized according to their mechanism of injury: thermal, chemical, electrical, or radiation. *Thermal* burns are caused by exposure to or contact with sources such as flames, hot liquids, steam, semisolids (tar), or hot objects.

Chemical burns are caused by tissue contact with or ingestion, inhalation, or injection of strong acids, alkalis, or organic compounds. Chemical burns can result from contact with certain household cleaning agents and various chemicals used in industry, agriculture, and the military.

Electrical burns are caused by heat that is generated by the electrical energy as it passes through the body. Electrical burns can result from contact with exposed or faulty electrical wiring, high-voltage power lines, or lightning.

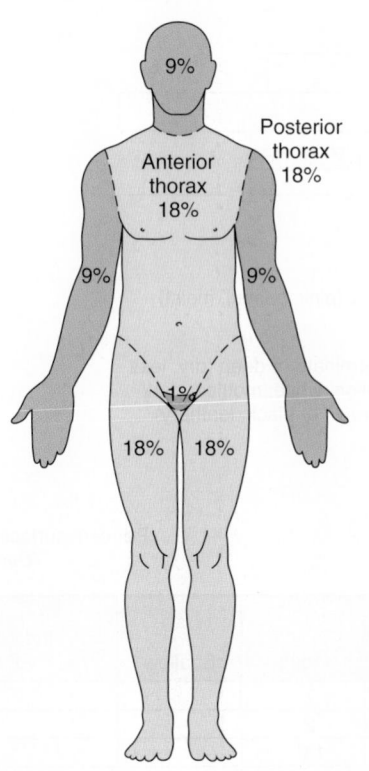

Figure 10-24

The rule of nines provides a quick method for estimating the extent of a burn injury.

Radiation burns are the least common burn injury and are caused by exposure to a radioactive source. These types of injuries have been associated with the use of ionizing radiation in industry or with therapeutic radiation sources in medicine. A sunburn from prolonged exposure to UV rays is also considered a type of radiation burn.

Risk Factors

Data collected from the National Burn Information Exchange indicate that 75% of all burn injuries result from the actions of the injured person, occurring most often in the home. Children younger than age 3 years and adults older than age 70 years are at the highest risk for burn injury.

Risk factors include inadequate adult supervision (in the case of children), psychomotor disorders (e.g., impaired judgment, impaired mobility, drug or alcohol use), rural location, mobile home residence, occupation, lack of smoke detectors, fireworks, and misuse of cigarettes.[26,113,115]

New data demonstrate a change in the epidemiology of burns from previous studies. These data point out the relationship between epileptic seizures and domestic scald injuries. Scald injuries are a major cause of burns in people with epilepsy and account for approximately 2% of all burn admissions.[81,180] Safety recommendations for prevention of burn injuries while showering have been made, including nonlever water handles, limited-temperature devices on water heaters, and curtains rather than cubicles for easy escape.[191]

Pathogenesis

Cutaneous Burns. The pathophysiologic changes that occur immediately following a cutaneous burn injury depend on the extent or size of the burn. For smaller burns, the body's response to injury is localized to the injured area. With more extensive burns (25% or more of the TBSA), the response is systemic, potentially affecting all major systems of the body. The systems more obviously affected include the cardiovascular, renal, GI, immune, and respiratory systems.

Cardiovascular changes occur immediately following a burn injury as vasoactive substances (catecholamines, histamine, serotonin, leukotrienes, and prostaglandins) are released from the injured tissue, causing an increase in capillary permeability.

Extensive burns result in generalized body edema in both burned and nonburned tissues and a decrease in circulating intravascular blood volume. Heart rate increases in response to catecholamine release and to the hypovolemia, but overall cardiac output falls. If the intravascular space is not replenished with IV fluids, hypovolemic (burn) shock and death may result.

Within 18 to 36 hours after the burn, capillary permeability decreases and continues to return to normal for several weeks following the injury. Cardiac output returns to normal and then increases approximately 24 hours after the injury to meet the hypermetabolic needs of the body. The body begins to reabsorb the edema fluid and excretes the excess fluid over the ensuing days and weeks. See also "Common Causes of Fluid and Electrolyte Imbalances" in Chapter 5.

The *renal* and *GI systems* are affected as the body responds initially by shunting blood from the kidneys and intestines, leading to oliguria (decreased urine output) and intestinal dysfunction, respectively, in clients with burns of greater than 25% of TBSA. *Immune system function* is depressed, increasing the risk of infection and life-threatening sepsis. The *respiratory system* may respond with pulmonary artery hypertension and decreased lung compliance, even when there has been no inhalation injury.

Smoke Inhalation. Smoke inhalation may result in injury secondary to inhalation of carbon monoxide, smoke poisoning from the inhalation of by-products of combustion, or direct thermal burns to the pulmonary airways. See "Noxious Gases, Fumes, and Smoke Inhalation" in Chapter 15.

Electrical and Chemical Burns. In electrical burns, heat is generated as the electricity travels through the body, resulting in internal tissue damage. However, entrance and exit wounds may be significant, distracting medical personnel from internal injuries.

Cutaneous burn injuries associated with electrical burns may be negligible, but soft tissue and muscle damage may be extensive, particularly in high-voltage electrical injuries. However, it is possible for electrical sources to ignite the person's clothes, causing thermal burns as well.

The voltage, type of current (direct or alternating), contact site, and duration of contact are important factors in the amount and type of damage sustained. Alternating current is more dangerous than direct and is often associated with cardiopulmonary arrest, ventricular fibrillation, and tetanic muscle contractions.

Other significant injuries, such as long-bone or vertebral compression fractures, spinal cord injury, or traumatic

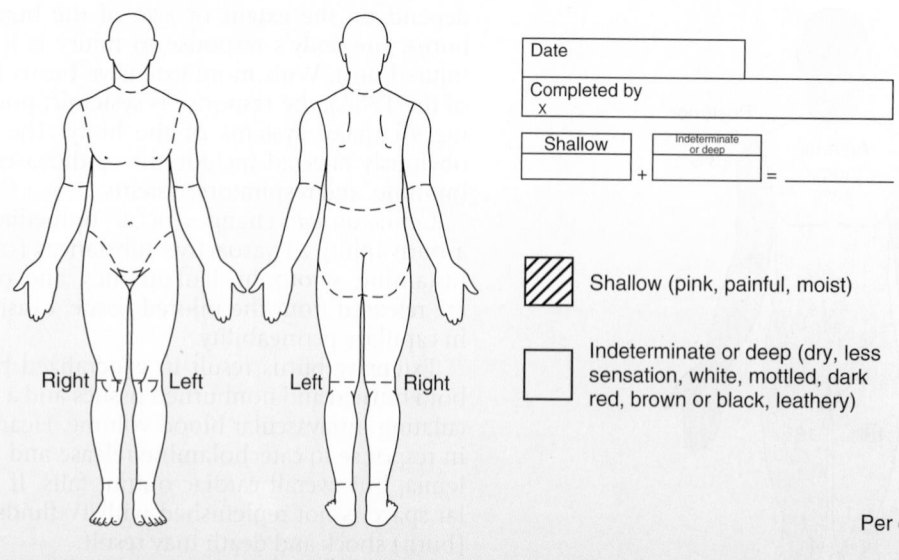

Per cent surface area burned
(Berkow formula)

Area	1 Year	1 to 4 Years	5 to 9 Years	10 to 14 Years	15 to 18 Years	Adult	Shallow	Indeterminate or deep
Head	19	17	13	11	9	7		
Neck	2	2	2	2	2	2		
Ant. trunk	13	13	13	13	13	13		
Post. trunk	13	13	13	13	13	13		
R. buttock	2½	2½	2½	2½	2½	2½		
L. buttock	2½	2½	2½	2½	2½	2½		
Genitalia	1	1	1	1	1	1		
R. U. arm	4	4	4	4	4	4		
L. U. arm	4	4	4	4	4	4		
R. L. arm	3	3	3	3	3	3		
L. L. arm	3	3	3	3	3	3		
R. hand	2½	2½	2½	2½	2½	2½		
L. hand	2½	2½	2½	2½	2½	2½		
R. thigh	5½	6½	8	8½	9	9½		
L. thigh	5½	6½	8	8½	9	9½		
R. leg	5	5	5½	6	6½	7		
L. leg	5	5	5½	6	6½	7		
R. foot	3½	3½	3½	3½	3½	3½		
L. foot	3½	3½	3½	3½	3½	3½		
Total								

Figure 10-25

A sample chart for recording the extent and depth of a burn injury using the Lund-Browder formula.

brain injury, can occur if the victim falls on electrical contact. Chemical burns are associated with systemic toxicity from cutaneous absorption. See also Chapter 4.

Clinical Manifestations

Appearance, sensation, and course of injury of superficial, partial-thickness, and full-thickness burns are outlined in Figure 10-23. Burn location influences injury severity in that burns of certain areas of the body are commonly associated with specific complications. For example, burns of the head, neck, and chest frequently have associated pulmonary complications.

Burns involving the face may have associated corneal abrasions. Burns of the hands (Fig. 10-27) and joints can result in permanent physical and vocational disability requiring extensive therapy and rehabilitation.

Circumferential burns of extremities may produce a tourniquet-like effect and lead to total occlusion of circulation (Fig. 10-28).

Theoretically, with a full-thickness burn the nerve endings have been destroyed and no pain should be associated with this type of injury. However, most full-thickness burns occur with superficial and partial-thickness burns in which nerve endings are intact and exposed. Excised eschar (dead tissue) and donor sites expose nerve fibers as well. As peripheral nerves regenerate, painful sensation returns. Consequently, people with burn injuries often experience severe pain that is related to the size and depth of the burn.

The clinical course of the (major) burn client can be divided into three phases: the emergent and resuscitation phase, the acute phase, and the rehabilitation phase. The *emergent period* begins at the time of injury and concludes

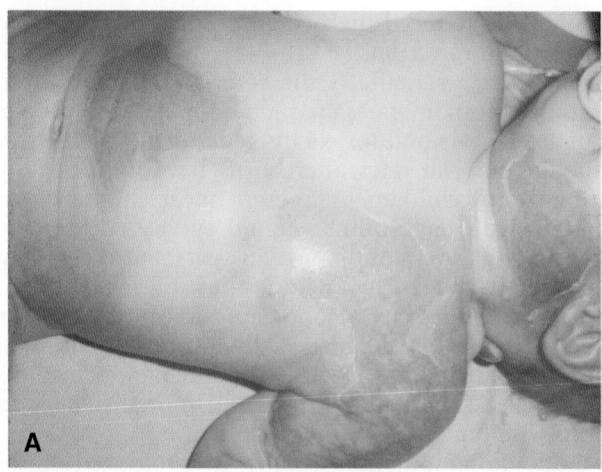

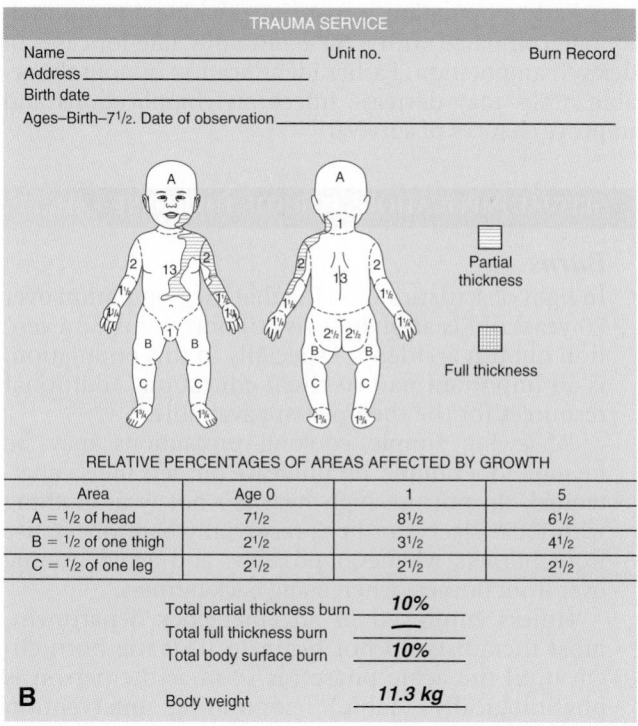

Figure 10-26

A, Pediatric scald burn. B, Corresponding Lund-Browder chart. (Courtesy Katherine S. Biggs, PT, Yale New Haven Hospital, New Haven, Conn.)

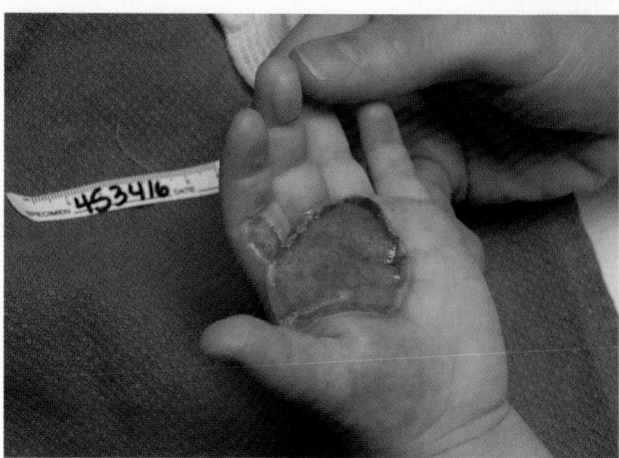

Figure 10-27

Pediatric burn of the hand. This 2-year-old grabbed a hot iron, sustaining a partial-thickness burn to her hand. An intact blister remains on her middle finger. (Courtesy Harriett B. Loehne, PT, DPT, CWS, FACCWS, Archbold Center for Wound Management & Hyperbaric Medicine, Thomasville, GA. Used with permission.)

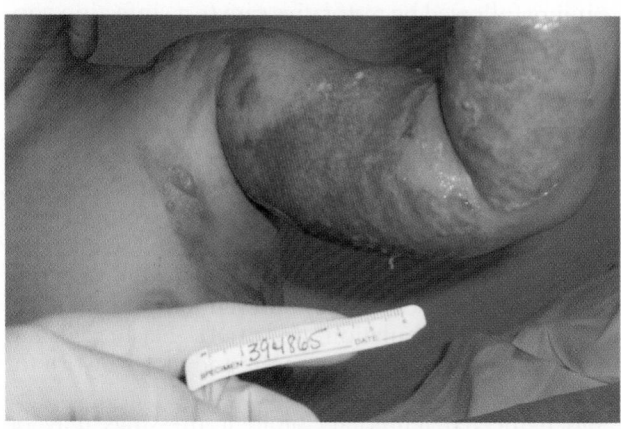

Figure 10-28

Circumferential burns of extremities may produce a tourniquet-like effect and lead to total occlusion of circulation. This 3-year-old child reached into the microwave oven and spilled macaroni in boiling water, resulting in a partial-thickness scald burn. (Courtesy Harriett B. Loehne, PT, DPT, CWS, FACCWS, Archbold Center for Wound Management & Hyperbaric Medicine, Thomasville, GA. Used with permission.)

with the restoration of capillary permeability, usually 48 to 72 hours following injury.

The *resuscitation period* begins with initiation of fluid resuscitation measures and ends when capillary integrity returns to near-normal levels and the large fluid shifts have decreased. The *acute phase* of recovery begins when the person is hemodynamically stable, capillary permeability is restored, and diuresis has begun, usually 48 to 72 hours after the initial injury occurred. The acute phase continues until wound closure is achieved.

The *rehabilitation phase* represents the final phase of burn care, often overlaps the acute care phase, and lasts well beyond the period of hospitalization. This phase focuses on gaining independence through achievement of maximal functional recovery.

Infection is the most common and life-threatening complication of burn injuries. Burn wound infections can be classified on the basis of the causative organism, the depth of invasion, and the tissue response.

Individuals with extensive burns and in whom wound closure is difficult to achieve are at greatest risk for infection and other complications. Inhalation injury with major burns and added staphylococcal septicemia are often fatal.[51] The multiple organ system response that occurs following a burn injury may result in the multiple organ dysfunction syndrome and death (see Chapter 5).

Hypertrophic scarring is a second complication that although not life-threatening is associated with considerable morbidity and potential lifelong disfigurement. Children and African Americans are at greatest risk for hypertrophic scarring, presumably because of the abundance of collagen in these groups. Aging white adults with wrinkled, loose skin have little to no hypertrophic scarring because of the absence of collagen.

MEDICAL MANAGEMENT

TREATMENT. The therapist may be involved in wound management for minor burns consisting of irrigation; removal of any damaging agents (e.g., chemicals, tar); debridement of loose, nonviable tissue; and application of topical antimicrobial creams or ointment and a sterile dressing. Blister management usually includes debridement of the blister (see the feature "Special Implications for the Therapist 10-1: Skin Lesions"). Although the blister fluid is theoretically sterile, most blisters break, and the fluid is an ideal medium for bacteria.[156]

Instructions for home care include observation for clinical manifestations of infection and active ROM exercises to maintain normal joint function, decrease edema formation, and decrease possible scar formation.

Treatment of major burns includes lifesaving measures (ABCs: *a*irway, *b*reathing, *c*irculation) immediately after the injury followed by restorative care (e.g., infection control, wound management, skin grafts, pain management) during the acute phase until wound closure is achieved. Therapists are closely involved early in the acute phase of recovery to maximize functional recovery and cosmetic outcome.

Therapeutic interventions include wound management—irrigation, debridement, advanced wound dressings, positioning, and immobilization following skin grafting to prevent unwanted movement and shearing of grafts, scar and contracture prevention and management, exercise, ambulation, and ADLs. Elasticized garments help reduce scar hypertrophy and may be worn for months to 2 years after hospitalization.

Bioengineered temporary biologic dressings may be used to minimize fluid and protein loss from the burn surface, prevent infection, and reduce pain. Types of temporary grafts include *allografts* (homografts), which are usually cadaver skin; *xenografts* (heterografts), which are typically pigskin; and *biosynthetic grafts*, which are a combination of collagen and synthetics. To treat a full-thickness burn, an *autograft* (the person's own skin) may be required.

The transplanted skin graft will be used intact over areas where appearance or joint movement is important, but the graft may be meshed (fenestrated) to cover up to three times its original size. Several new permanent skin substitutes are being utilized to aid in replacing dermal thickness and to assist in coverage of large surface area injuries.[140] Cultured skin is usually used in conjunction with allograft dermis. In addition, regenerative medicine may be promising for future of burn therapy.[114]

See "Skin Transplantation" in Chapter 21.

PROGNOSIS. Burn care has improved in recent years, resulting in a lower mortality rate for victims of burn injuries. Burn wound management with effective topical antimicrobials and early burn wound excision, have significantly reduced the overall occurrence of invasive burn wound infections.[142]

The client's age affects the severity and outcome of the burn. Mortality rates are higher for children younger than age 4 years and for clients older than age 65 years, although survival rates after burns have improved significantly for children. At present most children, even children with large burns, should survive.[167] Mortality rates among older adults (age 65 years and older) have decreased in the last two decades but still remain high.[4] Factors such as obesity, alcoholism, and cardiac disorders affecting general health, especially disorders that impair peripheral circulation, such as peripheral vascular disease, increase the complication and mortality rates for adults with burns.

Delay in amputation results in prolonged hospital stay, delayed rehabilitation, and a higher mortality rate. Early amputation is associated with a 14% mortality rate compared with a 50% mortality rate for cases of delayed amputation. Earlier identification of nonsalvageable limbs may decrease infectious complications and improve chances of survival.[203]

SPECIAL IMPLICATIONS FOR THE THERAPIST   10-16

Burns

In light of statistics showing that the population over 70 years old is at highest risk of burn injury, prevention of burn accidents, especially in this population, is an important part of client education. Additional resources for the therapist are available.[73,85,166]

Reviewing simple cooking precautions may be helpful; for example, do not leave burners in use unattended, do not use high heat, do not wear clothing with loose sleeves or belts (especially bathrobes), use front burners whenever possible, and avoid leaning over front burners when using back burners.

Unless employed in an emergency department, most therapists do not begin to treat the burn client until the acute phase (as soon as the person is physiologically stable), continuing intervention through much of the rehabilitation phase. However, initiating bedside intervention before the person is medically stable is ideal in reducing morbidity and functional loss.

The therapist will direct treatment intervention to encourage deep breathing and facilitate lung expansion; promote wound healing; reduce dependent edema formation and promote venous return; prevent or minimize deformities and hypertrophic scarring; increase ROM, strength, and function; increase independence in daily activities and self-care; and encourage emotional and psychologic well-being. Specific compression, lymphatic movement, debridement, and wound care procedures are beyond the scope of this book; the reader is referred to Chapter 13 more detailed information.

Throughout the acute and rehabilitation phases of burn care, the therapist must remain alert to the development of medical complications, such as ileus, gastric ulcers, respiratory distress, infection, and impaired circulation. Monitor vital signs (e.g., heart rate, blood pressure, oxygen saturation levels) to ensure the person can tolerate therapy. Notify the nursing staff of any new or unusual findings observed during assessment and intervention (Table 10-4).

Laboratory values will change with a burn, especially a full-thickness burn. It is important for the therapist to review the values prior to treatment interventions to be aware of response to treatment and possible mental status changes.

Clients with burns with acute renal failure and abnormal sodium, potassium, chloride, and magnesium values are candidates for hemodialysis. Abnormal BUN (blood urea nitrogen) can be a reflection of decreased renal function or fluid intake. A client may respond to physical therapy treatment with a decreased mental status. Because of the increased metabolism and catabolic state, clients will experience increased weakness.

Wounds will not heal optimally without addressing protein status, reflected in prealbumin, which will be affected by the catabolic state. Glucose must be monitored because of the same metabolic situation.

Regular inspection of the wound must be made; any change in wound appearance must be reported. The amount of body surface area exposed during wound care must be minimized to prevent hypothermia, because heat is lost in open wounds and after hydrotherapy by evaporation. Hydrotherapy treatment must be limited to 30 minutes or less with water temperature in the 98° to 102° F (36.7°-38.9° C) range if whirlpool is used. External heat shields or radiant heat lamps can provide a source of external heat.

Clients excluded from hydrotherapy are generally those who are hemodynamically unstable and those with new grafts. In recent years, hydrotherapy has been challenged, and alternative methods are being advocated (e.g., shower versus tub).[101] Pulsed lavage with suction (PLWS) (Fig. 10-29) is an ideal intervention for irrigation and debridement, allowing treatment in the Burn Unit of appropriate areas without disturbing new grafts.[101] See also the features "Special Implications for the Therapist 10-17: Pressure Ulcers" and "A Therapist's Thoughts: PLWS versus WP."

People with burns are at high risk of infection because of the significant loss of skin barrier and impaired immune response. Infection control techniques must be practiced carefully at all times (see Appendix A). Skin donor sites require the same care and precautions as other partial-thickness wounds in order to promote healing and prevent infection.

Arrange any therapy likely to elicit a painful response to coincide with medications (allow 30 minutes for oral, 10 minutes for intramuscular [IM], and 3-5 minutes for IV administration). Combining relaxation techniques, music therapy, distraction, and other techniques for pain modulation may be helpful. Burned areas must be maintained in positions of physiologic function within the limits imposed by associated injuries, grafting, and other therapeutic devices (see Table 10-5 for positioning recommendations).

Burned areas are prone to develop contractures requiring close assessment of ROM and muscle strength. Encourage active ROM exercises at least every 2 hours while the person is awake unless this is contraindicated by a recent grafting procedure.

Prolonged stretching is sometimes combined with splinting or orthoses to maintain motion. Splinting is sometimes controversial because of the lack of evidence validation, although most clinicians employ splints successfully to prevent contractures.[150]

Provide honest, positive reinforcement throughout intervention, being aware that each individual will progress through stages of denial, grief, and acceptance of injury and recovery. During the rehabilitation phase, chronic pain protocols may be helpful (see Box 3-15).

MISCELLANEOUS INTEGUMENTARY DISORDERS

Integumentary Ulcers

Integumentary ulcers can be caused by a variety of underlying disorders, including neuropathy, vascular insufficiency, radiation, SSc, vasculitis, and prolonged pressure. In keeping with the focus of this text of recognizing the underlying pathology for various conditions,

Table 10-4	Assessing Medical Complications in the Burn-Injured Adult
System	**Complications**
Urinary	Visible red or dark brown urine (catheter)
Respiratory	Signs of respiratory distress
	Restlessness
	Confusion
	Labored breathing
	Tachypnea (>24 respirations/min)
	Dyspnea
	PaO_2 <90 mm Hg; O_2 <95%
Peripheral vascular	Pulses absent on palpation
	Capillary refill (unburned area) >2 s
	Numbness or tingling
	Increased pain with active ROM exercises
	Increased edema, changes in skin color
Infection	Discoloration of wound periwound erythema, increased drainage, odor, delayed healing
	Headache, chills, anorexia, nausea
	Increased pain
	Change in vital signs
	Paralytic ileus, confusion, restlessness, hallucinations
Gastrointestinal	Paralytic ileus (painful, distended abdomen)
	Stress-induced gastric ulcer (epigastric pain, abdominal distention, loss of appetite, nausea)

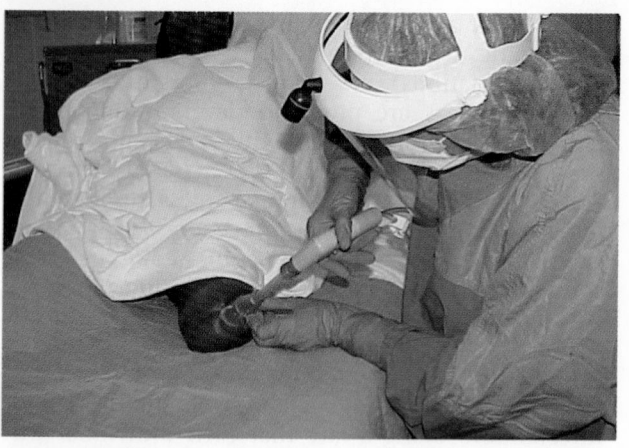

Figure 10-29

Personal protective equipment worn during treatment with pulsed lavage with suction. (Courtesy Harriett B. Loehne, PT, DPT, CWS, FAC-CWS, Archbold Center for Wound Management & Hyperbaric Medicine, Thomasville, GA. Used with permission.)

integumentary ulcers are discussed in individual sections according to the pathogenesis (e.g., diabetic ulcers, see "Diabetes Mellitus" in Chapter 11; arterial insufficiency ulcers, see "Peripheral Vascular Disease" in Chapter 12).

Pressure Ulcers

Definition and Overview

A pressure ulcer (formerly called *bed sore, decubitus ulcer*) is a lesion caused by unrelieved pressure resulting in damage to underlying tissue. Pressure ulcers usually occur over bony prominences, such as the heels, sacrum, ischial tuberosities, greater trochanters, elbows, and scapula, and are staged to classify the degree of tissue damage observed (Fig. 10-30; Box 10-12).

In 1975, a landmark paper was published describing a method of classifying pressure ulcers, defined by the anatomic depth of soft tissue damage[165] (see Fig. 10-30).

Table 10-5	Therapeutic Positioning for the Burn-Injured Client	
Burned Area	**Therapeutic Position**	**Positioning Techniques**
Neck		
Anterior	Extension	No pillow; small towel roll beneath cervical spine to promote neck extension
Circumferential	Neutral toward extension	No pillow
Posterior or asymmetric	Neutral	No pillow
Shoulder, axilla	Arm abduction to 90-110 degrees	Splinting; arms positioned away from body and supported on arm troughs; elbow splint
Elbow	Arm extension	Elbow splint; elbow(s) positioned in extension with slight bend at elbow (≤10 degrees of elbow flexion)
		Arms supported on arm troughs with the forearm in slight pronation
Hand		
Wrist	Wrist extension	Hand splint
Metacarpophalangeal (MCP) joints	MCP flexion at 90 degrees	Hand splint
Proximal or distal interphalangeal (PIP/DIP) joints	PIP/DIP extension	Hand splint
Thumb	Thumb abduction	Hand splint with thumb abduction
Web spaces	Finger abduction	Web spacers of gauze, foam, or thermoplastics to decrease webbing formation
Hip	Hip extension	Supine with the head of bed flat and legs extended
		Trochanter roll to maintain neutral rotation (toes pointing toward ceiling)
		Prone positioning
Knee	Knee extension	Supine with knees extended and toes pointing toward ceiling
		Prone with feet extended over end of mattress
		Sitting with legs extended and elevated
		Knee splint
Ankle	Neutral	Padded footboard
		Ankle-positioning devices (avoid position of ankle inversion or eversion)
		Suspend heels (lying and sitting) to prevent pressure ulcer

Modified from Carrougher GJ, Sandidge C: Management of clients with burn injury. In Black JM, Hawks JH, editors: *Medical-surgical nursing: Clinical management for positive outcomes*, ed 8, Philadelphia, 2008, Saunders, p 1262.

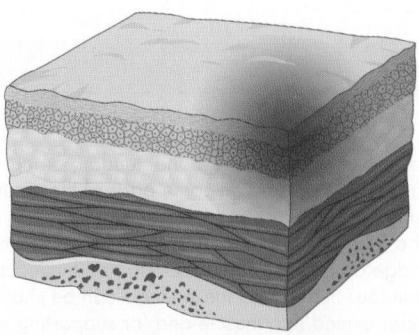

Stage I. Skin remains intact but with observable local changes in temperature (warmth or coolness), texture (firm or boggy feel), color (red in light skin; red, blue, or purple in darker skin), or sensation (pain or itching).

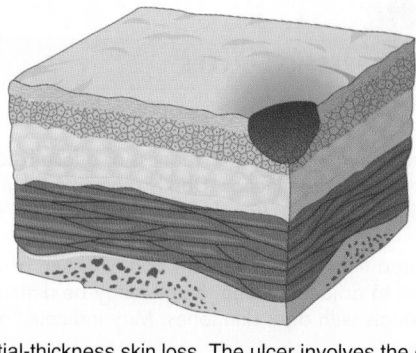

Stage II. Partial-thickness skin loss. The ulcer involves the epidermis, dermis, or both and is considered a partial-thickness skin loss. It is superficial and may look like an abrasion, blister, or shallow crater.

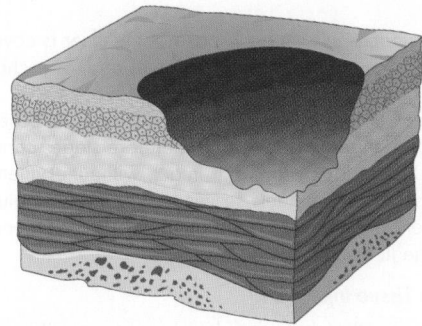

Step III. Full-thickness skin loss. The ulcer forms a deep crater. The adjacent tissue may be involved. There is damage to or necrosis of the subcutaneous tissue, which may extend down to the underlying fascia. The fascia is not affected.

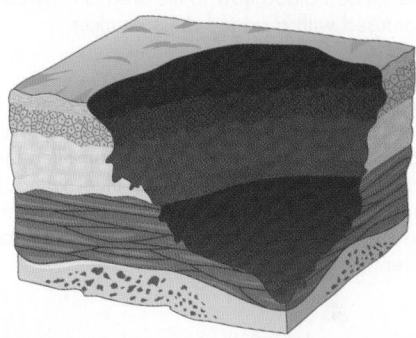

Step IV. Full-thickness skin loss accompanied by tissue necrosis or damage to muscle, bone, or supporting structures, such as tendon or joint capsule. There is extensive tissue destruction; sinus tracts may be present.

Figure 10-30

Staging pressure ulcers is based on the depth and type of tissue damage. This system was developed by the National Pressure Ulcer Advisory Panel (NPUAP). (From National Pressure Ulcer Advisory Panel, http://www.npuap.org/resources/educational-and-clinical-resources/pressure-ulcer-categorystaging-illustrations/.)

Since that time, the original staging system has been modified and developed into the current staging system adopted by the Agency for Health Care Policy and Research (AHCPR) Pressure Ulcer Guideline Panels and published in both sets of Pressure Ulcer Clinical Practice Guidelines.[15,75] The revised stage I definition adopted by the NPUAP in 1998 that is more inclusive of the range of skin pigmentation is included in Box 10-12. In 2007, the NPUAP added two new stages: Unstageable and Suspected Deep Tissue Injury (DTI).

Wounds cannot be backstaged. Once a pressure ulcer is designated as stage II, III, IV, Unstageable, or DTI, it will always remain classified the same for documentation. As the lesion fills with granulation tissue and closes with epithelial tissue, grafts, or flaps, it should be documented as *healing* stage II, III, or IV (still using the original deepest level noted). Nursing homes no longer are required to backstage pressure ulcers for reimbursement purposes.

It should be noted that this staging classification is only for pressure ulcers. Other types of ulcers, such as vascular (arterial, venous) are designated partial or full thickness. Neuropathic ulcers (see Table 12-20) are staged using Wagner classifications (Table 10-6). The term *neuropathic ulcer* is used interchangeably with

diabetic ulcer, but a diabetic ulcer is really a neuropathic ulcer in someone with diabetes. Neuropathic ulcers can occur in anyone with loss of sensation (e.g., alcoholic neuropathy, peripheral neuropathy).

Incidence

Each year, more than 2.5 million people in the United States develop pressure ulcers,[2] including 500,000 people in nursing homes and another 400,000 people with neuropathy.

According to the Agency for Healthcare Research and Quality (AHRQ), the number of hospitalizations involving individuals with pressure ulcers increased by almost 80% in the last 15 years. The AHRQ report uses statistics from the Nationwide Inpatient Sample.[159] More than 500,000 hospitalizations involving pressure ulcers were reported for 1 year. Pressure ulcers were the primary diagnosis in about 10% of those patients. The remaining pressure ulcers were a secondary diagnosis in patients admitted for pneumonia or infections.[159]

Pressure ulcers are viewed as high-volume, high-risk problems in most health care settings. In long-term care facilities, regulatory agencies have designated the development of pressure ulcers as an indicator of quality of care provided to clients.[46]

Box 10-12

STAGES OF PRESSURE ULCERS

Stage I*

Intact skin with nonblanchable redness of a localized area usually over a bony prominence. Darkly pigmented skin may not have visible blanching; its color may differ from the surrounding area.

The area may be painful, firm, soft, warmer, or cooler as compared to adjacent tissue. Stage I may be difficult to detect in individuals with dark skin tones. May indicate "at risk" persons.

Note: Reactive hyperemia will blanche when pressure is applied. Reactive hyperemia normally can be expected to be present for one-half to three-fourths as long as when the pressure-occluded blood flow to the area is restored; it should not be confused with a stage I pressure ulcer.

Stage II

Partial-thickness loss of dermis presenting as a shallow open ulcer with a red pink wound bed, without slough. May also present as an intact or open/ruptured serum-filled blister.

Presents as a shiny or dry shallow ulcer without slough or bruising. This stage should not be used to describe skin tears, tape burns, perineal dermatitis, maceration, or denudement.

Stage III

Full-thickness tissue loss. Subcutaneous fat may be visible but bone, tendon, or muscle is *not* exposed. Slough may be present but does not obscure the depth of tissue loss. *May* include undermining and tunneling.

The depth of a Stage III pressure ulcer varies by anatomic location. The bridge of the nose, ear, occiput, and malleolus do not have subcutaneous tissue and Stage III ulcers can be shallow. In contrast, areas of significant adiposity can develop extremely deep Stage III pressure ulcers. Bone/tendon is not visible or directly palpable.

Stage IV

Full-thickness tissue loss with exposed bone, tendon, or muscle. Slough or eschar may be present on some parts of the wound bed. Often include undermining and tunneling.

The depth of a Stage IV pressure ulcer varies by anatomic location. The bridge of the nose, ear, occiput, and malleolus do not have subcutaneous tissue, and these ulcers can be shallow. Stage IV ulcers can extend into muscle and/or supporting structures (e.g., fascia, tendon, or joint capsule) making osteomyelitis possible. Exposed bone/tendon is visible or directly palpable.

Note: Undermining and sinus tracts may also be associated with stage IV pressure ulcers.

Unstageable

Full-thickness tissue loss in which the base of the ulcer is covered by slough (yellow, tan, gray, green, or brown) and/or eschar (tan, brown, or black) in the wound bed.

Until enough slough and/or eschar is removed to expose the base of the wound, the true depth, and therefore stage, cannot be determined. Stable (dry, adherent, intact, without erythema or fluctance) eschar on the heels serves as "the body's natural (biological) cover" and should not be removed. These wounds are at least Stage III or Stage IV.

Suspected Deep Tissue Injury (DTI)

Purple or maroon localized area of discolored intact skin or blood-filled blister due to damage of underlying soft tissue from pressure and/or shear (Fig 10-31). The area may be preceded by tissue that is painful, firm, mushy, boggy, warmer or cooler as compared to adjacent tissue.

Deep tissue injury may be difficult to detect in individuals with dark skin tones. Evolution may include a thin blister over a dark wound bed. The wound may further evolve and become covered by thin eschar. Evolution may be rapid exposing additional layers of tissue even with optimal treatment.

Data compiled by Harriett B. Loehne, PT, DPT, CWS, FACCWS. Clinical Educator, Wound Management, Archbold Medical Center, Thomasville, Georgia.

Sources: U.S. Department of Health and Human Services: *Pressure ulcers in adults: prediction and prevention. Clinical Practice Guideline No. 3.* AHCPR publication no. 92-0047, Rockville, MD, 1992; National Pressure Ulcer Advisory Panel (NPUAP), 2007. NPUAP Pressure Ulcer Stages/Categories. Available at http://www.npuap.org/resources/educational-and-clinical-resources/npuap-pressure-ulcer-stagescategories/.

*The National Pressure Ulcer Advisory Panel redefined the definition of a pressure ulcer and the stages of pressure ulcers in 2007, including the original 4 stages and adding 2 stages on deep tissue injury and unstageable pressure ulcers.

Note: *Wounds cannot be backstaged (see text for explanation).*

Healthy People 2020 has set as an objective to reduce the number of pressure ulcer-related hospitalizations among older adults and the proportion of nursing home residents with current diagnosis of pressure ulcers.[69]

The target-setting method used by *Healthy People 2020* in conjunction with the NPUAP is based on a 50% reduction in prevalence and improvement over the baseline. *Incidence* refers to the rate at which new cases occur in a population over a given period of time, whereas *prevalence* refers to the number of both new and old cases at any one time in the population.

Etiologic and Risk Factors

Pressure ulcers are caused by unrelieved pressure that can result in damaged skin, muscle, and underlying tissue,

usually over bony prominences. The two causative factors for the development of pressure ulcers are interface pressure (externally) and pressure with shearing forces (two layers sliding against each other in opposite directions causing damage to the underlying tissues). Some of the risk factors for pressure ulcers are (1) friction (rubbing of the skin against another surface); (2) maceration (softening caused by excessive moisture); (3) decreased skin resilience (e.g., dehydration); (4) malnutrition; and (5) decreased circulation.

Pressure contributes to other types of ulcers (e.g., arterial, venous, neuropathic), and likewise, the underlying cause of the other types of ulcers can contribute to the development of pressure ulcers (see Table 12-20). However, pressure ulcers are a separate entity from these other types of ulcers. A systemic risk assessment

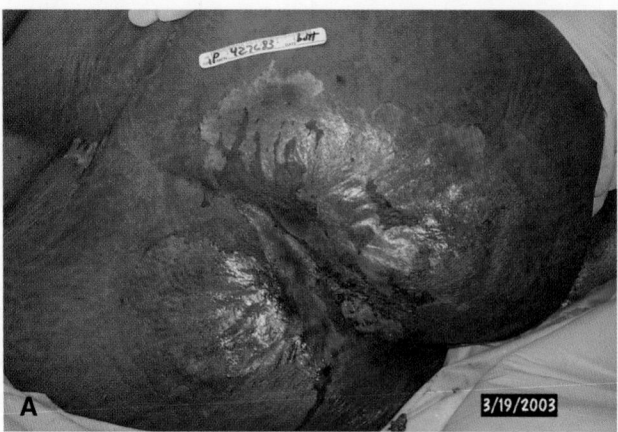
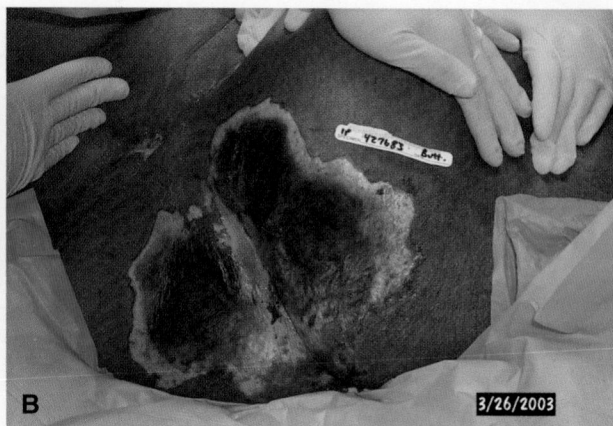

Figure 10-31

Deep tissue injury (DTI). A DTI pressure ulcer presents suddenly as a discolored or bruised-appearing area that quickly progresses to a deep wound regardless of any intervention. It is an unavoidable ulcer and usually occurs when other organs are shutting down. Because the skin is the largest organ in the body, necrosis of the skin will occur when circulation is significantly impaired. **A,** The DTI was discovered when an unstable patient in the intensive care unit was finally able to be turned over after 2 days. He had kidney failure, was on a ventilator, and had tenuous blood pressure. The wound presented as a discolored area with intact skin (formerly required to be staged as a stage I pressure ulcer). **B,** One week later it was solid eschar, which required sharp debridement because of purulent drainage at the margins and was necrosed to bone. The patient expired several days later. (Courtesy Harriett B. Loehne, PT, DPT, CWS, FACCWS, Archbold Center for Wound Management & Hyperbaric Medicine, Thomasville, GA. Used with permission.)

Table 10-6	Wagner Ulcer Grade Classification
Grade	**Characteristics**
0	Preulcerative lesions; healed ulcers; presence of bony deformity
1	Superficial ulcer without subcutaneous tissue involvement
2	Penetration through the subcutaneous tissue; may expose bone, tendon, ligament, or joint capsule
3	Osteitis, abscess, or osteomyelitis
4	Gangrene of digit
5	Gangrene of foot requiring disarticulation

This classification scheme for ulceration is used for neuropathic ulcers and does not represent pressure ulcers.
Data from Wagner REW: The dysvascular foot: a system for diagnosis and treatment, *Foot Ankle* 2:64-122, 1981.

evaluating both sensation and physiologic risk of pressure ulcers can be made using a validated risk assessment tool, such as the Braden Scale (Fig. 10-32) or the Norton Scale.

Intrinsic factors most commonly associated with pressure ulcer development include decreased sensation, impaired mobility or activity levels, incontinence, diaphoresis, impaired nutritional status, and altered levels of consciousness. Extrinsic factors include pressure, shear, friction, and moisture.

Bed- and chair-bound clients and those with impaired ability to reposition themselves should be assessed for additional factors that increase the risk of developing pressure ulcers. These factors include decreased mobility or immobility; hip or femoral fractures; contractures; increased muscle tone; loss of sensation; incontinence; obesity; nutritional factors; chronic disease accompanied by anemia, edema, renal failure, or sepsis; and altered level of consciousness.

Nutritional factors may include malnutrition or inadequate nutrition leading to weight loss and subsequent reduction of subcutaneous tissue and muscle bulk. The Agency for Health Care Policy and Research guidelines[15] for clinically significant malnutrition impairing wound healing include serum albumin less than 3.5 mg/dL and total lymphocyte count lower than $1800/mm^3$ (see Tables 40-5).

Prealbumin, which determines protein over the previous 48 hours, rather than over the previous 3 weeks as with albumin, is a better indicator of the current nutritional status of the client. Prealbumin should be more than 20 for optimal wound healing. It is considered the gold standard for monitoring nutritional progress, allowing for documentation and appropriate interventions.[28]

Pathogenesis

Pressure is the external factor causing ischemia and tissue necrosis. Continuous pressure on soft tissues between bony prominences and hard or unyielding surfaces compresses capillaries and occludes blood flow. Normal capillary blood pressure at the arterial end of the vascular bed averages 32 mm Hg.

When tissues are externally compressed, that pressure may be exceeded, reducing blood supply to, and lymphatic drainage of, the affected area.[74,75] Shearing (when the skin layers move in opposite directions) is the intrinsic factor that contributes to ripping or tearing of blood vessels, further damaging the integument.

If the pressure is relieved, a brief period of rebound capillary dilation (called *reactive hyperemia*) occurs and no tissue damage develops. If the pressure is not relieved,

Sensory Perception	Moisture	Activity	Mobility	Nutrition	Friction & Shear
1. Completely Limited: Unresponsive (does not moan, flinch or grasp) to painful stimuli, due to diminished level of consciousness or sedation. **OR** Limited ability to feel pain over most of body surface	**1. Consistently Moist:** Skin is kept moist almost constantly by perspiration, urine, etc. Dampness is detected every time patient is moved or turned.	**1. Bedfast:** Confined to bed.	**1. Completely Immobile:** Does not make even slight changes in body or extremity position without assistance.	**1. Very Poor:** Never eats a complete meal. Rarely eats more than 1/3 of any food offered. Eats 2 servings or less of protein (meat or dairy products) per day. Takes fluid poorly. Does not take liquid dietary supplement. **OR** Is NPO and/or maintained in clear liquids or IV's for more than 5 day.	**1. Problem:** Requires moderate to maximum assistance in moving. Complete lifting without sliding against sheets is impossible. Frequently slides down in bed or chair, requiring frequent repositioning with maximum assistance. Spasticity, contractures or agitation leads to almost constant friction.
2. Very Limited: Responds only to painful stimuli. Cannot communicate discomfort except by moaning or restlessness. **OR** Has a sensory impairment, which limits the ability to feel pain or discomfort over 1/2 of body.	**2. Very Moist:** Skin is often but not always moist. Linen must be changed at least once a shift.	**2. Chairfast:** Ability to walk severely limited or non-existent. Cannot bear own weight and/or must be assisted into chair or wheelchair.	**2. Very Limited:** Makes occasional slight changes in body or extremity position but unable to make frequent or slight changes independently.	**2. Probably Inadequate:** Rarely eats a complete meal and generally eats only about 1/2 of any food offered. Protein intake includes only 3 servings of meat or dairy products per day. Occasionally will take a supplement. **OR** Receives less than optimum amount of liquid diet or tube feeding.	**2. Potential Problem:** Moves feebly or requires minimum assistance. During a move skin probably slides to some extent against sheets, chair, restraints or other devices. Maintains relatively good position in chair or bed most of the time, but occasionally slides down.
3. Slightly Limited: Responds to verbal commands, but cannot always communicate discomfort or need to be turned. **OR** Has some sensory impairment, which limits ability to feel pain or discomfort in 1 or 2 extremities.	**3. Occasionally Moist:** Skin is occasionally moist, requiring an extra linen change approximately once a day.	**3. Walks Occasionally:** Walks occasionally during day, but for very short distances, with or without assistance. Spends majority of each shift in bed or chair.	**3. Slightly Limited:** Makes frequent though slight changes in body or extremity position independently.	**3. Adequate:** Eats over half of most meals. Eats a total of 4 protein (meat, dairy products) each day. Occasionally will refuse a meal, but will usually take a supplement if offered. **OR** TPN regimen, which probably meets most of nutritional needs.	**3. No Apparent Problem:** Moves in bed and chair independently and has sufficient muscle strength to lift up completely during move. Maintains good position in bed or chair at all times.
4. No Impairment: Responds to verbal commands. Has no sensory deficit, which would limit ability to feel or voice pain or discomfort.	**4. Rarely Moist:** Skin is usually dry, linen only requires changing at routine intervals.	**4. Walks Frequently:** Walks outside the room at least twice a day and inside the room at least once every 2 hours during waking hours.	**4. No Limitations:** Makes major and frequent changes in position without assistance.	**4. Excellent:** Eats most of every meal. Never refuses a meal. Usually eats a total of 4 or more servings of meat and dairy products. Occasionally eats between meals. Does not require supplementation.	

Used with Permission. If total is ≤ 18 and/or wound is present, initiate pressure ulcer prevention and/or wound treatment orders.

Total Score:_____

Identify Integumentary Integrity by placing appropriate letters on figure.

Key: □ ≤ 18: at risk for pressure ulcers   □ 15–18: low risk   □ 13–14: moderate risk   □ 10–12: high risk   □ < –9: Very high risk

☐ Skin Intact

E - Ecchymosis   A - Abrasion   RH - Rash   Er - Erythema   B - Blister   S - Scars (past 2 years)
L - Laceration   U - Ulcer   I - Incision   O - Open Wound   PU - Pressure Ulcer

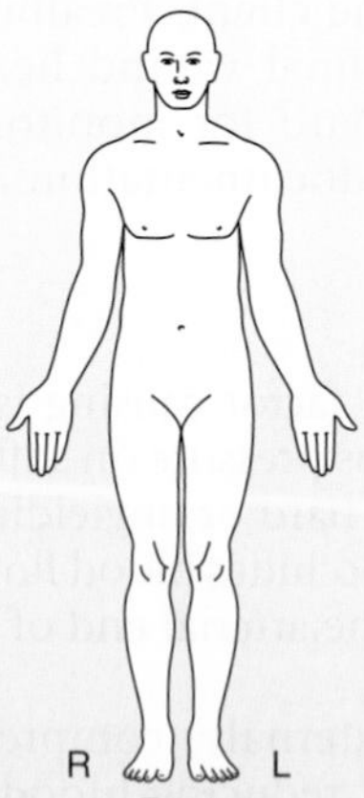

☐ IV Access

☐ Permanent Cath

Completed by:_____

Therapist's Signature

Date   Time

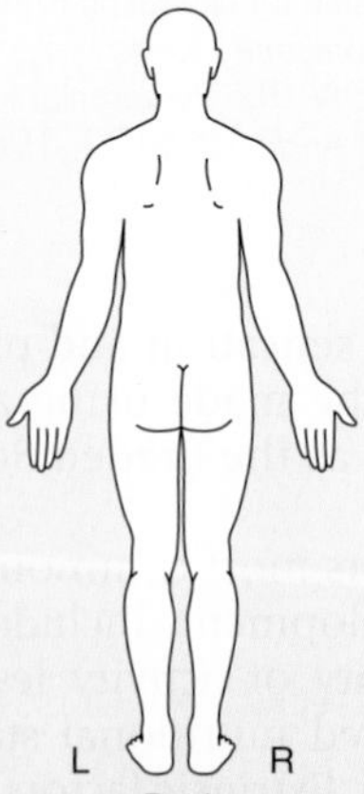

R   L
Front

L   R
Back

Figure 10-32

The Braden Scale for Predicting Ulcer Risk. NOTE: The question is often asked: Is there a score that should trigger a PT consult? We asked our panel of experts and received the following response: *It is advised that at all facilities (acute, in patient rehab, swing bed, nursing home) every patient/ resident should be scored on the Braden Scale. If a person scores <18, he/she should be placed on protocol orders for pressure ulcer prevention. The same is true if there is a wound or pressure ulcer, regardless of the Braden Score. There should be a place on the protocol sheet to order physical therapy for wound management as well as a consult for mobility, strengthening, etc. All physicians approved, and the nurse can place the order ASAP; the physician later signs it.* (Used with permission of Braden B. Frantz R: Selecting a tool to measure skin integrity. In Stromberg M, editor: *Instruments for clinical nursing research,* ed 2, Norwalk, CT, 1997. Appleton-Lange Publishing Co.)

Tissue load management

"Tip of the iceberg" effect

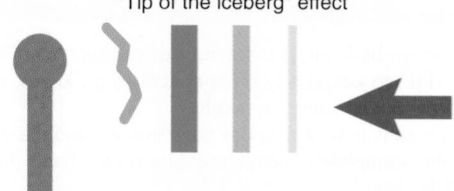

Figure 10-33

Evolving stages of a stage IV pressure ulcer. This diagram represents a trochanter partially surrounded by tendon, with subcutaneous, dermis, and epidermis layers *(vertical lines left to right)*. As pressure occurs from the outside *(arrow)*, the tendon becomes ischemic first, and then the subcutaneous layer is affected because it is less vascular than the dermis. The last tissue to become ischemic is the epidermis. The observer would initially identify the epidermal tissue change as a stage I pressure ulcer. Initially, the ischemic inner tissue layers would not be known. Only as the necrosis moves superficially will the full impact of tissue damage become observable, identifying the area as a stage IV pressure ulcer with extensive damage to the bone. (Courtesy Karen Kendall, PT, CWS, Medical Center for Continuing Education, Holiday, FL.)

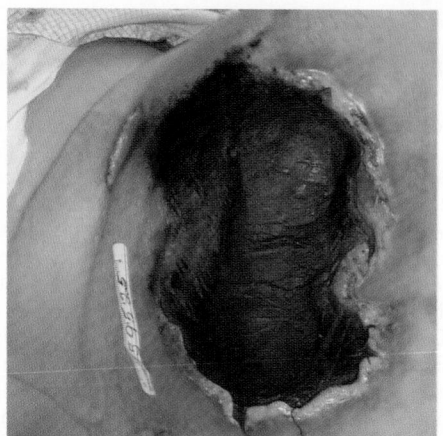

Figure 10-34

Unstageable (because of eschar) trochanteric pressure ulcer. (Courtesy Harriett B. Loehne, PT, DPT, CWS, FACCWS, Archbold Center for Wound Management & Hyperbaric Medicine, Thomasville, GA. Used with permission.)

the endothelial cells lining the capillaries become disrupted by platelet aggregation, forming microthrombi that occlude blood flow and cause anoxic necrosis of surrounding tissues. Necrotic tissue predisposes to bacterial invasion and subsequent infection, preventing healthy granulation. Muscle and tendon tissue can tolerate less pressure loading than skin before incurring ischemic damage (Fig. 10-33).[110]

In the case of neuropathic ulcers associated with diabetes, the primary pathogenesis is the absence of protective sensation combined with high pressure. The absence of protective sensation indicates a high risk for pressure ulcers on the feet and heels; diabetic ulcers are typically present on the soles of the feet (see "Diabetes Mellitus: Ulceration" in Chapter 11).

Clinical Manifestations

Pressure ulcers usually occur over bony prominences and often in a circular pattern shaped like an inverted volcano with the greatest tissue ischemia at the apex next to the bone, or they may assume the shape of objects causing the pressure, such as tubing or clamps. Irregular patterns indicate additional shearing forces or other contributing factors.

Sacral ulcers are often large, undermined, and deep to the bone because the tissue mass over the sacrum is thin and erodes easily to the deep tissues. Pressure ulcers are manifested at the surface as the deeper tissues die, so that a stage I ulcer can become a stage III or IV quickly without further injury.

The wounds (Fig. 10-34) can be described, measured, and categorized with respect to surface area, exudates, and type of wound tissue. Therapists may want to utilize the PUSH Tool to assess and document pressure ulcers. This tool is available from the NPUAP: www.npuap.org. When present, infection can be localized and self-limiting or can progress to sepsis. Proteolytic enzymes from bacteria and macrophages dissolve necrotic tissues and cause a foul-smelling discharge that appears to be, but is not, pus.

Necrosis associated with pressure ulcers is not painful, but the surrounding tissue can be painful in individuals who do not have loss of sensation from spinal cord trauma or neuropathy. Positioning is the first step, so that pressure is relieved if at all possible, or at least redistributed. Wound management interventions can be ameliorated by premedication. If needed, oral meds should be administered about 30 minutes before treatment, IM about 10 minutes, and IV immediately before treatment. An experienced physical therapist will carry out treatment with the least discomfort possible for the person.

Trauma to the tissues produces an acute inflammatory response with hyperemia, fever, and increased white blood cell count. Many individuals never initiate a significant acute inflammatory response because of the heavy bioburden from large amounts of necrotic tissue, but develop an unresolved chronic inflammation. Individuals who are immunosuppressed or who have diabetes mellitus are often unable to mount a sufficient inflammatory response to start the healing cascade and thus are at greater risk for infection.

MEDICAL MANAGEMENT

DIAGNOSIS. Prevention is the key to this condition (Box 10-13), starting with assessment of people at high risk for the development of pressure ulcers. In fact, risk prediction should be an ongoing assessment carried out by all health care professionals. In addition to the Braden Scale (see Fig. 10-32), laboratory data on hemoglobin, hematocrit, prealbumin, total protein, and lymphocytes should be assessed by all health care professionals involved.

The diagnosis is reached by looking at the location of the wound and the type of tissue response. The pressure ulcer is then staged (see Box 10-12 and Fig. 10-30). If there is evidence of infection, the wound is irrigated with isotonic saline and debrided if necrosis is present, and then viable tissue is cultured (not a swab specimen of the exudates or necrotic tissue).

Box 10-13

GUIDELINES FOR PREVENTION OF PRESSURE ULCERS IN ADULTS

- All clients at risk should have a systematic skin inspection at least once each day, paying particular attention to the bony prominences. Results of skin inspection should be documented (see Box 10-5).
- Cleanse skin at the time of soiling and at routine intervals. Individualize the frequency of skin cleaning according to need and client preference. Avoid hot water, and use a mild cleaning agent that minimizes irritation and dryness of the skin. During the cleaning or wound care process, minimize the force and friction applied to the skin. Ideal is the use of disposable perineal cloths, impregnated with dimethicone.
- Minimize environmental factors leading to skin drying, such as low humidity (<40%) and exposure to cold. Treat dry skin with moisturizers.
- Do NOT perform massage over reddened areas. Perform indirect soft tissue mobilization techniques or massaging the tissue around and toward the area with caution.
- Minimize skin injury caused by friction and shear forces through proper positioning, transferring, and turning techniques. Reduce friction injuries by the use of moisturizers, skin sealants, and protective padding.
- Maintain current activity level, mobility, and range of motion. Evaluate the potential for improving the person's mobility and activity status, and institute rehabilitation efforts.
- Monitor and document interventions and outcomes.
- If abnormal (<20 g/dl), order prealbumins one to two times weekly and have dietitian follow to optimize nutrition.
- Reposition any person in bed who is assessed to be at risk of developing pressure ulcers at least every 2 hours if consistent with overall treatment goals.

- For persons in bed, use positioning devices such as pillows or foam wedges to keep bony prominences (e.g., knees, ankles) from direct contact with one another.
- Provide persons in bed who are completely immobile with devices that completely relieve pressure on the heels (i.e., *suspend* the heels).
- Do not use doughnut-type devices.
- When side-lying position is used in bed, avoid positioning directly on the greater trochanter. A 30-degree tilt is efficacious.
- Maintain the head of the bed at the lowest degree of elevation (30-degree lateral incline; see Fig. 10-35) consistent with medical conditions and other restrictions, except at mealtimes. Limit the amount of time the head of the bed is elevated.
- Use lifting devices, such as a trapeze, hydraulic lift, slide board, or linen, to move (rather than drag) persons in bed who cannot assist during transfers and position changes.
- Place any person assessed to be at risk of developing pressure ulcers, when lying in bed, on a pressure-redistribution surface, such as foam, low air loss, or gel mattress.
- Avoid uninterrupted sitting in any chair or wheelchair for any person at risk of developing a pressure ulcer. Reposition the person, shifting the points under pressure at least every hour, or put him or her back to bed if consistent with overall management goals. Persons who are able should be taught to shift weight every 15 minutes.
- For chair-bound persons, use a pressure-redistribution device. Do not use doughnut-type devices.

Modified from Panel on the Prediction and Prevention of Pressure Ulcers in Adults: *Pressure ulcers in adults: prediction and prevention*. Clinical practice guidelines. CPR publication no. 92-0050, Rockville, MD, 1992, Agency for Health Care Policy and Research, U.S. Public Health Service.

The definition of infection is invasion into viable tissue. Cultures of the organisms that have invaded the tissue causing the infection must be determined following these procedures. Clinical practice of wound cultures must be careful to avoid culturing wound exudate contaminants, of which there are usually a minimum of three per wound.[87]

Sensitivity testing to identify infecting organisms and to help determine appropriate topical or systemic antibiotics may be needed. The AHCPR (No. 15) recommends blood cultures for ulcer-related sepsis to determine appropriate systemic antibiotics.

TREATMENT. Prevention and removing the causative factor are the first step in the treatment intervention for pressure ulcers. Preventing shear and friction forces requires education of the client and primary caretakers. The pressure ulcer is irrigated thoroughly. Healing will occur optimally when the ulcer is kept moist and the wound bed is prepared for appropriate healing cascade of acute versus chronic wounds, as discussed in Chapter 6.

Topical antimicrobials (e.g., Iodosorb, Iodoflex, silver dressings) can be effective on local infections without systemic involvement to control bacterial concentration, being mindful of allergic reactions. Neomycin and

bacitracin should not be used because of increasing episodes of allergic reactions. Antiseptics are not recommended because these are cytotoxic.

Some physicians continue to advocate the initial use of wet-to-dry dressing for debridement (application of open wet dressing, allowing it to dry on the ulcer, and mechanically debriding exudate by removal of the dressing). Because there is a risk of removing viable tissue, damaging new granulation tissue, as well as bleeding with this procedure, it is not acceptable for debridement if any viable tissue is evident and should be used only rarely. There are other more efficacious and safe methods of debridement. Wet-dry is not permissible as a dressing change order—only for debridement.[13,84]

The use of antiseptics such as hydrogen peroxide or povidone iodine (cadexomer iodine is an excellent antimicrobial dressing choice) is not recommended because these are cytotoxic and can be damaging to granulation tissue. Hyperbaric oxygen therapy (HOT) has not been approved for pressure ulcers except when osteomyelitis is present that has failed systemic antibiotic treatment or there are complications from a flap or graft.

Successful healing requires continued adequate redistribution of pressure (e.g., turning, positioning, support surfaces—including sitting) and absence of infection. The presence of necrotic tissue in a wound may provide an optimal environment for bacteria to grow, hence the importance of removing necrotic material from a wound as rapidly as possible.

Therapeutic intervention may include hydrotherapy (e.g., PLWS; see Fig. 10-29), electrical stimulation, ultrasound, debridement (autolytic, enzymatic, mechanical, sharp), or any combination of these. An appropriate wound dressing is then applied to provide an optimal wound environment.

Deep pressure ulcers may require sharp or surgical debridement of necrotic tissue and opening of deep pockets for drainage. A slower method of debridement is the use of enzymes. Collagenase enzymatic debrider is the only enzyme available now on the market; proteolytic enzymes are no longer available. A variety of skin-grafting techniques may be used if the wound requires surgical closure.

In stage III ulcers, undamaged tissue near the wound can be rotated to cover the ulcer. In stage IV ulcers, musculoskeletal flaps (a single unit of skin with its underlying muscle and vasculature), as well as a variety of other skin-grafting techniques, may be used effectively to close the wound.

Bioactive human dermal tissue capable of interacting with the wound bed is available commercially for use in pressure and neuropathic ulcer wound management.

These skin substitutes derived from living human tissue (human fibroblasts) represent an important advance in the treatment of burns and skin ulcers, including neuropathic foot ulcers, venous ulcers, and pressure ulcers. See "Skin Transplantation" in Chapter 21.

PROGNOSIS. Most clients have multiple complicating medical factors that contribute to poor wound closure. Each client responds differently to a course of therapy. Provided there is no infection, there is a good blood supply, the pressure has been eliminated or redistributed, and the client is not malnourished and has no medical complications, the wound should heal successfully. The presence of any of these factors alters the prognosis negatively.

Evolve Box 10-1 on the Evolve website presents a bibliography of selected references about pressure ulcers. Refer to this box for more in-depth information about pressure ulcers.

SPECIAL IMPLICATIONS FOR THE THERAPIST `10-17`

Pressure Ulcers

> **Note to Reader:** For a free continuing education course (2 contact hours) on Pressure Ulcer Prevention, go to http://edu.medbiopub.com. Instructions for accessing this program are provided on the Elsevier website in Evolve Box 10-2.

The therapist plays a pivotal role in the prevention and management of pressure ulcers. Not only is the therapist an expert in the delivery of therapeutic modalities, but also sharp debridement; appropriate dressing selection; education of patient, caregiver, and staff; appropriate positioning; management of tissue load (mechanical factors acting on the tissues); and good mobility which are essential to the success of the intervention.

High-risk clients should be identified using the Braden Scale (see Fig. 10-30), but all clients in the health care delivery system should be evaluated for risk levels and reassessed at least every month for changes in status (or when there is a change in medical status).

Anyone with a history of previous pressure ulcer is considered high risk requiring a prevention protocol immediately. Acute care clients should be reassessed daily, on transfer to another unit/floor, and with changes in medical status.

The high-risk client will need frequent position changes, at least every 2 hours in bed, and at least every hour while sitting, every 15 minutes if the client can move himself or herself. Utilizing all turning surfaces, position the client at a 35-degree oblique angle when side-lying (Fig. 10-35).

Elevate the head of the bed to no greater than 30 degrees when the client is supine (Fig. 10-36); if the head of the bed is elevated beyond 30 degrees (e.g., for eating, watching television, nursing care, or therapy intervention), the duration of this position needs to be limited to minimize both pressure and shear forces. A trapeze bar, turning sheet, or transfer board can be used to prevent shearing injury to the skin during movement or position change. Frequent shifting of body weight prevents ischemia by redistributing the weight and allowing blood to recirculate.

Static or dynamic pressure-redistribution devices using air, gel or water, foam, or other substances are commercially available, but the therapist must be aware that the material covering these devices can also create heat and friction contributing to pressure. Redistributing pressure on the skin must be accompanied by adequate fluid and nutrition intake (see also Box 10-13). Doughnut cushions never should be used, because they can cause tissue ischemia and new pressure ulcers.

The person who is incontinent presents an additional challenge to keeping the skin clean and dry. Stool or urine becomes an irritant and places the person at additional risk for skin breakdown. Contamination of an already existing wound by wound drainage, perspiration, urine, or feces is also a concern for the incontinent and immobile population.

Fecal containment products, both external and internal, are available for use in the case of acute diarrhea or fecal incontinence (see previous discussion of Incontinence-Associated Dermatitis in this chapter) when these conditions contribute to the development of ulcers. New products for urinary or fecal incontinence are available to help prevent skin maceration from backflow of urine or feces. These include skin barriers, ointments, and fecal incontinence systems.

Cleaning should be carried out using a mild agent that minimizes irritation and dryness of the skin. Avoid soaps, alcohol-based products that can cause vasoconstriction, tincture of benzoin (may cause painful erosions), and hexachlorophene (may irritate the central nervous system). During cleaning or wound care, the force and friction applied to the skin should be minimized. Ideal is the use of a disposable, no-rinse, perineal cloth that is impregnated with a barrier ingredient.

Anyone performing PLWS (see Fig. 10-29) must be aware of the potential for aerosolization of microorganisms from a wound during this intervention. Therapists and others in the room during PLWS should wear appropriate personal protective equipment to limit contact with infectious agents. To prevent possible exposure of other clients, PLWS should be performed in a private room or in a treatment room with walls and doors that close, not curtains.[102]

In 2004 and 2005, the FDA and CDC made recommendations for infection control that included the aforementioned plus cover any exposed supplies or client items in the room, cover any open areas not being treated (tubes, ports, etc.), consider masking the patient, observe Standard Precautions, dispose of disposables in appropriate waste stream, discard suction canister or liner after each treatment, do not reuse single-use-only items, and after treatment disinfect thoroughly all environmental surfaces.[48,111]

Concerns that high-pressure (output pressure of 70 psi) lavage may disseminate contaminants to surrounding tissues have not been substantiated. Until further research establishes safe levels of irrigation pressure in wound cleansing, therapists are advised to use the AHCPR guideline of irrigation pressures between 4 and 15 psi.[106] All wound management PLWS products provide a psi of 15 or less.

Note to Reader: Most therapists understand that the use of whirlpool for wound management is nearly obsolete and used on a very limited basis with select/appropriate patients. But to aid in "getting the word out," so to speak, we have asked Dr. Loehne to comment on this changing practice in our profession. Please also refer to her chapter on PLWS vs. WP.

(Loehne HB: In Sussman C, Bates-Jensen BM, eds: *Wound care: A collaborative practice manual for health professionals*, ed 4, Philadelphia, 2012, Lippincott, Williams and Wilkins.)

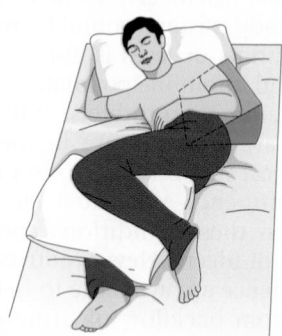

Figure 10-35

Following the "rule of 30s" (head of bed at ≤30 degrees; see Fig. 10-36, bed positioning should include side-lying with 30 degrees lateral inclined position to either side. (Pressure Ulcer Prevention Points©. Courtesy National Pressure Ulcer Advisory Panel, 2007.)

Pigmentary Disorders

Definition and Overview

Skin color or pigmentation is determined by the deposition of melanin, a dark polymer found in the skin, as well as in the hair, ciliary body, choroid of the eye, pigment layer of the retina, and certain nerve cells.

Melanin is formed in the melanocytes in the basal layer of the epidermis and is regulated (dispersion and aggregation) through the release of melatonin, a pineal hormone.

Hyperpigmentation is the abnormally increased pigmentation resulting from increased melanin production. *Hypopigmentation* is the abnormally decreased pigmentation resulting from decreased melanin production.

Pigmentary disorders (either hyperpigmentation or hypopigmentation) may be primary or secondary. Secondary pigmentary changes occur as a result of damage to the skin, such as irritation, allergy, infection, excoriation, burns, or dermatologic therapy, such as curettage, dermabrasion, chemical peels, or freezing with liquid nitrogen.

Etiologic and Risk Factors

The formation and deposition of melanin can be affected by external influences such as exposure to heat, trauma, solar or ionizing radiation, heavy metals, and changes in oxygen potential. These influences can result in hyperpigmentation, hypopigmentation, or both. Local trauma may destroy melanocytes temporarily or permanently, causing hypopigmentation, sometimes with hyperpigmentation in surrounding skin.

Other pigmentary disorders may occur from exposure to exogenous pigments, such as carotene, certain metals, and tattooing inks. Carotenemia occurs as a result of excessive carotene in the blood, usually from ingesting certain foods (e.g., carrots, yellow fruit, egg yolk). It may also occur in diabetes mellitus and in hypothyroidism. Exposure to metals such as silver can cause argyria, a poisoning marked by a permanent ashen grey discoloration of the skin, conjunctivae, and internal organs. Gold, when given long term for rheumatoid arthritis, can also cause pigmentary changes.

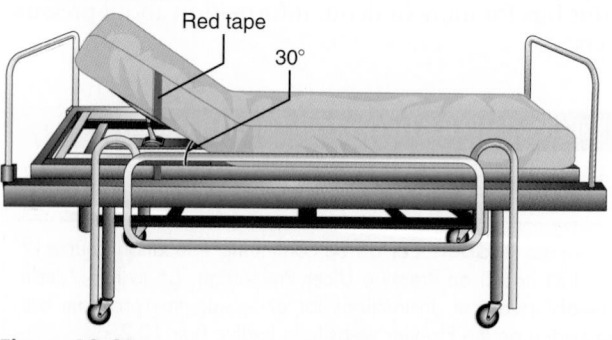

Figure 10-36

Head of bed at 30 degrees. Using a goniometer to determine a 30-degree angle, the therapist can mark the bed frame and raised headboard with colored tape to signify maximum inclination for pressure ulcer prevention. Client, family, and staff education and cooperation are vitally important and remain key intervention strategies. (Courtesy Anthony Stabler, Byron Health Center, Fort Wayne, IN. National Pressure Ulcer Advisory Panel, 2000.)

A THERAPIST'S THOUGHTS*
Pulsed Lavage with Suction (PLWS) Versus Whirlpool (WP)

For many years, physical therapists "treated" wounds by placing patients or their body parts in whirlpools (WPs), changing dressings, and returning them to their rooms or to home. It quickly became obvious that we needed to learn how to *manage* wounds, and that included not only appropriate dressings, sharp debridement, and other interventions, but also appropriate irrigation. When pulsed lavage with suction (PLWS) was developed, it provided the answer we needed for irrigation, and also a method of debridement.

With WPs, there is no way to know the pounds per square inch (psi) of the water against the wound. Treatment of tunnels, tracts, and undermining is not possible. There is no debridement taking place. Periwound maceration can occur. Often other open areas are in the water, increasing the risk for cross-over contamination/infection. Anyone with venous insufficiency should not have extremities placed in a dependent position in warm water, which is required if WP is used. A moist environment is contraindicated for nonnecrotic neuropathic and noninfected arterial wounds. Individuals who are unresponsive, have cardiopulmonary compromise, fever above a certain degree, and/or are incontinent, should not be placed in a full body WP. There actually are no references indicating the efficacy of WPs for wounds. The WP can be thought of as a glorified, very expensive, bath.

With PLWS, the PSI is between 4 and 15 (a known variable), and irrigation is usually with normal saline, making the treatment safe and efficacious. Numerous pulsatile tips are available for different wound contours. With a long, flexible tip, tunnels, tracts, and undermining can be treated effectively. An extra benefit is the ease of sharp debridement by the PT following PLWS, especially with the small splash shield, with hydration of the necrotic tissue. Granulation is not destroyed. There is no maceration of periwound tissue. Personal protective equipment is important for infection prevention because of aerosolization. Strict infection control policies must be adhered to; these are the same for treatment with either WP or PLWS.

As there are no known contraindications, those individuals with diagnoses and situations mentioned above can be treated with PLWS without difficulty. In addition, those for whom a WP is inaccessible or not optimal (even if it were an adequate treatment), can be treated with PLWS. Bedside treatment is an option and possible for individuals with contractures, ostomies, recently closed surgical incisions, IVs, skeletal traction, casted extremities, and morbid obesity exceeding the weight limit of stretchers/WP. Anyone who is combative/restrained, and those who are in ICU, IMCU, Burn Unit, or Isolation also can be treated bedside.

There are advantages with the use of PLWS, because of its ability to be used bedside. The patient does not have to be transferred to a stretcher and transported to the PT Department, placed in a WP, back on a stretcher and returned to his/her room—all with increased risk of pressure ulcers and decrease in comfort and safety. When the affected individual can be treated by the PT, there are cost savings because additional time and expenses incurred (e.g., operating room, physician, and staff) are saved. With PLWS rather than WP there is a cost savings with the elimination of WPs and thus water and maintenance, including staff time. Cross contamination is eliminated, reducing infection risks. For the PT the treatment is convenient, there is minimal clean-up, resulting in increased efficiency and increased productivity. For the facility there is a decreased length of stay because of the rapid rate of granulation and epithelialization with treatment with PLWS.

*Harriett B. Loehne, PT, DPT, CWS, FACCWS

Clinical Manifestations

Hyperpigmentation. Primary disorders in the hyperpigmentation category include pigmented nevi, mongolian spots, juvenile freckles (ephelides), lentigines (also called *liver spots*) from sun exposure, café au lait spots associated with neurofibromatosis, and hypermelanosis caused by increased melanocyte-stimulating hormone (e.g., Addison disease).

Secondary hyperpigmentation most commonly occurs after another dermatologic condition, such as acne (e.g., postinflammatory hyperpigmentation seen in darkskinned people). *Melasma*, a patterned hyperpigmentation of the face, can occur as a result of steroid hormones, estrogens, and progesterones, such as occurs during pregnancy and in 30% to 50% of women taking oral contraceptives. Secondary hyperpigmentation may also develop as a phototoxic reaction to medications, oils in perfumes, and chemicals in the rinds of limes, other citrus fruits, and celery.

Hypopigmentation and Depigmentation. The disorder most commonly seen by a therapist in the hypopigmentation/depigmentation category is vitiligo. Vitiligo is a common skin disorder affecting approximately 0.5% of the general population.[178] Melanocytes are destroyed resulting in small or large circumscribed areas of depigmentation often having hyperpigmented borders and enlarging

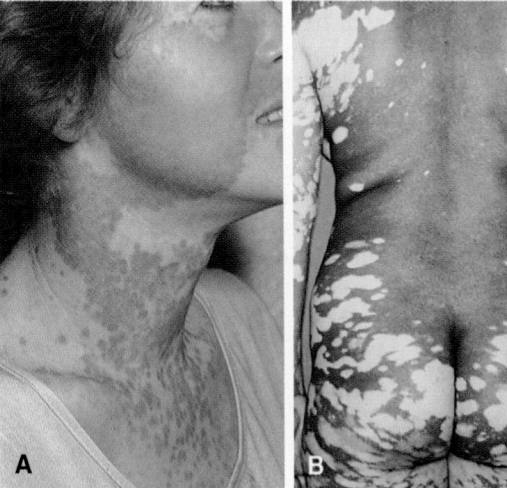

Figure 10-37

Vitiligo is a term derived from the Greek word for "calf," used to describe patches of light skin caused by loss of epidermal melanocytes. **A,** Note the patchy loss of pigment on the face, trunk, and axilla. **B,** This condition can affect any part of the face, hands, or body and can be very disfiguring, especially in dark-skinned individuals. (From Swartz MH: *Textbook of physical diagnosis,* ed 6, Philadelphia, 2009, Saunders.)

slowly (Fig. 10-37). The specifics of the etiopathogenic mechanisms are still poorly understood.[178] This condition may be associated with hyperthyroidism, hypothyroidism, pernicious anemia, diabetes mellitus, Addison disease, and carcinoma of the stomach. A quick summary of management of vitiligo is available online at http://www.medscape.org/viewarticle/769005?src=cmemp.

Hypopigmentation can also occur on African American skin from the use of liquid nitrogen. Intraarticular injections of high concentrations of corticosteroids may also cause localized temporary hypopigmentation.

Blistering Diseases

Definition, Incidence, and Etiologic Factors

On occasion, blistering diseases may be seen in a therapy practice when severe enough to warrant localized treatment intervention (wound management). Blisters occur on skin and mucous membranes in a condition called *pemphigus*, which is an uncommon intraepidermal blistering disease in which the epidermal cells separate from one another. This disease occurs almost exclusively in middle-aged or older adults of all races and ethnic groups.

The exact cause of blistering diseases is unknown, but they may occur as a secondary event associated with viral or bacterial infections of the skin (e.g., herpes simplex, impetigo) or local injury of the skin (e.g., burns, ischemia, dermatitis), or they may be drug induced (e.g., penicillamine, captopril). In other diseases, blistering of the skin occurs as a primary autoimmune event characterized by the presence of autoantibodies directed against specific adhesion molecules of the skin and mucous membranes.[53]

Paraneoplastic pemphigus, an autoantibody-mediated mucocutaneous disease associated with underlying neoplasm, is a syndrome that has a distinct clinical and histologic presentation. This form of pemphigus has a poor prognosis because of the underlying malignancy.

Clinical Manifestations

Blistering diseases are characterized by the formation of flaccid bullae, or blisters. These bullae appear spontaneously, often on the oral mucous membranes or scalp, and are relatively asymptomatic. Erosions and crusts may develop over the blisters, causing toxemia and a mousy odor. The lesions become extensive, and the complications of the disease, especially infection, can lead to great toxicity and debility. Disturbances of electrolyte balance are also common because of fluid losses through the involved skin in severe cases. See "Fluid and Electrolyte Balance" in Chapter 5.

MEDICAL MANAGEMENT

Medical management may include hospitalization (bed rest, IV antibiotics and feedings) when the disease is severe. For others, treatment may be with corticosteroids (e.g., prednisone) and local measures. The course of this disorder tends to be chronic in most people, and high-dose corticosteroids can mask the signs and symptoms of infection. If untreated, this condition is usually fatal within 2 months to 5 years as a result of infection. In the case of paraneoplastic pemphigus, early diagnosis and treatment of the underlying neoplasm are imperative.

Cutaneous Sarcoidosis

Sarcoidosis is a multisystemic disorder characterized by the formation of granulomas, inflammatory lesions containing mononuclear phagocytes usually surrounded by a rim of lymphocytes. These granulomas may develop in the lungs, liver, bones, or eyes (see Box 15-10) and may be accompanied by skin lesions (see Fig. 15-21).

Subcutaneous nodules around the knee and elbow joints may occur in association with pulmonary or cardiac involvement and resolve in response to systemic corticosteroids. In the United States, sarcoidosis occurs predominantly among African Americans, affecting twice as many women as men. Acute sarcoidosis usually resolves within 2 years. Chronic, progressive sarcoidosis, which is uncommon, is associated with pulmonary fibrosis and progressive pulmonary disability. See Chapter 15 for a complete discussion of this condition.

REFERENCES

To enhance this text and add value for the reader, all references are included on the companion Evolve site that accompanies this text book. The reader can view the reference source and access it online whenever possible.

CHAPTER 11

The Endocrine and Metabolic Systems

CATHERINE CAVALLARO GOODMAN • GINA PARISER

ENDOCRINE SYSTEM

The endocrine system is composed of various glands located throughout the body (Fig. 11-1). These glands are capable of synthesis and release of special chemical messengers called *hormones*, which are transported by the bloodstream to the cells and organs on which they have a specific regulatory effect (Table 11-1). The endocrine system and the nervous system control and integrate body function to maintain homeostasis. Whereas the nervous system sends its messages along nerve fibers, eliciting swift and selective neural responses, the endocrine system sends its messages in the form of hormones via the bloodstream.

Hormonal effects have a slower onset than neural effects, but they maintain a longer duration of action. The actions of the endocrine system may be localized to one area or generalized to all the cells of the body.[188] The endocrine system has the following five general functions:
1. Differentiation of the reproductive and central nervous system of the developing fetus.
2. Stimulation of sequential growth and development during childhood and adolescence.
3. Coordination of the male and female reproductive systems.
4. Maintenance of optimal internal environment throughout the life span.
5. Initiation of corrective and adaptive responses when emergency demands occur.[190]

The endocrine system meets the nervous system at the hypothalamic–pituitary interface. The hypothalamus, the main integrative center for the endocrine and autonomic nervous systems, controls the function of endocrine organs by neural and hormonal pathways. Although the communicative and integrative roles of the endocrine and nervous systems are similar, the precise ways in which each system functions differ.

Hypothalamic Control

Neural pathways connect the hypothalamus to the posterior pituitary (or neurohypophysis), providing the hypothalamus direct control over both the anterior and posterior portions of the pituitary gland (Fig. 11-2). Disorders of the hypothalamic–pituitary axis are manifested clinically, usually either by syndromes of hormone excess or deficiency or by visual impairment from optic nerve compression because of the location of the hypothalamus and pituitary.

Neural stimulation to the posterior pituitary provokes the secretion of two effector hormones: antidiuretic hormone (ADH) and oxytocin. The hypothalamus also exerts hormonal control at the anterior pituitary through releasing and inhibiting factors. Hypothalamic hormones stimulate the pituitary to release tropic (stimulating) hormones, such as adrenocorticotropic hormone (ACTH), thyroid-stimulating hormone (TSH), luteinizing hormone (LH), and follicle-stimulating hormone (FSH) (see Fig. 11-2). At the same time, effector hormones, such as growth hormone (GH) and prolactin, are released or inhibited, affecting the adrenal cortex, thyroid, and gonads. Endocrine pathology develops as a result of dysfunction of releasing, tropic, or effector hormones or when defects occur in the target tissue.

In addition to hormonal and neural controls, a negative feedback system regulates the endocrine system. The mechanism may be simple or complex. Simple feedback occurs when the level of one substance regulates the secretion of a hormone. For example, low serum calcium levels stimulate parathyroid hormone (PTH) secretion; high serum calcium levels inhibit it. Complex feedback loops occur through the hypothalamic–pituitary–target organ axis. For example, after an injury or major stress, secretion of the hypothalamic corticotropin-releasing hormone (CRH) releases pituitary ACTH, which in turn stimulates adrenal cortisol secretion. Subsequently, a rise in serum cortisol inhibits ACTH by decreasing CRH secretion (see Fig. 11-2).[328]

Steroid therapy disrupts the hypothalamic–pituitary–adrenal (HPA) axis by suppressing hypothalamic–pituitary secretion. Such treatment is necessary for some conditions but problems can occur when there is too rapid or abrupt of a withdrawal of exogenous steroid. The result can be life-threatening adrenal insufficiency, because the HPA axis does not have enough time to recover sufficiently to stimulate cortisol secretion.

Hormonal Effects

In response to the hypothalamus, the *posterior pituitary* secretes oxytocin and ADH. Oxytocin stimulates contraction of the uterus and is responsible for the milk letdown

471

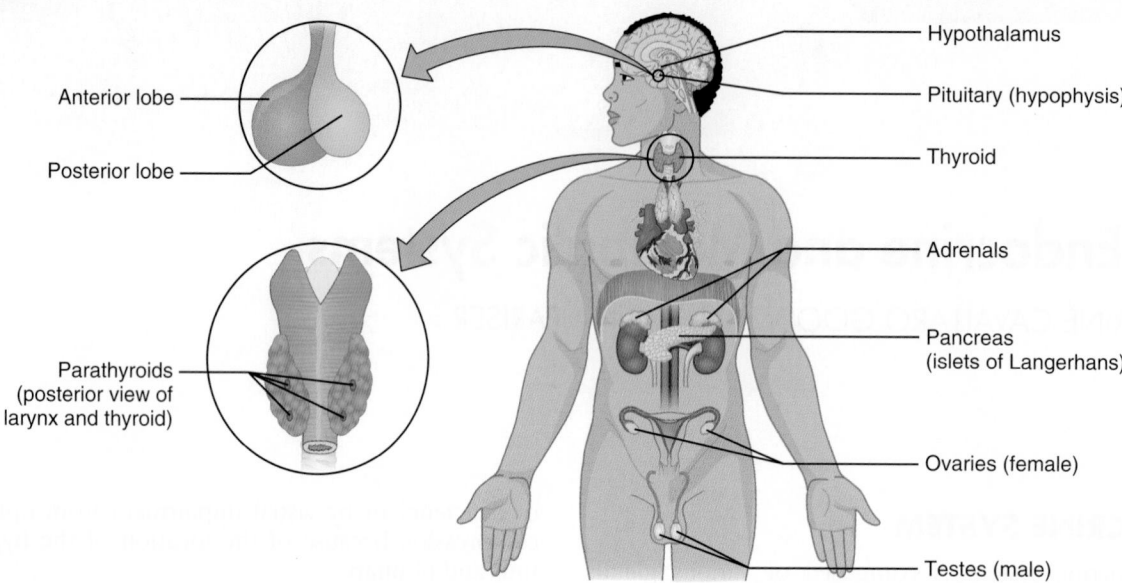

Figure 11-1

Endocrine glands; adipose not shown.

Table 11-1	Endocrine Glands: Secretion, Target, and Action		
Gland	**Hormone**	**Target**	**Basic Action**
Pineal	Melatonin	Melanocyte	Antioxidant, causes drowsiness, helps regulate sleep–wake cycle
Pituitary			
Anterior lobe	Somatotropin (growth hormone [GH])	Bones, muscles, organs	Stimulates growth and cell reproduction, releases insulin-like growth factor 1 from liver, retention of nitrogen to promote protein anabolism
	Thyroid-stimulating hormone (TSH)	Thyroid	Promotes secretory activity (T_3 and T_4)
	Follicle-stimulating hormone (FSH)	Ovaries, seminiferous tubules	Promotes development of ovarian follicle, secretion of estrogen (females), and maturation of sperm (males)
	Luteinizing hormone	Follicle, intestinal cell	Promotes ovulation and formation of corpus luteum, secretion of progesterone, and secretion of testosterone
	Prolactin (PRL; luteotropic hormone)	Corpus luteum, breast	Maintains corpus luteum and progesterone secretion; stimulates milk production; sexual gratification after sexual activity
	Adrenocorticotropic hormone (ACTH)	Adrenal cortex	Stimulates secretory activity, synthesis of corticosteroids
	Lipotropin (LPH)	Corticotropes (cells in anterior pituitary)	Breaks down fat (lipolysis); stimulates melanin production
	Melanocyte-stimulating hormone (MSH)	Melanotrope (cells in anterior pituitary)	Produces melanin in skin and hair
Posterior lobe	Antidiuretic hormone (ADH; vasopressin)	Distal tubules of kidney	Reabsorption of water (retention in kidneys), vasoconstriction, release ACTH in anterior pituitary
	Oxytocin (OXT)	Uterus	Stimulates contraction (cervix, vagina, orgasm), releases breast milk, regulates circadian rhythm (body temperature, sleep–wake cycle, activity level)
Thyroid	Thyroxine (T4) and Triiodothyronine (T3)	Widespread (heart, muscle, liver)	Regulate oxidation of body cells and growth metabolism, influence gluconeogenesis, mobilization of fats, and exchange of water, electrolytes, and protein synthesis, increase basal metabolic rate and sensitivity to catecholamines
	Calcitonin	Skeleton	Calcium and phosphorus metabolism; construct bone, reduce serum calcium

Table 11-1 Endocrine Glands: Secretion, Target, and Action—cont'd

Gland	Hormone	Target	Basic Action
Parathyroids	Parathyroid hormone (PTH)	Bone, kidney, intestinal tract	Essential for calcium and phosphorus metabolism and calcification of bone
Adrenal			
Cortex	Mineralocorticoids (aldosterone)	Widespread, primarily kidney	Maintains fluid/electrolyte balance; reabsorbs sodium chloride; secretes potassium
	Glucocorticoids (cortisol)	Widespread	Concerned with food metabolism and body response to stress; preserves carbohydrates and mobilizes amino acids; promotes gluconeogenesis; suppresses inflammation and immune function
	Sex hormone (testosterone, estrogen, progesterone)	Gonads	Ability to influence secondary sex characteristics
Medulla	Epinephrine (adrenaline)	Widespread	Fight-or-flight response[98]; cardiac; myocardial stimulation, increase heart rate, dysrhythmias; vasoconstriction with increased blood pressure; increased blood glucose via glycolysis; stimulates ACTH production
	Norepinephrine	Widespread	Vasoconstriction; other effects similar to epinephrine (see above)
Pancreas	Insulin	Widespread	Increased utilization of carbohydrate, decreased blood glucose
	Glucagon	Widespread	Hyperglycemic factor; increases blood glucose via glycogenolysis
	Amylin	Pancreatic beta cells	Slows down gastric emptying, inhibits digestive function and food intake
Gonads			
Ovaries	Estrogen	Widespread	Secondary sex characteristic; maturation and sexual function; multiple other functions affecting muscle, blood vessels, bone, platelets and coagulation, GI function, lung function
	Progesterone	Uterus, breast	Preparation for and maintenance of pregnancy
Testes	Testosterone (androgen)	Widespread	Secondary sex characteristics; maturation and normal sex function
Ovaries/Testes	Inhibin	Anterior pituitary	Inhibits production of FSH
Adipose tissue	Adiponectin leptin (LEP) Angiotensin	Widespread	Controls metabolism, hunger, and vasoconstriction

When considering each patient/client's current health and pathology and when reading lab values, it is important to know basic hormone functions or effects that may have an impact on therapy treatment. Over 50 different hormones have been identified, but only those most common to therapy clients are included here.

reflex in lactating women. ADH controls the concentration of body fluids by alteration of the permeability of the kidney's distal convoluted tubules and collecting ducts to conserve water. The secretion of ADH depends on plasma volume and osmolality as monitored by hypothalamic neurons. Circulatory shock and severe hemorrhage are the most powerful stimulators of ADH; other stimulators include pain, emotional stress, trauma, morphine, tranquilizers, certain anesthetics, and positive-pressure breathing.

The *anterior pituitary* secretes prolactin, which stimulates milk production, and human GH (HGH), which affects most body tissues. HGH stimulates growth by increasing protein synthesis and fat mobilization and by decreasing carbohydrate utilization. Hyposecretion of HGH results in dwarfism; hypersecretion causes gigantism in children and acromegaly in adults.

The *thyroid gland* secretes the iodinated thyroid hormones thyroxine (T_4) and triiodothyronine (T_3). (For reference values of thyroid hormone levels mentioned throughout this chapter, see Table 40-20.) Thyroid hormones, necessary for normal growth and development, act on many tissues to regulate our basal metabolism (i.e., the rate at which we convert food and oxygen into energy) and to increase metabolic activity and protein synthesis. T_4 is more abundant in the bloodstream than T_3, but T_3 is more active in directing the production of proteins vital to cell function.

Thyroid hormones influence renal development, kidney structure, renal hemodynamics, GFR, the function of many transport systems along the nephron, and sodium and water homeostasis. These effects of thyroid hormone are in part due to direct renal actions and in part are mediated by cardiovascular and systemic hemodynamic effects that influence kidney function. As a consequence, individuals with hypothyroidism or hyperthyroidism may experience clinically important alterations in kidney function.[182]

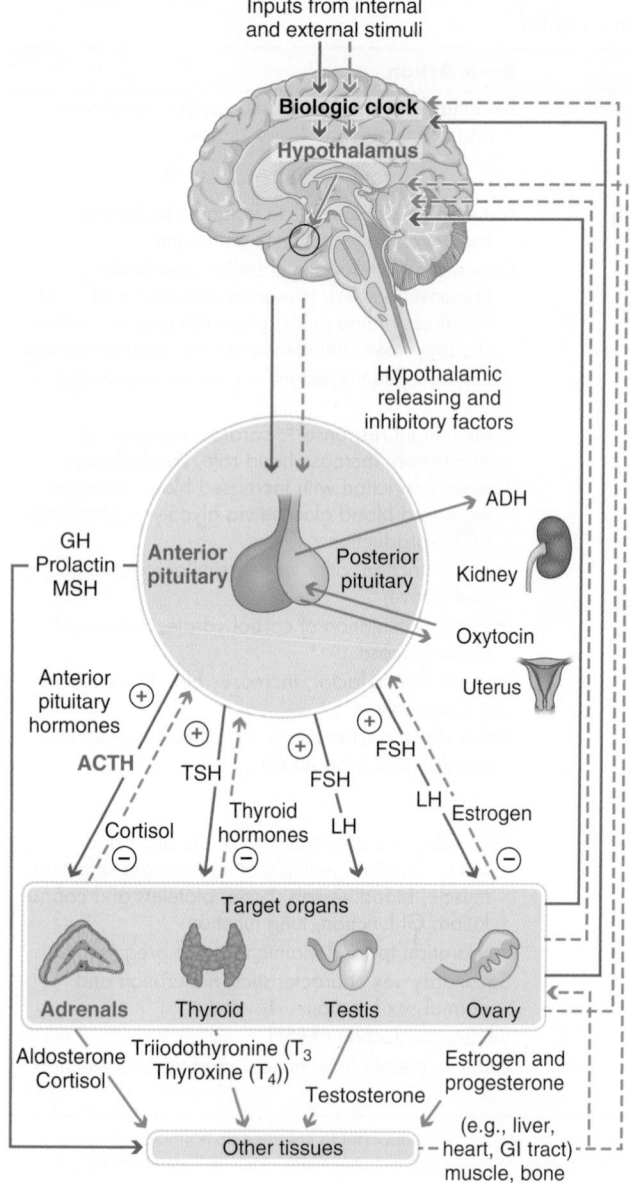

Inputs from internal
and external stimuli

Biologic clock

Hypothalamus

Hypothalamic
releasing and
inhibitory factors

GH
Prolactin
MSH

**Anterior
pituitary**

Posterior
pituitary

ADH

Kidney

Oxytocin

Uterus

Anterior
pituitary
hormones

(+)

ACTH

Cortisol

(+)

TSH

Thyroid
hormones

(−)

(+)

FSH

LH

(−)

(+)

FSH

LH

Estrogen

(−)

Target organs

Adrenals   **Thyroid**   **Testis**   **Ovary**

Aldosterone
Cortisol

Triiodothyronine (T₃)
Thyroxine (T₄))

Testosterone

Estrogen and
progesterone

(e.g., liver,
heart, GI tract)
muscle, bone

Other tissues

Excitatory responses +   Inhibitory responses −

Figure 11-2

Control of the endocrine system by the nervous system. One example
of the complex feedback loops described in the text is highlighted here.
The hypothalamus controls the pituitary gland through releasing and
inhibiting factors. The anterior lobe of the pituitary gland then releases
tropic (stimulating) hormones that act on target glands (thyroid, adrenals, gonads). Endocrine pathology occurs when dysfunction occurs in
releasing, tropic, or effector hormones, or when defects occur in the
target tissue.

Deficiency of thyroid hormone causes varying degrees
of hypothyroidism, from a mild, clinically insignificant
form to the life-threatening extreme, myxedema coma.
Congenital hypothyroidism causes a condition in children previously referred to as *cretinism* (now considered
an undesirable term).

Hypersecretion of thyroid hormone causes hyperthyroidism and in extreme cases, thyrotoxic crisis. Excessive
secretion of TSH from the pituitary gland causes thyroid

gland hyperplasia, resulting in goiter in chronic iodine
deficiency states. Other causes of goiter are discussed in
this chapter (see "Thyroid Gland" below).

The *parathyroid glands* secrete PTH, which regulates
calcium and phosphate metabolism. PTH elevates serum
calcium levels by stimulating resorption of calcium and
phosphate from bone, reabsorption of calcium and excretion of phosphate by the kidneys, and by combined
action with vitamin D, absorption of calcium and phosphate from the gastrointestinal (GI) tract.

Hyperparathyroidism results in hypercalcemia; hypoparathyroidism causes hypocalcemia. Altered calcium
levels also may result from nonendocrine causes such as
metastatic bone disease. Pathologic changes in calcium
affecting bone bring these conditions to the therapist's
attention.

The *endocrine pancreas* produces glucagon from the
alpha cells and insulin from the beta cells. Glucagon,
the hormone of the fasting state, releases stored glucose
to raise the blood glucose level. Insulin, the hormone
of the nourished state, facilitates glucose transport, promotes glucose storage, stimulates protein synthesis, and
enhances free fatty acid uptake and storage. Insulin deficiency causes diabetes mellitus (DM); insulin excess can
be exogenous (i.e., a person with diabetes may receive
more insulin than is required) or insulin excess may result
from a tumor of the beta cells called *insulinoma*. Whatever
the cause of excess insulin, hypoglycemia (abnormally
low level of glucose in the blood) is the result.

The *adrenal cortex* secretes mineralocorticoids, glucocorticoids, and sex steroids. Aldosterone, a mineralocorticoid, regulates the reabsorption of sodium and the
excretion of potassium by the kidneys and is involved
intimately in the regulation of blood pressure. An excess
of aldosterone (aldosteronism) can result primarily from
hyperplasia or from adrenal adenoma or secondarily
from many conditions, such as congestive heart failure or
cirrhosis. The *adrenal medulla* is an aggregate of nervous
tissue that produces the catecholamines epinephrine and
norepinephrine, which are involved in the fight-or-flight
response. (See "Neuroendocrine Response to Stress"
below.)

The *testes* and *ovaries* are also endocrine glands responsible for synthesizing and secreting hormones (see Chapters 19 and 20).

Adipose tissue can be classified as an endocrine gland
because it secretes several hormones responsible for
metabolism, hunger, vasoconstriction, and cellular
growth and development. The concept of adipose tissue
as an endocrine organ is quite new, but it is clear that
molecules secreted into the bloodstream by fat, such as
adiponectin and leptin, act on target organs at distant
sites (see "Adipose Tissue" below).

Endocrine Pathology

Dysfunctions of the endocrine system are classified as
hypofunction and hyperfunction. The source of hypofunction and hyperfunction may be inflammation or
tumor originating in the hypothalamus, the pituitary
gland, or in other endocrine glands. Inflammation may
be acute or subacute but is usually chronic, which results

Functions Affected	Physiologic Effects
Protein metabolism	Increases protein synthesis in the liver and depresses protein synthesis in muscle, lymphoid tissue, adipose tissue, skin, and bone; increases plasma level of amino acids
Carbohydrate and lipid metabolism	Diminishes peripheral uptake and utilization of glucose; increases output of glucose from the liver; enhances the elevation of blood glucose promoted by other hormones
Lipid metabolism	Breakdown of fat in the extremities (lipolysis) and produces/deposits fat in the face and trunk (lipogenesis)
Inflammatory effects	Decreases circulating eosinophils, lymphocytes, and monocytes; increases release of polymorphonuclear leukocytes from the bone marrow; decreases accumulation of leukocytes at the site of inflammation; delays healing; essential for vasoconstrictive action of norepinephrine
Digestive function	Promotes gastric secretion
Urinary function	Enhances urinary excretion
Connective tissue function	Decreases proliferation of fibroblasts in connective tissue (and thus delays healing)
Muscle function	Maintains normal contractility and maximal work output for skeletal and cardiac muscle
Bone function	Decreases bone formation
Vascular system and myocardial function	Maintains normal blood pressure; permits increased responsiveness of arterioles to the constrictive action of adrenergic stimulation; optimizes myocardial performance
Central nervous system function	Modulates perceptual and emotional functioning (mechanism unknown); essential for normal arousal and initiation of activity

Table 11-2 Physiologic Effects of Cortisol

in glandular hypofunction. Chronic endocrine abnormalities (e.g., deficiencies of cortisol, thyroid hormone, or insulin) are common health problems requiring lifelong hormone replacement for survival. Rarely, some endocrine gland tumors result in ectopic hormone production and may affect the musculoskeletal system.

Ectopic hormone production is the production and secretion of hormone or hormone-like substances from a source other than the normal source of the hormone. For example, some endocrine gland tumors can metastasize and produce excess hormone from new tumor sites (e.g., some types of thyroid, parathyroid, and adrenal cancers). Some nonendocrine cancers, particularly certain lung cancers, can secrete ACTH and GH. (See Chapter 9 for a discussion of paraneoplastic syndromes associated with this phenomenon.)

Neuroendocrine Response to Stress

The concept that stress of any kind (emotional, physical, psychological, or spiritual) may influence immunity and resistance to disease has been the foundation for psychoneuroimmunology for many years. The endocrine system, together with the immune system and the nervous system, mounts an integrated response to stressors; this is the subject of many past and current studies. Only a brief review of the neuroendocrine response to stress contributing to disease is presented in this section.

Hormones of the neuroendocrine system affect components of the immune system,[61] and mediators produced by immune components regulate the neuroendocrine response. The sympathetic nervous system is aroused during the stress response and causes the medulla of the adrenal gland to release catecholamines, such as epinephrine, norepinephrine, and dopamine, into the bloodstream. Simultaneously, the pituitary gland releases a variety of hormones, including ADH (from the posterior pituitary gland), prolactin, GH, and ACTH from the anterior pituitary gland.

Catecholamines

Catecholamines are organic compounds that play an important role in the body's physiologic response to stress. Their release at sympathetic nerve endings increases the rate and force of muscular contraction of the heart, thereby increasing cardiac output; constricts peripheral blood vessels, resulting in elevated blood pressure; elevates blood glucose levels by hepatic and skeletal glycogenolysis; and promotes an increase in blood lipids by increasing the catabolism (breakdown) of fats.

Glycogenesis is the splitting of glycogen, a starch stored primarily in the liver but also in the muscles, yielding glucose. The well-known metabolic effects of adrenal catecholamines prepare the body to take physical action in the fight-or-flight phenomenon. Stressors commonly associated with catecholamine release include exercise, thermal changes, and acute emotional states.

Cortisol

Cortisol is the principal glucocorticoid hormone released from the adrenal cortex and also known as *hydrocortisone* when synthesized pharmaceutically. Cortisol has multiple functions (Table 11-2), but it primarily regulates the metabolism of proteins, carbohydrates, and lipids to cause an elevation in blood glucose level. These effects on glucose level and fat metabolism result in increased blood glucose and plasma lipid levels and promote the formation of ketone bodies when insulin secretion is insufficient.

Cortisol is essential to norepinephrine-induced vasoconstriction and other physiologic phenomena necessary for survival under stress. The production of glucose promoted by cortisol provides a source of energy for body tissues (nerve cells in particular), and the pooling of amino acids from catabolized proteins may ensure amino acid availability for protein synthesis at sites where replacement is critical, such as muscle or cells of damaged tissue.

Another effect of cortisol is that of dampening the body's inflammatory response to invasion by foreign agents. This antiinflammatory protective mechanism helps preserve the integrity of body cells at the site of the inflammatory response and provides the basis for the major therapeutic use of this steroid. Cortisol also inhibits fibroblast proliferation and function at the site of an inflammatory response and accounts for the poor wound healing, increased susceptibility to infection, and decreased inflammatory response often seen in individuals with chronic glucocorticoid excess. Whether cortisol-induced effects are adaptive or destructive depends on the subsequent concentration and length of cortisol exposure.

Other Hormones

Other hormones, such as endorphins, GH, prolactin, and testosterone, may be released as part of the response to stressful stimuli. *Endorphins*, a term derived from *endogenous* and *morphine*, are a group of opiate-like peptides produced naturally by the body at neural synapses in the central nervous system. These hormones serve to modulate the transmission of pain perceptions by raising the pain threshold and producing sedation and euphoria.

As its name implies, *growth hormone* stimulates and controls the rate of skeletal and visceral growth by directly influencing protein, carbohydrate, and lipid metabolism. GH levels increase in the blood after a variety of physically or psychologically stressful stimuli such as surgery, fever, physical exercise, or the anticipation of exhausting exercise, cardiac catheterization, electroshock therapy, or gastroscopy.[183]

Prolactin stimulates the growth of breast tissue and sustains milk production in postpartum mammals. Prolactin levels in plasma increase with a variety of stressful stimuli, including such procedures as gastroscopy, proctoscopy, pelvic examination, and surgery, but they show little change after exercise. *Testosterone*, a hormone that regulates male secondary sex characteristics and sex drive (libido), decreases after stressful stimuli such as anesthesia, surgery, marathon running, and acute illness (e.g., respiratory failure, burns, or congestive heart failure). Decreased testosterone during these circumstances restrains growth and reproduction to preserve energy for protective responses.[183]

Aging and the Endocrine System[87,142]

The exact effects of aging on the endocrine system are not clear. In particular, the question of whether changes in endocrine function are a cause of aging or a natural consequence of aging remains unresolved. The endocrine system has not been implicated as the direct cause of aging. Coexisting age-related variables, such as acute and chronic nonendocrine disease, use of medications, alterations in diet, changes in body composition and weight, and changes in sleep–wake cycle affecting the endocrine system, confuse the picture. New analytical tools to evaluate the neuroregulation of the endocrine axes are predicted to yield important information in the next decade.

Age-associated declines in physiologic performance of the endocrine system are well documented, and it is accepted that the basis of this decline is a *failure of homeostasis*. The conventional view is that "normal" aging changes predispose to age-related disease and contribute

to the poor recovery of aging adults after illness or severe stresses such as surgery. Equilibrium concentrations of the principal hormones necessary to maintain homeostasis are not necessarily altered with age, but what may differ as we get older is the way we achieve equilibrium hormone levels, which points to changes in regulatory control.

Collectively, available clinical data suggest a general model of early neuroendocrine aging in the human (both males and females) with variable but predictable disruption in the time-delayed feedback and feedforward interconnections among neuroendocrine glands.[309] Thus with advancing age, significant alterations in hormone production, metabolism, and action are found.

The continuum of the age-related changes is highly variable and sex-dependent. Whereas only subtle changes occur in the pituitary, adrenal, and thyroid function, changes in glucose homeostasis, reproductive function, and calcium metabolism are more apparent. The role of the thyroid gland in the metabolism of the healthy older person remains unclear. No major defects are apparent in healthy individuals; however, during episodes of ill health, the thyroid's ability to maintain homeostasis is often limited.[87]

Aging is associated with a higher incidence of disorders or diseases of the endocrine system, including type 2 DM, hypothyroidism, and an increased incidence of atypical endocrine diseases during later life. Cellular damage associated with aging, genetically programmed cell change, and chronic wear and tear may contribute to endocrine gland dysfunction or alterations in responsiveness of target organs (as a result of changes with aging and disease, the target organs may lose their ability to respond to hormones).

Other endocrine changes that may be associated with aging and especially contribute to the age-associated failure in homeostasis include the *neuroendocrine theory of aging*. This theory attempts to explain the altered biologic activity of hormones, altered circulating levels of hormones, altered secretory responses of endocrine glands, altered metabolism of hormones, and loss of circadian control of hormone release. These changes are postulated to occur as a result of a genetic program encoded in the brain and then controlled and relayed to peripheral tissues through hormonal and neural agents.[190] This theory suggests that cells are programmed to function only for a given time.

Menopause as a result of programmed changes in the reproductive system is an example of this theory. Changes in the neuroendocrine system because of the loss of ovarian function at menopause have an important biologic role for women in the control of reproductive and nonreproductive functions and regulate mood, memory, cognition, behavior, immune function, the locomotor system, and cardiovascular functions.[241] It is thought that the temporal patterns of neural signals are altered during middle age, leading to cessation of reproductive cycles, and that the complex interplay of ovarian and hypothalamic/pituitary pacemakers becomes increasingly dysfunctional with aging, ultimately resulting in menopause.[241]

The relationship between aging and the structure and function of the endocrine system cannot be separated from the changes in the immune system and the central nervous system (CNS). Evidence is increasing in support of an immune–neuroendocrine homeostatic network in humans with the thymus gland playing a key role in the immunoregulation of the nervous and endocrine systems. The early onset of thymus involution may act as a triggering event that initiates the gradual decline in endocrine homeostasis, resulting in the aging process.[110]

Additionally, as the nervous system ages, a progressive reduction takes place in the body's capacity to maintain homeostasis in the face of environmental stress. The overall effect of the changes in aging in the neuroendocrine system is a progressive resistance to the inhibitory feedback of the end-organ hormonal secretion (see Fig. 11-2). Thus, although the initial response to a stressful stimulus may be appropriate, as the body ages, the response is more likely to be persistent and ultimately inappropriate or even harmful.[71]

Anatomic Changes with Aging

The *pituitary gland* undergoes both anatomic and histologic changes associated with aging. By age 80 years, the weight of the anterior pituitary lobe (adenohypophysis) is reduced approximately 75% from its peak during young adulthood. The blood supply is reduced, and a higher incidence of adenomas and cysts is described during later life.

The *thyroid gland* becomes relatively smaller and fibrotic, and its position becomes lower-lying and retrosternal with age. As with the pituitary gland, blood supply to the thyroid gland is decreased. Secretion of thyroid hormones may diminish with age.

The *parathyroid gland* demonstrates tissue changes with advancing age, but no major change is apparent in PTH levels. Hyperparathyroidism occurs primarily in persons older than 50 years and most commonly results from a single adenoma. It occasionally occurs with multiple adenomas or hyperplasia of two or more parathyroid glands. It is rarely caused by parathyroid carcinoma.

The *adrenal glands* have more fibrous tissue with aging, but because of compensatory feedback mechanisms, no relative alteration is apparent in functional cortisol levels. The most common cause of hypercortisolism occurs with the use of corticosteroids for medical conditions. As previously mentioned, because steroid use can suppress the pituitary–adrenal axis, adrenal insufficiency can occur after discontinuation of steroid therapy.

Changes in the *reproductive glands* have been shown clearly to have physiologic effects, most notably on the cardiovascular system and the skeleton (ovary) and muscle mass and libido (testis).[217] These effects are discussed elsewhere (see Chapters 19, 20, and 24).

Hormonal Changes with Aging

The female reproductive system undergoes changes as part of the normal aging process. Menopause leads to changes in the genitourinary tract and accelerates the loss of minerals from bone and leads to an alteration in the lipid composition in the mature woman. Male hormones have been linked to preservation of bone and muscle mass and to an increased tendency toward developing certain diseases (e.g., benign prostatic hypertrophy or liver disease) during later life.

Loss of body hair, changes in the skin's collagen content and thickness, an increase in the percentage of body fat, a decrease in lean body mass, a decrease in bone mass, and a decrease in protein synthesis are signs of endocrinopathy that may be associated with decreased GH levels.[142] With the decline of GH secretion, sleep cycles are disrupted, and the potential for sequelae associated with sleep deprivation (e.g., depression, fibromyalgia) is now recognized.[306]

As mentioned, interactions between the endocrine and immune systems also influence the aging process. Declining hormonal levels are accompanied by increased activity of tumor-suppressor genes in the aging population unless these genes have been mutated so that suppressor function is lost. In fact, the most common somatic mutation of human cancers is the loss of tumor suppressor genes as a result of exposures to a lifetime of mutagens. In the presence of decreased hormonal levels, loss of tumor suppressor genes accounts for the increased probability of tumors with advancing age, again demonstrating the link between the endocrine and immune systems.[142]

All of these changes have an increasing effect on humans because the average life span has increased, meaning a greater part of women's lives will be lived in an hypoestrogenic state. Men and women alike will experience a decline in GH secretion, increased exposure to mutagens, and a greater possibility of the loss of tumor suppressor genes.[241]

Musculoskeletal Signs and Symptoms of Endocrine Disease

Signs and symptoms of endocrine pathology vary, depending on the gland affected and whether the pathology is as a result of an excess (hyperfunction) or insufficiency (hypofunction) of hormonal secretions.[107] In a therapy setting, the most common signs and symptoms associated with endocrine pathology observed in the musculoskeletal system are presented here.

Growth and development of connective tissue structures are influenced strongly and sometimes controlled by various hormones and metabolic processes. When these processes are altered, structural and functional changes can occur in various connective tissues, producing musculoskeletal signs and symptoms in addition to other systemic signs and symptoms of endocrine dysfunction (Table 11-3).

The therapist must be aware that clients with an underlying but undiagnosed endocrine disorder may present initially with a musculoskeletal problem and that clients with established endocrine disorders are not cured by hormonal replacement or suppression. Rather, they may develop progression of musculoskeletal impairment in response to hormone fluctuations.

Rheumatoid arthritis can be an indicator of an underlying endocrine disease. Early rheumatic symptoms, such as myalgias and arthralgias, are seen commonly with a number of endocrine diseases. DM is associated with a variety of rheumatic syndromes such as the stiff-hand syndrome and limited joint motion syndrome. Although rheumatic symptoms can appear suddenly in people with an endocrine disorder, an insidious onset is much more common.

Table 11-3	Signs and Symptoms of Endocrine Dysfunction
Neuromusculoskeletal	**Systemic**
Rheumatic-like signs and symptoms	Excessive or delayed growth
Muscle weakness	Polydipsia
Muscle atrophy	Polyuria
Myalgia	Mental changes (nervousness, confusion, depression)
Fatigue	Changes in hair (quality and distribution)
Carpal tunnel syndrome	
Synovial fluid changes	Changes in skin pigmentation
Periarthritis	Changes in distribution of body fat
Adhesive capsulitis (diabetes mellitus)	Changes in vital signs (elevated body temperature, pulse rate, increased blood pressure)
Chondrocalcinosis	
Spondyloarthropathy	
Diffuse idiopathic skeletal hyperostosis (DISH)	Heart palpitations
	Increased perspiration
Osteoarthritis	Kussmaul respirations (deep, rapid breathing)
Osteoporosis	
Osteonecrosis	Dehydration or excessive retention of body water
Hand stiffness	
Arthralgia	
Pseudogout	

Muscle weakness, atrophy, myalgia, and *fatigue* that persist despite rest may be early manifestations of thyroid or parathyroid disease, acromegaly, diabetes, Cushing syndrome, or osteomalacia. In endocrine disease, most proximal muscle weakness is usually painless and may be unrelated to either the severity or the duration of the underlying disease. However, when true demonstrative weakness occurs (particularly in hyperthyroidism and hyperparathyroid disease), proximal muscle weakness is related to the severity and duration of the underlying endocrine problem. Any compromise of muscle energy metabolism aggravates and perpetuates trigger points such as are associated with myofascial pain syndrome (see Chapter 27) or tender points in muscle associated with fibromyalgia syndrome (see Chapter 7).

Carpal tunnel syndrome (CTS) (see discussion in Chapter 39) resulting from median nerve impairment at the wrist is a common finding in people with certain endocrine and metabolic conditions such as acromegaly, diabetes, pregnancy, and hypothyroidism (see Table 39-5). Any increase in the volume of contents of the carpal tunnel impinges on the median nerve (e.g., neoplasm, calcium, gouty tophi deposits, edema, or tenosynovitis).

In endocrine disorders, CTS is frequently bilateral, which is one characteristic that may distinguish it from overuse syndromes and other causes of CTS. Unreported tarsal tunnel syndrome may also occur, another distinguishing characteristic of an underlying systemic origin of symptoms when present along with CTS.

Tenosynovitis (inflammation of the tendon sheaths) occurs with some infectious processes and many musculoskeletal conditions. Fluid infiltrating the tunnel may soften the transverse carpal ligament, which can make the bony arch flatten and compress the nerve.[105] Thickening of the transverse carpal ligament also may occur with systemic disorders such as acromegaly or myxedema.

CTS in persons with diabetes represents one form of diabetic neuropathy caused by ischemia-related microvascular damage of the median nerve. This ischemia then causes increased sensitivity to even minor pressure exerted in the carpal tunnel area.[132] Vitamin B_6 deficiency, repetitive activities, and obesity may also be factors in the development of CTS for the person with diabetes.[4,75]

CTS occurring during pregnancy may be caused by extra fluid and/or fat, diabetes (gestational or previously diagnosed), vitamin deficiencies, or other causes unrelated to the pregnancy itself (e.g., rheumatoid arthritis or job-related biomechanical stress). The fact that many women develop CTS at or near menopause may suggest that the soft tissues about the wrist may be affected in some way by hormones.[51]

Periarthritis (inflammation of periarticular structures including the tendons, ligaments, and joint capsule) and *calcific tendinitis* occur most often in the shoulders of people who have endocrine disease. *Chondrocalcinosis* is the deposition of calcium salts in the joint cartilage; when accompanied by attacks of gout-like symptoms, it is called *pseudogout*. In 5% to 10% of people with chondrocalcinosis, an associated underlying endocrine or metabolic disease occurs such as hypothyroidism, hyperparathyroidism, or acromegaly.[94] People diagnosed with fibromyalgia also may have altered thyroid function[175] and present with shoulder impingement secondary to chondrocalcinosis (see "Fibromyalgia" in Chapter 7).

Spondyloarthropathy (disease of joints of the spine) and *osteoarthritis* occur in individuals with various endocrine or metabolic diseases, including hemochromatosis (disorder of iron metabolism with excess deposition in the tissues; also known as *bronze diabetes* and *iron storage disease*), ochronosis (metabolic disorder caused by alkali deposits, resulting in discoloration of body tissues), acromegaly, and DM.

Hand stiffness, hand pain, and arthralgias of the small joints of the hand may occur with endocrine and metabolic diseases. Flexor tenosynovitis with stiffness is a common finding in persons with hypothyroidism. This condition often accompanies CTS.[173]

SPECIAL IMPLICATIONS FOR THE THERAPIST   11-1

Overview of Endocrine and Metabolic Disease

Disorders of the endocrine and metabolic systems may present with recognizable clinical signs and symptoms (see Table 11-3). Clients with a variety of endocrine and metabolic disorders report symptoms of fatigue, muscle weakness, and occasionally, muscle or bone pain. Painless muscle weakness associated with endocrine and metabolic disorders usually involves proximal muscle groups. This muscle weakness and other symptoms, such as periarthritis and calcific tendinitis, may respond to treatment of the underlying endocrine pathology.

In most cases, the person who has received a diagnosis of an endocrine or metabolic disorder has undergone a combination of clinical and laboratory tests. This person may be in the care of a therapist for some other unrelated musculoskeletal problem that can be affected by symptoms associated with hormone imbalances.

Other clinical presentations of musculoskeletal symptoms, such as CTS, rheumatoid arthritis, or adhesive capsulitis, may be referred to the therapist without accurate diagnosis of the underlying endocrine pathology. The therapist always must remain alert to the client's report of systemic signs and symptoms (usually a constellation of symptoms, rather than an isolated few) preceding, accompanying, or developing along with the current musculoskeletal problems.

Additionally, the lack of progress in therapy should signal to the therapist the possibility of a systemic origin of musculoskeletal symptoms. Failure to recognize a metabolic cause of symptoms may result in prolonged, ineffective therapy; visits to a variety of therapists; and occasionally, one or more unsuccessful surgical procedures.

Any client who is taking diuretics must be monitored for signs or symptoms of potassium depletion or fluid dehydration (see Chapter 5) before initiating exercise and then throughout the duration of exercise. Cortisol suppresses the body's inflammatory response, masking early signs of infection. Any unexplained fever without other symptoms in the immunocompromised client must be reported to the physician.

SPECIFIC ENDOCRINE DISORDERS

Pituitary Gland

The pituitary gland, or hypophysis, is a small (1 cm in diameter), oval gland located at the base of the skull in an indentation of the sphenoid bone directly posterior to the sphenoid sinus (see Figs. 11-1 and 11-2). It is often referred to as the *master gland* because of its role in regulating other endocrine glands. It is joined to the hypothalamus by the pituitary stalk (neurohypophyseal tract) and is influenced by the hypothalamus through releasing and inhibiting factors. The pituitary consists of two parts: the anterior pituitary (adenohypophysis) and the posterior pituitary (neurohypophysis) lobes. The anterior pituitary secretes six different hormones (ACTH, TSH, LH, FSH, HGH, and prolactin) (see Fig. 11-2).

The posterior pituitary is a downward offshoot of the hypothalamus and contains many nerve fibers; it produces no hormones of its own. The hormones ADH (also called *vasopressin*) and oxytocin are produced in the hypothalamus and then stored and released by the posterior pituitary. These hormones pass down nerve fibers from the hypothalamus through the pituitary stalk to nerve endings in the posterior pituitary; they accumulate in the posterior pituitary during less active periods of the body. Transmitter substances, such as acetylcholine and norepinephrine, are thought to activate release of these substances by the posterior pituitary gland when they are stimulated by nerve impulses from the hypothalamus.[183]

Anterior Lobe Disorders

Disorders of the pituitary gland occur most frequently in the anterior lobe, most often caused by tumors, pituitary infarction, genetic disorders, and trauma. The three principal pathologic consequences of pituitary disorders are hyperpituitarism, hypopituitarism, and local compression of brain tissue by expanding tumor masses.[27]

Hyperpituitarism

Overview. Hyperpituitarism is an oversecretion of one or more of the hormones secreted by the pituitary gland, especially GH, resulting in acromegaly or gigantism. It is caused primarily by a hormone-secreting pituitary tumor, typically a benign adenoma. Other syndromes associated with hyperpituitarism include Cushing disease, amenorrhea, and hyperthyroidism.

Cushing disease is one form of Cushing syndrome and results from oversecretion of ACTH by a pituitary tumor, which in turn results in oversecretion of adrenocortical hormones (see "Cushing Syndrome" below). Pituitary tumors produce both systemic effects and local manifestations.

Systemic effects include the following:

1. Excessive or abnormal growth patterns, resulting from overproduction of growth hormone.
2. Hyperprolactinemia (increased prolactin secretion), resulting in amenorrhea, galactorrhea (spontaneous milk flow in women without nursing), and gynecomastia and impotence in men.
3. Overstimulation of one or more of the target glands, resulting in the release of excessive adrenocortical, thyroid, or sex hormones.

Local pituitary tumors produce symptoms as the growing mass expands within the bony cranium. Local manifestations may include visual field abnormalities (pressure on the optic chiasma where the optic nerve crosses over), headaches, and somnolence (sleepiness).

Gigantism and Acromegaly. Gigantism, an overgrowth of the long bones, and acromegaly, increased bone thickness and hypertrophy of the soft tissues, result from GH-secreting adenomas of the anterior pituitary gland. Although GH-producing tumors that cause these conditions are rare, they are the second most common type of hyperpituitarism. Gigantism develops in children before the age when the epiphyses of the bones close; people who develop gigantism may grow to a height of 9 feet. Gigantism develops abruptly, whereas acromegaly develops slowly.

Acromegaly is a disease of adults and develops after closure of the epiphyses; the bones most affected are those of the face, jaw, hands, and feet. In adults, acromegaly occurs equally among men and women and usually between ages 30 and 50 years.[27] Both conditions are characterized by the same skeletal abnormalities because hypersecretion of GH produces cartilaginous and connective tissue overgrowth, resulting in coarsened facial features; protrusion of the jaw (prognathism); thickened ears, nose, and tongue; and broad hands, with spade-like fingers (Fig. 11-3).

In gigantism, as the tumor enlarges and invades normal tissue, target organ functions are impaired by the loss of other tropic (stimulating) hormones such as TSH, LH, FSH, and ACTH. Clients with acromegaly may experience local manifestations, such as headache, diplopia, blindness, and lethargy, as the tumor compresses brain tissue.

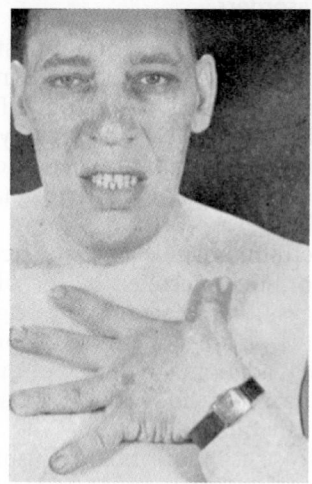

Figure 11-3

Acromegaly (hyperpituitarism). Acromegaly occurs as a result of excessive secretion of growth hormone after normal completion of body growth. The resulting overgrowth of bone in the face, head, and hands is pictured here. (From Jarvis C: *Physical examination and health assessment*, Philadelphia, 1992, WB Saunders.)

Acromegaly-induced myopathy with muscle weakness and reduced exercise tolerance may be more common than previously appreciated. The pathologic or physiologic reason for this weakness has not been determined. Alterations in muscle size and strength in individuals with acromegaly are an accepted association and may be multifactorial in origin. It could be the result of a combination of the direct effects of growth hormone on muscle, the metabolic and mechanical neuropathies present with the condition, the mechanical disadvantage occurring as a result of joint hypermobility, or restriction caused by articular changes and periarticular bone remodeling.[193]

MEDICAL MANAGEMENT

DIAGNOSIS, TREATMENT, AND PROGNOSIS. Increased mortality is linked with elevated GH and/or the target growth factor called insulin-like growth factor I (IGF-I).[82] Timely diagnosis and appropriate treatment are imperative in reducing this potentially disabling chronic and progressive condition.[82] Uncontrolled GH and IGF-I may accelerate the rate of bone turnover; in a small number of people, this long-term exposure may predispose the individual to malignant bone tumor.[169] Long-term follow-up of disease activity and comorbidities is recommended, with management rather than cure being the primary goal.[81] Quality of life is often below reference values for the normal population of the same age.[318] Diagnosis is established by documenting autonomous GH hypersecretion and by imaging of the pituitary gland. Pituitary tumors are treated usually by surgical removal, drug therapy, and/or external beam radiation therapy.

Drugs are now available that effectively normalize levels of growth hormone and prolactin and decrease pituitary tumor size.[81] Drug therapy has replaced surgery in most cases of prolactin-secreting adenomas, but surgery is still the treatment of choice for pituitary adenomas that cause acromegaly.

Some drug or radiation therapy may be required if levels of GH remain high after surgery. Radiation therapy is also useful when surgery is not curative.[210] Frequently, after pituitary surgery, pituitary function is lost and at that time, treatment with thyroid, cortisone, and hormone replacement may be necessary.

SPECIAL IMPLICATIONS FOR THE THERAPIST	11-2

Hyperpituitarism
Postoperative Care

Ambulation and exercise are encouraged within the first 24 hours after surgery. Coughing, sneezing, and blowing the nose are contraindicated after surgery, but deep breathing exercises are encouraged. Postoperatively, vital signs and neurologic status must be closely monitored. Any alteration in level of consciousness or visual acuity, falling pulse rate, or rising blood pressure may signal an increase in intracranial pressure resulting from intracranial bleeding or cerebral edema and must be reported immediately. Observe for signs of meningitis (e.g., severe headache, irritability, or nuchal [back of the neck] rigidity), a potential complication of surgery.

The nursing staff members monitor blood glucose levels often because GH levels fall rapidly after surgery, removing an insulin-antagonist effect in many people and possibly precipitating hypoglycemia (low blood glucose level). The therapist is advised to consult with nursing staff to determine the possible need for blood glucose monitoring during or after exercise. The therapist should be familiar with signs and symptoms and special implications of hypoglycemia (see "Hypoglycemia" below).

Tumors causing visual changes may require the therapist to consciously remain within the client's visual field. Unexpected mood changes can occur, requiring patience and understanding on the part of health care workers. Although surgical removal of the tumor and/or pituitary gland prevents permanent soft tissue deformities, bone changes already present do not change.

Orthopedic Considerations

Skeletal manifestations, such as arthritis of the hands and osteoarthritis of the spine, may develop with these conditions. Osteophyte formation and widening of the joint space as a result of increased cartilage thickening may be seen on x-rays. In late-stage disease, joint spaces become narrowed, and chondrocalcinosis occasionally may be present. CTS is seen in up to 50% of people with acromegaly and is thought to be caused by intrinsic and extrinsic factors (e.g., compression of the median nerve at the wrist from soft tissue hypertrophy, bony overgrowth, and hypertrophy of the median nerve).[194]

About half of individuals with acromegaly have thoracic and/or lumbar back pain. X-ray studies demonstrate increased intervertebral disk spaces and large osteophytes along the anterior longitudinal ligament. The therapist may be called on to provide a program that promotes maximum joint mobility, muscle strength, and functional skills. Assistance with activities of daily living may be an important aspect of intervention. Home health staff should assess the home to remove any obstacles and recommend necessary adaptive equipment or assistive devices.

Acromegaly

Anyone with acromegaly should be screened for weakness, changes in joint mobility, and poor exercise tolerance. Skeletal abnormalities associated with acromegaly are usually irreversible. Joint symptoms are controlled with aggressive medical intervention with surgery, pharmacologic treatment, and in some cases, pituitary irradiation trying to normalize hormonal levels. Improvement of joint pain, crepitus, and range of motion has been reported with the newer somatostatin analogues (drug therapy).[297] The role of physical therapy intervention in acromegaly has not been documented or validated.

Medical evaluation is necessary to rule out systemic causes of muscle weakness such as diabetes or thyroid or adrenal disorders. The therapist should refer clients with acromegaly who exhibit unusual muscle weakness for a complete workup for neuropathies and inflammatory myopathies to rule out any underlying causes that can be treated. Individuals with diabetes who have persistently elevated serum creatine kinase levels should be evaluated for acromegaly.[193]

Hypopituitarism

Hypopituitarism (also *panhypopituitarism* and *dwarfism*) results from decreased or absent hormonal secretion by the anterior pituitary gland. Panhypopituitarism refers to a generalized condition caused by partial or total failure of all six of the anterior pituitary's vital hormones (ACTH, TSH, LH, FSH, HGH, and prolactin).

Hypopituitarism and panhypopituitarism are rare disorders that occur as a result of the following:
1. Hypophysectomy (removal or destruction of the pituitary by surgery, irradiation, or chemical agents).
2. Nonsecreting pituitary tumors.
3. Postpartum hemorrhage (the fall in blood pressure and subsequent hypoxia after delivery causes necrosis of the gland).
4. Reversible functional disorders (such as starvation, anorexia nervosa, severe anemia, and GI tract disorders).

Clinical manifestations are dependent on the age at onset and the hormones affected (Box 11-1). More than 75% of the pituitary must be obliterated by tumors or thromboses before symptoms develop. Specific disorders resulting from pituitary hyposecretion include *GH deficiency*, with subsequent short stature, delayed growth, and delayed puberty; *secondary adrenocortical insufficiency* from diminished synthesis of ACTH by the pituitary gland, which in turn causes diminished secretion of adrenocortical hormones by the adrenal cortex; *hypothyroidism* (thyroid hormone is dependent on TSH secreted by the pituitary); and *sexual and reproductive disorders* from deficiencies of the gonadotropins (LH and FSH).

Box 11-1

CLINICAL MANIFESTATIONS OF HYPOPITUITARISM

Growth hormone deficiency
- Short stature
- Delayed growth
- Delayed puberty

Adrenocortical insufficiency
- Hypoglycemia
- Anorexia
- Nausea
- Abdominal pain
- Orthostatic hypotension

Hypothyroidism (see also Table 11-6)
- Fatigue
- Lethargy
- Sensitivity to cold
- Menstrual disturbances

Gonadal failure
- Secondary amenorrhea
- Impotence
- Infertility
- Decreased libido
- Absent secondary sex characteristics (children)

Neurologic signs (produced by tumors)
- Headache
- Bilateral temporal hemianopia
- Loss of visual acuity
- Blindness

Treatment for hypopituitarism involves removal (if possible) of the causative factor, such as tumors, and lifetime replacement of the missing hormones.

SPECIAL IMPLICATIONS FOR THE THERAPIST 11-3

Hypopituitarism

Although rarely encountered in a therapy setting, the client with hypopituitarism may report symptoms associated with hormonal deficiencies until hormone replacement therapy is complete. The therapist may observe weakness, fatigue, lethargy, apathy, and orthostatic hypotension (see "Special Implications for the Therapist 12-8: Orthostatic Hypotension" in Chapter 12). Nail beds and skin may demonstrate pallor associated with anemia (see "Special Implications for the Therapist 14-5: The Anemias" in Chapter 14).

Infection prevention requires meticulous skin care following the guidelines outlined in Box 12-14. Impaired peripheral vision associated with bilateral hemianopia (blindness in half of the visual field) requires special consideration. The therapist must be certain to stand where the affected individual can see others and to move slowly in and out of the client's visual field.

CAUSES OF DIABETES INSIPIDUS

- Intracranial or pituitary neoplasm
- Metastatic lesions (e.g., breast or lung cancer)
- Surgical hypophysectomy or other neurosurgery
- Skull fracture or head trauma (damages the neurohypophyseal structures)
- Infection (e.g., meningitis, encephalitis)
- Granulomatous disease
- Vascular lesions (e.g., aneurysm)
- Idiopathic
- Anorexia
- Autoimmune; heredity
- Drugs or medications (causing nephrogenic diabetes insipidus)
  - Lithium (most common)
  - Alcohol
  - Amphotericin B
  - Foscarnet
  - Aminoglycosides
  - Some chemotherapeutic agents

Data from pharmacotherapy update: Tisdale JE, Miller DA, eds: *Drug-induced diseases*, ed 2, Bethesda, MD, 2010, American Society of Health-System Pharmacists.

Posterior Lobe Disorders

Diabetes Insipidus. Diabetes insipidus, a rare disorder, involves a physiologic imbalance of water secondary to ADH deficiency or inaction. Injury or loss of function of the hypothalamus, the neurohypophyseal tract, or the posterior pituitary gland can result in diabetes insipidus (Box 11-2).

Because the major functions of ADH are to promote water resorption by the kidney and to control the osmotic pressure of the extracellular fluid, when ADH production decreases, the kidney tubules fail to resorb water. The end result is excretion of large amounts of dilute urine. Unlike urine in DM, which contains large amounts of glucose, urine in diabetes insipidus is dilute and contains no glucose. Other clinical manifestations include polydipsia (excessive thirst), nocturia (excessive urination at night), and dehydration (e.g., poor tissue turgor, dry mucous membranes, constipation, muscle weakness, dizziness, and hypotension) (see Box 5-8). Fatigue and irritability may develop secondary to sleep disruption and in association with nocturia.

If a person is conscious and able to respond appropriately to the thirst mechanism, hydration can be maintained. However, if a person is unconscious or confused and unable to take in necessary fluids to compensate for fluid loss, rapid dehydration, shock, and death can occur. Treatment is usually exogenous replacement of ADH with vasopressin or a synthetic derivative, such as Pitressin, along with administration of diuretics. When this condition is caused by tumor, resection of the tumor can effect a cure.

SPECIAL IMPLICATIONS FOR THE THERAPIST   11-4

Diabetes Insipidus

The therapist must be alert for possible serious side effects of any type of ADH administration. ADH stimulates smooth muscle contraction of the vascular system (causing increased blood pressure), the GI tract (causing diarrhea), and the coronary arteries (causing angina or myocardial infarction).[132]

Increases in blood pressure can cause additional serious problems in some people, particularly those with hypertension or coronary artery disease (CAD) and cerebrovascular disease. Additionally, after receiving vasopressin, clients must be assessed for signs and symptoms of water intoxication, which can lead to fluid overload (pulmonary crackles), cerebral edema, and seizures. (See also "Special Implications for the Therapist 5-10: Fluid Imbalances" and "Special Implications for the Therapist 5-11: Electrolyte Imbalances" in Chapter 5.)

Syndrome of Inappropriate Antidiuretic Hormone Secretion. Syndrome of inappropriate ADH (SIADH) is a disorder associated with excessive release of ADH, which disturbs fluid and electrolyte balance, resulting in a water imbalance. SIADH has a wide variety of causes, including pituitary damage resulting from infection or trauma, but the most common cause is ectopic ADH production by malignancies (e.g., oat-cell lung, pancreatic, brain, or prostate cancer; Hodgkin disease; thymoma).[248]

Tumors can cause unregulated production of ADH leading to severe hyponatremia (sodium depletion, less than 115 mEq/L) with resultant lethargy, nausea, anorexia, and generalized weakness. Mild hyponatremia (125-130 mEq/L) causes increased thirst, muscle cramps, and lethargy. Rapid onset of SIADH can result in coma, convulsions, or death.[293] SIADH can be triggered by the stress of surgery or many systemic disorders and response to certain medications, including chemotherapy medications such as vincristine and cyclophosphamide[230,293] (Box 11-3).

SIADH is the opposite of diabetes insipidus, so treatment of diabetes insipidus with vasopressin can lead to SIADH if excessive amounts are administered. In SIADH, instead of large fluid losses, water intoxication occurs as a result of fluid retention. Under normal circumstances, ADH regulates serum osmolality. Serum osmolality is a measure of the number of dissolved particles per unit of water in serum. In a solution, the fewer the particles of solute in proportion to the number of units of water (solvent), the less concentrated the solution. A low serum osmolality indicates a higher-than-usual amount of water in relation to the amount of particles dissolved in it.

In other words, serum osmolality provides a measure of hydration of cells. For example, a low serum osmolality accompanies overhydration (i.e., edema); an increased serum osmolality is present in a state of fluid volume deficit. Osmolality is proportional with dilutional or depletional states (true for water and sodium). The normal value for serum osmolality is 280 to 300 mOsm/kg of water.[47] When serum osmolality falls, a feedback mechanism causes inhibition of ADH, which promotes increased water excretion by the kidneys to raise serum

Box 11-3

CAUSES OF SYNDROME OF INAPPROPRIATE ANTIDIURETIC HORMONE SECRETION (SIADH)*

- Oat cell carcinoma (accounts for 80% of cases)
- Pulmonary disorders
  - Pneumonia
  - Tuberculosis
  - Lung abscess
  - Mechanical ventilation (e.g., positive pressure)
- Central nervous system disorders
  - Brain tumor or abscess
  - Cerebrovascular accident
  - Head injury
  - Guillain-Barré syndrome
  - Systemic lupus erythematosus
- Other neoplasms (e.g., pancreatic or prostatic cancer, Hodgkin disease, thymoma)
- Infection
- Stress (e.g., surgery) or trauma
- Medications with the strongest association with SIADH:
  - Selective serotonin reuptake inhibitors (SSRIs)
  - Serotonin-norepinephrine reuptake inhibitors
  - Chemotherapeutic agents (e.g., vinca alkaloids, cisplatin, cyclophosphamide)
  - Carbamazepine
  - Oxcarbazepine
- Myxedema
- Psychosis
- Porphyria

*Listed in descending order.

Data from pharmacotherapy update: Tisdale JE, Miller DA, eds: *Drug-induced diseases*, ed 2, Bethesda, MD, 2010, American Society of Health-System Pharmacists.

osmolality to normal. When this feedback mechanism fails and ADH levels are sustained, fluid retention results. Ultimately, serum sodium levels fall, resulting in hyponatremia and water intoxication.[132]

Although fluid retention is the primary symptom, edema is rare unless water overload exceeds 4 L; much of the free water excess is within cellular boundaries. Neurologic and neuromuscular signs and symptoms predominate and are directly related to the swelling of brain tissue and to sodium changes within neuromuscular tissues. CNS dysfunction, characterized by alterations in level of consciousness, seizures, and coma, can occur when serum sodium falls to 120 mEq/L or less. Hyponatremia can result in diminished GI function; this problem is complicated further by the need for fluid restriction.

Correction of life-threatening sodium imbalance is the first aim of treatment followed by correction of the underlying cause. If SIADH is caused by malignancy, success in alleviating water retention may be obtained by surgical resection, irradiation, or chemotherapy. Otherwise, treatment for SIADH is symptomatic and includes restriction of water intake, careful replacement of sodium chloride, and administration of diuretics. Other pharmaceuticals (e.g., demeclocycline and

tetracycline or lithium) also may be used to block the renal response to ADH.

SPECIAL IMPLICATIONS FOR THE THERAPIST   11-5

Syndrome of Inappropriate Antidiuretic Hormone Secretion

Anyone at risk for SIADH (see conditions listed in Box 11-3) should be monitored for sudden weight gain or fluid retention and changes in urination and fluid intake. Monitoring vital signs, oxygen saturation, and cardiac rhythm are important.

Throughout therapy, the client's cardiovascular status should be assessed regularly so that any unusual alterations can be noted immediately. (See also "Special Implications for the Therapist 5-10: Fluid Imbalances" in Chapter 5.) Observe for headache, lethargy, muscle cramps, restlessness, altered mental status, irritability, convulsions, or weight gain without visible edema (≥2 lb a day).

Continued need for sodium and fluid restrictions may be necessary for the person discharged to home or who is in a facility other than the acute care setting (hospital). People with unresolved SIADH should avoid the use of aspirin or nonsteroidal antiinflammatory agents (NSAIDs) without a physician's approval because these drugs can increase hyponatremia.

The role of the physical therapist has not been clearly defined for people with this condition. Clients with mild or moderate SIADH may benefit from physical therapy for intervention to improve mobility and prevent deconditioning, which can lead to further functional improvement and quality of life. Each individual must be evaluated individually to determine the most appropriate plan of care, ranging from bed mobility and transfers to range of motion to a program of strengthening and conditioning.[293]

In the acute care setting, fluid restrictions must be noted and followed. This may require some coordination and scheduling for anyone who may need water in association with his or her exercise program. Individuals on fluid restriction must also be monitored for urinary output. Physical therapists should coordinate with nursing staff to monitor fluid intake and output.[293] Any change in mental status, motor coordination, or energy level should be recorded and reported for consideration by the medical and nursing staff.

Thyroid Gland

The thyroid gland is located in the anterior portion of the lower neck, below the larynx, on both sides of and anterior to the trachea (see Fig. 11-1). The primary hormones produced by the thyroid are thyroxine (T_4), triiodothyronine (T_3), and calcitonin. Both T_3 and T_4 regulate the metabolic rate of the body and increase protein synthesis. Calcitonin has a weak physiologic effect on calcium and phosphorus balance in the body. Thyroid function is regulated by the hypothalamus and pituitary feedback controls and by an intrinsic regulator mechanism within the gland.[115]

Both thyroid hormones travel from the thyroid via the bloodstream to distant parts of the body, including the brain, heart, liver, kidneys, bones, and skin, where they activate genes that regulate body functions. When the hypothalamus senses that circulating levels have dropped, it signals the pituitary gland, which sends TSH to the thyroid to trigger the release of thyroid hormones.

Disorders of the thyroid gland may be functional abnormalities leading to hyperfunction or hypofunction of the gland or anatomic abnormalities such as thyroiditis, goiter, and tumor. Enlargement of the thyroid gland or neoplasm may or may not be associated with abnormalities of hormone secretion.

Susceptibility to thyroid disease is largely determined by the interaction of genetic makeup, age, and sex. Approximately 27 million Americans have been diagnosed with thyroid disease; many other people are undiagnosed because the signs and symptoms are so nonspecific. The risk of thyroid disease increases with age but is difficult to detect in adults older than age 60 because it typically masquerades as other illnesses such as heart disease, depression, or dementia. Women, particularly those with a family history of thyroid disease, are much more likely to have thyroid pathology than men. Although most thyroid conditions cannot be prevented, they respond well to treatment.

Thyroid hormone acts on nearly all body tissues, so excessive or deficient secretion affects various body systems. Alterations in thyroid function produce changes in nails, hair, skin, eyes, GI tract, respiratory tract, heart and blood vessels, nervous tissue, bone, and muscle.[115]

Women may notice disturbances in mood and in menstrual cycles. Menstrual irregularity, worsening premenstrual syndrome (PMS), new onset of depression later in life, postpartum depression (after pregnancy/birth), anxiety syndromes, and excessive fatigue have been reported by many women with thyroid dysfunction.

Both hyperthyroidism and hypothyroidism can adversely affect cardiac function. Sustained tachycardia in hyperthyroidism and sustained bradycardia with cardiac enlargement in hypothyroidism can result in cardiac failure. Both conditions affect the general rate of metabolism, the muscular system, the nervous system, the GI system, and as mentioned, the cardiovascular system.

Hyperthyroidism

Definition and Overview. Hyperthyroidism is an excessive secretion of thyroid hormone, sometimes referred to as *thyrotoxicosis*, a term used to describe the clinical manifestations that occur when the body tissues are stimulated by increased thyroid hormone. Excessive thyroid hormone creates a generalized elevation of body metabolism, the effects of which are manifested in almost every system.

The most common form of hyperthyroidism is the autoimmune condition known as Graves disease, which increases T_4 production and accounts for 85% of cases of hyperthyroidism. Like most thyroid conditions, hyperthyroidism affects women more than men (4:1), especially women between ages 20 and 40 years.

Rarely, a person with inadequately treated hyperthyroidism may experience what is called a *thyroid storm*. This potentially fatal condition is an acute episode of thyroid overactivity characterized by high fever, severe tachycardia, delirium, dehydration, and extreme irritability or agitation. Stress occurring in the presence of undiagnosed or untreated hyperthyroidism may precipitate such an event. Stressors may include surgery, infection, toxemia of pregnancy, labor and delivery, diabetic ketoacidosis (DKA), myocardial infarction, pulmonary embolus, and medication overdose.

Etiologic and Risk Factors. Hyperthyroidism may result from both immunologic and genetic factors. Graves disease, the most common form of hyperthyroidism, is most likely autoimmune in development, and although it is more common in women with family histories of thyroid abnormalities, major risk factors have not been identified. In addition, autoimmune hyperthyroid disease is present in people with other immune-related disorders such as Sjögren syndrome,[154] rheumatoid arthritis, and psoriatic arthritis.[187]

Hyperthyroidism also may be caused by the overfunction of the entire gland, such as in Graves disease, or less commonly, by hyperfunctioning of a single adenoma or multiple toxic nodules. Rarely, overtreatment of myxedema associated with hypothyroidism (see next section) may result in hyperthyroidism, and more rarely, thyroid cancer can cause glandular hyperfunction.

Pathogenesis. About 95% of people with Graves disease have circulating autoantibodies called thyroid-stimulating immunoglobulins (TSIs) that react against thyroglobulin (precursor for thyroid hormones). These autoantibodies may be the result of a defect in suppressor T-lymphocyte function that allows formation of TSIs. Evidently, TSIs in the serum of hyperthyroid Graves clients are autoantibodies that react against a component of the thyroid cell membranes, stimulating enlargement of the thyroid gland and secretion of excess thyroid hormone.

Because the action of thyroid hormone on the body is stimulatory, hypermetabolism results with increased sympathetic nervous system activity. The excessive amounts of thyroid hormone stimulate the cardiac system and increase the number of β-adrenergic receptors throughout the body. This excess thyroid hormone secretion, coupled with the increased secretion of catecholamines, leads to tachycardia, increased stroke volume, and increased peripheral blood flow. The increased metabolism also leads to a negative nitrogen balance, lipid depletion, and a resultant state of nutritional deficiency.

Clinical Manifestations. Because hyperthyroidism is caused by an excess secretion of thyroid hormone, the clinical picture of Graves disease is in many ways the opposite of that of hypothyroidism. The classic symptoms of Graves disease are mild symmetric enlargement of the thyroid (goiter), nervousness, heat intolerance, weight loss despite increased appetite, sweating, diarrhea, tremor, and palpitations. Hyperthyroidism may induce atrial fibrillation, precipitate congestive heart failure, and increase the risk of underlying CAD for myocardial infarction.

Exophthalmos (abnormal protrusion of the eyes) (Fig. 11-4) is considered most characteristic but is absent in many people with hyperthyroidism and may exacerbate after adequate treatment of the hyperthyroid state. Changes, such as swelling behind the eyes, are mediated by autoimmune production of antibodies to soft tissues (particularly the fibroblasts). Highly specialized ophthalmic surgery (surgical decompression) may be effective for correcting the severe exophthalmos when vision is impaired. Retroorbital radiation has also been shown to be effective.[317]

Many other symptoms are commonly present because this condition affects many body systems (Table 11-4). As mentioned, complications, such as thyroid storm and heart disease, can occur. Emotions are adversely affected by the increased metabolic activity within the body. Moods may be cyclic, ranging from mild euphoria to extreme hyperactivity or delirium and depression, which may persist even after successful treatment of hyperthyroidism.[37] Excessive hyperactivity may be associated with extreme fatigue.

Hyperthyroidism in older adults is notorious for presenting with atypical or minimal symptoms.[300] Signs and symptoms are not the usual ones and may be attributed to aging. Many older people actually appear apathetic instead of hyperactive. Cardiovascular abnormalities, as described previously, are much more common in older adults.

Neuromuscular Manifestations. Chronic periarthritis also is associated with hyperthyroidism. Inflammation that involves the periarticular structures, including the tendons, ligaments, and joint capsule, is termed *periarthritis.* This syndrome is characterized by pain and reduced range of motion. Calcification, whether periarticular or tendinous, may be seen on x-ray studies. Both periarthritis and calcific tendinitis can occur most often in the shoulder in clients who have undiagnosed, untreated, or inadequately treated endocrine disease. The involvement can be unilateral or bilateral and can worsen progressively to become adhesive capsulitis, or frozen shoulder. Acute calcific tendinitis of the wrist also has been described in

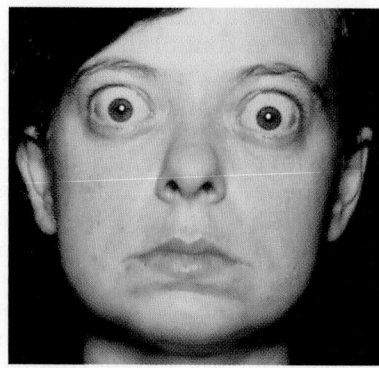

Figure 11-4

Exophthalmos, or protruding eyes. This is a forward displacement of the eyeballs associated with thyroid disease. Because the eyes are surrounded by unyielding bone, fluid accumulation in the fat pads and muscles behind the eyeballs causes protruding eyes and a fixed stare. Without treatment of the underlying cause, the client with severe exophthalmos may be unable to close the eyelids and may develop corneal ulceration or infection, eventually resulting in loss of vision. Note the lid lag; the upper eyelid rests well above the limbus (edge of the cornea where it joins the sclera), and white sclera is visible. This is evident when the person moves the eyes from up to down. Physical therapy is not recommended in these cases until after the endocrine problem is resolved. Then therapeutic intervention with ultrasound, joint mobilization, stretching, and strengthening may be indicated to treat any residual dysfunction. (From Seidel H et al: *Mosby's guide to physical examination,* ed 3, St Louis, 1995, Mosby.)

Table 11-4	Systemic Manifestations of Hyperthyroidism					
CNS effects	**Cardiovascular and Pulmonary Effects**	**Musculoskeletal Effects**	**Integumentary Effects**	**Ocular Effects**	**Gastrointestinal Effects**	**Genitourinary Effects**
Tremors Hyperkinesis (abnormally increased motor function or activity) Nervousness, irritability Emotional lability Weakness and muscle atrophy Increased deep tendon reflexes Fatigue	Increased pulse rate/tachycardia/palpitations Increased cardiac output Increased blood volume Arrhythmias (especially atrial fibrillation) Weakness of respiratory muscles (breathlessness, hypoventilation) Increased respiratory rate Low blood pressure Heart failure	Muscle weakness and fatigue Muscle atrophy Chronic periarthritis Myasthenia gravis	Capillary dilation (warm flushed, moist skin) Heat intolerance Onycholysis (separation of the finger nail from the nail bed) Easily broken hair and increased hair loss Hard, purple area over the anterior surface of the tibia with itching, erythema, and occasionally pain	Exophthalmos Weakness of the extraocular muscles (poor convergence, poor upward gaze) Sensitivity to light Spasm and retraction of the upper eyelids (bulging eyes), lid tremor	Hypermetabolism (increased appetite with weight loss) Increased peristalsis Increased frequency of bowel movements Diarrhea, nausea, and vomiting Dysphagia	Polyuria (frequent urination) Amenorrhea (absence of menses) Female infertility Increased risk of spontaneous miscarriage (first trimester) Gynecomastia (males)

Modified from Goodman CC, Snyder TE: *Differential diagnosis for physical therapists: screening for referral,* ed 5, Philadelphia, 2013, Saunders, p. 419.

such clients. Although antiinflammatory agents may be needed for acute symptoms, chronic periarthritis usually responds to treatment of the underlying hyperthyroidism.

Proximal muscle weakness (most marked in the pelvic girdle and thigh muscles) accompanied by muscle atrophy, known as *myopathy*, can occur in cases of undiagnosed, untreated, or inadequately treated hyperthyroidism. The therapist may first notice problems with coordination or balance or notice weakness of the legs, causing a client difficulty in ambulating, rising from a chair, or climbing stairs.[79]

Respiratory muscle weakness can present as dyspnea. The pathogenesis of the weakness is still a subject of controversy; muscle strength seems to return to normal in 6 to 8 weeks after medical treatment, with a slower resolution of muscle wasting. In severe cases, normal strength may not be restored for months.

The incidence of myasthenia gravis, which is also an antibody immune disease, is increased in clients with hyperthyroidism, which in turn can aggravate muscle weakness. If the hyperthyroidism is corrected, improvement of the myasthenia gravis usually follows.

Sudden, periodic paralysis while at rest characterized by recurrent episodes of motor weakness of variable intensity can occur in a selective population (more common among people of Asian origin). This phenomenon is precipitated by intracellular shifts of potassium triggered by thyroid overactivity and hyperinsulinemia after ingestion of carbohydrates and increased physical activity. Administration of potassium is required to prevent life-threatening arrhythmias.[207,238]

MEDICAL MANAGEMENT

PREVENTION. There is no way to prevent Graves disease. Early screening can help determine if someone is at risk. Two simple blood tests can be conducted, one to measure TSH and the second for antithyroid antibodies. Testing should be done by age 40 years (or perhaps earlier for women who intend to get pregnant), especially in the presence of a positive family history.

DIAGNOSIS. Diagnosis is based on clinical history, physical presentation, examination findings, and laboratory test results. Hyperthyroidism is almost always associated with suppressed TSH. The very rare exception is that of a TSH-secreting pituitary adenoma. In very mild hyperthyroidism the T_4 would be normal, but the measurement of T_3 usually would be elevated or at the upper range of normal. This is called T_3 *toxicosis* and almost always precedes Graves disease. Diagnostic tests, such as radioactive iodine uptake, can confirm the presence of hyperthyroidism and differentiate among causes of hyperthyroidism.[47] Radioactive iodine uptake studies are elevated in Graves disease and nodular thyrotoxicosis but are very low or negative in thyroiditis-caused hyperthyroidism. TSI is positive in almost all people with Graves disease. It is essential to distinguish hyperthyroidism caused by Graves disease and nodular thyrotoxicosis from thyroiditis because the treatment for each is different.[326]

TREATMENT. The three major forms of therapy are antithyroid medication, radioactive iodine (RAI), and surgery.

Most endocrine specialists would now recommend radioactive iodine as first-line therapy in anyone older than 18 years of age who is not pregnant. Some physicians treat as young as the age of 12 years because long-term studies have shown no increased incidence of thyroid cancer or leukemia in people receiving such treatment.[312]

Iodine-131 therapy takes several months before it is effective, so adrenergic-blocking agents are sometimes given in the interim to control the activity of the sympathetic nervous system. Once the RAI is administered, the iodine concentrates in the thyroid gland, disrupting hormone synthesis. Typically, everyone who receives RAI becomes hypothyroid and requires thyroid hormone replacement for the rest of their lives. Almost everyone treated with radioactive iodine is hypothyroid during the first year of therapy but eventually normalizes with replacement therapy.

Use of antithyroid drugs (propylthiouracil and methimazole) is also effective and is the usual choice of therapy during pregnancy and for children under the age of 12 years. Side effects from drug treatment include rheumatoid-like arthritis and agranulocytosis (serious and potentially fatal) and usually resolve after 10 days of discontinuing the drug. About half of the people treated with antithyroid drugs have a later recurrence of hyperthyroid activity. Again, adrenergic-blocking agents may be used with these drugs.[317]

Partial or subtotal thyroidectomy is an effective way to treat hyperthyroidism caused by Graves disease and single or multinodular thyrotoxicosis. The ideal surgical treatment leaves a small portion of the functioning thyroid gland to avoid permanent hormone replacement. Surgical treatment is effective in most cases, although surgical complications can develop such as vocal cord paralysis (resulting from laryngeal nerve damage) or hypoparathyroidism leading to hypocalcemia (resulting from inadvertent removal of parathyroid gland tissue).[27]

PROGNOSIS. Antithyroid drugs may be tapered and discontinued if remission is possible. Remission rates are higher in people with mild degrees of hyperthyroidism, small goiters, and for those who are diagnosed early. Even with remission, lifelong follow-up is recommended because many remissions are not permanent. Relapses are most likely to occur in the postpartum period.[326]

After radioiodine treatment, regular lifelong medical supervision is required. Frequently, hypothyroidism develops even as long as 1 to 3 years after treatment. Exophthalmos may not be reversed by intervention. In severe cases, the person may be unable to close the eyelids and must have the lids taped shut to protect the eyes. Without intervention, severe exophthalmos can progress to corneal ulceration or infection and loss of vision.

SPECIAL IMPLICATIONS FOR THE THERAPIST   11-6

Hyperthyroidism

Any time a therapist examines a client's neck and finds unusual swelling, enlargement with or without symptoms of pain, tenderness, hoarseness, or dysphagia (difficulty swallowing), a medical referral is required.

For the client requiring lifelong thyroid hormone replacement therapy, nervousness and palpitations may develop with overdosage. A small number of people experience fever, rash, and arthralgias as side effects of antithyroid drugs. The physician should be notified of these or any other unusual symptoms, because it may be possible to use an alternative drug.

Monitoring Vital Signs

Monitoring vital signs is important to assess cardiac function if the involved person is an older adult,[300] has CAD, or presents with symptoms of dyspnea, fatigue, tachycardia, and/or arrhythmia. If the heart rate is more than 100 beats/min, check the blood pressure and pulse rate and rhythm frequently. The person with dyspnea is most comfortable sitting upright or in a high Fowler position (head of the bed raised 18 to 20 inches. above a level position with the knees elevated).

Because clients with Graves disease may suffer from heat intolerance, they should avoid exercise in a hot aquatic or pool physical therapy setting. Exercise in a warm pool would be safe and would not be contraindicated as long as the person's temperature is monitored. True heat intolerance usually is associated with severe hyperthyroid states, such as thyroid storm, and probably would not occur in a nonhospitalized individual.

Postoperative Care

Postoperatively, observe for signs of hypoparathyroidism (muscular twitching, tetany, numbness and tingling around the mouth, fingertips, or toes), a complication that results from the accidental removal of the parathyroid glands during surgery. Symptoms can develop 1 to 7 days after surgery.

Any health care worker in contact with clients who have undergone radioiodine therapy must follow necessary precautions (see Chapter 5). Saliva is radioactive for 24 hours after iodine-131 therapy; health care professionals in contact with clients while they are coughing or expectorating must take precautions.

Side Effects of Radioiodine Therapy

Radioiodine therapy has few immediate side effects. Rarely, anterior neck tenderness may develop 7 to 10 days after therapy, consistent with radiation-induced thyroiditis.[262] The potential exists for worsening hyperthyroidism soon after radioiodine therapy, secondary to inflammation and release of stored thyroid in the bloodstream. Older adults and anyone with cardiac disease usually are pretreated with antithyroid agents before receiving radioiodine to prevent this occurrence.

The major adverse reaction from radioiodine is iatrogenic hypothyroidism. This development is so characteristic that it is considered an inevitable consequence of therapy rather than a side effect. Hypothyroidism develops in at least 50% of all cases treated with radioiodine therapy within the first year after therapy, with a gradual increased incidence thereafter. This complication necessitates lifelong follow-up with close monitoring of thyroid function.

For further discussion of radiation side effects and precautions for health care workers coming in contact with a person who has been irradiated, see Chapter 5.

Hyperthyroidism and Exercise

Hyperthyroidism is associated with exercise intolerance and reduced exercise capacity although the exact relationship is unknown. Cardiac output is either normal or enhanced (e.g., increased heart rate) during exercise in the hyperthyroid state and blood flow to muscles is augmented during submaximal exercise. However, proximal muscle weakness with accompanying myopathy is characteristic in individuals with Graves disease and may affect exercise capability.

Impaired cardiopulmonary function (more noticeable in older people with hyperthyroidism) also may affect exercise capacity. Thyrotoxicosis can aggravate preexisting heart disease; lead to atrial fibrillation, congestive heart failure, and worsening angina pectoris; and increase the risk for myocardial infarction. These factors must be considered in the overall discussion and planning of any exercise program for clients who are hyperthyroid.

Fatigue as a result of the hypermetabolic state and rapid depletion of nutrients may affect exercise capacity.[77] Using perceived exertion or exercise tolerance as a guide, exercise parameters (frequency, intensity, duration) remain the same for the person treated for hyperthyroidism as for anyone who does not have this condition. However, the therapist must remain alert for signs of subclinical hyperthyroidism (especially reduced VO_2max and other signs of impaired exercise performance) in the person receiving long-term TSH-suppressive therapy. These manifestations improve or disappear after careful tailoring of the medications.[197]

Ultrasound and Iontophoresis

The benefit of physical therapy intervention in the treatment of endocrine-induced calcific tendinitis has not been proved. Some experts advocate waiting until after the endocrine problem is resolved before initiating a plan of care. Therapeutic intervention with ultrasound, joint mobilization, stretching, and strengthening may be indicated to treat any residual dysfunction.

The limited research published on the subject of ultrasound in treating calcific tendinitis suggests that pulsed ultrasound, applied for 15 minutes at 2.5 W/cm^2 and at a frequency of 0.89 MHz, is associated with short-term clinical improvement in adults with calcific tendinitis when compared with sham treatment over a 6-week period of time. Decreased pain and improvement in quality of life were reported.[69]

Using acetic acid iontophoresis to promote a chemical reaction in which insoluble calcium carbonate molecules combine with acetic acid to form calcium acetate, which is more soluble, and therefore more easily dissolved within tendons and other soft tissues than calcium carbonate has not been proved effective.[49,50,321] This intervention does not appear to be effective in accelerating resorption of calcific lesions in tendons.[221] More study is needed to determine if duration of treatment makes a difference.

Table 11-5	Causes of Hypothyroidism

Primary	**Secondary**
Congenital defects	Pituitary tumor
Loss of thyroid tissue	Pituitary insufficiency
Radioiodine treatment of hyperthyroidism	Postpartum necrosis of the pituitary (Sheehan syndrome)
Surgical removal	
Radiation treatment for Hodgkin disease, lymphomas, cancer of the head and neck	
Defective hormone synthesis	
Chronic autoimmune thyroiditis (Hashimoto disease)	
Iodine deficiency	
Medications	
• Lithium	
• Interferon alpha and beta	
• Interleukin	
• Pharmaceutical overcorrection of hyperthyroidism	
• Amiodarone (rarely used)	

Data from pharmacotherapy update: Tisdale JE, Miller DA, eds: *Drug-induced diseases*, ed 2, Bethesda, MD, 2010, American Society of Health-System Pharmacists.

Hypothyroidism

Definition and Etiologic Factor. Hypothyroidism (hypofunction) refers to a deficiency of thyroid hormone in the adult that results in a generalized slowed body metabolism; it is the most common disorder of thyroid function in the United States and Canada. More than 50% of cases occur in families in which thyroid disease is present.

Like diabetes, hypothyroidism can be categorized as type I (hormone deficient) and type II (hormone resistant). The condition has traditionally been classified as either primary or secondary. *Type I/primary hypothyroidism* occurs as a result of reduced functional thyroid tissue mass or impaired hormonal synthesis or release. *Type II/secondary hypothyroidism* accounts for a small percentage of all cases of hypothyroidism and occurs as a result of inadequate stimulation of the gland because of pituitary or hypothalamic disease (failure to produce TSH and TRH, respectively) (Table 11-5). (See "Hashimoto Thyroiditis" below.)

In the United States and Canada, this disease commonly is caused by congenital autoimmune thyroiditis, thyroid ablation via surgery or RAI therapy, or medication with thiouracil or lithium; rarely, it is a result of subacute thyroiditis, iodine deficiency, dietary factors, congenital abnormalities in iodination, or pituitary failure.[325]

Incidence. Hypothyroidism is about four times more prevalent in women than in men. Although hypothyroidism may be congenital and therefore present at birth, the highest incidence is between ages 30 and 60 years. More than 95% of all people with hypothyroidism have the primary form of the disease.[132]

Pathogenesis. In type I/primary hypothyroidism, the loss of thyroid tissue leads to decreased secretion of thyroid hormone. In response to a decrease in thyroid hormone, TSH secretion is increased from the anterior pituitary gland as the body attempts to stimulate increased production of thyroid hormone. In the normal body, when hormone levels rise sufficiently, the pituitary slows TSH production. With hypothyroidism, the thyroid gland does not respond fully to TSH, so not enough T_3 and T_4 reach the body organs and body functions begin to slow. Whenever the body perceives an inadequate amount of thyroid hormone, the pituitary releases more and more TSH in an effort to stimulate thyroid hormone production. The result is an elevated TSH level in the blood when thyroid function is low.

Decreased levels of thyroid hormone lead to an overall slowing of the basal metabolic rate. This slowing of all body processes leads to bradycardia, decreased GI tract motility, slowed neurologic functioning, a decrease in body heat production, and achlorhydria (absence of hydrochloric acid from gastric juice). Lipid metabolism also is altered by hypothyroidism, with a resultant increase in serum cholesterol and triglyceride levels and a concomitant increase in arteriosclerosis and coronary heart disease. Thyroid hormones also play a role in the production of red blood cells with the potential for the development of anemia.

Type II/secondary hypothyroidism is most commonly the result of failure of the pituitary gland to synthesize and release adequate amounts of TSH.

Clinical Manifestations. As with all disorders affecting the thyroid and parathyroid glands, clinical signs and symptoms associated with hypothyroidism affect many systems of the body (Table 11-6). Typically, the early clinical features of hypothyroidism are vague and ordinary, so they escape detection (e.g., fatigue, mild sensitivity to cold, mild weight gain resulting from fluid retention [10-15 lb], forgetfulness, depression, and dry skin or hair).

As the disorder progresses, myxedema and its associated signs and symptoms appear. Myxedema is a result of an alteration in the composition of the dermis and other tissues, causing connective tissues to be separated by increased amounts of mucopolysaccharides and proteins. This mucopolysaccharide-protein complex binds with water, causing a nonpitting, boggy edema, especially around the eyes, hands, feet, and in the supraclavicular fossae. Thickening of the tongue, laryngeal and pharyngeal structures, hoarseness, and slurred speech occur as a result of myxedema.[325]

Other clinical manifestations associated with hypothyroidism may include decreasing mental stability; dry, flaky, inelastic skin; dry, sparse hair; hoarseness; upper eyelid droop; and thick, brittle nails. Cardiovascular involvement leads to decreased cardiac output, slow pulse rate, and signs of poor peripheral circulation. Other possible effects of hypothyroid function are anorexia, abdominal distention, menorrhagia,

| Table 11-6 | Systemic Manifestations of Hypothyroidism | | | | | | | |

CNS Effects	Musculoskeletal Effects	Cardiovascular Effects	Hematologic Effects	Respiratory Effects	Integumentary Effects	Gastrointestinal Effects	Genitourinary Effects
Slowed speech and hoarseness	Proximal muscle weakness	Bradycardia	Anemia	Dyspnea	Myxedema (periorbital and peripheral)	Anorexia	Infertility
Slow mental function (loss of interest in daily activities, poor short-term memory)	Myalgias	Congestive heart failure	Easy bruising	Respiratory muscle weakness	Thickened, cool and dry skin	Constipation	Menstrual irregularity, bleeding (menorrhagia)
Fatigue and increased sleep	Trigger points	Poor peripheral circulation (pallor, cold skin, intolerance to cold, hypertension)			Scaly skin (especially elbows and knees)	Weight gain disproportionate to caloric intake	
Headache	Stiffness	Severe atherosclerosis; hyperlipidemia			Carotenosis (yellowing of the skin)	Decreased protein metabolism (retarded skeletal and soft tissue growth)	
Cerebellar ataxia	Carpal tunnel syndrome	Angina			Coarse, thinning hair	Delayed glucose uptake	
Anxiety, depression	Prolonged deep tendon reflexes (especially Achilles)	Elevated blood pressure			Intolerance to cold	Decreased glucose absorption	
	Subjective report of paresthesias without supportive objective findings	Cardiomyopathy			Nonpitting edema of hands and feet		
	Muscular and joint edema				Poor wound healing		
	Back pain				Thin, brittle nails		
	Increased bone density						
	Decreased bone formation and resorption						

Modified from Goodman CC, Snyder TE: *Differential diagnosis for therapists: Screening for referral*, ed 5, Philadelphia, 2013, Saunders.

decreased libido, infertility, ataxia, intention tremor, and nystagmus.

Neuromuscular symptoms are among the most frequent manifestations of hypothyroidism seen in a therapy practice. Flexor tenosynovitis with stiffness can accompany CTS in persons with hypothyroidism. CTS arising from myxedematous tissue in the carpal tunnel area can develop before other signs of hypothyroidism become evident. Most people with CTS associated with hypothyroidism do not require surgical treatment because symptoms of median nerve compression respond to thyroid replacement.

A wide spectrum of rheumatic symptoms occurs in people with hypothyroidism. A subset of fibromyalgia with muscle aches and tender points may be seen early; replacement therapy with thyroid hormone eliminates the symptoms, which aids in the diagnosis of the underlying cause of this form of fibromyalgia. Most cases of fibromyalgia fall into the type II (hormone-resistant) category. It is likely acquired as a result of mutated receptors.[97]

An inflammatory arthritis indistinguishable from rheumatoid arthritis may be seen. The arthritis predominantly involves the small joints of the hands and apparently differs from the viscous noninflammatory effusions observed in large joints of individuals with hypothyroidism. In general, the arthritis resolves with normalization of the thyroid hormone levels.[143]

Proximal muscle weakness can occur in persons with hypothyroidism, sometimes accompanied by pain. Trigger points are frequently detected on examination, and diffuse muscle tenderness may be the major finding. Muscle weakness is not always related to either the severity or the duration of hypothyroidism; it can be present several months before a medical diagnosis of hypothyroidism is made. Deep tendon reflexes show delayed relaxation time (i.e., prolonged reflexes), especially in the Achilles tendon.[79]

MEDICAL MANAGEMENT

DIAGNOSIS. A substantial delay in diagnosis resulting from the vague onset of symptoms is not uncommon. Specific testing of TSH levels is the most sensitive indicator of primary hypothyroidism. TSH levels are always elevated in primary hypothyroidism. T_3 (triiodothyronine) levels do not change dramatically, even in severe hypothyroidism. T_4 (thyroxine) levels, however, decrease gradually until they are well below normal in advanced hypothyroidism.

Serum cholesterol, alkaline phosphatase, and triglyceride levels also can be significantly elevated in the presence of hypothyroidism. In addition, the presence of antithyroid antibodies documents the existence of autoimmune thyroiditis resulting in progressive destruction of thyroid tissue by circulating antithyroid antibodies.[161,330]

TREATMENT. The goals of treatment for hypothyroidism are to correct thyroid hormone deficiency, reverse symptoms, and prevent further cardiac and arterial damage. If treatment with lifelong administration of synthetic thyroid hormone preparations is begun soon after symptoms appear, recovery may be complete. There is some controversy over whether mild hypothyroidism (defined by an elevated serum TSH level with a normal free thyroxine level) should be routinely screened, identified, and treated. Treatment is safe and effective but the question is whether the clinical consequences are enough to justify screening and therapy.[161]

Proponents of early detection and treatment argue that they lower the risk of atherosclerotic cardiovascular disease (CVD) and prevent progression to overt hypothyroidism, especially in adults who are 65 or older. Older people with underlying heart disease (particularly underlying CAD) can be started on very low doses of thyroxine gradually increased in dosage to ultimately return the TSH to within the normal range. Cardiac complications can occur, including angina severe enough that intervention may be required. Only small doses should be initiated in anyone with preexisting heart problems.

Sometimes, individuals with diagnosed hypothyroidism and taking thyroid medication (e.g., Synthroid, Levothroid, Levoxyl, or Euthyrox) to regulate symptoms will have "normal" levels of TSH when tested but still experience lingering symptoms of the condition. Because there is a broad range of "normal," it is not always possible to find the exact dosage required for each individual.

Some physicians are reluctant to increase thyroid medication because of possible adverse side effects such as atrial fibrillation or osteoporosis. In some cases, a regimen of T_4 along with T_3 (Cytomel) works well along with lifestyle changes such as regular exercise and a healthy diet for gastrointestinal and other breakthrough symptoms.

Note to Reader: Although we present the standard medical practice here, you should be aware that some physicians and other health care professionals have published alternative opinions and recommend a slightly different approach.[245,249] For example: *Although many endocrinologists continue to debate the appropriate levels of TSH to use as boundaries for normal limits, we think that using TSH to assess thyroid function is counterproductive, particularly in those patients attempting to lose weight. From the published literature and our own clinical experience, we have come to understand that the set point for metabolism is adjusted downward in the hypocaloric state. The decrease in metabolism is often referred to as part of the "famine response." This metabolic response has been documented in several major vertebrate classes demonstrating its widespread importance in nature. In our current environment, the famine response limits the patient's ability to lose weight while consuming a hypocaloric diet and performing modest levels of exercise. Our own experience with the famine response is consistent with that found in the literature. Treating to normalize thyroid hormone levels and eliminate hypothyroid symptoms results in the suppression of TSH. This is understood as a normal part of treatment once we accept that the thyroid set point has been lowered. This is not an argument to use thyroid hormones to increase metabolism above normal to achieve weight loss. Our goal is to correct the hypothyroid response in a weight loss patient and return him/her to normal metabolism so that the patient feels normal and is better able to lose weight and maintain that loss.*

PROGNOSIS. Severely hypothyroid conditions accompanied by pronounced atherosclerosis (resulting from abnormal lipid metabolism) may cause angina and other symptoms of CAD. Treatment of hypothyroidism-induced angina can be difficult because thyroid hormone replacement increases the heart's need for oxygen by increasing body metabolism. This increase in metabolism then precipitates angina and aggravates the anginal condition. In severe hypothyroidism, psychiatric abnormalities can occur and are described as "myxedema madness" in the older literature.

Rarely, severe or prolonged hypothyroidism may progress to myxedema coma when aggravated by stress such as surgery, infection, or noncompliance with thyroid treatment. Myxedema coma can be fatal because of the extreme decrease in the metabolic rate, hypoventilation leading to respiratory acidosis, hypothermia, and hypotension.

SPECIAL IMPLICATIONS FOR THE THERAPIST   **11-7**

Hypothyroidism

In the case of myxedematous hypothyroidism, distinctive changes in the synovium can occur, resulting in a viscous noninflammatory joint effusion. Often the fluid contains calcium pyrophosphate dihydrate (CPPD) crystal deposits that may be associated with chondrocalcinosis (i.e., calcium salts in the synovium). When these hypothyroid clients have been treated with thyroid replacement, some have experienced attacks of acute pseudogout caused by the crystals in the periarticular joint structures (found in both the hyaline cartilage and fibrocartilage). Without medical treatment, this condition can lead to permanent joint damage.

Calcium pyrophosphate dihydrate crystal deposition disease (pseudogout) usually affects larger joints, but symptomatic involvement of the spine with deposition of crystals in the ligamentum flavum and atlantooccipital ligament can result in spinal stenosis and subsequent neurologic syndromes.[252] Effective treatment of pseudogout may include joint aspiration to relieve fluid pressure, steroid injection, and nonsteroidal antiinflammatories.[277] Although the synovium contains noninflammatory joint effusion, crystals may loosen, resulting in crystal shedding into the joint fluid, thereby causing an inflammatory response.

The role of the therapist is similar to the treatment of rheumatoid arthritis (see Chapter 27). Muscular complaints (aches, pain, and stiffness) associated with hypothyroidism are likely to develop into persistent myofascial trigger points. Clinically, any compromise of the energy metabolism of muscle aggravates and perpetuates trigger points. These do not resolve just with specific intervention by a therapist (e.g., trigger point therapy or myofascial release); they also require thyroid replacement.[271]

Hypothyroidism and Fibromyalgia

The correlation between hypothyroidism and fibromyalgia syndrome continues to be investigated.[23,176]

Despite the correlation between hypothyroidism and fibromyalgia syndrome, thyroid dysfunction is seen at least three times more often in women with rheumatoid arthritis than in women with similar demographic features with noninflammatory rheumatic diseases such as osteoarthritis and fibromyalgia.[187] Studies have shown an association between hypothyroidism and fibromyalgia. Persons with fibromyalgia syndrome may have a blunted response to a hypothalamic-releasing hormone (thyrotropin) that stimulates the anterior pituitary to secrete TSH, or, in some cases, a possible tissue-specific resistance may exist to thyroid hormone.[176]

Reduced high-energy phosphate in muscle, related to impairment of carbohydrate metabolism (glycolysis abnormalities), may explain the chronic fatigue that can approach lethargy; it is noticeable on arising in the morning and is usually worse during midafternoon. These clients are particularly weather conscious and have muscular pain that increases with the onset of cold, rainy weather.[277]

Acute Care Setting

Dry, edematous tissues associated with hypothyroidism are more prone to skin tears and breakdown. Prevention of pressure ulcers requires careful monitoring of the usual pressure points (e.g., sacrum, coccyx, scapulae, elbows, greater trochanter, heels, and malleoli).

Hypothyroidism and Medication

Clients with cardiac complications are started on small doses of thyroid hormone because large doses can precipitate heart failure or myocardial infarction by increasing body metabolism, myocardial oxygen requirements, and consequently, the workload of the heart. Carefully observe for any signs of aggravated CVD, such as chest pain and tachycardia. Report any signs of hypertension or congestive heart failure in the older adult. After thyroid replacement therapy begins, watch for symptoms of hyperthyroidism (e.g., restlessness, tremor, sweating, dyspnea, and excessive weight gain; see also Table 11-4).

All pharmaceuticals taken to replace thyroid hormone use the same synthetic T_4 but the inactive ingredients can vary. Altered absorption (increased or decreased) can occur, resulting in additional symptoms. If a client begins to report a change in thyroid symptoms, ask about a recent change in drug brand or name. Changes in symptoms, especially if occurring shortly after a switch to a generic form of the medication, should be reported to the treating physician.

Older adults (aged 70 or older, especially those who have been treated long-term with levothyroxine for hypothyroidism) are at increased risk of bone fractures. Older adults with hypothyroidism have lower requirements for levothyroxine replacement; if dosage is not changed and lowered appropriately, overtreatment can lead to iatrogenic hyperthyroidism.[302] The resulting chronic hyperthyroidism is associated with a higher risk of osteoporosis and an increase in bone fractures. An excess of thyroid hormone can also affect neuromuscular function and muscle strength, increasing the risk of arrhythmias and falls.[19,31,256] The physical therapist can be instrumental in making sure older adults are screened for aberrant vital signs, history of falls or falls risk, and osteoporosis and evaluated routinely for correct medication dosage.

Hypothyroidism and Exercise

Activity intolerance, weakness, and apathy secondary to decreased metabolic rate may require developing increased tolerance to activity and exercise once thyroid replacement has been initiated. Increased activity and exercise are especially helpful for the client who is constipated secondary to slowed metabolic rate and decreased peristalsis. Exercise-induced myalgia leading to rhabdomyolysis (disintegration of striated or skeletal muscle fibers with acute edema and excretion of myoglobin in the urine) has been reported in undiagnosed[84] or untreated hypothyroidism or in individuals who are noncompliant with treatment.[56] Rhabdomyolysis also could occur possibly as a result of poor drug compliance in combination with other aggravating factors such as exercise.[56,171,265]

Although they occur infrequently, the therapist should remain alert to any signs or symptoms of rhabdomyolysis (e.g., unexplained muscle pain and weakness) in exercising clients with hypothyroidism. Rhabdomyolysis can progress to renal failure. Reduction in stroke volume and heart rate associated with hypothyroidism causes lowered cardiac output, increased peripheral vascular resistance to maintain systolic blood pressure, and a variety of electrocardiogram (ECG) changes (e.g., sinus bradycardia, prolonged PR interval, and depressed P waves).

In animal models, exercise can affect skeletal and cardiac muscle systems independent of thyroid hormone replacement, which supports the role of exercise in improving muscle and cardiovascular function for the person with hypothyroidism.[64,143] Because changes in lipid and lipoprotein levels occur with exercise, an exercise program can improve the lipid profile. This is especially important for the person with altered lipid metabolism and associated cardiovascular complications (see "Clinical Manifestations" above). However, if the client is hypothyroid with lipid abnormalities, the thyroid deficit should be corrected first. After treatment, if any lipid abnormality remains, exercise should be instituted to treat it.

Goiter

Goiter, an enlargement of the thyroid gland, may be a result of lack of iodine, inflammation, or tumors (benign or malignant). Enlargement also may appear in hyperthyroidism, especially Graves disease. Goiter occurs most often in areas of the world in which iodine, which is necessary for the production of thyroid hormone, is deficient in the diet (Fig. 11-5). Factors that inhibit normal thyroid hormone production result in a negative feedback loop, with hypersecretion of TSH. The TSH increase results in the production and secretion of huge amounts of thyroglobulin (colloid) into the glandular follicles and the gland grows in size.

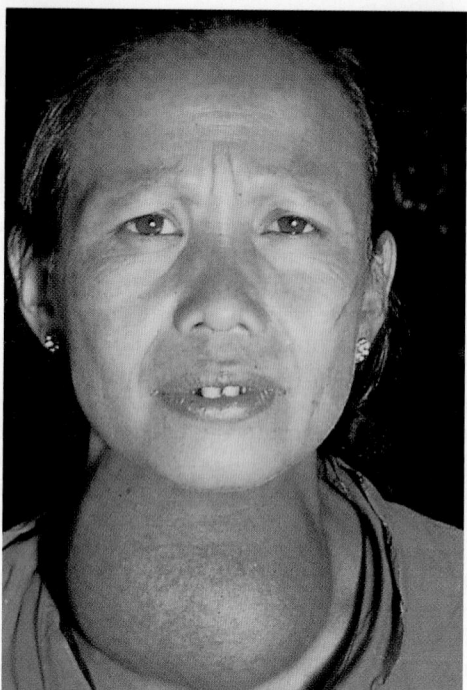

Figure 11-5

Goiter. The enlarged thyroid gland appears as a swelling of the anterior neck. This condition results from a low dietary intake of iodine and is rare in Canada and the United States but may be seen in other parts of the world. (From Thibodeau GA, Patton KT: *The human body in health & disease,* ed 4, St Louis, 2005, Mosby.)

Thyroglobulin is the large glycoprotein molecule in which thyroid hormones (T_3 and T_4) are produced in the presence of iodine. When iodine is absent, only the thyroglobulin is made by the gland in response to repeated TSH stimulation. Because the thyroglobulin molecule is large, its increased production causes rapid glandular growth and a marked increase in overall glandular mass occurs called a *colloid goiter.*[115] With the use of iodized salt and iodine-containing binders in commercial foods, this problem almost has been eliminated in the United States and Canada. Although the younger population in the United States may be goiter-free, aging adults may have developed goiter during their childhood or adolescent years and may still have clinical manifestations of this disorder.

Increased neck size may be observed, and when the thyroid increases to a certain point, pressure on the trachea and esophagus may cause difficulty breathing, dysphagia (difficulty swallowing), and hoarseness. Compression of the upper airway can be a fatal complication. Surgical intervention is essential when the trachea is compromised.

Thyroiditis

Thyroiditis, inflammation of the thyroid, may be classified as *acute suppurative* (pus forming and very rare), *subacute granulomatous* (uncommon), and *lymphocytic* or *chronic* (Hashimoto disease). Acute and subacute thyroiditis are uncommon conditions caused by bacterial (*Streptococcus pyogenes, Staphylococcus aureus,* and *Pneumococcus pneumoniae*) and viral agents, respectively. Infected

glands are painful and associated with systemic symptoms of fever and hyperthyroidism. Several varieties of related autoimmune causes of thyroiditis exist, such as Hashimoto (lymphocytic) thyroiditis and postpartum thyroiditis. These types of thyroiditis are generally painless, with only a rare case of Hashimoto causing pain. Only the most common form of Hashimoto thyroiditis is discussed further.

Hashimoto (chronic) thyroiditis affects women more frequently than it does men (10:1) and is most often seen in the 30- to 50-year-old age group. The disorder has an autoimmune basis, and genetic predisposition appears to play a role in the etiology. It is associated with HLA-DR3, which is also present in other autoimmune conditions (e.g., Graves disease, systemic lupus erythematosus, type 1 DM, pernicious anemia, myasthenia gravis, and rheumatoid arthritis).[187] Hashimoto thyroiditis causes destruction of the thyroid gland because of the infiltration of the gland by lymphocytes and antithyroid antibodies. This infiltration results in decreased serum levels of T_3 and T_4, thus stimulating the pituitary gland to increase the production of TSH.

The increased TSH causes hyperfunction of the tissue, and goiter formation (enlargement of the gland) results. In some cases, this increase in function helps maintain a normal hormonal level, but eventually, when enough of the gland is destroyed, hypothyroidism develops. Hashimoto thyroiditis is one of the most common causes of hypothyroidism in women older than age 50 years.

Signs of chronic thyroiditis usually include painless symmetric or asymmetric enlargement of the gland and an irregular surface, which occasionally causes pressure on the surrounding structures. This pressure may subsequently cause dysphagia or a more subtle "tight" sensation when swallowing, and respiratory distress.

Most clients are euthyroid (have a normally functioning thyroid), about 20% are hypothyroid, and fewer than 5% are hyperthyroid, with these people having combined Hashimoto and Graves disease caused by a genetic component.[132] The course of Hashimoto thyroiditis varies. Most people see a decrease in the size of the goiter and remain stable for years with treatment.

Treatment is directed toward suppressing the TSH to the lower end of the normal range to decrease TSH stimulation of the gland, and to correct hypothyroidism if present. Tablets containing thyroxine (T_4) can help regulate and maintain adequate levels of circulating hormones. Generally, long-term or permanent therapy is advised.

SPECIAL IMPLICATIONS FOR THE THERAPIST   **11-8**

Thyroiditis

Because the symptoms of thyroiditis are related to glandular function, and because the condition may be associated with hypothyroidism or hyperthyroidism, the therapist is referred to the sections relevant to client presentation (see "Special Implications for the Therapist 11-6: Hyperthyroidism" and "Special Implications for the Therapist 11-7: Hypothyroidism," above).

Thyroid Cancer

Overview. The thyroid gland contains two types of cells: follicular cells, which are responsible for the production of thyroid hormone, and C cells, which make calcitonin, a hormone that participates in calcium metabolism. There are four main types of thyroid cancer: papillary, follicular, medullary, and anaplastic thyroid cancer.[9]

Papillary thyroid cancer is the most common type of thyroid cancer. It develops from the follicular cells and grows slowly and is usually found in only one lobe; only 10% to 20% of papillary thyroid cancers appear in both lobes. **Follicular thyroid cancer** also develops from the follicular cells and is usually slow growing. It is less common than papillary thyroid cancer; both are curable, when found early and in people younger than 45. Together, papillary and follicular thyroid cancers make up about 90% of thyroid cancers.

Medullary thyroid cancer (MTC) accounts for 5% of thyroid cancers and develops in the C cells. It can be the result of a genetic syndrome called multiple endocrine neoplasia type 2 (MEN2). MTC accounts for about 5% of thyroid cancers. **Anaplastic thyroid cancer** is a rare, fast-growing, poorly differentiated thyroid cancer that accounts for only 2% of thyroid cancers.

Incidence and Etiology. Although malignant tumors of the thyroid are rare (less than 1% of Americans will be diagnosed in their lifetime), thyroid cancer makes up more than 90% of all endocrine cancers and accounts for 63% of deaths from endocrine cancer, with an increasing incidence worldwide.[29] In the United States, 33,550 new cases of thyroid cancer were diagnosed in 2007 with 1530 deaths reported the same year[136] with a significant increase to 60,220 new cases in 2013 and 1850 deaths.[268]

Thyroid cancer affects women more than men (2:1 ratio), mainly between the ages of 40 and 60 years. However, the presence of a thyroid nodule in a man is regarded with greater suspicion for cancer. A past medical history of radiation to the head, neck, or chest (e.g., for an enlarged thymus or tonsils, acne, or Hodgkin disease) or cumulative exposure over a lifetime is the most obvious risk factor. In other countries iodine deficiency and excess iodine have been linked with thyroid cancer.

Clinical Manifestations. The usual presentation of thyroid cancer is the appearance of a hard, painless nodule on the thyroid gland or a gland that is multinodular. Most palpable nodules of the thyroid are benign adenomas and rarely become malignant or grow to a significant size to cause pressure against the trachea. Red flag symptoms include vocal cord paralysis, ipsilateral cervical lymphadenopathy, and fixation of the nodule to surrounding tissues.[57,128]

MEDICAL MANAGEMENT

DIAGNOSIS, TREATMENT, AND PROGNOSIS. Thyroid cancer is diagnosed by fine-needle aspiration (FNA) biopsy. More advanced molecular techniques for the diagnosis of thyroid nodules are being developed.[195] Molecular diagnostic assays using tumor-specific markers may improve the sensitivity and accuracy of FNA, possibly reducing

the number of surgical procedures to remove lesions that later prove to be benign.[246]

Treatment usually involves removal of all or part of the thyroid. Neck resection of involved lymph nodes may be done for metastases to the neck. Radioactive ablation of remaining thyroid tissue is standard practice for most thyroid cancers. External radiation may be used in some situations. Major postoperative complications may involve damage to the laryngeal nerve, hemorrhage, and hypoparathyroidism.[216] Individuals treated for thyroid cancer require long-term follow-up to detect recurrent disease, which can present years after initial therapy.[161]

Most thyroid cancers are treatable; only about 5% of palpable nodules are malignant. Of the malignant nodules, most are a variety that seldom metastasize beyond regional lymph nodes of the neck, resulting in a good prognosis for most people. However, disease recurrence and metastasis may occur in as many as 20% of affected individuals.[29] Papillary and follicular thyroid cancers are very often curable, especially when diagnosed and treated early in adults younger than 45. Medullary thyroid cancer can be controlled if it is diagnosed and treated before it spreads. Anaplastic thyroid cancer grows very quickly, making it more difficult to treat successfully.[9]

SPECIAL IMPLICATIONS FOR THE THERAPIST   **11-9**

Thyroid Cancer

A thyroid neoplasm can be the incidental finding in persons being treated for a musculoskeletal condition involving the head and neck. Most thyroid nodules are benign, but as mentioned previously, any time a therapist examines a client's neck and finds an asymptomatic nodule or unusual swelling or enlargement (with or without symptoms of pain), hoarseness, dyspnea, or dysphagia (difficulty swallowing), a medical referral is required.

The therapist may become involved with clients who have developed radiation therapy–induced fibrosis contractures. Early intervention to prevent loss of motion, fibrosis, and lymphedema (e.g., self-manual lymphatic drainage techniques, see Chapter 13) is advised but studies have not been done to support this recommendation.

Individuals treated for head and neck cancers can present with complex, difficult to treat problems secondary to cancer treatment. Proper stretching to prevent loss of motion of the head, neck, and jaw is important, especially if fibrosis has impaired eating and swallowing. For clients with involvement of the head, neck, and jaw, baseline measurements should be taken to help document improvement. This can include mouth opening and tongue protrusion, as well as shoulder and neck active range of motion. Some clinicians advocate taking girth measurements circumferentially around the neck, as well as circumferentially around the head from the submandibular region to the hair line.[174]

Parathyroid Glands

Two parathyroid glands are located on the posterior surface of each lobe of the thyroid gland. These glands secrete PTH, which regulates calcium and phosphorus metabolism.

PTH exerts its effect by the following:

1. Increasing the release of calcium and phosphate from the bone (bone demineralization).
2. Increasing the absorption of calcium and excretion of phosphate by the kidneys.
3. Promoting calcium absorption in the GI tract.[132]

Disorders of the parathyroid glands may come to the therapist's attention because these conditions can cause periarthritis and tendinitis. Both types of inflammation may be crystal-induced, with formation of periarticular or tendinous calcification. Rarely, ruptured tendons resulting from bone resorption at the insertions occur in cases of primary hyperparathyroidism. These complications and problems are seen infrequently because most cases are diagnosed earlier with the advent of blood screening for identification of asymptomatic hypercalcemia.

Hyperparathyroidism

Definition and Incidence. Hyperparathyroidism is a disorder caused by overactivity of one or more of the four parathyroid glands that disrupts calcium, phosphate, and bone metabolism. Women are affected more than men (2:1), usually after age 60 years (postmenopausal). Hyperparathyroidism is frequently overlooked in the over-60 population. Symptoms in the early stages for this group are subtle and easily attributed to the aging process, depression, or anxiety. Eventually the symptoms intensify as the level of serum calcium rises, but this situation is accompanied by increased bone damage and other complications.

Etiologic and Risk Factors. Hyperparathyroidism is classified as primary, secondary, or tertiary. *Primary hyperparathyroidism* develops when the normal regulatory relationship between serum calcium levels and PTH secretion is interrupted. This occurs when one or more of the parathyroid glands enlarge, increasing PTH secretion and elevating serum calcium levels. The most common cause is a single adenoma of the parathyroid gland. Hyperplasia of the gland without an identifying injury and multiple adenomas are less common causes. Medications, such as thiazide diuretics for hypertension and lithium carbonate for psychiatric disorders, have also been implicated as a cause or factor that exacerbates hyperparathyroidism.

Secondary hyperparathyroidism occurs when the glands are hyperplastic from malfunction of another organ system. A hypocalcemia-producing abnormality outside the parathyroid gland results in a compensatory response of the parathyroid glands to chronic hypocalcemia. This is usually the result of renal failure (decreased renal activation of vitamin D), but it also may occur with osteogenesis imperfecta, Paget disease, multiple myeloma, carcinoma with bone metastasis, laxative abuse, and vitamin D deficiency.

Tertiary hyperparathyroidism is seen almost exclusively in dialysis clients who have long-standing secondary hyperparathyroidism. Hyperplasia occurs and the parathyroid glands ultimately become autonomous in function and unresponsive to serum calcium levels. Parathyroidectomy is required even after successful renal transplantation has resolved the cause of the secondary hyperparathyroidism.[88]

Pathogenesis and Clinical Manifestations. The primary function of PTH is to maintain a proper balance of calcium and phosphorus ions within the blood. PTH is not regulated by the pituitary or the hypothalamus and maintains normal blood calcium levels by increasing bone resorption and GI absorption of calcium. It also maintains an inverse relationship between serum calcium and phosphate levels by inhibiting phosphate reabsorption in the renal tubules.

Abnormal PTH production disrupts this balance; symptoms of hyperparathyroidism are related to this release of bone calcium into the bloodstream. Excessive circulating PTH leads to bone damage, hypercalcemia, and kidney damage (Table 11-7). In fact, hyperparathyroidism is the most common cause of hypercalcemia, which can lead to nervous system, musculoskeletal, metabolic, and cardiovascular problems. See Chapter 5 for further discussion of hypercalcemia.

Bone Damage. Oversecretion of PTH causes excessive osteoclast growth and activity within the bones. Osteoclasts are active in promoting resorption of bone, which then releases calcium into the blood, causing

Table 11-7	Systemic Manifestations of Hyperparathyroidism			

Early CNS Symptoms	Musculoskeletal Effects	Gastrointestinal Effects	Genitourinary Effects
Lethargy, drowsiness, paresthesias	Mild to severe proximal muscle weakness of the extremities	Peptic ulcers	Renal colic associated with stones
Slow mentation, poor memory	Muscle atrophy	Pancreatitis	Hypercalcemia (polyuria, polydipsia, constipation)
Depression, personality changes	Bone decalcification (bone pain, especially spine; pathologic fractures; bone cysts)	Nausea, vomiting, anorexia	Kidney infections
Easily fatigued	Gout and pseudogout	Constipation	Renal hypertension
Hyperactive deep tendon reflexes	Arthralgias involving the hands	Abdominal pain	
Occasionally glove-and-stocking distribution sensory loss	Myalgia and sensation of heaviness in the lower extremities		
	Joint hypermobility		

Modified from Goodman CC, Synder TE: *Differential diagnosis for physical therapists: Screening for referral*, ed 5, Philadelphia, 2013, Saunders.

hypercalcemia. This calcium loss leads to bone demineralization, and in time, the bones may become so fragile that pathologic fractures, deformity (e.g., kyphosis of the thoracic spine), and compression fractures of the vertebral bodies occur. If uncontrolled, osteoclast proliferation may cause lytic bone lesions (bone disintegrates, leaving holes).

Surgical treatment of hyperparathyroidism (parathyroidectomy) can be expected to result in biochemical cure and increased bone mineral density of the lumbar spine and femoral neck (areas rich in cancellous bone), in both symptomatic and asymptomatic clients. Cortical bone loss, however, is not as readily reversible in either group.[269] Early surgical treatment of hyperparathyroidism may assist in the prevention of spine and hip fractures in this population.

Hypercalcemia. As excessive PTH secretion results in bone resorption and hypercalcemia as just described, hypercalciuria (excessive calcium in the urine) eventually develops because the excessive filtration of calcium overwhelms this renal mechanism. High serum calcium levels also stimulate hypergastrinemia (excess gastrin, a hormone that stimulates secretion of gastric acid and pepsin in the blood), abdominal pain, peptic ulcer disease, and pancreatitis.

Kidney Damage. As serum calcium levels rise in response to excessive PTH levels, large amounts of phosphorus and calcium are excreted and lost from the body. Excretion of these compounds occurs through the renal system, leaving deposits of calcium phosphate within the renal tubules. This produces a kidney condition called *nephrocalcinosis*. Because calcium salts are insoluble in urine, kidney stones composed of calcium phosphate develop. Serious renal damage may not be reversible with parathyroidectomy.

Some people with hyperparathyroidism may be completely asymptomatic, but even seemingly asymptomatic clients with elevated serum and PTH levels have been found to have paresthesias, muscle cramps, and loss of pain and vibratory sensation in a stocking-glove distribution. Others suffer from a wide range of symptoms as a result of skeletal disease, renal involvement, GI tract disorders, and neurologic abnormalities.

MEDICAL MANAGEMENT

DIAGNOSIS. The diagnosis of hyperparathyroidism depends on measurement of PTH levels in persons found to be hypercalcemic (high serum levels of calcium). Serum calcium and PTH levels are elevated, serum phosphorus may be low normal or depressed, and urine calcium can range from low to high. Radiographic evidence of skeletal damage is important to measure in asymptomatic clients with mild hyperparathyroidism. Skeletal damage can be seen on x-ray as diffuse demineralization of bones, bone cysts, subperiosteal bone resorption, and loss of the laminae durae surrounding the teeth.

TREATMENT AND PROGNOSIS. Treatment for primary hyperparathyroidism is surgical removal (parathyroidectomy). Minimally invasive parathyroidectomy is advised even for individuals with mild elevation in calcium because of the risk for more serious complications of hyperparathyroidism such as renal failure, osteoporosis, and early death from CVD. Preoperative localization of the adenoma by scanning with technetium Tc 99m–labeled sestamibi allows for limited resection whenever possible.

The prognosis is good if the condition is identified and treated early. Untreated, hyperparathyroidism exacerbates many conditions among older adults such as osteoporosis and CAD. Emergency medical management of severe hypercalcemia includes use of drugs to lower serum calcium, such as hydration and loop diuretics, which promote calcium loss through the kidneys, and antiresorption agents, which inhibit calcium release from bone.

Long-term medical management of hypercalcemia with drugs is not as effective as parathyroid surgery, but if needed for short-term treatment, drugs, such as calcimimetics, bisphosphonates, estrogen, and calcitonin, can prevent progressive bone demineralization.[277]

SPECIAL IMPLICATIONS FOR THE THERAPIST / 11-10

Hyperparathyroidism

The therapist is likely to see skeletal, articular, and neuromuscular manifestations associated with hyperparathyroidism. Chronic low back pain and easy fracturing resulting from bone demineralization may be compounded by marked muscle weakness and atrophy, especially in the legs.[132]

Inflammatory erosive polyarthritis may be associated with chondrocalcinosis and calcium pyrophosphate dihydrate crystal deposits in the synovial fluid in some cases of hyperparathyroidism. This erosion, described as *osteogenic synovitis*, occurs as part of the bone destruction that can occur with hyperparathyroidism. When this complication develops, the Achilles, triceps, and obturator tendons are most commonly affected; other affected areas may include hands and wrists (CTS), shoulders, knees, clavicle, and axial skeleton. Because of better and earlier diagnosis, inflammatory erosive polyarthritis and chondrocalcinosis are much less common today than they were several decades ago. However, some older adults still experience these complications and may present with these problems. Concurrent illness and surgery (e.g., parathyroidectomy) are recognized inducers of acute arthritic episodes.

The therapist may be involved in treating the arthritis associated with this (or any other endocrine) condition, but unless the underlying cause is treated first, intervention for the arthritis will be frustrating and poorly effective. After medical treatment, the therapist's treatment of the residual arthritis is the same as for arthritis, regardless of the cause.

Acute Care

In the acute care setting, auscultate for lung sounds and listen for signs of pulmonary edema in the person receiving large amounts of intravenous (IV) saline solution, especially in the presence of pulmonary or cardiac disease. Monitor the person on digitalis carefully for any toxic effects produced by elevated calcium levels because clients with hypercalcemia are hypersensitive to digitalis and may quickly develop toxic symptoms (e.g., arrhythmias, nausea, fatigue, or visual changes) (see Table 12-5).

Clients with osteopenia are predisposed to pathologic fractures and must be treated with caution to minimize the risk of injury. Take every safety precaution, assisting carefully with walking, keeping the bed at its lowest position, raising the side rails, and lifting the immobilized person carefully to minimize bone stress. Schedule care to allow the person with muscle weakness recovery time and rest between all activities.

Postoperative Care

Postoperatively, after parathyroidectomy, the person should use a semi-Fowler position with support for the head and neck to decrease edema, which can cause pressure on the trachea. Observe for any signs of mild tetany, such as reports of tingling in the hands and around the mouth. These symptoms should subside quickly but may be prodromal signs of tetany resulting from hypocalcemia. Watch for increased neuromuscular irritability and other signs of severe tetany and report them immediately. Acute postoperative arthritis may occur secondary to gout or pseudogout.

Early ambulation (although uncomfortable) is essential, because weight bearing and pressure on bones speed up recalcification. The use of light ankle weights or light weight-resistive elastic for the lower extremities provides tension at the musculotendinous/ bone interface, accomplishing the same response. The physician first must approve the same type of exercise program for the upper extremities because care must be taken not to disturb the surgical site.

Home Health Care

For the person at home, fluids are important, and the use of cranberry or prune juice to increase urine acidity and help prevent stone formation may be recommended. Evaluate the living environment for any potential safety hazards that may predispose the client to injury, such as throw rugs, tub or shower stall without a rubber mat or decals to prevent slipping, missing hand and guard rails wherever necessary, and improper lighting. Encourage the use of a night-light in dark areas at all times.

Hypoparathyroidism

Definition. Hyposecretion, hypofunction, or insufficient secretion of PTH are ways to describe hypoparathyroidism.[27] Because the parathyroid glands primarily regulate calcium balance, hypoparathyroidism causes hypocalcemia and produces a syndrome opposite that of hyperparathyroidism with abnormally low serum calcium levels, high serum phosphate levels, and possible neuromuscular irritability (tetany) (Box 11-4).

Etiologic Factors and Incidence. Hypoparathyroidism is either iatrogenic, which is most common, or idiopathic. *Iatrogenic* (acquired) causes include accidental removal of the parathyroid glands during thyroidectomy or anterior

---

> **Box 11-4**
>
> ## CHARACTERISTICS OF HYPERPARATHYROIDISM AND HYPOPARATHYROIDISM
>
> *Hyperparathyroidism*
>
> - Increased bone resorption
> - Elevated serum calcium levels
> - Depressed serum phosphate levels
> - Hypercalciuria and hyperphosphaturia
> - Decreased neuromuscular irritability
>
> *Hypoparathyroidism*
>
> - Decreased bone resorption
> - Depressed serum calcium levels
> - Elevated serum phosphate levels
> - Hypocalciuria and hypophosphaturia
> - Increased neuromuscular activity, which may progress to tetany

---

neck surgery. Variations in location and color in addition to the minute size of parathyroid glands make identification difficult and may result in glandular damage or accidental removal during thyroid removal or anterior neck surgery. Other iatrogenic causes can include infarction of the parathyroid glands as a result of an inadequate blood supply to the glands during surgery, strangulation of one or more of the glands by postoperative scar tissue, and rarely, massive thyroid irradiation. Other secondary causes of hypoparathyroidism may include hemochromatosis, sarcoidosis, amyloidosis, tuberculosis, neoplasms, or trauma. Idiopathic causes affect children nine times as often as adults and affect twice as many women as men. Like Graves disease and Hashimoto thyroiditis, idiopathic hypoparathyroidism may be an autoimmune disorder with a genetic basis.

Pathogenesis. See "Pathogenesis and Clinical Manifestations" under "Hyperparathyroidism" above for a description of the regulation of calcium and phosphate by PTH and the parathyroid glands. PTH normally functions to increase bone resorption to maintain a proper balance between serum calcium and phosphate. When parathyroid secretion of PTH is reduced, bone resorption and GI tract absorption slow, serum calcium levels fall, and severe neuromuscular irritability develops. Calcifications may form in various organs such as the eyes and basal ganglia. Serum phosphate levels rise without sufficient PTH because fewer phosphorus ions are secreted by the distal tubules of the kidneys with decreased renal excretion of phosphorus.

Clinical Manifestations. Mild hypoparathyroidism may be asymptomatic, but it usually produces hypocalcemia and high serum phosphate levels that affect the CNS and other body systems (Table 11-8). The most significant clinical consequence of hypocalcemia associated with hypoparathyroidism is neuromuscular irritability. In people with chronic hypoparathyroidism, this neuromuscular irritability may result in tetany. Hypocalcemia resistant to PTH, called *pseudohypoparathyroidism*, is determined genetically and is associated with shortened metacarpals and metatarsals.[150]

Acute (overt) tetany begins with a tingling in the fingertips, around the mouth, and occasionally, the feet. This tingling spreads and becomes more severe,

Table 11-8	Systemic Manifestations of Hypoparathyroidism			
CNS Effects	**Musculoskeletal Effects***	**Cardiovascular Effects***	**Integumentary Effects**	**Gastrointestinal Effects**
Personality changes (irritability, agitation, anxiety, depression) Seizures	Hypocalcemia (neuromuscular excitability and muscular tetany, especially involving flexion of the upper extremity) Spasm of intercostal muscles and diaphragm compromising breathing Positive Chvostek sign	Cardiac arrhythmias Eventual heart failure	Dry, scaly, coarse, pigmented skin Tendency to have skin infections Thinning of hair, including eyebrows and eyelashes Fingernails and toenails become brittle and form ridges	Nausea and vomiting Constipation or diarrhea Neuromuscular stimulation of the intestine (abdominal pain)

Modified from Goodman CC, Synder TE: *Differential diagnosis for physical therapists: Screening for referral*, ed 5, Philadelphia, 2013, Saunders.
*The therapist should be aware of musculoskeletal and cardiovascular effects, which are the most common and important.

producing painful muscle tension, spasms, grimacing, laryngospasm, and arrhythmias. Trousseau sign (carpal spasm) and Chvostek sign (hyperirritability of the facial nerve, producing a characteristic spasm when tapped) are apparent on examination (see Figs. 5-8 and 5-9). In severe cases, a tracheostomy may be required to correct acute respiratory obstruction secondary to laryngospasm.

MEDICAL MANAGEMENT

DIAGNOSIS. Diagnosis of this condition is based on history, clinical presentation, examination, and laboratory values (low serum calcium, high serum phosphate, or low or absent urinary calcium). Radioimmunoassay for PTH demonstrates decreased PTH concentration.

TREATMENT. Acute hypoparathyroidism, with its major manifestation of acute tetany, is a life-threatening disorder. Treatment is directed toward elevation of serum calcium levels as rapidly as possible with intravenous calcium, prevention or treatment of convulsions, and control of laryngeal spasm and subsequent respiratory obstruction. Treatment of chronic hypoparathyroidism with pharmacologic management is accomplished more gradually than treatment for an acute situation. Surgical intervention is not appropriate and, in fact, is often the cause of this condition (see "Etiologic Factors" below).

PROGNOSIS. Full recovery from the effects of hypoparathyroidism is possible when the condition is diagnosed early, before the development of serious complications. Unfortunately, once formed, cataracts and brain (basal ganglion) calcifications are irreversible. Death can occur from respiratory obstruction secondary to tetany and laryngospasms if treatment is not initiated early in acute hypoparathyroidism.

SPECIAL IMPLICATIONS FOR THE THERAPIST   11-11

Hypoparathyroidism

Anyone experiencing acute tetany will be receiving acute medical care and will not be a likely candidate for therapy until the condition has resolved with treatment.

Chronic Hypoparathyroidism

For the person with chronic hypoparathyroidism, observe carefully for any minor muscle twitching or signs of laryngospasm because these may signal the onset of acute tetany. Chronic tetany is less severe, usually affects one side only, and may cause difficulty with gait and balance. Gait training and prevention of falls are key components of a therapy program. Hyperventilation may worsen tetany; focus on breathing during exercise is important.

Chronic hypoparathyroidism can lead to cardiac complications (e.g., arrhythmia, heart block, and decreasing cardiac output) that necessitate careful monitoring. Calcium in vitamin D preparations prescribed for this condition may result in hypercalcemia, which potentiates the effect of digitalis, thus requiring close monitoring for signs of digitalis toxicity and mild hypercalcemia (see Table 12-5). When one agent potentiates the effects of another agent, the enhancement is such that the combined effect is greater than the sum of the effects of the individual agents.

Home Health Care

Lifelong medication, dietary modifications, and medical care are required for the person with chronic hypoparathyroidism. Serum calcium levels must be checked by a physician at least three times a year to maintain normal serum calcium levels. If hypophosphatemia persists, cheese and milk should be omitted from the diet because they have a high calcium content. Other foods high in calcium but low in phosphorus are encouraged.

Adrenal Glands

The adrenals are two small glands located on the upper part of each kidney (see Fig. 11-1). Each adrenal gland consists of two relatively discrete parts: an outer cortex and an inner medulla. The outer cortex is responsible for the secretion of mineralocorticoids (steroid hormones that regulate fluid and mineral balance), glucocorticoids (steroid hormones responsible for controlling the metabolism of glucose), and androgens (sex hormones).

The centrally located adrenal medulla is derived from neural tissue and secretes epinephrine and norepinephrine, which exert widespread effects on vascular tone, the heart, and the nervous system, and affects glucose metabolism. Together, the adrenal cortex and medulla are major factors in the body's response to stress.

Glandular hypofunction and hyperfunction characterize the major disorders of the adrenal cortex. Underactivity of the adrenal cortex results in a deficiency of glucocorticoids, mineralocorticoids, and adrenal androgens. Overactivity results in excessive production of these same hormones.

Adrenal Insufficiency

Hypofunction of the adrenal cortex can originate from a disorder within the adrenal gland itself (primary adrenal insufficiency) or it may be due to hypofunction of the pituitary–hypothalamic unit (secondary adrenal insufficiency).[277] Adrenocortical insufficiency, whether primary or secondary, can be either acute or chronic.

Primary Adrenal Insufficiency (Addison Disease)

Definition and Overview. Addison disease is a condition that occurs as a result of a disorder within the adrenal gland itself, with insufficient cortisol release from the adrenal glands causing a wide range of problems. Addison disease was named for the physician who first studied and described the associated symptoms. Adrenal insufficiency affects about 4 adults in 100,000 each year in the United States. Both sexes are affected, but the incidence is slightly higher in women than men. Addison disease can occur anytime across the life span with a preponderance of cases during middle age (40-60 years).

Primary forms of adrenal insufficiency are uncommon; the therapist is most likely to see secondary adrenal insufficiency as a result of suppression of ACTH by steroid therapy or secondary to opportunistic infections related to human immunodeficiency virus (HIV).

Etiologic Factors. At one time, most causes of Addison disease occurred as a complication of tuberculosis, but now most cases are considered idiopathic or autoimmune. Because more than half of all people with idiopathic Addison disease have circulating autoantibodies that react specifically against adrenal tissue, this condition is considered to have an autoimmune basis.

Less frequent causes of primary insufficiency include bilateral adrenalectomy, adrenal hemorrhage or infarction, radiation to the adrenal glands, malignant adrenal neoplasm, and infections (e.g., histoplasmosis or cytomegalovirus). Destruction of the adrenal glands by chemical agents has been reported.[216] Medications, such as antifungals, adrenolytic agents, etomidate, rifampin, phenytoin, and phenobarbital, can also trigger Addison disease.

Risk Factors. Surgery (including dental procedures); pregnancy (especially with postpartum hemorrhage); accident, injury, or trauma; infection; salt loss resulting from profuse diaphoresis (hot weather or with strenuous physical exertion); or failure to take steroid therapy in persons who have chronic adrenal insufficiency can cause acute adrenal insufficiency.

Pathogenesis and Clinical Manifestations. This adrenal gland disorder results in decreased production of cortisol (a glucocorticoid) and aldosterone (a mineralocorticoid), two of the primary adrenocortical hormones. Glucocorticoid deficiency causes widespread metabolic disturbances. Consequently, when glucocorticoids become deficient, gluconeogenesis decreases, with resultant hypoglycemia and liver glycogen deficiency. The person grows weak, exhausted, hypotensive, and suffers from anorexia, weight loss, nausea, and vomiting. Emotional disturbances can develop, ranging from mild neurotic symptoms to severe depression. Glucocorticoid deficiency also diminishes resistance to stress.

In anyone who has previously been diagnosed with Addison disease, acute symptoms such as severe abdominal pain, low back or leg pain, severe vomiting, diarrhea, and hypotension may develop quickly in response to triggers such as trauma, infarction, or infection. The resulting condition, called *addisonian crisis*, can progress quickly to hypovolemic shock (e.g., hypotension, tachycardia, and loss of consciousness) from rapid fluid loss.

Chronic adrenal insufficiency with chronic cortisol deficiency results in a failure to inhibit anterior pituitary secretion of ACTH. The result is a simultaneous increase in ACTH secretion and melanocyte-stimulating hormone (MSH) (see Fig. 11-2); excessive MSH increases skin and mucous membrane pigmentation. Persons with Addison disease may have a bronzed or tanned appearance, which is the most striking physical finding with primary adrenal insufficiency (not present in all people with this disorder). This change in pigmentation may vary in the white population from a slight tan or a few black freckles to an intense generalized pigmentation. The change in pigmentation is most commonly observed over extensor surfaces such as the backs of the hands (metacarpophalangeal joints), elbows, knees, creases of the hands, lips, and mouth. Increased pigmentation of scars formed after the onset of the disease is common. Members of darker-skinned races may develop a slate-gray color that is obvious only to family members.

Aldosterone deficiency causes numerous fluid and electrolyte imbalances. Aldosterone normally promotes conservation of sodium and therefore conserves water and excretion of potassium. A deficiency of aldosterone causes increased sodium excretion, dehydration (see symptoms listed in Box 5-8), hypotension (low blood pressure causing orthostatic symptoms; see Chapter 12), and decreased cardiac output affecting heart size (decrease in size). Eventually, hypotension becomes severe and cardiovascular activity weakens, leading to circulatory collapse, shock, and death. Excess potassium retention (greater than 7 mEq/L) can result in arrhythmias and possible cardiac arrest.

Other clinical effects include decreased tolerance for even minor stress, poor coordination, fasting hypoglycemia (resulting from decreased gluconeogenesis), and a craving for salty food. Addison disease may also retard axillary and pubic hair growth in females, decrease the libido (from decreased androgen production), and in severe cases, cause amenorrhea (absence of menstruation).[324]

MEDICAL MANAGEMENT

DIAGNOSIS AND PROGNOSIS. Diagnosis of Addison disease depends primarily on blood and urine hormonal assays and cortisol response to synthetic ACTH administration. Decreased serum cortisol levels are the hallmark of Addison disease. An ACTH stimulation test can help identify the presence of Addison disease and the type. In an ACTH stimulation test, baseline measurements of blood and urine cortisol levels are measured. The individual receives an intramuscular injection or intravenous infusion of ACTH to stimulate cortisol secretion. Blood cortisol and aldosterone measurements are repeated 30 to 60 minutes later. These levels should be greater than baseline levels; with adrenal insufficiency, the levels do not rise or rise only slightly.

If the ACTH stimulation test is positive, a CRH stimulation test is conducted to determine if the adrenal insufficiency is primary or secondary. After injection of synthetic CRH, blood cortisol measurements are taken. A high ACTH level without increased cortisol signals primary adrenal insufficiency. An absent or delayed ACTH response without deficient cortisol level indicates secondary adrenal insufficiency.[125]

Complications from Addison disease such as hyponatremia, hypoglycemia, hyperkalemia, hypercalcemia, and metabolic acidosis will be apparent in the blood chemistry values obtained.

TREATMENT. Acute adrenal insufficiency is treated by replacing fluids, electrolytes, glucose, and cortisol while identifying the underlying cause of the problem. Medical management for chronic adrenal insufficiency is primarily pharmacologic, consisting of lifelong administration of synthetically manufactured corticosteroids and mineralocorticoids (fludrocortisone). If untreated, Addison disease is ultimately fatal. Adrenal crisis requires immediate hospitalization and treatment.

SPECIAL IMPLICATIONS FOR THE THERAPIST   11-12

Primary Adrenal Insufficiency (Addison Disease)

With pharmacologic therapy, listlessness and exhaustion should gradually lessen and disappear, making exercise possible. Stress (including physical stress) should be minimized with physical activity and exercise progressed very gradually per individual tolerance. Too much stress of any kind can put the client into an "addisonian crisis" as the body is unable to meet the cortisol demand caused by the extra "stress" of exercise.

Aquatic physical therapy may be contraindicated for anyone with Addison disease. The heat and humidity of the pool environment causes the body to require more cortisol so that blood vessels can respond in order to increase blood pressure and cool the body down. With adrenal insufficiency, the adrenal gland cannot produce enough cortisol for the demands on the individual.

The therapist should monitor vital signs in anyone with Addison disease, especially when initiating and progressing an exercise program. Even small changes in medication dose can create a medical emergency in people with Addison disease. Watch for any signs of an impending crisis such as dizziness, nausea, profuse sweating, elevated heart rate, and tremors or shaking.

Any signs of infection, such as sore throat or burning on urination (see Box 8-1), should be reported to the physician. The client may be directed by the physician to increase medication dosage during times of stress and self-limiting illnesses (e.g., colds and flu). The therapist may need to advise the person to check with the physician if illness or any of the listed risk factors develop at home or during outpatient care.

Individuals with known Addison disease who enter the hospital for orthopedic surgery are often administered increased doses of cortisol to adjust for the increased needs in stress situations. Clients with Addison disease should be assessed carefully for signs of hypercortisolism, which can result from excessive long-term cortisol therapy (see Tables 5-4 and 5-5). Assess for signs of sodium and potassium imbalance as well (see Table 5-10).

Steroid-induced psychosis can occur but often has some of the same symptoms as addisonian crisis. There can be personality changes as the affected individual becomes suspicious, confused, and irritable. Slurred speech and difficulty moving with poor motor planning and motor incoordination may be compounded by severe exhaustion. The therapist is encouraged to be sensitive to clients experiencing medication-induced psychosis; what may appear as a lack of motivation or poor/noncompliance may require compassion, understanding, and patience until the medical condition is under control and the client can begin to make progress. The therapist must monitor and help the client monitor fatigue or periods of adrenal insufficiency to avoid the return of psychotic symptoms. Working closely with the orthopedic surgeon and endocrinologist is very important for these individuals.

If steroid replacement therapy is inadequate or too high, changes in amounts of sodium and water are observed (see Tables 5-10 and 5-12). Persons receiving glucocorticoid alone may need mineralocorticoid therapy if signs of orthostatic hypotension or electrolyte abnormalities develop. Older adults may be more sensitive to the side effects of steroid therapy, such as osteoporosis, hypertension, and diabetes, when these conditions already exist. The therapist must not overlook the presence of these other conditions when providing treatment intervention.

Anyone with identified Addison disease should wear an identification bracelet and carry an emergency kit containing dexamethasone or hydrocortisone. Steroids administered in the late afternoon or evening may cause stimulation of the CNS and insomnia in some people. Anyone reporting sleep disturbances should be encouraged to discuss this with the physician.

Secondary Adrenal Insufficiency

Secondary adrenal insufficiency is caused by other conditions outside the adrenals, such as hypothalamic or pituitary tumors, removal of the pituitary, or other causes of hypopituitarism, or too-rapid withdrawal of corticosteroid drugs. Long-term exogenous corticosteroid stimulation suppresses pituitary ACTH secretion and results in adrenal gland atrophy. Untimely discontinuation of adrenocorticosteroid therapy results in acute adrenal insufficiency and can become a life-threatening emergency. Anyone receiving adrenocorticosteroid therapy should be identified through the use of a bracelet or necklace. Steroid therapy must be discontinued gradually so that pituitary and adrenal function can normalize.

Clinical manifestations of secondary disease are somewhat different from symptoms of primary adrenal insufficiency. Whereas most symptoms of primary adrenal insufficiency arise from cortisol and aldosterone deficiency, symptoms of secondary disease are related to cortisol deficiency only. Because the gland is still intact, aldosterone is secreted normally, but the lack of stimulation from ACTH results in deficient cortisol secretion. Arthralgias, myalgias, and tendon calcification can occur, which resolve with treatment of the underlying condition.

Hyperpigmentation is not part of the clinical presentation because ACTH and MSH levels are low. Additionally, because aldosterone secretion may continue at fairly normal levels in secondary adrenal hypofunction, this condition does not necessarily cause accompanying hypotension and electrolyte abnormalities.[183]

As with primary adrenal insufficiency, treatment involves replacement of ACTH and monitoring for fluid and electrolyte imbalances. Too much cortisol replacement can result in the development of Cushing syndrome (see next section).

Adrenocortical Hyperfunction

Hyperfunction of the adrenal cortex can result in excessive production of glucocorticoids, mineralocorticoids, and androgens. The three major conditions of adrenocortical hyperfunction are Cushing syndrome (glucocorticoid excess), Conn syndrome or aldosteronism (aldosterone excess), and adrenal hyperplasia (adrenogenital syndrome). This last condition is rare and congenital and is not discussed further in this text.

Cushing Syndrome

Definition and Overview. Hypercortisolism is a general term for an excess of cortisol in the body. This condition can occur as a result of hyperfunction of the adrenal gland (usually benign or malignant adenomas rarely a carcinoma), an excess of corticosteroid medication, or an excess of ACTH stimulation from the pituitary gland (or other sites). ACTH secreted by the pituitary has a key role in cortisol release. When the hypothalamus senses low ACTH levels in the blood, it sends CRH to the pituitary to stimulate ACTH secretion, which in turn stimulates the adrenal glands to release cortisol. When blood cortisol levels are adequate or elevated, the hypothalamus and pituitary release less CRH and ACTH.[3]

Hypercortisolism resulting from adrenal gland oversecretion or from hyperphysiologic doses of corticosteroid medications is called *Cushing syndrome.* When the hypercortisolism results from oversecretion of ACTH from the pituitary, the condition is called *Cushing disease.* The clinical presentation is the same for both conditions.[190]

A separate condition called *pseudo-Cushing syndrome* occurs when conditions such as depression, alcoholism, estrogen therapy, or eating disorders cause changes similar to those of Cushing syndrome. In pseudo-Cushing syndrome, the symptoms will go away when the cause is eliminated.

Etiologic Factors and Incidence. The primary causes of Cushing syndrome are hyperphysiologic doses of adrenocorticosteroids (exogenous cause) and adrenocortical tumors (endogenous cause). Cushing disease results from pituitary adenomas, which secrete an excess of ACTH causing overstimulation of a normal adrenal gland (70% of all cases are Cushing disease caused by pituitary tumor).[3]

Therapists are more likely to treat people who have developed medication-induced Cushing syndrome (exogenous steroid administration). This condition occurs after these individuals have received large doses of cortisol (also known as hydrocortisone) or cortisol derivatives. Exogenous steroids are administered in individuals who have received organ transplants and for a number of rheumatologic, pulmonary, neurologic, and nephrologic diseases. Noniatrogenic Cushing syndrome occurs mainly in women (5:1 ratio of women to men), with an average age at onset of 25 to 40 years, although it can be seen in people up to age 60 years.

Pathogenesis and Clinical Manifestations. Cushing syndrome occurs as a result of excess cortisol release from the adrenal glands or exogenously administered glucocorticoids. Cushing disease is usually due to an anterior pituitary tumor. When the normal function of the glucocorticoids becomes exaggerated, a wide range of physiologic responses can be triggered, including hyperglycemia, hypertension, proximal muscle wasting, and osteoporosis (Table 11-9; see also Table 5-4).

Cortisol has a key role in glucose metabolism and a lesser part in protein, carbohydrate, and fat metabolism. Cortisol also helps maintain blood pressure and cardiovascular function while reducing the body's inflammatory responses. Overproduction of cortisol causes liberation of amino acids from muscle tissue with resultant weakening of protein structures (specifically muscle and elastic tissue). The end result may include a protuberant abdomen (Fig. 11-6) with purple striae (stretch marks), poor wound healing, thinning of the skin, generalized (progressive) muscle weakness, and marked osteoporosis that is made worse by an excessive loss of calcium in the urine. In severe cases of prolonged Cushing syndrome, muscle weakness and demineralization of bone may lead to pathologic fractures and wedging of the vertebrae, kyphosis (Fig. 11-7), osteonecrosis (especially of the femoral head), bone pain, and back pain.

The effect of increased circulating levels of cortisol on the muscles varies from slight to marked. Muscle wasting can be so extensive that the condition simulates muscular dystrophy. Marked weakness of the quadriceps muscle often prevents affected people from rising out of a chair unassisted. Cortisone-induced myopathies are discussed in Chapter 5.

Whenever corticosteroids are administered, the increase in serum cortisol levels triggers a negative feedback signal to the anterior pituitary gland to stop its secretion of ACTH. This decrease in ACTH stimulation of the adrenal cortex results in adrenocortical atrophy during the period of exogenous corticosteroid administration. If these medications are stopped suddenly rather than

Table 11-9	Pathophysiology of Cushing Syndrome
Physiologic Effect	**Clinical Result**
Persistent hyperglycemia	"Steroid diabetes"
Protein tissue wasting	Weakness as a result of muscle wasting; capillary fragility resulting in ecchymoses; osteoporosis as a result of bone matrix wasting
Potassium depletion	Hypokalemia (Table 5-10), cardiac arrhythmias, muscle weakness, renal disorders
Sodium and water retention	Edema and hypertension
Hypertension	Predisposes to left ventricular hypertrophy, congestive heart failure, cerebrovascular accidents
Abnormal fat distribution	Moon-shaped face; dorsocervical fat pad; truncal obesity, slender limbs, thinning of the skin with striae on the breasts, axillary areas, abdomen, and legs
Increased susceptibility to infection; lowered resistance to stress	Absence of signs of infection; poor wound healing
Increased production of androgens	Virilism in women (e.g., acne, thinning of scalp hair, hirsutism or abnormal growth and distribution of hair)
Mental changes	Memory loss, poor concentration and thought processes, euphoria, depression ("steroid psychosis"; see Chapter 5)

reduced gradually, the atrophied adrenal gland will not be able to provide the cortisol necessary for physiologic needs. A life-threatening situation known as *acute adrenal insufficiency* can develop, requiring emergency cortisol replacement (see the discussion on addisonian crisis in "Primary Adrenal Insufficiency" below).[314]

MEDICAL MANAGEMENT

DIAGNOSIS. Although there is a classic cushingoid appearance in persons with hypercortisolism (see Fig. 11-6), diagnostic laboratory studies, including measurement of urine and serum cortisol, are used to confirm the diagnosis. If the initial laboratory tests are positive (elevated cortisol levels), then confirmatory tests (e.g., 2-day low-dose dexamethasone, low-dose DST-CRH testing, or late-night salivary cortisol) can be ordered.[144]

Serum ACTH levels help determine whether Cushing syndrome is ACTH-dependent (e.g., pituitary tumor, which technically makes it Cushing disease). Adrenal imaging can be used to assess for Cushing that is ACTH-independent (adrenal tumor). Further testing (pituitary contrast-enhanced magnetic resonance imaging [MRI] and abdominal computed tomographic [CT] scan) is determined on the basis of these results. X-rays or dual-energy x-ray absorptiometry scans may be needed to assess for fractures or to rule out osteopenia or osteoporosis, respectively. These tests may be conducted to obtain

a baseline measurement of bone density or they may be obtained in response to an individual's report of musculoskeletal symptoms such as bone pain or backache.[209]

TREATMENT AND PROGNOSIS. Treatment to restore hormone balance and reverse Cushing syndrome or disease may require pituitary irradiation, drug therapy, or surgery (e.g., adrenalectomy, resection of tumors) depending on the underlying cause. For individuals with muscle wasting or at risk for muscle atrophy, a high-protein diet may be prescribed. Lifelong glucocorticoid replacement is necessary when the pituitary is removed or destroyed and for individuals who undergo bilateral adrenalectomy.[3,222]

Prognosis depends on the underlying cause and the ability to control the cortisol excess. Surgical cure rates are approximately 80% with a 25% recurrence rate by 5 years. Prognostic factors include experience of surgeon, degree of postoperative hypocortisolism, and finding of a tumor at surgery.[26] The more rare adrenocortical carcinomas are associated with a 5-year survival rate of 30% or less.[3]

SPECIAL IMPLICATIONS FOR THE THERAPIST 11-13

Cushing Syndrome
See "Adverse Effects of Corticosteroids" in Chapter 5.

Conn Syndrome

Definition and Overview. Conn syndrome, or primary aldosteronism, occurs when an adrenal lesion results in hypersecretion of aldosterone, the most powerful of the mineralocorticoids. Its primary role is to conserve sodium, and it also promotes potassium excretion. The major cause of primary aldosteronism (an uncommon condition present most often in women aged 30 to 50 years) is a benign, aldosterone-secreting tumor called *aldosteronoma*.[95] Rarely, Conn syndrome develops as a consequence of adrenocortical carcinoma.

Secondary hyperaldosteronism also can occur as a consequence of pathologic lesions that stimulate the adrenal gland to increase production of aldosterone. For example, conditions that reduce renal blood flow (e.g., renal artery stenosis) or induce renal hypertension (e.g., nephrotic syndrome or ingestion of oral contraceptives) and edematous disorders (e.g., cardiac failure or cirrhosis of the liver with ascites) can cause secondary hyperaldosteronism.

Pathogenesis and Clinical Manifestations. Aldosterone affects the tubular reabsorption of sodium and water and the excretion of potassium and hydrogen ions in the renal tubular epithelial cells; an excess of aldosterone enhances sodium reabsorption by the kidneys. This leads to the development of hypernatremia (excess sodium in blood, indicating water loss exceeding sodium loss), hypervolemia (fluid volume excess, increase in the volume of circulating fluid or plasma in the body), hypokalemia (low blood levels of potassium), and metabolic alkalosis (see Chapter 5). With the hypervolemia and hypernatremia, the blood pressure increases, often to very high levels, and renin production is suppressed. This hypertension can lead to cerebral infarctions and renal damage.

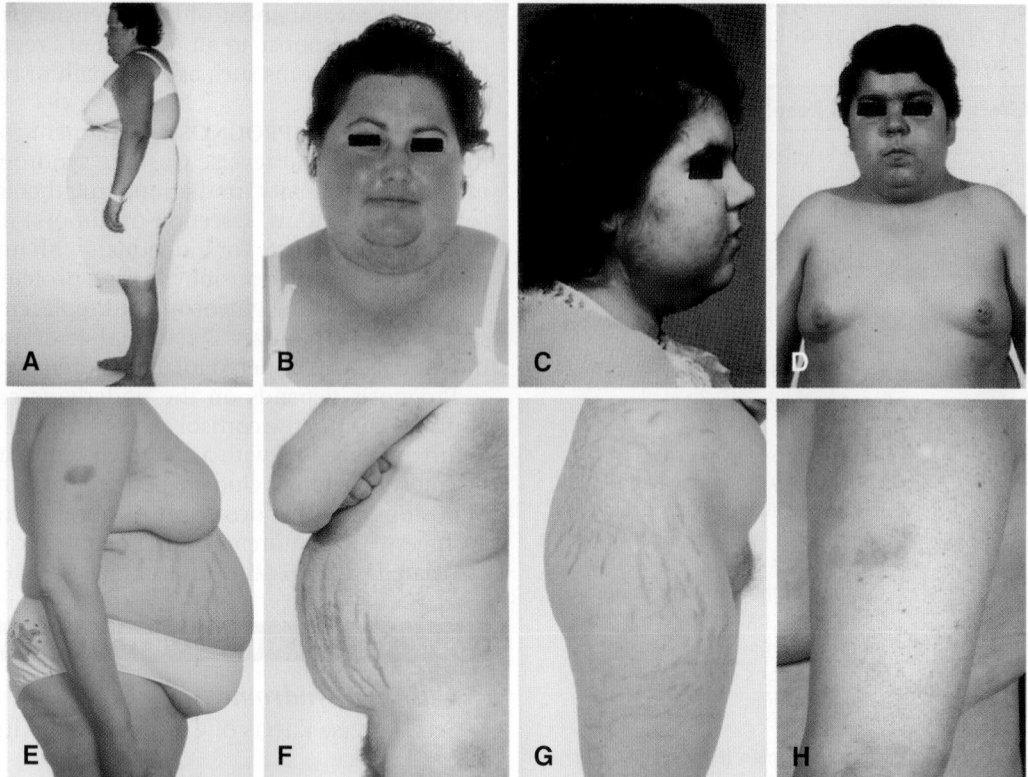

Figure 11-6

Clinical features of Cushing syndrome. **A,** Central and some generalized obesity and dorsal kyphosis in a 30-year-old woman with Cushing disease. **B,** Same woman as in **A,** showing moon facies (round face), hirsutism (hair growth), and enlarged supraclavicular fat pads. **C,** Facial rounding, hirsutism, and acne in a 14-year-old girl with Cushing syndrome. **D,** Central and generalized obesity and moon facies in a 14-year-old boy with Cushing syndrome. **E** and **F,** Typical central obesity with visible abdominal striae ("stretch marks") seen in a 41-year-old woman and 40-year-old-man with Cushing syndrome. **G,** Striae in a 24-year-old woman with congenital adrenal hyperplasia treated with excessive doses of dexamethasone as replacement therapy. **H,** Typical bruising and thin skin of Cushing syndrome. In this case, the bruising has occurred without obvious injury. (From Larsen RP: *Williams textbook of endocrinology,* ed 10, Philadelphia, 2003, WB Saunders.)

Without intervention, complications of chronic hypertension develop in the presence of hypertension, hypernatremia, and hypokalemia, heart failure, renal damage, and cerebrovascular accident. Hypokalemia results from excessive urinary excretion of potassium causing muscle weakness; intermittent, flaccid paralysis; paresthesias; or cardiac arrhythmias (see Table 5-10).

This excessive urinary excretion of potassium (hypokalemia) leads to polyuria and resulting polydipsia (excessive thirst). DM is common because hypokalemia interferes with normal insulin transport. Finally, hypokalemia leads to metabolic alkalosis, which can cause a decrease in ionized calcium levels, resulting in tetany and respiratory suppression. However, low serum potassium and alkalosis are not always present at the time of diagnosis.

MEDICAL MANAGEMENT

DIAGNOSIS, TREATMENT, AND PROGNOSIS. Diagnosis of primary hyperaldosteronism is based on elevations in serum and urine aldosterone studies and CT scanning of the abdomen for evidence of unilateral and sometimes bilateral adenomas of the adrenal gland.[95] Radiographic studies can reveal cardiac hypertrophy resulting from chronic hypertension. Radionuclide scanning techniques using radiolabeled substances allow visualization of any tumors present.

The goals of treatment are to reverse hypertension, correct hypokalemia, and prevent kidney damage. Surgical removal of the aldosterone-secreting tumor may also require adrenalectomy, which completely resolves the hypertension within 1 to 3 months. However, without early diagnosis and treatment, renal complications from long-term hypertension may be progressive. Pharmacologic treatment to increase sodium excretion and treat the hypertension and hypokalemia is a nonsurgical alternative.

SPECIAL IMPLICATIONS FOR THE THERAPIST   11-14

Conn Syndrome

The therapist treating someone with hyperaldosteronism, primary or secondary, may observe signs of tetany (muscle twitching and Chvostek sign; see Fig. 5-9) and hypokalemia-induced cardiac dysrhythmias, paresthesias, or muscle weakness. If these are encountered in an acute care setting, the medical team is usually well aware of such symptoms and is working to establish a fluid–electrolyte balance. When such signs and symptoms are observed in the outpatient setting, the client must seek medical attention.

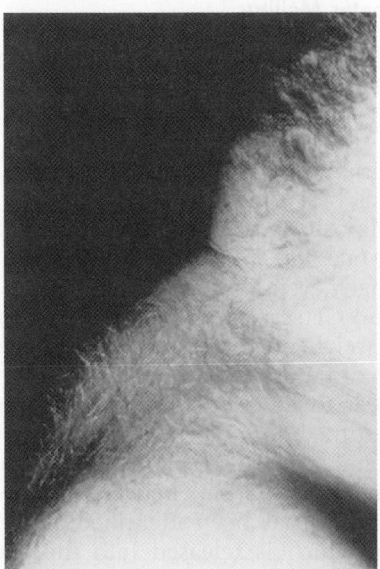

Figure 11-7

Buffalo hump and hypertrichosis (excessive hairiness; hirsutism) in a male with Cushing syndrome. This hump is a painless accumulation of fat that also may occur idiopathically in (usually) women. A familial pattern may exist (i.e., affected women report a similar anatomic change in their mothers). In the case of steroid-induced changes, this condition resolves when the individual stops taking the medication; in such cases, therapeutic intervention by the therapist has no permanent effect. Idiopathic fat deposits and underlying postural changes can be altered with postural correction and soft tissue and joint mobilization techniques. No studies have substantiated whether these changes are long-term. (From Callen JP, Jorizzo J: *Dermatological signs of internal disease*, ed 2, Philadelphia, 1995, WB Saunders.)

Adipose Tissue

One does not normally think of fat as endocrine tissue. In fact, adipose tissue can be classified as the largest endocrine organ in the body. This revelation was made only a few years ago. Before that time, fat was viewed as a storage site for energy, with little other function. Now it is clear that neurotransmitters and glucose (along with other molecules) directly act on adipocytes to induce the release of a number of different proteins collectively termed *adipokines* (or adipocytokines) that can act locally as autocrine hormones or through the bloodstream as endocrine hormones.[112] A large number of these mediators (adipokines) have been identified and studied (e.g., tumor necrosis factor alpha [TNF-α], leptin, adiponectin, resistin, chemerin, interleukin-6 [IL-6], visfatin).[45]

The role of adipocytes in the secretion of molecules that are transported in the blood has only recently been discovered and remains under investigation. Some of the factors released by adipocytes function to maintain the balance of energy. However, others have roles that are beyond the conservation of energy, including the induction of vasoconstriction (angiotensin), inflammation (leptin; see further discussion of inflammation below), or angiogenesis (vascular endothelial growth factor).

One of the reasons that the role of adipose tissue in health and disease has been difficult to describe is due to the fact that fat from different parts of the body functions in various ways. In mammals, adipose tissue is divided into two categories: brown and white. Brown fat is a very specialized tissue that is important in thermoregulation, converting energy from food into heat.[41] Infants have more brown fat; thus, they are more sensitive to temperature changes, especially the cold. The amount of brown fat decreases into adulthood, but some does remain in specific locations through the life span. The activity of the adipocytes in brown fat is closely regulated by the sympathetic nervous system.

White adipose tissue (white fat) is the classic adipose tissue responsible for storage of triglycerols to provide a long-term reservoir of energy for the body.[299] White adipose tissue is an important endocrine and secretory organ. Releasing a series of multiple-function mediators, white fat is involved in a wide spectrum of diseases, including not only cardiovascular and metabolic complications, such as atherosclerosis and type 2 diabetes, but also inflammatory- and immune-related disorders, such as rheumatoid arthritis and osteoarthritis.[45]

Important advances related to these proteins shed new insights into the pathophysiological mechanisms of many complicated diseases, although details of which remain unclear. Adiponectin, one of the most widely investigated adipokines, has been shown to possess both antiinflammatory and proinflammatory effects.

Another consideration is the association between obesity and accumulation of *ectopic fat*, defined as abnormal lipid droplets in nonfat cells such as the heart, pancreas, liver, and skeletal muscle. In obesity, fat cells themselves become insulin resistant and cannot uptake and store excess calories. As a consequence, ectopic fat accumulates in organs and skeletal muscle. Ectopic fat may cause skeletal muscle cell death and a decrease on lean body mass.[285] Excess adipose tissue has been found in skeletal muscles of individuals with obesity and diabetes and this has been associated with low muscle strength and impaired physical function.[124,184]

Obesity

(See complete discussion in Chapter 2). Obesity is the most common nutritional disorder in the Western world and has been categorized as a disease process by the U.S. Social Security Administration (SSA).[305] The SSA's policy ruling describes obesity as a "complex, chronic disease characterized by excessive accumulation of body fat."

Obviously there is a direct correlation with adipose cells and obesity—more adipose tissue results in a more obese person. However, obesity is a multifactorial problem related both to behavior and biology. The role of fat cells to send signals to the brain that are translated as feelings of hunger or satiation has only recently been uncovered.

Leptin, the first adipokine identified, acts on the hypothalamus to alter hunger, with increased levels of leptin acting as a hunger depressor. Leptin binds to neurons within the CNS that contain neuropeptide Y, thus confirming its action.[142] In humans and in animal models, the level of leptin highly correlates with the levels of adipose tissue.[177] Transgenic animals that lack the ability to make leptin are extremely obese and develop diabetes. If the animals are treated with leptin, there is a subsequent reduction in the animal's food intake and substantial weight loss.[219]

In human obesity, which has many causes, the role of leptin in hunger is not as clear. As a person becomes more obese, the leptin levels increase, which is the opposite of the expected result. It appears that the target receptors for leptin become less sensitive with increasing amounts of fat.[112]

It is now thought that leptin's role in appetite regulation is more important in reduced calorie situations. When calories are restricted and weight loss is occurring, leptin levels decrease. Historically, when humans had to gather their own food, this signal to the brain was important to stave off starvation. Leptin's role in hunger for persons that have sufficient calorie intake is unclear.

Obesity and Cancer. The link between obesity and cancer in humans has been apparent for years and continues to be borne out by statistics.[104,114] In a major study undertaken in Austria, obesity in men was associated with a high risk of colon cancer and pancreatic cancer. In women, there was a weak positive association between increasing body mass index (BMI) and all cancers combined and strong associations with non-Hodgkin lymphomas and uterine cancer.[239] In addition, the incidence of breast cancer was positively associated with high BMI but only after 65 years of age. Along with the greater risk of developing cancer in those individuals who have a BMI that places them in the obese category, the outcome for individuals who are obese and have cancer is significantly worse compared to the person with cancer who has a low BMI in terms of reoccurrence of the cancer, malignancy, and life span.[134,232]

Although the epidemiologic data strongly link some cancers with obesity, the physiologic mechanisms are only beginning to be elucidated. Leptin has been identified as a major adipokine linking prostate cancer with obesity.[21] Along with an increase in leptin levels in men who are obese, a decrease in the adiponectin levels is also associated with prostate cancer.[36]

In animal models that develop abdominal obesity, a high likelihood of hyperinsulinemia and precancerous changes in the colon have been observed.[59] In studies in men, low plasma adiponectin levels resulted in a higher risk of colorectal cancer.[319] At the cellular level, leptin has been shown to cause increased proliferation and precancerous changes in cultured colon epithelial cells.[85]

Obesity has been associated with an increased risk of breast cancer and a reduced survival rate in women with invasive breast cancer.[232] Obese women have higher levels of plasma leptin,[134] and high levels of leptin have been found in some types of breast cancer.[96] The exact mechanism by which leptin would induce breast cancer growth is unknown.

The number of newly identified adipokines continues to grow with the addition of apelin, visfatin, and others.[299] The field of adipose endocrinology is in its infancy and will expand our understanding of the dynamic role of fat in health and disease.

Type 2 Diabetes Mellitus

Although type 2 DM is discussed later in this chapter, the role of adipose tissue is presented here. Although excess white fat in any location may lead to the progression of diabetes, it is the fat surrounding the viscera and the hepatic circulation that is most important. Visceral adipose tissue is best defined as the collection of intraabdominal adipose deposits that includes omental and intrahepatic fat.[18]

Interestingly, even abdominal obesity has subcategories. MRI and CT scans indicate that some people carry abdominal weight in the subcutaneous region, but the distribution of fat around the organs is minimal. These people appear to have little insulin resistance. In contrast, when intraabdominal fat accumulates around the organs (visceral fat) (Fig. 11-8), insulin resistance quickly follows.[91] The molecular link between abdominal fat and insulin resistance has been identified as the adipokine adiponectin, which is released into the circulation by adipocytes.

Adiponectin increases insulin sensitivity in muscle and liver and increases free fatty acid oxidation in muscle tissues along with other cell types.[112] As the level of adiponectin decreases, the risk for insulin resistance increases. In overweight individuals, weight loss has been shown to increase adiponectin levels, and is associated with decreased insulin resistance.[285] The effect of exercise training on adiponectin levels is equivocal. In a systematic review of the effects of exercise on adiponectin, 38% of the randomized controlled trails demonstrated a small to moderate increase in adiponectin levels. Support in the literature for increasing adiponectin was favorable for moderate- to high-intensity long-term exercise programs and inconsistent for shorter-term programs (<12 weeks).[272] Several genetic mutations, including human polymorphisms, of the adiponectin gene are associated with reduced plasma adiponectin concentrations and an increased risk of insulin resistance and type 2 diabetes.[118,156] In addition, adiponectin inhibits the formation of atherosclerosis in the large vessels such as the coronary arteries.[284]

Other adipokines involved in inflammation have been linked to insulin resistance, including IL-6, IL-8, IL-10, Visfatin, and TNF-α.[310] These factors are increased with metabolic syndrome or prediabetes conditions.

Inflammation

An interesting observation led to the discovery of an additional role for adipose tissue. Obesity is associated with a systemic low-grade inflammation. This observation led to the idea that adipocytes released compounds into the blood to cause the inflammation. Eventually, it was determined that leptin activates many members of the inflammatory pathway, including CD4+/CD8+ T lymphocytes causing proliferation of the cells.[172]

Leptin can also activate natural killer cells.[330] Within the white fat of obese people, macrophages are known to infiltrate and produce local proinflammatory molecules like TNF-α and IL-6.[22] With weight loss, there is a decrease in the number of macrophages within adipose tissue and a decrease in the local inflammation. Thus, leptin works locally in the adipose tissue.

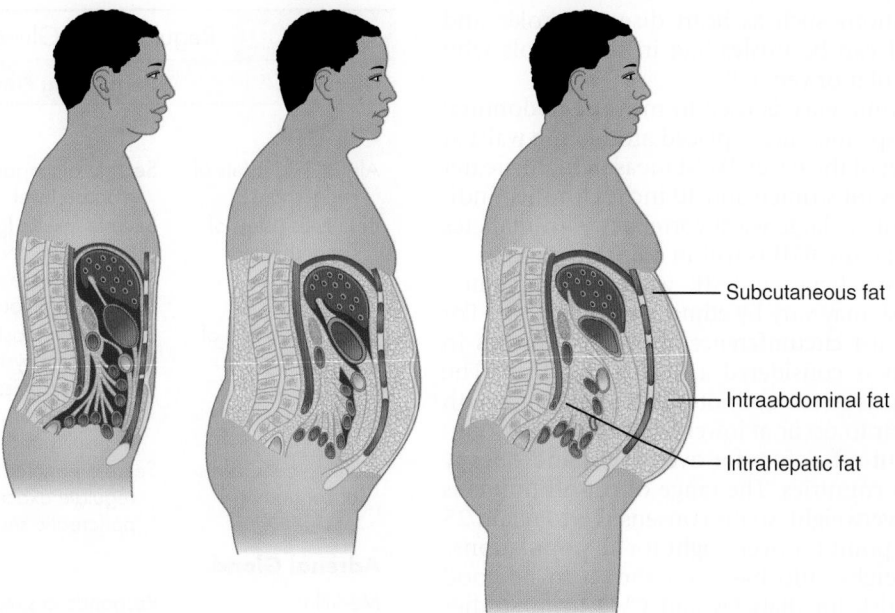

Subcutaneous fat

Intraabdominal fat

Intrahepatic fat

Figure 11-8

Abdominal adipose tissue (fat) can accumulate as subcutaneous, intraabdominal, or intrahepatic (fatty lobules throughout the liver). The body has an almost unlimited capacity to store fat. Central obesity has been linked with serious health consequences (e.g., cardiovascular disease, insulin resistance, diabetes mellitus).

However, it also has an effect on distant tissues. Leptin links the immune and inflammatory processes to the neuroendocrine system. In addition to playing a key role in modulating T cells, it also is important in autoimmune conditions such as autoimmune encephalomyelitis, type 1 diabetes, bowel inflammation, and rheumatoid arthritis.[215]

In obesity, leptin is not the only adipokine to induce widespread inflammation. White fat is characterized by an increased production and secretion of a wide range of inflammatory molecules including TNF-α and IL-6, which may have local and systemic effects. Visceral adipose tissue is again the site of much of the inflammatory secretion.

Adipocytes from visceral fat produce large amounts of monocyte chemoattractant protein 1, an adipokine directly involved in cellular remodeling of the heart. One study in women showed a strong correlation between visceral adipose tissue and monocyte chemoattractant protein 1, which resulted in inflammation of the heart and cardiac dysfunction as analyzed by echocardiograms.[179]

In contrast to leptin, adiponectin has an antiinflammatory action. It has been shown to be protective against atherosclerotic events in large vessels.[284] In addition, adiponectin levels may rise with long-term moderate- to high-intensity exercise along with a reduction in inflammatory mediators in the blood.[211] However, this antiinflammatory role may be tissue specific as evidence suggests that high adiponectin levels may be involved in the chronic inflammation associated with arthritis.[45,72,74,212]

SPECIAL IMPLICATIONS FOR THE THERAPIST   **11-15**

Adipose Tissue

Fat accumulated in the lower body (subcutaneous fat) results in a pear-shaped figure, whereas fat in the abdominal area (visceral fat) produces more of an apple shape. Specific genes have been identified that help dictate the number of fat cells and where they are located. This process is also influenced by hormonal production (decreased estrogen at menopause with increased ratio of androgens to estrogens).

Visceral fat produces cytokines (e.g., TNF or IL-6) that increase the risk of CVD by promoting insulin resistance and low-level chronic inflammation. Excess abdominal fat is considered a greater risk factor than overall obesity for cardiovascular disease and type 2 diabetes; it has also been linked to colorectal cancer, hypertension, and memory loss.[285] But the good news is that visceral fat can be reduced with diet and exercise. The therapist can offer education and guidance in this area of prevention and management.

Increasing physical activity and exercise to 1 hour daily may be ideal, but benefits have been observed with even 30 minutes of daily, moderate activity. Twice-weekly strength training has also been shown to prevent increases in body fat percentage and attenuate increases in abdominal fat in at least one study of overweight or obese women.[264]

The therapist can help individual clients assess BMI (see Table 2-3) and waist circumference. BMI helps identify people whose weight increases their risk for several conditions such as heart disease, stroke, and diabetes. BMI can be misleading in individuals who are very muscular or very tall.

Waist circumference is used to measure abdominal adiposity. A tape measure is placed around the waist at about the level of the navel. Waist measurement greater than 35 inches for women and 40 inches for men indicates rising risk. A large waist correlates with diabetes risk (even when the BMI is within a normal range).

Relationships between BMI, waist circumference, and health risk may vary by ethnic group.[166,251,327] For example, a waist circumference above 31.5 inches in Asian women is considered a health risk.[119,196] The WHO consensus statement notes that although health risks do appear to occur at lower BMIs for Asian populations, the cut-off points for overweight and obesity vary by Asian countries. The range of cut-off points is 22 to 25 for overweight, so the consensus is to retain 25 as the cut-off point for overweight for all populations.

Waist-to-height ratio has been shown to be good predictor of risk for diabetes and CVD from studies conducted in 14 different countries. Both waist circumference and waist-to-height ratios are stronger predictors than BMI. It has been suggested that "keep your waist circumference to less than half your height" may be a useful screening tool across cultures. For further discussion of commonly accepted measures to define obesity in adults, see "Obesity" in Chapter 2.[33]

Pancreas (Islets of Langerhans)

The pancreas lies behind the stomach, with the head and neck of the pancreas located in the curve of the duodenum and the body extending horizontally across the posterior abdominal wall (see Figs. 11-1 and 16-1). It has two functions, acting as both an endocrine gland (secreting the hormones insulin and glucagon) and an exocrine gland (producing digestive enzymes). The cells of the pancreas that function in the endocrine capacity are the islets of Langerhans.

The islets of Langerhans have three major functioning cells: (1) the alpha cells produce glucagon, which increases the blood glucose levels by stimulating the liver and other cells to release stored glucose (glycogenolysis); (2) the beta cells produce insulin, which lowers blood glucose levels by facilitating the entrance of glucose into the cells for metabolism; and (3) the delta cells produce somatostatin, which is thought to regulate the release of insulin and glucagon (Table 11-10).[132]

Diabetes Mellitus

Definition and Overview. DM is a chronic, systemic disorder characterized by hyperglycemia (excess glucose in the blood) and disruption of the metabolism of carbohydrates, fats, and proteins. Insulin, produced in the pancreas, normally maintains a balanced blood glucose level. DM is characterized as a group of metabolic diseases resulting from defects in the secretion of insulin, action of insulin, or both. The chronic hyperglycemia of DM is associated with long-term damage and dysfunction

Table 11-10	Regulation of Glucose Metabolism
Gland	**Regulating Function**
Pancreas	
Alpha cells (islets of Langerhans)	Secrete glucagon; increase blood glucose level
Beta cells (islets of Langerhans)	Secrete insulin (glucose-regulating hormone); decrease blood glucose level; release connecting or C-peptide in equal amounts to insulin
Delta cells (islets of Langerhans)	Secrete somatostatin (regulates endocrine system and affects neurotransmission and cell proliferation); regulate the release of insulin and glucagon
Gamma cells (islets of Langerhans)	Secrete pancreatic polypeptide (self-regulate exocrine and endocrine pancreatic secretion activities)
Adrenal Gland	
Medulla: Epinephrine	Responds to stress; epinephrine stimulates liver and muscle glycogenolysis to increase the blood glucose level
Cortex: Glucocorticoids	Increase blood glucose levels by promoting the flow of amino acids to the liver, where they are synthesized into glucose
Anterior Pituitary	
Adrenocorticotropic hormone (ACTH)	Increases blood glucose levels
Human growth hormone (GH)	Limits storage of fat; favors fat catabolism; inhibits carbohydrate catabolism, raising blood glucose levels
Thyroid	
T_3 and T_4	May raise or lower blood glucose levels

and impairment of tissues and organs, especially the eyes, kidneys, nerves, heart, and blood vessels.

The majority of cases of DM fall into two large categories: type 1 DM and type 2 DM, related to differences in etiology and pathogenesis of the disease. In type 1 DM (previously called *insulin-dependent DM [IDDM]* or *juvenile-onset DM*), the cause of hyperglycemia is an absolute deficiency of insulin production and secretion.

Most individuals with type 1 DM can be identified by serologic evidence showing an autoimmune process occurring in the islet cells of the pancreas along with specific genetic markers. People with type 1 DM are prone to ketoacidosis and specific metabolic derangements associated with hyperglycemia; they require exogenous insulin to maintain life.

Type 2 DM (previously called *non–insulin-dependent DM [NIDDM]* or *adult-onset DM*) is a much more prevalent form of diabetes, and the cause is a combination of cellular resistance to insulin action and an inadequate compensatory insulin secretory response. Individuals with type 2 DM are not as likely to exhibit the metabolic derangements common to the person with type 1 DM, and type 2 DM usually can be controlled with diet, exercise, and oral hypoglycemic agents. In some cases, however,

Table 11-11	Differences Between Types of Diabetes Mellitus	
Features	**Type 1 (Ketosis-Prone)**	**Type 2 (Not Ketosis-Prone)**
Age at onset	Usually <20 y	Usually >40 y; increasing number of cases in all ages, including children
Proportion of all cases	<10%	>90%
Type of onset	Abrupt (acute or subacute)	Gradual
Etiologic factors	Possible viral/autoimmune, resulting in destruction of islet cells	Obesity-associated insulin resistance
HLA association	Yes	No
Insulin antibodies	Yes	No
Body weight at onset	Normal or thin, obesity uncommon	Majority are obese (80%)
Endogenous insulin production	Decreased (little or none)	Variable (above or below normal)
Ketoacidosis	May occur	Rare
Treatment	Insulin, diet, and exercise	Diet, oral hypoglycemic agents, exercise, insulin, and weight control

Modified from Goodman CC, Snyder TE: *Differential diagnosis for physical therapists*, ed 5, Philadelphia, 2013, Saunders.

people with type 2 DM do require insulin replacement.[51] A comparison of the primary differences between the two types of diabetes is shown in Table 11-11.

In recent years, the lines between type 1 and 2 DM have begun to blur. An autoimmune type of diabetes that begins in middle to late adulthood has been identified. In addition, with increased obesity, type 2 DM is being diagnosed in younger and younger children.[234] Autoantibodies typical of type 2 diabetes have been identified in obese people with DM, previously labeled with type 2 DM. The exact classification of these "hybrid" types of diabetes is still being sorted out. Some have used the term *type 1.5*, or *maturity-onset diabetes of the young* (MODY). It is important to understand that the characteristics of type 1 and 2 diabetes are not mutually exclusive and should be considered along a spectrum of attributes of the disease.

Prediabetes. Prediabetes occurs when the body cannot utilize glucose the way it should. After ingesting food, carbohydrates are converted into glucose. The pancreas releases insulin to help move the glucose into the cells to be used for energy. In someone with prediabetes, this process is not completed because either the body cells do not recognize all of the insulin (decreased insulin sensitivity) or the cells stop responding to the action of insulin (increased insulin resistance).

With less glucose moving into the cells, the blood glucose levels start to rise. This is the beginning of a condition referred to as *prediabetes*. In prediabetes, the blood glucose levels are higher than normal but not quite high enough to be considered diabetes (Table 11-12). Many people with prediabetes have hypertension and dyslipidemia. The trio of comorbidities increases the risk of developing type 2 diabetes and heart disease. Most people diagnosed with prediabetes do, in fact, go on to develop diabetes. More than half have diabetes within 10 years.

According to the American Diabetes Association,[51] two categories of hyperglycemia classifications fall between normal and a true diagnosis of diabetes. *Impaired glucose tolerance* and *impaired fasting glucose* refer to intermediate metabolic stages that fall between normal glucose metabolism and diabetes. Elevated glucose levels on either test is defined as prediabetes.

Table 11-12	Blood Glucose Levels
Fasting Plasma Glucose Test	**Two-Hour Oral Glucose Tolerance Test**
Normal: <100 mg/dL	Normal: <140 mg/dL
Prediabetes: 100-125 mg/dL	Prediabetes: 140-199 mg/dL
Diabetes: >125 mg/dL	Diabetes: ≥200 mg/dL

Individuals with impaired glucose tolerance often manifest hyperglycemia only when challenged with the oral glucose load used in the oral glucose tolerance test, which is a measure of how well insulin clears glucose from the bloodstream. Impaired fasting glucose is diagnosed in people whose fasting plasma glucose levels are equal to or greater than 100 mg/dL but less than or equal to 125 mg/dL. (Normal plasma glucose as defined by the American Diabetes Association is less than 100 mg/dL.)[51]

The terms *prediabetes*, *borderline diabetes*, and *insulin resistance syndrome* are sometimes used interchangeably, and sometimes the terms *insulin resistance syndrome* and *metabolic syndrome* are used to describe the same condition. There are slight differences in these terms, with some overlap. For example, because prediabetes represents both a state of decreased insulin sensitivity and increased insulin resistance, it is not strictly the same thing as just insulin resistance syndrome. The test for insulin resistance syndrome, called the euglycemic clamp, is complicated and costly and therefore not used in most doctors' offices. If blood tests are indicative of prediabetes, insulin resistance syndrome is likely present. Although prediabetes can develop without metabolic syndrome, many people with prediabetes also have metabolic syndrome. Metabolic syndrome includes central obesity, insulin resistance (the "prediabetes component"), and dyslipidemia.

Borderline diabetes is not a label accepted by everyone; the issue can be explained as one of difficulty metabolizing sugar because of overloading the body with excess food. Labeling the condition as borderline diabetes can have a negative effect on employment and insurance.

Most people with prediabetes do not exercise adequately, do not control their weight or restrict fat and calories. The Diabetes Prevention Program Intervention Trial showed that diet and exercise can lower the incidence of type 2 diabetes by 58% over 3 years among those at high risk.[67] The American Diabetes Association recommends people with prediabetes lose 5% to 10% of body weight and increase physical activity to at least 150 minutes of moderate exercise each week.[53,247]

Other Types and Categories of Diabetes Mellitus

In addition to the main categories of type 1 and type 2 DM, other rare specific types of DM exist, which are associated with a variety of etiologies, including the following:
- Genetic beta-cell defects
- Genetic defects in insulin action
- Disorders of the exocrine pancreas such as injury, neoplasm, cystic fibrosis, or infection
- Other endocrinopathies that antagonize insulin secretion or action (e.g., increased growth hormone, cortisol, glucagons, or epinephrine)
- Drug or chemically induced DM (e.g., glucocorticoids, thiazides, thyroid hormone)
- Uncommon forms of immune or genetically associated syndromes (e.g., stiff-man syndrome, Down syndrome, Klinefelter syndrome, Turner syndrome, and Wolfram syndrome)
- Infections (certain viruses, including rubella, coxsackievirus B, cytomegalovirus, adenovirus, and mumps, have been associated with beta-cell destruction in people with existing genetic markers)
- Gestational DM

The final category, gestational DM, is defined as any degree of glucose intolerance recognized with the onset of pregnancy. Approximately 6 weeks or more after pregnancy ends, the woman should be reclassified into one of the other categories, depending on whether or not her glucose tolerance resolves. She could be reclassified as normal if no glucose intolerance remains after the pregnancy is completed. Gestational DM accompanies approximately 4% of all pregnancies.

Most women who have gestational DM return to normal glucose metabolism after pregnancy.[51] However, with time, these women will likely be diagnosed with type 2 DM.[287] In addition, children born to women with gestational DM generally have delayed fine and gross motor skills and a higher prevalence of inattention or hyperactivity compared to children born of women without gestational DM.[213]

Incidence and Prevalence. According to the American Diabetes Association, more than 14.6 million Americans have been diagnosed with diabetes, and approximately 6.2 million more people have undiagnosed cases. In addition to the 20.8 million Americans with diabetes (7% of the entire U.S. population), one fourth of U.S. adults are known to have prediabetes and are therefore at risk for developing type 2 diabetes, heart disease, and stroke. The prevalence of diagnosed diabetes is projected to be as high as one in three Americans by 2050.[30]

Diabetes, with its severe complications of heart disease, stroke, kidney disease, blindness, and loss of limbs, is the most common endocrine disorder, ranked as a leading cause of death from disease in the United States (mostly because of increased rates of CAD). It is the leading cause of blindness and renal failure in adults.[89,200]

Box 11-5

RISK FACTORS FOR TYPE 1 AND TYPE 2 DIABETES MELLITUS

Type 1 DM Risk Factors
- Presence of type 1 diabetes in a first-degree relative (sibling or parent)

Type 2 DM Risk Factors
- Positive family history (first-degree relative with diabetes mellitus)
- Ethnic origin: Black, Native American, Hispanic, Asian American, Pacific Islander
- Obesity (BMI >25)
- Increasing age (≥45 y)
- Habitual physical inactivity; sedentary lifestyle
- Previous history of gestational diabetes (GDM) or delivery of babies weighing more than 9 lb
- Presence of other clinical conditions associated with insulin resistance (e.g., polycystic ovary syndrome)
- History of vascular disease
- Previously identified impaired fasting glucose or impaired glucose tolerance
- Hypertension (≥140/90 mmHg in adults or on therapy for hypertension)
- HDL cholesterol level <35 mg/dL and/or triglyceride level ≥250 mg/dL
- Cigarette smoking

DM, Diabetes mellitus.

Black, Native, Hispanic, Mexican, and Asian Americans are 1.5 to 2 times more likely to develop DM than are white Americans, with increasing incidence associated with advancing age. Nearly one half of all Americans with DM are older than 60 years and nearly one fourth of the U.S. population older than age 65 have diabetes[58]; males and females are affected equally.

Approximately 90% of all cases of DM are type 2. Type 1 DM and secondary causes (e.g., medications, genetic disease, or hormonal changes) account for the remaining 10%. Since the mid-1970s, the incidence of diabetes has steadily increased as a result of prolonged life expectancy; increased incidence of obesity; and reduced mortality resulting in increased live births to people with type 1 DM, whose children are predisposed to future development of type 1 DM.

Etiologic and Risk Factors. Risk factors for type 1 and type 2 DM have been identified (Box 11-5). Additionally, lifestyle factors, such as watching 2 or more hours of television daily, skipping breakfast, drinking a daily carbonated beverage, and having a waist measurement larger than 35 inches for women and 40 inches (a sign of abdominal fat) for men, may be linked with type 2 diabetes.

More television (sedentary lifestyle) is often linked with less activity, which can lead to weight gain. Eating nonnutritious snacks while watching television and/or drinking soda pop adds extra empty calories, which can also result in weight gain. Eating fast food more than twice a week raises the risk of obesity and the likelihood of becoming resistant to insulin.

High stress can interfere with the body's ability to make insulin and process glucose; cortisol is a key factor in glucose metabolism and stress is linked with elevated cortisol levels. Stress can also interrupt sleep, and sleep disturbances may be linked with an increased risk of developing insulin resistance. Other lifestyle and risk factors under investigation for diabetes include consuming processed meat (e.g., bacon, hot dogs, and lunch meat[86]) and major depressive disorders.[292,308]

Type 1 Diabetes Mellitus

Type 1 DM results from cell-mediated autoimmune destruction of the beta cells of the pancreas and is a condition of absolute insulin deficiency. This autoimmune process is detectable because markers of cellular destruction called *autoantibodies* are specific to pancreatic beta cells. One and sometimes more of these autoantibodies are present and detectable in 85% to 90% of individuals with type 1 DM when the disease initially is diagnosed. People with autoimmune destruction of beta cells are also prone to other autoimmune disorders such as Graves disease, Hashimoto thyroiditis, Addison disease, vitiligo, autoimmune gastritis, and pernicious anemia.[163]

Certain human leukocyte antigens (HLA-DR3 and HLA-DR4) on specific chromosomes appear to predispose persons to the development of type 1 DM. For example, there is a fourfold increased prevalence of Down syndrome among people with type 1 diabetes, supporting the theory that genes on chromosome 21 may confer risk for type 1 diabetes.[24]

In type 1 DM, the rate of beta-cell destruction is rapid in some people (mainly infants and children) and slow in others (mainly adults). Even though immune-mediated diabetes commonly occurs in childhood and adolescence, it can occur at any age, even late in life. Both genetic and environmental factors are associated with autoimmune destruction of the beta cell, although the environmental relationship is still poorly defined.[51]

In about 10% of cases of type 1 DM, no definable etiology exists. Some individuals in this category (usually of African or Asian origin) have permanent hypoinsulinemia and are prone to ketoacidosis but have no evidence of autoimmunity. Their need for insulin replacement is usually inconsistent. Up to 20% of women with type 1 DM have some kind of eating disorder that predisposes them to further complications with glucose control. Binge eating and use of intense, excessive exercise are common in preteen, teenage, and young women with type 1 DM.[55,106] The emphasis on weight control, dietary habits, and food at a time when poor self-esteem, stress, and altered image occur in young women with type 1 DM may contribute to an increased risk for eating disorders.[181]

Individuals with type 1 DM and eating disorders are more likely to practice insulin omission and reduction, symptoms unique to DM and that increase the risk of DKA and microvascular complications, such as retinopathy, in this population group.[106]

Type 2 Diabetes Mellitus

Type 2 DM is a form of diabetes in which individuals have endogenous insulin production but have difficulty with effective insulin action at the cellular level. People with type 2 DM may not need insulin treatment to survive but need other forms of therapy to prevent hyperglycemia and its resulting complications. Although the specific etiologies of type 2 DM are not clear, autoimmune destruction of beta cells does not occur.

Type 2 DM is associated with obesity. In fact, obesity-dependent diabetes in childhood is now referred to as *diabesity* and is considered an inflammatory metabolic condition. Both insulin resistance and defective insulin secretion appear very prematurely in obese individuals, and both worsen similarly toward diabetes.[263]

Most people with type 2 DM are obese and sedentary; these two risk factors cause some degree of insulin resistance. At least 80% of all persons with type 2 DM are obese and the remaining 20%, who are not obese by traditional weight criteria, may have an increased percentage of body fat distribution, particularly in the abdominal area.[51]

Type 2 diabetes was originally called *late-* or *adult-onset diabetes* because it primarily occurred in people aged 60 years or older. Starting in the early 1990s, a trend toward the development of type 2 DM in children and adolescents was observed. Excess body fat and sedentary lifestyle are the key risk factors contributing to the development of type 2 DM in younger population groups. Type 2 DM susceptibility genes that lead to insulin resistance in humans have been identified.[257]

Cigarette smoking may also be a risk factor for developing type 2 DM. Smokers exhibit a significantly increased incidence of diabetes compared to people who have never smoked.[90]

People with this form of diabetes may have normal or elevated insulin levels, but the insulin produced is ineffective because the cells are resistant to attachment to their cellular receptors and subsequent action. Insulin secretion also is impaired, and the beta cells are unable to secrete increased amounts of insulin when needed. Ketoacidosis seldom occurs in this type of diabetes, but people with type 2 DM are at increased risk for developing macrovascular and microvascular complications. The risk of developing this form of diabetes increases with age, obesity, low cardiorespiratory fitness, and lack of exercise.[320] Type 2 DM occurs more frequently in women with prior gestational DM and in individuals with hypertension or dyslipidemia. Its frequency varies in different racial/ethnic groups (see Box 11-3).

Pathogenesis. Insulin is a hormone secreted by the beta cells of the pancreas that transports glucose into the cell for use as energy and storage as glycogen: it turns food into energy. It also stimulates protein synthesis and free fatty acid storage in the fat deposits. In DM, insulin is either insufficient in amount (type 1) or ineffective in action (type 2).

Insulin deficiency compromises the body tissues' access to essential nutrients for fuel and storage.[277] When glucose levels are elevated normally (e.g., after eating a meal), beta cells increase secretion of insulin to transport and dispose of the glucose into peripheral tissues, thereby lowering blood glucose levels and reestablishing blood glucose homeostasis. Defects in the pancreas, liver, or skeletal muscle, singularly or collectively, can contribute to abnormal glucose homeostasis when cells in each of these areas do not respond to insulin.

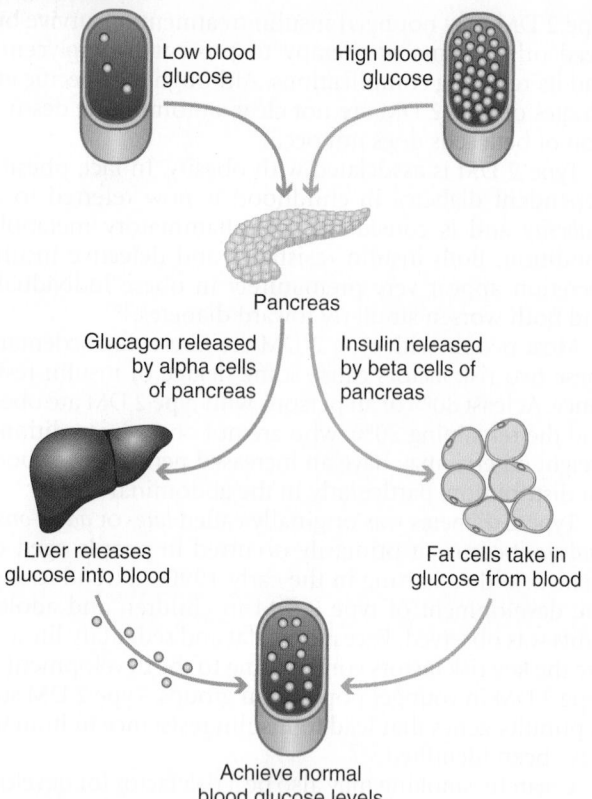

Figure 11-9

Endocrine function of the pancreas. Type 2 diabetes can promote excess sugar release from the liver, render the pancreas incapable of producing sufficient insulin, and dampen the effects of insulin on muscle and fat. Normally after intake of food, the stomach transforms food into glucose, which then enters the bloodstream. Rising blood glucose levels signal beta cells in the pancreas to release insulin. The insulin transports glucose into the cell and sets up a cascade of events (e.g., increased rate of glucose utilization and adenosine triphosphate [ATP] generation, conversion of glucose to glycogen, increase in protein and fat synthesis) that eventually results in a decline in blood glucose concentration and restoration of homeostasis. When the blood glucose levels drop (such as occurs in a hypoglycemic state or when fasting), alpha cells in the pancreas produce glucagon, which increases the blood glucose levels by stimulating the liver and other cells to release stored glucose (a process called *glycogenolysis*). The blood glucose concentration rises, thus restoring the proper balance and returning the body to a state of homeostasis. Either beta-cell dysfunction or insulin resistance can disrupt this process, resulting in decreased plasma insulin and ultimately hyperglycemia.

Normally, after a meal, the blood glucose level rises. The liver takes up a large amount of this glucose for storage or for use by other tissues such as skeletal muscle and fat. When insulin is deficient or its function is impaired, the glucose in the general circulation is not taken up or removed by these tissues; thus, it continues to accumulate in the blood, a condition called *hyperglycemia*. Because new glucose has not been deposited in the liver, the liver produces more glucose and releases it into the general circulation, which increases the already elevated blood glucose level (Fig. 11-9).[277]

When a true deficiency of insulin exists, such as that which occurs in type 1 DM diabetes, the following three major metabolic problems exist: (1) decreased utilization of glucose (as described), (2) increased fat mobilization,

and (3) impaired protein utilization. Cells that require insulin for transporting glucose inside the cell, such as in skeletal and cardiac muscle and adipose tissue, are affected most, whereas nerve tissue, erythrocytes, and the cells of the intestines, liver, and kidney tubules, which do not require insulin for glucose transport, are affected the least.

In an attempt to restore balance and normal levels of glucose, the kidney excretes the excess glucose, resulting in glucosuria (sugar in the urine). Glucose excreted in the urine acts as an osmotic diuretic and causes excretion of increased amounts of water. This process results in fluid volume deficit (see Chapter 5). The conscious person becomes extremely thirsty and drinks large amounts of water (polydipsia).

Increased fat mobilization occurs because the body can rely on fat stores for energy when glucose is not available. The process of fat metabolism leads to the formation of breakdown products called *ketones*, which accumulate in the blood and are excreted through the kidneys and lungs. Ketones can be measured in the blood and the urine to indicate the presence of diabetes. Ketones interfere with the acid–base balance by producing hydrogen ions. The pH can fall, and the affected person can develop metabolic acidosis (see Chapter 5).

After the renal threshold for ketones is exceeded, the ketones appear in the urine as acetone (ketonuria). When large amounts of glucose and ketones are excreted, osmotic diuresis becomes more severe and fluid and electrolyte loss through the kidneys increases. Sodium, potassium, and other critical electrolytes are lost in the urine, resulting in severe dehydration and electrolyte deficiency and worsening acidosis. When fats are used for a primary source of energy, the body lipid level can rise to five times the normal amount. This elevated level can lead to atherosclerosis and its subsequent cardiovascular complications (see Chapter 12).

Impaired protein utilization occurs because the transport of amino acids (the chief constituent of proteins) into cells requires insulin. Normally, proteins are constantly being broken down and rebuilt. Without insulin to transport amino acids, thereby contributing to protein synthesis, the balance is altered and protein catabolism increases. Catabolism of body proteins and resultant protein loss hamper the inflammatory process and diminish the tissue's ability to repair itself.

Because the person with type 2 DM continues to produce and use some amount of endogenous insulin, the metabolic problems associated with inappropriate use of fat and protein for energy do not occur as severely. People with type 2 DM are not prone to ketoacidosis and the metabolic derangements associated with type 1 DM. They are, however, still at great risk for hyperglycemic osmotic diuresis, dehydration, shock, and loss of electrolytes.[277]

Clinical Manifestations

Pathophysiology of Diabetic Complications. The long-term presence of DM affects the large blood vessels (macrovascular), small blood vessels (microvascular), and nerves throughout the body. The chronic hyperglycemia of diabetes results in the accelerated atherosclerosis that leads to macrovascular disease, affecting arteries that supply the heart, brain, and lower extremities. Insulin resistance has also been implicated in the macrovascular changes in diabetes.[103]

Diabetes is also associated with the development of diabetes-specific microvascular pathology in the retina, renal glomerulus, and peripheral nerve. As a result, diabetes is a leading cause of blindness, kidney failure, and a variety of debilitating neuropathies. The microvascular disease in the retina, glomerulus, and vasa nervorum has similar underlying pathophysiology.

Hyperglycemia causes abnormalities in blood flow and increased vascular permeability (caused by decreased activity of vasodilators, increased activity of vasoconstrictors, and abnormal production of extracellular matrix), and with time, microvascular cell loss and progressive capillary occlusion occur. In addition, hyperglycemia may also decrease production of trophic factors, which are required to maintain healthy endothelial and neuronal cells.

How does hyperglycemia cause these macrovascular and microvascular damages? Four main molecular mechanisms have been proposed: increased polyol pathway flux; increased advanced glycation end-product formation; activation of protein kinase C isoforms; and increased hexosamine pathway flux.[34,39] All four mechanisms seem to reflect a single hyperglycemia-induced process of overproduction of superoxide by the mitochondrial electron-transport chain. As an example, neuropathy in diabetes presumably results from the increased polyol pathway flux and is related to the accumulation in the nerve cells of sorbitol, a by-product of improper glucose metabolism. This accumulation then results in abnormal fluid and electrolyte shifts and nerve-cell dysfunction. The combination of this metabolic derangement and the diminished vascular perfusion to nerve tissues contributes to the severe problem of diabetic neuropathy. (See "Diabetic Neuropathy" in Chapter 39.)

Cardinal Signs and Symptoms. In type 1 diabetes, symptoms of marked hyperglycemia include polyuria, polydipsia, weight loss with polyphagia, and blurred vision (Table 11-13). These symptoms occur as a result of the inability of the body to use glucose appropriately and the resulting osmotic diuresis, dehydration, and starvation of body tissues. In type 1 DM, the utilization of fats and proteins for energy causes severe hunger, fatigue, and weight loss. The person with this type of diabetes may present initially in DKA.

People with type 2 diabetes also may have some of these cardinal signs and symptoms, but the aging population may not recognize the abnormal thirst or frequent urination as abnormal for their age. The person with type 2 diabetes frequently goes undiagnosed for many years because onset of type 2 DM is often gradual enough that the classic signs of hyperglycemia are not noticed. More commonly, they may experience visual blurring, neuropathic complications (e.g., foot pain), infections, and significant blood lipid abnormalities. Type 2 DM is commonly diagnosed while the client is hospitalized or receiving medical care for another problem. Frequently, the person presents with one of the long-term complications of DM such as CVD, neuropathy, retinopathy, or nephropathy.

Table 11-13	Cardinal Signs of Diabetes at Diagnosis
Clinical Manifestations	**Pathophysiologic Bases**
Polyuria (excessive urination, types 1 and 2)	Water is not reabsorbed from renal tubules because of osmotic activity of glucose in the tubules
Polydipsia (excessive thirst, types 1 and 2)	Polyuria causes dehydration, which causes thirst
Polyphagia (excessive hunger, type 1)	Starvation secondary to tissue breakdown causes hunger
Weight loss (type 1)	Glucose is not available to the cells; body breaks down fat and protein stores for energy; dehydration
Recurrent blurred vision (types 1 and 2)	Chronic exposure of the lenses and retina to hyperosmolar fluids causes blurring of vision
Ketonuria (type 1)	Fatty acids are broken down so ketones are present in urine
Weakness, fatigue, and dizziness (types 1 and 2)	Dehydration leads to postural hypotension; energy deficiency and protein catabolism contribute to fatigue and weakness
Often asymptomatic (type 2)	Physical adaptation often occurs because rise in blood glucose is gradual

Atherosclerosis. Because of the hyperglycemia and increased fat metabolism associated with type 1 DM, atherosclerosis begins earlier and is more extensive among people with diabetes than in the general population. Atherosclerotic changes in large blood vessels, caused by lipid accumulation and thickening of vessel walls, result in decreased vessel lumen size, compromised blood flow, and ischemia to adjacent tissues. As a consequence, people with diabetes have a much higher risk of myocardial infarction, stroke, and limb amputation.

Atherosclerosis and the accompanying large-vessel changes result in cardiovascular and cerebrovascular changes, skin and nail changes, poor tissue perfusion, decreased or absent pedal pulses, and impaired wound healing. Atherosclerosis combined with peripheral neuropathy and the subsequent foot deformities increases the risk for ulceration of skin and underlying tissues and limb amputation.

Individuals with undiagnosed type 2 DM are at significantly higher risk for CAD, stroke, and peripheral vascular disease than the population without diabetes. Screening of the type 2 at-risk population is essential in the prevention and treatment of diabetes-related complications. In addition, all individuals with diabetes should be aware of the strong and consistent data regarding the risks of smoking and the exacerbation of atherosclerosis-related diabetic complications.

Clients and families should be consistently and continuously counseled and encouraged in smoking cessation. The combination of smoking and diabetes dramatically increases the risks related to atherosclerotic vessel disease, impaired wound healing, and the associated morbidity and mortality rates.[7]

Cardiovascular Complications. CVD is the leading cause of mortality and morbidity in diabetes and accounts for approximately two-thirds of all deaths among the diabetic population.[51] People with diabetes have 1.5- to 4-fold increased risk of having CAD, stroke, and myocardial infarction.[51] Although diabetes has long been recognized as a potent and prevalent risk factor of ischemic heart disease caused by coronary atherosclerosis, diabetes has also become associated with left ventricular dysfunction independent of hypertension and CAD. This is a disease of a cardiac muscle itself and is called *diabetic cardiomyopathy*.[1,83,135]

Individuals with diabetic cardiomyopathy initially exhibit frequent left ventricular diastolic filling and relaxation abnormalities, later followed by systolic dysfunction, left ventricular hypertrophy, and left heart failure.[201] Diabetic cardiomyopathy is not fully explained by the cellular effects of hyperglycemia alone; the important mechanisms include metabolic disturbances, myocardial fibrosis, small vessel disease, cardiac autonomic neuropathy, and insulin resistance.[83,201] Because of the presence of autonomic neuropathy, people with diabetes may have what is called "silent ischemia" or silent heart attack. They do not experience typical pain because of the damage to nerves that occurs in diabetes.

The cardiovascular and renal systems are intricately connected and affected by diabetes. Low blood flow to the kidney causes a release of renin, which in turn triggers a cascade of events as angiotensin is converted to angiotensin I and then to angiotensin II, resulting in large increases in blood pressure. The risk of myocardial infarction and stroke increases as well.

Retinopathy and Nephropathy. Diabetic retinopathy is a highly specific vascular complication in persons with both type 1 and type 2 DM and its prevalence is correlated closely with duration and control of high blood glucose levels. After 20 years with DM, nearly all individuals with type 1 DM and more than 60% of type 2 DM have some degree of retinopathy.

Diabetic retinopathy poses a serious threat to vision. People with type 1 and type 2 diabetes should undergo yearly comprehensive eye exams. Underlying microvascular occlusion of the retina resulting in progressive areas of retinal ischemia and tissue death causes diabetic retinopathy. Studies have established that intensive management of blood glucose level control to consistent near-normal levels can prevent and delay the progression of diabetic retinopathy.[66]

Exercise may be protective against the development of macular degeneration, and individuals with diabetic retinopathy may benefit from low- to moderate-intensity aerobic and resistance exercise. However, individuals with proliferative or preproliferative retinopathy should be screened by a physician prior to beginning an exercise program. High-intensity exercise and high-impact activities, and head-down activities can greatly increase eye pressure and should be avoided.[153]

Diabetes is now the leading cause of end-stage renal disease, which is kidney failure requiring dialysis or transplantation, in the United States and Europe.[43] Hardening and thickening of the glomerular basement membrane, which result in eventual destruction of critical renal filtration structures, cause diabetic nephropathy. The presence of small amounts of albumin in the urine, called microalbuminuria, is the earliest clinical evidence of nephropathy. Approximately one of four people with type 2 diabetes have microalbuminuria that, if untreated, gradually worsens. Eventual destruction of the filtering ability of the kidney causes chronic renal failure and the need for permanent dialysis or renal transplantation.

Renal destruction, as with retinopathy, can be slowed significantly with early detection and monitoring, tight glucose control, early treatment of hypertension (particularly with angiotensin-converting enzyme [ACE] inhibitors), careful monitoring of dietary protein, and strong encouragement of cessation of smoking.[66,70,122] Hypertension is managed with ACE inhibitors initially and if blood pressure is not less than 130/85 mm Hg, a β-blocker may be added. However, combining a β-blocker with a diuretic can blunt awareness and symptoms of low glucose, so this combination usually is not recommended.

Infection. Chronic, poorly controlled diabetes mellitus can lead to a variety of blood vessel and tissue changes that result in impaired wound healing and markedly increased risk for infections. Impaired vision and peripheral neuropathy contribute to the decreased ability of the person with diabetes to feel or see breaks in skin integrity and developing wounds. Vascular disease contributes to tissue hypoxia, which further decreases healing ability.

In addition, once pathogens are inside the body, they multiply rapidly because the increased glucose content in body fluids and tissues fosters bacterial growth. Because the blood supply to tissues is already compromised, white blood cells are not mobilized to the affected areas efficiently or adequately. Diabetes results in higher incidences of skin, urinary tract, vaginal, and other types of tissue infections.[132]

Musculoskeletal Problems. Musculoskeletal complications are common, often involving the hands, shoulders, spine, and feet. Carpal tunnel syndrome, Dupuytren contracture, trigger finger (tenosynovitis), and adhesive capsulitis occur significantly more often in people with diabetes compared with those who do not have diabetes.[237] Available data show that more than 30% of people with type 1 or type 2 DM have some kind of hand or shoulder disease. More people with type 1 DM have musculoskeletal disorders than those with type 2 DM, and the degree of stiffness is greater with this type of diabetes. The exact mechanism by which the specific metabolic abnormalities of diabetes are linked to rheumatic manifestations remains unclear but appears to be linked to significantly higher A1c levels.[6,237]

Although these disorders are not life-threatening, they can add significant functional impairment to a person's life. See also the discussion of orthopedic problems that can develop secondary to sensory and motor neuropathy in "Sensory, Motor, and Autonomic Neuropathy" below.

Upper Extremity. In the hand, the syndrome of limited joint mobility (SLJM or LJM) and the stiff hand syndrome are unique to diabetes. SLJM is characterized by painless stiffness and limitation of the finger joints (Fig. 11-10). Flexion contractures typically progress to result in loss of dexterity and grip strength. The SLJM is an underdiagnosed complication of diabetes, largely because this type

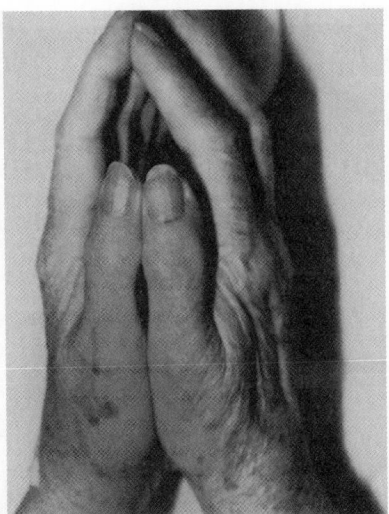

Figure 11-10

The prayer sign. The individual is unable to press the palms flat against each other, a diagnostic sign for the syndrome of limited joint mobility in diabetic persons. Other conditions also may result in loss of extension with a positive prayer sign. (From Kaye T: Watching for and managing musculoskeletal problems in diabetes. *J Musculoskelet Med* 11:25-37, 1994.)

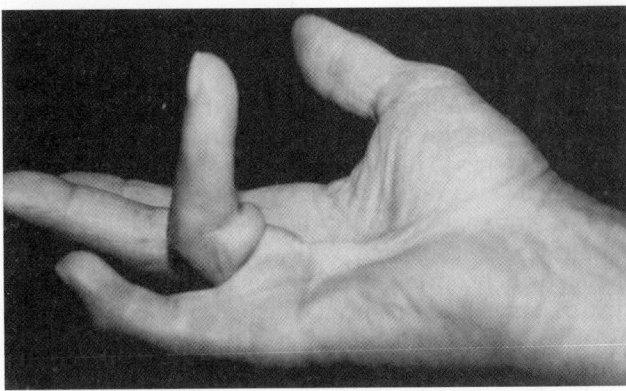

Figure 11-11

Dupuytren contracture. Painless nodules develop in the distal palmar crease, often in line with the ring finger, that slowly mature into a longitudinal cord that is readily distinguishable from a tendon. The skin overlying the nodules is usually puckered. The contracture may be symptomatic (painful), but with or without pain it results in impaired hand function. (From Kaye T: Watching for and managing musculoskeletal problems in diabetes. *J Musculoskelet Med* 11:25-37, 1994.)

of loss of hand range of motion is considered a common normal sign of aging.[107] The severity of this syndrome in diabetes is correlated with the duration of disease, duration and quantity of insulin therapy, and smoking. Joint contractures also may develop in larger joints, such as the elbows, shoulders, knees, and spine.

The stiff hand syndrome often is confused with or included in SLJM, but it has a distinct pathogenesis and clinical presentation. The stiff hand syndrome occurs uniquely with diabetes and is seen more frequently with type 1 DM and poor blood glucose control. Paresthesias, which eventually become painful, are accompanied by subcutaneous tissue changes such as stiffness and hardness. Vascular insufficiency may be the underlying cause or may be secondary to neuropathy, nodular tenosynovitis, and osteoarthritis.

Dupuytren contracture is characterized by the formation of a flexion contracture, palmar nodules, and thickening band or cord of palmar fascia (Fig. 11-11), usually involving the third and fourth digits in the population with diabetes (rather than the fourth and fifth digits in the population without diabetes). Pain and decreased range of motion are the primary presentation. Painless nodules develop in the distal palmar crease, often in line with the ring finger, which slowly mature into a longitudinal cord that is readily distinguishable from a tendon. The skin overlying the nodules is usually puckered.

In some cases, regression of symptoms does occur without intervention, although the underlying mechanism for this phenomenon remains unknown. Surgical excision has not been shown to be a reliable cure for the disease and is not recommended unless there is a contracture that is bothersome. It has been reported that if the disease recurs after surgical excision, the rate of progression may be faster.[242]

Flexor tenosynovitis (also called *chronic stenosing tenosynovitis*) is another rheumatologic condition seen more commonly in persons with diabetes. Tenosynovitis is caused by accumulation of fibrous tissue in the tendon sheath and can cause aching, nodularity along the flexor tendons, and contracture. Locking of the digit, called *trigger finger*, can occur in flexion or extension and may be associated with crepitus or pain. In the population with diabetes, tenosynovitis is found predominantly in women and affects the thumb, middle, and ring fingers most often.

Diabetes is the systemic disease most often seen in connection with peripheral neuropathy of the hand, including CTS. The clinical presentation of CTS is the same for the person with diabetes as for the person without diabetes, although in diabetes CTS can be either a neuropathic process or an entrapment problem. Both neuropathy and compression within the carpal tunnel may exist together.

Adhesive capsulitis (also known as *periarthritis* or *frozen shoulder*) is characterized by diffuse shoulder pain and loss of motion in all directions, often with a positive painful arc test and limited joint accessory motions. The pattern is slightly different from that of typical adhesive capsulitis, in which regional tightness in the antero-inferior joint capsule primarily compromises external rotation, followed by loss of abduction and less often, internal rotation and flexion.

The pattern in diabetes is one of significant global tightness with external and internal rotation equally limited in the dominant shoulder, followed by limitations in abduction and hyperextension. External rotation and hyperextension are most limited in the nondominant shoulder, followed by internal rotation and abduction. The pathogenesis of the capsular thickening and adherence to the humeral head remains unknown. The long head of the biceps tendon may become glued down in its tendon sheath on the anterior humeral head.[290]

Adhesive capsulitis may be accompanied by vasomotor instability of the hand previously referred to as reflex sympathetic dystrophy but now classified as the complex regional pain syndrome. This condition is characterized by severe pain, swelling, and trophic skin changes of the hand (e.g., thinning and shininess of the skin with loss of wrinkling, sometimes with increased hair growth).

Skin changes in diabetic hand arthropathy, in addition to changes caused by complex regional pain syndrome, may occur in association with adhesive capsulitis. Other skin changes associated with diabetes include scleroderma diabeticorum, an asymptomatic thickening of the skin that may lead to a peau d'orange appearance, which usually involves the posterior neck, upper back, and shoulders.[35] Skin and subcutaneous tissue atrophy and tendon flexion contractures develop. The natural history of this condition ranges from spontaneous remission to permanent loss of function. (See "Complex Regional Pain Syndrome" in Chapter 39.)

Tendinopathy with thickening of the plantar fascia and Achilles tendon and tendo-Achilles tightening occurs as glucose deposits in tendons and ligaments result in loss of flexibility and rigid foot. In the diabetic population, loss of Achilles tendon flexibility, especially when combined with a flatfoot, increases pressure under the foot, adding to the compressive forces that contribute to ulcer formation.[100]

Spine. Diffuse idiopathic skeletal hyperostosis (DISH; also known as *ankylosing hyperostosis* or *Forestier disease*) is a condition of the spine seen most often in people with type 2 DM, although it can occur in a person who does not have diabetes. In DISH, osteophytes develop into bony spurs, typically right-sided syndesmophytes that may join to form bridges (Fig. 11-12). The thoracic spine most commonly is involved. In contrast to ankylosing spondylitis, the sacroiliac joints are spared, and vertebral body osteoporosis is absent. Calcaneal and olecranon spurs may develop, and new bone may form around the hips, knees, and wrists.

People with DISH may be asymptomatic or they may experience back pain and stiffness without limitations in range of motion. Dysphagia may develop if extensive cervical spine involvement occurs. The pathogenesis of DISH is unknown, and apparently no correlation exists between the degree of diabetic control and the extent of hyperostosis.

Arthritis. Nearly half of people with diabetes also have arthritis. Moreover, the prevalence of arthritis-attributable activity limitations is significantly higher in adults with both diseases compared to adults with arthritis but not diabetes.[46] The prevalence of arthritis is higher with increased age, BMI, and physical inactivity. Both rheumatoid arthritis and osteoarthritis have been associated with diabetes, in different ways. Type 1 DM and rheumatoid arthritis are both autoimmune diseases. Levels of inflammatory markers, including C-reactive protein, IL-6, and TNF-α, high in people with rheumatoid arthritis, have also been found to be elevated in people with type 1 DM for longer than five years. The common connection between osteoarthritis and type 2 DM is obesity.[46]

Osteoporosis. Generalized osteoporosis usually develops within the first 5 years after the onset of DM and is more severe in persons with type 1 DM. It is hypothesized that bone matrix formation may be inadequate in

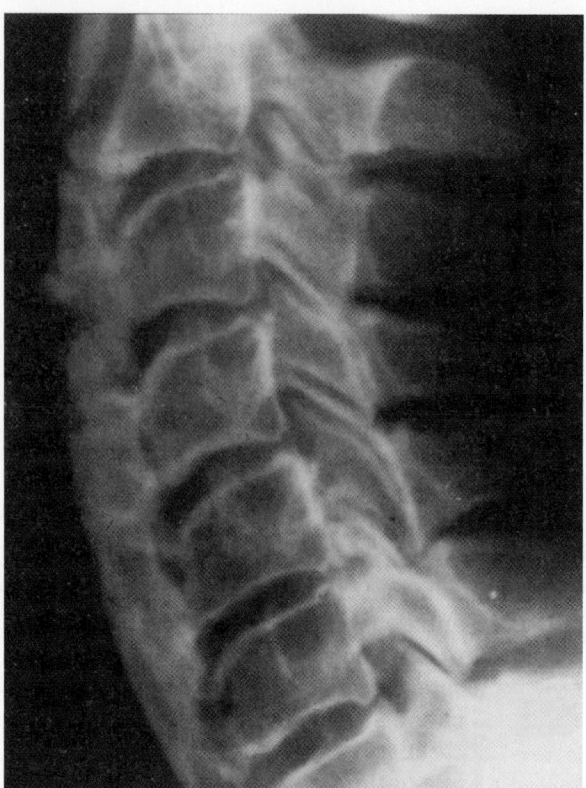

Figure 11-12

Diffuse idiopathic skeletal hyperostosis (DISH), or ankylosing hyperostosis, associated with type 2 diabetes mellitus (DM). DISH can occur with other conditions such as ankylosing spondylitis. Although the dense anterior bony bridging of the cervical vertebrae is pictured on this lateral roentgenogram, the thoracic spine most commonly is involved in diabetes. This type of DISH can be distinguished from ankylosing spondylitis by the preservation of sacroiliac joints, a site of typical involvement in ankylosing spondylitis. (From Kaye T: Watching for and managing musculoskeletal problems in diabetes. *J Musculoskelet Med* 11:25-37, 1994.)

the absence of normal circulating insulin levels. Results of bone density studies in persons with type 2 DM are conflicting, with some studies demonstrating decreased bone density and others indicating increased bone density. While bone mass may remain normal in people with type 2 DM, bone quality may be impaired. A class of oral diabetes medication, called glitazones, may promote bone loss and osteoporotic fractures in postmenopausal women.[116]

As in any case of osteoporosis, regardless of the underlying cause, this condition places the person at greater risk for fractures. With the additional loss of sensation associated with diabetes, minor trauma easily produces injury. Microfractures can occur in already weakened bone and cartilage and may remain unrecognized because of the lack of pain appreciation. A vicious circle is started, leading to further damage.

Sensory, Motor, and Autonomic Neuropathy. Sensory, motor, and autonomic neuropathy associated with DM is a common phenomenon with known risk factors (e.g., duration of diabetes, current A1c [glycated hemoglobin value], BMI, smoking, hypertension, and high triglycerides). The presence of CVD doubles the risk of neuropathy.[294]

Neuropathy may affect the CNS, peripheral nervous system, or autonomic nervous system (see Box 39-5). The most common form of diabetic neuropathy is a sensory polyneuropathy, usually affecting the hands and feet and causing symptoms that range from mild tingling, burning, numbness, or pain to a complete loss of sensation (usually feet) and foot drop. See further discussion of diabetic neuropathy in Chapter 39.

Sensory Neuropathy. Many people with diabetes suffer from *diabetic peripheral neuropathic pain* (DPNP) associated with nerve damage. Spontaneous pain, allodynia (painful response to benign stimuli), hyperalgesia, and other unpleasant symptoms are common with DPNP. Neuropathic pain often progressively increases in intensity throughout the day and is worse at night, significantly impairing sleep. Some individuals experience painful neuropathy called *insulin neuritis syndrome* at the beginning of therapy for diabetes; the feet are affected more often than the hands and it is usually self-limiting.[313]

The loss of sensation in diabetic neuropathy predisposes joints to repeated microtrauma and progressive, noninfectious joint destruction. Chronic progressive degeneration of the stress-bearing portion of a joint associated with loss of proprioceptive sensation in the joint produces a condition called *Charcot disease, Charcot arthropathy, neuroarthropathy,* or *neuropathic arthropathy.* Diabetes is the most common cause of neuropathic joints. Charcot neuroarthropathy presents in people with type 1 diabetes after an average duration of 20 to 24 years and in individuals with type 2 diabetes after only 5 to 9 years.[228]

Several stages of neuropathic arthropathy (Charcot foot) occur involving autonomic dysfunction of blood flow leading to bone destruction and absorption resulting in dislocation, deformity, and an unstable joint. Bone fragments and debris are deposited in the affected joint. Subluxation of the tarsal and metatarsal joints commonly results in a rocker-bottom foot deformity (see Fig. 23-9) and a redistribution of pressure on the plantar surface of the foot with progressive ulceration and possible infection. An acute neuropathic joint is swollen, warm, and edematous with bounding distal pulses. Pain may be minimal because of the underlying altered sensation but up to half of all affected individuals report some degree of pain.[32]

Left untreated, neuropathic changes can progress to complete destruction of the joint. The presence of autonomic neuropathy may hasten this process as the blood vessels are unable to respond appropriately (e.g., vasoconstrict) to even minor trauma. Prolonged and unregulated hyperemia in the foot may lead to excessive bone resorption resulting in decreased bone mineral density, further increasing the risk of bone and joint destruction.[307]

Joints with less movement transmit abnormal forces through the foot to injure already damaged joints. This is especially true during walking, when large forces are placed on the midtarsal and tarsometatarsal joints. Obesity further increases these forces, and in the presence of any preexisting gait abnormalities or deformities, both create additional stress that compounds the condition.

Assessment of the underlying problem is important in planning the appropriate treatment intervention. For example, improving circulation may be a goal with macrovascular or peripheral vascular disease, whereas foot care and orthoses are more appropriate treatments for microvascular-caused neuropathy. The underlying neurologic disorder should be treated but this has no effect on the existing arthropathy. Reduction of weight bearing, joint immobilization, and joint protection are important conservative treatment tools. Surgical fusion can be performed if all else fails, but joint replacement is contraindicated in this condition.[44,255]

Motor Neuropathy. Motor neuropathy is more common with long-standing disease and produces weakness and atrophy; bilateral but asymmetric proximal muscle weakness is called *diabetic amyotrophy.* Diabetic amyotrophy leads to bony deformities (e.g., claw toes, severe flatfoot with valgus of the midfoot, or collapse of the longitudinal arch) that contribute to biomechanical changes in foot function resulting in abnormal patterns of loading. Pain and erythema of the forefoot may constitute forefoot osteolysis, which is sometimes considered another form of neuropathy distinguished from cellulitis or osteomyelitis by laboratory values (leukocyte count) and roentgenographic appearance.

Autonomic Neuropathy. Autonomic neuropathy is sometimes referred to as *diabetic autonomic neuropathy* and affects nerves that innervate heart, lung, stomach, intestines, bladder, and reproductive organs. It may manifest itself through the loss of control of blood pressure, blood glucose levels, temperature, regulation of sweating (skin becomes dry and cracked with buildup of callus), and blood flow in the limbs. Skin changes such as these can create more openings for bacteria to enter. The combination of all three types of neuropathy can ultimately lead to gangrene and possible amputation, largely preventable with proper care (see "Special Implications for the Therapist 11-16: Diabetes Mellitus" and the subsection "Diabetes and Foot Care," below).

Cardiovascular autonomic neuropathy is manifested by the lack of heart rate variability in response to deep breathing and exercise, exercise intolerance, persistent sinus tachycardia, bradycardia, and postural hypotension. Stress testing should be considered before starting an exercise program, especially in the older adult.[10,12,53,127] Cardiovascular autonomic neuropathy may also result in reduced perception of ischemic pain, making a person with diabetes unaware of having a heart attack. This may delay appropriate medical treatment and lead to death.[312]

Diabetic autonomic neuropathy may lead to hypoglycemia without awareness because of loss of the warning signs of hypoglycemia such as sweating and palpitations. Being unaware of hypoglycemia and unresponsive to it are troublesome metabolic complications because they impair the person's ability to manage the disease and may result in death. Other forms of autonomic neuropathy include gastroparesis (decreased gastrointestinal motility accompanied by diarrhea and fecal incontinence), constipation, urinary tract infections (nerve damage can prevent the bladder from emptying completely, allowing bacteria to grow in the bladder and kidneys), urinary incontinence, and sexual (erectile) dysfunction.

Ulceration. Sensory neuropathy, occurring as a result of improper glucose metabolism and diminished vascular perfusion to nerve tissues, places the diabetic person at risk for the development of ulcers. Diabetic foot ulcers are caused primarily by repetitive stress on the insensitive skin with increased pressure and/or horizontal (shear) stress. Body weight and activity level increase the force that the foot must transmit, and this also may increase pressure and shear force, especially in the presence of an underlying bony prominence or foot imbalance. In addition, previously healed ulcers leave scars that transmit force to underlying tissues in a more concentrated manner and hold the fat pad locally so that it cannot function physiologically. As a result, it cannot transmit shear forces, and it becomes damaged easily.

The loss of autonomic nerve function eliminates the production of sweat, leaving the skin dry and inelastic. Changes in pressure and gait, fat atrophy, and muscle weakness are mechanical factors that, along with sensory neuropathy, influence the development of plantar skin abnormalities, especially ulceration.[28,276] Diabetes-induced changes in the skin are likely to contribute to ulceration because the collagen and keratin (a protein that is the principal constituent of epidermis, hair, and nails) may be glycosylated (saturated with glucose) with increased cross-linking, which makes the skin stiff. Keratin builds up in response to the increased pressure, covering the openings of unhealed ulcers, and cannot be removed as readily as normal keratin.

The areas most commonly affected by foot ulcers are the plantar areas of the metatarsal heads, the toes, and the plantar area of the hallux (Fig. 11-13). In the Charcot foot, the incidence of ulceration beneath the talus and navicular bones becomes more common because of the rigid rocker-bottom deformity.

Cognitive Function. Clearly, diabetes has deleterious effects on cardiovascular, renal, eye, peripheral nerve, and musculoskeletal function. The effects of diabetes on cognitive function are less well known. There is evidence that, in comparison to older adults without DM, older adults with DM may exhibit greater deficits in high-level cognitive processes responsible for planning, coordinating, and sequencing of cognitive operations. Impairments in these processes, collectively known as executive function, may contribute to balance and gait abnormalities, difficulty with activities of daily living, and increased risk of falls associated with diabetes.[250]

MEDICAL MANAGEMENT

PREVENTION. Prevention of obesity-related health problems, including prediabetes and subsequent type 2 diabetes, is a key focus of the medical community. Therapists play an important role in providing education on the beneficial effects of exercise combined with proper nutrition. Studies have clearly shown that people who incorporate physical activity and exercise into their daily lives are less likely to develop type 2 diabetes no matter what their initial weight. Adopting an activity program of 150 minutes weekly of moderate-intensity activity (e.g., brisk walking) similar to what the Surgeon General advises is a key prevention strategy.[157-159]

Studies using liposuction and studies using bariatric gastric bypass surgery in the overall treatment of obesity point to the possibility of this treatment option to disrupt the pathway that brings about insulin insensitivity in the obese individual and thus prevent diabetes from developing. Fat removal by liposuction and by bariatric surgery has been linked with modification of cardiovascular risk and vascular inflammatory markers in the obese individual, with beneficial effects on insulin resistance as well.[78,220,260]

SCREENING. The American Diabetes Association recommends universal screening for type 2 diabetes at age 45 and, if normal, repeat testing every three years. Testing should be considered in adults of any age who are overweight or obese (BMI >25 and who have one or more additional risk factors (see Box 11-5). Anyone who has been diagnosed with prediabetes should have their glucose monitored once a year.[96]

DIAGNOSIS. Diagnostic assessment may include a variety of testing procedures; fasting plasma glucose, oral glucose tolerance test, and A1c. A diagnosis of diabetes is confirmed by symptoms of hyperglycemia and blood and urine glucose and ketone abnormalities. Current defined criteria for definitive diagnosis of diabetes mellitus are the following[51]:

- Classic symptoms of diabetes (polyuria, polydipsia, and unexplained weight loss) plus a casual plasma glucose concentration ≥200 mg/dL. (*Casual* is defined as any time of day without regard to time since last meal.)

or

- Fasting plasma glucose (FPG) ≥126 mg/dL after no caloric intake for at least 8 hours.

or

- 2-hour postload glucose ≥200 mg/dL during an oral glucose tolerance test

or

- A1c ≥6.5%.

Obesity and type 2 diabetes are on the rise in children and adolescents. The American Diabetes Association recommends that children with body mass index ≥85th percentile for gender and age and two risk factors for DM (family history, race/ethnicity, signs/symptoms) be assessed for diabetes.[304]

GLUCOSE MONITORING. Individuals using multiple daily insulin injections or an insulin pump should perform self-monitoring of blood glucose (SMBG) three or more times a day. SMBG may also be useful for individuals using insulin injections that are less frequent, oral antidiabetes medications, or medical

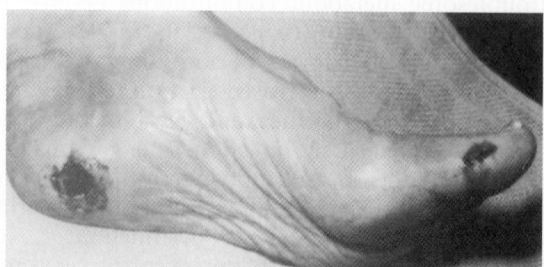

Figure 11-13

Neurotrophic ulcers associated with diabetic neuropathy. (From Callen JP, Jorizzo JL: *Dermatological signs of internal disease,* Philadelphia, 1995, WB Saunders.)

nutrition therapy. SMBG is also recommended when a new physical activity is introduced, such as occurs in an exercise or rehabilitation program and should be continued until the individual's response to the change is known and predictable in maintaining stable blood glucose levels.[80]

New insulins and easier blood glucose monitoring have improved the ability to obtain much tighter control of blood glucose levels with fewer fluctuations and reduced risk of hypoglycemia. There are two methods used to monitor glucose immediately and over time; direct blood sampling (fingersticks) and continuous glucose monitoring (CGM). CGM involves placement of a glucose sensor under the skin. The sensor measures glucose levels in the interstitial fluid and transmits this information to an electronic receiver (either an insulin pump or a pager-like device). CGM is considered to be useful for children and adults with type 1 diabetes and people who frequent hypoglycemia. CGM equipment is calibrated using fingersticks. Noninvasive technologies for SMBG such as near-infrared spectroscopy are under development. SMBG is an important management tool in the long-term treatment of this disease. Early screening and assessment of people at risk for diabetes are critical so that prevention and treatment of complications can be initiated before the onset of significant microvascular and macrovasular damage.

In addition to being a diagnostic tool, A1c level is used to monitor blood glucose control over time (Table 11-14). The A1c test should be performed at least two times per year in individuals with controlled diabetes and four times per year for those whose blood sugar levels are not well-controlled or who are on a new diabetes medication regimen. The American Diabetes Association recommends a target A1c level as 7% or less. A higher A1c target may be recommended for individuals who are older, have a history of severe hypoglycemic episodes, or

Table 11-14	Correlating A1c to Mean Plasma Glucose Levels	
A1c (%)	**Mean Plasma Glucose (mg/dL)**	
6	135	
7	170	
8	205	
9	240	
10	275	
11	310	
12	345	

Normal reference range for A1c is 4% to 6%. The goal for clients with diabetes is below 7% (target level is 6.5) but not everyone has the same target; it does depend on comorbidities, age, and duration of disease.[223] In general, higher levels are linked with greater risk of diabetes-related complications. A1c level of 7% correlates to an average daily plasma glucose level below 170 mg/dL. It is not used to diagnose diabetes and should not be measured too often in those who are using it to measure glucose control. Two measurements a year are sufficient in anyone who is meeting goals of treatment and who has stable control, and a maximum of 4 to 6 a year in people whose treatment has changed, or who are not meeting treatment goals.[179]

Data from: American Diabetes Association, 2012.

diabetes-related health complications.[80,291] According to the U.K. Prospective Diabetes Study, a 1% reduction of the A1c level reduces the risk of microvascular complications such as retinopathy and nephropathy by 25% and heart attack by 14% or more. People with A1c concentrations less than 5% had the lowest rates of CVD and mortality.[145]

TREATMENT. There is no widely available cure for diabetes. The goal of overall care for persons with diabetes is control or regulation of blood glucose. Many large-scale studies have shown that tight glucose control reduces the risk of vascular complications in both type 1 and type 2 diabetes. Tight control of blood pressure lowers the risk of strokes, heart attacks, and heart failure and slows the progression of diabetic kidney disease.[288] Early identification and intervention are strongly linked with risk reduction of late complications.[168] Three key standards and goals in the treatment and self-management of DM include the following:[80,133]

- A1c less than 7%
- Blood pressure less than 130/80 mm Hg
- Low-density lipoprotein (LDL) <100 mg/dL, high-density lipoprotein (HDL) cholesterol >50 mg/dL, and triglycerides <150 mg/dL.

Data from the National Center of Health Statistics show that only 7.3% of adults with diabetes have achieved all three targets.[258] To help people with diabetes reach these goals, the National Diabetes Education Program has started an education program called *Control the ABCs*, in which *A* is A1c, *B* is blood pressure, and *C* is cholesterol). Education materials are available in English and Spanish and for Asian Americans and Pacific Islanders.[206] A new position statement from the European Association for the Study of Diabetes and the American Diabetes Association have also published new recommendations (rather than guidelines) designed to approach each person with type 2 diabetes as an individual rather than prescribing to the singular idea of "one number fits all" (referring to the A1c target).[270] The position statement lists 7 key points related to glycemic targets; diet, exercise, and education; use of pharmaceuticals; consideration of individual preferences, needs, and values, and a clear focus on cardiovascular risk reduction. The reader is encouraged to read this document available online at http://care.diabetesjournals.org/content/35/6/1364.full. For details, see Inzucchi 2012.[133] Therapists can help reinforce all of the concepts presented in this section as part of their client education programs.

Data suggest that atherogenic and inflammatory mediators contributing to microvascular and macrovascular complications are elevated even before the onset of diabetes. There may even be a "metabolic memory" associated with these early changes. Comprehensive metabolic control instituted early may alter the natural history of diabetic complications by affecting this metabolic memory.[168]

Researchers continue to investigate drugs that would prevent the formation of fat cells, thereby reducing the problem of obesity before type 2 DM can develop. Studies of the use of gene therapy as a treatment for both types of diabetes are ongoing, utilizing a variety of approaches,

Table 11-15	Types of Insulin and Insulin Action			
Type	**Name**	**Onset of Action**	**Peak Response**	**Duration of Action**
Rapid-acting insulin	Insulin lispro (Humalog)	5 min	30-90 min	3-4 h
	Insulin aspart (NovoLog)	15 min	45-90 min	3-5 h
	Insulin glulisine (Apidra)	15 min	3-5 h	3-8 h
Short-acting or regular insulin	Insulin human regular (Humulin-R, Novolin-R)	30 min	2-3 h	3-8 h
Intermediate-acting insulin	NPH insulin (Humulin N, Novolin N)	1.5 h	4-12 h	Up to 18 h
Long-acting insulin	Insulin glargine (Lantus) Insulin detemir (Levemir)	1.5-4 h	No peak	Up to 24 h
Premixed insulins (combination of two types of insulin)	70/30 (%) (Humulin mix, Novolin mix) 50/50 (%) (Humalog mix) 75/25 (%) (Humalog mix) 70/30 (%) (NovoLog mix)	Depends on mixture; 5-30 min	Depends on mixture; 1-12 h	Up to 18 h

Onset of action is how long it takes before the insulin reaches the bloodstream and starts to lower glucose levels.
Peak response is the time at which the insulin exhibits maximum effectiveness.
Duration of action is how long the insulin continues to lower blood glucose.
Data from Micromedex Healthcare Series [Internet database]. Greenwood Village, CO, Thomson Reuters Healthcare Inc. Updated periodically.
Compiled by Tanner Higginbotham, PharmD, University of Montana Drug Information Service, 2012.

such as direct delivery of the insulin gene to non–beta cells, improving insulin secretion from existing beta cells, and implanting genetically modified cells.[101,102,141,329] Experimental research is under way in the development of a vaccine for type 1 DM that may help stop the immune system attack of the insulin-producing beta cells of the pancreas.[315,322] Research involving pancreatic islet cell and whole pancreas transplants for treatment of type 1 diabetes is also ongoing; immune rejection of the tissue remains problematic.[323]

Type 1 Diabetes Mellitus. Type 1 DM requires exogenous insulin administration and dietary management to achieve tight (near normal) blood glucose control. With no circulating endogenous insulin, the effect of aerobic exercise in providing increased glycemic control for the person with type 1 DM may be limited. To date, studies of the effect of aerobic exercise in type 1 DM have shown mixed results. Regardless, exercise should be taken into account as part of the total picture in order to minimize the complications associated with diabetes.

The insulin dosage schedule varies depending on the individual's age, level of compliance, and severity of diabetes (Table 11-15). Control over blood glucose levels dictates how "brittle" the diabetes is. *Brittle diabetes* (also known as *labile* or *unstable diabetes*) is a term used when a person's blood glucose level often swings quickly from high to low and from low to high. The individual with wide glucose excursions is considered very brittle.

Poorly controlled diabetes is ideally treated with more frequent administration of insulin (e.g., four times per day), whereas other individuals may receive insulin once or twice daily, sometimes mixing different types of insulin (e.g., rapid-acting [human analog; Humalog]; short-acting [regular] with intermediate-acting [NPH] insulin). Humalog (Lispro) is a type of insulin that has rapid action. It works faster than short-acting insulin and

must be taken with a meal to prevent hypoglycemia.[140] From a therapist's point of view, the client receiving more frequent dosages is less likely to develop hypoglycemia, especially when beginning an exercise program.

Insulin Pump. An insulin pump also known as *continuous subcutaneous insulin infusion* (CSII) is now available to deliver fixed amounts of regular insulin continuously, thereby more closely imitating the release of the hormone by the islet cells. This lightweight, pager-sized device is worn conveniently in a pocket or on a belt clip (Fig. 11-14); a waterproof design makes swimming possible.

The insulin pump offers many advantages such as flexible eating and exercising schedules, fewer episodes of severe hypoglycemia (especially at night and for teenagers who sleep longer hours), and convenience of taking insulin without the social consequences of public injections, to name a few.[54] Although this type of insulin administration provides better control, it has some disadvantages. It cannot detect and respond to changes in the blood glucose level so the individual must continue to monitor glucose levels and make dosage adjustments. There is no long-term backup supply of insulin such as is available with long-acting insulin injections. If the pump malfunctions and the person is unaware of it, blood glucose levels can rise quickly, potentially leading to ketoacidosis. The pump wearer must still monitor blood glucose levels at regular intervals.

It cannot be removed for more than 1 hour, reactions to the needle are common, bleeding can occur at the sensor insertion site, and like any other mechanical device, it is subject to malfunction. Insulin pump technology is improving every year; new "smart" features are added to the designs to simplify the tasks involved in delivering an insulin bolus. Implantable pump options that can dispense insulin in constant, steady pulses throughout the day are being tested. This type of pump would eliminate the need for an open needle site in the skin. Pen-like

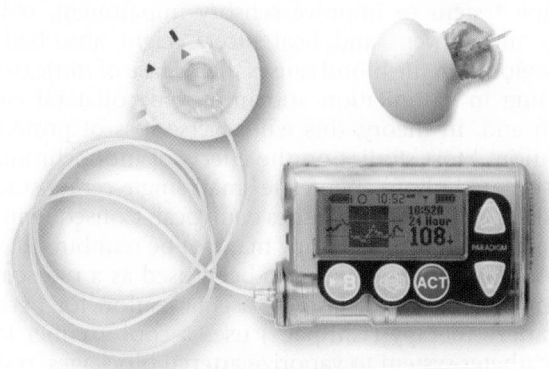

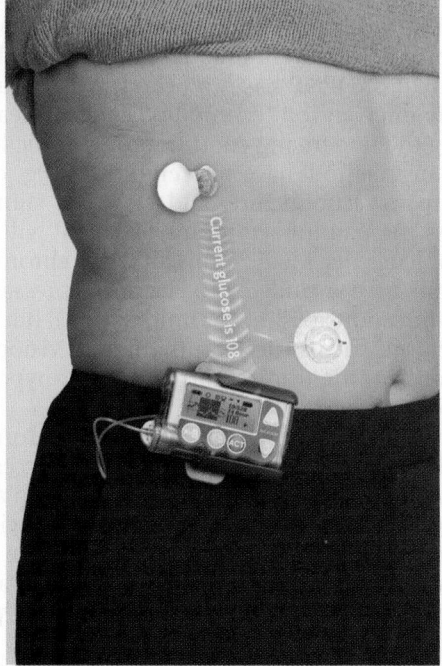

Figure 11-14

The programmable insulin pump delivery system. Compact and worn like a pager, the programmable insulin pump delivers fixed amounts of insulin continuously, based on continuous blood glucose levels determined by skin sensor. The device includes the pump itself (including controls, processing module, and batteries), a disposable reservoir for insulin (inside the pump), and a disposable infusion set, including a cannula for subcutaneous insertion (under the skin) and a tubing system to interface the insulin reservoir to the cannula. (Courtesy Medtronic Mini-Med Paradign Revel Insulin Pump, Medtronic, Northridge, CA, 2013; see YouTube demonstration available online at http://www.youtube.com/watch?v=AU78ETXSLjQ.)

injection cartridges also are in use.[151] Other methods for insulin delivery under investigation include nasal spray, suppositories, and iontophoresis. Pen-like injection cartridges also are in use.[151]

Type 2 Diabetes Mellitus

Type 2 DM is most often treated with diet and exercise, sometimes in conjunction with oral hypoglycemic drugs (OHDs); insulin may also be required. *Exercise* is a recognized therapy for the prevention of complications in type 2 DM. Numerous studies have shown a consistent positive effect of regular exercise training on carbohydrate metabolism and insulin sensitivity. Some of the beneficial effects include decreased need for insulin, prevention of CVD and obesity, management of hypertension, and reduction in very-low-density lipoprotein cholesterol.[51,191]

A plant-based *diet* is becoming more widely known for its potential effects and benefits in the prevention and treatment of type 2 DM. The use of whole-grain or traditionally processed cereals and legumes has been associated with improved glycemic control in individuals with diabetes and in individuals who are insulin-resistant. Long-term studies have shown that whole-grain consumption reduces the risk of both type 2 diabetes and CVD.[137]

The combination of diet and exercise is more powerful than either one alone and may be even more effective than drugs for preventing type 2 DM. A low-fat, low-calorie diet with moderate exercise (30 minutes 5 times a week) has been shown to reduce new diabetes cases by 58% over a 3-year period. By contrast, the drug metformin, which lowers blood sugar levels and boosts insulin sensitivity, reduced new cases by 31%.[152] The National Institutes of Health (NIH) is conducting a 12-year, 5000-patient study to further test the additive effects of diet and exercise on diabetes. See Evolve Box 11-1 on the Evolve website for more information on OHDs.

Another new class of drug for type 2 DM, incretin mimetics, is injected. Incretin mimetics, which include exanatide (Byetta), liraglutide (Victoza) and pramlintide (Symlin), mimic the action of GI hormones that increase secretion of insulin, like GLP-1, and slow the rate of digestion. This class of drug does not lead to weight gain and has been associated with weight loss in some people. Possible adverse effects include pancreatitis and pancreatic cancer.

Treatment of Long-Term Complications

Prevention of long-term complications is the goal for all clients with DM. Risk of complications is associated independently and additively with hyperglycemia and hypertension. Intensive treatment of both these risk factors is required to prevent and minimize the incidence of most complications.[286]

Medical treatment of long-term diabetic complications may include dialysis or kidney transplantation for renal failure and vascular surgery for large vessel disease. Currently, the American Diabetes Association advises that people with diabetes and increased cardiovascular risk take low-dose aspirin (75-162 mg) daily to help minimize risks such as heart attacks and strokes. This includes most men >50 years of age or women >60 years of age who have at least one additional major CVD risk factor. Prophylactic aspirin therapy is not recommended for adults with diabetes at low CVD risk because the potential adverse effects of gastrointestinal bleeding outweigh the potential benefits.[80]

New treatment guidelines from the American College of Physicians and the American Diabetes Association recommend lifestyle modifications focusing on diet, weight loss, and physical activity to help people with diabetes achieve and maintain a normal lipid profile. The use of statins (cholesterol-lowering drugs such as Crestor, Lipitor, Zocor, Mevacor, or Pravachol), regardless of baseline lipid levels, is recommended for adults with diabetes and CVD and adults without CVD who have one or more CVD risk factors. If lipid level targets (LDL < 100 mg/dL) are not reached with lifestyle modifications and statin therapy, other lipid-lowering medication may be considered.

Review of available data shows that statins reduced heart attacks and strokes by 22% to 44% in people with diabetes.[278] There is now evidence that statins are associated with increased risk of developing type 2 DM in some people. Likewise, there is controversy about the use of prophylactic statin therapy in adults, without diabetes, who are at moderate risk for developing CVD.[40,235]

Diabetic Ulcers. The therapist often is involved in prevention and wound care for diabetic ulcers, which may help prevent amputation. Early recognition and prompt management of wounds, ulceration, and Charcot foot can facilitate healing. For example, a CDC study showed that people with diabetes who wore proper shoe protection had only a 20% recurrence rate of ulceration compared with an 80% rate for those without offloading.[279]

A handheld, noninvasive, infrared thermometer can be used to measure and compare skin surface temperature for the purpose of identifying increased skin temperatures, intended as an early warning of inflammation, impending infection, and possible foot ulceration. Temperature difference of four or more degrees between the right and left foot is a predictive risk factor for foot ulcers; self-monitoring has been shown to reduce the risk of ulceration in high-risk individuals.[14,16,164,289]

Offloading or pressure reduction is a key component for healing ulcers and preventing recurrence. The normal response to damaged areas is to spare them from pressure because they are painful. However, in the insensitive foot of a person with diabetes, this normal alteration of weight-bearing surface, pressure, and duration does not take place, resulting in repetitive stress and injury with subcutaneous and cutaneous necrosis and skin breakdown.

A marked improvement in the rate of healing for plantar ulcers has been reported using a combination of total-contact cast and tendo-Achilles lengthening (percutaneous heel cord lengthening), as opposed to total-contact cast alone.[14,170,202,254]

The results of at least one study show tendo-Achilles lengthening should not be done in anyone with complete anesthesia of the heel pad; increased dorsiflexion can increase the risk of heel ulceration. This procedure is advised only in a multidisciplinary setting able to provide adequate nutrition, wound care, surveillance, treatment of complications and other biomechanical abnormalities and intervene early in any developing ulcerations.[126]

Other interventions include debridement, infection control, protective dressings, revascularization, proper nutrition, and client education. Active dressings, such as growth factors and living skin, are also in use. Topical application of growth factors on wounds without infection and with at least a minimal level of vascularization was introduced in the early 1990s and has progressed to include new techniques in skin transplantation.

Infrared light therapy, such as monochromatic near-infrared photo energy, has been applied using the anodyne therapy system to improve sensory impairment, reduce pain, and prevent and heal ulcers. Light absorbed by hemoglobin in the blood causes the release of nitric oxide, resulting in vasodilation and improved collateral circulation and, in theory, this will reverse loss of protective sensation. Most studies on the effects of monochromatic near-infrared photo energy are small single-center studies and the results of these studies equivocal. Consequently at the present time, this therapy may not be reimbursed.[208]

Cool laser therapy has also been used as a revascularization therapy. Cool laser revascularization for peripheral artery therapy (CliRpath) uses a cool excimer laser and catheter system to vaporize arterial blockages, restoring blood flow and promoting wound healing. Reduction in pain, improved circulation, and facilitation of wound healing may help prevent limb loss in this population.

Treatment of DPNP has not been successful using any one single intervention technique. The ideal treatment is correcting the underlying condition of chronic hyperglycemia. Many methods have been employed (e.g., capsaicin topical cream, acupuncture, and electrical stimulation) to address the painful symptoms of DPNP with limited and variable results. Medications aimed at chronic neuropathic pain have included tricyclic antidepressants (e.g., amitriptyline, nortriptyline, or imipramine), but anticholinergic effects, such as dry mouth, blurred vision, constipation, cardiac arrhythmias, and orthostatic hypotension, often limit their use.

Anticonvulsants, such as gabapentin (Neurontin) and pregabalin (Lyrica), have met with greater success. Selective serotonin reuptake inhibitors (SSRIs), such as duloxetine (Cymbalta), can be used by some individuals to treat painful DPNP. By inhibiting the reuptake of these neurotransmitters, descending inhibitory pathways in the spinal cord are activated and block ascending pain signals to the brain.[311] For individuals who fail to respond to nonnarcotic medications, narcotic analgesics, such as tramadol and oxycodone, may be considered as a second medication. More recently, in a large multicenter clinical trial, alpha-lipoic acid (an antioxidant) was found to decrease neuropathic pain and improve nerve conduction. Modest decreases in pain have also been reported with acetyl-L-carnitine, which may be deficient in neural fibers of people with type 2 DM.[160]

Transplantation. Research is being conducted on the use of transplanted pancreatic islet cells rather than the entire pancreas. The transplant recipient receives one or more infusions of pancreatic islet cells that include insulin-producing beta cells. High rates of insulin independence have been reported at 1 year in the leading islet transplant centers. Loss of insulin independence by 5 years occurs in the majority of recipients. Lifelong immunosuppression and its complications limit this treatment to candidates who have the most severe, unstable glycemic control despite optimal insulin therapy.[267]

Artificial pancreatic transplantation provide hope for future treatment without repeated injections for the person with type 1 diabetes. An artificial pancreas contains a reservoir for insulin (which must be filled by the affected individual, typically through a tube in the abdomen), and an internal glucose monitor that continuously determines the plasma glucose level, automatically releasing the appropriate amount of insulin. Several clinical trials are under way and such instruments are expected to reach the market shortly.[243]

Stem cell research may find a way for people to use their own stem cells to develop them into islet cells and allow infusions without cell-rejection complications and the need for lifelong immunosuppression.[25]

PROGNOSIS. Diabetes control depends on the proper interaction between the following three factors: (1) food, (2) insulin or oral medication to lower blood glucose, and (3) activity (e.g., sedentary or exertional) or exercise. When diabetes is regulated successfully, complications of hyperglycemia and hypoglycemia can be avoided with minimal disruption to a normal lifestyle. However, diabetes can be fatal even with medical treatment, or it can cause major permanent disabilities and seriously impair functional abilities.

Studies have shown that type 2 DM raises a person's risk of dying from heart disease by 2 to 3 times.[281] In fact, about 50% of myocardial infarctions and 75% of strokes are attributable to diabetes. Diabetes is the leading cause of new blindness and is a contributory cause to renal failure and peripheral vascular disease.

Regardless of the modality of treatment used for the person with type 1 or type 2 DM, studies have shown clearly that tight glucose control (plasma glucose levels consistently within normal limits, approximately 100 mg/dL) delays onset and progression of diabetic complications. The only apparent danger in maintenance of tight control is the greater possibility of hypoglycemia, particularly in those people with type 1 DM who receive frequent exogenous insulin administration.[51]

Diabetes Mellitus

Client education is the key to therapeutic, nonsurgical treatment of the neuromusculoskeletal complications associated with diabetes. Extensive self-management is the focus of the educational program. *Diabetes Self-Management* is an invaluable tool for anyone with diabetes, available online at http://www.diabetesselfmanagement.com.

Exercise is a key component of the overall intervention plan.[51] The client must be taught the importance of assessing glucose levels before and after exercise and to judge what carbohydrate and insulin requirements are suitable for the activity or workout. People with diabetes and peripheral neuropathy have a high incidence of injuries (e.g., falls, fractures, sprains, cuts, and bruises) during walking or standing and a low level of perceived safety. Suggested strategies for appropriate clinical intervention to reduce these complications are available.

Complications of Insulin Therapy

Hypoglycemia

Insulin therapy can result in hypoglycemia (low blood glucose, also called an *insulin reaction*)[60]; tissue

hypertrophy, atrophy, or both, at the site of injection; insulin allergy; erratic insulin action; and insulin resistance. Symptoms of hypoglycemia are related to two body responses: increased sympathetic activity and deprivation of CNS glucose supply (Table 11-16). The clinical picture may be varied, from a report of headache and weakness to irritability and lack of muscular coordination (much like drunkenness) to apprehension, inability to respond to verbal commands, and psychosis.

Symptoms can occur when the blood glucose level drops to 70 mg/dL or less, although this value varies among those with diabetes and can be lower than 70 mg/dL before symptoms are elicited. In diabetes, an overdose of insulin, late or skipped meals, or overexertion in exercise may cause hypoglycemic reactions. Immediately provide carbohydrates in some form (e.g., fruit juice, honey, hard candy, or commercially available glucose tablets or gel); a blood glucose test should be performed as soon as the symptoms are recognized. The unconscious person needs immediate medical attention; to prevent aspiration, fluids should not be forced. Hospitalization is recommended when the following occur:

- *The blood glucose is less than 50 mg/dL and/or the treatment of hypoglycemia has not resulted in prompt recovery of altered mental status.*
- *The individual has had seizures or is unconsciousness.*
- *A responsible adult cannot be with the person for the next 12 hours.*
- *A sulfonylurea drug causes the hypoglycemia; this type of drug reduces liver conversion of glycogen to glucose and prolongs the period of hypoglycemia.*

It is important to note that clients can exhibit signs and symptoms of hypoglycemia when their elevated blood glucose level drops rapidly to a level that is still elevated (e.g., 400-200 mg/dL). The rapidity of the drop is the stimulus for sympathetic activity–based symptoms; even though a blood glucose level appears elevated, affected individuals may still have symptoms of hypoglycemia.

When a person with diabetes mentions the presence of nightmares, unexplained sweating, and/or headache causing sleep disturbances, hypoglycemia may be

Table 11-16	Clinical Signs and Symptoms of Hypoglycemia
Sympathetic Activity (Increased Epinephrine)	**CNS Activity (Decreased Glucose to Brain)**
Pallor	Headache
Perspiration*	Blurred vision
Piloerection (erection of the hair)	Thickened speech
Increased heart rate (tachycardia)	Numbness of the lips and tongue
Heart palpitation	Confusion
Nervousness* and irritability	Emotional lability
Weakness*	Convulsion*
Shakiness/trembling	Coma
Hunger	

*Signs most often reported by clients.

indicated during nighttime sleep (most often related to the use of intermediate and long-acting insulins given more than once a day). These symptoms should be reported to the physician.

Erratic insulin action (i.e., low blood glucose followed by high blood glucose) can occur as a result of a variety of factors such as overeating, irregular meals, irregular exercise, irregular rest periods, chronic overdosage of insulin (Somogyi effect), emotional or psychologic stress, failure to administer insulin, or intermittent use of hyperglycemic or hypoglycemic drugs (e.g., aspirin, phenylbutazone, steroids, birth control pills, or alcohol).

The Somogyi effect occurs when the blood glucose level decreases to the point at which stress hormones (epinephrine, growth hormone, and corticosteroids) are released, causing a rebound hyperglycemia. Treatment consists of increasing the amount of food eaten and/or decreasing the insulin. The therapist may be a helpful source of education to help clients remember the many factors affecting their condition.

Lipogenic Effect of Insulin

Frequent injections of insulin at the same site can cause thickening of the subcutaneous tissues (hypertrophy or lipohypertrophy) and a loss of subcutaneous fat (atrophy or lipoatrophy), resulting in a dimpling of the skin that is lumpy and hard or spongy and soft. These abnormal tissue changes may cause decreased absorption of the injected insulin and poor glucose control.

The client usually is instructed to choose an injection site that is easily accessible (e.g., thighs, upper arms, abdomen, or lower back) and relatively insensitive to pain (away from the midline of the body). Sites of injection should be rotated, and rotation within each area is recommended. An individual can rotate within an area using 1 inch of the surrounding tissue at a time. The client who is going to exercise should avoid injecting sites or muscles that will be exercised heavily that day because exercise increases the rate of absorption. Following a definite injection plan can help avoid tissue damage.

Even with an insulin pump, the infusion site should be changed every 2 or 3 days or whenever the client's blood glucose is above 240 mg/dL for two tests in a row. Rotating insertion sites will help prevent infection and tissue damage.

Diabetic Ketoacidosis

The therapist must always be alert for signs of ketoacidosis (e.g., acetone breath, dehydration, weak and rapid pulse, and Kussmaul respirations) progressing to hyperosmolar coma (polyuria, thirst, neurologic abnormalities, and stupor). Immediate medical care is essential. If it is not clear whether the symptoms are the result of hypoglycemia or hyperglycemia (Table 11-17), the health care worker is advised to administer fruit juice or honey. This procedure does not harm the hyperglycemic person but could potentially save the hypoglycemic person. Everyone with diabetes should wear a medical alert identification tag.

Table 11-17	Comparison of Manifestations of Hypoglycemia and Hyperglycemia	
Variable	**Hypoglycemia**	**Hyperglycemia**
Onset	Rapid (minutes)	Gradual (days)
Mood	Labile, irritable, nervous, weepy	Lethargic
Mental status	Difficulty concentrating, speaking, focusing, coordinating	Dulled sensorium, confused
Inward feeling	Shaky, hungry, headache, dizziness	Thirst, weakness, nausea/vomiting, abdominal pain
Skin	Pallor, sweating	Flushed, signs of dehydration (see Box 5-8)
Mucous membranes	Normal	Dry, crusty
Respirations	Shallow	Deep, rapid (Kussmaul respirations)
Pulse	Tachycardia	Less rapid, weak
Breath odor	Normal	Fruity, acetone
Neurologic	Tremors; late: dilated pupils, convulsion	Diminished reflexes, paresthesias
Blood Values		
Glucose	Low: <50 mg/dL	High: ≥250 mg/dL
Ketones	Negative	High/large
pH	Normal	Low: ≤7.25
Hematocrit	Normal	High
Urine Values		
Output	Normal	Polyuria (early) to oliguria (late)
Glucose	Negative	High
Ketones	Negative/trace	High

From Ignativicius D, Workman M: *Medical-surgical nursing: Patient centered collaborative care,* ed 6, Saunders, 2010, Philadelphia.

Vitamin B Deficiency

Some individuals using metformin can develop vitamin B_{12} deficiency resulting in serious damage to the nervous system. Complications can be minimized with early detection and intervention. Anyone on metformin, especially high doses or a prolonged course of therapy, should be screened for the deficiency. The therapist can help monitor this with the client and recognize any early neurologic signs and symptoms.[295]

Diabetes and Exercise

An overwhelming body of evidence now exists that acute muscle contractile activity and chronic exercise improve skeletal muscle glucose transport and whole-body glucose homeostasis in the person with type 2 DM (Box 11-6).[53] High-intensity progressive resistance exercise has been shown to improve body composition, leading to better glucose control and less insulin resistance among older adults with type 2 diabetes.[189]

Exercise helps to increase insulin sensitivity, thus lowering blood glucose levels. Increased insulin

Box 11-6

DIABETES MELLITUS: KEY POINTS TO REMEMBER

General Guidelines

- Although "safe" blood glucose levels are between 100 and 250 mg/dL (i.e., the person is not likely to experience diabetic ketoacidosis), the goal of therapy may be toward tighter control (e.g., in a young person with type 1 DM, 90 to 130 mg/dL) or moderate control (e.g., in an adult with type 2 DM, up to 150 mg/dL). A measurement more than 120 mg/dL should still be monitored closely in any age group. Blood glucose levels between 250 and 300 mg/dL are considered in the "caution zone"; test urine for ketones and wait to exercise if there is a high level until blood sugar drops to a safe preexercise range.
- If the blood glucose level is ≤100 mg/dL, a carbohydrate snack should be given and the glucose retested in 15 minutes to ensure an appropriate level. Food eaten in response to blood glucose levels between 70 and 100 mg/dL is symptom dependent (i.e., if a person's blood glucose is 80 mg/dL but no signs or symptoms of hypoglycemia are present, no snack is necessary).
- Observe carefully for signs or symptoms of diabetic ketoacidosis: acetone breath, dehydration, weak and rapid pulse, Kussmaul respirations.
- *Avoid exercise* if blood glucose >250 mg/dL with evidence of ketosis; exercise is potentially permitted if blood glucose is up to 300 mg/dL without evidence of ketones in the urine.
- Administer fruit juice or honey to anyone with diabetes who is in a hypoglycemic state. If uncertain whether the person is hypoglycemic or hyperglycemic, provide juice or honey anyway.
- Exercise must be carefully planned in conjunction with food intake and administration of insulin or oral hyperglycemic agents.
- Do *not* exercise during peak insulin times. The peak activity of insulin occurs at different times depending on the type, dose, and time of the insulin injection (see explanation in text)
- When under stress, the person with diabetes has increased insulin requirements and may become symptomatic even though the disease is usually well-controlled in normal circumstances.
- Avoid exercising late at night if this has not been gradually and consistently incorporated into the overall lifestyle. Delayed hypoglycemic reactions can occur during sleep hours after heavy, unaccustomed exercise late in the evening.

Before Exercise

- Take at least 16 ounces of fluid before exercise (approximately two 8-oz glasses).
- Glucose levels must be monitored immediately before exercise
- Do not exercise when blood glucose levels are at or near 250 mg/dL with urinary ketones and use caution if glucose level is >300 mg/dL and no ketosis is present.[331]

- Do *not* exercise without eating at least 2 h before exercise (exercise about 1 h *after* a meal is best, but individual variations must be determined).
- Do *not* inject short-acting insulin in muscles or sites close to areas involved in exercise within 1 h of exercise because insulin is absorbed much more quickly in an active extremity.
- Clients with type 1 DM may have to reduce the insulin dose or increase food intake when initiating an exercise program.
- Ketosis can be checked by means of a urine test before exercise (e.g., if the blood glucose is close to 250 mg/dL). If the test is positive (i.e., showing large numbers of ketones in the urine), exercise should be delayed until the urine test shows negative or low numbers of ketones. The person should administer insulin. Delay exercise until glucose and ketones are under control.
- Do not use drugs that may contribute to exercise-induced hypoglycemia (e.g., beta blockers, alcoholic beverages, diuretics, estrogens, phenytoin).
- Menstruating women need to increase their insulin during menses, especially those who are inactive or who do not exercise on a regular basis.

During Exercise

- It is best to exercise regularly (5 times/wk or at least every other day) and consistently at the same time each day.
- Duration of exercise is optimal at 40 to 60 min, although as little as 20 to 30 min of continuous aerobic exercise is beneficial in improving glucose homeostasis.
- During prolonged activities, a readily absorbable carbohydrate snack (e.g., fruit) is recommended for each 30 minutes of activity. After exercise, a more slowly absorbed carbohydrate snack (e.g., bread, pasta, crackers) helps prevent delayed-onset hypoglycemia. Activities should be stopped with the development of any symptoms of hypoglycemia, and blood glucose tested.
- Replace fluid losses adequately.
- Monitor blood glucose every 30 min during prolonged exercise.
- Anyone with diabetes should not exercise alone. Health care workers, partners, teammates, and coaches must understand the possibility of hypoglycemia and how to manage it.

After Exercise

- Glucose levels must be monitored 15 min after exercise, especially if exercise is not consistent.
- Increase caloric intake for 12 to 24 h after activity, according to intensity and duration of exercise.
- Reduce insulin, which peaks in the evening or night, according to intensity and duration of exercise.

DKA, Diabetic ketoacidosis; *DM*, diabetes mellitus.

sensitivity allows the body to utilize the available blood glucose for the person with type 2 diabetes; an increase in insulin sensitivity can last 12 to 72 hours after exercise. A combination of both aerobic and resistance training (but not either one alone) has been shown to improve HbA1c levels[48,283] as well as produce greater benefit in some aspects of quality of life (e.g., bodily pain, mental health, vitality).[205]

There is a high prevalence of people with underlying skeletal muscle insulin resistance or impaired skeletal muscle glucose disposal such as occurs with inactivity, bed rest, limb immobilization, or denervation. Therapists must recognize, understand, and use the role of skeletal muscle in glucose homeostasis to address the needs of clients with any of these risk factors. For excellent, detailed reviews of the pathways of glucose transport into skeletal muscle and the pathophysiology of insulin action in skeletal muscle as it contributes to disturbances of whole-body glucose metabolism, refer to Turcotte and Fisher[301] and Sinacore and Gulve.[274]

A program of planned exercise, including all the elements of fitness (flexibility, muscle strength, and cardiovascular endurance) can benefit persons with diabetes, especially those with type 2 DM. Exercise increases carbohydrate metabolism (which lowers the blood glucose level); aids in maintaining optimal body weight; increases high-density lipoproteins (HDLs); and decreases triglycerides, blood pressure, and stress and tension (Table 11-18).

Exercise and physical activity (even leisure-time physical activity and activity on the job) have been shown to independently reduce the risk of total and cardiovascular mortality of adults with type 2 diabetes. Exercise capacity is reduced by diabetes-related CVD, but exercise training is an excellent therapeutic adjunct in the treatment of diabetic CVD.[191]

The favorable association of physical activity with longevity occurs regardless of BMI, blood pressure, smoking habits, and total cholesterol levels.[129,130] Once again, the therapist can be very instrumental in client education on the importance of exercise for a wide range of reasons and benefits to the individual with diabetes.

General Exercise Considerations

For anyone with diabetes, type 1 or type 2, the exercise prescription must take into account any of the complications present, especially cardiovascular changes, autonomic and sensory neuropathy, and retinopathy.[331] Muscle damage, with accompanying insulin resistance and impaired glucose uptake and disposal, can occur when untrained individuals begin to exercise.[274] For this reason, clients with diabetes must start any new activity at a well-tolerated intensity level and duration, gradually increasing over a period of weeks or even months.[331]

Some thought should be given to the specific type of exercise selected. The young individual, in good metabolic control, can safely participate in most activities. The therapist should always be aware of and screen for clients who may have eating disorders, especially those who engage in excessive, intense exercise as a means of controlling their weight. Specific screening methods and questions are available for the therapist.[108]

The middle-aged and older person with diabetes should be encouraged to be physically active, with consideration given to activity prescription, comorbidities, and age-related musculoskeletal changes.[53] These considerations are discussed in following sections, Specific recommendations for athletes and for adventure sports such as scuba diving are also described.

Exercise and Nephropathy

Aerobic and resistance exercise training has been found to delay progression of nephropathy in animals, but more research on humans is needed.[99] Increases in blood pressure during a single bout of physical activity may temporarily increase levels of microalbumin in urine. However, over the long run, the positive effects of exercise training on blood pressure control may help slow progression on nephropathy. Before initiating an exercise program individuals with nephropathy should be screened for CVD and possible abnormal vital sign responses to exercise. Exercise should be initiated at low intensity and volume and progressed to moderate intensity and volume per the person's capabilities. High-intensity exercise and the Valsalva maneuver should be avoided to prevent large increases in blood pressure.[139] Aerobic capacity, muscle strength, and physical function may be poor in people with diabetic nephropathy. Both supervised exercise programs during dialysis and home-based exercise programs have been shown to improve quality of life and physical function in people with kidney disease.[139]

Exercise Screening

As positive as exercise is in the prevention and control of diabetes, the therapist must keep in mind that diabetes is a metabolic disorder with cardiovascular and circulatory implications. Reduced blood flow to the skin and skeletal muscle can be further compromised by intense exercise, and recovery time is longer. All

Table 11-18	Benefits and Potential Risks of Exercise in People with Diabetes Mellitus

Benefits	Potential Risks*
Improves cardiovascular function	Hypoglycemia in people taking oral hypoglycemics or insulin
Improves maximum oxygen uptake	Worsening of hyperglycemia
Improves insulin binding and sensitivity	Cardiovascular disease, such as myocardial infarction, arrhythmias, excessive increases in blood pressure during exercise, postexercise orthostatic hypotension, or sudden death
Lowers insulin requirements (type 2 DM)	
Improves sense of well-being and quality of life	
Promotes other healthy lifestyle activities	Microvascular disease, such as retinal hemorrhage or increased proteinuria
Increases carbohydrate metabolism	Degenerative joint disease
Improves blood glucose control†	Orthopedic injury related to neuropathy
Reduces hypertension	
May help with weight reduction	
Improves lipid profile	
Reduces stress	

*These are potential risks over the long term. In general, the benefits of regular exercise outweigh the risks.
†Not confirmed for insulin-dependent diabetes mellitus (type 1 DM).
Data from: Hordern MD, Dunstan DW, Prins JB, Baker MK, Singh MA, Coombes JS: Exercise prescription for patients with type 2 diabetes and pre-diabetes: a position statement from Exercise and Sport Science Australia. *J Sci Med Sport* 15(1):25-31, 2012.
Colberg SR, Sigal RJ, Fernhall B, Regensteiner JG, Blissmer BJ, Rubin RR, Chasan-Taber L, Albright AL, Braun B; American College of Sports Medicine; American Diabetes Association: Exercise and type 2 diabetes: the American College of Sports Medicine and the American Diabetes Association: joint position statement executive summary. *Diabetes Care* 33(12):2692-6, 2010.

possible effects of exercise must be kept in mind when designing an exercise program to suit the individual's needs. Strenuous exercise can have some serious side effects for people with poorly controlled diabetes and related health complications.[167] However, with proper management of blood glucose and individualized evidence-based exercise plans, most people with diabetes can exercise in a safe and effective manner. Preexercise health screenings are useful for developing appropriate exercise plans. Current guidelines for preexercise screening are as follows:

- *A preexercise examination, conducted by a physician, is recommended for sedentary and older people prior to beginning exercise more vigorous than a brisk walk,*
- *A preexercise electrocardiogram (ECG) stress test may be indicated for people:*
  - *>40 years of age, with or without CVD risk factors in addition to diabetes*
  - *>30 years of age and*
    type 1 or type 2 diabetes >10 years

    one or more of the following CVD risk factors (hypertension, smoking, dyslipidemia)

    retinopathy

    nephropathy including microalbuminuria as well as advanced renal disease
  - *Any known or suspected cerebrovascular or peripheral artery disease*
  - *Autonomic neuropathy*
- *A preexercise electrocardiogram (ECG) stress test may not be necessary for people with controlled diabetes at low risk of coronary artery disease.*

Preexercise evaluation should include screening for the presence of macrovascular and microvascular complications and musculoskeletal conditions that may be worsened by the exercise program.[53]

Exercise in Type 1 Diabetes Mellitus

The person with type 1 DM tends to be thin, may be poorly nourished, and because of the islet cell deficiency, always needs exogenous insulin for adequate control of blood glucose. Exercise can increase strength and facilitate maintenance of weight and provide other important benefits (see Table 11-18), but unfortunately exercise has not been proven to provide increased glycemic control for the person with type 1 DM.

Glycemic Response to Exercise

In individuals without diabetes, plasma insulin levels decrease during exercise and insulin counterregulatory hormones (glucagon and epinephrine) promote increased hepatic glucose production, which matches the amount of glucose used during exercise. As a result, during exercise in individuals without diabetes, blood glucose levels remain normal.

The glycemic response to exercise in people with type 1 DM as well as people with type 2 DM who require insulin therapy, insulin secretagogue therapy, or both is influenced by several factors. Plasma insulin levels may not fall during exercise in persons who are not insulin deficient and whose insulin levels are dependent exclusively or predominately upon medication. Insulin concentrations may even increase if exercise occurs within 1 hour of insulin injection. These sustained insulin levels during exercise enhance peripheral glucose uptake and stimulate glucose oxidation by exercising muscle. For this reason, insulin should not be injected into muscles or at sites close to areas involved in exercise within 1 hour of exercise. Insulin pump infusion sites must be subcutaneous and not intramuscular.

Hypoglycemia During Exercise

Moderate periods (30-45 minutes) of moderate-intensity exercise provide beneficial effects, but longer periods may result in hypoglycemia. Lack of adequate glycogen stores (i.e., decreased glycogen stores in the liver and to a lesser extent, in skeletal muscle) leads to impaired aerobic exercise endurance when compared with the nondiabetic person. Watch for symptoms of hypoglycemia such as sweating, shakiness, nausea, headache, and difficulty concentrating. The greatest risk of severe hypoglycemia occurs 6 to 14 hours after strenuous exercise. Strategies for avoiding hypoglycemia following exercise include (a) reducing insulin dose taken prior to exercise, (b) injecting insulin distant from exercising limbs, and (c) ingesting carbohydrate before and/or during exercise. People who have a tendency for hypoglycemia should consult with their physician to develop a diabetes and exercise plan of action. It is also important that muscle and hepatic glycogen be restored during periods of rest. Insulin and caloric intake must be adjusted after strenuous exercise to avoid severe nocturnal hypoglycemia.

Hyperglycemia

Hyperglycemia may result from high-intensity aerobic exercise in persons with and without diabetes. This can be challenging, particularly for people requiring insulin or insulin secretagogues. During high-intensity exercise, catecholamine (epinephrine and norepinephrine) levels increase significantly more than in moderate-intensity exercise. The change in catecholamines increases liver glucose production to levels exceeding muscle glucose uptake, resulting in hyperglycemia.

After high-intensity exercise, in people without diabetes and people with diabetes not requiring insulin, liver glucose production declines at a faster rate than declines in muscle glucose uptake, with blood glucose levels returning to normal within 1 to 2 hours. Postexercise hyperglycemia may persist and become problematic in people who use insulin and decrease their exercise insulin dose prior to exercise. Lower levels of insulin during recovery (attributed to reduction in dosing) slows the decline in hepatic glucose production and muscle glucose uptake.

When too little insulin is available, the cells are sensing starvation so increased release of glucagon and catecholamines persists. These hormones further increase glucose mobilization into the bloodstream and significantly increase an already high level of glucose and ketones. If the hyperglycemia and ketosis is high enough and/or if the person is dehydrated, DKA can be precipitated.[51,113] Alternating bouts of high-intensity with low-intensity activity (interval training) does not appear to lead to less of a tendency for both hypoglycemia and hyperglycemia and therefore may be a good strategy for exercise prescription for people requiring insulin to control diabetes.[51,113]

Sports Participation

Managing diabetes is very challenging for competitive athletes. The National Athletic Trainers' Association Position Statement on this topic and the Diabetes Exercise and Sports Association are helpful resource for therapists, trainers, and athletes.[138] In the past, people with diabetes, dependent on insulin, were discouraged from participating in adventure sports such as scuba diving and rock climbing. However, guidelines now exist that, if followed, may allow for safe participation in adventure sport activities.[231]

Exercise in Type 2 Diabetes Mellitus

In contrast to Type 1 DM (discussed in previous section), people with type 2 DM are often obese, and exercise is a major contributor in controlling hyperglycemia. Exercise can improve short-term insulin sensitivity and reduce insulin resistance, making it possible to prevent type 2 DM in those persons at risk and to improve glycemic control in those with diabetes. These effects disappear a few days after exercise is discontinued.

Consequently, for exercise to be an effective means of controlling diabetes there should be no more than 2 days between exercise bouts. Regular physical activity, a healthy diet, and weight loss of at least 7% to 10% in people who are overweight are cornerstones to management of type 2 DM.[53,127]

Hypoglycemia is not as common a problem for the person with type 2 DM who do not require insulin or insulin secretagogues because endogenous insulin levels usually can be maintained. However, individuals with type 2 DM who receive insulin or sulfonylureas may have a risk for hypoglycemia similar to that of people with type 1 DM.[51,113] Many people with type 2 DM are obese, sedentary, and have additional health comorbidities that need to be considered in exercise prescription. Box 11-6 includes key considerations for exercise and blood glucose control for people with type 1 and type 2 DM. Another helpful resource is American Physical Therapy Association's (APTA's) Physical Fitness and Type 2 Diabetes Pocket Guide (http://www.apta.org/PFSP/). General guidelines for exercise prescription follow and considerations for exercising with diabetes and health comorbidities, such as peripheral neuropathy and retinopathy, are discussed in subsequent sections.

General Guidelines for Exercise Prescription

For blood glucose control, people with type 2 DM should perform at least 150 minutes of moderate- to vigorous-intensity aerobic exercise spread out over at least 3 days, with not more than 3 consecutive days between bouts of exercise. In addition to aerobic exercise, moderate to vigorous resistance training (50%-80% of 1 repetition maximum) 2 to 3 days per week is advised. Each resistance training session should include 5 to 10 exercises covering all major muscle groups and one to three sets of 10 to 15 repetitions per exercise. Resistance exercise improves bone health, increases muscle mass, and benefits blood glucose control.[185]

Low-intensity exercise and interval training, alternating low–moderate aerobic exercise with resistance exercise may also reduce hyperglycemia. These types of exercise are better tolerated by people with poor exercise capacity, increasing the likelihood that they will regularly achieve the recommended amount of physical activity.[180]

For anyone with diabetes, exercise should not be initiated if the blood glucose is 70 mg/dL or less. Because one effect of exercise is the transfer of glucose in the cells, glucose levels should be checked again 2 hours after exercise. However, anyone with blood glucose levels at or near 300 mg/dL and with positive ketone levels should *NOT* exercise because vigorous activity also can raise the blood glucose level by releasing stored glycogen. Exercise or therapy sessions should be scheduled to avoid peak insulin times (see Table 11-15) and to avoid periods of fasting (e.g., missed meal or just before the next meal). Vigorous exercise should not be undertaken within 2 hours before going to sleep at night because this is when exercise-induced hypoglycemia can occur with potentially fatal consequences.

Exercise in the morning is recommended to avoid hypoglycemia resulting from fluctuations in insulin sensitivity caused by factors such as diurnal variations in growth hormone. Growth hormone levels remain low in the afternoon, and less gluconeogenesis occurs. Vigorous or intense exercise late in the day or evening can lead to delayed hypoglycemia during sleep, which is dangerous.

Balancing Insulin, Food, and Exercise

As mentioned, insulin should be injected in sites away from the part of the body involved in exercising. Because glucose can enter the cells without insulin during exercise, food should be eaten if the person is exercising more than usual. Conversely, when exercising less often, a lighter diet or more insulin is required.

Glucose levels should be monitored before and after exercise (or therapy activities), remembering that the effect of exercise can be felt up to 12 to 24 hours later. Those clients taking insulin should have their own glucose-monitoring devices (fingerstick or laser punctures).

After exercise, available glucose is important for the replenishment of muscle glycogen stores. Bouts of hypoglycemia can be delayed until hours after completion of exercise. The insulin-dependent person must regulate activity so that the rate of energy expenditure balances the amount and type of insulin and food intake (Table 11-19). Women who are menstruating may need to increase their insulin during menses.

Table 11-19 Making Food Adjustments for Exercise: General Guidelines

Type of Exercise and Examples	If Blood Glucose Is*	Increase Food Intake By	Suggestions of Food to Use
Exercise of short duration and low- to-moderate intensity (walking half mile or leisurely bicycling for <30 min)	<100 mg/dL ≥100 mg/dL	10-15 g of carbohydrate per hour of exercise not necessary to increase food	1 fruit or 1 starch/bread exchange
Exercise of moderate intensity (1 h of tennis, swimming, jogging, leisurely bicycling, golfing)	<100 mg/dL	25-50 g of carbohydrate before exercise, then 10-15 g per hour of exercise	½ meat sandwich with a milk or fruit exchange
	100-179 mg/dL	10-15 g per hour of exercise	1 fruit or 1 starch/bread exchange
	180-300 mg/dL	Not necessary to increase food	
	≥300 mg/dL	Do not begin exercise until blood glucose is under better control	
Strenuous activity or exercise (about 1-2 h of football, hockey, racquetball, or baseball games; strenuous bicycling or swimming; shoveling heavy snow)	<100 mg/dL	50 g carbohydrate; monitor blood glucose carefully	1 meat sandwich (2 slices of bread) with a milk and fruit exchange
	100-179 mg/dL	25-50 g carbohydrate, depending on intensity and duration	½ meat sandwich with a milk or fruit exchange
	180-300 mg/dL	10-15 g carbohydrate	1 fruit or starch/bread exchange
	≥300 mg/dL	Do not begin exercise until blood glucose is under control	

*100 mg/dL = 100 mL. The 100 mg/dL is a general guideline. Wide individual variations occur in this area. The timing of food intake may be symptom-dependent. Some individuals may experience symptoms of hypoglycemia when the blood glucose is 150 mg/dL, others not until the level is below 80 mg/dL and so on.

Exercise and the Insulin Pump

The normal metabolic response to exercise in a person who does not have diabetes is to decrease the release of insulin as muscles contract, causing the transport of more blood glucose into cells without insulin. A small amount of circulating insulin remains available during exercise to counterbalance the release of glucose-raising hormones (e.g., catecholamines, glucagon, growth hormone, and cortisol).

CSII therapy brings the exercising individual with diabetes a response as close to normal as possible. But anyone with diabetes who uses an insulin pump must make frequent insulin adjustments to mimic the normal metabolic response, thereby maintaining a more normal glycemic control, especially during periods of higher intensity or longer duration exercise.[54] Most people using an insulin pump have type 1 (insulin-dependent) DM, although anyone with type 2 DM who uses insulin can also wear a pump.

Time of day, exercise intensity, and elevated starting blood glucose levels appear to affect the metabolic response and can result in hyperglycemia instead of the more usual hypoglycemia for several hours after exercise. Metabolic control can deteriorate with intense exercise even in people who have tightly controlled blood glucose levels. It is suggested that 30 minutes of mild to moderate exercise is possible 2 or 3 hours after breakfast when using insulin pumps. The insulin level can be adjusted to minimize circulating free insulin levels and the risk of hypoglycemia during and after activity.[54,282]

One of the disadvantages of an insulin pump is that it can malfunction or become displaced without the person knowing it. Exercise can exacerbate the situation when insulin delivery has been unknowingly disrupted and hypoinsulinemia is developing. The therapist should always be alert to any signs of DKA in clients using an insulin pump. Teach the client to be vigilant during exercise to maintain the integrity of the infusion site and to pay attention to any symptoms of impending DKA (e.g., thirst, nausea, weakness, or excessive urination).

Before the advent of the insulin pump, anyone with type 1 diabetes whose blood glucose was less than 100 mg/dL was instructed to consume a carbohydrate snack before starting or continuing the activity. With CSII, pump users can simply reduce or suspend insulin during the activity. Insulin reduction and carbohydrate intake are determined by the intensity and duration of the exercise activity. For example, a change in either insulin or carbohydrate intake may compensate for shorter, less intense activities but not in the case of intense, aerobic exercise.[54]

Diabetic Autonomic Neuropathy

Many people with diabetes may not be able to exercise intensely to a calculated heart rate because of preexisting heart conditions, deconditioning, age, neuropathies, arthritis, or other joint problems. Exercise may be contraindicated in anyone with a severe form of autonomic neuropathy (Box 11-7), especially anyone with vasomotor instability, angina, and a history

Box 11-7

CONTRAINDICATIONS TO EXERCISE IN DIABETES MELLITUS

- Poor control of blood glucose levels
- Unevaluated or poorly controlled associated conditions:
  - Retinopathy
  - Hypertension
  - Neuropathy (autonomic or peripheral)
  - Nephropathy
- Recent photocoagulation or surgery for retinopathy
- Dehydration
- Extreme environmental temperatures (hot or cold)

Data from Hordern MD, Dunstan DW, Prins JB, Baker MK, Singh MA, Coombes JS: Exercise prescription for patients with type 2 diabetes and pre-diabetes: a position statement from Exercise and Sport Science Australia, *J Sci Med Sport* 15(1):25-31, 2012; Colberg SR, Sigal RJ, Fernhall B, Regensteiner JG, Blissmer BJ, Rubin RR, Chasan-Taber L, Albright AL, Braun B; American College of Sports Medicine; American Diabetes Association: Exercise and type 2 diabetes: the American College of Sports Medicine and the American Diabetes Association: joint position statement executive summary, *Diabetes Care* 33(12):2692-6, 2010.

of myocardial infarction.[51] The therapist is advised to communicate and collaborate with the client and physician when considering an exercise program for anyone with this problem.

Generally, individuals with autonomic neuropathy have a poor ability to perform aerobic exercise because of decreased maximal heart rate and increased resting heart rate. Postexercise heart-rate recovery is lower and may even be a sensitive enough screening test for individuals needing a clinical autonomic evaluation.[253] Persons with a generalized form of autonomic neuropathy may have hypotensive episodes after exercising, especially those who are deconditioned. They also demonstrate a predisposition toward dehydration in the heat and poor exercise tolerance in cold environments.

People with diabetic autonomic neuropathy may have a higher resting heart rate but lower maximal heart rate, making exercise at safe levels more difficult. It may be better to use the percentage of heart rate reserve (% HRR), which is the difference between resting heart rate and maximum heart rate, as a valid measure in prescribing exercise intensity instead of the rating of perceived exertion (RPE) scale, which relies on self-assessment of exertion.[52]

When using % HRR to determine an appropriate exercise intensity, maximal HR should be directly measured using an exercise stress test rather than estimated from age for better accuracy. The American College of Sports Medicine (ACSM) recommends that individuals with diabetic autonomic neuropathy be screened and receive physician approval before initiating exercise and that exercise intensity levels for clients with diabetic autonomic neuropathy should remain in the 40%-75% HRR span.[6,53,127]

Some people with autonomic neuropathy may have silent myocardial infarctions without angina. The first symptom may be shortness of breath resulting from congestive heart failure. Decrease in nerve innervation to the heart associated with this type of neuropathy may prevent a normal increase in heart rate with stress or exercise, requiring careful observation and monitoring of vital signs during exercise. Blood pressure regulation is altered with autonomic neuropathy; exercise can further stress the impaired system. Clients with autonomic neuropathy are prone to hypothermia, dehydration, and hypotension or hypertension.

Diabetes is associated with reduced tolerance to heat. Autonomic neuropathy may also include changes in thermoregulation with a decreased or altered ability to perspire. Exercise with a concomitant increase in core body temperature can lead to heat stroke.[225] Impairment of sweating has been demonstrated even with isometric exercise.[227] Proper hydration is essential, and precautions should be taken to avoid heat stroke. The Valsalva maneuver should be avoided.

Diabetes and Neuromusculoskeletal Complications

The treatment of musculoskeletal problems does not differ from treatment for these same conditions in the nondiabetic population. Early aggressive therapy for the adhesive capsulitis usually results in restoration of functional motion, even though full range of motion may not be achieved.

Hand function can be maintained and disease progression delayed with hand therapy, especially for the stiff hand syndrome. SLJM does not always benefit from therapy, but treatment intervention should be tried. For all neuromusculoskeletal conditions, the therapist must pay attention to elevated A1c levels as these have been linked with the presence of neuropathy and upper limb impairments.[237] The client must understand the importance of monitoring and maintaining control of the A1c levels. A self-directed exercise program established by the therapist can help prevent recurrence of symptoms and maintain functional outcomes.

Intervention for CTS must take into account the neuropathic and the entrapment components in the person with diabetes; surgical decompression may not be beneficial because of the neuropathic component. Nonsurgical efforts should be the focus of treatment. In conditions such as adhesive capsulitis and complex regional pain syndrome, a successful outcome is more likely with early medical and therapeutic intervention.

Diabetes and Foot Care

Disorders of the feet constitute a source of increasing morbidity associated with diabetes. Foot problems are a leading cause of hospital admission in people with diabetes, and diabetes is the most common reason for lower limb amputation. Half of those cases are preventable with proper foot care.[276,313] Treatment of the underlying diabetes has little effect on any joint disease already present. The most beneficial intervention includes stabilizing the joint, minimizing trauma, maintaining muscular strength, and performing daily foot care.

The therapist must teach each person with diabetes proper foot and skin care (see Box 12-14). Regular foot checks after exercise using a mirror to inspect all surface areas and between the toes is advised. Having the therapist demonstrate and consistently carry this out with the client is a helpful educational tool. Any areas of warmth, erythema, swelling, or skin changes must be evaluated carefully and immediately. The therapist is advised to reinforce client education at each and every session.

Diabetic Peripheral Neuropathy

Assess for risk factors for amputation (e.g., previous ulcer or amputation) and for signs of diabetic neuropathy (e.g., numbness or pain in hands or feet or foot-drop; see Table 12-21 and discussion of neuropathic [diabetic] ulcers). Scarborough[259] includes an excellent summary of assessment (tests and measures) for the foot and lower extremity. Vinik and Mehrabyan also offer an excellent review of diabetic neuropathies that will be of interest to any clinician working with this problem.[313]

Keep in mind that ankle-brachial index (ABI) measurements used to assess arterial circulation may have limited value in anyone with diabetes because calcification of the tibial and peroneal arteries may render them noncompressible.[38]

Provide clients with a monofilament for self-testing (Fig. 11-15). For a description of an easy and reliable method to test for protective sensation using the Semmes-Weinstein monofilaments, see the reference section.[65,203] This test is an easily used clinical indicator for identifying people who are at risk for developing foot ulcers and requiring subsequent amputations. It can clearly demonstrate physiologic changes in peripheral nerve function. If the person cannot feel the monofilament when applied with slight pressure against the skin, there is an increased risk of ulceration. The results of this test provide a definitive idea of who can benefit most from preventive care, education, and prescription of appropriate therapeutic footwear.[203]

Decreased sensation in the feet associated with diabetic neuropathy can affect both the timing and quality of gait, requiring retraining of the somatosensory and vestibular systems to help compensate for the somatosensory deficit.[121,226] Gait and strength training are important in the management of large-fiber neuropathies when impaired vibration, depressed tendon reflexes, and shortening of the Achilles tendon occur.[313] Diabetes gait may occur independent of sensory impairment. Increased joint movement, wider stance, and slower pace demonstrated in some individuals with type 2 diabetes may be neurologic in origin and not related to muscle weakness or loss of sensation in the feet.[224]

Anyone with peripheral neuropathy is advised to avoid soaking the feet. There is a danger of burns, and prolonged exposure to warm water leaves the skin susceptible to fungal infections. Whirlpools are contraindicated and baths are not advised (showering may be best). Bathing and soaking remove the protective barrier from the skin and can lead to other infections,

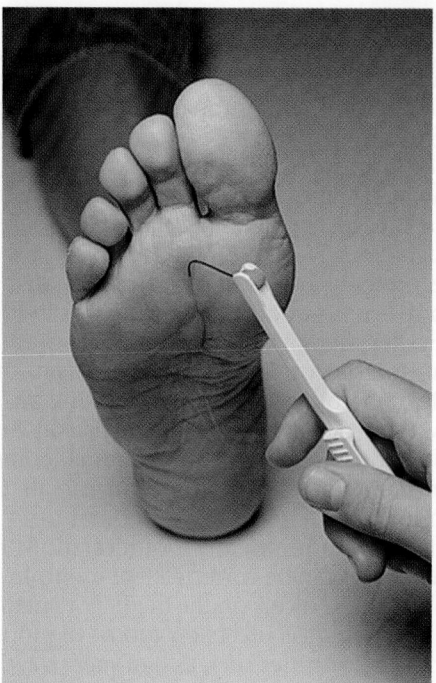

Figure 11-15

Semmes-Weinstein monofilament testing for protective sensation. Performed if the client is suspected of having peripheral neuropathy or known diabetes with possible peripheral neuropathy. The 5.07 monofilament (calibrated to apply 10 grams of force) has been adopted for screening in the diabetic population. The monofilament is applied perpendicular to the test site with enough pressure to bend the monofilament for 1 second. Abnormal response: client does not perceive the monofilament. Do not test over calloused areas. An initial foot screen should be performed on anyone with diabetes and at least annually thereafter. Anyone who is at risk should be seen at least four times a year to check their feet and shoes to help prevent foot problems from occurring. (From Seidel HM: *Mosby's physical examination handbook,* ed 6, St Louis, 2006, Mosby.)

especially if there are fissures from dry skin caused by decreased circulation.

The first Consensus Guidelines for DPNP developed by the American Society of Pain Educators (ASPE) are now available.[11] Having a standard of care is important in the treatment of pain associated with DPNP. Improved safety and quality of care may result in fewer amputations and potentially better compliance with recommendations for physical activity and exercise with subsequent decreased secondary complications associated with poor glycemic control.

Moderate-intensity aerobic exercise may help prevent the onset of peripheral neuropathy. Exercise guidelines for people with diabetes and peripheral neuropathy have been changed to allow moderate-intensity weight-bearing exercise for individuals with peripheral neuropathy but no foot ulcers. Recent studies indicate that walking at moderate intensity does not increase risk of foot ulcer, including reoccurrence of ulcers in people with peripheral neuropathy.[167,303]

Neuropathic (Diabetic) Ulcers

All people with diabetes should have an annual comprehensive foot examination to identify risk factors predictive of neuropathic ulcers. The most common cause for neuropathic (diabetic) ulcers is excessive plantar pressure in the presence of sensory neuropathy and foot deformity. Neuropathic foot ulcers can occur at any areas where pressure or shear force is applied to the foot (top, sides, or bottom). Many occur beneath the metatarsal heads and are the result of painless trauma caused by excessive plantar pressures during walking.[204]

The presence of corns or calluses is an indication that footwear fits poorly and should be carefully evaluated by the therapist. Additionally, cartilage requires insulin for glucose uptake, metabolism of carbon dioxide, and collagen synthesis. Lacking an adequate supply, the articular cartilage in the person with diabetes does not tolerate repetitive trauma, compression, and motion, making proper footwear all the more important.[233]

Note the location of any foot ulcerations for possible causes that can be corrected. For example, ill-fitting shoes may cause ulcers on the medial or lateral borders of the feet, whereas ulcers on top of the foot may be caused by deformities such as hammer (claw) toes.

The risk of ulceration and poor wound healing in the diabetic population underscores the importance of therapists providing nonsurgical alternatives for these problems. Although the management of the diabetic foot (Charcot joint) sometimes requires surgery to restore osseous alignment, regain stability, and prevent ulceration,[162] most people can be treated with appropriate cast, shoe, orthotic devices, or other therapeutic footwear. When a neuropathic joint is detected early, offloading the joint and avoiding weight bearing for 8 weeks may prevent progression of disease.

The presence of a previous history of plantar ulceration may alert the therapist to the need to teach the client how to control activity levels to lessen shear forces on scars from previous ulcers.[35] Orthoses are often used to redistribute or move pressure away from a blister or other area of pressure. Soft, moldable orthoses are preferred to the rigid orthoses used by clients with other types of foot problems. An excellent review of various offloading techniques for the treatment of neuropathic ulcers is available.[266]

Total-contact cast is an effective intervention for neuropathic plantar ulcers. The cast encases the entire foot and ankle, with all major bony prominences padded with foam or felt and reduces total loads on the foot by about one-third of the normal load. Frequent cast changes are made as the swelling goes down and to avoid ulceration in the cast. Monitoring of foot problems through the use of skin temperature changes using dermal thermography may provide valuable information to the clinician in the detection, treatment, and prevention of neuropathic foot problems.[15]

Total contact inserts and metatarsal pads can be used to reduce excessive plantar stresses, thereby preventing skin breakdown and ulceration. The total contact insert reduces excessive pressures at the metatarsal heads by increasing the contact area of weight-bearing forces. Metatarsal pads act by compressing the soft tissues proximal to the metatarsal heads and relieving compression at the metatarsal heads.[204]

The prevention of foot problems before they begin is always the most effective method in offsetting the development of foot ulceration and infection and their potentially devastating effects. The use of proper footwear, proper cleaning and lubrication of the feet, safe removal of corns or calluses, and removal of mechanical sources of foot pressure are critical components in the prevention of foot problems. Client education is a key component in the monitoring and detection of potential difficulties.[233]

Delayed Wound Healing

Because wound healing (surgical and nonsurgical) is impaired in the diabetic foot, surgery can be accompanied by increased risks of poor healing and infection. Sympathectomy, arthrodesis, and joint immobilization have not been proved helpful. Organ transplantation in someone with diabetes is also a risk factor for delayed wound healing because of the long-term immunosuppression required.[273]

The detrimental effects of cigarette smoking on wound healing and peripheral circulation are well documented (see "Substance Abuse" in Chapter 3). Smoking increases insulin resistance, worsens diabetes complications, and has a negative effect on prognosis. People with diabetes who smoke have a higher all-cause mortality rate than those who do not smoke.[280]

Smoking cessation is one of the two most important ways to reduce macrovascular complications in adults with diabetes. Control of hypertension is the other. The American Diabetes Association recommends that all health care providers routinely identify the smoking (tobacco use) status of clients with diabetes and offer cessation support and education.[8]

Substance abuse of any kind can impair or slow the rehabilitation process, especially delaying wound healing. Client education in this area is an important aspect of treatment. Despite strong evidence that clinician support of smoking cessation is effective for smokers who have diabetes, only about half report that their physician ever advised them to stop or cut down on their smoking (or substance use).[178]

The U.S. Public Health Service Clinical Guideline[296] suggests health care providers use the 5 A's: ask, assess, advise, assist, and arrange. A brief nonconfrontational discussion of smoking cessation may help move the smoker to the next level of readiness. The clinician can help clients think about what will be better if they quit; moving the person to the contemplation stage (ready to quit in the next 6 months) doubles the chance of quitting during that time.[229,236]

Diabetes and Physical Agents

Numerous studies from the 1980s and continued ongoing research have documented the large interindividual and intraindividual variability in subcutaneous insulin absorption, a major contributing factor in the variability of blood glucose. The therapist must be aware of these factors and plan intervention accordingly.

Specifically, insulin absorption is impaired or altered by smoking, injection site, thickness of skinfold (adipose tissue), exercise, subcutaneous edema, local subcutaneous blood flow, ambient and skin temperature, and local massage.[13,123]

The application of heat causes local vasodilation and hyperemia (excess blood to an area), necessitating burn precautions in this population. In a therapy practice, heat application may take the form of hot packs, paraffin, hydrotherapy, fluidized therapy, infrared radiation, ultrasound, or aquatic (pool) physical therapy.

Heat from the use of hot baths, whirlpools, saunas, or sun beds has been shown to accelerate the absorption of subcutaneous injections of insulin, by increasing skin blood flow. To reduce the risk of hypoglycemia, local application of heat to the site of a recent insulin injection should be avoided. The use of cryotherapy (cold) with its effects of vasoconstriction and decreased skin blood flow would be expected to slow or delay insulin absorption from the injection site.

Diabetes and Menopause

As life expectancy increases, women are living a greater proportion of their lives in the postmenopausal phase, a time when the prevalence of type 2 diabetes also increases. The therapist should be aware that the consequences of CVD, osteoporosis, and cancer are more pronounced in women who have type 1 or type 2 diabetes, especially in women who have metabolic syndrome followed by the development of type 2 diabetes.

The transition from premenopause to postmenopause estrogen-deficient status is associated with the emergence of many features of the metabolic syndrome, such as central obesity (intraabdominal body fat), insulin resistance, and dyslipidemia, which are also known to be risk factors for CVD. The prevalence of the metabolic syndrome increases with menopause and may partially explain the apparent acceleration of heart disease after menopause.[41]

Women with type 1 diabetes frequently go through menopause at an earlier age than women who do not have diabetes. Premature or early menopause may be considered an unstudied complication of type 1 diabetes.[68] Risk factor assessment for any of these comorbidities throughout the life cycle is especially important for any woman who has diabetes.

As the woman with diabetes approaches menopause, changes in estrogen and progesterone affect how cells respond to insulin and therefore blood glucose levels. Menopause symptoms can mimic low blood glucose levels (e.g., moodiness or short-term memory loss).

Sleep disturbance and weight gain associated with menopause make it harder to control blood glucose levels. There is an increased risk of urinary tract infection, especially for the menopausal/postmenopausal woman on insulin and/or who has had diabetes for 10 or more years.[20] During the postmenopause years when female hormone levels remain low, insulin sensitivity may increase with a drop in the expected blood glucose levels.[244]

There are conflicting reports on the role of hormone replacement therapy for postmenopausal women who have type 2 DM. Whether hormone replacement therapy improves glycemic control or worsens insulin sensitivity remains unproved. Results may vary according to the type of hormone replacement therapy, age of the woman, and route of administration.[109,146,192]

Polycystic ovary syndrome (PCOS) is an endocrine disorder characterized by multiple ovarian cysts and insulin resistance syndrome. Clinical signs include menstrual irregularities, infertility, acne, and obesity. PCOS affects about 10% of women. However, its prevalence may increase commensurate with current trends in increasing obesity, insulin resistance syndrome, and type 2 diabetes. Exercise and a healthy diet may appear to be important components in treatment of PCOS (see further discussion of PCOS in Chapter 20).[298]

Diabetes and Psychosocial Behavior

The therapist should keep in mind the psychologic and behavioral aspects of diabetes with regard to improving clinical outcomes. Most people with diabetes experience a high degree of emotional distress that continues throughout their lives but is rarely addressed by professionals.[275]

Common psychologic problems known to complicate diabetes management include depression, poor self-esteem, impact on the family dynamics, family and social support, compliance and motivation, eating disorders (particularly compulsive overeating), quality of life, and so on. Twenty percent to 40% of people with diabetes experience some level of depression, twice the rate of depression in people without diabetes.[76] Depression can negatively impact diabetes self-care. Exercise may help relieve depression.[165] It is also important to remember that symptoms of poor glycemic control, such as lethargy, look like symptoms of depression.

A team approach that includes close collaboration between diabetologists, psychologists, and physical therapists is important.[2] A good resource for information on depression and on eating disorders for both therapists and patients/clients is the Behavioral Diabetes Institute (http://behavioraldiabetesinstitute.org). Motivational interviewing and cognitive behavioral strategies including empowerment-based strategies have been proposed to improve metabolic and psychosocial outcomes. The therapist can be instrumental in helping the client formulate a personal self-management plan that incorporates experimentation and exploration to find what the stumbling blocks may be and what works best for achieving consistency in results and attaining goals.[93,111]

Diabetes and Aquatic Physical Therapy

See also Appendix B: Guidelines for Aquatic Physical Therapy.

The Aquatics Section of the APTA has an annotated bibliography with relevant articles related to pool therapy, including the use of aquatics with medical conditions such as diabetes mellitus. This document is available through the Aquatics Section of the APTA.

Swimming may be a good choice to offer the individual with diabetes to improve exercise capacity and muscle function, especially those who have cardiovascular disease and peripheral complications that may hamper many types of conventional exercises.[17] The physical therapist can be very instrumental in providing education about providing meticulous foot care. Wearing boat shoes (specially designed shoes for water wear available in many local stores) can help prevent scraping the feet along the sides or bottom of the pool. Care must be taken to gently dry the feet, especially between the toes, after swimming to prevent infection. Anyone with abrasions or open sores should not enter a swimming pool environment.

A rise in ambient (surrounding) temperature such as a client might experience in an indoor, warm, and humid pool setting also causes an increase in insulin absorption from subcutaneous injection sites. The insulin disappearance rate may be as much as 50% to 60% greater with an increase of 15° in ambient temperature.[155]

Additionally, the ease of movement in the water allows increased activity without the same perceived intensity of exertion for the same amount of work performed outside the water. The combination of increased temperatures and increased activity can result in hypoglycemia. The therapist and client must work closely together to maintain a balance of activity, food intake, and insulin dosage.

When a client with diabetes begins aquatic physical therapy, both the time in the water and the intensity of exercise should be systematically progressed and monitored, with one of the parameters being increased with each session according to the client's tolerance. Before pool therapy, the client must not miss any meals or snacks and must measure blood glucose levels.

A snack or beverage, such as orange juice, should be readily available throughout the therapy session for anyone developing symptoms of hypoglycemia. Glucose testing should be performed after completion of the pool program. Exercise can have a positive effect in reducing blood glucose levels in persons with type 2 DM, but sudden drops in blood glucose levels after exercise should be avoided.

With careful management, the individual should be able to adjust food intake and exercise tolerance to avoid having to increase insulin dosage. Throughout the pool program, the therapist must closely monitor each individual with diabetes for any signs of hypoglycemia (see Table 11-16). The affected individuals must be cautioned to carry out self-monitoring and to respond to the earliest perceived symptoms.

Insulin Resistance Syndrome

Insulin resistance refers to the phenomenon of having high levels of both circulating insulin and glucose in the bloodstream, but the insulin molecules cannot bind properly to the insulin receptor sites on the surface of the cell to allow glucose to enter the cells and be used for energy. A syndrome of insulin resistance has been proposed to explain the frequent association of hypertension, carbohydrate intolerance, abdominal obesity, dyslipidemia, and accelerated atherosclerosis associated with type 2 DM.

Although a primary insufficiency of insulin secretion is the pathology in the development of type 2 DM, obesity is a major risk factor for the development of this type of DM, caused in part by the associated insulin resistance. In 1988, the combination of hypertension, glucose intolerance, hyperinsulinemia, and dyslipidemia was called *syndrome X*, and later renamed *metabolic syndrome*, by Gerald Reaven, MD, a diabetes expert who predicted an increased incidence of coronary heart disease and type 2 diabetes.[240] Since then, several organizations have proposed definitions of metabolic syndrome in an attempt to define the syndrome more precisely, in a manner useful for clinicians and research groups.

The merit of each of the different definitions of metabolic syndrome is still being debated. In consideration of this, in 2009, a consensus definition was released by a group of professional organizations (e.g., American Heart Association, International Diabetes Federation, National Heart, Lung and Blood Institute) identifying specific criteria for the clinical diagnosis of metabolic syndrome (see Box 12-2). Criteria for metabolic syndrome in this consensus definition include the presence of three of these five measurements: abdominal obesity (waist circumference); elevated triglyceride levels, and low HDLs, hypertension, and elevated fasting glucose.

Recently, it has been suggested that other conditions such as proinflammatory states, should be added to the definition of metabolic syndrome, increasing its complexity. In contrast, the American Diabetes Association and the European Association for the Study of Diabetes object to the manner in which the metabolic syndrome is characterized as a risk factor for heart disease or diabetes. They argue that there is no need to diagnose someone with this syndrome; emphasis should be placed on aggressively treating the individual risk factors.[5] See Chapter 12 for further discussion of metabolic disorder.

Regardless of the criteria used to define metabolic syndrome, prevalence estimates are high and rising in all societies, probably as a result of the obesity epidemic. Most agree that obesity is the single modifiable factor that sets off the cascade. The syndrome is associated with alterations in the abdominal fat cells. With increased fat storage, these cells become distorted in shape, and the receptor site for insulin becomes "warped" or out of proper alignment, so the insulin molecule "key" no longer fits in the receptor. Insulin resistance makes it more difficult to lose weight because the cells are not getting enough fuel and the individual perceives hunger when adequate amounts of circulating glucose exist. The affected individual may develop elevated blood pressure and problems with reactive hypoglycemia. When the excess insulin is suddenly used, glucose rushes into the cells and the blood glucose drops suddenly. This sequence creates intense sweet cravings, and the cycle repeats itself with increasing insulin resistance.[314]

The term *insulin resistance syndrome* (IRS) was suggested by the American College of Endocrinology and the American Association of Clinical Endocrinologists to more aptly describe the prediabetic state.[73] Although IRS has many of the same characteristics of metabolic syndrome, diagnosis is based on a fasting glucose level (100 mg/dL < IRS < 126 mg/dL). Insulin resistance, a generalized metabolic disorder in which the body cannot use insulin efficiently, appears to play a key role in metabolic syndrome. Although not everyone with insulin resistance has metabolic syndrome, most people with metabolic syndrome are also resistant to the action of insulin.

Insulin resistance, a generalized metabolic disorder in which the body cannot use insulin efficiently, appears to play a key role in metabolic syndrome. Although not everyone with insulin resistance has metabolic syndrome, most people with metabolic syndrome are also resistant to the action of insulin.

The most important implications of recent research indicate that a diagnosis with a syndrome is not necessary in order to treat the individual risk factors. At this prediabetic stage, changes in lifestyle will have the greatest impact on halting any disease progression. In fact, it may be the only time in the disease progression when changes in daily activity levels and nutritional status may have an impact.

SPECIAL IMPLICATIONS FOR THE THERAPIST   11-17

Insulin Resistance Syndrome/Metabolic Syndrome

Physical therapists have a unique opportunity to address IRS/metabolic syndrome through reasonable dietary advice and carefully prescribed exercise counseling. After assessment, physical therapists should guide individuals toward an activity program that includes near-daily exercise that is progressive to a weekly expenditure exceeding 1200 kilocalories of aerobic activity.[131]

The therapist can provide education regarding the importance of weight loss, exercise, and dietary changes needed to help control dyslipidemia and hypertension. With appropriate lifestyle changes, people can reduce their risk of CVD, prediabetic states, and diabetes.

Studies have not yet determined the ideal exercise program for IRS/metabolic syndrome. Moderate aerobic exercise three times/week based on the ACSM guidelines increases insulin activity in non-obese, nondiabetic subjects despite the fact that there were no changes in weight, BMI, waist-to-hip ratio, lipid profile, or oxygen consumption after 2 months of exercise.[53,120] The mechanisms responsible for the improvement in insulin sensitivity after exercise training have been studied extensively but are not fully understood. Research focusing on insulin resistance in skeletal muscle and in particular its relation to changes in aerobic fitness in type 2 diabetes is ongoing.[214,261,301]

Hyperglycemia

Two primary life-threatening metabolic conditions, DKA and hyperosmolar hyperglycemic state (HHS), can develop if uncontrolled or untreated DM progresses to a state of severe hyperglycemia (greater than 300 mg/

dL).[149] Between DKA and HHS is a continuum of metabolic abnormalities.

Diabetic Ketoacidosis

Definition and Overview. DKA is most commonly seen in type 1 diabetes when complications develop from severe insulin deficiency. About one-half of the people who require hospitalization for DKA develop this hyperglycemic emergency secondary to an acute infection or failure to follow their prescribed dietary or insulin therapy.[316]

Most episodes of DKA occur in persons with previously diagnosed type 1 DM. However, the condition may occur in new cases of type 1 and in persons with type 2 DM (under stressful conditions in the latter such as during a myocardial infarction). It is characterized by the triad of hyperglycemia, acidosis, and ketosis.[277]

Etiologic Factors. Any condition that increases the insulin deficit in a person with diabetes can precipitate DKA. Causes of DKA commonly include taking too little insulin; omitting doses of insulin; failing to meet an increased need for insulin because of surgery, trauma, pregnancy, stress, puberty, or infection; and development of insulin resistance caused by insulin antibodies. Other precipitating causes are listed in Box 11-8.

The most common precipitating factor is infection, which occurs in up to half of all cases and may seem like a trivial condition such as mild cellulitis or upper respiratory tract infection. Omission of insulin, either because of noncompliance or because people mistakenly believe that insulin is not required on sick days when they are not eating well, is another important and preventable cause of DKA.

In young individuals with type 1 DM, psychologic problems complicated by eating disorders may be a contributing factor in 20% of recurrent ketoacidosis. Factors that may lead to insulin omission in younger people include fear of weight gain with improved metabolic control, fear

Box 11-8

PRECIPITATING CAUSES OF DIABETIC KETOACIDOSIS*

- Inadequate insulin under stressful conditions
- Infection
- Missed insulin doses
- Trauma
- Medications
  - Beta blockers
  - Calcium-channel blockers
  - Pentamidine (NebuPent, Pentam)
  - Steroids
  - Thiazides (diuretics)
- Alcohol abuse (inability to manage insulin because of mentation change; alcoholic ketoacidosis)
- Hypokalemia
- Myocardial ischemia
- Surgery
- Pregnancy
- Pancreatitis
- Renal failure
- Stroke

* Listed in descending order.

of hypoglycemia, rebellion from authority, and stress of chronic disease. In approximately 15% to 30% of cases, no identifiable cause of DKA can be determined.[277]

Pathogenesis. The initiating metabolic defect in DKA is an insufficient or absent level of circulating insulin. Insulin may be present, but not in a sufficient amount for the increase in glucose resulting from the stressor (see Box 11-8). Inadequate insulin creates a biologic state of starvation, which triggers the excess secretion of counterregulatory hormones, particularly glucagon, in an attempt to get more glucose to the cells and tissues. The abnormal insulin-to-glucagon ratio, with excess circulating catecholamine, cortisol, and GH levels, initiates a host of complex metabolic reactions, leading to hyperglycemia, acidosis, and ketosis.

When the body lacks insulin and cannot use carbohydrates for energy, it resorts to fats and proteins. The process of catabolizing fats for fuel gives rise to incomplete lipid metabolism, dehydration, metabolic acidosis, and electrolyte and acid–base imbalances. (See more complete discussion in "Diabetes Mellitus: Pathogenesis" above.)

Clinical Manifestations. The signs and symptoms of DKA vary, ranging from mild nausea to frank coma (Table 11-20). Common symptoms are thirst, polyuria, nausea, and weakness that have progressed over several days. This condition also may develop quickly, with symptoms progressing to coma over the course of only a few hours. Other symptoms may include dry mouth; hot, dry skin; fruity (acetone) odor to the breath, indicating the presence of ketones; overall weakness, possible paralysis; confusion, lethargy, or coma; and deep, rapid respirations (Kussmaul respirations). Fever is seldom present even though infection is common, primarily a result of peripheral vasodilation. Severe abdominal pain, possibly accompanied by nausea and vomiting, easily mimics an acute abdominal disorder.

MEDICAL MANAGEMENT

DIAGNOSIS, TREATMENT, AND PROGNOSIS. Prevention of DKA through client education is the key to avoiding this serious condition. Once DKA is suspected, the diagnosis must be established quickly, with immediate treatment after diagnostic confirmation (blood glucose level >300 mg/dL [>250 with serum ketones], pH <7.3, and bicarbonate level <18 mEq/L).

Treatment includes fluid administration, insulin therapy, and correction of metabolic abnormalities (potassium, bicarbonate, and phosphate), in addition to correction of any underlying illnesses (e.g., infection). Before the discovery of insulin in the 1920s, DKA was almost universally fatal. This complication is still potentially lethal, with an average mortality rate between 5% and 10%.

SPECIAL IMPLICATIONS FOR THE THERAPIST | 11-18

Diabetic Ketoacidosis

The therapist will be an active member of the health care team, emphasizing to anyone with type 1 DM the need for regular, daily self-monitoring of blood glucose, adherence to the diabetes management program, and early recognition of and intervention for mild ketosis. The therapist also must be able to recognize early signs and symptoms of DKA in addition to signs of infection, a major cause of DKA (see Box 8-1). The first sign of an infection in a foot or leg or an upper respiratory, urinary tract, or vaginal infection should be reported immediately to the physician.

DKA can cause major potassium shifts accompanied by muscular weakness that can progress to flaccid

---

Table 11-20	Clinical Symptoms of Life-Threatening Glycemic States		
	Hyperglycemia		**Hypoglycemia**
Diabetic Ketoacidosis (DKA)	**Hyperosmolar, Hyperglycemic Syndrome (HHS)**		**Insulin Shock**
Gradual onset*	Gradual onset		Sudden onset
Headache	Extreme thirst (may disappear over time)		Pallor
Thirst (very dry mouth)	Polyuria leading quickly to decreased urine output		Perspiration
Hyperventilation	Volume loss from polyuria leading quickly to renal insufficiency		Piloerection
Fruity odor to breath	Severe dehydration		Increased heart rate
Lethargy/confusion/coma	Lethargy/confusion		Palpitations
Abdominal pain and distention	Seizures		Irritability/nervousness
Dehydration	Hallucinations, coma		Weakness
Polyuria, ketones in urine	Blood glucose level >600 mg/dL		Hunger
Flushed face	Arterial pH >7.30		Shakiness
Elevated temperature			Headache
Blood glucose level >300 mg/dL (250-300 is the "caution zone")			Double/blurred vision
Arterial pH <7.30			Slurred speech
			Fatigue
			Numbness of lips/tongue
			Confusion
			Convulsion/coma
			Blood glucose level <70 mg/dL

*Less gradual than HHS.
Modified from Goodman CC, Snyder TE: *Differential diagnosis for physical therapists: screening for referral*, ed 5, Philadelphia, 2013, Saunders.

quadriparesis. The weakness is initially most prominent in the legs, especially the quadriceps, and then extends to the arms with involvement of the respiratory muscles. (See Chapter 5 for further discussion of hypokalemia in addition to a discussion of the other conditions associated with DKA, such as dehydration, metabolic acidosis, and electrolyte and acid–base imbalances.)

Hyperosmolar Hyperglycemic State. HHS is another acute complication of diabetes, a variation of DKA. HHS is characterized by extreme hyperglycemia (800-2000 mg/dL), mild or undetectable ketonuria, and the absence of acidosis. It is seen most commonly in older adults with type 2 DM.[149,168]

The precipitating factors of HHS may be similar to those for DKA such as infections, inadequate fluid intake, medications (see Box 11-8), or stress. HHS may be the first indication of undiagnosed diabetes, and it may occur in the case of someone who is receiving total parenteral nutrition (hyperalimentation) or who is on renal dialysis and receiving solutions containing large amounts of glucose.

The major difference between HHS and DKA is the lack of ketosis with HHS. Because some residual ability exists to secrete insulin in type 2 DM, the mobilization of fats for energy is avoided. When adequate insulin is lacking, blood becomes concentrated with glucose. Because glucose molecules are too large to pass into cells, osmosis of water occurs from the interstitial spaces and cells to dilute the glucose in the blood. Osmotic diuresis occurs, and eventually the cells become dehydrated. If not treated promptly, the severe dehydration leads to vascular collapse and death.

Clinical manifestations of HHS are polyphagia, polydipsia, polyuria, glucosuria, dehydration, weakness, changes in sensorium, coma, hypotension, and shock (see Table 11-20). Lactic acidosis also can develop if tissue perfusion is compromised.

Treatment is with short-acting insulin, electrolyte replacement, and careful fluid replacement to avoid congestive heart failure and intercerebral swelling in older adults, who often have other cardiovascular or renal disorders.

SPECIAL IMPLICATIONS FOR THE THERAPIST 11-19

Hyperosmolar Hyperglycemic State
The therapist should be alert to any signs of HHS in the aging adult who may have a previous diagnosis of type 2 DM. Early recognition and treatment to restore fluid and electrolyte balance are important for a good prognosis in this condition. (See also "Special Implications for the Therapist 11-16: Diabetes Mellitus.")

METABOLIC SYSTEM

As noted earlier, the endocrine system works with the nervous system to regulate and integrate the body's metabolic activities. Metabolism is the physical and chemical (physiologic) processes that allow cells to utilize food to continually rebuild body cells and transform food into energy. Metabolism is broken down into two phases: the anabolic (tissue-building) and catabolic (energy-producing) phases. The *anabolic phase* converts simple compounds derived from nutrients into substances the body cells can use, whereas the *catabolic phase* is a consumptive phase when these organized substances are reconverted into simple compounds with the release of energy necessary for the proper functioning of body cells.[115]

The body gets most of its energy by metabolizing carbohydrates, especially glucose. A complex interplay of hormonal and neural controls regulates the homeostasis of glucose metabolism. Hormone secretions of five endocrine glands dominate this regulatory function (see Table 11-10). The rate of metabolism can be increased by exercise, elevated body temperature (e.g., high fever or prolonged exertional exercise), hormonal activity (e.g., thyroxine, insulin, or epinephrine), and increased digestive action after the ingestion of food.

Fluid and Electrolyte Balance (see also discussion, Chapter 5)

Fluid and electrolyte balance is a key component of cellular metabolism. Homeostasis, maintaining the body's chemical and physical balance, involves the proper functioning of body fluids to preserve osmotic pressure, acid–base balance, and anion–cation balance. The goal of metabolism and homeostasis is to maintain the complex environment of body fluid that nourishes and supports every cell.

Body fluids, classified as intracellular and extracellular, contain two kinds of dissolved substances: those that dissociate (separate) in solution (electrolytes) and those that do not. For example, when dissolved in water, glucose does not break down into smaller particles but sodium chloride dissociates into sodium cations (positively charged) and chloride anions (negatively charged).

The composition of these electrolytes in body fluids is electrically balanced, so the positively charged cations (sodium, potassium, calcium, and magnesium) equal the negatively charged anions (chloride, bicarbonate, sulfate, phosphate, and carbonic acid). Although these particles are present in relatively low concentrations, any deviation from their normal levels can have profound physiologic effects.

Because many situations in the body cause both normal and abnormal fluid shifts, it is important to have a clear understanding of fluid compartments. The recognition of pathologic conditions, such as edema, dehydration, ketoacidosis, and various types of shock, can depend on the understanding of these concepts.

In the healthy body, fluids and electrolytes are constantly lost or exchanged between compartments. This balance must be maintained for the body to function properly. The amount used in these functions depends on such factors as humidity; body and environmental temperature; physical activity; metabolic rate; and fluid loss from the GI tract, skin, respiratory tract, and renal system. Normal balance is achieved through fluid intake and dietary consumption. Alterations in fluid and electrolyte balance are discussed more completely in Chapter 5.

Acid–Base Balance

The proper balance of acids and bases in the body is essential to life. The body maintains the pH of extra-cellular fluid (fluid found outside cells) between 7.35 and 7.45 through a complex chemical regulation of carbonic acid by the lungs and base bicarbonate by the kidneys. The pH is essentially a measure of hydrogen ion concentration in body fluid. Nutritional deficiency or excess, disease, injury, or metabolic disturbance may interfere with normal homeostatic mechanisms and cause a lowering of pH called *acidosis* or a rise in pH called *alkalosis*.

Various bodily functions operate to keep the pH at a relatively constant level. Acid–base regulatory mechanisms include chemical buffer systems, the respiratory system, and the renal system. These systems interact to maintain a normal acid–base ratio of 20:1 bicarbonate to carbonic acid. The consequences of an acid–base metabolism disorder can result in many signs and symptoms encountered by the therapist. These conditions are discussed more completely in Chapter 5.

Aging and the Metabolic System

Aging as measured by loss of physiologic function has not yet been defined precisely, so the distinction between usual, normal, and ideal metabolic changes remains undetermined. Studies of the aging population have shown that several physiologic parameters, such as body weight, basal metabolism, renal clearance, and cardiovascular function, decline with age. Protein-calorie nutritional status has pervasive effects on metabolic regulatory systems; nutritional status often declines with age, which contributes to metabolic dysfunction.[142]

Because the respiratory and renal systems are largely responsible for maintaining acid–base balance, changes in these systems associated with aging also have an impact on metabolic function. A common measure for metabolic loss in tissues is the decline in VO_2max, the maximum oxygen extraction capacity of the lungs.

Loss of muscle mass associated with aging can affect stroke volume capacity and oxidative metabolism.[218] The low-level metabolic acidosis that appears to occur in many people with advancing age may play a role in age-associated bone loss, a factor that has received little attention from those who study bone loss and aging.[186]

Oxidative stress has been implicated in the pathogenesis of a number of diseases and has been labeled the *free radical theory of aging* (discussed in Chapters 2 and 6); studies indicate that protection from the consequences of excess metabolic activity results in a slowing of the aging process, particularly in the postreproductive period of life.[42,92] Links between oxidative stress and aging focus on mitochondria in a theory called the *mitochondrial theory of aging*. Mitochondria, the principal site of adenosine triphosphate (ATP) synthesis (also containing DNA and RNA), is the cellular site of energy production from oxygen and the principal site of free radical damage.[62]

Free radical derivatives of oxygen are generated as a result of normal metabolic activity, producing destructive oxidation of membranes, proteins, and DNA. These free radicals (unstable oxygen molecules robbed of electrons) attempt to replace their missing electrons by scavenging the body and taking electrons from healthy cells, causing a chain reaction called *oxidation* (see Fig. 6-2).

The formation of free radicals can be triggered by many exogenous (outside) factors such as cigarette smoke, air pollution, anticancer drugs, ultraviolet lights, pesticides and other chemicals, uncontrolled diabetes, radiation, and emotional stress. The major defenses against these destructive byproducts of normal metabolism are the protective enzymes, which remove the free radicals and remove, repair, and replace cell constituents.

Impairment of cellular function and metabolism occurs as proteins and DNA (which turn over slowly or not at all) are damaged over time.[71] The use of antioxidants found naturally in fruits and vegetables or ingested as a nutritional supplement to counteract this process is thought to increase longevity but remains under scientific investigation.[198,199]

Signs and Symptoms of Metabolic Disease

Clinical manifestations of metabolic disorders vary, depending on the specific pathology present. Fluid and electrolyte disorders, disorders of acid–base metabolism leading to metabolic (nonrespiratory) alkalosis or acidosis, and their associated signs and symptoms are discussed in Chapter 5.

SPECIFIC METABOLIC DISORDERS

Metabolic bone disease is discussed in Chapter 24, and *disorders of purine and pyrimidine metabolism* resulting in gout and pseudogout are discussed in Chapter 27.

Metabolic Bone Disease

Metabolic disorders involving the connective tissue may result in pathologic loss of bone mineral density, such as occurs in osteomalacia or osteoporosis, or acceleration of both deposition and resorption of bone, as seen in Paget disease. These disorders differ in pathogenesis and treatment and are discussed in Chapter 24.

Metabolic Neuronal Diseases

Metabolic neuronal diseases are rare and are not likely seen in a therapy practice. Phenylketonuria (PKU), Wilson disease, and porphyrias are the three most often encountered and are briefly discussed in this section.

Phenylketonuria

PKU is an autosomal recessive disease resulting from a genetic defect in the metabolism of the amino acid phenylalanine (Phe). This condition is transmitted recessively through apparently healthy parents, who show signs of the disease only on testing. The lack of an enzyme (phenylalanine hydroxylase) necessary for the conversion of the amino acid Phe into tyrosine results in an accumulation of Phe in the blood with excretion of phenylpyruvic acid in the urine. If untreated, the condition results in mental retardation and other manifestations such as tremors, poor muscular coordination, excessive perspiration, mousy odor (resulting from skin and urinary excretion of phenylpyruvic acid), and seizures.

Although PKU cannot be cured, a simple screening test for PKU can be administered to newborns and is required by law in most states in the United States and in all provinces in Canada. Currently, between 160 and 400 of the 4 million babies born in the United States each year are affected. The practice of discharging newborns in 24 hours is resulting in an increase in the number of babies at risk of PKU.

Treatment is primarily through Phe restriction of the infant's diet to control the effects of PKU and is prescribed on an individual basis with the additional administration of a dietary protein substitute. The start of newborn screening for PKU during the early 1970s has given rise to an increasing number of people who have been identified and successfully treated for the disease in childhood. Initiation of nutritional therapy before conception for women assures a successful pregnancy outcome.[147] A need remains for maternal screening before pregnancy to identify undiagnosed maternal PKU and subsequent prophylactic treatment to prevent maternal PKU syndrome.[117]

The prognosis for people with PKU has improved greatly with early institution of treatment after birth. However, hyperphenylalaninemia can cause white matter abnormalities, psychiatric illness, and decreased performance on neuropsychologic tests for people with PKU compared with subjects without PKU. It has been shown that the diet necessary to reduce Phe levels cannot be terminated after adolescence without elevation of plasma levels resulting in poor neuropsychologic performance.[63]

Wilson Disease

Wilson disease, also known as *hepatolenticular degeneration*, is a progressive disease inherited as an autosomal recessive trait (both parents must carry the abnormal gene). This condition produces a defect in the metabolism of copper, with accumulation of copper in the liver, brain, kidney, cornea, and other tissues. Although the pathogenesis of Wilson disease is still uncertain, it seems likely that defective biliary excretion of copper is involved.

The disease is characterized by the presence of Kayser-Fleischer rings around the iris of the eye (from copper deposits), cirrhosis of the liver (see Chapter 17), and degenerative changes in the brain, particularly the basal ganglia. Liver disease is the most likely manifestation in the pediatric population, and neurologic disease is most common in young adults. Cerebellar intoxication from deposition of copper in the brain results in athetoid movements and an unsteady gait.

Other CNS symptoms may include pill-rolling tremors in the hands, facial and muscular rigidity, dysarthria, and emotional and behavioral changes. Musculoskeletal effects occur in severe disease and may include muscle atrophy and wasting, contractures, deformities, osteomalacia, and pathologic fractures.[277]

Treatment is pharmacologic (e.g., lifetime administration of vitamin B_6 and D-penicillamine) and is aimed at reducing the amount of copper in the tissues by promoting its urinary excretion. Managing hepatic disease is also important; if left untreated, Wilson disease progresses to fatal hepatic failure.

SPECIAL IMPLICATIONS FOR THE THERAPIST   11-20

Wilson Disease

For the person with Wilson disease, physical or vocational rehabilitation may be required. In the advanced stage of this disease, self-care is promoted to prevent further mental and physical deterioration. An exercise schedule is essential to encourage consistent focus on rehabilitation. Sensory deprivation or overload should be avoided and prevention of integumentary and musculoskeletal injuries that could occur as a result of neurologic deficits is important (see Box 12-14).

Porphyrias

Porphyrias are a group of hereditary and sometimes acquired diseases characterized by enzymatic abnormalities in biosynthesis of the heme molecule. Normally, porphyrins and their precursors are necessary for the synthesis of the heme molecule. In porphyrias, because of enzyme deficiencies, an accumulation of excessive amounts of porphyrins and their precursors occurs. This accumulation results in generalized clinical symptoms.

Neurologic abnormalities, acute abdominal pain, skin fragility, and photosensitivity and psychiatric problems are symptoms that characterize the porphyrias. Various drugs and chemicals can cause porphyria (e.g., large amounts of alcohol, hemodialysis, or other chemical toxins) or can trigger acute, potentially life-threatening attacks in susceptible individuals. Diagnosis is suspected when clinical symptoms are combined with substantial increases in porphyrins or porphyrin-precursors in the blood and urine.[47]

REFERENCES

To enhance this text and add value for the reader, all references are included on the companion Evolve site that accompanies this textbook. The reader can view the reference source and access it online whenever possible.

CHAPTER 12

The Cardiovascular System

IRINA V. SMIRNOVA

The cardiovascular system functions in coordination with the pulmonary system to circulate oxygenated blood through the arterial system to all cells in the body. The deoxygenated blood is then collected from the venous system and delivered to the lungs for reoxygenation (Fig. 12-1).

Pathologic conditions of the cardiovascular system are varied, multiple, and complex. This chapter presents cardiovascular diseases according to how they affect structure and function of individual components of the cardiovascular system, including diseases of the heart muscle and heart vessels, cardiac nervous system, heart valves, pericardium, and blood vessels.

Influence of aging on cardiovascular system components and function is discussed with emphasis on positive effects of physical exercise. Gender differences are described as they relate to the cardiovascular system and diseases. Whenever possible, ethnicity as it relates to cardiovascular diseases is included in each section. Ethnic differences are an area just coming under closer review, and the knowledge available is limited at this time.

Other factors, such as surgery, pregnancy, cardiogenic shock, and complications from other pathologic conditions (e.g., acquired immunodeficiency syndrome [AIDS], cancer treatment, collagen vascular diseases [now more commonly referred to as diffuse connective tissue diseases]) can also adversely affect the normal function of the cardiovascular system. Discussion of these additional factors is limited in this chapter (see specific chapters for each subject).

PREVALENCE OF CARDIOVASCULAR DISEASE AND RISK FACTORS

Cardiovascular disease (CVD) causes one in three deaths reported each year in the United States.[390] The leading risk factors for CVD include hypertension, high serum cholesterol levels, and smoking.[146] Of these, at least one risk factor is present in nearly half (47%) of the adult population age 20 years and older.[158] Sedentary lifestyle and unhealthy dietary pattern leading to overweight and obesity add to the risk factors.[84]

Middle-age adults (in their 40s and 50s) who have no CVD risk factors have a significantly lower risk of death through the age of 80 years than do middle-age adults who have two or more risk factors for CVD.[53] This implicates the importance of addressing CVD risk factors in the young

population so that they remain risk-free, or with low risk, into their middle age and beyond, and for the middle-age adults with risk factors to help control their effects. Evaluation of family history improves cardiovascular risk assessment leading to better and earlier prevention options.[369]

CARDIOVASCULAR DISEASE PREVENTION STRATEGIES

With 80 million U.S. adults affected by the CVD,[275] its prevention is of utmost importance. *Primary prevention* is aimed at reducing chances of the first adverse cardiovascular event and is possible to achieve only through lifestyle and environmental changes. *Secondary prevention* encompasses approaches to decrease the recurrent cardiovascular events and reduce death resulting from CVD. Beyond primary and secondary prevention, *primordial prevention* is a more far-reaching idea. It includes "ensuring that the ideal levels of cardiovascular risk factors are observed in healthy children" and "are preserved into adulthood."[84] The American Heart Association supports the primordial prevention concept as a critical strategy in maintaining cardiovascular health in U.S. population.[289]

SIGNS AND SYMPTOMS OF CARDIOVASCULAR DISEASE

Cardinal symptoms of cardiac disease usually include chest, neck, or arm pain or discomfort; palpitations; dyspnea; syncope (fainting); fatigue; cough; and cyanosis. Edema and leg pain (claudication) are the most common symptoms of the vascular component of cardiovascular pathologic conditions. Symptoms of cardiovascular involvement should be reviewed by system as well (Table 12-1).

Chest pain or discomfort (e.g., tightness, pressure sensation) is a common presenting symptom of CVD and must be evaluated carefully. Chest pain of systemic origin may be cardiac or noncardiac and may radiate to the neck, jaw, upper trapezius, upper back, shoulder, or arms (most commonly the left arm). Radiating pain down the arm is in the pattern of ulnar nerve distribution. Noncardiac chest pain can be caused by an extensive list of disorders and is not covered in this text.

Cardiac-related chest pain may arise secondary to ischemia, myocardial infarction (MI), pericarditis, endocarditis, mitral valve prolapse, or aortic dissection with or

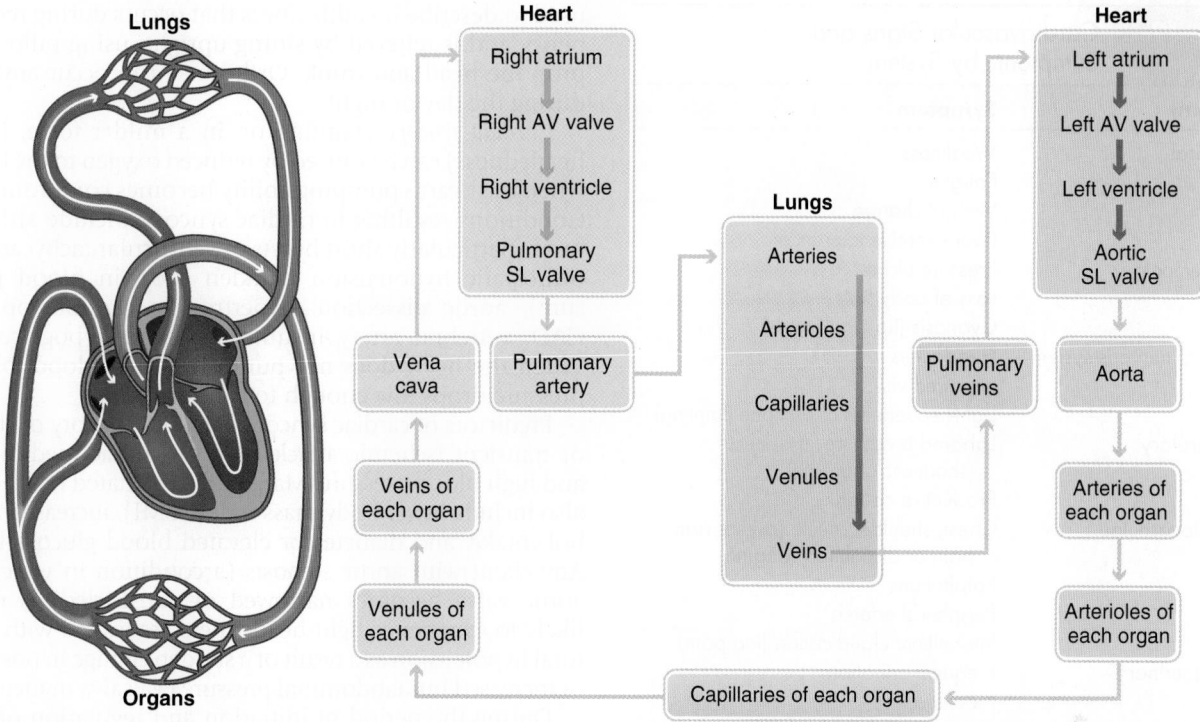

Figure 12-1

Structure and circulation of the heart. Blood flows from the superior and inferior venae cavae into the right atrium through the tricuspid valve to the right ventricle. The right ventricle ejects the blood through the pulmonic valve into the pulmonary artery during ventricular systole. Blood enters the pulmonary capillary system, where it exchanges the carbon dioxide for oxygen. The oxygenated blood then leaves the lungs via the pulmonary veins and returns to the left atrium. From the left atrium, blood flows through the mitral valve into the left ventricle. The left ventricle pumps blood into the systemic circulation through the aorta to supply all the tissues of the body with oxygen. From the systemic circulation, blood returns to the heart through the superior and inferior venae cavae to begin the cycle again. (From Thibodeau and Patton: *The human body in health and disease,* ed 6, St Louis, Mosby, 2014.)

without aneurysm. Location and description (frequency, intensity, duration) vary according to the underlying pathologic condition (see each individual condition).

Chest pain is often accompanied by associated signs and symptoms, such as nausea, vomiting, diaphoresis, dyspnea, fatigue, pallor, or syncope. Cardiac chest pain or discomfort can also occur when coronary circulation is normal, as in the case of anemia causing lack of oxygenation of the myocardium (heart muscle) during physical exertion, although this situation is uncommon.

Angina (see "Angina Pectoris" below for more details) is a chest pain or discomfort occurring when a heart muscle does not get enough oxygen. It is a symptom of coronary artery disease (CAD). It usually starts behind the breastbone, but it may project in the arm, shoulder, neck, jaw, throat, and back. It is described as pressure, squeezing, or tightness in the chest. Some people may mistake it for indigestion. Shortness of breath, weakness, lightheadedness, and sweating may occur.

Palpitations, the presence of an irregular, fast, or "extra" heartbeat, may also be referred to as arrhythmias or dysrhythmias, which may be caused by a relatively benign condition (e.g., mitral valve prolapse, caffeine, anxiety, exercise, athlete's heart [increase in left ventricular mass as a result of intensive training])[354] or a severe condition (e.g., CAD, cardiomyopathy, complete heart block, ventricular aneurysm, atrioventricular valve disease, mitral or aortic stenosis).

Palpitations may occur as a response to the bursts of adrenaline that occur with drops in estrogen levels, as a response to excess or erratic production of adrenaline-type compounds associated with panic disorder, or as a result of hyperthyroidism through other mechanisms. Up to one third of heart transplant recipients are aware of their resting heartbeat, despite the absence of cardiac innervation.[43]

Palpitations have been described as a bump, pound, jump, flop, flutter, butterfly, or racing sensation of the heart. Associated symptoms may include light-headedness or syncope. Palpated pulse may feel rapid or irregular, as if the heart has skipped a beat. Some people report fluttering sensations in the neck rather than in the chest or thoracic area.

Dyspnea, also referred to as breathlessness or shortness of breath, can be cardiovascular in origin, but it may also occur secondary to pulmonary pathologic conditions (see also Chapter 15), trauma, fever, certain medications, or obesity. Early onset of dyspnea may be described as a sensation of having to breathe too much or as an uncomfortable feeling during breathing after exercise or exertion. Shortness of breath with mild exertion (dyspnea on exertion) can be caused by an impaired left ventricle that is unable to contract completely. The result is an abnormal accumulation of blood in the pulmonary circulation. Pulmonary congestion and shortness of breath then ensue. With severe compromise of the cardiovascular or pulmonary system, dyspnea may occur at rest.

Dyspnea may be a predictor of death from cardiac or other causes. In a large study of more than 17,000 adults undergoing myocardial perfusion single-photon emission computed tomography during stress and at rest,

Table 12-1	Cardiovascular Signs and Symptoms by System

System	Symptom
General	Weakness
	Fatigue
	Weight change
	Poor exercise tolerance
Integumentary	Pressure ulcers
	Loss of body hair
	Cyanosis (lips, nail beds)
Central nervous system	Headaches
	Impaired vision
	Light-headedness or syncope (fainting)
Respiratory	Labored breathing, dyspnea (shortness of breath)
	Productive cough
Cardiovascular	Chest, shoulder, neck, jaw, or arm pain or discomfort (angina)
	Palpitations
	Peripheral edema
	Intermittent claudication (leg pain)
Genitourinary	Frequent urination
	Nocturia
	Concentrated urine
	Decreased urinary output
Musculoskeletal	Muscular fatigue
	Myalgias
	Chest, shoulder, neck, jaw, or arm pain or discomfort
	Peripheral edema
	Intermittent claudication (leg pain, cramping, or discomfort)
Gastrointestinal	Nausea and vomiting
	Abdominal distention (caused by ascites)
	Abdominal pain (abdominal angina)

those with no history of CAD who presented with dyspnea had four times the risk of sudden death from cardiac causes compared to asymptomatic individuals. They also had twice the risk compared to participants already diagnosed with typical angina.[2]

The severity of dyspnea is determined by the extent of disease; the more severe the heart disease, the more readily episodes of dyspnea occur. More extreme dyspnea includes paroxysmal nocturnal dyspnea and orthopnea. *Paroxysmal nocturnal dyspnea* is sudden, unexplained episodes of shortness of breath that, at night awaken a person sleeping in a supine position. The person feels like they do not have enough air to breeze and they have to sit upright and/or open a window. Moving to the upright position brings relief because the amount of blood returning to the heart and lungs from the lower extremities decreases in this position. This type of dyspnea frequently accompanies congestive heart failure (CHF).

During the day, the effects of gravity in the upright position and the shunting of excessive fluid to the lower extremities permit more effective ventilation and perfusion of the lungs, keeping the lungs relatively fluid free, depending on the degree of CHF. *Orthopnea* is the term used to describe breathlessness that occurs during recumbency and is relieved by sitting upright, using pillows to prop the head and trunk. Orthopnea can occur anytime during the day or night.

Cardiac syncope (fainting or, in a milder form, lightheadedness) can be caused by reduced oxygen to the brain when the heart's pumping ability becomes compromised. Conditions resulting in cardiac syncope include arrhythmias (particularly short bursts of ventricular tachycardia), orthostatic hypotension (sudden drop in blood pressure), aortic dissection, hypertrophic cardiomyopathy, CAD, vertebral artery insufficiency, and hypoglycemia. When the heart does not pump as much blood, blood pressure drops low enough to cause fainting.

Predictors of cardiac syncope include a history of stroke or transient ischemic attacks, use of cardiac medication, and high blood pressure. Marginally associated risk factors also include lower body mass index (BMI), increased alcohol intake, and diabetes or elevated blood glucose level. Any client with aortic stenosis (a condition in which an aortic valve becomes narrowed or constricted) is more likely to experience light-headedness associated with postural hypotension as a result of a sudden change in position or increased intraabdominal pressure (Valsalva maneuver).

During the period of initiation and regulation of cardiac medications (e.g., vasodilators), side effects such as orthostatic hypotension may occur. Implantable loop recorders are available to assess falls associated with syncope of unknown cause. Implantable recorders allow for continuous electrocardiogram (ECG) monitoring for recurrent but infrequent syncope.

Noncardiac conditions, such as anxiety and emotional stress, migraine headaches, seizures, or psychiatric conditions, can cause hyperventilation and subsequent light-headedness.

Vasovagal syncope is a term that is used for persons who have a very strong parasympathetic response that leads to vasodilation throughout the body. It can occur after a prolonged period of sitting or standing. Normally, in such a situation, blood tends to pool in the legs, requiring a heart rate and vasoconstriction sufficient to push the blood back to the heart, but when vasovagal syncope occurs, it is because the heart rate slows and vessels dilate, causing hypotension and cerebral hypoperfusion with subsequent fainting and/or falling.

The individual has a vagal response to the vascular system and passes out but regains consciousness right away (after being recumbent). Some individuals may experience this type of parasympathetic reaction when having blood drawn for testing or when donating blood. This type of syncope is not as serious as cardiac syncope (except as a potential source of injury from falling).

Fatigue provoked by minimal exertion indicates a lack of energy that may be cardiac in origin (e.g., CAD, aortic valve dysfunction, cardiomyopathy, myocarditis), or it may occur secondary to neurologic, muscular, metabolic, or pulmonary pathologic conditions. Often fatigue of a cardiac nature is accompanied by associated symptoms, such as dyspnea, chest pain, palpitations, or headache.

Cough (see also Chapter 15) is usually associated with pulmonary conditions but may occur as a pulmonary complication of a cardiovascular pathologic condition.

Left ventricular dysfunction, including mitral valve dysfunction as with resulting pulmonary edema, may result in a cough when aggravated by exercise, metabolic stress, supine position, or paroxysmal nocturnal dyspnea. The cough is often hacking and dry when associated with left ventricular dysfunction and failure. Cough may be productive of large amounts of frothy, blood-tinged sputum in full-blown pulmonary edema. In the case of CHF, cough develops because a large amount of fluid is trapped in the pulmonary tree, irritating the lung mucosa. A persistent, dry cough can develop as a side effect of some cardiovascular medications (e.g., angiotensin-converting enzyme [ACE] inhibitors) (see Table 12-5).

Cyanosis is a bluish discoloration of the lips and nail beds of the fingers and toes in the white population that accompanies inadequate blood oxygen levels (reduced amounts of oxygenated hemoglobin). Look for gray color tones (instead of pink/red) along the gum line (buccal mucosa) in the mouths of African Americans, Hispanics, or other dark-skinned individuals. Although cyanosis can accompany cardiac, pulmonary, hematologic, or central nervous system (CNS) disorders, visible cyanosis most often accompanies cardiac and pulmonary problems.

Peripheral edema is the hallmark of right ventricular failure; it is usually bilateral and dependent and may be accompanied by jugular venous distention (see Fig. 12-13), cyanosis (of lips, appendages), and abdominal distention from ascites (see Fig. 17-5). Right upper quadrant pain, described as constant, aching, or sharp, may occur secondary to an enlarged liver with this condition. Right-sided heart failure and subsequent edema can also occur as a result of cardiac surgery, venous valve incompetence or obstruction, or cardiac valve stenosis. Noncardiac causes of edema include pulmonary hypertension and lung dysfunction resulting in right-sided heart failure, as well as kidney dysfunction, cirrhosis, burns, infection, lymphatic obstruction, and allergic reaction.

Claudication, sometimes described as cramping or leg pain, is brought on by a consistent amount of exercise or activity. It develops as a result of peripheral vascular disease (PVD), arterial or venous, often occurring simultaneously with CAD.[90] Claudication can be more functionally debilitating than other associated symptoms, such as angina or dyspnea, and may occur in addition to these other symptoms. The presence of pitting edema along with leg pain is usually associated with venous disease. Pitting edema leaves a dent on the skin after the area has been pressed with a thumb for several seconds. This happens as a result of an excess of interstitial fluid collected in the tissue. The dent will slowly fill back.

Other noncardiac causes of leg pain (e.g., sciatica, anterior compartment syndrome, gout, peripheral neuropathy, pseudoclaudication) must be differentiated from pain associated with PVD. Low-back pain associated with *pseudoclaudication* often indicates spinal stenosis. The typical person affected is approximately 60 years old and bothered less by back pain than by a discomfort occurring in the buttock, thigh, or leg that (like true claudication) is brought on by walking but (unlike true claudication) can also be elicited by prolonged standing. The discomfort associated with pseudoclaudication is frequently bilateral and improves with rest or with flexion of the lumbar spine.

SPECIAL IMPLICATIONS FOR THE THERAPIST 12-1

Signs and Symptoms of Cardiovascular Disease
Evaluation and Monitoring

As part of the evaluation, the physical therapist assesses cardiac signs and symptoms, assesses the degree of risk of an adverse cardiac event, assesses the type and degree of impairment (dysfunction at the level of the tissue, organ or organ system, and circulation), and assesses the level of disability (difficulty performing activities of daily life) and functional limitations (restrictions in the ability to perform specific actions).[122]

Older adults with cardiac impairment should be examined by a physician. Exercise testing to diagnose the specific level of pathology and impairment aids the therapist in prescribing an individual exercise program with specific parameters (mode, intensity, duration, frequency) determined based on the results of examination and testing.[151]

In some cases, monitoring individuals closely and minimizing risk of an adverse event are a priority (e.g., the person with oxygen transport impairment with or without symptoms). If the individual is symptomatic, recommendations are given to minimize life-threatening risks; interventions are directed at the underlying impairments whenever possible.

As a general guideline, the therapist monitors the unstable cardiac client (whether or not an initial ECG readout is available) during initial exercise to keep intensity lower than the threshold at which cardiac symptoms appear. In other cases, when the degree of risk is low, the need for monitoring may be reduced accordingly and treatment can be less conservative.[122]

The evaluation and intervention strategies for clients with the cardiac symptoms described go beyond the scope of this text, and the physical therapist is referred to any of the specific cardiopulmonary texts available. Special implications included in this chapter should be supplemented by other such materials.

Signs and Symptoms

Cervical disk disease and arthritic changes can mimic atypical *chest pain* requiring screening for medical disease. Pain of cardiac origin can be experienced in the shoulder because the heart (and diaphragm) are supplied by the C5 to C6 spinal segment, which refers visceral pain to the corresponding somatic area. Chest pain attributed to trigger points and other noncardiac causes is discussed in detail elsewhere.[180]

Palpitations lasting for hours or occurring in association with pain, shortness of breath, fainting, or severe light-headedness or dizziness require medical evaluation. Palpitations in any person with a personal history of cardiac disease or a family history of unexplained sudden death require medical referral. Clients describing palpitations or similar phenomena may not be experiencing symptoms of heart disease.

Palpitations can be considered physiologic (i.e., fewer than six occurring per minute may be considered within the normal function of the heart), or they may occur as a result of an overactive thyroid, secondary to caffeine sensitivity, as a side effect of some medications, during menopause when estrogen levels decline, and through the use of drugs, such as cocaine.

Encourage the client to report any such symptoms to the physician if this has not already been brought to the physician's attention. ECG monitoring of the heart's electrical impulses along with a diary of symptoms while wearing the monitor is most often used to identify the underlying condition. (See also "Arrhythmias: Disturbances of Rate or Rhythm" below.)

Before referring the client to the physician, the therapist can help the client characterize the symptom or symptoms by asking a series of questions: Is the sensation long-lasting or transient? Palpitations that begin and end abruptly are more often true sustained arrhythmias. Episodes that gradually appear and disappear tend to be normal alterations in heart rhythm.

Does anything precipitate the symptom or symptoms? Eliminating possible triggers (e.g., caffeine) one at a time may reduce or eliminate palpitations. Is there an association between hormonal status and palpitations (e.g., onset or change in frequency associated with ovulation or start or stop of menstruation)? If exercise brings on the palpitations, ventricular tachycardia may be the underlying cause.

On the other hand, sometimes starting an exercise program reduces the frequency of palpitations. Some people find that deep breathing, coughing, or relaxation can stop the symptom when it begins. If fainting occurs with the palpitations and there is a family history of sudden death, there may be an inherited cardiomyopathy or primary arrhythmia. For the experienced clinician, auscultation may provide additional useful information. Gathering this type of information for the physician's consideration can be very helpful in making the medical diagnosis.

Dyspnea may be a sign of poor physical conditioning, obesity, or asthma or allergies. Anyone who cannot climb a single flight of stairs without feeling moderately to severely winded or who awakens at night or experiences shortness of breath when lying down should be evaluated by a physician. Anyone with known cardiac involvement in whom progressively worse dyspnea develops must also notify the physician of these findings.

Dyspnea relieved by specific breathing patterns (e.g., pursed-lip breathing) or by specific body positions (e.g., leaning forward on arms to lock the shoulder girdle) is more likely to be pulmonary than cardiac in origin. Because breathlessness can be a terrifying experience, any activity that provokes the sensation is avoided, which quickly reduces functional activities. Pulmonary rehabilitation can favorably influence both exertional and clinically assessed dyspnea. The therapist is a key in preventing this vicious circle and in delaying decline of function in the cardiopulmonary population. Specific measures for the determination of dyspnea are available.[120]

Syncope without any warning period of light-headedness, dizziness, or nausea may be a sign of heart valve or arrhythmia problems but rarely occurs as a result of myocardial ischemia. Dizziness or syncope can occur shortly after stopping exercise can occur as a result of decreased venous return to the heart in a normal, healthy adult but should always be evaluated in light of the whole person and context of the situation.[15] Syncope under any circumstance should not be ignored as sudden death can occur; therefore medical referral is recommended for any unexplained syncope, especially in the presence of heart or circulatory problems or if the client has any risk factors for heart attack or stroke.

Physical therapy orthopedic examination of the cervical spine may include vertebral artery tests for compression of the vertebral arteries that can contribute to the development of syncope. Specific test procedures are available.[37,283,386] Traditionally, if signs of eye nystagmus, changes in pupil size, or report of visual disturbances and symptoms of dizziness or light-headedness occurred, this was considered an indication of vertebral artery compromise requiring special care with any subsequent intervention. However, the effect of these tests (known as the vertebral basal artery test, vertebral artery compression test, Wallenberg test, or de Kleyn hanging head test) on blood flow velocity has come under question. For example, the extension-rotation test as a valid clinical screening procedure to detect decreased blood flow in the vertebral artery has been reviewed with variable results. Although one study found it to be a useful test of the adequacy of collateral circulation,[387] it has been suggested that other factors, such as individual sensitivity to extreme head positions, age, and vestibular responsiveness, could affect the results of this test for vertebral artery compression.[471] Larger studies are needed to determine whether subjects testing positive significantly differ from those testing negative.

Athletes may experience neurocardiogenic syncope (neurally mediated hypotension; also known as vasodepressor syncope, vasovagal attack), a benign noncardiac cause of fainting in athletes. This disorder of autonomic cardiovascular regulation (i.e., blood pressure control system) is precipitated by prolonged standing after exertion, a warm environment, or stress, or it may occur during or after exercise, and is not life-threatening. Fainting during exertion, however, should always be evaluated by medical personnel.

Fatigue beyond expectations during or after exercise, especially in a client with a known cardiac condition, must be closely monitored. It should be remembered that β-blockers prescribed for cardiac problems can also cause unusual fatigue symptoms. For the client experiencing fatigue without a prior diagnosis of heart disease, monitoring vital signs may indicate a failure of the blood pressure to rise with increasing workloads.

Such a situation may indicate inadequate cardiac output to meet the demands of exercise. Cardiac output is the amount of blood that the heart is able to pump per minute and is directly affected by stroke volume (the amount the ventricle pumps out with each heartbeat) and the heart rate (the number of heart beats per minute). However, poor exercise tolerance is often the result of deconditioning, especially in the older adult population. Further testing (e.g., exercise treadmill test) may be helpful in determining whether fatigue is related to cardiac problems.

Peripheral edema in the form of a 3-lb or greater weight gain in 24 hours or gradual, continuous gain over several days with swelling of the ankles, abdomen, and hands, and shortness of breath, fatigue, and dizziness may be a red flag symptom of CHF. When such symptoms persist despite rest, medical referral is required. Edema of a cardiac origin may require ECG monitoring during exercise or activity (the physician may not want the client stressed when extensive ECG changes are present), whereas edema of peripheral origin requires medical treatment of the underlying cause.

Claudication is always accompanied by diminished peripheral pulses in the presence of vascular disease, usually accompanied by skin discoloration and trophic changes (e.g., thin, dry, hairless skin). Core temperature, peripheral pulses, and skin temperature should be assessed. Cool skin is more indicative of vascular obstruction; warm to hot skin may indicate inflammation or infection. Sudden worsening of intermittent claudication may be a result of thromboembolism and must be reported to the physician immediately.

If persons with intermittent claudication have normal-appearing skin at rest, exercising the extremity to the point of claudication usually produces marked pallor of the skin over the distal one third of the extremity. This postexercise cutaneous ischemia occurs in both upper and lower extremities and is caused by selective shunting of the available blood to the exercised muscle and away from the more distal parts of the extremity.

AGING AND THE CARDIOVASCULAR SYSTEM

CVD, especially coronary atherosclerosis, is the most common cause of hospitalization and death in the older population in the United States. With the aging of America, by the year 2030 nearly 50% of all Americans will be 45 years old or older. By that time the number of people 65 years and older will more than double and the population 85 years and older is expected to triple.[91] With this increase in the number of older persons, CVD is likely to be even more of a major health problem in the future, as it accounts for greater than 80% of cardiovascular deaths in people age 65 years and above.[254]

Specific Effects of Aging

Aging of the heart is associated with a number of typical morphologic, histologic, and biochemical changes, although not all observed changes with age are associated with deterioration in function. The high prevalence of hypertension and ischemic heart disease makes distinction between normal aging changes and the effects of underlying CVD processes difficult.

Disease-independent changes in the aging heart associated with a reduction in function include (1) reduction in the number of myocytes and cells within the conduction tissue, (2) the development of cardiac fibrosis, (3) a reduction in calcium transport across membranes, (4) lower capillary density, (5) decreases in the intracellular response to β-adrenergic stimulation (sometimes referred to as blunted β-adrenoceptor responsiveness), and (6) impaired autonomic reflex control of heart rate.[254]

Other characteristic changes, such as epicardial fat deposition and "brown atrophy" caused by intracellular lipofuscin deposits, appear to be signs of the aging process but without any obvious effects on function. The hearts of older persons, even fit, healthy, and active adults, pump less blood to the skin; and the heart of the older person has to work much harder under the same circumstances (e.g., exercise in warm environments) than that of a younger person.

Although the specific organ changes associated with aging are discussed here, disease and lifestyle may have a greater impact on cardiovascular function than aging. Research now shows that even children need to control their modifiable risk factors for heart disease.

Postmortem heart studies of adolescents and young adults demonstrate that heart disease begins earlier than formerly expected. Cholesterol deposits and blood vessel changes have been demonstrated in early adolescence with substantial changes observed by age 30 years in some people. More recent studies of overweight and obese children and teens have confirmed their arteries are as stiff and thick as those of middle-aged adults.[93,371,453]

As the arteries age, increased collagen and calcium content and progressive deterioration of the arterial media combined with atherosclerotic plaque formation result in stiff arterial walls and narrowed lumen. Combination of increased systolic blood pressure and increased fatigue of arterial walls, all of which accelerate arterial damage, produce a self-perpetuating cycle. Age-related changes in aorta vary by anatomic region rather than occurring uniformly along its length. With aging, the greatest difference in aortic stiffness is found in the abdominal region followed by the thoracic-descending region, the mid-descending region, and aortic arch,[204] and coinciding with the greatest degree of calcium deposition in the abdominal region.[297] The mechanical properties of the descending thoracic aorta, including tensile strength and the ability to stretch, decline with age, falling abruptly after age 30 years.[189]

Comprehensive explanation of the effects of aging on aorta and microvessels is provided by the Vascular Aging Continuum[335]; according to this document, arterial aging leads not only to cardiac failure, major stroke, and death, but also to microvascular disease in highly perfused organs, such as brain and kidney, resulting in end-stage cerebral or renal disease, and death.

Effects of Aging on Function

None of the changes described earlier has clinical relevance at rest but may have considerable consequences during cardiovascular stress, such as occurs with increased flow demand (e.g., exercise, postoperative), demand for acute autonomic reflex control (e.g., change in posture), or severe disease (e.g., uncontrolled hypertension, tachyarrhythmias, myocardial ischemia). Physiologic aging is accompanied by a progressive decline in resting organ function. Consequently, the reserve capacity to compensate for impaired organ function, heat, drug metabolism, and added physiologic demands is impaired, and functional disability will occur more quickly and take longer to resolve.[339]

According to experts at the National Institute on Aging, age is the greatest risk factor for CVD.[254,318] The heart also undergoes some changes associated with advanced age in individuals who do not exercise and who have risk factors for cardiac disease. Moderate thickening of the left ventricular wall (exaggerated in hypertensive clients) and increased left atrial size occur as a result of myocyte enlargement (hypertrophy) or replacement by fibrous tissue. Decreased ventricular filling compensated by increased systolic blood pressure occurs as a result of the changes in the ventricular wall. Left ventricular functioning is compromised in the presence of stress such as vigorous exercise or disease. Arrhythmia or hypertension may occur as a result.

The vasculature changes with aging as the arterial walls stiffen with age and the aorta becomes dilated and elongated. The incidence and severity of atherosclerosis do increase with aging, and this contributes to changes in vasculature function.

Calcium deposition and changes in the amount of and loss of elasticity in elastin and collagen most often affect the larger and medium-sized vessels. The unpredictable interaction between age-related and disease-associated changes in all organ functions (including the heart) and the altered neurohormonal response to various forms of stress in the aging older adult may result in atypical clinical presentations of disease that delay diagnosis and medical intervention.[271,339]

There is some evidence that age-related decline in steroid hormones, particularly the sex hormones (estrogen, progesterone, testosterone, dehydroepiandrosterone [DHEA], pregnenolone) triggers a feedback loop to elevate cholesterol concentrations. This mechanism allows the body to maintain levels of vital hormones needed for tissue repair, maintenance, and respond to physiologic stresses. But age-impaired hormone synthesis does not allow the elevated cholesterol to actually restore hormones to the optimum levels, thus resulting in damaging, elevated cholesterol levels leading to coronary heart disease and stroke. Based on this paradigm, there are some experts who suggest that cholesterol-lowering drugs do not restore physiologic function and are not the answer to the problem.[135,136]

Resting cardiac function (e.g., cardiac output, heart rate) shows minimal age-related changes. Changes in functional capacity are more apparent during exercise than at rest. The maximal heart rate, or the highest heart rate during exercise, does decline with age, possibly because of a decreased cardiovascular response to catecholamines. This decline in maximal heart rate is reflected in the target zone heart rates for exercising senior citizens. See Appendix B for calculation of target heart rates for sedentary and physically fit older adults. The effect of the Frank-Starling mechanism is unaltered with age and is used effectively during exercise to maintain cardiac output through a higher stroke volume.

The Frank-Starling law states that the greater the myocardial fiber length (or stretch), the greater will be its force of contraction. The more the left ventricle fills with blood, the greater will be the quantity of blood ejected into the aorta. This is like a rubber band: the more it is stretched, the more strongly it recoils or snaps back. Thus a direct relationship exists between the volume of blood in the heart at the end of diastole (the length of the muscle fibers) and the force of contraction during the next systole.

Exercise and Age-Associated Changes in the Heart

It is commonly accepted that a decline in maximal oxygen uptake, heart rate, and reduced maximal cardiac output with aging occurs during exercise, even in older athletes. These cardiovascular alterations parallel changes that occur with deconditioning or disuse, including the decrease in maximal oxygen intake and maximal cardiac output. These functions normalize with increased activity, and exercise can reverse some of the age-associated changes in the heart at least partially,[254] supporting the hypothesis that age-related cardiovascular changes are simply the result of inactivity.

In older people, aerobic exercise training lowers heart rate at rest, reduces heart rate and levels of plasma catecholamine at the same absolute submaximal workload, improves heat tolerance,[446] and, at least in men, improves left ventricular performance during peak exercise.[407] It may be that the effect of training is relatively greater in older subjects.

Finally, although the benefits of physical activity and exercise among older persons are becoming increasingly clear, the role of exercise stress testing and safety monitoring for older people who want to start an exercise program is unclear. Current guidelines regarding exercise stress testing may not be applicable to the majority of adults age 75 years or older who are interested in restoring or enhancing their physical function through a program of physical activity and exercise.

Recommendations and precautions to minimize the risk of adverse cardiac events among previously sedentary older adults who do not have symptomatic CVD and are interested in starting an exercise program are available.[174] The therapist is very instrumental in conducting an examination and performing exercise testing to identify the specific level of pathology, impairment, disability and/or functional limitations.[48] An individual exercise prescription is made (mode, intensity, duration, frequency) based on the results of the examination and testing.[151,261]

GENDER DIFFERENCES AND THE CARDIOVASCULAR SYSTEM

Interest in gender differences in all of medicine but especially the cardiovascular system has come to the forefront in the new millennium. Only a small, representative portion of the new information now available can be presented here; the reader is referred to other, more complete sources.[266,267,312]

Female hearts not only are smaller than male hearts but also are constructed differently and respond to age and hypertrophic stimuli differently. Structural differences in the mitral valve may explain why women are more prone to mitral valve prolapse than men. At puberty, a young woman's QT interval lengthens, and the woman with a long QT interval is at greater risk for a serious form of ventricular arrhythmia (known as *torsades de pointes*) and sudden cardiac death, especially when taking drugs that prolong the QT interval.[51]

The QT interval is a measure of the duration of ventricular depolarization and repolarization. A prolonged period of time for depolarization prolongs the suprathreshold period of an action potential and upsets the critical influx and efflux of electrolytes during action potential activity that may predispose a person to ventricular tachycardia.

Left ventricular mass increases with age in healthy women but remains constant in men. Under increased cardiac loading conditions (e.g., hypertension, aortic stenosis) this disparity between genders is even more obvious, especially in adults older than 50 years.[201] The risk for drugs other than cardiac and psychotropic ones to cause prolongation of the QT interval has been recognized. Women also have a three times greater risk of potentially fatal arrhythmias from some cardiac and psychotropic medications. It is anticipated that the list of drugs known to produce such effects will grow.[405] Complications from antiarrhythmic drug use are most common during the first 3 days or after a dosage increase.

Women tend to have a higher incidence of bleeding episodes from thrombolytic agents (see Table 12-5). Women also have different outcomes with surgery and percutaneous transluminal coronary angioplasty (PTCA), with more repeat procedures of PTCA, possibly because of smaller arteries, more advanced disease compared to men, or different tolerance to medications.[259] Women, in contrast to men, with premature coronary disease are at higher risk of developing vascular and ischemic complications after percutaneous coronary intervention.[258]

Many studies have suggested that women with acute MI receive less-aggressive therapy than men and have a poorer outcome when treatment is received. Until recently, women in all age groups have been less likely to undergo diagnostic catheterization than men, and this difference was especially pronounced among older women (older than age 85 years). Women have been less likely than men to receive preventive care (drug treatment for lipid management; risk factor management through exercise, nutrition, and weight reduction), invasive treatments (revascularization procedures), and thrombolytic therapy within 60 minutes of heart attack (or stroke).[163,477] Now that these facts are recognized, there is hope that this equal-opportunity disease will become an equally treated disease. A new generation of physicians trained to recognize differences between men and women will help.

Women delay longer than men before seeking help for symptoms of acute MI, referred to as *decision delay*, further compromising effective treatment and improved outcomes.[395] This is especially true given the evidence that first heart attacks in women may be more severe and that women are more likely to die in the first weeks and months after a heart attack. The Women's Ischemia Syndrome Evaluation (WISE) study has provided detailed evaluation of gender-related risk factors for ischemic heart disease.[417]

Increased rate of mortality is reported in middle-age women with new-onset atrial fibrillation.[112] The increased risk of death is attributed to increased heart failure, stroke and MI. Aggressive treatments are suggested, including anticoagulants and hypertension medications in order to reduce the incidence of stroke and mortality risk.

For many years, women and minorities were underrepresented in studies conducted on heart disease and stroke, but this has changed over the last decade along with concomitant expansion of prevention and educational outreach programs for heart attack, stroke, and other CVDs in women.[312] The use of noninvasive testing in women was controversial because of a perception of diminished accuracy, limited female representation, and technical limitations.

Large observational studies now report marked improvements in the accuracy of results for women undergoing exercise treadmill, echocardiography, and nuclear testing as a result of expanding risk parameters in the test interpretations and improved diagnostic accuracy of such tests.[304] New heart rate estimates for women based on a modified formula are also being incorporated (peak heart rate = 206 − [age × 0.88]).[190] For further discussion, see Appendix B.

Because of technologic advances, improved surgical techniques, greater awareness of gender differences in heart disease, and increased funding for gender-based research, these trends are improving, and women now seem to do as well as men after surgical (revascularization) procedures to restore blood flow to the heart.

Although the American Heart Association reports a decline in death rates in women for CAD and stroke, women are still twice as likely as men to die within 1 year of having a heart attack, and women are at greater risk for second heart attacks and for disability because of heart failure. In 2007 in the United States, CVD was responsible for approximately one death per minute in women.[390] The death rate among black women is 33.7% higher for stroke and 69% higher for heart disease than that of white women. At the same time, black women have significantly lower awareness of heart disease and stroke compared to white women.[311,390] Not surprising, almost half of all women do not realize the necessity of clinical care in case of acute cardiovascular event. Only 53% of women would call 911 if they suspected they were having the event.[311] The need for education and increasing awareness of CVD risk factors of women and their families is obvious.

In 2011, the American Heart Association updated its guidelines on prevention of CVD in women transforming them from evidence-based into effectiveness-based, stressing the effectiveness (benefits and risks derived from clinical practice) of preventive therapies versus efficacy (benefits derived from clinical research).[312]

Coronary Artery Disease in Women

It was long believed that CAD was a more benign process in females, but this has been soundly disproved. A woman presenting with angina postmenopausally has the exact same mortality as a man presenting with angina in his sixties. CAD is the single leading cause of death and a significant cause of morbidity among women in the United States.

Certain characteristics and clinical conditions may place women at higher risk of CAD development or progression, such as depression, being black, menopausal status, age, type 2 diabetes mellitus, and thyroid function. In addition, female gender may adversely influence the relative benefits of some risk modification interventions in older adults (e.g., cholesterol lowering, sedentary behavior, smoking cessation).[223,470]

Many women die of CAD without any warning signs, and by age 65 years one in four women has heart disease (the same proportion as in men). CAD claims the lives of nearly 250,000 women annually in the United States,[304] compared with 40,200 for breast cancer and 63,000 for lung cancer. Despite these statistics, misperceptions still exist that CVD is not a real problem for women and that, despite the fact that some risk factors for CAD can be prevented, CAD is not curable. For these reasons, education and prevention[329] are vitally important to reduce risk of heart disease.

Underrecognition and underdiagnosis of CAD in women contribute to the high mortality rate,[304] and underuse of guideline-based preventive and therapeutic strategies for women probably contributes to their less-favorable CAD outcomes.[477] Researchers are actively studying specific risk factors for women.

A new predictive model for women that combines newer risk markers with traditional risk factors and family history is being investigated. A family history of heart attack prior to age 60 years has been added to the list of risk factors of which women should be aware. The Reynolds Risk Score could help target women who could benefit from more aggressive preventive treatment, including diet, exercise, hormone therapy, nutriceuticals,[137] and possibly a statin or other cholesterol-lowering medication.[384] You can calculate your own score if you are a woman, or help your female clients do so, at www.reynoldsriskscore.org.

Coronary Artery Surgery and Women

The number of women undergoing coronary artery bypass graft (CABG, pronounced "cabbage") continues to increase. Women may experience more chest wall discomfort as a common side effect of CABG than men; it is most often reported in those women who had an internal mammary artery graft.

Women undergoing bypass surgery have a death rate about twice as high as that of men; the difference is more evident in younger women (younger than 50 years old).[56,483] This has been attributed to the fact that women generally have smaller bodies, meaning smaller coronary arteries on which it may be technically more difficult to operate. Data from the WISE study also suggest that women may have both CAD and unrecognized microvascular disease, in which case, opening the arteries is not sufficient.

As a result, a variation of CABG surgery has been developed, known as off-pump coronary artery bypass, which

has reduced the death rate among women and brought about greater equalization in outcomes between men and women.[139,396] Off-pump coronary artery bypass is less invasive because the procedure does not require a cardiopulmonary bypass, which stops the heart during surgery and directs the blood outside the body.[74,359] However, even with this procedure, gender differences remain as women still experience more postoperative complications.[140]

Coronary Microvascular Dysfunction

A "stealth" form of heart disease called *coronary microvascular dysfunction or disease* (previously called syndrome X) has been identified in women. This type does not show up on angiograms. Classic signs of reduced blood flow to the heart (ischemia) are not present. Instead there are false-positive stress test results (significantly abnormal results on the stress test but clear arteries on an angiogram). It may be that the tiny blood vessels to the heart become constricted, reducing blood flow.

Scientists suspect ischemia may have different effects on women compared to CAD (Table 12-2). It was previously thought that women with chest pain but clear arteries had an aggravating case of coronary microvascular syndrome but it was not considered harmful.

Research in the WISE study, a federally funded investigation into ischemic heart disease in women, is ongoing to explain this phenomenon.[41,370,416,417] Autopsy comparisons of women and men have shown that women who die of heart attacks are more likely to have plaque buildup uniformly around the inside of the blood vessel, possibly as a result of chronic inflammation. Inflammation may not be the only cause of coronary microvascular dysfunction. Risk factors such as anemia and polycystic ovarian syndrome have been identified as well.[197] Women with this type of heart disease are at increased risk for heart attack, stroke, and reduced quality of life.

Hormonal Status

Influence of Hormones on Coronary Artery Disease

Estrogen has been considered to have a cardioprotective benefit for women via a variety of mechanisms. It stimulates the formation of high-density lipoprotein (HDL), the good cholesterol, which carries plaque away from the artery wall and back to the liver to be broken down and excreted, while also stimulating low-density lipoprotein (LDL) receptors in the liver and possibly the blood vessel walls. These receptors bind the LDL, the bad cholesterol, and remove it from the circulation, preventing its damaging effects in plaque formation.

Estradiol acts as a calcium channel blocker to relax artery walls, which helps dilate the arteries, improves blood flow throughout the brain and body, and helps to reduce blood pressure. Estrogen maintains the normal balance of prostacyclin and thromboxane, two chemicals that regulate clot formation. Estrogen increases arterial wall production of prostacyclin, which improves blood flow and reduces platelet aggregation. Estrogen receptors locate different regulatory molecules that attract and

Table 12-2   Ischemic Heart Disease

	Coronary Artery Disease	**Coronary Microvascular Disease**
Clinical presentation	Chest pain often described as "crushing" radiating to the left arm, jaw, upper back; can present differently in women (see Figs. 12-7 and 12-11) Cold sweat, nausea	Diffuse discomfort Extreme fatigue Depression Dyspnea Older adult: confusion or increased confusion
Pathology	Plaque build-up extending in toward the blood vessel lumen	Microvascular constriction (narrowing of smaller coronary arteries) *plaque deposited uniformly around inside of the artery walls*
Diagnosis	Stress test, coronary angiography	Stress test*, functional vascular imaging (e.g., multidirectional CT scan of the heart, stress echocardiography, SPECT)
Treatment	Surgery (angioplasty, CABG) Medication (statins)	Medication (antihypertensives, antiinflammatories, statins)

CABG, Coronary artery bypass graft; CT, computed tomography (serves as a noninvasive angiogram; moves around the heart generating a three-dimensional image of the heart and coronary arteries); SPECT, single-photon emission computed tomography (injects a radioactive tracer into bloodstream to chart the flow of blood in the heart and coronary vessels).

*Stress echocardiography uses ultrasound to produce images of the heart after an exercise stress test.

Data from Bonow RO: *Braunwald's heart disease—a textbook of cardiovascular medicine*, ed 9, Philadelphia, 2011, WB Saunders.

bind to estrogen in the cells of the smooth muscle layer of blood vessels. Atherosclerosis may develop because blood vessel cells cannot extract needed estrogen from the blood without the necessary receptors.

Another possible mechanism by which estrogen protects against heart disease before menopause is the release of endothelium-derived relaxing factor (thought to be nitric oxide), a chemical stimulated by estrogen and responsible for dilating blood vessels to maintain normal pressure and flow. As women lose the biologically active estradiol, gender differences become gender similarities and the incidence of CVD increases dramatically, matching the incidence among men within 10 years of menopause without hormone replacement therapy.

Myocardial ischemia may be more easily induced when estrogen concentrations are low, a finding that may be important for timing the assessment and evaluating treatment in women with CAD. The early follicular phase, when estradiol and progesterone concentrations are low, may be associated with poor exercise performance as measured by onset to myocardial ischemia. These findings are preliminary and have not been reproduced or confirmed.

Hormone Replacement for Postmenopausal Women

The use of hormones for cardioprotection has been under investigation for many years. Because heart attacks tend to occur 10 years later in women than in men, it was assumed that the protective effect of estrogen was responsible. Exogenous (externally administered) estrogen has been reported to improve serum lipid profiles, carbohydrate metabolism, and vascular reactivity, but surprisingly, hormonal therapy does not alter the progression of CAD or protect against MI or coronary death. The Heart and Estrogen/Progestin Replacement Study (HERS) failed to demonstrate cardioprotection and even showed an early adverse outcome in women with documented CAD who received daily hormone replacement therapy (HRT). Several large randomized clinical trials for primary and secondary prevention showed mixed results.[467]

Fifty percent of all women who have had a hysterectomy (without removal of the ovaries) and all women who have an oophorectomy (ovary removal) become endocrinologically menopausal by 3 years after surgery, regardless of age. Their heart disease risk increases when they become menopausal regardless of their age or the means by which menopause occurs.

Oral Contraceptives

Studies show that women smokers older than age 35 years who use oral contraceptives are much more likely to have a heart attack or stroke than nonsmokers who use birth control pills. In the last 20 years, cardiovascular complications in all women taking oral contraceptives have become less common because current contraceptives contain the lowest dose of estrogen possible without breakthrough bleeding.

At this dose, the risk of thromboembolic disease is reduced to about 40 events per 100,000 women per year, approximately the same risk as in the general population.[77] However, much debate continues about the use of so-called third-generation (newest) oral contraceptives containing low doses of estrogen and a type of progestin known as *desogestrel*. Women taking this contraceptive are twice as likely to develop superficial venous blood clots compared to women taking second-generation oral contraceptives containing progestins, such as levonorgestrel and norethindrone. It is estimated that 425 ischemic strokes can be attributed to oral contraceptive use each year in the United States, even with the newer low-estrogen preparations.[175]

Hypertension in Women

More women than men eventually develop hypertension in the United States because of their higher numbers and greater longevity. White coat hypertension (rise in blood pressure when being evaluated by a physician or other health care worker) is more prevalent among women, and black women are more likely to have white coat hypertension than black men. There is some indication that white coat hypertension is really caused by the physician or other health care provider asking the patient/client questions right before blood pressure readings. Dialogue (the communicative factor) increases blood pressure. Individuals who rely on sign language to communicate have similar blood pressure responses when trying to communicate.[278]

Recent study of conventional and 24-hour ambulatory measurements of blood pressure indicated that the 24-hour monitoring and especially nighttime blood pressure was a very important predictor of outcomes in women, when compared to men, with hypertension.[59] In this study, conventional monitoring indicated that more men than women had hypertension and cardiovascular outcomes, leading to a misleading conclusion that the absolute risk was higher in men than it was in women. In another study, hypertension was significantly more prevalent among women who reported frequent symptoms of restless legs syndrome.[44] Of women with restless legs syndrome, 80% displayed leg movement in sleep that was associated with periodic fluctuations in blood pressure, allowing speculation about the possible role for restless legs syndrome in the pathogenesis of hypertension.

Alcohol, obesity, and oral contraceptives are important causes of rise in blood pressure among women. Alcohol is known to have specific toxic effects on heart muscle fibers, and excessive alcohol consumption is increasing in women; yet women are less likely than men to be identified as alcohol abusers at early stages of the illness and are less often referred for alcohol treatment until later stages of abuse, when cardiac and other severe complications have occurred.[462]

Women with left ventricular hypertrophy are at greater risk of death than men. ACE inhibitors and angiotensin receptor blockers are contraindicated in pregnancy and should be avoided in women with childbearing potential.[373] Infants who were exposed to the ACE inhibitors during the first trimester were found to be at increased risk of major congenital malformations that affected the cardiovascular and nervous systems.[115]

In the WISE study, early onset of high systolic blood pressure or pulse pressure (the difference between systolic and diastolic blood pressures) has been linked with a higher risk of having significant CAD.[41]

Cholesterol Concerns for Women

Total cholesterol is broken into HDL, or good cholesterol, which carries cholesterol away from the cells, and LDL, or bad cholesterol, which carries cholesterol to the cells. A helpful way to remember the function of these is to think of HDL as "Healthy" or beneficial cholesterol and LDL as "Lousy" or detrimental cholesterol. Lipoproteins are complexes of fat and proteins that help dissolve, transport, and utilize the cholesterol molecule.

The National Heart, Lung, and Blood Institute estimates that more than half of all women older than age 55 years need to lower their blood cholesterol. Reference guides for cholesterol testing and recommendations based on

lipid levels have not been standardized for women with the exception of the HDL. The recommended level for initiating treatment in women is less than 50 mg/dL and for men is less than 40 mg/dL. Whether the current established guidelines on other lipids (based on data derived from studies of men) are most appropriate for women remains unknown.

After menopause, women have higher concentrations of total cholesterol than men do, but the significance of this finding remains unknown. Research results at this time suggest that women need higher levels of the good cholesterol (HDL) for protection against heart disease and that other blood markers, such as triglycerides and C-reactive protein (CRP), may play more meaningful roles in defining women's heart disease risk. Low levels of HDL cholesterol are predictive of CAD in women and appear to be a stronger risk factor for women older than 65 years than for men of the same age.[312]

DISEASES AFFECTING THE HEART MUSCLE

Ischemic Heart Disease, Coronary Heart Disease, Coronary Artery Disease

Coronary arteries carry oxygenated blood to the myocardium. When these arteries become narrowed or blocked, the areas of the heart muscle supplied by that artery do not receive sufficient amount of oxygen and become ischemic and injured, and infarction may result. Major disorders of the myocardium owing to insufficient blood supply are collectively known as ischemic heart disease, coronary heart disease (CHD), or CAD.

Despite improved clinical care, heightened public awareness, and widespread use of health innovations, atherosclerotic diseases (resulting in narrowing of arteries) and their thrombotic complications remain the number one cause of mortality and morbidity in the United States (see Table 2-1).

An estimated 12 million persons in the United States have CAD. Of the 1.1 million CAD events that occurred during 2001, approximately 650,000 were first events and 450,000 were recurrences. Each year approximately 220,000 fatal CAD events occur suddenly among unhospitalized people. Eleven million Americans who are alive today have a history of angina pectoris, MI, or both, and an estimated 2 million middle-aged and older adults (more than 75 years) have silent myocardial ischemia.[92]

Although CAD death rates in the United States have decreased since reaching a peak during the late 1960s (146.2 cases per 100,000 in 1948 with a peak of 220.3 in 1963 to 87 cases per 100,000 in 1996), a decline in the incidence of coronary disease has not been achieved. In 1940, the rate of CAD was 26.4 per 100,000 people compared to 113.6 in 2010.[18]

The declining mortality rate does not apply to those adults with diabetes and has been attributed to improvements in lifestyle (e.g., reduced smoking in men, improved treatment for lipid lowering, improved coronary care), whereas the increased incidence may be related to the increasing number of people who are surviving past age 65 years.

Nonatherosclerotic causes of coronary artery obstruction and subsequent ischemic heart disease are uncommon (Box 12-1). For example, mediastinal radiotherapy for left-sided breast cancer, Hodgkin lymphoma, or non–Hodgkin lymphoma may be an independent risk factor in the development of ischemic heart disease.

Radiotherapy causes cardiac perfusion defects 6 months after treatment in most people, but it remains unknown if these changes are transient or permanent. Improvements in radiation technique have reduced complications, especially late cardiac deaths. At the present time, the benefit of treatment for operable breast cancer for individuals who may be cured of the disease appears to outweigh the risks of long-term cardiac sequelae.[496] Researchers continue to investigate the need to optimize adjuvant radiotherapy for early breast cancer by considering the dose both to the cancer and to the heart.

Arteriosclerosis

Arteriosclerosis represents a group of diseases characterized by thickening and loss of elasticity of the arterial walls, often referred to as hardening of the arteries. Arteriosclerosis can be divided into three types: (1) *atherosclerosis*, in which plaques of fatty deposits form in the inner layer or intima of the arteries; (2) *Mönckeberg arteriosclerosis*, involving the middle layer of the arteries with destruction of muscle and elastic fibers and formation of calcium deposits; and (3) *arteriolosclerosis* or *arteriolar sclerosis*, characterized by thickening of the walls of small arteries (arterioles). All three forms of arteriosclerosis may be present in the same person but in different blood vessels. Frequently, the terms *arteriosclerosis* and *atherosclerosis* are used interchangeably, although technically atherosclerosis is the most common form of arteriosclerosis.

Atherosclerosis

Atherosclerosis, defined as thickening of the arterial wall through the accumulation of lipids, macrophages, T lymphocytes, smooth muscle cells, extracellular matrix, calcium, and necrotic debris, can affect any of the arteries in a condition known as CVD.

When the arteries of the heart are affected it is referred to as CAD or CHD; when the arteries to the brain are affected, cerebrovascular disease develops. Atherosclerosis of blood vessels to other parts of the body can result in PVD, aneurysm, and intestinal infarction. Atherosclerosis as it affects the heart vessels is discussed in this section. The effect of atherosclerosis on other blood vessels is discussed individually elsewhere.

Etiologic and Risk Factors

In 1948, the U.S. government decided to investigate the etiologic factors, incidence, and pathologic findings of CAD by studying residents of a typical small town in the United States: Framingham, Massachusetts. In 1971, a second generation of adult children and their spouses of the original participants were added. Results from this ongoing research have identified important modifiable and nonmodifiable risk factors associated with death caused by CAD.

Modifiable risk factors that can be controlled are referred to now as "risk factors for which dintervention has been shown to *reduce* incidence of CAD"; other risk factors that can be managed are now referred to as "risk factors for which intervention is *likely to reduce* incidence of CAD" or "risk factors for which intervention *might reduce* incidence of CAD." Some risk factors cannot be altered (nonmodifiable), such as age, gender, family history of heart disease, ethnicity, and exposure to infectious agents (Table 12-3).

As the Framingham study continues to gather and analyze new data, results are reported that help modify existing health risk appraisal models relating risk factors to the probability of developing CAD. With these new models, blood lipid levels, diabetes, and, in women, systolic blood pressure and cigarette smoking are emphasized once again as independent predictors of risk.

The Framingham study is engaged in quantifying the independent contributions of plasma homocysteine (an amino acid by-product of protein metabolism); lipoprotein (a) (Lp[a]), a cholesterol-rich plasma lipoprotein that encourages overgrowth of cells in the artery walls; insulin resistance; small, dense LDL; CRP, a producer of inflammation; fibrinogen; and genetic determinants of CVD.[236]

In a national sample of older women and men (65-84 years), black and Mexican American women and black men were at the greatest risk for CVD. These findings parallel a previously documented increased risk of CVD among younger ethnic minority populations. Differences in socioeconomic status (as measured by educational level and family income) do not explain the higher prevalence of CVD risk factors in these ethnic minority groups.[435]

Higher prevalence of certain risk factors in black women, particularly diabetes and obesity, may explain their increased risk of CAD, but ethnic differences in CAD for Hispanics remain unknown. The Newcastle Thousand Families Study confirms that adult lifestyles are more important than socioeconomic variables,[255] but further

| Table 12-3 | Coronary Artery Disease Risk Factors |

MODIFIABLE RISK FACTORS			NONMODIFIABLE RISK FACTORS	NEWER PREDICTORS OF RISK FACTORS
Risk Factors for Which Intervention Has Been Shown to Reduce Incidence of CAD	**Risk Factors for Which Intervention Is Likely to Reduce Incidence of CAD**	**Risk Factors for Which Intervention Might Reduce Incidence of CAD**		**Risk Factors Under Investigation**

Cigarette smoking
Elevated total serum cholesterol level
Elevated LDL cholesterol level
Hypertension
	Obesity
	Physical inactivity
	Diabetes or impaired glucose tolerance; insulin resistance
	Low HDL
	• Men <40 mg/dL
	• Women <50 mg/dL
	Hormonal status; oral contraceptives; hysterectomy or oophorectory; menopause without hormone replacement (especially before age 40 yr)
	Thrombogenic factors
		Psychologic factors and emotional response to stress
		Discriminatory medicine*
		Oxidative stress
		Excessive alcohol consumption or complete abstinence
		Elevated triglycerides
		Sleep-disordered breathing
		Poor nutrition
			Age
			• Women >55 yr
			• Men >45 yr
			Male gender
			Family history; genetic determinants
			Ethnicity
			Infection (viral, bacterial)
				Elevated homocysteine (>15 µmol/L)
				C-reactive protein (CRP)
				• Below 1 mg/dL: low risk
				• 1-3 mg/dL: moderate risk
				• Above 3 mg/dL: high risk
				Fibrinogen
				Lipoprotein (a) or Lp(a) (>30 mg/dL)†
				Troponin T
				Plasminogen activator inhibitor (marker for recurrence of MI)
				D-dimer (fibrin)
				Dermatologic indicators
				  Graying of the hair
				  Thoracic hairiness
				  Earlobe creases
				Male erectile dysfunction (impotence)
				Ankle/brachial blood pressure index (see Box 12-15)

CAD, Coronary artery disease; LDL, low-density lipoprotein; HDL, high-density lipoprotein; MI, myocardial infarction.
*Discriminatory medicine is not technically a risk factor for CAD but rather results in a different natural history for some individuals.
†Applies to whites and Asians but not to blacks.

research to identify ethnic differences in CVD risk factors is needed.

Modification of Risk Factors That Reduce Incidence of Coronary Artery Disease. *Cigarette smoking* remains the leading preventable cause of CAD. Products of tobacco burning increase heart rate and blood pressure; decrease the oxygen-carrying capacity of blood; increase poisonous gases and elements of the blood such as carbon monoxide, cyanide, formaldehyde, and carbon dioxide; cause narrowing of blood vessels; and increase the work of the heart.

Nicotine enhances the process of atherosclerosis by a direct effect on the blood vessel wall, increasing the circulating levels of fibrinogen and predisposition for plaque formation in the coronary arteries. Nicotine also increases the expression of LDL receptors on smooth muscle cells lining the plaque, priming the cells for the entry of LDL cholesterol particles. By-products of tobacco smoking in the blood act as potent oxidizing agents. This oxidation damages the intimal lining of the arterial walls, exposes collagen, and accelerates platelet aggregation. People who quit smoking will reduce their risk of CAD by half after 1 year and equalize their risk of CAD to that of a nonsmoker in 15 years (see Table 3-12).

Elevated total serum cholesterol levels (>200 mg/dL) place a person at greater risk for heart disease; this risk doubles when cholesterol levels exceed 240 mg/dL and the ratio of total cholesterol to HDL cholesterol is more than 4.5 (Table 12-4). However, control of high LDL in the United States remains below 35%.[95] It is now well known that therapy to lower LDL levels can stabilize, reduce, or even reverse the progression of atherosclerotic plaques and coronary stenosis and reduce recurrent cardiac episodes. Cholesterol levels are influenced by heredity, diet, exercise, alcohol consumption,[121,250] obesity, medications, menopausal status, thyroid function, and smoking. Impaired thyroid function is a cause of elevated cholesterol and arterial stiffness, especially in women older than 50 years who smoke.[338,463]

Hypertension, or high blood pressure, causes the heart to work harder and may injure the arterial walls, making them prone to atherosclerosis. Epidemiologic studies document a strong association between high levels of both systolic and diastolic blood pressure and risk of CAD (and stroke) in both men and women.

Hypertension is aggravated by obesity and is associated with diabetes and regular alcohol use. It can be initiated or aggravated by the use of oral contraceptives, especially in women who smoke. Women who have undetected or uncontrolled hypertension are five times more likely to experience angina, heart attack, or sudden death than women with normal blood pressure. Weight reduction, dietary interventions, and pharmacologic intervention have important roles in the prevention and treatment of hypertension.

Modification of Risk Factors That Are Likely to Reduce Incidence of Coronary Artery Disease. Physical inactivity, sedentary lifestyle, and obesity are parallel, interrelated epidemics in the United States that contribute to increased risk of CAD.

Obesity (see discussion in Chapter 2) alone can lead to CAD, because the excess weight makes the heart work harder to pump blood throughout the body. Obesity is commonly associated with diabetes mellitus, high blood

Table 12-4	Heart Disease Prevention Target Measurements*

Risk Factors	Targets
Body Measurements	
• Body mass index (BMI): multiply your weight in pounds by 700, then divide that number by the square of your height in inches	18.5-24.0 (see also Table 2-3)
• Waist-to-hip ratio (WHR): divide your waist measurement in inches by your hip measurement in inches	≤0.8
Lipids, Lipoproteins	
• Total cholesterol	<200 mg/dL
• HDL cholesterol	≥40 mg/dL (men)[†]
	≥50 mg/dL (women)[†]
• LDL cholesterol	≤129 mg/dL (optimal: 100 mg/dL; <70 mg/dL for women at high risk for heart attack or stroke)
	≤200 mg/dL (<150 mg/dL)[†]
• Triglycerides	<4.5
• Total cholesterol/HDL ratio	See Table 12-8
Blood Pressure	

*These target measures are for healthy adults without evidence of heart disease.

[†]The current standard for all adults is set at ≥35 mg/dL. Proposed targets of ≥40 mg/dL for men and ≥50 mg/dL for women are the guidelines from the American Heart Association[284] and are developed for adults and children older than age 2 years (no upper age limit). Some experts recommend 55 mg/dL or higher for women.

Fletcher B, Berra K, Ades P, et al: Council on Cardiovascular Nursing; Council on Arteriosclerosis, Thrombosis, and Vascular Biology; Council on Basic Cardiovascular Sciences; Council on Cardiovascular Disease in the Young; Council on Clinical Cardiology; Council on Epidemiology and Prevention; Council on Nutrition, Physical Activity, and Metabolism; Council on Stroke; Preventive Cardiovascular Nurses Association. Managing abnormal blood lipids: a collaborative approach. *Circulation* Nov 15;112(20):3184-3209, 2005.

pressure, and high serum lipid (triglycerides and cholesterol) levels. The prevalence of obesity has increased among both men and women in the United States in the past decade. More than half of adult Americans are overweight or obese, and more than half of this population is overweight with associated medical conditions.[322]

The U.S. Department of Health and Human Services reports that one of every five children is obese, and the obesity rates have increased 147% from 1971 to 1994 among children ages 6 to 11 years.[91] Table 12-4 lists target body measurements (adults) for the prevention of heart disease. Increasing research and knowledge related to nutrition have led to identification of several dietary factors that influence CAD risk. The epidemiologic evidence confirms that diets low in saturated fat and high in fruits, vegetables, whole grains, and fiber are associated with a reduced risk of CAD.

Physical inactivity is a major risk factor equal to cholesterol, cigarette smoking, and high blood pressure. Because a higher proportion of U.S. adults lead a sedentary lifestyle (60%) than have hypertension (10%), have hypercholesterolemia (excessive cholesterol in the blood) (10%), or smoke one pack or more of cigarettes per day (18%), increasing the general population's physical activity level may have a greater effect on reducing the incidence of CAD than the modification of the other three risk factors.

Regular aerobic exercise lowers resting pulse rate and blood pressure, improves the ratio of good to bad cholesterol, and helps prevent and control diabetes and osteoporosis. The risk of heart attack and death from heart disease declines steadily as the frequency of vigorous exercise increases. Occasional exercise (one or two times per week) reduces the risk of heart attack by 36%, moderate exercise (three or four times per week) reduces it by 38%, and regular, vigorous exercise (five or more times per week) reduces it by 46%. The benefit of habitual

exercise toward reducing heart attack was greatest among those who worked out for 11 to 24 minutes and did not change or increase further after 24 minutes of exercise.[7]

Impaired glucose metabolism (e.g., insulin resistance, hyperinsulinemia, glucose intolerance) is reported to be atherogenic. Diabetes mellitus, impaired glucose tolerance, and high-normal levels of glycated hemoglobin are powerful contributors to atherosclerotic cardiovascular events in the Framingham study.[488]

The association is complex, and the pathways by which elevated insulin adversely affects both CAD risk factors and the risk of developing CAD remain unknown. The risk for CAD in participants younger than age 65 years was double in men and triple in women with diabetes compared with their nondiabetic counterparts. Individuals with type 2 diabetes mellitus have a risk of MI equivalent to that of someone without diabetes who has had a previous MI.

Diabetes confers the same risk of CVD as aging 15 years.[60] Kidney disease accompanied by hypertension is a serious complication affecting the cardiovascular system among people with diabetes. More than 80% of persons who have diabetes die of some form of CVD. Bypass surgery provides significantly better survival than angioplasty for individuals with diabetes in some subgroups. This may be attributed to the more extensive CAD among people with diabetes and the greater tendency for their arteries to restenose after angioplasty.

Low levels of HDL cholesterol (and high levels of triglycerides) produce twice as many cases of CAD as any other lipid abnormality; this effect is exaggerated in women (see Table 12-4). *Hormonal status* in the menopausal or postmenopausal woman is now known to be a likely contributing risk factor in the development of CAD. The mechanism through which a protective effect is mediated by estrogen has not been explained completely (see previous discussion in this chapter: "Influence of Hormones on Coronary Artery Disease").

Modification of Risk Factors That Might Reduce Incidence of Coronary Artery Disease. *Psychologic factors and emotional stress* (e.g., depression, anxiety, anger, personality factors and character traits, social isolation, chronic life stress including job stress) contribute significantly to the pathogenesis and expression of CAD. Job stress in particular takes a toll: women who worry about losing their jobs have an increased risk of heart disease, including heart attacks and the need for coronary artery surgery compared with less-stressed age and gender-matched individuals.[319,423]

People who are negative, insecure, and distressed (type D personality) are three times more likely to experience a second heart attack than non–D types.[126] Possible mechanisms linking type D personality to cardiovascular events include hypothalamic–pituitary–adrenal axis hyperreactivity, autonomic disturbance, inflammatory dysregulation, and increased oxidative stress.[127]

Other personality traits likely to affect the heart are free-floating hostility associated with anger and a sense of time urgency (two major components of the type A personality). People who have antagonistic personality have higher risk of MI or stroke. Studies showed that they have thicker carotid artery walls than people who are more agreeable.[438]

The long-held belief that anger can increase the risk of acute MI and can be an immediate trigger of heart attacks has been verified.[485] Modifying type A behaviors (pressured, rapid, intense behavior with rapid, breathless speech patterns and interrupting others) can make a difference in terms of heart health.[278]

The relationship between these entities and CAD can be divided into behavioral mechanisms, whereby psychosocial conditions contribute to a higher frequency of adverse health behaviors such as poor diet and smoking, and direct stress-induced pathophysiologic mechanisms, which contribute to neuroendocrine activation, hemodynamic and catecholamine responses, and platelet activation.[430] Personality traits are more difficult to change than other psychologic risk factors, such as depression or anxiety.[126]

About one in four people experience symptoms of depression after a heart attack or coronary bypass surgery. Individuals with depression are more likely to have another acute event in the year after their heart attack, and have an increased likelihood of death in the following years European Society of Cardiology.[316] Thus, treating depression is an important step in preventing disability and premature death in people with CAD.

Research demonstrates that acute mental or emotional stress triggers myocardial ischemia, promotes arrhythmogenesis, stimulates platelet function, and increases blood viscosity through hemoconcentration. Moderate to severe depression is associated with altered cardiac autonomic modulation, including elevated heart rate, elevated norepinephrine, and reduced heart rate variability, known risk factors for cardiac morbidity and mortality.

In the presence of atherosclerosis in people with CAD, acute stress also causes coronary vasoconstriction. Hypersensitivity of the sympathetic nervous system to perceived adversity (manifested by exaggerated heart rate and blood pressure responses to psychologic stimuli) is an intrinsic characteristic among these individuals; in addition, the calming response of the parasympathetic nervous system is diminished in persons who are hostile and the parasympathetic counterbalance does not stop the effects of adrenaline on the heart.

Whereas negative emotions trigger the stress response, increasing blood pressure and heart rate and altering platelet function, positive emotions and laughter can lower the risk of cardiovascular events. One of the mechanisms involves changes in endothelial function and blood flow. In one study, people who watched movies that elicited laughter had their blood flow increased 22% compared to the baseline values. In contrast, those who watched stressful movies had blood flow reduced by 35%.[306] Joyful music increased blood flow, whereas music eliciting anxiety reduced it.[307] The magnitude of positive effects of joyful music on endothelial vasoreactivity was comparable to that observed with aerobic activity or statin therapy.

Cognitive behavior therapy was able to increase HDL cholesterol levels in acute-MI patients who previously had undergone CABG surgery or percutaneous coronary intervention.[316] In addition, as these individual's depression level was reduced, they were better at managing their anger and anxiety and showed significant improvements in self-rated health. Increasing evidence suggests that cognitive behavioral therapy and anger management may benefit cardiac clients by improving medical outcome. (See also "Special Implications for the Therapist 2-5: Stress, Coping, and Self-Efficacy" in Chapter 2.)

Discriminatory medicine, the idea that women (and minorities) are treated less aggressively than men for heart problems, has been strongly debated. On the one hand, it has been suggested that a woman's symptoms are more likely to be misinterpreted, overlooked, or dismissed as psychosomatic and that women are less likely to undergo diagnostic procedures. On the other hand, lower rates of cardiac catheterization among women may be related to women's lower rate of positive exercise test results and older age at the time of symptomatic presentation rather than bias based on gender. As mentioned earlier in this chapter, there is evidence to suggest that this trend is changing toward improved gender equity. Research to understand ethnic differences remains limited.

Oxidative stress, or the oxidation of LDL particles as part of the atherosclerotic formation, is under active investigation. Oxidative stress is considered a significant risk factor for CVD. However, antioxidant nutrients failed to provide benefits for CVD in several human trials.

This apparent paradox between the role of antioxidants in reducing oxidative stress and the failure of many antioxidant supplementations warrants further research. Meanwhile, according to the current American Heart Association scientific statement, antioxidant vitamin supplements to prevent CVD are not recommended.[272] See further discussion of the oxidation process in Chapter 6.

Moderate alcohol consumption decreases the risk of heart disease in some people. In fact, when light to moderate alcohol drinkers were compared with nondrinkers, the lowest risk of CHD mortality occurred with one to two drinks a day.[391] This is attributed to alcohol's beneficial effects on hemostasis, including platelet aggregation, coagulation factors, and fibrinolytic system.[397] Alcohol intake increases activity of an enzyme called *tissue-type plasminogen activator (tPA)* that helps to keep blood flowing smoothly by initiating dissolving of clots (fibrinolysis). The highest levels of endogenous tPA have been found among daily consumers of red wine, and the lowest levels have been found among subjects who never (or rarely) consume alcohol.[3]

Although a small amount of alcohol taken daily with meals may elevate levels of HDL cholesterol and the bioflavonoids in red wine reduce atherosclerosis, most researchers oppose recommending drinking as a public health measure to fight heart disease and stress that no one, particularly people with a personal or family history of alcohol abuse, should drink alcohol to improve cholesterol. It should always be remembered that heavy alcohol consumption and binge drinking increase risk of blood clot formation, cardiac arrhythmia, elevated blood pressure, and CVD. Dietary supplements containing flavonoids and antioxidants are now available without the sugar in grape juice or the alcohol in wine.

The cardioprotective benefits appear to be effective only in men older than age 45 years and women older than age 55 years when limited to one or two drinks per day.[207] Greater concentrations of alcohol cause direct coronary artery constriction, which may explain the relationship between ethanol and sudden coronary ischemia that is seen clinically. In addition, the depressive effect of excessive alcohol on the function of myocardial cells decreases myocardial contractility and can be very disabling. Chronic abuse of alcohol is also related to a higher incidence of hypertension, which places greater stress on a heart already compromised by CAD. Chemical dependency is also associated with increased stress on the diseased heart.

In addition, several epidemiologic studies suggest that *sleep-disordered breathing* is a risk factor for CVD, particularly hypertension, stroke, and heart failure.

Nonmodifiable Risk Factors. The risk of CVD or CAD increases with *increasing age,* and the person older than 40 years is more likely to become symptomatic. *Gender* as a nonmodifiable risk factor is reflected in the fact that heart disease is more prevalent among men; women generally experience heart attacks 10 years later than men, possibly because of the biologic protection factor provided premenopausally by estrogen.

By age 45 years, heart disease affects one woman in nine. By age 65 years, this ratio becomes one in three, more closely approximating rates among men. These statistics represent the outcome when no HRT is initiated, but as previously mentioned, the effectiveness of HRT in reducing morbidity and mortality associated with CAD is still under investigation.

A *family history* of CVD (i.e., one or more members of the immediate family with the disease) is associated with increased incidence of heart disease. It is proposed that a mix of environmental and genetic factors leads to atherosclerosis of the coronary arteries in a complex, unpredictable, and unknown series of interactions. For selected individuals, genetic predisposition, especially abnormalities in lipoprotein metabolism, can

play a very important role in their risk of developing atherosclerosis.

Current research is exploring the possibility of "candidate genes" that may be associated with an increased risk of CAD. One example is familial hypercholesterolemia affecting 1 in 300 to 500 individuals in some populations. A majority of this population (80%-85%) has a mutation in the gene for the LDL receptor. Approximately 5% to 10% of people with the condition have mutations in the apolipoprotein B gene that results in an abnormality that prevents interaction with the LDL receptor. In familial hypercholesterolemia, serum LDL levels are double what are considered normal levels. The National Lipid Association Expert Panel on Familial Hypercholesterolemia recently issued a clinical guidance[178] calling for universal screening in all individuals, regardless of family history, beginning at the age of 9 years.

Another example of a gene associated with an increase in LDL and total cholesterol is apolipoprotein E-4 *(apoE-4)*, one of three forms of a gene involved in clearing cholesterol from the body. Another candidate gene *(DSCAM)*, present in individuals with Down syndrome and CAD, has been identified, and a mutation in the *ABC-1* (*a*denosine triphosphate [ATP]–*b*inding *c*assette transporter-1) protein involved in lipoprotein metabolism can disrupt normal transport and processing of cholesterol. In the future, inherited markers in combination with traditional risk factor assessment will be used first to prevent and then to manage vascular disease through better utilization of diagnostic testing and individualized pharmacologic intervention.

Modern technology and information from the Human Genome Project now allow linkage in family studies to be supplemented with accurate localization of a disease-causing or susceptibility (candidate) genes in the whole genome (our entire set of genes). In order to identify genomic changes leading to development of different diseases, genome-wide association studies are conducted that involve scanning complete genomes of many people to find genetic variations associated with a particular disease. This approach proved to bring considerable success. After the completion of the Human Genome Project in 2003, more than 1000 genome-wide association studies have been performed that revealed association in more than 200 different human diseases (including diabetes, obesity, heart disease, and hypertension[324]) and nondisease traits.

Although a person's genetic make-up was always considered a nonmodifiable risk factor of CVD, recent evidence suggests that common variations in genes responsible for HDL levels may be affected by physical activity levels.[5] Although exercise has been known for increasing the good cholesterol (HDL) levels, researchers have identified genes related to maintenance of HDL level that are influenced by exercise. Depending on what variants of HDL-related genes an individual has, the individual may need to exercise more or less to achieve the same increase in HDL levels.[5]

Ethnicity is a risk factor, and certain ethnic groups have a higher rate of heart disease. The risk of heart disease is highest among blacks, who are three times more likely to have extremely high blood pressure, a major risk factor for CAD, and who have a higher prevalence of other risk factors, such as diabetes mellitus, obesity, and cigarette smoking.

Native Americans have an unusually high rate of diabetes and obesity, although lower total and LDL cholesterol levels appear to offset the difference. Conflicting comparisons of CAD mortality between Mexican Americans and non-Hispanic whites have been reported. Despite their adverse cardiovascular risk profiles, especially a greater prevalence of diabetes, Mexican Americans are reported to have lower mortality rates from CAD. However, when death certificates are more carefully examined and coded, Mexican Americans have rates equal to or higher than those of non-Hispanic whites.[343] Hispanics are less likely than whites to receive catheterization and angioplasty procedures.[153]

Infections (bacterial and viral) as a cause of atherosclerosis and thereby CAD in some people have been supported by experimental and clinical data. This discovery came about as researchers identified the presence of a common virus (cytomegalovirus) in arterial plaque as a contributing factor to angioplasty failure. Atherosclerosis, now recognized as an inflammatory process, and injury to the inner layer of the artery may be triggered by acute or chronic infection, particularly in more susceptible disease states such as diabetes.

Epidemiologic studies have suggested a link between chronic *Helicobacter pylori* infection[353] or prior infection with *Chlamydia pneumoniae* and ischemic heart disease, but this idea is speculative, and research results have been correspondingly conflicting. Although *C. pneumoniae* infection is associated with the initiation and progression of atherosclerosis, results of clinical trials investigating antichlamydial antibiotics as adjuncts to standard therapy in individuals with CAD are inconsistent,[30] and evidence available to date does not demonstrate an overall benefit of antibiotic therapy in reducing mortality or cardiovascular events in adults with CAD. More recently, human papillomavirus was added to the list of infectious agents associated with MI or stroke in women.[253]

Newer Predictors. Investigators may have identified markers for heart disease present in apparently healthy people, that is, components of blood or other factors that can help identify risk of CAD before symptoms develop (see Table 12-3). Serum cholesterol has been used for a long time, but many more potential predictors of risk are being examined. *Homocysteine*, an amino acid that is generated as the body metabolizes another amino acid, methionine (found in animal-derived foods), occurs naturally in blood and tissues and is more common in people with CAD. Elevated levels of homocysteine may be as much of a risk factor as high cholesterol or smoking.

CRP, an acute-phase reactant that reflects low-grade systemic inflammation, is produced by the liver in response to trauma, tissue inflammation, and infection, and seems to predict hypertension, diabetes, heart attacks, and strokes before they occur.[383] People with even slightly elevated blood levels of CRP appear to be at increased risk for CAD and its complications regardless of age, gender, general health, or the presence of other CAD risk factors (see Table 12-3).

Cigarette smokers have elevated levels of CRP, and individuals experiencing a heart attack who have high levels of CRP have a slower than normal response to antithrombotic medication. Preliminary data suggest that the relative effectiveness of secondary preventive therapies, such as cholesterol-lowering drugs and aspirin, may depend on an individual's baseline CRP level.[8]

Fibrinogen, a blood protein essential for proper clotting, may predict first heart attacks (and strokes) in people with unstable CAD and is a risk factor for future cardiovascular problems in those who have not yet developed CAD.

Lp(a), an LDL cholesterol particle with an additional protein attached, slows the breakdown of blood clots. People with high levels of Lp(a) are at greater risk for MI than those with lower levels of Lp(a).

Pulse pressure (<60 mm Hg), a measure of arterial stiffness *(systolic blood pressure minus diastolic blood pressure)*, has been investigated as an independent predictor of CHD risk. Pulse pressure does predict risk for cardiovascular events in men; this association has not been well established in women. Results of postmenopausal women with CAD evaluated in the HERS showed that pulse pressure has a predictive value for heart failure and stroke, but is not associated with mortality associated with CAD.[317]

Dermatologic indicators of coronary risk, such as graying of the hair, hair loss (baldness), thoracic hairiness, and diagonal ear lobe crease are additional but weak risk indicators of CAD in men younger than age 60 years, independent of age and other established coronary risk factors. Short stature may also be an early indicator of heart disease risk. Available data on the mentioned skin conditions as markers for elevated coronary disease risk have come under question.[40,192]

Erectile dysfunction (impotence) is a hemodynamic event that can warn of ischemic heart disease in some men. Researchers may eventually call impotence a "penile stress test" that can be as predictive as a treadmill exercise stress test.[334]

Metabolic syndrome has received increased attention within the last few years (see also discussion in Chapter 11). Several terms were proposed previously for it: the "deadly quartet," syndrome X, insulin-resistance syndrome, and hypertriglycemic waist.[187] The term *metabolic syndrome* is most commonly used now.[240]

Metabolic syndrome can be viewed as an aggregation of multiple cardiovascular risk factors of endogenous origin in one individual. It is a complex group of interrelated factors of metabolic origin—*metabolic risk factors*—that appear to directly promote the development of the atherosclerotic CVD. Another group of factors, the *underlying risk factors*, can precipitate the metabolic syndrome. The rising prevalence worldwide of this problem is largely due to increasing obesity and sedentary lifestyles.[9] Anyone with metabolic syndrome is twice as likely to develop CVD over the next 5 to 10 years as individuals without the syndrome and five times more likely to develop type 2 diabetes mellitus.[9]

Metabolic risk factors include dyslipidemia (elevated serum levels of triglycerides, apolipoprotein B, and LDL; low level of HDL cholesterol), elevated blood pressure (hypertension), elevated blood glucose level (hyperglycemia), and abdominal obesity.[9] The most important *underlying risk factors* are abdominal obesity and insulin resistance; other associated conditions include physical inactivity, aging, hormonal imbalance, and genetic or ethnic predisposition.[128] Excess visceral fat is considered more strongly associated with the metabolic syndrome than any other adipose tissue compartment.[88,214]

In 2001 the National Cholesterol Education Program (NCEP) Adult Treatment Panel III (ATPIII)[320] proposed a set of diagnostic criteria based on common clinical measures, including waist circumference, triglycerides, HDL, blood pressure, and fasting blood glucose level (Box 12-2). Abnormalities in any three of these five measures constitute a diagnosis of the metabolic syndrome. The definition of metabolic syndrome and diagnostic criteria was modified and published in 2009 but with considerable debate regarding what constitutes abdominal obesity and cut off points for waist measurements among different population (United States vs. Europe) and ethnic groups.[9]

Most of the time, metabolic syndrome is manifested in the presence of some degree of obesity and physical inactivity. In addition to the lifestyle changes (exercise, smoking cessation), drug therapy for risk factors may be required.

The primary goal of clinical management of the metabolic syndrome is to reduce the risk for atherosclerotic CVD. When encountering clients presenting with abdominal obesity, physical therapists should appreciate that waist circumference may be associated with lipid abnormalities.[214]

A possible link has been demonstrated between psychosocial stressors from everyday life and the metabolic syndrome. Employees with chronic work stress have more than double the odds of the syndrome compared with those without the stress.[99]

Pathogenesis

The exact mechanism by which the development of CVD/CAD can be explained has yet to be determined. Even the understanding of cholesterol's role in plaque formation is being reexamined. Viewing different types of cholesterol as "good" (HDL) and "bad" (LDL) is much too simplistic. For example, HDL cholesterol is a complex substance from a family of different particles (not just a single particle). Different cholesterol types have more than just one function and can be protective or destructive depending on how the molecules are chemically altered by stress, oxidation, exercise, tobacco use, hormonal influences, nutrition, and other factors.

Additionally, clinical and laboratory studies have shown that inflammation plays a major role in the initiation, progression, and destabilization of atheromas and has gained a much more central focus in the investigation of this disease. CRP has been found in a variety of CVDs. An excess of CRP in the bloodstream signals a steady, low-grade inflammatory response that accompanies atherosclerosis, a key contributor to CVD.

Mutations in the PCSK9 gene (chromosome 1) are linked with naturally high levels of LDL in some people. Other PCSK9 variations cause naturally *low* levels of LDL

Box 12-2

CRITERIA FOR CLINICAL DIAGNOSIS OF METABOLIC SYNDROME

Any three of these five components constitute a diagnosis of metabolic syndrome:
- Elevated waist circumference (in the United States: waist size of more than 40 inches [102 cm] in men and 35 inches (88 cm) in women; lower values are recommended for Asian, Middle Eastern, South American, and African groups)
- Reduced levels of HDL (good or "healthy" cholesterol): less than 40 mg/dL in men and 50 mg/dL in women
- Increased blood pressure of 130/85 mm Hg or greater
- Elevated fasting blood glucose level of 100 mg/dL or greater
- Elevated serum triglyceride levels of 150 mg/dL or greater

Data from Alberti KG, Eckel RH, Grundy SM, et al: Harmonizing the Metabolic Syndrome. Joint Interim Statement of the International Diabetes Federation Task Force on Epidemiology and Prevention; National Heart, Lung, and Blood Institute; American Heart Association; World Heart Federation; International Atherosclerosis Society; and International Association for the Study of Obesity. *Circulation* 120:1640–1645, 2009.

---

by increasing the number of LDL receptors in the liver, making the liver better able to attract excess LDL.[108]

Many new studies emphasize the fact that cholesterol deposits are only one of many mechanisms through which acute CAD develops. New information points to the endothelium as a modulating factor in the pathogenesis of CAD through the production of nitric oxide and angiotensin II, which maintain the homeostatic environment influencing the progression of CAD. This imbalance tends to promote CAD in individuals who have multiple risk factors.

Endothelium-derived nitric oxide is an important mediator of exercise-induced changes in skeletal muscle blood flow. This molecule is responsible for the natural dilation of blood vessels.

Nitric oxide is an antilipid that provides a nonstick coating to the lining of blood vessels, much like Teflon. These two effects have helped explain how nitric oxide might prevent heart attacks and strokes and why nitroglycerin works—nitroglycerin is converted to nitric oxide inside vascular tissue, where it relaxes smooth muscle in arteries and causes blood vessels to dilate.

In the normal artery, the endothelial lining is tightly packed with cells that allow the smooth passage of blood and act as a protective covering against harmful substances circulating in the bloodstream. The normal endothelium presents a nonreactive surface to blood, but injury triggers the thrombotic process.

In the earliest stage of atherosclerosis, damage to arteries arises from a combination of factors. In some cases, the initial damage comes from LDL cholesterol that has been modified by free radicals (see Fig. 6-2). Free radicals are abundant in people who smoke and who have high blood pressure or diabetes. In other cases, high levels of homocysteine or bacteria may contribute to early damage of arterial linings.

In general, most current theories include the following major events in the development of an atherosclerotic plaque (Fig. 12-2): Arterial wall damage occurs either from injury caused by harmful substances in the blood or by physical wear and tear as a result of high blood pressure. This injury to the blood vessel wall permits the infiltration of macromolecules (especially cholesterol) from blood through the damaged endothelium to the underlying smooth muscle cells. Naked collagen acts like flypaper for platelets, causing them to aggregate at the site of injury and plug up the wound.

The core of a coronary thrombus (clot) is composed of platelets, forming a so-called white thrombus. Early-stage plaque formations known as fatty streaks consist of foam cells (white blood cells coated with LDL particles, smooth muscle cells that move in from deeper layers of the artery wall, and platelets).

Cholesterol-filled plaques can take decades to form, sitting snugly in an artery wall for years. What makes a plaque break open and leak its contents into the bloodstream, causing a clot that can block an artery supplying the heart or brain, remains unknown. Experts speculate it could be a spike of high blood pressure or a surge of chemical messages that accompany anger, stress, or other intense emotion. It could be the result of cholesterol crystallization inducing cap rupture and/or erosion.[1,280]

Although platelet activation is a normal response to injury, in atherosclerosis, once the platelets adhere, they also release chemicals that alter the structure of the blood vessel wall, so that what starts out as a small erosion in the wall can end up a swollen mound of platelets, muscle cells, and fibrous clots, a process called *proliferation* that obstructs the flow of blood through the vessel.

After a thrombus forms and causes static or reduced blood flow in the vessel, the clot fibrin is stabilized by crosslinking. This is commonly referred to as a *red thrombus* because of the presence of entrapped red blood cells. Within the thrombus is thrombin, which remains active and can activate platelets. Platelets also release plasminogen activator inhibitor-1 (PAI-1), a potent natural inhibitor of fibrinolysis, and vasoactive amines that can lead to vessel spasm, further platelet aggregation, and thrombus formation or reocclusion. This cycle of injury, platelet activation, and lipid deposition can lead to complete blockage of a vessel and result in ischemia and necrosis of tissue supplied by the obstructed blood vessel.

Newer evidence shows that even small plaques can rupture and cause problems. These vulnerable plaques are covered by a thin cap rather than the thick, fibrous one shown in Figure 12-2. Inflammation and cellular changes weaken and degrade the think cap until it ruptures, exposing its fatty core, which is made up of cholesterol, inflammatory T cells, and white blood cells.

Clinical Manifestations

Atherosclerosis by itself does not necessarily produce symptoms. For manifestations to develop, there must be a critical deficit in blood supply to the heart or other structures supplied by affected blood vessels. For example, symptoms of CAD may not appear until the lumen of the coronary artery narrows by 75%. Then, pain and dysfunction referable to the region supplied by an occluded artery may occur.

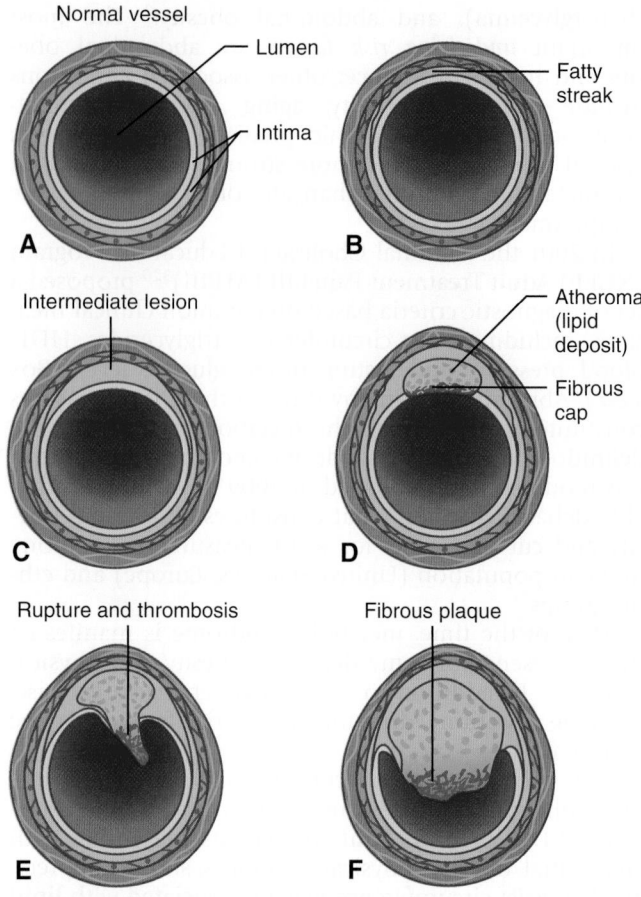

Figure 12-2

Updated model of atherosclerosis. Atherosclerosis begins with an injury to the endothelial lining of the artery (intimal layer) that makes the vessel permeable to circulating lipoproteins. New technology using intravascular ultrasound shows the entire atherosclerotic plaque and has changed the way we view things. The traditional model held that an atherosclerotic plaque in the blood vessel, particularly a coronary blood vessel, kept growing inward and obstructing flow until it closed off and caused a heart attack. This is not entirely correct. It is more accurate to say that in the normal vessel **(A),** penetration of lipoproteins into the smooth muscle cells of the intima produces fatty streaks **(B)** and the start of a coronary lesion forms. **C** and **D,** The coronary lesion grows outward first in a compensatory manner to maintain the open lumen. This is called *positive remodeling.* The blood vessel tries to maintain an open lumen until it can do so no longer. A little roof or "fibrous cap" separates the plaque from the inside of the lumen. A blood clot called an *intraplaque thrombosis* can form inside the plaque; the clot may never leave the plaque. **E,** The plaque (atheroma) begins to build up, gradually pressing inward into the lumen with obstruction of blood flow and possible rupture and thrombus potentially leading to myocardial infarction or stroke. Capped plaques are not as likely to rupture as the softer type packed with viscous cholesterol and white blood cells but only capped with a thin layer of collagen. **F,** Vascular disease today is considered a disease of the wall. Some researchers like to say the disease is in the donut, not the hole of a donut, and that is a new concept. (From Goodman CC, Snyder TE: *Differential diagnosis for physical therapists: screening for referral,* ed 5, Philadelphia, 2013, WB Saunders. Data from Horn HR: Insulin resistance, diabetes, and vascular disease: the rationale for prevention. Available online at http://www.medscape.com/viewarticle/466799_2. Accessed April 2007.)

When atherosclerosis develops slowly, collateral circulation develops to meet the heart's needs. Complications from atherosclerosis occur because it is a progressive disorder that results in more severe cardiac disease if it is not prevented or untreated. Common sequelae of atherosclerosis affecting coronary arteries include angina pectoris, MI or heart attack, and sudden death.

Men experience angina as the first symptom of CAD in one third of all cases and heart attack or sudden death in the majority of cases, whereas half of all women experience angina and remain asymptomatic or present with atypical symptoms in the remaining cases.

Atypical symptoms of angina in women include breathlessness, pain in the left chest, upper abdominal pain, and back or arm pain (more rarely, isolated pain in the right biceps muscle) in the absence of substernal chest pain. The pain may be more diffuse and is described as sharp or fleeting, unrelated to exercise, unrelieved by rest or nitroglycerin but relieved by antacids, and characterized by palpitations without chest pain. The pain may be repeated and prolonged. Chest pain in women with chronic stable angina is more likely to occur during rest, sleep, or periods of mental stress.

MEDICAL MANAGEMENT

PREVENTION. Overwhelming evidence indicates that CVD and CAD are largely preventable; therefore whenever possible, prevention of CVD and CAD is the goal for everyone. And atherosclerosis is not a disease of middle to old age; it begins in adolescence and young adulthood and develops slowly but progressively throughout the body.

Preventing heart disease means controlling LDL before atherosclerosis gets a chance to do much damage. Reduction in the serum level of LDL (at or below 100 mg/dL) throughout the life span through the use of diet, exercise, and statins or other cholesterol-lowering drugs is one way experts propose to do this.[108] Others suggest a multimodal method of treating many conditions (e.g., migraines, fatigue, menopause, erectile dysfunction, elevated cholesterol) that appear to be unrelated but represent underlying hormonal and physiologic imbalances that contribute to the development of CAD and CVD. This treatment approach, referred to as *restorative medicine*, uses hormones and nutraceuticals to achieve stabilization of physiologic homeostasis.[135,137]

Healthy People 2020[202] has identified the following goals for heart disease and stroke: improvement of cardiovascular health and quality of life through the prevention, detection, and treatment of risk factors; early identification and treatment of heart attacks and strokes; and prevention of recurrent cardiovascular events. An excellent guide to evidence-based primary prevention of CVD and similar recommendations for prevention of cerebrovascular disease (i.e., stroke) are available.[182,188,203,351,352]

Health perceptions, health care–seeking behavior, and willingness to participate in long-term preventive therapies are significantly influenced by age, cultural, and socioeconomic factors. Many physicians underestimate the life expectancy in older adults. For example, the average 65-year-old can expect to live an additional 15 to 20 years and function independently for more than 70% of this time.

Adults older than 80 years can expect to live 7 to 10 more years and function independently for half of that time. Older individuals are less likely to be referred to cardiac rehabilitation and exercise-training programs, and less likely to attend, than younger adults. Therefore, preventive cardiology, including primary and secondary preventive efforts directed at the older adult, is important.[262]

Primary and secondary prevention programs are needed that are modified for the language, cultural, and medical needs of people of all age groups and ethnic backgrounds but especially for older ethnic minorities who are at increased risk for CVD.[435] Ethnic comparisons of health behaviors and prevalence of risk factors among teenagers support the need for health promotion intervention among urban ethnic teenagers.[145]

Women are less likely than men to receive health care advice on risk reduction while they are still healthy (i.e., before a significant cardiac event), even though they are more likely to die with the first heart attack. For this reason, new guidelines for prevention of heart disease in women were published in 2007 and updated in 2011.[312]

The bottom line is that even for people with a strong genetic component, modifying risk factors can slow the growth and spread of atherosclerotic plaque and reduce the risk of heart attack or stroke. The goal is to prevent cholesterol-filled plaque from rupturing, a key event that leads to the formation of blood clots that can block a coronary or carotid artery. Many people with significant nonmodifiable risk factors for heart disease but who follow a heart-healthy lifestyle live longer and in better health with better quality of life compared with those individuals who do not follow a heart-healthy plan.

Modification of Risk Factors. Modifying risk factors whenever possible can decrease the risk of CVD/CAD. This includes cessation of cigarette smoking, management of diabetes and hypertension, body weight reduction, lipid management, preventing excessive blood clotting, and annual influenza vaccination.[425]

Changing dietary habits by reducing fat intake can result in regression and disappearance of fatty streaks consisting of lipid-laden macrophages, T lymphocytes, and smooth muscle cells before these components progress to form a fibrous plaque.

Dietary changes are recommended for everyone, including children and adults, as it is now recognized that blood vessel changes associated with heart disease begin as early as 15 years of age and the progression of the lesions is strongly influenced by the same risk factors that predict risk of clinically manifest coronary disease in middle-age adults.[431,497] In addition, at least one third of all Americans younger than age 19 years are overweight or obese.[469]

There is a need for early and aggressive control of all risk factors in young persons for long-range prevention of CAD and related diseases. The Unified Dietary Guidelines have been published as nutritional guidelines by experts from the American Heart Association, American Cancer Society, American Dietetic Association, American Academy of Pediatrics, and National Institutes of Health.[123]

In addition, an excellent guide to risk reduction outlining goals, screening, and recommendations for lifestyle factors and pharmacologic interventions is available.[188, 272, 425] The National Heart, Lung, and Blood Institute also has a validated health risk appraisal instrument (ATPIII scale) that is easy to use.[323]

Exercise and Physical Activity. Exercise and physical activity according to recommendations from the Centers for Disease Control and Prevention (CDC) (i.e., moderate-intensity exercise for at least 30 minutes on most days of the week) have been shown to reduce the risk for coronary events,[425] ischemic stroke,[210] metabolic syndrome and insulin resistance, and diabetes mellitus for men and women.[289,464]

The American College of Sports Medicine's position on the quantity and quality of exercise for developing and maintaining cardiorespiratory and muscular fitness and flexibility in healthy adults recommends aerobic endurance training at least 2 days/wk at 50% or higher VO_2 and for at least 10 minutes.

VO_2 is a measure of oxygen uptake sometimes described as aerobic capacity, ventilatory uptake, or physical working capacity. Maximal oxygen consumption is referred to as VO_{2max}. This measurement reflects the integration of three components of the delivery system that transports O_2 from the outside air to the working muscles: pulmonary ventilation, blood circulation, and muscle tissue. It is a measure of the maximum amount of oxygen being delivered and consumed by the body during exercise in a given period of time.

In recent years, the view that physical activity has to be vigorous to achieve a reduction in risk of CAD has been under question. Substantial evidence supports the benefit of continued regular physical activity that does not need to be strenuous or prolonged and includes daily leisure activities, such as walking or gardening. Taking up regular light or moderate physical activity in middle or older age confers significant benefit for CVD.[463] The U.S. Department of Health and Human Services stipulation that "some physical activity is better than none"[454] has been supported by a quantitative study on the association of the intensity of physical activity and CAD risk.[399] Exercising for 300 min/wk lowered the risk of CAD by 20% while exercising for 150 min/wk or only 75 min/wk reduced the risk by 14%. The benefit of exercise was more pronounced in women whose risk for CAD was 1.5 times lower than in men exercising for the same duration of time.

Newer evidence shows that exercise helps keep the inner lining of the arteries healthy and less prone to injuries that lead to plaque formation. Regular expansion and contraction of arteries during exercise is thought to keep the vessels "in shape," maintaining endothelial function and limiting attachment of plaque to the arterial walls. This movement of the arterial walls inhibits clot formation by making platelets less "sticky" and promoting the release of enzymes that break down clots.[196] For individuals with CAD, moderate exercise (3 hr/wk), in combination with low-fat diet and stress management, improved endothelial function and reduced inflammatory markers associated with atherosclerosis.[132]

The National Runners' Health Study reports that substantial health benefits occur (in men) at exercise levels that exceed the CDC guidelines, suggesting that intense exercise offers one set of benefits whereas lengthy exercise provides another.[486] Other studies report the benefits of shorter periods of physical activity in decreasing the risk of CAD as being equal to one longer, continuous session of exercise, as long as the total caloric expenditure is equivalent.[183]

Heart rate recovery, a prognostic indicator and predictor of mortality, can be improved by exercise. Individuals with abnormal (slowed) heart rate recovery after 12 weeks of aerobic exercise performed 3 times per week for 30 to 50 minutes per session, were able to normalize it and had mortality levels similar to persons with normal heart recovery rate.[228] Heart rate recovery is defined as a delayed decrease in heart rate during recovery after exercise to less than or equal to 12 beats per minute after the first minute while walking in recovery.[15]

The effect of exercise on cholesterol has been documented, but it remains unclear which component of exercise is the underlying beneficial mechanism. Exercise frequency may be more important than intensity in improving HDL cholesterol and cholesterol ratios,[246] and resistive exercise training has been reported to raise HDL cholesterol levels, but studies in these areas have been limited.[179,356] Even so, many health benefits from physical activity can be achieved in shorter bouts at less intensity.[16] Regular exercise has been shown to raise HDL by an average of 4.6%; for every 1% increase in HDL, risk of death from heart disease goes down by 3.5%.[196]

More studies are required to identify the ideal prescriptive exercise. Interestingly, endothelial damage has been reported after intense aerobic exercise, raising additional questions about exercise for athletes with cardiovascular risk factors.[52] At the same time, exercise has been shown to improve skeletal muscle capillary density in middle-age adult women, thus improving exercise capacity.[134] It is likely that in the future, different exercise regimens for specific heart disease risk factors will be individually prescribed.

The benefits of strength training for people with heart disease have generated debate on both sides. In the past, there was some concern that abrupt surges of blood pressure could increase the risk of plaque disruption. But new recommendations from the American Heart Association suggest that resistance training can be safe and beneficial for individuals with heart disease at low risk. This would include people who do not have heart failure, symptoms of exercise-induced angina, or severe heart arrhythmias.

Exercise alone independent of weight loss or diet changes can have significant beneficial effects on cardiovascular risk factors in overweight people with elevated cholesterol levels.[72] Exercise is the one single intervention with the ability to influence the greatest number of risk factors (e.g., aids in smoking cessation, alters cholesterol levels, reduces blood pressure, helps control blood glucose levels, reverses the effects of a sedentary lifestyle, contributes to weight loss, helps in managing stress-induced increases in heart rate and blood pressure).

In fact, researchers at the University of Texas using real-time three-dimensional (RT3D) echocardiography to compare the effects of medications with the effects of exercise on coronary artery perfusion declare exercise to be "the most powerful drug available in preventing cardiac events."[102] Exercise can lessen depression, anger, and stress, which frequently interfere with recovery, and heart attack survivors who follow the CDC exercise guidelines reduce their risk of a fatal second episode by up to 25%.[225]

Pharmacotherapy and Chemoprevention. Chemoprevention is an established method in the primary and secondary prevention of cardiovascular (and cerebrovascular) disease. Clinical trials have proven conclusively that both fatal and nonfatal coronary events and strokes can be prevented.[456] Pharmacologic management is used to reduce the risk of clotting, to treat hypertension, and to decrease serum cholesterol level when it exceeds 200 mg/dL.

Medications such as 3-hydroxy-3-methylglutaryl coenzyme A (HMG-CoA) reductase inhibitors (better known as "statins") are proven effective not only in lowering LDL levels and raising HDL levels (primary prevention), but also in reducing cardiovascular events (secondary prevention) in specific populations, for instance, in people with ischemic heart disease.

Recent observational study of MI patients who already had low LDL levels (below 70 mg/dL) at the time of MI showed that these patients had reduced cardiac death and improved cardiac revascularization a year after the discharge on statins versus those patients who were not taking statins.[265] Use of statins in other populations, including patients with heart failure remains controversial.[279] Some statin effects seem to be gender specific. Although statins are effective for both genders in secondary prevention, they do not reduce stroke or all-cause mortality in women versus men.[193]

Table 12-4 lists target measurements to reduce risk factors developed by the American College of Cardiology and the American Heart Association. The routine use of low-dose aspirin (75-162 mg/day) is recommended in everyone with CAD, unless there are contraindications.[425] The American Heart Association now recommends low-dose aspirin therapy of 81 mg/day or 100 mg every other day for all women age 65 years or older. Studies show that aspirin will not prevent heart attacks in individuals with diabetes who have no evidence of CVD, and routine use of low-dose aspirin is not recommended for healthy women younger than age 65 years, but it may still be considered for all women at risk for stroke who are not at increased risk of bleeding and whose blood pressure is controlled.[312]

DIAGNOSIS. Current national guidelines advise everyone older than age 20 years to have his or her cholesterol checked to establish a baseline with follow-up (retesting) once every 5 years (more often for those with risk factors for heart disease).

Advances in technology are rapidly changing the diagnostic tools available to physicians for diagnosing and evaluating CAD. Coronary angiography (angiogram or arteriogram; x-ray examination of the arteries with dye injection) has been the most widely used anatomic test to assess the degree of obstructive coronary disease and left ventricular contractility.

Angiograms are limited by their inability to detect which plaques represent vulnerable sites for rupture, and all forms of chest pain in women are associated with a lower prevalence of positive findings on angiography, making the diagnosis challenging. Tests using ultrasound or nuclear agents are less reliable in women because signals are blocked by breast tissue. Angiography is much more accurate than echocardiography; echocardiography improves the diagnostic accuracy of stress tests.

Echocardiography is a group of interrelated applications of ultrasound imaging (including Doppler, contrast, stress, and RT3D echocardiography). Advances in echocardiography have expanded its use in assessment of regional myocardial function, analysis of diastolic function, and quantification of regional myocardial function in different pathologic conditions, including ischemic heart disease.

Echocardiography has the potential to image myocardial perfusion along with wall motion and wall thickening. Stress echocardiography showing responses of the heart can be performed during or after a number of different physical stressors. This is important, because responses of the heart to stressors are probably even more important than how the heart functions at rest.

Until this technology is available everywhere, exercise treadmill testing to record symptoms and the electrical activity of the heart under stress continues to offer a means of assessing risk of future cardiac events in most groups (obese, sedentary, middle-aged or older men and women; studies among ethnic groups are under way).[181]

Heart rate recovery after submaximal exercise has been confirmed as a predictor of mortality. This measurement is routinely obtained during exercise testing; it is determined by subtracting the heart rate 2 minutes after exercise from the heart rate at the end of exercise. Abnormal heart rate recovery is defined as a reduction of 12 beats/min or less from the heart rate at peak exercise as compared to the heart rate measured 2 minutes after exercise cessation.

People with an abnormal heart rate recovery are four times as likely to die as those with a normal heart rate recovery. This screening tool can be used with healthy adults as well as with those who have known heart disease.[109,110] A delay in decline of systolic blood pressure after graded exercise is another independent correlate of CAD.

Other diagnostic test procedures available include ultrafast computed tomography (fast CT; "heart scan"), which allows for a computer image accommodating for the heart's pumping cycle. Multidirectional or multidetector CT (also referred to as the "new angiogram") generates up to 64 slice-like images of the heart. A computer then reconstructs these slices to create a detailed 3D image of the heart and coronary arteries. Although less expensive, this new technology is not yet considered a replacement for angiography as it exposes people to increased doses of radiation compared to a traditional coronary angiogram.

Magnetic resonance angiography (MRA) uses a powerful cylinder-shaped magnet that is able to vibrate in distinctive ways to create a signal that is translated into a picture. This technique is also synchronized to the heart cycle and is able to detect plaques. High-speed rotational angiography may be the next technologic diagnostic technique. It is a newly available angiographic modality that gives a dynamic multiple-angle perspective of the coronary tree during a single contrast injection.[282]

With a standard angiogram, the camera is placed at different angles and takes a series of pictures of the heart. Dye is injected with each angle photographed. High-speed rotational angiography allows the camera to sweep across the heart in an arc, taking all the (digital) pictures with one injection. The digital component allows the cardiovascular surgeon to stop and look at each frame.

In the future, advanced technology may be able to determine which plaques are most likely to rupture. Thermography using probes to check the temperature of arteries may also reveal vulnerable plaques that are at risk for rupture, because these will be inflamed with elevated temperatures. The routine measurement of newer predictors, such as Lp(a) and CRP, is not recommended at this time for prognostic use and will be delayed until the clinical benefits of altering these concentrations are made available.

TREATMENT. Medical management is directed toward the specific blood vessel occlusion and depends on complications, for example, occlusive disease of the peripheral vasculature, arterial disease in diabetic clients, occlusive cerebrovascular disease, or visceral artery insufficiency (intestinal ischemia) (see discussion of each individual complication).

Surgery. Surgical management of atherosclerosis of the coronary arteries may include PTCA (Fig. 12-3), CABG (Fig. 12-4), and coronary stents (Fig. 12-5). The current generation of drug-coated stents are bare metal covered with a polymer (plastic) coating that holds and releases a drug to inhibit the growth of endothelial cells. Several companies are working on polymers that are more compatible with the body and less likely to trigger clots. Others are testing polymers that dissolve and disappear after some time.

Angioplasty is performed 10 times more often than bypass surgery; angioplasty combined with a stent reduces the incidence of restenosis, especially for people with diabetes who have a high restenosis rate when treated by standard balloon angioplasty.[457] Antiplatelet treatment with aspirin (Table 12-5) is a standard pharmacologic regimen after coronary artery stenting for the prevention of thrombosis (*thrombosis* is the formation of a clot; *thrombus* is the clot).

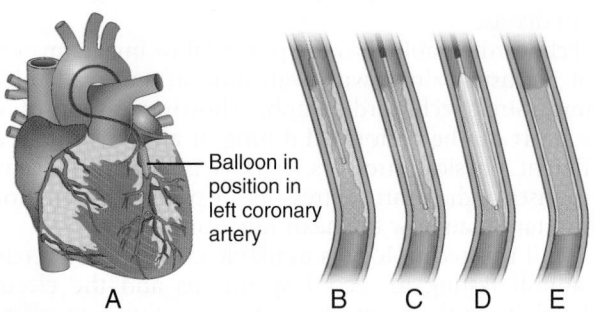

Balloon in position in left coronary artery

A   B   C   D   E

Figure 12-3

PTCA can open an occluded coronary artery without opening the chest, an important advantage over bypass surgery. A, Once coronary angiography has been performed to determine the presence and location of an arterial occlusion, a guide catheter is threaded through the femoral artery (groin) or the radial artery (wrist) into the left coronary artery. **B,** When the angiography shows the guide catheter positioned at the site of occlusion, the uninflated balloon is centered in the obstruction. **C,** A smaller double-lumen balloon catheter is inserted through the guide catheter. **D,** The balloon is inflated, compressing the plaque against the arterial wall and deflated until the angiogram confirms a reduced pressure gradient in the vessel. **E,** The balloon is removed, and the artery is left unoccluded.

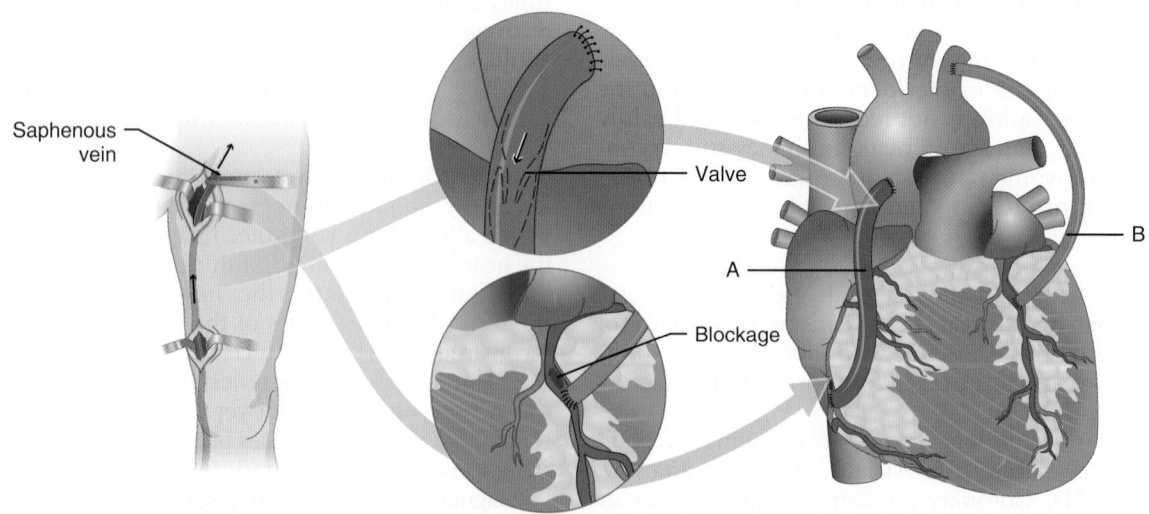

Saphenous vein

Valve

A

B

Blockage

Figure 12-4

CABG. This procedure involves taking a portion of a vein or artery from the leg, chest, or arm and grafting it onto the coronary artery. In this illustration, a section of the saphenous vein *(A)* is used as a graft to route blood around areas of blockage. Bypassing the clogged vessel provides an alternative route *(B)* for blood to reach the heart muscle. The internal mammary artery and, more recently, radial or brachial arteries can be used as an alternate graft site. CABG has been a major surgery requiring a sternotomy but is being refined to possibly become an off-pump bypass grafting through a partial sternotomy. It is considered most effective in individuals who have several severely blocked coronary arteries and a previously damaged heart muscle or when repeated revascularization has failed. (From Black JM, Hawks JH, Keene AM: *Medical-surgical nursing: clinical management for positive outcomes,* ed 6, Philadelphia, 2001, WB Saunders.)

For the person with significant coronary and carotid artery disease, the importance of treating symptomatic stenosis of the carotid artery as a means of stroke prevention is now widely accepted. Carotid artery angioplasty and stenting constitute a procedure that is an alternative to carotid endarterectomy, especially for people considered at high risk for postoperative complications.

Blockages that are heavily calcified and that involve long stretches of coronary artery are difficult to treat successfully with angioplasty or stenting. In such cases, rotational atherectomy can be accomplished using a device called a *rotoblator* (catheter tipped with a tiny rotary blade). This procedure makes sharp cuts in plaque, shaving away the blockage and producing a relatively smooth luminal surface.

Other surgical techniques, such as mechanical thrombectomy using a device (AngioJet System) that removes blood clots in the coronary (or carotid) arteries before

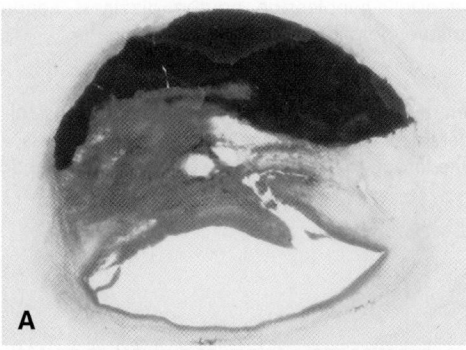

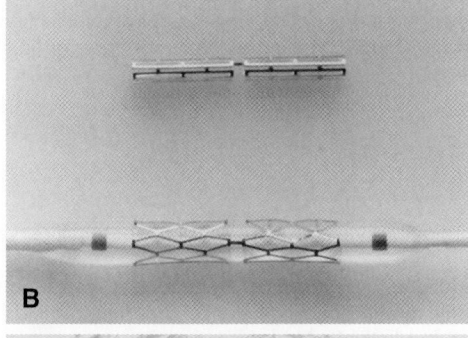

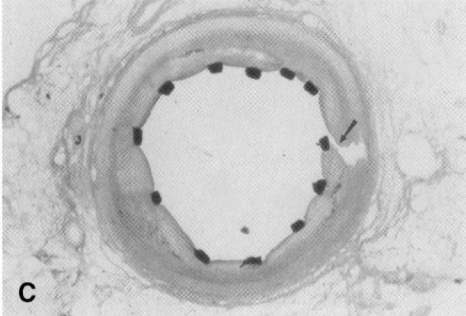

Figure 12-5

Application of the coronary stent. A, Cross-section of a severely occluded coronary artery. **B,** Blocked coronary artery can be held open using a balloon-expandable device called a *coronary stent.* **C,** Stent shown here is in place to maintain opened vessel, allowing blood to pass through freely. Biodegradable stents are under development to reduce or eliminate problems associated with metal stents.[493] Delivery of drugs or gene therapy to inhibit intimal hyperplasia and prevent post-angioplasty restenosis is under investigation.[117,150] (Courtesy Thomas Jefferson University, Philadelphia.)

angioplasty are viable options in some cases, but carry a higher rate of major complications, especially for women.

Intravascular ultrasound, a technology that combines echo with catheterization, may eventually allow diagnosis and therapy to be combined as the cardiologist uses a camera on the tip of a catheter to precisely target atherosclerotic blockage. In keeping with the new data on the time of day that cardiac events occur (i.e., thrombus formation is more likely to occur in the morning hours), researchers are now investigating the possibility that postoperative complications are related to the time the procedure takes place.[443]

Although surgical intervention has been a mainstay for the treatment of CAD, researchers are questioning the necessity of heart surgery and studying the benefits of pharmacologic intervention combined with exercise and lifestyle changes. The role of exercise in the prevention of atherosclerosis has been discussed, but the role of exercise as a treatment modality is equally important.

Cardiac Rehabilitation. The Science Advisory and Coordinating Committee of the American Heart Association has recommended that health care providers implement a coordinated effort to promote outpatient cardiac rehabilitation to eligible individuals. Home health nurses and physical therapists are specifically highlighted as valuable agents in facilitating referral and enrollment and bridging the gap between acute care and outpatient status.[87]

Cardiac rehabilitation exercise training consistently improves objective measures of exercise tolerance, without significant cardiovascular complications or other adverse outcomes. Appropriately prescribed and conducted exercise training is recommended as an integral component of the treatment of atherosclerosis and CAD.[4] See further discussion in "Special Implications for the Therapist 12-2: Ischemic Heart Disease, Coronary Heart Disease, Coronary Artery Disease" below.

Results from the Stanford Coronary Risk Intervention Project conducted over 4 years demonstrate that intensive multifactor risk reduction favorably alters the rate of luminal narrowing in coronary arteries of men and women with CAD and decreases hospitalizations for clinical cardiac events. In cases of low-risk, stable CAD, aggressive lipid-lowering therapy is at least as effective as angioplasty in reducing the incidence of ischemic events.[73]

Numerous other trials (e.g., Leiden Intervention Trial, Heidelberg Diet and Exercise Study, St. Thomas's Atherosclerosis Regression Study, Cholesterol Lowering Atherosclerosis Study) have focused on the effect of diet-induced reductions in LDL cholesterol and the resultant changes in CAD. Restricting the intake of saturated fat and cholesterol has a favorable result in changing the course of coronary atherosclerosis.

In addition, dietary and lifestyle interventions slowed CAD progression, decreased the incidence and severity of angina, and reduced the number of cardiac events. Anyone with CAD, a family history of CAD, or other risk factors should read the American Heart Association scientific statement "Diet and Lifestyle Recommendations Revision 2006"; as of this writing, this document has not been updated since its release.[272] Exercise-based cardiac rehabilitation is effective in reducing cardiac deaths, but the effect of exercise alone without a comprehensive cardiac rehabilitation intervention has not been evaluated.[227]

Table 12-5	Common Cardiovascular Medications

Medications: Trade Names (Generic Names)	Indications and Side Effects*
α-Adrenergic Receptor Agonists	
Aldomet (methyldopa) Catapres (clonidine) Proamatine (midodrine) Tenex (guanfacine) Wytensin (guanabenz)	**Indication:** midodrine treats symptomatic orthostatic hypotension; clonidine, guanabenz, methyldopa, and guanfacine treat hypertension **Side effects:** Midodrine: hypertension, piloerection, dysuria, severe hypertension[†]; Clonidine: contact dermatitis, erythema, xerostomia, dizziness, headache, sedation, somnolence, fatigue; Guanabenz: xerostomia, asthenia, sedation, somnolence; Methyldopa: asthenia, dizziness, headache, sedation, erectile dysfunction (impotence), reduced libido; Guanfacine: orthostatic hypotension, abdominal pain, constipation, xerostomia, dizziness, headache, somnolence, hypotension,[†] syncope[†]
α-Adrenergic Receptor Antagonists	
Cardura (doxazosin) Hytrin (terazosin) Minipress (prazosin)	**Indication:** hypertension **Side effects:** edema, orthostatic hypotension, nausea, dizziness, headache, somnolence, vertigo, fatigue, palpitations, asthenia, syncope[†]
Angiotensin-Converting Enzyme (ACE) Inhibitors	
Accupril (quinapril) Altace (ramipril) Capoten (captopril) Lotensin (benazepril) Prinivil (lisinopril) Vasotec (enalapril) Zestril (lisinopril)	**Indications:** heart failure, hypertension, ventricular dysfunction post-MI **Side effects:** dry and persistent cough, fatigue, headaches, dizziness, syncope,[†] swelling of the throat, face or lips or swelling of feet or abdomen[†]
Angiotensin II Receptor Blockers (ARBs)	
Atacand (candesartan) Avapro (irbesartan) Benicar (olmesartan) Cozaar (losartan) Diovan (valsartan) Edarbi (azilsartan) Micardis (telmisartan)	**Indications:** heart failure, hypertension, ventricular dysfunction post-MI **Side effects:** diarrhea, heartburn, headache, upper respiratory infection, fatigue, dizziness, diarrhea, cough, swelling of the throat, face, or lips,[†] muscle pain or tenderness[†]
β-Adrenergic Receptor Antagonists (β Blockers)	
Blocadren (timolol) Bystolic (nebivolol) Coreg (carvedilol) Corgard (nadolol) Inderal (propranolol) Lopressor (metoprolol tartrate) Sectral (acebutolol) Tenormin (atenolol) Toprol XL (metoprolol succinate) Trandate (labetalol) Visken (pindolol) Zebeta (bisoprolol)	**Indications:** angina, cardiac arrhythmias, hypertension, heart failure, ventricular dysfunction post-MI **Side effects:** dizziness, fatigue, bradyarrhythmia, headache, depression, peripheral edema, erectile dysfunction, somnolence, diarrhea, asthma,[†] bronchospasm,[†] heart failure,[†] arrhythmias[†]
Antiarrhythmics	
Cordarone (amiodarone) Lanoxin (digoxin) Multaq (dronedarone) Quinaglute (quinidine) Rythmol (propafenone) Tambocor (flecainide) Tikosyn (dofetilide)	**Indications:** cardiac arrhythmias, heart failure **Side effects:** chest pain, diarrhea, headache, hypotension, photosensitivity, visual disturbances, dyspnea, taste disturbances, nausea, vomiting, abnormal gait, dizziness, fatigue, arrhythmias[†]
Direct Renin Inhibitors	
Tekturna (aliskiren)	**Indication:** hypertension **Side effects:** diarrhea, dizziness, headache, cough, swelling of the throat, face, and lips[†]

Table 12-5	Common Cardiovascular Medications—cont'd

Medications: Trade Names (Generic Names)	Indications and Side Effects*

Calcium-Channel Blockers

Adalat (nifedipine)
Calan (verapamil)
Cardene (nicardipine)
Cardizem (diltiazem)
Isoptin (verapamil)
Norvasc (amlodipine)
Plendil (felodipine)
Procardia (nifedipine)
Tiazac (diltiazem)
Verelan (verapamil)

Indications: angina, hypertension, cardiac arrhythmias
Side effects: palpitations, peripheral edema, flushing, nausea, vomiting, dizziness, headache, cough, bradyarrhythmia, fatigue, somnolence, constipation, gastroesophageal reflux, angina[†]

Anticoagulants

Argatroban
Arixtra (fondaparinux)
Coumadin (warfarin)
Heparin, unfractionated
Low-molecular-weight heparins (LMWHs)
  Fragmin (dalteparin)
  Lovenox (enoxaparin)
Pradaxa (dabigatran)
Refludan (lepirudin)
Xarelto (rivaroxaban)

Indications: treatment and prevention of clot formation and emboli in the deep veins, heart, lungs, and extremities
Side effects: fever, diarrhea, nausea, hematoma, gastritis (dabigatran), gastroesophageal reflux disease (dabigatran), major bleeding/hemorrhage,[†] anemia,[†] syncope (rivaroxaban)[†]

Antiplatelets

Brilinta (ticagrelor)
Ecotrin (aspirin)
Effient (prasugrel)
Persantine (dipyridamole)
Plavix (clopidogrel)
Ticlid (ticlopidine)

Indication: prevention of clot formation and emboli in the deep veins, heart, and brain
Side effects: abdominal discomfort, diarrhea, nausea, dizziness, headache, hypertension (prasugrel), backache (prasugrel), cough (ticagrelor), dyspnea (ticagrelor), severe bleeding/hemorrhage,[†] angina,[†] syncope,[†] arrhythmias (prasugrel),[†] swelling of the throat, face, and lips (prasugrel)[†]

Hemostatics

Amicar (aminocaproic acid)
Cyklokapron (tranexamic acid)

Indications: excessive bleeding, hemorrhage
Side effects: aminocaproic acid: nausea, vomiting, dizziness, headache, bradycardia, myopathy[†]; tranexamic acid: abdominal pain, arthralgia, backache, cramp, musculoskeletal pain, headache, nasal sinus problems, anemia,[†] visual disturbance[†]

Cholesterol-Modifying Agents

Crestor (rosuvastatin)
Lipitor (atorvastatin)
Livalo (pitavastatin)
Lopid (gemfibrozil)
Loscol (fluvastatin)
Mevacor (lovastatin)
Nia-Bid (niacin)
Niacor (niacin)
Nicobid (niacin)
Pravachol (pravastatin)
Questran (cholestyramine)
Zetia (ezetimibe)
Zocor (simvastatin)

Indications: prevention and treatment of coronary heart disease, dyslipidemias, hypercholesterolemia, hypertriglyceridemia, atherosclerosis
Side effects: diarrhea, abdominal pain, nausea, indigestion, arthralgia, pain in extremities (except cholestyramine), headache, flushing (niacin), myalgia (except cholestyramine),[†] rhabdomyolysis (except cholestyramine),[†] increased risk of myopathy (80 mg simvastatin)

Antidiuretics

DDAVP (desmopressin)

Indication: central diabetes insipidus
Side effects: headache, rhinitis

Continued

Table 12-5	Common Cardiovascular Medications—cont'd
Medications: Trade Names (Generic Names)	**Indications and Side Effects***

Diuretics

Aldosterone antagonists
- Aldactone (spironolactone)

Carbonic anhydrase inhibitors
- Diamox (acetazolamide)

Loop diuretics
- Bumex (bumetanide)
- Demadex (torsemide)
- Lasix (furosemide)

Potassium-sparing diuretics
- Dyrenium (amiloride)
- Inspra (eplerenone)
- Midamor (triamterene)

Thiazide/thiazide-like diuretics
- Diuril (chlorothiazide)
- Hydrodiuril (hydrochlorothiazide)
- Hygroton (chlorthalidone)
- Lozol (indapamide)
- Zaroxolyn (metolazone)

Indications: heart failure, hypertension, edema
Side effects: diarrhea, nausea, vomiting, headache, lethargy, fatigue, erectile dysfunction (impotence), increased urination, cough (eplerenone), gynecomastia (spironolactone), increased hair growth (spironolactone), electrolyte abnormalities,[†] orthostatic hypotension[†]

Phosphodiesterase Inhibitors

Revatio (sildenafil)

Indication: pulmonary arterial hypertension
Side effects: flushing, indigestion, headache, visual disturbance, nasal congestion and bleeding, rhinitis, priapism[†]

Vasodilators

Apresoline (hydralazine)
Imdur (isosorbide mononitrate)
Isordil (isosorbide dinitrate)
Loniten (minoxidil)
Nitro-Bid (nitroglycerin)
Nitrostat (nitroglycerin)
Sorbitrate (isosorbide dinitrate)

Indications: angina; hydralazine and minoxidil are used for hypertension
Side effects: nitroglycerin: dizziness, headache, flushing, severe hypotension[†]; isosorbide mononitrate and dinitrate: dizziness, headache, bradycardia; hydralazine: headache, palpitations, diarrhea, nausea, vomiting, chest pain[†]; minoxidil: hirsutism, edema, cardiac conduction abnormalities[†]

MI, Myocardial infarction.

*The therapist is more likely to see potential side effects that develop when the person is physically challenged and that are not otherwise present. Any unusual signs or symptoms and potential side effects should be documented and reported to the prescribing physician.

[†]Document and contact physician.

Data from: DiPiro JT, Talbert RL, Yee GC, et al, editors: *Pharmacotherapy: a pathophysiologic approach,* ed 8, New York, 2011, McGraw Hill; Brunton LL, Chabner BA, Knollmann BC, editors: *Goodman & Gilman's the pharmacological basis of therapeutics,* ed 12, New York, 2011, McGraw Hill; *Micromedex Healthcare Series* [Internet database]. Greenwood Village, CO: Thomson Reuters (Healthcare) Inc. Updated periodically. Drug Facts and Comparisons: *Facts & Comparisons eAnswers* [online]. 2012. Available from Wolters Kluwer Health, Inc.

Because pharmaceutical agents, surgery, and lifestyle changes, including diet and exercise, have been unable to maintain blood flow without restenosis in some people, new technologic approaches to intervention are being investigated. Emerging treatments for reclosure (restenosis) include antiproliferative (drug)–coated stents and photoangioplasty.

Drug-coated stents resist colonization of the stent (smooth muscle cells cover the surface) and prevent restenosis but can lead to the formation of blood clots. The drugs that prevent the accumulation of scar tissue around the stent also delay healing over the stent site. When tissue does not heal quickly, blood collects and thickens around the stent site, causing a stent-related thrombosis that can cause a heart attack. People with drug-coated stents often take antiplatelet medication (e.g., Plavix [clopidogrel] in combination with aspirin) to prevent this from happening.

Photoangioplasty uses a photosensitive drug that selectively accumulates in atheromatous plaque and remains inactive until exposed to an endovascularly delivered far-red light that reduces or destroys the deposits without damage to the normal vessel wall.[199]

Gene Therapy. Gene therapy (i.e., gene transfer–based antirestenosis therapy) is one strategy with the potential to prevent some of the sequelae after arterial injury, induce growth of new vessels, or remodel preexisting vessels.[150] Several groups have injected a gene that makes a protein called *vascular endothelial growth factor.* When injected directly into the heart, this gene prompts the heart to sprout tiny new blood vessels to bypass the blocked vessels, a process referred to as *therapeutic angiogenesis* or *biologic revascularization.*[329,497]

Alternatively, endothelial stem cells derived from bone marrow and injected into the region bordering an infarction have been shown to regenerate new myocardium or new blood vessels in animal studies. The increase in oxygen and nutrients accompanying this new tissue formation has the potential of preventing death of myocardial cells, reducing myocardiac remodeling and scarring, and improving heart function by levels of 30% to 40%.[160,336]

Genetic approaches will continue to identify genes and pathways involved in the predisposition to and pathophysiology of atherosclerosis. Targets for therapeutic intervention based on gene profiling continue to be the focus of research at this time.[305]

Complementary and Integrative Medicine. The role of complementary and alternative or integrative medicine, sometimes referred to as mind–body therapies, is increasing as more people seek out self-management techniques.[490] At the same time there is more evidence now to support the effects of these therapies on heart disease, blood pressure, lipid levels, morbidity, and mortality.[365]

Examples of these techniques include prayer or meditation and/or religious attendance at church, synagogue, or other services[47,100]; yoga, Tai Chi, and other forms of martial arts; BodyTalk, reiki, and acupuncture; social support and/or support groups; cognitive-behavioral therapy; imagery; hypnosis; physiologic quieting; relaxation techniques; music therapy; and others (Table 12-6).

PROGNOSIS. The American Heart Association reports compelling scientific evidence that comprehensive risk factor interventions in people with cardiovascular heart disease extend overall survival, improve quality of life, decrease the need for interventional procedures, and reduce the incidence of subsequent MI. Even so, despite the well-documented benefit of preventive measures and cardiac rehabilitation, compliance with recommendations for reducing risk factors and utilization rates of rehabilitation programs remain low, especially among women.[312a]

Prognosis depends on the site and extent of myocardial necrosis, but nearly 500,000 deaths each year in the United States are attributable to CAD/CHD. Fatality rates for CAD remain low before age 35 years, but these figures increase exponentially until age 75 years, with men generally experiencing mortality at approximately twice the rate of women until age 65 years. Total CAD mortality in women after age 65 years now exceeds that of men. Of the nearly 20,000 persons eligible for heart transplants, only 10% receive a new heart each year. Advanced atherosclerosis is usually fatal if vessels to the brain or heart are affected, but new technology and new surgical intervention may reduce mortality in the decade ahead.

Surgical procedures are considered safe, and although complications can occur, the rates of complications (e.g., reintervention or repeat procedures, reexploration for bleeding) following CABG surgery have declined substantially in the last 15 years despite higher client risks. In the case of angioplasty, the risks of failure, reoperative procedures, and operative mortality are higher with advanced age, female gender, diabetes mellitus, elevated serum cardiac enzymes following the procedure, and impaired left ventricular dysfunction.[428]

PTCAs are associated with greater rates of restenosis, especially among women, who are at greater risk for complications and have a higher mortality rate. Most studies attribute the higher mortality rate to the fact that women more often undergo the surgery during an emergency, they are usually older at the time of diagnosis than men, they are more likely to have other complicating conditions (e.g., hypertension, diabetes), and they may have smaller, more delicate coronary arteries, making surgery more difficult.

The higher rates of morbidity and mortality associated with angioplasty have resulted in the use of the balloon-expandable stent, which is associated with a low restenosis rate and a favorable clinical outcome with event-free survival rate at 1 year. The need for repeat revascularization has also been significantly reduced.

SPECIAL IMPLICATIONS FOR THE THERAPIST 12-2

Ischemic Heart Disease, Coronary Heart Disease, Coronary Artery Disease
(See also "Stroke" in Chapter 32.)

Other practice patterns may be necessary depending on the clinical manifestations and disease outcomes (see discussion of each specific disease). Physical therapists can be very instrumental in guiding individuals through a preoperative wellness program, including client education, risk factor reduction, and exercise program. The physical therapist is one of the health care professionals whose clinical judgment should assist a physician in selecting the most beneficial therapeutic approach for individuals with CVD.[35]

In the inpatient setting, physical therapists assessing patients' functional capacity and determining discharge placement may dramatically improve referral to outpatient cardiac rehabilitation.[35] This approach, referred to as a "paradigm shift,"[35] may be especially beneficial for CVD people who demonstrate severe disability at discharge. Specifically, individuals with CAD who completed cardiac rehabilitation had reduced risk of death and hospitalization.[294]

Prescriptive Exercise

The known benefits of regular physical activity and exercise in both primary and secondary prevention of CVD have been thoroughly documented (and discussed in this section; see "Prevention"). Exercise training increases cardiovascular functional capacity and decreases myocardial oxygen demand at any level of physical activity in apparently healthy people as well as in most people with CVD.

Regular dynamic exercise is considered adjunctive therapy for lipid management along with dietary management and reduction of excess weight but must be maintained in order to sustain the training effects. Both short- and long-term endurance exercise can contribute to an improvement in blood lipid abnormalities.[392]

Although exercise and physical training have been shown to improve exercise capacity and recovery of the autonomic nervous activity,[441] there is an increased risk that exercise may precipitate cardiovascular complications and silent symptoms of ischemia, arrhythmias, or abnormal blood pressure. Heart responses to exercise and fatigue necessitate special considerations for the formulation and execution of physical conditioning programs. Determining how heart rate and blood

Table 12-6   Medical Management of Cardiovascular Conditions

Coronary Artery Disease/Myocardial Infarction	Angina Pectoris	Hypertension	Congestive Heart Failure	Arrhythmias
Lifestyle changes (see text)	Lifestyle changes	Lifestyle changes	Lifestyle changes	Cardioversion (electrical or pharmacologic)

Prescriptive exercise Medications:
 	
• Morphine
• β-Adrenergic blockers
• Angiotensin-converting enzyme (ACE) inhibitors
• Angiotensin II receptor blockers (ARBs)
• Statins
• Nitrates
• Calcium channel blockers
• Antiplatelets
• Anticoagulants
• Thrombolytics
• Aldosterone antagonists
• Aldosterone receptor blockers
	Prescriptive exercise Medications:
	
	• β-Adrenergic blockers
	• ACE inhibitors
	• Statins
	• Nitrates
	• Calcium channel blockers
	• Antiplatelets
	• Anticoagulants
		Prescriptive exercise Medications (frequent combination therapy):
		• ACE inhibitors
		• ARBs
		• Diuretics
		• β-Adrenergic blockers
		• Calcium channel blockers
		• α_1-Adrenergic blockers
		• Central α_2-adrenergic agonists
		• Peripheral adrenergic blockers
		• Vasodilators
		• Aldosterone receptor blockers
		• Direct renin inhibitors
			Prescriptive exercise Medications (frequent combination therapy):
			• Hydralazine
			• ACE inhibitors
			• ARBs
			• β-Adrenergic blockers
			• Diuretics
			• Calcium channel blockers
			• Nitrates
			• Aldosterone antagonists
			• Aldosterone receptor blockers
				Medications:
				
				• Aspirin
				• Warfarin
				• Antiarrhythmics:
				  • Class I: Block sodium and potassium channels
				  • Class II: β-Adrenergic blockers (used as antiarrhythmics drugs)
				  • Class III: Block potassium channels
				  • Class IV: Calcium channel blockers (used as antiarrhythmics drugs)

Surgery: • Percutaneous transluminal coronary angioplasty (PTCA) • Coronary bypass graft (CABG) • Coronary stent • Implantation • Atherectomy • Mechanical thrombectomy • Transmyocardial revascularization (TMR) • Photo angioplasty • Intraaortic balloon pump (IABP) • Transplantation	Surgery: • Revascularization procedures for unstable angina; see CAD/MI, this table • TMR	Surgery: • Transplantation	Surgery: • Revascularization procedures (see CAD/MI, this table) • IABP • Left ventricular assistive device (see Chapter 21) • Cardiac resynchronization therapy (CRT) • Implantable cardioverter defibrillator (ICD) • Transplantation	Surgery: • Maze procedure (surgical or catheter) • Pacemaker • ICD • Ventricular resynchronization therapy
Gene therapy	Enhanced external counterpulsation (EECP)		EECP	
Stem cell therapy				

The term *blocker* is synonymous with *antagonist*.

Combination medication therapy is frequently used in all of these cardiovascular conditions.

Antiplatelets, anticoagulants, and thrombolytics are used to treat overactive clotting but have distinct uses and mechanisms of action. Antiplatelets block platelet aggregation and platelet-induced clotting, anticoagulants inhibit the synthesis of clotting factors, and thrombolytics facilitate clot breakdown after the formation of a clot.

*The use of complementary-integrative therapies in the adjunctive treatment of each of these conditions is under investigation at this time (see text discussion in "Atherosclerosis: Treatment"). Research centered on pharmacologic and surgical approaches to these conditions is changing rapidly. This information represents a broad overview and may not include every option available.

Data from: Susan Queen, PT, PhD, University of New Mexico, Albuquerque, NM (with permission); DiPiro JT, Talbert RL, Yee GC, et al, editors: *Pharmacotherapy: a pathophysiologic approach*, ed 8, New York, 2011, McGraw Hill.

pressure respond to exercise (e.g., at what point symptoms of oxygen deprivation occur) forms the basis for an exercise prescription.

Frequent premature ventricular contractions are considered a contraindication to exercise unless approved by the physician (e.g., as in the case of automatic implantable cardioverter-defibrillators). Indications for stopping an exercise test can be used as precautions during therapy or exercise (see Box 12-4; see also Box 12-8). Therapists in all settings are encouraged to read the complete American Heart Association Exercise Standards[391] and the Guidelines for Cardiac Rehabilitation and Secondary Prevention Programs developed by the American Association of Cardiovascular and Pulmonary Rehabilitation.[12] Risks associated with resistance exercise in older adults and recommended guidelines for resistance exercise prescription in this population of cardiac rehabilitation clients are also available.[64]

Monitoring During Exercise

More than half of all ischemic episodes are not accompanied by angina. Ask any client with identified CAD risk factors or diagnosed CAD to report all unusual sensations, not just episodes of chest pain or discomfort. Exercise testing should be performed before beginning an exercise program, but if this has not been accomplished and baseline measurements are unavailable for use in planning exercise, use pulse oximetry (a noninvasive and cost-effective method of measuring heart rate and the percentage of blood [hemoglobin] saturated with oxygen; it can be used continuously to help provide clinicians with insight into a patient's oxygenation status at rest as well as during activity); monitor the heart rate and rhythm, respiratory rate, and blood pressure; and note any accompanying symptoms before, during, and after exercise (see Appendix B). This type of monitoring can be modified for each individual and is recommended throughout therapy intervention. Documentation of vital signs can be an excellent way to demonstrate evidence-based outcomes of intervention.

Side effects of cardiovascular medications may not appear until the cardiovascular system is challenged, such as occurs during therapy intervention. Monitoring for drug-related problems is essential, and a basic understanding of how these medications work is helpful (see Table 12-5). Striking a balance between the benefits of cardiovascular medications and acceptable or tolerable side effects can be a challenge, and the therapist must keep in mind when documenting and reporting drug-related effects that these medications often produce physiologic responses that increase the effectiveness of physical therapy. A more comprehensive discussion of this topic is available.[105]

Several drugs used in the treatment of CAD are known to alter the heart rate. For example, β-adrenergic blocking agents used in the treatment of angina and hypertension cause a reduction in resting and exercise heart rate. Anyone taking these medications may not be able to achieve a target heart rate above 90 beats/min; therefore, using symptoms (e.g., angina, diaphoresis,

shortness of breath, dizziness, pallor, isolated [arm or leg] or overall fatigue) and rating perceived exertion may be a more appropriate means of monitoring. Avoid increases of more than 20 beats/min over the resting rate for individuals taking these medications.

Conservative limits postoperatively include a maximal heart rate of 130 beats/min, 120 beats/min for medically managed cases, or an increase of 30 beats/min for surgical cases and 20 beats/min for medical cases. A safe rate of exercise will allow the heart rate to return to the resting level within 5 minutes after stopping exercise.

Almost all antihypertensive agents, including diuretics that may have a dual action of peripheral dilation and volume depletion, can have a profound effect on postexercise blood pressure. In some healthy people, when exercise is terminated abruptly, precipitous drops in systolic blood pressure can occur owing to venous pooling. Some people with CAD have higher levels of systolic blood pressure that exceed peak exercise values; a proper cool-down after vigorous exercise is important to prevent such an occurrence.

More detailed information on the effects of various drugs on the exercise response during training in clients with CAD can be found in *Guidelines for Exercise Testing and Prescription* by the American College of Sports Medicine.[15]

Postoperative Considerations

Cardiac rehabilitation (phases I to IV) is an important component of intervention for anyone treated medically for CHF, arrhythmias, unstable angina, CAD, MI, valvular disease, or heart transplantation. This multidisciplinary program of education and exercise is designed to promote the development of and maintenance of a desirable level of physical, social, and psychologic function in those individuals with an acute cardiovascular illness.

Specific goals of cardiac rehabilitation include stratifying risk, improving emotional well-being and psychologic factors, reducing CAD risk factors, and decreasing symptoms. In addition, older adults often have reduced functional capacity and quality of life scores compared with younger CAD clients, making this an important goal for those individuals.[260,262]

Implementation of phase I cardiac rehabilitation is carried out by exercise physiologists in many locations. Consultation with a physical therapist may only be requested when there are postoperative complications or preexisting conditions that limit phase I (e.g., amputation, cerebrovascular accident, polio, spinal cord injury). Supervision by a physical therapist may not be needed once the individual is safe with ambulation that does not require skilled therapy.

Phase I begins 1 to 3 days following CABG (or other) surgery or an MI. Primary emphasis is on postsurgical mobilization; client education is essential given the presence of comorbidities and the need for individualized prescriptive exercise.

During this phase the therapist uses and teaches the client sternal precautions (Box 12-3; see also "The Cardiac Client and Surgery" below) and adjusts the

Box 12-3

STERNAL PRECAUTIONS

Limited amount of evidence exists for using sternal precautions and many precautions may be overly restrictive and limit the person's mobility and function (see "Special Implications for the Therapist 12-2: Ischemic Heart Disease, Coronary Heart Disease, Coronary Artery Disease" for more details). Below, sternal precautions are listed that are used in practice; these are likely to be revised as more evidence is gained on their restrictive nature that may impede the process of functional recovery. These precautions vary from center to center and sometimes from surgeon to surgeon based on the surgical procedure performed.

It is important to know whether the procedure was with a traditional sternotomy and if the chest has been closed; the skin may be sutured, but the underlying chest structures may not be closed versus a minimally invasive procedure (possibly affecting only one side).

- To evaluate chest wall stability at rest, the therapist places his or her hands on the client's chest and asks the client to cough. Observe chest movement; any type of asynchronous movement between the two chest sides is a sign of an unstable chest requiring sternal precautions that usually include the following:
  - No pulling up in bed during acute care is allowed; client must roll into side-lying position and use the top (or unaffected) arm to assist in pushing up while allowing the feet to drop off the side of the bed as a pendulum type of assist. Head of bed may be raised to assist with this transfer.
  - Handheld assistance during mobilization may be required initially in place of assistive devices, such as walkers or canes.
  - Cough with splinting (use of heart pillow is popular for this).
  - No pushing, pulling, or lifting more than 10 lb (some precautions list 5 lb) for 5 to 8 weeks postoperatively is allowed; this includes vacuuming, lifting pets (or walking pets on a leash), furniture, bowling balls, doors, children, or anything that weighs more than 1 gallon of milk (see comments in the text).

- Avoid using armrests of chairs to push up (arms abducted) from sit-to-stand; encourage placement of hand on knees (arms adducted) to create compressive rather than distraction load across the sternum.
- No driving motorized vehicles (e.g., automobile, golf cart, or other similar large conveyance) for 4 weeks postoperatively (some centers require 6-8 weeks) is permitted; during this time, person should not sit in the front seat of any vehicle and especially vehicles equipped with airbags.
- Full neck, shoulder, and torso range of motion may be permitted as long as the sternum is stable but not if a sternectomy with skin or muscle flap is present; presence of a flap may limit range of motion to 90 degrees (flexion or abduction) or until the point of movement at the chest wall or rib cage.
- Avoid shoulder horizontal abduction with extreme external rotation; some surgeons advise against reaching behind or backwards (e.g., when dressing or reaching into back pocket).
- Unilateral movements and forces are best avoided; bilateral movements producing a symmetrical load are better for sternal healing[452]
- Progression is based on client tolerance and signs of wound healing; once the incision is fully healed, scar mobilization is permissible. The usual precautions for scar mobilization apply, including mobilizing the tissue in the direction of the scar before using any cross-transverse techniques and mobilizing toward the scar rather than away from the scar to avoid overstretching the healing tissue.
- Use of the more conservative precautions is advised with anyone who has diabetes mellitus, severe osteoporosis, or other equally compromising comorbidities.
- Woman with larger breasts are at higher risk for dehiscence post sternotomy.
- Sternal support or harness may be useful to treat pain associated with sternotomy wounds especially while coughing.[300]

---

intensity of mobilization to optimize recovery from surgery and tissue injury, thereby minimizing length of stay without compromising the client.[218]

Sternal Precautions

Although sternal precautions are widely used their origin is not known. Moreover, there is limited amount of evidence for using sternal precautions and many of them may be overly restrictive and limit the patient's mobility and ability to perform activities of daily living. In addition, person's functional recovery is impeded. For these reasons, the use of sternal precautions has recently been called into question along with their impact on patient recovery.[83,452] In fact, it is speculated whether the term "precautions" should be replaced with "restrictions."[83] Nevertheless, if properly prescribed, they can be beneficial, especially for individuals with increased risk of complications or mortality.[478] Patient-specific precautionary, rather than restrictive, approach focused on function is likelier to facilitate the recovery.[83]

After the surgery, it is important to know whether the chest has been closed, because the skin may be closed, but the chest may not be. Mobility status might need to be reviewed in the light of their sternal closure; assistance from the therapist (rather than the use of walking aids) may be required at first.

For sternal instability, dehiscence, and mediastinitis, risk factors include obesity, chronic obstructive pulmonary disease, bilateral internal mammary artery grafts, diabetes, smoking, prolonged mechanical ventilation, previous thoracotomy, and number of transfused units. Other contributing factors include large breast size in women, longer hospital stay, the use of staples for skin closure, and poor compliance with sternal precautions.[83]

Upper extremity precautions are determined by the physician according to the surgery that was performed and the status of the incision. When the chest is closed, shoulder flexion and abduction can proceed until the point of movement at the chest wall or rib cage. This rotation can cause a torque, and further motion may need to be limited.

Pushing activities may have to be limited. For sit-to stand activities, patients are instructed to keep hands on knees with the arms adducted against the body; the

Box 12-4

INDICATIONS FOR DISCONTINUING OR MODIFYING EXERCISE*

Symptoms

- New-onset or easily provoked anginal chest pain
- Increasing episodes, intensity, or duration of angina (unstable angina)
- Discomfort in the upper body, including chest, arm, neck, or jaw; chest pain unrelated to chest incision
- Fainting, light-headedness, dizziness
- Sudden, severe dyspnea
- Severe fatigue or muscle pain
- Nausea or vomiting
- Back pain during exercise
- Bone or joint pain or discomfort during or after exercise
- Severe leg claudication

Clinical Signs

- Pallor; peripheral cyanosis; cold, moist skin
- Staggering gait, ataxia
- Confusion or blank stare in response to inquiries
- Resting heart rate >130 beats/min or <40 beats/min
- >6 Arrhythmias (irregular heartbeats; palpitations) per hour
- Frequent premature ventricular contractions
- Uncontrolled diabetes mellitus (blood glucose level >250 mg/dL)
- Oxygen saturation <90% (98% is normal); some variability (individual and geographic)
- Acute infection or fever >37.8° C (100° F)
- Persistent drainage or change in drainage from any incision
- Increased swelling, tenderness, and redness around any incision site
- Inability to converse during activity
- Blood pressure (BP) abnormalities
  - Fall in systolic BP with increase in workload; specifically, a decrease of 10 mm Hg or more below any previously recorded BP accompanied by other signs or symptoms
  - Rise in systolic BP above 250 mm Hg or diastolic BP above 115 mm Hg
- Signs of CNS involvement (e.g., confusion or delirium, cognitive decline, encephalopathy, seizure, stroke)

Other

- Person indicates need or desire to stop
- Recent myocardial infarction (within 48 hours)

*Not all signs and symptoms require immediate cessation of exercise or intervention. The therapist is advised to document any clinical signs or symptoms observed or reported along with any modifications made in the intervention and notify the physician accordingly.
Adapted from Fletcher GF: Exercise standards for testing and training: a statement for healthcare professionals. From the American Heart Association, *Circulation* 104:1694–1740, 2001.

Box 12-5

DISCHARGE INSTRUCTIONS AFTER CARDIOVASCULAR SURGERY

- **Showers:** Permitted 2 days after surgery or hospitalization. Avoid tub baths or soaking in water until incisions are healed; avoid extremely hot water.
- **Incisions:** The incision should be kept dry but can be gently washed with mild soap and warm water (directly over the tapes); lotions, creams, oils, or powders are not permitted until the wound is completely healed unless prescribed by the physician.
- **Care of surgical leg** (for bypass graft involving the leg): Avoid crossing the legs, which impairs circulation; avoid sitting in one position or standing for prolonged periods. Elevate the involved leg when sitting or lying down. Swelling in the grafted leg is common until collateral circulation develops. Swelling should decrease after leg elevation but may recur when standing. Progressive edema must be reported to the physician.
- **Compression stockings:** Worn for at least 2 weeks after discharge during the daytime and removed at bedtime.
- **Rest:** A balance of rest and exercise is an essential part of the recovery process. Resting between activities and short naps are encouraged. Resting may include sitting quietly or reading for 20 to 30 minutes; loss of appetite is common for the first 2 weeks and may contribute to fatigue.
- **Walking:** Walking increases circulation throughout the body and to the heart muscle and is encouraged. Activity must be increased gradually, but frequent walks of short duration are recommended initially. Pacing of activities throughout the day, combined with energy conservation, is important.
- **Stairs:** Climbing stairs is permitted unless the physician indicates otherwise.
- **Sexual relations:** Sexual relations can be resumed when the client feels physically comfortable (usually 2-4 weeks after discharge; see also text discussion).
- **Sternal precautions:** See Box 12-3.
  Stop any activity immediately if dyspnea, palpitations, chest pain or discomfort, or dizziness or fainting develops. Notify the physician if symptoms do not subside with rest within 20 minutes.

intention is to transfer compressive forces across the sternum rather than creating distraction. Patients are encouraged to avoid using chair armrests with upper extremities in a position of abduction, which can potentially create distraction across sternum. Use of the arms overhead may be allowed if it does not cause excessive pain or a feeling of movement within the sternum. Lifting of heavy objects is prohibited; each physician sets the maximum limit (usually no more than 10 pounds).[83]

This limitation on weight lifting seems to have no evidence and in fact many activities of daily living individuals commonly perform postoperatively without restriction involve heavier weights or produce higher force in comparison to lifting 10 pounds.[346,452] In fact, cough produces more force on the median sternotomy incision than lifting a 40-pound weight.[346] Heart pillows are used for bed mobility and coughing. Transfers from side-lying to sitting are initiated with the head of the bed elevated until discharge planning is begun.

Resistive elastic or small weights and aerobic training are introduced between 4 and 6 weeks postoperatively. Pushing or pulling activities and lifting more than 10 pounds have traditionally been contraindicated in the first 4 to 6 weeks because of a suspected but not proven link between the use of the upper extremities and sternal instability/dehiscence. The American College of Sports Medicine advises that upper extremity range of motion and exercise is permissible during the first 5 to 8 weeks when there is no evidence of sternal instability (e.g., sternal movement, pain, pulling sensation, cracking, popping).[15]

In the past, airway clearance techniques were recommended routinely for persons who had abdominal or cardiothoracic surgery, but their efficacy for reducing complications after coronary artery surgery has been repeatedly studied and never been proven. With advances in surgical techniques, smaller incisions, reduced postoperative pulmonary dysfunction, and earlier mobilization, airway clearance techniques such as postural drainage and manual techniques now are limited to clients who are very acutely ill and cannot participate in early mobilization.[106]

Postoperative brachial plexus injury can occur following cardiac surgery that requires a sternotomy when prolonged sternal separation or asymmetric traction of the sternal halves causes nerve compression or overstretching. Uncomplicated cases are usually transient and do not require intervention by a therapist. In rare cases, peripheral neuropathy will persist, resulting in impaired function and disability. As cardiac operative techniques continue to improve and move toward noninvasive methods, this type of injury will become obsolete.

Home monitoring of symptoms for the first weeks after surgery is essential following the guidelines in Box 12-4. The physician should be notified if the client experiences one or more of the signs and symptoms outlined. Transfusion is no longer a standard part of open heart surgery, so hematocrit levels are usually low (25%-29%) following this procedure, requiring modification of exercise guidelines (see Table 40-8) unless directed otherwise by the physician. Carotid artery disease is a risk factor for CNS complications after CABG surgery, requiring close monitoring for signs and symptoms of CNS involvement.

Discharge instructions for the cardiovascular surgical population may vary according to physician and institution, but some general guidelines apply (Box 12-5). The therapist can be helpful in teaching about unexpected symptoms and ways to manage them. For example, women experiencing postoperative chest discomfort can be reassured that this is not uncommon, will subside over time, and may be minimized by wearing a snug all-cotton undershirt under loose clothing to decrease friction. Women with large breasts are likely to benefit from wearing a supportive bra. However, more research is needed on using supportive undergarments to reduce sternal skin stress.[219]

Reassurance and education are extremely important for clients who are emotionally distressed. Although these people are successful in improving their functional status and physical capacity, they are more likely to experience angina during activities of daily living and during exercise and to be less successful in returning to work.

Postoperative Exercise

People recovering from cardiac surgery, despite an excellent hemodynamic result, may be disabled by persistent left ventricular hypertrophy and years of presurgical restricted activity and deconditioning. Exercise rehabilitation is an important part of the recovery process. Easy fatigability related to muscular weakness lessens with increased physical activity. Exercise-induced symptoms of angina and light-headedness or syncope disappear immediately after surgery with a successful result.

New guidelines developed by the American College of Cardiology Foundation and the American Heart Association emphasize for the first time the importance of participating in a cardiac rehabilitation program after a heart attack or bypass surgery.[425] The exercise capacity of clients soon after MI and bypass surgery is determined by the same parameters as in healthy individuals or for other cardiac problems, including time since MI, age, physical training status, and amount of myocardial dysfunction that occurs with exercise. CNS dysfunction is a common consequence of otherwise uncomplicated CABG surgery that may affect exercise capacity. The exact cause of this neurologic phenomenon remains unknown, but it may be the result of preoperative intracranial or extracranial carotid artery disease contributing to compromised hemodynamics and cerebral hypoperfusion.

Heart rate variability (HRV; analysis of beat-to-beat heart rate variability) may be altered (decreased) after PTCA. HRV is a simple, reproducible, and noninvasive method for quantitatively assessing cardiac autonomic regulation. The alteration in HRV can be transient or may remain for 6 months or more. A high variability in heart rate is a good sign of adaptability, implying that the autonomic nervous system control mechanisms are functioning well. Beneficial effects of exercise training in restoring HRV after coronary angioplasty have been documented.[451]

A program to increase the strength and flexibility of the pectoral and leg muscles is usually recommended. During this time, elastic stockings are usually worn to prevent fluid accumulation at the site of the leg incisions. Special exercises are prescribed to improve chest wall function, facilitate breathing, and prevent adhesive capsulitis, a common finding 6 to 12 weeks after a CABG or other open chest procedure.

Data to support the need for early range of motion (ROM) to prevent loss associated with surgery are limited. One small study of the effect of shoulder ROM exercises after CABG surgery reported that ROM exercises do not ameliorate the early loss of ROM associated with surgery, as the loss is a function of the surgical procedure and not lack of ROM challenge.[415] The delay in presentation of adhesive capsulitis suggests other variables may be present during the time when clients are enrolled in phase I (inpatient) and phase II (outpatient) cardiac rehabilitation programs to account for this development.

Side Effects of Medication

As shown in Table 12-5, there is a wide range of commonly prescribed cardiovascular medications with an equally wide variety of potential side effects. The therapist must make note of medications used by each client and observe for any of the common adverse effects.

Although simvastatin is usually the first statin to be prescribed because of availability of a generic form and low cost, an 80-mg dose of this drug is linked to an increased risk of myopathy,[432] resulting in a warning issued by the U.S. Food and Drug Administration (FDA) in June 2011.

Of particular note is the potential for muscle pain from statins. Less than 5% of the adult population who take statins develop this problem. A more serious form of this side effect associated with statins (cholesterol-lowering medications) is called *rhabdomyolysis*, the rapid breakdown of skeletal muscle.

Myalgia as a result of taking a statin medication usually occurs within a few weeks of starting the drug. Any unexplained muscle pain, cramps, stiffness, spasm, or weakness in an adult taking a statin should be reported to the physician. This is especially true if there are any predictive risk factors. Risk factors for this particular effect include older than 80 years, small body frame or frail health, presence of kidney disease, and polypharmacy. For anyone experiencing adverse muscular effects from statin therapy alternative approaches are recommended such as using a different dose of the same statin or using another drug from the statin group and using vitamin D and coenzyme Q10 supplements.[376]

Individuals taking some forms of statins (e.g., Zocor [simvastatin], Lipitor [atorvastatin], and Pravachol [pravastatin]) are warned to avoid drinking grapefruit juice while taking statins because grapefruit juice contains inhibitors of the enzyme responsible for statin metabolism (breaking down). Inhibition of the enzyme may lead to drug accumulation in the body and resulting toxicity.

Angina Pectoris

Definition and Incidence

As blood vessels become obstructed by the formation of atherosclerotic plaque, the blood supply to tissues supplied by these vessels becomes restricted. When the cardiac workload exceeds the oxygen supply to myocardial tissue, ischemia occurs, causing temporary chest pain or discomfort, called *angina pectoris*. The exact incidence of angina is unknown, although it is considered common, especially in people age 65 years and older; it occurs more often in men.

Overview

There are several types of anginal pain (Box 12-6). *Chronic stable angina*, classified as classic, exertional angina, occurs at predictable levels of physical or emotional stress and responds promptly to rest or to nitroglycerin. No pain occurs at rest; and the location, duration, intensity, and frequency of chest pain are consistent over time (60 days). *New-onset angina* describes angina that has developed for the first time within the last 2 weeks and is also considered unstable. *Nocturnal angina* may awaken a person from sleep with the same sensation experienced during exertion and is usually caused by increased heart rate associated with dreams or in response to underlying CHF.

Box 12-6

TYPES OF ANGINA PECTORIS

- Chronic (stable) angina; classic exertional angina
- New-onset (unstable) angina
- Nocturnal angina
- Postinfarction angina
- Preinfarction angina (unstable); progressive, crescendo angina
- Prinzmetal (variant) angina; vasospastic
- Resting angina (decubitus)
- Metabolic syndrome; microvascular angina

Postinfarction angina occurs after MI when residual ischemia triggers an episode of angina. *Preinfarction angina* or *unstable angina*, also known as progressive angina or crescendo angina, is unpredictable and is characterized by an abrupt change (increase) in the intensity and frequency of symptoms or decreased threshold of stimulus. This angina lasts longer than 15 minutes and is a symptom of worsening cardiac ischemia.

Prinzmetal, vasospastic, or *variant angina* produces symptoms similar to those of typical angina, but it is caused by abnormal or involuntary coronary artery spasm rather than directly by build-up of plaque from atherosclerosis. These spasms periodically squeeze arteries shut and keep the blood from reaching the heart. About two thirds of people with Prinzmetal angina have severe coronary atherosclerosis in at least one major vessel. The spasm usually occurs very close to the blockage. The pattern of Prinzmetal angina is typically characterized by early morning occurrence, frequently at the same time each day, and it occurs at rest (i.e., it is unrelated to exertion).

Prinzmetal angina is more common in women younger than 50 years; it is often associated with various types of arrhythmias or conduction defects. It is not a benign condition, but is less likely to lead to a heart attack than angina caused by atherosclerosis, because most heart attacks are caused by the rupture of an atherosclerotic plaque.

Decubitus or *resting angina* is considered atypical; it occurs most often when at rest and frequently occurs at the same time every day. This type of anginal chest pain is atypical in that it is paroxysmal in nature, not brought on by exercise, and not relieved by rest, but it is reduced when the person sits or stands up.

It is more prevalent among women, particularly those who have undergone hysterectomy. Microvascular angina associated with insulin resistance syndrome affects the microcirculatory system, a network of tiny blood vessels that branch from the large coronary vessels and that provide oxygen to each of the millions of myocardial cells. Why these vessels spasm and cause decreased blood flow remains undetermined; the cause may be a decrease in estrogen during menopause or a specific trigger from within the heart. Long-term survival rates are not reduced in women with this syndrome.

Etiologic and Risk Factors

Any condition that alters the blood (oxygen) supply or demand of the myocardium can cause ischemia

Table 12-7   Causes of Myocardial Ischemia

Decreased Oxygen Supply	Increased Oxygen Demand
Vessels	
Atherosclerotic narrowing	Hyperthyroidism
Inadequate collateral circulation	Arteriovenous fistula
Spasm caused by smoking, emotion, or cold	Exercise or exertion
Coronary arteritis	Emotion or excitement
Hypertension	Digestion of large meal
Hypertrophic cardiomyopathy	
Circulatory Factors	
Arrhythmias (decreased blood pressure)	
Aortic stenosis	
Hypotension	
Bleeding	
Blood Factors	
Anemia	
Hypoxemia	
Polycythemia	

Data from Bonow RO: *Braunwald's heart disease—a textbook of cardiovascular medicine*, ed 9, Philadelphia, 2011, WB Saunders; Goldman L, Schafer AI: *Goldman's Cecil medicine*, ed 24, Philadelphia, 2012, WB Saunders.

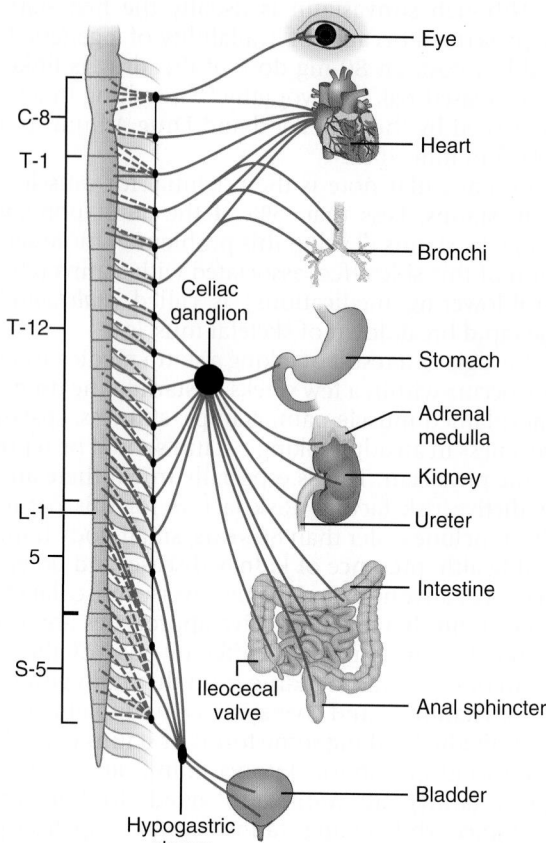

Figure 12-6

Diagram of the autonomic nervous system. The visceral afferent fibers mediating cardiac pain travel with the sympathetic nerves and enter the spinal cord at multiple levels (C3 to T4). This multisegmental innervation results in a variety of pain patterns associated with myocardial ischemia and infarction.

(Table 12-7). Increased oxygen needs of the heart, increased cardiac output, or reduced blood flow to the heart can cause angina. CAD accounts for 90% of all cases of angina, although other conditions affecting normal vessels can also cause angina. Disorders of circulation, such as relative hypotension secondary to spinal anesthesia, antihypertensive drugs, or blood loss, can also result in decreased blood return to the heart and subsequent ischemic pain.

Onset of angina may be triggered by physical exertion or exercise, especially involving thoracic or upper extremity muscles or walking rapidly uphill; increase in pulse rate or blood pressure (e.g., psychologic or emotional stress); or vasoconstriction. The threshold for angina is often lower in the morning or after strong emotion; the latter can provoke attacks in the absence of exertion. Angina may also occur less commonly during sexual activity, at rest, or at night during sleep. In the case of Prinzmetal or variant angina, episodes can be triggered by cocaine, amphetamines, migraine medication, and herbal supplements such as ephedra or bitter orange.

Pathogenesis

Angina is a symptom of ischemia usually brought on by an imbalance between cardiac workload and oxygen supply to myocardial tissue usually secondary to CAD (see previous discussion on pathogenesis of atherosclerosis). Disruption of a formed plaque with sudden total or near-total arterial occlusion may bring on unstable angina. Rupture leads to the activation, adhesion, and aggregation of platelets and the activation of the clotting cascade,

resulting in the formation of an occlusive thrombus. If this process leads to complete occlusion of the artery, then MI occurs. If the process leads to severe stenosis but the artery remains open, then unstable angina occurs.

Metabolites within the ischemic segment of the myocardium (e.g., histamines, bradykinin, prostaglandins) and buildup of lactic acid or abnormal stretching of the myocardium irritate myocardial fibers, resulting in myocardial pain. Afferent sympathetic fibers of the autonomic nervous system enter the spinal cord from levels C3 to T4 (Fig. 12-6), accounting for the varied locations and radiation patterns of anginal pain. The effects of temporary ischemia are reversible; if blood flow is restored, no permanent damage to or necrosis of the heart muscle occurs.

Clinical Manifestations

Angina is characterized by temporary pain or, more often, discomfort that starts suddenly in the chest (substernal or retrosternal) and sometimes radiates to other parts of the body, most commonly to the left shoulder and down the ulnar border of the arm to the fingers. Pain or discomfort may also be referred to any dermatome from C3 to T4, presenting at the back of the neck, lower jaw, teeth, left upper back, interscapular area, abdomen occasionally, and possibly down the right arm (Fig. 12-7).

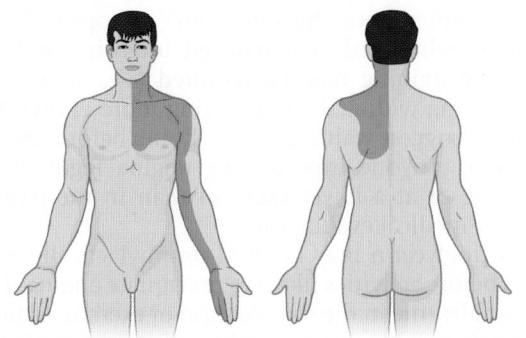

Figure 12-7

Pain patterns associated with angina. *Left,* Area of substernal discomfort projected to the left shoulder and arm over the distribution of the ulnar nerve. Referred pain may be present only in the left shoulder or in the shoulder and along the arm only to the elbow. *Right,* Occasionally, anginal pain may be referred to the back in the area of the left scapula or the interscapular region. See Figure 12-11 for pain pattern associated with myocardial ischemia or infarction experienced by some women (see text for complete description).

The sensation described is often referred to as squeezing, burning, pressing, heartburn, indigestion, or choking. It is usually mild to moderate (rarely reported as severe); it usually lasts 1 to 3 minutes, sometimes 3 to 5 minutes, but can persist up to 15 to 20 minutes. Symptoms are usually relieved by rest or nitroglycerin; in women, symptoms may be relieved by taking an antacid.

Recognizing symptoms of myocardial ischemia in women is more difficult, as the symptoms are less reliable and do not follow the classic pattern described. Many women describe the pain in ways consistent with unstable angina, suggesting that they first become aware of their chest discomfort or have it diagnosed only after it reaches more advanced stages. Some experience a sensation similar to that of inhaling cold air, rather than the more typical shortness of breath. Other women note only weakness and lethargy, and some have observed isolated pain in the midthoracic spine or throbbing and aching in the right biceps muscle.

MEDICAL MANAGEMENT

DIAGNOSIS. The diagnosis of angina pectoris is strongly suspected by history and is supported if sublingual nitroglycerin shortens an attack and if prophylactic nitrates permit greater exertion or prevent angina entirely. Medical evaluation includes examination for signs of diseases that may produce angina or contribute to or accompany atherosclerotic disease (see "Clinical Manifestations" above).

Early and accurate triage to assess risk (low, intermediate, high) can help identify those people for whom medical therapy will probably fail and lead to better outcomes through a more appropriate management strategy. ECG is normal in approximately 25% to 30% of people with angina, so the exercise tolerance test is a more useful noninvasive procedure for evaluating the ischemic response to exercise in the client with angina. Diagnostic testing continues as for CAD (see "Atherosclerosis: Diagnosis" above and "Myocardial Infarction: Diagnosis" below).

PREVENTION AND TREATMENT. Prevention of attacks is the first step after the acute attack subsides. Treatment of underlying disorders such as hypertension is essential. The client is also encouraged to avoid situations and stressors that precipitate angina. This usually requires modifying all possible risk factors through changes in lifestyle and modifications of lifelong habits.

Short-acting sublingual nitroglycerin is the drug of choice for the acute attack, usually relieving symptoms within 1 to 2 minutes. Nitroglycerin oral spray is also available in a metered delivery system, which is especially useful for anyone having difficulty handling or swallowing pills. The spray is also easy to use in the dark and is more rapidly acting. Long-acting nitrates (e.g., oral sustained-release nitroglycerin, transdermal nitroglycerin patches, nitroglycerin ointment) are especially useful for people for whom sudden drop in blood pressure associated with taking nitroglycerin is not desirable (i.e., people with hypotension).

Pharmacologic therapy may include other vasodilators, such as β-blockers (i.e., β-adrenergic receptor blockers) and calcium channel blockers (see Table 12-5). Intravascular thrombosis is a key element in the pathophysiology of unstable angina and its progression to MI. Anticoagulation therapy using aspirin and/or heparin is an important part of treatment for unstable angina.[492]

Anticoagulants, such as aspirin and heparin, slow down or prevent clot formation, whereas thrombolytic agents, such as tPA, urokinase and streptokinase, facilitate break down of clots that have already formed. Both anticoagulants and thrombolytics are antithrombotics. Aspirin blocks platelet cyclooxygenase, preventing the formation of thromboxane A_2, thereby inhibiting platelet aggregation. Heparin binds to an enzyme inhibitor, antithrombin III, enabling it to inactivate clotting factors such as thrombin or factor X. tPA, urokinase, or streptokinase do not break clot themselves, but each can activate plasminogen to plasmin that lyses the clot.

Second-line alternatives to aspirin (sometimes referred to as "clot busters" or "super aspirins"; e.g., Ticlid [ticlopidine], clopidogrel) are more effective than aspirin in preventing platelet aggregation and thereby reducing the combined risk of ischemic stroke, MI, or death from vascular disease, and may be useful in preventing coronary stent thrombosis.

Revascularization procedures are recommended for persons who do not become ischemia free on medical therapy, especially clients with progressive unstable angina. Surgical intervention, such as PTCA, has been shown to relieve angina, but it does not halt the progress of atherosclerosis. CABG can diminish the probability that ischemia will lead to necrosis and lethal infarction.

For people who are not good candidates for any of the proven procedures or whose angina persists despite angioplasty or bypass surgery, transmyocardial revascularization (TMR) may be recommended. In TMR, a computer-controlled laser drills tiny channels through the wall of the left ventricle while the chamber is filled with oxygenated blood. In theory, this allows blood to flow through the channels to the oxygen-deprived tissue, relieving angina. The openings on the heart's surface scar over quickly, but it is not known how long the channels stay open on the inside of the heart; long-term results remain unknown.

TMR is still considered experimental and may not be available in all centers, but studies consistently report success in relieving severe angina that has been refractory to medical and surgical intervention.[230] This procedure is performed through a 4-inch incision between the ribs and does not require a bypass machine; efforts to develop noninvasive techniques for TMR using fiberoptic catheters are under investigation.

PROGNOSIS. Myocardial ischemia leaves the heart vulnerable to arrhythmias and MI, which can be fatal. About one third of all people who experience angina pectoris die suddenly from MI or arrhythmias. Prognosis depends primarily on left ventricular function (i.e., ejection fraction) but is influenced by type of angina, ability to prevent angina, and severity of underlying disease, such as hypertension or atherosclerosis.

SPECIAL IMPLICATIONS FOR THE THERAPIST **12-3**

Angina Pectoris

Identifying Angina

Referred pain from the external oblique abdominal muscle and the pectoral major muscle can cause the sensation referred to as heartburn in the anterior chest wall, which mimics angina. When active trigger points are present in the left pectoralis major muscle, the referred pain is easily confused with that from coronary insufficiency. Physical therapy to eliminate the trigger points can aid in the diagnostic process.

Anterior chest wall syndrome with localized tenderness of intercostal muscles, Tietze syndrome with inflammation of the chondrocostal junctions, intercostal neuritis, and cervical or thoracic spine disease involving the dorsal nerve roots can all produce chest pain that mimics angina. Evaluation of range of motion, palpation of soft-tissue structures, and analysis of relieving or aggravating factors usually differentiate these conditions from true angina.[122] Likewise, heartburn from indigestion, hiatal hernia, peptic ulcer, esophageal spasm, and gallbladder disease can also cause angina-like symptoms that require a medical evaluation for an accurate medical diagnosis.

The development of unstable angina also requires immediate medical referral and may be reported as the onset of angina at rest, occurrence of typical angina at a significantly lower level of activity than usual, changes in the typical anginal pattern (e.g., symptoms occurring more frequently), or changes in blood pressure (decrease) or heart rate (increase) with levels of activity previously well tolerated. Educating the public about reducing delays and getting to an emergency department at the earliest signs of heart attack is essential. Reperfusion therapy within the first 60 to 70 minutes of a heart attack can make a significant difference in outcome.

Nitroglycerin

A person experiencing angina should reduce the pace of or, if necessary, stop all activity and sit down for a few minutes until the symptoms disappear. Exercise can be reinitiated at a reduced intensity, and interval-type training may be required (i.e., slow activity alternating with activity requiring more effort). Some experts suggest waiting several hours before resuming exercise. Anyone experiencing angina regularly with exercise or at a lower exertion than in the past may need a medical evaluation.

Nitroglycerin may be used prophylactically 5 minutes before activities likely to precipitate angina. This is especially true in the intervention or exercise setting for the person with chronic, stable, exertional angina. The use of nitroglycerin must be by physician order and cannot be decided solely by the therapist and client.

Clients must be reminded that they are not to alter their prescribed drug schedule without consulting their health care provider and that nitroglycerin should be taken as prescribed. For example, taking sublingual nitroglycerin orally markedly decreases its effectiveness. Clients should be seated when taking nitroglycerin to avoid syncope and falls. For anginal pain or discomfort that is not relieved by rest or relieved by up to three nitroglycerin doses in 10 to 15 minutes (i.e., the initial dose followed by a second dose 5 minutes later and a third dose 5 minutes after the second dose), the physician should be contacted. Until the angina is controlled and coronary blood flow reestablished, the client is at risk of myocardial damage from myocardial ischemia.

Nitroglycerin tablets are inactivated by light, heat, air, and moisture, and they should be stored in the refrigerator in an amber container with a tight-fitting cover. Nitroglycerin has a short shelf life and needs to be replaced about every 3 months. A potent nitroglycerin tablet should produce a burning sensation under the tongue when taken sublingually (if it does not, check the expiration date).

Orthostatic Hypotension

Orthostatic hypotension (see more complete discussion of orthostatic [postural] hypotension later in this chapter) is one of the most common side effects of prophylactic medications for angina. Caution on the part of the therapist is required when exercising or ambulating clients who take these medications. If the person becomes hypotensive, have the person assume a supine position with legs elevated to increase venous return and to ensure cerebral blood flow.

Extra caution must be taken when placing anyone with orthostatic hypotension and CHF supine with legs elevated because this may overload an already stressed ventricle. Keeping the head elevated and monitoring carefully are required in this circumstance. Vascular support hose may be recommended, and the person should be reminded to change positions slowly to minimize the effects of orthostatic hypotension. Headache, weakness, increasing pulse, or other unusual signs or symptoms should be reported to the physician. In a home health setting, the home should be evaluated for potentially hazardous conditions. All clients should be encouraged to avoid hazardous activities until their condition is stabilized by medication, especially in the presence of dizziness.

Monitoring Vital Signs

Exercise testing should be performed before a client begins an exercise program, but if this has not been accomplished and baseline measurements are unavailable for use in planning exercise, monitor the heart rate and blood pressure and note any accompanying symptoms during exercise (see Appendix B). All factors and patient variables must be considered, including cognitive function, resting blood pressure, heart rate response to rest after physical activity and exercise, gait speed during ambulation, medications (especially antihypertensives), the presence of other comorbidities that can affect vital signs, and so on.

Exercise and activity should be performed below the anginal threshold. The therapist must document heart rate and blood pressure when the ischemia began (as evidenced by symptoms of angina) to establish these parameters. Angina occurring after an MI is not considered normal and should be reported to the physician. Exercise testing is recommended before a client resumes an exercise program.

Hypertensive Cardiovascular Disease

Hypertensive CVD includes hypertensive vascular disease and hypertensive heart disease. Other conditions affecting the heart caused by an underlying pulmonary pathologic condition (e.g., pulmonary hypertension, pulmonary heart disease) are discussed in Chapter 15.

Hypertension (Hypertensive Vascular Disease)

Definition and Overview. Blood pressure is the force exerted against the walls of the arteries and arterioles; diastolic pressure (bottom number) is the pressure in these vessels when the heart is relaxed between beats, and systolic pressure (top number) is the pressure exerted in the arteries when the heart contracts. Between ages 55 and 60 years, diastolic blood pressure often begins to plateau and may even decline, whereas systolic blood pressure often starts to rise.

Hypertension, or high blood pressure, is defined by the World Health Organization (WHO) as a persistent elevation of diastolic blood pressure (higher than 90 mm Hg), systolic blood pressure (higher than 140 mm Hg), or both measured on at least two separate occasions at least 2 weeks apart (i.e., sustained elevation of blood pressure).

Recent evidence supports a systolic blood pressure threshold of 140 mm Hg for even "low-risk" individuals. In high-risk persons, there is evidence for lower thresholds.[338] The Centers for Disease Control and Prevention has recently added "reported current use of blood pressure lowering medication" to the definition of hypertension.[94] Based on epidemiologic data from the Framingham Heart Study, the development of hypertension is neither inevitable nor beneficial; both systolic pressure and diastolic pressure are important determinants of cardiovascular sequelae. Even small increased increments in blood pressure increase risks of cardiovascular events.

Hypertension can be classified according to type (systolic or diastolic), cause, and degree of severity.

Table 12-8	Classification of Blood Pressure for Adults	
	Systolic Blood Pressure (mm Hg)	**Diastolic Blood Pressure (mm Hg)**
Normal	<120	<80
Prehypertension	120-139	80-89
Stage 1 hypertension	140-159	90-99
Stage 2 hypertension	≥160	≥100

From Chobanian AV: National High Blood Pressure Education Program Coordinating Committee: The seventh report of the Joint National Committee on Prevention, Detection, Evaluation, and Treatment of High Blood Pressure, *JAMA* 289:2560–2571, 2003.

Classification of Blood Pressure for Children and Adolescents

Normal	<90th percentile; 50th percentile is the midpoint of the normal range
Prehypertension	90th–95th percentile or if blood pressure is greater than 120/80 mm Hg (even if this figure is <90th percentile)
Stage 1 hypertension	95th–99th percentile + 5 mm Hg
Stage 2 hypertension	>99th percentile + 5 mm Hg

The relationship between blood pressure (BP) and risk of coronary vascular disease (CVD) events is continuous, consistent, and independent of other risk factors. The higher the BP, the greater the chance of heart attack, heart failure, stroke, and kidney disease.

For individuals 40 to 70 years of age, each 20 mm Hg incremental increase in systolic BP (SBP) or 10 mm Hg in diastolic BP (DBP) doubles the risk of CVD across the entire BP range from 115/75 to 185/115 mm Hg.

From National Heart, Lung, and Blood Institute (NHLBI): Fourth report on the diagnosis, evaluation, and treatment of high blood pressure in children and adolescents, *Pediatrics* 114(2):555–576, 2004.

Hypertension can also be classified based on risk according to the most recent guidelines (Table 12-8).[104]

Primary (or essential) *hypertension* is also known as idiopathic hypertension and accounts for 90% to 95% of all cases of hypertension. *Secondary hypertension* accounts for only 5% to 10% of cases and results from an identifiable cause. Intermittent elevation of blood pressure interspersed with normal readings is called *labile hypertension* or borderline hypertension. *Malignant hypertension* (also known as hypertensive crises) is a syndrome of markedly elevated blood pressure (diastolic blood pressure >125 mm Hg) with target organ damage (e.g., retinal hemorrhages, papilledema, heart failure, encephalopathy, renal insufficiency, stroke). The elevation of systolic blood pressure independently of change in the diastolic blood pressure is now recognized as a medical condition referred to as *isolated systolic hypertension*.

Incidence. Worldwide, more than 1 billion people have hypertension.[217] The incidence of hypertension varies considerably among different groups in the American population, but it is estimated that one in three adult Americans (70+ million) have high blood pressure. One of every two adults older than age 60 years has isolated systolic hypertension. Not surprisingly, hypertension contributes to every seventh death and nearly half of all

CVD-related deaths in the United States.[94] Hypertension is twice as prevalent and more severe among blacks than whites. This phenomenon has been attributed to heredity, greater environmental stress, and greater salt intake or salt sensitivity (i.e., responsiveness to changes in sodium balance and extracellular fluid and volume status), although the actual cause is not clear; reduced access to health care increases the prevalence of untreated hypertension.

The population that has the lowest prevalence of blood pressure control are adults 18 to 39 years of age.[94] Blood pressure control rates vary in minority populations and are lowest in Mexican Americans and Native Americans.[104] Socioeconomic factors and lifestyle may be important barriers to blood pressure control in some minority individuals.

Hypertension control goals in *Healthy People 2020* include the following: (1) reduce the proportion of adults with high blood pressure from the current incidence (29.9%) to 26.9% (10% improvement) and (2) reduce the proportion of children and adolescents (ages 8-17 years) with high blood pressure from current rates of 3.5% to a target rate of 3.2% (10% improvement).[202]

Etiologic and Risk Factors. *Primary (essential) hypertension* has no established etiology but is probably related to genetics and other risk factors, such as smoking, obesity, high cholesterol levels, and being of black descent. In the recent past, hypertension research shifted strongly in the direction of molecular genetics.

A familial association with hypertension has been documented, possibly attributable to common genetic background, shared environment, or lifestyle habits. Using the candidate gene approach, allelic variants in the genes for angiotensinogen, β_2-adrenergic receptor, mutation in the β subunit of the epithelial sodium channel, and several others have been identified, but the mechanisms by which these contribute to hypertension have not been identified.[290]

Recently, a large genome-wide association study of systolic and diastolic blood pressure was conducted involving 200,000 individuals of European descent.[217] Twenty-nine genomic loci containing genes that control blood pressure physiology were identified. Based on these findings, a genetic risk score was associated with hypertension, left ventricular wall thickness, stroke and CAD, but not kidney disease or kidney function. Such findings are extremely important in providing new insights into the genetics and biology of blood pressure, and suggesting potential novel therapeutic pathways for the disease prevention.

Small arteries branching from the aorta, called arterioles, regulate blood pressure. Any condition that can narrow the opening of these arterioles can increase the blood pressure in the arteries. A variety of specific diseases or problems, such as chronic renal failure, renal artery stenosis, or endocrine disease, can cause *secondary hypertension* (Box 12-7). The risk for CVD in adults with hypertension is determined not only by the level of blood pressure but also by the presence or absence of target organ damage or factors such as smoking, dyslipidemia, and diabetes. *Isolated systolic hypertension* has very distinct causes, often not directly vascular and often related to a specific organ or tissue, such as anemia, malfunctioning aortic valve,

---

Box 12-7

CAUSES OF SECONDARY HYPERTENSION

- Coarctation of the aorta
- Alcohol abuse
- Pregnancy induced
- Thyrotoxicosis
- Increased intracranial pressure from tumors or trauma
- Collagen disease
- Endocrine disease
  - Acromegaly
  - Cushing disease
  - Diabetes
  - Hypothyroidism
  - Hyperthyroidism
  - Pheochromocytoma (rare catecholamine- secreting tumor)
- Chronic kidney disease (most common cause in the general population: vascular renal disease)
- Drug induced or drug related (e.g., oral contraceptives, corticosteroids, cyclosporine, cocaine, anabolic steroids, amphetamines)
- Acute stress
  - Surgery
  - Psychogenic hyperventilation
  - Alcohol withdrawal
  - Burns
  - Pancreatitis
  - Sickle cell crisis
- Neurologic disorders
  - Brain tumor
  - Respiratory acidosis
  - Encephalitis
  - Sleep apnea
  - Guillain-Barré syndrome
  - Quadriplegia
  - Lead poisoning

Data from Chobanian AV, Bakris GL, Black HR, et al: The seventh report of the Joint National Committee on Prevention, Detection, Evaluation, and Treatment of High Blood Pressure: the JNC 7 report, *JAMA* 289:2560–2571, 2003.

---

obstructive sleep apnea, kidney disease, or overactive thyroid.

Risk factors for hypertension may be modifiable or nonmodifiable (Box 12-8). The risk of hypertension increases with age as arteries lose elasticity and become less able to relax. Hypertension occurs slightly more often in men than in women and at an earlier age, but after age 50 years, hypertension begins to develop in more women than men. In all groups the incidence of hypertension increases with age, with a poorer prognosis for people whose hypertension begins at a young age.

Although hypertension mostly affects older people (65 years and older), most hypertension trials have upper age limits or do not present age-specific results. Considering that by 2040, 75 million Americans will be 65 years of age and older, representing more than 20% of the U.S. population, the first official recommendations on hypertension therapy in elderly adults issued by the American College of Cardiology Foundation and American Heart Association[36] are very timely and contain a wealth of information on the subject. Hypertension is the most important risk factor for CVD in older Americans, with

Box 12-8

RISK FACTORS OF PRIMARY (ESSENTIAL) HYPERTENSION

Modifiable

- High sodium intake (causes water retention, increasing blood volume)
- Obesity (associated with increased intravascular volume)
- Insulin resistance and metabolic abnormalities
- Diabetes mellitus
- Hypercholesterolemia and increased serum triglyceride levels
- Smoking (nicotine restricts blood vessels)
- Long-term abuse of alcohol (increases plasma catecholamines)
- Continuous emotional stress (stimulates sympathetic nervous system)
- Personality traits (hostility, sense of hopelessness)
- Sedentary lifestyle
- White coat hypertension (see explanation in text)
- Hormonal status (menopause, especially before age 40 years and without HRT; hysterectomy/oophorectomy)

Nonmodifiable

- Positive family history of cardiovascular disease
- Age (>55 years)
- Gender (male <55 years; female >55 years)
- Ethnicity (African American*, Hispanic)

*From a pathogenetic point of view, recent research findings have suggested that β-adrenergic receptor downregulation is characteristic of hypertension in whites, whereas heightened vascular α-receptor sensitivity or early vascular hypertrophy may be a feature of hypertension in African Americans.[418] African Americans demonstrate somewhat reduced blood pressure responses to monotherapy with β-blockers, ACE inhibitors, or angiotensin receptor blockers compared with diuretics or calcium channel blockers. These differential responses are largely eliminated by drug combinations.[32,103]

69% of patients with incident MI, 77% with incident stroke, and 74% with incident heart failure having antecedent hypertension.[36]

Similar to other anxiety-provoking situations that cause raise in blood pressure, white coat hypertension increases the risk of heart disease. Personality traits such as hopelessness and hostility are important factors in CVD, including hypertension; research is under way to identify the neuroendocrine and CNS mechanisms underlying these associations and to identify other possible risk-associated personality traits.[141] Hypertension itself represents a significant risk factor for the development of CAD, stroke, CHF, and renal failure, preceding heart failure in 90% of all cases and increasing in all other associated conditions.

The influence of nonsteroidal antiinflammatory drugs (NSAIDs) on blood pressure in normotensive and hypertensive persons remains in question. At the very least, it has been determined that there is always the potential for NSAIDs to interact with antihypertensive agents, most notably diuretics, β-receptor antagonists, and ACE inhibitors.

Given the high prevalence of NSAID use by older adults, especially for conditions such as arthritis, gout, and similar problems, the association between this drug use and blood pressure must be observed carefully (see "Medications" in "Special Implications for the Therapist 12-4: Hypertension (Hypertensive Vascular Disease)" below). Alcohol is estimated to be responsible for as many as 10% of all cases of hypertension and may be the actual unknown cause of "essential" hypertension.[159]

Blood pressure is linked to salt intake and modulated by the "salt gene" (angiotensinogen) in some people. Those who are salt sensitive (including those who do not yet have high blood pressure) may have an increased risk of death. Salt sensitivity is a measure of how blood pressure responds to sodium and is independent of other risk factors (including elevated blood pressure) for death from CVD.

Inadequate sleep has been identified as a risk factor for hypertension among adults in their fourth to sixth decades who sleep less than 5 hours each night. Short sleep duration activates the hormones leptin and ghrelin, which affect appetite, making sleep deprivation a risk factor for obesity, as well as for diabetes, two conditions commonly linked with hypertension. Men are more likely than women to report getting fewer than 6 hours of sleep, although women are more likely to have trouble falling asleep or getting back to sleep after waking up early.[138,165]

Some experts suggest that "communicative fitness" is every bit as important as physical fitness and diet in achieving normal blood pressure and optimal cardiovascular health. Toxic talk (abusive language), the inability to engage in conversation without negative physiologic effects, communicative isolation because of school failure, depression, and loneliness contribute to this concept referred to as poor communicative fitness. A hidden risk factor (communicative difficulties) increases peripheral vasoconstriction while the heart ejects blood against that system, causing increased surges in blood pressure while talking. The effect of human companionship on heart disease and death rates and the role of love and interpersonal relationship to cardiovascular health have been documented.[278]

Pathogenesis. Blood pressure is regulated by two factors: blood flow and peripheral vascular resistance. Blood flow is determined by cardiac output (strength, rate, rhythm of heartbeat; blood volume). The resistance to flow is primarily determined by the diameter of blood vessels and, to a lesser degree, by the viscosity of blood.

Increased peripheral resistance as a result of the narrowing of the arterioles is the single most common characteristic of hypertension. Constriction of the peripheral arterioles may be controlled by two mechanisms, each with several components: (1) sympathetic nervous system activity (autonomic regulation) and (2) activation of the renin–angiotensin system.

In the case of the sympathetic nervous system, norepinephrine is released in response to psychogenic stress or baroreceptor activity. The blood vessels constrict causing an increase of peripheral resistance. At the same time, epinephrine is secreted by the adrenal medulla, resulting in increased force of cardiac contraction, increased cardiac output, and vasoconstriction.

With prolonged hypertension, the elastic tissue in the arterioles is replaced by fibrous collagen tissue. The thickened arteriole wall becomes less distensible, offering even greater resistance to the flow of blood. This process leads to decreased tissue perfusion, especially in the target organs of high blood pressure (i.e., heart, kidneys, brain). Atherosclerosis is also accelerated in persons with high blood pressure.

Within the renin–angiotensin system, vasoconstriction results in decreased blood flow to the kidney. Whenever blood flow to the kidney diminishes, renin is secreted and angiotensin is formed, causing vasoconstriction within the renal system and increased total peripheral resistance. Angiotensin also stimulates the secretion of aldosterone, which promotes sodium and water retention by the kidney tubules, causing an increase in intravascular volume. All these factors increase blood pressure.

Evidence from animal, clinical, and epidemiologic studies points to an association between high blood pressure and abnormal calcium metabolism, leading to increased calcium loss, secondary activation of the parathyroid gland, increased movement of calcium from bone, and increased risk of urinary tract stones and osteoporosis.[85]

Clinical Manifestations. Hypertension is frequently asymptomatic; this creates a significant health care risk for affected people. When symptoms do occur, they may include headache (usually occipital and present in the morning, worse on waking, and slowly improving with activity), vertigo, flushed face, spontaneous epistaxis, blurred vision, and nocturnal urinary frequency. Elevated blood pressure when measured, especially in the early stages, may be the only sign of hypertension.

Sleep-disordered breathing is also associated with systemic hypertension in middle-age and older individuals of both genders and different ethnic backgrounds.[328] Progressive hypertension may be characterized by cardiovascular symptoms (dyspnea, orthopnea, chest pain, and leg edema) or cerebral symptoms (nausea, vomiting, drowsiness, confusion, and fleeting numbness or tingling in the limbs). Hypertensive encephalopathy, a neurologic syndrome that occurs as a result of a sudden sustained rise in blood pressure, may be accompanied by nonspecific neurologic symptoms, such as confusion, headache, nausea, and even coma. It is also well recognized that end-stage renal disease is associated with accelerated and malignant hypertension; hypertension is associated with increased urinary calcium excretion and subsequent bone loss and osteoporosis, especially at the femoral neck.[55]

MEDICAL MANAGEMENT

PREVENTION. The American Society of Hypertension recommends that everyone, regardless of age, know his or her blood pressure (the actual numbers). An annual blood pressure check is important for everyone; more frequent blood pressure measurements should be taken in anyone with risk factors or known hypertension. Elevated blood pressure in an adult younger than age 50 years can cause long-term accumulated damage that is irreversible by age 50 or 60 years; therefore, any elevation in blood pressure at any age must be addressed.

The most important prevention factor is physical activity and exercise; other key variables include weight control; limitations on salt, sugar, and alcohol intake; and modification of other risk factors present (see Box 12-8).

Combining a low-sodium diet with the DASH (Dietary Approaches to Stop Hypertension) diet (high intake of fruits, vegetables, and low-fat dairy foods) helps reduce blood pressure more than the DASH diet alone, both for healthy people and for those with high blood pressure. Reducing salt intake also lowers the risk of osteoporosis and possible fracture, as a high salt intake increases urinary calcium excretion and hypertension is associated with bone loss.

DIAGNOSIS. In the past, hypertension was diagnosed primarily on the basis of the diastolic measurement, which was considered a better representation of the overall condition of the circulatory system. The rise of systolic pressure with age was considered to be normal and therefore not a risk factor. Today, it is recognized that although diastolic hypertension (higher than 90 mm Hg) is common and usually controllable, systolic hypertension (higher than 140 mm Hg) is the most common in older adults and the most powerful risk factor for stroke and is strongly linked with heart attack, heart failure, and kidney failure, even when the diastolic blood pressure is within normal limits. Systolic pressure measures the maximal strain on the heart and blood vessels and is a more precise measure of future damage to the system.

Blood pressure varies over the course of any single day depending on exertion, emotional state, ingestion of food, medications, and the presence of risk factors described previously. Thus it is important that blood pressure be measured at several different times and under consistent circumstances before a diagnosis of hypertension is made. Twenty-four–hour blood pressure monitoring using a portable device that automatically takes blood pressure readings at regular intervals is available and especially helpful in mapping out labile hypertension.

The individual maintains a log of activities and emotions corresponding to the times when readings are taken; this information is compared with the computer-generated map of blood pressures generated from the data collected by the measurement device. No other tests are specific for essential hypertension.

Studies used in the routine evaluation of hypertension may include a complete blood count; urinalysis; serum potassium, serum cholesterol, and creatinine assays; fasting blood glucose level; ECG; and chest radiography. Other more specific tests may be needed for secondary hypertension, and more complete cardiac assessment may be required for selected individuals.

TREATMENT. Once diagnosed, hypertension requires ongoing management (see Table 12-6) despite the absence of symptoms. According to the Joint National Committee,[103] the goal is to achieve and maintain the lowest safe arterial blood pressure (without side effects); the intended target goal is to reduce blood pressure to less than 140/90 mm Hg for people younger than 60 years of age and people with diabetes or kidney disease, and to less than 150/90 mm Hg in adults 60 years of age and older,[103] and a systolic blood pressure of 140–145 mm Hg if tolerated in adults age 80 years and older.[36]

The decision to treat and the method and intensity of intervention are based on the concept of total risk, not just blood pressure measurements. This approach takes into account cardiovascular risk factors in people with hypertension (see Box 12-8) and the presence of target organ damage or clinical CVD (e.g., prior coronary revascularization, MI, stroke, peripheral arterial disease, retinopathy).

The WHO has published guidelines for the management of hypertension that review the management of risk factors in detail and prognosis based on risk stratification.[482] In addition, a comprehensive list of recommendations on the treatment of hypertension in the prevention and management of ischemic heart disease is available from the American Heart Association.[394]

Management of hypertension may begin with a "stepped care" approach including smoking cessation and other nonpharmacologic interventions through lifestyle modification as initial therapy for primary hypertension (including those with blood pressure on the high side of normal or a family history of hypertension). This approach has been shown effective in lowering blood pressure and can reduce other cardiovascular risk factors.

Even when lifestyle modifications alone are not adequate in controlling hypertension, they may reduce the dosage of medication needed to manage the condition.[104] This program may include weight reduction; smoking cessation; a regular program of aerobic exercise; moderation of alcohol, dietary fat, caffeine, and dietary sodium; administration of nutritional supplements (e.g., potassium, calcium, magnesium); and behavioral cognitive therapy for those with hypertension associated with certain personality traits. See "Atherosclerosis: Treatment" above.

If nonpharmacologic measures fail to produce the desired results or if the blood pressure is very high at the time of diagnosis, blood pressure–lowering medications are prescribed starting with the lowest effective dose (to avoid intolerable side effects) and modified accordingly. A large number of antihypertensive medications is currently available and they can be classified by mode of action as listed in Table 12-6.

Only 30% of cases of hypertension can be controlled with one drug. Blood pressure control in more than two-thirds of individuals with hypertension cannot be done with one medication but requires a combination of two or more medications from different classes.[103] Combination of drugs allow to achieve greater blood pressure reduction at lower drug dose and thus with fewer side effects. Diuretics, alone or combined with drugs from other classes, are recommended as the first step in the pharmacologic management of uncomplicated hypertension. In high-risk conditions, medications from other classes, specifically ACE inhibitors, are recommended to use initially.[103] Because diuretics decrease plasma volume and cause potassium depletion and renal complications, the use of other classes of antihypertensive drugs is required.

Direct renin inhibitors such as aliskiren (Tekturna) are a new class of antihypertensive medication that can be used as a single treatment or in combination with other antihypertensive drugs. Aliskiren blocks the action of renin, a key kidney enzyme that helps regulate blood pressure. The blocking action takes place at the beginning of the renin–angiotensin–aldosterone system by directly inhibiting the renin released from the kidneys, thereby preventing renin-catalyzed conversion of angiotensinogen to angiotensin I. This is different from most other antihypertensive medications, which take action later in the renin–angiotensin–aldosterone system.

African Americans have a greater need for combination therapy to control blood pressure as they are generally more responsive to calcium antagonists and diuretics than to β-blockers, ACE inhibitors, or angiotensin receptor blockers. Older adults with hypertension are generally equally responsive to all classes of antihypertensive medications, but they have an increased likelihood of side effects. Pharmacologic therapy is individualized, matching the individual's clinical presentation with medications available.

More aggressive early treatment of people with diabetes and elevated blood pressure is recommended. Hypertensive people who tend to be hostile may be told to take their medication at bedtime to avoid the sharp rises in blood pressure in the early morning hours associated with heart attacks. The use of home monitoring devices is an important part of the management program both to monitor the blood pressure and to evaluate the effect of antihypertensive medication.

Home monitoring can also distinguish between sustained hypertension and white coat hypertension and improves program compliance. In individuals with hypertension, the blood pressure readings taken in a clinic setting tend to be 5 to 10 mm Hg higher than measurements taken at home. Recommended frequency of readings is twice daily (morning and evening) on work and nonwork days for anyone newly diagnosed or in whom antihypertensive medication has recently been initiated or changed. Anyone with stable hypertension can take blood pressure reading several days per week.

Obesity has long been associated with hypertension and is an independent risk factor for CVD and CAD. Regular exercise enhances weight loss and reduces blood pressure independent of weight loss. (For further discussion see "Special Implications for the Therapist 12-4: Hypertension (Hypertensive Vascular Disease)" and the sections on exercise below.)

Older individuals, black people, and hypertensive individuals are more sensitive to change in dietary sodium chloride than are other individuals. A reduction of sodium intake alone may be enough to control blood pressure in persons with mild hypertension and may reduce the medication requirements in those who require drug therapy.

It is also recommended that individuals with high blood pressure limit their intake of alcohol to 2 oz of liquor, 10 oz of red wine, or 24 oz of beer per day. Women and lighter-weight men should limit alcohol intake to half of these amounts per day.[104]

Dietary potassium deficiency may have a role in increasing blood pressure; individuals may also become hypokalemic from increased urinary magnesium excretion during diuretic therapy and require additional potassium. Magnesium and calcium influence vascular tone because magnesium acts to relax blood vessels and calcium assists in blood vessel contraction.

A proper balance of these two ions is essential, as they compete for entry into the cell. When magnesium is low, an abnormally large amount of calcium enters the cells so that blood vessels begin to lose their ability to relax. Progressive vasoconstriction and subsequent spasms result in elevated blood pressure and eventual ischemia. Muscle weakness with depressed tendon reflexes may accompany this condition. A fall in serum potassium level also enhances the effects of cardiac glycoside digoxin, increasing the risk of digoxin toxicity (see Table 12-5). Although digoxin is an inhibitor of sodium-potassium pump in heart muscle, it competes with potassium ions for binding to the pump.

PROGNOSIS. Hypertension is a major risk factor for atherosclerosis, implicating hypertension as a common cause of death in the United States. Among black Americans, hypertension is also the most common fatal familial disease. More than half of persons with angina pectoris, sudden death, stroke, and thrombotic occlusion of the abdominal aorta or its branches have hypertension.

Three fourths of people with CHF, dissecting aortic aneurysm, intracerebral hemorrhage, or rupture of the myocardial wall also have elevated blood pressure. If it is untreated, nearly 50% of people with hypertension die of heart disease, 33% die of stroke, and 10% to 15% die of renal failure.

When a person with hypertension achieves the target blood pressure, it must be emphasized that blood pressure control does not equal cure. Adherence to treatment and follow-up monitoring must be continued on an ongoing basis. Unfortunately, the cost of antihypertensives, side effects, and lack of symptoms sometimes lead to poor compliance with treatment. Treatment prolongs life, and antihypertensive medications have dramatically reduced the mortality rate associated with hypertension. (See also "Atherosclerosis: Prognosis" [especially regarding pulse pressure as the newest predictor of mortality] above.)

SPECIAL IMPLICATIONS FOR THE THERAPIST   **12-4**

Hypertension (Hypertensive Vascular Disease)

It is estimated that hypertension remains undiagnosed in nearly half of the 60 million Americans who have it. It is possible that many people in a therapy practice will be hypertensive without knowing it. Cardiac pathology may be unknown, requiring the therapist to remain alert for risk factors that require medical screening. For anyone with identified risk factors, a baseline blood pressure measurement should be taken on two or three separate occasions, and any unusual findings should be reported to the physician.

The role of the therapist in screening to identify conditions such as hypertension is important, as an essential early component of intervention for this condition includes exercise. The therapist has an important role in helping to identify people with undiagnosed hypertension and referring them for medical evaluation and treatment. Patient education includes emphasizing the importance of adherence to the medical treatment (i.e., taking medication as prescribed; not discontinuing medications without the medical doctor's approval) and follow-up, and teaching them how to identify signs and symptoms of stroke or MI that can occur as a result of a hypertensive crisis. The therapist is also instrumental in reviewing modifiable risk factors and encouraging clients to lose weight if necessary, stop smoking, and exercise appropriately.

Anyone with hypertension is at risk for a hypertensive crisis (severe elevation of blood pressure with target organ damage), especially anyone who discontinues prescribed hypertensive medications without physician approval or those individuals who have longstanding essential hypertension that has not been managed optimally.[461] Elevated blood pressure with any symptoms of target organ damage (e.g., epistaxis, chest discomfort, back pain, headache, visual disturbances, shortness of breath, confusion or other sign of altered mental state) is a red flag requiring immediate medical attention.

The potential for osteoporosis and subsequent hip fractures in older adults (especially women) with hypertension points to the importance of osteoporosis screening and prevention in this population. The physical therapist has an important role in the primary prevention of impairments and functional limitations in people with hypertension. A sudden increase in blood pressure such as occurs with any increase in intraabdominal pressure (e.g., Valsalva maneuver; see also Box 16-1) during exercise or stabilization exercises can be dangerous for already hypertensive persons. The therapist must alert individuals with hypertension to this effect and teach proper breathing techniques during all activities.

Medications

People with CAD taking NSAIDs for pain relief may also be at risk for a myocardial event during times of increased myocardial oxygen demand (e.g., exercise, fever). In addition, older adults taking NSAIDs and antihypertensive agents must be monitored carefully. Regardless of the NSAID chosen, it is important to check blood pressure within the first few weeks after therapy or exercise is initiated and periodically thereafter.

A 2007 statement from the American Heart Association indicates that NSAIDs may cause an increased risk of serious cardiovascular thrombotic events, MI, stroke, heart failure, and hypertension.[33] Individuals with a prior history of CVD or with risk factors for CVD may be at greater risk. Specifically, a warning was issued for using selective inhibitors of cyclo-oxygenase-2.[33] Cyclooxygenase is an enzyme involved in production of prostanoids, biologic mediators of inflammation with a variety of functions. In the cardiovascular system, they regulate interactions between platelets and the vessel wall. As with all medications, a balance should be considered between the risks and benefits of NSAIDs.

Whenever a health care provider knows that a client has been prescribed antihypertensive medications, appropriate follow-up questions as to whether the client is taking the medication and taking it as prescribed must be addressed. Many people take the medication only when symptoms are perceived and are at risk for the complications described previously (especially during an exercise program, when oxygen demands of the myocardium increase).

Obtain as much information as possible about a client's medications so that potential side effects can be anticipated and intervention planned accordingly. Any side effects noted may indicate that a medication adjustment is needed and should be brought to the physician's attention (see Table 12-5).

The following brief description of the impact of various drug classes (all of which dilate blood vessels) on exercise may assist the therapist in prescribing activities for those who require pharmacologic agents and provide insight into therapeutic decisions for active hypertensive individuals. Antihypertensive medications reduce resting blood pressure levels and may influence blood pressure changes during submaximal and maximal exertion, which affects exercise capacity.

Vasodilators such as nitroglycerin and other nitrates act as a prophylactic for angina by dilating the coronary arteries and improving collateral cardiac circulation, increasing oxygen to the heart muscle, and decreasing the blood pressure, thereby decreasing symptoms of angina.

The β-adrenoreceptor antagonists (β-blockers) selectively inhibit an increase in heart rate. Clinically, this means that when the person increases his or her activity or exercise level, the normal physiologic response of increased heart rate is blunted. This requires a longer warm-up and cool-down period. Sudden changes in position (e.g., supine to standing) should be avoided to prevent dizziness and falls associated with the resulting orthostatic hypotension (see "Special Implications for the Therapist 12-8: Orthostatic Hypotension" below).

The β-blockers diminish catecholamine-induced elevations of heart rate, myocardial contractility, and blood pressure. These effects reduce myocardial oxygen requirements during exertion and stress, thereby preventing angina and allowing the person to exercise for longer periods before the onset of angina. The intended action of β-blockers may prevent normal blood pressure and heart rate responses to exercise; therefore, using heart rate as an index for monitoring response to exercise is not recommended. Although β-blockers are effective antihypertensives, most of them adversely alter aerobic capacity so that exercise capacity is reduced.

An exercise prescription should be based on exercise stress test results using recommended guidelines.[15] Side effects of β-blockers include bronchospasm, which causes difficulty breathing, and chest tightness, which mimics angina; orthostatic hypotension; syncope; headache; and fatigue and weakness.

Diuretics have been first-line antihypertensive agents for many years, but few studies have observed the effect of diuretic therapy on exercise performance. Existing evidence reveals that peak blood pressures induced by physical activity may not always be controlled with diuretics. Diuretic therapy can result in hypokalemia accompanied by muscular cramps and skeletal muscle fatigue (see also Chapter 5).

Potassium-sparing diuretics may cause hyperkalemia, which can, in turn, cause ventricular arrhythmias. Exercise tolerance may be reduced with arrhythmias because of a decrease in left ventricular filling time. Prolonged exercise in the heat is not recommended for people taking diuretics because of the cumulative effects of heat, exercise, and diuretics on blood volume and electrolytes. The length of time an individual who is taking a diuretic can safely exercise in the heat varies with the heat index and the physical condition of the person.

Calcium plays a role in the electrical excitation of cardiac cells and in the mechanical contraction of the myocardial and vascular smooth muscle cells. Calcium channel antagonists inhibit calcium ion influx across the cell membrane during cardiac depolarization, relax coronary vascular smooth muscle, dilate coronary and peripheral arteries, and increase myocardial oxygen delivery in people with vasospastic angina. This class of vasodilators decreases peripheral vascular resistance at rest and during physical activity, thereby altering exercise tolerance by affecting heart rate and blood pressure during exercise.

During exercise, calcium channel antagonists have been observed to reduce systolic and diastolic pressure at submaximal loads, but higher systolic blood pressures measured during maximal exercise are not lowered. Side effects of calcium antagonists (e.g., drowsiness, dizziness, headache, peripheral edema, tachycardia or bradycardia) may interfere with a client's ability to participate in an exercise program.

ACE inhibitors reduce blood pressure by lowering peripheral vascular resistance and are considered the first line of treatment by many physicians. They are readily available as generic drugs (less expensive). One of the side effects of ACE inhibitors is chronic dry cough[368] that may vary in intensity, from tolerable to debilitating. Contrary to expectation, the aerobic exercise capacity of patients was found to be greater with the lower dose of lisinopril, suggesting that therapy with ACE inhibitors for heart failure may require tailoring the doses to the individual to optimize functional benefits.[114]

Use of calcium channel antagonists and ACE inhibitors in hypertension increased dramatically in the 1990s, whereas the use of less-expensive agents, such as diuretics and β-blockers, declined.

Exercise and Blood Pressure

The benefits of resistive or dynamic exercise in people with and without CVD are well known and available for review.[363] A regular program of aerobic exercise, introduced gradually, facilitates cardiovascular conditioning, may assist in weight reduction, and may provide some benefit in reducing blood pressure. Exercising using primarily the lower extremities (e.g., cycling, walking) can also reduce blood pressure.

Postexercise hypotension (lowered blood pressure in response to exercise) in mildly hypertensive individuals has been observed for up to 7 hours after exercise independent of other variables.[357] Diastolic blood pressure reduction seems to be related to the duration of the exercise program (i.e., the longer the program, the more likely the hypotensive effect). Blood pressure reduction has occurred after just several weeks to 6 months of regular training.[195] On the other hand, blood pressure will return to its previous elevated level if training is discontinued.

Heavy isometric exercises and heavy weightlifting may be harmful, because the blood pressure often rises because of vasovagal reflexes that occur. During fatiguing isometric exercise, the rate and rise of systolic blood pressure appear to be higher in hypertensive individuals, but studies in this area are limited. Generally, antihypertensive drugs have not been found to affect the blood pressure response to isometric exertion. However, the use of isometric exercise to lower blood pressure has not been studied in hypertensive individuals; a fall in resting blood pressure has been observed in normotensive individuals after repetitive isometric contractions equal to 30% of maximal capacity.[483]

Exercise and Malignant Hypertension

There is always a concern for a stroke (cerebrovascular accident [CVA]) or recurrent stroke in anyone with uncontrolled, malignant hypertension. Therapists in the acute care setting must monitor vital signs closely in individuals with a history of hypertension-induced CVA. With malignant hypertension, the set point for cerebral autoregulation (i.e., ability of tissues/organs to remain evenly perfused with fluctuating blood/perfusion pressures) is higher, which means blood pressure must be higher to prevent hypoperfusion of the brain.

The question becomes, what are the outside parameters of acceptable blood pressure values during treatment? There are no evidence-based guidelines, only therapists' reports from the field of how this is handled by their neurosurgeons, cardiologists, and neurologists. For example, with ischemic (not hemorrhagic) CVA and malignant hypertension, systolic blood pressure is maintained anywhere between 160-180 and 210-220 mm Hg (depending on individual factors) with diastolic limits up to 110 mm Hg.

These higher levels are needed to maintain adequate blood perfusion. Until researchers can answer the question of blood pressure parameters in this population, the therapist must identify physician preference for each individual and report any deviation from the acceptable range or large jumps in pressures (e.g., going from 120/80 mm Hg to 220/110 mm Hg).

Exercise Training Guidelines

The intensity of exercise required to produce health benefits and decrease blood pressure has been confused with the level of exercise necessary to improve physical fitness. Health benefits can be achieved without large gains in fitness. Encouraging people to increase their level of total energy expenditure is the key to increasing activity levels, rather than emphasizing physical

fitness. The type, intensity, duration, and frequency of training, as well as progression, should be assessed regularly.

A preexercise evaluation and exercise testing may be prescribed by the physician. This information is helpful in establishing submaximal and maximal blood pressure responses. Monitoring vital signs before, during, and after exercise or activity is essential. Any person with an exaggerated systolic blood pressure response (higher than 250 mm Hg) or failure to reduce diastolic pressure (to less than 90 mm Hg) should be referred to the physician for reevaluation.

Training intensity does not need to be high, and it appears that low-intensity activity (65%-70% of maximal heart rate) three times per week is as effective as high-intensity activity in blood pressure reduction. Training intensity should be based on maximal heart rate using the calculated formulas (see Appendix B) or measured during a maximal exercise test. After 12 to 16 weeks, if the blood pressure is adequately controlled, the physician may reduce the antihypertensive medication slowly to determine the long-term effect of training on blood pressure. Several resources are available for determining the appropriate exercise program for the hypertensive client, whether symptomatic or asymptomatic.[14,63]

Monitoring During Exercise

Therapists often treat people who are diagnosed with conditions that are highly correlated with hypertension, such as stroke, obesity, diabetes mellitus, alcoholism, CAD, and pregnancy (see Box 12-7). Monitoring tolerance to exercise by observing for unusual symptoms and measuring blood pressure before, during, and after therapy are important steps in identifying a potential cardiovascular event. Many factors can cause an increase in blood pressure (see Appendix B).

Hypertensive Heart Disease

Definition and Overview. The term *hypertensive heart disease* is used when the heart is enlarged as a result of persistently elevated blood pressure (hypertension) (see previous discussion). Left ventricular hypertrophy and diastolic dysfunction are found in 10% to 30% of the adult population with chronic hypertension, and it may present with many of the signs and symptoms of CHF. Both the prevalence and the severity of the disease are greater in blacks than in whites. In all adults, it increases progressively with age.

MEDICAL MANAGEMENT

DIAGNOSIS, TREATMENT, AND PROGNOSIS. Cardiac enlargement and left ventricular hypertrophy, best viewed with echocardiography, are diagnostic of hypertensive heart disease. Treatment is as for hypertension unless heart failure develops, in which case treatment is as for heart failure (see the sections on each of these conditions for more discussion). The most common cause of death in hypertensive heart disease is CHF, accounting for 40% of all deaths from hypertension.

SPECIAL IMPLICATIONS FOR THE THERAPIST   **12-5**

Hypertensive Heart Disease

See "Special Implications for the Therapist: Ischemic Heart Disease, Coronary Heart Disease, Coronary Artery Disease" above; "Special Implications for the Therapist 12-4: Hypertension (Hypertensive Vascular Disease)" above; and "Special Implications for the Therapist 12-7: Congestive Heart Failure" below.

Myocardial Infarction

Definition and Incidence

MI, also known as a heart attack or referred to as a "coronary," is the development of ischemia with resultant necrosis of myocardial tissue. Any prolonged obstruction depriving the heart muscle of oxygen can cause an MI. MI occurs in 1.5 million persons each year and represents the leading cause of death (500,000 deaths annually) in the adult American population. See "Ischemic Heart Disease, Coronary Heart Disease, Coronary Artery Disease" above.

Etiologic and Risk Factors

Etiologic and risk factors are the same as for all forms of CVD, especially angina pectoris associated with CAD (see "Angina Pectoris" above). Eighty percent to 90% of MIs result from coronary thrombus at the site of a preexisting atherosclerotic stenosis. New cases of MI occur in many people with only a borderline risk profile or even lack of known risk factors, suggesting other unidentified risk factors.

Other causes may include cocaine use (causes vasoconstriction of the coronary arteries), vasculitis, aortic stenosis, or aortic root or coronary artery dissection. Smokers have more than twice as many heart attacks as nonsmokers, and sudden cardiac death occurs two to four times more frequently in smokers. After an infarction, smokers have a poorer chance of recovery than nonsmokers. People with single-vessel CAD, compared to those with triple-vessel CAD, have higher risk of exertion-related MI, which may include weakness or shortness of breath while working with the arms extended overhead in habitually inactive people. It is the presence of the thrombus in a large atherosclerotic coronary artery in single-vessel disease that is associated with the exertion-related MI.[176]

It is a well-established fact that heart attacks occur more frequently in the early morning hours. This peak incidence is attributed to an increase in catecholamines with the resultant increased blood pressure, increased workload of the heart, as well as increased clotting factors in the early morning. Heart attacks also occur in a seasonal pattern with an increased incidence between Thanksgiving and New Year's Day across all ages, in both genders, and across geographic regions. Whether this can be attributed to mood changes, weather, circadian rhythms, large quantities of food consumed, or some other mechanism remains unknown.

Upper respiratory tract illnesses are associated with an increased risk of ischemic heart disease and stroke, especially during the flu season, in adults 65 years old and older who have not received a flu shot. Studies show a reduction in the risk of hospitalization and mortality for heart disease, as well as for cerebrovascular disease, pneumonia, and influenza, among elderly adults receiving flu vaccine.[326,327]

The association between periodontal disease (e.g., gingivitis, periodontitis) and acute MI is under investigation. There is a definite association between common forms of periodontal disease and CVD and stroke, but the causal relations have not been identified.[361]

Researchers have found that bacteria in the mouth spill into the bloodstream and can be found in the walls of major arteries. Recent research showed that intensive periodontal treatment may reverse atherosclerosis by improving elasticity of the arteries, or endothelial function,[448] suggesting that periodontal treatment may reduce cardiovascular risk.

Acute respiratory tract infections, such as the common cold, flu, and bronchitis, may also increase the risk of a heart attack's occurring within 2 weeks of a first heart attack and may account for some cases of MI, although researchers point out that early symptoms of heart attacks may be mistaken for acute upper respiratory tract infection.[299]

Silent ischemia is highly prevalent among people with diabetes; increased PAI-1 activity has been identified as a risk factor for MI in persons with diabetes as well as for postmenopausal women not receiving HRT. PAI-1 is a naturally occurring substance that inhibits another natural substance, tPA. tPA is an enzyme released endogenously as part of the body's defense against thrombosis; it lyses polymerized fibrin and dissolves the blood clot (thrombus). The effect of PAI-1 on tPA is to *prevent* clot destruction in the bloodstream.

Research now shows that diabetic clients have higher PAI-1 activity than nondiabetic clients, both at hospital admission for acute MI and at follow-up 1 year later. Raised PAI-1 activity may predispose diabetic clients to MI and may also impair pharmacologic and spontaneous reperfusion after acute MI, contributing to the poor outcome in this population.[440]

Ratio of waist-to-hip measurements may provide one of the best predictors of heart attack risk. Higher waist measurements relative to hip measurements increases heart attack risk even if BMI is within the acceptable range (85% or higher ratio for women and 90% or higher for men increases the risk). Fat cells in the abdomen affect pancreas and liver, increasing heart attack risk.[495]

Pathogenesis

The myocardium receives its blood supply from the two large coronary arteries and their branches (Fig. 12-8; Table 12-9). One or more of these blood vessels may become occluded by a clot that forms suddenly when an atheromatous plaque ruptures through the sublayers of a blood vessel or when the narrow, roughened inner lining of a sclerosed artery becomes completely filled with thrombus. In most cases, infarcts result from an occlusive thrombus superimposed on an atherosclerotic plaque.

Researchers have found that plaque most likely to rupture (vulnerable plaque) is comprised of the soft form of cholesterol (cholesteryl ester) and is vulnerable to mechanical forces such as occur with the increase in

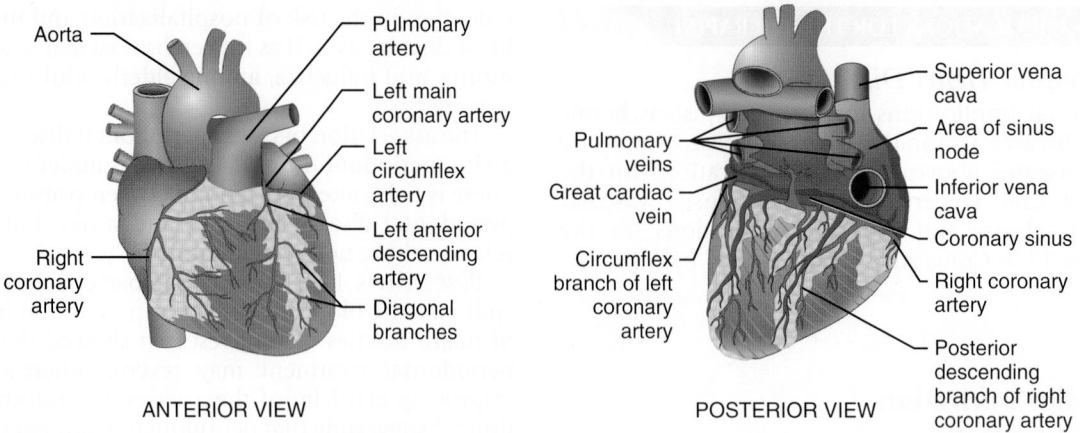

ANTERIOR VIEW   POSTERIOR VIEW

Figure 12-8

Areas of myocardium affected by arterial insufficiency of specific coronary arteries. The right and left coronary arteries branch off the aorta just above the aortic valve and normally supply the myocardium with oxygenated blood. Table 12-9 lists the most commonly affected arteries and the area of myocardium supplied.

Table 12-9	Blood Supply to the Myocardium
Area of Myocardium*	**Supplied By**
Anterior	Left coronary artery
	Left anterior descending branch[†]
Posterior	Right coronary artery
Inferior	Right coronary artery
Anteroseptal	Left coronary artery
	Left anterior descending branch
High Lateral	Circumflex artery
	Left coronary artery
	Diagonal branch
Apical	Usually left coronary artery
	Left anterior branch
	Sometimes right coronary artery
	Posterior descending branch

*Most commonly affected arteries and the area of myocardium supplied are listed in order of deceasing occurrence.

[†]Often referred to as the "widow maker" untreated blockage of the left anterior descending branch leads to permanent heart damage if the individual does not die first.

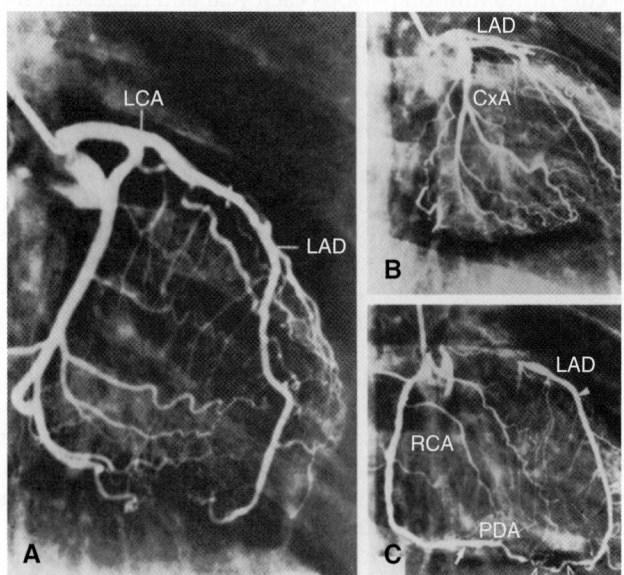

Figure 12-9

A, Angiogram of a normal left coronary artery (LCA). **B,** Angiogram of a totally obstructed left anterior descending (LAD) coronary artery. **C,** Angiogram of the right coronary artery (RCA) and its major branch, the posterior descending artery (PDA) (same heart as in **B**). The LAD is seen because of collateral vessels connecting the LAD and the RCA system. (From Boucek R, Morales A, Romanelli R, et al: *Coronary artery disease: pathologic and clinical assessment,* Baltimore, 1984, Williams & Wilkins, pp. 4, 9.)

hormones early in the morning or even the vibration of the heartbeat.

Rupturing plaque does not always result in an MI. It is likely that plaque breaks off frequently without triggering a heart attack, and the large plaques visible on angiograms are often the healed-over and more stable plaques. Although these plaques occlude the coronary vessels, resulting in obstruction, ischemia, and angina, they are not as likely to cause rupture and sudden death as happens with the soft, smaller, and usually undetected plaques.

The most common site involved is the left ventricle, the chamber of the heart with the greatest workload. Thrombosis of the anterior descending branch of the left coronary artery is the most common cause of infarction and affects the anterior left ventricle (Fig. 12-9).

Occlusion of the left circumflex artery produces anterolateral or posterolateral infarction. Right coronary artery thrombosis leads to infarction of the posteroinferior portion of the left ventricle and may involve the right ventricular myocardium and interventricular septum. The arteries supplying the atrioventricular node and the sinus node more commonly arise from the right coronary artery; thus atrioventricular block at the nodal level and sinus node dysfunction occur more frequently during inferior infarctions.

Myocardial ischemia/reperfusion injury is accompanied by an inflammatory response involving three major components: (1) molecular oxygen, (2) cellular blood

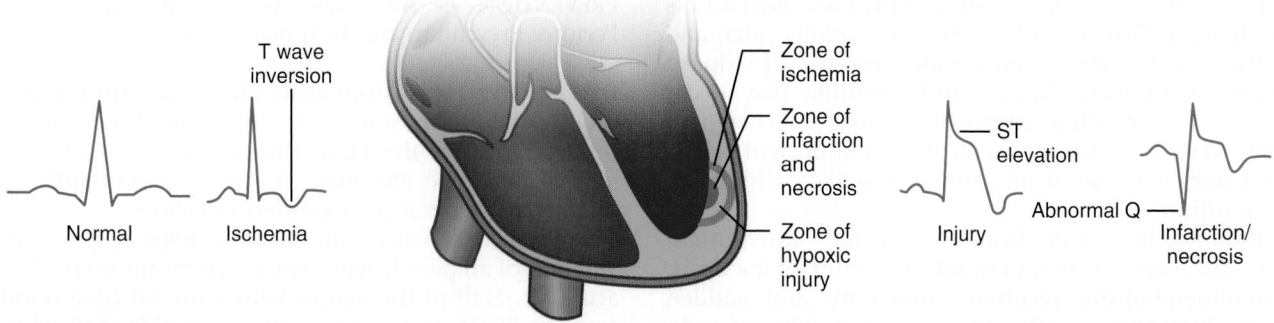

Figure 12-10

Electrocardiographic (ECG) alterations associated with the three zones of myocardial infarction (MI).

elements (especially neutrophils), and (3) activated complement system. When the myocardium has been completely deprived of oxygen, cells die and the tissue becomes necrotic in an area called the *zone of infarction* (Fig. 12-10; see also Figs. 6-8 and 6-9). In response to this necrosis, leukocytes aid in removing the dead cells, and fibroblasts produce fibrotic proteins, mostly collagens, and form a fibrous scar within the area of infarction. The remaining heart muscle cells enlarge to compensate for the loss in heart pump function (see "Cell Injury" in Chapter 6; a complete discussion of the role of oxidative stress and complement activation in heart disease is available[97,130]). Usually the formation of fibrous scar tissue is complete within 6 to 8 weeks (Table 12-10; see Fig. 6-9).

Immediately surrounding the area of infarction is a less-seriously damaged area of injury called the *zone of hypoxic injury*. This zone is able to return to normal, but it may also become necrotic if blood flow is not restored. With adequate collateral circulation, this area may regain its function within 2 to 3 weeks. Adjacent to the zone of hypoxic injury is another reversible zone called the *zone of ischemia*. Ischemic and injured myocardial tissues cause characteristic ECG changes; as the myocardium heals, the ST segment and T waves gradually return to normal, but abnormal Q waves may persist.

Oxygen deprivation is accompanied by electrolyte disturbances, particularly cellular loss of potassium, calcium, and magnesium. Myocardial cells deprived of necessary oxygen and nutrients lose contractility, thereby diminishing the pumping ability of the heart. Normally the myocardium takes up varying quantities of catecholamines (epinephrine, norepinephrine), which are released when significant arterial occlusion occurs. Released catecholamines predispose the individual to serious imbalances of sympathetic and parasympathetic function, irregular heartbeats (arrhythmia), and heart failure.

Clinical Manifestations

The most notable symptom of MI is a sudden sensation of pressure, often described as prolonged crushing chest pain, occasionally radiating to the arms, throat, neck

Table 12-10	Tissue Changes After Myocardial Infarction
Time After MI	**Tissue Changes**
6-12 hr	No gross changes; healing process has not begun
18-24 hr	Inflammatory response; intercellular enzyme release
2-4 days	Visible necrosis; proteolytic enzymes remove debris; catecholamines, lipolysis, and glycogenolysis elevate blood glucose and increase free fatty acids to assist depleted myocardium recovery from anaerobic state
4-10 days	Debris cleared; collagen matrix laid down
10-14 days	Weak, fibrotic scar tissue with beginning revascularization; area vulnerable to stress
6 wk	Scarring usually complete; tough, inelastic scar replaces necrotic myocardium; unable to contract and relax like healthy myocardial tissue

Modified from McCance KL, Huether SE: *Pathophysiology: the biologic basis for disease in adults and children*, ed 7, St Louis, 2013, Mosby.

(as high as the occipital area), and back (Fig. 12-11). The pain is constant, lasting 30 minutes up to hours, and may be accompanied by pallor, shortness of breath, and profuse perspiration. Catecholamine release resulting in sympathetic stimulation may produce diaphoresis and peripheral vasoconstriction that cause the skin to become cool and clammy. Angina pectoris pain can be similar, but it is less severe, does not last for hours, and is relieved by cessation of activity, rest, or nitrates.

Symptoms do not always follow the classic pattern, especially in women. Two major symptoms in women are shortness of breath, sometimes occurring in the middle of the night, and chronic, unexplained fatigue. Atypical presentation may include continuous pain in the midthoracic spine or interscapular area, neck and shoulder pain, stomach or abdominal pain, nausea or indigestion as the only symptom, unexplained anxiety, or heartburn that is not altered by antacids. Women are more likely than men to have symptoms unrelated to chest pain such as aching, heaviness, or weakness in one or both arms, heat or flushing sensation, or racing heart.

Silent attacks (painless infarction without acute symptoms) are more common among nonwhites, older adults (more than 75 years), all smokers, and adults (men and women) with diabetes, presumably because of reduced sensitivity to pain. Nausea and vomiting may occur because of reflex stimulation of vomiting centers by pain fibers. Fever may develop in the first 24 hours and persist for a week because of inflammatory activity within the myocardium.

Postinfarction complications include arrhythmias, CHF, cardiogenic shock, pericarditis, rupture of the heart, thromboembolism, recurrent infarction, and sudden death. Arrhythmias, affecting more than 90% of individuals, are the most common complication of acute MI and are caused by ischemia, hypoxia, autonomic nervous system imbalances, lactic acidosis, electrolyte imbalances, drug toxicity, or alterations of impulse conduction pathways or conduction defects.

MEDICAL MANAGEMENT

PREVENTION. See "Atherosclerosis: Prevention" and "Angina Pectoris: Prevention and Treatment" above.

DIAGNOSIS. Diagnosis of acute MI and determination of the site and extent of necrosis rely on the clinical history, interpretation of the ECG, and measurement of serum levels of cardiac enzymes. Diagnostic uncertainty frequently arises because of a variety of factors.

Many people with acute MI have atypical symptoms, and half of all people with typical symptoms do not have acute MI. Half of the people with acute MI have nondiagnostic ECGs, and some people are unable to provide a history. Biochemical markers of cardiac injury are commonly relied on to diagnose or exclude acute MI. These laboratory tests dramatically reduce the cost of treating

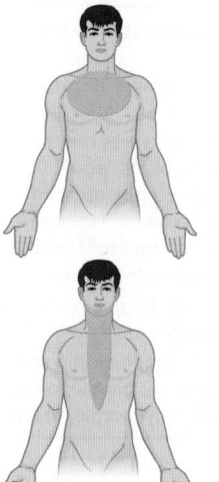
Localized just under breastbone; or in larger area of mid-chest; or entire upper chest

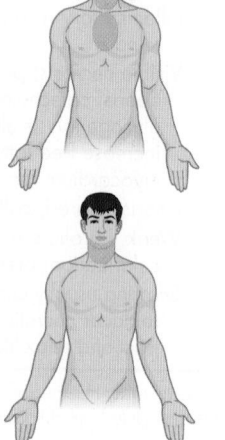
Common combination: mid-chest, neck and jaw

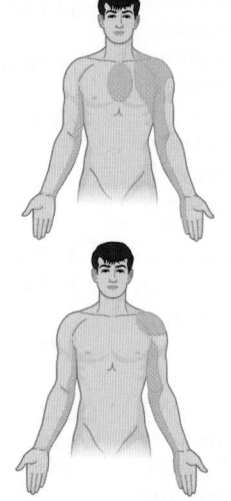
Mid-chest and inside arms. Left arm and shoulder more frequent than right

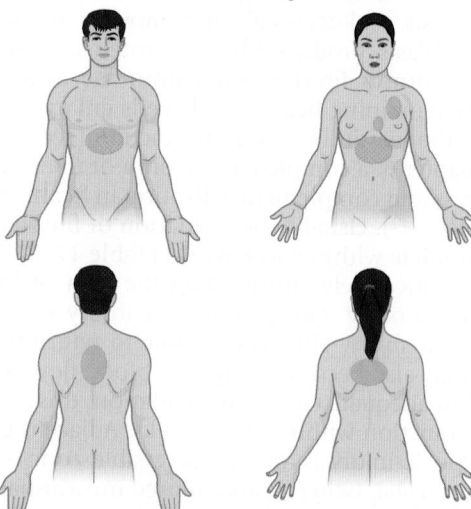
Upper abdomen–where most often mistaken for indigestion

Larger area of chest, neck, jaw and inside arms

Lower center neck, to both sides of upper neck; and jaw from ear to ear

Inside right arm from armpit to below elbow; inside left arm to waist. Left arm and shoulder more frequent than right

Between shoulder blades

Most common warning signs of heart attack	Atypical, less common warning signs (especially women)
• Uncomfortable pressure, fullness, squeezing or pain in the center of the chest (prolonged) • Pain that spreads to the throat, neck, back, jaw, shoulders, or arms • Chest discomfort with lightheadedness, dizziness, sweating, pallor, nausea, or shortness of breath • Prolonged symptoms unrelieved by antacids, nitroglycerin, or rest	• Unusual chest pain (quality, location, e.g., burning, heaviness; left chest), stomach or abdominal pain • Continuous midthoracic or interscapular pain • Continuous neck or shoulder pain • Pain relieved by antacids; pain unrelieved by rest or nitroglycerin • Nausea and vomiting; flu-like manifestation without chest pain/discomfort • Unexplained intense anxiety, weakness, or fatigue • Breathlessness, dizziness

Figure 12-11

Early warning signs of a heart attack. Multiple segmental nerve innervation shown in Figure 12-6 accounts for the varied pain patterns possible. A woman can experience any of the various patterns described but is more likely to develop atypical symptoms of pain as depicted here. (Modified from Goodman CC, Snyder TE: *Differential diagnosis for physical therapists: screening for referral*, ed 4, Philadelphia, 2007, WB Saunders.)

heart attacks by allowing physicians to quickly discharge people with noncardiac chest pain.

Newer biochemical markers of myocardial injury are making it possible to tailor treatment to individual differences and needs. Biomarkers are hormones or other substances released by organs under stress and can point to inflammation of the arteries; stretching, injury, or lack of oxygen to cells; damage to the collage matrix that connects cells; and toxic damage from free radical formation.

This personalized, biologically driven approach to care utilizes biomarkers such as cardiac troponin I (TnI) and cardiac troponin T (TnT) (regulatory proteins that help the heart muscle contract), are now being used instead of or along with the standard markers, such as the myocardial isoenzyme of creatine kinase (CK-MB). TnT is quite specific for myocardial ischemia and necrosis. It remains elevated 5 to 7 days after an MI and is a predictor of cardiovascular mortality.

TnI is a better cardiac marker than CK-MB for MI because it is more sensitive and more specific to myocardial injury; TnT is a better predictor of cardiovascular mortality (as well as all-cause mortality). Both TnI and TnT are useful markers for myocardial injury that help determine the prognosis in people who have unstable angina but no evidence of CK-MB elevation. (See also "Cardiac Enzymes and Markers" in Chapter 40; see Tables 40-15 and 40-16.)

Researchers are continuing to investigate other hemostatic markers based on the knowledge that coronary thrombosis involves both coagulation and fibrinolysis cascades. For example, increases of fibrinogen and D-dimer, a circulating marker of fibrin turnover, are significantly higher in people with acute ischemic events such as MI and unstable angina than in nonischemic individuals, but it has not been determined to what extent this is causal. Other tests may include nuclear scanning, coronary angiography, echocardiography, CT, cardiac magnetic resonance stress testing, and MRA. Serum cholesterol must be determined because of its importance as a modifiable risk factor. See "Angina Pectoris: Diagnosis" and "Atherosclerosis: Diagnosis" above.

Other cardiac markers include homocysteine, Lp(a), and CRP. Although these have not become "standard" laboratory values, they can be used as independent predictors of future coronary events in apparently healthy men and women. For example, elevated plasma homocysteine is a risk factor for atherosclerosis and endothelial dysfunction, and CRP may be used as a marker of subclinical atherosclerosis and cardiovascular risk specifically linked to MI and sudden death.

Infarcted tissue is electrically silent and does not contribute to the ECG. Most clients with acute infarction have ECG changes, although this test provides only a crude estimate of the magnitude of infarction. When diagnosis by ECG and enzymes is not possible (e.g., when people seek medical attention after MI), scintigraphic studies (radionuclide imaging) can show areas of necrotic myocardium and diminished perfusion. These tests, which use radiotracers, do not distinguish old damage from recent infarction, and false-positive results can occur.

Other test procedures may include echocardiography, which is useful in assessing the ability of the heart walls to contract and relax, and transesophageal echocardiography (TEE), an ultrasonic technique that provides a clearer image of the heart, including the posterior wall, valvular anatomy, and thoracic aortic structure, providing identification of structural heart diseases. Newer technology, such as RT3D imaging, has the potential to improve evaluation of heart function (especially ventricular) with TEE.

Magnetic resonance imaging (MRI) to evaluate structural defects of the heart and positron emission tomography to evaluate cardiac physiology and metabolism and assess tissue perfusion have contributed significantly to the understanding of the pathophysiology of the ischemic heart.

Another new technique being investigated is the use of a contrast agent called EchoGen, used in conjunction with an ultrasound procedure. This agent infiltrates healthy heart muscle but not muscle that has been deprived of blood or oxygen. Existing contrast agents only image the heart chambers, which provides information about the flow of blood through the chamber but not about the structure of the heart muscle itself.

TREATMENT. The goal of treatment is reestablishing the flow of blood in blocked coronary arteries. Pharmacologic intervention is used to provide pain relief (essential because angina is evidence of ongoing ischemia), limit infarction size, reduce vasoconstriction, prevent thrombus formation, and augment repair. MI caused by intracoronary thrombi can be relieved by infusion of thrombolytic agents (e.g., streptokinase, urokinase, tPA) that dissolve clots, promote vasodilation, and reduce infarct size.

PAI-1 is a naturally occurring substance that inhibits another natural substance, tPA; tPA is an enzyme released endogenously as part of the body's defense against thrombosis; it promotes degradation of fibrin leading to dissolving of blood clots. tPA is now a genetically engineered drug used in thrombolytic therapy.

This intervention initiated within 70 minutes of symptom onset is associated with improved outcome.[468] After a thrombolytic agent is administered, intravenous (IV) heparin therapy is usually given with adjunctive drug therapy during and after MI, because platelet inhibitors and other cardiovascular medications (see Table 12-5) are known to further reduce mortality when administered during the acute phase.

Right now, only a small portion of heart attack victims receive reperfusion therapy within that crucial first hour after symptom onset, primarily because people delay (sometimes by hours) coming to the emergency department. This points out the extreme importance of early intervention and education of the general population (and especially for those with known risk factors, such as hypertension, previous heart attack, diabetes, smoking, or hyperlipidemia) as to the importance of getting to an emergency department at the earliest sign of heart attack. Educating the public about the less common or atypical warning signs and symptoms is essential. Information about public education, reducing delays at home or at work, and the National Heart Attack Alert Program is available.[118,321]

Other treatment interventions, including identification and modification of risk factors, angioplasty, stenting, atherectomy, angiogenesis, tissue engineering, gene therapy, stem cell transplantation, and cardiac rehabilitation utilizing exercise programs, have been previously discussed in detail (see "Atherosclerosis: Medical Management" and "Hypertension: Medical Management" above).

A study to determine whether early, rapid use of cholesterol-lowering therapy can reduce recurrent ischemic events in acute coronary syndromes is under way through the Myocardial Ischemia Reduction with Aggressive Cholesterol Lowering (MIRACL) program. The study showed that lipid-lowering therapy with 80 mg/day of atorvastatin, initiated during acute coronary syndrome, reduces recurrent ischemic events in patients in the first 16 weeks.[404,489]

Exercise has been recommended as a means of increasing pain tolerance, increasing the threshold of the stimulus required to induce angina, alleviating depression, reducing anxiety, and inducing collateral circulation. Increasing evidence suggests that combining a low-fat diet and intensive exercise training can improve myocardial perfusion by regression of coronary atherosclerosis. Exercise training may be contraindicated for some people (Box 12-9; see also Box 12-4). Medical clearance must be obtained for entry into an exercise training program.

Exercise testing is the most useful tool to establish guidelines for exercise training in apparently healthy adults and is mandatory for people with known or suspected CVD.[151,261] The majority of exercise testing can be done within 3 days of MI with a very low incidence of complications. Criteria for testing usually include clients who are off IV nitroglycerin with no angina at rest, uncontrolled cardiac failure, or arrhythmias. Early testing can lead to early triage and potential cost savings.

Box 12-9

CONTRAINDICATIONS TO EXERCISE AFTER MYOCARDIAL INFARCTION

- Acute MI (<1 or 2 days after an MI without physician approval)
- Unstable angina; easily provoked angina
- New ECG with abnormalities
- Signs and symptoms of MI (e.g., nausea, dyspnea, light-headedness, chest pain)
- Pao_2 <60 mm Hg
- O_2 saturation <85%
- Hemoglobin <8 g/dL; hematocrit <26%
- Severe aortic outflow obstruction
- Suspected or known dissecting aneurysm
- Acute myocarditis or pericarditis
- Uncontrolled complex arrhythmias
- Active severe CHF; resting respiratory rate >45 breaths/min
- Recent pulmonary embolism or thrombophlebitis
- Untreated third-degree heart block
- Severe systemic hypertension unresponsive to medication
- Uncontrolled diabetes
- Acute infections
- Digoxin toxicity (see Table 12-5)

Modified from Bonow RO: *Braunwald's heart disease—a textbook of cardiovascular medicine*, ed 9, Philadelphia, 2011, WB Saunders.

PROGNOSIS. The size and anatomic location of the infarction, together with the amount of damage from previous infarctions, determine the acute clinical picture, the early complications, and the long-term prognosis. The first 24 hours after onset of symptoms is the time of highest risk for sudden death. The sooner someone reaches the hospital, the better the prognosis. Of those experiencing an acute MI, 80% survive the initial attack when transported to a coronary care unit. Substantial reductions in post-MI death have occurred over the last 5 decades because of improved intervention.

Factors negatively affecting prognosis include age (clients older than 80 years have a 60% mortality); evidence of other CVDs, respiratory diseases, or uncontrolled diabetes mellitus; anterior location of MI (30% mortality rate); and hypotension (clients whose systolic blood pressure is less than 55 mm Hg have a 60% mortality rate). The risk of reinfarction is increased in women, people with elevated blood pressure, and people with elevated serum cholesterol. As MI survivors with longstanding hypertension live longer, cardiac failure has become an increasingly important long-term sequela of MI.

Prognostic testing predictive of cardiac events includes standard exercise testing such as functional capacity and heart rate recovery[151] and imaging using single-photon emission computed tomography with contrast agents (e.g., thallium-201, technetium-99m sestamibi). In the imaging studies, a radioisotope is taken up by adequately perfused tissue, allowing detection of myocardial perfusion defects at rest and during exercise (areas of infarction appear as regions of diminished isotope activity or no activity, referred to as *cold spots*).

Study of the prognostic value of treadmill exercise testing in older persons shows that workload (measured in metabolic equivalents) is the only treadmill exercise testing predictive of death both in younger persons and in adults older than 65 years of age.[181] An abnormal exercise test result is a more powerful predictor of risk in those people with conventional risk factors than in those without such risk factors.

SPECIAL IMPLICATIONS FOR THE THERAPIST   12-6

Myocardial Infarction
Early Postmyocardial Infarction Considerations

Although the myocardium must rest, bed rest puts the client at risk for development of hypovolemia (low blood volume), hypoxemia (hypoxia), muscle atrophy, and pulmonary embolus (see also "The Cardiac Client and Surgery" below). Developing a program of progressive physical activity with adequate pacing and rest periods begins within 24 hours for the acute care client in uncomplicated cases. Evidence-based standards for mobility after administration of tPA remain lacking. Many institutions hold therapy until 24 hours after tPA because of issues of perfusion, bleeding risks, or because of multiple other medical diagnostic procedures ordered (e.g., CT scans, echocardiograms).

Even if mobility is limited, therapeutic interventions are not; the therapist must use clinical expertise and critical thinking skills to formulate an appropriate plan-of-care. For example, gentle movement exercises, deep breathing, and coughing can begin immediately as prophylactic measures. Incisional pain or discomfort from cardiac surgery may cause a person to exhibit rapid, shallow respirations in an attempt to ease the discomfort. If analgesics are prescribed to prevent severe discomfort, the drug can be administered before therapy to better enable the person to carry out breathing exercises. This problem is of limited duration and usually resolves when the incision heals. The therapist must be aware that analgesics also mask pain response, making it possible for the client to overexert.

Early therapeutic exercise helps prevent cardiopulmonary complications, venous stasis, joint stiffness, and muscle weakness. Relaxation is often promoted with low-intensity activity. Activities that increase intrathoracic or intraabdominal pressure, such as breath holding and Valsalva maneuvers (see Box 16-1), can precipitate bradycardia followed by increased venous return to the heart, causing possible cardiac overload. For this reason, these actions are contraindicated and should not be performed in any stage of the rehabilitation program.[122]

During the first 6 weeks post-MI, the client is cautioned to avoid saunas, hot tubs, whirlpools, and excessively warm swimming pools. Early rehabilitation lasting 2 to 3 weeks is often followed by exercise testing, at which time water therapy may be permissible per physician approval (see "Guidelines for Aquatic Therapy" in Appendix B). Specific aspects of cardiac rehabilitation and postoperative care are beyond the scope of this text. Other more specific texts are available to guide the therapist in this area.[157,205,220] See also the Agency for Health Care Policy and Research's clinical guidelines for cardiac rehabilitation.[4]

Monitoring Vital Signs

The therapist must continually monitor for signs of impending infarction, including generalized or localized pain anywhere over the thorax, upper limbs, and neck; palpitations; dyspnea; light-headedness; syncope; sensation of indigestion; hiccups; and nausea (see Fig. 12-11). Pain medications, such as morphine, used to minimize discomfort initially may also depress the respiratory drive.

The coronary care unit therapist must monitor corresponding vital signs. The home health therapist must monitor pulse and blood pressure measurements for hypotension because of the side effects precipitated by antihypertensive medications, vasodilators, and other antianginal agents. (See also "Special Implications for the Therapist 12-3: Angina Pectoris" above.) Initial ambulation and activities at home should be roughly equivalent to levels achieved at the hospital at the time of discharge, depending on the client's physiologic response to the transition from hospital to home.

The client must increase activities gradually to avoid overtaxing the heart as it pumps oxygenated blood to the muscles. The metabolic equivalent system provides one way of measuring the amount of oxygen needed to perform an activity as a measure of the intensity of an activity. One metabolic equivalent of the task (MET) equals 3.5 mL of oxygen per kilogram of body weight per minute; 1 MET is approximately equivalent to the oxygen uptake a person requires when resting. At 2 METs, the individual is working at twice the individual's resting metabolic rate.

Early mobilization activities after acute MI should not exceed 1 to 2 METs (e.g., brushing teeth, eating). By comparison, people who can exercise to 8 or more METs (oxygen uptake of 28 mL/kg/min or more) can perform most daily physical activities. In general, 3 to 6 METs is considered the equivalent of moderate exercise. Activities with METs higher than 6 include singles tennis, cycling more than 10 mph, walking more than 4 mph, and cross-country skiing.

The MET system may not be as accurate for overweight, obese, or older adults. For example, because maximal aerobic capacity usually declines with age,[16] even when working at the same MET level as a younger person, the older individual's relative exercise intensity will usually be greater.[16] In addition, research shows that using the MET system underestimates the energy used for an activity in overweight or obese individuals who may end up working at a level too high for them. The therapist is advised to use the rate of perceived exertion (RPE; see Table 12-13) instead for these population groups.[154]

As activity level increases, the therapist must monitor heart rate, blood pressure, and fatigue, keeping in mind that METs can vary as a result of abnormal hemodynamic responses requiring adjustment of activity level accordingly. During phase I (acute hospital) care, the heart rate should not rise more than 25% above resting level, and blood pressure must not rise more than 25 mm Hg above resting level.

When systolic blood pressure falls or fails to increase as the intensity of exercise increases, exercise intensity should be immediately reduced. A drop in systolic blood pressure during exercise below the rest value as measured in the standing position is associated with increased risk of lethal arrhythmia in clients with a prior MI or myocardial ischemia.

Supplemental oxygen may be used to supply the myocardium with oxygen when the demand exceeds supply, thereby reducing myocardial stress and eliminating dyspnea. Caution must be exercised as too much oxygen can be deleterious for clients with acute MI.[479] Even though supplemental oxygen can increase arterial oxygen level in MI, it reduces cardiac output, increases blood pressure, and increases resistance to blood flow. Only clients with low oxygen levels should be administered oxygen and only to the extent that it does not cause hyperoxia.[479,221]

In addition, excessive oxygen may provoke oxidative stress damaging tissues. Blood gas analysis in clients is usually performed within 1 hour of initiating oxygen therapy to establish a baseline of arterial saturation. By monitoring blood gases, oxygen dose can be altered to regulate blood gases and acid–base balance. The therapist must monitor oxygen saturation levels (see Table 40-18) during exercise or intervention, because these activities may increase myocardial oxygen demand.

The client with chronic obstructive pulmonary disease (COPD) who receives oxygen therapy may develop hypercapnia (high levels of CO_2 in blood caused by hypoventilation; see Chapter 15) or experience its worsening and must be monitored very closely for symptoms of decreased ventilation, such as headache, giddiness, tinnitus (ringing in the ears), nausea, weakness, and vomiting. Elevated CO_2 levels in the COPD client eliminate the drive to breathe normally that is initiated by rising levels of CO_2. The only drive to breathe in the COPD client is hypoxia (reduced oxygen levels), and when the normoxic state is reached the hyperoxic drive becomes depressed. Appropriately prescribed oxygen is vital for the individual with COPD, whereas administration of excessive oxygen to a person with CO_2 retention can further depress the respiratory drive, resulting in death. Of importance, evidence shows that physical activity is a powerful drive that counteracts respiratory depression even in people with COPD who retain CO_2.

Exercise After Myocardial Infarction

As little as 20 years ago, exercise was avoided following a heart attack, but research shows that a reasonable amount of regular exercise is the best way to strengthen the heart and control blood pressure, improve cholesterol status, manage diabetes, and control weight. Survivors who exercise usually require less medication, are less likely to need future invasive procedures (e.g., angioplasty, bypass graft), and are less likely to die of a second heart attack than those who remain sedentary.

Traditionally, isometric exercises have been contraindicated, and resistance training or weightlifting has been excluded from the cardiac client's program. Recently, the approach was revised and clients post-MI are advised to use different types of exercise to increase their aerobic capacity, endurance, and muscle strength, so as to increase their ability to perform activities of daily living.

It is now recommended that individuals with a history of MI combine aerobic exercise (at least 3 days per week; 20-40 minutes each session; at 40%-80% of VO_{2max}; RPE of 11-15 on scale of 20), resistance training (2-3 days per week; 1-3 sets of 10-15 repetitions of 8-10 exercises; 40%-50% maximal voluntary contraction [avoid Valsalva maneuver]), and flexibility exercise aimed at static stretching of the upper and lower body (2-3 days per week; hold for 10-30 seconds).[14, 372] However, for some people, use of a cane or walker is an isometric use of muscles that can increase heart rate; therefore, careful monitoring of vital signs and indications of perceived exertion are required. This is especially critical for high-risk cardiac clients. Special care for clients who receive thrombolytic agents, to reduce their blood-clotting ability, is necessitated to avoid tissue trauma during exercise therapy.

In general, heart attack survivors are often people who have never exercised before and need sound advice and careful supervision by a physical therapist. Exercise may induce cardiac arrhythmias during diuretic and digoxin therapy, and recent ingestion of caffeine may exacerbate arrhythmias. Exercise-induced arrhythmias are generated by enhanced sympathetic tone, increased myocardial oxygen demand, or both. The immediate postexercise period is particularly dangerous because of high catecholamine levels associated with a generalized vasodilation. Sudden termination of muscular activity is accompanied by diminished venous return and may lead to a reduction in coronary perfusion while heart rate is elevated. A careful cooldown period is required with continued monitoring of vital signs after exercise.[492]

Sexual Activity

People with cardiac disease, both men and women, are prone to sexual dysfunction. Often their concerns are voiced to the therapist. The link between CVD and erectile dysfunction in men has been the subject of recent studies. Erectile dysfunction is an early predictor of CAD and should be medically evaluated.[393,447]

Problems may be caused by medications, anxiety, depression, or limited physical capacity. Hypertensive medications are the most common drugs to cause sexual dysfunction (e.g., loss of sexual desire or ability to reach orgasm).

Marijuana increases myocardial oxygen consumption and heart rate and results in decreased testosterone levels and decreased libido. Cocaine can hinder erection, ejaculation, and orgasm; it may also cause coronary artery vasoconstriction and resulting chest pain and fatal MI.

Fear of death during sexual intercourse, fear of another infarction caused by sexual activity, and diminished sexual ability caused by illness and aging may occur. The sexual partner may have many similar fears and may want to be included in any information provided about return to sexual function. The relative risk of triggering an MI by sexual activity is less than 1%.[315,270]

Sexual activity is considered a reasonable activity for most people with CVD. Before engaging in sexual activity, a comprehensive physical examination is recommended for anyone who has concerns or who is at risk for triggering an MI with sexual activity. A scientific statement from the American Heart Association provides general recommendations for individuals with specific CVD conditions, following angioplasty and stenting, and after a heart attack.[270]

Sexual intercourse with orgasm is physiologically equivalent to activities such as a brisk walk or climbing a flight of stairs. It has been equated to 5 METs of work on an exercise stress test; preorgasmic and postorgasmic phases require about 3.7 METs. Advice to clients should be based on consultation with the physician.

Some general guidelines include the following: (1) When the client can sustain a heart rate of 110 to 120 beats/min with no shortness of breath or anginal pain, the client can resume sexual activity; (2) sexual activity should be resumed gradually and only after activities such as walking moderate distances (equivalent to 3 or 4 miles on a level treadmill) or climbing stairs comfortably have been accomplished; (3) sexual activity causes the least amount of stress when it occurs in familiar surroundings with the usual partner in a comfortable environment; (4) gradual foreplay helps the heart prepare for coitus; less strenuous sexual activities, such as cuddling, kissing, touching, and hugging, can be engaged in without sexual intercourse; (5) positions requiring isometric contractions should be avoided; (6) eating a large meal or drinking alcohol 1 to 3 hours before sexual activity should be avoided; (7) anal stimulation and anal intercourse should be avoided, because this stimulates the vagus nerve and may cause chest pain and slows down the heart rate and rhythm, impulse conduction, and coronary blood flow[296]; and (8) the physician should be asked about whether the client should take prophylactic nitroglycerin before intercourse.[247]

Congestive Heart Failure

Definition and Overview

CHF is a condition in which the heart is unable to pump sufficient blood to supply the body's needs. Backup of blood into the pulmonary veins and high pressure in the pulmonary capillaries lead to subsequent pulmonary congestion and pulmonary hypertension. Failure may occur on both sides of the heart or may predominantly affect the right or left side. Heart failure is not a disease, but rather represents a group of clinical manifestations caused by inadequate pump performance from either the cardiac valves or the myocardium. It may be chronic over many years, requiring management by oral medications, or it may be acute and life-threatening, requiring more dramatic medical management to maintain an adequate cardiac output.

Four distinct types of CHF are recognized: (1) systolic heart failure (caused by contractile failure of the myocardium), (2) heart failure with preserved ejection fraction (HFpEF), formerly known as diastolic failure (occurs when increased filling pressures are required to maintain adequate cardiac output despite normal contractile function), (3) left-sided heart failure (occurs when the left ventricle can no longer maintain a normal cardiac output), and (4) right-sided heart failure (right-sided ventricular dysfunction secondary to either left-sided heart failure or to pulmonary disease).

Strictly classified, left ventricular failure is referred to as CHF; acute right ventricular failure, seen almost exclusively in association with massive pulmonary embolism, is labeled cor pulmonale. Cor pulmonale is heart disease, but it arises from an underlying pulmonary pathologic condition; consequently, it is discussed in Chapter 15. Right-sided heart dysfunction secondary to left-sided heart failure, vascular dysfunction, or congenital heart disease is excluded in the definition of cor pulmonale (see "Cor Pulmonale" in Chapter 15).

Incidence

CHF is a common complication of ischemic and hypertensive heart disease, occurring most often in the older adult and, in its chronic form, referred to as a cardiogeriatric syndrome. Because the heart muscle is damaged during a heart attack, many heart attack survivors develop CHF. In the United States, heart failure develops in an estimated 550,000 individuals annually: it is the most common cause for hospitalization in people older than 65 years, with an estimated 5 million men and women living with CHF in the United States today. This condition is on the increase as the population ages and more people survive heart attacks.

Etiologic and Risk Factors

Many cardiac conditions predispose individuals to CHF, but hypertension is one of the most prevalent (Table 12-11). People with preexisting heart disease are at greatest risk for the development of CHF, because when the heart is stressed, compensatory mechanisms may be inadequate. For example, a faster redistribution of blood volume and increased demand for oxygen by the myocardium occur with increased activity, such as exercise, resulting in heart failure.

Pulse pressure appears to be the best single measure of blood pressure for predicting mortality in older people and helps explain apparently discrepant results for low diastolic blood pressure. Pulse pressure is more predictive than even systolic blood pressure alone. Each elevation of 10 mm Hg between systolic and diastolic blood pressure increases the risk of CHF by 14%.[96,177,342] Although the literature supports the use of pulse pressure as a significant prognostic indicator, day-to-day clinical use is not common.

CHF occurring during middle age as distinguished from CHF at advanced age includes an increasing proportion of women, a shift from CHD to hypertension as the most common etiology, and intact left ventricular systolic function.[379] Women tend to have more risk factors and concurrent medical problems, such as hypertension, diabetes, or renal insufficiency. In addition, there may be other gender differences contributing to the development

Table 12-11	Etiologic and Risk Factors Associated with Congestive Heart Failure
Etiologic Factors	**Risk Factors***
Hypertension	Emotional stress
Coronary artery disease	Physical inactivity
Myocardial infarction	Obesity
Valvular heart disease	Diabetes mellitus
Congenital heart disease	Nutritional deficiency
Endocarditis	(vitamin C, thiamin)
Pericarditis	Fever
Myocarditis	Infection
Cardiomyopathy	Anemia
Chronic alcoholism	Thyroid disorders
Atrioventricular malformation	Pregnancy
Thyrotoxicosis (arrhythmia)	Paget disease
Chronic anemia	Pulmonary disease
	Medications (e.g., steroids, NSAIDs)
	Drug toxicity
	Renal disease

NSAIDs, nonsteroidal antiinflammatory drugs.
*Risk factors for new onset or exacerbation of previous CHF.

of CHF in women, such as differences in myocardial distensibility (the degree to which muscle fibers stretch) or hormonal differences as yet undetermined.

Paget disease causes vascular proliferation in the bones. When the disease involves more than one third of the skeleton, a high cardiac output state exists and may tax the compromised heart. Medications such as steroids or NSAIDs and drug toxicity are also risk factors. For the person with chronic, stable heart failure, acute exacerbations may occur caused by alterations in therapy, client noncompliance with therapy, excessive salt and fluid intake, arrhythmias, excessive activity, pulmonary embolisms (PEs), infection, or progression of the underlying disease.

Recently, human immunodeficiency virus (HIV) infection was identified as a risk factor for heart failure in the absence of CAD.[78] Specifically, individuals with ongoing viral replication had higher risk of developing heart failure.

Pathogenesis and Clinical Manifestations

Over the last 15 years, major advances have occurred in our understanding of heart failure, involving the complex interactions that take place among the adrenergic nervous system, the renin–angiotensin axis, the immune system, the peripheral circulation, and other vasoactive substances in response to impaired cardiac function.

The pathophysiology involves structural changes such as loss of myofilaments, apoptosis (programmed cell death), disturbances in calcium homeostasis, and alteration in receptor density, signal transduction, and collagen synthesis. A neurohormonal hypothesis has replaced the hemodynamic model focusing on the neuroendocrine activation of a progressive disorder of left ventricular remodeling. This cascade of events occurs as a result of a cardiac event (e.g., MI) that develops into a clinical syndrome characterized by impaired cardiac function and circulatory congestion.[156]

CHF is a complex event involving one or both ventricles. This discussion is based on left ventricular failure. See "Cor Pulmonale" in Chapter 15 for a complete discussion of right-sided heart failure. When the heart fails to propel blood forward normally (such as occurs with left ventricular failure), the body uses three neurohormonal compensatory mechanisms; these are effective for a short time but eventually become insufficient to meet the oxygen needs of the body.

First, the failing heart attempts to maintain a normal output of blood by enlarging its pumping chambers so that they can hold a greater volume of blood. This lengthening of the muscle fibers, called *ventricular dilation*, increases the amount of blood ejected from the heart. This compensatory mechanism has limits, because contractility of ventricular muscle fibers ceases to increase when they are stretched beyond a certain point.

During this *first compensatory phase*, the right ventricle continues to pump more blood into the lungs. Congestion occurs in the pulmonary circulation with accumulation of blood in the lungs. The immediate result is shortness of breath (most common symptom), and if the process continues, actual flooding of the air spaces of the lungs occurs, with fluid seeping from the distended blood vessels; this is called *pulmonary congestion* or *pulmonary edema*. Congestion in the vascular system interferes with the movement of body fluids in and out of the various fluid compartments, resulting in fluid accumulation in the tissue spaces and progressive edema.

During the *second compensatory phase*, the sympathetic nervous system responds to increase the stimulation of the heart muscle, causing it to pump more often. In response to failing contractility of the myocardial cells, the sympathetic nervous system activates adaptive processes that increase the heart rate and increase its muscle mass to strengthen the force of its contractions. This results in ventricular hypertrophy and a need for more oxygen.

Eventually, the coronary arteries cannot meet the oxygen demands of the enlarged myocardium, and the person may experience angina pectoris owing to ischemia. Secondary compensatory mechanisms activate the sympathetic nervous system and release endothelin from vascular linings, vasopressin (antidiuretic hormone) from the pituitary gland, and atrial natriuretic hormone from the heart.

The *third compensatory phase* involves activation of the renin–angiotensin–aldosterone system. With less blood coming from the heart, less blood passes through the kidneys. The kidneys respond by retaining water and sodium in an effort to increase blood volume, which further exacerbates tissue edema. The expanded blood volume increases the load on an already compromised heart. These mechanisms are responsible for the symptoms of diaphoresis, cool skin, tachycardia, cardiac arrhythmias, and oliguria (reduced urine excretion).

When the combined efforts of these three compensatory mechanisms achieve a normal level of cardiac output, the client is said to have compensated CHF. Ultimately, however, the body's efforts to compensate may backfire and produce higher blood volume, higher blood pressure, and more stress on the already weakened heart. The heart's ongoing failure to supply the body with blood compels the body to keep compensating in ways that further burden the heart, and the cycle perpetuates itself. When these mechanisms are no longer effective and the disease progresses to the final stage of impaired heart function, the client has decompensated CHF.

Decompensated CHF ranges from mild congestion with few symptoms to life-threatening fluid overload and total heart failure (Table 12-12). Symptoms usually develop very gradually so that many people do not recognize or report signals of serious disease. The older adult, in particular, may wrongly associate early symptoms with a lack of fitness or consider them a sign of aging. Confusion and impaired thinking can characterize heart failure in older adults.

Left-Sided Heart Failure. Failure of the left ventricle (Fig. 12-12) prevents the heart from pumping enough blood through the arterial system to meet the body's metabolic needs and causes either pulmonary edema or a disturbance in the respiratory control mechanisms. The degree of respiratory distress varies with the client's position, activity, and level of emotional or physical stress, but any of the symptoms listed under "Pulmonary Edema" in Chapter 15 may occur.

Table 12-12	Clinical Manifestations of Heart Failure

Left Ventricular Failure	Right Ventricular Failure
Progressive dyspnea (exertional first)	Dependent edema (ankle or pretibial first)
Paroxysmal nocturnal dyspnea	Jugular vein distention
Orthopnea	Abdominal pain and distention
Productive spasmodic cough	Weight gain
Pulmonary edema	Right upper quadrant pain (liver congestion)
Extreme breathlessness	Cardiac cirrhosis
Anxiety (associated with breathlessness)	Ascites
Frothy pink sputum	Jaundice
Nasal flaring	Anorexia, nausea
Accessory muscle use	Cyanosis (nail beds)
Crackles (formerly called rales)	Psychologic disturbances
Tachypnea	
Diaphoresis	
Cerebral hypoxia	
Irritability	
Restlessness	
Confusion	
Impaired memory	
Sleep disturbances	
Fatigue, exercise intolerance	
Muscular weakness	
Renal changes	

Dyspnea is subjective and does not always correlate with the extent of heart failure; exertional dyspnea occurs in all clients to some degree. Time for dyspnea to subside is an indication of progress or deterioration in a client's status, and it can be measured for documentation. Paroxysmal nocturnal dyspnea resembles the frightening sensation of awakening with suffocation. Once the client is in the upright position, relief from the attack may not occur for 30 minutes or longer. The client often assumes a three-point position, sitting up with both hands on the knees and leaning forward. In severe heart failure, the client may resort to sleeping upright in a chair or recliner. Other sleep disturbances may occur from central sleep apnea present in approximately 40% of all adults with heart failure.

Fatigue and *muscular weakness* are often associated with left ventricular failure because dyspnea develops along with weight gain and a faster resting heart rate, which decrease the person's ability to exercise. Inadequate cardiac output leads to decreased peripheral blood flow and blood flow to skeletal muscle. The resultant tissue hypoxia and slowed removal of metabolic wastes cause the person to tire easily. Disturbances in sleep and rest patterns may aggravate fatigue; muscle atrophy is common in advanced CHF.

Renal changes can occur in both right- and left-sided heart failure, but they are more evident with left-sided failure. During the day, the client is upright, decreased cardiac output reduces blood flow to the kidneys, and the formation of urine is reduced (oliguria). Sodium and water not excreted in the urine are retained in the vascular system, adding to the blood volume.

Diminished blood supply to the renal system causes the kidney to secrete renin, stimulating production of angiotensin, which causes vasoconstriction, thereby causing an increase in peripheral vascular resistance, increasing blood pressure and cardiac work, and resulting in worse heart failure. Renin secretion also indirectly stimulates the secretion of aldosterone from the adrenal gland. Aldosterone acts on the renal tubules, causing them to increase reabsorption of sodium and water, further increasing fluid volume. At night, urine formation increases with the recumbent position as blood flow to the kidney improves. *Nocturia* may interfere with effective sleep patterns, which contributes to fatigue as mentioned.

Right-Sided Heart Failure. Failure of the right ventricle (see Fig. 12-12) to adequately pump blood to the lungs results in peripheral edema and venous congestion of the organs. Symptoms result from congestion in the heart's right side and throughout the venous system (see Table 12-12; see also "Cor Pulmonale" in Chapter 15).

Dependent edema is one of the early signs of right ventricular failure, although significant CHF can be present in the absence of peripheral edema. In CHF, fluid is retained because the baroreceptors of the body sense a decreased volume of blood as a result of the heart's inability to pump an adequate amount of blood. The receptors subsequently relay a message to the kidneys to retain fluid so that a greater volume of blood can be ejected from the heart to the peripheral tissues. Unfortunately this compounds the problem and makes the heart work even harder, which further decreases its pumping ability, causing a sense of weakness and fatigue.

The retained fluid commonly accumulates in the extracellular spaces of the periphery. The resultant edema is usually symmetric and occurs in the dependent parts of the body, where venous pressure is the highest. In ambulatory persons, edema begins in the feet and ankles and ascends up the lower legs (pretibial areas). It is most noticeable at the end of a day and often decreases after a night's rest. In the recumbent person, pitting edema may develop in the presacral area and, as it worsens, progress to the medial thighs and genital area.

Jugular venous distention also results from fluid overload. The jugular veins empty unoxygenated blood directly into the superior vena cava. Because no cardiac valve exists to separate the superior vena cava from the right atrium, the jugular veins give information about activity on the right side of the heart. As fluid is retained and the heart's ability to pump is further compromised, the retained fluid backs up into both the lungs and the venous system, and the jugular veins reveal this. Jugular venous pulsations are examined by inspecting the silhouette of the neck with the person reclining at a 45-degree angle (Fig. 12-13). The right internal jugular vein is recommended because the left internal jugular may be falsely elevated in some people.

As the liver becomes congested with venous blood it becomes enlarged, and *abdominal pain* occurs. If this occurs rapidly, stretching of the capsule surrounding the liver causes severe discomfort, and the person may notice either a constant aching or a sharp *right upper quadrant pain*. In chronic CHF, longstanding congestion of the liver with venous blood and anoxia can lead to ascites (see Fig. 17-5) and jaundice, which are symptoms of liver damage. Anorexia, nausea, and bloating develop secondary

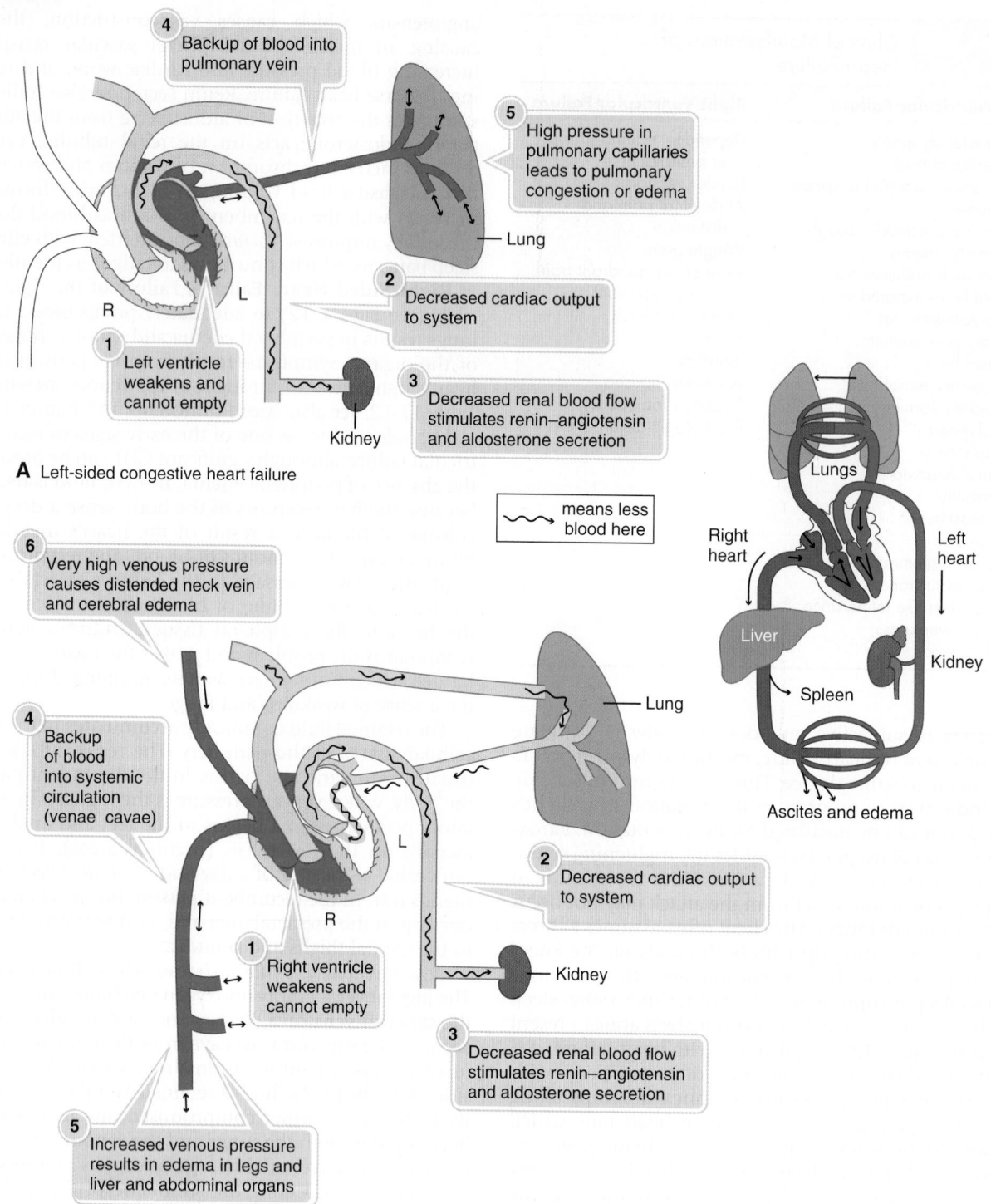

4 Backup of blood into pulmonary vein

5 High pressure in pulmonary capillaries leads to pulmonary congestion or edema

— Lung

R   L

2 Decreased cardiac output to system

1 Left ventricle weakens and cannot empty

Kidney

3 Decreased renal blood flow stimulates renin–angiotensin and aldosterone secretion

A Left-sided congestive heart failure

means less blood here

6 Very high venous pressure causes distended neck vein and cerebral edema

— Lung

4 Backup of blood into systemic circulation (venae cavae)

L

2 Decreased cardiac output to system

1 Right ventricle weakens and cannot empty

R

— Kidney

3 Decreased renal blood flow stimulates renin–angiotensin and aldosterone secretion

5 Increased venous pressure results in edema in legs and liver and abdominal organs

B Right-sided congestive heart failure

Lungs

Right heart

Left heart

Liver

Kidney

Spleen

Ascites and edema

Figure 12-12

Pathophysiologic mechanisms of congestive heart failure. A, Left-sided heart failure leads to pulmonary edema (see text description). **B,** Right ventricular failure causes peripheral edema that is most prominent in the lower extremities. *Inset,* Integration of the pulmonary and systemic circulation. When the heart contracts normally, it pumps blood simultaneously into both loops, but pump failure causes circulatory or pulmonary problems, depending on the underlying pathologic mechanism. (A and B from Gould B: *Pathophysiology for the health professions,* ed 2, Philadelphia, 2002, WB Saunders, p. 286; inset from Damjanov I: *Pathology for the health-related professions,* ed 3, Philadelphia, 2006, WB Saunders.)

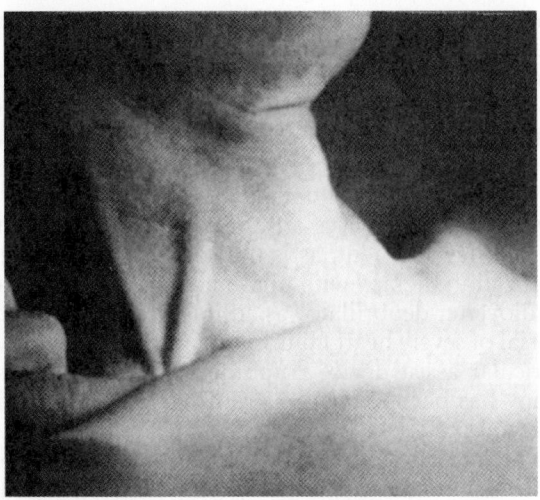

Figure 12-13

Jugular venous distention occurs bilaterally if there is a cardiac cause such as congestive heart failure; a unilateral distention indicates a localized problem. (From Daily EK, Schroeder JP: *Techniques in bedside hemodynamic monitoring,* ed 2, St Louis, 1981, Mosby.)

to venous congestion of the gastrointestinal (GI) tract. Anorexia and nausea may also result from digoxin toxicity, which is a common problem because digoxin is usually prescribed for CHF.

Cyanosis of the nail beds appears as venous congestion reduces peripheral blood flow. Clients with CHF often feel anxious, frightened, and depressed. Fears may be expressed as frightening nightmares, insomnia, acute anxiety states, depression, or withdrawal from reality.

Heart Failure with Preserved Ejection Fraction. HFpEF is characterized by a heart that is normal in size but with stiffness of the heart muscle both when relaxed and when contracting. These changes interfere with the diastole (filling) phase of heart function and present with symptoms of dyspnea, coughing, wheezing, and fatigue. If left untreated, pulmonary and peripheral edema can develop suddenly. Triggers for the development of this type of "flash" pulmonary edema include sudden surge of emotion or activity, high-fat meals, sudden excessive exercise, or forgetting to take prescription cardiovascular medications. Symptoms of heart failure but with an ejection fraction of 50% or greater defines HFpEF.

MEDICAL MANAGEMENT

DIAGNOSIS. Diagnosis is based on the clinical picture and depends on where symptoms are on the continuum of mild to severe. Because the two sides of the heart serve different functions, distinguishing the symptoms of left-sided heart failure from those of right-sided heart failure is critical in both diagnosis and treatment. Equally important is consideration of systolic and diastolic dysfunction, both of which indicate a functional or structural defect in the ventricles.

An echocardiogram is the main diagnostic tool; noninvasive cardiac tests such as ECG and chest radiography are secondary tools that can determine left ventricular size and function well enough to confirm the diagnosis. Cardiac catheterization is not routinely performed, but it

may be useful in certain cases (e.g., atherosclerotic heart disease, which is potentially correctable). Arterial blood gases are measured to evaluate oxygen saturation. Liver enzymes (e.g., aspartate transaminase, alkaline phosphatase) are often elevated (see Tables 40-5 and 40-18); liver involvement with hyperbilirubinemia commonly occurs, resulting in jaundice.

A new screening tool for individuals with suspected heart failure was introduced. Biomarkers, molecules that can be detected in blood of individuals with specific conditions (although they are undetectable or present at lower levels in healthy state), became an important supplement for confirming a diagnosis. Measuring B-type natriuretic peptide, a protein secreted from the cardiac atria in response to wall tension and pressure overload, can reliably predict the presence or absence of heart failure, even helping to identify when dyspnea is associated with heart failure or some other underlying pathologic condition.[285] In addition to the natriuretic peptides, assessment of other biomarker types may be useful in people with heart failure. The candidate biomarkers may indicate myocyte stretch or necrosis, oxidative stress and systemic inflammation, and other processes in the diseased heart.[458]

PREVENTION AND TREATMENT. Managing heart failure begins with treatment of the underlying cause whenever possible. Nonpharmacologic interventions such as diet and exercise that alter interactions between the heart and the periphery are now accepted therapeutic approaches.

Alterations in lifestyle reduce symptoms and the need for additional medication. There is an urgent need to develop more effective strategies for the prevention and treatment of this increasingly common disorder. Multiple comorbidities in older clients require a multidisciplinary approach to management. Persons with CHF are placed on a sodium-restricted diet, sometimes with limited fluid intake. Emotional and physical rest during the initial phases of intervention is also important in diminishing the workload of the heart.

Activity and Exercise. Traditionally, the diagnosis of CHF was a contraindication for participation in exercise training because of concerns that further decline in cardiac function would occur. It is now clear that activity restriction is no longer appropriate, because exercise programs have proved to quantitatively achieve results similar to those attained with most effective drug therapies. These findings have shifted attention away from treating the heart toward exercising the muscles.

Whenever possible, physical activity and exercise are prescribed per client tolerance. Physical training for clients with CHF results in an increase in muscular strength and better adaptation to effort owing to the effect of training on skeletal muscles (e.g., decreased vascular resistance in the muscles, delay in the onset of anaerobic metabolism). Determined to be a safe therapy for individuals with CHF,[244] exercise training also improves exercise and functional capacities,[216,362] reduces symptoms, improves health[244] and psychosocial status, and provides a modest reduction for future cardiac events.[244] Resistance training combined with short or long bouts of aerobic exercise is also beneficial for people with CHF.[82]

Pharmacotherapy. Pharmacologic therapy is now responsive to the updated understanding of CHF as a cascade of neurohormonal events centered on ventricular remodeling. Pharmacologic agents are used to reduce the heart's workload, increase muscle strength and contraction, and inhibit neuroendocrine responses to heart failure (see Tables 12-5 and 12-6).

ACE inhibitors have become standard therapy for heart failure because of their ability to block the renin–angiotensin–aldosterone system, increasing renal blood flow and decreasing renal vascular resistance, thereby enhancing diuresis. ACE inhibitors reduce left ventricular filling pressure and moderately increase cardiac output. Vasodilator therapy in combination with ACE inhibitors prolongs life in persons with moderate to severe heart failure.

Diuretics are used to control fluid buildup and prevent congestion, and digoxin may be added to stimulate the heart's pumping action if symptoms persist despite treatment with ACE inhibitors and diuretics. Angiotensin II receptor antagonists have been added to function as an antihypertensive and enhance the clearance of sodium and water.

The β-blockers, once rarely considered in the treatment of CHF, are effective in reducing symptoms, improving clinical status, reducing hospitalizations, and reducing the risk of death. Combining β-blockers with ACE inhibitors can produce additive effects on two neurohormonal systems (renin–angiotensin system and sympathetic nervous system).

Surgery. Surgical intervention may include CABG (see Fig. 12-4) for underlying myocardial ischemia and infarction; reconstruction of incompetent heart valves; ventricular remodeling or heart reduction (e.g., Batista procedure, in which a piece of the heart tissue is removed and the heart muscle is sutured back together, making a smaller, tauter heart with a stronger heartbeat); internal counterpulsation (Fig. 12-14) or external counterpulsation, which uses an external pump or balloon to adjust the aortic blood pressure; temporary ventricular assistive devices for people unable to come off bypass (see Chapter 21); and use of an artificial heart or cardiac transplantation.

The implantation of skeletal muscle (removed from the individual's thigh and multiplied in the laboratory) into the postinfarction scar after infarction in the case of severe ischemic heart failure has been shown experimentally to improve heart function.[301] A review of surgical innovations for chronic heart failure in the context of cardiopulmonary rehabilitation for the therapist is available.[215] (See also "Atherosclerosis: Treatment" above and "Heart Transplantation" in Chapter 21.)

Cardiac transplantation is now more common for treatment of heart failure. Transplantation is successful for selected individuals, usually those who are treated early in the course of heart failure, before advanced symptoms develop. Reform of the selection process is recommended to identify people who, although not critically ill, will not survive without early transplantation. See further discussion in Chapter 21.

A pacemaker-like device designed to deliver electrical stimulation to the ventricles (biventricular pacing) in an effort to improve the heart's overall cardiac efficiency by coordinating the heart's contractions (both ventricles pump at the same time, making the heart pump more forcefully) has been approved by the FDA. This technique, referred to as cardiac resynchronization therapy, is available on a limited basis for selected individuals with severe heart failure. The results are promising for people who because of age criteria or lack of donor hearts are not able to undergo cardiac transplantation.

Other similar devices are under continued investigation and development, as is the combined use of resynchronization therapy with pharmacologic therapy and/or a cardioverter-defibrillator as adjunct treatment for CHF. Reversal of severe heart failure with a continuous-flow left ventricular assist device combined with pharmacologic therapy has been shown to produce significant myocardial recovery.[54]

Self-care. American Heart Association has issued a scientific statement on promoting self-care for individuals with heart failure,[385] advocating for self-care as a method of improving outcomes from heart failure. Self-care is defined as a "naturalistic decision-making process that patients use in the choice of behaviors that maintain physiological stability (symptom monitoring and treatment adherence) and the response to symptoms when they occur".

Specific self-care behavior include medication adherence, symptom monitoring, dietary adherence, fluid and alcohol restriction, weight lost, exercise, smoking cessation, preventive behaviors (personal hygiene, dental health, immunizations etc.), and nonprescription medication taking. There is a variety of factors that make self-care difficult, including comorbid conditions, depression, anxiety, age-related issues, impaired cognition, sleep disturbances, poor health literacy, and problems with the health care system. Skill development, behavioral changes, and family support are recognized interventions that promote self-care. Poor quality of life and early mortality in individuals with heart failure may be reduced if the people are actively engaged in consistent self-care.[385]

PROGNOSIS. Treatment of CHF remains difficult, and the prognosis is poor, even with recent advances in pharmacologic therapy. Annual mortality rates range from 10% in stable clients with mild symptoms to greater than 50% in people with advanced, progressive symptoms. Approximately 40% to 50% of clients with heart failure die suddenly, probably owing to ventricular arrhythmias.

To achieve the maximal benefit from drug therapy, symptoms must be recognized as early as possible and intervention initiated. Because this condition often develops gradually, intervention is delayed, full resolution is not usually possible, and CHF becomes a chronic disorder.

Exercise capacity was the most powerful predictor of survival in CHF, but a new test that measures swings in heart rate during the day has been developed that can identify individuals who are at the highest risk of dying from CHF. The test measures the amount by which the heart rate changes from slow rates to fast rates in one 24-hour period. The less the heart rate varies over 24 hours, the more likely a person is to die of CHF.[330]

Other signs of poor prognosis include severe left ventricular dysfunction, severe symptoms and limitation of

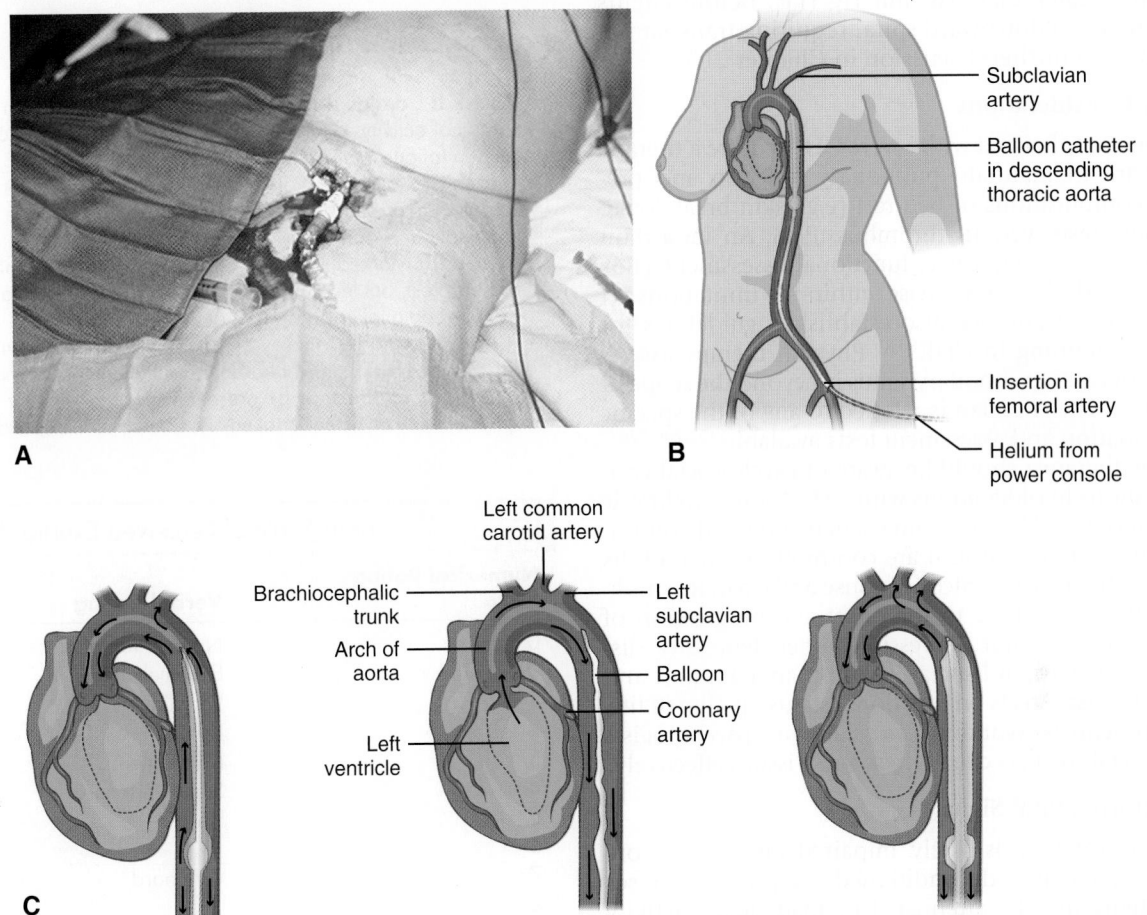

Figure 12-14

The intraaortic balloon pump is a common type of cardiac assist device that is used to improve myocardial oxygen supply–demand for individuals with deteriorating hemodynamics or ongoing ischemia, as evidenced by rest pain or electrocardiographic changes in the region of the infarct. The primary functions of balloon counterpulsation are to reperfuse the coronary arteries at the end of systole and reduce the left ventricular afterload (the amount of work the ventricle must do), thereby decreasing myocardial oxygen consumption and improving cardiac output. These intravascular catheter-mounted counterpulsation devices are traditionally used for cases of cardiogenic shock following cardiac surgery or an acute myocardial infarction as well as for people who have chronic end-stage heart failure and who are not candidates for long-term ventricular assistive device support. The rationale for intraaortic balloon pump counterpulsation in this latter situation is to maintain systemic perfusion and preserve end-organ function until cardiac transplantation occurs. **A,** The catheter is usually placed through the femoral artery, and the balloon is moved up the iliac artery to the descending aorta, where it is then placed, **B,** above the renal arteries and below the subclavian artery. This position is critical in order to prevent ischemia to the upper extremities or kidneys. **C,** When the heart contracts (systole), the balloon is deflated, creating a decline in aortic pressure. After the heart contracts (during diastole), the balloon is filled with air, causing the blood to regurgitate back toward the root of the aorta, thereby perfusing the coronary arteries. When the left ventricle is ready to pump, the balloon is deflated (cardiac systole again), reducing ventricular afterload. (**A,** courtesy Chris Wells, PT, MS, PhD, University of Pittsburgh Medical Center, 2001. **B,** from Black JM, Hawks JH, Keene AM: *Medical-surgical nursing: clinical management for positive outcomes,* ed 7, Philadelphia, 2005, WB Saunders. **C,** from Lewis SL, Heitkemper MM, Dirksen SR: *Medical surgical nursing: assessment and management of surgical problems,* ed 7, St Louis, 2007, Mosby.)

exercise capacity, secondary renal insufficiency, and elevated plasma catecholamine levels.

SPECIAL IMPLICATIONS FOR THE THERAPIST   12-7

Congestive Heart Failure

Therapists have a unique role in the prevention, medical management, and rehabilitation of people with heart failure. Physical therapists can provide programs that profoundly improve the exercise tolerance and functional status of individuals with CHF.

Medical intervention can be more objectively implemented by using information obtained during physical therapy assessments and interventions. Tests such as the 6-minute walk test may be helpful in predicting peak oxygen consumption and early survival, as well as in implementing a proper exercise conditioning program for people with advanced heart failure.[59]

Education of physicians and other health care professionals about the role of the physical therapist in defining prescriptive exercise is important.[35] Consideration for the complex pathologic conditions and comorbidities of people in this population is an important contribution to cardiac rehabilitation from the physical therapist's training. Clients should be referred to rehabilitation before the VO_{2max} drops below 14 mL/kg/min and when the wedge pressure is still greater than 16 mm Hg (i.e., before clients progress in a downward spiral requiring transplantation). (See further discussion in Chapter 21.)

Early Considerations

Clients hospitalized with severe CHF require a therapy program to maintain pulmonary function and prevent complications of bed rest (e.g., skin breakdown, venous stasis, venous thrombus, PEs). An important aspect of intervention is functional assessment (Box 12-10) and physical exercise within the limitations set by the physician. See also established guidelines for exercise training in CHF.[80,81] Physical therapy assessment of cardiopulmonary status is beyond the scope of this text. The clinician is referred to any of the specific examination and assessment texts available.[157,206,220]

The therapist should be aware of psychosocial considerations in older adults with CHF. Neuropsychiatric conditions such as Alzheimer's dementia and complications such as delirium are common in older adults with CHF. Persistent alcohol abuse and cigarette smoking often contribute to the onset and progression of heart failure. Major depression, other depressive disorders, anxiety, and social isolation are common and have adverse effects on functional status, quality of life, and prognosis. Working as a team with psychologists and social workers can address these issues effectively.

Monitoring Vital Signs

Aerobic capacity is likely impaired and even more so if the client is deconditioned; adaptive responses to activity may be attenuated or inadequate; activity may exacerbate cardiovascular pump dysfunction; and signs of fatigue and shortness of breath are common. The downward cycle of disease, deconditioning, decreased activity, and disability necessitates the monitoring of vital signs.[71] Progressing activities from bed rest to transfers or ambulation requires vital sign assessment immediately after the major activity and 3 minutes later to assess for return to baseline. Oxygen can be assessed through pulse oximetry and/or blood gas analysis and the amount needed can be determined by the therapist in consultation with the patient's physician. Oxygen may be administered by mask or cannula; team members should consult respiratory therapy staff to determine appropriate oxygen levels during exercise.

Monitor the client for signs of increasing peripheral edema by assessing jugular neck vein distention, peripheral edema in the legs or sacrum, and any report of right upper quadrant pain. In the outpatient or home health setting, the client is advised to call the nurse or physician if shoes, belt, or pants become too tight to fasten, usual activities of daily living or tasks become difficult, extra sleep is needed, or urination at night becomes more frequent.

Monitoring blood pressure is essential to detect heart failure; observe for decreasing blood pressure and report any change in status to the nurse or physician immediately. Observe for flat or falling systolic blood pressure in response to activity indicative of

---

NEW YORK HEART ASSOCIATION'S FUNCTIONAL CLASSIFICATION OF HEART DISEASE

- **Class I:** Cardiac disease present but no limitation on physical activity. Ordinary physical activity does not cause undue fatigue, palpitation, dyspnea, or anginal pain.
- **Class II:** Slight limitation on physical activity. Comfortable at rest, but ordinary physical activity results in fatigue, palpitation, dyspnea, or anginal pain.
- **Class III:** Marked limitation of physical activity. Comfortable at rest, but less than ordinary physical activity causes fatigue, palpitation, dyspnea, or anginal pain.
- **Class IV:** Unable to carry on any physical activity without discomfort. Symptoms of cardiac insufficiency or of the anginal syndrome may be present even at rest. If any physical activity is undertaken, discomfort is increased.

Table 12-13 Borg Scale of Perceived Exertion*

Numerical Rating Scale	Verbal Rating
0	No exertion at all
0.5	Extremely light
1	Very light
2	Light
3	Moderate
4	Somewhat hard
5	Hard
6	
7	Very hard
8	
9	
10	Very, very hard
—	Maximal exertion

*Using a perceived exertion scale is a useful approach to activity prescription. The individual is asked to identify a desirable rating of perceived exertion and uses that level of intensity as a daily guideline for activity. A suggested rating of perceived exertion for most healthy individuals is 3 to 5 (moderate to hard on the scale); for the compromised person, a more moderate level of perceived exertion may be recommended by the physician.

Modified from Borg GA: Psychosocial bases of perceived exertion, *Med Sci Sports Exerc* 472:194–381, 1982.

---

inadequate pump function (a linear increase of systolic blood pressure with increased activity should be seen). Exaggerated increases in heart rate may be observed as the heart attempts to maintain adequate cardiac output. Observe for dyspnea at rest and/or with activity, and auscultate for changes from baseline during activity.[71] (See also Appendix B.)

Continuous supervision and frequent monitoring of blood pressure are necessary when starting an exercise program for someone with CHF. RPE should range from 11 to 14 (light to somewhat hard; Table 12-13). Anginal symptoms should not exceed 2 on the 0 to 4 angina scale (moderate to bothersome), and exertional dyspnea should not exceed a rating of mild, some difficulty with activity. Initially, full resuscitation equipment should be available.[62]

Positioning

Positioning is important, and the client is taught to use a high Fowler position (head of the bed elevated at least 20 inches above the level position) or chair to reduce pulmonary congestion, facilitate diaphragmatic expansion and ventilation, and ease dyspnea.

The legs are maintained in a dependent position as much as possible to decrease venous return. Range of motion to decrease venous pooling and monitoring for the development of thrombophlebitis (e.g., unilateral swelling, calf pain, pallor) are required.

Activity in the upright position is preferred (again because of increased venous return in the supine position); this guideline should apply during pool activities as well. Monitoring vital signs is important as these individuals can deteriorate at any time. Extra caution is advised if the systolic blood pressure is less than 80 mm Hg and resting heart rate is less than 50 beats/min or more than 100 beats/min. Worsening orthopnea may be suspected if the individual requires more and more pillows in the upright position.

Exercise and Congestive Heart Failure

The best guideline is to customize initial exercise intensity for each individual,[476] keeping in mind the individual's goals and expected outcomes (e.g., preparation for transplantation, improved functional daily living, perceived quality of life). This point cannot be over emphasized. Exercise should be avoided immediately after eating or after taking vasodilator medication. Using an interval training approach is helpful with those individuals who demonstrate marked exercise intolerance.

The American College of Sports Medicine's guidelines[17] suggest that CHF clients entering an exercise program should start with moderate-intensity exercise (40%-60% VO_{2max}) for a duration of 2 to 6 minutes, followed by 2 minutes of rest. Blood pressure and heart rhythm should be routinely monitored at rest, during peak exercise, and after cool-down. The goal is to gradually increase the intensity and duration of exercise.

Others advocate starting CHF clients at a low to moderate exercise intensity (less than 40% VO_{2max}) with a shorter duration of exercise initially and a shorter rest period of less than 2 minutes). Recommendations for interval exercise training (following work phases of 30 seconds by recovery phases of 60 seconds) have also been reported.[302]

Symptoms and general fatigue level serve as a guideline to determine frequency, and warm-up/cool-down periods should be longer than normal for observation of possible arrhythmias. This is especially important for anyone with heart failure with preserved ejection fraction as they are prone to atrial fibrillation and subsequent risk of blood clots and stroke. These individuals are also prone to a condition called *chronotropic incompetence*, difficulty getting the heart rate to increase during exercise.[403]

For anyone with heart failure, determination of appropriate exercise intensity based on 40% to 60% VO_{2max} is recommended (rather than based on heart rate peak) because the response to exercise is frequently abnormal. Alternatively, the initial exercise intensity should be 10 beats below any significant symptoms, including angina, exertional hypotension, arrhythmias, and dyspnea.

Rehabilitation personnel must observe for symptoms of cardiac decompensation during exercise, including cough or dyspnea, hypotension, light-headedness, cyanosis, angina, and arrhythmias. Exercise progression following these recommendations is available in detail[62]; see also "Monitoring Vital Signs" above. Endurance exercise training modifies neuroendocrine activation in heart failure and may have a long-term beneficial impact.[63]

The therapist should keep in mind that some older CHF clients are unable to increase their exercise intensity or duration despite starting very slowly. These people do not achieve the goal of increased endurance and often leave the program owing to increased symptoms and exercise intolerance. Maintaining or even improving functional activities and independence at home may be more appropriate goals for this group. An excellent review of exercise assessment, exercise training, and exercise training guidelines in heart failure for all clients is available.[79,80]

Medications

Diuretics can produce mild to severe electrolyte imbalance requiring special consideration (see Chapter 5). A small drop in the serum potassium level can precipitate digoxin poisoning (digoxin toxicity) and serious arrhythmias, as a consequence of digoxin competing with potassium ions for binding to its target, sodium-potassium pump. This situation is a life-threatening condition and may present with systemic or cardiac manifestations. In the past it occurred in one of every five people. The occurrence of digoxin toxicity has decreased over the years because of less usage, lower doses, and better monitoring, and today occurs in approximately 1% to 4% of patients.[6,164] Any sign or symptom of digoxin toxicity (see Table 12-5) should be reported to the physician.

Digoxin toxicity may occur at therapeutic levels (less than 2.0 ng/mL); however, it usually occurs when plasma levels are greater than 2 ng/mL. Side effects from digoxin can occur when digoxin levels are within the therapeutic range, but the serum albumin level is low (less than 3.5 g/dL; see Table 40-5) because digoxin binds to albumin in the serum. If the serum albumin level is low, digoxin may not be bound to albumin and will be circulating as "free" digoxin producing toxic effects. It is possible, however, for the digoxin toxicity to occur when digoxin blood levels are in therapeutic range and albumin levels are normal. Albumin levels are not always abnormal when side effects occur.

Digoxin toxicity can cause a dip in the ST segment on ECG; whenever possible, the ECG should be monitored during exercise. Activity should not increase the magnitude of the altered ST segment. A physical therapist should watch for a low, irregular pulse (less than 60 beats/min); the heart rate normally increases to compensate for CHF, but in the presence of digoxin, heart rate decreases.

NSAIDs, including nonprescription drugs such as ibuprofen, increase fluid retention independently and significantly blunt the action of diuretics and other cardiovascular drugs (especially ACE inhibitors), exacerbating preexisting CHF and causing isolated lower extremity edema. The major consideration for exercise in clients taking ACE inhibitors is the possibility of hypotension and accompanying arrhythmias. These problems should be reported to the physician and can be addressed by maintaining proper hydration and by altering dosages and the simultaneous use of other medications.

Orthostatic (Postural) Hypotension

Definition and Overview

The term *orthostatic (postural) hypotension* signifies a decrease of 20 mm Hg or greater in systolic blood pressure or a drop of 10 mm Hg or more in both systolic and diastolic arterial blood pressure with a concomitant pulse increase of 15 beats/min or more on standing from a supine or sitting position.

Orthostatic hypotension may be acute and temporary or chronic. Orthostatic hypotension occurs frequently in older adults and occurs in more than one half of all frail, older adults, contributing significantly to morbidity from syncope, falls, vital organ ischemia (e.g., MI, transient ischemic attacks), and mortality among older adults with diabetic hypertension. It is highly variable over time but most prevalent in the morning when supine blood pressure is highest and on first arising.

Etiologic Factors

Orthostatic hypotension is recognized in all groups as a cardinal feature of autonomic nervous dysfunction as well as other nonneurogenic etiologies (Box 12-11). In young adults, orthostatic intolerance and tachycardia may be associated with norepinephrine transporter deficiency.

Box 12-11

CAUSES OF ORTHOSTATIC HYPOTENSION

- Volume depletion (e.g., burns, diabetes mellitus, sodium or potassium depletion)
  - Side effects of alcohol and other drugs that cause volume depletion (e.g., antidepressants, antihypertensives, diuretics, ACE inhibitors, vasodilators)
- Venous pooling (e.g., pregnancy, varicosities of the legs)
- Prolonged immobility
- Starvation, malnutrition, alcoholism, eating disorders
- Performing Valsalva maneuver
- Sluggish normal regulatory mechanisms (e.g., anatomic variation, altered body chemistry)
- Autonomic nervous system dysregulation (e.g., diabetes mellitus, Parkinson disease, aging, fibromyalgia syndrome, chronic renal failure)

Data from Bonow RO: *Braunwald's heart disease—a textbook of cardiovascular medicine*, ed 9, Philadelphia, 2011, WB Saunders.

A single gene coding a protein that clears norepinephrine does not function in some individuals, pointing to a genetic etiology.

Postural reflexes are slowed as part of the aging process for some, but not all, persons. Normal aging is associated with various changes that may lead to postural hypotension. Cardiac output falls with age; in the older adult with hypertension, it is even lower. When subjects older than age 65 years are put under passive postural stress (60-degree upright tilt), their stroke volume falls even further. These normal changes obviously predispose the aging adult to postural hypotension from any process that further reduces fluid volume or vascular integrity. For example, pooling of blood after eating may lead to profound hypotension, called *postprandial hypotension*.

In addition, as systolic pressure rises from atherosclerosis, baroreceptor sensitivity and vascular compliance are reduced further, increasing the likelihood of postural hypotension. In the older adult with hypertension and CVD receiving vasoactive drugs, the circulatory adjustments to maintain blood pressure are disturbed, leaving the person vulnerable to postural hypotension.[243]

Drugs are a major cause of orthostatic hypotension in the aging adult. Many have effects on the autonomic nervous system, both centrally and peripherally, and on fluid balance. Diuretics, calcium channel blockers, nitrates, and L-dopa have hypotensive effects. Antidepressants are a common, overlooked cause of orthostasis, even though this is a known side effect of these medications. A general result of treatment for hypertension may be hypotension. In addition, many older adults with systolic hypertension have postural hypotension that may require management before the hypertension is addressed.

Chronic orthostatic hypotension may occur secondary to a specific disease, such as endocrine disorders, metabolic disorders, nephropathy, or neurogenic disorders affecting the autonomic or central nervous systems. Alcohol and drugs such as vincristine used in the treatment of cancer can cause autonomic neuropathy.

Pathogenesis

Orthostasis is a physiologic stress related to upright posture. When a normal individual stands up, the gravitational changes on the circulation are compensated for by several mechanisms, including the circulatory and autonomic nervous systems. On standing, the force of gravity in the vertical axis causes venous pooling in the lower limbs, a sharp decline in venous return, and reduction in filling pressure of the heart, which increase further on prolonged standing because of shifting of water to interstitial spaces and hemoconcentration.

These mechanical events can cause a marked reduction in cardiac output and consequent fall in arterial blood pressure. In healthy people, cardiac output and blood pressure regulation are maintained by powerful compensatory mechanisms involving a rise in heart rate. Blood pressure is maintained by a rise in peripheral resistance. These compensatory mechanisms are initiated by the baroreceptors located in the aortic arch and carotid bifurcation. Orthostatic hypotension results from failure of the arterial baroreflex, most commonly because of disorders of the autonomic nervous system.[243]

In people with autonomic failure or dysreflexia (e.g., Parkinson disease, aging, diabetes, fibromyalgia), orthostatic hypotension results from an impaired capacity to increase vascular resistance during standing. This dysfunction leads to increased downward pooling of venous blood and a consequent reduction in stroke volume and cardiac output that exaggerates the orthostatic fall in blood pressure.

Approximately 80% of the blood pooled in the lower limb is contained in the upper leg (thighs, buttocks) with less pooling in the calf and foot. The location of the additional venous pooling has not been clearly identified, but present data suggest the abdominal compartment and perhaps leg skin vasculature. The pooled blood in the veins of the feet and calves is arterial in origin in that it arises as a result of decreased venous drainage of that region.

In contrast, the blood pooled in the thighs, buttocks, pelvis, and abdomen arises primarily from venous reflux. The pooled blood is not actually stagnant; its mean circulatory time through the dependent region is merely increased by changes in the pressure gradient across the vascular bed and by increases in venous volume. The identification of venous pooling may offer insights for intervention techniques in the future.

Clinical Manifestations

Orthostatic hypotension is often accompanied by dizziness, blurring or loss of vision, and syncope or fainting. There are three main modes of presentation in the older adult: (1) falls or mobility problems, (2) acute or chronic mental confusion, and (3) cardiac symptoms.

A common clinical picture is the person whose legs give way when attempting to stand, usually after prolonged recumbency, after physical exertion, or in a warm environment. These episodes may be accompanied by confusion, pallor, tremor, and unsteadiness. Loss of consciousness may cause frequent falls and additional injuries that can be quite serious. Ischemic neck pain in the suboccipital and paracervical region is often reported by individuals with autonomic failure and orthostatic hypotension.[58]

Other reported ischemic symptoms of orthostatic hypotension are nonspecific, such as lethargy, weakness, low backache, calf claudication, and angina. Some older adults may experience unexpected and unexplained falls associated with orthostatic hypotension. The cause of such falls may be circulatory impairment that results in a drop in blood pressure on standing upright quickly. Orthostatic hypotension may be an early sign of some other illness or the effects of medication.

MEDICAL MANAGEMENT

There are several general and specific approaches to the management of orthostatic hypotension but no curative intervention for orthostatic hypotension of unknown cause. Prevention is important, and whenever the underlying disorder causing hypotension is corrected, symptoms cease. Nonneurogenic causes, such as diminished intravascular volume, are treated specifically. In orthostatic hypotension caused by autonomic failure there are considerable difficulties in reestablishing sympathetic or parasympathetic efferent activity.

Tilt study or tilt-table testing may be used to assess hypotension by monitoring blood pressure and pulse while tilting a person from horizontal supine to 60 degrees upright. This test has proved very valuable in determining the cause of dizziness or syncope and can reveal irregularities in the vascular regulating system. A combination of general measures and pharmacologic measures is needed in the management of neurogenic postural hypotension.[186]

SPECIAL IMPLICATIONS FOR THE THERAPIST ▸ 12-8

Orthostatic Hypotension

Many medications used to treat hypertension can result in hypotension, especially when combined with interventions or exercise that result in vasodilation. Of particular concern are heat modalities, such as the whirlpool or Hubbard tank. In addition, moderate to vigorous exercise of large muscle groups can produce significant vasodilation and can result in hypotension. This is particularly true following exercise, when venous return diminishes as exercise abruptly ceases. A cool-down period is essential, and safety measures must be employed.[466] Aerobic conditioning is an important part of treatment for orthostatic hypotension resulting from autonomic insufficiency, perhaps best accomplished through aquatic exercise therapy.[186]

Stationary standing, as is performed in many activities of daily living, can produce hypotension, especially among those individuals with autonomic failure. With autonomic failure, symptoms of postural hypotension are increased on standing after exercise. The therapist can instruct the individual in protective measures that reduce excessive orthostatic blood pooling, including avoidance of precipitating factors.

Anyone with orthostatic hypotension, especially persons taking antihypertensive agents, should be instructed to rise slowly from the bed or chair after a long period of recumbency or sitting to avoid loss of balance and prevent falls. Dorsiflexing the feet (ankle pumps), raising the arms overhead with diaphragmatic breathing, and abdominal compression before standing often promote venous return to the heart, accelerate the pulse, and increase blood pressure.

The use of abdominal binders and elastic stockings may also help with venous return. Stockings should not be taken off at night to avoid falls when getting up to go to the bathroom or when getting out of bed in the morning. Elevating the head of the bed 5 to 20 degrees prevents the nocturnal diuresis and supine hypertension caused by nocturnal shifts of interstitial fluid from the legs to the rest of the circulation. Eating small meals may help to avoid postprandial (after eating) hypotension.

The person who becomes hypotensive should assume a supine position with legs elevated to increase venous return and to ensure cerebral blood flow. As previously mentioned, this position must be monitored carefully for anyone with orthostatic hypotension and CHF, possibly requiring modifying the position to include slight head and upper body

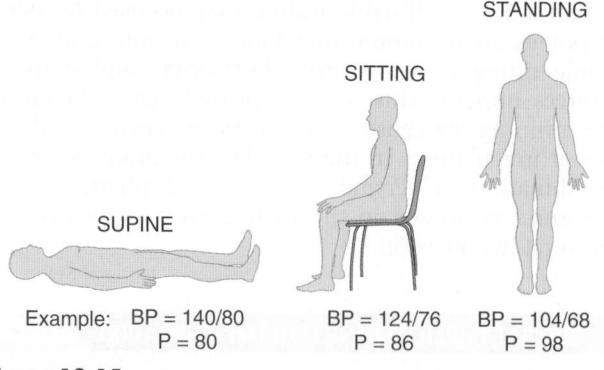

STANDING

SITTING

SUPINE

Example: BP = 140/80   BP = 124/76   BP = 104/68
           P = 80   P = 86   P = 98

Figure 12-15

Assessing postural hypotension. After measuring the blood pressure (BP) and pulse (P) in the supine position, leave the blood pressure cuff in place and assist the person in sitting. Remeasure the blood pressure within 15 to 30 seconds. Assist the person in standing, and measure again. A drop of more than 20 mm Hg systolic and more than 10 mm Hg diastolic accompanied by a 10%-20% increase in heart rate (pulse) indicates postural hypotension. Sample measurements are given. (From Black JM, Hawks JH, Keene AM: *Medical-surgical nursing: clinical management for positive outcomes,* ed 7, Philadelphia, 2005, WB Saunders.)

elevation. Crossing the legs, which involves contraction of the agonist and antagonist muscles, also has been shown to increase cardiac output, thereby increasing blood pressure.[424]

The physician should be notified if the person remains symptomatic after these measures have been taken. Anyone who is considered borderline hypotensive when tested in the supine position should have blood pressures measured and pulses counted in a sitting position with the legs dangling. If no change occurs when this is done, repeat the measurements with the person standing, if possible. A drop in systolic pressure of 10 to 20 mm Hg or more that is associated with an increase in pulse rate of more than 15 beats/min suggests depleted intravascular volume (Fig. 12-15). Some normovolemic persons with peripheral neuropathies or those taking antihypertensive medications may demonstrate an orthostatic fall in blood pressure but without an associated increase in pulse rate.

Myocardial Disease

Myocarditis

Myocarditis is a relatively uncommon acute or chronic inflammatory condition of the muscular walls of the heart (myocardium). It has now been reclassified by the American Heart Association as an acquired (inflammatory) cardiomyopathy.[292]

It is most often a result of bacterial or viral infection, but it also includes those inflammatory processes related to infectious and noninfectious causes of ischemic heart disease. Other possible causes of myocarditis include chest radiation for treatment of malignancy, sarcoidosis, and drugs, such as lithium, interleukin-2, and cocaine.

The therapist is most likely to treat the person with systemic lupus erythematosus (SLE; see Chapter 7) who may have a type of myocarditis called *lupus carditis* (see also "The Heart in Collagen Vascular Diseases: Lupus Carditis" below). SLE is a multisystem autoimmune disease characterized by a release of autoantibodies into the circulation, with a subsequent inflammatory process that can target the heart and vasculature.

Myocarditis typically evolves through active, healing, and healed stages that are characterized by inflammatory cell infiltrates leading to interstitial edema and focal myocyte necrosis with replacement fibrosis over time. Ventricular tachyarrhythmias develop as a result of the pathologic changes' creating an electrically unstable environment.[292]

Clinical evidence of cardiac involvement is found in up to 50% of all people with SLE. Clinical manifestations may include mild continuous chest pain or soreness in the epigastric region or under the sternum, palpitations, fatigue, and dyspnea; and onset may follow a viral upper respiratory tract illness in the population at large as well as in persons with SLE. Complications include heart failure, arrhythmias, dilated (congestive) cardiomyopathy (see next section), and sudden death.

Myocarditis usually resolves with treatment of the underlying condition or cause; specific antimicrobial therapy is prescribed if an infectious agent can be identified. Viral myocarditis is treated with medications that improve cardiac output and reduce arrhythmias, if present.

Management of myocarditis in SLE is usually with corticosteroids, but immunosuppressive agents may be required. Myocarditis that progresses to dilated cardiomyopathy with heart failure is frequently fatal without heart transplantation.

SPECIAL IMPLICATIONS FOR THE THERAPIST   12-9

Myocarditis

Active myocarditis is considered a contraindication for therapy, because this condition can progress very quickly and stress must be avoided; each case is evaluated by the physician. Athletes in whom myocarditis is suspected or diagnosed should discontinue all sports for 6 months after onset of symptoms. Preparticipation evaluation of cardiac function is essential before resuming sports activities. An athlete can resume competing when ventricular function and cardiac dimensions return to normal and clinically significant arrhythmias are absent on ambulatory monitoring.[124]

If an impairment of myocardial contractility is present, diastolic blood pressure may be elevated to maintain stroke volume. Disruptions leading to lethal cardiac arrhythmias cannot be predicted. (See also "Special Implications for the Therapist 12-14: Infective Endocarditis" and "Special Implications for the Therapist 12-15: Rheumatic Fever and Heart Disease.")

Cardiomyopathy

Definition and Overview. Cardiomyopathy is actually part of a group of conditions affecting the heart muscle itself, so that contraction and relaxation of

Table 12-14	AHA Classification of Cardiomyopathies

Primary*	Secondary†
Genetic	**Infiltrative**
• Hypertrophic cardiomyopathy	Amyloidosis
• Arrhythmogenic right ventricular cardiomyopathy/dysplasia (rare)	Gaucher disease (genetic/familial)
• Left ventricular noncompaction	Hurler disease (genetic/familial)
• Conduction defects	Hunter disease (genetic/familial)
• Ion channel disorders	**Storage**
Mixed (genetic and nongenetic)	Hemochromatosis
• Dilated cardiomyopathy	Glycogen storage disease
• Restrictive (nonhypertrophied; rare)	Niemann-Pick disease (genetic/familial)
Acquired	**Toxicity**
• Myocarditis (inflammatory cardiomyopathy)	Drugs, heavy metals, chemical agents
• Stress-induced	**Endomyocardial fibrosis**
• Peripartum/postpartum (rare)	**Inflammatory** (sarcoidosis)
• Infants of mothers with insulin dependent diabetes mellitus	**Endocrine**
	Diabetes
	Hyperthyroidism
	Hypothyroidism
	Hyperparathyroidism
	Pheochromocytoma
	Acromegaly
	Neuromuscular/neurologic
	Friedrich ataxia disease (genetic/familial)
	Muscular dystrophy (genetic/familial)
	Neurofibromatosis (genetic/familial)
	Tuberous sclerosis
	Nutritional deficiencies
	Autoimmune
	• Systemic lupus erythematosus
	• Dermatomyositis
	• Rheumatoid arthritis
	• Scleroderma
	• Polyarteritis nodosa
	Electrolyte imbalance
	Cancer treatment (chemotherapy, radiation therapy)

*Predominantly involves the heart.

†Myocardial changes occur as part of a generalized systemic disorder affecting many organs; previously referred to as "specific cardiomyopathies." Only the most common diseases associated with cardiomyopathies are listed.

Data from Maron BJ: Contemporary definitions and classification of the cardiomyopathies: an American Heart Association Scientific Statement from the Council on Clinical Cardiology, Heart Failure and Transplantation Committee; Quality of Care and Outcomes Research and Functional Genomics and Translational Biology Interdisciplinary Working Groups; and Council on Epidemiology and Prevention, *Circulation* 113(14):1807–1816, 2006.

myocardial muscle fibers are impaired. The original definition of *cardiomyopathy* stated that this condition was not caused by other heart or systemic disease, which excluded structural and functional abnormalities caused by valvular disorders, CAD, hypertension, congenital defects, and pulmonary vascular disorders.

The American Heart Association expert consensus panel in its 2006 document proposed the following definition for cardiomyopathy, which reflects the idea that many cardiomyopathies have an underlying etiology, with ischemia from CAD as probably being the most common.

Cardiomyopathies are a heterogeneous group of diseases of the myocardium associated with mechanical and/or electrical dysfunction that usually (but not invariably) exhibit inappropriate ventricular hypertrophy or dilation and are the result of a variety of causes that frequently are genetic. Cardiomyopathies either

are confined to the heart or are part of generalized systemic disorders, often leading to cardiovascular death or progressive heart failure–related disability.[292]

The classification of cardiomyopathies is problematic. There was much confusion using the former classification of dilated, hypertrophic, and restrictive categories because of overlap when the same disease could appear in two different categories. And sometimes cardiomyopathy progresses from one category to another during the natural history of the disease, making classification difficult. As new knowledge of the pathogenesis of cardiomyopathy has unfolded and as new cardiomyopathies have been defined, the old classification scheme has been replaced with a new (but probably not final) classification.[292]

Cardiomyopathies are classified as *primary* and *secondary*, based on predominant organ involvement. Primary cardiomyopathies include genetic, mixed (genetic and nongenetic), and acquired (Table 12-14). They are confined to the heart muscle.

Genetic cardiomyopathies include hypertrophic and arrhythmogenic right ventricular cardiomyopathies, left ventricular noncompaction, conduction system disease, and ion channelopathies. In general, these congenital or familial types of cardiomyopathies are fairly uncommon individually, but a growing number of different types caused by mutations in genetic encoding have been identified.

Mixed cardiomyopathies included dilated and primary restrictive nonhypertrophied cardiomyopathies. An example of an acquired cardiomyopathy is myocarditis. Considerable overlap can occur among the primary classifications within the same person (see "Pathogenesis" below).

Secondary cardiomyopathies involve myocardial pathology as part of a large number and variety of generalized systemic disorders that affect the heart along with other organs at the same time.

Incidence and Risk Factors. Cardiomyopathy can affect any age group and is often seen in young adults in the second and third decades. The actual incidence is unknown, but the disease may be more common than was previously realized.

This increase in incidence may be attributed to two important variables: (1) improved technology, which has allowed for more accurate evaluation of ventricular dimensions and ventricular wall movement; and (2) an increased incidence of myocarditis, an important precursor to cardiomyopathy, as a result of a wide variety of pathogens, toxins, and autoimmune reactions.

Delayed-onset cardiotoxic effects of chemotherapeutic agents may appear as chronic cardiomyopathy. Risk factors for the development of this type of cardiomyopathy include increasing doses of chemotherapeutic agents and previous mediastinal radiation.[465] Adriamycin (doxorubicin hydrochloride) and Cerubidine (daunorubicin hydrochloride) are the two agents recognized most often in association with dilated cardiomyopathy.

Dilated cardiomyopathy occurs most often in black men between the ages of 40 and 60 years. About half of the cases of dilated cardiomyopathy are idiopathic, and the remainder result from some known disease process (e.g., rheumatic fever, myasthenia gravis, progressive muscular dystrophy, hemochromatosis, amyloidosis, sarcoidosis). Risk factors for dilated cardiomyopathy may include obesity, long-term alcohol abuse, systemic hypertension, cigarette smoking, infections, and pregnancy.

Peripartum cardiomyopathy is a rare but very serious disease that results in heart failure. It may appear for no apparent reason during the last month of pregnancy or shortly after delivery; incidence is higher among multiparous women older than 30 years, particularly those with malnutrition or preeclampsia. Estimates vary, but the occurrence may be 1 in every 1300 to 4000 deliveries. Maternal death from CHF, blood clots, infection, and stillbirth can occur. Symptoms of orthopnea, cough, palpitations, and high blood pressure may not occur until several weeks after delivery.

Hypertrophic cardiomyopathy appears to be genetically transmitted as an autosomal dominant trait on chromosome 14; currently 11 mutant genes have been linked

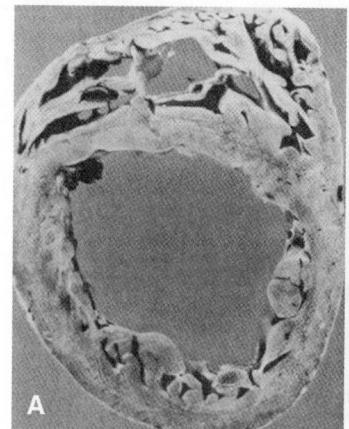
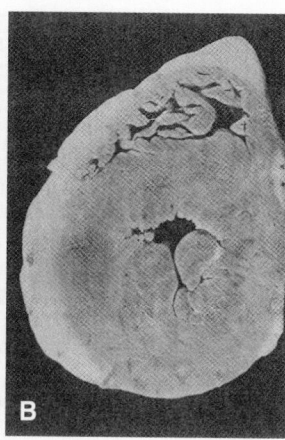

Figure 12-16

A, Cross-sectional view of dilated cardiomyopathy. **B,** Hypertrophied heart. (From Kinney M: *Comprehensive cardiac care,* ed 7, St Louis, 1991, Mosby, pp. 346, 349.)

with hypertrophic cardiomyopathy. It is still the most frequently occurring cardiomyopathy and the most common cause of sudden cardiac death in the young (including trained athletes).[42,292]

Restrictive cardiomyopathy occurs as a result of myocardial fibrosis (e.g., amyloidosis, sarcoidosis, hemochromatosis), hypertrophy, infiltration, or defect in myocardial relaxation.

Pathogenesis. The exact pathogenesis of cardiomyopathy is unknown; the risk factors mentioned previously seem to lower the threshold for the development of cardiomyopathy. For example, heavy consumption of alcohol is thought to cause dilated cardiomyopathy through three mechanisms: direct toxic effect of alcohol or of its metabolites; effects of nutritional deficiencies, especially thiamine deficiency; and toxic effects of beverage additives, such as cobalt.

Obesity produces an increase in total blood volume and cardiac output because of the high metabolic activity of excessive fat. In moderate to severe cases of obesity, this may lead to left ventricular dilation, increased left ventricular wall stress, and left ventricular diastolic dysfunction.

Regardless of the underlying cause, dilated cardiomyopathy results from extensively damaged myocardial muscle fibers and is characterized by cardiac enlargement. The heart ejects blood less efficiently than normal, so that a large volume of blood remains in the left ventricle after systole, which results in ventricular dilation with enlargement and dilation of all four chambers and eventually leads to CHF (Figs. 12-16 and 12-17).

Hypertrophic cardiomyopathy is distinguished by inappropriate and excessive left ventricular hypertrophy (thickening of the interventricular septum) and normal or even enhanced cardiac muscle contractile function. Over time, the overgrowth of the wall leads to rigidity in the myocardium. The result is decreased diastolic functioning, because the rigid myocardium cannot relax during the diastolic phase, reducing the amount of blood flowing into the ventricles. Restrictive cardiomyopathy is the least common form; it is identified by marked endocardial scarring (fibrosis) of the ventricles, and the resulting rigidity impairs diastolic filling.

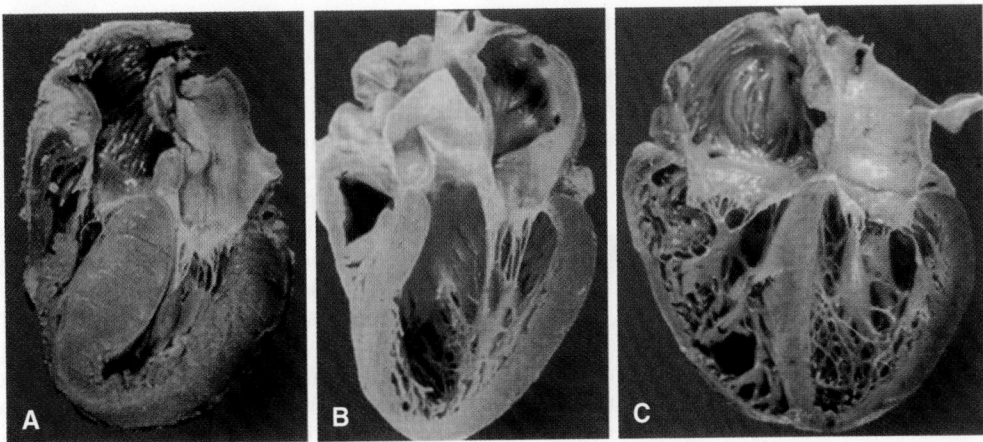

Figure 12-17

Gross pathologic specimens of the cardiomyopathies. A, Hypertrophic cardiomyopathy, showing a marked increase in myocardial mass and preferential hypertrophy of the interventricular septum. **B,** Normal heart, with normal left ventricular dimensions and thickness. **C,** Dilated cardiomyopathy, showing marked increase in chamber size. Atrial enlargement is also evident in both cardiomyopathies (**A** and **C**). (From Seidman JG, Seidman C: The genetic basis for cardiomyopathy: from mutation identification to mechanistic paradigms, *Cell* 104:557, 2001.)

Clinical Manifestations. Generally, the symptoms of cardiomyopathy are the same as for heart failure (e.g., dyspnea, orthopnea, tachycardia, palpitations, peripheral edema, distended jugular vein).

Dilated cardiomyopathy is characterized by fatigue and weakness; chest pain (unlike angina) may occur. Blood pressure is usually normal or low.

Hypertrophic cardiomyopathy is frequently asymptomatic, sudden death being the presenting sign; in fact, hypertrophic cardiomyopathy is the most common cause of sudden death in young competitive athletes. The most common symptom is dyspnea caused by high pulmonary pressures produced by the elevated left ventricular diastolic pressure; symptoms are often exacerbated during strenuous exercise.

Restrictive cardiomyopathy causes clinical manifestations related to decreasing cardiac output. As cardiac output falls and intraventricular pressures rise, signs of CHF appear. The earliest manifestations may include exercise intolerance, fatigue, and shortness of breath followed by other symptoms such as peripheral edema and ascites.

MEDICAL MANAGEMENT

DIAGNOSIS AND TREATMENT. Diagnosis requires exclusion of other causes of cardiac dysfunction, especially causes of CHF and arrhythmias. Catheterization to assess arteries and valves, echocardiography, chest radiography, blood chemistries, genetic mutation analysis (for hypertrophic cardiomyopathy), and ECG are specific tests that are performed. Researchers continue to investigate ways to monitor people with heart failure and to devise noninvasive diagnostic techniques. Comprehensive practice guidelines are available for the diagnosis and treatment of hypertrophic cardiomyopathy.[171]

The specific treatment of cardiomyopathy is determined by the underlying cause and may include physical, dietary, or pharmacologic interventions; mechanical circulatory support; or surgical intervention, including transplantation. Cardiac resynchronization therapy, the use of a pacemaker-like device to electrically stimulate both ventricles simultaneously (biventricular pacing), has been approved for use in CHF and is under investigation for use with dilated cardiomyopathy.

Alternatively, a cardiac support device called a "heart jacket" is under investigation for use in the United States for cardiomyopathy. This specially designed polyester material is stitched into place around the heart to prevent diseased heart muscle from further enlargement. Clinical safety trials are under way at the University of Pennsylvania.

Idiopathic dilated cardiomyopathy has no known cause; therefore, there is no specific therapy. In contrast to the other forms of cardiomyopathy, the progression of myocardial dysfunction in dilated cardiomyopathy may be stopped or reversed if alcohol consumption is reduced or stopped early in the course of the disease.

The β-blockers have an important immunoregulatory role in modifying the dysregulated cytokine network and reducing myocardial contractility and workload.[333] Calcium channel blocking agents (see Table 12-5) may be used to relieve symptoms and reduce exercise intolerance. Restrictive cardiomyopathy has no specific treatment interventions. The goal is to control CHF through the use of diuretics, vasodilators, and salt restriction.

PROGNOSIS. Seventy-five percent of persons diagnosed with idiopathic dilated cardiomyopathy die within 5 years after the onset of symptoms, because diagnosis does not usually occur until advanced stages. Persons with hypertrophic cardiomyopathy can lead long, relatively asymptomatic lives; some people have a history of gradually progressive symptoms, but others experience sudden death, especially during exercise, as the initial diagnostic event. Restrictive cardiomyopathy may cause sudden death as a result of arrhythmia, or a more progressive course may occur, with eventual heart failure. Intervention rarely results in long-term improvement.

Many persons with various types of cardiomyopathy experience stabilization or even an improvement in symptoms, but the end result of cardiomyopathy is sudden death or a fatal progression toward heart failure. No cure exists, outside of cardiac transplantation. Heart transplantation shows a 1-year survival rate of greater than 80% and a 3-year survival rate of 70% for dilated cardiomyopathy. The 1-year survival rate without transplantation is 5%.

SPECIAL IMPLICATIONS FOR THE THERAPIST `12-10`

Cardiomyopathy

Sudden death can occur, but the incidence is rare. It occurs more often in younger people who have cardiomyopathy, and it may be avoided by eliminating strenuous exercise (e.g., running, competitive sports) when a diagnosis has been established. Rest improves cardiac function and reduces heart size.

During the early stages of the disease, many people find it difficult to accept activity restrictions and need encouragement to follow guidelines for activity restriction. Clients should avoid poorly tolerated activities; combine rest with activity; understand that physical stress and emotional stress exacerbate the disease; learn correct breathing techniques, as the Valsalva maneuver decreases the inflow of venous blood and impairs outflow and should be avoided; and understand that alcohol depresses myocardial contractility and should be eliminated.

The therapist can provide valuable information regarding energy conservation techniques (see Box 9-8) to assist persons with continued independence in activities of daily living and possibly even with improvement of activity tolerance. This is especially true for the person awaiting a cardiac transplant. The therapist involved with athletes (of all ages) is advised to follow the American Heart Association's guidelines for preparticipation screening and identifying athletes at risk for sudden cardiac death.[124,292,293] Baman has written an excellent review of sports participation for athletes with cardiovascular conditions.[42]

Cardiomyopathy associated with cardiotoxicity following chemotherapy is often clinically silent because of the clients' low levels of physical activity. An evaluation to screen for potential cardiopulmonary dysfunction is essential with these clients.

The evaluation should include an assessment of current physical activity levels and exercise tolerance and monitoring of heart rate and rhythm, blood pressure, respiratory responses, and any other signs and symptoms of exercise intolerance (e.g., dyspnea, fatigue, light-headedness or dizziness, pallor, palpitations, chest discomfort).[465] A scale that rates perceived exertion (see Table 12-13) is often useful during the evaluation and for establishing initial exercise guidelines toward improving endurance.

For the person who has been hospitalized and has not ambulated yet, the therapist will need to assess tolerance to activities in bed before ambulating. During activities, monitor pulse, oxygen saturation, respirations, blood pressure, and color. The heart rate, systolic blood pressure, and respiratory rate normally increase in proportion to the exercise (movement) intensity, whereas the diastolic blood pressure changes minimally (±10 mm Hg).

Improved activity tolerance may be demonstrated by minimal change in pulse or blood pressure during activities with minimal fatigue after the activity. Pulse, respirations, and blood pressure should return to a normal range within 3 minutes of the end of the activity. Discontinue any activity that results in chest pain, severe dyspnea, cyanosis, dizziness, hypotension, or sustained tachycardia.

Abnormal responses include either blunted or excessive rises in heart rate or systolic blood pressure, excessive increases in diastolic blood pressure or respiratory rate, a fall in systolic blood pressure with increasing activity, or increasing irregularity of the pulse. These signs may be the result of cardiopulmonary toxicity or simply the result of deconditioning. Increasing irregularity in the pulse with pairs or runs of faster beats or more than six isolated irregular beats per minute must be reported to the physician.[465] If the person is receiving diuretics, monitor for signs of too-vigorous diuresis (e.g., muscle cramps, orthostatic hypotension). If the person becomes hypotensive, use a supine position with legs elevated to increase venous return and to ensure cerebral blood flow.

Trauma

Nonpenetrating

Any blunt chest trauma, which is especially common in steering wheel impact from an automobile accident, may produce myocardial contusion, resulting in myocardial hemorrhage with little if any myocardial scar once healing is complete. Large contusions may lead to myocardial scars, cardiac rupture, CHF, or formation of aneurysms.

The chest pain of myocardial contusion is similar to that of MI and is often confused with musculoskeletal pain from soft-tissue consequences of chest trauma. Myocardial contusion is usually treated similarly to MI, with initial monitoring and subsequent progressive ambulation and cardiac rehabilitation (see "Special Implications for the Therapist 12-6: Myocardial Infarction" above).

Penetrating

Penetrating cardiac injuries are most often caused by external objects, such as bullets or knives, and sometimes from bony fragments secondary to chest injury. Iatrogenic causes of cardiac penetrating injury include perforation of the heart during catheterization and cardiac trauma from cardiopulmonary resuscitation. Complications include arrhythmias, aneurysm formation, death from infection (e.g., bacterial endocarditis or infection from a retained foreign body), a form of pericarditis associated with this type of injury, ventricular septal defects, and foreign body embolus.

Myocardial Neoplasm

Primary cardiac tumors are rare, with an autopsy frequency of 0.001 to 0.030%.[77] Malignant cardiac tumors account for 25% of primary cardiac tumors, with 95% of these tumors being sarcomas arising from connective tissue (e.g., angiosarcoma, rhabdomyosarcoma, mesothelioma, fibrosarcoma) and the remaining 5% being lymphomas.

Some of these sarcomas are limited to the myocardium, replacing functional cardiac tissue with cancerous cells without any intracavity extension. These tumors may produce no cardiac symptoms or may present with arrhythmias and conduction disturbances.

Tumors projecting into a cardiac cavity may present with progressive CHF, precordial pain, pericardial effusion tamponade, arrhythmias, conduction disturbances, and sudden death. Because these tumors occur more frequently in the right side of the heart, right-sided heart failure is more common (jugular venous distention, ascites, systemic edema). People with sarcomas face a rapid functional decline, with death occurring from a few weeks to 2 years after onset of symptoms. These tumors proliferate rapidly, invading and damaging not only the myocardium but contiguous structures such as the venae cavae and tricuspid valve as well.[77]

Benign primary cardiac tumors occur approximately three times more often than malignant primary tumors, with myxomas accounting for nearly 50% of these primary benign tumors. Myxomas arise most often from the endothelial surface of the left atrium, causing mechanical interference with cardiac function including intracardiac obstruction.[65] Tumors located in other cardiac chambers account for 10% of myxomas.[77] Other benign cardiac tumors (also rare) include lipoma, papilloma, fibroelastoma, rhabdomyoma, and fibroma.

Signs of obstruction can include right-sided heart failure, pulmonary edema, orthopnea, and dyspnea. Constitutional symptoms include fatigue, fever, weight loss, arthralgia, and myalgia. Embolization caused by fragments from the tumor can also occur in these individuals. If the tumor is in the left side of the heart, the emboli result in infarction damage to the viscera, including the heart, limbs, kidneys, and CNS.[377] Because these tumors often lie in the atrial cavity they can (if large enough) cause damage to the mitral valve or even block the orifice of this valve, leading to sudden death. Tumors found in the right side of the heart infrequently lead to pulmonary hypertension and PEs.

Metastases to the heart and pericardium are much more common, occurring 100 to 1000 times more often than primary cardiac tumors.[77,388] Melanoma has the highest frequency of metastasis to the heart, with metastases also possible from carcinomas of the lung, breast, and esophagus and malignant leukemia and lymphoma.[378]

Tumor may involve the heart by one of four metastatic pathways: retrograde lymphatic extension, hematogenous spread, direct contiguous extension, or transvenous extension. Metastatic involvement of the heart and pericardium may go unrecognized until autopsy. Impairment of cardiac function occurs in approximately 30% of cases and is usually attributed to pericardial effusion. The clinical presentation includes shortness of breath, cough, anterior thoracic pain, pleuritic chest pain, or peripheral edema. Cardiac neoplasms come to the attention of a therapist when (1) progressive interference with mitral valve function results in exercise intolerance or exertional dyspnea; (2) embolus causes a stroke; or (3) systemic manifestations occur, including muscle atrophy, arthralgias, malaise, or Raynaud phenomenon.

Diagnosis of myxomas and other cardiac neoplasms is usually made by echocardiography followed by imaging studies, with MRI being of greater value in delineating cardiac tumors.[388] There are no specific physical or laboratory tests for metastatic heart disease, and diagnosis is difficult as these tumors can masquerade as other cardiac defects. ECG is nonspecific, chest radiography may reveal an enlarged cardiac silhouette, and radionuclide angiography is helpful in diagnosing intracavity tumors. Two-dimensional echocardiography is the method of choice to detect cardiac metastases.[378]

Treatment of choice for myxomas is usually resection of the tumor, which in most cases is curative. Cardiac rehabilitation may be required according to the individual's postoperative cardiovascular condition. Recurrence is rare and appears to be the result of incomplete resection of the tumor or intraoperative dislocation of tumor material. The presence of cancer cells in more than one area of the myocardium (multifocal genesis) may also lead to recurrence despite treatment.[377]

In most cases, cardiac metastases are treated with palliative care because advanced disease is present at the time of diagnosis. Radiation is not typically used to treat cardiac neoplasms, which means that radiation heart disease occurs secondarily to radiation therapy for tumors in the area of the heart (e.g., mediastinum, breast, head and neck, and thyroid). A history of such tumors should alert the therapist to the possibility that cardiac defects may be present.

Congenital Heart Disease

Overview and Incidence

Congenital heart disease is an anatomic defect in the heart that develops in utero during the first trimester and is present at birth in approximately 1% of births in the United States.[358] Over the past 3 decades, major advances have been made in the diagnosis and treatment of congenital heart disease, resulting in many more children who have survived to adulthood with surgically corrected or uncorrected anomalies. Today, there are more than 1 million adults with congenital heart conditions. Congenital heart disease affects about 8 of every 1000 babies born in the United States, making this the most common category of congenital structural malformation. Other than prematurity, it is the major cause of death in the first year of life. Children with congenital heart disease are also more likely to have extracardiac defects, such as tracheoesophageal fistula, diaphragmatic hernias, and renal abnormalities.

There are two categories of congenital heart disease: cyanotic and acyanotic (Table 12-15). In clinical practice this system of classification is problematic, because children with acyanotic defects may develop cyanosis, and those with cyanotic defects may be pink and have more clinical signs of CHF.

Cyanotic defects result from obstruction of blood flow to the lungs or mixing of desaturated blue venous blood

Table 12-15	Congenital Heart Disease		
Defect	**Incidence**	**Clinical Manifestations**	**Prognosis**
Cyanotic			
Transposition of the great vessels	16%*; 3:1 male-to-female ratio	Depends on size and type of defects; cyanosis; CHF (newborn)	Improved surgical treatment provides excellent long-term outcome
Tetralogy of Fallot	10%-15%	*Infants:* acutely cyanotic at birth or progressive cyanosis first year *Children:* hypoxic events with tachypnea, increasing cyanosis, digital clubbing; poor growth and development; seizures, loss of consciousness, death possible *Adults:* dyspnea, limited exercise tolerance	At risk for sudden lethal arrhythmias; mild obstruction progresses with age; reduced life expectancy
Tricuspid atresia	<1%; relatively rare	Newborn cyanosis; tachycardia; dyspnea digital clubbing (older child)	Unreported; depends on success of treatment
Acyanotic			
Ventricular septal defect	25%; single most common CHD; 25%-40% close spontaneously by age 2 yr; 90% close by age 10 yr	Asymptomatic with small defect; CHF (age 1-6 mo); history of frequent respiratory infections; poor growth and development; dyspnea, fatigue and exercise intolerance (older child)	No physical restrictions
Atrial septal defect	10% children; 2:1 female-to-male ratio Accounts for 33% of all congenital heart disease cases surviving to adulthood	*Older child:* asymptomatic; growth failure; CHF *Adult:* fatigue or dyspnea on exertion	No physical restrictions if corrected; frequent complications in adults
Coarctation of the aorta	6%; 3:1 male-to-female ratio	High systolic blood pressure and bounding pulses in arms; weak or absent femoral pulses; cool lower extremities with lower blood pressure *Infants:* CHF *Children:* headaches, fainting, epistaxis (hypertension); exercise intolerance, easy fatigability *Adults:* asymptomatic or signs of hypertension (headache, epistaxis, dizziness, palpitations)	No physical restrictions if corrected; frequent complications in adults
Patent ductus arteriosus	12%; spontaneous closure in normal term infants by day 4; common in children born to mothers affected by rubella during first trimester; increased incidence in infants born at high altitudes (higher than 10,000 ft); present in 20%-60% of premature infants weighing <1500 g	*Children:* asymptomatic; CHF *Adult:* if symptomatic: fatigue, dyspnea, palpitations	Closure may occur up to age 2 yr; normal life expectancy with small defect; aneurysm and rupture can occur; poor prognosis for large defect without transplantation
Aortic stenosis	5% of all congenital heart disease	Asymptomatic; exercise intolerance, dizziness, and chest pain with prolonged standing	Good with early detection and surgical treatment; exercise testing recommended before participation in athletics

CHD, Congenital heart disease; CHF, congestive heart failure.
*Figures account for percentage of all congenital heart disease.

with fully saturated red arterial blood within the chambers of the heart. Most *acyanotic* defects involve primarily left-to-right shunting through an abnormal opening.

Etiologic Factors

Many congenital heart diseases have genetic causes with well-known chromosomal anomalies (e.g., trisomy 13, 18, 21; Turner syndrome). Approximately 10% of all congenital heart defects are known to be associated with a single identified mutant gene or chromosomal abnormalities; for the remainder, the causes are either unknown or involve multiple factors, such as alcohol consumption, viruses, maternal rubella infection during the first trimester, maternal pregestational diabetes, and drugs such as thalidomide.[358] In fact, the CDC's National Birth Defects Prevention Study identified the increased risk for congenital heart defects as associated with maternal obesity,[173] diabetes,[116] and smoking.[287]

Major cyanotic defects

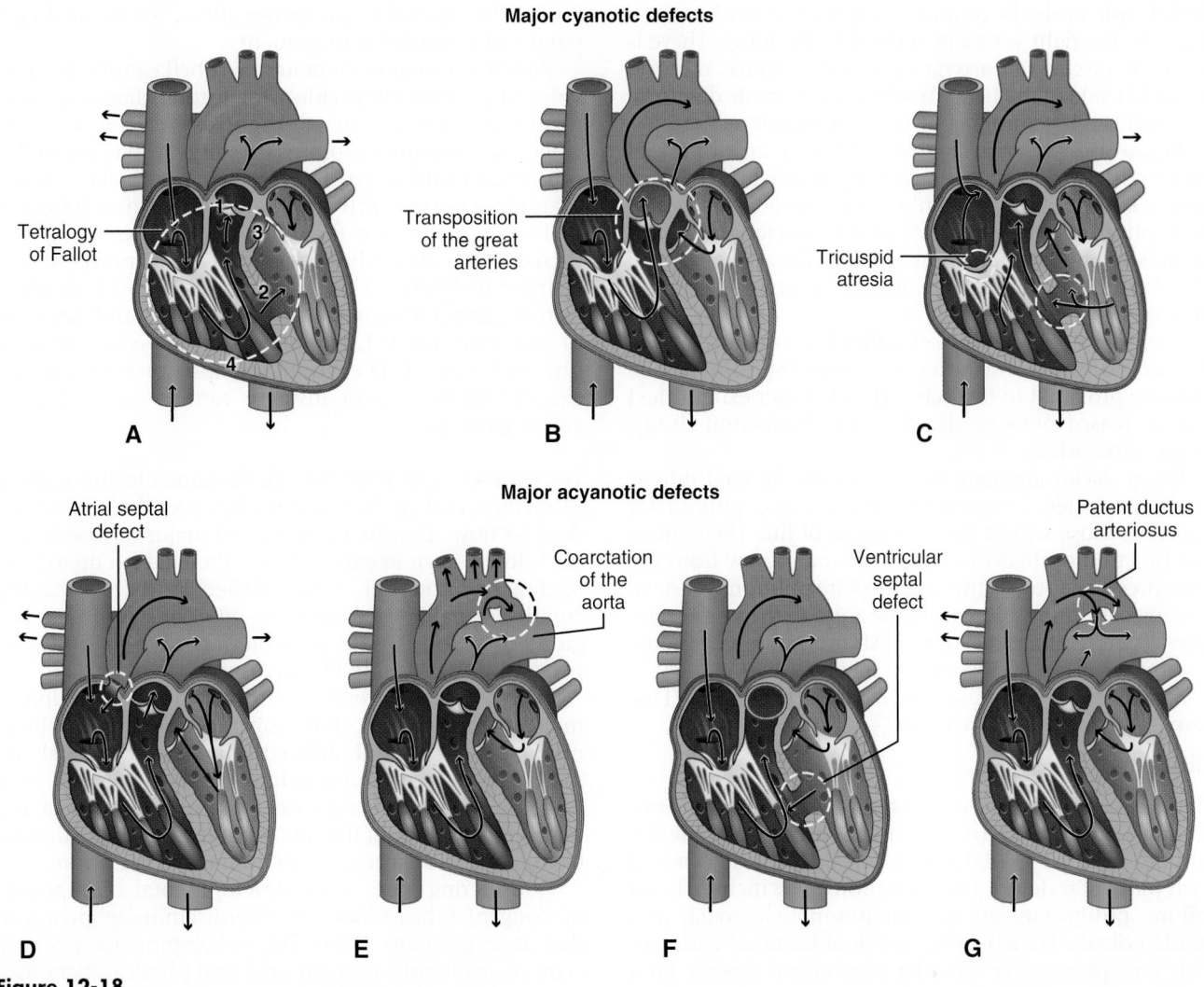

Figure 12-18

Major cyanotic defects (see Fig. 12-1 for normal structure and circulation of the heart). A, *Tetralogy of Fallot* has four defects: (1) pulmonary stenosis: narrowing at or just below the pulmonary valve; (2) ventricular septal defect (VSD): hole between the two bottom chambers (ventricles) of the heart; (3) aorta is positioned over the ventricular septal defect instead of in the left ventricle; (4) right ventricle is more muscular than normal. **B,** *Transposition of the great arteries:* systemic venous blood returns to the right atrium and then goes to the right ventricle and on to the aorta instead of going to the lung via the pulmonary artery. **C,** *Tricuspid atresia:* failure of the tricuspid valve to develop with a lack of communication from the right atrium to the right ventricle. Major acyanotic defects: **D,** *Atrial septal defect:* blood from the pulmonary vein enters the left atrium, and some blood crosses the atrial septal defect into the right atrium and ventricle. **E,** *Coarctation of the aorta:* severe obstruction of blood flow in the descending thoracic aorta. **F,** *Ventricular septal defect:* when the left ventricle contracts, it ejects some blood into the aorta and some across the ventricular septal defect into the right ventricle and pulmonary artery. **G,** *Patent ductus arteriosus:* some of the blood from the aorta crosses the ductus arteriosus and flows into the pulmonary artery.

In the case of atrial septal defect, most result from spontaneous genetic mutations, although some are inherited. Patent ductus arteriosus occurs in pregnancies complicated by persistent perinatal hypoxemia or maternal rubella infection and among infants born at high altitude or prematurely.[68]

Pathogenesis

The heart begins to form from a tube-like structure during the fourth week after conception. As development progresses, the tube lengthens and forms chambers, septa, and valves. Anything that interferes with this developmental process during the first 8 to 10 weeks of pregnancy can result in a congenital defect (Fig. 12-18).

Cyanotic. In *transposition of the great vessels,* no communication exists between systemic and pulmonary circulations, so that the pulmonary artery leaves the left ventricle and the aorta exits from the right ventricle. For the infant with this condition to survive, there must be communication between the two circuits. In approximately one third of all cases, another associated defect occurs that permits intracardiac mixing (e.g., atrial septal defect, ventricular septal defect, patent ductus arteriosus), but two thirds of cases have no other defect present and severe cyanosis develops.[69]

Tetralogy of Fallot consists of four classic defects: (1) pulmonary stenosis, (2) large ventricular septal defect, (3) aortic communication with both ventricles, and (4) right ventricular hypertrophy. *Tricuspid atresia* is a failure of the tricuspid valve to develop, with a lack of communication from the right atrium to the right ventricle. Blood flows through an atrial septal defect or a ductus arteriosus to the left side of the heart and through a ventricular septal defect to the right ventricle and out to the lungs. There is complete mixing of unoxygenated and oxygenated blood in the left side of the heart, resulting in systemic desaturation and varying amounts of pulmonary obstruction.

Acyanotic. *Ventricular septal defect* is an abnormal opening between the right and left ventricles that may vary in size from a small pinhole to complete absence of the septum, resulting in a common ventricle. *Atrial septal defect* is an abnormal opening between the atria, allowing blood from the higher-pressure left atrium to flow into the lower-pressure right atrium.

Coarctation of the aorta is a localized narrowing near the insertion of the ductus arteriosus, resulting in increased pressure proximal to the defect (head, upper extremities) and decreased pressure distal to the obstruction (body, lower extremities).

Patent ductus arteriosus is a failure of the fetal ductus arteriosus (artery connecting the aorta and pulmonary artery) to close within the first weeks of life. The continued function of this vessel allows blood to flow from the high-pressure aorta to the low-pressure pulmonary artery, causing continuous flow from the aorta to the pulmonary artery (referred to as left-to-right shunting). A patent ductus arteriosus rarely closes spontaneously after infancy.

Aortic stenosis is discussed later in this chapter in "Diseases Affecting the Heart Valves."

Clinical Manifestations

The most common signs and symptoms include cyanosis and signs of CHF (e.g., dyspnea, pulmonary edema, fatigue). See Table 12-15 for clinical manifestations of each particular defect. Complications may include heart failure, pulmonary edema, pneumonia, hypoxia, and sudden death. There is often a risk of bacterial endocarditis and pulmonary vascular obstructive disease later in life.

It is important to recognize the presence of neurodevelopmental disabilities seen in those with congenial heart disease. As these children reach school age, they have a two to three times higher incidence of neurodevelopmental disabilities and 10% to 15% incidence of behavioral disorders (anxiety, mood changes) than seen in the general population of children the same ages. It is possible that both congenital heart disease and abnormal brain development may be influenced by genetic contributions causing a developmental delay in both.

MEDICAL MANAGEMENT

PREVENTION AND DIAGNOSIS. As whole genome sequencing continues to develop, identification of genetic mutations predisposing to congenital heart disease may allow preventive measures by modulation of secondary genetic or environmental factors.[427] Until then, most forms of congenital heart disease can potentially be detected in utero with the routine use of ultrasonography.

The prenatal diagnosis of a major cardiac malformation requires further assessment for extracardiac and chromosomal disorders. Conversely, diagnosis of Down syndrome (prenatally or postnatally) requires early cardiologic assessment for cardiac anomalies, most commonly atrioventricular and ventricular septal defects. Prenatal knowledge of cardiac anomalies allows for optimal perinatal and postnatal management.

Prenatal screening for maternal rubella antibodies provides important information for further diagnostic testing. In cases where prenatal diagnosis does not occur and when there are no symptoms initially, cardiac anomalies can remain undetected for years and even decades. For example, a person with atrial septal defect may have normal sinus rhythm for the first three decades of life and then develop atrial fibrillation (AF) and supraventricular tachycardia (SVT).[69] Clinical diagnosis begins with detection of signs and symptoms, auscultation, and detection of heart murmur. TEE, Doppler color-flow echocardiography, and now RT3D echocardiography provide a definitive diagnosis without invasive cardiac catheterization and angiography.

TREATMENT AND PROGNOSIS. Remarkable innovations in medical and surgical approaches over the past several decades now allow for correction of major cardiac defects in children, even in early infancy. Prenatal (in utero) correction has not been accomplished as yet. Postnatally, curative or palliative (providing relief of symptoms) surgical correction is now available for more than 90% of persons with congenital heart disease.

There is a clear trend toward complete correction of malformations rather than staged procedures to obtain initial palliation and delayed correction. The risk for most surgical procedures is low (between 1% and 5%). Gene transfer to create a patent ductus arteriosus in animal studies may lead the way for additional gene transfer techniques to be successful in humans in the future.

Considering the neurodevelopmental component in congenial heart disease, interdisciplinary neurocardiac care program (involving developmental pediatricians, neurologists, occupational and physical therapists, speech and language pathologists, social workers, nurses, and dietitians) should be beneficial at improving the outcomes for these children.[101]

SPECIAL IMPLICATIONS FOR THE THERAPIST 12-11

Congenital Heart Disease

Therapists need to be alert to signs of CHF in children with congenital heart disease and in infants with suspected congenital heart disease. Signs of CHF indicate a worsening clinical condition; the earlier these are detected, the sooner intervention can be initiated. (See also "Special Implications for the Therapist 12-7: Congestive Heart Failure" above).

The surgical procedures associated with the repair of congenital heart disease (e.g., bypass, deep hypothermia) are associated with an increased incidence of neurologic abnormalities. Neurodevelopmental deficits resulting from surgical repair of cardiac defects may include choreoathetosis, cerebral palsy, or hemiparesis.[172]

Gross motor development can be negatively impacted by prolonged hospitalization, deficiencies in cardiovascular status, surgical techniques used to minimize blood loss, or any combination of these factors. The more complex the defect or defects and the more numerous the open heart surgeries required, the greater the risk for neurologic impairment.[442]

Most children with significant heart defects will have had heart surgery before they start school. In addition to a developmental assessment, the therapist should evaluate for soft-tissue restriction at the site of the healed scar (either sternal or thoracic), which may affect breathing capacity.

Physiologic response to therapy intervention can be assessed by observing skin color, respiratory effort, and behavioral response. Oxygen saturation monitors may not be helpful, because these children have abnormally low readings as their baseline level.[442] Data on exercise capacity after specific types of surgical procedures are available.[422]

In general, anyone who has had successful surgery is allowed unrestricted sports activity. Young children with unrepaired tetralogy of Fallot instinctively learn to squat, getting into the flat-footed baseball catcher's stance when they are fatigued. This posture increases the tension in the leg muscles, reduces blood flow to the leg muscles, and raises peripheral resistance and blood pressure.

Twenty or 30 years ago, diagnosis of congenital defects was much more difficult, and many anomalies went undetected. Adults with undiagnosed congenital defects may develop exercise intolerance, shortness of breath, palpitations, blood pressure irregularities, or symptoms of CHF, which should alert the therapist to the need for medical referral.

Care of pregnant women with congenital heart disease requires understanding of the specific congenital defect, the nature of previous surgical correction, and the presence of any complications or sequelae.[111] Exercise recommendations for children and adolescents with congenital malformations are available.[124] Therapists who work with children in Special Olympics should be aware of any cardiac issues in athletes with Down syndrome, especially with activities requiring greater levels of physical exertion than normal daily activities.

DISEASES AFFECTING THE CARDIAC NERVOUS SYSTEM

Arrhythmias: Disturbances of Rate or Rhythm

Definition and Overview

The heart rhythm and the number of times the heart beats (rate) are generated and regulated by the sinoatrial (SA) node, the internal pacemaker located in the upper right portion of the heart. The signal from the SA node travels through the cardiac conduction system, first through the walls of the atria and then through the walls of the ventricles, causing the atrial (supraventricular) and ventricular chambers of the heart to contract and relax at regular rates necessary to maintain circulation at different levels of activity. An arrhythmia (dysrhythmia) is a disturbance of heart rate or rhythm caused by an abnormal rate of electrical impulse generation by the SA node or the abnormal conduction of impulses.

Arrhythmias can be classified according to their origin as ventricular or supraventricular (atrial), according to the pattern (fibrillation or flutter), or according to the speed or rate at which they occur (tachycardia or bradycardia).

Several types of AF are now recognized, including first-detected-episode AF (may or may not be symptomatic; may self-resolve), recurrent paroxysmal AF (two or more episodes that resolve spontaneously), persistent AF, and permanent AF. Persistent AF is sustained for more than 7 days. It can occur after a first-detected-episode AF or after recurrent paroxysmal AF. Permanent AF, also known as chronic AF, occurs when sinus rhythm cannot be sustained after cardioversion (normal heart rhythm returns spontaneously) or when the decision has been made to let AF continue without efforts to restore normal sinus rhythm.[161]

Arrhythmias vary in severity from mild, asymptomatic disturbances that require no intervention (e.g., sinus arrhythmia, in which the heart rate increases and decreases with respiration) to catastrophic ventricular fibrillation, which requires immediate resuscitation. The clinical significance depends on the effect on cardiac output and blood pressure, which is partially influenced by the site of origin.

Etiologic Factors and Incidence

Arrhythmias may be congenital or may result from one of several factors, including hypertrophy of heart muscle fibers secondary to hypertension, previous MI, valvular heart disease, or degeneration of conductive tissue that is necessary to maintain normal heart rhythm (called *sick sinus syndrome*).

Chronic alcohol use and binge drinking have been linked with disturbances in cardiac rhythm, even in individuals without underlying heart disease. *Holiday heart syndrome* is the term used to describe acute arrhythmia (usually SVT) triggered by excessive alcohol intake in an otherwise healthy person. The affected individual experiences intermittent or continuous palpitations with dyspnea, dizziness, or chest pain often mentioned.

The prevalence of AF doubles with each advancing decade of age beginning at age 50 to 59 years, with a statistically significant increase among men ages 65 to 84 years, although this gap closes with advancing age and remains unexplained.[237,303]

BMI appears to correlate strongly with the risk of AF.[133] With each unit increment of BMI the risk of AF increases 3%. A person who is obese has approximately a 34% greater risk of AF when compared to a person with normal BMI. Moreover, people in the heaviest BMI category have 2.3 times the risk. Improved cardiac care has increased the number of survivors of cardiac incidents who may experience subsequent complications, such as arrhythmias.

Cardiac arrhythmias are very common in the setting of heart failure, with atrial and ventricular arrhythmias often present in the same person. Arrhythmias can occur when a portion of the heart is temporarily deprived of oxygen, disturbing the normal pathway of the heartbeat. Toxic doses of cardioactive drugs (e.g., digoxin and other cardiac glycosides), phenylpropanolamine found in some decongestants, alcohol and caffeine consumption, high fevers, and excessive production of thyroid hormone (hyperthyroidism) may also lead to arrhythmias. In many cases, particularly in younger people, there is no known or apparent cause.

Pathogenesis and Clinical Manifestations

Rate. The adult heart beats an average of 60 to 100 beats/min; an arrhythmia is considered to be any significant deviation from the normal range. Whether change in heart rate (number of contractions of the cardiac ventricles per period of time) produces symptoms at rest or on exertion depends on the underlying state of the cardiac muscle and its ability to alter its stroke output to compensate.

Rate arrhythmias are of two basic types: tachycardia and bradycardia. Tachycardia occurs when the heart beats too fast (more than 100 beats/min). Tachycardia develops in the presence of increased sympathetic stimulation, such as occurs with fear, pain, emotional stress, exertion, or exercise; or with ingestion of artificial stimulants, such as caffeine, nicotine, and amphetamines.

Tachycardia is also found in situations in which the demands for oxygen are increased, such as fever, CHF, infection, anemia, hemorrhage, myocardial injury, and hyperthyroidism. Usually the individual with tachycardia perceives no symptoms, and medical intervention is directed toward the underlying cause.

Bradycardia (less than 50 beats/min) is normal in well-trained athletes, but it is also common in individuals taking β-blockers, those who have had traumatic brain injuries or brain tumors, and those experiencing increased vagal stimulation (e.g., from suctioning or vomiting) to the physiologic pacemaker.

Organic disease of the sinus node, especially in older people and those with heart disease, can also cause sinus bradycardia. Bradycardia is usually asymptomatic, but when it is caused by a pathologic condition, the person may experience fatigue, dyspnea, syncope, dizziness, angina, or diaphoresis (profuse perspiration). Medical intervention is not usually required unless symptoms interfere with function or are drug or angina induced; atropine or a mechanical pacemaker can be used to reestablish a more normal heart rate.

Rhythm. Arrhythmias as variations from the normal rhythm of the heart (especially the heartbeat) are detected when they become symptomatic or during monitoring for another cardiac condition. Abnormalities of cardiac rhythm and electrical conduction can be lethal (sudden cardiac death), symptomatic (syncope or near syncope, dizziness, chest pain, dyspnea, palpitations), or asymptomatic. They are dangerous because they reduce cardiac output so that perfusion of the brain or myocardium is impaired, or they tend to deteriorate into more serious arrhythmias with the same consequences.

The many different types of abnormal cardiac rhythms are usually classified according to their origin (atrial, ventricular), but only the most common ones are included here. Complete discussion of all other cardiac arrhythmias is available.[206]

Sinus arrhythmia is an irregularity in rhythm that may be a normal variation in athletes, children, and older people or may be caused by an alteration in vagal stimulation. Sinus arrhythmia may be respiratory (increases and decreases with respiration) or nonrespiratory and associated with infection, drug toxicity (e.g., digoxin, morphine), or fever. Treatment for the respiratory type of sinus arrhythmia is not necessary; all other sinus arrhythmias are treated by providing intervention for the underlying cause.

AF is the most common type of SVT or chronic arrhythmia. SVT is also called paroxysmal SVT or paroxysmal atrial tachycardia. It is characterized by rapid, involuntary, irregular muscular contractions of the atrial myocardium—quivering or fluttering instead of contracting normally. Consequently, blood remains in the atria after they contract and the ventricles do not fill properly. The heart races, but blood flow may diminish, creating a drop in oxygen levels that results in symptoms of shortness of breath, palpitations, fatigue, and, more rarely, fainting. AF occurs most often as a secondary arrhythmia associated with rheumatic heart disease, dilated cardiomyopathy, atrial septal defect, hypertension, mitral valve prolapse, recurrent cardiac surgery, and hypertrophic cardiomyopathy (conditions that affect the atria).

Secondary AF can also occur in people without cardiac disease but in the presence of a systemic abnormality that predisposes the individual to arrhythmia (e.g., hyperthyroidism, medications, diabetes, obesity, pneumonia, or alcohol intoxication or withdrawal). People with AF are prone to blood clots because blood components that remain in the atria aggregate and attract other components, triggering clot formation. The effect rarely occurs before 72 hours of the first abnormal contraction. AF can result in CHF, cardiac ischemia, and arterial emboli that can result in an ischemic stroke.

Ventricular fibrillation is an electrical phenomenon that results in involuntary uncoordinated muscular contractions of the ventricular muscle; it is a frequent cause of cardiac arrest. Treatment is directed toward depolarizing the muscle, thus ending the irregular contractions and allowing the heart to resume normal regular contractions.

Heart block is a disorder of the heartbeat caused by an interruption in the passage of impulses through the heart's electrical system. This may occur because the SA node misfires or the impulses it generates are not properly transmitted through the heart's conduction system. Heart blocks are differentiated into three types determined by ECG testing: first-degree, second-degree, and third-degree (complete) heart block. Causes include CAD, hypertension, myocarditis, and overdose of cardiac medications (e.g., digoxin, calcium channel blockers, β-blockers). Depending on the degree of the heart block, it can cause fatigue, dizziness, or fainting. Heart block can affect people at any age, but this condition primarily affects older people. Mild cases do not require intervention; medication and pacemakers are the two primary forms of management for symptomatic cases.

Sick sinus syndrome, or brady-tachy syndrome, is a complex cardiac arrhythmia and conduction disturbance that is associated with advanced age, CAD, or drug therapy (e.g., digoxin, calcium channel blockers, β-blockers, antiarrhythmics). Sick sinus syndrome as a result of degeneration of conductive tissue necessary to maintain normal heart rhythm occurs most often among older people. A variety of other heart diseases and other conditions (e.g., cardiomyopathy, sarcoidosis, amyloidosis) also may result in sinus node dysfunction. Sick sinus syndrome is characterized by bradycardia alone, bradycardia alternating with tachycardia, or bradycardia with atrioventricular block resulting in cerebral manifestations of light-headedness, dizziness, and near or true syncope.

Sinus node dysfunction is suspected in the older adult experiencing episodes of syncope or near syncope, especially in the presence of heart palpitations. An accurate diagnosis is made with ECG, often requiring a 24-hour Holter monitor to document the arrhythmias described.

Treatment for the symptomatic person varies according to the specific arrhythmia manifestations and may include antiarrhythmic agents alone or combined with a permanent-demand pacemaker or withdrawal of agents that may be responsible.

Holiday heart syndrome may occur when the heart responds to the increase in catecholamines (epinephrine, norepinephrine) brought on by excessive alcohol intake. Alcohol metabolites may also cause conduction delays. The toxic effects of alcohol can also cause a rise in the level of free fatty acids, contributing to the onset of this condition.

MEDICAL MANAGEMENT

DIAGNOSIS. ECG is the most common test procedure to document arrhythmias, but if the person is not experiencing symptoms, the heartbeat may look normal. Tape-recorded ambulatory ECG may be used to document arrhythmias. The individual may use continuous monitoring (external cardiac monitoring; Holter monitoring; Fig. 12-19) recording all cardiac cycles over a prescribed

period of time (usually 24-48 hours) or cardiac event monitoring recording ECG just when symptoms are perceived.

Monitoring is especially helpful in recording sporadic arrhythmias that an office or stress test ECG might miss. Monitoring may also be used by persons recovering from MIs, receiving antiarrhythmic medications, or using pacemakers. New pocket-sized devices to allow home monitoring are available; readings may be stored, and the device can be hooked up to the physician's ECG or diagnostic computer or transmitted over the telephone. For symptoms that occur rarely (e.g., once every 6 months), an insertable loop recorder can be used. This small device is implanted under the skin in the chest using a local anesthetic. Monitoring units do not replace an ECG and should not be used without a physician's approval.

TEE imaging study using an ultrasonic transducer mounted on the tip of a flexible instrument is used to detect cardiac emboli before medications are initiated to control rate and rhythm. If a serious arrhythmia is suspected, an electrophysiologic study can be performed. This test is an invasive study that uses wires placed via catheterization to electronically stimulate the heart in an attempt to reproduce the arrhythmia.

TREATMENT. The goal of treatment is to control ventricular rate, prevent thromboembolism, and restore normal sinus rhythm if possible. Normal heart rhythm returns spontaneously (called *cardioversion*) almost immediately in some cases, especially if there is no underlying heart disease. When conversion to normal rate and rhythm does not occur, there are two major approaches to cardioversion: electrical and pharmacologic.

The electrical method employs the use of a device called a *defibrillator* and is usually most effective and may require several weeks (or longer) of anticoagulant therapy (warfarin) to reduce stroke risk. Anyone who has been in AF less than 48 hours but is hemodynamically unstable

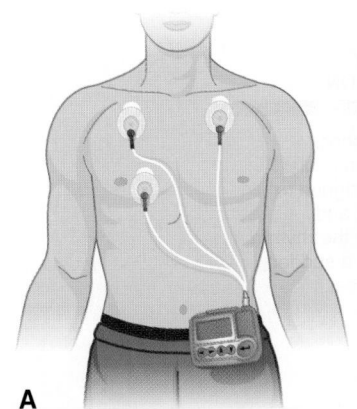
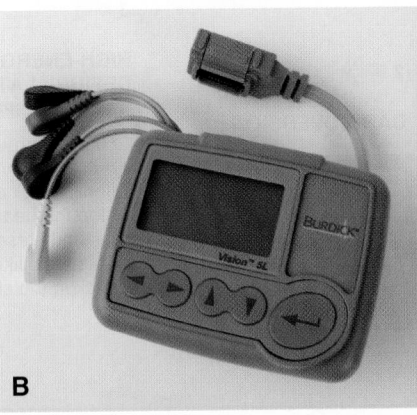
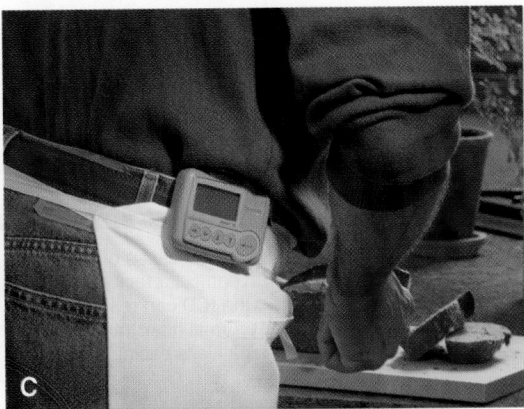

A **B** **C**

Figure 12-19

A, External cardiac monitoring (a form of telemetry, also called ambulatory electrocardiography [ECG] or Holter monitoring) uses a tape recorder that is attached to the skin by ECG electrodes. It is able to record the heart rhythm over a 24-hour period. Any symptoms experienced while wearing the unit should be recorded by the individual wearing the device. The recording is then analyzed. It may detect changes in heart rhythm or changes in the ECG that might indicate a lack of blood supply to the heart. **B,** Any number of electrodes up to 12 leads can be used. The standard three-electrode system in **A** consists of positive electrode, negative electrode, and ground electrode. **C,** The unit is small and convenient and can be clipped to the belt or waistband or slipped into a pocket. (Courtesy Cardiac Science Corporation, Bothell, WA. Used with permission.)

with serious signs and symptoms related to AF will need immediate electrical cardioversion. Low-voltage electric shocks interrupt the irritable foci of the heart, letting the SA node resume its role as a primary pacemaker.[389]

Pharmacologic treatment may include agents prolonging depolarization and/or other cardiovascular medications (see Table 12-5). If successful, cardioversion restores sinus rhythm, and drug therapy is used to maintain normal heart rate and rhythm. Even with successful electrical cardioversion, long-term antiarrhythmic and anticoagulation drug therapy is used to sustain normal sinus rhythm.

Some tachycardias can be treated with radiowave ablation, a nonsurgical but invasive technique that uses catheterization to thread wires into the heart through which radio waves can be aimed at the heart tissue where the arrhythmia originates. The catheter-delivered quick bursts of current destroy the specific areas of heart muscle that are generating the abnormal electrical signals causing the arrhythmia. One complication of this technique is the potential destruction of the conducting system (the heart's own internal pacemaker), which necessitates surgical implantation of an artificial pacemaker for some people.

Pacemakers, implants designed to replace the heartbeat by delivering a battery-supplied electrical stimulus through leads attached to electrodes in contact with the heart, may be used in cases of bradycardia, heart block, or refractory tachycardia. Refractory tachycardia is a condition in which the heart is beating very quickly, but only a portion of those beats are functional; many more beats just echo or make a beat but without contractile force behind the blood flow. Functionally, the heartbeat is actually very slow.

Pacemakers initiate the heartbeat when the heart's intrinsic conduction system fails or is unreliable. In the case of life-threatening arrhythmias (e.g., ventricular tachycardia, ventricular fibrillation) that do not respond to other types of intervention, a device called an implantable cardioverter-defibrillator may be implanted (Fig. 12-20). The cardioverter-defibrillator monitors the heart rhythm, and if the heart starts beating abnormally, it generates an electric shock to restore the normal sinus (heart) rhythm.

For people whose arrhythmias are resistant to pharmacologic therapy, another surgical intervention is available called the *maze procedure*. This procedure can now be done with a scope, catheter, and robotics to make a series of mazelike cuts in the atria, which are then sewn back together. The scar tissue that forms during the healing process blocks faulty circuits, preventing AF. Many people

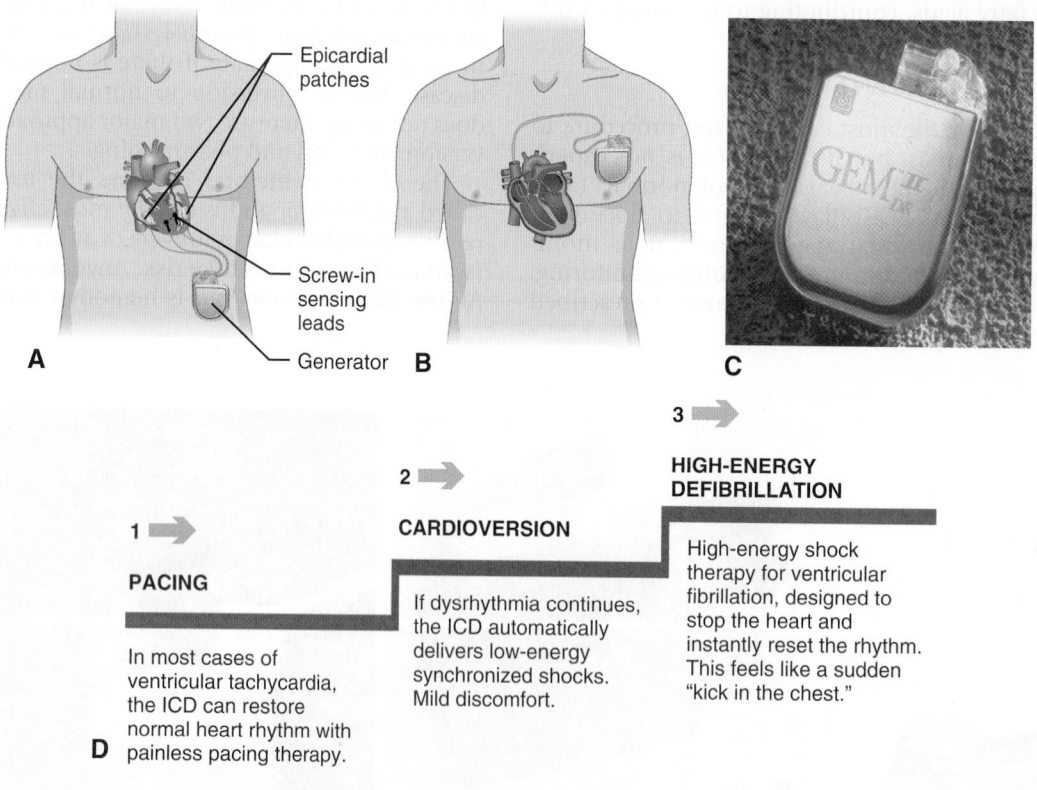

Figure 12-20

A, Placement of an implantable cardioverter defibrillator (ICD) and epicardial lead system. The generator is placed in a subcutaneous "pocket" created in the left upper abdominal quadrant. The epicardial screw-in sensing leads monitor the heart rhythm and connect to the generator. If a life-threatening dysrhythmia is sensed, the generator can pace-terminate the dysrhythmia or deliver electrical cardioversion or defibrillation through the epicardial patches. With this system, the leads/patches must be placed during open chest surgery. **B,** Transvenous lead system. Open chest surgery is not needed to place this unit. The pacing/cardioversion/defibrillation functions are all contained in a lead (or leads) inserted into the right atrium and ventricle. New generators are small enough to place in the pectoral region. **C,** An example of a dual-chamber ICD (Medtronic Gem II DR) with tiered therapy and pacing capabilities. **D,** Tiered therapy is designed to use increasing levels of intensity to terminate ventricular dysrhythmias. (From Urden LD: *Thelan's critical care nursing: diagnosis and management,* ed 5, St Louis, 2006, Mosby. Courtesy Medtronic Inc., Minneapolis, MN.)

still need a pacemaker and drug therapy to maintain normal rate and rhythm. A more refined version of this procedure (catheter maze) takes a percutaneous, nonsurgical, noninvasive approach using radiofrequency ablation to destroy tissue.

A more recently developed treatment intervention called *ventricular resynchronization therapy* is gaining recognition for the treatment of intraventricular conduction disturbances associated with CHF. This redesigned pacemaker resynchronizes the right and left ventricles so they pump at the same time, making the heart pump more forcefully instead of pumping faster (as occurs with a typical pacemaker or in the case of CHF when the heart beats faster to compensate for a weak pumping mechanism).[460]

PROGNOSIS. About half of all individuals with AF will spontaneously convert to normal sinus rhythm within 24 to 48 hours; this is less likely to occur in people whose AF has lasted longer than 7 days.[484]

Sudden cardiac arrest (sudden death) is responsible for 300,000 deaths annually and is often preceded by fatal heart dysrhythmias in people who have no prior history of heart disease. In fact, new data from the Framingham Heart Study indicate that AF is independently associated with a substantially increased risk for death in both men and women, even after adjustment for age and associated factors, such as hypertension, CHF, and stroke.

Defibrillation within the first few minutes of cardiac arrest can save up to 50% of lives; by comparison, an estimated 5% of sudden cardiac arrest victims in the United States survive without this treatment. Early defibrillation is the key to survival, and toward that end, emergency medical teams are using portable automatic external defibrillator units that use a computer program to sense whether a defibrillatory shock is warranted and will initiate the shock.[366]

The most appropriate and effective drug or drug combination remains unknown, and side effects of long-term rate and rhythm control intervention (e.g., organ toxicity of the lung, liver, and thyroid; aggravation of a preexisting arrhythmia or development of a new arrhythmia instead of preventing it) may prevent long-term use of drug therapy. Approximately 10% of affected individuals continue to have episodes despite treatment, and half of those who are treated have a recurrence within 6 months.

SPECIAL IMPLICATIONS FOR THE THERAPIST 12-12

Arrhythmias

Any time a person's pulse is abnormally slow, rapid, or irregular, especially in the presence of known cardiac involvement, documentation and notification of the physician are necessary. Early detection and treatment of AF can be critical in reducing the client's risk of stroke and hemodynamic compromise.

Predisposing factors for arrhythmias include fluid and electrolyte imbalance (see Chapter 5) and drug toxicity (see Table 12-5 and "Special Implications for the Therapist 12-10: Cardiomyopathy" above).

To prevent postoperative cardiac arrhythmias, therapist should determine client's blood oxygen level using pulse oximetry and/or blood gas analysis and, in consultation with the physician, provide adequate oxygen during activities that increase the heart's workload.

Individuals experiencing exercise intolerance as a result of palpitations, fatigue, and shortness of breath should be assessed further. Keep in mind that people with arrhythmias can be completely asymptomatic. And it is possible that clients describing palpitations or similar phenomena may not be experiencing symptoms of arrhythmic heart disease at all.

Palpitations can occur as a result of an overactive thyroid, secondary to caffeine sensitivity, as a side effect of some medications, from decreased estrogen levels, and through the use of drugs such as cocaine. Encourage the client to report any such symptoms to the physician if this has not already been brought to the physician's attention. See "Special Implications for the Therapist 12-1: Signs and Symptoms of Cardiovascular Disease" above.

It is the position of the American Physical Therapy Association that properly trained physical therapists should be authorized to perform advanced cardiac life support procedures, including cardiac monitoring for arrhythmia recognition and cardiac defibrillation.[24]

Physical therapists exercise many people with a history of personal or family heart disease or known risk factors for cardiac disease potentially necessitating cardiopulmonary resuscitation. Make sure to have advanced cardiac life support equipment available in case of emergency.

Public access to emergency defibrillation was signed into law (Cardiac Arrest Survival Act; HR 2498) in 2000 placing automatic external defibrillators in federal buildings and providing nationwide Good Samaritan protection that exempts from liability anyone who renders emergency treatment with a defibrillator to save a life. Also signed into law was the Rural Access to Emergency Devices Act (SF 2528) authorizing $25 million in federal funds to help rural communities purchase automatic external defibrillators and train people to use them. Clinics offering physical and occupational therapy services should have an automatic external defibrillator on site at all times.[366]

Performing an assessment of falls for individuals with cardiac disease, especially for anyone with a personal or family history of arrhythmias, is highly recommended. Screening for syncope, assessing balance and fall risk, and falling prevention programs are important components of a therapist's evaluation. If the individual is also on anticoagulation therapy, the individual should be monitored (and taught how to self-monitor) for signs and symptoms of bleeding; in the acute care setting, the therapist can monitor international normalized ratio. Evaluations of specific assessment and screening tests are available.[98,143,442,459]

Exercise and Arrhythmias

Individuals with a history of atrial fibrillation should be encouraged to maintain as normal and active a lifestyle as possible. They should be informed that exercise can increase arrhythmias because of the increase in activity of the sympathetic nervous system and the increase in circulating catecholamines. Exercise may induce cardiac arrhythmias under several specific conditions, including diuretic and digoxin therapy, or following recent ingestion of caffeine. Avoiding triggers such as caffeine, alcohol, or overeating can help and should be encouraged. Good nutrition, tobacco cessation for those who use tobacco, and regular physical activity and exercise are key components of the management program.

Exercise-induced arrhythmias are generated by enhanced sympathetic tone, increased myocardial oxygen demand, or both. The therapist can be involved in preparticipation screening of all athletes for conditions that put them at risk for sudden cardiac death (see "Special Implications for the Therapist 12-10: Cardiomyopathy" above). At times, the arrhythmias may disappear with exercise and increased perfusion. Exercise recommendations for athletes with selected arrhythmias are available.[124]

Medications that are effective in controlling arrhythmias at rest may not be effective during exertion or stress. In addition, side effects of antiarrhythmic agents may be more apparent during exercise. For example, decreases in either exercise performance or blood pressure during exercise may occur. Because of their effects on the electrophysiologic characteristics of cardiac cells, these medications have the potential to cause abnormal rhythms. The effect of slowing the impulse through the myocardium may manifest itself during exercise as a partial or complete heart block.

Individuals with known arrhythmias and clients who are taking antiarrhythmic medications may need to be evaluated under conditions of graded exercise to ensure that the arrhythmia remains under control during activity. Monitoring heart rate and blood pressure during activity and palpation of peripheral pulses are essential in the absence of ECG.

Continued monitoring and observation during the recovery period are also important, because arrhythmias often occur during recovery rather than during peak exercise. If the exercise is stopped abruptly and the individual remains upright, pooling of blood in the lower body occurs. The decreased venous return and subsequent decreased blood flow to the heart may facilitate an irregular rhythm. By continuing to exercise at a low intensity during recovery, a sudden decrease in venous return is avoided.

For the client who is wearing or has worn a cardiac monitor (Holter, event, loop), the therapist must obtain the interpretation of the results to determine if modifications are needed in the person's activities. Anyone with life-threatening arrhythmias should not begin physical therapy activity until intervention for the arrhythmia is initiated and the condition is stabilized. Increasing frequency of arrhythmias developing with activity must be evaluated by the physician.[205]

Pacemaker

For the client wearing a pacemaker, the first weeks after surgery may be characterized by fatigue, during which time activity restrictions apply. Most people can drive, but strenuous activities using the arms (e.g., housework, golf, tennis, lifting more than 10 lb) are contraindicated. Once the incision is fully healed and the pacemaker is stable, scar mobilization is permissible. The usual precautions for scar mobilization apply, including mobilizing the tissue in the direction of the scar before using any cross-transverse techniques and mobilizing toward the scar rather than away from the scar to avoid overstretching the healing tissue.

Problems with pacemakers are uncommon, but any unusual deviation from the set heartbeat expected or the development of unusual symptoms, such as dyspnea, dizziness or light-headedness, and syncope or near syncope, must be reported immediately to the physician. It is important that the therapist understand the underlying problem as well as the type of pacemaker the client is using before monitoring the client's response to an exercise program. More detailed information regarding types of pacemakers and pacemaker implantation is available[206]; see also information from pacemaker manufacturers.

It should be noted that MRIs and prolonged exposure to electromagnetic waves are contraindicated in anyone who is pacemaker dependent. Most exposures to electromagnetic interference are transient and pose no threat to people with pacemakers and implantable cardioverter-defibrillators. Concerns that cellular telephone radiation is linked to pacemaker or implantable cardioverter-defibrillator disruption have not been substantiated or proven clinically important.

Heart rate is limited to the programmed level, and individuals with fixed-rate ventricular synchronous devices require monitoring by blood pressure and perceived exertion scales, with close attention to symptoms of cerebral ischemia. Newer, improved pacemakers produce the cardiac output needed for exercise, making it possible for individuals with pacemakers to be physically active at work and during recreation. Exercise may be limited only by the underlying heart disease and left ventricular function. If the pacemaker recipient has undergone exercise testing safely, aerobic conditioning and endurance training can be initiated, although precaution is still advised regarding vigorous upper-body activities.

In some individuals who have suffered cardiac arrest and now have a pacemaker (or other implantable device), the response to surviving cardiac arrest has been compared to posttraumatic stress disorder that can occur after a person experiences a traumatic event that is outside the realm of usual human experience. Depression, anxiety, difficulty concentrating, negative health beliefs, and increased somatic complaints may be present with or without persistent emotional disability and maladaptation to the event. The therapist should refer anyone suspected of having persistent depression or anxiety to the physician or mental health professional.

DISEASES AFFECTING THE HEART VALVES

Heart problems that occur secondary to impairment of valves may be caused by infections such as endocarditis, congenital deformity, or disease (e.g., rheumatic fever, coronary thrombosis). Valve deformities are classified as functional (e.g., stenosis, insufficiency) or anatomic (e.g., prolapse; congenital deformities; deformities caused by rheumatic fever, trauma, infection, ischemia) (Fig. 12-21).

Stenosis is a narrowing or constriction that prevents the valve from opening fully and may be caused by scars or abnormal deposits on the leaflets. Valvular stenosis causes obstruction to blood flow, and the chamber behind the narrow valve must produce extra work to sustain cardiac output.

Insufficiency (also referred to as *regurgitation*) occurs when the valve does not close properly and causes blood to flow back into the heart chamber. The heart gradually dilates in response to the increased volume of work; severe degrees of incompetence are possible in the absence of symptoms. *Prolapse* affects the mitral or tricuspid valve and occurs when enlarged leaflets bulge backward into the atrium.

Valve conditions increase the workload of the heart and require the heart to pump harder to force blood through a stenosed valve or to maintain adequate flow if blood is seeping back. Initially the cardiovascular system compensates for the overload and the person remains asymptomatic, but eventually as stenosis or insufficiency progresses, cardiac muscle dysfunction and accompanying symptoms of heart failure (breathlessness, dyspnea) develop.

Over the past 15 years, advances in surgical techniques and a better understanding of timing for surgical intervention have brought tremendous improvement in the clinical outcome of people with valvular heart disease, extending survival rates with less overall morbidity.[86]

The presence of CAD in clients with either mitral or aortic valve disease is a negative prognostic indicator; ischemic mitral regurgitation carries the worst prognosis, with higher operative mortality and lower long-term survival compared with nonischemic cases.[86]

Heart transplantation may be necessary when the risk of surgery is prohibitively high in some cases of valvular disease. Continued advances in noninvasive assessment (e.g., RT3D echocardiography) and noninvasive treatment (e.g., gene therapy, valves grown from blood vessel cells, and even valve self-repair with tissue-engineering techniques) should improve the outlook for anyone with valvular heart disease in the years to come.

Mitral Stenosis

Etiologic Factors and Pathogenesis

Mitral stenosis is a sequela of rheumatic heart disease that primarily affects women. Often a history of rheumatic fever is absent. Because the mitral valve is thickened, it opens in early diastole with a snap that is audible on auscultation and then closes slowly with a resultant murmur.

The anterior and posterior leaflets are fixed like a funnel with an opening in the center, and they move together, rather than in opposite directions. When the valve has narrowed sufficiently, left atrial pressure rises to maintain normal flow across the valve and to maintain a normal cardiac output. This results in a pressure

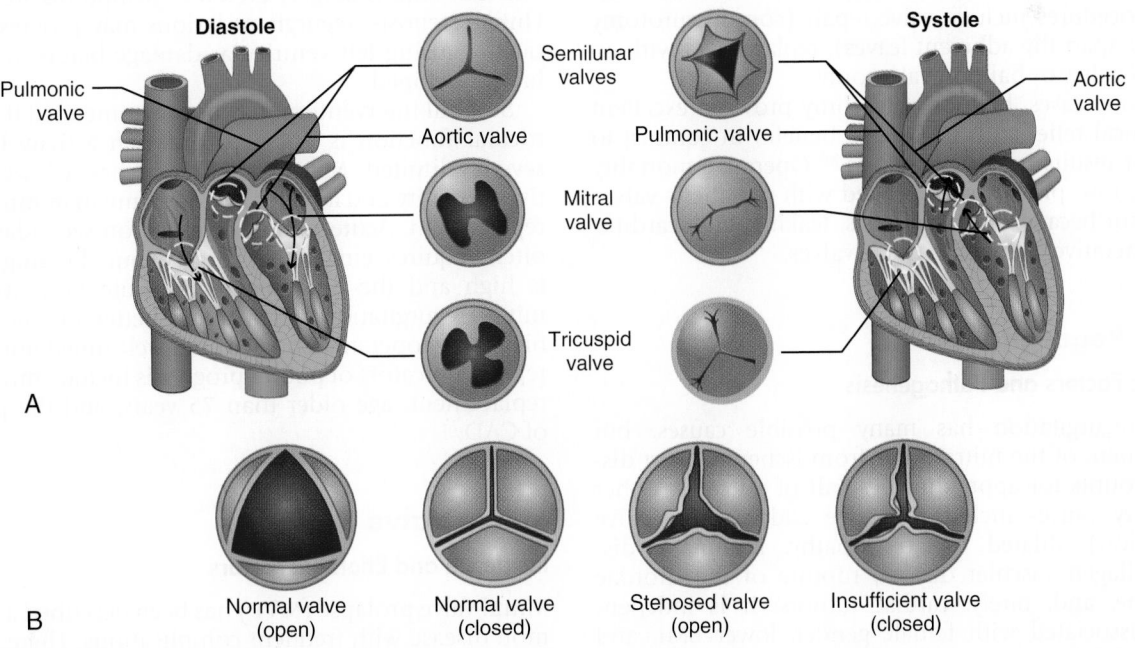

Figure 12-21

Valves of the heart. A, The pulmonic, aortic, mitral, and tricuspid valves are shown here as they appear during diastole (ventricular filling) and systole (ventricular contraction). **B,** Normal position of the valve leaflets, or cusps, when the valve is open and closed; fully open position of a stenosed valve; closed regurgitant valve showing abnormal opening into which blood can flow back.

difference between the left atrium and the left ventricle during diastole.

Clinical Manifestations

In mild cases, left atrial pressure and cardiac output remain normal, and the person is asymptomatic, perhaps until pregnancy or the development of AF, when dyspnea and orthopnea develop. In moderate stenosis, dyspnea and fatigue appear as the left atrial pressure rises and mechanical obstruction of filling of the left ventricle reduces cardiac output.

With severe stenosis, left atrial pressure is high enough to produce pulmonary venous congestion at rest and reduce cardiac output, with resulting dyspnea, fatigue, and right ventricular failure. Lying down at night further increases the pulmonary blood volume, causing orthopnea and paroxysmal nocturnal dyspnea.

MEDICAL MANAGEMENT

DIAGNOSIS, TREATMENT, AND PROGNOSIS. Echocardiography is the most valuable technique for assessing mitral valve stenosis and providing information about the condition of the valve and left atrial size. Doppler techniques (measuring blood flow using ultrasound) can be used to determine the severity of the problem.

Because mitral stenosis may be asymptomatic, intervention is delayed until symptoms develop. Mitral stenosis may be present for a lifetime with few or no symptoms, or it may become severe in a few years. The onset of AF accompanied by more severe symptoms may be treated pharmacologically (digoxin, antiarrhythmic agents, anticoagulants).

Surgery may be indicated in the presence of uncontrollable pulmonary edema, severe dyspnea limiting function, pulmonary hypertension, arrhythmia, or systemic emboli uncontrolled by anticoagulation treatment. Surgical procedures include valve repair (commissurotomy to break apart the adherent leaves), replacement with an artificial valve, or balloon valvotomy.

In many cases, balloon valvotomy provides excellent mechanical relief with prolonged benefit, in contrast to the poor results in aortic stenosis.[86] Operative mortality rates are low; problems associated with prosthetic valves may occur because of thrombosis, leaking, endocarditis, or degenerative changes in tissue valves.

Mitral Regurgitation

Etiologic Factors and Pathogenesis

Mitral regurgitation has many possible causes, but involvement of the mitral valve from ischemic heart disease accounts for approximately half of all cases. Other secondary causes include infective endocarditis (valve perforation), dilated cardiomyopathy, rheumatic disease, collagen vascular disease, rupture of the chordae tendineae, and, rarely, cardiac tumors. It is independently associated with female gender, lower BMI, and older age. Evidence suggesting that mitral regurgitation may be induced by appetite-suppressant medications has resulted in new research investigating the relationship of mitral regurgitation to obesity.[229]

During left ventricular systole, the mitral leaflets do not close normally, and blood is ejected into the left atrium as well as through the aortic valve. In acute regurgitation, left atrial pressure rises abruptly, possibly leading to pulmonary edema. When regurgitation is a chronic condition, the left atrium enlarges progressively; the degree of enlargement usually reflects the severity of regurgitation.

Clinical Manifestations

Unfortunately, people with mitral regurgitation lack early warning signs and may remain asymptomatic until severe and often irreversible left ventricular dysfunction occurs. For many years the left ventricular end-diastolic pressure and the cardiac output may be normal at rest, even with considerable increase in left ventricular volume. Eventually, left ventricular overload may lead to left ventricular failure. People with mitral regurgitation experience exertional dyspnea (because of increased left atrial pressure) and exercise-induced fatigue (because of reduced cardiac output). AF may also develop.

MEDICAL MANAGEMENT

DIAGNOSIS, TREATMENT, AND PROGNOSIS. The diagnosis is primarily clinical (auscultation), but it can be confirmed and quantified by color Doppler echocardiography. Other testing procedures may include cardiac catheterization to assess the regurgitation, left ventricular function, and pulmonary artery pressure; coronary arteriography to determine the cause of the lesion and for preoperative evaluation; and nuclear medicine techniques to measure left ventricular function and estimate the severity of regurgitation.

Persons with chronic lesions who are asymptomatic require careful monitoring for left ventricular function and may require surgery even if no symptoms are present. Unlike stenosis, regurgitant lesions may progress insidiously, causing left ventricular damage before symptoms have developed.

Surgical intervention may be recommended if left ventricular function is impaired or when activity becomes severely limited. Mitral valve repair has a lower operative mortality and a better late outcome than mitral valve replacement. Acute mitral regurgitation secondary to MI often requires emergency surgery, but the surgical risk is high and the outcome poor. Acute non–MI-related mitral regurgitation has a much better prognosis with higher postoperative survival after well-timed mitral valve repair. Indicators of poorer prognosis include mitral valve replacement, age older than 75 years, and the presence of CAD.[86]

Mitral Valve Prolapse

Incidence and Etiologic Factors

Mitral valve prolapse (MVP) has been described as a common disease with frequent complications. There is some dispute about the incidence of MVP. According to data from the Framingham Heart Study, MVP is not as prevalent as previously reported (2.4% compared to previously reported 10% or higher).

The American Heart Association and other sources report that MVP occurs in approximately 2% to 6% of "normal" adults, especially young women and is detected most often during pregnancy.[19,88] Other researchers report that MVP is equally common in men and women, although men seem to have a higher incidence of complications.[200]

MVP is characterized by a slight variation in the shape or structure of the mitral (left atrioventricular) valve. This structural variation has many other names, including floppy valve syndrome, Barlow syndrome, myxomatous mitral valve syndrome, and click-murmur syndrome. Barlow syndrome is a controversial clinical syndrome that may have as its only manifestation MVP without regurgitation.

The cause remains unknown, although there may be a genetic component involving the angiotensin receptor gene resulting in autonomic or neuroendocrine dysfunction.[439] Results of family studies of people with MVP favor an autosomal dominant pattern of transmission for primary MVP with nearly 100% gene expression by females.[128] This condition usually occurs in isolation; however, it can be associated with a number of other conditions, such as Marfan syndrome, rheumatic fever, endocarditis, myocarditis, atherosclerosis, SLE, muscular dystrophy, acromegaly, adult polycystic kidney disease, and cardiac sarcoidosis.

Pathogenesis

MVP is a pathologic, anatomic, and physiologic abnormality of the mitral valve apparatus affecting mitral valve leaflet motion. Normally, when the lower part of the heart contracts, the mitral valve remains firm and prevents blood from leaking back into the upper chambers. In MVP, the slight variation in shape of the mitral valve allows one part of the valve, the leaflet, to billow back into the left atrium during contraction of the ventricle. One or both of the valve leaflets may bulge into the left atrium during ventricular systole. Usually the amount of blood that leaks back into the left atrium is not significant, but in a small number of people, it develops into mitral regurgitation. MVP is the most common cause of isolated mitral regurgitation.

The presence of symptoms linked to neuroendocrine dysfunctions or to the autonomic nervous system has led to the recognition of a pathologic condition known as *mitral valve prolapse syndrome (MVPS)*. Usually diagnosed by chance in asymptomatic individuals during routine tests, MVPS (prolapse with or without mitral regurgitation) has a high clinical incidence of neuropsychiatric symptoms (e.g., anxiety disorder, panic attacks, depression), as well as symptoms of autonomic dysfunction (e.g., postural hypotension, palpitations, cold hands and feet, shortness of breath, chest pain).

As the autonomic nervous system is being formed in utero, the mitral valve is also being formed. If there is a slight variation in the structure of the heart valve, there is also a slight variation in the function or balance of the autonomic nervous system. The importance of recognizing that MVP may occur as an isolated disorder or with other coincident findings has led to the use of both terms.

Clinical Manifestations

More than 50% of all people with MVP are asymptomatic, another 40% experience occasional symptoms that are mildly to moderately uncomfortable, and only 1% suffer severe symptoms and lifestyle restrictions. Although the malformation occurs during gestation, it usually remains unnoticed until young adulthood. The person usually becomes aware of symptoms suddenly, and there does not appear to be any correlation between the severity of symptoms and the severity of the prolapse.

The most common triad of symptoms associated with MVP is profound fatigue that cannot be correlated with exercise or stress, palpitations, and dyspnea. Fatigue may not be related to exertion, but deconditioning from prolonged inactivity may develop, further complicating the picture.

The therapist is more likely to see the individual with MVP associated with connective tissue disorders or the MVPS with autonomic dysfunction. Frequently occurring musculoskeletal findings in clients with MVPS include joint hypermobility, temporomandibular joint syndrome, pectus excavatum, mild scoliosis, straight thoracic spine, and myalgia. The increased joint mobility that has been identified in a small proportion of persons with MVP does not appear to lead to either severe arthritis or frequent joint dislocations.[129]

Other symptoms associated with MVPS may include tremors, swelling of the extremities, sleep disturbances, low back pain, irritable bowel syndrome, excessive perspiration or inability to perspire, rashes, muscular fasciculations, visual changes or disturbances, difficulty in concentrating, memory lapses, and dizziness.

Chest pain or discomfort may occur as a result of autonomic nervous system dysfunction (dysautonomia). The autonomic nervous system imbalance results in inadequate relaxation between respirations and eventually causes the chest wall muscles to go into spasm. The chest pain is sharp, lasts several seconds, and is usually felt to the left of the sternum. It is intermittent pain that may occur frequently for a few weeks and then disappear completely, only to return again some weeks later.

MEDICAL MANAGEMENT

DIAGNOSIS, TREATMENT, AND PROGNOSIS. MVP is often discovered during routine cardiac auscultation or when echocardiography is performed for another reason. It is characterized by a symptomatic clinical presentation and clicking noise on auscultation in late systole, with or without sounds of valvular leak (murmur).

The mitral valve begins to prolapse when the reduction of left ventricular volume during systole reaches a critical point at which the valve leaflets no longer coapt (edges approximate together); at that instant, the click occurs and the murmur begins. Complete diagnostic (major and minor) criteria have been outlined elsewhere.[66] Echocardiography may be used to confirm the diagnosis, and ECG, event, or Holter monitoring (see Fig. 12-19) to show arrhythmias may be used.

Management includes reassurance; β-blockers to control arrhythmias; an exercise program to improve overall cardiovascular function; counseling to eliminate caffeine, alcohol, and cigarette use; and administration of antibiotics before any invasive procedure (including dental work, sigmoidoscopy) as prophylaxis against endocarditis.

Rarely, surgical replacement of the valve may be recommended when severe structural problems are present that contribute to reduced activity or deterioration of left ventricular function from progression of MVP to mitral regurgitation.

MVP or MVPS is a benign condition in the vast majority of people. It is not life-threatening and only rarely does it result in complications or significantly alter a person's lifestyle. Progressive mitral regurgitation with gradual increase in left atrial and left ventricular size, AF, pulmonary hypertension, and the development of CHF occur in 10% to 15% of people with both murmurs and clicks. Men older than 50 years are most often affected.[66]

According to new data available, people with MVP or MVPS are not at greater risk for heart failure, other forms of heart disease, or early death from stroke as was once thought.

Aortic Stenosis

Etiologic Factors and Pathogenesis

Aortic stenosis is a disease of aging that is likely to become more prevalent as the proportion of older people in our population increases. It is most commonly caused by progressive valvular calcification either superimposed on a congenitally bicuspid valve or, in the older adult, involving a previously normal valve following rheumatic fever.

Other risk factors for aortic stenosis are the same as those for heart disease and include obesity, a sedentary lifestyle, smoking, and high cholesterol. Factors affecting the progression of the disease remain uncertain. More than 80% of affected persons are men, and when women are affected, differences are noted (e.g., women with aortic stenosis have thicker ventricular walls reducing wall stress and higher ejection fractions) that require different postoperative management (e.g., low cardiac output requiring volume expansion rather than the use of pressor agents).[86] Ejection fraction is the amount of blood the ventricle ejects; the normal ejection fraction is approximately 60% to 75%. A decreased ejection fraction is a hallmark finding of ventricular failure.

Although the deformed valve is not stenotic at birth, it is subjected to abnormal hemodynamic stress, which may lead to thickening and calcification of the leaflets with reduced mobility. The orifice of the aortic valve narrows, causing increased resistance to blood flow from the left ventricle into the aorta.

Outflow obstruction increases pressure within the left ventricle as it tries to eject blood through the narrow opening, causing decreased cardiac output, left ventricular hypertrophy, and pulmonary vascular congestion. Preschool and school-age children are more likely to have a bicuspid valve; teenagers and young adults present with three leaflets, but these are partially fused.

Clinical Manifestations

In adults, aortic stenosis is usually asymptomatic until the sixth (or later) decade. Characteristic sounds may be heard on auscultation, but cardiac output is maintained until the stenosis is severe and left ventricular failure, angina pectoris, or exertional syncope develops. The origin of exertional syncope in aortic stenosis remains controversial; it is perhaps caused by an exercise-induced decrease in total peripheral resistance, which is uncompensated because cardiac output is restricted by the stenotic valve. The most common sign of aortic stenosis is a systolic ejection murmur radiating to the neck (usually heard best in the aortic area). Aortic stenosis can lead to symptoms such as fatigue, chest pain, dizziness, and shortness of breath (breathlessness). Sudden death may occur, even in previously asymptomatic individuals.

MEDICAL MANAGEMENT

DIAGNOSIS, TREATMENT, AND PROGNOSIS. The clinical assessment of aortic stenosis can be difficult, especially in the older person. Echo Doppler (echocardiography with Doppler ultrasonography) is diagnostic in most cases. ECG may show left ventricular hypertrophy, and x-ray or fluoroscopy may show a calcified aortic valve. Coronary angiography may be necessary in older adults at risk for coronary disease before valve replacement.

Pharmacologic therapy has limited use in this condition. Surgical intervention is usually required for the symptomatic person and should be strongly considered for the asymptomatic person because of the risk of sudden death.

Surgical procedures may include valve replacement with a mechanical prosthesis or bioprosthesis (made with biologic material) or use of the pulmonary valve in place of the aortic valve and replacement of the pulmonary valve with a homograft (Ross procedure). Homografts have been shown to have a superior durability compared to xenogenic biologic prostheses. Approximately 40% were still in place 20 years after implantation in the aortic position. Their low rate of thromboembolic events made life-time anticoagulative therapy unnecessary, and their hemodynamics may be superior to that of all other heart valve prostheses.[191]

A new technique for replacing failing aortic valves without open heart surgery, called transcatheter aortic valve replacement, is now available. The new valve is delivered to the heart through catheter inserted through an artery in the groin. This procedure is currently reserved for individuals with severe aortic valve stenosis who are considered unsuitable for traditional open-heart surgery.[277] Transcatheter aortic valve replacement is not without risk of serious complications and remains under investigation.[245,325]

Adults with aortic stenosis who are asymptomatic have a normal life expectancy; they should receive prophylactic antibiotics against infective endocarditis. Once symptoms appear, the prognosis is poor without surgery but excellent with valve replacement even in the older adult, especially in the absence of coexisting illnesses.[86]

The onset of angina, exercise-induced syncope, or cardiac failure indicates a poor prognostic outcome resulting in death. Mortality rises to 10% after age 80 years. Bioprostheses may develop degenerative changes, requiring replacement in 2 to 20 years. This is quite variable and depends on the person's age at the time of implantation.

Aortic Regurgitation (Insufficiency)

Etiologic Factors and Pathogenesis

In the past, aortic regurgitation occurred secondary to rheumatic fever, but antibiotics have reduced the number of rheumatic fever–related cases. Nonrheumatic causes account for most cases today, including congenitally bicuspid valves, infective endocarditis (valve destruction by bacteria), and hypertension. Aortic regurgitation may also occur secondary to aortic dissection with or without aortic aneurysm (see Fig. 12-28), ankylosing spondylitis, Reiter syndrome, collagen vascular disease, syphilis, and Marfan syndrome.

When cardiac systole ends, the aortic valve should completely prevent the flow of aortic blood back into the left ventricle. A leakage during diastole is referred to as *aortic regurgitation* or *aortic insufficiency*. When aortic regurgitation develops gradually, the left ventricle compensates by both dilation and enough hypertrophy to maintain a normal wall thickness/cavity ratio, thereby preventing development of symptoms. Eventually the left ventricle fails to stand up under the chronic overload, and symptoms develop.

Clinical Manifestations

Longstanding aortic regurgitation may remain asymptomatic even as the deformity increases, causing enlargement of the left ventricle. The large total stroke volume in aortic regurgitation produces a wide pulse pressure and systolic hypertension, resulting in exertional dyspnea, fatigue, and excessive perspiration with exercise as the most frequent symptoms; paroxysmal nocturnal dyspnea and pulmonary edema may also occur. Angina pectoris or atypical chest pain may be present, but this is uncommon in the absence of CAD.

MEDICAL MANAGEMENT

DIAGNOSIS, TREATMENT, AND PROGNOSIS. Once aortic regurgitation is suspected on physical examination, echocardiography with Doppler examination of the aortic valve can help estimate its severity. Aortography during catheterization helps confirm the severity of the disease. Scintigraphic studies can quantify left ventricular function and functional reserve during exercise and provide a useful predictor of prognosis.

Acute aortic regurgitation may lead to left ventricular failure; surgical reconstruction or replacement of the valve (Ross procedure; see "Aortic Stenosis" above) is advisable before onset of permanent left ventricular damage (usually before ejection fraction falls below 55%), even in asymptomatic cases. Chronic regurgitation carries a poor prognosis without surgery when significant symptoms develop. Medical therapy may include vasodilators to reduce the severity of regurgitation and diuretics and digoxin to stabilize or improve symptoms.

Tricuspid Stenosis and Regurgitation

Tricuspid stenosis may be congenital or rheumatic in origin and is uncommon. Exercise testing and rehabilitation do not occur until after valve surgery. Tricuspid regurgitation may occur secondary to carcinoid syndrome, SLE, or infective endocarditis among injection drug users, and in the presence of mitral valve disease. Surgical repair is more common than valvular replacement for tricuspid valve disease.

SPECIAL IMPLICATIONS FOR THE THERAPIST   **12-13**

Valvular Heart Disease

People with mild valvular malfunction have no symptoms and can usually exercise vigorously and take part in intense sports activities without adverse effects. Although exercise will not improve the mechanical function of a valve, improvement in submaximal cardiac capacity can occur. Exercise is usually stopped for the same reason as it is in healthy adults (i.e., when respiratory distress is obvious or when the person expresses a desire to stop).

Involvement of more than one valve is not uncommon in people with rheumatic valvular disease and in people who develop valvular regurgitation as a result of ventricular dilation. Usually symptoms and clinical course are determined by the predominant pathologic condition. When two valves are affected equally, symptoms are determined by the most proximally located valve. The combination of aortic regurgitation with mitral valve regurgitation is the most common, but the combination of mitral valve disease (either regurgitation or stenosis) with aortic stenosis is the most problematic.[414]

Exercise

Exercise testing for most people with valvular disease is of limited value. For example, there is poor correlation between the degree of mitral stenosis and the duration of symptom-limited treadmill exercise. However, exercise echocardiography performed while the individual is on a stationary cycle can be a valuable means for determining left ventricular function in people during exercise.

Prescriptive exercise must be individualized based on the underlying pathologic condition, medical intervention, and condition of the person. General guidelines include exercise a minimum of 3 days per week with alternate days of rest to allow for maximum recuperation. Walking, biking, and swimming are acceptable exercise modalities, but weight training may be considered contraindicated in anyone who is symptomatic with shortness of breath or chest pain or discomfort.

A perceived exertion between light and somewhat hard (rate of perceived exertion of 11-14; see Table 12-13) is the goal, but the individual will usually begin with a much lighter workout and progress over time to this level.[414] Tolerance to symptoms and current exercise habits are important determinants in progressing an exercise program.

Some people with valvular disease avoid physical activity as much as possible and never exercise to the point of developing any symptoms of dyspnea, fatigue, or muscular discomfort. These symptoms develop at light loads in people unaccustomed to any physical activity, regardless of the severity of the valvular disease. Other people force themselves to ignore mild (or even moderate to severe) symptoms to stay on the job or finish a task started.

Fatigue, weakness, and pallor are signs of an inadequate cardiac output for the demands of the exercise. These signs and symptoms are partly subjective, and it is a clinical decision as to how far to allow these people to continue exercising. Chest pain may indicate myocardial ischemia or pulmonary hypertension, or it may be a noncardiac symptom arising from the chest wall.

Follow precautions for angina pectoris. Exercise should be stopped immediately when any signs of reduced cerebral blood flow develop, such as severe facial pallor, confusion, dizziness, heart palpitations, or unsteady gait (see also Boxes 12-4 and 12-9).

Pulmonary edema can be produced by exercising beyond a certain point in people with valvular disease, especially those with mitral stenosis. Pulmonary congestion induced by exercise may cause coughing rather than dyspnea, and exercise should be stopped if coughing becomes significant. Heart failure may occur secondary to chronic, progressive valvular disease. Slight puffiness of the ankles at the end of the day, nocturia, mild nocturnal dyspnea, unexpected weight gain, or more than the usual amount of fatigue can be minor symptoms that are passed over unless specifically sought. Such symptoms must be reported to the physician. (See also "Special Implications for the Therapist 12-7: Congestive Heart Failure" above.)

The status of the myocardium is another important variable in exercise impairment relative to valvular heart disease. Severe aortic regurgitation is well tolerated for many years until myocardial weakness occurs. In all forms of heart disease, the healthy myocardium can compensate and maintain the systemic blood flow at or near normal levels for an extended period of time. For the client with valvular disease and myocardial disease or associated CAD, this compensation is not possible, and a lower exercise capacity results.

Stenosis

Valvular stenosis develops or progresses gradually, and because the normal valve orifice is larger than is necessary, stenosis is usually severe before exercise symptoms occur (i.e., a normal valve is larger than is needed for normal functioning and therefore has excess capacity). Stenosis only becomes symptomatic when the condition encroaches on the critical cross-sectional diameter of the opening so that a doubling of the blood flow (from activity or exertion) across the valve quadruples the atrial pressure. When the atrial pressure exceeds 25 mm Hg, dyspnea develops. The intensity of exertion associated with dyspnea does correlate with the magnitude of atrial pressure, providing a good indicator of the severity of stenosis. However, some people do not complain of dyspnea from lung congestion, only muscular fatigue on exertion as a result of a low cardiac output.

Stress testing may be performed before initiation of an exercise program; with or without those test results, clients should be monitored closely, possibly using the perceived exertion or dyspnea scales mentioned earlier in this chapter. Because of reduced cardiac output, muscle perfusion is reduced and lactate is produced at low workloads. Maximal heart rate may be reduced when dyspnea is the cause of premature termination of exercise. Exercise systolic blood pressure may reach only 130 mm Hg because of low output. Exercise capacity in clients with mitral stenosis can be improved by slowing heart rate and prolonging the diastolic filling period with the use of β-blocking agents.

In the case of symptomatic aortic stenosis, clients are not candidates for exercise programs because of the danger of sudden death. Persons who are asymptomatic must be carefully screened before increasing their physical activity, and for most, exercise intensity should be mild. In people with impaired left ventricular function, cardiac output fails to increase normally with exercise, causing fatigue. Angina with exercise is a common symptom when the aortic stenosis is severe.

Regurgitation

Exercise capacity may be unaffected in cases of mild regurgitation. Mitral regurgitation increases when aortic blood pressure is increased, such as occurs during isometric contractions. Light to moderate rhythmic and repetitive exercise reduces peripheral resistance and is recommended in place of isotonic exercise, which increases the heart rate. Persons with aortic regurgitation caused by weakening of the aortic wall (Marfan or Ehlers-Danlos syndrome) must avoid all strenuous exercise.[125,340]

Prolapse

Most people with MVP can participate in all sports activities, including intense competitive sports. Exercise is a key component in the management of MVP (not to alter function of the prolapsed valve but to improve overall cardiovascular function), and although many clients are referred to an exercise physiologist, the physical therapist may also encounter requests for conditioning and exercise programs. Many times, symptoms of fatigue and dyspnea cause a person to limit physical activity, leading to deconditioning and contributing to a cycle of even more fatigue and shortness of breath.

Caution is advised in the use of weight training for the client with MVP; gradual buildup using light weights and increased repetitions is recommended. Some people with MVPS are prone to exercise-induced arrhythmias, which can (rarely) result in sudden death. Any time tachycardia develops in someone with known MVP, immediate medical referral is necessary.

Postoperative Considerations

Postoperative considerations are the same as for people who have had abdominal or cardiothoracic surgery (see "The Cardiac Client and Surgery" below; see also Boxes 12-3 and 12-4). After uncomplicated valve ballooning, a return to normal activities is possible within 5 to 7 days. Gradual walking programs can be initiated at home for most people 10 days after surgery, or the client may enroll in a structured cardiac rehabilitation program.

Cardiac rehabilitation postoperatively in people with valvular heart disease is similar to that in post-CABG clients. Care should be taken to avoid high-impact exercises or exercises with a risk of trauma in people who are receiving anticoagulation therapy to avoid hemarthrosis and bruising (see Tables 40-8 and 40-9).[414]

Exercise outcomes differ after aortic, mitral, and mitral/aortic valve surgery. The degree of improvement in exercise capacity depends on the degree of residual dysfunction, presence or absence of arrhythmia, age of the subject, and the effort made to improve exercise capacity. Functional capacity is substantially increased following aortic valve surgery but limited following mitral and mitral/aortic surgery, possibly because of differences in oxygen uptake. As mentioned, for people with mitral stenosis, exercise provides an early warning system, because the onset of dyspnea with strenuous exercise signals the beginning of clinical deterioration.[414]

People with mechanical prosthetic valves receive lifelong anticoagulant therapy (not required for bioprostheses) and may not tolerate vigorous, weight-bearing activities. Mechanical prostheses have fixed openings that place some limitation, at least theoretically, on cardiac performance during maximal effort.[239] Because stress testing results can be normal, exercise Doppler echocardiography has been used to help prescribe physical activity in clients with prosthetic valves.

Infective Endocarditis

Infective, or bacterial, endocarditis is an infection of the endocardium, the lining inside the heart, including the heart valves; it most commonly damages the mitral valve, followed by the aortic, tricuspid, and pulmonic valves. Bacterial endocarditis may involve normal valves but more often affects valves that have been damaged by some other previous pathologic process (e.g., rheumatic disease, congenital defects, cardiac surgery).

Endocarditis is categorized as either acute or subacute, depending on the clinical course, organisms, and condition of the valves. Endocarditis can occur at any age but rarely occurs in children; half of all clients diagnosed are older than 60 years. Older adults may be at greater risk of endocarditis because valvular endocardial disruption is more common, immunity is impaired, and nutrition is poor. Endocarditis is more prevalent among men than women.

Etiologic and Risk Factors

Endocarditis is frequently caused by bacteria (particularly streptococci or staphylococci) normally present in the mouth, respiratory system, or GI tract or as a result of abnormal growths on the closure lines of previously damaged valves (e.g., rheumatic disease).

In addition to those with previous valvular damage, persons with prosthetic heart valves, injection drug users, immunocompromised clients (including individuals receiving treatment for cancer), women who have had a suction abortion or pelvic infection related to intrauterine contraceptive devices, and postcardiac surgical clients are at high risk for developing endocarditis. Congenital heart disease and degenerative heart disease, such as calcific aortic stenosis, may also cause endocarditis.

Hospital-acquired infective endocarditis has become more common as a result of iatrogenic endocardial damage produced by surgery, intracardiac pressure-monitoring catheters, ventriculoatrial shunts, and hyperalimentation lines that reach the right atrium. Portals of entry for microorganisms are also provided by wounds, biopsy sites, pacemakers, IV and arterial catheters, indwelling urinary catheters, and intratracheal airways.

Pathogenesis

As an infection, endocarditis causes inflammation of the cardiac endothelium with destruction of the connective tissue. As these bloodborne microorganisms adhere to the endocardial surface, destruction of the connective tissue occurs as a result of the action of bacterial lytic enzymes. The surface endocardium becomes covered with fibrin and platelet thrombi that attract even more thrombogenic material.

The result is the formation of wart-like growths called *vegetations*. These vegetations, consisting of fibrin and platelets, can break off from the valve, embolize, and cause septic infarction in the myocardium, kidney, brain, spleen, abdomen, or extremities. These thromboemboli contain bacteria that not only cause ischemic infarcts but also form new sites of infection transforming into microabscesses. Bacteria may further invade the valves, causing intravalvular inflammation, destroying portions of the valves, and causing valve deformities.

Splinter hemorrhages of the nail beds may be caused by distal vasospasm, embolic events, or other local factors promoting engorgement and bleeding of the capillaries that lie right below the nail. The cause of digital clubbing is unclear, but perhaps platelet clumps lodge in the nail bed capillaries of the fingers and toes and release platelet-derived growth factor, resulting in the pathologic changes of clubbed digits.

Petechiae (small, red, nonblanching macules on the conjunctivae, palate, buccal mucosa, heels, shoulders, arms, legs, and upper chest) are thought to involve microemboli, but some have also suggested that immune complex vasculitis is the primary process.[235] Infective endocarditis of the right-side heart valves occurs commonly in injection drug users. Although a variety of hypotheses have been put forward to explain this phenomenon, no single explanation has been proven.

Clinical Manifestations

Endocarditis can develop insidiously, with symptoms remaining undetected for months, or it can cause symptoms immediately, as in the case of acute bacterial endocarditis. Clinical manifestations can be divided into many groups (Table 12-16). It causes varying degrees of valvular dysfunction and may be associated with manifestations involving any number of organ systems, including lungs, eyes, kidneys, bones, joints, and CNS. The mitral, aortic, tricuspid, and pulmonic valves can be affected (descending order); more than one valve can be infected at the same time. Neurologic signs and symptoms are predominant in about one third of all cases in those people older

Table 12-16	Clinical Manifestations of Infective Endocarditis			
Systemic Infection	**Intravascular Involvement**	**Immunologic Reaction**	**Musculoskeletal**	**Neurologic**
Fever	Chest pain	Arthralgia	Arthralgia	Confusion
Chills	Congestive heart failure	Proteinuria	Myalgias	Abscess
Sweats	Cold and painful extremities	Hematuria	Low-back pain	Cerebritis
Malaise	Clubbing	Acidosis		Meningitis
Weakness	Petechiae	Arthritis		Stroke (embolic or
Anorexia	Splinter hemorrhages			hemorrhagic)
Weight loss	Osler nodes			
Cough				
Dyspnea				
Hemoptysis				

than 60 years. The classic findings of fever, cardiac murmur, and petechial lesions of the skin, conjunctivae, and oral mucosa are not always present.

Up to 50% of people with infective endocarditis initially have musculoskeletal symptoms, including arthralgia (most common), arthritis, low back pain, and myalgia. Half of these people will have only musculoskeletal symptoms without other manifestations of endocarditis. The early onset of joint pain and myalgia as the first sign of endocarditis is more likely if the person is older and has had a previously diagnosed heart murmur.

Proximal joints are most often affected, especially the shoulder, followed by knee, hip, wrist, ankle, metatarsophalangeal and metacarpophalangeal joints, and acromioclavicular joints (order of declining incidence). Most often one or two joints are painful, and symptoms begin suddenly, accompanied by warmth, tenderness, and redness. Symmetric arthralgia in the knees or ankles may lead to a diagnosis of rheumatoid arthritis, but as a rule, morning stiffness is not as prevalent in clients with endocarditis as in those with rheumatoid arthritis or polymyalgia rheumatica.

Bone and joint infections are particularly common among injection drug users. The most common sites of osteoarticular infections are the vertebrae, wrist, and sternoclavicular and sacroiliac joints, often with multiple joint involvement.[398]

Almost one third of clients with endocarditis have low back pain, which may be the primary symptom reported. Back pain is accompanied by decreased range of motion and spinal tenderness. Pain may affect only one side, and it may be limited to the paraspinal muscles. Endocarditis-induced back pain may be very similar to that associated with a herniated lumbar disk, as it radiates to the leg and may be accentuated by raising the leg or by sneezing, coughing, or laughing; however, neurologic deficits are usually absent in persons with endocarditis.

Endocarditis may produce destructive changes in the sacroiliac joint characterized by pain localized over the sacroiliac, probably as a result of seeding of the joint by septic emboli. Widespread diffuse myalgia may occur during periods of fever, but this is not appreciably different from the general myalgia seen in clients with other febrile illnesses. More commonly, myalgia is restricted to the calf or thigh. Bilateral or unilateral leg myalgias occur in approximately 10% to 15% of all persons with endocarditis.

The cause of back pain and leg myalgia associated with endocarditis has not been determined. Concurrent aseptic meningitis is a possible hypothesis; a role for emboli that break off from the infected cardiac valves is supported by biopsy evidence of muscle necrosis or vasculitis in clients with endocarditis. Rarely, other musculoskeletal symptoms, such as osteomyelitis, tendinitis, hypertrophic osteoarthropathy, bone infarcts, and ischemic bone necrosis, may occur.

MEDICAL MANAGEMENT

DIAGNOSIS, TREATMENT, AND PROGNOSIS. Infective endocarditis is often difficult to diagnose because it can present with a wide array of signs and symptoms, as well as a confusing clinical picture. Blood cultures to identify specific pathogens in the presence of septicemia are required to determine appropriate antibiotic therapy, which is the primary medical intervention.

Other laboratory test results indicative of infectious endocarditis include elevated erythrocyte sedimentation rate, proteinuria, and hematuria. Echocardiography may be used to confirm the diagnosis and is useful in showing underlying valvular lesions and quantifying their severity. This test is not as useful in older adults, because it is common to find echogenic areas around and on degenerative valves that are impossible to distinguish from the infective vegetations seen in infective endocarditis. Large masses on valves are much more diagnostic.

Although it is easily prevented (for the at-risk person) by taking antibiotics before and after procedures such as dental cleaning, genitourinary instrumentation, and open cardiovascular surgery, endocarditis is difficult to treat and can result in serious heart damage or death. Potential complications are many, including CHF and arterial, systemic, or PEs. Therapy with antibiotics may be prolonged, and without complete treatment, relapse can occur up to 2 or more weeks after medical intervention. Surgical valve replacement may be necessary, depending on the response to treatment, sites of infection, recurrent infection, or infection of a prosthetic valve.

SPECIAL IMPLICATIONS FOR THE THERAPIST 12-14

Infective Endocarditis
Physical exertion beyond normal activities of daily living is usually limited for the person receiving antibiotic therapy for endocarditis and during the following weeks of recovery. The therapist is not likely to treat a

person diagnosed during this acute phase of endocarditis. However, because early manifestations of endocarditis may be primarily peripheral (musculoskeletal or cutaneous) in nature, the therapist may be the first to recognize signs and symptoms of a systemic disorder.

Splinter hemorrhages (dark red linear streaks resembling splinters under the nail bed), clubbing (see Fig. 15-4), petechiae, purplish red subcutaneous nodes on the finger and toe pads, and lesions on the thenar and hypothenar eminences of the palms, fingers, and sometimes the soles are present in up to 50% of affected individuals.[235]

For any client with known risk factors or a recent history of endocarditis, the therapist must be alert for signs of endocarditis, indications of complications (easy fatigue associated with heart failure or peripheral emboli), lack of response to therapy intervention, or signs indicating relapse. Often, the client thinks the symptoms are recurrent bouts of the flu.

Rheumatic Fever and Heart Disease

Overview, Incidence, and Etiologic Factors

Rheumatic fever is one form of endocarditis (infection), caused by streptococcal group A bacteria, that can be fatal or may lead to rheumatic heart disease (10% of cases), a chronic condition caused by scarring and deformity of the heart valves (Figs. 12-22 and 12-23). It is called rheumatic fever because two of the most common symptoms are fever and joint pain.

The infection generally starts with strep throat in children between ages 5 and 15 years and damages the heart in approximately 50% of cases. The aggressive use of specific antibiotics in the United States had effectively reduced the incidence of rheumatic fever to around 0.5 cases per 100,000 school-age children and removed it as the primary cause of valvular damage.

However, between 1985 and 1987, a series of epidemics of rheumatic fever were reported in several widely diverse geographic regions of the continental United States, affecting children, young adults aged 18 to 30 years, and, occasionally, middle-aged persons. Currently, the prevalence and incidence of cases have not approximated the 1985 record, but they have remained above previous levels.

Pathogenesis

The exact pathogenesis is unclear, but rheumatic fever produces a diffuse, proliferative, and exudative inflammatory process in the connective tissue of certain structures. The bacteria adhere to the oral and pharyngeal cells and then release their degradation products. Antigens to streptococcal cells bind to receptors on the heart, brain cells, muscles, and joints, which begins the autoimmune response; thus rheumatic fever is classified as an autoimmune disease. In the case of the heart valves, the inflammatory products cross-react with cardiac proteins, affecting cardiac valve tissue and myocardium. All layers of the heart (epicardium, endocardium, myocardium,

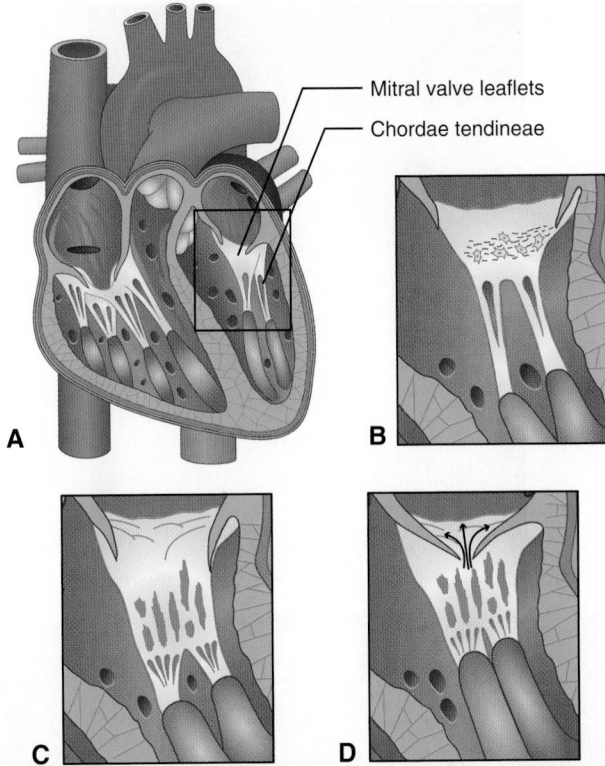

Mitral valve leaflets

Chordae tendineae

A **B**

C **D**

Figure 12-22

Cardiac valvular disease caused by rheumatic fever. A, Inflammation of the membrane over the mitral (and aortic) valves may cause edema and accumulation of fibrin and platelets on the chordae tendineae. **B,** This accumulation of inflammatory materials produces rheumatic vegetations that affect the support provided by the chordae tendineae to the atrioventricular valves. **C,** In this view, the mitral valve leaflets have become thickened with scar tissue and calcified. The chordae tendineae often fuse. **D,** As a result, the scarred valve fails to close tightly (mitral stenosis) and regurgitation or backflow of blood into the atrium develops. Prolonged, severe stenosis with mitral regurgitation leads to symptoms of congestive heart failure. (Modified from Goodman CC, Snyder TE: *Differential diagnosis in physical therapy,* ed 3, Philadelphia, 2000, WB Saunders, p. 110.)

pericardium) (Fig. 12-24) may be involved, including the valves.

Endocardial inflammation causes swelling of the valve leaflets, with secondary erosion along the lines of leaflet contact. Small, bead-like clumps of vegetation containing platelets and fibrin are deposited on eroded valvular tissue and on the chordae tendineae; the mitral and aortic valves are most commonly affected.

Chordae are the tendinous cords connecting the two atrioventricular valves (the tricuspid valve between the right atrium and right ventricle and the mitral valve between the left atrium and left ventricle) to the appropriate papillary muscles in the heart ventricles; the chordae tendineae in effect anchor the valve leaflets. This support to the atrioventricular valves during ventricular systole helps prevent prolapse of the valve into the atrium.

Over time, scarring and shortening of the involved structures occur, and the leaflets adhere to each other as the valves lose their elasticity. As many as 25% of clients will have mitral valvular disease 25 to 30 years later, with fibrosis and calcification of valves, fusion of commissures

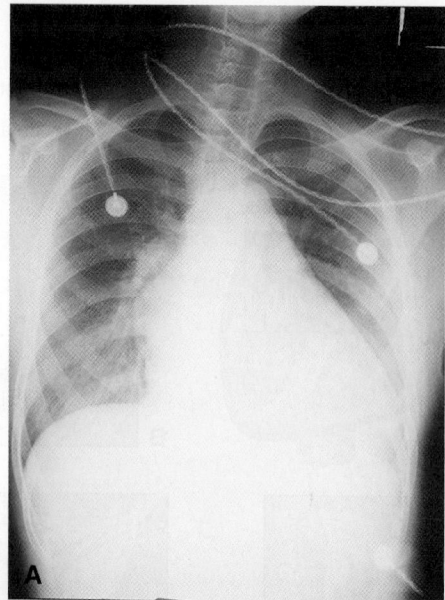

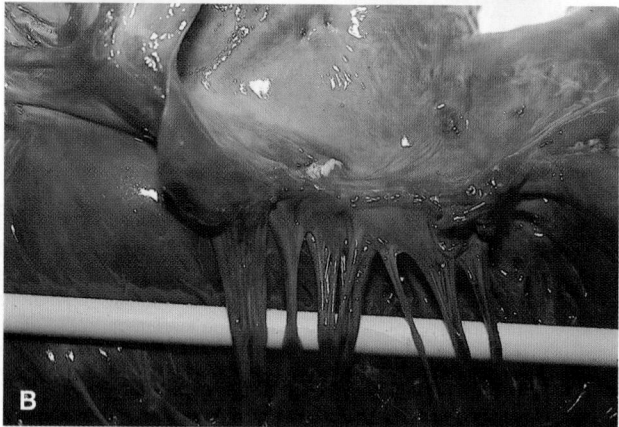

Figure 12-23

A, Chest radiograph of a 15-year-old boy who had multiple occurrences of acute rheumatic fever, showing gross cardiac enlargement and failure. He had mitral regurgitation and stenosis, and aortic regurgitation and stenosis. **B,** Postmortem cardiac examination of the same boy, showing thickened, shortened mitral valve cusps with calcific vegetation and thickened chordae tendineae. Chordae are the tendinous cords connecting the two atrioventricular (AV) valves (the tricuspid valve between the right atrium and right ventricle and the mitral valve between the left atrium and left ventricle) to the appropriate papillary muscles in the heart ventricles; the chordae tendineae in effect anchor the valve leaflets. This support to the AV valves during ventricular systole helps prevent prolapse of the valve into the atrium. (From Cohen J, Powderly WG: *Infectious diseases*, ed 2, St Louis, 2004, Mosby. Courtesy Professor Bart Currie, Darwin, NT, Australia.)

(union or junction between adjacent cusps of the heart valves) and chordae tendineae, and mitral stenosis with fish-mouth deformity (Fig. 12-25).

Clinical Manifestations

Although strep throat is the most common manifestation of the streptococcal virus, streptococcal infections can also affect the skin and, less commonly, the lungs. In some cases of strep throat, the initial triggering sore throat or pharyngitis does not cause extreme illness, if any discomfort at all.

However, the major manifestations of acute rheumatic fever are usually carditis, acute migratory polyarthritis, and chorea, which may occur singly or in combination. In the acute, full-blown sequelae, shortness of breath and increasing nocturnal cough also occur. A ring- or crescent-shaped rash with clear centers on the skin of the limbs or trunk (erythema marginatum) is present in fewer than 2% of persons in an acute episode. Subcutaneous nodules may occur over bony prominences and along the extensor surfaces of the arms, heels, knees, or back of the head, but these do not interfere with joint function.

Carditis is most likely to occur in children and adolescents. Mitral or aortic semilunar valve dysfunction (see "Pathogenesis" above) may result in a previously undetected murmur. Chest pain caused by pericardial inflammation and characteristic heart sounds may occur. *Polyarthritis* may develop in a child or young adult with acute rheumatic fever 2 to 3 weeks after an initial cold or sore throat. Sudden or gradual onset of painful migratory joint symptoms in knees, shoulders, feet, ankles, elbows, fingers, or neck; fever (37.2°-39.4° C [99°-103° F]); palpitations; and fatigue are present. Malaise, weakness, weight loss, and anorexia may accompany the fever.

The migratory arthralgias usually involve two or more joints simultaneously or in succession and may last only 24 hours, or they may persist for several weeks. In adults, only a single joint may be affected. Joints that are sore and hot and contain fluid completely resolve, followed by acute synovitis, heat, synovial space tenderness, swelling, and effusion present in a different area the next day. The persistence of swelling, heat, and synovitis in a single joint or joints for more than 2 to 3 weeks is extremely unusual in acute rheumatic fever.

Rheumatic *chorea* (also called Sydenham chorea or St. Vitus dance) occurs in 3% of cases 1 to 3 months after the streptococcal infection and is always preceded by polyarthritis. Chorea in a child, teenager, or young adult is almost always a manifestation of acute rheumatic fever. Other causes of chorea are SLE, thyrotoxicosis, and cerebrovascular accident, but these are uncommon and unlikely in a child.

The chorea develops as rapid, purposeless, nonrepetitive movements that may involve all muscles except the eyes. This pattern of movement may last for 1 week, several months, or even several years without permanent impairment of the CNS.

MEDICAL MANAGEMENT

DIAGNOSIS AND TREATMENT. Late diagnosis can have serious consequences requiring immediate antibiotic and antiinflammatory treatment. Jones criteria are used as the basis for diagnosis (Table 12-17), and results of throat culture for group A streptococci are usually positive. Echocardiography combined with Doppler technology provides reliable hemodynamic and anatomic data in the assessment of rheumatic heart disease.

Aspirin may be used to treat the joint manifestations and as a general antiinflammatory agent. Corticosteroids are used when there is clear evidence of rheumatic carditis. Children with acute chorea are generally treated with some form of CNS depressant, such as phenobarbital. Commissurotomy and prosthetic valve replacement

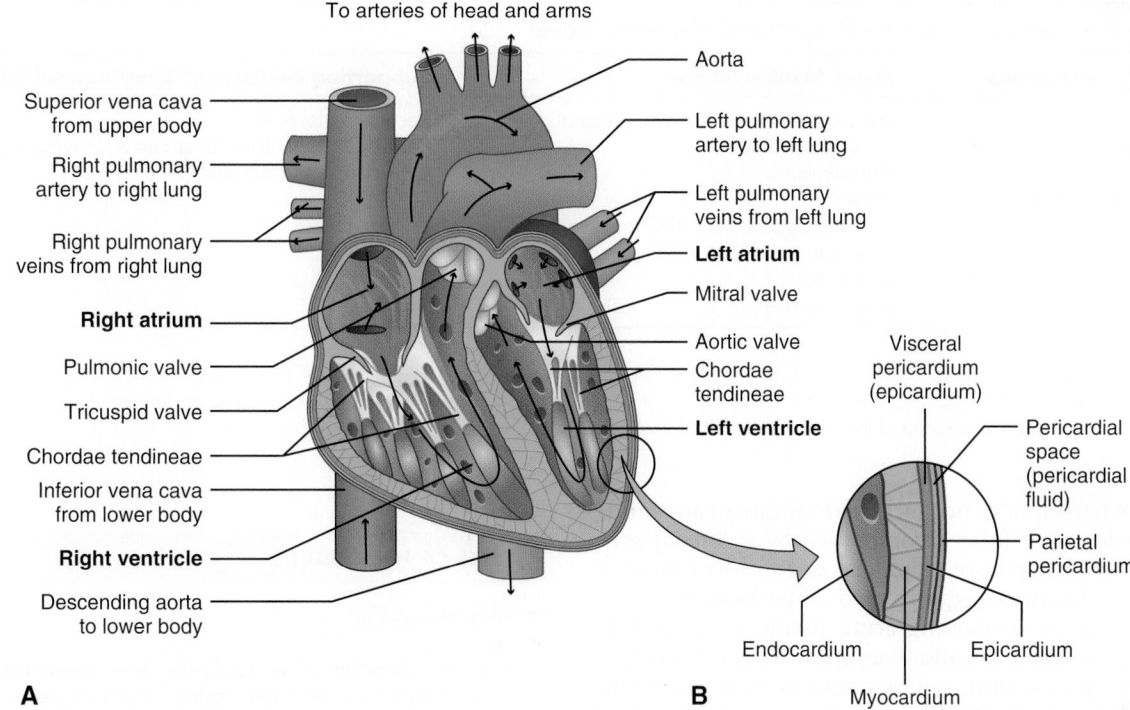

To arteries of head and arms

Aorta

Superior vena cava from upper body

Left pulmonary artery to left lung

Right pulmonary artery to right lung

Left pulmonary veins from left lung

Right pulmonary veins from right lung

Left atrium

Right atrium

Mitral valve

Pulmonic valve

Aortic valve

Tricuspid valve

Chordae tendineae

Chordae tendineae

Left ventricle

Inferior vena cava from lower body

Right ventricle

Visceral pericardium (epicardium)

Pericardial space (pericardial fluid)

Parietal pericardium

Descending aorta to lower body

Endocardium

Epicardium

A

B

Myocardium

Figure 12-24

A, Structure and circulation of the heart. Blood flows from the superior and inferior venae cavae into the right atrium through the tricuspid valve to the right ventricle. The right ventricle ejects the blood through the pulmonic valve into the pulmonary artery during ventricular systole. Blood enters the pulmonary capillary system, where it exchanges the carbon dioxide for oxygen. The oxygenated blood then leaves the lungs via the pulmonary veins and returns to the left atrium. From the left atrium, blood flows through the mitral valve into the left ventricle. The left ventricle pumps blood into the systemic circulation through the aorta to supply all the tissues of the body with oxygen. From the systemic circulation, blood returns to the heart through the superior and inferior venae cavae to begin the cycle again. **B,** Sagittal view of the layers of the heart wall.

may be necessary for valvular dysfunction associated with chronic rheumatic disease.

PROGNOSIS. Initial episodes of rheumatic fever last weeks to months, but 20% of children affected have recurrences within 5 years; relapses increase the risk of heart damage that leads to rheumatic heart disease, with mitral or aortic stenosis or insufficiency caused by progressive valve scarring. Mortality for acute rheumatic fever is low (1%-2%), but persistent rheumatic activity with complications (enlarged heart, AF, arterial embolism, heart failure, pericarditis) is associated with long-term morbidity and mortality.

SPECIAL IMPLICATIONS FOR THE THERAPIST 12-15

Rheumatic Fever and Heart Disease

The increased incidence of infection with streptococcal group A bacteria in the adult population may result in cases of sudden or gradual onset of painful migratory joint symptoms affecting the knees, shoulders, feet, ankles, elbows, fingers, or neck. Any time an adult presents with intermittent or migratory joint symptoms, the client's temperature must be taken.

The therapist should ask about recent exposure to someone with strep throat and a recent history or presence of rash anywhere on the body, sore throat, or cold. The sore throat or cold symptoms may be mild enough

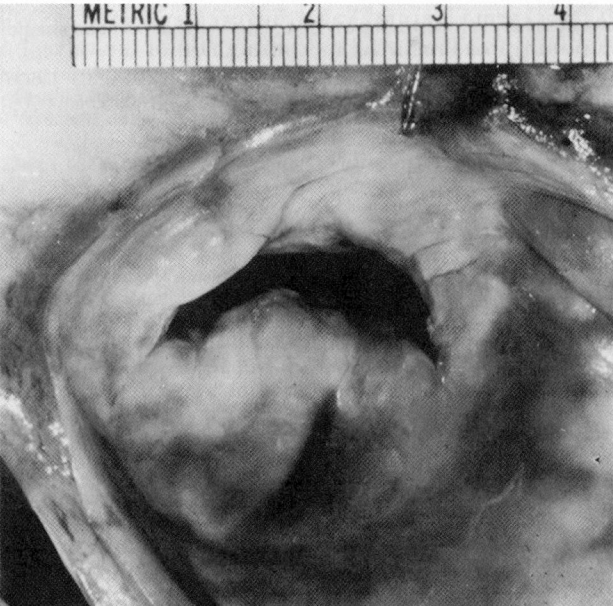

Figure 12-25

When viewed from the atrial aspect, a severely stenotic mitral valve has a narrowed orifice that has the appearance of a classic fish-mouth deformity. (From Kissane JM, ed: *Anderson's pathology,* St Louis, 1990, Mosby.)

Table 12-17	Jones Criteria for Diagnosis of Rheumatic Fever		
Major Manifestations	**Minor Manifestations**		**Supporting Evidence of Streptococcal Infection**
Carditis	Previous rheumatic fever or rheumatic		Recent scarlet fever
Polyarthritis	heart disease		Positive throat culture for group A *Streptococcus*
Chorea	Arthralgia		Other positive laboratory tests
Erythema marginatum	Fever		
Subcutaneous nodules	Elevated appearance of C-reactive		
	protein (see Table 12-3)		
	Leukocytosis		
	ECG changes		

ECG, Electrocardiogram.
Data from Dajani AS, Ayoub A, Burman FZ, et al: American Heart Association Medical/Scientific Statement: guidelines for the diagnosis of rheumatic fever: Jones criteria, 1992 update, *Circulation* 87:302–307, 1993. Jones criteria have been reviewed and remains valid per the Jones Criteria Working Group. In Ferrieri P: Proceedings of the Jones Criteria Workshop, *Circulation* 106:2521–2423, 2002.

that the person does not seek medical care of any kind. The presence of fever accompanied by a clinical presentation of migratory arthralgias or a history of recent illness as described requires medical evaluation.

The risk of developing acute rheumatic fever following untreated tonsillopharyngitis is only 1% in the pediatric population, but as many as 25% of people affected by rheumatic fever develop mitral valve dysfunction 25 to 30 years later. Adults who experience exercise intolerance or exertional dyspnea of unknown cause and who have a previous history of childhood rheumatic fever may be experiencing the effects of MVP. Dyspnea associated with MVP is most commonly accompanied by fatigue and palpitations. This history in combination with this triad of symptoms requires evaluation by a physician.

In the case of a confirmed diagnosis of rheumatic fever–related mitral valve involvement, exercise will not improve the mechanical function of the valve, but improvement in cardiovascular function can occur. (See "Special Implications for the Therapist 12-13: Valvular Heart Disease" above.)

DISEASES AFFECTING THE PERICARDIUM

The pericardium consists of two layers: the inner visceral layer, which is attached to the epicardium, and an outer parietal layer (see Fig. 12-24).

The pericardium stabilizes the heart in its anatomic position despite changes in body position and reduces excess friction between the heart and surrounding structures. It is composed of fibrous tissue that is loose enough to permit moderate changes in cardiac size but that cannot stretch fast enough to accommodate rapid dilation or accumulation of fluid without increasing intracardiac pressure.

The pericardium may be a primary site of disease and is often involved by processes that affect the heart; it may also be affected by diseases of the adjacent tissues. Pericardial diseases are common and have multiple causes. Three conditions primarily affect the pericardium: acute pericarditis, constrictive pericarditis, and pericardial effusion. These

Box 12-12

CAUSES OF PERICARDITIS

- Idiopathic (85%)
- Infections
  - Viral (Coxsackie, influenza, Epstein-Barr, hepatitis B, HIV, cytomegalovirus, varicella zoster, herpes simplex)
  - Bacterial (tuberculosis, *Staphylococcus*, *Streptococcus*, meningococcus, pneumonia, *Salmonella*, *Neisseria gonorrhoeae*, *Pseudomonas*)
  - Parasitic
  - Fungal
- Myocardial injury
  - MI
  - Cardiac trauma: instrumentation; blunt or penetrating pericardium; rib fracture
  - Postcardiac surgery
- Hypersensitivity
  - Collagen diseases: rheumatic fever, scleroderma, SLE, rheumatoid arthritis
  - Drug reaction
  - Radiation or cobalt therapy
- Metabolic disorders
  - Uremia
  - Myxedema
- Chronic anemia
- Neoplasm
  - Lymphoma, leukemia, lung or breast cancer
- Aortic dissection
- Graft-versus-host disease

Data from Bonow RO: *Braunwald's heart disease—a textbook of cardiovascular medicine*, ed 9, Philadelphia, 2011, WB Saunders.

three diseases are grouped together for ease of understanding in the following section.

Pericarditis

Definition and Overview

Pericarditis or inflammation of the pericardium, the double-layer membrane surrounding the heart, may be a primary condition or may be secondary to a number of diseases and circumstances (Box 12-12). It may occur as a single acute event, or it may recur and become a chronic condition called *constrictive pericarditis* (uncommon).

Incidence and Etiologic Factors

The most common types of pericarditis encountered by the therapist will be drug induced or those present in association with autoimmune diseases (e.g., connective tissue disorders such as SLE, rheumatoid arthritis), after MI, in conjunction with renal failure, after open heart surgery, and after radiation therapy.

Other types encountered less often include viral pericarditis (e.g., Epstein-Barr, hepatitis, HIV) and neoplastic pericarditis (from spread to the pericardium of adjacent lung cancer or invasion by breast cancer, leukemia, Hodgkin lymphoma). Isolated cases of constrictive pericarditis as a manifestation of chronic graft-versus-host disease after peripheral stem cell transplantation have been reported.[420]

Pathogenesis

Many causes of pericarditis affect both the pericardium and the myocardium (myopericarditis) with varying degrees of cardiac dysfunction. Constrictive pericarditis is characterized by a fibrotic, thickened, and adherent pericardium that is compressing the heart. The heart becomes restricted in movement and function (cardiac tamponade). Diastolic filling of the heart is reduced, venous pressures are elevated, cardiac output is decreased, and eventual cardiac failure may result.

When fluid accumulates within the pericardial sac it is referred to as *pericardial effusion*. Blunt chest trauma or any cause of acute pericarditis can lead to pericardial effusion. Rapid distention or excessive fluid accumulation from this condition can also compress the heart and reduce ventricular filling and cardiac output.

Clinical Manifestations

The presentation and course of pericarditis are determined by the underlying etiology. For example, pericarditis may occur 2 to 5 days after infarction as a result of an inflammatory reaction to myocardial necrosis, or it may occur within the first year after radiation initiates a fibrinous and fibrotic process in the pericardium. Often there is pleuritic chest pain that is made worse by lying down and by respiratory movements and is relieved by sitting upright or leaning forward. The pain is substernal and may radiate to the neck, shoulders, upper back, upper trapezius, left supraclavicular area, or epigastrium, or down the left arm.

Other symptoms may include fever, joint pain, dyspnea, or difficulty swallowing. Auscultation of the lower left sternal border where the pericardium lies close to the chest wall will produce a pericardial friction rub, a high-pitched scratchy sound that may be heard at end expiration. This sound is produced by the friction between the pericardial surfaces that results from inflammation and occurs during heart movement. Symptoms of constrictive pericarditis develop slowly and usually include progressive dyspnea, fatigue, weakness, peripheral edema, and ascites. Constrictive disease can lead to diastolic dysfunction and eventual heart failure.

MEDICAL MANAGEMENT

DIAGNOSIS. Clinical examination, including clinical presentation, auscultation, and client history, may be diagnostic. A classic sign of pericarditis is the pericardial friction rub heard on auscultation. Other diagnostic tools include chest x-ray (showing enlarged cardiac shadow), characteristic ECG changes (showing evidence of an underlying inflammatory process), and laboratory studies (e.g., elevated sedimentation rate or elevated white blood count [nonspecific indicators of inflammation] and elevated cardiac enzymes [post-MI]). CT, MRI, and echocardiography are modalities used for imaging the pericardium and pericardial disease.

TREATMENT. New treatments for pericardial diseases are being developed as a result of modern imaging, new understanding of molecular biology, and immunologic techniques. Comprehensive and systematic implementation of new techniques of pericardiocentesis, pericardial fluid analysis, pericardioscopy, and epicardial and pericardial biopsy, as well as the application of new techniques for pericardial fluid and biopsy analyses, have permitted early specific diagnosis, creating foundations for etiologic intervention in many cases. In cases of recurrent pericarditis resistant to conventional intervention and in the case of neoplastic pericarditis, intrapericardial application of medication has been proposed.[284]

Conventional treatment remains twofold, directed toward prevention of long-term complications and the underlying cause. For example, while any underlying infection is treated when possible (antibiotics for bacterial pericarditis), symptomatic treatment is provided for idiopathic, viral, or radiation pericarditis; antiinflammatory drugs are given for severe, acute pericarditis or pericarditis associated with connective tissue disorders; chemotherapy is given for neoplastic pericarditis; and dialysis is performed for uremic pericarditis. Analgesics may be prescribed for the pain and fever. Pericardiocentesis (surgical drainage with a needle catheter through a small subxiphoid incision) may be performed if cardiac compression from pericardial effusion does not resolve.

Treatment for constrictive pericarditis is both medical and surgical, including digoxin preparations, diuretics, sodium restriction, and pericardiectomy (surgical excision of the damaged pericardium).

PROGNOSIS. The prognosis in most cases of acute viral pericarditis is excellent when there is no (or only minimal) myocardial involvement, because this is frequently a self-limited disease. Without medical intervention, shock and death can occur from decreased cardiac output with cardiac involvement. Constrictive pericarditis is a progressive disease without spontaneous reversal of symptoms. Most people become progressively disabled over time. Surgical removal of the pericardium is associated with a high mortality rate when progressive calcification in the epicardium and dense adhesions or fibrosis between the pericardial layers are present.

SPECIAL IMPLICATIONS FOR THE THERAPIST **12-16**

Pericarditis

Pericardial pain can masquerade as a musculoskeletal problem, presenting as just upper back, neck, or upper trapezius pain. In such cases, the pain may be diminished by holding the breath or aggravated by swallowing or neck or trunk movements, especially side bending or rotation.

Pain is also aggravated by respiratory movements, such as deep breathing, coughing, and laughing. The therapist must screen for medical disease by assessing aggravating and relieving factors and by asking the client about a history of fever, chills, upper respiratory tract infection (recent cold or flu), weakness, heart disease, or recent MI (heart attack).

Special precautions depend on the underlying cause of the pericarditis. Mild cases require intervention per client tolerance, and the therapist observes for any symptoms of CHF. A mild pericarditis can quickly progress to a severe condition that requires medical evaluation. The clinician is referred to each individual section in this text representing the etiology of pericarditis for precautions.

DISEASES AFFECTING THE BLOOD VESSELS

Diseases of blood vessels observed in a therapy setting can include intestinal infarction, aneurysm, PVD, vascular neoplasm, and arteriovenous malformation; only intestinal infarction will not be discussed here.

Aneurysm

Definition and Overview

An aneurysm is an abnormal stretching (dilation) in the wall of an artery, a vein, or the heart with a diameter that is at least 50% greater than normal. When the vessel wall becomes weakened from trauma, congenital vascular disease, infection, or atherosclerosis, a permanent sac-like formation develops. A false aneurysm (pseudoaneurysm) can occur when the wall of the blood vessel is ruptured and blood escapes into surrounding tissues, forming a clot (Fig. 12-26; see also Fig. 12-28). Dissection is the disruption of the tunica media layer of the vessel wall with bleeding occurring within and along the wall that results in the separation of the wall layers.[208]

Aneurysms are of various types (either arterial or venous) and are named according to the specific site of formation (Fig. 12-27). The most common site for an arterial aneurysm is the aorta, forming a thoracic aneurysm (which involves the ascending, transverse, or first part of the descending portion of the aorta) or an abdominal aneurysm (which generally involves the aorta between the renal arteries and iliac branches).

Thoracic aortic aneurysms located above the diaphragm account for approximately 10% of all aortic aneurysms and occur most frequently in hypertensive men between the ages of 40 and 70 years. Men are more likely to have thoracic or abdominal aneurysms. Thoracic aortic aneurysms occur less often than other types but tend to be more life-threatening.

Abdominal aortic aneurysms located below the diaphragmatic border occur about four times more often than

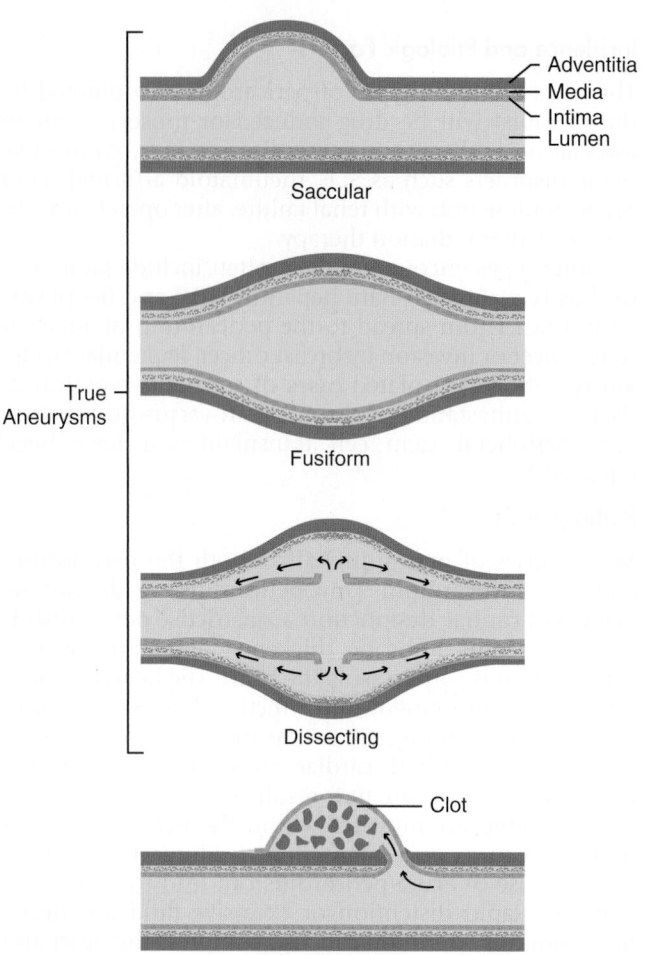

Figure 12-26

Longitudinal sections showing types of aneurysms. In a true aneurysm, layers of the vessel wall dilate in one of the following ways: saccular, a unilateral outpouching; fusiform, a diffuse dilation involving the entire circumference of the artery wall; or dissecting, a bilateral outpouching in which layers of the vessel wall separate, with creation of a cavity. In a false aneurysm, the wall ruptures, and a blood clot is retained in an outpouching of tissue.

thoracic aneurysms, most likely because the aorta is not supported by skeletal muscle at this location. The incidence of abdominal aortic aneurysm is increasing, probably because of the increasing number of adults over 65 years of age.

Peripheral arterial aneurysms affect the femoral and popliteal arteries.

Intracranial (cerebral) aneurysms affect cerebral arteries or veins. Unruptured intracranial aneurysms occur in 1% to 5% of the general population.[70] Fifty percent to 80% of all intracranial aneurysms do not rupture in the course of a person's lifetime.

Incidence and Etiologic Factors

According to the Society for Vascular Surgery, approximately 200,000 people in the United States are diagnosed annually with aortic aneurysm and 15,000 of those aneurysms are severe enough to rupture, causing a medical emergency.[426]

ANEURYSMS

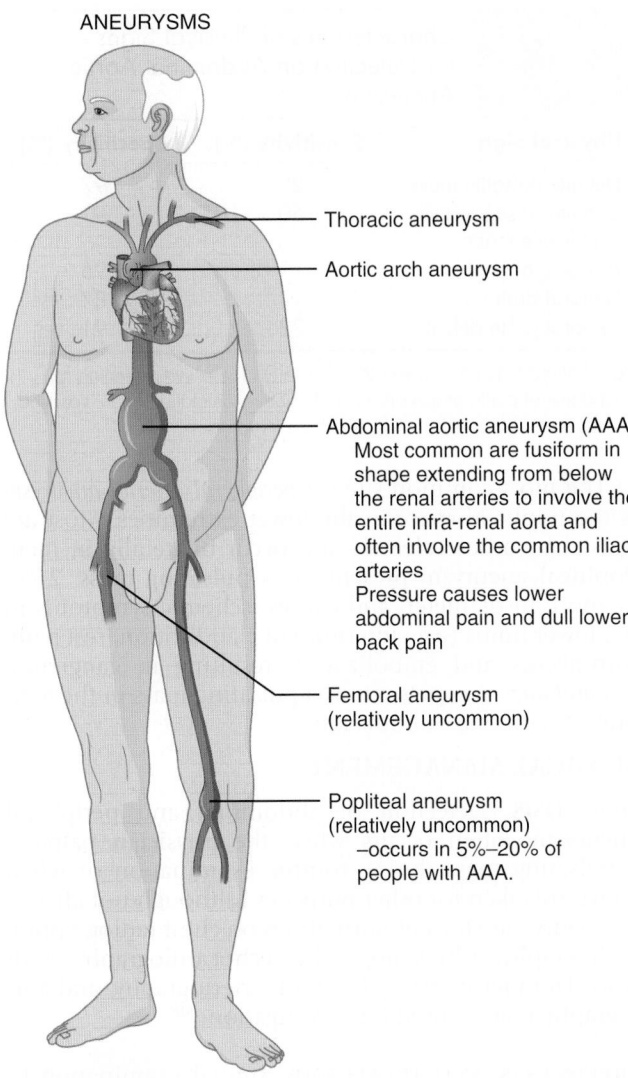

Thoracic aneurysm

Aortic arch aneurysm

Abdominal aortic aneurysm (AAA)
Most common are fusiform in
shape extending from below
the renal arteries to involve the
entire infra-renal aorta and
often involve the common iliac
arteries
Pressure causes lower
abdominal pain and dull lower
back pain

Femoral aneurysm
(relatively uncommon)

Popliteal aneurysm
(relatively uncommon)
—occurs in 5%–20% of
people with AAA.

Figure 12-27

Aneurysms are named according to the specific site of formation.
Abdominal aortic aneurysms are the most common type; more than
95% of abdominal aortic aneurysms are located below the renal arter-
ies and extend to the umbilicus, causing low back pain. (From Jarvis C:
Physical examination and health assessment, ed 5, Philadelphia, 2008,
WB Saunders.)

Aneurysms occur much more often in men than
in women, and half of affected persons are hypertensive. Incidence increases with increasing age, usually
beginning after age 50 years, presumably as a result
of chronic inflammatory cellular changes resulting in
atherosclerosis. However, someone without evidence
of atherosclerosis can develop an aneurysm, especially
in the presence of congenital weakness of the blood
vessel walls.

Family members (parent, adult child, or sibling) of
anyone with an aneurysm have a fourfold increased risk
of aneurysm, and gene defects on chromosomes 11[485]
and 15[245] are identified with some of the connective tissue disorders associated with aneurysm. A mutation in
a specific protein, transforming growth factor β receptor, is responsible for causing aneurysms.[276] Recently,
a genome-wide association study identified a gene for

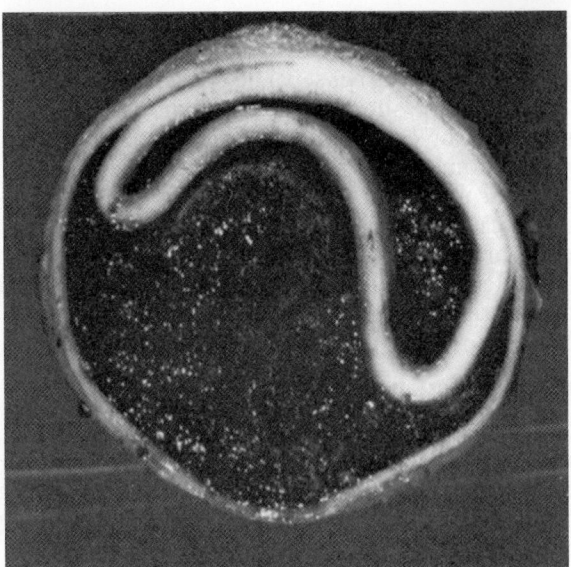

Figure 12-28

Dissecting aneurysm. Cross-section of the aorta with dissecting aneurysm showing true aortic lumen (*above and right*) compressed by dissecting column of blood that separates the media and creates a false
lumen. (From Kissane JM, ed: *Anderson's pathology*, St Louis, 1990,
Mosby.)

fibrillin 1 (the one implicated in Marfan syndrome) as
susceptible for the development of thoracic aortic aneurysms and aortic dissections.[263] This is exciting news as it
allows physicians to employ strategies used in individuals with Marfan syndrome to prevent or treat aortic aneurysms and dissections.

Atherosclerosis or any injury to the middle or muscular layer of the arterial wall (tunica media) is responsible
for most arterial aneurysms. Hypertension is an added
risk factor. Other, less-common causes of aneurysm
include trauma (blunt or surgical), Marfan disease (congenital defects of the arterial wall) and other hereditary
abnormalities of connective tissue, and inflammatory diseases and infectious agents (bacterial infection, syphilis,
polyarteritis).

The emergence of HIV has been associated with a dramatic increase in the incidence of syphilis. Because syphilitic aortitis generally presents between 10 and 30 years
after the primary infection, there may be an increased
incidence of associated aneurysms in the coming years.
Hypertension seems to enhance aneurysm formation.

Pathogenesis

The vessel wall weakens as a result of the decrease or loss
of elastic fibers that are replaced with nonstretchable proteoglycans, and loss of smooth muscle cells in the tunica
media.[208] Increased levels of possessing elastolytic activity
matrix metalloproteinases detected in the media of aortic
aneurysms are associated with degradation of elastin.[208]
Atherosclerotic plaques and inflammatory processes may
contribute to thinning and weakening of the wall.[208]

Plaque formation erodes the vessel wall, predisposing
the vessel to stretching of the inner and outer layers of the
artery and formation of a sac. When a dissection occurs,
the innermost layer of the aorta tears, creating a false

channel that allows blood to flow into the middle layer. With each heartbeat, the dissection can extend, causing the aortic wall to further separate or dissect.

With time, the aneurysm becomes more fibrotic, but it continues to bulge with each systole, thus acting as a reservoir for some of the stroke volume. In the case of thoracic aortic aneurysms, the sheer force of elevated blood pressure causes a tear in the intima with rapid disruption and rupture of the aortic wall. Subsequent hemorrhage causes a lengthwise splitting of the arterial wall, creating a false vessel (Fig. 12-28), and a hematoma may form in either channel (i.e., the false or true lumen).

Clinical Manifestations

Aneurysms may be asymptomatic; when they do occur, manifestations depend largely on the size and position of the aneurysm and its rate of growth. Persistent but vague substernal, back, neck, or jaw pain may occur as enlargement of the aneurysm impinges adjacent structures.

Aortic dissection may be experienced as extreme, sharp pain felt at the base of the neck or along the back into the interscapular areas. When pressure from a large volume of blood is placed on the trachea, esophagus, laryngeal nerve, lung, or superior vena cava, symptoms of dysphagia; hoarseness; edema of the neck, arms, or jaw and distended neck veins; and dyspnea and/or cough may occur, respectively.

Other signs and symptoms may be present in the case of *acute aortic dissection* as a result of compression of branches of the aorta. These include acute MI, reversible ischemic neurologic deficits, stroke, paraplegia, renal failure, intestinal ischemia, and ischemia of the arms and legs. Acute chest pain may also result from a nondissecting hematoma of the aorta or erosion of a penetrating atherosclerotic ulcer.[251]

In the case of an untreated *abdominal aortic aneurysm* expansion and rupture can occur in one of several places, including the peritoneal cavity, the mesentery, the retroperitoneum, into the inferior vena cava, or into the duodenum or rectum. Rupture refers to a tearing of all three tunicae (tunica adventitia, tunica media, tunica intima) with bleeding into the thoracic or abdominal cavity. The most common site for an abdominal aortic aneurysm is just below the renal arteries, and it may involve the bifurcation of the aorta (see Fig. 12-27).

Most abdominal aortic aneurysms are asymptomatic, but intermittent or constant pain in the form of mild to severe mid-abdominal or lower back discomfort is present in some form in 25% to 30% of cases. Groin or flank pain may be experienced because of increasing pressure on other structures.

Early warning signs of an impending rupture may include abdominal heartbeat when lying down or a dull ache (intermittent or constant) in the mid-abdominal left flank or lower back. Rupture is most likely to occur in aneurysms that are 5 cm or larger, causing intense flank pain with referred pain to the back at the level of the rupture. Pain may radiate to the lower abdomen, groin, or genitalia. Back pain may be the only presenting symptom before rupture occurs. Table 12-18 lists the sensitivity and specificity of some physical signs for detecting of an abdominal aortic aneurysm.[264]

Table 12-18	Characteristics of Physical Signs for Detecting an Abdominal Aortic Aneurysm	
Physical Sign	**Sensitivity (%)**	**Specificity (%)**
Definite pulsatile mass	28	97
Definite or suggestive pulsatile mass	50	91
Abdominal bruit	11	95
Femoral bruit	17	87
Femoral pulse deficit	22	91

Data from Lederle FA, Walker JM, Reinke DB: Selective screening for abdominal aortic aneurysms with physical examination and ultrasound, *Arch Intern Med* 148:1753, 1988.

The most common site for *peripheral arterial aneurysm* is the popliteal space in the lower extremities. Most are caused by atherosclerosis and occur bilaterally in men. Popliteal aneurysm presents as a pulsating mass, 2 cm or more in diameter, and causes ischemic symptoms in the lower limbs (e.g., intermittent claudication, rest pain, thrombosis and embolization resulting in gangrene). *Femoral aneurysm* presents as a pulsating mass in the femoral area on one or both sides.

MEDICAL MANAGEMENT

DIAGNOSIS. Detection of abdominal and peripheral aneurysms often occurs when the physician palpates a pulsating mass during routine examination or when x-rays are taken for other purposes (although not all aortic aneurysms show abnormalities on chest radiography). Radiography, ultrasonography, echocardiography with color Doppler imaging, CT, MRI, arteriography, and aortography may be used for investigation.[208]

PREVENTION AND TREATMENT. Annual examination to ensure early identification is recommended for family members (parent, adult child, or sibling) of anyone who has previously been diagnosed with an aortic aneurysm. Anyone with a family risk or signs of diseased arteries should take preventive measures, including smoking cessation, regular exercise, blood pressure control, and cholesterol management.[208]

Treatment is determined based on the size of the bulge, how fast it is expanding, and the individual's clinical presentation. The goal in managing dissecting aneurysms is to prevent further dissection and minimize the damage to organs that may not have received enough blood flow.[309]

For small aneurysms of any type, watchful waiting is often advised. Watchful waiting and preventive pharmacology (e.g., statin to lower cholesterol; β-blocker or ACE inhibitor to control blood pressure and prevent the aneurysm from getting larger or bursting) may be advised depending on individual factors. As a less-invasive alternative to open surgery, an endovascular treatment is used for some types of thoracic aortic aneurysm and dissection.[144] It involves insertion of an endovascular stent graft,[208] a fabric tube supported by a metal mesh.

For peripheral aneurysms, open or endovascular repair techniques are recommended.[392] Surgical intervention before rupture provides a good prognosis; at 5.5 cm distention in diameter (about 2 inches), the risk of rupture exceeds the risk of repair. A less invasive endovascular repair procedure known as *endoluminal stent-graft* may offer an alternative to traditional open abdominal surgery with better survival rates even for older, sicker adults. Guided by angiographic imaging, a catheter is inserted through the femoral or brachial artery to the aneurysm. A balloon within the catheter is then inflated, pushing open the stent graft, which attaches with tiny hooks to healthy arterial wall above and below the aneurysm. This creates a channel for blood flow that bypasses the aneurysm.[288]

PROGNOSIS. The standard open surgical approach to replace the diseased aorta is steadily improving but is still associated with high morbidity and substantial mortality rates. MI, respiratory failure, renal failure, and stroke are the principal causes of death and morbidity after surgical procedures performed on the thoracic aorta.

At the same time, the endoluminal stent-graft comes with its own set of complications, including fever, breakdown or migration of the device, leaks, and unknown durability. Further studies to improve treatment are ongoing. Aneurysm rupture is associated with a high mortality; frequently, aneurysms are discovered only at autopsy.

SPECIAL IMPLICATIONS FOR THE THERAPIST   12-17

Aneurysm

Because the prevalence of all diseases of the aorta increases with age and because the population in the United States is aging, it is expected that aortic aneurysm will be encountered with increasing frequency. Knowledge of the natural history, familial history, and clinical features of this disorder may alert the therapist to the need for medical intervention.

For the person who has had a surgically repaired aneurysm (open or endovascular repair), activities are restricted and are only gradually reintroduced. The therapist may be involved in bedside exercises and early mobility, which are especially important to prevent thromboembolism as a result of venous stasis during prolonged bed rest and immobility.

Because of the invasiveness of open abdominal surgery, anyone undergoing this procedure is at high risk for pulmonary complications. In fact, anyone with complications associated with an aneurysm is also at risk for pulmonary complications. Even with less-invasive endovascular repair, traditional manual muscle testing (or other activities involving isometric contraction) can significantly increase arterial blood pressure.[493] The therapist must be careful in documenting deficits in strength, endurance, and balance without overtly increasing blood pressure, especially in the early stages of rehabilitation.[360]

Incisional pain and the use of abdominal musculature in coughing discourage the person from full inspirations as well as effective forceful huffing or coughing. The acute care therapist will utilize clinical techniques to assist with cough with pillows or towel rolls at the incisional site and forceful huffing (see description in Chapter 15).[206]

Proper lifting techniques should be reviewed before discharge, even though the client will not be able to provide a return demonstration. Activities that require pushing, pulling, straining, or lifting more than 10 lb are restricted for 6 to 10 weeks postoperatively.

Anterior or abdominal soft tissue mobilization for persons with back pain who have postoperative abdominal scars may require indirect techniques. This precaution is especially true for the person with a previous abdominal aneurysm, the person with a known nonoperative aneurysm (less than 5 cm), or the person with a family history of aneurysm or an undiagnosed aneurysm.

The therapist must always palpate the abdomen for a pulsating mass before performing anterior or abdominal therapy. It is possible to palpate the width of the pulse beginning at the abdominal midline and progressing laterally. The pulse should be characterized by a uniform width on either side of the abdominal midline until the umbilicus is reached, at which point the aortic bifurcation results in expansion of the pulse width. Throbbing pain that increases with exertion should alert the therapist to the need to monitor vital signs and palpate pulses.

Peripheral Vascular Disease

Although PVD is usually thought to refer to diseases of the blood vessels supplying the extremities, in fact, PVD actually encompasses pathologic conditions of blood vessels supplying the extremities and the major abdominal organs, most often apparent in the intestines and kidneys.

PVD is organized based on the underlying pathologic finding (e.g., inflammatory, arterial occlusive, venous, or vasomotor disorders) (Box 12-13). Although the terms *peripheral arterial disease* (PAD) and *peripheral vascular disease* (PVD) are often used interchangeably, PVD is a broader, more encompassing grouping of disorders of both the arterial and venous blood vessels, whereas PAD only refers to arterial blood vessels. PVD typically affects the legs more often than the arms, but upper extremity involvement is not uncommon.

Approximately 8 million Americans older than age 60 years are affected by PVD, with 20% of those people older than age 70 years. Like CAD and cerebrovascular disease, arterial occlusive forms of PVD are most common as a result of atherosclerosis. Intermittent claudication is the classic symptom of PAD. Like angina associated with CAD, intermittent claudication associated with PAD is predictable and nearly always develops after the same amount of exertion (e.g., walking a specific distance), generally occurs in the calves and less commonly in the thighs and buttocks,[90] and usually improves rapidly with rest.[332]

Data from the Framingham Heart Study and other population studies indicate that intermittent claudication sharply increases in late middle age and is somewhat higher among men than women. In fact the true prevalence of PAD is at least five times higher than expected based on the reported prevalence of intermittent claudication.[117] Specific symptoms of the various forms of PVD depend on the underlying pathologic condition, the blood vessels involved (arteries or veins), and the location of the affected blood vessels; each form is discussed individually in the following sections.

Box 12-13

PERIPHERAL VASCULAR DISEASES

Inflammatory Disorders

- Vasculitis (see also Table 12-19)
- Polyarteritis nodosa
- Arteritis
- Allergic or hypersensitivity angiitis
- Kawasaki disease
- Thromboangiitis obliterans (Buerger disease)

Arterial Occlusive Disorders

- Arterial thrombosis/embolism
- Thromboangiitis obliterans
- Arteriosclerosis obliterans

Venous Disorders

- Thrombophlebitis
- Varicose veins
- Chronic venous insufficiency

Vasomotor Disorders

- Raynaud disease
- Complex regional pain syndrome (formerly reflex sympathetic dystrophy)

Inflammatory Disorders

Inflammatory conditions of the blood vessels are often discussed as immunologic conditions, because inflammation and damage to large and small vessels result in end-stage organ damage. Vasculitis (e.g., arteritis, such as polyarteritis nodosa and giant cell arteritis, Kawasaki disease) is the most commonly encountered inflammatory blood vessel disease in a therapy practice.

Vasculitis is actually a group of disorders that share a common pathogenesis of inflammation of the blood vessels involving arteries, veins, or nerves, resulting in narrowing or occlusion of the lumen or formation of aneurysms that can rupture. Vascular inflammation is a central feature of many rheumatic diseases, especially rheumatoid arthritis and scleroderma. (See also "Rheumatoid Vasculitis" in Chapter 5.)

Vasculitis. Vasculitis can involve blood vessels of any size, type, or location, and can affect any organ system, including the nervous system; classification is usually according to the size of the predominant vessels involved (Table 12-19). Vasculitis may be acute or chronic with varying degrees of involvement. The distribution of lesions may be irregular and segmental rather than continuous.

Neurologic manifestations of vasculitis can occur in conjunction with any of the vasculitides listed, affecting the peripheral nervous system or the CNS. Vasculitis may occur as an isolated peripheral nerve vasculitis (localized vasculitis). Numerous vasculitic diseases have been reported in association with HIV disease. The primary

---

Table 12-19 Vasculitis

Vessels Involved	Vasculitides	Organ Systems Involved
Small vessels (arterioles, capillaries, venules)	Inflammatory bowel disease vasculitis Hypersensitivity vasculitis; drug-induced vasculitis Vasculitis associated with infections or other diseases Immune-complex small vessel vasculitis associated with autoimmune conditions (paraneoplastic vasculitis)	Skin, viscera, heart, synovium, GI tract According to underlying cause and involved structures
Medium-size and small vessels	Vasculitis associated with malignancy Thromboangiitis obliterans (Buerger disease) Kawasaki disease (muscular arteries, rarely veins) Polyarteritis nodosa Vasculitis in rheumatic disease and connective tissue disorders Angiitis of the CNS Wegener granulomatosis (uncommon)	Determined by site of malignancy Arteries and veins of digits and limbs Cardiac, iliac, renal, internal mammillary Aorta and its primary and secondary branches, renal and visceral arteries, muscle, testes, nerves Synovium, skin, nail beds CNS Local: nasal structures Systemic: lungs (upper and lower respiratory tracts), renal (glomerulonephritis), any organ can be involved
Large and medium-size vessels	Takayasu arteritis (rare) Giant cell (temporal) arteritis	Aorta and its primary branches, renal and visceral arteries Extracranial arteries of the head and neck; any other artery but less common
Peripheral nervous system	Localized vasculitis	Vasa nervosum at the level of the epineural arteries (i.e., blood vessels supplying the neural arch in the spinal axis)

GI, Gastrointestinal; CNS, central nervous system.

target organ involvement is usually muscle and nerve, skin, testicle, kidney, and, less often, the CNS.

Immune (antibody–antigen) complexes to each disorder are deposited in the blood vessels, resulting in varying symptoms depending on the organs affected. In the case of vasculitic neuropathy, the formation of antibody–antigen complexes activates the complement cascade with generation of C3a and C5a (chemotactic agents that recruit polymorphonuclear leukocytes to the vessel walls).

Phagocytosis of the immune complexes takes place, and release of free radicals and proteolytic enzymes disrupts cell membranes and damages blood vessel walls. The complement cascade generates the formation of complement membrane attack complex that also contributes to endothelial damage. The resulting damage to endothelial cells results in thickening of the vessel wall, occlusion, and ischemia of the affected nerves with axonal degeneration and the resultant neuropathy.

Polyarteritis Nodosa.

Overview and Etiologic Factors. Polyarteritis nodosa refers to a condition consisting of multiple sites of inflammatory and destructive lesions in the arterial system; the lesions are small masses of tissue in the form of nodes or projections (nodosum). The cause of polyarteritis nodosa is unknown, although hepatitis B is present in 50% of cases, and polyarteritis occurs more commonly among IV drug abusers and other groups who have a high prevalence of hepatitis B (see "Hepatitis B" in Chapter 17). Any age can be affected, but it is more common among young men.

Clinical Manifestations. Polyarteritis nodosa affects small and medium-sized blood vessels, resulting in a variety of clinical presentations depending on the specific site of the blood vessel involved. Some of the more likely symptoms include abrupt onset of fever, chills, tachycardia, arthralgia, and myositis with muscle tenderness.

Any organ of the body may be affected, but most often involved are the kidneys, heart, liver, GI tract, muscles, and testes. Abdominal pain, nausea, and vomiting are common with GI tract involvement. Pericarditis, myocarditis, arrhythmias, and MI reflect cardiac involvement. Complications may include aneurysm, hemorrhage, thrombosis, and fibrosis leading to occlusion of the lumen. Multiple asymmetric neuropathies (motor and sensory distribution) can occur when vasculitis affects the arteries of the peripheral nerves (vasa nervorum). Paresthesias, pain, weakness, and sensory loss occur, involving several or many peripheral nerves simultaneously.

MEDICAL MANAGEMENT

DIAGNOSIS, TREATMENT, AND PROGNOSIS. Diagnosis is made by characteristic laboratory findings, biopsy of symptomatic sites (especially muscle or nerve), and, possibly, visceral angiography. When CNS vasculitis is suspected, angiography is necessary, because MRI and CT do not provide sufficient evidence to confirm the diagnosis.

Prolonged use of corticosteroids is necessary to control fever and constitutional symptoms while vascular lesions are healing. Immunosuppressants may be used in conjunction with steroids to improve survival; withdrawal from drugs is often followed by relapse. Treatment of

polyarteritis nodosa associated with hepatitis B is more complicated, because cytotoxic drugs used to treat the vasculitis can exacerbate the hepatic disease. Prognosis is poor without intervention, with a 5-year survival rate of only 20%. Pharmacologic therapy with corticosteroids increases survival to 50%, and steroids combined with immunosuppressive drugs have improved 5-year survival to 90%.

Arteritis.

Overview and Incidence. Arteritis, sometimes called giant cell arteritis (GCA) or cranial or temporal arteritis, is a vasculitis primarily involving multiple sites of temporal and cranial arteries (i.e., arteries of the head and neck and sometimes the aortic arch).

It is the most common vasculitis in the United States and affects older people; the incidence increases with age after 50 years. Postmenopausal women are affected twice as often as men, especially those individuals who have an arthritis-related disease called *polymyalgia rheumatica* (PMR). Other risk factors identified in women include heart murmurs and smoking.

Etiologic Factors and Pathogenesis. Most studies show an association of GCA with a specific human leukocyte antigen allele, and tumor necrosis factor appears to influence the susceptibility to both GCA and PMR. There may be an infectious origin, but additional studies are necessary to clarify the genetic influence on susceptibility to these conditions. The molecular pathogenesis of GCA involves interleukin-1, intercellular adhesion molecules, and other factors, but the exact pathogenesis remains unknown. The possible role of female sex hormones requires further investigation.

Immunologic research indicates an antigen-driven disease with local T-cell and macrophage activation in vessel walls with calcified atrophic media. The middle layer (tunica media) of the large and medium-size arteries, particularly those blood vessels supplying blood to the head, is inflamed, causing the arteries to swell and obstruct blood flow (stenosis); ischemic complications and secondary thrombosis may occur. Healing produces fibrosis of the arterial wall and the affected blood vessel becomes cord-like, thickened, and nodular, which can be observed externally when the temporal artery is involved.

Clinical Manifestations. The onset of arteritis is usually sudden, with severe, continuous, unilateral, throbbing headache and temporal pain as the first symptoms, with flu-like symptoms or visual disturbances. The pain may radiate to the occipital area, face, or side of the neck. Visual disturbances range from blurring to diplopia to visual loss. Irreversible blindness may occur anywhere in the course of the disease from involvement of the ophthalmic artery.

Other symptoms may include enlarged, tender temporal artery; scalp sensitivity; and jaw claudication (i.e., pain in response to chewing, talking, or swallowing) when involvement of the external carotid artery causes ischemia of the masseter muscles; the pain is relieved by rest.

Approximately 40% of cases present with nonclassic symptoms of respiratory tract problems (most often dry cough), fever of unknown origin, painful paralysis of a shoulder (mononeuritis multiplex), or claudication of the arm with cold hands, arm weakness, and absent radial pulses.[242] Left untreated, the condition may lead to blindness and occasionally to a stroke, heart attack, or aortic dissection.

MEDICAL MANAGEMENT

DIAGNOSIS. Early diagnosis is important to prevent blindness caused by obstruction of the ophthalmic arteries. Diagnosis is made by recognition of the presenting symptoms, and in some cases, arteritis follows PMR, a similar condition. Although GCA and PMR may occur as separate entities, most epidemiologic surveys group these two conditions together as one disorder. These may be two forms of a common pathophysiologic process characterized by varying degrees of synovitis and arteritis. They may actually represent two points along a single disease continuum.

Biopsy of the temporal artery may be performed, but results are often negative given the focal (segmental) nature of the disease. Color ultrasonography of the temporal arteries detects characteristic signs of vasculitis with a high sensitivity and specificity even in the absence of clinical signs of vascular inflammation (helpful in diagnosing temporal arteritis in people with previously diagnosed PMR).

People with extracranial GCA present with occlusive arterial lesions that may be detected with multiple imaging modalities: arteriography, IV digital subtraction angiography, CT scanning, and MRA. However, inflammation of the arterial wall cannot be detected by these means.

Standard CT imaging with contrast enhancement and certain magnetic resonance sequences, as well as ultrasound, permit identification of the edema and inflammation of the vessel wall. This is an important marker for active disease. Laboratory findings include elevated erythrocyte sedimentation rate, reflective of the underlying inflammatory process.

TREATMENT AND PROGNOSIS. Treatment of arteritis to prevent blindness and other vascular complications is with oral antiinflammatory drugs (usually a corticosteroid such as prednisone), providing symptomatic relief in 3 to 5 days. Visual loss can be permanent if allowed to persist for several hours without adequate intervention. With proper intervention, arteritis is a self-limiting disease, usually resolving within 6 to 12 months. Approximately 30% of affected individuals relapse in the first year of treatment during dose tapering. Alternative therapies of combined pharmacology with corticosteroids and methotrexate may be more effective in controlling disease with fewer complications.[233]

Hypersensitivity Angiitis. Hypersensitivity angiitis, a form of vasculitis, can occur at any age, but it most commonly affects children and young adults. The etiology is unknown, but the disease often follows an upper respiratory tract infection, and allergy or drug sensitivity plays a role in some cases. It is usually localized to the small vessels of the skin, first appearing on the lower extremities in a variety of possible lesions.

A classic triad of symptoms occurs in 80% of cases that includes purpura (bruising and petechiae or round purplish red spots under the skin), arthritis, and abdominal pain. Inflammation and hemorrhage may occur in the synovium and CNS. Medical management (diagnosis, treatment, prognosis) is the same as for the other forms of vasculitis already discussed.

Kawasaki Disease.

Overview and Etiologic Factors. Kawasaki disease, also known as mucocutaneous lymph node syndrome, is an acute febrile illness associated with systemic (multiorgan) vasculitis. It can occur in any ethnic group but seems most prevalent in Asian populations (especially Japanese, with equal incidence in Japan and in the United States among Japanese or Japanese descendants).

Children younger than age 5 years comprise 80% of all cases, and 20% develop cardiac complications that can be fatal. The etiology is unknown, but because seasonal and geographic outbreaks appear to occur, an infectious cause is suspected. Current etiologic theories center on an immunologic response to an infectious, toxic, or antigenic substance.[269]

Pathogenesis. Substantial evidence suggests that immune activation has a role in the pathogenesis of Kawasaki syndrome. The principal area of pathologic findings is the cardiovascular system. Kawasaki disease progresses pathologically and clinically in stages. During the acute stage of the illness (first 2 weeks) vascular inflammation and immune activation within the arterioles, venules, and capillaries occur, which later progress (stage 2, weeks 2-4) to include the main coronary arteries, the heart, and the larger veins.

The acute phase is also associated with the appearance of circulating antibodies that are cytotoxic against vascular endothelial cells; the presence of elevated anticardiac myosin autoantibodies may be involved in the myocardial damage that occurs in this phase. In the final stage the vessels develop scarring, intimal thickening, calcification, and formation of thrombi. If death occurs as a result of this disease (rare), it is usually the result of aneurysm, coronary thrombosis, or severe scar formation and stenosis of the main coronary artery.

Clinical Manifestations. Clinical manifestations present in three phases: acute phase, subacute phase, and convalescent phase. In the *acute phase*, a sudden high fever (lasting over 5 days) that is unresponsive to antibiotics and antipyretics is followed by extreme irritability.

During the *subacute phase* (lasting approximately 25 days), the fever resolves, but the irritability persists along with other symptoms, such as anorexia, rash (exanthema) of the trunk and extremities with reddened palms and soles of the hands and feet, and subsequent desquamation (skin scales off) of the tips of the toes and fingers, peripheral edema of the hands and feet, cervical lymphadenopathy (usually unilateral), bilateral conjunctival infection without exudate, and changes in the oral mucous membranes (e.g., erythema, dryness and cracks or fissures of the lips, reddening or strawberry tongue).

In one third of all cases, children develop arthralgias and GI tract symptoms, typically lasting about 2 weeks. Joint involvement may persist for as long as 3 months. During this subacute phase, the person is at risk for cardiac involvement, especially the development of myocarditis, pericarditis, and arteritis that predisposes to the formation of coronary artery aneurysm in nearly 25% of cases not treated within 10 days of fever onset.

The *convalescent phase* occurs 6 to 8 weeks after onset of Kawasaki disease and is characterized by a resolution of all clinical signs and symptoms. However, during this phase the blood values have not returned to normal. At the end of the convalescent phase, all values return to normal and the child has usually regained his or her usual temperament, energy, and appetite.

MEDICAL MANAGEMENT

DIAGNOSIS, TREATMENT, AND PROGNOSIS. Early recognition and prompt management of the acute syndrome are critical. Diagnosis is made on the basis of clinical manifestations and associated laboratory tests (there are no specific laboratory tests for Kawasaki disease). Echocardiograms are useful in providing a baseline and for monitoring myocardial and coronary artery status.

The introduction of high-dose IV immune globulin in combination with aspirin therapy to reduce fever and control inflammation and aneurysm formation has significantly reduced the prevalence of coronary artery abnormalities. The exact mechanism by which this treatment intervention reduces the vasculitis of acute Kawasaki syndrome has not been determined.

Prognosis is good for recovery with intervention, although serious cardiovascular problems (e.g., coronary thrombosis, aneurysm) may occur later in persons with cardiac sequelae. Giant aneurysms (diameter exceeding 8 mm) have the worst prognosis, because these are unlikely to regress or resolve, with death common in this subgroup population. Occasionally, severe ischemic heart disease requires cardiac transplantation.[269]

Thromboangiitis Obliterans (Buerger Disease).

Overview and Pathogenesis. Thromboangiitis obliterans, also referred to as Buerger disease, is a vasculitis (inflammatory and thrombotic process) affecting the peripheral blood vessels (both arteries and veins), primarily in the extremities. The cause is not known, but it is most often found in men younger than 40 years who smoke heavily, although the incidence in women is increasing. There has been some suggestion that unrecognized cocaine use may masquerade as Buerger disease.[290]

The pathogenesis of thromboangiitis obliterans is unknown; general inflammatory concepts apply. The inflammatory lesions of the peripheral blood vessels are accompanied by thrombus formation and vasospasm occluding and eventually obliterating (destroying) small and medium-size vessels of the feet and hands.

Recent studies have linked elevated levels of homocysteine to Buerger disease. Homocysteine has many potential effects: it limits the bioavailability of nitric oxide, impairs endothelium-dependent vasorelaxation, increases oxidative stress, stimulates smooth muscle cell proliferation, alters the elastic properties of vessel walls, and generates a prethrombotic state through the activation of factor V.

Clinical Manifestations. Clinical manifestations of pain and tenderness of the affected part are caused by occlusion of the arteries, reduced blood flow, and subsequent reduced oxygenation. The symptoms are episodic and segmental, meaning that the symptoms come and go intermittently over time and appear in different asymmetric anatomic locations. The plantar, tibial, and digital vessels are most commonly affected in the lower leg and foot. Intermittent claudication centered in the arch of the foot or the palm of the hand is often the first symptom.

When the hands are affected, the digital, palmar, and ulnar arteries are most commonly involved. Pain at rest occurs, with persistent ischemia of one or more digits. Other symptoms include edema, cold sensitivity, rubor (redness of the skin from dilated capillaries under the skin), cyanosis, and thin, shiny, hairless skin (trophic changes) from chronic ischemia. Paresthesias, diminished or absent posterior tibial and dorsalis pedis pulses, painful ischemic ulceration, and eventual gangrene may develop (see Fig. 12-30). Inflammatory superficial thrombophlebitis is common.

MEDICAL MANAGEMENT

DIAGNOSIS, TREATMENT, AND PROGNOSIS. Arteriography may be used in the diagnosis, but definitive diagnosis of thromboangiitis obliterans is determined by histologic examination of the blood vessels (microabscesses in the vessel wall) in a leg amputated for gangrene. Given the new findings that cocaine use may present very much like Buerger disease, laboratory screening for drug use may be appropriate in some cases.[290]

Intervention should begin with cessation of smoking and avoidance of any environmental or secondhand smoke inhalation. All other treatment techniques are aimed at improving circulation to the foot or hand, including pharmacologic intervention (e.g., vasodilators, pain relief) and physical or occupational therapy (see also "Atherosclerosis: Medical Management" above).

Regional sympathetic ganglionectomy may produce vasodilation, ulcerations require wound care, and amputation (sometimes multiple) may be required when the individual is unable to quit smoking or when conservative care fails. With the recent finding of elevated levels of plasma homocysteine associated with Buerger disease, screening for hyperhomocysteinemia and treatment of this condition have been recommended, especially to assess which clients may eventually require amputation.

Thromboangiitis is not life-threatening, but it can result in progressive disability from pain and loss of function secondary to amputation. Cessation of smoking is the key determinant in prognosis.

SPECIAL IMPLICATIONS FOR THE THERAPIST   **12-18**

Inflammatory Disorders

Peripheral neuropathy is a well-known and frequently early manifestation of many vasculitic syndromes. The pattern of neuropathic involvement depends on the extent and temporal progression of the vasculitic process that produces ischemia. A severe, burning dysesthetic pain in the involved area is present in 70% to 80% of all cases.

Other symptoms may include paresthesias and sensory deficit; severe proximal muscle weakness and muscular atrophy can occur secondary to the neuropathy. In the early phase, one nerve is affected and causes symptoms in one extremity (mononeuritis multiplex), but other nerves can become involved as the disorder progresses.

The therapist should watch for anyone with neuropathy who exhibits constitutional symptoms, such as fever, arthralgia, or skin involvement. This may herald a possible vasculitic syndrome and requires medical referral for accurate diagnosis. Early recognition of vasculitis can help prevent a poor outcome. With no treatment or with a poor outcome to intervention, CNS involvement (e.g., encephalopathy, ischemic and hemorrhagic stroke, cranial nerve palsy) can occur late in the course of vasculitis.

When corticosteroids (e.g., prednisone alone or sometimes in combination with other medications) are used (e.g., in the case of vasculitic neuropathy), the therapist must be aware of the need for osteoporosis prevention and attend to the other potential side effects from the chronic use of these medications (see "Corticosteroids" in Chapter 5).

Alternative methods of pain control may be offered in a rehabilitation setting, such as biofeedback, transcutaneous electrical nerve stimulation, and physiologic modulation (e.g., using a handheld temperature sensor to control autonomic nervous system function; see "Fibromyalgia" in Chapter 7).

Vasculitis (Inflammatory Disease of Arteries and Veins)

The therapist's role in management of vasculitis may be primarily for relief of painful muscular and joint symptoms when present and in the prevention of functional loss in the case of neuropathies. For the client with thromboangiitis obliterans (Buerger disease), exercise must be graded to avoid claudication and the client must be instructed in a home program for preventive skin care (see Box 12-14). Gangrene can occur as a result of prolonged ischemia from vessel obliteration; clients are typically treated for wound care and postoperatively after amputation. (See "Arteriosclerosis Obliterans" below.)

Often a client with some other primary orthopedic or neurologic diagnosis has also been medically diagnosed with vasculitis (see "Rheumatoid Vasculitis" in Chapter 5 and the "Special Implications for the Therapist" boxes for clients with associated cardiovascular involvement, such as atherosclerosis, myocarditis, pericarditis, or aneurysm).

Arteritis

Early recognition and referral can prevent the serious complications associated with arteritis. Older adults who experience sudden or unexplained headaches, lingering flu-like symptoms such as muscle aches (myalgia) and fatigue, persistent fever, unexplained weight loss, jaw pain when eating, or visual disturbances must be referred to their physicians. This is especially true for anyone with a previous diagnosis of PMR.

The use of corticosteroids can result in side effects such as osteoporosis and bone fractures, weight gain, diabetes, and high blood pressure (see complete discussion in Chapter 5). The client must be advised regarding an osteoporosis prevention program (see discussion in Chapter 24) and how to handle an increase in appetite. Remaining physically active and exercising are key components for both these issues.

Arterial Occlusive Diseases

Occlusive diseases of the blood vessels are a common cause of disability and usually occur as a result of atherosclerosis. Other causes of arterial occlusion include trauma, thrombus or embolism, vasculitis, vasomotor disorders such as Raynaud disease or phenomenon and complex regional pain syndrome (formerly reflex sympathetic dystrophy), arterial punctures, polycythemia, and chronic mechanical irritation of the subclavian artery as a result of compression by a cervical rib. For each individual case, see the discussion of the underlying cause of the occlusion to understand etiologic and risk factors and pathogenesis.

Atherosclerotic occlusive disease can also affect other vessels throughout the body other than the cardiac blood vessels. For example, occlusive disease affecting the intestines results in acute intestinal ischemia or ischemic colitis (see Chapter 16), depending on the location of the occlusion.

Occlusive cerebrovascular disease (see Chapter 32) as a result of atherosclerosis accounts for many episodes of weakness, dizziness, blurred vision, or sudden cerebrovascular accident or stroke. Extracranial arterial ischemia (e.g., common carotid bifurcation, vertebral artery) accounts for more than half of these types of strokes.

Arterial Thrombosis and Embolism. Occlusive diseases may be complicated by arterial thrombosis and embolism (Fig. 12-29). Chronic, incomplete arterial obstruction usually results in the development of collateral vessels before complete occlusion threatens circulation to the extremity. Arterial embolism is generally a complication of ischemic or rheumatic heart disease, with or without MI.

Signs and symptoms of pain, numbness, coldness, tingling or changes in sensation, skin changes (pallor, mottling), weakness, and muscle spasm occur in the extremity distal to the block (Fig. 12-30). Treatment may include immediate or delayed embolectomy, anticoagulation therapy (e.g., heparin), and protection of the limb.

Thromboangiitis Obliterans (Buerger Disease). Thromboangiitis obliterans is discussed as a vasculitis in an earlier section (see Inflammatory Disorders) but is mentioned here as an occlusive disorder because the inflammatory lesions of the peripheral blood vessels are accompanied by thrombus formation and vasospasm, occluding blood vessels.

Arteriosclerosis Obliterans (Peripheral Arterial Disease).

Definition and Overview. Arteriosclerosis obliterans, defined as arteriosclerosis in which proliferation of the intima has caused complete obliteration of the lumen of the artery, is also known as atherosclerotic occlusive disease, chronic occlusive arterial disease, obliterative

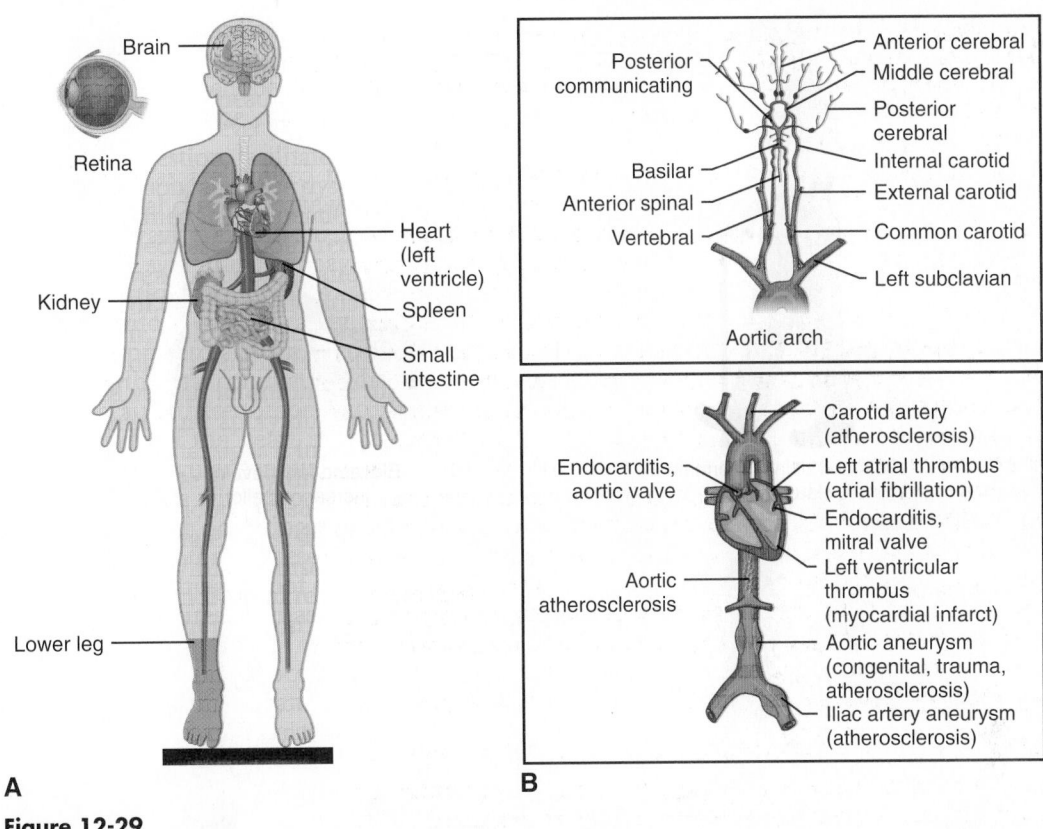

Figure 12-29

A, Common sites of infarction from arterial emboli. **B,** Sources of arterial emboli.

arteriosclerosis, and PAD. It is the most common arterial occlusive disease and accounts for approximately 95% of cases. It is a progressive disease that causes ischemic ulcers of the legs and feet and is most often seen in older clients, associated with diabetes mellitus.

Etiologic and Risk Factors. Atherosclerosis as the underlying cause of occlusive disease, with its known etiologic and associated risk factors, is discussed earlier in the chapter. PAD correlates most strongly with cigarette smoking and either diabetes or impaired glucose tolerance. Other risk factors include male gender, hypertension, low levels of HDL cholesterol, and high levels of triglycerides, apolipoprotein B, Lp(a), homocysteine, fibrinogen, and blood viscosity.

It has been reported that PAD is more prevalent in women than generally appreciated, but estimates vary greatly according to the diagnostic criteria applied. Prevalence and incidence rates do not differ significantly by gender, although incidence rates in women lag behind those in men in a pattern similar to that for CAD.[312]

Individuals with PAD are more likely to have CHD and cerebrovascular disease than those without PAD.[117] There has been a debate as to usefulness of screening for PAD, and a conclusion has been made that targeted screening is likely to reduce heart attack, stroke, and death in individuals with asymptomatic PAD.[45]

Pathogenesis. See also "Atherosclerosis: Pathogenesis" above.

Because peripheral disease is one expression of atherosclerosis, understanding the pathogenesis of atherosclerosis is important. The arterial narrowing or obstruction that occurs as a result of the atherosclerotic process reduces blood flow to the limbs during exercise or at rest. Muscular reactivity is also adversely affected in PAD. Prostacyclin and nitric oxide usually activate vascular relaxation. In PAD, these relaxation factors are reduced and constrictive factors such as endothelin increase. This imbalance of vascular reactivity contributes to decreased blood flow.[402]

Clinical Manifestations. In peripheral vessels, claudication symptoms appear when the diameter of the vessel narrows by 50%. PAD affecting the lower extremities is primarily one of large and medium-size arteries and most frequently involves branch points and bifurcations. Symptoms of arterial occlusive disease usually occur distal to the narrowing or obstruction. Acute ischemia may present with some or all of the classical symptoms, such as pain, pallor, paresthesia, paralysis, and pulselessness. However, arteries can become significantly blocked without symptoms developing, a phenomenon referred to as *silent ischemia.*

Even though silent ischemia is not associated with symptoms, it poses the same long-term sequelae and complications as overt ischemia and must be treated. It is strongly suspected when systolic blood pressure is lower at the ankle than at the arm (see further discussion of ankle/brachial index in this section).

Occlusive disease of the distal *aorta* and *iliac arteries* usually begins just proximal to the bifurcation of the common iliac arteries, causing changes in both lower extremities (Fig. 12-31; Table 12-20). Bilateral, progressive, intermittent claudication (pain, ache, or cramp in the muscles causing limping) is almost always present in

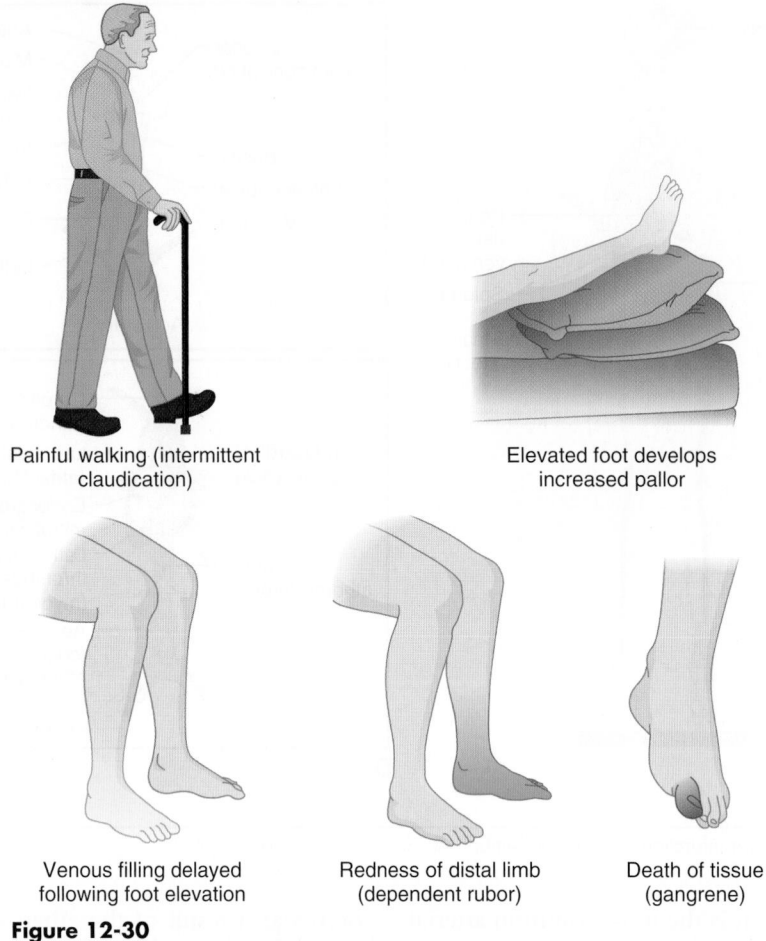

Painful walking (intermittent claudication)

Elevated foot develops increased pallor

Venous filling delayed following foot elevation

Redness of distal limb (dependent rubor)

Death of tissue (gangrene)

Figure 12-30

Signs and symptoms of arterial insufficiency.

the calf muscles and is usually present in the gluteal and quadriceps muscles presenting as buttock, thigh, and calf pain.

The distance a person can walk before the onset of pain indicates the degree of circulatory inadequacy (e.g., 2 blocks or more is mild; 1 block is moderate; 0.5 block or less is severe). The primary symptom may only be a sense of weakness or tiredness in these same areas; both the pain and weakness or fatigue are relieved by rest.

Occlusive disease of the *femoral and popliteal arteries* usually occurs at the point at which the superficial femoral artery passes through the adductor magnus tendon into the popliteal space. Occlusion of these regions is also marked by intermittent claudication of the calf and foot that may radiate to the ipsilateral popliteal region and lower thigh. Although symptoms occur ipsilateral to the occlusion anywhere distal to the bifurcation of the aorta, most people have bilateral disease and therefore bilateral symptoms. There are definite changes of the affected lower leg and foot as listed in Table 12-20.

Occlusive disease of the *tibial* and *common peroneal arteries*, as well as the pedal vessels and small digital vessels, occurs slowly and progressively over months or years. The eventual outcome depends on the vessels that are occluded and the condition of the proximal and collateral vessels. Arterial ulcers may develop as a result of

ischemia, usually located over a bony prominence on the toes or feet (e.g., metatarsal heads, heels, lateral malleoli). The skin is shiny and atrophic, and fissures and cracks are common.

Pain at rest indicates more severe involvement, which may mimic deep vein thrombosis (DVT), but relief from the occlusive disease can sometimes be obtained by dangling the uncovered leg over the edge of the bed. This dependent position would increase symptoms of DVT, which is usually treated by leg elevation. Exercise may cause pedal pulses to disappear in some people. Sudden occlusion of the arteries, usually at the level of one of these smaller branches, results in gangrene. The necrotic tissue may become gangrenous and infected, requiring surgical intervention.

Occlusive arterial disease for the person with diabetes is further complicated by very slow healing, and healed areas may break down easily. In the case of diabetes mellitus, diabetic neuropathy with diminished or absent sensation of the toes or feet often occurs, predisposing the person to injury or pressure ulcers that may progress because of poor blood flow and subsequent loss of sensation (Table 12-21) (see "Diabetes" in Chapter 11). Amputation rate in people with diabetes is markedly higher than for those individuals with PAD without diabetes mellitus.

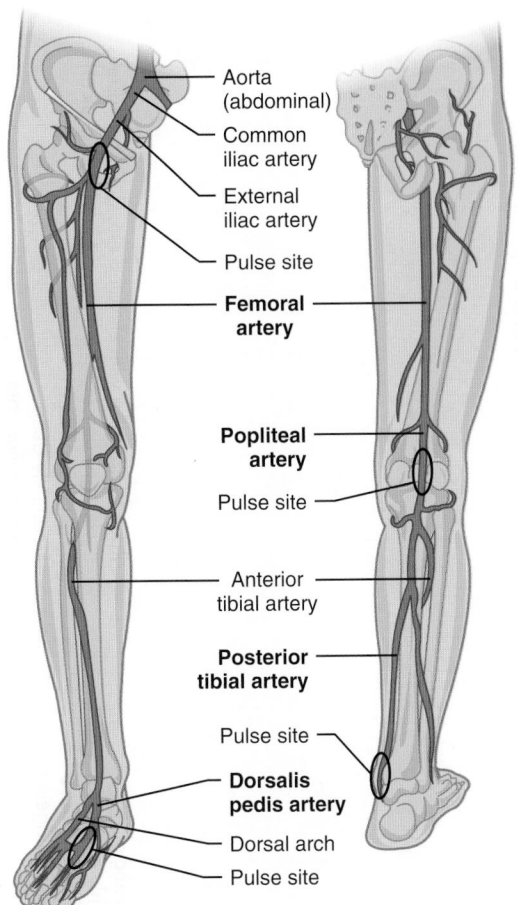

Figure 12-31

Arteries in the leg. The abdominal aorta branches (aortic bifurcation) into the right and left common iliac arteries. These arteries pass through the pelvic cavity and under the inguinal ligament to become the major arteries supplying the leg, called the femoral arteries. Each femoral artery travels down the thigh until, at the lower thigh, it courses posteriorly, where it becomes the popliteal artery. Below the knee, the popliteal artery divides into the anterior tibial artery and posterior tibial artery. The anterior tibial artery travels down the front of the leg onto the dorsum of the foot, where it becomes the dorsalis pedis artery. In the back of the leg, the posterior tibial artery travels down behind the malleolus and forms the plantar arteries in the foot. (From Jarvis C: *Physical examination and health assessment*, ed 5, Philadelphia, 2008, WB Saunders.)

Table 12-20	Arterial Occlusive Disease
Site of Occlusion	**Signs and Symptoms**
Aortic bifurcation	Sensory and motor deficits • Muscle weakness • Numbness (loss of sensation • Paresthesias (burning, pricking) • Paralysis Intermittent claudication (lower back, gluteal muscles, quadriceps, calves; relieved by rest) Cold, pale legs with decreased or absent peripheral pulses
Iliac artery	Intermittent claudication (buttock, hip, thigh; relieved by rest) Diminished or absent femoral or distal pulses Erectile dysfunction in males
Femoral and popliteal artery	Intermittent claudication (calf, foot; may radiate) Leg pallor and coolness Dependent rubor Blanching of feet on elevation No palpable pulses in ankles and feet Gangrene
Tibial and common peroneal artery	Intermittent claudication (calves; feet occasionally) Pain at rest (severe disease); possibly relieved by dangling affected leg Same skin and temperature changes in lower leg and foot as described above Pedal pulses absent; popliteal pulses may be present

MEDICAL MANAGEMENT

DIAGNOSIS. Diagnosis is based on client history and clinical examination. Diagnostic tools may include noninvasive vascular tests (e.g., ankle/brachial index, segmental limb pressures, pulse volume recordings, duplex ultrasonography) or, if invasive tests are required, arteriography with contrast or with MRI. An in-depth discussion of the diagnosis and intervention strategies for chronic arterial insufficiency of the lower extremities is available.[392]

PREVENTION AND TREATMENT. Prevention is the key to reducing the incidence of PAD caused by atherosclerosis. The American College of Cardiology Foundation and American Heart Association have recently updated their guideline for the management of people with PAD.[392]

Risk factor reduction and lifestyle measures are the first steps, with smoking cessation (or not ever starting) as the single most effective prevention tool. A conservative approach to care that includes a program of dietary management to decrease cholesterol and fat, pain control, and daily physical training and exercise[89] therapy to improve collateralization and function has been uniformly endorsed by experts in vascular disease.[392] Careful attention must be given to preventive skin care (Box 12-14) to avoid even minor injuries, infections, or ulcerations.

Recommendations for antiplatelet and antithrombotic drugs[392] include administering of aspirin in a wide range of doses (75-325 mg) as an antiplatelet agent. As an alternative to aspirin therapy, clopidogrel can be given. Combination antiplatelet therapy with aspirin plus clopidogrel can be used for certain high-risk individuals with PAD who are not considered at increased risk of bleeding. Oral anticoagulation therapy (such as warfarin) in addition to antiplatelet therapy is not recommended for prevention of cardiovascular events among people with PAD.[392]

Surgical intervention (revascularization procedures such as bypass graft or angioplastic treatment; Fig. 12-32) is indicated if blood flow is compromised enough to produce symptoms of ischemic pain at rest, if tissue death has occurred, or if claudication interferes with essential activities or work.[90] This decision is usually made after exercise therapy combined with risk factor modification

Table 12-21 Comparison of Arterial, Venous, and Neuropathic Ulcers

	Arterial Ulcer	Venous Ulcer	Neuropathic (Diabetic) Ulcer
Etiology*	Arteriosclerosis obliterans Atheroembolism Large- or medium-vessel atherosclerosis Raynaud disease Diabetes mellitus Collagen disease Vasculitis	Valvular incompetence History of DVT Venous insufficiency accompanied by hypertension Peripheral incompetence; varicose veins	Diabetes mellitus; combination of arterial disease and peripheral neuropathy Repetitive unrecognized trauma
Location	Anywhere on leg or dorsum of foot or toes Bone prominences (anterior tibial) Lateral malleolus	Medial aspect of distal one third of lower extremity Behind medial malleolus	Same areas in which arterial ulcers appear, especially toes Areas where peripheral neuropathy occurs (pressure points on plantar aspect of foot, toes, heels)
Clinical Manifestations	Painful, especially with legs elevated Pulses poor quality or absent Intermittent claudication (exertional calf pain) Rest pain or nocturnal aching of foot or forefoot relieved by dependent dangling position Integumentary (trophic) changes Hair loss Thin, shiny skin Ischemia: pale, white skin color Areas of sluggish blood flow: Red-purple mottling Hypersensitivity to palpation History of minor nonhealing trauma	Can be very painful; venous insufficiency can cause aching pain; more comfortable with legs elevated Normal arterial pulses Eczema or stasis dermatitis Edema Venous perimound (dark pigmentation) is called hemosiderin or staining; leakage of hemosiderin is due to blood that cannot return because of vascular incompetence	Classic symmetric ascending stocking-glove distribution of sensory loss (begins in feet and ascends to knees, then symptoms begin in the hands) May not be painful because of loss of sensation (e.g., neuropathic ulcers are painless or insensate when palpated) Some people experience unpleasant sensations (tingling or hypersensitivity to normally painless stimuli) Loss of vibratory sense and light touch Pulses may be present or diminished (arteries become calcified) Neuropathic foot is warm and dry Loss of vascular tone increases arteriovenous shunting and impairs blood flow necessary for wound healing; sepsis common Altered biomechanics and weight bearing
Wound Appearance	Minimal exudate with dry necrosis Blanched wound base and periwound tissue	Superficial Highly exudative Red wound base Irregular edges	Round, craterlike with elevated rim; diabetes hastens changes described in figure at left (arterial ulcer) Minimal drainage Frequently deep High infection rate

DVT, deep vein thrombosis.
*Ulceration may also occur as a result of lymphatic disorders (see Chapter 10), metabolic abnormalities, and vasculitis (see Table 12-18).

Box 12-14

GUIDELINES FOR SKIN CARE AND PROTECTION

Temperature Protection

- Nicotine causes vasoconstriction of the small vessels in the hands and feet; avoid all tobacco products.
- Recognize and avoid other triggers that cause vasoconstriction (e.g., emotional distress, caffeine, cold or cough remedies that contain a decongestant).
- Wear layers of clothing made of natural fibers, such as cotton, to draw moisture away from the skin; in cold weather, wear a hat and scarf because heat is lost through the scalp; silk is a good insulator, consider it for socks and long underwear.
- Wear thick mittens, which are warmer than gloves, and socks purchased from an outdoor clothing or ski shop designed to wick moisture away while retaining body heat.
- Avoid air conditioning; wear warmer clothes, layer light clothing, or wear a sweater or jacket in air conditioning; be careful when going into an air-conditioned environment after being out in the heat or vice versa.
- Test water temperature before bathing or showering or have a member of the family test first; use other portion of the body to test if insensitivity exists in hand or foot.
- Use a heating pad, hot water bottle, or an electric blanket to warm the sheets of your bed before getting into bed, but do not apply these directly to the skin and do not sleep with any electric device left on; if necessary wear light socks and mittens or gloves to bed. Do not soak hands or feet in hot water.
- Keep household temperatures at a constant, even, and comfortable level.
- Keep protective covering available at all times, even in the summer.
- Avoid contact with extremes of temperature, such as oven, dishwasher (hot dishes), refrigerator, or freezer; wear thick oven mitts whenever reaching into the oven. Keep mittens or warm gloves by the refrigerator and freezer to prevent symptoms when reaching into it.
- Wear rubber gloves whenever cleaning, washing dishes, or rinsing or peeling vegetables under water.
- Avoid holding ice, ice-cold fruit, hot or cold drinks, or frozen foods; wear protective gloves whenever making contact with any of these items.

Skin Care

- Take care of your skin, and give your hands and feet extra care and protection; examine hands and feet daily; at the first sign of bruising, skin changes (e.g., cracking, calluses, blisters, redness), swelling, infection, or ulcer, immediately contact a member of your health care team (e.g., nurse, physical therapist, physician). If vision is impaired, have a family member or health care professional inspect your hands and feet.
- Circulation problems tend to create dry skin and delay healing; keep your skin clean and well-moisturized; wash with a mild, creamy, or moisturizing liquid soap or gel; clean carefully between fingers and toes; do not soak them.
- Avoid perfumed lotions, and do not put lotion on sores or between toes.
- Observe carefully for any activities that might put pressure on your fingertips, such as using a manual typewriter, playing a musical instrument (e.g., guitar, piano), and doing crafts or needlework.

- Do not go barefoot indoors or outdoors; this includes getting up at night; avoid wearing open-toed shoes, pointy-toed shoes, high heels, or sandals; always wear absorbent socks or socks that wick perspiration away from skin; avoid nylon material (including pantyhose material); avoid stockings with seams or with mends; change socks or stockings daily.
- Make sure shoes provide good support without being too tight, avoid shoes that cause excessive foot perspiration, and alternate shoes throughout the week (i.e., do not wear the same shoes every day). Do not wear shoes without socks or stockings.
- Avoid hot tubs and prolonged baths; dry carefully between toes; water temperature should be between 32.2° and 35° C (90° and 95° F).
- Use heel protectors, sheepskin, and other protective devices whenever recommended.

Other Tips

- For Raynaud disease or phenomenon, avoid situations that precipitate excitement, anxiety, or feelings of fear; teach yourself how to recognize early signs of these emotions and use relaxation techniques to reduce stress.
- For Raynaud disease or phenomenon, when you have an attack, gently rewarm fingers or toes as soon as possible; place your hands under your armpits, wiggle fingers or toes, or move or walk around to improve circulation; if possible, run warm (not hot) water over the affected body part until normal color returns.
- Do not use razor blades; use electric razors.
- Avoid medications and substances (e.g., nicotine; caffeine in chocolate, tea, coffee, and soft drinks) that can cause blood vessels to narrow; discuss all medications with your physician.
- Maintain good circulation; do not stay in one position for more than 30 minutes; use breathing and stretching exercises whenever confined to a desk, chair, car, or bed for more than 30 minutes.
- Do not wear constricting or tight clothing, especially tight socks; avoid elastic around wrists or ankles.
- Do not wear jewelry, such as watches or bracelets, to bed at night.
- Leave a night light on in dark areas; turn on lights in dark areas and hallways.
- Do not sit with legs crossed because this can cause pressure on the nerves and blood vessels.
- Avoid sunburn.
- Do not scratch insect bites; do not scratch areas of itchy skin.
- Do not do bathroom surgery on corns or calluses; do not use chemical agents for the removal of corns or calluses; see your physician.

Care of Nails

- Use clippers, not scissors; do not use razor blades; cut toenails straight across, but file fingernails in a rounded fashion to the tips of your fingers.
- Take care of your nails; use cuticle softener or moisturizing cream or lotion around cuticles; push the cuticles back very gently with a cotton swab soaked in cuticle remover; do not push cuticles back with a sharp object and do not cut the cuticles with scissors or nail clippers.
- Use lamb's wool between overlapping toes.

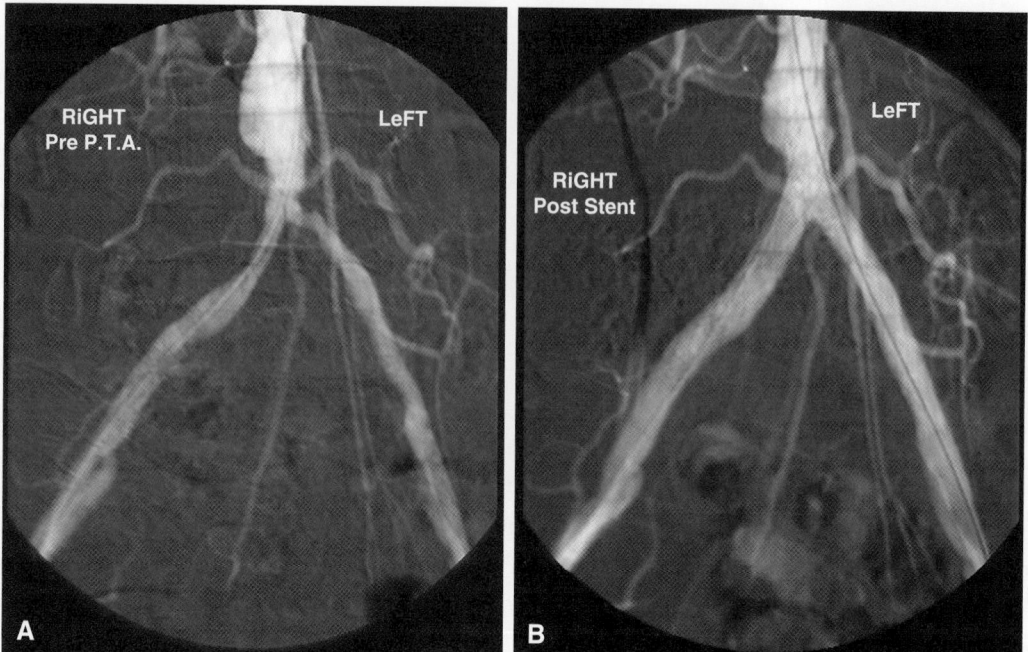

Figure 12-32

Percutaneous transluminal angioplasty (PTA) may be used in peripheral vascular disease. A, Significant narrowing of the aortic bifurcation and both common iliac arteries. The narrowing in both iliac arteries was successfully treated by angioplasty, and bilateral stents were inserted to maintain patency. **B,** The client had presented with bilateral calf claudication, which was relieved by this procedure. (From Forbes CD, Jackson WF: *Color atlas and text of clinical medicine,* ed 3, London, 2003, Mosby.)

has been unsuccessful in preventing this level of impairment and subsequent disability.

Cessation of smoking may be required by the physician before surgery is considered. Persons with localized occlusions of the aorta and iliac arteries less than 10 cm in length, with relatively normal vessels proximally and distally, are good candidates for angioplasty or stenting (see Figs. 12-3 and 12-5). Conversely, people with multisegmented arterial disease with more involved symptoms are at greater risk of amputation. Endovascular and open surgical treatment are recommended for limb salvage in patients with critical limb ischemia.[8] The endovascular intervention includes a variety of catheter-based surgical techniques that are being improved by laser techniques.

Statins, used for the prevention of CVD because of their antithrombotic properties, have been shown effective in reducing the risk of DVT and may become useful in the primary and secondary prevention of DVT.[375]

PROGNOSIS. Arterial occlusive diseases are not life-threatening, but people with symptoms such as intermittent claudication often have a decreased quality of life because of mobility limitations. Symptoms of chronic arterial insufficiency progress slowly over time, so that progressive disability from pain, ulceration, gangrene, and loss of function or limbs is more likely to occur than death as a result of peripheral occlusive diseases.

On the other hand, because people with either asymptomatic or symptomatic PAD have widespread arterial disease, they have a significantly increased risk of stroke, MI, and cardiovascular death. Twenty percent of all individuals with PVD have a heart attack or stroke, and 30%

of those have a 5-year mortality rate that climbs to 62% in men and 33% in women in 10 years.[226]

SPECIAL IMPLICATIONS FOR THE THERAPIST   12-19

Arteriosclerosis Obliterans (Peripheral Arterial Disease)

See also "Special Implications for the Therapist 12-24: Peripheral Vascular Disease" below.

Note to Reader: There seems to be a lack of consensus between different guidelines for PAD screening.[148]

Arterial Tests and Measures

Until recently, exercise testing using a 12-degree grade at a preset speed of 2 mph was the current practice to assess for claudication associated with PAD, but limited reproducibility and limited sensitivity to change in exercise performance were serious problems. Graded treadmill protocols have been developed to test people with PAD that give highly reproducible results and are able to evaluate change in exercise performance.

Two widely used graded protocols maintain a walking speed of 2 mph, one with grade increases of 3.5% every 3 minutes, the other with grade increases of 2% every 2 minutes. As the individual walks on the treadmill, time to pain and maximal walking time are recorded. All people limited by claudication are reproducibly brought to maximal levels of discomfort using either of these protocols.[17]

Venous filling time provides a reasonable assessment of the general state of perfusion but requires patent venous valves to be a valid measure. Have the client assume a recumbent position and elevate the legs to facilitate venous drainage. When the veins have collapsed below the level of the skin, quickly bring the person to a sitting position with the legs hanging in a dependent position. The time necessary for the veins to fill to skin level is the venous filling time. A filling time greater than 25 seconds implies an increased risk of ulceration, infection, and poor wound healing.

The ankle-brachial index (ABI) (Box 12-15) is another measure of arterial perfusion at the level measured available to therapists for use in documenting the need for and benefit of a prescriptive exercise program. The ABI is a simple, inexpensive, and noninvasive tool that correlates well with angiographic disease severity and functional symptoms. It is well established as an independent predictor of cardiovascular morbidity and mortality.[308]

Blood pressures are measured both in the arm (brachial blood pressure) and the ankle with the client in a supine position for both measures. The ankle blood pressure may be auscultated using the dorsalis pedis pulse or posterior tibialis artery with the cuff placed above the ankle or using Doppler if available. The systolic ankle pressure is divided by the brachial systolic pressure.

With increasing degrees of arterial narrowing, there is a progressive fall in systolic blood pressure distal to the sites of involvement. If both pressures are measured with the person in the supine position and the vessels are unobstructed, the ratio of ankle to brachial pressures should be 1.0.[402]

If flow to the lower extremity is decreased, the ratio will be less than 1.0. The reference standard of ABI less than 0.90 at rest or less than 0.85 after exercise in adults older than 65 years, or older than 50 years with a history of smoking or diabetes, indicates PAD.[392] ABI measurements may be of limited value in anyone with diabetes, because calcification of the tibial and peroneal arteries may render them noncompressible.[392] ABI below 0.9 (0.8 in some facilities) at rest may exclude individuals from early ambulation and compression in the acute care setting as part of a DVT protocol decision-making algorithm regarding ambulation and compression.

ABI can be measured before and after exercise to assess the dynamics of intermittent claudication. This can be accomplished by leaving the ankle pressure cuffs in place during the exercise. Once the walk is completed or pain develops, the person rapidly assumes a supine position and the ankle pressures are measured.

At modest workloads, the healthy adult can maintain ankle systolic pressures at normal levels. If the exercise is strenuous, there may be a transient fall in systolic pressure that rapidly returns to baseline levels. In people with intermittent claudication, a different response is seen, even at low workload. If the person walks to the point of claudication, ankle systolic pressure falls precipitously, often to unrecordable

---

Box 12-15

ANKLE–BRACHIAL INDEX*

- ≥1.1: Suspicious for arterial calcification; blood vessels do not compress (e.g., diabetes)
- 1.0: Adequate blood supply; compression acceptable
- <1.0: Inadequate blood supply; impaired wound healing; requires medical evaluation; prescriptive exercise beneficial
- 0.5-0.9: Indicates arterial occlusion; prescriptive exercise may be beneficial; delayed wound healing; light compression acceptable
- <0.5: Severe arterial occlusive disease; may require surgical revascularization procedure; wound healing unlikely; rarely compress; DVT protocol: excluded from early ambulation and compression

*Values vary slightly from institution to institution and geographically from one area of the United States to another. Consider these values a general guideline and check the standard used at your current facility/location.

---

levels, and will not return to baseline levels for several minutes.

It is not necessary (and may be misleading) to measure arm systolic pressure after exercise, because this will increase by an amount related to the workload, and the most important variable is the extent to which ankle pressure falls and the time it takes to recover (i.e., the period of postexercise ischemia). In general, if ankle pressure falls by more than 20% of the baseline value and requires more than 3 minutes to recover, the test result is considered abnormal.[392,345]

However, a difference of 10 to 15 (or more) points in systolic blood pressure between the arms may signal peripheral vascular disease and warrants further vascular assessment.[107]

Prescriptive Exercise

Supervised exercise programs are more effective than nonsupervised programs in improving treadmill walking distances for individuals with intermittent claudication.[75,49] In prescribing an exercise program for someone with claudication secondary to occlusive disease, exercise tolerance must be determined. A training heart rate should be based on the exercise tolerance test, because persons with PVD frequently have CAD as well. Frequently, symptoms of claudication occur before training heart rate is reached, but the heart rate should be monitored and should not exceed the training heart rate, even in the absence of symptoms. Anginal chest pain is a red flag to decrease intensity.

A progressive conditioning program, including walking for fixed periods, is essential, even if the initial length of walking time is only 1 minute. Exercise can protect against atherothrombotic events by elevating tPA[491]; improving peripheral circulation[168]; improving ambulatory function; increasing endothelial progenitor cells (cells that line the blood vessels capable of blood vessel repair),[411] endothelial-dependent dilation, and calf blood flow[67]; and favorably altering cardiovascular risk factor profile (e.g., improved lipid profile, reduced blood pressure), an important element in the management of PAD.[222]

The greatest improvement occurs with intermittent exercise to near-maximal pain progressing to a long-term (6 months or longer) program of structured walking for at least 30 minutes three times weekly.[169] The most effective program includes brisk treadmill walking at a pace that is comfortable for the individual until claudication begins, followed by immediate rest and continued walking when the pain subsides.

The therapist can direct the client to progress quickly to levels of exercise at maximal tolerable pain in order to obtain optimal symptomatic benefit over time. This pattern is repeated starting with intervals as short as 1 to 5 minutes, alternating with rest periods of sufficient duration to eliminate pain (usually 2-10 minutes). Without complicating factors, the individual is usually able to complete at least a 30- to 45-minute walk without pain or rest breaks within 6 to 8 weeks.

Claudication is influenced by the speed, incline, and surface of the walk and should be modified whenever possible to improve exercise tolerance. Impairment measures, functional measures, quality-of-life assessment, and specific walking parameters are outlined in detail elsewhere.[402] Supervised exercise and social support are recommended to improve both physical function and quality of life in people with PAD and intermittent claudication.[401]

Altered gait pattern has been documented with PAD,[167] with less time spent in the swing phase of the gait cycle and more time in double stance. This ambulatory pattern favors greater gait stability at the expense of greater walking speed and can be improved with exercise rehabilitation. People with intermittent claudication associated with PAD are also functionally limited by dorsiflexion weakness, impairing their ability to perform tasks requiring distal lower extremity strength.[406]

After exercise, numbness in the foot as well as pain in the calf may occur. The foot may be cold and pale, which is an indication that the circulation has been diverted to the arteriolar bed of the leg muscles. Many people with claudication are already receiving β-blockers for angina or hypertension (see also "Special Implications for the Therapist 12-3: Angina Pectoris" and "Special Implications for the Therapist 12-4: Hypertension [Hypertensive Vascular Disease]" above).

The main factor limiting success of exercise therapy is lack of client motivation. For this reason, the most successful programs combine regular, supervised outpatient sessions with home exercise programs; regularity rather than intensity should be stressed.

Comorbid diseases, such as CAD or diabetes mellitus, and severity and location of arterial occlusive disease do not preclude successful response to prescriptive exercise. Unstable cardiopulmonary conditions require more careful consideration and collaboration with the health care team.[392]

Precautions

When arterial thrombosis or embolism is suspected, the affected limb must be protected by proper positioning below the horizontal plane and protective skin care provided. Heat or cold application and massage are contraindicated, and family members must also be notified of these restrictions. The home health therapist must be alert to the possibility of hot water bottles, heating pads, electric blankets, and hot foot soaks being used by the client without physician approval. This precaution is especially true for people with diabetes-associated peripheral neuropathies and for people with paraplegia.

Encourage the person with vascular disease to prevent becoming chilled by keeping the thermostat at home set at 21.1° to 22.2° C (70°-72° F) and to avoid prolonged exposure to cold outdoors (e.g., by prewarming the car, dressing properly in layers, especially protecting hands and feet).

In addition, many people with PVD and diabetes mellitus have peripheral sensory neuropathy and are at greater risk for skin breakdown on the foot from weight-bearing activities such as walking or running (see Box 12-14). These individuals should participate in alternative forms of exercise (e.g., bicycling, swimming/aquatics) even though these exercises may not improve walking ability as much as a structured walking program.[313]

VENOUS DISEASES

James W. Farris, PT, PhD, and John Heick, PT, DPT

Venous disease can be acute or chronic; acute venous disease includes thrombophlebitis, and chronic venous disease includes varicose vein formation and chronic venous insufficiency.

Thrombophlebitis. Thrombophlebitis is swelling of a vein because of vein wall inflammation (phlebitis) occurring as a result of thrombus (blood clot) deposition in the vein. Depending on the depth location of the affected veins, there are two different types: DVT and superficial thrombophlebitis.[367]

Deep Vein Thrombosis and Pulmonary Embolism. (See also discussion of PE in Chapter 15.)

Definition and Overview. Vein thrombosis is a partial occlusion (mural thrombus) or complete occlusion (occlusive thrombus) of a vein by a thrombus (clot) with secondary inflammatory reaction in the wall of the vein (thrombophlebitis). A venous thrombus is an intravascular collection of fibrin network, platelets, erythrocytes and leukocytes, the end result of the activation of the clotting cascade with the potential to produce significant morbidity and mortality.[10]

Together, DVT and PE are referred to as venous thromboembolism (VTE). The presence of a VTE in the venous system is divided by depth and proximity. In the lower extremity, the superficial system is comprised of the great (long) and small (short) saphenous veins (Fig. 12-33). The deep veins are divided into distal and proximal. The distal deep veins include the anterior tibial, posterior tibial, and peroneal veins. The proximal deep veins include the popliteal, superficial femoral, deep femoral, common femoral and external iliac veins.

A DVT is classified as distal if it is below the knee and proximal if it is located in the popliteal vein or above.[149]

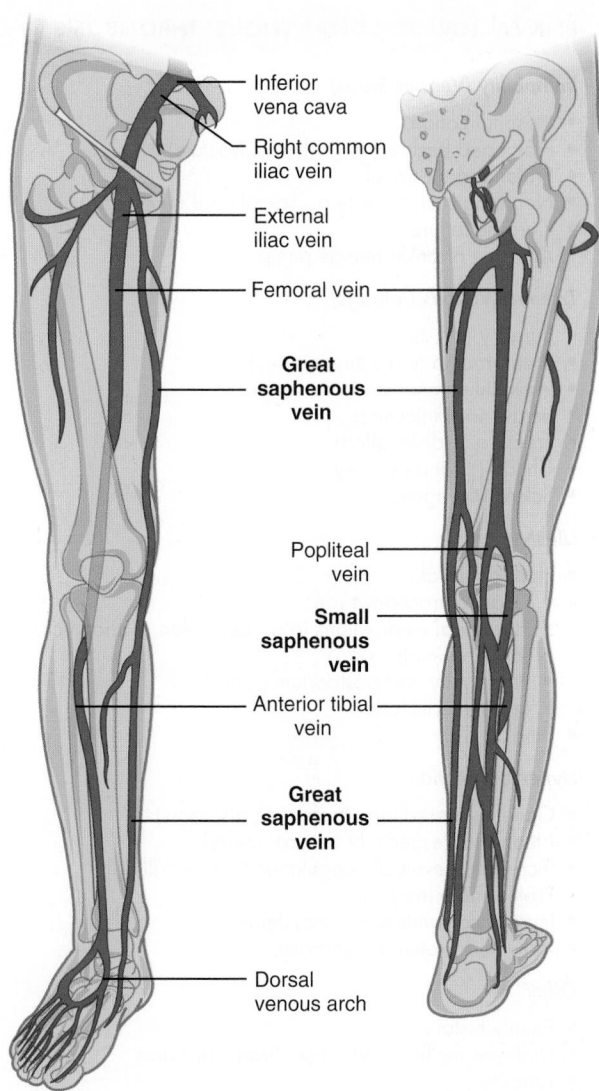

Figure 12-33

Veins in the leg. The legs have three types of veins: deep veins (femoral and popliteal) coursing alongside the deep arteries to conduct most of the venous return from the legs; superficial veins, the great and small saphenous veins; and perforators (not pictured), the connecting veins that join the two sets and route blood from the superficial into the deep veins. The great saphenous vein starts at the medial side of the dorsum of the foot and ascends in front of the medial malleolus, crossing the tibia obliquely and ascending along the medial side of the thigh. The small saphenous vein starts on the lateral side of the dorsum of the foot and ascends behind the lateral malleolus and up the back of the leg, where it joins the popliteal vein. (From Jarvis C: *Physical examination and health assessment,* ed 5, Philadelphia, 2008, WB Saunders.)

The most common superficial vein thrombosis occurs in the saphenous vein in the lower extremity (see Fig. 12-33); and the most common DVT occurs in the femoral or iliac veins.

A PE can occur when part of a thrombus (embolus) in DVT breaks loose and travels through the right side of the heart into the pulmonary artery. Embolus lodged in a pulmonary artery or one of its branches, occludes blood flow to that part of the lung and impairs gas exchange.

If a thrombus occludes a major vein (e.g., femoral, ena, axillary), the venous pressure and volume rise dis-lly. However, if a thrombus occludes a deep small vein (e.g., tibial, popliteal), collateral vessels develop and relieve the increased venous pressure and volume. This is why the majority of PEs come from proximal DVTs.

Incidence, Etiology, and Risk Factors. The number of people affected by VTE (DVT and PE combined) is unknown; estimates are wide-ranging because there is not an organized national surveillance system[374] and variable presentations lead to diagnostic challenges.[149]

The proportion of hospitalized patients with PE is increasing but whether this represents more admissions with PE or more diagnoses made in hospitalized individuals is uncertain. The number of hospitalized patients with DVT has also increased significantly.[429] Because of the increasing awareness of the seriousness of the public health burden from VTE, recommendations have been made for the development of a national systematic surveillance system to monitor the prevalence and annual incidence of DVT and PE.[374]

Estimates of the prevalence and incidence of VTE have been based on specific population reports, hospital discharge and health insurance claim databases from inpatient and outpatient records.[61,185,344,374] Prevalence of VTE is estimated to be 8.7 per 1000[185] with 300,000 to 900,000 people being affected each year in the United States.[46,374]

The annual incidence of VTE is estimated to be between 1.0 and 1.5 per 1000 adults, with DVT accounting for approximately two thirds of VTE. This is the equivalent of approximately 160,000 to 240,000 new cases of symptomatic DVT per year, with the true incidence thought to be at or above the upper end of this range.[185] Mortality figures for VTE-related deaths range from 60,000 to 300,000 people per year.[46,374]

VTE has become such a significant health problem that the Surgeon General has called for increased awareness by all stakeholders and the use of screening, prevention, diagnostic, and treatment methods that are evidence-based.[455] VTE is considered to be the most preventable cause of hospital-related death and is among the top causes of pregnancy-related death.[46]

Approximately 30% to 60% of all people (women more than men) undergoing major general surgical procedures or having common pathologies such as cerebrovascular accidents develop clinical manifestations of DVT up to 4 weeks after the operation or incident (Fig. 12-34).[10,480]

VTE is the most common reason for hospital readmission and death after total hip and total knee arthroplasty.[273] High-risk surgical candidates have a history of recent VTE or have undergone extensive pelvic or abdominal surgery for advanced malignancy, CABG, renal transplantation, splenectomy, or major orthopedic surgery to the lower limbs (e.g., hip or knee arthroplasty, surgery for fractured hip, tibial osteotomy).

Emboli can be formed of other substances besides a blood clot. Air bubbles, fat droplets, amniotic fluid, clumps of parasites, or tumor cells can lead to a VTE. Fat embolism syndrome from fat thromboembolic phenomenon is a well-known consequence of femoral total hip replacement arthroplasty. Intravasation of fat into the bloodstream during prosthetic implantation has

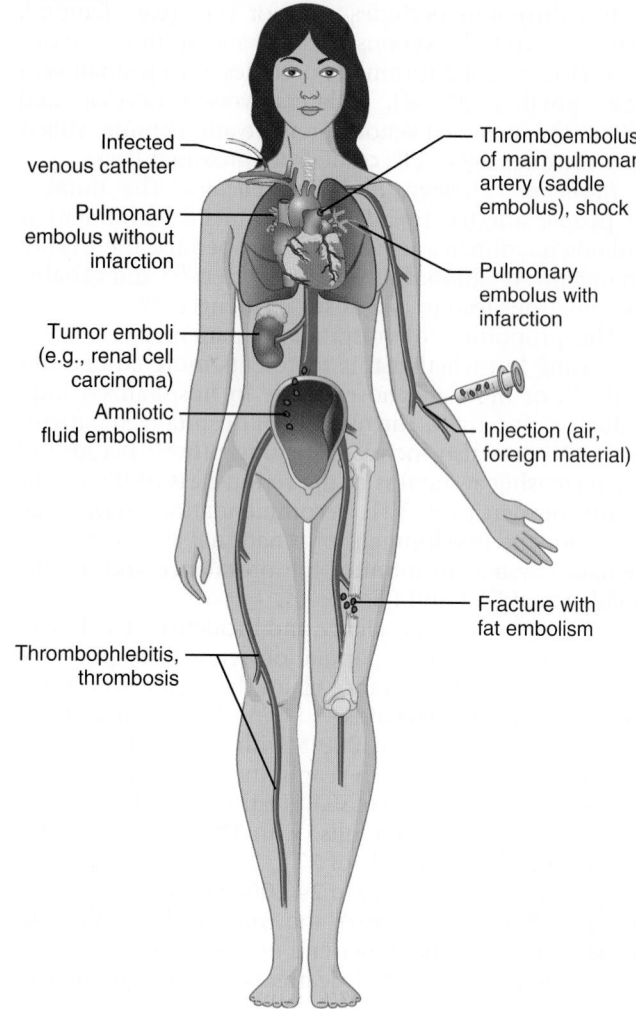

Infected venous catheter

Pulmonary embolus without infarction

Tumor emboli (e.g., renal cell carcinoma)

Amniotic fluid embolism

Thrombophlebitis, thrombosis

Thromboembolus of main pulmonary artery (saddle embolus), shock

Pulmonary embolus with infarction

Injection (air, foreign material)

Fracture with fat embolism

Figure 12-34

Sources and effects of venous emboli.

Box 12-16

RISK FACTORS FOR DEEP VENOUS* THROMBOSIS

Immobility (Venous Stasis)

- Hospitalization
- Prolonged bed rest (e.g., burns, fracture)
- Prolonged air travel
- Neurologic disorder (e.g., spinal cord injury, stroke)
- Cardiac failure
- Absence of ankle muscle pump

Trauma (Venous Damage)

- Surgery
- Local trauma (e.g., direct injury)
- Indwelling venous access devices
- Intravenous injections
- Fracture or dislocation
- Childbirth and delivery
- Sclerosing agents

Lifestyle

- Hormonal status
  - Oral contraceptive use
  - Hormonal medications (e.g., tamoxifen, Adriamycin [doxorubicin])
  - Pregnancy and postpartum period
  - In vitro fertilization
- Smoking

Hypercoagulation

- Genetics (hereditary thrombotic disorders)
- Neoplasm (especially viscera, ovary)
- Increasing levels of coagulation factors (VIII, XI)
- Prothrombin mutation
- Increasing levels of homocysteine
- Activated protein C syndrome

Other

- Family history
- Diabetes mellitus and other chronic diseases
- Obesity
- Previous DVT
- Buerger disease
- Age >60 years
- Idiopathic (50% of all DVT cases)

*The terms *venous* and *vein* are used interchangeably in the literature and in this text.

been linked with postoperative confusion and cognitive decline. The risk of fat embolism syndrome is four times greater with simultaneous bilateral total knee or total hip replacements.[249,257,382] Changes have been made in the arthroplasty surgical technique that may result in a reduced incidence of this complication.

Brain microemboli from cardiac surgery with subsequent neurologic dysfunction have also been reported. The major source of the microemboli is lipid droplets of the patient's fat that drip into the blood in the surgical field. The lipid-laden blood is aspirated and returned to the patient via the cardiopulmonary bypass apparatus.[433]

Substantial evidence indicates that the pathologic processes of venous (and arterial) thromboembolism involve both genetic and lifestyle influences. Scientific progress over the past decade has revealed a growing number of genetic factors present in more than 1% of the population that increase the relative risk of vein thrombosis between two-fold and seven-fold. Several of these factors have been demonstrated to interact adversely with lifestyle influences, such as oral contraceptives and smoking.

Thrombus formation is usually attributed to venous stasis, hypercoagulability, or injury to the venous wall, although other risk factors may be present (Box 12-16). It is commonly held that at least two of these three conditions must be present for thrombi to form. Fifty percent of all DVT cases are viewed as idiopathic.[46]

What were previously considered to be idiopathic causes of thrombosis are now identified as abnormalities associated with thrombophilia, such as elevated levels of coagulation factors VIII and XI, a particular prothrombin mutation (e.g., prothrombin G20210A), elevated levels of homocysteine, and a syndrome of activated protein C resistance.[147] Acquired resistance to the anticoagulant action of activated protein C may be associated with the increased risk of vein thrombosis associated with pregnancy, HRT, the use of oral contraceptives, and possibly even in vitro fertilization.[119]

Pathogenesis. Any trauma to the endothelium of the vein wall exposes subendothelial tissues to platelets and clotting factors in the venous blood, initiating thrombosis. Platelets adhering to the vein wall attract the deposition of fibrin, leukocytes, and erythrocytes, forming a thrombus that may remain attached to the vessel wall.

Clinical Manifestations. In the early stages, approximately half of the people with DVT are asymptomatic for any signs or symptoms in the affected extremity. The lower extremities appear to be affected most often (more than 90%) but upper extremity venous thrombi can also develop.[29]

Lower-Extremity Vein Thrombosis. When symptoms occur in the lower extremity, the client may report a dull ache, a tight feeling, or pain in the calf, often misdiagnosed as some other cause of leg pain. In 80% of the cases with symptoms, the DVT is proximal, above the trifurcation of the popliteal vein. It is important to realize that proximal DVTs more often lead to severe consequences of DVT, and that at the time of diagnosis more than 50% of the affected individuals already have PE.[26,381]

Signs are often absent; when present but taken alone, they may be variable and unreliable. Signs and symptoms include leg or calf swelling, pain or tenderness, dilation of superficial veins, and pitting edema. The skin of the leg and ankle on the affected side may be relatively warmer than on the unaffected side (check for temperature changes with the backs of the fingers or a skin thermometer). If venous obstruction is severe, the skin may be cyanotic.

Any of these symptoms can occur without DVT, possibly associated with other vascular, inflammatory, musculoskeletal, or lymphatic conditions that produce signs and symptoms similar to those of DVT.[444]

PEs (see Chapter 15), most often from the large, deep veins of the pelvis and legs, are the most devastating complication of DVT and can occur without apparent warning ending in sudden death. Signs and symptoms of PE are dependent on the size and location of the PE[209,381] and may include the following[180]:

- Pleuritic chest pain
- Diffuse chest discomfort
- Tachypnea
- Tachycardia
- Hemoptysis
- Anxiety, restlessness, apprehension
- Dyspnea
- Persistent cough

Upper-Extremity Vein Thrombosis. Venous thrombosis of the upper extremity accounts for up to 10% of all cases of DVT most often affecting the subclavian vein, axillary vein or both with occurrences less often affecting the internal jugular and brachial vein.[412] Primary upper-extremity DVT is either idiopathic or associated with strenuous physical activity (effort-induced thrombosis). Secondary upper-extremity DVT is usually associated with infection, a systemic illness (e.g., malignancy), the use of an indwelling peripherally inserted central catheter (PICC) lines or central venous catheters (CVCs) (e.g., used in the treatment of cancer, parenteral nutrition), malignancy, or, less often, hemodialysis.[224,231,256,291,449]

In the case of upper-extremity superficial vein thrombosis, dull pain and local tenderness in the region of the involved vein may be accompanied by signs of superficial induration (firm or hard cord) and redness.

Upper-extremity *superficial* vein thrombosis is self-limiting and does not cause PE, because the blood flow to deeper veins is through small perforating venous channels. Iatrogenic superficial vein thrombosis is often secondary to prolonged IV catheter use. Upper-extremity *deep* vein thrombosis is not as common as in the lower extremity, but, again, incidence may be on the rise as a consequence of the increasing use of PICC lines or CVCs.

CVCs are frequently used in people with hematologic/oncologic disorders to administer drugs, stem cell infusions, blood products, parenteral alimentation, and blood sampling. Other risk factors include blood clotting disorders,[274] clavicle fracture,[232] insertion of pacemaker wires, and arthroscopy of the shoulder or reconstructive shoulder arthroplasty.[166,487]

Unfortunately, the first clinical manifestation of *deep* thrombosis may be PE, and as a consequence of upper extremity DVT it can be fatal.[487] Symptoms (when present) are similar to those for the lower extremity. The therapist should be aware of the presence of any risk factors and watch for pain and pitting edema or swelling of the entire (usually upper) limb and/or an area of the limb that is 2 cm or more larger than the surrounding area indicating swelling requiring further investigation.

Other symptoms include numbness, heaviness, redness or warmth of the arm, dilated veins, or low-grade fever possibly accompanied by chills and malaise. Bruising or discoloration of the area or proximal to the thrombosis has been observed in some cases.[256] Swelling can contribute to decreased neck or shoulder motion. Severe thrombosis can cause superior vena cava syndrome; symptoms include edema of the face and arm, vertigo, and dyspnea.[162] In addition to any of the signs and symptoms listed here, the individual with a PICC line may also report pain or tenderness at or above the insertion site.

Chronic venous insufficiency or postthrombotic syndrome are possible sequelae to upper extremity DVT.[256,337]

MEDICAL MANAGEMENT

PREVENTION. Primary prevention of DVT/VTE through the use of early mobilization for low-risk individuals and prophylactic use of anticoagulants (see Table 12-5) in people considered at moderate to high risk for DVT is important. Mobilization and compression stockings following acute DVT reduce the risk of postthrombotic syndrome.[347,364,434] Although such interventions reduce the risk of DVT, it must be understood that even people receiving anticoagulant therapy can still develop DVT. The highest incidence of DVT occurs with abdominal, thoracic, pelvic, hip, or knee surgical procedures[286]; neurologic or other conditions leading to paresis or paralysis; and prolonged immobilization, cancer, and CHF.

Routine use of knee elastic stockings in all postoperative clients has been adopted in most hospitals, and many facilities use pneumatic pressure devices with on/off cycles applied for the first few hours after major surgery to mimic the calf pump. Once the person is able, ankle pumping is added, because this is effective in increasing average peak venous velocity (flow) from the lower extremity with dorsiflexion of the ankle by greater than 200%, thereby reducing DVT while the person is immobilized.[481]

Evidence-based clinical practice guidelines for the prevention of thrombosis in orthopedic surgery with antithrombotic therapy have been published by the American Academy of Orthopaedic Surgeons[149] and are also available online at http://www.aaos.org/research/gui delines/VTE/VTE_full_guideline.pdf.

DIAGNOSIS. The diagnosis of a DVT has been aided by the inclusion of Clinical Decision Rules (CDRs), or more currently named as Risk Assessment Tools.[429] One such tool is the use of the Wells Risk Assessment,[472,475] which has been shown to be a reliable and valid tool for clinical assessment for predicting the risk of DVT in the lower extremity.[27,28,252,471,473,474] A simple model to predict upper-extremity DVT has also been proposed and remains under investigation.[113] The best available test for the diagnosis of upper-extremity DVT is contrast venography; color Doppler ultrasonography may be preferred for some people because it is noninvasive.[131]

Use of the Wells Risk Assessment has been specifically shown to be valid with orthopedic outpatients[380] and iterations of the Wells have been proposed for other settings, such as the inpatient hospital setting, primary care setting,[474,486] and for specific populations, such as the elderly[419] and individuals with diagnosed cancer.[238] Utilization of the Wells CDR in anyone with suspected DVT clusters signs, symptoms, and risk factors and classifies the person's likelihood of having DVT as low, moderate, or high (Table 12-22). The CDR is a reliable and valid tool for clinical assessment for predicting the risk of DVT in the lower extremity.[27,28,252,471,473,474] The CDR has been specifically shown to be valid with orthopedic outpatients.[380] One study has shown that physical therapists often underestimate the likelihood of DVT in high-risk individuals and frequently do not refer to a physician when they should.[381]

At-risk clients as assessed by history and clinical examination with the CDR receive a D-dimer blood test (checking for fibrin breakdown products released from a thrombus) to determine the DVT risk level. Moderate-to high-risk individuals (D-dimer level above 500 ng/mL) receive Doppler duplex ultrasonography as a rapid screening procedure to detect thrombosis. Venous duplex ultrasonographic scanning has replaced contrast venography as the primary diagnostic test for DVT because it allows noninvasive real-time visualization of the vein while simultaneously providing information on venous flow.

It is recognized that often other calf muscle strain or contusion may be difficult to differentiate from vein thrombosis; further diagnostic testing may be required to determine the correct diagnosis. Occasionally, a ruptured Baker cyst may produce unilateral pain and swelling in the calf. A history of arthritis in the knee of the same leg and the disappearance of the popliteal cyst at the time symptoms develop are clues the physician can use to make the differentiation. Although the Homans sign was once used for differential diagnosis of acute DVT, it is no longer considered a sensitive or specific test for ruling in or out DVT.

Table 12-22	Wells Clinical Decision Rule for DVT*	
Clinical Presentation		**Score**
Active cancer (within 6 months of diagnosis or receiving palliative care)		1
Paralysis, paresis, or recent immobilization of lower extremity		1
Bedridden for more than 3 days or major surgery in the last 4 weeks		1
Localized tenderness in the center of the posterior calf, the popliteal space, or along the femoral vein in the anterior thigh/groin		1
Entire lower-extremity swelling		1
Unilateral calf swelling (more than 3 mm larger than uninvolved side)		1
Unilateral pitting edema		1
Collateral superficial veins (nonvaricose)		1
An alternative diagnosis is as likely (or more likely) than DVT (e.g., cellulitis, postoperative swelling, calf strain)		-2
Total Points		

Key:
-2 to 0: Low probability of DVT (3%)
1 to 2: Moderate probability of DVT (17%)
≥3: High probability of DVT (75%)
Medical consultation is advised in the presence of low probability; medical referral is required with moderate or high score.
*For Wells Clinical Decision Rule for Pulmonary Embolism, see Chapter 15.
See also Clinical Decision Rule for PE and DVT available online at: http://www.med.unc.edu/im/files/internal-medicine-clinic-documents/clinical%20decision%20rule%20for%20PE%20and%20DVT.pdf.
From Wells PS, Anderson DR, Bormanis J. Value of assessment of pretest probability of deep-vein thrombosis in clinical management. *Lancet* 350:1795–1798, 1997. Used with permission.

TREATMENT. The goals of DVT management are to prevent progression to PE, limit extension of the thrombus, limit damage to the vein, and prevent another clot from forming. Current therapy is to administer anticoagulants such as low-molecular-weight heparins (LMWHs) Fragmin (dalteparin) and Lovenox (enoxaparin); or Arixtra (fondaparinux), followed by long-term oral anticoagulants (Coumadin [warfarin]) (see Table 12-5). Anticoagulation therapy for acute DVT prevents enlargement of the thrombus and allows for further attachment of the thrombus to the vessel wall, thereby reducing the likelihood of PE.[444] Anticoagulants facilitate the dissolution of clots, whereas thrombolytics accelerate the process. The rate of clot lysis in individuals treated with anticoagulants is slow and it can take up to several months in some cases for the clot to completely resolve.[241]

Management of DVT changed dramatically with the introduction of LMWHs used as a bridge to warfarin. The LMWHs are more effective than the previously used unfractionated heparin, has fewer major bleeding complications, and does not require laboratory monitoring of coagulation test results to adjust medications, allowing for earlier hospital discharge or treatment at home. However, anticoagulation therapy does not effectively address the need to restore venous function in the thrombosed veins.

Elastic stockings must be worn whenever the person is ambulating or in the upright position. The standard of care for DVT is moving toward the following protocol: inject with LMWH, discharge to home with additional doses the client can use to inject at home over the next week while taking warfarin. Return for follow-up evaluation of activated partial thromboplastin time, prothrombin time, and/or international normalized ratio, depending on the time of discharge in relation to initiation of anticoagulation therapy. Clients are advised to remain active but avoid any straining maneuvers.

For cases of massive DVT, thrombolysis, thrombectomy, and embolectomy (often performed in an interventional angiography laboratory) are being used with increasing skill and improved outcomes. New research is leading to the next generation of antithrombotic compounds, such as direct coagulation factor inhibitors and tissue factor pathway inhibitors; the use of statins[375]; and gene therapy.

Gene therapy as an antithrombotic strategy can involve a number of different approaches, such as overexpression of anticoagulant factors or modulation of endothelial biology to make thrombus formation or propagation unfavorable.

Other investigators are looking at the systemic administration of recombinant tissue factor pathway inhibitor to decrease intimal hyperplasia after vascular injury and to suppress systemic mechanisms of blood coagulation and thrombosis.[498]

PROGNOSIS. DVTs that are not diagnosed can lead to life-threatening consequences, such as PE. With appropriate intervention and in the absence of complications, a return to normal health and activity can be expected within 1 to 3 weeks for the person with an upper-extremity or calf DVT and within 6 weeks for the person with thigh or pelvic DVT.

Prognosis depends on the size of the vessel involved, the presence of collateral circulation, and the underlying cause of the thrombosis (e.g., spinal cord injury, stroke, or neoplasm may prevent return to former health). Recurrence occurs in 5% of DVT cases and 1% of PE cases and may be related to risk factors listed in Box 12-16 or too short a time on anticoagulants.

It remains uncertain whether anticoagulant therapy should be extended for longer periods (more than 3 months), whether lower intensity should be recommended during this extension (i.e., with a target international normalized ratio of less than 2.0), or if the benefits of extended anticoagulant therapy outweigh the risk of bleeding complications.

A potential long-term complication of DVT is venous stasis or insufficiency (postthrombotic syndrome) when permanent damage to the vein has occurred (see "Chronic Venous Insufficiency" below). Between 25% and 30% of people who had DVT treated with anticoagulants will develop some form of postthrombotic syndrome in the first 10 years following DVT.

The National Institutes of Health are investigating the combined use of anticoagulants and thrombolytics to preserve the patency of the veins, thereby reducing the frequency of postthrombotic syndromes compared to anticoagulation therapy alone. Previously, the prohibitive cost, need for hospitalization, and procedural complications associated with thrombolytic therapy have prevented their use in proximal DVT.

| SPECIAL IMPLICATIONS FOR THE THERAPIST | 12-20 |

Vein Thrombosis and Pulmonary Embolism

(See also "Special Implications for the Therapist 15-23: Pulmonary Embolism and Infarction.")

Evolve Box 12-1 on the Evolve website presents a case example for DVT.

Risk Assessment

Populations at risk (see Box 12-16), especially postoperative, postpartum, and immobilized clients, should be identified by the medical staff and observed carefully. Risk factor assessment scales (e.g., Autar DVT scale, Wells' Clinical Decision Rules for DVT or PE) for use in a therapy practice are available.[38,39,444,170] Using seven risk categories (i.e., increasing age, BMI, immobility, special DVT risk, trauma, surgery, high-risk disease), the therapist can accurately predict and categorize each person's risk for VTE disease as no risk (less than 10%), low risk (10%), moderate risk (11%-40%), or high risk (greater than 41%).[444]

The person at risk for DVT secondary to fracture and subsequent immobility involving a lower-extremity cast should be carefully evaluated when the cast is removed. Normally, calf muscle atrophy is easily observed when the cast is removed. Normal calf size (less than 1 cm difference between left and right) without atrophy on cast removal may signal swelling associated with DVT.

For the client with diagnosed thrombophlebitis, the therapist should monitor and report any signs of PE, such as chest pain, hemoptysis, cough, diaphoresis, dyspnea, and apprehension. Clients with a history of DVT may develop chronic venous insufficiency even years later and therefore must be monitored periodically for life.

Precautions During Anticoagulation Therapy

Anyone receiving anticoagulant therapy (e.g., warfarin) must be monitored for manifestations of bleeding, as evidenced by blood in the urine, in the stool, or along the gums or teeth; subcutaneous bruising; or back, pelvic, or flank pain. The presence of any of these signs or symptoms must be reported to the physician immediately.

The risk for bleeding is increased with alcohol use, especially if there is concomitant liver disease, as alcohol also can potentiate warfarin. Many herbs have natural anticoagulant effects that can potentiate the effect of warfarin, and others can counteract its effect. Ginkgo biloba, garlic, dong quai, dan shen, and ginseng (herbs commonly ingested in supplemental form) should not be used or taken at the same time as warfarin. Anyone using these products should be encouraged to discuss medication dosage with the prescribing physician.

Eating large quantities of vitamin K–rich foods can also interfere with the drug's anticoagulant effects, requiring careful monitoring of food intake while on warfarin.

Bleeding under the skin and easy bruising in response to the slightest trauma can occur when platelet production is altered. This condition necessitates extreme care in the therapy setting, especially any intervention requiring soft tissue mobilization, manual therapy, or the use of any equipment, including any modalities and weight-training devices. (See the section on platelets in Chapter 40; see also Tables 40-8, 40-9, and 40-12.) Rarely, skin necrosis associated with the use of warfarin occurs, presenting as large hemorrhagic blisters on the breasts, buttocks, thighs, and penis requiring wound management.

Prevention and Intervention

Prevention is the key to treatment of thrombophlebitis, both preventing thrombus formation and preventing thrombi from becoming emboli. Preventive therapy can be tailored to the individual's level of risk and focuses on physical activity, exercise, and compression. The activity and exercise protocol may include active and passive range-of-motion exercise, early ambulation for brief but regular periods whenever possible, coughing and deep-breathing exercises, and proper positioning.

After thrombosis of a deep calf vein, elastic support hose should be worn for at least 6 to 8 weeks or longer if risk assessment is moderate or high. Helping the client find easier ways to put the hose on and explaining the purpose may increase compliance in using the hose consistently and correctly.

The use of TED (antiembolism) hose should be restricted to individuals who are nonambulatory for short periods of time. They do provide compression in the range of 13 to 18 mm Hg but are not intended for use while ambulating. A light gradient compression stocking of 20 to 30 mm Hg (available off-the-shelf) is advised to prevent blood clot formation when medically necessary in individuals who are upright, active, or ambulatory. (This would be a much better choice for orthopedic patients postoperatively once they are ambulatory.)

Support pantyhose may be an acceptable alternative for some people who have trouble putting on the compressive stockings or who live in very hot climates. The rationale for the use of compressive or elastic stockings is that the compressive force applied by the stocking causes the vessel wall to become applied to the thrombus, thereby keeping the thrombus in its location and preventing movement inside the blood vessel. Without the external compressive force of the stocking, once the person stands, increased hydrostatic pressure causes venous distention and permits the thrombus to become free floating inside the vessel.[444]

The American College of Chest Physicians recommends that anyone flying or sitting in a motor vehicle for more than 8 hours avoid wearing constrictive clothing around the waist or legs, stay hydrated, and perform frequent ankle pumps or other foot and leg exercises.[170]

Regarding positioning, the person at risk must be taught the importance of avoiding one position for prolonged periods and avoiding pillows under the legs postoperatively to facilitate venous return. At the same time, elevation of the legs just above the level of the heart aids blood flow by gravitational force and prevents venous stasis as a contributing factor to the formation of new thrombi.

Placing the foot of the bed in the Trendelenburg position (6-inch elevation with slight knee bend to prevent popliteal pressure) decreases venous pressure and helps relieve pain and edema. Prolonged sitting in a chair in the early postoperative period should be avoided.

DVT and Ambulation

(See also "Activity and Ambulation for Anyone with PE" in Chapter 15.)

Before anticoagulants, symptomatic intervention included bed rest for 3 to 5 days to prevent emboli and pressure fluctuations in the venous system that occur with walking; elevation of the leg with the knee flexed until the edema and tenderness subsided; and continuous local application of mild heat to relieve venospasm, produce analgesia, and promote resolution of inflammation. Ambulation (while wearing elastic stockings) was permitted if local tenderness and swelling had resolved (usually after 7 days for calf thrombosis and 10-14 days for thigh or pelvic thrombosis).

Today, routine practice is to authorize ambulation in all cases of DVT after an adequate anticoagulant has been administered if local symptoms and general condition permit. The concern in an acute care or rehabilitation setting is the increased risk of PE in clients who are aggressively mobilized too soon after a diagnosis of a DVT and before adequate anticoagulation has been administered. Bed rest (up to 24 hours) may be advised before returning a person with acute DVT to ambulation and physical therapy.

However, there is a concern that bed rest promotes venous stasis and the risk of PE increases as the DVT is allowed to increase with continued inactivity. Current evidence supports encouraging patients to resume activity (e.g., ambulate) with appropriate compression as soon as they are therapeutic on anticoagulation. The American College of Chest Physicians recommends ambulation as tolerated with a newly diagnosed DVT.[13]

Several randomized controlled trials and large registry trials have shown no increased risk of PE in the mobilized (ambulation with compression) group as compared to the immobilized (strictly bed rest) group.[57,234,348–350,450] Of significant importance, there is evidence that ambulation and compression does not cause new PEs; in fact, ambulation and compression reduces stasis and thrombus formation with faster relief of pain and swelling and reduced frequency and severity of postthrombotic syndrome.[57,347]

Knowledge of the evidence and current practice guidelines allows therapists to collaborate with physicians and make the most appropriate decisions for our patients, potentially avoiding unnecessary and detrimental bed rest/immobility. Of interest is a recent report from an International Compression Club meeting discussing dogmas and controversies in compression therapy where evidence-based findings rather than "common sense" were provided to substantiate indications for using compression and application of compression techniques.[152]

The standard 24-hour hold policy after injection of enoxaparin or LMWH has been called into question because these pharmacologic agents reach a maximum therapeutic dose in 3 to 5 hours. Some facilities practice a 5-hour hold on patients receiving enoxaparin. Others initiate mobility as soon as 1 hour after administration of a LMWH for newly diagnosed extremity DVT. With other types of heparin (unfractionated heparin), activity can be resumed when the activated partial thromboplastin time is therapeutic; some clinical settings use the heparin anti–factor Xa level of 0.3 to 0.7. Waiting for the prothrombin time/international normalized ratio (INR) to reach therapeutic levels is only necessary when there is no other form of anticoagulation (e.g., LMWH) being used. Compression along with anticoagulation when mobilizing remains the standard practice.[350]

In the absence evidence-based clinical guidelines, a team approach is advocated. Protocols may be established but each individual should be evaluated carefully taking all risk factors into consideration when establishing the plan of care.

DVT and Laboratory Values

Therapists need to know what anticoagulant medication patients are taking and how to determine if the medication is therapeutic. Warfarin is monitored by INR and unfractionated heparin is monitored by partial thromboplastin time. LMWH is therapeutic almost immediately after given and, unlike the others, does not require a lab value to determine achievement of a therapeutic range.

The INR is a measure of coagulability and was developed to provide results that would not vary between laboratories. Individuals receiving anticoagulation therapy because of history of DVT, coronary artery disease, cerebrovascular disease, atrial fibrillation, and other reasons are usually anticoagulated to an INR of 2 to 3.[32]

As INR increases, however, the risk of bleeding with minor trauma increases and excessive bleeding may occur during surgery, as well as spontaneous bleeding. Therapists must keep INR levels in mind when working with clients. An INR between 2.0 and 3.0 is considered "therapeutic" for anticoagulation. Guidelines have not been published for levels above which physical activity would be contraindicated.

As with any clinical decision, the individual being considered would be evaluated taking factors such as medical history; symptoms related to activity; type of activity (bed exercises or out of bed activities); size, location, and number of thrombi; clinical presentation (e.g., obvious signs of severe swelling, redness, warmth, tenderness; evidence of PE), and cognitive function in following directions.

A THERAPIST'S THOUGHTS*

Mobility and Activity after Anticoagulation Therapy

Note to Reader: I consulted with numerous experts in the medical and pharmacologic fields as to the need for holding therapy or minimizing mobility after the initiation of anticoagulation in the hospital setting. The compilation of thoughts and ideas may prove useful to you in your clinical decision-making.

To date, there has been no evidence that holding therapy achieves anything useful. The question has been raised, "What is achieved when doses are 'therapeutic'?" It is erroneous to talk about this as if the clot or thrombus magically disappears as soon as the dose is therapeutic. Even the discussion of the therapeutic dose does not mean much because people can still coagulate (or bleed) at different values no matter what test is chosen.

A peak response in 3 to 5 hours indicates that Lovenox [generic name enoxaparin] reaches its greatest ability to prevent clot formation at about 3 to 5 hours after injection. The medication prevents clot formation but does not break down the clots. In other words, if there is an already existing thrombus, the enoxaparin should help in keeping it from getting bigger, but it will not help reduce the size of the clot. There is evidence that it can take months for the clot to break down; the LMWH does not speed up this process.[241]

The coagulation system is much too complex to boil down to a single value regardless of what anticoagulant is used. As health care practitioners, we must not become dependent on single lab values but rather use lab values in conjunction with clinical judgment and collaborative communication with the other health care team members.

Because immobility is a contributor to coagulation, bed rest is a risk factor for anyone with excess coagulation/thrombosis. Everyone involved with the patient must watch closely for signs of a pulmonary embolus as well as consider any other risk factors present.

The pharmacology consultant for this text commented that holding activity/physical therapy for a few hours is not a recommendation given by pharmacologists to individuals receiving LMWH for the treatment of a DVT. There are still many institutions that follow the guideline of patient mobilization when they are 4 hours post first enoxaparin dose.

Lymphedema therapists encourage orders for edema therapy right away when seeing someone with a new DVT of the upper or lower extremity. Stockings are fitted 24 hours after the start of anticoagulation and ambulation is encouraged as soon as compression is in place.

*Catherine C. Goodman, MBA, PT, CBP

Monitoring all vital signs while paying attention to signs of PE (e.g., chest pain, shortness of breath, dizziness, tachycardia, apprehension) is always advised. Heart rate greater than 100 beats per minute with an O_2 sat less than 90%, especially in the presence of any of these other symptoms requires a nursing or medical consult.

Varicose Veins.

Definition and Incidence. Varicose veins are an abnormal dilation of veins, usually the saphenous veins of the lower extremities, leading to tortuosity (twisting and turning) of the vessel, incompetence of the valves, and a propensity to thrombosis. Women are affected with leg varicosities more often than men (secondary to pregnancy) until age 70 years, when the gender difference disappears. Forty-one percent of women ages 40 to 50 years and 72% of women ages 60 to 70 years have varicose veins.[198]

This condition most often develops between the ages of 30 and 50 years for all persons. A separate but similar condition called *spider veins* or *telangiectasia* (broken capillaries) results in fine-lined networks of red, blue, or purple veins, usually on the thighs, calves, and ankles. The veins may form patterns resembling a sunburst, a spider web (see Fig. 10-3), or a tree with branches but can also appear as short, unconnected, or parallel lines.

Etiologic and Risk Factors. Varicose veins may be an inherited trait, but it is unclear whether the valvular incompetence is secondary to defective valves in the saphenous veins or to a fundamental weakness of the walls of the vein leading to dilation of the vessel.

Periods of high venous pressure associated with heavy lifting or prolonged sitting or standing are risk factors. Hormonal changes (e.g., pregnancy, menopause, hormonal therapy) often contribute to the development of this condition by relaxing the vein walls.

Other risk factors include pressure associated with pregnancy or obesity, heart failure, hemorrhoids, constipation, esophageal varices, and hepatic cirrhosis. Risk factors for spider veins are similar (age, hormones, familial predisposition) but also include local injury (past or present).

Pathogenesis. Blood returning to the heart from the legs must flow upward through the veins, against the pull of gravity. This blood is milked upward, principally by the massaging action of the muscles against the veins. To prevent the blood from flowing backward, the veins contain one-way valves located at intervals, which operate in pairs by closing to stop the reverse movement of the blood.

The vessels most commonly affected by varicosities are located just beneath the skin superficial to the deep fascia and function without the kind of support deep veins of the legs receive from surrounding muscles. As the one-way valves become incompetent or the veins become more elastic, the veins engorge with stagnant blood and become pooled.

Any condition accompanied by pressure changes places a strain on these veins, and the lack of pumping action of the lower leg muscles causes blood to pool. Other sites involved include the hemorrhoidal plexus of the rectum and anal canal (either inside or outside the anal sphincter), submucosal veins of the distal esophagus, and the scrotum (varicocele).

The weight of the blood continually pressing downward against the closed venous valves causes the veins to distend and eventually lose their elasticity. When several valves lose their ability to function properly, the blood collects in the veins, causing the veins to become swollen and distended. During pregnancy, the uterus may press against the veins coming from the lower extremities and prevent the free flow of returning blood. More force is required to push the blood through the veins, and the increased back-pressure can result in varicose veins.

Clinical Manifestations. The clinical picture is not directly correlated with the severity of the varicosities; extensive varicose veins may be asymptomatic, but minimal varicosities may result in multiple symptoms. The development of varicose veins is usually gradual; the most common symptom reported is a dull, aching heaviness, tension, or feeling of fatigue brought on by periods of standing. Cramps of the lower legs may occur, especially at night, and elevation of the legs often provides relief. Itching from an associated dermatitis may also occur above the ankle.

The most visible sign of varicosities is the dilated, tortuous, elongated veins beneath the skin, which are usually readily visible when the person is standing (Fig. 12-35). Varicosities of long duration may be accompanied by secondary tissue changes, such as a brownish pigmentation of the skin and a thinning of the skin above the ankle. Swelling may also occur around the ankles.

Untreated, the veins become thick and hard to the touch; impaired circulation and skin changes may lead to ulcers of the lower legs, especially around the ankles (see Table 12-21). (See also "Esophageal Varices" in Chapter 16.) One of the most important distinctions between

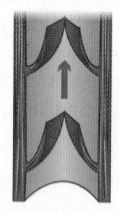
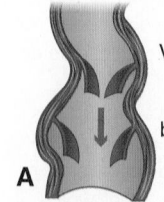
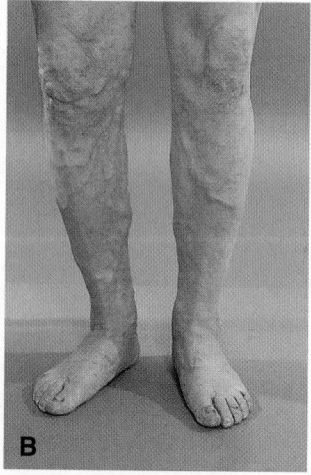

NORMAL VEINS
Functional valves aid in flow of venous blood back to heart

VARICOSE VEINS
Failure of valves and pooling of blood in superficial veins

A   **B**

Figure 12-35

A, Diagrams of normal *(top)* and varicose *(bottom)* veins. **B,** Person with varicose veins. (A, from O'Toole M, ed: *Miller-Keane encyclopedia and dictionary of medicine, nursing, and allied health,* ed 6, Philadelphia, 1997, WB Saunders, p. 1702. B, from Forbes CD, Jackson WF: *Color atlas and text of clinical medicine,* ed 3, London, 2003, Mosby.)

varicose veins and spider veins is that, in some cases, varicose veins can result in thromboses (blood clots) and phlebitis (inflammation of the vein) or venous insufficiency ulcers, whereas spider veins are merely a cosmetic issue with no adverse effects.

MEDICAL MANAGEMENT

DIAGNOSIS. The physician must distinguish between the symptoms of arteriosclerotic PVD, such as intermittent claudication and coldness of the feet, and symptoms of venous disease, because occlusive arterial disease usually contraindicates the operative management of varicosities below the knee. When the two conditions coexist, the reduced blood flow caused by the atherosclerosis may even improve the varicosities by reducing blood flow through the veins.

Visual inspection and palpation identify varicose veins of the legs, and Doppler ultrasonography or the duplex scanner is useful in detecting the location of incompetent valves. Endoscopy or radiographic diagnosis identifies esophageal varices, rectal examination or proctoscopy is used to diagnose hemorrhoids, and palpation identifies varicocele (scrotal swelling).

TREATMENT. Treatment of mild varicose veins is conservative, consisting of periodic daily rest periods with feet elevated slightly above the heart. Client education as to the importance of promoting circulation is stressed, including instructions to make frequent changes in posture, a daily exercise program, and the appropriate use of properly fitting elastic stockings.

When varicosities have progressed past the stage at which conservative care is helpful, surgical intervention and compression sclerotherapy may be considered. In the past, surgical treatment of varicose veins consisted of removing the varicosities and the incompetent perforating veins (ligation and stripping), a procedure sometimes referred to as *stripping the veins* or *miniphlebectomy*.

Other procedures for varicose veins have been developed, including radiofrequency ablation (radio waves used to seal off the vein), sclerotherapy (injections of a hardening, or sclerosing, solution; over several months' time, the injected veins atrophy and blood is channeled into other veins), and laser therapy (noninvasive use of near-infrared wavelengths).

Radiofrequency and laser treatments were found comparable with respect to the venous occlusion rates at 3 months after treatment with the former procedure accompanied with less pain, lower analgesia levels and reduced bruising.[331] Ligation and stripping of the great saphenous vein prevent its use as a source for future CABGs, motivating researchers to develop effective intervention techniques that salvage large veins.

Oral dietary supplementation has been adopted by some individuals as an addition to traditional management of varicose veins. The loss of vascular integrity associated with the pathogenesis of both hemorrhoids and varicose veins may be aided by several botanical extracts shown to improve microcirculation, capillary flow, and vascular tone while strengthening the connective tissue of the perivascular substrate.[281]

PROGNOSIS. Good results with relief of symptoms are usually possible in the majority of cases. Early conservative care for varicose veins during initial stages may help prevent the condition from worsening, but advanced disease may not be prevented from recurring, even with surgical intervention or sclerotherapy. Although surgery for varicose veins can improve appearance, it may not reduce the physical discomfort, suggesting that most lower limb symptoms may have a nonvenous cause. A high mortality is associated with ruptured, bleeding esophageal varices (see Chapter 16).

SPECIAL IMPLICATIONS FOR THE THERAPIST   12-21

Varicose Veins

The therapist can be very instrumental in developing prescriptive exercise and preventive measures for anyone at risk for, or already diagnosed with, varicose veins. Because excessive sitting or standing contributes to this condition, the therapist can individualize a program to help the person avoid static postures and utilize quick stretch or movement breaks coordinated with deep-breathing exercises.

Nonprescription pantyhose should be replaced with special compressive hose that do not constrict behind the knee, upper leg, waist, or groin. These should be worn as much as possible during the daytime hours (including during exercise for some people) but may be removed at night. After exercise and at the end of the day, instruct the individual to elevate the legs in a supported position above the level of the heart for 10 to 15 minutes.

Encourage the person to practice good breathing techniques during this time. Aerobic exercise, strength training, or resistive exercises are encouraged, but high-impact activities, such as jogging or step aerobics, should be avoided. Brisk walking, cycling, cross-country skiing or Nordic track, rowing, and swimming are all good alternatives to high-impact activities.

Chronic Venous Insufficiency

Definition and Incidence. Chronic venous insufficiency (CVI), also known as postphlebitic syndrome and venous stasis, is defined as inadequate venous return over a long period of time. This condition follows most severe cases of DVT, although it is possible to develop CVI without prior episodes of DVT. CVI may also occur as a result of leg trauma, varicose veins, and neoplastic obstruction of the pelvic veins. The long-term sequelae of CVI may be chronic leg ulcers, accounting for the majority of vascular ulceration; incidence is expected to continue rising with the aging of America.[91]

Etiologic Factors and Pathogenesis. CVI occurs when damaged or destroyed valves in the veins result in decreased venous return, thereby increasing venous pressure and producing venous stasis. Without adequate valve function and in the absence of the calf muscle pump, blood flows in the veins bidirectionally, causing high ambulatory venous pressures in the calf veins (venous hypertension). Superficial veins and capillaries dilate in response to the venous hypertension. Red blood cells, proteins, and fluids leak out of the capillaries into interstitial spaces, producing edema and the reddish brown pigmentation characteristic of CVI.

Chronic pooling of blood in the veins of the lower extremities prevents adequate cellular oxygenation and removal of waste products. Any trauma, especially pressure, further lowers the oxygen supply by reducing blood flow into the area. Cell death occurs, and necrotic tissue develops into venous stasis ulcers. The cycle of reduced oxygenation, necrosis, and ulceration prevents damaged tissue from obtaining necessary nutrients, causing delayed healing and persistent ulceration. Poor circulation impairs immune and inflammatory responses, leaving venous stasis ulcers susceptible to infection.

Other contributing factors may include poor nutrition, immobility, and local trauma (past or present). A previous history of burns requiring skin grafts predisposes the individual to venous insufficiency. The area of the graft usually lacks superficial veins, properly functioning capillaries, or both, resulting in blood pooling in these areas. As a result previously burned areas and skin grafts in the lower extremity are susceptible to vascular ulceration.

Clinical Manifestations. CVI is characterized by progressive edema of the leg; thickening, coarsening, and brownish pigmentation of skin around the ankles; and venous stasis ulceration (see Table 12-21). Venous insufficiency ulcers constitute approximately 80% of all lower extremity ulcers, occurring most often above the medial malleolus where venous hypertension is greatest.

These ulcers characteristically are shallow wounds with a white creamy to fibrous slough over a base of good granulation tissue. They can be very painful with a moderate to large amount of drainage. The wounds typically have irregular borders and are partial to full thickness, often with signs of reepithelialization (e.g., pink or red granulation base). Frequently, moderate to severe edema is present in the limb; in longstanding cases, this edema becomes hardened to a dense, woody texture. The skin of the involved extremity is usually thin, shiny, dry, and cyanotic. Dermatitis and cellulitis may develop later in this condition.

MEDICAL MANAGEMENT

The physician will differentiate between CVI and other causes of edema and ulceration of the lower extremities using client history, clinical examination, and diagnostic tests to rule out or confirm superimposed acute phlebitis. Arterial and venous insufficiency may coexist in the same person.

Treatment goals and techniques are as for varicose veins (increase in venous return, reduction of edema). Conventional methods of compression and rest and elevation (e.g., more frequent periods of leg elevation above the level of the heart are encouraged throughout the day with the foot of the bed elevated 6 inches at night) have been augmented by surgical intervention.

Rapid progress in endovascular procedures with angioplasty and stenting has made it possible for the development of techniques to relieve obstruction and repair reflux in the deep veins. Venous stasis ulcers require ongoing treatment, usually involving the therapist (e.g., primary intervention for edema reduction and topical ulcer and wound care).

More detailed information is available.[211,248,436,437] Researchers are developing bioengineered skin, a living human dermal replacement for the management of venous ulcers. See "Skin Transplantation" in Chapter 21.

The prognosis is poor for resolution of CVI, with chronic venous stasis ulcers causing loss of function and progressive disability. Recurrent episodes of acute thrombophlebitis may occur, and noncompliance with the treatment program is common.

SPECIAL IMPLICATIONS FOR THE THERAPIST   12-22

Chronic Venous Insufficiency

The therapist can be very instrumental in providing clients with venous insufficiency with education and prevention to avoid complications that can occur with vascular ulceration and chronic wounds. Formulating an exercise prescription; collaborating with a nutritionist; and understanding the underlying etiology, hemodynamics, comorbidities, and principles of tissue repair are essential in developing a plan of care.

Compression therapy (e.g., bandages, gradient compression stockings, pumps) is the gold standard for treatment of venous insufficiency, especially when venous leg ulcers are present. The goal is to promote venous return from peripheral veins to central circulation. The therapist may also use layered gradient compression wraps (see Fig. 10-9, C). Antiembolism TED hospital stockings are not an effective treatment for vein disease. They do offer mild equalized compression for individuals who are bedridden, but they cannot support the vein walls for individuals who are upright. The presence of CHF is considered a precaution to the use of external compression and requires close collaboration between the physician and therapist.

Before initiating compression therapy the ankle-brachial index (ABI) should be measured. ABI is determined using a noninvasive arterial Doppler study to assess the level of circulation. Compression may not be tolerated and/or may have to be modified if arterial circulation is compromised. Arterial obstruction in the presence of venous insufficiency may not be readily recognized.

The ABI is the result of a vascular diagnostic test comparing the systolic blood pressure between the ankle and brachial pulses. ABI results should be reported with noncompressible values defined as greater than 1.40, normal values 1.00-1.40, borderline 0.91-0.99, and abnormal 0.90 or less.[31,392]

An index result of 1.0 indicates an adequate arterial blood supply; an index less than 1.0 indicates insufficient blood flow to the distal regions for healing to occur (see Box 12-15, which includes acceptable values for compression therapy). ABIs can be higher than 1.0 in individuals with diabetes as the vessels do not compress because of arterial calcification.[392]

Assessing ABI is also warranted if wounds associated with CVI do not demonstrate healing within 2 weeks of beginning wound care. An assessment of the legs should be performed frequently to observe for insufficiency (stasis) ulcers, skin changes (e.g., color, texture, temperature), impaired growth of nails, and discrepancy in size of extremities, including observations and measurements for edema.

In the home health setting, the client or family should be instructed to contact a member of the medical team if any edema or change in the condition of the extremity occurs. When a stasis ulcer of any size is detected, treatment is initiated. A wound care specialist (usually a physical therapist or a nurse) is a vital part of the health care team in the management of stasis ulcers. Information on specific wound care management is available elsewhere.[211,248,436,437]

Whirlpool beyond an initial one or two treatments is contraindicated, because the increased blood volume and dependent position (underlying causes of wound) can make the edema worse. When pulsatile debridement devices are unavailable, limited hydrotherapy (maximal temperature 26.7° C [80° F]) may be indicated to remove loose debris, and antiseptics may be indicated to moisten dried exudate or to facilitate debridement.

The client should be advised to avoid prolonged standing and sitting; crossing the legs; sitting too high for feet to touch the floor or too deep, causing pressure against the popliteal space; and wearing tight clothing (including girdles, elastic waistbands, or too-tight jeans) or support hose or stockings that extend above the knee, which act as a tourniquet at the popliteal fossa. Elastic stockings are recommended, but they must be worn properly to avoid bunching behind the knee or uneven compression in the popliteal fossa.

Vasomotor Disorders

Vasomotor disorders of the blood vessels causing headaches and complex regional pain syndrome (complex regional pain syndrome; formerly reflex sympathetic dystrophy) are discussed in Chapters 37 and 39, respectively).

Raynaud Disease and Raynaud Phenomenon

Definition and Overview. Intermittent episodes of small artery or arteriole constriction of the extremities causing temporary pallor and cyanosis of the digits (fingers more often than toes) and changes in skin temperature are called *Raynaud phenomenon*. These episodes occur in response to cold temperature or strong emotion, such as anxiety or excitement. When this condition is a primary vasospastic disorder it is called (idiopathic) *Raynaud disease* or *primary Raynaud*. If the disorder is secondary to another disease or underlying cause, the term *Raynaud phenomenon* or *secondary Raynaud* is used.

Incidence and Etiologic Factors

Raynaud Disease. Eighty percent of persons with Raynaud disease are women between the ages of 20 and 49 years. The exact etiology of Raynaud disease remains unknown, but it appears to be caused by hypersensitivity of digital arteries to cold, release of serotonin, and genetic susceptibility to vasospasm. Raynaud disease accounts for 65% of all people affected by this condition. Raynaud disease is usually experienced as more annoying than medically serious.

Raynaud Phenomenon. Epidemiologists estimate that Raynaud phenomenon is a problem for 10% to 20% of the general population; it affects women 20 times more frequently than men, usually between the ages of 15 and 40 years. Risk factors for Raynaud phenomenon are different between men and women. The Framingham Offspring Study reports that age and smoking are associated with Raynaud phenomenon in men only, whereas an association with marital status and alcohol use was observed in women only. These findings suggest that different mechanisms influence the expression of Raynaud phenomenon in men and women.[155]

Raynaud phenomenon as a condition secondary to another disease is often associated with Buerger disease or connective tissue disorders (collagen vascular diseases), such as Sjögren syndrome, scleroderma, polymyositis and dermatomyositis, mixed connective tissue disease, SLE, and rheumatoid arthritis (see Box 12-17). Raynaud phenomenon can be a sign of occult (hidden) neoplasm, especially suspected when it presents unilaterally.

Raynaud phenomenon may also occur with change in temperature, such as occurs when going from a warm outside environment to an air-conditioned room. In addition, Raynaud phenomenon may be associated with occlusive arterial diseases and neurogenic lesions, such as thoracic outlet syndrome, or with the effects of long-term exposure to cold (occupational or frostbite), trauma, or use of vibrating equipment such as jackhammers. Injuries to the small vessels of the hands may produce Raynaud phenomenon. The trauma can be a result of repetitive stress that comes from using crutches for extended periods, typing on a computer keyboard, or even playing the piano.

Several medications (e.g., β-blockers, ergot alkaloids prescribed for migraine headaches, antineoplastics used in chemotherapy) have also been implicated. Because nicotine causes small blood vessels to constrict, smoking can trigger attacks in persons who are predisposed to this phenomenon.

Pathogenesis and Clinical Manifestations. Scientists theorize that Raynaud phenomenon is associated with a disturbance in the control of vascular reflexes. Although the causes differ for Raynaud disease and Raynaud phenomenon, the clinical manifestations are the same, based on a pathogenesis of arterial vasospasm in the skin.

It begins with the release of chemical messengers that cause blood vessels to constrict and remain constricted. The flow of oxygenated blood to these areas is reduced, and the skin becomes pale and cold. The blood in the constricted vessels, which has released its oxygen to the tissues surrounding the vessels, pools in the tissues, producing a bluish or purplish color.

In the case of fibromyalgia-associated Raynaud phenomenon, symptoms may be the result of cold-induced spasms of the arteries caused by a problem in the autonomic nervous system control of the blood supply to the extremities. Altered or reduced numbers of β_2-adrenergic receptors on the platelets correlate with Raynaud phenomenon in fibromyalgia-associated Raynaud.[50] These receptors are involved in the functioning of the autonomic nervous system. This could explain why the cold-induced pain is significant but without skin color changes in this population.

In most cases, the skin color progresses from blue to white to red. First, ischemia from vasospastic attacks causes cyanosis, numbness, and the sensation of cold in the digits (thumbs usually remain unaffected). The affected tissues become numb or painful. For unknown reasons, the flow of chemical that triggered the process eventually stops. The vessels relax, and blood flow is restored. The skin becomes white (characterized by pallor) and then red (characterized by rubor) as the vasospasm subsides and the capillaries become engorged with oxygenated blood. Oxygen-rich blood returns to the area, and as it does so, the skin becomes warm and flushed. The person may experience throbbing, paresthesia, and slight swelling as this occurs.

Sensory changes, such as numbness, stiffness, diminished sensation, and aching pain, often accompany vasomotor manifestations. Initially, no abnormal findings are present between attacks, but over time, frequent, prolonged episodes of vasospasm causing ischemia interfere with cellular metabolism, causing the skin of the fingertips to thicken and the fingernails to become brittle.

In severe, chronic Raynaud phenomenon, the underlying condition may have produced scars in the vessels, reducing the vessel diameter and therefore blood flow. When attacks occur, they are often more severe, resulting in prolonged loss of blood to fingers and toes, which can produce painful skin ulcers; rarely, gangrene may develop. Episodes of Raynaud disease are often bilateral, progressing distally to proximally along the digits. Raynaud phenomenon may be unilateral, involving only one or two fingers, but this clinical presentation warrants a physician's differential diagnosis, as it can be associated with cancer (Fig. 12-36).

MEDICAL MANAGEMENT

DIAGNOSIS AND PROGNOSIS. Diagnosis is usually made by clinical presentation and past medical history. Raynaud disease is diagnosed by a history of symptoms for at least 2 years with no progression and no evidence of underlying

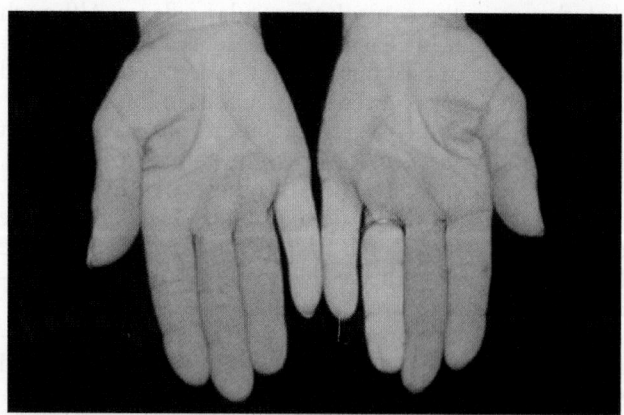

Figure 12-36

Raynaud disease or phenomenon. White color (pallor) from arteriospasm and resulting deficit in blood supply may initially involve only one or two fingers, as shown here. Cold and numbness or pain may accompany the pallor or cyanosis stage. Subsequent episodes may involve the entire finger and may include all the fingers. Toes are affected in 40% of cases. (From Jarvis C: *Physical examination and health assessment*, ed 4, Philadelphia, 2004, WB Saunders.)

cause. Raynaud disease must be differentiated from the numerous possible disorders associated with Raynaud phenomenon. Untreated and uncontrolled Raynaud may damage or destroy the affected digits. Rarely, necrosis, ulceration, and gangrene result. Even with intervention, the person with Raynaud disease or phenomenon may experience disability and loss of function.

PREVENTION AND TREATMENT. Treatment for *Raynaud disease* is limited to prevention or alleviation of the vasospasm because no underlying cause or condition has been discovered, although pharmacologic agents for primary and secondary Raynaud are under investigation. Clients are encouraged to avoid stimuli that trigger attacks, such as cool or cold temperatures, changes in temperature, and emotional stress, and to eliminate use of nicotine, which has a constricting effect on blood vessels.

Physical or occupational therapy is often prescribed and should include client education about managing symptoms through protective skin care and cold protection (see Box 12-14), biofeedback, stress management and relaxation techniques, whirlpool or other gentle heat modalities, and exercise. Large movement arm circles in a windmill fashion can restore circulation in some people. The individual will have to experiment with the speed at which to move the arms; some people benefit from slow, gentle movement, whereas others find greater success with fast rotations.

Evidence now exists that calcium channel blockers are an effective pharmacologic treatment of secondary Raynaud.[212] Administration of iloprost, both oral and IV, is also effective.[212] The drug, a prostacyclin analogue, improves circulation by dilating blood vessels and reducing blood cell clumping. Pharmacologic management may also include nonaddicting analgesics for pain. Therapists can be instrumental in teaching physiologic modulation starting with hand warming. A handheld device to measure fingertip temperature combined with self-guided or audio-guided relaxation can be very effective and is available.[213]

When conservative care fails to relieve symptoms and the condition progresses clinically, sympathetic blocks followed by intensive therapy may be helpful. Sympathectomy may be necessary for persons who only temporarily benefit from the sympathetic blocks.

Treatment for *Raynaud phenomenon* consists of appropriate treatment for the underlying condition or removing the stimulus causing vasospasm. The clinical care described for Raynaud disease may also be of benefit. In addition, the use of antioxidants as an effective treatment of Raynaud phenomenon as well as the role of therapeutic angiogenesis (regeneration of vessels) remains under investigation.

SPECIAL IMPLICATIONS FOR THE THERAPIST	12-23

Vasomotor Disorders
Raynaud Disease and Phenomenon

Prevention of episodes of Raynaud is important. The affected individual must be encouraged to keep warm, avoid air conditioning, and dress warmly in the winter (e.g., protect the extremities as well as the head, chest, and back to maintain overall body temperature).

Aquatic therapy is often helpful in diminishing symptoms, but again, the individual must be careful when moving from place to place with extreme temperature changes (e.g., from outside winter temperatures into a warm pool area and back outside). The use of antihypertensives for Raynaud can result in postural hypotension; the physician should be notified of these findings to alter the dosage.

SPECIAL IMPLICATIONS FOR THE THERAPIST   12-24

Peripheral Vascular Disease

Even though Special Implications for the Therapist boxes for each individual disease making up PVD have been presented, a brief overview or summary of PVD as a whole seems warranted and a reminder that because of the prevalence of atherosclerotic disease in anyone with PVD, heart rate and blood pressure should be monitored during the evaluative process and during initial interventions. This is especially important in those with diabetes mellitus, and for anyone who has undergone an amputation, which implies severe disease.

Notably, people with PAD may exhibit precipitous rises in blood pressure during exercise owing to the atherosclerotic process present and the diminished vascular bed.[465] Examination of the pedal pulses should be part of the physical examination for all clients older than 55 years, and measurement of the ABI is recommended for those who have diminished or nonpalpable pedal pulses but who do not have diabetes.[392]

For the client with back pain, buttock pain, or leg pain of unknown or previously undiagnosed cause, screening for medical disease, including assessment of risk factors, past medical history, and special tests and measures (e.g., bicycle test, palpation of pulses), is essential.[180,184]

PVD can be confusing, with the wide range of diseases affecting veins and arteries, the etiology of which is sometimes occlusive, sometimes inflammatory, and, occasionally, as in the case of Buerger disease, both occlusive and inflammatory. The basic point to keep in mind is how arterial disease differs (significantly) from venous disease in clinical presentation, pathogenesis, and management.

Focusing on the underlying etiologic factors is the key to choosing the most appropriate and effective intervention. For example, in the case of acute arterial disease, the tissues are not oxygenated, and ischemia can result in local trauma or burns; gangrene can develop quickly. The goal is to increase oxygen without increasing demand or need for oxygen. Claudication occurs when the activity causes increased oxygen demand in an already compromised area.

During the acute phase of arterial ischemia rehabilitation, intervention and movement are minimized, heat and massage are contraindicated, and the person is instructed in the use of positions that will increase blood flow to the tissues involved (e.g., head elevated with legs slightly lower than the heart).

Chronic arterial disease can be treated by the therapist by concentrating on improving collateral circulation and increasing vasodilation. The role of exercise in PAD (especially in reducing claudication) is well documented[202] (see also "Arterial Occlusive Diseases" above). There is a suggestion that supervised exercise may be more beneficial than nonsupervised exercise.[268]

In venous disorders, the tissues are oxygenated but the blood is not moving, and stasis occurs. With venous occlusion, the skin is discolored rather than pale (ranging from angry red to deep blue-purple), edema is prominent, and pain is most marked at the site of occlusion, although extreme edema can render all the skin of the limb quite tender.

The goal of therapy is to create compressive pumping forces to move fluid volume and reduce edema. For this reason, heat or cold, compressive stockings, massage, and activity (e.g., ankle pumps, heel slides, quad sets, ambulation) are part of the treatment protocol.

Further guidelines for exercise in the management of PVD are outlined elsewhere.[17,194] See also "Arteriosclerosis Obliterans (Peripheral Arterial Disease)" above. Modifying cardiovascular risk factors, improving exercise duration and decreasing claudication, preventing joint contractures and muscle atrophy, preventing skin ulcerations, promoting healing of any pressure ulcers, and improving quality of life are part of the therapy plan of care. In the case of lower-extremity amputation, the use of unweighted ambulation to reduce the physiologic demands of walking during early rehabilitation has been reported.[314]

For people with vascular ulcers, improving the arterial supply or venous return will lessen pain, increase mobility, and allow ulcers to heal. Whenever ulcers are present, understanding the type of ulcer and underlying etiology will point to the best intervention. The assessment of and therapeutic intervention for vascular wounds are beyond the scope of this text; the reader is referred to other, more appropriate texts.[248,436,437]

Vascular Neoplasms

Malignant vascular (i.e., involving the blood vessels) neoplasms are extremely rare and include angiosarcoma, hemangiopericytoma, and Kaposi sarcoma. *Angiosarcomas* (hemangiosarcomas) can occur in either gender and at any age, most commonly appearing as small, painless, red nodules on the skin, soft tissue, breast, bone, liver, and spleen. Almost one half of all people with angiosarcoma die of the disease.

Hemangiopericytoma arises from the smooth muscle cells that are external to the walls of capillaries and arterioles. Most commonly located on the lower extremities and retroperitoneum (space between the peritoneum lining the walls of the abdominal and pelvic cavities and the posterior abdominal wall), these tumors are composed of spindle cells with a rich vascular network. Metastasis to the lungs, bone, liver, and lymph nodes occurs in 10% to 50% of cases, but the majority of hemangiopericytomas are removed surgically without having invaded or metastasized.

Kaposi sarcoma in association with AIDS most likely occurs as a result of loss of immunity. One form of the tumor resembles a simple hemangioma with tightly packed clusters of capillaries, most often visible on the skin. Although Kaposi sarcoma is malignant and may be widespread in the body, it is not usually a cause of death.

Arteriovenous Malformations

Arteriovenous malformations (AVMs) are congenital vascular malformations of the cerebral vasculature. AVMs are the result of localized maldevelopment of part of the primitive vascular plexus consisting of abnormal arteriovenous communications without intervening capillaries. There is a central tangled mass of fragile, abnormal blood vessels called the *nidus* that shunts blood from cerebral feeding arteries directly into cerebral veins. The loss of the normal capillary network between the high-pressure arterial system and the low-pressure venous system results in a faster flow and elevated pressure within the delicate vessels of the AVM. The lack of a gradient pressure system predisposes the lesion to rupture.

AVMs vary in size, ranging from massive lesions that are fed by multiple vessels to lesions too small to identify. Perfusion to adjacent brain tissue may be impaired because blood flow is diverted to the AVM, a phenomenon referred to as *vascular stealing*. AVMs may occur in any blood vessel, but the most common sites include the brain, GI tract, and skin. Approximately 10% of cases present with aneurysms. Small AVMs are more likely to bleed than large ones, and once bleeding occurs, repeated episodes are likely.

Clinical presentation depends on the location of the malformation and may relate to hemorrhage from the malformation or an associated aneurysm or to cerebral ischemia caused by diversion or stasis of blood. Seizures, migraine-like headaches unresponsive to standard therapy, and progressive neurologic deficits may develop.

Diagnostic testing and planned intervention rely on cerebral angiography to show the AVM size, location, feeding vessels, nidus, and venous outflow vessels. Other tests may include MRI, x-rays, ultrasound, electroencephalogram, and arteriogram. Treatment options are individualized depending on the size and location of the lesion, as well as any other surgical risks present.

In the last 15 years, endovascular embolization and stereotactic radiosurgery (delivery of extremely precise doses of radiation to destroy abnormal blood vessels) have increased survival outcomes, especially for lesions previously considered inoperable or in cases of high surgical risk factors. Prognosis is guarded, as there is a 2% to 4% chance of hemorrhage with the concomitant risk of permanent neurologic deficit or even death.

SPECIAL IMPLICATIONS FOR THE THERAPIST 12-25

Arteriovenous Malformations

Generally, the individual with a known AVM is advised to avoid activities and exercise that can increase intracranial or blood pressure (see Box 16-1). Weight

training and contact sports are contraindicated, and some physicians advise against high-aerobic exercise, including running.

Postoperative complications can include hemorrhage, seizures, nausea, vomiting, or headache, and symptomatic perilesional edema can occur up to 1 year after the procedure. Neurologic deficits vary but are usually transient; radiation-induced brain injury is rare. The radiation's effect begins immediately, but complete obliteration of the lesion can take up to 3 years, during which time the affected individual must continue to maintain a normal blood pressure.

OTHER CARDIAC CONSIDERATIONS

Despite the success of new immunosuppressive regimens and better results with transplantation, few people who are dying of heart failure will actually have the opportunity to receive a heart transplant. The mechanical technology may eventually allow selected persons to receive long-term (permanent) support as a substitute for cardiac transplantation. The recipient is often home in 6 weeks with follow-up home health care. In the future, studies may be done to determine the efficacy of removing the cardiac assistive device after prolonged heart rest provides cardiac recovery. Survival with the natural recovered heart may be possible in some people.

Researchers are actively pursuing tissue engineering to replace transplantation and mechanical devices (e.g., artificial heart, implanted cardiac assistive devices or other bridges to transplantation) to help keep people alive while they await heart transplant or as a replacement intervention for transplantation.

The Cardiac Client and Surgery

Postsurgical complications following cardiac surgery can include myocardial injury, blood loss, superficial incisional infections, AF, pneumonia, cognitive impairments, brachial plexus injuries, and subxiphoid incisional hernias. Complications associated with a cardiopulmonary bypass machine can include AF, altered cognition and/or memory associated with systemic inflammation, cerebral hypoperfusion, atheromatous debris, and microemboli (e.g., platelet aggregates, red blood cell fragments, air bubbles).[83]

Persons with previously diagnosed cardiac disease undergoing general or orthopedic surgery are at risk for additional postoperative complications. Anesthesia and surgery are often associated with marked fluctuations of heart rate and blood pressure, changes in intravascular volume, myocardial ischemia or depression, arrhythmias, decreased oxygenation, and increased sympathetic nervous system activity. In addition, changes in medications, surgical trauma, wound healing, infection, hemorrhage, and pulmonary insufficiency may overwhelm the diseased heart. All these factors place an additional stress on the cardiac client during the perioperative period.

Cardiac surgery via traditional median sternotomy requires a longitudinal incision and disruption of the sternum. During the operative procedure, the bone is rewired with stainless steel wire and fixed with low separation strength and security of closure approximately 5% of normal (this increases to 90% of normal strength at 6 weeks for most people).[295]

Complications following a sternotomy include mediastinitis, poor wound healing, chronic pain, posttraumatic stress disorder, and, more rarely, brachial plexus injury. Risk factors for these complications may include obesity, osteoporosis, diabetes or other comorbidities, large breasts in women (the weight of both breasts puts additional traction on sutures), and client noncompliance or poor compliance.

Less invasive means of performing cardiac surgery are now possible with advances in technology, especially videoscopic visualization and the ability to provide myocardial protection. More and more surgeons are using minimally invasive techniques such as a partial upper sternotomy or small right thoracotomy instead of the traditional median sternotomy in hopes of reducing operative stress, postoperative pain, and postoperative recovery time.

A minithoracotomy or "keyhole" thoracotomy via a small incision allows surgeons to operate on a beating heart. These alternative surgical techniques involve passing instruments through small incisions in the skin and muscle and between the ribs. Surgeons can suture bypass vessels around blocked coronary arteries without shutting down the heart and rerouting the blood through a bypass machine.

Cardiac transplantation procedures are described in Chapter 21.

SPECIAL IMPLICATIONS FOR THE THERAPIST   12-26

The Cardiac Client and Surgery
Noncardiac Surgery

Therapy for people with CVD undergoing noncardiac (orthopedic, neurosurgery) surgery is only altered by the need for more deliberate and careful monitoring of the person's response to activity and exercise. Comprehensive guidelines for perioperative and postoperative care for such patients are available.[11]

Postoperative rehabilitation may take longer because of the underlying cardiac condition and any complications that may arise as a result of cardiovascular compromise. Careful observation for DVT must be ongoing during the first 1 to 3 weeks postoperatively. Anyone with polycythemia or thrombocytopenia is at increased risk for hemorrhage, necessitating additional special precautions (see Chapter 14).

Physical therapy initiated in the intensive care unit focuses on restoring mobility, increasing strength, and improving balance and reflexes; heel slides, ankle pumps, and bedside standing are included in the early postoperative protocol. Airway clearance techniques (formerly, chest physical therapy, pulmonary physical therapy, pulmonary hygiene) and breathing exercises are essential to prevent atelectasis (particularly left lower lobe atelectasis), especially in the case of implantation of an artificial heart, because of the location of the device. Frequent, slow, rhythmic reaching, turning, bending, and stretching of the trunk and all extremities many times throughout the day help alleviate the surgical pain-tension cycle and facilitate pulmonary function.

Cardiac Surgery

(See also discussion of "Postoperative Considerations" in "Special Implications for the Therapist 12-2: Ischemic Heart Disease, Coronary Heart Disease, Coronary Artery Disease" above).

Individuals undergoing cardiothoracic procedures have some unique challenges to overcome. The damaged heart is subjected to the stress of paralysis and reinitiation of function when cardiopulmonary bypass is part of the procedure. Trauma from the cardiac event, combined with trauma from the cardiac surgery, alter the heart's ability to resume a normal working load immediately after surgery. Physical activity must be titrated or applied in a dosing fashion to load the heart according to each individual's hemostatic status and tolerance.

Progressive ambulation can be initiated as soon as the client can transfer. In the case of open heart surgery, sternal precautions are standard postoperative orders (see Box 12-3; see also "Special Implications for the Therapist 12-2: Ischemic Heart Disease, Coronary Heart Disease, Coronary Artery Disease" above and "Special Implications for the Therapist 21-4: Heart Transplantation" in Chapter 21).

When the client can ambulate 1000 feet, the treadmill (1 mile/hr) or exercise cycle (0.5 rate of perceived exertion) can be used (see Table 12-13), usually around the fourth postoperative day if there are no complications. Whether to use the treadmill or bicycle is generally an individual decision made by the client based on personal preference; presence of orthopedic problems must be taken into consideration.

Chest (and in women, breast) discomfort, shortness of breath, upper quadrant myalgia (chest, arms, neck, upper back), palpitations, low activity tolerance, mood swings, and localized swelling in the case of grafts taken from the leg are all commonly reported in the early days and weeks after cardiac surgery. These clinical manifestations are minimized but not completely eliminated with the less invasive keyhole (minithoracotomy) surgery performed in some facilities.

Exercise

The use of lower-extremity–derived aerobic exercise to improve hemodynamics, normalize heart rate, improve oxygen uptake and delivery, and decrease diastolic blood pressure has been well documented and discussed earlier in this chapter. Many of these individuals have not exercised in years and demonstrate balance deficits, deconditioning, significant endurance limits (fatigue), and/or are fearful of exercise. Those who walk into their scheduled surgery may not have endurance limits from longstanding disease so exercise and physical activity recommendations are less limited.

The therapist must firmly encourage active participation in a program of physical activity and exercise for anyone who has given up and chosen to remain sedentary.

Exercise tolerance must be monitored closely during the early weeks after surgery. Periodic and multiple episodes of mobility and activity is advised until a moderate to somewhat hard level of exertion is reached (e.g., 12-14 on the Rate of Perceived Exertion scale or 4 out of 10 on the modified Borg scale). For all cardiac patients, the therapist is encouraged to use perceived exertion scales, such as the dyspnea index or Borg Scale (see Table 12-13), monitor changes in diastolic pressure, and rely on measurements of oxygen uptake to set exercise limits.

In the case of median sternotomy, altered pulmonary function and movement impairments of the chest and abdomen may be present. Posture is important, especially for anyone with a kyphotic posture for any reason. Optimizing capacity and increasing activity intensity depends on an upright posture to enhance rib mobility, chest movement, and lung expansion.

Psychosocial Considerations

Psychologic and emotional recovery from cardiac surgery is not always addressed or discussed. Recent research has documented that cardiac surgery is often accompanied by significant cognitive decline, especially memory loss (verbal and visual) and decline in task planning ability (visuoconstruction) and psychomotor speed.

Additional research is needed to determine if the observed cognitive decline is related to the surgery itself (e.g., effects of anesthesia, hypoperfusion associated with use of the heart-lung bypass machine, disruption of atherosclerotic plaque-forming emboli), normal aging in a population with cardiovascular risk factors, or a combination of these and other factors.[408-410]

Depression is commonly reported after CABG and after cardiac surgery in general. The majority of people who are depressed after cardiac surgery were depressed before surgery. There does not appear to be any correlation between depressed mood and cognitive decline after cardiac surgery, which suggests that depression alone cannot account for the cognitive decline.

Because cardiac surgery is increasingly performed in older adults with more comorbidities, identifying people at risk for adverse neurocognitive outcomes is helpful in protecting them by modifying the surgical procedure or by more effective medical therapy.[298,408-410]

Cardiogenic Shock

Shock is acute, severe circulatory failure associated with a variety of precipitating conditions. Regardless of the cause, shock is associated with marked reduction of blood flow to vital organs, eventually leading to cellular damage and death. See Table 14-1 for categories and causes of shock.

The therapist may see a client in one of three stages of shock. *Stage 1*, compensated hypotension, is characterized by reduced cardiac output that stimulates compensatory mechanisms that alter myocardial function and peripheral resistance. During this stage, the body tries to maintain circulation to vital organs such as the brain and the heart and clinical symptoms are minimal. Blood pressure may remain normotensive.

In *stage 2*, compensatory mechanisms for dealing with the low delivery of nutrients to the body are overwhelmed, and tissue perfusion is decreased. Early signs of cerebral, renal, and myocardial insufficiency are present. Cardiogenic shock (inadequate cardiac function) may result from disorders of the heart muscle, valves, or electrical pacing system. Shock associated with MI or other serious cardiac disease carries a high mortality rate. The therapist is only likely to see this type of client in a coronary care unit setting.

Stage 3 is characterized by severe ischemia with damage to tissues by toxins and antigen–antibody reactions. The kidneys, liver, and lungs are especially susceptible; ischemia of the GI tract allows invasion by bacteria with subsequent infection.

Clinical manifestations of shock may include (in early stages) tachycardia, increased respiratory rate, and distended neck veins. In early septic shock (vascular shock caused by infection), there is hyperdynamic change with increased circulation, so that the skin is warm and flushed and the pulse is bounding rather than weak.

In the second phase of shock (late septic shock) hypoperfusion (reduced blood flow) occurs with cold skin and weak pulses, hypotension (systolic blood pressure of 90 mm Hg or less), mottled extremities with weak or absent peripheral pulses, and collapsed neck veins. This phase is usually irreversible; the client is unresponsive, and cardiovascular collapse eventually occurs. The therapist should be aware that some healthy adults may have blood pressure levels this low without ill effects or with only minor symptoms of orthostatic hypotension when changing positions quickly.

Treatment is directed toward both the manifestations of shock and its cause.

SPECIAL IMPLICATIONS FOR THE THERAPIST 12-27

Cardiogenic Shock

The therapist in an acute care or home health setting may be working with a client who is demonstrating signs and symptoms of impending shock. Careful monitoring of vital signs and clinical observations will alert the therapist to the need for medical intervention (see early signs of shock listed in "The Cardiac Client and Surgery" above). The client in question may demonstrate normal mental status or may become restless, agitated, and confused.

For the acute care therapist, people hospitalized with shock are critically ill and are usually unresponsive. Cardiopulmonary and musculoskeletal function as well as prevention of further complications will be the focus of the therapist. Treatment for the immobile person in shock, which is directed toward positioning, skin care, and pulmonary function, must be short in duration but effective, to avoid fatiguing the person.

The Cardiac Client and Pregnancy

Normal physiologic changes during pregnancy can exacerbate symptoms of underlying cardiac disease, even in previously asymptomatic individuals. The most common cardiovascular complications of pregnancy are peripartum cardiomyopathy, aortic dissection, and pregnancy-related hypertension.

Peripartum cardiomyopathy or cardiomyopathy of pregnancy is discussed briefly earlier in the chapter (see "Cardiomyopathy" above). Pregnancy predisposes to aortic dissection, possibly because of the accompanying connective tissue changes. Dissection usually occurs near term or shortly postpartum in the arteries (including coronary arteries) or the aorta, and special implications are the same as for aneurysm.

The Heart in Collagen Vascular Diseases

Collagen vascular diseases (now more commonly referred to as diffuse connective tissue disease) (Box 12-17) often involve the heart, although cardiac symptoms are usually less prominent than other manifestations of the disease.

Lupus Carditis

SLE is a multisystem clinical illness (see Chapter 7) characterized by an inflammatory process that can target all parts of the heart, including the coronary arteries, pericardium, myocardium, endocardium, conducting system, and valves. Lupus cardiac involvement may include pericarditis, myocarditis, endocarditis, or a combination of the three. Cardiac disease can occur as a direct result of the autoimmune process responsible for SLE or secondary to hypertension, renal failure, hypercholesterolemia (excess serum cholesterol), drug therapy for SLE, and, more rarely, infection (infective carditis).

Pericarditis is the most frequent cardiac lesion associated with SLE, presenting with the characteristic substernal chest pain that varies with posture, becoming worse in recumbency and improving with sitting or bending forward. In some people, pericarditis may be the first manifestation of SLE.

Myocarditis (see also "Myocardial Disease" above) is a serious complication reported to occur in less than 10% of people with SLE. The simultaneous involvement of cardiac and skeletal muscle may occur more commonly than previously suspected. More sensitive diagnostic techniques now make early detection of occult myocarditis possible. Myocarditis in association with SLE occurs

most often as left ventricular dysfunction and conduction abnormalities with varying degrees of heart block.

Lupus *endocarditis* occurs in up to 30% of persons affected by SLE. Major lesions associated with lupus endocarditis include the formation of multiple noninfectious wartlike elevations (verrucae) around or on the surface of the cardiac valves, most commonly the mitral and tricuspid valves. Other types of valvular disease associated with SLE include mitral and aortic regurgitation or stenosis.

Rheumatoid Arthritis

On rare occasions, the heart is involved as a part of rheumatoid arthritis, a chronic, systemic, inflammatory disorder that can affect various organs but predominantly involves synovial tissues of joints (see Chapter 27). When the heart is affected, rheumatoid granulomatous inflammation with fibrinoid necrosis may occur in the pericardium, myocardium, or valves. Involvement of the heart in rheumatoid arthritis does not compromise cardiac function.

Ankylosing Spondylitis

Ankylosing spondylitis is a chronic, progressive inflammatory disorder affecting fibrous tissue primarily in the sacroiliac joints, spine, and large peripheral joints (see Chapter 27). A characteristic aortic valve lesion develops in as many as 10% of persons with longstanding ankylosing spondylitis. The aortic valve ring is dilated, and the valve cusps are scarred and shortened. The functional consequence is aortic regurgitation (see "Aortic Regurgitation [Insufficiency]" above).

Scleroderma

Scleroderma or systemic sclerosis is a rheumatic disease of the connective tissue characterized by hardening of the connective tissue (see Chapter 10). Involvement of the heart in persons with scleroderma is second only to renal disease as a cause of death in scleroderma. The myocardium exhibits intimal sclerosis (hardening) of small arteries, which leads to small infarctions and patchy fibrosis. As a result, CHF and arrhythmia are common. Cor pulmonale may occur secondary to interstitial fibrosis of the lungs, and hypertensive heart disease may occur as a result of renal involvement.

Polyarteritis Nodosa

Polyarteritis refers to a condition of multiple sites of inflammatory and destructive lesions in the arterial system; the lesions consist of small masses of tissue in the form of nodes or projections (nodosum) (see previous discussion of polyarteritis nodosa in this chapter). The heart is involved in up to 75% of cases of polyarteritis nodosa. The necrotizing lesions of branches of the coronary arteries result in MI, arrhythmias, and heart block. Cardiac hypertrophy and failure secondary to renal vascular hypertension occur.

Box 12-17

COLLAGEN VASCULAR DISEASES

- Ankylosing spondylitis
- Dermatomyositis
- Localized (cutaneous) scleroderma
- Mixed connective tissue disease
- Polyarteritis nodosa
- Polymyalgia rheumatica
- Polymyositis
- Rheumatoid arthritis
- Sjögren syndrome
- SLE
- Systemic sclerosis (scleroderma)
- Temporal arteritis

SPECIAL IMPLICATIONS FOR THE THERAPIST **12-28**

Collagen Vascular Diseases

Treatment of the collagen vascular diseases described must take into consideration the possibility of cardiac involvement. The physician has usually diagnosed concomitant cardiac disease, but complete health care records are not available to the therapist. If the therapist identifies signs or symptoms of cardiac origin, the client may be able to confirm previous diagnosis of the condition. In such cases, careful monitoring may be all that is required. However, the alert therapist may be the first health care provider to identify signs or symptoms of underlying dysfunction during onset, necessitating medical referral. (See each collagen vascular disease for discussion of individual implications.)

Cardiac Complications of Cancer and Cancer Treatment[310,413]

Many treatments for cancers are also known to be cardiotoxic. People with cancer experience all the usual cardiac problems that occur in the general population in addition to complications of cancer and its therapy. Tumor masses can cause compression of the heart and great vessels resulting in pericardial effusions and tamponade. Certain tumors can cause arrhythmias and may secrete mediators that are directly toxic to the heart. Pericardial effusions and tamponade can follow surgery, radiation, or chemotherapy.

Cardiac toxicity may occur following chest irradiation, especially when combined with the administration of many chemotherapeutic agents. Chest radiation for any type of cancer (e.g., Hodgkin disease, non-Hodgkin lymphoma, esophageal cancer, lung cancer, breast cancer) exposes the heart (and lungs) to varying degrees and doses of radiation. Previous mediastinal radiation and increasing cumulative doses of chemotherapy or irradiation are known risk factors for the development of cardiotoxicity.

Radiation exposure can cause considerable scarring within the subendocardial adipose tissue, endocardial thickening, and interstitial fibrosis.[388] Collectively, the latter three defects would make the heart less capable of expanding during systole. Pericardial effusion is the most common manifestation of radiation heart disease, but coronary arteries are known to become fibrotic and undergo luminal narrowing, resulting in hypertension, angina, and MI.

Adriamycin (doxorubicin) was identified as being cardiotoxic during the early drug trials in the 1970s, but it took 5 to 6 years of actual use for the full extent of cardiac damage to become obvious. Today, cumulative doses of doxorubicin are limited to approximately 500 mg/m^2 because the drug can cause fatal CHF in doses above this amount.[413,421] Often these effects are not seen until years or decades after treatment with the drug has been completed. Many other chemotherapeutic agents are cardiotoxic, but not to the extent of doxorubicin, and these effects tend be more acute than chronic.[494]

Chemotherapy agents may prompt acute and chronic heart failure (e.g., anthracycline antibiotics, including doxorubicin, mitoxantrone, and doxorubicin, combined with paclitaxel used in the treatment of breast cancer)[355] or coronary spasm leading to angina, MI, arrhythmias, or sudden death (e.g., 5-fluorouracil). Anthracycline effects on the heart reduce exercise tolerance. Endocarditis also

occurs in cancer clients with vascular access devices and immune compromise.

Recombinant DNA technology has resulted in the development of biologic response modifiers, including the interferons, interleukins, and tumor necrosis factor, which also have some adverse cardiovascular effects. Hypotension and tachycardia are the most common problems, although there have been some reports of myocardial ischemia and infarction. These adverse effects appear to be caused by significant alterations in fluid balance rather than any dysrhythmic or cardiotoxic properties of the drugs. Fortunately, many of the cardiac complications associated with chemotherapeutic agents and biologic response modifiers are transient and reversible.[206]

The most common manifestations of cardiotoxicity are cardiac arrhythmias or acute or chronic pericarditis. Other cardiac problems that may develop include blood pressure changes, thrombosis, ECG changes, myocardial fibrosis with a resultant restrictive cardiomyopathy, conduction disturbances, CHF, accelerated and radiation-induced CAD, and valvular dysfunction. These may occur during or shortly after treatment or within days or weeks after treatment; or they may not be apparent until months and sometimes years after completion of chemotherapy.[341]

Chemotherapy induced cardiotoxicity develops on average in 28% to 36% of cancer patients.[413] (See Chapter 5 for further discussion.) A number of risk factors may predispose someone to cardiotoxicity, including total daily dose, increasing cumulative dose, schedule of administration, concurrent administration of cardiotoxic agents, prior chemotherapy, mediastinal radiation, age (younger than 18 years or older than 70 years), female gender, history of preexisting cardiovascular disorders or other comorbidities such as diabetes, and presence of electrolyte imbalances (e.g., hypokalemia, hypomagnesemia).[341]

Early detection of cardiotoxicity in cancer treatment is essential as it allows to identify individuals who need to be protected with heart medications in order to continue the cancer treatment or to seek alternative therapies.[400] The American Society of Echocardiography has issued recommendations to use echocardiography in clinical trials to assess cardiotoxicity in cancer patients after chemotherapy and radiation.[25]

SPECIAL IMPLICATIONS FOR THE THERAPIST   12-29

Cardiac Complications of Cancer Treatment

Any client referred to therapy who has completed oncologic treatment should be assessed for potential cardiac (and pulmonary) dysfunction, including questions about previous and current activity levels, evaluation of exercise tolerance or endurance, monitoring of heart rate and rhythm, blood pressure, and respiratory responses.

Any symptoms of exercise intolerance (shortness of breath, light-headedness or dizziness, fatigue, pallor, palpitations, chest pain or discomfort) must be noted. (See also "Special Implications for the

Therapist 12-10: Cardiomyopathy" and "Special Implications for the Therapist 12-16: Pericarditis" above.)

Clients may be asymptomatic, with the only manifestation being ECG changes. Ideally, the oncology and cardiac team will recommend continuous cardiac monitoring with baseline and regular ECG and echocardiographic studies and measurement of serum electrolytes and cardiac enzymes for those individuals with risk factors or a history of cardiotoxicity.

Specific exercise guidelines have also been outlined for the inclusion of gradual endurance training as a part of the treatment plan for anyone with cardiotoxicity secondary to oncologic treatment.[465] (See also "Radiation Injuries" in Chapter 5 and "Cancer and Exercise" in Chapter 9.)

Cardiotoxicity can be prevented by screening and modifying risk factors, aggressively monitoring for signs and symptoms as chemotherapy is administered, and continuing follow-up after completion of a course or the entire treatment. Cardioprotective agents are being developed with approval by the FDA, such as dexrazoxane for anthracycline chemotherapy.[341]

REFERENCES

To enhance this text and add value for the reader, all references are included on the companion Evolve site that accompanies this textbook. The reader can view the reference source and access it online whenever possible.

CHAPTER 13

The Lymphatic System

BONNIE LASINSKI

The lymphatic system develops embryologically from the venous system. Two major theories exist of the embryologic origin of the lymphatic system: the *centrifugal*, or venous budding, theory and the *centripetal* theory. The centrifugal theory states that the lymphatic endothelium develops from the venous endothelium; the centripetal theory states that both systems (venous and lymphatic) develop from undifferentiated (stem type) mesenchymal cells. Advances in lymphangiogenesis research may clarify which theory is correct; this information will have a great impact on genetic research and the eventual molecular treatment of lymphangiodysplasias.[156]

The interstitial fluid that remains after the extracellular fluid is resorbed via the veins is taken up by the initial lymphatic vessels, into larger collecting vessels, into lymphatic trunks, and back into the right side of the heart via the lymphatic ducts that empty into the subclavian veins in the neck. This is a regional system that moves fluid from the periphery to the central circulation. It is designed to help maintain fluid balance in the tissues, fight infection, and assist in the removal of cellular debris and waste products from the extracellular spaces. In many ways, it functions like the "sanitation" system of a major city. It is largely ignored and goes unnoticed until it is disrupted and the "garbage" (in the form of lymphedema) piles up. This drainage system is separate from the general circulatory system but is the conduit for returning tissue fluids to the circulatory system.[55,151]

The cardiovascular system is a one-cycle system of vessels with a pump (the heart) to move the fluid (blood) through arteries, capillaries, and cells and then back to the heart via the veins. Fluid that leaves the arterial side of the capillary bed in a process called *ultrafiltration* nourishes the tissues and cells.

Of the fluid volume that perfuses the tissues, up to 90% reenters the circulation via the venous capillary network (*reabsorption*) because of differences in concentration of fluid and protein in the tissues and in the venous end of the capillary network. The remaining volume of extracellular tissue fluid (this can be greater than 10% depending on circumstances) and plasma proteins in the interstitial spaces must be returned to the heart via the lymphatic system.[86]

Most protein molecule diameters are too large to pass through openings in the endothelium of the venous capillaries. A small amount of protein, if broken down into smaller molecules by macrophages, can pass through the open junctions in the venous endothelium. However, the majority of extracellular protein must be transported via the lymphatic system.

The lymphatic system is a pressure-driven system based on the principles of osmotic diuresis. If the normal lymphatic transport mechanisms are disrupted (e.g., by scar tissue or reduced muscle pumping), significant accumulations of water and protein can remain in the tissue spaces, resulting in latent, acute, or chronic lymphedema. This protein is a result of cellular metabolism and is not related to protein ingested from food.

The dynamics of fluid exchange in the tissues are controlled by the microcirculation unit consisting of the arterial and venous capillaries, the tissue channels, the proteolytic cells (macrophages) in the tissues, and the initial lymphatics (see the description of initial lymphatics in "Anatomy and Physiology of the Lymphatic System" below).

MICROCIRCULATION UNIT: PRINCIPLES OF FLUID DYNAMICS AND EXCHANGE

Starling's Hypothesis

A brief discussion of Starling's theory of fluid dynamics is helpful to understand the microcirculation unit. In 1897, Starling proposed the mechanism governing fluid flow out of the blood capillaries into the tissues and back into the capillaries again. There are four pressures that are important in the Starling Law: (1) *plasma hydrostatic pressure*, the pressure inside the capillaries that decreases as fluid passes from the arterial to the venous side of the capillary loop; (2) *tissue hydrostatic pressure*, the pressure of fluid in the tissue channels (usually negative or less than atmospheric pressure) that tends to pull fluid from the capillaries into the tissues*; (3) *plasma colloidal osmotic pressure*, caused by plasma proteins, this pressure creates a siphon effect and pulls fluid into the capillaries; and (4) *tissue colloidal osmotic pressure*, the pressure caused by plasma proteins in the tissues that causes a net movement of fluid into the tissues. All of these pressure

---

*However, in edema, it can become positive and tend to keep fluid out of the tissues. This is the one "safety factor" that controls lymphedema (i.e., the fibrous tissue actually helps to increase tissue hydrostatic pressure and control the size of the limb to some extent).

systems determine how much fluid moves and where it moves within the body.

Fluid Dynamics

The laws of basic fluid dynamics dictate that fluid flows from an area of high pressure to an area of lower pressure until equilibrium is reached. The Starling Law simplified means that fluid at the arterial end of the capillary will tend to flow into the tissue spaces because plasma (blood) hydrostatic pressure is higher at the arterial end compared with the tissue hydrostatic pressure of the tissues.

If all else is "normal," when the fluid reaches the venous side of the capillary, the plasma hydrostatic pressure will be lower than the plasma colloid (protein) osmotic pressure, and the fluid will be forced back into the venous side of the capillary, which accounts for up to approximately 90% of the fluid on the venous end of the capillary.

Ten percent (or more) of net ultrafiltrate must return to the central circulation via the lymphatics. If all is normal there, the initial lymphatics will take up that fluid, move it to the collecting lymphatics and larger lymphatic trunks, through regional lymph nodes, and eventually into the right lymphatic duct or the thoracic duct, and back into the vena cava (see Fig. 13-8).

Although 10% (or more) of the total fluid volume seems small, it can amount to 2 to 8 L/day, a large proportion of which can be absorbed by small vessels in the lymph nodes. This revision of the basic Starling principle assigns the lymphatic system a greater role in maintaining fluid balance.[85,86]

In the presence of lymphatic dysfunction, some part or all of the 10% of fluid volume and the proteins will remain trapped in the tissue spaces and cause lymphedema. With lymphedema, the challenge for the therapist is to effectively move that fluid back into functioning lymphatics and then into the central circulation. This model is a very gross simplification but can be helpful in understanding the basics of fluid dynamics in the capillary loop. Many other factors affect the tissues in addition to those mentioned previously.[27,86,154]

ANATOMY AND PHYSIOLOGY OF THE LYMPHATIC SYSTEM

The lymphatic system is composed of superficial and deep lymph vessels and nodes. Other lymphatic organs and tissues include the thymus, bone marrow, spleen, tonsils, and Peyer patches of the small intestine. These perform important immune functions discussed in Chapter 7. Superficial vessels rely on an interaction of oncotic and hydrostatic pressures, muscle contraction, arterial pulsation, and gentle movement of the skin to move lymph fluid, whereas the deeper vessels, which generally parallel the venous system, contain smooth muscle and valves and help prevent backflow.[26,81]

Lymph Vessels

The lymphatic vessel network is an intricate one-way vessel system that serves to drain the excess tissue fluid volume and plasma proteins that remain in the interstitium after normal capillary perfusion/filtration has taken place and return it to the central circulation via the large veins in the neck. All lymph fluid eventually passes through lymph nodes before emptying into the right lymphatic duct and the thoracic duct. The fluid is then returned to the bloodstream via the left and right subclavian veins.[55,81,151]

The anatomy of the lymphatic vessel system can be compared in some ways to the vein system on the leaves and stems of trees. The smallest vessels, or veins, are at the periphery of the tissues (leaves), and the diameter of these vessels gradually increases in the stem of the leaf as the system progresses into larger and larger vessels (corresponding to deeper tissues) and continues to progress to larger stems and branches of the tree until the trunk is reached.

Initial Lymphatics

The smallest of lymphatic vessels (diameter 20-40 µm), called *lymphatic capillaries* or *precollectors*, begin as blind-ended sacs of endothelium just under the epidermis.[26,46,55] These are referred to as the *initial lymphatics* and are in close proximity with the venous and arterial capillaries (Fig. 13-1).

The vessel walls of these initial lymphatics are 1 cell thick, formed by overlapping endothelial cells with many loose junctions between cells opening and closing (Fig. 13-2). This action allows for movement of water and proteins into the vessel and prevents the escape of protein into the interstitium during the compression of the initial lymphatics.

These cells are also in direct contact with the microfilaments of the surrounding connective tissues. They are connected to the tissue matrix by anchoring filaments that act as "guidewires" to pull the cell junctions open when the tissue pressure rises as a result of increased extracellular fluid volume (Fig. 13-3).[26,81] These vessels are arranged in a mesh-like plexus; for every square millimeter of tissue, 7 mm of lymphatics are available to drain it.[26]

The initial lymphatics function as force-pumps powered by variations in total tissue pressure caused by movement, muscular contraction, respiration, and variations in external pressure caused by massage, gravity, change in position, and other similar factors. Without changes in total tissue pressure, these force-pumps cannot function, and fluid will accumulate in the interstitium, leading to edema.

Lymph Vessel Network

Deeper in the dermis are *precollectors* (Fig. 13-4), which flow into *collecting lymphatics* located in the subcutaneous tissue (Fig. 13-5). The true collecting vessels have valves to prevent backflow and some muscle tissue in their walls to further enhance their pumping action.[26,154] Extrinsic muscle contraction or lymphatic drainage massage also increases this pumping action.

Collecting lymphatics do not form a plexus, but there can be connections between them. Their diameter gradually increases in size to form the *lymph trunks*, which lie near the deep fascia. Each segment of collecting lymphatic vessels between valves is called a *lymphangion* (Fig. 13-6). The muscle in the collecting lymphatic walls contracts

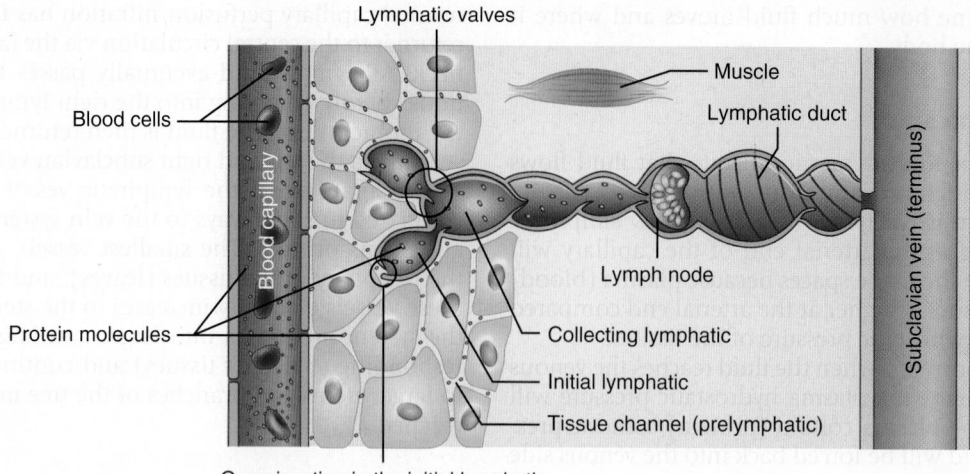

Figure 13-1

Anatomy of the lymphatic vessel system (schematic). This diagram shows the passage of protein *(dots)* in normal tissue from the blood capillary, through the tissue channels, into and through the lymphatic system, back to the venous system, and eventually emptying into the subclavian vein. Terminology has changed over the years; the reader should be aware that initial lymphatic and lymphatic capillary refer to the same structure. Note that the protein molecules are not on the venous side of the diagram because for the most part, these molecules are too large to pass through the openings in the venous endothelium. Also note that this is a schematic diagram and not drawn to scale; the lymphatic duct depicted emptying into the venous system (subclavian vein) is much deeper (under the fascia) than this two-dimensional illustration can portray. Various malfunctions are illustrated in Figure 13-15. (From Casley-Smith JR, Casley-Smith JR: *Modern treatment for lymphoedema,* ed 5, Adelaide, Australia, 1997, Lymphoedema Association of Australia.)

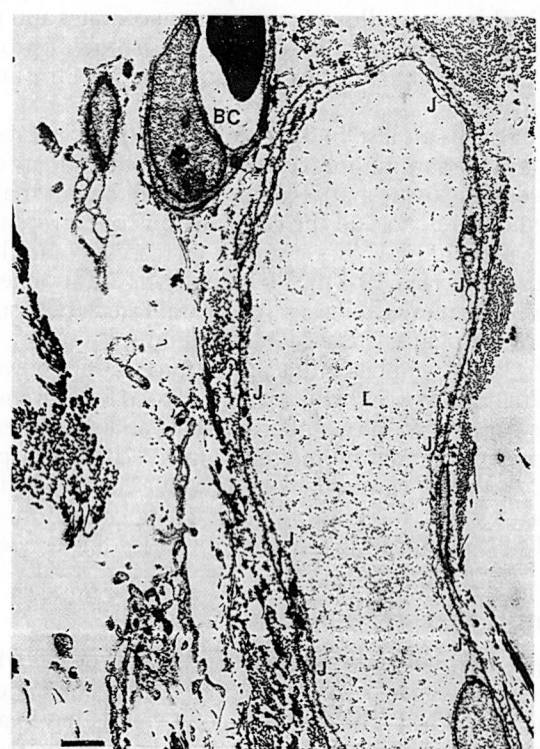

Figure 13-2

An initial lymphatic *(L)* **in a quiescent (at rest or inactive) tissue.** Many closed (narrow or tight) junctions *(J)* are evident. A blood capillary *(BC)* is shown for comparison of size, endothelial opacity, and other characteristics. The bar at the lower left (1 µm) is provided to give the viewer size perspective. (From Casley-Smith JR, Casley-Smith JR: *Modern treatment for lymphoedema,* ed 5, Adelaide, Australia, 1997, Lymphoedema Association of Australia. Modified from Casely-Smith JR: Endothelial permeability. II. The passage of particles through the lymphatic endothelium of normal and injured ears. *Br J Exp Pathol* 46:35-49, 1965.)

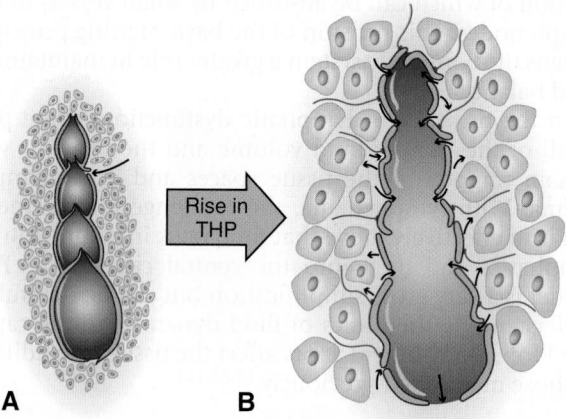

Figure 13-3

Effects of elevated tissue hydrostatic pressure *(THP)* on initial lymphatic functioning. A, Normal lymphatic vessel at a fairly low THP and normal lymphatic drainage. **B,** Tissue response to a tremendous increase in THP (represented by the *large arrow*). The swelling in the interstitial tissues pulls on the anchoring filaments, pulling and holding open the initial lymphatic endothelial junctions *(thin arrows* pointing outward), allowing fluid to pour into the initial lymphatic in an attempt to reduce edema. In this way, in place of a few widely open junctions, there are many slightly open ones, through which fluid is forced *(thicker arrows* directed inward) down a hydrostatic pressure gradient. (From Casley-Smith JR, Casley-Smith JR: *Modern treatment for lymphoedema,* ed 5, Adelaide, Australia, 1997, Lymphoedema Association of Australia.)

rhythmically. Smooth muscle cells around the endothelial cell layer face the lumen of the vessel. These are innervated by the autonomic nervous system and contract on the average of 5 to 10 times per minute.[157] This "lymphangiomotoricity" combines with the contraction of the lymphangion itself, which is triggered by distention of the vessel wall.

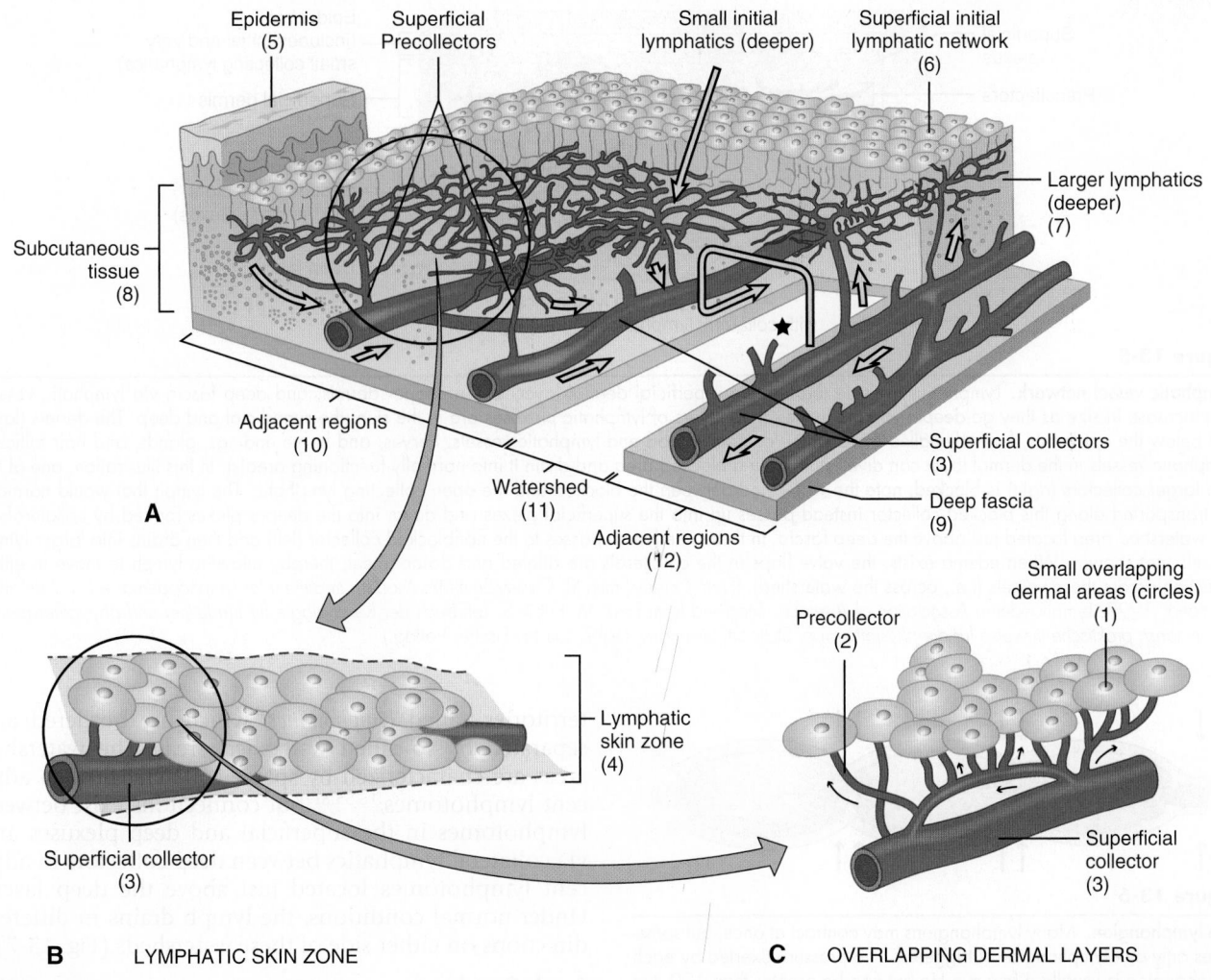

Figure 13-4

Overview of the lymphatic drainage system. A, Overview of the lymphatic drainage paths from a skin region. The epidermis *(5)* is superficial to a superficial initial lymphatic network *(6)*, which sends blindly ending vessels into the dermis and which is linked to the deep dermal plexus of larger initial lymphatics *(7)*, in the subcutaneous tissue *(8)*, by many connections. The superficial collecting lymphatics *(3)*, which discharge into the larger ones (not shown), lie next to the deep fascia *(9)*. A watershed *(11)* lies between two adjacent regions *(10* and *12)*, which drain in opposite directions *(medium arrows)*. One of these is obstructed *(red vessels)*. The deep and superficial initial lymphatic plexuses overlap across this watershed. These groups of cross-connections provide collateral drainage and are enlarged by manual massage. The large, *U-shaped arrow (*)* shows this path. **B,** Lymphatic skin zone *(4)* that extends along the length of a superficial collector *(3)*. Certain areas of the skin drain into a specific superficial collector, which accounts for the clinical observation of lymphedema in portions of an extremity (e.g., pockets of extra swelling or asymmetric edema). When a specific superficial collector is blocked (or if the deep collector into which it drains is blocked), the result is edema at that site. **C,** Small overlapping dermal areas *(1, circles)*, which drain into networks of initial lymphatics (not shown), which drain into small collecting lymphatics called precollectors *(2)* and then to larger superficial collectors *(3)*. (From Casley-Smith JR, Casley-Smith JR: *Modern treatment for lymphoedema*, ed 5, Adelaide, Australia, 1997, Lymphoedema Association of Australia. Modified from Földi M, Kubik S: *Lehrbuch der lymphologie fur mediziner und physiotherapeuter mit anhang: praktische linweise fur die physiotherape*, Stuttgart, Germany, 1989, Gustav Fischer Verlag.)

The greater the stretch the greater the force of the contraction. If many lymphangions contract at once and outflow is obstructed (e.g., by scarred or radiated lymph nodal areas), pressure inside the vessel can reach 100 mm Hg or more.

High intravascular pressure fatigues the muscle wall, leading to ineffective smooth muscle contraction and, ultimately, to vessel failure. The walls dilate, preventing closure of valve flaps, and a backflow of lymph distal to the site of obstruction occurs, causing lymphedema. This is one plausible explanation for the fact that many individuals with a "limb at risk" develop lymphedema months or even years after their original surgery. For a time, the remaining lymphatics function marginally without evidence of clinical lymphedema, but these units become overtaxed, eventually the walls fatigue, and latent lymphedema progresses to acute and then to chronic lymphedema.

The lymph trunks in the extremities join into the larger lymph vessels of the trunk, which join to form the *thoracic duct* and the *right lymphatic duct* that pump the lymph into the central circulation at the left and right subclavian veins in the root of the neck. The lymphatic vessels are embedded in fatty tissue and accompany the chains of lymph nodes along the blood vessels.[46] This explains why injury to blood vessels in an area implies injury to lymphatic vessels in that area, too, regardless of whether it is "unexpected" or "controlled" trauma, as in surgery.

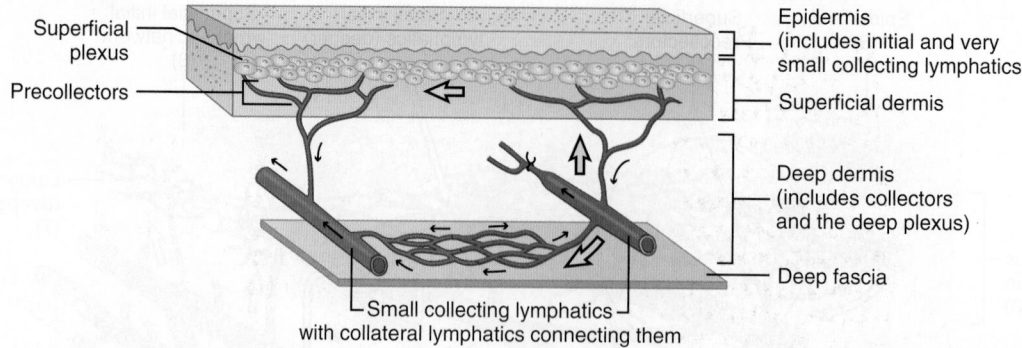

Figure 13-5

Lymphatic vessel network. Lymphatics traverse through the superficial dermal layer, to the deeper dermis, and deep fascia via lymphatic vessels that increase in size as they go deeper into the tissues. Two layers of lymphatic plexuses are in the skin: the superficial and deep. The dermis (layer just below the epidermis, formerly called the corium), contains blood and lymphatic vessels, nerves, and nerve endings, glands, and hair follicles. Lymphatic vessels in the dermal layer can divert fluid from a blocked area and drain it into normally functioning area(s). In this illustration, one of the two larger collectors (right) is blocked; note the watershed between the blocked and the open collecting lymphatic. The lymph that would normally be transported along this blocked collector instead passes up into the superficial plexus and down into the deeper plexus formed by collaterals in the watershed area located just above the deep fascia. In these, the lymph passes to the nonblocked collector (left) and then drains into larger lymph vessels (not shown). When edema exists, the valve flaps in the collaterals are dilated and do not meet, thereby allowing lymph to move in either direction across these vessels (i.e., across the watershed). (From Casley-Smith JR, Casley-Smith JR: *Modern treatment for lymphoedema*, ed 5, Adelaide, Australia, 1997, Lymphoedema Association of Australia. Modified from Földi M, Kubik S: *Lehrbuch der lymphologie fur mediziner und physiotherapeuter mit anhang: praktische linweise fur die physiotherape*, Stuttgart, Germany 1989, Gustav Fischer Verlag.)

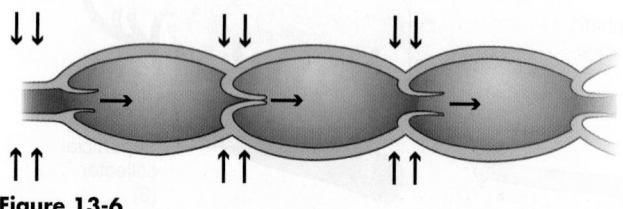

Figure 13-6

The lymphangion. Many lymphangions may contract at once, but sometimes only one lymphangion is triggered. The pressure exerted by each lymphangion is usually a few mm Hg but can be greater than 100 mm Hg if outflow is obstructed and many units are contracting at once. Contraction is triggered by distention (i.e., greater filling creates greater force) but can be modified by humoral (including medications) and nervous factors. Pumping is greatly aided by varying total tissue pressure (e.g., from adjacent muscles, respiration, or manual lymphatic drainage), as previously mentioned in the text. (From Casley-Smith JR, Casley-Smith JR: *Modern treatment for lymphoedema*, ed 5, Adelaide, Australia, 1997, Lymphoedema Association of Australia.)

As lymph flows from the periphery to the root of the limbs to the center of the body, it passes through many *lymph nodes*, which act as filters to cleanse the lymph of waste products and cellular debris. Vessels distal to nodes are called *afferent lymph vessels*. Vessels leaving lymph nodes for more proximal points are called *efferent lymph vessels.*

Lymph nodes also produce lymphocytes and macrophages, which are critical for immune function; destroy foreign bacteria, harmful viruses, and cancer cells; and filter waste products. Lymph nodes offer 100 times the normal resistance to flow of lymph within the lymphatic vessels themselves, which explains why they are often the sites of obstruction in lymphatic dysfunction.[26,54,55,154]

Lymphatic Territories and Watersheds

The anatomy of the lymphatic system is a regional one. The body is divided into a series of lymph drainage territories called *lymphotomes*, which are bordered and separated by so-called watershed areas. The watershed areas are characterized by sparse collateral flow to adjacent lymphotomes,[18,55,81] but connections exist between lymphotomes in the superficial and deep plexuses and via collateral lymphatics between deep collectors in adjacent lymphotomes located just above the deep fascia. Under normal conditions, the lymph drains in different directions on either side of these watersheds (Fig. 13-7).

Trunk Quadrants

The trunk can be divided into four quadrants: the left and right thoracic lymphotomes and the left and right abdominal lymphotomes. The left and right thoracic lymphotomes drain into the ipsilateral axilla, as do the left and right upper extremities. Some individuals possess an auxiliary drainage pathway from the lateral aspect of the upper arm called the *deltoid-pectoral* or *cephalic chain*. This pathway drains directly into the ipsilateral subclavian nodal area, bypassing the axilla entirely. If present, an individual may be less likely to develop upper-extremity lymphedema secondary to axillary disruption (surgical or by radiation), as this pathway may provide sufficient lymph transport capacity for the upper extremity. This pathway can be disrupted by supraclavicular radiation therapy sometimes used to treat recurrent cancer of the chest wall.[82]

The left and right abdominal lymphotomes drain into the left and right superficial inguinal nodes, respectively. Each leg and corresponding half of the lumbar, gluteal, and genital region drains to the ipsilateral superficial inguinal nodes. From there, fluid drains into the deep inguinal, pelvic, and abdominal nodes, into the cisterna chyli, the thoracic duct, and to the left subclavian vein (Fig. 13-8).[55] Most of the lower leg drains via the femoral trunks, which run on the anterior thigh to the inguinal nodes, also draining the medial and lateral thigh

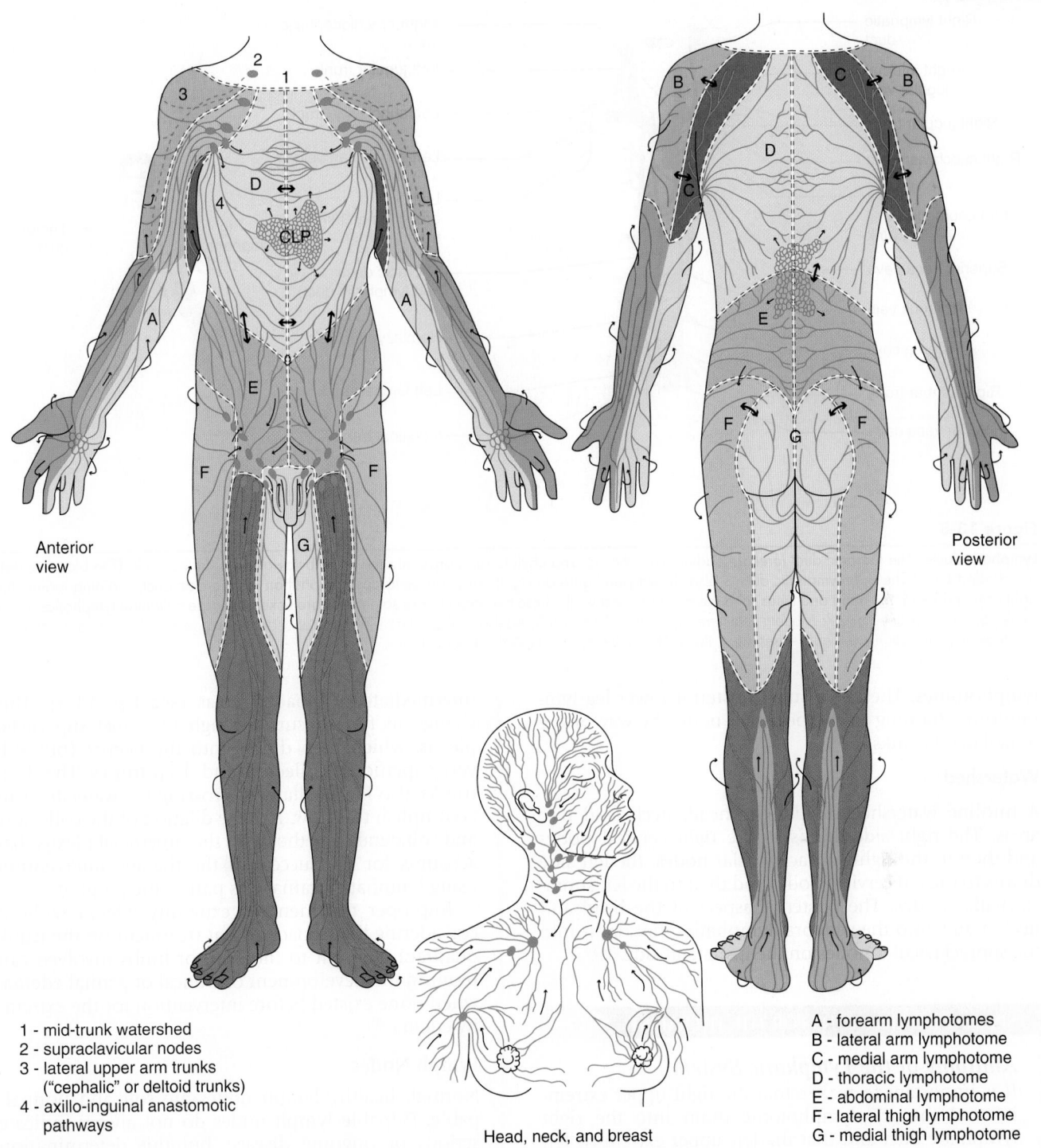

1 - mid-trunk watershed
2 - supraclavicular nodes
3 - lateral upper arm trunks
    ("cephalic" or deltoid trunks)
4 - axillo-inguinal anastomotic
    pathways

Anterior view

Posterior view

Head, neck, and breast

A - forearm lymphotomes
B - lateral arm lymphotome
C - medial arm lymphotome
D - thoracic lymphotome
E - abdominal lymphotome
F - lateral thigh lymphotome
G - medial thigh lymphotome

Figure 13-7

Regional lymphatic system. The dermal and subcutaneous lymph territories (lymphotomes are indicated by different shadings) of the lymphatic system are separated by watersheds (marked by = = = =). *Arrows* indicate the direction of the lymph flow. Normal drainage is away from the watershed, but collaterals cross the watershed *(thick double arrows)*. When the main drainage paths from each of these regions are blocked, lymph *(thick single arrows)* has to be carried across the watersheds via collaterals and the plexuses. The cutaneous lymphatic plexus *(CLP)* is shown in the center of the chest only. It is filled from the tissues and covers the entire body; this is not shown to avoid confusion. These initial lymphatics fill superficial collectors, which drain into deep ones and then into the lymphatic trunks *(small arrows)*. The lymphotome of the external genitals and perineum is shown but unlabeled. (From Casley-Smith JR, Casley-Smith JR: *Modern treatment for lymphoedema*, ed 5, Adelaide, Australia, 1997, Lymphoedema Association of Australia. Modified from Földi M, Kubik S: *Lehrbuch der lymphologie fur mediziner und physiotherapeuter mit anhang: praktische linweise fur die physiotherapie*, Stuttgart, Germany, 1989, Gustav Fischer Verlag.)

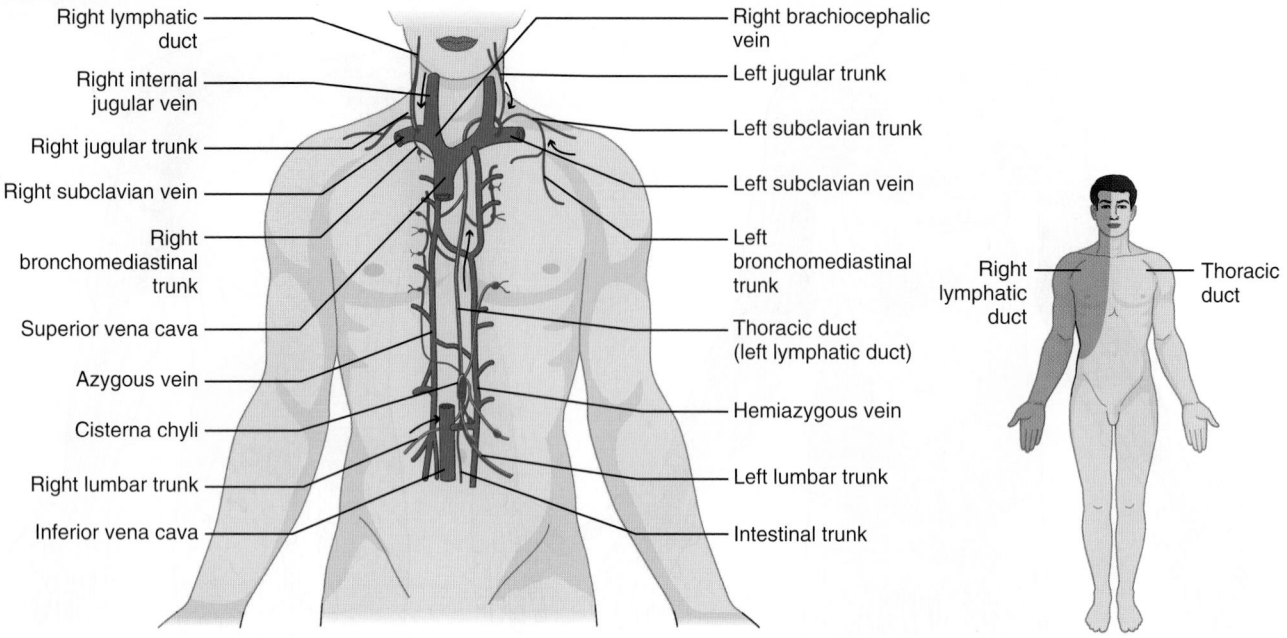

Figure 13-8

Lymphatic ducts. The thoracic duct *(green),* leading from the cisterna chyli to discharge into the left subclavian vein, in the neck. (The blood vessels are shaded *blue.*) The right lymphatic duct is also shown (see figure on right). This carries far less lymph than the thoracic duct, draining mainly the right arm and head, the heart and lungs, and the anterior chest wall. These two main trunks sometimes are linked by large collateral lymphatics. (From Casley-Smith JR, Casley-Smith JR: *Modern treatment for lymphoedema,* ed 5, Adelaide, Australia, 1997, Lymphoedema Association of Australia. *Inset,* Jarvis C: *Physical examination and health assessment,* ed 6, Philadelphia, 2011, WB Saunders.)

lymphotomes. There is a small posterior lower leg lymphotome draining to the popliteal nodes by way of the dorsolateral trunks.

Watersheds

A midline watershed divides the head, neck, and face areas. The right side drains to the right cervical nodes and then to the right supraclavicular nodes; the left side drains to the left cervical nodes and then to the left supraclavicular nodes. The posterior aspect of the head and neck drains into the vertebral lymphatics that drain into the supraclavicular nodes on the ipsilateral side.[26,55]

SPECIAL IMPLICATIONS FOR THE THERAPIST 13-1

Anatomy of the Lymphatic System
It is important to realize that the right upper extremity and thoracic lymphotome drain into the right lymphatic duct and that the left upper extremity, left thoracic lymphotome, and both lower extremities, external genital areas, and abdominal lymphotomes drain into the left subclavian vein via the thoracic duct. Lymphatic obstruction or impairment affects the trunk quadrants and extremities. In addition to extremity edema, individuals may develop lymphedema of the breast, lateral trunk, abdomen, genitals, suprapubic area, or buttocks.

Collateral Lymph Flow
Drainage can be changed from one lymphotome to another by expelling lymph from an overloaded one toward a normal one, even across two or three

intermediate overloaded areas (see Fig. 13-5). This change in flow occurs through the most superficial plexus, which then drains into the deeper (but still very superficial) collectors and deep trunks. The deep trunks also have collaterals crossing the watersheds to accomplish this flow. It is the dilation of the collectors and collaterals together with the superficial plexus that accounts for the success of the therapy intervention using lymphatic drainage as part of the program.

Improper treatment of extremity edema without considering the impact of that treatment on the trunk quadrant adjacent to the limb or limbs involved can result in the development of truncal or genital edema, when none existed before intervention for the extremity edema.[20]

Lymph Nodes
Normal, healthy lymph nodes are soft and nonpalpable. Palpable lymph nodes do not always indicate serious or ongoing disease, but this determination requires an evaluation by a physician. Therapists may identify suspicious palpable lumps in a client who has already been examined by a physician. However, the therapy profession offers greater opportunity for identification of suspicious nodes, given the specificity of palpatory skills and techniques practiced by a therapist. For this reason, the therapist should not hesitate to return a client to the referring or primary physician for further evaluation.

Past medical history is extremely helpful in determining the urgency of referral. A suspicious, palpable node in the presence of a previous history of cancer warrants immediate medical referral. Supraclavicular and inguinal nodes are common metastatic sites for cancer. Nodes involved with metastatic cancer are usually hard and fixed to the underlying tissue.

Lymphadenopathy

In acute infections (lymphadenitis), nodes are tender asymmetrically, enlarged, and matted together, and the overlying skin may be red and warm (erythematous). Changes in size (greater than 1 cm), shape (matted together), and consistency (rubbery or firm) of lymph nodes in more than one area or the presence of painless enlarged lymph nodes must be reported to the physician.

In the case of recent pharyngeal or dental infections, minor, residual enlargement of cervical nodes may be observed. Intraoral infection may also cause an inflamed cervical node. The therapist may first be alerted to this condition by a spasm of the sternocleidomastoid muscle causing neck pain.

Palpation may appear to aggravate a primary spasm, as if the spasm were originating in the muscle, when, in fact, a lymph node under the muscle is the source of symptoms. In such cases, the past history is the key to quickly identifying the need for medical referral or follow-up care.

Lymphadenopathy in certain anatomic areas, such as preauricular or postauricular (in front of or behind the ear), supraclavicular, deltopectoral, and pectoral regions, is viewed by the medical community with greater suspicion because these areas are not usually enlarged as a result of local subclinical infections or trauma.[144]

INFLAMMATION AND INFECTION IN THE LYMPHATIC SYSTEM

Disorders of the lymphatic system may result from *lymphangitis* (inflammation of a lymphatic vessel), *lymphadenitis* (inflammation of one or more lymph nodes), *lymphedema* (an increased amount of lymph fluid in the soft tissues), or *lymphadenopathy* (enlargement of the lymph nodes). Lymph nodes act as defense barriers and are secondarily involved in virtually all systemic infections and in many neoplastic disorders arising elsewhere in the body.

The specific node, or nodes, affected in an infectious disease depends on the location of the infection, the nature of the invading organism, and the severity of the disease. For example, infections involving the pharynx, salivary glands, and scalp often cause tender enlargement of the neck nodes, referred to as *reactive cervical lymphadenopathy*. *Generalized lymphadenopathy*, enlargement of two or three regionally separated lymph node groups, is usually a result of inflammation, neoplasm, or immunologic reactions.

These two types of lymphadenopathy are normal reactions to infection that result in large and tender lymph nodes, but the node is not necessarily infected (warm or reddened, as with lymphadenitis). The presence of lymphadenopathy is usually more significant in people

older than 50 years; lymphadenopathy in people younger than age 30 is usually from benign causes, but this must be medically determined.

Lymphedema

Definition

Lymphedema is a swelling of the soft tissues that results from the accumulation of protein-rich fluid in the extracellular spaces. It is caused by decreased lymphatic transport capacity and/or increased lymphatic load and is most commonly seen in the extremities but can occur in the head, neck, abdomen, and genitalia.

Classification of Lymphedema

Lymphedema is divided into two broad categories: primary (idiopathic) and secondary (acquired) lymphedema. In the past, primary lymphedema was classified as connatal if it appeared at birth, praecox if it appeared at puberty, or tarda if it developed after age 35 years. The term *connatal* (present from birth) applies to most primary lymphedemas that are present at birth, rather than the term *congenital*, which implies a specific genetic abnormality. The severity of lymphedema is graded using the scale from the International Society of Lymphology: Stage 0 (latent lymphedema), Stage I, Stage II, and lymphostatic elephantiasis (Stage III) (Box 13-1).[13,67-69]

In *Stage 0* (or *latent lymphedema*), lymph transport is impaired, but there is no clinical evidence of swelling. Stage 0 may last months or years before any obvious lymphedema occurs. Understanding the concept of latent lymphedema is critical in providing guidance to individuals at risk, as well as in recognizing the early signs and

---

Box 13-1

STAGES OF LYMPHEDEMA

Stage 0 (Latent Lymphedema)
- Lymph Transport capacity is reduced; no clinical edema is present

Stage I
- Accumulation of protein-rich, pitting edema
- Reversible with elevation; area affected may be normal size upon waking in the morning
- Increases with activity, heat, and humidity

Stage II
- Accumulation of protein-rich, nonpitting edema with connective scar tissue
- Irreversible; does not resolve overnight; increasingly more difficult to pit
- Clinical fibrosis is present
- Skin changes present in severe Stage II

Stage III (Lymphostatic Elephantiasis)
- Accumulation of protein-rich edema with significant increase in connective and scar tissue
- Severe nonpitting fibrotic edema
- Atrophic changes (hardening of dermal tissue, skin folds, skin papillomas, hyperkeratosis)

symptoms of progression from Stage 0 to Stage I. These may include a sensation of heaviness, fatigue, ache, or pain in the limb at risk.[8]

Stage I lymphedema is soft, pits on pressure, and reverses with elevation. In the early stages, there is a chronic inflammatory response to the excessive protein in the interstitium.[3,106] The subcutaneous tissues begin to fibrose, progressing the lymphedema from Stage I to Stage II. In fact, a lymphedematous limb may be Stage II in the foot and ankle and Stage I in the thigh.

Stage II lymphedema is nonpitting and does not reduce on elevation of the limb, and clinical fibrosis is present. Skin changes, such as eczema, warts, papillomas, and lymph fistulae, are common in severe Stage II lymphedema. Chronic inflammation can lead to recurrent bacterial and fungal infections.

The most severe, *Stage III lymphedema*, is referred to as lymphostatic elephantiasis. This is characterized by severe nonpitting, fibrotic edema with atrophic skin changes such as thickened, leathery, keratotic skin, skin folds with tissue flaps, warty protrusions, papillomas, and leaking lymph fistulae. Lymphangiomas (form of lymphangiectasia) may also be present.

Incidence and Risk Factors

The exact incidence of primary lymphedema is unknown because many people remain undiagnosed or if diagnosed, treatment or follow-up care does not occur, and the condition remains unreported.[83]

Primary Lymphedema. Approximately 15% of primary lymphedemas are present at birth (formerly called *connatal*). The most common form of primary lymphedema occurs from adolescence to midlife and accounts for 75% of primary lymphedema in a 4:1 ratio of females to males (formerly called *lymphedema praecox*). Of all primary lymphedema, 10% to 20% appears abruptly after age 35 years (formerly called *lymphedema tarda*).[31] A small percentage of primary lymphedemas occur in association with rare genetic syndromes, such as Milroy (appears at birth) and Meige (develops anywhere from early childhood to puberty) diseases, accounting for approximately 2% of primary lymphedemas.

Secondary Lymphedema. The incidence of secondary lymphedema also remains an approximate figure. Lymphatic filariasis affects more than 120 million people in 80 countries throughout the tropics and subtropics of Asia, Africa, the Western Pacific, and parts of the Caribbean and South America. Currently, more than 1.3 billion people in 72 countries are at risk. Approximately 65% of those infected live in the World Health Organization (WHO) South-East Asia Region, 30% in the African Region, and the remainder in other tropical areas.[158] Presently, no detailed maps are available of the geographical distribution of secondary lymphedema caused by filariasis, but distribution may be governed by climate, with an estimated 420 million people exposed to this infection in Africa in the year 2013.[89] The WHO estimates 700,000 people in the Americas are affected today (including 400,000 in Haiti and 100,000 in the Dominican Republic).

Clinical reports on the incidence of secondary lymphedema from other causes vary depending on the criteria used to define lymphedema, the measurement tool used, and the length of time individuals are followed posttreatment, with an estimated 3 million new cases in the United States each year.

Incidence Associated with Cause

Medical Procedures—Upper Extremity. There is a reported incidence of 0% to 3% of lymphedema after lumpectomy alone, and up to 70% after modified radical mastectomy with axillary lymph node dissection and radiation.[130] Eighty percent to 90% of women who are going to develop breast cancer–related lymphedema will develop it within 3 years of treatment.[105] However, the risk persists even years later. Individuals at risk have a 50% risk of developing lymphedema by 20 years posttreatment.[112] The incidence increases after surgery and radiation when these procedures are combined.[30,37,94,100]

Many individuals who undergo lumpectomy receive axillary lymph node dissection (ALND) and radiation therapy, too; these are the very factors that multiply an individual's risk of developing lymphedema. It has been reported that a 3% incidence of lymphedema after sentinel lymph node biopsy (SLNB) alone increased to 17% when the client required an axillary dissection following the SLNB.[128] These numbers increase exponentially when radiation to the axilla is added.[130]

A 2005 report on surgical complications of SLNB in 5500 cases cited a 6.9% incidence of "proximal upper extremity lymphedema" (change from baseline arm circumference of greater than 2 cm when compared to the contralateral arm).[155] After ALND and axillary radiation to treat melanoma of the upper extremity, a 53% incidence of lymphedema has been reported.[122]

Bevilacqua et al[14] created validated nomograms to assist in predicting risk of breast cancer–related lymphedema after ALND for breast cancer. The authors collected data from a prospective cohort of 1054 women with unilateral breast cancer, defining lymphedema as a 200-mL difference between arms at 6 months or more after surgery. Risk factors included age, body mass index, ipsilateral arm chemotherapy infusions, level of ALND, location of radiation field, development of postoperative seroma, infection, and early edema.

Another study followed 102 women treated for breast cancer, defining lymphedema as a greater than a 2-cm difference between measurement sites, and recorded lymphedema in 43.3% of women who underwent ALND alone, 22.2% of those who underwent SLNB alone, and 25% of those with combined SLNB and ALND.[94] Overall, the proportion of women experiencing increased arm size, numbness, or firmness/tightness in the limb on their operative side was higher in the ALND group than in the SLNB group.[5] Researchers are looking at evidence comparing long-term outcomes from SLNB versus ALND, debating whether there may be a subset of women who may not need axillary surgery if treated with systemic therapy (chemotherapy or radiation).

Armer and colleagues[8] followed 236 breast cancer survivors at risk for lymphedema for 60 months postoperatively. Limb volumes were assessed preoperatively and participants were followed every 3 months for 12 months and then every 6 months, for a total of 60 months. Limb volume changes were assessed with perometry, by circumference at 4-cm intervals, and subjectively by symptom experience through interview. At 60 months posttreatment, lymphedema incidence ranged from 43% to 94% with symptom assessment associated with the lowest incidence at 43% and the 2-cm difference between arms being the highest incidence at 94%. Ten percent limb volume change (which is a definition used by some researchers) and self-report of heaviness and swelling scored the lowest incidence of 41% and 45%, respectively.[8] This study highlights the importance of ongoing assessment of individuals at risk for lymphedema well beyond the initial 12-month period, as well as the inclusion of symptom assessment in addition to limb volume change as an indicator of lymphedema.

According to Armer, "perhaps in part because of differences in measurement and diagnosis, the reported incidence of lymphedema varies greatly among persons treated with surgery and radiation for breast cancer. Through increased measurement accuracy, lymphedema incidence and prevalence following current therapeutic approaches for breast cancer treatment, cancer will be better understood, and more informed decisions about risk factors, treatment interventions, and recovery will be made."[4]

Investigations into predictive factors for lymphedema after breast cancer surgery have identified the following: individuals with lymphedema are more likely to be overweight (body mass index [BMI] ≥25), to have had axillary radiation, mastectomy versus lumpectomy, more positive lymph nodes, chemotherapy, fluid aspirations after surgery, and active cancer.[145]

Risk and severity of lymphedema may be associated with postoperative infection on the side of the surgery, BMI equal to or greater than 25 kg/m^2, and the amount of hand use on the operative side.[136] Controlling the predisposing risk factors has a significant effect on the probability of developing lymphedema. Individuals with low risk for lymphedema may be more prone to develop it if they have high BMI, a postoperative infection, or prefer to use their at-risk hand for most activities.[136]

The effect of weight reduction on lymphedema has been studied in a small number of women with breast cancer–related lymphedema. Weight reduction with a corresponding decrease in BMI reduced the volume of affected limbs more than twice that of the unaffected limb. Several possible explanations for the greater volume loss in the affected limbs include improvement in lymph drainage because of fat loss, the actual change in composition of the tissues in the limb with reduced fat, and loss of fat allowing improved function of elastic compression garments.[132] Body weight is one significant risk factor that the person can be empowered to impact by exercise and dietary modification.[11]

Medical Procedures—Lower Extremity. The incidence of lower-extremity lymphedema after inguinal lymph node dissection to treat melanoma has been reported to be 30%.[39] The average reported incidence of lower-extremity lymphedema after treatment for prostate cancer has been reported to be 4%, with the range being 1% to 18%. The overall risk of lymphedema in individuals with prostate cancer after pelvic node dissection has been reported to be 8%, rising to 16% after radiation treatment.[39]

Gould et al found lower-extremity lymphedema in 30% of individuals undergoing inguinal lymph node dissection in the treatment of vulvar cancer.[63] Zhang et al reported only 3% lower-extremity lymphedema after inguinal node dissection (during surgery to treat vulvar cancer) when they were able to preserve the saphenous vein, compared to 32% lymphedema incidence in those people who underwent inguinal node dissection and saphenous vein ligation.[160]

Etiologic Factors

Primary Lymphedema. The exact cause of *primary lymphedema* is unknown and cannot be linked to any significant traumatic event (Table 13-1). Primary lymphedema is most likely the result of lymphangiodysplasias or malformations of the lymphatic vessel present at birth (Fig. 13-9) but sometimes delayed in symptomatic presentation. Although a small percentage of primary lymphedemas are linked to genetic causes (e.g., Milroy disease and Meige syndrome), most cases are not genetically linked and are more likely the result of some developmental abnormality in the fetus. A family history of lymphedema is present in only 10% to 20% of all people with primary lymphedema.[31]

Klippel-Trénaunay-Weber syndrome is a rare occurrence in embryonic development and is associated with numerous anomalies. These can include varicose veins, cavernous hemangioma of the skin, and hypertrophy of bones and soft tissues in one or several extremities. In addition, dysplasia of the lymphatic system and neurogenic and visceral vascular malformations can occur. The dysplasia of the lymphatics can result in lymphedema in the involved extremities (Fig. 13-10).[23,154]

Malformations of the lymphatic vessels associated with primary lymphedema can be divided into three types: aplastic, hypoplastic, and hyperplastic. *Aplasia* occurs when the lymphatic collectors are so few that they are considered "absent." Aplasia may also involve the absence of lymph capillaries that render the adequate collectors less functional. Aplasia is most often combined with hypoplasia; complete aplasia would result in tissues unable to support life.

Hypoplasia refers to less than the normal expected number of lymph collectors in the affected region and may also occur when collectors present are unable to function as transport vessels. Hypoplasia represents the most common cause of primary lymphedema, occurring in 75% of the cases. *Hyperplasia* accounts for 15% of primary cases and is characterized by grossly dilated and enlarged lymphatics that can become varicose. Hyperplasia can occur in the lymphatics of the superficial plexus of the skin or in the main lymph trunks. As a result of the overdilation of the vessels, the intralymphatic valve flaps do not seal, and a reflux of lymph occurs.

When this occurs in the mesenteric and intestinal lymphatics, a reflux of chyle to distal areas also takes place—that is, to the skin of the genitals, buttocks, and thighs, or

Table 13-1	Etiology and Risk Factors for Lymphedema

Primary	Secondary*
Unknown	Filariasis
Hereditary	Primary or metastatic neoplasm (benign or
Developmental	malignant)
abnormality	Surgery (lymph node dissection or removal;
• Aplasia	other surgery: see text)
• Hypoplasia	Radiation treatment
• Hyperplasia	Chemotherapy
	Severe infection
	Lipedema
	Chronic venous insufficiency
	Liposuction
	Crush injury
	Compound fracture
	Severe laceration
	Degloving skin injury
	Burns
	Obesity
	Multiparity
	Paralysis
	Medications
	• Prolonged systemic use of cortisone
	(cortisone skin)
	• Tamoxifen/Adriamycin
	• HIV/AIDS
	Air travel (may be a "trigger" for those at
	risk; see Table 13-2)

*Listed in approximate descending order.

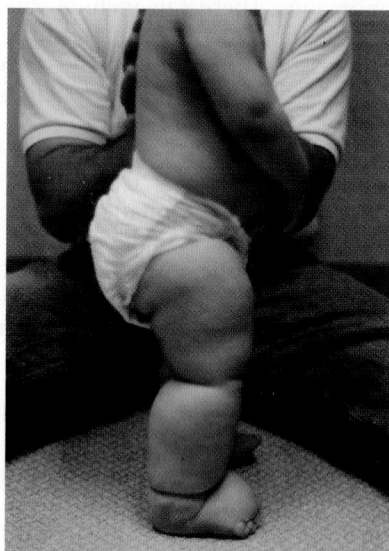

Figure 13-9

A 13-month-old with primary lymphedema of the right lower extremity, right buttock, and genital area since birth. (Courtesy Lymphedema Therapy, Woodbury, NY.)

to the knee joint (Fig. 13-11). Chyle is the protein-rich, milky fluid taken up by the intestinal lymphatics during digestion, consisting of lymph and triglyceride fat in a stable emulsion, and transported by the thoracic duct to the venous system.

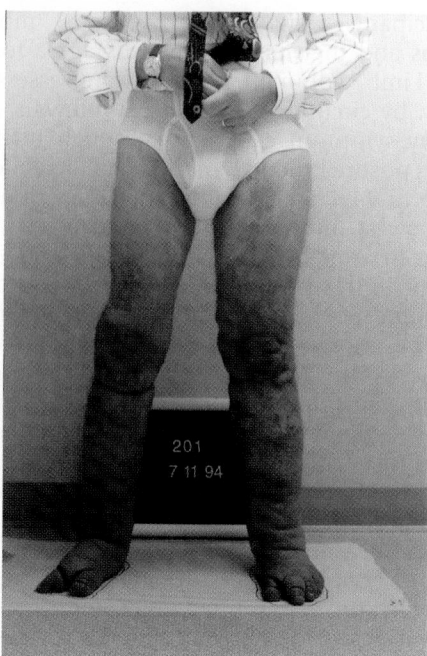

Figure 13-10

A 50-year-old man with Klippel-Trénaunay-Weber syndrome, a lymphangiodysplasia that caused lymphedema in both lower extremities. Note the skeletal abnormalities of the toes, the large hemangioma on the left thigh, and the venous varicosities in the lower legs. (Courtesy Lymphedema Therapy, Woodbury, NY.)

Lymphangiectasia refers to lymphatic hyperplasia in a deeper organ or localized area of a limb. Lymphangiomas and lymph cysts are forms of lymphangiectasia.[31,55]

Secondary Lymphedema. Secondary lymphedema occurs as the result of damage to otherwise normal lymphatic vessels or nodes from a known entity. The most common cause of secondary lymphedema worldwide is *filariasis*. Filariasis is a parasitic infection carried by mosquitoes in endemic regions, often found in tropical climates (Africa, South America, India, and Malaysia). The larvae of the worm are injected into the dermis with the mosquito bite. They pass into the initial lymphatics and larger collecting lymphatics and can grow to 20 cm in length and 1 to 2 cm in diameter as they mature into the adult worm forms. The adult male has a long tail that whips back and forth, which can damage the fragile lymphatic walls.

The greatest damage, however, is done after the worm dies, often 5 to 10 years after the initial infection. At that time, foreign proteins from the worm body cause severe local inflammatory reactions that lead to severe fibrosis and scarring of the tissues, totally blocking the larger lymph collectors. This total blockage results in massive swelling distal to that collection site.[58,119,154]

In the United States and other regions of the world where the filaria parasite does not exist or has been eradicated, the most common cause of secondary lymphedema is invasive procedures used in the diagnosis and treatment of cancer. *Regional lymph node dissection* for diagnostic staging and eradication of tumor sites disrupts the lymphatic system. Radiation therapy, reconstructive or other surgical procedures, or the combination of these

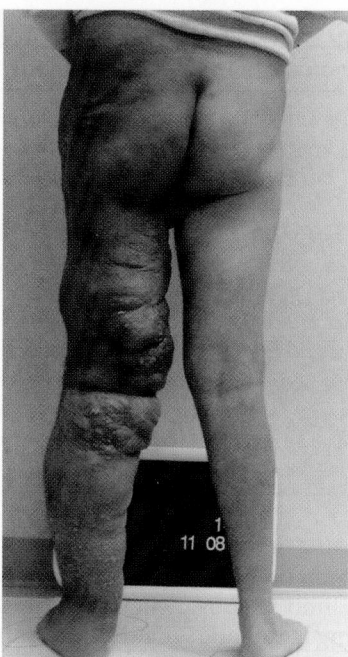

Figure 13-11

A 19-year-old male with primary lymphedema of the left lower extremity (onset at age 8 years). Lymphedema progressed to involve the buttocks and genitalia after prolonged pneumatic compression pump usage. This young man had three microsurgical procedures (lymphovenous and lympholymphatic anastomoses) in an attempt to reduce the genital and extremity edema. In addition, he had two debulking surgeries, which also were unsuccessful in reducing the lymphedema. He developed chylous reflux and eventually had sclerotherapy to his leaking abdominal lymphatics, which was very successful in stopping the severe leakage of chyle from his scrotum, medial thigh, and buttock. The chyle-filled papules are visible on the posterior aspect of the thigh and calf. Notice the abnormal bulges and skin folds on the posterior thigh, which result when the debulked areas fill in with edema fluid. (Courtesy Lymphedema Therapy, Woodbury, NY.)

procedures are well-known contributing factors to the development of lymphedema.

Local radiation treatment after surgery for cancer increases the incidence of secondary lymphedema three times that of surgery alone, probably a result of the increase in local tissue fibrosis that further impairs lymph flow through the remaining functioning lymphatic vessels.[26,81] If there is significant burning and blistering of the skin during radiation treatment, the risk of lymphedema is increased because of the decreased elasticity of the skin and subcutaneous tissues.[121]

Other causes of secondary lymphedema include bacterial or viral infection; multiple abdominal surgeries, particularly in the obese individual; any trauma or surgery that impairs the lymphatics; or repeated pregnancies (see Table 13-1). Liposuction done for cosmetic reasons to enhance appearance, when performed on an individual with an asymptomatic but marginal lymphatic system, can trigger lymphedema in the operative limb.

Crush injuries, compound fractures, or severe lacerations or degloving injuries to the skin can significantly impair lymph flow. These types of injuries are also usually associated with damage to blood vessels. The damaged blood vessels leak fibrinogen, blocking the tissue

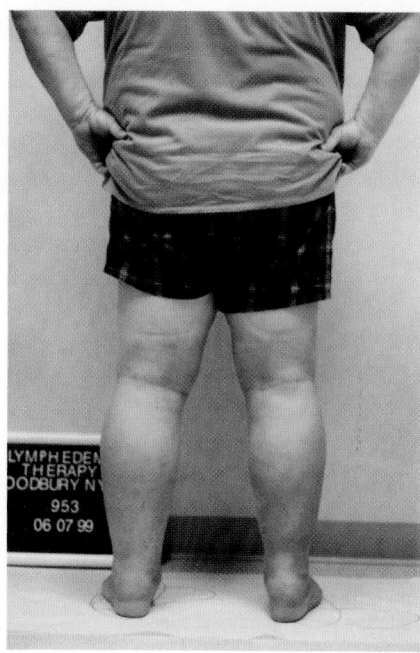

Figure 13-12

A 63-year-old man with lymphedema of both lower extremities, left greater than right. The swelling developed in the left leg 1 year after a coronary artery bypass graft (CABG) procedure in which veins were harvested from the left leg. The swelling began in the right leg, worsened in the left leg, and progressed into the abdomen after radium seed implantation for prostate cancer. This man's marginal lymphatic system was overwhelmed by the "trauma" caused by the CABG procedure and the radium seed implantation procedure. (Courtesy Lymphedema Therapy, Woodbury, NY.)

channels and initial lymphatics and thus contributing to the development of lymphedema. Other known causes that have been reported as associated with secondary lymphedema include paralysis, lipedema, skin thinned by cortisone (sometimes referred to as *cortisone* or *steroid skin*), and acquired immunodeficiency syndrome (AIDS), particularly if Kaposi sarcoma is present.[27]

Some medications used in the treatment of breast cancer (e.g., tamoxifen or Adriamycin) are associated with peripheral thrombophlebitis. These medications can cause blood clots resulting in deep vein thrombosis, venous insufficiency, and eventual secondary lymphedema.

Surgery is "controlled trauma," but it is trauma nevertheless; the more extensive the procedure, the more extensive is the trauma. Surgery in individuals with a marginal lymphatic system (where the lymph transport capacity equals the normal lymph load) can cause enough of an overload to trigger lymphedema. For example, an individual undergoing a triple coronary artery bypass graft procedure with donor veins taken from the legs may develop chronic leg edema that is often misdiagnosed as venous insufficiency or "cardiac related." This is particularly true in the older, obese individual who has poor functional mobility. If the diagnosis of lymphedema is delayed or never made and is not addressed, the individual may not be able to succeed in postoperative rehabilitation (Fig. 13-12).

In the past, most health care professionals knew about upper-limb lymphedema secondary to axillary dissection

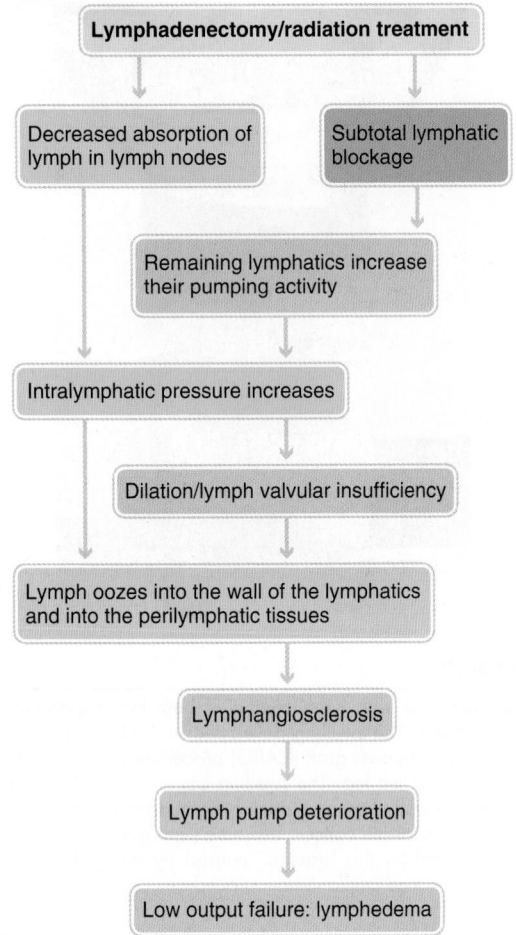

Figure 13-13

Pathogenesis of lymphedema. This flow chart follows the progression from an "at-risk" or latent phase of lymphedema to acute lymphedema after lymphadenectomy and/or radiation treatment to the nodal area. (Courtesy Dr. Michael Földi, June 1999.)

flow. At the same time, increased lymph production from the enlarging limb may overwhelm the capacity of a normal functioning lymphatic system to move and remove the fluid from the extremity.[64]

Pathogenesis

Lymphedema by definition is a low-flow edema that occurs when the lymph transport capacity is inadequate to transport the normal volume of lymph. It is a failure of the safety valve mechanisms (Fig. 13-13). This can occur when the lymph load is normal, but the lymph transport capacity is inadequate (*decreased absorption of lymph in lymph nodes*) or when there is an increase in the lymphatic load (e.g., fluid entering the tissues) and the transport capacity is inadequate (*subtotal lymphatic blockage*).

In reality, the body adjusts the load if the capacity alters in response to changes in tissue hydrostatic pressure and other changes in homeostasis (*remaining lymphatics increase their pumping activity*), and conversely, the capacity can be adjusted if the load alters (*intralymphatic pressure increases*). When the safety valve mechanisms are no longer effective or become overwhelmed, the body's normal compensation is not enough, and lymphedema develops.

The puzzle of why some individuals develop lymphedema post lymph node dissection and some do not begs to be solved. It has been found that muscle lymph flow is higher in both arms of women who ultimately develop lymphedema compared with those who do not. Higher fluid filtration in the upper extremity may be a predisposing factor for lymphatic failure after lymphatic obstruction occurs.[138]

Higher arterial blood flow and lower amplitude venous blood flow pulse have been observed in women with lymphedema.[98] Stout et al studied segmental limb volume changes over time from preoperation to 12 months postoperation in 46 women who were at risk for breast cancer–related lymphedema.[141,142] Segmental volume increases were found in two segments in the affected forearm before the onset of lymphedema. This study highlights the importance of prospective surveillance in individuals at risk to develop lymphedema.[141,142]

Lymphedema causes the lymphatic vessels to dilate; the valve flaps become incompetent (*dilation/lymph*

for breast cancer, but many were not aware that an individual who had a coronary artery bypass graft procedure; inguinal node dissection for melanoma of the foot, testicular cancer, or prostate cancer; or pelvic/abdominal node dissection for gynecologic cancer was at risk for lymphedema of the leg and possibly the genitals, buttocks, or abdomen.

Anyone with postoperative leg edema after a fracture or total hip or knee replacement would not have been routinely evaluated for lymphedema 10 years ago. The combination of venous edema and lymphedema is often overlooked in the management of edema secondary to trauma. Many cases of chronic edema with recurrent infection and skin ulcerations are treated as pure venous edemas with poor results because the lymphatic component of the edema is not addressed.

Obesity may be a cause of lower-extremity lymphedema.[64] There may be a threshold above which lymphatic flow becomes impaired. Proximal transport of lymphatic fluid from the extremity depends on normal clearance function of the lymphatic vasculature. Anything that can increase the volume of lymph produced by the tissues increases the load. With increased adipose tissue there can be increased compression on the lymphatic vessels reducing lymphatic

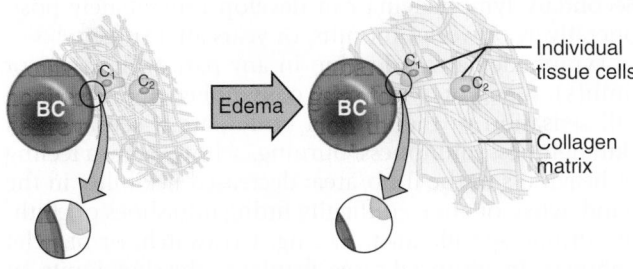

Figure 13-14

Reduction of gas (oxygen) exchange. Even a relatively minor amount of edema, which moves the fibers and individual tissue cells *(C1, C2)* apart by only a small amount, can cause a great increase in the resistance to diffusion of gases (and other small lipid-soluble molecules) between the cells and the blood capillaries *(BC)*. The magnified view of the distance between the BC and the tissue cell (representing the cell's oxygen supply) is greatly increased in the edematous state. The greater distance for oxygen to diffuse to nourish the cells will eventually lead to a hypoxic state. (From Casley-Smith JR, Casley-Smith JR: *Modern treatment for lymphoedema*, ed 5, Adelaide, Australia, 1997, Lymphoedema Association of Australia.)

valvular insufficiency), and the protein-rich lymphatic fluid refluxes to the tissue spaces *(perilymphatic tissues)*. At first, a proliferation of initial lymphatic vessels occurs as the system tries to cope with the accumulation of lymphatic load. Lymph vessels can rejoin, or collateral lymphatics can develop to bypass the damaged area.

Chronic Inflammation. In lymphedematous tissue, a state of chronic inflammation exists.[107] This chronic inflammation leads to progressive tissue fibrosis, resulting in a state of relative hypoxia in the tissues, further impeding tissue oxygenation and contributing to a cycle of chronic inflammation and increased risk of infection.

Infection or Delayed Wound Healing. In either primary or secondary lymphedema, infection or delayed wound healing (the latter can be directly related to the low oxygen state caused by edema) will add to the high-protein edema. Infection in the tissues (cellulitis) or infection in the lymph vessels (lymphangitis) can cause progressive tissue fibrosis and/or scarring in the lymph vessels *(lymphangiosclerosis)*. Although some recanalization and collateralization of lymph vessels take place, lymphatic function remains compromised. An increase in the size of the tissue channels occurs with an increase in the distance for the oxygen to diffuse from the capillaries to the cells (Fig. 13-14). Gas exchange and metabolism of cellular waste products are impaired.

Lymph Pump Deterioration. Although the number of macrophages increases, their activity is decreased in the lymphedema fluid for reasons not clearly understood. Some theories suggest that the chronic lack of essential nutrients (e.g., oxygen) or perhaps a toxic factor produced by the stagnant proteins or the damaged tissues contribute to the deterioration of macrophages.[30,33] In chronic lymphedema, the muscle wall of the collecting lymphatics hypertrophies, reducing the effective pumping power of these vessels *(lymph pump deterioration)*.

Impaired Transport Mechanism. The effect of lymphedema on the blood vessels causes a proliferation of new small blood vessels and the development of arteriovenous anastomoses. These new small vessels may leak

as a result of abnormal changes in total tissue pressure in the lymphedematous region, further overloading the area. Proteins, fats, cellular waste products, and the 10% (or more depending on the situation) of tissue fluid volume that is not directly transported by the venous system have no alternative transport pathway from the interstitium to the venous system except via the lymphatic system. When this transport mechanism is impaired, lymphedema develops (Fig. 13-15, *A*). The impairment can be structural or functional.

Structural Impairment. Aging or damaged blood vessels are associated with structural impairment as fibrin physically narrows or blocks tissue channels (Fig. 13-15, *B*). Hypoplasia of the collecting lymphatics is also associated with the pathogenesis of structural lymphedema (Fig. 13-15, *C*). Primary lymphedema that manifests itself in puberty with a growth spurt and increase in tissue mass causes the body to outgrow or outstrip the capacity of the lymphatic system. The functioning vessels become overwhelmed, the walls fail, dilate, and result in valvular incompetence, causing increased peripheral intralymphatic pressures and peripheral lymphedema.

Structural lymphedema may also occur when the flaps of incompetent valves of the collecting lymphatics (Fig. 13-15, *D*) no longer meet, allowing reflux of lymph to regions distal to the blockage. The initial lymphatics eventually dilate as well, their endothelial junctions remain open, and lymph refluxes to the tissues.

Other causes of structural lymphedema include gaps and tears in the initial lymphatic walls associated with trauma and inflammation (Fig. 13-15, *E*), physical obstruction of collecting lymphatics (Fig. 13-15, *F*) associated with fibrosis, radiation therapy, tumor growth, surgical excision of lymphatics during tumor removal, and torn anchoring filaments (Fig. 13-15, *G*) associated with sudden acute edema. The latter may occur secondary to massive trauma or infection and can tear the microfilaments that connect the initial lymphatics to the interstitial tissues, resulting in the collapse of the initial lymphatics because of the high total tissue pressure.[31]

In the case of lymphedema caused by filariasis, damage to lymph vessels can occur from the whip-like action of the constantly motile adult worms and the toxic effects of parasite secretory and excretory products. When the worm dies, the toxins released stimulate a granulomatous reaction with infiltration of plasma cells, eosinophils, and giant cells, further damaging the vessel and surrounding tissue as severe inflammation develops. Over time, repeated limb bacterial infections in previously damaged vessels may superimpose additional lymphatic damage.[23,119]

Functional Impairment. Anything that causes a lack of variation in total tissue pressure may cause lymphedema. Bed rest, paralysis, or prolonged immobility can severely limit changes in total tissue pressure. It is this variation that contributes to a pressure gradient between the interstitial tissues and the intralymphatic pressure. Normally, this pressure gradient stimulates the lymphangions to contract, which enhances the flow of lymph from the periphery to the center of the body. When the tissue pressure does not change or vary, the force pumps remain inactive.

Other factors contributing to functional impairment of the lymphatic system may include spasm of collecting lymphatics (e.g., lymphangiospasm caused by inflammation stimulating sympathetic nerves); paralysis of the collecting lymphatics (e.g., prolonged distention leading to fatigue and ultimately, failure); and impaired contraction of the collecting lymphatics caused by physical obstruction of fibrotic tissue surrounding lymphatic vessels. This type of functional impairment is common in severe Stage II lymphedema and Stage III lymphostatic elephantiasis. If collectors cannot pump, lymph refluxes peripherally, causing overdilation of the collecting lymphatics, valvular incompetence, lymphatic failure, and, ultimately, lymphedema.[31,55,154]

Clinical Manifestations. Primary or secondary lymphedema is characterized by clinical signs and symptoms caused by the effects of lymphedema on the lymphatics, body tissues, and blood vessels. Lymphedema resulting from filariasis is reversible in its early stages; secondary lymphedema can be transient if damage is minor.

Secondary lymphedema can develop immediately postoperatively or weeks, months, or years after surgery.[8]

Lymphedema can develop in any part of the body or limb(s). Signs or symptoms of lymphedema include a full sensation in the affected body part; a sensation of skin tightness; numbness, burning, aching, pain; a feeling of heaviness in the limb/area; decreased flexibility in the hand, wrist, or ankle; difficulty fitting into shoes or clothing in one specific area; or ring, wristwatch, or bracelet tightness. In advanced cases, fistulas to the skin, joints, or gut may develop; these are portals of entry for bacteria to invade the skin and cause recurrent infection.

Physical impairments caused by lymphedema can include increased circumferential limb girth; postural changes; tremendous discomfort (heavy, aching, or bursting sensations); neuromuscular deficits; and integumentary complications. These physical impairments can

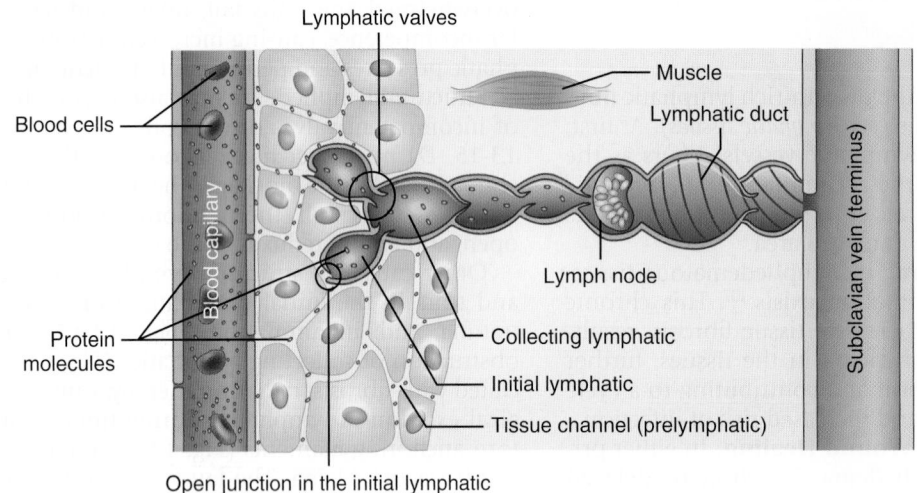

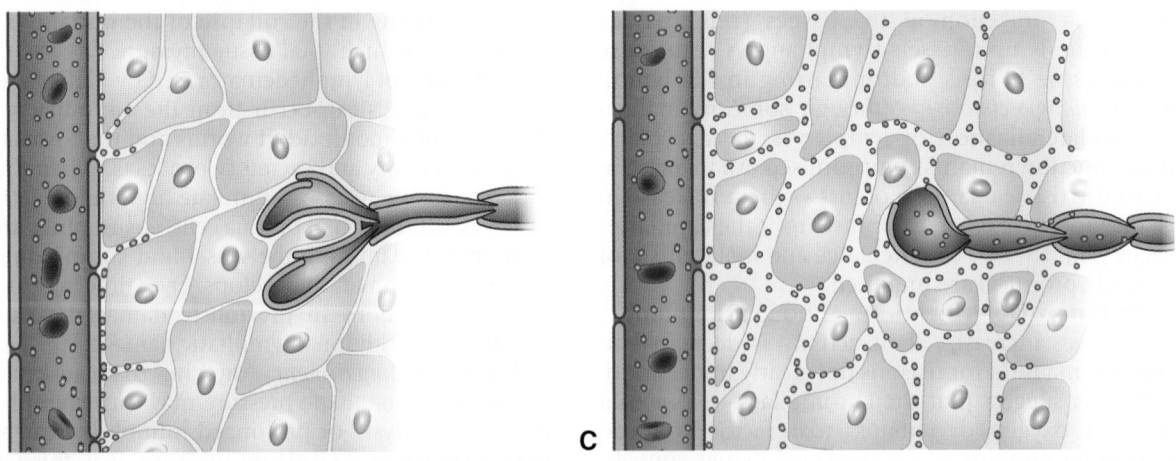

Figure 13-15

Low-flow, high-protein lymphedema caused by structural impairment. A, "Normal" tissue for comparison showing the passage of protein (dots) in normal tissue from the blood capillary, through the tissue channels, into and through the lymphatic system, and back to a vein. **B,** Altered interstitial tissue (e.g., too few or too narrow tissue channels). Notice that the prelymphatic channels are much narrower than in the normal tissue and the protein molecules are stacked up on the arterial side, unable to move easily through the narrow tissue channels, causing impaired lymph flow (and eventual tissue fibrosis). Inlet valves are closed because the endothelial cell junctions cannot open properly in fibrosed tissues, contributing to poor lymph drainage. **C,** Abnormally few initial lymphatics. This may occur developmentally or because some of the vessels become blocked (e.g., by fibrin). In this case, too few initial lymphatics are evident. Notice the dilation of the prelymphatic channels, the greater concentration of protein molecules in the tissue channels, and the malformed inlet valve. Low-flow, high-protein lymphedema caused by structural impairment.

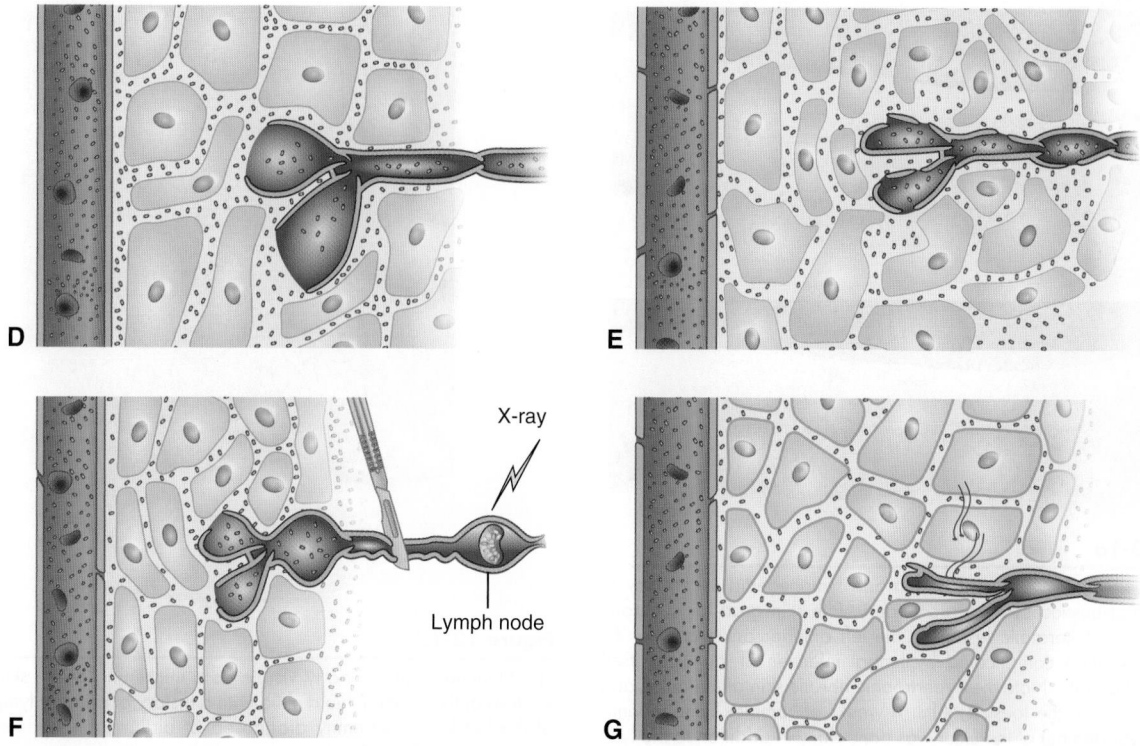

Figure 13-15, cont'd

D, Malformations of the initial lymphatics preventing their inlet valves from sealing; the prelymphatic tissue channels are dilated, a high-protein concentration exists there, and the tissue channels become dilated and stretched. This can happen in both primary and secondary lymphedema; in secondary lymphedema, it occurs after prolonged lymphostasis from a more proximal blockage. **E,** Injuries to the walls of the very fragile initial lymphatics. Lymph refluxes into the tissue channels, causing them to dilate. The high concentration of protein in the extracellular tissues causes a chronic inflammatory response and greater risk of infection. Note the larger spaces between the tissues. This results in a larger distance for oxygen to diffuse and leads to tissue hypoxia. **F,** Iatrogenic factors (e.g., surgery, radiation, tumor growth) that damage the lymphatic ducts or larger vessels impair lymph flow from the periphery. When movement of lymph from the tissue channels into the initial lymphatics is impaired, the tissue channels dilate, lymph stasis occurs, and there is a high-protein concentration in the tissues with subsequent chronic inflammation, increased risk of infection, and progressive swelling of the limb. **G,** Anchoring filaments tearing away from the interstitial tissue. This occurs in severe edema from other causes (e.g., rapid swelling from acute lymphedema as a result of trauma can tear the anchoring filaments from the surrounding tissues). The initial lymphatics can no longer function as conduits, as they would normally. The lymphostasis this produces worsens the existing edema. (From Casley-Smith JR, Casley-Smith JR: *Modern treatment for lymphoedema,* ed 5, Adelaide, Australia, 1997, Lymphoedema Association of Australia.)

lead to functional limitations and disability along with the potential for psychosocial morbidity (e.g., social isolation, depression, or suicide).[10,73] Healing time is increased, and all of this is occurring in a heavy, painful, and clumsy limb that is more prone to injury because of its abnormally large size and decreased functional mobility. Risk of injury is increased, whereas oxygenation and metabolism of waste and cellular debris are decreased. This is a most dangerous environment.

As the lymphedema progresses, atrophic skin changes can occur as a result of the low oxygen state, including loss of hair and sweat glands, formation of keratotic patches on the skin, and the development of papillomas (blister-like outpocketings of the skin) that sometimes leak lymphatic fluid. Angiosarcoma (Stewart-Treves syndrome) is a rare malignancy that can develop in an advanced, chronic lymphedema that is left untreated.[154]

Primary Lymphedema. Primary lymphedema is more common in females and affects the lower extremities most often. However, it is also seen in males and in the upper extremities.[24] Primary lymphedema can be present in many parts of the body, and if it is present from birth, the deep internal organs can be affected. Clinical cases of primary

lymphedema of the lower extremities may involve the buttocks, genitals, and intestines with reflux of intestinal chyle (chylous reflux/protein-losing enteropathy) through fistulae on the genitals, buttocks, and thighs (see Fig. 13-23).

This protein-losing enteropathy is a medical emergency. Severe protein loss can occur from this leakage of protein-rich chyle from the intestinal lymphatics. Individuals with primary lymphedema who complain of abdominal bloating, chronic diarrhea, or intolerance of fatty foods may also experience fluid accumulation in the abdomen and genitals from the pressure of the fluid leaking from the intestinal lymphatics into the abdomen. In some cases, these clients are treated medically or surgically with sclerotherapy to seal off these leaking lymphatics in an attempt to halt the reflux of this fluid into the abdomen.

Secondary Lymphedema. Surgical dissection and radiation therapy involving the cervical, supraclavicular, or mandibular lymph nodes can cause secondary head and neck edema. Significant edema of the head and neck can cause severe functional impairments in speech, swallowing, and respiration, in addition to the pain and psychologic trauma from cosmetic disfigurement. Disruption of any regional lymph node basin (i.e., axillary, inguinal, pelvic,

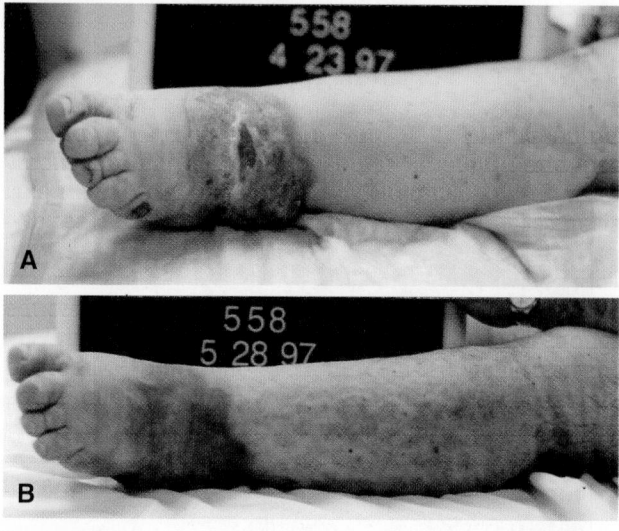

Figure 13-16

A 30-year-old male with spina bifida and lymphedema secondary to paralysis and unsuccessful plastic surgery with skin graft for a chronically itchy, 2-cm keratotic lesion on the left anterior ankle crease. **A,** Chronic ulceration complicated by fungal infection of the ulcer itself and the foot or toes. Note the hypertrophic fibrotic skin at the ankle and warty changes on the toes. **B,** After 4 weeks of complex lymphedema therapy (debridement of the ulcer was done daily in addition to the lymphatic drainage, compression bandaging, and other skin care). Exercise was not possible because of paralysis; deep abdominal breathing exercises and modified self-lymphatic drainage were taught and then practiced daily. Note that the wound healed completely and the infection resolved. (Courtesy Lymphedema Therapy, Woodbury, NY.)

abdominal) can cause secondary lymphedema in the body part/region that drains to that regional nodal area.

Complications of Lymphedema. As lymphedema progresses, the dermal layer of the skin thickens, the skin itself dries and cracks, and ulcerations often develop. These ulcers may not heal because of the tension on the tissues from the edema and the decreased oxygen state, coupled with the subcutaneous fibrosis and chronic inflammation. As the skin and tissues stretch, skin folds and tissue flaps can develop. These folds and flaps become breeding grounds for fungal and bacterial infections that further damage skin integrity, creating new portals of entry for the bacteria as the skin macerates and cracks.

Chronic fungus (tinea) is common on the foot and toes of anyone with lymphedema of the legs, as well as in the groin and under the breast. This fungus can be difficult, if not impossible, to treat topically. If this tinea is not addressed during treatment, a successful outcome is not possible (Fig. 13-16).[31]

The progressive increase in girth and weight of the affected areas contributes to pathologic alterations in the gait pattern and decreases in functional range of motion and strength caused by fatigue and inactivity. Coupling this with impairments in shoulder mobility caused by tightness of the pectoralis major and minor muscles secondary to radiation treatment for breast cancer and there is a risk for development or worsening of shoulder impingement or rotator cuff problems.[84,131] With increasing edema and subcutaneous fibrosis, tactile sensation and kinesthetic awareness are impaired, increasing the risk of injury to the affected areas.

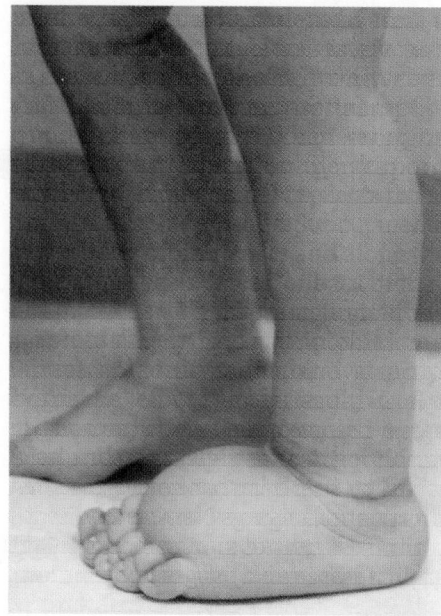

Figure 13-17

The Stemmer sign is clearly visible as a thickening of the skin folds of the toes of this 22-month-old child with a history of primary lymphedema of the left lower extremity diagnosed at birth. (Courtesy Lymphedema Therapy, Woodbury, NY.)

If the edema progresses into the trunk quadrant adjacent to the lymphedematous limb, a further loss of trunk strength and function can occur. Some individuals, for example, must sleep in a recliner chair to prevent losing their independence, as they can no longer mobilize themselves and their heavy limbs in bed. A vicious cycle develops with decreasing mobility and loss of strength leading to joint contractures, further increasing the risk to the already impaired skin integument.

The limbs may be painful and hypersensitive, and the adjacent trunk quadrants may ache and throb. Balance may be impaired, and the individual may no longer be able to shower or bathe independently, as a result of the fear of falling or inability to move the heavy limbs over the bath or shower ledge. Hygiene becomes a problem, further increasing the risk for fungal and bacterial infections.[95,102]

MEDICAL MANAGEMENT

Remarkable progress has occurred in diagnosis and management of lymphedema in the United States since 1990. Ironically, this has occurred despite the incorrect prediction for those with breast cancer that the advent of breast-conserving lumpectomy would eliminate the upper-extremity lymphedema so commonly seen in individuals postmastectomy.

DIAGNOSIS

Primary Lymphedema. An easy-to-perform clinical test for determining primary lower-extremity lymphedema is the Stemmer sign, a thickened cutaneous fold of skin over the second toe, typically present in the early and differential diagnosis of a primary ascending lymphedema without false-positive findings. It appears in the late stages of the descending lymphedema (Fig. 13-17).[139] It is possible

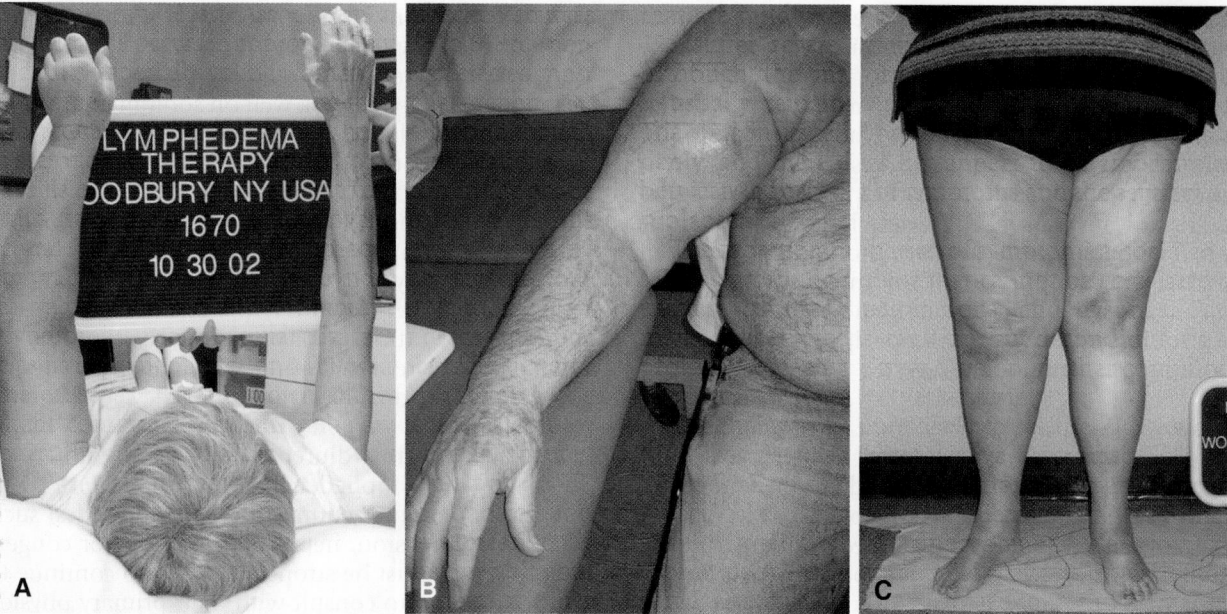

Figure 13-18

A, Malignant lymphedema left upper extremity; edema is more marked in the upper arm. Note dusky color and shiny quality of the skin. Note obvious weakness in the left shoulder—the patient is unable to elevate the left arm as far as the right. She is status postlumpectomy and radiation treatment for breast cancer 2 years prior to sudden onset of painful proximal limb swelling with progressive weakness of the left shoulder. Recurrence of cancer in the axilla was diagnosed and she was treated with chemotherapy. Lymphedema treatment was recommended in consultation with her oncologist and primary care provider to reduce pain and improve quality of life. **B,** Malignant lymphedema right upper extremity secondary to recurrent melanoma right axilla. Note varices right upper arm and the extension of the swelling into the right anterior axillary line and into the right chest wall. **C,** Malignant lymphedema both lower extremities, right greater than left. Edema is more marked in the thigh than in the lower leg. Note dusky color and shiny quality of the skin of the right leg. This woman had recurrence of her ovarian cancer with severe pain in the right hip/groin/genital areas with marked genital edema. What you don't see in this photo are the proximal varices that were present in the right proximal thigh extending over the inguinal crease—a sign that is frequently seen with recurrent cancer in the pelvis/abdomen. (In the case of malignant lymphedema of the upper extremity, there are often varices seen in the proximal aspect of the upper arm extending into the chest wall.) (Courtesy Lymphedema Therapy, Woodbury, NY.)

to have primary lymphedema without a Stemmer sign present.

Secondary Lymphedema. The clinical diagnosis of secondary lymphedema is fairly straightforward in a limb at risk, when there is known disruption to the regional lymphatics (e.g., after axillary dissection/radiation for breast cancer or after inguinal node dissection/radiation for melanoma of the leg). A detailed medical history, including all surgical procedures and their chronology relative to the onset or worsening of the edema, is the cornerstone of a successful lymphologic evaluation. In secondary lymphedema, most often no other diagnostic tests are needed to confirm the diagnosis.

A venous Doppler study of the edematous limb is often done to rule out a thrombus as the cause of the swelling. It is crucial to have recurrence of cancer firmly ruled out as the causative factor before initiating treatment for the lymphedema. Many oncologists will request a magnetic resonance imaging (MRI) or computed tomography (CT) scan of the chest for upper-extremity swelling or the pelvis and abdomen for lower-extremity swelling before initiating a referral for treatment of the lymphedema.

Lymphedema may be the first sign of cancer recurrence even years after cancer treatment. The prospect of recurrent disease is a frightening one, but it must be ruled out. Malignant lymphedema (i.e., directly resulting from neoplasm blocking a major nodal region or lymph vessel) is usually more severe and progresses more rapidly than

nonmalignant secondary lymphedema. Typically, malignant lymphedema is more severe in the proximal portion of the limb and alterations in skin color and texture are common (Fig. 13-18).

It is often associated with severe pain and/or sensorimotor deficits, particularly in the upper extremity when the brachial plexus is involved. These symptoms must be differentiated from the pain and weakness of radiation plexopathy, which sometimes progresses more slowly, but causes the same type of functional deficits.

Diagnostic Tests. In cases of unexplained swelling, particularly in the lower extremities when no known trauma or surgery is evident, the clinical examination and history may not provide a definitive medical diagnosis. Although the MRI and CT scan will clearly show edema fluid in a limb or region, these tests do not give a description of lymphatic function. This type of information is obtained from a lymphoscintigram, a sophisticated nuclear medicine test (with cost comparable to the MRI or CT scan) that outlines the major lymphatic trunks in a region and provides a functional description of how much tracer material is moved, how far, and in what unit of time, compared with the "normal" values of a person of similar height and weight.

The test involves subcutaneously injecting a small amount of radioactive tracer in the web spaces of the first and second digits of either the hands or feet. The client then performs a set of standard movements for a specific time period and serial radiographs are taken. The amount of exposure from all the radiographs is approximately equal to one x-ray.

As the tracer is taken up by the lymphatics, it will outline the major lymph trunks and show the volume of tracer moved per unit of time. The presence of tracer reflux that moves back down a limb is called *dermal backflow* and gives an indication of more proximal obstruction in the deeper lymphatic collectors. When the etiologic factors of edema are unclear, this test clearly shows the functional deficits in the lymphatics. It can be helpful in ruling out secondary lymphedema in cases of lipedema with questionable lymphedema of the legs.

TREATMENT. The primary focus in a case of lymphedema triggered by a new or metastatic cancer is to treat the cancer first and then manage the lymphedema. Input on how to minimize exacerbation of the lymphedema during the cancer treatment is often well received, if given with the intent to provide comfort and function.

Individuals are encouraged to undergo the cancer treatment that they wish to pursue, without guilt or fear that it will worsen the lymphedema. They need to know the possibilities and risks, but should not be frightened from necessary treatment for the cancer by a well-meaning health care professional.

On the other hand, the lymphedema should not be ignored. Management of the lymphedema must be coordinated with the medical team (e.g., medical oncologist, surgeon, and radiation oncologist) and the client. This communication can avoid further overloading the person with additional appointments and adding more to their daily activities than they can handle.

Medications. No clear-cut pharmaceutical drug is available to treat lymphedema, although there is hope for a safe, effective medication that will lyse the protein accumulating in the obstructed area and speed the healing process. Clinical studies show that the benzopyrones (Coumarin, Venalot, Daflon, and their natural counterparts, the bioflavonoids, rutin, horse chestnut, and grapeseed extract)* have some effect on increasing proteolysis and increasing macrophage activity (remember that the macrophages become inactive in the lymphedema fluid and unable to perform their immune functions). However, these substances also raise some health risks, specifically liver toxicity. Further randomized clinical trials are needed to assess efficacy and dosing.

This increased proteolysis helps to reduce the interstitial protein concentration, signaling the body to reabsorb more extracellular fluid, thereby reducing the lymphedema. These substances have been shown to soften fibrotic tissue and increase the healing of chronic ulcerations and

---

*The benzopyrones have not been approved by the Food and Drug Administration (FDA) in the United States, and the oral Coumarin was decertified in Australia because of several cases of death associated with liver problems. Other oral benzopyrones are still available in Switzerland, France, and Germany. Topical Coumarin powder and ointment is still available through compounding pharmacists in the United States. Bioflavonoid liquid and tablets have been available in U.S. health food stores for years. They are combined with various other compounds (known as bioflavonoid complex) and necessitate taking a larger dose of the complex to receive the desired amount of bioflavonoid.

bacterial infections in Stage III lymphedema, probably a result of the activity of the macrophages, stimulating the immune response.[23,27,31,34,54,55,90,99,111,148]

Diuretics. Diuretics work well on sodium retention edemas but do not help lymphedema, yet they continue to be prescribed. Although it is true that taking large doses of diuretics will reduce total body fluid volume, these medications do not address the cause of the lymphedema (i.e., that the lymph load is exceeding the reduced lymph transport capacity). Furthermore, diuretics may move the "water" component of the lymphatic fluid, further concentrating the extracellular protein in the tissues increasing fibrosis. Moreover, chronic use of high-dose diuretics leaves the individual at great risk for developing electrolyte disturbances and renal impairments.

Experts agree that diuretics may be indicated in cases of malignant lymphedema. Individuals with comorbid conditions that require the use of diuretics, such as arterial hypertension, nephritic syndrome, or congestive heart disease, must be strongly advised to continue their medication and to consult with their primary physician/specialist with questions regarding their prescription.[23,55]

Medications That Can Cause or Worsen Edema. Some nonsteroidal antiinflammatory drugs (NSAIDs) that are cyclooxygenase-2 (COX-2) inhibitors (e.g., Celebrex) have a warning in the package insert about leg edema being a possible side effect. This has been clinically reported in several cases with lymphedema and arthritis; the individual with arthritis may experience an increase in edema when taking these drugs.[17]

Other commonly prescribed drugs, such as Norvasc (used to treat hypertension) and Avandia (used to treat diabetes), can cause leg edema. Lyrica (pregabalin) and Requip, drugs prescribed for neuropathy (used with diabetic neuropathy and shingles) and restless leg syndrome, may cause heart failure and limb edema.

Many people do have neuropathy from chemotherapy (e.g., docetaxel [Taxotere]) that is permanent and take these medications to manage the symptoms of neuropathy. Therapists must be aware of this possible side effect in any of these medications and not assume that increased edema is a result of, for example, behavioral nonadherence or a problem with fit of a compression garment.

Clients may experience similar problems as new drugs for other conditions are introduced into the market. Even if the package does not warn of edema as a possible side effect, the therapist and client must observe carefully for any early signs or symptoms associated with the use of a new prescription.

SURGERY. Surgery has been used to "treat" severe lymphedema in the past with limited success. It is still done today if an individual receives no benefit from conservative treatments or does not have access to these treatments. Numerous surgical approaches have been proposed to treat chronic lymphedema of the extremity.

Microsurgery. Microsurgical procedures attempt to anastomose a lymph vessel or node with a vein or with another functioning lymph vessel or lymph node. The morbidity and mortality from these procedures can be significant. These procedures may fail soon after the surgery, leaving the individual with more superficial scarring that further blocks collateral lymph flow from the obstructed limb. Animal and cadaver studies continue investigating surgical techniques to resect tumors, reconstruct breast tissue, or perform liposuction[59,62] that will prevent venous occlusion and subsequent lymphatic dysfunction.

Tissue transfer procedures involve transplanting lymph nodes or lymphatic tissue from a distant site to an area where lymphatics are obstructed. Some studies have demonstrated beneficial effects for select individuals.[88] Most of the published reports, however, are based on small numbers of people, use different tools to measure lymphedema, and lack long-term follow-up. The risk of developing lymphedema at the sites distal to the harvest site is not reported.[40]

Debulking. Debulking procedures (e.g., the Charles operation) seek to physically remove the excess fibrosclerotic connective tissue. (These procedures are rarely done in the United States except in extreme cases; debulking is still done in other countries.) These operations create extensive longitudinal scars on the involved extremities. Long incisions are made in the skin and subcutaneous tissues are removed down to the muscle and bone; the skin flaps are reapposed and sutured in place.

Although these procedures attempt to address the severely impaired cosmesis in the affected individuals, they do not address the cause of the impairment, which is decreased lymph transport capacity. This problem is unchanged by these procedures; over time, without maintaining continuous compression on the limbs with compression bandages or garments, the limbs begin to swell again, often with disfiguring asymmetrical tissue flaps, large lymph cysts called *papillomata* (up to 8 cm in diameter), or warty protrusions on the skin (see Fig. 13-11).[31,55]

Brorson, in Sweden, has reported successful maintenance of limb volume reduction following liposuction to reduce chronic, fibrotic lymphedema.[22] The majority of his cases have been breast cancer–related lymphedema and he emphasizes that these individuals must commit to wearing compression garments 24 hours daily to avoid such complications.[22]

Reconstructive Breast Surgery. Lymphedema can develop as a complication of breast reconstructive surgery. Many different procedures are available from the insertion of a tissue expander, followed later by the insertion of a permanent saline implant to the more extensive myocutaneous tissue flap procedures (i.e., transverse rectus abdominal muscle [TRAM] flap, free latissimus [LAT] flap, deep inferior epigastric artery perforator [DIEP] flap, gluteal artery perforator [GAP] flap, transverse upper gracilis [TUG] flap) involving transplanting flaps of muscle and skin or tissue and skin, with blood vessels to the breast area to form a more "natural" breast.[134] See complete discussion in Chapter 20.

The TRAM flap transplants the contralateral rectus abdominis muscle by tunneling it across the abdomen and up to the breast area. The DIEP flap transplants soft tissue and skin to the breast area leaving the abdominal muscles intact. These procedures usually consist of two other minor procedures, performed separately to tattoo the areola and create a nipple.

These procedures involve extensive scarring in the suprapubic area extending from hip to hip, in addition to the individual scars on the breast area. The horizontal hip-to-hip scar effectively blocks a large area of collateral lymph flow from the ipsilateral thoracic lymphotome through the abdominal lymphotome to the superficial inguinal nodes. This area of collateral lymph drainage is important for the treatment of ipsilateral upper-extremity lymphedema that can develop after axillary dissection and mastectomy.

In some cases, abdominal lymphedema develops after these procedures. This should not be confused with *asymmetric edema*, which may really be a hernia of the abdominal contents on the contralateral side where the abdominal muscle was removed in the TRAM flap technique. This occurs on rare occasions, but it must be medically diagnosed and surgically corrected.[134]

The LAT flap procedure also creates a long transverse scar on the ipsilateral posterolateral thorax, effectively blocking a large area of collateral lymph drainage from the upper extremity to the ipsilateral superficial inguinal nodes. This lymphatic pathway may be needed to treat an upper-extremity lymphedema secondary to axillary dissection or radiation. These procedures may lead to truncal lymphedema, which is often not recognized, sometimes discounted as psychosomatic, and can cause considerable disability, impairment of function, and psychosocial distress.[50]

The scar from the GAP flap, which transfers tissue and skin from the buttock is concealed in the gluteal fold and does not obstruct any lymphatic pathways for the upper extremity. The TUG flap transfers the small adductor gracilis muscle and skin leaving a scar on the medial aspect of the proximal thigh. Although the scars from these procedures do not obstruct collateral lymphatic pathways, these procedures remove tissue bulk from one side of the body (buttock and the medial thigh) that may require tissue reduction on the contralateral side to obtain acceptable cosmetic symmetry.[134]

PROGNOSIS. Thanks to advances in surgery and chemotherapy and the emphasis on early detection, many more individuals are surviving cancer for many years, living and functioning well with "limbs at risk" for lymphedema. Refinement in measurement tools, as well as the inclusion of self-reported symptoms, which may be present well before a 2-cm difference between measurement sites can be recorded, will hopefully lead to earlier diagnosis and management of lymphedema.[6,12]

Left untreated, lymphedema is a progressive disease; current surgical and pharmacologic approaches do not bring about a "cure." Lymphedema is a life-long, chronic condition, but one that can be managed effectively with proper intervention, client education, and regular follow-up care.

When scarring and lymphatic dysfunction are severe, treatment, such as manual lymphatic drainage, cannot always restore normal cosmesis; however, it can successfully reduce some of the edema, leading to improved function. For example, in individuals with severe edema of the throat and neck after surgery and radiation for tongue cancer, lymphatic drainage can reduce the swelling enough to allow the person to discontinue use of a tracheotomy tube previously considered permanent. Some clients are able to eat solid foods again; others with severe periorbital and lower facial edema may be able to open their eyes and read and watch television again. Although these are not "cures," they are great improvements in function that are important to individual quality of life.

SPECIAL IMPLICATIONS FOR THE THERAPIST   13-2

Lymphedema

It is critical to advise those who are at risk for lymphedema of the signs and symptoms of lymphedema and to educate them on risk-reduction strategies (http://www.lymphnet.org/resources/position-paper-lymphedema-risk-reduction-practices) to minimize stress on their marginal lymphatic systems (Table 13-2). Great care must be taken to avoid further overloading an already compromised area by the application of various modalities or therapeutic exercises.

Stout et al proposed a prospective surveillance model to monitor and screen clients at risk for breast cancer–related lymphedema.[142] They followed two groups of women. The prospective surveillance model (PSM) group were assessed preoperatively (range of motion, muscle strength, limb volume, body mass index, functional status, and level of physical activity). Subjects received education in lymphedema risk reduction and advice on postoperation activity. They returned for follow-up assessment of the above in 3-month intervals postoperation for 1 year. Lymphedema onset would be identified at an early stage, potentially requiring less intensive treatment to manage it at the earlier stage.

The other group, the traditional model of care (TMC), assumed that the physician would identify women with lymphedema at the same average incidence rate (one third of women over a 1-year period) and refer those women for treatment. Costs for treatment for each model were estimated, and the savings in the PSM group were considerable: the treatment cost was $636.19 in the PSM compared to $3,124.92 in the TMC group. Early identification and treatment minimize progression of lymphedema to a more advanced stage, potentially necessitating fewer treatment visits at a considerable cost savings.[133,142]

For clients who are free of lymphedema but receiving radiation therapy, the radiated area must be observed carefully and consistently for any signs such as blistering, discoloration, erythema (redness), or increased skin temperature changes. Any of these can be indications of developing lymphedema.

Many people do not "report" edema unless it is severe. This is common during the interview and history taking during patient/client consults. The individual's legs can be four times the size of their normal leg, yet they will say the swelling "just started" or "only just started to bother me" or "never swelled like this." When asked if they ever noticed even a little swelling in the foot or ankle, a mark when they removed socks or shoes, or swelling when it was hot or when they stood for a long time, clients often report all of these events have occurred for years "but it never bothered me" or "it was not really bad," and so on. This behavior is particularly common in the heavier clients who do not have a perception of how overweight they are or really cannot see or reach their feet.

Lymphodynamic insufficiency is a concern when treating lymphedema. Clients, particularly those with primary lymphedema of the lower extremities, should be evaluated for abdominal and genital edema before undergoing any treatment to reduce the extremity lymphedema to avoid the complication of moving more fluid into an already overloaded abdominal area.

Throughout the episode of care, observe the areas adjacent to the lymphedematous limb or region (the ipsilateral buttock, suprapubic/genital areas, ipsilateral breast/lateral trunk, or the contralateral lower extremity in a case with pelvic/abdominal node obstruction) to ensure that treatment of the peripheral lymphedema does not create lymphedema in adjacent lymph drainage areas.

An increased risk of this fluid movement may occur when using gradient compression pump therapy (intermittent pneumatic compression [IPC]) to treat extremity lymphedema. See "Intermittent Pneumatic Compression (IPC) - Compression Pumps" and "A Therapist's Thoughts" below related to IPC.

Orthopedic Lymphedema

Postsurgical lymphedema may occur after total knee or total hip replacement.[38] If the individual is poorly mobile and had some degree of "swelling" in the legs preoperatively (often attributed to arthritis), the increase in edema postoperatively is often considered the normal sequelae for the procedure. Important loss of time in rehabilitation occurs for these people who are in pain and experience decreased range of motion and strength because of the increasing edema.

When the edema is properly reduced and maintained, rehabilitation can progress quite well, provided that the therapist remembers the concept of limiting lymph load so as not to exceed the individual lymph transport capacity.

This clinical skill comes with experience and constant monitoring in the early stages of activity to assess which activities increase the person's subjective feeling of "congestion and fullness" in the affected areas. Heat modalities will increase superficial vasodilation and ultrafiltration, increasing edema, and therefore should be used with great caution. Electrical stimulation, particularly waveforms and intensities that produce sustained tetanic muscle contractions, should be used cautiously. Prolonged sustained tetanic muscle contractions (as opposed to rhythmic, reciprocal muscle contractions) can impair lymph flow in the area of skin overlying the muscle group, causing a retrograde edema distal to that site.

A past history of multiple abdominal or thoracic surgeries, vein stripping or sclerotherapy, and liposuction in the legs should remind the evaluating therapist to carefully assess signs and symptoms of lymphedema. A limb that was perceived as "less than perfect" can become a severely swollen, distorted limb, psychologically devastating the individual whose appearance was of paramount importance.

Table 13-2	Lifelong Precautions for Clients with Lymphedema

Risk	Activity
Infection	Maintain clean and dry skin; keep the skin supple by applying oil or bland cream; perfumed or fragranced lotions and creams can be irritating. A mild cleansing lotion such as Cetaphil or Alpha Keri Oil is recommended. Moisturizers with a high petroleum content (i.e., first ingredient listed is mineral oil or petrolatum) will damage the rubber/latex fibers of compression garments; check with therapist/garment manufacturer regarding safe products to use under garments.
	When drying, be gentle but thorough. Make certain to dry in any creases and between the digits. Watch for moist, cracking skin between the toes as a sign of fungal infection that must be treated.
	If possible, avoid needle sticks, injections, vaccinations, acupuncture, electrolysis, or blood drawing on the involved extremity. If a technician is unsuccessful obtaining blood from the uninvolved arm, use legs or feet for blood drawing (unless these are at risk). If the affected limb must be used, ask for an experienced phlebotomist who should be able to draw blood without using a tourniquet using a small butterfly needle.[16]
	Immediate treatment with cleansing, antibiotic ointment, and/or bandaging for all wounds no matter how minor (e.g., insect bites, paper cuts, hangnail, blister, burn); check often for signs of infection.
	Protect hands and feet at all times (e.g., socks and supportive footwear, rubber gloves for cleaning, long oven mitts, garden gloves for any outdoor work, thimble for sewing).
	Avoid harsh chemicals and abrasive compounds.
	Use extreme caution when cutting fingernails, toenails, or cuticles; creams are sometimes recommended for removing cuticles, but these are still chemicals and should not be used; use vegetable oil and gently push back cuticles with the pad of your finger, do *not* use a stick or nail file.
	Use electric razor to remove unwanted hair. A razor blade can cut the skin and infection could develop.
Circulatory compromise	Avoid blood pressure measurements on the involved extremity if possible. If blood pressure (BP) must be taken on the affected or at risk limb, request it be taken manually so that the cuff is only inflated to a level slightly above your "usual" blood pressure. Automatic BP machines usually inflate the cuff to excessively high pressures that are usually far above typical systolic BP.
	Avoid constricting jewelry and clothing, especially tight underwear, underwire brassieres, socks, or stockings; avoid elastic around neck, upper arm, wrists, fingers, ankles, and toes.
	Avoid lifting or carrying heavy objects with the involved extremity; no heavy handbags with over-the-shoulder straps; be extremely cautious when lifting children, as they can make sudden and unexpected movements.
	Avoid repetitive limb movements against resistance (e.g., pushing, pulling, rubbing, scraping, or scrubbing) that could cause sudden, rapid blood flow through muscle and tissue. Pace work and activity, gradually building your endurance.
	Maintain an ideal body weight with proper nutrition and low-salt, low-caffeine diet; avoid smoking, using recreational or illicit drugs, and drinking alcoholic beverages.
	Changes in pressure gradient during air travel require use of compression garments and low-salt diet.
	Avoid prolonged automobile travel; if travel is necessary, take frequent breaks and exercise other precautions (e.g., elevation, hydration, loose clothing, proper nutrition, compressive garment or bandages when recommended).
	Avoid overheating local body parts or rise in core body temperature: use pyrogenic medications, even with low-grade fever; avoid saunas, hot tubs, hot pads, hot packs, or tanning booths; close monitoring is required during extensive exercise or marathon running.
	Avoid sunburn; keep the limb protected from the sun; avoid tanning booths.
	Chemicals such as those used in the application of artificial fingernails may cause an edematous response in some people
Stress to impaired lymphatic system	Avoid heavy breast prostheses after a mastectomy; too much pressure on the supraclavicular lymph nodes can slow and interrupt the lymphatic pathways.
	Do not overtire a limb at risk. If it starts to ache, lie down with it elevated. If your leg is involved, avoid prolonged sitting. It is better to lie down with the affected leg elevated than to sit with the leg elevated. Prolonged sitting can prevent lymphatic drainage through the gluteal region.
	As previously mentioned, avoid tight jewelry and clothing on the affected limb, especially if some swelling is present. Underpants, brassieres, jeans, shoes, or any other article of clothing with straps must be loose around the waist, thighs, and crotch. *No* redness or indentation should be evident upon removal.
	Compression stockings/sleeves must not leave a compressive band at the ankle, knee, groin, or waist. It should not chafe at any point. If it does, obtain help from the therapist.

Note: For additional resources, see Box 13-2.
For more detailed information for individuals at risk for lymphedema go to http://www.lymphnet.org/pdfDocs/nlnriskreduction.pdf.
Modified from Boris M, Weindorf S, Lasinski B: Managing lymphedema: risk reduction strategies, Lymphedema Ther, New York, 2012, Woodbury.

A THERAPIST'S THOUGHTS

Risk Reduction Strategies

Although there have been no double-blind studies published that prove that these strategies are effective in reducing risk of developing lymphedema, the guidelines in Table 13-2 follow the common sense application of the anatomic and physiologic principles of lymphatic function.

Lymphedema specialists report countless numbers of cases in which individuals report lymphedema was triggered from a sunburn; an infection in the limb at risk; a strain or sprain injury in the limb at risk; exposure to excessive heat or overuse while cooking holiday meals; a fungal infection around the nails; repetitive lifting and scrubbing associated with spring cleaning; packing to move from one home to another; shopping, carrying, and wrapping heavy holiday packages; a bee sting on the limb at risk; or exercising without proper warm up or progression and grading of the exercise program.

Caution is advised in anyone with all three major risk factors for lymphedema: ALND (or any regional lymph nodal dissection), radiation therapy, and obesity. There is only anecdotal evidence that taking blood pressures (BPs) on a limb that is healed after ALND increases the risk of lymphedema. However, the therapist must remember tissue healing (not postoperative) requires a minimum of 6 weeks in the absence of multiple risk factors; indeed any risk is deemed unacceptable.[113]

It is likely that these anecdotal cases were in (1) persons not healed, (2) individuals at high risk of inflammation (e.g., comorbidity of autoimmune tissue disease or other inflammatory process affecting the limb), (3) obese persons who may have undergone radiation therapy, and (4) individuals who could have sustained trauma from improper BP measurement leading to inflammation.[113]

Blood Pressure Assessment as a Potential Trigger

Although there is no proof that taking BP measurements on the limb at risk will trigger lymphedema, it is logical to consider that applying the BP cuff and inflating it to 200 mm Hg will compress veins and lymphatics under the area of the cuff.

For those who argue that compression is part of the treatment for lymphedema, it should be pointed out that there is a difference between gradual, gradient compression applied with the most compression distally on the limb involved, gradually decreasing proximally, and a sustained, high level of compression at a single site proximally on the involved limb.[35]

If those lymphatics were the only vessels that are functional in the limb at risk (because others were damaged or excised during regional lymph node dissection/radiation), then it would make sense to avoid further compromise of their function. If the limb at risk must be used, it is helpful to avoid inflating the cuff to more than the person's average systolic pressure. This would limit the compression of the local lymphatics as much as possible.

Individuals who are obese are more likely to be hypertensive, requiring inflation of the BP cuff to higher pressure to get the baseline measure. Because obesity and weight gain during treatment are primary risk factors for lymphedema, this subset of the breast cancer population may warrant more caution; again, no data support clinical practice guidelines at this time.[35,113]

Do not apply the BP cuff above an intravenous (IV) line where fluids are infusing or an arteriovenous shunt on the same side where breast or axillary surgery has been performed, or when the arm or hand has been traumatized or diseased. Until research data support a change, it is recommended that clients who have undergone ALND avoid having BP measurements taken on the affected side if possible.

Although it is recommended that anyone who has had bilateral ALND should have BP measurements taken in the leg, this is not standard clinical practice across the United States.[109] Leg pressures can be difficult to assess and inaccurate. Some oncology staff advise taking BPs in the arm with the least amount of nodal dissection. For clients who have had a mastectomy without ALND (i.e., prophylactic mastectomy), blood pressure can be obtained in either arm.[87]

Venipuncture as a Potential Trigger

Although venipuncture is done with "sterile" technique, the reality is that the degree of "sterility" varies greatly and depends on where and in what type of facility the puncture is done and who is doing it. There is still a risk of introducing bacteria with the needle stick, as well as potential damage to the local veins and lymphatics, depending on the degree of compression under the tourniquet and how many times the person has to be punctured to get a full sample.

Again, it makes sense to err on the side of caution and to avoid using the limb at risk for venipuncture unless there is no other option. For people who have had bilateral axillary dissection this poses a problem. Many laboratories do not have anyone who is competent in venipuncture on the leg or foot. Some physicians feel that the risk of deep venous thrombosis in the leg is too great and will not recommend using the leg or foot to draw blood. It has been suggested to try to minimize tourniquet time or to eliminate the use of the tourniquet during venipuncture to reduce the risk of damaging lymphatics.

Guidelines and Precautions

There are no absolutes, and these "guidelines" are just that—guidelines for clients to discuss with their physicians. Many of the other "precautions" are common sense recommendations. For example, if you knew that you had sensitive skin, you would avoid exposing that skin to harsh chemicals like those in household cleaning solutions—petroleum, ammonia, and lye-based products.

In the same way, if you have never exercised in the past, you would not begin to weight train with 5-lb weights—you would build up from no weight gradually to whatever weight you could tolerate comfortably without causing muscle ache and a feeling of tightness in the limb at risk. The evidence supporting this "common sense" recommendation (cited in the third edition of this book) is now reported in the literature.[65,124-126]

Another example is gardening, as garden soil contains rocks, insects, sharp roots, bacteria, fungus, and possibly pesticides. Wearing gloves when one gardens just makes sense to avoid the risk of getting a cut, insect bite, or exposure to some bacteria or fungus. It is important to remember that the skin on the limb at risk needs to be protected from anything that threatens the integrity of that skin.

Currently, there is no cure for lymphedema. Any strategy that might delay the onset of this condition is worth pursuing. Individuals with a limb at risk should be educated about these risk-reduction strategies so that they can incorporate some or all of them into their daily activities if they so choose. It is the clients' right to choose, but they need to have appropriate information to make an informed choice.[60,103]

A THERAPIST'S THOUGHTS
On Infection

Understanding the risk for infection is critical when evaluating and educating individuals with or at risk for lymphedema. These individuals are extremely prone to local infection from even a minor trauma, abrasion, or insect bite and must be educated in risk reduction and proper skin care to minimize their risk for recurrent infections. Ryan eloquently explains the rationale behind meticulous skin care[120]: "The epidermis and adipose tissues...are likely factories of growth factors and mediators of inflammation....[C]ytokines manufactured by the epidermis...are perhaps also responsible for recurrent inflammatory episodes....[A]pplication of external emollients that are antiinflammatory...should be looked upon as being proactive in the management of lymphedema."

Minor irritations, local areas of redness of the skin, and minor dermatitis reactions must be observed and treated aggressively to avoid progression to a major infection. In a therapy department, the treatment environment and all equipment must be meticulously cleaned.

In a therapy setting, careful thought must be given even to everyday procedures. For example, a woman with mild Stage I upper-extremity lymphedema secondary to axillary dissection developed cellulitis in her involved extremity after receiving a week of treatment for her lymphedema. Treatment involved a skin care program using moisturizer. During treatment, the jar of moisturizing cream was always open on the counter, and the therapist dipped into the jar with a bare hand, applying the cream to the client's skin, returning to the jar several times with the same bare hand that had rubbed the cream on her arm. Although the skin on the arm was intact, the client was concerned that a possible link existed between her infection and the cream that was used on others, some of whom she noted had open wounds. Although no direct proof of the connection between this clinical practice and the client's infection is available, it is a reminder of the need to improve our infection control on *all* clients, regardless of their "level" of risk. (See "Infectious Diseases" in Chapter 8 and "Standard Precautions" in Appendix A.)

Many people with lymphedema are unaware of the increased risk of infection or are lulled into complacency by health care professionals who tell them "not to worry" because antibiotics are available if an infection develops. Any infection further stresses the already overloaded regional lymphatic system, possibly scarring some of the remaining functioning lymphatic vessels and ultimately contributing to progressive and chronic lymphedema.

Any infection in a lymphedematous limb, even local, must be medically treated immediately without delay. Individuals must be instructed to contact the physician immediately or go to the emergency department, and they must advise the staff of the lymphedema diagnosis and the impending infection requiring antibiotics. Making this pronouncement firmly can save precious time, eliminating the need to request a referral from the infectious diseases department or obtaining cultures while the bacteria are multiplying and increasing in strength.

Evaluation

When evaluating an individual with suspected lymphedema (or the individual with unexplained edema of an extremity or extremities, trunk, or head and neck), cardiac, renal, hepatic, thyroid, and arteriovenous disease must be ruled out medically. The results of specific tests used to diagnose the edema should be reviewed.

Venograms and lymphangiograms involve cutdowns, and the injection of dyes into the vessels (these have been known to sclerose and damage vessels) is no longer recommended by lymphologists. Lymphoscintigrams, which are useful to differentiate between venous edema, lipedema, and lymphedema, have already been discussed. Remember that a combination of these conditions can coexist. Cases complicated by genetic lymphangiodysplasias need the intervention of an experienced lymphologist.[23,54,55,90]

Importance of Past Medical History

A detailed history must be taken, including past medical history, especially cancer; information about swelling; onset and progression; tests conducted to evaluate and diagnose the condition; chronology of all surgeries; vein stripping; bypass stents; and insertion or removal of ports for administration of chemotherapy, especially biological response modifiers, as these tend to cause high levels of fluid retention and metabolic dysfunction.

An accurate history of infections in the affected areas, how these were treated, and how they responded to treatment is also critical. A chronologic review of the person's previous treatments and/or interventions for lymphedema and the response to treatment is important.

It is essential to keep in mind that secondary lymphedema can be the result of an orthopedic surgery or trauma that further disrupted marginal lymphatics. Individuals with extensive acute or chronic edema after trauma or surgery should be evaluated for lymphedema. Early intervention and management of this type of lymphedema can significantly minimize the complications of advanced, untreated lymphedema mentioned earlier.

In the case of a known history of cancer, lymphedema that does not respond to proper treatment may be caused by metastases blocking lymphatic flow. In such a case, treatment may result in proper lymphatic drainage, but the results would be temporary and the lymph fluid would begin to build up again. The therapist must remain alert to this possibility.

Clinical Assessment

Clinical evaluation includes a detailed description of skin integrity, using body diagrams, both anterior-posterior and lateral, to draw unusual body contours. This description also includes the presence of edema or fibrosis on the trunk quadrants, the head and neck, as well as on the limbs; location and condition of scars, fibrotic areas, and open wounds; evidence of healed ulcerations; and the location of papillomas, warts, leaking edema, and/or subcutaneous fibrosis, folliculitis, and palpable nodes in the axillary or inguinal areas.

The presence of toenail fungus, presence or absence of pitting and subcutaneous fibrosis, presence or history of folliculitis, and palpable nodes in the axilla or inguinal areas should be noted.

Signs and symptoms of cording or axillary web syndrome may be present in individuals after axillary dissection (see Figs. 20-19 and 20-20). The therapist may palpate a firm cord-like structure extending from the axilla to the forearm or even to the wrist. These cords limit mobility of the shoulder and can significantly impair activities of daily living.[56,129,150]

Experts debate whether these are venous or lymphatic in origin or a combination of both structures, possibly caused by contracture of these vessels after being resected during axillary dissection.[159] The presence or absence of pain, paresthesias, or other sensory impairments is documented. Using a visual analogue scale of 0 to 10 is the easiest documentation for this assessment.

Role of Photography in Documentation

Photographs are helpful to detail changes in skin color and texture. If a digital camera is not available, high-speed film without flash is preferable to avoid distortion of color and shadows. Accurate circumferential measurements taken at fixed intervals with standardized positioning noted are often more helpful describing the limb segments than volumetric measurements that give a total difference in overall volume of the entire limb. Volumetric measurements are particularly helpful in cases of bilateral extremity edema when no "normal" limb can be used for comparison. There are no standardized measurement tools for truncal or head and neck lymphedema.

Photographs taken in fixed positions from a standardized height and distance are helpful to detail asymmetry. Hemi-circumferences of the trunk taken at intervals measured from the floor to specific heights can give a relative difference in volume if the swelling is unilateral. There are some reports of individual measurement strategies used to document head and neck edema.[47]

Documenting Functional Impairments

Careful documentation of the individual's functional impairments related to the lymphedema is key to evaluating the outcome of any treatment that is recommended.[48] Many individuals with chronic lymphedema have "learned to live with it" and often do not consider lymphedema as a "limitation." Tactful questioning can uncover the many compensating mechanisms employed to get through the day.[61]

Lymphedema and lymphedema treatment impact quality of life in many domains other than functional including psychologic, economic, and social. Therapist and client need to collaborate as a team to develop a strategy that affords the client the best outcome in all domains.[9,80,116,117]

Early Recognition of Lymphedema

A preoperative screening evaluation should record baseline measurements of both operative and non-operative extremities. Circumferential measurements taken with a flexible tape measure are the easiest, most economic measures to take. These measurements do assess the shape and contour of a limb more accurately than a volumetric measure; but volumetric measures are a more precise measure of total volume of a limb.

Volumes from circumferential measurements have a high validity when compared with volumes from water displacement, but they were slightly larger.[149] Tissue texture, unusual limb asymmetries or contours, skin color, strength, and functional range of motion are recorded.

Perometry, tonometry, and bioimpedance also have been utilized to quantify lymphedema. The perometer, an optoelectric device, calculates limb volume with infrared light that transects the limb every 3 mm. It can measure any part of a limb or limb segment and accurately calculate changes in volume in seconds. It is a valuable but expensive measurement tool. The tonometer measures tissue compliance, and the degree of compression provides an assessment of tissue fibrosis.[25]

Bioimpedance is another noninvasive technique that measures total body fluid and extracellular fluid in extremities by measuring the resistance of various tissues to the flow of an electrical current. It detects very small differences in the extracellular volumes of arms, suggesting that this technique may be able to diagnose lymphedema in its first stage, prior to the onset of visible swelling and discomfort.[42,44,135]

There is still no consensus on what amount of limb volume change defines lymphedema. However, lymphedema is not only defined by a change in limb volume. Sensations of limb heaviness, tightness, soreness, fatigue, and pain accompany subtle changes in limb volume that may or may not be readily detectable in the early stages of lymph stasis that occur on the continuum from latent lymphedema (Stage 0) to where obvious pitting edema is present in Stage I.

Further study needs to be done to examine these factors and their relationship to the progression of lymphedema.[6,7,61,116] Any sensory abnormalities or neurologic impairments are noted. Risk-reduction strategies with emphasis on proper skin hygiene and recognition of the early signs of lymphedema and secondary infection are reviewed with the individual.

A list of resources, including whom to contact should a problem arise (and when available), is provided to the individual. Discussion of individual activities of daily living and brief task analysis of job and home can point to possible problem areas that may need to be modified to reduce the risk of triggering lymphedema from "overuse" of the postoperative extremity or reduce potential exposure to trauma, chemicals, excessive heat, or repetitive tasks.

Physical Therapist's Intervention

Regardless of the training approach to lymphedema, several overall components of the following interventions may be modified, according to each individual client:

- *MLD*
- *Compression bandaging (CB)*
- *Exercise*
- *Compression garments*
- *Compression pumps (IPC)*
- *Education (e.g., basic anatomy, skin and nail care, self-MLD, self-bandaging, garment care, infection management)*
- *Psychologic and emotional support*

These components make up a treatment approach referred to as *comprehensive lymphedema management* that is the same for all the combined manual lymphatic therapies and is carried out in two distinct phases: the initial intensive intervention phase and the optimization phase. Different countries use different acronyms for this treatment approach; comprehensive lymphedema management is sometimes referred to as *complete decongestive therapy* (CDT); *combined decongestive physiotherapy* (CDP); *complex lymphedema/lymphatic therapy* (CLT); *decongestive lymphatic therapy* (DLT); or *complex physical therapy* (CPT). In the United States, the more common usage is CDT or CLT.

Initial Intensive Intervention Phase

During this phase of treatment, daily intervention requiring maximum adherence is often necessary to disperse lymph fluids through the superficial lymphatic vessel network and to prevent congestion of fluid in areas proximal to the compression bandages. Components of treatment include the following:

1. Meticulous skin care and treatment of any infections that may also include debridement of ulcers and wound care.
2. MLD: variations exist in specific stroke and pressure techniques such as Vodder, Leduc, Földi, Casley-Smith; however, all schools of thought work to decongest the trunk quadrants first before addressing the lymphedematous extremity/areas, decongesting the proximal portions of the limb first and progressively working distally to the end of the limb with the direction of flow always toward the trunk. Special strokes are available for fibrotic areas.
3. The affected limb or limbs are then bandaged with short-stretch compression bandages during the initial treatment phase and fitted with a compression garment at the completion of treatment.
4. Each individual is instructed in specific self-care, self-MLD techniques, and exercises that are modified for the individual. The basic principle is to enhance the lymphatic pumping and collateral lymph flow from the involved or impaired areas into adjacent, normally functioning areas and eventually into the trunk with return to the central circulation via the right lymphatic duct and the thoracic duct.[18,19,56,81]

Optimization Phase

During this second phase, the individual home program is finalized, continuing with the components of comprehensive lymphedema management from the initial intervention phase now modified for each person according to the clinical presentation and individual needs. During this phase, customized pressure gradient elastic support garments may replace compression bandaging when the limb is normal or close to normal. There are also inelastic compression garments with Velcro closures that are an option for night compression or for individuals who cannot manage elastic compression garments or prefer the ease of Velcro for donning and doffing.[80]

Components of Comprehensive Lymphedema Therapy

Considerable advances were made in the treatment of lymphedema after Kubik's detailed description of the regional anatomy of the lymphatic system published in 1985 (see Fig. 13-7). Földi and Földi reported the successful results of their techniques, referred to as CDP, documenting 50% reductions in lymphedema after a 4-week course of daily CDP. Of those individuals, 50% maintained that reduction by adhering to a home program of self-MLD; exercises; and continuous compression on the affected limb using compression garments or bandages.[52,53]

Casley-Smith and Casley-Smith presented results of another conservative treatment, referred to as CPT, reporting reductions of more than 60% in 618 lymphedematous limbs.[31]

Manual Lymph Drainage

Von Winiwarter first introduced the concepts of MLD in 1882. These techniques were improved by Vodder in the 1930s, but were originally applied to improve the functioning of normal lymphatics.[157] Moreover, the reductions in edema obtained with MLD in those early years could not be maintained because of a lack of adequate compression bandages and garments. The Vodder techniques were modified by Asdonk and Leduc and later by Földi and Casley-Smith.[29]

These major contributors have developed training programs to teach their methods; however, no standards are available in the United States for lymphedema training programs. The Lymphology Association of North America, a nonprofit organization composed of physicians, nurses, physical and occupational therapists, massage therapists, and researchers who specialize in lymphedema management, has developed standards for lymphedema therapists in the United States. This will help ensure access to adequate treatment for all individuals living with lymphedema.

The Education Committee of the International Lymphoedema Framework (www.lympho.org) continues to work with partner countries to determine core concepts in lymphology critical in health professional education both at the basic and advanced levels. The United States has representation on this committee by members of the American Lymphedema Framework (for more information visit http://www.alfp.org).

MLD, a gentle, manual treatment technique consisting of several basic strokes, is designed to improve the activity of intact lymph vessels by providing mild mechanical stretches on the wall of the lymph collectors. Some proponents of MLD advise against the use of the word *massage* (e.g., manual lymphatic massage or lymphatic drainage massage) because the term *massage* means "to knead." MLD does not have kneading elements and is generally applied suprafascially, whereas massage is usually applied to subfascial tissues.[55]

Compression Bandaging

Short-stretch Compression Bandages

Short-stretch compression bandages applied to the lymphedematous extremity after lymphatic drainage help maintain the edema reduction achieved through the lymph drainage (Fig. 13-19). Short-stretch

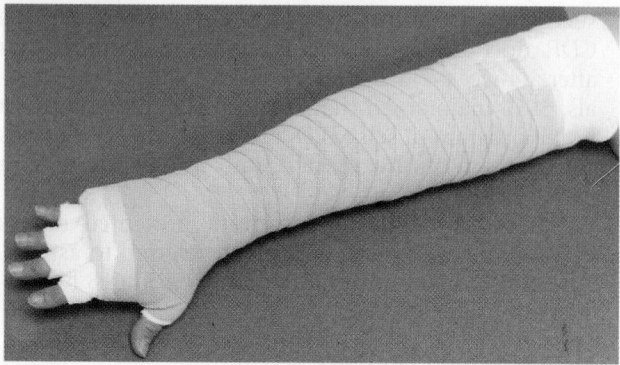

Figure 13-19

An example of multilayer short-stretch compression bandaging of the upper extremity. (Courtesy Lymphedema Therapy, Woodbury, NY.)

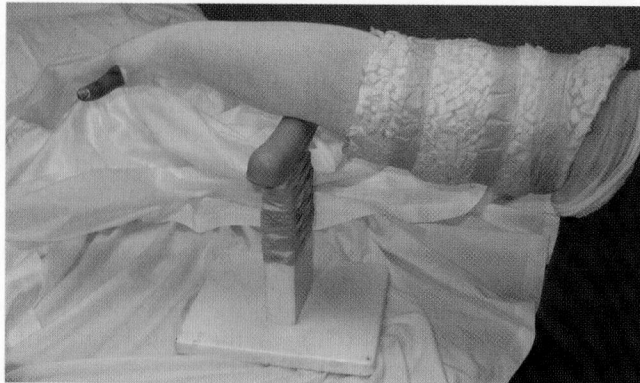

Figure 13-20

Example of therapist-made custom foam chip pads that are placed under the compression layer to soften fibrosis and reshape the limb. (Courtesy Lymphedema Therapy, Woodbury, NY.)

bandages have minimal recoil and only stretch 70% of their "unstretched" length. They have a low resting pressure (i.e., when the bandaged limb is at rest, they exert minimal pressure on the skin), avoiding any skin ischemia or breakdown.

Conversely, they have a high working pressure. When the muscles in the bandaged limb contract against the short-stretch bandage, the bandage provides a semirigid force, creating an increase in interstitial tissue fluid pressure, an increase in lymph uptake, and increased pumping of the collecting lymphatics. Consequently, these bandages are comfortable when the limb is at rest and greatly increase the transport of lymph when the limb is in motion.[45]

The effects of low-stretch compression bandaging alone and in combination with MLD can create an additional 11% reduction in arm lymphedema when MLD is added to compression bandaging.[70] An additional 20% limb volume reduction has been demonstrated in a group of women with breast cancer–related lymphedema when MLD was added to compression bandaging.[72] The same benefit was reported in a randomized controlled trial of 50 women with breast cancer–related lymphedema.[96]

Long-stretch Compression Bandages

Long-stretch compression bandages have a low working pressure and a high resting pressure; that is, they are not very effective in increasing the transport of lymph when the bandaged limb is moving and they can become dangerously tight when the limb is at rest, creating a tourniquet effect on the limb at rest. These are not the bandages of choice for the individual with lymphedema.

Proper bandaging techniques, using sufficient padding materials over bony prominences and to even out unusual limb contours, ensure that a gradient of pressure is achieved. This gradient must be greatest at the most distal point of the involved limb, gradually decreasing as the bandage layers reach the proximal portion of the limb. This gradient is particularly critical in limbs where large, balloon-like areas separated by a deep skinfold or ridge occur at a joint such as the ankle, knee, wrist, or elbow.

Maintaining a Proper Compression Gradient

According to the Laplace law, the pressure applied by the bandage is inversely proportional to the radius of the limb segment bandaged; that is, the smaller the radius of the limb segment, the greater is the pressure applied by the bandage. For example, when bandaging an upper extremity with significant edema in the dorsum of the hand but a narrow wrist relative to the hand and forearm, the wrist area must be sufficiently padded to increase the radius (of the wrist limb segment) to be larger than the radius of the hand. If this is not done, the bandaging may actually cause an increase in the edema in the dorsum of the hand.[32]

A proper compression gradient achieved with short-stretch bandages can increase tissue pressure, improve the activity of the lymphangion, and increase the efficiency of the muscle pump in the involved limb. It not only maintains the reduction in the involved limb that was achieved through lymph drainage; it can actually increase that reduction by enhancing the muscle pump during activity.[93]

In addition, the application of varying densities of foam pieces or "chips," encased in adhesive gauze, stockinet, or fabric may be applied under the compression bandages (Fig. 13-20).

Compression bandaging is usually worn 24 hours during the initial intensive phase of treatment, removed only for bathing and lymph drainage, and immediately reapplied. After the initial treatment phase, the individual is able to maintain adequate compression during the day with a compression garment. Getting the individual to understand that they must maintain some form of nighttime compression is the key to success in the optimization phase of the program.[19,74,75,80]

The short-stretch bandages, because of their low resting pressure and "customized" fit, provide the optimal nighttime compression. The drawback to these bandages is that self-bandaging is time consuming and difficult for the less mobile or obese individual or person with a very large, heavy limb.

Several "compression alternatives" are now available for this purpose that use various fabric "sleeves/leggings" with foam padding and Velcro closures for easier application. Results of one clinical study reported that individuals who wore their compression garments day and night maintained their reductions during the optimization phase.[19]

No skin problems or tissue breakdown resulted from wearing the garments to bed. It should be noted, however, that most of the involved individuals had custom-made, low-elastic garments that were not measured and fitted until the involved limbs were fully reduced (plateau in reduction).[19]

Exercise Guidelines

Lymph transport capacity can be impaired in 27% to 49% of individuals after breast cancer treatment.[77] The exact pathology and etiology of breast cancer–related lymphedema is thought to be multifactorial and not as simple as a "stop-cock" effect. The stop-cock effect is like putting a cork in a bottle. Various factors, such as cutting lymph vessels and nodes, have the stop-cock effect of impairing flow of lymph fluid. Likewise, venous impairment/impingement, the action of inflammatory mediators, and tissue changes related to late effects of radiation are other factors that may contribute to the development of breast cancer–related lymphedema because of this effect. Exercise helps mediate this effect.

Impairment in venous circulation from surgery and/or radiation treatment may contribute significantly to impaired fluid transport in the at-risk or affected limb.[77,138] Szuba et al[147] found clinically relevant venous stasis (on evaluation of 35 radiocontrast venograms) in 5 of 7 subjects with edema of the upper extremity and venous occlusion in 2 of 7 subjects with upper-extremity edema in a cohort of 365 subjects with lymphedema and suspected presence of mixed lymphatic and venous edema.[147] Again, exercise can be beneficial in facilitating decompression.

Exercise activates muscle groups and joints in the affected extremity. Combining a specific exercise program for each individual with the use of sufficient compression facilitates the process of decongestion by using the natural pumping effect of the muscles to increase lymph flow while preventing limb refilling.[36]

Most clinicians experienced in lymphedema treatment agree on basic guidelines for exercise. Any exercise program for the individual with lymphedema must follow the basic concepts of the combined approach—that is, work the trunk muscles first, followed by the limb girdle muscles, working from proximal to distal on the limb and finishing with trunk exercises and deep abdominal breathing to enhance flow through the thoracic duct.

Exercise should be performed with a compression garment or compression bandages on the involved limb(s) to enhance the variation in total tissue pressure to facilitate increased lymph flow. An increase in limb volume in individuals with lymphedema who are exercising with a compression sleeve has been observed in comparison with when exercise is performed without the sleeve.[71] The small increases in volume were measured immediately after exercise, and limb volume returned to baseline when measured again in 24 hours.[71]

In addition, therapists must remember that lymph load must not exceed lymph transport capacity or the exercise or activity will increase the lymphedema or possibly trigger lymphedema in a client with limbs at risk for lymphedema.[65,124–126]

Certain activities are considered higher risk for exacerbating lymphedema, such as running, jogging, stair climbing machines, sports involving ballistic type movements of the involved limbs such as tennis and racquetball, and activities with risk of traumatic sprain or strain injuries (e.g., karate, soccer, football, hockey, and downhill skiing). Activities such as brisk walking, cycling, swimming, cross country skiing, and tai chi are thought to be lower-risk activities.

Weight Training

Although weight training is not contraindicated, the progression of the program must be carefully monitored to avoid overload of the limbs or trunk, causing lymph congestion and subsequent exacerbation of the lymphedema.[65,124–126]

Ahmed et al found no increase in severity of lymphedema and no onset of lymphedema in 45 breast cancer survivors who participated in a program of weight training twice a week for 6 months.[1] These results suggest that participating in a resistive exercise program does not increase the risk for developing lymphedema or worsening lymphedema already present, although the follow-up of only 6 months is a very short time to conclude with certainty that individuals at risk would not develop lymphedema thereafter. Hayes et al conducted a pilot study on 32 subjects with breast cancer related lymphedema and found that after 6 months (3 months after the 12-week combined aerobic and resistance exercise intervention) the exercise did not exacerbate lymphedema.[65]

Participants received proper instruction in small groups to ensure that they performed proper warm-up, weight-training exercise, cool-down, and stretching exercises. Throughout the course of the study, participants exercised with constant access to fitness trainers when needed. The importance of individualized instruction and proper progression of any exercise program cannot be overemphasized.

Schmitz et al followed 141 breast cancer survivors (previously diagnosed with lymphedema) who participated in a supervised, twice-weekly weight-lifting program for 1 year.[126] Participants all wore compression garments on their affected arm and hand during the trial. Lymphedema did not worsen with the exercise, and participants reported improvement in arm and hand symptoms, reduction in exacerbations of their lymphedema, and improved upper-extremity strength.[124,126,137]

The follow-up study to this was published in 2010, following 154 breast cancer survivors (from 1 to 5 years postoperation) at risk for lymphedema who participated in a similar supervised weight-lifting exercise program. The reported incidence of lymphedema during the trial period was no greater for the exercise group than for the control group (11% vs. 17% and in women with ≥5 lymph nodes removed 7% exercise group vs. 22% control

A THERAPIST'S THOUGHTS
Exercise and Activity

Simply stated, the greater the intensity of the exercise, the greater the oxygen demand. With increased oxygen demand comes increased blood flow to the muscles, which provides the oxygen to do the work. Signs of limb "overload" are aching; congested, full feeling; discomfort in the proximal lymph nodal area (axilla or inguinal areas); pain; throbbing; or change in skin color. If any of these signs or symptoms occurs, the activity should be discontinued and the limb should be elevated and a cold compress applied. Deep breathing exercises and some self-lymph drainage may help decongest the trunk and limbs and reduce the discomfort.[101] The individual must learn to "listen" to his or her body and grade future activity accordingly to avoid overloading the system.[123]

group). This suggests that weight lifting does not increase the risk for breast cancer–related lymphedema.[125]

Turner et al followed 10 women after breast cancer treatment for 3 months after they participated in a moderate intensity exercise program consisting of mild strengthening exercises and cardiovascular exercises.[152] Participants reported a decrease in fatigue and improved quality of life with no precipitation or exacerbation of lymphedema.[152] Courneya et al conducted a multisite randomized controlled trial in Canada of 242 individuals treated for breast cancer who were beginning adjuvant chemotherapy.[43] One group (n = 82) received standard care, another (n = 82) supervised resistance exercises, and a third group (n = 78) supervised aerobic exercise for the 17 weeks that they were undergoing the chemotherapy. Cancer-related fatigue, quality of life, and lymphedema were measured. Neither aerobic nor resistance exercise was shown to trigger lymphedema in the study groups.[43] Further studies are needed in this area.[76]

Compression Garments

Compression garments were never designed to "treat and reduce" lymphedema but rather were meant to "hold" a limb that had already been reduced. Because lymphedema damages the elastic fibers of the skin, compression of the affected area is necessary to prevent reaccumulation of the lymphatic fluid.

Originally, compression garments were engineered to treat venous edema and were meant to be applied to the edema-free extremity before the individual got out of bed after a night of limb elevation. The same premise should apply to the lymphedematous extremity—that is, the edema must be reduced for the garment to work effectively.

Care must be given to the fit and function of the myriad of fabrics, compression grades, and styles available, with proper instruction given in donning and doffing. In addition, realistic expectations concerning these garments are a must to achieve client success and comfort.[19,27,50,54,91]

Clients need to understand that blood moves into the affected extremity with each beat of the heart approximately 60 to 70 times/min, 60 min/hr, 24 hr/day. When there is obstruction to lymph flow back to the central

circulation at a regional lymph node basin, the only way to assist that flow is to apply external pressure over the skin of the affected extremity on a continuous basis.

Compression garments are a means to achieve this, but they are only one component of a total self-care program. However, they are an essential component. For example, a client with lymphedema in the fingers, hand, and arm will not achieve good control of the lymphedema by wearing a wrist-to-axilla compression sleeve without a glove. In fact, wearing a compression sleeve without a glove in the presence of significant finger and hand edema will actually worsen that edema. Removing the compression sleeve may allow some of the hand swelling to shift into the forearm and make the hand appear "better" but that is not a solution to the problem—a well-fitting compression glove designed to wear with the compression sleeve is a more effective solution.

Designing, measuring, and fitting compression garments is as much art as it is science. What works for one client may be inappropriate for another. Experience and honest client/therapist communication lead to the best outcomes. Regular follow-up to evaluate the efficacy of the compression garments is important to determine when modifications in style or compression are needed to optimize client adherence.

Education and Home Program

Education begins on the first day of therapy intervention and is an absolutely essential part of both phases of the program. Remember the analogy to lanes on the highway in the "Pathogenesis" section of this chapter? Using this visualization (or others you may develop yourself), the clients gain an understanding of the physiologic reasons why they are doing what they are doing for each component of therapy. It is this understanding that helps them carry through on discharge into their home program. The success of any combined lymphedema treatment program hinges on adherence with the home maintenance program.[117]

Client education includes instruction in the basic anatomy and physiology of the lymphatic system, the pathophysiology of the individual's particular lymphedema, individual self-drainage pathways to follow during the exercise program, basic principles of the individual exercise program, the risk of infection and how to reduce that risk, wear and care instruction for compression bandages or garments, and individual skin care regimens.

Hands-on instruction in self-bandaging techniques requires practice and patience but is essential for the individual to master. In the home maintenance phase after initial intensive, treatment, skin care, and risk reduction and management of infection are three of the most important components of the home program. Psychologic support, including support groups, is another critical component of a comprehensive lymphedema management program.

Importance of Compliance

Maintaining reductions of lymphedema has been documented with adherence to a home program of skin

A THERAPIST'S THOUGHTS

Common Sense Explanations to Facilitate Adherence to Compression Garments and Exercise/Self-MLD

Lymphedema results when lymph load (the amount of lymph fluid to be moved) exceeds the ability of the system to move that fluid (lymph transport capacity). Lymph transport capacity can be impaired by damage or removal of lymph vessels and or nodes (as in secondary lymphedema) or by maldevelopment of lymph vessels or nodes (as in primary lymphedema).

To expand on the analogy of lymph fluid being like cars on a highway where the lanes/toll booths are the lymph vessels/nodes mentioned earlier in the chapter, consider this next idea. If the client imagines that 3 of 6 toll booths are suddenly shut down, the same number of cars have to pass through so traffic (lymph) backs up. Once the initial backlog is cleared, traffic may start to move again, but very slowly, inching along (lymphedema is decreased by treatment and compression garments are worn). Now someone jams on their brakes (compression garment is removed) and traffic (lymph) backs up again. The only way to keep traffic moving is to keep that slow flow going consistently (wear compression garment and perform self-MLD daily) so that lymph load does not exceed lymph transport capacity.

Once traffic backs up, it takes a long time to get it going again, and sometimes it never gets back to normal (an exacerbation of lymphedema related to infection, injury, recurrent malignant disease, or non-adherence to self-care may not resolve). Modi et al showed this in individuals who had breast cancer–related lymphedema.[97] They applied a blood pressure cuff to the affected arms and showed that when they decreased the pressure in the cuff, the lymph did not begin to flow in the affected arm until much later and at a lower pressure than their unaffected arm. When the affected arm is constricted and flow is stopped, it takes a lot longer for the flow to begin again once the constriction is removed. Lymphedema not only worsens but when the constriction is removed, resumption of flow is slow so more interstitial fluid is building up and not moving out of the tissues, again because the resumed flow is so slow.

So, even if some of the toll booths open again (collateral lymph flow; person does self-MLD and puts compression bandages or garment back on) the signal person does not let the cars start to drive through again for another few minutes so more cars (lymph) back up even though some lanes have reopened—so more of a back-up than before and longer for the traffic (lymph flow) to get back to its "normal" flow, which, in the case of a limb with lymphedema, is slow to begin with. Clients who understand this concept have an easier time adhering to their self-care program of exercise and compression garment wear because they know how it affects their lymphedema.

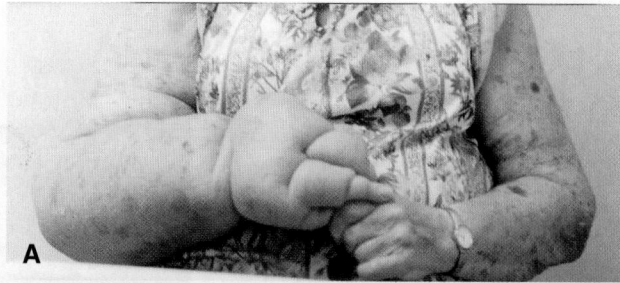
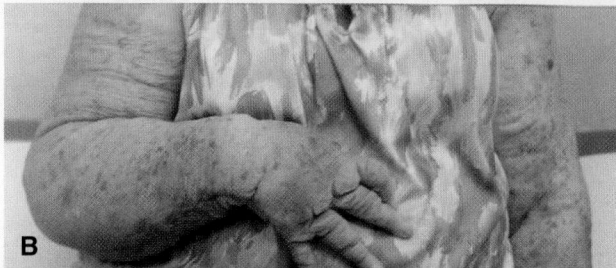
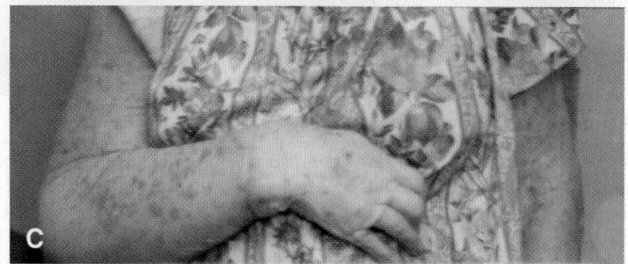

Figure 13-21

A, Before treatment, an 84-year-old woman with severe, elephantitic lymphedema of her right upper extremity for 20 years, secondary to surgery and radiation treatment for breast cancer 30 years ago. Her right hand was essentially nonfunctional. She needed assistance in all areas of activities of daily living (ADLs). **B,** After 20 complete decongestive therapy (CDT) treatments, she has achieved a 77% reduction in the lymphedema in her right upper extremity and has begun to use her right hand functionally again. **C,** Four years after CDT treatment. She follows through with a home exercise program, skin care, and compression garment wear. She has not had any additional treatments other than the initial 20, and she has improved her reduction to almost 100% in the years after treatment. She is more independent in ADLs and can even don her compression glove and sleeve with minimal assistance. (Courtesy Lymphedema Therapy, Woodbury, NY.)

Intermittent Pneumatic Compression–Compression Pumps

Historically in the United States, a person with lymphedema was given a prescription for a compression garment and range-of-motion exercises. In some cases, treatment with a pneumatic compression pump (also known IPC) was prescribed as the edema progressed. The degree and intensity of this treatment varied greatly because of the lack of verified, long-term scientific studies proving the efficacy of one treatment form over another.

Treatment with pneumatic compression consisted of placing the involved limb into a rubber sleeve that inflated with air from the pump, squeezing the limb, and moving fluid proximally toward the trunk. Olszewski et al studied the effect of applying intermittent pneumatic compression on the movement of lymph

care, exercise with self-lymphatic drainage, and compression garment wear. Significant decreases in microlymphatic hypertension (measured by fluorescence microlymphography and lymph capillary pressure measurement), decreases in extremity lymphedema, and improvements in lymphoscintigraphic findings have been reported after a course of CDT.[57,66] Individuals with less than 100% adherence with their home program lose a portion of their reductions (Figs. 13-21, 13-22, and 13-23).[19,75,79]

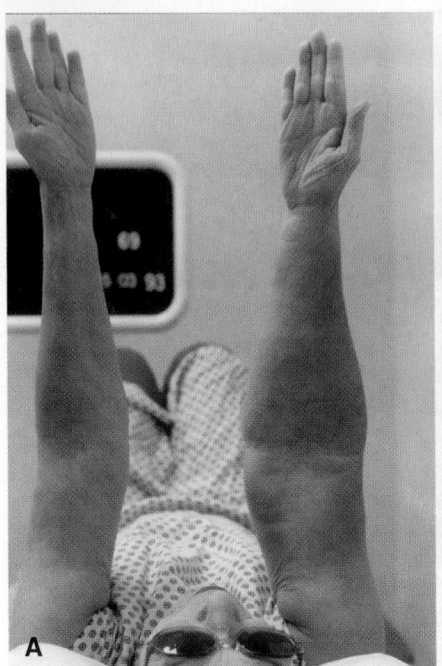
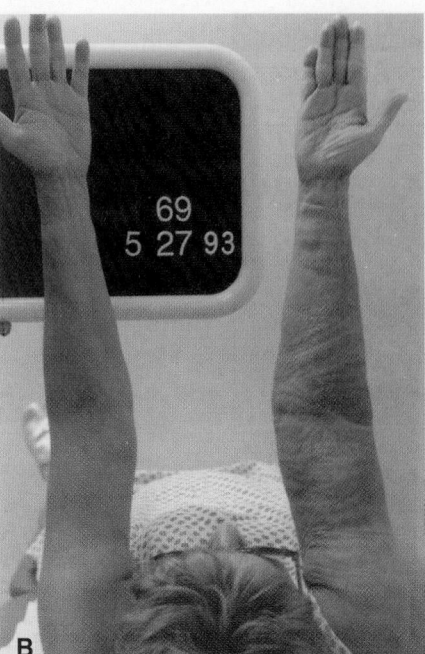
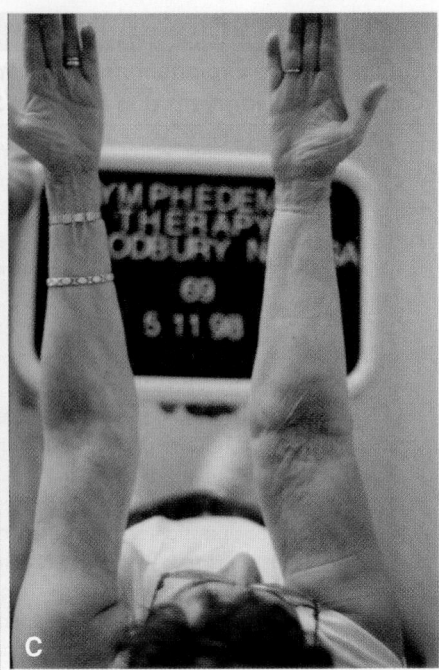

Figure 13-22

A, Before treatment, a 69-year-old woman with Stage II lymphedema of the right upper extremity of 20 years' duration, secondary to breast cancer surgery and treatment. For the past few years, she has had recurrent cellulitis infections in the right arm with hospitalization several times per year to receive IV antibiotics. **B,** After 18 complete decongestive therapy (CDT) treatments, she achieved a 57% reduction in the lymphedema in the right upper extremity. The wrinkling in her forearm and upper arm is from the compression bandaging, which was removed shortly before taking this photograph. These wrinkles are only temporary. Note the significant reduction in lymphedema. **C,** Five years after CDT treatment. She has improved the reduction in the lymphedema of her right upper extremity to 64%. She has had no additional treatment for her lymphedema, but she follows her home program of self-massage, exercise, skin care, and compression garment wear. She has had only two cellulitis infections in the past 5 years that were treated successfully with only oral antibiotics. Note the reshaping of the forearm and upper arm since previous photos were taken. (Courtesy Lymphedema Therapy, Woodbury, NY.)

in 15 individuals with lower-extremity lymphedema caused by obstruction.[108] They found that IPC moved an isotope in lymph that remained in functioning lymphatics and in tissue fluid in the interstitial spaces toward the inguinal region but lymph did not cross the inguinal crease into the pelvis/abdomen. It collected at the proximal thigh.[108] Pumps available in single or multichamber models can apply pressures from 10 to 100 mm Hg; the walls of the superficial lymphatics may collapse with greater than 60 mm Hg pressure.[20,28,49,51]

Significant discrepancies have been found between target pressures set on the compression device control dial (30, 60, 80, or 100 mm Hg), and the actual pressures measured inside the cuff chamber (54, 98, 121, or 141 mm Hg). It has been recommended that the devices be set at much lower target pressures (<30 mm Hg) than those typically applied in clinical practice.[127]

Newer devices have added a truncal appliance that provides programmable compression to the trunk and lymph node basins at the root of the treated limb to prepare the trunk to receive fluid from the treated limb.

Skin Care

Generally, for most people, an hour a day spent on exercise and garment care is reasonable for this condition. It is reasonable to spend 20 minutes twice daily on exercise and self-massage and another 20 minutes on skin care and washing or caring for compression garments. The better the individual understands the pathophysiology of the lymphedema, the greater the adherence.

Instruction in skin care includes the use of low pH or neutral pH soaps, cleansers, and moisturizers; the proper care of nails on finger and toes (see Table 13-2 and Box 12-14); use of topical antibiotic or antifungal preparations; and instruction in skin hygiene and compression garment/bandage washing for good hygiene.

The normal pH of healthy skin is acidic (less than 7.0) and accounts for the waterproof barrier of the skin surface. Repeated use of alkaline soaps and cleansers on the skin will result in the loss of this waterproof property, drying the skin and causing microscopic cracks in the skin surface, increasing the likelihood of bacterial invasion.

The elements of a personal first aid kit, including oral and topical nonprescription or prescription antibiotics, adhesive bandages, and alcohol wipes, are discussed. The client is instructed to carry this kit whenever traveling. For older adults, poorly mobile individuals, or the visually impaired person, a caregiver can be instructed in how to inspect the lymphedematous limb or area daily for signs of skin irritation or infection. A large magnifying mirror on a long handle

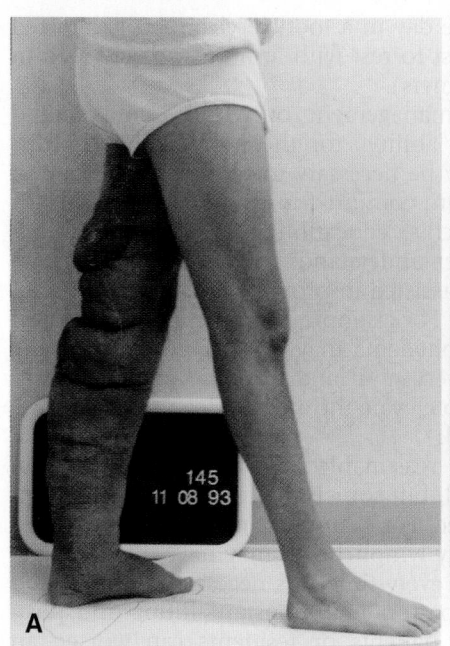
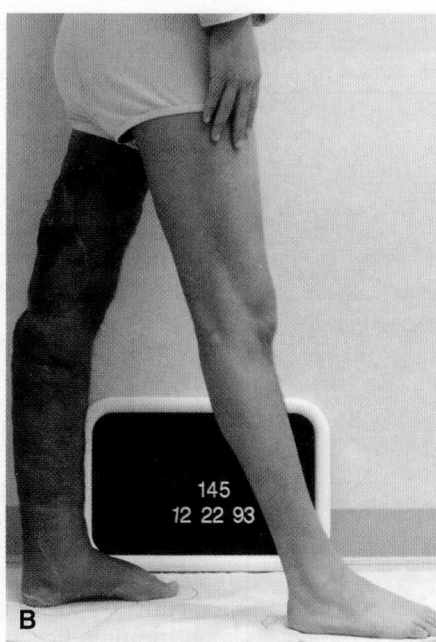
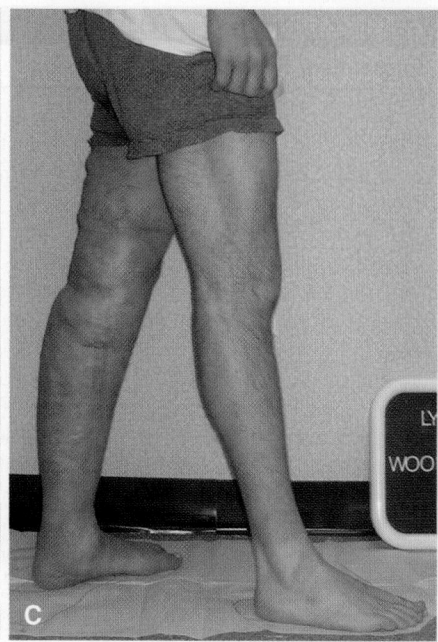

Figure 13-23

A, Before treatment, a 19-year-old male with severe Stage II primary lymphedema of the left lower extremity, progressing to the left buttock and genitals, with chylous reflux to the scrotum, buttock, and thigh. The onset of the edema was at age 8 years (see Fig. 13-11). He spent most of his high school years in and out of the hospital. In the 24 months before treatment, he was hospitalized 22 times for cellulitis in the left lower extremity and placed in the intensive care unit (ICU) with septic shock three times. **B,** After one course of complete decongestive therapy (CDT) of 30 treatments interrupted by a 2-week hospitalization (1 week in ICU) for cellulitis of the left leg and buttock with severe chylous leakage from the scrotum, buttock, and thigh. This individual went into septic shock and needed hyperalimentation to treat the hypoproteinemia (that resulted from the chylous leakage) via a central venous line. Despite the massive increase in swelling and open areas on the posterior left thigh and buttock resulting from the cellulitis, he achieved a 67% reduction in the lymphedema of his left lower extremity with reductions in the abdominal, suprapubic, and genital swelling as well. **C,** Twelve-and-a-half years after CDT. Note that some increase in the girth of the left lower extremity has occurred, particularly in the areas just proximal and distal to the knee, where the tissues are lax from the original debulking surgery. These areas fill in quickly without compression. Some of the girth increase is due to weight gain, now that he no longer has recurrent cellulitis and the chylous reflux is under control. This young man, having spent his high school years in and out of the hospital, was able to complete his college degree and is now a registered nurse working in an emergency department. Since his CDT treatment, he has made his lymphedema management home program a priority in his life and continues to maintain a 60% reduction in the lymphedema in his left lower extremity. (Courtesy Lymphedema Therapy, Woodbury, NY.)

or a full length wall mirror can assist clients to inspect the back of their limbs/torso/side of body for signs of impaired skin integrity.

No absolute dos and don'ts are available, but people must be cautioned to prevent lymph overload in their work and home activities. Each individual must weigh the risk level of each activity and learn what is safe for him or her. Typically, most time is spent teaching the client self-massage, exercise, and bandaging techniques.

Although consistency in using these techniques is very important, many people suffer exacerbation of the lymphedema from an infection or skin problem, necessitating removal of the compression garment. These incidents can be minimized if the individual knows what to look for and how to proceed when an infection occurs. Knowing the procedure for an emergency visit, who to contact, and how to advocate for their own care within the medical system should be discussed and reviewed at the time of discharge and at subsequent follow-up visits.[78]

If an infection develops, a decision must be made whether to remove compression garments or bandages, discontinue any lymphatic drainage, and discontinue exercise until the infection is under control.

When an infection is diagnosed in the very early stages (e.g., minor erythema may be present without pain or fever), the physician may recommend continuing use of the compression garments if tolerated to avoid any significant increase in limb size.

Every situation is individual and unique and requires consultation with the physician and the therapist before making any changes in the management program. Any sign or symptom of infection always requires immediate medical attention.

Guidelines for Job and Lifestyle Modifications

The same principles for exercise also apply to pacing and modifying work activities and activities of daily living to avoid overload. Affected individuals do not necessarily have to give up a job just because lymphedema has been diagnosed. Cooperative discussion may be helpful between the therapist, the client, and the client's supervisor to implement simple task modifications ensuring client safety and comfort at work.

Some work requirements may have to be reduced, modified, or eliminated, and the supervisor should be aware of any special needs the employee may have (e.g., the need to wear compression garments and to protect them with constant changes of vinyl gloves

A THERAPIST'S THOUGHTS

Intermittent Pneumatic Compression

Not all IPC devices are the same. It is important for the clinician to be familiar with the specific parameters and pressures provided by each unit to determine what unit best fits the individual goals of a client's treatment plan.[92,93]

In the presence of soft-tissue injury, vigorous massage or the use of compression pumps at pressures higher than 60 mm Hg can cause severe damage to the walls of the initial lymphatic vessels (possibly by tearing the anchoring microfilaments mentioned earlier). This collapse of the initial lymphatic walls impairs lymphatic transport capacity and results in lymphedema and extravasation of lymphedema into an adjacent trunk quadrant.[20]

Atrophy or hypertrophy of the skin can further compromise lymphatic function as a result of the loss of elasticity. A network of collagen and elastin fibers surrounding the lymphatic system helps the skin respond to movement so any variable that can damage the lymph system of the skin (e.g., aging, chronic sun exposure, or prolonged use of systemic steroids) compromises the response of the tissues to movement caused by massage or pneumatic compression.

The resultant injury to the blood vessels and lymphatics causes fluid and protein to leak from the damaged vessels, setting up a chronic inflammatory response potentially leading to permanent fibrosclerotic changes.[121] These fibrosclerotic changes further compromise oxygen perfusion in the tissues, resulting in a repetitive cycle of hypoxia and chronic inflammation,[3,106] which is the perfect environment for bacterial and fungal infections to flourish. In addition, IPC treatment protocols require daily use for hours per day, physically and psychologically restricting the person who is "tied to the machine" for hours at a time.

Although IPC can be helpful in early Stage I lymphedema, when simple elevation overnight usually reduces the edema, they may be less helpful in Stage II fibrotic lymphedema. Although the pumps increase the reabsorption of water by the venous system, they do not move the extracellular protein because these molecules are too large to enter the venous fenestrae. Proteins must be transported via the lymphatics.

This is a situation that may trigger more fluid to filter into the tissue spaces, diluting the concentrated protein and ultimately increasing the edema. The higher protein concentration remaining in the tissues also causes the chronic inflammatory response discussed earlier, triggering the development of more subcutaneous fibrosis. The vicious cycle of lymphedema repeats itself. The chronic inflammatory response increases the individual's risk of developing secondary infections (cellulitis/lymphangitis).

Therapists should monitor truncal measurements in addition to full limb measurements when treating individuals with IPC. Excessive shear on the skin of a lymphedematous limb or a limb at risk from vigorous massage or from a compression pump exceeding 60 mm Hg compression may tear the fragile anchoring microfilaments and collapse the initial lymphatic walls, advancing a preexisting lymphedema or triggering lymphedema in a limb at risk.

IPC used at lower pressures may be effective for immobile individuals who sit for prolonged periods with their legs in the dependent position, provided they don't have comorbid conditions that contraindicate the use of IPC such as congestive heart failure, active infection, malignant disease in the limb to be treated, or deep vein thromboses.[110]

throughout the day in a food service job or the need for a hair stylist to rest with arm or arms elevated in between customers).

Successful management of lymphedema should mean greater "ability" for the individual, not "disability." It may be necessary to modify a workstation to provide more comfort for the individual with leg edema. Interactive education is the key to success. If the employer understands the problem of lymphedema and is assisted in providing a simple solution, everyone wins. For example, an individual with lower extremity lymphedema may need to get up from the workstation every hour and walk around for 5 minutes. A place to elevate the affected leg under the desk may be needed.

Requesting reasonable accommodations is an important goal, but sometimes, certain job tasks cannot be modified. For example, a nurse with significant upper-extremity lymphedema may have difficulty getting assistance every time it is necessary to move and lift a patient or resident. Constant lifting and positioning heavy patients or residents can worsen an upper-extremity lymphedema. In such cases, the decision rests with the individual whether a job change is needed or whether it will be necessary to stay and make the best of things.

Psychosocial Considerations and Quality of Life

Great emphasis has been given to the myriad of physical symptoms and resulting impairments associated with lymphedema. Little is reported on the psychologic distress these individuals must suffer on a daily basis. People are curious about the change in size and shape of the affected limb.

Individuals are faced with tremendous alterations in body image, often deal with chronic pain and impaired mobility/function and many feel embarrassed. Some are scorned by a public perception that they are deformed or distorted. Some feel that their job security may be threatened because of their appearance or the perception that they "cannot do the job."[41,61] Those with severe leg lymphedema with chronic infections and ulcerations may leak lymphatic fluid from their limbs and experience public humiliation when people turn away from them in fear and ignorance.

Affected individuals become prisoners in their own homes, too embarrassed or afraid to go out in public. Many are judged by others who do not understand "how this could happen" and why it was not "taken care of." Individuals living with lymphedema have experienced tremendous guilt and self-doubt in the past.

Many people were told by numerous medical professionals, "There is nothing to be done; just learn to live with it." Even today, there are some physicians and therapists in this country who still tell individuals with lymphedema that not much can be done except to "elevate the limb and wear loose long sleeves or long pants."

Clinicians and researchers are realizing that individuals with lymphedema need tremendous psychologic support to cope with the problems associated with living with such a chronic condition.[96,105] Today,

---

Box 13-2

IMPORTANT RESOURCES IN THE TREATMENT OF LYMPHEDEMA*

- American Cancer Society
  In 1998, the American Cancer Society sponsored an international meeting on breast cancer–related lymphedema in New York City. Lymphologists from all over the world met and discussed current diagnosis, treatment, management, resources, professional education, and advocacy. The results from that meeting are published in Lymphedema: results from a workshop on breast cancer, treatment-related lymphedema, and lymphedema resource guide, *Cancer* 83:2775–2890, 1998. Available from the American Cancer Society: (800) 231-5355.
  www.cancer.org
- American Lymphedema Framework Project (ALFP)
  www.alfp.org
- American Physical Therapists Association (APTA): Oncology Section—Lymphedema Special Interest Group (SIG)
  www.oncologypt.org
- Casley Smith International (CSI)
  www.casleysmithinternational.org
- International Lymphoedema Framework Project (ILF)
  www.lympho.org
- International Society of Lymphology (ISL)
  The University of Arizona
  College of Medicine
  University Medical Center
  1510 North Campbell Avenue
  Tucson, AZ 85724
  (520) 626-6118
  FAX: (520) 626-0822
  www.u.arizona.edu/~witte/ISL.htm
  A quarterly journal is available on international research on lymphedema.
- Lymphoedema Association of Australia (LAA)
  www.lymphoedema.org.au.
- Lymphology Association of North America (LANA)
  www.clt-lana.org
- The Lymphatic Education & Research Network
  40 Garvies Point Road (Suite D)
  Glen Cove, New York 11542
  (516) 625-9675
  FAX (516) 625-9410
  www.lymphaticresearch.org.
  e-mail contact: lfr@lymphaticresearch.org
- Lymphovenous Canada
  Lymphovenous News is published by Lymphophenous Association of Ontario.
  Available at http://www.lymphovenous-canada.ca/treatont.htm.
- National Lymphedema Network, Inc.
  116 New Montgomery Street, Suite 235
  San Francisco, CA 94105
  Hotline: (800) 541-3259
  Direct: (415) 908-3681
  FAX: (415) 908-3813
  www.lymphnet.org.
  A quarterly newsletter is available.

*The listing of any particular program or the omission of others does not denote support or preference for one method of lymphedema intervention over another. This list of resources is meant to guide the interested therapist to further information.

---

innovative lymphedema treatment programs offer support groups (Box 13-2). The National Lymphedema Network, an advocacy organization, hosts a biannual educational conference offering workshops and an opportunity to network with other affected individuals and health care providers who specialize in lymphology (the study of the lymphatic system). Patient advocates supported by lymphedema specialists offer online education and outreach to individuals who may not have access to specialty care in their communities (visit http://www.stepup-speakout.org).

Radina and Armer studied women's coping strategies and found that "the potential 'pile up' of stressors leading to vulnerability after breast cancer treatment lymphedema reported by participants included modification of daily household and work-related tasks, living with a constant reminder of the cancer, and feelings of abandonment by medicine." They state that "resiliency. . .is characterized as adjustment, adaptation, or crisis" and suggest that practitioners "need to serve the patient and the family."[114] This is particularly true for the older adult cancer survivor. Older adults may have multiple medical comorbidities that cause chronic impairments in mobility and function that affect their ability to undergo an intensive treatment program, as well as to adhere to an ongoing self-care program for lymphedema.[9]

Great strides are being made in recognizing lymphedema as a condition that deserves to be acknowledged and treated early and aggressively. Theoretically, all clinicians know that psychologic support is crucial to success in managing a chronic illness or condition. However, having the practical applications in place to help the individual takes a tremendous commitment in personal time and financial resources. Nevertheless, a successful lymphedema treatment program must offer ongoing support and follow-up care.

Lymphadenitis

Infections elsewhere in the body can lead to lymphadenopathy as described previously. When the lymph node becomes overwhelmed by the infection, the lymph node itself can become infected; this is called *lymphadenitis.* Lymphadenitis can be classified as acute or chronic; acutely inflamed lymph nodes are most common locally in the cervical region in association with infections of the teeth or tonsils or in the axillary or inguinal regions secondary to infection of the extremities.

In acute lymphadenitis, the lymph nodes are enlarged, tender, warm, and reddened. In the case of chronic lymphadenitis, longstanding infection from a variety of sources results in scarred lymph nodes with fibrous connective tissue replacement. The nodes are enlarged and firm to palpation but not warm or tender. The management of lymphadenitis is treatment of the underlying disorder.

Lymphangitis and Cellulitis

Lymphangitis, an acute inflammation of the subcutaneous lymphatic channels, usually occurs as a result of hemolytic streptococci or staphylococci (or both) entering the lymphatic channels from an abrasion or local trauma, wound, or infection (usually cellulitis; see further discussion of cellulitis in Chapter 10). The involvement of the lymphatics is often first observed as a red streak under the skin (referred to in layperson terms as *blood poisoning*), radiating from the infection site in the direction of the regional lymph nodes.

The red streak may be very obvious, or it may be very faint and easily overlooked, especially in dark-skinned people. The nodes most commonly affected are submandibular, cervical, inguinal, and axillary, in that order. Involved nodes are usually tender and enlarged (greater than 3 cm).

Systemic manifestations may include fever, chills, malaise, and anorexia. Other symptoms may present in association with the underlying infection located elsewhere in the body. Bacteremia from any cause can result in suppurative arthritis (inflammatory with pus formation), osteomyelitis, peritonitis, meningitis, or visceral abscesses.

When cellulitis results in lymphangitis, throbbing pain occurs at the site of bacterial invasion, and the client presents with a warm, edematous extremity (or possible scrotal lymphedema in males and occasionally vulvar lymphedema in females).

MEDICAL MANAGEMENT: INTACT LYMPHATIC SYSTEM

DIAGNOSIS. Lymphangitis may be confused with superficial thrombophlebitis, but the erythema associated with lymphangitis is first seen as a red streak under the skin radiating toward the regional lymph nodes (usually ascending proximally), whereas the erythema associated with thrombosis is usually over the thrombosed vein with local induration and inflammation.

However, suppurative thrombophlebitis may develop if bacteria are introduced during IV therapy, especially when the needle or catheter is left in place for more than 48 hours. The physician also needs to differentiate cellulitis from soft-tissue infections (e.g., gangrene or necrotizing fasciitis) that may require early and aggressive incision and resection of necrotic infected tissue.

Anyone with a history of vascular disease taking anticoagulant medication should have a Doppler ultrasound to rule out deep vein thrombosis before being treated. Laboratory tests are often not required but may include blood culture (often positive for staphylococcal or streptococcal species) and culture and sensitivity studies on the wound exudate or pus.

TREATMENT AND PROGNOSIS. Prompt parenteral antibiotic therapy is mandatory because bacteremia and systemic toxicity develop rapidly once organisms reach the bloodstream via the thoracic duct. Antibiotic treatment may be accompanied by general measures such as heat, elevation, immobilization of the infected area, and analgesics for pain.

Appropriate wound care may include drainage of the pus from an infected wound when it is clear that an abscess is associated with the site of initial infection. An area of cellulitis should not be excised because the infection may be spread by attempted drainage when pus is not present. Treatment as described should be effective against invading bacteria within a few days.

MEDICAL MANAGEMENT: INFECTIONS WITH IMPAIRED AND AT-RISK LYMPHATIC SYSTEM AND LYMPHEDEMA

DIAGNOSIS. Confusion of cellulitis or lymphangitis with thrombophlebitis in the individual with lymphedema or at risk for lymphedema is common and has a disastrous impact on the severity of the lymphedema. An episode of cellulitis or lymphangitis often triggers the development of lymphedema in the individual who is at risk but has no clinical signs of edema. Improper, inadequate treatment of these infections can lead to chronic infection or inflammation and progression of the lymphedema.

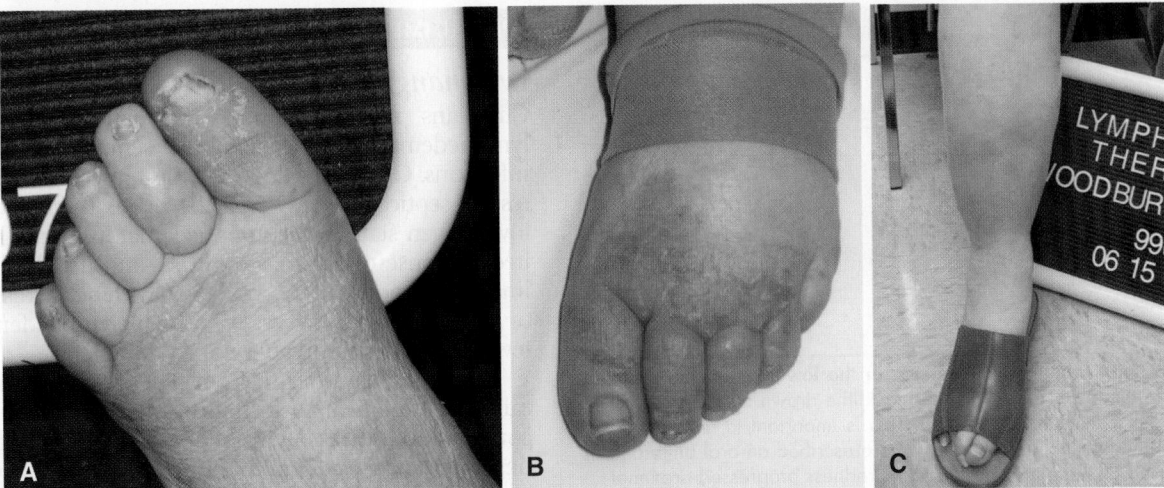

Figure 13-24

A, Cellulitis of the left great toe/forefoot secondary to an ingrown toenail in a man with diabetes and lymphedema in the lower extremities secondary to chronic venous insufficiency. **B,** Cellulitis of the left toes/foot in a woman with primary lymphedema of the left-lower extremity. This young woman often worked double shifts as a waitress. Her foot would swell and the skin would become irritated/blistered in her shoe causing recurrent infections of the left foot/leg accompanied by fever, chills, malaise and pain. A change in footwear resulted in a marked reduction in frequency of the infections. **C,** Cellulitis right lower leg secondary to an insect bite in a woman with lymphedema secondary to pelvic lymph node dissection and radiation to treat cervical cancer. (Courtesy Lymphedema Therapy, Woodbury, NY.)

The individual who has had regional lymph node dissection and/or radiation has an impaired immune response in the areas that drain to that regional nodal area. Consequently, infection can spread rapidly in those regions and any delay in treatment while awaiting blood cultures and vascular tests can cause progression of the infection.

The combination of the impaired nodal area and the inactivity of the macrophages in the lymphedematous region allows the bacteria to multiply rapidly, feeding on the high protein lymphedema fluid. It is not uncommon for a person to develop a high fever with shaking chills (40.5° C [105° F]) within 30 minutes of "feeling ill" or "feeling an ache or pain" in the lymphedematous region. It is not acceptable for these people to "wait and see" and call their physician in a day or two. They must be seen and evaluated by a physician immediately to rule out thrombosis versus cellulitis or lymphangitis and initiate appropriate treatment immediately.

The more insidious onset of local infection (cellulitis) may manifest with an area of redness on the skin that looks like a rash or sunburn. The area may be warm to touch but not initially painful, and the individual may not develop any pain or fever. In fact, cellulitis is often mistaken for an allergic reaction, thought to be a reaction to an insect bite, or a local reaction to a sprain or strain, even when these triggers were not present (Fig. 13-24).

Individuals with advanced Stage II and Stage III lymphedema may develop recurrent cellulitis that is mistaken for "normal" skin changes associated with chronic lymphedema (Fig. 13-25).

TREATMENT AND PROGNOSIS. Treatment of cellulitis or lymphangitis in the individual with lymphedema or at risk for lymphedema differs from treatment of these conditions in the individual with an intact lymphatic system. In a healthy individual, cellulitis and lymphangitis

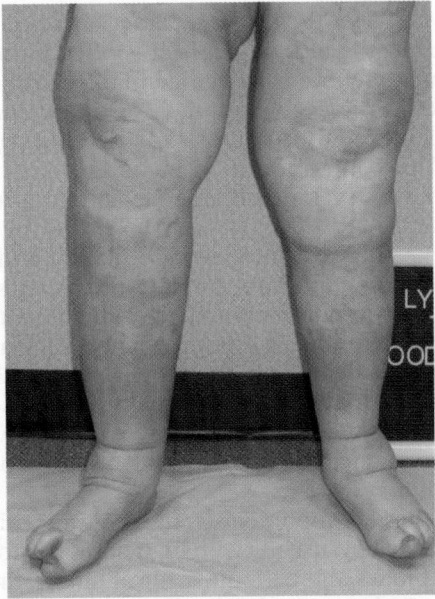

Figure 13-25

This individual had suffered from pain, increased swelling, and itching of the skin on both legs for months. She had suffered from swollen ankles and feet as a teen and the swelling had worsened as she aged. She had seen a vascular surgeon who performed Doppler studies and ruled out deep vein thrombosis but had no diagnosis for her problem. She had seen a dermatologist who diagnosed a contact dermatitis and prescribed topical cortisone cream. Luckily, her podiatrist referred her to a lymphedema specialist who promptly diagnosed primary lymphedema of both legs, complicated by cellulitis. (Courtesy Lymphedema Therapy, Woodbury, NY.)

are relatively rare. Many cases of primary lymphedema are missed in young individuals who present with unexplained recurrent cellulitis in the absence of injury or trauma. Recurring cellulitis does not develop unless some underlying pathology is causing it (usually primary lymphedema).

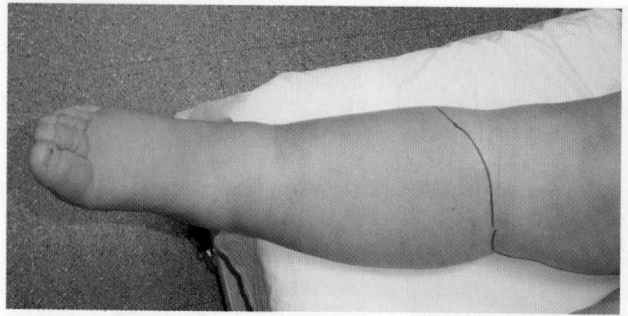

Figure 13-26

Individual with primary lymphedema in the lower extremities with cellulitis in the lower leg. Note the black line drawn by the therapist to mark the extent of the infection. This is important to monitor the course of the infection. The person was prescribed an oral antibiotic and advised by the physician that if the redness progressed proximal to the black line, she must go to the emergency room and be assessed for intravenous antibiotics. Note the severity of the swelling and fibrosis of the toes. Examination of the skin between her toes revealed that she had a fungal infection that caused the skin to macerate and crack. Bacteria can then enter the broken skin and cause a secondary bacterial infection. This is a common problem in people with lymphedema of the lower extremities. (Courtesy Lymphedema Therapy, Woodbury, NY.)

In the healthy individual, heat is often prescribed as an adjunct to relieve pain in the inflamed area, whereas heat should *never* be applied to individuals with lymphedema or those at risk for developing lymphedema. This contraindication includes those individuals who have developed lymphedema after orthopedic surgeries.

Local heating will increase vasodilation and ultrafiltration of more fluid into the interstitial spaces, further overloading the decompensated lymphatic transport capacity, exacerbating the existing lymphedema, or possibly triggering lymphedema in the limb at risk, where no clinical lymphedema existed before the onset of the infection. Rest and immobilization of the involved areas are recommended measures. Cold can be applied to relieve pain.

Experienced lymphologists initiate immediate oral antibiotic therapy, usually with high doses of broad-spectrum antibiotics and periodic medical monitoring in the first 48 to 72 hours to observe the area for spread of the infection. It is imperative that the original area of redness be outlined with indelible marker to check on the progress or regression of the infection (Fig. 13-26).

If a poor response to the oral antibiotics is evident, hospitalization for IV antibiotics may be necessary. A local infection can progress to septic shock if not treated effectively. A common cause of recurrent cellulitis or lymphangitis is poor, inadequate treatment of a previous infection. A common complaint is recurrent infection in the same area of the same limb every 2 to 3 weeks. In fact, this is more likely the same infection that was never eradicated the first time. Cases like this often have a common history of administration of too short (3 to 5 days) or inadequate doses of oral antibiotics to treat the cellulitis or lymphangitis associated with lymphedema.

SPECIAL IMPLICATIONS FOR THE THERAPIST   13-3

Lymphangitis and Cellulitis

Clinicians must remember the pathophysiology of lymphedema to understand the seriousness of these infections. Obviously, not every local infection will progress to septicemia. However, the risk is there, given the low oxygen state in the lymphedematous area, the limited response of the macrophages, and the diminished immune response in the individual with nodal dissection or irradiation, or in the case of primary lymphedema, too few, fibrosed, or poorly developed nodes.

At the first sign of infection, the affected individual must seek medical consultation immediately and discontinue all current lymphedema treatment modalities, including manual lymphatic drainage, pumps, bandaging, and garments, until the physician determines it is safe to resume.

If the infection is treated early, some physicians may allow resumption of bandaging or garments as tolerated to avoid the limb ballooning out of control as the infection is resolving. This is determined on a case-by-case basis by the physician who is familiar with the individual, follows the individual's care closely, and provides emergency treatment as needed for that person.

Lipedema

Overview and Etiologic Factors

The term *lipedema* was first used by Allen and Hines to describe a symmetrical "swelling" of both legs, extending from the hips to the ankles, caused by deposits of subcutaneous adipose tissue.[2] The underlying etiologic factors of these fat deposits remain unknown. Although lipedema is not a disorder of the lymphatic system per se, it is often confused with bilateral lower-extremity lymphedema, thus the reason for discussing it in this chapter. It occurs almost exclusively in women, may have an associated family history (20% of cases), and is usually accompanied by hormonal disorders.[143] If present in a man, it is accompanied by massive hormonal disorder.

Fat in the lower extremities extends to the malleoli, often with flaps of tissue hanging over the foot. The feet are not affected; occasionally, lipedema is found in the arms. Typically, fatty bulges are in the medial proximal thigh and the medial distal thigh, just above the knee. Clinically, the affected individuals complain of pitting edema as the day progresses, which is relieved by prolonged elevation of the leg or legs overnight.[27,115,118]

Stages of Lipedema

In Stage I, the skin is still soft and regular, but nodular changes can be felt on palpation (Fig. 13-27). No color changes occur in the skin, and the subcutaneous tissues have a spongy feel, like a soft rubber doll. In Stage II, the subcutaneous tissue becomes more nodular and tough. Large fatty lobules begin to form on the medial distal and proximal thighs and medial and lateral ankles just above the malleoli (Fig. 13-28). Pitting edema is

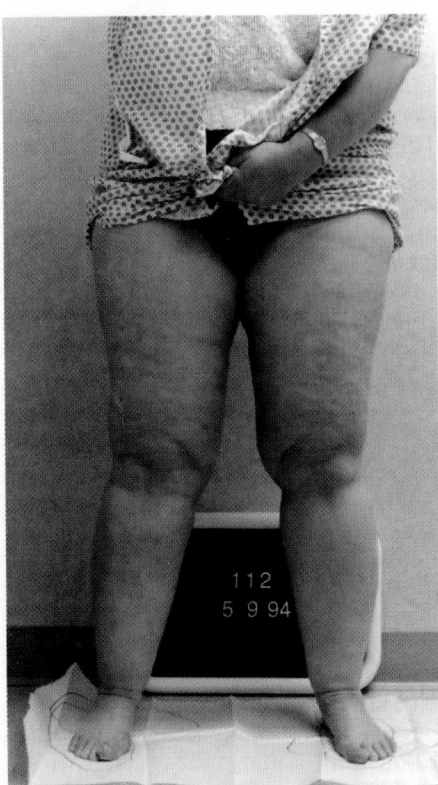

Figure 13-27

Stage I lipedema. Note that the feet are free of edema and the ankles and lower legs have pitting edema. Fatty nodules are beginning to appear on the distal thighs. (Courtesy Lymphedema Therapy, Woodbury, NY.)

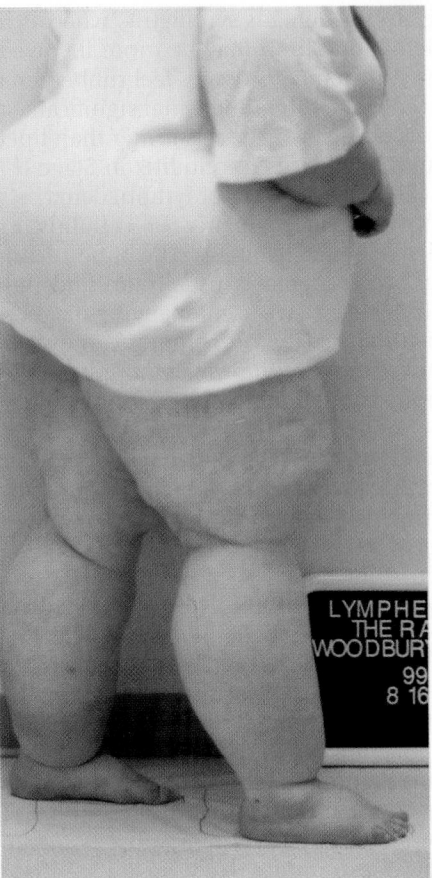

Figure 13-28

Stage II lipedema. Note that obvious pitting edema on the dorsum of the feet is evident, and the tissues are beginning to hang over the medial and lateral ankles and above the knees. The discoloration at the anterodistal left lower leg is from a resolving cellulitis, secondary to the lymphedema that developed secondary to the lipedema. (Courtesy Lymphedema Therapy, Woodbury, NY.)

common, increasing as the day progresses. The individual may report hypersensitivity over the anterior tibial area. Skin color changes occur in the lower leg, indicative of secondary lymphedema, which often occurs in later-stage lipedema.

Pathophysiology of Lipedema[143]

Many histologic and physiologic changes occur in lipedema. A decrease in the elasticity of the epidermis and subcutis also occurs. The basement membrane of vessels is thickened, and disturbances in vasomotion take place. The venoarterial reflex is disturbed, causing decreased vascular resistance, increased skin perfusion, and increased capillary filtration. Under normal circumstances, the venoarterial reflex is an important mechanism for the regulation of microcirculation and interstitial fluid exchange. It is measured as a ratio between skin perfusion in the supine versus the standing position using a laser Doppler flowmeter.

Increased venous or blood capillary pressure causes increased ultrafiltration. These changes, combined with the decreased efficiency of the calf muscle pump, result in both the dependent pitting edema seen in Stage I and the secondary lymphedema that often complicates lipedema in its later stages.[55]

Histologic changes seen in lipedema include a thinning of the epidermal layer, thickening of the subcutaneous tissue layer, fibrosis of arterioles, tearing of elastic fibers, dilated venules and capillaries, and hypertrophy

and hyperplasia of fat cells. Clinical studies show enlargement of the prelymphatic channels[140] and defects in capillary perfusion.[153] Some authors have reported no alteration in lymphatic transport,[21] whereas others[15] have reported decreased lymph outflow in those individuals with lipedema. Földi and Földi reported an increase in fat cell growth during lymphostasis.[54]

MEDICAL MANAGEMENT

DIAGNOSIS. The diagnosis of lipedema is difficult if the clinician is unfamiliar with this condition. Often, those affected are told that they are "fat" and should just lose weight to resolve the problem. For reasons still unknown, the fatty tissue accompanying this condition cannot be significantly decreased by diet. It is not uncommon for a diagnosis of primary lymphedema to be made. This results in frustration for the person who then seeks out lymphedema therapy, with poor results.

Several significant clinical differences exist between lipedema and bilateral primary lymphedema. The feet are not involved in lipedema; although they are edematous with a positive Stemmer's sign in lymphedema, Stemmer's sign is absent in lipedema (see Fig. 13-17). The "swelling" in lipedema is symmetric, whereas in primary lymphedema, one limb may be more involved than the other. The subcutaneous tissues feel rubbery in lipedema. In advanced Stage II lymphedema, significant subcutaneous fibrosis occurs, which feels firmer than lipedema.

Although incidences of cellulitis in Stage II lipedema, usually with a component of lymphedema as well, have been reported, the frequency of cellulitis in Stage II lymphedema is much higher. The time of onset of the "swelling" in lipedema is usually around puberty, and 90% of these cases have accompanying diagnoses of hormonal disturbance (thyroid, pituitary, or ovarian). This is usually not the case with primary lymphedema.

A lymphoscintigram may be helpful to differentiate between lymphedema and lipedema; however, results can be conflicting, because lymphedema often occurs to some degree in the later stages of lipedema, probably a result of impairment of lymph flow caused by the pressure of fatty tissue.

In fact, clinical cases of bilateral lower extremity lymphedema in the morbidly obese individual are seen; the onset of the lymphedema occurs after body weight exceeds 350 to 400 lb. It is plausible to suspect that the pressure of a large apron of abdominal fat can effectively block lymph flow through the inguinal area, causing the lymphedema, but the difference between these cases and lipedema is that obesity does not cause lipedema.

Lipedema is caused by a hormonal imbalance resulting in excessive deposition of adipose tissue, most often in the lower extremities (see Figs. 13-27 and 13-28), although it can occur in the upper extremities, too.

TREATMENT AND PROGNOSIS. No effective medical treatment for lipedema is available, and the prognosis is guarded; however, significant functional improvements are possible with good program adherence and therapy intervention. Medical management involves treating the hormonal disturbance as effectively as possible and providing nutritional guidance to avoid additional weight gain. Many of these individuals have endured years of ridicule because of their physical appearance and become recluses in their homes, further limiting their activity level.

As lipedema progresses and the hypersensitivity increases, they feel less inclined to walk or exercise because of the pain. They inevitably gain more weight as a result of the inactivity and depression, often finding food their only comfort.

SPECIAL IMPLICATIONS FOR THE THERAPIST 13-4

Lipedema

The primary goal of therapy intervention in the person with lipedema is symptomatic relief and realistic improvement of trunk and lower extremity function. Application of the combined lymphedema treatments has shown some success in relieving the pain and hypersensitivity in the lower legs and improving general mobility.[146] Usually, a lower level of compression is needed to support a lipedematous limb, compared with a lymphedematous limb of the same size and girth. This guideline applies to the compression garments, too.

These individuals often require more padding under the compression bandages, particularly in the anterior tibial area. They do not tolerate the heavier, denser compression fabrics and usually require a lower class of compression garment than someone with uncomplicated lymphedema. The therapist must remember, however, that later-stage lipedema is often accompanied by lymphedema, too, and that treatment includes compression garments, often of a higher compression class.

The main goals of intervention are to decrease pain and hypersensitivity, decrease the lymphedematous component of the disease, and assist the individual in maintaining and/or reducing adipose tissue through exercise and nutritional guidance. The compression garments can help decrease the adipose tissue with exercise and weight loss. The most difficult task is fitting the compression garments. They must be custom-made because of the large size of the individual and are often uncomfortable at the waist, particularly when sitting.

It may be more functional to compromise with compression ending just below the knee if that is all that the individual can tolerate. Compression garments can be designed in two pieces, one from the toes to just below the knee and a second layer from below the knee to the waist in a lighter fabric that can be removed if needed, leaving the lower leg garment intact.

Making the radical change in daily activity level is most challenging for these individuals. Providing continued support and encouragement is important. Networking is helpful and is facilitated by offering a support group, even when held on an irregular, informal basis. An hour-long educational meeting, even if only offered three or four times per year, can provide a neutral meeting place for people to begin networking.

Nothing can compare with the encouragement and hope that an individual with lipedema or lymphedema can derive from seeing and talking with someone else living with the same problem and hearing how others cope on a day-to-day basis. Therapists can receive some of the best guidance on exercise and coping with compression garments in a group like this.

REFERENCES

To enhance this text and add value for the reader, all references are included on the companion Evolve site that accompanies this textbook. The reader can view the reference source and access it online whenever possible.

CHAPTER 14

The Hematologic System

CELESTE PETERSON • CATHERINE CAVALLARO GOODMAN

Hematology is the branch of science that studies the form, structure, and function of blood and blood-forming tissues. Two major components of blood are examined: plasma and formed elements (erythrocytes, or red blood cells [RBCs]; leukocytes, or white blood cells [WBCs]; and platelets, or thrombocytes).

Delivery of these formed elements throughout the body tissues is necessary for cellular metabolism, defense against injury and invading microorganisms, and acid–base balance. The formation and development of blood cells, which usually take place in the bone marrow, are controlled by hormones (specifically erythropoietin) and feedback mechanisms that maintain an ideal number of cells.

The hematologic system is integrated with the lymphatic and immune systems; for a complete understanding of these systems, see Chapters 7 and 13. The lymph nodes are part of the lymphatic system but also part of the hematopoietic (blood-forming) system and the lymphoid system, which consists of organs and tissues of the immune system.

Lymph fluid passes through these nodes, or valves, which are located in the lymph channels at 1- to 2-cm intervals. As the fluid passes through the nodes, it is purified of harmful bacteria and viruses. Networks of the lymphatic system are situated in several areas of the body and may be considered primary (thymus and bone marrow) or secondary (spleen, lymph nodes, tonsils, and Peyer patches of the small intestine).

All the lymphoid organs link the hematologic and immune systems in that they are sites of residence, proliferation, differentiation, or function of lymphocytes and mononuclear phagocytes (mononuclear phagocyte system: macrophage and monocyte cells capable of ingesting microorganisms and other antigens).

Lymphocytes are any of the nonphagocytic leukocytes (WBCs) found in the blood, lymph, and lymphoid tissues that make up the body's immunologically competent cells. They are divided into two classes: B and T lymphocytes (see "Leukocytosis" below and Chapter 7). For example, in the hematologic system, the lymphocytes of the spleen produce approximately one-third of the antibody available to the immune system.

SIGNS AND SYMPTOMS OF HEMATOLOGIC DISORDERS

Disruption of the hematologic system results in circulatory disorders as well as signs and symptoms noted in the hematologic tissues themselves. The circulatory disorders can be characterized by edema and congestion, infarction, thrombosis and embolism, lymphedema, bleeding and bruising, and hypotension and shock (Box 14-1).

Edema is the accumulation of excessive fluid within the interstitial tissues or within body cavities. *Congestion* is the accumulation of excessive blood within the blood vessels of an organ or tissue. The forms of lymphedema include cerebral edema, inflammatory edema, peripheral dependent edema, and pulmonary edema. Congestion may be localized, as with a venous thrombosis, or generalized, as with heart failure (e.g., congestive heart failure [CHF]), which results in congestion in the lungs, lower extremities, and abdominal viscera.

Infarction is a localized region of necrosis caused by reduction of arterial perfusion below a level required for cell viability. Such a situation occurs as a result of arterial obstruction caused by atherosclerosis, arterial thrombosis, or embolism, when oxygen supply fails to meet the oxygen requirements of organs with end arteries, such as the gastrointestinal (GI) tract, the heart, and, less often, the kidneys and spleen. Cerebral cortical neurons (cerebral infarction) and myocardial cells (myocardial infarction) are most vulnerable to ischemia, although protective collateral blood flow develops in the heart through anastomoses.

A *thrombus* is a solid mass of clotted blood within an intact blood vessel or chamber of the heart. An *embolus* is a mass of solid, liquid, or gas that moves within a blood vessel to lodge at a site distant from its place of origin (see Fig. 12-29). Most emboli are thromboemboli. Thrombosis (development of a thrombus or clot) results from pathologic activation of the hemostatic mechanisms involving platelets, coagulation factors, and blood vessel walls. Endothelial injury, alteration in blood flow (stasis and turbulence), and hypercoagulability of the blood (e.g., protein abnormalities either primary or associated with cancers) promote thrombosis and thromboembolism.

MOST COMMON SIGNS AND SYMPTOMS OF HEMATOLOGIC DISORDERS

- Edema
  - Lymphedema
  - Cerebral edema
  - Inflammatory edema
  - Peripheral dependent edema
  - Pulmonary edema
- Lymphadenopathy
- Congestion
- Infarction (brain, heart, GI tract, kidney, spleen)
- Thrombosis
- Splenomegaly
- Embolism
- Bleeding and bruising
- Shock
  - Rapid, weak pulse (late phase)
  - Hypotension (systolic blood pressure <90 mm Hg)
  - Cool, moist skin (late phase)
  - Pallor
  - Weak/absent peripheral pulses

Lymphedema, or chronic swelling of an area from accumulation of interstitial fluid (edema), occurs in hemolymphatic disorders secondary to obstruction of lymphatic vessels or lymph nodes. Obstruction may be of an inflammatory or mechanical nature from trauma, regional lymph node resection or irradiation, or extensive involvement of regional nodes by malignant disease.

Women who have been treated surgically for breast cancer with lymph node dissection, mastectomy, and/or radiation therapy are at double the risk of developing lymphedema of the arm and/or chest wall (see Chapter 13). When the obstruction that slows the lymph fluid exceeds the pumping capacity of the system, the fluid accumulates in the tissues in the extremity, causing edema in one or more limbs. This accumulation of fluid may become a source for bacterial growth, leading to infection, fibrosis, and possible loss of functional limb use.

Bleeding and bruising can occur from trauma of various types and are normal consequences of injury. However, when bleeding and bruising are elicited with minor trauma (e.g., brushing teeth) or bleeding continues longer than normal, there is more concern for a disorder of the blood. These symptoms are often a result of platelet abnormalities (function or quantity) such as idiopathic thrombocytopenic purpura, thrombotic thrombocytopenic purpura, or von Willebrand disease.

Purpura is a hemorrhagic condition that occurs when not enough normal platelets are available to plug damaged vessels or prevent leakage from even minor injury to normal capillaries. Purpura is characterized by movement of blood into the surrounding tissue (extravasation), under the skin, and through the mucous membranes, producing spontaneous ecchymoses (bruises) and petechiae (small, red patches) on the skin. When accompanied by a decrease in the circulating platelets, it is called *thrombocytopenic purpura*. In the acute form, bleeding can occur from any of the body orifices such as hematuria, nosebleed, vaginal bleeding, and bleeding gums.

Shock occurs when the circulatory system (heart as well as arteries) is unable to maintain adequate pressure in order to perfuse organs. Common clinical signs include tachycardia, tachypnea, cool extremities, decreased pulses, decreased urine output, and an altered mental status. Hypotension is typically present but may be initially absent. The end result is hypoxia to end-organ tissues, particularly the kidneys, brain, and heart.

Diagnosis as to the cause of shock should include an evaluation of the heart and the peripheral arteries (systemic vascular resistance). Myocardial infarction and heart failure are problems that make it difficult for the heart to pump an adequate amount of blood to the body. Decreased blood volume (hypovolemia) from hemorrhaging or severe volume depletion (e.g., nausea, vomiting, and diarrhea) also reduces the body's ability to perfuse tissue.

Disorders that cause a decrease in the arterial pressure include sepsis (infection from any source), liver failure, severe pancreatitis, anaphylaxis, and thyrotoxicosis. The three most common classes of shock therefore are cardiogenic (heart related), hypovolemic, and causes related to reduced systemic vascular resistance, although many overlap (Table 14-1).

Lymphadenopathy is the abnormal enlargement of a lymph node(s). Lymph nodes filter lymph as it returns to the heart. Infectious organisms (e.g., Epstein-Barr virus [EBV] and tuberculosis) and autoimmune disorders (e.g., rheumatoid arthritis [RA] and systemic lupus erythematosus [SLE]) can cause an inflammatory expansion and enlargement of lymph nodes. Malignant diseases, such as lymphoma, chronic lymphocytic leukemia, and Hodgkin lymphoma, can also cause enlarged lymph nodes.

Lymph nodes are typically "rubbery" in feel, unattached to surrounding tissue (mobile), and small (usually less than 1 cm). Inflammatory nodes may be tender to the touch, warm, and enlarged but usually remain mobile and soft. Malignant nodes are often not tender or mobile; they are firm and enlarged. Most cases of lymphadenopathy are not malignancy related, although all instances of abnormal adenopathy should be investigated.

Enlargement of the spleen, or *splenomegaly*, is present in many hematologic diseases. The spleen is normally involved in removing old or deformed erythrocytes, producing antibodies, and removing antibody-laden bacteria or cells. When the spleen exceeds normal function in one of these areas, it becomes enlarged. For example, if a client has hereditary spherocytosis and forms abnormally shaped erythrocytes, the spleen attempts to remove all these cells, thereby increasing in size to accomplish this task.

Splenomegaly is often noted in people with infectious mononucleosis or malignancies such as Hodgkin lymphoma (where the spleen is infiltrated by disease). If the bone marrow is unable to produce cells (because of an infiltrative process), the spleen often assumes that role and becomes enlarged (extramedullary hematopoiesis).

Table 14-1	Etiologic Factors of Shock
Category of Shock	**Causes**
Hypovolemic	Hemorrhage (loss of blood, shock)
	Vomiting
	Diarrhea
	Dehydration secondary to:
	• Decreased fluid intake
	• Diabetes mellitus (diuresis during diabetic ketoacidosis or severe hyperglycemia)
	• Diabetes insipidus
	• Inadequate rehydration of long-distance runner
	Addison disease
	Burns
Cardiogenic	Arrhythmias
	Acute valvular dysfunction
	Acute myocardial infarction
	Severe congestive heart failure
	Cardiomyopathy
	Obstructive
	Septic
	Neurogenic
	Obstructive valvular disease (aortic or mitral stenosis)
	Cardiac tumor (atrial myxoma)
Reduced system vascular resistance	Bacteremia; overwhelming infections
	Spinal cord injury
	Pain
	Trauma
	Vasodilator drugs
	Burns
	Thyrotoxicosis
	Pancreatitis
	Anaphylaxis
	Liver failure

SPECIAL IMPLICATIONS FOR THE THERAPIST 14-1

Hematologic Disorders

Hematologic conditions alter the oxygen-carrying capacity of the blood and the constituents, structure, consistency, and flow of the blood. These changes can contribute to hypocoagulopathy or hypercoagulopathy, increased work of the heart and breathing, impaired tissue perfusion, and increased risk of thrombus.

Hematologic abnormalities require that the results of the client's blood analysis and clotting factors be monitored so that therapy intervention can be modified to minimize risk.[68] Precautions and interventions for the client with lymphedema are discussed in Chapter 13 (see Table 13-2).

Platelet disorders require special consideration by the therapist during exercise. Decreased platelets are associated with the risk of life-threatening hemorrhage; physical therapy intervention must be tailored to the individual's platelet levels. For example, platelet levels between 40,000 and 60,000 µL face an increased risk of postsurgical or traumatic bleed. Low-load resistance exercise is permitted with 1- to 2-lb weights. Safe exercise includes walking, stationary bicycling with light resistance, and minimal activities of daily living.

For clients with platelet levels in the 20,000 to 40,000 range, low-intensity exercise with no weights or resistance up to 2 lb is permitted but with no resistance during stationary biking. Activity and exercise restriction is even more stringent when platelet levels are below 20,000. Below 10,000, spontaneous central nervous system, GI, and/or respiratory tract bleeding may occur.[374] In all cases, clients are monitored carefully for any signs of bleeding. Guidelines vary from one geographic region to another and even from center to center within a single geographic location.

Splenomegaly

Because splenomegaly is often associated with conditions characterized by rapid destruction of blood cells, it is important to follow the usual precautions for anyone with poor clotting abilities (e.g., see "Special Implications for the Therapist 14-5: The Anemias" below).

The client must be taught proper breathing techniques in conjunction with ways to avoid activities or positions that could traumatize the abdominal region or increase intracranial, intrathoracic, or intraabdominal pressure.

The person with a small or absent spleen is more susceptible to streptococcal infection, which calls for prevention techniques such as good handwashing (see Boxes 8-4 and 8-5 and Appendix A).

Exercise and Sports

Exercise training can induce blood volume expansion immediately (plasma volume) and over a period (erythrocyte volume) and is associated with healing, improved quality of life, and improved exercise capabilities in cases of anemia from hemorrhage, trauma, renal disease, and chronic diseases. The reestablishment of erythropoiesis through exercise and effects of exercise on blood volume in other groups remain unknown but are a potential area for further investigation and consideration in the clinical setting.[93,299]

Improvements in athletic performance with exogenous erythropoietin (referred to as "blood doping") have been documented as improvements in running time and maximal oxygen uptake. However, these effects are not without risk for increased blood viscosity and thrombosis, with potentially fatal results. Until a definitive test is developed for detection of exogenous erythropoietin, the therapist must remain aware of this potential problem.[314,315]

Monitoring Vital Signs

Clients in whom shock develops may exhibit orthostatic changes in vital signs. A drop in systolic blood pressure of 10 to 20 mm Hg or more, associated with an increase in pulse rate of more than 15 beats/min, may indicate a depleted intravascular volume.

The therapist is unlikely to see a client with acute hypovolemia; hypovolemia is more likely the result of dehydration, as in the case of the long-distance runner or the client with severe diarrhea or slow GI tract bleeding. The aging population is especially vulnerable to development of unknown slow intestinal bleeding, especially with the use of aspirin or nonsteroidal anti-inflammatory drugs.

Clients with peripheral neuropathies or clients taking medications such as certain antihypertensive drugs may be normovolemic and experience an orthostatic fall in blood pressure but without associated increase in pulse rate. If any doubt exists, the client should be placed in the supine position with legs elevated to maximize cerebral blood flow. The Trendelenburg position, in which the head is lower than the rest of the body, is no longer used because of the increased difficulty of breathing in this position.

AGING AND THE HEMATOPOIETIC SYSTEM

Although blood composition changes little with age, the percentage of the marrow space occupied by hematopoietic (blood-forming) tissue declines progressively. The percentage of bone marrow fat is equal to the person's age, reaching a plateau at around age 50 years.

Other changes include decreased total serum iron, total iron-binding capacity, and intestinal iron absorption but with increased total body and bone marrow iron; increased fragility of plasma membranes; a rise in fibrinogen and increased platelet adhesiveness; red cell rigidity; and early activation of the coagulation system. Platelet morphology (form and structure) does not appear to change with age, but platelet count and function have been found to vary from normal to increased or decreased.

The cumulative effect of these changes appears in the form of disturbed blood flow in older subjects, leading to the development or aggravation of various circulatory disorders, especially hypertension, stroke, and diabetes. In addition, correlations found between hematologic changes and changes in behavioral patterns and some cognitive functions suggest that hematologic changes contribute to other changes associated with aging as well.[7]

Age-related changes in the peripheral blood include slightly decreased hemoglobin and hematocrit, although levels remain within the normal adult range. Low hemoglobin levels noted in aging adults can be caused by iron deficiency (usually via blood loss such as ulcer, telangiectasia, colon polyps, or cancer) or can be associated with a longstanding condition such as rheumatologic conditions often seen in a therapy practice (referred to as *anemia of chronic disease*). Vitamin B_{12}, which is required to produce blood cells, and the subsequent development of anemia (resulting from a B_{12} deficiency) with its hematologic, neurologic, and GI manifestations, are discussed later in this chapter.

Aging is also associated with a decreased number of lymph nodes and diminished size of remaining nodes, decreased function of lymphocytes, and decline in cellular immunity owing to altered T-cell function (see "Effects of Aging on the Immune System" in Chapter 7). The effect of aging on quantity, form, and structure of lymphocytes is not well documented.

BLOOD TRANSFUSIONS

Advances in treating hematologic/immunologic disorders through blood transfusions and hematopoietic cell transplantation (HCT) have provided new success in long-term treatment and a cure for some previously fatal disorders (see Chapter 21). Modern blood banking and transfusion medicine have developed techniques to administer only the blood component needed by the client, such as packed RBCs for anemia, plasma for people with coagulation deficiencies, or cryoprecipitate for bleeding disorders such as hemophilia.

Clients in a therapy setting who have undergone numerous surgical procedures (e.g., traumatic injuries) or elective orthopedic or cardiac procedures may also receive autologous blood transfusions (i.e., reinfusion of a person's own blood) when significant blood loss may be a complication and a transfusion may be anticipated.

The development of recombinant human erythropoietin (rHuEpo, EPO, or Epogen), with its ability to stimulate erythropoiesis (bone marrow production of red cells) and elevate RBCs, has reduced the need for blood transfusion in a variety of clinical situations (e.g., chronic renal disease, hematologic malignancies, cancer-related anemia, and surgical procedures, especially joint arthroplasty and cardiac procedures).

Reaction to Blood and Blood Products
Febrile Nonhemolytic Reaction

Because blood products are most often donated from another person, reactions may occur. The most common transfusion-related reaction is a febrile, nonhemolytic reaction (occurring in 0.5%-1% of erythrocyte transfusions and 30% of platelet transfusions). The condition is characterized by an increase in temperature by more than 0.6° C (1° F) during or soon after the transfusion. These reactions are usually a result of donor-derived cytokines to recipient-derived leukoreactive antibodies.

Treatment includes stopping the transfusion, checking the blood for a direct hemolytic process (in the laboratory), and administering antipyretics. Symptoms are usually transient, and the removal of donor leukocytes from the blood (leukocyte reduction) can reduce the risk of another similar reaction (Box 14-2).

Transfusion-Related Acute Lung Injury

Transfusion-related acute lung injury occurs in as many as 1 in every 5000 transfusions and is the most common cause of transfusion-related death (mortality rate of 5%). Transfusion-related acute lung injury occurs as a consequence of antibodies in donor plasma directed against recipient neutrophil antigens. Once the antibodies bind the antigen, leukocytes are recruited and inflammation ensues. This reaction typically presents within 6 hours of the transfusion. Common findings include fever, hypotension, and pulmonary edema. Unlike adult respiratory distress syndrome, improvement can be seen

Box 14-2

SIGNS AND SYMPTOMS OF REACTIONS TO BLOOD AND BLOOD PRODUCTS

Febrile, Nonhemolytic Transfusion Reaction

- Fever/chills
- Headache
- Nausea/vomiting
- Hypertension
- Tachycardia

Transfusion-Related Acute Lung Injury

- Pulmonary edema
- Acute respiratory distress
- Severe hypoxia

Acute Hemolytic Transfusion Reaction

- Fever/chills
- Nausea/vomiting
- Flank, abdominal pain
- Headache
- Dyspnea
- Hypotension
- Tachycardia
- Red urine

Delayed Hemolytic Transfusion Reaction

- Unexplained drop in hemoglobin—anemia
- Increased bilirubin level—jaundice
- Increased lactate dehydrogenase level

Allergic Reactions

- Hives/rash
- Wheezing
- Mucosal edema

Anaphylaxis

- Abrupt hypotension
- Edema of the larynx
- Difficulty breathing
- Nausea
- Abdominal pain
- Diarrhea
- Shock
- Respiratory arrest

Septic Reactions

- Fever/chills
- Hypotension
- Headache
- Back, chest, abdominal pain
- Shortness of breath

Circulatory Overload

- Red face
- Shortness of breath
- Tachycardia
- Orthopnea
- Hypertension
- Headache
- Seizures

within days. With appropriate respiratory intervention, most people recover without permanent pulmonary damage.[283]

Acute Hemolytic Transfusion Reaction

Less common (only 1 in every 25,000 transfusions) but the most feared complication is the acute hemolytic transfusion reaction. This is caused by ABO incompatibility: Typically, a mistake is made by giving the wrong blood to a person or blood is mislabeled. Symptoms begin soon after the transfusion is begun (see Box 14-2). Erythrocytes are destroyed intravascularly with resultant red plasma and red urine.

The mortality rate is high, ranging from 17% to 60%. The transfusion is immediately terminated and the client given cardiovascular support. Renal failure, disseminated intravascular coagulation, and severe hypotension may occur.

Delayed Hemolytic Transfusion Reaction

Delayed hemolytic transfusion reactions occur as a consequence of an amnestic response of an erythrocyte alloantigen after reexposure to an erythrocyte antigen. Symptoms develop 5 to 10 days after the transfusion. These reactions are often asymptomatic and are noted only because the hemoglobin does not rise as predicted following the transfusion.

Allergic Reaction

Mild allergic reactions (such as urticaria) are common, particularly in clients who have received multiple transfusions. The allergy is usually caused by donor plasma proteins and often does not recur. More severe respiratory symptoms may occur, such as wheezing, shortness of breath, and mucosal edema. Pretreatment with antihistamines and washing of the cellular blood products can prevent the allergic symptoms.

Anaphylaxis

True anaphylaxis is rare (approximately 1 in 20,000-50,000 transfusions) and may occur with or without allergic reactions. It is usually caused by immunoglobulin (Ig) A deficiency or from the presence of anti-IgA antibodies. Symptoms include acute onset of hypotension and edema of the larynx with associated difficulty breathing. Nausea, abdominal pain, and diarrhea may accompany the reaction. This reaction can be severe and fatal and is associated with shock, respiratory failure, and vascular collapse. The earlier the symptoms occur, the more severe the reaction. Treatment consists of immediately discontinuing the transfusion, administering epinephrine and corticosteroids, and providing cardiovascular and respiratory support. All subsequent transfusions require washing of all blood products. Plasma products must be obtained from IgA-deficient donors.

Septic Reactions

Rarely, septic reactions can occur secondary to bacterial contamination of blood products, principally platelets (they are not stored at cold temperatures). In March 2004, all blood banks began to routinely screen platelets for bacterial contamination with a subsequent reduction in septic reactions. Symptoms of such reactions include fever/chills; hypotension; headache; back, chest, and abdominal pain; and shortness of breath. Culture of the product and appropriate antibiotics and cardiovascular support are the mainstays of treatment.

Transfusion as a source for hepatitis (B and C) has been reduced since the initiation of donor screening for the hepatitis antibody. People with hemophilia who received coagulation factor concentrates before 1984 have been at highest risk among transfusion recipients because of exposures to pooled blood products prepared from thousands of donors. The availability of nonhuman plasma factors has virtually eliminated the transmission of viruses among people with hemophilia.

The risk of HIV infection by transfusion is low overall, calculated at 1 in 1 million transfusions. The risk of HIV transmission by blood transfusion has been continually reduced through the elimination of high-risk individuals from blood donor pools and the use of more sensitive screening. Acquired immune deficiency syndrome (AIDS) has developed in a small percentage of people receiving transfusion of RBCs, platelets, or commercial coagulation factor concentrates. AIDS has also been reported in infants after neonatal exchange, but the majority of pediatric cases were associated with maternal transmission from mothers with HIV.

Blood Transfusions

As a general rule, people are not usually exercising or being treated by the physical therapist during a blood transfusion. There are no published guidelines for this protocol and it is not a hard and fast rule. Each case can be evaluated on its own merits person by person.

The therapist must consider why a person is receiving a blood product, what is the underlying medical condition and the goals of therapy for that day/week. Consideration should be given for what is in the best interest of the individual's health and safety. In other words, will mobilizing the person during a blood transfusion be beneficial or detrimental? Can treatment be held (postponed) until a later time either later in the transfusion process or later in the day or the next day?

In some facilities, cautious therapy can be carried out during blood transfusions for those individuals who can tolerate it. Movement and gentle exercise or range-of-motion is not advised until the nursing staff approves it.

The reasons for holding physical therapy during blood transfusion are not always physiologic. Sometimes it is more a matter of logistics. For example, during the transfusion procedure, nothing the therapist does should compromise (dislodge) the intravenous line. The policy of physical therapists working with individuals receiving blood transfusions varies from region to region and even within the same facility. Perhaps it is more a matter of how routine the procedure is for the health care staff. For example, nurses in the intensive care units are often more comfortable getting people mobilized with multiple lines and while watching unstable hemodynamics. On the orthopedic floors, where multiple lines are not standard, nurses may wait for very stable hemodynamics before mobilizing postoperative patients.

On the orthopedic floor, therapists may only do supine therapeutic exercise with individuals receiving transfusion, when in fact there is no reason to withhold treatment. In reality, blood transfusions through an intravenous line are no different than any other fluid administered in the same way. Monitor vital signs, observe for tolerance to treatment, and carry on as usual.

Most blood transfusion reactions occur during the actual transfusion and are not of consequence to the therapist unless working with the individual during the actual transfusion. Exercise or therapy of any kind is not advised during the first 30 minutes (possibly up to 60 minutes) of the transfusion. This allows the nurses to evaluate how the patients are responding to the blood while monitoring for any adverse reactions. Most adverse reactions occur during the first 15 minutes (e.g., fever, chills, urticaria, acute respiratory distress, transfusion-related acute lung injury). Once the therapist begins working with the individual being transfused, then it is important to monitor for signs of adverse reactions to the transfusion and signs of orthostatic hypotension.

There may be some question as to the appropriateness of physical therapy treatment for individuals receiving a blood transfusion for anemia. If the person is anemic enough to need a blood transfusion, is the person able to tolerate therapeutic exercise?

If the person is asymptomatic, the IV site is stable, and activity or movement is tolerated, then therapeutic exercise may be prescribed. When autologous transfusion is unavailable or inappropriate, the therapist must be alert for any signs of adverse reaction. Among the most common transfusion reactions are febrile, non-hemolytic transfusion reactions and delayed hemolytic transfusion reactions. Clinical symptoms from these reactions are typically mild and can usually be prevented on subsequent transfusions.

One of the most severe, but uncommon, reactions is the acute hemolytic transfusion reaction. This is a result of antigen–antibody reactions resulting from blood type incompatibility with clumping of cells, hemolysis, and release of cellular elements into the serum. Box 14-2 lists the signs and symptoms indicating such a reaction.

Occasionally, a client may develop an allergic reaction observed as dyspnea or hives; the latter may be brought to the therapist's attention after local modality intervention. The therapist may also be the first to recognize early signs of hepatitis (jaundice), especially changes in sclerae or skin color or reported changes in urine (dark or tea colored) and stools (light colored or white).

Bloodless Medicine and Surgery

Karen Wilk, PT, DPT

Bloodless medicine and surgery, the use of technological and pharmaceutical techniques to minimize blood loss and avoid the use of allogeneic blood transfusions, has advanced in recent years into the concept of patient blood management.[310] Patient blood management uses evidence-based medicine to develop an individualized plan for each person to minimize or eliminate the need for transfusions. This is based on three main principles applied to medical and surgical patients: manage anemia, minimize blood loss, and optimize hemostasis.[309,344]

Why has there been a movement away from transfusions? For generations blood transfusions have been viewed by the medical community and recipients as a lifesaving treatment. A number of factors are moving the medical community in this direction. One is the community of Jehovah's Witnesses who seek medical care but decline the use of most forms of transfusions. Rather than refuse to treat these individuals without the use of transfusions, some physicians worked to find techniques that were compatible with the religious beliefs of this group.[309]

Second, although the blood supply can be considered safer than ever as a result of donor prescreening and post-donation testing, new infectious agents are possible and donor history of HIV and/or hepatitis have made some people caution in accepting blood transfusions.[308,311]

Finally, there is a growing body of evidence that there are risks to receiving a transfusion. Risks of receiving transfusions include infections, increased length of stay in ICU and hospital, increased renal and cardiac events, acute respiratory distress syndrome, cancer recurrence, and death.[308,311,344] Despite safeguards in place, human error cannot be eliminated from the transfusion process, and currently mistransfusion is the greatest risk of mortality from transfusion.[311,344] For these reasons, individuals whose religious beliefs are incompatible with transfusions are seeking bloodless alternatives.

Objectives

The first objective of patient blood management is the control of anemia. Anemia is related to the decreased production or increased destruction of blood cells or a combination of both. In trauma patients, the rapid loss of blood may require the use of transfusions. For the nontrauma patient the identification and treatment of anemia is critical.

For surgical patients adequate timely screening is needed. It is important to review personal or family history of anemia prior to surgery. The presence of undetected anemia must be discovered and treated prior to surgical intervention. Treatment of preoperative anemia can include iron, recombinant human erythropoietin and folic acid with the goal of normal range hemoglobin by the time of surgery.[308,309,311,344]

Some patients consider the predonation of their own blood preoperatively. Blood donated in this way must be timed well with the surgical date and is therefore subject to the same changes all blood undergoes during cold storage including changes to the RBCs. Also, some people who predonate their own blood face issues of anemia in the preoperative phase and may need treatment for anemia.[309,311]

Minimizing Blood Loss

During surgery steps can be taken to minimize blood loss. These measures can include positioning the individual to elevate the area of blood loss, use of a tourniquet, and gentle handling of tissues.[309,311] Instruments that minimize blood loss include the harmonic scalpel, argon beam and radiofrequency assisted thermal ablation.[311] There are also topical and systemic agents that contain collagen, thrombin and fibrinogen to promote coagulation.[309]

Acute normovolemic hemodilution can be used when blood loss is expected. Just before surgery several units of blood are removed and replaced with a crystalloid or colloid solutions so blood volume is maintained. Any fluid lost during surgery contains fewer RBCs and clotting factors are preserved. At the conclusion of the surgery the blood is reinfused to the patient. The entire process is completed through a closed circuit.[307,311]

Another way to impact blood loss in the operating room is to avoid hypothermia. Hypothermia can impede platelet function resulting in increased blood loss.[309,325] During surgery blood that is lost can be suctioned and saved. It is collected, mixed with anticoagulants, filtered and reinfused to the patient. The use of cell salvage can continue into the postoperative phase through the use of drains.[309,311] Anyone diagnosed with cancer cannot use this technique because of concerns about cancer spread.

Postoperative Concerns

Postoperatively, continuing steps to minimize blood loss should be taken. If there is postoperative bleeding, the patient may need to return to the operating room. Postoperatively phlebotomy should be minimized and microsampling techniques used, as routine blood draws can cause anemia.[356]

Clinician acceptance of lower hemoglobin levels is essential. It is not uncommon for surgical patients to experience a drop in postoperative hemoglobin levels. Monitoring to ensure it is in the range of acceptability is prudent.[325] Research shows there is a hemoglobin reserve that allows individuals to tolerate lower hemoglobin levels than previously thought if tissue perfusion is maintained. Hemoglobin levels alone should not be a trigger for transfusion, rather the individual should be looked at as a whole.

The number of bloodless medicine and surgery programs is growing, allowing an increasing number of patients access to these techniques for surgeries, including Whipple procedure for pancreatic cancer, joint replacements, and coronary artery bypass.

SPECIAL IMPLICATIONS FOR THE THERAPIST | 14-3

Bloodless Medicine and Surgery

Therapists who work in acute care, surgical, and postoperative settings need to have an awareness of the impact of lower hemoglobin levels on the patient's ability to participate in therapy. The therapist should review blood work results prior to each therapy session, looking specifically at hemoglobin levels. Routine vital signs including pulse oximetry must be monitored throughout the session. Watch and talk to the patient and monitor how the patient is tolerating the activity level. There are no studies looking at hemoglobin levels and safe activity levels, but individuals participating in bloodless medicine programs tolerate therapy sessions well with hemoglobin levels in the 6.5 to 9.0 range. Practice guidelines for blood management are published by the Society of Thoracic Surgeons (STS) and updated every 3 years. The most recent update may be of interest to therapists working in settings where blood conservation is employed. For the full text of this and other STS Practice Guidelines, visit http://www.sts.org/resources-publications at the official STS Web site (www.sts.org).[99]

DISORDERS OF IRON ABSORPTION

Hereditary Hemochromatosis

Hemochromatosis is an autosomal recessive hereditary disorder characterized by excessive iron absorption by the small intestine. The genetic susceptibility is seen in 1 in 250 people[274] of Northern European descent;

however, only 10% of these people develop the full expression of the disease.[18] Although the genetic mutation is fairly common, the full expression of the disorder is not common. Hemochromatosis is present at birth but remains asymptomatic until the development of iron overloading and onset of symptoms between ages 40 and 60 years (sometimes as early as age 30 years). The prevalence is equal among men and women, but men experience symptoms 5 to 10 times more often than do women (menstruation and pregnancy help to slow progression of the disorder).

Pathogenesis

Hemochromatosis can be caused by mutations in the genes of any of the proteins that regulate the entry of iron into the blood, including alterations in the hepcidin and ferroportin genes, and iron regulatory proteins, such as human hemochromatosis protein (HFE), hemojuvelin, and transferrin receptor 2.

The most common inherited form of the disease is caused by abnormalities of the *HFE* gene located on chromosome 6.[17] The product of the *HFE* gene interacts with other receptors and proteins to regulate hepcidin production. Hepcidin is produced by the liver and decreases iron absorption from the gut and inhibits the release of iron from macrophages.

The severity of the disease depends on several factors including how many and which genes are affected. For example, 85% of people with clinical hemochromatosis have homozygous mutations for C282Y[18]; yet even among people with this type of mutation, they are only predisposed for the disease and there is significant variability in the clinical manifestation.[69] Those with mild iron overload may be homozygous for H63D but heterozygotes for C282Y and H63D (one gene of each affected). But people who are heterozygotes for C282Y rarely develop the disease. Environmental factors are also thought to play a role in the clinical manifestations of the disease, such as blood loss, alcohol intake, coexistence of chronic hepatitides B and C, and nonalcoholic fatty liver disease.[271,276]

Clinical Manifestations

The body typically absorbs iron at a rate equal to body requirements. But in hemochromatosis, there is an uncoupling between absorption and body needs. Excess iron is slowly deposited in cells, particularly in the liver, pancreas, heart, and, to a lesser extent, other endocrine glands (e.g., the pituitary gland).

Signs and symptoms can include weakness, chronic fatigue, myalgias, joint pain (particularly the hands and wrists),[347] abdominal pain, hepatomegaly, elevated hemoglobin, and elevated liver enzymes. Continued iron overload leads to tissue damage. The liver is the most commonly affected organ, and clients may present with hepatomegaly without liver enzyme abnormalities. If the disease progresses without treatment, cirrhosis and liver cancer may ensue.

Other complications of untreated hemochromatosis include diabetes mellitus, cardiac myopathy (with associated CHF) and arrhythmias, "bronzing" of the skin (from iron deposition in the dermis and increase of melanin), destructive arthritis, and impotence (men) or decreased libido (women) and sterility.

MEDICAL MANAGEMENT

DIAGNOSIS. Diagnosis can best be made through blood tests. The most sensitive test is the measurement of transferrin saturation. Levels higher than 60% in men and 50% in women are suggestive of the disease (a cutoff of transferrin saturation of more than 45% is often used).[18] If the client has a family history of the disease, genetic testing may be diagnostic. Ferritin levels greater than 1000 ng/mL (without evidence of inflammation) also suggest an iron overload state.

A liver biopsy with measurement of iron stores should be performed in some cases to detect the presence or absence of fibrosis and cirrhosis for treatment purposes; however, positive results from the genetic and blood tests may be sufficient for diagnosis. In families where hemochromatosis has been previously diagnosed, all first-degree blood relatives should be genetically screened for hemochromatosis. Careful monitoring of affected family members can be done through blood tests. MRI is being used more often to diagnose elevated hepatic iron stores.[348] Monthly monitoring is required for those with known hemochromatosis.

TREATMENT. Treatment should begin early in the disease process, when iron levels exceed normal values and prior to the deposition of iron in tissue.[253] Medical intervention consists of weekly to twice-weekly therapeutic phlebotomy. This is performed until iron stores are at normal levels, with ferritin levels less than 50 ng/mL (for some clients this may take 1-2 years), after which maintenance therapy is done as needed to maintain appropriate levels (about once every 3 months).

Chelating agents (i.e., agents that bind iron) may be given parenterally in cases where anemia or protein loss is severe.[236] Phlebotomy, however, is less expensive and safer. Affected individuals are instructed to avoid ingesting alcohol because it increases the risk of developing cirrhosis nearly tenfold.

PROGNOSIS. The prognosis is good, with improved life expectancy as long as the iron levels remain in the normal range and the disease has not caused organ damage. With treatment malaise, fatigue, abdominal pain, and liver function improves, cardiac failure may be reversed, skin color lightens, and approximately 40% of clients with diabetes mellitus have improved glycemic control. Cirrhosis does not improve with therapy and 30% of clients go on to develop hepatocellular carcinoma. Hypogonadism and arthropathy typically do not improve with treatment, and joint symptoms may actually progress despite therapy.[18]

SPECIAL IMPLICATIONS FOR THE THERAPIST   14-4

Hemochromatosis

Arthropathy occurs in 40% to 60% of individuals with hemochromatosis and can be the first manifestation of the disease.[152] The arthropathy associated with hemochromatosis is not reversible and often continues to progress even with effective medical intervention.

Osteoarthritic manifestations are diverse, with minimal joint inflammation at first. The affected individual may report twinges of pain on flexing the small joints of the hand, especially the second and third metacarpophalangeal joints. Involvement of these joints often helps to distinguish hemochromatosis-related arthropathy from osteoarthritis.

Acute joint presentation can occur with progression that involves the large joints, including the hips, knees, and shoulders, accompanied by destruction to the joint, severe impairment, and resulting disability. Hemochromatosis may be associated with calcium pyrophosphate dihydrate deposition disease. This presents as an acute inflammatory arthritis.[320]

Therapeutic intervention is essential in providing flexibility, strength, and proper alignment to promote function, prevent falls, and prevent the loss of independence in activities of daily living. The therapist can be very helpful in evaluating the need for assistive devices, orthotics, and splints toward these goals.

DISORDERS OF ERYTHROCYTES

The Anemias

Definition

Anemia is a pathologic state resulting in a reduction of the oxygen-carrying capacity of the blood from an abnormality in the quantity or quality of RBCs. The World Health Organization (WHO) has defined anemia in terms of the level of hemoglobin: less than 14 g/dL for men and less than 12 g/dL for women. Different ranges exist for men and women, infants and growing children, and different metabolic and physiologic states.

These normal values must be evaluated on an individual basis; normal levels may be inadequate if tissue oxygen delivery is impaired by pulmonary insufficiency, cardiac disorders, or an increase in hemoglobin oxygen affinity.

Overview

Anemia is not a disease entity in itself; rather, it is a symptom of many other diseases, such as dietary deficiency (anemia caused by folate or vitamin B_{12} deficiency); acute or chronic blood loss (iron deficiency); congenital defects of hemoglobin (sickle cell diseases); exposure to industrial poisons; diseases of the bone marrow; chronic inflammatory, infectious, or neoplastic disease; or any other disorder that upsets the balance between blood loss through bleeding or destruction of blood cells and production of blood cells. Anemia may be classified into three main pathophysiologic states and results from either (1) blood loss, (2) decreased production of erythrocytes, or (3) peripheral destruction of erythrocytes (Box 14-3). Anemias are also described according to cellular morphology (form/structure) (Box 14-4). Descriptions of anemias based on erythrocyte morphology refer to the size and hemoglobin content of the RBC. In some

Box 14-3
CAUSES OF ANEMIA

Excessive Blood Loss (Hemorrhage)
- Trauma, wound
- GI cancers
- Angiectasia
- Bleeding peptic ulcer
- Excessive menstruation
- Bleeding hemorrhoids
- Varices, diverticulosis

Destruction of Erythrocytes (Hemolytic)
- Mechanical (e.g., microangiopathic hemolytic anemia; damage by a mechanical heart valve)
- Autoimmune hemolytic anemia
- Hemoglobinopathies (e.g., sickle cell diseases)
- Enzyme defects (e.g., glucose-6-phosphate dehydrogenase deficiency)
- Parasites (e.g., malaria)
- Hypersplenism
- Cell membrane abnormalities (e.g., hereditary spherocytosis)
- Thalassemias

Decreased Production of Erythrocytes
- Chronic diseases (e.g., rheumatoid arthritis, tuberculosis, cancer)
- Nutritional deficiency (e.g., iron, vitamin B_{12}, alcohol abuse, folic acid deficiency)
- Cellular maturational defects (e.g., thalassemias, cytotoxic or antineoplastic drugs)
- ↓ Bone marrow stimulation (e.g., hypothyroidism, decreased erythropoietin production)
- Bone marrow failure (e.g., leukemia, aplasia)
- Bone marrow replacement (myelophthisis; neoplasm)
- Myelodysplastic syndromes (sideroblastic anemia)

Box 14-4
ANEMIA CLASSIFIED BY MORPHOLOGY

- Normocytic (normal size)
- Macrocytic (abnormally large)
- Microcytic (abnormally small)
- Normochromic (normal amounts of hemoglobin)
- Hyperchromic (high concentration of hemoglobin)
- Hypochromic (low concentration of hemoglobin)
- Anisocytosis (various sizes)
- Poikilocytosis (various shapes)

anemias, variations occur in size (e.g., anisocytosis) or shape (e.g., poikilocytosis) of erythrocytes.

Etiologic Factors and Pathogenesis

Anemia results from (1) excessive blood loss, (2) increased destruction of erythrocytes, or (3) decreased production of erythrocytes. Anemia is the most common hematologic abnormality; only the anemias most commonly observed in rehabilitation or therapy settings are discussed here, using the three etiologic categories from Box 14-3 as a guideline.

The underlying pathogenesis can be multifactorial and depends on the condition causing the anemia. A number of physiologic compensatory responses to anemia occur, depending on the rapidity of onset and duration of anemia and the condition of the individual.

The production of erythrocytes is controlled by the hormone erythropoietin. When the kidneys detect hypoxia, hypoxia induced factors are released. These act as transcription factors to increase the production of erythropoietin, a hormone produced by the kidney. Erythropoietin then stimulates the maturation and release of RBCs from the bone marrow, and, depending on the severity of the anemia, the spleen and liver.[267] Other factors are also required for making a RBC, including iron, cobalamin, folate, and a healthy bone marrow.

In acute-onset anemia with severe loss of intravascular volume, peripheral vasoconstriction and central vasodilation occur to preserve blood flow to the vital organs.

If the anemia persists, small-vessel vasodilation will provide increased blood flow to ensure better tissue oxygenation. These vascular compensations result in decreased systemic vascular resistance, increased cardiac output, and tachycardia, resulting in a higher rate of delivery of oxygen-bearing erythrocytes to the tissues. Other compensatory mechanisms include an increase in plasma volume to maintain total blood volume and enhance tissue perfusion and stimulation of erythropoietin production to increase new erythrocyte production.

Excessive Blood Loss. Excessive blood loss, such as occurs with GI bleeding in the client with a history of aspirin or nonsteroidal antiinflammatory drug (NSAID) use, is a cause of anemia seen in a therapy practice. Slow, chronic GI blood loss from medication or any GI disorder (e.g., peptic and duodenal ulcers, gastritis, GI cancers, hemorrhoids, diverticulosis, ulcerative colitis, and colon polyps) can result in iron-deficiency anemia.

Destruction of Erythrocytes. Destruction of erythrocytes (hemolysis) can occur as a result of congenital or acquired disorders caused by congenital RBC membrane abnormalities, lack of necessary enzymes needed for normal metabolism, autoimmune processes, or infection. All but the autoimmune processes are discussed elsewhere in this chapter.

Autoimmune hemolytic anemia (AIHA) is caused by an autoantibody that attaches to the RBC, leading to its destruction. AIHA is classified according to the temperature at which the antibodies optimally bind to the RBC. The most common form of AIHA is warm antibody-mediated, an IgG autoantibody that binds to erythrocyte Rh antigens at body temperature. Macrophages are attracted to the attached autoantibody and release enzymes that begin to destroy the cell membrane. The resultant spherical cells are removed by the spleen.

Cold agglutinin disease is another autoimmune hemolytic process caused by IgM autoantibodies that bind to erythrocytes at temperatures less than 37° C (98.6° F) and trigger complement fixation and clumping of erythrocytes. These complement-laden erythrocytes may be destroyed intravascularly or removed by the liver. Hemolytic anemia can be idiopathic or a result of collagen vascular diseases (e.g., SLE), lymphoproliferative diseases (e.g., chronic lymphocytic leukemia or lymphoma), or other malignancies. Medications such as dapsone, penicillin, quinidine, quinine, and methyldopa can also cause AIHA.

Decreased Production of Erythrocytes. Anemias resulting in the underproduction of RBCs usually stem from either a lack of erythropoietin, a hormone produced in the kidney that helps the body produce oxygen carrying RBCs (as seen in chronic kidney disease), or an inability of the bone marrow to respond to erythropoietin. Hyporesponsiveness of the bone marrow may be a result of a nutrient deficiency or a chronic disease such as RA, SLE, tuberculosis, or cancer.

Nutritional deficiency as a cause of anemia can occur at any age. Iron, vitamin B_{12}, and folate are among the most important vitamins and minerals in the production of hemoglobin and the formation of erythrocytes. Iron is necessary for DNA synthesis, oxygen transport, and respiration. Iron deficiency can occur secondary to blood loss (RBCs are the principal site of iron storage), malabsorption, normal growth, and pregnancy. Menstruating women, pregnant women, growing children, lower socioeconomic groups, and older adults (as a result of economic constraints, lack of interest in food preparation, and poor dentition) are the most common groups to develop iron-deficiency anemia.

Vitamin B_{12} (cobalamin) is required for DNA synthesis. Deficiency of the vitamin may infrequently occur because of a lack in the diet (the body is very efficient at retaining cobalamin), but most often develops because of an absence of intrinsic factor (IF). Normally, after cobalamin is ingested it combines with R-binders in the stomach, which then is transferred to IF in the small intestine. IF is produced by gastric parietal cells and is required for cobalamin absorption in the terminal small bowel. Without IF, cobalamin is not absorbed.

Pernicious anemia is an anemia caused by a loss of IF. Antibodies against the membrane of gastric parietal cells cause an atrophy of these cells, resulting in a lack of IF production. Destruction of IF production sites may also occur with gastrectomy (see "Aging and the Gastrointestinal System" in Chapter 16).

Other causes of vitamin B_{12} deficiency include bacterial overgrowth in the lumen of the intestine (competes for vitamin B_{12}), surgical resection of the ileum (eliminates the site of vitamin B_{12} absorption), pancreatic insufficiency, achlorhydria (lack of acid in the stomach), severe Crohn disease, and, more rarely, dietary deficiency (e.g., strict vegetarian diet) and tapeworm infection. Crohn disease can cause sufficient destruction of the ileum to retard vitamin B_{12} absorption.

Folic acid deficiency is a common cause of decreased production of erythrocytes. Folic acid deficiency has many causes, but it usually results from inadequate dietary intake, chronic alcoholism, malabsorption syndromes, medications (triamterene or phenytoin), anorexia, and disorders associated with increased cell turnover. In anemia caused by folic acid deficiency associated with alcoholism, not only is the diet poor in folate, but alcohol inhibits the enzyme needed to absorb folate. The common occurrence of folic acid deficiency during the growth spurts of childhood and adolescence and during the third trimester of pregnancy is explained by the increased demands for folate required for DNA synthesis in these circumstances. Pregnant women need twice the normal amount of folic acid to meet the needs of the developing fetus.

Inflammatory anemia, previously called anemia of chronic disease, is very common in the therapy setting. It is characterized by a modest reduction in hemoglobin (9-11 g/dL), the presence of inflammation, and decreased responsiveness of the bone marrow to erythropoietin. Illnesses associated with this type of anemia include infections (i.e., tuberculosis, osteomyelitis), malignancies, and collagen vascular diseases. Many diseases associated with inflammation have accompanying elevated levels of cytokines (including interleukin [IL]-6), which lead to altered erythropoietin responsiveness. Erythropoietin production is inhibited and the erythroid precursor's response to erythropoietin is blunted. IL-6 induces the production of hepcidin, a protein synthesized by the liver, which regulates iron absorption. Hepcidin both inhibits the absorption of iron from the gut and the release of iron from macrophages for bone marrow use. Clients with an underlying chronic illness usually do not need iron, and anemia of chronic disease does not respond to iron.

Anemia also results from chronic kidney disease with subsequent decreased erythropoietin production. Most dialysis clients respond to erythropoiesis-stimulating agents.

Bone marrow disorders constitute another source of anemia caused by decreased production of erythrocytes in a therapy practice. Aplastic anemia, marrow replacement with fibrotic tissue or tumor, acute leukemia, and infiltrative disease (e.g., lymphoma, myeloma, and carcinoma) fall into this etiologic category.

Anemias of radiation-induced bone marrow failure occur because the bone marrow stem cells are destroyed and mitosis (cell division) is inhibited, preventing the synthesis of RBCs. Antimetabolites used in cancer therapy also cause bone marrow failure by blocking the synthesis of purines or nucleic acids required for synthesis of DNA within the cell. Aplastic anemia may result from either damage to the stem cells or immune-mediated destruction of the stem cells.

Clinical Manifestations

Signs and symptoms associated with anemia are related to the severity of anemia and the amount of time over which the erythrocytes were lost. Mild anemia often causes only minimal and usually vague symptoms such as fatigue until hemoglobin concentration is significantly reduced. As the anemia progresses, general signs and symptoms caused by the inability of anemic blood to supply the body tissues with enough oxygen may include weakness, dyspnea on exertion, easy fatigue, pallor, tachycardia, increased angina in people with preexisting heart disease, leg ulcers (sickle cell), and, occasionally, koilonychia (Fig. 14-1). Signs and symptoms indicative of hemolysis include jaundice, caused by the hemolysis of hemoglobin, splenomegaly, and gallstones.

Pallor in dark-skinned people may be observed by the absence of the underlying red tones that normally give brown or black skin its luster. The brown-skinned individual demonstrates pallor with a more yellowish-brown color, and the black-skinned person appears ashen or gray.

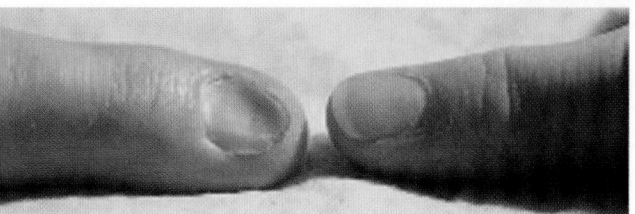

Figure 14-1

Normal nail *(right)* compared with nail referred to as koilonychia and sometimes called spoon-shaped nails or spoon nails *(left)*. They are thin, depressed nails with lateral edges turned up and are concave from side to side. They may be idiopathic, congenital, or a hereditary trait and are occasionally caused by iron-deficiency anemia. (Reprinted from Swartz MH: *Textbook of physical diagnosis*, ed 5, Philadelphia, 2006, WB Saunders.)

Mild iron deficiency may produce symptoms of irritability, lack of exercise tolerance, and headaches. Uncommonly, more substantial iron deficiency can lead to the tendency to eat ice, clay, starch, and crunchy materials (pica).

Neuropsychiatric complications such as dementia, ataxia, psychosis, and peripheral neuropathies can develop in cases of B_{12} deficiency. These abnormalities are caused by lesions in the spinal column, the cerebrum, and peripheral nerves. The lack of cobalamin initially leads to demyelination of the nerves followed by axonal degeneration. Axonal death may result if cobalamin deficiency persists.

Reversal of symptoms may be possible if treatment is initiated before permanent damage to the nerves. The findings typically consist of a symmetric sensory neuropathy that begins in the feet and lower legs, although rarely it may involve the upper extremities, especially fine motor coordination of the hands. This upper-extremity neuropathy may clinically manifest as problems with deteriorating handwriting.

Affected individuals may also describe moderate pain or paresthesias of the extremities, especially the feet. Individuals may interpret the neuropathy as difficulty with locomotion when, in fact, they are experiencing the loss of proprioception. The affected individual may need to hold on to the wall, countertops, or furniture at home due to difficulties maintaining balance. An associated positive Romberg sign may be present. Loss of motor function is a late manifestation of B_{12} deficiency.

Although a symmetrical neuropathy is the usual pattern, B_{12} deficiency occasionally presents as a unilateral neuropathy and/or bilateral but asymmetrical neuropathy. Central nervous system (CNS) manifestations range from mild cognitive changes to dementia to frank psychosis. Clients may present with personality changes and/or inappropriate behavior.

Complications depend on the specific type of anemia; severe anemia can cause heart failure and hypoxic damage to the liver and kidney with all the signs and symptoms associated with either of those conditions. Anemia in the presence of a coronary obstruction precipitates cardiac ischemia and is a risk factor for heart attack.

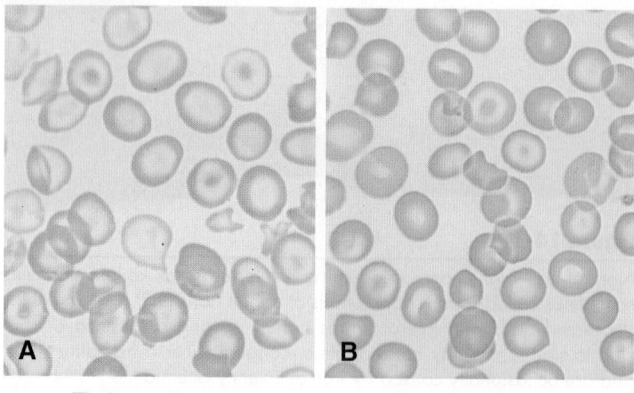

Thalassemia major   Thalassemia minor

Figure 14-2

Thalassemia is a hemolytic hemoglobinopathy anemia characterized by microcytic, short-lived RBCs caused by deficient synthesis of hemoglobin polypeptide chains. Classification of type depends on the chain involved (α-thalassemia, β-thalassemia). β-Thalassemia occurs in two forms: **(A)** thalassemia major and **(B)** thalassemia minor. Characteristic bull's-eye or target cells are shown here in both forms. (Reprinted from Damjanov I, Linder J: *Pathology: a color atlas*, St Louis, 2000, Mosby.)

MEDICAL MANAGEMENT

DIAGNOSIS. Anemia in the early stages often goes unnoticed because symptoms may not be recognized until hemoglobin concentration is reduced. Once symptoms become pronounced or noted on routine laboratory tests, the diagnosis is most often made by blood tests.

A complete blood count (CBC) gives the percentage of blood volume composed of erythrocytes, the concentration of hemoglobin, the erythrocyte count, and RBC indices. Included in the RBC indices is the size (reported as mean corpuscular volume), the shape, and size distribution (RBC distribution width). The normal hemoglobin for men is 14 to 17 g/dL (androgen effect), whereas for women it is 12 to 16 g/dL (depending on menses).

The RBC indices indicate if the RBCs are normal (normocytic), larger than normal (macrocytic, as seen with B_{12} and folate deficiency), or smaller than normal (microcytic, as seen with thalassemias and iron deficiency). The peripheral smear may reveal structural characteristics, which give clues to the underlying cause of the anemia. For example, target cells (bull's-eye erythrocytes) are often associated with thalassemia (Fig. 14-2) and microspherocytes can be seen in warm antibody-induced hemolysis, whereas sickled erythrocytes are noted with sickle cell disease (Fig. 14-3). Tear-drop cells suggest bone marrow fibrosis, whereas schistocytes (pieces of RBCs) are indicative of a microangiopathy (thrombotic thrombocytopenic purpura, hemolytic uremic syndrome, and disseminated intravascular coagulation [DIC]) or hemolysis.

A reticulocyte count is often very telling; underproduction anemias tend to have low reticulocyte counts (the bone marrow is unable to compensate), whereas anemias resulting from blood loss or peripheral destruction have a high reticulocyte count. Laboratory values indicative of hemolysis include an elevated indirect bilirubin and lactate dehydrogenase (LDH), decreased haptoglobin, and a positive direct Coombs test.

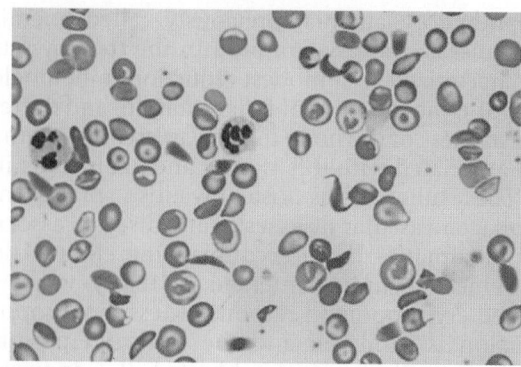

Figure 14-3

Target and sickle cells typical of sickle cell anemia (×200). (Reprinted from Goldman L: *Cecil textbook of medicine*, ed 22, Philadelphia, 2004, WB Saunders. Courtesy Jean Shafer.)

Personal and family history may point to congenital anemia, and a physical examination may elicit signs of primary hematologic diseases such as lymphadenopathy, hepatosplenomegaly, skin and mucosal changes, stool positive for blood, or bone tenderness.

Following these initial tests, more specific laboratory tests can be done to verify the diagnosis. These may include an iron profile, serum ferritin (low in iron deficiency), haptoglobin, B_{12} level, methylmalonic acid and homocysteine (both are elevated in cobalamin deficiency but only homocysteine is elevated in folate deficiency), folate level, and LDH (high in hemolysis).

TREATMENT. Treatment of anemia is directed toward alleviating or controlling the causes, relieving the symptoms, and preventing complications. It is critical that the underlying cause of anemia is determined so that appropriate treatment can be given. For example, endoscopy to identify the source of GI blood loss for a client with a long-term history of NSAID use would indicate the need to stop taking the medication and prescribe the use of proton pump inhibitors.

Treating the underlying cause can include the replacement of deficient vitamins and minerals (e.g., vitamin B_{12}, folate, or iron) or corticosteroids for warm-antibody AIHA. The anemia of cold agglutinin disease is typically mild, requiring only a warm environment, whereas bone marrow transplantation may be required for malignancies.

PROGNOSIS. The prognosis for anemia depends on the etiologic factors and potential treatment for the underlying cause. For example, the prognosis is good for anemia related to nutritional deficiency but poor for lymphoproliferative diseases. Likewise, treatment is aimed at correcting the underlying pathogenesis.

Untreated or misdiagnosed B_{12} deficiency can be progressive, resulting in irreversible neurologic damage. Anemia in the older adult (age 85 years or older) is associated with an increased risk of death. Although anemia was once considered a normal consequence of aging, it is now recognized as a sign of other disease in the older adult (e.g., hip fracture, RA, erosive gastritis, peptic ulcer, malnutrition, cirrhosis, ulcerative colitis) requiring further assessment.[159]

The Anemias

Anemia of chronic disease (also known as *anemia of inflammation*) is very common in the therapy setting.[108] It is characterized by a modest reduction in hemoglobin (7-12 g/dL), the presence of inflammation (secondary to inflammation, infection, and some malignancies), and decreased responsiveness of the bone marrow to erythropoietin. Chronic illness or inflammation signals the immune system to release a steady supply of inflammatory proteins that interfere with the production of red blood cells.

Bone marrow disorders constitute another source of anemia caused by decreased production of erythrocytes in a therapy practice. Aplastic anemia, marrow replacement with fibrotic tissue or tumor, acute leukemia, and infiltrative disease (e.g., lymphoma, myeloma, and carcinoma) fall into this etiologic category.

Exercise and Anemia

The impact of anemia on functional recovery in the acute care or rehabilitation setting and the theoretical risk of increased morbidity and mortality during prescribed therapeutic exercise have not been thoroughly investigated. Further study is indicated to examine the implications for anemia on functional recovery and cardiopulmonary complications during rehabilitation.[77]

The following guidelines should be used until proven protocols are developed. Exercise prescription for any anemic person should be reviewed with the physician.

Diminished exercise tolerance may be expected in anyone with anemia along with easy fatigability, depending on the cause of the anemia. Increased physical activity increases the demand for oxygen, which may not be adequately available in the circulating blood. Pacing and training that distribute the intensity of the workload over time can be used to promote physiologic recovery.[68]

Progress slowly for anyone with decreased exercise tolerance and monitor vital signs closely. For the sedentary aging adult, decreased activity can mask exercise intolerance; observe carefully for any changes in mental status.

The prevalence of iron-deficiency anemia is likely to be higher in athletic populations and groups, especially in younger female athletes, than in sedentary individuals. In anemic individuals, iron deficiency decreases athletic performance and impairs immune function, leading to other physiologic dysfunction.

Although it is likely that blood losses secondary to exercise, such as foot-strike hemolysis or iron loss through sweat, may contribute to anemia, nonathletic causes must also be considered. Dietary choices explain much of a negative iron balance, but the GI and genitourinary systems must be evaluated for blood loss.[315]

Evidence also exists for increased rates of RBC iron and whole-body iron turnover. The young female athlete may want to consult with medical or dietary consultants about the use of low-dose iron supplements during training.[22,377]

Research shows that people with chronic renal failure who have severe anemia are able to exercise but must do so at a lower intensity than the normal population. The maximum oxygen consumption (VO_2max) for the anemic client is at least 20% less than that for the normal population. Exercise testing and prescribed exercise(s) in anemic clients must be initiated with extreme caution and should proceed gradually to tolerance and/or perceived exertion levels.[85,262]

Precautions

Knowing the underlying cause of the anemia may be helpful in identifying red flag symptoms indicating the need for alteration of the program or medical referral. For example, GI blood loss associated with NSAID use may worsen suddenly, precipitating a crisis in a therapy setting. After major noncardiac surgery (e.g., orthopedic procedures), even mild anemia is associated with increased morbidity and mortality. Rates of postoperative conditions such as sepsis and venous thromboembolism can be much higher associated with anemia.[233]

It is not uncommon for clients to present with both anemia and cardiovascular disease, precipitating angina. Studies show that the amount of oxygen-carrying hemoglobin (Hb) circulating in the blood of older women is an independent risk factor for mobility problems. Hb perceived as mildly low and even low-normal (12 g/dL) in women at least 70 years old increases the likelihood of difficulty performing daily tasks by 1.5 times.[51,52]

The therapist may identify older adults who have a difficult time with general mobility, such as walking more than one block, climbing a flight of stairs, or doing housework. When they have difficulty, they become more sedentary, resulting in a decline in independence. The condition of mildly low Hb is no longer considered clinically benign as mortality risk has been shown to be lower with higher Hb levels.[53] It may be appropriate to request assessment of Hb levels and/or communicate with the physician about the potential harm of low-normal Hb levels.

Bleeding under the skin and easy bruising in response to the slightest trauma often occur when platelet production is altered (thrombocytopenia) secondary to hypoplastic or aplastic anemia. This condition necessitates extreme care in the therapy setting, especially any intervention requiring manual therapy or the use of any equipment, including modalities and weight-training devices. Splenomegaly associated with some types of anemia requires precautions in performing soft tissue techniques in the left upper quadrant, especially up and under the rib cage; indirect techniques away from the spleen are indicated.

Decreased oxygen delivery to the skin results in impaired healing and loss of elasticity as well as delaying wound healing and healing of other musculoskeletal injuries. If the anemia is caused by vitamin B_{12} deficiency (e.g., pernicious anemia, pregnancy, hyperthyroidism), the nervous system is affected.

Alteration of the structure and function of the peripheral nerves, spinal cord (myelin degeneration), and brain may occur. Paresthesias, especially numbness mimicking carpal tunnel syndrome; gait disturbances; extreme weakness; spasticity; and abnormal reflexes can result. Permanent neurologic damage unresponsive to vitamin B_{12} therapy can occur in extreme cases when intervention has been delayed.

Monitoring Vital Signs

Many individuals who are anemic are asymptomatic. Careful monitoring is required. Tachycardia may be the first change observed when monitoring vital signs, usually accompanied by a sense of fatigue, generalized weakness, loss of stamina, and exertional dyspnea. Systolic blood pressure may not be affected, but diastolic pressure may be lower than normal, with an associated increase in the resting pulse rate.

Resting cardiac output is usually normal in people with anemia, but cardiac output increases with exercise more than in nonanemic people. As the anemia becomes more severe, resting cardiac output increases and exercise tolerance progressively decreases until dyspnea, tachycardia, and palpitations occur at rest.

A THERAPIST'S THOUGHTS*

Anemia

Anemia may be defined differently from region to region, hospital to hospital, and even physician to physician. Hemoglobin less than 8 g/dL is no longer a complete contraindication to physical therapy intervention.

A general guideline is to review and possibly modify or restrict activity and exercise when hemoglobin is less than 8 with a hematocrit level less than 25. This is especially applicable to individuals who are not critically ill or who are in the intensive care unit with acute coronary syndromes. Some institutions use less than 7 as a guideline for individuals in intensive care who have stable cardiac disease.

Low-impact and low-intensity aerobics (e.g., stationary bicycle) may be tolerated by individuals with anemia and hemoglobin levels between 10 and 12 g/dL. Isometrics and resistive exercise can also be incorporated slowly and carefully in this population group. Hemoglobin levels between 8 and 10 g/dL may be a contraindication to aggressive therapeutic strengthening and endurance training. Use the guidelines offered here to guide your thinking for each individual.

Remember to look at the *trend* an individual's hemoglobin levels over the last few days and try to understand what is going on with that particular person. Consider the past medical history as well as the current medical and physical (conditioning) status.

Look for acute blood loss (even with normal or near-normal hemoglobin levels) versus chronic anemia. Engage in discussion with the medical staff to more fully understand the person's physiologic status. A person who is chronically anemic (e.g., chronic kidney disease) will probably be better able to withstand exercise at a lower hemoglobin level compared with an individual who is at the same level but has had an acute drop in hemoglobin.

*Eva Gold, PT

DISORDERS OF LEUKOCYTES

Alterations in blood leukocyte (WBC) concentration and in the relative proportions of the several leukocyte types are recognized as measures of the reaction of the body to infection, inflammation, tissue damage, or degeneration. In many instances, these alterations give useful indications of the nature of the pathologic process and may be seen in association not only with acute infections but also with many chronic ailments treated by the therapist.

Leukocytes may be classified in three main groups: granulocytes (basophils, eosinophils, neutrophils), monocytes, and lymphocytes. *Granulocytes* (granular leukocytes) contain lysing agents within their granules that are capable of digesting various foreign materials. The main type of granulocyte is the neutrophil, also called the *polymorphonuclear leukocyte*; these are usually not found in normal "healthy" tissue and are referred to as the first line of hematologic defense against invading pathogens.

Granulocytes are also involved in the pathophysiology of organ damage in ischemia/reperfusion, trauma, sepsis, or organ transplantation. Basophils and eosinophils are involved with allergic reactions and respond to parasitic and fungal infections.

Monocytes are the largest circulating blood cells and represent an immature cell until it leaves the blood and travels to the tissues. Once migrated, monocytes form macrophages when activated by foreign substances, such as bacteria. Monocytes/macrophages participate in inflammation by synthesizing numerous mediators and eliminating various pathogens.

Lymphocytes are further divided into B and T cells. B lymphocytes are responsible for the humoral portion of the immune system and are known to secrete antibodies that react with antigens and initiate complement-mediated destruction or phagocytosis of foreign pathogens, particularly bacteria. T lymphocytes are in control of cell-mediated immunity and are able to recognize and destroy cells altered by viruses.

These cells are also responsible for coordinating the immune response through the release of lymphokines and inflammatory modulators, creating a cell-to-cell communication with B cells and monocytes. The exact role or function of leukocytes during inflammatory processes remains the subject of considerable investigation.

Leukocytosis

Definition and Etiology

Leukocytosis, defined as an increase in the number of leukocytes in the blood, may occur as a result of a variety of causes (Box 14-5) and may also occur as a normal protective response to physiologic stressors such as strenuous exercise, emotional changes, temperature changes, anesthesia, surgery, pregnancy, some drugs, toxins, and hormones.

Leukocytosis develops within 1 or 2 hours after the onset of acute hemorrhage and is greater when the bleeding occurs internally (e.g., into the peritoneal cavity, pleural space, or joint cavity, or as a result of a skull fracture

Box 14-5

CAUSES OF LEUKOCYTOSIS

- Acute hemorrhage
- Infection (viral, bacterial, or fungal)
- Malignancies (leukemia, lymphoma, non–small cell lung cancer, multiple myeloma)
- Myeloproliferative disorders
- Glucocorticosteroid therapy
- Trauma (burns)
- Tissue necrosis (infarction)
- Inflammation (autoimmune-mediated such as myositis or vasculitis)

with associated intracranial bleed or subarachnoid hemorrhage) than when the bleeding is external.

Leukocytosis is a common finding in and characterizes many infectious diseases recognized by a count of more than 10,000 WBCs/mm^3 (see Table 40-7). An elevated WBC count (greater than 50,000/mm^3, with the majority of cells being neutrophils and neutrophil precursors) in response to a serious underlying process is referred to as a leukemoid reaction (see Box 14-5).

Leukocytosis frequently results from an increase in circulating neutrophils (neutrophilia), recruited in large numbers in the course of infections and in the presence of some rapidly growing neoplasms (e.g., leukemia, non–small cell lung cancer, renal cell carcinoma, and gastric carcinoma). The counts may be especially high in tumors with significant necrosis. Some tumors can also release hormone-like substances that cause leukocytosis.

Clinical Manifestations

Clinical signs and symptoms of leukocytosis are usually associated with symptoms of the conditions listed in Box 14-5 and may include fever, headache, shortness of breath, symptoms of localized or systemic infection, and symptoms of inflammation or trauma to tissue.

MEDICAL MANAGEMENT

DIAGNOSIS, TREATMENT, AND PROGNOSIS. Major leukocyte functions are accomplished in the tissues so that the leukocytes in the blood are in transit from the site of production or storage to the tissues, even in normal people. Variations in the blood concentrations of each leukocyte type may be of brief duration and easily missed or may persist for days or weeks. Laboratory tests for detecting leukocyte abnormalities include total leukocyte count, leukocyte differential cell count (see Chapter 40), peripheral blood morphology, and bone marrow morphology.

Treatment is directed toward the underlying cause of the change in leukocytes and control of any infections. Prognosis depends on the etiology of the leukocytosis.

SPECIAL IMPLICATIONS FOR THE THERAPIST 14-6

Leukocytes

It is important for the therapist to be aware of the client's most recent leukocyte (WBC) count before and during episodes of care if that person is immunosuppressed.

At that time, the client is extremely susceptible to opportunistic infections and severe complications.

The importance of good handwashing (see Boxes 8-4 and 8-5) and hygiene practices cannot be overemphasized when treating immunocompromised clients. Some centers recommend that people with a WBC count of less than 1000/mm^3 or a neutrophil count of less than 500/mm^3 wear a protective mask. Therapists should ensure that these people are provided with equipment that has been disinfected according to standard precautions.

Leukopenia

Definition and Etiology

Leukopenia, or reduction of the number of leukocytes in the blood below 5000/mL (see Chapter 40), can be caused by a variety of factors such as HIV (or other viral infection, such as hepatitis), alcohol and nutritional deficiencies, drug-induced condition, and connective tissue disorders (e.g., SLE). It can occur in many forms of bone marrow failure, such as that following antineoplastic chemotherapy or radiation therapy or in overwhelming infections.

People with leukemia, lymphoma, myeloma, and Hodgkin lymphoma have serious underlying WBC abnormalities that contribute to the risk of infection associated with leukopenia. Unlike leukocytosis, leukopenia is never beneficial. As the leukocyte count decreases, the risk for various infections increases.

The risk of infection from leukopenia after bone marrow radiation has been reduced with continued improvements in medical treatment. The use of naturally occurring glycoproteins to help collect blood stem cells administered after chemotherapy reduces the duration of blood cell reduction and prevents the serious problems encountered in the past.

These glycoproteins are hematopoietic growth factors called colony-stimulating factors or, more specifically, granulocyte colony-stimulating factor, or filgrastim (Neupogen). Growth factors move the stem cells from the bone marrow into the peripheral blood and can result in a temporary 10-fold to 100-fold increase in the numbers of circulating stem cells at the time of bone marrow recovery. Filgrastim not only increases the number but also the function of granulocytes.

Clinical Manifestations

Leukopenia may be asymptomatic (and detected by routine tests) or associated with clinical signs and symptoms consistent with infection such as sore throat, cough, high fever, chills, sweating, ulcerations of mucous membranes (e.g., mouth, rectum, vagina), frequent or painful urination, or persistent infections.

MEDICAL MANAGEMENT

DIAGNOSIS AND TREATMENT. As with leukocytosis, diagnosis is by laboratory testing for leukocyte abnormalities. Treatment is directed toward elimination of the cause of the reduced leukocytes and control of any infections.

Pharmacologic therapy includes the use of antibiotics, antifungal agents, and colony-stimulating factor drugs such as filgrastim (Neupogen). This drug markedly assists in decreasing the incidence of infection in people who have received bone marrow–depressing antineoplastic agents.

Basophilia

Basophilia refers to a condition where the number or proportion of basophils to other leukocytes in the blood or tissue is increased. Basophilia is primarily associated with myeloproliferative disorders, particularly chronic myeloid leukemia. Basophils are the least common subtype of leukocytes accounting for 0.5% of all leukocytes. They are often involved in parasitic infections and inflammatory and allergic reactions.[336] Basophils express multiple types of receptors (cytokine, chemokine, complement, immunoglobulin, and prostaglandin). Basophils mature in the bone marrow and circulate in the periphery. They have a half-life of only a few days. Although basophils are typically not found in tissue, they are able to infiltrate to inflamed tissue such as seen in asthma and atopic dermatitis.[165,334]

Aggregation of immunoglobulin Fc receptor (expressed by the surface of the basophil) bound by antigen to IgE results in basophil activation and granule and mediator release. Other cytokines and chemokines activate basophils or prime basophils for activation. Mediators that are released include histamine, complexed with chondroitin sulfates, heparin (less than mast cells contain), cytokines (such as IL-4), and leukotrienes (potent bronchorestrictors and increase vascular permeability).

Eosinophilia

Eosinophilia is the increased number of eosinophils in tissue or blood. Eosinophils are a prominent feature of helminthic infections, allergy, asthma, and pulmonary and GI disorders. Eosinophils mature in the bone marrow and are stimulated to differentiate and develop by IL-5, which is produced in areas of inflammation. Once mature, they are released into the circulation and migrate into tissue. These tissues are in areas that have contact with the external environment, such as the skin, GI tract, and lungs. Eosinophils express a wide variety of cell surface receptors (immunoglobulin IgG and IgA, chemokines, cytokines, complement, and adhesion molecules) and can be activated by various antibodies and interleukins and stimulated to release proinflammatory mediators (such as chemokines, growth factors, cytokines, peroxidase, and other modulating proteins).

An elevation in the number of eosinophils in the blood, eosinophilia (eosinophil count greater than 500/mm^3) is seen most often in mild atopic asthma, allergic reactions to drugs (aspirin, sulfonamides, penicillins), helminthic reactions, and hypereosinophilic syndromes. Hypereosinophilia syndromes (6 subtypes; >1500/mm^3) are associated with marked, persistent, eosinophilia with/without end-organ damage and exclusion of other known causes of eosinophilia. Allergic diseases such as allergic rhinitis, atopic asthma, and atopic dermatitis, may have a mild eosinophilia, but the number of eosinophils in tissues is typically more significantly elevated than the blood.[334]

Neutrophilia

Granulocytes assist in initiating the inflammatory response, and they defend the body against infectious agents by phagocytosing bacteria and other infectious substances. Generally, the neutrophils (the most plentiful of the granulocytes) are the first phagocytic cells to reach an infected area, followed by monocytes; neutrophils and monocytes work together to phagocytose all foreign material present.

Granulocytosis (an excess of granulocytes in the blood) or *neutrophilia* (increased number of neutrophils in the blood) are terms used to describe the early stages of infection or inflammation. The capacity of corticosteroids or alcohol to diminish the accumulation of neutrophils in inflamed areas may be due to their ability to reduce cell adherence.

The many potential causes of neutrophilia include inflammation or tissue necrosis (e.g., after surgery from tissue damage, severe burns, myocardial infarction, pneumonitis, rheumatic fever, RA); acute infection (e.g., *Staphylococcus*, *Streptococcus*, *Pneumococcus*); drug- or chemical-induced causes (e.g., epinephrine, steroids, heparin, histamine); metabolic causes (e.g., acidosis associated with diabetes, gout, thyroid storm, eclampsia); and neoplasms of the liver, GI tract, or bone marrow. Physiologic neutrophilia may also occur as a result of exercise, extreme heat/cold, third-trimester pregnancy, and emotional distress.

Neutropenia

Neutropenia is the condition associated with a reduction in circulating neutrophils (less than 2500/µL). Causes are either acquired or congenital. Acquired neutropenias are typically a result of toxicity to neutrophil precursors in the bone marrow. This may be from drugs (e.g., NSAIDs, sulfonamides, penicillins, anticonvulsants) or infectious agents (e.g., hepatitis B, cytomegalovirus, EBV, HIV). Other drugs can cause an autoimmune-related peripheral destruction of neutrophils, leading to neutropenia.

Other causes of neutropenia include carcinoma of the lung, breast, prostate, and stomach and malignant hematopoietic disorders that can occupy enough of the bone marrow to cause global marrow failure with resultant pancytopenias (all cell lines are decreased in number). Congenital causes usually come to attention early in life and are much less common than acquired causes.

The longer an individual exists without neutrophils, the higher the risk for significant infection. Drug-induced neutropenia generally resolves in 10 to 12 days; administration of granulocyte colony-stimulating factor may shorten the time to resolution.

Lymphocytosis/Lymphocytopenia

Lymphocytosis occurs most commonly in acute viral infections, especially those caused by EBV. Other causes include endocrine disorders (e.g., thyrotoxicosis, adrenal insufficiency) and malignancies (e.g., acute and chronic lymphocytic leukemia).

Lymphocytopenia may be acquired or congenital. Acquired lymphocytopenias can be attributed to abnormalities of lymphocyte production associated with neoplasms and immune deficiencies and destruction of lymphocytes by drugs, viruses, or radiation.

Other causes include corticosteroid therapy, severe systemic illnesses (e.g., military tuberculosis), SLE, sarcoid, or severe right-sided heart failure. For individuals with AIDS, lymphocytopenia can be a major problem, increasing their susceptibility to viral illnesses, malignancies, and fungal infections.

Monocytosis

Monocytosis, an increase in monocytes, is most often seen in chronic infections, such as tuberculosis and subacute endocarditis, and other inflammatory processes, such as SLE and RA. Monocytosis is present in more than 50% of people with collagen vascular disease (see Box 12-17).

Clients with sarcoid or other granulomatous processes may also have elevated monocytes. Monocytosis also exists as a normal physiologic response in newborns (first 2 weeks of life). Although not common, monocytes can go through a transformation, becoming leukemia, or an elevation of normal monocytes can be seen in malignancies such as Hodgkin and non-Hodgkin lymphoma. Monocytosis can be indicative of bone marrow recovery following a drug-induced loss of granulocytes.

NEOPLASTIC DISEASES OF THE BLOOD AND LYMPH SYSTEMS

Hematologic malignancies include diseases in any hematologic tissue (e.g., bone marrow, spleen, thymus) that arise from changes in stem cells or clonal (genetically identical cells) proliferation of abnormal cells. The primary hematologic disorders that result from stem

cell abnormalities include the myeloproliferative neoplasms (e.g., polycythemia vera, essential thrombocythemia, chronic myeloid leukemia, and myelofibrosis with myeloid metaplasia) and acute myeloid leukemia. Myelofibrosis is the replacement of hematopoietic bone marrow with fibrous tissue such as fibroblasts and collagen.

Multiple myeloma and plasma cell diseases arise from clonal proliferation of abnormal plasma cells. Lymphoid malignancies are also a clonal proliferation of malignant cells and can be categorized according to the malignant cell type: B-cell, T-cell/natural killer cell, and Hodgkin lymphoma. For ease of discussion, the leukemias are presented together.

Hematopoietic Stem Cell Transplantation

Hematopoietic stem cell transplantation (HSCT or HCT) is often a treatment choice for many of the neoplastic diseases of the blood and lymph systems. Technical explanations of HSCT are found in Chapter 21.

The Leukemias

Leukemia is a malignant neoplasm of the blood-forming cells that replaces the normal bone marrow with a malignant clone (genetically identical cell) of lymphocytic or myelogenous cells. The disease may be acute or chronic based on its natural course; acute leukemias have a rapid clinical course, resulting in death in a few months without treatment, whereas chronic leukemias have a more prolonged course. The four major types of leukemia are acute or chronic lymphocytic and acute or chronic myeloid leukemia (Table 14-2).

When leukemia is classified according to its morphology (i.e., the predominant cell type and level of maturity), the following descriptors are used: *lympho-*, for leukemias involving the lymphoid or lymphatic system; *myelo-*, for leukemias of myeloid or bone marrow origin involving

Table 14-2	Overview of Leukemia			
	Acute Lymphocytic Leukemia (ALL)	**Chronic Lymphocytic Leukemia (CLL)**	**Acute Myelogenous Leukemia (AML)**	**Chronic Myelogenous Leukemia (CML)**
Incidence (% of all leukemias)	20%	25%	40%	15%-20%
Adults	30%	100% (common)	80% (most common)	95%-100%
Children	65%-70% (most common	NA	20%	2%
Age (yr)	Peak: 3-7	50+	Mean age: 63; incidence increases with age from 45-80+	Average age 66 (mostly adults)
Etiologic factors	? Unknown; chromosomal abnormalities; Down syndrome (high incidence)	Chromosomal abnormalities; slow accumulation of CLL lymphocytes	Benzene; alkylating agents; radiation; myeloproliferative disorders; chromosome abnormalities	Philadelphia chromosome; radiation exposure
Prognosis	Adults: 40% survival Children: 80% survival	Poor cytogenetics: median 8 yr Good cytogenetics: median 25 yr Median survival: 10-14 yr	Adults: • Poor cytogenetics: 10% • Intermediate cytogenetics: 40% • Good cytogenetics: 60%	Moderately progressive with new treatment; current survival rate unknown

hematopoietic stem cells (see Fig. 21-6); -*blastic*, for leukemia involving large, immature (functionless) cells; and -*cytic*, for leukemia involving mature, smaller cells. If classified immunologically, T-cell/natural killer cell and B-cell leukemias are described.

Acute leukemia is an accumulation of neoplastic, immature lymphoid or myeloid cells in the bone marrow and peripheral blood. It is defined as more than 30% blasts in the bone marrow (the WHO classification accepts 20% as the definition of leukemia).

Chronic leukemia is a neoplastic accumulation of mature lymphoid or myeloid elements of the blood that usually progresses more slowly than an acute leukemic process and permits the production of greater numbers of more mature, functional cells. With rapid proliferation of leukemic cells, the bone marrow becomes overcrowded with abnormal cells, which then spill over into the peripheral circulation. Crowding of the bone marrow by leukemic cells inhibits normal blood cell production.

The three main symptoms that occur as a consequence of this infiltration and replacement process are (1) *anemia* and reduced tissue oxygenation from decreased erythrocytes, (2) *infection* from neutropenia as leukemic cells are functionally unable to defend the body against pathogens, and (3) *bleeding tendencies* from decreased platelet production (thrombocytopenia) (Fig. 14-4).

Leukemia is not limited to the bone marrow and peripheral blood. Abnormalities in the CNS or other organ systems can result from the infiltration and replacement of any tissue of the body with nonfunctional leukemic cells or metabolic complications related to leukemia.

Leukemia is a complex disease that requires careful identification of the subtype for appropriate treatment. Molecular probes can be used to establish a morphologic diagnosis of the type of leukemia, which then determines treatment and prognosis. These analyses are sufficiently sensitive to detect one leukemic cell among 100,000 or even in 1 million normal cells. Because of this extreme sensitivity, molecular markers have generally been used to determine the presence or absence of a few leukemic cells remaining after intensive therapy, so-called residual disease.

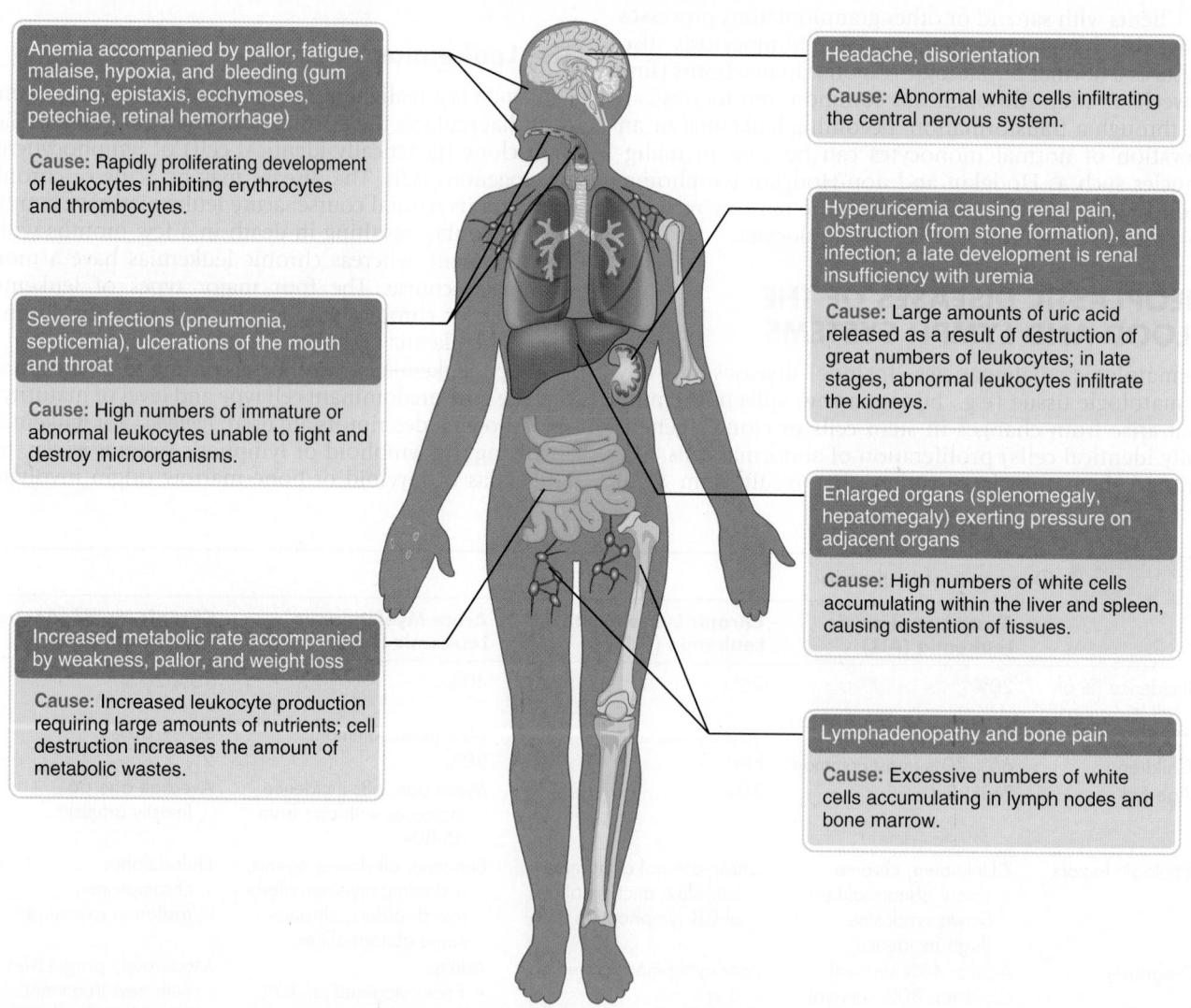

Figure 14-4

Pathologic basis for the clinical manifestations of leukemia. (Modified from Black JM, Matassarin-Jacobs E, editors: *Luckmann and Sorensen's medical-surgical nursing*, ed 4, Philadelphia, 1993, WB Saunders.)

Over the last 30 years, death rates for leukemia have been falling significantly (57% decline) for children and more modestly for adults younger than age 65 years. These declines in mortality reflect the advances made in the biologic and pathologic understanding of leukemia, technologic advances in medical care, and subsequent treatment that is more specifically targeted at the molecular level.

The aim of treatment is to bring about complete remission, or no evidence of the disease, with return to normal blood and marrow cells without relapse. For leukemia, a complete remission that lasts 5 years after treatment often indicates a cure. Future clinical and laboratory investigation will likely lead to the development of new, even more effective treatments specifically for different subsets of leukemia. The development of new chemotherapeutic and biologic agents combined with refined dose and schedule and stem cell transplantation has already contributed to the clinical success of treatment.

Acute Leukemia

Acute leukemia is a rapidly progressive malignant disease that results in the accumulation of immature, functionless cells called *blast cells* in the bone marrow and blood that block the development of normal cell development.

The two major forms of acute leukemia are *acute lymphoblastic leukemia* (ALL) and *acute myelogenous leukemia* (AML). Lymphocytic leukemia involves the lymphocytes (B or T lymphoblasts) and lymphoid organs, and myelogenous leukemia involves hematopoietic stem cells that differentiate into myeloid cells (monocytes, granulocytes, erythrocytes, and platelets).

Acute Myelogenous Leukemia

Incidence and Risk Factors. AML is the most common leukemia in adults, constituting 80% of adult acute leukemias. Only 6% of individuals with AML are children. AML remains an uncommon disease, with more than 13,000 cases in 2012.[151]

The incidence of AML increases with each decade of life, with the median age at onset of 66 years.[151] Most cases of AML develop for unknown reasons, whereas some cases occur following treatment for another cancer (chemotherapy or radiation induced), from a preexisting myelodysplastic syndrome, or a bone marrow failure syndrome (such as aplastic anemia).[362]

Two predominant types of treatment-related AML (t-AML) are described. The first typically occurs 5 to 10 years following exposure to an alkylating agent (i.e., cyclophosphamide, cisplatin) and/or radiation and is often heralded by a dysplastic phase. The other appears shortly after exposure to a topoisomerase II inhibitor (approximately 1 year) and lacks a dysplastic phase. Abnormalities in chromosome 5 and/or 7 are often seen in treatment-related AML and carry a worse prognosis than those cases that are idiopathic.[115,296]

Other risk factors for AML include previous radiation exposure and chemical/occupational exposure (e.g., benzene, herbicides, pesticides, cigarette smoking). Persons with uncommon genetic disorders, such as Down syndrome or Fanconi syndrome, also have a higher incidence of developing acute leukemia than the general population.

Pathogenesis. AML is a heterogeneous group (not all the same) of neoplastic myeloid cells. Myeloid stem cells have the capability of differentiating into granulocytes, monocytes, erythrocytes, and platelets; neoplastic changes can occur along any line, resulting in many subtypes of AML.

Current techniques allow for cytogenetic analyses that can reveal specific chromosomal abnormalities where portions of a chromosome translocate (move) and fuse with another gene, creating a fusion gene. It is these successive abnormalities that lead to the development of leukemia, either allowing the cell to divide without regulation or failing to undergo programmed cell death (apoptosis).[114]

Clinical Manifestation. Initial clinical indications of AML are related to pancytopenia (reduction in all cell lines), reflecting leukemic cell replacement of bone marrow. Clients often have infections because of a lack of neutrophils or bleeding secondary to platelet deficiency (thrombocytopenia).

Spontaneous bleeding or bleeding with minor trauma often occurs in the skin and mucosal surfaces, manifested as gingival bleeding, epistaxis, mid-cycle menstrual bleeding, or heavy bleeding associated with menstruation (see Fig. 14-4). Petechiae (small, purplish spots caused by intradermal bleeding) are common clinical manifestations of thrombocytopenia particularly noted on the extremities after prolonged standing or minor trauma.

Fatigue, loss of energy, and shortness of breath with physical exertion are common because of anemia. Leukemia cells may infiltrate the skin (known as leukemia cutis), seen most often in the acute monocytic or myelomonocytic subtypes of AML. Leukemia cutis may present as multiple purplish papules or as a diffuse rash (Fig. 14-5). Uncommonly, AML cells may also form masses in the skin, tissue, or bone.

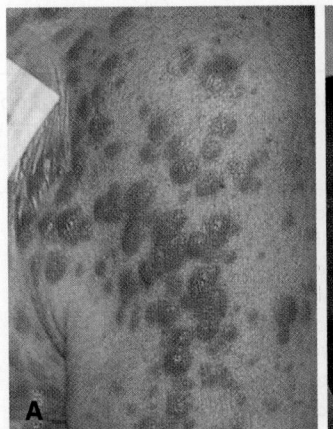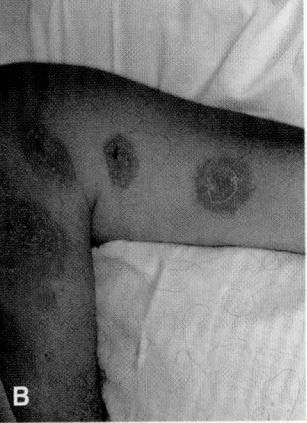

Figure 14-5

A, Leukemia cutis in an individual with monoblastic leukemia. **B,** Another example of leukemia cutis in the form of erythematous nodular tumors. (A, Reprinted from Hoffman R: *Hematology: basic principles and practice*, ed 4, Philadelphia, 2005, Churchill Livingstone. **B,** Reprinted from Noble J: *Textbook of primary care medicine*, ed 3, St Louis, 2001, Mosby.)

Modest splenomegaly is seen in 50% of clients with AML, whereas lymphadenopathy is uncommon. Discomfort in the bones, especially of the sternum, ribs, and tibia, caused by expanded leukemic marrow may occur. In the older adult, the disease can present insidiously with progressive weakness, pallor, a change in sense of well-being, and delirium.

CNS involvement is uncommon, occurring in only 1% to 2% of adults presenting with AML.[23] These people present with symptoms similar to meningitis (e.g., headache, stiff neck, and fever). Some clients may develop cerebral bleeding or meningitis because of pancytopenia. In a small number of cases, AML may be more subtle, presenting at first with progressive fatigue and normal blood counts.

MEDICAL MANAGEMENT

DIAGNOSIS. Initial blood tests often reveal an elevated leukocyte count with an excessive amount of immature cells although low counts may be seen, especially in the elderly. Uncommonly initial counts may be normal. Sometimes Auer rods (linear groupings of primary granules) are seen on peripheral blood smear, which are indicative of AML, rather than ALL. Diagnosis usually requires a bone marrow biopsy and aspiration in order to view bone marrow architecture and perform further tests such as cytogenetics, immunophenotyping, and flow cytometry. The diagnosis of AML is made when more than 20% of blasts are detected in the bone marrow.

Because most AML does not involve the CNS, lumbar punctures are not needed unless clinically indicated. Treatment is determined by lineage, and AML treatment differs from ALL treatment. AML can be subdivided into various subtypes or classifications, and each subtype may receive varying initial therapy. The FAB system (French-American-British classification, first published in 1976) describes eight subdivisions classifying AML according to cell morphology and according to how the cells react to various stains (Table 14-3).

The WHO has provided a revised classification of AML, using cytogenetic information (chromosomal abnormalities) and clinical information. The categories include AML with recurrent genetic abnormalities, AML with myelodysplasia related changes, therapy-related AML, and AML not otherwise specified (which is similar to the FAB classification system).[354]

Some of the more common genetic abnormalities include a translocation between chromosomes 8 and 21 (which is a favorable mutation); a translocation or inversion in chromosome 16 (favorable mutation); changes in chromosome 11; and a translocation between chromosomes 15 and 17 (favorable mutation). The latter translocation, known as acute promyelocytic leukemia, is important to identify, because it is treated differently from other AML subtypes and carries a better prognosis.

Other abnormalities that have been identified include mutations of the *FLT3* gene (found in approximately 30% of AML cases and associated with a poor prognosis) and *NPM1* mutation, which is associated with a better prognosis. Pretreatment cytogenetics often prognosticate outcomes (favorable, intermediate, and high risk for recurrence) and influence therapy.[40,124]

TREATMENT. The diagnosis of acute leukemia is a medical emergency, especially if the WBC count is high (greater than 100,000/mL), placing the person at risk for cerebral hemorrhage caused by leukostasis (obstruction of and damage to blood vessels plugged with rigid, large blasts). Clients with high a WBC prior to receiving chemotherapy are at risk for tumor lysis syndrome (see "Acute Lymphoblastic Leukemia [Acute Lymphocytic Leukemia]" below).

Treatment decisions are based on the subtype of AML and cytogenetics. Most induction (initial) treatment protocols utilize aggressive combination chemotherapy (typically cytarabine and an anthracycline) in order to eradicate the neoplastic cells and restore normal hematopoiesis. Supportive care, including fluids, blood product replacement, and prompt treatment of infection with broad-spectrum antibiotics, is frequently needed during the 3- to 4-week hospitalization required for bone marrow recovery. Significant complications occur during this period, with a death rate of 5% to 10%.[20]

Table 14-3	Revised Classification of Acute Myelogenous Leukemia		
FAB Classification		**Incidence**	**Prognosis Compared to Average AML**
M0	Acute myeloblastic leukemia Minimal differentiation	5%	Worse
M1	Acute myeloblastic leukemia Without maturation	15%	Average
M2	Acute myeloblastic leukemia With maturation	25%	Better
M3	Acute promyelocytic leukemia	10%	Best
M4	Acute myelomonocytic leukemia	20%	Average
M4eos	Acute myelomonocytic leukemia with eosinophilia	5%	Better
M5	Acute monoblastic leukemia	10%	Average
M6	Acute erythroleukemia	5%	Worse
M7	Acute megakaryoblastic leukemia	5%	Worse

AML, acute myelogenous leukemia; FAB, French-American-British.

Data from Learn About Cancer. American Cancer Society. Available at http://www.cancer.org/cancer/leukemia-acutemyeloidaml/detailedguide/leukemia-acute-myeloid-myelogenous-classified. Accessed March 25, 2013.

Induction chemotherapy is followed by consolidation chemotherapy, which is intended to maintain a complete remission and eradicate residual disease. Consolidation treatment is administered in 3 to 4 courses.

People who are young with cytogenetics consistent with a good prognosis can undergo consolidation therapy. Individuals at high risk for recurrent disease should consider allogeneic HSCT or HCT after induction chemotherapy. Older people with favorable-to-intermediate cytogenetics typically receive an abbreviated consolidation treatment. Elderly clients with high-risk disease and comorbidities may not be able to tolerate aggressive therapy, in which case they are offered supportive care. This usually consists of transfusions, antibiotics, and low-dose chemotherapy (such as hydroxyurea) to control leukocytosis.

The discovery of mutations and translocations that may be causing leukemia has led to the development of targeted therapeutic agents. One example is all-*trans*-retinoic acid. It is used against acute promyelocytic leukemia along with chemotherapy and targets the promyelocytic leukemia–retinoic acid receptor-α fusion transcript of the t(15,17) translocation.

PROGNOSIS. If left untreated, all leukemias are fatal. Adverse prognostic features include older age (often have more chromosome abnormalities and comorbidities), history of myelodysplastic syndrome or myeloproliferative disorder, previous exposure to chemotherapy and/or radiation, or chromosome abnormalities associated with a poor prognosis. With induction treatment, approximately 60% to 70% of clients younger than 60 years achieve a remission. The rate of remission decreases as age increases over 60 years.[13]

On average, clients older than 60 years of age have a 5-year disease-free survival of 5% to 10%,[117] whereas those younger than 60 years have a 5-year disease-free survival of 30%. Current research is focused on cytogenetics and targeted therapies in hopes of improving long-term survival.

Acute Lymphoblastic Leukemia (Acute Lymphocytic Leukemia)

Incidence and Risk Factors. In contrast to AML, ALL is diagnosed more frequently in children. Of the 4000 cases of ALL identified each year, two-thirds occur in children, whereas only one-third are diagnosed in adults.[151] Yet of the 1500 annual deaths, almost two-thirds occur in adults. Unfortunately, the incidence of ALL has slowly increased over the past 25 years.[306]

Like AML, most ALL cases develop for unknown reasons. A few risk factors have been identified including previous exposure to chemotherapy and/or radiation and infection with HTLV-1 (human T-cell lymphoma/leukemia virus). Persons with genetic disorders such as Down syndrome also have an increased risk.

Questions have arisen as to whether electromagnetic fields, such as those generated in high-voltage power lines, increase the risk of developing ALL. Studies are still ongoing, but show either a modest or no increase in risk.[164,224,305]

Pathogenesis. Abnormal cytogenetics or translocations and mutations are frequently seen in ALL cases.

These genetic changes lead to an inability to differentiate or mature. These various abnormalities are associated with poor or good prognosis. For instance, leukemic cells with more than 50 chromosomes (hyperdiploidy), particularly trisomies of chromosomes 4, 10, and 17,[133] and the *ETV6-RUNX1* fusion t(12,21) have a good prognosis. Leukemic cells with less than 45 chromosomes are difficult to treat and carry a poor prognosis.[235] Rearrangements of the *MLL* gene and the presence of the Philadelphia chromosome t(9;22) also have a poor prognosis.

Clinical Manifestations. ALL exhibits clinical signs and symptoms resulting from an abnormal bone marrow that is unable to engage in normal hematopoiesis. Fever and frequent infections indicate a lack of normal neutrophils, whereas easy bleeding and bruising are indicative of thrombocytopenia. Clients are often tired as a result of anemia.

ALL is more likely than AML to have leukemic cells spread to extramedullary sites. Although symptoms are not typically present at diagnosis, the CNS is frequently involved, and can cause headache, weakness, seizures, vomiting, difficulty with balance, radiculopathy, cranial nerve palsy, and blurred vision.[12] Testicles in males and ovaries in females commonly harbor leukemic cells and are difficult to reach with chemotherapy agents.

Bone and joint pain from leukemic infiltration or hemorrhage into a joint may be the initial symptoms (more common finding in children than adults). Involvement of the synovium may lead to symptoms suggestive of a rheumatic disease, especially in children.

Hepatosplenomegaly and lymphadenopathy (particularly in the mediastinum) are frequently encountered along with an enlarged thymus. If thymic swelling is significant, the client may exhibit difficulty breathing or upper extremity swelling from increased pressure on the bronchus or superior vena cava (superior vena cava syndrome), which requires immediate attention.

Tumor lysis syndrome is common at diagnosis or shortly after the instigation of chemotherapy. This life-threatening condition occurs when there is a high turnover rate of cells (seen in acute leukemias) or chemotherapy agents lyse significant numbers of cells, resulting in high levels of potassium, phosphate, calcium, and uric acid. Complications such as acute renal failure and DIC may also occur. Prevention of tumor lysis syndrome is accomplished with hydration and the use of allopurinol or rasburicase. For serious cases, dialysis may be required. See also discussion of tumor lysis syndrome in chapter 9.

MEDICAL MANAGEMENT

DIAGNOSIS. The diagnosis of ALL is similar to that of AML (see "Diagnosis" in "Acute Myelogenous Leukemia" above). The peripheral blood smear is examined, and additional special tests are performed using peripheral blood and bone marrow. A bone marrow biopsy and aspirate are needed for many of these tests. Diagnosis requires at least 25% of lymphoblasts on bone marrow examination.

Bone marrow is used to perform flow cytometry/immunophenotyping to determine if the leukemic cells are myeloid or lymphoid in origin (rarely there are cells that express features of both). Cytogenetic studies are performed to aid in prognosis and assist in determining subsequent treatment.

Because ALL commonly involves the CNS, a lumbar puncture is done to collect cerebral spinal fluid for analysis. As with AML, ALL is a heterogenous group of lymphoid leukemias with varying prognoses.

The FAB classification of ALL is no longer used as it lacked prognostic significance. The WHO classifies ALL as either T-lymphoblastic or B-lymphoblastic leukemia.[338] Prior to the WHO classification, B-lymphoblastic leukemia was referred to as precursor B-lymphoblastic leukemia in order to differentiate it from mature B-lymphoblastic leukemia or Burkitt leukemia. This terminology is still frequently used.

TREATMENT. ALL treatment protocols vary depending on age (adult or child), subtype of ALL, and genetic abnormalities associated with risk of recurrence. Some centers treat ALL on a risk-based assessment (i.e., age, morphology, cytogenetics).[304] All therapy is given in phases. Initial treatment is called remission-induction therapy and consists of aggressive chemotherapy (an anthracycline, vincristine, L-asparaginase, and a corticosteroid).

Clients with CNS involvement receive intrathecal chemotherapy periodically throughout their treatment, and those at high risk for CNS relapse may receive cranial radiation. Intensification therapy (consolidation) is administered following successful remission-induction treatment. This consists of a reinduction treatment (a readministration of induction agents) followed by cyclic use of other chemotherapy agents over a period of 2 years or longer, termed continuation therapy or maintenance therapy.

Selection of these agents is based on risk of recurrence, age, and subtype. Drugs, dosages, and scheduling can be individualized. For ALL subtypes at high risk of recurrence, allogeneic HSCT is offered. Adults frequently require transplantation and can achieve long-term survival rates of approximately 26% to 49%.[345]

Ninety-eight percent of children and 85% of adults achieve a complete remission following remission-induction therapy. With such favorable results, efforts are being made to reduce toxicities associated with aggressive combination chemotherapy, especially in children with standard risk of ALL with favorable cytogenetics.

Studies show that children who survive cancer go on to develop significant long-term medical problems, including other cancers, heart disease, learning disabilities, cognitive dysfunction, joint replacement, short stature, and hearing/vision loss.[257,286] Some of the strategies being implemented in protocols include a dose reduction of vincristine in infants, the omission of cranial irradiation in girls and young children, and a dose reduction of methotrexate in clients with Down syndrome.

Another strategy is to provide targeted agents referred to as "smart bombs" because they work at the molecular level within the cancer cells. Tyrosine kinase inhibitors, such as imatinib mesylate (Gleevec[350]), dasatinib, and nilotinib are available for the treatment of cancers with the Philadelphia chromosome t(9;22) translocation. The use of targeted drugs reduces toxicity and alleviates the requirement of adjuvant agents.

PROGNOSIS. Children with ALL do better than adults (the older the client, typically the worse the prognosis) and the survival rate has been improving; for children and adolescents, the 5-year survival rate is approximately 90%[153] with a cure rate of greater than 80%. Infants (younger than 1 year) have a poor prognosis and often die as a consequence of complications of therapy.[275] Although 80% to 90% of adults achieve a remission following remission-induction therapy, about half will relapse, resulting in a 30% to 40% cure rate.

Continuing research into the cytogenetics has provided significant prognostic information regarding various abnormalities. Good prognostic features include T-cell lineage, quick response to initial treatment, and favorable risk cytogenetics (12,21 gene translocation). Features indicative of a poor prognosis are B-cell lineage, advanced age, a high circulating WBC at diagnosis (greater than 30,000/μL), CNS involvement,[35] and the presence of the Philadelphia chromosome [t(9;22)] or translocations of the *MLL* gene.[158]

Chronic Leukemia

Chronic leukemia is a malignant disease of the bone marrow and blood that progresses slowly and permits numbers of more mature, functional cells to be made. Chronic leukemia has two major groups: chronic myeloid leukemia (CML) and chronic lymphocytic leukemia (CLL), each with several subtypes.

These are entirely different diseases and are presented separately. CML is also known as chronic myelogenous leukemia or chronic myelocytic leukemia. Other less-common forms include prolymphocytic leukemia (terminal transformation of CLL) and hairy cell leukemia (accounting for only 1%-2% of adult leukemias).

Chronic Myeloid Leukemia

Incidence and Etiologic Factors. CML is a neoplasm of the hematopoietic stem cell. The genetic abnormalities created in the stem cell are the result of acquired injury to the DNA and passed on to all related cell lines, resulting in increases in myeloid cells and clonal anomalies in erythroid cells and platelets. This leads to abnormal cells in peripheral blood and marked hyperplasia in the bone marrow.

CML accounts for 15% of all leukemias, with approximately 5400 cases diagnosed per year. The average age at diagnosis is 64 years, with an incidence of 1.6 cases per 100,000 people.[151] This type of leukemia occurs mostly in adults, with only 2% developing in children. Although the exact etiologic factors are unknown, the incidence of CML is increased in people with severe radiation exposure. No chemical or other environmental risk factors are known to cause CML.

Pathogenesis. CML originates in the hematopoietic stem cell (i.e., this cell has the ability to develop into any one of several blood cells; see Fig. 21-6) and involves overproduction of myeloid cells. The genetic defect detected in CML cells is called the Philadelphia chromosome. This translocation [t(9;22)] was the first consistent chromosomal anomaly identified in a cancer and is now detected in all cases of CML and known to be the cause of CML.

The abnormal chromosome develops from the accidental translocation and fusion of the *BRC* gene on chromosome 22 and the *ABL* gene on chromosome 9, creating a unique gene *(BRC-ABL)*. The *BRC-ABL* gene encodes for an abnormal protein product that acts as a tyrosine kinase, resulting in a dysregulated proliferation signal.

Tyrosine kinase is an enzyme that is necessary for normal cell growth. In normal cells the enzyme turns on and off as it should, but in people with CML this enzyme appears to be in the permanent "switched on" state, eliminating the normal checks and balances on proliferation.

Unlike AML, CML permits the development of mature WBCs that generally function normally. This important distinction from acute leukemia accounts for the less-severe early course of the disease.[291]

Clinical Manifestations. Presenting signs and symptoms are often quite nonspecific. The most typical symptoms at presentation are fatigue, anorexia, and weight loss, although approximately 40% of affected individuals are asymptomatic. Sweats, malaise, and shortness of breath during physical activity are also reported.

Splenomegaly is present in 50% of all cases with corresponding complaints of left upper quadrant pain and early satiety. Thrombocytosis is also very common. The natural history of CML is a progression (over years) from a proliferative phase (chronic phase), into an accelerated phase (more symptoms but not acute leukemia), to an aggressive acute leukemia (blast crisis) that can be rapidly fatal within months.

MEDICAL MANAGEMENT

DIAGNOSIS. Early in the disease process, only vague symptoms or routine blood analysis may herald the disease. Peripheral blood counts and smears often demonstrate an abnormal leukocytosis, which leads to further testing. The peripheral blood smear will often reveal a wide range of cells in a variety of stages. Basophilia may also be seen. The appearance of both mature and immature cells in the peripheral blood is suggestive of CML but must be differentiated from other myeloproliferative diseases.

The diagnosis is made by detecting the BCR-ABL fusion by routine cytogenetics or fluorescence in situ hybridization or by polymerase chain reaction. Cytogenetic testing and bone marrow evaluation determine the phase of the disease.

TREATMENT AND PROGNOSIS. All people diagnosed with CML require treatment, even those who are asymptomatic. Recent research has significantly changed the treatment and prognosis of CML. Knowledge that the cause of the disease was an abnormal *BCR-ABL* gene led to the development of the drug imatinib mesylate (Gleevec), designed to target and inhibit tyrosine kinase. In clients with chronic-phase disease, treatment with imatinib led to an overall survival of 89% at 5 years. However, with time most people develop resistance to imatinib, requiring further treatment. Nilotinib and dasatinib, more potent tyrosine kinase inhibitors, are second-line therapies with similar results to imatinib.[295]

The overall 5-year survival rate is approximately 60% but improving for some individuals treated with new treatment options.[151] For those individuals with CML who are not responsive to these new treatments (or for those who are unable to tolerate tyrosine kinase inhibitors), chemotherapy can control the symptoms for a time. HSCT continues to be an option that may provide a cure. This procedure is for select people with resistant disease (regardless of phase) or with accelerated or blast-phase disease.

Chronic Lymphocytic Leukemia

Incidence, Etiologic Factors, and Risk Factors. CLL is the most common type of leukemia in adults, accounting for 25% to 30% of all leukemias, with almost 17,000 cases per year. The incidence of CLL increases with advancing age, with the median age of presentation being 72 years[151]; 90% are older than 50 years, and men are affected more often than women.

The cause of CLL is also unknown but a few environmental factors are implicated, such as farming pesticides and the chemical warfare herbicide Agent Orange, although conclusive evidence is lacking. Some groups of people may have a genetic predisposition, including persons with a first-degree family member with CLL.[373]

Pathogenesis. The cell type responsible for more than 95% of the cases of CLL is the B cell (T-cell CLL is uncommon). When a normal B cell is stimulated by an antigen, it enters a proliferative phase, creating clones able to fight infection. It is during this stage that a cell may develop a mutation and predispose it to become cancerous.[106] Despite the common name for this type of leukemia, there are many types of genetic changes and expression of the disease.[370] The most common mutation is the deletion of 13q, seen in approximately 50% of clients with CLL. This genetic abnormality carries a more benign prognosis, with slowly progressive disease.

Another abnormality, noted in 15% of people with CLL, is trisomy 12 and usually associated with progressive disease. A deletion in chromosome 17 (17p13) is significant for aggressive disease, shorter remission, and decreased overall survival. Studies also reveal an overexpression of the proto-oncogene *bc12*. This is a regulatory gene known to suppress apoptosis, allowing cells to live longer. Two genes, located at 13q14, normally encode for regulatory RNA, which breaks down messenger RNA or blocks the transcription of messenger RNA.[131] With the deletion of these genes, the downstream regulation of other genes, such as the *bc12* gene, is lost and become overexpressed. This is seen in 70% of CLL cases.[91] Zeta-associated peptide (ZAP-70) is another genetic abnormality that is associated with a poor prognosis. ZAP-70 is believed to decrease the threshold for signaling *bc12*.

Clinical Manifestations. In the early stages of the disease, most clients remain asymptomatic or complain of vague, nonspecific symptoms such as fatigue or enlarged lymph nodes (seen in 87% of symptomatic people). Depending on the mutations present in the abnormal clone, clients may experience a prolonged, indolent course with few symptoms.

Those people with more aggressive CLL develop pancytopenia (with accompanying symptoms of infections, hemorrhage, and significant fatigue) and decreased immunoglobulin levels. The most common opportunistic infections include *Pneumocystis jiroveci*, cytomegalovirus, and herpes simplex virus. With progression of the disease, clients may develop lymphadenopathy, splenomegaly, hepatomegaly, weight loss, bone pain, and bone marrow infiltration. Approximately 10% of clients develop the complication of AIHA,[266] and immune thrombocytopenia occurs in 2% of cases.[36] Approximately 10% of people with CLL develop a rapidly progressive large-cell lymphoma called Richter transformation, requiring more aggressive therapy.

MEDICAL MANAGEMENT

DIAGNOSIS AND STAGING. Examination of the peripheral blood smear, CBC, and flow cytometry are performed to make a diagnosis. Bone marrow examination is not required but may be helpful. Staging is established according to the Rai and Binet systems.

The Rai system recognizes stages conferring a low (stage 0), intermediate (I, II), and high (III, IV) risk of progression. This staging determines which clients should receive treatment and when, but this staging system does not provide reliable prognostic information. The Binet system uses hemoglobin, platelet count, and number of involved lymph node groups, classifying the disease into stages A, B, and C.

TREATMENT. CLL is difficult to treat and typically is without a cure. Better understanding of the pathogenesis of CLL is leading to improved treatments,[171] but most initial treatments are based on clinical staging and symptoms.

Low-risk clients require careful monitoring and frequent examinations with treatment initiated when symptoms worsen or if there is evidence of rapidly progressive leukemia. Treatment prior to the presence of symptoms has not been shown to be of benefit.[28,39] Clients with symptoms or rapidly progressive disease are treated with chemotherapy (fludarabine and chlorambucil) often accompanied by monoclonal antibodies.[19] Alemtuzumab is an approved monoclonal antibody for the treatment of CLL, although rituximab is frequently used because of its better side-effect profile.

Immunomodulating agents (such as lenalidomide) are currently being studied and may prove to be beneficial as an adjuvant therapy.[48,227] The use of HSCT for the treatment of CLL has increased recently, but remains a successful option in a limited number of cases because of high morbidity and mortality.[226]

PROGNOSIS. CLL continues to be a fatal disease with a significant impact on life expectancy, but in the last few years a trend toward an improvement in overall survival has taken place.[184]

Because CLL is a heterogenic disease, prognosis varies greatly at diagnosis. Prognostic information includes stage of disease at diagnosis and the presence or absence of biologic markers.

People without ZAP-70 or CD38 appear to live longer, with an average life expectancy of 10 years, whereas those with more aggressive disease with biologic markers have a shorter survival. Clients who present in Rai stages III–IV have an average life expectancy of 5 years, whereas those with less-aggressive leukemia may never require treatment (depending on the age at diagnosis). Approximately 70% of people with CLL eventually require treatment.[168]

As mutations are discovered, studies are underway to correlate them to prognosis. As previously discussed, CLL that displays ZAP-70+ or CD38 mutations has a poor prognosis, whereas mutations in the immunoglobulin heavy-chain variable region have a good prognosis (median survival of 25 years).

SPECIAL IMPLICATIONS FOR THE THERAPIST	14-7

Leukemia

Like all cancers, medical innovations in the treatment of leukemia are increasing the affected individual's life span while increasing the likelihood of treatment side effects. Strengthening and energy-enhancing programs during cancer treatment can significantly improve symptoms of fatigue and depression, increase cardiovascular endurance, and maintain quality of life.[89]

Many more research studies are available now on the role of exercise specifically during the medical management of pediatric and adult leukemias. Significant improvement in health-related quality of life, fitness, mental health, and reduced symptom interference on daily life activities have been reported.[10,116,161] Observational studies also report low physical activity levels among survivors of leukemias with the potential for adverse health effects as a result.

There is a growing body of literature with evidence to support the idea that regular physical activity is safe and has potential benefits for both adult and pediatric hematologic cancer survivors.[366] The physical therapist working with this group of individuals can be very instrumental in client education and supervised exercise programs to potentially improve muscle strength, physical function, and cardiorespiratory fitness while reducing fatigue and improving overall quality of life.[366]

Precautions

The period after chemically induced remission is critical for each client, who is now highly susceptible to spontaneous hemorrhage and defenseless against invading organisms. The usual precautions for thrombocytopenia, neutropenia, and infection control must be adhered to strictly. The importance of strict handwashing technique (see Boxes 8-4 and 8-5) cannot be overemphasized. The therapist should be alert to any sign of infection and report any potential site of infection, such as mucosal ulceration, skin abrasion, or a tear (even a hangnail). Precautions are as for anemia, outlined earlier in this chapter (see "The Anemias.").

Anticipating potential side effects of medications used in the treatment of leukemia can help the therapist better understand client reactions during the episode of care. Drug-induced mood changes, ranging from feelings of well-being and euphoria to depression and irritability, may occur; depression and irritability may also be associated with the cancer. Exercise intensity and duration and activity modifications are necessary for clients with anemia.

Clients with a history of prolonged corticosteroid use should be assessed for muscle weakness and avascular necrosis of the hips and shoulders.

Joint Involvement

Arthralgia or arthritis occurs in approximately 12% of adults with chronic leukemia, 13% of adults with acute leukemia, and up to 60% of children with ALL. Articular symptoms are the result of leukemic infiltrates of the synovium, periosteum, or periarticular bone or of secondary gout or hemarthrosis. Asymmetrical involvement of the large joints is most commonly observed. Pain that is disproportionate to the physical findings may occur, and joint symptoms are often transient.

Children with Leukemia

Because of increasing survival rates for children with ALL and the extensive side effects of the treatments, the therapist must pay attention to specific measures of cognition, function, activity, and participation when planning an appropriate intervention program. All components are needed in a comprehensive program.[215]

Short- and long-term impairments can affect any or all of these components. Decreased hemoglobin levels, osteonecrosis, joint range of motion, strength, gross and fine motor performance, fitness, and attendance or absence from school are all factors to consider.[215]

Long-term effects of treatment and CNS prophylaxis can include peripheral neuropathies, neuropsychologic disorders, problems with balance, decreased muscle strength, and obesity. CNS prophylaxis includes intrathecal chemotherapy (injection of drugs into the spinal fluid) and cranial irradiation. Cranial irradiation and obesity are significant predictors of impaired balance.[369]

Preschool children with immature nervous systems may be more sensitive to the neurotoxicity of radiation and chemotherapy, placing them at a greater risk for CNS damage than children with fully developed neurologic systems.[228] Learning difficulties, cognitive deficits, attention problems, and lack of participation in physical activities can be sequelae of medical treatment.[369]

Personal factors such as a family's cultural belief system may influence how children and their parents perceive rehabilitation and specific interventions. Health-related quality of life and goals may be driven by family and cultural values that are not necessarily what the therapist perceives as in the best interest of the child's function and fitness.

The therapist should try to match the program with the family's cultural expectations, ability to participate, and emotional and financial resources. Expecting from the family only what they can succeed at and providing support and education where they are needed to help the family grow and care for their child with medical needs will create the best therapeutic environment for the child to thrive in.

Malignant Lymphomas

Lymphoma is a general term for cancers that develop in the lymphatic system. Lymphomas are divided into two groups: Hodgkin lymphoma (HL; also known as Hodgkin disease) and non-Hodgkin lymphoma (NHL). With the extensive progression in cytogenetic research that has occurred over the past 5 years, this distinction is beginning to obscure.

It is becoming more useful to categorize lymphomas according to their clinical behavior—indolent or aggressive—and their chromosome features. Currently HL is distinguished from other lymphomas by the presence of a characteristic type of cell known as the Reed-Sternberg cell. All other types of lymphoma are called NHL.

Hodgkin Lymphoma

Definition and Overview. HL is a lymphoid neoplasm with the primary histologic finding of giant Reed-Sternberg cells in the lymph nodes. These cells are of B-cell linage and have twin nuclei and nucleoli that give them the appearance of owl eyes (Fig. 14-6).

Although this malignancy originates in the lymphoid system and primarily involves the lymph nodes, it can spread to other sites such as the spleen, liver, and bone marrow. There are two groups of HL: classic HL (further divided into four categories) and nodular lymphocyte-predominant HL (LPHL). LPHL is uncommon and represents only 4% to 5% of HL cases.

Incidence and Risk Factors. Classic HL can occur in both children and adults but peaks at two different ages: between the ages of 15 and 35 years and after the age of 55 years. Children younger than 5 years rarely develop this disease, and only 10% of HL cases occur in children 16 years old and younger. LPHL typically has only one peak incidence around the fourth decade. It is estimated that 1950 new cases of HL were diagnosed in 2014 with 1180 deaths.

Although the exact cause of HL remains under investigation, certain risk factors have been identified. One

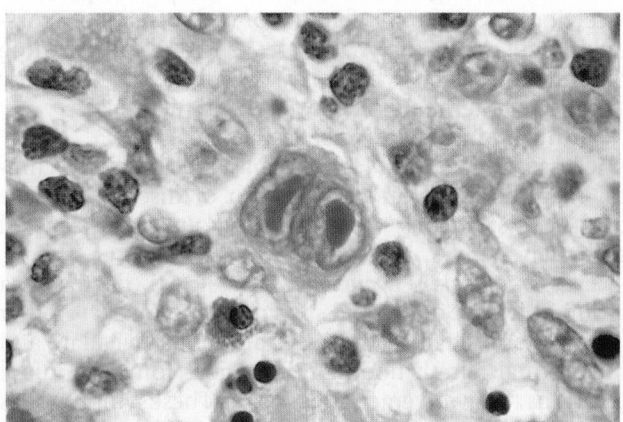

Figure 14-6

Reed-Sternberg cell. Named for Dorothy M. Reed, American pathologist (1874–1964), and Karl Sternberg, Austrian pathologist (1872–1935). This is one example of the large, abnormal, multinucleated reticuloendothelial cells in the lymphatic system found in Hodgkin lymphoma. The number and proportion of Reed-Sternberg cells identified are the basis for the histopathologic classification of Hodgkin lymphoma. (Reprinted from Kumar V, Cotran RS, Robbins SL: *Basic pathology,* ed 6, Philadelphia, 1997, WB Saunders. Courtesy Dr. Robert W. McKenna, University of Texas Southwestern Medical School, Dallas.)

factor that has been related to HL is previous infection with EBV. The DNA of this virus has been found in the Reed-Sternberg cells of approximately 30% to 50% of clients with classic HL.

Pathogenesis. The pathologic cell of HL is the Reed-Sternberg cell, which is a clonal lymphoid cell, and usually is of B lineage.[187] These cells are surrounded by reactive cells—granulocytes, lymphocytes, and plasma cells. The reason for the transformation from a normal B cell to a malignant cell is still under investigation, but significant progress has been made. Most likely there are various causes that account for the bimodal distribution of the disease (i.e., younger people may develop HL caused by a different etiology than older people). Recent evidence suggests that an infection or inflammation may be involved. As just discussed, genes from EBV are found in one-third to one-half of all HL cases in the industrialized world. Yet, other factors in concert with EBV infection, such as an abnormal antibody response to EBV,[195,231] are likely required for malignant transformation.[139]

Many cytokines, particularly interleukins, are involved in producing an environment where the Reed-Sternberg cells thrive. For example, some interleukins attract inflammatory cells (eosinophils, monocytes, and mast cells), which aid in the survival of the cell.[9,140] In the laboratory, if these inflammatory cells are not surrounding the Reed-Sternberg cells, they do not survive.

Other interleukins expressed by the Reed-Sternberg cells inhibit the activation of T cells, which normally destroy abnormal cells. This inhibition creates an area of local immunosuppression and allows the Reed-Sternberg cell to evade detection. Some interleukins act as growth factors, encouraging proliferation, metastasis, and angiogenesis. Another protein induced by nuclear factor kappa B, termed c-FLIP, is incorporated into a complex that signals cell death but is not functional in that capacity, thereby evading apoptosis and making the cell immortal.[176]

Reed-Sternberg cells also express multiple receptors for receiving signals from inflammatory cells, creating "cross-talking" between the malignant cells and surrounding inflammatory cells, which may contribute to the ability of the Reed-Sternberg cells to grow and metastasize.

Clinical Manifestations. See Figure 14-7.

Classic HL and LPHL present with different clinical manifestations and progression of disease. Because of these distinctions, these two subgroups are discussed separately.

Classic Hodgkin Lymphoma. Classic HL begins in a group of lymph nodes and spreads contiguously to other lymph node chains. The cervical, supraclavicular, and mediastinal lymph nodes are the most common initial locations for involvement (Fig. 14-8). These lymph nodes are typically nontender and firm.[79]

Nodular sclerosing HL typically presents with supradiaphragmatic lymph node involvement, whereas mixed cellularity classic HL (MCHL) often exhibits smaller involved lymph nodes in a subdiaphragmatic location or involves organs. Clients who have disease below the diaphragm, MCHL, or "B" symptoms (fever, night sweats, weight loss) are more likely to develop splenic involvement. Splenic involvement is seen in 30% to 40% of people with HL, but detection is often difficult. An enlarged spleen does not necessary indicate involvement, and a normal-size spleen does not rule out involvement. HL in the liver is uncommon and seen with splenic involvement and "B" symptoms.[79]

Bone marrow involvement occurs in less than 10% of newly diagnosed cases. If lymph nodes become large and bulky, they can lead to further symptoms, such as tracheal or bronchial compression (with accompanying shortness of breath) or obstruction of the GI tract. Lymph nodes may grow and enlarge and finally perforate the lymph node capsule, continuing to grow and invade into adjacent tissue or organs. This can occur in the lung, pericardium, pleura, chest wall, gut, or bone.[79]

Effusions (collections of fluid) may also develop in the lung, heart, or abdominal cavity. Tumor can spread not only from lymph node to adjacent lymph node, but via the bloodstream to lung, liver, bone marrow, and bone. Involvement in these areas is often indicative of extensive disease. As bone marrow is replaced, infections, anemia, and thrombocytopenia result.[79]

Primary involvement of the CNS is rare, and dissemination of disease to the CNS is uncommon.[25] Occasionally spinal cord involvement may occur in the dorsal and lumbar regions, and compression of nerve roots of the brachial, lumbar, or sacral plexus can cause nerve root pain. Epidural involvement (also uncommon) causes back and neck pain with hyperreflexia. Extremity involvement is characterized by pain, nerve irritation, and obliteration of the pulse.

A significant number of people (25%-35%) present with "B" symptoms. The fever associated with HL is intermittent and occurs with drenching night sweats. Clients may also complain of fatigue, pruritus, and pain associated with drinking alcohol.

Lymphocyte-Predominant Hodgkin Lymphoma. LPHL typically presents with one-node involvement rather than groups of involved lymph nodes. This occurs in peripheral lymph nodes such as the cervical, axillary, or inguinal lymph node chains. Unlike classic HL, LPHL does not follow an orderly pattern of spread, but can be found in lymph nodes distant from the original node of disease. LPHL infrequently involves the bone marrow, spleen, or thymus. "B" symptoms rarely occur. LPHL has an indolent clinical course with long disease-free intervals. Relapse is common but responds well to treatment.[277]

Special Problems

Pregnancy and Hodgkin Lymphoma. As the mean age at diagnosis of HL is 32 years, it is not uncommon for women to develop HL while pregnant. Diagnostic staging can be accomplished safely with ultrasound or magnetic resonance imaging (MRI) because it does not use ionizing radiation[252]; it has no adverse impact on the natural course of HL; and HL has no effect on the course of gestation, delivery, or the incidence of prematurity or spontaneous abortions. The risk of metastatic involvement of the fetus by HL is negligible.[93]

The management of HL during pregnancy must be individualized. Many women have been successfully treated while pregnant without adverse effects on the fetus.[97,157] In cases of disease onset early in pregnancy, the recommendation may be made to consider a therapeutic abortion. Women presenting in later pregnancy are

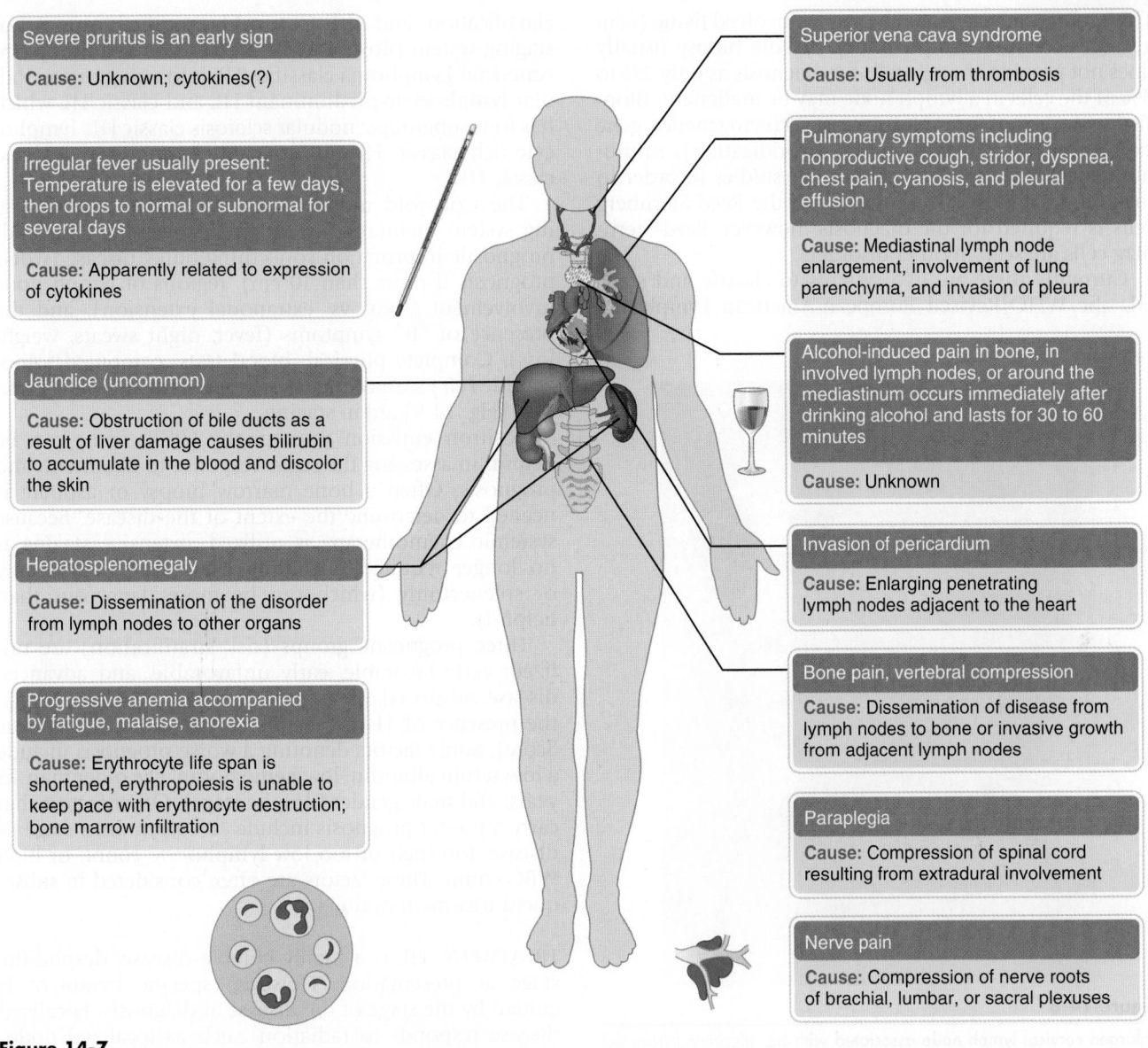

Severe pruritus is an early sign

Cause: Unknown; cytokines(?)

Irregular fever usually present: Temperature is elevated for a few days, then drops to normal or subnormal for several days

Cause: Apparently related to expression of cytokines

Jaundice (uncommon)

Cause: Obstruction of bile ducts as a result of liver damage causes bilirubin to accumulate in the blood and discolor the skin

Hepatosplenomegaly

Cause: Dissemination of the disorder from lymph nodes to other organs

Progressive anemia accompanied by fatigue, malaise, anorexia

Cause: Erythrocyte life span is shortened, erythropoiesis is unable to keep pace with erythrocyte destruction; bone marrow infiltration

Superior vena cava syndrome

Cause: Usually from thrombosis

Pulmonary symptoms including nonproductive cough, stridor, dyspnea, chest pain, cyanosis, and pleural effusion

Cause: Mediastinal lymph node enlargement, involvement of lung parenchyma, and invasion of pleura

Alcohol-induced pain in bone, in involved lymph nodes, or around the mediastinum occurs immediately after drinking alcohol and lasts for 30 to 60 minutes

Cause: Unknown

Invasion of pericardium

Cause: Enlarging penetrating lymph nodes adjacent to the heart

Bone pain, vertebral compression

Cause: Dissemination of disease from lymph nodes to bone or invasive growth from adjacent lymph nodes

Paraplegia

Cause: Compression of spinal cord resulting from extradural involvement

Nerve pain

Cause: Compression of nerve roots of brachial, lumbar, or sacral plexuses

Figure 14-7

Pathologic basis for the clinical manifestations of HL.

often able to have therapy delayed until after delivery or can undergo modified or standard combination chemotherapy and radiation therapy.[93,290]

Antiretroviral treatment and prophylaxis for opportunistic infection may also be administered for HIV-positive women.[180] With the increased use of ABVD therapy (Adriamycin [doxorubicin], bleomycin, vinblastine, and dacarbazine) and reduced reliance on radiation therapy, the use of radiation can be avoided. However, with appropriate shielding, the estimated fetal dose of radiation can be reduced by 50% or more in most cases if required.[123] In nonpregnant women, to further reduce any risk, it is advisable to delay pregnancy for 12 months after completion of radiation therapy.[97]

Although men who survive HL have a good chance of preserving fertility,[330] long-term semen banking is available for men whose future fertility may be compromised by aggressive treatment. Banking of a single ejaculate

before chemotherapy or radiotherapy treatment may preserve potential fertility without compromising the oncology treatment.[150]

Hodgkin Lymphoma in HIV. Although HL does not occur as frequently in HIV-positive clients as does NHL, people with HIV are still at increased risk of developing HL.[26] When it occurs, the histology is usually MCHL or lymphocyte-depleted HL associated with aggressive, disseminated disease and systemic symptoms. Since the introduction of highly active antiretroviral therapy (HAART), the incidence of HL in clients with HIV has not changed significantly, but there has been an improvement in mortality rate, particularly as a result of HAART and reduced AIDS-related deaths.[109,135,144]

MEDICAL MANAGEMENT

DIAGNOSIS AND STAGING. The diagnosis of HL is made through the evaluation of an affected lymph node.

This requires an excisional biopsy of involved tissue (usually an accessible lymph node). Needle biopsy usually does not provide enough cells for diagnosis as only 2% to 3% of the cells in a lymph node may be malignant. Biopsied tissue is sent for molecular testing (cytogenetics, gene expression, fluorescence in situ hybridization), immunophenotyping, and histopathologic studies in order to make the diagnosis. The presence of the Reed-Sternberg cells is required for the diagnosis; however, Reed-Sternberg cells are seen in other disorders.

Currently there are two systems to classify and stage HL: the WHO/Revised European-American Lymphoma classification and the Cotswold modified Ann Arbor staging system (Box 14-6). The WHO/Revised European-American Lymphoma classifies HL into two groups: nodular lymphocytic-predominant HL and classic HL which has four subgroups: nodular sclerosis classic HL, lymphocyte-rich classic HL, MCHL, and lymphocyte-depleted classic HL.

The Cotswold modification of the Ann Arbor staging system maintains the original stages I–IV but adds prognostic information concerning bulky disease (worse prognosis if more than 10 cm), regions of lymph node involvement (local vs. extranodal extension), and the presence of "B" symptoms (fever, night sweats, weight loss). Complete physical, blood tests, computed tomographic (CT) scan of the chest, abdomen, and pelvis, and MRI (Fig. 14-9) aid in staging.

Positron emission tomography (PET) scans can be helpful in assessing the stage, response to treatment, and prognosis. Often a bone marrow biopsy or aspirate is needed to determine the extent of the disease. Because systemic chemotherapy is utilized, extensive staging is no longer required, including exploratory laparotomy or splenectomy (which can be more dangerous than helpful).

Three prognostic groups (risk stratification) are utilized: early favorable, early unfavorable, and advanced disease. Advanced disease is further stratified according to the presence of 11 risk factors (International Prognostic Score). Some factors denoting a worse prognosis include a low serum albumin, low hemoglobin, age older than 45 years, and male gender (despite stage). Other factors that carry a poorer prognosis include "B" symptoms, stage IV disease, too high or too low lymphocyte count, or high WBC count. These factors are often considered in subsequent treatment options.

TREATMENT. HL is a highly curable disease, despite the stage at presentation. However, specific treatment is guided by the stage of the disease at diagnosis. Localized disease responds to radiation, such as localized nodular LPHL, and may or may not require short courses of chemotherapy. But as a result of long-term side effects,

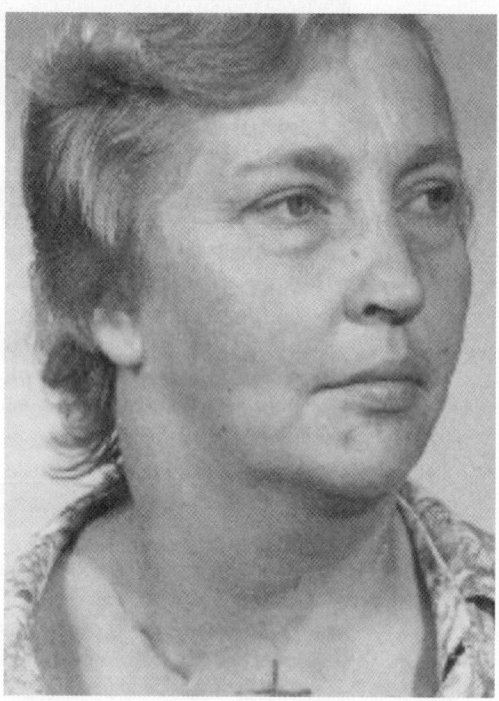

Figure 14-8

Enlarged cervical lymph node associated with HL. (Reprinted from del Regato J, Spjut HJ, Cox JD: *Cancer: diagnosis, treatment, and prognosis*, ed 6, St Louis, 1985, Mosby–Year Book.)

Box 14-6

COTSWOLD MODIFICATION OF THE ANN ARBOR STAGING CLASSIFICATION FOR HODGKIN LYMPHOMA*

Stage I	Involvement of a single lymph node, group of nodes, or a single extralymphatic site IE** (e.g., spleen, thymus, Waldeyer ring) except liver and bone marrow
Stage II	Involvement of two or more lymph node regions on the same side of the diaphragm or an extralymphatic site and its regional lymph nodes with or without other lymph nodes on the same side of the diaphragm
Stage III	Involvement of lymph node regions or structures on both sides of the diaphragm; may include spleen or localized extranodal disease
Stage IV	Multiple extranodal sites or lymph nodes with extranodal disease
X	Disease bulk >10 cm
E	Extranodal extension or single, isolated site of extranodal disease
A/B	B symptoms: weight loss >10%, fever, night sweats

*For all stages: A, asymptomatic; B, constitutional or systemic symptoms.
From Hoffmann R: *Hematology: basic principles and practice*, ed 5, Philadelphia, 2009, Churchill Livingstone.
**IE is used to designate a single lymphatic nodal involvement (I) and the E designates that it is extralymphatic (outside the lymphatic system such as in the spleen as designated here) involvement.

attempts are made to limit the use of radiation and expose only diseased tissue (involved field radiation).[16,88]

Standard treatment involves combination chemotherapy consisting of six cycles of ABVD, with or without radiation.[223] Unlike NHL, HL subtypes are treated in a similar manner, with the exception of lymphocytoid-predominant HL, where rituximab is added to the chemotherapy regimen. Other regimens include Stanford V and BEACOPP (bleomycin, etoposide, doxorubicin, cyclophosphamide, vincristine, procarbazine, and prednisone); all have significant toxicities and varying effectiveness.[78,113]

After two to three cycles of treatment, many oncologists are utilizing PET scans to determine the effect of treatment as well as long-term outcomes. For example, people who had a complete response to treatment after two cycles of treatment, at 2 years follow-up, 95% had disease free PET scans. Yet of people without a complete response to two treatments, only 13% remained disease free at 2 years. PET scans can also aid in avoiding unnecessary treatment. PET scans are also used to determine if there is any residual disease upon completion of therapy.

HSCT is offered to people who do not respond to therapy or have relapsed disease. Autologous HSCT is the procedure of choice because of the more-severe complications of allogeneic HSCT. If an autologous HSCT fails, allogeneic HSCT remains an option.

People with LPHL may be treated with radiation, a combination of radiation and chemotherapy, or chemotherapy alone. Rituximab may also be added. Radiation does appear to be an important component to long-term disease survival.[54]

Survivors of HL have a 1% risk per year for 30 years for developing a secondary malignancy.[103] Clients who received radiation to the chest also have a higher risk of fatal myocardial infarction (presumed to be caused by damage to the intimal lining of the coronary arteries), which persists for 25 years.[338] The risk of stroke or transient ischemic attack also increases in survivors of HL (two to three times greater than the general population). This is most likely related to radiation to the neck and chest.[67]

ABVD has not been shown to cause subfertility in men or women, as do the older alkylating agents previously used.[142] Because of the increased long-term complications, the use of radiation has been limited to only areas in field and lower doses are being used, particularly in children. The combination therapy of ABVD appears to be a better long-term choice for treatment.[82] Treatment options have attempted to balance toxicities with high cure rates.[170,178]

PROGNOSIS. HL is now considered one of the most curable forms of cancer, and death rates have decreased 60% since the early 1970s. Prognosis depends on the staging and presence of risk factors at presentation including: age older than 45 years, male sex, leukocyte count greater than 15,000/μL, serum albumin level less than 4 g/dL, and hemoglobin level less than 10.5 g/dL. For clients without risk factors, the 5-year survival rate is 90%,[87] whereas those with five risk factors have a reduced 5-year survival of 56%.

The cause of death in the majority of cases prior to 15 years is recurrent disease. After 15 years, most die of other causes, including secondary neoplasms derived from HL therapy, such as NHL, leukemia, lung, colorectal, and breast cancer.

SPECIAL IMPLICATIONS FOR THE THERAPIST   14-8

Hodgkin Lymphoma

The therapist may palpate enlarged, painless lymph nodes during a cervical, spine, shoulder, or hip examination. Lymph nodes are evaluated on the basis of size, consistency, mobility, and tenderness. Lymph nodes up to 2 cm in diameter, soft consistency, freely and easily moveable, tender to palpation, and transient are considered within normal limits but must be followed carefully.

Lymph nodes greater than 2 cm in diameter that are firm in consistency, nontender to palpation, fixed, and hard are considered suspicious and require evaluation. Enlarged lymph nodes associated with infection are more likely to be tender than slow-growing nodes associated with cancer.

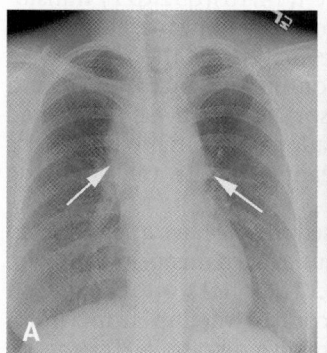
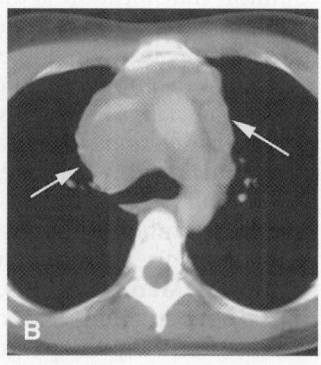
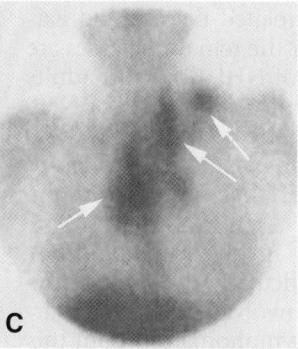
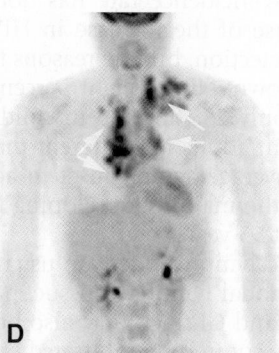

Figure 14-9

HL as seen on chest radiograph (**A**); CT scan of the chest (**B**); gallium scan of the head, neck, and chest (**C**); and positron emission tomography (PET) scan (**D**). The *arrows* indicate sites of diseases. Note that PET and CT scans provide more detailed information compared with chest radiograph and gallium scan. (Reprinted from Goldman L: *Cecil textbook of medicine*, ed 22, Philadelphia, 2004, WB Saunders.)

Changes in size, shape, tenderness, and consistency should raise a red flag. The physician should be notified of these findings and the client advised to have the lymph nodes evaluated by the physician; in someone with a history of cancer, immediate medical referral is necessary.

The therapist's role in lymphoma includes, but is not limited to, assessing and/or addressing (1) quality-of-life issues, including emotional and spiritual needs; (2) impairments, functional limitations, and disabilities; and (3) physical conditioning and deconditioning.

Generalized weakness, decreased endurance, impaired mobility, altered kinesthetic awareness and balance, including unstable gait; respiratory impairment; involvement of the lymphatic system (lymphedema); and pain are only a few of the identified signs and symptoms of impairment common with this group of people.

Requirements for infection control and treatment subsequent to the cytotoxic effects on the CNS are outlined previously in the section on the leukemias. Additionally, side effects of radiation and/or chemotherapy must be considered (see Chapter 5 and Table 9-7).

Depending on the results of the therapist's examination and evaluation, intervention strategies may include client and family education, pain management, mobility and gait training, therapeutic exercise, balance training, aerobic conditioning, respiratory rehabilitation, and lymphedema management.

Monitoring vital signs is important, as is daily evaluation of laboratory values (e.g., hemoglobin, platelets, WBCs, hematocrit). See Tables 40-8 and 40-9 for planning or carrying out a therapy program.[21]

Non-Hodgkin Lymphomas

Overview and Incidence. NHL comprises a large group (about 30 specific types described) of lymphoid malignancies that present as solid tumors arising from cells of the lymphatic system. More than 65,000 people develop NHL per year, making it the most common hematologic malignancy and the sixth most common cancer in the United States. NHL is five times more common than HL.

The incidence rate has doubled since 1970, in part because of the increase in HIV-related disease and earlier detection, but the reasons for the remaining cases are unknown. Ninety-eight percent of NHL occurs in adults and only 2% develop in children; yet the types of NHL seen in adults are different than those seen in children. The average age of onset in adults is about 66 years,[151] with the majority developing NHL being older than the age of 55 years.

The lymph nodes are usually involved first, and any extranodal lymphoid tissue, particularly the spleen, thymus, and GI tract, may also be involved. The bone marrow is commonly infiltrated by lymphoma cells, but this is rarely the primary site of a lymphoma.

There are several classification systems. The Working Formulation, first proposed in 1982, grouped lymphomas as low, intermediate, and high grade. Lymphomas classified according to the Revised European-American Lymphoma/WHO system rely on the histochemical, genetic, and cytologic features are either B-cell or T/natural killer (NK)-cell. Approximately 85% of NHL are B-cell lymphomas, whereas only 15% are of T-cell or NK-cell origin. The clinical course for each of the NHLs, even subtypes, is variable.

The most common lymphoma is diffuse large B-cell lymphoma (DLBCL), which comprises 33% of all NHLs. It is an aggressive, fast-growing tumor. The second most common is follicular lymphoma. It is an indolent, slow growing tumor with a median survival of 8 to 10 years.

Etiologic and Risk Factors. Some studies have linked benzene (found in cigarette smoke, gasoline, and industrial pollution) and polychlorinated biphenyls to the development of NHL. More research is still needed to solidify this causal association. People that have been previously exposed to chemotherapy and/or radiation also have a higher risk of developing NHL.

A wide variety of autoimmune diseases (RA and SLE), immunosuppressive states, and immunodeficiency disorders are associated with an increased incidence of lymphomas. This phenomenon may reflect a decrease in the host's surveillance mechanism against transformed cells or be from prolonged exposure to oncogenic agents, such as EBV, as a consequence of failure to mount an adequate immune response.

In people with HIV, the risk of developing NHL is significantly elevated compared with noninfected people. Hepatitis C is also associated with certain subtypes of NHL, including lymphoplasmacytic lymphoma. The presence of *Helicobacter pylori* (bacteria) in the stomach lining is associated with the development of gastric mucosa-associated lymphoid tissue lymphomas, but this comprises a very small proportion of cases.

Pathogenesis. Although the exact cause of NHL is unknown, studies using techniques of molecular biology have provided some clues to the pathogenesis. Malignant lymphomas develop from the accumulation of genetic abnormalities affecting protooncogenes or tumor suppressor genes, leading to the clonal expansion of a neoplastic lymphocyte that is arrested at a specific stage of B- or T/NK-lymphoid cell differentiation. Oncogenes can be activated by chromosomal translocations. The most common translocation is the t(14;18)(q32;q21) translocation, seen in 85% of follicular lymphomas. The 8q24 translocation leads to dysregulation of the *c-Myc* gene and noted in Burkitt and non-Burkitt small noncleaved lymphoma. Tumor suppressor genes can be inactivated by genetic deletions or mutations. Eventually these cells crowd out healthy cells, creating tumors and enlarging lymph nodes.

Because immunosuppressed people have a greater incidence of the disease, an immune mechanism is suspected.

Clinical Manifestations. The NHLs are variable in clinical presentation and course, varying from indolent disease to rapidly progressive disease. NHLs can be loosely grouped together corresponding to presentation and clinical behavior according to the Working Formulation classification of disease as low grade, intermediate grade, and high grade. Low-grade lymphomas present with peripheral lymphadenopathy that is painless and slowly progressive. Occasionally there is spontaneous regression of disease.

Extranodal disease and "B" symptoms (fever, weight loss, and sweats) are not usually seen at diagnosis, unless the disease is advanced. The bone marrow is frequently involved resulting in cytopenias.[376] The intermediate and high-grade lymphomas vary in presentation and progression, yet most display lymphadenopathy. Only one-third of people exhibit extranodal disease; the most common sites being bone marrow, skin, thyroid, CNS, GI/genitourinary tracts, and sinuses. "B" symptoms are common and noted in 30% to 40% of clients. Splenomegaly is noted in approximately 40% of people with NHL.

Lymphoblastic lymphoma, a high-grade lymphoma, can present with lymph node enlargement in the chest, leading to compression of the trachea or bronchus, causing shortness of breath and coughing. Development of the superior vena cava syndrome can occur secondary to compression of the superior vena cava by enlarged nodes; this causes edema of the upper extremities and face. superior vena cava syndrome is life threatening and requires immediate attention. This type of lymphoma may also cause cranial nerve palsies as a result of leptomeningeal involvement.

Clients with Burkitt lymphoma may present with bowel obstruction caused by large abdominal masses or obstructive hydronephrosis from bulky lymph nodes obstructing the ureters.

Primary CNS lymphomas are restricted to the nervous system and are typically large cell lymphomas or immunoblastomas. Presenting symptoms may include headache, confusion, seizures, extremity weakness/numbness, personality changes, difficulty speaking, and lethargy. These lymphomas result from immunodeficiencies (HIV, genetic immunodeficiencies, posttransplantation).[98] Prior to the spread of HIV, this type of lymphoma was rare.

HIV and Non-Hodgkin Lymphoma. NHL is more common in clients with HIV than is HL and is an AIDS-defining illness. Typically, lymphomas that occur in clients with HIV are aggressive, fast-growing tumors. The two major subtypes of lymphomas are CNS and systemic lymphomas (with or without CNS involvement).

Two rare lymphomas seen more frequently in people with HIV are primary effusion lymphoma and plasmablastic lymphoma of the oral cavity, but the most common types are DLBCL and Burkitt lymphoma. Tumor is frequently diffusely spread at the time of diagnosis, with extranodal involvement common.

As discussed above, many illnesses that are accompanied by a reduced immune system demonstrate an increased incidence of NHL. Prior to aggressive HIV therapy (i.e., HAART), lymphomas in persons with HIV were associated with a very poor prognosis.

Currently the use of HAART has significantly reduced the risk of developing NHL and also improved tolerance for chemotherapy once diagnosed with NHL. This reduction is based on higher CD4 counts and improving the immune system. It appears that if HAART therapy is not effective, people with AIDS still have the same increased risk of developing NHL.[197] The improved immune status derived from HAART has increased treatment options for HIV-related lymphoma. Clients are now treated with the intent to cure, receiving chemotherapy, immune modulators, and HSCT.

MEDICAL MANAGEMENT

STAGING/DIAGNOSIS. Clinical staging of NHL is according to the modified Ann Arbor system, ranging from stage I to stage IV (see Box 14-6). Compared with HL, NHLs are more likely to present in an extranodal site, and the progression of the NHL does not follow the orderly anatomic progression from one lymph node to the next. Stages I and II NHLs are uncommon because the disease is much more likely to be disseminated at the time of diagnosis.

Accurate diagnosis is important because other clinical conditions can mimic malignant lymphomas (e.g., infection, tuberculosis, SLE, lung and bone cancer). Molecular genetic techniques that take advantage of the clonal nature of this malignancy are now being applied to better characterize and diagnose the lymphomas. However, at the present time a biopsy is still required to establish a definitive diagnosis.

CT scans of the chest, abdomen, and pelvis are helpful in staging, whereas MRI is used to image the brain and spinal cord. Bone marrow may be examined for staging and peripheral blood may be tested, but blood abnormalities are not present until the disease is in an advanced stage. If clinical symptoms warrant, a lumbar puncture for spinal fluid may be performed. Immunohistochemistry, flow cytometry, or cytogenetic testing is often done to distinguish one type of NHL from another.

The gallium scan (scintigraphy) using radiotracer (gallium-67) uptake is 85% to 90% accurate to predict residual disease after chemotherapy and is able to differentiate between active tumor tissue and fibrosis (uptake only occurs in viable lymphoma tissue, not in fibrotic or necrotic tissue). PET imaging is becoming more widespread and can be performed to aid in the initial diagnosis and help ascertain if a lymph node is malignant or benign. PET is also used following chemotherapy (frequently along with CT) to determine if the lymphoma is reduced in size and the treatment is effective.

Recently, the chemokine CXCL-13 was found to be elevated years prior to diagnosis of HIV-associated NHL. This may, in the future, serve as a biomarker for early detection.[154]

TREATMENT. Treatment varies for NHL depending on the stage, bulkiness of disease, phenotype (B or T/NK type), tumor grade (low, intermediate, high grade), age, and presence of comorbidities. NHL is often clinically separated into two general prognostic groups: indolent and aggressive.

In general, fast-growing tumors can be cured but require aggressive treatment. Slow-growing tumors often cannot be cured, particularly in advanced stages, but the clinical course is chronic and therapy is often reserved until symptoms develop, such as for follicular lymphoma. Localized disease (stage I or II) may be treated with radiation, whereas disseminated disease requires radiation and chemotherapy. The most common chemotherapy combination is CHOP (cyclophosphamide, doxorubicin, vincristine, and prednisone), but multiple regimens are used.

Because many risk factors for NHL are associated with a reduced immune system, immune modulators, such as interferon and monoclonal antibodies, have been employed to combat NHL. Combining the monoclonal antibody rituximab (Rituxan) with chemotherapy has produced high rates of response and is the treatment of choice for many NHLs, including DLBCL.[64,174] Clinical studies suggest that the immune modulator rituximab may alter the sensitivity of B-cell lymphoma to chemotherapy, as well as induce apoptosis and cause the lysis of B cells.

HSCT/HCT may be used for individuals who relapse or do not completely respond to treatment (which often occurs with aggressive lymphomas). Combined with intensive chemotherapy, HSCT/HCT (autologous or allogeneic) can be curative.[206] Nonmyeloablative (i.e., the doses of chemotherapy are not high enough to ablate the bone marrow) transplants can be performed for older clients who normally cannot tolerate high-dose chemotherapy, but graft-versus-host complications are problematic.

For some lymphomas, chemotherapy becomes palliative because of drug resistance; attempts at overcoming specific drug-resistance mechanisms have had limited success. Other strategies involve the use of antigen-presenting cells for taking up, processing, and presenting tumor protein in a vaccine strategy. This may provide a new immune mode to eradicate lymphoma, particularly tumor cells that persist following therapy.[49,209] Researchers have found an experimental vaccine for follicular lymphoma that nearly doubles the time before disease recurs. In the future, more tumor-specific vaccines may extend disease-free survival for all subtypes of NHL.[289]

Radioimmunotherapy, radioactive labeling of a monoclonal antibody, is also under investigation to provide targeted therapy and provide tumor-free grafts for transplant.[23,42,365]

The optimal management of women with NHL who are pregnant requires special considerations because of the poor prognosis without treatment. Treatment during the first trimester is associated with significant risk to the developing fetus and should be avoided. Treatment during the second or third trimester should include standard chemotherapy despite the potential risk to the developing fetus.[282]

PROGNOSIS. Good prognostic features include age younger than 60 years, limited disease at diagnosis (stage I or II), lack of extranodal disease, and a normal LDH level. Individuals with NHL survive for long periods when involvement is only regional. The presence of diffuse disease reduces survival time.

In general the 5-year survival rate of NHL is 50% to 60%, with a 30% cure rate for aggressive lymphomas. The indolent lymphomas are usually systemic and widespread and cure cannot be achieved, whereas intermediate- and

fast-growing lymphomas are more likely to present as treatable and even curable localized disorders but require aggressive therapy. The 5-year overall survival rate for intermediate and aggressive lymphomas in low-risk clients is 73%, whereas the rate significantly decreases for high-risk clients to 26%.

Traditionally high-grade NHL associated with AIDS was associated with an extremely poor prognosis. But with the advent of antiretroviral therapy for HIV and a multidisciplinary approach to complex AIDS cases involving malignancy, return to functional health has become possible for many individuals. Although survival rates have improved, clients with HIV still experience a higher mortality rate compared to those without HIV.[59,75,76,197,198,293]

Survivors of NHL are approximately 15% more likely to develop secondary malignancies as a result of treatment, particularly those who were diagnosed at younger ages.

SPECIAL IMPLICATIONS FOR THE THERAPIST　14-9

Non-Hodgkin Lymphoma

See "Special Implications for the Therapist 14-8: Hodgkin Lymphoma" above.

Although uncommon, the association between the use of methotrexate in RA and the development of lymphoma has been reported.[30,66] Any time an individual receiving methotrexate for RA complains of back pain accompanied by constitutional symptoms and/or GI symptoms and/or the therapist palpates enlarged lymph nodes at any of the nodal sites, a medical referral is warranted.

Multiple Myeloma

Definition and Overview. Multiple myeloma (MM) is a primary malignant neoplasm of plasma cells arising in the bone marrow. This tumor initially affects the bones and bone marrow of the vertebrae, ribs, skull, pelvis, and femur. Progression of the disease causes damage to the kidney, leads to recurrent infections, and damages bone and nerves. The extent, clinical course, complications, and sensitivity to treatment vary widely among affected people depending upon specific genetic alterations.

Several disorders and malignancies develop from the proliferation of monoclonal plasma cells and have to be distinguished from MM, such as monoclonal gammopathy of undetermined significance (MGUS) (which frequently leads to MM), AL amyloidosis (a disease involving the precipitation of proteins that results in end-organ damage), and Waldenström macroglobulinemia (a lymphoplasmacytic malignancy).

MM cells secrete monoclonal proteins (called M-proteins). They may be intact immunoglobulins with a heavy chain (IgA, IgG, IgD) and light chain (κ or λ), or free light chains (16% of cases), or, uncommonly, may not secrete proteins.

Incidence and Etiologic Factors. The incidence of MM has doubled in the past 2 decades, with an annual incidence rate of 5.3 cases per 100,000 people based on data obtained between 2005 and 2009. For the same time period, the death rate was 3.4 per 100,000 persons per year.[151] Because more people are living longer, much of this increase is owing to the occurrence of MM in people older than age 85 years.

MM occurs less often than the most common cancers (e.g., breast, lung, or colon), accounting for 1% of cancers, but is the second most common cause of hematologic cancers (13%).[151,263] This disease can develop at any age, but is most commonly seen in older people. The median age of diagnosis is 69 years of age; only 4% of people diagnosed with MM are younger than 44 years,[151] whereas almost 10% are older than age 85.

Black men are affected twice as often as white men, and MM is slightly more common in men than in women.[151] Risk factors and causes of MM are not clearly identifiable, but exposure to ionizing radiation may be linked. Certain occupational hazards found in the petroleum, leather, lumber, and agricultural industries may also increase the risk for developing MM as well. Each year, approximately 1% of people with monoclonal gammopathy of unknown significance (MGUS) go on to develop MM.[189]

Pathogenesis. MM is caused by multiple genetic abnormalities and microenvironmental changes that lead to the transformation of plasma cells to cancerous cells.

The normal maturation process of plasma cells is tightly controlled and begins with the differentiation of a hematopoietic stem cell in the bone marrow that becomes committed to the B-cell lineage through transcription factors. These transcription factors aid in the rearrangement of the immunoglobulin heavy chain (IgH) genes of pro-B cells creating the precursor (pre) B-cell. These transcription factors aid in the rearrangement of the immunoglobulin heavy chain (IgH) genes of pro-B cells creating the precursor (pre) B-cell. Pre B-cells express developing MM and continue the maturation process through transitional stages T1 and T2. Cells again undergo a selection process before becoming mature cells in the T2 stage.

Some cells remain in the spleen, whereas most mature cells leave the spleen and circulate between lymph nodes, bone marrow, and spleen until they encounter an antigen or die. It is at this point of antigen exposure that B cells develop into plasma cells. This may occur in the spleen, lymph node, or the bone marrow. Postexposure B cells, with the aid of T cells and follicular dendritic cells, can form germinal centers in follicles. Secretion of cytokines and other proteins leads to continued maturation and proliferation of the B cells with class-switch recombination of immunoglobulin, specific to antigens.

Plasma cells and memory B cells then leave the germinal center. These plasma cells express a transcription repressor (among other factors) termed BLIMP1, which results in the inability to divide or form germinal centers while inducing immunoglobulin secretion.[312] Whereas plasma cells undergo apoptosis (controlled cell death) in the spleen after a few weeks, plasma cells in the bone marrow continue to secrete antibodies for up to a year.

MM develops when genetic aberrations acquired during proliferation and maturation of the plasma cell, closely linked to microenvironmental changes, promote and sustain the growth and migration of these malignant

cells. Early, initial genetic changes in the IgH chain or the formation of trisomies can lead to both MGUS and MM. Furthermore, secondary chromosomal abnormalities are seen in MM, but rarely in MGUS (such as MYC [8q24], MAFB [20q12], and IRF [6p25]), whereas additional mutations are specific to MM but not MGUS, including MYC dysregulation, deletion in p18, and TP53 mutations.

Genetic changes determine the characteristics of the disease, which result in a heterogeneity of tumor growth, progression of disease, and resistance to therapy.[263] Myeloma cells, caused by genetic mutations, alter the expression of adhesion molecules that change the interaction between the malignant myeloma cells and the surrounding stromal cells and extracellular matrix proteins. When myeloma cells adhere to hematopoietic and stromal cells there is a resultant release of cytokines and growth factors (principally IL-6, vascular endothelial growth factor, IL-10, insulin-like growth factor 1, members of the tumor necrosis factor family, and transforming growth factor β1). Response to growth stimuli is also altered, leading to the production of apoptotic proteins; other abnormalities include the induction of blood vessel formation (angiogenesis).[263] It is also these adhesion molecules that attract malignant plasma cells together, forming plasmacytomas or masses of plasma cells.

An imbalance in the function of bone cells, osteoclasts (break down bone) and osteoblasts (bone building), results in the characteristic lytic bone lesions. One pathway, the Wnt pathway, is inhibited, thereby suppressing osteoblasts. Stromal cells are induced to increase production of the RANK (receptor activator of nuclear factor-kappa B) ligand that binds to osteoclasts thereby stimulating bone destruction. RANK ligand also leads to the inhibition of osteoclastic apoptosis (programmed cell death).[210]

Clinical Manifestations. MM is categorized as either asymptomatic (smoldering) or symptomatic, depending on the presence of signs and/or symptoms of organ or tissue dysfunction. The onset of MM is usually gradual and insidious. Common presenting features include fatigue, bone pain, neurologic symptoms, renal insufficiency, hypercalcemia, and recurrent infections. Fatigue is a frequent problem that is caused by anemia and elevated levels of cytokines. Anemia, caused by bone marrow infiltration and/or renal insufficiency, is present in 73% of people presenting with MM. Bony lesions were noted in 80% of newly diagnosed MM clients, whereas 58% reported bone pain.[263] Renal insufficiency is seen in approximately 20% to 40% of clients at presentation. Hypercalcemia is present in 13%,[190] whereas elevated creatinine levels are noted in 48% of newly diagnosed individuals.

The risk for infections is increased prior to treatment and with refractory disease, particularly with gram-negative organisms (60% of infections).[255] However, this risk decreases with response to therapy. Sinopulmonary infections are the most common. MM in older adults (older than 75 years) is the same as that reported in younger people except for a higher rate of infection in the older population.[292] These malignant plasma cells can also form large masses known as plasmacytomas, which can grow in bones and soft tissues.

Musculoskeletal. Most people with MM develop bone pain and other bone-related problems as bone marrow expands and bone is destroyed. Bone pain is seen particularly in the ribs, pelvis, spine, clavicles, skull, and humeri. Bone loss, the major clinical manifestation of MM, often leads to pathologic fractures, spinal cord compression, and bone pain.

Initially, the bone pain may be mild and intermittent, or may occur acutely as severe pain in the back, rib, leg, or arm, often the result of an abrupt movement or minor effort that results in a spontaneous (pathologic) bone fracture. The pain is often radicular and sharp to one or both sides and is aggravated by movement. Symptoms associated with bone pain usually subside within days to weeks after initiation of systemic chemotherapy, but if the disease progresses there is associated progression of bone destruction. Bone destruction can lead to hypercalcemia, seen in 30% to 40% of people with MM, which can be life-threatening. Symptoms of hypercalcemia may include confusion, increased urination, loss of appetite, abdominal pain, constipation, and vomiting (see "Hypercalcemia" in Chapter 5).

Muscular weakness and wasting affect nearly half of all individuals with cancer and contribute to the cause of cancer-related fatigue. Muscle wasting occurs as a result of disuse, pathology, anemia, nutritional imbalances, or decreased rates of muscle protein synthesis.

Neurologic. Neurologic complications of MM stem from bone loss or tumor invasion or are protein related. As bone is destroyed in the vertebrae, collapse of the bone with subsequent compression of the nerves can occur. Clients may complain of back pain, numbness, tingling, or loss of strength.

Large plasmacytomas (particularly in the spinal canal or skull) can compress nerves, leading to spinal cord or cranial nerve compressions. Spinal cord compression is usually observed early or in the late relapse phase of the disease. Presenting symptoms include back pain with radiating numbness/tingling, muscle weakness or paralysis of the lower extremities, and loss of bowel or bladder control. Spinal cord compression is a medical emergency requiring immediate attention.

High concentrations of protein are also neuropathic. Amyloidosis (deposits of insoluble fragments of a protein) develops in approximately 10% of people with MM. These deposits cause tissues to become waxy and immobile and may affect nerves, muscles, and ligaments, especially the carpal tunnel area of the wrist. Carpal tunnel syndrome with pain, numbness, or tingling of the hands and fingers may develop.

Renal. Renal impairment is a common complication of MM.[155] The pathogenesis is multifactorial including toxic effect of the excess proteins on the renal tubules, dehydration, nephrotoxic drugs, and hypercalcemia. The large amount of monoclonal light chains secreted by the malignant plasma cells can form large casts in the tubules of the kidneys, causing dilation and atrophy, which leads to the inability of the nephron to function and interstitial nephritis.

Hypercalcemia occurs from increased bone destruction and absorption of calcium into the blood. In an effort to rid the body of the excess calcium, the kidneys increase the output of urine, which can lead to serious

Table 14-4	International Myeloma Working Group Diagnostic Criteria		
Diagnosis	**M Protein (g/dL)**	**Bone Marrow Plasma Cell Percentage by Biopsy**	**Tissue or Organ Dysfunction Caused by MM**
MGUS	<3 g/dL	<10%	No
Asymptomatic MM	≥3 g/dL	≥10%	No
Symptomatic MM	present	≥10%	Yes

MGUS, monoclonal gammopathy of undetermined significance; MM, multiple myeloma.

Data from International Myeloma Working Group: Criteria for the classification of monoclonal gammopathies, multiple myeloma and related disorders: a report of the International Myeloma Working Group, *Br J Haematol* 121(5):749–757, 2003; and Kyle RA, Rajkumar SV: Criteria for diagnosis, staging, risk stratification and response assessment of multiple myeloma, *Leukemia* 23(1):3-9, 2009.

dehydration and result in further kidney damage if intake of fluids is inadequate.

Calcium can also be deposited in the kidney, creating another source of interstitial nephritis. Hypercalcemia is a common presenting feature but is less common after adequate chemotherapy. Recurrent urinary tract infections are also common and detrimental to the kidneys.

Many medications are nephrotoxic, including some antibiotics, radiographic dyes, and chemotherapy agents. NSAIDs can reduce blood flow to the kidneys, causing further damage. Because of the many factors that can cause injury to the kidneys, nephrotoxic medications should be avoided or used with caution in clients with MM as renal dysfunction and renal failure can occur.

MEDICAL MANAGEMENT

DIAGNOSIS. The diagnosis of MM is determined by clinical and laboratory factors as well as bone marrow examination. Because other diseases also present with an elevated monoclonal gammopathy (i.e., MGUS and AL amyloidosis), criteria have been developed by the International Myeloma Working Group to aid in the diagnosis and distinction of these plasma cell dyscrasias so as to provide appropriate treatment (Table 14-4).[62,122] The principal difference is the involvement of tissue and organs in persons with MM, which may include hypercalcemia, renal insufficiency, anemia, and lytic bone lesions.

Clients with a serum M-protein less than 3 g/dL, a clonal plasmacytosis in the bone marrow of less than 10%, and no evidence of organ or tissue involvement are categorized as having MGUS. Those with M-protein levels greater than 3 g/dL, a clonal plasmacytosis greater than 10%, and no evidence of organ or tissue involvement are considered as having smoldering or asymptomatic MM. MM is diagnosed if M-protein is present, the bone marrow exhibits a monoclonal gammopathy or plasmacytoma, and there is evidence of organ or tissue involvement. Approximately 40% of people with MM display less than 3 g/dL of M-protein and 5% have less than 10% bone marrow plasmacytosis.

The International Staging System was developed for MM to stage the severity of disease. It defines three risk groups based on the serum β_2-microglobulin albumin levels: Stage 1: serum β_2-microglobulin is less than 3.5 mg/L and serum albumin greater or equal to 3.5 g/dL; Stage 2 demonstrates values between stages 1 and 2; Stage 3 has a serum β_2-microglobulin greater than or equal to 5.5 mg/L. The diagnosis must already be made and the usefulness of the system may vary with the use of newer drugs.[122]

Tests performed to determine if criteria are met for the diagnosis of MM include a bone marrow biopsy and aspiration, measurement of M-protein in the blood and urine (serum protein electrophoresis and urine protein electrophoresis, respectively, or more sensitive tests such as immunoelectrophoresis and immunofixation), and biopsy of any suspect mass.

Other tests that are helpful in providing prognostic information include LDH, β_2-microglobulin, plasma cell labeling index (a measurement of the proliferative capacity of the myeloma cells), and quantitative measurement of immunoglobulins and free light chains. Other standard laboratory tests include chemistries (assessing calcium and kidney function), CBC, and peripheral blood smear (rouleaux are often noted).

A radiographic skeletal survey is necessary to determine bone involvement. MRI is recommended if plain radiographs are normal or suggest a plasmacytoma[81]; if spinal cord compression is suspected, an emergent MRI or CT should be performed. PET scans are being used more frequently, particularly to determine the extent of the disease at the time of diagnosis, and contributing to more accurate staging.[31]

TREATMENT. Current chemotherapy drugs have improved the disease-free survival of people with MM. The center of treatment of MM includes the immunomodulatory drugs thalidomide and lenalidomide, the proteasome inhibitor bortezomib, and the alkylating agent melphalan. Therapy is related to age and ability to tolerate toxic regimens. For those who are younger than 65 years of age and without significant heart, lung, renal, or liver dysfunction, induction with thalidomide, lenalidomide, or bortezomib plus a hematopoietic stem-cell transplantation is the principal therapy. Autologous stem-cell transplantation with a less-toxic medical regimen can be considered for older clients or those with comorbidities.

Conventional therapy combined with thalidomide, lenalidomide, or bortezomib can be offered to older people who cannot tolerate stem-cell transplantation.[263] Biologic age, however, should be the main consideration over chronologic age when a therapy and drug dose are selected. Consolidation and maintenance therapy is given following stem-cell transplantation. MM is currently incurable and relapsed disease is often treated with lenalidomide- or bortezomib-based regimens.

Thalidomide and lenalidomide are teratogenic agents and increase the risk for thrombosis. Clients on these medications should be monitored carefully during times of immobility and proper precautions instituted. Constipation, peripheral neuropathy, and somnolence are often seen with thalidomide. Lenalidomide and melphalan cause myelosuppression, whereas bortezomib may cause thrombocytopenia and peripheral neuropathy.

Early treatment of asymptomatic MM does not improve survival and should not be instituted until criteria are met for MM with associated evidence of tissue/organ dysfunction.[190] Clients should be carefully followed in order to receive treatment once disease does progress to MM.

Advances have also been made in correcting symptoms caused by the myeloma and surrounding cells. Bone pain is one of the most significant problems faced by clients with MM. Pathologic fractures are treated with surgery and pain control. Kyphoplasty can improve pain from vertebral-body compression fractures. Lytic lesions often require radiation for pain relief along with opioids. Radiation may be all that is needed to decrease pain and stabilize the cervical spine when metastases occur. In some cases radiation has been shown to stop and even reverse bone destruction.[107]

The bisphosphonates pamidronate and zoledronic acid reduce vertebral fractures, skeletal related events, and pain.[225] Because of side effects (i.e., renal insufficiency, jaw osteonecrosis), other methods of treating bone disease in MM are under investigation.[200]

Hypercalcemia is treated with hydration, corticosteroids, and bisphosphonates. Anemia improves with myeloma treatment, but the use of erythropoietin can speed up recovery of erythrocyte production following chemotherapy.

Oncologists are looking toward individualizing treatment depending on the types of mutations present in the myeloma cells. Treatments attempt to disrupt the abnormal signaling pathways that support the uncontrolled growth and migration of malignant plasma cells. They also endeavor to stimulate apoptotic pathways and disrupt abnormal cell adhesion and angiogenesis.

PROGNOSIS. Current medications for MM have extended overall survival but it remains an incurable disease. The 5-year survival rate is approximately 67% in cases that were diagnosed with local disease. For those with distant disease, the 5-year survival is reduced to 40% with an overall 5-year survival rate of 41%.[151] In people who develop MM before the age of 60 years, the 10-year survival is approximately 30%.[32]

The risk of asymptomatic (smoldering) MM progressing to MM or a related disorder during the first 5 years after diagnosis is 10% per year. Over the next 5 years the risk is 3% per year, whereas over the next 10 years the risk decreases to 1% to 2% per year.[189]

A poorer prognosis is seen in persons with any chromosomal abnormality. Specific translocations in the IgH chain (such as t(4;14), deletion 17p13, and chromosome 1 abnormalities) are also associated with a poor prognosis. Much research has been done and continues in order to profile each client's genetic mutations to determine prognosis and best treatment.[263]

If untreated, unstable MM can result in skeletal deformities, particularly of the ribs, sternum, and spine. Diffuse osteoporosis develops, accompanied by a negative calcium balance. Prognosis is affected by the presence of renal failure (poorer prognosis if present at the time of diagnosis), hypercalcemia, or extensive bony disease; infection and renal failure are the most common causes of death.

Multiple Myeloma

MM can have severe and devastating effects on the musculoskeletal system. Fatigue and skeletal muscle wasting can result in a weak and debilitated individual who is at risk for falls and subsequent musculoskeletal injuries. Bone pathology with fracture can also be very painful and disabling, affecting function and quality of life. The therapist may be instrumental in early detection and referral to minimize detrimental secondary effects.[166]

Multiple Myeloma and Exercise

Therapists can assist individuals with MM to manage both the disease and treatment-related symptoms, improve overall quality of life, and prevent further complications associated with decreased activity and exercise.

The therapist may play an important role in various stages of the progression of this disease, including prevention and management of skeletal muscle wasting, cancer-related fatigue, and pathologic fractures.[166] Individualized exercise programs for individuals receiving aggressive treatment for MM may be effective for decreasing fatigue and mood disturbance and for improving sleep.[58]

Symptoms such as fatigue can be so overwhelming at times that some people have even said that they would rather just die than continue suffering the extremes of fatigue and malaise.[63] The National Comprehensive Cancer Network continues to recommend exercise in their updated clinical practice guidelines for the management of cancer-related fatigue.[238,239]

The guidelines suggest referral to physical therapy for fitness assessment and exercise recommendations with emphasis on getting clients to gradually increase their activity level to avoid sustaining an injury or becoming discouraged. Short, low-intensity exercise programs may be helpful at first. The key is to get the individual to implement and maintain the program.

Individuals with MM have a number of intrinsic and extrinsic factors that can challenge their ability to engage in an exercise program. Intrinsic factors include a belief that exercise will help, a commitment to one's health, creation of personal goals, and a plan to reach them. Extrinsic factors include a good support system and adequate medical care (e.g., prophylactic epoetin alfa used to treat anemia).[60]

The therapist's ability to implement falls assessment and prevention programs can be a lifesaving intervention for the individual at risk for pathologic fractures. Exercise interventions to improve function and decrease muscle wasting and cancer-related fatigue during and after cancer treatment for MM have been shown effective. Suggested exercise protocols for MM are available.[335]

Complications

Specific examination and evaluation can provide early recognition of complications such as hypercalcemia and spinal cord compression. Any symptoms of hypercalcemia (see "Clinical Manifestations" above)

must be reported to the physician; the client should seek immediate medical care as this condition can be life-threatening. (For the client with anemia, or renal failure, see the "Special Implications for the Therapist 14-5: The Anemias and 18-5: Chronic Kidney Disease".) Adequate hydration and mobility help minimize the development of hypercalcemia.

The client with MM who develops signs of cord compression must be referred to the physician. Emergency MRI is required to locate the area of cord compression. A laminectomy may be required when spinal cord compression occurs, but immediate radiation and high-dose glucocorticoid therapy usually relieve the compression, avoiding the need for surgical intervention.

Spinal instability may be a problem. Orthopedic back braces may help with pain management and reduce the risk of further trauma but are often poorly tolerated; newer lightweight supports with hook-and-loop fasteners may be more useful. Vertebroplasty and kyphoplasty procedures may help improve spinal stability; cement injected into the collapsed vertebrae reinforces the bone. In the case of kyphoplasty, vertebral height is restored.[101]

Weight Bearing

There is little clinical evidence to guide the therapist in choosing a safe amount of weight bearing through cancer-lysed metastatic bone during exercise, transfers, ambulation, or other activities of daily living skills.[61] Some general guidelines based on radiographic findings have been suggested for individuals with bone metastases[110]:

>50% (cortical metastatic involvement)	Non–weight bearing with crutches or walking; touch down permitted
25%-50%	Partial weight bearing; avoid twisting or stretching
0%-25%	Full weight bearing; avoid lifting or straining

These recommendations must be used with caution, taking into consideration the client's age, general health, overall level of fitness, and level of pain. Through careful assessment, the therapist guides the client in maintaining mobility as much as possible while preventing fracture. Continual monitoring of symptoms to detect developing or new fracture is imperative. The affected individual must be taught what to look for and when to seek medical attention if signs and symptoms of new fracture appear.

Supportive and Palliative Care

In preterminal and terminal stages, attention to supportive therapy and palliation are integral and can make a great impact on the individual and family's quality of life. The role of the therapist increases in late stages when immobility and renal failure complicate the clinical picture.[284]

Myeloproliferative Neoplasms (Myeloproliferative Disorders)

Myeloproliferative disorders are a group of diseases of the bone marrow in which excess cells are produced. There is a transformation of hematopoietic stem cells that allows the cells to mature and function, yet there is uncontrolled production. Myeloproliferative disorders also share other characteristics, including a hypercellular bone marrow, tendency toward thrombosis and hemorrhage, and an increased risk of evolving into acute leukemia over time.[44] Myeloproliferative neoplasms are related to (and may transform into) myelodysplastic syndrome, a common blood cancer of the elderly that can progress to AML.

The four classic myeloproliferative neoplasms include CML, polycythemia vera (PV), essential thrombocythemia, and primary myelofibrosis. Even though all of these disorders can exhibit elevations in all cell lines, each disease has a main cell line that is affected. As a result of specific molecular abnormalities being discovered in association with these disorders, the WHO has revised the diagnostic criteria for these conditions and the term chronic myeloproliferative disorders has been changed to myeloproliferative neoplasms.[341]

Polycythemia vera is an uncontrolled production of erythrocytes. Essential thrombocythemia is characterized by an elevated platelet count. Excessive fibrosis of the marrow is a dominant feature of primary myelofibrosis. Myelofibrosis and other more rare diseases are not covered in this text. CML is discussed with the leukemias.

Polycythemia Vera

Definition, Overview, and Etiologic Factors. PV is a myeloproliferative neoplasm of bone marrow stem cells affecting the production of erythrocytes. The term *polycythemia* means an elevated RBC mass that may be primary or secondary.

Secondary polycythemia is typically acquired as a result of decreased oxygen availability to the tissues; the body attempts to compensate for the reduced oxygen by producing more erythrocytes (e.g., smoking, high altitudes, and chronic heart and lung disorders). However, PV is a primary cause of polycythemia and results from a genetic abnormality that allows for the uncontrolled production of erythrocytes from a neoplastic hematopoietic stem cell.

The prevalence of PV is approximately 22 cases per 100,000.[205] It typically occurs in older people between the ages of 50 and 75 years with approximately 5% diagnosed younger than the age of 40, with a slightly higher incidence in men than in women. The etiologic factors of PV are attributed to benzene and other occupational exposures, including radiation.

Pathogenesis. PV results from the mutation of a hematopoietic stem cell. Not only does this cell produce RBCs, but often develops into leukocytes and platelets. More than 95% of people with PV have a mutation in the Janus kinase 2 (*JAK2*) gene, where valine is replaced for phenylalanine at position 617 (JAK2 V617F). Normally, once induced by erythropoietin, the *JAK2* gene produces a kinase that is responsible for intracellular communication and ultimately leads to cell production.[352]

This gene normally exerts a negative effect in that it controls signals and the production of cells. But with this mutation cellular production occurs despite the lack of binding erythropoietin and cytokines (cells become cytokine independent), leading to many of the problems seen in myeloproliferative neoplasms, including PV.

Other genetic abnormalities are also described, and several genetic modifications are most likely required for cellular transformation.[14] There is also an increased risk of PV evolving into AML over time. Although the mechanisms are not understood, clients without the JAK2 mutation can develop AML, demonstrating that other mutations may be the source.

Clinical Manifestations. PV clinical manifestations are often categorized by phases: latent, proliferative, and spent phases. Latent refers to early disease that is asymptomatic. The proliferative phase is related to uncontrolled proliferation of cells leading to symptoms. The symptoms of PV are often insidious in onset and characterized by vague complaints such as irritability, general malaise and fatigue, backache, and weight loss. Diagnosis may not be made until a secondary complication, such as stroke or thrombosis, occurs.

Symptoms are related to hyperviscosity, hypervolemia, and hypermetabolism. The increased concentration of erythrocytes may cause hypertension or neurologic symptoms such as headache, blurred vision, feeling of fullness in the head, disturbances of sensation in the hands and feet, dizziness, ringing in the ears, or vertigo. Bone pain may develop from increased production of cells.

Blockage of the capillaries supplying the digits of either the hands or feet may cause a peripheral vascular neuropathy with decreased sensation, burning numbness, or tingling. This same small blood vessel occlusion can also contribute to the development of cyanosis and clubbing of the digits. Other symptoms include increased skin coloration (e.g., ruddy complexion of face, hands, feet, ears, and mucous membranes), and on physical exam splenomegaly is common. Dyspnea may develop secondary to hypervolemia. Abnormal interactions among erythrocytes, leukocytes, platelets, and the endothelium lead to thrombosis (e.g., splenic infarctions and Budd-Chiari syndrome,[319] which is a thrombosis of the hepatic vein) or bleeding (e.g., easy bruising, GI bleeding, and epistaxis).

Gout and uric acid stones may develop because of hypermetabolism or increased turnover of RBCs. Intolerable pruritus (itching), especially after bathing in warm water, may be prominent and is characteristic of PV.

The spent phase describes a phase of the disease where the bone marrow fills with fibroblasts and hematopoiesis is transferred to the liver and spleen. This results in progressive hepatosplenomegaly and associated cytopenias. Clients may require transfusions.

MEDICAL MANAGEMENT

DIAGNOSIS. PV is frequently asymptomatic and is often detected from a laboratory value obtained for another reason. Diagnosis is established by history, examination, and laboratory analysis. The erythrocyte count is greater than 60% of normal for men and 56% for women (without the presence of secondary polycythemic factors).

WBC and platelet count are often elevated in people with PV and are normal in most people with secondary polycythemia.

The presence of the JAK2 mutation can be identified by polymerase chain reaction and other sensitive tests of molecular markers. A positive JAK2 (seen in 95% of people with PV), low erythropoietin level, and appropriate clinical factors may be enough information to make the diagnosis.

However, because not all cases of PV express the JAK2 abnormality, other tests can be performed, including labeling RBCs with chromium to distinguish between absolute polycythemia (increased RBC mass) and relative polycythemia (normal RBC mass but decreased plasma volume), growing cells to verify erythropoietin independence, bone marrow biopsy with cytogenetic studies, and performing an ultrasound of the spleen to demonstrate splenomegaly.

TREATMENT. Treatment goals are to reduce erythrocytosis and blood volume, control symptoms, and prevent thrombosis. Repeated phlebotomy is the most common treatment that is used to maintain a stable hemoglobin (less than 45% in men and 42% in women) by causing iron deficiency.

Low-dose aspirin, if no contraindications exist, has been found to be beneficial to all people with PV in reducing the risk of thrombotic events, although overall mortality and cardiovascular mortality rates are not significantly reduced.[192]

For clients who do not respond to aspirin and phlebotomy, alternative medications include the antimetabolite hydroxyurea (particularly helpful for people at high risk for thrombosis), and interferon alpha (often used in younger people or women of childbearing age).

With the recent discovery of mutant alleles contributing to altered cellular signaling pathways in the pathogenesis of myeloproliferative neoplasms, research is now focused on finding targeted therapies for these disorders.

PROGNOSIS. The prognosis for PV is good with those who are properly treated and monitored living near-normal life expectancy. The risk for stroke, myocardial infarction, and thromboembolism is high for people with this condition (27%-31%)[329]; thrombosis or hemorrhage is the major cause of death. Mortality rate increases with age starting at age 50 years.[352] Late in the course of this disease, bone marrow may be replaced with fibrous tissue (myelofibrosis) or be transformed into AML (10%-15%),[328] which are the most serious complications of PV and account for many deaths.[186,207]

SPECIAL IMPLICATIONS FOR THE THERAPIST   14-11

Polycythemia Vera

Thrombosis occurs more often in clients with PV, which requires the therapist to be alert to any possible signs of Budd-Chiari syndrome (abdominal pain, ascites, and liver function abnormalities) and deep vein thrombosis or stroke (e.g., weakness, numbness, inability to speak, visual changes, headache; see

"Thrombophlebitis" in Chapter 12). Older age (greater than 60 years) and a previous history of thrombosis are standard risk factors for thrombosis. Risk may increase for those who are hypertensive, smoke or use other tobacco products, have diabetes, or hyperlipidemia.[352]

GI bleeding, bruising, and epistaxis are also common. Watch for other complications, such as dyspnea and splenomegaly. If the person has symptomatic splenomegaly, follow precautions for soft-tissue techniques required in the left upper quadrant, especially up and under the rib cage. These procedures must be secondary or indirect techniques away from the spleen.

Essential Thrombocythemia

Overview and Etiology. Essential thrombocythemia (ET) is categorized as one of the myeloproliferative neoplasms. It is defined as a disease with a platelet count greater than 600,000/µL without secondary causes for an elevated number of platelets.

ET is a primary thrombocytosis disorder resulting from a transformation of a hematopoietic stem cell and occurs most frequently in middle-aged to older adults (average age of onset is between 50 and 60 years). There may be more of a predisposition for women to develop the disease than men. The incidence has significantly increased over the last decade due to the use of JAK2 gene testing and the ability to diagnose the disease earlier.[112] Approximately 6000 cases are diagnosed in the United States each year.

Secondary causes of thrombocytosis occur as a result of conditions such as acute bleeding, iron deficiency, infection (e.g., tuberculosis), chronic inflammatory disease (e.g., RA), and malignancy, and resolve with treatment of the underlying pathology.[300] Secondary thrombocytosis may also be seen following splenectomy because platelets that normally would be stored in the spleen return to the circulating blood.

Pathogenesis. Approximately 50% of clients with ET demonstrate the JAK2 mutation, linking it with other myeloproliferative neoplasms (see "Polycythemia Vera" above). The JAK2 mutation is known to significantly increase the activity of the JAK2 gene, induce cytokine-independent signaling, and activate downstream communications.[346] Thrombosis, a serious problem seen in ET, may develop as a result of an abnormal interaction among leukocytes, platelets, and vascular endothelium; although leukocytosis may be a better indicator of thrombosis risk than absolute platelet count.[92] Other genetic abnormalities are most likely responsible for the remaining cases that do not exhibit the JAK2 mutation.

Clinical Manifestations. The most prominent feature is a platelet count elevation above 600,000/µL. Many people with ET also exhibit splenomegaly (50%) and episodes of bleeding (40%) and/or thrombosis (30%), such as microvascular thrombi causing digital ischemia.

Visual disturbances, headache, burning sensation of the feet and hands accompanied by redness (secondary to vasodilation; erythromelalgia), and skin changes (livedo reticularis; Fig. 14-10) develop with increasing platelet counts. The most serious complications bleeding and thrombosis, occur secondary to a qualitative

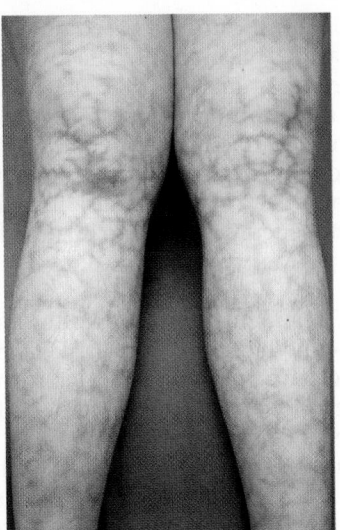

Figure 14-10

Livedo reticularis associated with thrombocythemia (elevated platelet count). The classic fishnet pattern is shown. (Reprinted from Piccini JP, Nilsson KR: *The Osler medical handbook*, ed 2, Baltimore, 2006, Johns Hopkins University.)

platelet dysfunction. Although major bleeding is uncommon, the likelihood increases as platelet counts exceed 1,500,000/μL. Unlike PV, ET rarely progresses to AML.

MEDICAL MANAGEMENT

DIAGNOSIS. Because most people are asymptomatic at diagnosis, the disease is usually identified from incidental laboratory tests. Causes of secondary thrombocytosis need to be eliminated in order to diagnose ET. Approximately 50% of people with ET exhibit a mutation in the *JAK2* gene. The presence of this mutation may portend a more aggressive course of disease. A sustained, elevated platelet count; the JAK2 mutation; splenomegaly; and abnormal bone marrow are features indicative of ET.

TREATMENT. The treatment of ET depends on the age and symptoms of the person. Asymptomatic, young clients (age younger than 65 years) with a platelet count less than 1,500,000/μL may not require treatment. Hydroxyurea with low-dose aspirin is used for people who are older than 65 years with a history of a thrombotic event to reduce the platelet count to less than 400,000/μL. This therapy significantly reduces the risk bleeding or another thrombotic event.

Anagrelide reduces platelet counts in persons who are able to tolerate it. Side effects include arrhythmias, palpitations, hypotension, fluid retention, and heart failure. It should not be used in elderly persons with heart problems. Interferon-α, low-dose, may also be beneficial.[318]

Persons who develop acute ischemic events and have a platelet count greater than 1,500,000/μL can receive immediate plateletpheresis. If surgery is required, the platelet count should be brought to near-normal levels to reduce the risk of bleeding and thrombosis perioperatively.

PROGNOSIS. Most people with ET have near-normal life expectancies. ET carries a small (less than 1%) risk of

transforming into acute leukemia, and rarely develops into myelofibrosis.[183] Bleeding and thrombotic events are the most serious complications and can be life-threatening. Better understanding of the mutations resulting in ET may lead to improved treatment (i.e., JAK2 inhibitors[346]) and prophylaxis against bleeding and thrombotic complications.

SPECIAL IMPLICATIONS FOR THE THERAPIST   14-12

Thrombocythemia

The therapist may recognize this condition when the client presents with livedo reticularis accompanied by reports of headache, burning sensation in the hands and feet, and visual disturbances. Medical referral is required if the person has not been previously evaluated.

In cases of known thrombocythemia, the therapist must maintain surveillance for arterial and venous thrombotic episodes and educate the client about what to watch for and when to seek medical assistance immediately. Signs and symptoms of arterial emboli include pain, numbness, coldness, tingling or changes in sensation, skin changes (pallor, mottling), weakness, and muscle spasm occurring in the extremity distal to the block (see Table 12-19).

With venous occlusion, the tissues are oxygenated but the blood is not moving and stasis occurs. The skin is discolored rather than pale (ranging from angry red to deep blue-purple), edema is present, and pain is most marked at the site of occlusion, although extreme edema can render all the skin of the limb quite tender.

Myelodysplastic Syndrome

Overview. Myelodysplastic syndrome (MDS) is a heterogeneous group of disorders resulting from the clonal expansion of a malignant hematopoietic stem cell. MDS was previously categorized as a preleukemic disorder, but in the year 2000, the WHO changed the categorization to malignant.[104] In comparison to myeloproliferative disorders, MDS typically presents with anemia and cytopenias. MDS can have a significant impact on quality of life and survival[100]; it also progresses at a variable rate to AML.

MDS has been underdiagnosed and underrecognized in the past. In 1995, only 1500 cases were reported, whereas between 2001 and 2004 there were about 10,000 new cases per year. MDS is more common in older people,[237] with an incidence rate of about 75 per 100,000 in people 65 years of age and older.[57] Approximately 86% of people with MDS were 60 years of age or older, whereas only 6% were younger than age 50.[203] White men have the highest incidence of MDS.

As awareness of the disease improves, the incidence rate will most likely increase in the future.

Etiology. Some established risk factors associated with MDS include ionizing radiation and chemotherapy from a previous malignancy treatment; exposure to benzene (such as cigarette smoking)[268]; genetic disorders (i.e., Down syndrome); and the congenital diseases (i.e., Fanconi anemia). MDS that results from previous cancer treatment is termed secondary MDS and carries a poorer prognosis. The number of secondary cases has significantly increased most likely because of the increase in people who have survived previous malignancies. Other factors that may be related include pesticides, alcohol consumption, and increased body mass index.[204]

Pathogenesis.[94,196] A variety of genetic abnormalities are associated with MDS. The final common pathway of these abnormalities is a hematopoietic stem cell that is unable to effectively mature and develop, and which undergoes premature apoptosis.[121]

Clinical Manifestations. Because the malignant cells are unable to effectively differentiate, they eventually undergo apoptosis. This results in ineffective hematopoiesis in the bone marrow, leading to various cytopenias. Clinical manifestations of MDS vary depending on the presence and severity of the cytopenias. Many people remain asymptomatic and MDS is only suspected by laboratory values obtained for other clinical symptoms. Anemia (usually macrocytic) is the most common laboratory manifestation, noted in 80% to 85% of people presenting with MDS.[327] Clients typically exhibit fatigue or exacerbation of underlying comorbidities such as CHF or chronic obstructive pulmonary disease. Neutropenia is seen in 40% of newly diagnosed individuals, whereas thrombocytopenia is noted in 30% to 45% of clients.[100,327] Pancytopenia is found in approximately 50% of cases. People with MDS may be more prone to infections (some unexplainable) or bleeding. MDS should be suspected in any elderly client with unexplained anemia and progressive cytopenias.

MEDICAL MANAGEMENT

DIAGNOSIS. Because MDS previously was thought to be rare, a primary care provider should have a high suspicion for MDS when evaluating older persons with anemia. Although anemia is common in the elderly, it is not an expected result of normal aging.[127] When taking a history, particular attention should be given to past cancer treatment, occupational exposures, tobacco use, or congenital/genetic disorders. Symptoms of fatigue, infection, and bleeding should be addressed.

For clients with one or more cytopenias and suspected MDS, the National Comprehensive Cancer Network guidelines[240] recommend a thorough history and exam; a bone marrow biopsy and aspiration with iron staining and cytogenetics; a serum erythropoietin level; RBC folate and vitamin B_{12} levels; a CBC with reticulocyte count; a peripheral blood smear; and a serum ferritin level. The peripheral blood smear may demonstrate hypolobulated, hypogranulated neutrophils and nucleated erythrocytes.

MDS is difficult to diagnose. Often other entities that present with anemia and dysplasia of blood cells must be excluded. This is particularly true in people who have early disease or mild dysplasia. The minimum diagnostic criterion for MDS is dysplasia in ≥10% of any of the myeloid linages or cytogenetics suggestive of MDS.[342]

Several classification systems and prognostic models are used to aid in the diagnosis and stratification of clients according to determining risk for progression to AML. The FAB classification is based on cell morphology and bone marrow blast count. The WHO classification recognizes seven variants of MDS, taking into account cytogenetics and immunophenotypic characteristics in addition to the FAB classification.[208,353] The International Prognostic Scoring System utilizes bone marrow blast percentage, number of cytopenias, transfusion dependence, and cytogenetics as features that tend to determine outcome.[120]

TREATMENT. Treatment of MDS is often determined by classification, whether high or low-risk for progression to AML, life expectancy, or ability to tolerate medications or HSCT. People at low-risk for developing AML can use the "watch and wait" approach.

Symptomatic anemia can be treated with transfusion, although this leads to iron overload and must be carefully monitored. Iron chelation therapy may be considered for those clients with a ferritin level of 1000 ng/mL. Bleeding may require platelet transfusions and infections are treated with appropriate antibiotics. Attempts at avoiding chronic transfusion dependence are essential and may include the use of erythrocyte-stimulating agents, epoetin and darbepoetin alfa, granulocyte colony-stimulating factor, or granulocyte-macrophage colony-stimulating factor.

Medications that have improved MDS treatment include lenalidomide (an immunomodulating agent), azacitidine and decitabine (hypomethylating agents), and antithymocyte globulin and cyclosporine (for clients with an immune component).

Those at high risk for progression to AML should receive treatment immediately. Because allogeneic HSCT is potentially the only cure for MDS, treatment decisions must be made with this in mind. Good candidates for HSCT include age younger than 55 (although performance status if more important), good performance status, high-risk MDS, and suitable donor.

PROGNOSIS. Because MDS is a heterogenic group of related disorders, the progression and prognosis vary substantially between variants. Data from the Surveillance, Epidemiology, and End Results program from 2001–2008 indicate the observed 3-year survival rate is 42% and the 5-year survival rate is 29%.

DISORDERS OF HEMOSTASIS

Hemostasis is the arrest of bleeding after blood vessel injury and involves the interaction among the blood vessel wall, the platelets, and the plasma coagulation proteins. Normal hemostasis is divided into two separate and independent processes: primary and secondary.

Primary hemostasis involves the formation of a platelet plug at the site of vascular injury. When a vessel is disrupted, collagen fibrils and von Willebrand factor (vWF) in the subendothelial matrix of the blood vessel become exposed to blood. The vWF (which is usually coiled when inactive) in the plasma and the subendothelium becomes uncoiled and binds the collagen fibrils to the platelets via special receptors on the platelets. This ultimately leads to the formation of a platelet plug.

Secondary hemostasis is triggered when vascular damage exposes tissue factor. Tissue factor is found in places not normally exposed to blood flow, where the presence of blood is pathologic. It is present in significant amounts in the brain, subendothelium, smooth muscle, and epithelium. Tissue factor is not found in skeletal muscle or synovium, the usual locations for spontaneous bleeding in people with hemophilia.

Tissue factor then binds clotting factor VII, which, in turn, activates factors X and IX. This eventually leads to the formation of thrombin, which cleaves fibrinogen into fibrin, creating a fibrin clot at the site of injury.

Normal primary hemostasis requires normal number and function of platelets and vWF. Persons who have abnormalities in primary hemostasis have defects in either the number or function of platelets or a deficiency or dysfunction of vWF.

A decrease in the number of platelets, called *thrombocytopenia*, can prevent hemostasis. An exceptionally high number of platelets, called thrombocytosis, may cause bleeding, thrombosis, or both Persons with a deficiency or dysfunction in vWF have von Willebrand disease (vWD).

Bleeding caused by platelet disorders or vWD is characterized by mucosal or skin bleeding. Normal secondary hemostasis necessitates the presence of clotting factors. Defects in secondary hemostasis result from clotting factor deficiencies or dysfunction, such as those seen in hemophilias A and B. Persons with abnormalities in secondary hemostasis tend to have more serious bleeding such as deep muscle hematomas and spontaneous hemarthrosis.

von Willebrand Disease

> **Note to Reader:** Anyone treating individuals with vWD will likely want to pursue additional information. The National Hemophilia Foundation (www.hemophilia.org) is a good place to start. Additional materials that may be beneficial include:
> - Federici AB: *Von Willebrand disease: basic and clinical aspects*, Hoboken, NJ, 2011, Wiley-Blackwell.
> - U.S. Department of Health and Human Services, National Institutes of Health: *The diagnosis, evaluation, and management of von Willebrand Disease*. Full Report. NIH Publication No. 08-5832, 2007.

Definition and Overview

vWD is the most common inherited bleeding disorder. It affects both genders and is caused by a lack (deficiency) or dysfunction of vWF. The prevalence of this illness may be as high as 2% of the population (based on population screening studies) with 500,000 or more Americans with this disorder (many of whom do not know they have it).

vWF is a plasma protein that mediates the initial adhesion of platelets at sites of bleeding injuries; it bind and stabilizes blood clotting factor VIII in the circulation. Defects in vWF can cause bleeding by impairing platelet adhesion or by reducing the concentration of factor VIII. vWF binds collagen fibrils and platelets in areas of vascular injury to create a platelet plug. It also stabilizes factor VIII and prevents it from being inactivated and cleared from the plasma during times of bleeding.[349]

vWD represents a range of genetic diseases with the clinical manifestation of mucocutaneous bleeding, generally milder than hemophilia. vWD is classified into three main subtypes: types 1, 2, and 3. Type 1 is the most common subtype and accounts for 60% to 80% of clients with vWD. Persons with this subtype have 5% to 30% of the normal amount of vWF, leading to mild to moderate symptoms. Type 1 is inherited in an autosomal dominant fashion.[160]

Type 2 is less common and seen in only 10% to 30% of vWD cases. It is caused by a dysfunction in vWF rather than a reduction in quantity of vWF. Because the severity of the abnormality can vary, this subtype is further divided into types 2A, 2B, 2M, and 2N. This subtype is also inherited in an autosomal dominant manner.

The rarest (and most severe) form of vWD subtypes is type 3, which makes up only 1% to 5% of cases. Persons affected with this form have less than 1% of the normal plasma levels of vWF (levels may be undetectable) and very low levels of functional clotting factor VIII. Because these clients are lacking both vWF and factor VIII, their symptoms are more severe and resemble hemophilia A. Inheritance is autosomal recessive.[96]

Pathogenesis

vWF was first identified as an adhesive glycoprotein involved in hemostasis in the early 1970s. vWF plays a vital role in platelet adhesion, platelet binding to collagen, and factor VIII protection. Recent studies have implicated vWF as a regulator of angiogenesis, smooth muscle cell proliferation, tumor cell metastasis, and crosstalk in the immune system.[202]

vWF is produced from a gene located on chromosome 12. Many factors are involved in determining inheritance of the disease, yet often only one mutation on one chromosome leads to minor bleeding problems, whereas abnormalities on both genes (homozygous) have more serious problems, with defects in both platelet plug and fibrin formation.[339]

vWD occurs because of a qualitative lack of vWF or because of an abnormally functioning vWF (although vWF is produced, a mutation causes a malformation in the function of the proteins). Significant investigation has been placed into the discovery of the genetic abnormalities associated with vWD, and more than 250 mutations of multiple types have been documented.[169,302]

Clinical Manifestations

Symptoms experienced by clients with vWD vary depending on the subtype and severity of the abnormality. Clients with type 1 experience bleeding consistent with a primary hemostasis defect. This most frequently involves mucosal and skin bleeding such as petechiae, nose bleeds, blood in the stool, and/or prolonged oozing of blood after minor trauma or surgery.

Other common problems include epistaxis, gum bleeding, and GI bleeding. Symptoms associated with type 2 depend on the severity of the mutation and the quantity of functional vWF. It is estimated that 10% to 20% of women with menorrhagia (excessive menstruation) have vWD. Menorrhagia is a common presenting symptom yet is frequently overlooked and undiagnosed because gynecologists only rarely (less than 1%) perform tests to confirm or exclude a bleeding disorder.[47,70,80] Women also experience significant postpartum hemorrhaging and endometriosis.

Type 3 clients present not only with symptoms of mucosal and skin bleeding but also more frequent and severe symptoms, including hemarthrosis and muscular hematomas (similar to hemophilia A). Women with type 3 vWD are particularly vulnerable to bleeding problems associated with their menstrual cycle, resulting in anemia and fatigue. Pregnancy places these women at risk for early trimester miscarriage or prolonged bleeding during delivery and postpartum.

MEDICAL MANAGEMENT

DIAGNOSIS. Diagnosis relies on the triad of a personal history of excessive mucocutaneous bleeding, laboratory tests consistent with vWF, and a positive family history of the condition. In the laboratory, measurement of vWF antigen and function continue to be the most important diagnostic studies. The most common screening laboratory tests used to assess coagulation are the activated partial thromboplastin time and the prothrombin time.

Despite available tests, many clinicians find making the diagnosis very difficult—particularly for clients with mild disease. Test results are often normal in clients with vWD. vWD cannot be diagnosed with just one laboratory test; the clinician relies on many tests to aid in the diagnosis: a platelet function test, vWF antigen and propeptide test, ristocetin cofactor activity, factor VIII coagulant activity level,[160] and collagen binding.[105] Because of the fluctuation of vWF from stress, exercise, estrogen, inflammation, and bleeding, testing may need to be repeated.

Because of the increased frequency of menorrhagia and other bleeding problems related to obstetrics and gynecology, guidelines have been developed that may lead to improved diagnosis and treatment of women with bleeding disorders, particularly vWD.[3,70]

TREATMENT AND PROGNOSIS

> **Note to Reader:** The National Hemophilia Foundation has a document summarizing recommendations for the pharmacologic treatment of bleeding disorders including vWD (MASAC Recommendations Concerning Products Licensed for the Treatment of Hemophilia and Other Bleeding Disorders).

The treatment of vWD centers on the replacement of vWF and/or factor VIII as needed during times of bleeding or prophylactic administration during pregnancy or prior to an invasive procedure.[213] Long-term prophylaxis is not done as routinely as in hemophilia; who might benefit from prophylaxis and optimal dosing are areas currently under study.[24] Most clients with vWD (especially type 1) do not require treatment except during times of surgery or trauma or after delivery of a baby.

Those persons exhibiting more serious complications, such as hemarthrosis or frequent GI bleeding (type 3 or some type 2), may require scheduled prophylactic treatment. People with types 2 and 3 vWD often require concentrates of factor VIII/vWF for spontaneous bleeding, surgery, or trauma. If synthetic concentrates are not available, other plasma replacements can be used. Fresh-frozen plasma contains both vWF and factor VIII but is accompanied by a large volume, and multiple bags can cause volume overload. Cryoprecipitate contains both proteins in a smaller, concentrated volume yet has the potential of being infectious (although rare with current screening).

Desmopressin is the principal drug of choice for treating most cases of vWD. It is a synthetic antidiuretic-hormone derivative that induces the secretion of vWF and factor VIII from storage. This medication can be given intravenously, subcutaneously, or intranasally. A new-generation of plasma-derived concentrate of vWF (factor VIII) is commercially available in Europe and the United States, but remains under investigation.[188,272] Other available medications, which are used for dental or minor mucosal bleeding, include antifibrinolytic agents. Along mucosal linings of the body there is fibrinolytic activity, which prevents fibrin from forming a clot. Antifibrinolytic amino acids can be given to inhibit this activity. Frequently, they are used as adjuvant medications along with concentrates and desmopressin during major and minor surgery.[213]

Despite advancement in treatment, clients with type 3 vWD still face the challenge of developing inhibitors to available treatment. These inhibitors are typically antibodies that clear vWF from the plasma. Further use of concentrates with vWF can lead to anaphylaxis. Concentrates of factors VIII and VII have been used to aid with clot formation with success (and antibodies do not form to pure factor VIII concentrates), although factor VIII has a short half-life without vWF. Research is ongoing to determine strategies for overcoming these issues.[273]

Women with severe symptoms can suppress menstruation with the use of oral contraceptives or receive concentrates when needed for menorrhagia. Studies are pending that may provide better information concerning best treatment options for women with bleeding disorders.

vWF and factor VIII levels do rise with pregnancy, but pregnant clients often still require ongoing self-infusion with vWF as prophylaxis during pregnancy and the postpartum period. They must be followed very carefully; concentrates and desmopressin are routinely used at birth and during the immediate postpartum period. Care must also be taken when treating the newborn as the baby may have vWD as well. Intramuscular injections, surgery, and circumcision should be avoided in babies with a high risk of a bleeding disorder until an adequate diagnosis is made.[3,70]

Clients with minor bleeding manifestations have problems that can often be avoided with proper care. Individuals with more serious symptoms and complications have significant alterations in quality of life; surgery and trauma can be life threatening. Orthopedic surgery is possible for these individuals but requires a multidisciplinary approach with careful planning and communication among all concerned.[214]

Recombinant activated factor VII is a concentrate that can be used for vWD and for clients with vWD who have developed inhibitors to routine medications and concentrates.[102] The cytokine IL-11 has been noted to increase both factor VIII and vWF levels, and studies are underway to determine efficacy and safety.[72] Recombinant and other biologic therapies are currently undergoing clinical trials and may significantly change the way vWD is managed in the future.[95]

Hemophilia

> **Note to Reader:** Anyone treating individuals with hemophilia will want to pursue more information. The National Hemophilia Foundation (www.hemophilia.org) is a good place to start. Additional materials that may be beneficial include:
> - Rodriguez-Merchan E: *Current and future issues in hemophilia care.* Hoboken, NJ, 2011, Wiley-Blackwell.
> - Lee CA: *Textbook of hemophilia*, ed 2, Hoboken, NJ, 2010, Wiley-Blackwell.

Overview

Hemophilia is a bleeding disorder inherited as a sex-linked autosomal recessive trait. The two primary types of hemophilia are *hemophilia A*, or classic hemophilia, and *hemophilia B*, or Christmas disease. Hemophilia A results from a lack of the clotting factor VIII and constitutes 80% of all cases of hemophilia. Hemophilia B is less common, affecting approximately 15% of all people with hemophilia, and is caused by a deficiency of factor IX. Other, less-common deficiencies, such as deficiencies of clotting factors I, II, V, VII, X, or XIII, are rare and are not fully discussed in this text. Unless otherwise noted, *hemophilia* refers to both hemophilia A and hemophilia B in this text.

Factors VIII and IX are required in secondary hemostasis (in contrast to vWF, which is needed in primary hemostasis). These clotting factors are activated and result in the production of thrombin, which cleaves fibrinogen to fibrin, creating a stable clot.

The level of severity of the disease depends on the defect in the clotting factor gene and is classified according to the percentage of clotting factor present in plasma (determined through blood tests): mild (6%-30%), moderate (1%-5%), and severe (less than 1%). Normal concentrations of coagulation factors are between 50% and 150%.

For people with *mild* hemophilia (25% of all cases), spontaneous hemorrhages (bleeding that occurs with no apparent cause) are rare, and joint and deep muscle bleeding are uncommon. Surgical, dental, or other injury or trauma precipitates symptoms that must be treated the same as for severe hemophilia.

For those people with *moderate* hemophilia (15% of all people with hemophilia), spontaneous hemorrhage is not usually a problem, but major bleeding episodes can occur after minor trauma. There is a considerable subset of individuals with moderate hemophilia with more severe bleeding patterns who will need prophylactic treatment.[71]

People with *severe* hemophilia make up 60% of people with hemophilia and may bleed spontaneously or with only slight trauma, particularly into the joints and deep muscle.

Incidence

Hemophilia affects 1 in 5000 male births. About 400 babies are born with hemophilia each year. Hemophilia primarily affects males without bias for race or socioeconomic group. The exact number of people living with hemophilia in the United States is not known. A Centers for Disease Control and Prevention study conducted in six states in 1994 estimated that about 17,000 people had hemophilia at that time. Currently, the number of people with hemophilia in the United States is estimated to be about 20,000, based on expected births and deaths since 1994.[46,321]

Etiologic Factors

The gene responsible for codes for factors VIII and IX are located on the X chromosome, making hemophilia a gender-linked recessive disorder. Because females normally carry two X chromosomes, they only develop hemophilia if both genes are affected, if the normal X gene is inactivated, or if they only have one X chromosome (i.e., Turner syndrome), making hemophilia rare in females.

Males, on the other hand, only inherit one X chromosome and therefore develop hemophilia because they lack another normal X chromosome to provide these clotting factors (such as most females do). Thus females are the carriers of the abnormality, whereas males present with the disease (Fig. 14-11).

Every carrier has a one in four chance of having a child with hemophilia. Men with the mutation will pass this on to their daughters (making them carriers), yet their sons will only inherit a normal Y chromosome and not develop hemophilia. Although in two-thirds of the cases of hemophilia a known family history is evident, this disorder can occur in families (approximately one-third) without a previous history of blood-clotting disorders because of spontaneous genetic mutation. The remaining rare clotting factor deficiencies are inherited in an autosomal recessive manner.

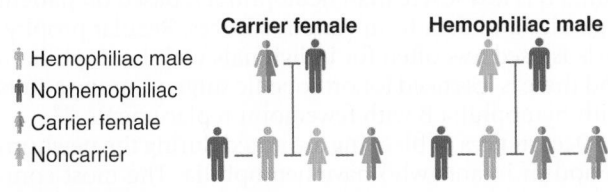

Figure 14-11

Inheritance patterns in hemophilia for all family members. A woman is definitely a carrier if she is (1) the biologic daughter of a man with hemophilia; (2) the biologic mother of more than one son with hemophilia; or (3) the biologic mother of one hemophilic son with at least one other blood relative with hemophilia. A woman may or may not be a carrier if she is (1) the biologic mother of one son with hemophilia; (2) the sister of a male with hemophilia; (3) an aunt, cousin, or niece of an affected male related through maternal ties; or (4) the biologic grandmother of one grandson with hemophilia. (Reprinted from Beare PG, Myers JL: *Adult health nursing*, ed 3, St Louis, 1998, Mosby.)

Pathogenesis

At least 10 proteins called *clotting factors* in the blood must work in a precise order to make a blood clot. Hemophilia A is caused by a deficiency of the protein clotting factor VIII (antihemophilic factor), whereas hemophilia B is caused by a lack of factor IX. These clotting factors are produced by the liver and released into the blood. Factor VIII, once in the plasma, combines with vWF (as previously discussed). Factors VIII and IX are necessary for the formation of thrombin, which converts fibrinogen into fibrin, generating a clot. Clients with these factor deficiencies are unable to produce thrombin and clot.

The genetic pattern of hemophilia is quite different from that of disorders such as sickle cell disease, in which every affected individual has the identical genetic defect. The presence of such variable defects in the same gene accounts for the differences in severity of hemophilia.

Many different genetic lesions cause factor VIII deficiency, such as gene deletions, with all or part of the gene missing, or missense and nonsense mutations, which cause the clotting factor to be made incorrectly or not at all. Not all mutations are inherited; 25% to 30% of cases are caused by new mutations. Hundreds of different mutations have been discovered. Most of these mutations are nucleotide substitutions (missense) or small deletions; however, one common mutation noted in more than 40% of people with severe hemophilia A is a partial inversion. An Internet database is available that documents the mutations in the factor VIII gene.[221]

Although uncommon, a woman who is a carrier of hemophilia can have very low levels of factors VIII or IX. This is because in every cell of the body either the normal X chromosome or the affected X chromosome is randomly inactivated (turned off) in a process called *lyonization*. If the majority of the inactivated chromosomes are the normal X, then the levels of clotting factors may be very low, and such carriers may experience excessive bleeding.

Clinical Manifestations

Clinically, hemophilia A and hemophilia B present with the same symptoms and can only be distinguished by specific factor assay tests. Unlike most clients with vWD, those with hemophilia manifest delayed and joint and deep muscle bleeding. There is some evidence that hemophilia B is less severe than hemophilia A based on patient registries and data from various sources. Regular prophylaxis is used less often for individuals with hemophilia B and there is less need for orthopedic surgery among adults with hemophilia B with fewer joint replacements.[212]

Occurrences of bleeding are noted during the newborn period in infants who have hemophilia. The most common instances include immunizations, heel sticks, blood draws, and circumcision. If a child is born to a known carrier, circumcision should not be performed until appropriate tests are completed. As the child grows, bleeding problems will continue to be manifested.

Hematoma formation may result from injections or after firm holding (such as occurs when a child is held under the arms or by the elbow and lifted), excessive bruising from minor trauma, delayed hemorrhage (hours to days after injury) after a minor injury, persistent bleeding after tooth loss, and recurrent bleeding into muscles and joints.

Bruising, bleeding from the mouth or frenulum, intracranial bleeding, hematomas of the head, and hemarthrosis (bleeding into the joints) can occur during early ambulation. By age 3 to 4 years, 90% of children with severe hemophilia have had an episode of persistent bleeding not seen in mild cases.

Clients with severe hemophilia often display episodes of spontaneous bleeding (into the joints, muscles, and internal organs) along with severe bleeding with trauma or surgery. Those persons affected with mild to moderate hemophilia do not commonly have spontaneous bleeding but exhibit excessive bleeding with trauma and surgery.

Women with Hemophilia. Women with hemophilia experience excessive uterine bleeding during their menstrual cycle, with possible oozing from the ovary after ovulation mid-cycle. Heavy menstrual flow is often the symptom that initiates a coagulation evaluation or more often is reported but not adequately diagnosed.

Cases have occurred in which a female carrier of the hemophilia gene has abnormal bleeding when the level of clotting factor is low enough to cause significant problems with coagulation, especially after trauma or surgery. Abnormal bleeding from bruising, dental extractions, abortion or miscarriage, complications of pregnancy (e.g., placenta not delivered completely, episiotomy or tearing, prolonged postpartum hemorrhage), nosebleeds, and minor trauma (such as cuts with prolonged oozing) may be overlooked because of the misconception that hemophilia does not occur in women.

Joint. Bleeding into the joint spaces (hemarthrosis) is one of the most common clinical manifestations of hemophilia (occurring during the first year after birth), significantly affecting synovial joints. The knee is the most frequently affected joint, followed by the ankle, elbow, hip, shoulder, and wrist. Bleeding in the synovial joints of the feet, hands, temporomandibular joint, and spine is less common.

Joints with at least four bleeds in 6 months are called target joints, and in children with severe hemophilia, this can occur as a toddler. When blood is introduced into the joint, the joint becomes distended, causing swelling, pain, warmth, and stiffness. The synovial membrane responds by producing an increased number of synovial villi and undergoing vascular hyperplasia in an attempt to reabsorb the blood. Blood is an irritant to the synovium, which releases enzymes that break down RBCs and the cell byproducts (e.g., iron). This process causes the synovium to become hypertrophied, with formation of fingerlike projections of tissue extending onto the articular surface.

The mechanical trauma of normal weight-bearing motion may then impinge and further injure the inflamed synovium. Iron in the form of hemosiderin is deposited in the synovium, which impairs the production of synovial fluid. A vicious cycle is established as the synovium attempts to cleanse the joint of blood and debris, becoming more hypertrophic and susceptible to still further bleeding.[15] Erosive damage of the cartilage follows these changes in the synovium with narrowing of the joint space (Fig. 14-12), erosions at the joint margins,

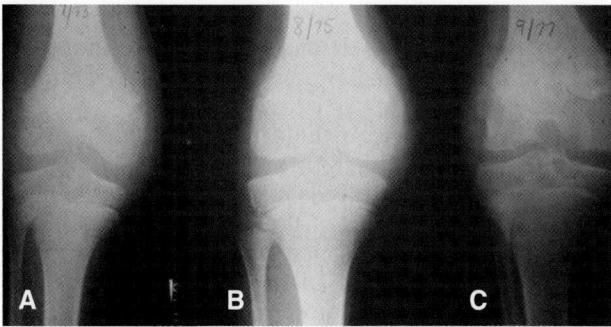

Figure 14-12

Stages of hemophilic arthropathy according to the Arnold-Hilgartner scale. A, Stage I (1973). **B,** Stage III (1975). **C,** Stage IV (1977). (Courtesy Mountain States Regional Hemophilia Center, Colorado State Treatment Program, Denver, 1995.)

Box 14-7

ARNOLD-HILGARTNER HEMOPHILIC ARTHROPATHY STAGES

Staging scheme to classify joint changes seen on x-ray:

0   Normal joint

I   No skeletal abnormalities; soft-tissue swelling

II   Osteoporosis and overgrowth of epiphysis; no erosions; no narrowing of cartilage space

III   Early subchondral bone cysts, squaring of the patella; intercondylar notch of distal femur and humerus widened; cartilage space remains preserved

IV   Finding of stage III more advanced; cartilage space narrowed significantly; cartilage destruction

V   End stage; fibrous joint contracture, loss of joint cartilage space, marked enlargement of the epiphyses, and substantial disorganization of the joints

Data from Arnold WD, Hilgartner MW: Hemophilic arthropathy, *J Bone Joint Surg Am* 59:287–305, 1977.

Table 14-5   Pettersson Radiologic Classification of Hemophilic Arthropathy

Type of Change	Finding	Score*
Osteoporosis	Absent	0
	Present	1
Enlarged epiphysis	Absent	0
	Present	1
Irregular subchondral surface	Absent	0
	Slight	1
	Pronounced	2
Narrowing of joint space	Absent	0
	<50%	1
	>50%	2
Subchondral cyst formation	Absent	0
	1 Cyst	1
	>1 Cyst	2
Erosions at joint margins	Absent	0
	Present	1
Incongruence between joint surfaces	Absent	0
	Slight	1
	Pronounced	2
Joint deformity (angulation and/or displacement between articulating bones)	Absent	0
	Slight	1
	Pronounced	2

A joint scoring system based on radiographic findings used to classify and monitor joint changes and damage.

*Note: Possible total joint score is 0 to 13 points.

From Anderson A, Holtzman TS, Masley J: *Physical therapy in bleeding disorders,* New York, 2000, National Hemophilia Foundation.

---

and subchondral cyst formation. Collapse of the joint, joint sclerosis, and eventual spontaneous ankylosis may occur.

In later stages of joint degeneration, chronic pain, severe loss of motion, muscle atrophy, crepitus, and joint deformities occur. Despite advances in medical management, target joints can progress to advanced arthropathy. This is most commonly seen in people with severe hemophilia. The articular cartilage softens, turns brown (from hemosiderin), and becomes pitted and fragmented. The inflamed synovium is thick and highly vascularized and can grow over the joint surfaces, becoming pannus.

Eventually, lesions in the deeper layers of cartilage result in subchondral bone breakdown and the formation of subchondral cysts. Osteophyte formation occurs along the edges of the joint (Box 14-7 and Table 14-5). With the destruction of the cartilage, little to no joint space is left.

This bone-on-bone contact can lead to significant pain, limitation of motion, joint malalignment, muscle atrophy, functional impairment, and disability.

At this point joint bleeds are rare. For the child, recurrent bleeds into the same joint can lead to growth abnormalities. The epiphyses, where bone growth takes place, are stimulated to grow in the presence of hyperemia caused by bleeding. Postural asymmetries may develop (e.g., leg length differences, angulatory deformities, bony enlargement at the affected joint).[15]

Classification of Hemophilic Arthropathy. Several different classification scales are used to identify progression of hemophilic arthropathy. The Arnold-Hilgartner and Pettersson score classification scales have been in use for many years. With the Arnold-Hilgartner scale, the arthropathy is divided into stages that are assumed to be progressive. With the Pettersson score, a number of specific findings are evaluated and the additive sum of the assigned points is calculated.

In addition, there is now some MRI information being used for classification as well. With improvements in hemophilia care, evaluation of subtle joint changes not readily apparent with conventional radiography has become increasingly important. MRI can visualize effusion, hemarthrosis, synovial hypertrophy and/or hemosiderin deposition, subchondral cysts and/or surface erosions, and loss of cartilage (Fig. 14-13).

Different MRI methods for joint scoring use either a progressive or additive scoring strategy. Using proposed

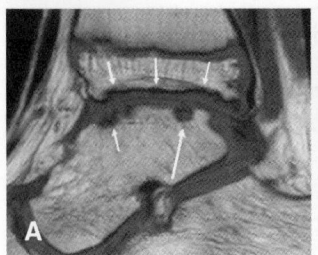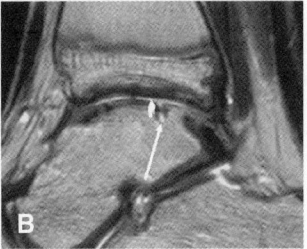

Figure 14-13

MRI of hemophilic arthropathy. **A,** Left ankle of a 9-year-old boy with moderate hemophilia. Sagittal spin echo (SE) T1-weighted sequence. **B,** Sagittal turbo spin echo (TSE) T2-weighted sequence. Cortical irregularity (best seen on T1-weighted image, *small arrows*) is the hallmark of surface erosions. Different types of subchondral cysts have different signal characteristics. In this joint a cyst is discerned in the dorsal part of the talar dome (intermediate signal on T1-weighted image and bright signal on T2-weighted image, *large arrows*), and a focal defect in the overlying cartilage is revealed (joint fluid in defect is bright on T2-weighted image). (Courtesy Bjorn Lundin, MD, University Hospital of Lund, Sweden.)

MRI scoring methods, imaging specialists can detect and monitor early joint changes, assess therapeutic outcomes, and further define the pathophysiology of hemophilic joint disease. An in-depth discussion of these techniques is available for readers interested in the specifics.[201]

Physical therapists in the United States, Canada, Sweden, and The Netherlands are working collaboratively on an international joint evaluation scale to identify and quantify the early changes seen in hemophilia joint disease. The 11-item scoring tool for assessing joint impairment in boys with hemophilia from 4 to 18 years of age (Hemophilia Joint Health Score) was designed for use in a 10-year prospective study of two types of aggressive treatment in young children with severe hemophilia. Reliability testing of the scoring tool has been published[138]; validity testing is underway.

Muscle. Muscle hemorrhages can be more insidious and massive than joint bleeding, and although they can occur anywhere, muscle hemorrhages most often involve the flexor muscle groups (e.g., iliopsoas, gastrocnemius, forearm flexors). Intramuscular hemorrhage that is visible in superficial areas such as the calf or forearm will also result in pain and limitation of motion of the affected part. Less-obvious intramuscular hemorrhage such as occurs in the iliopsoas may result in groin pain, pain on extension of the hip, and reflexive flexion of the hip and thigh (see Figs. 16-14 and 16-15).

Other signs and symptoms may include warmth, swelling, palpable hematoma, and neurologic signs such as numbness and tingling. A large iliopsoas hemorrhage can cause displacement of the kidney and ureter and can compress the neurovascular bundle, including the femoral nerve with subsequent weakness; decreased sensation over the thigh and knee in the L2, L3, and L4 distribution; decreased or absent knee reflexes; temperature changes; and even permanent impairment. Iliopsoas bleeds are considered a medical emergency requiring immediate referral to a physician.

Nervous System. In general, compression of peripheral nerves and blood vessels by hematoma may result in severe pain, anesthesia of the innervated part, loss of perfusion, permanent nerve damage, and even paralysis. The femoral, ulnar, and median nerves are most commonly affected.

CNS hemorrhage may include intracranial hemorrhage and, rarely, intraspinal hemorrhage. Intracranial hemorrhages (ICHs), or head bleeds inside the skull, in a newborn can occur regardless of the severity of hemophilia and may have long-term consequences such as paralysis, seizures, cerebral palsy, and other neurologic deficits.

Although signs and symptoms of ICH may be dramatic (e.g., seizures, paralysis, apnea, unequal pupils, excessive vomiting, or tense and bulging fontanelles), they are often vague (e.g., crankiness or lethargy, feeding difficulty), leading to a delay in diagnosis. The lifetime risk of ICH is approximately 2% to 8%, although many are asymptomatic and unreported.[181] ICH in clients with hemophilia carries a mortality rate of up to 30% when it occurs, making it one of the most common causes of death after HIV.

Inhibitors. With the production of safer factor concentrates, the development of antibody inhibitors (antibodies that destroy the infused factor) poses the most serious complication to hemophilia treatment. Inhibitors occur infrequently, approximately two cases per 1000 person years, but can be serious, causing complications in 20% to 33% of persons who develop an inhibitor.[90,172] Individuals affected most often are children who have severe hemophilia A; the phenomenon occurs during the first 50 days of exposure to factor concentrate.[249]

The risk of developing an inhibitor does not remain the same during the lifetime of a person with hemophilia, and the appearance of antibodies can be transient or low titers. Factors that increase the risk for developing inhibitors are still under investigation, including significant exposure to factor VIII concentrates (continuous infusion)[313] or the type of factor VIII product used. Clients with high titers of inhibitors, which decrease therapy efficacy, may receive factor IX concentrates or undergo immune tolerance therapy (frequent infusions of factor VIII).

Transmissible Diseases. Individuals, primarily those with severe hemophilia, who were treated before current purification techniques for factor concentrates (before 1986) may have been exposed to hepatitis B or C and/or HIV. Approximately 50% of people with hemophilia during this period became infected with HIV. No other at-risk group had such a high prevalence. Currently, approximately 10% to 15% of people with hemophilia have HIV, but since 1986 no further HIV transmission has occurred.

Transmission of hepatitis is equally serious, and approximately 70% to 90% of people with hemophilia who received clotting factor before the mid-1980s test positive for hepatitis C.[230] Current improved methods of viral inactivation of factor concentrates through pasteurization and solvent treatment and monoclonal and recombinant technology have resulted in safer products.

Improved screening methods to identify donors with hepatitis have also reduced the risk of hepatitis transmission. As of 1997, there have been no reports of hepatitis A, B, or C transmission through clotting factor treated with these improved processes.[147] Up to one-third of individuals with a bleeding disorder and hepatitis C were coinfected with HIV, and everyone who was infected with HIV also contracted hepatitis C.[243]

The transmission of hepatitis A and parvovirus B19 has also been reduced in plasma-derived products, but hepatitis A can now be prevented by immunization with a vaccine. All newborns with hemophilia now receive the hepatitis B vaccination series, but older clients often have hepatitis B along with its long-term sequelae.

MEDICAL MANAGEMENT

DIAGNOSIS. Effective treatment of hemophilia is based on an accurate diagnosis of the deficient clotting factor and its level in the blood. Diagnosis is not always straightforward, as a variety of factors can confound the test results (e.g., blood type; factor levels can be elevated by stress, hyperthyroidism, and pregnancy, yet decreased in hypothyroidism).

Additionally, cord blood sample at birth may have physiologically low levels of factor IX that only reach adult values by 3 to 6 months of age. Blood tests include assays for clotting factors, CBC (differential and platelets), and activated partial thromboplastin time. Other tests may be added depending on individual variables. It is also important for female relatives of those with hemophilia to identify their carrier status through factor level analysis and DNA testing.

If possible, genetic studies to determine carrier status should be completed before pregnancy. However, prenatal diagnosis of hemophilia A and B is possible if a specific mutation has been found or if linkage studies have provided enough information about carrier status in the family. If one of these two criteria has been met, prenatal diagnosis can be performed, analyzing DNA for specific mutations.

The most common method is through chorionic villus sampling at 10 to 12 weeks, gestation. Ultrasound at 14 to 16 weeks' gestation to determine the gender of the unborn child, amniocentesis at approximately 16 weeks' gestation, percutaneous umbilical blood sampling at 18 weeks' gestation, and preimplantation genetic diagnosis (involving polar body, blastomere, and blastocyst biopsy) are other methods of diagnosis. The advantages and disadvantages of these tests as well as management issues are reviewed in the literature.[185]

Once the diagnosis has been made, distinguishing pain, warmth, and swelling caused by joint bleeding versus arthritis or synovitis is important. Hemarthrosis triggers hemophilic arthropathy because bleeding starts synovitis immediately, damages cartilage, and leads to loss of function and disability. To prevent this sequelae, but also to avoid over- or undertreating with clotting factor (based on patient/client perception), rapid, high-resolution joint ultrasound is recommended. Objective imaging should be done within 24 hours of reported onset of joint pain to avoid treatment on the basis of patient/client perception.[74,222]

TREATMENT

Currently no known cure or prenatal treatment for hemophilia exists. Until a medical cure is developed, primary goals for intervention in the case of bleeding

Note to Reader: The National Hemophilia Foundation has written a document summarizing recommendations for the pharmacologic treatment of bleeding disorders, including vWD, available online at http://www.hemophilia.org/NHFWeb/Resource/StaticPages/menu0/menu5/menu57/masac190.pdf.[244]

episodes are to stop any bleeding that is occurring as quickly as possible and to infuse the missing factors until the bleeding stops.

Treatment for severe forms of hemophilia is recommended to take place in specialized hemophilia treatment centers across the United States and its territories. In these centers the specialized care required can be provided through a multidisciplinary team approach with appropriately trained and experienced health care providers. Treatment at a hemophilia treatment center has been shown to minimize disability, morbidity, and mortality rates.[47,322]

Factor replacement therapy, given intravenously, is currently the mainstay of hemophilia treatment. Treatment with infusion of the missing factor at a 25% to 30% plasma factor level is recommended for minor bleeding; at least a 50% level is recommended before minor surgery and dental extractions or in case of minor injury, and it may be recommended before physical or occupational therapy interventions. Infusion at 75% to 100% may be recommended before major surgery or in the case of life-threatening bleeding.

Permanent prophylaxis of recombinant factors for severe hemophilia (i.e., factor infusion given on a regularly scheduled basis) to maintain blood factor levels in the moderate range is now widely accepted. Most clients should receive infusions on at least a weekly basis, although questions remain of when to initiate prophylaxis (first joint bleed vs. early age).[1] Prophylaxis therapy is very expensive, but treatment of target joints can increase the cost as much as twofold.[173] Uncertainty exists as to whether prophylaxis helps prevent joint disease, and studies are pending completion that would help answer these questions. Difficulties associated with prophylactic treatment include frequent venipuncture or the need to use central venous lines, which can lead to thrombosis and infection. Efforts are being made to develop a long-lasting recombinant factor protein that would require less frequent injections.

Most factor VIII concentrates are produced using recombinant techniques to provide virus-free products. Current third-generation products do not contain animal or human plasma proteins in either the cell culture medium or the final product. Methods used prior to the availability of recombinant technology to manufacture factor VIII concentrates utilized plasma pooled from thousands of donors that was then purified for factor VIII. This purified concentrate was treated to deplete viruses (heating in an aqueous solution, treated by a solvent detergent, or immunoaffinity purification). Although this type of product is still available and there have been no reports of clients being infected with hepatitis B or C or HIV, the risk remains that these pooled-plasma products could possibly lead to viral transmission. This possible increased risk of transmitting a virus makes recombinant concentrates the recommended treatment of choice.

Persons with mild hemophilia can use the drug desmopressin when possible (see information about desmopressin in above section "vWD: Treatment and Prognosis"). If this medication does not provide adequate hemostasis or the client is pregnant or younger than 2 years, factor VIII concentrates should be utilized.

Hemophilia B. Treatment for clients with hemophilia B consists of factor IX concentrates. Recombinant factor IX concentrates do not use animal or human plasma proteins in the purification process, making the product safe from viruses. Pooled plasma–derived factor IX products are available, and like the factor VIII concentrates from pooled plasma, undergo a viral-depletion step. However, because of the safety factor of recombinant technology, recombinant factor IX concentrate is the medication of choice. Although treatment for hepatitis B is available, liver transplantation may be required. Liver transplantation is successful in people who have hemophilia with advanced liver disease but is often unavailable.

Hemophilia and Hepatitis. For those clients who developed chronic hepatitis C from the use of blood products prior to the mid-1980s, progression and treatment response appear to be similar to those people without hemophilia.[193,230] Treatment and prognosis for hepatitis are discussed in Chapter 17. Administration of the hepatitis A and hepatitis B vaccines is recommended for anyone with chronic hepatitis C because of the potential for increased severity of acute hepatitis superimposed on existing liver disease. Younger children are now vaccinated against hepatitides A and B, but no vaccine is available for hepatitis C at this time.

Pain Control. Comprehensive medical management of hemophilia may involve the use of drugs to control pain in acute bleeding and chronic arthropathies. People with hemophilia cannot use the common pain relievers aspirin or ibuprofen because these agents inhibit platelet function. More precisely, platelets do form an initial clot, but factor VIII or IX is unavailable to stabilize the clot. Some medications contain derivatives of aspirin and must be used cautiously. Corticosteroids are used occasionally for the treatment of chronic synovitis. Acetaminophen (Tylenol) is a suitable aspirin substitute for pain control, especially in children. Most centers use opioid medications to treat chronic pain for select individuals. Currently, there are no clinical practice guidelines on pain management in people with hemophilia who experience acute, disabling pain from hemarthroses and chronic arthropathy.[118,148]

Gene Therapy. Gene therapy is still in experimental stages but appears very promising. When successful, gene therapy will deliver a normal (unaffected) copy of a gene into a target cell that contains a defective gene. Human trials are underway for hemophilias A and B using a variety of different delivery techniques. In fact, hemophilia is considered a model disease for treatment with gene therapy because it is caused by a single malfunctioning gene, and only a small increase in clotting factor could provide a great benefit.[211]

PROGNOSIS. Years ago most males with hemophilia died in their youth. For the past 50 years, the care for individuals with hemophilia has improved significantly to the point that a newborn with hemophilia living in a developed nation can expect to have a normal life span and a high quality of life. Currently, the majority of deaths in persons with hemophilia are viral related (hepatitides B and C, HIV).[372]

Tremendous improvement has been made in carrier detection and prenatal diagnosis to provide early treatment and prevent complications. Gene therapy for hemophilias A and B holds promise of a cure, but whether gene therapy will be sufficiently safe and cost-effective to eventually replace factor-replacement therapy remains to be seen.[137,288,361] Additionally, home infusion therapy provides immediate treatment with clotting factor for joint and muscle bleeds recognized early. Early treatment has significantly reduced the morbidity formerly associated with hemophilia.

Medical treatment prolongs life and improves quality of life associated with improved joint function, but HIV and hepatitis can significantly reduce longevity and quality of life. Fortunately, improvements in blood screening tests, more stringent donor exclusion criteria, improved viral inactivation methods, and the introduction of recombinant hemophilia therapies have combined to dramatically reduce the rate of new bloodborne viral infections among people with hemophilia, especially those children born in the last decade.

During the period 1979–1998, the death rate of persons with hemophilia A and HIV decreased 78%.[55] Much of this decrease was related to improved HIV therapy. With the advent of safer factor concentrates, there is a trend of increased life expectancy for people with hemophilia. Those people with hemophilia but without HIV or hepatitis have a life expectancy near normal.

ICH still remains a deadly complication of hemophilia, but prophylaxis treatment and improved understanding of the signs and symptoms associated with ICH may help to improve outcomes. Long-term effects of prophylaxis may present additional challenges in terms of safety, efficacy, and pharmacokinetics and remain the focus of research efforts. And with the normalization of lives as a result of improved treatment, new comorbidities are developing, including obesity, diabetes, cancer, and osteoporosis.[372] Changes in medical and psychosocial challenges facing today's individuals with hemophilia are referred to as transitional issues. The need for a well-developed transition plan from birth to adulthood for individuals with hemophilia will force the way care is delivered from total dependence on caregivers to complete independence by the time the individual reaches 18 years of age.[371]

SPECIAL IMPLICATIONS FOR THE THERAPIST 14-13

Hemophilia

Note to Reader: Only a brief discussion of treatment for the adult or child with hemophilia can be included in this text. For a more detailed examination, evaluation, and interventions, the reader is referred to other more specific publications by the National Hemophilia Foundation endorsed by the Medical and Scientific Advisory Committee (MASAC).[15,38,136,219,220,232,242,245–248]

Physical therapy intervention has been effective in reducing the number of bleeding episodes through protective strengthening of the musculature surrounding affected joints, muscle reeducation, gait training, and client education. Physical therapy is used during episodes of acute hemorrhage to control pain and additional bleeding and to maintain positioning and prevent further deformity.

Physical therapy intervention for individuals with hemophilia has undergone a drastic change. Two decades ago, everyone in the hemophilia community had joint disease in varying degrees of severity. Today treatment protocols are more aggressive, with more frequent infusions given at younger ages, resulting in less joint damage.[56] Many children with hemophilia are growing up without having a single joint bleed. The focus has shifted from rehabilitation to prevention; therapists are an important health care professional in helping these individuals lead normal, active lives.[56]

Hemophilia, Physical Activity, and Exercise

A regular exercise program, including appropriate sports activities, resistance training, cardiovascular/aerobic training, and therapeutic strengthening and stretching exercises for affected extremities, is an important part of the comprehensive care of the individual with hemophilia.[324] In fact, regular physical activity and exercise can be considered a nonpharmacologic treatment used in conjunction with conventional treatment.[324]

The therapist can help individuals with hemophilia identify, seek out, and enjoy physical activity, exercise, and sport participation that provide benefits that outweigh the risks.[136] Patient/client education is key here because many people with bleeding disorders participate minimally in exercise[250] and have even expressed fear of exercise-induced bleeding, pain, or physical impairment.[232] But as Mulvany et al demonstrated, with an individualized and supervised exercise program, benefits gained are measurable and significant, especially for those individuals with the most severe joint damage and coexisting illness.[232] The therapist can present the individual with evidence that refraining from exercise results in decreased strength, range-of-motion, function, and quality of life (see Mulvany et al[232] for details).

Specific protocols for prescriptive exercise based on evidence are not yet available leaving the physical therapist to design a program for each individual relying on an understanding of tissue healing, best practice, expert opinions, and clinical judgment. Physical therapists may find a review of reference-based global recommendations and suggestions from clinicians with specialized training in the management of hemophilia valuable as provided by the Adult Bleeding Disorders Clinic in Canada.[27]

Vigorous physical activity may be transiently associated with a moderate relative risk of bleeding but the absolute risk of bleeds is small.[33] Physical activity and exercise not only promote physical wellness in the form of improved work capacity, it protects joints, enhances joint function, and is beneficial for decreasing the frequency of bleeds and has been shown to temporarily increase the levels of circulating clotting factor in individuals with a factor VIII deficiency.[251] Immobilization of joints can lead to deterioration of muscles, which, in turn, leads to joint instability and repeated bleeding and premature development of arthropathy.[229,333]

Growing evidence suggests that exercise, coupled with a healthy diet, may boost the immune system of people with hemophilia who also have HIV and/or are living with hepatitis C.[363] The therapist can be instrumental in helping the person with hemophilia to individualize an exercise or sports activity plan with specific but realistic goals and a schedule with alternating exercises (cross-training).

Although many factors related to joint bleeding are fixed, one risk factor that can be modified by the therapist is the body mass index. Clients with more severe disease develop joint problems earlier with accompanying range-of-motion problems. An increased body mass index also increases the risk of limited joint range-of-motion and may be a modifiable risk factor in clients with hemophilia.[323]

An overall therapy program includes client education early on for family, client, school personnel, and coaches for prevention, conditioning, and wellness. Specific guidelines are available including all age levels from infants, toddlers, and preschoolers to adults, including sports safety information and the categorization of sports and activities by risk.[15,242]

For older children and adolescents, selecting a sport with a good chance of success and adequate preparation (e.g., stretching and flexibility, conditioning including strength and weight training, endurance including an aerobic component, and possibly infusion before participation) for the sport are crucial. There is some early evidence that high-intensity exercise can increase endogenous factor VIII in individuals with mild to moderately severe hemophilia A. Further evidence is needed before promoting high-intensity activity to reduce bleeding risk prior to participation in sports.[125]

The National Hemophilia Foundation has mapped out categories of activity that are safe to participate in for anyone with hemophilia along with precautions for some forms of exercise and contraindications to others (Table 14-6).

Category 1 involves primarily aerobic activities that are considered "safe" for most individuals with hemophilia. Category 1 activities build muscles to protect joints and help decrease the frequency of bleeds. Gaining flexibility and core strength through category 1 activities is a prerequisite for anyone with hemophilia before participating in category 2 activities.

Category 2 activities include sports and recreational activities in which the physical, social, and psychologic benefits of participation outweigh the risks. Individuals with severe hemophilia may have to avoid category 2 activities. Category 3 activities should be avoided by anyone with hemophilia; they are dangerous even for

Table 14-6	Categories of Activities Based on Risk	
Category 1 (Safest)	**Category 2 (Moderately safe)**	**Category 3 (Potentially dangerous)**
Archery	Baseball	All-terrain vehicle
Badminton	Basketball	Boxing
Bicycling	Bowling	High diving (competitive)
Dancing	Cross-country skiing	Football
Fishing	Diving (recreational)	Hockey
Frisbee	Dog sledding	Lacrosse
Golfing	Gymnastics	Motorcycling
Hiking	Horseback riding	Racquetball/ handball
Ping pong	Ice skating	Rock climbing/ rappelling
Snowshoeing	Jogging	Rugby
Swimming	Martial arts	Wrestling
Tai Chi/yoga/ qi gong	Mountain biking	Power lifting; competitive weight lifting
Walking	River rafting	
Low-impact workout machines	Roller skating/blading	
	Rowing/crew	
	Running	
	Skiing (downhill or cross-country)	
	Snowboarding	
	Snowmobiling	
	Soccer	
	Tennis	
	Track and field	
	Volleyball	
	Water skiing	
	Weight lifting	

This is not an exhaustive list of possible activities but provides a guideline to use when assessing activities for safety.
Data from Playing It Safe: *Bleeding Disorders, Sports, and Exercise*. National Hemophilia Foundation, 2012. Available online at http://www.hemophilia.org/sites/default/files/document/files/PlayingItSafe.pdf. Accessed July 9, 2014.

people without hemophilia. The risks outweigh the benefits.

Although it is obvious that some bleeding may result from participation in a sport, fewer bleeding episodes occur when children engage in physical activities on a regular basis than when they are sedentary. When a particular sport or activity is often followed by bleeding, then that activity should be reevaluated. A joint that requires multiple infusions to stop bleeding, remains symptomatic, or has persistent synovitis is not likely to withstand the stresses of a sport that relies on that joint.[242] Breakthrough bleeding despite prophylaxis occurs more often than previously recognized and should be part of a daily surveillance program.

As orthopedic problems occur, a problem-oriented program is developed specific to the pathology. Generally, a therapy program includes exercises to strengthen muscles and improve coordination; methods to prevent and reduce deformity; methods to influence abnormal muscle tone and pathologic patterns of movement; techniques to decrease pain; functional training related to everyday activities; special techniques such as manual traction and mobilization; massage; and physiotechnical modalities such as cold, heat (including ultrasound), and

electric modalities. Orthotics may improve participation in activities and have been shown to reduce joint pain.[199,285]

Aquatic therapy is an excellent modality, especially for chronic arthropathy to improve physical functioning and quality of life.[167,359] The buoyancy of the water allows for ease of active movements across joints without the compressive force induced by gravity, thus decreasing pain. Water's density creates a resistive force to allow muscle strengthening, and the hydrostatic pressure can help reduce swelling.[15,167]

Guidelines to Strength Training

In the past people with bleeding disorders were told to avoid strenuous exercise and any kind of weight training to avoid the risk of bleeding episodes. Today we know that a well-planned, supervised exercise program (Box 14-8) can be extremely beneficial to all individuals with a bleeding disorder.[232] Weight training is still approached with caution as overly strenuous free-weight lifting can still cause micro-tears in the muscles and intramuscular bleeds.[8,218]

Strength training, also known as resistance training, builds muscle, increases strength, stabilizes joints, improves circulation, and potentially reduces the risk of injury and spontaneous bleeding episodes. It is not body building, power lifting, or competitive weightlifting; these activities should be avoided.

The importance of warm-up and cool-down periods should be emphasized. Little or no weight is used until the individual can complete 10 to 15 repetitions with proper form. Weight or resistance can be gradually increased by 5% to 10% when the first phase of 10 to 15 repetitions is easy. The client should be reminded never to attempt to lift maximal weight.[8,11]

As with all strength training, it is best to utilize full pain-free range of motion slowly and with good breathing throughout the cycle of contraction and relaxation. Maintain adequate hydration at all times. Adolescents must especially be reminded that pain is a red flag to stop and seek help. Most injuries result from improper form and performing the exercise too fast. Any time an individual of any age with hemophilia experiences joint trauma or injury, strength training may have to be discontinued and gradually reintroduced after healing occurs.[8]

Maintaining Joint Range of Motion

The therapist and client must be alert to recognize any signs of early (first 24-48 hours) bleeding episodes (Table 14-7). Providing immediate factor replacement to stop the bleeding and following the RICE (rest, ice, compression, and elevation) principle (Table 14-8) to promote comfort and healing are two goals for treating an acute joint (hemarthrosis) or muscle bleed (intramuscular hemorrhage).

The joint range of motion can be measured during this acute episode in the pain-free range but should not be strength tested. Elastic wraps, splints, slings,

Box 14-8

SUPERVISED EXERCISE PROGRAM FOR PEOPLE WITH BLEEDING DISORDERS AND HEMOPHILIC ARTHRITIS

Strength Training Protocol and Progression

1. Progression to next level only if no adverse reaction to previous week of exercise.
2. Prophylaxis: Factor infusion recommended for people with severe hemophilia; people with mild and moderate hemophilia to have medications available, if needed.
3. Intensity: percent of isometric Nicholas dynamometry muscle test to assess pounds of weight to use or color of Thera-Band exercise band. The Hygenic Corporation* reports correspondence of colors to weight resistance as the following: yellow = 2.5 lb, red = 4.5 lb, green = 5.0 lb, blue = 7.5 lb, black = 9.0 lb, and silver = 15 lb.
4. Repetitions: to be done only in pain-free range.
5. Rate: 5-10 seconds concentric with exhale; 5-10 seconds eccentric with inhale.

Level 1: Prescribed for the most fragile joints, target joints, previously injured muscle, and joints with painful active range of motion, passive range of motion, or weight bearing. No acute swelling or bleeding within past 2 weeks.

	Progression Intensity	No. of Repetitions	No. of Sets
Week 1	40%	10	1
Week 2	45%-50%	10-20	2
Week 3	50%-60%	10-20	3
Week 4	55%-65%	10-20	3
Week 5	60%-70%	10-20	3
Week 6	65%-75%	10-20	3

Level 2: Prescribed for joints and muscles with history of bleeding and chronic, mild-to-moderate impairment. No bleeding in past 6 months.

	Progression Intensity	No. of Repetitions	No. of Sets
Week 1	50%	10	1
Week 2	55%-60%	10-20	2
Week 3	60%-70%	10-20	3
Week 4	65%-75%	10-20	3
Week 5	70%-75%	10-20	3
Week 6	75%	10-20	3

Level 3: Prescribed for joints and muscles with minimal history of bleeding and no signs of impairment.

	Progression Intensity	No. of Repetitions	No. of Sets
Week 1	60%	10-20	1
Week 2	65%-70%	10-20	2
Week 3	70%-75%	10-20	3
Week 4	75%	10-20	3
Week 5	75%	10-20	3
Week 6	75%	10-20	3

Example

Participant 4, a 23-year-old man with severe hemophilia.

Right elbow = level 1: Target joint; had six episodes of bleeding over past 2 months. Active and passive range of motion painful at end range of flexion and extension. No acute swelling, no bleeding within past 2 weeks. Right biceps: isometric Nicholas dynamometry muscle test = 5 lb.

Left elbow = level 3: Only two episodes of bleeding in past. Last episode of bleeding was 2 years previously. Pain-free motion, no swelling or crepitus. Normal end-feel.

Left biceps: isometric Nicholas dynamometry muscle test = 30 lb.

Week 1:

Right elbow flexion: 40% of 5 lb = 2 lb or use yellow Thera-Band for 1 set of 10 repetitions in pain-free range.

Left elbow flexion: 60% of 30 lb = 18 lb or double thickness of black Thera-Band for 1 set of 10-20 repetitions in pain-free range.

*The Hygenic Corporation, 1245 Home Ave, Akron, OH 44310.

From Mulvany R, Zucker-Levin AR, Jeng M, et al: Effects of a 6-week, individualized, supervised exercise program for people with bleeding disorders and hemophilic arthritis, *Phys Ther* 90:509–526, 2010. Used with permission American Physical Therapy Association.

and/or assistive devices may be necessary and a tolerance and/or weaning schedule established.[15] Static or dynamic night splints may be used to apply a low-load stretch to a muscle shortened because of an underlying condition such as synovitis or articular contracture.

A static splint made of plaster, synthetic casting materials, or thermoplastic splinting materials holds the joint in a single position. The material is molded to the extremity, then hardens, and straps are applied to keep it in place on the extremity. A static splint does not bend or straighten the joint. It must be remolded or remade as the individual gains range of motion.[163]

A dynamic splint applies a small amount of pressure (1-2 lb) to stretch a joint over a long period. The individual can still bend and straighten the joint and the therapist can adjust the amount of load applied as needed. There is less irritation and fewer bleeds with the dynamic splint.

Repeated bleeds in the same area can cause a muscle to shorten, limiting joint range of motion. Individuals with inhibitors or limited access to treatment are at

Table 14-7	Clinical Signs and Symptoms of Hemophilia Bleeding Episodes		
Acute Hemarthrosis	**Muscle Hemorrhage**	**Gastrointestinal Involvement**	**Central Nervous System Involvement**
Aura, tingling, or prickling sensation Stiffening into the position of comfort (usually flexion) Decreased range of motion Pain/tenderness Swelling Protective muscle spasm Increased warmth around joint	Gradually intensifying pain Protective spasm of muscle Limitation of movement at the surrounding joints Muscle assumes a position of comfort (usually shortened) Loss of sensation	Abdominal pain and distention Melena (blood in stool) Hematemesis (vomiting blood) Fever Low abdominal/groin pain from bleeding into wall of large intestine or iliopsoas muscle Hip flexion contracture due to spasm of the iliopsoas muscle secondary to retroperitoneal hemorrhage	Impaired judgment Decreased visual and spatial awareness Short-term memory deficits Inappropriate behavior Motor deficits: spasticity, ataxia, abnormal gait, apraxia, decreased balance, loss of coordination

Modified from Goodman CC, Snyder TE: *Differential diagnosis for the physical therapist: screening for referral*, ed 5, Philadelphia, 2013, WB Saunders.

Table 14-8	Management of Joint and Muscle Bleeds		
Joint: Acute Stage	**Joint: Subacute Stage**	**Muscle**	
Factor replacement RICE Pain-free movement; non (or minimal) weight-bearing Pain medication; splinting and support as appropriate	Factor replacement (if indicated) Progressive weight-bearing, movement, and exercises Wean from splints and slings	Factor replacement RICE Progressive movement; appropriate weight-bearing status Bed rest for iliopsoas bleed	

RICE, rest, ice, compression (applying pressure to the area for at least 10-15 minutes), and elevation (immobilization and elevating the body part above the heart level while applying the ice).
Modified from Anderson A, Holtzman TS, Masley J: *Physical therapy in bleeding disorders*, New York, 2000, National Hemophilia Foundation. See also *Physical Therapy Practice Guidelines for Persons with Bleeding Disorders: Joint Bleeds*. Available online at http://www.hemophilia.org/sites/default/files/document/files/ptJointBleedGuidelines.pdf. Accessed July 11, 2014.

increased risk for this type of problem. Night splints may be a good option for people who have muscle contractures that are not responding to other treatment interventions. The desired effect can be obtained in 6 to 8 weeks for individuals who do not have an inhibitor. For those clients with inhibitors, night splinting can take much longer (6 months to 1 year).[163] Serial casting may be a better choice for clients with longstanding problems; either splinting or casting should be used before resorting to surgery.[111,294]

The therapist must watch for leg length discrepancy as a long-term result of joint arthropathy. Even minor discrepancies can affect standing posture and gait mechanics and contribute to low back pain and other lower quadrant impairments. Shoe lifts in conjunction with appropriate prophylactic therapy and exercise can be effective.[128,162]

Specific Exercise Guidelines

Initiation of exercise after a bleed must be delayed, and rehabilitation progress is typically slower for individuals with factor VIII and factor IX deficiency who develop factor inhibitors. Prognosis for full return of function is diminished in such cases. In all cases of joint bleed, the use of heat is contraindicated; if used, hydrotherapy or aquatic intervention must be performed in comfortable but not hot temperatures to avoid blood vessel dilation.

When active bleeding stops, isometric muscle exercise should be initiated to prevent muscular atrophy. This exercise is especially critical with recurrent knee hemarthroses to prevent the visible atrophy of the quadriceps femoris muscle. As pain and edema diminish, the client should begin gentle active range-of-motion exercises followed by slowly progressing strengthening exercises when the joint is pain free through its full range. In the case of an iliopsoas bleed, when ambulation is resumed, crutches and toe-touch weight bearing are initiated. Active movement should be performed in a pain-free range and progressed very slowly.[15]

For all muscles, as the strengthening program is progressed, strengthening aids such as elastic bands or tubing and cuff weights can be used before transitioning to weight equipment. Preadolescents should avoid using high–weight lifting machines.

Postbleed exercise should also take into consideration any damage that may have occurred to the joint, such as ligamentous or capsular stretching. Closed chain and other exercises to restore proprioception should be incorporated into the rehabilitation program.[15]

As a prophylactic measure, clients with severe hemophilia generally need to infuse with clotting factor when participating in a strengthening program. With careful supervision and progression of the exercise program, the individual can progress to aerobic activities.

In some individuals, increased stress levels result in increased frequency of spontaneous bleeding. Biofeedback may be considered especially helpful for these clients who experience spontaneous bleeding during emotional upsets and periods of depression. Biofeedback can also be used for muscle retraining or relaxation techniques to control muscle spasm and allow range of motion.

Psychosocial Aspects of Hemophilia

Psychosocial factors have a significant impact on quality of life for individuals with chronic diseases such as hemophilia. Physical therapists have an important role in supporting the psychosocial needs of affected individuals as well as their families. Providing information and assistance, answering questions, and teaching coping strategies to minimize the impact of disabilities, may help to maximize functional outcomes and improve quality of life for the individual and their families.[45]

The physical therapist can be helpful in encouraging consistent adherence to prophylaxis, an essential part of the treatment program to prevent and control bleeding episodes and their debilitating complications.[298,303] Technology such as web-based and mobile tools can help track bleeding episodes and infusions to assist individuals in managing this disease. The first tool available for this purpose (called ATHNadvoy) was developed in 2001 and donated to the American Thrombosis & Hemostasis Network in 2010. More information is available online at http://www.athn.org/content/tracking-your-bleeds-and-infusions.

A recent review of the literature[45] in this area showed that quality of life is reduced in persons with hemophilia, with a potential impact on education, employment and career, interpersonal relationships, family dynamics, and lifestyle decisions.[126,256] These findings were especially true when prophylactic treatment was not available. Carrier status in women may have a psychosocial impact and affect reproductive choices. There is a need for more international, multifaceted research to explore and quantify the social and psychological aspects of life with hemophilia.[45]

Depression is known to increase in individuals of all ages with chronic illnesses and early childhood trauma. Adults with hemophilia who also have life-threatening comorbidities associated with hemophilia (e.g., hepatitis C and/or HIV) are especially at risk for depression. The physical therapist may need to screen for depression (or suggest screening to the multidisciplinary team); a comprehensive treatment program that includes treatment for depression may improve overall health outcomes.[156]

The Older Adult with Hemophilia

Life expectancy has increased dramatically with modern treatment for hemophilia extending life expectancy to nearly that of the general population.[177,331] Adults with hemophilia are reaching older age and experiencing various age-related health conditions never before seen in this population.[177] Consequently, they are not spared from other health care concerns such as diabetes, heart disease, stroke, or cancer. The management of comorbidities may be complicated even more by the bleeding disorder. Age-related orthopedic comorbidities include degenerative joint changes, osteoporosis,

muscle atrophy or sarcopenia, muscle weakness and disturbance of gait and balance. Increased pain, muscle weakness and atrophy along with an increased risk of falling are key features of advanced hemophilic arthropathy and aging.[331]

Although today's treatments have reduced the number and severity of joint bleeds, middle-aged and older adults with hemophilia did not have the benefit of powdered concentrates and prompt home care earlier on in their lives.

As children they were hospitalized and/or bed bound with casts, packed in ice while whole blood was administered slowly by intravenous drip. It took days for their levels to go up. Before factor replacement, it could take weeks to get a joint bleed under control. The consequence of this type of treatment was contracted joints and severe arthritis.[43]

Today's older adult still may not have quick and easy access to factor replacement. Mobility impairments can make it difficult, if not impossible, to get to a hemophilia treatment center. Loss of fine motor control or the onset of tremors makes self-care at home equally problematic.

The therapist can begin education about long-term planning with middle-aged clients. Introducing the idea of home modifications to improve accessibility should begin early. The importance of staying active cannot be overemphasized. All older adults find that recovery time and rehabilitation take longer as they advance through the decades. Resuming normal activities after injury, surgery, or health conditions that set them back is extremely important.[43]

It is also important to keep educating young clients who are noncompliant with their treatment and ignore recommendations. These individuals likely will have problems in the future similar to those experienced by today's older adult population, who did not have the benefit of modern treatment interventions.

The same is true for young adults during the college years or transitioning from living at home with adult supervision during high school to living on their own independently. For many people with bleeding disorders, this is the first time they will assume "ownership" of their disease.[218] Maintaining physical fitness at every stage of life is a key part of management for hemophilia.

Orthopedic, Surgical, and Medical Interventions

Whereas factor replacement can be used to control bleeding associated with surgery, any operative or invasive medical procedure can create complications for individuals with hemophilia, especially those who develop inhibitors. For example, deep venous thromboses are a concern for individuals with bleeding disorders who require central venous catheters. According to one study,[61] central venous catheter–related deep venous thrombosis is common in children with inherited bleeding disorders and likely occurs earlier than previously thought.

Sometimes, even with optimal infusion therapy and aggressive hemophilia care, a joint becomes a chronic problem. In such cases orthopedic or surgical intervention may be indicated to alleviate pain and deformity and to restore the joint to a more functional state. This may include prescription for an orthosis or a splint or serial casting to increase range of motion. Joint replacement (arthroplasty) is now a treatment option as well.

Synovectomy (removal of the joint synovium) is recommended to stop a target joint from its cycle of bleeding. This procedure is not usually done to improve range of motion or to decrease pain, but rather to reduce the rate of destruction and prevent further damage to the joint caused by bleeding. Arthroscopic synovectomy is best performed before joint degeneration has progressed beyond stage II on the Arnold-Hilgartner scale (see Box 14-7).

Injection of a radioactive isotope (referred to as *isotopic synovectomy* or *synoviorthesis*, usually phosphorus-32 in the United States), which causes scarring to the synovium to arrest bleeding, is an option. This procedure has unique advantages and disadvantages and may be more appropriate for one type of client than another.[83,84]

Arthroplasty (joint replacement) is indicated when a joint shows end-stage damage and has become extremely painful. Client age, range of motion, and level of pain and function are determinants as to the timing of this procedure. Knees, hips, and shoulders are most commonly helped through arthroplasty, with restoration of pain-free joint movement.

The benefits of a 6-week preoperative physical therapy program (prehabilitation) combined with 6 weeks of postoperative rehabilitation have been demonstrated. An individually tailored and supervised program to increase range of motion and muscle strength enables rapid mobilization and recovery of function while minimizing the risk of bleeding.[332]

Long-term results of joint replacement are still under investigation. Mechanical survival of the implant is reported as good or excellent for 80% of knees, but complication rates are higher than in the nonhemophilic population and the incidence of late infection (months to years later) resulting in implant failure remains high (16%).[254,317,364]

With anyone with a bleeding disorder, the question of thromboembolic prophylaxis comes up. Although the American College of Chest Physicians and the American Academy of Orthopaedic Surgeons have set guidelines for thromboembolic prophylaxis in the general population, no such standard of care is in place for individuals with hemophilia. The risk of thrombosis in people with hemophilia following joint replacement (hip and knee) is thought to be lower, but cases have been reported of pulmonary embolism and deep vein thrombosis in these individuals.[329]

Arthrodesis (joint fusion) may be performed in a joint with advanced, painful arthropathy untreatable by arthroplasty. Joint fusion can relieve or eliminate pain to provide improved quality of life, but it also causes permanent loss of joint motion. Arthrodesis can be a very effective way to provide the individual a more stable base for weight-bearing activities.

Osteotomy (removal of a section of bone) may be done to correct angular deformities in a joint and may be considered before arthroplasty to reduce the stresses placed on a joint caused by poor alignment. Other, less-common interventions may include excision of a hemophilia pseudotumor or removal of cysts or exostoses.

The Person with Hemophilia and HIV

It is important for anyone with both hemophilia and HIV to maintain optimal care of their musculoskeletal systems during and between bleeding episodes. It is especially important in the presence of chronic arthropathy and HIV or AIDS to maintain joint function through nonsurgical means, especially exercise.

Surgery may be contraindicated if the risk of infection is too great (e.g., when the CD4 cell count is less than 200). Activities such as tai chi and yoga provide stretching, strengthening (including weight bearing), and a mild aerobic component. Aquatics or swimming must be approached with caution because of the potential for transmission of *Cryptosporidium* oocysts, which cause infection in immunocompromised individuals.[15]

THROMBOCYTOPENIA. Thrombocytopenia, a decrease in the platelet count below 150,000/mm^3 of blood, is caused by inadequate platelet production from the bone marrow, increased platelet destruction outside the bone marrow, or splenic sequestration (entrapment of blood and enlargement in the spleen). Thrombocytopenia is a common complication of leukemia or metastatic cancer (bone marrow infiltration) and aggressive cancer chemotherapy (cytotoxic agents). Thrombocytopenia may also be a presenting symptom of aplastic anemia (bone marrow failure); Box 14-9 lists other causes.

Mucosal bleeding is the most common event and occurs by simply blowing the nose or brushing the teeth. Other sites of mucosal bleeding may include the uterus, GI tract, urinary tract, respiratory tract, and brain (ICH). Symptoms include epistaxis (frequent and difficult to stop), petechiae and/or purpura in the skin (especially the legs) and oropharynx, easy bruising, melena, hematuria, excessive menstrual bleeding, and gingival bleeding.

Diagnosis requires laboratory examination of blood and perhaps bone marrow (if clinically indicated) to confirm the diagnosis. Treatment depends on the precipitating cause (e.g., treatment of underlying leukemia or cessation of cytotoxic drugs until platelet count elevates).

Other treatment methods for immune-related thrombocytopenia (e.g., immune thrombocytopenic purpura) may include use of corticosteroids (e.g., prednisone); intravenous immune globulin and Rho(D); splenectomy; monoclonal antibody agents (e.g., rituximab); and plasmapheresis, a procedure that removes blood from the body, separates the portion containing the antiplatelet antibodies, and then returns the cleansed blood to the body. Newer drugs, thrombopoietic agents, are being tested to provide medications with fewer adverse events.[37]

Box 14-9

CAUSES OF THROMBOCYTOPENIA

Increased Platelet Destruction

- Immune thrombocytopenia purpura
- Drug-induced (immune-related) (heparin, sulfa drugs)
- Thrombotic microangiopathy (thrombotic thrombocytopenic purpura)
- Disseminated intravascular coagulation
- Vasculitis
- Bypass during heart surgery
- Mechanical heart valve
- Splenic sequestration
- von Willebrand disease

Decreased Platelet Production

- Bone marrow infiltration (metastatic neoplasms, leukemia, lymphoma, myeloma)
- Bacterial infections (mycobacteria)
- Viral infections (HIV, cytomegalovirus, hepatitis C)
- Nutritional deficiencies (folate, vitamin B_{12})
- Aplastic anemia
- Myelofibrosis
- Drug-induced (non–immune-related) (alcohol, chemotherapy agents, chloramphenicol)

Transfusions with platelets are avoided in clients with immune thrombocytopenic purpura unless severe bleeding occurs. However, clients with a secondary cause for thrombocytopenia (e.g., acute leukemia treatment and severe complications of chemotherapy agents that cause thrombocytopenia) may require platelet transfusions for bleeding and/or counts less than 15,000/mm³.

The prognosis is variable depending on the underlying cause; it is poor when associated with leukemia or aplastic anemia but good with conditions amenable to treatment.

SPECIAL IMPLICATIONS FOR THE THERAPIST | 14-14

Thrombocytopenia

Thrombocytopenia can cause bleeding into the muscles or joints, and the therapist may encounter the severe consequences of this condition. The therapist must be alert for obvious skin or mucous membrane symptoms of thrombocytopenia such as severe bruising, external hematomas, and the presence of petechiae.

Such signs usually indicate a platelet level below 150,000/mm³. Instruct the client to watch for signs of thrombocytopenia and when noted to immediately apply ice and pressure to any external bleeding site. They should avoid aspirin and aspirin-containing compounds without a physician's approval because of the risk of increased bleeding.

Strenuous exercise or any exercise that involves straining or bearing down could precipitate a hemorrhage, particularly of the eyes or brain. See Table 40-9 for specific exercise guidelines for thrombocytopenia. Exercise prescription is highly individualized and should take into account intensity, duration, and frequency appropriate for the individual's condition, age, and previous activity level.

Blood pressure cuffs and similar devices must be used with caution. When used, elastic support stockings must be thigh high, never knee high. Mechanical compression with a pneumatic pump and soft-tissue mobilization are contraindicated unless approved by the physician. Practice good handwashing (see Boxes 8-4 and 8-5) and observe carefully for any signs of infection (see Box 8-1). (See also "Special Implications for the Therapist 14-5: The Anemias" above.)

Effects of Aspirin and Other Nonsteroidal Antiinflammatory Drugs on Platelet Function

Acquired disorders of platelet function can occur through the use of aspirin and other NSAIDs that inactivate platelet cyclooxygenase. This key enzyme is required for the production of thromboxane A_2, a potent inducer of platelet aggregation and constrictor of arterial smooth muscle.

A single dose of aspirin can suppress normal platelet aggregation for 48 hours or longer (up to 1 week) until newly formed platelets have been released. Platelets are anucleated, and once aspirin irreversibly inhibits cyclooxygenase, the platelet is unable to synthesize new enzyme and remain inactive for the rest of its life span.

NSAIDs have less-potent antiplatelet effects than aspirin because they reversibly inhibit cyclooxygenase. Symptoms from this phenomenon are mild and may consist of easy bruising and bleeding, usually confined to the skin. The use of aspirin or NSAIDs is usually contraindicated before any surgical procedure. Prolonged oozing following dental procedures or surgery may occur.

Disseminated Intravascular Coagulation

Definition and Overview

DIC, sometimes referred to as *consumption coagulopathy*, is a thrombotic disease caused by overactivation of the coagulation cascade (i.e., normal coagulation gone awry).

It is an acquired disorder with diffuse or widespread coagulation occurring within arterioles and capillaries all over the body. DIC is actually a paradoxic condition in which clotting and hemorrhage occur simultaneously within the vascular system.

Uncontrolled activation occurs in both the coagulation sequence, causing widespread formation of thromboses (clots) in the microcirculation, and the fibrinolytic system, leading to widespread deposition of fibrin in the circulation. Hemorrhage may occur in the kidneys, brain, adrenals, heart, and other organs.

Incidence and Etiologic Factors

DIC is common, particularly after shock, sepsis, obstetric/gynecologic complications, cancer (e.g., acute leukemia, colon cancer, pancreatic carcinoma), and massive trauma. The oncology client may develop this syndrome as a result of either the neoplasm itself, the treatment for the neoplasm, or complication (such as sepsis). DIC may occur as a result of a variety of predisposing conditions that activate the clotting mechanisms (see Fig. 6-17).

Pathogenesis

In the normal steady state there is a balance between the procoagulant and the anticoagulant factors, which keeps blood flowing. When DIC occurs there is serious disruption of this system, increasing the procoagulant factors but decreasing the anticoagulant factors.

Typically a stimulus causes a disruption of a vessel, resulting in the release of cytokines and chemokines, which activate systemic coagulation and inflammation. The best-studied activator of DIC is the lipopolysaccharide endotoxin of gram-negative bacteria. The activation of coagulation and inflammation inhibits anticoagulants, fibrinolytics, and antiinflammatory pathways. Microvascular thrombi begin to form in the vasculature, which can become extensive, leading to dysregulation of coagulation and ultimately multiorgan failure.[149]

When overwhelming coagulation occurs, these anticoagulant factors are reduced, allowing for unregulated coagulation. Sepsis, for example, lowers the levels of anticoagulants such as protein C, protein S, and antithrombin III, further reducing the body's ability to respond to the coagulation process. The following three pathogenetic steps are observed and illustrated in Figure 6-14. Hemostasis is initiated by (1) endothelial or tissue injury (exposure of tissue factor), (2) activation of factor XII, and (3) direct activation of factor X. *Damage to the endothelium* (e.g., from sepsis, hypoxia, cardiopulmonary arrest) can precipitate DIC by activating the intrinsic clotting pathway, whereas *tissue injury* (e.g., obstetric complications, malignant neoplasm, infection, burns) can precipitate DIC by activating the extrinsic pathway. *Release of factor XII* in the circulation facilitates the *activation of factor X* (proteolytic effect).

Once either clotting cascade (intrinsic or extrinsic) is stimulated, widespread coagulation occurs throughout the body, leading to thrombotic events within the vasculature. The normal inhibitory mechanisms become overwhelmed so that clotting can occur unrestricted. As a result of the widespread clotting that occurs, platelets and clotting factors become used up and hemorrhage ensues. This leads to the two primary pathophysiologic alterations of DIC: thrombosis in the presence of hemorrhage.

Clinical Manifestations

DIC may be mild to severe with either thrombotic or hemorrhagic symptoms or both. The tendency toward excessive bleeding can appear suddenly, with little warning, and can rapidly progress to severe or even fatal hemorrhage. Thrombosis may occur in various sites distant to the tumor or its metastases.

Signs of DIC include continued bleeding from a venipuncture site, occult and internal bleeding, and, in some cases, profuse bleeding from all orifices. Other, less-obvious and more easily missed signs are generalized sweating, cold and mottled fingers and toes (caused by capillary thrombi and hypoxia), and petechiae.

MEDICAL MANAGEMENT

DIAGNOSIS, TREATMENT, AND PROGNOSIS. Diagnosis is made based on clinical presentation in combination with client history; laboratory blood tests can aid in the diagnosis (e.g., elevated D-dimer test, coagulation tests, low fibrinogen, presence of schistocytes (red cell fragments) on peripheral blood smear).

Treatment is always directed toward the underlying cause and must be highly individualized according to the person's age, nature and origin of DIC, site and severity of hemorrhage or thrombosis, and other clinical parameters. The hemorrhagic or thrombotic symptoms may be alleviated by appropriate blood product replacement or anticoagulants, but the coagulopathy will continue until the causative process is reversed. Supportive methods include platelet, fresh frozen plasma, and clotting factor transfusions for people who are hemorrhaging.[194] Heparin may be considered in cases where thrombotic features are dominant.[360]

Researchers are investigating strategies aimed at inhibiting coagulation activation with protein C, antithrombin, and tissue factor pathway inhibitor.[375]

The mortality rate for DIC is no longer high with early recognition and treatment, but DIC does contribute to significant morbidity and some mortality as it occurs often with sepsis and cancer. Acute DIC can be fatal depending on the response to treatment.

SPECIAL IMPLICATIONS FOR THE THERAPIST 14-15

Disseminated Intravascular Coagulation

Clients with DIC are treated by the therapist in oncology or intensive care units. DIC is either the consequence of malignancy or the end result of multisystem organ failure after trauma affecting multiple systems (e.g., severe trauma or burns).

Clients are in critical condition and require bedside care. Care must be taken to avoid dislodging clots and cause new onset of bleeding. Monitor the results of serial blood studies, particularly hematocrit, hemoglobin, and coagulation times prior to any intervention. To prevent injury, bed rest during bleeding episodes is required.

When monitoring vital signs, watch for hypotension and tachycardia. Regularly assess for signs and symptoms of bleeding such as bleeding gums, bruising, petechiae, nose bleeds, reports of melena or hematuria, headaches, or changes in mental status. Assess the skin for necrosis and hematomas.

Hemoglobinopathies

Several diseases result from an abnormality in the formation of hemoglobin (Hb). Because Hb is essential for life, anomalies in the shape, size, content, or oxygen-carrying capacity can lead to severe problems. Sickle cell disease and thalassemia are two hemoglobinopathies with potential for serious complications and are discussed further.

Hereditary spherocytosis, hereditary elliptocytosis, hereditary stomatocytosis, and pyropoikilocytosis are rare diseases that occur because of defects in the erythrocyte membrane that cause premature clearance of RBCs (hemolysis). Glucose-6-phosphate dehydrogenase deficiency also leads to hemolysis. Discussions of these diseases can be found elsewhere.

Sickle Cell Disease

Overview and Incidence. *Sickle cell disease* (SCD) is an autosomal recessive disorder characterized by the presence of an abnormal form of Hb, called hemoglobin S (Hb S), within the erythrocytes. This irregular form of Hb is the result of a single mutation in the β-Hb chain where the amino acid glutamic acid at position 6 is substituted with valine.

The presence of Hb S can cause RBCs to change from their usual biconcave disk shape to a crescent or sickle shape once the oxygen is released (deoxygenated). SCD occurs when two sickle cell genes are inherited (one from each parent) or one sickle cell gene and another abnormal Hb is inherited, so that almost all of the Hb is abnormal.

Homozygous Hb SS occurs when an individual inherits two sickle cell genes. *Heterozygous Hb SC* is the result of inheriting one sickle cell gene and one gene for another abnormal type of Hb called C. Persons with this type of abnormality have fewer complications than those with homozygous Hb S, but they exhibit more ophthalmologic and orthopedic complications, because individuals with heterozygous Hb SC have increased blood viscosity.

Heterozygous *Hb S β-thalassemia* is the result of inheriting one sickle cell gene and one gene for a type of thalassemia, another inherited anemia. β-Thalassemias are caused by genetic mutations that abolish or reduce production of the β-globin subunit of Hb.[269]

The sickle cell trait refers to people who carry only one *Hb S* gene and is discussed at the end of this section. Hb F, or fetal Hb, is found in infants. Although most infants switch to making α- and β-Hb, some continue to make Hb F, termed hereditary persistence of Hb F. For those people who inherit one sickle gene and the hereditary persistence of Hb F abnormalities, they make $\alpha_2\gamma_2$ Hb and do not develop the severe symptoms of SCD.

Although exact numbers are not available, the Centers for Disease Control and Prevention estimates that 1 of every 500 black or African American newborns and 1 of every 36,000 Hispanic Americans has SCD. It is further estimated that 90,000 to 100,000 Americans have SCD.[241] It is a worldwide health problem, affecting many races, countries, and ethnic groups, and is the most common inherited hematologic disorder. The WHO estimates that each year more than 300,000 babies are born worldwide with severe Hb disorders.[368] The disease is particularly common among people whose ancestors come from sub-Saharan Africa, India, Saudi Arabia, and Mediterranean countries.[367]

The two primary pathophysiologic features of sickle cell disorders are chronic hemolytic anemia and vasoocclusion resulting in ischemic injury. Children with SCD are at increased risk for severe morbidity and mortality, especially during the first 3 years of life.

When a sickled cell reoxygenates the cell resumes a normal shape, but after repeated cycles of sickling and unsickling the erythrocyte is permanently damaged and hemolyzes. This hemolysis is responsible for the anemia that is a hallmark of SCD. A brief discussion of the related sickle cell syndromes is presented, but only the most severe disorder, sickle cell anemia, is fully discussed in this text.

Etiologic Factors. The cause of SCD and its worldwide incidence is the result of several factors. The sickle cell trait may have developed as a single genetic mutation that provided a selective advantage against severe forms of falciparum malaria.

Anyone who carries the inherited trait for SCD but does not have the actual illness is more resistant against this form of malaria. In countries with malaria, children born with sickle cell trait survived and then passed the gene for SCD to their offspring. As populations migrated (including the slave trade), the sickle cell trait and SCD moved throughout the world.

Several theories purport to explain the origination of SCD, but its actual origin is unknown. Four separate haplotypes are known; each is related to the severity of illness and each is associated with a different geographic location, including different locations in Africa, eastern Saudi Arabia, and India.

Risk Factors. Because SCD is inherited as an autosomal recessive trait, both parents of an offspring must have the Hb S gene. When both parents have sickle cell trait, they have a 25% chance with each pregnancy of having a child with sickle cell anemia. If one parent has sickle cell trait and the other has a β-thalassemic disorder, they are at the same risk for having a child with a sickle β-thalassemia syndrome.

In couples in which one individual has sickle cell trait and one has Hb C trait, the chance of having a child with Hb SC disease is also 25% with each pregnancy. If one parent has SCD and the other has the sickle cell trait, the risk of having a child with SCD is 50% (Fig. 14-14).

Individuals with sickle cell trait can receive nondirective genetic counseling (given objective information without personal bias and without provision of specific recommendations) after Hb electrophoresis and other measurements have been performed on each prospective parent.

Risk factors likely to induce symptoms or episodes (episode is now the preferred term over crisis; however, clinicians may find that some affected individuals prefer the term crisis) are factors that cause physiologic stress, resulting in sickling of the erythrocytes. Stress from viral or bacterial infection, hypoxia, dehydration, extreme temperatures (hot or cold), alcohol consumption, or fatigue may precipitate an episode.

Additionally, episodes may be precipitated by the presence of acidosis; exposure to low oxygen tensions as a result of strenuous physical exertion, climbing to high altitudes, flying in nonpressurized planes, or undergoing anesthesia without receiving adequate oxygenation; pregnancy; trauma; and fever. Any of these factors may increase the body's need for oxygen, increasing the percentage of erythrocytes that deoxygenate, thereby precipitating an episode.

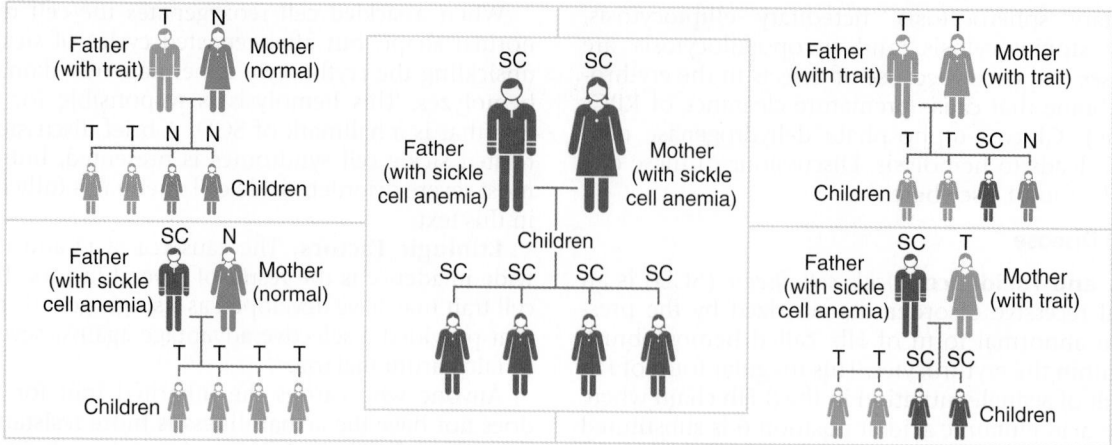

Figure 14-14

Statistical probabilities of inheriting sickle cell anemia. (Reprinted from O'Toole MT: *Miller-Keane encyclopedia and dictionary of medicine, nursing, and allied health,* rev ed, Philadelphia, 2005, WB Saunders.)

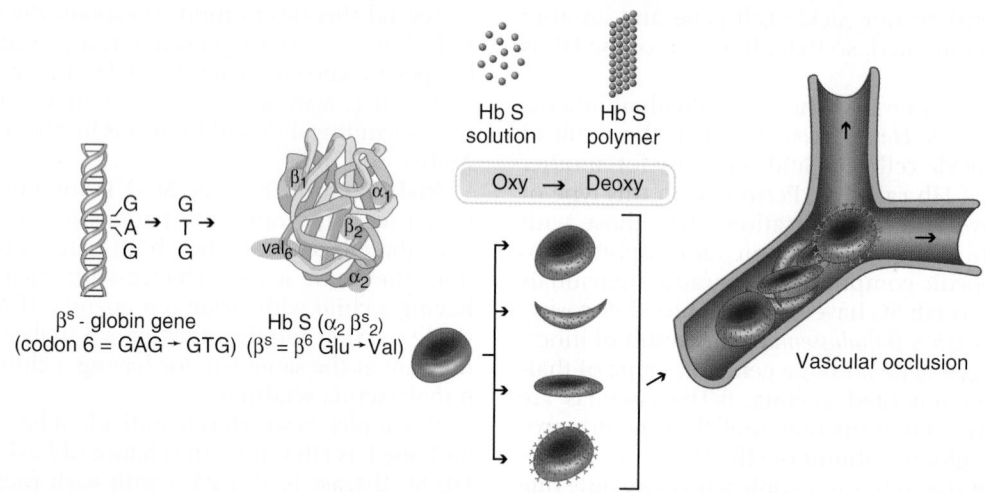

Figure 14-15

Schematic view of the pathophysiologic characteristics of SCD. The double-stranded DNA molecule on the *left* represents a β-globin gene in which a GAG→GTG substitution in the sixth codon has created the sickle cell gene. Valine is substituted for glutamic acid as the sixth amino acid, creating a mutant Hb tetramer (Hb S). A tetramer is a protein with four subunits (tetrameric). Hb S loses solubility and polymerizes when deprived of oxygen. Upon deoxygenation, most sickle cells lose deformability. Some cells sickle; a fraction becomes dehydrated, irreversibly sickled, and poorly deformable; a few become highly adherent. Vasoocclusion *(right)* is initiated by adherent cells sticking to the vascular endothelium, thereby creating a nidus that traps rigid cells and facilitates linking together in a chain formation, a process called polymerization. (Reprinted from Goldman L: *Cecil textbook of medicine,* ed 22, Philadelphia, 2004, WB Saunders.)

Pathogenesis. The sickle cell defect occurs in Hb, the oxygen-carrying constituent of erythrocytes. Hb contains four chains of amino acids, the compounds that make up proteins. Two of the amino acid chains are known as *α-globin chains*, and two are called *β-globin chains*.

In normal Hb, the amino acid in the sixth position on the β-globin chains is glutamic acid. In people with SCD, the sixth position is occupied by another amino acid, valine (Fig. 14-15). DNA recombinant technology has identified the genetic locus for the β-globin on chromosome 11.

This single-point mutation of valine for glutamic acid results in a loss of two negative charges that causes surface abnormalities. The sickle Hb transports oxygen normally, but after releasing oxygen, those Hb molecules that contain the β-globin chain defect stick to one another instead of remaining separate. The Hb then polymerizes (change molecular arrangement), forming long, rigid rods or tubules inside RBCs.

The higher the concentration of deoxygenated sickle Hb molecules and the lower the blood pH, the faster the polymerization occurs.[280] The rods cause the normally smooth, doughnut-shaped RBCs to take on a sickle or curved shape and to lose their vital ability to deform and squeeze through tiny blood vessels (Fig. 14-16).

For a time, this sickling is reversible because the cells are reoxygenated in the lungs; however, eventually the change becomes irreversible. In the process of sickling and unsickling, the erythrocyte membrane becomes damaged and the cells are removed (hemolyzed).

The sickled cells, which become stiff and sticky, clog small blood vessels, depriving tissue from receiving an

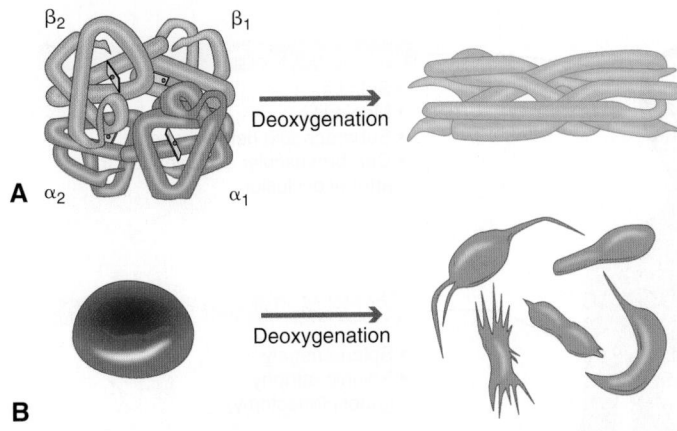

Figure 14-16

A, The molecular structure of Hb contains a pair of α polypeptide chains and a pair of α chains, each wrapped around a heme group (an iron atom in a porphyrin ring). The quaternary structure of the Hb molecule enables it to carry up to four molecules of oxygen. In the folded β-globin chain molecule, the sixth position contacts the α-globin chain. The amino acid substitution at the sixth position of the β-globin chain occurring in sickle cell anemia causes the Hb to aggregate into long chains, altering the shape of the cell (Hb S). **B,** The change of the RBC from a biconcave disk to an elongated or crescent (sickle) shape occurs with deoxygenation.

adequate blood supply. Under stress, tissues experience increased oxygen requirements, which causes more Hb to release its oxygen, leading to increased numbers of deoxygenated and polymerized cells.

Deoxygenation of sickle cells induces potassium (followed by water) efflux, which increases cell density and the tendency of Hb S to polymerize. The sickle cell also has a chemical on the cell surface that binds to blood vessel walls, leading to endothelial cell activation. As a result, these sickle-shaped, rigid, sticky blood cells cannot pass through the capillaries, blocking the flow of blood.[269]

Occlusion of the microcirculation increases hypoxia, which causes more erythrocytes to sickle; thus a vicious cycle is precipitated. This accumulation of sickled erythrocytes obstructing blood vessels produces tissue injury. The organs at greatest risk are those with sluggish circulation, low pH, and a high level of oxygen extraction (spleen and bone marrow) or those with a limited terminal arterial supply (eye, head of the femur). No tissue or organ is spared from this injury. The higher the concentration of deoxygenated cells, the more severe (clinically) the complications.

Average sickle RBCs last only 10 to 20 days (normal is 120 days). The RBCs cannot be replaced fast enough, and anemia is the result. Although significant injury occurs in the microvasculature as a result of sickling, the most severe complication of SCD is a cerebral infarct, which occurs in the large blood vessels, where blood is moving rapidly and the diameter is wide.

Research has shown that not only are the Hb cells abnormal, but so are the blood vessel walls. This is likely a product of sickle cells adhering to and damaging endothelium, which leads to an inflammatory response of WBCs, cytokines, chemoattractants, and procoagulants. Over time, smooth muscle cells migrate into the wall, where they proliferate and narrow the lumen of the vessel.[278]

Significantly narrowed or stenotic arteries can further collect sickled cells, thereby occluding the lumen, resulting in stroke. Further complicating stroke and pulmonary hypertension is the lack of nitric oxide production. Normally, when hypoxia is present, nitric oxide is produced to cause local vasodilation, inhibit endothelial damage, and prevent proliferation of vascular smooth muscle.[357] But the hemolysis of erythrocytes and release of Hb inhibits the production of nitric oxide, thus blocking the beneficial effects of nitric oxide.

Clinical Manifestations. Sickled erythrocytes lead to hemolytic anemia and tend to occlude the microvasculature, resulting in both acute and chronic tissue injury. Intravascular sickling and hemolysis can begin by 6 to 8 weeks of age, but clinical manifestations do not usually appear until the infant is at least 6 months old, at which time the postnatal decrease in Hb F, which inhibits sickling, and increased production of Hb S lead to the increased concentration of Hb S.

Acute clinical manifestations of sickling, called *crises* or *episodes*, usually fall into one of four categories: vasoocclusive or thrombotic, aplastic, sequestration or, rarely, hyperhemolytic (Fig. 14-17).

Pain caused by the blockage of sickled RBCs (thrombosis) is the most common symptom of SCD, occurring unpredictably in any organ, bone, or joint of the body, wherever and whenever a blood clot develops. The symptoms and frequency, duration, and intensity of the painful episodes vary widely (Box 14-10). Some people experience painful episodes only once a year; others may have as many as 15 to 20 episodes annually. The vasoocclusive episodes causing ischemic tissue damage may last 5 or 6 days, requiring hospitalization and subsiding gradually. Older clients more often report extremity and back pain during vascular episodes.

Chest Syndrome. Two life-threatening thrombotic complications associated with SCD include acute chest syndrome and stroke. Acute chest syndrome results from the inability of sickled cells to become reoxygenated in the lungs. Sickled cells then adhere to lung endothelium cells, resulting in further inflammation, occluding vessels, and resulting in infarction. The most common precipitants are infection, fat emboli (from infarcted bone marrow), and infarction.

Symptoms include chest pain, shortness of breath, fever, wheezing, and cough (Box 14-11). Chest radiographs typically demonstrate an infiltrate, sometimes days after the symptoms began. Prognosis for this complication is poor and is one of the most common causes of death.[280]

Pulmonary hypertension can be a severe consequence of repeated microthrombotic events in the lung even without a history of acute chest syndrome. Autopsy studies suggest that more than one-third of people with SCD develop this complication (although the real incidence is probably higher). Chronic intravascular damage from

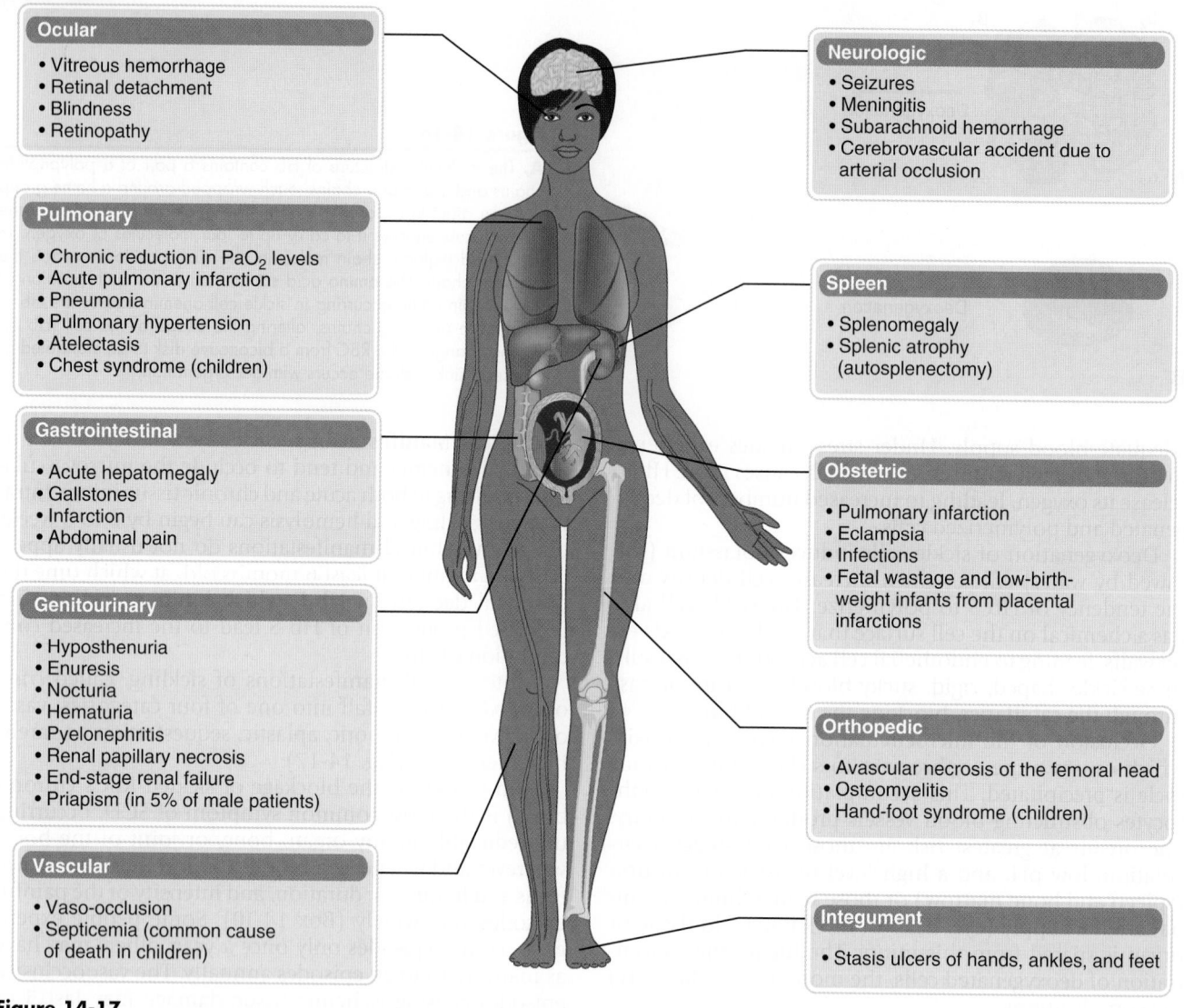

Ocular

- Vitreous hemorrhage
- Retinal detachment
- Blindness
- Retinopathy

Pulmonary

- Chronic reduction in PaO_2 levels
- Acute pulmonary infarction
- Pneumonia
- Pulmonary hypertension
- Atelectasis
- Chest syndrome (children)

Gastrointestinal

- Acute hepatomegaly
- Gallstones
- Infarction
- Abdominal pain

Genitourinary

- Hyposthenuria
- Enuresis
- Nocturia
- Hematuria
- Pyelonephritis
- Renal papillary necrosis
- End-stage renal failure
- Priapism (in 5% of male patients)

Vascular

- Vaso-occlusion
- Septicemia (common cause of death in children)

Neurologic

- Seizures
- Meningitis
- Subarachnoid hemorrhage
- Cerebrovascular accident due to arterial occlusion

Spleen

- Splenomegaly
- Splenic atrophy (autosplenectomy)

Obstetric

- Pulmonary infarction
- Eclampsia
- Infections
- Fetal wastage and low-birth-weight infants from placental infarctions

Orthopedic

- Avascular necrosis of the femoral head
- Osteomyelitis
- Hand-foot syndrome (children)

Integument

- Stasis ulcers of hands, ankles, and feet

Figure 14-17

Clinical manifestations and possible complications associated with SCD. These findings are a consequence of infarctions, anemia, hemolysis, and recurrent infections.

sickled cells leads to a reduction in nitric oxide (a potent vasodilator), which allows for continual vasoconstriction. Eventually, these small vessels become thickened and blocked by thrombin and fibrous tissue with the loss of the vascular bed. This process often proceeds without clinical symptoms until the person is short of breath, at which time the damage is irreversible. Affected persons exhibit symptoms of right heart failure (i.e., edema, renal insufficiency). Pulmonary hypertension increases the risk of sudden death and is a common cause of death in people with SCD.

Stroke. Stroke, or cerebral infarction, is another serious thrombotic complication of SCD. By the age of 45 years, 24% of people with SCD will have experienced a stroke.[355] Stroke occurs in 11% of SCD clients younger than age 20 years, causing death or severe disability.[259] Large vessels can become stenosed through chronic injury to the endothelium. Once the diameter of an affected artery is significantly narrowed, acute occluding of the vessel can occur (by a clot made of sickle and normal

cells, WBCs, platelets, and thrombin), causing a cerebral infarct.[278]

Ischemic reperfusion injury occurs encompassing endothelial cell damage, platelet clumping, release of cytokines, and the attraction of granulocytes, macrophages, T-cells and NK T-cells to the site.[29,279] The acute obstruction and resulting inflammation lead to further hypoxia and acidosis and a vicious cycle of continued sickling.[355]

Symptoms are similar to strokes in people without SCD, including paralysis, weakness, speech difficulties, seizures, and tingling/numbness of extremities. Infarcts can occur in the microvasculature as well. MRI and magnetic resonance angiography of the head and neck may show more extensive changes than are seen clinically, suggesting that silent strokes are not uncommon.

Additionally, many cognitive effects from these microvasculature strokes result in learning problems. Children demonstrate problems with memory, attention, visual–motor performance, and academic or social skills; neuromotor delays; mild hearing loss and auditory

Box 14-10

CLINICAL MANIFESTATIONS OF SICKLE CELL ANEMIA

Pain

- Abdominal
- Chest
- Headaches

Bone and Joint Episodes

- Low-grade fever
- Extremity pain
- Back pain
- Periosteal pain
- Joint pain, especially shoulder and hip

Vascular Complications

- Cerebrovascular accidents
- Chronic leg ulcers
- Avascular necrosis of the femoral head
- Bone infarcts

Pulmonary Episodes

- Hypoxia
- Chest pain
- Dyspnea
- Tachypnea

Neurologic Manifestations

- Seizures
- Hemiplegia

- Dizziness
- Drowsiness
- Coma
- Stiff neck
- Paresthesias
- Cranial nerve palsies
- Blindness
- Nystagmus
- Transient ischemic attacks

Hand-Foot Syndrome

- Fever
- Pain
- Dactylitis

Splenic Sequestration Episodes

- Liver and spleen enlargement, tenderness
- Hypovolemia

Renal Complications

- Enuresis
- Nocturia
- Hematuria
- Pyelonephritis
- Renal papillary necrosis
- End-stage renal failure (older adult population)

Modified from Goodman CC, Snyder TE: *Differential diagnosis for the physical therapists: screening for referral*, ed 5, Philadelphia, 2013, WB Saunders.

Box 14-11

COMPLICATIONS ASSOCIATED WITH PEDIATRIC SICKLE CELL ANEMIA

Chest Syndrome

- Severe chest pain
- Fever of ≥38.8° C (≥102° F)
- Very congested
- Cough
- Dyspnea
- Tachypnea
- Sternal or costal retractions
- Wheezing

Stroke

- Seizures
- Unusual or strange behavior
- Inability to move an arm and/or a leg
- Ataxia or unsteady gait (do not assume these are guarding responses to pain)
- Stutter or slurred speech
- Distal muscular weakness in the hands, feet, or legs
- Changes in vision
- Severe, unrelieved headaches
- Severe vomiting

processing disorders; and failed speech and language screening.[6,146,179,326]

Other Complications. For most people with SCD, the incidence of complications can be reduced by simple protective measures such as prophylactic penicillin in children (until about age 5 years),[217] maintaining current vaccinations (to pneumococcus, meningococcus, *Haemophilus influenzae* type b, hepatitis B virus, and an annual vaccination against influenza virus), avoidance of excessive heat or cold and dehydration, and contact as early as possible with a specialist center. These precautions are most effective if susceptible infants are identified at birth.

Other thrombotic complications include *hand-and-foot syndrome* (dactylitis), which occurs when a microinfarction (clot) occludes the blood vessels that supply the metacarpal and metatarsal bones, causing ischemia; it may be an infant's first problem caused by SCD. It presents with low-grade fever and symmetric, painful, diffuse, nonpitting edema in the hands and feet, extending to the fingers and toes (Fig. 14-18). This is a fairly common phenomenon seen almost exclusively in the young infant and child. Despite radiographic changes and swelling, the syndrome is almost always self-limiting, and bones usually heal without permanent deformity (Fig. 14-19).

Priapism is also a thrombotic complication and requires immediate medical attention. Repeated and prolonged episodes can lead to impotence. The kidneys exhibit thrombotic complications and slowly lose function; end-stage renal disease can occur.

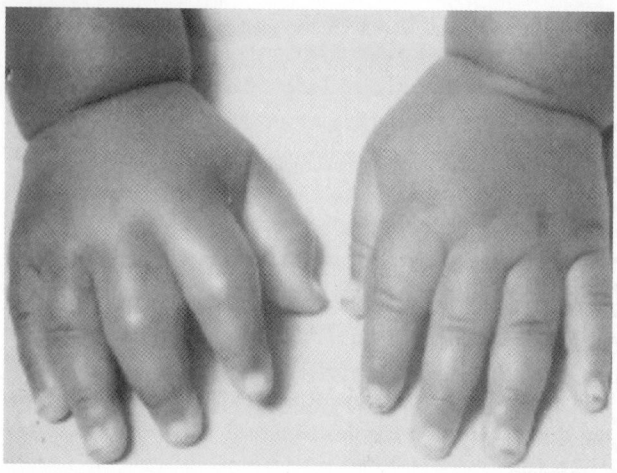

Figure 14-18

Dactylitis. Painful swelling of the hands or feet can occur when a clot forms in the hands or feet. This problem, known as hand-and-foot syndrome, occurs most often in children affected by SCD. (Reprinted from Gaston M: *Sickle cell anemia*, NIH Pub No 90-3058, Bethesda, MD, 1990, National Institutes of Health.)

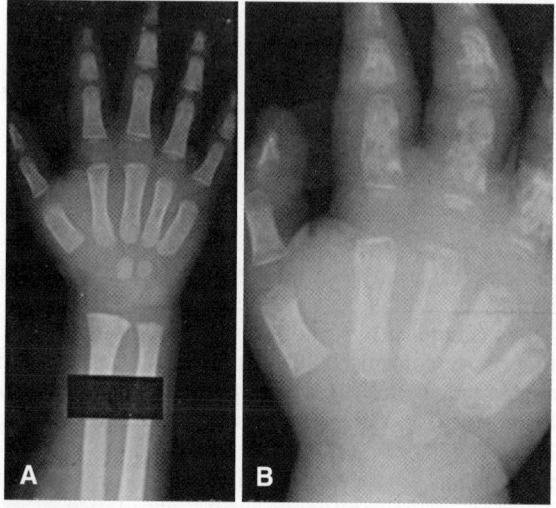

Figure 14-19

Radiographs of an infant with sickle cell anemia and acute dactylitis. A, The bones appear normal at the onset of the episode. **B,** Destructive changes and periosteal reaction are evident 2 weeks later. (Reprinted from Behrman RE: *Nelson textbook of pediatrics*, ed 17, Philadelphia, 2004, WB Saunders.)

Jaundice is another common manifestation of SCD. Sickled cells do not live as long as normal cells and therefore die more rapidly than the liver can filter them. Bilirubin from these broken down cells builds up in the system, causing jaundice.

Anemia is a constant feature of SCD, with a Hb concentration of around 8 g/dL; acute, severe anemia, termed an aplastic crisis or episode, can occur when erythropoiesis abruptly stops. Clinical manifestations are pallor, fatigue, and jaundice. This is typically a result of parvovirus B19 infection.

Folate deficiency is another cause of severe anemia (often because of noncompliance in taking folate supplements). Anemia can also be worsened by renal insufficiency (decreased levels of erythropoietin) secondary to thrombosis.

Some of the complications associated with SCD are treated with transfusions, resulting in iron overload. *Hyperhemolysis* develops in some clients as a consequence of the formation of alloimmune responses to erythrocyte antigens, resulting in a delayed transfusion reaction with significant acute hemolysis of erythrocytes.

The spleen is an organ that is very susceptible to thrombotic occlusions (i.e., low blood flow, low oxygen tension, and low pH). In sequestration episodes, large numbers of cells undergo sickling in the spleen, leading to ischemia, acute hemolysis, and necrosis of the spleen.

Hypovolemic shock can occur, particularly in children, accompanied by a tender spleen and splenomegaly. Sequestration episodes may be precipitated by infection and can be fatal in the pediatric population. Over time the spleen is severely damaged and becomes completely fibrotic, which is called *autosplenectomy*.

The spleen is destroyed in most children with SCD. In children, sickle-shaped RBCs often become trapped in the spleen, leading to a serious risk of death before the age of 7 years from a sudden, profound anemia associated with rapid splenic enlargement or because lack of splenic function permits an overwhelming infection.

Sequestration can occur in the liver but less frequently than splenic sequestration. Children with severe manifestations of sickle cell anemia have low bone mineral density and possess significant deficits in dietary calcium and circulating vitamin D, which complicates growth. Most children have growth retardation by the age of 2 years (weight more than height), which leads to osteoporosis and other bone abnormalities.[191]

MEDICAL MANAGEMENT

PREVENTION. SCD can be prevented. Couples at risk of having affected children can be identified by inexpensive and reliable blood tests; chorionic villus sampling from 9 weeks' gestation can be performed for prenatal diagnosis.

Adoption of such measures goes hand in hand with health education. However, prenatal diagnosis can raise ethical questions that differ from one culture to another. Experience has clearly shown that genetic counseling, coupled with the offer of prenatal diagnosis, can lead to a large-scale reduction in births of affected children.

The risk of having affected children can be detected before marriage or pregnancy; however, to do so requires a carrier screening program. There is extensive experience with such programs in low- and high-income countries. For example, in the case of thalassemia prevention, unmarried people in Montreal (Canada) and the Maldives are offered screening. Premarital screening is a national policy in Cyprus and the Islamic Republic of Iran, and prereproductive screening is emphasized in Greece and Italy.

The WHO recommends these approaches be practiced in conformity with the three core principles of medical genetics: the autonomy of the individual or the couple, their right to adequate and complete information, and the highest standards of confidentiality.[367]

DIAGNOSIS. It is required in every state that all infants be screened for SCD regardless of race or ethnic background (universal screening). This recommendation is based on the following factors: (1) although SCD is more prevalent in certain racial and ethnic groups, it is not possible to define accurately an individual's heritage by physical appearance or surname; and (2) prophylactic penicillin and pneumococcal vaccination reduce both morbidity and mortality from pneumococcal infections in infants with sickle cell anemia and sickle thalassemia.

Screening targeted to specific racial and ethnic groups will therefore miss some affected infants, subjecting them to an increased risk of early mortality. Universal screening is the best, most reliable, and most cost-effective screening method to identify affected infants.[264] The cord blood of newborns is tested in the United States.

The diagnosis of sickle cell trait or any of the other sickle syndromes depends on the demonstration of sickling under reduced oxygen tension. A sickle turbidity test (Sickledex, Streck, Inc., Omaha, NE) can confirm the presence of Hb S in peripheral blood, and Hb electrophoresis (separation and identification of Hb under the influence of an applied electric field) is used to determine the amount of Hb S in erythrocytes.

Electrophoresis is used to screen blood for sickle cell trait and will also detect SCD and heterozygosity (carrier state) for other Hb disorders, such as Hb C. Because the Hb S and Hb C amino acid substitutions change the electrical charge of the protein, the migration patterns of the Hb with electrophoresis result in distinct diagnostic patterns.[269]

New tests are being developed to use in developing countries that would distinguish SCD from sickle cell trait.[287]

Safe, accurate methods for performing prenatal diagnosis for SCD are possible as early as 10 weeks' gestation. Analyses of DNA from fetal cells obtained by amniocentesis or chorionic villus sampling can be performed at 16 weeks' gestation. The sickle and Hb C genes can be detected directly in fetal DNA samples, as can most Hb S β-thalassemia genes.

TREATMENT. Supportive care is essential for all pain crises and complications (e.g., rest, pain medication [opioid and nonopioid], oxygen, administration of intravenous fluids, electrolytes, and antibiotics, and physical and occupational therapy for joint and bone involvement). Routine health maintenance is required including updating vaccinations, regular ophthalmologic care, screening for proteinuria, and pulmonary hypertension. The medication hydroxyurea has been shown to reduce the number of painful episodes and hospitalizations; it is recommended for clients with repeated painful crises, acute chest syndrome, and symptomatic anemia.[50]

Acute stroke is managed with exchange transfusions to reduce the amount of Hb S to less than 30% while keeping the total Hb (through transfusions) at 10 g/dL. Because sickle cells function best at lower viscosities, blood is exchanged rather than just transfused.

The likelihood of a second stroke is increased, and prophylactic transfusions (this inhibits their own erythropoiesis of Hb S) have been shown to help decrease the risk of stroke and reduce the stenosis of arteries.[4,5] Complications with iron overload are common and can have significant long-term problems as well as alloimmunization (creating antibodies against "foreign" transfused cells). Chelating therapy is available but is often difficult for children to tolerate.

Acute chest syndrome is treated with oxygen, antibiotics, pain medication, and avoidance of overhydration. Incentive spirometry may improve atelectasis, whereas bronchodilators aid in reactive airway symptoms. Erythrocyte transfusion or exchange transfusion may be required if hypoxia continues despite supplemental oxygen.

Optimal treatment for pulmonary hypertension requires more research. Hydroxyurea has not been shown to be beneficial; care is usually supportive and treated similarly to primary pulmonary hypertension.

Acute aplastic episodes can be treated with a transfusion if the anemia is severe and the reticulocyte count is low. Most often this is self-limiting and erythropoiesis resumes in a few days. Splenic or hepatic sequestration requires aggressive rehydration and transfusion.

Transfusions are used in specific situations: stroke, symptomatic anemia, acute chest syndrome, and surgical interventions. Exchange transfusions are indicated for stroke, acute chest syndrome with significant hypoxia, and multiorgan failure/hepatopathy. Best treatments are under investigation for splenic sequestration, particularly for children younger than age 2 years.[34]

Prenatal and neonatal screening can identify this disorder and significantly reduce morbidity and mortality through the use of prophylactic antibiotics. Infants with documented SCD (sickle cell anemia or Hb S β-thalassemia) should be started on twice-daily oral prophylactic penicillin as soon as possible but no later than 2 months of age. Children who have experienced pneumococcal sepsis should remain on prophylactic penicillin indefinitely.

The use of inhaled nitrous oxide to treat SCD is also under investigation because of its ability to prevent pulmonary hypertension and endothelial damage. The onset of peripheral neuropathy associated with nitric oxide use in this population has delayed the final development of treatment protocols incorporating nitric oxide.[258,337]

Researchers are continuing to investigate the use of fetal Hb as a treatment possibility. Fetal Hb is produced during fetal development and for the first 6 months after birth. Hb F has some ability to prevent sickling and reduce hemolysis; some adults with SCD who naturally make substantial amounts of Hb F have less pain and better spleen function than others with SCD who do not have elevated levels of Hb F.

Other researchers are investigating drugs to reverse cellular dehydration (dehydration increases the rate of polymerization) and fetal cord blood transplantation (see Chapter 21).

HSCT has been shown to help, and possibly cure, individuals with SCD.[65] Matched related donors are best, providing an overall survival of 93%. People who receive cells from unrelated donors have lower overall survival of 75%. HSCT is often used for individuals with early complications and at high risk for early death.[316] It can provide long-term protection from stoke, acute chest syndrome, and other serious complications of SCD.

PROGNOSIS. Historically, SCD has been associated with high mortality in early childhood from overwhelming bacterial infections, acute chest syndrome, and stroke. In the mid-1970s the average life expectancy was only 14.3 years. By 1994 the life expectancy had increased to 42 years for men and 48 years for women with sickle cell anemia.[281,367] Between 1999 and 2002, the mortality rate for blacks and African Americans younger than age 4 years fell by 42%. This dramatic drop is thought to be secondary to the introduction of the pneumococcal vaccine.[241]

SCD remains a devastating condition with recurrent episodes leading to early death. The complications of SCD can be life-threatening depending on their location. Recovery may be complete in some cases, but serious neurologic damage is more likely to occur, and repeated cerebrovascular accidents may lead to increased neurologic involvement, permanent paralysis, or death. Permanent damage from blood clots to the heart, kidney, lungs, liver, or eyes (blindness) can occur.

SPECIAL IMPLICATIONS FOR THE THERAPIST 14-16

Sickle Cell Disease

It is important for the therapist to recognize signs of complications, especially signs of acute chest syndrome, stroke, and neurodevelopmental impairment (see Box 14-11). Providing client education is also an important role. Clients should be taught about risks and risk prevention, including the importance of physical activity and/or mobility, prevention of pulmonary complications using breathing and incentive spirometry, and the importance of remaining well hydrated. Screening for referral to other rehabilitation or behavioral services is also part of the therapist's intervention. Be aware, too that A1C lab values can be altered in individuals with sickle hemoglobin, an important finding in the long-term management of diabetes.[134]

Stroke is a relatively infrequent complication in the young infant; the median age for occurrence of stroke in children is 7 years. Splenic sequestration (entrapment of blood and enlargement in the spleen) can occur in children younger than 6 years with homozygous Hb S and at any age with other types of SCD. Circulatory collapse and death can occur in less than 30 minutes.

Any signs of weakness, abdominal pain, fatigue, dyspnea, tachycardia accompanied by pallor, and hypotension require emergency medical attention. Client and family education should emphasize the importance of regularly scheduled medical evaluations for anyone receiving hydroxyurea. The risk of developing an undetected toxicity that can result in severe bone marrow depression must be explained. Outward signs of drug complications are rarely evident.

Neurodevelopment

SCD is a blood disorder; however, the CNS is one of the organs frequently affected by the disease.[145,301] Brain disease can begin early in life and often leads to neurocognitive dysfunction.

Approximately one-fourth to one-third of children with SCD have some form of CNS effects from the disease, which typically manifest as deficits in specific cognitive domains and academic difficulties.

The impact of the disease on families shares many features similar to other neurodevelopmental disorders; however, social-environmental factors related to low socioeconomic status, worry and concerns about social stigma, and recurrent, unpredictable medical complications can be sources of relatively higher stress in SCD.

Greater public awareness of the neurocognitive effects of SCD and their impact on child outcomes is a critical step toward improved treatment, adaptation to illness, and quality of life.

Exercise

Multiple factors contribute to exercise intolerance in individuals with sickle cell anemia, but little information exists regarding the safety of maximal cardiopulmonary exercise testing or the mechanisms of exercise limitation in these clients.

For example, low peak VO_2, low anaerobic threshold, gas exchange abnormalities, and high ventilatory reserve comprise a pattern consistent with exercise limitation due to pulmonary vascular disease in this population group. Low peak VO_2, low anaerobic threshold, no gas exchange abnormalities, and a high heart rate reserve reflect peripheral vascular disease and/or myopathy. Low peak VO_2, low anaerobic threshold, no gas exchange abnormalities, and a low heart rate reserve are best explained by anemia.[41] These kinds of cardiopulmonary factors must be considered when prescribing exercise for this population.[261]

During a sickle cell episode, the therapist may be involved in nonpharmacologic pain control or management. Precautions include avoiding stressors that can precipitate an episode, such as overexertion, dehydration, smoking, and exposure to cold or the use of cryotherapy for painful, swollen joints. (See "Special Implications for the Therapist 14-1: Hematologic Disorders" above.)

Fear of movement (kinesophobia) has been reported among individuals with sickle cell disease; greater kinesophobia is associated with greater pain and psychologic distress.[270] Addressing anxiety and fear and the effects of these emotions on pain, movement, and disability may help the individual remain active and able to participate in physical activity and exercise. Should a person with SCD experience an isolated musculoskeletal injury (e.g., sprained ankle) in the absence of any sickle cell episodes, careful application of ice can be undertaken.

Pain Management

People with SCD suffer both physically and psychosocially. They may describe feelings of helplessness against the disease and fear a premature death. Frequent hospitalizations and consequent job absences often result in stressful financial constraints.

Depression is a common finding in this group of people. A program offering holistic treatment focuses on pharmacologic and nonpharmacologic strategies, offering the client multiple self-management options. The sickle cell pain can be successfully managed using whirlpool therapy at a slightly warmer temperature (38.9°-40° C [102°-104° F]), facilitating muscle relaxation through active movement in the water.

The therapist should teach the client alternative methods of pain control, such as the appropriate application of mild heat to painful areas or the use of visualization or relaxation techniques. Combined use of medications, psychologic support, relaxation techniques, biofeedback, and imagery is a useful intervention to lessen the effects of painful episodes.[141] Cognitive-behavioral therapy can be helpful in the management of sickle pain because of the high level of psychologic stress people with SCD experience.[343]

Joint effusions in SCD can occur secondary to long bone infarctions with extension of swelling and septic arthritis. Clients with SCD may also have coexistent rheumatic or collagen vascular disease or osteoarthritis, necessitating careful evaluation to determine the presence of marked inflammation or fever before initiating intervention procedures.

Teaching joint protection is important and may include assistive devices, equipment, and technology and pain-free strengthening exercises. Persistent thigh, buttock, or groin pain in anyone with known SCD may be an indication of aseptic necrosis of the femoral head. Blood supply to the hip is only adequate, even in healthy people, so the associated microvascular obstruction can leave the hip especially vulnerable to ischemia and necrosis. Up to 50% of sickle cell cases develop this condition.

Total hip replacement may be indicated in cases in which severe structural damage occurs; sickle cell–related surgical complications most commonly include excessive intraoperative blood loss, postoperative hemorrhage, wound abscess, pulmonary complications, and transfusion reactions.[358]

Tolerance, Dependence, and Addiction

It is helpful if the client, family, and clinician understand the differences among tolerance, dependence, and addiction as they relate to the individual with SCD receiving or needing narcotic medications. Tolerance and dependence are both involuntary and predictable physiologic changes that develop with repeated administration of narcotics; these terms do not indicate the person is addicted.

Tolerance occurs when, after repeated administration of a narcotic, larger doses are needed to obtain the same effect. *Dependence* has occurred if withdrawal symptoms emerge when the narcotic is stopped abruptly. In either case, this means that once the medication is no longer needed, the dosage will have to be tapered down to avoid withdrawal symptoms.

Addiction, although also based on physiologic changes associated with drug use, has a psychologic and behavioral component characterized by continuous craving for the substance. Addicted people will use a drug to relieve psychologic symptoms even after the physical pain is gone.

The chronic use of narcotics for pain relief may lead to addictive use in vulnerable individuals, but even if someone is addicted, the pain should still be treated and narcotics should not be withheld if they are the drugs of choice for the pain condition. Ironically, undertreating the pain because of fear of fostering addiction actually encourages a pattern of drug-seeking and drug-hoarding behaviors.[119]

Sickle Cell Trait

Sickle cell trait is not a disease but rather a heterozygous condition in which the individual has the mutant gene from only one parent (β^s gene), and the normal gene (β^A globin gene), resulting in the production of both Hb S and Hb A, with a predominance of Hb A (60%) over Hb S (40%). One in 12 African Americans has the sickle cell trait,[241] and many other races and nationalities also carry the genetic defect. The gene has persisted because heterozygotes gain slight protection against falciparum malaria.

Under normal circumstances, sickle cell trait is rarely symptomatic; symptoms may occur with conditions associated with marked hypoxia and at high altitudes. No increased risk is evident for individuals with sickle cell trait who undergo general anesthesia, and a normal life expectancy is predicted. It was previously reported that no increased risk of sudden death was evident for those who participate in athletics, but a small number of cases have now been reported. However, it remains controversial whether the pathogenesis of these exercise-related deaths involved microvascular obstruction by sickled erythrocytes because sickling can occur postmortem. The recommendations are that athletes with sickle cell trait adhere to compliance with general guidelines for fluid replacement and acclimatization to hot conditions and altitude.[315]

In 2010, the National Collegiate Athletic Association (NCAA) recommended all players be screened for sickle cell trait as a prerequisite prior to participation in athletics.[340] The American Society of Hematology, however, does not support this recommendation, commenting that it could harm the student athletes and the sickle cell community because all athletes should adhere to rules for hydration and avoiding adverse conditions, like any other athlete.[2,182] More research needs to be completed to substantiate this policy.[132]

The Thalassemias

Definition. The thalassemias are a group of inherited disorders of Hb synthesis with abnormalities in one or more of the four globin genes. Hb is composed of four protein chains: two α-globin chains and two β-globin chains (see Fig. 14-16). These four proteins are attached to heme (iron and protoporphyrin), which allows a molecule of oxygen to reversibly bind to this complex molecule.

Depending on which globin chain is affected, people may have β-thalassemia or α-thalassemia. α-Thalassemia is common among people from Africa, the Mediterranean (*thalassa* is Greek for "sea," referring to early cases of SCD reported around the Mediterranean), the Middle East, and Asia. β-Thalassemia is most prevalent in the Mediterranean, Southeast Asia, India, and Pakistan.

Overview and Pathogenesis. The thalassemias are characterized by abnormalities in the globin genes leading to incomplete or abnormal formation of Hb. This results in ineffective erythropoiesis and chronic hemolysis. Because there are four α-globin genes, several diseases can occur.

Clients who lack only one α gene (−α/αα) manifest no clinical symptoms and are carriers of the disorder. If two α genes are deleted (−,α or −α/−α), this condition is termed α-thalassemia trait and results in mild anemia. Hb H disease is characterized by three α gene deletions (−,−α) and results in severe anemia, CHF, and death. Fetal death occurs when all four of the α genes are deleted (hydrops fetalis).

Whereas α-thalassemia occurs with gene deletions, β-thalassemia is a heterogenous group of disorders caused by various genetic anomalies (usually point mutations), resulting in defects in the production of β-globin chains.

Thalassemia major (β°, also called Cooley anemia) results from significant genetic defects in both β-globin genes, leading to a lack of β-globin chain synthesis. β-Thalassemia intermedia is caused by a mutation in each of the β-globin genes, with one mutation being mild, allowing for more β-globin chains to be produced with improved function compared with β-thalassemia major.

β-Thalassemia trait (β+) is characterized by only one gene having a mutation. Normally, the α- and β-globin chains are produced in an even ratio. When thalassemia occurs, there is a mismatch of globin chains produced. In persons affected with severe mutations, there are five to six times the number of normal precursor erythrocytes and 15 times the number of cells in apoptosis (programmed cell death) in the bone marrow as the body attempts to compensate for anemia. The cells that are released from the bone marrow may be rigid and unable to adapt to the size of the small capillaries or cleared by the immune system, resulting in hemolysis.[297]

Clinical Manifestations. α-Thalassemia is not as common as β-thalassemia. The clinical manifestations of β-thalassemia vary depending on the severity and number of mutations. The clinical manifestations of thalassemia are primarily attributable to (1) defective synthesis of Hb (ineffective erythropoiesis), (2) structurally impaired RBCs, and (3) hemolysis or destruction of the erythrocytes.

β-Thalassemia major exhibits the most severe complications of the β-thalassemias as a result of significant genetic mutations. Most of these complications are a result of severe anemia and iron overload (from blood transfusions and increased absorption from the gut).

Clients with β-thalassemia major require frequent and regular transfusions beginning in infancy. Anemia and iron overload lead to endocrinopathies, cardiomyopathy, and cirrhosis of the liver. The endocrinopathies can be severe, including diabetes mellitus, hypoparathyroidism, hypopituitarism, delayed puberty, testicular and ovarian failure, and hypothyroidism.

These endocrine problems along with the anemia result in decreased bone mineral density, bone deformities,

and osteoporosis (increasing the risk for pathologic fractures).[130] Even with appropriate management (i.e., well-transfused and iron-chelated individuals with thalassemia major), osteoporosis affects 40% to 50% of all affected children and adults.[130]

As a reaction to the anemia, the body attempts to compensate by making erythrocytes in extramedullary locations, including the spleen and liver (causing hepatosplenomegaly). Because the bone marrow is filled with more cells than normal, there is bone expansion (often noted on the skull).

Multiple and frequent transfusions place the client at risk for all complications related to transfusions, although cardiomyopathy is the most common cause of death.[297] Clients with thalassemia intermedia exhibit mild to moderate anemia. Transfusion requirements are less than that received by clients with thalassemia major, but depending on the severity of the mutations, clients may still develop splenomegaly, iron overload, and bone deformities. Persons with the thalassemia trait typically have mild or no anemia. Their erythrocytes may be very small, but splenomegaly and bone deformities do not develop.

MEDICAL MANAGEMENT

DIAGNOSIS. Diagnosis is by laboratory testing. The peripheral blood smear may demonstrate target cells (RBCs that appear like a target), fragments of erythrocytes (because of hemolysis), and very small RBCs (see Fig. 14-2). The serum bilirubin and fecal and urinary urobilinogen levels may be elevated due to the severe hemolysis of abnormal cells. Electrophoresis is usually diagnostic for all types of thalassemia except α-thalassemia trait (requires a reference laboratory for gene deletion studies).

TREATMENT. The anemia associated with thalassemia intermedia may range from mild (not requiring transfusions) to more moderate, requiring occasional transfusions. The goal is to maintain an Hb level of 9 to 10 g/dL, which allows for more normal development and growth and reduces the incidence of hepatosplenomegaly and bone deformities. Clients requiring more frequent transfusions can develop clinical manifestations as described above.

Treatment for thalassemia major consists of optimizing transfusions, providing chelation therapy for iron overload, and implementing hormone replacement as needed. Splenectomy can decrease transfusion requirements. Thalassemia major requires lifelong transfusion, which places these persons at risk for transfusion-related infectious diseases. HSCT is a possible curative treatment option, although long-term complications can be significant.[175]

The blood supply in the United States is rigorously tested, resulting in a significantly decreased incidence of hepatitides B and C and HIV, although transmission of these viruses can still occur. Most blood is also leukodepleted (WBCs removed) to reduce the problems of transfusion reactions and cytomegalovirus transmission.

Chelators remove iron from the bloodstream, and routine use in these clients has led to a doubling of life expectancy.[143] Deferoxamine is the most common agent given, although intravenous dosing and side effects make its use difficult. Newer oral chelating agents are being developed, including deferiprone and deferasirox. These drugs also have several significant adverse effects, although it does provide the advantages of oral administration. An experimental approach is to combine the two drugs to provide intracellular chelation along with good plasma chelation. Progressive disease (or in clients who do not respond to chelation therapy) often requires hormone replacement. Clients can receive growth hormone, hormone replacement for testicular and ovarian failure, insulin for diabetes, levothyroxine for hypothyroidism, and calcium and vitamin D (and perhaps bisphosphonates) for osteoporosis.

Other experimental treatments include agents that increase fetal Hb production, such as histone deacetylase inhibitors, 5-azacytidine, and hydroxyurea, although transfusion decreases the responsiveness of the bone marrow to these agents.[234,260]

Human recombinant erythropoietin and antioxidants may aid in treatment, but guidelines and study results are still pending. Gene therapy has been successful in animal (mice) studies, but enormous hurdles need to be crossed to be clinically feasible.[86,216,351]

PROGNOSIS. Thalassemia trait does not affect life expectancy, but clients who carry the mutation need genetic counseling. Until recently the outlook for clients with thalassemia major has been poor, with lethal, severe hemolytic anemia and subsequent iron overload and dysfunction of almost all organ systems.

Children are significantly delayed in growth and development; delay of puberty is universal and many die before puberty. Treatment with blood transfusion and early chelation therapy has improved life expectancy from early puberty to early adulthood. Death from *hydrops fetalis* occurs in homozygous α-thalassemia and consistently results in stillbirth or death in utero.

SPECIAL IMPLICATIONS FOR THE THERAPIST 14-17

β-*Thalassemia Syndromes*

Intervertebral disc degeneration is also possible caused by transfusional iron overload or the use of deferoxamine.[130] Back pain is common secondary to osteoporosis, compression fractures, and disc degeneration.[73] Spinal asymmetry and scoliosis are also common in this group of individuals. Progression of deformity is less than reported in individuals with idiopathic scoliosis and is mainly attributed to anemia, hemosiderosis, iron chelation therapy, and associated endocrinologic disorders. In some cases (smaller curves), the curve resolves spontaneously. Optimal treatment for any of the musculoskeletal effects (osteoporosis, degenerative disc disease, scoliosis) remains an area for future investigation.[265]

Individuals with β-thalassemia syndromes may develop soft-tissue masses in many areas, but especially along the paraspinal region. Neural compression can result in back pain, lower extremity pain, paresthesia, abnormal proprioception, exaggerated or brisk deep tendon reflexes, Babinski response, Lasègue sign, ankle clonus, urgency of urination, and bowel incontinence.[129] For an excellent review of spine involvement in individuals with this condition, the reader is referred to Haidar.[130]

REFERENCES

To enhance this text and add value for the reader, all references are included on the companion Evolve site that accompanies this textbook. The reader can view the reference source and access it online whenever possible.

CHAPTER 15

The Respiratory System

LORA PACKEL

OVERVIEW

Anatomically, the respiratory system can be divided into three main portions: the upper airway, the lower airway, and the terminal alveoli (Fig. 15-1). The upper airway consists of the nasal cavities, sinuses, pharynx, tonsils, and larynx. The lower airway consists of the conducting airways, including the trachea, bronchi, and bronchioles (Fig. 15-2). The alveoli, or air sacs, at the end of the conducting airways in the lower respiratory tract are the primary lobules, sometimes called the *acini*, of the lung.

Physiologically, lung function is comprised of ventilation and respiration. *Ventilation* is the ability to move the air in and out of the lungs via a pressure gradient. *Respiration* is the gas exchange that supplies oxygen to the blood and body tissues and removes carbon dioxide. Pathology or impairment of the airways, lungs, chest wall, and diaphragm will affect ventilation. Pathology of the lungs and cardiovascular system, as well as peripheral tissues, will affect respiration.

Major Sequelae of Pulmonary Disease or Injury

Hypoxemia is the most common condition caused by pulmonary disease or injury. *Hypoxemia*, deficient oxygenation of arterial blood, may lead to *hypoxia*, a broad term meaning diminished availability of oxygen to the body tissues. Prolonged hypoxia will cause tissue damage or death. Hypoxemia is caused by respiratory alterations (Table 15-1) or cardiovascular compromise, whereas hypoxia may occur anywhere in the body caused by alterations of other systems and may not be related to changes in the pulmonary system.

Signs and symptoms of hypoxemia vary, depending on the level of oxygenation in the blood (Table 15-2). Exercise testing may be performed to determine the degree of oxygen desaturation and/or hypoxemia that occurs on exertion. This testing requires analysis of arterial blood samples drawn with the subject at rest and at peak exercise. Continuous noninvasive measurement of arterial oxyhemoglobin saturation is usually determined by pulse oximetry.

Oxygen Transport Deficits in Systemic Disease

Although this chapter focuses on primary pulmonary impairment, pathologic conditions of every major organ system can have secondary effects on pulmonary function and on the oxygen transport pathway (which includes the cardiovascular system). Such effects are of considerable clinical significance given that they can be life-threatening and that therapy interventions usually put additional demands on the oxygen transport system. The resulting secondary effect may include a large range of pulmonary impairments such as altered ventilation, perfusion, and ventilation–perfusion matching; reduced lung volumes, capacities, and flow rates; atelectasis; reduced surfactant production and distribution; impaired mucociliary transport; secretion accumulation; pulmonary aspiration; impaired lymphatic drainage; pulmonary edema; impaired coughing; and respiratory muscle weakness or fatigue.[141]

When assessing signs and symptoms of pulmonary disease, the therapist must consider the possibility that these are secondary effects and should investigate the nature of the underlying etiologic factors. Making as specific a physical therapy diagnosis as possible enables the therapist to identify and implement the most effective interventions.

Signs and Symptoms of Pulmonary Disease

Pulmonary disease is often classified as acute or chronic, obstructive or restrictive, infectious, or oncologic and is associated with many common signs and symptoms. The most common of these are cough and dyspnea. Other manifestations include chest pain, abnormal sputum, hemoptysis, cyanosis, digital clubbing, and altered breathing patterns (Box 15-1 and Table 15-3).

Cough

As a physiologic response, cough occurs frequently in healthy people, but a persistent dry cough may be caused by a tumor, congestion, or hypersensitive airways (allergies). A productive cough with purulent sputum (yellow

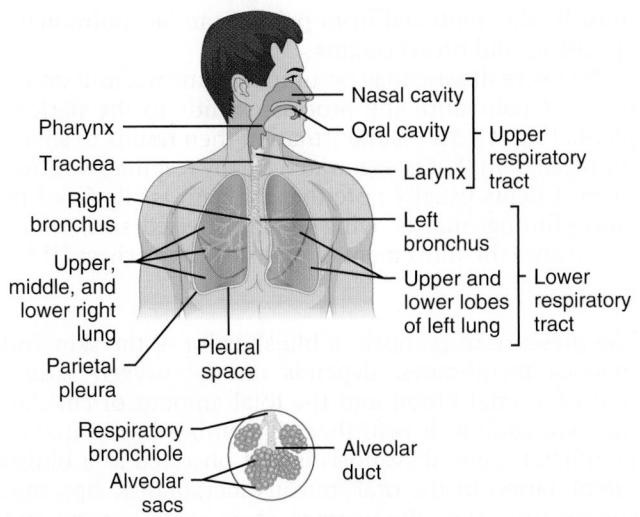

Figure 15-1

Structures of the upper and lower respiratory tracts. The upper respiratory tract consists of the nasal cavity, pharynx, and larynx; the lower respiratory tract includes the trachea, bronchi, and lungs. The circle shows the acinus, the terminal respiratory unit, which consists of the respiratory bronchioles, alveolar ducts, and alveolar sacs. This is the portion of the lungs where oxygen and carbon dioxide are exchanged.

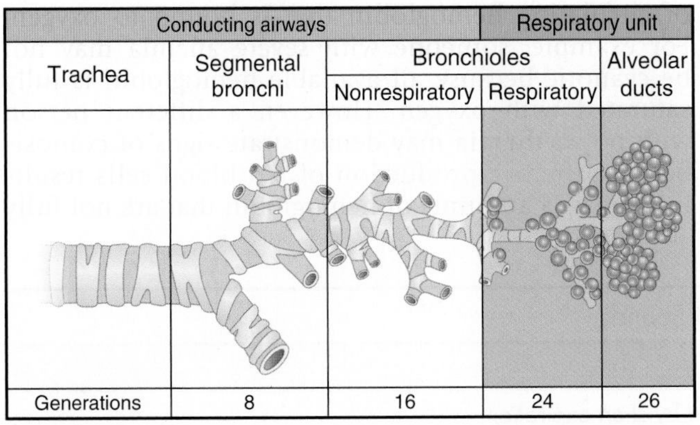

	Conducting airways			Respiratory unit
Trachea	Segmental bronchi	Bronchioles		Alveolar ducts
		Nonrespiratory	Respiratory	
Generations	8	16	24	26

Figure 15-2

Structures of the lower airway. The first 16 generations of the airways branching in human lungs are purely conducting; transitional airways lead into the final respiratory zone consisting of alveoli where gas exchange takes place.

or green) may indicate infection, whereas a productive cough with nonpurulent sputum (clear or white) is nonspecific and indicates airway irritation. Hemoptysis (coughing and spitting blood) indicates a pathologic condition—infection, inflammation, abscess, tumor, or infarction. Rust-colored sputum can be a sign of pneumonia.

Dyspnea

Shortness of breath (SOB), or dyspnea, usually indicates hypoxemia but can be associated with emotional states, particularly fear and anxiety. Dyspnea is usually caused by diffuse and extensive rather than focal pulmonary disease, pulmonary embolism being the exception. Factors contributing to the sensation of dyspnea include increased work of breathing (WOB), respiratory muscle fatigue,

Table 15-1	Causes of Hypoxemia
Mechanism	**Common Clinical Cause**
Ventilation–perfusion mismatch	Asthma Chronic bronchitis Pneumonia
Decreased oxygen content	High altitude Low oxygen content Enclosed breathing space (suffocation)
Hypoventilation	Lack of neurologic stimulation of the respiratory center • Oversedation • Drug overdose • Neurologic damage Chronic obstructive pulmonary disease
Alveolocapillary diffusion abnormality	Emphysema Fibrosis Edema
Pulmonary shunting	Acute respiratory distress syndrome (ARDS) Hyaline membrane disease (ARDS in newborn) Atelectasis

Modified from McCance KL, Huether SE, editors: *Pathophysiology: the biologic basis for disease in adults and children*, ed 3, St Louis, 1998, Mosby-Year Book.

Table 15-2	Signs and Symptoms of Hypoxemia
PaO$_2$ (mm Hg)	**Signs and Symptoms**
80-100	Normal
60-80	Moderate tachycardia, possible onset of respiratory distress, dyspnea on exertion
50-60	Malaise Light-headedness Nausea Vertigo Impaired judgment Incoordination Restlessness
35-50	Marked confusion Cardiac arrhythmias Labored respiration
25-35	Cardiac arrest Decreased renal blood flow Decreased urine output Lactic acidosis Lethargy Loss of consciousness
<25	Decreased minute ventilation* secondary to depression of the respiratory center

PaO$_2$, Partial pressure of arterial oxygen.
*The total expired volume of air per minute.
Modified from Frownfelter DL, Dean E: *Principles and practice of cardiopulmonary physical therapy*, ed 4, St Louis, 2006, Mosby-Year Book, p. 234.

increased systemic metabolic demands, and decreased respiratory reserve capacity. Dyspnea when the person is lying down is called *orthopnea* and is caused by redistribution of body water. Fluid shift leads to increased fluid in the lung, which interferes with gas exchange and leads to orthopnea. In supine and prone, the abdominal contents also exert pressure on the diaphragm, increasing the WOB and often limiting vital capacity.

Chest Pain

Pulmonary pain patterns are usually localized in the substernal or chest region over involved lung fields. However, pulmonary pain can radiate to the neck, upper trapezius, costal margins, thoracic area of the back, scapulae, or shoulder. Shoulder pain caused by pulmonary involvement may radiate along the medial aspect of the arm, mimicking other neuromuscular causes of neck or shoulder pain. Musculoskeletal causes of chest (wall) pain must be differentiated from pain of cardiac, pulmonary, epigastric, and breast origins.

Extensive disease may occur in the lung without occurrence of pain until the process extends to the parietal pleura (Fig. 15-3). Pleural irritation then results in sharp, localized pain that is aggravated by any respiratory movement. Clients usually note that the pain is alleviated by autosplinting, that is, lying on the affected side, which diminishes the movement of that side of the chest.[444,463]

Cyanosis

The presence of cyanosis, a bluish color of the skin and mucous membranes, depends on the oxygen saturation of arterial blood and the total amount of circulating hemoglobin. It is further differentiated as central or peripheral. Central cyanosis is best observed as a bluish discoloration in the oral mucous membranes, lips, and conjunctivae (i.e., the warmer, more central areas) and is most often associated with cardiac right-to-left shunts and pulmonary disease. Peripheral cyanosis is associated with decreased perfusion to the extremities, nail beds, and nose (i.e., the cooler, exposed areas) and is commonly caused by cold external temperature, anxiety, heart failure, or shock.

Clinically detectable cyanosis depends not only on oxygen saturation but also on the total amount of circulating hemoglobin that is bound to oxygen. For example, someone with severe anemia may not be cyanotic because all available hemoglobin is fully saturated with oxygen. However, a different person with polycythemia may demonstrate signs of cyanosis because the overproduction of red blood cells results in increased amounts of hemoglobin that are not fully

---

Box 15-1

MOST COMMON SIGNS AND SYMPTOMS OF PULMONARY DISEASE

- Cough
- Dyspnea
- Abnormal sputum
- Chest pain
- Hemoptysis
- Cyanosis
- Digital clubbing
- Altered breathing patterns

Table 15-3   Descriptions of Altered Breathing Patterns and Sounds

Breathing Pattern or Sound	Description
Apneustic	Gasping inspiration followed by short expiration
Biot respiration (ataxia)	An irregular pattern of deep and shallow breaths; fast, deep breaths interspersed with abrupt pauses in breathing
Cheyne-Stokes respiration	Repeated cycle of deep breathing followed by shallow breaths or cessation of breathing
Crackles/rales	Discontinuous, low pitched sounds, predominantly heard during inspiration and indicate secretions in the peripheral airways[138]
Hyperventilation	Abnormally prolonged and deep breathing
Hypoventilation	Reduction in the amount of air entering the pulmonary alveoli, which causes an increase in the arterial CO_2 level
Kussmaul respiration	A distressing dyspnea characterized by increased respiratory rate (>20/min), increased depth of respiration, panting, and labored respiration typical or air hunger
Lateral-costal breathing	Chest becomes flattened anteriorly with excessive flaring of the lower ribs (supine position); minimal to no upper chest expansion or accessory muscle involvement with outward flaring of the lower rib cage instead; the person breathes into the lateral plane of respiration (gravity eliminated) because the weakened diaphragm and intercostal muscles cannot effectively oppose the force of gravity in the anterior plane; used to focus expansion in areas of the chest wall that have decreased expansion (e.g., spinal cord injury with atelectasis or pneumonia, asymmetric chest expansion with scoliosis)*
Paradoxical breathing (sometimes referred to as reverse breathing)	All or part of the chest wall falls in during inspiration; may be abdominal expansion during exhalation, can lead to a flattened anterior chest wall or pectus excavatum
Stridor	A shrill, harsh sound heard during inspiration in the presence of laryngeal obstruction
Wheezing	High pitched, continuous whistling sound, usually with expiration and related to bronchospasm or other constriction of the airways

*From Massery M: Personal communication.

saturated with oxygen. In some instances, however, such as in carbon monoxide poisoning, hemoglobin is bound with a substance other than oxygen. Cyanosis is not present because the hemoglobin is fully bound, but because the hemoglobin is not bound to oxygen, there is inadequate tissue oxygenation and potential tissue death.

Arterial saturation in central cyanosis is usually decreased, whereas arterial saturation may be normal in peripheral cyanosis. In the case of peripheral cyanosis,

vasoconstriction with decreased blood supply and perfusion rather than unsaturated blood is the underlying cause of symptoms.

Clubbing

Thickening and widening of the terminal phalanges of the fingers and toes result in a painless club-like appearance recognized by the loss of the angle between the nail and the nail bed (Fig. 15-4). Conditions that chronically interfere with tissue perfusion and nutrition

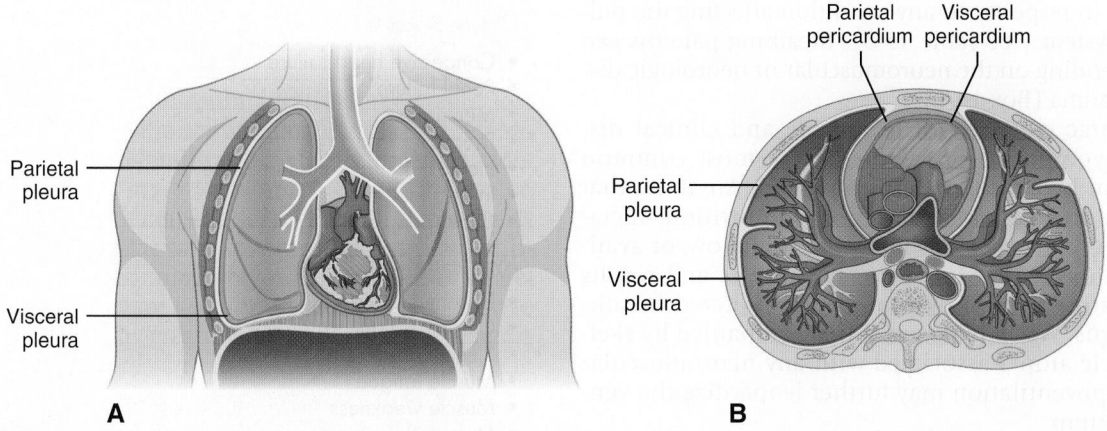

Figure 15-3

Chest cavity and associated structural linings shown in anterior **(A)** and cross-sectional **(B)** views. For instructional purposes the layers are depicted larger than actually found in the human body.

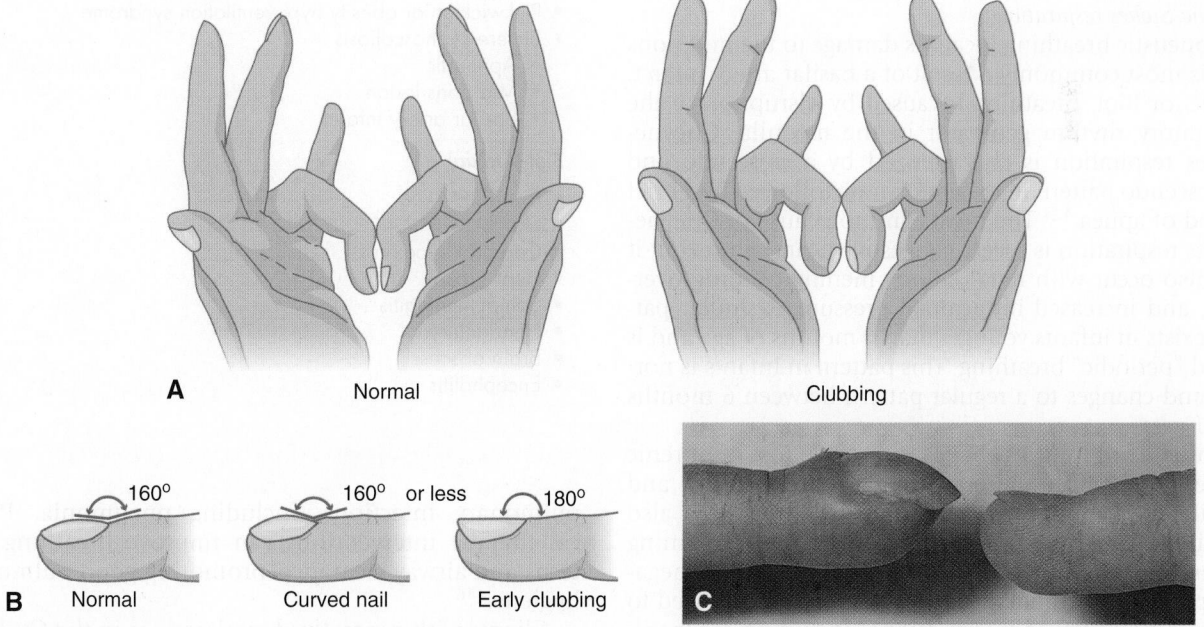

Figure 15-4

A, Assessment of clubbing by the Schamroth method. The client places the fingernails of opposite fingers together and holds them up to a light. If a diamond shape can be seen between the nails, there is no clubbing. **B,** The profile of the index finger is examined, and the angle of the nail base is noted; it should be approximately 160 degrees. The nail base is firm to palpation. Curved nails are a variation of normal with a convex profile and may look like clubbed nails, but the angle between the nail base and the nail is 160 degrees or less. In early clubbing, the angle straightens out to 180 degrees and the nail base feels spongy to palpation. **C,** Photograph of advanced clubbing of the finger *(left)* compared with normal finger *(right)*. (A and B, from Swartz MH: *Textbook of physical diagnosis: history and examination,* Philadelphia, 1989, WB Saunders; C, from Swartz MH: *Textbook of physical diagnosis: history and examination,* ed 6, Philadelphia, 2009, WB Saunders.)

may cause clubbing, including cystic fibrosis (CF), chronic obstructive pulmonary disease (COPD), lung cancer, bronchiectasis, pulmonary fibrosis, congenital heart disease, and lung abscess. Although 75% to 85% of clubbing is caused by pulmonary disease and resultant hypoxia (diminished availability of blood to the body tissues), clubbing does not always indicate lung disease. It is sometimes present in heart disease, peripheral vascular disease, and disorders of the liver and gastrointestinal tract.

Altered Breathing Patterns

Changes in the rate, depth, regularity, and effort of breathing occur in response to any condition affecting the pulmonary system (see Table 15-3). Breathing patterns can vary, depending on the neuromuscular or neurologic disease or trauma (Box 15-2).

In a large cross-section of people and clinical disorders, hypoventilation is one of the most common changes in breathing patterns observed. Anything that can cause hypoxemia (e.g., fever, malnutrition, metabolic disturbance, loss of blood or blood flow, or availability of oxygen) reduces energy supplies and results in respiratory muscle dysfunction and altered breathing patterns. When hypoxemia is accompanied by skeletal muscle atonia associated with any neuromuscular cause, hypoventilation may further jeopardize the ventilatory pump.

Breathing pattern abnormalities seen with head trauma, brain abscess, diaphragmatic paralysis of chest wall muscles and thorax (e.g., generalized myopathy or neuropathy), heat stroke, spinal meningitis, and encephalitis can include *apneustic breathing*, *ataxic breathing*, or *Cheyne-Stokes respiration*.

Apneustic breathing localizes damage to the mid pons and is most commonly a result of a basilar artery infarct. Ataxic, or Biot, breathing is caused by disruption of the respiratory rhythm generator in the medulla. Cheyne-Stokes respiration is characterized by a crescendo and decrescendo pattern in respiratory rate followed by a brief period of apnea.[424] The most common cause of Cheyne-Stokes respiration is severe congestive heart failure, but it can also occur with renal failure, meningitis, drug overdose, and increased intracranial pressure. A similar pattern exists in infants younger than 6 months of age and is called "periodic" breathing. This pattern in infants is normal and changes to a regular pattern between 6 months and 1 year.

Spinal cord injuries above C3 result in loss of phrenic nerve innervation, necessitating a tracheostomy and ventilatory support. Upper thoracic injuries may also require ventilatory support depending on the remaining respiratory muscles' ability to generate adequate negative pressure for inhalation. *Ventilatory support* is used to refer to a variety of interventions, including mechanical ventilation via endotracheal intubation, noninvasive ventilatory support with continuous positive airway pressure, positive end-expiratory pressure (PEEP), and bilevel positive airway pressure. Those with lower thoracic injuries or incomplete injuries may also have altered breathing mechanics. These altered mechanics may place the person with spinal cord injury at risk for

---

Box 15-2

BREATHING PATTERNS AND ASSOCIATED CONDITIONS

Hyperventilation

- Anxiety
- Acute head injury
- Hypoxemia
- Fever

Kussmaul

- Strenuous exercise
- Metabolic acidosis

Cheyne-Stokes

- Congestive heart failure
- Renal failure
- Meningitis
- Drug overdose
- Increased intracranial pressure
- Infants (normal)
- Older people during sleep (normal)

Hypoventilation

- Fibromyalgia syndrome
- Chronic fatigue syndrome
- Sleep disorder
- Muscle fatigue
- Muscle weakness
- Malnutrition
- Neuromuscular disease
  - Guillain-Barré
  - Myasthenia gravis
  - Poliomyelitis
  - Amyotrophic lateral sclerosis
- Pickwickian or obesity hypoventilation syndrome
- Severe kyphoscoliosis
  - Apneustic
  - Mid pons lesion
  - Basilar artery infarct

Biot (Ataxia)

- Exercise
- Shock
- Cerebral hypoxia
- Heat stroke
- Spinal meningitis
- Head injury
- Brain abscess
- Encephalitis

---

pulmonary infections, including pneumonia. Physical therapy interventions can improve breathing patterns and airway clearance, promoting good pulmonary hygiene.[446]

Clients with generalized weakness, as in the Guillain-Barré syndrome, some myopathies or neuropathies, or incomplete spinal cord injuries, may show a tendency toward a specific breathing pattern called *lateral-costal breathing* (see Table 15-3). Others who are experiencing failure of the ventilator system may demonstrate a paradoxical breathing pattern where the abdomen moves "inward" during inspiration instead of expanding.

SPECIAL IMPLICATIONS FOR THE THERAPIST   `15-1`

Signs and Symptoms of Pulmonary Disease

Many people with neuromusculoskeletal conditions, as well as people with primary or secondary pulmonary pathology, have the potential for oxygen transport deficits, impaired ventilation, and altered breathing patterns. For each type of condition, the therapist must identify those steps in the oxygen transport pathway that are affected so that intervention targets the specific underlying problem.

Monitoring the cardiopulmonary status is important because many of the interventions provided by a therapist elicit an exercise stimulus and stress the oxygen transport system. Because impairment can result from diseases other than cardiopulmonary conditions, therapists in all settings need expertise in anticipating and detecting pulmonary dysfunction in the absence of primary pulmonary disease.[141,181]

Recognizing abnormal responses to interventions is important in identifying the client who needs additional intervention or who needs to be referred to another health care professional. For an excellent review of the oxygen transport deficits concept and more detailed implications by system, see reference 143.

Clinical observation of the client as the client breathes is important (Box 15-3) and can alert the therapist to respiratory pathologic conditions. Therapists should assess the muscle groups (abdominal and intercostal muscles, accessory muscles, and the diaphragm) involved in normal ventilatory function. Techniques to improve ventilation can enhance motor performance and improve a client's functional level. The reader is referred to more specific texts for information about intervention techniques.[181,236]

High blood pressure in the pulmonary circulation (pulmonary hypertension) can cause pain during exercise that is often mistaken for cardiac pain (angina pectoris). For the therapist, musculoskeletal causes of chest pain must be differentiated from pain of cardiac, pulmonary, epigastric, and breast origins before treatment intervention begins.[207] The therapist involved in performing airway clearance techniques and pulmonary rehabilitation must recognize precautions for and contraindications to therapy interventions in the medical client (Table 15-4).

AGING AND THE RESPIRATORY SYSTEM

Aging affects not only the physiologic functions of the lungs (ventilation and respiration) but also the ability of the respiratory system to defend itself. More than any other organ, the lung is susceptible to infectious processes and environmental and occupational pollutants (see "Environmental and Occupational Diseases" below). These factors, combined with the normal aging process, contribute to the decline of lung function.

Box 15-3

CLINICAL INSPECTION OF THE RESPIRATORY SYSTEM

- Respiratory rate, depth, and effort of breathing
  - Tachypnea
  - Dyspnea
  - Gasping respirations
- Breathing pattern or sounds (see also Table 15-3)
  - Cheyne-Stokes respiration
  - Hyperventilation or hypoventilation
  - Kussmaul respiration
  - Upper chest breathing
  - Diaphragmatic breathing
  - Lateral-costal breathing
  - Paradoxical breathing
  - Prolonged expiration
  - Pursed-lip breathing
  - Wheezing/rhonchi
  - Crackles (formerly called rales)
- Cyanosis
- Pallor or redness of skin during activity
- Clubbing (toes, fingers)
- Nicotine stains on fingers and hands
- Retraction of intercostal, supraclavicular, or suprasternal spaces
- Use of accessory muscles
- Nasal flaring
- Tracheal tug
- Chest wall shape and deformity
  - Barrel chest
  - Pectus excavatum
  - Pectus carinatum
  - Kyphosis
  - Scoliosis
- Cough
- Sputum: clear or white (normal) frothy; red-tinged, green, or yellow (pathologic)

Age-related alterations in the respiratory system are based on structural changes that lead to functional impairment of gas exchange.[471,554] Chest wall compliance decreases with aging because of changes in joints of the ribs and spine, as well as alterations in collagen. This increased stiffness affects the volume of air moved and the WOB. Elastic recoil also is decreased by intermolecular collagen crosslinks. Alveolar walls flatten, surface area is reduced, and the small airways more readily collapse and trap air, reducing the capacity for gas exchange.[181,265] Thus diminished gas exchange is primarily due to increased physiologic dead space.

Many changes that occur with aging affect the lower airway, but in the upper airway the movement of the cilia slows and becomes less effective in sweeping away mucus and debris. This reduced ciliary action combined with the other changes noted predisposes the older client to increased respiratory infections.

Reduction in respiratory muscle strength and endurance and subsequent increase in the WOB requiring greater muscle oxygen consumption at any workload are observed with increasing age.[65,181] The respiratory muscles show reduced calcium transport in the sarcoplasmic reticulum and decreased production of myosin

Table 15-4	Considerations for and Contraindications to Airway Clearance Techniques in the Medical Client

Considerations	Contraindications
Hemoptysis	Untreated tension
Fragile ribs (e.g., metastatic bone cancer, osteoporosis, flail chest. Rib fractures, osteomyelitis of the ribs)	Pneumothorax; treat when chest tube has been inserted and client is stable
Burns, open wounds, skin infections in thoracic area	Unstable
Pulmonary edema, congestive heart failure	Cardiovascular system
Large pleural effusion	Hypotension
Pulmonary embolism (controversial)	Uncontrolled hypertension
Symptomatic aneurysm or decrease in circulation of the main blood vessels	Acute myocardial infarction
Platelet count between 20,000 and 50,000/mm^3	Arrhythmias
Postoperatively	Conditions prone to hemorrhages (platelet count <20,000/mm^3 must have physician approval)
Neurosurgery (positioning may cause increased intracranial pressure; can begin gentile breathing exercises)	Unstabilized head and neck injury
Esophageal anastomosis (gastric juices may affect suture line)	Intracranial pressure >20 mm Hg
Orthopedic clients who are limited in positioning	
Recent spinal fusion	
Surgical complications (e.g., pericardial sac tear)	
Recent skin grafts or flaps	
Resected tumors (avoid tumor area)	
Recently placed pacemaker	
Older or nervous clients who become agitated or upset with therapy	
Acute spinal injury or recent spinal surgery such as laminectomy (precaution: log-roll and position with care to maintain vertebral alignment)	

chains that contribute to weakness. Moreover, because of airway hyperinflation, the respiratory muscles are at a mechanical disadvantage.[394] Respiratory muscle strength is measured by maximum inspiratory pressure and maximum expiratory pressure. These measurements have been correlated with spirometry, nutritional status, and grip strength. Loss of respiratory muscle strength can lead to dyspnea and, ultimately, to ventilatory pump failure.

Normal minute ventilation of older adults is comparable to that of younger people, although tidal volumes are smaller and rate is higher. There is a significant blunting of response to hypoxia and hypercapnia from both the respiratory and cardiovascular systems, particularly at rest. The hypercapnia response during exercise is greater in older adults, contributing to more dyspnea for a given workload even in the absence of oxygen desaturation or metabolic acidosis.

Most adults attain maximal lung function (as measured by forced expiratory volume [FEV]) during their early 20s, but with increasing age, especially after age 55 years, there is an overall decrease in the functional ability of the lungs to move air in and out. This decline peaks by age 75 years, falling to approximately 70% of our maximum. Aging reduces the reserve capacity of virtually all pulmonary functions regardless of lifestyle, although a sedentary lifestyle accelerates the decline in functional capacity.[300] With age, there are decrements in inspiratory capacity, vital capacity and increases in functional residual capacity, and residual volume. Total lung capacity stays about the same if changes in height that occur with aging are considered.[394]

All of these changes contribute to the increased WOB, meaning that the older adult works harder for the same air exchange as the younger person. These changes are influenced by lifestyle and environmental factors, respiratory disease, and body size. The effects of age are not nearly as influential as the effects of smoking in causing

a premature decline in lung function and in limiting the ability to exercise.

Pulmonary complications during anesthesia and the postoperative period are significantly increased in older adults with preexisting diseases. Loss of an effective cough reflex contributes to an increased susceptibility to pneumonia and postoperative atelectasis in the older population. Other contributing factors to the loss of an effective cough reflex include conditions more common in older age such as reduced consciousness, use of sedatives, impaired esophageal motility, dysphagia, and neurologic diseases.

SPECIAL IMPLICATIONS FOR THE THERAPIST	15-2

Aging and the Respiratory System

The therapist practicing in a geriatric setting needs to be knowledgeable about the normal consequences of aging to be able to identify the origin of and differences between impairments of aging and pathology. The ability to measure and discriminate between the process of aging and the sequelae of pathologic conditions (including consideration of the impact of comorbidities) is essential in the management of impairment and prevention of functional decline. Descriptions of the normal progressive decline of the respiratory system and the physiologic effects of pathologic conditions (both acute and chronic) as these conditions relate to the aging adult are available.[65,181,364] Appropriate test measures are available for this type of differential assessment.[215]

Pulmonary Capacity and Exercise

Although ventilatory and respiratory functions of older adults undergo a process of change related to aging that begins in early adulthood, it does not appear that healthy older people are limited by these changes in exercise capacity for activities that require moderate levels of oxygen consumption (VO_2).

On the other hand, clients with obstructive lung disease have a significant loss of vital capacity and may experience SOB at relatively low exercise intensities. In fact, the older person with obstructive lung disease may self-limit exercise because of dyspnea as opposed to exercise limitation by reduced cardiovascular capacity. The normal anatomic and physiologic changes associated with aging that reduce the pulmonary reserve capacity of older adults combine with COPD pathology to exaggerate the pulmonary symptoms associated with aging.

Exercise capacity or exercise tolerance does decrease in the older adult as the PaO_2 (measure of oxygen in arterial blood) decreases. Daily physical activity can be assessed using the following categories: sedentary; sedentary with some daily activity; active through occupation or recreational activity; and trained athlete. A higher level of habitual physical activity is one factor favorably influencing oxygen delivery.

The ability to deliver oxygen to the tissues is called *maximal* VO_2 (VO_{2max}) and reflects the functioning of the oxygen transport pathway. Age-associated reductions in cardiac output may compromise the ventilation/perfusion balance, and the PaO_2 (and thus oxygen delivery) may be reduced even more.

Regular exercise can substantially slow the decline in VO_{2max} delivery caused by cardiovascular deconditioning related to age or lowered levels of habitual physical activity. Decreases in respiratory muscle strength and endurance occurring with age can be enhanced with exercise, although much of the improved ventilatory efficiency has been attributed to peripheral changes (decreased carbon dioxide production and blood lactate).[525] In other words, peripheral conditioning improves function but does not make changes in the lung parenchyma.

Weight loss appears to alter static lung volumes, suggesting that some of the changes in lung function associated with aging may be a result of the development of obesity and therefore modifiable with diet and exercise.[539] A sedentary lifestyle contributes to the normal loss of muscle mass that occurs with aging. This loss of muscle mass contributes to reduced exercise capacity and deconditioning. These changes can be slowed by exercise training.

INFECTIOUS AND INFLAMMATORY DISEASES

Pneumonia

Overview and Etiologic Factors

Pneumonia is considered an acute lung injury (ALI) where an inflammatory process affects the parenchyma of the lungs. Pneumonia can be caused by (1) a bacterial, viral, fungal, or mycoplasmal infection (organisms that have both viral and bacterial characteristics); (2) inhalation of toxic or caustic chemicals, smoke, dusts, or gases; or (3) aspiration of food, fluids, or vomitus. It may be primary or secondary, and it often follows influenza. The common feature of all types of pneumonia is an inflammatory pulmonary response to the offending organism or agent. This response may involve one or both lungs at the level of the lobe (lobar pneumonia) or more distally at the bronchioles and alveoli (bronchopneumonia).

Routes of Infection

The major routes of infection are airborne pathogens, circulation, sinus or contiguous infection, and aspiration. Nosocomial infections have twice the mortality and morbidity of non–hospital-acquired infections.[374]

Incidence

Pneumonia is a commonly encountered disease with more than 4 million cases diagnosed each year. It is a leading cause of death in the United States, claiming the lives of approximately 52,000 Americans annually. Approximately 30% of pneumonias are bacterial and especially prevalent in the older adult. Viral pneumonia, accounting for nearly half of all cases, is not usually life-threatening, except in the immunocompromised person. The remaining 20% of all cases are caused by *Mycoplasma*.

Risk Factors

Infectious agents responsible for pneumonia are typically present in the upper respiratory tract and cause no harm unless resistance is lowered by some other factor. Many host conditions promote the growth of pathogenic organisms, but cigarette smoking (more than 20 cigarettes/day) is highly correlated with community-acquired pneumonia.[11] Pneumonia is also a frequent complication of acute respiratory infections such as influenza and sinusitis.

Other risk factors include chronic bronchitis, poorly controlled diabetes mellitus, uremia, dehydration, malnutrition, and prior existing critical illnesses such as chronic renal failure, chronic lung disease, or acquired immunodeficiency syndrome (AIDS). In addition, the stress of hospitalization, confinement to an extended care facility or intensive care unit, surgery, tracheal intubation, treatment with antineoplastic chemotherapy or immunosuppressive drugs, and urinary incontinence promotes rapid colonization of pathogenic organisms.

Infants, older adults, people with profound disabilities or who are bedridden, and persons with altered consciousness (e.g., caused by alcoholic stupor, head injury, seizure disorder, drug overdose, or general anesthesia) are most vulnerable. Inactivity and immobility cause pooling of normal secretions in the airways that creates an environment promoting bacterial growth.

People with severe periodontal disease, those who have difficulty swallowing, those who have an inability to take oral medications, or those whose cough reflexes are impaired by drugs, alcohol, or neuromuscular disease are at increased risk for the development of pneumonia as a result of aspiration.

Pathogenesis

Although a common disease, pneumonia is relatively rare in healthy people because of the effectiveness of the respiratory host defense system and the fact that healthy lungs are generally kept sterile below the first major bronchial divisions. In the compromised person, the normal release of biochemical mediators by alveolar macrophages as part of the inflammatory response does not eliminate invading pathogens. The multiplying microorganisms release damaging toxins stimulating full-scale inflammatory and immune responses with damaging side effects.

Endotoxins released by some microorganisms damage bronchial mucous and alveolocapillary membranes as well as damage type II cells which produce surfactant.[418] Inflammation and edema cause the acini and terminal bronchioles to fill with infectious debris and exudate so that air cannot enter the alveoli and gas exchange is impaired, leading to ventilation–perfusion abnormalities and dyspnea. With the appearance of an inflammatory response, clinical illness usually occurs. Production of interleukin (IL)-1 and tumor necrosis factor by alveolar macrophages can contribute to many of the systemic effects of pneumonia such as fever, chills, malaise, and myalgias.

Resolution of the infection with eventual healing occurs with successful containment of the pathogenic microorganisms. When there is only mild or moderate damage to the epithelium, types I and II cells grow and restore the alveolar capillary membrane. In some with severe injury, inflammation is followed by laying down of fibroblasts and lead to pulmonary fibrosis and gas exchange abnormalities.[418]

Aspiration Pneumonia. The risk of aspiration pneumonia occurs when anatomic defense mechanisms are impaired such as occurs with seizures; a depressed central nervous system (CNS) inhibiting the cough reflex; recurrent gastroesophageal reflux; neuromuscular disorders, especially with suck-swallow dysfunction; anatomic abnormalities (laryngeal cleft or tracheoesophageal fistula); and debilitating illnesses. Chronic aspiration often causes recurrent bouts of acute febrile pneumonia. Although any region may be affected, the right side, especially the right upper lobe in the supine person, is commonly affected because of the anatomic configuration of the right main-stem bronchus.

Fungal Pneumonia. Pneumonia caused by fungi may present with mild symptoms, though some people become very ill. The three most common types, *histoplasmosis*, *coccidioidomycosis*, and *blastomycosis*, are generally specific to a limited geographic area. Other fungal lung infections primarily affect people with compromised immune systems. Diagnosis is made by culturing sputum samples.

Viral Pneumonia. Viral pneumonia is usually mild and self-limiting, often bilateral and panlobular but confined to the septa rather than the intraalveolar spaces as is more likely with bacterial pneumonia. Viral pneumonia can be a primary infection creating an ideal environment for a secondary bacterial infection, or it can be a complication of another viral illness such as measles or chickenpox. The virus destroys ciliated epithelial cells

and invades goblet cells and bronchial mucous glands. Bronchial walls become edematous and infiltrated with leukocytes. The destroyed bronchial epithelium sloughs throughout the respiratory tract, preventing mucociliary clearance.

Bacterial Pneumonia. Destruction of the respiratory epithelium by infection with the influenza virus may be one mechanism whereby influenza predisposes people to bacterial pneumonia. The lung parenchyma, especially the alveoli in the lower lobes, is the most common site of bacterial pneumonia. When bacteria reach the alveolar surfaces, most are rapidly ingested by phagocytes.

Once phagocytosis has occurred, intracellular lysis proceeds but at a slower rate for bacteria than for other particles. As the condition resolves, neutrophils degenerate and macrophages appear in the alveolar spaces, which ingest the fibrin threads, and the remaining bacteria in the respiratory bronchioles are then transported by lung lymphatics to regional lymph nodes. The infection is usually limited to one or two lobes.

Clinical Manifestations

Most cases of pneumonia are preceded by an upper respiratory infection, frequently viral. Signs and symptoms of pneumonia include sudden and sharp pleuritic chest pain aggravated by chest movement and accompanied by a hacking, productive cough with rust-colored or green purulent sputum. Other symptoms include dyspnea, tachypnea accompanied by decreased chest excursion on the affected side, cyanosis, headache, fatigue, fever and chills, and generalized aches and myalgias.

Older adults with bronchopneumonia have fewer symptoms than younger people, and 25% remain afebrile[381,382] because of the changes in temperature regulation as part of the normal aging process. Associated changes in gas exchange (hypoxia and hypercapnia) may result in altered mental status (e.g., confusion) or loss of balance and may lead to falls.

Most cases of pneumonia are relatively mild and resolve within 1 to 2 weeks, although symptoms may linger for 1 or 2 more weeks (more typical of viral or *Mycoplasma* pneumonia). If the infection develops slowly with a fever so low as to be unnoticeable, the person may have what is referred to as "double pneumonia" (both lungs involved) or "walking pneumonia." This form tends to last longer than any other form of pneumonia. Complications of pneumonia can include pleural effusion (fluid around the lung), empyema (pus in the pleural cavity), and, more rarely, lung abscess.

MEDICAL MANAGEMENT

DIAGNOSIS. The clinical presentations of pneumonias caused by different pathogenic microorganisms overlap considerably, requiring microscopic examination of respiratory secretions in making a differential diagnosis. Gram stain, color, odor, and cultures are part of the sputum analysis. A blood culture may help identify the bacteria, but bacterial counts are only positive in approximately 10% of bacterial pneumonias; 90% of bacterial pneumonias do not show a positive bacterial count.

The U.S. Food and Drug Administration (FDA) has approved a simple, quick urine test (urinary antigen testing) for detecting *Streptococcus pneumoniae* that provides results in 15 minutes. Immediate test results allow specific treatment to begin right away, thus controlling antibiotic overuse and antibiotic resistance with cost-effective targeted antibiotics. Results of the urine test should be confirmed with a culture, as there are false negatives with the urine test. Polymerase chain reaction testing) to determine the microbiologic etiology of pneumonia allows for quicker diagnosis but is not widely available.

Other diagnostic procedures may include chest films showing infiltrates that may involve a single lobe (lobar pneumonia from staphylococci) or may be more diffuse as in the case of bronchopneumonia (usually streptococci). Physical examination, including percussion and auscultation of the chest, may reveal signs of lung consolidation such as dullness, inspiratory crackles, or bronchial breath sounds.

TREATMENT. The primary treatment for bacterial and mycoplasmic forms of pneumonia is antibiotic therapy along with rest and fluids. Treatment with specific antibiotics is based on the history; whether the pneumonia was community-acquired, hospital-acquired, or extended-care facility–acquired; and on the medical status and overall condition of the client (e.g., otherwise healthy or debilitated). Airway clearance techniques (formerly, chest physical therapy, pulmonary physical therapy, and pulmonary hygiene) may aid in clearing purulent sputum.

Fungal pneumonia is treated with antifungal drugs. Viral pneumonia is treated symptomatically unless secondary bacterial pneumonia develops. Hospitalization may be required for the immunocompromised client.

A vaccine is recommended for everyone age 65 years or older; for people with chronic disorders of the lungs, heart, liver, or kidneys; for individuals with poorly controlled diabetes mellitus; and for those with a compromised immune system or confined to a long-term care facility. Immunization can provide protection from pneumococcal disease for a period of 3 to 5 years in more than 80% of vaccinated persons. A pneumococcal conjugate vaccine for routine use in infants and in high-risk children that is effective against invasive pneumococcal disease and, to a lesser degree, against otitis media and pneumonia, is licensed for use in the United States.[363,459]

The pneumonia vaccine has been successful in reducing penicillin-resistant *S. pneumoniae* in infants and in the elderly. Because pneumonia is a common complication of the flu, the U.S. Centers for Disease Control and Prevention (CDC) recommends annual flu vaccinations.

PROGNOSIS. Community-acquired pneumonia remains a common and serious clinical problem despite the availability of potent antibiotics and aggressive supportive measures. Hospital-acquired pneumonia has an even higher mortality rate. Pneumonia ranks eighth[296] among the causes of death in the United States, and currently accounts for almost 40% of hospital deaths; 90% of those fatalities occur in people older than age 65 years, largely as a result of coexisting medical problems that weaken the immune system. In adults, there is a mortality rate from influenza and pneumonia of 17 per 100,000 people.

In people 65 years or older, the mortality rate surges to 117.1 per 100,000.[91]

Highly effective prevention and treatment methods can improve survival and reduce the likelihood of developing pneumonia, but 59% of older adults do not get vaccinations that could cut the death rate in half.[522] The *Healthy People 2020* Objective 1-9c is to reduce hospitalization for immunization-preventable pneumonia to 8 per 10,000 in persons age 65 years or older.

SPECIAL IMPLICATIONS FOR THE THERAPIST | 15-3

Pneumonia

The CDC recommends adherence to standard precautions for clients with pneumonia. At the very least, careful hand hygiene by all personnel involved is essential for reducing the transmission of infectious agents (see Appendix A). Adequate hydration and airway clearance techniques, including deep breathing, coughing, and ventilation–perfusion matching should be instituted in all clients hospitalized with pneumonia. Ventilatory support and supplemental oxygen may be needed to maintain adequate gas exchange in severely compromised clients.

Preventive measures are important and include early ambulation in postoperative clients and postpartal women unless contraindicated. Proper positioning to prevent aspiration during the postoperative period and for all people who are immobilized or who have a poor gag reflex is important. Reducing rates of catheter-related and ventilator-associated pneumonia can be done following guidelines published by CDC and with appropriate hand hygiene.[56]

Occasionally, a lower-lobe infection can irritate the diaphragmatic surface so that pain referred to the shoulder is the presenting symptom. For the client with a known diagnosis of pneumonia, the breathing pattern and the position assumed in bed can indicate the client's discomfort, reveal tachypnea, and demonstrate splinting of the chest to minimize pleuritic pain (i.e., lying on the affected side reduces the pleural rubbing that often causes discomfort).

Lobes affected by pneumonia will remain vulnerable to further infection for some time, especially in the bedridden, debilitated, or in those with neuromuscular compromise. However, the client, family, or caretakers should be instructed in breathing exercises and a positional rotation program with frequent positional changes to prevent secretions from accumulating in dependent positions and to optimize ventilation–perfusion matching.

Pneumocystis carinii Pneumonia

Definition, Etiology, and Risk Factors

Pneumocystis carinii pneumonia (PCP) is a fungal pneumonia that affects people with altered immunity. The variety that infects humans is the *P. carinii*. The origin of the organism is unknown. It is possibly acquired from the environment, infected humans, or animals, fungi, or protozoa. People at risk for the development of PCP include anyone who is immunosuppressed for organ transplantation, by chemotherapy for lymphoma or leukemia, by steroid therapy, or by malnutrition. Moreover, those who take immunosuppressant medications for autoimmune diseases are also at risk.[85]

Previously, the majority of people with AIDS developed PCP during the course of their illness, but this is much less common now with pharmacologic prophylaxis. PCP has been shown to be the first indicator of conversion from human immunodeficiency virus (HIV) infection to the designation of AIDS. In a retrospective 10-year analysis of people with PCP, 6 of 18 patients were HIV-positive.[252]

Pathogenesis and Clinical Manifestations

PCP is thought to be transmitted as aerosolized particles.[85] The mechanism of spread is not fully known, but recently attention has been given to theories that point toward an infection in early childhood that either resurfaces in adulthood in immunosuppressed states or primes the host to re-acquire the infection in adulthood.[85]

PCP is mostly a disease that affects the lungs, but can occasionally spread to other organs. Infection begins with the attachment of the *Pneumocystis* trophozoite (the feeding stage of a sporozoan parasite) to the alveolar lining cell. The trophozoite feeds on the host cell, enlarges, and transforms into the cyst form that ruptures (excystment) to release new trophozoites, repeating the cycle. The cell wall of PCP also elicits a brisk inflammatory response in the host and can contribute to respiratory failure in those with a significant pneumonia.[85] If the process is uninterrupted by the immune system or antibiotic therapy, the affected alveoli progressively fill with organisms and proteinaceous fluid until consolidation disrupts gas exchange, slowly causing hypoxia and death.

The physiologic response to PCP includes fever, impaired gas exchange, and altered respiratory function. Symptoms of PCP develop slowly in those with HIV and present as fever and progressive dyspnea, accompanied by a nonproductive cough. Fatigue, tachypnea, weight loss, and other manifestations of underlying immunosuppressive disease may be present and worsened as a result of the increased metabolic demands. In those who are immunocompromised without HIV, the presentation is more rapid, with significant SOB and fever.[85]

MEDICAL MANAGEMENT

DIAGNOSIS, TREATMENT, AND PROGNOSIS. PCP must be considered in the differential diagnosis in individuals with immune dysfunction or suppression. Diagnosis is made based upon clinical symptoms, chest radiographs, and microscopic examination of the infectious agent. Specimens are acquired through bronchioalveolar lavage, tissue sampling, or sputum cultures.[85]

PCP is primarily treated with antibiotics, although some people also receive corticosteroids. While pulmonary disease remains a major problem for people with HIV, prophylaxis against opportunistic infection in people with HIV has cut the number of those infected with PCP by 91%.[85] Prophylaxis with antibiotics is now recommended for those who are immunosuppressed including those on steroids, certain people undergoing treatment for cancer, and those who are undergoing solid or liquid transplantation.

PCP is fatal if untreated and is a common cause of death in those with HIV. The mortality rates have decreased over the past 10 years, but still remain high. In those with HIV, hypotension, low PaO_2, and low CD4 count are associated with higher mortality rates.[519]

SPECIAL IMPLICATIONS FOR THE THERAPIST 15-4

Pneumocystis carinii Pneumonia

Carefully adhere to standard precautions to prevent contagion. Teach the client energy conservation techniques (see Box 9-4), as well as deep-breathing exercises. Expiratory airflow reductions that persist after the acute infection resolves have been documented in cases of PCP (and bacterial pneumonia) in HIV-infected individuals. The clinical implications of these changes are unknown but may contribute to prolonged respiratory complaints and compromise in HIV-infected individuals who have had PCP.[359] See also "Special Implications for the Therapist 15-3: Pneumonia" above.

Pulmonary Tuberculosis

Definition

Tuberculosis (TB), formerly known as consumption, is an infectious, inflammatory systemic disease that affects the lungs and may disseminate to involve lymph nodes and other organs. TB is caused by infection with *Mycobacterium tuberculosis* and is characterized by granulomas, caseous (resembling cheese) necrosis, and subsequent cavity formation. Latent infection is defined as harboring *M. tuberculosis* without evidence of active infection; active infection is based on the presence of clinical and laboratory findings.

Overview

When exposed to TB, the body can sometimes completely eradicate it through normal immune defenses. Other times, the TB will cause a primary TB infection, while in others the body walls off the particles temporarily controlling the disease. This is referred to as a latent infection that can become reactivated later in life in approximately 5% to 10% of people.[447]

TB may be primary or secondary. The first or primary infection with the tubercle bacillus is usually asymptomatic and almost always (99%) remains quiet after the development of a hypersensitivity to the microorganism. The primary infection usually involves the middle or lower lung area with lesions consisting of exudation in the lung parenchyma. These lesions quickly become caseous and spread to the hilum, where they gain access to the bloodstream and predispose the person to the subsequent development of chronic pulmonary and extrapulmonary TB at a later time.

Secondary TB develops as a result of either endogenous or exogenous reinfection by the tubercle bacillus. This is the most common form of clinical TB. Reactivated TB usually causes abnormalities in the upper lobes of one or both lungs. In the United States, development of secondary TB is almost always the result of endogenous reinfection that occurs when the primary lesion becomes active as a result of debilitation or lowered resistance.

Incidence

Despite improved methods of detection and treatment, TB remains a global health problem with an estimated 2 billion people latently infected worldwide and 2 million deaths annually from active TB.[340] The highest rates are reported from Southeast Asia, sub-Saharan Africa, and Eastern Europe (new cases 200-400 per 100,000 population).[102] Before the development of anti-TB drugs in the late 1940s, TB was the leading cause of death in the United States. Drug therapy, along with improvements in public health and general living standards, resulted in a marked decline in incidence. However, recent influxes of immigrants from developing third world nations, rising homeless populations, prolonged life spans, and the emergence of HIV led to an increase in reported cases in the mid-1980s, reversing a 40-year period of decline.

After years of rising TB infection rates, the United States has started to see a decrease in the annual number of cases (current incidence is 4.2 cases per 100,000 U.S.-born individuals, which is the lowest rate recorded since national reporting began in 1953).[340]

Foreign-born persons and racial/ethnic minorities continue to bear a disproportionate burden of TB disease in the United States. The TB rate in foreign-born persons in the United States is 10 times higher than in U.S.-born individuals. The greatest rates of racial disparity are between U.S.-born blacks and U.S.-born whites: blacks have seven times the rate of whites.[92,417] Cases of multidrug-resistant TB have continued to rise annually, and there remains a huge reservoir of individuals who are infected.

Multidrug-resistant TB has emerged as a major infectious disease problem throughout the world. The infected individual begins taking the prescribed medication, feels better, and discontinues taking the drugs that are normally required to be taken for 6 to 9 months. The disease flares up months later and is now resistant to the medications, and the infected person passes it along as a new drug-resistant strain characterized by mutations in existing genes.[180]

The AIDS pandemic, the increased incidence of TB in populations without easy access to anti-TB medications (e.g., homeless people and economically disadvantaged people), the deterioration of the public health infrastructure, interruptions in the drug supply, and inadequate training of health care providers in the epidemiology of TB are some factors contributing to the increased incidence of multidrug-resistant TB.

Risk Factors

Although TB can affect anyone, certain segments of the population have an increased risk of contracting the disease, particularly those with HIV infection and people age 65 years and older. The latter constitute nearly 50% of the newly diagnosed cases of TB in the United States and most cases of reactivation of dormant mycobacteria.

Other groups at risk include (1) economically disadvantaged or homeless people living in overcrowded conditions, frequently ethnic groups such as Hispanics, Native Americans, and Asian/Pacific Islanders; (2) immigrants from Southeast Asia, Africa (high HIV incidence), Eastern Europe, Mexico, and Latin America; (3) clients dependent on injection drugs, alcohol, or other drugs associated with malnutrition, debilitation, and poor health; (4) infants and children younger than age 5 years; (5) current or past prison inmates; (6) people with diabetes mellitus; (7) people with end-stage renal disease; (8) others who are immunocompromised (not only those who are HIV infected but also those who are malnourished, organ transplant recipients, anyone receiving cancer chemotherapy or prolonged corticosteroid therapy); and (9) women who are pregnant.

The Institute of Medicine estimates that more than half of all TB cases in the United States are attributable to foreign-born residents. The Institute of Medicine published a report calling for TB screening of all U.S. immigrants to prevent a predicted resurgence of the disease in the United States.[258]

Limited access to health care because of socioeconomic status or illegal alien status and sociocultural differences contribute to delays in seeking care and influence adherence to treatment, contributing to the rise in TB among ethnic groups, especially along the U.S.–Mexican border.[358]

Risk associated with processing contaminated medical waste has been reported,[275] and the first documented case of cadaver-to-embalmer (mortician) TB has occurred, possibly by exposure to infectious aerosols generated during the aspiration of blood and other body fluids from the cadaver.[472]

Staff members of laboratories and necropsy rooms are estimated to be between 100 and 200 times more likely than the general public to develop TB by the inhalation of the bacilli in aerosols or dried material, by injuries (e.g., cuts and accidental inoculations with infected instruments), and by contact with infected materials and surfaces. Necropsies on individuals who had undiagnosed TB while alive present a potential hazard to pathologists, technicians, and medical students involved in postmortem examinations.[116]

Environmental factors that enhance transmission include contact between susceptible persons and an infectious person in relatively small, enclosed spaces (e.g., evidence of limited transmission during extended airline, train, or bus travel has been documented)[289]; inadequate ventilation that results in insufficient dilution or removal of infectious droplet nuclei (e.g., older buildings such as hospitals, prisons, government buildings, universities); and recirculation of air containing infectious droplet nuclei. Adequate ventilation is the most important measure to reduce the infectiousness of the environment. Mycobacteria are susceptible to ultraviolet irradiation (i.e., sunshine), so outdoor transmission of infection rarely occurs.

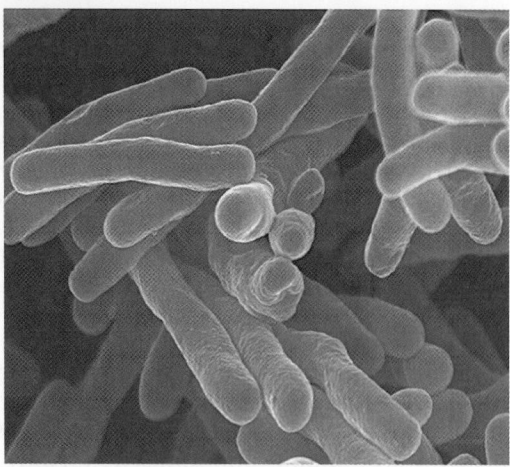

Figure 15-5

Tuberculosis bacteria. (Courtesy National Institute of Allergy and Infectious Diseases, National Institutes of Health, Bethesda, MD, 2001.)

Etiologic Factors

The causative agent is the tubercle bacillus (Fig. 15-5), commonly transmitted in the United States by inhalation of infected airborne particles, known as droplet nuclei, which are produced when the infected persons sneeze, laugh, speak, sing, or cough. The mycobacterium that infect humans are *M. tuberculosis, Mycobacterium bovis,* and *Mycobacterium africanum.*[210]

Casual contact or brief exposure to a few bacilli will not result in transmission of sufficient bacilli to infect a person. Rather, prolonged exposure in an enclosed space is required for transmission. Genetic factors determining susceptibility and resistance to the infection are suspected but have not been proven. In some other parts of the world, bovine TB carried by unpasteurized milk and other dairy products from tuberculous cattle is more prevalent.

The tubercle bacillus is capable of surviving for months in sputum that is not exposed to sunlight. Within the body it becomes encapsulated and can lie dormant for decades and then become reactivated years after an initial infection. This secondary TB infection (endogenous reinfection) can occur at any time the person's resistance is lowered (e.g., alcoholism, immunosuppression, silicosis, advancing age, or cancer).

The older people of today were children when transmission of tubercle bacilli occurred more often. Now, reactivation of the disease is developing in their later years because an increasing portion of older adults who were previously not infected are acquiring new infections in extended care facilities.

Pathogenesis

Once a susceptible person inhales droplet nuclei containing *M. tuberculosis* and bacilli become established in the alveoli of the lungs, a proliferation of epithelial cells surrounds and encapsulates the multiplying bacilli in an attempt to wall off the invading organisms, thus forming a typical tubercle.

Two to 10 weeks after initial human infection with the bacilli, acquired cell-mediated immunity usually limits further multiplication and spread of the TB bacilli.

Although the TB bacilli are walled off inside a tubercle, the bacilli are not necessarily destroyed; they can remain alive but dormant inside the structure.

No one yet knows how the TB bacterium does its damage. *M. tuberculosis* has no known endotoxins or exotoxins so there is no immediate host response to the infection. The organisms grow for 2 to 12 weeks until they reach a number sufficient to elicit a cellular immune response that can be detected by a reaction to the tuberculin skin test.

The organisms tend to be localized or focused at sites of infection. In persons with intact cell-mediated immunity, collections of activated T cells and macrophages form granulomas that limit multiplication and spread of the organism, rendering the infection inactive, or *latent.* The tubercles stay intact as long as the immune system is maintained.

For the majority of individuals with an intact immune system, latent infection is clinically and radiographically undetected; a positive tuberculin (purified protein derivative) skin test result is the only indication that infection has taken place. Individuals with latent TB infection but not active disease are not infectious and cannot transmit the organism. When residual lesions are visible on chest radiograph these sites remain potential lesions for reactivation.

If, however, the infection is not controlled by the immune defenses, the person develops symptoms of progressive primary TB. The granulomas become necrotic in the center and eventually produce fibrosis and calcification of the tissues.

Tubercle bacilli can spread to other parts of the body by way of the lymphatics to the hilar lymph nodes and then through the bloodstream to more distant sites, producing a condition called *miliary* (evenly distributed small nodules) *TB,* which is most common in people age 50 years or older and in very young children with unstable or underdeveloped immune systems.

Erosion of blood vessels by the primary lesion can cause a large number of bacilli to enter the circulatory system, where they are carried to all areas of the body and may lodge in any organ, especially the lymph system, spine and weight-bearing joints, urogenital system, and meninges. Untreated, these tiny lesions spread and produce large areas of infection (e.g., TB pneumonia, tubercular meningitis). The same pharmacologic treatment is used for extrapulmonary and pulmonary TB, although the duration may be extended for some neurologic or skeletal infections.[203]

Researchers have identified a segment of deoxyribonucleic acid (DNA) that allows the TB organism to invade macrophages, where they lie dormant for years before leaving the macrophage cells to invade the lungs or other parts of the body. Finding this genetic fragment may provide information needed to block the microorganisms from entering human cells. The DNA fingerprint identified probably represents only one of several mechanisms that permit the TB transmission and invasion.[230] Using DNA, scientists are developing faster and more accurate diagnostic tests for TB. Earlier detection improves treatment effectiveness.[271]

Clinical Manifestations

Most symptoms associated with TB do not appear in the early, most curable stage of the disease, although a skin

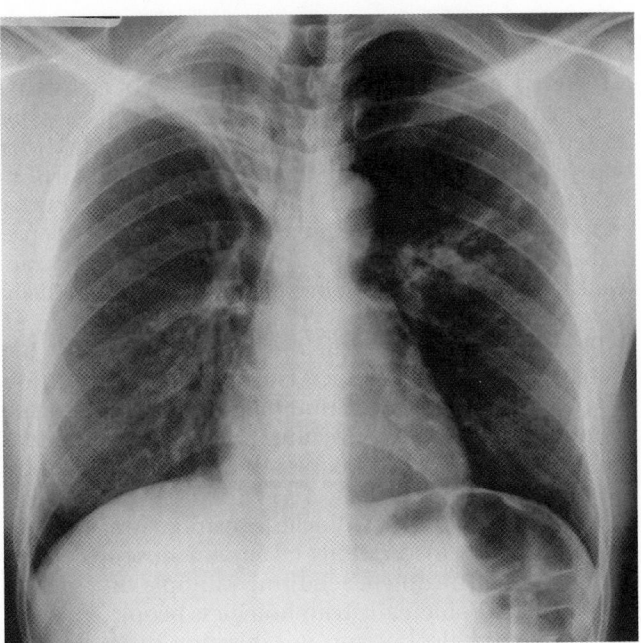

Figure 15-6

Segmental consolidation in tuberculous bronchopneumonia. The right upper lobe is grossly collapsed, scarred, and bronchiectatic. It had remained stable for many years until segmental nodular and linear consolidation appeared in the left mid zone, signaling reactivation. The segmental lesion was thought to be secondary to aspiration of bacteria from the right upper lobe. (From Grainger RG, Allison D: *Grainger and Allison's diagnostic radiology: a textbook of medical imaging,* ed 4, Philadelphia, 2001, Churchill Livingstone. Used with permission.)

test administered would be positive. Often symptoms are delayed until 1 year or more after initial exposure to the bacilli. Symptoms suggestive of TB include productive cough of more than 3 weeks' duration, especially when accompanied by other symptoms such as weight loss, fever, night sweats, fatigue, malaise, and anorexia. Rales may be heard in the area of lung involvement, as well as bronchial breath sounds, if there is lung consolidation.

Complications associated with TB can include bronchopleural fistulae, esophagopleural fistulae, pleurisy with effusion, tuberculous pneumonia or laryngitis, and sudden lung atelectasis, indicating that a deep tuberculous cavity in the lung has perforated or created an opening into the pleural cavity, allowing air and infected material to flow to it (Fig. 15-6).

Extrapulmonary involvement (e.g., abdominal, pericardial, genitourinary, lymph node, CNS, or skeletal TB) increases in frequency in the presence of declining immunocompetency. Extrapulmonary TB occurs alone (i.e., without pulmonary involvement) in one-third of HIV-infected persons and in another one-third of HIV-infected persons with pulmonary involvement.[19]

Tuberculous involvement of the brain and spinal cord (extrapulmonary TB) is a common neurologic disorder in developing countries and has recently shown resurgence when associated with HIV. In tuberculous meningitis the process is located primarily at the base of the brain, and symptoms include those related to cranial nerve involvement, as well as headache, decreased level of consciousness, and neck stiffness. Tuberculous meningitis is associated with high morbidity and mortality. Tuberculous spondylitis (Pott disease), a rare complication of extrapulmonary TB, is discussed in Chapter 25.

MEDICAL MANAGEMENT

PREVENTION. In 2007, the CDC issued revised technical instructions for TB screening and treatment for children and adults applying for immigration to the United States. More comprehensive diagnostic testing among applicants and treatment before entry into the United States may help reduce the number of TB cases contributed by foreign-born persons. The CDC is also conducting studies to find ways to reduce TB in blacks.[417]

Preventing the transmission of TB is essential and can be done by using such simple measures as covering the mouth and nose with a tissue when coughing and sneezing, reducing the number of organisms excreted into the air. However, preventive and therapeutic interventions must address not only the bacillus but also the financial, nutritional, and employment status of those people at risk.

Adequate room ventilation and preventing overcrowding such as in homeless shelters and prisons are well-known preventive measures, but preventing this infection in many high-risk groups is complicated. For example, should control efforts among the poor emphasize the amelioration of social problems or merely the ingestion of appropriate dose and duration of antibiotic therapy?

Involuntary isolation is no longer acceptable, and directly observed therapy (i.e., the client receives the antibiotics under the supervision of an outreach worker) may be a violation of civil rights. How are individuals' civil liberties and the public health best balanced? How should health professionals address the problem of the noncompliant individual? The complex issues surrounding TB in the United States remain an ongoing challenge.

The term *preventive drug therapy* has been changed to *treatment of latent TB infection.* The failure of vaccination with bacille Calmette-Guérin (BCG), a freeze-dried preparation of a live-attenuated strain of *M. bovis,* to control the global TB epidemic and the spread of multidrug resistance has resulted in renewed research efforts to develop a better vaccine.

Preventing TB disease by treating those with latent TB infection is now the most current strategy for TB elimination. This new regimen, referred to as the "12-dose regimen," reduces treatment from 270 doses given daily for 9 months to 12 once-weekly doses given for 3 months using a combination of isoniazid and rifapentine. Directly observed therapy is recommended for this regimen, and monthly clinical monitoring is advised, including inquiries about side effects and a physical assessment for signs of adverse effects.[101,473]

The 12-dose regimen is recommended as an equal alternative to other treatments for otherwise healthy persons, 12 years of age and older, who have latent TB infection and factors that are predictive of progressing to TB disease. Such factors include recent exposure to a person with infectious TB disease, or persons who have a positive tuberculin skin test or a positive blood test for TB infection. The 12-dose regimen is also an option for HIV-infected persons who are otherwise healthy and not taking antiretroviral medicines.[88]

This new regimen is not recommended for children younger than 2 years of age or for HIV-infected persons taking antiretroviral medicines, pregnant women, women who expect to become pregnant during treatment, and persons who have latent TB infection with strains presumed to be resistant to isoniazid or rifapentine. These persons should be treated with other available regimens.

The choice between the 12-dose regimen and other approved latent TB infection treatment regimens depends on several factors, including the feasibility of providing directly observed therapy, drug availability, patient monitoring, expectation of treatment completion, and the preferences of the patient and the prescribing physician.

DIAGNOSIS. Recent advances in DNA molecular techniques for the diagnosis of TB have improved the accuracy and speed of laboratory diagnosis in symptomatic people. Fortunately, some of these improved tools are appropriate for low-income settings and may help integrate new diagnostic tools into national TB control programs.[270,395]

Diagnostic measures for identifying TB currently include history, physical examination, tuberculin skin test, chest radiograph, and microscopic examination and culture of sputum. The tuberculin skin test determines whether the body's immune response has been activated by the presence of the bacillus. The skin and other tissue become sensitized to the protein part of the tubercle bacilli. A positive reaction causes a swelling or hardness at the site of infection and develops 3 to 10 weeks after the initial infection. A positive skin test reaction indicates the presence of a TB infection but does not show whether the infection is dormant or is causing a clinical illness. Other diagnostic methods, such as sputum analysis, bronchoscopy, or biopsy, may be indicated in some cases.

Because of the dormant properties of the tubercle bacillus, anyone infected with TB should have periodic TB testing performed. In the case of someone with known TB, the skin test will always be positive, requiring periodic screening with chest x-ray studies. Previously an annual examination was recommended, but currently, screening is based on symptomatic presentation (if asymptomatic, testing is not required) and job exposure (i.e., those health care workers treating persons with active TB or AIDS or HIV infection are at increased risk of exposure).

Before 2001 the tuberculin skin test was the only practical method to test for infection with *M. tuberculosis* in the absence of active TB. Newer methods using interferon-gamma (IFN-γ) release assays have been approved by the FDA as aids in diagnosing *M. tuberculosis* infection, both latent infection and infection manifesting as active TB.[340]

The new test has higher sensitivity and specificity (fewer false-negative and false-positive tests) than the old TB purified protein derivative skin test and the former QuantiFERON TB Gold-in-Tube test, which used purified protein derivative as the incubating agent. The peptide-sensitizing agents used in the test are absent from all BCG vaccine strains and most commonly encountered non-TB mycobacteria. The client only needs one appointment for the test.

TREATMENT. The American Thoracic Society and the CDC[20] have published guidelines for the treatment of TB infection. These guidelines should contribute to improved TB control worldwide and to TB elimination in the United States. Once diagnosed, all cases of active disease are treated, and certain cases of inactive disease are treated prophylactically, although it is unclear that preventive treatment is helpful in people with latent TB.[179] Treatment may be initiated with only a positive skin test even if chest film and sputum analyses show no evidence of the disease. In this way, the disease is less likely to reactivate later in life when the immune system is more likely to be compromised.

Pharmacologic treatment through medication is the primary treatment of choice and renders the infection noncontagious and nonsymptomatic. These agents work by inhibiting cell wall biosynthesis, but the intracellular response that occurs is complex and poorly understood at this time.

Drug treatments now include combinations of all primary anti-TB medications taken in 1 dose to replace the traditional treatment requiring multiple drugs daily. Treatment is problematic with homeless people and people who abuse alcohol and use injection drugs because this population is often noncompliant with the recommended 6- to 9-month treatment regimen. Children are usually treated with isoniazid and rifampin for 6 months. Multidrug-resistant TB has further complicated treatment. Treatment of resistant mycobacteria or the complications of TB frequently requires pneumonectomy.

Chemotherapy using a variety of chemical agents may be used, and often two or more drugs are used simultaneously to prevent the emergence of drug-resistant mutants. Immune amplifiers, such as IFN-γ, IL-2, and IL-12, are being tested as possible treatment alternatives. Treatment regimens do not differ for pulmonary and extrapulmonary TB.

PROGNOSIS. Pulmonary TB is a major cause of morbidity and mortality worldwide, resulting in the greatest number of deaths from any one single infectious agent. This trend is partly a result of increasing numbers of individuals infected with both HIV and TB. Untreated, TB is 50% to 80% fatal, and the median time period to death is 2.5 years. HIV-related death from TB represents 12% of all adult AIDS-related deaths.[282] Noncompletion of treatment (especially among inner-city residents and homeless people) is the primary factor in multidrug-resistant TB. Mortality from multidrug-resistant TB is high in both persons infected with HIV and persons free of HIV. The presence of meningitis and disseminated tubercular disease are two negative predictive risk factors associated with poor outcomes.[340]

SPECIAL IMPLICATIONS FOR THE THERAPIST   15-5

Pulmonary Tuberculosis

Health care workers should be alert at all times to the need for preventing TB transmission when cough-inducing procedures are being performed, but especially in cases of known TB or HIV infection. Isolation measures for anyone who may be dispersing *M. tuberculosis* must be taken both in the acute care setting and in outpatient areas. Inpatient rooms must be posted with airborne/acid-fast bacilli precautions.

If there is a high degree of suspicion or proved TB, clients should be cared for in negative-pressure isolation rooms while undergoing assessment and/or treatment. Procedures that may generate infectious aerosols should be carried out in similarly ventilated rooms. Precautions must be followed by all health care personnel having contact with clients diagnosed with TB (Box 15-4; see also Appendix A).

Therapists may be asked to assist individuals with a weak cough to generate a stronger one, either to improve ventilation or sometimes to obtain a sputum sample without undergoing the more invasive bronchoscopy. In such cases, the therapist should always check to see if the person has ever been diagnosed with pulmonary TB or had a recent TB test. When in doubt, the therapist should practice self-protective measures such as wearing a high-efficiency particulate air (HEPA) respirator or a protective mask. Training in the use of the mask and the proper sizing for the therapist are important when using these devices.

For the therapist evaluating a client with pulmonary TB, a thorough chest assessment and musculoskeletal evaluation should be performed. Chest expansion may be decreased because of diffuse fibrotic changes in progressive disease. Tracheal deviation may be present if there is a significant loss of volume in the upper lobes. Postural adaptations may have developed in late stages of the disease because of poor breathing patterns.[187] Other areas of assessment should include overall posture, gait, muscle strength, balance, and functional mobility. The therapist is referred to the *Guide to Physical Therapist Practice* for examination guidelines, as well as considerations for evaluation and plan of care.

People with TB typically have a poor nutritional status and a progressive weight loss that may have secondary effects on the musculoskeletal system such as postural defects and trigger point irritability. The effects of isolation result in disuse atrophy and cardiopulmonary and physical deconditioning, including progressive dyspnea.

Finding the balance between exercise and clinical limitations is challenging and there is little evidence that exercise is effective in people with active TB. Specific guidelines for evaluation of medical status during exercise are offered by Galantino and Bishop.[187] Exercise training for individuals with post-TB lung disorders has been shown to be effective in improving oxygen uptake, dyspnea, functional outcomes, and timed walking distance.[22,549]

Side effects of the medication can lead to peripheral neuritis that may be brought to the attention of the therapist. This and any other complication, such as hepatitis, hemoptysis, optic neuritis, or purpura, should be reported to the physician. Isoniazid-induced liver injury may present with excess fatigue, nausea, vomiting, and abdominal pain mimicking the flu. All health care workers should be alert to these symptoms in anyone taking this medication. Early diagnosis and treatment can affect outcomes considerably.[452]

Box 15-4

GUIDELINES FOR THERAPISTS FOR PREVENTING TRANSMISSION OF TUBERCULOSIS

All TB control recommendations for inpatient facilities apply to hospices and home health services and outpatient settings.

All facilities should have a supervisor in charge of infection control compliance.

All new employees (and student therapists) should be screened with the two-step tuberculin skin test or Blood Assay M. tuberculosis test (BAMT).

Doors to airborne infection isolation rooms must be kept closed.

Clients infected with TB must cover mouth and nose with tissues when coughing, sneezing, or laughing.

Cough-inducing procedures should not be performed on TB clients unless absolutely necessary; such procedures should be performed using local exhaust, in a high-efficiency particulate air (HEPA)–filtered booth or individual TB isolation room. After completion of treatment, such persons should remain in the booth or enclosure until the cough subsides.

Clients must wear a mask when leaving the room.

Anyone entering the room must wear a gown and protective mask, called a HEPA respirator, properly.

Therapists must be adequately trained in the use and disposal of masks and should use a particulate respirator (PR; a special mask)* whenever the client is undergoing cough-inducement or aerosol-generating procedures.

- The therapist must check the condition of both the face piece and face seal each time the PR or HEPA respirator is worn.
- Gloves are used for Standard Precautions
- Disinfect the stethoscope between treatment sessions.
- Staff and employees are screened for TB yearly or more if working with high-risk populations.
- Hand washing is required before and after contact with the client.
- Isolation precautions must be continued until a clinical and bacteriologic response to medical treatment has been demonstrated.
- Environmental surfaces (e.g., walls, crutches, bed rails, walkers) are not associated with transmission of infections; only routine cleaning of such items is required.
- Therapists with current pulmonary or laryngeal TB should be excluded from work until adequate treatment is instituted, cough is resolved, and sputum is free of bacilli on three
- consecutive smears.
- Home health personnel can reinforce client education about the importance of taking medications as prescribed.

*There are several types of face masks designated as particulate respirators; all National Institute for Occupational Safety and Health (NIOSH)–certified respirators are acceptable protection for health care workers against *Mycobacterium tuberculosis*. The respiratory protection standard set by the Occupational Safety and Health Administration (OSHA) requires a NIOSH-certified respirator; when such a respirator is used, the law requires that a training and fit-test program be present.

From Jensen PA, Lambert LA, Iademarco MF, Ridzon R; CDC: Guidelines for preventing the transmission of *M. tuberculosis* in health-care facilities, *MMWR Recomm Rep* 54(RR-17):1–141, 2005.

Extrapulmonary TB is much less common than pulmonary TB but occurs in 50% of individuals with concurrent HIV. Musculoskeletal and nervous system lesions are prevalent in extrapulmonary TB cases. Treatment of Pott disease follows the same chemotherapy regimen, with prompt response. Immobilization and avoidance of weight bearing may be required to relieve pain, with attention to maintaining strength and range of motion (see further discussion in Chapter 25).

For the Health Care Worker

Health care workers now take a two-step purified protein derivative test to screen for TB. The skin test is given on two separate occasions to reduce the likelihood of a false reading. For the health care worker who is exposed to TB and develops active disease, treatment will yield a "cure" if the appropriate pharmacologic intervention is followed for the full course prescribed, usually a minimum of 6 months. A cure simply means the active TB will not likely recur, but the person can be reexposed and reinfected. Treatment failure (not taking enough medication or for long enough duration) is a more likely outcome than reinfection because treatment compliance (i.e., noncompliance) is a much bigger problem.

A person with active disease who misses 2 weeks of treatment must restart the entire course and risks the development of drug-resistant infection. After 2 weeks on effective medication, more than 85% of people with positive sputum cultures convert to a noninfectious status. Although the individual is no longer considered infectious, a minimum of 6 months is required before the disease is considered cured.

If the health care worker is exposed and infected but does not develop active disease (approximately 90% of all cases), there is a 10% lifetime risk that active disease can develop; half of that risk takes place in the first 2 years. That 10% risk can be reduced to approximately a 1% risk if a single prophylactic medication is taken properly for 6 months.

In such cases, the individual is considered a "TB reactor" and will always skin test positive for TB. These individuals will require TB clearance in order to work in health care settings, schools, or other similar settings. Clearance is provided via medical documentation of treatment and with a letter from the attending physician.

The TB bacterium must be inhaled and cannot be transmitted by physical contact with extrapulmonary sites unless the organism is expelled, aerosolized, and then inhaled. Although unusual, this type of situation may be encountered during wound care involving the integument and should be approached with appropriate standard precautions.

Lung Abscess

Definition

Lung abscesses are a thick-walled cavity with purulent exudate within the lung. An abscess usually develops as a complication of pneumonia, especially aspiration and staphylococcal pneumonia. This can occur when bacteria are aspirated from the oropharynx along with foreign material or vomitus, or it can occur from septic embolus from a heart valve. Septic pulmonary emboli from staphylococcal endocarditis of the tricuspid or pulmonary valves are most often a complication of the use of illicit injection drugs. An abscess may also form when a neoplasm becomes necrotic and contains purulent material that does not drain from the area because of partial or complete obstruction. Abscesses may also occur in those who are immunosuppressed or who have CF.[368]

Risk Factors

Aspiration associated with alcoholism is the single most common condition predisposing to lung abscess. Other predisposed persons include those with altered levels of consciousness because of drug or alcohol use as mentioned, seizures, general anesthesia, lung cancer, or CNS disease; impaired gag reflex as a result of esophageal disease or neurologic disorders; poor dentition and periodontal care; bronchiectasis, and tracheal or nasogastric tubes, which disrupt the mechanical defenses of the airways.

Pathogenesis and Clinical Manifestations

As with all abscesses, a lung abscess is a natural defense mechanism in which the body attempts to localize an infection and wall off the microorganisms so these cannot spread throughout the body. As the microorganisms destroy the local parenchymal tissue (including alveoli, airways, and blood vessels), an inflammatory process causes alveoli to fill with fluid, pus, and microorganisms (consolidation). Death and decay of consolidated tissue may progress proximally until the abscess drains into the bronchus, spreading the infection to other parts of the lung and forming cavities (cavitation).

Clinical signs and symptoms of abscess include cough, fever, night sweats, and pleuritic chest wall pain. Of people with abscess, 50% present with a cough and foul-smelling sputum.[547] Affected individuals may present acutely or have a history of these symptoms for 2 to 3 weeks before presenting to the physician.

MEDICAL MANAGEMENT

DIAGNOSIS. The radiographic appearance of a thick-walled solitary cavity surrounded by consolidation suggests lung abscess but must be differentiated from other possible lesions. Cavitary lesions in the apex of the upper lobes are frequently caused by TB rather than bacterial abscess. CT may also be used to rule out malignancy or pleural effusion.[547] Bronchioalveolar lavage may be used to determine the exact microbes in the abscess.

TREATMENT AND PROGNOSIS. Treatment includes a 3- to 6-week course of antibiotics and good nutrition. If antibiotics are unsuccessful, surgical drainage will be considered. Airway clearance techniques may be helpful if the abscess communicates with the mainstem bronchi; percussion helps promote drainage of associated secretions. Other measures are similar to the treatment of pneumonia. Bronchoscopy may be used to drain the abscess. Percutaneous drainage has also been deemed to be effective and safe for refractory lung abscess.[517]

Prognosis is good if antibiotics can treat the underlying cause, leaving only a residual lung scar. However, mortality remains in the range of 10% to 20% and is influenced by the severity of the primary disease that initially caused consolidation, low albumin levels, anemia, and infection by particular microbes.[367,547]

Pneumonitis

Pneumonitis, an acute inflammation of lung tissue usually caused by infections, is discussed in this chapter (see "Environmental and Occupational Diseases" below) under its most common presentation as hypersensitivity pneumonitis. Other causes of pneumonitis include lupus pneumonitis associated with systemic lupus erythematosus (SLE), aspiration pneumonitis associated with inspiration of acidic gastric fluid, obstructive pneumonitis associated with lung cancer, and interstitial pneumonitis associated with AIDS. Consolidation with impaired gas exchange may occur in the involved lung tissue, but with successful inactivation of the infecting agent, resolution occurs with restoration of normal lung structure.

Acute Bronchitis

Acute bronchitis is an inflammation of the trachea and bronchi (tracheobronchial tree) that is of short duration (1-3 weeks) and self-limiting with few pulmonary signs. It may result from chemical irritation, such as smoke, fumes, or gas, or it may occur with viral infections such as influenza, measles, chickenpox, or whooping cough. These predisposing conditions may become apparent during the therapist's interview with the client.

Symptoms of acute bronchitis include the early symptoms of an upper respiratory infection or a common cold, which progress to fever; a dry, irritating cough caused by transient hyperresponsiveness; sore throat; possible laryngitis; and chest pain from the effort of coughing. Later, the cough becomes more productive of purulent sputum, followed by wheezing. There may be constitutional symptoms, including moderate fever with accompanying chills, back pain, muscle pain and soreness, and headache.

Clients with viral bronchitis present with a nonproductive cough that frequently occurs in paroxysms and is aggravated by cold, dry, or dusty air. Bacterial bronchitis (common in clients with COPD) causes retrosternal (behind the sternum) pain that is aggravated by coughing.

Acute bronchitis should be differentiated from chronic bronchitis, pneumonia, whooping cough, rhinosinus conditions, and gastrointestinal reflux disease before treatment begins.[70] Treatment is conservative and symptomatic with rest, humidity, and nutrition and hydration.

Seasonal vaccination of people with recurrent bouts of bronchitis reduces the number and severity of exacerbations over the winter months.[178] Bronchodilators are not indicated and the use of antibiotics for acute bronchitis is not recommended.[70,524]

Prognosis is usually good with treatment, and although acute bronchitis is usually mild, it can become complicated in people with chronic lung or heart disease and in older adults because they are more susceptible to secondary infections. Pneumonia is a critical complication.

OBSTRUCTIVE DISEASES

Chronic Obstructive Pulmonary Disease

Definition

COPD refers to chronic progressive airflow limitation that is not fully reversible and includes chronic bronchitis and emphysema.[199] In COPD, an inflammatory process attempts to repair injury to the airways, however the repair process is altered resulting in structural changes to the airways and a perpetuation of the inflammatory response.[199]

Incidence and Risk Factors

COPD is second only to heart disease as a cause of disability in adults younger than 65 years of age. It is the fourth leading cause of death in the United States, predicted to be the third leading cause of death by 2020. Fourteen million people were diagnosed with COPD in 2009 with an estimated 12 million people who had COPD but were undiagnosed.[371]

In 2009, an estimated 14,800,000 people in the United States were living with COPD.[371] There were approximately 124,000 deaths from COPD in 2007.[142] In the years 1999 to 2006, death rates from COPD declined in men, but no significant changes were seen for women.[99] The burden from COPD is expected to increase over the next few decades as a consequence of the aging population and chronic exposure to risk factors.[199]

COPD is almost always caused by exposure to environmental irritants, especially smoking, which is the most common cause of COPD; this condition rarely occurs in nonsmokers. As with all chronic diseases, the prevalence of COPD is strongly associated with age and usually presents at age 55 to 60 years. More men are affected than women, but the incidence in women is increasing as a result of an increase in smoking by women. Morbidity and mortality rates for COPD increase with the effects of repeated or chronic exposure to irritating gases, dusts, allergens and pollution in urban environments. Other contributing factors include chronic respiratory infections (e.g., sinusitis), periodontal disease,[443] the aging process, heredity, exposure to fuels used in cooking, and genetic predisposition.

Pathogenesis and Clinical Manifestations

The characteristics of COPD pathology include airway obstruction, air trapping, gas exchange abnormalities, mucus secretion, pulmonary hypertension, and systemic features.[199] Clients will present with varying degrees of these pathophysiologic changes, depending on the severity and location of their disease.

In COPD, structural airway changes with inflammation cause airway narrowing and decrements in expiratory flow as measured by spirometry. The air that can't escape during expiration is trapped and results in hyperinflation and an increase in functional residual capacity.

Increases in functional residual capacity reduce the volume of air available for inspiration during activities and exercise resulting in dyspnea. Air trapping and hyperinflation also result in an increased anterior-posterior diameter of the thoracic cage and a flattening of the diaphragm. These two thoracic cage changes decrease the efficiency of the respiratory muscles which also contributes to dyspnea with activity. COPD is also associated with an upregulation of circulating inflammatory cytokines which are implicated in COPD related muscle atrophy.

Common presenting signs of COPD include some or all of the following: dyspnea, sputum production, and chronic cough. Dyspnea is often described as having difficulty breathing, heaviness, and having "air hunger."[199] Dyspnea tends to be progressive over time and is worse with exercise. The chronic cough experienced by people with COPD may be productive or unproductive. It is often the cough that brings person into the physician for evaluation. People with COPD may also experience neurocognitive dysfunction as a result of chronic hypoxia and systemic inflammation.[288] There

is no correlation between Global Initiative Chronic Obstructive Lung Disease (GOLD) stage of COPD and quality of life or exercise tolerance, indicating that there is a varied experience of COPD within each disease category.[515]

The pathogenesis and clinical manifestations of each component of COPD are discussed separately in their respective sections. Figure 15-7 provides a broad overview of COPD. The person with COPD often develops a characteristic look with shoulders raised and muscles tensed from SOB and the increased WOB (Fig. 15-8).

MEDICAL MANAGEMENT

The GOLD is a joint project of the National Heart, Lung, and Blood Institute and the World Health Organization that recently updated guidelines on the diagnosis and management of COPD. The 2011 GOLD standards discuss treatment strategies noting the level of evidence to support their recommendations.

DIAGNOSIS. Physical examination and airflow limitation on pulmonary function testing (see Table 40-22)

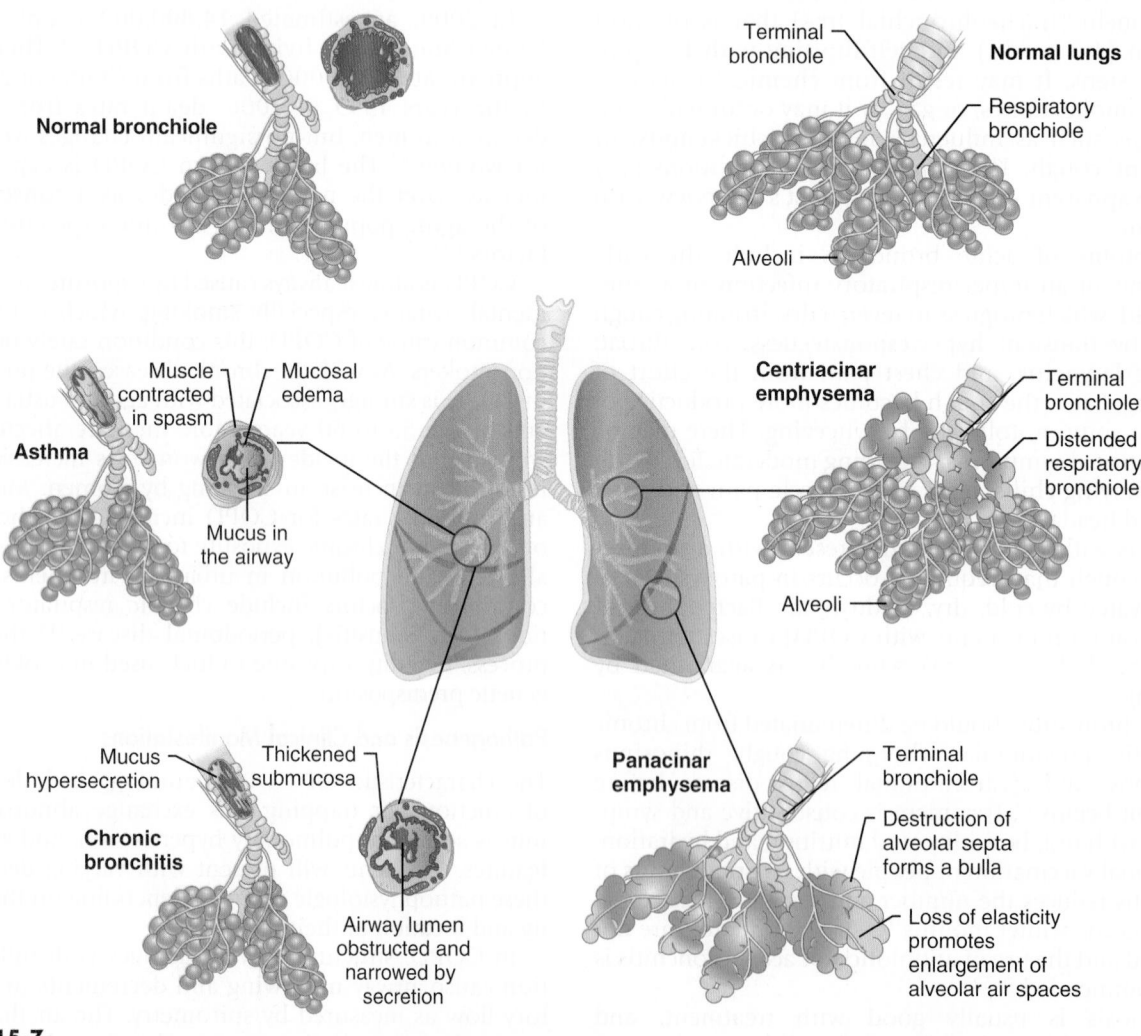

Figure 15-7

What happens in chronic obstructive lung disease/chronic airflow limitation.

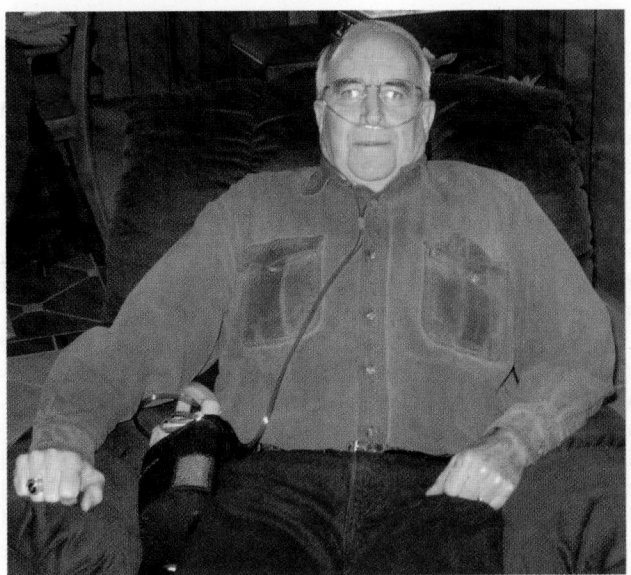

Figure 15-8

Characteristic look of chronic obstructive pulmonary disease (COPD) with shoulders raised and muscles tensed from shortness of breath (SOB) and the increased work of breathing (WOB). This man had a 30-year history of smoking 1.5 packs/day combined with asthma, eventually leading to stage IV emphysema and COPD. The effects of asthma and emphysema weakened the heart, resulting in congestive heart failure. Symptoms of SOB, productive cough, fatigue, dizziness, and muscular pain (caused by lack of oxygen) result in disability and reduced quality of life. Use of portable oxygen is required at all times. (Courtesy William T. Cannon, Missoula, MT. Used with permission.)

are assessment tools used to determine the presence and extent of COPD. COPD should be considered in anyone age 40 years or older with any of the following symptoms; progressive dyspnea that is worse with exercise, chronic cough, intermittent or persistent sputum production, exposure to risk factors, or a family history of COPD).[199]

Spirometry is the most basic and frequently performed test of pulmonary (lung) function. The spirometer measures how much air the lungs can hold and how well the respiratory system is able to move air into and out of the lungs (Table 15-5).

History, clinical examination, x-ray studies, and laboratory findings usually enable the physician to distinguish COPD from other obstructive pulmonary disorders, such as bronchiectasis, adult CF, and central airway obstruction. High-resolution computed tomography (CT) scan is used to diagnose and quantify emphysema. Most cases of emphysema involve a history of cigarette smoking, chronic cough with sputum production, and dyspnea.

Laboratory analysis may include blood gas measurements and blood pH to indicate the presence of hypoxemia or hypercapnia (excess carbon dioxide in blood) and acid–base balance, and sputum culture to identify the presence of immunoglobulin E (IgE) antibodies against specific allergens. Skin testing for allergens that trigger attacks is most useful in young clients with extrinsic allergic asthma.

Table 15-5   Classification of Severity of Airflow Limitation in COPD

Classification (For Individuals Whose FEV_1/FVC Is <0.70)	Categories of Severity	Symptoms	Measurement
GOLD (Stage) 1	Mild COPD	Minimal shortness of breath (SOB); may or may not have cough; lung function may appear normal unless tested	FEV_1 ≥80% normal (or predicted)
GOLD (Stage) 2	Moderate COPD	Moderate to severe SOB on exertion; may or may not have cough or sputum; often first stage the individual seeks medical attention	FEV_1 50%-79% normal
GOLD 3 (Stage) 3	Severe COPD	More severe SOB; may or may not have cough; reduced exercise capacity; presence of fatigue; quality of life impaired	FEV_1 30%-49% normal
GOLD (Stage) 4	Very severe COPD	Severe SOB with multiple exacerbations of dyspnea, cough, sputum production that reduce quality of life	FEV_1 <30% normal FEV_1 <50% normal with chronic respiratory failure usually requiring long-term oxygen therapy

The Global Initiative for Chronic Obstructive Lung Disease (GOLD) is a collaboration between the National Institutes of Health and the World Health Organization. The GOLD COPD staging uses these four categories of severity for COPD, based on the degree of airflow limitation (measured by FEV_1, a test of pulmonary function).

FEV_1 is the forced expiratory volume in 1 second (volume of air expelled in the first second of forced expiration). When blowing out forcefully, people with normal lungs can exhale most of the air in their lungs in 1 second. Normal lung function is defined by a FEV_1 that is at least 70% of the forced vital capacity (FVC).

Because of lung damage, people with COPD take longer to blow air out. This impairment is called obstruction or airflow limitation. An FEV_1 less than 70% of FVC contributes to the diagnosis of COPD in someone with compatible symptoms and history. As COPD progresses, FEV_1 tends to decline (i.e., the lower the FEV_1, the worse the airflow limitation).

Adapted from the Global Strategy for the Diagnosis, Management and Prevention of COPD, Global Initiative for Chronic Obstructive Lung Disease (GOLD) 2011. Available online at http://www.goldcopd.org/.

A THERAPIST'S THOUGHTS*
Spirometry

Because spirometry is based on a maximal forced exhalation, the accuracy of its results are highly dependent on the person's understanding, cooperation, and best efforts. Spirometry differs from peak flow readings in that spirometry records the entire forced breathing capacity against time, and peak flow records the largest breathing flow that can be sustained for 10 milliseconds. Both are often used to assess results in the management of asthma.

The spirometer measures the expired airflow rate and volume in a specific time period. COPD is diagnosed when the FEV_1/FVC ratio is <0.70 after a bronchodilator has been given. In the past, FEV_1 was used to diagnose COPD, with predicted values based on age, height, gender, and body weight. Using the fixed ratio of FEV_1/FVC to diagnose COPD eliminates the need for reference values. This is important, as there weren't validated reference values for all races and ethnicities.

Other spirometry measures such as FEV_1 still require the use of reference values and are reported as a percentage of predicted values. Individuals with similar decrements in FEV_1 can experience a variety of symptoms and also a varied impact on their quality of life. It is important to assess the impact that COPD has on the person's function, as spirometric values are insufficient to capture this aspect of health.

*Lora Packel, MS, PT, CCS, PhD

TREATMENT. The successful management of COPD requires a multifaceted approach that includes smoking cessation, pharmacologic management, airway clearance as needed, exercise (aerobic, strength, flexibility, posture, and breathing), control of complications, avoidance of irritants, psychologic support, and dietary management.

The main goals for the client with COPD are to improve oxygenation, decrease carbon dioxide retention and maximize quality of life. These are accomplished by (1) reducing airway edema secondary to inflammation and bronchospasm (asthma) through the use of bronchodilator medication, (2) facilitating the elimination of bronchial secretions, (3) preventing and treating respiratory infection, (4) increasing exercise tolerance, (5) controlling complications, (6) avoiding airway irritants and allergens, (7) relieving anxiety and treating depression, which often accompany COPD, and (8) exercising to improve muscle oxidative capacity.

Common classifications of medications used in the treatment of COPD include oral or inhaled bronchodilators (β_2 agonists or anticholinergics), antiinflammatory agents, antibiotics, mucolytic expectorants, mast cell membrane stabilizers, and antihistamines (Table 15-6). Combining bronchodilators helps to reduce exacerbations and improves lung function.[154] Systemic corticosteroids are of some help in acute exacerbations of COPD but have some immediate side effects, such as hyperglycemia and hypertension[543] and osteoporosis and proximal muscle weakness (steroid myopathy), without producing any long-term benefits.[376]

Pneumococcal vaccination for the person with COPD decreases mortality rates and hospitalizations and is recommended for former smokers, current smokers, and all people with COPD.[304] Annual prophylactic vaccination against influenza is also recommended.

Long-term oxygen treatment, defined as longer than 15 hours per day,[199] reduces morbidity and extends life in clients with significant daytime hypoxemia.[123,288] People with PaO_2 of 55 or less, or a resting oxygen saturation of 88% or less, measured at two time periods 3 weeks apart (see Table 15-2), are considered for long-term oxygen therapy.[199] Oxygen therapy is also considered for those who desaturate during sleep or exercise although the present research does not show a survival advantage for oxygen therapy in those with mild daytime hypoxia or nocturnal hypoxia.[288]

Surgical treatment for COPD may include lung-volume reduction surgery (LVRS) requiring thoracotomy or minimally invasive bronchoscopic lung-volume reduction techniques (endobrachial valves, airway bypass) for appropriate individuals. In surgical LVRS, large bullae or overdistended nonfunctional alveoli are removed, enabling compressed lung tissue to reexpand, thereby reducing overall dead space. LVRS is most successful in those with upper lobe disease who have a postrehabilitation low exercise capacity, and has been shown to reduce hyperinflation, improve respiratory mechanics, and reduce morbidity.[89,199,237]

Endobronchial valve procedures place stents designed to block air from entering diseased lung tissue during inhalation but allowing air to exit during exhalation. This type of device is intended to provide one-way airflow in segmental or subsegmental bronchi in individuals with pulmonary conditions complicated by air leaks or hyperinflation.[500]

Exhale airway bypass, a catheter-based bronchoscopic procedure creates new (very small) passageways into the lung to bypass the collapsed airways, thus enabling trapped air to exit the lungs. Small stents are then inserted to keep the new pathways from closing. This procedure is also designed to allow the flow of air and secretions out of the targeted portion of the lung but prevent return flow. These pathways could potentially provide a way for the trapped air to escape when the patient exhales. If the amount of air trapped in the lungs is reduced then it should be easier for the person to breathe.[453]

Lung transplantation, both single and double, is appropriate for clients with severe COPD when FEV_1 is less than 24% predicted and/or the partial pressure of arterial carbon dioxide ($PaCO_2$) is equal to or greater than 55 mm Hg.

Pulmonary rehabilitation is a multidimensional program that utilizes exercise, group education, smoking cessation, and nutritional guidance to improve symptoms and function in those with respiratory diseases. Pulmonary rehabilitation improves exercise performance, quality of life, and feelings of dyspnea, and reduces the number of hospitalizations.[13,199,301] It is recommended for those with stable COPD and for those who are recovering from an exacerbation.

PROGNOSIS. The prognosis for chronic bronchitis and emphysema is poor because these are chronic, progressive, and debilitating diseases. In the period 1980 to 2000, the death rate from COPD increased by 67%. The death rate in men from 1999 to 2006 declined in the United States, with no significant changes in mortality rates for women.[99]

Table 15-6	Pharmacotherapy for Chronic Obstructive Pulmonary Disease and Asthma

	COPD	Asthma

Maintenance	**Inhaled Bronchodilators**
	
	β_2-Adrenergic agonists
	• Short-acting
	  • Albuterol
	  • Levalbuterol
	• Long-acting
	  • Salmeterol
	  • Formoterol
	  • Arformoterol
	Anticholinergics
	• Short-acting
	  • Ipratropium
	• Long-acting
	  • Tiotropium
	
	Oral Bronchodilators
	
	• Methylxanthines
	  • Theophylline
	  • Aminophylline
	
	Inhaled Corticosteroids
	
	• Fluticasone
	• Budesonide
		Inhaled Bronchodilators
		
		β_2-Adrenergic agonists
		• Short-acting
		  • Albuterol
		  • Levalbuterol
		• Long-acting
		  • Salmeterol
		  • Formoterol
		
		Oral Bronchodilators
		
		• Methylxanthines
		  • Theophylline
		  • Aminophylline
		
		Inhaled Corticosteroids
		
		• Fluticasone
		• Budesonide
		• Mometasone
		
		Oral Corticosteroids
		
		• Methylprednisolone
		• Prednisone
		• Prednisolone
		
		Leukotriene Modifiers
		
		• Montelukast
		• Zafirlukast
		• Zileuton
		
		Mast Cell Stabilizers
		
		• Cromolyn
		
		Anti-IgE Antibodies
		
		• Omalizumab

Acute exacerbations	**Inhaled Bronchodilators**
	
	β_2-Adrenergic agonists
	• Short-acting
	  • Albuterol
	  • Levalbuterol
	Anticholinergics
	• Short-acting
	  • Ipratropium
	
	Oral and Intravenous Corticosteroids
	
	• Methylprednisolone
	• Prednisone
	• Prednisolone
	
	Antibiotics
	
	• Macrolides
	• Cephalosporins
	• Fluoroquinolones
	• Doxycycline
		Inhaled Bronchodilators
		
		β_2-Adrenergic agonists
		• Short-acting
		  • Albuterol
		  • Levalbuterol
		Anticholinergics
		• Short-acting
		  • Ipratropium
		
		Oral and Intravenous Corticosteroids
		
		• Methylprednisolone
		• Prednisone
		• Prednisolone

Sources for pharmacotherapy updates: Global Initiative for Chronic Obstructive Lung Disease, Inc. Global initiative for chronic obstructive lung disease. *Global strategy for the diagnosis, management, and prevention of chronic obstructive pulmonary disease* (12/2011). Available at: http://www.goldcopd.org/uploads/users/files/GOLD_Report_2011_Feb21.pdf. Accessed July 17, 2012; and National Heart, Lung, and Blood Institute. *National asthma education and prevention program. Expert panel report 3: guidelines for the diagnosis and management of asthma. Full report 2007* (8/28/2007). Available at: http://www.nhlbi.nih.gov/guidelines/asthma/asthgdln.pdf. Accessed July 18, 2012.

COPD is largely preventable, and many believe that early recognition of small airway obstruction with appropriate treatment and cessation of smoking may prevent disease progression. Early treatment of airway infections and vaccination against influenza and pneumococcal disease have an effect on morbidity and mortality of individuals with COPD as do public health campaigns that address environmental toxins.

There is no cure for COPD, but smoking cessation increases the survival rate. Pulmonary rehabilitation also increases survival,[18] improves quality of life, decreases hospitalizations, and decreases incidence of COPD exacerbations.[18,66,451]

SPECIAL IMPLICATIONS FOR THE THERAPIST | 15-6

Chronic Obstructive Pulmonary Disease
Pulmonary Rehabilitation

Pulmonary rehabilitation (PR) is effective in reducing the risk of hospitalization, reducing mortality, improving health-related quality of life, and increasing exercise capacity.[420] The PR model is a multidimensional approach to improving quality of life and includes airway clearance techniques, exercise, smoking cessation, nutrition and weight control, psychosocial support, lifestyle modification, and optimal medical care.[181]

Treatment of COPD includes breathing exercises, airway clearance techniques, physical training, a program to improve posture, and conditioning of respiratory musculature. For the motivated child with asthma, breathing exercises and controlled breathing are of value in preventing overinflation, improving the strength of respiratory muscles and the efficiency of the cough, and reducing the WOB.

People with COPD often adopt a sedentary lifestyle, which leads to progressive deconditioning. Deconditioning will lead to progressive deterioration in limb and respiratory muscle function that could adversely affect exercise capacity. A focus on education is key in helping clients with COPD make important lifestyle changes (e.g., increasing physical activity, reducing smoking), taking medications as prescribed, and seeking care early on for any signs of new onset upper respiratory infection.[269]

Although there is little evidence that rehabilitation efforts can result in improved pulmonary function or arterial blood gases, there is strong and growing evidence that programs that include exercise retraining can result in significant benefits, such as reduced hospitalizations, increased exercise tolerance, reduced dyspnea, improved skills in using inspiratory muscle training devices, increased independent activities of daily living skills, and increased sense of well-being and quality of life.[426]

Exercise

Exercise limitation is a common and disturbing manifestation of COPD. The skeletal muscle dysfunction seen in COPD is associated with increased mortality, reduced exercise capacity, and increased use of health care resources.[288] Muscle weakness is caused by a combination of factors, including deconditioning, chronic hypoxia, and systemic inflammation.[288] Hypoxia is implicated as the initiating factor for systemic inflammation as well as for an increase in oxidative stress, which causes muscle weakness and decreased aerobic capacity. Exercise tolerance can be improved despite the presence of fixed structural abnormalities in the lung. This suggests that factors other than lung function impairment (e.g., deconditioning and peripheral muscle dysfunction) play a predominant role in limiting exercise capacity in people with COPD.

Muscle weakness in stable COPD does not affect all muscles the same. For example, proximal upper limb muscle strength may be impaired more than distal upper limb muscle strength, peripheral muscle may be limited mainly by endurance capacity, and the diaphragm muscle may be altered structurally (e.g., changes in muscle length and configuration affecting the mechanical force and action)[86] and limited in strength capacity.

Clients with COPD must be encouraged to remain active, with specific attention directed toward activities they enjoy. Training in pacing and energy conservation (see Box 9-4) allows even those with limited exercise tolerance to increase their daily activities. Exercise testing, individualized to the specific client's needs and goals, is used to determine the person's baseline and for prescribing a training regimen. Oximetry, heart rate, respiratory rate, and blood pressure are routinely monitored, and blood gases or expired gases may be used to assess response to testing. Respiratory muscle strength testing is measured as maximum inspiratory and expiratory pressures.[181]

Pursed-lip breathing helps slow the respiratory rate and prevent airway collapse during exhalation. The client is instructed to inhale through the nose and exhale with the lips pursed in a whistling or kissing position. Each inhalation should take about 4 seconds and each exhalation about 6 seconds.

Effective coughing techniques can help to improve inspiratory volume for secretion mobilization and collateral ventilation and expiratory techniques can improve expectoration of secretions. Diaphragmatic breathing may be helpful to those with mild disease, but is not indicated in those with moderate or severe COPD as the result of structural changes in the shape of the diaphragm from hyperinflation. Respiratory muscle training with resistive loads is controversial in PR, with studies both supporting and refuting its role.

People with chronic airflow obstruction report disabling dyspnea when performing seemingly trivial tasks (e.g., activity with unsupported arms). Some muscles of the upper torso and shoulder girdle share both a respiratory and a positional function for the arms, resulting in functional limitations in many clients with lung disease during unsupported upper extremity activities.

Simple arm elevation results in significant increases in metabolic and ventilatory requirements in clients with long-term airflow limitations. PR that includes upper extremity training (progressive resistance exercises) reduces metabolic and ventilatory requirements for arm elevation. This type of program may allow clients with COPD to perform sustained upper extremity activities with less dyspnea.[193]

Lower-extremity training should be included routinely in the exercise prescription. The choice of type and intensity of training should be based primarily on the individual's baseline functional status, symptoms, needs, and long-term goals. Continuous walking is the most common form of exercise for COPD although more recent evidence supports the use of high-intensity interval training. This type of training utilizes the overload principle, but because of the rest breaks, elicits a lower lactate response and lower ratings of perceived exertion.[301] Swimming is a preferred exercise option for clients with bronchial asthma (see next discussion).

When tolerated, high-intensity (continuous or interval), short-term training may lead to greater improvements in quality of life and aerobic fitness than low-intensity training of longer duration, but it is not absolutely necessary to achieve gains in exercise endurance.[66,184] Therapists working with these clients should encourage them to maintain hydration by drinking fluids (including before, during, and after exercise) to prevent mucous plugs from hardening and to take medications as prescribed.

Exercise tolerance may improve after exercise training (including weight training)[142] because of gains in aerobic fitness or peripheral muscle strength,[112a,331] enhanced mechanical skill and efficiency of exercise, improvements in respiratory muscle function, breathing pattern, or lung hyperinflation. Exercise improves muscle oxidative capacity and recovery in individuals with COPD.[419]

Exercise training can also reduce anxiety, fear, and dyspnea previously associated with exercise in the deconditioned person. Exercises for flexibility, posture, and motor control can improve mechanical and kinetic efficiency and thus can reduce oxygen demand during daily activities and exercise.

Gains made in exercise tolerance, peripheral and respiratory muscle strength, and quality of life can last up to 2 years after a limited duration (6- to 12-week) rehabilitation program.[66,495] The optimal duration for an exercise program remains unknown; a 7-week course provides greater benefits than a 4-week course in terms of improvements in health status. Further studies in this area are needed.[211] Intensity varies in the literature, but the recommended minimal training zone is 60% of max heart rate achieved on a symptom limited exercise test.[199]

Monitoring Vital Signs

Using a pulse oximeter can help the therapist and client observe for a decrease in oxygen saturation before hypoxemia occurs. Oxygen saturation is generally kept at 90% or above by adjusting supplemental oxygen levels, adjusting activity level, and practicing physiologic modulation or Physiologic Quieting.[254] Altering physiologic responses using principles of self-induced biofeedback and breathing techniques may be able to help some clients self-regulate oxygen saturation levels (see reference 259 for a description of these techniques). It is important to note that oxygen is a drug and can only be titrated in emergencies or when there is a physician order allowing therapists to change oxygen dose.

Some people with COPD retain carbon dioxide and have a depressed hypoxic drive requiring low oxygen levels to stimulate the respiratory drive. In such cases the upward adjustment of supplemental oxygen levels must be monitored very carefully; increasing total oxygen administered via nasal canula higher than 1 to 2 L requires careful monitoring of the respiratory system (e.g., respiratory rate and breathing pattern), documentation, and consultation with other members of the PR team. Clinical judgment is used judiciously here. Some pulmonologists suggest it is acceptable to increase supplemental oxygen delivered when activity level increases as the individual with COPD will "blow it off." Studies to confirm this idea are needed.

Blood pressure and pulse should be observed at rest and in response to exercise, especially in anyone with COPD and cardiac arrhythmias. Most people with COPD who have mild arrhythmias at rest do not tend to have increased arrhythmias during exercise. See also "Exercise and Arrhythmias" in Chapter 12.

In people with expanded lung volumes because of air trapping,[114] such as occurs in COPD (especially emphysema), the first heart sound is best heard under the sternal area (put the scope in the client's left epigastric area) rather than the apical or mitral area. The hyperinflation of the lungs causes the heart to elongate, displacing the left ventricle downward and medially.

Lung sounds are also changed because the loss of interstitial elasticity and the presence of interalveolar septa lead to air trapping with increased volume of air in the lungs. Air pockets are poor transmitters of vibrations; thus vocal fremitus (the client whispers "99, 99, 99"), breath sounds, and the whispered and spoken voice are impaired or absent on auscultation.

This absence of the vesicular quality of lung sounds is distinctive and may be heard before radiographic evidence of COPD. On the other hand, when there is fluid in the lung or lungs, consolidation, or collapse (e.g., atelectasis), whispered words are heard perfectly and clearly. This is the earliest sign of atelectasis.

A peak flowmeter, a home monitoring device to measure fast expiratory flow (a reflection of bronchorestriction), can be used to determine how compromised a client with asthma or reactive airways may be compared to the normal values for that person. This may be a useful measure in determining response to therapy intervention and documenting measurable outcomes.

Exercise and Medication

The majority of pulmonary medications are used to promote bronchodilation and improve alveolar ventilation and oxygenation and are delivered as an aerosol spray through a device called a *metered-dose inhaler*. Although newer medications can be given in powder form, in either the powder form or the metered-dose inhaler, older adults sometimes have difficulty using the device because of hand weakness or poor coordination.

Proper technique is important to ensure delivery of the medication to the desired location (Box 15-5).[67] When medications are properly used, their effects should improve an individual's ability to exercise and

IMPORTANT CONCEPTS IN THE USE OF A METERED-DOSE INHALER

The therapist should observe the client self-administer the medication at least one time. Schedule the use of the metered-dose inhaler (MDI) for 15-20 minutes before exercise so as to maximize ventilation.

- MDIs are used to deliver medication to the lungs, avoiding deposition of the medication on the tongue and back of the throat. For this to occur, users must take in a slow deep breath over the course of 10 seconds while maintaining a good seal on the device.
- Each manufacturer has specific use instructions as well as cleaning instruction. Refer to the user manual for the specifics of each device.
  - Be sure to note directions for use, including cleaning and the need for priming the MDI.
- A therapist should evaluate the ability of the child or adult to adequately press on the device to release medication and to coordinate this with inhalation.
- A spacer may be used in conjunction with the MDI. With a spacer, the medication is released into the chamber and the user can slowly take a deep breath in without having to focus on coordinating the pressing of the device with inhalation.
  Instructions for the use of different inhalers and video demonstrations are available online. When appropriate, the therapist should review proper administration with each individual based on the type of inhaler used.

more effectively obtain the benefits of training. However, the many side effects of pulmonary medications may interfere with normal adaptations to habitual exercise so that exercise tolerance and conditioning may not occur.[82]

For example, corticosteroids mask or impede the beneficial effects of exercise. Anyone with pulmonary disease taking prolonged corticosteroids may develop steroid myopathy (see Chapter 5) and muscular atrophy not only in the peripheral skeletal muscles but also in the muscle fibers of the diaphragm. Animal studies also suggest that severe undernutrition causes a decrease in muscle energy status, which contributes to diaphragmatic fatigue.[297]

Chronic Bronchitis

Definition and Overview

Chronic bronchitis is clinically defined as a condition of productive cough lasting for at least 3 months (usually the winter months) per year for 2 consecutive years. Chronic bronchitis can exist alone in people with normal spirometry, or in combination with airway obstruction.[7,199] Having chronic bronchitis increases one's risk of developing COPD.[171]

Risk Factors and Pathogenesis

Chronic bronchitis is characterized by inflammation and scarring of the bronchial lining. This inflammation may obstruct airflow to and from the lungs and increases mucus production. Irritants, such as cigarette smoke, long-term dust inhalation, or air pollution, cause mucus hypersecretion and hypertrophy (increased number and size) of mucus-producing glands in the large bronchi. Epithelial atrophy, changes in squamous cells, and hypertrophy of smooth muscle cells occur.[484]

The swollen mucous membrane and thick sputum obstruct the airways, causing wheezing and a subsequent cough as the person tries to clear the airways. In addition, impaired ciliary function reduces mucous clearance and increases client susceptibility to infection. Infection results in even more mucus production with bronchial wall inflammation and thickening. If airway collapse is present, air is trapped in the distal portion of the lung, causing reduced alveolar ventilation, hypoxia, and acidosis. This downward spiral continues since the client now has an abnormal ventilation/perfusion ($\dot{V}/\dot{Q}$) ratio and resultant decreased PaO_2.

As compensation for the hypoxemia, polycythemia (overproduction of erythrocytes) occurs. Cyanosis results from insufficient arterial oxygenation and peripheral edema from right ventricular failure. Pulmonary vascular resistance caused by inflammation and loss of capillary beds will contribute to cor pulmonale (right-sided congestive heart failure).

Clinical Manifestations

The symptoms of chronic bronchitis are persistent cough and sputum production (worse in the morning and evening than at midday). The increased secretions from the bronchial mucosa and obstruction of the respiratory passages interfere with the flow of air to and from the lungs. The result is SOB, prolonged expiration, persistent coughing with expectoration, and recurrent infection. Infection may be accompanied by fever and malaise.

If the person goes on to develop COPD, reduced chest expansion, wheezing, cyanosis, and decreased exercise tolerance may occur. In addition, the obstruction present results in decreased alveolar ventilation and increased $PaCO_2$. Hypoxemia leads to polycythemia and cyanosis. If not reversed, pulmonary hypertension leads to cor pulmonale. Severe disability or death is the final clinical picture.

MEDICAL MANAGEMENT

In stable conditions, reducing irritants and using a combination of bronchodilators is effective. There is no evidence for use of antibiotics, oral corticosteroids, expectorants, or postural drainage. In significant acute exacerbations of chronic bronchitis, antibiotics and oral or IV corticosteroids can be effective.[71] See also "Medical Management" and "Special Implications for the Therapist 15-6: Chronic Obstructive Pulmonary Disease" above.

Emphysema

Definition and Overview

Emphysema is defined as an enlargement of the air spaces beyond the terminal bronchiole, and is associated with a loss of elasticity in the distal airways, airway collapse, and gas trapping.[287] There are three types of emphysema (see Fig. 15-7). Centrilobular emphysema, the most common type, produces destruction in the bronchioles of the upper lung regions. Inflammation develops in the bronchioles, but usually the alveolar sac (distal to respiratory bronchioles) remains intact. Centrilobular emphysema is the most common type in smokers.[287]

Panlobular emphysema destroys the air spaces of the entire acinus and most commonly involves the lower lung. Panlobular is common in those with α_1-antitrypsin deficiency. Paraseptal (panacinar) emphysema destroys the alveoli in the lower lobes of the lungs, resulting in isolated blebs along the lung periphery. Paraseptal emphysema often occurs alongside of centrilobular in chronic smokers. Paraseptal emphysema is believed to be the likely cause of spontaneous pneumothorax.

Etiologic Factors

Cigarette smoking is the major etiologic factor in the development of emphysema and has been shown to increase the numbers of alveolar macrophages and neutrophils in the lung*, enhance protease release†, and impair the activity of antiproteases. However, other factors, such as heredity, must determine susceptibility to emphysema because less than 10 to 15% of people who smoke develop clinical evidence of airway obstruction.

In many cases, emphysema occurs as a result of prolonged respiratory difficulties, such as chronic bronchitis that has caused partial obstruction of the smaller divisions of the bronchi. Emphysema can also occur without serious preceding respiratory problems as in the case of a defect in the elastic tissue of the lungs or in older persons whose lungs have lost their natural elasticity.

Approximately 1% to 5% of people with early onset of COPD have an inherited deficiency of (low levels or absent) α_1-antitrypsin, a protective protein.[157,499] α_1-Antitrypsin is made primarily in the liver, but also in lung cells, monocytes, and intestinal epithelial cells.[499] The role of this protein is to dampen inflammation, control protease activity, and to inhibit cell apoptosis. When absent or in low quantities, people with this inherited mutation are at risk for developing COPD in the third to fifth decade of life.[499]

Those with α_1-antitrypsin who are also smokers have accelerated COPD and die approximately 10 to 20 years earlier than nonsmokers. Systemic effects of α_1-antitrypsin include low bone mineral density, increased aortic stiffness, and low lean muscle mass.[157] These effects may be amenable to the risk reduction provided by pulmonary rehabilitation.

Pathogenesis

Inhaled particles impair the mucociliary escalator and induce inflammation and damage of the airways. This can lead to increased compliance of the airways, chronic inflammation, airway trapping and chronic sputum production.

---

*Neutrophils, the most numerous type of leukocytes (white blood cells), increase dramatically in number in response to infection and inflammation. However, neutrophils not only kill invading organisms but also may damage host tissues when there are too many.

†Proteases, or proteolytic enzymes, are enzymes that destroy cells and proteins. The airway goblet cells and serous cells of bronchial glands normally secrete a protein called *secretory leukoprotease inhibitor*, which is capable of inhibiting neutrophils. The cellular interactions associated with smoking result in inactivation of protease inhibitors. This results in an imbalance between proteases and antiproteases (in favor of proteases), allowing even more cellular destruction than warranted by the inflammatory process already present.

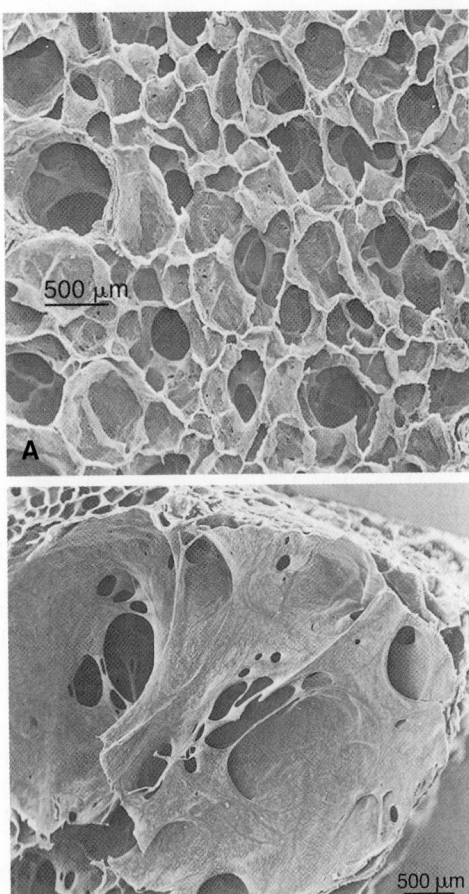

Figure 15-9

Effects of emphysema seen in these scanning electron micrographs of lung tissue. A, Normal lung with many small alveoli. **B,** Lung tissue affected by emphysema. Notice that the alveoli have merged into larger air spaces, reducing the surface area for gas exchange. (From Thibodeau GA, Patton KT: *Structure and function of the body*, ed 14, St Louis, 2012, Mosby. Used with permission.)

In emphysema, there is destruction of elastin protein in the lung that normally maintains the strength of the alveolar walls which leads to permanent enlargement of the acini. It is suspected that an interaction of accelerated cellular apoptosis, inflammation, and proteolysis causes the tissue destruction associated with emphysema.[484]

Eventually the loss of elasticity in the lung tissue causes narrowing or collapse of the bronchioles so that inspired air becomes trapped in the lungs. During exercise, this air trapping is worsened, with inhalation occurring before full expiration resulting in stacking of breaths and dynamic hyperinflation of the lungs.[287] Obstruction results from changes in lung tissues, rather than from mucus production and swelling as in chronic bronchitis.

The permanent overdistention of the air spaces with destruction of the walls (septa) between the alveoli is accompanied by partial airway collapse and loss of elastic recoil. Pockets of air form between the alveolar spaces (blebs) and within the lung parenchyma (bullae). This process leads to increased ventilatory dead space, or areas that do not participate in gas exchange diminishing $\dot{V}/\dot{Q}$ matching (Fig. 15-9).[288]

The WOB is increased as a result of ventilatory drive from hypoxemia and hypercapnia, increased effort during exhalation (normally passive recoil), and flattening of the diaphragm caused by hyperinflation. As the disease progresses, there is increasing dyspnea and risk of pulmonary infection. Pulmonary hypertension develops from capillary loss and vessel intimal thickening, and this eventually leads to cor pulmonale (right-sided heart failure).

In centrilobular emphysema the destruction of the lung is uneven and originates around the airways. The membranous bronchioles are thicker, narrower, and more reactive than in panlobular emphysema. Lung compliance is low or normal and does not relate to the extent of the emphysema (i.e., not to the losses of elastic recoil), but rather the decrease in airflow is related mainly to the degree of airway abnormality.

In contrast, panlobular emphysema is characterized by even destruction of the lung and the small airways appear less narrowed and less inflamed than in centrilobular emphysema. Lung compliance is increased and is related to the extent of the emphysema; the decrease in airflow is primarily associated with the loss of elastic recoil rather than with the abnormalities in the airways.[118]

At the molecular and microvascular levels, protease–antiprotease (associated with α_1-antitrypsin disease [AATD] emphysema) and oxidant–antioxidant theories continue under investigation as theories relate to impaired reparative mechanisms in the causation of emphysema. Oxidative damage by free radicals, which is the basis for the free radical theory of aging (see discussion in Chapter 6), identifies cigarette smoke as the main source of oxidants contributing to epithelial damage associated with smoking-induced emphysema. Determining the mechanisms regulating the antioxidant responses is critical to understanding the role of oxidants in the pathogenesis of smoking-induced lung disease and to developing future strategies for antioxidant therapy.[451]

Muscle wasting in emphysema and COPD is linked to increased tumor necrosis factor-α production. Respiratory muscle atrophy can lead to deterioration of lung function and increased WOB.[484]

Clinical Manifestations

At first, symptoms may be apparent only during physical exertion, but eventually marked exertional dyspnea progresses to dyspnea at rest. This occurs as a result of the irreversible destruction reducing elasticity of the lungs and increasing the effort to exhale trapped air. Cough is uncommon, with little sputum production. The client is often thin, has tachypnea with prolonged expiration, and must use accessory muscles for ventilation. To increase lung capacity and use of accessory muscles, the client often leans forward with arms braced on the knees supporting the shoulders and chest. The combined effects of trapped air and alveolar distention change the size and shape of the client's chest, causing a barrel chest and increased expiratory effort appearance (Fig. 15-10).

Nocturnal hypoxemia is another clinical manifestation of emphysema. During sleep (especially rapid eye movement stage) there is a decrease in the sensitivity of chemoreceptors, decreased firing of the intercostal muscles, and increased airway resistance. These changes can be significant for the person with emphysema and worsen $\dot{V}/\dot{Q}$ matching leading to nocturnal hypoxia.[288] This may be worsened in people who also have obstructive sleep apnea. Persons with emphysema have three times the rate of anxiety as the general public. This anxiety is associated with dyspnea or fear of dyspnea. Antianxiety medications, particularly selective serotonin reuptake inhibitors, and cognitive behavioral therapy have been shown to be helpful, although more research is needed.[73]

The most common signs and symptoms of AATD include dyspnea, wheezing, cough, chronic allergies (year round), asthma that does not respond to treatment, and liver problems. A high prevalence of wheezing to allergen and irritant exposures with symptoms of atopy suggests that asthma is common in AATD but is usually associated with COPD. Individuals with AATD who are susceptible to asthma require allergy evaluation and aggressive anti-inflammatory management.[159]

MEDICAL MANAGEMENT

DIAGNOSIS AND TREATMENT. Diagnosis is made on the basis of history (usually cigarette smoking), physical examination, chest film, and pulmonary function tests. The most important factor in the treatment of emphysema is cessation of smoking. Human lungs benefit no matter when someone quits smoking (see Table 3-12); quitting smoking is the most effective way of preventing lung function decline caused by emphysema (and chronic bronchitis).

Pursed-lip breathing causes resistance to outflow at the lips, which in turn maintains intrabronchial pressure and improves the mixture of gases in the lungs. This type of

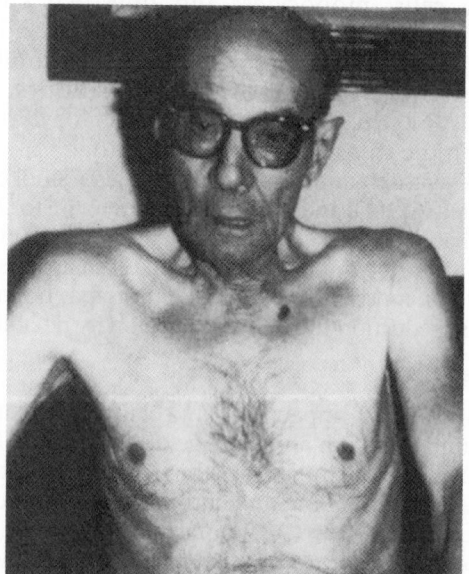

Figure 15-10

The person with emphysema presents with classic findings. Use of respiratory accessory (intercostal, neck, shoulder) muscles and cachectic appearance (wasting caused by ill health) reflect two factors: (1) shortness of breath, the most disturbing symptom, and (2) the tremendous increased work of breathing necessary to increase ventilation and maintain normal arterial blood gases. (From Kersten LD: *Comprehensive respiratory nursing*, Philadelphia, 1989, WB Saunders.)

breathing should be encouraged to help the client get rid of the air trapped in the lungs. Diaphragmatic breathing may benefit some clients in the early stages of emphysema. Methods to examine diaphragmatic movement and the potential for success with diaphragmatic breathing are available.[82] Pulmonary rehabilitation and supplemental oxygen are critical aspects of management of COPD.[89]

Lung transplantation is an established treatment for individuals with advanced emphysema. Double-lung transplantation may help avoid complications following single-lung transplantation, including native lung hyperinflation. However, single-lung transplantation is done more often because of limited donor organ availability.[536]

LVRS (surgically removing damaged areas of the lung) may help improve breathing, ventilation, and survival.[6] Studies are underway to help predict who can benefit the most from this treatment approach.[536] Substantial information regarding the role of LVRS in severe emphysema has come from the National Emphysema Treatment Trial (NETT).[122]

The NETT was not a crossover trial and therefore was able to examine the effects of optimal medical management and LVRS on short- and long-term survival, as well as lung function, exercise performance, and quality of life. The NETT generated multiple insights into the preoperative, perioperative, and postoperative management of patients undergoing thoracotomy; described pain control techniques that were safe and effective; and emphasized the need to address nonpulmonary issues to optimize surgical outcomes. After the NETT, newer investigation has focused on other less invasive techniques to achieve lung reduction.[121]

In the case of AATD, serum testing to measure the levels of α_1-antitrypsin is required to identify this problem. Underrecognition of AATD is common with diagnostic and treatment delays documented.[476] AATD is treated with weekly intravenous augmentation therapy to slow down or halt the destruction of lung tissue. Home infusion is available for some people.

Infusion of purified α_1-antitrypsin from pooled human plasma raises the concentration in serum and epithelial-lining fluid above the protective threshold. Although evidence suggests this treatment slows the decline of lung function and may reduce infection rates while enhancing survival, the cost-effectiveness has been questioned.[475] Only nonsmokers can benefit from this treatment regimen; smoking increases neutrophils, which, in turn, inhibit α_1-antitrypsin.

PROGNOSIS. Prognosis for individuals with symptomatic AATD is poor, with a high incidence of transplantation for liver and lung disease and even more on a transplant waiting list.[477] See also "Medical Management" under "Chronic Obstructive Pulmonary Disease" and "Special Implications for the Therapist 15-6: Chronic Obstructive Pulmonary Disease" above.

Asthma

Definition and Overview

Asthma is defined as a reversible obstructive lung disease characterized by inflammation and increased reactivity

Table 15-7	Types of Asthma
Classification	**Triggers**
Extrinsic	Immunoglobulin E–mediated external allergens • Foods; sulfite additives (wines) • Indoor and outdoor pollutants, including ozone, smoke, exhaust • Pollen, dust, molds • Animal dander, feathers
Intrinsic	Unknown; secondary to respiratory infections
Adult-onset	Unknown
Exercise-induced	Alteration in airway temperature and humidity; mediator release
Aspirin-sensitive (associated with nasal polyps)	Aspirin and other nonsteroidal antiinflammatory drugs
Allergic bronchopulmonary aspergillosis	Hypersensitivity to *Aspergillus* species
Occupational	Metal salts (platinum, chrome, nickel) Antibiotic powder (penicillin, sulfathiazole, tetracycline) Toluene diisocyanate Flour Wood dusts Cotton dust (byssinosis) Animal proteins Smoke inhalation (firefighters) Latex-induced (see Boxes 4-4 and 4-5) Emotional stress

of smooth muscle of the airways to various stimuli. It is a chronic condition with acute exacerbations and characterized as a complex disorder involving biochemical, autonomic, immunologic, infectious, endocrine, and psychologic factors. This condition can be divided into two main types according to causative factors: extrinsic (allergic) and intrinsic (nonallergic), but other recognized categories include adult-onset, exercise-induced, aspirin-sensitive, *Aspergillus*-hypersensitive, and occupational asthma (Table 15-7).

Incidence and Prevalence

Asthma accounts for almost 500,000 hospitalizations annually in the United States. More than 34.1 million people in the United States have been diagnosed with asthma, with 9 million diagnosed in childhood.[15] Between 2001 and 2009, the prevalence of asthma across all ages increased from 7.3% to 8.2%.[514] In the last 5–10 years, the incidence of asthma has begun to level off.[104] Asthma is the most common chronic disease of childhood, affecting 9.4% of all children.[90] Puerto Ricans have the highest incidence, followed by non-Hispanic blacks and Native Americans.[62,372]

Risk Factors

The environment, including air pollution and exposure to other environmental toxins (including pesticides),[195,246] homes that are airtight, exposure to pets, and windowless offices may also be risk factors contributing to the significant rise in incidence. The *hygiene hypothesis* of asthma blames lack of exposure to stimulants or overexposure to cleaning agents.[334,436]

Large families, early exposure to pets, early infections, having older siblings, and attending daycare may protect against allergic sensitization.[502] Asthma can occur at any age, although it is more likely to occur for the first time before the age of 5 years. Antibiotic exposure during infancy appears to be a risk factor for developing childhood asthma. In childhood, it is three times more common and more severe in boys; however, after puberty, girls are more likely to be diagnosed.[168]

Children with lower birth weight (less than 5.5 lb at birth) and prematurity (more than 3 weeks premature) are more susceptible to the effects of ozone (air pollution) compared with children who are born full term or full weight.[360] It is estimated that asthma goes unrecognized as an adverse factor affecting performance in 1 in 10 adolescent athletes.

Asthma is found most often in urban, industrialized settings; in colder climates; and among the urban disadvantaged population (areas of poverty). Asthma is more prevalent and more severe among black children, but this may not be a result of race or low income per se but rather of demographic location because all children living in an urban setting are at increased risk for asthma.[8] The number of African American boys with asthma increased in 2001–2004, whereas the incidence remained stable for African American girls and white children of both sexes.[335]

Overcrowded living conditions with repeated exposure to cigarette smoke, dust, cockroaches, and mold and where the use of a gas stove or oven is used for heat may be contributing factors.[311] Alcoholic drinks, particularly wines, appear to be important triggers for asthmatic responses. Sensitivity to the sulfite additives and salicylates present in wine seems likely to play an important role in these reactions.[504]

There is a relationship between obesity and asthma. Data from the Nurses' Health Study II show that obesity increases women's risk of developing adult-onset asthma possibly as a result of estrogen stored in adipose tissue. The higher the body mass index (BMI), the greater the risk of developing asthma.[83] One study demonstrated reduced respiratory function in 32% of obese children whereas only 3% of children with a normal BMI demonstrated respiratory dysfunction.[501]

Inflammatory mediators are produced by adipose tissue and may represent an immunologic connection between asthma and obesity. Increased leptin secretion may enhance airway inflammation while reduced adiponectin (an antiinflammatory agent) secretion affects modulation of inflammation. Comorbidity of asthma and obesity may complicate the treatment of either condition and appropriate asthma treatment may help with exercise and weight loss. Prevention of obesity and/or weight loss should be encouraged for all persons with asthma.[415]

Etiologic Factors

Asthma occurs in families, which indicates that it is an inherited disorder. Asthma is influenced by two genetic tendencies: one associated with the capacity to develop allergies (atopy) and the other with the tendency to develop hyperresponsiveness of the airways independent of atopy. Seventy percent of childhood asthma occurs in children with allergies.[104] Environmental factors interact with inherited factors to cause attacks of bronchospasm. Asthma can develop when predisposed persons are infected by viruses or exposed to allergens or pollutants.

Extrinsic asthma, also known as atopic or allergic asthma, is the result of an allergy to specific triggers; usually the offending allergens are environmental antigens suspended in the air in the form of pollen, dust, molds, smoke, automobile exhaust, or animal dander. In this type of asthma, mast cells, sensitized by IgE antibodies, degranulate and release bronchoactive mediators after exposure to a specific antigen. More than half of the cases of asthma in children and young adults are of this type.

Intrinsic asthma, or nonallergic asthma, has no known allergic cause or trigger, has an adult onset (usually older than 40 years of age), and is most often secondary to chronic or recurrent infections of the bronchi, sinuses, or tonsils and adenoids. This type of asthma may develop from a hypersensitivity to the bacteria, or more commonly, viruses causing the infection. Other factors precipitating intrinsic asthma include drugs (aspirin and β-adrenergic antagonists), environmental irritants (occupational chemicals and air pollution), cold dry air, exercise, and emotional stress.

Occupational asthma is defined as variable narrowing of airways, causally related to exposure in the working environment to specific airborne dusts, gases, acids, molds, dyes, vapors, or fumes. Many of these substances are very common and not ordinarily considered hazardous. Only a small proportion of exposed workers develop occupational asthma, but it has received considerable attention recently as the most frequent occupational lung disease worldwide.

New substances and processes used in manufacturing have increased dramatically in the last 2 decades, and there is little information about "safe" levels of exposure that protect all workers.[37] High-risk occupations for asthma include farmers, animal handlers, and agricultural workers; painters; plastics and rubber workers; cleaners and homemakers (especially if cooking is done with a gas stove); textile workers; metal workers; and bakers, millers, and other food processors. Exposure to biologic dusts and gases and fumes can cause a 30% to 50% increase in risk of asthma.

Pathogenesis

Asthma is characterized by chronic airway inflammation and intermittent attacks of bronchospasm caused by airway hyperresponsiveness to allergens or irritants. The airways are the site of an acute inflammatory response consisting of cellular infiltration, epithelial disruption, mucosal edema, and mucous plugging (Fig. 15-11). The release of inflammatory mediators produces bronchial smooth muscle spasm; vascular congestion; increased vascular permeability; edema formation; production of thick, tenacious mucus; and impaired mucociliary function.

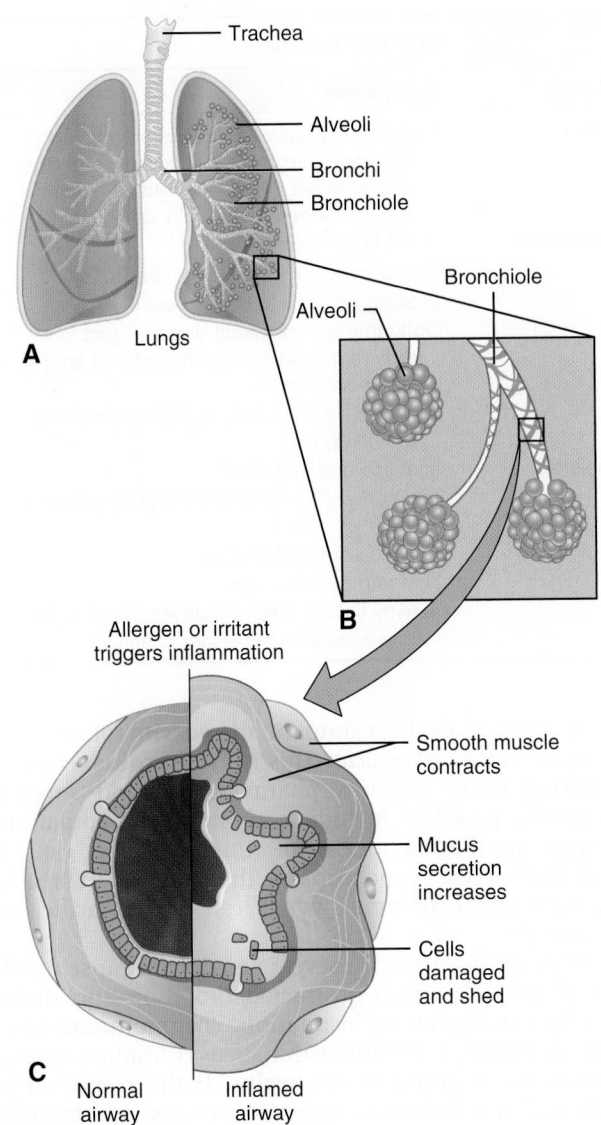

Figure 15-11

Bronchiole response in asthma. A, Air is distributed throughout the lungs via small airways called *bronchioles*. **B,** Healthy bronchioles accommodate a constant flow of air when open and relaxed. **C,** In asthma, exposure to an allergen or irritant triggers inflammation, causing constriction of the smooth muscle surrounding the bronchus (bronchospasm). The airway tissue swells; this edema of the mucous membrane further narrows airways with production of excess mucus also interfering with breathing.

Chronic inflammation can lead to airway remodeling with permanent structural changes in the airways associated with progressive loss of lung function. Several mediators cause thickening of airway walls and increased contractile response of bronchial smooth muscles. These changes in the bronchial musculature, combined with the epithelial cell damage caused by eosinophil infiltration, result in the airway hyperresponsiveness characteristic of asthma.

Once the airway is in spasm and airways are swollen, mucous plugs the airway, trapping distal air. $\dot{V}/\dot{Q}$ mismatch, hypoxemia, obstructed expiratory flow, and increased workload of breathing follow. Most attacks of asthmatic bronchospasm are short-lived, with freedom

from symptoms between episodes, although airway inflammation is present, even in people who are asymptomatic.

Excessive airway narrowing occurs when the smooth muscle shortens (not necessarily to an abnormal degree). The relationship between the mechanical and contractile properties of smooth muscle and lung volume and how these interact to determine smooth muscle length are the subject of new research. The relative importance of smooth muscle area and mechanical properties, altered airway structure, and airway inflammation in asthma is not yet determined.[264]

Although definitive causes of asthma have not been determined, there is much known about the immune system mechanisms that lead to allergic airway obstruction. T-helper cells secrete cytokines, which contribute to inflammation that is mediated by IgE. IgE is present on mast cells and other airway cells. After repeated contact with antigens, these cells break down and release toxins, particularly leukotrienes, which cause bronchospasm and hypersecretions.[41]

Researchers are also investigating the possibility of underlying neurogenic mechanisms that may contribute to the pathogenesis and pathophysiology of asthma.[109,401,429] Investigations include determination of the linkages among psychosocial factors and behavioral, neural, endocrine, and immune processes in the role of asthma. It has been shown that health-related behaviors, demographic factors, and psychosocial factors influence susceptibility to and severity of exacerbation of asthma.[290,462]

Clinical Manifestations

Clinical signs and symptoms of asthma differ in presentation (Box 15-6), degree (Table 15-8), and frequency among clients. Although current symptoms are the most important concern of affected people, they reflect the present level of asthma control more than underlying disease severity.[260]

During full remission, clients are asymptomatic and pulmonary function tests are normal. Over time, repeated attacks cause airway remodeling, chronic air trapping, proliferation of submucosal glands, and hypertrophied smooth muscle. This may progress to irreversible changes and COPD.

At the beginning of an attack, there is a sensation of chest constriction described as "chest tightness" or a sense of suffocation caused by the constriction of the smooth muscle in the respiratory tract and the inflammatory response in the lungs. Inspiratory and expiratory wheezing occurs when the airways narrow; prolonged expiration is seen in a 1:3 or 1:4 ratio (instead of the normal inspiratory-to-expiratory ratio of 1:2).

Nonproductive coughing fails to mobilize secretions and can intensify an attack as well as interfere with sleep. Production of yellow or green sputum requires medical evaluation for infection. Other symptoms may include tachycardia, tachypnea, fatigue, a tickle in the back of the throat accompanied by a cough in an attempt to clear the airways, and nostril flaring (advanced). Decreased oxygen saturation (hypoxemia; less than 90%) can occur quickly. Oxygen saturation level can be measured and monitored

Box 15-6

CLINICAL MANIFESTATIONS OF BRONCHIAL ASTHMA

Cough

- Hacking, paroxysmal, exhausting, irritative, involuntary, nonproductive
- Becomes rattling and productive of frothy, clear, gelatinous sputum
- Main or only symptom
- Tickle in the back of the throat accompanied by a cough

Respiratory-Related Signs

- Shortness of breath; may occur at rest
- Prolonged expiratory phase
- Audible wheeze on inspiration and expiration or on expiration only; never on inspiration only
- Often appears pale
- May have a malar flush and red ears
- Lips deep dark red color
- May progress to cyanosis of nail beds, mouth, and lips
- Restlessness
- Apprehension
- Anxious facial expression
- Itching around nose, eyes, throat, chin, scalp
- Sweating may be prominent as attack progresses
- May sit upright with shoulders in a hunched-over position, hands on the bed or chair, and arms braced (older children)
- Speaks with short, panting broken phrases

Chest

- Coarse, loud breath sounds (may become quiet or silent if severe)
- Prolonged expiration
- Generalized inspiratory and expiratory wheezing; increasingly high-pitched
- Loss of breath sounds with severe cases

With Repeated Episodes

- Barrel chest
- Elevated shoulders
- Use of accessory muscles of respiration
- Skin retraction (clavicles, ribs, sternum)
- Facial appearance: flattened malar bones, circles beneath the eyes, narrow nose, prominent upper teeth, nostrils flaring

Modified from Wong DL: *Whaley and Wong's essentials of pediatric nursing*, ed 5, St Louis, 1997, Mosby-Year Book.

Table 15-8	Stages of Asthma
Stage	**Symptoms**
Mild	Symptoms reverse with cessation of activity; daytime symptoms ≤2 times/wk; nighttime symptoms ≤2 times/mo; inhaled medication as needed (not usually daily)
Moderate	Audible wheezing
	Use of accessory muscles of respiration
	Leaning forward to catch breath
	Daily (but not continual) daytime symptoms requiring short-acting inhalant and long-term treatment
	Episodes ≥2 times/wk; nighttime symptoms ≥ 4 times/mo
Severe	Blue lips and fingernails
	Tachypnea (30-40 breaths/min) despite cessation of activity
	Cyanosis-induced seizures
	Skin and rib retraction
	Activity limited; frequent daytime and nighttime episodes, sometimes continual

An acute attack that cannot be altered with routine care is called *status asthmaticus*. This is a medical emergency requiring more vigorous pharmacologic and support measures, possibly including mechanical ventilation. Despite appropriate treatment, this condition can be fatal. With severe bronchospasm, the workload of breathing increases 5–10 times, which can lead to acute cor pulmonale.

When air is trapped, a severe paradoxical pulse develops as venous return is obstructed; blood pressure drops over 10 mm Hg during inspiration. Pneumothorax occasionally develops. If status asthmaticus continues, hypoxemia worsens and acidosis begins. If the condition is untreated or not reversed, respiratory or cardiac arrest will occur.

MEDICAL MANAGEMENT

PREVENTION. Heavier emphasis on teaching self-management and especially prevention for anyone with asthma is recommended by the American Academy of Allergy, Asthma, and Immunology. *Healthy People 2020* has identified 11 objectives specifically related to this condition, including increasing the proportion of people with asthma who receive formal education as part of their management program (see *Healthy People 2020*: http://health.gov/healthypeople/). People with asthma must take an active role in preventing an asthma attack and treating it appropriately when one occurs. Each child and adult with asthma should utilize a peak flow meter to monitor their flow rates. This peak flow reading should be a part of their asthma action plan (Fig. 15-12) and this should be given to school nurses and any health care professional caring for a person with asthma.[14]

DIAGNOSIS. Pulse oximetry, pulmonary function studies, bronchial challenge test with methacholine, skin prick tests, arterial blood gas analysis, serum IgE and blood eosinophil counts, induced sputum cell counts, exhaled

in order to respond quickly to changes in SpO_2. The individual may become agitated, restless, anxious, and hypertensive with tachycardia, tachypnea, and diaphoresis.

The person usually assumes a classic sitting or squatting position to reduce venous return, leaning forward so as to use the accessory muscles of respiration. The skin is usually pale and moist with perspiration, and in a severe attack there may be cyanosis of the lips and nail beds. In the early stages of the attack coughing may be dry, but as the attack progresses, the cough becomes more productive of a thick, tenacious mucoid sputum. The nocturnal worsening of asthma is a common feature of this disease and may affect daytime alertness, even in children.[148] Rhinitis, chronic cough, snoring, and apnea may be responsible for sleep disturbance.

Asthma Action Plan

For: _____ Doctor: _____ Date: _____

Doctor's Phone Number _____ Hospital/Emergency Department Phone Number _____

GREEN ZONE

Doing Well

- No cough, wheeze, chest tightness, or shortness of breath during the day or night
- Can do usual activities

And, if a peak flow meter is used,

Peak flow: more than _____
(80 percent or more of my best peak flow)

My best peak flow is: _____

Take these long-term control medicines each day (include an anti-inflammatory).

Medicine	How much to take	When to take it
_____	_____	_____
_____	_____	_____
_____	_____	_____

Before exercise	□ _____	□ 2 or □ 4 puffs _____	5 minutes before exercise

YELLOW ZONE

Asthma Is Getting Worse

- Cough, wheeze, chest tightness, or shortness of breath, or
- Waking at night due to asthma, or
- Can do some, but not all, usual activities

-Or-

Peak flow: _____ to _____
(50 to 79 percent of my best peak flow)

First **Add: quick-relief medicine—and keep taking your GREEN ZONE medicine.**

_____ □ 2 or □ 4 puffs, every 20 minutes for up to 1 hour
(short-acting beta₂-agonist) □ Nebulizer, once

If your symptoms (and peak flow, if used) return to GREEN ZONE after 1 hour of above treatment:
□ Continue monitoring to be sure you stay in the green zone.

-Or-

Second **If your symptoms (and peak flow, if used) do not return to GREEN ZONE after 1 hour of above treatment:**
□ Take: _____ □ 2 or □ 4 puffs or □ Nebulizer
(short-acting beta₂-agonist)

□ Add: _____ mg per day For _____ (3–10) days
(oral steroid)

□ Call the doctor □ before/ □ within _____ hours after taking the oral steroid.

RED ZONE

Medical Alert!

- Very short of breath, or
- Quick-relief medicines have not helped, or
- Cannot do usual activities, or
- Symptoms are same or get worse after 24 hours in Yellow Zone

-Or-

Peak flow: less than _____
(50 percent of my best peak flow)

Take this medicine:

□ _____ □ 4 or □ 6 puffs or □ Nebulizer
(short-acting beta₂-agonist)

□ _____ mg
(oral steroid)

Then call your doctor NOW. Go to the hospital or call an ambulance if:
- You are still in the red zone after 15 minutes AND
- You have not reached your doctor.

DANGER SIGNS	■ Trouble walking and talking due to shortness of breath	▶ ■ Take □ 4 or □ 6 puffs of your quick-relief medicine AND
	■ Lips or fingernails are blue	■ Go to the hospital or call for an ambulance _____ NOW!
		(phone)

See the reverse side for things you can do to avoid your asthma triggers.

Figure 15-12

Asthma Action Plan. (From National Heart, Lung, and Blood Institute. NIH Publication No. 07-5251, April 2007. Available online at: http://www.nhlbi.nih.gov/health/public/lung/asthma/asthma_actplan.pdf.)

nitric oxide (marker for eosinophilic inflammation),[491] questionnaires, exercise tests followed by spirometry, and chest films may be used in assessing for both the presence and the severity of asthma (see Chapter 40 for a description of and reference values for these tests). The methacholine challenge test is a valuable diagnostic measure. There are strong correlations with this test and some symptoms.[553] Inexpensive but reliable spirometer testing can be used to obtain evidence of the bronchial hyperreactivity associated with asthma.

Diagnosis may be delayed in older clients who have other illnesses that cause similar symptoms or who attribute their breathlessness to the effects of aging and respond to the onset of asthma by limiting their activities to avoid eliciting symptoms. The diagnosis of occupational asthma is usually based on history of a temporal association between exposure and the onset of symptoms and objective evidence that these symptoms are related to airflow limitation. Sputum induction and analysis may be helpful in confirming occupational asthma.[196]

TREATMENT. Identifying specific allergens for each individual and avoidance of asthma triggers, combined with the use of two classes of medications (bronchodilators and antiinflammatory agents; see Table 15-6), has been recommended in the management of asthma.

Treatment of asthma depends on the frequency and severity of symptoms. Those who have intermittent symptoms of two days or less in a week and no physical activity limitations are treated with a short-acting β-agonist as needed.[104]

Most people require bronchodilator therapy to control symptoms by activating β-agonist receptors on smooth muscle cells in the respiratory tract, thereby relaxing the bronchial muscle and opening the airways; those with mild symptoms may use metered-dose inhalers to administer sympathomimetic bronchodilators on an as-needed basis (see Box 15-5).

People who experience moderate-to-severe asthma may require daily administration of antiinflammatory agents, such as corticosteroids, to prevent asthma attacks. Corticosteroids dampen the entire immune system response. Antiinflammatory drugs have a preventive action by interrupting the development of bronchial inflammation. It is now clear that asthma attacks are actually episodic flare-ups of chronic inflammation in the lining of the airways necessitating the use of inhaled antiinflammatories to suppress the underlying inflammation and allow the airways to heal.

It is important that people with asthma know the difference between medications that must be taken daily to prevent asthma symptoms and medications that relieve symptoms once they begin. Low-dose corticosteroid inhalants are recommended to reduce the risk of side effects (e.g., psychiatric problems, reduced growth in children, ocular effects, death, osteoporosis, or alopecia and hirsutism) from prolonged use.[140,479] Leukotriene-receptor antagonists inhibit inflammation and have been shown to be safe and effective in adults with asthma and allergic rhinitis (see further discussion in Chapter 6).[512]

Oxygen metabolites (free radicals) may play a direct or indirect role in the modulation of airway inflammation. Excessive superoxide and hydroxyl radical production accompanied by significantly lower free radical scavengers in asthma (the latter even during rest) endorses the correlation between disease severity and oxygen radical production in people with asthma.[455]

Low dietary intake and blood levels of vitamins C and E, selenium, and flavonoids are seen in people with asthma.[353,402,457] Although some researchers suggest that antioxidant nutrients (especially when obtained from food sources such as fruits and vegetables) appear helpful in asthma treatment,[341,351,373,402] others report that people with asthma may have a diminished capacity to restore the antioxidant defenses, making the use of supplemental antioxidants questionable in this population.[407]

Many complementary treatments have been used to ameliorate asthma symptoms though there has been minimal research to validate most of these claims. There is minimal but growing evidence to support the use of acupuncture.[324] Spinal manipulation and other manual therapy have been deemed to be ineffective in the treatment of asthma.[165,245] In one study of 65 people, yoga was found to have no effect on asthma.[438] Complementary treatments are still being studied for benefits and adverse effects.[58]

Genetic treatment is under investigation. For example, gene transfer into the airway cells to block mediator proteins (signal transducer activator of transcription [STAT]) from setting off an immune response or too strong an immune response in the asthma pathway is the subject of several studies.[166,441] Recombinant monoclonal antibodies prevent IgE from binding to mast cells and other effector cells, preventing inflammation.[518]

PROGNOSIS. The outlook for clients with *bronchial asthma* is excellent despite the recent increase in the death rate.

Childhood asthma may disappear, but only about one-quarter of the children with asthma become symptom-free when their airways reach adult size. Factors that predict adult asthma include gender (males are more likely to outgrow asthma), smoking, allergy to dust mites, degree of airway hyperresponsiveness, and early age of onset.[448,490]

Adults with asthma are 12 times more likely to progress to COPD, but studies indicate that the majority of people with asthma do not experience a decline in pulmonary mechanics or appear to be at risk for reduced life expectancy.[216,343] The risk of lung cancer, however, is two times greater in people with asthma compared with those who do not have a history of asthma.[4]

Attention to general health measures and use of pharmacologic agents permit control of symptoms in nearly all cases. In some people, chronic inflammation can lead to airway remodeling with permanent structural changes in the airways associated with progressive loss of function. For these individuals, remodeling is not fully reversed by current therapy.

Status asthmaticus can result in respiratory or cardiac arrest and possible death (see previous discussion). If ventilation becomes necessary, prognosis for recovery is poor.

SPECIAL IMPLICATIONS FOR THE THERAPIST   15-7

Asthma
Exercise-Induced Bronchospasm (Formerly Exercise-Induced Asthma)

Exercise-induced bronchospasm (EIB) does not represent a unique syndrome but rather an example of the airway hyperactivity common to all persons with asthma. EIB is an acute, reversible, usually self-terminating airway obstruction that develops 5 to 15 minutes after vigorous intensity exercise. During exercise, a person increases their respiratory rate and humidification is lost. Moreover, the airways become dehydrated and cooled which triggers the release of mast cells and inflammatory markers (Osmotic Theory). These cells trigger bronchoconstriction and the symptoms of an asthma attack.[529] EIB lasts 15 to 60 minutes after the onset.

EIB is often diagnosed with an exercise test followed immediately with spirometry. The person with EIB demonstrates a 10% to 15% or greater drop in FEV_1* when they reach at least 80% of maximum heart rate for at least 4 minutes.[474,529] The recommended treatment focuses on prophylaxis, with the affected individual taking a short-acting β-agonist 5 minutes prior to exercise and having an adequate warm-up period.

Because physical therapists prescribe and observe exercise, they may be the first to recognize symptoms of undiagnosed asthma. Coughing is the most common symptom of EIB, but other symptoms include chest tightness, wheezing, and SOB. The affected (but undiagnosed) individual may comment, "I am more out of shape than I thought." This should be a red flag for the therapist to consider the possibility of asthma and need for medical diagnosis and intervention.

If an asthma attack should occur during therapy, first assess the severity of the attack. Place the person in the high Fowler position and encourage diaphragmatic and pursed-lip breathing. If the client has an inhaler available, provide whatever assistance is necessary for that person to self-administer the medication. Help the person relax while assessing their response to the medication.

Usually the episode subsides spontaneously in 30 to 60 minutes. The severity of an attack increases as the exercise becomes increasingly strenuous. Warm-up exercise can ameliorate the inflammatory process by affecting platelet-eosinophil/neutrophil reactions.[520] The problem is rare in activities that require only short bursts of energy (e.g., baseball, sprints, gymnastics, or skiing) compared with those that involve endurance exercise (e.g., soccer, basketball, distance running, or biking).

Swimming, even long-distance swimming, is well tolerated by people with EIB, partly because they are breathing air fully saturated with moisture, but the type of breathing required may also play a role. Exhaling under water, which is essentially pursed-lip breathing, is beneficial because it prolongs each expiration and increases the end-expiratory pressure within the respiratory tree.

Effect of Exercise

There are many barriers to exercise for people with asthma, including lack of motivation, time constraints, weather conditions, and belief that exercise is not good for this condition.[332] To prevent secondary complication of a sedentary lifestyle and because obesity can contribute to the inflammatory process associated with asthma, exercise and education about exercise should be part of any treatment program.

There is strong evidence to support physical training for cardiovascular training in this population.[421] There is inadequate evidence for a positive effect of breathing exercises and inspiratory muscle training in individuals who have asthma.[244,422]

Exercise and Medication

EIB is often treated with short-acting β_2-agonists given 5 minutes before the exercise bout. However, people can develop tolerance to short-acting β_2-agonists, in which case their medication regimen must be altered. Those with EIB should also be evaluated for control of their underlying disease, as EIB may indicate inadequate control.[529]

Bronchospasm can occur during exercise (especially in EIB) if the person with asthma has a low blood oxygen level before exercise. For this reason, it is helpful to take bronchodilators by metered-dose inhaler 20 to 30 minutes before exercise, performing mild stretching and warm-up exercises during that time period to avoid bronchospasm with higher workload exercise. Increased exercise should be accompanied by good bronchodilator coverage to promote bronchodilation and improve alveolar ventilation and oxygenation. Exercise guidelines for adults with asthma can be modified from recommendations for children with asthma (Table 15-9).

Many clients have found that using their inhalers in this way before exercise permits them to exercise without onset of symptoms. Proper administration of an metered-dose inhaler is essential (see Box 15-5). The first dose induces dilation of the larger, central bronchial tubes, relaxing smooth muscles in the airways; the second dose dilates the bronchioles (smaller airways).

Table 15-9	Exercise Guidelines for Children With Asthma
Recommendation	**Benefit**
General exercise, school-based physical education	Maintains motor control, flexibility, strength, cardiovascular fitness, and prevents or reverses side effects of medication (e.g., corticosteroids)
	Raises threshold for strenuous exercise before mouth breathing and EIB occur
Low-impact exercise (aerobics, weight training, stationary bike)	Permits exercise without increased bronchospasm
Warm-up before aerobic activity	Helps control airway reactivity; gradually desensitizes mast cells, reducing release of bronchoconstrictive mediators
Exercise in a trigger-free environment (i.e., avoid cold, pollution, or increased pollen outdoors; exercise indoors; avoid tobacco smoke; swimming program is ideal)	Prevents bronchospasm; controls symptoms
Take prescribed medication properly before exercise or activity producing bronchospasm	Prevents bronchospasm
Monitor FEV$_1$/FVC ratio before, during, and after physical activity*	Determines whether shortness of breath is caused by intensity of exercise or by diminished airflow as a result of bronchospasm
Decrease of 10% requires slowing activity	
Drop of 15%-20% from initial measurement requires cessation of exercise	

EIB, Exercise-induced bronchospasm; FEV$_1$/FVC, ratio of forced expiratory volume in 1 second to forced vital capacity.
*Peak flowmeters can be used to obtain this information. Determine the child's normal range of lung function by having the child blow in the meter in the morning and evening for 1 week. The average level measured varies from person to person and is influenced by gender and height. Testing should establish a peak flow protocol against which lung function can be compared to determine if deterioration has occurred.

Metabolism of certain drugs administered can be altered by exercise, tobacco, marijuana, or phenobarbital (all of which increase drug metabolism). Cimetidine (Tagamet), erythromycin, or the presence of a viral infection may decrease drug metabolism.

If a client develops signs of asthma or any bronchial reactivity during exercise, the physician must be informed. Medication dosage can then be altered to maintain optimal physical performance. Excessive use of inhaled β-adrenergic agents (using three or more full canisters monthly) requires physician referral for further evaluation.

Common manifestations of drug-induced (theophylline) toxicity include nausea, vomiting, tremors, anxiety, tachycardia and arrhythmias, and hypotension. The use of nonsteroidal antiinflammatory drugs, including aspirin, in older people with asthma should be avoided if possible because the drug interactions can cause increased bronchospasm in susceptible individuals.

Some athletes do not achieve the control needed for the performance demands of competition. The effectiveness of short-acting medications and medications in general for asthma varies widely among people with asthma while exercising. The preventive benefits of each medication dose may wane after taking a new drug for several weeks. Any athlete with asthma who cannot perform at the levels desired or expected because of asthma symptoms should be advised to review medications and medication use with the physician.

Medication and Bone Density

Long-term use of inhaled corticosteroids in the management of moderate-to-severe asthma is associated with decreased bone mineral density and associated increased risk of fractures and a high occurrence of asymptomatic vertebral fractures, particularly in high-risk postmenopausal women (i.e., those not receiving hormone replacement therapy).[23,432,540] African American children may be afforded some protection from osteoporosis as compared to white children using high-dose inhaled corticosteroids.[212]

All people receiving glucocorticoid therapy (e.g., prednisolone) at doses of 7.5 mg/day or more for 6 months or longer should discuss with their physician the use of low-dose inhaled corticosteroids, assessment of bone mineral density, and preventive therapies (e.g., bisphosphonates, calcium supplementation, or vitamin D).[378] The physical therapist can be very instrumental in providing education for the prevention and intervention for the treatment of osteopenia and osteoporosis. See "Osteoporosis" in Chapter 24.

Monitoring Vital Signs

Monitoring vital signs can alert the therapist to important changes in bronchopulmonary function. Developing or increasing tachypnea may indicate worsening asthma or drug toxicity. Other signs of toxicity, such as diarrhea, headache, and vomiting, may be misinterpreted as influenza. Hypertensive blood pressure readings may indicate asthma-related hypoxemia.

Auscultate the lungs frequently, noting breath sounds including the degree of wheezing and the quality of air movement. In this way, any change in respiratory status will be more readily perceived. If the client does not have a productive cough in the presence of wheezing/rhonchi (rattling or snoring sound in the bronchial tube), teach effective coughing techniques.

Status Asthmaticus

Therapy can augment the medical management of the client with status asthmaticus. In coordination with the individual's medications, the therapist helps to remove secretions; promotes relaxed, more efficient breathing; enhances $\dot{V}/\dot{Q}$ matching; reduces hypoxemia; and teaches the client to coordinate relaxed breathing with general body movement.

Caution needs to be observed to avoid stimuli that bring on bronchospasm and deterioration (e.g., aggressive percussion, forced expiration maneuvers, aggressive bag ventilation, or manual hyperinflation with an intubated individual). Certain body positions may have to be avoided because of client intolerance or exacerbation of symptoms in those positions.[141]

Immediate medical care is recommended for anyone with asthma who fails to have a response to 3 doses of a short-acting β_2-agonist within 1 to 2 hours, tachypnea despite 3 doses of a short-acting β_2-agonist, subcostal retractions, cyanosis, inability to drink or speak because of SOB, or oxygen saturation on room air below 92%.[548]

*FEV_1 is the forced expiratory volume, a measure of the greatest volume of air a person can exhale during forced expiration; the subscript is added to indicate the percentage of the vital capacity that can be expired in 1 second. FVC is forced vital capacity, a measure of the greatest volume of air that can be expelled when a person performs a rapid, forced expiratory maneuver. This usually takes about 5 seconds.

Bronchiectasis

Definition

Bronchiectasis is a progressive condition with irreversible destruction and dilation of airways. Abnormal and permanent dilation of the bronchi and bronchioles develops when the supporting structures (bronchial walls) are weakened by chronic inflammatory changes associated with secondary infection.

Incidence and Etiologic and Risk Factors

The incidence of bronchiectasis is rising, possibly as a consequence of the use of high-resolution chest CT, which is helping physicians to identify cases in their early stages.[202] The most common cause of bronchiectasis is chronic inflammation that occurs after a pulmonary infection. Common infections that can cause bronchiectasis include TB, flu, *Pseudomonas*, and pertussis.[202] The most common congenital issue associated with bronchiectasis is primary ciliary dyskinesia. In primary ciliary dyskinesia, ineffective clearance of secretions increases the risk of chronic or recurrent respiratory infections that precipitate bronchiectasis. Bronchiectasis also develops in people with immunodeficiencies involving humoral immunity, and recurrent aspiration.

CF causes about half of all cases of bronchiectasis. Rheumatoid arthritis, sinusitis, dextrocardia (heart located on right side of chest), Kartagener syndrome (alterations in ciliary activity), defective development of bronchial cartilage (Williams-Campbell syndrome), and endobronchial tumor predispose a person to bronchiectasis. Bronchiectasis may also affect those with COPD, worsening the dyspnea and lung function as compared to those without bronchiectasis.[202] Bronchiectasis can also occur in those with ulcerative colitis, even when the disease is medically stable.

Pathogenesis

Although bronchiectasis has been viewed as a progressive disease of destruction and dilation of the medium and large airways, there is now evidence of the importance of the small airways in the pathogenesis of this condition. Bronchiectasis is characterized by chronic infection, inflammation, and airway dilation. The airways in those with bronchiectasis are often beleaguered with pathogens that stimulate an inflammatory response.

Chronic inflammation of the bronchial wall by mononuclear cells is common to all types of bronchiectasis, with the inflammatory process often continuing after the infection has been cleared.[202] Abnormal bronchial dilation is the result of enzymatic degradation of the airway's connective tissue. Infection, inflammation of the airways and dilation cause an increase in mucus production, airway plugging, and bronchospasm (Fig. 15-13).[497] People with bronchiectasis demonstrate a decline in FEV_1, with more significant decreases in those with systemic inflammation and more frequent and severe exacerbations.[202]

In response to these changes, large anastomoses develop between the bronchial and pulmonary blood vessels to increase the blood flow through the bronchial circulation. $\dot{V}/\dot{Q}$ mismatch causes hypoxia and hypercapnia.

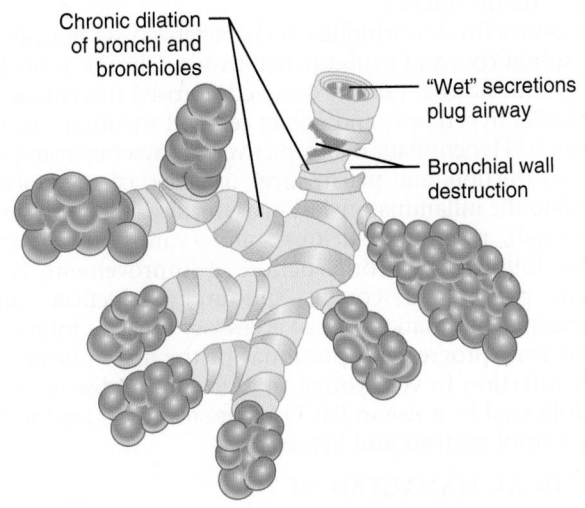

Chronic dilation of bronchi and bronchioles

"Wet" secretions plug airway

Bronchial wall destruction

Figure 15-13

Airway pathology in bronchiectasis.

Damage to these anastomoses is responsible for the hemoptysis present in persons with bronchiectasis.

Clinical Manifestations

There is a varied presentation and symptom experience in those with bronchiectasis. The most common symptoms of bronchiectasis include persistent coughing, with large amounts of purulent sputum production (worse in the morning). Chest pain, rhinosinusitis, dyspnea, fatigue, weight loss, and exercise intolerance may also occur. Clubbing may occur, and the breath and sputum may become foul-smelling with advanced disease. Heart failure may occur as a result of the vascular fibrosis. There is a known correlation between bronchiectasis and rheumatoid arthritis, but the exact mechanism remains unknown.

MEDICAL MANAGEMENT

DIAGNOSIS. Bronchiectasis is diagnosed through a combination of sputum culture, CT imaging, and pulmonary function testing. Underlying conditions that may contribute to the development of bronchiectasis are also evaluated, including tests for CF, inflammatory bowel disease, and ciliary dysfunction.[202]

Bronchiectasis is diagnosed by CT if the airway diameter is greater than the adjacent blood vessel and there is wall thickening. The degree of bronchiectasis is determined by the extent of the dilation, the severity of mucous plugging, and the extent of airway dysfunction.

TREATMENT. Treatment interventions differ for those with CF related bronchiectasis versus non-CF bronchiectasis. In those with CF, airway clearance techniques (chest physical therapy, Active Cycle of Breathing) are recommended to aid secretion removal. The evidence to support the role of airway clearance in non-CF bronchiectasis is sparse, however it is still a recommended treatment intervention. Bronchiectasis exacerbations are treated with antibiotics and bronchodilators. Other strategies include education about smoking cessation and vaccination for influenza virus. Hydration is important, and oxygen may be administered. Surgical resection is reserved for the few clients with localized bronchiectasis and adequate pulmonary function who fail to respond to conservative management or for the person with massive hemoptysis.

PROGNOSIS. The morbidity and mortality associated with bronchiectasis have declined markedly in industrialized nations, but prevalence remains high in Pacific and Asian countries. A recent study noted survival rates of 91% at 4 years after diagnosis, 83.5% at 8.8 years after diagnosis, and 68.3% at 12 years after diagnosis.[321] Lower life expectancy was associated with increased age, lower activity scores as measured by the St. George Respiratory Questionnaire, infection by *Pseudomonas aeruginosa*, and reduced lung function.[321] Complications of bronchiectasis include recurrent pneumonia, lung abscesses, metastatic infections in other organs (e.g., brain abscess), and cardiac and respiratory failure. Good pulmonary hygiene and avoidance of infectious complications in the involved areas may reverse some cases of bronchiectasis.

Bronchiectasis

The effects of bronchopulmonary airway clearance techniques (formerly referred to as *hygiene physical therapy, chest therapy, chest physical therapy*) to improve pulmonary function in bronchiectasis remain inconclusive because of insufficient research.[276,277] The beneficial effects of airway clearance techniques to mobilize secretions and improve pulmonary clearance (e.g., sputum production or radioaerosol clearance) in the treatment of bronchiectasis have been documented in one small study.[277]

In many settings, postural drainage and percussion for the person with bronchiectasis is administered routinely on the basis of diagnosis rather than specific clinical criteria. Further research to clarify outcomes of airway clearance techniques is necessary and may provide the therapist with clinical goals other than secretion mobilization. In non CF-bronchiectasis, there was a small, but positive effect on quality of life and exercise performance with twice daily use of an oscillatory positive expiratory pressure device.[365]

The selection of techniques to include in an airway clearance regimen varies among institutions as well as among practitioners and may include positioning, oscillatory positive expiratory pressure and high-frequency chest wall oscillation, postural drainage, and chest percussion of involved lobes performed several times per day. Family members can be instructed in how to provide this care at home.

Directed coughing and breathing exercises to promote good ventilation and removal of secretions should follow positional or percussive therapy. The best times to do this are early morning and several hours after eating the final meal; performing these techniques just before bedtime may result in increased coughing and prevent the person from sleeping. An excellent review of the use of airway clearance techniques in the acute care setting is available.[181]

Inspiratory muscle training appears to have an effect on exercise endurance, but insufficient evidence exists to support other types of physical training.[69] However, a recent randomized control study demonstrated improvement in exercise tolerance with pulmonary rehabilitation.[68]

Bronchiolitis

Definition and Overview

Bronchiolitis refers to several morphologically distinct pathologic conditions that involve the small airways. Acute bronchiolitis is a commonly occurring, diffuse, and often severe inflammation of the lower airways (bronchioles) in children younger than age 2 years that is caused by a viral infection. Acute adult onset is related to infections, asthma, aspiration, or bronchiectasis.[10]

Bronchiolitis was once classified as a type of chronic interstitial pneumonia and referred to as *small airways disease*. Progress in pathology has provided more specific etiology-directed diagnoses that reflect the individual reaction patterns observed. Constrictive bronchiolitis, diffuse panbronchiolitis, and airway-centered fibrosis are also forms of bronchiolitis.

Bronchiolitis obliterans in the adult is now called constrictive bronchiolitis. It is now classified as acute or chronic, with identification of these special forms (e.g., obliterative, eosinophilic bronchiolitis in asthma, necrotizing bronchiolitis in viral infection, or toxic fume bronchiolitis after exposure to noxious gases and the development of chemical pneumonitis).[283,513] Constrictive bronchiolitis is the most important clinical complication in heart-lung and lung transplant recipients and may represent a form of allograft rejection; it is a rare complication of allogeneic (human-to-human) bone marrow transplantation. Circulating fibroblast precursors from bone marrow may be implicated in transplant recipients with bronchiolitis.[75]

Constrictive bronchiolitis may occur in association with rheumatoid arthritis, polymyositis, and dermatomyositis. Penicillamine therapy has been implicated as a possible cause of constrictive bronchiolitis in clients with rheumatoid arthritis.

Incidence and Etiologic Factors

Constrictive bronchiolitis in adults usually occurs with chronic bronchitis; bronchiolitis in children is associated with pulmonary infections, such as respiratory syncytial virus (RSV), parainfluenza viruses, adenoviruses, or pertussis (whooping cough), or associated with measles. Primarily present in winter and spring, it is easily spread by hand-to-nose or nose-to-eye transmission. Exudative bronchiolitis, which is inflammation of the bronchioles with exudation of gray tenacious sputum, is often associated with asthma.

Pathogenesis and Clinical Manifestations

Variable degrees of obstruction occur in response to infection as the bronchiolar mucosa swells and the lumina fill with mucus and exudate. Depending on the type, these changes occur as the walls of the bronchi and bronchioles are infiltrated with inflammatory cells, increased goblet cells, and fibroblasts.

Constrictive bronchiolitis is characterized by fibrosis of the submucosa and peribronchial tissues. Chronic bronchiolitis with fibrosis (airway centered fibrosis) presents with epithelial hyperplasia and goblet cell and squamous metaplasia.[513] Hyperinflation, obstructive emphysema from partial obstruction, and patchy areas of atelectasis may occur distal to the inflammatory lesion as the disease progresses.

Cough, respiratory distress, and cyanosis occur initially, followed by a brief period of improvement. Dyspnea, paroxysmal cough, sputum production, and wheezing with marked use of accessory muscles follow as the disease progresses. Apnea may be the first indicator of RSV infection in very young infants. Severe disease may be followed by a rise in $PaCO_2$ (hypercapnia), leading to respiratory acidosis and hypoxemia.

MEDICAL MANAGEMENT

PREVENTION. Currently there is no vaccine for RSV. The outcome of infection depends on host and viral genetics.

A better understanding of RSV molecular biology and pathogenesis will help facilitate an effective vaccine and molecular targets for new drug treatment. Understanding RSV disease mechanisms in order to develop a vaccine is difficult because there is a wide range of RSV disease phenotypes in humans and disparities in RSV disease phenotypes among the animal models used in research.[357]

Frequent handwashing and not sharing items, such as cups, glasses, and utensils, with persons who have RSV illness can decrease the spread of virus to others. Excluding children with colds or other respiratory illnesses (without fever) who are well enough to attend childcare or school settings may not decrease the transmission of RSV, as it is often spread in the early stages of illness. In a hospital setting, RSV transmission can and should be prevented by strict attention to contact precautions such as meticulous hand hygiene and wearing gowns and gloves.

DIAGNOSIS AND TREATMENT. Diagnosis is made on the basis of clinical findings, age, the season, and the epidemiology of the community. On chest radiographs, this condition is difficult to differentiate from bacterial pneumonia. RSV can be positively identified using an enzyme-linked immunosorbent assay from direct aspiration of nasal secretions. Early diagnosis in transplant recipients may be facilitated by using CT.[139]

There is no specific treatment for bronchiolitis, and medical therapy is controversial. Treatment modalities may include steroids, humidified air, hydration, and airway clearance techniques such as postural drainage, coughing, and deep-breathing exercises. Antibiotics may be used initially when a bacterial cause of illness has not been ruled out or for secondary infections. Mist therapy combined with oxygen by hood or tent to alleviate dyspnea and hypoxia may be used with children.

Corticosteroids should be used with caution because there is a relationship between levels of cortisol and severity of the disease.[410] Heliox therapy (combination of oxygen and helium) has been shown to have a positive effect on wheezing and respiratory distress by improving gas flow through high-resistance airways and decreasing the WOB.[318]

PROGNOSIS. The acute disease lasts about 3 to 10 days, and the majority of cases can be managed at home with a good prognosis. Hospitalization may be necessary for anyone with complicating conditions such as underlying lung or heart disease, associated debilitated states, poor hydration, or questionable care at home. Some children deteriorate rapidly and die within weeks; others may follow a more long-term course. Onset before the age of 1 year may be related to allergies or asthma, but there appear to be adverse long-term pulmonary consequences.[485] In the adult, the acute form usually has a good prognosis, but the prognosis for chronic constrictive bronchiolitis is poor.

SPECIAL IMPLICATIONS FOR THE THERAPIST   15-9

Bronchiolitis

RSV is the most common cause of pediatric acute bronchiolitis and pneumonia (see the section on RSV in

Chapter 8). For this reason, any staff member with evidence of upper respiratory infection serves as a potential reservoir of RSV and should be excluded from direct contact with high-risk infants. All persons who come within 3 feet of an RSV client must wear a gown and mask with an eye shield and keep hands away from the face, especially the eyes, nose, and mouth. Hands must be washed before and after caring for any client and after handling potentially contaminated client care equipment. Standard Precautions (see Appendix A) must be strictly carried out.

Because RSV is readily transmitted by close contact with personnel, families, and other children both by direct contact (especially lifting or holding) and through contact with objects handled by the child, precautions against cross-infection are important. The primary routes of inoculation for the organisms are large-droplet inhalation through the nose and eyes. When contact is made with mucous discharge or drainage from the eye, nose, or mouth, the therapist is reminded to wear an exterior hospital gown and to discard the gown (or change clothing) when leaving.

Pregnant female personnel or visitors should be advised of the risk of potential physical defects in the developing embryo from contact with RSV. Immunoprophylaxis to prevent RSV in high-risk infants is effective, and prevention of RSV may be possible in the future with active maternal immunization during pregnancy providing passive immunity of infants.[198,510]

Sleep-Disordered Breathing

Definition

Sleep-disordered breathing comprises a collection of syndromes characterized by breathing abnormalities during sleep that result in intermittently disrupted gas exchange and sleep interruption. Sleep-disordered breathing includes Cheyne-Stokes respiration, hypoventilation syndromes with and without chronic lung disease, heavy snoring with daytime sleepiness (upper airway resistance syndrome), and sleep apnea. The most common sleep apnea syndrome, and the only one discussed here, is defined as significant daytime symptoms (e.g., sleepiness) in conjunction with evidence of sleep-related upper airway obstruction and sleep disturbance.[53,399]

There are three types of sleep apnea: central, obstructive, and mixed. *Central sleep apnea* is caused by altered chemosensitivity and cerebral respiratory control. In this type of apnea, the brain intermittently fails to send the appropriate signals to the respiratory muscles to initiate breathing and there is no diaphragmatic movement and no airflow. This is seen in infants younger than 40 weeks' gestational age and in people with neurologic disorders (e.g., tumors, brain infarcts, diffuse encephalopathies).

The most dramatic presentation is the person with repetitive apneas during sleep, accompanied by extreme daytime sleepiness. *Obstructive sleep apnea* (OSA), the most commonly diagnosed form of sleep apnea, is characterized by repetitive episodes of arrest of breathing for

10 seconds or longer with ventilation measured as 50% or less of normal[399] because of transient upper airway obstruction. *Mixed sleep apnea* is a central apnea that is immediately followed by an obstructive event.

Incidence

In a landmark study from the Wisconsin Sleep Cohort, the prevalence of sleep disorders was reported as affecting 24% of men and 9% of women.[551] The Centers for Disease Control and Prevention report an estimated 70 million people in the United States have some kind of sleep problem.[344] An estimated 12 million to 18 million adults in the United States have untreated breathing disorders associated with sleep, a number that is expected to rise with the country's epidemic of obesity. Gender differences in upper airway collapse have not been observed, although there appears to be a relationship to testosterone levels.[434,555,556] It is estimated that 1% to 3% of children have OSA.[9]

Forty percent of obese people have OSA, and 70% of people with sleep apnea are obese. OSA in children without neurologic impairment is most commonly caused by adenotonsillar hypertrophy, although obesity is positively correlated with this disorder in children as well.[26] Children with Down syndrome are particularly vulnerable to OSA and should be tested at age 3 to 4 years.[461]

Etiologic and Risk Factors

OSA is caused by partial or complete pharyngeal collapse during sleep, leading to either reduction (hypopnea) or cessation (apnea) of breathing. Relaxation of the musculature of the pharynx and tongue during sleep obstruct ventilation. The main cause in adults is upper body obesity (BMI ≥30).[164] A neck circumference greater than 16 inches for a woman or greater than 17 inches in a man correlates with an increased risk for this disorder.[260]

People with craniofacial abnormalities (e.g., anatomically narrowed upper airways, such as occur in micrognathia; macroglossia (large tongue); and adenoid, uvula, elongated soft palate, or tonsillar hypertrophy), are predisposed to the development of OSA. Fat deposits or swelling in any or all of these tissues causes further obstruction.

Medical conditions that are associated with OSA include cardiovascular disease (hypertension, coronary artery disease, heart failure, dysrhythmias), cerebrovascular disorders (stroke, dementia, transient ischemic attacks), hypothyroidism,[428] depression, and erectile dysfunction.[399]

Other risk factors include history of snoring, history of excessive daytime sleepiness and complaints of fatigue or nonrestorative sleep. Increasing age; genetic factors (sleep-disordered breathing clusters in families); allergic rhinitis, neurologic disorders; smoking; and chronic bronchitis, are additional risk factors for OSA. Alcohol or sedatives before sleeping may precipitate or worsen the condition.

In children, risk factors include adenoid and tonsillar hypertrophy, craniofacial abnormalities, allergic rhinitis, and neurologic disorders such as Down syndrome, cerebral palsy, and myotonias.[9]

Pathogenesis and Clinical Manifestations

There are several hypotheses as to the pathogenesis of OSA syndrome. Collapse or obstruction of the airway may occur with the inhibition of muscle tone that characterizes some phases of non–rapid eye movement sleep, and rapid eye movement sleep.[316] During inspiration, the negative pressure generated by the respiratory muscles triggers a reflex in pharyngeal muscles that causes upper airway dilation. This reflex is dampened during sleep, causing those with OSA syndrome to have partial or complete collapse of the upper airway. When the airway is obstructed, there is a drop in oxygenation and a concomitant increase in carbon dioxide. In addition to a decrease in upper airway tone during sleep, there is also a drop in the sensitivity of chemoreceptors, further exacerbating loss of upper airway tone.[316]

By definition, apnea is a complete cessation of ventilation and therefore is precipitated by complete pharyngeal collapse, whereas hypopnea results from partial pharyngeal closure and is manifested by a substantial reduction in, but not a cessation of, breathing.

The cycle of recurrent pharyngeal collapse with subsequent arousal from sleep as the brain signals the person to wake up in order to breathe leads to the primary symptoms of daytime somnolence and an increase in the sympathetic drive.[176,316] Activation of the sympathetic nervous system fight-or-flight response increases heart rate, blood pressure, respiratory rate, and glucose levels. Over time, the loss of deep or restful sleep from repeated apneic episodes results in hypertension,[240] daytime sleepiness, fatigue, and difficulty concentrating.[307]

Research efforts to find the genes that are responsible for sleeping and waking are underway. Finding the gene that carries the signal that shuts down connections in the brain during sleep could help advance understanding and treatment of this problem.[78,111]

Bed partners usually report loud cyclic snoring with periods of silence (breath cessation), restlessness, frequent episodes of waking up gasping, and often thrashing movements of the extremities during sleep.

Neurocognitive effects may include personality changes; irritability, hyperactivity, judgment impairment, difficulty concentrating, poor school or work performance, automobile accidents; and memory loss.[112,235] Neurocognitive effects of apnea may also cause a mood disorder leading to an erroneous diagnosis of dysthymia (depressive mood disorder); treatment with standard antidepressant medications may exacerbate the condition.[283]

Fragmented sleep with its repetitive cycles of snoring, airway collapse, and arousal may cause hypertension in some people.[240] Sleep-disordered breathing is also a risk factor for cardiovascular involvement, including angina pectoris, acute myocardial infarction, cardiac arrhythmias, and ischemic stroke.[239]

The primary symptom in children is hyperactivity, not daytime somnolence. OSA syndrome in children is associated with impaired growth, inattention, depression, and an increased risk for cardiovascular conditions.[9]

MEDICAL MANAGEMENT

DIAGNOSIS. Diagnosis may be made using sleep monitoring devices, radiologic imaging, laboratory assays, questionnaires (e.g., Epworth Sleepiness Scale; http://epworthsleepinessscale.com),[273] and clinical signs and symptoms. An in-home system for diagnosing OSA is available, but the most reliable test to confirm the diagnosis is overnight polysomnography (i.e., monitoring the subject during sleep for periods of apnea and lowered blood oxygen saturation). Severity is classified as mild (5-14 episodes of apnea/hypopnea per hour), moderate (15-30 episodes), or severe (more than 30 episodes).[399]

The physician must differentiate sleep apnea syndrome from seizure disorder, narcolepsy, or psychiatric depression. A hemoglobin level is obtained, and thyroid function tests are performed. Several clinical diagnostic predictive formulas are being studied.[396] Diagnosis criteria for children have not been standardized, although it is recognized that they should be different from adult criteria.[425]

TREATMENT. Obstructive and mixed types of sleep apnea syndrome can be treated. Because many clients with sleep apnea are overweight, weight loss is recommended. Weight loss may be curative, but only a small percentage of people maintain their weight loss and symptoms return with weight gain. Bariatric surgery may be an acceptable alternative. The most common treatment for OSA is positive airway pressure (continuous, bilevel, or autopositive) used during sleep. The positive pressure from the pumps stents opens the airway, preventing or minimizing obstruction.

In adults, positive airway pressure is more effective than no treatment and treatment with oral appliances in reducing apnea, decreasing blood pressure, and improving quality of life.[194] An oral appliance may be inserted into the mouth at bedtime and used to hold the jaw forward, thus preventing pharyngeal occlusion. Surgery is recommended if an airway obstruction can be determined as the cause of the sleep apnea. Maxillomandibular surgery to correct anatomic factors is invasive with potential complications but can be very successful in alleviating OSA for carefully selected individuals.[350]

Neurogenic causes of sleep apnea are more difficult to control. There is insufficient evidence to draw any conclusions about the effectiveness of medication. Medication has been directed at improving tone in the upper airway, increasing ventilatory drive, reducing rapid eye movement sleep, and reducing airway resistance or surface tension. Alcohol and hypnotic medications should be avoided. In children, tonsillectomy/adenoidectomy is effective in a majority of cases.[425,458]

PROGNOSIS. Evidence indicates that OSA may be associated with increased long-term cardiovascular and neurophysiologic morbidity. Cardiac and vascular morbidity may include systemic hypertension, cardiac arrhythmias, pulmonary hypertension, cor pulmonale, left ventricular dysfunction, stroke, and sudden death. In fact, the death rate for people with untreated sleep apnea is three times higher than for those who do not have this problem.[550]

Recognition and appropriate treatment of OSA and related disorders will often significantly enhance the client's quality of life, overall health, productivity, and safety on the highway and job.

SPECIAL IMPLICATIONS FOR THE THERAPIST | **15-10**

Sleep-Disordered Breathing: Apnea

Therapists should be aware that OSA increases with age and know the risk factors. Individuals with risk factors should be referred to a sleep center. Sleep position can affect the tongue's position. Individuals with sleep-aid devices, such as continuous positive airway pressure, often report noncompliance with use when asked; the therapist can encourage individuals to use these pumps routinely in order to improve function. Any devices placed inside the mouth that are designed to hold the lower jaw in a forward position can put strain on the temporomandibular joint and affect jaw movements. The therapist should evaluate and monitor these potential adverse effects of these appliances.

Therapists can also work with individuals to find comfortable sleep positions that minimize the anatomical effects contributing to this problem. For example, raising the head of the bed with a wedge, or using a hospital bed can help bring the tongue forward and reduce symptoms of reflux at the same time. Using pillows to elevate the head should be discouraged if it causes increased cervical flexion and/or increased intraabdominal pressure.

There is increasing research on the effects of exercise on persons with sleep apnea. Small studies show improved sleep quality and reduction of obstructive severity with moderate-intensity aerobic activity.[12,294] The incidence of OSA in people scheduled for elective total joint arthroplasty may be higher than previously appreciated. Many are undiagnosed prior to surgery and may develop complications postoperatively. Obesity is a strong risk factor for both OSA and knee arthritis. Studies document a prevalence of 6.7% to 8.7% of previously diagnosed and undiagnosed OSA in this population undergoing joint replacement.[45,55,226] The therapist is advised to observe individuals with diagnosed OSA and obese individuals carefully after surgery for respiratory compromise. Transition to a step-down or transitional care unit may be necessary before discharge to home.[226]

Pulmonary rehabilitation may be an effective adjunct intervention to improve quality of life and cardiovascular fitness and to assist with weight loss. Because of the possible cardiovascular complications associated with clients who have OSA, vital signs should be monitored before, during, and after submaximal or maximal exercise. The client should not be left in the supine position for prolonged periods of time, even while awake.

There are some reports of sleep apnea in association with cervical lesions (e.g., osteophytes caused by diffuse idiopathic skeletal hyperostosis),[327] as well as after anterior cervical spine fusion.[217] Individuals with rheumatoid arthritis complicated with temporomandibular joint destruction and cervical involvement can also develop OSA.[393] Physical therapy may be explored in developing treatment protocols when the musculoskeletal structures of the mandible contribute to the problem.

Restrictive Lung Disease

Overview

Restrictive lung disorders are a major category of pulmonary problems, including any condition that reduces chest wall movement and lung volume. Pulmonary function tests are characterized by a decrease in total lung capacity. There are many causes of restrictive lung disease that are covered in other sections of this chapter or book. More than 100 identified interstitial lung diseases can cause restrictive lung disease.

Extrapulmonary causes may include neurologic or neuromuscular disorders (e.g., head or spinal cord injury, amyotrophic lateral sclerosis, myasthenia gravis, Guillain-Barré syndrome, muscular dystrophy, or poliomyelitis), musculoskeletal disorders (e.g., ankylosing spondylitis, kyphosis or scoliosis, or chest wall injury or deformity), postsurgical conditions, particularly involving the abdomen or thorax, obesity, and collagen vascular diseases (scleroderma, systemic lupus, rheumatoid arthritis).

Clinical Manifestations

Clinical presentation varies according to the cause of the restrictive disorder. Generally, clients exhibit a rapid, shallow respiratory pattern. Chronic tachypnea (fast rate) occurs in an effort to overcome the effects of reduced lung volume and compliance.

Exertional dyspnea progresses to dyspnea at rest because of the loss of inspiratory reserves. As the disease progresses, respiratory muscle fatigue may occur, leading to inadequate alveolar ventilation and carbon dioxide retention. Decreased chest wall movement and increased use of accessory muscles of ventilation are accompanied by the characteristic rapid, shallow breathing. Hypoxemia with digital clubbing is a common finding, especially in the later stages of restrictive disease.

MEDICAL MANAGEMENT

TREATMENT AND PROGNOSIS. The management of restrictive lung disease is based in part on the underlying cause, but is also guided by the severity of the disease. Treatment goals are oriented toward adequate oxygenation, maintaining an airway, and obtaining maximal function. For example, persons with spinal deformities may be helped with corrective surgery and obese persons may experience improved breathing after weight loss.

Corticosteroids may help control inflammation and reduce further impairment, but previously damaged alveolocapillary units cannot be regenerated or replaced. Some clients with end-stage disease may be candidates for heart/lung transplantation. Most restrictive lung diseases are not reversible, and the disease progresses to include

pulmonary hypertension, cor pulmonale, severe hypoxia, and eventual ventilatory or cardiac failure.

SPECIAL IMPLICATIONS FOR THE THERAPIST 15-11

Restrictive Lung Disease

Restrictive lung disease is less prevalent than many of the other conditions discussed in this chapter. Most of the guidelines offered in other sections apply here as well. Exercise testing (6-Minute Walk Test or other submaximal exercise evaluation) plays an important role in determining the extent of the disease and assessing outcomes. Many residual effects of pulmonary pathology are neuromuscular in nature and can be addressed by appropriate physical therapy.[336]

A primary problem for clients with restrictive lung disease secondary to generalized weakness and neuromuscular disease is ineffective cough. Airway clearance techniques to facilitate cough and effective dislodging of secretions to the central airways may be exhausting for the client. Rest periods must be incorporated in the treatment.

A person with restrictive lung disease will be more adversely affected by the restriction of lung function in the recumbent position, emphasizing the importance of routine positioning for immobile clients and active or active-assisted movements whenever possible. Extrapulmonary causes of restriction are most amenable to physical therapy intervention. Consider manual therapy for improving chest wall compliance with injury or after surgery, as well as flexibility exercises. Assess and address muscle weakness, impaired mobility, and difficulty with self-care. Educate the client to watch for and report adverse effects of medications.

Pulmonary Fibrosis

Definition and Overview

Pulmonary fibrosis (also known as interstitial lung disease) is a general term that refers to a variety of disorders in which ongoing epithelial damage leads to progressive scarring (fibrosis) of the lungs, predominantly fibroblasts and small blood vessels that progressively remove and replace normal tissue.[380] Affected individuals commonly present with progressive dyspnea and a nonproductive cough. Pulmonary function tests show a decreased total lung capacity, forced vital capacity, and FEV_1.[249] Incidence appears to be increasing, though in many cases, the etiology remains uncertain.[173]

Etiologic and Risk Factors

Two-thirds of cases of pulmonary fibrosis are idiopathic pulmonary fibrosis (IPF), in which the cause is unknown. In the remaining one-third, fibrosis in the lung is caused by healing scar tissue after active disease, such as TB, systemic sclerosis, CF, or adult respiratory distress syndrome (ARDS). IPF is often diagnosed between 50 and 70 years of age, with a median age at diagnosis of 66.[249,292]

Other risk factors include smoking, exposure to metal dust, sand, and livestock.[386] Additionally, some infections and connective tissue diseases, such as rheumatoid arthritis or SLE, certain drugs (particularly some chemotherapy agents), and, in rare cases, genetic or familial predisposition, increase the risk for developing pulmonary fibrosis.

Thoracic radiation (e.g., postmastectomy radiation of the chest wall and regional lymphatics in clients with breast cancer) may result in pericarditis and pneumonitis, which can progress to pulmonary fibrosis weeks, or even months, after radiation treatments have ended (see "Radiation Lung Disease" in Chapter 5). In addition, some chemotherapies can cause pulmonary fibrosis.[391]

Pathogenesis and Clinical Manifestations

Fibroblast proliferation (fibrosis) irreversibly distorts and shrinks the lung lobe at the alveolar level and causes a marked loss of lung compliance. The lung becomes stiff and difficult to ventilate with decreased diffusing capacity of the alveolocapillary membrane, causing hypoxemia. There does not appear to be an inflammatory process but rather abnormal wound healing in response to multiple, microscopic sites of ongoing alveolar epithelial injury and fibrosis.[380,450] Apoptosis of the alveolar epithelial cells, imbalance of oxidants and antioxidants in the lung, and alterations in telomerase activity have all been implicated in the etiology of IPF.[249] The course of pulmonary fibrosis varies, with early symptoms such as SOB and a dry cough potentially progressing to further complications.

MEDICAL MANAGEMENT

DIAGNOSIS. Diagnosis of IPF is made by high-resolution CT combined with clinical presentation and the exclusion of other possible lung disorders. If the CT is borderline, a lung biopsy may be performed.[386] Clinical assessment, pulmonary function tests, and radiographic studies support the pathologic findings.

TREATMENT AND PROGNOSIS. Exacerbations of IPF are treated with steroids and antibiotics.[292] If the person also has pulmonary hypertension, treatment is targeted to address this issue as it is associated with increased mortality. Patients may also be referred to pulmonary rehabilitation to improve peripheral muscle function and to learn to improve breathing efficiency.

Other approaches to treat IPF include immunomodulatory, immunosuppressive, or antifibrotic agents.[136] Novel approaches target growth factors, angiogenesis (formation of new capillaries), cytokines, apoptosis (programmed cellular death), epithelial regeneration, and oxidative stress.[24] These treatments, alone and in combination, require much further study to determine their effectiveness in slowing or curing this disease.

Lung transplantation may be indicated for those with severe IPF with a 5-year survival rate of approximately 44%.[292] The clinical course of people with pulmonary fibrosis and rheumatoid arthritis is chronic and progressive. Response to treatment is unpredictable, and the overall prognosis is poor, with median survival time of less than 4 years.[39,411]

| SPECIAL IMPLICATIONS FOR THE THERAPIST | 15-12 |

Pulmonary Fibrosis

One of the most common late effects of chest irradiation is pulmonary fibrosis, which may not occur for months to years after radiation to the thorax. The total dose of radiation and the size of the treatment portal determine the severity of this condition. The changes in pulmonary function are usually a progressive decline in lung volumes and a decrease in lung compliance and diffusing capacity. As doses increase, the frequency of pulmonary fibrosis increases, but with improved dosage fractionation, most people die from the cancer before these complications develop.

Early identification of IPF may improve morbidity. Identifying and referring anyone who has unusual SOB or progressive decrease in exercise tolerance may help with early diagnosis. Physical therapy intervention depends on clinical presentation and may focus on peripheral conditioning and motor control for more efficient oxygen utilization. Pulmonary rehabilitation including exercise training has been shown to improve both exercise capacity, endurance (decreased fatigue), and health-related quality of life in small studies involving individuals with idiopathic pulmonary fibrosis,[481] especially early on when the disease is mild.[243,379]

Systemic Sclerosis Lung Disease

Definition

Systemic sclerosis (SSc), or scleroderma, is an autoimmune disease of connective tissue characterized by excessive collagen deposition in the skin and internal organs, particularly the kidneys and lungs. This condition is discussed in detail in Chapter 10.

Incidence

Clinically, more than half of all people with SSc die of pulmonary disease.[469] The presence of pulmonary arterial hypertension is a major prognostic factor in mortality. The lungs, as a result of a rich vascular supply and abundant connective tissue, are a frequent target organ (second to the esophagus in visceral involvement). Skin changes generally precede visceral alterations, and lung involvement rarely presents symptoms at first, but pulmonary symptoms develop after an average of 7 years.[51]

Pathogenesis and Clinical Manifestations

Three pathways produce organ damage. First, inflammation is caused by T cells and cytokines, resulting in alveolitis before fibrosis. Second, severe thickening and obstruction of vessels occurs, resulting in pulmonary hypertension and renal failure. Third, cutaneous fibrosis occurs.[468] Immunosuppressive therapy may delay onset of symptoms by up to 4 years.[51]

Oxidative stress contributes to disease progression by a rapid degeneration of endothelial cell function in SSc. Daily episodes of hypoxia-reperfusion injury produce free radicals (see Fig. 6-2) that cause endothelial damage, intimal thickening, and fibrosis along with inactivation of antioxidant enzymes.[185]

Studies have determined that the balance between fibrotic and inflammatory mediators may be important to developing pathology.[234] Lung biopsy of early lesions shows capillary congestion, hypercellularity of alveolar walls, increased fibrous tissue in the alveolar septa, and interstitial edema with fibrosis. As a result, initial symptoms of dyspnea on exertion and nonproductive cough develop. As fibroblast proliferation and collagen deposition progress, fibrosis of the alveolar wall occurs and the capillaries are obliterated. Clinically, the client demonstrates more severe dyspnea and has a greater risk of deterioration in pulmonary function.

MEDICAL MANAGEMENT

DIAGNOSIS. Traditional tests, such as pulmonary function tests and chest radiographs, are insensitive and not predictive of outcome. Thin-section CT is very sensitive for early diagnosis of SSc lung involvement. Bronchoalveolar lavage and serum markers (surfactant protein D and LK-6) give some indication of the disease process.[234]

TREATMENT. Successful treatment of SSc pulmonary disease remains an area for further development. Pharmacologic treatments include corticosteroids and immunosuppressive agents. Steroids reduce inflammation as well as reduce fibrosis. Monoclonal antibodies are also being investigated although at the time of this writing their effectiveness remains to be seen.[79] Identifying the cycle of oxidative stress and antioxidant inactivation may result in treatment by supplementation of antioxidants and different kinds of drugs with antioxidant properties.[185,471]

Investigations conclude that lung transplantation is a viable option for carefully selected individuals with scleroderma-related lung disease. Single-lung transplantation may be indicated in those without significant visceral dysfunction. Survival rates are equivalent to lung transplant recipients with other disorders with a 2-year survival rate of 64%.[185,337]

PROGNOSIS. SSc lung disease is unpredictable and may be a mild, prolonged course, but as the pulmonary fibrosis advances and causes pulmonary hypertension, cor pulmonale characterized by peripheral edema may develop, progressing rapidly to respiratory failure and death. Lung disease is the most frequent cause of death from SSc. Morbidity and mortality of adults older than 75 years were worse than that of younger adults, in part related to late diagnosis.[147]

SPECIAL IMPLICATIONS FOR THE THERAPIST   15-13

Systemic Sclerosis Lung Disease
The effectiveness of a pulmonary rehabilitation program with SSc lung disease remains unknown and warrants research investigation. Therapy implications and interventions should be based on general principles regarding pulmonary involvement and specific clinical presentation.

Chest Wall Trauma or Lung Injury

Blunt Chest Trauma

Chest or thoracic trauma ranges from superficial wounds such as contusions and abrasions to life-threatening tension pneumothorax. Flail chest occurs as a result of sternum or multiple rib fracture. By definition, a flail chest consists of fractures of four or more adjacent ribs on the same side, and possibly the sternum, with each bone fractured into two or more segments.[377] The fractured rib segments are detached (free-floating) from the rest of the chest wall. The integrity of the thorax is compromised, and the inspiratory force of the diaphragm causes inward (paradoxical) movement of the fractured ribs. The number of rib fractures is directly correlated with lung-related complications, and the presence of six or more rib fractures significantly increases mortality from nonpulmonary causes.[174]

Early identification improves outcomes, particularly in children in whom chest trauma is the second leading cause of death.[442] Complex soft tissue injury can occur in the absence of chest wall fractures.[2] Cough-induced rib fractures occur primarily in women and can occur in persons with normal bone density.[222] These fractures are typically lateral, in the middle ribs, and do not cause flail chest.

Clinical Manifestations. It is common for a fractured rib end to tear the pleura and lung surface, thereby producing hemopneumothorax. This causes the lung to collapse from the loss of negative pressure. Fractured ribs can also lacerate abdominal organs, the brachial plexus, and blood vessels.

In flail chest, the paradoxical chest motion impairs movement of gas in and out of the lungs (Fig. 15-14), promotes atelectasis, and impairs pulmonary drainage. Other clinical manifestations of flail chest include excruciating pain, severe dyspnea, hypoventilation, cyanosis, and hypoxemia, potentially leading to respiratory failure without the appropriate intervention.

MEDICAL MANAGEMENT

DIAGNOSIS. Rib fractures and/or flail chest are diagnosed by clinical examination, radiograph, and chest CT. Because blunt trauma may also involve significant soft tissue injury, multidetector CT is recommended to more accurately determine the extent of injury.[352]

TREATMENT. Initial treatment follows the ABCs (airway, breathing, and circulation) of emergency treatment to treat the pneumothorax, thereby enabling the person to breathe deeply and to effectively clear secretions. A chest tube removes both air and blood in the pleural cavity after chest trauma, which helps restore the negative pressure in the pleural space so that the lungs can remain inflated. The tube is usually positioned in the sixth intercostal space in the posterior axillary line. Continuous positive airway pressure or PEEP may be used to enhance lung expansion.[38]

In those with flail chest, treatment involves pain management via epidural, chest physical therapy, mechanical ventilation as needed, and the consideration for surgical stabilization.[158,377] The use of surgical fixation remains controversial, as most with rib involvement and no pulmonary contusion recover with mild impairments.

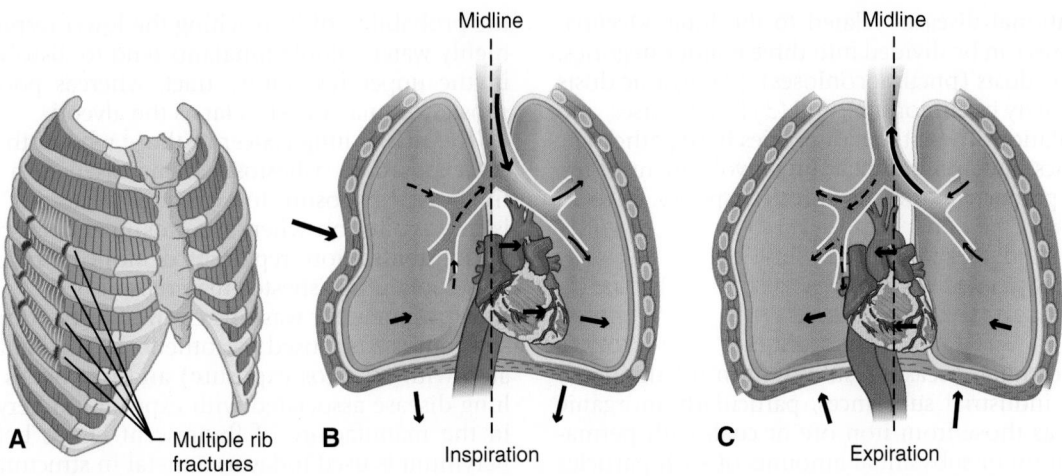

Figure 15-14

Flail chest. *Arrows* indicate air movement or structural movement. **A,** Flail chest consists of fractured rib segments that are detached (free-floating) from the rest of the chest wall. **B,** On inspiration, the flail segment of ribs is sucked inward. The affected lung and mediastinal structures shift to the unaffected side. This compromises the amount of inspired air in the unaffected lung. **C,** On expiration, the flail segment of ribs bellows outward. The affected lung and mediastinal structures shift to the affected side with the diaphragm elevated on that side (not shown). Some air within the lungs is shunted back and forth between the lungs instead of passing through the upper airway.

Whenever pulmonary function is adequate, intubation is avoided to help reduce infection, the most common complication associated with morbidity and mortality in clients with flail chest.

Pharmacologic treatment may include muscle relaxants or musculoskeletal paralyzing agents to reduce the risk of separation of the healing costochondral junctions. Those with flail chest and pulmonary contusion have been found to have ongoing chest wall pain, dyspnea and reduced functional residual capacity.[158] Morbidity and mortality information from chest wall trauma is difficult to decipher as many of these people have other injuries, such as brain injury, that contribute to mortality.

Chest Wall or Lung Injury

See also "Pneumothorax" and "Special Implications for the Therapist 15-26: Pneumothorax" below.

The emergency room therapist is the most likely therapist to evaluate and treat someone with a flail chest, although this varies by geographic region. Transcutaneous electrical nerve stimulators have been shown to be more effective than nonsteroidal antiinflammatory drugs for controlling pain associated with rib fractures.[387] This is important because pain can further compromise pulmonary function.[284]

Once the person has been stabilized and moved to the acute care setting, therapists may come into contact with patients who experience chest wall injuries. Manual techniques for secretion removal may be used, but the presence of a lung contusion directs medical intervention more toward drainage or aspiration of any blood pooled in the area.

Airway clearance techniques may have a role in facilitating chest tube drainage, but must be used carefully in the presence of any rib fractures. Percussion

and vibration techniques are contraindicated directly over fractures, but can be used over other lung segments. Rib or chest taping and ultrasound over the site of the fracture should not be used. Once the fractures have healed, rib mobilization and soft tissue mobilization for the intercostals may be necessary to restore normal respiratory movements.

It should be noted that airway clearance techniques can cause rib fractures and that infants are particularly vulnerable to rib fractures.[103] Frequent turning and position changes, as well as deep-breathing and coughing exercises, are important. A semi-Fowler position may help with lung reexpansion necessary to prevent atelectasis.

In the case of flail chest from injury, simultaneous cardiac damage (myocardial contusion) may have occurred, necessitating the same care as for a person who has suffered a myocardial infarction (see "Special Implications for the Therapist 12-6: Myocardial Infarction" in Chapter 12).

Scapular fractures are often overlooked when only supine chest radiographs are performed. The therapist may recognize a suspicious clinical presentation (e.g., loss of scapular–humeral motion, symptoms disproportionate to the injury, or development of previously undocumented large hematomas) suggesting the need for more definitive medical diagnosis. In the case of all fractures, once the fracture is healed the therapist may become involved in restoration of movement and strength.

ENVIRONMENTAL AND OCCUPATIONAL DISEASES

The relationship between occupations and disease has been observed, studied, and documented for many years. An in-depth discussion of this broad topic is included in Chapter 4. This chapter discusses only environmental and occupational diseases related to the lung. Occupational diseases can be divided into three major categories: (1) inorganic dusts (pneumoconioses); (2) organic dusts (hypersensitivity pneumonitis); and (3) fumes, gases, and smoke inhalation. These three categories have pathologic characteristics in common, including involvement of the pulmonary parenchyma with a fibrotic response.

Pneumoconiosis

Overview

Any group of lung diseases resulting from inhalation of particles of industrial substances, particularly inorganic dusts, such as those from iron ore or coal, with permanent deposition of substantial amounts of such particles in the lung, is included in the generic term *pneumoconiosis* (dusty lungs). Clinically, common pneumoconioses include coal workers' pneumoconiosis, silicosis, and asbestosis. Other types of pneumoconiosis include talc, beryllium lung disease (berylliosis), aluminum pneumoconiosis, cadmium workers' disease, and siderosis (inhalation of iron or other metallic particles). Farmers in dry climate regions exposed to respirable dust (inorganic agricultural dusts) during farming activities (e.g., plowing and tilling) and toxic gases (e.g., from animal confinement) may develop chronic bronchitis, hypersensitivity pneumonitis, and pulmonary fibrosis.

Incidence and Etiologic Factors

Obviously occurring in occupational groups, pneumoconiosis is most common among miners, sandblasters, stonecutters, asbestos workers, insulators, and agriculture workers. There is an increasing incidence with age because of cumulative effects of exposure, but overall incidence of diseases caused by mineral dust has declined recently in postindustrial countries. Instead, there is a rise in occupational asthma and illnesses caused by exposure in new office buildings and hospitals.[48]

Silicosis, formerly called *potters' asthma, stonecutters' cough, miners' mold,* and *grinders' rot,* is most likely to be contracted in today's industrial jobs involving sandblasting in tunnels, hard-rock mining (extraction and processing of ores), and preparation and use of sand. It can occur in anyone habitually exposed (usually over a period of 10 years) to the dust contained in silica, and any miner is subject to it. Usually, silicosis is associated with extensive or prolonged inhalation of free silica (silicon dioxide) particles in the crystalline form of quartz.

Risk Factors

Higher-risk workplaces are those with obvious dust, smoke, or vapor or those in which there is spraying, painting, or drying of coated surfaces. Heavier exposure occurs when there is friction, grinding, heat, or blasting; when very small particles are generated; and in enclosed spaces.

Not all clients exposed to occupational inhalants will develop lung disease. Harmful effects depend on the (1) type of exposure, (2) duration and intensity of exposure, (3) presence of underlying pulmonary disease, (4) smoking history, and (5) particle size and water solubility of the inhalant. The larger the particle, the lower the probability of its reaching the lower respiratory tract; highly water-soluble inhalants tend to dissolve and react in the upper respiratory tract, whereas poorly soluble substances may travel as far as the alveoli.

The risk of lung cancer in those who both smoke and are exposed to asbestosis is increased in a multiplicative way.[60] Exposure to significant amounts of asbestos is most common when asbestos materials are disturbed during renovation, repair, or demolition of older buildings containing asbestos materials.

Exposure while washing clothes soiled with these toxic substances has caused mesothelioma (malignancy associated with asbestos exposure) and berylliosis (beryllium lung disease associated with exposure to beryllium used in the manufacture of fluorescent lamps before 1950). Beryllium is used today as a metal in structural materials employed in aerospace industries, in the manufacture of industrial ceramics, and in atomic reactors, so exposure is still possible.

Pathogenesis

Dust particles (indestructible mineral fibers) that are not filtered out by the nasociliary mechanism or mucociliary escalator may be deposited anywhere in the respiratory tract and lungs, especially the small airways and alveoli. Each disease has its own pathogenesis, but in general the most dangerous dust particles measure 2 μm or less and are deposited in the smallest bronchioles and the acini (see Fig. 15-2).

The particles are ingested by alveolar macrophages, and most of the phagocytosed particles ascend to the mucociliary lining and are expectorated or swallowed. Some migrate into the interstitium of the lung and then into the lymphatics. These indestructible mineral fibers can actually pierce the lung cells. In response to the continued presence of these fibers and to the cell damage, activated macrophages secrete fibroblast-stimulating factor, which in turn mediates excessive fibrosis (i.e., the thickening and scarring of lung tissue that occur around the mineral fiber).

In *coal workers' pneumoconiosis*, ingestion of inhaled coal dust by alveolar macrophages leads to the formation of coal macules, which appear on the radiograph as diffuse small opacities (or white areas) in the upper lung. Anthracite or hard coal is associated with a higher incidence of black lung than is bituminous or soft coal.

In the pathogenesis of silicosis, groups of silicon hydroxide on the surface of the particles form hydrogen bonds with phospholipids and proteins, an interaction that is presumed to damage cellular membranes and thereby kill the macrophage. The dead macrophages release free silica particles and fibrogenic factors. The released silica is then reingested by macrophages, and the process is amplified.

Between 10 and 40 years after initial exposure to silica, small rounded opacities called *silicotic nodules* form throughout the lung. These fibrotic nodules scar the lungs and make them receptive to further complications (e.g., TB, bronchitis, or emphysema).

Asbestosis is characterized by inhalation of asbestos fibers, a fibrous magnesium and calcium silicate nonburning compound used in roofing materials, insulation for electric circuits, brake linings, and many other products that must be fire resistant. As with the other pneumoconioses, asbestos particles are engulfed by macrophages. Once activated, macrophages then release inflammatory mediators resulting in nodular interstitial fibrosis that can be seen on radiographs along with thickened pleura.

After an interval of 10 to 20 years between exposure and further complications, calcified pleural plaques on the dome of the diaphragm or lateral chest wall develop. The lower portions of the lungs are more often involved than the upper portions in asbestosis.

How asbestos causes mesothelioma is unclear; the formation of oxygen free radicals by macrophages can be a cause of chromosomal damage, or there may be a growth factor that governs individual susceptibility to mineral fiber–induced mesothelioma. Other mechanisms of oncogenesis have been proposed but remain unconfirmed.[87,425]

Clinical Manifestations

Symptoms of pneumoconioses from dust exposure include progressive dyspnea, chest pain, chronic cough, and expectoration of mucus containing the offending particles. In rare cases, rheumatoid arthritis coexisting primarily with coal workers' pneumoconiosis but also with silicosis and asbestosis causes Caplan syndrome, a condition characterized by the presence of rheumatoid nodules in the periphery of the lung. Long-term exposure to acid and other substances produces ulceration and perforation of the septum, whereas nickel and certain wood dusts cause nasal carcinoma.

Work-related asthma can be an exacerbation of asthma that was previously subclinical or in remission (work-aggravated asthma), a new onset of asthma caused by a sensitizing exposure (asthma with latency), or asthma that results from a single heavy exposure to a potent respiratory irritant (referred to as asthma without latency, irritant asthma, or reactive airways dysfunction syndrome). Symptoms are as discussed in "Asthma" above.

Simple silicosis is usually asymptomatic and has no effect on routine pulmonary function tests. As the disease progresses, mucus tinged with blood, loss of appetite, chest pain, and general weakness may occur. In complicated silicosis, dyspnea and obstructive and restrictive lung dysfunction occur.

Asbestosis is characterized by dyspnea, inspiratory crackles (on auscultation), and sometimes clubbing and cyanosis. As in the case of the other pneumoconioses, the simple or uncomplicated form of coal workers' pneumoconiosis is uncommon, but the chronic form is often associated with chronic bronchitis and infections.

MEDICAL MANAGEMENT

PREVENTION. Prevention is the first line of defense against occupational diseases. Workplace-based education, pre-employment screening, yearly physical examinations, surveillance and exposure reduction, and elimination of the pathogen are essential components of a strategy to prevent occupational lung disorders. Precautions, such as the use of face masks, protective clothing, and proper ventilation, are essential. Regular chest films are recommended for all workers exposed to silica, as a means of early detection.

In 1971, asbestos became the first material to be regulated by the U.S. Occupational Safety and Health Administration. The Environmental Protection Agency (EPA) has classified asbestos as a Group A human carcinogen, causing both lung cancer and mesothelioma. It is still unclear if lung cancer can occur as result of exposure to asbestos without the presence of asbestosis.[232] The EPA maintains the Integrated Risk Information System database on health effects of exposure to various substances. This agency also controls the National Emission Standards for Hazardous Air Pollutants (http://www.epa.gov).

DIAGNOSIS. Identifying a workplace-related cause of disease is important because it can lead to cure and to prevention for others. The recognition of occupational causes can be difficult because of the latency period, delayed responses that occur at home either after work or years after exposure. Diagnosis is by history of exposure (which may be minimal with asbestosis and far removed in time from the onset of disease; the person may even be unaware of the exposure), sputum cytology, lung biopsy, chest film showing nodular or interstitial fibrosis, and pulmonary function studies.

Other pulmonary imaging techniques used in conjunction with the initial chest radiograph include conventional CT, high-resolution CT, and gallium scintigraphy. High-resolution CT scanning is the best imaging method to differentiate different origins of pneumoconiosis as presentation varies with the stimulus (silica, coal dust, iron dust, or asbestos). Magnetic resonance imaging (MRI) is helpful to distinguish progressive fibrosis from lung cancer (see "Diagnosis" under "Lung Cancer" below).[108,333] Imaging alone is inadequate to make most diagnoses; clinical presentation of symptoms and lung function are also important.[431] Genetic susceptibility may be associated with beryllium-induced disease and may play a role in mediating other types of pneumoconiosis.[177]

TREATMENT. There is no standard treatment for these diseases. The dust deposits are permanent so treatment is directed toward relief of symptoms. Corticosteroids may produce some improvement in silicosis. Although there is no cure for any of the pneumoconioses, the complications of chronic bronchitis, pulmonary hypertension, and cor pulmonale must be treated. When lung neoplasm occurs, surgical removal and therapeutic modalities, such as radiotherapy or chemotherapy, may be employed.

PROGNOSIS. The devastating feature of pneumoconioses is that there may be no obvious symptoms until the disease is in an advanced state. Once fully developed, prognosis is poor for most occupational lung diseases, with progressive and disabling results. Simple silicosis is not ordinarily associated with significant respiratory dysfunction unless complicated by emphysema and chronic bronchitis from cigarette smoking.

Although now uncommon, acute silicosis resulting from heavy exposure to silica rarely responds to treatment and progresses rapidly over a few years when it occurs. The increased incidence of TB among people with silicosis presents an additional negative factor to the prognosis.

Exposure to asbestos, radon, silica, chromium, cadmium, nickel, arsenic, and beryllium may result in neoplasm. Crystalline silica is a known human carcinogen, but this link is not defined and may be overestimated.[306,405] Both bronchogenic carcinoma and mesotheliomas of the pleura and peritoneum have been linked to asbestos. The exposure typically occurs 20 years before the development of bronchogenic carcinoma and approximately 30 to 40 years before the appearance of mesothelioma. The disease culminates in the sixth decade, with few cases occurring before age 40 years. Although progress has been made, mesothelioma still has a 5-year survival rate of only 9%. New chemotherapy drugs have increased the life expectancy but are not curative.

Coal workers' pneumoconiosis was once thought to cause severe disability, but it is now clear that black lung causes minor impairment of pulmonary function at its worst. When coal miners have severe airflow obstruction, it is usually from smoking.

SPECIAL IMPLICATIONS FOR THE THERAPIST | 15-15

Pneumoconioses

New materials are being introduced into the workplace at a faster rate than their potential toxicities can be evaluated despite the fact that many have a pathologic effect on the pulmonary system. The possibility of occupational lung disease should be considered whenever a working or retired person has unexplained respiratory illness.

The ventilatory equivalent for O_2 (VE/VO_2) during exercise is more predictive of clinical dyspnea than airway obstruction in pneumoconiosis. VE is minute ventilation or the total amount of air inhaled or exhaled by the lungs each minute; VO_2 refers to oxygen consumption per minute per kg of body weight. This ratio documents the degree of $\dot{V}/\dot{Q}$ mismatch and can be useful for therapists in prescribing exercise programs for this patient population.[46]

Steam inhalation and airway clearance techniques, such as controlled coughing and segmental bronchial drainage with chest percussion and vibration, help clear secretions. Exercise tolerance must be increased slowly over a long period beginning with increasing regular activities of daily living. Daily activities should be planned carefully to conserve energy (see Box 9-4), to decrease the WOB, and to afford frequent rest periods.

Graded progression from increasing tolerance for daily activities to a conditioning program may precede or replace an aggressive exercise program. In severe cases, oxygen may be necessary for any increase in activity level or exercise and the person may not progress beyond self-care skills.

Hypersensitivity Pneumonitis

Exposure to organic dusts may result in hypersensitivity pneumonitis, also called extrinsic allergic alveolitis. The alveoli and distal airways are most often involved as a result of inhalation of organic dusts and active chemicals. Most of the diseases are named according to the specific antigen or occupation and involve organic materials such as molds (e.g., mushroom compost, moldy hay, sugar cane, or logs left unprotected from moisture), fungal spores (e.g., stagnant water in air conditioners and central heating units), plant fibers or wood dust (particularly redwood and maple and cotton), cork dust, coffee beans, bird feathers, and hydroxyurea (cytotoxic agent).

Gram-bacterial endotoxins may be more to blame than dust in causing pneumonitis in cotton textile workers.[521] Mycobacteria have also been shown to be responsible for hypersensitivity pneumonitis in industrial metal grinding and in "hot tub lung."[5,224]

Regardless of the specific antigen involved in the pathogenesis of hypersensitivity pneumonitis, the pathologic alterations in the lung are similar. A combination of immune complex–mediated and T-cell–mediated hypersensitivity reactions occurs, although the exact mechanism of these processes is still unknown.

Symptoms usually develop after years of exposure and common complaints are fever, dyspnea, coughing and weight loss.[238] Diagnosis is made through clinical history, radiograph, pulmonary function tests, bronchioalveolar lavage, and high-resolution chest CT. The bronchioalveolar lavage often shows increased white blood cells, largely an increase in lymphocytes. Moreover, the CD4:CD8 ratio may be less than 1, with a normal ratio of 1.8. On chest CT, there is the presents of bilateral ground glass opacities, centrilobular nodular opacities, and air trapping.[238]

Initially, symptoms may be reversed by removing the worker from the exposure (the only adequate treatment), modifying the materials-handling process, or using protective clothing and masks. The symptoms typically remit within 24 to 48 hours but return on reexposure and with time and in some people, may become chronic. If severe, treatment may include high-dose steroids to dampen inflammation.[238]

Hypersensitivity pneumonitis may present as acute, subacute, or chronic pulmonary disease depending on the frequency and intensity of exposure to the antigen. Chronic pulmonary impairments differ depending on the offending agent; however, many people will only have mild airflow obstruction or have complete resolution with avoidance of the offending antigen.

Noxious Gases, Fumes, and Smoke Inhalation

Exposure to toxic gases and fumes is an increasing problem in modern industrial society. Any time oxygen in the air is replaced by another toxic or nontoxic agent, asphyxia (deficient blood oxygen and increased carbon dioxide in blood and tissues) occurs. Such is the case when products manufactured from synthetic compounds are heated at high temperatures, releasing fumes. For example, workers who use heating elements to seal meat in plastic wrappers and workers involved in the manufacture of plastics and packaging materials made of polyvinyl chlorides are exposed to these fumes. Workers exposed to the artificial butter flavoring for popcorn, diacetyl, have developed significant respiratory obstruction.[303]

The most common mechanism of injury is local irritation, the specific type and extent depending on the type and concentration of gas and the duration of exposure. For example, highly soluble gases, such as ammonia, rapidly injure the mucous membranes of the eye and upper airway, causing an intense burning pain in the eyes, nose, and throat. Insoluble gases, such as nitrogen dioxide, encountered by farmers cause diffuse lung injury.

Metal fume fever is a systemic response to inhalation of certain metal dusts and fumes such as zinc oxide used in galvanizing iron, the manufacture of brass, and chrome and copper plating. Symptoms include fever and chills, cough, dyspnea, thirst, metallic taste, salivation, myalgias, headache, and malaise. Welding fumes create exposure to multiple hazardous agents and cause varied respiratory and systemic pathology.[349] *Polymer fume fever*, associated with heating of polymers, may cause similar symptoms. With brief exposures, the symptoms associated with these two syndromes are self-limiting, but prolonged exposure results in chronic cough, hemoptysis, and impairment of pulmonary function associated with a wide range of lung pathologic conditions.

Chemical pneumonitis can result from exposure to toxic fumes. The acute reaction may produce diffuse lung injury characterized by air space disease typical of pulmonary edema. In its chronic form, constrictive bronchiolitis develops.

Smoke inhalation injury produces direct mucosal injury secondary to hot gases, tissue anoxia caused by combustion products, and asphyxia as oxygen is consumed by fire. Thermal injury seen in the upper airway is characterized by edema and obstruction. Incomplete combustion of industrial compounds produces ammonia, acrolein, sulfur dioxide, and other substances in today's fires.

Environmental tobacco smoke (ETS), or exposure to secondhand smoke among nonsmokers, is widespread. The home is the largest exposure source for children.[256] A total of 15 million children are estimated to be exposed to secondhand smoke in their homes annually. ETS increases the risk of heart disease and respiratory infections in children, increases the incidence of otitis media, increases the risk of lung cancer by a factor of 2 to 3, and is a major risk factor for sudden infant death syndrome.[317] ETS also increases the risk for neurobehavioral problems such as attention-deficit hyperactivity disorder and decreased school performance.[256]

Infants born to women exposed to ETS during pregnancy have an increased chance of decreased birth weight and intrauterine growth retardation.[233] Prenatal exposure to mainstream smoke from the mother and even to ETS from the mother has been shown to change fetal lung development and cause airflow obstruction, promote airway hyperresponsiveness and early development of asthma and allergy, and double the odds of future attention-deficit hyperactivity disorder.[261,309] The effects of prenatal ETS can last through adolescence and beyond.[256]

Newborns, infants, and children younger than age 2 years are at high risk for cardiovascular effects if they are exposed to household ETS during this time. Endothelial cells of the blood vessels damaged as a result of exposure to passive smoking can be measured during the first decade of life. ETS over a period of more than 10 years changes the intima-to-media ratio by enhancing the thickness of the vessel wall. There is also early lipid accumulation in the coronary arteries and aorta.[256] Other effects of involuntary smoking among children may include middle ear disease, upper and lower respiratory infections, and asthma.[262,489]

Children are highly susceptible to ETS because of their proximity to parents while the parents are smoking, surface-area-to-body-weight ratio, and immaturity of their systems to metabolize ETS.[256]

Adults are also exposed to ETS; however, this exposure is declining as a consequence of new laws regarding smoking in public places. Approximately 88 million nonsmokers in the United States were exposed to ETS in 2007–2008, whereas 53.6% of children between 3 and 11 years old were exposed.[385] Nonsmoking adults who are exposed to ETS increase cardiovascular risk by up to 30% and increase lung cancer risk by the same amount according to the CDC Office on Smoking and Health.

Third-hand smoke (THS) is also emerging as a risk factor for disease. THS refers to the constituents of tobacco smoke that are left on surfaces such as carpets and drapes or in the air after the THS has moved into the gas phase.[339] THS may remain on surfaces for weeks to months after smoking.[339] Research on the acute and long-term effects of THS is in its infancy at the time of this writing.

DROWNING

Definition

Near drowning was a term previously used to describe an episode of drowning with survival, but the term "drowning" is now preferred. Drowning involves immersion or submersion in a liquid with or without survival (survival means >24 hours). Submersion causes hypoxemia and acidosis. Drowning occurs in three forms: (1) dry drowning, inhalation of little or no fluid with minimal lung injury because of laryngeal spasm (10%-15% of cases); (2) wet drowning, aspiration of fluid with asphyxia or secondary changes caused by aspiration (85%); and (3) recurrence of respiratory distress secondary to pneumonia or pulmonary edema within 1 to 2 days after a drowning incident. Recovery is rapid if respiration and circulation are restored before permanent neurologic damage occurs. Death may occur from asphyxia secondary to reflex laryngospasm and glottic closure.

Incidence and Risk Factors

Unintentional drowning is the leading cause of injury death among children ages 4 years and younger[94,313]; it is the second leading cause of death by injury in those ages 5 to 15 years, and the third leading cause of accidental death among all age groups. The death rate for males is nearly four times that for females, which is generally attributed to their choice of higher-risk activities, overestimation of swimming ability, and use of alcohol.[313] Alcohol consumption while swimming or boating is involved in approximately 25% to 50% of adolescent and adult deaths associated with water recreation and is a major contributing factor in up to 50% of drownings among adolescent boys.[93]

Other risk factors include epilepsy, intellectual developmental disorder, heart attack, head or spinal cord injury at the time of the accident, failure to use personal flotation devices, increased use of hot tubs and spas, and lack of proper swimming training or overestimation of endurance by those who can swim, according to the National Center for Injury Prevention and Control.[313]

Pathogenesis

For every child younger than 15 years who drowns, five require medical care for drowning injuries. The complications of drowning fall into two categories: the effects of prolonged anoxia on the brain and kidney, which as end organs may experience complications that are irreversible (determining the final prognosis), and ALI from aspiration of fluids. When aspiration accompanies drowning, severe pulmonary injury often occurs, resulting in persistent arterial hypoxia and metabolic acidosis even after ventilation has been restored.

In the past, a distinction was made between the effects of saltwater and freshwater drowning (e.g., cardiovascular function and changes in blood volume and serum electrolyte concentrations), but it is now known that hypoxia is the most important determinant of survival in human drowning, regardless of the type of water involved.

The duration of submersion and the water temperature determine the pathologic events. Hypoxia results in global cell damage; different cells tolerate variable lengths of anoxia. Neurons, especially cerebral cells, sustain irreversible damage after 4 to 6 minutes of submersion. The heart and lungs can survive up to 30 minutes.

The extent of CNS injury tends to correlate with the duration of hypoxia, but hypothermia accompanying the incident is associated with changes in neurotransmitter release (glutamate, dopamine) and may reduce the cerebral oxygen requirements and help reduce CNS injury. For a detailed review of cold-water submersion, its mechanisms, and its effects the reader is referred to other sources.[191,225]

Clinical Manifestations

The clinical features in drowning are variable, and the person may be unconscious, semiconscious, or awake but apprehensive. Pulmonary and neurologic symptoms predominate, with cough, tachypnea, and possible development of ARDS (see section: "Acute Lung Injury and Acute Respiratory Distress") with progressive respiratory failure.

Other pulmonary complications include pulmonary edema, bacterial pneumonia, pneumothorax, or pneumomediastinum secondary to resuscitation efforts. Fever occurs in the presence of aspiration during the first 24 hours, but can occur later in the presence of infection.

Early neurologic manifestations include seizures, especially during resuscitative measures, and altered mental status, including agitation, combativeness, and coma. Speech, motor, or visual abnormalities may occur, improve gradually, and resolve over several months.

MEDICAL MANAGEMENT

PREVENTION. Prevention of drowning and drowning events is a vital part of education. The CDC recommends mandating and enforcing legal limits for blood alcohol levels during water recreation activities, public education about the danger of combining alcohol (and other substances) with water recreation, restricting the sale of alcohol at water recreation facilities, and eliminating advertisements that encourage alcohol use during boating. Additional safeguard techniques for prevention of drowning among children are available.[93,98]

TREATMENT. Improved training in cardiopulmonary resuscitation has resulted in survival of the majority of drowning victims who live long enough to receive hospital care. Restoration of ventilation and circulation by means of resuscitation at the scene of the accident is the primary goal of treatment to restore oxygen delivery and prevent further hypoxic damage. Other treatment is largely supportive, with antibiotics for pulmonary infection, maintenance of fluid and electrolyte balance, possible transfusion for significant anemia, and management of acute renal failure.

Comatose drowning victims frequently have elevated intracranial pressure caused by cerebral edema and loss of cerebrovascular autoregulation. Reduction of cerebral blood flow adds ischemic injury to already damaged brain tissue. To reserve cerebral function in such cases, cerebral resuscitation (controlled hyperventilation, deliberate hypothermia, or use of barbiturates, glucocorticoids, and diuretics) may be utilized.

PROGNOSIS. The prognosis depends in large part on the extent and duration of the hypoxic episode. People have survived as long as 70 minutes of immersion with complete recovery, but up to 20% of all drowning victims will have permanent sequelae, many of which are ultimately fatal. If laryngospasm is finally overcome and the person aspirates water or if aspiration of vomitus occurs during resuscitative measures, prognosis is worse than without these complications.

Other unfavorable prognostic indicators include first blood pH values below 7, low rectal temperature on admission to the hospital, abnormal electroencephalogram, deterioration of room air oxygen saturation, and degree of electroencephalogram disturbance.

Coincident head trauma or subdural hematoma presents an additional prognostic complication. Neurologic injury is the most serious and least reversible complication in those persons successfully resuscitated. Little, if anything, has been shown to help, and it carries a grave prognosis.

SPECIAL IMPLICATIONS FOR THE THERAPIST   15-16

Drowning

All drowning victims should be admitted to a hospital inpatient setting for observation over 24 to 48 hours because of the possibility of delayed drowning syndrome with confusion, substernal pain, and adventitious breath sounds (crackles or wheezing/rhonchi). The therapist is often involved early on in the case management, providing bedside care much the same as for a person with traumatic brain injury or spinal cord injury. It is not uncommon for a drowning accident to be associated with either traumatic brain injury or spinal cord injury.

Evaluate cardiopulmonary status, monitor vital signs, and observe respirations. Airway clearance techniques may be necessary. To facilitate breathing, elevate the head of the bed slightly if possible; observe for signs of infection (see Box 8-1); and check for any areas of skin pressure or factors precipitating pressure ulcers. Provide passive or active-assistive exercise according to the person's functional abilities, and progress as quickly as possible given the medical status.

In the rehabilitation setting, large doses of steroids are administered early in the treatment of some cases of spinal cord injury to control cerebral or spinal cord edema. Suppression of the inflammatory reaction in persons receiving large doses of steroids may be so complete as to mask the clinical signs and symptoms of major diseases, perforation of a peptic ulcer, or spread of infection. See also "Corticosteroids" in Chapter 5.

CONGENITAL DISORDERS

Cystic Fibrosis

Karen von Berg, PT

Definition and Overview

CF is an inherited disorder of ion transport (sodium and chloride) in the exocrine glands affecting the hepatic, digestive, reproductive (the vas deferens is functionally disrupted in nearly all cases; decreased fertility in both sexes), and respiratory systems (Fig. 15-15). The basic genetic defect predisposes to chronic bacterial airway infections, and almost all persons develop obstructive lung disease associated with chronic infection that leads to progressive loss of pulmonary function.

CF was previously thought to be a multisystem disease that manifests either at birth (with intestinal obstruction) or in infancy/early childhood (with growth failure and recurrent sinopulmonary symptoms). It is now recognized that a broad spectrum of conditions are associated with mutations in the CF transmembrane conductance regulator (CFTR) gene. This includes older children and adults presenting with manifestations in one organ, including sinopulmonary diseases, pancreatitis, or obstructive azoospermia. In many of these individuals, a diagnosis of CF is difficult to establish or exclude.[388]

Incidence

CF is the most common inherited genetic disease in the white population, affecting approximately 30,000 children and young adults (equal gender distribution) in the United States. More than 800[131] new cases are diagnosed each year. The disease is inherited as an autosomal recessive trait, meaning that both parents must be carriers so that the child inherits a defective gene from each one. In the United States, 5% of the population, or 12 million people, carry a single copy of the defective (CF) gene. Each time two carriers conceive a child, there is a 25% chance (1:4) that the child will have CF, a 50% (1:2) chance that the child will be a carrier, and a 25% chance (1:4) that the child will be a noncarrier.

Ten percent of new cases are diagnosed in those older than 18 years of age.[126] The severity of the disease is strongly correlated with socioeconomic status and access to health care.[445]

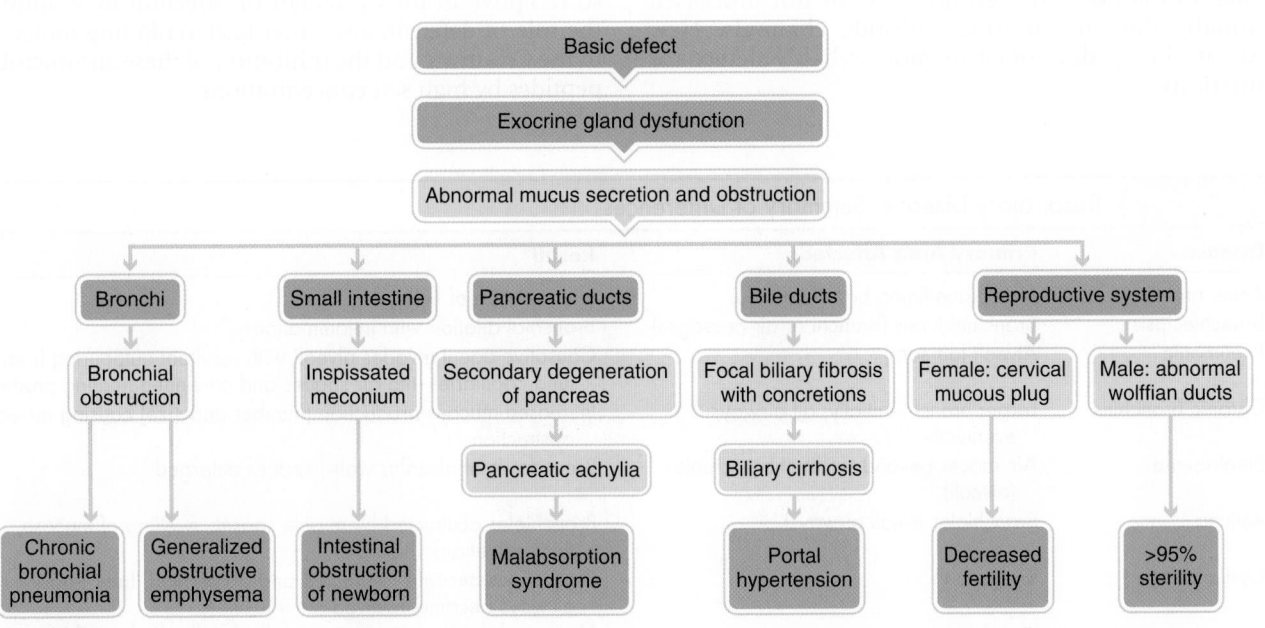

Figure 15-15

Various effects of exocrine gland dysfunction in cystic fibrosis. (From Wong DL: *Whaley and Wong's essentials of pediatric nursing,* ed 4, St Louis, 1993, Mosby.)

Etiologic Factors

In recent years, there have been major advances in understanding the underlying genetic factors related to this disease. In 1985, the CF gene was located on the long arm of chromosome 7. In 1989, the gene for CF was cloned and abnormalities in the CFTR protein were attributed to CF. Clones are identical copies of genes used to study the DNA sequence that allows scientists to determine the nature and function of the protein encoded by the gene. Cloning opens up the possibility of gene therapy for a disorder. It should be noted that the CFTR genotype is not a good predictor of disease severity, and a modifier gene has yet to be identified.[125]

In healthy people, this CFTR protein provides a channel by which chloride (a component of salt) can pass in and out of the plasma membrane of many epithelial cells, including those of the kidney, gut, and conducting airways. People with CF have a defective gene that produces a mutant protein that interferes with cells' ability to manage chloride. There are several classes of abnormalities ranging from no production of the protein to just accelerated degeneration of it.

At least two gating mechanisms of CFTR are now known; one relies on hydrolysis and the second depends on stable adenosine triphosphate binding.[224] There are complex relationships between CFTR, the epithelial sodium channel, and mucociliary clearance, which are currently being examined.[250] The loss of CFTR function appears to be as important as the defective transport channel.[50]

More than 1900 mutations in the CFTR gene have been identified.[133] The most common CFTR mutation is F508del, which results in production of a misfolded protein that does not reach the cell surface. In some mutations, the CFTR protein is synthesized to a lesser degree or not synthesized at all. In others, CFTR is made, but is not activated normally or not processed normally due to abnormal chloride channels. New tests are being developed to more reliably detect for mutations.[280]

Inflammation plays a role in lung damage associated with CF unrelated to the genetic defect.[138] The role of polymorphism (individual variation) of a gene that regulates protection from lung injury (by producing a substance called *glutathione*) has strong association with the severity of CF lung disease.[345]

Pathogenesis

Much about the complex pathogenesis of CF is still unknown, but it does appear that this impermeability of epithelial cells to chloride results in (1) dehydrated and increased thickening of mucous gland secretions, primarily in the lungs, pancreas, intestine, and sweat glands; (2) elevation of sweat electrolytes (sodium chloride); and (3) pancreatic enzyme insufficiency. The dehydration results in thickened dry and gooey secretions that cause the mechanical obstruction responsible for the multiple clinical manifestations of CF.

In the pancreatic ducts, the flow of digestive enzymes is blocked. As a result, absorption of food becomes increasingly difficult, particularly fat. Because of this effect, children with CF fall below norms for weight and height. Bronchial and bronchiolar obstruction by the abnormal mucus predisposes the lung to infection and causes patchy atelectasis with hyperinflation. The disease progresses from mucous plugging and inflammation of small airways (bronchiolitis) to bronchitis, followed by bronchiectasis, pneumonia, fibrosis, and the formation of large cystic dilations that involve all bronchi. Table 15-10 summarizes the differences among these various respiratory diseases.

New data on the structure of CFTR, including the size and shape of the channel through which the chloride must pass, how to stabilize the channel and increase the time it stays open, and the life cycle of this protein, are being used to provide scientists with ideas for new treatments.

Other researchers are investigating why the CF lung is so receptive to the onslaught of infection by examining the role of defensin and other bacteria-killing molecules in the CF airway and the inhibition of these antimicrobial peptides by high salt concentrations.

Table 15-10	Respiratory Disease: Summary of Differences	
Disease	**Primary Area Affected**	**Result**
Acute bronchitis	Membrane lining bronchial tubes	Inflammation of lining
Bronchiectasis	Bronchial tubes (bronchi or air passages)	Bronchial dilation with inflammation
Pneumonia	Alveoli (air sacs)	Causative agent invades alveoli with resultant outpouring from lung capillaries into air spaces and continued healing process
Chronic bronchitis	Larger bronchi initially; all airways eventually	Increased mucous production (number and size) causing airway obstruction
Emphysema	Air spaces beyond terminal bronchioles (alveoli)	Breakdown of alveolar walls; spaces enlarged
Asthma	Bronchioles (small airways)	Bronchioles obstructed by muscle spasm, swelling of mucosa, thick secretions
Cystic fibrosis	Bronchioles	Bronchioles become obstructed and obliterated; later larger airways become involved
		Mucous plugs cling to airways walls, leading to bronchitis, bronchiectasis, atelectasis, pneumonia, or pulmonary abscess

From Goodman CC, Snyder TE: *Differential diagnosis for the physical therapist*, ed 4, Philadelphia, 2007, Saunders.

Clinical Manifestations

The consistent finding of abnormally high sodium and chloride concentrations in the sweat is a unique characteristic of CF. Parents frequently observe that their infants taste salty when they kiss them. Almost all clinical manifestations of CF are a result of overproduction of extremely viscous mucus and deficiency of pancreatic enzymes. Box 15-7 gives a complete list of clinical manifestations by organ and in order of progression. Recurrent pneumothorax, hemoptysis, pulmonary hypertension, and cor pulmonale are serious and life-threatening complications of severe and diffuse CF pulmonary disease.

Pancreas. Approximately 90% of clients have pancreatic insufficiency with thick secretions blocking the pancreatic ducts and causing dilation of the small lobes of the pancreas, degeneration, and eventual progressive fibrosis throughout. The blockage also prevents essential pancreatic enzymes from reaching the duodenum, thus impairing digestion and absorption of nutrients. Clinically, this process results in greasy, bulky, frothy (undigested fats because of a lack of amylase and tryptase enzymes), and foul-smelling stools (decomposition of proteins producing compounds such as hydrogen sulfide and ammonia).

As the life expectancy for people with CF has improved, the incidence of glucose intolerance and CF-related diabetes has increased because pancreatic damage can eventually affect the β cells. Approximately 50% of adults with CF eventually develop CF-related diabetes. Hyperglycemia may adversely influence nutritional status and weight, pulmonary function, and development of late microvascular complications.[535]

Gastrointestinal. The earliest manifestation of CF, *meconium ileus* (sometimes referred to as distal intestinal obstruction syndrome), is present in approximately 10% to 15% of newborns with CF; the small intestine is blocked with thick, putty-like tenacious meconium. Prolapse of the rectum is the most common gastrointestinal complication associated with CF, occurring most often in infancy and childhood.

Box 15-7

CLINICAL MANIFESTATIONS OF CYSTIC FIBROSIS

Early Stages

- Persistent coughing
- Sputum production
- Persistent wheezing
- Recurrent pulmonary infection
- Excessive appetite, poor weight gain
- Salty skin and sweat
- Bulky, foul-smelling stools

Pulmonary
Initial

- Wheezy respirations
- Dry, nonproductive cough

Progressive Involvement

- Increased dyspnea
- Decreased exercise tolerance
- Paroxysmal cough
- Tachypnea
- Obstructive emphysema
- Patchy areas of atelectasis
- Nasal polyps, chronic sinusitis

Advanced Stage

- Barrel chest
- Kyphosis
- Pectus carinatum
- Cyanosis
- Clubbing (fingers and toes)
- Recurrent bronchitis
- Recurrent bronchopneumonia
- Pneumothorax
- Hemoptysis
- Right-sided heart failure secondary to pulmonary hypertension

Gastrointestinal

- Voracious appetite (early)
- Anorexia (late)
- Weight loss

- Failure to thrive or grow; protein-calorie malnutrition
- Distended abdomen
- Thin extremities
- Sallow (yellowish) skin
- Acute gastroesophageal reflux
- Intussusception

Distal Intestinal Obstruction Syndrome (Meconium Ileus)

- Abdominal distention
- Colicky, abdominal pain
- Vomiting
- Failure to pass stools (constipation)
- Rapid development of dehydration
- Anemia

Liver

- Cirrhosis
- Portal hypertension

Pancreatic

- Large, bulky, loose, frothy, foul-smelling stools (pancreatic enzyme insufficiency)
- Fat-soluble vitamin deficiency (vitamins A, D, E, K)
- Recurrent pancreatitis
- Iron-deficiency anemia
- Malnutrition
- Diabetes mellitus

Genitourinary

- Male urogenital abnormalities
- Delay in sexual development
- Sterility (most males); infertility (some females)

Musculoskeletal

- Marked tissue wasting, muscle atrophy
- Myalgia
- Osteoarthropathy (adult)
- Rheumatoid arthritis (adult)
- Osteopenia/osteoporosis (adult)

People of all ages with CF are susceptible to intestinal obstruction from thickened, dried, or impacted stools (inspissated meconium). Advances in investigative techniques have led to increasing reports of Crohn disease and ischemic bowel disease in persons with CF. Prolonged administration of excessive doses of pancreatic enzymes is associated with the development of fibrosing colonopathy. To avoid this complication, current recommendation for a daily dose of pancreatic enzymes for most people with CF is below 10,000 units of lipase per kilogram per day.

Currently, there are four pancreatic enzyme products prepared from porcine pancreases approved by the FDA. Liprotamase is another pancreatic enzyme replacement, not derived from animal sources. Phase 3 clinical trials with liprotamase, which are complete, found that this product is safe and leads to improved fat absorption.

A higher BMI in people with CF correlates with better lung function.[465] Although this data does not demonstrate a causal relationship, it reinforces the importance of maintaining adequate nutrition and striving to maintain a normal BMI.

Pulmonary. Chronic cough and purulent sputum production are symptomatic of lung involvement. The individual is unable to expectorate the mucus because of its increased viscosity. This retained mucus provides an excellent medium for bacterial growth, placing the individual at increased risk for infection. Common bacteria are *Staphylococcus aureus* and *P. aeruginosa*. Approximately 80% of people with CF become infected with *P. aeruginosa*.[131] Reduced oxygen–carbon dioxide exchange causes variable degrees of hypoxia, clubbing (see Fig. 15-4), cyanosis, hypercapnia, and resultant acidosis. Chronic pulmonary infection and hyperinflation lead to secondary manifestations of barrel chest, pectus carinatum, and kyphosis.

The most common complication of CF is progressive decline of lung function with episodes of acute worsening of respiratory symptoms, often referred to as "pulmonary exacerbations." Although a generally applicable definition of a pulmonary exacerbation has not been developed, clinical features of an exacerbation have been described (Box 15-8).[208] Pulmonary exacerbations require medical and physical therapy intervention, but can still have an adverse impact on the individual's quality of life and a major impact on the overall cost of care.[175] Respiratory failure is a frequent complication of severe pulmonary disease in persons with CF and is the most common cause of CF-related deaths.

Liver. Liver involvement in CF is much less frequent than both pulmonary and pancreatic diseases, which are present in 80% to 90% of individuals with CF. Liver disease affects only one-third of the CF population; however, because of the decreasing mortality from extrahepatic causes, its recognition and management are becoming a relevant clinical issue.[117]

Recent observations suggest that clinical expression of liver disease in CF may be influenced by genetic modifiers; their identification is an important issue because it may allow recognition of people at risk for the development of liver disease at the time of diagnosis of CF and early institution of prophylactic strategies.[117]

Genitourinary. Genitourinary manifestations are primarily related to reproduction; infertility once thought to be universal in men and common in women can be treated successfully with new techniques for in vitro fertilization. The vas deferens may be absent bilaterally, or if present, it is obstructed so that although sperm production is normal, blockage or fibrosis of the vas deferens prevents release of the sperm into the semen (azoospermia). Delayed puberty and amenorrhea due to malnutrition are common in females with CF. Women experience decreased fertility because thick mucus in the cervical canal prevents conception.

Musculoskeletal. By the 1990s, the majority of children with CF were living long enough to reach skeletal maturity.[221] Musculoskeletal dysfunctions can impair the person's ability to support the function of the lungs, thus contributing to the overall morbidity and mortality of the disease.[200] The muscles of respiration and posture are one and the same. As the WOB increases, the postural role of the trunk muscles is compromised.[338] Clinically, this is seen as altered spinal alignment (scoliosis, kyphosis) and abdominal muscle (low back pain) and pelvic floor muscle weakness (stress urinary incontinence).

Decreased bone mineral density and bone mineral content are common at all ages in CF and attributed to multifactorial causes (e.g., nutrition, exposure to glucocorticoid therapy, gonadal dysfunction, age, body mass, or activity). Spinal consequences of bone loss include excessive kyphosis and neck and back pain.

Hypertrophic pulmonary osteoarthropathy occurs with increasing frequency with increasing age and severity of disease in 2% to 7% of affected individuals. This condition is accompanied by clubbing of the fingers and toes; arthritis; painful periosteal new bone formation (especially over the tibia); and swelling of the wrists, elbows, knees, or ankles. The periostitis is observed radiographically in

---

Box 15-8

SIGNS AND SYMPTOMS OF PULMONARY EXACERBATION IN CYSTIC FIBROSIS

- Increased cough
- Increased sputum production and/or a change in appearance of sputum
- Fever
- Weight loss
- School or work absenteeism (because of illness)
- Increased respiratory rate and/or work of breathing
- New findings on chest examination (e.g., wheezing, crackles)
- Decreased exercise tolerance
- Decrease in FEV_1 of 10% or more from baseline value within past 3 months
- Decrease in hemoglobin saturation of 10% or more from baseline value within past 3 months
- New finding(s) on chest x-ray

FEV_1, forced expiratory volume in 1 second.
For further information, see Flume PA: Cystic fibrosis pulmonary guidelines: treatment of pulmonary exacerbations, *Am J Respir Crit Care Med* 180(9):802–808, 2009. Available online at http://www.cff.org/UploadedFiles/treatments/CFCareGuidelines/Respiratory/CF-Care-Guidelines-Pulmonary-Exacerbations.pdf

the diaphysis of the tubular bones and may be a single layer or a solid cloaking of the bone.

Separately and usually without association with other manifestations of CF, attacks of episodic arthritis accompanied by severe joint pain, stiffness, rash, and fever may occur intermittently but repeatedly. Also related to CF are rheumatoid arthritis, spondyloarthropathies, sarcoidosis, and amyloidosis, which are caused by coexistent conditions and drug reactions.[64] Muscle pain is reported and may be alleviated with proper nutrition and exercise, although this is based on anecdotal information and has not been verified in studies.

MEDICAL MANAGEMENT

DIAGNOSIS. Now that the gene responsible for CF has been identified, prenatal diagnosis and screening of carriers are possible as part of genetic counseling. The test is more than 99% accurate when positive. A negative genetic screening test is not as accurate because there are some rare mutations not yet identified. Prepregnancy genetic testing that involves DNA analysis of oocytes is available for couples at risk for having children with CF.

In 2004, the CDC issued a recommendation that all newborns should be screened for CF and currently all 50 states and the District of Columbia do routine screening. Newborn screening is not a diagnostic test to confirm CF but will lead to other tests that can confirm or rule out CF: sweat test, genotype analysis, and nasal potential difference.

CF is traditionally diagnosed using pilocarpine iontophoresis, also known as the sweat test; a positive test occurs when the sodium chloride concentration is greater than 60 mEq/L for anyone younger than 20 years (reference value: 40 mEq/L) and above 80 mEq/L for those older than 20 years.[468]

Although elevated sweat electrolytes are associated with other conditions, a positive sweat test coupled with the clinical picture usually confirms the diagnosis. The test should be performed at an accredited CF center and repeated a second time. Alternatively, CF can be diagnosed by genotype analysis (performed prenatally or postnatally). Testing of the most common 23 mutations in the United States will detect greater than 90% of whites with CF. CF can be diagnosed on DNA alone. Nasal potential difference measures salt transport in the nasal epithelial cells. Nasal potential difference is very sensitive at detecting abnormalities and can be used to diagnose CF, but is only available at a limited number of CF research centers.[354]

The age at presentation can vary, and some people are not diagnosed until adulthood. However, now that CF is included in newborn screening, in future years fewer cases will be diagnosed later in life. Diagnosis of CF in adulthood is generally attributable to a milder presentation of the disease and has a more favorable prognosis. Adults with unexplained chronic respiratory infections, bronchiectasis, pancreatitis, or absence of vas deferens should be screened for CF.[375,468]

Clinical Screening Tests. Pancreatic elastase-1 (EL-1), a marker of exocrine pancreatic insufficiency in CF, can be measured in feces. EL-1 is a specific human protease synthesized by the acinar cells of the pancreas and is a reliable test of pancreatic sufficiency in newborns older than age 2 weeks. Fecal elastase has good sensitivity and specificity and predictive values for severe cases of pancreatic insufficiency. This test can be used to confirm the need for pancreatic enzymes and for annual monitoring of pancreatic-sufficient individuals to detect the onset of pancreatic insufficiency. Pulmonary function tests are performed in affected individuals from the age of 6 years and up to measure and monitor lung function over time (see Table 40-22). These tests are used to classify the severity of baseline lung disease. Almost all measures are based on the flow of air into and out of the lungs in a given period of time.

The two most common lung function measures are FEV_1 and FVC (forced vital capacity). These tests should be performed at least four times each year for adults to assess the effectiveness of treatment; pulmonary function declines with progressive lung disease.

Several scoring systems have been developed to assess disease severity, measure acute changes, and evaluate appropriateness for lung transplantation. The most reliable and useful are the modified Shwachman and modified Huang scores. There is a need for a longitudinal assessment tool to follow individuals with milder CF.[218] High-resolution CT scans are more sensitive than FEV_1 at detecting changes in people with mild disease, but introduce a risk of radiation exposure. Lung clearance index, obtained via a breath test, may be sensitive (and safer than high-resolution CT)[31] at detecting mild disease, in the presence of normal FEV_1.

CF-related diabetes mellitus should be identified early by annual screening with a glucose tolerance test from the age of 10 years and treated with insulin, dietary management, and exercise from the time of diagnosis of diabetes. Symptoms of CF-related diabetes are often confused with pulmonary infection. Diabetes significantly impacts the course of CF leading to worse nutrition, lower lung function, more hospitalizations, and worse mortality.[467]

Bone mineral density should be monitored routinely in people with CF. By the age of 18 years, all people with CF should have a dual-energy X-ray absorptiometry (DEXA) scan to detect osteopenia or osteoporosis. A repeat scan is recommended every 1 to 5 years, based on the DEXA results as well as other factors, such as FEV_1 and BMI.

TREATMENT. A multidisciplinary approach must be taken in treating CF toward the goal of promoting a normal life for the individual. Everyone should be followed at an accredited CF center where all of the disciplines are present and work together. The treatment of CF depends on the stage of the disease and which organs are involved. Some care teams take an aggressive approach from a young age, prior to onset of clinical symptoms. Medical management is oriented toward managing and preserving lung function and includes the use of antibiotics, antiinflammatories, aggressive pulmonary therapy with drugs (mucolytics) to thin mucous secretions, airway clearance techniques, and supplemental oxygen. Adequate hydration and pancreatic enzymes administered with meals will enhance nutritional outcomes.

Pharmacotherapy. Drug therapy for CF is primarily directed at preventing accumulation of thick, sticky

Table 15-11	Inhaled Pharmacotherapy for Cystic Fibrosis
Type of Therapy	**Medication**
Bronchodilator therapy	AccuNeb (albuterol)
	ProAir HFA (albuterol)
	Proventil HFA (albuterol)
	Ventolin HFA (albuterol)
Mucus clearance therapies	HyperSal (sodium chloride solution)
	Pulmozyme (dornase alfa)
Antibiotic therapies	Tobi (tobramycin)
	Coly-Mycin M (colistimethate)*
	Cayston (aztreonam)

*Colistimethate is available as a solution for injection and must be diluted appropriately for nebulization.
Courtesy Tanner Higginbotham, PharmD, Drug Information Specialist, Skaggs School of Pharmacy, Department of Pharmacy Practice, University of Montana, Missoula, Montana.

mucus, managing infection, and preserving lung function. Discussion here is in the order in which medications are typically administered (e.g., bronchodilator, saline, dornase alfa, antibiotic, steroid).

Pharmacologic treatment may include sympathomimetics to control bronchospasm, parasympatholytics to offset smooth muscle constriction and bronchodilation, mucolytics to thin mucous secretions, aerosolized antibiotics (e.g., tobramycin), and inhaled antiinflammatory agents to decrease the amount of inflammation in the airways (Table 15-11).

A combination of treatments can result in fewer flareups and faster recovery.[162] First, a bronchodilator is administered to open the airways and improve mucociliary clearance. Inhaled bronchodilators are effective in individuals who have bronchial hyperresponsiveness.[220] Next, hypertonic saline, an inexpensive, "low-tech" intervention is inhaled. Saline, with a high concentration of salt (typically 7%) rehydrates the airway secretions, replenishes the airway surface liquid, and often induces a cough. Recombinant human deoxyribonuclease (rhDNase), known as dornase alfa or Pulmozyme, a mucolytic, is effectively used to reduce sputum viscosity and increase mucociliary clearance.[480]

Hypertonic saline improves airway clearance but is not as effective as DNase in longer-term lung improvement.[524] Historically, it has been recommended to administer DNase 30 minutes prior to performing airway clearance techniques. However, a 2011 systematic review[146] suggests the timing of DNase in relation to airway clearance should be based largely on the individual's preference.

Tobramycin (Tobi) is an aminoglycoside antibiotic that works by stopping the growth of *P. aeruginosa*. It can be given intravenously or via nebulizer. Nearly 80%[131] of people with CF are infected with *P. aeruginosa* by adulthood. Another common antibiotic in CF care is aztreonam (Cayston), a monobactam. When inhaled, antibiotics should be administered after the person performs airway clearance techniques. Many individuals who require frequent courses of intravenous antibiotics may have an implantable venous intravenous access device

put in place. The risks of mechanical failure, sepsis, and thrombosis have made this device more successful when inserted and cared for at a CF center.[25,166,283]

High-dose ibuprofen (the generic name for the drug found in Advil, Motrin, and Nuprin) may be used to slow the deterioration of the lungs by reducing inflammation and breaking the cycle of mucus buildup, infection, and inflammatory destruction. Neutrophils are responsible for much of the inflammatory response and are unresponsive to traditional chemotherapeutic treatment. Investigations are currently underway to determine inflammatory response in CF with docosahexaenoic acid (an omega-3 fatty acid) and N-acetylcysteine (an antioxidant).[132]

Pharmacologic intervention with microencapsulated pancreatic enzymes is critical when pancreatic involvement is severe. Aggressive nutritional management is needed to ameliorate the effects of malabsorption and the side effects of therapeutic intervention. Calcium supplements are warranted because of the high incidence of osteopenia and fractures.[29] Deficiency of vitamin D is common in individuals with CF and is associated with decreased bone mass in children, osteoporosis in adults and may impact other comorbidities common in CF. Vitamin D_3 (cholecalciferol) is recommended for all individuals with CF to achieve and maintain serum 25-hydroxyvitamin D levels of at least 30 ng/mL.[487]

Supplemental oxygen may improve exercise endurance and peak performance. Mild hypercapnia (too much carbon dioxide in the blood) can occur with exercise and during sleep. More research is needed to assess the benefits of oxygen therapy.[330] Several medications to address CF-associated liver disease are in clinical trials. However, no therapies have been proven to impact long-term prognosis in individuals with CF-associated liver disease.[231] Injected insulin and insulin pumps may be used to control CF-related diabetes.

Gene Therapy. The identification of the mutated CF gene in 1989 was followed by the first phase of gene therapy in 1993 to correct the basic defect in CF cells, rather than relying on treatment of the symptoms. Finding a way to deliver the normal copy of the gene into the lung or intrahepatic biliary epithelial cells with adequate gene expression remains a challenge. Obstacles include vector toxicity and ineffective transgene expression.[160]

It is possible that delivery through an aerosolized technique will incorporate sufficient quantities of the CFTR gene into the cells without toxicity and stimulating an immune response.[145] The expectation is that the normal CFTR will reverse the physiologic defect in CF cells.

In the future, current therapeutic measures, such as intravenous antimicrobial treatment, will be improved by the additional delivery of new drugs to the bronchial tree by aerosol. Antibiotics, as well as protease inhibitors delivered by aerosol, should help to prevent damage by infection and inflammation and increase the probability of successful somatic gene therapy in this disease.[137]

In 2012, Kalydeco, the first drug to target the underlying cause of CF was approved by the FDA. Approximately 1200 people with CF (4.6%) have the G551D mutation. With the G551D mutation, the defective protein gets to the cell surface, but acts like a locked gate, preventing the flow of sodium and chloride. Kalydeco unlocks the gate and restores the function of the CFTR protein. Clinical trials have shown dramatic improvements in lung function, sweat chloride levels, and nutritional status.[129]

Transplantation. Double-lung transplantation is required to treat people with CF. Transplantation is not a cure for CF, but a bridge to allow people to live longer with a better quality of life. In the United States, the United Network for Organ Sharing has addressed perceived inequities in organ distribution by allocating organs by illness severity rather than time on the waiting list. A lung allocation score ranks severity for potential recipients 12 years of age and older for transplantation based on variables, including lung function, oxygen and ventilatory needs, diabetes, weight, and physical performance.[320]

Liver transplantation should be offered to anyone with CF and progressive liver failure and/or with life-threatening sequelae of portal hypertension, who also have mild pulmonary involvement that is expected to support long-term survival.[117,257]

Long-term survival has yet to be determined, but improved quality of life has been achieved. The new lungs do not acquire the CF ion-transport abnormalities but are subject to the usual posttransplantation complications. CF problems in other organ systems persist and may be worsened by some of the immunosuppressive regimens.[546]

CNS complications occur more frequently in CF transplant recipients than in other lung transplant recipients.[205] Criteria for lung transplantation are published, and early referral and continuous monitoring are required to anticipate decline as a result of the long waiting period.[197]

PROGNOSIS. Using its innovative CF patient registry, which tracks information on more than 26,000 clients who receive care through the CF Foundation's Care Center Network, researchers have analyzed the numbers and continue to assess trends in the health status of registered individuals. When first distinguished from celiac disease in 1938, life expectancy with CF was approximately 6 months.[138]

The natural history of CF lung disease has been one of chronic progression with intermittent episodes of acute worsening of symptoms frequently called acute pulmonary exacerbations. These exacerbations typically warrant medical intervention.[175] But data shows that the prognosis has steadily improved over the past 30 years with a gradual increase in longevity; at the time of this publication the median survival had risen to 38.3 years. Cases of adults with CF living into the ninth decade (early eighties) have been recorded.[131]

More than 50% of children with CF live into adulthood. The new median age of survival is based on 2010[131] data that includes date of birth, date of death, gender, and date of diagnosis. A detailed CF Foundation Annual Patient Registry Data Report is available.

Improvement in both the length and quality of life for adults with CF is primarily the result of newborn screening to identify and treat affected individuals before pulmonary or nutritional problems arise. Standardization of care, implementation of best practices, continuous multidisciplinary care provided by specialists in CF centers, improved CF therapies, and improved nutrition and

pulmonary function are two main prognostic factors for improved survival.[328]

Children whose presenting symptoms were gastrointestinal at diagnosis have a good clinical course; those whose initial symptoms at diagnosis were pulmonary frequently demonstrate subsequent clinical deterioration. Pulmonary failure is still the most common cause of death. Males have a more favorable prognosis than females. New agents and gene therapy may substantially change the morbidity and mortality of this disease with continued improved survival time.

Lung disease is the primary cause of death for 80% for individuals with CF. Lung transplantation is an important therapeutic option for this group, comprising the third largest group of transplant recipients receiving lung transplantation (after people with chronic obstructive lung disease and IPF). The primary goal of transplantation has always been to treat individuals with CF with end-stage lung disease for whom medical therapies have failed. The secondary goal has been to improve quality of life.[320]

Since the first lung transplant for CF in 1983, survival rates have improved. Refinements in surgical technique, medications, and improved selection criteria have gradually improved postsurgical survival.[320] Individuals with CF who are listed for lung transplantation may require mechanical ventilatory support before transplantation. Pretransplantation mechanical ventilation increases short-term morbidity and mortality in pediatric clients.[161] Besides ventilator dependence, other negative predictive factors for prognosis after transplantation include *Burkholderia cepacia* infection, young age, and arthropathy.[320]

The 3-year predicted survival rate after lung transplantation was reported as 55% at centers that performed more than 10 transplants. The 5-year rate was 53% in 2010 and expected to continue to improve over time.[389] The 1-year survival rate after liver transplantation for this population is approximately 80%, with beneficial effects on lung function, nutritional status, body composition, and quality of life in most cases.[117]

Improved quality of life after lung transplantation remains tightly linked to survival and is difficult to evaluate. Current information suggests that quality of life increases after lung transplantation for survivors but that it decreases with time and complications such as constrictive bronchiolitis.[320]

SPECIAL IMPLICATIONS FOR THE THERAPIST 15-17

Cystic Fibrosis

> **Note to Reader:** There is a document written by physical therapists that presents the scope of physical therapy practice for cystic fibrosis in the United States, available through the Cystic Fibrosis Foundation.[482]

Airway Clearance Techniques

The therapist must always be aware that anyone with CF is susceptible to infections, in particular *Burkholderia cepacia*. Care must be taken to avoid transmission via equipment, other people, or oneself. Hand hygiene is essential, and high alcohol hand rubs may be more effective.[201] The therapist will be involved with airway clearance techniques (ACTs) carried out several times per day or as often as the person is able to tolerate it without undue fatigue. It is generally recommended for individuals to perform ACTs twice daily, for maintenance, when healthy and increase frequency to at least three to four times per day during an exacerbation. Airway clearance techniques should not be performed before or immediately after meals, so treatment must be scheduled to avoid mealtimes for those who experience nausea, vomiting, or any other type of discomfort during treatment.

Aerosol therapy to deliver medication to the lower respiratory tract should be administered just before airway clearance techniques to maximize the effectiveness of both treatments. Breathing exercises, improving posture, mobilizing the thorax through active exercise, and manual therapy are part of promoting good breathing patterns and improving inspiratory muscle endurance.

Routine airway clearance is recommended for all individuals with CF. However, there is not one airway clearance technique proven to be more beneficial than the others, so the prescribed ACTs should be tailored for each individual. Specifics of ACTs for this population are beyond the scope of this text; the reader is referred to the more detailed materials available.[127,128,354]

The many difficulties surrounding percussion and postural drainage (e.g., gastroesophageal reflux, decrease in oxygen saturation, poor compliance, time consuming, and requiring the assistance of a trained individual) have resulted in the development of alternative airway clearance techniques that can be accomplished without the assistance of another caregiver and without adverse side effects.

A THERAPIST'S THOUGHTS*

Tipping

Postural drainage using traditional head-down positions can have detrimental effects, as mentioned above. This has been well documented in infants and the current standard of practice is to perform modified postural drainage (no head down; positions angled up to 30 degrees) when treating infants.[80,310] However, there is limited evidence for the older child and adult populations. Some therapists feel strongly and avoid Trendelenburg positioning in treatment of all ages. Other therapists argue that the benefits (improved ventilation and perfusion as well as secretion clearance) outweigh the risks. Therapists should consider that many adults with CF have diagnosed reflux, while others may have undiagnosed or silent reflux and aspiration. Each person should be assessed individually and alternative treatments or modified positions should always be considered, even in an ICU setting.

*Karen von Berg, PT

Each of these techniques (e.g., autogenic drainage, active cycle breathing, positive expiratory pressure [PEP], and high-frequency chest wall oscillation [HFCWO, also known as high-frequency chest compression or oscillatory PEP]) requires a certain level of compliance, motivation, understanding, neuromuscular function, and breath control. The therapist is very instrumental in evaluating each individual's needs, motivation, abilities, resources, and preferences in determining the best intervention or interventions to use.

Autogenic drainage, active cycle breathing, and PEP help the individual to move the mucus up to the larger airways where it can be expectorated more easily. Autogenic drainage comprises a series of sequential breathing exercises designed to clear the small, medium, and large airways in that order. The PEP device maintains pressure in the lungs, keeping the airways open and allowing air to get behind the mucus (Fig. 15-16). Examples of low pressure PEP devices include PARI PEP, TheraPEP, acapella, Quake, RC Cornet, and the Flutter. These devices have been shown to be effective in increased sputum production, improved lung function, and improved oxygenation.[135]

Current practice is to use one of the devices followed by a forced expiratory technique. The total treatment time is about 15 minutes and can be carried out independently by some children and most adolescents and adults who can follow the directions and control their breathing.

Assisted autogenic drainage and active cycle of breathing can be administered to infants and to older adults with more severe disease who are not capable of performing these techniques independently. Younger children may enjoy "Bubble PEP" (see Fig. 15-16), which can be made from common items at home or in the hospital. The individual can blow through respiratory tubing to make bubbles in a jug. Tubing diameter and depth of water will determine the amount of expiratory resistance and PEP created.

A HFCWO device can provide another alternative airway clearance technique and can be used throughout the life span, beginning as early as about the age of 1 year (although the cost may seem prohibitive, it is less than a single hospitalization for a pulmonary exacerbation). The device consists of an inflatable jacket attached to an air pulse generator (Fig. 15-17). The generator, a compressor-like device, rapidly inflates and deflates the vest, gently compressing and releasing the chest wall to create airflow within the lungs. This device treats all lobes simultaneously for the duration of the time it is activated. This process moves mucus toward the larger airways where it can be cleared by coughing. Pressure and frequency settings are adjustable. Currently, three companies offer HFCWO devices: The Vest (Hill-Rom, Batesville, IN), the inCourage System (RespirTech, St. Paul, MN), and the SmartVest (Electromed, New Prague, MN).

HFCWO alters the properties of mucus by thinning secretions and improving the ciliary beat.[329] HFCWO is a reliable ACT alternative.[411] An advantage to using an HFCWO device is that it is independent of position and technique. However, when possible, it should not be a passive treatment. The individual should take normal-large volume breaths and incorporate a forced expiratory technique intermittently to enhance the treatment effects.

All ACTs should incorporate a forced expiratory technique, also known as a "huff." The huff creates increases in expiratory airflow and mobilizes mucus

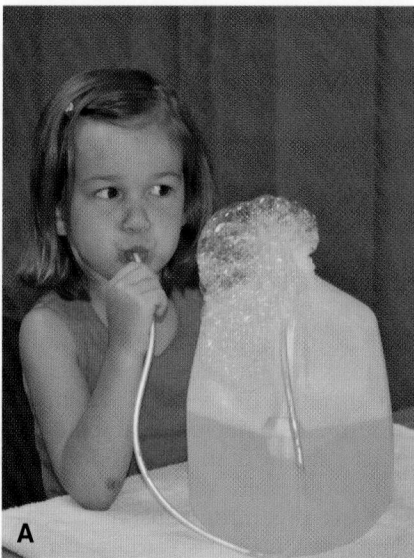

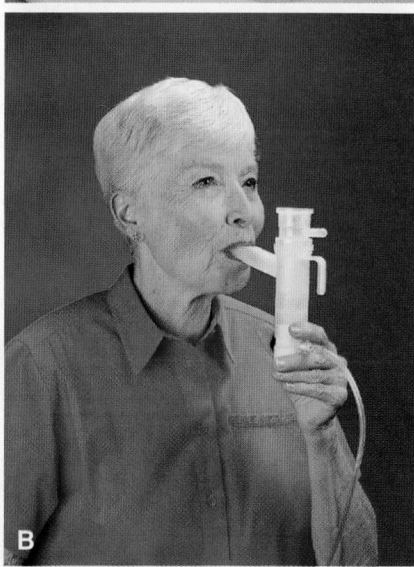

Figure 15-16

PARI PEP. The positive expiratory pressure (PEP) device maintains pressure in the lungs, keeping the airways open and allowing air to get behind the mucus to improve airway clearance, lung volume capacity, and oxygenation. The device can be used by children **(A)** and adults **(B)**. Bubble PEP as seen in **(A)** can make breathing treatments fun for young children. They can begin to learn breathing control while getting the benefits of PEP therapy. Amount of expiratory resistance can be adjusted as needed for individuals by changing the amount of water and diameter of the tubing. (Courtesy Karen von Berg. Used with permission. PARI PEP is a registered trademark of PARI GmbH. Used with permission. Please note: the authors have no commercial gain from inclusion of this product.)

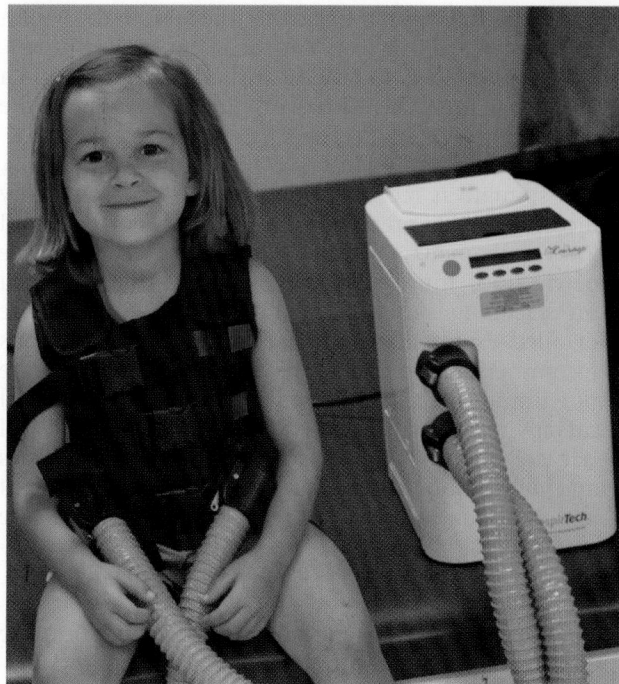

Figure 15-17

High-frequency chest wall oscillation (HFCWO) vest. A 5-year-old using the RespirTech inCourage system to assist with airway clearance therapy. During a hospital stay, some form of airway clearance is performed at least three times per day. HFCWO settings (frequency, pressure and time) should be monitored and adjusted as needed to increase treatment effectiveness. Huffs are performed at regular intervals. The home program is adjusted accordingly. Any changes are documented and communicated with the outpatient CF team. (Courtesy Karen von Berg. Used with permission.)

A THERAPIST'S THOUGHTS*
Airway Clearance

Traditionally, ACT was the main role of physical therapists involved in CF care. At many hospitals today ACT is performed by respiratory therapists. However, the physical therapist should still be involved in the care of all individuals with CF. Early intervention will detect musculoskeletal changes and improve outcomes. Many people with CF have spine and rib mobility restrictions that when mobilized will improve breathing mechanics, secretion clearance, pain and quality of life. Combining breathing exercises (active cycle of breathing technique, forced expiration technique) with stretches and manual therapy can enhance treatment sessions. Individuals with cystic fibrosis often feel much better after these sessions than they do after ACT or exercise alone.

*Karen von Berg, PT.

Musculoskeletal and Neuromuscular Complications

As people with CF are living longer, the role of the physical therapist in CF care is evolving. Musculoskeletal and neuromuscular complications are becoming more prevalent. Changes in posture and decreases in bone mineral density are seen in grade-school-age

from the small, distal airways to the larger, central airways where it can then be expelled with a cough. The huff is a forced, but not harsh or violent expiration. Volume of inspiration can be varied to optimize secretion clearance from the different generations of airways. Affected individuals are encouraged to huff (two or three times) intermittently throughout the ACT session (i.e., after each lung segment during postural drainage, after every 10-15 breaths with PEP, every 5-10 minutes with HFCWO).

children. It is much easier to prevent, rather than correct, musculoskeletal and neuromuscular impairments. Therefore, the physical therapist should be a part of the interdisciplinary care team throughout the life span.

Annual screening for posture, range of motion, and strength is recommended. Because stress urinary incontinence is present in up to 49%[151] of girls and 73% of women[509] with CF, screening should include pelvic floor muscle health. Any impairments noted on screening should be followed up with a more detailed examination with appropriate interventions recommended. Interventions should include, but are not limited to: neuromuscular reeducation, manual therapy (i.e., spine and rib mobilizations, myofascial release), and therapeutic exercise for trunk, extremities and pelvic floor musculature. For further assessment and treatment options, the reader is referred to a case study by Mary Massery.[338]

Nutrition

Malnutrition and deterioration of lung function are closely interrelated and interdependent in the person with CF. Each affects the other, leading to a spiral decline in both. The occurrence of malnutrition during childhood seems to be associated with impaired growth and repair of the airway walls. In children, when growth in body length occurs, good nutrition is associated with better lung function. When adequate nutrition is combined with physical training and aerobic exercise, improved body weight, respiratory muscle function, lung function, and exercise tolerance occur with increases in both respiratory and other muscle mass.[229] Current guidelines recommend children with CF maintain a BMI greater than 50%. In those older than age 18 years, greater than 23% is ideal for males, and at least 22% for females.[131]

Exercise

Increasingly, exercise and sport are being advanced as core components of treatment for individuals with CF of all ages. A large portfolio of exercise literature has already established that supervised exercise programs enhance fitness (and thereby improve survival), increase sputum clearance, delay the onset of dyspnea, delay declines in pulmonary function, prevent decrease in bone density,[527] enhance cellular immune response,[63] and increase feelings of well-being, thereby potentially improving self-image,[398] self-confidence, and quality of life for the person with CF (Fig. 15-18). Both short- and long-term aerobic and anaerobic training have positive effects on exercise capacity, strength, and lung function.[68]

Reduced systemic oxygen extraction is an important factor, limiting exercise in many individuals with CF, but the specific parameters of this limitation remain unknown and probably vary from person to person.[361,384] Even unsupervised programs produce a training effect and pulmonary benefits.[356] Inspiratory muscle training alone in individuals with CF has shown improved lung function and increased work capacity, as well as improved psychosocial status.[143,163]

Exercise is an important adjunct to airway clearance. Although physical activity can increase expiratory airflow (shears mucus from the airway walls) and minute ventilation (opens previously collapsed airways), there is no evidence to support exercise as a sole form of airway clearance.

The therapist can be very instrumental in providing client and family education about the importance of combining good nutrition and exercise/activity. Use of a field exercise test is beneficial to determine exercise guidelines. The Modified Shuttle Walk Test, 3-Minute Step Test, and 6-Minute Walk Test are examples of endurance tests that have been studied in the CF population. The therapist helps each individual develop an exercise routine that includes strengthening, stretching, aerobic, and endurance components with special attention to breathing exercises to aerate all areas of the lungs. Use of gaming console exercise is gaining in popularity and provides cardiovascular demand[305] similar to treadmill or other more traditional modes of exercise.

Weight loss with exercise is of special concern in this population, especially for the individual with CF and diabetes mellitus. Energy expenditure is higher than usual for individuals with CF and diabetes during periods of recovery from mild exercise or activity because of increased WOB consistent with higher ventilatory

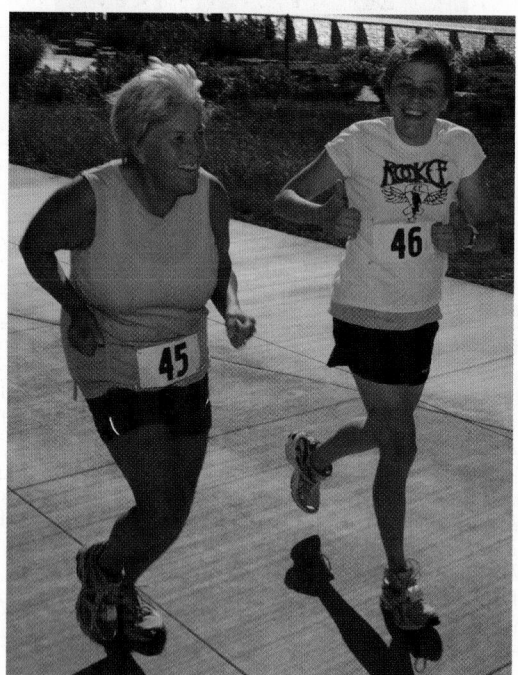

Figure 15-18

Value of exercise for individuals with cystic fibrosis. The 30-year-old woman on the right reports this photo was taken during her sixth half marathon. She reports that within 3 months of starting to run and train for a 5K marathon she noticed that her lung function improved measurably. This motivated her to keep gradually increasing her level of exercise. She says, "To me exercise is now just as important as the other treatments that I do each day. Everyone is different so starting slow and setting real goals is very important. I couldn't run a block 5 years ago when I started, so it does take time to build up and reach your goals." (Courtesy Emily Schaller. Used with permission.)

requirements.[523] This requires careful collaboration among client/family, therapist, and nutritionist/dietician. In addition, systemic inflammatory response to exercise may be greater for individuals with CF, potentially exacerbating the disease.[259]

Individuals with CF awaiting a transplant must remain as active as possible; whenever possible, the therapist can design a safe but effective exercise program. If significant oxygen desaturation or severe breathlessness limits activity, then exercise on a treadmill, stationary bike, or even a stationary device for seated pedaling is recommended with supplemental oxygen supplied at sufficient flow to match minute ventilatory requirements.[527]

Studies of exercise performance in lung transplant recipients with end-stage CF report that exercise performance improves after transplantation but remains well below normal.[384] In a study of 12 individuals 8 to 95 months after lung transplant, the diaphragm and abdominal muscle strength was preserved relative to healthy controls, but quadriceps strength was significantly diminished and affected exercise performance. Corticosteroid use partly contributed to this strength deficit.[409]

Athletes with Cystic Fibrosis

For those individuals who are able and interested in participating in sports (Fig. 15-19), special considerations must be addressed. Calorie intake and maintaining weight, nutrition, and fluid and electrolyte balance are major concerns. Each individual must be assessed, evaluated, and monitored carefully. The therapist, family, and nutritionist/dietician can work together to minimize exercise and nutrition-induced complications. The information presented here is only a general guideline and may need to be modified for individual needs, metabolism, personal health, level and type of sports participation, and so on.

To maintain weight during the off-training season, the individual (especially children and adolescents) will need to eat 1.5 times the protein and calories of an athlete who does not have CF. During the sport season, calorie intake must be increased with the goal of maintaining weight.

Hyponatremia (deficiency of sodium in the blood; see discussion in Chapter 5) can be a serious problem for athletes with CF, who excrete three to five times the sodium (in sweat) of an athlete without CF during sports participation. This situation combined with increased intake of water further dilutes the sodium levels in the body. Sodium loss combined with losses of potassium and magnesium can result in life-threatening situations for these individuals.

Some guidelines for these athletes include weighing before and after exercise and considering the loss as a loss of fluids accompanied by electrolytes; replacing fluid loss with electrolytes (e.g., drinks such as Gatorade or Recharge) instead of water; and eating a meal with sodium-, potassium-, and magnesium-rich foods.

Sporting activities should not be undertaken during infective exacerbations. Sports that carry a medical risk for people with CF (e.g., bungee and parachute jumping, skiing, or scuba diving) should be avoided. Infection control is a concern with contact sports such as wrestling. Individuals with CF who have portal hypertension with significant enlargement of the spleen and liver should be advised against contact sports, such as rugby and football, in addition to bungee and parachute jumping.

Skiing for anyone with CF who is already hypoxic is not advised; episodes of acute right-sided heart failure brought on by a combination of altitude and

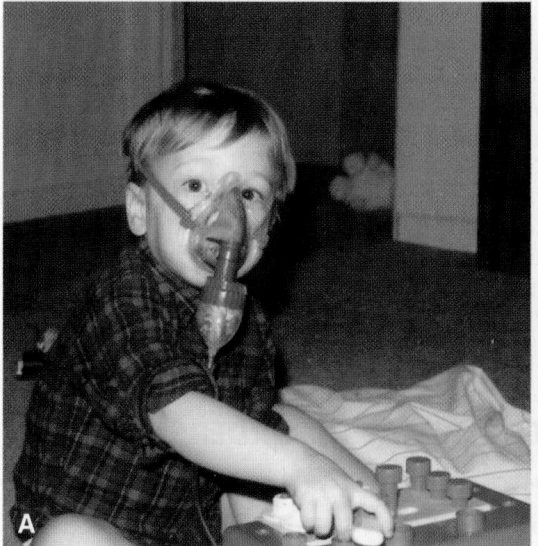
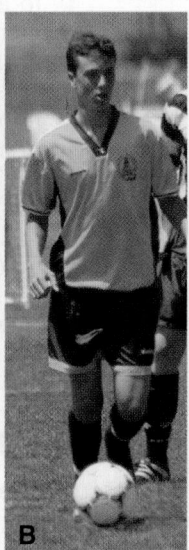
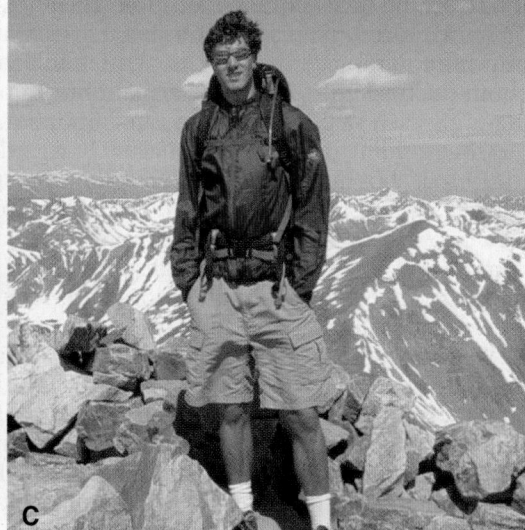

Figure 15-19

A, An 18-month-old boy shortly after diagnosis; the face mask is a nebulizer (device designed to create and throw an aerosol) that is delivering albuterol (bronchodilator). **B,** This same individual in 1999 at age 15 years (6 feet tall; 145 lb) competing in a regional soccer tournament. **C,** Same young man at 23 years (6 feet 2 inches, 175 lb), still actively hiking, cycling, running, and playing intramural sports, while enrolled in graduate school. (Courtesy Kevin Hanson, Helena, MT, 2007. Used with permission.)

unaccustomed strenuous anaerobic and aerobic exercise have been reported. Scuba diving is contraindicated for anyone with lung disease if there is any evidence of air trapping. On ascent, the air expands, increasing the risk of developing a pneumothorax.[527]

Transition to Adult Care

CF centers and other centers providing life-long care for clients with CF have realized the need for a transition phase between pediatric and adult care and the provision of counseling for parents and the young adult with CF to assist them with this marked change in approach to the young adult's care.

The physical therapist can and should have an integral role in preparing families and clients for various phases in care from pediatrics to adolescent care to a more independent model of adult care. If such a program does not exist in your current facility, materials and resources are available to help get such a program started and established.[52,106,342,498]

Many families receive care for their child for years at a pediatric center and develop life-long relationships with health care agencies and staff. Every effort should be made to accomplish a smooth transition for the client and the family, as the move from the well-established pediatric facility to a new facility or medical team can be a stressful transition for all.

Families in rural settings or who travel distances to benefit from centralized services in CF clinics or centers have some unique needs that should be addressed as well. For example, maintaining a complete medical record in more than one facility is not always possible. Without a good systems coordinator, gaps in the medical record from one clinic to another become all too common.

Transition to adult care should be a planned process over time. Every effort should be made to avoid an abrupt transfer. The pediatric team has the responsibility to "set the stage" for the transition. The process can be started early with expectations for an eventual adult transition reinforced in intervals. Written information about the transition, setting an actual time frame, and planning each step in the process are important.[342]

Three guiding principles are suggested, regardless of the format chosen for transition. First, there must be an adult team that is both interested and able to provide care. Second, there needs to be a very well planned, coordinated approach to the transition. Third, there must be excellent communication and interaction between the pediatric and adult teams.[342]

Transition programs should be flexible enough to meet the needs of a wide range of young people, health conditions, and circumstances. The actual transfer of care should be individualized to meet the specific needs of young people and their families.[430] Family involvement, including parents, guardians, and/or partner and the client, is essential to the success of any transition phase. The omission of any key people from the transition team can result in frustration, feelings of abandonment, and miscommunication, which could ultimately lead to compromised care for the individual with CF.

Adults With Cystic Fibrosis

As individuals with CF survive longer into adulthood, the unique needs of this population group are being considered. Health care in the adult setting encourages independence and increased self-reliance.[546] Achieving an ideal nutritional status is an integral part of management of people with CF, but how these requirements change as the individual ages remains unknown. Emphasis is continually placed on dietary intake and weight; the effects of this on eating behavior and self-perceptions are under investigation.[1,496,534]

Other concerns include the effects of long-term use of pancreatic enzymes, CF-related diabetes, osteoporosis associated with late-stage CF and its complications of increased fracture rates and severe kyphosis,[28,29,228] the effects of hormonal changes in relation to the menstrual cycle on lung function,[270] psychosocial-spiritual issues,[241] and infertility issues.[253]

The origin of bone disease in CF is multifactorial and not completely understood. However, glucocorticoid therapy, delayed pubertal maturation, malabsorption of vitamin D, poor nutritional status, inactivity, and hypogonadism are all potential contributing factors.[130] In addition, chronic pulmonary inflammation causes increased circulating levels of cytokines that augment bone resorption and suppress bone formation. Decreases in bone mineral density resulting from these factors can lead to osteoporosis, fragility fractures, and possible exclusion from lung transplant candidacy.[130]

Although a number of therapeutic options are now available for osteoporosis, it is likely that prevention, prompt recognition, and early treatment will be far more effective in achieving bone health than intervention at later stages of the problem. An in-depth discussion of bone health and disease in CF is available.[27]

Stress urinary incontinence has also been shown to affect many girls and women and some boys and men with CF, probably caused by the forceful and prolonged coughing bouts characteristic of the disease.[416,509] Interventions aimed at improving pelvic floor muscle strength and coordination may be appropriate for these individuals (see Chapter 27).

Life events such as attending college and/or starting a career, starting a family (including the pregnant patient) and emerging issues of aging with CF all require individualized plans from the coordinated CF team. These challenges are expected to increase as life span for CF increases.

PARENCHYMAL DISORDERS

Atelectasis

Definition

Atelectasis is the collapse of normally expanded and aerated lung tissue at any structural level (e.g., lung parenchyma, alveoli, pleura, chest wall, bronchi) involving all or part of the lung. Most cases are categorized as obstructive-absorptive or compressive.

Etiologic Factors and Pathogenesis

The primary cause of atelectasis is obstruction of the bronchus serving the affected area. If a bronchus is obstructed (e.g., by tumors, mucus, or foreign material), atelectasis occurs as air in the alveoli is slowly absorbed into the bloodstream with subsequent collapse of the alveoli. Atelectasis can also develop when there is interference with the natural forces that promote lung expansion (e.g., hypoventilation associated with decreased motion or decreased pulmonary expansion such as occurs with paralysis, pleural disease, diaphragmatic disease, severe scoliosis, or masses in the thorax). Failure to breathe deeply postoperatively (i.e., because of muscular guarding and splinting from pain or discomfort with an upper abdominal, chest, or sternal incision), oversedation, immobility, coma, or neuromuscular disease can also interfere with the natural forces that promote lung expansion, leading to atelectasis.

Insufficient pulmonary surfactant, such as occurs in respiratory distress syndrome, anesthesia, high concentrations of oxygen, lung contusion, aspiration of gastric contents or smoke inhalation, or increased elastic recoil as a result of interstitial fibrosis (e.g., silicosis, asbestosis, radiation pneumonitis), can also interfere with lung distention. When atelectasis is caused by inhalation of concentrated oxygen or anesthetic agents, quick absorption of these gases into the bloodstream can lead to collapse of alveoli in dependent portions of the lung.

Although atelectasis is usually caused by bronchial obstruction, direct compression can also cause it. The compressive type is due to air (pneumothorax), blood (hemothorax), or fluid (hydrothorax) filling the pleural space. Abdominal distention that presses on a portion of the lung can also collapse alveoli, causing atelectasis. *Right middle lobe syndrome* refers to atelectasis secondary to compression of the bronchus to the right middle lobe by lymph nodes containing metastatic cancer.

Clinical Manifestations

When sudden obstruction of the bronchus occurs, there may be dyspnea, tachypnea, cyanosis, elevation of temperature, drop in blood pressure, substernal retractions, or shock. In the chronic form of atelectasis, the client may be asymptomatic with gradual onset of dyspnea and weakness. The physical therapist may hear crackles in dependent lung bases in the postsurgical or immobile patient. Low oxygen saturations and shallow respirations may also be noted.

MEDICAL MANAGEMENT

DIAGNOSIS. Atelectasis is suspected in penetrating or other chest injuries. X-ray examination may show a shadow in the area of collapse. If an entire lobe is collapsed, the radiograph will show the trachea, heart, and mediastinum deviated toward the collapsed area, with the diaphragm elevated on that side (see Figs. 15-14 and 15-24). Chest auscultation demonstrating absent breath sounds, diminished breath sounds, or crackles, and physical assessment add to the clinical diagnostic picture. Blood gas measurements and pulse oximetry may show decreased oxygen saturation.

TREATMENT AND PROGNOSIS. Once atelectasis occurs, treatment is directed toward removing the cause whenever possible. Suctioning or bronchoscopy may be employed to remove airway obstruction. Airway clearance techniques are helpful to remove secretions and promote segmental inflation after the obstruction has been removed. Breathing techniques that employ a breath hold to allow for cross-ventilation between alveoli are also used to improve alveolar expansion.

Surfactant has been used to resolve atelectasis in infants with respiratory distress syndrome, meconium aspiration, and other pathologies.[172] Antibiotics are used to combat infection accompanying secondary atelectasis. Reexpansion of the lung is often possible, but the final prognosis depends on the underlying disease.

SPECIAL IMPLICATIONS FOR THE THERAPIST 15-18

Atelectasis

Atelectasis is a postoperative complication of thoracic or high abdominal surgery. Left lower lobe atelectasis can occur following cardiac surgery. Within a few hours after surgery, atelectasis becomes increasingly resistant to reinflation. This complication is exacerbated in people receiving narcotics. Although there has not been sufficient research to support its use, one of the goals of acute care therapy is to prevent atelectasis in the high-risk client.[400]

Diminished respiratory movement as a result of postoperative pain is often addressed by the therapist. Frequent, gentle position changes, deep breathing, coughing, and early ambulation help promote drainage of all lung segments. Deep breathing and effective coughing enhance lung expansion and prevent airway obstruction. Deep breathing is beneficial because it promotes the ciliary clearance of secretions, stabilizes the alveoli by redistributing surfactant, and permits collateral ventilation of the alveoli, through the Kohn pores in the alveolar septa.

The Kohn pores, which open only during deep breathing, allow air to pass from well-ventilated alveoli to obstructed alveoli, minimizing their tendency to collapse and facilitating removal of the obstruction. To minimize postoperative pain during deep-breathing and coughing exercises, teach the client to hold a pillow firmly over the incision.

There is evidence that vigorous airway clearance techniques are as effective in resolving atelectasis from mucous plugs as bronchoscopy.[302] Bronchoscopy has the adverse effect of temporarily lowering oxygen saturation and further irritation of lung tissue.

Pulmonary Edema

Definition and Incidence

Pulmonary edema or pulmonary congestion is an excessive fluid accumulation in the lungs that develops in the interstitial tissue, air spaces (alveoli), or both. The fluid is a barrier to gas exchange. Pulmonary edema is a common complication of many disease processes. It occurs at any age but with increasing incidence in older people with left-sided heart failure.

Etiologic and Risk Factors

Most cases of pulmonary edema are caused by left ventricular failure (see Fig. 12-12, *A*), acute hypertension, or mitral valve disease, but noncardiac conditions, especially kidney or liver disorders that cause sodium and water retention, can also produce pulmonary edema. These causes of pulmonary edema include intravenous narcotics, increased intracerebral pressure, brain injury, high altitude, diving and submersion, sepsis, medications, inhalation of smoke or toxins (e.g., ammonia), blood transfusion reactions, shock, and disseminated intravascular coagulation.[44,114,186]

Other risk factors include hyperaldosteronism, Cushing syndrome, use of glucocorticoids, and use of hypotonic fluids to irrigate nasogastric tubes. Pulmonary edema itself is a major predisposing factor in the development of pneumonia that complicates heart failure and ARDS.

Pathogenesis

Pulmonary edema occurs when the pulmonary vasculature fills with fluid that leaks into the alveolar spaces, decreasing the space available for gas exchange. Normally the lung is kept dry by lymphatic drainage and a balance among capillary hydrostatic pressure, capillary oncotic pressure, and capillary permeability.

Pulmonary edema develops as a result of (1) fluid overload, (2) decreased serum and albumin, (3) lymphatic obstruction, and (4) disruption of capillary permeability (tissue injury or immunoresponse) (Fig. 15-20). New studies show that loss of sodium transport capacity may be a factor in the development of some types of pulmonary edema.[537]

Fluid Overload. When the filling pressures on the left side of the heart increase, this increased pressure is transmitted "upstream" to the left atrium and then the pulmonary vasculature. If it surpasses the oncotic pressure that holds fluid in the capillaries, fluid is drawn from capillaries in the interstitial space and then into the alveoli.[397] Normally, the lymphatic system removes this fluid from the lungs, but if the flow of fluid into the interstitium exceeds the ability of the lymphatic system to remove it, fluid overload and consequently pulmonary edema develops.* When osmotic pressure in the venous end of the capillary exceeds

---

*A brief review of this concept may be necessary for an understanding of many pulmonary conditions. For an in-depth discussion the reader is referred to Guyton AC, Hall JE: *Textbook of medical physiology*, ed 12, Philadelphia, 2011, WB Saunders. Fluid movement in the lung (as in all vessels) is governed by vascular permeability and the balance of the hydrostatic and oncotic pressures across the capillary endothelium as described by Starling's equation. Hydrostatic forces favor fluid filtration, whereas oncotic pressure promotes reabsorption. Normally, filtration forces dominate and fluid continuously moves from the vascular space into the interstitium. Extravascular water does not accumulate because the lung lymphatics effectively remove the filtered fluid and return it to the circulation. When the capacity of the lymphatic system is exceeded, if the rate of fluid filtration exceeds its functional capabilities, water accumulates in the loose interstitial tissues around the airways, pulmonary arteries, and eventually, the alveolar walls (alveolar edema).

interstitial pressure, fluid cannot return to the bloodstream and peripheral and pulmonary edema may result. Fluid overload may also occur from decreased sodium and water excretion associated with renal disorders.

Pulmonary edema is commonly seen when the left side of the heart is distended and fails to pump adequately (e.g., myocardial ischemia or infarction or mitral or aortic valve damage). Increased left atrial pressure may also result from inadequate emptying of the atria as occurs with atrial fibrillation. This increases left atrial pressure, which is then transmitted to the pulmonary vasculature, eventually disrupting fluid homeostasis and causing the alveoli to flood. In right-sided heart failure, the increased pressures are transmitted from the right ventricle to the right artery and then to the systemic circulation causing peripheral edema. Untreated or severe left-sided heart failure can also lead to right-sided failure so both pulmonary and peripheral edema may exist simultaneously.

In high-pressure acute heart failure, there may be inflammatory and oxidative induced damage to the alveolar-capillary interface leading to increased permeability and edema.[397] In chronic heart failure, the alveolar–capillary interface may have increased collagen deposition leading to decreased diffusion of gasses.

Decreased Serum and Albumin. In the case of liver cirrhosis, the serum protein and albumin levels are reduced in the vascular fluids. Thus less fluid reabsorption from the tissue spaces occurs, which results in pulmonary and peripheral edema and ascites.

Lymphatic Obstruction. When lymphatic channels are obstructed, tissue oncotic pressure rises and results in edema. This obstruction can occur as a result of tumor infiltration but most often occurs in association with cardiogenic causes of pulmonary edema. When hemodynamic alterations (changes in the movement of blood and the forces involved) in the heart increase the perfusion pressure in the pulmonary capillaries, effective lymphatic drainage is blocked.

Tissue Injury. Disruption of capillary permeability is the cause of pulmonary edema in ALI associated with ARDS, inhalation of toxic gases, aspiration of gastric contents, viral infections, and uremia. In these conditions, destruction of endothelial cells or disruption of the tight junctions between them alters capillary permeability. Transfusion reactions are caused by leukocyte antibodies and result in increased capillary permeability.[124]

Clinical Manifestations

Clinical manifestations of pulmonary edema occur in stages. During the initial stage, clients may be asymptomatic or they may complain of restlessness and anxiety and the feeling that they are developing a common cold. Other common clinical complaints are dyspnea on exertion, decreases in physical activity, and orthopnea.[149] Signs include a persistent cough, and crackles. If the pulmonary edema worsens or occurs rapidly, respirations increase in rate, and there may be audible wheezing. If the edema is severe, the cough becomes productive of frothy sputum tinged with blood, giving it a pinkish hue. If the condition persists, the person becomes hypoxic, less responsive, and may lose consciousness.

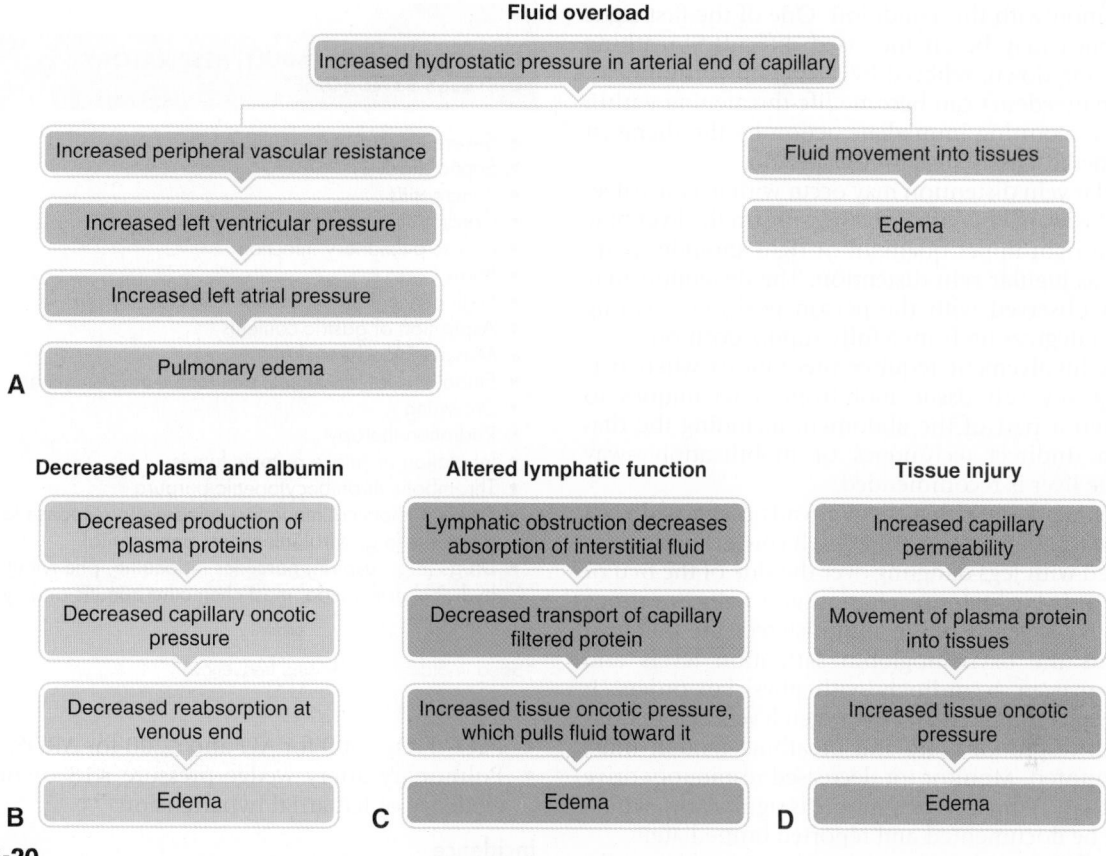

Figure 15-20

Mechanisms of pulmonary edema formation. A, Fluid overload. **B,** Decreased serum and albumin. **C,** Lymphatic obstruction. **D,** Tissue injury. (From Black JM, Hawks JH, eds: *Medical-surgical nursing,* ed 7, St Louis, 2005, WB Saunders.)

MEDICAL MANAGEMENT

PREVENTION. Prevention is a key component with persons at increased risk for the development of pulmonary edema. Preventive measures may be as simple as lowering salt intake or pharmacologic treatment such as the use of digoxin and diuretics. Refer to Chapter 12 for a discussion on heart failure.

DIAGNOSIS. Pulmonary edema is usually recognized by its characteristic clinical presentation. Cardiogenic pulmonary edema is differentiated from noncardiac causes by the history and physical examination. An underlying cardiac abnormality can usually be detected clinically or by the electrocardiogram (ECG), chest film, cardiac CT, or echocardiogram. A chest film may show increased vascular pattern; increased opacity of the lung, especially at the bases; and pleural effusion.

There are no specific laboratory tests diagnostic of pulmonary edema; when the condition progresses enough to cause liver involvement the physician may observe the hepatojugular reflex (positional or palpatory pressure on the liver results in distention of the jugular vein). Auscultation reveals distinct abnormal breath sounds with crackles or rales. Blood gas measurements indicate the degree of functional impairment, and sputum cultures may indicate accompanying infection. B-type natriuretic peptide may be measured, with elevated levels indicating pulmonary edema from a cardiac cause.

TREATMENT. Once pulmonary edema has been diagnosed, treatment is aimed at enhancing gas exchange, reducing fluid overload, and strengthening and slowing the heartbeat. Oxygen by mask, continuous positive airway pressure, or through ventilatory support is used along with diuretics, diet, and fluid restriction to remove excess alveolar fluid.

Morphine to relieve anxiety and reduce the effort of breathing may be used for people who do not have narcotic-induced pulmonary edema. Other pharmacologic-based treatment may be used to help dilate the bronchi and increase cardiac output, strengthen contractions of the heart, and increase cardiac output.

PROGNOSIS. The prognosis depends on the underlying condition. The presence of pulmonary edema is a medical emergency requiring immediate intervention to prevent further respiratory distress and death. It is often reversible with clinical management.

SPECIAL IMPLICATIONS FOR THE THERAPIST 15-19

Pulmonary Edema

Signs and symptoms of pulmonary edema that may come to the therapist's attention include engorged neck and hand veins (because of peripheral vascular fluid overload), pitting edema of the extremities, adventitious breath sounds, and paroxysmal nocturnal dyspnea so common with this condition. One of the first signs of dyspnea may be an increased difficulty breathing when lying down, relieved by sitting up (orthopnea). Pulmonary edema can become life-threatening within minutes, requiring immediate action by the therapist to get medical assistance for this person.

Jugular vein distention may occur with liver involvement. Positional or palpatory pressure on the liver may result in right upper quadrant or right shoulder pain, as well as jugular vein distention. The distention may be best observed with the person positioned sitting 30 to 45 degrees up from a fully supine position.

Liver involvement requires precautions when performing any soft tissue mobilization techniques to the anterior part of the abdomen, including the diaphragm. Indirect techniques or mobilization away from the liver is recommended.

When working with a client already diagnosed with pulmonary edema, the sitting (high Fowler) position is preferred with legs dangling over the side of the bed or plinth. This facilitates respiration and reduces venous return. If oxygen is being administered, the therapist monitors the oxyhemoglobin saturation levels and titrates oxygen accordingly with physician orders. It may be necessary to increase oxygen levels before exercise, but respiratory rate and breathing pattern must be monitored. Monitor for decreased respiratory drive (fewer than 12 breaths per minute is significant), which should be documented and reported immediately.

The client may be taking nitroglycerin sublingually, which will further increase vasodilation and decrease ventricular preload. Monitor blood pressure closely, and observe for signs of hypotension because nitroglycerin can drop blood pressure dangerously. The therapist should consult with nursing or respiratory staff for any special considerations for each individual client.

Gradual exercise intolerance usually occurs as the dyspnea progresses. The client may comment about weight gain or difficulty fastening clothes. Check for peripheral edema in the immobile or bedridden client. In this group of people, edema can occur in the sacral hollow rather than in the feet and legs because the sacrum is the lowest place on the trunk. Care must be taken to prevent pressure ulcers in this area.

Acute Lung Injury and Acute Respiratory Distress Syndrome

Definition

ALI/ARDS is a form of acute respiratory failure after a systemic or pulmonary insult. It is also called *ARDS, shock lung, wet lung, stiff lung, hyaline membrane disease (adult or newborn), posttraumatic lung,* or *diffuse alveolar damage.* It is a syndrome and not a specific diagnosis; often a fatal complication of serious illness (e.g., sepsis), trauma, or major surgery. ALI/ARDS is defined by the American-European Consensus conference Committee as:

- Acute onset of diffuse bilateral pulmonary infiltrates on radiograph;

Box 15-9

CAUSES OF ACUTE (ADULT) RESPIRATORY DISTRESS SYNDROME*

- Severe trauma (e.g., multiple bone fractures)
- Septic shock
- Pancreatitis
- Cardiopulmonary bypass surgery
- Diffuse pulmonary infection
- Burns
- High concentrations of supplemental oxygen
- Aspiration of gastric contents
- Massive blood transfusions
- Embolism: fat, thrombus, amniotic fluid, venous air
- Drowning
- Radiation therapy
- Inhalation of smoke or toxic fumes
- Thrombotic thrombocytopenic purpura
- Indirect: chemical mediators released in response to systemic disorders (e.g., viral infections, pneumonia)
- Drugs (e.g., aspirin, narcotics, lidocaine, phenylbutazone, hydrochlorothiazide, most chemotherapeutic and cytotoxic agents)

*Listed in order of decreasing frequency.

- $PaO_2/FiO_2 \leq 300$ for ALI and ≤ 200 for ARDS; and
- Pulmonary artery wedge pressure ≤ 18 or no clinical evidence of left atrial hypertension.[274]

Incidence

ALI/ARDS has an incidence of about 200,000 and kills upwards of 50,000 people in the United States each year (more than breast cancer). ALI/ARDS mortality rates have declined since the mid 1990s but still carries a relatively high mortality rate of 29% to 42%, depending on comorbidities and risk factors.[274]

Risk Factors

ALI/ARDS can affect anyone at any time regardless of gender, age, or health status. Factors that increase the risk of ALI/ARDS include increasing age, sepsis, pneumonia, aspiration, trauma, pancreatitis, blood transfusions, and smoke inhalation (Box 15-9).[274] Those with ALI/ARDS caused by underlying sepsis have the highest mortality rate. Why some people develop this condition and others do not is unknown. The presence of too much inflammation or the lack of immune cells necessary to resolve inflammation are two possibilities that may be linked to genetic and molecular risk factors.[152]

Pathogenesis

ALI/ARDS results from three primary issues in the lung; acute injury to the alveolar–capillary membrane, inflammation, and increased permeability of the alveolar–capillary membrane leading to pulmonary edema.[274] The alveolar–capillary membrane becomes injured, causing protein-rich fluid to leak into the interstitium. When this volume exceeds the ability of the lymphatics to remove it, the edema moves into the airspaces impacting gas exchange.

Second, neutrophils become activated and begin to erode the basement membrane of the alveoli.

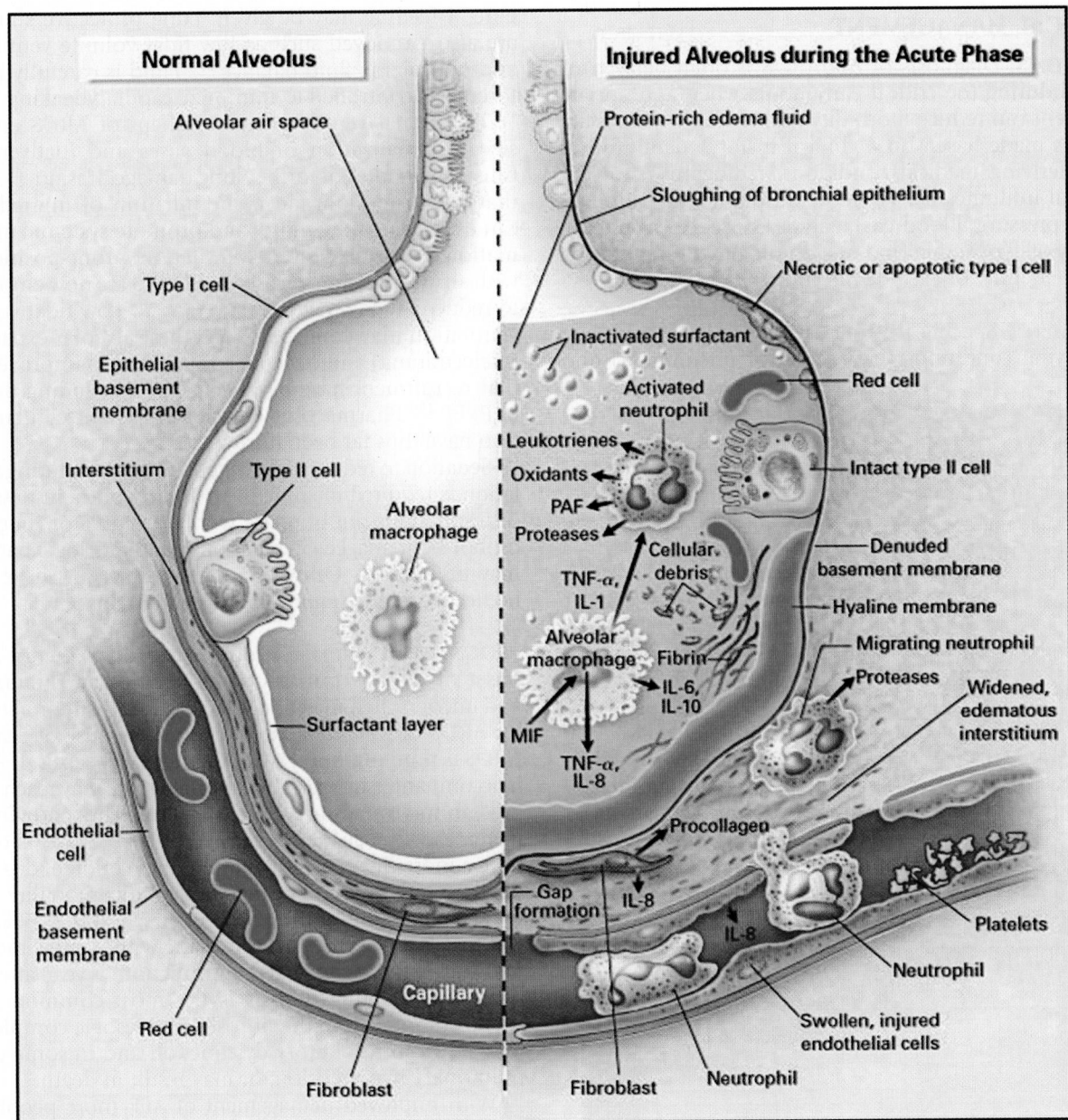

Figure 15-21

Figure demonstrates both a normal alveolus and one with ALI/ARDS.

Moreover, neutrophils release mediators that are pro-inflammatory and contribute to cell apoptosis. Finally, there is also damage to type II alveolar cells which produce surfactant. Reduction of surfactant contributes to alveolar collapse, increased compliance, and impaired gas exchange. Type II cells also have a role in repairing the epithelium, so when destroyed, remodeling can be affected and fibrosis or scarring ensues, adding to the problem.[274]

Figure 15-21 demonstrates both a normal alveolus and one with ALI/ARDS.

These are only the pulmonary manifestations of what is now recognized as a more systemic process called *multiple organ dysfunction syndrome* (MODS), formerly called *multiple organ failure*. See Chapter 5 for a discussion of MODS.

Clinical Manifestations

The clinical presentation is relatively uniform regardless of cause and occurs within 12 to 48 hours of the initiating event. The earliest sign of ARDS is usually an increased respiratory rate characterized by shallow, rapid breathing. Pulmonary edema, atelectasis, and decreased lung compliance causing dyspnea, hyperventilation, and the changes observed on chest radiographs (Fig. 15-22).

As breathing becomes increasingly difficult, the individual may gasp for air and exhibit intercostal, clavicular, or sternal retractions and cyanosis. Unless the underlying disease is reversed rapidly, especially in the presence of sepsis (toxins in the blood), the condition quickly progresses to full-blown MODS, involving kidneys, liver, gut, CNS, and the cardiovascular system.

MEDICAL MANAGEMENT

DIAGNOSIS. Diagnosis of ALI/ARDS is often delayed or missed during the critical early hours when appropriate treatment can reduce morbidity and mortality. The diagnosis is made based on a clinical history, identification of underlying medical conditions, radiograph showing bilateral infiltrates, PaO_2/FiO_2, and pulmonary capillary wedge pressure. Blood gas analysis is used to assess the severity of hypoxemia, and microbiologic cultures may be used to identify or exclude infection.

TREATMENT. Specific treatment is administered for any underlying conditions (e.g., sepsis or pneumonia) and

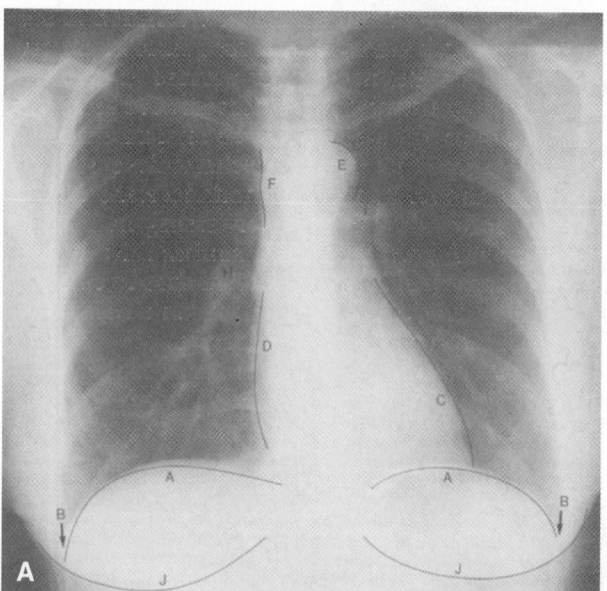

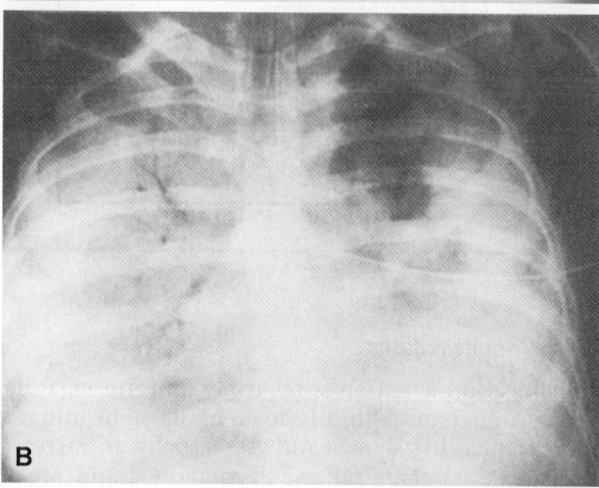

Figure 15-22

A, Normal chest film taken from a posteroanterior view. The backward L in the upper right corner is placed on the film to indicate the left side of the chest. Some anatomic structures can be seen on the x-ray study and are outlined: A, diaphragm; B, costophrenic angle; C, left ventricle; D, right atrium; E, aortic arch; F, superior vena cava; G, trachea; H, right bronchus; I, left bronchus; J, breast shadows. **B,** This chest film shows massive consolidation from pulmonary edema associated with acute (adult) respiratory distress syndrome after multisystem trauma. (A, from Black JM, Hokanson Hawks, J, editors: *Medical-surgical nursing*, ed 7, St Louis, 2005, WB Saunders; B, from Fraser RG, Paré JA, Paré PD, et al: *Diagnosis of diseases of the chest*, ed 3, Philadelphia, 1990, WB Saunders.)

enteral feeding may be given. Lung protective strategies are also employed such as low tidal volume ventilation and optimizing fluid balance.[274] Fluid is carefully monitored and controlled to minimize capillary leaking.[439]

Traditional ventilator management of ARDS emphasized normalization of blood gases and inadvertently caused high rates of further lung damage. It is now known that overdistention and cyclic inflation of injured lung can exacerbate lung injury and promote systemic inflammation. Low tidal volume ventilation, prone positioning with airway pressure release ventilation are now employed to reduce lung damage.[274,439,440,507,508] Low tidal volume ventilation may contribute to cyclical alveolar expansion (atelectrauma) and collapse so strategies to improve alveolar recruitment have been developed including the use of PEEP.[439] Pharmacologic strategies to reduce inflammation have thus far been unsuccessful.[274]

Sedation to reduce anxiety and restlessness during ventilation is required in some cases. If tachypnea, restlessness, or respirations out of phase with the ventilator (bucking) cannot be managed by sedation, pharmacologic paralysis may be induced. Other pharmacologic agents have been ineffective in altering morbidity or mortality.[3,262]

PROGNOSIS. The final outcome is difficult to predict at the onset of disease, but associated multiorgan dysfunction and uncontrolled infection contribute to the mortality rate for ARDS of 29% to 42%.[274] The major cause of death in ARDS is nonpulmonary MODS, often with sepsis. If ARDS is accompanied by sepsis, the mortality rate may reach 90%. Median survival in such cases is 2 weeks. The mortality rate increases with age, and clients older than 60 years of age have a mortality rate as high as 90%. In children, degree of hypoxia and multiple organ failure predict mortality. Mortality rates for children range between 8% and 27.5%.[439]

Most survivors are asymptomatic within a few months and have almost normal lung function 1 year after the acute illness. Lung fibrosis is the most common post-ARDS complication; the fibrosis may resolve completely; may result in respiratory dysfunction and in some cases, pulmonary hypertension; or may result in death.

With improved management of ALI, more people are surviving than ever before. Newer evidence is pointing to persistent impairments in physical functioning and possibly cognitive and mood disturbances (depression, anxiety, posttraumatic stress disorder) as well.[59,247] Risk factors for post-ALI mood disorder include obesity, hypoglycemia, alcohol dependence, female sex, younger age, and cognitive dysfunction..[33] The research in this area is in its infancy and early investigations highlight that it is difficult to tease out ALI/ARDS related issues from general ICU issues such as myopathy, fatigue, neuropathy, and cognitive decline.

SPECIAL IMPLICATIONS FOR THE THERAPIST   15-20

*Acute (Adult) Respiratory Distress Syndrome**
Assessment and Monitoring

ALI/ARDS requires careful monitoring and supportive care. Timely physical therapy interventions improve gas

---

*There is a case study on this topic available on the Evolve site (Box 15-1).

exchange and reverse pathologic progression, thereby curtailing or avoiding artificial ventilation.[541] The application of an early intervention, including peripheral muscle training, in tracheotomized patients admitted to a respiratory ICU can help recovery from immobility, dysfunction, and overmedication (such as with sedatives), which are typical in patients transferred from the ICU.[493]

Assess the client's respiratory status frequently, and observe for retractions on inspiration, the use of accessory muscles of respiration, and developing or worsening dyspnea. On auscultation, listen for adventitious (crackles/rales or wheezing/rhonchi) or diminished breath sounds and report any clear, frothy sputum that may indicate pulmonary edema.

Closely monitor heart rate and blood pressure watching for arrhythmias (see "Special Implications for the Therapist 12-12: Arrhythmias" in Chapter 12) that may result from hypoxemia, acid–base disturbances, or electrolyte imbalance.

Critical illness polyneuropathy is a possible neurologic complication of ARDS, multiple organ failure, and other trauma (see discussion of this polyneuropathy in Chapter 5). Therapists should be alert for signs of motor or sensory changes in clients with ARDS.[4] Using an explicit protocol, manual muscle testing is a highly reliable method for assessing strength following ARDS.[110] A standardized clinical examination can be completed with mechanically ventilated patients who can tolerate sitting upright in bed and are able to follow two-step commands.[169] A video demonstration of the protocol for manual muscle testing is available at http://www.jove.com/video/2632. Each muscle is tested with specific techniques for positioning, stabilization, resistance, and palpation.

Positioning

$\dot{V}/\dot{Q}$ mismatch is common in ARDS and can be altered by position changes that can facilitate lung expansion and redistribute fluid in the lungs. Oxygenation in clients with ALI/ARDS may sometimes be improved by turning them from the supine to the prone position, dramatically reducing pulmonary dead space and improving aeration.[167] This change takes the weight off (and improves ventilation in) the posterior regions of the lungs while promoting perfusion in the anterior aspects. The net result is improved oxygenation, expansion of atelectatic alveoli, and increased functional residual lung capacity.

Caregivers may be reluctant to use the prone position. The therapist can be very instrumental in providing education on proper technique and rationale. Selection criteria for this type of positioning may include individuals receiving ventilatory support at an oxygen concentration greater than 50%, with poor arterial blood gas levels and PEEP of 10 to 15 mm Hg or higher. Prone positioning should be considered if routine ventilator management has not been enough to improve the ventilatory status in an individual who is already pharmacologically immobilized or sedated (sedation is a requirement for prone positioning).

The client should be turned as far as possible on the abdomen; a 270-degree turn can improve oxygenation in some individuals, but the full prone position is optimal. The person can be turned almost fully prone and supported with two or three pillows to help protect the airway, permit visualization, and allow suctioning as necessary. The better the person responds to the prone position, the longer that position can be maintained, although tolerance may build up with repeated use of the position. It is the repeated change from supine to prone positioning that redistributes pulmonary fluid and improves aeration and oxygenation overall.

Before turning, identify all invasive lines and bring them above the person's waist and over the head; lines inserted in the groin area can be moved over to the side that will remain nondependent. Taking these precautions will reduce the chances that the lines will get kinked or dislodged. One person should be in charge of the person's airway during the turning, supporting the client's head and watching the intravenous lines. Any side-port line of a pulmonary artery catheter must be monitored especially carefully because it is closest to the client and more likely to kink. When the turn is completed, this same clinician turns the client's head to one side, making sure the airway is visible and open. Extra pillows or foam/gel pads may be needed to make room for the airway and increase comfort level. The dependent shoulder should be positioned with the elbow directly to the side and the hand facing up toward the head to prevent dislocation. A pad around the mouth to absorb bronchial secretions will decrease the potential for eye contamination.

The prone position promotes secretion removal by propelling secretions toward the upper airways. It also makes it easy to perform back care and help maintain sacral and heel skin integrity. Disadvantages include the potential for facial skin irritation (especially on the forehead), loss of important vascular accesses, and difficulty performing cardiopulmonary resuscitation if required. Blood pressure may drop after the turn but should stabilize within a few minutes; unstable blood pressure will necessitate returning the person to the supine position. Other indicators of poor position tolerance include a decline in Sao_2, SVO_2, or the tidal volume over time.[150,167]

Survivors of ALI/ARDS

Survivors of acute respiratory distress syndrome (ARDS) and other causes of critical illness often have generalized weakness, reduced exercise tolerance, and persistent nerve and muscle impairments after hospital discharge.[110] The role of the therapist in reversing disability and restoring health status has been documented with improved long-term outcomes reported for mechanically ventilated patients.[113,209]

Postoperative Respiratory Failure

Postoperative respiratory failure can result in the same pathophysiologic and clinical manifestations as ARDS but without the severe progression to MODS (see previous discussion of ARDS). Risk factors include surgical procedures of the thorax or abdomen, limited cardiac reserve, chronic renal failure, chronic hepatic disease, infection, period of hypotension during surgery, sepsis, and smoking, especially in the presence of preexisting lung disease. In the pediatric population, a difficult respiratory course may result in necrotizing enterocolitis, a postoperative gastrointestinal complication related to ischemia of the bowel. This condition occurs when oxygen depletion in the heart or brain causes blood to be shunted away from less vital organs, such as the intestine.

The most common postoperative pulmonary problems include atelectasis, pneumonia, pulmonary edema, and pulmonary emboli. Prevention of any of these problems involves frequent turning, deep breathing, humidified air to loosen secretions, antibiotics for infection as appropriate, supplemental oxygen for hypoxemia, and early ambulation.

If respiratory failure develops, mechanical ventilation may be required, and treatment is very similar to that for ARDS.

Sarcoidosis

Definition

Sarcoidosis is a systemic disease of unknown cause involving any organ and is characterized by noncaseating granulomas present diffusely throughout the body. Its primary effects are seen in the lung and lymphatic tissues.[414] Technically, this condition could have been discussed earlier in the "Infectious and Inflammatory Diseases" section, but without a better sense of the underlying etiology, it remains here under diseases that affect the lung parenchyma. The granulomas consist of a collection of macrophages surrounded by lymphocytes taking a nodular form. In fact, granulomatous inflammation of the lung is present in 90% of clients with sarcoidosis. Secondary sites include the skin, eyes, liver, spleen, heart, and small bones in the hands and feet.

Incidence

Sarcoidosis occurs predominantly in the third and fourth decades (between the ages of 20 and 40 years) and has a slightly higher incidence in women than men. It is present worldwide with some interesting differences in prevalence among ethnic groups. It is more prevalent in African Americans and Puerto Ricans.[314] Socioeconomic, environmental, and genetic factors appear to influence the occurrence.[120]

Etiologic Factors and Pathogenesis

The etiologic factors and pathogenesis of sarcoidosis are unknown, but there appears to be an exaggerated cellular immune response on the part of the helper T lymphocytes to a foreign antigen whose identity remains unclear. Increasing evidence points to a triggering agent that may be genetic, infectious (bacterial or viral), immunologic, or toxic. Abnormalities of immune function, as well as autoantibody production, including rheumatoid factor and antinuclear antibodies, are seen in sarcoidosis and in connective tissue diseases, suggesting a common immunopathogenetic mechanism.

IFN-γ, tumor necrosis factor, and IL-2, IL-6, and IL-8 all have a part in the granulomatous process.[383] A series of interactions between the excessive accumulation of T lymphocytes and monocytes and macrophages leads to the formation of noncaseating (i.e., do not undergo necrotic degeneration) granulomas in the lung and other organs characteristic of the disease. Granuloma formation may regress with therapy or as a result of the disease's natural course but may also progress to fibrosis and restrictive lung disease.

Clinical Manifestations

Sarcoidosis can affect any organ, including bones, joints, muscles, and vessels. Lungs and thoracic lymph nodes are most often involved with acute or insidious respiratory problems sometimes accompanied by symptoms affecting the skin, eyes, or other organs. The diverse manifestations of this disorder lend support to the hypothesis that sarcoidosis has more than one cause. The clinical impact of sarcoidosis is directly related to the extent of granulomatous inflammation and its effect on the function of vital organs.

Pulmonary sarcoidosis has a variable natural course from an asymptomatic state to a progressive life-threatening condition. Signs and symptoms may develop over a period of a few weeks to a few months and include dyspnea, nonproductive cough, fever, malaise, weight loss, skin lesions (Fig. 15-23), erythema nodosum (multiple, tender, nonulcerating nodules) and fatigue.[144]

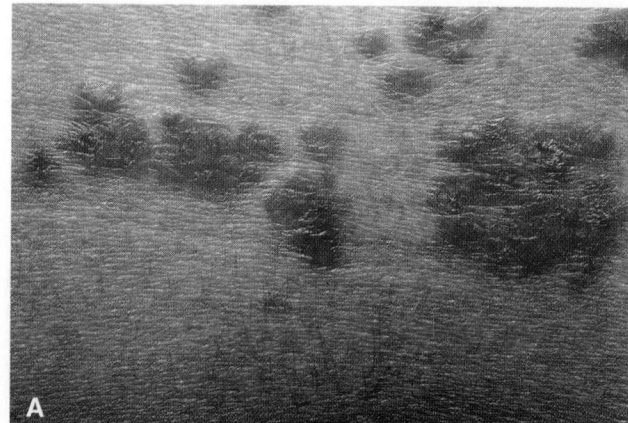

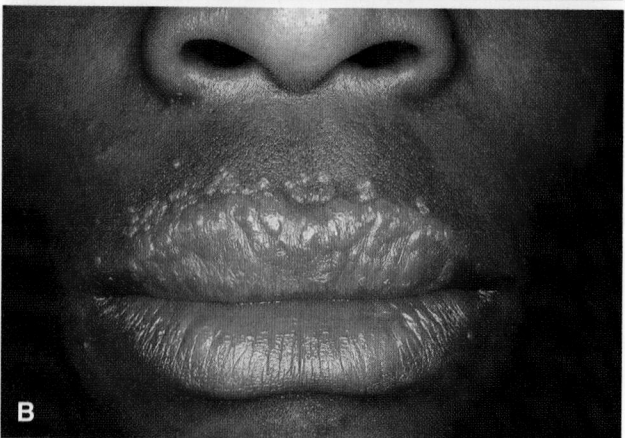

Figure 15-23

Sarcoidosis. A, Cutaneous sarcoidosis usually consists of papules and plaques with a typical reddish-brown color. **B,** Lesions often favor the lips and perioral region. (From Bolognia JL, Jorizzo JL, Rapini RP: *Dermatology,* St Louis, 2003, Mosby. Courtesy Jean Bolognia, MD. Used with permission.)

This condition may be entirely asymptomatic, presenting with abnormal findings on routine chest radiographs. Respiratory symptoms of dry cough and dyspnea without constitutional symptoms (symptoms of systemic illness, including fatigue, weakness, malaise, weight loss, sweating, and fever) occur in more than half of all people with sarcoidosis, and up to 15% develop progressive fibrosis. Chest pain, hemoptysis, or pneumothorax may be present.

Sarcoidosis may present with extrapulmonary symptoms referable to bone marrow, skin, eyes, cranial nerves or peripheral nerves (neurosarcoidosis), liver, or heart (Box 15-10). Sarcoid arthritis with arthralgia, myopathy, chronic tissue swelling, tenosynovitis and other periarthritic inflammatory changes occur less often but bring the affected individuals to the therapist's attention.[454] Neurosarcoidosis is an uncommon but severe, and sometimes life-threatening, manifestation of sarcoidosis occurring in 5% to 15% of cases. Sarcoidosis appears to be associated with a significantly increased risk for cancer in affected organs (e.g., skin, liver, lymphoma, or lung). Chronic inflammation is the mediator of this risk.[30]

MEDICAL MANAGEMENT

DIAGNOSIS. There is no specific test other than history for sarcoidosis so diagnosis is based on clinical examination, chest CT, pulmonary function and laboratory test findings, and biopsy of easily accessible granulomas (e.g., skin lesions, salivary gland, or palpable lymph nodes). When lung involvement is suspected, further testing may be required and new imaging techniques improve detection. Other granulomatous diseases (e.g., TB, berylliosis, lymphoma, carcinoma, and fungal disease) must be ruled out.

CNS involvement in sarcoidosis poses a difficult diagnostic problem. Although neurologic involvement may occur long before the onset of symptoms, contrast-enhanced CT does not always reveal parenchymal and meningeal involvement.

TREATMENT. Treatment may not be required, especially in those clients who are asymptomatic and have an FVC >70% predicted.[279] A combination of chest CT findings indicating active inflammation and decrements in FVC help determine if a watch-and-wait strategy will be used or if medication will be employed. Short-term (less than 6 months) use of inhaled steroids may improve symptoms especially in people who mainly have cough. The long-term use of corticosteroids is the treatment of choice for those clients who have impaired lung function with pulmonary granulomas.

Corticosteroids are quite effective in reducing the acute granulomatous inflammation as seen on radiograph, but their efficacy in improving lung function and altering the long-term prognosis is unproven. It has been suggested that those who receive corticosteroids have a higher rate of relapse, possibly due to a decrease in ability of the body to clear the offending antigen.[279]

People with sarcoidosis who smoke are encouraged to quit because smoking aggravates impaired lung function and promotes osteoporosis. Management of osteoporosis in this population requires special attention because there is often an underlying disorder in calcium metabolism that results in hypercalciuria and hypercalcemia.

Prolonged exposure to direct sunlight should be avoided because vitamin D aids absorption of calcium, which can contribute to elevated serum and urinary calcium levels and the formation of kidney stones. Bronchoscopy may be required if fibrosis or swelling leads to stenosis of the airways.[312]

In cases of end-stage sarcoidosis, lung transplantation has been proven successful.[312] Selection of clients with pulmonary sarcoidosis for transplantation requires that medical therapy, including the use of corticosteroids and alternative medications, has been exhausted and that other contraindicated variables are not present (see "Lung Transplantation" in Chapter 21). Sarcoidosis frequently recurs in the allograft but rarely causes symptoms or pulmonary dysfunction.[278]

PROGNOSIS. The prognosis is usually favorable, with complete resolution of symptoms and chest radiographic changes within 1 to 2 years. Most clients do not manifest clinically significant sequelae. However, because sarcoidosis is a multisystem disease that can cause complex problems, it can have a variable prognosis ranging from spontaneous remissions to progressive lung disease with pulmonary fibrosis in active sarcoidosis. In such cases, respiratory insufficiency and cor pulmonale may

---

Box 15-10

CLINICAL MANIFESTATIONS OF SARCOIDOSIS

Pulmonary

- Asymptomatic with abnormal chest film
- Sinusitis
- Gradually progressive cough and shortness of breath
- Interstitial pneumonitis
- Pulmonary fibrosis with pulmonary insufficiency
- Laryngeal and endobronchial obstruction
- Necrotizing sarcoid granulomatosis

Extrapulmonary

- Löfgren syndrome: fever, arthralgia, bilateral hilar adenopathy, erythema nodosum
- Heerfordt syndrome (uveoparotid fever): fever, swelling of parotid gland and uveal tracts, seventh cranial nerve palsy
- Erythema nodosum
- Peripheral lymphadenopathy/splenomegaly
- Lymphoma
- Eyes: excessive tearing, swelling, uveitis, iritis, glaucoma, cataracts
- Integument: nodules or skin plaques (see Fig. 15-21); skin cancer
- Nervous system: peripheral and/or cranial nerve palsies (cranial neuropathy), subacute meningitis, diabetes insipidus, spinal myelopathy
- Joints: polyarticular and monarticular arthritis
- Skeletal: osteolytic lesions in phalangeal and metacarpal bones
- Cardiac: paroxysmal arrhythmias, conduction disturbances, pericarditis, myocarditis, congestive heart failure, sudden death
- Renal: hypercalcemia with nephrocalcinosis or nephrolithiasis, interstitial cystitis
- Liver: granulomatous hepatitis, liver cancer

eventually occur. In 65% to 70% of cases, there are no residual manifestations, 20% are left with permanent lung or ocular changes, and 10% of all cases die. Active sarcoidosis responds well to the administration of corticosteroids. Overall, sarcoidosis has a mortality rate of 1% to 6%.[144]

SPECIAL IMPLICATIONS FOR THE THERAPIST   15-21

Sarcoidosis

There is a distinct arthritic component associated with sarcoidosis, variously reported in 10% to 35% of people who develop extrapulmonary involvement. Arthralgia has been reported in up to 70% of individuals with this disease; often predating other manifestations of sarcoidosis.[454] The knees or ankles are the most common sites of acute arthritis. Distribution of joint involvement is usually polyarticular and symmetric, and the arthritis is commonly self-limiting after several weeks or months. Occasionally, the arthritis is recurrent or chronic, but even then, joint destruction and deformity are rare.

Treatment of arthritis in sarcoidosis is usually as for any other form of arthritis. The arthritic symptoms may develop early as the first manifestation of the disease or late in the disease and are usually accompanied by erythema nodosum. When further complicated by bilateral hilar adenopathy (enlargement of hilum or roots of the lung where the main bronchi enter the lungs), this triad of symptoms is called Löfgren syndrome. Recurrent Löfgren syndrome is extremely rare and is usually self-limiting.

Therapists should be alert to any presenting signs or symptoms of increased disease activity associated with sarcoidosis as medical vigilance with attention to new symptoms is important in the management of sarcoidosis. Serious visceral complications (e.g., cardiac disease) may present suddenly and silently with arrhythmia. Taking vital signs routinely is especially important with this disease. Palpitations, chest pain, or progressing dyspnea require medical evaluation.

This disease presents in many and diverse patterns, but observe especially for exertional dyspnea that progresses to dyspnea at rest, chest pain, joint swelling, or increased fatigue and malaise, reducing the client's functional level or ability to participate in therapy. Muscle involvement and bone involvement are frequently underdiagnosed. Symptoms of muscle weakness, aches, tenderness, and fatigue, often accompanied by neurogenic atrophy, may indicate sarcoid myositis.[40]

Cranial nerve palsies (especially facial palsy), multiple mononeuropathy, and less commonly, symmetric polyneuropathy may all occur. Symmetric polyneuropathy can affect either motor or sensory fibers solely or both disproportionately. An unusual combination of neurologic deficits affecting the CNS or peripheral nerves (or both) suggests sarcoidosis and should be evaluated medically. Improvement of neurologic function may occur with the use of corticosteroids.

For clients receiving steroid therapy, increased side effects of the medication should be reported to the physician. For example, long-term use of steroids lowers resistance to infection, may induce diabetes and myopathy, and is associated with weight gain, loss of potassium in the urine, and gastric irritation (see "Corticosteroids" in Chapter 5 and Tables 5-4 and 5-5).

Lung Cancer

Overview

Lung cancer, a malignancy of the epithelium of the respiratory tract, is the most frequent cause of cancer death in the United States and the most common type of cancer worldwide (excluding nonmelanoma skin cancer). The term *lung cancer*, also known as bronchogenic carcinoma, excludes other pulmonary tumors such as sarcomas, lymphomas, blastomas, hematomas, and mesotheliomas.

Types of Lung Cancer

At least a dozen different types of tumors are included under the broad heading of lung cancer. Clinically, lung cancers are classified as small cell lung cancer (SCLC; 10%-15% of all lung cancers), and non–SCLC (NSCLC; 85%-90% of all lung cancers). Within these two broad categories, there are four major types of primary malignant lung tumors: SCLC includes small cell carcinoma (oat cell carcinoma); NSCLC includes squamous cell carcinoma, adenocarcinoma, and large cell carcinoma. Table 15-12 summarizes the characteristics of these four lung cancers.

Adenocarcinoma, the most common form of lung cancer in the United States, tends to arise in the periphery, usually in the upper lobes at different levels of the bronchial tree. An individual tumor may reflect the cell structure of any part of the respiratory mucosa from the large bronchi to the smallest bronchioles. Because of this, adenocarcinoma refers to a heterogeneous group of neoplasms that have in common the formation of gland-like structures.

Adenocarcinoma is further subdivided into four categories: acinar, papillary, bronchioloalveolar, and solid carcinoma. Increasing incidence of adenocarcinomas is currently attributed to changes in smoking patterns (e.g., deeper and more intense inhalation) in response to reduced tar and nicotine in cigarettes. Presumably, the excess volume inhaled to satisfy addictive needs for nicotine delivers increased amounts of carcinogens and toxins to the peripheral areas of the lungs.[471]

Large cell carcinomas are so poorly differentiated that they cannot be classified with the other three categories above and require special diagnostic testing procedures to differentiate from other lung pathologic conditions.

Incidence

Lung cancer remains the leading cause of cancer death in the United States, with an estimated 158,248 deaths in 2010.[96,299] It is one of the world's leading causes of preventable death.[268] More people die of lung cancer than of colon, breast, and prostate cancer combined. In 1987, lung cancer overtook breast cancer to become the most

Table 15-12 | Characteristics of Lung Cancer

Tumor Type	Growth Rate	Metastasis	Treatment
Small Cell Lung Cancer			
Small cell (oat cell)	Very rapid	Very early; to mediastinum or distal area of lung	Combination chemotherapy; surgical resectability is poor
Non–Small Cell Lung Cancer			
Squamous cell (epidermal)	Slow	Localized metastasis not common or occurs late, usually to hilar lymph nodes, adrenals, liver	Surgically, resectability is good if stage I or II Chemoradiation therapy is considered
Adenocarcinoma	Slow to moderate	Early; metastasis throughout lung and brain or to other organs	Surgical resectability is good if localized stage I or II Chemotherapy or chemoradiation and surgery may be combined for stage III
Large cell (anaplastic)	Rapid	Early and widespread metastasis to kidney, liver, adrenals	Surgical resection is poor if involvement is widespread; better prognosis if stage I or II Chemotherapy of limited use, radiation therapy is palliative

*A major histologic change has occurred over the last 3 decades as the most common cell type has shifted from squamous cell to adenocarcinoma. This shift appears to be the result of physiochemical changes in late 20th century smoke (e.g., increased levels of tobacco-specific nitrosamines, increased use of filtered cigarettes).[32]

common cause of death from cancer among women in the United States.

The incidence of lung cancer has declined in men by approximately 2% from 1998 to 2007. The incidence in women remained level.[299] Mortality has mirrored the trends in incidence, with a reduction amongst men and a leveling off in women.[299]

Black males have the highest death rate and Asian/Pacific Islanders, American Indian/Alaska natives, and Hispanic males have the lowest death rate. Among women, whites and African Americans have the highest mortality, whereas Asian/Pacific Islander and Hispanic females have the lowest death rate from lung cancer.[267]

Risk Factors

Risk factors for lung cancer include environment (smoking, secondhand smoke, occupational exposure, and air pollution), nutrition, and genetic factors (enzymes for carcinogen metabolism, enzymes that detoxify, and the capacity to repair DNA damage).[293] Age, family history, and medical history, especially lung disease, also influence occurrence, morbidity, and mortality.

Cigarette Smoking. Cigarette smoking (more than 20 cigarettes per day) remains the greatest risk factor for lung cancer, accounting for 90% of all lung cancer deaths in men who smoke, and 80% of all lung cancer deaths in women. Of all lung cancers, 85% to 90% occur in smokers, although, remarkably, fewer than 20% of cigarette smokers develop this disease. The relative risk of lung cancer increases with the number of cigarettes smoked per day and the number of years of smoking. The people at highest risk are those who begin smoking in their teens, inhale deeply, and smoke at least one-half pack per day. However, occasional smoking or lower numbers of cigarettes smoked each day also elevates risk for lung cancer.[9] Approximately 19.1% of the adult population smoke cigarettes, with a slightly higher prevalence in men than women.[96] The highest smoking rates are seen in the American Indian/Alaska Native population, followed by non-Hispanic whites and blacks.[96] Among high school students, 19.5% smoke; among middle-school students, 5.2% smoke.[93,96]

The number of pack-years is calculated by multiplying the packs of cigarettes consumed per day by the number of years of smoking. Lung cancer risk is increased as the amount of packs smoked per year increases, as well as longer breath holds, and size of puff. The risk for dying of lung cancer is 20 times higher amongst people who smoke two or more packs of cigarettes per day than among those who do not smoke.

Smoking increases the risk for heart disease, stroke, lung cancer, and chronic obstructive lung disease (CDC Fact Sheet: Health Effects of Smoking), (http://www.cdc.gov/tobacco/data_statistics/fact_sheets/health_effects/effects_cig_smoking/). Smoking also increases the risk for other types of cancer, such as acute myeloid leukemia and cancers of the bladder, cervix, esophagus, larynx, mouth, pharynx, stomach, and kidney. Moreover, smoking and exposure to smoke is associated with infertility, preterm delivery, low birth weight, and sudden infant death syndrome.[97] For other effects of smoking, see "Tobacco" in Chapter 3.

Former smokers have about half the risk for dying from lung cancer than do current smokers (see Table 3-12). Compared with current smokers, the risk for lung and bronchus cancer among former smokers declines as the duration of abstinence lengthens, but it takes more than 20 years to reach the risk level of people who never smoked.[293] These statistics support the fact that lung cancer is the most preventable of all cancers. The elimination of cigarette smoking would virtually eradicate SCLC. Smoking cessation also appears to slow the rate of progression of carotid atherosclerosis and other vascular diseases. Smoking cessation also significantly reduces the risk for heart disease and stroke.

There are approximately 50 known carcinogens found in tobacco smoke; the major causal agents of lung cancer are the polynuclear aromatic hydrocarbons (PAHs) and tobacco-specific *N*-nitrosamines (nicotine). Tobacco smoking also results in increased exposure to ethylene oxide, aromatic amines, and other agents that cause damage to DNA.[406] For this reason, the risk of lung cancer is increased in a smoker who is also exposed to other carcinogenic agents, such as radioactive isotopes, polycyclic aromatic hydrocarbons and arsenicals, vinyl chloride, metallurgic ores, and mustard gas.

Marijuana. Marijuana is similar to tobacco smoke in that it contains many of the same organic and inorganic compounds that are carcinogens, cocarcinogens, or tumor promoters. Marijuana produces inflammation, edema, and cell injury in the tracheobronchial mucosa of smokers and contributes to oxidative stress, which is a precursor for DNA mutations.[483] However, cannabinoids modulate and minimize free radical production and inhibit tumor angiogenesis. In addition, cannabinoid receptors are not found in the lung epithelial cells.[348] Cannabinoids have been shown to inhibit certain breast, lung, and brain cancers,[298] although other studies have shown an increase in head, neck, and lung cancers.[219]

The risk of marijuana smoking is difficult to ascertain as people often smoke both tobacco and marijuana. It is known that cannabis causes large airway inflammation, increased mucous production, increased airway resistance, and lung hyperinflation.[315] For those with low or occasional use of marijuana, early studies show little effect on FEV_1. However, decrements are seen in flow rates with long-term and high-volume usage.[412] The relationship between smoking marijuana and lung cancer is still controversial at the time of this writing.[248,315]

Environmental Tobacco Smoke. In 1992, the EPA declared secondhand smoke or ETS to be a group A human carcinogen. ETS increases the relative risk for lung cancer about 1.5-fold and there are 3000 lung cancer deaths each year from ETS.[95] This exposure increases the risk for the children and partners of smokers and becomes an occupational hazard in individuals working in bars, restaurants, or other places that are not smoke-free. See previous section on "Environmental Tobacco Smoke."

Occupational Exposure. Studies on whether occupational factors increase the risk of cancer development in the nonsmoker are limited in number but confirm that certain occupational exposures are associated with an increased risk for lung cancer among both male and female nonsmokers.[413] The inhalation of asbestos fibers is associated with higher cancer risks for both smokers and nonsmokers, although the rate is considerably higher for smokers.

The rate of lung cancer in people who live in urban areas is 2.3 times greater than that of those living in rural areas, possibly implicating air pollution as a risk factor in lung cancer. The exact role of air pollution is still unknown, but carcinogens with known genotoxicity continue to be released into outdoor air from industrial sources, power plants, and motor vehicles; epidemiologic research provides evidence for an association between air pollution and lung cancer.[115,511]

Indoor exposure to radon, which is a colorless, odorless gas that is a product of uranium and radium produced from the decomposition of rocks and soil, is a known carcinogen and the second leading cause of lung cancer. Concentrations vary geographically (more in the northern United States), and radon gas levels are highest in basements, nearest the soil.[182] Other sources of radon exposure include radioactive waste and underground mines; exposure to tobacco smoke multiplies the risk of concurrent exposure to radon.

Other occupational or environmental risk factors associated with lung cancer include diesel exhaust, coal tar fumes, untreated mineral oils, mustard gas, vinyl chloride, benzopyrenes, silica, formaldehyde, copper, chromium, cadmium, arsenic, alkylating compounds, sulfur dioxide, and ionizing radiation.

Previous Lung Disease. The presence of other lung diseases, such as pulmonary fibrosis, scleroderma, and sarcoidosis, may increase the risk of developing lung cancer. COPD, or fibrosis of the lungs, inhibits the clearance of carcinogens from the lungs, thereby increasing the risk of alteration of DNA with resultant malignant cell growth.

Nutrition. Other risk factors may include low consumption of fruits and vegetables,[206] reduced physical activity, increased dietary fat (especially diets high in saturated or animal fat and cholesterol), and high alcohol intake. There is limited evidence that some foods are protective (e.g., selenium, nonstarchy vegetables, foods containing quercetin).[544]

Studies show no beneficial effect of vitamin E (α-tocopherol), beta-carotene, and retinol, and several studies have determined that beta-carotene supplementation in smokers increases the risk for lung cancer. The mechanism for this carcinogenic action remains unknown.[435]

Genetic Susceptibility. Several published studies suggest that lung cancer can aggregate in some families, and it has been hypothesized that the defect in the body's ability to defend against the carcinogens in tobacco smoke may be inherited.[542] Although some of the familial risk could be from ETS exposure, a shared genetic risk is strongly suggested. Regardless, the independent effect on lung cancer risk is strongly amplified by cigarette smoking.[84,119]

Pathogenesis

As mentioned, there is a clear relationship between cigarette smoking and the development of SCLC. The effects of smoking include structural, functional, malignant, and toxic changes. DNA-mutating agents in cigarettes produce alterations in both oncogenes and tumor-suppressor genes, as well as genes that detoxify and assist with DNA repair. Normal polymorphism (variations in genes) also plays a role in the development of or resistance to cancer. Lung cancer in nonsmokers is on the rise, accounting for 10% to 25% of lung malignancies.[528]

The understanding of the molecular pathology of lung cancer is advancing rapidly, with several specific genes and chromosomal regions having been identified. Lung cancer appears to require many mutations in both dominant and recessive oncogenes before they become invasive. Several genetic and epigenetic changes are common to all lung cancer histologic types, whereas others appear to be tumor-type specific. The sequence of changes remains unknown.[293] There appears to be an interaction between estrogen receptors and epidermal growth factor in the lung that plays a role in women's susceptibility to lung cancer.[156]

There are two main genetic lesions in NSCLC that are being explored; mutations in the epidermal growth factor receptor (EGFR) and the KRAS genes.[528] Overexpression of EGFR can be found in 62% of people with NSCLC and contributes to angiogenesis, metastasis, and inhibition of apoptosis.[528] Mutations in the RAS genes can be found in 10% to 50% of NSCLC and leads to rapid cellular proliferation.[528]

All lung cancers are thought to arise from a common bronchial precursor cell, with differentiation then proceeding along various histologic pathways from poorly differentiated small cell cancer to the more intermediate undifferentiated large cell tumors, to the more differentiated adenocarcinomas and squamous cell tumors. Perhaps the histologic changes (thickening of bronchial epithelium, damage to and loss of protective cilia, mucous gland hypertrophy and hypersecretion of mucus, and alveolar cell rupture) that occur more frequently in long-term smokers than nonsmokers predispose the lungs to changes. This results in a multistep process involving the development of hyperplasia, metaplasia, dysplasia, carcinoma in situ, invasive carcinoma, and metastatic carcinoma. As the details of the carcinogenic process are unraveled, one goal is to identify intermediate (preneoplastic) markers of exposure and inherent predisposition that will help assess the risk of lung cancer and allow for early detection.

Small Cell Lung Cancer. When the cells become so dense that there is almost no cytoplasm present and the cells are compressed into an ovoid mass, the tumor is called small cell carcinoma or oat cell carcinoma. SCLC develops most often in the bronchial submucosa, the layer of tissue beneath the epithelium, and tends to be located centrally, most often near the hilum of the lung. These tumors can produce hormones that stimulate their own growth and the rapid growth of neighboring cells causing bronchial obstruction and pneumonia with early intralymphatic invasion. Lymphatic and distant metastases are usually present at the time of diagnosis.

Non–Small Cell Lung Cancer. Squamous cell carcinomas arise in the central portion of the lung near the hilum, projecting into the major or segmental bronchi. Although these tumors tend to grow rapidly, they often remain located within the thoracic cavity, making curative treatment more likely compared with other NSCLC types. These tumors may be difficult to differentiate from TB or an abscess because they often undergo central cavitation (formation of a cavity or hollow space).

Clinical Manifestations

Symptoms of early stage localized lung cancer do not differ much from pulmonary symptoms associated with chronic smoking (e.g., cough, dyspnea, and sputum production), so the person does not seek medical attention. Often times, lung cancer may be an incidental finding on a routine chest x-ray. Symptoms may depend on the location within the pulmonary system, whether centrally located, peripheral, or in the apices of the lungs. Systemic symptoms, such as anorexia, fatigue, weakness, and weight loss, are common, especially with advanced disease (metastases) and are associated with a poor prognosis.[49]

Pain associated with bone metastasis is common; other symptoms resulting from metastases depend on the site of involvement (e.g., hepatomegaly and jaundice with liver metastasis and seizures, headaches, confusion, or focal neurologic signs with brain metastasis).

Other signs and symptoms of disease include recurring bronchitis or pneumonia; productive cough with hemoptysis; wheezing; poorly defined persistent chest pain; difficulty swallowing or hoarseness; orthopnea; nerve involvement (phrenic, laryngeal, brachial plexus, or sympathetic ganglion); and vascular (superior vena cava), cardiac, and esophageal compression as a result of local tumor invasion.[49,183,415]

Small Cell Lung Cancer. Signs and symptoms of SCLC depend on the size and location of the tumor and the presence and extent of metastases. Because SCLCs most commonly arise in the central endobronchial location in people who are almost exclusively long-term smokers, typical symptoms are a result of obstructed airflow and consist of persistent, new, or changing cough, dyspnea, stridor, wheezing, hemoptysis, and chest pain.[74]

Intercostal retractions on inspiration and bulging intercostal spaces on expiration indicate obstruction. As obstruction increases, bronchopulmonary infection (obstructive pneumonitis) often occurs distal to the obstruction. Centrally located tumors cause chest pain with perivascular nerve or peribronchial involvement that can refer pain to the shoulder, scapula, upper back, or arm.

SCLC is (more often than NSCLC) associated with several paraneoplastic syndromes, including ectopic hormone production such as with Cushings syndrome (adrenocorticotropic hormone), production of hormones by tumors of nonendocrine origin, or production of an inappropriate hormone (antidiuretic hormone) by an endocrine gland. Neuroendocrine cells containing neurosecretory granules exist throughout the tracheobronchial tree. This phenomenon is important because resulting signs and symptoms may be the first manifestation of underlying cancer. See "Special Implications for the Therapist 15-22: Lung Cancer" below; see also "Paraneoplastic Syndromes" in Chapter 9.

Non–Small Cell Lung Cancer. The less common peripheral pulmonary tumors (large cell) often do not produce signs or symptoms until disease progression produces localized, sharp, and severe pleural pain increased on inspiration, limiting lung expansion; cough and dyspnea are present. Pleural effusion may develop and limit lung expansion even more.

Tumors in the apex of the lung, called *Pancoast tumors*, occur both in squamous cell and adenocarcinomatous cancers. Symptoms do not occur until the tumors invade the brachial plexus (see "Special Implications for the Therapist 15-22: Lung Cancer" below). Destruction of the first and second ribs can occur. Paralysis, elevation of the hemidiaphragm, and dyspnea secondary to phrenic nerve involvement can also occur.

Other manifestations may include digital clubbing, skin changes, joint swelling associated with hypertrophic pulmonary osteoarthropathy (see discussion of this condition in "Cystic Fibrosis" above), decreased or absent breath sounds on auscultation, or pleural rub (inflammatory response to invading tumor).

Metastasis

The rich supply of blood vessels and lymphatics in the lungs enables the disease to metastasize rapidly. Lung cancers spread by direct extension, lymphatic invasion, and through the vasculature. Tumors spread by direct invasion in the bronchus of origin; others may invade the bronchial wall and circle and obstruct the airway. Intrapulmonary spread may lead to compression of lung structures other than airways such as blood or lymph vessels, alveoli, and nerves.

Direct extension through the pleura can result in spread over the surface of the lung, chest wall, or diaphragm. Carcinomas of the lung of all types metastasize most frequently to the regional lymph nodes, particularly the hilar and mediastinal nodes. Supraclavicular, cervical, and abdominal channels may also be invaded. Tumors originating in the lower lobes tend to spread through the lymph channels.

Lung cancer generally has a widespread pattern of hematogenous metastases. This is caused by the invasion of the pulmonary vascular system. After tumor cells enter the pulmonary venous system, they can be carried through the heart and disseminated systemically. Tumor emboli can become lodged in areas of organ systems where vessels become too narrow for their passage or where blood flow is reduced.

The most frequent site of extranodal metastases is the adrenal gland. Lung cancer can also metastasize to the brain, bone, and liver before presenting symptomatically. Brain metastases constitute nearly one-third of all observed recurrences in people with resected NSCLC of the adenocarcinoma type. Metastases to the brain usually result in CNS symptoms of confusion, gait disturbances, headaches, or personality changes.

Tumor spread intrathoracically to the mediastinum and beyond can produce superior vena cava (SVC) syndrome, with swelling of the face, neck, and arms, and neck and thoracic vein distention more common in the early morning or after being recumbent for several hours. SVC syndrome is usually a sign of advanced disease. If left untreated, SVC syndrome results in cerebral edema and possible death. Increased intracranial pressure, headaches, dizziness, visual disturbances, and alteration in mental status are signs of progressive compression. Cardiac metastasis can occur and result in arrhythmias, congestive heart failure, and pericardial tamponade.

As a form of secondary malignancy, the lungs are the most frequent site of metastases from other types of cancer. Any tumor cell dislodged from a primary neoplasm can find its way into the circulation or lymphatics, which are filtered by the lungs. Carcinomas of the kidney, breast, pancreas, colon, and uterus are especially likely to metastasize to the lungs.

MEDICAL MANAGEMENT

PREVENTION. Prevention is the key to reducing the need for treatment of lung cancer. Targeted state and federal antitobacco programs have contributed to significant drops in cigarette consumption.

Healthy People 2020 has set a goal of reducing the lung cancer mortality rate from 50.6 per 100,000 population (1998 figure) to 45.4 per 100,000 population, representing a 10% improvement. *Healthy People 2020* has outlined a systematic approach to health improvement that includes methods for lung cancer prevention through prevention of tobacco use and tobacco addiction in all age, ethnic, and socioeconomic groups. *Healthy People 2020* is available online at http://www.health.gov/healthypeople/.

Another strategy for lung cancer prevention is chemoprevention. Chemoprevention involves the administration of drugs, nutraceuticals or nutritional supplements in those with early stages of cancer aimed at absorbing free oxygen radicals and blocking or reversing carcinogenesis. Reducing exposures to workplace toxins, such as asbestos, arsenic, chromium, nickel, radon, and tar, is also another risk-reduction strategy.[369]

Other strategies for lung cancer prevention include eliminating arsenic in drinking water (the need to do so applies to smokers only), adopting a diet high in fruits and vegetables, foods high in carotenoids, and reduction of ETS.

DIAGNOSIS. Many lung cancers are detected on routine chest film in clients presenting for unrelated medical conditions without pulmonary symptoms, although 90% of the people with lung cancer are symptomatic at diagnosis. Many people mistake the signs of lung cancer with other common issues such as a cold, flu, or aging. Unfortunately, chest radiographs are not sensitive enough to show tumors when they are small and operable and routine screening is not supported by evidence.

A chest scan called low-dose spiral or helical CT detects tumors too small to be seen on radiographs. There are some concerns with low-dose spiral CT such as cost, false-positive findings, unnecessary biopsies of small benign tumors, and a small risk of death from procedures that result from a (+) finding.

The National Lung Screening Trial attempted to determine the benefits of spiral CT one time per year for 3 years as compared to standard radiograph for screening purposes.[370] This trial did indicate that there may be a benefit for those at high risk for NSCLC, such as those with a 30 pack-year history who are current smokers or who have quit in the past 15 years.[263] A 20% reduction in deaths from lung cancer among current and former heavy smokers screened with this type of CT (compared with chest radiograph) was reported.[34] For most people, screening to detect early lung cancer is not recommended.[16]

Despite the above limitations, a chest radiograph is usually the first diagnostic tool employed. If there is a high suspicion before the radiograph or as a result of the radiograph, physicians may order a CT scan which can visualize smaller tumors. If there is suspicion of metastasis to the spinal cord, an MRI may be indicated. Physicians may also utilize a positron emission tomography (PET) scan to detect metastatic spread. In a PET scan, a radioactive sugar substance (fluorodeoxyglucose) is injected. Cancer cells are quite metabolically active and therefore readily take up fluorodeoxyglucose, which can then be visualized in a PET scanner.

Once a tumor is found, a biopsy via bronchoscopy or fine-needle aspiration may be used to capture cells for histology. Efforts are underway to find a simple blood test to detect lung cancer and reduce the need for invasive biopsies, unnecessary surgery, and repeated imaging tests.[390,503]

Other routine procedures include evaluation of serum chemistry values to look for electrolyte abnormalities (see Chapter 5), especially those associated with paraneoplastic syndrome (see Chapter 9), evaluation of renal and hepatic function, hematologic profiles, and ECG analysis.

STAGING. The seventh edition of the American Joint Committee on Cancer's *Cancer Staging Manual*, put forth new staging guidelines in 2010. Staging of lung cancer uses the TNM or tumor, nodes, metastasis system (see explanation in Chapter 9). In the new classification, tumor size has been adjusted and there is a system to indicate additional nodules in the same lobe or in ipsilateral lobes. Metastatic disease has been divided into local metastasis and extrathoracic metastasis.[423] Tumors confined to the lung without any metastases, regional or distant, are classified as stage I, and tumors associated with only hilar or peribronchial lymph node involvement (N1) are classified as stage II. Locally advanced tumors with mediastinal or cervical lymph node metastases and those with extension to the chest wall, mediastinum, diaphragm, or carina are classified as stage III tumors. Finally, tumors presenting with distant metastases (M1), or have malignant pleural or pericardial effusions are classified as stage IV.

SCLC is usually not considered a surgical disease requiring staging but rather is designated as limited or extensive disease. Limited disease is defined by involvement of one lung, the mediastinum, and either or both ipsilateral and contralateral supraclavicular lymph nodes (i.e., disease that can be encompassed in a single radiation therapy port). Spread beyond the lung, mediastinum, and supraclavicular lymph nodes is considered extensive disease.

TREATMENT. Awareness of the influence of growth factors, oncogenes, and tumor suppressor genes, as well as signal transduction and angiogenesis pathways on the natural history of cancer cells, has led to attempts to develop new molecular-based strategies directed at interrupting tumor cell growth. Treatments using monoclonal antibodies, inhibitors, antiangiogenic substances, and gene transfer and alteration are still under investigation.[77]

In the meantime, current treatment with new agents used in combination, as well as when combined with radiation and hormones, has led to an improved response rate in the treatment of some lung cancers.[76] Photodynamic therapy is used successfully with tumors in the airways. Photochemical sensitization of the tumor precedes laser therapy that causes necrosis of the cancer.[355] Chemotherapy approaches are numerous and address different targets. Newer agents that inhibit EGFRs are showing promise alone and in combination with other drugs.[492]

Small Cell Lung Cancer. Surgical resection in the treatment of SCLC is not usually considered. For those with early stage SCLC who receive combination chemotherapy, surgery may be considered and results in high response rates (65%-85%).[286] For clients with more advanced disease, surgery causes unnecessary risk and stress, with no valid benefits. Laser therapy is a surgical treatment used when the tumor mass is causing nonresectable bronchial obstructions and when accessible by bronchoscope.

SCLC is quite sensitive to radiation therapy, which, in conjunction with chemotherapy, is now routinely administered to those with limited disease.[57] Individuals with extensive disease usually receive combination chemotherapy initially. Other treatment options depend on the clinical manifestations and client needs (e.g., radiation therapy may be administered to the brain, bone, spine, or other sites of metastasis). In the future, tumor growth may be halted by replacement or substitution of mutated tumor suppressor gene functions or biochemical modulation of oncogene products. New forms of immunotherapy may also be targeted specifically toward mutant oncogenes in cancer cells.

Non–Small Cell Lung Cancer. The standard treatment for stages I and II lung cancer includes surgical resection (lobectomy, segmentectomy, pneumonectomy). Anyone with positive surgical margins and mediastinal lymph node disease may also get radiation therapy and chemotherapy. Those who are poor surgical candidates receive radiotherapy or stereotactic body radiotherapy or radiofrequency ablation.[423]

For stage III NSCLC, surgery may be offered. Many tumors at this stage are unresectable or have metastasized, necessitating a combined chemoradiation approach.[423] The present regimens include platinum based chemotherapies that have a significant side-effect profile, including neuropathy. Multimodal treatments can cure up to 20% of individuals with locally advanced lung cancer.[423] Approach to stage IV disease is palliative and depends on location and extent of disease and clinical manifestations. For example, clients who develop spinal cord compromise secondary to metastatic disease can be palliated effectively with short-course external-beam radiotherapy.

SVC obstruction can also be ameliorated by chemotherapy and radiotherapy as well as the placement of stents.[433] Short-term radiotherapy can also reduce some lung symptoms.[325] Chemotherapy has also been useful in improving palliation and increasing survival in stage IV disease.[464]

As the understanding of lung cancer improves, so do the interventions. Targeted therapies are being evaluated to address the abnormal pathways/mutations discussed earlier such as upregulation of EGFR and KRAS.

PROGNOSIS. The curability of lung cancer remains poor because by the time lung cancer is detected, invasion and metastasis have already occurred in many people. Prognosis is considerably better in cases of NSCLC than in cases of SCLC. The overall prognosis is influenced by the stage of the disease at presentation, the cell type, the treatment that can be given, and the status of the client at the time of diagnosis (e.g., people who are ambulatory respond to treatment better than those who are confined to bed more than 50% of the time). Prognosis is poor in general, but it is considerably better in cases of NSCLC than in cases of SCLC.

Other factors associated with poor prognosis include weight loss of more than 10% of body weight in 6 months, generalized weakness, male gender, age older than 70 years, prior chemotherapy, elevated serum lactic dehydrogenase levels, low serum sodium, and elevated alkaline phosphatase levels (see Tables 40-14 and 40-15).

Mortality rates for men have declined approximately 2% from 1998 to 2007, but remained the same for women during the same time period.[299] Currently, with treatment, only 5% of people with lung cancer survive beyond 5 years after diagnosis. However, if caught early, the 5-year survival rate is approximately 50% for NSCLC.[528] The 5-year survival rate for stage II disease is approximately 30%, 5% to 14% for stage III, and approximately 1% for stage IV NSCLC.[17]

For SCLC, the 5-year survival rate for stage I is approximately 31%, dropping to 2% in stage IV. Survival without treatment is rarely possible, and most untreated persons die within 1 year of diagnosis, with a median survival of less than 6 months. Curative treatment requires effective control of the primary tumor before metastasis occurs. Chemotherapy is usually combined with surgery or irradiation for more advanced tumors.

Overall 5-year survival rate among older blacks with NSCLC is significantly lower compared with whites, largely explained by lower rates of surgical treatment.[35] Although women appear to be more susceptible to lung cancer, they have higher survival rates, suggesting the potential role of hormones. Women with NSCLC are 60% more likely to die of the disease if they take combined hormone-replacement therapy than if they do not.[107]

SPECIAL IMPLICATIONS FOR THE THERAPIST 15-22

Lung Cancer

The effective management of short- and long-term side effects from lung cancer and its treatment is essential for rehabilitation. The American College of Chest Physicians has developed recommendations for improving quality of life in end-of-life care.[214] Increasing the therapist's knowledge of psychosocial–spiritual effects in these cases assists the therapist in planning appropriate intervention programs and promoting the optimal use of resources. If clients and their families can overcome treatment barriers, they will be more motivated toward achieving increased and sustained independence and quality of life.

The therapist can be very helpful in teaching clients with lung cancer nonpharmacologic means of pain relief and energy conservation techniques while providing an optimal activity program in accordance with the degree of pulmonary involvement. Effective breathing and coughing techniques should be taught and reinforced. There is some evidence to support noninvasive treatment to improve quality of life for people with cancer. For example, studies of preoperative pulmonary rehabilitation for lung cancer show a decrease in hospitalization complications.[54]

Metastasis

Metastatic spread of pulmonary tumors to the long bones and to the vertebral column, especially the thoracic vertebrae, is common, occurring in as many as 50% of all cases. Local metastases by direct extension may involve the chest wall and may even erode the first and second ribs and associated vertebrae, causing bone pain and paravertebral pain associated with involvement of sympathetic nerve ganglia. Subsequently, chest, shoulder, arm, or back pain can be the presenting symptom but usually with accompanying pulmonary symptoms.

The client may not associate the musculoskeletal symptoms with the pulmonary symptoms, so the therapist must always remember to screen for medical disease. Cases of individuals with lung cancer and shoulder pain for which no local cause could be found have been reported, and in each case, radiotherapy to the ipsilateral mediastinum eliminated symptoms. Pain referred from intrathoracic involvement of the phrenic nerve was the suspected underlying pain generator.[291] Any time a mechanical cause is not found or the client fails to progress or improve in therapy, return to the physician is recommended for further diagnostic evaluation.

Spinal cord compression from extradural metastases of lung cancer usually occurs from direct extension of vertebral metastases or through venous spread. Tumors often invade the vertebral body first, followed by the pedicles, often in the thoracic vertebra.[326] Back pain is often the first sign and may occur as progressive back pain 6 months before the diagnosis is made. The pain may be constant and aggravated by Valsalva maneuver, sneezing or coughing, movement, and lying down, and diminished by sitting up. Weakness, sensory loss, and a positive Babinski reflex may be observed.

Radiation is usually the treatment of choice for epidural metastases from lung cancer. Neurosurgical intervention may be indicated if the area of compression has been previously irradiated to maximal tolerance. Surgical decompression may also be indicated if neurologic deterioration occurs during the initiation of radiation therapy. The treatment field extends two vertebral bodies above and below the level of blockage. Corticosteroids are prescribed to reduce swelling and inflammation around the cord.[192]

Brain metastases also occur in people with lung cancer. Presenting symptoms may be headache, seizures, balance dysfunction, or focal deficits. Treatment is first aimed at reducing swelling and preventing seizures, followed by surgery and/or radiation therapy.[192]

Apical (Pancoast) tumors do not usually cause symptoms while confined to the pulmonary parenchyma, but once they extend into the surrounding structures, the brachial plexus (C8 to T2) may become involved, presenting as a form of thoracic outlet syndrome. This nerve involvement produces sharp pleuritic pain in the axilla, shoulder (radiating in an ulnar nerve distribution down the arm), and subscapular area of the affected side, with atrophy and weakness of the upper extremity muscles and hand intrinsics. Invasion of the cervical sympathetic plexus may cause *Horner syndrome* with unilateral miosis, ptosis, and absence of sweating on the affected side of the face and neck.

Treatment for these two conditions may involve chemoradiation followed by surgical resection. The brachial plexus can withstand some radiation; however radiation is difficult to deliver to posterior tumors. Individuals with distant metastasis, positive mediastinal nodes, and brachial plexus involvement above T1 are not surgical candidates.[403] Local anesthetics administered through an axillary catheter placed in the brachial plexus for intractable neuropathic pain have also been reported; this approach is reversible and may be preferable to destructive procedures, such as cordotomy.[516] Therapy intervention for the thoracic outlet syndrome is an important part of the palliative treatment for this condition (see also "Thoracic Outlet Syndrome" in Chapter 39).

Trigger points of the serratus anterior muscle also mimic the distribution of pain caused by C8 nerve root compression and must be ruled out by palpation, lack of neurologic deficits, and possible elimination with appropriate trigger point therapy. Pancoast tumors may also masquerade as subacromial bursitis.

Paraneoplastic Syndrome

Paraneoplastic syndromes (remote effects of a malignancy; see discussion in Chapter 9) occur in 10% to 20% of lung cancer clients, more commonly in SCLC, and may have an autoimmune origin. This syndrome may also result from the secretion of hormones by the tumor acting on target organs producing a variety of symptoms, most commonly fluctuating weakness, fatigue, and neuropathy.[192] Hypercalcemia, digital clubbing, osteoarthropathies, or rheumatologic disorders, such as polymyositis, lupus, and dermatomyositis, may also be present.

Occasionally, symptoms of paraneoplastic syndrome occur before detection of the primary lung tumor or as the first sign of recurrence presenting as a neuromusculoskeletal condition. Treatment may involve corticosteroids, immunoglobulin therapy, and treatment for the primary malignancy.

DISORDERS OF THE PULMONARY VASCULATURE

Pulmonary Embolism and Infarction

James W. Farris, PT, PhD, and John Heick, PT, DPT

Definition and Incidence

Pulmonary embolism (PE) is the lodging of a blood clot in a pulmonary artery with subsequent obstruction of blood supply to the lung parenchyma. Although a blood clot is the most common cause of occlusion, air, fat, bone marrow (e.g., fracture), foreign intravenous material, vegetations on heart valves that develop with endocarditis, amniotic fluid, and tumor cells (tumor emboli) can also embolize and occlude the pulmonary vessels.

PE is common, and in the United States from 1992–2006, the incidence of PE in hospitalized patients increased 2.5 times, from 33 per 100,000 population to 83 per 100,000 population.[470] It is the most common cause of sudden death in the hospitalized population.

Etiologic and Risk Factors

The most common cause of PE is deep vein thrombosis (DVT) originating in the proximal deep venous system primarily of the lower extremity, but 20% come from the upper extremity (see further discussion in DVT section of Chapter 12). PE encompasses embolism from many sources, including air, bone marrow, arthroplasty cement, amniotic fluid, tumor, and sepsis. Before the introduction of routine prophylaxis with heparin (now low-molecular-weight heparin [LMWH]) or warfarin sodium (Coumadin), the incidence of DVT after hip fracture, total hip replacement, or other surgeries involving the abdomen, pelvis, prostate, hip, or knee was extremely high.

Three major physiologic risk factors linked with PE are (1) blood stasis (e.g., immobilization caused by prolonged trips including air travel or spinal cord injury; bed rest, such as with burn cases, pneumonia, or obstetric and gynecologic clients; fracture care with casting or pinning; and older or obese populations); (2) endothelial injury (local trauma) secondary to surgical procedures (as late as 1 month postoperatively), trauma, or fractures of the legs or pelvis; and (3) hypercoagulable states (e.g., oral contraceptive use, cancer, and hereditary thrombotic disorders).

Major clinical risk factors for PE (DVT) include immobility; abdominal/pelvic surgery; hip/knee replacement; late pregnancy; cesarean section; lower-limb fractures; malignancy of pelvis or abdomen; and previous PE. Minor risk factors include congenital heart disease; congestive heart failure; hypertension; superficial venous thrombosis; indwelling catheter; COPD; oral contraceptives; hormone replacement therapy; neurologic disability; long distance travel; obesity; and smoking.[308]

Pathogenesis

In DVT, clots form in the popliteal or iliofemoral arteries (50%) and deep calf veins (5%) or subclavian vein (up to 20%). Part or all of the clot may embolize, traveling through the venous system, the right side of the heart, and into the lungs. Each embolus is a mass of fresh or organizing thrombus comprised of alternating bands of red cells, fibrin strands, and leukocytes with a rim of fibroblasts at the periphery. Any level of the pulmonary artery, from the main trunk to the distal branches, is a site for emboli to lodge. This causes an area of blockage and ischemic necrosis to the area perfused by that vessel.

PE ranges from peripheral and clinically insignificant to massive embolism and sudden death. PE may lead to $\dot{V}/\dot{Q}$ mismatch, which leads to hypoxia. PE and DVT should be considered part of the same pathologic process, and in fact, studies showed that a large percentage of people with DVT but no symptoms of PE also had evidence of PE on lung scanning. Conversely, people with PE often have abnormalities on ultrasonographic studies of leg veins.[204]

In addition to the loss of capillary beds, pulmonary emboli cause vasoconstriction as a result of vasoactive mediators released by activated platelets, increased pulmonary vascular resistance, pulmonary hypertension, and right ventricular failure (in severe cases).

Clinical Manifestations

Clients may be asymptomatic in the presence of small thromboemboli or sustain cardiac arrest, depending on the size and location of the embolus and the individual's preexisting cardiopulmonary status. Common symptoms in people with PE include dyspnea (84%) or deterioration of existing dyspnea, pleuritic chest pain (74%), apprehension (59%), and cough (53%). Common signs include tachypnea greater than 16 breaths/min (92%), rales (58%), accentuated S2 gallop (53%), tachycardia (44%), and fever (43%).

Other signs and symptoms may include hemoptysis, diaphoresis, S3 or S4 gallop, lower-extremity edema, cardiac murmur, and cyanosis.[308] Many of the symptoms and signs detected in people with acute PE are also common among individuals without PE, emphasizing the need for additional evaluation.

Individuals undergoing primary total hip arthroplasty or total knee arthroplasty have exhibited rates of symptomatic PE as high as 20% and 8%, respectively, when no prophylaxis has been administered.[456]

MEDICAL MANAGEMENT

DIAGNOSIS. PE is difficult to diagnose because the signs and symptoms are nonspecific. Diagnosing PE clinically is problematic because its symptoms overlap with those of other conditions and because there are numerous causes of postoperative hypoxia (e.g., hypoventilation, narcotic effects, fluid overload, and postoperative atelectasis).[32]

Clinical screen and need for further testing are conducted using Wells criteria and nonimaging laboratory tests (especially D-dimer, which is a by-product of fibrin crosslinks). Huisman and Klok (2013) recommend the Wells test and the Revised Geneva score and they provide revised algorithms. Negative clinical assessment and D-dimer test may limit the need for further testing. Arterial blood gases are not helpful in the physician's differential diagnosis.

Using combinations of additional tests to rule out or rule in PE to make the diagnosis is optimal. $\dot{V}/\dot{Q}$ scans can rule out PE if it is normal in the presence of normal x-ray and with no other cardiopulmonary disease.[308]

Alveolar dead space evaluation in combination with D-dimer created a false-negative response of less than 1%. Echocardiogram can detect PE in 80% of cases. Conventional angiogram has potential for serious side effects and has poor reliability. Compression ultrasonography is used for the detection of DVT, but a negative result should not rule out DVT. Huisman & Klok (2013) report that

multi-row computed tomographic pulmonary angiography (CTPA) are the imaging tests of choice in patients with clinically suspected acute PE; these diagnostic tests are readily available in most hospitals.[258]

PREVENTION AND TREATMENT. The management of DVT and PE has changed dramatically in the last few years. Given the mortality of PE and the difficulties involved in its clinical diagnosis, prevention of DVT and PE is crucial. Primary prevention of DVT through the prophylactic use of anticoagulants is important for persons undergoing total hip replacement, major knee surgery, abdominal or pelvic surgery, prostate surgery, and neurosurgery. In fact, anyone hospitalized should be evaluated for risk of PE and placed on prophylaxis as appropriate.

LMWH (anticoagulant now replacing unfractionated heparin) is the most common agent for prophylaxis because it prolongs the clotting time and allows the body time to resolve the existing clot, thereby preventing further development of the thrombus; it does not reduce the immediate embolic risk or enhance clot lysis. LMWHs have fewer major bleeding complications and do not require laboratory monitoring of coagulation tests to adjust medications.

The FDA has approved outpatient treatment of DVT with the LMWH enoxaparin as a bridge to warfarin. Warfarin (Coumadin), an oral anticoagulant, is used simultaneously with heparin or during the transition from intravenous to oral anticoagulant with a targeted activated partial thromboplastin time of 1.5 to 2.5 times the baseline value and an international normalized ratio of 2 to 3 (see discussion in Chapter 40).

Prophylaxis and treatment with these medications for PE and DVT are different (see further discussion in "Thrombophlebitis" in Chapter 12). The direct thrombin inhibitors fondaparinux, idraparinux, and ximelagatran, are at least as effective as LMWH and well tolerated.[362]

Thrombolytic therapy (a controversial, expensive treatment used with massive embolism) to lyse pulmonary thromboemboli in situ is accomplished through the use of thrombolytic agents, such as streptokinase, urokinase, recombinant tissue plasminogen activator, and newer agents, such as reteplase, saruplase, and recombinant staphylokinase, that enhance fibrinolysis by activating plasminogen, generating plasmin.

Plasmin directly lyses thrombi both in the pulmonary artery and in the venous circulation and has a secondary anticoagulant effect. Successfully utilized, PE thrombolysis reverses right-sided heart failure rapidly and safely. There is limited evidence that thrombolytics are better than heparin for PE,[153] but moderate evidence that they are effective in reducing postthrombotic syndrome and maintaining vessel patency.[526]

Implantation of Filter in Inferior Vena Cava.
Pat Hoover, PT

Surgical implantation of a filter in the inferior vena cava (IVC) may be used to prevent PE. The indication to use an IVC filter should be carefully evaluated in each individual case, based on a clear understanding of the objectives of filter insertion and consideration of alternatives. IVC filters are often inserted for unproven and inappropriate reasons.[189]

The generally accepted indication for IVC filter insertion is the presence of a recently diagnosed proximal DVT plus an absolute contraindication to therapeutic anticoagulation. Contraindications to therapeutic anticoagulation include:

- Current or recent active major bleeding that cannot be treated acutely.
- Frank intracranial bleeding in the past 5 days.
- Need for a major surgical procedure in the next 2 weeks.
- Severe, prolonged thrombocytopenia.[189]

As a general rule, the use of an IVC filter does not change the need for or duration of anticoagulation. Because most (or all) individuals who have IVC filters inserted have a proximal DVT, therapeutic anticoagulation should be instituted as soon as it is considered safe to do so (usually within a few days after insertion). Although IVC filters may reduce the risk of PE in individuals with DVT, they do not prevent extension of DVT, including extension through the filter. The duration of anticoagulation is the same as for individuals with DVT but without a filter.[189]

To better achieve the desired performance goals of IVC filters, it is crucially important to adhere to established criteria in selecting candidates for filter insertion. Selection criteria is clearer for the use of permanent filters as opposed to retrievable ones. A variety of both permanent and retrievable filters are available in the interventionists' armamentarium.[392] It would be important for the physician to be familiar with the particular characteristics of each device and have knowledge of comparative advantages and disadvantages.

The filter itself is a potential focus of thrombosis. IVC filters are viewed as a temporizing measure for preventing life-threatening PE.

As indicated in the case of proximal DVT, concomitant anticoagulation after filter placement is desirable when there are no contraindications, so as to prevent early IVC filter thrombosis. In the case of filter thrombosis, PE can occur either through collateral pathways or by means of propagation of caval clots through the filter. *Caval clot* is the term used to refer to an inferior vena cava filter occluded by a thrombosis.

The diagnosis of IVC filter thrombosis is based on radiologic investigations. IVC thrombosis appears to be one of the more frequent and major complications of filter placement.[488]

Inferior vena cava syndrome (IVCS) is a result of obstruction of the IVC. It can be caused by invasion or compression by a pathologic process (enlarged aorta [abdominal aortic aneurysm], the gravid uterus [aortocaval compression syndrome], and abdominal malignancies such as colorectal cancer) or by thrombosis in the vein itself. Thrombosis at the insertion site is a common complication for filter placement.[478]

IVCS presents with a wide variety of signs and symptoms, making a clinical diagnosis difficult. Primary symptoms may include edema of the lower extremities and tachycardia. Other symptoms of IVC obstruction include progressive ascites and scrotal edema.[466]

Occlusion of the IVC is considered life-threatening. Because the IVC is not centrally located, there are some asymmetries in drainage patterns. The gonadal veins and suprarenal veins drain into the IVC on the right side, but into the renal vein on the left side, which, in turn, drains into the IVC.

In one study, placement of IVC filter in individuals with advanced cancer denoted a direct correlation between the onset of kidney failure or hydronephrosis with placement of IVC filter. The elevated pressure from obstruction may ultimately damage the kidney and can result in loss of its function.[408] It is noted that blood return with an "absent" IVC is inadequate, despite adequate collaterals, resulting in chronic venous hypertension in the lower extremities and causing venous stasis that precipitates thrombosis. "Absent" refers to a blocked or obstructed IVC (in this case caused by thrombosis under the filter, i.e., caval clot).

Essentially, the IVCS (blockage under the IVC filter) causes fluid to leak into surrounding tissue. This hypovolemia in the central circulatory system will lead to hypotension (low blood pressure), which presents significant problems for individuals with cardiac problems especially anyone with congestive heart failure.

Inferior Vena Caval Thrombosis and Treatment. Both surgical and medical options are available to treat IVC thrombosis depending on the underlying pathophysiology. Surgical therapy of IVC thrombosis encompasses caval interruption and thrombectomy. Currently, both of these modalities are being used less frequently.[170]

The goals of drug therapy center on managing the primary impact of the DVT and the impact of embolization. Medical management can include anticoagulation and thrombolytic agents.[170] However, there is the risk in use of thrombolytic agents to cause iatrogenic tear of IVC and internal bleeding.

Prognosis with Inferior Vena Cava Filter. Studies tend to confirm that IVC filter thrombosis is not a rare event, the frequency of which is probably underestimated. In a study[488] performed over an 8-year period, IVC thrombosis was demonstrated in 30 patients. In the group of patients as a whole, the mean delay between the diagnosis of filter occlusion and its placement was 20.8 months. However, in 15 of 30 patients (50%), filter thrombosis occurred during the first 6 months after filter placement, with the remaining 50% developing clots by the end of 20 months (100% thrombosis rate). Other symptoms were PE alone in three cases, acute bilateral edema and/or acute lumbar pain in six cases, and recent collateral abdominal circulation in three cases.[488]

Knowledge of the prognosis of IVC filter is limited. This device was designed to eliminate DVT. However, with the pending complications of IVC thrombosis and the likelihood of collateral vascularization, there is still a risk of developing DVT. In addition, even with placement of the IVC filter there is still the possibility of a proximal DVT that will not be addressed with the filter. Anticoagulation remains a therapy with placement of IVC filter. Complications of IVCS include bilateral lower-extremity edema, which may lead to compartment syndrome.[460] Hypotension as a result of hypovolemia (secondary to fluid leak into surrounding tissue) remains a cardiac complication. Circulatory impedance leads to organ death.

A THERAPIST'S THOUGHTS*
IVC Filter

An IVC filter placement may attempt to address the problem of DVT, but the complications associated with this treatment potentially outweigh the benefits. In other words, placement of an IVC filter does not prolong an individual's life and, in most cases, it may shorten that life.

I hope that medical physicians will begin to evaluate the efficacy of and use of the IVC filters and weigh the pros and cons of instituting the use of this device.

Collateral vascularization around a caval clot under the IVC will increase the risk of DVT formation. In addition, the stagnation of fluid under a caval clot promotes blood to the clot and further exposure of DVT thru collateralization around caval clot. Disruption of circulation will promote compromised kidney function and organ disruption, with possible organ death as a result of the lack of appropriate circulation. Complications created by the device, such as hypotension, can prove to be detrimental in a cardiac client.

Before placement of an IVC filter in a person who may present with a cardiac condition, a physician may consider a simple BNP (B-type natriuretic peptide) blood test. This test measures the level of the BNP hormone in the blood. The heart's pumping chambers (ventricles) produce extra BNP when they cannot pump enough blood to meet the body's needs. If the BNP level is high, the risk of heart failure is much higher. This would be good to know before placement of an IVC filter. BNP is a very useful and simple blood test to rule out the presence of a cardiac condition.

In addition, it is important to understand the necessity of continued use of anticoagulation therapy after IVC filter. There is no such thing as "all or none" in this situation. The person will need to continue a therapeutic dose of anticoagulation therapy in an "attempt" to avoid formation of caval clot. Taking anticoagulation medication does not guarantee that a clot will not form under the filter.

It is also important to understand that the device is not retrievable in most cases, and the complication of caval clot formation is life-threatening. Treatment for caval clot includes medications that promote clot embolization. These drugs can cause perforation of the IVC, which is a life-threatening situation. This alone may be a reason to carefully reconsider the use of this device.

The IVC filter has not been proven to increase a persons' life. Reviewing the objectives of the device and the exposure to potential medical complications will likely deem this device inappropriate for many individuals.

*Pat Hoover, PT

PROGNOSIS. PE is the primary cause of death for as many as 100,000 people each year (perhaps double that amount) and a contributory factor in another 100,000 deaths annually. Approximately 10% of victims die within the first hour, but prognosis for survivors (depending on underlying disease and on proper diagnosis and treatment) is generally favorable. Clients with PE who have cancer, congestive heart failure, atrial arrhythmias, or chronic lung disease have a higher risk of dying within 1 year than do clients with isolated PE.

Small emboli resolve without serious morbidity, but large or multiple emboli (especially in the presence of severe underlying cardiac or pulmonary disease) have a poorer prognosis. PE may recur despite LMWH therapy, most commonly in people with massive PE or in whom anticoagulant therapy has been inadequate. PE is the leading cause of pregnancy-related mortality in the United States.

SPECIAL IMPLICATIONS FOR THE THERAPIST   15-23

Pulmonary Embolism and Infarction

Paget-Schroetter syndrome is a DVT of the upper extremity primarily caused by weight lifting; it results in compression and subsequent stenosis of the subclavian vein. Therapists should be aware of this syndrome and other causes of DVT discussed in Chapter 12 because early detection can prevent PE and other complications.[72]

A careful review of the client's medical history may alert the therapist to the presence of predisposing factors for the development of a DVT or PE. For further information on assessment of DVT, see Chapter 12. If a PE is suspected, the *simplified* Wells criteria can be used to determine likelihood. A score of 2 or more requires a medical consult[190,505]; a score of 0 or 1 suggests PE is unlikely. The original Wells clinical decision rule for PE was published in 1997; it was later modified and more recently simplified even more as shown here[155,531-533]:

- Clinical symptoms of DVT (leg swelling, pain with palpation) (1 point)
- Other diagnoses less likely than PE (1 point)
- Heart rate greater than 100 beats/min (1 point)
- Immobilization 3 or more days or surgery in previous 4 weeks (1 point)
- Previous DVT/PE (1 point)
- Hemoptysis (1 point)
- Malignancy (1 point)

The Wells criteria also outlines seven factors that constitute the PE rule-out criteria (PERC). Combining information from this list with the PE score can help the therapist recognize low versus high priority for medial consultation.[505] The PERC approach has a high negative predictive value and sensitivity when combined with a low probability of PE using the Wells criteria, but a low positive predictive value and specificity. In other words, low-risk individuals who have all of the PERC are highly unlikely to have PE, but the absence of one or more of the PERC does not mean that a PE exists.[538]

- Age younger than 50 years
- Heart rate less than 100 beats/min
- Oxyhemoglobin saturation equal to or greater than 95%
- No hemoptysis
- No estrogen use
- No prior DVT or PE
- No unilateral leg swelling
- No surgery or trauma requiring hospitalization within the past 4 weeks

Frequent changing of position, exercise, the use of graduated-compression stockings, devices that provide intermittent pneumatic compression, and early ambulation are necessary to prevent thrombosis and embolism; sudden and extreme movements should be avoided.

The use of TED (antiembolism) hose should be restricted to individuals who are nonambulatory for short periods of time. They do provide compression in the range of 13 to 18 mm Hg but are not intended for use while ambulating. Intermittent compression devices (Venodyne) are also commonly used in ICU and other settings where patients are likely to be less mobile.

A light gradient compression stocking of 20 to 30 mm Hg (available off-the-shelf) is advised when medically necessary to prevent blood clot formation in anyone who is upright, active, or ambulatory. All postsurgical patients should be taught to do ankle pumps hourly. Under no circumstances should the legs be massaged to relieve muscle cramps, especially when the pain is located in the calf and the person has not been up and about.

Restrictive clothing, crossing the legs, and prolonged sitting or standing should be avoided. Elevating the legs, bending the bed at the knees, or propping pillows under the knees can produce venous stasis and should be done with caution to avoid severe flexion of the hips, which will slow blood flow and increase the risk of new thrombi.

After a PE or in the case of joint replacement, treatment with anticoagulation continues for those at high risk of recurrence. Venous thromboembolism with the additional risk of pulmonary embolism is the most common reason for hospital readmission and death after total hip or total knee arthroplasties.[272]

Anyone taking anticoagulants should be monitored carefully for signs of bleeding such as bloody stool, blood in urine, vaginal bleeding, bloody gums or nose, or large ecchymoses. Extended chemoprophylaxis is usually recommended for 3 to 6 weeks after surgery. Anyone still taking anticoagulants past this time without medical follow-up should be advised to see their doctor for a reevaluation.[404] If the person mentions any suspicious symptoms to the therapist, the client should be instructed to contact the physician immediately. Anyone with room air pulse oximetry readings less than 95% at the time of diagnosis are at increased risk of in-hospital complications, including respiratory failure, cardiogenic shock, and death.[295]

Medications should not be changed without the physician's approval; the use of additional medications, especially nonprescription preparations for colds, headaches, rheumatic pain, or any other reason must be approved by the physician. See also "Special Implications for the Therapist 12-24: Peripheral Vascular Disease" in Chapter 12.

Activity and Ambulation for Anyone with Pulmonary Embolism

See also "DVT and Ambulation" in Chapter 12.

Therapists around the country report variable activity and ambulation protocols for in-patients with a PE. Some physicians prefer early activity and ambulation with no restrictions. The most common standard of practice has been to hold physical therapy for 48 hours status post PE, but this is being reviewed and revised based on current evidence-based literature. Some physicians say that waiting until the person is therapeutic (i.e., acceptable international normalized ratio levels) increases the risk of another PE.

The timing of activity after PE may depend on individual's acuity and physician/provider's willingness to provide clear activity orders. According to a systematic review, the clinical benefits of mobility and the lack of significant differences for risk of developing a PE or development and progression of a new DVT between ambulation and bed rest suggest therapists should be confident in prescribing ambulation in this population.[21]

Pulmonary Arterial Hypertension

Definition and Incidence

PAH is high blood pressure in the pulmonary arteries defined as a mean pulmonary artery pressure greater than 25 mm Hg with a normal pulmonary capillary wedge pressure.[346]

In 2008 at the fourth World Symposium on PAH, a new classification system created (Dana System) five main categories for PAH.[346] Category one refers to PAH that is idiopathic, genetic, drug-induced (largely weight-loss drugs), congenital, or as a result of HIV. Category two refers to PAH that stems from left heart disease; category three refers to hypertension as a result of lung disease or hypoxia; category four refers to thromboembolic disorders; and category five refers to pulmonary hypertension that has a multifactorial etiology involving systemic conditions.[346]

Primary PAH is rare, that is, 1 or 2 cases per 1 million population in the United States. PAH in neonates occurs in 1.9/1000 live births from a variety of conditions.[213] PAH occurs most commonly in young and middle-aged women with a mean age at onset of 37 years (pregnant women have the highest mortality).[346] It has no known cause (idiopathic), although familial disease (defects in the bone morphogenetic protein receptor type II gene and the transforming growth factor β have been found)[486] accounts for approximately 10% of cases.

Pathogenesis

PAH is characterized by diffuse narrowing of the pulmonary arterioles caused by hypertrophy of smooth muscle in the vessel walls and formation of fibrous lesions in and around the vessels. The underlying cause of these changes is unknown, but looking beyond simple pulmonary vasoconstriction, it is now recognized that defects in endothelial function, pulmonary vascular smooth muscle cells, and platelets may all be involved in the pathogenesis and progression of PAH. It is likely that a combination of genetic and environmental factors contribute to this condition.[36,346]

Endothelial cell injury may result in an imbalance in endothelium-derived mediators. Impaired endothelium release may account for reduced production of nitrous oxide (N_2O), a vasodilator, from the airways resulting in vasoconstriction.

Defects in ion channel activity in smooth muscle cells in the pulmonary artery also may contribute to vasoconstriction and vascular proliferation.[255] These changes create increased resistance to the right side of the heart, which can eventually cause heart failure (cor pulmonale).

Secondary pulmonary hypertension is caused by any respiratory or cardiovascular disorder that increases the volume or pressure of blood entering the pulmonary arteries; narrows, obstructs, or destroys the pulmonary arteries; or increases the pressure of blood leaving the heart (pulmonary veins).

Increased volume or pressure overloads the pulmonary circulation whereas narrowing or obstruction elevates the blood pressure by increasing resistance to flow within the lungs. For example, COPD destroys alveoli and associated capillary beds thus increasing pressure through the remaining vasculature. Left-sided heart failure causes blood to "back up" and thus resistance is increased.

With persistent PAH, there is an increase in the afterload on the right ventricle, resulting in hypertrophy. This compensation is only temporary, and often progresses to right ventricular dilation, reduced right ventricular ejection fraction, and, ultimately, cor pulmonale. Because the pediatric heart is better able to withstand this afterload, there is a better prognosis for the pediatric population.[346]

Clinical Manifestations

Signs and symptoms of secondary pulmonary hypertension are difficult to recognize in the early stages when the symptoms of the underlying disease are more prominent. People may attribute their symptoms to a known underlying cardiopulmonary disorder, therefore delaying physician evaluation.

The most common symptoms of primary or secondary pulmonary hypertension are typical cardiorespiratory symptoms, such as fatigue, weakness, chest discomfort or pain, syncope, peripheral edema, abdominal distention, and unexplained SOB, beginning with exercise and later occurring with minimal activity or at rest.[43] In children, the most typical presentation includes dyspnea on exertion and syncope.[42]

MEDICAL MANAGEMENT

DIAGNOSIS. PAH can be difficult to diagnose, and there is usually a delay of 1 to 2 years between onset of symptoms and diagnosis. Sometimes the first indication of pulmonary hypertension is seen incidentally on a chest radiograph or ECG. The x-ray study may show rib scalloping (erosion of the inferior aspect of the ribs) from dilation of the arteries supplying the ribs. Standard assessment should include heart and lung auscultation and observation and palpation for jugular vein distention, hepatomegaly, and peripheral edema. Chest x-ray, ECG, and Doppler echocardiogram are also part of the screening.

If PAH is suspected, then additional testing is done to determine severity and to choose appropriate treatment. Essential testing should include pulmonary function tests; oximetry; chest CT; blood tests, including complete blood count, HIV, and antinuclear antibody tests; test for exercise capacity (usually the 6-Minute Walk Test); and right-heart catheterization (with and without vasodilator).[43] Additional tests, such as spiral CT or angiography, may be needed. Right-heart catheterization is needed to confirm the diagnosis.

TREATMENT. First-line treatment for PAH includes anticoagulation, diuretics to manage cor pulmonale, and digoxin.[346] Oxygen may also be prescribed to keep S_aO_2 greater than 90%. Those without right-heart failure may be prescribed calcium channel blockers to facilitate vasodilation. Synthetic prostacyclin and prostacyclin analogues (vasodilators) are effective in improving tolerance to exercise and hemodynamics. Inhaled prostacyclins show some promise with short-term improvement and may be beneficial in early stages of PAH.[134]

Endothelin-1 receptor antagonists work to counteract the vasoconstriction caused by overproduction of endothelin-1. Investigational oral drug therapy used to treat pulmonary hypertension (e.g., bosentan or ambrisentan) has shown promise in improving exercise capacity and hemodynamics. The phosphodiesterase 5 inhibitor, sildenafil, causes vasodilation and improvement of symptoms, although more research needs to be done with this medication.[188,281]

Inhaled N_2O (not nitric oxide, which is NO), a vasodilator, has not been shown to be effective in treatment of PAH in children and has potential toxicity.[61] Calcium channel blockers have been effective in children in high doses. Balloon atrial septostomy and lung transplantation are used in end-stage PAH, and heart–lung transplants may be more beneficial because of cor pulmonale.

Other treatment approaches under investigation include gene therapy and focus on pathogenetic factors outside the pulmonary endothelium (e.g., potassium channel defect favoring vasoconstriction and cell proliferation, role of elastase, and circulating blood factors contributing to blood thrombosis). In secondary PAH, it is essential to treat the underlying cause.

PROGNOSIS. The progression of PAH varies for each affected individual, but prognosis is poor without heart–lung transplantation. Some individuals may live 5 to 6 years from the time of diagnosis, but most people have a downhill course over a shorter period of time (2-3 years) with a fatal outcome.

The cause of death is usually right ventricular failure or sudden death; sudden death occurs late in the disease process. Mortality rates in the United States have increased notably since 1979, possibly attributable to increased awareness of PAH. Survival time has improved in PAH with the advent of treatment with prostacyclin.[100] Some portion of this reported increase may be related to improvements in diagnostic recognition, and some data suggest that the disease may be more common in the older population than has been previously recognized and reported.[319]

Secondary PAH can be reversed if the underlying disorder is successfully treated. If the hypertension has persisted long enough for the medial smooth muscle layer to hypertrophy, secondary PAH is no longer reversible.

SPECIAL IMPLICATIONS FOR THE THERAPIST   15-24

Pulmonary Hypertension

Impairment of exercise performance is associated with PAH because pulmonary vascular resistance and pulmonary artery pressure increase dramatically with exercise. There may be impaired heart rate kinetics during exercise with corresponding impaired cardiac output response and slow recovery of the heart.[427] For these reasons, clients with PAH must be closely monitored when participating in activities or therapy that requires increased physical stress. See Appendix B and Table 40-17.

Maintenance of adequate systemic blood pressure is essential, and the therapist must be familiar with the medications used and potential side effects, especially if blood pressure is altered pharmacologically. A drop in blood pressure can indicate heart failure. Inhaled N_2O or prostacyclin, which are endogenous vasodilators, increase oxygen consumption at the same workload during exercise, thereby improving exercise capacity. N_2O use is diminishing as a result of its toxicity and cost.[322]

Secondary PAH may occur in clients with connective tissue diseases, such as scleroderma, because the disease affects the vasculature of several organs, including the lungs (pulmonary fibrosis) and kidneys. The arterioles usually demonstrate intimal proliferation with progressive luminal occlusion. The development of hypertension often indicates the onset of an accelerated scleroderma renal crisis. Medical treatment is toward control of the blood pressure.

Cor Pulmonale

Definition and Incidence

Cor pulmonale, also called *pulmonary heart disease*, is the enlargement of the right ventricle secondary to the pulmonary hypertension that occurs in diseases of the thorax, lung, and pulmonary circulation. It is a term that describes the pathologic effects of lung dysfunction as it affects the right side of the heart. Right-sided heart dysfunction secondary to left-sided heart failure, vascular dysfunction, or congenital heart disease is excluded in the definition of cor pulmonale.

Chronic cor pulmonale occurs most frequently in adult male smokers, although the incidence in women is increasing as heavy smoking in females becomes more prevalent. The actual prevalence of cor pulmonale is difficult to determine because cor pulmonale does not occur in all cases of chronic lung disease and because routine physical examination and laboratory tests are relatively insensitive to the presence of pulmonary hypertension. It has been estimated that cor pulmonale accounts for 5% to 10% of organic heart disease.

Etiologic and Risk Factors

Pulmonary vascular diseases and respiratory diseases (e.g., emphysema or chronic bronchitis) are the primary causes of cor pulmonale. Emphysema and chronic bronchitis cause more than 50% of cases of cor pulmonale in the United States. When a PE has been sufficiently massive to obstruct 60% to 75% of the pulmonary circulation, acute cor pulmonale can occur. Cor pulmonale is frequently the cause of death in COPD.[530]

Cor pulmonale can also develop under conditions of sustained elevations in intrathoracic pressure associated with mechanical ventilation (and PEEP). The intrathoracic vessels narrow, leading to reduced cardiac output and possible cor pulmonale. Chronic widespread vasculitis, such as occurs in association with the collagen vascular disorders (e.g., rheumatoid arthritis, SLE, dermatomyositis, polymyositis, Sjögren syndrome, CREST [*c*alcinosis cutis, *R*aynaud phenomenon, *e*sophageal dysfunction, *s*clerodactyly, and *t*elangiectasis] syndrome accompanying scleroderma), can also cause chronic cor pulmonale. Occasionally, widespread radiation pneumonitis can be the underlying cause.

Other (uncommon) causes include pneumoconiosis, pulmonary fibrosis, kyphoscoliosis, pickwickian syndrome, lymphangitic infiltration from metastatic carcinoma, and obliterative pulmonary capillary changes that cause vasoconstriction and later, hypertension. The feature common to all these conditions that predisposes to cor pulmonale is hypoxia, which leads to vasoconstriction.[530]

Pathogenesis

Sustained elevation in pulmonary arterial hypertension can be mediated through persistent vasoconstriction, abnormal vascular structural remodeling, or vessel obliteration (see "Pulmonary Arterial Hypertension" above). Cor pulmonale develops as these factors increase pulmonary vessel pressure and overload in the right ventricle. Normally, the ventricle is a thin-walled (heart) muscle able to meet an increase in volume and pressure, but long-term pressure overload from hypertension causes the tissue to hypertrophy. In the case of acute cor pulmonale caused by emboli from DVT, the thrombus breaks loose and lodges at or near the bifurcation of the main pulmonary artery. Whether caused by vascular abnormalities or embolic obstruction, there is a marked fall in pressure necessary to drive blood through the compromised vascular bed because the right ventricle is compromised.

Clinical Manifestations

Evidence of cor pulmonale may be obscured by primary respiratory disease and appear only during exercise testing. The heart appears normal at rest, but with exercise, cardiac output falls and the ECG shows right ventricular hypertrophy. The predominant symptoms are related to the pulmonary disorder and include chronic productive cough, exertional dyspnea, wheezing respirations, easy fatigability, and weakness.

With a large pulmonary embolus, sudden severe, central chest pain can occur, caused by acute dilation of the root of the pulmonary artery and secondary to ischemia. The person may collapse, often with loss of consciousness, and death may occur within minutes if the thrombus is large and does not dislodge. If the thrombus is small or moves more peripherally in response to pounding on the chest or chest compression during resuscitation, acute cor pulmonale develops rather than sudden death.

Low cardiac output causes pallor, sweating, hypotension, anxiety, impaired consciousness, and a rapid pulse of small amplitude. The specific signs associated with cor pulmonale include exercise-induced peripheral cyanosis, clubbing (see Fig. 15-4), distended neck veins, and bilateral dependent edema. Hypoxia can cause pulmonary vasoconstriction and worsen symptoms.

MEDICAL MANAGEMENT

DIAGNOSIS. Diagnosis is made on the basis of physical examination, radiologic studies, and ECG or echocardiogram, sometimes both. Echocardiogram can effectively detect right ventricular enlargement, as well as excessive right ventricular afterload.[266] Pulmonary function tests usually confirm the underlying lung disease. Laboratory findings may include polycythemia present in cor pulmonale secondary to COPD. ECG and chest film may not be diagnostic in the early stages of cor pulmonale.

TREATMENT. The primary goal of medical treatment is to reduce the workload of the right ventricle. This is accomplished by lowering pulmonary artery pressure, as in the treatment of pulmonary hypertension (see "Pulmonary Arterial Hypertension" above). Oxygen administration, salt and fluid restriction, and diuretics are essential, as well as treatment of the underlying chronic pulmonary disease, while at the same time relieving the hypoxemia, hypercapnia, or acidosis.

Surgical removal of embolic material is a controversial procedure performed only when a confirmed diagnosis of massive PE with accessible thrombus in the main pulmonary artery or its branches is available. There is no specific surgical treatment available for most causes of chronic cor pulmonale. Heart–lung transplantation for clients with PAH is valuable in late-stage disease.

PROGNOSIS. Because cor pulmonale generally occurs late during the course of COPD and other irreversible disease, the prognosis is poor. Once congestive signs appear, the average life expectancy is 2 to 5 years, but survival is significantly longer when uncomplicated emphysema is the cause. Although cor pulmonale can be caused by obstructive and restrictive lung diseases, restrictive lung diseases have a lower life expectancy once they reach the stage of cor pulmonale.

SPECIAL IMPLICATIONS FOR THE THERAPIST 15-25

Cor Pulmonale

Diaphragmatic and pursed-lip breathing exercises should be reviewed for anyone with COPD and used with appropriate individuals; more details about this are available.[81]

Teach the client (or family member) how to detect edema in the lower extremities, especially the ankles, by pressing the skin over the shins for 1 to 2 seconds, looking for a lasting finger impression. Watch for signs of digitalis toxicity (see Table 12-5), such as complaints of anorexia, nausea, vomiting, or yellow halos around visual images.

Because pulmonary infection exacerbates COPD and cor pulmonale, all health care workers must practice careful hand hygiene and follow standard precautions (see Appendix A). Early signs of infection (e.g., increased sputum production, change in sputum color, chest pain or chest tightness, or fever) must be reported to the physician immediately. Watch for signs of respiratory failure such as change in pulse rate; deep, labored respirations; and increased fatigue produced by exertion.

Collagen Vascular Disease

Collagen vascular diseases, now more commonly referred to as diffuse connective tissue diseases (see Box 12-17), are often associated with pulmonary manifestations, including exudative pleural effusion, pulmonary nodules, rheumatoid nodules in association with coal workers' pneumoconiosis (Caplan syndrome), interstitial fibrosis, and pulmonary vasculitis. All of these pulmonary conditions are associated with rheumatoid arthritis; all except the nodules and pleural effusion have been seen with SLE; and pleuritis and pneumonitis have been observed in Sjögren syndrome, polymyositis, and dermatomyositis.

Pulmonary fibrosis or pulmonary hypertension, or both, are commonly part of the clinical picture associated with scleroderma. Polymyalgia rheumatica and temporal arteritis may demonstrate granulomatous inflammation of the pulmonary parenchyma. Approximately half of clients with SLE develop lung disease, primarily pleuritis, pleural effusion, or acute pneumonitis. Pulmonary involvement may not be evident clinically, but pulmonary function tests reveal abnormalities in many persons with SLE.

Lupus pneumonitis causes recurrent episodes of fever, dyspnea, and cough. Interstitial pneumonitis leading to fibrosis occurs in a small proportion of people with SLE; the inflammatory phase may respond to treatment, whereas the fibrosis does not. Occasionally, pulmonary hypertension develops. Rarely are ARDS and massive intraalveolar hemorrhage fatal pulmonary complications.

Interstitial lung disease can develop before joint involvement becomes evident in rheumatoid arthritis, particularly in men. People with rheumatoid arthritis who are receiving treatment with methotrexate or gold may develop interstitial lung disease that represents a drug hypersensitivity. Penicillamine therapy in clients with rheumatoid arthritis has been implicated in causing constrictive bronchiolitis.

Bilateral upper lobe fibrosis may develop late in ankylosing spondylitis. Lung involvement varies in SSc, but there is radiographic evidence of pulmonary disease in a majority of clients. Cutaneous scleroderma can involve the anterior chest wall and abdomen, causing restrictive lung function.

General dryness and lack of airway secretions cause the major problems of hoarseness, cough, and bronchitis in Sjögren syndrome, and interstitial lung disease is possible. Only 5% to 10% of clients with polymyositis and dermatomyositis develop interstitial lung disease, but weakness of respiratory muscles contributing to aspiration pneumonitis is common.

DISORDERS OF THE PLEURAL SPACE

Pneumothorax

Definition

Pneumothorax is an accumulation of air or gas in the pleural cavity caused by a defect in the visceral pleura or chest wall. The result is collapse of the lung on the affected side. Pneumothorax is classified as spontaneous or traumatic. Primary spontaneous pneumothorax develops with no underlying lung pathology. Secondary spontaneous pneumothorax is typically a result of blebs or bullae that occur in COPD, CF, or other lung disorders. Traumatic pneumothoraces are iatrogenic or noniatrogenic (Fig. 15-24).[47]

Incidence and Risk Factors

Although pneumothorax can develop at any age, spontaneous pneumothorax is especially common in tall, slender boys and men between the ages of 10 and 30 years. Smoking appears to increase the risk of primary spontaneous pneumothorax in men by as much as a factor of 20 in

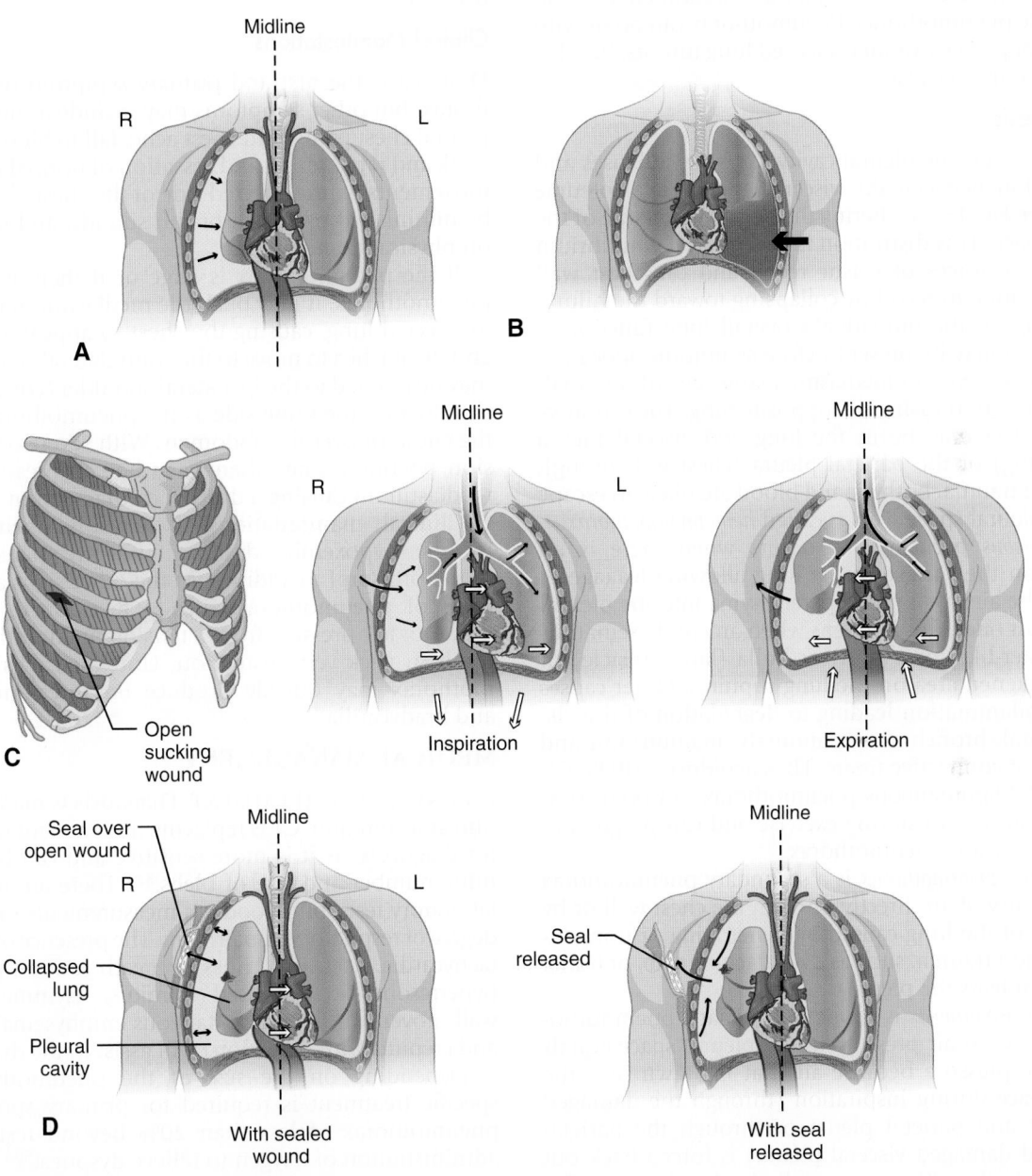

Figure 15-24

A, Pneumothorax. Lung collapses as air gathers in the pleural space between the parietal and visceral pleurae. **B,** Massive hemothorax, blood in the pleural space *(arrow)* below the left lung, causing collapse of lung tissue. **C,** Open pneumothorax (sucking chest wound). Air movement *(solid arrows)* and structural movement *(open arrows)*. A chest wall wound connects the pleural space with atmospheric air. During inspiration, atmospheric air is sucked into the pleural space through the chest wall wound. Positive pressure in the pleural space collapses the lung on the affected side and pushes the mediastinal contents toward the unaffected side. This reduces the volume of air in the unaffected side considerably. During expiration, air escapes through the chest wall wound, lessening positive pressure in the affected side and allowing the mediastinal contents to swing back toward the affected side. Movement of mediastinal structure from side to side is called mediastinal flutter. **D,** Tension pneumothorax. If an open pneumothorax is covered (e.g., with a dressing), it forms a seal, and tension pneumothorax with a mediastinal shift develops. A tear in lung structure continues to allow air into the pleural space. As positive pressure builds in the pleural space, the affected lung collapses, and the mediastinal contents shift to the unaffected side. Tension pneumothorax is corrected by removing the seal (i.e., dressing), allowing air trapped in the pleural space to escape.

a dose-dependent manner (i.e., chances increase as number of cigarettes smoked increases).[437] The incidence of primary spontaneous pneumothorax is 7.4 to 18 per 100,000 in males and 1.2 to 6 per 100,000 in females.[323]

The most common causes of iatrogenic pneumothorax are transthoracic needle lung biopsy, subclavian vein catheterization, thoracentesis, transbronchial lung biopsy, and positive pressure ventilation. Surgical procedures that involve the chest wall and abdomen also can precipitate pneumothorax. Pneumothorax can occur with a variety of primary or metastasized lung tumors, but this is an uncommon cause.

Pathogenesis

When air enters the pleural cavity the lung collapses and a separation between the visceral and parietal pleurae occurs (see Fig. 15-3), altering the negative pressure of the pleural space. This disruption in the normal equilibrium between the forces of elastic recoil and the chest wall causes the lung to recoil by collapsing toward the hilum. Depending on the individual's overall lung function, a loss of 40% may be present before symptoms appear.[437] The result is SOB and mediastinal shift toward the unaffected side, compressing the opposite lung. The causative pleural defect may be in the lung and visceral pleura (lung lining) or the parietal pleura (chest wall lining). After chest trauma, both air and blood are likely to escape into the pleural space. This is called *hemopneumothorax*.

Spontaneous pneumothorax occurs when there is an opening on the surface of the lung allowing leakage of air from the airways or lung parenchyma into the pleural cavity. Most often this happens when an emphysematous bleb (blister-like formation) or bulla (larger vesicle) or other weakened area on the lung ruptures. Other causes include inflammation leading to degradation of the visceral pleural, bronchial tree anomaly, malnutrition and disorders of connective tissue, TB, sarcoidosis, ARDS, CF, and PCP.[323] Spontaneous pneumothorax can occur during sleep, at rest, or during exercise and can progress to become a tension pneumothorax.

Traumatic pneumothorax is a secondary pneumothorax with the entry of air directly through the chest wall or by laceration of the lung caused by penetrating or nonpenetrating chest trauma, such as a rib fracture, stab, or bullet wound that tears the pleura.

Open pneumothorax is a type of traumatic pneumothorax occurs when air pressure in the pleural space equals barometric pressure because air that is drawn into the pleural space during inspiration (through the damaged chest wall and parietal pleura or through the parietal pleura and damaged visceral pleura) is forced back out during expiration. This can rapidly lead to hypoventilation and hypoxia.

Iatrogenic pneumothorax develops as a result of direct puncture or laceration of the visceral pleura during attempts at central line placement, percutaneous lung aspiration, thoracentesis, or closed pleural biopsy. Direct alveolar distention can occur with anesthesia, cardiopulmonary resuscitation, or mechanical ventilation with PEEP.

Tension pneumothorax can result from any type of pneumothorax and is life-threatening. In tension pneumothorax, the site of pleural rupture acts as a one-way valve,

permitting air to enter on inspiration but preventing its escape by closing up during expiration. Under these conditions, continuously increasing air pressure in the pleural cavity may cause progressive collapse of the lung tissue. Air pressure in the pleural space pushes against the already recoiled lung, causing compression atelectasis, and against the mediastinum, compressing and displacing the heart and great vessels. Venous return and cardiac output decrease.[545]

Clinical Manifestations

Dyspnea is the first and primary symptom of pneumothorax, but other symptoms may include a sudden sharp pleural chest pain, mild chest ache, fall in blood pressure, weak and rapid pulse, and cessation of normal respiratory movements on the affected side of the chest.[323] There will be diminished or absent breath sounds, and tachycardia on physical examination.

If the pneumothorax is large or if there is a tension pneumothorax, it may push the mediastinum toward the unaffected lung, causing the chest to appear asymmetric and the trachea to move to the contralateral side. The pain may be referred to the ipsilateral shoulder (corresponding shoulder on the same side as the pneumothorax), across the chest, or over the abdomen. With severe or large tension pneumothorax, there may be compression of the mediastinum causing a drop in cardiac output.

Clinical manifestations of tension pneumothorax include hypoxemia, dyspnea, and hypotension (low blood pressure) in addition to the other signs and symptoms of pneumothorax already mentioned. Increased intrathoracic pressure from a tension pneumothorax may result in neck vein distention. Untreated tension pneumothorax may quickly produce life-threatening shock and bradycardia.

MEDICAL MANAGEMENT

DIAGNOSIS AND TREATMENT. Diagnosis is made by chest film at inspiration. CT is replacing the standard radiograph for diagnosis, as it is more sensitive and can help determine number and size of blebs.[323] There are no specific laboratory tests, but blood gas measurements indicate the degree of respiratory impairment. The presence of dyspnea, tachycardia, decrease or loss of breath sounds, percussive hyperresonance, decreased fremitus, asymmetric chest wall movement, and subcutaneous emphysema (swelling and crepitus with palpation) will assist in the diagnosis.

Depending on the size of the pneumothorax, no specific treatment is required for primary spontaneous pneumothorax of less than 20% beyond rest and the administration of oxygen to relieve dyspnea.[506] However, recurrences are frequent and associated with increased mortality in secondary spontaneous pneumothorax.

For large pneumothorax or recurrent pneumothorax, video-assisted thoracic surgery procedures are performed or aspiration with drainage from a catheter or chest tube. In a video-assisted thoracic surgery procedure, blebs are resected and attempts are made to seal the pleural space through pleurodesis.[323] Placement of a chest tube is standard procedure for traumatic pneumothoraces.[47]

Pneumothorax is an unwanted sequela to respiratory distress syndrome in premature infants. The use of prophylactic surfactant significantly reduces the incidence of pneumothorax in this population.[468]

It is not a good idea to travel by airplane (because of air pressure changes) or to have pulmonary function tests performed (e.g., CF) for at least 2 weeks after a pneumothorax has healed. Encouraging smoking cessation is essential. In CF, airway clearance techniques that include positive expiratory pressure (oscillatory positive expiratory pressure) are usually held during pneumothorax and recovery as well.

PROGNOSIS. There is a low mortality rate with idiopathic pneumothorax, but a corresponding 15% mortality rate for pneumothorax associated with underlying lung disease. From 30% to 50% of affected persons experience a recurrence, and after one recurrence, subsequent episodes are much more likely. The physiologic events associated with tension pneumothorax are life-threatening, requiring immediate treatment.

SPECIAL IMPLICATIONS FOR THE THERAPIST | **15-26**

Pneumothorax

In the case of trauma (e.g., motor vehicle accident, assault, or traumatic falls) the presence of undiagnosed nondisplaced rib fractures or rib fragments must be considered when getting a person up for the first time. The client's movements and the action of parasternal intercostal muscles can displace the rib, causing puncture of the lung or penetrating aortic injury.

When getting someone up for the first time, monitor vital signs, especially blood pressure and pulse, and request emergency medical help immediately anytime someone with this type of history demonstrates sudden shoulder or chest pain, altered breathing pattern, or drop of blood pressure accompanied by weak and fast pulse, pallor, dyspnea, or extreme anxiety.

Anyone with a history of secondary spontaneous pneumothorax should also be monitored closely during treatment because of the chance for recurrence and complications. See also "Special Implications for the Therapist 15-14: Chest Wall or Lung Injury" above.

Pleurisy

Definition and Etiologic Factors

Pleurisy (pleuritis) is an inflammation of the pleura caused by viral or bacterial infection, injury (e.g., rib fracture), or tumor (particularly malignant pleural mesothelioma). It may be a complication of lung disease, particularly of pneumonia, but also of TB, lung abscesses, influenza, SLE, rheumatoid arthritis, or pulmonary infarction.

Clinical Manifestations

The symptoms develop suddenly, usually with a sharp chest pain that is worse on inspiration, coughing, sneezing, or movement associated with deep inspiration. Other symptoms may include cough, fever, chills, and rapid shallow breathing (tachypnea). The visceral pleurae are

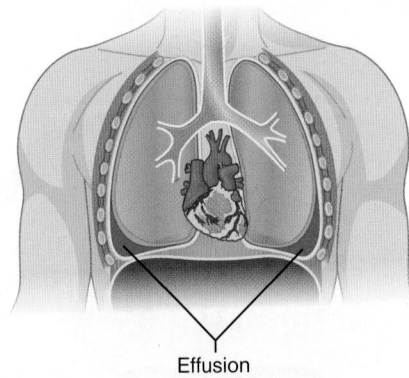

Figure 15-25

Pleural effusion, a collection of fluid in the pleural space between the membrane encasing the lung and the membrane lining the thoracic cavity, as seen on upright x-ray examination. Pleurisy (pleuritis) is an inflammation of the visceral and parietal pleurae. When there is an abnormal increase in the lubricating fluid between these two layers, it is called pleurisy with effusion.

insensitive; pain results from inflammation of the parietal pleurae. Because the latter is innervated by the intercostal nerves, chest pain is usually felt over the site of the pleuritis, but pain may be referred to the lower chest wall, abdomen, neck, upper trapezius muscle, and shoulder. If the pleura near the diaphragm is inflamed, pain may be referred to the ipsilateral shoulder.[285] On auscultation, a pleural rub can be heard (sound caused by the rubbing together of the visceral and costal pleurae).

Pathogenesis

There are two types of pleurisy: wet and dry. The membranous pleura that encases each lung is composed of two close-fitting layers; between these layers is a lubricating fluid. If the fluid content remains unchanged by the disease, the pleurisy is said to be dry. If the fluid increases abnormally, it is a wet pleurisy, or pleurisy with effusion (Fig. 15-25). Inflammation of the part of the pleura that covers the diaphragm is called diaphragmatic pleurisy and occurs secondary to pneumonia.

When the central portion of the diaphragmatic pleura is irritated, sharp pain may be referred to the neck, upper trapezius muscle, or shoulder. Stimulation of the peripheral portions of the diaphragmatic pleura results in sharp pain felt along the costal margins, which can be referred to the lumbar region by the lower thoracic somatic nerves (Fig. 15-26).

Wet pleurisy is less likely to cause pain because there usually is no chafing. The fluid may interfere with breathing by compressing the lung. If the excess fluid of wet pleurisy becomes infected with formation of pus, the condition is known as *purulent pleurisy* or *empyema*. Pleurisy causes pleurae to become reddened and covered with an exudate of lymph, fibrin, and cellular elements and may lead to pleural effusion. In dry pleurisy, the two layers of membrane may become congested and swollen and rub against each other, which is painful. Although only the outer layer causes pain (the inner layer has no pain nerves), the pain may be severe enough to require the use of a strong analgesic.

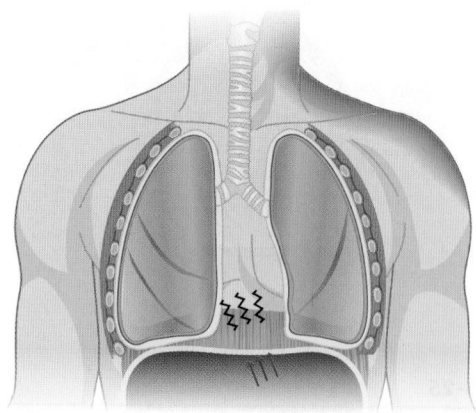

Figure 15-26

Diaphragmatic pleurisy. Irritation of the peritoneal (outside) or pleural (inside) surface of the central area of the diaphragm refers sharp pain to the neck, supraclavicular fossa, and upper trapezius muscle. The pain pattern is ipsilateral to the area of irritation. Irritation to the peripheral portion of the diaphragm refers sharp pain to the costal margins and lumbar region (not shown).

MEDICAL MANAGEMENT

Physical examination may reveal a pleural rub or diminished breath sounds. Other pathologies should be ruled out when considering pleurisy. Most important is the evaluation for pulmonary embolus, pneumothorax, and myocardial infarction.[285] Diagnostic work-up may include chest radiograph or CT, ECG if cardiac origin is suspected, and evaluation of the pleural fluid through thoracentesis.[285] Treatment is usually with nonsteroidal antiinflammatory drugs for pain management and treatment of the underlying condition. Sclerosing therapy for chronic or recurrent pleurisy may be recommended.

Pleural Effusion

Definition

Pleural effusion is the collection of fluid in the pleural space (between the membrane encasing the lung and the membrane lining the thoracic cavity) where there is normally only a small amount of fluid to prevent friction as the lung expands and deflates (see Fig. 15-25). Pleural fluid normally seeps continually into the pleural space from the capillaries lining the parietal pleura and is then reabsorbed by the visceral pleural capillaries and lymphatics.

Incidence and Etiologic Factors

The causes of pleural effusions are best considered in terms of the underlying pathophysiology: transudates caused by abnormalities of hydrostatic or osmotic pressure (e.g., congestive heart failure, cirrhosis with ascites, nephrotic syndrome, or peritoneal dialysis) and exudates resulting from increased permeability or trauma (e.g., infection, primary or secondary malignancy, PE, trauma including surgical trauma [e.g., cardiotomy]). In children, the most common causes of pleural effusion are congenital heart abnormalities, and pneumonia.[552]

An exudate is a fluid with a high content of protein and cellular debris that has escaped from blood vessels and has been deposited in tissues or on tissue surfaces, usually as a result of inflammation. A transudate is a fluid substance that has passed through a membrane or has been forced out from a tissue; in contrast to an exudate, a transudate is characterized by high fluidity and a low content of protein, cells, or solid matter derived from cells. (See discussion of "Inflammation and Chronic Inflammation" in Chapter 6 and Figs. 6-11 and 6-12.)

Any condition that interferes with either the secretion or drainage of this fluid will lead to pleural effusion. Pleural effusion is common with heart failure and lymphatic obstruction caused by neoplasm. Less common causes include drug-induced effusion, pancreatitis, collagen vascular diseases (SLE or rheumatoid arthritis), intraabdominal abscess, or esophageal perforation. A person of any age can be affected, but it is more common in the older adult because of the increased incidence of heart failure and cancer.

Pathogenesis

The most common mechanism of pleural effusion is migration of fluids and other blood components through the walls of intact capillaries bordering the pleura. When stimulated by biochemical mediators of inflammation, junctions in the capillary endothelium separate slightly, enabling leukocytes and plasma proteins to migrate out into affected tissues. Rupture of a blood vessel or leakage of blood from an injured vessel causes a form of pleural effusion called hemothorax (see Fig. 15-25).

Malignant pleural effusions occur in 50% of individuals with widespread cancer, largely from breast or lung cancers. Malignant pleural effusions produce exudative fluid from seeding of the cancer in the pleural space, and are associated with a medial life expectancy of 3 to 12 months.[552] The effusion can be a local effect of the tumor such as lymphatic obstruction or bronchial obstruction with pneumonia or atelectasis. Lymphatic blockage from any cause can result in drainage of the contents of lymphatic vessels into the pleural space. It can also be a result of systemic effects of tumor elsewhere, but in either case, malignant cells in the pleural effusion of a person with lung cancer indicate an inoperable situation.

Clinical Manifestations

Clinical manifestations of pleural effusion will depend on the amount of fluid present and the degree of lung compression. A small amount of effusion may be discovered only by chest x-ray examination. Large effusions cause clinical manifestations related to their volume and the rate at which they accumulate in the pleural space causing restriction of lung expansion. Clients usually present with dyspnea on exertion that becomes progressive. They may develop nonspecific chest discomfort; sometimes the chest pain is pleuritic, which is a sharp, stabbing pain exacerbated by coughing or breathing and changes in position. Other symptoms characteristic of the underlying cause of pleural effusion may be the primary clinical picture (e.g., weight loss and fever with TB or cancer or signs of heart failure). Tachycardia, distant heart sounds, fixed jugular venous distention, edema of the extremities, and a paradoxical pulse may be part of the developing clinical picture.

MEDICAL MANAGEMENT

DIAGNOSIS. Diagnosis begins with a chest radiograph or CT followed by aspiration of pleural fluid. The pleural fluid is evaluated for pH; specific gravity; protein; stains and cultures for bacteria, TB, and fungi; eosinophilia count; and glucose concentration to aid in the differential diagnosis.[449] Chest pain must be differentiated from pain of pericardial or musculoskeletal origin.

TREATMENT. Pleural effusions, if symptomatic, are a medical emergency requiring immediate attention.[219] Treatment is different for transudative fluid as compared to exudative.[552] Transudative pleural effusions may resolve with antibiotics and treatment of the underlying medical condition. Exudative effusions, large transudative effusions, infected effusions (empyema), malignant effusions, and hemothorax require drainage. Drainage options include thoracentesis with drainage by a small- or large-bore catheter or chest tube. Those with recurrent effusions or malignant effusions may be treated with pleurodesis (sclerosing substance introduced into the pleural space to create an inflammatory response that scleroses tissues together).

PROGNOSIS. Without treatment of the symptomatic client, cardiac function declines as venous return to the heart becomes limited by the effusion; it is essentially a restrictive heart disease. Ultimately, these individuals can go into complete circulatory shutdown. Prognosis for pleural effusion depends on the underlying cause. Those with malignant pleural effusions have a median life span of 3 to 12 months. Those with empyema or recurrent pleural effusion may have long-term changes which mimic restrictive lung disease.

SPECIAL IMPLICATIONS FOR THE THERAPIST   15-27

Pleural Effusion

After transthoracic aspiration, encourage deep-breathing exercises to promote lung expansion and watch for respiratory distress or pneumothorax (sudden onset of dyspnea or cyanosis). In the presence of a chest tube, prevent kinking by carefully coiling the tubing on top of the bed and securing it to the bed linen, leaving room for the client to turn.

Position changes must be performed carefully to avoid disturbing the surgical site or the chest tube. The therapist may apply firm support with both hands to the surgical site and chest tube area to help lessen

---

muscle pull and pain as the client coughs. If the person has open drainage through a rib resection or intercostal tube, use hand and dressing precautions.

Small pleural effusions (greater than 500 mL) frequently have minimal findings on physical exam. Effusions with 500 to 1500 mL demonstrate dullness to percussion, diminished breath sounds, and reduced tactile and vocal fremitus over the involved hemithorax. Effusions greater than 1500 mL will present with concomitant atelectasis, demonstrate bronchial or tracheal breath sounds, and sound like the bleating of a goat on auscultation (referred to as egophony) with inspiratory lag on the affected side.

Pleural Empyema

Pleural empyema (infected pleural effusion) is an accumulation of pus that occurs occasionally as a complication of pleurisy or some other respiratory disease, usually pneumonia. It is a normal response to infection but may also occur after external contamination (penetrating trauma, chest tube placement, or other surgical procedure) or esophageal perforation. Symptoms include dyspnea, coughing, ipsilateral pleural chest or shoulder pain, malaise, tachycardia, cough, and fever. In addition to chest films, transthoracic aspiration biopsy may be done to confirm the diagnosis and determine the specific causative organism.

The condition is treated with intercostal chest tube drainage or pig-tail catheter drainage. Long-term antibiotics are generally needed, and attention must be paid to the person's nutritional status.[105] Intrapleural fibrinolytic agents may have some use reducing need for surgery in people with empyema.[494] See "Special Implications for the Therapist 15-27: Pleural Effusion" above.

Pleural Fibrosis

Pleural fibrosis may follow inflammation (especially from asbestos), hemorrhagic effusion, and infection of the pleurae. It can present as localized plaques or diffuse. There appears to be a complex interaction of inflammatory cells, coagulation, profibrotic mediators, and growth factors in this process.[366] Early use of corticosteroids may decrease the incidence but is not effective in reducing established fibrosis. Surgical decortication can be effective in resolving symptoms.[251]

REFERENCES

To enhance this text and add value for the reader, all references are included on the companion Evolve site that accompanies this textbook. The reader can view the reference source and access it online whenever possible.

CHAPTER 16

The Gastrointestinal System

CELESTE PETERSON • CATHERINE CAVALLARO GOODMAN

The gastrointestinal (GI) tract consists of upper and lower segments with separate functions. The upper GI tract includes the mouth, esophagus, stomach, and duodenum, and aids in the ingestion and digestion of food. The lower GI tract includes the small and large intestines (Fig. 16-1). The small intestine accomplishes digestion and absorption of nutrients, whereas the large intestine absorbs water and electrolytes, storing waste products of digestion until elimination.

The enteric nervous system has become the focus of new research and discoveries in a new area of study referred to as *psychoneuroimmunology* with a subspecialty of clinical gastroenterology called *neurogastroenterology*. There are as many nerve cells in the human small intestine as there are in the human spinal cord, and the enteric nervous system can function completely independently of the central nervous system. The enteric nervous system is sometimes referred to as the "brain in the bowel."

Insight into the connections among emotions, brain function, and GI function has revolutionized our thinking about the so-called mind–body connection. New information is being discovered about the sensory functions of the intestine and how neural, hormonal, and immune signals interact. More than 30 chemicals of different classes (neuropeptides, neurotransmitters) transmit instructions to the brain, and all these chemicals are represented in the enteric nervous system.

Representatives of all the major categories of immune cells are found in the gut or can be recruited rapidly from the circulation in response to an inflammatory stimulus. The constant presence of these neurotransmitters and neuromodulators in the bowel suggests that emotional expression or active coping generates a balance in the neuropeptide-receptor network and physiologic healing beginning in the GI system. In fact, it has been suggested that because the enteric nervous system can function on its own, it is possible that the brain in the bowel can have its own psychoneuroses, such as the functional bowel syndromes discussed in this chapter (see "Irritable Bowel Syndrome" section).[98]

Scientists continue to study influences of the nervous system on immune and inflammatory responses in the mucosal surfaces of the intestines along with the innervation of the immune system and the molecular communication pathways as these relate to emotions and thoughts and the GI system.[148]

The gut immune system has 70% to 80% of the body's immune cells, and the protective blocking action of the secretory response in the gut is crucial to the integrity of the GI tract immune function and host defense. Studies suggest that the development and expression of the regional immune system of the GI tract is independent of systemic immunity. Nutrients have fundamental and regulatory influences on the immune response of the GI tract and therefore on host defense.

Reduction of normal bacteria in the gut after antibiotic treatment or in the presence of infection may interfere with the nutrients available for immune function in the GI tract. New understanding of intestinal disorders and new approaches to the management of these disorders are expected in the next decade.

SIGNS AND SYMPTOMS OF GASTROINTESTINAL DISEASE

Clinical manifestations of GI disease can be caused by a variety of underlying conditions or disorders. The primary condition may be of GI origin, but some GI symptoms are part of a collection of systemic symptoms called *constitutional symptoms* and may be associated with any systemic condition (Table 16-1).

Nausea occurs when nerve endings in the stomach and other parts of the body are irritated and usually precedes vomiting. Intense pain in any part of the body can produce nausea as a result of the nausea-vomiting mechanism of the involuntary autonomic nervous system. Nausea can be caused by strong emotions and may accompany psychologic disorders, a variety of systemic disorders (e.g., acute myocardial infarction, diabetic acidosis, migraine, hepatobiliary and pancreatic disorders, Ménière syndrome, and GI disorders), and drugs such as morphine, codeine, excess alcohol, anesthetics, and anticancer drugs.

Vomiting may be caused by anything that precipitates nausea. Complications of vomiting include fluid and electrolyte imbalances, pulmonary aspiration of vomitus, gastroesophageal mucosal tear (Mallory-Weiss syndrome), malnutrition, and rupture of the esophagus.

Diarrhea (abnormal frequency or volume of stools) results in poor absorption of water and nutritive elements and electrolytes, fluid volume deficit, and acidosis as a result of bicarbonate depletion (see Tables 5-10 and 5-13 and corresponding text, "Electrolyte Imbalances, Fluid

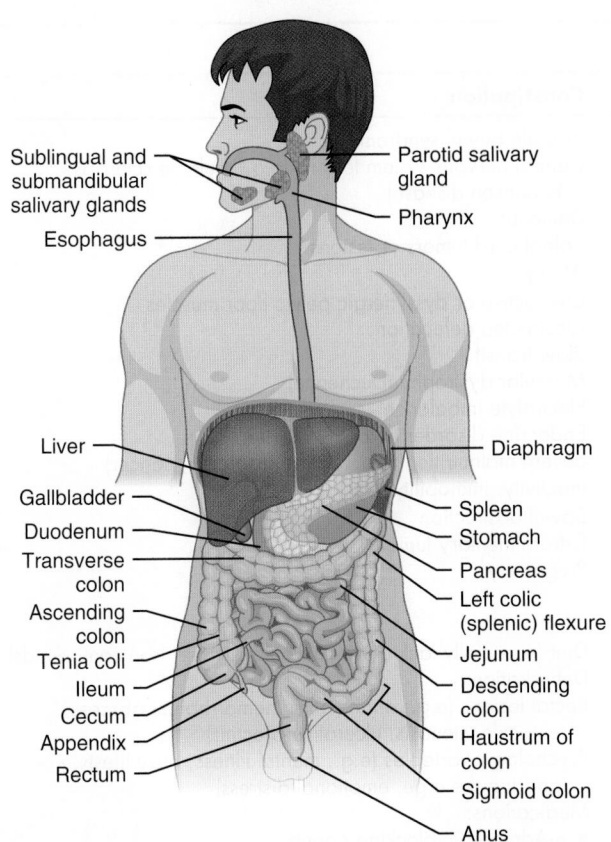

Figure 16-1

The digestive system.

Labels: Sublingual and submandibular salivary glands, Esophagus, Parotid salivary gland, Pharynx, Liver, Diaphragm, Gallbladder, Spleen, Duodenum, Stomach, Transverse colon, Pancreas, Ascending colon, Left colic (splenic) flexure, Tenia coli, Jejunum, Ileum, Descending colon, Cecum, Appendix, Haustrum of colon, Rectum, Sigmoid colon, Anus

Table 16-1	Clinical Manifestations of Gastrointestinal Disease	
GI Signs and Symptoms	**Constitutional Symptoms**	**GI Signs and Symptoms Associated with Strenuous Exercise**
Nausea and vomiting	Nausea	Fecal urgency; diarrhea
Diarrhea	Vomiting	Abdominal cramps
Anorexia	Diarrhea	Belching
Constipation	Malaise	Nausea and vomiting
Dysphagia	Fatigue	Heartburn
Achalasia	Fever	
Heartburn	Night sweats	
Abdominal pain	Pallor	
GI bleeding:	Diaphoresis	
Hematemesis	Dizziness	
Melena		
Hematochezia		
Fecal incontinence		

and Electrolyte Imbalances" and Acid-Base Balances"). Other systemic effects of prolonged diarrhea are dehydration, electrolyte imbalance, and weight loss. The causes of diarrhea are many and varied (Table 16-2). Drug-induced diarrhea, most commonly associated with antibiotics, may not develop until 2 to 3 weeks after first ingestion of an antibiotic, but if the onset of diarrhea coincides with the use of drugs, it may resolve when the drug is discontinued.

Anorexia, diminished appetite or aversion to food, is a nonspecific symptom often associated with nausea, vomiting, and sometimes diarrhea. It may be associated with disorders of other organ systems, including cancer, heart disease, and renal disease. It is the major component of eating disorders such as anorexia nervosa.

Anorexia-cachexia, a systemic response to cancer, occurs as a result of increased metabolic rate caused by the tumor cells and metabolites produced and released by tumor cells into the bloodstream. These effects of tumor cells stimulate the satiety center in the hypothalamus and produce appetite loss, gross alterations of metabolic patterns, and a profound systemic condition referred to as anorexia-cachexia. A downward spiral of symptoms occurs with appetite loss leading to malnutrition, weight loss, muscular weakness, and a negative nitrogen balance that contributes to the development of cachectic wasting.

Constipation is a common condition affecting up to one-quarter of the American population, and is especially prevalent in women and people older than age 65 years.[118] Constipation occurs when fecal matter is too hard to pass

easily or when bowel movements are so infrequent that discomfort and other symptoms interfere with daily activities. Because constipation is so common and occurs as part of disorders, standard criteria have been developed in order to better define it. The Rome III diagnostic criteria for *functional constipation* includes two or more of the following, present for the last 3 months, and symptom onset at least 6 months prior to diagnosis[190]:

- Straining during at least 25% of defecations
- Lumpy or hard stools in at least 25% of defecations
- Sensation of incomplete evacuation for at least 25% of defecations
- Sensation of anorectal obstruction/blockage for at least 25% of defecations
- Manual maneuvers to facilitate at least 25% of defecations (e.g., digital evacuation, support of the pelvic floor)
- Fewer than 3 defecations per week
- Loose stools are rarely present without the use of laxatives
- There are insufficient criteria for irritable bowel syndrome

Constipation may occur as a result of many factors such as diet, dehydration (including lack of fluid intake), side effects of medication, acute or chronic diseases of the digestive system, inactivity or prolonged bed rest, emotional stress, personality, and lack of exercise (see Table 16-2).

Although constipation often is described as a condition of old age, there is some controversy over this assumption. Research shows that colorectal functions (colonic transit times and motility) are not significantly different in healthy older adults compared to younger healthy adults.[110] It is thought that an increase in constipation is caused by an increase in constipation-promoting factors, not changes in the intestinal organ itself. Constipation is multifactorial, caused more often by lifestyle factors than by physiologic decline. Lifelong bowel habits, current diet, lack of fluid intake, and immobility are likely causes of constipation in the adult older than 65 years.[68] Constipation may be the

Table 16-2	Causes of Diarrhea and Constipation	
	Diarrhea	**Constipation**
Neurogenic	Irritable bowel syndrome Diabetic enteropathy Hyperthyroidism Caffeine	Irritable bowel syndrome Central nervous system lesions (e.g., multiple sclerosis, Parkinson disease) Dementia Spinal cord tumors or lesions Atomy
Muscular	Pelvic floor muscle weakness Electrolyte imbalance Endocrine disorder	Overactive or dyssynergic pelvic floor muscles Obstructed defecation Slow transit Muscular dystrophy (Duchenne) Electrolyte imbalance Endocrine disorder (hypothyroidism) Severe malnutrition (e.g., eating disorders, cancer) Inactivity; immobility; back injury/pain
Mechanical	Incomplete obstruction (e.g., neoplasm, adhesions, stenosis) Postoperative effect (e.g., gastrectomy, ileal bypass, intestinal resection, cholecystectomy) Diverticulitis	Bowel obstruction Extraalimentary tumors Pregnancy
Other	Diet (including food allergy, lactose intolerance, food additives) Supplements (creatine) Malabsorption Infectious/inflammatory disorders (including pelvic inflammatory disease) Strenuous exercise Medications: • Antibiotics • Nonprescription drugs • Laxative abuse • Magnesium (often found in antacids) • Antihypertensive medication • Nonsteroidal antiinflammatory drugs • Proton pump inhibitors • Antiarrhythmics	Diet (especially lack of dietary bulk or fiber, iron compounds) Dehydration Rectal lesions (e.g., anal fissure, hemorrhoids, abscess, rectocele, stenosis, ulcerative proctitis) Psychologic variables (e.g., mental illness, busy lifestyle or ignoring the urge, emotional distress) Medications: • α-Adrenergic blocking agents • Angiotensin-converting enzyme inhibitors • Antacids with calcium carbonate or aluminum hydroxide • Antiarrhythmics • Anticholinergics • Antiseizure drugs • Antihistamines • Antilipidemics • Antiparkinson agents • Antipsychotics • Benzodiazepines • Calcium channel blockers • Nonsteroidal antiinflammatory drugs • Opioids • Antidepressants • Diuretics

Modified from DiPiro JT, Talbert RL, Yee GC, Matzke GR, Wells BG, Posey LM (eds): *Pharmacotherapy: a pathophysiologic approach*, ed 8, New York, 2011, McGraw Hill.

result of underlying organic disease or may be caused by lesions or structural abnormalities within the colon that narrow the intestines and/or rectum, slow-transit alimentary canal, and defecatory disorders.[111]

People with mechanical low back pain may develop constipation as a result of muscle guarding and splinting that causes reduced bowel motility. Pressure on sacral nerves from stored fecal content may cause an aching discomfort in the sacrum, buttocks, or thighs.[103] Individuals with a herniated disc and taking narcotic medications can be constipated resulting in bearing down (Valsalva), which has the potential to make the herniation worse.

Constipation is typically divided into two groups: slow transit constipation and obstructed defecation.[111] Slow transit constipation is a decrease in peristalsis so

physical therapy intervention will have little effect on this condition.

Constipation associated with obstructed defecation is the result of pelvic floor or anal sphincter dysfunction, including pelvic floor dyssynergia, spastic pelvic floor syndrome, and anismus. Unlike slow transit constipation, obstructed defecation does respond well to muscle retraining. In cases of obstructed defecation, the external anal sphincter contracts and tightens rather than relaxing and opening during defecation. Individuals with this type of constipation often strain to defecate and experience incomplete bowel emptying.[176]

Dysphagia (difficulty swallowing) produces the sensation that food is stuck somewhere in the throat or chest (esophagus). Dysphagia may be a symptom of many other disorders, including neurologic conditions (e.g., stroke, Alzheimer disease, Parkinson disease), local trauma and muscle damage (including physical assault), or mechanical obstruction. Obstruction may be *intrinsic*, originating in the wall of the esophageal lumen (e.g., tumors, strictures, outpouchings called *diverticula*), or *extrinsic*, outside the esophageal lumen, such as a tumor or swelling that prevents the passage of food. Dysphagia caused by swelling can occur as a side effect of certain types of drugs such as antidepressants, antihypertensives, and asthma medications.

Achalasia is a failure to relax the smooth muscle fibers of the GI tract. This especially occurs as a result of failure of the lower esophageal sphincter (LES) to relax normally with swallowing. The affected person reports a feeling of fullness in the sternal region and progressive dysphagia.

Although the cause of achalasia is not known, the loss or absence of ganglion cells in the myenteric plexus of the esophagus appears to be a part of the cause. The myenteric plexus is the nerve plexus lying in the muscular layers of the esophagus, stomach, and intestines. Anxiety and emotional tension aggravate the condition and precipitate the attacks. Progression of the condition results in dilation of the esophagus and loss of peristalsis in the lower two-thirds of the esophagus.

Heartburn, dyspepsia, pyrosis, or indigestion, a burning sensation in the esophagus usually felt in the midline below the sternum in the region of the heart, is often a symptom of gastroesophageal reflux and occurs when acidic contents of the stomach move backward or regurgitate into the esophagus. The presence of a hiatal hernia, drugs such as alcohol and aspirin, and movements such as lifting, stooping, or bending over after a large meal may bring on heartburn. Indigestion also may be a potential manifestation of angina associated with coronary artery disease.

Certain foods act as muscle relaxants and can also bring on heartburn. For example, chocolate contains four substances that can relax the LES: caffeine, theobromine, theophylline, and fat. Fat-rich foods lower sphincter muscle pressure by release of cholecystokinin from the upper intestinal mucosa. Fat also delays emptying of the stomach, giving more opportunity for this effect to occur. Other implicated foods include spicy and highly seasoned foods, onions, alcohol, peppermint, and spearmint.

Emotional stress can stimulate the vagus nerve, which controls the secretory and motility functions of the stomach. Stimulation of this cranial nerve causes the stomach to churn, increases the flow of various gastric juices, and causes contraction and spasm of the pylorus (opening of the stomach into the duodenum). Heartburn can occur if some of the stomach contents are displaced into the esophagus during this nervous activity.

Abdominal pain accompanies a large number of GI diseases and may be mechanical, inflammatory, ischemic, or referred. *Mechanical pain* occurs because of stretching of the wall of a hollow organ or the capsule of a solid organ. *Inflammatory pain* occurs via the release of mediators such as prostaglandins, histamine, and serotonin or bradykinin that stimulate sensory nerve endings.

Ischemic pain occurs as tissue metabolites are released in an area of diminished blood flow. Ischemic pain may originate from decreased blood flow to organs or the abdominal muscles. Abdominal muscle trigger points can mimic pain from organ disease and can intensive visceral dysfunctions.[291] Abdominal muscle trigger points respond to physical therapy treatment.[249,296]

Referred pain usually is well localized and may be associated with hyperalgesia and muscle guarding. Pain from the spine also can be referred to the abdomen, usually as a result of nerve root irritation or compression. This type of neuromusculoskeletal pain referred to the abdomen is characteristically associated with hyperesthesia over the involved spinal dermatomes and is intensified by motions such as coughing, sneezing, or straining.

GI bleeding may be characterized by coffee-ground emesis (vomiting of blood that has been in contact with gastric acid), hematemesis (vomiting of bright red blood), melena (black, tarry stools), or hematochezia (bleeding from the rectum, or maroon-colored stools), depending on the location of the lesion. Bleeding may not be clinically obvious to the client and may be diagnosed only by further testing.

The major causes of upper GI bleeding in the therapy population are erosive gastritis common in (1) severely ill people with major trauma or systemic illness, burns, or head injury; (2) peptic ulcers; (3) use of nonsteroidal antiinflammatory drugs (NSAIDs) such as aspirin or ibuprofen; and (4) chronic alcohol use. Drugs such as warfarin, heparin, and aspirin, used as anticoagulants in the treatment of pulmonary emboli, venous thrombus, or valvular abnormalities, can contribute to or exacerbate gastric erosion and subsequent bleeding.

Accumulation of blood in the GI tract is irritating and increases peristalsis, causing nausea, vomiting, or diarrhea with possible referred pain to the shoulder or back. The digestion of proteins originating from massive upper GI bleeding is reflected by an increase in blood urea nitrogen (see Table 40-2). Other complications include fatigue, postural hypotension, tachycardia, weakness, or shortness of breath on exertion. Slow, chronic blood loss may result in iron-deficiency anemia.

Fecal incontinence (inability to control bowel movements) has both psychologic and physiologic contributing factors. Psychologic factors include anxiety, confusion, disorientation, and depression. The most commonly observed physiologic causes seen in a therapy practice are neurologic sensory and motor impairment (e.g., stroke and spinal cord injury); anal sphincter damage secondary to traumatic childbirth, sexual assault, hemorrhoids, and hemorrhoidal surgery; altered levels of consciousness; and severe diarrhea. External anal sphincter damage is a form of underactive pelvic floor and can be improved with focused exercises.

SPECIAL IMPLICATIONS FOR THE THERAPIST   16-1

Signs and Symptoms of Gastrointestinal Disease
Fluid and Electrolyte Imbalance

Body fluid loss associated with weight loss, excessive perspiration, or chronic diarrhea and vomiting may cause an imbalance in the body chemistry (electrolyte imbalance) and may cause orthostatic changes in blood pressure (i.e., postural drops in blood pressure).

Electrolyte changes often include decreased potassium, which alters the sodium-potassium pump necessary for normal muscle function (contraction and relaxation). Muscle cramping occurs, which increases a person's risk for musculoskeletal injury during exercise.

The client with chronic diarrhea who is taking antidiarrheal agents containing bismuth subsalicylate, such as Pepto-Bismol, Bismatrol, Pink Bismuth, or Kaopectate, may report darkened or black stools. The client's tongue may also appear black.

Significant postural hypotension often reflects extracellular fluid volume depletion as occurs with excessive body fluid loss. The maintenance of arterial pressure during upright posture depends on adequate blood volume, an unimpaired venous return, and an intact sympathetic nervous system. Monitoring vital signs and observing for accompanying symptoms promote safe and effective exercise for anyone with the potential for electrolyte imbalance. See Chapter 5 and Appendix B: Guidelines for Activity and Exercise.

In a screening interview, the therapist should always ask clients if there are any other symptoms of any kind to report. Remember to ask about the use of nutritional or other supplements (especially among athletes) as these can have adverse GI effects on some people. For example, creatine used to improve athletic performance can cause loss of appetite, diarrhea, dizziness, and cramps, presumably from dehydration.

Pelvic Floor Muscle Rehabilitation

The physical therapist can assist individuals with constipation associated with defecatory disorders involving the skeletal muscle of the pelvic floor. Pelvic floor muscle strength, tone, endurance, coordination, and breathing patterns can be assessed. Fecal incontinence related to underactive or weak pelvic floor muscles responds to pelvic floor muscle strength training.[114] In fact, a systematic review concluded that pelvic floor muscle training represents an appropriate treatment for women with persistent postpartum fecal incontinence.[114] Retraining pelvic floor muscle function during evacuation is a key part of the rehabilitation process.[111]

Clients with overactive or dyssynergia pelvic floor muscles can be trained to relax their external anal sphincter and learn to coordinate abdominal contractions to assist stool propulsion into the rectum. Toileting techniques to avoid straining during a bowel movement may help decrease the risk of developing pudendal nerve dysfunction. The therapist can be helpful in identifying ways to incorporate scheduled toileting with transfer, strength, and balance training.[111] Bathroom and safety modifications can also be made.

Exercise and Gastrointestinal Function

Slow-transit constipation as a result of decreased neuromuscular function of the colon can be improved with aerobic exercise.[211] Strengthening exercises can also improve GI transit time.[162] The therapist has a key role in client education helping people understand the benefit of exercise and activity in promoting better bowel transit time and potentially relieving constipation. Older adults who are constipated do not want to exercise or engage in activity. They must understand that refusal to increase activity can aggravate the constipation. On the other hand, individuals with diarrhea can exercise but may have to take intermittent rest breaks to conserve energy and curtail activity during acute diarrhea in order to decrease gut motility.

During an upper quadrant screening, the therapist usually inquires whether the client has difficulty swallowing. Forward head posture or anterior disk protrusion may be a possible cause of difficulty swallowing, but a pathologic condition of the esophagus may also be the cause.

The therapist can instruct anyone with dysphagia who does not have cervical disk disease in an isometric/isotonic head lift exercise that may restore normal swallowing, thereby helping some individuals to eat normally and keep food or liquids from being aspirated into the lungs (Fig. 16-2).[188] This effect is attributed to strengthening of the suprahyoid muscles, as evidenced by comparison of electromyographic changes in muscle fatigue before and after 6 weeks of exercise.[209]

This exercise strengthens these muscles that open the upper esophageal sphincter, the "gate" that allows food or drink to slide down the esophagus to the stomach. This exercise works best for people with weak or ineffective upper esophageal sphincter but may prove useful for other types of swallowing problems. Performance of the exercise is associated with mild muscle discomfort that resolves spontaneously after a couple of weeks.[77]

Studies document the physiologic changes in the GI system and the onset of GI symptoms during and after strenuous exercise. Intensity and duration of exercise are important factors, and lower GI symptoms predominate.[340] On the other hand, GI bleeding can be reduced with regular exercise, and people with limited physical activity (e.g., physical disability) are at greater risk for ulceration and GI bleeding.

Referred Pain Patterns

An acute ulcer can present as thoracolumbar junction pain. Back pain and/or shoulder pain caused by GI bleeding and perforation associated with an ulcer of longstanding may cause painful biomechanical changes in muscular contractions and spinal movement.[103,266] The clinical presentation may be one with objective musculoskeletal findings to support a diagnosis of back or shoulder dysfunction when, in fact, the symptoms may be associated with GI bleeding. See also "Special Implications for the Therapist 14-5: Anemias" in Chapter 14.

Pain in the left shoulder caused by free air or blood in the abdominal cavity is called the *Kehr sign* and may occur with perforation of viscus (e.g., stomach ulcer, diverticular disease), after laparoscopy (lasting 24–48 hours), or after rupture of the spleen.

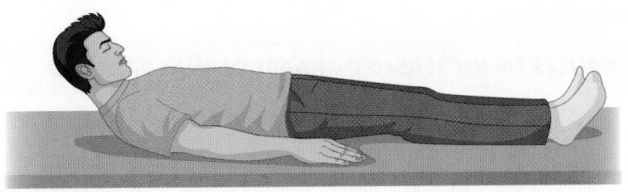

Figure 16-2

The Shaker head-lifting exercise to strengthen the upper esophageal sphincter muscle. The affected person lies in the supine position keeping the feet, back, and shoulders and arms down. The person raises the head until the toes can be seen, pauses but does not hold the head lift, then lowers the head back down. This movement is repeated 30 times (isokinetic exercise) using a relatively constant speed of movement. The person rests for 1 minute, then raises the head and looks at the feet for 1 minute, pauses 1 minute, and repeats the long look and long rest twice more (isometric exercise). The entire sequence should be completed three times daily. These exercises can be used by anyone with dysphagia or other swallowing problems in addition to hiatal hernia and gastroesophageal reflux disease (GERD). (Exercise developed by R. Shaker, MD, Medical College of Wisconsin, Milwaukee, 1998.)

AGING AND THE GASTROINTESTINAL SYSTEM

Age-related changes in GI function begin before the age of 50 years. Constipation, incontinence, and diverticular disease are the GI problems most commonly seen in older adults, but each of these disorders has many different underlying causes, and the specific pathogenesis dictates treatment.

Oral changes may include tooth enamel and dentin wear and increasing tooth decay, causing periodontal disease and subsequent tooth loss. Sensory changes may include decreased taste buds and diminished sense of smell resulting in altered sense of taste. These oral and sensory changes eventually depress the appetite and make eating less pleasurable. Salivary secretion decreases, contributing to dry mouth, and when it is complicated by tooth decay or loss, chewing food and swallowing become more difficult.

The alimentary organs (esophagus, stomach, small intestine, and colon), like all muscular structures, lose some tone with age but still manage to perform almost as well in age as in youth. Changes within the alimentary tract can include oropharyngeal muscular dysmotility with associated difficulty in swallowing (dysphagia) and reduced esophageal peristalsis combined with LES pressure, which may lead to gastroesophageal reflux. Gastric motility and emptying, as well as small intestinal motility, remain normal. Slowing of the large intestine does occur with aging, leading to constipation. The stomach exhibits a decrease in acid secretion contributing to ulcer formation while pancreatic secretions are also reduced.[105] Proteins, fats, minerals including iron and calcium, and vitamins are absorbed more slowly and in lesser amounts, and carbohydrates are absorbed more slowly.

A decline in the production of intrinsic factor, a substance that promotes vitamin B_{12} absorption in the stomach, frequently occurs after middle age. B_{12} is required to produce blood cells and to maintain the integrity of the nervous and GI systems. B_{12} deficiency can lead to

pernicious anemia with its hematologic and neurologic manifestations and GI symptoms (e.g., diarrhea, constipation, weight loss).

In advanced age, the prevalence of such problems associated with B_{12} deficiency increases to 90% for those age 90 years and older. Other causes of B_{12} deficiency with aging include low dietary intake of B_{12}, gastric atrophy (gradual loss of stomach lining with decreased hydrochloric acid), and atrophic gastritis. As these conditions progress, intrinsic factor is lost and, with it, the ability to extract B_{12} from food.

Atrophic gastritis may be the result of many possible variables, including normal aging, nutritional deficiency (e.g., iron, folate, ascorbate), autoimmune mechanisms, endocrine insufficiency (e.g., thyroid, adrenal, pancreatic), or infection (usually with *Helicobacter pylori*).[140] *H. pylori* is a Gram-negative spiral bacterium that lives in the gastric mucosal layer of humans and induces a chronic inflammatory response that can result in both peptic ulceration and gastric neoplasms. It greatly reduces the bioavailability of vitamin C, which may play a role in the development of stomach cancer.[91]

Further research is needed regarding the basic mechanisms in neuromuscular dysfunction with aging, including studies of physical characteristics of the colonic wall, pelvic floor function, and neurohormonal control of motility and sensation. Insights on the pathophysiology and mechanisms of neural injury and aging may lead to more specific treatments in the future (e.g., serotonergic agents and neurotrophins).[38]

In addition to the effects of aging on the GI system, changes in other organ systems (e.g., endocrine, cardiovascular, and nervous systems) also can affect GI structure and function, producing many variations in presentation of illness. Extraintestinal disorders, such as diabetes and the neurologic and vascular changes that occur with age, have a greater effect on the GI tract than the natural process of aging.

THE ESOPHAGUS

Hiatal Hernia

Definition and Incidence

A hiatal or diaphragmatic hernia occurs when the cardiac (lower esophageal) sphincter becomes enlarged, allowing the stomach to pass through the diaphragm into the thoracic cavity (Fig. 16-3). Hernias are either *congenital*, resulting from a failure of formation or fusion of the multiple developmental components of the diaphragm, or *acquired*. There are several theories as to how they develop.[350] One suggests that increased intraabdominal pressure forces the gastroesophageal junction through the diaphragm. Another states that fibrosis or excessive vagal stimulation shortens the esophagus, thereby pulling the gastroesophageal junction above the diaphragm. The final theory implies there is a loosening of the diaphragmatic hiatus as a result of changes in the tissue. The development may also be secondary to trauma or surgery. Most likely, hiatal hernias are multifactorial in origin.

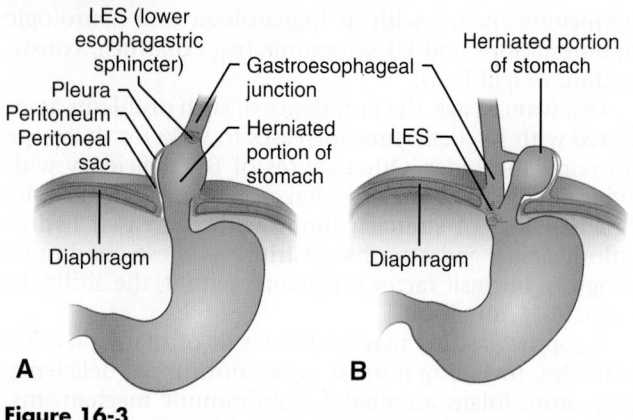

Figure 16-3

Hiatal hernia. A, Sliding hiatal hernia. Approximately 90% of esophageal hiatal hernias are sliding hernias. The stomach and gastroesophageal junction are displaced upward into the thorax (i.e., the stomach and gastroesophageal junction slide up into the thoracic cavity, following the usual path of the esophagus through an enlarged hiatal opening in the diaphragm). **B,** Rolling hiatal hernia. The remaining hiatal hernias are rolling or paraesophageal hernias. The gastroesophageal junction stays below the diaphragm, but all or part of the stomach pushes through into the thorax.

Hiatal hernia (symptomatic or asymptomatic) is common, and the incidence is estimated as 5 per 1000 people. The incidence increases with age and may be as high as 60% in people older than 60 years of age. Women are affected more often than men, and children may have the sliding type, but do not usually exhibit symptoms until they reach middle age.

Etiologic and Risk Factors

As an acquired condition, multiple causes and risk factors exist for the development of hiatal hernia. Anything that weakens the diaphragm muscle or alters the hiatus (the opening in the diaphragm for the passage of the esophagus) and increases intraabdominal pressure can predispose a person to hiatal hernia. Muscle weakness can be congenital or caused by aging, trauma, surgery, or anything that increases intraabdominal pressure (Box 16-1).

Pathogenesis and Clinical Manifestations

As part of the stomach herniates through a weakness in the diaphragm, regurgitation and motor impairment cause the major clinical manifestations associated with this type of hernia. There is evidence for its origin in esophageal longitudinal muscle dysfunction, indicating that this condition could originate from alterations in nerve innervation, alteration in the viscoelastic properties of distal esophagus, or increased strength of unopposed longitudinal muscle layers.[52,53]

Symptoms vary depending on the type of hernia present and increase in the presence of tight, constrictive clothing, or if the person is in a recumbent position. A sliding hernia may produce heartburn 30 to 60 minutes after a meal, especially if the person is lying down or sleeping in the supine position. Large sliding hernias with reflux may be associated with substernal pain. Rolling hernias are not subject to altered pressure or the resulting

---

reflux, but the person may complain of difficult and painful swallowing.

MEDICAL MANAGEMENT

DIAGNOSIS, TREATMENT, AND PROGNOSIS. Hiatal hernias may be diagnosed by endoscopy or barium swallow, although barium swallow may not provide more information than without this type of invasive diagnostic testing.[181]

The primary treatment remains symptomatic control through the use of proton pump inhibitors and other measures used to treat gastroesophageal reflux disease (GERD) (see "Gastroesophageal Reflux Disease" below). The prognosis is good overall with recurrences expected. Surgery or laparoscopic surgery is performed if medical management of GERD is not achieved.

SPECIAL IMPLICATIONS FOR THE THERAPIST 16-2

Hiatal Hernia

For any client with a known hiatal hernia, the flat supine position and any exercises requiring the Valsalva maneuver (which increases intraabdominal pressure) should be avoided during therapy intervention. Before discharge, the client must be warned against activities that cause increased intraabdominal pressure and given safe lifting instructions.

A slow return to function over the next 6–8 weeks is advised. Postoperatively (after surgical repair of the hernia using the thoracic approach), the client may have chest tubes in place requiring careful observation of the tubes during turning and repositioning and chest physical therapy to prevent pulmonary complications.

Gastroesophageal Reflux Disease

Definition

GERD may be defined as the consequences from the reflux (backward flow) of gastric contents into the esophagus accompanied by a failure of anatomic and

Table 16-3 | Causes of GERD

Decreased Pressure of LES or Alteration in Esophageal Acid Clearance	Gastric Contents Near Junction
Foods: chocolate, peppermint, fatty foods, citrus products (including tomatoes), spicy foods, garlic, onions	Recumbency Increased intraabdominal pressure
Beverages: coffee (including decaf), carbonated drinks, alcohol	
Caffeine	
Nicotine or cigarette smoke	
Central nervous system depressants (e.g., morphine, diazepam)	
Other medications (e.g., calcium channel blockers, nitrates, aspirin and other nonsteroidal antiinflammatory drugs, dopamine, theophylline, tricyclic antidepressants)	
Estrogen therapy	
Nasogastric intubation	
Scleroderma	
Prolonged vomiting	
Surgical resection (destroys sphincter)	
Position (right side-lying; sitting)	
Pregnancy (last trimester: increased progesterone relaxes sphincter)	

physiologic mechanisms to protect the esophagus. Gastroesophageal reflux occurs in most people on a routine basis. The disease occurs when this physiologic process causes significant symptoms or complications. GERD can occur without visible damage to the esophagus, termed nonerosive GERD, or injury can occur causing complications (such as esophagitis, strictures, Barrett esophagus, or gastric cancer), and is called erosive GERD.

Incidence and Etiologic Factors

GERD is one of the most common disorders seen in clinics. Approximately 10% to 20% of American adults have this disorder, seen equally in men and women.[225] Prevalence is often an estimate and data vary, depending on whether symptoms (i.e., heartburn) or visual inspection (i.e., via endoscopy) is used. Although any age can be affected, this condition has an increasing incidence with increasing age; older people are more likely to develop severe disease.[142,247]

It is estimated that nearly two-thirds of U.S. adults will experience significant symptoms of GERD sometime in their lives and that 15% or more of the population has daily symptoms of GERD and as much as one third of the population has monthly symptoms.

A wide range of foods and lifestyle factors can contribute to GERD (Table 16-3),[229] particularly obesity and smoking. Hiatal hernia and medications are other risk factors for developing GERD.

Obesity is linked to GERD,[134] which may account for the recent increase in prevalence at a time when peptic ulcer disease is decreasing. Hospitalizations (primary or secondary) because of GERD increased significantly between 1998 and 2005 (216%), particularly for infants and small children.[361] The cost in 2005 alone was $622 million.

Controversy exists as to whether *H. pylori* is protective of GERD (*H. pylori* decreases the amount of acid produced in the stomach), yet more recent studies have found no relation between *H. pylori* treatment and the development of GERD.[264]

Pathogenesis

Three factors are involved in aiding the esophagus to remain healthy: anatomic barriers between the stomach and the esophagus; mechanisms to clear the esophagus of stomach acid; and maintaining stomach acidity and acid volume. People without GERD have episodes of reflux, but do not develop disease because of normal functioning of these mechanisms.

The most important anatomic barrier between the stomach and the esophagus is the LES. Most reflux is secondary to transient relaxation of the LES that is not related to swallowing, allowing for acid to pass into the esophagus. Persons with severe disease are often found to have consistently low pressure of the LES. Hiatal hernias, where the LES and part of the stomach are above the diaphragm, create a change in the configuration of the LES increasing susceptibility to reflux.

The esophagus utilizes several mechanisms to neutralize and clear acid volume. Saliva, as well as the alkaline secretions from esophageal epithelium, serve to neutralize acid. Peristalsis and gravity help move acid out of the esophagus. Medications, cigarette smoking, esophageal dysmotility disorders, and xerostomia ("dry mouth") can all lead to increased acid exposure (by increasing the amount of time the esophagus is exposed and/or increasing the volume of acid), thereby causing GERD. Any of the predisposing factors listed in Table 16-3 may alter the pressure of the LES or alter protective mechanisms, resulting in reflux.

Several complications, such as esophagitis, strictures, Barrett esophagus, and adenocarcinoma can occur with significant GERD.[144] Esophagitis is the necrosis of the esophageal epithelial lining that leads to erosions and ulcers. Subsequent granulation of tissue causes scarring that frequently develops into esophageal strictures that narrow the esophagus, making swallowing difficult. Barrett esophagus is a precancerous change in the type of cells that line the lower end of the esophagus (columnar cells replace squamous cells). Adenocarcinoma is a cancer of the esophagus.

Clinical Manifestations

Heartburn is the principal symptom of reflux. It is described as a burning sensation beginning at the stomach and rising up the chest. It may radiate to the chest, throat, or back. Other common symptoms include chest pain, acid regurgitation, belching, dysphagia, nausea, vomiting, early satiety, and painful swallowing.[100] Heartburn most often occurs 30 to 60 minutes after a large meal or meal with alcohol, spicy foods, fats, and citrus. Lying down may worsen symptoms, making the night a common time to experience reflux.

Children and infants can be affected by GERD. For children, symptoms are similar to those experienced by adults; however, the diagnosis in infants can be difficult.

Crying, fussiness, irritability, refusal to feed, and regurgitation are common symptoms in this age group and not specific for GERD.[191] Persistent GERD has been linked to developmental problems. Neurologic disorders and GERD can have overlapping symptoms, such as irritability associated with arching, neck extension, and abnormal muscle tone with spastic movements.

Adults older than 70 years are more likely to have atypical symptoms such as dysphagia, vomiting, respiratory difficulties, weight loss, anemia, and anorexia with or without heartburn or acid regurgitation. The elderly may also present with more severe disease because of long-standing disease with few symptoms.[142]

Extraesophageal Manifestations. Up to one-third of people evaluated for heartburn will also exhibit symptoms separate from the esophagus.[159] The three main extraesophageal manifestations include asthma, cough, and laryngitis.[17,275] GERD is thought to cause asthma because of microaspirations of reflux material and/or vagally mediated esophagobronchial reflex. It is estimated that 30% to 90% of people diagnosed with asthma also have reflux symptoms.[158] Unfortunately, asthma does not respond as well as GERD to proton pump inhibitor (PPI) medications.[205,303]

GERD accounts for approximately 13% of chronic cough cases, defined as longer than 8 weeks' duration.[246] Cough can develop from two different mechanisms. The first is a direct reflux of gastroduodenal contents (inflammation of the larynx can be seen endoscopically). The second is from an indirect vagal stimulation (inflammation is not visible). It is estimated that 35% to 75% of people with GERD-related cough do not exhibit classical symptoms.[83,175] They may describe cough during the day, while upright, and/or eating. Because of the expense and discomfort of testing, a trial of PPIs is given in order to diagnose and treat.[46] Those who do not have improvement of chronic cough may undergo esophagogastroduodenoscopy (EGD) and/or 24-hour pH monitoring of the esophagus.

GERD is an important cause of laryngitis. Associated symptoms include hoarseness, difficulty swallowing, repeated throat clearing, sensation of having something caught in the throat, cough, excessive phlegm, voice fatigue, and heartburn.[275]

MEDICAL MANAGEMENT

DIAGNOSIS. The diagnosis of GERD is principally by symptoms, often defined as troublesome heartburn occurring two or more times per week and/or complications associated with reflux. Unfortunately, frequency and severity of heartburn do not predict the severity of esophageal damage. Diagnostic tools include history, endoscopy, barium radiography, and *H. pylori* and esophageal pH monitoring with or without impedance (quantifying acid and reflux events with a correlation with symptoms). A full diagnostic evaluation is not always required when history and current symptoms clearly point to GERD. A diagnosis is often made by a trial of medication (PPIs) that relieves symptoms. Other tests are utilized when warning signs (e.g., weight loss, anemia) or atypical symptoms are present in order to evaluate for possible complications or another disease.

TREATMENT. The goals of treatment are to alleviate symptoms, heal esophagitis if present, maintain remission of the disease, and manage any complications. Treatment options consist of medications, surgery when needed, or endoscopic therapy.

Lifestyle Modifications. Lifestyle modifications are recommended,[13,145] including avoiding aggravating foods such as citrus, tomatoes, spicy foods, fatty or fried foods, chocolate, mint, and caffeine. Chewing sugarless gum after a meal helps promote salivation and may aid in reducing reflux.[215] Eating more frequent and smaller meals may be beneficial. Keeping a food diary and recording any symptoms may help each individual determine personal triggers and which foods to avoid.

Clients should be aided in smoking cessation and encouraged to reduce alcohol consumption. Avoid medications that alter protective mechanisms. People with GERD should remain upright for at least 3 hours after meals[93] and should avoid meals near bedtime or naptime. Elevating the head of the bed or lying in the left lateral decubitus position can be helpful for persons with nighttime symptoms. Obese clients should wear loose-fitting clothes and lose weight.

Medications. Many people will initially use nonprescription antacids to treat symptoms. Antacids work principally by buffering gastric acid for a short period of time. Other nonprescription medications include H_2-blockers (e.g., cimetidine, ranitidine, famotidine). These medications block histamine, which normally induces parietal cells via gastrin to secrete acid. Unfortunately, these are most effective for nighttime symptoms rather than meal-induced symptoms and are less effective in healing esophagitis and other complications.

The most effective therapy is the use of acid suppression with PPIs (e.g., Prilosec, Aciphex, Prevacid, Nexium). These medications reduce nighttime and meal-induced acid production, although they do not completely shut off all acid production. PPIs are superior to H_2-blockers in relieving symptoms and healing esophagitis (both nonerosive and erosive). PPIs are well tolerated and have as their main side effects diarrhea and headaches. Omeprazole can interfere with warfarin.

PPIs may often be given for long periods of time for people with daily symptoms, erosive esophagitis, and/or complications. Many clients with mild to moderate disease can consider a step-down approach once a PPI has healed the esophagitis and relieved symptoms. This may include a switch to an H_2-blocker or prokinetics.[131] Younger clients and more severe disease predicted the need for PPI maintenance therapy. PPIs may increase the risk for community-acquired pneumonia[170] and enteric infections[178]; they may also interfere with calcium absorption (leading to osteoporosis), particularly when high doses of PPIs were used.[327] Evidence also suggest an interaction between PPIs and clopidogrel, leading to an increase in cardiovascular events.

Individuals should avoid prolonged and regular use of antacids as this can reduce the body's phosphate levels, with resultant fatigue and loss of appetite. Aluminum hydroxide tends to produce constipation, whereas magnesium hydroxide can cause loose stools or diarrhea in some individuals.

Surgery. Surgical procedures (e.g., antireflux surgery) are available for carefully selected individuals when conservative (nonoperative care) has failed to control symptoms.[307] Surgery attempts to reconstruct the normal anatomic and physiologic function of the diaphragmatic hiatus and eliminate the need for medications. Minimally invasive surgery is done laparoscopically. Experienced surgeons in a hospital with a high volume of procedures should perform this type of surgery.

Postoperative complaints occur in approximately 25% of people,[241] and include gas bloating, dysphagia, and diarrhea. Antireflux surgery does reduce the need for stricture dilation but has no effect on the development of Barrett esophagus.[59] Many clients may still require medication following the surgery. Gastric bypass surgery may be the treatment of choice when the underlying problem is morbid obesity.[257,307] Not everyone is a good candidate for surgical intervention and relapse rates are still higher than hoped.[307,324]

Endoscopic Therapy. Endoscopically delivered techniques for the treatment of GERD include radiofrequency therapy to the gastroesophageal junction, implantation of a bioprosthesis into the LES or endoscopic injection of bulking agents into the LES, suture plication of proximal gastric folds (gastroplication), transoral incision less fundoplication, and a staple system that creates a partial fundoplication.[135] Data to establish long-term efficacy of these techniques have not been established nor have certain guidelines been given for when endoscopic therapy is indicated.[85] Most procedures have not been shown to be superior to available surgical and medical treatments.

PROGNOSIS. The prognosis is good for GERD symptom resolution and reduction of complications. GERD can be a long-term disease, particularly with clients who have severe symptoms, severe esophagitis, or chronic low LES pressure. Six months after discontinuation of therapy, GERD frequently returns. GERD can contribute to asthma and vocal cord inflammation, and people who have uncontrolled acid reflux are at increased risk of developing esophageal cancer, which has a poor prognosis.[84,106]

SPECIAL IMPLICATIONS FOR THE THERAPIST | 16-3

Gastroesophageal Reflux Disease

Clients with GERD are often treated in a therapy practice or rehabilitation setting for orthopedic and other conditions. Occasionally, GERD presents with atypical head and neck symptoms (e.g., sensation of a lump in the throat) without heartburn.

Exercise and Gastroesophageal Reflux Disease

Exercise is important for anyone with GERD who is overweight. Excess abdominal fat puts pressure on the stomach; even moderate weight loss can reduce symptoms. However, people with GERD may have trouble exercising because some types of physical activity can worsen symptoms. In fact, GERD induced by strenuous exercise is extremely common among athletes. The degree of reflux is greater in activities with more body agitation (e.g., running, aerobics) than in swimming or biking.

Strenuous exercise inhibits both gastric and small intestinal emptying, which may contribute to GERD. This, combined with the potential for relaxation of the gastroesophageal sphincter, suggests the importance of avoiding high-calorie meals or fatty foods (or other triggers) immediately before exercising to avoid or minimize exercise-related GERD.[340]

The therapist can be instrumental in providing education and encouragement, essential to the lifestyle modifications necessary to this condition, and assist the person to implement changes related to diet and exercise.

Positioning

Any intervention requiring a supine position should be scheduled before meals and avoided just after eating. Modification of position toward a more upright posture may be required if symptoms persist during therapy. Consider a trial of the exercises to strengthen the muscles around the esophageal sphincter (see Fig. 16-2).

For nocturnal reflux, encourage the individual to sleep on the left side with a pillow in place to maintain this position. Right side lying makes it easier for acid to flow into the esophagus because of the effect of gravity on the esophagus (the lower esophagus bends to the left and this straightens out with right side lying).[157] See "Special Implications for the Therapist 16-2: Hiatal Hernia" above. Activities that increase intraabdominal pressure, constipation, which often accompanies back pain and other conditions (see Table 16-2), and tight clothing must be avoided.

The presence of GERD requires careful positioning to promote drainage of secretions without causing reflux. This is more readily accomplished when the stomach is empty. Positioning clients with GI dysfunction for breathing control and coughing maneuvers requires special attention to minimize the risk of aspiration. Although head-up positions minimize reflux by reducing intraabdominal pressure, they can promote aspiration of pharyngeal contents. Side-lying positions (especially left side lying) prevent regurgitation and aspiration and promote oropharyngeal accumulations and ease of suctioning.[70]

Other Considerations

Polypharmacy (the use of multiple medications for a single disorder or for comorbidities) can result in significant toxicity and drug interactions when taken with medications for acid-related diseases. Any new or unusual symptoms reported to the therapist should be documented with physician notification. Fracture risk increases with prolonged use of PPIs in adults with osteoporosis. The therapist can instruct anyone taking PPIs over a long period of time in an osteoporosis prevention program.[326,358]

With postoperative complications, airway clearance techniques (formerly, chest physical therapy, pulmonary physical therapy, and pulmonary hygiene) may be indicated. In addition, coughing and bronchospasm can result from a vagally mediated reflex secondary to refluxed acid contents in the esophagus. The therapist also may observe reflux in clients who have chronic bronchitis, asthma, and pulmonary fibrosis.

Esophageal Cancer

Overview and Incidence

Histologically, two types of esophageal cancer exist: squamous cell and adenocarcinoma. Squamous cell is typically develops in the middle of the esophagus, whereas adenocarcinoma is more often located in the distal portion of the esophagus. Worldwide, more than 90% of all esophageal cancers are squamous cell carcinomas. In the West, however, there has been a decline in the frequency of squamous cell carcinoma and a dramatic rise in the frequency of adenocarcinoma of the esophagus,[72] with adenocarcinoma being more common.

Esophageal cancer is relatively uncommon, accounting for only 6% of GI cancers, but the incidence of adenocarcinoma is rising. For the year 2012, the estimated number of cases was 17,460, whereas the number of deaths was 15,070.[294] Men are significantly more likely to develop esophageal cancer than women. The median age at diagnosis in the United States between 2001 and 2005 was 69 years.

Etiologic and Risk Factors

Esophageal cancer is known for its marked variation by geographic region, ethnic background, and gender. In the United States, adenocarcinoma of the esophagus most frequently affects middle-aged white men and often develops from Barrett esophagus, whereas squamous cell cancer is more common in blacks and is associated with alcohol and tobacco use.[36,61]

Other risk factors for developing squamous cell esophageal cancer include exposure to nitrosamine, corrosive injury to the esophagus (burning from chemicals), achalasia, vitamin deficiencies (vitamins C, E, and B_6, niacin, selenium, and zinc), and human papillomavirus infection.[108,173,200,321]

Adenocarcinoma is highly correlated with Barrett esophagus, gastroesophageal reflux, tobacco use, and obesity. Approximately 5% to 15% of people with GERD will develop Barrett esophagus.[290]

Pathogenesis

Both adenocarcinoma and squamous cell carcinoma develop through a stepwise process that allows cells to grow unchecked accompanied with uncontrolled cell death. Several growth factors allow for autonomous growth, such as epidermal growth factor and transforming growth factor-α. Disordered apoptosis (cell death) is seen in most esophageal cancers, with an alteration in genes which usually regulate apoptosis.[280] Cancer cells, most often seen in adenocarcinoma associated with Barrett esophagus, have an increased expression of telomerase that allows for unlimited cellular replication. Esophageal cancer also exhibits factors that promote neo-angiogenesis (new blood vessel formation), invasion, and metastasis.[192]

Barrett esophagus is a complication of GERD that can lead to adenocarcinoma. It occurs when the normal epithelial cells of the lower esophagus are replaced with columnar cells, typically seen in the intestine. This process is termed *metaplasia*. One hypothesis is that stem cells are either located in the esophagus or migrate from the bone marrow in order to repair damage from reflux. The repeated need to repair cells would result in mistakes in the DNA (genomic instability) and eventually develop a cell that is cancerous.[163]

Persons with Barrett esophagus are at a 30- to 40-fold increase risk for developing cancer.[300] People who are diagnosed with Barrett esophagus are screened and placed on a surveillance program.[345]

Clinical Manifestations

Presenting symptoms for both squamous cell and adenocarcinoma of the esophagus are similar. The most common symptom is dysphagia, initially with solids and progressing to involve liquids. Weight loss occurs in 90% of affected people. Other symptoms include odynophagia (pain with swallowing), cough, hoarseness, chest pain, and regurgitation. Odynophagia is frequently associated with an ulcerated tumor. Most clients with early esophageal tumors are asymptomatic. Symptoms are often associated with progressive disease, such as recurrent pneumonia from the formation of an esophagorespiratory fistula or chest pain from tumor invasion into periesophageal structures.

MEDICAL MANAGEMENT

PREVENTION. Preventing GERD and Barrett esophagus is the major method of reducing rates of esophageal adenocarcinoma.[44] Despite this knowledge, the rates of esophageal adenocarcinoma are increasing. There are many possible reasons for this, but the exact reason(s) remains unclear. It is possible that GERD is underreported and undertreated in many adults, especially those older than age 65 years. Many people with GERD may have few or no symptoms, so that progression of the condition to Barrett disease and transformation to adenocarcinoma goes unnoticed until it is too late.[348]

Whereas early screening and detection can reveal dysplasia (atypical, precancerous cells), there is no evidence that such screening programs actually reduce morbidity or mortality associated with this condition.[304] Studies also show that suppression of reflux does not protect from developing esophageal cancer. Targeted surveillance of high-risk people may be beneficial.[99]

Studies suggest that 40% of individuals with esophageal adenocarcinoma have no history of GERD symptoms.[130] This means that screening only individuals with known GERD will leave out a significant portion of adults who may be affected. And there are reports of incurable malignancies developing despite endoscopic surveillance programs.[313]

Research is underway to identify a biomarker or better guidelines for the surveillance of esophageal cancer in high-risk people. Primary prevention for squamous cell esophageal cancer centers on modifiable risk factors, such as excessive alcohol intake and smoking.[81]

DIAGNOSIS AND STAGING. Diagnosis is made by endoscopy with cytology and biopsy. Following a diagnosis, staging of the disease is performed by endoscopic ultrasonography, with chest and abdominal computed tomographic (CT) scanning, positron emission tomography scanning, laparoscopy, and video-assisted thoracoscopy to determine the presence of metastatic lesions and the most appropriate treatment.[325] The American Joint Committee on Cancer (AJCC) TNM (tumor, node, metastasis) system is used to stage both types of esophageal cancer.[262]

TREATMENT. Esophageal cancer is classified as resectable with curative intent, resectable but not curable, and not resectable and not curable. As with other solid tumors, surgery is preferred for cure. Endoscopic therapy can be utilized for early disease but not for more advanced disease. The presence of distant metastases, invasion of the mediastinal muscularis or pleural invasion, or distant lymph node involvement excludes a curative resection. Curative surgery consists of tumor removal with esophageal reconstruction.

The use of preoperative chemotherapy with radiation (neoadjuvant chemoradiation) has been controversial, although a more recent trial has shown neoadjuvant chemoradiation to be beneficial for both types of esophageal cancer.[337]

Individuals with unresectable disease, metastatic disease, or poor operative candidates may receive radiation therapy, which provides short-term relief of symptoms. Other options include esophageal brachytherapy, external beam radiation, stent placement, targeted antibodies,[255] and chemotherapy. The use of brachytherapy appears to be associated with severe toxicity[217] and fewer complications are noted with radiation given after stent placement[137] for obstructive disease.

PROGNOSIS. Endoscopic surveillance can detect esophageal adenocarcinomas when they are early and curable, but most, approximately 50%,[330] of these neoplasms are detected at an advanced stage. Carcinoma of the esophagus has a high morbidity and mortality with 5-year survival rate for stage I is approximately 80%; for stage II, it is approximately 50%; for stage III, it is approximately 10%; and for stage IV it is 0%.[323]

The first symptoms of esophageal cancer are not usually apparent until the tumor involves the entire esophageal circumference. More importantly, by that time the tumor has often invaded the deeper layers of the esophagus and adjacent structures and is unresectable. Esophageal cancer metastasizes rapidly, and given the continuous nature of lymphatic vessels in the area, removal of lymph nodes with the tumor is difficult, contributing to the poor prognosis.

| SPECIAL IMPLICATIONS FOR THE THERAPIST | 16-4 |

Esophageal Cancer

Lymphatic vessels of the esophagus are continuous with mediastinal structures and drain to the lymph nodes from the neck of the celiac axis. Metastasis is via this lymphatic drainage, with tumors of the upper esophagus metastasizing to the cervical, internal jugular, and supraclavicular nodes. During an upper quarter screening examination the therapist may identify changes in lymph nodes, requiring medical referral.

The usual precautions regarding clients with cancer apply to those with neoplasms of the GI system. The primary concern is the side effects of chemotherapy-induced bone marrow suppression. An exercise regimen including aerobic exercise at a minimal level enhances the immune system and is incorporated whenever possible. See also "Cancer and Exercise" in Chapter 9.

Radical surgery for thoracic esophageal cancer is highly invasive and often leads to respiratory complications; thoracoscopic surgery is a less-invasive alternative, but may still result in respiratory decline. Airway clearance techniques discussed in Chapter 15 may be needed postoperatively for anyone undergoing surgery for this condition.[222]

Esophageal Varices

Esophageal varices are dilated veins in the lower third of the esophagus immediately beneath the mucosa. Dilation occurs in the presence of portal hypertension, usually secondary to cirrhosis of the liver. All the blood from the intestine drains via the portal vein to the liver before passing into the general circulation. Therefore, any disease of the liver or portal vein that obstructs the flow of blood will cause expanding force pressure.

The normal anatomic reaction to this condition is to decompress the portal venous system by opening up bypass veins (collaterals), most commonly around the lower esophagus and stomach. When blood flow can no longer be counterbalanced by the variceal wall tension, the dilated veins (varices) rupture and bleed.

Variceal bleeding usually presents with painless but massive hematemesis with or without melena. Associated signs range from mild postural tachycardia to profound shock, depending on the extent of blood loss and degree of hypovolemia (decreased amount of blood in the body).

Diagnosis requires differentiation from peptic ulcer, gastritis, and other bleeding sources, often concurrent conditions in people with cirrhosis secondary to alcoholism. Diagnosis is made by endoscopy. Bleeding varices constitute one of the most common causes of death in people with cirrhosis and other disorders associated with portal hypertension; therefore, prevention and treatment are very important to prevent and replace blood loss and maintain intravascular volume.

Treatment aims to either reduce portal hypertension or act in another fashion to relieve the pressure in the esophageal vessels. Splanchnic vasoconstrictors, such as vasopressin or somatostatin, and nonselective β-blockers act to constrict vessels. Endoscopic interventions such as band ligation,[18] tissue adhesions, or sclerotherapy (the injection of hardening agents) are available to obliterate the vessel, although varices eventually recur. For acute bleeds, temporizing measures include balloon tamponade and placement of an expandable stent.[125] About half of all episodes of variceal hemorrhage cease without intervention, although a high risk of rebleeding exists.

For bleeding not controlled with these methods, a stent may be placed between the hepatic vein and the intrahepatic portion of the portal vein (transjugular intrahepatic portosystemic shunt).[94,116] This procedure provides a means of lowering portal pressure. Liver transplantation may be considered in cases unresponsive to treatment.[104]

SPECIAL IMPLICATIONS FOR THE THERAPIST   16-5

Esophageal Varices

The primary concerns in therapy are to avoid causing rupture of varices and proper handling of clients with known GI bleeding. Carefully instruct the client in proper lifting techniques and avoid any activities that will increase intraabdominal pressure (see Box 16-1). See also "Special Implications for the Therapist 14-5: The Anemias" in Chapter 14 and "Portal Hypertension" in Chapter 17.

For the client with known esophageal varices, observe closely for signs of behavioral or personality changes. Report increasing stupor, lethargy, hallucinations, or neuromuscular dysfunction. Watch for asterixis (involuntary jerking movements), a sign of developing hepatic encephalopathy.

To assess fluid retention, inspect the ankles and sacrum for dependent edema. To prevent skin breakdown associated with edema and pruritus, caution the client and family members caring for that person to avoid using soap when bathing the client and to use moisturizing cleansing agents instead. Precautions must be taken to handle the client gently, turning and repositioning often to keep the skin intact. Rest and good nutrition will conserve energy and decrease metabolic demands on the liver.

Congenital Conditions

Esophageal Atresia and Tracheoesophageal Fistula

Overview. Esophageal atresia and tracheoesophageal fistula (TEF) are the most common esophageal anomalies and common congenital defects, occurring in approximately 1 in 4000 live births with equal gender distribution. Esophageal atresia develops when the esophagus fails to develop as a continuous passage (recanalize) and TEF forms when the lung bud fails to separate completely from the foregut, forming an abnormal communication between the lower portion of the esophagus and trachea. Esophageal atresia occurs as an isolated defect in only 7% of cases; it is accompanied by TEF for the remaining cases (Fig. 16-4).[71]

TEF are typically two types, a distal-type (89%) and an H-type fistula (3%). There are other types of TEF but they are much more rare. In isolated esophageal atresia, the esophagus ends in a blind pouch and the lower esophagus connects to the stomach. Esophageal atresia with a distal-type TEF exhibits an upper esophageal blind pouch and communication with the trachea and the lower esophagus. Other associated conditions include congenital heart disease, prematurity, and the VACTERL (*v*ertebral, *a*nal, *c*ardiac, *t*racheal, *e*sophageal, *r*enal, and *l*imb) complex. Specific abnormalities include imperforate anus, patent ductus arteriosus, and cardiac septal defects.

Etiologic Factors and Pathogenesis. Because esophageal atresia and TEF are congenital malformations, the

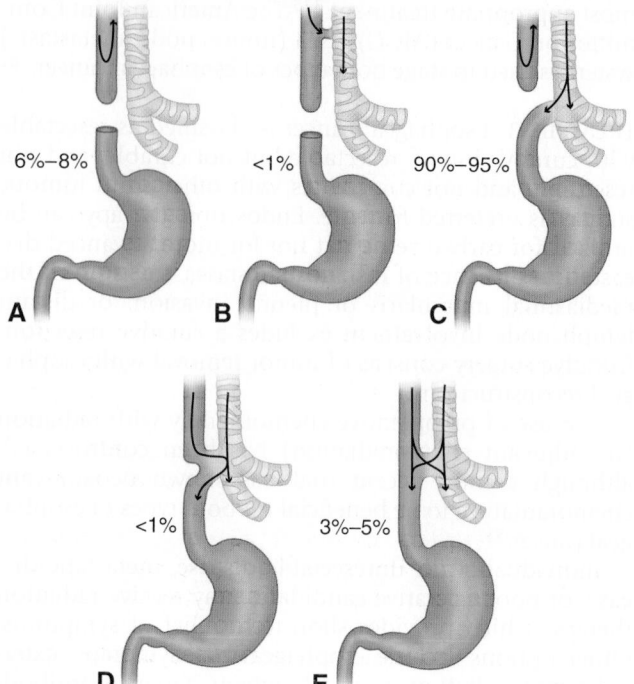

Figure 16-4

Five types of esophageal atresia and tracheoesophageal fistula. A, Simple esophageal atresia. Proximal and distal esophagus end in blind pouches. Nothing enters the stomach; regurgitated food and fluid may enter the lungs. **B,** Proximal and distal esophageal segments end in blind pouches, and a fistula connects the proximal esophagus to the trachea. Nothing enters the stomach; food and fluid enter the lungs. **C,** Proximal esophagus ends in a blind pouch, and a fistula connects the trachea to the distal esophagus. Air enters the stomach; regurgitated gastric secretions enter the lungs through the fistula. **D,** Fistula connects both proximal and distal esophageal segments to the trachea. Air, food, and fluid enter the stomach and lungs. **E,** Simple tracheoesophageal fistula between otherwise normal esophagus and trachea. Air, food, and fluid enter the stomach and lungs. Between 90% and 95% of esophageal anomalies are type C; 6% to 8% are type A; 3% to 5% are type E; and less than 1% are type B or D.

cause is unknown, but abnormalities are postulated to arise from genetic defects which prevent the trachea from separating from the esophagus during the fourth to sixth weeks of embryonic development. Defective growth of endodermal cells leads to atresia (closure or absence of a normal body opening or tubular structure).

Clinical Manifestations. The blind end of the proximal esophagus has a capacity of only a few milliliters, so as the infant with esophageal atresia swallows oral secretions, the pouch fills and overflows into the pharynx, resulting in excessive drooling and, occasionally, aspiration. It can often be seen prenatally as polyhydramnios, because of the fetus' inability to swallow fluid.

If a fistula connects the trachea with the distal esophagus, the abdomen fills with air and becomes distended, potentially interfering with breathing. If the fistula connects the proximal esophagus to the trachea, the first feeding after birth will signal a problem. As the infant swallows, the blind end of the esophagus and the mouth fill with fluid that is aspirated into the lungs when the infant tries to take a breath. This triggers a protective cough and the choke reflex with intermittent cyanosis. Coughing, choking, and cyanosis are called the three Cs of TEF and may occur, especially, with the H-type fistula, which may not be diagnosed for weeks to months after birth.

MEDICAL MANAGEMENT

DIAGNOSIS, TREATMENT, AND PROGNOSIS. Esophageal anomalies are usually diagnosed at birth on the basis of clinical manifestations, but new technology is making in utero diagnosis more readily available. Occasionally this condition escapes detection until adulthood, when recurrent pulmonary infections call attention to it. Confirmation of the non–H-type fistula is made by passing a catheter into the esophagus with radiographs of the chest and abdomen taken with the tube in place to show the level of the blind pouch. Fluoroscopy using radiopaque fluid also may be used to establish the diagnosis. Esophagography and bronchoscopy are often helpful in determining configuration of the defects.

Surgical treatment to restore esophageal continuity and eliminate the fistula usually is performed shortly after birth. Surgical procedures may be performed in stages for infants who are premature, have multiple anomalies, or are in poor health. Antibiotics are instituted early owing to the certainty of aspiration pneumonia.

Without early diagnosis and treatment this condition is rapidly fatal. Early detection prevents feedings until the problem is corrected; feeding can cause aspiration and its complications. The long-term survival rate is nearly 90%.

THE STOMACH

Gastritis

There is currently no universally recognized classification or definition for gastritis. Gastritis is not a single disease but represents a group of the most common stomach disorders. These disorders have in common disease limited to the mucosa and not extended beneath the muscularis mucosae. Based on clinical features, gastritis can be classified as *acute* or *chronic*.

Other classifications may be made according to clinical, endoscopic, radiographic, or pathologic criteria. *Acute gastritis* may be hemorrhagic or acute erosive, reflecting the presence of bleeding from the gastric mucosa. Gastric erosions and sites of hemorrhage may be distributed diffusely throughout the gastric mucosa or localized to the body of the stomach.

Chronic gastritis has three forms: *H. pylori* gastritis, multifocal atrophic gastritis (MAG), and autoimmune metaplastic atrophic gastritis. *H. pylori* gastritis is typically in the antral portion of the stomach and is caused by the bacteria *H. pylori*. Multifocal atrophic gastritis is often related to *H. pylori* as well, but is patchy, involving the body and antrum. Autoimmune metaplastic atrophic gastritis is the autoimmune destruction of the body of the stomach and accounts for less than 5% of cases of chronic gastritis. As a result of the destruction of cells and the absence of gastric acid, pernicious anemia develops. *H. pylori* may also be associated with autoimmune metaplastic atrophic gastritis.[250]

Many other types of gastritides exist, including infectious gastritis, granulomatous gastritis, and reactive gastritis. Infectious gastritis may be caused by bacteria, viruses, and rarely fungi and parasites. The most common bacterium, of course is *H. pylori*. Other bacteria are much less commonly involved in gastritis. Cytomegalovirus frequently affects the entire GI tract, particularly in immunocompromised people.

Reactive gastritis, or acute erosive gastritis, includes medications and toxins, alcohol, portal hypertensive gastropathy, cocaine, stress, radiation, bile reflux, and aging gastropathy.

Aspirin and NSAIDs are the most common cause of reactive gastritis. Chemotherapy drugs are also known to cause an acute, hemorrhagic/erosive gastritis.

Acute erosive gastritis associated with physiologic stress, often referred to as *stress-induced gastritis*, is associated with hospitalization for severe life-threatening disease, central nervous system injury, or trauma (particularly burns but also renal failure, mechanical ventilation, sepsis, and hepatic failure).

Most people with gastritis are asymptomatic. Of those with symptoms, the most noticeable is epigastric pain with a feeling of abdominal distention, loss of appetite, and nausea. Pain is much less common with erosive gastritis than with ulcer disease. Other symptoms relate to the cause of the gastritis, such as heartburn, low-grade fever, and vomiting. Occult (no visible evidence) GI bleeding commonly occurs, especially in cases of trauma and in people taking aspirin or other NSAIDs. Chronic gastritis may be asymptomatic, or pain may occur after eating accompanied by indigestion.

The diagnosis of gastritis may be made by a careful history, but confirmation is made by upper endoscopic examination, possibly including biopsy, because epigastric pain may be caused by peptic ulcer, gastroesophageal reflux, gastric cancer, biliary tract disease, food poisoning, and viral gastroenteritis.

Management of gastritis requires treatment of the underlying problem.

SPECIAL IMPLICATIONS FOR THE THERAPIST   16-6

Gastritis

Half of all clients receiving NSAIDs on a long-term basis have acute gastritis (often asymptomatic). The therapist should continue to monitor clients for any symptoms of GI involvement indicating need for medical referral. For the client with known chronic GI bleeding, urge the client to seek immediate attention for recurring symptoms such as hematemesis, nausea, or vomiting.

Urge the client to take prophylactic medications as prescribed by the physician. Steroids should be taken with milk, food, or antacids to reduce gastric irritation; antacids can be taken between meals and at bedtime. Aspirin-containing compounds should be avoided unless specifically recommended by the physician. See also "Special Implications for the Therapist 16-1: Signs and Symptoms of Gastrointestinal Disease" above, and "Special Implications for the Therapist 14-5: The Anemias" in Chapter 14.

Peptic Ulcer Disease

Definition and Overview

Peptic ulcer disease (PUD) is an erosion or an ulcer of the stomach or duodenum owing to a number of different causes. Pepsin, an enzyme that is active in acid, is often the final cause of the lesion, despite the inciting event or organism. Acute lesions of the mucosa that do not extend through the muscularis mucosae are referred to as *erosions*. Chronic ulcers involve the muscular coat, destroying the musculature and replacing it with permanent scar tissue at the site of healing. Ulcers extending to the muscularis mucosae damage blood vessels, causing hemorrhage (Fig. 16-5).

Two kinds of peptic ulcer exist, although they are collectively referred to as PUD: the *gastric ulcer*, which affects the lining of the stomach, and the *duodenal ulcer*, which occurs in the duodenum. Approximately 95% of duodenal ulcers occur in the duodenal bulb or cap. Approximately 60% of benign gastric ulcers are located at or near the lesser curvature and most frequently on the posterior wall (Fig. 16-6).

Stress ulcers, or stress-related mucosal disease, occur in response to significant physiologic stress (e.g., severe trauma, surgery, extensive burns, brain injury). For example, gastric mucosal changes develop within 72 hours in 80% of clients with burns over more than 35% of the body. The mechanism causing stress ulcers is unknown but probably involves ischemia of the gastric mucosa, which has large oxygen requirements and low gastric pH (high acidity). Stress ulcers differ pathologically and clinically from peptic ulcers with very few symptoms and are painless until perforation and hemorrhage occur. Controversy currently exists as to which clients need prophylactic therapy,[6] what type (such as intravenous PPIs), and the role of enteral feeding in reducing the risk.[199]

Incidence

PUD affects approximately 6 million people per year in the United States,[87] with a prevalence rate of around 3.3% and a lifelong prevalence of 13.8%.[297] The incidence and prevalence have been decreasing over the past decade, presumed to be related to the treatment of *H. pylori*.[318] PUD equally affects both men and women.

Etiologic and Risk Factors

NSAIDs, low-dose aspirin, and *H. pylori* bacterial infection[284] are the most common causes of peptic ulcers, accounting for approximately 90% of peptic ulcers. Other causes include Crohn disease, acid hypersecretion states (such as Zollinger-Ellison syndrome), cancer, viral infections (cytomegalovirus), and drugs (cocaine). As more people are being treated for dyspepsia-related *H. pylori*, the incidence of *H. pylori*–related PUD has decreased, with other medications, such as NSAIDs and low-dose aspirin, increasing in prevalence,[220] particularly in the elderly population.

Psychologic stress, diet, caffeine, tobacco use, and alcohol consumption may have some role in causing PUD, although many studies were done prior to the discovery of *H. pylori*, and have subsequently been found to play less of a role than once thought. Corticosteroids alone do not increase the risk for PUD,[203] although they have been found when used with NSAIDs to increase the risk.

Pathogenesis

In the upper GI tract, there is a balance between mucosal insults and mucosal defenses. If there is an imbalance, an ulcer can form. Gastric acid is made by parietal cells in the stomach. There are three types of receptors on the parietal cell which stimulate production of acid: gastrin, acetylcholine, and histamine. Gastric acid production is inhibited by somatostatin and prostaglandins. Defenses include a mucous and bicarbonate layer, an epithelial barrier, and adequate blood flow. Ulcers develop when this balance is changed.

Prostaglandin deficiency can lead to the formation of ulcers. Cyclooxygenase types 1 and 2 (COX-1 and COX-2) are responsible for the production of prostaglandins.

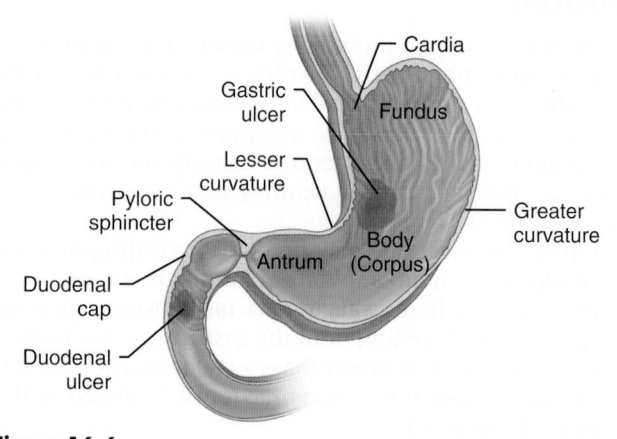

Figure 16-6

Most common sites of peptic ulcers.

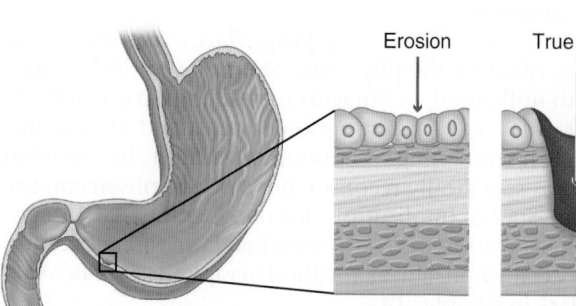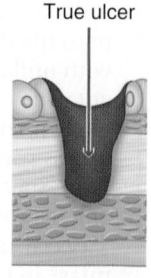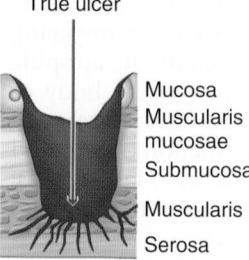

Figure 16-5

Lesions caused by peptic ulcer disease.

NSAIDs are known to lead to a deficiency of prostaglandin production through inhibiting COX-1 and/or COX-2. This then allows for enhanced gastric motility, increased mucosal permeability, neutrophils to infiltrate, and the production of oxyradicals. This eventually leads to the formation of gastric lesions and ulceration.[322] (For further discussion of the systemic effects of NSAIDs, see Chapter 5; see also Table 5-1 for a list of commonly used NSAIDs).

Although *H. pylori* has been proven to cause PUD, the mechanism is not completely understood. It may be the result of a direct effect on the parietal cell, causing an increased production of gastrin,[150,207] or through an indirect mechanism secondary to inflammation and the production of cytokines. *H. pylori* is also a known carcinogen and involved in the development of gastric cancer and mucosa-associated lymphoid tissue (MALT) lymphoma. It is also evident that not all people who are infected with *H. pylori* go on to develop a disease (only approximately 20%).[319] Specific genes the bacteria carry may correlate not only to disease but to drug resistance.

Other drugs may cause ulcers, including methamphetamines and cocaine. It is presumed to be secondary to restricted blood flow and ischemia in the stomach.

Clinical Manifestations

There are no symptoms or physical findings specific or sensitive for PUD. In fact, many people with NSAID-induced PUD do not have pain at diagnosis. They are often discovered because of bleeding or noted on an EGD exam. The classic symptom of PUD, when present, is epigastric pain described as burning, gnawing, cramping, or aching near the xiphoid, coming in waves that last several minutes. Pain may radiate to the back.

Many people report symptoms outside the classic presentation of PUD. Some people are asymptomatic until complications occur; this is especially typical in the older adult as weakened abdominal muscles and diminished pain perception mask early symptoms or present as nonspecific indicators such as mental confusion.

A family history of GI cancer in the presence of symptoms that are worrisome for malignancy associated with ulcer disease include unintentional weight loss, iron deficiency and bleeding, persistent vomiting, jaundice, or left supraclavicular lymphadenopathy. Endoscopy should be performed on individuals with these symptoms.

Complications. Bleeding from a peptic ulcer is a serious complication, requiring hospitalization and causing deaths every year. Approximately 15% of people with PUD will develop bleeding, mostly in the older population. One study found that 68% of people who presented with bleeding secondary to PUD were older than age 60 years.[228] Bleeding may be manifested by hematochezia (bleeding per rectum), hematemesis (vomiting blood), coffee-ground emesis, or melena (dark, tarry stools secondary to blood). The elderly tend to have more episodes and more severe bleeding secondary to higher use of aspirin, NSAIDs, antiplatelet medications, and other comorbidities.[146]

Perforation of the stomach or duodenum may occur, presenting with sudden severe pain (thoracic spine from T6 to T10 with radiation to the right upper quadrant), associated with hemodynamic compromise. Fever may be present; bowel sounds may be absent with guarding of the abdomen. This requires immediate surgical attention.

Gastric outlet obstruction (rare) may occur because of scarring of the prepyloric region from healed ulcerations or a neoplastic process. Affected individuals may exhibit nausea, vomiting, early satiety, and weight loss.

MEDICAL MANAGEMENT

DIAGNOSIS. Ulcers are diagnosed on the basis of symptoms, history, and laboratory/endoscopic testing. Because upper GI symptoms are common in clinical practice, it is not practical to perform endoscopy on all individuals with symptoms consistent with PUD. A "test and treat"[174] method allows for the testing for *H. pylori* in people who are likely to have the organism and do not have worrisome symptoms (see above).

Tests can be performed to diagnose *H. pylori* that do not require endoscopy, such as antibody testing (serum or whole blood), enzyme-linked immunosorbent assay, stool antigen test, or urea breath test. If positive, treatment for the eradication of *H. pylori* can be given. As the prevalence of *H. pylori* decreases, alternative treatment models will need to be addressed, such as prescribing PPIs. Upper endoscopy is the test of choice for diagnosing PUD. Not only does endoscopy determine the site of ulceration, but biopsies can be obtained to evaluate for cancer and aid in diagnosing *H. pylori*.

Tests performed on endoscopically obtained specimens include urease test, culture, and polymerase chain reaction. The serum antibody test, stool antigen, urea breath test, and urease test have comparable sensitivity and specificity. The urea breath test and stool antigen test are able to detect active infection and are reliable at least 4 weeks posttreatment to confirm eradication. As resistance rates increase, eradication testing may become more common.

Contrast radiography of the upper GI tract can be used to display an ulcer; although less expensive than endoscopy, it is not used as frequently because of the inability to obtain biopsies.

PREVENTION AND TREATMENT. Treatment of PUD is oriented toward the cause. If a client is taking an NSAID, it should be discontinued and an alternative analgesic implemented, if needed. PPI therapy aids in the healing of the ulcer. If *H. pylori* is present, therapy should be toward the eradication of the organism, although the addition of a PPI can aid in the healing of complicated gastric ulcers. For those needing an NSAID or low-dose aspirin to reduce stroke or acute coronary events, evidence shows that a PPI with aspirin reduces the risk of peptic ulcer bleeding.[124] NSAIDs should be taken at the lowest, effective dose. Misoprostol can also be taken concurrently with an NSAID to reduce the risk of developing PUD.[268] However, some studies show that a subset of people who concomitantly use the antiplatelet medication clopidogrel and a PPI have a greater incidence of acute coronary events. Although the concomitant use of clopidogrel and PPIs does not need to be completely avoided, care must be taken in determining which clients are best suited and further testing may need to be done.[226]

Treatment regimens are 70% to 90% effective in the eradication of *H. pylori* and the treatment of PUD secondary to *H. pylori*.[12] Most treatment regimens include antibiotics and a PPI for 7 to 14 days (triple therapy) (Table 16-4). The "sequential regimen" has been shown to be highly effective (5 days of one set of drugs, followed by 5 more days of another set of drugs).[363] Following the eradication of *H. pylori*, maintenance therapy with a PPI is usually not warranted.[90] Follow-up endoscopy should only be performed when ulcers are large or complicated or when initial biopsies were inadequate or had suspicious biopsy results. Reinfection with *H. pylori* following initial eradication is low; even so, researchers are working on vaccine development[107] to prevent recurrence.

Bleeding peptic ulcers are most often treated endoscopically. Injection, clipping, bipolar electrocoagulation, or heater probe therapy are options, depending on what is seen endoscopically.[171] Nearly all cases of perforation require surgical intervention/consultation. Outlet obstruction caused by scarring of the duodenum or caudal portion of the stomach typically needs endoscopic or surgical treatment.

PROGNOSIS. Because of improved medical treatment of PUD, including treatment of *H. pylori* and the availability of PPIs, the hospitalization rate for PUD has significantly decreased (by 21% between 1998 and 2005).[87] There has also been a significant reduction in mortality, except in the older population.[301,302] Prognosis is usually good and medical management can adequately control ulcers unless massive hemorrhage or perforation occurs, which carries a high mortality. In the elderly, the mortality of a perforated ulcer is 3 to 5 times higher (up to 50%) than in younger people.[23] Mortality from a bleeding ulcer, around 5%, is also increased in the elderly.[172,183]

Well-controlled, double-blind studies show that curing *H. pylori* usually results in curing PUD, although treatment failure is not uncommon. More research is needed in determining the optimal treatment for non–*H. pylori*-, non–NSAID-related PUD, a class of PUD that is now increasing.[11]

SPECIAL IMPLICATIONS FOR THE THERAPIST   **16-7**

Peptic Ulcer Disease
Monitoring Symptoms and Vital Signs

Ulcer presentation without pain occurs more frequently in older, aging adults and in persons taking NSAIDs for painful musculoskeletal conditions, especially arthritis. Anyone with this type of medical history should be monitored for signs and symptoms of bleeding. Observe color (pallor), activity or exercise tolerance, and fatigue level.

Vital signs should be monitored for systolic blood pressure less than 100 mm Hg, pulse rate greater than 100 beats/min, or a 10-mm Hg or greater drop in diastolic blood pressure, with position changes accompanied by increased pulse rate, which may signal bleeding. Any client complaining of GI symptoms should be encouraged to report these findings to the client's physician.

Referred Pain Patterns

Peptic ulcers located on the posterior wall of the stomach or duodenum can perforate and hemorrhage, causing back pain as the only presenting symptom. Occasionally, ulcer pain radiates to the midthoracic back and right upper quadrant, including the right shoulder. Right shoulder pain alone may occur as a result of blood in the peritoneal cavity from perforation and hemorrhage.

When back pain appears to be the only presenting symptom, a careful history may reveal alternating or concomitant GI symptoms such as vomiting of bright red blood or coffee-ground vomitus. Back pain relieved by antacids is an indication of GI involvement and must be reported to the physician, as well as any other indication of shoulder or back pain with accompanying GI involvement.

Table 16-4	Common Types of Medications Used for GERD		
Medication	**Common Examples (Generic [Brand])**	**Mechanism**	**Common Side Effects**
Proton pump inhibitor (PPI)	Lansoprazole (Prevacid) Omeprazole (Prilosec) Esomeprazole (Nexium) Rabeprazole (Aciphex) Pantoprazole (Protonix)	Blocks acid pump and prevents stomach acid production	Headache Constipation or diarrhea Abdominal pain Nausea and vomiting
Histamine₂-receptor blocker	Cimetidine (Tagamet) Ranitidine (Zantac) Famotidine (Pepcid)	Reduces acid produced by the stomach	Headache Nausea Constipation or diarrhea Dizziness Abdominal pain
Antacid	Calcium carbonate (Tums) Calcium carbonate-magnesium hydroxide (Mylanta, Rolaids) Magnesium-aluminum hydroxide (Maalox)	Neutralizes and reduces stomach acid	Loss of appetite Constipation or diarrhea

Data from pharmacotherapy update: DiPiro JT, Talbert RL, Yee GC, Matzke GR, Wells BG, Posey LM (eds): *Pharmacotherapy: a pathophysiologic approach*, ed 8, New York, 2011, McGraw Hill; Micromedex Healthcare Series [Internet database]. Greenwood Village, CO: Thomson Reuters (Healthcare) Inc. Updated periodically.

Musculoskeletal symptoms may recur after discontinuing the NSAIDs, owing to the masking effects of these drugs. Once the drug is discontinued, painful symptoms may return in the presence of continued underlying ulcer disease. Medical follow-up is required in such situations.

Exercise and Peptic Ulcer Disease

Researchers have reported that exercise at least three times a week greatly reduces the risk of GI bleeding. More strenuous forms of exercise such as swimming and bicycling do not provide greater protection from GI bleeding than do more moderate exercises such as walking.[48,231]

For the competitive athlete, during the acute episode, anxiety and nervousness may increase gastric secretions. This effect in combination with poor nutrition (often the athlete has not eaten at all) requires careful monitoring and maximizing the use of medications and food intake with the performance schedule. For the average adult uninvolved in competitive sports, regular exercise as part of stress reduction is essential during remission.

Gastric Cancer

Primary Gastric Lymphoma

Primary gastric lymphoma is a type of non-Hodgkin lymphoma that frequently arises from lymphoid tissue in the mucosa of the stomach. There are various histologic types of primary gastric lymphoma with the most common types being diffuse large B-cell lymphoma and marginal zone B-cell lymphoma, also known as MALT or MALT lymphoma. Gastric lymphoma is a rare cancer, accounting for only 2% to 8% of all primary gastric cancers.[4] It is most commonly seen in men 50 years of age or older. Epigastric pain, early satiety, nausea, vomiting, and fatigue characterize clinical symptoms.

H. pylori is associated with MALT lymphoma and eradication of the organism can result in varying degrees of regression in 70% to 80% of affected people.[50,364] Treatment for clients with disease that either does not respond to *H. pylori* eradication or is not *H. pylori*–related can be treated with surgery, radiation, or chemotherapy.

Prognosis varies depending upon the staging and histologic type (40%-70% survival at 5 years),[120,230] but is better than gastric carcinoma or GI lymphoma because the cancerous cells remain localized longer. Research is also underway to find biomarkers in order to better stage, treat, and determine prognosis.[4]

SPECIAL IMPLICATIONS FOR THE THERAPIST 16-8

Primary Gastric Lymphoma

Special considerations relate to any complications present with this condition, such as anemia from intestinal bleeding or complications associated with chemotherapy and radiation therapy. See "Special Implications for the Therapist 9-1: Oncology/Cancer" in Chapter 9.

Gastric Adenocarcinoma

Definition and Incidence. Gastric adenocarcinoma, a malignant neoplasm arising from the gastric mucosa, constitutes more than 90% of the malignant tumors of the stomach. Gastric cancer is the second most common cause of cancer death in the world,[235] with almost a million new cases worldwide in 2008.[356] In the United States, for the year 2014, 22,200 new cases are estimated and 10,990 deaths.[10]

Gastric cancer is divided into two types: tumors of the cardia (the upper part of the stomach adjoining the esophagus) and noncardia (lower part of the stomach). Noncardia tumors have been declining while the incidence of cardia tumors has increased. Gastric cancer can also be classified by histologic subtypes: intestinal type and diffuse type. The intestinal type is related to environmental and dietary risk factors and is most often seen in areas with a high incidence of gastric cancer. The diffuse type is typically seen in younger people and carries a worse prognosis.

Etiologic and Risk Factors. In the United States, *H. pylori* infection is associated with noncardia type cancer. Epstein-Barr virus, another infective agent that has been found in noncardia gastric tumors, may also cause gastric cancer.[218] Smoking has been linked to both cardia and noncardia types of gastric cancer.[169] Lifestyle choices that increase the risk of stomach cancer include dietary factors such as low intake of fruits and vegetables,[91] ingestion of salt[347] and salt-preserved foods, and consumption of smoked fish and meat containing nitrates.[57,136] Obesity may also be a risk factor for cardia-related gastric cancer.[51] Other nonenvironmental risk factors include individual susceptibility, pernicious anemia, which causes atrophy of the gastric mucosa,[232] blood group A (may be related to the blood antigen or genes in close proximity), previous gastric resection, and gastric polyps.

Men are twice as likely as women to have stomach cancer during their lifetime. Asian individuals have a higher rate of stomach cancer than persons of other races.[234] The most likely age group affected is adults 65 years and older.

Pathogenesis. The development of the intestinal type of gastric cancer is thought to begin with a series of changes to the mucosa. The first change is chronic inflammation (gastritis), followed by intestinal metaplasia (change in normal gastric epithelial cells to an intestinal type), then dysplasia (significant cellular abnormalities), ending with invasive carcinoma.[60]

H. pylori infection appears to play a major causal role in the development of gastric cancer, particularly in the noncardia portion of the stomach. *H. pylori* has been deemed a group 1 carcinogen (definitely carcinogenic to humans) and is the leading cause of gastric carcinoma worldwide. Several genes have been located in the *H. pylori* genome that may contribute to the cancerous changes of the gastric cells.[270]

The most common site for adenocarcinoma appears to be the glands of the stomach mucosa located in the distal portion of the stomach on the lesser curvature of the pre-pyloric antrum (see Fig. 16-6).

Clinical Manifestations. The most common clinical manifestations are weight loss and abdominal pain. Other symptoms include early satiety (feeling full despite small food intake), nausea, gastric outlet obstruction (tumors near the pyloric sphincter), or occult bleeding. Most clients remain asymptomatic until the disease is advanced (80%), which results in a poorer prognosis. Typically only 50% of people are candidates for surgical resection and cure. Peptic ulcers commonly harbor gastric cancers, making biopsies of ulcers important. Paraneoplastic syndromes are rare clinical manifestions of gastric cancer (discussed in Chapter 9).

MEDICAL MANAGEMENT

PREVENTION. At the present time, the best advice for reducing the risk of stomach cancer is to alter lifestyle-related risk factors, such as avoiding foods that may be related to an increased risk, quit smoking, and lose weight if obese. There is conflicting data as to whether eradication of *H. pylori* would reduce the risk and trials are ongoing.[204,265] In families or areas with a high incidence of gastric cancer, screening endoscopy can be performed.[216]

DIAGNOSIS. Diagnosis may be delayed because of a lack of symptoms or by because symptomatic relief can be obtained from using nonprescription medications. Endoscopy is typically the first test performed with biopsies of suspicious lesions. Staging is accomplished with CT, which can appropriately determine if metastases are present, and endoscopic ultrasonography, which assesses depth of invasion.

TREATMENT. Surgical therapy is still the treatment of choice for primary gastric adenocarcinoma. Unfortunately, only 50% of people diagnosed with gastric cancer are candidates for resection. Of these people, approximately 50% will have micrometastases at the time of surgery and have a return of the disease. Clients who are candidates for surgery may receive neoadjuvant chemotherapy (preoperatively) and combined adjuvant chemotherapy and radiation therapy. Persons who are not surgical candidates may receive palliative chemotherapy and stent placement for obstruction of the pylorus, but the disease is incurable. Endoscopic therapies are available for people with early disease.[299]

PROGNOSIS. Prognosis depends on the degree of gastric wall penetration, the presence of lymph node involvement, and the location of the primary site. People with localized disease who successfully undergo surgery have a 5-year survival rate of 47%,[96] which is improved to 55% with chemotherapy. Overall, there is 5-year survival rate of approximately 20%, principally as a result of late stage detection.[62,112]

| SPECIAL IMPLICATIONS FOR THE THERAPIST | 16-9 |

Gastric Cancer

Epigastric or back pain, possibly relieved by antacids, is a frequent complaint that the physician must differentiate from PUD. In general, the first manifestations of carcinoma are caused by distant metastasis when the condition is quite advanced. The therapist may palpate

the left supraclavicular (Virchow) lymph node, or the client may point out an umbilical nodule.

After surgery, position changes every 2 hours, deep breathing, coughing, and incentive spirometry (use of a handheld device to provide visual feedback for voluntary maximal inspiration) may be used to prevent pulmonary complications. The semi-Fowler position (head of the bed raised 6-12 inches with knees slightly flexed) facilitates breathing and drainage after any type of gastrectomy.

Congenital Conditions

Pyloric Stenosis

Definition and Overview. Pyloric stenosis (PS) is an obstruction at the pyloric sphincter (the sphincter at the distal opening of the stomach into the duodenum) that occurs in 1 in 1000 live births. The pyloric sphincter is a ring of muscles that serve to close the opening from the stomach into the intestine (Fig. 16-7). Obstruction occurs as a congenital condition, or in adults the most common causes are ulcer disease or cancer. Treatment of GERD has greatly reduced the number of acquired PS cases. When present as a congenital condition, it is known as *hypertrophic PS*, which is caused by hypertrophy of the sphincter and is one of the most common surgical disorders of early infancy.

Incidence and Etiologic Factors. The cause of congenital hypertrophy of the pyloric sphincter is unknown. White males are affected more commonly than females in a 4:1 ratio. It is more likely to occur in a full-term infant than in a premature infant, especially the first-born child. Siblings, offspring of affected persons, and fathers and sons are at increased risk of developing PS (genetic predisposition). Prophylactic administration of erythromycin to newborns exposed to neonatal pertussis has been reported to have a possible causal role in infantile PS.[45,195] The role of *H. pylori* as a cause of infantile hypertrophic PS is under investigation.[65,236,292]

Increased third-trimester maternal gastric secretion associated with maternal stress-related factors increases the likelihood of PS in the infant. PS may also be associated with other congenital conditions such as Turner syndrome, trisomy 18, intestinal malrotation, esophageal and duodenal atresia, and anorectal anomalies.

The incidence of adult idiopathic PS is unknown, but it is considered rare. Although many physicians think this condition is secondary to local disease, others think the condition in adults is the same entity as that observed in infants and children, but in a milder form and later in appearance.

Pathogenesis. The histologic and anatomic abnormalities in adult PS are indistinguishable from those in the infantile form. Individual fibers of the pyloric sphincter thicken or hypertrophy, so the entire sphincter is grossly enlarged and inelastic.

Hyperplasia of the pyloric muscle occurs because of the extra peristaltic effort required to force the gastric contents through the narrow opening into the duodenum. This hypertrophy and hyperplasia form a palpable nodule severely narrowing the pyloric canal between the stomach and the duodenum, causing partial obstruction.

Over time, inflammation and edema further reduce the size of the lumen, progressing to complete obstruction preventing food from passing from the stomach to the small intestine. Progressive obstruction results in complications of malnutrition and fluid and electrolyte abnormalities.

This may be the result of a lack of localized nitric oxide synthase, associated with smooth muscle relaxation, or from decreased muscle neurofilaments.[161]

Clinical Manifestations. Projectile vomiting is the most common and dramatic early symptom and may occur at birth. *Projectile vomiting* describes forcible vomiting that ejects vomitus 1 foot or more when in a supine position and 3 to 4 feet when in an upright or side-lying position.

Overall, the age of onset and pattern of vomiting vary, but usually regurgitation or occasional projectile vomiting develops around the second to fourth week after birth. Projectile vomiting quickly leads to dehydration and lethargy with rapid progression to complete obstruction and the accompanying complications of malnutrition, weakness, wasting, weight loss, and fluid and electrolyte imbalances.

The palpable nodule is firm, moveable, about the size of an olive, and felt in the right upper quadrant in approximately 80% of all infants with PS. Persistent or episodic symptoms in some adults may extend from infancy, with nausea and vomiting, epigastric pain, early satiety, epigastric pain, weight loss, and anorexia most commonly present. In contrast to congenital PS in the infant, the abdominal mass that occurs in adult PS is too small to be palpable.

MEDICAL MANAGEMENT

DIAGNOSIS, TREATMENT, AND PROGNOSIS. In infancy, diagnosis is usually by history and recognition of the clinical presentation. Ultrasound imaging is so accurate for the diagnosis of PS that it has replaced the upper GI series.

Some infants are treated with antispasmodic drugs to relax the pylorospasm and nutritional management,

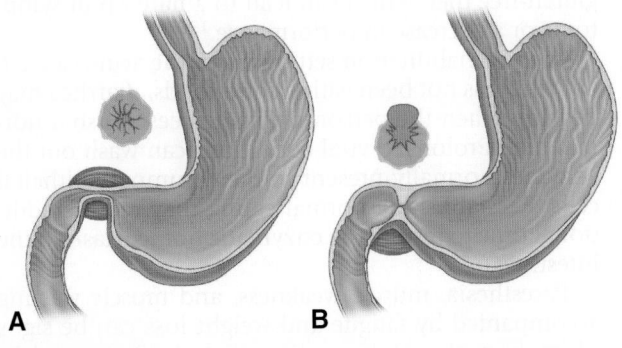

Figure 16-7

Hypertrophic pyloric stenosis. A, Enlarged muscular area nearly obliterates the pyloric channel. **B,** Longitudinal surgical division of muscle down to the submucosa or the placement of an expandable stent (not shown) establishes an adequate passageway.

including refeeding the infant after vomiting, waiting to see if the pylorus spontaneously opens by 6 to 8 months of age (although not usually done in the United States). Pyloromyotomy (local resection of the involved region of the pylorus), often performed laparoscopically, is typically the procedure of choice. Endoscopic balloon dilations, and pyloroplasty have been successfully utilized, but the recurrence rate is high. Placement of a stent at the site of obstruction is gaining popularity as an alternative intervention procedure for adults with unresectable cancer.

Postoperative vomiting is not uncommon in the pediatric population, especially during the first 24 to 48 hours. Prognosis is very good following surgery with infants able to resume normal growth and development. Complications include persistent pyloric obstruction; partial, superficial, or total wound separation (dehiscence); or in the case of stent implantation, stent migration.

THE INTESTINES

Malabsorptive Disorders

There are myriad diseases that have malabsorption of nutrients as a consequence. These diseases typically affect the small intestine where most nutrients are absorbed. The most common disease is celiac disease. Other malabsorptive disorders include infectious causes; short-gut syndrome secondary to surgery; structural defects such as strictures/fistulas; or a deficiency of digestive enzymes seen in pancreatic insufficiency. Celiac disease is covered here because it is the most common malabsorptive disorder.

Celiac Disease

Definition and Overview. Celiac disease is an immune-mediated disorder triggered by the exposure of the digestive tract to gluten in people who are susceptible. Celiac disease was once thought to be rare, but with improved methods of detection and understanding of clinical manifestations, it has become one of the most common disorders in westernized countries. It currently affects approximately 1% of the population and the incidence is increasing.[338] With westernizing of diets, more of the world will also become affected in the future.

Risk Factors. Celiac disease is more common in people with other autoimmune diseases, immunoglobulin (Ig) A deficiency, some genetic syndromes (e.g., Down, Turner), with a family history of celiac disease, type 1 diabetes, and thyroiditis.

Etiologic Factors. This disorder occurs in people with a genetic predisposition. It is strongly associated with the genes *HLA-DQ2* (95%) and *HLA-DQ8*. Approximately 30% of whites carry the DQ2 gene, although this does not mean they will develop the disease. Several other genes contribute to the development of the disease,[128] with more yet to be detected. Chronic inflammation and malabsorption of nutrients appear to be responsible for most of the complications seen in celiac disease.[40]

Pathogenesis. Celiac disease is caused by the exposure of the small intestine to gluten, a compound found in wheat, rye, and barley. This triggers an immune response to the gluten, with the aggregation of T cells into the mucosa of the small intestine. This inflammatory response leads to the destruction of intestinal cells.[210] Celiac disease also is linked to a higher risk for cancer, probably because of chronic inflammation. Skin manifestations, particularly dermatitis herpetiformis (Fig. 16-8), develop secondary to autoantibodies (the same that cause bowel inflammation).[30]

Clinical Manifestations. People with celiac disease manifest a broad array of symptoms that range from no symptoms to life-altering symptoms, making the diagnosis at times difficult. The disorder is typically characterized by diarrhea (can be severe), bloating, indigestion, flatulence, weight loss, and abdominal cramping. Malabsorption and malnutrition often accompany the disease, depending on the time of diagnosis (early vs. late) with associated complications. Nutrient deficiencies include folate, iron,[80] fat-soluble vitamins, and vitamin B_{12}.[95] Clients diagnosed with celiac disease should be evaluated for nutritional deficiencies, which should be corrected.[95]

A skin manifestation often linked to celiac disease is dermatitis herpetiformis,[41] characterized by erythema, urticarial plaques, papules, grouped vesicles (blisters), and associated with an intense itch.[41] Long-term complications include osteoporosis,[26] infertility, coagulation abnormalities, anemia, and neurologic problems.[261] Cancer is a known complication, although it is not as prevalent as once thought.[92] Thyroid cancer,[343] small intestine adenocarcinoma, esophageal squamous cell carcinoma, and T-cell lymphoma are all linked with celiac disease. The risk can be eliminated or partially reduced by following the appropriate diet.[92]

MEDICAL MANAGEMENT

DIAGNOSIS. Serologic testing is available to diagnose celiac disease. The laboratory test for IgA antibodies to tTG (anti-tTG) is the recommended initial test. If positive, the confirmatory test is the IgA anti-EMA. Another test identifying deamidated gliadin peptides, for the IgG class is comparable and can be used in persons with IgA deficiency.[182,274] A small intestine biopsy is recommended to histologically prove the diagnosis. This is

typically performed by EGD. On pathology, celiac disease demonstrates an infiltration of lymphocytes, elongation of the crypts, and atrophy of the villous. A "four out of five" rule has been suggested for the confirmation of the diagnosis[43]:

- Typical symptoms of celiac disease
- Positivity of serum IgA class autoantibodies at a high titer
- HLA-DQ2 and/or HLA-DQ8 genotypes
- Celiac enteropathy found on small bowel biopsy
- Response to a gluten free diet

TREATMENT. Although other treatments are under investigation, the most practical consists of a diet free of gluten.[256] Rice, corn, quinoa, tapioca flour, potato starch, millet, and sorghum are other grain substitutes.[223] If the diagnosis is delayed or the diet not adhered to, there are many complications of celiac disease caused by chronic inflammation.

PROGNOSIS. Most people can live asymptomatic lives if they follow the strict diet. Because celiac disease has become more common and the public more aware of it, more restaurants and stores are offering special food products to accommodate people with celiac disease. Many complications of the disease can be avoided with rapid diagnosis and treatment.

SPECIAL IMPLICATIONS FOR THE THERAPIST   16-10

Malabsorptive Disorders

Athletes with prolonged unexplained illnesses may have a malabsorptive disorder, such as gluten intolerance, or the full-blown celiac disease. Celiac disease can present with a number of different symptoms with a delay in diagnosis. A multidisciplinary approach in helping the newly diagnosed athlete with celiac disease is important to the successful treatment of the disease. Athletes with celiac disease often have problems with iron absorption (leading to anemia) and/or vitamin D and calcium absorption (leading to osteoporosis and poor bone health). Even athletes with known and longstanding celiac disease need additional care and supervision in ensuring there is no disruption in their gluten-free diet, which can lead to a flare-up of symptoms or a decrease in performance.[196]

In the rehabilitation setting or for the acute care client who has not been eating solid foods, diarrhea may develop when the person begins to reestablish a normal diet. Prolonged viral conditions can wash out the enzymes normally present in the columnar epithelial cells. Reestablishing normal eating may require additional time to restore the enzymatic homeostasis in the intestines.

Paresthesia, muscle weakness, and muscle wasting accompanied by fatigue and weight loss can be signs of malnutrition (e.g., eating disorders) or malabsorbed fat, protein, or carbohydrates. Malabsorption of calcium, vitamin D, magnesium, and potassium can cause paresthesia, tetany, and positive Trousseau and Chvostek signs (see Figs. 5-8 and 5-9).

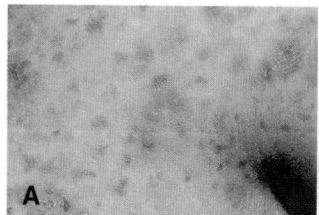
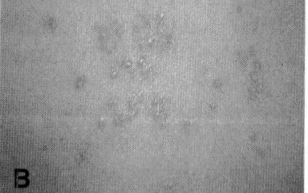

Figure 16-8

A and **B**, Dermatitis herpetiformis. Typical grouped pruritic papulovesicles associated with skin reaction from gluten sensitivity. This skin manifestation usually appears on the buttocks, elbows, or knees. It can affect children but is more common in adults between the ages of 30 and 40 years. It is almost always a sign of celiac disease and will usually resolve in 3 to 6 months with a gluten-free diet. (A, from Feldman M: *Sleisenger and Fordtran's gastrointestinal and liver disease*, ed 8, Philadelphia, 2006, WB Saunders. Courtesy of Dr. Timothy Berger, San Francisco. B, from Noble J: *Textbook of primary care medicine*, ed 3, St Louis, 2001, Mosby. Courtesy James C. Shaw, MD.)

The Trousseau sign is an indication of tetany seen as carpal spasm elicited by compressing the upper arm (as occurs when taking a blood pressure measurement). The Chvostek sign is a spasm of the facial muscles elicited by tapping the facial nerve in the region of the parotid gland; it is seen in tetany.

Other effects of malabsorptive disorders possibly seen in a therapy setting include muscle spasms caused by electrolyte imbalance (especially low calcium) and pregnancy, easy bleeding or bruising as a result of a vitamin K deficiency, and generalized swelling caused by protein depletion (Table 16-5).

Malabsorption of calcium, vitamin D, and protein can cause osteoporosis, bone pain with pathologic (compression) fractures, and skeletal deformities. In fact, 20% of osteoporosis is osteomalacia secondary to decreased absorption of vitamin D associated with malabsorptive conditions.[289]

On the other hand, excessive absorption of vitamin D and calcium through the use of calcium carbonate for acid indigestion should be evaluated by a physician; these antacids may be used by women to obtain the daily 1500-mg calcium requirement as protection against osteoporosis. The therapist can direct education and intervention toward prevention and treatment of these related conditions.

Physicians may recommend vitamin B_{12} or other vitamin B supplements for people with carpal tunnel syndrome. Malabsorption of these essential vitamins alters the structure and disrupts the function of the peripheral nerves, spinal cord, and brain and can cause numbness and tingling and permanent neurologic damage unresponsive to vitamin B_{12} therapy in extreme cases.

Vascular Diseases

Blood is supplied to the bowel by the celiac and superior and inferior mesenteric arteries. These arteries have anastomotic intercommunications at the head of the pancreas and along the transverse bowel. Obstruction of blood flow can occur as a result of atherosclerotic occlusive lesions or embolism.

Intestinal Ischemia

Intestinal ischemia results from decreased blood supply to the bowel. Ischemia can be categorized as acute mesenteric ischemia, chronic mesenteric ischemia or colonic ischemia.

Acute mesenteric ischemia is life-threatening and must be treated emergently. It results from occlusions of the visceral branches of the abdominal aorta. The most common vessel involved is the superior mesenteric artery, which accounts for approximately 50% of cases. Left ventricular or atrial thrombi associated with atrial fibrillation often leads to acute mesenteric ischemia.

The principle symptom is abdominal pain. Occult blood in the stool is common, although overt bleeding is rare. Symptoms seen later in the course include nausea, vomiting, fever, back pain, and shock. Most people with acute mesenteric ischemia are older than 50 years of age; the elderly may have atypical symptoms, including mental status changes. Acute mesenteric ischemia can also occur in response to hypovolemia (nonobstructive). In this situation, an initially protective vasoconstrictive process occurs secondary to an event, such as a myocardial infarction, hypovolemia, cirrhosis, renal failure, cardiac bypass surgery,[153] or sepsis. However, if the event continues or progresses without hemodynamic improvement, ischemia can ensue. Key to diagnosis is a high suspicion. Pain is often initially disproportionate to the physical exam.

Angiography, CT angiography, and/or magnetic resonance angiography are used to diagnose the involved vessel in occlusive disease. Treatment is to correct the underlying problem and give appropriate resuscitation. Persons with thrombotic/embolic disease or who display peritoneal signs should undergo exploratory surgery. During surgery necrotic tissue and perforated bowel can be removed, thrombectomy with repair of artery performed, and the abdomen lavaged. For people without peritoneal signs, thrombolytic agents can be considered. Papaverine, a nonspecific vasodilator, is frequently utilized in nonobstructive disease to reverse the vasoconstriction.[153] If unsuccessful, exploratory surgery may still be warranted. Mortality for acute mesenteric ischemia is high.

Chronic mesenteric ischemia, also known as intestinal angina, occurs in the setting of diffuse atherosclerotic disease of the splanchnic arteries. This leads to abdominal pain, particularly after meals (30 minutes to 3 hours), when an increased blood supply is needed during digestion, but not able to adequately flow. Magnetic resonance and CT angiography are the tests of choice to make the diagnosis. Bypass surgery is the preferred treatment, although percutaneous angioplasty and stenting procedures are alternative treatments.

Colonic ischemia is a spectrum of ischemic injury ranging from transient colitis to fulminant colitis. Unlike acute mesenteric ischemia, mortality is low. It is also more common. Factors known to contribute to colonic

Table 16-5	Symptoms Associated With Malabsorptive Disorders
Symptoms	**Malabsorbed Nutrients**
Muscle weakness, muscle wasting, paresthesia	Generalized malnutrition; fat, protein, carbohydrates
Osteomalacia	Fat, protein, carbohydrates, iron, water; vitamins A, D, K
Tetany, paresthesias, Trousseau sign, Chvostek sign	Calcium, vitamin D, magnesium, potassium
Numbness and tingling; neurologic damage	Vitamin B_{12}, vitamin B
Bone pain, fractures, skeletal deformities	Calcium, vitamin D, protein
Muscle spasms	Electrolyte imbalance, calcium, pregnancy
Easy bleeding or bruising	Vitamin K
Generalized swelling	Protein
Dermatitis herpetiformis (see Fig. 16-8)	Gluten induced

ischemia include aortic or cardiac bypass surgery, any event that results in hypotension, medications (oral contraceptives), drugs (cocaine), hypercoagulable states, and prolonged physical activity. The descending, sigmoid, and splenic flexure are the most commonly involved portions of the colon.

People older than age 60 years are most frequently affected. Symptoms include left, lower quadrant abdominal pain, urgency to defecate, and red or maroon rectal bleeding. Diagnosis is by colonoscopy and treatment includes intravenous fluids, correcting the underlying process, if able, review and stop offending medications, and surgery if needed.

SPECIAL IMPLICATIONS FOR THE THERAPIST 16-11

Intestinal Ischemia

Intestinal angina as a result of atherosclerotic plaque–induced ischemia can result in intermittent back pain (usually at the thoracolumbar junction) with exertion. Clinical presentation combined with past medical history, the presence of coronary artery disease risk factors (see Table 12-3), and the presence of peripheral vascular disease may alert the therapist to the need for a medical referral if the client has not been medically diagnosed.

Inflammatory Bowel Disease

Overview and Definition

Inflammatory bowel disease (IBD) collectively refers to two inflammatory conditions: Crohn disease and ulcerative colitis (Table 16-6). Although the two are separate entities with their own unique pathophysiology, there are many overlapping similarities. *Crohn disease* (CD) is a chronic, lifelong, inflammatory disorder that can affect any segment of the intestinal tract, although most commonly it affects the ileum or colon. It can affect all layers of the intestine and is characterized by diseased areas of intestine with normal intestine between ("skip" areas) with periods of exacerbation and remission. CD is also referred to as *regional enteritis, regional ileitis, terminal ileitis,* depending on the location of the inflammation.

Ulcerative colitis (UC) is a chronic inflammatory disorder of the mucosa of the colon, typically involving the rectum, which can then advance proximally in a continuous manner to involve the entire colon. Depending on which portion of the colon is affected, it may be more specifically referred to as *ulcerative proctitis* (involving the rectum only) or *pancolitis* (involving the entire colon).

Incidence

Both CD and UC are bowel disorders of unknown cause involving genetic and immunologic influences on the GI tract. These two conditions can occur in all age groups

---

Table 16-6 Comparison of the Characteristics of Crohn Disease and Ulcerative Colitis

Characteristics	Crohn Disease	Ulcerative Colitis
Incidence		
Age at onset	Any age; 10-30 yr most common	Any age; 10-40 yr most common
Family history	20%-25%	20%
Gender (prevalence)	Equal in women and men	Equal in women and men
Cancer risk	Increased; early detection best means of prevention	Increased; preventable with bowel resection
Pathogenesis		
Location of lesions	Any segment; usually small or large intestine	Rectum and left colon
Skip lesions	Common	Absent
Inflammation and ulceration	Entire intestinal wall (all layers) involved	Mucosal layers involved; submucosal involvement only in severe cases
Granulomas	Typical	Uncommon
Thickened bowel wall	Typical	Uncommon
Narrowed lumen and obstructed	Typical	Uncommon
Fissures and fistulas	Common	Absent; rare
Clinical Manifestations		
Abdominal pain	Mild to severe; common	Mild to severe; less frequent
Diarrhea	May be absent; moderate	Typical; often severe; chronic
Bloody stools	Uncommon unless colon is involved	Typical
Abdominal mass	Common; right lower quadrant	Uncommon
Anorexia	Can be severe	Mild or moderate
Weight loss	Can be severe	Mild to moderate
Skin rashes	Common, mild	Common, mild
Joint pain	Common, mild to moderate	Common, mild to moderate
Growth retardation (pediatric)	Often marked	Usually mild
Clinical course	Remissions and exacerbations	Remissions and exacerbations
Complications	Cancer uncommon	Cancer fairly common

and affect both genders equally; incidence peaks between the ages of 15 and 30 years, but CD can occur in later decades, usually after age 50. UC has a higher incidence and prevalence than CD, with an incidence rate of 1.2 to 20.3 cases per 100,000 persons/year and a prevalence of 7.6 to 246 cases per 100,000 persons/year. CD's incidence rate is 0.03 to 15.6 cases and a prevalence of 3.6 to 214 cases per 100,000 persons/year.[186] There are between 1 and 1.5 million people with IBD[149] in the United States. IBD is found most frequently in Northern Europe and North America; Asia sees the fewest cases.

Etiology and Pathogenesis

Although great strides have been made in the understanding of IBD on a molecular basis, many important questions remain. IBD appears to be a polygenic disease with complex interactions between gut microbiota, host immunity, and intestinal mucosal response. Multiple genes have been located that are associated with IBD. Variants in genes are specific for either CD or UC, found in both CD and UC, or associated with IBD and other immune-related diseases.[66] Several genes are associated with increased susceptibility to IBD, particularly in regards to developing CD.[74] Other genes are implicated in epithelial-barrier dysfunction or in causing cellular apoptosis (cell death), whereas abnormalities in other genes may lead to defects in transcriptional regulation.

Interactions between the host and microorganisms in the gut appear to play a crucial role in the development of IBD. Colonic health appears to depend upon tolerance of the gut immune system to the large load of microorganisms in the colon. It is hypothesized that a breakdown of tolerance may lead to IBD,[194] although evidence is currently lacking. It is known that the density of microorganisms is greater in people with UC or CD than in healthy controls.[276] However, treatment with antibacterial medication has no clinical effect upon UC, whereas in persons with CD, antibiotics can provide some benefit.[248] People with CD also exhibit a higher titer of antibacterial antibodies than those with UC.

Another key aspect of IBD involves the response of the intestinal mucosa. As stated above, for the colon to remain healthy, there must be a controlled response to microorganisms. This control is hypothesized to be maintained through toll-like receptors and nucleotide-binding oligomerization domain–like receptors on epithelial and immune cells.[1] It is suggested that these receptors contribute to tolerance. For example, several abnormalities in genes that normally code for proteins that mediate recognition of bacteria, are linked to CD.[109] Another example comes from the knowledge that less-developed countries have fewer cases of IBD than more-developed countries. One hypothesis is that the presence of intestinal parasitic worms may change intestinal immunity, leading to greater tolerance. Studies show that these parasites may activate toll-like receptors, and thereby allow for tolerance.[316]

People with IBD also have a much higher production of inflammatory cytokines (e.g., interleukin-1 and tumor necrosis factor) than those without IBD. IgM, IgA, and IgG levels are all increased in IBD, with IgG$_1$ disproportionately increased in UC. Abnormalities are seen in both

UC and CD in adaptive immunity. In UC, natural killer T cells that secrete interleukin-3 are present, which mediates epithelial-cell cytotoxicity, apoptosis, and epithelial-barrier dysfunction. CD has an increase in the production of interferon.

Because UC is typically limited to the colon, the production of antibodies to colonic cells is implicated in the pathogenesis. People with UC often express an autoantibody termed *perinuclear antineutrophil cytoplasmic antibody*. Another antibody seen in UC is an IgG$_1$ antibody against a colonic epithelial antigen that is shared with the skin, eye, joints, and biliary epithelium. This autoantibody may be responsible for the extraintestinal disease seen in people with UC.[24]

Clinical complications are principally related to the overproduction of proinflammatory cytokines (such as tumor necrosis factor-α and interleukin-1β) and fibrogenic cytokines (such as transforming growth factor-β).[279] This leads to ulceration, fistula formation, and strictures.

Pathologically, the inflammation associated with CD involves all layers of the bowel wall, referred to as *transmural inflammatory disease*, and the inflammatory process is discontinuous, so that segments of inflamed areas are separated by normal tissue in a skip pattern. Granulomatous lesions, one of the classical differences between the two diseases, are seen in CD but not UC, although granulomas aren't always seen on biopsies of CD (Fig. 16-9). A combination of the granulomas, ulceration, and fibrosis results in a cobblestone appearance of the mucosal surface of the colon (Fig. 16-10). Inflammation of the mucosa associated with UC results in small erosions and

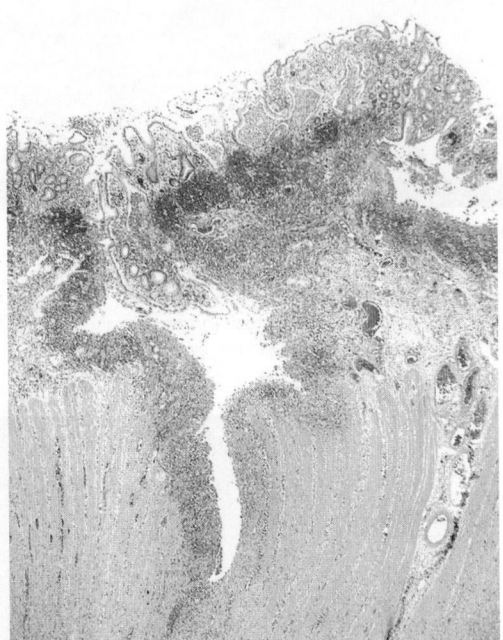

Figure 16-9

Crohn disease of the colon. A deep fissure extending into the muscle wall and a second, shallow ulcer *(upper right)*. Abundant lymphocyte aggregates are present, evident as blue patches of cells at the interface between the mucosa and submucosa. (From Kumar V: *Robbins and Cotran: pathologic basis of disease,* ed 7, Philadelphia, 2007, WB Saunders.)

subsequent ulcerations with eventual abscess formation and necrosis (Figs. 16-11 and 16-12).

Clinical Manifestations

IBD presents most often with diarrhea, abdominal pain, GI bleeding, and weight loss. The hallmark of UC is bloody diarrhea with or without mucus.[66] UC typically presents gradually often with periods of spontaneous improvement followed by relapse of disease. Severity and location of disease often dictate symptoms. Because inflammation begins in the rectum, clients often exhibit bloody diarrhea with fecal urgency, although constipation is not uncommon.

Other frequent symptoms include fever, abdominal pain, malaise and weight loss. Symptoms associated with CD depend upon the location of disease (e.g., mouth, small intestine); however, many symptoms of CD are shared with UC. CD typically begins as inflammation, but with time, most people develop fistulas and strictures. Watery diarrhea is more often seen in CD, whereas bloody diarrhea is more frequently noted in UC. For comparison of specific signs and symptoms, see Table 16-6.

Complications. Complications can be categorized as acute and chronic. The most serious acute problems seen in UC include severe blood loss and toxic megacolon. Colon cancer is the most serious long-term complication.

Risk factors for developing colon cancer associated with UC include duration of disease, degree of involvement (i.e., the greater the involvement, the more likely to develop cancer), young age at onset, severe inflammation, family history of colorectal cancer, and presence of primary sclerosing cholangitis.[66]

CD is associated with significant complications including severe bleeding; abscess formation (spontaneous and fistula associated); bowel obstruction; fistula formation with the bladder, skin, intestine, and vagina; impaired growth in children; nutritional deficiencies; and inflammation of the joints. Fistulas are seen in approximately 50% of people with CD and cause significant morbidity and quality of life changes (particularly the perianal fistulas).[341] Fistulas also carry a high risk of abscess formation.

Extraintestinal Manifestations. Studies demonstrate that certain antibodies have a cross-reaction with the colon and other organs of the body. This may account for

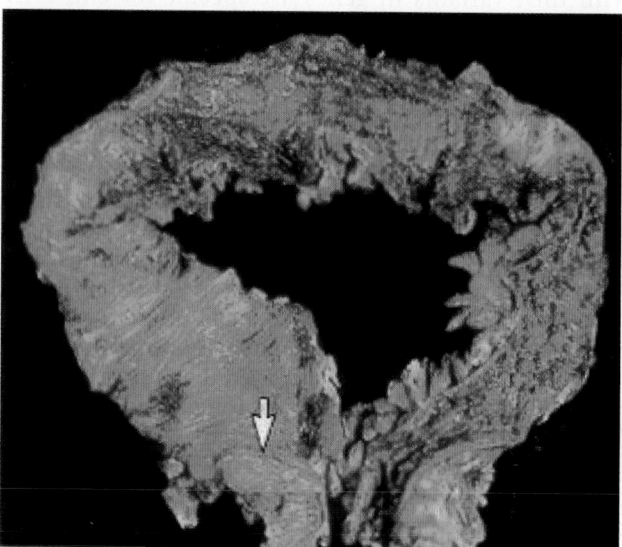

Figure 16-12

Total colectomy specimen from an individual with ulcerative colitis. The colon shows diffuse mucosal inflammation that extends proximally from the rectum without interruption to the transverse colon. The mucosal pattern in the terminal ileum and cecum (arrow) is normal. The distal mucosa is erythematous and friable with many ulcers and erosions. (From Feldman M: *Sleisenger and Fordtran's gastrointestinal and liver disease,* ed 8, Philadelphia, 2006, WB Saunders. Courtesy of Feldman's GastroAtlas online, Current Medicine Group Ltd.)

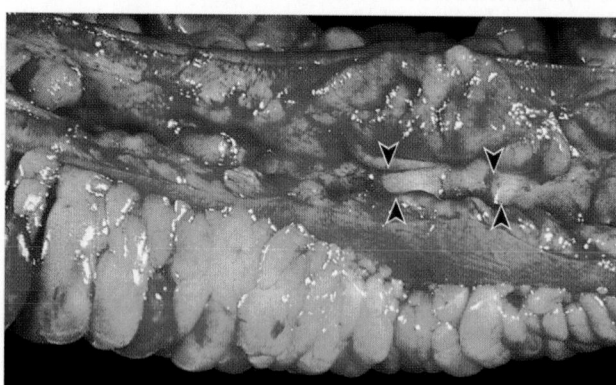

Figure 16-10

Crohn disease of the ileum, showing narrowing of the lumen, bowel wall thickening, serosal extension of mesenteric fat ("creeping fat"), and linear ulceration of the mucosal surface (arrows). (From Kumar V: *Robbins and Cotran: pathologic basis of disease,* ed 7, Philadelphia, 2007, WB Saunders.)

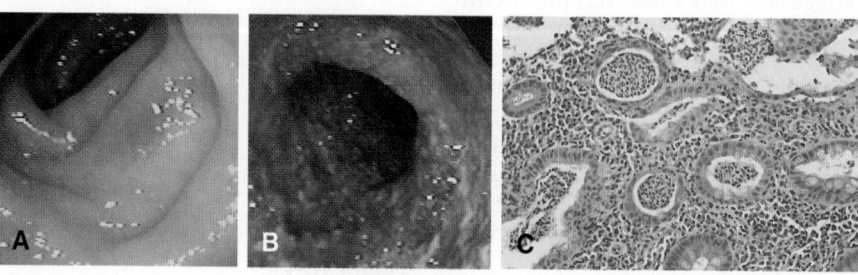

Figure 16-11

Spectrum of severity of ulcerative colitis. A, Colonoscopic findings in mild ulcerative colitis demonstrating edema, loss of vascularity, and patchy subepithelial hemorrhage. **B,** Colonoscopic findings in severe ulcerative colitis with loss of vascularity, hemorrhage, and mucopus. **C,** Histologic specimen showing a severe acute and chronic inflammatory process with multiple abscesses. (From Feldman M: *Sleisenger and Fordtran's gastrointestinal and liver disease,* ed 8, Philadelphia, 2006, WB Saunders.)

extraintestinal involvement of the joints (arthritis), eyes (uveitis), skin (erythema nodosum or pyoderma gangrenosum), lungs, biliary tree (primary sclerosing cholangitis), and the blood (anemia and thromboembolism), although studies are lacking.

Joint involvement ranging from arthralgia to acute arthritis is the most common extraintestinal finding in IBD (in 16%-33% of clients with IBD). Arthritis associated with IBD is usually continuous and symmetrical. Arthropathies associated with IBD (a subdivision of seronegative spondyloarthropathies) are divided into peripheral and axial involvement.[14,33] Persons with IBD may have both types.

Peripheral arthritis can be divided into type 1 and type 2. Type 1 is an oligoarthritis with five or fewer painful/inflamed joints, typically involving the larger joints of the lower extremity. Type 1 is usually self-limited, correlating with bowel disease activity, resolving within several months as the underlying disease is treated and without permanent sequelae or joint deformities. Type 2 is more often polyarticular, symmetrical, and involving more than five joints, particularly in the small joints of the hands (metacarpophalangeal joints). Type 2 can be chronic, but like type 1, it is usually nondeforming. Type 2 may not parallel bowel disease. Axial arthritis often occurs independent of bowel disease activity and may include inflammatory back pain, sacroiliitis, or ankylosing spondylitis. Pathologic evaluation of the synovial fluid is nonspecific without crystals or evidence of infection. Tests for specific forms of arthritis (e.g., rheumatoid factor and antinuclear antibody) usually give negative results; test results for HLA-B27 can be positive (see explanation of human leukocyte antigen [HLA] in Chapter 7; see also Table 40-20).

MEDICAL MANAGEMENT

DIAGNOSIS. The diagnosis of IBD typically requires both endoscopy and biopsy. Because biopsies only include the mucosa and not full thickness of bowel, often no distinction can be made between UC and CD. Endoscopy or colonoscopy reveals the pattern of disease and often is able to make the diagnosis between the two disorders.

TREATMENT. Therapy for both UC and CD is principally medical with surgery required less frequently. Treatment is directed toward obtaining remission of disease then beginning a maintenance therapy with the goal of keeping inflammation and symptoms under control.

Treatment for UC consists of sulfasalazine and 5-aminosalicylates (5-ASAs; mesalamine, olsalazine, and balsalazide) given orally or rectally (suppository or enema) or both. Glucocorticoids may be added either orally, rectally, or for severe disease, intravenously. If an appropriate response is not obtained, a monoclonal antibody (infliximab) or immunosuppressant (azathioprine) can be used. Infrequently, colectomy may be needed for uncontrollable disease. In the case of UC, surgery can be curative, unlike CD. Time of surgery is determined based on lab values and symptoms.[14] Maintenance therapy is initiated once disease is in remission. Multiple medications can be used, although glucocorticoids should be strictly avoided. Drugs are often selected according to their side-effects profile. Probiotics may have a role in maintenance therapy for UC, unlike CD.[164]

There are multiple indications for surgery in the treatment of UC. Among these are failure of medical therapy, toxic megacolon, intestinal perforation, uncontrollable bleeding, intolerable side effects of medications, strictures that cannot be managed endoscopically, cancer, and growth retardation in children.[54] The current surgical option of choice is a total proctocolectomy with ileal pouch–anal anastomosis, as this type of surgery preserves anal sphincter function. The most significant complication following surgery is the development of pouchitis. This is thought to be a nonspecific inflammation of the newly formed pouch caused by antibodies toward the microflora.[357] Symptoms include increased stool frequency, urgency, incontinence, and abdominal discomfort/perianal discomfort.

CD is most often treated medically with surgery offered when needed for complications or severe, unresponsive disease. Some nonprescription medications can improve symptoms such as fiber supplements and loperamide for diarrhea. NSAIDs can make symptoms worse and should be avoided. Prescription medications of choice for mild to moderate disease include 5-ASAs given orally or rectally. Glucocorticoids are often added for treatment of moderate to severe disease. Azathioprine and 6-mercaptopurine are used for moderate to severe disease. Biologic agents, such as infliximab, adalimumab, certolizumab, and natalizumab, are given when other agents are unable to control symptoms and inflammation.[64]

Indications for surgery include severe bleeding, failure to grow (children), symptomatic fistulas, bowel obstruction, abscesses, or strictures of the intestine. Modified approaches to therapy of CD may include "deep remission" (verifying that all tissue is healed endoscopically) instead of solely clinical improvement of symptoms. This may reduce the need for hospitalization and surgery. Ensuring adequate initial therapy may also lead to less involvement of tissue and less destruction of tissue.[233]

Some resistance has been noted in treating CD with biologic agents, and measuring antibodies to these agents may be helpful as well as drug levels.[221] New modalities of treatment are targeted to improve the epithelial barrier or modulate bacterial recognition/tolerance, such as toll-like receptor agonists. Other avenues of treatment include reducing inflammation using biologic agents, such as alternative anti–tumor necrosis factor-α agents[259]; antibodies that prevent leukocytes from homing to the intestine[86]; or cytokine blocking agents.[198]

Chemoprevention and routine screening colonoscopy are advised for the prevention of colorectal cancer associated with longstanding IBD. Several agents have been used as chemoprotective agents, although none have been shown to indisputably protect against the development of cancer. However, 5-ASAs and thiopurine analogues have been shown to be beneficial by reducing inflammation and are often already used in maintenance therapy.[315]

For UC, colonoscopy should be performed every 1 to 2 years after 8 to 10 years of disease with a specific biopsy protocol. Unfortunately, the cancers associated with IBD can be flat, unlike sporadic colorectal carcinoma, which are typically polypoid. Flat lesions are difficult to see endoscopically and can be missed. Currently, precise biomarkers able to detect colonic dysplasia are lacking but research is underway.[132]

PROGNOSIS. IBD is a chronic and sometimes debilitating disease with a known increased risk of intestinal cancer. The risk for colorectal cancer is related to severity, extent of disease and duration of disease.[271] People with UC have a 2% incidence of cancer after 10 years, a 9% incidence after 20 years, and an 18% incidence after 30 years of disease.[333,352]

CD also increases a person's risk for cancer, with a cumulative risk of 2.9% at 10 years and 8.3% at 30 years.[39] Risk factors for colorectal cancer include younger age at diagnosis of CD, duration of disease (longer duration increases risk), and greater interval between exams.[21] Resection of disease does not prevent the development of cancer in other portions of the bowel, so screening is important.[20,56] Colorectal cancer is responsible for 20% of IBD-related mortality.

Persons with UC have a good prognosis during the first decade after diagnosis, with a low rate of colectomy as a consequence of improved medical treatment. Approximately 85% of clients with UC have mild to moderate intermittent disease managed without hospitalization. The remaining 15% demonstrate a full-blown course involving the entire colon, severe diarrhea, and systemic signs and symptoms. Approximately 30% will undergo surgery at some point to control inflammation, whether emergently, urgently, or electively.

CD is a chronic disease without cure and most clients have an intermittent disease course. Only 13% will have an unremitting disease course and 10% maintain a prolonged remission. Less than half of people require corticosteroids at any time, but 60% to 80% of people require at least one surgical resection in their lifetime.[42,187]

SPECIAL IMPLICATIONS FOR THE THERAPIST   16-12

Inflammatory Bowel Disease
Musculoskeletal Involvement

When terminal ileum involvement in CD produces periumbilical pain, referred pain to the corresponding low back is possible. Pain of the ileum is intermittent and perceived in the lower right quadrant with possible associated iliopsoas abscess or ureteral obstruction from an inflammatory mass, causing buttock, hip, thigh, or knee pain, often with an antalgic gait. Specific objective tests are available to rule out systemic origin of hip, thigh, or knee pain (Figs. 16-13 and 16-14; see also Fig. 16-19).

Psoas abscesses most commonly result from direct extension of intraabdominal infections such as appendicitis, diverticulitis, and CD. Clinical manifestations of a psoas abscess include fever, lower abdominal pain, or referred pain as described. Flexion deformity of the hip may develop from reflex spasm with a positive psoas sign as shown. Symptoms are exacerbated by hip extension. A tender or painful mass may be palpated in the groin.

Approximately 25% of all clients with IBD present with migratory arthralgia, monarthritis, polyarthritis, or sacroiliitis. The joint problems and GI disorders may appear simultaneously, the joint problems may manifest first (sometimes even years before bowel symptoms), or intestinal symptoms present along with articular symptoms but are disregarded as part of the whole picture by the client.

Any time a client presents with low back, hip, or sacroiliac pain of unknown origin, the therapist must screen for medical disease by asking a few simple questions about the presence of accompanying intestinal symptoms, known personal or family history of IBD, and possible relief of symptoms after passing stool or gas.[103] Joint problems usually respond to treatment of the underlying bowel disease but in some cases require separate management. Interventions for the musculoskeletal involvement follow the usual protocols for each area affected.

People with IBD are known to have low bone mineral content and a high prevalence of osteoporosis. The pathogenesis is not completely understood but is considered multifactorial at this time, including possible genetic factors,[286] malabsorption, corticosteroid use, and deficiency of fat-soluble vitamins, among them vitamin K necessary for calcium binding to bone.[283]

Low bone mineral density may be more characteristic of CD than of UC, but no consistent differentiation has been made between CD and UC in this regard.[282] The therapist can provide osteoporosis education and prevention for clients with IBD. See "Osteoporosis" in Chapter 24.

The therapist must always know what medications clients are taking so that the first sign of possible side effects will be recognized and the physician alerted. Corticosteroids are an important and effective drug for treating moderate and severe IBD but carry with them all of the complications of prolonged high-dose steroid therapy (see Table 5-4).

Dehydration

Hydration and nutrition are always long-term concerns with clients who have UC or CD. The client must be observed for any signs of dehydration (e.g., dry lips, dry hands, headache, brittle hair, incoordination, disorientation; see Box 5-8), in addition to any increase or pathologic change in symptoms. Any increase in painful symptoms or increased stool output or stool frequency must be reported to the physician.

Psychologic Issues

Psychologic factors and the autonomic nervous system are implicated in the pathogenesis of IBDs.[240] The chronic nature of IBD affecting persons in the prime of life often results in feelings of anger, anxiety, and possibly depression. These emotions are important factors in the client's well-being and response to treatment and in modifying the overall course of the disease.[208]

The therapist can be instrumental in acknowledging the client's feelings, validating the effects of the disease, and prescribing an exercise program to match the needs of the individual. Exercise can help moderate depression, boost immune system function, combat the effects of long-term corticosteroid use, and help improve body image.

The therapist can help individuals develop positive coping strategies and management techniques to deal with the disruptions that can occur with intermittent and unexpected bouts of diarrhea and abdominal pain. Stress management, relaxation techniques (e.g., Physiologic Quieting, autogenic breathing, guided imagery)

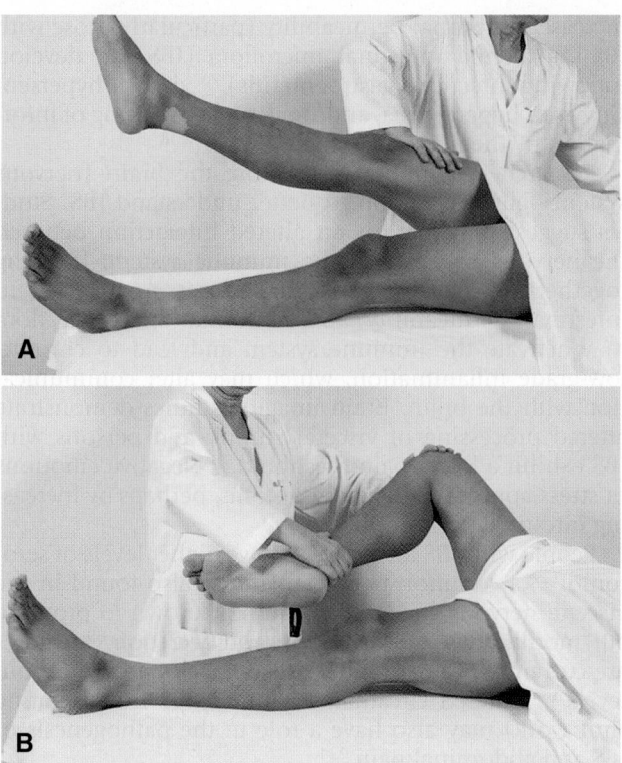

Figure 16-13

Muscle tests. A, Iliopsoas muscle test. With the client supine, instruct the client to lift the right leg straight up; apply resistance to the distal thigh as the client tries to hold the leg up. When the test result is negative, the client feels no change; when the test result is positive (i.e., the iliopsoas muscle is inflamed or abscessed), pain is felt in the right lower quadrant. **B,** Obturator muscle test. With the client supine, perform active assisted motion, flexing at the hip and knee; hold the ankle and rotate the leg internally and externally. A negative or normal response is no pain; a positive test result for inflamed obturator muscle is right lower quadrant (abdominal) pain. The physical therapist trained in internal palpation can also assess obturator dysfunction by palpating the muscle inside the vagina or rectum. (**A** from Jarvis C: *Physical examination and health assessment*, ed 6, Philadelphia, 2012, WB Saunders; **B** from Jarvis C: *Physical examination and health assessment*, ed 4, Philadelphia, 2004, WB Saunders, p. 586.)

can help with visceral pain and discomfort. The therapist can help individuals find ways to improve activity and participation, not just deal with impaired body structures and functions.

A THERAPIST'S THOUGHTS*

IBD and Pelvic Floor Activity

According to Van der Velde and colleagues, the pelvic floor muscles contract in normal subjects in response to situations perceived as threatening.[336] The data support the idea of a general defense reaction as a mechanism of involuntary pelvic floor muscle activity. The Van der Velde study was clearly looking at skeletal muscle response. It would be interesting to know which muscle they were testing—external or internal anal sphincter. This determines whether it would be treated with physical therapy or behavioral cognitive therapy.

*Beth Shelly, PT, DPT, WCS, BCB-PMD

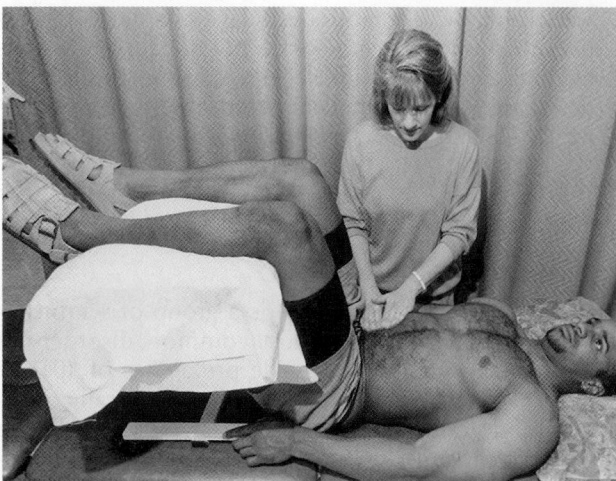

Figure 16-14

Palpating the iliopsoas muscle. In addition to assessing the McBurney point, the examiner may also palpate the iliopsoas muscle by placing the client in a supine position with the hips and knees both flexed 90 degrees and with the lower legs resting on a firm surface (a traction table stool works well for this; pillows under the lower legs may be necessary to obtain the full position). Palpate approximately one-third the distance from the anterior superior iliac spine toward the umbilicus; it may be necessary to ask the client to initiate hip flexion on that side to help isolate the muscle and avoid palpating the bowel. Palpation may produce back pain or local muscular pain from a shortened or tight muscle, indicating the need for soft tissue mobilization and stretching of the iliopsoas muscle. A positive test result for iliopsoas abscess is right lower quadrant (abdominal) pain; manual therapy (e.g., soft tissue mobilization) in this area would be contraindicated in the presence of any abdominal or pelvic inflammatory process involving the iliopsoas muscle until the infection has been treated with complete resolution.

Antibiotic-Associated Colitis

For further discussion of this topic, see Chapter 8.

| SPECIAL IMPLICATIONS FOR THE THERAPIST | 16-13 |

Antibiotic-Associated Colitis

The primary concern with any client experiencing excessive watery diarrhea is fluid and electrolyte imbalance. See special implications for fluid and electrolyte imbalances previously discussed in Chapter 5 (Special Implications for the Therapist 5-10, 5-11, and 5-12). Because the onset of this condition may occur up to 1 month after the antibiotic has been discontinued, the client may not recognize the association between current GI symptoms and previous medications. Anytime someone taking antibiotics or recently completing a course of antibiotics develops GI symptoms, especially with joint and/or muscle involvement, encourage physician notification.

Reactive arthritis occurring after *Clostridium difficile* infection is most common with colitis associated with antibiotic therapy. *Reactive arthritis* is defined as the occurrence of an acute, aseptic, inflammatory arthropathy arising after an infectious process, but at a site remote from the primary infection.

The arthritis typically involves the large and medium joints of the lower extremities and first manifests 1 to 4 weeks after the infectious insult (see Chapter 25). Reactive arthritis may include some, but not all, of the three features associated with Reiter syndrome and is often designated incomplete Reiter syndrome.

Irritable Bowel Syndrome

Definition and Incidence

Irritable bowel syndrome (IBS) is a group of symptoms that represent one of the most common disorders of the GI system, with a worldwide prevalence of 10% to 15%.[73,206] These symptoms include chronically reoccurring abdominal pain or discomfort associated with altered bowel habits[34] in the absence of structural, inflammatory, or biochemical abnormalities. Because there are no detectable organic causes, it is referred to as a "functional" disorder. IBS is separated into four categories depending on predominant symptoms as established by the Rome III criteria: diarrhea-predominant IBS (IBS-D), constipation-predominant IBS (IBS-C), mixed-symptom IBS, and unsubtyped (Box 16-2).[305]

Women are affected twice as often than men,[353] typically between the ages of 20 and 40 years. Onset of symptoms after the age of 50 years is uncommon. Many other pain syndromes and functional disorders are associated with IBS, such as fibromyalgia, chronic fatigue syndrome, temporomandibular joint disorder, and chronic pelvic pain. Psychologic conditions, such as anxiety and somatization,[287] are also seen more frequently in people with IBS. A correlation exists between IBS and a history of early adverse life events, such as physical and/or emotional abuse or sexual abuse,[32] as well as increased stress.

IBS is costly, with direct and indirect costs estimated at $20 billion,[126] and affected people use at least 50% more health care resources than matched controls.[213]

Etiologic Factors and Pathogenesis

IBS is considered a "functional" disorder because the symptoms currently cannot be attributed to any identifiable abnormality of the bowel (structural or biochemical). Current theories as to the cause of IBS include: altered GI motor activity (IBS-C affected clients have a slower transit time that increases abdominal distention and bloating),[3]

Box 16-2
SUBTYPING IRRITABLE BOWEL SYNDROME BY THE PREDOMINANT STOOL PATTERN FOLLOWING ROME III CRITERIA

1. IBS with constipation (IBS-C): ≥25% of stools are hard or lumpy and <25% of stools are loose or watery.
2. IBS with diarrhea (IBS-D): >25% of stools are loose or watery and <25% of stools are hard or lumpy.
3. Mixed IBS (IBS-M): >25% of stools are hard or lumpy and >25% of stools are loose or watery.
4. Unsubtyped IBS (IBS-U): Insufficient abnormality of consistency of stool to meet criteria of other types.

Data from Spiller R: Clinical update: irritable bowel syndrome, *Lancet* 369:1586–1588, 2007.

---

increased intestinal permeability (particularly those with IBS-D), altered intestinal microflora (IBS can develop following infectious gastroenteritis),[76] visceral hypersensitivity or hyperalgesia, and/or altered processing of information by the nervous system.[5,79,88,227,258]

Researchers continue to explore the brain (nervous system)–gut connection to better understand IBS. Studies suggest that there is an altered interaction between the nervous system and the immune system, bringing together many of the above hypothesis. An increase in intestinal permeability and abnormal intestinal flora may activate the immune system and lead to chronic, low-grade inflammation, which may alter communication with the brain. Brain imaging studies demonstrate altered processing of visceral stimuli and persons with IBS exhibit a lower pain theshhold.[79] Negative emotions or stress appear to worsen symptoms, perhaps by increasing intestinal permeability.[7]

People with IBS are noted to have higher levels of serotonin,[122] a common neurotransmitter also found in the visceral nervous system. Serotonin is known to promote gut motility, visceral sensation and secretion.[69] Studies are currently evaluating the cause for elevated serotonin levels.[166] Altered circadian rhythms (e.g., from rotating shift work) may also have a role in the pathogenesis of IBS and abdominal pain.[224]

Clinical Manifestations

Symptoms of IBS usually begin in young adulthood and persist intermittently throughout life with variable periods of remission (see specific signs and symptoms in "Diagnosis" below).

For some people, IBS symptoms are annoying but manageable. Approximately 25% of Americans have symptoms consistent with IBS, but do not seek medical attention. For others, IBS significantly affects quality of life and daily function.

Pain may be steady or intermittent, and there may be a dull, deep discomfort with sharp cramps in the morning or after eating. Often there is relief with evacuation of the bowels. The typical pain pattern consists of lower left quadrant abdominal pain accompanied by constipation and/or diarrhea. Other symptoms may include nausea and vomiting, anorexia, sour stomach, and flatus. Symptoms of IBS tend to disappear at night when the affected individual is asleep. Nocturnal GI symptoms suggest a diagnosis other than IBS.[193]

MEDICAL MANAGEMENT

DIAGNOSIS. Diagnosis is based on history, as there are currently no definitive tests. Symptom-based criteria have been developed for the diagnosis of IBS[189,252] known as the Rome III criteria[113] (Box 16-3). In conjunction with the history, inquiries must be made concerning possible "alarm" symptoms or objective findings (e.g., rectal bleeding, use of antibiotics or weight loss) that could be indications of another disease.

Extensive studies should not be undertaken if the history is consistent with IBS. However, laboratory studies that may confirm another suspected disease may be helpful. Because anemia is an alarm sign, a complete blood count is often beneficial. For subtypes IBS-D and

ROME III DIAGNOSTIC CRITERIA FOR IRRITABLE BOWEL SYNDROME

Recurrent abdominal pain for discomfort (abdominal sensation not described as pain) at least 3 days a month in past 3 months (with onset greater than 6 months prior) associated with two or more of the following:

- Improvement with defecation
- Onset associated with change in frequency of stool
- Onset associated with change in form (appearance) of stool
  Alarm indicators that suggest other diseases:
- Age >50 years
- Short history of symptoms
- Documented weight loss
- Nocturnal symptoms
- Family history of colon cancer
- Rectal bleeding
- Recent antibiotic use

Modified from Spiller R: Clinical update: irritable bowel syndrome, *Lancet* 369:1586–1588, 2007.

mixed-symptom IBS, testing for celiac disease or lactose intolerance may be appropriate. Colonoscopy should only be performed if an alarm symptom or a symptom relating to another diagnosis is present. Research is underway to identify biomarkers that are more able to reliably make the diagnosis of IBS.[156,306]

TREATMENT. As the cause of IBS is unknown, treatment is aimed at relieving symptoms. Dietary changes, medications, exercise, stress reduction, and cognitive behavioral treatment have been advocated. Although many people with IBS believe there is a connection between food and IBS symptoms, there is no clear evidence that food intolerance plays a significant role in the production of IBS symptoms.[78] Affected individuals often avoid specific foods, potentially causing nutritional deficiencies. Several studies demonstrate that dietary guidance improves both health and symptoms.[78] Elimination diets or food allergy testing should not be done unless there is clear evidence that symptoms are triggered by specific food.

Because people with IBS-C can have a slower intestinal transit time resulting in constipation, the use of fiber supplements such as polycarbophil (FiberCon) or psyllium seed (Metamucil) has been advocated, although studies are conflicting.[269,332] There is good evidence that antispasmodics, which act as GI smooth muscle relaxants, are effective for the treatment of IBS. Examples include dicyclomine, hyoscyamine and peppermint oil. Antidepressants, particularly selective serotonin receptor inhibitors and tricyclic antidepressants, improve abdominal pain and improve other IBS symptoms.[332] Loperamide improves bowel movement frequency and consistency in clients with IBS-D, although it had no effect on other IBS symptoms.

Although not completely understood, there has been a link with bacterial overgrowth and IBS symptoms. The use of an unabsorbable antibiotic, such as rifaximin, has produced significant improvement in symptoms, particularly diarrhea.[245] The efficacy of probiotics is still under investigation,[214] although *Bifidobacterium infantis* has shown some efficacy in symptom improvement.[354]

A stress-reduction program[360] with a regular program of relaxation techniques and exercise in conjunction with cognitive-behavioral therapy[185] and biofeedback training may be effective for some people. Behavioral therapy is focused on identifying and reducing or eliminating triggers and reducing negative self-talk. Hypnotherapy (hypnosis) and biofeedback therapy (relaxation training) can give some control over the muscle activity of the GI tract and the gut's sensitivity to stress and other influences.[355]

Physical activity and exercise has also shown to be of benefit in reducing symptoms[49,139] and can be implemented with other treatment modalities.[15,49]

PROGNOSIS. IBS is not a life-threatening disorder, and prognosis is good for controlling symptoms through diet, medication, regular physical activity, and stress management. Future research looks to unlock the pathophysiology of IBS in order to treat it more effectively.

SPECIAL IMPLICATIONS FOR THE THERAPIST   16-14

Irritable Bowel Syndrome

Regular physical activity helps relieve stress and assists in bowel function, particularly in people who experience constipation. It may be necessary to avoid exercises that result in jarring or jumping as this can increase pain related to abdominal organ dysfunction. The therapist should encourage anyone with IBS to continue with the prescribed rehabilitation intervention program during symptomatic periods.

Therapists must be alert to the person with IBS who has developed breath-holding patterns or hyperventilation in response to stress. Teaching proper breathing is important for all daily activities, especially during exercise and relaxation techniques.

Diverticular Disease

See also "Meckel Diverticulum" below.

Definition and Incidence

Diverticular disease is the term used to describe diverticulosis and diverticulitis. Diverticulosis refers to the presence of outpouchings (diverticula) in the wall of the colon or small intestine, a condition in which the mucosa and submucosa herniate through the muscular layers of the colon to form outpouchings (Fig. 16-15). Diverticulitis is defined as inflammation/infection of the diverticula(um) with possible complications such as perforation, abscess formation, obstruction, fistula formation, and bleeding.

This acquired deformity of the colon is rarely reversible and usually asymptomatic. The most common site in Western countries is the sigmoid colon (85% of cases), but any segment of the colon may be involved. In Asian countries, diverticular disease tends to be on the right side.

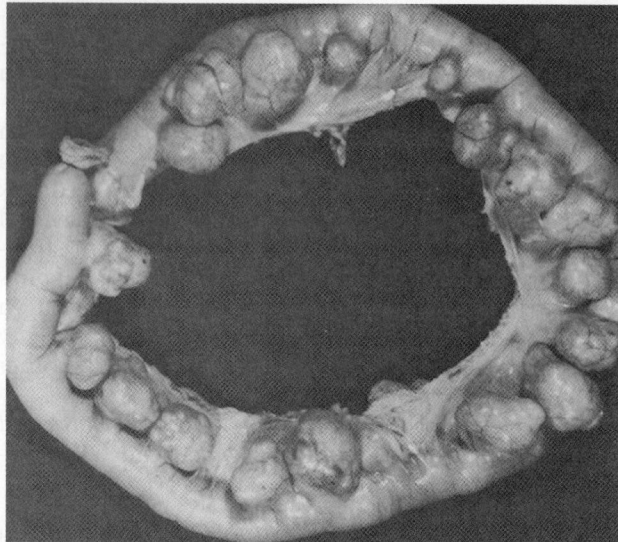

Figure 16-15

Multiple diverticula in resected section of the colon. Weak spots in the muscle layers of the intestinal wall permit the mucosa to bulge outward (herniate) into the pelvic cavity. (From Rosai J: *Ackerman's surgical pathology*, ed 7, St Louis, 1989, Mosby.)

Diverticular disease is common and increasing in incidence in westernized countries. The disease is most common in persons older than 60 years of age, although the average age has been decreasing.[82] Between the years 1998 and 2005, persons in age groups 18 to 44 and 45 to 64 years had the greatest increase in incidence, whereas the incidence in the age group 65 to 74 years remained stable. Younger people frequently have more aggressive disease and often require surgery after an initial episode.[237] Diverticula are present in as many as half of all adults older than 60 years of age,[349] with 10% to 25% developing complications, including diverticulitis.[351] Diverticular disease is more common in men younger than age 50 years, but is seen more frequently in women in older age groups.[349]

Etiologic and Risk Factors

It is well known that Western countries have a much higher incidence of diverticular disease than developing countries or countries where the diet is high in fiber. A lack of fiber was once thought to be the principal cause of diverticular disease; however, new studies provide conflicting data in which a diet high in fiber was not found to be protective.[238,334]

Risk factors associated with the development of diverticulosis include constipation, physical inactivity, red meat, obesity, smoking, and NSAID use.[119,133,311] Several connective tissue disorders also have a link with diverticular disease, including Ehlers-Danlos syndrome, Marfan syndrome, and scleroderma.[288] Genetics may also play a role as some people are born with diverticula, probably resulting from an inherited defect in the muscular wall of the intestines. The majority of people who have diverticulosis develop it with age, indicating that both heredity and lifestyle play a role.

Clients on chronic steroids and immunosuppressants are at a higher risk for developing diverticulitis.[344]

Foods such as nuts and corn were once thought to lead to diverticulitis, however recent studies have not substantiated this.[311] Fruits and vegetables, including those with small seeds, are good sources of fiber and should not be avoided.[310,328]

Pathogenesis

Diverticular disease is a multifactorial process related to diet, structural changes in the colonic wall (alterations in musculature, collagen, elastin), as well as functional changes in the bowels (intestinal motility). As discussed above, a lack of dietary fiber was traditionally believed to cause diverticula. It was thought that a low-fiber diet produced small stool volumes and decreased stool transit time. This then resulted in increased intraluminal pressure which forced the mucosa and submucosa through the weakened colonic wall. However, current studies provide conflicting results and more studies will need to be done in order to understand the role of fiber in the causality of diverticular disease.

Diverticula form at weak points in the colon wall, usually where arteries penetrate the muscularis. Changes in the muscular portion of the intestinal wall have been documented. The longitudinal muscle, taeniae coli, becomes thickened from aberrant deposition of elastin; the muscle cells themselves remain normal. There is also an increased production of collagen.[29] The circular portion of muscle, plicae circulares, which controls peristalsis, also thickens, narrowing the lumen and increasing the intraluminal pressure.[342] These changes progress as a person ages and ultimately lead to a weakened colonic wall.

Changes in intestinal motility are also associated with diverticular disease. Based on manometric catheters, clients with diverticular disease have elevated pressures compared to persons without the disease. This is postulated to occur because the colon contracts in segments, rather than a continuous tube. This increases the pressure in each fold or segment. There are documented alterations in the enteric nervous system as well, which may account for some of the abnormal motility (imbalance in excitatory vs. inhibitory influences) and research is currently underway to determine if neurotransmitters play a role in diverticular disease.[31,138]

There is also controversy regarding the pathophysiology of diverticulitis. Diverticulitis is speculated to be secondary to fecal obstruction of the diverticulum, which then causes increased pressure within the diverticulum, resulting in local ischemia. As this process continues, ulcerations and perforations form, confounded by bacterial overgrowth. This process is similar to what occurs in appendicitis. Another more recent theory attributes diverticulitis to microperforations rather than fecal obstruction of the diverticulum.[344]

In diverticulosis, for unknown reasons, there can be weakening of blood vessels, predisposing to bleeding. Bleeding is uncommon in diverticulitis and is unrelated to infection. Recurrent diverticulitis can result in increased scarring and narrowing of the bowel lumen, potentially leading to obstruction. Perforated diverticula provide an opening through which bacteria can enter, leaving the bowel at risk for a bacterial invasion into the diverticulum with subsequent abscess formation.

Clinical Manifestations

Diverticular disease is asymptomatic in 80% of affected people. Persons with diverticula that are not inflamed may exhibit mild, nonspecific, episodic pain. Symptoms may overlap with those of IBS such as bloating, cramping, irregular bowel movements, and flatulence.

When diverticula become inflamed, diverticulitis develops. Approximately 75% of diverticulitis cases are uncomplicated. Persons experience episodic or constant abdominal pain located in the left quadrant (if the sigmoid is involved) or midabdominal region, often with extension into the back. Other common symptoms include fever, change in bowel habits, nausea, vomiting, and anorexia. Bleeding is uncommon in uncomplicated diverticulitis. Approximately 10% to 15% of people will have urinary symptoms related to the close proximity of the bladder. Eating and increased intraabdominal pressure can increase pain (see Box 16-1), whereas temporary partial or complete relief may follow a bowel movement or passage of flatus.

Another entity related to diverticular disease is segmental colitis associated with diverticula. This appears to be inflammation involving tissue surrounding the diverticulum but not inside the diverticulum itself. Clinical symptoms include chronic abdominal pain (usually left-sided) associated with hematochezia (bleeding per rectum). Examination of tissue displays features similar to IBD and some affected people have been treated with drugs used in IBD therapy.[293]

MEDICAL MANAGEMENT

DIAGNOSIS. When the history and physical are suggestive of diverticulitis, the diagnosis of can be confirmed by CT of the abdomen/pelvis. Laboratory evaluation will often demonstrate an elevated white blood cell count (in approximately 50% of cases). CT of the abdomen/pelvis can also reveal complications including fistula formation, abscess, and obstruction. Colonoscopy in the acute setting of diverticulitis is avoided because of the increased risk of perforation with air entering the abdominal cavity.

PREVENTION AND TREATMENT. Asymptomatic diverticular disease requires no treatment. The mainstay of treatment for uncomplicated diverticulitis is bowel rest (or clear liquids), antibiotics, and pain control.[351] Antibiotic treatment may be given on an outpatient basis for 7 to 10 days for persons with stable vital signs, absence of fever, and no significant laboratory or CT abnormalities.

Prevention of diverticulosis is accomplished primarily through lifestyle changes, although evidence is lacking. Adherence to a high-fiber diet, decreased red meat intake, prevention of constipation with adequate fluid and fiber intake, encourage smoking cessation, and exercise during periods of remission may decrease the risk.

Approximately one-third of people will have another acute bout of diverticulitis following an initial episode. In the past, surgery (elective sigmoidectomy) was recommended after the second episode of diverticulitis. Currently, surgery is laparoscopically performed on a case-by-case basis[272] with good outcomes.[160,254]

Hospitalization is suggested for persons with diverticular disease with radiographic abnormalities, fever, and leukocytosis. Symptoms should improve over 2 to 3 days' time, when diet may be advanced. Failure to improve should prompt reevaluation with CT and other appropriate laboratory tests. Surgical consult should be obtained where needed. Four to 6 weeks after resolution of the initial attack, colonoscopy should be performed to verify the presence of disease and exclude colorectal cancer.

Approximately 25% of people with diverticulitis will also develop a complication.[147] Abscesses form when a perforation is contained.[308] People with an abscess less than 3 cm can often be treated with antibiotics and bowel rest alone. Larger abscesses (greater than 3 cm) frequently require CT-guided percutaneous drainage and antibiotics. Surgery is often required once the infection is controlled.

Fistulas may form, most commonly between the colon and the bladder or vagina. This complication requires surgical management. Recurrent diverticulitis frequently leads to scarring and narrowing of the lumen with resultant obstruction. Temporary endoscopic dilation with stent placement can be performed for temporary relief until surgery is accomplished.[155] Frank perforation and peritonitis are uncommon complications but carry a high mortality (as high as 25%). Immediate surgery is required with resuscitative efforts.

PROGNOSIS. Prognosis is good for the person with known diverticular disease, particularly as most people remain asymptomatic. Diverticulitis can have significant complications, but the mortality remains low, except in cases of frank perforation and peritonitis. Suspicion for diverticular disease should be entertained in young people because the incidence is increasing in this age group.

SPECIAL IMPLICATIONS FOR THE THERAPIST 16-15

Diverticular Disease

Exercise is an important treatment component during periods of remission. Physical activity may have a protective effect on the gastrointestinal system.[202] Data from a large prospective cohort suggests that vigorous physical activity lowers the risk of diverticulitis and diverticular bleeding.[312] The therapist is instrumental in helping establish an appropriate exercise program. Throughout all activity and exercise, clients with diverticular disease must be careful to avoid activities that increase intraabdominal pressure (see Box 16-1) to avoid further herniation. The therapist can provide valuable information regarding appropriate body mechanics and techniques to reduce intraabdominal pressure for all activities.

Back pain can occur as a symptom of this disease. Anyone with back pain of nontraumatic or unknown origin must be screened for medical disease, including possible GI tract involvement. If infection occurs and penetrates the pelvic floor or retroperitoneal tissues (i.e., those organs outside the peritoneum such as the kidneys, pancreas, colon, and pancreas), abscesses may result, causing isolated referred hip or thigh pain.

A variety of objective test procedures may be employed by the therapist to assess for iliopsoas abscess formation, including palpation of the McBurney point (see Fig. 16-19), assessment of the pinch-an-inch test (see Fig. 16-21), the iliopsoas muscle test, the obturator test, and palpation of the iliopsoas muscle (see Figs. 16-13 and 16-14).

Neoplasms

Intestinal Polyps

A growth or mass protruding into the intestinal lumen from any area of mucous membrane can be termed a *polyp*. Polyps are either *neoplastic* or *nonneoplastic*. Two of the more common types of nonneoplastic polyps are hyperplastic and inflammatory. Adenomatous polyps, a neoplastic type of polyp, usually develop during middle age, and more than two-thirds of the population older than 65 years old have at least one polyp. Until a polyp becomes large enough to obstruct the intestine, no symptoms are discernible. Early symptoms may be lower abdominal cramping pain, diarrhea with rectal bleeding, and passage of mucus.

Adenomatous polyps may develop into adenocarcinoma (colorectal cancer); therefore, regardless of the clinical manifestations, adenomatous polyps are removed (by polypectomy, usually performed through a sigmoidoscope or colonoscope; large polyps may require removal by laparotomy). Hyperplastic polyps do not progress to become cancerous.

Benign Tumors

The most common benign tumors of the small intestine are adenomas, leiomyomas, and lipomas. Benign tumors of the small intestine rarely become malignant and may be symptomatic or may be incidental findings at operation or autopsy.

Malignant Tumors

The most common malignant tumors of the small intestine are metastatic through direct extension from adjacent organs (e.g., stomach, pancreas, colon). Adenocarcinoma and primary lymphoma account for the majority of bowel malignancies. Other types of tumors found in the colon, including melanoma, fibrosarcoma, and other types of sarcoma, are rare and are not discussed further in this book.

Colorectal Cancer.

Overview and Incidence. Colorectal cancer (cancer of the colon and/or rectum) is the third leading cause of cancer among American men and women with an estimate of 143,000 new cases in 2012.[295] It is also the third leading cause of cancer death in both men and women in the United States with an estimate of 51,000 deaths in 2012.[8] Overall incidence and mortality rates are on the decline, possibly indicating that screening is leading to earlier detection with improved survival rates. Incidence increases with age, starting at 40 years, and the disease occurs slightly more often in men and in populations of high socioeconomic status, possibly owing to dietary factors. African Americans have the highest incidence of colorectal cancer among all racial groups, with death rates approximately 30% higher than for whites. This disparity is most likely a result of differences between African Americans and whites in screening rates, early detection, and intervention.[9,247,260]

Etiologic and Risk Factors. The cause of colon cancer is unknown, although a number of environmental and familial factors have been considered. Genetic syndromes are more likely to occur before age 40 years and make up less than 6% of all colorectal cancers. Approximately 75% of all colorectal cancer occurs in people with no known predisposing factors; for such individuals, the lifetime risk of developing this type of cancer is approximately 5%.

Known factors associated with increased risk of colonic cancer include increasing age, male gender, a personal history of adenomatous polyps, IBD (UC, CD), family history of colon cancer or familial adenomatous polyposis, and obesity. Cigarette smoking and excessive alcohol consumption may possibly increase risk.[167] Anyone who has first-degree relatives diagnosed with colon or rectal adenoma is twice as likely to develop colon cancer as those with no history of such cancer in the immediate family. The risk is even higher if the relative was younger than 50 years of age at the time of diagnosis.

Geographic distributions of highest incidence coincide with regional diets low in fiber and high in animal fat, sugar, and protein; people who emigrate tend to acquire the risk characteristics of their new environment. Eating large amounts of red or processed meat over a long period of time can increase colorectal cancer risk, but the risk from obesity and lack of exercise (inactivity) is even greater.[47]

Pathogenesis. The development of colorectal cancer is a slow process. The disease begins as a benign adenomatous polyp (adenomatous refers to the type of cells in the polyp). These cells then develop into an adenoma with high-grade dysplasia (dysplasia is changes seen in the cell which indicate abnormalities that may become cancer). It finally progresses into an invasive cancer (uncontrolled growth and cell death).[201] Colorectal cancer is not caused by one mutation, rather multiple changes, accumulation of mutations, and pathway interruptions. The goal of colorectal treatment in the future is to determine in each case why the cancer developed, ascertain what drives the progression and growth, and determine the response to certain treatments.

The development of colorectal cancer often begins with genomic instability. This may be from abnormalities in chromosome copy number and structure.[177] Some cancers display the inability to repair DNA defects or have mutations in tumor suppressor genes. Cancer progression also involves interruption of signaling pathways and activating pathways which are oncogenic (genes which promote growth and replication) or enhance growth factors.

Clinical Manifestations. Colon carcinoma has few early warning signs, as is the case with esophageal and stomach cancers. Common symptoms include occult blood loss (with resultant anemia and iron deficiency), melena, hematochezia, abdominal pain, weight loss, and change in bowel habits. Bright red blood from the rectum is a cardinal sign of colon cancer, particularly rectal cancer, but must be differentiated from diverticulosis, anal fissures, and hemorrhoids, which are also common causes of bright red blood. Many cases of colon cancer are asymptomatic until metastasis has occurred, which may manifest as right upper quadrant pain (liver metastases), abdominal bloating, and early satiety. Complications include intestinal obstruction, GI bleeding, perforation, anemia, ascites, and distant metastases, to the liver most commonly but also to the lungs, bone, and brain.

MEDICAL MANAGEMENT

SCREENING/PREVENTION. Because colorectal cancer is slow growing (approximately 10-15 years for a polyp to become a cancer), screening is very effective. Evidence exists that reductions in colorectal cancer morbidity and mortality can be achieved through screening,[16,117,179,197] early detection,[281] and removal of polyps.[359] Unfortunately, approximately 22 million Americans between the ages of 50 and 75 years do not receive screening of any type, and 25,000 lives could be saved.[115] Many types of tests are available with advantages and disadvantages.[180] The least-expensive laboratory tests identify blood in the stool; they are the guaiac fecal occult blood tests (cards) and fecal immunochemical test, which can be done at home and tested in the health care provider's office. People are often more likely to comply with these tests, rather than invasive procedures.[253] These tests, however, are not highly sensitive (guaiac test has a sensitivity of 50%-75% and the immunochemical test has a sensitivity of 60%-85% with three samples) and require annual screening.

A colonoscopy is required if the test is positive for blood. Fecal samples may be collected at home and tested for DNA specific for mutations seen in colorectal cancer. This test is costly and sensitivity is poor for advanced adenomas. CT colonography (virtual colonoscopy) is a newer test that involves inflating the colon via a rectal tube and then CT scans are taken of the colon in both supine and prone positions. It has a high sensitivity (95%)[244] for lesions larger than 1 cm[141] and is less invasive than colonoscopy. Its ability to decrease the incidence and mortality of colorectal cancer is not known and many questions regarding follow-up, capacity to identify flat lesions, etc., remain to be answered.

Sigmoidoscopy and colonoscopy are very sensitive (colonoscopy is 90%) in finding lesions larger than 1 cm. Sigmoidoscopy reduces the incidence by 26% and mortality by 50%.[281] Colonoscopy reduces the incidence of colorectal cancer by 67% and reduces the mortality by 65%.[143] Sigmoidoscopy is sensitive for finding lesions in the descending colon, but will miss proximal lesions. Both colonoscopy and sigmoidoscopy are invasive with risk of adverse outcomes (i.e., perforation).

Alternatively, technology has made it possible to use a tiny camera that can be swallowed for a virtual endoscopy that is less invasive but may not be as complete, because the camera's field of view is only 140 degrees, leaving some portions of the GI tract in blind spots. Food and other debris also can obscure lesions from view. In rare cases, the vitamin-sized capsule may get obstructed by strictures or other problems within the intestines,

requiring surgical removal. This technology currently is not standard of care.

Colonoscopy should be performed every 10 years for persons 50 years of age and older at average risk for colorectal cancer (more frequently if abnormalities are found). For those with special risk (e.g., UC, familial adenomatous polyposis, hereditary nonpolyposis colorectal cancer), screening should be more frequent and each disorder has a suggested schedule.

The U.S. Preventive Services Task Force recommends routine screening end at the age of 75 years and does not recommend screening for persons older than age 85.[251] For people between the ages of 75 and 85 years, decisions can be made on a case-by-case basis, particularly if they have had no prior exam.

Environmental and dietary factors have been linked to colorectal cancer, either as preventative agents or as risk factors in contributing to the development of colorectal cancer. Diets high in fruits, vegetables, and dietary fiber appear to be preventative.[129] Diets high in fat and red meat show an increased risk. An increased intake of calcium, folate, vitamin D, vitamin C, and selenium is associated with a decreased risk.[317] Obesity and a sedentary lifestyle are also associated with a higher risk for colorectal cancer.[22]

Colorectal cancer has been extensively studied in relation to physical activity, with consistent findings that adults who increase their physical activity (frequency, intensity, or duration) can reduce their risk of developing colorectal cancer by 30% to 40%, relative to those who are sedentary (regardless of age or body mass index). The greatest risk reduction occurs in those who are most active. The protective effect appears greatest with high-intensity activity. Optimal exercise levels and duration have not yet been determined. Likewise studies show that moderate exercise (e.g., walking 2-3 miles in 1 hour 6 days per week) decreases the risk of colorectal cancer recurrence by 50%.[212] Smoking and increased alcohol intake have been consistently connected with an increased risk of colorectal cancer recurrence.[273]

Individuals at increased risk for colorectal cancer should talk with their physicians about the preventive use of aspirin and NSAIDs.[37,335]

DIAGNOSIS AND STAGING. Carcinoma of the colon should be suspected in anyone older than age 40 years who presents with occult blood in the stool, iron-deficiency anemia, overt rectal bleeding, weight loss, or alteration in bowel habits, especially if associated with abdominal discomfort or any of the risk factors mentioned earlier. Diagnostic procedures include rectal examination, colonoscopy with biopsy of lesions, and CT scan. CT colonography also known as virtual colonoscopy, is a series of CT images of the intestine that has advanced enough to become sensitive and accurate enough for use with many, but not all, people.[243] Endoscopic ultrasound is more accurate than CT for determining the staging of rectal cancer.

Laboratory tests may include evaluation for anemia, liver function tests, and screening for fecal blood. A blood test for carcinoembryonic antigen (CEA), detected in some individuals with colorectal carcinoma is one of the most widely used tumor markers, primarily in GI cancers, especially colorectal malignancy. It is of little use in screening for colorectal cancer, but high preoperative concentrations of CEA correlate with adverse prognosis, and serial CEA measurements can detect recurrent cancer in asymptomatic clients.[75]

The tumor-node-metastasis (TNM) staging system of the American Joint Committee on Cancer (AJCC) is the standard for colorectal cancer and has replaced the Dukes classification.[298] The TNM system incorporates both clinical and pathologic staging approaches and can be applied to the preoperative evaluation of affected individuals.[58] Features associated with a risk of recurrence include obstruction or perforation at presentation, tumor adherence to adjacent organs, positive margins on the surgical specimen, pathology consistent with a poorly differentiated tumor, and the presence of lymphovascular or perineural invasion.

TREATMENT. Surgical removal of the tumor is the mainstay of colorectal cancer treatment. For some clients, this may be laparoscopically performed.

Using the AJCC TNM staging, stage 0 disease requires local or regional excision of the tumor with wide margins. Stage 1 cancer is treated the same way, but the individual may need bowel resection and anastomosis. Stage 2 may be treated surgically or with surgery combined with adjuvant chemotherapy (depending on risk factors present predicting potential recurrence; e.g., high-grade tumor, absence of clear margins, metastases). Stage 3 disease requires surgical excision and removal and biopsy of regional lymph nodes. Regional metastasis has occurred at this stage, requiring additional regimens of chemotherapy and/or radiation therapy. Stage 4 cancer is accompanied by systemically metastasized disease requiring a more comprehensive treatment regimen to address local, regional, and systemic disease.[97]

Adjuvant chemotherapy (postoperative) and/or neo-adjuvant therapy (preoperative) may be administered, depending on the results of the staging process for both colon and rectal cancer, in order to eradicate the micrometastases and improve postsurgical survival. Adjuvant chemotherapy does improve survival for resectable cancers.[25] The benefit for stage 2 is controversial but stage 3 receives survival benefit with adjuvant chemotherapy.[101,242,362] Even clients with limited metastatic disease can have significant improvement in their prognosis with surgical resection of metastases and adjuvant chemotherapy.

In treating rectal cancer, radiation therapy may be given before surgery (neoadjuvant therapy) to reduce the tumor size and/or after surgery to improve local control. Rectal tumors are located in a retroperitoneal position and their location in the pelvis makes resection with wide margins difficult. Tumors in the distal rectum may require resection of the entire rectum with subsequent colostomy (a 2-cm margin is needed to perform sphincter-saving surgery).

Targeted (biologic) therapy with monoclonal antibodies (MABs such as cetuximab [Erbitux], bevacizumab [Avastin], panitumumab [Vectibix]) has been developed for the treatment of cancers. These MABs bind to either epidermal growth factor receptors (cetuximab and panitumumab) or vascular endothelial growth factor receptors (bevacizumab) (which are overexpressed in these tumors). Bevacizumab can prevent the formation of new blood vessels (angiogenesis) supplying a tumor, thus effectively starving tumor cells. Even though significant controversy surrounds these agents in treating colorectal cancer, they are utilized for the treatment of metastatic colorectal cancer. Although designed to be given as monotherapy or accompanying chemotherapy/radiation,[239] MABs are principally given with chemotherapy. More research is needed to determine the optimal uses.[263,331,346] Alternately, MABs may also assist surgeons in finding occult disease at the time of surgery in order to better identify tumor margins.[267]

PROGNOSIS. The 5-year survival for all stages combined is 64%; local (early) stages have a 90% 5-year survival; regional stages carry a 69% 5-year survival; and metastatic disease (late stages) has only a 12% 5-year survival.[123] Most often death from rectal cancer is from local recurrence rather than from distant metastasis.

Colorectal cancer survival is related closely to the clinical and pathologic stage of the disease at diagnosis. The depth of tumor penetration into the bowel wall is an important prognostic indicator. The deeper it penetrates, the worse the prognosis. Involvement of local lymph nodes is also associated with a worse prognosis. Stage-for-stage, rectal carcinoma has a poorer prognosis compared to colon cancer, due to the location of the tumor.

CEA is a marker for recurrent tumor and should be monitored every 3 to 6 months for 2 years and every 6 months for the subsequent 3 years. Follow-up colonoscopy is recommended at year 1, with a repeat in 1 year if abnormal or 3 years if no lesions or polyps are present. Screening colonoscopy can then be done every 5 years. CT of the chest, abdomen, and pelvis are recommended every year for 3 years after surgery for people who exhibited perineural invasion or poorly differentiated tumors. CT is able to detect liver metastases, which, if limited and resected, can improve mortality rate by 25%. Approximately 25% of people present with evidence of hematogenous spread and 50% will develop metastatic disease. As with most solid cancers, early detection is the key to cure.

SPECIAL IMPLICATIONS FOR THE THERAPIST   16-16

Colorectal Cancer

The physical therapist's involvement may vary depending on individual comorbidities and clinical presentation. For example, the client who has a history of corticosteroid therapy, or the woman who has had surgically induced menopause prematurely, may be at risk for skeletal demineralization.[97]

Impaired posture can occur as a result of adaptive shortening of the abdominal musculature as a result of extensive surgical disruption and pain contributing to a stooped posture and inability to lie completely supine. Such a condition can place increased stress on the muscles of the lower back and alter body mechanics, placing the individual at increased risk for injury during lifting and risk of decreased function in other activities.[97]

The removal of lymph nodes from the abdominal/pelvic area can put a client at increased risk of lymphedema. The therapist can be instrumental in providing education regarding lymphedema risk and prevention.

Many individuals are deconditioned before beginning cancer treatment. The benefits of exercise in general and especially for those recovering from cancer treatment have been reported in the literature and are summarized in Chapter 9.

Metastases

Tumors of the rectum can spread through the rectal wall to the prostate in men and the vagina in women. Prostate involvement can cause dull, vague, aching pain in the sacral or lumbar spine regions. See "Special Implications for the Therapist: Prostate Cancer" in Chapter 19. Pelvic, hip, or low back pain may occur with extension to the vagina in women.

Systemic and pulmonary metastases occur through the hemorrhoidal plexus, which drains into the vena cava. Subsequent chest, shoulder, arm, or back pain can occur, usually accompanied by pulmonary symptoms; see also "Special Implications for the Therapist 15-22: Lung Cancer" in Chapter 15.

Liver metastasis occurs after invasion of the mesenteric veins from the left colon or the superior veins from the right colon, which empty into the portal circulation; see also "Hepatic Encephalopathy" in Chapter 17. Any time a person with low back pain reports simultaneous or alternating abdominal pain at the same level as the back pain, or GI symptoms associated with back pain, a medical referral is required.

Anemia caused by intestinal bleeding associated with colon cancer requires special consideration. See "Special Implications for the Therapist 14-5: The Anemias" in Chapter 14.

Rehabilitation

Many factors can influence whether an individual with colorectal cancer will be referred to rehabilitation services. The client's tolerance to pain, ability to recover, presence of other comorbidities, and even the physician's perception of physical debilitation may play a role in the decision to refer.[63]

Complications and side effects arising from comprehensive treatment can produce impairments for which physical therapy intervention can improve quality of life, tolerance of cancer treatment, and recovery of function.[97]

The therapist may be involved in the rehabilitation of some clients with (colorectal) cancer to improve function and mobility after abdominal surgery or other medical treatments.[55]

Individuals who have had laparoscopic surgery may be able to tolerate a more aggressive approach to rehabilitation and recovery of function.[151]

Movement to stimulate the gastric system and help the flow of the abdominal contents may begin as early as the same day as surgery, with ambulation every 4 to 6 hours on the first day.[67] The therapist may be called upon to evaluate the client's needs and to instruct the staff and family in ambulation if assistance is needed.

Many people who have a colectomy without a colostomy bag have to relearn bowel control, because the pelvic floor muscles are often manipulated and weakened during surgery. A program of pelvic floor rehabilitation, possibly including biofeedback and electrical stimulation, can help restore pelvic floor function.[35]

For an example of how rehab might flow for someone with extensive involvement at various stages of disease based on the natural history following surgery, chemotherapy, and radiation therapy, see Evolve Box 16-1 on the book's Evolve website.

Obstructive Disease

Obstruction can occur in either the small or large intestines. Small intestinal obstruction is more common because of the narrower diameter of the lumen. Hernias, intestinal adhesions, intussusception, and volvulus account for 80% of mechanical obstructions. Tumors and infarction account for another 10% to 15%.

Mechanical Obstruction

Adhesion. Adhesions are the most common cause of small and large intestine obstruction. Adhesions are caused by fibrous scars formed as a consequence of previous surgery, infections (resulting in peritonitis), endometriosis, and the like. These fibrous bands of scar tissue create bridges through which intestine can slide and become trapped, or by creating an axis around which the bowel can twist (volvulus).

Intussusception. Intussusception is a telescoping of the bowel into itself; that is, one part of the intestine propels into the lumen of an immediately adjacent section (Fig. 16-16). Once trapped inside the next section, continuing peristalsis forces the attached mesentery along. If left untreated, these segments compress the mesenteric vessels and can become ischemic, with resulting infarction and obstruction. There is an association between the rotavirus vaccine and intussusception in infants and young children (small increased risk).[219,329] In adults, the leading point of an intussusception is often a lesion in the bowel wall, such as Meckel diverticulum.

Volvulus. Volvulus is a torsion of a loop of intestine, frequently redundant loops of sigmoid colon, twisted on its mesentery, kinking the bowel and interrupting the blood supply (Fig. 16-17). The cause of this phenomenon is usually a congenital abnormality, such as a malrotation

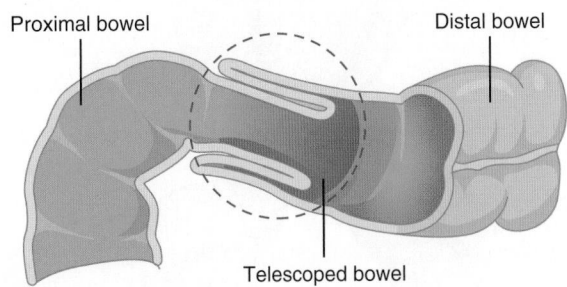

Figure 16-16

Intussusception. A portion of the bowel telescopes into adjacent (usually distal) bowel.

of the bowel that allows excess mobility of the bowel loops and predisposes the intestine to volvulus. Nonsurgical methods are initially undertaken to detorse the intestine. It is seen in all ages, but is rare.

Clinical manifestations include abdominal pain and distention, nausea and vomiting, constipation, and obstipation (a more significant clinical feature for obstruction). Complications include ischemia and subsequent necrosis, perforation, peritonitis, and sepsis. Usually, diagnostic testing includes rectal examination, abdominal radiography, and CT. Surgical intervention, either open procedure or by laparoscope, exploratory or therapeutic, is often required. The goal is to intervene prior to significant loss of tissue to ischemia. The prognosis for children and adults with this condition is good if treated.

Hernia.

Definition and Incidence. A *hernia* is defined as a weakness of the abdominal wall through which part of the bowel pushes, forming the hernia. A hernia is caused by a weakness in the peritoneal cavity through which peritoneum can slide through and form a serosa-lined sac or bulge, followed by protrusion of part of an organ or tissue in the groin, abdomen, and navel (often the intestine). About 5 million Americans of all ages have some type of abdominal hernia. Hernias can occur at any age in men or women, and most frequently occur in the abdominal cavity as a result of a congenital or acquired weakness of abdominal musculature.

Weakness can occur as part of the aging process, contributing to acquired hernias. As people age, muscular tissues become infiltrated by adipose and connective tissues, resulting in weakness. The most common types of hernias are inguinal (direct and indirect), femoral, umbilical, and incisional or ventral (Fig. 16-18). See "Hiatal Hernia" above for further discussion.

Etiologic and Risk Factors. When muscular weakness (congenital or acquired) is accompanied by obesity, pregnancy, heavy lifting, coughing, surgical incision, or traumatic injuries from blunt pressure, the risk of developing a hernia increases. Often, herniation is the result of a multifactorial process involving one or more of these factors. Many possible combinations of risk factors exist (Table 16-7).

Structural abnormalities account for most congenital hernias, but congenital factors do not explain the increased incidence of hernias (e.g., the direct inguinal type) in advancing age groups. Sudden stress, as occurs in abdominal trauma or industrial accidents, also may contribute to the development of a hernia with or without an underlying congenital defect.

Predisposing factors are equally important, such as physical stress (e.g., repetitive local trauma, strenuous physical activities), degenerative changes associated with increased abdominal pressure, the wear and tear of living, multiparity (women), and altered collagen synthesis in middle age.

Pathogenesis. Structural and biochemical abnormalities and abnormalities of local collagen metabolism have been proposed as factors in the eventual appearance of a hernia. Weakness of the tissues around the *inguinal* canal leads to tears and separation of the tissues. The inguinal canal is formed by fascia to the abdominal muscles on one side and the internal oblique abdominal muscle on the other. Inside the canal is the spermatic cord in men and the round ligament in women.

Other biologic factors can affect the balance between collagen synthesis and lysis, eventually leading to the development of herniation. For example, any condition such as renal failure, diabetes mellitus, malnutrition, vitamin or mineral deficiencies, underlying systemic disease, altered immunity, or resistance to infection that can impair a person's ability to generate the proteinaceous constituents of collagen can alter collagen metabolism.

Inguinal hernias account for approximately 75% of all hernias and will affect approximately 25% of men in the United States sometime during their lifetime. Women, too, can have inguinal hernias. Indirect hernias occur in infants as the result of a congenital patency of the processus vaginalis. In adults, there is a weakening and widening of the internal ring. A peritoneal sac is then able to slip into the ring. The indirect inguinal hernia is most common in infants, young people, and males, in the last because it follows the tract that develops when the testes descend into the scrotum before birth. A wide space at the inguinal ligament also can contribute to the development of an inguinal hernia.

Direct hernias, the second most common type of hernia, occurs most often as a result of a deficient number of transverses abdominis aponeurotic fibers at a site called the *Hesselbach triangle,* the area between the pubic ramus and the musculofascial components in the lower abdominal wall. The direct inguinal hernia is more common in older adults, especially in an area that is congenitally weak because of a deficient number of muscle fibers.

Femoral hernia is a protrusion of a loop of intestine into the femoral canal, a tubular passageway into the thigh that carries nerves and blood vessels. The pathologic anatomy present is an enlarged femoral ring with a correspondingly narrowed transverses abdominis aponeurosis. This type occurs more often in multiparous women, acquired as a result of increased intraabdominal pressure gradually forcing more and more preperitoneal fat into the femoral canal, enlarging the femoral ring. Femoral hernias are uncommon and the diagnosis is often difficult to make.

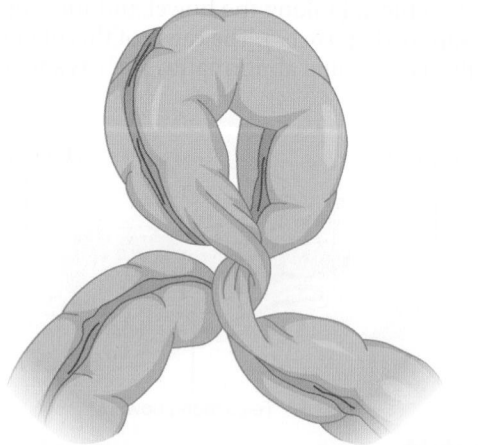

Figure 16-17

Volvulus. The intestine twists, causing obstruction and ischemia.

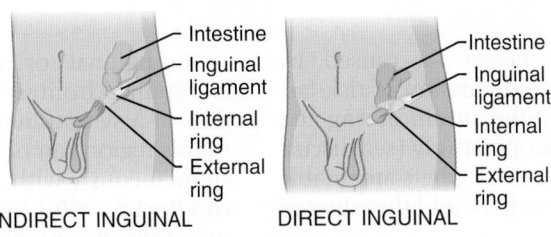

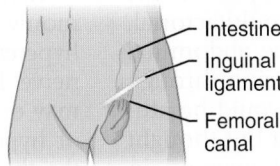

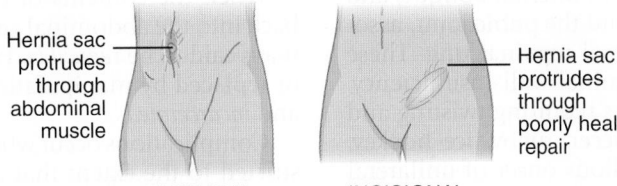

	Indirect Inguinal	Direct Inguinal	Femoral	Umbilical	Incisional
Location	Sac herniates through internal inguinal ring; can remain in canal or pass into scrotum (men), can extend to the labia (women)	Directly behind and through external inguinal ring, above inguinal ligament; rarely enters scrotum	Through femoral ring and canal, below inguinal ligament, more often on right side	Through umbilical ring; congenital defect in abdominal muscle	Through inadequately healed surgical site
Clinical signs and symptoms	Pain with straining; soft swelling that increases with increased intraabdominal pressure; may decrease when lying down	Usually painless; round swelling close to the pubis in area of internal inguinal ring; easily reduced when supine	Pain may be severe, may become strangulated	Firm bulge that increases with increased neuralgic pain possible (see text)	Usually painless
Frequency	Most common; 60% of all hernias; more common in infants <1 yr and in males age 16 to 20 yr	Less common, occurs most often in men >40 yr, rare in women	Least common, 4% of all hernias; more common in women	More common in women	Affects men and women
Cause	Congenital or acquired	Acquired weakness; deficient posterior inguinal wall brought on by heavy lifting, muscle atrophy, obesity, chronic cough, or ascites	Acquired; due to increased abdominal pressure, muscle weakness, or frequent stooping	Increased abdominal pressure; obesity; multiparous women	Postoperative complications such as infection, inadequate nutrition, extreme distention, or obesity

Figure 16-18

Hernias. (Modified from Jarvis C: *Physical examination and health assessment*, ed 3, Philadelphia, 2000, WB Saunders, p. 779.)

Table 16-7	Risk Factors for Hernias		
Inguinal	**Femoral**	**Umbilical**	**Incisional**
Advanced age	Pregnancy (multiparous)	Infancy	Poor wound healing
Prematurity		Low birth weight	Infection
Positive family history		African descent	Inadequate nutrition
Abdominal wall defects		Congenital hypothyroidism	Abdominal distention
Undescended testis		Mucopolysaccharidoses	Obesity
Connective tissue disorders		Down syndrome	Prolonged use of steroids
Cystic fibrosis		Obesity	Advanced age
Shunt for hydrocephalus		Pregnancy	Immunosuppression
Ascites		Ascites	Postoperative pulmonary complications (coughing, straining)
			Type of incision (vertical)

The pathology of *umbilical hernias* is caused by increased abdominal pressure (see discussion of risk factors) exerted against a thinning of the umbilical ring and fascia. *Incisional hernia* occurs postoperatively (see discussion of risk factors) when the transected fibers are unable to form collagen links strong enough to hold the edges of the wound together.

Sports hernia is a term used to describe pain in the pubic joint of athletes and is probably multifactorial. The name is misleading as it is not a true abdominal hernia as it does not involve bowel protrusion through the abdominal wall; a more correct term would be athletic pubalgia. The pathogenesis is not clear but thought to begin initially as tendinosis (adductor longus origin or the rectus abdominis insertion), this progresses to involve muscles (rectus abdominis, internal oblique, and transverse abdominis muscles) and the pubic joint, associated with dilation of the external inguinal ring. These changes are called posterior inguinal wall insufficiency. Athletes who participate in sports requiring twisting and turning at high speeds (e.g., soccer, rugby, ice hockey, tennis) are at greatest risk. Insidious onset of unilateral groin pain is the most common symptom of this type of hernia.[154]

Clinical Manifestations. The most common manifestation of a hernia of any type is an intermittent or persistent bulge, accompanied by intermittent or persistent pain. Inguinal hernia usually begins as a small, marble-size soft lump under the skin. At first it is painless and can be reduced by pushing it back in place. As pressure from the abdominal contents pushes against the weak abdominal wall, the size of the lump formed by the hernia increases, requiring surgical repair (herniorrhaphy).

The pain associated with simple hernias depends on the involved structures and whether these are compressed or irritated. The pain usually is localized and sharp, aggravated by changes in position, by physical exertion, during a bowel movement, or by any activity causing the Valsalva maneuver (bearing down with increased intraabdominal pressure such as during coughing or sneezing), and relieved by cessation of the physical activity that precipitated it.

Inguinal hernias are often more noticeable after a heavy meal or long period of standing. Sports hernias are aggravated by sudden movements, acceleration, twisting and turning, cutting, kicking, resisted sit-ups, or any activity that stretches or stresses the abdominal muscles.

Pain may radiate from the groin to the testicles (males), ipsilateral thigh, flank, or hypogastrium (lowest middle abdominal region). In the female, painful symptoms may be aggravated by the onset of menstruation. Sports hernia in females is often characterized by tenderness at the site of the superficial inguinal ring.[154]

The ilioinguinal nerve penetrates the abdominal wall cranially and somewhat laterally to the deep inguinal ring, passing the transverse and internal oblique muscles stepwise. Neuralgic pain may occur when the dull inguinal hernial pain causes a local reflex increase of tone in the internal oblique and transverse muscles of the abdomen. As the nerve passes these muscles in steps, it may be exposed to pressure, giving rise to pain of the neuralgic type.

Ilioinguinal or femoral neuritis caused by nerve entrapment from sutures, adhesions, or the actual formation of a symptomatic neuroma after section of a nerve in this region can occur. These conditions usually resolve spontaneously without specific treatment, but therapy in conjunction with local nerve blocks may be indicated if symptoms persist after the first postoperative month.

Genitofemoral neuralgia (causalgia) occurs less commonly but results in severe pain and paresthesia (or hyperesthesia) in the distribution of the genitofemoral nerve. Radiation of pain to the genitalia and upper thigh may occur, and pain is aggravated by walking, stooping, or hyperextending the hip. Recumbency and flexion of the thigh may relieve painful symptoms. This condition requires neurectomy for pain relief.

When the contents of the hernial sac can be pushed back into the abdominal cavity by manipulation, the hernia is said to be *reducible*. Hernias that cannot be reduced or replaced by manipulation are referred to as *irreducible* and *incarcerated*.

Complications occur when the protruding organ is constricted to the extent that circulation is impaired (strangulated hernia) or when the protruding organs encroach on and impair the function of other structures. When a hernia contains incarcerated or strangulated structures, the pain becomes persistent and often is associated with systemic signs or symptoms such as elevated temperature, tachycardia, vomiting, and abdominal distention.

MEDICAL MANAGEMENT

DIAGNOSIS. History and physical examination remain the most important aspects of diagnosis for all types of hernia; there may be a past history of hernia. Inguinal hernias are most frequently diagnosed by noting the bulge in the inguinal canal. The diagnosis of umbilical hernia is usually obvious because of protrusion of the umbilicus confirmed by palpation of the involved structures.

Radiographic investigations (plain films and CT) are important in diagnosing sports hernias, especially to identify osteitis pubis, adductor tenoperiosteal lesions, and symphyseal instability, and to rule out hip osteoarthritis and tumors.

MRI may be used to diagnose bone marrow edema about the pubic symphysis (a sign of osteitis pubis), stress fractures, avascular necrosis, labral hip tears, and articular cartilage defects that can accompany a sports hernia.[320]

TREATMENT. Various supports and trusses are available to contain hernias, but these offer only a temporary solution and may not prevent the hernia from getting bigger with associated complications. The use of strapping techniques is not recommended, because the tape used may lead to ulceration of the thin skin covering the hernia and eventual rupture.

Watchful waiting is an acceptable treatment approach for minimally symptomatic *inguinal* hernias. Delaying surgical repair until symptoms increase is considered safe because acute hernia incarcerations rarely occur.

Surgical repair is the only curative treatment, but it is no longer recommended as watchful waiting does not increase morbidity or mortality for asymptomatic inguinal hernias. Often the size and location determine need for surgery. For example, large ventral hernias often do not require surgery because tissue does not become incarcerated/strangulated. Inguinal hernias should be repaired when exam and pain consistent with a hernia are documented. Complications of herniorrhaphy, such as cutaneous nerve injury, bleeding, wound infection, chronic pain, and recurrence, have led to a rethinking of surgical correction for asymptomatic hernias. Further studies are needed to identify the natural history of inguinal hernias and to identify the best treatment plan.[89,314]

When surgical repair is indicated, there are now several methods of correction, depending upon the size and location of the hernia. When repairing an inguinal hernia, choices include type of procedure open/laparoscopic and use of mesh (many products available). Each type of procedure has different operative complications, recurrence rates, postoperative pain, and recovery time.[27] One method frequently utilized to repair an inguinal hernia is strengthening the tissue with a mesh repair. This mesh can be fixed into place with staples or fibrin sealant (glue) laparoscopically. Staples may result in an increase in chronic inguinal pain; both have similar recurrence rates.[152] Ventral or incisional hernia repairs can be repaired through an open surgical procedure or laparoscopically, although the latter method requires further long-term studies.[277] Laparoscopic repair appears to reduce the risk of incisional wound infection and may reduce hospital stay.

PROGNOSIS. Prognosis varies with the type of hernia and accompanying complications. The incidence of incarceration is approximately 10% in indirect inguinal hernia and 20% in femoral hernia. Umbilical hernia in adults has a high morbidity and mortality associated with incarceration. Open and laparoscopic repairs produce excellent results; the laparoscopic procedure allows earlier return to play for athletes.

SPECIAL IMPLICATIONS FOR THE THERAPIST 16-17

Hernia
Prevention, Screening, and Referral for Hernia

Congenital muscle weakness complicated by the additional risk factors of obesity and increased intraabdominal pressure should be identified and treated. Educate clients in proper lifting techniques and precautions to avoid heavy lifting and straining, which reduce intraabdominal pressure as an additional risk factor for the development of hernias and aid in preventing worsening of an already existing hernia. The mouth-open position as a reminder to breathe properly and to prevent increased intraabdominal pressure is essential during all lifting procedures. Obesity as a cause of increased intraabdominal pressure may be addressed by weight control through exercise (see "Special Implications for the Therapist 2-3: Obesity" in Chapter 2).

Early diagnosis is important in preventing bowel incarceration and strangulation. Any client experiencing chronic cough, pregnancy, or back, hip, groin, or sacroiliac pain should be asked, "Have you ever been told you have a hernia, or do you think you have a hernia now?"

Any person (especially an older client) with a known hernia complaining of pain, nausea, vomiting, or other new symptom in the anatomic vicinity of the hernia should report these symptoms to the physician to rule out a systemic condition unrelated to the herniation.

Any time a person chooses to wear a truss without prior physician evaluation, the therapist is advised to encourage that client to seek medical advice. The therapist should be aware of two complications that may occur in a client wearing a truss. In the client with a small hernia, the pressure of the overlying truss on a protruding hernial mass enhances the chances of strangulation by obstructing lymphatic and venous drainage. In a person with a large direct inguinal hernia, the constant overlying pressure of the truss pad on the margins of the hernial defect can lead to atrophy of the fascial aponeurotic structures, enlarging the hernial opening, and promoting growth of the hernia, thus making subsequent surgical repair more difficult.

Although uncommon, psoas abscess still can be confused with a hernia. The therapist may perform evaluative tests to rule out a psoas abscess, but the physician must differentiate between an abscess and a hernia; see the iliopsoas and obturator muscle tests (see Fig. 16-13), iliopsoas palpation (see Fig. 16-14), and the McBurney point (see Fig. 16-19). Psoas abscess is often softer than a femoral hernia and has ill-defined borders, in contrast to the more sharply defined margins of the hernia. The major differentiating feature is the fact that a psoas abscess lies lateral to the femoral artery, not medial to it, as is the case for the femoral hernia.

Postoperative Recovery

For most clients recovering from surgical repair of a hernia, heavy lifting and straining should be avoided for 4 to 6 weeks after surgery. This guideline may vary depending on the specific type of hernia and surgical procedure used. The therapist should read the medical record to identify these two features before beginning a postoperative rehabilitation program.

Substance abusers and cigarette smokers have an additional risk factor for delayed wound healing and dehiscence. Transient anesthesia of the skin beneath the hernial incision is a possible postoperative phenomenon. Whether in the presence of an uncorrected hernia or postoperatively, the client should avoid activities and positions that produce painful symptoms associated with the hernia.

Whereas most people do well after surgical repair, some have persistent postoperative pain or discomfort. If a person has had a previous inguinal hernial repair and now presents with painful groin or thigh pain, the physician must differentiate between ilioinguinal nerve entrapment and neuroma of a branch of the nerve severed previously.

Although most hernia surgeries are done laparoscopically, for those individuals who have an open procedure, special care must be taken when there is a vertical incision. When a vertical incision transects fascial aponeurotic fibers, the incision is made perpendicular to the direction of those fibers. Simple muscle contraction, as in coughing, straining, or turning over in bed, tends to distract the wound edges. Laparoscopic repair will likely eliminate this type of surgical incision.

Postoperative Rehabilitation

For the most part, the guidelines for postoperative rehabilitation of herniorrhaphy presented in the literature are not evidence based.[320] Research in this area is needed. It has been suggested that postoperative rehabilitation of the athlete with an uncomplicated sports hernia can begin with isometric abdominal and adductor exercises as early as the first day after minimally invasive surgery. Progression to concentric and eccentric strengthening progresses after the end of the first week. Walking can begin during the first week after surgery.[154] The safety of these recommendations has not been verified by randomized controlled trials.

The same authors suggest that the client can be progressed to jogging by day 10 if approved by the surgeon. Straight-line sprinting begins around day 21, with sport-specific exercises introduced gradually after that. Athletes may expect to return to full sports participation 6 to 8 weeks after open surgery (much sooner after minimally invasive surgery) unless comorbid muscle strains or unrepaired tears exist; recovery from complicated injuries can take 3 months or more. The therapist should address all aspects of pelvic flexibility, strength, and stability.[154]

Other retrospective studies report that most athletes return to their normal sports level within 3 months after surgery.[339] A structured rehabilitation program including client education on proper posture and body mechanics, core and pelvic stabilization strengthening exercises, eventually progressing to sport-specific drills is suggested as a means of maximizing the benefits of surgery, but there are no empirical data to support this recommendation.[165]

Congenital Conditions

Intestinal atresia and stenosis, although rare, are the most frequent causes of neonatal intestinal obstruction. Either condition is diagnosed on the basis of persistent vomiting of bile-containing fluid during the first 24 hours after birth. Surgical correction is usually successful, but coexistent anomalies often are seen and complicate treatment.

Stenosis and Atresia. *Stenosis* is a narrowing of a canal, in this case the small intestine. Intestinal atresia refers to defects caused by the incomplete formation of a lumen, in this case the tubular portion of the intestine. Many hollow organs originate as strands and cords of cells, the centers of which are programmed to die, thus forming a central cavity or lumen.

Most cases of intestinal atresia are characterized by complete occlusion of the lumen, which was not fully established in embryogenesis. Meconium ileus (accumulation of meconium in the small intestine causing neonatal intestinal obstruction) accounts for 25% of all cases, and cystic fibrosis accounts for another 10%. Intestinal atresia may have several forms: multiple intestinal occlusions giving the appearance of a string of sausages, disconnected blind ends, blind proximal and distal sacs joined by a cord, or a thin transluminal diaphragm across the opening. All forms require surgical intervention with good prognosis for recovery.

Meckel Diverticulum. Meckel diverticulum is an outpouching of the bowel located at the ileum of the small intestine, about 2 feet from the ileocecal valve. It occurs because of failure of destruction of the vitelline duct, an embryonic communication between the midgut and the yolk sac. Meckel diverticulum is the most common congenital malformation of the GI tract, present in 2% of the population. Males are affected more often than females in a 3:1 ratio, with accompanying complications in the same ratio.

Meckel diverticulum may be asymptomatic or produce symptoms that include abdominal pain similar to that in other conditions such as appendicitis, CD, and PUD. Meckel diverticulum has several associated complications. The most common includes painless bleeding or hemorrhage from peptic ulceration from acid produced by ectopic (out-of-place) gastric cells in the Meckel diverticulum. The second is intestinal obstruction that may occur from a herniation, volvulus, or intussusception. Diverticulitis occurs secondary to chronic inflammation and can mimic appendicitis. Perforation may also occur and is caused by peptic ulceration in the diverticulum.

Diagnosis is made usually during the first 2 years, but the condition may go undetected into adulthood when it is discovered on autopsy or during laparotomy for an unrelated condition. The diagnosis is made usually based on history, physical examination, and the Meckel scan. Prognosis is good with surgical resection to remove the diverticulum.

THE APPENDIX

Appendicitis

Definition and Incidence

Appendicitis is an inflammation of the vermiform appendix that often results in necrosis and perforation with subsequent localized or generalized peritonitis. On the basis of operative findings and histologic appearance, acute appendicitis is classified as simple, gangrenous, or perforated.

It is the most common disease of the appendix, occurring at any age, with the peak incidence between the ages of 15 and 19 years, with men more often affected than women. The lifetime risk of acute appendicitis in the United States is approximately 9% for males and 7% for females.[127] A general decrease in incidence was seen until the year 2000, when a slight increase was noticed, although a certain trend is not seen.[184]

Etiologic Factors

Approximately half of all cases of acute appendicitis have no known cause. At least one-third are caused by obstruction that prevents normal drainage. Obstruction may occur as a result of tumor, foreign body such as fecal material (fecalith) lodged in the lumen of the appendix, parasites (e.g., intestinal worms), or lymphoid hyperplasia.

Because the appendix is chiefly lymphatic tissue, an infection that produces enlarged lymph nodes elsewhere in the body also can increase the glandular tissue in the appendix and obstruct its lumen. Other causes include CD of the terminal ileum, UC when it spreads to the mucosa of the appendix, and tuberculous enteritis.

Pathogenesis

Classically, appendicitis is thought to develop primarily from obstruction of the lumen and secondarily from bacterial infection. When the long, narrow appendiceal lumen becomes obstructed, inflammation begins in the mucosa, with swelling and hyperemia of the vermiform appendix. As mucous distends the obstructed appendix, the intraluminal pressure rises and eventually exceeds the venous pressure, causing ischemia, necrosis, and perforation.

Another hypothesis considers infection to be the principle source with bacteria or virus (such as cytomegalovirus) infiltrating mucosa resulting in ulceration. Pathology specimens have supported this. This may also indicate why the number of appendicitis cases had decreased over time with improved hygiene and sanitation.[19]

Clinical Manifestations

The presenting symptoms of acute appendicitis occur in a classic sequence of abdominal (epigastric, periumbilical, or right lower quadrant) pain accompanied by anorexia, nausea, vomiting, and low-grade fever in adults. High fevers in adults can be indicative of perforation. Children tend to have higher fevers. Infants and children often seem withdrawn with a nonspecific presentation.[127] Women may experience acute pelvic pain that must be differentiated from other causes of pelvic pain (e.g., ectopic pregnancy, diverticulitis, incarcerated hernia, kidney stones).

Pain associated with appendicitis is constant and may shift within 12 hours of symptom onset to the right lower quadrant with point tenderness over the site of the appendix at the McBurney point, a point between 1.5 and 2 inches superomedial to the anterior superior iliac spine, on a line joining that process and the umbilicus (Fig. 16-19). Signs and symptoms of perforation include a white blood cell count of 20,000/mm^3 or greater; a tense or rigid abdomen; and elevated temperature (39° C [102° F]).

Aggravating factors include anything that increases intraabdominal pressure (see Box 16-1), such as coughing, walking, laughing, and bending over. Older adults frequently have few or no symptoms with minimal fever and only slight tenderness until perforation occurs. Confusion or increased confusion may be the first and only presenting symptom among older adults. Although appendicitis is rare in older adults, half of all people who die from a ruptured appendix are 70 years old or older.[309]

Atypical Appendicitis. An atypical presentation occurs in 40% to 50% of cases. Many cases of appendicitis are atypical because of the position of the appendix (Fig. 16-20), the person's age, or the presence of associated

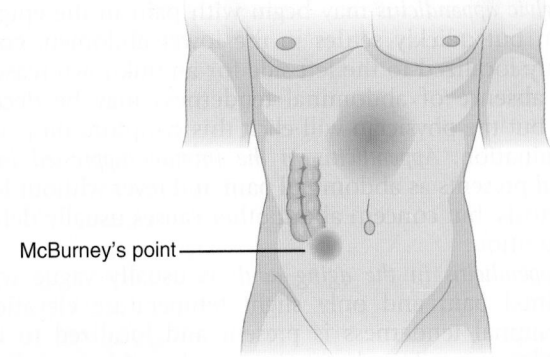

Figure 16-19

Pain areas associated with appendicitis, including the McBurney point. Tenderness upon palpation of this point is indicative of appendicitis. With the client supine and legs extended, isolate the anterior superior iliac spine and the umbilicus, then gently palpate approximately half the distance between those two points. A positive test produces painful symptoms in the right lower quadrant. (Modified from O'Toole M, editor: *Miller-Keane encyclopedia and dictionary of medicine, nursing, and allied health,* ed 6, Philadelphia, 1997, WB Saunders, p. 119.)

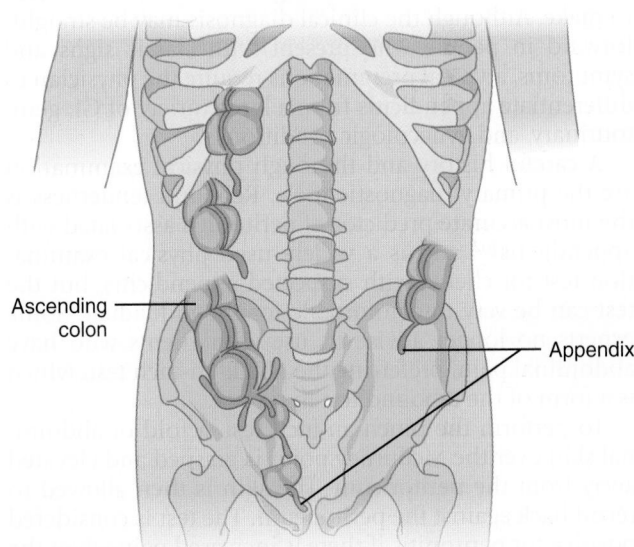

Figure 16-20

Variations in the location of the vermiform appendix. Negative test results for appendicitis using the McBurney point may occur when the appendix is located somewhere other than at the end of the cecum. (From Goodman CC, Snyder TE: *Differential diagnosis for physical therapists: screening for referral,* ed 5, Philadelphia, 2013, WB Saunders.)

conditions, especially in people who are pregnant or who are immunocompromised or have AIDS. The person may not recognize the need for medical attention but may report symptoms to the therapist. Early recognition of the need for medical evaluation is imperative.

Retrocecal appendicitis and *retroileal appendicitis* may occur when the inflamed appendix is shielded from the anterior abdominal wall by the overlying cecum and ileum. The pain seems less intense and less localized, and less discomfort occurs with walking or coughing. The pain may not shift as expected from the epigastrium to the right lower quadrant.

Pelvic appendicitis may begin with pain in the epigastrium but quickly settles in the lower abdomen, commonly localized to the left side for an unknown reason. The absence of abdominal tenderness may be deceptive, but the physician will elicit this symptom on pelvic examination. *Appendicitis in the immunosuppressed individual* presents as abdominal pain and fever without leukocytosis, but concern about other causes usually delays recognition.

Appendicitis in the aging adult is usually vague with minimal pain and only slight temperature elevation. Abdominal tenderness is present and localized to the right lower quadrant but is deceptively mild. *Appendicitis in pregnancy* does not present a diagnostic problem in the first trimester but later in gestation may be confused with an obstetric condition. Displacement of the appendix by the enlarged uterus may result in tenderness in the right subcostal area or adjacent to the umbilicus.

MEDICAL MANAGEMENT

DIAGNOSIS. Acute appendicitis must be diagnosed early to prevent perforation, abscess formation, and postoperative complications, but the diagnosis is not always easy to make. Although the clinical diagnosis may be straightforward in people who present with classic signs and symptoms, atypical presentations require the physician to differentiate appendicitis from a large variety of GI, genitourinary, and gynecologic conditions.

A careful history and thorough physical examination are the primary diagnostic tools. Rebound tenderness is the most accurate predictor of peritonitis associated with appendicitis[102] and is a widely used physical examination test for clients with suspected appendicitis, but the test can be very uncomfortable for the individual. Some experts no longer advise its use with clients who have abdominal pain, preferring the pinch-an-inch test, which is a form of the rebound test in reverse.

To perform the pinch-an-inch test, a fold of abdominal skin over the McBurney point is grasped and elevated away from the peritoneum. The skin is then allowed to recoil back against the peritoneum. The test is considered positive for peritonitis if there is increased pain when the skin fold strikes the peritoneum (Fig. 16-21).[2]

An elevated white blood cell count (more than 20,000/mm^3; leukocytosis) suggests a ruptured appendix and peritonitis. Urinalysis reveals abnormalities in up to 40% of individuals tested.[127] Abdominal CT is more diagnostic than ultrasound, but is usually only done when a diagnosis cannot be made.[127] Histologic examination of the resected appendix is used to confirm the diagnosis.

TREATMENT. Appendectomy, or surgical removal of the vermiform appendix, is performed as soon as possible, either by open procedure or laparoscopically; both are safe and effective in nonperforated appendicitis. Each method has pros and cons associated with it.[278] Antibiotics are administered preoperatively to decrease the incidence of postoperative wound infection and intraabdominal abscess.[127] With accurate diagnosis and early surgical removal, mortality and morbidity rates are less than 1%.

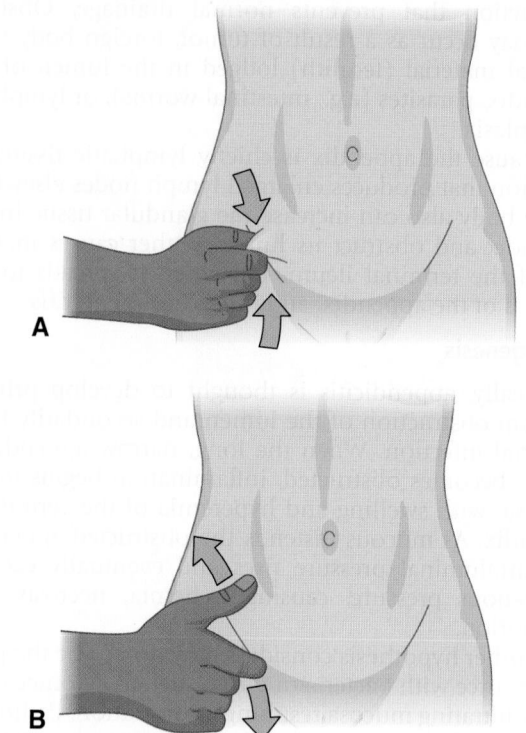

Figure 16-21

Pinch-an-inch test.[2] To avoid the discomfort of the traditionally used (and sometimes inaccurate) rebound test, the pinch-an-inch test was developed as an alternative test for peritonitis associated with appendicitis. **A,** Gently grasp and lift 2 to 3 inches of skin from over the McBurney point on the left side of the abdomen. The individual with a low threshold of pain may report pain during the initial pinch. The clinician must assess this response accordingly. **B,** Quickly release the skin. A positive sign occurs if increased pain is reported when the skin returns to its position against the abdominal wall.

PROGNOSIS. Prognosis is good unless diagnosis is delayed and perforation occurs (usually more than 24 hours after initial symptoms begin). Perforation is associated with complications such as peritonitis, hypovolemia, and septic shock, and carries a mortality rate of 1% to 4%, with a complication rate of 12% to 25% (such as abscess formation). Perforation is more likely in infants younger than 2 years of age and in adults older than 60 years. In up to 20% of individuals who undergo emergency appendectomy, pathologic examination of the tissue shows a normal appendix.[121]

SPECIAL IMPLICATIONS FOR THE THERAPIST   16-18

Appendicitis

When appendicitis is atypical the client may not recognize the need for medical attention but may report the symptoms to the therapist. Early recognition of the need for medical referral is important. In an athletic training or physical therapy setting, appendicitis may present with symptoms of right thigh pain, groin (testicular) pain, pelvic pain, or referred pain in the hip.

In addition to screening for the presence of constitutional symptoms, a variety of objective test procedures may be employed by the therapist. Ask the client to cough: localization of painful symptoms to the site of the appendix is typical.

Perform the iliopsoas muscle test and the obturator muscle test (see Fig. 16-13), palpate the iliopsoas muscle (see Fig. 16-14), palpate the McBurney point (see Fig. 16-19), and perform the pinch-an-inch test (see Fig. 16-21). If the result of any of these tests is positive for reproduction of symptoms in the right lower quadrant, a medical referral is necessary.

If appendicitis is suspected, medical attention must be immediate. The client should be instructed to lie down and remain as quiet as possible, taking nothing by mouth (including water); heat is contraindicated.

THE PERITONEUM

Peritonitis

Overview

Peritonitis, or inflammation of the serous membrane lining the walls of the abdominal cavity, is caused by a number of situations that introduce microorganisms into the peritoneal cavity. Peritonitis that occurs spontaneously is called *primary peritonitis*. Peritonitis as a consequence of trauma, surgery, or peritoneal contamination by bowel contents (e.g., perforated duodenal ulcer or appendix) is referred to as *secondary peritonitis*.

Etiologic Factors

Specific causes of peritonitis are many and varied. Primary peritonitis is associated with ascites and chronic liver disease, called spontaneous bacterial peritonitis. Secondary peritonitis occurs as a result of inflammation of abdominal organs, irritating substances from a perforated gallbladder or gastric ulcer, rupture of a cyst, or irritation from blood, as in cases of internal bleeding.

Secondary peritonitis may be classified as bacterial, chemical, or metastatic. *Bacterial peritonitis* is caused by bacterial infection (*Escherichia coli, Bacteroides, Staphylococcus, Streptococcus, Pneumococcus, Gonococcus, Mycobacterium tuberculosis*) introduced most commonly by perforation of a viscus. Such perforation can occur in the case of appendicitis, an ulcer, a bowel infarct, colonic diverticulum, long-term peritoneal dialysis at the site of catheter exit, and urinary infection. These bacterial organisms spread quickly throughout the abdominal cavity and may enter the bloodstream from the peritoneum, causing life-threatening septicemia.

Chemical peritonitis is a noninfectious inflammation caused by bile leakage, usually from a perforated gallbladder but sometimes from a needle biopsy of the liver, or any breach in the GI tract wall that allows GI tract contents to spill into the abdominal cavity. Once bacteria enter the abdominal cavity, then chemical peritonitis progresses quickly and develops into bacterial peritonitis.

Other causes include substances such as gastric acid, blood, or foreign material introduced by surgery (e.g., talc), and acute pancreatitis, which releases and activates lipolytic and proteolytic enzymes. *Metastatic peritonitis* occurs when neoplasm perforates the viscus of the stomach and tumor cells infiltrate the peritoneum.

Pathogenesis

The GI tract normally contains bacteria, but the peritoneum is sterile. Inflammation and perforation of the GI tract from appendicitis, diverticulitis, perforated gallbladder, or a peptic ulcer allow bacteria to invade the peritoneum.

Once the inflammatory process has begun, a fibrinopurulent exudate covers the peritoneal surface. The exudate becomes organized and fibrotic, forming adhesions and causing obstruction. Usually infection in the peritoneal cavity is localized as an abscess.

When a perforation drains contaminants into the peritoneal cavity, however, the ability of the peritoneum to combat the inflammatory process can be overpowered. The entire surface of the peritoneum may be involved (generalized peritonitis) or only specific sites (localized). When the pelvic peritoneum is involved, pelvic peritonitis (also called *pelvic inflammatory disease*) occurs.

Peritonitis creates severe systemic effects. Circulatory alterations, fluid shifts, and respiratory problems can cause critical fluid and electrolyte imbalances. The circulatory system undergoes great stress from several sources. The inflammatory response shunts extra blood to the inflamed area of the bowel to combat the infection. Peristaltic activity of the bowel ceases, leading to bowel obstruction. Fluids and air are retained within its lumen, raising pressure and increasing fluid secretion into the bowel; circulating volume diminishes.

Clinical Manifestations

Peritonitis commonly decreases intestinal motility and causes intestinal distention with gas. At first the affected individual may feel vague, generalized abdominal pain. As the peritonitis progresses, the client presents with an acute abdomen and severe abdominal pain. The abdomen becomes rigid (involuntary guarding) and sensitive to touch, with rebound tenderness. Pain is severe, increasing with movement and respirations, and can be referred to the shoulder or thoracic area. Nausea, vomiting, and high fever follow.

Without treatment, peritonitis can lead to paralytic ileus (diminished to absent peristalsis), sepsis, or multiple organ dysfunction syndrome. A peritoneal abscess develops if the perforation becomes self-encased or walled off. Antibiotic therapy may mask or delay the recognition of signs of abscess.

In persons with underlying ascites, the signs and symptoms of peritonitis may be more subtle, with fever as the only manifestation of infection, or possibly nausea, vomiting, nonspecific abdominal pain, or altered mental status.

MEDICAL MANAGEMENT

DIAGNOSIS, TREATMENT, AND PROGNOSIS. Abdominal films, CT, and an abdominal tap may be used in the differential diagnosis of peritonitis. Peritonitis should be treated immediately to control infection; preserve the barrier to further microbial invasion; minimize the effects of paralytic ileus; and correct fluid, electrolyte, and nutritional disorders.

If peritonitis is advanced and surgery is contraindicated because of shock and circulatory failure, oral fluids are prohibited and intravenous fluids are necessary for replacement of electrolyte and protein losses. A long intestinal tube is inserted through the nose into the intestine to reduce pressure within the bowel. Once the infection has become walled off and the client's condition improves, surgical drainage and repair can be attempted.

Despite treatment with antibiotics, surgical drainage and debridement, and supportive measures, generalized peritonitis is still associated with a high mortality rate and is especially dangerous in the older adult.

SPECIAL IMPLICATIONS FOR THE THERAPIST   **16-19**

Peritonitis

Special considerations associated with peritonitis are related to the underlying cause (e.g., liver or kidney disease, postoperative state, cancer) and resultant complications (e.g., fluid and electrolyte imbalance, pulmonary compromise). The client with peritonitis usually is hospitalized and undergoing medical treatment. The therapist should be familiar with implications associated with the underlying cause and any complications present.

Vital signs should be regularly monitored (see Appendix B) and a semi-Fowler position used to help the client breathe deeply with less pain to prevent pulmonary complications. Position changes must be accomplished with extreme caution, because the slightest movement intensifies the pain. Watch for signs of dehiscence (separation of layers of a surgical wound), such as the person's reporting that something broke loose or gave way inside. Follow all safety measures such as keeping the side rails up on the bed if fever and pain disorient the client.

THE RECTUM

Rectal Fissure

A rectal or anal fissure is an ulceration or tear of the lining of the anal canal. An acute fissure occurs as a result of excessive tissue stretching or tearing, such as childbirth or passage of a large, hard bowel movement through the area. The most common cause of an anal fissure in an atypical location is CD. Anal fissures are thought to develop as a result of ischemia and spasm of the anal area, followed by trauma. The skin tear is very fragile and tends to reopen easily with the next bowel movement, prompting the person to avoid going to the bathroom for days. Neglecting the "call of the stool" can result in constipation and further exacerbation of the problem, especially in the presence of risk factors for constipation (see "Constipation" above).

Sharp pain, followed by burning, accompanies defecation. Bleeding may be noted by blood on toilet paper. Other symptoms include spasms, mucus, an external skin tag at the anus (sentinel pile), and itching. Anal fissures frequently heal within a month or two when treated with a combination of bran and bulk laxatives or stool softeners, sitz baths, and emollient suppositories.[168] Injections with botulism toxin or use of diltiazem ointment may help relieve spasm and ultimately aid in healing. Chronic fissures may require surgery if other therapies have failed.

Hemorrhoids

Hemorrhoids, or piles, are varicose veins of a pillow-like cluster of veins that lie just beneath the mucous membranes lining the lowest part of the rectum and anus. They can be internal or external. Hemorrhoids are fairly common, affecting about 1 million people.[28,285] Hemorrhoids are vascular tissue in the anal canal which are sinusoids because they have no muscle.[285] Hemorrhoids contribute to anal sphincter continence and may act to protect the sphincter during defecation.

Symptomatic hemorrhoids occur when these vessels pathologically dilate. This may result from vascular congestion or mucosal prolapse. Vascular congestion can occur from prolonged straining or increased intraabdominal pressure (ascites, obesity, or pregnancy) (see Box 16-1).

Common symptoms include burning, itching, and bleeding. In approximately 20% of cases, anal fissures are concomitantly seen with hemorrhoids. Bleeding from internal hemorrhoids is typically painless, with red blood surrounding normal stool. Other types of bleeding need immediate evaluation. Pain is not usually associated with hemorrhoids unless thrombosis has occurred, particularly in external hemorrhoids. External hemorrhoids are formed in nerve-rich tissue outside the anal canal. Internal hemorrhoids may prolapse with straining and are classified according to the degree of prolapse.

Diagnosis is made by examination. Digital, anoscopic, and sigmoidoscopic examinations may be required. Painful, thrombosed hemorrhoids should be removed. Most other hemorrhoids should be medically managed. Conservative treatment consists of local application of topical medications, sitz baths, high-fiber diet, and avoidance of constipation and other causes of increased intraabdominal pressure. A stool softener or psyllium preparation may be used when a modified diet is unsuccessful in eliminating constipation. Local topical preparations for hemorrhoids are used to reduce pain or itching. In addition, moderate aerobic exercise such as brisk walking 20 to 30 minutes daily can help stimulate bowel function.

Hemorrhoids that fail medical treatment may require rubber band ligation, sclerosing, laser surgery, or cryosurgery to destroy the affected tissue. In the case of advanced chronic hemorrhoids, recurrent bleeding and anemia may necessitate surgery (hemorrhoidectomy, stapled hemorrhoidopexy, ultrasonic scalpel hemorrhoidectomy and the bipolar sealing and cutting device).

The Rectum

Therapists may work with individuals who have an overactive external anal sphincter and pain. These individuals experience severe muscle spasm of the sphincter, resulting in groin or pelvic pain and trigger points in the pelvic floor and gluteal muscles. Any anorectal symptoms (e.g., change in bowel habits, rectal pain, bleeding) that have not been reported to the physician or are changing in pattern must be evaluated by a physician.

Clients involved in any activity requiring increased abdominal support or causing increased intraabdominal pressure should be questioned as to the presence of hemorrhoids. For clients with hemorrhoids postoperatively, prone positioning or side lying supported with pillows between the knees and ankles is preferred.

Supine positioning and sitting for brief periods can be accomplished with a rubber air ring under the buttocks for support. Movement, exercise, drinking plenty of fluids, and heeding the call of nature are important in the prevention of constipation-induced hemorrhoids.

In some cases the healed fissure, fistula, or surgical scar can become painful and contribute to further overactive paradoxical pelvic floor muscle contractions. Both painful scars and overactive anal sphincter tightens can be treated by specialized physical therapy.

REFERENCES

To enhance this text and add value for the reader, all references are included on the companion Evolve site that accompanies this textbook. The reader can view the reference source and access it online whenever possible.

CHAPTER 17

The Hepatic, Pancreatic, and Biliary Systems

CATHERINE CAVALLARO GOODMAN • CELESTE PETERSON

The *liver* has more than 500 separate digestive, endocrine, excretory, and hematologic functions. It is the sole source of albumin and other plasma proteins and also produces 500 to 1500 mL of bile each day. Conversion and excretion of bilirubin (red bile pigment, which is an end-product of heme from hemoglobin in red blood cells) take place in the liver. Other important functions of the liver include production of clotting factors and storage of vitamins. The liver and gut are the key organs in nutrient absorption and metabolism; nutrients bind to toxins in this pathway and aid in eliminating these toxins from the body.

The liver contributes to a functional immune system by reducing the amount of toxins that could impair the gut lining, which in turn helps prevent the entry of bacteria and viruses into the system. Bile acids, drugs, chemicals, and toxins undergo extensive enterohepatic circulation during the processes of metabolism. The liver also filters all of the blood from the gastrointestinal (GI) system and is therefore the primary organ for metastasis of intestinal cancer.

The *pancreas* is both an exocrine and an endocrine gland. Its primary function in digestion is exocrine secretion of digestive enzymes and pancreatic juices, transported through the pancreatic duct to the duodenum. Proteins, carbohydrates, and fats are broken down in the duodenum, aided by pancreatic and other secretions, which also help to neutralize the acidic substances passed from the stomach to the duodenum. The endocrine function involves the secretion of glucagon and insulin by islet of Langerhans cells for the regulation of carbohydrate metabolism. Pancreatic disease may result in a variety of clinical presentations, depending on whether the exocrine or endocrine function has been impaired.

The *gallbladder*, acting as a reservoir for bile, stores and concentrates the bile during fasting periods and then contracts to expel the bile into the duodenum in response to the arrival of food. Bile helps in alkalinizing the intestinal contents and plays a role in the emulsification, absorption, and digestion of fat. The signal for the gallbladder to contract comes from the release of cholecystokinin, a hormone released into the bloodstream from the wall of the duodenum and upper small intestine.

SIGNS AND SYMPTOMS OF HEPATIC DISEASE

Primary signs and symptoms of liver diseases vary and can include GI symptoms, edema/ascites, dark urine, light-colored or clay-colored feces, and right upper abdominal pain (Box 17-1). Impairment of the liver can result in *hepatic failure* when either the mass of liver cells is sufficiently diminished or their function is impaired as a result of cirrhosis, liver cancer, or infection and/or inflammation. Hepatic failure does not refer to one specific morphologic change but rather to a clinical syndrome that includes hepatic encephalopathy, renal failure (hepatorenal syndrome), endocrine changes, and jaundice.

Dark urine and *light stools* occur in association with jaundice (yellow pigmentation of skin, sclerae, and mucous membranes) (see "Jaundice [Icterus]" below) when the serum bilirubin level increases from normal (0.1-1.0 mg/dL) to a value of 2 or 3 mg/dL. Any damage to the liver impairs bilirubin metabolism from the blood. Normally, bile converted from bilirubin causes brown coloration of the stool. Light-colored (almost white) stools and urine the color of tea or cola indicate an inability of the liver or biliary system to excrete bilirubin properly.

Skin changes associated with the hepatic system include jaundice, pallor, and orange or green skin. When bilirubin reaches levels of 2 to 3 mg/dL, the sclera of the eye takes on a yellow hue. When bilirubin level reaches 5 to 6 mg/dL, the skin becomes yellow. The changes described here in urine, stool, or skin color may be caused by hepatitis, gallbladder disease, pancreatic cancer blocking the bile duct, hepatotoxic medications, or cirrhosis. Other skin changes may include bruising, spider angiomas, and palmar erythema.

Spider angiomas (arterial spider, spider telangiectasis, or vascular spider) are branched dilations of the superficial capillaries, which may be vascular manifestations of increased estrogen levels (hyperestrogenism) (see Fig. 10-3). Spider angiomas and palmar erythema both occur in the presence of liver impairment as a result of increased estrogen levels normally metabolized by the liver. *Palmar erythema* (warm redness of the skin over the palms, also called *liver palms*) especially affects the hypothenar and thenar eminences and pulps of the finger. The soles of the feet may be similarly affected. The person may complain of throbbing, tingling palms.

Box 17-1

MOST COMMON SIGNS AND SYMPTOMS OF HEPATIC DISEASE

- Gastrointestinal symptoms (see Table 16-1)
- Edema/ascites (see Fig. 17-5)
- Dark urine
- Light- or clay-colored stools
- Right upper quadrant abdominal pain
- Skin changes
  - Jaundice
  - Bruising
  - Spider angioma
  - Palmar erythema
- Neurologic involvement
  - Confusion
  - Sleep disturbances
  - Muscle tremors
  - Hyperreactive reflexes
  - Asterixis (see Fig. 17-1)
- Musculoskeletal pain (see text for sites)
- Hepatic osteodystrophy

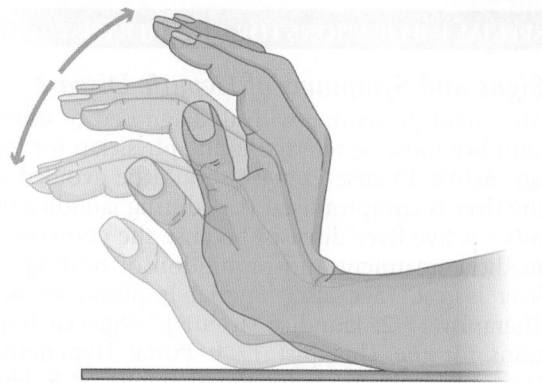

Figure 17-1

Flapping tremor. The flapping tremor elicited by attempted wrist extension while the forearm is fixed is the most common neurologic abnormality associated with liver failure. It can also be observed in uremia, respiratory failure, and severe heart failure. The tremor is absent at rest, decreased by intentional movement, and maximal on sustained posture. It is usually bilateral, although one side may be affected more than the other. (From Sherlock S, Dooley J: *Diseases of the liver and biliary system,* ed 9, Oxford, 1993, Blackwell Scientific Publications.)

Neurologic symptoms, such as confusion, sleep disturbances, muscle tremors, hyperreactive reflexes, and asterixis (see following discussion), may occur. When liver dysfunction results in increased serum ammonia and urea levels, the accumulation of neurotoxins can result in impaired peripheral nerve function. Ammonia from the intestine (produced by protein breakdown) is normally transformed by the liver to urea, glutamine, and asparagine, which are then excreted by the renal system. When the liver does not metabolize and detoxify ammonia, ammonia is transported to the brain, where it reacts with glutamate (excitatory neurotransmitter) to produce glutamine. The reduction of brain glutamate impairs neurotransmission, leading to altered central nervous system (CNS) metabolism and function.

Asterixis and numbness or tingling (misinterpreted as carpal tunnel syndrome) can occur as a result of this ammonia abnormality, causing intrinsic nerve pathology. Asterixis, also called *flapping tremors* or *liver flap,* is a motor disturbance; specifically, it is the inability to maintain wrist extension with forward flexion of the upper extremities. A test for asterixis is asking the client to extend the wrist and hand with the rest of the arm supported on a firm surface or with the arms held out in front of the body. Observe for quick, irregular extensions and flexions of the wrist and fingers (Fig. 17-1). Altered neurotransmission, in the form of impaired inflow of joint and other afferent information to the brainstem reticular formation, causes the movement dysfunction.

Musculoskeletal locations of pain associated with the hepatic and biliary systems include thoracic pain between scapulae, right shoulder, right upper trapezius, right interscapular, or right subscapular areas. Sympathetic fibers from the biliary system are connected through the celiac and splanchnic (visceral) plexuses to the hepatic fibers in the region of the dorsal spine. These connections account

for the intercostal and radiating interscapular pain that accompanies gallbladder disease. Although the innervation is bilateral, most of the biliary fibers reach the cord through the right splanchnic nerves, producing pain in the right shoulder.

Hepatic osteodystrophy, abnormal development of bone, can occur in all forms of cholestasis (bile flow suppression) and hepatocellular disease, especially in the alcoholic. Bone pain may occur especially in the presence of osteomalacia or more often, osteoporosis. Hepatic osteoporosis is secondary to osteoblastic dysfunction rather than to excessive bone resorption. The pathogenesis is probably complex, and factors include calcium malabsorption, alcohol, corticosteroid therapy, estrogen deficiency in the postmenopausal woman, and vitamin D deficiency with secondary hyperparathyroidism.

Vertebral wedging, vertebral crush fractures, and kyphosis can be severe; decalcification of the rib cage and pseudofractures occur frequently. Pseudofractures or Looser zones are narrow lines of radiolucency (areas of darkness on x-ray film) usually oriented perpendicular to the bone surface. This may represent a stress fracture that has been repaired by the laying down of inadequately mineralized osteoid, or these sites may occur as a result of mechanical erosion caused by arterial pulsations, as arteries frequently overlie sites of pseudofractures.

Osteoporosis associated with primary biliary cirrhosis and primary sclerosing cholangitis parallels the severity of liver disease rather than the duration. Painful osteoarthropathy may develop in the wrists and ankles as a nonspecific complication of chronic liver disease.

Portal hypertension, ascites, and *hepatic encephalopathy* are three other major complications of liver disease that are discussed in greater depth in this chapter as distinct clinical conditions.

Signs and Symptoms of Hepatic Disease

Any client presenting with undiagnosed or untreated jaundice must be referred to the physician for follow-up. Active, intense exercise should be avoided when the liver is compromised (i.e., during jaundice or any other active liver disease) because the cornerstone of medical treatment and promotion of healing of the liver is rest. (See also "Special Implications for the Therapist 17-2: Jaundice (Icterus)," "Special Implications for the Therapist 17-4: Portal Hypertension," "Special Implications for the Therapist 17-5: Hepatic Encephalopathy," and "Special Implications for the Therapist 17-6: Ascites" below.)

The physical therapist can be instrumental in helping the affected individual to organize self-care, pace activities, and practice relaxation techniques such as Physiologic Quieting or other forms of biofeedback. At the same time, steps must be taken to prevent the potential complications of reduced activity or immobility. Identify individuals at-risk for pressure ulcers and implement prevention strategies such as skin care, optimal nutrition, and hydration, teaching the client and family pressure-reducing or -relieving positions and turning strategies. Referral to a nutrition specialist may be needed.

An increased risk of coagulopathy (decreased clotting ability) also occurs with liver disease, necessitating precautions. Easy bruising and bleeding under the skin or into the joints in response to the slightest trauma can occur when coagulation is impaired. This condition necessitates extreme care in the therapy setting, especially with any intervention requiring manual therapy or the use of any equipment, including modalities, resistive exercise or weight-training devices, and potentially the use of gait belts.

The most common neurologic abnormality associated with liver failure (liver flap or asterixis) (see Fig. 17-1) also can be observed in uremia, respiratory failure, and severe heart failure. The rapid flexion extension movements at the metacarpophalangeal and wrist joints often are accompanied by lateral movements of the digits. Sometimes movement of arms, neck, and jaws; protruding tongue; retracted mouth; and tightly closed eyelids are involved, and the gait is ataxic. The tremor is absent at rest, decreased by intentional movement, and maximal on sustained posture. It is usually bilateral, although not bilaterally synchronous, and one side may be affected more than the other. It may be observed by gentle elevation of a limb or by the client's gripping the therapist's hand. In coma, the tremor disappears.

AGING AND THE HEPATIC SYSTEM

Of all the organ systems, the liver appears to be relatively protected from age-related deficits, instead it continues its remarkable ability to regenerate its mass following partial hepatectomy. However, the liver does slowdown in its ability to regenerate quickly and it does decrease in size and weight with advancing age, requiring more time to process substances, medications, and alcohol.[205] The decreased liver weight is accompanied by diminished blood flow. This combination of decreased liver mass and blood flow may account for some changes in drug elimination observed in the older adult. And with comorbidity and polypharmacy so prevalent in the aging adults, age-related changes in pharmacokinetics and pharmacodynamics have become an increasingly important area of research.[210]

Other studies are bringing to light the effects of physiologic age-related changes in the hepatic system, such as the significance of growth hormone synthesis by the hepatic system responsible for maintaining various body tissues (e.g., bones, muscles, cardiovascular system, immune system, and CNS). Researchers are particularly interested in examining whether treatment with exogenous growth hormone can retard or reverse hepatic age-related changes in body structure and function.[13,205]

Drug Distribution and Metabolism

In the past, adjusting dosage downward based on hepatic function related to aging has not been considered necessary. However, emerging data on the use of pharmacologic agents in the older population suggest that the administration of many agents (especially chemotherapeutic agents) may be affected by physiologic changes occurring with age.[142] Dose adjustments to compensate for pharmacokinetic and pharmacodynamic changes that occur in the older adult are being studied and adjustments for specific drugs presented.[118,149,183]

Modification of drug distribution may be required as we age because of a decrease in serum albumin and to accommodate for modifications of body composition (increase in the proportion of fat mass and decrease of lean mass).[107] In older adults, changes in the response to drugs can develop, affecting the CNS (increased sensibility to any neurologic effect of drugs), the cardiovascular system, and the renal management of water and electrolytes. The incidence of renal failure increases with age; the accompanying changes in glomerular filtration rate requires that doses of drugs having significant renal elimination must be adjusted.[107]

Immune Function and Metabolism

The liver is an important immune system organ as it contains a large number of immunologically active cells (e.g., T and B lymphocytes, Kupffer cells, liver-adapted natural killer cells (pit cells), natural killer cells expressing T-cell receptor, stellate cells, and dendritic cells). The liver is the major site of production of proteins that are associated with acute inflammatory reactions. Kupffer cells have an important role in the phagocytosis that presents a barrier to invasion of pathogenic organisms from the intestine.[172] The hepatic natural killer cells and natural killer cells expressing T-cell receptor are important in resistance to tumor cell invasion.

Age-related changes in sinusoids result in substantial alterations in many immunologic functions.[172]

Sinusoidal endothelial cells of the liver aid in disposal of waste molecules generated through inflammatory, immunologic, or general homeostatic processes. Loss of these cells allows a build-up of toxins within the liver that negatively impacts immune system function. For example, on autopsy, a buildup of brown pigment is seen, which is a result of accumulated unexcretable metabolic residue (end-stage metabolic products of lipids and proteins) acquired over a lifetime. No apparent physiologic significance has been identified with this pigment.

Excessive fat accumulation in the liver (a condition called *hepatic* steatosis) occurs with aging and increases the risk and likelihood of changes in hepatic function and metabolism as we get older.[68] These changes have been associated with metabolic abnormalities (e.g., central obesity, insulin resistance, type 2 diabetes, and dyslipidemia—all risk factors for cardiovascular diseases and cancer).[65] And, of course, the role of the hepatic system in cholesterol formation and whole-body cholesterol metabolism and hepatic-induced lipid profiles (also as these factors relate to cardiovascular health) are under intense scientific scrutiny.[65,139]

The pancreas undergoes structural changes, such as fibrosis, fatty acid deposits, and atrophy, but the pancreas has a large reserve capacity, and 90% of its function would have to be lost before any observable dysfunction occurs. Much remains unknown about the gallbladder in the aging process, but aging apparently has little effect on gallbladder size, contractility, or function. The gallbladder releases less bile into the liver, allowing more time for gallstones to develop. There is some evidence that moderate and vigorous physical activity enhances the function of the gallbladder as measured by reduced risk of gallbladder removal in physically active women.[112]

Lab Tests

Liver function test results (see Chapter 40), such as levels of aspartate transaminase (AST), alanine transaminase (ALT), γ-glutamyl transpeptidase, alkaline phosphatase (ALP), and total serum bilirubin, remain unchanged and within normal limits established for the adult. However, these tests often measure hepatic damage rather than overall function; abnormal values for these tests in older adults reflect disease rather than the effects of aging.

LIVER

Liver Disease Complications

As a result of the extraordinary number of vital functions the liver performs, severe complications result when the liver has been damaged or is no longer functioning. Jaundice is a symptom that occurs with many types of diseases and disorders (both acute and chronic). End-stage complications occur most often because of cirrhosis and include portal hypertension, hepatic encephalopathy, ascites, and the hepatorenal syndrome. Any illness, toxin, or infection that leads to end-stage liver disease can display these complications.

Jaundice (Icterus)

Jaundice (icterus) is not a disease, but is a common symptom of many different diseases and disorders (Box 17-2). It is clinically characterized by yellow discoloration of the skin, sclerae, and mucous membranes. Jaundice occurs either as a result of an overproduction of bilirubin, defects in bilirubin metabolism (in uptake by the liver or conjugation), the presence of liver disease, or obstruction of bile flow.

In the normal breakdown of hemoglobin, the end product is bilirubin. In this metabolic process, the heme portion of hemoglobin is converted into biliverdin and then to bilirubin in the bone marrow and the spleen. Bilirubin is released into the bloodstream, where it binds to albumin, and is then taken up by hepatocytes to be conjugated with glucuronic acid. Once it is conjugated, it is then released into the bile. A small percentage of conjugated bile returns to the plasma and is excreted into the kidneys. In the terminal ileum and colon, conjugated bilirubin is deconjugated and excreted as colorless urobilinogen. Diseases that result in ineffective erythropoiesis (abnormal formation of erythrocytes) produce large amounts of bilirubin as a result of chronic hemolysis or destruction of cells.

Some diseases, such as Gilbert syndrome, have defects in the liver's ability to conjugate bilirubin. Drugs, such as rifampin, may compete with bilirubin for uptake by the liver, decreasing the quantity of bilirubin the liver

---

Box 17-2

CLASSIFICATION OF JAUNDICE

Diseases Associated with Overproduction of Bilirubin

- Hemolysis
  - Thalassemia, sickle cell anemia
  - Autoimmune hemolytic anemia
- Reabsorption of hematoma
- Blood transfusion

Decreased Uptake or Conjugation in Bilirubin Metabolism

- Gilbert syndrome
- Jaundice of newborns
- Medications

Hepatocyte Dysfunction

- Hepatitis
  - Viral
  - Alcohol-related
  - Autoimmune
  - Toxic/medication-induced
  - Ischemia
- Chronic Hepatic Disease
  - Wilson disease
  - Hemochromatosis

Impaired Bile Flow

- Cholelithiasis
- Primary sclerosing cholangitis
- Pancreatic cancer
- Pancreatitis

can process. Diseases, toxins, infections, and ischemia can cause generalized liver disease (acute and chronic), which reduces the capability of the liver to function normally and process bilirubin. Finally, bile ducts can be obstructed by diseases, tumors, and stones, leading to an elevation in bilirubin that has been conjugated.

As mentioned, jaundice is not clinically evident (particularly in the sclera of the eyes) until the plasma level reaches 3 mg/dL. Once the level reaches 5 to 6 mg/dL, the skin becomes a yellow color. Urine turns a darker color and stool is light in color. Signs and symptoms of liver disease may also be present.

Laboratory testing can aid in the specific diagnosis of jaundice. Bilirubin can be reported as conjugated or unconjugated, which provides a more accurate measurement than direct and indirect. Direct refers to the capability of the laboratory to directly measure conjugated bilirubin, whereas the indirect bilirubin refers to the unconjugated portion of bilirubin, which cannot be directly measured in the laboratory, and must be subtracted from the total bilirubin present in the blood.

Conjugated and direct are not always equivalent, particularly in disorders of bilirubin metabolism. In clients with jaundice, an elevation in the conjugated bilirubin is more common than unconjugated. Elevations in liver transaminases (AST and ALT) suggest that liver disease is involved. Many other tests are available for the specific diagnosis of jaundice, depending on the suspected process, and are included in the specific disease sections in this chapter.

SPECIAL IMPLICATIONS FOR THE THERAPIST   17-2

Jaundice (Icterus)

With successful treatment of the underlying cause, jaundice usually begins to resolve within 4 to 6 weeks. After this time, activity and exercise can be resumed or increased per individual tolerance, depending on the overall medical condition and presence of any complications. The return of normal stool and urine colors is an indication of resolution. (See also "Special Implications for the Therapist 17-1: Signs and Symptoms of Hepatic Disease" above.)

Cirrhosis

Cirrhosis is the final common pathway of chronic, progressive inflammation of the liver. It is characterized pathologically by a progressive loss of normal tissue that is replaced with fibrosis and nodular regeneration. There are many diseases, medications, and toxins that can damage the liver and ultimately lead to cirrhosis, but the most common in the United States include alcohol abuse and hepatitis C virus (HCV).

Overall, in the United States, cirrhosis is the 12th leading cause of death, accounting for about 28,000 deaths a year.[7] Cirrhosis of the liver occurs when inflammation (from disease or toxin) causes liver tissue damage and/or necrosis. With continued cycles of inflammation and healing, fibrous bands of connective tissue replace normal liver cells. These fibrous bands eventually constrict

and partition the liver into irregular nodules. Once 80% to 90% of the liver is replaced with scar tissue, there is also significant loss of function, associated with decompensation of homeostasis.

The signs and symptoms of cirrhosis (Figs. 17-2 and 17-3) are multiple and varied, representing interference with major functions of the liver, and include processing dietary amino acids, carbohydrates, lipids, and vitamins; metabolizing cholesterol, hormones, vitamins, medications, and toxins; producing clotting factors and other plasma proteins; and storing glycogen.

Clients with cirrhosis exhibit fatigue, weight loss, jaundice, coagulopathies, loss of ability to metabolize drugs, and hypoalbuminemia (the remaining serious complications are discussed later). History, physical examination, laboratory tests, and imaging tests aid in diagnosing the specific cause. Once cirrhosis has developed, it is usually not reversible, although each disease may have a specific therapy to reduce the risk of developing cirrhosis.

Typically, complications are treated on an individual basis and transplantation provides the best therapy for long-term survival. Despite improvements in medical care for individuals with cirrhosis, mortality from infection, renal failure, hepatic encephalopathy, and hepatocellular carcinoma remains high.[63] The life expectancy of individuals with cirrhosis who develop uncomplicated ascites is reportedly 50% for 3 years.[217]

SPECIAL IMPLICATIONS FOR THE THERAPIST   17-3

Cirrhosis

One of the most common symptoms associated with cirrhosis is ascites, an accumulation of fluid in the peritoneal cavity surrounding the intestines. The distention often occurs very slowly over a number of weeks or months and may be associated with bilateral edema of the feet and ankles. The client may be unable to put on a pair of shoes, preferring to leave the shoes unlaced or to wear slippers. In a home health or inpatient hospital setting, this change in dress may not be as noticeable as it would be in a private practice or outpatient clinic. It is always important to remain alert to these potential signs of fluid retention and to ask about any changes in health status or weight gain.

Detection of blood loss in the form of hematemesis, tarry stools, bleeding gums, frequent and heavy nosebleeds, or excessive bruising must be reported to the physician. Preventing increased intraabdominal pressure (see Box 16-1) and preventing injury owing to falls require client education regarding safety precautions.

Alcohol causes whole-body and tissue-specific changes in protein metabolism. Chronic alcohol use increases nitrogen excretion and reduces skeletal muscle protein synthesis with concomitant loss of lean tissue mass. Loss of skeletal collagen contributes to alcohol-related osteoporosis. The loss of skeletal muscle protein (i.e., chronic alcoholic myopathy) occurs in up to two-thirds of all chronic alcohol users. Protein turnover changes in organs such as the heart have important implications for cardiovascular function and morbidity. Most clients with cirrhosis have

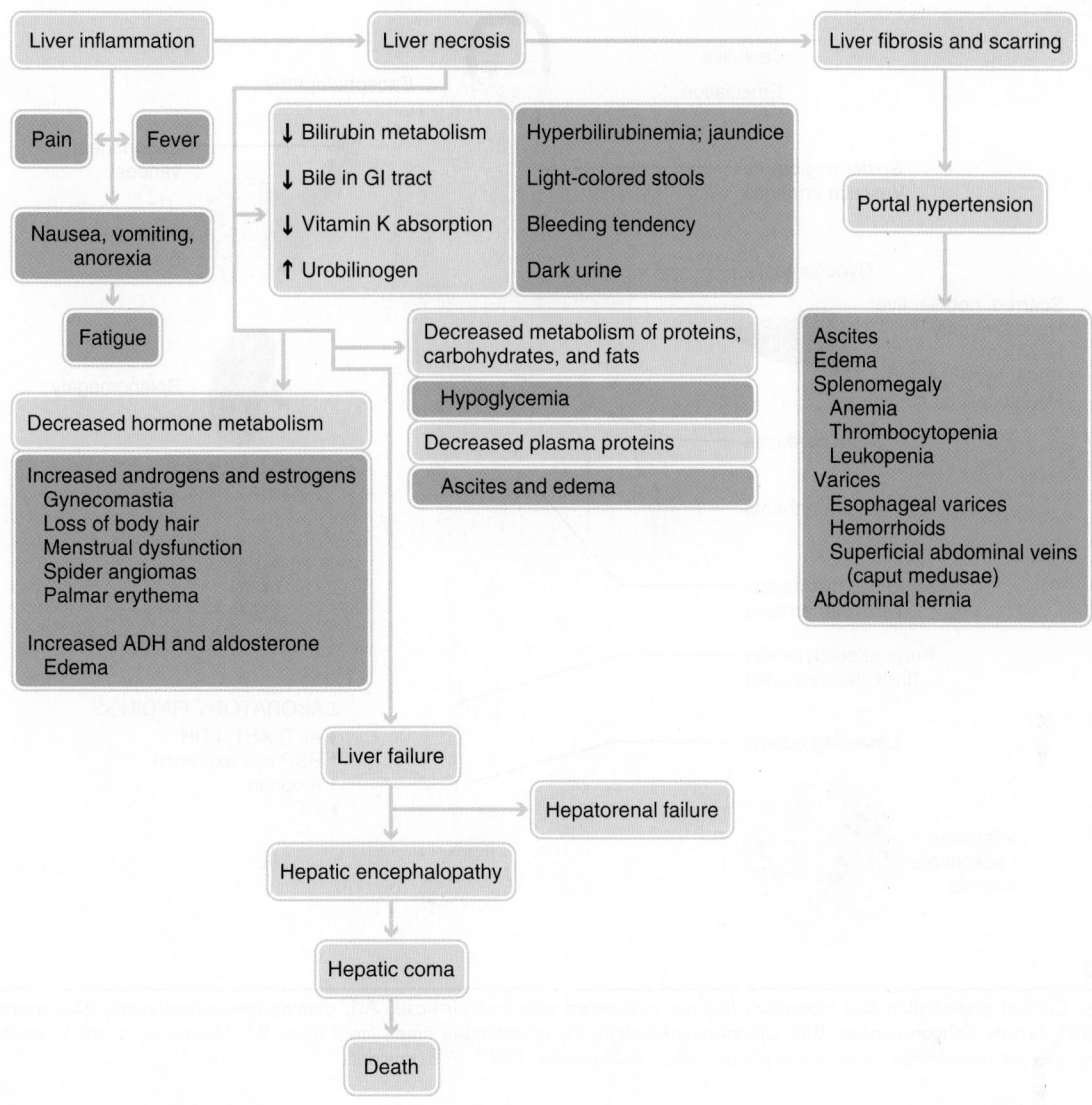

Figure 17-2

Pathologic basis *(yellow boxes)* and resultant clinical manifestations *(green boxes)* associated with cirrhosis of the liver.

significantly reduced aerobic capacity, although the exact mechanism for this has not been proved.[56,185]

Rest to reduce metabolic demands on the liver and to increase circulation often is recommended for clients with cirrhosis. Frequent rests during therapy and avoiding unnecessary fatigue are also important. Exercise limitation in cirrhosis is typically attributed to cirrhotic myopathy without impaired oxygen utilization. Chronic alcoholic myopathy affecting the proximal muscles is usually mild and results in muscle atrophy and measurable decrease in muscle strength. The therapist must remain alert to any potential medical complications in any client, regardless of the physical therapy diagnosis.

Portal Hypertension

Portal hypertension is defined as an increase in hepatic sinusoidal (sinuses in the liver where blood flows) pressure greater than 6 mm Hg. Portal refers to the area where blood vessels enter into the liver. Venous blood returning from the stomach, large and small intestine, pancreas, and spleen is transported via the portal vein to the liver (the splanchnic circulation). Most cases of portal hypertension are related to cirrhosis. Other causes include thrombus, tumor, or infection, or may be idiopathic. With the development of cirrhosis, hyperdynamic vascular responses and mechanical factors prevent the flow of blood, resulting in increased pressure and resistance in the portal circulatory system (Fig. 17-4).

A reduction in nitric oxide release from liver endothelial cells and production of endothelin-1 leads to intrahepatic vasoconstriction, whereas increased blood flow from the portal vein and splanchnic circulation further increases the pressure. Fibrosis, nodularity, and abnormal liver architecture combine to form mechanical barriers to blood flow and increase the resistance.

As a result of this increased portal pressure, blood that normally flows to the portal vein is reversed and blood

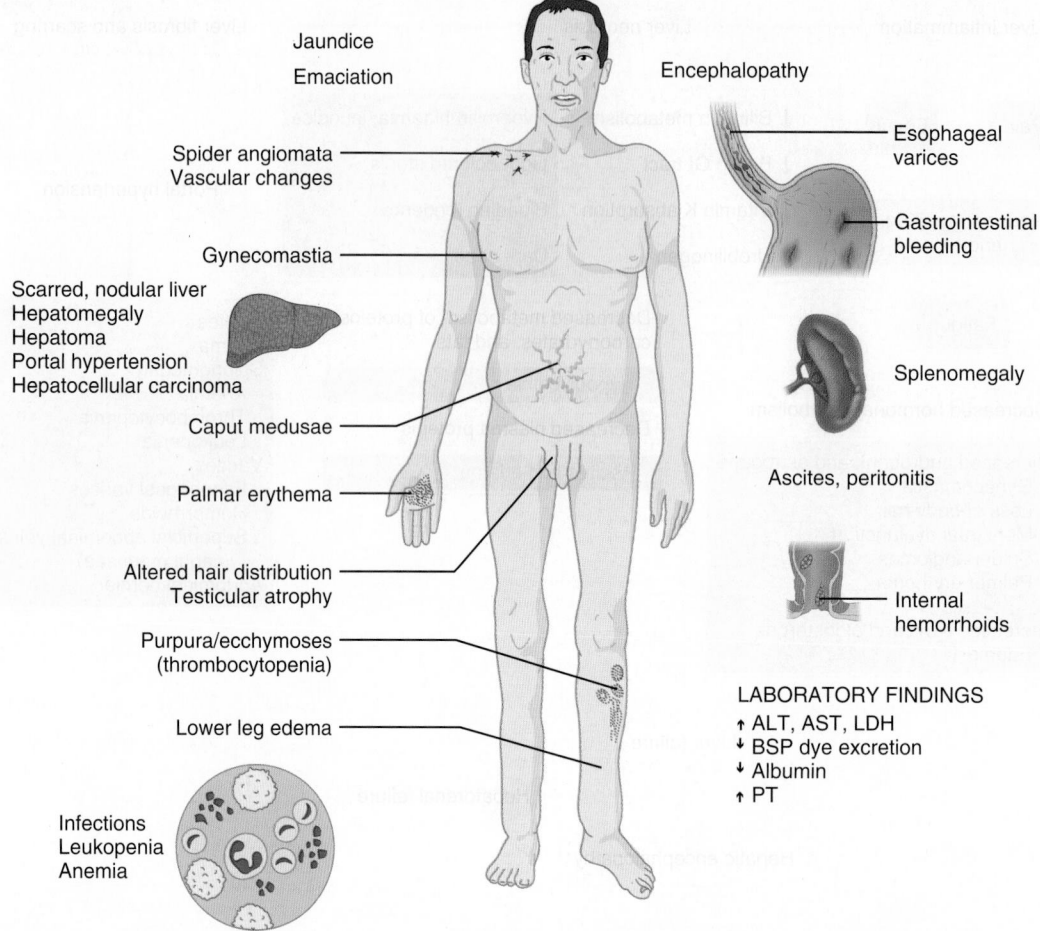

Jaundice
Emanciation

Encephalopathy

Esophageal
varices

Gastrointestinal
bleeding

Spider angiomata
Vascular changes

Gynecomastia

Scarred, nodular liver
Hepatomegaly
Hepatoma
Portal hypertension
Hepatocellular carcinoma

Caput medusae

Palmar erythema

Splenomegaly

Ascites, peritonitis

Altered hair distribution
Testicular atrophy

Purpura/ecchymoses
(thrombocytopenia)

Lower leg edema

Internal
hemorrhoids

LABORATORY FINDINGS
↑ ALT, AST, LDH
↓ BSP dye excretion
↓ Albumin
↑ PT

Infections
Leukopenia
Anemia

Figure 17-3

Liver cirrhosis. Clinical presentation and laboratory findings associated with liver cirrhosis. ALT, alanine aminotransferase; AST, aspartate aminotransferase; LDH, lactate dehydrogenase; BSP, sulfobromophthalein; PT, prothrombin time. (From Black JM, Matassarin-Jacobs E, editors: *Medical-surgical nursing: clinical management for continuity of care*, ed 5, Philadelphia, 1997, WB Saunders.)

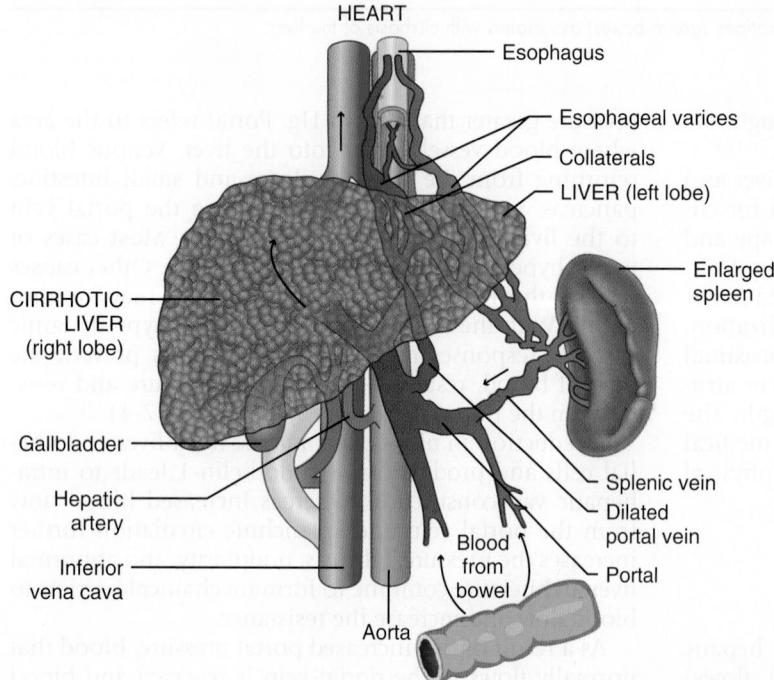

HEART

Esophagus

Esophageal varices

Collaterals

LIVER (left lobe)

Enlarged
spleen

CIRRHOTIC
LIVER
(right lobe)

Gallbladder

Hepatic
artery

Inferior
vena cava

Splenic vein

Dilated
portal vein

Blood
from
bowel

Portal

Aorta

Figure 17-4

Portal hypertension. Normally, in the portal venous system (consisting of the portal veins, sinusoids, and hepatic veins), the portal veins carry blood from the GI tract, gallbladder, pancreas, and spleen to the liver. Veins collecting from these sites form the splenic vein and superior and inferior mesenteric veins, which, in turn, merge to create the portal vein. Portal hypertension occurs when portal venous pressure exceeds the pressure in the nonportal abdominal veins (e.g., inferior vena cava) by at least 6 mm Hg. As portal pressure rises, increased resistance to blood flow causes blood pooling in the spleen and the development of collateral channels formed in an effort to equalize pressures between these two venous systems. These collateral vessels or varices bypass the liver and cause large, tortuous veins, especially in the esophagus *(esophageal varices).*

begins to flow back to the stomach, esophagus, umbilicus, and rectum. This system is normally small with modest blood flow. However, in the cirrhotic state, blood flow increases in these vessels, causing dilation and expansion. These engorged vessels give rise to rectal varices, prominent vessels around the umbilicus (caput medusae), and gastroesophageal varices. The collateral veins of the stomach and esophagus are the most likely to bleed because of a lack of communicating vessels.

Gastroesophageal varices are one of the most serious complications of portal hypertension, occurring in 40% of people with cirrhosis. Endoscopy should be performed in all clients with cirrhosis to screen for varices. Follow-up endoscopy is scheduled, depending on the presence and severity of varices. Clinical manifestations of gastroesophageal bleeding include hematemesis or melena (or both). The blood is usually dark red in color. More than half of bleeds stop spontaneously and more than 90% of bleeds can be controlled with therapy. But serious bleeding can quickly result in hypovolemia, shock, and death. Treatment is aimed at preventing bleeding by decreasing portal blood flow and intrahepatic pressure.

Nonselective β-blockers aid in preventing bleeding and rebleeding, whereas vasopressin, octreotide, and somatostatin are used to decrease splanchnic flow. Nitrates may relieve intrahepatic vasoconstriction. Endoscopic sclerotherapy can be used prophylactically or in clients who do not tolerate medications; variceal band ligation can be utilized in acute esophageal bleeding and to prevent rebleeding. Surgical shunts or more commonly, placement of a transjugular intrahepatic portacaval shunt can divert blood around the liver and away from the collateral systems.

Prognosis is poor for clients with repeated esophageal varices, and liver transplantation should be pursued.

SPECIAL IMPLICATIONS FOR THE THERAPIST 17-4

Portal Hypertension

Portal pressure in individuals is dynamic, with highest pressures during the night, after eating, and in response to coughing, sneezing, and exercise. Such variations may combine with local factors in vessel walls to contribute to a pressure surge that can lead to a variceal bleed. The therapist can teach the individual how to modify and reduce pressure, especially anything that increases intraabdominal pressure (see Box 16-1), such as coughing, straining at stool, or improper lifting. Any therapy program for a client with known varices must take this factor into account when presenting active or active-assisted exercises, or unsupported gait training.[66]

Hepatic Encephalopathy

Definition and Overview. Hepatic encephalopathy or portosystemic encephalopathy is a complex neuropsychiatric syndrome with symptoms ranging from subtle neuropsychiatric and motor disturbances to deep coma and death. It is a potentially reversible, decreased level of consciousness in people with severe liver disease. This complication can occur with both acute and chronic liver disease.[167]

Clinical Manifestations. There is consensus that hepatic encephalopathy is characterized as a spectrum of neuropsychiatric symptoms in the absence of brain disease, ranging from overt hepatic encephalopathy to minimal hepatic encephalopathy.[98] People with chronic end-stage liver disease often have an insidious onset; initially there are mild changes in ability to concentrate and complete complex tasks. Subtle signs of hepatic encephalopathy (e.g., difficulty with executive decision making and/or decreased psychomotor speed) are observed in nearly 70% of adults with cirrhosis.[250]

As the hepatic encephalopathy progresses, mental status changes become more obvious. The classification system used most often with hepatic encephalopathy is the West Haven Criteria with scores ranging from zero (minimal hepatic encephalopathy) to 4 (being in a coma), depending on the severity of neurologic involvement (Table 17-1).

Etiology and Pathogenesis. Although the pathologic mechanisms of hepatic encephalopathy are not well understood, they are thought to involve increased levels of ammonia and inflammation, which lead to low-grade cerebral edema.[98] Shunting of blood away from the hepatic portal system (because of cirrhosis) to the vena cava contributes to encephalopathy. Ammonia with increased formation of glutamine (inhibitory neurotransmitter affecting brain function) plays a central role in the development of hepatic encephalopathy,[221] but is not likely the sole cause.

Research is beginning to show how elevated ammonia and other metabolic abnormalities (including changes in neurotransmitters in the brain and circulating amino acid levels) combine to result in encephalopathy. For example, the role of γ-aminobutyric acid– or glutamate-mediated neurotransmission in the pathophysiology of hepatic encephalopathy, and the involvement of other neurotransmitters (e.g., serotonin, dopamine, adenosine, and histamine) and neurosteroids or endogenous benzodiazepines also have been suggested.[167]

Ammonia is created by bacteria in the colon from the metabolism of protein and urea. Ammonia is absorbed into the portal blood system and is 5 to 10 times higher there than in the general circulatory system. The liver is typically able to metabolize ammonia, but with liver disease and shunting of blood away from the liver (particularly to the brain), ammonia levels rise. The kidneys are also a source of ammonia, which is increased in the face of diuretic use and hypokalemia. Muscles aid in ammonia removal but cirrhosis is often accompanied by muscle wasting. In the brain, ammonia appears to directly alter the function and signaling of nerve cells.

MEDICAL MANAGEMENT

DIAGNOSIS, TREATMENT, AND PROGNOSIS. The development of hepatic encephalopathy warrants a careful evaluation and correction of the cause. Serious and common causes include bleeding, infection (particularly spontaneous bacterial peritonitis), hypovolemia, or electrolyte abnormalities (hypokalemia). Other common factors that may precipitate or severely aggravate hepatic encephalopathy include constipation, diuretics, increased

Table 17-1   Grades of Hepatic Encephalopathy

Grade 0*	Grade 1	Grade 2	Grade 3	Grade 4
Nearly asymptomatic Normal level of consciousness No detectable personality or behavior changes Minimal changes in memory and concentration (e.g., mildly forgetful or confused) Minimal changes in intellectual function	Slight personality changes, mood swings (irritability, restless) Short attention span Mild confusion Bilateral numbness/tingling Muscular incoordination Apraxia Tremor; asterixis may be observed with clinical testing (see Fig. 17-1) Impaired handwriting Sleep disorders (inverted sleep patterns[202])	Tremor progresses to asterixis Resistance to passive movement Myoclonus; hypoactive deep tendon reflexes Lethargy or apathy Unusual behavior (abusive, violent, noisy) Apraxia Ataxia Slow or slurred speech	Hyperventilation Marked confusion, amnesia Incoherent speech Asterixis (liver flap) Muscle rigidity Hyperreactive deep tendon reflexes Positive Babinski sign Sleeps most of the time but can be aroused Disorientation to time and place Disinhibited (inappropriate) behavior	Comatose; unresponsive to verbal or noxious stimuli No asterixis Positive Oculocephalic (doll's-eye) reflex Decerebrate posturing Dilated pupils Lack of response to stimuli

*Previously known as subclinical hepatic encephalopathy.
The West Haven Classification reflected in this table is used most often to grade hepatic encephalopathy.[25,194]

dietary protein, and CNS-depressant drugs, such as alcohol, benzodiazepines (e.g., Librium, Valium, Dalmane, and Tranxene), and opiates.

Because protein can precipitate or worsen encephalopathy, many of the symptoms can be improved by eliminating or reducing sources of protein (i.e., stopping any internal bleeding and restricting dietary protein to 60 g/day). Lactulose (or lactitol) is a first-line pharmacologic therapy that decreases nitrogenous compounds from being absorbed from the gut and increases transit time through the intestine (the goal is 2-4 bowel movements a day). Ammonia-lowering therapy in suspected encephalopathy cases can be beneficial even when the ammonia level is normal, as the production is tied to other toxins.

Neomycin is an antibiotic that decreases the bacterial count in the intestine but carries nephrotoxicities and ototoxicities as a result of systemic absorption. The new medication rifaximin (a nonabsorbable antibiotic) has been shown in preliminary studies to be effective in hepatic encephalopathy.[136] Flumazenil is a benzodiazepine-receptor antagonist that may block the γ-aminobutyric acid receptor complex, reversing inhibition. It has been shown to improve hepatic encephalopathy in the short term but has no effect on survival.[4]

Reversal of hepatic encephalopathy is typically successful when a source is identified, corrected, and treated appropriately. Altered mental status caused by hepatic encephalopathy is a negative prognostic factor.[187] *Without intervention, mortality is high, as the person's condition progresses into coma.* Similar to most complications of end-stage liver disease, liver transplantation provides the best long-term treatment.

SPECIAL IMPLICATIONS FOR THE THERAPIST   17-5

Hepatic Encephalopathy

The inpatient or homebound client with hepatic encephalopathy has difficulty ambulating and is extremely unsteady. Protective measures must be taken against falls. The home health therapist must be alert for any report of GI bleeding that will result in protein accumulation in the GI tract, exacerbating this condition (e.g., blood in stools or black or tarry stools). The client should be following a low-protein diet.

The physician may prescribe lactulose in the prevention and treatment of hepatic encephalopathy,[243] but diarrhea is a side effect. The client experiencing prolonged diarrhea should be encouraged to report this information to the physician for possible follow-up. A reduced dosage may be required to prevent further electrolyte imbalance. (See "Electrolyte Imbalance" in Chapter 5.)

The immobile client who lacks reflexes is vulnerable to numerous complications requiring attention to the prevention of pneumonia and skin breakdown. Skin breakdown in a client who is malnourished from liver disease and is immobile, jaundiced, and edematous can occur in less than 24 hours. Careful attention to skin care, passive exercise, and frequent changes in position are required.

Rest between activities is advocated, and strenuous exercise is to be avoided. The therapist should watch for (and immediately report) signs of anemia (e.g., reduced hemoglobin, weakness, dyspnea on exertion, easy fatigability, skin pallor, or tachycardia; see "Anemia" in Chapter 14), infection (see Box 8-1), and GI bleeding (e.g., melena, hematemesis, easy bruising).

Minimal hepatic encephalopathy (grade 0) in cirrhosis is associated with impaired driving skills and increased risk of motor vehicle accidents.[18] In earlier stages of hepatic encephalopathy, health care providers may identify subtle changes in mental status with impaired ability to drive. Assessments of psychometric and neurophysiologic techniques are often used to test for minimal hepatic encephalopathy in order to prevent driving accidents.[97] In one study, clients with cirrhosis but no evidence of hepatic encephalopathy underwent psychomotor testing; 60% were found unfit to drive and 25% displayed questionable driving skills.[207] Other studies have shown similar results.[19]

A more recent review of driving fitness among people with chronic health conditions[134] concluded there is not enough evidence that clinical and neuropsychologic screening tests would lead to a reduction in motor vehicle crashes involving chronic disabled drivers. The authors of that report state: "It seems necessary to develop tests with proven validity for identifying high-risk drivers so that physicians can provide guidance to their patients in chronic conditions, and also to medical advisory boards working with licensing offices." Until standardized driver simulation tests are available to screen effectively for individuals with cirrhosis, driving must be assessed on a case-by-case basis[134]; the therapist should keep in mind that appropriate referral for currently available testing may be needed sooner than later.

Ascites

Ascites is the abnormal accumulation of fluid within the peritoneal cavity.[70] Ascites is most often caused by decompensated liver cirrhosis (85% of cases[217]), but other diseases associated with ascites include heart failure, abdominal malignancies, nephrotic syndrome, infection, and malnutrition.

The mechanism for the accumulation of fluid in the case of cirrhosis is principally a result of portal hypertension. High pressure in the vessels attempting to pass blood through the cirrhotic liver leads to vasodilation of the splanchnic vessels (vessels to the gut or viscera), which, in turn, decreases the filling of the vessels going to the kidney. The renin–angiotensin–aldosterone system is activated, resulting in sodium and water retention. However, because of the high pressure in the liver and splanchnic vessels, excessive lymph (protein-rich fluid) is produced that leaks into the tissues and eventually into the abdominal cavity.[12]

Ascites becomes clinically detectable when more than 500 mL has accumulated, causing weight gain, abdominal distention, increased abdominal girth, and, eventually, peripheral edema (Fig. 17-5). Dyspnea with increased respiratory rate occurs when the fluid displaces the diaphragm.

Diagnosis of ascites is usually based on clinical manifestations in the presence of liver disease. Paracentesis is used as the initial test in people with new-onset ascites to determine the cause. Fluid is sent to the laboratory for chemical and microscopic evaluation. Abdominal ultrasonography can aid in locating pockets of ascitic fluid that may be loculated (formed or divided into small cavities or compartments).

In people with established cirrhosis, paracentesis can be diagnostic and therapeutic. Large-volume paracentesis with administration of albumin is the treatment of choice for tense ascites (i.e., when a person is no longer able to breathe or eat comfortably), followed by the use of diuretics to reduce reaccumulation of fluid.

Treatment of mild-to-moderate ascites includes sodium restriction accompanied by diuretic use.[197] Fluid restriction is appropriate when the serum sodium decreases to less than 120 to 125 mEq/L. The development of refractory

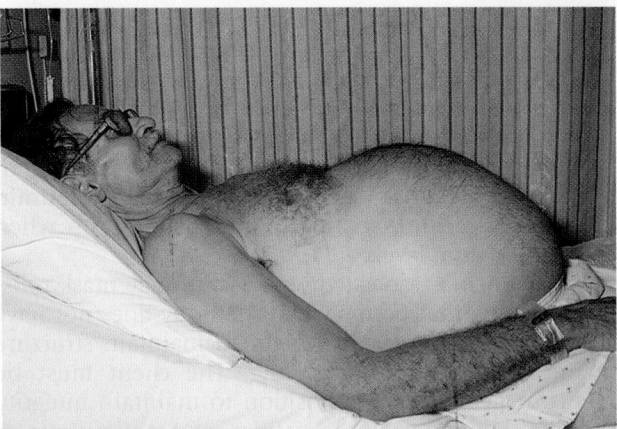

Figure 17-5

Ascites in an individual with cirrhosis. Distended abdomen, dilated upper abdominal veins, and inverted umbilicus are classic manifestations. Peripheral edema associated with developing ascites may be observed first by the therapist. (From Swartz MH: *Textbook of physical diagnosis*, ed 5, Philadelphia, 2006, WB Saunders.)

ascites affects 10% of individuals with advanced cirrhosis[21]) and is associated with a poor prognosis.[217] Serial large-volume paracentesis or transjugular intrahepatic portacaval shunt alleviates pressure in the portal area, but may induce hepatic encephalopathy caused by bypassing the liver (see "Hepatic Encephalopathy" above). Liver transplantation provides the best treatment option but is not always readily available.

Over a 10-year period, 50% of individuals with previously compensated cirrhosis develop ascites. Ascites is a sign of hepatic decompensation and, therefore, associated with a poor prognosis, with only a 56% survival 3 years after onset. In addition, morbidity is increased because of the risk of additional complications, such as spontaneous bacterial peritonitis and hepatorenal syndrome.[70]

The microbial source of infection of the ascitic fluid is the gut, where organisms (typically *Escherichia coli*, streptococci [mostly pneumococci], and *Klebsiella*) are translocated into lymph nodes and then into the ascitic fluid. Bacterial peritonitis is symptomatic in the majority of cases (fever, chills, abdominal pain, mental status changes, and tenderness), but symptoms can often be subtle. Without diagnosis by paracentesis and then antibiotic treatment, the infection can be fatal.[70]

SPECIAL IMPLICATIONS FOR THE THERAPIST　**17-6**

Ascites

Most people with ascites are more comfortable in a high Fowler position (head of the bed raised 18-20 inches above the level with the knees elevated). Breathing techniques are important to maintain adequate respiratory function and to prevent the development of atelectasis or pneumonia. The homebound person who has ascites should be monitored for the possible development of bacterial peritonitis. Onset of fever, chills, abdominal pain, and tenderness should be reported to the physician.

Decreases in serum albumin associated with the development of ascites are accompanied by a parallel decrease in oncotic pressure in blood vessels causing peripheral edema. Persons with serum albumin levels between 2.5 and 3.5 g/dL are at moderate risk of malnutrition, and those whose levels are 2.5 g/dL or less are at great risk (see Table 40-5). Because albumin binds to calcium, serum albumin levels drop when serum calcium levels are low.

The edema associated with ascites may mask muscle wasting that occurs when the body does not have an adequate intake of protein to maintain structure and facilitate wound healing. The client must be encouraged to change position to maintain integrity of the skin and promote circulation. Small pillows or folded towels can be used to support the rib cage and the bulging flank while the client is lying on his or her side.

The abdominal distention associated with ascites may develop very slowly over a number of weeks or months and may be accompanied by bilateral edema of the feet and ankles. The client may be unable to put on a pair of shoes, preferring to leave the shoes unlaced or to wear slippers. In a home health, inpatient hospital, or nursing home setting, this change in dress may not be as noticeable as it would be in a private practice or outpatient clinic. It is always important to remain alert to these potential signs of fluid retention and to ask about any changes in health status or weight gain.

Aldosterone-antagonist diuretics or potassium-sparing diuretics may be prescribed to decrease fluid retention, thus slowing the development of ascites and reducing the workload of the heart. Sometimes these diuretics lose their effectiveness. Loop diuretics may be prescribed instead. The therapist must be alert to the development of this phenomenon. Symptoms of fluid overload, such as weight gain, hypertension, peripheral edema, dyspnea, tachypnea, orthopnea, neck vein distention, or pulmonary crackles, must be reported to the physician. Conversely, when diuretic therapy works too well, volume depletion (hypovolemia) may present with signs and symptoms of dehydration (e.g., hypotension, tachycardia, flat neck veins, poor skin turgor, thirst). Recognizing medical complications of this type and getting the person the necessary medical care can reduce morbidity and mortality for these individuals.[141]

Fluid intake and output are usually carefully measured and restricted, so in any setting the therapist is encouraged to know the individual's limits and to participate in reporting measurements. This is especially important because clients frequently ask the therapist for fluids in response to perceived exertion or increased exertion after exercise or ambulation. The person who is noncompliant or in denial requests fluids because of the false belief that fluids provided but not recorded do not count. For the homebound client who is receiving diuretics, the bedroom should be close to the bathroom.

Hepatorenal Syndrome

Hepatorenal syndrome is a severe complication of advanced cirrhosis with ascites associated with poor survival.[8,251] Hepatorenal syndrome develops as a result of abnormal hemodynamics, leading to splanchnic (liver) and systemic vasodilation, but renal vasoconstriction.[131,188,251] Approximately 7% to 15% of people with end-stage cirrhosis develop this syndrome, which portends a poor prognosis.

This vasodilation leads to underfilling of the arteries and a low blood pressure elsewhere in the body, which particularly affects the blood pressure in the kidney (which is very sensitive to blood pressure). Because the blood pressure the kidney "sees" is low, there is an activation of the renin–angiotensin–aldosterone system in an attempt to constrict the blood vessels. This leads to constriction of the vessels in the limbs and to the brain, as well as the kidneys. The total effect is that the vasoconstrictors have a greater effect than the vasodilators, and kidney dysfunction develops. [225]

Criteria defining the diagnosis of hepatorenal syndrome were established by the International Ascites Club and include the presence of advanced liver disease with portal hypertension; serum creatinine of greater than 1.5 mg/dL; urine protein of less than 500 mg/dL; and, most importantly, the absence of other causes for kidney involvement. Efforts are underway to identify novel biomarkers to predict kidney involvement leading to hepatorenal syndrome; such renal biomarkers could allow early diagnosis and targeted treatment.[235]

Common illnesses found in people with cirrhosis that can cause renal insufficiency include infection (particularly spontaneous bacterial peritonitis), shock, medications, bleeding, and fluid losses. Renal obstruction should be "ruled out" by ultrasonography. The presence of these features, along with the failure to improve after diuretics are removed and 1 to 1.5 L of saline given, suggests the diagnosis of hepatorenal syndrome.

Hepatorenal syndrome is classified into two types. Type 1 is rapid (1-2 weeks) both in onset and progression to renal failure and carries a poor short-term prognosis. Type 2 is more insidious in onset with slower progression over months; ascites is often the key feature of this type. Because of the intense vasoconstriction, treatment centers around the use of vasodilators and albumin, which aid in increasing blood flow to the kidneys; this type of treatment is only 50% effective.[84] Transjugular intrahepatic portosystemic shunts may also be of benefit.[251]

Optimal treatment consists of liver transplantation, which provides a 5-year posttransplant survival rate of 70%. Although many people will improve with medical treatment, liver transplantation should be pursued because of poor long-term prognosis. Hemodialysis may be required to bridge treatment until a transplant is available.

Hepatitis

Hepatitis is an acute or chronic inflammation of the liver caused by a virus, a chemical, a drug reaction, or alcohol abuse. Classifications of hepatitis discussed in this text are listed in Box 17-2. Six different identifiable hepatitides viruses (A, B, C, D, E) are responsible for more than 95% of all viral-induced cases worldwide. The letter *F* was not skipped; it represents the sixth form of hepatitis, the fulminant form, a term for any rapidly progressing form of liver inflammation resulting in hepatic encephalopathy within a few weeks of developing infection. Fulminant hepatitis is not strictly viral induced but can develop as a result of any form of hepatitis (see further discussion this chapter: "Fulminant Hepatitis [Acute Liver Failure]").

Other viral causes of hepatitis include Epstein-Barr virus (mononucleosis), herpes simplex virus types I and II, varicella-zoster virus, measles, and cytomegalovirus. Hepatitis from any cause produces very similar symptoms and usually requires a careful client history to establish the diagnosis.

People with mild-to-moderate acute hepatitis rarely require hospitalization. The emphasis is on preventing the spread of infectious agents and avoiding further liver damage when the underlying cause is drug-induced or toxic hepatitis. Persons with fulminant hepatitis (which has a severe, sudden intensity and is sometimes fatal) require special management because of the rapid progression of the disease and the potential need for urgent liver transplantation.

Chronic Hepatitis

Chronic hepatitis comprises several diseases that are grouped together because they have common clinical manifestations and are all marked by chronic necroinflammatory injury that can lead insidiously to cirrhosis and end-stage liver disease. The disease is defined as chronic with evidence of ongoing injury for 6 months or more.

Previously, chronic hepatitis was classified as either chronic persistent hepatitis or chronic active hepatitis, but advances in understanding of the causes and natural history of this type of liver injury have led to the elimination of these terms. Now chronic hepatitis is described in diagnostic terms that include the etiology, degree of active inflammation and injury (i.e., grade: mild, moderate, severe, or I, II, III), and the degree of scarring or how advanced the process is (i.e., stage: I, II, or III; IV represents cirrhosis). Stages of disease are usually irreversible.

Chronic hepatitis has multiple causes, including viruses, medications, metabolic abnormalities, and autoimmune disorders. Despite extensive testing, some cases cannot be attributed to any known cause and are probably the result of as yet unidentified viruses. Hepatitis B (HBV), with or without hepatitis D (HDV), HCV, and GB virus (GBV) can progress to chronic hepatitis.

Most people with chronic hepatitis are asymptomatic, and when symptoms occur, these are nonspecific and mild, with fatigue, malaise, loss of appetite, polyarthralgias, and intermittent right upper quadrant discomfort. Some people report sleep disturbances or difficulty in concentrating. Symptoms of advanced disease or an acute exacerbation include nausea, poor appetite, weight loss, muscle weakness, itching, dark urine, and jaundice. Once cirrhosis is present, weakness, weight loss, abdominal swelling, edema, easy bruising, muscle wasting and

weakness, GI bleeding, and hepatic encephalopathy with mental confusion may arise.

The diagnosis of chronic viral hepatitis is based on serologic testing. The strict definition of chronic hepatitis (from any cause) is based on histologic features of hepatocellular necrosis and chronic inflammatory cell infiltration in the liver, but the diagnosis can usually be made from clinical features and blood test results alone.

Liver biopsy is important to assess the severity of underlying liver disease (grade and stage) and to determine the need for antiviral treatment. The treatment for chronic viral hepatitis has improved substantially in the last decade and depends on the underlying cause and grade and stage of disease. With the advances currently being made in the fields of antiviral and immunomodulatory therapeutics, it is anticipated that the considerable progress made in treating these diseases over the past decade will continue in the future.

The prognosis in chronic hepatitis is variable depending on the development of cirrhosis and other complications such as hepatocellular carcinoma (HCC). Male gender, moderate-to-severe alcohol consumption, and other coexistent liver disorders are the factors that increase the rate of progression to cirrhosis. The 5-year survival rate for compensated cirrhosis is greater than 90%, but the prognosis and survival rate for decompensation (characterized by development of variceal bleeding, ascites, and hepatic encephalopathy) are extremely poor.[93] Progression of chronic hepatitis to decompensated cirrhosis is an indication for liver transplantation.

Fulminant Hepatitis (Acute Liver Failure)

Fulminant hepatitis or *fulminant hepatic failure* is the generic term for any rapidly progressing form of liver inflammation without prior liver disease or cirrhosis.[111] It develops in 1 to 2 weeks (some cases involve up to 6 months) and results in hepatic encephalopathy (complex neuropsychiatric condition characterized by confusion, stupor, coma, and possible death; see "Hepatic Encephalitis" above for further discussion). According to the American Association for the Study of Liver Diseases, the term *acute liver failure* is preferred over fulminant hepatic failure and fulminant hepatitis or necrosis for conditions lasting 26 weeks or less.[177]

This type of hepatitis is rare, occurring in less than 1% of persons with acute viral hepatitis (approximately 2000 cases annually in the United States[111]), but can be fatal. The most common causes are acetaminophen hepatotoxicity (50% of all cases of fulminant hepatitis[111]); idiosyncratic drug reaction; infections such as hepatitis A (HAV) and HBV, Epstein-Barr virus, cytomegalovirus, varicella-zoster virus, or herpes simplex virus; and hepatic ischemia.[226]

Encephalopathy (mental alteration) may progress to cerebral edema, which is the most serious complication and most common cause of death. Release of neurotoxins (e.g., ammonia) from the GI system (no longer cleared by the now dysfunctional liver) accumulate in the systemic circulation and are transported to the brain where they cause brain cell swelling and disruption of the blood–brain barrier leading to cerebral edema and irreversible neurologic damage.

In addition to liver failure, numerous complications can occur, including infection, hypoglycemia, coagulation defects (international normalized ratio [INR] equal to or greater than 1.5), lactic acidosis, ascites, GI hemorrhage, electrolyte disturbances, and renal insufficiency.

Diagnosis is made in the presence of a combination of hepatic encephalopathy, acute liver disease (elevated serum bilirubin and transaminase levels), and liver failure. Treatment has improved from just supportive to the possibility of recovery with early antiviral treatment (e.g., lamivudine therapy) and/or liver transplantation.[226,238]

Prognosis is determined in part by the cause of the condition (toxic agents vs. infectious disorders) and availability of liver transplantation. If the prognosis is deemed poor and no contraindications to transplantation are present, the person should be immediately considered for transplantation. Short-term prognosis without liver transplantation is very poor, and the mortality rate is extremely high (often exceeding 90%[111]). Despite the poor prognosis, there is a 60% survival rate with transplantation as a result of liver cell regeneration with recovery of liver function.

Viral Hepatitis

Note to Reader: Additional information about viral hepatitis is available at http://www.cdc.gov/hepatitis. Information regarding viral hepatitis is also available from The Institute of Medicine http://www.iom.edu. (Use the search window to type in hepatitis for a wide range of information on this topic.) Information about the World Hepatitis Alliance is available at http://www.worldhepatitisalliance.org.

Overview. Each of the recognized hepatitis viruses belongs to a different virus family, and each has a unique epidemiology. Table 17-2 presents the characteristics of these strains of viruses. The identification of the specific virus is made difficult by the fact that a long incubation period often occurs between acquisition of the infection and development of the first symptoms. The incubation period for HAV is 15 to 50 days, 1 to 6 months for HBV, and 1 week to 6 months for HCV. Not all causative agents have been identified, and because hepatitis can be easily spread before symptoms appear, morbidity is high in terms of loss of time from school or work. More than half and possibly as many as 90% of all cases go unreported because symptoms are mild or even subclinical.

HAV, formerly known as *infectious hepatitis*, is transmitted by the fecal–oral route. The fecal–oral route of transmission is primarily from poor or improper handwashing and personal hygiene, particularly after using the bathroom and then handling food for public consumption. This route of transmission also may occur through the shared used of oral utensils such as straws, silverware, and toothbrushes.

Major outbreaks of HAV occur when people consume contaminated water or food. HAV most commonly affects children, men who have sex with men, and people who live or travel in underdeveloped countries (Table 17-3). HAV is rarely transmitted through transfused blood, and little placental transmission occurs, although the antibody is often detected in infants of infected mothers.

HAV is highly contagious, with the peak time of viral excretion and contamination occurring during the 2-week period *before* the onset of jaundice. Thus the greatest danger of infection is during the incubation period, when a person is unaware that the virus is present. The illness can last from 4 to 8 weeks; it generally lasts longer and is more severe in persons older than 50 years or in people with chronic, underlying liver disease.[61]

HBV is transmitted percutaneously (i.e., puncture of the skin) or through mucosal contact. HBV is highly infectious: 100 times more infectious than human immunodeficiency virus (HIV) and 10 times more infectious than HCV. Because HBV can be transmitted through heterosexual or homosexual intercourse, it is considered a sexually transmitted disease. The average incubation period is 90 days (with a range of 60-150 days) with symptoms occurring around 60 days.[137]

HCV, formerly posttransfusion non-A, non-B hepatitis associated with blood transfusion, is now most commonly associated with injection-drug use. As with HAV, the period of infectivity begins before the onset of symptoms, and the person may become a lifetime carrier of this virus. Clinically, HCV is very similar to HBV and often is asymptomatic; the acute HCV infection is usually mild. Chronic HCV varies greatly in its course and outcome from asymptomatic with normal liver function to mild degree of liver injury and overall good prognosis to severe symptomatic HCV with complications of cirrhosis and end-stage liver disease.

HDV, or delta virus, is a defective single-stranded RNA that presents as a coinfection or superinfection of HBV. This virus requires hepatitis B surface antigen (HBsAg) for its replication, so only individuals with HBV are at risk for HDV. Risk factors and transmission mode are the same as for HBV; parenteral drug users have a high incidence of HDV. The symptoms of HDV are similar to those of HBV except that clients are more likely to have fulminant hepatitis and to develop chronic active hepatitis and cirrhosis.

Hepatitis E virus (HEV), previously known as enteric non-A, non-B hepatitis, is transmitted by contaminated water via the fecal–oral route and clinically resembles HAV. Hepatitis E has been considered to be a travel-associated, acute, self-limiting liver disease that causes fulminant hepatic failure in specific high-risk groups only. HEV genotype 3 infection can be transmitted via pigs and rodents.[240] It is thought to be nonfatal, although it has been clearly associated with liver damage. A 20% to 25% mortality rate exists in pregnant women from fulminant hepatitis.[3] This virus tends to occur in poor socioeconomic conditions, primarily occurs in developing countries (contaminated waste water and sewage), and is rare in the United States. No specific treatment is available for HEV, but ensuring clean drinking water remains the best preventive strategy.

Hepatitis G virus (HGV) seems to be an incorrect term and has fallen out of favor; the accepted term is now GBV-A and GBV-B[258] (GBV-C is a subset of GBV-B). GBV is most prevalent in African countries although it has been found in people worldwide. GBV has been identified as the causative agent of approximately 20% of posttransfusion hepatitis cases and approximately 15% of community-acquired hepatitis cases that are not caused by HAV. However, studies fail to show conclusive evidence of

Table 17-2 Types of Viral Hepatitis

	Hepatitis A	Hepatitis B	Hepatitis C	Hepatitis D	Hepatitis E
Incidence	Overall reduced incidence with introduction of hepatitis vaccine A; 1670 reported cases in 2010 but an estimated 7000 of actual cases and a total of 17,000 new infections	1.5 million carriers; 3374 cases reported in 2010 but an estimated 9000 actual new cases; total of 38,000 new acute cases	Transfusion-related cases decreasing with blood screening but increased incidence expected related to risk behaviors in the 1960s and 1970s; 3.2 million chronically infected; 853 reported cases in 2010 but an estimated 2800 actual cases with a total of 38,000 new acute cases	Uncommon in United States; most common in injection-drug users, sexually active young adults, individuals receiving multiple blood transfusions	Epidemic in developing countries; rare in United States; risk greatest to persons traveling to endemic regions
Morbidity	Results in acute infection only; does not progress to chronic hepatitis or cirrhosis; small risk of fulminant hepatitis; lifetime immunity	Most common cause of chronic hepatitis and liver cancer; second major cause of cirrhosis in the United States after alcohol abuse	Accounts for 60%-70% of all chronic hepatitis; 30% of chronic cases progress to cirrhosis; associated with liver cancer	Coinfection of HBV and HDV leads to more severe acute disease (fulminant hepatitis 2%-20%) but low risk of chronic disease Superinfection (acquire HDV after HBV) has high risk of severe chronic disease (70%-80%[58])	Causes acute self-limiting infection; does not progress to chronic hepatitis; high mortality in pregnant women, 10% mortality
Transmission	Fecal–oral route; spread by feces, saliva, and contaminated food and water	Parenteral Sexual contact Vertical Unidentified exposure	Parenteral Unidentified exposure	Parenteral Sexual contact (Same as B) Perinatal rare requires coinfection with HBV to reproduce	Same as A; fecal–oral (contamination of water) specifies type of fecal-oral transmission
Treatment	Immune globulin before or within 2 weeks of exposure; supportive; most people recover within 4-8 weeks	α-Interferon and antiviral agents for chronic HBV; HBIG for exposed, unvaccinated persons	Combination therapy (interferon, ribavirin) in select cases	Interferon alfa-2b can inhibit HDV replication but effect ends when therapy ends	None; preventive measures
Diagnosis	Blood test to identify antibody; IgM; anti-HAV	Blood tests to identify antigen and antibodies; HBsAg; HBeAg; HBcAg (see text under diagnosis)	Blood test to identify antibody; does not distinguish between current and past infection; anti-HCV Limited use of nucleic acid test (polymerase chain reaction)	Blood test to detect antigen and antibody; anti-HDV	Blood test to detect anti-HEV IgM antibodies
Vaccine	Vaccine available; combined HAV and HBV vaccine available	Vaccines available (see text)	None available	Immunization against HBV can prevent HDV infection	Recombinant vaccine (rHEV vaccine) IgM antibodies under investigation

HBIG, hepatitis B immune globulin; HBcAg, hepatitis B core antigen; HBeAg, hepatitis B early antigen; HBsAg, hepatitis B surface antigen; HEV, hepatitis E virus; IgM, immunoglobulin M.

From Centers for Disease Control and Prevention (CDC): National Center for Infectious Diseases (last updated 2012). Available online at: http://www.cdc.gov/ncidod/diseases/submenus/sub_hepatitis.htm

clinical hepatitis after infection with GBV; this potential form of hepatitis remains under investigation.

Incidence and Risk Factors. Each year, approximately 500,000 Americans are infected with some form of hepatitis virus; annually about 15,000 persons die from its complications. HAV is the predominant type of hepatitis, causing 40% to 60% of acute viral hepatitis

cases. An estimated 3.5 million to 5.3 million people are living with viral hepatitis in the United States, and many more are at risk for infection.[229]

Because HAV is transmitted via the fecal–oral route, one risk factor for acquiring the virus is working at a daycare center; children who attend daycare centers are also at higher risk. Because of the HAV vaccine, the infection

Table 17-3	Risk Factors for Hepatitis			
HAV	**HBV**	**HCV**	**HDV**	**HEV**
Household contacts or sexual contacts of infected persons	Injection drug use	Current or previously used injected illegal drugs (even if only 1 or 2 times years ago); intranasal cocaine use with shared equipment	Same as B	Same as A
Unprotected homosexual/ bisexual activity	Unprotected homosexual/bisexual activity; persons with multiple sex partners or diagnosis of sexually transmitted disease			
Injection/noninjection illegal drug users (regional outbreaks reported)	Incarceration in correctional facilities—adults and youth (drug use, unsafe sexual practices)	Received blood transfusion or organ transplant before July 1992 or blood clotting products made before 1987		
Living in areas with increased rates of HAV (children at greatest risk)	Certain ethnic groups and adoptive families with adoptees from these areas: Asia, South America, South Africa, Mexico, Eastern and Mediterranean Europe			
Travel in areas where HAV is epidemic	Travel to high-risk areas			
Tattoo inscription or removal; body or ear piercing with shared or unsterile needles	Occupational risk*: morticians, dental workers, emergency medical technicians, firefighters, health care workers in contact with body fluid or blood	Tattooing has been linked as a risk factor for HCV[31]		
	Liver transplant recipient	Evidence of liver disease, liver transplant recipient		
	Infants born to mothers with HBV	Infants born to HCV-infected mothers (low risk; 5%)		
	Immunocompromised individuals; receiving/administering chronic kidney dialysis (clients/staff)	Long-term kidney dialysis (clients/staff)		
Blood clotting factor disorder (no new cases between 1998 and 2002)	Multiple blood product or blood transfusions before July 1992			

*HBV can also survive in dried blood for at least 1 week.

From Centers for Disease Control and Prevention (CDC): National Centers for Infectious Diseases (updated 2012). Available online at: http://www.cdc.gov/ncidod/diseases/submenus/sub_hepatitis.htm

rate in this population has improved; this may change the prevalence of the disease, with more cases being reported in adults (adults display a more severe clinical course than children).[48] Another risk factor for HAV is visiting or living in an underdeveloped country where the rate is high.

In the United States, among the estimated 38,000 persons newly infected with HBV, the highest rate was reported among persons aged 25 to 44 years, and the majority of these infections were among at-risk adults.[33] Prevalence of HBV infection has significantly decreased in most ethnic populations except blacks, who continue to demonstrate an elevated prevalence of three times that of other racial/ethnic populations.[137] Prevalence varies most according to risk factors for acquisition, so for parenterally transmitted hepatitis (B, C, and D), the highest rates are among persons with direct percutaneous blood exposures such as injection-drug users.

Common risk factors for HBV include sexual relations, injection-drug use, sharing needles, needlesticks, and perinatal (vertical) transmission from mother to child. Injection-drug use and intimate contact with another person with HBV are the two most frequent sources of HBV in the United States. Transfusion-related HBV is rare, because the initiation of donor screening for HBV and the HBV vaccine have improved the incidence in dialysis clients and workers.

In the past, HCV infection was commonly acquired through blood transfusion. Currently, because of donor screening, the incidence of HCV from transfusion is uncommon. The number of people with chronic HCV is significant: approximately 3% of the world's population is infected with HCV with more than 170 million chronic carriers who are at risk for developing liver cirrhosis and/or liver cancer.[47] The Centers for Disease Control and Prevention (CDC) estimates that persons born during 1945–1965 account for three-fourths of all HCV infections in the United States.[34,219] They account for 73% of HCV-associated mortality and are at greatest risk for HCC and other HCV-related liver disease.[219]

The reason this group of people have the highest rates of HCV is unknown. Risk factors for HCV include exposures to contaminated blood or blood products (e.g., injectable-drug use with needle sharing, intranasal cocaine use with sharing of straws or other paraphernalia, those who received blood from infected donors, persons with hemophilia, people on hemodialysis, individuals with high-risk sexual behaviors, sexual and household contacts of persons with HCV infection). Up to one-third of individuals with a bleeding disorder are coinfected with HIV and persons with a bleeding disorder who were infected with HIV also contracted HCV (before screening for HCV was made available). Vertical transmission is not common in HCV but occurs occasionally. See Table 17-3 for other risk factors but keep in mind that 45% of infected individuals have no known risk factor.[32]

The number of cases of people who developed HBV/HCV infection from dialysis or work-related exposure has become low. People undergoing chronic hemodialysis are at risk for HBV/HCV infection because the process of hemodialysis requires vascular access for prolonged periods. In an environment where multiple clients receive dialysis concurrently, repeated opportunities exist for person-to-person transmission of infectious agents, directly or indirectly via contaminated devices, equipment and supplies, environmental surfaces, or hands of personnel. Furthermore, individuals receiving hemodialysis are immunosuppressed, which increases their susceptibility to infection, and they require frequent hospitalizations and surgery, which increases their opportunities for exposure to nosocomial infections.[190]

HBV is relatively stable in the environment and remains viable for at least 7 days on environmental surfaces at room temperature. HBsAg has been detected in dialysis centers on clamps, scissors, dialysis machine control knobs, and doorknobs. Thus blood-contaminated surfaces that are not routinely cleaned and disinfected represent a reservoir for HBV transmission. Dialysis staff members can transfer virus to clients from contaminated surfaces by their hands or gloves or through use of contaminated equipment and supplies.[190]

HEV is most common in developing countries. On the basis of serologic tests, an estimated one-third of the world's population has been infected with HEV. In India, the lifetime prevalence is more than 60%.[213]

Pathogenesis. The viruses associated with hepatitis are not typically cytopathic (destroy cells), yet the body's reaction to the virus often creates significant inflammation; the intensity of the disease depends on the degree of immune response.[28,191] Initially, cytokines (interferons) and natural killer cells are employed to remove virus from the body. Later, antigen-specific T cells (matured in the lymph tissue) enter the liver to aid in the removal of virus; antibodies prevent spread of virus and provide immunity against further infection. In adults with intact immunity, this response is able to clear the virus. However, in infants, young children, and the immunosuppressed, the immune system is unable to mount an adequate defense and the virus continues to replicate and reside in the liver, leading to a chronic state. In these people, there is a weak response with few antigen-specific T cells.

In HCV, the virus is able to bypass the immune system in most cases. Current theories include T-cell exhaustion, T-cell dysfunction, viral escape mutations, or rapid T-cell deletion in the liver.[159] Antibodies are not produced soon after infection with HCV and in some cases do not develop at all.

Clinical Manifestations. Most cases of acute viral hepatitis are asymptomatic and never reported (for HAV, HBV, and HCV). Up to 70% of children younger than age 6 years remain asymptomatic with HAV infection.[61] Infants, children younger than age 5 years, and immunosuppressed adults typically have no symptoms associated with acute HBV infection, whereas most cases of HCV infection are subclinical and not reported.

Classic symptoms of acute hepatitis are often the same, regardless of the responsible virus. Most individuals present with malaise, fatigue, mild fever, nausea, vomiting, anorexia, right upper quadrant discomfort, and occasionally diarrhea. Jaundice, dark urine, and clay-colored stools may also be observed, particularly with acute HAV, HDV, HEV, and frequently in HBV (30% of cases).

Acute HCV usually does not present with jaundice. In more than 95% of adults with normal immunity, infection with HBV is self-limited; but in 5% of adults, 30% of children (younger than the age of 5), 90% of infants, and those with immunodeficiencies, the infection becomes chronic. Most people who acquire HCV remain asymptomatic but become chronic carriers of the disease (60%-85%).

Some people may develop extrahepatic manifestations (more frequent in HCV than in HBV) such as essential mixed cryoglobulinemia, porphyria cutanea tarda, lichen planus, rheumatoid arthritis, Hodgkin lymphoma, and diabetes mellitus. Rheumatologic (arthralgias, myalgias, sicca syndrome, sensory neuropathy, paresthesias) and skin manifestations (pruritus) are the most common. Individuals with acute HBV may also demonstrate extrahepatic symptoms including rash, arthralgias, and arthritis.

HDV is a highly pathogenic virus that causes acute, often fulminant hepatitis, as well as a rapidly progressive form of chronic viral hepatitis, leading to cirrhosis in 70%-80% of the cases.[59]

MEDICAL MANAGEMENT

PREVENTION. Prevention takes place at three levels: primary, secondary, and tertiary. Primary prevention involves primary immunization (HAV, HBV, and HEV), education regarding food preparation and proper handwashing, avoiding needle punctures by contaminated needles (or other similar infective material), and practicing protective sex or avoiding sexual contact during the period of HBsAg positivity.

Secondary prevention involves passive immunization following exposure to HAV or HBV, travel precautions when visiting areas where hepatitis is endemic (e.g., avoid drinking unbottled water or beverages served with ice; avoid eating foods rinsed in contaminated water, such as fruits and vegetables; and avoid eating shellfish).

Tertiary prevention involves education to those infected about preventing possible infectivity to others and self-care during active infection (e.g., avoid strenuous activity and ingestion of hepatotoxins, such as alcohol and acetaminophen; some advocate alternative treatment such as herbs, acupuncture, and dietary measures).

Hepatitis A. Preventive measures include HAV vaccine, standard precautions, and immunoglobulin, which is a preparation of antibodies against HAV. Immunoglobulin can be used before infection and provides passive immunity for 3 to 5 months or can be given to household and intimate contacts of people with HAV. When given after exposure, immunoglobulin is 80% to 90% effective in preventing HAV infection. The sooner immunoglobulin is given after exposure, the more efficacious it is.[61] People who have received the HAV vaccine at least 1 month before exposure do not require immunoglobulin.

HAV vaccine is recommended (before exposure) for persons 1 year of age and older (as a standard childhood vaccination), adults wishing to obtain immunity, or anyone who is at risk for infection (e.g., persons traveling to areas with intermediate to high rates of endemic HAV, persons living in communities with high endemic rates or periodic outbreaks of HAV infection, men who have sex with men or who are bisexual and their partners of either gender, and clients with chronic liver disease). HAV vaccine confers 97% to 100% protection in children and 94% to 100% in adults.

Hepatitis B. HBV is a preventable disease achieved by administering a HBV vaccine. Currently, two vaccines are available as single-antigen vaccines: Recombivax HB and Engerix-B. Three are available as combination vaccines: Twinrix (for HAV and HBV in adults), Comvax (for HBV and *Haemophilus influenzae* type B in children), and Pediarix (for HBV, diphtheria and tetanus toxoids, pertussis, and poliovirus in children). The vaccine is given in three doses over a period of 6 months.

Life-long protective immunity develops in more than 90% of healthy adults. In the unvaccinated person, hepatitis B immunoglobulin is used for postexposure prophylaxis and should be administered soon after the exposure, followed by the HBV series at 0, 1, and 6 months. Effectiveness of postexposure prophylaxis decreases with time between exposure and treatment. Postexposure prophylaxis should be given in less than 7 days from exposure for needlesticks and in less than 14 days for sexual exposure. Immunity to HBV also confers immunity to HDV; consequently, HBV vaccination is recommended for preexposure immunization prophylaxis for HDV.

Once individuals begin to engage in behaviors associated with high-risk groups, they may become infected before vaccine can be given. A major obstacle in eliminating HBV is identifying persons and vaccinating them before they become infected. For this reason, in the United States, it is now recommended that all infants, health care workers, and persons in the high-risk category for HBV receive the HBV vaccine.

According to the Occupational Safety and Health Administration Bloodborne Pathogen Standard (1991), HBV vaccination must be offered to all employees within 10 days of employment. Records related to this vaccination must be maintained. Employees who decline vaccination must sign a standardized declination form.

Children younger than 5 years of age, if infected, have a high risk of becoming HBV carriers. Testing to identify pregnant women who are HBsAg-positive and providing their infants with immunoprophylaxis effectively prevents HBV transmission during the perinatal period. The HBsAg is a core protein antigen of the HBV present in the nuclei of infected cells. Presence of HBsAg in the blood usually indicates the individual is infectious. HBc antibodies appear during the acute infection but do not protect against reinfection.

The World Health Organization (WHO) has recommended that all countries integrate HBV vaccination into their national immunization programs, and much progress has been made toward the goal to control, eliminate, and eradicate hepatitis in the coming generations.[234]

Hepatitis C. Currently, no vaccine is available to prevent HCV because of the rapidity of HCV mutations in adaptation to the environment[110] and no immunoglobulin (Ig) is effective in treating exposure. The only means of preventing new cases of HCV are to screen the blood supply, encourage health care professionals to take precautions when handling blood and body fluids, and educate people about high-risk behaviors (particularly injection-drug users and those involved with multiple sex partners). Anyone at risk for HCV should be tested. The CDC has recommended that all adults born in the United States between 1945 and 1965 should be tested for exposure to hepatitis C because of the risk of liver disease, including liver cancer.[32] Early diagnosis is the key to preventing serious life-threatening liver diseases. Readers can preassess risk by taking the Hepatitis Risk Assessment offered by the CDC: http://www.cdc.gov/hepatitis/RiskAssessment/

Hepatitis D. Universal HBV vaccination programs have led to a significant decline in incidence in Western countries; however, HDV is not a vanishing disease. Immigration poses a threat of HDV resurgence; it has been recommended that continuous efforts should be made to improve its prevention and treatment.[59]

Hepatitis E. A new recombinant protein vaccine has been developed and shown effective in preventing HEV in high-risk populations.[213] The vaccine is a good option to prevent this infection that affects a large number of people in deprived geographical areas but unfortunately it is not universally available.[174]

DIAGNOSIS. In addition to the history and clinical examination, serologic and molecular testing help provide an accurate diagnosis. Serology is the standard for diagnosis of viral hepatitis (see Table 17-2). People with a positive IgM HAV have acute disease, whereas IgG HAV is present at the onset of disease and remains in the blood for life. IgG HAV signifies previous exposure, whereas IgM HAV signifies only acute infection.

Serology relating to HBV changes as the disease progresses or is contained. HBV has an acute phase, a convalescent phase, and a chronic phase. Early in HBV infection, the serologic marker HBsAg is positive, but the antibodies are negative until an immune response has been mounted by the body. Acute infection is demonstrated by a positive HBsAg and the presence of antibodies total anti-HBc (anti-HBc refers to the antibody to the hepatitis B core antigen) and IgM anti-HBc (IgM is an acute antibody). Resolving infection has eliminated the HBsAg, and antibodies remain present (anti-HBsAg, or the antibody to the surface antigen, may also be present). A serologic pattern positive for anti-HBc and anti-HBs demonstrates past infection and existing immunity.

Chronic infection is marked by the presence of HBsAg and anti-HBc. Vaccinated people display a positive anti-HBsAg. Hepatitis B e antigen appears early in the acute infection and continued presence in the chronic state suggests increased infectivity, greater number of virus replication, and the need for antiviral therapy.

HBV deoxyribonucleic acid (DNA) can be detected in persons with chronic infection by polymerase chain reaction techniques[126]; this information is useful in treatment and prognosis. None of the serodiagnostic tests are able to determine the current extent of liver damage; a liver biopsy provides information about the severity of disease and establishes grading and degree of fibrosis but is only necessary in the case of chronic hepatitis.

One-time testing for HCV is now recommended for all adults born in the United States between 1945 and 1965[221]; further testing to identify active HCV infection may be advised if tests for anti-HCV are positive. Liver biopsy is not mandatory but may be helpful for assessing liver damage associated with chronic hepatitis C (HCV) infection.[47,78] Liver function tests (see Table 40-5) can indicate coinfection with HBV or HIV, drug toxicity, or alcoholic hepatitis. Screening for alcohol abuse, drug abuse, or depression is recommended.[47]

TREATMENT. Treatment options have expanded and prevention methods are available for two of the six viruses although no cure is available for the viruses that are responsible for chronic liver disease. The development of direct acting antiviral agents that inhibit steps in the viral replication process is under investigation.[242] Any hepatic irritants, such as alcohol, medications, or chemicals (e.g., occupational exposure to carbon tetrachloride), must be avoided in all types of hepatitis.

Hepatitis A. Treatment for HAV is primarily symptomatic and supportive. Good sanitation and hygiene practices should be followed. Hospitalization may be required for excessive vomiting and subsequent fluid and electrolyte imbalance.

Hepatitis B. Treatment for acute HBV is symptomatic. Only clients with chronic disease receive treatment, which depends on the severity of the disease. People with normal liver enzyme values, an HBV DNA level of less than 10^{21} copies/mL, and findings on biopsy that are normal are considered "inactive carriers." Their prognosis is good and compares favorably with people who are not infected with HBV. People with abnormal liver enzymes (elevated AST), HBV DNA levels greater than 10^{21} copies/mL, and architecture on liver biopsy consistent with active disease require treatment. Pegylated interferon and lamivudine, adefovir, and entecavir (nucleoside analogues) are current therapies available. Interferon is expensive and has many side effects, but therapy duration is limited and maintenance therapy is not required.

Nucleoside analogues can be given orally, cost less than interferon, and have few side effects but require continued treatment to maintain response. The newest of these drugs for chronic HBV infection, telbivudine (Tyzeka) is an oral medication that reduces the viral load by inhibiting HBV reverse transcriptase and HBV replication. It is indicated for adults with evidence of viral replication and either persistent elevations in serum aminotransferases or histologically active HBV. Combination therapy is frequently used. Because people with cirrhosis and HBV are at high risk for the development of HCC, ultrasonography of the liver every 6 to 12 months is advisable.

Hepatitis C. Because the majority of complications occur in clients who develop cirrhosis from HCV, treatment is provided to those at risk of developing cirrhosis. This includes people with a history of alcohol abuse, people who contracted HCV at a young age, and those with active disease by liver biopsy. Because people with genotypes 2 and 3 (subtypes of HCV) have a high likelihood of responding to therapy, a liver biopsy is often not required before therapy.

Treatment of acute HCV includes 6 months of interferon therapy. In 2011, the first generation of direct-acting antiviral agents was licensed in the United States for the treatment of the most common HCV genotype. Other HCV treatments with protease and polymerase inhibitors that attack the virus are expected to change treatment recommendations as new medications become available for use.[219] Surveillance by ultrasonography every 6 to 12 months is recommended to detect HCC. Administration of HAV and HBV vaccine is recommended for anyone with chronic HCV because of the potential for increased severity of acute hepatitis superimposed on existing liver disease.[214]

For individuals coinfected with HCV and HIV with compensated cirrhosis, pegylated interferon plus ribavirin significantly reduces the incidence of liver-related decompensations and overall mortality.[147]

PROGNOSIS. Prognosis varies with each type. Chronic HBV or HCV infection is associated with increased risk of death, particularly from liver- and drug-related causes.[236] A substantial proportion of HBV morbidity and mortality that occurs in the health care setting can be prevented by vaccinating health care workers against HBV. In addition, health care workers must practice infection control measures (see Appendix A). Other prophylactic strategies are based on avoidance of high-risk behavior and use of immunoglobulin.

Hepatitis A. HAV is almost always a self-limited disease and rarely leads to fulminant hepatitis requiring transplantation (approximately 0.3%-0.6% of cases). It does not lead to chronic hepatitis or cirrhosis. Most people recover fully and become immune to HAV.

Hepatitis B. In adults with normal immune status, most (94%-98%) recover completely from newly acquired HBV infections, eliminating virus from the blood and producing neutralizing antibody that creates immunity from future infection. In immunosuppressed persons (including hemodialysis clients), infants, and young children, most newly acquired HBV infections result in chronic infection.

Although the consequences of acute HBV can be severe (1% die from acute hepatitis), most of the serious sequelae associated with the disease occur in persons in whom chronic infection develops. Approximately 15% of people who acquire the disease as adults and 25% of people who acquired HBV as a child die prematurely from cirrhosis or liver cancer.[137]

Despite reinfection rates, orthotopic liver transplantation for cirrhosis caused by HBV provides the best treatment. Continued treatment of the virus with the administration of hepatitis B immunoglobulin (intravenously or intramuscularly) used in combination with lamivudine has been found to be efficacious, making liver transplantation outcomes successful.

Hepatitis C. Infection with HCV is usually not self-limiting and ends up becoming a chronic infection in up to 80% of people infected.[26] HCV infection increases the risk of HCC and other HCV-related liver disease.[93] HCV-associated disease is the leading risk factor for HCC and the main reason for liver transplantation in the United States.[36,93] The majority of disease sequelae (e.g., leading to cirrhosis) develop within 20 years of disease onset in individuals with chronic disease.[160] Approximately 25% of all cases of HCV progress to cirrhosis, but newer therapies now available can clear the body of HCV infection and are expected to reduce HCV-related morbidity and mortality.[219,233]

The progression of HCV is accelerated if a person is also coinfected with the acquired immunodeficiency syndrome virus acquired by transfusion, causing cirrhosis and HCC more quickly and twice as often.[71,222] HIV/HCV coinfection among individuals with bleeding disorders results in mortality; more than 5000 people have died, and the numbers continue to climb.[156]

Hepatitis D. HDV by itself appears to be relatively harmless, but it has a high morbidity and mortality rapidly leading to hepatic failure and cirrhosis when it accompanies HBV.

Hepatitis E. HEV is typically a self-limited acute hepatitis, usually lasting 1 to 4 weeks. Severity of symptoms increases with age. It does not progress to chronic disease. When it occurs in epidemics, it can cause substantial rates of death and complications, especially in pregnant women. The overall fatality rate is estimated to be 3%; pregnant women who develop the infection have the highest risk of acute hepatic failure.[213]

SPECIAL IMPLICATIONS FOR THE THERAPIST `17-7`

Viral Hepatitis

Any direct contact with blood or body fluids of clients with HBV or HCV requires the administration of immunoglobulin, a preparation of antibodies, in the early incubation period. Therapists at risk for contact with HBV because of their close contact with the blood or body fluids of carriers should receive active immunization against HBV. All therapists should follow standard precautions at all times to protect themselves and must wear personal protective equipment whenever appropriate. Such gear should never be worn in the car or laundered at home to avoid contamination of those sites.

Enteric precautions are required when caring for individuals with type A or E hepatitis. Any therapist working in dialysis units or providing wound care should review infectious control guidelines available.[190] For the therapist who has been diagnosed with viral hepatitis, recommendations and work restrictions for health care workers are discussed in Chapter 8; see Table 8-5.

Studies dealing with the natural history of acute hepatitis have provided perspective on the frequency of skin and joint manifestations. More than a third of the adults studied had joint pains during the course of the illness. The frequency of arthralgia as a symptom associated with hepatitis increases with age. Joint pains affected only 18% of children, compared with 45% of adults older than 30 years.

No known studies have been published regarding the benefit of physical therapy in providing symptomatic joint relief until these symptoms resolve as the person recovers from the underlying pathology. In the case of a client with undiagnosed hepatitis presenting with joint symptoms, the systemically derived arthralgia will not respond to therapy. Any time intervention fails to provide symptomatic relief or resolution of symptoms, the results must be reported to the physician for further follow-up evaluation.

Overall, in the recovery process, adequate rest to conserve energy is important. The affected individual is encouraged to gradually return to levels of activity before illness. Fatigue associated with the anicteric phase of hepatitis may interfere with activities of daily living and may persist even after the jaundice resolves. A careful balance of activity is important to avoid weakness secondary to prolonged bed rest; a reasonable activity level is more conducive to recovery than is enforced bed rest. Whenever possible, rehabilitation intervention or increased activity should not be scheduled right after meals.

Affected individuals are advised by all health care professionals to avoid alcohol and to talk with a physician or pharmacist before taking any medications or nutraceuticals (herbal products, supplements).

Watch for signs of fluid shift, such as weight gain and orthostasis; dehydration; pneumonia; vascular problems; and pressure ulcers and any signs of recurrence. After the diagnosis of viral hepatitis has been established, the affected individual should have regular medical checkups for at least 1 year and should avoid using any alcohol or nonprescription drugs during this period.

α-Interferon (antiviral used in the treatment of some hepatitides) has bone marrow–suppressive effects requiring careful monitoring of platelet or neutrophil count (see Tables 40-8 and 40-9). Other side effects of combination therapy may include increased fatigue, increased muscle pain and potential inflammatory myopathy, headaches, local skin irritation (site of injection), irritability and depression, hair loss, itching, sinusitis, and cough. These symptoms usually subside in the first few weeks of treatment; prolonged or intolerable side effects must be reported to the physician.

Hepatitis B

Nosocomial transmission of HBV is a serious risk for health care workers. The risk of acquiring HBV infection from occupational exposure is dependent on the degree of exposure to blood and the presence of HBV e antigen (HBeAg) from the source. An approximate 22% to 31% chance exists of acquiring HBV after percutaneous (needlestick) contact with a hepatitis surface antigen (HBsAg) and HBeAg seropositive source.[88,246]

HBV can be transmitted to health care workers via percutaneous injuries or by direct or indirect contact with blood from an infected client. Blood contains the highest amount of infected particles and is the most efficient means of transmission. HBV in blood is able to survive up to 1 week on environmental surfaces. The incubation period is 45 to 180 days (average: 60-90 days).

Preexposure HBV vaccination of health care workers who are at risk (e.g., those who work in an area likely to have contact with blood and body fluids) is strongly recommended and can prevent acquisition of HBV (see Table 8-4).[40] Once a health care worker has been exposed, the HBsAg status of the person and vaccination and vaccine-response status of the exposed health care worker must be determined. Postexposure prophylaxis should then be given if the health care worker is unvaccinated or nonresponsive to previous vaccine and the source is HBsAg-positive.

The Occupational Safety and Health Administration bloodborne pathogen standard mandates that HBV vaccine and hepatitis B immunoglobulin be made available, at the employer's expense, to all health care workers with potential occupational exposure. In addition, strict adherence to handwashing and standard precautions (see Appendix A) is critical in prevention of the transmission of hepatitis-contaminated body fluids. Transmission is also prevented by use of barriers during sexual activity and by not sharing personal or other items that may have blood on them.

For the health care worker who is positive for HIV, HBV, or HCV, the CDC guidelines are based on the assumption that the risk of transmission to others is greatest during invasive procedures that include (for the therapist) sharp debridement or digital palpation of a needle tip (or other sharp instrument) in a poorly visualized or highly confined anatomic site.

Any therapist performing such procedures should determine his or her own HIV, HBV DNA serum levels (rather than hepatitis B e-antigen status previously recommended), and HCV antigen status to monitor infectivity. HBV DNA less than 1000 IU/mL is considered "safe" for practice. Those who are infected should not perform the procedures unless they have obtained guidance from an expert panel about when and how they may safely do so. The CDC does not mandate restricted practice, and according to the updated guidelines, prenotification of patients/clients of a healthcare professional's HBV status is not required.[88] For a complete summary of the current recommendations, see Holmberg et al[88] (available online at http://www.cdc.gov/mmwr/preview/mmwrhtml/rr6103a1.htm?s_cid=rr6103a1_e).

Hepatitis and the Athlete

Great concern is often expressed over the possibility of contagion among athletes in competitive sports, particularly sports with person-to-person contact. Infectious agents, such as HIV and other viruses, bacteria, and even fungi, have been examined. No cases of HIV or HCV transmission resulting from sports participation have been reported, but two cases of HBV transmission through exposure to blood during sports participation have been documented.

For most of the infections considered, the athlete is more at risk during activities off the playing field than while competing. The main pathways of transmission of bloodborne infections in athletes are similar to those experienced in the general population. The greatest risk to the athlete for contracting any bloodborne pathogen infection is through sexual activity and parenteral drug use, and not in the sporting arena.[206] One report specific to the risk of transmission among climbing athletes suggests that the transmission risk in climbing is even smaller compared to contact sports.[206]

Inclusion of immunizations against measles and HBV as a prerequisite to participation would eliminate these two diseases from the list of dangers to athletes (and all individuals). Education, rather than regulations, is the best approach in considering the risks to athletes from contagious diseases.[52,204]

Although the risk of bloodborne pathogen infection during sports is exceedingly small, good hygiene practices concerning blood are still important. The American Academy of Pediatrics has made recommendations to minimize the risk of bloodborne pathogen transmission in the context of athletic events and has issued safety precautions. The therapist in this type of setting is encouraged to review these guidelines.[6]

No evidence has been reported that intense, highly competitive training is harmful for the asymptomatic HBV-infected person, whether the disease is acute or chronic. Therefore, the presence of HBV infection does not contraindicate participation in sports or athletic activities; decisions regarding play are made according to clinical signs and symptoms such as fatigue, fever, or organomegaly. Chronic HBV infection with evidence of organ impairment requires reduction in intensity and duration of activity.

Hepatitis C

HCV is the most common etiologic agent in cases of non-A, non-B hepatitis in the United States. Seroprevalence studies among health care workers have shown a significant association between acquisition of disease and health care employment, specifically client care or laboratory work. Accidental percutaneous injuries (needlesticks or cuts with sharp instruments) are the highest risk vehicle for transmission to health care workers from people with acute or chronic HCV.

The incubation period for HCV is 6 to 7 weeks, and nearly all individuals with acute infection will have chronic (more than 3-6 months' duration) HCV infection with persistent viremia and the potential for transmission to others over an extended period.

Serologic assays to detect HCV antibodies (not protective antibodies) are available and are used to determine source and health care worker status after exposure. More than 75% of all people with HCV develop chronic hepatitis, and cirrhosis may develop in up to 25% of those with chronic HCV. A risk of developing hepatocellular carcinoma (approximately 3% to 5% per year) exists, and a small percentage of people with HCV may progress to fulminant liver failure.[166]

Currently no vaccine against HCV is available, and no postexposure prophylaxis can be recommended. Postexposure prophylaxis with immunoglobulin or antiviral agents does not appear to be effective in preventing HCV infection.[246] Follow-up HCV testing should be performed to verify if seroconversion occurs.

Strict adherence to handwashing and standard precautions (see Appendix A) is critical in prevention of transmission of hepatitis-contaminated body fluids. Transmission is also prevented by use of barriers during sexual activity and by not sharing personal or other items that may have blood on them.

Drug-Related Hepatotoxicity

Overview and Incidence

Injury to the liver can be caused by many drugs or toxins. More than 600 medicinal agents, chemicals, and herbal remedies are recognized as producing hepatic injury.[117] For example, herbal products, such as chaparral, comfrey, germander, Jin Bu Huan, mistletoe, nutmeg, ragwort, sassafras, senna, or tansy, can cause liver-related complications (ranging from acute hepatitis and jaundice to cirrhosis and death from liver failure) in anyone with an underlying liver disease.

Although nonprescription and prescription medications are often thought to be the only agents to cause liver injury, complementary or alternative medications, such as chaparral, germander, pennyroyal oil, Jin Bu Huan, and Sho-saiko-to, are also known to be hepatotoxic.[228]

Chemicals, such as carbon tetrachloride, trichloroethylene, derivatives of benzene and toluene, vinyl chloride, and organic pesticides, can also lead to liver injury. Carbon tetrachloride was the most common industrial chemical considered an occupational inhalation poison until it was banned in most countries. Ingestion of poisonous mushrooms, including *Amanita phalloides* and related species (rare in the United States but more common in Europe), can lead to fulminant liver failure.

Although uncommon, drugs are currently the most common cause of acute liver failure.[165] A study of the WHO database demonstrated acetaminophen, troglitazone, valproate, stavudine, and halothane to be the five drugs most frequently associated with hepatotoxicity and death (particularly acetaminophen).[24,108]

The incidence of hepatotoxicity as a result of these noninfectious agents is difficult to determine because many cases may be subclinical (i.e., mild symptoms) or misdiagnosed, leading to underreporting. One French study demonstrated a rate of 14 cases/100,000 people in the general population; 12% required hospitalization, and 6% died as a result of acute liver failure.[208] Hepatotoxicity has also been the principal reason for removing several new drugs from the market.[73]

Drugs or chemicals typically cause either predictable (or dose-related) or unpredictable (or idiosyncratic) liver injury (Box 17-3). Drugs that cause predictable liver damage are dose-related (i.e., a specific toxic dose most likely will cause damage) and result in injury soon after ingestion. Acetaminophen is the most common example of predictable drug-related liver disease. Unpredictable reactions occur without warning, are unrelated to dose, and may occur days to months after ingestion.

Etiologic Risk Factors

A host of factors may enhance susceptibility to drug-induced liver disease, including age (adults more so than children), gender (women have a higher risk than men), obesity, malnutrition, pregnancy, concurrent medication use, history of drug reactions, and genetic variability (probably the most important factor). Preexisting liver diseases and comorbidities appear to alter the rate of recovery rather than affect the risk of developing hepatotoxicity.[198]

Box 17-3

CAUSES OF CHEMICAL AND DRUG-INDUCED HEPATITIS

Dose-Related (Predictable)

- Acetaminophen* (Tylenol) (analgesic; suicide attempt)
- Alcohol
- *Amanita phalloides* (poisonous mushroom)
- Anabolic steroids
- Aspirin
- Benzene, toluene
- Carbon tetrachloride
- Chloroform (anesthetic)
- Methotrexate (antineoplastic agent)
- Oral contraceptives
- Organic pesticides
- Penicillin
- Tetracyclines (antibiotic)
- Trichloroethylene
- Vinyl chloride

Idiosyncratic (Unpredictable)

- α-Methyldopa (antihypertensive)
- Halothane (anesthetic)
- Isoniazid (antitubercular)
- Minocycline (antibiotic)
- Monoamine oxidase inhibitors (antidepressant)
- Nitrofurantoin
- Phenytoin (Dilantin) (anticonvulsant)
- Rifampin (antitubercular)
- Quinidine (antiarrhythmic)
- Sulfonamides (antibiotic)
- Sulindac (NSAID)†
- Valproate (anticonvulsant)

NSAID, nonsteroidal antiinflammatory drug.

* Acetaminophen is Tylenol and is not an NSAID. It has no antiinflammatory properties, only analgesic and antipyretic uses. It has no relationship to ibuprofen.

† NSAIDs as a class have the potential to cause liver injury.

Data from pharmacotherapy update: Tisdale JE, Miller DA, editors. *Drug-induced diseases*, ed 2, Bethesda, MD, 2010, American Society of Health-System Pharmacists; Goldman L, Schafer A, editors, *Goldman's Cecil medicine*, ed 24, Philadelphia, 2012, Elsevier Saunders.

Alcohol use and fasting may increase the likelihood of acetaminophen-related hepatotoxicity.[256]

Pathogenesis

Drugs and toxins can result in liver injury via numerous mechanisms.[96] Some of these mechanisms include programmed cell death (apoptosis) as a result of tumor necrosis factor (TNF); binding of drug to cellular proteins, which causes an immunologic response, leading to cell death[194]; inhibiting metabolism of drugs; and mitochondrial dysfunction with formation and accumulation of reactive oxidative species.[175]

The pattern of injury is often drug-dependent. Patterns of liver injury include hepatocellular, cholestatic, mixed, hypersensitivity (or immunologic), and mitochondrial injury. Hepatocellular injury is defined by inflammation of the hepatocytes, breakup of the hepatic lobule (comprised of the central vein, the portal vein, hepatic artery, bile duct, and hepatic cords), and hepatocellular necrosis.

Isoniazid is an example of a drug that can cause this type of injury. Cholestatic injury is demonstrated by mild bile duct injury with pooling of bile in the hepatocytes. Amoxicillin-clavulanic acid is one drug that can cause this type of injury. Mixed patterns exhibit both hepatocellular and cholestatic patterns. Hypersensitivity reactions often show an eosinophilic infiltration of the portal triad; phenytoin can lead to this type of response. Mitochondrial injury is demonstrated by small droplets of fat (or microvesicular steatosis) within the hepatocyte. Valproic acid has been known to cause this type of cellular change.

Clinical Manifestations

The manifestations of drug-related liver disease can range from mild symptoms to fulminant liver failure. Vague symptoms, including fatigue, nausea, and right upper quadrant pain or discomfort, may be the first indications of hepatotoxicity. Other symptoms associated with liver injury are jaundice, pruritus, and dark urine. Fever and rash are often present with a hypersensitivity reaction. As discussed, drugs often cause a specific pattern of injury. The most readily identifiable patterns are hepatocellular and cholestatic.

Hepatocellular liver disease frequently presents with abdominal discomfort/pain, fatigue, and jaundice; the clinical course is acute and can be severe. Cholestatic liver disease is manifested clinically by jaundice and pruritus. In contrast to the hepatocellular pattern, cholestatic disease is often less acutely serious, but healing may be prolonged and chronic, taking weeks to months.

MEDICAL MANAGEMENT

DIAGNOSIS. Because drug-induced hepatotoxicity is uncommon, people who present with symptoms consistent with liver disease should have a complete evaluation to avoid missing more common causes. This includes laboratory testing for viral hepatitis, autoimmune liver diseases, Wilson disease, hemochromatosis, and α_1-antitrypsin deficiency. Ultrasonography, computed tomography (CT) scanning, magnetic resonance imaging (MRI), or endoscopic retrograde cholangiopancreatography (ERCP) are useful to identify biliary obstruction. A history of heavy alcohol consumption may be consistent with alcohol-related hepatitis.

A review of medications taken, remembering to question exposures to chemicals, herbals, and nonprescription medications, may point toward drug-related liver disease. Although many drugs have more immediate effects, unpredictable injury may not exhibit symptoms for months.

Tests used to detect liver injury include ALT, bilirubin, and ALP. ALT values that are at least three times normal are suggestive of liver injury, whereas ALP values of two times normal are considered abnormal. A bilirubin more than twice the upper limit of normal and associated with an abnormal ALT or ALP suggests disease. An elevation in the ALT value, with minimal changes in ALP, is consistent with hepatocellular damage, whereas a predominantly elevated ALP is associated with cholestatic disease.

Significant elevations in these laboratory values are not predictive of prognosis because the liver has the prodigious ability to heal. Function is often a better indicator of prognosis. Several laboratory tests indicate how well the liver is functioning. Prothrombin/INR and albumin demonstrate the liver's ability to synthesize proteins, and total bilirubin and conjugated bilirubin reflect the liver's ability to move bilirubin from the blood into bile.[157]

The liver also has the ability to adapt to some medications. This ability is demonstrated when the introduction of a drug leads to transient elevations in liver enzyme tests, but there is no progression of injury. In these cases, the drug does not have to be stopped. For example, isoniazid often causes a transient, minor increase in liver enzymes but is permanently stopped in only 1 in 1000 affected clients.[161]

TREATMENT AND PROGNOSIS. Treatment for drug-related hepatotoxicity most often consists of removal of the causative agent and providing supportive care. Two exceptions include the usage of N-acetylcysteine soon after toxic ingestion of acetaminophen and intravenous carnitine for valproate-induced hepatotoxicity. Reexposure or rechallenge of the offending agent should be avoided, particularly if the drug has an unpredictable liver toxicity and the hepatotoxicity was immune-related. Reexposure could lead to an even more severe and serious reaction.

Liver injury accompanied by increases in liver enzyme levels may worsen for days to weeks before improvement. In some severe cases, improvement of liver enzyme levels suggests liver failure rather than healing of injury caused by severe necrosis and loss of hepatocytes. In this setting, laboratory values indicative of liver function (such as prothrombin time/INR and albumin) and symptoms (such as encephalopathy) are better indicators of hepatic function.

Chronic liver disease can also develop; up to 6% of drug-induced liver disease can become chronic (principally with a cholestatic pattern of injury). Methyldopa, minocycline, and nitrofurantoin are drugs that have been associated with this problem. A poor prognosis is seen in clients who develop jaundice, impaired liver function, and encephalopathy within 26 weeks of the onset of symptoms.[176] Prognosis is the most serious and poor for those people with hepatocellular damage accompanied by jaundice, with a mortality of 10% to 50% (known as the *Hy law*). This type of injury is more likely than others to require liver transplantation.[23]

SPECIAL IMPLICATIONS FOR THE THERAPIST `17-8`

Drug-Related Hepatotoxicity

Therapists should be alert to the possibility of drug toxicity or drug reactions in clients taking multiple medications or reactions in people who are combining prescription medications or nonprescription medications with complementary or alternative medications. Many people do not consider nonprescription drugs as medications and may take the same drug with different names or combine nonprescription drugs with prescription medications. People with memory loss or short-term memory deficits may take multiple doses in a short amount of time because they cannot remember when or whether they took their medication. Other guiding principles for the recovery process are as mentioned for viral hepatitis.

Autoimmune Hepatitis

Overview and Incidence

Autoimmune hepatitis is a chronic progressive, inflammatory disorder of the liver of unknown cause. It occurs in adults and children and is characterized by the presence of abnormal liver histology, autoantibodies, elevated levels of serum immunoglobulins, and frequent association with other autoimmune diseases. Autoimmune hepatitis is one of the three major autoimmune liver diseases, along with primary biliary cirrhosis and primary sclerosing cholangitis. Variant forms of autoimmune hepatitis have been termed *overlap syndromes* because they share features of several liver diseases.

The International Autoimmune Hepatitis Group has classified two types of autoimmune hepatitis: type 1 and type 2.[5] Both forms are more common among women than men and have similar clinical and serum biochemical features. Type 2 is rare and most often seen in childhood and in young adulthood; it is associated with more severe and advanced disease at presentation. Autoimmune hepatitis is seen worldwide and in various ethnic groups, although type 2 is uncommon in North America.

Etiologic Factors and Pathogenesis

The cause and pathogenesis of autoimmune hepatitis are not known. The disease appears to occur among genetically predisposed individuals on exposure to as-yet unidentified environmental agents, triggering a cascade of T-cell–mediated events directed at liver antigens.[104]

Purported triggering agents include viruses (such as measles, hepatitis, cytomegalovirus, and Epstein-Barr viruses) and drugs (such as methyldopa, nitrofurantoin, diclofenac, interferon, pemoline, minocycline, and atorvastatin). It is uncertain if drugs actually trigger autoimmune hepatitis or merely cause a drug-mediated hepatitis with features similar to autoimmune hepatitis. Most

people with autoimmune hepatitis, however, have no identifiable trigger. Factors that predispose an individual to autoimmune hepatitis are not certain, but specific human leukocyte antigen (HLA) genes have been linked to the development of autoimmune hepatitis and probably play a major role.

Type 1 is associated with HLA-DR3 and HLA-DR4. Studies show that HLA-DR3–associated disease correlates to earlier onset, particularly in girls and young women, and more severe disease, whereas HLA-DR4 is associated with milder disease (although extrahepatic findings are more common) and better response to treatment.[104] HLA-DR2 may be protective.[50]

Autoreactive T cells and their proinflammatory response appear to cause the liver destruction seen in autoimmune hepatitis. Research continues to identify the antigens that are targeted by T cells, but one possibility is the asialoglycoprotein receptor, which is a liver membrane protein found in hepatocytes.

Continued T-cell response with chronic liver damage may ensue because of a failure of CD4+CD25+ regulatory T cells to regulate the response of CD8+ and CD4+CD25 cells (autoreactive T cells). Normally, regulatory T cells control the adaptive immune response of CD8+ and CD4+CD25– T cells by suppressing the proliferation and function of these T cells, which allows for self-tolerance maintenance. In autoimmune hepatitis, the low number and defective function of regulatory T cells leads to a change in cytokine production, proliferation, and apoptosis of autoreactive T cells.[124]

Antibodies are also produced and vary, depending on the type of autoimmune hepatitis. Antinuclear antibodies, smooth-muscle antibodies, atypical perinuclear antineutrophilic cytoplasmic antibodies, and antiactin antibodies are seen with type 1 autoimmune hepatitis. Type 2 is associated with liver-kidney microsome 1 and liver cytosol 1 antibodies. Although present in the serum, there is little evidence to support the theory that these autoantibodies cause the disease.[104] Yet measurement of these antibodies can be helpful in the diagnosis of autoimmune hepatitis.

Clinical Manifestations

Autoimmune hepatitis is represented by a wide spectrum of clinical manifestations. Although most clients present with nonspecific, mild, or chronic liver symptoms, up to 40% present with acute symptoms of hepatitis, including fulminant hepatitis with cirrhosis and liver failure. Autoimmune hepatitis is usually progressive and chronic, although a minority of cases are characterized by a fluctuating course.

The most common presenting symptoms are fatigue (85%), jaundice (46%), anorexia (30%), myalgias (30%), and diarrhea (28%). Other symptoms include abdominal pain, arthralgias (particularly small joints), and malaise. Weight loss is uncommon and should prompt an evaluation for another disorder.

The presence of another autoimmune disorder, such as thyroiditis, ulcerative colitis, type 1 diabetes, rheumatoid arthritis, and celiac disease,[1] is seen in one-third of affected individuals. Physical examination may be normal, but 78% of clients present with hepatomegaly.

Individuals with fulminant hepatitis often have profound jaundice.

Complications of autoimmune hepatitis are similar to other chronic liver diseases, particularly the development of cirrhosis. Although occurring less frequently than hepatitis associated with a virus, another serious complication is the development of HCC.

MEDICAL MANAGEMENT

DIAGNOSIS. The diagnosis of autoimmune hepatitis can be difficult as no one test is diagnostic for the disease. The diagnosis is based on a synthesis of clinical, biochemical, and histologic information. Laboratory findings consistent with autoimmune hepatitis include elevated aminotransferase values, hypergammaglobulinemia, elevated bilirubin and ALP values, and the presence of autoantibodies. At presentation aminotransferase values are typically between 150 U/L and 500 U/L, but people with severe disease at presentation can have significantly elevated aminotransferase values in the thousands.

More than 80% of affected people have hyperbilirubinemia, although this is typically mild with values less than 3 mg/dL. Serum ALP values are usually elevated, but values twice the upper limit of normal are likely indicative of another disease. Serum globulins are elevated up to three times normal, particularly gammaglobulin and IgG.

As discussed, autoantibodies are produced and can be helpful in making the diagnosis of autoimmune hepatitis, but 10% of cases do not exhibit autoantibody production. The most common autoantibodies seen in type 1 are antinuclear and smooth muscle. Titers of at least 1:80 in adults are considered a positive value.[104] Anti–liver-kidney microsome 1 and anti–liver cytosol 1 antibodies are more specific to type 2.

The magnitude of the elevations of aminotransferase and gammaglobulin does not necessarily correlate with the extent of liver damage, making liver biopsy important. Although histologic appearance of autoimmune hepatitis is similar to chronic hepatitis (can also be seen in other liver diseases), there are characteristic findings of autoimmune hepatitis that include a mononuclear-cell infiltrate of the interface around the portal triad, particularly with plasma cells. Fibrosis is another common finding.

TREATMENT. The mainstay of therapy is immunosuppression. More than 80% of clients achieve remission with prednisone or prednisone plus azathioprine. Serum aminotransferases and gammaglobulin levels can be used to monitor response to treatment. Therapy can be withdrawn once in remission, although relapse is high, occurring in 50% to 85% of affected people, particularly during the first 6 months.

Therapy for relapsed disease is the same as that used for the initial treatment and can successfully induce remission of the disease. Individuals who experience repeated relapses tend to have a poorer prognosis.[152] Maintenance therapy with azathioprine is often needed and life-long maintenance therapy is frequently used in persons with type 2 disease or cirrhosis at diagnosis.

Liver transplantation may be required for clients who develop end-stage liver disease because of intolerance to therapy (and have progression of the disease) or who have progression of the disease while receiving adequate therapy. Five-year survival rates after liver transplantation are 80% to 90%, and the 10-year survival rate is approximately 75%.[54] Autoimmune hepatitis reoccurs in approximately 40% of clients who undergo liver transplantation,[189] although this is often mild and related to the immunosuppressive medications used after transplantation.

PROGNOSIS. Prognosis depends on the stage of disease at the time of diagnosis and initiation of therapy, but 10-year survival rates (meaning not requiring liver transplantation or causing death) surpass 90%, whereas 20-year survival rates are probably less than 80%. People who respond to treatment often have life spans similar to healthy persons.[44] Individuals who present with cirrhosis have 20-year survival rates of only 40%.

SPECIAL IMPLICATIONS FOR THE THERAPIST	17-9

Autoimmune Hepatitis

Management of a client who has an autoimmune disease with liver involvement is a challenge. Energy conservation and maintaining quiet body functions during active liver disease must be balanced by activities to prevent musculoskeletal deconditioning with accompanying loss of strength, flexibility, and/or mobility.

Alcohol-Related Liver Disease

Overview, Incidence, and Risk Factors

Alcoholic liver disease, ranging from steatosis to cirrhosis to HCC, remains a major cause of liver-related mortality in the United States and worldwide. Alcohol-related problems result in significant morbidity and mortality; more than 40% of deaths from cirrhosis are alcohol-related and 30% of HCC cases are a result of alcohol-related liver disease.[64]

More men than women acquire liver disease, but women develop the disease after a shorter exposure to alcohol and while consuming lower quantities of alcohol as compared to men. In men, 6 to 8 alcohol-containing beverages daily (60-80 g/day) over a 5-year period can lead to liver disease, whereas only 3 to 4 drinks/day are needed to cause the same effect in women.

Women are more vulnerable to the effects of alcohol than men. Women produce substantially less of the gastric enzyme alcohol dehydrogenase, which breaks down ethanol in the stomach. As a result, women absorb 75% more alcohol into the bloodstream. Other effects and gender differences are discussed further in Chapter 2.

Approximately 90% of heavy drinkers develop fat accumulation in the liver (the first sign of alcohol abuse), yet although many persons are heavy drinkers for long periods of time, only a minority progress to develop alcoholic hepatitis and alcoholic cirrhosis. Research suggests that genetics may play an important role in preventing liver damage despite chronic alcohol exposure.

Alcohol-related liver disease encompasses alcoholic hepatitis and alcoholic cirrhosis. Alcoholic hepatitis occurs in only 10% to 35% of heavy drinkers and is the precursor for the development of alcoholic cirrhosis. People with alcoholic hepatitis are nine times more likely than people with fatty liver infiltration to develop cirrhosis.[119]

Some cofactors that may predispose to cirrhosis include coexisting HCV, smoking, and obesity. Although much progress has been made in understanding potential causes, many questions remain such as determining which factors lead to severe liver damage and the mechanisms that protect other heavy drinkers.

Pathogenesis

The initial physiologic change observed in the liver with alcohol exposure is the accumulation of fat, which is reversible with abstinence. In some people, with continued exposure to alcohol, there is a progression of damage to the liver consisting of inflammation, necrosis of individual cells, and early fibrosis, termed *alcoholic hepatitis*. With continued heavy drinking, micronodular fibrosis (small bands of fibers) can develop and eventually progress to large bands of fibrosis, creating large nodules of fibrotic liver tissue (macronodular cirrhosis). Once cirrhosis has developed, HCC may result.

Research has demonstrated that heavy quantities of alcohol can have significant detrimental effects. Many mechanisms have been described that may be responsible for liver injury caused by alcohol consumption. Damage most likely requires several of these processes to be present, and genetic factors probably play a role in prevention or progression of liver injury. A few of these mechanisms include the toxic buildup of acetaldehyde, inflammatory reaction of immune cells, overproduction of reactive oxidative species and reduction of antioxidants, mitochondrial dysfunction, and abnormal metabolism of methionine and *S*-adenosylmethionine (SAMe).

Acetaldehyde is an intermediate product in the metabolism of alcohol. Typically, alcohol is converted to acetaldehyde by the enzymes alcohol dehydrogenase and cytochrome P450 2E1; acetaldehyde is, in turn, metabolized to acetate by aldehyde dehydrogenase. When the metabolism process is overwhelmed by alcohol, acetaldehyde can build up. Acetaldehyde is a reactive molecule and is able to modify proteins. These altered proteins are then not only unable to function appropriately in the hepatocyte but may also elicit an immune response, bringing inflammatory leukocytes into the liver and contributing to cellular injury.

Alcohol can also alter the balance between pro-oxidants and antioxidants, causing oxidative stress and liver injury. The enzyme cytochrome P450 2E1 leaks electrons when it is activated. These electrons create reactive species (such as superoxide anions), which then react with proteins, lipids, and DNA, or deplete antioxidants, leading to the inability of the hepatocyte to function. Reactive molecules can also signal other pathways, such as activating transcription factors, to produce TNF. Hepatocytes can be very sensitive to the damaging effects of TNF as a result of the abnormally increased level of acetaldehyde.[123]

Another factor contributing to oxidative stress is alcohol-related mitochondrial dysfunction. Mitochondria utilize oxygen and produce reactive oxidative species, but are protected from oxidative stress by glutathione (which is transported from the cytosol). In the presence of alcohol, hepatic mitochondria produce increased amounts of superoxide molecules, but the transport of glutathione into the mitochondria does not function, leaving the mitochondria to the damaging effects of reactive oxidative species.

Alcohol also interrupts the important metabolism of methionine to SAMe. The enzyme responsible for this conversion is methionine adenosyltransferase, which is depressed by alcohol.[140] SAMe is a necessary molecule, donating methyl groups in many enzymatic reactions involving DNA, RNA, phospholipids, and proteins. SAMe is the precursor of glutathione and may be hepatoprotective; the depletion of SAMe can result in abnormal functioning of hepatocytes and sensitization of hepatocytes to destructive cytokines.

Clinical Manifestations

The initial histologic change noted in heavy drinkers is fatty liver infiltrate. This is often asymptomatic and detected only on laboratory evaluation. Even clients with alcoholic hepatitis and/or cirrhosis may be asymptomatic. Others may present with nausea, vomiting, abdominal pain, jaundice, anorexia, fever, and weight loss.

The most common sign in people with fatty liver or alcoholic hepatitis is hepatomegaly; 60% of all people with alcohol-related liver disease exhibit jaundice and ascites (typically in clients with severe disease). Splenomegaly is more common as the disease worsens and hepatic encephalopathy can exist in varying degrees, ranging from mild cognitive impairment to coma. Clients with alcoholic hepatitis or cirrhosis often display spider angiomata, liver tenderness, and edema.[144]

MEDICAL MANAGEMENT

DIAGNOSIS. The diagnosis of alcoholic hepatitis is made using the appropriate history of heavy drinking, consistent laboratory values, and no evidence of other diseases that could cause liver injury. Because alcohol can worsen preexisting diseases, such as viral hepatitis, the diagnosis of alcohol-related liver disease should not be made without a thorough evaluation.

A history of heavy drinking may not be present because of client denial. Only 50% of clients who abuse alcohol are identified by their physician. Elevated levels of aminotransferases (AST and ALT) are the most common abnormalities seen in alcohol-related liver disease. The AST is rarely greater than 300 to 500 U/L, whereas the ALT is typically only slightly elevated, giving an AST:ALT ratio of greater than 2. Serum ALP and bilirubin can range from normal to 1000 U/L and 20 to 40 mg/dL, respectively.

Often, despite advanced disease, laboratory levels may be only mildly elevated. Alcohol-related liver disease is usually accompanied by malnutrition and is evident in the low albumin levels and elevated prothrombin time. Erythrocyte count is often low (anemia) and thrombocytopenia may be present; the white blood cell count frequently is elevated. Because the diagnosis of alcohol-related liver disease can competently be made using history, physical, and laboratory information, liver biopsy is rarely needed.

TREATMENT AND PROGNOSIS. Treatment of alcoholic hepatitis centers on cessation of alcohol drinking, nutritional support and education, and prevention of the complications of end-stage disease. Corticosteroids can be used for severe cases of alcoholic hepatitis, whereas SAMe, an antioxidant, may reduce mortality and decrease the need for liver transplantation.[64,138]

Steroid therapy in people with moderate-to-severe alcoholic hepatitis is being used more often now. "Off-label" use of various pharmacotherapies aimed at the underlying mechanisms of injury (e.g., cytokine dysregulation, endotoxin translocation, and oxidative stress) are under investigation.[64] Alcoholic hepatitis carries a poor prognosis if the person continues to drink alcohol. Frequently, the disease will stabilize if the person stops drinking.

Clients who develop cirrhosis (but are asymptomatic) and are able to abstain from alcohol have a prognosis of 80% at 5 years. Liver transplantation is offered to clients who have end-stage liver disease and are able to stop drinking, typically for at least a period of 6 months. This often allows for sufficient improvement to the point of not requiring a liver transplant. Outcomes of transplantation for alcohol-related liver disease are similar to other groups requiring transplantation,[193] with a 7-year survival of 60%.

Prognosis depends on the severity of disease, other coexisting illnesses (e.g., HCV), nutritional status, the client's ability to abstain from alcohol, and the presence of end-stage liver disease. The prognosis and severity of disease can be determined using the discriminant function equation; the model for end-stage disease predicts survival and is often used in allocating livers for transplantation.[55] People with a discriminant function score greater than 32 have a 50% mortality within 30 days.

SPECIAL IMPLICATIONS FOR THE THERAPIST 17-10

Alcohol-Related Liver Disease

Follow the same guidelines regarding liver protection as are discussed in "Special Implications for the Therapist 17-7: Viral Hepatitis" above. Increased susceptibility to infections requires careful handwashing before treating this client. (See also "Special Implications for the Therapist 17-3: Cirrhosis" above.) The presence of coagulopathy requires additional precautions. (See the discussion "Special Implications for the Therapist 17-1: Signs and Symptoms of Hepatic Disease" above.)

Nonalcoholic Fatty Liver Disease

Nonalcoholic fatty liver disease (NAFLD) is now the most prevalent chronic liver disease in the United States.[10,37] It is a condition related to systemic insulin resistance associated with obesity and diabetes (the two major risk factors for this disease) characterized by an abnormal accumulation of fat within the liver cells.[51] There is a reported prevalence of 30%,[43] coinciding with increased rates of obesity and insulin resistance. This condition may be a liver manifestation of metabolic syndrome; it is expected to be the main reason for liver transplantation in the coming decade.

NAFLD can be mild but can develop into a more progressive form, called nonalcoholic steatohepatitis (NASH) in which inflammation occurs in liver tissue. The amount of inflammation does not appear to be correlated with the amount of fat in the liver cells. The chronic form causes damage in the liver tissue, decreased blood flow, and involves diminished ability in the gut to process nutrients, hormones, medications, and toxins.[11] The eventual result is cirrhosis, liver cancer, and liver-related death.[248] Risk factors for progression from NAFLD to NASH include age (45 years old or older), type 2 diabetes, obesity, and hyperlipidemia. There may be genetic factors as well as not all people with NASH have these risk factors and not all people with these risk factors develop NASH.[257]

Symptoms of NAFLD (when present; usually asymptomatic) include right upper abdominal pain, fatigue, and increased levels of liver enzymes in the blood. NAFLD may be asymptomatic and only detected incidentally by blood liver function tests or imaging performed for other reasons. Mortality rate is higher in individuals with this condition compared to the general population. There is also an increased risk of developing cardiovascular disease and diabetes in the future.[83,220]

Because NAFLD is likely related to diabetes and insulin resistance, lifestyle changes (dietary and exercise) are the key approaches to prevention and treatment.[35] Exercise is considered a "rescue" treatment—restoring adipose tissue insulin sensitivity and thereby rescuing the liver from lipotoxicity.[43] Moderate- to high-intensity exercise and resistance training linked with behavioral therapy is recommended three to five times each week.[35,89] Individuals at risk and with this condition should be advised to increase all forms of physical activity (e.g., taking the stairs, walking whenever possible) as well as engage in strength training of all major muscle groups at least twice a week.[60]

Alcohol consumption should be limited for anyone with NAFLD and eliminated for anyone with NASH. Some experts recommend avoiding herbal supplements (even those specific for promoting liver health) as they may be toxic to the already compromised liver. Efforts are being made to find a signalling pathway that regulates bile acid metabolism and glucose homeostasis in order to provide more direct intervention.[9]

Primary Biliary Cirrhosis

Overview and Incidence

Primary biliary cirrhosis (PBC) is a chronic, progressive liver disorder with uncertain cause. Similar to autoimmune hepatitis, PBC has an autoimmune basis, but unlike autoimmune hepatitis, the areas of destruction involve the small bile ducts. The incidence of PBC has been stable over time, although the prevalence has been increasing, which is most likely a result of earlier diagnosis and prolonged survival. PBC occurs most frequently in women (80%-90% of cases) between the ages of 40 and 60 years.

PBC is a slowly progressive (irreversible), chronic liver disease that causes inflammatory destruction of the small intrahepatic bile ducts, decreased bile secretion, cirrhosis, and, ultimately, liver failure. An autoimmune attack against the bile duct is probably an important pathogenetic element, but the precipitating event and contribution of genetic and environmental factors are uncertain. The disease is associated with other autoimmune disorders, including scleroderma, Sjögren syndrome, thyroiditis, pernicious anemia, and renal tubular acidosis. Although it is most common in whites from North America and Europe, cases have occurred in all races.

Etiologic Factors and Pathogenesis

The underlying cause of PBC has a basis in aberrant autoimmunity. People affected with PBC express antimitochondrial antibodies (90%-95% of cases). These are specifically targeted toward large enzyme complexes associated with oxidative phosphorylation (pyruvate dehydrogenase complex-E2).[67]

Although these enzymes occur throughout the body, only the epithelial cells of the small bile ducts in the liver are affected. This may be related to how a bile duct epithelial cell processes glutathione once the bile duct cell undergoes apoptosis.[95] Autoreactive T cells then respond to these antibodies, causing inflammation. As the ducts are destroyed, toxic substances build up in the liver, intensifying the damage. Chronic inflammation leads to fibrosis, cirrhosis, and eventually, without treatment, liver failure.

Research has also been investigating factors that lead to the production of antimitochondrial antibodies. Several hypotheses are centered on molecular mimicry.[95] Evidence suggests that antibodies made against bacteria have similarities to the pyruvate dehydrogenase complex-E2 in mitochondrial cells, thus producing antibodies that target bile duct cells. Some of the bacteria proposed to play a role in this process are *E. coli*, *Novosphingobium aromaticivorans*, lactobacilli, and *Chlamydia*.[95] Other possible environmental factors include chemicals, such as halogenated hydrocarbons found in pesticides and detergents, but more research is needed to verify this association.[29,114]

Clinical Manifestations

Most people with PBC are asymptomatic (50%-60%) at diagnosis; the remainder may present with symptoms ranging from minor annoyances to advanced disease. The most common presenting symptom is fatigue, which is noted in more than 20% of affected clients at diagnosis. With progression of the disease, fatigue becomes more significant, occurring in approximately 80% of people,[62] and may be disabling.[181]

Pruritus is frequently present (20%-70%), particularly in the perineal area and the palmar and plantar surfaces of the hands and feet, although it can be diffuse. Pruritus often worsens at night or when the environment is warm. Contact with fibers, such as wool, can also aggravate the pruritus. Less commonly noted is the presence of right upper quadrant pain (approximately 10%).

Other symptoms of the disease include hyperlipidemia, osteopenia, and the presence of other autoimmune diseases (e.g., Sjögren and scleroderma).[116,244] In the later stages of the disease, clients may exhibit portal hypertension, malabsorption, fat-soluble vitamin deficiencies, and steatorrhea (the result of impairment of excretion of bile into the intestine). Complications from advanced liver disease include ascites, bleeding from esophageal varices, and hepatic encephalopathy.

The physical examination is typically normal in asymptomatic people, but skin manifestations often occur as the disease progresses. Pruritus frequently leads to excoriations of the skin, and spider nevi, thickening of the skin, and increased skin pigmentation are often detected with advancement. Xanthelasmas are seen in 5% to 10% of persons with the disease (Fig. 17-6). Hepatomegaly is noted in 70% of clients, yet splenomegaly is uncommon at presentation, often developing only near the end stages of PBC. Jaundice is observed later in the illness, often months to years after diagnosis. Muscle wasting, edema, and ascites often herald liver failure.

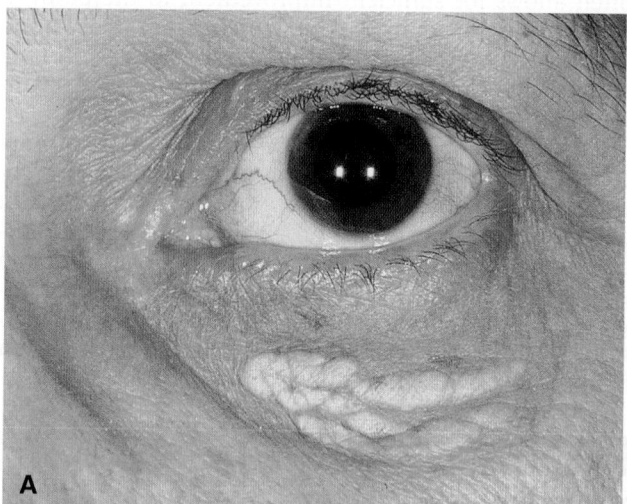

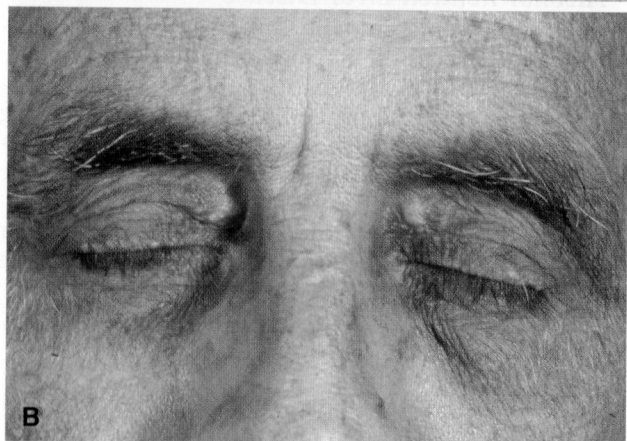

Figure 17-6

Xanthelasma. Multiple, soft yellow plaques involving the eyelid (lower and upper). Lipid-laden foam cells seen in the dermis tend to cluster around blood vessels. Lipid deposits can also be seen along the extensor surfaces of the body (not shown) such as the heels, elbows, and dorsum of the hands. (A, From Yanoff M: *Ophthalmology*, ed 2, St. Louis, 2004, Mosby; B, from Rakel RE: *Textbook of family medicine*, ed 7, Philadelphia, 2007, WB Saunders.)

MEDICAL MANAGEMENT

DIAGNOSIS. The diagnosis of PBC is based on a triad of criteria: presence and elevation of antimitochondrial antibodies (titer 1:40 or greater), elevated levels of serum liver enzymes (particularly serum ALP and γ-glutamyltransferase) for more than 6 months, and liver biopsy histology consistent with PBC. A probable diagnosis of PBC can be made with only the presence of antimitochondrial antibodies and elevated liver enzymes, but a definite diagnosis requires a liver biopsy. A liver biopsy may be beneficial for several reasons. First, the stage of the disease can be defined since the magnitude of the elevation of antimitochondrial titers is not indicative of the severity of the disease. Second, 5% to 10% of clients with PBC do not manifest antimitochondrial antibodies. Third, liver biopsy gives a baseline with which to compare response to treatment.

The histology of PBC is divided into four successive stages, referred to as stages 1 to 4, as seen on evaluation of the liver biopsy. As the liver is affected asymmetrically, a biopsy may not give a complete picture of the disease process. If more than one stage is observed on biopsy, the stage assigned is the highest of those seen. The hallmark of PBC is asymmetric inflammation and destruction of the bile duct within the portal triads. In stage 1 the damage is confined to the portal triad. Stage 2 is characterized by a reduction in the number of bile ducts and an inflammatory involvement of the surrounding parenchyma. Stage 3 disease demonstrates fibrosis, which connects the affected portal triads, whereas stage 4 manifests frank cirrhosis with regenerative nodules and accompanying liver failure.

The clinical course of the disease is variable and early diagnosis is important in order to initiate therapeutic measures before the development of advanced disease.

TREATMENT. Most people with PBC are now treated with ursodeoxycholic acid (UDCA), or ursodiol, a bile acid taken in capsules. It is currently the only drug approved by the Food and Drug Administration (FDA) for the treatment of PBC. Twenty-five percent to 30% of clients will have a complete response with UDCA,[115] which can reduce serum liver enzymes, cholesterol, and IgM; it also reduces pruritus.[171]

UDCA has also been shown to reduce the risk of death or need of liver transplantation after 4 years of therapy and can be effective for up to 10 years.[179,183] It appears to be safe and has few adverse effects. If used in clients with early-stage disease, it may delay the development of hepatic fibrosis and esophageal varices, with survival rates slightly lower than that seen in an age–sex–matched control population.[40,41,180]

UDCA has little effect in clients with advanced disease, and better options are still needed for this subgroup. Clients who have a complete response to UDCA require indefinite therapy. Progression, however, occurs in many people, requiring additional medical treatment or liver transplantation. Colchicine and methotrexate are two drugs that are often utilized when UDCA is no longer efficacious; other drugs are under investigation.[132]

Liver transplantation is considered for clients with end-stage liver disease (i.e., hepatorenal syndrome, diuretic-resistant edema, bleeding esophageal varices, and hepatic encephalopathy), unacceptable quality of life caused by intractable symptoms, or anticipated death in less than 1 year.[129]

Many laboratory values and factors are followed to aid in determining the appropriate time for liver transplantation such as the bilirubin, AST:ALT ratio, serum albumin, prothrombin time, and presence of complications from portal hypertension. Clients who receive a liver transplant often have difficulty weaning from immunosuppressants, and evidence of recurrent disease appears in 15% of clients at 3 years and 30% at 10 years.[158]

Complications of PBC, such as fatigue, pruritus, osteoporosis, fat-soluble vitamin deficiencies, portal hypertension, and hyperlipidemia, also receive treatment. Fatigue is difficult to treat and can be debilitating. One preliminary study showed some improvement in daytime drowsiness with the use of modafinil in people who were able to tolerate the drug.[92]

Cholestyramine and rifampin are the principal drugs used to relieve pruritus, although side effects may not be tolerable. PBC-associated osteoporosis occurs in up to one-third of clients with PBC, but severe bone disease (i.e., with multiple fractures) is uncommon except in more advanced disease. Treatment with alendronate may increase bone mineral density, but long-term studies are needed to demonstrate efficacy.[81]

Liver transplantation leads to an initial worsening of osteopenia, but bone mineral density typically returns to baseline after 1 year and can subsequently continue to improve. Because of a lack of bile acid secretion, the fat-soluble vitamins D, A, and K are not absorbed in the intestine. This typically occurs in the later stages of the disease and clients can be given supplements as needed.

Many clients with PBC have significantly elevated serum lipids, yet they appear not to be at increased risk for cardiovascular complications, usually making treatment with a cholesterol-lowering agent unnecessary.[125] People with PBC may have early esophageal bleeding, which cause portal hypertension leading to later esophageal bleeds.

Treatment consists of placement of a distal splenorenal shunt by endoscopic rubber-band ligation. If this is not successful, a transjugular intrahepatic portosystemic stent-shunt is placed. Survival is not significantly altered by treatment and many people are stable for years without requiring liver transplant.

PROGNOSIS. Clients who are diagnosed with stage 1 or 2 disease typically have a better response to treatment. In one study, people with stage 1 or 2 disease who were treated with UDCA for a mean average of 8 years demonstrated a survival rate similar to healthy controls. However, in this same study, those people with stage 3 or 4 disease were at significantly higher risk of requiring a liver transplant.[41]

Liver transplantation offers persons with liver failure improved survival. The survival rate at 1 year is 92%, and the 5-year rate is 85%. Clients with an elevated bilirubin level above 10 mg/dL have an average life expectancy of 2 years without liver transplantation. Death is usually a result of hepatic failure or complications of portal hypertension associated with cirrhosis.

Primary Biliary Cirrhosis

The most significant clinical problem for PBC clients is bone disease characterized by impaired osteoblastic activity and accelerated osteoclastic activity. Calcium and vitamin D should be carefully monitored and appropriate replacement instituted. Physical activity after an osteoporosis protocol should be encouraged but with proper pacing and energy conservation. (See also "Special Implications for the Therapist 17-1: Signs and Symptoms of Hepatic Disease" above, and "Special Implications for the Therapist 21-5: Liver Transplantation", "Special Implications for the Therapist 24-1: Osteoporosis," and "Special Implications for the Therapist 24-2: Osteomalacia".)

Occasionally, sensory neuropathy (xanthomatous neuropathy) of the hands and/or feet may occur as a result of increased serum cholesterol levels and an abnormal lipoprotein X. Cholesterol-laden macrophages accumulate in the subcutaneous tissues and create local lesions, termed xanthomas, around the eyelids and over skin, tendons, nerves, joints, and other locations. Treatment and precautions are as listed for this condition associated with diabetes mellitus or other etiologies (see "Special Implications for the Therapist 11-16: Diabetes Mellitus" in Chapter 11).

Pregnancy-Related Liver Diseases

Liver disorders occurring during pregnancy include hyperemesis gravidarum; intrahepatic cholestasis; preeclampsia; hemolysis, elevated liver enzymes, and low platelets (HELLP syndrome); acute kidney injury (secondary to hyperemesis gravidarum or septic abortion[128]); and acute fatty liver of pregnancy. Liver diseases associated with pregnancy have unique presentations, but it can be difficult differentiating these from liver diseases that just happen to occur during pregnancy.[169] Symptoms of liver involvement during pregnancy vary depending on the cause but can include pruritus (itching), nausea, vomiting, epigastric pain, jaundice, and polyuria-polydipsia.[16]

Intrahepatic cholestasis (sluggish or interrupted bile flow out of the liver) of pregnancy leads to raised bile salts (bile acids). The condition is characterized by pruritus and cholestatic jaundice; it usually occurs in the last trimester of each pregnancy and promptly resolves after delivery.[16] Most women present with pruritus; clinical jaundice is evident in only a minority of women. Abnormal liver tests with elevated serum bile acids are common.[15]

Of the women who develop pregnancy-induced intrahepatic cholestasis, up to 50% have other family members who have experienced jaundice during pregnancy or after the use of oral contraceptives. Women who have experienced cholestatic jaundice of pregnancy should avoid contraceptives because of a high risk of disease recurrence.

Cholestasis of pregnancy is most likely related to the inhibitory effect estrogen has on bile formation in susceptible women. Maternal health is unaffected by this condition, but the effects on the unborn child can be serious, including fetal distress, fetal anoxia, stillbirth, prematurity, and an increased risk of intracranial hemorrhage during delivery.[15,143] UDCA can be used to relieve symptoms and is well tolerated by both mother and fetus, but it is uncertain if it reduces perinatal morbidity and mortality.[143,249] No significant effects are apparent on the liver of the mother, although the risk of developing gallstones is increased.

HELLP syndrome is a rare but life-threatening complication of pregnancy. It represents a severe manifestation of preeclampsia (hypertension and proteinuria). Rupture of hepatic hematomas created by this condition is associated with high mortality for both mother and child despite early diagnosis and treatment with corticosteroids and hepatic artery embolization.[74,253]

Acute fatty liver of pregnancy is a rare, potentially fatal complication that occurs in the third trimester (between weeks 30 and 38) or in the early postpartum period. Usually the acute fatty liver of pregnancy symptoms start and 1 to 2 weeks later the woman presents with nausea, emesis, general uneasiness, jaundice, epigastric pain and other symptoms. A careful history and physical examination, in conjunction with compatible laboratory and imaging results, are often sufficient to make the diagnosis, and liver biopsy is rarely indicated. The maternal outcome has improved considerably during the last decade. Prognosis of acute fatty liver of pregnancy has been radically transformed by early diagnosis, early delivery by cesarean section, and treating complications.[17,241]

Vascular Disease of the Liver

Congestive heart failure is the major cause of liver congestion, especially in the Western world, where ischemic heart disease is so prevalent. Backward congestion of the liver and the decreased perfusion of the liver secondary to decline in cardiac output result in abnormal liver function tests. Hepatic encephalopathy may contribute to the altered mentation seen with severe congestive heart failure. Decreased cerebral perfusion, hypoxemia, and electrolyte imbalance are usually the major contributors to the confused state that can be seen in people with severe congestive heart failure.

Portal vein obstruction can be the result of thrombosis, infection, constriction, or invasion. Thrombosis of the portal system is typically caused by a hypercoagulable state or secondary to inflammation, cirrhosis, trauma, or cancer. Inflammatory diseases that affect thrombosis of the portal vein include pancreatitis and inflammatory bowel disease. HCC and pancreatic cancer are the two most common malignancies to cause thrombosis; they also lead to constriction and invasion of the vein.

Ischemic hepatitis or hypoxic hepatitis results when tissue of the liver does not receive adequate oxygen. This may occur in any disease process that reduces blood flow (cardiac failure), reduces oxygen supply (respiratory failure), or increases oxygen requirements (sepsis).

The Budd-Chiari syndrome is an uncommon disease manifested by a thrombosis in and on the hepatic veins where the veins open into the inferior vena cava.

Symptoms include pain, ascites, and impaired liver function. Hypercoagulable states, cancer, and infections are the most common causes.

Liver Neoplasms

Hepatic neoplasms can be divided into three groups: benign neoplasms, primary malignant neoplasms, and metastatic malignant neoplasms. Cancer arising from the liver itself is called *primary*; liver cancer that has spread from somewhere else is labeled *secondary* or *metastatic*.

Primary liver tumors may arise from hepatocytes, connective tissue, blood vessels, or bile ducts and are either benign or malignant (Table 17-4). Primary malignant cancer is almost always found in a cirrhotic liver and is considered a late complication of cirrhosis. Benign and malignant neoplasms can also occur in women taking oral contraceptives. A few rare tumors arise from the bile ducts within the liver and are associated with certain hormonal drugs and cancers. *Cholangiocarcinomas* are discussed later in this chapter (see "Malignant Neoplasms").

Benign Liver Neoplasms

Cavernous Hemangioma. Approximately 7% of autopsied livers contain hemangiomas, making this lesion the most common benign liver tumor. It is of unknown etiology and occurs in all age groups, more commonly among women. The pathology is similar to that of hemangiomas anywhere in the body; it is a blood-filled mass of variable size and can be located anywhere in the liver. Multiple lesions are observed in approximately 10% of cases. Areas of thrombosis are common, and older lesions may begin to calcify. The end stage is a fibrous scar.

Most hepatic hemangiomas are asymptomatic until they become large enough to cause a sense of fullness or upper abdominal pain. Hepatomegaly or an abdominal mass is the most common physical finding. Approximately 10% of clients with clinically detectable lesions are febrile. Hepatic hemangiomas are often discovered coincidentally on CT scan, by MRI, or during laparotomy; otherwise the diagnosis is made by contrast-enhanced serial CT, MRI (particularly if small), or single-photon emission CT. Needle aspiration or biopsy is avoided because of the risk of hemorrhage.

Treatment is not usually recommended because most hepatic hemangiomas have a benign course with negligible risk of malignancy and minimal chance of spontaneous hemorrhage. Surgical resection may be performed if the hemangioma is consistently symptomatic, producing pain or fever, or if the tumor is large enough for traumatic rupture to be considered a risk (e.g., a palpable lesion in an athlete). Other methods, such as radiofrequency ablation, arterial embolization, and systemic glucocorticoids, have had limited success.

SPECIAL IMPLICATIONS FOR THE THERAPIST 17-12

Cavernous Hemangioma

Most liver hemangiomas are small and found incidentally and require no special precautions. In the case of a known large liver hemangioma, the client must be cautioned to avoid activities and positions that will increase intraabdominal pressure to avoid risk of rupture (see Box 16-1). For the same reason, throughout therapy and especially during exercise, the client must be instructed in proper breathing techniques.

Liver Adenomas. Liver cell adenomas occur most commonly in the third and fourth decades, almost exclusively in women. The incidence of adenomas before the marketing of oral contraceptives was very low. Although it remains low in men, oral contraceptives have significantly increased the incidence in women. Most remain asymptomatic, although with growth, right upper quadrant abdominal pain may be present. Although classified as benign tumors, they are highly vascular and carry a risk for rupture and subsequent hemorrhage. The clinical presentation is often one of acute abdominal disease because of necrosis of the tumor with hemorrhage. Pain, fever, and circulatory collapse occur in the presence of hemorrhage. Most adenomas are evaluated with hepatic angiography, MRI, or CT. Liver function test results are usually within normal limits. Because of the risk of rupture and rarely, malignant transformation to HCC, resection is usually recommended. Affected women should refrain from taking oral contraceptives.

SPECIAL IMPLICATIONS FOR THE THERAPIST 17-13

Liver Adenomas

The therapist is most likely to see this client postoperatively after the danger of rupture and hemorrhage has passed. Standard postoperative protocols are usually sufficient.

Malignant Liver Neoplasms

Primary Hepatocellular Carcinoma

Overview and Incidence. HCC is the is the second leading cause of death from cancer worldwide and the fifth leading cause of cancer deaths among males in the United States[130]; it is also the most common primary liver cancer, constituting approximately 90% to 95% of primary liver cancers in adults.[215] The geographic locations with the highest incidence include China and sub-Saharan Africa. In Western countries, HCC is linked to cirrhosis, particularly HBV- and HCV-related cirrhosis. HCC is seen three times more often in men than women. Incidence has tripled since 1975, largely attributable to the increasing incidence of HCV infection[163]; HCC incidence also increases with age.[216] Hispanics and Asians have the

Table 17-4	Classification of Primary Liver Neoplasms	
Origin	**Benign**	**Malignant**
Hepatocytes	Adenoma	Hepatocellular carcinoma
Connective tissue	Fibroma	Sarcoma
Blood vessels	Hemangioma	Hemangioendothelioma
Bile ducts	Cholangioma	Cholangiocarcinoma

highest incidence and death rates (two times higher than among non-Hispanic/non-Asian whites).[216]

Etiologic and Risk Factors. Epidemiologic and laboratory studies have firmly established a strong and specific association between HCC and chronic infection with HBV and HCV. More than 80% of HCC is related to chronic HBV in Africa and China, whereas HCV is causal for 80% of HCC in Japan, Italy, and Spain. In the United States, HCV is emerging as a principal cause of HCC, particularly when associated with alcohol. Cirrhosis is typically prerequisite for HCC development in association with HCV.

Alcohol is a major risk factor for liver cancer. Reactive metabolites of alcohol are carcinogenic, DNA mutations are less efficiently repaired in the presence of alcohol, and alcohol acts as a solvent enhancing penetration of other carcinogenic molecules into cells. Heavy drinkers often have diets low in essential nutrients making tissues even more susceptible to carcinogenesis. Tumor promotion has been linked to inflammation in the liver through alcohol-associated fibrosis and hepatitis. Even moderate amounts of alcohol increase the levels of circulating HCV in carriers of this infection.[252]

In all parts of the world, there is a strong correlation between HCC and cirrhosis (of any cause). Another risk factor is dietary exposure to aflatoxin B$_1$, derived from the fungi *Aspergillus flavus* and *Aspergillus parasiticus* and a contaminate of cereals (grains) and legume stored in hot, wet conditions. This is a major concern in Africa and Asia. Up to 45% of individuals with hemochromatosis (an iron overload disease) can develop HCC. Although the tumor is more likely to arise with the development of cirrhosis, it is not necessarily true (i.e., HCC can develop in the absence of cirrhosis).

Other diseases, such as NAFLD[248], Wilson disease, and α_1-antitrypsin deficiency, also display an increased risk with the development of cirrhosis and subsequent HCC. Epidemiologic studies have demonstrated an increase risk with the long-term use of oral contraceptives,[39] although the number of cases involved is extremely small.

Pathogenesis and Clinical Manifestations. The exact events leading to malignant transformation of the hepatic cell remain unknown. The liver is a common site for metastasis of tumors originating in other organs.

In primary liver cancer, HBV appears to be an oncogenic virus that can integrate its viral DNA sequences into the cellular genome. Whether this integration is a necessary step for the mentioned transformation is still uncertain; but it does appear that HBV is both directly and indirectly carcinogenic. Likewise, the metabolic product of aflatoxin B1 is formed in the liver and known to be genotoxic, directly damaging DNA.

Indirect carcinogenic effects are the result of the chronic necroinflammatory hepatic disease. Continuous turnover of cells with cycles of inflammation and regeneration can lead to tumor formation. HCV does not integrate into human DNA but appears to be directly oncogenic. Aflatoxin appears to cause HCC by inactivating a tumor suppressor gene.

Most people who develop HCC are unaware of it until advanced stages. Right upper abdominal pain (60%-95%) and weight loss (35%-70%) are the most common initial symptoms. Other symptoms include weakness, fatigue, poor appetite, early satiety, fullness of the abdomen, diarrhea, and constipation. Jaundice is observed in only 5% to 25% of cases. Metastases occur to the bone and lungs, resulting in back pain and cough. Physical examination may demonstrate an enlarged liver, ascites, or splenomegaly. Unfortunately, many of these signs and symptoms may already be present because of cirrhosis and not distinguished as HCC.

Rarely, paraneoplastic syndromes (a result of a bioactive substance produced by the tumor) can be associated with this tumor. Hypoglycemia, caused by the defective processing of a precursor to insulin-like growth factor II, can occur early in the disease process and may be the presenting symptom. Polycythemia (an increase in erythrocytosis) occurs in less than 10% of cases of HCC but may warn of the presence of the tumor.

Uncommon complications include rupture of tumor with associated hemoperitoneum, thrombosis of portal or hepatic vein, and tumor embolism.

MEDICAL MANAGEMENT

DIAGNOSIS. Changes in liver transaminases are not helpful in distinguishing HCC from cirrhosis or other masses. One tumor marker that can be useful is serum α-fetoprotein. In high-risk populations, an elevation in α-fetoprotein is 80% to 90% sensitive and 90% specific.

Ultrasonography and contrast-enhanced CT scans or MRIs are the most commonly used imaging tests and have largely replaced percutaneous liver biopsy to avoid risks associated with needle biopsy (bleeding, tract seeding).[130] CT most often is able to reveal tumor size and extent (tumor often involves the portal blood vessels). Definitive diagnosis is based on histologic findings in resected hepatic tumors or biopsy specimens.

PREVENTION AND TREATMENT. The use of vaccination to prevent infection with HBV is expected to reduce the incidence of HCC associated with HBV. This is the only malignancy for which an effective prophylactic immunization is available. In the meantime, early screening of high-risk populations using α-fetoprotein and ultrasonography remains the key to successful treatment of this malignancy.

Surgical resection (partial or total hepatectomy) has been the primary treatment if no nodal involvement or distant spread is present; but only 15% of cases are feasibly resectable at presentation. Liver transplantation is the most effective method to treat both the cancer and the underlying liver disease. This option is possible if fewer than three lesions are present (with the largest being less than 3 cm) or one lesion that is less than 5 cm. This may be the optimal therapy for individuals with cirrhosis who cannot tolerate resection.[130] Some transplantation centers have broadened eligibility criteria but only when doing so does not compromise cancer-specific survival for that individual.

Newer liver-directed treatment techniques take advantage of the fact that intrahepatic tumors derive their blood supply from the hepatic artery. Transarterial chemoembolization (angiography to embolize the tumor arterial supply associated with chemotherapy or chemotherapy eluting beads) for unresectable HCC can reduce the size of large tumors. This type of hepatic-artery based therapy may provide superior survival rates but studies have not confirmed this.[130]

Percutaneous ethanol injection (alcohol injection into the tumor) or radiofrequency thermal ablation are beneficial in connection with small tumors with a 5-year survival rate of 40% to 50% (rarely curative for small tumors). Tyrosine kinase inhibitors and antiangiogenic agents are newer agents currently undergoing clinical trials.[122]

Several radioembolization techniques are being employed; yttrium-90 microspheres or iodine-131– or rhenium-188–labeled lipiodol is injected into the hepatic artery. Holmium-166–loaded[173] poly(L-lactic acid) microspheres have also been developed.[24] This method of treatment targets the tumor with radiation while decreasing radiation dose to the body. Criteria are currently lacking on which clients benefit most from this type of therapy, and more study is required to determine optimal dosing in individuals with cirrhosis.[203]

Stereotactic body radiation therapy, a type of targeted radiation therapy that uses computer modeling to minimize the treatment area can be used with single lesions or up to three tumors if smaller than 3 cm. Chemotherapy alone or in combination with liver-directed therapies and internal radiation are also being used in individuals with advanced metastatic HCC. Early results show a 3-month survival advantage over nontreated groups.[2,135]

PROGNOSIS. Symptomatic HCC has a very poor prognosis, especially in clients with multiple tumor nodules. Five-year survival rate has improved from 10% to 26%, which is attributed to improved surveillance in high-risk individuals (those with hepatitis B and C). Factors affecting the prognosis favorably include early detection (potentially curative at this stage[94]), tumor size (less than 5 cm), tumor location, presence of a tumor capsule, well-differentiated tumor, lack of vascular invasion, and absence of cirrhosis. Successful treatment with liver resection or transplantation has also contributed to increased 5-year survival rates but tumor recurrence is very frequent. Tumor resection in the presence of cirrhosis is accompanied by risk of tumor recurrence or death from the remaining underlying liver dysfunction. If treatment fails to eradicate the tumor process, the expected survival is no more than 4 to 6 months.

SPECIAL IMPLICATIONS FOR THE THERAPIST   17-14

Primary Hepatocellular Carcinoma

Liver tumors that cause elevation of the diaphragm can cause right shoulder pain or symptoms of respiratory involvement. Peripheral edema associated with developing ascites may be observed first by the therapist (see "Ascites" above). As the tumor grows, pain may radiate to the back (midthoracic region). Paraneoplastic syndromes (see Chapter 9) resulting from ectopic hormone may occur, including polycythemia, hypoglycemia, and hypercalcemia. (See "Special Implications for the Therapist 9-1: Oncology/Cancer" in Chapter 9).

Metastatic Malignant Tumors

The liver is one of the most common sites of metastasis from other primary cancers (e.g., colorectal, stomach, pancreas, esophagus, lung, breast, melanoma, Hodgkin disease, and non-Hodgkin lymphoma). Metastatic tumors occur 20 times more often than primary liver tumors and constitute the bulk of hepatic malignancy.

As with other types of cancers, secondary liver cancer can occur as a result of local invasion from neighboring organs, lymphatic spread, spread across body cavities, and spread via the vascular system. The liver filters blood from anywhere else in the body, but because all blood from the digestive organs passes through the liver before joining the general circulation, the liver is the first organ to filter cancer cells released from the stomach, intestine, or pancreas.

Metastatic tumors to the liver originating in some organs (e.g., stomach or lung) never give rise to hepatic symptoms, whereas others produce hepatic symptoms or jaundice with less than 60% replacement of the liver. Certain tumors (colon, breast, or melanoma) typically replace 90% of the liver before jaundice develops. Melanomas are associated with such minimal tissue reaction that almost complete hepatic replacement occurs before hepatic symptoms develop.

Clinical manifestations, diagnosis, and treatment are the same as for the primary (original) neoplasm. Experimental and clinical data show evidence of a correlation between elevated blood levels of carcinoembryonic antigen (CEA) and the development of liver metastases from colorectal carcinomas. A cause–effect relationship between these two observations has not been identified. Investigations continue to explore the use of tumor markers and the clinical usefulness of CEA throughout the different stages of management in both animal and human studies.

Treatment is the same as for unresectable liver cancer; see "Primary Hepatocellular Carcinoma" above. In liver metastases from colorectal cancer, liver resection results in 5-year survival rates of 25% to 50% and 10-year survival rates of 20% to 26% with potential cure. The most common site for disease recurrence after surgical resection is the residual liver.[227]

Other ongoing research is investigating the use of a totally implantable pump for hepatic arterial infusion therapy for those with unresectable hepatic metastases and for posthepatic resection. This enables oncologists to give much higher doses of chemotherapy directly into the blood supply of the tumors, as well as use a continuous infusion schedule. This approach may offer more successful treatment of people with metastatic colorectal carcinoma to the hepatic system.[100,103]

Liver Abscess

Liver abscess most often occurs among individuals with other underlying disorders. Most common underlying causes include *bacterial cholangitis* secondary to obstruction of the bile ducts by stone or stricture; *portal vein bacteremia* secondary to bacterial seeding via the portal vein from infected viscera following bowel inflammation or organ perforation; *liver flukes*, a parasitic infestation; or *amebiasis*, an infestation with amebae from tropical or subtropical areas.[254] *Klebsiella pneumoniae* is an emerging pathogenic cause of liver abscess resulting in an invasive syndrome characterized by liver abscesses and metastatic complications including bacteremia, meningitis, and necrotizing fasciitis.[218]

Other predisposing factors are diabetes mellitus, infected hepatic cysts, metastatic liver tumors with secondary infection, and diverticulitis. Pyogenic (pus-filled) abscesses may be single or multiple; liver cirrhosis is a strong risk factor for single pyogenic liver abscess, and multiple abscesses often arise from a biliary source of infection.

Clinical manifestations are commonly right-sided abdominal and shoulder pain, nausea, vomiting, rapid weight loss, high fever, and diaphoresis. The liver's close proximity to the base of the right lung may contribute to the development of right pleural effusion. Complications of hepatic abscess relate to rupture and direct spread of infection. Pleuropulmonary involvement from the rupture of an abscess through the diaphragm and peritonitis from leakage into the abdominal cavity can occur.

Diagnosis is accomplished by a variety of possible tests, including liver function tests, chest x-ray, contrast-enhanced CT scan of the abdomen, ultrasonography of the right upper quadrant, liver scan, and arteriography. Treatment may consist of antimicrobial therapy alone or percutaneous needle aspiration or catheter drainage of the abscess with antimicrobial therapy.[90] Surgery may be required to relieve biliary tract obstruction and to drain abscesses that do not respond to percutaneous drainage and antibiotics.

Unrecognized and untreated, pyogenic liver abscess is universally fatal. The mortality from hepatic abscess in treated cases remains high, ranging from 40% to 80%. Amebic abscesses are an exception; when treated, the mortality rate is less than 3%. Early diagnosis and aggressive treatment can significantly reduce the mortality in some cases. Specific antibiotics are required whenever abscess is caused by amebic infestation.

SPECIAL IMPLICATIONS FOR THE THERAPIST 17-15

Liver Abscess

Clients with liver abscess are very ill and usually are seen only by the therapist assigned to an intensive care unit team. In such situations, vital signs are assessed regularly to detect high fever and rapid pulse, which are early signs of sepsis (a common complication). Movement, coughing, and deep breathing are important to prevent or limit pulmonary complications related to hepatic abscess, and skin care in the presence of high fever is essential. Careful disposal of feces and careful handwashing to avoid transmission are required when abscess is caused by amebic infestation.

Liver Injuries

Toxic liver injury can occur as a result of drugs or from occupational exposure to chemicals and toxins. Hepatotoxic chemicals produce liver cell necrosis, a consequence of the metabolism of the compound by the oxidase system of the liver. Agents responsible for toxic liver injury include yellow phosphorus, carbon tetrachloride, phalloidin (mushroom toxin), and acetaminophen (analgesic). Reye syndrome in children may be related to aspirin toxicity. In addition to jaundice, other symptoms of liver toxicity may occur (e.g., cholestasis or chronic hepatitis).

Toxic liver injury produces toxic hepatitis (discussed earlier in this chapter (see "Hepatitis")). The prognosis is usually good if the toxin is withdrawn and never reintroduced. Whatever drug is responsible, it is well documented that liver toxicity becomes more severe with advancing age.

Liver injury by trauma may be either penetrating or blunt, leading to laceration and hemorrhage. Penetrating injuries are usually knife or missile wounds (gunshot). A knife wound leaves a sharp clear incision, whereas gunshot wounds enter and exit with greater damage. Blunt trauma from a fall or from hitting a steering wheel has varying effects, from small hematomas to large lacerations as a result of severe impact forces.

SPECIAL IMPLICATIONS FOR THE THERAPIST 17-16

Liver Injuries

The therapist will likely be treating clients with liver injury secondary to trauma postoperatively in the trauma unit. The common postoperative problems include pulmonary infections and abscess formation. Clients are assessed postoperatively for manifestations of infection (e.g., fever, chills, or difficulty breathing). Physical therapy intervention is focused on prevention of respiratory complications, especially pneumonia and provision of skin care and extremity movement, until the client can begin progressive transfer and mobility skills.

PANCREAS

Diabetes Mellitus

The pancreas has dual functions, acting as both an endocrine gland in secreting the hormones insulin and glucagon and as an exocrine gland in producing digestive enzymes. The cells of the pancreas that function in the endocrine capacity are the islets of Langerhans, constituting 1% to 2% of the pancreatic mass. Defective endocrine function of the pancreas resulting in ineffective insulin (whether deficient or defective in action within the body) characterizes diabetes mellitus (see Chapter 11).

Pancreatitis

Pancreatitis is a potentially serious inflammation of the pancreas that may result in autodigestion of the pancreas by its own enzymes. Pancreatitis may be acute or chronic; the acute form is brief, usually mild, and reversible, whereas the chronic form is recurrent or persisting. Because the hormones and enzymes provided by the pancreas perform many vital functions, acute pancreatitis causes systemic problems and complications that affect the entire body. Approximately 15% of all cases of acute pancreatitis develop into chronic pancreatitis.

Acute Pancreatitis

Incidence and Etiologic Factors. Acute pancreatitis is an inflammatory process of the pancreas that can involve surrounding organs, as well as cause a systemic reaction. Pancreatitis can arise from a variety of factors and conditions (Box 17-4) or as a result of an unknown cause (10% of cases). The most common cause is gallstones, followed by chronic alcohol consumption. Other causes include hypertriglyceridemia (levels greater than 1000 mg/dL), trauma, duct obstruction (neoplasms), and medications. The incidence has increased over the past few decades, but the mortality rate has remained fairly constant at 7%.

Pancreatitis can involve only the interstitium of the pancreas, termed *interstitial pancreatitis*, or have necrosis of pancreatic tissue, called *necrotizing pancreatitis*. Interstitial pancreatitis accounts for 80% of cases and has a milder course and few complications, whereas necrotizing pancreatitis occurs in 20% of cases and can result in significant complications and higher mortality.

Pathogenesis. Acute pancreatitis is thought to result from the inappropriate activation of trypsinogen within acinar cells to the enzyme trypsin. Trypsin is the principal enzyme responsible for activating other pancreatic enzymes. The buildup of pancreatic enzymes can trigger pancreatic autodigestion. In the development of pancreatitis, the conversion of trypsinogen to trypsin occurs in sufficient quantities to overwhelm the normal mechanisms of eliminating trypsin from the cells. The release of enzymes leads to acinar cell and vascular damage, resulting in a disproportionate inflammatory response with associated edema and inflammation.[246]

Box 17-4

CONDITIONS ASSOCIATED WITH ACUTE PANCREATITIS

- Alcohol abuse*
- Autoimmune diseases
- Cystic fibrosis
- Gallstones*
- Hereditary (familial) pancreatitis
- Hypercalcemia
- Hyperlipidemia (hypertriglyceridemia)
- Infection (bacterial, viral)
- Ischemia
- Medications (oral estrogens, antibiotics, AZT, thiazide diuretics, corticosteroids)
- Neoplasm (pancreatic tumors)
- Peptic ulcers
- Post endoscopic retrograde cholangiopancreatography
- Postoperative inflammation
- Pregnancy (third trimester)
- Toxins
- Blunt or penetrating trauma (including ischemia/perfusion that occurs during some surgical procedures)
- Vasculitis
- Unknown

* Most common causes.

Pancreatitis becomes severe when cytokines (interleukins 1, 6, and 8, TNF, and platelet-activating factor) and free radicals mediate a systemic response,[22,200] leading to multiorgan failure and, occasionally, death. Severe ischemia and inflammation can disrupt the ducts, resulting in the leakage of pancreatic fluid and the formation of fluid collections and pseudocysts. A pseudocyst is a liquefied collection of necrotic debris and pancreatic enzymes surrounded by a rim of pancreatic tissue or adjacent tissues; it contains no true epithelial lining. Complications of pseudocysts include infection, bleeding, and rupture into the peritoneum.

Infection can occur secondary to the breakdown of normal barriers in the gut because of hypoperfusion of the colon. Multiple genes are also under investigation, which, coupled with the appropriate environmental conditions, may be responsible for the development of pancreatitis.[247]

Clinical Manifestations. Symptoms in clients presenting with acute pancreatitis can vary from mild, nonspecific abdominal pain to profound pain accompanied by systemic symptoms. Most people with mild-to-moderate disease present with pain, nausea, anorexia, and vomiting. Abdominal pain, the cardinal symptom of acute pancreatitis, may be dull at first but can increase in quality and intensity to sharp and severe.

Quality of pain can vary, depending on the cause and severity of disease, but often involves the entire upper abdomen. Right upper quadrant pain with radiation to the back may be more prevalent with gallstones. The pain is typically steady and at maximal intensity within 10 to 20 minutes. Pain can be triggered or made worse by eating fatty meals or drinking alcohol. Position changes usually do not alleviate the discomfort. Nausea and vomiting occur in 90% of people with pancreatitis and can be severe.

A minority of cases develops into severe pancreatitis with serious complications. Symptoms that warn of worsening condition include tachycardia, hypoxia, tachypnea, and changes in mental status. Complications of pancreatitis include pancreatic fluid–filled collections (57% of cases), pseudocysts, and necrosis. These fluid collections can enlarge, leading to worsening pain. Bacteria can infect these collections and necrotic areas, resulting in pain, leukocytosis, fever, hypotension, and hypovolemia. Often the first sign of a complication is the failure to improve followed by unexpected deterioration. Ascites and pleural effusions are rare complications.

MEDICAL MANAGEMENT

DIAGNOSIS. Diagnosis is based on clinical presentation, laboratory tests, and imaging studies. Early in the disease process (within 24-72 hours), pancreatic enzymes released from injured acinar cells result in elevated serum amylase and lipase levels, which are diagnostic for acute pancreatitis. The amylase level is typically three times the upper limit of normal, whereas lipase increases proportionately with the amylase level. Amylase rises early (within 2 hours of symptom onset), but decreases quickly (within 36 hours). Amylase levels may not be very helpful unless the person seeks medical attention very early on.

Lipase levels are more specific to acute pancreatitis, rising in 4 to 8 hours, peaking around 24 hours, and staying elevated for at least 14 days. Lipase levels at least three times the normal range (10-140 U/L) indicate acute pancreatitis.[87] An elevated ALT is suggestive of pancreatitis caused by gallstones (where alcohol abuse is not a factor).

Other tests may demonstrate hypertriglyceridemia or hypercalcemia. Imaging studies include an abdominal CT scan to evaluate the pancreas (possibly serial examinations if symptoms fail to resolve with treatment) and transabdominal ultrasound to evaluate the gallbladder and cystic duct for possible gallstones. The CT is also able to demonstrate necrotizing pancreatitis, which provides management and prognostic information.

In clients who have contraindications for ERCP, CT, or MRI with contrast, magnetic resonance cholangiopancreatography (MRCP), a noninvasive procedure that allows visualization of the biliary tree and pancreatic ducts without the use of contrast media, can be performed, which can reveal necrosis when present. If gallstones in the common bile duct are suspected but are not seen on CT scan, endoscopic ultrasonography (EUS) or MRCP can be employed.

TREATMENT. For most persons (approximately 80% of cases), acute pancreatitis is a mild disease that subsides spontaneously within several days. Treatment for mild pancreatitis is largely symptomatic and designed to preserve normal pancreatic function while preventing complications and includes intravenous fluids for hydration, analgesics for pain control, and eating nothing by mouth to allow the pancreas to rest. If after 2 to 3 days, there is no improvement, a CT scan should be obtained to determine whether complications are present.[20]

Clients are allowed to return home once the pain is under control and they are able to eat, drink, and take oral analgesics. Food intake progresses from clear liquids for 24 hours to small, low-fat meals with a slow increase in quantity over several days as tolerated.[246] If pancreatitis is secondary to gallstones, laparoscopic cholecystectomy can be performed before discharge from the hospital (if pancreatic fluid collections or other complications are not present).

If fluid collections are present, surgery should be delayed until they have resolved. If after 6 weeks the collections have not resolved, laparoscopic cholecystectomy with fluid collection drainage can be performed.[109] ERCP with endoscopic sphincterotomy may be performed postoperatively if common bile duct stones are present or for clients who are not surgical candidates.

Severe pancreatitis is defined by the presence of organ failure, local complications, or both. It is important to identify clients with severe pancreatitis at admission to provide aggressive care and close observation for complications. The Acute Physiology and Chronic Health Evaluation score (APACHE II) is an accurate predictor of severity of disease, complications, and death. An elevated C-reactive protein value, elevated hematocrit (above 44%), and obesity (body mass index greater than 30) are factors that predict severe disease.

People admitted to the hospital with severe pancreatitis require admittance to an intensive care unit, aggressive intravenous hydration, and pain control. Enteral nutrition (within 2-3 days) is preferred to parenteral feeding in most cases of severe pancreatitis because it decreases infectious complications.[133] Evidence fails to show a benefit of medications designed to improve the course of severe pancreatitis; some of these medications include inhibitors of platelet-activating factor, somatostatin, and protease inhibitors.[91,246]

Severe pancreatitis can be accompanied by significant complications, including the formation of pancreatic fluid collections, pseudocysts, necrosis, bacterial cholangitis, and infected fluid collections and necrotic areas. Fluid collections should be followed by serial CT scans to verify improvement.

ERCP with sphincterotomy should be performed early in the course of severe pancreatitis caused by bile duct stones. This procedure decreases the risk for complications.[14] If the person's medical condition allows, surgery should be avoided in cases of severe pancreatitis because there is a high rate of death if done within the first few days of onset.[231]

Fluid collections that are infected can be treated with antibiotics and drained; necrotic areas that are not infected can be watched. If necrotic areas become infected, a necrosectomy can be performed or the area can be drained percutaneously once the client is stable.[109] Prophylactic antibiotics are controversial for severe pancreatitis.

PROGNOSIS. Prognosis of acute pancreatitis depends on the severity of the condition. Individuals with mild pancreatitis (80% of cases) have a better outcome than those with necrotizing or severe disease. The clinical course of mild disease follows a self-limiting pattern, resolving within 2 weeks of onset. The risk of dying from severe pancreatitis is between 10% and 30%, and is the result of complications such as infection. Yet most people who experience severe pancreatitis are able to recover (recovery may take up to 2 months) and at 6 years, approximately 65% of people are able to work full time. Recurrences and the development of diabetes mellitus are common in alcoholic pancreatitis, particularly with continued drinking of alcohol.

SPECIAL IMPLICATIONS FOR THE THERAPIST `17-17`

Acute Pancreatitis

The therapist is most likely to see acute pancreatitis either when the early presentation is back pain (undiagnosed) or when acute respiratory distress syndrome develops as a complication, necessitating assisted respiration and pulmonary care. Pancreatic inflammation and scarring occurring as part of the acute pancreatic process can result in decreased spinal extension, especially of the thoracolumbar junction. This problem is difficult to treat and requires the therapist to make reasonable goals (e.g., maintain function and current range of motion), especially when the pancreatitis is in an active, ongoing phase.

Even with client compliance with treatment intervention and the subsiding of inflammation, the residual scarring is difficult to reach or affect with mobilization techniques and continues to reduce mechanical motion. Back pain associated with acute pancreatitis may be accompanied by GI symptoms such as diarrhea, pain after a meal, anorexia, and unexplained weight loss. The client may not see any connection between GI symptoms and back pain and may not report the additional symptoms.

The pain may be relieved by heat initially (decreases muscular tension); preferred positions include leaning forward, sitting up, or lying motionless on the left side in a fetal-flexed position. Promoting comfort and rest as part of the medical rehabilitation process may necessitate teaching the client positioning (side-lying, knee-chest position with a pillow pressed against the abdomen, or sitting with the trunk flexed may be helpful) and relaxation techniques.

For the client who is restricted from eating or drinking to rest the GI tract and decrease pancreatic stimulation, even ice chips can stimulate enzymes and increase pain. In such cases, the therapist must be careful not to give in to the client's repeated requests for food, water, or ice chips unless approved by nursing or medical staff. Clients with acute pancreatitis are allowed to resume oral intake when all abdominal pain and tenderness have resolved. (See also Chapter 5 for care of the client with fluid or electrolyte imbalance.)

Monitoring Lab Values

Monitor the individual with acute pancreatitis for signs and symptoms of bleeding; alert the health care team about bruising or prolonged bleeding. With acute pancreatitis, expect to see increased white blood cell count (inflammation), elevated hematocrit (associated with dehydration secondary to pancreatic necrosis), decreased hemoglobin when there is internal bleeding, tachycardia, and fever due to the inflammatory process. Mild confusion and hypoxemia are also common, so monitor pulse oximetry and ask about the need for supplemental oxygen if indicated. Monitor pain intensity levels using the same rating scale to determine changing patterns of pain and evaluate the individual's response to treatment.

Chronic Pancreatitis

Overview, Incidence, and Etiology. Chronic pancreatitis is characterized by the development of irreversible changes in the pancreas secondary to chronic inflammation. The principal causes are chronic alcohol consumption, a history of severe acute pancreatitis, autoimmune, hereditary, and idiopathic. In Western industrialized nations, the most common cause of chronic pancreatitis is alcohol abuse, accounting for more than 50% of cases.[255]

Incidence and prevalence of chronic pancreatitis are low but increasing over time.[255] The typical person with alcohol-related chronic pancreatitis is male, between the ages of 35 and 45 years, and has consumed large quantities of alcoholic beverages (150 g or more) for more than 6 years. Hereditary pancreatitis is found in clients who have two or more relatives with the disease, including cystic fibrosis.

Several mutations have been discovered that are associated with the disease although the specific pathogenesis is under investigation. The *PRSS1* and *R122H* are cationic trypsinogen genes,[42] the *PST1/SPINK1* are pancreatic secretory trypsin inhibitor genes, and the *CFTR* gene is a cystic fibrosis transmembrane conductance regulator gene.

Autoimmune chronic pancreatitis occurs most frequently in the Far East and is associated with an elevated IgG level, diffuse involvement of the pancreas, a mass in the pancreas, an irregular main pancreatic duct, and the presence of autoantibodies.[164] It is occasionally related to other autoimmune diseases such as Sjögren syndrome, ulcerative colitis, and systemic lupus erythematosus.

Pathogenesis. Several hypotheses have been published to explain the development of chronic pancreatitis. Most are directed toward alcohol-related chronic pancreatitis but have some applicability to other types. The first one suggests that alcohol consumption leads to release of pancreatic fluid that is high in protein but low in volume and bicarbonate. These characteristics result in the precipitation of protein, creating plugs in the pancreatic ducts, which may calcify and produce pancreatic stones. Plugs and stones can obstruct the ducts, causing an increased pressure and damage to pancreatic tissue and ducts. Pancreatic stones are seen in several types of chronic pancreatitis, although damage is noted in areas without obstruction.

A second hypothesis proposes that alcohol or one of its metabolites acts as a direct toxin on pancreatic tissue or sensitizes the acinar cells to the effects of pathologic stimuli. Alcohol may also stimulate the release of cholecystokinin, which, in the presence of alcohol, leads to the transcription of inflammatory enzymes.[170]

A third hypothesis explains that after repeated bouts of acute pancreatitis, areas of necrosis heal with the formation of scar tissue or fibrosis. In persons without a history of acute episodes, the pathogenesis of chronic pancreatitis may relate to persistent necrosis and insidious scarring, similar to the progression of cirrhosis of the liver. Several genetic mutations have also been implicated; many occur in the trypsinogen gene, which renders trypsin resistant to inactivation.[57] Theories continue to evolve, and the pathogenesis most likely depends on both genetic and environmental factors.

Clinical Manifestations. Most clients with chronic pancreatitis present with abdominal pain, which is also the most significant problem. Chronic pain often leads to an abuse of opioids, decreased appetite, weight loss, and poor quality of life; it is also the most common reason for surgery in people with this disease. Pain is typically epigastric in location, often with radiation to the back. It is made worse with meals but can be relieved by bringing the knees to the chest or bending forward. Nausea and vomiting are often associated with the pain. Pain during the course of the disease varies; many people will experience acute attacks followed by periods of feeling well. As the number of attacks increases and occurs more frequently, pain becomes more chronic in nature. Others have continual pain, which gradually increases in intensity.

Chronic destruction of pancreatic tissue contributes to the loss of pancreatic function, resulting in diarrhea, steatorrhea, and diabetes mellitus. Once the production of lipase is reduced to less than 10% of normal, fat maldigestion occurs, producing bulky, foul-smelling, oily stools (steatorrhea). This complication is seen in late stages of the disease, signifying the destruction of most of the acinar cells.

Diabetes is also seen later in the course of the disease, particularly after surgical removal of the pancreas. Unlike type 1 diabetes, there is destruction of both β cells (which produce insulin) and α cells (which produce glucagon). This can lead to severe and prolonged hypoglycemia with the use of insulin.

History is often significant for alcohol abuse; other clients may have a history of pancreatitis or family history of chronic pancreatitis. Physical examination is usually significant for abdominal tenderness, with few other findings.

MEDICAL MANAGEMENT

DIAGNOSIS. The diagnosis of chronic pancreatitis may be difficult to make, particularly in the early stages of the disease when the pancreas lacks significant functional or structural changes. Routine laboratory tests, such as lipase and amylase, are often not elevated except during an acute episode of pancreatitis. Bilirubin may only be abnormal if there is significant compression of the bile duct by a pseudocyst or fibrosis.

More specialized functional tests are available, which either directly measure pancreatic enzymes produced by the pancreas or indirectly measure a product from the action of a pancreatic enzyme or its presence in the serum or stool (such as stool fat or serum trypsinogen). These functional tests are not well tolerated and not widely available.

Imaging tests can demonstrate structural changes. Some of the changes seen in chronic pancreatitis include dilated pancreatic ducts (both large and small), strictures, pancreatic stones, lobularity, and atrophy. *Large duct disease*, which is disease characterized by involvement of the large pancreatic duct by imaging) is often seen with alcohol abuse and is associated with functional problems as well. *Small duct disease* is often difficult to diagnose, and the cause is often idiopathic. Various imaging modalities can be used to diagnose chronic pancreatitis. Often the least invasive test is utilized such as transabdominal ultrasonography or CT.

Other tests are used as needed, such as EUS, ERCP, or MRCP/MRI.

TREATMENT. The treatment of chronic pancreatitis is directed toward prevention of further pancreatic injury, pain relief, and replacement of lost endocrine/exocrine function. Cessation of alcohol intake is essential in the management of chronic pancreatitis in clients with alcohol-related pancreatitis. Smoking has also been linked with increased risk of mortality in people with alcohol-related pancreatitis and should be avoided.[127]

Pain can be initially treated with nonnarcotics and advanced to narcotics as needed. Narcotics are useful for persons with established chronic pancreatitis, but the risk for addiction is approximately 10% to 30%. High-dose pancreatic enzyme therapy can reduce pain in some people with small duct disease but not for large duct disease. Nerve blocks can also aid in the reduction of pain.

Treatment of a dominant stricture in the pancreatic duct with stents and pancreatic duct sphincterotomy improves pain in over half of the clients with large duct disease[196]; yet the long-term management of stents is controversial. Surgical drainage for persistent pseudocysts, as well as surgical intervention to eliminate obstruction of pancreatic ducts, may be indicated for severe pain, although the pain often returns.

A pancreatectomy may be performed as a last means of relieving refractory pain. People who undergo pancreatectomy can consider islet cell autotransplantation,[38] which has been successful in a small group of clients. Oral enzyme replacements are taken before, during, and after meals to correct enzyme deficiencies and to prevent malabsorption. Insulin may be required in the case of islet cell dysfunction but used with care secondary to the loss of glucagon-producing cells.

PROGNOSIS. Complications include the development of large pseudocysts, bleeding from pseudoaneurysms, splenic vein thrombosis, and fistula formation. Pancreatic cancer develops in approximately 3% to 4% of people with chronic pancreatitis and is often difficult to distinguish from chronic changes of pancreatitis. Chronic pancreatitis is a serious disease, often leading to chronic disability. Alcohol-related chronic pancreatitis has a poor prognosis without alcohol cessation and increases the risk of mortality by 60%. Overall, the 10-year survival of chronic pancreatitis is 70%, and the 20-year survival rate is 45%.[127]

SPECIAL IMPLICATIONS FOR THE THERAPIST   17-18

Chronic Pancreatitis

Back pain in the upper thoracic area or pain at the thoracolumbar junction may be the presenting symptom for some individuals with chronic pancreatitis, but past medical history including the presence of pancreatitis should raise a red flag and suggest that careful screening is required in these cases. People with alcohol-related chronic pancreatitis often have peripheral neuropathy.

The clinical presentation with aggravating and relieving factors (e.g., alcohol consumption, food intake, or positional changes noted) or failure to improve with therapy intervention adds additional red flag symptoms.[69] The person with known pancreatitis and/or pancreatectomy may need monitoring of vital signs and/or blood glucose levels depending on complications present. Education about the effects of malabsorption and associated osteoporosis should be included. See also "Special Implications for the Therapist 16-10: Malabsorptive Disorders" in Chapter 16.

Pancreatic Cancer

Overview and Incidence

Pancreatic cancer represents the fourth leading cause of cancer mortality in the United States, with more than 45,000 deaths each year.[215] It also has the lowest 5-year survival rate after diagnosis (3%-5%) of any type of cancer, being responsible for 6% of all cancer-related deaths.

Most pancreatic neoplasms (90%) arise from exocrine cells and are *adenocarcinoma* (75% in the proximal or head of the pancreas, 15%-20% in the pancreas body, and 5%-10% in the tail[53]). The remaining primary pancreatic neoplasms include cystic neoplasms, intraductal papillary mucinous tumors, and neuroendocrine tumors. Adenocarcinoma, the most aggressive type of pancreatic malignancy is the focus of this discussion.

Pancreatic cancer is more common in black men and women than in whites, occurs in the Western world most often, and has a peak incidence in the seventh and eighth decades.

Etiologic and Risk Factors

Although the specific cause of pancreatic cancer is unknown, many genes are under investigation as possibly linked to its development. Approximately, 40% of pancreatic cancer cases are sporadic, that is, caused by spontaneous rather than inherited mutations. The K-*ras* mutation has been found in more than 90% of tested pancreatic adenocarcinomas. K-*ras* is thought to be an oncogene, along with AKT2. Genes that inactivate tumor-suppressor genes include *p16*, *p53*, and *DPC4*, whereas *hMLH1* and *hMLH2* are defective DNA repair genes. Mutations in the epidermal growth factor receptor have also been described,[106] with investigations into epidermal growth factor receptor–targeted agents.[195]

Clear evidence of increased risk of pancreatic cancer has been shown related to advancing age with most people in their 70s and 80s before diagnosis. Pancreatic adenocarcinoma is rare in people younger than age 45 years; however, the risk increases after the age of 50 years. Approximately 5% to 10% of people with pancreatic adenocarcinoma have a family history or some genetic predisposition to developing the disease.[77] Other genetic syndromes with an increased risk include adenomatous polyposis, Peutz-Jeghers syndrome, and von Hippel-Lindau syndrome.

Tobacco use (smoking and smokeless tobacco) accounts for 30% of cases of pancreatic cancer and increases the risk up to five times that of nontobacco users. Exposure to certain chemicals (such as benzidine), diets high in fats and red or processed meat,[105,162] history of familial chronic pancreatitis, history of nonfamilial chronic pancreatitis, and a history of partial gastrectomy are also risk factors.[105] The presence of adult-onset diabetes mellitus and impaired glucose tolerance (especially in women), increases the risk of developing pancreatic cancer twofold.[155] Obesity (especially abdominal fat), sedentary lifestyle, and physical inactivity (linked with abnormal glucose metabolism) are associated with increased risk of pancreatic cancer.

No support exists for any direct effect from exposure to radiation, socioeconomic status, alcohol intake, or coffee consumption, although these risk factors remain under investigation.[120,252] Chronic pancreatitis from alcohol consumption is associated with a much higher incidence and an earlier age of onset of pancreatic carcinoma.[245]

Pathogenesis

As mentioned, molecular genetics of pancreatic cancer (e.g., mutations in the K-*ras* gene, mutations or deletions in the *CDKN2* gene, mutations in the *p53* gene) account for a large proportion of these tumors.[82,209,223] The ductal cells in the head of the pancreas are exposed to pancreatic secretions, as well as bile, and environmental carcinogens can reach these cells through those fluids or in the blood.

Microscopically, adenocarcinomas contain infiltrative glands of various sizes and shapes surrounded by dense, reactive fibrous tissue. Many adenocarcinomas infiltrate into vascular spaces, lymphatic spaces, and perineural spaces. Pancreatic cancer appears to progress from flat ductal lesions to papillary ductal lesions without irregularities then with irregularities (atypia) and finally to infiltrating adenocarcinoma. The existence of such a progression suggests that it may be possible to detect a curable precursor lesion and early cancer with a molecular test in the future.[120]

Clinical Manifestations

The clinical features of pancreatic cancer are initially nonspecific and vague or subtle in onset (e.g., anorexia, malaise, nausea, fatigue, pruritus), which contribute to the delay in diagnosis. Most clients are seen for abdominal pain (80%-85%), weight loss (60%), and jaundice (47%). These symptoms suggest advanced disease. Typically, people with significant pain have tumor in the body or tail of the pancreas, whereas jaundice and weight loss are more suggestive of tumor in the head of the pancreas.

Pain is a common symptom of pancreatic carcinoma because of invasion of tumor into nerves. In later stages of the disease, pain may be intractable. Pain (especially night pain) is often epigastric in location, radiating to the back (thoracic or lumbar regions). Jaundice accompanied by pruritus, dark urine, and acholic stools occurs caused by compression of the biliary tree by tumor. Obstruction of the portal vein results in the presence of ascites, enlarged liver, and palpable abdominal mass.

Pancreatitis may also develop from obstruction of the pancreatic duct. In some people, pancreatitis may be the first sign of the disease. Diabetes within the previous year of symptom presentation is not uncommon.[53] Deep venous thrombosis can occur as a result of tumor presence. In one-third of people with pancreatic adenocarcinoma, the gallbladder may be palpable on physical examination.

Metastasis. Pancreatic adenocarcinomas metastasize first to regional lymph nodes then via the hematologic and lymphatic systems to the liver, peritoneum, lungs and pleura, and adrenal glands. These metastasized tumors may grow by direct extension, causing further involvement of the duodenum, stomach, spleen, and colon. Tumors of the body and tail of the pancreas are twice as likely to metastasize to the peritoneum compared with tumors in the head of the pancreas. Palpable metastatic cervical nodes may be present behind the medial end of the left clavicle (called the *Virchow node*) and other areas of the cervical spine.[53] Metastasis to the bone is uncommon.[53]

MEDICAL MANAGEMENT

PREVENTION. At the present time, the best advice to reduce the risk of pancreatic cancer is to avoid tobacco use, maintain a healthful weight, remain physically active, and eat five or more half-cup servings of vegetables and fruits each day.[105] Foods containing folate are probably protective. Folate is important in the synthesis and repair of DNA. Although the risk of pancreatic cancer decreases with increased activity, there is no clear dose-response relationship.[252]

DIAGNOSIS. Pancreatic cancer is difficult to diagnose in its early stages. Spiral CT with intravenous contrast of the abdomen is the most common test in the assessment of pancreatic adenocarcinoma, with 90% sensitivity and 95% specificity. These CT scans also provide staging information that aids in determining resectability. One common sign noted on CT scan is the "double duct" sign, which occurs secondary to obstruction of both the bile and pancreatic ducts. EUS is helpful in viewing pancreatic tumors that may not be seen on CT and is accurate in detecting local lymph nodes.

If a tumor is thought to be resectable by CT and is in the body or tail of the pancreas, laparoscopy may be performed with washing samples, as CT is unable to discern small liver and peritoneal metastases in 20% to 30% of cases (false negative).[199] Biopsy is not required for the diagnosis, but in some cases is helpful. This can be done percutaneously but EUS-guided fine-needle aspiration may cause less seeding of tumor.[146]

Laboratory tests can be abnormal, including elevated bilirubin level if biliary tree obstruction is present and evidence of malnutrition (low serum albumin or cholesterol level). The serum tumor markers CA19-9 antigen and CEA may be increased, but these are nonspecific for pancreatic cancer and should not be solely relied on as diagnostic. This marker can be useful, however, in monitoring treatment.

The TNM staging system (*tumor, node, metastases*) (see Chapter 9) classifies pancreatic carcinoma according to tumor size, extent of local invasion, presence or absence of regional lymph node metastases, and presence or absence of distant nonnodal metastatic disease based on high-quality cross sectional imaging. Preoperative staging provides information required for determining surgical resectability and prognosis.[99]

TREATMENT. Treatment of pancreatic adenocarcinoma is based on the stage of the tumor and is often divided into three broad categories: resectable (15%-20%), locally advanced (often encasing major blood vessels) (40%-45%), and metastatic (40%-45%). Surgical resection before the tumor invades nearby blood vessels or spreads to other areas of the body provides the only curative therapy, yet this is only appropriate for a minority of clients because even in what appears to be early-stage disease, micrometastases has already occurred.

Chemoradiation can be provided to people with locally advanced disease and chemotherapy for those with metastatic disease. Neoadjuvant therapy (given before surgery) consists of chemoradiation and can be given for local tumors that have a high probability of not being entirely resectable (microscopic tumor is often seen at the margins of the surgical incision or tumor in the tail of the pancreas). The goal is to reduce tumor size to increase the likelihood of complete resection at surgery. Chemoradiation may be administered after surgery to improve survival.[86] Research is also focused on finding drugs tailored to the genetics of pancreatic cancer and novel ways to deliver those drugs into tumors. A pancreatic cancer vaccine is being investigated. Cancer recurrence may be possible when a vaccine makes it possible for immune-surveillance cells to seek out and destroy pancreatic cancer cells for years. Johns Hopkins medical oncologists Elizabeth Jaffee, M.D., and Daniel Laheru, M.D., have developed a pancreas cancer vaccine currently being tested in clinical trials. Additional information about clinical trials for vaccine therapy for pancreatic cancer is available at the National Cancer Institute website: http://www.cancer.gov/clinicaltrials/search/results?protocolsearchid=7232381.

Much of the therapy offered to clients with pancreatic carcinoma is palliative to improve quality of life. Pain control is a significant part of therapy. Long-lasting opioids and celiac plexus neurolysis can substantially improve quality of life. Pancreatic enzyme replacement aids clients with malabsorption and steatorrhea problems. For clients who experience jaundice and will receive neoadjuvant therapy or may not be a candidate for surgery, ERCP-guided stent placement in the biliary ducts can help relieve obstruction or biliary bypass surgery can be performed.

Return of hepatic function after relief of obstruction is variable. Bile secretion may return to normal within hours; immunologic dysfunction may take weeks to normalize; jaundice characteristically improves dramatically within the first several days but may not disappear for weeks, and some of the other symptoms, such as pruritus, loss of appetite, and malaise, correct within hours or days after relief of the obstruction.

PROGNOSIS. Surgical resection is currently the only treatment that provides long-term survival; yet only 20% of people with tumor deemed to be resectable are alive at 5 years; this is most likely related to microfoci of tumor still present outside the main mass. For clients with locally advanced or metastatic disease, long-term survival is rare and the mortality rate is nearly 100%. Chemoradiation therapy can prolong survival to a median of 1 year for people with locally advanced disease, whereas chemotherapy offers clients with metastatic disease approximately 6 months.

Factors associated with a more favorable outcome include tumor size less than 3 cm, lymph nodes without tumor, surgical margins free of tumor, and pathology consistent with a well-differentiated tumor.

SPECIAL IMPLICATIONS FOR THE THERAPIST   17-19

Pancreatic Cancer

Like all health care professionals, the physical therapist has a role in primary prevention of pancreatic cancer through patient/client education as smoking is the most significant reversible risk factor for this condition.

Vague back pain may be the first symptomatic presentation, and cervical lymphadenopathy (called the Virchow node) may be the first sign of distant metastases. The therapist is most likely to palpate an enlarged supraclavicular lymph node (usually left-sided), a finding that should always alert the therapist to the need to screen for medical disease.

Paraneoplastic syndrome (see Chapter 9) associated with pancreatic carcinoma may present as neuromyopathy, dermatomyositis, or thrombophlebitis associated with abnormalities in blood coagulation (coagulopathy). The presence of coagulopathy represents a precaution in the administration of certain therapeutic interventions. See "Special Implications for the Therapist 17-1: Signs and Symptoms of Hepatic Disease" above.

The therapist is most likely to be involved with the client with diagnosed pancreatic cancer who experiences intractable back pain. Referral to chronic pain clinics or hospice centers likely includes physical therapy services. Repeated nerve blocks may be performed after a reasonable effort to manage pain through the use of transcutaneous electrical nerve stimulation, biofeedback, analgesics, or other pain control techniques. Indwelling infusion pumps implanted to deliver analgesics directly to the site of visceral afferent nerves in the epidural or intrathecal spaces may be used for short periods (i.e., 1-3 months).

Cystic Fibrosis

Cystic fibrosis is a disease of the exocrine glands that results in the production of excessive, thick mucus that obstructs the digestive and respiratory systems. When the disease was first being differentiated from other conditions, it was given the name cystic fibrosis of the pancreas, because cysts and scar tissue on the pancreas were observed during autopsy. This term describes a secondary rather than primary characteristic (in-depth discussion of this disorder is found in Chapter 15).

BILIARY

See Table 17-5.

Cholelithiasis (Gallstone Disease)

Overview, Definition, and Incidence

Cholelithiasis, or gallstone disease, is one of the most common GI diseases in the United States, occurring in an estimated 20 million people (about 14 million women and 6 million men). Most gallstones are asymptomatic and are only detected on radiologic examinations performed for other reasons. Yet, in approximately 25% of cases, significant symptoms and complications develop because of the presence of gallstones, requiring surgery or other treatment. Age appears to play a role in the development of cholelithiasis so that gallstones are present in 20% to 35% of people by age 55 years.

Cholelithiasis occurs when stones form in the bile. These gallstones form in the gallbladder as a result of changes in the normal components of bile. Two types are classified according to composition: 80% consist primarily of cholesterol (cholesterol stones), whereas 20% are composed of

Table 17-5	Biliary Tract Terminology
Term	**Definition**
Chole-	Pertaining to bile
Cholang-	Pertaining to bile ducts
Cholangiography	Radiographic study of bile ducts
Cholangitis	Inflammation of bile duct
Cholecyst-	Pertaining to the gallbladder
Cholecystectomy	Removal of gallbladder
Cholecystitis	Inflammation of gallbladder
Cholecystography	Radiographic study of gallbladder
Cholecystostomy	Incision and drainage of gallbladder
Choledocho-	Pertaining to common bile duct
Choledocholithiasis	Stones in common bile duct
Choledochostomy	Exploration of common bile duct
Cholelith-	Gallstones
Cholelithiasis	Presence of gallstones
Cholescintigraphy	Radionuclide imaging of biliary system
Cholestasis	Stoppage or suppression of bile flow

Box 17-5

RISK FACTORS ASSOCIATED WITH GALLSTONES

- Age (increasing incidence with increasing age)
- Genetic factors
  - Deficiency in ABCG5/G8
  - Pima women
  - Sickle cell anemia
- Decreased physical activity
- Pregnancy
- Obesity
- Diabetes mellitus
- Hypertriglyceridemia/low high-density lipoprotein cholesterol
- Rheumatoid arthritis
- Diseases of the terminal ileum
- Total parenteral nutrition
- Rapid weight loss
- Liver disease
- Biliary strictures
- Drugs
  - Clofibrate
  - Estrogen
  - Octreotide

bilirubin salts (e.g., calcium bilirubinate and other calcium salts), called *pigment stones* (black and brown). Symptoms occur when these stones block bile flow in any of the ducts, the most common being the cystic duct.

Etiologic and Risk Factors

Many risk factors are associated with the development of gallstones (Box 17-5). Advancing age is a significant risk factor. Older people experience an increase in cholesterol secretion into bile with a simultaneous decrease in bile salt production. Genetics plays a role in gallstone formation; in some ethnic populations the risk for gallstone disease is high. For example, 70% of the Native American women in the Pima tribe in Arizona develop gallstones by the age of 25 years. Alternately, African Americans have less than half the rate of white Americans.

Obesity is a well-known risk factor, particularly in women. One study demonstrated a linear increase in the incidence of cholelithiasis as the body mass increased.[224] Women are also more than twice as likely to develop gallstones as men. This trend is seen until the fifth decade when the risk for women approaches that of men, suggesting estrogen may be the principal factor.

Because of the prevalence of gastric bypass surgery and other methods of extreme weight loss, rapid weight loss has emerged as a risk for cholelithiasis. One study demonstrated the development of gallstones in up to 50% of people within the first 6 months of gastric bypass surgery; 40% became symptomatic.[211]

People who receive total parenteral nutrition (TPN) often develop cholelithiasis; after 3 to 4 months of TPN, approximately 45% of people form gallstones. Pregnancy is another common factor in cholelithiasis. As pregnancy progresses, the bile is more lithogenic (i.e., more prone to stone formation); up to 2% of pregnant women develop gallstones.

Many drugs contribute to the formation of gallstones. Estrogen is the most studied (i.e., oral contraceptives [excluding newer, low-dose products], estrogen replacement therapy),[232] but reports show that ceftriaxone, clofibrate, and octreotide are also lithogenic.

Pathogenesis

Gallstones are caused by changes in the composition of bile, especially bile salts, phospholipids, bilirubin, and cholesterol. When these solids become supersaturated in the gallbladder, gallstones may form. There are three types of gallstones: (1) soft, yellow-green stones (most common type) formed from cholesterol supersaturation in bile just mentioned; (2) small, brittle, black stones formed from high concentrations of calcium bilirubinate, carbonate, and phosphate, usually caused by hemolytic disorders (e.g., sickle cell disease, hereditary spherocytosis) or end-stage liver disease or pancreatitis; and (3) soft, mushy, brown stones formed from calcium bilirubinate and bacterial cell bodies secondary to a bacterial infection that causes bile stasis.

In the formation of cholesterol gallstones, the cholesterol is obtained principally from the diet (only 20% is synthesized by the liver). Some of the common mechanisms associated with cholesterol gallstone formation include stasis of bile in the gallbladder (gallbladder hypomotility), changes in mucin glycoproteins in the gallbladder, or processes that may increase the amount of cholesterol or reduce the amount of bile salts or phospholipids that are secreted into the bile.

Gallbladder hypomotility is presumed to occur when insoluble or supersaturated cholesterol is absorbed into the gallbladder wall, making it difficult for the smooth muscle of the gallbladder to contract.[239] This is seen during pregnancy, after a period of rapid weight loss, in rheumatoid arthritis clients, and when a person is receiving TPN.[80,168]

Environmental, as well as genetic, factors most likely affect the amount of biliary cholesterol. There are several genes that code for transporters of biliary lipids and receptors for lipoproteins. A deficiency in one of these, such as the ABCG5/G8 transporter protein, may be responsible for excess cholesterol secretion into bile.[79,80]

Excess dietary cholesterol consumption may lead to an increase in the amount absorbed into the liver from the blood, but studies are conflicting.[101,148] Obese people may express an overactive enzyme required for cholesterol synthesis (3-hydroxy-3-methylglutaryl coenzyme A [HMG-CoA] reductase), leading to excessive cholesterol production. Because of elevated levels of estrogen, pregnancy can also increase the amount of cholesterol secreted into bile and reduce bile acid production.

Clinical Manifestations

The majority of gallstones remain asymptomatic once formed in the gallbladder. Only a minority (approximately 25%) cause painful symptoms. This occurs when the stone attempts to pass down the ducts leading to the duodenum, becoming wedged. The most common location of obstruction is the cystic duct (Fig. 17-7). This causes abdominal pain (often referred to as *biliary colic*). Obstruction of the cystic duct distends the gallbladder while the muscles in the duct wall contract, trying to expel the stone. The pain of biliary colic may be intermittent or steady; it is usually severe and is located in the right upper quadrant just below or slightly to the right of the sternum with abdominal tenderness and muscle guarding. In more severe cases, rebound pain may be present. Painful symptoms are frequently related to meals, although not exclusively postprandial. The pain often radiates to the right shoulder and upper back (60% of cases) and is associated with nausea and vomiting. Radiating pain to the midback and scapula occurs as a result of splanchnic (visceral) fibers synapsing with adjacent phrenic nerve fibers (major branch of the cervical plexus innervating the diaphragm).

Episodes can last from 20 minutes to several hours and may develop daily or as infrequently as once every few years. Complicated cases often feature jaundice, fever, nausea and vomiting, and leukocytosis.

Other symptoms are vague, including heartburn, belching, flatulence, epigastric discomfort, and food intolerance (especially for fats). Gallstones in the older adult may not cause pain, fever, or jaundice; instead, mental confusion may be the only manifestation of gallstones.

Serious complications occur in 20% of cases when a stone becomes lodged in the lower end of the common bile duct, causing inflammation (cholangitis) leading to bacterial infection and jaundice (indicating the stone is in the common bile duct). Sometimes acute pancreatitis develops when the duct from the pancreas that joins the common bile duct also becomes blocked (see Fig. 17-7). Approximately 15% of clients with gallstones also have stones in the common bile duct (choledocholithiasis).

MEDICAL MANAGEMENT

DIAGNOSIS. Diagnosis is based on history, physical examination, and radiographic evaluation. Physical examination often reveals tenderness to palpation in the right upper quadrant of the abdomen. The radiologic test of choice is the transabdominal ultrasound. Ultrasonography reveals gallstones in more than 95% of cases (when 1.5 mm or greater in size). Ultrasound can also provide information concerning the gallbladder and ducts and can aid in predicting possible technical difficulties during surgery.[178]

EUS can be used to detect stones too small for typical transabdominal ultrasound, and functional ultrasonography (gallbladder volumes with fasting and postprandial)

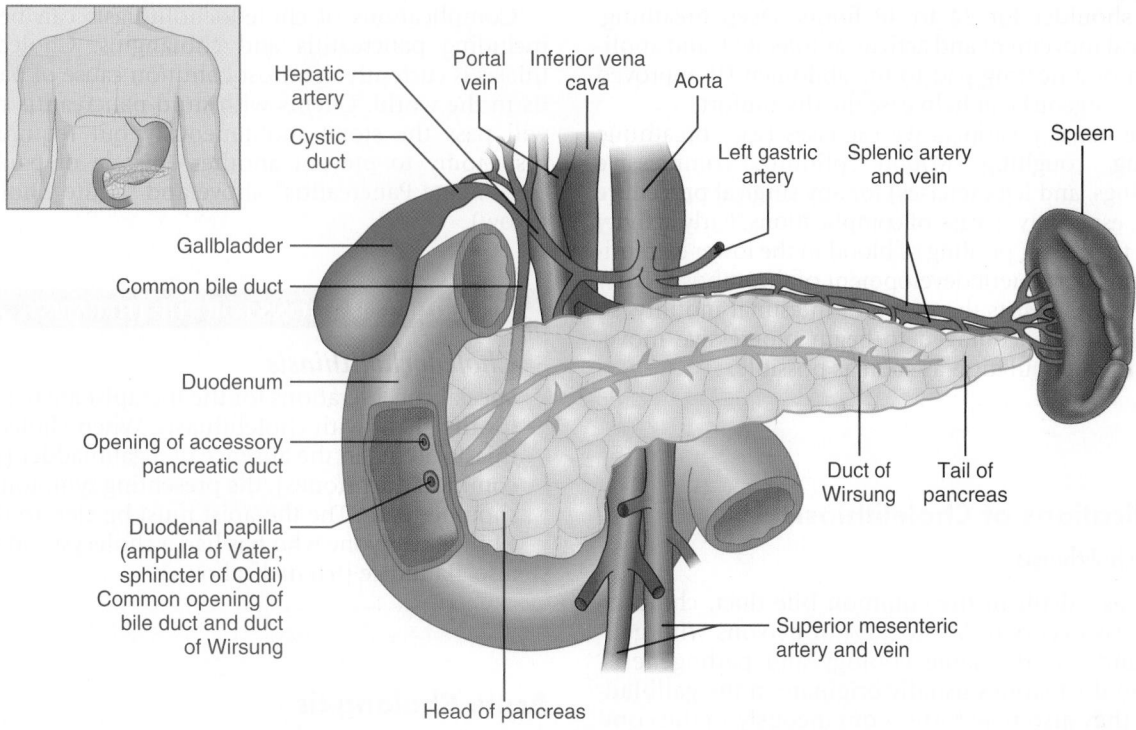

Figure 17-7

The pancreas. The pancreas (located behind the stomach) and gallbladder are anterior to the L1-L3 vertebral bodies. Attaching to the duodenum to the right, the pancreas extends horizontally across to the spleen in the left abdomen, coming in contact with the duodenum, kidneys, liver, and spleen. Obstruction of either the hepatic or common bile duct by stone or spasm blocks the exit of bile from the liver, where it is formed, and prevents bile from ejecting into the duodenum. (From Black JM, Matassarin-Jacobs E, editors: *Luckmann and Sorensen's medical–surgical nursing,* ed 4, Philadelphia, 1993, WB Saunders.)

is used to assess gallbladder motility. These latter tests are not routinely employed because transabdominal ultrasound is frequently sufficient for diagnosis. Other tests are available to detect the location of stones if they are not in the cystic duct and are discussed in the next section.

TREATMENT AND PROGNOSIS. Asymptomatic gallstones typically do not require treatment, except in populations at high risk, such as the women of the Pima tribe or people with sickle cell anemia. Prophylactic cholecystectomy may be recommended in these cases. Other groups requiring prophylactic treatment include those experiencing rapid weight loss or receiving TPN. People who experience rapid weight loss can receive prophylactic UDCA,[212] and those needing prolonged TPN can be treated with cholecystokinin-octapeptide.

Once gallstones cause pain, there is a 1% to 2% annual risk of developing complications, and 50% of people with symptomatic cholelithiasis will have a recurrent episode. Consequently, cholecystectomy is recommended for most symptomatic clients. Laparoscopic cholecystectomy is the preferred surgical approach because the complication rate is decreased when compared to an open procedure. When the gallbladder is removed, bile drains directly from the liver into the intestine, eliminating the opportunity for stone formation.

Medical treatment is used only in select clients and consists of oral dissolution with UDCA, with or without extracorporeal shockwave lithotripsy. Characteristics that deem a client a candidate for medical therapy include presence of small cholesterol stones; reversible cause of gallstone formation (such as medication use); infrequent, mild pain attacks; functioning gallbladder; and a patent cystic duct for the passage of stones. Even with successful medical treatment, 30% to 50% of stones recur within 5 years.

SPECIAL IMPLICATIONS FOR THE THERAPIST   17-20

Cholelithiasis (Gallstone Disease)

Physical activity may play an important role in the prevention of symptomatic gallstone disease in up to a third of all cases. Based on a limited number of studies, increasing exercise to 30 minutes of endurance-type training five times per week is recommended.[112,113] When the gallbladder has been removed (or is blocked by a stone) a small amount of less-concentrated bile is still secreted into the intestine. The loss of a gallbladder itself does not appear to have an impact on physical activity and exercise.

In the past, gallbladder removal required a significant incision with muscle disruption, scarring, and, frequently, postoperative back pain associated with the formation of deep scar tissue. Now the closed procedure (laparoscopic cholecystectomy) can be performed as outpatient (day) surgery without these complications.

Air introduced into the abdomen during this operative technique is removed after the procedure, thereby reducing the postoperative abdominal pain. However, many individuals still experience referred pain to the right shoulder for 24 to 48 hours. Deep breathing, physical movement and activity as tolerated, and application of a heating pad to the abdomen (if approved by the surgeon) can help ease the discomfort.

The usual postoperative exercises (e.g., breathing, turning, coughing, wound splinting, compressive stockings, and leg exercises) for any surgical procedure apply, especially in case of complications. Early activity helps to prevent pooling of blood in the lower extremities and subsequent development of thrombosis. Early activity also assists the return of intestinal motility, so the client is encouraged to begin progressive movement and ambulation as soon as possible.

Complications of Cholelithiasis

Choledocholithiasis

Defined as calculi in the common bile duct, choledocholithiasis occurs in 5% to 10% of persons with gallstones and has the same etiology and pathogenesis. Common duct stones usually originate in the gallbladder, but they also may form spontaneously in the common duct and can, therefore, occur after a person has had a cholecystectomy (10%-15%). Stones that occur in the absence of a gallbladder are referred to as *primary common duct stones*. Approximately 30% to 40% of duct stones are asymptomatic; they are typically small enough to pass through without causing an obstruction. When symptomatic, duct stones produce right upper quadrant pain often with radiating pain to the shoulder and/or back (see "Clinical Manifestations" under "Cholelithiasis [Gallbladder Disease]" above). Liver enzymes are frequently elevated; in some cases the values can be similar to those seen in hepatitis. Serum aminotransferase, ALP, and bilirubin values are usually elevated at least twofold.

Diagnosis is based on clinical picture and radiologic or endoscopic evidence of dilated bile ducts, ductal stones, or impaired bile flow. Although transabdominal ultrasonography is very sensitive for identifying stones in the gallbladder, it is the least-sensitive method for detecting stones in the common bile duct (identifying only 30%-50%).

Helical CT has a sensitivity nearing 80% in imaging common bile duct stones, whereas EUS has a sensitivity of greater than 90%. But ERCP is very sensitive and provides the means to extract the stone during the procedure.[59] ERCP consists of introduction of radiopaque medium into the biliary system by percutaneous puncture of a bile duct to provide x-ray examination of the bile ducts. ERCP is the test of choice for clients with choledocholithiasis associated with cholangitis or pancreatitis but may be contraindicated in clients who have had GI reconstructive surgery (such as a Billroth II procedure) or stones greater than 1 cm or those who have a biliary stricture. Laparoscopic transcystic bile duct exploration can detect and remove common bile duct stones in greater than 90% of clients, and laparoscopic choledochotomy can be performed if transcystic bile duct exploration is not successful.

Complications of choledocholithiasis can be severe, including pancreatitis and cholangitis. Choledocholithiasis is currently the most common cause of pancreatitis in the world. Clients with mild pancreatitis typically will pass the stone spontaneously but require cholecystectomy to prevent another episode of pancreatitis (see "Acute Pancreatitis" above and "Acute Cholangitis" below).

SPECIAL IMPLICATIONS FOR THE THERAPIST   17-21

Choledocholithiasis

Special considerations for the therapist are the same as for the client with cholelithiasis. When choledocholithiasis occurs in the absence of a gallbladder (primary common duct stones), the presenting symptom can be shoulder pain. The therapist must be alert to this possibility in anyone who has had a cholecystectomy. (See also "Jaundice [Icterus]" above.)

Acute Cholangitis

In 6% to 9% of cholelithiasis cases, obstruction and stasis of bile leads to a suppurative infection of the biliary tree, termed *acute cholangitis*. Acute cholangitis symptoms include those of cholelithiasis plus fever and jaundice. These three symptoms—pain, fever, and jaundice—are referred to as the Charcot triad and are noted in 50% to 100% of people with cholangitis.

The Reynolds pentad (seen in only 14% of cases) includes the Charcot triad plus hypotension and mental confusion. The presence of the Reynolds pentad is an ominous sign, with mortality approaching 100% unless there is emergent decompression of the biliary tree. Acute cholangitis can be categorized into three stages: mild grade I (responds to medical therapy), moderate grade II (no organ dysfunction but does not respond to initial medical treatment), and severe grade III (at least one new organ dysfunction).[237]

The total bilirubin is typically elevated greater than two times normal, although it may be in the normal range early in the infection process. Bacteria are isolated in the bile in more than 80% of cases and in the blood in anywhere from 20% to 80% of cases (reports vary widely). Aerobic and anaerobic gram-negative bacilli and enterococci are the most common organisms isolated.

CT scans and ultrasonography can aid in discerning cholecystitis from cholangitis, as well as identify possible abscesses in the liver. EUS can identify stones in the common bile duct.

Treatment is given according to the grade of illness. Grade 1 is mild and can typically be treated with appropriate antibiotics with subsequent laparoscopic cholecystectomy. Clients with grade II disease are treated with antibiotics and early biliary drainage. Once stable, this therapy is followed by open or laparoscopic cholecystectomy. Stage III disease requires appropriate intensive care support with urgent endoscopic or percutaneous transhepatic biliary drainage once the person's hemodynamics are stable. Endoscopic biliary drainage can be achieved with either endoscopic nasobiliary drainage or tube stent placement. There is no significant difference in the success rate, effectiveness, and morbidity between the two procedures. Percutaneous transhepatic biliary drainage has a lower success rate with more complications reported as compared to endoscopic methods.[230]

The decision to perform endoscopic sphincterotomy is made based on the person's condition and the number and diameter of common bile duct stones,[153] although this method has demonstrated higher rates of hemorrhaging and pancreatitis. As the client improves, delayed elective cholecystectomy can be performed.[150]

A complication of cholangitis and biliary drainage includes biliary peritonitis. This can occur because of perforation of the gallbladder with leakage of bile into the abdominal cavity. This requires immediate cholecystectomy and/or drainage.

Cholecystitis

Cholecystitis is the most common complication of gallstone disease, with 700,000 cholecystectomies performed in the United States each year.[121] Cholecystitis, or inflammation of the gallbladder, may be acute or chronic and occurs most often as a result of impaction of gallstones in the cystic duct (see Fig. 17-7), causing obstruction to bile flow and painful distention of the gallbladder.

Acute cholecystitis caused by gallstones accounts for the majority of cases, and acalculous cholecystitis (i.e., gallstones not present) makes up the remaining 10%. Acute cholecystitis from stones is most common during middle age (particularly in women), whereas the acute acalculous form is most common among older adult men and carries a worse prognosis.

Some of the causes for acalculous cholecystitis include ischemia; chemicals that enter biliary secretions; motility disorders associated with drugs; infections with microorganisms, protozoa, and parasites; collagen disease; and allergic reactions. Acute acalculous cholecystitis is associated with a recent operation, trauma, burns, multisystem organ failure, and TPN.[102]

Gallbladder attacks are usually caused by gallbladder and/or cystic duct distention as the stone causes obstruction to the flow of bile. The increased pressure and stasis of bile leads to damage of the mucosa with subsequent release of inflammatory enzymes. Gallbladder inflammation causes prolonged pain characterized as steady right upper quadrant abdominal pain with abdominal tenderness, muscle guarding, and rebound pain. Upper quadrant pain often radiates to the upper back (between the scapulae) and into the right scapula or right shoulder. The Murphy sign (interruption of deep breathing with deep palpation under the right costal arch) is a fairly sensitive and specific sign for gallbladder disease. Accompanying GI symptoms usually include nausea, anorexia, and vomiting and there may be signs of visceral or peritoneal inflammation (e.g., pain worse with movement and locally tender to touch).

Diagnosis is made on the basis of clinical history, examination, laboratory findings, and imaging. The white blood cell count is usually elevated (12,000-15,000/mL). Total serum bilirubin, serum aminotransferase, and ALP levels are often elevated in the acute disease, but they are normal or minimally elevated in the chronic form. X-ray films of the abdomen show radiopaque gallstones in only 15% of cases. Abdominal ultrasonography often shows stones, thickened gallbladder wall, and pericholecystic fluid.

Biliary scintigraphy (hepatoiminodiacetic acid scan) is useful in demonstrating an obstructed cystic duct. The client swallows a long thin, lighted flexible tube connected to a computer and a monitor. A special dye is injected that stains the bile ducts, making them more visible. If the isotope fills the gallbladder and the gallbladder is visualized, acute cholecystitis is unlikely. But failure to visualize the gallbladder suggests cholecystitis.

Any stone detected can be removed immediately. The same information can be obtained by passing a thin needle into the abdominal wall through which dye is injected into the ducts, a procedure called *percutaneous transhepatic cholangiography*.

Laparoscopic cholecystectomy (gallbladder resection) is the treatment and procedure of choice, because it is less invasive than an open procedure and healing and hospital time are reduced.[27] It is often performed during the first hospitalization for acute cholecystitis, although the exact timing depends on the surgeon's judgment; the presence of complications may delay surgery.

Prognosis for both acute and chronic cholecystitis is good with medical intervention. Acute attacks may resolve spontaneously, but recurrences are common, requiring cholecystectomy. Complications can be serious and usually are associated with cholangitis. The mortality of acute cholecystitis is 5% to 10% for clients older than 60 years with serious associated diseases.

An infrequent complication of laparoscopic cholecystectomy is injury to the bile duct (0.4%-0.6% of all cases), causing leakage of bile into the abdomen. Symptoms postoperatively include fever, abdominal pain, ascites, nausea, elevated bilirubin levels, and rarely, frank jaundice. Intraperitoneal bile fluid collections can be seen on ultrasonography, CT scanning, or hepatoiminodiacetic acid scan. ERCP can be used to detect the site of injury and treat the obstruction. Prompt repair requires less treatment than delayed diagnosis, which often requires a more complex reconstruction.

SPECIAL IMPLICATIONS FOR THE THERAPIST 17-22

Cholecystitis

Special considerations for the therapist are the same as for the client with cholelithiasis (see also "Jaundice [Icterus]" above). It is possible for a person to develop a cholelithiasis cholecystitis, or inflammation of the gallbladder without gallstones. The therapist may see a clinical picture typical of gallbladder disease, including mid-upper back or scapular pain (below or between the scapulae) or right shoulder pain associated with right upper quadrant abdominal pain. Close questioning may reveal accompanying associated GI signs and symptoms.

The person may have been evaluated for gallbladder disease, but ultrasonography does not always show small stones. Unless further and more elaborate testing has been performed to examine gallbladder function, the individual may end up in therapy for treatment of the affected musculoskeletal areas. Lack of results from therapy and/or progression of symptoms corresponding to progression of disease requires further medical follow-up.

Primary Biliary Cirrhosis

See "Primary Biliary Cirrhosis," above, under "Liver."

Primary Sclerosing Cholangitis

Sclerosing cholangitis is a chronic cholestatic disease of unknown etiologic origin characterized by progressive destruction of intrahepatic and extrahepatic bile ducts. It has been linked to altered immunity, toxins, ischemia, and infectious agents, in people who are genetically susceptible. Approximately two-thirds of cases occur in clients 20 to 40 years of age and the incidence is thought to be rising; it is seen more commonly in men than women (3:1 ratio). Eighty percent of clients with primary sclerosing cholangitis also have inflammatory bowel disease, most frequently ulcerative colitis, yet only 5% of people with ulcerative colitis develop primary sclerosing cholangitis (PSC).[145]

The inflammatory process associated with this disease results in hepatitis, fibrosis, and thickening of the ductal walls. This fibrosing process narrows and eventually obstructs the intrahepatic and extrahepatic bile ducts; the basic mechanisms of disease pathogenesis in PSC remain unknown.

More than 40% of people are asymptomatic at the time of diagnosis. But with the progression of disease, symptomatic presentation usually includes pruritus and jaundice accompanied by abdominal pain, fatigue, anorexia, and weight loss. Complications associated with the disease include bacterial cholangitis, pigmented bile stones, steatorrhea, malabsorption, and metabolic bone disease; severe complications involve the development of cirrhosis and portal hypertension, and the risk of developing cholangiocarcinoma (10%-30% lifetime risk), HCC, and colon cancer.[184]

Diagnosis is made on the basis of clinical, laboratory, and radiologic findings. ALP is typically three to five times normal accompanied by a mild elevation in bilirubin. The diagnosis is confirmed by ERCP or MRCP, which demonstrate the characteristic "beads on a string" appearance of the bile ducts (strictures and dilation of the ducts). Liver biopsy is performed for staging rather than diagnosis. Causes of secondary sclerosing cholangitis (such as chronic bacterial cholangitis, biliary neoplasms, and drug-induced bile duct injury) should also be excluded.

Medical therapy is based on managing symptoms, correcting dominant strictures, and treating bacterial cholangitis when it occurs. Pruritus can be treated with bile acid–binding resins and dominant duct strictures can be endoscopically treated (by dilation or placement of stents). Clients should receive vitamin D and calcium supplements, although select people may require bisphosphonates.

UDCA improves biliary secretion and laboratory parameters but has not been shown to significantly improve survival. Currently, liver transplantation is the only therapeutic option for people with end-stage liver disease resulting from this disorder.[85,201] Many clinical trials of medical therapy have been conducted, but none have demonstrated significant efficacy compared to liver transplant. The results of transplantation for PSC are excellent, with 1-year survival rates of 90% to 97% and 5-year survival rates of 80% to 86%.[75] Optimal timing for liver transplantation is still not well defined, but the goal of therapy is to treat people as early as possible to prevent progression to the advanced stages of this disease or the development of cancer. Recurrence of PSC after liver transplantation occurs in approximately 4% of clients per year but appears to have little effect on survival.[76] Clients who develop cholangiocarcinoma and undergo liver transplant have a poor prognosis.[72]

SPECIAL IMPLICATIONS FOR THE THERAPIST   17-23

Primary Sclerosing Cholangitis

Special considerations for the therapist are the same as for the client with cholelithiasis (see also "Jaundice [Icterus]" above).

Neoplasms of the Gallbladder and Biliary Tract

Benign Neoplasms

Biliary neoplasms, whether benign or malignant, are rare. Most nonmalignant tumors of the gallbladder and biliary tree are polyps. These polyps can be adenomas, pseudotumors, or hyperplastic inflammatory lesions and most are found incidentally by ultrasonography or during cholecystectomy (for gallstone symptoms). Adenomas may be premalignant and have been associated with carcinoma in situ and invasive adenocarcinomas. Because polyps that are 1 cm or larger have a greater potential to be malignant, treatment consists of cholecystectomy.

Malignant Neoplasms

Cancers of the biliary tract are divided into gallbladder cancer, cholangiocarcinoma, and adenocarcinoma of the ampulla of Vater. *Gallbladder cancer* is the sixth most common GI cancer, causing about 3230 deaths per year, and is the most common cancer of the biliary tree.[215] Adenocarcinoma of the gallbladder is the most common type of gallbladder cancer (greater than 90% of cases), with squamous cell and small cell carcinoma accounting for the remaining cases.

Risk factors for gallbladder cancer include age (two-thirds of all cases occur in people age 65 years and older), female gender (women are three times more likely to develop gallbladder cancer), and gallstones (80%-90% of people with gallbladder cancer have gallstones). Other factors include obesity, gallbladder wall calcification (porcelain gallbladder), chronic typhoid carriers, and gallbladder polyps. In elderly adults, gallbladder polyps larger than 10 mm are more likely to be malignant whereas smaller polyps can be followed. However, despite these known risk factors, many cases of gallbladder cancer occur in people without obvious risk factors.[46]

The pathogenesis of gallbladder cancer is not well understood, partly because it is often diagnosed at a late state. The associated inflammation with gallstones decreases the speed at which bile empties from the gallbladder; the risk of cancer is proportional to the size of the gallstones. Toxins from diet, smoke inhalation, and metabolic products from environmental sources are excreted and concentrated in the bile and likely contribute to the risk of gallbladder cancer. Early stages of the disease include plaque-like lesions and small ulcerations in the mucosal lining of the gallbladder that progress to carcinoma in situ and then to invasive tumors. The process likely takes 20 years or more.[252]

Clinical presentation of malignant gallbladder diseases depends on the stage of disease and the location and extent of the lesion, but it is often insidious. By the time the tumor becomes symptomatic, it is often incurable.

Symptoms most often mimic gallstone disease (acute and chronic cholecystitis). Right upper quadrant pain radiating to the upper back is the most common symptom (80% of cases), with weight loss, progressive (obstructive) jaundice (30% of cases), anorexia, fatty food intolerance, and right upper quadrant mass (in advanced disease).

Pruritus and skin excoriations are commonly associated with the presence of jaundice. Gallbladder cancer is usually found either as an incidental finding at surgery, as a suspected tumor (because of symptoms) with the prospect of resectability, or as advanced unresectable disease.

Ultrasonography is the most common initial test for diagnosis, although CT and MRI can detect the extent of disease. CT scans and cholangiography are used preoperatively to determine resectability of the tumor. Disease can be metastatic to lungs and bones and usually involves the liver. Simple cholecystectomy is appropriate only for stages 0 and 1; the remainder require extended or radical cholecystectomy (with removal of lymph nodes, adjacent hepatic tissue, and/or portions of the extrahepatic biliary tree).[49]

For clients with unresectable disease and jaundice, a biliary bypass (hepaticojejunostomy) can be performed to relieve obstruction. Overall prognosis is poor with a 5-year survival rate of 5% to 10%. Cures are only obtained when all detectable tumor is surgically removed in the early stages of the disease. Stage I tumors have an overall survival rate of 100% and nearly 50% for node-negative stage II and stage III disease. Chemotherapy and radiation provide little benefit.

Cholangiocarcinoma, or cancer of the bile ducts, is a rare tumor. Historically, the term *cholangiocarcinoma* referred only to tumors of intrahepatic bile ducts; however, it now encompasses intrahepatic, perihilar, and distal extrahepatic tumors of the bile ducts.[46] Cholangiocarcinoma occurs more frequently in people between the ages of 50 and 70 years; other risk factors include PSC, ulcerative colitis, recurrent bacterial cholangitis, bile duct adenomas and papillomas, intraductal gallstones, certain infectious diseases (such as the liver fluke *Clonorchis sinensis*), and exposure in the past to the radiologic contrast agent thorium dioxide (Thorotrast).

Most tumors are located near the porta hepatis (60%-80%), although 20% are in the distal bile duct and less than 5% are intrahepatic. Affected persons most often present with jaundice secondary to obstruction of the bile duct (90% of cases) with associated acholic stool (light colored) and pruritus. Other symptoms include weight loss, anorexia, and fatigue.

On physical examination, hepatomegaly or a palpable gallbladder (the Courvoisier sign) may be present with advanced disease. Laboratory values are consistent with biliary obstruction with an elevated bilirubin and ALP. CA19-9 and CEA are elevated but nonspecific. CT scans or MRCP can detect the disease, and ERCP with brushings or biopsy may be diagnostic and relieve obstruction (a presurgical histologic diagnosis is often difficult to obtain).

Resectability is determined by a lack of metastatic disease, local invasion of the vascular structures around the liver, or the ability to completely resect the tumor. Laparoscopic surgery may be done initially to determine whether metastatic disease is present (metastatic disease is found in 25% of cases that were thought to be resectable by imaging studies). A pancreaticoduodenectomy is performed for tumors in the distal portion of the biliary tree. However, because most cholangiocarcinomas are near the liver and large vessels, surgery must be tailored to the location of the tumor, with 35% actually resectable.

Radiation therapy may be of some survival benefit. Endoscopic or percutaneous stent placement for biliary decompression often relieves symptoms for clients with nonresectable disease. Cure is obtained by complete surgical resection of tumor. Survival rates are determined by extent of disease and involvement with large vessels and structures around the liver. In one study, 56% of the perihilar tumors were resectable, and the overall 5-year survival rate was 11%.[154] Improved survival rates of 21% to 56% are associated with aggressive hepatic resection to remove all tumors with negative resection margins.[30,151] Distal bile duct tumor has a 5-year survival of 28% after successful surgical treatment.

Adenocarcinoma of the ampulla of Vater is a rare, distal bile duct tumor. The ampulla of Vater is a small area (about 1 cm in diameter) located at the common opening of the pancreatic and bile ducts into the duodenum (see Fig. 17-7). This cancer has an incidence of 2.9 cases per million people in the United States.

Risk factors include people with Peutz-Jeghers syndrome and familial adenomatous polyposis syndrome. Because of its location, this tumor causes obstructive jaundice early in the disease process (80% of cases). Abdominal pain (50%), weight loss (75%), and occult GI bleeding (30%) are other common symptoms.

Diagnosis is made by EUS, CT scan, and ERCP. Surgical resection, typically a pancreaticoduodenectomy, is the treatment of choice, with no clear benefit to chemoradiation. Resection is feasible in over 85% of cases with a 5-year survival of up to 45%.[45,186]

SPECIAL IMPLICATIONS FOR THE THERAPIST　17-24

Gallbladder and Biliary Tract Neoplasm

Special considerations for the therapist are the same as for the client with cholelithiasis. See also "Jaundice [Icterus]" above and "Special Implications for the Therapist 9-1: Oncology/Cancer" in Chapter 9.

REFERENCES

To enhance this text and add value for the reader, all references are included on the companion Evolve site that accompanies this textbook. The reader can view the reference source and access it online whenever possible.

CHAPTER 18

The Renal and Urologic Systems

MICHAEL S. CASTILLO • JANICE T. DINGLASAN • BETH SHELLY • KATHLEEN L. ALLEN

The structures associated with the excretion of urine are (1) the kidneys and ureters, comprising the *upper urinary tract*, and (2) the bladder and urethra of the *lower urinary tract* (Fig. 18-1). The kidneys serve as both an endocrine organ and a target of endocrine action, with the aim of controlling mineral and water balance. The kidneys' main function is to filter waste products and remove excess fluid from the blood. Every day the kidneys filter 200 quarts of fluid; about 2 quarts leave the body in the form of urine, and the remainder is retained in the body.

These filtration and storage functions associated with excretion expose the kidney and bladder to carcinogens for extended periods, increasing the risk of cancer's developing in these organs compared with the other urinary tract structures. In addition, the urethra of females lies close to the vaginal and rectal openings, allowing for relative ease of bacterial transport and increased risk of infection. The shorter urethra in females also contributes to the increased incidence of urinary tract infections (UTIs) in females.

Therapists have an important role on the medical team for primary intervention for a number of renal/urinary tract disorders such as urinary incontinence (UI) and for those on dialysis or having a renal transplant. UI afflicts a significant percentage of the geriatric population, and UTIs rank second only to upper respiratory tract infections in incidence of bacterial infections. Therapists encounter these two disorders often as common comorbidities in the clinical arena.

The presence of a UTI increases the risk of infections developing elsewhere. This could occur while the therapist is treating someone for a knee injury or after cerebral vascular accident. Recognizing clinical signs and symptoms of renal/urologic problems (Box 18-1) will facilitate medical referral. Understanding how these diseases and the prescribed medical treatment can influence rehabilitative efforts is essential to help ensure a positive functional outcome.

AGING AND THE RENAL AND UROLOGIC SYSTEMS

Aging is accompanied by a gradual reduction of blood flow to the kidneys, coupled with a reduction in nephrons (the units that extract wastes from the blood and concentrate them in the urine; see Fig. 18-6). As a result the kidneys become less efficient at removing waste from the blood, and the volume of urine increases somewhat with age. A tendency toward greater renal vasoconstriction in the older adult is evident, as compared with young individuals. This occurs as a result of mental stress, in physiologic circumstances such as physical exercise, or in disease manifestations such as the effective circulatory volume depletion that develops in heart failure.[280] Physiologic changes in renal aging is associated with altered activity and responsiveness to vasoactive stimuli, such that responses to vasoconstrictor stimuli are enhanced, whereas vasodilatory responses are impaired.[291]

Renal system changes that occur with aging cause alterations in the functional balance of fluid and electrolytes so that sodium regulation is not as effective. Mild hyponatremia is the most common electrolyte imbalance in the older population, affecting the musculoskeletal system.[148] Changes typical of the aging kidney are also accelerated when hypertension overlaps the physiologic renal process, because both aging and hypertension affect the same structure (i.e., the glomeruli).

A reduction in bladder capacity increases the number of times an individual urinates in a day and the urinary timetable also changes (i.e., length of time between episodes of bladder emptying). Although the kidneys produce most of the urine during the day in young people, a shift to night production over time makes one or two nocturnal trips to the bathroom commonplace after age 60 years.

Although specific age-related anatomic changes are not associated with urinary tract disease, certain age groups (e.g., older adults) are at significant risk of developing a variety of disorders. Hormonal changes in women, combined with the aging properties of the connective tissues, fascia, or collagen fibers, contribute to pelvic floor muscle dysfunction. Transient ischemic attacks and strokes may result in mild to severe deficits or fluctuations in muscle tone affecting the pelvic floor muscles.

The effect of multiple medications, conditions such as benign prostatic hyperplasia and pelvic floor muscle dysfunction, and the incidence of pelvic surgeries and catheterization in the older population all increase the risk of developing urinary tract problems. A large number of adults older than age 60 years are incontinent, and many older adults require alternative living situations because of this disorder. Considering the percentage of

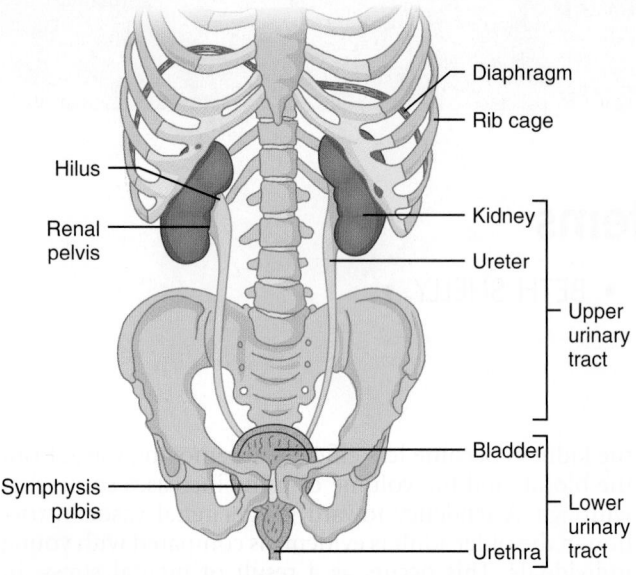

Figure 18-1

Structure and function of the renal and urologic systems. The kidneys are located in the posterior upper abdominal cavity in the retroperitoneal space (behind the peritoneum) at the vertebral level of T12 to L2. The upper portion of the kidney is in contact with the diaphragm and moves with respiration. The lower urinary tract consists of the bladder and urethra. The bladder, a membranous, muscular sac, is located directly behind the symphysis pubis and is used for storage and excretion of urine. From the renal pelvis, urine is moved by peristalsis to the ureters and into the bladder. The urethra serves as a channel through which urine is passed from the bladder to the outside of the body. (From Goodman CC, Snyder TE: *Differential diagnosis in physical therapy*, ed 3, Philadelphia, 2000, WB Saunders.)

Box 18-1

MOST COMMON SIGNS AND SYMPTOMS OF URINARY TRACT PROBLEMS

- Urinary frequency
- Urinary urgency
- Urinary incontinence
- Nocturia
- Pain (shoulder, back, flank, pelvis, lower abdomen)
- Costovertebral tenderness
- Fever and chills
- Hyperesthesia of dermatomes
- Dysuria
- Hematuria
- Pyuria
- Dyspareunia

---

the rehabilitation population made up by the older adult, therapists will continue to be involved in the treatment of renal/urologic disorders.

INFECTIONS

Urinary Tract Infections

UTIs are very common, affecting men, women, and children. Any portion of the urinary tract can become infected, although the bladder (cystitis) and urethra (urethritis) are usually involved. Bacteria may also spread to the upper portion of the urinary tract and involve the kidneys, causing a more serious infection referred to as *pyelonephritis.*

UTIs can be defined as either uncomplicated or complicated, and relapsed or recurrent. Complicated infections develop in persons with factors that can make diagnosis and treatment difficult—including diabetes, history of stroke, pregnancy, immunosuppression, structural abnormalities, or functional abnormalities of the urinary tract. The presence of such complications often requires longer treatment and further testing.[258]

Generally, UTIs in men, pregnant women, children, and clients who are hospitalized or in a long-term care setting can be considered complicated. Uncomplicated UTIs lack these factors and are more easily diagnosed and treated. UTIs may relapse or, more commonly, recur. Relapsed infections are infections that persist with the original organism without completely clearing. Recurrence of UTIs is considered a different infection that occurs after successful treatment of the initial infection, although it may be with the same organism because of repeated contamination.[258]

Incidence and Prevalence

UTIs are among the most common bacterial infections acquired in the community and in hospitals. In individuals without anatomical or functional abnormalities, UTIs are generally self-limiting, but have a propensity to recur.[90] UTIs frequently occur in the general population, although women and older adults comprise the majority of cases. UTIs affect more than 11.3 million women per year,[89] or up to 5% of all females. Five percent to 30% of the older adult population is also affected.[91] By age 24 years, one-third of women will have had at least one physician-diagnosed UTI that is treated with prescription medication.

For those living in skilled nursing facilities, assisted living arrangements, or extended care facilities, the prevalence of infection is even higher: 25% for women and 20% for men.[12] UTIs affect children, involving approximately 7% of girls and 2% of boys before the age of 6 years.[180] Recurrent UTIs can be problematic for many people, occurring in 3% to 5% of women[129] and 80% of children who previously experienced an uncomplicated infection. The cost is substantial at more than $1.6 billion per year (diagnosis, treatment, and management cost). UTIs also result in restrictions in daily activities and lost days of work.

Etiologic and Risk Factors

Most UTIs occur in adult women. The urethra in females is shorter, compared to that in males, and also close to the entrances to the vagina and rectum. The bacteria that result in most UTIs are acquired from the large bowel (fecal flora). The urethral meatus is close to the fecal reservoir and rectum.

Young, sexually active women are at higher risk of developing UTIs because it is thought that sexual intercourse can influence the movement of bacteria in the direction of the bladder. This again is because of the

RISK FACTORS FOR URINARY TRACT INFECTIONS

- Age
- Immobility/inactivity (impaired bladder emptying)
- Instrumentation and urinary catheterization
- Frequently catheterized neurogenic bladder
- Atonic bladder (spinal cord injury; diabetic neuropathy)
- Increased sexual activity
- Spermicide associated in use with diaphragm or condoms
- Uncircumcised penis (first year of life)
- Obstruction
  - Renal calculi
  - Prostatic hyperplasia
  - Malformations or urinary tract abnormalities
- Constipation
- Women greater than men (see explanation in text)
  - Anatomic variations
  - Surgical or natural menopause without hormone replacement therapy
  - Pregnancy
- Kidney transplantation
- Diabetes mellitus
- Partners of Viagra (sildenafil citrate) users*
- Sexually transmitted disease (urethritis)

*This is most likely the result of increased frequency of intercourse in women older than age 35 years who are more likely to also experience vaginal dryness.

proximity of the urethral meatus and vagina. There are numerous risk factors for UTIs (Box 18-2) that depend upon the characteristics of the person affected. For example, risk factors for an acute, uncomplicated UTI in a premenopausal woman may be different than those for a postmenopausal woman in a long-term care setting.

For young women, the most common risk factors include a history of a previous UTI, frequent or recent sexual activity, or the use of a spermicidal agent.[82,92] UTIs are also more common during pregnancy. The increased risk is from dilation of the upper urinary system, reduction of the peristaltic activity of the ureters, and displacement of the urinary bladder, which moves to a more abdominal position, thus further affecting the ureteral position.

In older women who are in a long-term care setting, the most frequently noted risk factors are advancing age and debilitation associated with conditions that impair voiding or cause poor perineal hygiene, such as dementia or stroke.[81] Healthy, community-dwelling postmenopausal women share risk factors seen in both young and older women. Sexual activity and a previous history of UTI are common risk factors for both young and postmenopausal women, while incontinence is an additional risk factor in these older women.[131] The effects of estrogen decline (dry mucosa and vaginitis) may contribute to increased risk of infection because of the change in vaginal flora, but study findings remain unclear.

People with diabetes receiving treatment are also more prone to UTIs as a consequence of immunologic impairments; the presence of glycosuria, which provides a fertile medium for bacterial growth; and voiding difficulties resulting from diabetic neuropathy (detrusor paresis).[26,103]

Another significant and common risk factor for UTI is indwelling catheterization. Placement of a urinary catheter is a leading cause of infection in the hospital setting, accounting for 40% of health care–associated infections. The reasons are clearly related to the introduction of a foreign body that provides a direct pathway for bacteria to travel from the perineum to the bladder.

Less commonly, a client may display a structural or functional abnormality that leads to a UTI. Contributing structural problems may be kidney stones, cystocele, or prostatic hyperplasia. Examples of functional problems include reflux of urine from the bladder to the kidney and neurogenic bladder from diabetes, spinal cord injury, or multiple sclerosis. Neurologic conditions that can result in low bladder tone and urine retention contributing to UTI include Parkinson disease, multiple systems atrophy, multiple sclerosis, sacral lesions, lower motor nerve conus lesions, disc disease, trauma following pelvic surgery, and diabetes mellitus.

Overactive pelvic floor muscle and interstitial cystitis can mimic symptoms of UTI.[99,244] Therapists should encourage patients to have urine tested and avoid automatic prescription of antibiotics especially with recurrent UTI and in the presence of other pelvic pain syndromes.[99,244]

Pathogenesis

The bacteria most often responsible for UTI are fecal-associated gram-negative organisms, with *Escherichia coli* accounting for approximately 80% of urinary tract pathogens. *Staphylococcus saprophyticus* causes 5% to 15% of UTIs, while *Enterococcus*, *Klebsiella*, and *Proteus* make up the remaining common organisms.

Hospitalized clients are more likely to become infected with *Enterobacter*, *Klebsiella*, *Proteus*, *Pseudomonas*, enterococci, and staphylococci bacteria than outpatients with UTI. *Candida* species can be seen in persons who have undergone invasive instrumental investigations or catheterizations and in children with urogenital abnormalities.

These common urinary tract pathogens are able to adhere to the urinary tract mucosa, colonize, and cause infection. Several subtypes of bacteria contain genes that allow for greater virulence and ability to colonize urothelium than other organisms, making them uropathogenic. Uropathogens have specialized characteristics, such as the production of adhesins, siderophores and toxins that enable them to colonize and invade the urinary tract. The most common route of entry of bacteria into the urinary tract is ascending up the urethra into the bladder.[90] Although infrequent in occurrence, infections may be bloodborne (bacteria in the bloodstream) or acquired via the lymphatic system.

Clinical Manifestations

Classic features of UTIs are evident in older children and adults and include frequency, urgency, dysuria, nocturia, and, in children, enuresis. Fever, chills, and malaise may also be present. The individual may notice cloudy, bloody, or foul-smelling urine and a burning or painful sensation during urination or intercourse. Pain may be noted in the suprapubic, lower abdominal, groin, or flank areas, depending on the location of the infection.

In the case of kidney involvement, the diaphragm may become irritated, resulting in ipsilateral shoulder or lumbar back pain. The clinical manifestations in frail, older adults can be varied, often with malaise, anorexia, and mental status changes (especially confusion or increased confusion) as the most prominent features. Flank pain, fever, and chills often indicate an upper UTI or pyelonephritis.

Asymptomatic bacterial urine infections occur in approximately 10% of women in early pregnancy[158] (and 25%-50% in residence of long-term care facilities).[202] In elderly adults, new-onset confusion or delirium may be a sign of UTI.[77,78] Physical therapists are in a unique position to recognize this and should encourage consultation with the physician in these circumstances.

MEDICAL MANAGEMENT

PREVENTION. UTIs can be prevented in some cases by drinking at least eight 8-oz glasses of water each day; urinating soon after sexual intercourse; for females, wiping from the front to back after urination so that bacteria from the anal area are not pushed into the urethra; changing sanitary pads often during menstruation; and washing the genital area with warm water before sexual activity to minimize the chance that bacteria can be introduced. The use of spermicidal agents with a diaphragm is associated with an increased risk for UTIs. The use of another form of birth control may be warranted if repeated UTIs become problematic.

Certain foods may also be preventative. Berry juices and products containing fermented milk may be helpful in reducing the occurrence of UTIs, although further studies are needed to verify this relationship.[154] The use of cranberry juice in the prevention and treatment of UTIs has been controversial, with different studies showing positive and negative effects of cranberry juice as a preventive or therapeutic agent.[11,55] A recent randomized controlled trial showed that cranberry juice did not significantly reduce UTI risk compared with placebo in premenopausal women with a history of recent UTI.[260] More studies are needed to determine efficacy, dose, and appropriate candidates for this dietary treatment. The use of probiotics to increase normal vaginal flora may be of benefit.[259] Preliminary studies are encouraging, although only certain types of Lactobacillus have had promising results.[80,259]

There has also been debate as to whether hormone therapy can prevent UTIs in postmenopausal women. Recent studies indicate that oral as well as vaginal hormone therapy is not preventative[29,137,230] for UTIs, but its believed detrimental effects to cardiovascular health have been closely scrutinized. Further analysis of the Women's Health Initiative shows that when started earlier in the menopausal period, some significant benefits, including protection from heart disease, reduced risk of colon cancer, and reduced risk of osteoporotic fractures, can be achieved with hormone therapy.[21,126,262]

Instrumentation and, particularly, placement of urinary catheters frequently lead to UTI. However, if a catheter is needed, intermittent catheterization is recommended. Condom catheters may reduce the risk of causing UTI compared to indwelling catheters and should be considered.[46] Preliminary studies also suggest that use of catheters coated with an antimicrobial agent may reduce the risk, but further investigations are needed.[140]

DIAGNOSIS AND TREATMENT. The diagnosis of a UTI is typically made based on history and urinalysis results. A bacterial count of greater than 100,000 organisms/mL of urine is a commonly accepted criterion for diagnosis. Besides the bacterial count, the urine leukocyte count (more than 10 leukocytes/mm^3 of urine collected midstream), and presence of leukocyte esterase, nitrates, and protein are also helpful.

Many people demonstrate pyuria (leukocytes in the urine) without infection, and corroborating clinical and laboratory information must be evident to diagnose an infection. In clients who are healthy and without complicating features, empiric treatment with antibiotics is effective and urine cultures are not required.

Acute UTIs in healthy, nonpregnant clients are typically treated with antibiotics, as recommended by the Infectious Diseases Society of America guidelines. Because of rising resistance to antibiotics with regional differences, initial treatment must take into account local resistance patterns as well as the health of the client. For individuals with complicating features, treatment failure could lead to severe morbidity and mortality.

Women who experience recurrent infections have several options for treatment depending upon the clinical situation and compliance of the client. They may take antibiotics prophylactically (typically as a daily dose), they may self-treat as they recognize typical symptoms,[113,260] or in the case of sexual intercourse as a precipitating factor, women may be advised to take antibiotics just after sex. Increased fluid intake may also help relieve symptoms and signs and is often used as an adjunct to pharmacologic treatment. Lactobacillus acidophilus, a probiotic supplement of live, active organisms, may be recommended for anyone taking antibiotics to replace the naturally occurring bacteria in the intestines and to prevent candidiasis (yeast growth). A vaccine to prevent recurrent urinary infections of the bladder has proved successful in mice and is currently being tested in clinical trials.

For clients who develop UTIs as a result of structural or functional problems, further testing is needed to correct the abnormality. Ultrasound, radiographs, computed tomographic (CT) scans, and renal scans may be used to identify contributing factors such as obstruction. Postvoid residual and more complex tests, such as voiding cystourethrography (upper urinary system) and urodynamic testing with and without fluoroscopy determination, may be recommended for anyone at risk for urinary retention. Whenever possible, ultrasound assessment, rather than urinary catheterization, is recommended for measuring the postvoid residual.

Urinary Tract Infections

Depending on the severity of the infection, the person with a UTI may not be able to participate fully in a rehabilitation program until the disease is brought under control. If the client begins to complain of nausea or vomiting, or has a fever greater than 39° C (102° F), or the therapist notes a change in mental status (most often confusion), immediate contact with the client's physician is warranted. These may be indications for hospital admission.

Awareness of the symptoms and signs associated with this disease may allow the therapist to recognize the onset of infection in its early stages. The initial symptoms may be subtle enough that the client is not alarmed to the point that the client visits a physician. Early detection and treatment of this disorder are important to prevent possible permanent structural damage. In the case of insidious onset of back or shoulder pain, onset of confusion, or increased confusion, especially with a recent history of any infection, a medical screening examination may be warranted.

UTIs also increase the risk of development of infection elsewhere in the body, including osteomyelitis, pleurisy, and pericarditis. Therapists should also always be aware of their role in infection prevention and minimize their involvement as a risk factor (see Chapter 8).

Appropriate catheter care involves minimizing risks of infection. These may include: maintaining unobstructed urine flow, keeping the catheter and collecting tube free from kinking, and having the collecting bag below the level of the bladder at all times. Do not rest the bag on the floor. Changing indwelling catheters or drainage bags at routine, fixed intervals is not recommended. Rather, it is suggested to change catheters and drainage bags based on clinical indications such as infection, obstruction, or when the closed system is compromised.[107]

Pyelonephritis

Overview and Incidence

Pyelonephritis can be either an infectious process involving the kidneys (acute pyelonephritis) or a chronic inflammatory disease involving the kidney parenchyma and renal pelvis (chronic pyelonephritis). Acute pyelonephritis occurs in over 250,000 people per year, causing over 100,000 hospitalizations. The direct and indirect costs are estimated at $2.14 billion.[31] It typically results from bacteria ascending from the bladder to infect the kidneys.[130] Similar to UTIs, acute pyelonephritis occurs more frequently in women than men, although men have a higher complication rate.[93]

Chronic pyelonephritis is a tubulointerstitial disorder characterized by specific changes in the kidney (cortical scarring and deformation of the calices). These alterations can be a result of several diseases that can lead to renal insufficiency. Chronic pyelonephritis may be responsible for up to 25% of the population with end-stage renal disease (ESRD).

Etiologic and Risk Factors

The majority of acute pyelonephritis cases are associated with ascending UTIs (see Box 18-2) and are caused most commonly by *E. coli* (up to 85%).[246] A smaller proportion are caused by other gram-negative organisms such as *Proteus*, *Klebsiella*, *Enterobacter*, and *Pseudomonas* species.

Risk factors associated with increased risk for pyelonephritis in healthy, nonpregnant women include frequent sexual activity, recent UTI, recent spermicide use, diabetes, and recent incontinence.[246] There may be a genetic component for increased susceptibility to these infections; a history of upper respiratory infection in female relatives is strongly and consistently associated with UTI recurrence and pyelonephritis.[245]

In other cases, pyelonephritis can stem from blood-borne pathogens associated with infection elsewhere. People with bacterial endocarditis and miliary tuberculosis are susceptible to kidney involvement. In addition, immunocompromised people are at risk for bacterial and fungal seeding of the kidney with subsequent abscess formation.

Chronic pyelonephritis is the term that describes specific, abnormal renal findings. Several diseases or processes can lead to chronic pyelonephritis, such as vesicoureteral reflux (urine is forced from the urinary bladder into the ureters and kidneys), urinary obstruction, analgesic nephropathy, or bacterial infection superimposed on a structural/functional abnormality. The most common cause of chronic pyelonephritis is vesicoureteral reflux, although the renal insufficiency associated with this is most often referred to as *reflux nephropathy*.

Pathogenesis

Although urine is typically sterile, the distal end of the urethra is commonly colonized by bacterial flora. As described under "Etiologic and Risk Factors" above, bacteria can be transported to the urinary bladder in many ways. After urination, the subsequent passage of sterile urine from the kidneys to the bladder dilutes any bacteria that may have entered the bladder. If the residual urine volume is increased, as with an atonic bladder, an accumulation of insufficiently diluted bacteria can occur. Bacteria in the bladder urine typically do not gain access to the ureters for a variety of anatomic reasons. However, people with an abnormally short passage of the ureter within the bladder muscle wall and an angle of ureter insertion into the bladder wall that is more perpendicular are at risk for reflux of urine into the ureter itself. This reflux can be of sufficient force to carry the urine and the accompanying bacteria into the renal pelvis and calices.

Chronic pyelonephritis is defined by scarring with deformity of the calices. Processes that continually cause inflammation in the kidney can lead to chronic changes. Only a few processes can cause these changes, and they can be divided into three main groups: reflux, obstruction, and idiopathic.

Clinical Manifestations

The onset of symptoms and signs associated with acute pyelonephritis is usually abrupt. The complaints may include fever, chills, malaise, headache, and flank pain. The person may also complain of tenderness over the costovertebral angle (Murphy sign). Symptoms of bladder irritation may be present (including dysuria, urinary frequency, and urgency) but are not required for the diagnosis.

Symptoms associated with chronic pyelonephritis vary depending upon the causative process; however, symptoms may not be present. The diagnosis is made more often by laboratory detection of kidney function changes.

MEDICAL MANAGEMENT

DIAGNOSIS, TREATMENT, AND PROGNOSIS. The presence of suggestive symptoms for acute pyelonephritis warrants laboratory testing and treatment. Urinalysis typically reveals pyuria, bacteriuria, and varying degrees of hematuria. A urine culture should always be obtained and often will result in the growth of the offending bacteria or fungus. In addition, the blood count usually demonstrates leukocytosis.

If the infection is severe enough or if complicating factors are present, hospital admission may be required for intravenous antibiotics and hydration. Typically, however, the condition is treated with an appropriate antibiotic medication. Symptoms typically begin disappearing within several days. If the person does not show improvement within 48 to 72 hours, contact with the physician is warranted.

If the process associated with chronic pyelonephritis continues to progress, creating worsening scarring, the result may be ESRD requiring dialysis or transplantation.

RENAL DISORDERS

Cancer

Renal Cell Carcinoma

Overview and Incidence. Adult kidney neoplasms account for approximately 3% to 4% of all cancers.[255] During the past 2 decades, the incidence of these cancers has increased by approximately 2% each year.[233]

Renal cell carcinoma (RCC) is the most common adult renal neoplasm, accounting for more than 90% of renal tumors, and its incidence is rising (although the death rate is not). RCC occurs more frequently in males than females (about a 1.6:1 ratio). Risk increases with age with a peak incidence between 60 and 70 years. In the United States, rates are higher among Blacks than in whites.

Most adult kidney cancers are sporadic RCCs, which can be divided into two main types. The conventional (or clear cell) type accounts for 75%; 12% of cases are the papillary form, which are less likely to metastasize. In 60% of conventional carcinomas there is a mutation in the von Hippel-Lindau tumor-suppressor gene.

Chromophobe RCC and collecting duct RCC account for a small number of cases, 4% and 1%, respectively.

Etiologic and Risk Factors. RCC is linked to several hereditary diseases, including von Hippel-Lindau disease (a rare autosomal dominant familial cancer syndrome related

to clear cell RCC),[191] hereditary papillary renal carcinoma (an autosomal dominant disorder related to papillary RCC), and the Birt-Hogg-Dubé syndrome (a rare autosomal dominant disorder related to chromophobe RCCs or mixed chromophobe RCCs–oncocytomas). These hereditary disorders are rare and only account for a small percentage of RCCs. Risk factors that can lead to the development of sporadic RCC include tobacco smoking, moderate to heavy drinking (alcohol),[168] obesity, hypertension,[57] barbecued meat,[66] occupational exposure to substances such as dust,[144] organic solvents and asbestos, and acquired cystic kidney disease associated with ESRD.[50,60]

Pathogenesis. Urine contains many waste products from food, beverages, and other environmental sources; some of these are potential carcinogens and may play a role in the pathogenesis of kidney cancer. Body fat directly affects levels of many circulating hormones, such as insulin, insulin-like growth factors, and estrogens, creating an environment that encourages carcinogenesis and discourages apoptosis. It also stimulates the body's inflammatory response, which may contribute to the initiation and progression of cancer. The evidence of tobacco and greater body fatness contributing to kidney cancer is convincing.[4]

As for other cancers, genetic mechanisms are now being discovered for RCC, which better explain the causes and aid in the treatment. Because RCC is seen in a few hereditary diseases, scientists have been able to locate specific genetic abnormalities. von Hippel-Lindau disease has several characteristic abnormalities, including the development of RCC (clear cell type). The von Hippel-Lindau tumor-suppressor gene *(VHL)* is located on chromosome 3.

Of interest, this same abnormality has been detected in 60% to 80% of people with sporadic clear cell RCC. The product of the *VHL* gene normally suppresses genes that, in the presence of hypoxia, cause endothelial growth, cell growth, and glucose uptake, and affect acid–base balance.[56] When this gene is altered, cell proliferation occurs unchecked. Another gene linked to RCC is the *MET* protooncogene. This abnormal gene, located on chromosome 7, is duplicated in approximately 75% of sporadic papillary RCC cases. If the *FH* gene (which encodes for the Krebs cycle enzyme fumarate hydratase) is inactivated, the result is another hereditary disorder known as hereditary leiomyomatosis and renal cell cancer syndrome.

Clinical Manifestations. The classic triad of symptoms related to RCC is flank pain, hematuria, and a palpable abdominal mass. Yet about half of all cases are discovered incidentally on a radiographic examination, such as a CT scan.[56] Kidney cancers are generally silent, particularly in the early stages, although nonspecific symptoms may develop such as malaise, anemia, or unexplained weight loss. Hematuria is the single most common presenting finding, occurring in up to 50% of cases, yet it is frequently intermittent and microscopic.

Symptoms associated with metastasis can be the initial manifestation; approximately 25% to 30% of clients have metastatic disease at the time of diagnosis.[163] Metastases most often occur in the lungs (75%), regional lymph nodes (65%), bones (40%), and liver (40%).[304] The client may develop a cough or bone pain secondary to metastasis to the lungs or bone, respectively.

Potentially confusing the clinical presentation of this condition is the fact that RCCs are associated with ectopic hormone production and paraneoplastic symptoms, including fever, hypertension, hepatic dysfunction, and hypercalcemia. Hormones produced by the tumors include parathyroid-like hormone, gonadotropins, renin, erythropoietin, glucagon, and insulin.

As discussed earlier, several hereditary syndromes predispose to the development of RCC. Each of these disorders has its own unique clinical manifestations other than RCC. For example, von Hippel-Lindau disease is associated with retinal angiomas, hemangioblastomas of the central nervous system, pheochromocytomas, and clear cell RCCs. These distinguishing features lead to the diagnosis and allow regular monitoring and surveillance for RCC.

MEDICAL MANAGEMENT

DIAGNOSIS. The primary feature of RCC is the renal parenchymal mass, which can be detected by a variety of imaging modalities (Fig. 18-2). The widespread availability of abdominal ultrasound (Fig. 18-3), magnetic resonance imaging (MRI), and CT scanning has increased the diagnosis of incidental renal tumors.

Determining whether the mass is benign or malignant can be difficult, often requiring surgical removal before a definitive diagnosis can be made. If hematuria is present, intravenous pyelography (IVP) may be the initial procedure to identify renal abnormalities. IVP is a radiographic test that allows for evaluation of the kidneys, ureters, and bladder. A dye injected into the bloodstream is filtered and secreted by the renal tubules. The IVP provides information including renal size, function, position, the presence of calculi, masses, and congenital variants.

Ultrasonography can be used to further evaluate the renal parenchyma and detect small tumors (less than 1 cm). The advantage of the CT scan is that the greatest renal anatomic detail is obtained and details of

neighboring organs such as the liver, colon, spleen, and lymphatics will also be available.

STAGING. The American Joint Committee on Cancer (AJCC) and the University of California, Los Angeles (UCLA) Integrated Staging Systems are currently used to stage this disease. The AJCC utilizes the TNM (tumor, node, metastasis) system defining stages I through IV (Fig. 18-4). The UCLA Integrated Staging System employs the Eastern Cooperative Oncology Group (ECOG) performance status scale and the Fuhrman nuclear grade to determine both stage and prognosis. Clients are classified

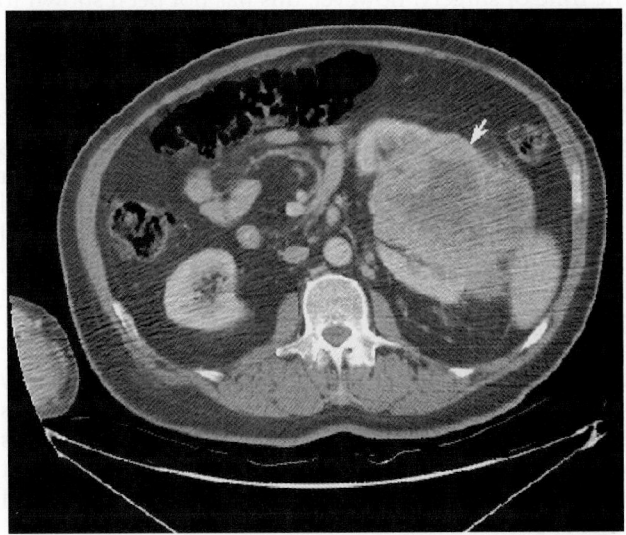

Figure 18-3

CT scan of abdomen demonstrating a large left renal mass *(arrow)* consistent with renal cell carcinoma. (From Townsend CM: *Sabiston textbook of surgery*, ed 17, Philadelphia, 2004, WB Saunders.)

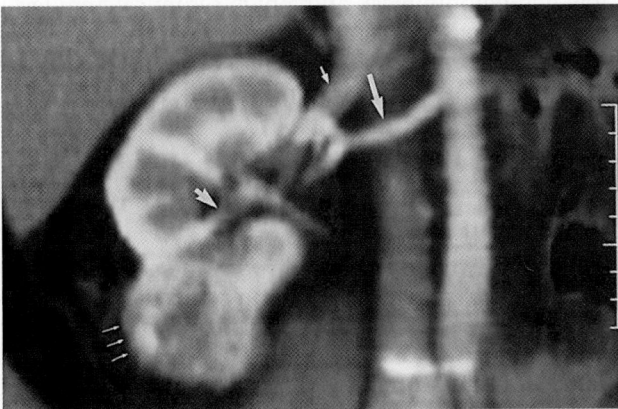

Figure 18-2

Renal cell carcinoma on CT scan. A reconstructed image in the coronal plane of section shows vascular anatomy by demonstration of the renal artery *(large arrow)*, renal vein *(small arrow)*, excretion into the pelvicaliceal system, which is not obstructed *(arrowhead)*; and renal cell carcinoma arising from the lower pole of the right kidney *(thin arrows)*. The cancer is confined to the cortex; therefore, partial nephrectomy can be performed. (From Brenner BM: *Brenner and Rector's the kidney*, ed 7, Philadelphia, 2004, WB Saunders.)

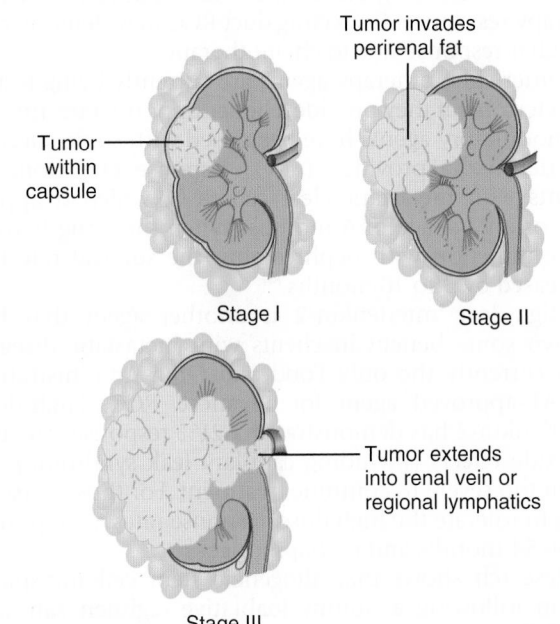

Figure 18-4

Renal cell carcinoma stages. Not shown: stage IV, distant metastases.

into low-, intermediate-, and high-risk groups. This staging system also provides risk categories for those with metastatic disease.

TREATMENT. Surgery is the principal treatment for RCC. Traditionally, a radical nephrectomy (removal of the kidney, the Gerota fascia [a fibroareolar tissue surrounding the kidney and perirenal fat], the adrenal gland, and regional lymph nodes) has been preferred, although less-aggressive methods are being investigated. Nephrectomy may also be beneficial for clients with metastatic disease, as combined surgical and medical therapy has slightly improved survival. Metastatic lesions may be removed at the time of surgery; however, this has not been shown to improve survival.

A partial nephrectomy may be appropriate for clients with a small mass (less than 4 cm), a solitary kidney, masses in both kidneys, renal insufficiency, or the presence of a hereditary disorder related to RCC. This approach, however, carries a 3% to 6% risk of tumor recurrence.[203] Laparoscopic nephrectomy has gained acceptance as a method for reducing hospital stay and postoperative pain, and providing a faster recovery. Partial nephrectomy is challenging and often requires an open procedure.

Newer, less-invasive methods for treating RCC include percutaneous thermal ablation using radiofrequency heat ablation or cryoablation. These types of procedures are best for small tumors (less than 3 cm) and in clients with comorbidities that can increase surgical risk. Further investigations are required, although the complication rates appear to be low.[56]

Medical treatment, adjuvant to surgery, is offered for more locally advanced or metastatic disease. Response rates to standard medical modalities have not been good. Only 4% to 6% of clients respond to chemotherapy[300]; clear cell and papillary RCC may express a protein that transports the drug out of the cells, leading to chemotherapy resistance. Collecting duct RCC may demonstrate a higher response rate to chemotherapy.

Other chemotherapy agents are currently being tested to determine if they provide a better response rate. Immunomodulatory agents have been used with some success. Interferon-alfa provides a 14% response rate alone in clients with metastatic clear cell RCC, which is apparent for an average of 6 months. When this drug is used in conjunction with nephrectomy, the survival rate has increased by 3 to 10 months.[86]

High-dose interleukin-2 is another agent that has shown some benefit in clients with metastatic disease; it is currently the only Food and Drug Administration (FDA)–approved agent for advanced RCC. High-dose interleukin-2 has demonstrated a 21% response rate, but the side effects (including capillary leak syndrome) are often too severe to continue treatment. For those persons able to tolerate the high dose, response rates are reported to be 54 months and perhaps longer.[97]

Research shows that allogeneic stem cell transplantation following a nonmyeloablative regimen can successfully create a graft-versus-tumor effect, which in initial studies demonstrated a 44% response (although continued studies have been less successful).[49] Two

difficulties encountered with transplantation include the life-threatening problem of graft-versus-host disease and the requirement of a matched sibling donor.

Other areas of ongoing research include tumor vaccines and tumor-specific targeting agents (i.e., targeting specific pathways with an antibody or blocking blood vessel formation). Angiogenic agents are able to block the receptors of vascular endothelial growth factor and platelet-derived growth factor, thus decreasing the blood supply to the tumor.[195,218,234]

PROGNOSIS. The prognosis of RCC depends upon the type and staging. Sporadic papillary RCC has a 5-year survival rate of almost 90% and is known to have a lower incidence of metastasis compared to clear cell RCC. However, individuals with metastatic papillary RCC have a lower survival rate than those with metastatic clear cell RCC.

Most chromophobe RCCs will have a favorable postsurgical course providing the tumor size is small and the grade low. Collecting duct RCC is an aggressive tumor with a poorer prognosis. The survival rates according to the AJCC system of tumor size demonstrate a 5- and 10-year survival of 95% and 91%, respectively, for T1-stage tumors; of 80% and 70% for T2 tumors; and of 66% and 53% for T3a tumors.

Utilizing the UCLA Integrated Staging System, the 5-year survival rate for the low-risk group is 91%, while the intermediate- and high-risk groups have an 80% and 55% survival rate, respectively. Unfortunately, 40% of locally removed renal cell tumors return.[213]

People with renal cancer often develop a second malignancy (prostate, bladder, and bowel for men; breast, gynecologic organs, thyroid, and bladder for women) but this does not appear to impact prognosis or limit surgical treatment for the renal cancer.[7]

Factors that portend a poor prognosis for metastatic RCC include a low performance score (Karnofsky performance status score), a high lactate dehydrogenase level, a low hemoglobin level, and a high serum calcium level. Metastatic disease has a much worse prognosis than localized tumor, with a 5-year survival of 0% to 7% for clients with multiple metastatic lesions.[229]

SPECIAL IMPLICATIONS FOR THE THERAPIST 18-2

Renal Cell Carcinoma
Therapists working primarily with the geriatric population need to be aware of the symptoms and signs of this disease. Questions in the history related to hematuria, unexplained weight loss, fatigue, fever, and malaise are important, regardless of the reason for the physical therapy care.

Awareness of new onset of unexplained abdominal, flank, or back pain; cough; or other signs of pulmonary involvement should raise concern on the therapist's part and warrants communication with a physician. In addition, RCC is the most common metastatic tumor to the sternum. An onset of sternal pain or a mass in someone with a history of RCC should be brought to the physician's attention.

The extensive abdominal and thoracic surgical sites may produce scarring that affects the client's posture and ability to move, increasing mechanical stress on the musculoskeletal system. Myofascial and soft-tissue mobilization of the abdominal and thoracic regions may be of benefit to these people. If a history of abnormal renal function in addition to the cancer is evident, additional precautions may need to be taken by the therapist. See the section on chronic renal failure later in this chapter.

Persons undergoing targeted therapies for renal cancer may experience the familiar side effects of cancer treatment such as: headache, fatigue, hypertension, sore mouth and taste changes, diarrhea, nausea, and even nose bleeds. It is important that health professionals familiarize themselves with the potential side effects of the drug treatments and methods for managing these side effects.[147]

Wilms Tumor

Overview, Incidence, and Risk Factors. Wilms tumor, or nephroblastoma, is the most common malignant kidney neoplasm in children. Approximately 500 new cases are reported annually in the United States. Age is the primary risk factor. The disease most commonly occurs during the first 6 years of life, with approximately 75% of cases occurring in children younger than age 5 years. The peak incidence is between the ages of 3 and 4 years, and the tumor occurs slightly more often in African Americans and girls. Wilms tumors occur bilaterally in 5% of cases.

There are several hereditary syndromes that can predispose children to the development of Wilms tumor. The three most common include the WAGR syndrome (*W*ilms, *a*niridia, *g*enitourinary malformation, mental *r*etardation), the Beckwith-Wiedemann syndrome, and the Denys-Drash syndrome.

Etiologic Factors and Pathogenesis. Although the majority of cases are sporadic, approximately 1% to 3% have a family history of Wilms tumor, and up to 10% are seen in hereditary syndromes. Molecular genetics plays an important role in the cause of Wilms tumor. The biologic signaling pathways determining the origin of Wilms tumor are complex, and several genes at several loci may be involved.

The most well-known and studied gene of Wilms tumor is the *WT1* suppressor gene, a complex protein that is an essential regulator of kidney development; mutations in this gene result in the formation of tumors in approximately 10% of Wilms tumor cases.[170] These genes also are implicated in the formation of many other cancers.

Other genetic alterations, such as *WT2* and familial genetic alterations termed *FWT1* and *FWT2*, have also been located. Significant investigations are ongoing to determine how these genes and their products interact in order to understand the mechanisms in the development of Wilms tumor and provide improved therapy.

Clinical Manifestations. Wilms tumors can be difficult to discover early because the tumor can grow to a large size before causing symptoms. Fortunately, despite large tumor size, most Wilms tumors do not metastasize. An abdominal mass, most often detected by the parents, is the most common presenting sign. Up to 30% of children may complain of abdominal pain, malaise, loss of appetite, or nausea/vomiting. Hematuria may occur in up to 30% of cases and hypertension in up to 25% of affected children. Congenital abnormalities may be present, particularly those associated with hereditary syndromes with a predilection for Wilms tumor (13%-28%).

MEDICAL MANAGEMENT

STAGING AND DIAGNOSIS. Staging is performed according to the National Wilms Tumor Study Group (NWTSG) staging system. Tumors are staged into five groups (stages I to V), depending on tumor size and growth into surrounding structures. Histologic features are also important. Histologically, tumors can be classified as having favorable histology or unfavorable histology (anaplastic features). Approximately 40% of tumors are discovered while in stage I, whereas only 5% of cases are at stage V. Most adults with Wilms tumors are diagnosed unexpectedly following nephrectomy for presumed RCC.[250]

Abdominal ultrasonography helps define the cystic or solid nature of the mass and helps determine whether the renal vein or vena cava is involved. CT scan of the abdomen is helpful in determining the extent of the tumor but can be difficult to perform with small children. A chest radiograph and CT of the chest are used to determine the presence of metastases to the lung. MRI may also be beneficial in determining the extent of the disease.

TREATMENT. Surgical resection of the tumor is the primary treatment regardless of the stage of the disease. A radical nephrectomy is the most common procedure, although a nephron-sparing procedure may be performed in clients who have lesions in both kidneys. Regional lymphadenectomy may be carried out, as lymph node involvement strongly affects the prognosis. Chemotherapy is also used for all stages of the disease, sometimes preoperatively, with radiation therapy being added to the treatment regimen for stages III and IV disease and for tumors with unfavorable histologic findings. (See Chapter 9 for the side effects associated with chemotherapy and radiation therapy.)

There are no standard treatments available for adults. A standardized approach for the management of adult Wilms tumors is proposed with the aim to limit treatment delay after surgery and encourage a uniform approach for this rare disease and thereby improve survival.[250]

PROGNOSIS. Prognosis depends on the histologic appearance of the lesion, stage of the disease, and age of the child. But the overall 5-year survival is very good at 90%.[141] Multimodality therapy with surgery, whole-abdomen radiotherapy, and three-drug chemotherapy delivered according to the NWTS-4 and -5 protocols resulted in excellent abdominal and systemic tumor control rates.[141]

With the development of successful treatment, emphasis is now being placed on limiting significant long-term side effects while maintaining the high cure rate in tumors with favorable histology. All children should be monitored in long-term surveillance programs for the early detection and management of therapy-related toxicities.[141] Further treatment options are needed for advanced tumors with unfavorable histology. Wilms tumor may recur years after the initial diagnosis.

Wilms tumor occurs rarely in adults; outcome for adults is inferior compared with children, although better results are reported when treated within pediatric trials. Multiple factors, including the unfamiliarity of adult oncologists and pathologists with Wilms tumors, lack of standardized treatment and consequent delays in initiating the appropriate risk-adapted therapy, may contribute to the poor outcome.

Renal Cystic Disease

Overview

A renal cyst is a cavity filled with fluid or renal tubular elements making up a semisolid material. The presence of these cysts can lead to degeneration of renal tissue and obstruction of tubular flow. Renal cysts vary considerably in size, ranging from microscopic to several centimeters in diameter, and can be single or multiple, unilateral or bilateral.

Cysts in the kidney are rather common and can be classified into six categories of cystic diseases: (1) polycystic kidney disease (PKD), (2) cystic diseases of the renal medulla, (3) acquired cystic disease, (4) single cysts, (5) cystic renal dysplasia, and (6) miscellaneous renal cystic disorders.

The formation of simple cysts is the most common cystic disorder of the kidney. Simple cysts are usually less than 1 cm in diameter and do not often produce symptoms or compromise renal function. Acquired cysts may develop secondary to dialysis, diabetes mellitus, or glomerulonephritis. PKD is a leading cause of ESRD, frequently requiring dialysis and renal transplantation. Because of the seriousness and fairly common occurrence of PKD, this section principally discusses PKD. The remaining disorders constitute less-common causes of renal cysts.

Incidence

PKD is manifested as either an autosomal dominant (ADPKD) or autosomal recessive (ARPKD) disorder. Although PKD can occur spontaneously, most cases are hereditary. ADPKD is one of the most common hereditary disorders in the United States, affecting more than 600,000 Americans (about 1 in every 500 to 1 in every 1000 persons). ARPKD is rare.

Persons with ADPKD may not manifest symptoms until the third or fourth decade of life, whereas ARPKD is evident at birth and can cause death early in life. ADPKD affects people from all races and ethnic groups. Most people with ADPKD will exhibit evidence of the disease by the age of 80 years, but only half progress to ESRD. ADPKD is the fourth leading cause of ESRD and accounts for 10% of all cases of ESRD.

Risk Factors

Even though there is currently no way of determining which people with ADPKD will develop ESRD, there are a few risk factors that have been linked to a more rapid progression. These factors include hypertension, multiple pregnancies, male gender, and the expression of the genetic mutation PKD1.

Etiology and Pathogenesis

Most renal cysts form from the epithelium of a preexisting renal tubule. These epithelial cells typically exhibit a reabsorptive function, but have secretory capabilities. In the case of cyst formation, epithelial cells with genetic mutations begin to secrete fluid into the tubule once stimulated by endocrine, paracrine, and autocrine regulating proteins. Such proteins may also play a role in the size and rate of growth of the cyst.

As a cyst grows, it detaches from the nephron (approximately 75% detach completely). The epithelial cells then continue to proliferate and fibrosis develops. With time, the pressure created by the expanding, multiple cysts interrupts the function of neighboring nephrons, leading to apoptosis of noncystic nephrons. Although normal nephrons enlarge in an attempt to compensate for the loss of nephrons, this is unsuccessful in half of people with PKD.

In ADPKD, there have been several genes linked to the development of cysts. These abnormalities are located on chromosomes 16 and 4 and are called PKD1 and PKD2. Other genes are likely involved as well. These genes code for proteins that function in transferring signals from the extracellular matrix into the cell to promote cellular proliferation and differentiation. Both genes need to be affected before there is the resultant development of disease.

Approximately 85% of persons with ADPKD express a mutation in PKD1; only 15% demonstrate a mutation in PKD2. A small percentage has a mutation in another gene. Although clinical manifestations are similar for people with PKD1 and PKD2, clients who exhibit the PKD2 mutation progress to end-stage renal failure about 10 years later than those with the PKD1 mutation.

Mutations to the gene coding for a large protein called fibrocystin on chromosome 6 lead to ARPKD. Further studies are needed in order to clearly define the role of these genes and their products in the formation of PKD.

Clinical Manifestations

Although PKD is a hereditary disorder, only 60% of people are able to give a familial history of PKD, suggesting that spontaneous mutations occur frequently. For those families with a history of PKD, individuals can be monitored. In people who lack a familial history, cysts often are asymptomatic and found incidentally on routine urographic examination.

Symptoms associated with autosomal dominant disease may include pain, hematuria, fever, and hypertension. Abdominal or flank pain is the most common symptom in ADPKD. It can be associated with bleeding, growth of cysts, stones, infection, or, rarely, tumor. Most of these clients will have significantly enlarged kidneys that are palpable abdominally.

Associated hematuria may be gross or microscopic. Rupture of a cyst usually accounts for incidents of gross hematuria. Fever can be related to an infected cyst secondary to pyelonephritis. Hypertension is hypothesized to occur as a result of sodium and water retention because of damage to the tubules.[166,228] Hypertension also hastens the development of fibrosis and is linked with accelerated progression to ESRD.

Liver cysts are also common in clients with ADPKD; about half have liver cysts at diagnosis. Unlike the kidney cysts, liver cysts rarely lead to problems such as liver failure or portal hypertension. People with ADPKD may also be affected with other genetic abnormalities, such as thoracic and abdominal aortic aneurysms, cerebral aneurysms, mitral and aortic valve prolapse, colonic diverticular disease, and pancreatic cysts.

MEDICAL MANAGEMENT

DIAGNOSIS. Ultrasonography is used to screen for PKD. People younger than 30 years of age should demonstrate at least two cysts in *one* kidney in order for PKD to be diagnosed. Persons between the ages of 30 and 59 years should have at least two cysts in *each* kidney, and people older than 60 years should demonstrate four cysts per kidney. Genetic tests can be performed to corroborate radiographic information. Simple cysts are uncommon in clients with PKD; the simultaneous presence of both large and small cysts is the norm.

CT is a useful radiographic test, distinguishing between solid and fluid-filled masses and displaying the presence of cysts of varied sizes. CT can also reveal the presence of hepatic cysts, making the diagnosis of PKD more likely. Prognostic information can also be obtained from the contrast-enhancing portion of a CT. Only the normal renal tubules will have contrast in them, revealing the degree of functioning nephrons.

MRI is often a better choice, especially for children or persons with renal dysfunction or who are in the early stages of the disease. Urinalysis may detect hematuria and proteinuria, or the clinical examination may reveal enlarged, palpable kidneys. As appropriate, other causes of renal cysts should be addressed. Occasionally, tissue biopsy or surgical exploration is necessary to make the definitive diagnosis.

TREATMENT. Because hypertension is a known risk factor for progression to ESRD, blood pressure should be monitored and controlled, particularly if a family history is present and the disease is diagnosed in young adults. Stimulation of the renin-angiotensin system was thought to be the cause of hypertension in ADPKD, but this has been questioned and other causes postulated. For this reason, angiotensin-converting enzyme (ACE) inhibitors and angiotensin receptor blockers (ARBs) have not been more successful than other blood pressure medications in preventing the progression of ADPKD.[180] Studies suggest that by keeping blood pressure at a normotensive level there is a slowing of progression to ESRD.[41,42,247]

Pain can be controlled through analgesics or treatment of the underlying cause (i.e., treating infections with antibiotics). Percutaneous aspiration of cystic fluid followed by injection of a sclerosing agent has helped some clients with pain from expanding cysts. Surgery and laparoscopic surgery can be performed to remove or unroof large cysts for pain relief. Infections can be difficult to treat, since the infection may be isolated in the cyst or an abscess may

form. Possible associated findings, such as cerebral aneurysms, should be screened for and monitored.

SPECIAL IMPLICATIONS FOR THE THERAPIST   18-3

Renal Cystic Disease

When treating a client with a history of renal cystic disease, therapists should be aware of symptoms and signs suggesting that the condition is worsening. The presence of any of these clinical findings warrants referral to a physician. An awareness that this population is at risk for hypertension and UTI and at increased risk of developing cerebral and aortic aneurysms and mitral valve problems is also necessary. The presentation of any symptoms or signs suggestive of the presence of these conditions again warrants referral to a physician. Lastly, the fact the kidneys may be enlarged can account for atypical findings on palpation.

Renal Calculi

Overview

Urinary stone disease, or nephrolithiasis, is the third most common urinary tract disorder, exceeded only by infections and prostate disease. Although a majority of the stones develop in the kidneys, once they move into the ureter, they are referred to as ureteral stones (bladder stones are considered a separate disorder).

The stones, also called calculi, are crystalline and range from popcorn kernel shapes to jagged starbursts, and can cause urinary obstruction and severe pain. Urinary obstruction typically occurs at one of the following three sites: (1) the ureteropelvic junction, (2) where the ureter crosses over the iliac vessels, and (3) at the ureterovesical junction (Fig. 18-5). The four basic types of stones are calcium (oxalate and phosphate), struvite, uric acid, and cystine.

Calcium stones are by the far the most common (70% to 85%). Struvite stones are related to recurrent bacterial UTIs with organisms that produce urease. Uric acid stones (5%-10% of nephrolithiasis cases) occur as the result of an increased level of urate in the blood and uric acid crystals in the urine, which is common in persons with gout. Cystine stones are uncommon (accounting for approximately 1% of all cases of nephrolithiasis) and caused by a hereditary disorder, cystinuria. Affected persons are unable to absorb cystine, and large amounts are excreted in the urine.

Incidence

Nephrolithiasis occurs in approximately 5% of adults, with men being affected more frequently than women (6% vs. 4%, respectively).[257] Because of the severe and debilitating pain associated with kidney stones, cost is significant, including doctor visits, hospitalizations, and lost work. In 2000, than 2 million doctor visits annually and 177,496 hospital stays have been reported resulting from kidney stones, costing $2.07 billion.[174,265] The primary

The renal and urologic systems

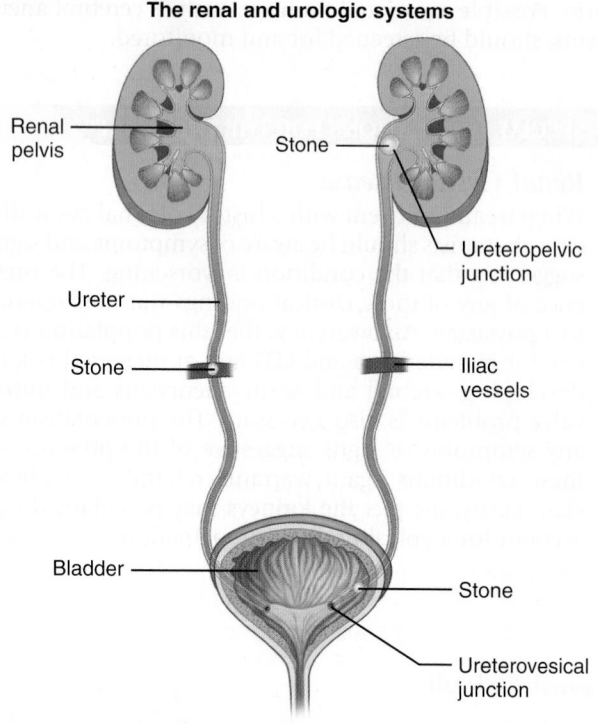

Figure 18-5

The three most common sites of urinary obstruction secondary to renal calculi.

age span for the initial presentation of the disease is 30 to 60 years of age for men, and 20 to 30 years for women. A higher incidence of renal calculi occurs in industrialized countries and areas noted for high temperatures and humidity. The incidence of this disease is highest in the hot summer months.

Etiologic and Risk Factors

With an understanding of the factors and mechanisms that lead to stone formation, risk factors are more evident and modifiable. Disorders that lead to an overexcretion and hypersaturation of calcium or oxalate can lead to stone formation. These include illnesses such as idiopathic hypercalciuria, renal tubular acidosis, primary hyperparathyroidism, and hyperoxaluria.

It is also known that low quantities of citrate (which typically binds calcium, thereby acting as an inhibitor to stone formation) can lead to nephrolithiasis. Uric acid crystals are sensitive to urine pH, coming out of solution in an acidic pH; thus an acidic urine pH can lead to uric acid stones.[253] Gout is a disorder in which excess urate is excreted into the urine, leading to a supersaturation of uric acid crystals. Chronic dehydration can lead to stone formation because of a decreased fluid content compared to crystals.

Other risk factors have been identified by epidemiologic studies but the mechanism remains unclear. For example, among persons with recurrent stone formation, it is often on one side only (unilateral). Some investigators have hypothesized that sleep posture (i.e., consistently sleeping on one side) may promote stone formation on the one side.[252] Obesity is associated with an increased incidence of urinary stone episodes in women but not in men.[225]

Excess intake of supplemental calcium, sodium, sucrose, and animal protein have been dietary risk factors implicated in stone formation. A lack of sufficient calcium and potassium in the diet can also increase risk for kidney stones.[62] Following a DASH (Dietary Approaches to Stop Hypertension)-style diet is associated with a reduced risk of kidney stones.[270]

Pathogenesis

Several factors lead to the formation of stones—saturation, nucleation, crystal growth and aggregation, and cell/crystal interactions. Saturation refers to the amount of dissolved crystal (such as calcium oxalate or calcium phosphate) in the urine compared to volume.

Crystals are able to stay dissolved in the urine until it becomes oversaturated. Factors such as the amount of calcium, oxalate, and water excretion determine saturation. With oversaturation, crystals come out of solution (or out of the urine) into a solid and begin to grow around a particle, or nucleus. It is uncommon for urine to become so oversaturated that a new nucleus of calcium oxalate or calcium phosphate is formed. Most often, a small particle, bacteria (small nanobacteria), or other crystal already present in the urine acts as a nucleus for the crystals to grow around (i.e., stones may have a nucleus of one crystal type, but surrounded by another crystal type).

Crystals then grow at a rate depending on the saturation of the urine. The more supersaturated, the more quickly larger stones form. These stones also require enough time to enlarge, since normal flow is often sufficient to move small stones through the urinary tract. It is proposed that the growing crystal aggregate becomes attached to the urinary tract epithelium and transported into the cell membrane. Here, the cell membrane may also act as a nucleus. Investigations are ongoing to determine the significance of cell/crystal interactions.

Clinical Manifestations

Clinical symptoms are the same for the various types of stones. The classic presentation of a kidney stone is acute "colicky" flank pain radiating to the groin or perineal areas (including the scrotum in males and labia in females) with hematuria. The pain is severe; most people are unable to find a comfortable position.

The location of the pain may vary depending on where the stone is lodged in the ureter. Abdominal pain with radiation to the groin may be more pronounced if the stone is higher in the abdomen, while a stone at the ureterovesical junction may give rise to lower quadrant abdominal pain radiating to the tip of the urethra.

Symptoms consistent with a UTI such as urinary urgency and frequency and dysuria are often present. Hematuria is present in more than 90% of cases, although the absence of hematuria does not mean nephrolithiasis is not the diagnosis.[25] Nausea and vomiting may also be manifested.

MEDICAL MANAGEMENT

PREVENTION. Stone disease is a highly prevalent condition associated with substantial cost and morbidity. The cost-effectiveness of a primary prevention strategy has been calculated.[174] Although preventive strategies cost more than no prevention, these strategies are at least 50% effective in preventing stones.[174]

Recurrence of calculi is common in up to 50% of people within 5 years if preventive steps are not taken. A metabolic evaluation should be performed in clients who are willing to comply with tests and prophylactic methods (only 36%-70% of people with recurrent stones comply long-term with recommended measures).[215,282] Tests and appropriate preventive measures vary depending on the type of stone passed. Common tests include 24-hour urine collection for calcium, oxalate, uric acid, phosphate, citrate, pH, potassium, and creatinine; serum calcium; serum blood urea and creatinine; and parathyroid hormone (PTH). If a specific disorder, such as hyperparathyroidism, is identified, treatment reduces the risk for further stones.

Adequate fluid intake is essential to the prevention of stones and recurrences by reducing the saturation of stone-forming crystals. Clients should be encouraged to drink enough fluid to maintain clear-colored urine. Other dietary modifications are made according to stone type. Urinary uric acid can be reduced by decreasing the amount of protein ingested. Urine citrate can be increased by consuming more fruits and vegetables and decreasing the amount of acid-producing food (such as animal protein).[269,271] A restriction of calcium is not recommended and may be harmful.[24,64]

Medications can be helpful in certain situations if dietary means alone are insufficient to prevent stone formation. Thiazide diuretics (which increase calcium excretion), alkali, such as potassium citrate (beneficial in increasing urine citrate excretion), and allopurinol (prevents the precipitation of uric acid crystals) may be useful. Further research is needed to determine the efficacy of specific dietary changes and the best means to prevent kidney stones.

DIAGNOSIS. A variety of tests are used to diagnose this disease. Noncontrast helical CT scanning is the first-line imaging test for renal colic. Once a stone has been visualized on CT, a plain radiograph can help determine the type of stone. Approximately 90% of calculi are radiopaque, making them visible on an abdominal radiograph. These types of stones are composed of calcium or other minerals, whereas uric acid stones are not visible on a plain radiograph. Other traditional imaging tests (e.g., ultrasonography and IVP) can also help in the management of stone disease. Hematuria, infection, the presence of stone-forming crystals, and urine pH can be determined on urinalysis.

TREATMENT. The mainstay of treatment for acute nephrolithiasis includes intravenous fluids and medications to relieve nausea/vomiting and pain (narcotics or nonsteroidal antiinflammatory drugs [NSAIDs]). The α-blockers and calcium channel blockers are commonly used to treat hypertension, but both drugs also appear to flush out kidney stones by relaxing the ureter and increasing liquid pressure. Some physicians prefer α-blockers because they have fewer side effects. Most clients can be watched; however, some require immediate intervention to remove the stone.

Characteristics requiring urgent care include the presence of high-grade obstruction, anuria (no passage of urine), obstruction plus infection proximal to the stone, impending renal function deterioration, unresponsive pain or vomiting, or a solitary or transplanted kidney.[272] In these situations, percutaneous nephrostomy or ureteral stenting can be performed. Intravenous antibiotics are given for infection; E. coli is the most common organism.

A majority of stones less than 5 mm in diameter (a little smaller than the width of a pencil eraser) will pass spontaneously; the stones that do pass on their own do so within 4 weeks. The urine should be strained to retrieve any stones so they can be analyzed for crystal content.

Persons waiting for stones to pass should continue drinking fluid (enough to produce about 2 L/day of urine or keep the urine clear-colored instead of yellow). Fluids with sodium should be avoided; lemonade may be helpful because it increases urinary citrate and decreases calcium oxalate supersaturation.[251] A follow-up CT 3 to 4 weeks after the initial episode will verify the passage of the stone or the need for intervention if the stone is unmoved.

Clients who have kidney stones of less than 1 cm in the proximal ureter can receive shockwave lithotripsy.[287] Shockwave lithotripsy uses the transmission of shock waves (a type of sound wave) to break the calculi into fragments. Because the soft tissues of the body have similar densities, the shock waves pass through these structures with low attenuation. When the shock wave encounters a boundary between substances of differing acoustic density (i.e., a calculus in the ureter), high compressive forces are generated, causing a breakdown of the stone. The goal is to reduce the diameter to the point where spontaneous passage of the stone occurs.

Stones larger than 1 cm (and in the proximal ureter) benefit from ureteroscopy. Ureteroscopy involves passing a scope through the urethra and bladder into the ureter until the stone is reached. Then a laser is passed through the scope, the tip of the laser is placed on the stone, and the laser is discharged, producing photothermal lithotripsy.[284]

Stones located in the distal portion of the ureter can be treated with either method or with medical expulsive therapy, such as tamsulosin, the most commonly used agent, at a much lower cost.[15]

Uric acid stones are unique in their treatment. Because these stones dissolve in acid, the urine of affected clients can be acidified with potassium citrate or sodium citrate to increase the urine pH to at least 6.5. Stones are frequently not composed purely of uric acid, and further intervention may be required.

| SPECIAL IMPLICATIONS FOR THE THERAPIST | 18-4 |

Renal Calculi

If the classic symptoms are present, the renal colic associated with the calculi will not be confused with muscular or joint pain. The condition, however, may be manifested by symptoms that are intermittent and not severe. Depending on the location of the obstruction, the condition may be manifested solely by unilateral back pain, ranging from the thoracolumbar junction to the iliac crest. The therapist needs to be vigilant for complaints of urinary dysfunction and risk factors associated with this disease. The Murphy percussion test can be performed to determine the need for medical referral.

If working with someone who is concurrently being treated conservatively for renal calculi, the therapist must be vigilant for complaints of fever, chills, or sweats. An onset of these symptoms warrants immediate communication with the physician.

Chronic Kidney Disease

Overview

Chronic kidney disease (CKD) is defined as the alteration of kidney function or structure for a duration of 3 months or longer.[75] CKD can be attributed to a variety of conditions that lead to a loss of kidney function. The three most common causes are diabetes (44%), hypertension (27%), and glomerulonephritis (8%). Cystic kidney disease and other urologic diseases account for approximately 5%, while other conditions (such as excessive aspirin or acetaminophen use) account for the remaining few percent.

ESRD is the final stage of CKD, with the loss of kidney function accompanied by symptoms requiring either dialysis or kidney transplant. The loss of kidney function is devastating, resulting in significant systemic effects, reduced quality of life, increased morbidity and mortality, and costing more than $23 billion per year.[139,231,297]

Incidence

The incidence of CKD continues to increase in the United States, with more than 20 million people currently affected. The number of persons with ESRD also continues to rise, with a prevalence of more than 500,000.[198] Recent data show a significant leap in the number of people with ESRD requiring treatment (dialysis or transplant) from 1994 to 2004. In 1994, the number of people who started dialysis or received a renal transplant was 68,757; in 2004 this number had increased to 102,356.[101] Much of this increase was reported in persons with diabetes, with 26,848 cases reported in 1994 and 44,953 cases in 2004.

The incidence of ESRD from diabetes, hypertension, and glomerulonephritis is higher in African Americans compared to the general population. The rate of ESRD caused by hypertension was three times higher in African Americans compared to the general population. Encouraging data from 2004, however, showed that the incidence of CKD decreased in the Native American population, although prevalence has tripled among Hispanic Americans.[200]

ESRD carries a high mortality rate, particularly in the older population. In 2004, people older than age 65 years who received dialysis had a mortality rate seven times that of equivalent-age people not on dialysis.[101] People older than age 60 years who start dialysis have a life expectancy of only 5 years, whereas a 60-year-old without ESRD can expect to live 20 more years.

Etiologic and Risk Factors

The presence of a number of diseases can account for destruction of nephrons, but diabetes mellitus (principally type 2 causes diabetic nephropathy), high blood pressure, and glomerulonephritis are the leading causes of CKD. Other disorders contributing to the development of kidney failure include PKD, urinary tract obstruction, repeated infection, hereditary defects of the kidneys, toxicities, and systemic lupus erythematosus.

An increased risk of renal damage and ESRD is also associated with excessive nonprescription analgesic drug use, called *analgesic nephropathy*. This association was first noted with phenacetin-containing analgesics,[109] but is also noted with the drugs acetaminophen, aspirin, and combination analgesics (i.e., combining analgesics with codeine or caffeine).[88,124]

Heavy average intake or high cumulative intake of analgesics may increase the likelihood of developing ESRD, particularly in older people with a disorder already affecting the kidneys.[104] NSAIDs, both selective and nonselective, have significant short-term effects on the kidney, yet data have been inconsistent with regard to the risk for ESRD from NSAID use.[63,249] More research is needed to answer this question, but it may be that moderate use of NSAIDs in healthy individuals does not put them at significant increased risk for ESRD.[232]

Pathogenesis

The basic functioning unit of the kidney is the nephron. It is composed of the glomerulus, the renal tubules, and the collecting duct (Fig. 18-6). The glomerulus is a small bundle of capillaries, surrounded by a capsule that allows fluid and electrolytes to pass through the membrane and into the tubules. The renal tubules transport electrolytes or create a gradient for fluid and electrolytes to become balanced, while the collecting tubule is responsible for the final regulation of electrolytes and water under the influence of the hormone aldosterone.

As discussed earlier, many disease processes can result in CKD. Diabetes, for example, induces kidney damage through hyperglycemia. Angiotensin II is also released, which causes vasoconstriction of the arterioles and arteries (both in the glomerulus and systemically) in an attempt to keep the pressure adequate for filtration.

Angiotensin II release also leads to the attraction of inflammatory cells, which release cytokines and growth factors (which change the structure of the glomerulus). These changes result in mesangial expansion (a layer of cells around the glomerular capillaries), enlargement of the glomerulus, and ultimately interstitial fibrosis and glomerular sclerosis.

These processes slowly reduce the amount of surface area available for filtration to occur, thereby reducing the glomerular filtration rate (GFR). With the gradual loss of nephron function, the kidneys are unable to adequately regulate fluid, electrolytes, and pH balance or remove metabolic waste products from the blood.

The rate of nephron destruction can vary considerably, depending on the disease process. Typically, five stages mark the progression of chronic renal failure; each stage is defined by the level of the GFR (measured

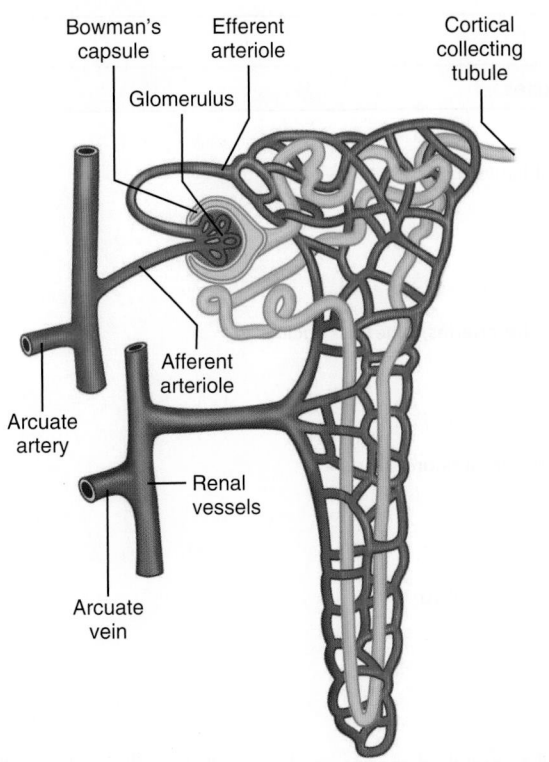

Figure 18-6

Components of the nephron. The afferent arteriole carries blood to the glomerulus for filtration through the Bowman capsule and the renal tubular system.

in milliliters per minute): (1) kidney damage with normal or increased GFR (90 mL/min or more), (2) kidney damage with mildly decreased GFR (60-89 mL/min), (3) moderately decreased GFR (30-59 mL/min), (4) severely decreased GFR (15-29 mL/min), and (5) kidney failure (ESRD; GFR of less than 15 mL/min). Systemic complications typically develop once stage 4 CKD is reached, when the GFR is less than 30 mL/min.

Clinical Manifestations

In stage 1 of CKD, the GFR is normal or increased (hyperfiltration). No overt symptoms of impaired renal function are typically evident. Depending on the health of the person, the kidneys have tremendous adaptive and compensatory capabilities, accounting for the delay in symptoms. The unaffected nephrons undergo structural and physiologic hypertrophy in an attempt to make up for those nephrons that are no longer functioning. Results of blood tests which are indicative of kidney function such as blood urea nitrogen (BUN) and creatinine are typically normal.

The onset of symptoms is usually very gradual and subtle with the continued loss of nephrons and reduction in GFR, often resulting in a delay in diagnosis. Early clinical manifestations include hypertension and anemia. Abnormalities in laboratory values include an increase in BUN and creatinine, or protein detected in the urine. Stage 1 is reversible for some people (e.g., those with diabetes who benefit from early detection and proper glycemic control). Some individuals remain in stage 1 indefinitely, whereas others progress.

During stage 2, the damaged capillaries allow small amounts of albumin to be excreted in the urine. Individuals may remain in this stage for several years with proper control of hypertension and blood glucose levels. Stage 3 is more noticeable as albumin levels increase in the urine and decrease in the blood, resulting in noticeable edema. During this stage, levels of creatinine and BUN increase, resulting in an accumulation of waste products in the blood called *azotemia*.[78]

In the final stages of CKD (stages 4 and 5, with stage 5 being ESRD), the kidney is unable to function and a multitude of complications appear with accompanying symptoms and signs. Proteinuria is the hallmark of stage 4; the kidneys are no longer able to excrete toxins, so there is a progressive increase in BUN and creatinine levels. Most people in stage 4 are hypertensive because of an increased production of renin. Hypertension accelerates the progression to stage 5 (ESRD) when the kidneys have failed to function.

Stage 5 or ESRD is heralded by a cluster of symptoms referred to as *uremia*.[217] The kidneys cannot excrete toxins; maintain fluid, pH, and electrolyte balances; or secrete important hormones (e.g., renin, vitamin D, erythropoietin). Uremia develops when poorly identified toxins are not removed from the blood. Uremia is characterized by nausea, vomiting, anorexia, lethargy, pruritus (itching), sensory and motor neuropathy, pericarditis, impaired heart function, asterixis, and seizures. Asterixis is an intermittent inability to sustain a posture, often noted when holding up the hand with the wrist flexed, creating a small "flapping-like" motion.

Dialysis or kidney transplant improves these symptoms. Hematologic, cardiovascular, gastrointestinal, musculoskeletal, and neurologic complications become more common in stages 4 and 5. Table 18-1 summarizes the systemic effects associated with CKD and ESRD.

Hematologic. Anemia is a significant hematologic problem associated with CKD. The hormone erythropoietin, primarily produced by the interstitial cells of the kidneys, has the principal function of controlling the production of red blood cells in the bone marrow. CKD leads to decreased erythropoietin production, reduced red blood cell life span, and reduced iron absorption, resulting in a subsequent decrease in red blood cells and anemia.

Anemia associated with CKD occurs most frequently in clients with a GFR of less than 60 mL/min and in persons 75 years of age or older.[5] However, a lack of erythropoietin is not the only factor causing anemia in clients with CKD. Other causes, such as gastrointestinal bleeding, iron or folate deficiency, or hemolysis, may play a role and should be evaluated.

Anemia in CKD can cause significant fatigue and reduced quality of life. Another important result of anemia is the stress it places on the heart. Anemia is an independent risk factor for cardiovascular disease and should be treated aggressively (see Chapter 14 for additional information regarding anemia).[278] ESRD also leads to white blood cell dysfunction and bleeding problems caused by impaired platelet function.

Cardiovascular. Cardiovascular diseases often occur in people with CKD and are the leading cause of death in

Table 18-1 | Systemic Manifestations of Kidney Failure

Systemic Symptoms	Probable Causes
Urinary System	
Decreased urinary output	Damaged renal tissue
Abnormal urinary constituents (blood cells, protein, casts)	
Abnormal blood serum level, such as elevated BUN and creatinine	
Cardiopulmonary	
Coronary artery disease	Calcification of the arteries, other risk factors
Hypertension	
Congestive heart failure	Fluid overload
Pulmonary edema	
Dyspnea	
Pericarditis	Uremic toxins irritate pericardial sac
Gastrointestinal Tract	
Bleeding	Platelet changes
Nausea and vomiting	
Uremic breath	Uremic toxins change saliva
Anorexia	
Nervous System	
Central	
Headache	
Irritability	Effect of electrolyte and fluid changes on brain cells (usually resolves with
Impaired judgment	dialysis treatment)
Inability to concentrate	
Seizures	
Lethargy/coma	
Sleep disturbances	
Peripheral	
Loss of vibratory sense and deep tendon reflexes	Effect of uremic toxins on peripheral nerves
Impairment of motor nerve conduction velocity	
Burning, tingling, paresthesias	
Tremors	
Muscle cramps, muscle twitching	Electrolyte imbalances (calcium, sodium, potassium)
Foot drop	
Weakness	
Integumentary (Skin)	
Pruritus (itching)/excoriation (scratching)	Skin calcifications related to calcium/phosphorus imbalances
Hyperpigmentation	Retained uremic pigments
Pallor	Anemia
Bruising	Platelet dysfunction
Eyes	
Band keratopathy	Corneal calcifications related to calcium/phosphorus imbalance
Visual blurring	
Dry eyes	Conjunctival calcifications related to calcium/phosphorus imbalance
Red eyes	
Endocrine	
Fertility and sexual dysfunction	Effect of uremic toxins on menstrual cycles, ovulation, and sperm production
Hyperparathyroidism	Result of calcium/phosphorus imbalance
Hematopoietic	
Anemia	Decreased production of erythropoietin by kidney; destruction of red blood cells by dialysis
Platelet dysfunction	Uremic toxins interfere with platelet aggregation
Skeletal	
Renal osteodystrophy (demineralization of bones)	Related to decreased calcium absorption and resultant calcium/phosphorus imbalance
Joint pain	Joint calcifications
Myopathy	

From Goodman CC, Snyder TE: *Differential diagnosis in physical therapy,* ed 3, Philadelphia, 2000, WB Saunders.

persons with ESRD. As the GFR decreases, the risk for cardiovascular disease increases in a graded fashion.[102,157,277] Many of the risk factors that cause CKD, such as diabetes and hypertension, also contribute to cardiovascular disease. Diseases common in clients with CKD include coronary artery disease, left ventricular hypertrophy, and congestive heart failure. Persons with CKD often have hyperlipidemia, another risk factor for coronary artery disease.

Symptoms may include chest pain (although many often have atypical or no pain), nausea, shortness of breath, and sweating. Excess fluid volume, sodium retention, and anemia associated with ESRD lead to left ventricular hypertrophy, a thickening of the left ventricle of the heart, which predisposes to congestive heart failure.

Associated clinical features include lower extremity edema and shortness of breath. Hypertension often appears early in the course of this disease because of increased angiotensin II production. Clients in stage 3 of CKD often need two or more medications to control blood pressure. Clients with CKD also have a higher incidence of stroke, peripheral vascular disease, arrhythmias, pericarditis, and heart valve abnormalities.

Gastrointestinal. Gastrointestinal system complaints occur often once the later stages of ESRD are reached. Azotemia (high levels of urea and other toxins in the blood) causes nausea, vomiting, and anorexia. The resultant depressed appetite contributes to malnutrition, fatigue, weakness, and malaise. Malnutrition has a high prevalence in those with advanced kidney disease, partly as a result of the therapeutic restriction on calories and proteins but also because of the metabolic reactions typical with this disease. Other clinical manifestations include gastritis, duodenitis, pancreatitis, hiccups (often difficult to control), and ascites.

Musculoskeletal. The skeletal changes associated with CKD are common and can occur early in the disease secondary to abnormalities in calcium, phosphate, and vitamin D metabolism. With the impairment of GFR, the body is unable to excrete phosphate or synthesize 1,25-dihydroxyvitamin D (a vitamin D derivative called *calcitriol*). Higher blood levels of phosphate lead to low ionized calcium levels. Calcitriol normally regulates calcium absorption from the gut and inhibits the parathyroid gland. But with low levels of calcitriol, hypocalcemia and increased PTH secretion result. A drop in serum calcium signals a cascade of events starting with the release of PTH, which signals the body to increase calcium resorption from bone to make up for the perceived loss (Fig. 18-7).

Several skeletal abnormalities result from varying types of bone turnover, collectively referred to as renal osteodystrophy. Renal osteodystrophy is a type of rickets formerly called renal rickets, and sometimes referred to as azotemic osteodystrophy. Although uncommon at one time, the incidence has risen with increased survival of people with renal disease on dialysis.

Renal osteodystrophy is characterized by varying degrees of osteomalacia, osteitis fibrosa, and adynamic bone disease. Osteomalacia occurs secondary to low bone turnover caused by aluminum deposition in the bones with resultant increased nonmineralized bone

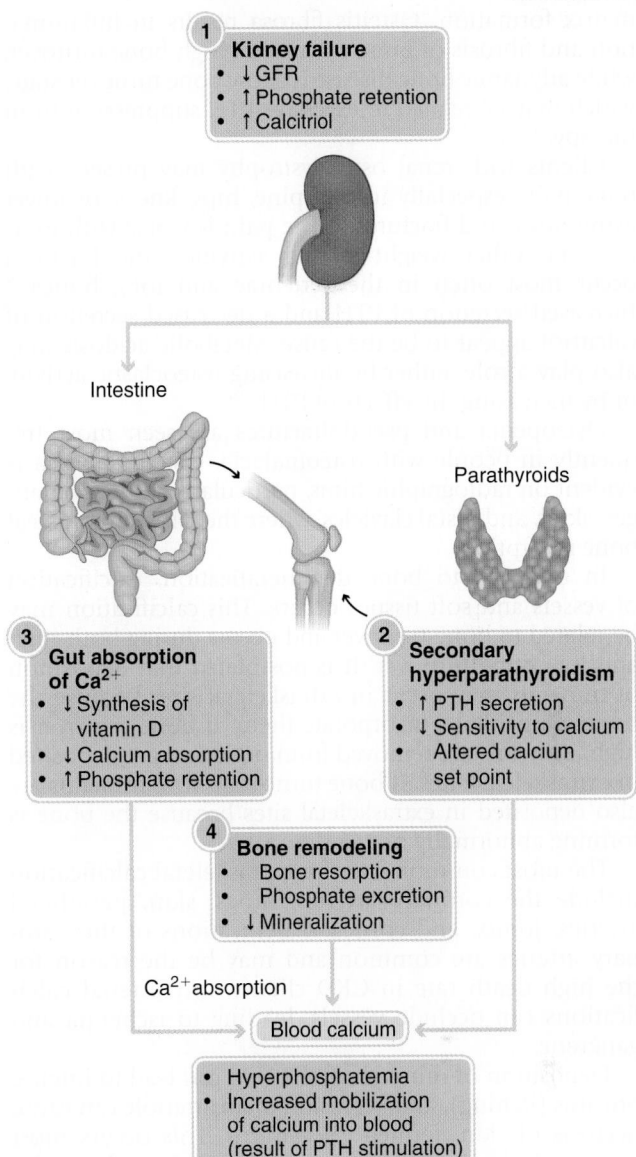

Figure 18-7

Mechanisms of altered bone turnover. (1) Renal osteodystrophy can be viewed as the result of a vicious cycle that begins with moderate to severe renal failure. As the glomerular filtration rate (GFR) decreases, phosphate excretion decreases, and calcium elimination increases. (2) The body attempts to compensate for the loss of calcitriol and reduced calcium absorption by increasing parathyroid hormone (PTH) secretion. PTH mobilizes calcium from the bones (bone reabsorption) and facilitates phosphate excretion. This release of calcium and phosphate into the blood results in hyperphosphatemia and hypercalcemia. (3) As kidney failure progresses, the damaged kidneys can no longer convert vitamin D to its active form and without active vitamin D, calcium absorption in the intestines is decreased and paradoxically facilitates phosphate retention. (4) Thus the normal process of bone mineralization with calcium and phosphate is impaired. Demineralization of the bone frees more calcium and phosphorus into the blood. As the disease progresses even more, the parathyroid gland may become unresponsive to the normal feedback system and continue to produce PTH, causing acceleration of renal osteodystrophy.

matrix formation. Osteitis fibrosa results in inflammation and fibrosis of bone because of high bone turnover, while adynamic bone disease is a low bone turnover state, which may be related to excessive PTH suppression from therapy.[76]

Clients with renal osteodystrophy may present with bone pain, especially in the spine, hips, knees, or lower extremities, and fractures.[76] The pain is worse with exercise and other weight-bearing activities; the fractures occur most often in the vertebrae and long bones.[78] Increased secretion of PTH and a decreased secretion of calcitriol appear to be the cause. Metabolic acidosis may also play a role, either by increasing osteoclastic activity or by increasing the effects of PTH.[290]

Osteopenia and pseudofractures are seen most frequently in people with osteomalacia. Osteitis fibrosa is evident on radiographic films, particularly in the phalanges, skull, and distal clavicles, where there is subperiosteal bone resorption.

In addition to bone demineralization, calcification of vessels and soft tissues occurs. This calcification may be related to bone turnover and occurs during both high and low bone turnover. It is postulated that deposition of minerals may occur in extraskeletal sites because the bone is unable to incorporate them. If bone turnover is high, minerals are removed from bone and are deposited in extraskeletal sites. If bone turnover is low, minerals are also deposited in extraskeletal sites because the bone is forming abnormally or at a slow rate.

The most common sites for extraskeletal calcification include the coronary arteries, lungs, skin, peripheral arteries, joints, and cornea. Calcifications of the coronary arteries are common and may be the reason for the high death rate in CKD clients. Intraarterial calcifications can occlude vessels, leading to ischemia and gangrene.

Deposition of minerals in the skin can lead to intense pruritus (itching), and occlusion of an arteriole can cause necrosis of skin, termed *calciphylaxis*. This occurs most commonly in the lower extremities, trunk, or buttocks. Articular cartilage and joints can become calcified, causing pseudogout and arthritis symptoms.

Calcification of a tendon may lead to spontaneous rupture with minimal stress. The quadriceps tendon may rupture simply by walking, tripping, or going down stairs. Tendon ruptures can lead to pain, deformity, and disability. Other areas of commonly observed ruptures in this population include the triceps and extensor tendons of the fingers.[78] Hyperparathyroidism and metabolic acidosis are responsible for the abnormal collagen that results in weak tendons.[51,290]

Calcifications are frequently found on the cornea and conjunctiva but are typically asymptomatic. Clients who have kidney disease characterized by a slow decline in function may have more severe cases of both renal osteodystrophy and calcification of vessels and soft tissue. (Although cardiovascular manifestations were discussed earlier in this section, in view of the information here on calcification, it should be noted that vascular calcification of the arteries resulting in vascular insufficiency has been observed in nearly all individuals with ESRD by age 50 years. In fact, most people with CKD actually die from cardiovascular disease, rather than progress to the final stages of ESRD.[143,227])

Myopathy can occur with proximal muscle weakness affecting the muscles of the shoulder and pelvic girdles, leading to functional disabilities. The gluteus medius, hamstring, and psoas muscles are affected first and most severely, resulting in gait impairments and difficulty rising from low seats or accomplishing functional activities such as getting in and out of a bathtub. As the condition progresses, activities of daily living, such as combing the hair, brushing the teeth, or household tasks, become more difficult to manage independently.

Neurologic. Alteration of central nervous system and peripheral nervous system function often occurs in association with ESRD. Early central nervous system changes include sleeping disturbances (both getting to sleep and staying asleep) followed by daytime sleepiness and personality changes.

Uremic encephalopathy occurs when the GFR is less than 10 mL/min and is manifested by recent memory loss, inability to concentrate, perceptual errors, confusion, asterixis, and decreased alertness. These symptoms abate once dialysis is instituted. Without treatment, seizures, lethargy, obtundation, and coma develop.

The peripheral neuropathy associated with uremic toxins is characterized by a dying back of the axons of both sensory and motor nerves. These neurologic changes are typically symmetrical (stocking-glove distribution) and similar to those of any other polyneuropathy with a stocking-glove distribution. Clients can also exhibit restless leg syndrome, which occurs in up to 40% of uremic clients.[112] Like central nervous system manifestations of uremia, peripheral nervous system symptoms improve with dialysis.

MEDICAL MANAGEMENT

PREVENTION. Everyone should be screened for hypertension and diabetes with early intervention when present. The ultimate goal and mission of the National Kidney Foundation is the eradication of diseases of the kidney. Toward that end, *Healthy People 2020* has identified several goals related to kidney failure, including (1) reduce kidney failure resulting from diabetes; (2) increase the proportion of people with chronic kidney failure who receive a transplant within 3 years of registration on the waiting list; (3) increase the proportion of people with chronic kidney failure who receive counseling on nutrition, treatment choices, and cardiovascular care 12 months before the start of renal replacement therapy; (4) reduce deaths from cardiovascular disease in persons with chronic kidney failure; and (5) reduce the rate of new cases of ESRD.

Because diabetic nephropathy is the leading cause of kidney failure in the United States, prevention strategies and risk factor modification related to improving glycemic control, preventing hypertension, preventing coronary artery disease, increasing physical activity, and reducing or eliminating tobacco-related behaviors (e.g., smoking) are a large part of the prevention of renal disease. In the future, pancreas transplantation may become a part of diabetes prevention and therefore ESRD prevention.

DIAGNOSIS. As discussed earlier, the early stages of CKD are often without symptoms. Because of the significant morbidity and mortality associated with CKD, early detection is emphasized, with the goal of slowing progression or reversing the disease if possible. People with diabetes, hypertension, or a family history of kidney disease are at high risk for kidney disease and should be monitored for early indications of kidney disease.

Because there are many causes for CKD, multiple tests may be required to determine the cause and severity. Several laboratory tests are helpful in detecting and following progression of CKD and ESRD. Persons with diabetes should routinely be tested for microprotein in the urine (an indication of early kidney disease). GFR, BUN, and creatinine are blood tests that can indicate kidney dysfunction (GFR is actually calculated using laboratory results).

In the presence of CKD, GFR will be the first laboratory indicator of renal damage, followed by increases in BUN and creatinine with continued kidney damage. GFR not only characterizes the stage of kidney disease but also demonstrates disease progression. Urine tests may show protein or casts (abnormal protein "castings" of the tubules). For those persons with known CKD or ESRD, intact PTH (or N-terminal PTH molecule) levels should be monitored in an attempt to avoid renal osteodystrophy.

Imaging modalities may demonstrate obstruction, masses, or bilateral small kidneys (which is consistent with ESRD from a chronic disease). A kidney biopsy may be needed to confirm specific kidney pathology (such as a glomerulonephritis).

TREATMENT. Following the diagnosis of CKD, a referral to a nephrologist should be made. Although best outcomes occur when a referral is made early in the course of CKD, up to 40% are not referred until 3 months prior to initiating dialysis.[281] Delayed referrals lead to an increase in morbidity and mortality.

The goals of treating CKD include treating the underlying disease, modifying risk factors for cardiovascular disease, and preventing further loss of kidney function. For some diseases, treating the principal disease may involve immunosuppressive agents, such as with the treatment of membranous nephropathy. Renal artery stenosis may require angioplasty with stenting. Diabetes requires tight glycemic control.

Cardiovascular complications are common and require risk factor modification and treatment. Clients with CKD should lose weight, exercise, eliminate smoking, and modify their diet. Dyslipidemia treatment involves lifestyle modifications, and medication may be needed. Blood pressure should be strictly controlled in order to reduce cardiovascular risk and prevent further loss of renal function (although the exact range is disputed, a systolic blood pressure between 120 mm Hg and 130 mm Hg should be the goal).[169]

Measures that help prevent further loss of kidney function include avoidance of nephrotoxic drugs and radiocontrast agents; treatment of anemia; strict blood pressure control; and the use of ACE inhibitors or ARBs.[169]

For the predialysis stage, data are lacking to establish the optimal hemoglobin level to begin erythropoietin therapy. But a more recommendation has been published to suggest initiation of subcutaneous erythropoietin when the hemoglobin drops below 10 g/dL, after verification of adequate iron stores and exclusion of other causes of anemia.[72] Studies demonstrate that the use of an ACE inhibitor or ARB is renoprotective beyond the ability of just lowering blood pressure.

The treatment of clients who develop ESRD continues with many of the same measures used to treat the other stages of CKD, such as blood pressure control and anemia treatment. Dietary modifications are necessary, including low-potassium, low-sodium, and low-protein diets. Excess protein can increase urea levels, and clients should not consume more than 1 g/kg per day of protein. Dietitian referrals are important, since malnutrition may occur with strict dietary regulation. Fluid intake is restricted, and diuretics are needed to maintain fluid balance.

Prevention of renal osteodystrophy necessitates monitoring of calcium–phosphate balance and PTH levels. The goal is to maintain calcium at less than 9.5 mg/dL and phosphate at less than 5.5 mg/dL. This has typically been accomplished using calcium-binding agents and vitamin D sterols.

New questions have been raised, however, concerning calcification of vessels (principally the coronary arteries) and calcium/phosphate metabolism. The traditional methods of lowering calcium and phosphate may still leave levels too high to reduce calcification of the coronary arteries. A new calcimimetic agent, recently approved by the FDA, called cinacalcet, appears to treat secondary hyperparathyroidism and maintain normal calcium and phosphate levels. Further use of this drug in a larger population will determine efficacy in preventing renal osteodystrophy and cardiovascular complications.

Renal replacement therapy (dialysis or transplantation) is the treatment of choice for ESRD. The decision is based on the client's age, general health, donor availability, and personal preference. Dialysis can take the form of hemodialysis (HD) or peritoneal dialysis (PD) (also referred to as *continuous ambulatory peritoneal dialysis [CAPD]* and *continuous cycling peritoneal dialysis [CCPD]*). The main difference between these methods of dialysis is in their exchange schedules (daytime vs. nighttime, length of time required).

HD typically requires three sessions per week for 3 to 4 hours per session. The blood flows from an artery through the dialysis machine chambers and then back to the body's venous system, with the waste products and excess fluid and electrolytes diffusing into the dialyzing solution. HD can be done at home, although this requires specialized training, or the client can travel to a renal center. Although it is common practice that the person remains relatively immobile throughout the session, studies show that appropriately prescribed low- to moderate-intensity exercise programs done during the first 2 hours of dialysis can improve physical health, quality of life, and dialysis efficacy.[43,44,196,206,217,263] Only 1% of dialysis clients receive home HD, while 85% receive in-center treatment.

Approximately 10% of dialysis clients use PD. PD relies on the same principles as HD, it can be done independently at home whereas individuals on home HD must have a care partner to assist them. A catheter is implanted in the peritoneal cavity, and sterile dialyzing solution is instilled and then drained over a specific period. This process is completed four times daily or at night while the individual sleeps. With CAPD/CCPD, fewer dietary restrictions and fewer of the dramatic symptom swings associated with HD occur. Potential complications of PD include infection, catheter malfunction, dehydration, hyperglycemia, and hernia. Peritonitis occurs about once every 3 years in those undergoing PD and is the most serious potential complication. The majority of affected people are successfully treated with intraperitoneal antibiotics.

The steady improvement in the outcome of renal allografts has made kidney transplantation the treatment of choice for many people with ESRD. Transplantation is less expensive than long-term dialysis, but donor availability limits the number of transplants performed. The current contraindications for transplant include active substance abuse or noncompliance, metastatic cancer, severe arterial disease involving the iliac arteries, active infection, active ischemic cardiac and cerebrovascular disease, advanced dementia, and debility.

In adults, the renal graft is placed extraperitoneally in the iliac fossa through an oblique lower abdominal incision. In small children, the graft is located retroperitoneally with a midline abdominal incision. Complications of the procedures include renal artery thrombosis, urinary leak, and lymphocele.

PROGNOSIS. Despite significant advances in technologic and pharmacologic interventions, the current annual mortality rate of people with ESRD in the United States is approximately 24% compared to the general population.[10] Cardiovascular diseases remain the number one cause of death in those with all categories of renal disease, including persons with CKD, those with ESRD on dialysis, and renal transplant recipients. This is most likely a result of the presence of multiple cardiovascular risk factors (e.g., hypertension, abnormal lipids, smoking, dietary factors).[175] Individuals with diabetes and ESRD have higher morbidity and mortality rates than individuals with ESRD only.[199]

Nephrogenic Systemic Fibrosis

Michael S. Castillo, PT, MHS, MPA, GCS, NCS

Nephrogenic systemic fibrosis (NSF), also earlier known as nephrogenic fibrosing dermopathy, is an illness recently described in individuals with kidney disease presenting with firm, erythematous, indurated plaques of the skin associated with subcutaneous edema.[237]

Once believed to affect only the skin (hence the previous name), further testing revealed it affects several structures and organs. Postmortem autopsy of affected individuals showed fibrosis and calcification of the psoas muscle, renal tubules, testes, and diaphragm, to name a few.[114] People with this condition present with skin thickening on their arms, legs, and torso; similar skin lesions are absent from the face. The skin lesions are typically symmetrical and distributed bilaterally and seem to fuse

together to form hyperpigmented plaques that resemble the "skin of an orange" (also known as peau d'orange).[114] These areas are described as pruritic with concomitant burning pain sensation.

The first incidence of NSF was observed in 1997 in renal transplantation centers worldwide among individuals receiving HD. The majority were kidney transplant recipients who are or were rejecting the donor organ. The occurrence in this population initially led some investigators to think of possible infection or contamination during dialysis.

Medical practitioners were quick to note its similarity to scleromyxedema and were calling it "scleromyxedema-like cutaneous disease during dialysis." It was later differentiated from scleromyxedema by the absence of paraproteinemia and the absence of pools of dermal mucin and plasma cell infiltrates.[67]

The probable etiology of NSF remained unknown until 2006 when several people developed NSF within weeks of receiving gadolinium for magnetic resonance angiography or contrast-enhanced MRI. Scientists found a strong correlation between exposure to a gadolinium-based contrast agent and NSF in individuals with kidney disease, particularly in the presence of a proinflammatory process such as major surgery, infection, or a vascular thromboembolic event.[110,237]

It was hypothesized that the high doses of free gadolinium ions may have caused a toxic reaction. In the same year, the FDA issued a health advisory stating that for at-risk kidney individuals, alternative imaging is indicated to avoid exposure to gadolinium-based contrast agents.[27,177] However, because not all people who develop NSF can be traced to an exposure to a gadolinium-based contrast agent,[276] more studies are needed to search for a definitive answer.

There is still no known cure for NSF. Some cases resolve after renal transplantation and others after plasmapheresis. Treatment options being considered include oral and topical corticosteroids, photophoresis, ultraviolet therapy, and high dose immunoglobulin therapy.[27] The majority of affected individuals develop complications such as decreased joint mobility, flexion contractures, and resulting muscle weakness. Physical therapy is highly recommended for this population.[150] NSF is a debilitating disease and is proving to be an unwelcome burden to an already physically fragile group. Further research is needed to its cause, management and most importantly, prevention.

A THERAPIST'S THOUGHTS*
NEPHROGENIC SYSTEMIC FIBROSIS

People with kidney disease or injury are an especially challenging population when it comes to exercise prescription. They have varying sensitivities to medications, nutrition, and physical activity. Depending on the severity of their condition, these persons can have diminished activity tolerance and strength, resulting to impaired mobility status relative to comparable age-groups.[22,36,123] Their weakened condition can easily tip toward a vulnerable state.

Nephrogenic systemic fibrosis is a crippling condition that is afflicting this population. NSF manifestations include thickening of the skin and connective tissue, which can lead to muscle tightness and contractures. The trunk and the extremities can be equally

A THERAPIST'S THOUGHTS—cont'd
NEPHROGENIC SYSTEMIC FIBROSIS

involved. Afflicted individuals have also complained of sharp joint pains, as well as deep bone pain on the hips and ribs. These symptoms can result in progressive weakness and loss of function. It is imperative that prompt intervention is provided in order to avoid further deconditioning. Physical therapy should be instituted and be part of a comprehensive treatment program.

These individuals may benefit from joint manipulation with connective tissue mobilization and massage. Distal joints such as those of the hands can utilize paraffin wax treatments to increase flexibility and range of motion. Manual stretching of affected joints and skin can relieve the feeling of restricted movement. Therapeutic pool exercises and swimming has been found to be beneficial for this group. Individuals may need an assessment and instruction on the use of an assistive device or an ambulatory aid in order to continue their level of mobility. Both the individual and the individual's caregivers should be educated about the condition and instructed on a program so as to extend the management to the home setting. The physical therapist should consider all possibilities so as to prevent inactivity and to maintain the individual's quality-of-life.

As a result of the accompanying complaints of pain, a formal pain management program conducted by a physician-led team should be established. A special consideration brought about by the thickened skin is the difficulty in finding venous access in the extremities. Any current and potential access should be identified and kept patent for intravenous use.

Perhaps more importantly than the support and treatment to affected individuals is the prevention of the condition itself. Each health professional in every setting should be vigilant about possibly exposing at-risk individuals to gadolinium-based agents, and should advise on its potential for causing NSF. There may be other causes for the development of NSF and it is our priority to avert any occurrence. This can only be consistently done by consciously staying informed and current on research.

*Michael S. Castillo, PT, MHS, MPA, GCS, NCS

SPECIAL IMPLICATIONS FOR THE THERAPIST 18-5

Chronic Kidney Disease

Therapists must be aware that several specific renal syndromes may be induced by the interaction of NSAIDs and other analgesics (see Table 5-1) on renal function. Although the nephrotoxicity is relatively low, the increased availability of these medications as nonprescription products and the concentration of people taking NSAIDs/analgesics in a rehabilitation setting are factors contributing to the fact that a larger percentage of these people come into contact with a therapist. Anyone with renal failure who is a regular user of acetaminophen and aspirin is at up to 2.2 times higher risk of developing CKD.[88] Analgesic nephropathy is still a real risk, but has dramatically declined as a result of the removal of phenacetin from the analgesic market, although mixed analgesics containing paracetamol, the main metabolite of phenacetin, remain popularly used.[185,186]

Older adults are especially susceptible and more likely to use these agents. Additionally, NSAID-related renal involvement is probably underrecognized, and

with the FDA approval of nonprescription sale of NSAIDs (e.g., naproxen sodium, ketoprofen, ibuprofen), incidence may increase in the coming years.[178] Any time a client reports a history of prolonged and regular NSAID/analgesic use and renal symptoms, medical evaluation is required. In general, clinicians are advised to consider the risk and benefits on a case-by-case basis, with determination and consideration of the affected individual's CKD status and use of NSAIDs. The potential risk of CKD progression maybe outweighed by the individual's improved quality of life.[224]

Physical therapy care of people with CKD has increased significantly in the past 20 years. Treating people with a diagnosis of CKD can be extremely challenging because of malnutrition, side effects of medications, complications from dialysis, and the number of body systems involved. The decreased alertness, inability to concentrate, and short-term memory deficits interfere with following instructions, including transfers, exercises, body mechanics, and so on.

Musculoskeletal changes occur because of abnormalities in calcium, phosphate, and vitamin D metabolism, resulting in osteomalacia, osteoporosis, and soft-tissue calcification. Spontaneous tendon ruptures have been reported in the ESRD population, especially those individuals with hyperparathyroidism. Their risk is increased when treated with quinolone antibiotics and/or steroids.[13] Neuromuscular effects of CKD include both central and peripheral nervous system disorders. Kasinskas and Piazza offer consideration for a clinical pathway for clients with CKD using the *Guide to Physical Therapist Practice* that is worth reviewing for any therapist working with this population group.[4,145]

Adverse effects of some of the medications used for renovascular hypertension may include angioedema (i.e., swelling around the face, mouth, or throat), requiring immediate medical attention. Clients should be taught to rise slowly, dangling the legs and feet before standing, and to report any unusual swelling.

Reliance on the assistance of family and other health care providers is often necessary. The fatigue and general weakness may dictate that the therapist provide rest periods during a rehabilitation session. The potential osteodystrophy requires modification of evaluation and intervention techniques, including osteoporosis education and prevention (see "Special Implications for the Therapist 24-1: Osteoporosis" in Chapter 24).

A number of potential renal transplantation complications that the therapist should be aware of are hypertension, lipid disorders, hepatitis, cancer, tendinopathies, and osteopenia (see "Transplantation" in Chapter 21). Lastly, corticosteroids appear to be the primary factor in the impaired bone formation found in graft recipients (see Chapter 5).

Dialysis

Complications of dialysis are multiple and varied. Fluid shifts during dialysis can contribute to adverse neuromuscular and hemodynamic consequences that must be reported so that adjustments can be made in the dialysis fluid (dialysate). Symptoms of increased thirst and weight gain are common, and the weight gain and abdominal distention, especially with CAPD/CCPD, may cause extreme distress in the individual.

Depression among people on dialysis may be more common than is currently recognized, often masquerading as functional impairment, anorexia, or noncompliance. It has been suggested that approximately 20% to 30% of the ESRD population suffer from depression.[48] Impaired libido, impotence, infertility, dysfunctional uterine bleeding, amenorrhea, and anovulation are very common. Altered platelet function results in bleeding tendencies in anyone with uremia, and the therapist is advised to follow the precautions listed in Tables 40-8 and 40-9.

People on dialysis have increased susceptibility to infection by various pathogens because they are immunosuppressed, and the dialysis process requires vascular access for prolonged periods of time. Infection of the vascular access site is a major concern, because signs and symptoms of local infection are often absent early on. Careful monitoring for infection or inflammation is warranted, with early medical referral. Standard precautions are essential for the individual in a dialysis unit, for those individuals dialyzing and handling the equipment at home, and for the treating therapist.

Contact transmission can be prevented by hand hygiene (i.e., handwashing or use of a waterless hand rub), glove use, and disinfection of environmental surfaces. Of these, hand hygiene is the most important. In addition, nonsterile disposable gloves provide a protective barrier for workers' hands, preventing them from becoming soiled or contaminated, and reduce the likelihood that microorganisms present on the hands of personnel will be transmitted to clients. It is important to remember to use the hand rub prior to reaching for the gloves so as to prevent contaminating the gloves in the process of putting them on. However, even with glove use, handwashing is needed, because pathogens deposited on the outer surface of gloves can be detected on hands after glove removal, possibly because of holes or defects in the gloves, leakage at the wrist, or contamination of hands during glove removal.[39]

During progressive renal failure, catabolism and anorexia lead to loss of lean body mass, but concurrent fluid retention and weight gain can mask the loss of body mass. Malnutrition, anemia, and this loss of body mass can result in significant losses in muscle strength, requiring careful assessment and rehabilitation. The mixed sensory and motor peripheral neuropathy common in people with uremia often improves symptomatically with adequate dialysis. Muscle mass will also improve with consistently good dialysis and nutrition.

Fluid retention also results in hypertension at the beginning of dialysis; alternatively, dialysis can result in dialysis hypotension when fluid is removed too quickly or too much is removed causing a nervous system response to the drop in blood volume. Dialysis hypotension affects up to 50% of individuals who receive this treatment. It is defined as a decrease in systolic blood pressure by more than 20 mm Hg or a decrease in mean arterial pressure by 10 mm Hg associated with any of the following signs and symptoms: abdominal discomfort, yawning, sighing, nausea, vomiting, muscle cramps, restlessness, dizziness or fainting, and/or anxiety.[214]

The therapist should ask the client about the dialysis schedule and encourage the individual not to miss any treatment. Younger clients and those who have recently started dialysis are more likely to miss treatments. This may be reflected in rising blood pressure and elevated pulse rate. Monitoring vital signs and laboratory values is essential throughout the rehabilitative process.

Chest and back pain can occur during the early days of dialysis, referred to as *first-use syndrome*. Delayed hypersensitivity reactions with mild itching and urticaria may be reported to (or observed by) the therapist. Maintaining the dialysis access site is critical, but is often difficult secondary to recurrent thromboses. Extreme caution must be given to the access site during any rehabilitation or exercise intervention. Ischemia of the arm (or leg, depending on the location of the fistula) may be the first indication of thrombosis and subsequent stenosis. Any of these signs and symptoms should be reported to the renal staff.

Exercise Considerations for Individuals with Chronic Kidney Disease

For the individual with CKD, myopathies, neuropathies, and reduced muscle mass, carrying and lifting the bag of dialysate can be difficult. Strength training, balance, and mobility are key components of a home exercise program for the person using CAPD/CCPD.

Gains in strength and mobility are possible but may require a mildly to moderately intense rehabilitation program of longer duration than expected.[153,182,223] What may seem like a short-term goal for the average, healthy adult can be a long-term goal for someone with CKD, especially the client with end-stage kidney disease.

Exercise can be performed before, during, or after dialysis. Finding the best schedule may take a period of trial and error. For some people, functional tolerance may be lowest the day before the first and second dialysis sessions of the week. Establishing a plan of care that takes into account day-to-day differences in energy, function, and motivation may have a chance for better outcomes.[274]

Compliance can be a big issue if the therapist is unable to convey to the client the importance of exercise and how an exercise program can really benefit that individual. Focusing on greater function and independence in day-to-day activities and gaining an increased sense of well-being or quality of life may be more important to the client than riding a bicycle 10 minutes twice each day.

Living with CKD usually involves management of other chronic conditions such as diabetes or hypertension. The changes required in lifestyle can create a profound sense of loss, depression, and emotional fatigue for some individuals.[275] They often report memory loss and a decreased ability to stay on task.

When exercise is performed after dialysis, blood chemistry levels will be at their optimum, although fatigue may be a factor. Exercise during dialysis may be an option for some and usually improves the efficiency of dialysis because of better mobilization of dependent fluids and improved solute removal,[69] but most people do not choose this option.

The limited research available has shown that impaired oxygen transport plays a role in limiting exercise in anyone with CKD, especially once dialysis begins.[187,239] Adults with CKD have low cardiorespiratory capacity with maximum oxygen consumption (VO_2max) at one-third to one-half the normal rates for age-matched sedentary but healthy adults without kidney disease. They often show signs and symptoms of anemia, fatigue, wasting, and reduced work capacity with concomitant findings of reduced cardiac performance and muscle mass.[138,295]

Functional capacity in people on dialysis is typically more than two standard deviations below the age- and gender-predicted norm and is often far lower, sometimes barely enough to carry out activities of daily living. A prescriptive program of regular activity and exercise can improve physical functioning, exercise tolerance, and health-related quality of life.[190,210,213] Fatigue severity does respond with low-level exercise during dialysis, but the exercise must continue to maintain the effect.[295]

Exercise Prescription

Low- to moderate-intensity exercise can increase exercise capacity and possibly improve blood pressure for individuals with CKD.[212] Individuals with CKD benefit from stationary bicycle exercise protocols requiring exercise three times a week at intensities of 40% to 70% of the target heart rate.

Exercise can be done on dialysis days as well as on nondialysis days. Some people may find it more difficult to exercise on dialysis days or even during dialysis due to decrease in blood pressure and muscle cramping. Both are common side effects of dialysis.[296]

Clients who exercise both during dialysis and on nondialysis days have greater improvements in exercise tolerance and peak VO_2max compared to individuals who exercise only during dialysis or only on nondialysis days.[72]

Exercise protocols consisting of gentle stretching and warm-up followed by an aerobic phase beginning at intensities of 50% to 60% of the target heart rate, followed by a low-intensity cool-down and relaxation phase can increase exercise tolerance.[118]

The beneficial effects of regular aquatic exercise on cardiorespiratory function, renal lipids, and oxidative stress have been studied in a group of individuals with mild to moderate renal failure. Low-intensity aerobic exercises in the pool for 30 minutes twice a week over a period of 12 weeks led to improvement in cardiorespiratory function, improved resting blood pressure, and enhanced GFR.[100]

Exercise Considerations for Individuals with End-Stage Renal Disease

ESRD is characterized by compromised autonomic function associated with cardiac mortality; this is particularly prevalent in people with diabetes. Autonomic dysfunction may limit maximal age-predicted heart rates by as much as 20 to 40 beats/min. Therefore, when prescribing exercise intensity, the perceived exertion rating may be a better choice for monitoring exercise.[167]

Exercise has been identified as a factor associated with improved autonomic cardiac function in ESRD.[37,38] Exercise prescription for anyone with chronic disease and/or disability must take these factors into consideration. For anyone with CKD and diabetes, glucose levels must also be taken into consideration when planning, monitoring, and, when possible, progressing an exercise program.

A timely and effective rehabilitation program can improve quality of life, endurance, and functional abilities toward greater independence. For the individual on dialysis, the most important independent quality-of-life predictor is the usual level of exercise activity. The person's perception of physical functioning as it relates to quality of life is important, because these variables can be the focus for intervention strategies to prevent early deterioration in dialysis.[159-161]

The individual's clinical condition (and response to exercise) provides the greatest guidance in determining exercise or physical activity mode, intensity, frequency, and duration. With numerous medical problems associated with ESRD, a major concern before initiating an exercise program is physiologic stability.

Exercise testing before starting an exercise program is usually not recommended for this population group. Muscle fatigue limits testing procedures, and the results do not really offer any new information. General exercise guidelines for individuals with ESRD are for exercise four to six times each week; low exercise capacity may direct the therapist toward establishing an interval training program to start. The goal is to exercise for longer periods of time, with 30 minutes as the final desired outcome. Intensity is kept low, especially on days the individual undergoes dialysis. The rate of perceived exertion (RPE) scale can be used to monitor intensity.[78]

Many of the risks of exercise are related more to exacerbation of comorbid conditions (e.g., arthritis, diabetes, hypertension) than to the kidney disease itself. Exercise might cause a potassium efflux from exercising muscles and may elevate blood levels, although the possibility of exercise-induced hyperkalemia and resultant cardiac arrhythmias is small. Serum potassium levels must be controlled before exercise and should not be greater than 5 mEq/L. Individuals with uncontrolled blood chemistries should avoid weight training.

Reviews of specific prescription principles, including weight-training guidelines, for individuals with chronic disease and specifically renal disease are available.[14,74,167,190] Some sources recommend exercise during dialysis[211,212] (see discussion in next section) and the day after dialysis, as the chance of instability is greater before dialysis (PD is usually done daily and is easiest with an empty abdomen for mechanical reasons).

Exercise may help control blood pressure, especially in those individuals who are hypertensive. Blood pressure should be monitored in the arm opposite the arteriovenous shunt before exercise. If blood pressure is greater than 200/100 mm Hg, the individual should not exercise. Exercise can also improve lipid levels and glucose metabolism, and increase hematocrit and hemoglobin levels. Psychosocial effects, such as improved mood and quality of life, are also possible.[139,209,210]

Anyone with diabetes should be monitored for hypoglycemia or sudden drops in blood glucose levels. In addition, the kidney is essential in the production of vitamin D, which is necessary for calcium absorption. Exercise training ameliorates the enhanced muscle protein degradation associated with chronic renal failure.

Anyone undergoing dialysis will be monitored for bone disease; strengthening exercises can help bone density, and bone density studies can provide outcome-based evidence of the value of exercise in these clients. In the case of polycystic kidney disease, moderate exercise in animal models was considered safe but did not alter bone mineral density. Additional research in this area is needed, as other benefits may be derived from exercise in this and other kidney-diseased populations.[68]

Exercise During Hemodialysis
Janice T. Dinglasan, PT, MPT

Although advancements in hemodialysis treatment have done well to expand the life span, this does not ensure preservation of quality of life. Persons with CKD and, subsequently, end-stage renal disease, are plagued with associated musculoskeletal, vascular, cardiac, immunologic, and various physiologic complications.[217,297]

Compared to healthy age- and sex-matched counterparts, those with CKD show a 50% reduced physical work capacity.[217] This corresponds to approximately 3 to 5 metabolic equivalents of the task (METs; 1 MET is equal to energy expenditure at rest; activities of daily living require 1.5-5 METs). Ultimately, this can lead to a sedentary lifestyle, decreased independence, and decreased quality of life—all of which can be improved by appropriately prescribed exercise training.[40,139]

The time spent during hemodialysis treatment, whether in an inpatient or outpatient setting, is typically viewed as a time of inactivity and exercise treatments are deferred. However, studies to verify the effectiveness of low- to moderate-intensity exercise programs done during the first 2 hours of hemodialysis have provided evidence-based protocols (see Evolve Table 18-1: Summary of Exercise Protocols, which is found on the book's Evolve website).[45,189,196,206,217]

Both resistive strengthening exercises and aerobic training done intradialytically have shown to be safe, practical, effective, and preferable[153,196,217] in improving muscle strength,[43,44,206,263] physical performance,[40,45,217,263] cardiopulmonary function,[153,263] quality of life/psychologic well-being,[44,45,206] and dialysis efficacy.[44,217]

Exercise protocols included strength interventions that were done in a seated, semi-recumbent or supine position directly from the dialysis chair. Interventions consisted of open- and closed-chain hip and knee exercises with or without resistance at a submaximal individually determined intensity,[45,206] or were done isokinetically.[196] Duration of the exercise varied from 2 to 3 sets of 8 to 15 repetitions.

Aerobic interventions were also performed at submaximal rates of 50% to 60% of VO$_2$peak using a cycle ergometer or weighted stepper.[40,189,196,206,217,263] Intensities were individually determined (based on RPE, target heart rate, subjective symptoms, or work rates [Watts] determined by a peak study), duration ranged from 5 to 30 minutes with 60 minutes of cumulative cycling being the maximum. Cycling was done intermittently or continuously based on individual tolerance. Blood pressure, heart rate, subjective symptoms, and RPE were continuously monitored.

Adverse reactions were minimized when exercise was performed within first 2 hours of hemodialysis, when cardiovascular response is stable. After 3 hours, cardiovascular decompensation precluded exercise and resulted in increased incidences of hypotension and muscle cramping.[189]

Intradialytic exercise also provides an easy means for medical supervision and can facilitate increased compliance and good habit forming for this cohort.[40,153] Careful consideration must be given to inclusion/exclusion criteria to reduce potential risks or complications.

Ideal candidates will be compliant with their current dialysis, medication, and diet regimens and will have received clearance from their doctor to participate. Significant cardiovascular, neurologic, or orthopedic complications may also limit full participation. It is important to note that development of such a program in any setting requires a multidisciplinary effort. Collaboration among nephrologists, physical therapists, nurses, and dialysis technicians should occur prior to program implementation.

Routine exercise is important for this population as many have comorbid medical conditions that restrict physical and psychologic aspects of life. International studies indicate that routine exercise is associated with better outcomes for this population. Furthermore, patients at hemodialysis facilities that offer exercise programs show higher odds of exercising.[273]

Individuals on dialysis who routinely exercise show increased physical fitness and psychological function; both contribute to improved quality of life. Intradialytic exercise can be an intervention that provides a means to enhance quality of life as the CKD life span has been lengthened through improvements in care.[40]

A THERAPIST'S THOUGHTS*
EXERCISE DURING HEMODIALYSIS

Because exercise during hemodialysis presents a nontraditional approach to treatment, there is no formal exercise protocol that is standardized for this population. Consequently, this section should neither be viewed as if the information is complete nor as if it was

A THERAPIST'S THOUGHTS—cont'd
EXERCISE DURING HEMODIALYSIS

written to convey that this approach must be integrated as routine treatment; although, we may get there in the future.

The intent of the exercise during hemodialysis section is to provide general guidelines for exercise protocols and inclusion/exclusion criteria based on an informal review of current research. The section was written with the mindset to introduce a physical therapist to this topic and to challenge the therapist's stance on current treatment strategies, possibly leading to further research.

The exercise protocols were not exclusively performed or supervised by physical therapists. However, physical therapists are uniquely qualified to develop and supervise such programs because of our ability to understand principles of exercise physiology and how they relate to pathology. For a population that is stricken by comorbid conditions that limit exercise capacity, physical therapists may be the ideal health care professionals to oversee such a program. Regardless of when the exercise is performed for this population, physical therapists must continue with their roles as educators, motivators, and facilitators for maximizing function and independence.

*Janice T. Dinglasan, PT, MPT

Laboratory Values

Renal failure causes metabolic waste products to accumulate in the blood, which can be measured to assess renal function. The two most commonly measured waste products are serum creatinine and BUN. Changes in creatinine and BUN levels do not usually contraindicate physical or occupational therapy intervention, but other test measures are important. Depressed serum albumin levels reflect poor nutritional status and these laboratory values should be monitored whenever available (see "Renal Function Tests" in Chapter 40 and Table 40-2).

People with ESRD often have low levels of hemoglobin associated with anemia and poor exercise tolerance due to excessive fatigue. Dyspnea at rest or on exertion, increased fatigue, and chest pain with exertion may be signs of low hematocrit levels. Exercise guidelines based on laboratory values provided in Chapter 40 can be used with clients who have ESRD. Keep in mind that hemoglobin and hematocrit levels are usually lower for people with ESRD; potassium, creatinine, and BUN levels will be higher than normal.

GLOMERULAR DISEASES
Overview

Glomerular diseases are a group of conditions that damage the kidney's filtering units (glomeruli). Glomerulonephritis is also a group of diseases that affect the glomeruli but specifically manifest with hematuria. Glomerulonephritis is a glomerular disease, but not all glomerular diseases are termed *glomerulonephritis*. Glomerular diseases are the most common cause of ESRD worldwide, while glomerulonephritis is the third leading cause of end-stage kidney disease in the United States.

The glomeruli are tufts of capillaries connecting the afferent and efferent arterioles of the nephron (see Fig. 18-6). The capillaries are supported by a stalk made up of mesangial cells and a basement membrane and are arranged in lobules. The circulating blood is filtered in the glomeruli, with the urine filtrate being an end-product. Glomerular damage produces two types of syndromes: the nephrotic syndrome and the nephritic syndrome.

Nephrotic syndrome is not a specific kidney disease but rather occurs as a result of any disease that causes damage to the kidney-filtering units. Nephrotic syndrome is principally associated with proteinuria, which occurs with such diseases as diabetes, amyloidosis, and membranous glomerulopathy. *Nephritic syndrome* is correlated with hematuria. Glomerular diseases that result in a nephritic syndrome include lupus nephritis, immunoglobulin A (IgA) nephropathy, and acute diffuse proliferative glomerulonephritis. Overlap of the two syndromes is common, and a precise diagnosis often requires a kidney biopsy.

Etiologic Factors

Most cases of nephritic syndrome and some cases of nephrotic syndrome have an immune origin and are part of a systemic process, such as lupus nephritis or membranoproliferative glomerulonephritis. Two different mechanisms have been proposed to account for the pathologic changes seen in glomerular diseases. The first is a result of the deposition of a circulating antigen–antibody complex into some portion of the glomerulus (the glomerular basement membrane [GBM], mesangium), followed by an inflammatory response and damage. Injury is caused via the second mechanism when an antigen is deposited into the glomerulus with subsequent antibody interaction with the antigen, followed by an inflammatory response. Antigens may be exogenous, as seen in poststreptococcal glomerulonephritis, or endogenous, as noted with lupus nephritis.

Risk Factors

The presence of a variety of disorders can increase the risk of glomerular damage. Diabetes, principally type 2 diabetes, is a significant risk factor for CKD and the development of nephrotic syndrome. Age is another factor in the development of some diseases associated with nephrotic syndrome. For example, minimal change glomerulopathy is seen in children younger than age 10 years and accounts for more than 80% of cases of nephrotic syndrome in children. Race is also a factor in the development of glomerular disease. Focal segmental glomerulosclerosis is the most common cause of nephrotic syndrome in African Americans, whereas membranous nephropathy is seen more commonly in whites. Focal segmental glomerulosclerosis is also seen more often in persons who are obese.

Pathogenesis

Damage to the glomerular epithelial cells or the GBM allows larger molecules, such as protein, to escape out of the circulation and into the urine, causing nephrotic syndrome. Rupture of a capillary wall or proliferation of mesangial cells leads to hematuria and nephritic syndrome. The processes that cause this damage vary depending on the underlying glomerular disease.

Nephritic syndromes are caused by antibody–antigen complexes. Damage and clinical manifestations depend on where these complexes are deposited in the glomerulus. IgA nephropathy results when circulating antibodies (IgA antibodies) complex with an antigen (currently not defined) but are not able to be filtered through the glomerulus. These complexes stimulate an inflammatory response, accompanied by the release of cytokines and growth factors. Mesangial cell proliferation and glomerular scarring result.

Poststreptococcal glomerulonephritis occurs when antigen (streptococcal) is deposited between the glomerular epithelial cells and the GBM, resulting in an antibody response and damage to the GBM. This disruption of the GBM results in proteinuria as well as nephritis. Lupus nephritis can result from either antigen deposition followed by antibody reaction or the deposition of antibody/antigen complexes. These depositions can also occur in several locations. Those found in the mesangium result in proliferation of mesangial cells. Complexes placed in the GBM cause proteinuria, while deposition in the subepithelial space leads to nephrosis-range proteinuria. If the antigen is chronically produced, the recurrent inflammatory reactions lead to chronic glomerulonephritis. These changes adversely affect the glomerular filtration mechanism and alter capillary permeability.

Although the nephritic syndrome results most often from depositions of immune complexes, causes of nephrotic syndrome vary, with many not well understood. For example, minimal change disease shows very few abnormalities on microscopic or electron microscopic inspection. This disease may result from damage created by a lymphocyte product. Causes of other diseases, such as membranous nephropathy, are better understood. Antigen is initially deposited in the GBM with subsequent antibody interaction and inflammatory response. These immune complexes also trigger the complement system, causing further damage to the GBM and allowing large amounts of protein to escape from the plasma.

Clinical Manifestations

Glomerular disease causing a nephrotic syndrome produces proteinuria (greater than 3 g in 24 hours), hypoalbuminemia, hyperlipidemia, lipiduria, and edema. The significant loss of protein from the kidney accounts for the hypoalbuminemia, which, in turn, reduces the plasma oncotic pressure in the vessels. Fluid flows to areas of greater protein concentration, which in this instance is outside the blood vessel, causing edema. The kidney perceives a loss in volume and retains both fluid and sodium, thus increasing the edema. Edema is the principal symptom that brings affected people to the physician's office. The edema can be severe enough to be disabling.

The loss of protein also stimulates the liver to produce cholesterol, leading to hypercholesterolemia (cholesterol can be as high as 300-400 mg/dL). High cholesterol not only increases atherosclerosis of the coronary arteries but also worsens existing kidney disease. Other clinical manifestations include coagulation abnormalities from the loss of coagulation proteins, resulting in a venous thrombotic event (i.e., pulmonary embolism, deep venous thrombosis, or renal vein thrombosis). Hypothyroidism may occur secondary to the loss of thyroxine, and anemia may develop because of the loss of transferrin and erythropoietin.

The nephritic syndrome is characterized by hematuria, but oliguria, hypertension, and renal insufficiency often accompany this syndrome. The urine typically contains abnormally shaped erythrocytes (sometimes called "Mickey Mouse cells"), which distinguishes the hematuria of nephritic syndromes from that of urinary or bladder sources (normally shaped erythrocytes).

Proteinuria may be present, depending on which part of the glomerulus is affected. Hematuria may be asymptomatic, as with IgA nephropathy, or clinically apparent, as with anti-GBM antibody disease. Proliferation of mesangial cells may occur. If less than 50% of the glomeruli are affected, the disease may be asymptomatic. If greater than 50% of glomeruli are involved, hematuria and proteinuria are more profound. Renal insufficiency may be mild or may lead to a rapid loss in function. This depends on the percentage of kidney involved and the severity of the disease. Epithelial crescents form when the disease involves the Bowman space. Crescent formation or extracapillary proliferation is caused by the accumulations of macrophages, fibroblasts, proliferating epithelial cells, and fibrin within the Bowman space. *Crescentic glomerulonephritis* defines a disease process that results when more than 50% of the glomeruli have crescents. Progressive disease can result in ESRD.

MEDICAL MANAGEMENT

DIAGNOSIS. The diagnosis of glomerular disease requires analysis of urine, looking for protein, casts (protein, erythrocyte, or lymphocyte "castings" of the tubules), and erythrocytes. The erythrocytes are often misshaped, demonstrating the damage acquired while going through the glomerulus. A 24-hour urine collection may be required to assess the amount of proteinuria. Blood pressure is often elevated, and anemia may develop. A kidney biopsy is frequently needed to make the precise diagnosis.

TREATMENT. Treatment depends on the specific cause of the glomerular disease, but there are several features that may be shared and the treatment may be similar. Diseases causing nephrotic syndrome are treated with an ACE inhibitor or ARB to control blood pressure and to reduce proteinuria.

Hypercholesterolemia is usually treated with a hydroxymethylglutaryl–coenzyme A reductase inhibitor (statin). Erythropoietin can be employed if anemia is symptomatic, and vitamin D sterols may be needed to prevent a deficiency in vitamin D. Fluid is restricted, and diuretics are often used to reduce edema. Diseases with immune-associated injury often require treatment with prednisone, cyclosporine, or cytotoxic agents. Others, such as membranoproliferative glomerulonephritis, improve with treatment of the underlying disorder (i.e., treating hepatitis C–induced disease with interferon-alfa-2 with ribavirin). Some diseases progress and require dialysis or transplantation.

Glomerular Diseases

Therapists working with clients with a diagnosis of diabetes, systemic lupus erythematosus, vasculitis, and hypertension need to be aware of the association of glomerulonephritis with these disorders. Being vigilant for the clinical manifestations of glomerulonephritis (e.g., edema, hypertension, hematuria, oliguria) is important, and their presence warrants referral of the client to a physician.

An awareness of the side effects associated with diuretics is also important. Potential side effects include muscle weakness, fatigue, muscle cramps, headaches, increased frequency of urination with possibility of incontinence, and depression, all of which can interfere with the rehabilitation program. (See Chapter 5 for additional information regarding diuretics; see also Table 12-5.) The onset of any of these complaints also warrants communication with a physician. Finally, many clients with glomerulonephritis progress to chronic renal failure.

DISORDERS OF THE BLADDER AND URETHRA

Bladder Cancer

Overview and Incidence

The bladder is lined with transitional cells and in some places, such as at the trigone, epithelial cells. Transitional cell carcinoma is the most common type of bladder cancer, accounting for 90% of all cases. Transitional cell bladder cancer is a heterogeneous group of cancers with a wide spectrum of aggressiveness and clinical manifestations. Squamous cell carcinoma of the bladder is unusual, accounting for 8% of all cases, typically resulting from chronic inflammation. A rarer form, adenocarcinoma, accounts for the remaining 2% of cases and is thought to arise from remnants of the embryologic urachus (ligaments).

There are approximately 73,500 cases of bladder cancer each year in the United States.[255] As the fourth leading cause of cancer in men and eighth leading cause of cancer death in the United States, bladder cancer is more common than is generally appreciated.[255] Overall, the incidence of bladder cancer is increasing in industrialized countries, although the survival rate is improving. Though it is more prevalent in men, women lose more years of life and a greater fraction of their life expectancy to bladder cancer.[248,255]

Etiology and Risk Factors

The specific cause of bladder cancer is unknown, but multiple risk factors are linked with the development of bladder cancer (Box 18-3). The strongest and most significant risk factor is *smoking*. Sixty-five percent to 75% of all individuals with bladder cancer have a strong smoking history. Cigarette smokers are twice as likely as nonsmokers to develop bladder cancer.

> **Box 18-3**
> ### RISK FACTORS FOR BLADDER CANCER
>
> - Cigarette smoking
> - Occupational exposures to chemicals and other toxins
>   - Truck drivers (diesel exhaust)
>   - Painters
>   - Leather workers
>   - Metal workers
> - Male gender
> - Age 55 years and older
> - Previous treatment with cyclophosphamide or iphosphamide (chemotherapy)
> - Previous pelvic radiation (e.g., ovarian cancer treatment)
> - European descent
> - Chronic inflammation:
>   - History of chronic bladder infections (such as with spinal cord injury, stroke)
>   - Kidney or bladder stones
>   - Long-term catheterization (e.g., dementia, Alzheimer disease, neurologic impairment)
>   - Infection with parasite causing schistosomiasis
> - Neurogenic bladder
> - History of previous bladder cancer
> - Family history or retinoblastoma gene inheritance
> - Under investigation:
>   - Gene–environment interaction
>   - Coffee
>   - Fluid intake
>   - Bacon consumption
>   - Gonorrhea infection

Occupational exposures are also related to bladder cancer, particularly exposure to β-naphthylamine, 4-aminobiphenyl (ABP), and benzidine, used in the dye and rubber tire industries. Although these chemicals have been banned, others are currently being investigated for possible association, and those in many occupations appear to be at risk for the development of bladder cancer, such as painters, metalworkers, and truck drivers.[20,96,261] It is estimated that up to 20% of bladder cancer is caused by an occupational exposure.[149]

More than 90% of cases occur in people older than 55 years, making *age* another risk factor. *Whites* are twice as likely as African Americans to develop the disease, and *men* develop bladder cancer four times more often than women. A previous history of bladder cancer; previous treatment with high doses of the chemotherapy drugs cyclophosphamide or iphosphamide; and radiation to the pelvis also place people at higher risk.

Decreased fluid intake may be a risk factor as the more concentrated the urine, the more toxic irritants come in contact with the bladder mucosa. Conversely, increased fluid intake may decrease the risk of bladder cancer, leading to speculation that a more frequent urine flow decreases the time of contact between carcinogens and the bladder epithelium.[235,303]

There is evidence that food, nutrition or physical activity are not significant factors in the development of bladder cancer. However, as to prevention, copious fruit consumption may reduce the risk for smokers by as much as 50%.[3,33] The relationship between coffee and bladder cancer remains controversial despite decades of research.[240,268,301,302] Recent studies are adding to the continued controversy by suggesting that this relationship may be a consequence of the differential confounding effect of coffee consumption with tobacco smoking—smoking being the major risk factor for bladder cancer.[219,220,286] Individuals with some chromosomal mutations who smoke cigarettes may be at further increased risk of bladder cancers.[172]

Chronic inflammation may also contribute to an increased risk of bladder cancer. The mechanism may be chronic irritation and inflammation cause transitional cells to undergo metaplasia and transform into malignant cells. This may also occur in areas already epithelialized with squamous cells, such as at the trigone. Chronic inflammatory irritation, such as from recurrent UTIs, kidney or bladder stones, or the parasite causing schistosomiasis, increase the risk for the development of squamous cell carcinoma of the bladder.

Long-term catheterization (e.g., in spinal cord injury) was previously thought to be a risk factor for squamous cell bladder cancer because of chronic inflammation. However, new research shows that indwelling catheters may not be the only source of increased incidence of squamous cell cancer in spinal cord patients, but the very presence of a neurogenic bladder may be a contributing factor.[142] This may be because of the interaction of the bladder mucosa with a high volume of urine commonly seen in neurogenic bladders. Whatever is the main cause, it is recommended to perform an annual cystoscopy for screening of neoplasms in this high-risk group.

Rare risk factors include uncommon birth defects such as exstrophy (where there is a defect in the abdominal wall), inheritance of the retinoblastoma gene, or a family history of bladder cancer.[65,87]

Pathogenesis

Tumors of the urinary collecting system can arise from epithelial, mesenchymal, or hematopoietic tissues, but the majority of bladder cancers arise from the epithelium. Approximately 90% of these cancers are transitional cell carcinomas, with squamous cell carcinomas and adenocarcinomas making up the remainder. Bladder cancer is believed to develop through reversible premalignant stages followed by irreversible steps, ending in invasive cancer that can give rise to distant metastases. Variations in the clinical course suggest that different forms of bladder cancer develop along different molecular pathways, leading to tumor presentations of various malignant potential.[294]

The systemic absorption of environmental carcinogens, including cigarette smoke, followed by storage in the bladder exposes the urinary epithelium to concentrated levels of the agents for prolonged periods. This interaction of urine-soluble carcinogens with the epithelium is known as contact chemical carcinogenesis. The precise molecular events leading to the formation of bladder cancer are not known, but several genes appear to be involved. One includes the 9p21 locus (chromosome 9), which contains the CDKN2A/ARF tumor-suppressor gene.[16] Another factor may be the inability to repair deoxyribonucleic acid (DNA) following damage from carcinogens.[238] Further research is needed to determine which genes are involved and how risk factors interact in the development of bladder cancer.

Clinical Manifestations

Painless hematuria is the most common sign of bladder cancer. Gross hematuria is present in up to 85% of people with this condition, and microscopic hematuria is present in a majority of the remainder. The onset of hematuria is often sudden, and the hematuria is frequently intermittent; the degree of hematuria is not related to the volume of tumor or its stage.[71] Clots may form and cause urethral blockage with resultant bladder enlargement and painful spasms. The intermittent pattern of bleeding can result in a delay in diagnosis.

Other signs of voiding dysfunction may also be present, including frequency, urgency, and dysuria. Overactive bladder with or without hematuria (blood in the urine) may be a presenting symptom. This symptom is 10 times more common in women than men despite the fact that bladder cancer is more common in men than women.[292]

Lymphedema of the lower extremities may occur secondary to locally advanced masses or pelvic lymph node involvement. Obstruction of the ureter can lead to hydroureter or hydronephrosis. In the presence of advanced disease, back pain secondary to metastases to the vertebral bones may occur. Metastatic disease may also lead to liver or pulmonary symptoms.

MEDICAL MANAGEMENT

PREVENTION. Although there is no specific way to prevent bladder cancer, modification of risk factors may help. Smoking cessation is the number one prevention strategy for bladder cancer. Reducing exposure to industrial or occupational carcinogens would also lower the incidence of this type of malignancy. Large total fluid intake may reduce the risk of bladder cancer by reducing the time of contact between carcinogens and the bladder epithelium.[32,183]

Vitamins and increasing consumption of fruits and vegetables initially showed benefit in reducing the risk for bladder cancer, but larger studies have not supported this relationship.[127,184]

Currently, screening of the general population for bladder cancer is not recommended, principally due to a lack of evidence for its effectiveness (large studies have not been continued for more than 10 years). But there is evidence to suggest that screening people at high risk (i.e., smokers, people with an occupational exposure) may be beneficial.[181] Early detection of bladder cancer when still superficial can reduce mortality.

The best specific tests to use to screen for bladder cancer have not been determined, but in high-risk individuals, a urine dipstick test, evaluating for the presence of hematuria, and urine cytology are economical and noninvasive. Even with the presence of intermittent symptoms, these screening tests may miss many tumors. Some experts suggest cystoscopy, which visualizes the bladder and has an increased ability to detect tumors that are intermittently symptomatic. Cystoscopy, however, is more invasive and expensive. It is probably best done for the high risk groups such as chronic heavy smokers or individuals with spinal cord injuries. Further research is needed to determine the most appropriate candidates and tests to screen for bladder cancer.

The majority of bladder cancers are low-grade, superficial carcinomas that do not tend to metastasize. However, 50% to 90% of bladder cancers will recur, depending on the grade and stage. With recurrence, 10% to 50% will progress in stage or grade. Regular follow-up for early detection of cancer recurrence is important for anyone with a previous history of bladder cancer.

DIAGNOSIS. Bladder cancer is seldom recognized in its preclinical stage but rather is detected once symptoms present, usually hematuria. Younger people with hematuria most often have a benign cause, such as a UTI or kidney or bladder stones.

Evaluation usually consists of a history, physical examination, urinalysis, and urine culture. If the cause is not determined with these measures, further evaluation should be done. For people older than age 50 years with hematuria (gross or microscopic), a history, physical examination, urinalysis, urine cytology, and cystoscopy should be performed. It is important to note risk factors the client may have for bladder cancer.

Cystoscopy allows the urologist to view the bladder for tumor and take a biopsy and cytology washings for evaluation. The cytology samples improve the ability to detect smaller tumors (especially if they are flat), as they are difficult to distinguish from normal bladder tissue.

If tumor is noted in the biopsy specimen, depth of involvement can be determined, which aids in determining staging and treatment. Staging of the tumor may involve ultrasound, CT scan, bone scan, or other tests. A number of urine-based markers, including telomerase and nuclear matrix protein 22 (NMP22), are under investigation for their potential usefulness in diagnosing transitional cell cancer and in monitoring for recurrence.[111,151,242]

STAGING. The TNM staging system is a staging scheme based on the progressive depth of invasion of tumor into the bladder wall that has been used to assign treatment, assess outcomes, and predict prognosis. Cancer cells that are present along the surface of the bladder mucosa but have not yet invaded, also called in situ carcinomas, do not yet have the potential for metastasis and are classified as Tis.

Tumors that have penetrated the basement membrane and invaded into the submucosa/lamina propria but not the muscularis propria are categorized as T1. T2 tumors invade the muscularis propria, whereas T3 tumors invade through the wall into perivesical tissue. T4 tumors invade other organs and structures, such as the prostate, uterus, vagina, pelvic wall, or abdominal wall (Fig. 18-8).

Once tumor is invasive, it has the capacity to metastasize and commonly first reaches lymph nodes near the bladder. The presence of lymph node involvement, number of lymph nodes affected, and distance of involved lymph nodes from the bladder determine the N categorization (N0 for no involvement, N1 for nodes near the bladder, and N2 for nodes further away). Distant sites of metastasis include the liver, lung, and bone. The stage is determined by combining the T, N, and M status (e.g., stage 1 is T1, N0, M0). Approximately 74% of bladder cancer is diagnosed as T1 or T2 tumors; 19% is T3; and 3% is T4.

TREATMENT. Treatment of bladder cancer is determined on the basis of the stage of the tumor and the person's general health. Surgery is the principal treatment for invasive bladder cancer. The optimal treatment for noninvasive disease is not clear; more aggressive approaches including cystectomy, systemic chemotherapy, or radiotherapy have been shown to reduce mortality.[194] Transurethral resection, surgery completed through the urethra using a rigid cystoscope called a resectoscope, is performed for early and superficial tumors. After the removal of the lesion, the tumor bed is treated either with a high-beam laser or fulguration (electric current used to destroy tumor tissue). Most clients can return home the same day or the next day. Complications include bleeding

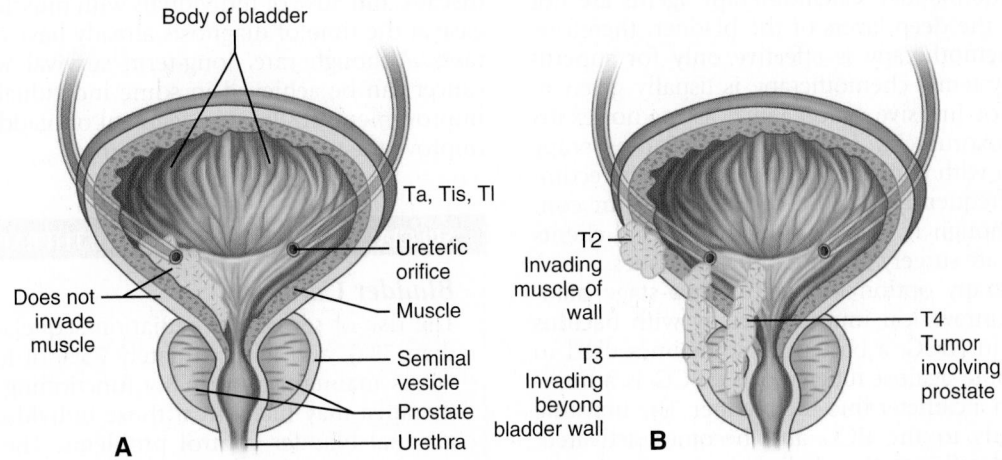

Figure 18-8

Bladder cancer staging using the TNM method. A, In Ta, Tis, and T1 tumors, cells do not invade muscle. **B,** If the muscle is involved, the tumor is staged as T2. T3 tumors invade beyond the bladder wall but do not involve other organs. T4 tumors are locally invasive to outside structures such as the prostate as shown or systemically with distant metastases (not shown).

and discomfort. Long-term effects of repeated transurethral resection include fibrosis of the bladder and loss of continence.

Cystectomy is performed for invasive bladder cancer. If the tumor is small, a partial cystectomy may be performed in order to salvage functioning bladder tissue.[79] This approach is controversial, with some urologists preferring cystectomy even for selected clients with small tumor mass. A radical cystectomy is the surgery of choice for larger, invasive tumors or multiple tumors. This procedure removes the bladder and adjacent lymph nodes. The prostate is removed in men, and the uterus, ovaries, and a portion of the vagina are removed in women.

Following cystectomy, reconstructive surgery is performed to create a urine drainage system to compensate for the loss of the bladder. A urostomy procedure allows drainage of urine into a bag outside the abdomen. This is the least-preferred long-term method of draining urine. The surgery that uses a short piece of small or large intestine to create a pouch or conduit from the ureters to the outside of the body is called an ileal conduit procedure.

Another surgical option is the creation of a continent diversion. In this procedure, the reserve pouch (intestine) has a valve. This valve allows urine to be stored until a catheter is placed to drain the urine. Newer reconstructive methods create a "neobladder" from intestine, which is then attached to the urethra. This surgery allows clients the ability to urinate normally, using a Valsalva maneuver (increasing intraabdominal pressure). The surgical complications from these types of procedures include infection, urine leakage, and obstruction. Sexual side effects are common, particularly for men. Impotence has been an issue with radical cystectomies in the past, but newer techniques have reduced the risk of nerve damage. If impotence does occur, function can improve with time. Generally, younger men (younger than age 60 years) are more likely to regain function than older men.

Chemotherapy is administered in two ways: intravesically or systemically. Intravesical chemotherapy is given through a catheter into the bladder, directly affecting the lining of the bladder. Chemotherapy agents are not absorbed into the deep layers of the bladder; therefore, intravesical chemotherapy is effective only for superficial cancers. Systemic chemotherapy is usually given in combination for invasive cancer (such as methotrexate, vinblastine, doxorubicin, and cisplatin). Radiotherapy in conjunction with concurrent chemotherapy is recommended less frequently because of the long-term consequences, although it is an option for treating clients unable to tolerate surgery because of health issues.

Another therapy option for treating low-stage bladder cancer is intravesical immunotherapy with bacillus Calmette-Guérin (BCG; a bacterium sometimes used to immunize people against tuberculosis). BCG is administered through a catheter into the bladder. The immune system responds to the BCG and becomes activated. These activated cells are then believed to recognize the cancer cells as foreign and destroy them. BCG is typically administered on a weekly basis for 6 weeks. BCG may reduce the risk of recurrence by as much as 50%. Side effects include flu-like symptoms and a burning sensation

in the bladder. Rarely, the bacterium can spread into the bloodstream, causing sepsis.

Stages 0 and 1 tumors are treated with transurethral resection followed by intravesical BCG. If the tumor does not respond to the BCG, intravesical chemotherapy is administered, although either BCG or intravesical chemotherapy can be used first.[98] However, more than half of the people with stage 1 tumors will have a recurrence, and 20% to 30% will have a cancer that is invasive.

Stage 2 is treated with a radical cystectomy, with or without lymph node removal. Selected people may undergo a partial cystectomy with fulguration. Systemic chemotherapy may be given prior to or after surgery to treat any small micrometastases not seen during the staging process. A radical cystectomy is also the treatment for stage 3.

Chemotherapy may be added prior to surgery (neoadjuvant) to improve survival, but further investigations are needed to determine the appropriate timing for chemotherapy.[136] Stage 4 therapy focuses on quality of life and slowing tumor growth. A radical cystectomy may be performed with chemotherapy if there are no distant metastases. Various combinations of therapy may be employed when distant metastases are present.

PROGNOSIS. Despite the continued increase in the number of new cases occurring each year, the mortality attributed to bladder cancer has remained fairly stable. Stage and grade of the tumor are prognostic indicators for local failure. The 5-year survival rates with treatment are 84% for white males, 71% for black males, 76% for white females, and 51% for black females (most likely reflecting delay in diagnosis and inadequate care because of socioeconomic issues). Individuals with T1 tumors have a 90% 5-year survival, whereas for those with muscle-invasive tumors survival at 5 years is 50%; those with deep muscle invasion will go on to have metastatic disease within 2 years.[9]

Bladder cancer is sensitive to chemotherapy and immunotherapy but also has a high incidence of local recurrence, usually within the first 2 years. In approximately 30% of cases metastasis develops during the course of the disease, and 50% of individuals with muscle-invasive disease at the time of diagnosis already have distant metastases. Although rare, long-term survival with recurrent cancer can be achieved in some individuals. Continued improvements in the management of bladder cancer will improve the prognosis in the future.

SPECIAL IMPLICATIONS FOR THE THERAPIST   18-7

Bladder Cancer

The risk of severe late radiation sequelae is low (less than 5%), and approximately 75% of long-term survivors maintain a normally functioning bladder. The therapist may likely treat those individuals who have residual bladder control problems. The high rate of cancer recurrence requires therapists to be vigilant in observing for the onset or return of symptoms and signs suggestive of urogenital system disease or metastatic spread. Anyone reporting visible blood in the urine must be evaluated further by a physician.

Surgical management of muscle-invasive neoplasms may involve radical cystectomy (gold standard) with adjuvant chemotherapy.[2,59] Incisional considerations, pain and reaction to medications should be considered during mobility activities. Pelvic physical therapists may be involved in the retraining of voiding patterns and pelvic floor muscle coordination for individuals after neobladder procedures. See "Pelvic Floor Muscle Dysfunction" in Chapter 27.

Urinary Incontinence

See also "Pelvic Floor Muscle Dysfunction" in Chapter 27.

Normal Bladder Function

Understanding the basics of normal bladder function will be helpful in understanding UI. The process of micturition and continence involves a complex interplay of nerves, smooth muscle and skeletal muscle. Proper functioning of these structures is needed for normal voiding to occur. Normal urination involves nerve signals from the cortex of the brain, through the pons, spinal cord, peripheral autonomic system, sensory afferent innervation of the lower urinary tract, and finally to the bladder itself.

Neural control begins in the cortex with cognitive awareness and decision making. The pontine micturition reflex center is located in the brainstem. The efferent (exiting) neurons travel down the spinal cord in the reticulospinal tract to the skeletal pelvic floor muscle and the detrusor muscle of the bladder. Parasympathetic nerves originate in the spinal cord at the level of S2, S3, and S4, and innervate the bladder wall via the pelvic nerve.

Preganglionic sympathetic nerves have their origin in the spinal cord at the levels of T10 through L2 and travel through the sympathetic chain ganglion to the bladder neck and fundus of the bladder. The bladder neck contains the internal urethral sphincter (involuntary smooth muscle). The external urethral sphincter, part of the pelvic floor muscles (PFM) (voluntary skeletal muscle) is innervated by the pudendal nerves, which originate in the spinal cord at the level of S2 through S4.

These nerve signals result in coordination of the smooth muscle of the detrusor and internal urethral sphincter and the skeletal muscle of the external urethral sphincter of the PFM. Bladder patterns in asymptomatic individuals vary greatly. Normally, the bladder is designed to hold a pint of urine for several hours. As it fills, the detrusor muscle remains relaxed to allow the bladder to stretch and accommodate more urine; the internal urethral sphincter remains contracted to prevent urine from escaping through the urethra.

Voluntary PFM support the base of the bladder and compress the urethra, further blocking the flow of urine. When the bladder is full, a message to get to the bathroom is received; the person makes their way to the toilet. When positioned appropriately, urination is initiated with voluntary relaxation of the PFM. This is followed by relaxation of the internal urethral sphincter and

contraction of the detrusor muscle to squeeze the urine out of the bladder.

Coordinated detrusor smooth muscle contraction with relaxation of the smooth muscle internal urethral sphincter and skeletal muscle of the external urethral sphincter is necessary to empty effectively.

Normal voiding interval is a minimum of 2 hours (often in the elderly) and usually 3 to 5 hours between voids for others. Urinating more than eight times a day is a symptom of urinary frequency. Most people feel bothersome nocturia is voiding two or more times per night. Bladder training can be used to restore normal bladder pattern and function.

Definition and Overview

UI may be defined as a "complaint of involuntary urine loss."[117] There are currently eight categories of UI.[117] The two most common categories used to classify UI are:

1. *Stress urinary incontinence* (SUI): complaint of involuntary loss of urine on effort or physical exertion, or on sneezing or coughing. This occurs during activities that increase intraabdominal pressure.
2. *Urgency urinary incontinence* (UUI): complaint of involuntary loss of urine associated with urgency. Urgency is the report of a sudden compelling desire to urinate that is difficult to defer. UUI is often related to detrusor instability, a condition in which the bladder contracts at small volumes often in response to triggers such as running water or arriving home. Overactive bladder syndrome (older terms include hyperreflexive bladder, or detrusor hyperreflexia) is defined as "urinary urgency, usually accompanied by frequency and nocturia, with or without UUI, in the absence of UTI or other obvious pathology."[117]

Many people have more than one type of incontinence (most often SUI and UUI together), known as *mixed* UI.

UI is common, particularly in older adults. Approximately 10% to 35%[134] of community-dwelling and 50% to 60% of nursing home adults have incontinence. Yet the condition is poorly understood, underdiagnosed, and often inadequately treated. Many people are embarrassed to acknowledge that they are incontinent. Only 20% to 50% of incontinent adults seek medical care.[289] Others regard incontinence as part of the normal aging process.

The economic price tag associated with UI is estimated to be greater than $26 billion per year in the United States,[131a] approaching the cost of treatment for osteoporosis, Alzheimer disease, and arthritis.[6] Incontinence can be a significant contributory factor related to falls in older adults,[30] pressure sores, skin breakdown, UTIs, institutionalization, depression, and isolation. Data from the Canadian Community Health Survey indicates 15.5% prevalence of depression in women with UI compared to 9.2% without UI.[285] Social isolation, limited work opportunities, and decreased exercise participation are also reported in association with UI.

Prevalence

UI is more prevalent in women than men and in the aging over the young. Overall prevalence of UI in women in 2008 was 51.1% and in men 13.9%.[179] The prevalence of UI was first reported in 1988 at the National Institutes of Health Consensus Conference on Adult Urinary Incontinence. At that time, an estimated 10 million adults in the United States experienced incontinence, including 15% to 30% of community-dwelling older adults and more than 50% of nursing home residents.[58] More current estimates suggest as many as 25 million individuals experience problematic incontinence.[179] Other groups who report a higher prevalence include athletes (e.g., gymnasts, athletes competing on trampolines) and men after prostate surgery.

Since the first consensus conference, there has been an increased awareness of and focus on the problem of UI. Until recently, the impact of UI on working women employed full time, a population generally characterized as healthy, has not been the focus of research. One survey at a large university center reported that 21% of the women surveyed (age 18 years and older) reported UI at least monthly.[85]

Risk Factors

A wide range of factors can contribute to the increased risk of developing UI (Box 18-4).[264] Some risk factors are more likely to lead to one type or another or several types of incontinence. The literature varies widely as to which risk factors are significant for different population groups.

Research constantly shows elevated body mass index is a major risk factor for UI. Obesity is a common condition among women in developed countries and is believed to have a major impact on stress incontinence. The proposed mechanisms for this association includes the increased intraabdominal pressures that adversely stress the urethra, bladder, and pelvic floor, and the effect of obesity on the neuromuscular function of the genitourinary tract.[61] Obesity is also associated with overactive bladder, and weight loss has been shown to decrease UUI symptoms.[266,298a]

Advancing age plays a significant role in the development of all forms of UI.[264] As older adults lose their mobility and manual dexterity secondary to a multitude of ailments, getting to the bathroom or commode in a timely fashion and manipulating clothing become increasingly difficult. The presence of two or more diseases significantly increases the likelihood of developing UI. Common illnesses associated with UI include diabetes, stroke, hypertension, cognitive impairment, parkinsonism, arthritis, and hearing and visual impairments.

Women are more likely than men to develop UI. This is related to structural differences, several factors associated with childbirth, and gynecologic surgery. Women who have had multiple pregnancies and deliveries (whether cesarean section or vaginal birth) have a higher incidence of UI. Hysterectomy, the presence of a cystocele, and uterine prolapse may also increase a woman's risk.

Medications commonly prescribed for other illnesses can also increase the risk of incontinence. These pharmacologic agents can interfere with conscious inhibition of voiding, induce a quick diuresis (diuretics),[188] or reduce urethral resistance to the point of stress incontinence. Tranquilizers and sedatives may impair awareness of the usual cues related to urinary urgency and may also depress the cerebral corticoregulatory tract, affecting detrusor

---

Box 18-4

RISK FACTORS FOR URINARY INCONTINENCE

- Obesity and elevated body mass index
- Age
- Pregnancy/multiple pregnancies; childbirth/delivery (vaginal or cesarean section); episiotomy; large gestational weight
- Cystocele or uterine prolapse
- Any pelvic surgery including hysterectomy for women, prostatectomy for men
- Diabetes mellitus
- Depression
- Constipation, fecal impaction
- Tobacco use
- Medications
  - α-Adrenergic blockers (antihistamines, decongestants)
  - Antihypertensives
  - Antiparkinson agents
  - Antipsychotics
  - Diuretics
  - Narcotic analgesics
  - Tranquilizers, sedatives
  - Tricyclic antidepressants
- History of recurrent urinary tract infections
- Bladder irritation (low fluid intake, caffeine, and possibly alcohol)*
- Loss of activities of daily living skills for toileting, decreased or impaired mobility
- Impaired cognitive function
- Race (white)
- Neurologic disorder (e.g., myelomeningocele, multiple sclerosis, brain injury, Parkinson disease, cerebral palsy, spinal cord injury, stroke)
- Psychogenic (e.g., childhood and/or adult sexual trauma for both males and females, negative sexual experiences, emotional stress)
- Frequent high impact exercise[204,254]

* Bladder irritants are not likely to cause urinary incontinence without other contributing actors.

Source used for pharmacotherapy update: DiPiro JT, Talbert RL, Yee GC, Matzke GR, Wells BG, Posey LM, eds: *Pharmacotherapy. A pathophysiologic approach*, ed 8, New York, 2011, McGraw Hill.

---

muscle activity.[164] Laxatives, estrogen, and antibiotics are also associated with an increased risk for UI.[83,128,241]

Findings regarding the role of hormonal changes contributing to UI are inconsistent.[264] Estrogen deficiency results in changes in the urethra, which seems to predispose women to UI. Hormone replacement, including estrogen plus progestin, in healthy postmenopausal women has been linked with incontinence.[108,236] Topical estrogen can be used if incontinence is caused by atrophic vaginitis or severe vaginal atrophy.

High caffeine intake (more than 400 mg/day) can also contribute to the development of urge incontinence, while studies involving alcohol consumption have reported mixed results.[95,243] Constipation and other bowel problems increase the risk of UI, which may be related to pelvic organ prolapse.[47]

Recurrent UTI is also an independent risk factor for developing UI. Race and socioeconomic class may also play roles in the development of UI. It appears that white women are more likely to have UI than African American women, while women from a higher socioeconomic class have an increased risk of UI. Smoking is an independent risk factor for UI.

Pathogenesis and Clinical Manifestations

Incontinence, as discussed earlier, is categorized depending on the cause and pathophysiology. Each type of UI has associated clinical manifestations. *UUI* is often caused by involuntary bladder (detrusor) spasms (also called detrusor overactivity) and is associated with both increased frequency and urgency. The pathophysiology of detrusor overactivity is not fully understood and may be related to irritated sensory signals from overactive PFM, bacteria of UTI, fear of leaking, and other psychologic factors.

Urge incontinence is characterized by leakage (sometimes large-volume accidents) after a sudden precipitant desire to urinate or by events such as trying to insert a key in the door, running hands under water (or hearing running water), thinking about going to the bathroom, or passing by a bathroom.

Some clinicians use the term *functional incontinence* to describe the consequence of chronic impairments of physical or cognitive function that make toileting in a timely fashion difficult (e.g., difficulty getting to the toilet on time, inability to manage pant zippers, forgetting how to get on and off the toilet).

SUI results from weakness or loss of tone in the PFM, internal urethral sphincter failure, hypermobility of the ureterovesical junction, or damage to the pudendal nerve (e.g., infection, tumor, childbirth) (see Figs. 20-6 and 20-7). It is accompanied by leakage that is coincident with increases in intraabdominal pressure (e.g., coughing, sneezing, laughing, bending, high-impact physical activity or exercise). Someone with mixed UI will exhibit signs of both UUI and SUI.

Other clinical manifestations of UI depend on the type of incontinence and underlying pathology, but may include constant dribbling, frequency, urgency, nocturia, hesitancy, weak stream, or straining to void. Prolapsed bladder, uterus, and/or bowel may accompany or contribute to leakage, especially when caused by multiple pregnancies and deliveries.

MEDICAL MANAGEMENT

SCREENING AND PREVENTION. Preventive education may decrease the occurrence of incontinence. Many health care professionals advocate early education on proper PFM contraction for adolescent girls and young women before they become pregnant. Prepartum and postpartum PFM training has been shown to have immediate and long-term effects in preventing incontinence, improving quality of life, and improving sexual dysfunction.[18,19,192,193,]

Modifying risk factors is also suggested. This might include losing weight, stopping smoking, avoiding provocative medications if possible, avoiding irritating fluids like caffeine and alcohol, and avoiding constipation through proper nutrition, adequate hydration, and responding to the need to toilet.

The therapist can be very instrumental in establishing screening programs for all ages to assess for risk factors for UI or for the presence of incontinence.

All therapists can teach proper lifting techniques to minimize unnecessary increase in intraabdominal pressure, which could contribute to the occurrence of SUI and pelvic organ prolapse. Patients should be taught to contract the PFM before increased abdominal pressure (e.g., lifting, laughing, coughing, sneezing, vomiting). Anyone experiencing leaking during exercise needs a prescriptive PFM exercise program and modification of the exercise that precipitates the leaking.

DIAGNOSIS. Because UI is related to a wide variety of disorders and factors, a detailed investigation may be necessary to determine the cause(s). An important part of this investigation is a bladder diary to determine the frequency, timing, and amount of voiding and to assess the numerous other risk factors potentially associated with UI. Bladder dairies are reliable and reproducible and provide a great deal of valuable information for development of treatment strategies.[28]

A careful history will investigate medication usage, prescribed and nonprescription; past and current illnesses; and surgical and birth histories. There are many validated quality of life and symptom indexes used to quantify symptoms associated with UI and bladder dysfunction. Physical examination should include a pelvic, genitourinary, and rectal examination to evaluate for the presence of prolapse, fecal impaction, atrophic vaginitis, cystocele, PFM dysfunction, masses, prostate hypertrophy, and prostate nodule (in men).

Urinalysis may reveal hematuria or infection. In order to differentiate between UUI and urinary retention, a postvoid residual should be obtained. With a normal postvoid residual, the bladder should contain less than 50 to 100 mL of urine after voiding. Many cases of incontinence can be diagnosed without significant invasive techniques and treated by modifying reversible risk factors. The mnemonic DIAPPERS summarizes the reversible causes of incontinence: *D* for delirium, *I* for infection, *A* for atrophic urethritis/vaginitis, *P* for pharmaceutical, *P* also for psychologic disorders, *E* for excessive urine output (associated with congestive heart failure or hyperglycemia), *R* for restricted mobility, and *S* for stool impaction.[283]

Clients who have abnormal physical or laboratory findings may require further workup, particularly if surgery is planned or the diagnosis is in doubt. Cystoscopy is beneficial in the presence of hematuria to assess for bladder cancer. Urodynamic evaluation is used in select clients who may have nonspecific symptoms or for whom a more precise diagnosis of obstruction is needed.

Urodynamic studies include uroflowmetry, cystometry, urethral pressure studies, pressure-flow micturition studies, electrophysiologic studies, and video urodynamic studies. All or a portion of these tests can be performed as appropriate. One component of the urodynamic study, cystometry is used to assess bladder capacity, sensation, voluntary control, and contractility. Cystometry consists of filling the bladder with water and recording changes in intravesicular pressure, abdominal pressure and PFM activity.

When stress incontinence is suspected, provocative stress testing is carried out. The client is asked to cough vigorously during cystometry while the examiner observes for urine loss. The test is initially done in the lithotomy position but if the result is negative, the test is repeated in a standing position.[81] Dynamic MRI is being investigated to study specific structural aspects of PFM dysfunction such as avulsion, which may be associated with stress incontinence.[17,122]

TREATMENT. Management of UI depends on the type of incontinence and the person's age and general health but usually falls into one of three categories: conservative, pharmacologic, and surgical. Conservative intervention is considered the first line of treatment for UI and includes a combination of:

- Education: lifestyle, dietary changes, fluid modifications, treatment of constipation, weight loss, instruction in proper lifting and exercising techniques to avoid excessive increased intra-abdominal pressure, toilet position especially for children and elderly.
- Bladder training, behavioral modification, and urge deferment
- Prescriptive exercises including general pelvic stability exercises, specific transversus abdominal exercise, PFM exercises, with or without facilitation (see discussion in Chapter 27), and vaginal weight training
- Environmental modifications to increase accessibility and functional mobility training to increase timely access to bathroom facilities.
- Modalities such as pelvic floor electrical stimulation, biofeedback therapy
- Support devices such as pessaries

Pessaries are devices inserted into the vagina that are designed to support the bladder and bladder neck reducing pelvic organ prolapse and compressing the urethra to decrease UI. These devices come in a variety of shapes and sizes and are made of flexible or rigid silicone, latex, or acrylic. Some pessaries can stay in the vagina for up to 3 months before being removed, cleaned, and replaced; others are used just during exercise or sexual intercourse. A properly fitted pessary should not interfere with bowel or bladder function and should not be uncomfortable.

Physical and occupational therapists can often help improve mobility skills. For example, if physical impairments make mobility difficult, thus affecting the client's ability to reach a bathroom, appropriate devices (i.e., bedside commode) and therapy can be provided. Clothing should be easy to remove.

Stress Urinary Incontinence. SUI can be treated by the conservative methods listed above and surgical methods. Cochrane reviews report PFM training to be effective for the treatment of SUI or mixed incontinence.[73,119,120,125] Electrical stimulation shows only slight improvement over placebo, while the use of vaginal weights shows no significant benefit over PFM exercises alone.[118,120,125] See further specific discussion of PFM training in Chapter 27.

There are many surgeries that may be used to correct pelvic floor laxity including an open retropubic colposuspension, bladder neck needle suspension, and suburethral sling procedure. The suburethral sling is the most often used technique and results in 80% to 90% success.[256] Surgical correction of pelvic organ prolapse may improve symptoms of UI. Periurethral injections with a bulking agent (such as collagen) may be administered to increase sphincter resistance in women and in men who have internal sphincter deficiency. Artificial urinary sphincters can be considered but have a cure rate of approximately 50% with high morbidity.[100]

Urgency Urinary Incontinence. Various interventions are used to treat UUI, with the primary focus being behavioral modification[267] and pharmacotherapy. Biofeedback and PFM training, along with bladder training, can significantly improve UUI.[298] Bladder training consists of scheduled voiding (trying to increase time between each void) and urge-suppression techniques. For clients with cognitive impairment, prompted voiding can be beneficial and decrease incontinent episodes (remind every 2 hours to toilet). Clients should also be encouraged to manage constipation and avoid bladder irritants such as caffeine, alcohol, nicotine, and carbonated soft drinks.

Pharmacologic therapy is frequently used in conjunction with behavioral modifications. First-line drug therapy for UUI is the use of anticholinergics or muscarinic antagonists, which inhibit involuntary detrusor contractions.[121,165,197] The most common side effect is dry mouth. Other adverse effects include drowsiness, cognitive impairment, delirium, and hallucinations. These side effects are more likely to occur in older adults than younger clients.

Other medications have shown some benefit but are not as effective as the anticholinergics/muscarinic antagonists or have off-label usage. In the past estrogen has been used to treat UI, although there is little data to support their use, and oral hormone therapy has been associated with increased incidence of incontinence. In men with symptoms of UUI and prostatic hypertrophy, α-adrenergic antagonists can be used initially. If these agents do not alleviate symptoms, obstruction should be ruled out before starting an anticholinergic agent.[208]

SPECIAL IMPLICATIONS FOR THE THERAPIST 18-8

Urinary Incontinence

See "Pelvic Muscle Dysfunction" in Chapter 27.

Therapists have an important direct role in the assessment and treatment intervention of UI. Physical therapy guides the rehabilitation of muscle imbalance and pelvic alignment and promotes pelvic muscle awareness and function through biofeedback, therapeutic exercise, neuromuscular reeducation, and a behavioral management approach.[23,34,35,105,106,156]

The pelvic rehabilitation program is designed to prevent recurrence of the impairment and to restore bowel, bladder, sexual, and supportive muscle functioning.[226]

To All Physical Therapists

Many adults think that UI is an inevitable part of aging or disease and do not report the problem. *Everyone* should be asked if they have urinary incontinence, but especially the perimenopausal or postmenopausal woman, any woman who has been pregnant, anyone (male or female) older than age 60 years (earlier if prostate or bladder infection or cancer is evident), and any person with multiple risk factors.

Anyone with onset of UI with concomitant cervical spine pain (even without a history of trauma or known cause) may be experiencing cervical disc protrusion, requiring additional screening and evaluation. Additionally, the possibility of genitourinary disorders as a result of sexual abuse or assault exists and requires careful assessment.

The generally positive rapport that develops between client and therapist may facilitate the acknowledgment that UI exists and uncover the potential underlying risk factors. Specific questions should be included in the intake history for *all* individuals to help bring this information to light, such as the following:

- *Do you leak urine when you lift, cough, sneeze, or stand up?*
- *Do you get up at night to urinate? How often?*
- *Do you go to the bathroom more often than every 2 to 3 hours?*
- *How much water do you drink in a waking day?*
- *Are you constipated?*

The therapist may be in a position to direct the person to the appropriate physician for evaluation. Successful intervention in UI may enhance rehabilitation efforts geared to improve the client's physical and social activity level. It is helpful for physical therapists to have handouts or other resources for patients/clients to refer to. The National Association for Continence (http://www.nafc.org) offers a wide variety of information and is a very supportive organization for affected individuals, caregivers and professionals. The Section on Women's Health of the American Physical Therapy Association (APTA) offers a broad range of information for patients and therapists on this topic as well.

Some physical therapists seek advanced postgraduate education and training in comprehensive treatment of PFM and pelvic dysfunction. See section on PFM dysfunction (Chapter 27) for more on evaluating and training this skeletal muscle.

Understanding the use of medications and potential side effects for these conditions is essential; many of the same medications used to treat incontinence can also cause incontinence if used inappropriately. Medications to treat other conditions can have side effects that cause incontinence. A concise listing of this information is available.[133]

Fracture Risk and Prevention

An episode of UUI at least once a week increases the risk of fractures by 34% related to falls at night.[30,132] Early diagnosis and appropriate treatment of UUI may decrease the risk of fracture.[30] The therapist can be very instrumental in performing a home assessment for the older adult with urge incontinence. Placing strategically located night lights near the bed, hallway to the bathroom, and bathroom and removing objects along the path (e.g., throw rugs) are essential preventive steps to take.

For the individual with incontinence and postural orthostatic hypotension, low blood pressure (or even use of hypertensives with the potential for hypotension as a side effect) and rising from bed quickly at night can also result in falls. Assessing for this complication and teaching prevention measures are recommended (see "Orthostatic [Postural] Hypotension" in Chapter 12).

Physical Therapist Intervention for Urinary Incontinence

PFM exercises can be performed to retrain and strengthen the pelvic floor musculature. Please refer to Chapter 27 for a complete review of PFM training. Weighted vaginal cones and electrical stimulation can also be used to rehabilitate the pelvic floor muscles. Continence requires the ability to suppress uninhibited detrusor contractions especially in individuals with overactive bladder. Pelvic floor rehabilitation specifically using PFM exercises may help suppress the desire to void by reducing detrusor pressure and increasing urethral pressure, resulting in suppression of the micturition reflex.

Bladder training involves teaching the bladder to respond to a specific voiding schedule. Clients void at scheduled intervals to increase bladder capacity and decrease urinary frequency. The initial retraining interval is determined by the bladder dairy and is usually 60 minutes. The voiding intervals are increased by 15- to 30-minute extensions using urge-suppression techniques.

Normal bladder pattern varies greatly; however, success is usually marked by voiding at 3- to 4-hour intervals, continence (perhaps measured by number of pads used), minimal sensory symptoms, and functional capacity (minimum of 300 mL of urine). Biofeedback (visual, or auditory, electromyographic or pressure) for general relaxation and physiologic quieting (e.g., diaphragmatic breathing) can also be used to train the client to reduce detrusor pressure.[289] Physiologic quieting, including hand warming, diaphragmatic breathing, and body/mind quieting can be used to normalize bladder function and autonomic nervous system innervation of bladder and bowel.[133]

Neurogenic Bladder Disorders

Overview

Voiding dysfunction associated with neurologic pathology is termed a *neurogenic bladder disorder*. There are many types of voiding dysfunction that can interfere with normal urine storage and coordinated, voluntary release.

Voiding dysfunction associated with neurologic pathology can be classified using one of many descriptive systems available. Each categorization scheme has advantages and disadvantages. For example, the Bors-Comarr Classification is well suited for clients with voiding dysfunction secondary to spinal cord injury but not as useful for clients with other problems.

There is no one accepted scale or categories for neurogenic bladder. Urodynamic classification correlates urodynamic findings and symptoms, while the International Continence Society Classification (ICSC) separates storage and voiding abnormalities and expands many of the urodynamic classification categories. The ICSC is the classification most physical therapists use now. *The Lapides Classification is well known and helpful to nonurologists, so it will be used as the classification system for this section. It correlates cystometry findings with clinical symptoms.*

This classification system separates voiding dysfunction into five categories: (1) sensory neurogenic bladder, (2) motor paralytic bladder or motor neurogenic bladder, (3) uninhibited neurogenic bladder, (4) reflex neurogenic bladder, and (5) autonomous neurogenic bladder Box 18-5. This system provides a framework for understanding neurogenic bladder disorders, particularly for the nonurologist, but applies only to those disorders with a neurologic basis for pathology. Many clients may demonstrate a mixture of sensory and motor abnormalities, and symptoms may overlap between categories.

Prevalence

Voiding dysfunction is a common problem associated with many types of neurologic diseases. In the United States, more than 91,000 people are released from the hospital each year with a neurologic disease or spinal cord injury.[54] Voiding dysfunction is costly and leads to significantly decreased quality of life, particularly in the older adult when long-term care is often considered for this problem in an otherwise healthy adult. The following gives some idea of the general prevalence of voiding dysfunction by condition[299]:

Cerebral palsy, 36%
Dementia, 30% to 100%
Parkinson's 37% to 70%
Multiple systems atrophy, 73%
Multiple sclerosis, 37% to 72%
Spinal stenosis, 61% to 62%
Spinal surgery, 38% to 60%
Disc disease, 28% to 87%
Diabetes mellitus, 25% to 87%
Radical hysterectomy, 8% to 57%
Guillain-Barré, 25%

Etiologic Factors

The common disorders that can result in neurogenic bladder dysfunction include cerebrovascular accident, dementia, Parkinson disease, multiple sclerosis, and brain tumors. Neurogenic bladder dysfunction can also occur secondary to spinal cord lesions such as spinal cord injury, herniated intervertebral disc, vascular lesions, spinal cord tumors, and myelitis.

Pathogenesis

Damage to nerves involved in micturition can result in different types of voiding dysfunction. Voiding dysfunction in neurological conditions varies greatly but usually falls into three categories: hyperreflexic bladder or neurogenic detrusor overactivity, detrusor sphincter dyssynergia, and areflexic or hypotonic bladder.

Cerebral injury (above the pontine micturition reflex center) leads to loss of voluntary inhibition of voiding

---

Box 18-5

TYPES OF NEUROGENIC MICTURITION PATHOLOGY

- *Sensory neurogenic bladder* occurs when there is a disruption of the nerves between the bladder and the spinal cord or the afferent nerves to the brain. Diabetes, tabes dorsalis (from syphilis), and pernicious anemia (vitamin B_{12} deficiency) are the most common causes. Initial changes include an abnormal sensation to bladder distention. Affected people will not recognize the need to void and unless frequent voiding is instigated, the bladder becomes chronically distended. This eventually leads to bladder hypotonicity with urine retention.

- *Motor paralytic bladder* results from the destruction of the parasympathetic motor nerves that innervate the bladder. This may occur with extensive pelvic surgery or trauma. Clinical symptoms can initially vary, ranging from a mild inability to initiate or maintain a urine stream to painful urine retention. Like sensory neurogenic bladder, with chronic bladder overdistention, motor paralytic bladder results in a distended bladder with large volume urine retention.

- *Uninhibited neurogenic bladder* (may also be known as neurogenic detrusor overactivity) refers to damage of the "corticoregulatory tract." This nomenclature is somewhat outdated; the term is no longer used to classify bladder dysfunction but still may be found in the literature. It was presumed that the regulatory site for reflex bladder control was located in the sacral spinal cord or the micturition reflex center. If there was damage to the corticoregulatory tracts, there was, in turn, a disinhibition of the micturition center, leading to incontinence. Conditions classified as leading to this type of neurogenic bladder included cerebrovascular accidents, brain or spinal cord tumors, Parkinson disease, demyelinating diseases, and brain tumors. Clinical symptoms included frequency, urgency, and urge incontinence.

Bladder sensation is normal but involuntary contractions occur at low volumes. Voluntary contractions can be initiated by the affected person but the capacity to store urine is decreased.

- *Reflex neurogenic bladder* describes the condition of the bladder following a spinal cord injury or "post spinal shock." This occurs when there is a complete disruption between the sacral spinal cord and the brainstem, as seen with traumatic spinal cord injury or transverse myelitis.

Other disorders or disease processes that cause significant demyelination of the spinal cord can also lead to reflex neurogenic bladder. The bladder lacks sensation and the person is unable to determine when the bladder is distended. Affected people also are unable to initiate micturition (voiding) and develop sphincter dyssynergia incontinence (the external sphincter tightens during micturition as the detrusor muscle is contracting, resulting in increased intravesicular pressure and vesicoureteral reflux).

- *Autonomous neurogenic bladder* refers to the complete separation of sensory and motor nerves of the bladder to the spinal sacral cord. Damage to the sacral roots or cord or the pelvic nerves can lead to this type of voiding dysfunction. Clients with this problem are unable to initiate voiding and there is no bladder sensation, leading to large volume bladder capacity and distention.

This type of voiding dysfunction can be seen in clients with spinal shock. Initial cystometric findings can be similar to the late stages of motor or sensory paralytic bladder (large capacity with low bladder pressure), but with continued inflammation and nerve damage, the bladder can lose capacity and compliance.

and a hyperreflexic bladder, but coordinated sphincter function is retained. This results in UUI related to urgency without urinary retention or incomplete empting. This can be seen in brain tumors, cerebral palsy, cerebrovascular accidents, dementia, Parkinson disease, pernicious anemia, and Shy-Drager syndrome.

Lesions in the spinal cord may take on qualities of hyperreflexic bladder seen in cerebral injuries or areflexic bladder seen in lower spinal injuries. The most dangerous dysfunction in patients with spinal cord injury is detrusor sphincter dyssynergia. In this dysfunction the sphincter remains closed while the bladder contraction occurs resulting in urinary retention and incomplete voiding. High bladder pressure and ureteral reflux can lead to kidney damage. Diseases that can result in this type of voiding problem include anterior spinal cord lesions, ischemia, multiple sclerosis, myelodysplasia, and trauma.

This type of injury also involves the sympathetic nerves and loss of sympathetic inhibition, leading to systemic sympathetic symptoms such as hypertension, facial flushing, perspiration, and headache. Because the vagal nerve is intact, bradycardia accompanies this syndrome.

Spinal cord lesions at the level of S2 and below usually lead to bladder *areflexia* and underactive PFM dysfunction. In this situation, both the bladder and PFM are weak. In some conditions (sacral lesions and some disc disease), the smooth muscle internal urethral sphincter is overactive; in other cases (conus lesions), the internal sphincter is underactive. The most common result is urinary retention, which usually manifests as SUI as the bladder is so full a small increase in intraabdominal pressure will cause overflow leakage. Acute transverse myelitis, diabetes, Guillain-Barré syndrome, herniated intervertebral disc, myelodysplasia, pelvic surgery, tabes dorsalis (syphilis), and trauma can cause this type of neurogenic bladder.

Diabetic bladder neuropathy occurs in 43% to 87% of people with type 1 diabetes mellitus and 60% to 75% of people with type 2 diabetes.[94,146] The actual neurologic damage and symptoms vary among clients with diabetes and include diabetic cystopathy (impaired bladder sensation, increased postvoid residuals, increased bladder capacity, and decreased bladder contractility), detrusor overactivity, bladder outlet obstruction (seen in men), and urge and stress incontinence. Diabetic bladder neuropathy occurs when other diabetic complications are apparent (e.g., diabetic retinopathy, microalbuminuria).

Clinical Manifestations

Neurogenic bladder dysfunction is manifested by partial or complete urinary retention, incontinence, urgency, suprapubic pain, or frequent urination. Common complications include UTIs, kidney stones, and deterioration in renal function.

In urinary retention the bladder fills and becomes overdistended, the pressure inside the bladder finally exceeds the maximal urethral pressure and urine "overflows." Incontinence related to urinary retention often manifests with symptoms of stress and urge incontinence and is characterized by frequent or constant dribbling, inability to completely empty the bladder, hesitancy, weak stream, need to strain to void, bladder distention,

and urinary urgency and frequent urination. Anticholinergics, narcotics and α-adrenergic agonists can worsen these symptoms.

MEDICAL MANAGEMENT

DIAGNOSIS. Numerous tests can be used to assess the anatomic and physiologic status of the bladder, associated structures, and nervous system. Urodynamic testing is frequently performed to categorize abnormalities and determine cause and most appropriate treatment in individuals with neurological deficits.

Many diseases lead to voiding dysfunction, and a complete history and physical can often reveal the cause. Other tests can be performed as needed to diagnose these disease processes. If spinal cord or brain abnormalities are suspected, an MRI is beneficial.

TREATMENT. The most important goals of treatment include preventing bladder overdistention, UTIs, and renal damage. Management of UI is also important to avoid skin damage and maximize quality of life. Treatment modalities include catheterization, pharmacologic agents, bladder training, and surgery.

Catheterization. Clean intermittent catheterization is a commonly employed intervention to avoid bladder overdistention in cases of urinary retention. It is usually performed at 4-hour intervals and aids in reducing the risk for vesicourethral reflux and kidney damage. Permanent indwelling catheters are used only in specific medical situations, and alternatives should be used as possible.

Indications for short-term indwelling urinary catheter include the following: (1) for accurate monitoring of urine output, (2) for relief of urinary obstruction, (3) for prevention of obstruction from large clots when hematuria is present, (4) for surgical procedures involving general or spinal anesthesia, and (5) for incontinence when pressure ulcers are present.

Although a medical necessity in certain situations, permanent indwelling catheters carry a risk. UTIs, urethral irritation, epididymoorchitis, pyelonephritis, renal calculi, and cancer are all associated with the use of permanent indwelling catheters in people with spinal cord injury.[70,293] Although associated with fewer adverse effects, intermittent catheterization can lead to reduced quality of life.[205]

Catheterization is frequently used in conjunction with medications. Anticholinergic agents are used to treat voiding dysfunctions that include detrusor hyperactivity. These agents relax the bladder, reduce high pressures, and increase bladder capacity. Side effects include dry mouth, gastrointestinal disturbances, drowsiness, cognitive impairment, hallucinations, and delirium.

Botox Injections. Although a relatively new treatment, botulinum toxin A injections into the detrusor muscle appear to reduce involuntary bladder contractions in people with neurogenic detrusor overactivity.[8,176,221] Long-term studies are needed to determine appropriate frequency, duration and efficacy of treatment.

Bladder Training. Bladder training methods are designed to enhance bladder function and prevent complications. Patients are often encouraged to attempt urination every 2 hours. Establishing a bladder pattern can result in less UI. Sitting position on the toilet is also important for full empting. Full relaxation of the legs (particularly the adductors and gluteals) can improve PFM relaxation and decrease residual urine. Patients may also be encouraged to double void (stand and sit immediately after voiding to allow a chance for more urine to be released). Adequate fluid intake is important for the prevention of infection and over concentrated urine. With a hyperreflexive bladder or detrusor–sphincter dyssynergia the abnormally concentrated urine can stimulate afferent nerve endings, exacerbating the bladder disorder. This could increase vesicular pressures, vesicoureteral reflux, and overflow urine leakage. Conversely, excessive fluid intake can exacerbate bladder over distention.

Biofeedback. Biofeedback techniques using electromyography can help the individual learn better voluntary control of PFM sphincters in conditions with incomplete nerve damage. Complete relaxation of the PFM is necessary for full bladder empting.

Surgery. A variety of surgical interventions for neurogenic bladder exist, although because of the invasive nature of the surgery, surgical intervention is often utilized after more conservative methods have failed. Procedures include bladder augmentation cystoplasty (colon, ileus, stomach, or ureter can be used); cystectomy with or without continent diversion; ureteral and bladder neck suspension; artificial urinary sphincter implantation[162]; ileovesicostomy, ileal conduit, or placement of suprapubic catheters; denervation procedures and electrostimulation (for complete lesions); and sacral nerve neuromodulation (for incomplete lesions).

SPECIAL IMPLICATIONS FOR THE THERAPIST	18-9

Neurogenic Bladder Disorders

Therapists provide care for many people who have sustained spinal cord injuries and cerebrovascular accidents or who have myelomeningoceles, multiple sclerosis, or brain tumors. Neurogenic bladder disorders are usually only one of the complications associated with these conditions, but familiarity with this complication is important. The potential for UTIs, renal calculi, and renal damage is high in those with neurogenic bladder disorders.

The development of any of these comorbidities can interfere with the rehabilitation process. Several medical conditions such as UTI, diabetes, congestive heart failure, bladder cancer, and enlarged prostate can be mistaken for a bladder control problem. Familiarity with the signs and symptoms associated with these potential diseases is a necessity. Detection of any of these symptoms warrants communication with a physician.

Incontinence associated with any of the bladder conditions discussed here can be greatly improved and even eliminated in many people through a program of exercise and behavioral intervention. Therapists should work on maximizing functional mobility, relaxed sitting position on the toilet, and the ability to relax the adductors. Therapists in the rehabilitation facility will need to work within established bladder schedule in scheduling therapy sessions. Coordination with nursing helps to establish a routine that allows for health bladder and bowel scheduling.

Interstitial Cystitis/Painful Bladder Syndrome

Overview and Incidence

Painful bladder syndrome (PBS) is a term introduced in 2002 by the International Continence Society (ICS) and defined as "complaint of suprapubic pain related to bladder filling accompanied by other symptoms such as increased daytime and night-time frequency in the absence of proven urinary infection or other obvious pathology."[1]

Interstitial cystitis (IC) is a subgroup of PBS. The terms PBS and IC are often used interchangeably; however, IC is a specific diagnosis and requires confirmation by typical cystoscopic and histologic features.[116] Chronic prostatitis/chronic pelvic pain syndrome in men (discussed more fully in Chapter 19; see section on "Chronic Prostatitis") are terms used to describe a symptoms complex characterized by pelvic pain and voiding dysfunction without infection or obvious pathology very similar to PBS/IC. Some practitioners think they may share similar etiology.

Exact figures on the incidence of PBS/IC are unavailable because of a lack of uniform definitions and inconsistent terminology. Many individuals go undiagnosed for years.[135] Current estimates show 2.7% to 6.5% of women in the United States report symptoms consistent with PBS/IC.[152] Most are women[53,201] but some practitioners believe the occurrence in men is even more severely underreported.

Etiologic and Risk Factors

The etiology of PBS/IC has not been identified. Some genetic components have been reported.[279,288] Risk factors for PBS/IC have not been identified; however, there are a number of conditions that have been found to be coexistent with PBS/IC, including gastritis, child abuse, fibromyalgia, anxiety disorder, headache, esophageal reflux, unspecified back disorder, depression, allergic reactions, vulvodynia, and irritable bowel syndrome.[52,77,116,279]

Pathogenesis

The pathophysiology of PBS/IC is unclear and appears to be related to several factors including altered permeability of the bladder wall, overactive PFM and visceromuscular reflex, and hypersensitivity and neurologic irritation. Studies show overactive PFM in 70% to 90% of individuals with PBS/IC.[171,201,222] Hunner lesions are superficial hemorrhages of the bladder wall seen on hydrodistention with cystoscopy. The lesions are only seen in 4% of cases and in those with severe presentation.[207]

Clinical Manifestation

PBS/IC is a symptoms complex with many variations. The most common symptoms are urinary urgency and frequency (in some cases up to four times per hour).[216] Several groups of researchers are documenting subgroups of PBS/IC with very different patterns, suggesting the possibility of different etiologies.[173] Other symptoms include nocturia, pain in the bladder, urethra, or vagina, suprapubic pain, and dull low back pain are common. There may also be difficulty emptying the bladder, pressure, burning, "electric shocks," spasm, and a stabbing sensation. Symptoms may increase with physical/emotional stress, acid foods, travel, or intercourse.

MEDICAL MANAGEMENT

DIAGNOSIS, TREATMENT, AND PROGNOSIS. Initial assessment is focused on ruling out other causes of the symptoms with history, physical, cystoscopy, and urinalysis with cytology. Voiding diaries and symptom indexes also help to identify impairments. Optional investigations include cystoscopy with hydrodistention to look for Hunner lesions, potassium sensitivity test to check for bladder wall permeability, urodynamics, pelvic ultrasound, and intravenous pyelogram.[201]

Medical treatment is focused on symptom relief. Complete resolution is rare. Types of treatment may include: medications, hydrodistention with or without intravesical therapy, neuromodulation, or in rare cases removal of the bladder with stoma placement.

SPECIAL IMPLICATIONS FOR THE THERAPIST 18-10

Interstitial Cystitis
Physical therapists are playing a larger role in conservative management of PBS/IC.

The current American Urological Association guidelines for treatment of interstitial cystitis and bladder pain syndrome list patient education, stress management, and self-help as first-line treatments.[115] Manual therapy including soft-tissue mobilization inside the vagina or rectum is a second-line

treatment.[84] Relaxation training of the pelvic floor muscle and treatment of any orthopedic dysfunctions of the pelvis are also offered to treat overactive PFM.

Intervention by a physical therapist will address any deficits in the musculoskeletal system as noted by the evaluation, postural dysfunction, increased or decreased range of motion, and decreased strength. A crucial aspect to evaluation and intervention is the condition of the soft tissue, especially in the lower quadrant and inside the vagina and rectum.

Restrictions are commonly found in people with interstitial cystitis involving the muscles that attach to the pelvis (e.g., adductors, gluteals, obturator internus and externus, piriformis, abdominals, and iliopsoas). A trigger point evaluation is essential in determining the presence of somatovisceral responses contributing to frequency and urgency.

Specific passive and active stretching exercises and muscle reeducation activities are progressed according to the individual's response to the soft tissue interventions. Modalities such as biofeedback, ultrasound, and electrical stimulation externally and internally along with behavioral techniques (e.g., for reducing frequency and urgency) may be employed.[155]

REFERENCES
To enhance this text and add value for the reader, all references are included on the companion Evolve site that accompanies this textbook. The reader can view the reference source and access it online whenever possible.

CHAPTER 19

The Male Genital/Reproductive Systems

LISA A. MASSA • BETH SHELLY

The male genital or reproductive system is made up of the testes, epididymis, vas deferens, seminal vesicles, prostate gland, and penis (Fig. 19-1). These structures are susceptible to inflammatory disorders, neoplasms, and structural defects. Unless treating individuals with urinary incontinence or pelvic pain, therapists do not typically treat people for primary reproductive system disease, but because of the incidence and nature of these disorders, an understanding of their clinical presentation is essential.

Prostate cancer is the most common cancer in males in the United States, and testicular cancer, although relatively rare, is on the rise and the most common cancer in males aged 15 to 35 years. Benign prostatic hyperplasia (BPH) is one of the most common disorders of the aging male population. Because of the high incidence of these diseases, therapists will see clients with such a history, and the disorder or prescribed medical treatment could have a profound effect on the client's clinical presentation and response to treatment.

The initial presenting symptom for some of these disorders could be urinary dysfunction or back or groin pain, the latter being musculoskeletal conditions for which physical therapy care is often sought. An awareness of other symptoms besides pain and signs associated with urogenital system diseases may alert the therapist to other origins of the back pain. The presence of such symptoms warrants communication with a physician regarding the client's status.

Therapists have long been taught to ask clients with back pain questions regarding sexual function, the concern being the possible presence of cauda equina syndrome. An awareness of the more probable causes of sexual dysfunction helps the therapist determine the relevance and potentially urgent nature of a client's complaints. The disorders discussed in this chapter are those of the highest incidence or of greatest implications for therapists.

AGING AND THE MALE REPRODUCTIVE SYSTEM

The reproductive system undergoes degenerative changes associated with aging that can affect sexual function. The testes become smaller, with thickening of the seminiferous tubules impeding sperm production; the prostate gland enlarges, potentially affecting urine outflow; and sclerotic changes occur in the local blood vessels, possibly resulting in sexual dysfunction (erectile dysfunction [ED]/impotence).

The age-related decrease in male sex hormone levels (androgen deficiency) also has significant local and systemic effects. Protein synthesis, salt and water balance, bone growth, and homeostasis and cardiovascular function are all under the influence of these hormones. A decline in bioavailable testosterone has been clearly correlated with age-related memory changes; decreasing sexual interest; and physical changes, including decreased strength, body mass, and bone density.[97,109,162]

Arteriosclerosis of the blood vessels resulting in peripheral vascular disease can also affect the vessels supplying the penis. While decreases in testosterone levels, penile rigidity, and ejaculation volume are all common age-relate changes in male sexual function, sexual (erectile) dysfunction can be an indicator of ischemic heart disease and should not be ignored as a symptom requiring medical evaluation.

DISORDERS OF THE PROSTATE

Prostatitis

Overview

Clinically, the diagnosis of "prostatitis" refers to multiple disorders that cause pelvic pain and discomfort ranging from acute bacterial infection to complex conditions that may not necessarily be caused by prostatic inflammation or infection. Because the traditional etiologic-based classification system did not always correlate symptoms with what worked in treatment, the National Institutes of Health (NIH)/National Institute of Diabetes and Digestive and Kidney Diseases devised a new classification of prostatitis (Table 19-1).[82] Inflammation of the prostate gland can be acute bacterial, chronic bacterial, chronic prostatitis/chronic pelvic pain syndrome, or asymptomatic inflammatory prostatitis.

Acute bacterial prostatitis (category I) is the least common of the four types but also the easiest to diagnose and treat effectively. Men with this disease often have chills, fever, hypotension (a finding that may help explain low

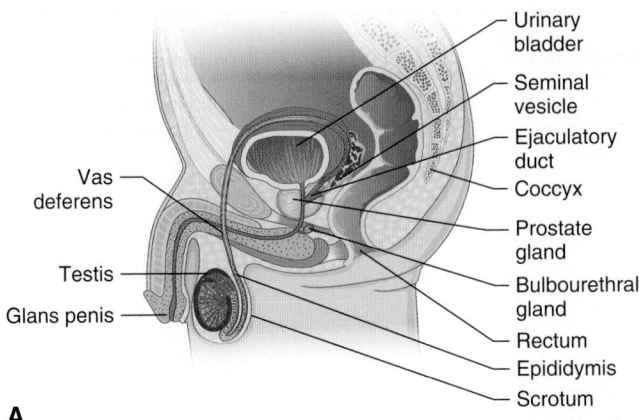

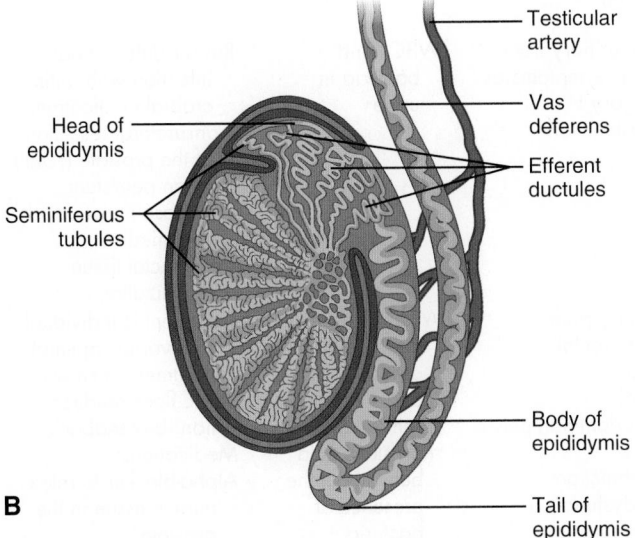

Figure 19-1

A, The male reproductive system. **B,** Internal structure of the testis and relationship of the testis to the epididymis. Note the tunica vaginalis, the serous covering or pouch folded around the testis. The inner or visceral layer of the tunica vaginalis covers the testis, epididymis, and lower portion of the spermatic cord. The outer or parietal layer of the tunica vaginalis lines the walls of the scrotal pouch and is attached to the fascial coverings of the testis. A small amount of fluid is normally present between these two layers, especially between the testicle and epididymis. **C,** Anatomy of the prostate, rectum, bladder, dorsal vein complex, striated urethral sphincter, pelvic plexus, and neurovascular bundle. (A, modified from Bloom V, Fawcett DW: *Textbook of histology*, ed 10, Philadelphia, 1975, WB Saunders; B, redrawn from Guyton AC: *Anatomy and physiology*, Philadelphia, 1985, Saunders College Publishing.)

blood pressure in some men), pain in the lower back and genital area, urinary frequency and urgency often at night, burning or painful urination, body aches, and a demonstrable infection of the urinary tract as evidenced by white blood cells and bacteria in the urine. The treatment is an appropriate antibiotic.[112]

Chronic bacterial prostatitis (category II), also relatively uncommon, is acute prostatitis associated with an underlying defect in the prostate, which becomes a focal point for bacterial persistence in the urinary tract. During a symptomatic infection, the bladder is also involved.[2,108] Effective treatment usually requires identifying and removing the defect and then treating the infection with antibiotics. However, antibiotics often do not cure this condition.[112]

Chronic prostatitis/chronic pelvic pain syndrome (CP/CPPS), also known as noninflammatory sometimes called *prostatodynia* (and previously known as *nonbacterial prostatitis*), is classified as category III and the most common (more than 90% of cases) but least understood form of prostatitis.

> **Note to Reader:** The term *chronic pelvic pain syndrome* (CPPS) may be used to describe conditions of males or females in whom pain is located in the pelvic region without other pathology. These conditions often involve the musculoskeletal system. This is a diagnosis of exclusion when other potential life conditions could have or should have been ruled out. CP/CPPS is a term specific to males.

CP/CPPS is found in men of any age, its symptoms go away and then return without warning, and it may be inflammatory or noninflammatory. In the inflammatory form (category IIIA), urine, semen, and other fluids from the prostate show no evidence of a known infecting organism but do contain the kinds of cells the body usually produces to fight infection. The consensus definition identifies genitourinary pain as the primary component of this syndrome. It also includes several exclusion criteria including active urethritis, urogenital cancer, urinary tract disease, urethral stricture or neurological disease affecting the bladder. Urinary symptoms and sexual dysfunction are often prevalent with this syndrome.[2]

In the noninflammatory form (category IIIB), no evidence of inflammation, including white blood cells, is present in the semen.[112] An α-blocker may be used to relax the muscle tissue in the prostate. No single solution works for everyone with this condition.[112]

Asymptomatic inflammatory prostatitis (category IV) is the diagnosis when the man does not complain of pain or discomfort but has white blood cells in his semen. Doctors usually find this form of prostatitis when looking for causes of infertility or when testing for prostate cancer.[112]

These conditions are typically preceded by lower urinary tract infections (UTIs) (see Chapter 18). Therapists are least likely to encounter problems associated with acute prostatitis because the symptoms are usually severe enough that physician contact is initiated by the client (or family), and rehabilitation is typically placed on hold until the antibiotic therapy is successful.

> **Note to Reader:** Prior to 1995, prostatitis was classified into four categories: acute bacterial prostatitis, chronic bacterial prostatitis, nonbacterial prostatitis, and prostatodynia. In 1995, the U.S. National Institutes of Health (NIH) developed a new classification scheme. The first two categories—acute and chronic bacterial prostatitis—remained the same.[81] Nonbacterial prostatitis and prostatodynia were combined as category III (i.e., chronic abacterial prostatitis/chronic pelvic pain syndrome [CPPS]). Category III was further subdivided into IIIa, inflammatory CPPS, and IIIb, noninflammatory CPPS. Category IV encompasses asymptomatic inflammatory prostatitis. Recent documentation by Hanno (2012) has confirmed this is still the recommended categorization.[62a]

Table 19-1	**Prostatitis Classification***				
Category	**NIDDK Classification**	**Description**	**Clinical Manifestation**	**Lab Findings**	**Treatment**

I	Acute bacterial prostatitis; least common	Bacterial infection of the prostate gland as a result of a bacteria, virus, or STD	Sudden onset of fever, chills, hypotension
			Malaise, myalgia
			Arthralgia
			Pain:
			  Low back
			  Sacral
			  Groin/pelvis (genital area)
			  Rectal
			Urinary symptoms:
			  Frequent and painful urination; urgency
			  Weak stream when urinating
			  UTI
				WBCs and bacteria in urine	Antimicrobial medications

II	Chronic bacterial prostatitis; uncommon	Recurrent infection associated with anatomic defect of the prostate	Intermittent urinary tract infections; symptoms as for category I Erectile dysfunction	WBCs and bacteria in urine	Repair defect; treat infection with antimicrobial medications Transurethral resection of the prostate (TURP) when persistent disease is not cured with medications Deep rectal tissue mobilization

IIIA	Inflammatory chronic prostatitis/chronic pelvic pain syndrome (CP/CPPS)	No demonstrable infection	Genitourinary pain:
			  Perineum, rectal
			  Testicular
			  Penis (tip)
			  Lower abdominal/pelvic
			  Low back
			Sexual dysfunction
			  Erectile dysfunction
			  Painful ejaculation
			  Disturbed quality of life
			Urologic symptoms may be present:
			  Frequency
			  Urgency
			  Dysuria
			  Decreased force of urine stream
			  Nocturia
				WBCs and other infection-fighting cells may be present in urine, semen, and prostatic fluid but without the presence of bacteria	Treatment is individual and varies; optimal treatment unknown
					Pelvic floor reeducation; biofeedback
					Medications:
					Alpha-blocker to relax muscle tissue in the prostate
					Neuropathic pain medications
					Herbal treatments (see text)

IIIB	Noninflammatory CP/CPPS	Previously known as chronic nonbacterial prostatitis	Same as IIIA	None	Same as for CP/CPPS in IIIA
IV	Asymptomatic inflammatory prostatitis		No symptoms	WBCs in semen and prostate fluid	None

STD, sexually transmitted disease; UTI, urinary tract infection; WBCs, white blood cells.
*Note: These are possible symptoms; not all men will have all symptoms.

On the other hand, therapists are likely to encounter chronic bacterial prostatitis, which is a much more subtle disorder, and complete resolution with treatment is often difficult to obtain. CP/CPPS is common and may benefit from pelvic floor reeducation with a specialized physical therapist.[20]

Incidence and Risk Factors

Prostatitis affects millions of men. In the United States, 8.2% of men will experience prostatitis.[3,130] The prevalence is highest among men in their forties; older men especially prone to UTI develop prostatitis, but this condition can affect men of all ages. UTIs are among the more common infections, afflicting the male population secondary to bladder outlet obstruction associated with BPH. As the infection ascends through the urogenital system, the prostate can become involved. UTIs generally occur with much higher frequency in women than men, but men can still be affected and should not view UTI as a "woman's disease."

Besides a history of UTI and BPH, recent urethral catheterization or instrumentation, history of sexually transmitted infections, and multiple sexual partners increase the risk of developing prostatitis. Some men find that stress, emotional factors, alcohol, spicy foods, or caffeine triggers episodes. Poorly controlled diabetes mellitus increases the risk of UTI and prostatitis developing because the increased urine glucose provides the substrate for bacterial growth.

Etiologic Factors and Pathogenesis

The etiology of prostatitis appears to be multifactorial. The etiology of the most common form of prostatitis, CP/CPPS, is poorly understood. Despite the assumption that there is an infectious or inflammatory process, this theory has not been proved. It has also been suggested that CP/CPPS may not be an organ-specific syndrome. Instead it may be a urogenital manifestation of regional or systemic abnormalities.[5,124] Some hypothesize that the process may begin with an initial infection or trauma that affects the prostate, pelvic floor, bladder, or perineum. If not effectively treated in the early stages it may lead to central sensitization. Autoimmunity may play a role in chronic prostatitis, because up to one-third of men with prostatitis have elevated levels of specific molecules that regulate the inflammatory response. Another hypothesis is that many of the men affected have overactive pelvic floor muscle and trigger points of the pelvic floor muscle mimicking prostatitis.[65,168,174] In the Zermann (1999) study,[173] 88% of the men with CP/CPPS had pelvic floor muscle trigger points and 52% had dyssynergia.[174] The NIH is funding several prostatitis studies to examine this further.

Some evidence of the relationship of CP/CPPS to muscle spasms, trigger points, and overactive pelvic floor muscle exists. It is also postulated that CP/CPPS may have a similar mechanism as vulvodynia in women, fibromyalgia, and other central sensitization syndromes.[65,174]

The most commonly found pathogens associated with chronic bacterial infections are the gram-negative enterobacteria such as *Escherichia coli*, *Proteus mirabilis*, *Klebsiella pneumoniae*, and *Pseudomonas aeruginosa*. The pathogens associated with acute prostatitis include *E. coli*, pseudomonads, staphylococci, and streptococci. Although controversial, other infectious agents, such as gonococci, *Ureaplasma* species, chlamydiae, and mycoplasmata, are possible etiologic factors.

Clinical Manifestations

Table 19-1 contains a summary of symptoms associated with the four categories of prostatitis. Acute prostatitis occurs suddenly with severe symptoms. Fever, chills, and UTI are typical, along with pelvic discomfort. Blood in the urine, urinary retention, and urinary blockage are frequent, and there may be a steep rise in prostate-specific antigen (PSA), a marker for prostate cancer.

If not treated, acute prostatitis may become chronic. Men who experience chronic prostatitis are plagued by persistent low-grade symptoms with flare-ups of pelvic pain, voiding problems, and sexual dysfunction (e.g., erectile dysfunction, ejaculatory pain, and a decline in emotional well-being).[131] The pelvic pain is usually located behind the scrotum or in the perineum, the area between the rectum and testicles. This pain is usually made worse by sitting down and may be relieved or increased by ejaculation. Pain in the tip of the penis may be experienced.

MEDICAL MANAGEMENT

DIAGNOSIS. Urinalysis, analysis of an expressed prostatic specimen, and when appropriate, a digital rectal examination (DRE), in which the physician palpates manually for prostate changes or enlargement, are used to establish a diagnosis of prostatitis. Point of clarification: a DRE is *not* performed if category I prostatitis is suspected because it can further spread an infection.

> **Note to Reader:** Although we could not find any published evidence to support this statement, this point was brought to our attention and confirmed by several urologists.

The DRE may reveal a swollen, tender, and warm prostate. Computed tomography (CT) and transrectal ultrasonography (TRUS) provide anatomic details often needed in the evaluation of these individuals. Urodynamic testing may help identify voiding dysfunction, especially in men with pelvic or perineal pain and voiding symptoms.[35]

Prostatitis is differentiated in part from BPH and prostate cancer by the presence of pain (rarely present in BPH or cancer) and by age (more than half of all men with prostatitis are younger than 45 years of age). Current NIH guidelines, which stratify prostatitis into the four categories of prostatitis, advise using the NIH Chronic Prostatitis Symptom Index (NIH-CPSI)[113] to assess symptoms and plan treatment. The CPSI assesses the severity of symptoms and quality of life in men with CP/CPPS.[20,89,113] Because there is no gold standard diagnostic test for CP/CPPS, it remains a diagnosis of exclusion for the most part.

TREATMENT. Treatment depends on the type of prostatitis present. Acute prostatitis (category I) is treated with antibiotics. For men who are unable to empty their bladders, suprapubic drainage is preferred over an indwelling urethral catheter.

Treatment of category II (chronic bacterial) prostatitis also involves antibiotics to eliminate the organism producing the infection. Men with frequent recurrences may be placed on antibiotic prophylaxis for 3 to 6 months and have their clinical course reassessed. Treatment of bladder outlet obstruction, which may impair bladder emptying, is also important.

Treatment of chronic bacterial prostatitis can be difficult, as the antibiotic agents have difficulty penetrating the chronically inflamed prostate. Drug therapy of 4 to 6 months' duration may be used in an attempt to treat this infection. Transurethral resection of the prostate (TURP) may be indicated if the disease is not cured with medications.

Optimal treatment for CP/CPPS is unknown. Multimodal treatment may be best with biofeedback, pelvic floor reeducation, and α-blocker therapy (to relax smooth muscle of the prostate and at the base of the bladder). Newly diagnosed cases or those who have not been treated before are more likely to respond to α-blocker therapy compared to chronic refractory cases. Longer courses of treatment (4-6 months) seem to work better than shorter courses.[85]

Because the cause of nonbacterial prostatitis is unknown, treatment is often given to simply provide symptom control and relief. Antiinflammatory medications are administered. Antibiotics, fluoroquinolone, and antifungal agents may also be given. For unknown reasons, about half of men with nonbacterial prostatitis respond to antibiotics; antibiotics are used to treat bacterial prostatitis.

Other treatments for CP/CPPS range from medications to treat neuropathic pain, anticholinergic medications, phytotherapies (e.g., herbal treatment with quercetin or bee pollen), physical therapy, and in rare cases, surgery to treat bladder neck obstruction. For category IV prostatitis, no treatment is recommended.[108]

SPECIAL IMPLICATIONS FOR THE THERAPIST   19-1

Prostatitis

When treating people at risk for developing prostatitis, therapists need to be vigilant for the onset of symptoms listed in Table 19-1. The symptoms may be subtle initially or difficult to ascertain because of communication difficulties common in the aging adult. The fact that therapy may extend over a number of weeks may allow the therapist to detect the subtle changes and initiate contact with the primary physician.

In young people with back pain, visceral disease is rarely the first thought as a cause of back pain. Prostatitis can be the cause of back pain of unknown origin in young males. The presence of any of the symptoms listed in Table 19-1, along with the onset of back pain, should raise concern.

When rehabilitating someone with a history of chronic prostatitis, therapists need to be aware of symptoms associated with UTIs. Many of these men experience recurrent UTIs as the prostatic bacteria continue to invade the bladder. The waxing and waning of symptoms may interfere with the client's compliance with a rehabilitation program. Reassurance that prostatitis is not a warning sign of cancer may be helpful. Bicycle seats can aggravate prostatitis; thus, a recumbent bicycle is recommended because it puts less pressure on the groin.

Physical therapy to correct musculoskeletal imbalances of the pelvis can result in decreased pain in men with CP/CPPS. All therapists are encouraged to perform a complete musculoskeletal examination and provide treatment of impairments found. Biofeedback and neuromuscular reeducation for pelvic floor muscle dysfunction provided by specialized physical therapists are also beneficial. Several researchers have documented improvement in CP/CPPS with electrical stimulation,[74] biofeedback,[9,84] and rectal deep tissue mobilization.[9]

Benign Prostatic Hyperplasia

Overview

BPH is an age-related nonmalignant enlargement of the prostate gland. It is defined as a prostate volume (PV) greater than 30 mL.[7,41]

Incidence and Risk Factors

Of men age 50 years and older, 75% experience symptoms of prostate enlargement.[142] The disease is rarely noted in men under age 40 and tends to become symptomatic after age 50 years. Besides age, geography and ethnicity are important factors in the incidence of this disease. BPH is found most often in the United States and western Europe and least often in the Far East. The incidence of BPH is also higher in blacks than in whites. Drinking moderate amounts (one or two alcoholic drinks per day) is associated with a reduced risk of BPH. Cigarette smoking increases the risk for BPH-like symptoms, possibly because bladder irritation caused by cigarette smoke may heighten the urgency and frequency of urination.

Dietary risk factors are under investigation. Milk and dairy products have been related to an increase in BPH, but not all studies confirm this association; fruit has been reported to have a protective effect against this condition. Other food groups, including meat and vegetables, have been analyzed in relation to BPH, but the results have been inconsistent. More frequent consumption of prepared cereals, bread, eggs, and poultry may be a risk factor.[25] Markers to assess risk of progression include the following: (1) age greater than 50 years, (2) PSA greater than 1.4 ng/mL, (3) prostate volume (PV) greater than 30 mL, and (4) International Prostate Symptom Score (available online at http://www.urospec.com/uro/Forms/ipss.pdf) greater than 8. These parameters are used to determine which individuals would benefit from medical therapy and possibly avoid surgery.[13,16]

Pathogenesis

The prostate gland, a muscular part of the male reproductive system, is normally about the size and shape of a walnut, normally weighing about 20 g. It is located in front of the rectum and just below the bladder (see Fig. 19-1). It consists of five lobes that surround the urethra and produces seminal fluid to nourish and transport semen. Throughout life, the body constantly replaces old, dying prostate cells with new ones. For reasons still not completely clear, as men age, the ratio of new prostate cells to old prostate cells shifts in favor of lower cell death. By age 70 years, the hypertrophic prostate can weigh up to 200 g, resulting in significant urethral obstruction, decreased urine storage capability, and difficulty emptying the bladder.

Although the cause is unknown, changes in hormone balance associated with aging may be responsible for the development of BPH. The condition is commonly referred to as *benign prostatic hypertrophy*, but the pathologic changes are marked by *hyperplasia*, not hypertrophy. Multiple prostatic nodules develop, resulting from the proliferation of epithelial cells, smooth muscle cells, and stromal fibroblasts of the gland. These nodules initially develop in the periurethral region of the prostate as opposed to the periphery of the gland (Fig. 19-2). The enlargement of the prostate increases smooth muscle tone at the bladder neck and prostatic capsule leading to increased resistance. These effects narrow the prostatic urethra and thus diminish urinary flow.

Both androgens and estrogens contribute to the hyperplasia of this condition. Dihydrotestosterone (DHT), the biologically active metabolite of testosterone, is thought to be the primary mediator of hyperplasia, whereas estrogens sensitize the prostatic tissue to the growth-producing effects of DHT. The increased levels of estrogen that occur with aging may enhance the action of androgens at this point in the life cycle.

Clinical Manifestations

The clinical presentation of BPH is related to secondary involvement of the urethra. As men age, the prostate slowly grows larger. If it becomes too large, urine flow can become restricted. Lower urinary tract symptoms (LUTS) occur when men experience disturbances to the urinary flow. LUTS can occur in two forms: storage and voiding (urinary retention) symptoms. Storage symptoms include nocturia, frequency, or urgency. Voiding symptoms include hesitance, intermittency, or weakened stream.[14,48] These symptoms can lead to an overactive bladder.

Overactive bladder is defined as the inability to hold increasing volumes of urine and increased sensations of urgency and frequency. It is often associated with uninhibited detrusor contractions. The affected individual experiences urinary urgency, usually accompanied by frequency and nocturia, with or without urgency urinary incontinence, in the absence of urinary tract infection or other obvious pathology.

Quality of life and emotional function can be adversely affected by fatigue, micturition problems, and sleeping disturbances.[43] As the urethral obstruction progresses, the risk of developing UTIs, marked bladder distention with destructive bladder wall changes, hydroureter, and hydronephrosis increases (Fig. 19-3).

Hydroureter refers to the ureteral wall as it becomes severely stretched secondary to the bladder outflow obstruction, which increases the pressure in a retrograde direction. The ureteral wall can become stretched to the point where it loses the ability to undergo peristaltic contractions. With hydronephrosis, urine-filled dilation of the renal pelvis and calices occurs; destruction of renal tissue may occur.

Ultimately, renal failure and death may occur if treatment is not initiated. Other urinary symptoms associated with the later stages of the disease include urge incontinence, terminal urinary dribbling, urgency, hematuria, and dysuria.

MEDICAL MANAGEMENT

PREVENTION. There has been some controversy over the use of saw palmetto, lycopene, and tomato products as possible antioxidant prevention of BPH. The general consensus is that these natural products will not do any harm but they may not help either.

DIAGNOSIS. Correlation of the history, palpation findings (digital rectal exam [DRE]), and urodynamic test results (flow rate and force of stream) typically give rise to the diagnosis of BPH and indicate the choice of treatment. Regarding palpation, the bladder may be palpable as urinary retention progresses. In addition, a smooth, rubbery enlargement of the prostate may be noted

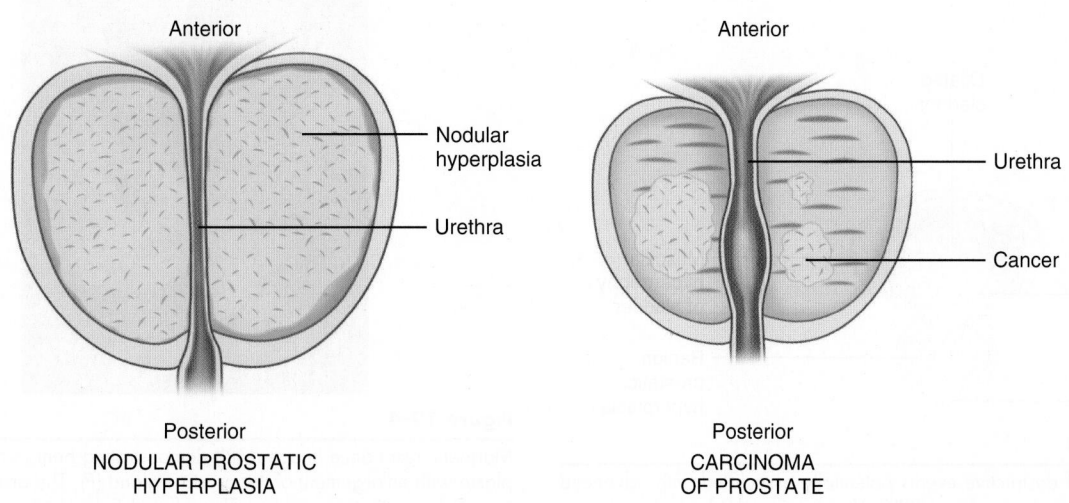

Figure 19-2

In benign prostatic hyperplasia (BPH), the nodules initially develop in the periurethral region, compressing the urethra. Cancer of the prostate typically develops initially in the periphery of the gland.

during DRE, although the perceived size of the prostate does not always correlate with the degree of urethral compression.

Prostate-specific antigen (PSA), a measure of protein in the bloodstream secreted by cells in the prostate gland, is an additional blood test that helps predict the natural course of BPH. Higher levels of PSA are linked with a greater risk of future prostate growth and subsequent complications. Urinalysis is usually done to check for hematuria and UTI. The most commonly employed urodynamic test for the assessment of BPH is uroflowmetry. The urine flow rate and the force of the urine stream are measured. It is generally agreed that a peak urine flow rate of less than 10 mL/sec is suggestive of obstruction.

Uroflowmetry by itself is a screening modality, not diagnostic, because the urinary obstruction could be occurring at sites other than at the prostate gland. In addition, diagnostic ultrasound, magnetic resonance imaging (MRI), and abdominal radiographs may be used to evaluate the size and length of the urethra, the size and configuration of the prostate, and the bladder capacity (Fig. 19-4). The American Urological Association has also developed a self-administered screening tool (International Prostate Symptom Score; available online at: http://www.urospec.com/uro/Forms/ipss.pdf) used to determine the frequency and severity of urinary symptoms.

TREATMENT. If symptoms related to BPH are mild, the condition is often just monitored because the clinical status of the disorder may stabilize or even improve. Aggressive treatment is indicated, when the condition progresses to a more advanced stage. Symptoms suggesting advanced disease include urine retention, incontinence, hematuria, and chronic UTIs. The goals of treatment include providing client comfort and avoiding serious renal damage. For those with moderate to severe symptoms, the two medical treatment approaches for BPH are pharmacologic and surgical.

Medication. In most cases, symptoms associated with BPH can be controlled with medications. One trial, the Medical Therapy of Prostatic Symptoms (MTOPS), found that combining medications produces better results than administering only one drug (monotherapy).[76]

Three main pharmacologic agents are used to treat BPH: (1) medications to shrink glandular tissue (5-α-reductase inhibitors); (2) drugs to relax smooth muscle tissue of the prostate, bladder neck, and urethra (α-adrenergic blockers); and (3) antimuscarinics to address overactive bladder symptoms. The 5-α-reductase inhibitors address the hormonal causes of BPH by preventing the enzyme 5-α-reductase from converting testosterone into DHT (DHT prompts glandular tissue to develop). As a result, the prostate shrinks by as much as 20%. This is a gradual process that can take up to a year to obtain maximum benefit.

The α-adrenergic receptors are located in the muscle fibers of the adenoma and prostate capsule. The resultant smooth muscle relaxation decreases pressure on

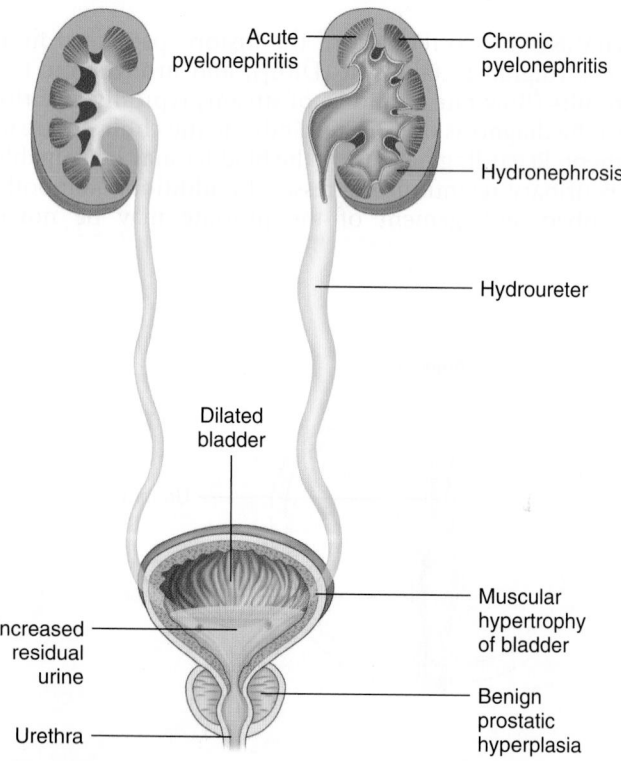

Figure 19-3

A cascade of destructive events potentially associated with advanced benign prostatic hyperplasia (BPH). Viewing Fig. 19-1, *A*, the relationship of the prostate located at the base of the bladder, surrounding a part of the urethra, can be visualized. As the prostate enlarges, the urethra becomes obstructed, interfering with the normal flow of urine.

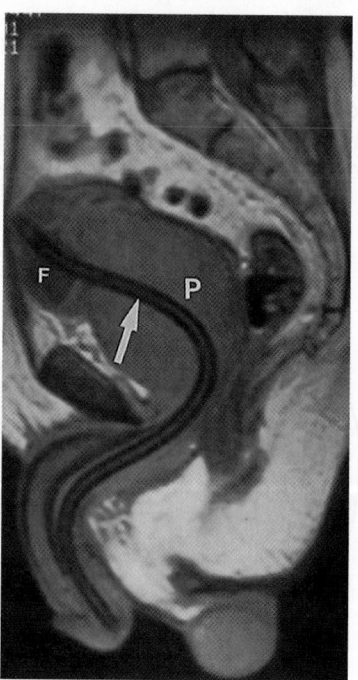

Figure 19-4

Magnetic resonance image (MRI) demonstrating benign nodular hyperplasia with enlargement of the prostate gland (*P*). The arrow is pointing to a Foley catheter in place. The inflated Foley balloon (*F*) indicates the level of the bladder neck. (From Grainger RG: *Grainger & Allison's diagnostic radiology: a textbook of medical imaging,* ed 4, Philadelphia, 2001, Churchill Livingstone.)

the urethra, enhancing urinary flow. Antimuscarinics block cholinergic receptors in the bladder wall to prevent bladder spasms. Antimuscarinics have demonstrated to improve bladder capacity, increased volume at first detrusor contraction, and maximum cytometric capacity.[1,18] Phytopharmaceuticals (e.g., substrates from the saw palmetto plant) used for the management of BPH represent up to 80% of all prescriptions in many European countries.[81] Earlier studies in the United States showed significant effects of saw palmetto on epithelial contraction, urinary flow rates, and improved symptoms compared with placebos,[56,93] but more recent studies have shown mixed results and a lack of convincing evidence.[17,138,148] Presently, the American Urologic Association does not recommend any dietary supplement for the management of BPH.

Androgen suppression drug therapy can also be used to block the synthesis and action of testosterone, including DHT. A 20% to 30% reduction in prostate volume can be noted. This can result in a lessening of the severity of symptoms and improvement in the objective criteria related to urinary obstruction although this can take 3 to 6 months.

Surgery. Not everyone with BPH responds adequately to medications. In such cases, BPH can progress to the point where surgery is required. The goal of surgical intervention is to alleviate the obstruction to urine flow. Presently the AUA recommends surgery for men who report the following conditions: recurrent gross hematuria of prostatic origin, recurrent UTI, renal insufficiency secondary to BPH, bladder stones, or LUTS refractory to other therapies. TURP is considered the gold standard in surgical treatments for BPH. A long tube with a miniature camera on the tip is threaded up the urethra into the bladder, allowing visual inspection of both of these structures. When the excess prostate tissue is identified, a surgical instrument is threaded through this tube, and resection of excess prostate tissue is performed to enlarge the urinary channel.

TURP is very successful in relieving symptoms and improving quality of life, but some drawbacks are evident (e.g., requires a general anesthetic and hospital stay and may be accompanied by side effects such as bleeding, incontinence, ED/impotence, or retrograde ejaculation [in which an ejaculation goes back into the bladder]). An alternative technique is transurethral incision of the prostate (TUIP). In the case of TUIP, incisions in the muscle wall of the prostate and bladder neck allow for an outward expansion of the gland, relieving some of the pressure on the urethra. TURP is preferable when there is a large gland, severe and recurrent gross hematuria, and prostatitis; the goal is to remove infected tissue and calculi.

Thermotherapy by either transurethral microwave therapy (TUMT), such as Prostatron, or laser surgery through laser-induced thermotherapy, such as Green Light laser or indigo laser, has been developed over the past 10 years to provide effective alternatives to surgical management. Lasers are used for rapid incision and vaporization of the prostate with minimal bleeding. This treatment procedure is indicated in the case of small-size BPH and in the presence of risk factors, such as heart disease or anticoagulation therapy, or for men who do not tolerate medications well. This modality restores spontaneous urine flow by destroying diseased prostate tissue.

Results of long-term studies are not available at this time, but short-term results demonstrate that laser therapy is at least as safe and effective in relieving BPH symptoms as TURP and may provide reduced morbidity.[55] The potential advantages of these procedures over TURP and TUIP are shorter operative time, usually without hospitalization; minimal bleeding; and decreased incidence of postoperative retrograde ejaculation and bladder neck contracture.

Potential disadvantages of laser treatment include postoperative urinary retention, no tissue being available for histologic study, and less than optimal prospects for treating large lesions. This technique may be associated with a high recurrence rate requiring additional treatment.[158] In the case of laser, the larger the lesion, the more passes are required, increasing the associated risks.[161] The introduction of an integrated system of computer, robotics, and laser technology for prostate resection may be the intervention of the future.[66]

Other. Other procedures include water-induced thermotherapy. Heated water is injected into a balloon inserted into the urethra. The heat destroys excess prostate tissue. The procedure is done on an outpatient basis, but a catheter must be worn for 1–3 weeks afterward. Water-induced thermotherapy is not advised for men who have had previous prostate, pelvic, or rectal surgery. A past history of pelvic radiation for prostate cancer is another exclusion factor.

Transurethral ethanol ablation of the prostate (TEAP) involves injecting ethanol (a type of alcohol) through the urethra into the prostate to destroy excess prostate tissue. Both of these procedures are designed to improve peak flow rate, but long-term data are not yet available.

Botulinum toxin (BTX, or Botox), has been used successfully in the treatment of BPH. Botulinum toxin injected directly into the prostate has been shown to reduce lower urinary tract symptoms and improve erectile function. The mechanism by which BTX can reduce prostate volume and intravesicular resistance remains unclear.[12] Promising preliminary results have been reported in studies combining medications with BTX.[34,153] The use of botulinum neurotoxin in the prostate is currently considered Food and Drug Administration (FDA) off-label use.

PROGNOSIS. BPH can contribute to chronic problems with lower urinary tract symptoms, ED, and decreased quality of life. Treatment is reserved for symptomatic presentation, but there is considerable risk of progression with possible development of prostate cancer.

SPECIAL IMPLICATIONS FOR THE THERAPIST 19-2

Benign Prostatic Hyperplasia

BPH often results in obstructed voiding with symptoms of urgency, frequency, hesitancy, intermittency, nocturia, and weak stream. Therapists conducting a medical history with men over the age of 50 years can easily include a series of four questions to help identify the presence of obstructed voiding:

- Do you urinate more than every 2 hours, or more than once during the night?
- Do you have trouble starting or continuing your urine?
- Do you have weak flow of urine or interrupted urine stream?
- Does it feel like your bladder is not emptying completely?

A *yes* answer to any of these questions warrants further medical evaluation. Painful urination; blood in the urine; or unexplained lower back, pelvis, hip, or upper thigh pain in the presence of any of these symptoms requires medical referral. Men over the age of 40 years should be encouraged to get regular check-ups in order to prevent complications from delayed diagnosis of BPH.

Surgical procedures for BPH carry the risk of complications, such as ED/impotence, urinary leakage, and retrograde ejaculation; venous thromboembolism is a potential complication of open prostatectomy. Unexplained reports of sexual dysfunction warrant communication with a physician. Frequent monitoring of sexual function (or screening for sexual dysfunction) may be warranted, i.e., if the person notes sexual dysfunction and has a history of the previously mentioned procedures, the therapist can ask about changes in sexual function. If there appears to be a worsening, communication with a physician would again be warranted.

Physical therapy management may be appropriate for men with BPH who are experiencing urinary incontinence, urgency, and/or frequency. The physical therapist can offer strength training for underactive pelvic floor muscles related to BPH procedures. Bladder training for overactive bladder is also helpful for symptoms of urgency and frequency.

Pharmacologic agents used to treat BPH are associated with numerous side effects, which the therapist should be aware of and watch out for. These include general muscle weakness, ED (inability to achieve an erection), loss of libido, gynecomastia, drowsiness, dizziness, tachycardia, and postural orthostatic hypotension. The therapist can advise clients about the possibility of falls from dizziness and loss of balance associated with these medications and take steps to institute a falls prevention program when appropriate (see "Special Implications for the Therapist 12-8: Orthostatic Hypotension" in Chapter 12). Any change or new onset of symptoms should be reported to the physician.

A THERAPIST'S THOUGHTS*

Screening Questions for Everyone

The questions provided above in this section are adequate for screening for BPH. It is recommended *all* clients of physical therapy should be screened for any type of pelvic floor disorder with the following questions:

- Do you ever leak urine or feces (stool)?
- Do you ever wear a pad because of leakage?

- Do you have pain associated with intercourse?
- Do you routinely experience genital and/or pelvic pain?
- Do you have difficulty emptying your bladder completely?
- Do you have problems with constipation?

People who answer yes to any of these questions may still be appropriate for physical therapy intervention but further evaluation is warranted and a decision made for medical referral, treat, or treat and refer.

*Beth Shelly, PT, DPT, WCS, BCB-PMD

Prostate Cancer

Overview

Adenocarcinoma of the prostate arises from the glandular cells and accounts for 98% of primary prostatic tumors. Ductal and transitional cell carcinomas make up the remainder of the tumors. Prostate cancer usually starts in the outer portion of the prostate and spreads inwardly and then beyond the gland, with metastases in more advanced stages.

Incidence

Prostate cancer, the most frequently diagnosed visceral malignancy in American men, is the second most common cause of male death from cancer. One in six American men will develop prostate cancer. According to the National Cancer Institute, approximately 241,740 men were newly diagnosed in 2012 (up from 189,000 in 2002) and 28,170 men died.[19,139]

The number of new cases of prostate cancer in the last decade represents an increase of 200%.[73] However, the evidence suggests the use of PSA screening as a means of early detection may be the reason for the increased incidence. With PSA testing, more than 90% of prostate cancers are found early when they are highly curable. Widespread implementation of prostate cancer screening in the United States has led to more cancers being detected but at an earlier stage with fewer cases of metastases at diagnosis and a decrease in mortality rate. Autopsy studies indicate that occult prostate cancer is present in 25% of men age 60 to 69 years, in 40% of men age 70 to 79 years, and in more than 50% of men age 80 years and older.[132] Men less than 50 years of age make up less than 1% of those with prostate cancer. Prostate cancer incidence and mortality vary strikingly among ethnic and national groups, with a particular propensity for African Americans.[50]

In the United States, the incidence of prostate cancer is approximately 60% higher in African American men than in European American men; the mortality rate from the disease is more than twice as high among African Americans.[125] Screening rates for African American men with a positive family history of prostate cancer are significantly lower than in Caucasians, especially in older men ages 60 to 70 years.[106]

Risk Factors

Box 19-1 lists risk factors related to prostate cancer. Prostate cancer is a disease of the aging male, but evidence exists that genetic, environmental, and social factors

Box 19-1

RISK FACTORS FOR PROSTATE CANCER

- Age >50 years
- African American
- Geography (United States and Scandinavian countries)
- Family history; inherited gene mutation
- Environmental exposure to cadmium
- High-fat diet
- Alcohol consumption

Box 19-2

GLEASON SCORE

The Gleason scale score, or Gleason grading system, is used to evaluate the prognosis of men with prostate cancer. Scores are assigned based on cytologic examination and range from 2 to 10, based on how the cancerous cells look compared to normal prostate cells. The higher the Gleason score, the more likely the cancer cells will grow and spread rapidly. Pathologists often identify the two most common patterns of cells in the tissue (majority of the tumor and minority of the tumor), assign a Gleason grade from 1 to 5 to each, and add the two grades. The result is a number between 2 and 10. A Gleason score of less than 6 indicates a less aggressive cancer. A grade 7 or higher is considered more aggressive.

Score	Interpretation
2-4	Unlikely to spread, good prognosis
5-6	Mildly aggressive
7	Moderately aggressive
8-10	Highly aggressive, poor prognosis

Data from Gleason DF: The Veteran's Administration Cooperative Urologic Research Group: histologic grading and clinical staging of prostatic carcinoma. In Tannenbaum M, ed, *Urologic pathology: the prostate*, Philadelphia, 1977, Lea and Febiger, pp. 171–198.

jointly and in combination contribute to observed differences in various populations. Geographically, the highest frequencies of prostate cancer are found in the United States and northwestern Europe (Scandinavian countries), whereas the lowest are found in Mexico, Greece, and Japan. As mentioned, African Americans have twice the risk of non-Hispanic whites, which is attributed to traditional socioeconomic, clinical, and pathologic factors.[67]

Although no genetic marker has been found, a familial history of prostate cancer is a risk factor. A significant increase in risk has been estimated for men who have both a first- and second-degree relative with the disease.[144] If a close relative has prostate cancer, a man's risk of the disease doubles; with two relatives, his risk increases fivefold; and with three close relatives, the risk is about 97%.[114] In addition, mortality from prostate cancer is thought to be three times greater in relatives of men with prostate cancer compared with those without such a family history.

Exposure to cadmium through welding, electroplating, alkaline battery production, farming, typesetting, and ship fitting places men at higher risk of prostate cancer. High levels of dietary fat and calcium have been correlated with prostate cancer,[57,117] with a protective effect from higher intake of tomato sauce and physical activity.[58,59] Other risk factors still under investigation include having a vasectomy, eating red meat,[141] vitamin deficiency (vitamins D and E),[80] and frequency of ejaculations. The role of frequency of ejaculations (either through sexual intercourse or masturbation) in developing prostate cancer has been questioned, but results of a study involving 30,000 men suggest that ejaculation frequency is not related to increased risk of prostate cancer.[86]

One study[11] demonstrated evidence of an association between exercise and prostate cancer risk as well as tumor grade in men scheduled to undergo prostate biopsy. In this study of 190 men who underwent prostate biopsy, it was noted that men who reported 9 or more metabolic equivalent task hours (MET) per week of exercise were significantly less likely to have a malignant tumor and were associated with a lower risk of more advanced disease (Gleason score 7 or greater; see explanation of Gleason scoring/staging and Box 19-2 below).[11] Regular exercise has been demonstrated to be a stimulator of endogenous antioxidant pathways, promoting immune function and reducing systemic inflammation and proinflammatory factors.[15,33,96] Because of the strength of this evidence, the American Cancer Society has endorsed regular physical exercise for cancer survivors. The American College of Sports Medicine issued guidelines of 150 minutes per week of moderate to vigorous physical activity for cancer survivors (see further discussion of cancer and exercise, Chapter 9).

Etiologic Factors

Although the precise cause of prostate cancer is unknown, a strong endocrine system link is theorized. Androgens in particular have been implicated based on the androgenic control of normal growth and development of the prostate and the fact that males castrated before puberty do not develop prostate cancer or BPH. In addition, the responsiveness of prostate cancer to surgical castration and estrogen therapy supports this theory.[126] The higher incidence of cancer in African Americans is correlated with a 15% higher serum testosterone level in this same population.[47]

Environmental factors, especially dietary factors, may be linked with inflammation associated with the development of prostate cancer.[110]

The development of prostate cancer reflects a complex sequence of biologic and molecular events. Even though it is difficult to identify genes that predispose to prostate cancer because of late age at diagnosis, several inheritable and somatic genetic changes have been identified, including a prostate cancer susceptibility locus with linkage to a locus on chromosome 17p.[160] However, this gene is only responsible for between 2% and 5% of all prostate cancers, suggesting that additional genes contribute to this disease.[116,150] The EphB2 gene has been implicated as a prostate cancer tumor suppressor gene, with somatic inactivating mutations occurring in approximately 10% of sporadic tumors. This may be an important factor in African American men with a positive family history of prostate cancer.[78,129]

A newly identified retrovirus, called *XMRV*, previously thought to be associated with the development of prostate cancer in genetically susceptible men has been disproved. XMRV is closely related to a virus that causes leukemia in mice and is a newly identified infectious agent in humans. At first, researchers theorized that XMRV could be sexually transmitted, leading to chronic inflammation and cancer similar to how human papillomavirus triggers cervical cancer.[42] But there is sufficient evidence (and a lack of biological evidence) now to discredit this theory.[68,99]

Pathogenesis

Most prostatic adenocarcinomas are characterized by small- to moderate-size disorganized glands that infiltrate the stroma of the prostate. The tumors are more likely to develop initially in the periphery of the prostate, unlike BPH, in which the pathologic changes typically originate close to the urethra (see Fig. 19-2). Growth factors such as IGF and androgens have been implicated in prostate cancer. High levels of testosterone promote cell differentiation, which could protect against the development of prostate cancer. Declining levels of this hormone in older age may contribute to the increased incidence of prostate cancer with aging.

The cancer invades adjacent local structures, such as the seminal vesicles and urinary bladder, and spreads to the musculoskeletal system, particularly the axial skeleton, and lungs. Lymphatic metastasis may involve the obturator, iliac, and periaortic lymph nodes, extending up through the thoracic duct (see Fig. 13-8).

The mechanism underlying the *organ-specific* metastasis of prostate cancer cells to the bone is still poorly understood. Whether the cells only invade the bone and proliferate there or whether they invade many tissues but survive mainly in the bone is unclear; this concept is referred to as *seed and soil.*

Research suggests that osteonectin, a small protein found in bone marrow, attracts prostate cancer cells to bone and, once attracted, stimulates the cells to invade bone. These findings suggest that antibodies to osteonectin could reduce the invasiveness of prostate cancer (and breast cancer) and offer a potential way of preventing the spread of prostate cancer to the bone.[72]

Clinical Manifestations

The clinical presentation of prostate cancer is extremely variable and may be completely asymptomatic until the disease is advanced. In many men, the disease is noted incidentally on DRE or discovered in fragments of prostatic tissue removed through TURP for BPH. Depending on the size and location of the lesion, the initial presenting symptom could be related to urinary obstruction, onset of pain, or constitutional symptoms such as fatigue and weight loss.

The urinary obstruction symptoms associated with cancer are similar to those associated with BPH but typically present in later stages of the disease compared with BPH. Cancer originating in the subcapsular region of the prostate as opposed to the periurethral area would account for this difference. The obstructive symptoms include urinary urgency, frequency, hesitancy, dysuria, hematuria, difficulty initiating or continuing the urine stream, and decreased urine stream. Blood in the ejaculate may also be noted.

Bony metastasis occurs via lymphatics to adjacent structures and pelvic nodes in the majority of people with metastatic disease; the spinal column is the most common site.[127,169] Of the primary tumors that metastasize to the spine, prostate lesions rank fourth behind breast, lung, and myeloma. Prostate cancer can also metastasize to the lungs and liver. Metastases to the axial skeleton occur more often than to the appendicular skeleton, especially the spine, ribs, sternum, femur, and pelvis. Prostate cancer is unique in that bone is often the only clinically detectable site of metastasis, and the resulting tumors tend to be osteoblastic (bone forming) rather than being osteolytic (bone lysing).[90]

Pain complaints associated with prostate cancer can vary tremendously. A dull, vague ache may be noted in the rectal, sacral, or lumbar spine region, and the individual may have difficulty walking. The sacral and lumbar pain is typically associated with bony metastasis. Pain may be noted in the thoracic and shoulder girdle areas secondary to lymphatic spread of the disease or again secondary to local bony metastasis. Symptoms such as fatigue, weight loss, anemia, and dyspnea have all been attributed to metastatic spread of the disease.

MEDICAL MANAGEMENT

PREVENTION. Prostate cancer has a long latency period between appearance of premalignant lesions and clinically evident cancer, making it a type of cancer susceptible to chemoprevention (the use of agents to slow progression of, reverse, or inhibit carcinogenesis). There is some evidence that this cancer may be preventable with a nontoxic oral agent such as vitamin E, selenium, soy,[115,164] or other dietary or nutritional supplement.[51,155]

In 2003, the Prostate Cancer Prevention Trial (PCPT) became the first phase III clinical trial of prostate cancer prevention. Started in 1993, this landmark study ended early because of the 24.8% reduction of prostate cancer prevalence over a 7-year period in men taking finasteride (Proscar), a 5-α-reductase inhibitor. Other ongoing phase III clinical trials of prostate cancer chemoprevention include the REDUCE study using dutasteride (Avodart) and the SELECT study using vitamin E and selenium.[155]

The relationship between dietary intake of selenium and lycopene and the risk of prostate cancer has been investigated, with mixed results reported. Vitamin and lycopene supplementation (and other antioxidants) may be a form of effective chemoprevention but there is insufficient evidence to support or refute the use of these products; these antioxidants remain under investigation.[53,70,71,79,166]

Prostate cancer growth is known to depend on androgen, making this another area of study in chemoprevention of this particular type of cancer. Data support the use of antiandrogens to block androgens at the cellular level in the prevention of prostate cancer, although the toxicity of these agents (gynecomastia and gastrointestinal disturbance) poses concerns for the current application in all men.[24] Studies of predictive factors, biomarkers for chemoprevention, or agents, such as calcitriol, that can interrupt the development of prostate cancer are under investigation.[75,157]

A review of the literature suggests a strong link between physical activity and exercise and decreased prostate cancer risk.[58,59,173] Average risk reduction from physical activity and exercise is between 10% and 30%. Exercise may modulate hormone levels and can prevent obesity while enhancing immune function and reducing oxidative stress as possible mechanisms for risk reduction.[156]

SCREENING. The U.S. Preventive Services Task Force (USP-STF) recommends against screening men for prostate cancer with the PSA test (http://www.cancer.gov/cancertopics/factsheet/Detection/PSA).[107] The Task Force's 2008 recommendation advised only against screening men aged 75 and older; the update has extended that guidance to include all men regardless of age. The recommendation does not apply to PSA testing to monitor prostate cancer progression after diagnosis or treatment. Based on some of the responses to the recommendation, it appears that the debate about the value and appropriate use of PSA screening is likely to continue for some time.[111]

Some questions have been raised about how long to continue PSA screening in older men with limited life expectancy. There is some evidence that the potential immediate harms (e.g., false positive tests leading to additional procedures, psychologic distress, and morbidity associated with treating clinically insignificant prostate cancer) outweigh the potential benefits.[163]

The American Urological Society is currently revising their clinical guidelines but these have not been published as of this date. The reader is advised to check the AUS website for the executive summary of the AUS recommendations regarding PSA screening.

The PSA is a blood test that measures an enzymatic protein manufactured only in the prostate gland. An elevated value (usually 4.0 ng/mL or higher) may be caused by BPH, prostatitis, or cancer. Some medications (e.g., finasteride [Proscar] for BPH and Propecia for hair loss) can depress PSA levels.[152] PSA as a biomarker has some limitations. Its specificity ranges from 20% to 40% and its sensitivity from 70% to 90%.[26,34] One of the reasons for the poor sensitivity is that several noncancerous events can elevate the level of the PSA. New biomarkers that are being developed now include PCA3 (prostate cancer antigen 3), TMPRSS-ERG, and prostatic-derived exosomes.

PSA may be age-specific, but the exact values for each age remain under investigation.[8,77] PSA normally rises with age but remains in the 0 to 4 ng/mL range. The level should not rise more than 0.75 ng/dL per year. A level of 4 to 10 increases the risk of prostate cancer by 25%; a level greater than 10 ng/mL has a 50% higher risk of prostate cancer.

The optimal upper limit of the normal range for PSA is unknown; approximately 15% of men with PSA levels of 4 ng/mL or less have prostate cancer (some even aggressive tumors).[154] However, lowering the PSA threshold below 4.0 ng/mL would dramatically increase the number of men subjected to prostate biopsy without any evidence that the mortality rate would be lowered. There is some question that screening and early detection has any effect on mortality rate. This remains an area of controversy and debate.[10,100]

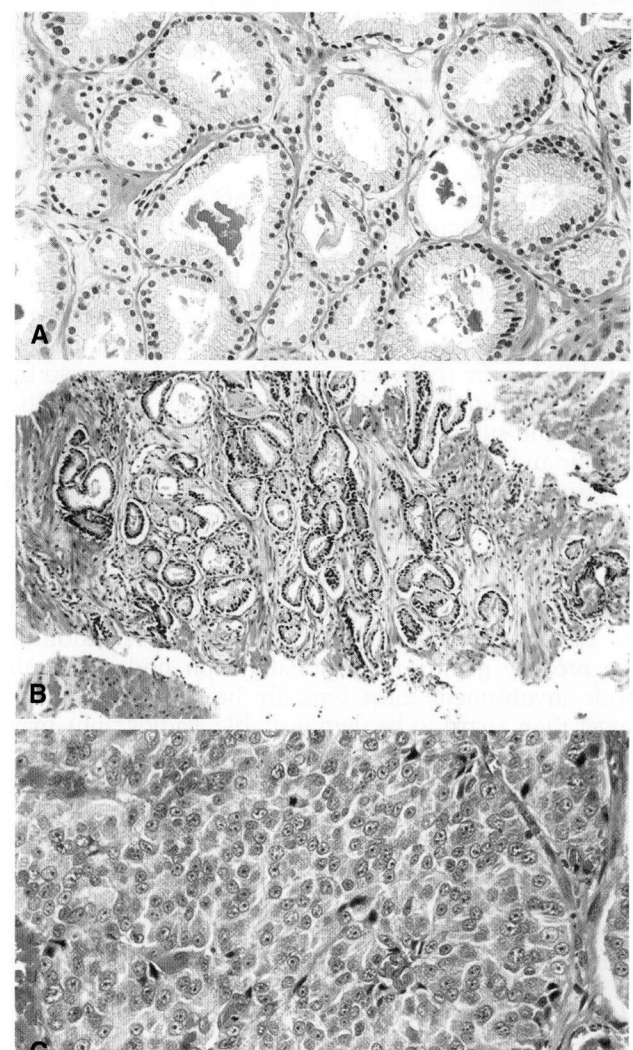

Figure 19-5

A, Low-grade (Gleason score 2) prostate cancer consisting of back-to-back, uniformly sized, well-differentiated (resembling normal cells) malignant glands. **B,** Variably sized, more widely dispersed glands of moderately differentiated adenocarcinoma (Gleason score 6). The higher the Gleason score, the more abnormal and poorly differentiated the cells, the more aggressive the tumor is likely to be. **C,** Poorly differentiated adenocarcinoma composed of sheets of malignant cells (Gleason score 10). (From Kumar V: *Robbins and Cotran: pathologic basis of disease*, ed 8, Philadelphia, 2010, WB Saunders.)

DIAGNOSIS. The diagnosis of prostate cancer is made by a variety of tests, including DRE, transrectal ultrasound, serum PSA assay (see previous comments regarding the use of this test), and radiographic imaging modalities. Tissue biopsy is performed to confirm the diagnosis, usually when PSA is elevated for unexplained reasons. The Gleason score is used to grade prostate cancer cells on how they appear under a microscope (Fig. 19-5) and predict the likelihood of metastases (Box 19-2).

The DRE may reveal a hardened, fixed structure or a diffusely undulated gland. A limitation to this procedure is that typically only the posterior and lateral aspects of the prostate can be palpated. TRUS can be performed by inserting a small ultrasound probe into the rectum. The sound waves emitted by the probe produce a video or photographic image of the prostate. These images help guide a thin needle through the rectum to the gland for a biopsy and staging (TRUS-guided biopsy). The use of positron emission tomography (PET) as a non-invasive means of detecting prostate cancer is under investigation.[84]

Experts suggest that prostate cancer cannot be diagnosed by PSA alone. The PSA assay may offer some diagnostic information, but this remains under investigation. The average prostatic cancer produces approximately 10 times the PSA a normal prostate gland does. However, PSA values bounce around on a daily basis and an elevated PSA assay (between 4 and 10 ng/mL) may also be related to prostatitis, BPH, prostatic infarcts, and prostatic biopsy and surgery. Therefore, an elevated PSA is organ-specific and has some predictive value but is not diagnostic by itself. The PSA may be false negative in up to 30% of cases with localized prostate cancer. Observing PSA velocity (how fast a man's PSA values rise over time) may be a better measure of the presence of cancer.

Radiographic imaging modalities are also utilized for staging of the disease. MRI allows for evaluation of the prostate gland and regional lymph nodes. Lymph node involvement must typically be advanced (nodes larger than 1 cm) to be demonstrable. Radiographs may detect metastatic lesions, but the radionuclide bone scan, though not diagnostic, is a more sensitive modality for detection of a metabolically active lesion.

Another testing method, known as reverse transcription–polymerase chain reaction (RT-PCR), is capable of testing tiny markers that cancer cells carry when they spread to lymph nodes. This test is able to detect cancer previously undetected with standard tests and may also be able to assist in the detection of cancer cells in the surgical margins after radical prostatectomy.[63,175]

STAGING. The Whitmore-Jewett staging system is a commonly used method of staging for prostate cancer. With this system, the spread of prostate cancer has been divided into four stages: A through D (Fig. 19-6). The stage of the disease at the time of the diagnosis helps dictate the course of treatment. Alternately, the Gleason score may be used to determine the aggressiveness of the cancer tumor and the suitability of treatment (see Box 19-2).

TREATMENT. The medical treatment of prostate cancer depends on the man's age and health, the stage of the disease, speed at which the PSA is doubling, and personal preferences. Many uncertainties surround the issue of treating prostate cancer because of the inability to differentiate tumors that will progress from those that will remain unchanged. More men appear to die *with* prostate cancer than *from* it.[64]

No randomized controlled trials have demonstrated the superiority of one treatment over another in terms of survival, although differences in complications vary. The American Urologic Association advocates a presentation of all options for the individual to consider. Once the cancer treatment has begun, most clients are reevaluated every 3 to 6 months. At follow-up visits, symptoms of urinary obstruction and pain are investigated. DRE and a PSA assay are carried out, and prostatic acid phosphatase

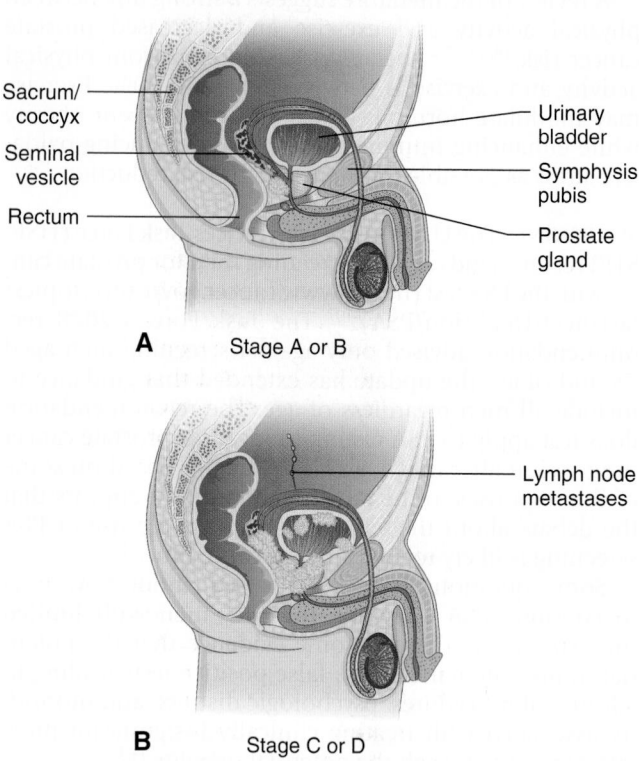

Sacrum/coccyx

Seminal vesicle

Rectum

Urinary bladder

Symphysis pubis

Prostate gland

A Stage A or B

Lymph node metastases

B Stage C or D

Figure 19-6

Prostate cancer: clinical staging using the Whitmore-Jewett staging system. **A,** The tumor has not spread beyond the gland's capsule in stages A and B. **B,** In stage C the tumor has spread into adjacent tissues; in stage D the disease has spread into the lymphatic system and beyond.

levels are measured. Other tests may be routinely ordered depending on the individual's status.

The most commonly used effective treatments include observation, radical prostatectomy, radiation (external-beam or brachytherapy), and hormonal therapy. Unless relatively young, men with early stage A disease (see Fig. 19-6) may be simply monitored because prostate cancer can be an indolent disease. These cancers rarely progress during the initial 5 years after diagnosis but do progress in 10% to 25% of clients 10 years after diagnosis.[21,49] In general, however, men with a life expectancy of 10 years or more and with disease diagnosed in later stage A or B undergo radical prostatectomy and possibly radiation therapy.

Surgery. Surgery is an option for men at any stage of prostate cancer (Fig. 19-7). The primary surgical option is a prostatectomy. This surgery can be done as an open procedure or robotically. There are two approaches to this surgery: retropubic and perineal. Both approaches will remove the prostate, seminal vesicles and bladder cuff neck en bloc. There are two significant differences between these two approaches: (1) a pelvic lymph node dissection is not done with the perineal approach, and (2) there is a lower incidence of bladder neck contractures with the perineal approach.[20,143] There is also a lower incidence of bladder neck contractures in robotic radical prostectomies versus open radical prostectomies.[21,165] Bladder neck contractures can lead to leakage due to urinary retention

Before

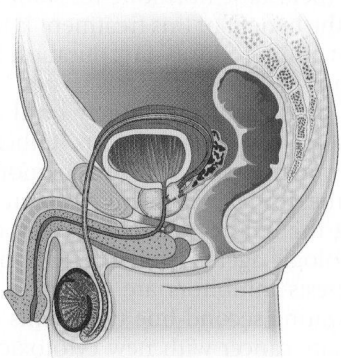

After

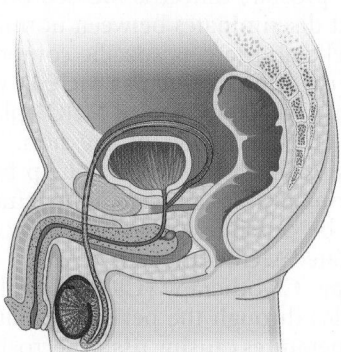

Figure 19-7

Before and after prostatectomy: view of male anatomy with removal of the prostate, reattachment of the urethra, and the importance of the external sphincter for continence.

(previously referred to as overflow incontinence, which is no longer considered an acceptable term). Even with these surgical advancements, there is still a fairly high incidence of erectile dysfunction. This may be because of fibrosis that builds in the soft tissue of the penis or injury to the vascular bed after the surgery.[22,135]

It should also be noted that the internal urethral sphincter can be sacrificed during a prostatectomy. The loss of this sphincter places greater importance on the pelvic floor muscles to maintain urinary continence. In addition to surgery to remove the tumor, a pelvic lymph node dissection will be done to see if the cancer cells have left the prostate and possibly traveled elsewhere to the body. The lymph node dissection does not have any known direct impact on the pelvic floor function but may result in lower limb lymphedema.

The primary postoperative complications with conventional surgery are infection; urinary incontinence (UI); ED/impotence; excessive bleeding; and rectal injury with fecal incontinence. Potency may return gradually over the course of a year; however, after these procedures, as many as one-third of men have incontinence or urinary frequency beyond 1 year and an even greater number continue to experience ED.

In selected individuals with prostate cancer metastases to the spine, aggressive surgical decompression and spinal

reconstruction is a useful treatment option. The results show that on average, neurological outcome is improved and use of analgesics is reduced.[169]

Radiation. Radiation therapy may be used to treat localized prostatic lesions as an adjunctive treatment after radical prostatectomy or for palliative effects in the presence of widespread disease. Relief of pain and improvement in symptoms associated with urethral obstruction are possible benefits of this treatment modality. Potential side effects of radiation therapy include urinary frequency, burning with urination, rectal pain or burning, and diarrhea. Some men never experience these problems, but if they do, they are usually transient and clear up within days to weeks after therapy.

Sexual dysfunction (erectile dysfunction or impotence) is a possible long-term complication and occurs in up to 50% of men treated with radiation. Age and comorbidities, such as diabetes or heart disease, can also increase this risk. Pharmacologic treatment for ED in this population is usually successful.

Palliative radiation therapy may be used for sites of pain secondary to bone lesions from bone metastases in men who have failed hormonal therapy. Metastases to the spine with or without spinal cord compression can be treated with external-beam radiation. Benefit has been demonstrated even for men with neurologic changes. Surgery may be combined with radiation for spinal cord compression.[123]

Radiation therapy is most often used with stage C disease because many men have occult pelvic lymph node metastases. The radiation therapy can be administered daily by external-beam radiation over a number of weeks (usually up to 2 months). External-beam radiation makes it easier to focus and shape the radiation beam (intensity modulation) so that it is less likely to hit other organs, thereby reducing rectal and bladder toxicity.

Examples of external-beam radiation include three-dimensional conformal radiation therapy, which conforms to the shape of the tumor, or intensity-modulated external-beam radiation therapy that directs thousands of pencil-thin radiation beams of varying intensities at the tumor from many different angles. Intensity-modulated radiation therapy beam intensity is highest in the thicker, middle portion of the prostate and much lower in thinner, outer parts of the gland, which minimizes the risk of postradiation bladder and bowel problems.

For men with small, nonaggressive tumors, brachytherapy may be the preferred treatment.

Brachytherapy. Brachytherapy, a specific type of radiotherapy is the delivery of tiny, rice-sized radioactive seeds by a single injection directly into the prostate. This treatment provides a constant, highly concentrated, yet confined dose of radiation to the tissue in and immediately around the tumor. Once in place, the seeds deliver radiation 24 hours a day for several months; they remain in place after they lose their radioactivity.

Brachytherapy is also indicated for men with medical problems that put them at increased risk for any type of surgery or for men who do not feel comfortable with the idea of losing their prostate if there is another option. Small tumors in men with a Gleason score of 6 or less and a pretreatment PSA level of less than 10 may be the best candidates for this type of treatment. Difficulty with urination may preclude brachytherapy because the procedure increases the risk of developing a sudden inability to urinate after undergoing the procedure.

The prostate absorbs almost all of the radiation so that nerves and other tissues of the surrounding structures of the rectum, bladder, and urethra are spared, with fewer complications with ED or incontinence.[122] In one retrospective review, it was noted that quality of life scores for urinary continence and erectile function were still diminished up to 2 years after they received brachytherapy treatment.[23,146]

With technologic advances, brachytherapy now has similar cure rates for localized cancer as radiation and radical prostatectomy.

Hormone Therapy. Hormone therapy is the treatment of choice in the presence of Jewett-Whitmore stage D disease (see Fig. 19-6); the goal of treatment is androgen deprivation. Testosterone stimulates prostate cancer growth, so by blocking its production, hormone therapy shrinks or slows the progression of prostate tumors. Because the testes produce 95% of the circulating testosterone, orchiectomy is the primary method of manipulating hormone levels.

There are three options for hormone therapy. An orchiectomy is the removal of the testicles and eliminates the major source of testosterone in the body. Luteinizing hormone–releasing hormone agonists cause castration levels of testosterone in the body by decreasing testosterone production. Antiandrogens prevent the binding of testosterone to an androgen receptor. A generalized reduction in muscle mass is not uncommon with hormone therapy. Loss of muscle mass in pelvic floor can lead to weakness, which can cause or exacerbate urinary incontinence.

In recent years, there has been an increase in the use of hormone therapy at all stages of prostate cancer. The extensive use of androgen-deprivation therapy (ADT) has raised concerns about potential adverse effects such as hot flashes, osteoporosis, sexual dysfunction (e.g., loss of libido or ED/impotence), reduced body mass, insulin resistance, hyperlipidemia, and psychologic effects (e.g., depression, mood swings, or memory loss).[60]

Another option, estrogen therapy, is used less often because of adverse effects, including gynecomastia, loss of libido and ED/impotence, bloating, and pedal edema. Hormone therapy is not usually advocated for newly diagnosed, locally contained prostate cancer because of its adverse effects (e.g., bone deterioration, decreased libido, mood changes, and anemia). Additionally, serious cardiovascular disease, including stroke, heart attack, and deep venous thrombosis, can be associated with estrogen therapy in anyone at high risk.

Chemotherapy. Chemotherapy may be advised for men with androgen-independent prostate cancer, also known as *hormone refractory prostate cancer*, whose PSA doubling time is less than 6 months, especially if there is a positive bone scan. These men have advanced, metastatic prostate cancer and have relapsed after initial treatment with hormone therapy. In the majority of men with prostate cancer, androgen-independent prostate cancer occurs after a median time of 18 months of hormone deprivation.[134] They are resistant to further hormone manipulation.[103]

Docetaxel chemotherapy is now the standard of care for men with metastatic hormone-resistant prostate cancer; however, the benefit of this treatment is limited. Optimal treatment timing, dose, and duration have not yet been established.[92,105,122]

Some men are treated indefinitely until unacceptable toxicity or disease progression occurs. Others are treated using an intermittent approach with chemotherapy interrupted after the initial response.[88] Research is focused on improving the efficacy of docetaxel by combining it with novel biologic agents; studies combining docetaxel with angiogenesis inhibitors are underway. Other studies are investigating second-line treatments of hormone-resistant prostate cancer with new cytotoxic agents (e.g., satraplatin and ixabepilone).[40]

Immunotherapy. Targeted immunotherapy for control of metastatic prostate cancer is focused on designing an antibody that discriminates between normal and adenocarcinoma cells and targets specific components within tumor cells (e.g., mucins such as MUC1) with toxins or radionuclides. Overexpression of MUC1 plays an important role in prostate cancer progression. Targeting this particular glycosylated protein may help prevent and/or control micrometastases and hormone refractory disease. It may even be possible to develop a vaccine targeting tumor-associated MUC1 antigen.[87]

Cryotherapy. Cryotherapy (CRYO) involves the insertion of needles through the perineum that can produce freezing temperatures causing tissue necrosis and destruction of the cancer cells. With this type of focal treatment, the goal is to destroy the cancer cells with less impact on the urinary function and sexual potency of the individual. Cryotherapy is recommended only for localized low-risk disease or as treatment for local recurrent prostate cancer. It is considered an intermediate management technique between radical approaches (radical prostatectomy, external beam radiation, and brachytherapy) and watchful waiting to manage some early-stage prostate cancers.[12,24]

Vaccine. Clinical trials are under way to investigate the development of a vaccine that fights prostate cancer by a variety of immunomodulation techniques.[95,155] For example, a dendritic cell–based cancer vaccine for prostate cancer has moved from the laboratory to human clinical trials. Dendritic cells are antigen-presenting (immune system) cells. They initiate and shape an adaptive immune response by capturing, processing, and presenting antigen material to T and B cells. Early results of dendritic cell vaccinations are being reported.[101,153] Research continues to focus on improving patient selection, vaccine delivery methods, immune monitoring, and vaccine manufacturing.

In other areas of research, scientists are able to trick the human immune system into recognizing cancerous prostate cells as foreign invaders by genetically engineering the individual's own cells and injecting them back into the body. This is done by harvesting prostate cancer cells, irradiating them, treating them with autologous granulocyte-macrophage colony–stimulating factor (GM-CSF), and reintroducing them into the body.[17] Results so far indicate that both T-cell and B-cell immune responses to human prostate cancer can be generated.[52,140]

Researchers are also combining vaccines with cytokines or immune modulators, which can foster dramatic antitumor responses. A variety of immunotherapeutic approaches have been followed through to phase III trials for other types of cancer. There is hope that this type of immune therapy can be developed for prostate cancer treatment as well.[10,104,141]

PROGNOSIS. Multiple sources of data show that prostate cancer incidence rates rose after the introduction of PSA testing. The average age at diagnosis has fallen, the proportion of advanced-stage tumors has declined, the proportion of moderately differentiated tumors has increased, and a decline in mortality began in the United States in 1991.[100] Data show that 93% of men diagnosed with prostate cancer survive at least 10 years, and 77% survive at least 15 years, but it is still the second most common cause of cancer deaths among American men.[138] Earlier detection has given men more choices and better treatment, resulting in improved morbidity and mortality rates.[7]

Men with small or nonaggressive tumors are more likely to be cancer free than men with large or aggressive tumors. Seed implants are more successful for men whose pretreatment level of PSA is below 10 ng/mL. Without any treatment at all, men with the least aggressive prostate cancers face only a 4% to 7% risk of dying from prostate cancer within 15 years of diagnosis.[6]

The rate of relapse in men with pathologic evidence of pelvic lymph node involvement is high (more than 50%, although some studies report as high as 90%) within 5 years of local treatment. Lymph node involvement occurs in 15% to 20% of men with localized prostate cancer that exhibits high-risk features (as defined by tumor size, serum PSA level, and Gleason score).[50]

Prostate cancer is sometimes referred to as a "two-decade disease" because it often returns 10 to 20 years after successful local therapy, which is one reason why some physicians advocate radical prostatectomy. Even with radical prostatectomy, recurrence is reported in up to 40% of men. One-third of those men progress to incurable metastatic disease.[153] Metastatic prostate cancer remains a lethal disease, although new treatment strategies discussed earlier are being developed and incorporated into clinical trials that may improve survival rates.

Men with advanced, metastatic prostate cancer who have relapsed after hormone therapy often have disease extending to the skeleton, which is associated with severe pain and disability. The prognosis for this group of individuals is poor at this time (median survival is between 10 and 20 months),[133] but improved overall survival demonstrated in studies with chemotherapy for these individuals shows promising results.[102]

Incidence of urinary incontinence after radical prostatectomy has been reported in ranges from 2% to 66%. Erectile dysfunction has been reported between 79% and 85%.[132] There has been a considerable amount of research regarding the efficacy of the pelvic floor exercise programs for prostate cancer. One study noted that compared with regular care, an early pelvic rehabilitation program after radical prostatectomy would result in additional 107 cases of continence per 1000 treated men.[137] Another study reviewed 11 randomized controlled trials that provided level II evidence using pelvic floor muscle training in men with urinary incontinence, post micturition dribble, and erectile dysfunction.[2] Postoperatively, after radical prostatectomy, incontinence is 100% when the catheter is removed; this is very upsetting for most men. However, urinary control is regained for many men within the first 6 to 8 weeks. Men can speed recovery of urinary function and reduce the likelihood of remaining incontinent with pelvic floor exercises.[158,159] Any incontinence 12 months or more after surgery and rehabilitation may require additional medical intervention such as collagen injection (a sclerosing agent to "tighten up" the sphincter) or placement of an artificial urinary sphincter (AUS).

Besides the complications of radiation therapy already discussed, rectal cancer is another potential serious complication, especially for men treated with older forms of radiation therapy 10 years ago before the development of more modern tissue-sparing techniques. Men who have had radiation therapy for prostate cancer should be followed and screened regularly for rectal cancer.

SPECIAL IMPLICATIONS FOR THE THERAPIST   19-3

Prostate Cancer

Screening for Referral

Considering the number of aging adult men seen in a rehabilitative setting and the incidence of prostate disease, therapists are seeing a number of clients with preexisting prostate conditions. Investigating the symptoms or signs associated with any prostate condition provides the therapist with the baseline information needed to monitor the client's status. For example, if the client experiences difficulty with initiating the urine stream, continuing the stream of flow, urinary frequency, painful urination, or dribbling or continuous leaking, the therapist should periodically ask if there has been a change regarding the urinary dysfunction.

Pain is often the primary or only symptom associated with prostate disease. If the pain is located in the thoracic, lumbar, or sacral area, the client may seek care from a therapist, thinking the pain has a mechanical origin. Metastatic spread of the disease to the axial skeleton or the periaortic lymph nodes may account for these complaints. If the back pain does not present in a mechanical fashion (based on history and physical examination findings) or if the person notes urologic dysfunction, referral to a physician is warranted.

A previous history of prostate cancer in any man with current reports of shoulder, back, groin, or hip pain of unknown cause must be screened for medical disease. Age over 50 years, past history of cancer, and unknown cause of musculoskeletal pain or symptoms are three red flags that warrant further medical investigation.

Pelvic Physical Therapy
Beth Shelly, PT, DPT, WCS, BCB-PMD

Preoperative pelvic floor muscle training is advocated and several randomized controlled studies have shown quicker return to continence after surgery in groups who started the exercises preoperatively.[27,28,31]

Pelvic floor rehabilitation is aimed at both the rhabdosphincter (external urethral sphincter) that maintains resistance and the levator ani muscles that can tighten quickly to prevent leakage during increased intraabdominal pressure (e.g., laughing, coughing, and lifting) (see Box 16-1).

Pelvic floor reeducation with and without biofeedback has been shown effective in returning men to being functional or complete continence after radical prostatectomy and should be recommended as a first-line option.[15,26,35,50,68,102,120,158,167]

Postoperative biofeedback-enhanced pelvic floor exercises initiated 6 weeks after radical prostatectomy to prevent urinary incontinence has been studied with mixed results.[54] Studies with similar biofeedback methods that began exercises immediately after catheter removal seem to be more effective. Current literature suggests that the time period toward continence after radical prostatectomy can be shortened if pelvic floor reeducation is initiated directly after catheter removal.[36,121] More study is needed to confirm these results.[51]

Pelvic floor electrical stimulation has been shown in some studies to have benefit in restoring continence after radical prostectomy.[103,168] But the addition of biofeedback and pelvic floor electrical stimulation has not been shown to provide greater effectiveness compared with muscle training alone.[61,175] A 2012 Cochrane analysis evaluating conservative management of postprostatectomy UI was unable to show which treatment (or combinations of treatment) would be most effective for this problem. Most trials were not high-quality and some approaches (e.g., lifestyle changes) were not included.[29]

One study of ball-assisted pelvic floor exercises did report that men regained bladder control significantly sooner compared with men who did not do the exercises. However, the treatment had little benefit for men who were still incontinent 4 months or more after surgery; it is likely that their bladder problems resulted from surgical damage.[121]

Although pelvic floor exercises help men regain continence faster, the rates of continence at the end of 1 year have been reported equal between the exercise group and control group. There is still a potential cost savings and improved quality of life with earlier return to continence.[69,121,168]

If continuous urinary incontinence persists months after the surgery, "stove pipe urethra" (intrinsic sphincter deficiency) may be diagnosed, and medical intervention is required. Medical intervention may include injection of bulking agents at the sphincter or surgical implantation of an artificial sphincter. If urine flow is difficult to initiate or flow is weak, an overactive pelvic floor muscle, a stricture, or decreased bladder contractions may be evident. Exercise, biofeedback, and medication are treatment options to relax the pelvic musculature; however, surgical intervention may be necessary if urethral stricture is the major cause of urinary obstruction.

If no improvement has taken place with an appropriate rehabilitation program or if the symptoms are getting worse, the client should be referred to the physician who is managing the prostate condition. Knowledge of other potential symptoms associated with prostate conditions provides the basis for a screening checklist the therapist could use periodically while treating the individual. Once again, if the onset of new symptoms is noted, referral to the physician is warranted.

Metastases to the pelvic lymph nodes can cause lumbar plexopathy and swelling caused by compression of veins and/or lymphatics. The development of lymphedema may be related to smoking, stage of cancer, and radiation therapy. The therapist has an important role in screening men for risk of lymphedema and early recognition/intervention of this condition.[38]

Complications of Medical Treatment

Important implications exist related to the commonly employed treatment approaches to the various prostate conditions. Complications associated with radical prostatectomy procedures include infection, incontinence, and sexual dysfunction. If the therapist is seeing someone who has undergone such a procedure, being vigilant for symptoms associated with infection is necessary for months after the surgery. If the client reports malaise, fever, chills, sweats, or sudden worsening of symptoms, communication with the physician is warranted.

The surgery may account for the individual's complaints of incontinence and ED/impotence. Postoperative ED occurs in 70% of men who undergo retropubic prostatectomy as a result of compromise of the neurovascular bundle that provides circulation and nerve supply to the penis. Potency can be spared in 70% to 80% with nerve sparing in young men.

Although reduced in recent years, delayed complications of radiation therapy can occur with increasing problems from 6 to 24 months postradiation.[64] Diarrhea, gastrointestinal or urinary bleeding, irritative voiding symptoms, ED, and tenesmus (painful spasm of the anal sphincter with straining) are all possible complications. The presence of these problems could interfere with a rehabilitation program, slowing progress. A recent onset or worsening of any of these complications should be brought to the physician's attention.

Multiple potential side effects are associated with endocrine or hormonal manipulation (Box 19-3). Decrease in bone mass and increase in bone turnover with a concomitant increased risk of fracture has been documented in men receiving ADT (antiandrogen deprivation therapy).[67,145] Significant loss of bone mineral density occurs within 12 months of starting therapy and continues indefinitely while treatment continues; there is no recovery after treatment is stopped.[67]

Exercise and fracture prevention is an important feature of treatment for anyone on androgen deprivation therapy. Up to 20% of men surviving at least 5 years after diagnosis of prostate cancer have a fracture if treated with ADT compared with 12.6% of men not receiving ADT. Vitamin D deficiency exacerbates the development of osteoporosis. Treatment with bisphosphonates in men on ADT has been shown to prevent bone loss and increase bone mineral density, but it does not prevent fractures in this population group.[67]

Many men on ADT for prostate cancer are not being screened or treated for osteoporosis.[149] The therapist can assess for additional risk factors and institute an osteoporosis education and prevention plan for anyone receiving this treatment. As with the complications associated with surgical procedures and radiation therapy, these problems may interfere with rehabilitation, altering the prognosis. Knowing the individual is being treated with endocrine manipulative therapy and being familiar with the side effects can lessen alarm on the therapist's part if the client reports any of these symptoms.

Exercise and Prostate Cancer

The role of physical activity and exercise in reducing the risk of prostate cancer were discussed earlier in this chapter (see "Risk Factors" under "Prostate Cancer" above). Exercise and physical activity may be able to counter some of these side effects of ADT (e.g., fatigue, functional decline, increased body fat, loss of lean body tissue, insulin resistance, and decreased quality of life associated with these physical changes) by reducing fatigue, elevating mood, building muscle mass, and reducing body fat. This form of exercise may be an important component of supportive care for these men.[4,136,172]

The question of whether it is more efficacious to commence exercise therapy at the same time as initiating androgen deprivation is being studied.[83,117] The intent is to immediately attenuate or perhaps even prevent treatment-induced adverse effects. This is in contrast to the implementation of a rehabilitative exercise program 90 days or more after the start of ADT, by which time many of the physical and psychologic problems have developed.

Moderate intensity exercise has also proven effective in reducing radiation-induced fatigue and other treatment-induced complications in men with prostate cancer.[169] Both resistance and aerobic exercise have been shown to mitigate fatigue, increase strength, and improve quality of life in men with prostate cancer receiving radiotherapy in the short term (6 months).[135]

The overall role of exercise with individuals who have cancer is discussed in Chapter 9. If symptoms or signs of myocardial infarct, cerebral vascular accident, or deep venous thrombosis develop, immediate referral to a physician is warranted (see Chapter 12).

DISORDERS OF THE TESTES

Orchitis

Overview and Etiologic Factors

Orchitis is inflammation of the testis, can be acute or chronic, and is often associated with epididymitis. Gram-negative bacteria and *Chlamydia trachomatis* are the usual infectious agents.

Incidence and Risk Factors

Anyone with primary infections of the genitourinary tract or infections in other body regions (e.g., pneumonia or scarlet fever) is at risk of developing orchitis. Sexually active males with multiple partners are at higher risk of

---

Box 19-3

SIDE EFFECTS OF HORMONAL MANIPULATION

- Muscle atrophy
- Decreased bone density, osteoporosis
- Loss of libido
- Erectile dysfunction/impotence
- Hot flashes
- Gynecomastia
- Bloating and pedal edema
- Nausea and vomiting
- Diarrhea
- Weight gain/redistribution
- Myocardial infarction, cerebrovascular accident, deep venous thrombosis

---

developing genitourinary infections. Males 10 years of age and older who have parotitis (mumps) are also at risk of developing orchitis. The incidence of orchitis in this group can be as high as 25% to 33%.[56] Men with indwelling catheters are also at higher risk of developing orchitis secondary to genitourinary tract infection.

Pathogenesis and Clinical Manifestations

Orchitis is often secondary to UTIs. The bloodstream and lymphatics are then the route of spread from other body areas to the testes. An insidious onset will often be suggestive of infection, whereas a sudden onset should raise suspicions of testicular torsion, which is considered a medical emergency.[26,144] Systemic infections, such as pneumonia, scarlet fever, and parotitis, use the same routes to spread to the testes. Orchitis is marked by testicular pain and swelling. Pain usually presents as unilateral scrotal pain that may radiate to the groin. Inquiry about recent change in sexual partners or urethral discharge can further clarify this diagnosis. Fever and malaise can be present, but symptoms of urinary dysfunction are usually absent.

MEDICAL MANAGEMENT

DIAGNOSIS. Physical examination reveals a tender and swollen testicle. Laboratory tests revealing an elevated white blood cell (WBC) count and urinalysis are an important component of the diagnostic process. Presence of an enlarged or erythematous scrotum may be present.

TREATMENT. See "Epididymitis" (next section) and "Special Implications for the Therapist 19-4: Testicular Torsion" below.

Epididymitis

Overview and Risk Factors

Epididymitis is an inflammation of the epididymis (Fig. 19-8, *A*). The two primary types of epididymitis are sexually and nonsexually transmitted infections. Males typically under the age of 40 years who are sexually active with multiple partners are at higher risk of developing genitourinary disease that can lead to epididymitis. Iatrogenic sources of infection include cystoscopy and indwelling catheters. In the older male population, this condition can be precipitated by prostatitis and UTIs.

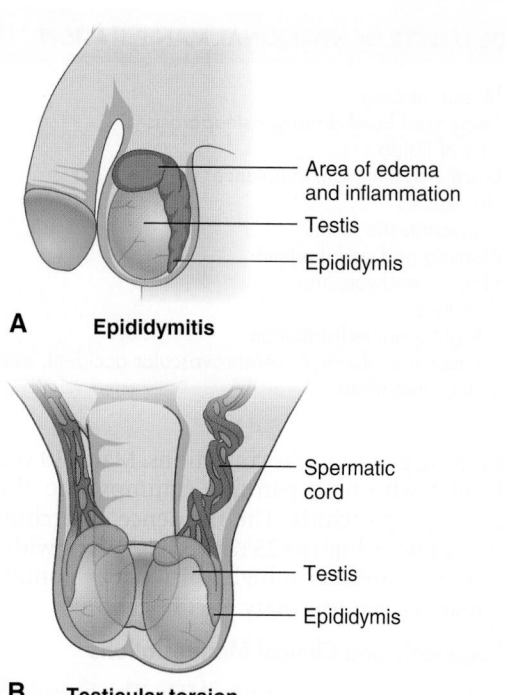

A   **Epididymitis**

B   **Testicular torsion**

Figure 19-8

A, Epididymitis: Inflammation or infection of the epididymis, the tube that holds the testicle in place. The epididymis is found along the posterolateral aspect of each testis. The tail of the epididymis becomes the vas deferens as it ascends superiorly out of the scrotum. The spermatic cord suspends the testis in the scrotum and consists of arteries, veins, nerves, lymphatics, and the vas deferens. Sperm made in the testis is stored in the epididymis, then transferred to the seminal vesicle through the vas deferens for ejaculation. **B,** Testicular torsion: Testis twists on its spermatic cord cutting off blood supply to the testis. The spermatic cord suspends the testis in the scrotum and consists of arteries, veins, nerves, lymphatics, and the vas deferens.

Pathogenesis and Etiologic Factors

Epididymitis is typically caused by bacterial pathogens. The sexually transmitted infections leading to epididymitis are associated with urethritis. In the nonsexually transmitted infections, urine containing pathogens may be forced up the ejaculatory ducts, through the vas deferens, and into the epididymis. Pressure associated with voiding and physical strain can force the urine from the urethra. Infection originating elsewhere in the body can spread to the epididymis via the lymphatics of the spermatic cord. Congenital urinary tract abnormalities can lead to epididymitis in children. Recent urinary tract infections and transurethral instrumentation (e.g., cystoscopy) are risk factors, especially in older men.

Clinical Manifestations

Epididymitis may be associated with gradual onset of pain over a 24-hour period accompanied by urinary dysfunction, fever, chills, and urethral discharge. Unilateral scrotal pain is common, but pain may also be noted in the lower abdominal, flank, groin, or hip adductor muscle areas. Elevating the scrotum usually relieves the pain.

When bacteriuria is present, urinary frequency and urgency and dysuria can occur. When the epididymitis is related to sexually transmitted disease, urethritis and urethral discharge are present concurrently. Local scrotal erythema and swelling are associated with epididymitis.

MEDICAL MANAGEMENT

DIAGNOSIS. In addition to the findings noted under the section on Clinical Manifestations, urinalysis, urethral smear, and urine culture are important for the diagnosis of epididymitis. A negative urinalysis does not rule out this condition. An elevated WBC count is also usually present.

TREATMENT. During the acute phase, treatment includes bed rest, limiting physical activities and strain (including sexual intercourse), scrotal elevation and support, ice packs to the affected area, sitz baths, nonsteroidal antiinflammatory drugs (NSAIDs), or antibiotics. Hospitalization may be necessary if signs of sepsis or abscess formation are present or if the pain is severe. Spermatic cord block may be used to help relieve pain in severe cases. Once treatment has been initiated, a significant decrease in pain should be noted within a week, but the scrotal edema may be present for 2 to 3 months. (See "Epididymitis" and "Testicular Torsion.")

Testicular Torsion

Overview

Testicular torsion is an abnormal twisting of the spermatic cord as the testis rotates within the tunica vaginalis (Fig. 19-8, *B*). The torsion can occur intravaginally or extravaginally, but intravaginal torsion is the more common. This condition is a surgical emergency. Early diagnosis and treatment is imperative to save the testis.

Etiologic Factors

Torsion of the spermatic cord is often associated with congenital abnormalities. These include absence of the scrotal ligaments, incomplete descent of the testis, and a high attachment of the tunica vaginalis. Increased mobility of the testis and epididymis within the tunica vaginalis facilitate twisting of the spermatic cord. Testicular torsion can also occur after heavy physical activity.

Incidence and Risk Factors

Intravaginal torsion most often occurs in males 8 to 18 years of age. The condition is rarely seen after age 30 years. The extravaginal torsions occur primarily in neonates. A firm, painless scrotal mass is discovered shortly after birth.

Pathogenesis

Normally the testes are held in a fixed position in the scrotum by the tunica vaginalis, a serous membrane that partially surrounds the testes and prevents the spermatic cord from twisting. The spermatic cord contains the vas deferens and the nerve and blood supply for the scrotal contents. Congenital abnormalities account for the majority of cases of testicular torsion. These anomalies allow for rotation of the testis around the spermatic cord, or the torsion may occur between the testis and epididymis. Extravaginal torsion occurs most often during the fetal descent of the testes, before the tunica adheres to the scrotal wall. This allows the testis and fascial tunica to rotate around the spermatic cord above the level of the tunica vaginalis.

Clinical Manifestations

An abrupt onset of severe unilateral testicular and scrotal pain followed by swelling suggests testicular torsion. In most cases, only one testis is affected; bilateral torsion is possible but rare. The pain may extend up into the inguinal area. Cremasteric reflex (retraction of the scrotum and testicle as the skin on the same side of the inner thigh is lightly stroked) is almost always absent because nerve compression occurs when the testicle twists on its spermatic cord. There are no urinary symptoms and no fever. Nausea, vomiting, tachycardia, and lightheadedness may be present, possibly because of the severity of the pain. If the torsion is severe enough to occlude the arterial supply, blood supply to the testicle and surrounding scrotal structures can be compromised. With prolonged or complete loss of blood supply, tissue ischemia and necrosis can develop, making this condition a medical emergency.

MEDICAL MANAGEMENT

DIAGNOSIS. Diagnosis can be difficult and misdiagnosis of epididymitis can delay treatment, resulting in testicular loss.[94] Physical examination reveals a firm, tender testis that is often positioned high in the scrotum. Erythema and scrotal edema may be present. The absence of the cremasteric reflex is diagnostic. Color and power Doppler sonography make it possible to identify the absence of perfusion in the affected testis. Scintigraphy (radionuclide scanning) may be ordered to assess testicular blood flow. A urinalysis is performed to help rule out infection.

TREATMENT. Testicular torsion is considered a urologic emergency. Once the diagnosis of testicular torsion is made, emergency surgery is performed. The procedure includes detorsion, and if the testis is deemed nonviable, then an orchiectomy is performed. The duration of the torsion is critical regarding salvage of the testis. If the surgery is performed within 3 hours of onset, a greater than 80% salvage rate occurs. The salvage rate drops to 20% if more than 12 hours passes before the surgery.

| SPECIAL IMPLICATIONS FOR THE THERAPIST | 19-4 |

Testicular Torsion
Pain extending into the groin and scrotum can occasionally be referred from muscle or joint structures, but if a client notes the onset of scrotal pain, immediate communication with a physician is warranted. Ask the client if he has noted scrotal swelling or tenderness; feels feverish or nauseated; has any difficulties with urination, including urgency, frequency, or dysuria; or has noted any urethral discharge. If the scrotal or groin pain is associated with musculoskeletal dysfunction, it can be expected that the therapist could alter the symptoms by mechanically stressing the involved component of the musculoskeletal system. Structures to test include the genitofemoral nerve as is courses through

the abdominal wall, pudendal nerve in its relationship to the obturator internus and Alcock's canal, pelvic floor muscles, adductor, and iliopsoas muscles, and the connective tissue of the scrotum and perineum in relation to scaring and adhesions.

Testicular Cancer

Overview

Testicular cancer occurs when cells in one or both testicles become malignant. Primary testicular tumors are divided into two histogenetic categories: seminoma and nonseminoma. Germ cell tumors (origin in the primordial germ cells) make up more than 95% of testicular tumors, whereas the remaining neoplasms are mostly tumors of stromal or sex cord origin (sex cords develop from the gonadal ridge in embryology and later become the testis cords in males). Metastatic tumors to the testis from primary neoplasm elsewhere in the body are uncommon, although involvement by lymphoma may occur in older men.

Incidence

Although relatively rare, testicular cancer is the most common solid organ tumor in young men. According to the National Cancer Institute in 2011, there were 8590 new cases and 360 deaths from testicular cancer.[138] There are considerable geographic and ethnic variations in the global incidence of testicular cancer. The disease mainly affects Western populations, with an increasing incidence since the middle of the 20th century.[55] Average rates in developed areas of the world are six times higher than those in developing areas.[25]

Testicular cancer is the most common cancer in the 15- to 35-year-old male age group and second most common malignancy from age 35 to 39 years, with a white-to-black incidence ratio of 5 : 1.

Etiologic and Risk Factors

The etiology of testicular cancer is not well understood. Although the cause is unknown, hormonal balance at various life stages appear to be related. Congenital and acquired factors have been associated with the development of testicular cancer; familial clustering has been observed particularly among siblings.[42,53]

The first susceptibility gene for testicular cancer has been located and named TGCT1 on the long arm of chromosome X, inherited from the mother; its presence increases a man's risk of testicular cancer by up to 50 times.[127] There is some evidence that cancer stem cells are derived from normal stem cells that have gradually accumulated various genetic defects; a group of tumor-specific antigens known as cancer/testis antigens (CTAs) may be expressed at early stages during embryogenesis in germ cell precursors eventually leading to testicular cancer.[37]

The most significant factor in testicular cancer is the association of cryptorchidism (the testes not descending into the scrotum). The incidence of testicular cancer is

35 times higher in males with a cryptoid testis. There is now strong evidence that prenatal or postnatal environmental estrogen exposures (e.g., endocrine-mimicking environmental pollutants, pesticides, industrial chemicals, or chemical contaminants in drinking water) contribute to testicular cancer; this remains under further investigation.[39,59]

Other risk factors still under investigation may include mothers who took exogenous estrogen during pregnancy (diethylstilbestrol)[147,148]; scrotal trauma[99]; exposure to high levels of radiofrequency/microwave radiation in radar technicians[128]; first-born sons[167]; and nonidentical twins.

Men with Klinefelter syndrome (a sex chromosome disorder characterized by low levels of male hormones, sterility, breast enlargement, and small testes) are also at greater risk of developing testicular cancer. Lifestyle and occupational exposures occurring later in life may play a role in promoting the disease, but they are not likely involved in the initiation of the cancer development.[55]

A previous history of testicular cancer and a history of infertility and poor semen quality or infection have been associated with an increased risk of developing testicular cancer. A causal relationship has not been established between infertility and infection and testicular cancer.[91]

Pathogenesis

Because germ cell tumors make up the vast majority of testicular cancers, the following discussion focuses solely on such tumors. Carcinoma in situ usually becomes an invasive germ cell tumor in a median period of approximately 5 years.[23] The neoplastic transformation of a germ cell results in either a seminoma, an undifferentiated tumor, or a nonseminomatous tumor composed of embryonal carcinoma teratoma, choriocarcinoma, or yolk-sac carcinoma (endodermal-sinus tumor). Seminomas are the most common testicular cancers, accounting for approximately 40% to 50% of germ cell tumors and most often appearing in the fourth decade of life. Seminomas appear as a solid, grey-white growth and are rarely necrotic or cystic. The entire testis can be replaced by the tumor.

The incidence of nonseminomas peaks in the third decade of life, and hemorrhage, necrosis, or cystic changes are more common. Yolk-sac tumors are the most common germ cell tumors of infants. These tumors result in enlarged testes, which appear grossly as poorly defined lobulated masses. Focal areas of hemorrhage are common.

Clinical Manifestations

The most common initial sign of testicular cancer is enlargement of the testis with diffuse testicular pain, swelling, hardness, or some combination of these findings. The condition may go undetected if no pain is experienced and the male is not periodically performing testicular self-examination. The enlargement may be accompanied by an ache in the abdomen or scrotum or a sensation of heaviness in the scrotum. Metastasis, although with little or no local change, is noted in the scrotum.

Retroperitoneal primary tumors may present with back pain and/or groin or pelvic pain (psoas muscle invasion).

Metastatic testicular cancer can present as back pain (may be the primary presenting complaint), abdominal mass, hemoptysis, or neck or supraclavicular adenopathy. Up to 21% of men with testicular germ cell cancer have back pain as the primary presenting symptoms.[30] A significant delay occurs in diagnosis of testicular cancer in these men compared with men who also had symptomatic unilateral testicular enlargement.

Pain may be the sole presenting symptom in metastasis to the retroperitoneal, cervical, and supraclavicular lymphatic chains. Because the testis embryologically originates in the genital ridge and descends during fetal life through the abdomen and inguinal canal into the scrotum, the primary lymphatic and vascular drainage of the testis is to the retroperitoneal lymph nodes and the renal or great vessels, respectively. Approximately 20% of all cases have involved lymph nodes.[23] Bone metastasis is a late event, often combined with metastasis to the retroperitoneal lymph nodes, lung, and liver. Symptomatic, solitary bone lesions are responsive to chemotherapy and local radiation therapy.

Occurring during the prime of life for most men and potentially affecting sexual and reproductive capabilities, testicular cancer has a major emotional impact and can affect overall quality of life.

MEDICAL MANAGEMENT

PREVENTION. No known preventive strategies exist but teaching and promoting testicular self-examination as a technique for early detection of this disease is recommended.[35] Because survival is dependent on early detection, men should be encouraged to practice testicular self-examination at least every 6 months. For optimal effect, health education programs need to take into account complexities such as cultural diversity, if men are to heed vital and, in some cases, life-sustaining advice.

DIAGNOSIS. A thorough urologic history and physical examination are the basis for making a diagnosis of testicular cancer. A painless testicular mass is highly suggestive of testicular cancer. Transillumination of the scrotum may also reveal a testicular mass. Serum tumor markers (e.g., alpha-fetoprotein, human chorionic gonadotropin, and lactate dehydrogenase) are increased in 40% to 60% of all cases and may be used to guide treatment and follow-up.

Testicular ultrasound is used to differentiate a variety of scrotal disorders besides cancer (e.g., epididymitis, orchitis, hydrocele, or hematocele). The modalities used to assess metastatic spread include CT scans and MRI. MR lymphography may replace the currently used tomography scanning or MRI used to noninvasively stage retroperitoneal lymph nodes.[18] Biopsy with microscopic examination of testicular tissue by a pathologist is the best way to make a definitive diagnosis.

STAGING. Clinical staging is based on the TNM classification system: stage I, or tumor confined to the testis, epididymis, or spermatic cord; stage II, which has spread to the retroperitoneal lymph nodes and divided into A, B, and C according to the size of the nodes; and stage III, which is distant metastasis or high serum tumor–marker values.

TREATMENT. Management of testicular cancer has changed substantially in the last 20 years, primarily because of the ability of cisplatin-containing combination chemotherapy to cure advanced disease. Even over the last 5 years, the management of stage I testis cancer has changed tremendously.[5]

Organ-sparing surgery has become an accepted approach to treat malignant and nonmalignant tumors of a single testis. Combined with adjuvant radiotherapy to the retroperitoneal and ipsilateral pelvic lymph nodes, this approach has proven as effective as orchidectomy. Nerve-sparing retroperitoneal lymph node dissection is an integral part of testis cancer management strategies for both early and advanced-stage disease.[71] Nerve-sparing techniques help preserve sexual function and prevent incontinence. As many as 50% of men with clinical stage I testis cancer can be treated with close surveillance instead of immediate adjuvant treatment.[5]

Testicular-sparing management of testicular masses is an alternative to radical orchiectomy and allows for preservation of sperm and hormonal function without endangering survival rates.[120] Sperm collection and cryopreservation before the initiation of therapy is an available reproductive technology. Only a few sperm are needed for successful in vitro fertilization.[171]

Chemotherapy is used in all stages of seminoma and non-seminoma. The most common chemotherapeutic drugs that would be used include carboplatin, bleomycin, etoposide, and cisplatin. Carboplatin and cisplatin are known to cause peripheral neuropathy and bleomycin can cause pulmonary fibrosis. These are the consensus guidelines on testicular cancer management.[170] The recommendation of which therapies to include is based on pathologic findings from the orchiectomy and results of the CT and MRI procedures. Second-line conventional-dose or high-dose chemotherapy with stem cell rescue may cure 25% to 50% of men with recurrent testicular tumors.

PROGNOSIS. With early detection, more than 95% of men with newly diagnosed germ-cell tumors are cured. It is estimated that with adequate diagnostics and treatment, 100% of men with stage I testis cancer will survive in the future.[5] Delay in diagnosis correlates with a higher stage at presentation for treatment.[23] One confounding factor related to the diagnosis being delayed is the potential lack of perceptible testicular changes while the disease spreads. Men who have had testicular cancer have an increased likelihood of developing cancer in the remaining testicle.

Long-term sequelae of cisplatin use may include leukemia, cardiovascular events, and reports that circulating cisplatin can be detected in the plasma as long as 20 years after treatment.[97,119] The most serious long-term complications of chemotherapy or radiotherapy are cardiovascular toxicity and second malignancies; each has a 25-year risk of approximately 16%.[47]

Chemotherapy-related cardiovascular toxicity may be the result of both direct endothelial damage induced by cisplatin and indirect hormonal and metabolic changes. There is an increased incidence of metabolic syndrome in long-term survivors that is most likely caused by the lower testosterone levels.[47]

Current therapeutic regimens have significantly improved survival but often adversely affect fertility[120]; cisplatin-based chemotherapy results in 30% to 50% infertility rates in men with testicular cancer who are treated with chemotherapy.[82] Options to maintain fertility after testicular cancer and its treatment are discussed in detail elsewhere.[139]

Other chemotherapy-induced complications include chronic neurotoxicity (50%), permanent ototoxicity and renal function impairment (30%), pulmonary fibrosis (5%-10% when treated with bleomycin), and late relapse.[47]

SPECIAL IMPLICATIONS FOR THE THERAPIST 19-5

Testicular Cancer

Therapists need to be aware of the potential signs and symptoms related to this disease because clients may be seen by the therapist for other conditions before the cancer is diagnosed. The most likely scenario is someone with thoracic or lumbar pain secondary to undiagnosed lymph node adenopathy or someone with low lumbar pain that radiates around the iliac crest to the groin.

Low lumbar and iliac crest pain may be secondary to biomechanical dysfunction, whereas the groin pain could be secondary to the cancer. Correlation of findings from the history and physical examination and the client's response to treatment may raise suspicion, warranting communication with a physician.

An awareness of the location of superficial lymph nodes is also important for the therapist (see Fig. 13-7). Observation of a mass or even a filling-in of the concavity normally found in the left supraclavicular region should alert the therapist to palpate this area. Palpation of a nodule or a positive iliopsoas sign (see Figs. 16-13 and 16-14) requires medical referral.

Surgical treatment of testicular cancer also holds implications for the therapist. Postoperatively, lymph node dissection can result in compromised lymphatic flow and resultant lymphedema (see Chapter 13). The surgical scars related to orchiectomy and retroperitoneal lymph node dissection may affect the person's posture or movement mechanics of the trunk, pelvis, and hip regions.

Other potential adverse effects of the surgery include infertility associated with sexual dysfunction, such as occurs with retrograde ejaculation or failure to ejaculate. Serious adverse effects of combination chemotherapy include neuromuscular toxic effects, death from myelosuppression, pulmonary fibrosis, and Raynaud syndrome. See "Treatment and Special Implications for the Therapist 19-3: Prostate Cancer" and Chapter 5 for a description of the side effects of radiation and chemotherapy.

PENILE CANCER

Overview and Incidence

Penile cancer is a relatively rare malignancy, with approximately 1500 new cases and 300 deaths each year. It is more common in Asia, Africa, and South America than in the United States. The 5-year survival rate for all men affected by this type of cancer is approximately 50%. This ranges from 66% survival rate for individuals with node negative disease, 25% to 30% for men with positive inguinal lymph nodes, and approaches 0% for men with pelvic node metastases.

Risk Factors[16]

The majority of men diagnosed with penile cancer (85%) are 50 years or older, with a median age of 68 years.[110] Penile cancer is far more common in uncircumcised men. Phimosis is strongly associated with increased risk for penile cancer. Phimosis is a congenital narrowing of the opening of the foreskin so that it cannot be retracted. Presence of HPV, HIV, cigarette smoking, heavy alcohol use, lichen sclerosis, phototherapy for psoriasis, and a high number of sexual partners are other risk factors for penile cancer. Interestingly, penile cancer is also more common in men who do not have health insurance.[110]

Pathogenesis

Histopathology reveals that 59% of penile cancers are squamous cell carcinomas, 15% papillary carcinomas, 10% basaloid carcinomas, 7% warty, 3% verrucous, and 3% sarcomatoid. Basaloid and sarcomatoid tumors carry the worst prognosis.

Clinical Manifestations

Signs and symptoms of penile cancer can include the following: a visible lesion on the penis, foul odor, pain, discharge, or bleeding. There may also be a report of swelling or mass in inguinal node region. Because of the significantly poorer prognosis once the cancer has reached the lymph nodes, it is important to have any of these signs/symptoms addressed by a physician promptly.

MEDICAL MANAGEMENT

DIAGNOSIS. Men should be screened for the presence of phimosis. Most common locations include the glans penis and prepuce. These two regions account for greater than 50% of all penile cancers. After a thorough history and physical examination are performed by a physician, a biopsy and inguinal lymph node dissection is required to determine a proper diagnosis. CT scans can be used in obese men or men who have had previous inguinal surgery.

TREATMENT. Treatment is divided into three categories based on staging of the tumor: superficial (Tis, Ta, T1a), invasive (T1b, T2), and deeply invasive (T3, T4). For superficial penile cancers, topical 5-fluorouracil cream, laser therapy, Moh surgery, and local excision with or without circumcision are all viable options for treatment. For invasive cancers, a glansectomy or partial penectomy is recommended. Radiation therapy can be considered as an organ-sparing option; however, this can lead to considerable fibrosis of the soft tissue, which can impact both urinary and erectile function. The goal for all of the male genital cancers is sometimes referred to the "trifecta."

The trifecta consists of cancer control, urinary continence, and erectile function.

Deeply invasive cancers require a radical penectomy with perineal urethrostomy in conjunction with chemotherapy and palliative radiation treatment. Bilateral superficial inguinal lymph node dissection is recommended for tumors staged as high-grade T1 stage or higher. Chemotherapy regimens include cisplatin, bleomycin, and methotrexate. These medications can cause peripheral neuropathy and pulmonary fibrosis. The goal of all treatment is organ preservation, with cancer eradication whenever possible.

SPECIAL IMPLICATIONS FOR THE THERAPIST 19-6

Penile Cancer

Men with penile cancer may report pain and swelling in pelvis, genitals, and legs. It is important for a therapist to be able to discern if the pain arises from a musculoskeletal, neuromuscular, or visceral origin. If a therapist is able to discern that the problem arises from the pelvic floor muscles, it is important to initiate an appropriate exercise program for these muscles.

It would be prudent for physical therapists to advocate for individuals with early stage testicular and penile cancer to engage in an exercise program to try to mitigate some of the effects of their treatment. Remember as previously stated, the goal for all of the male genital cancers is the trifecta consisting of cancer control, urinary continence, and erectile function. In order to attain cancer control, urinary incontinence and erectile dysfunction often occur. A pelvic floor exercise program could improve the quality of life for the cancer survivor.

ERECTILE DYSFUNCTION

Overview

Erectile dysfunction (ED), also referred to as *impotence*, is a general term that refers to the inability to achieve, keep, or sustain an erection sufficient for satisfactory sexual performance for both partners and may include a problem with libido, penile erection, ejaculation, or orgasm. The degree of erectile dysfunction may be graded according to the number of satisfactory attempts out of 10 (mild: 7-8, moderate: 4-6, and severe: 0-3).

Incidence and Risk Factors

The prevalence of ED in various community studies has varied from as low of 7% to as high as 52% and has a definite correlation with increasing age. There are an estimated 30 million men in the United States and 152 million men worldwide with ED.[3] Epidemiologic studies of ethnic groups in the United States are not available at this time.

Risk factors for ED include age-related testosterone deficiency; certain medications; chronic diseases, particularly coronary artery disease, neurologic conditions, and diabetes mellitus; alcohol use; mental or emotional

Box 19-4

RISK FACTORS FOR ERECTILE DYSFUNCTION

- Age
- Smoking
- Medical history
  - Diabetes mellitus
  - Coronary heart disease
  - Peripheral vascular disease
  - Hypothyroidism
  - Hypopituitarism
  - Hypertension
  - Hyperlipidemia
  - Chronic uremia
  - Neuromuscular disease
  - Psychiatric disorders
  - Multiple sclerosis
  - Chronic alcoholism
  - Kidney or liver disease
  - Obesity
- Surgical history
  - Transurethral procedures
  - Aortoiliac procedures
  - Proctocolectomy
  - Abdominoperineal resection
  - Prostatectomy
- Adverse reaction to Medications
  - Antihypertensives*
  - Antipsychotics
  - Amphetamines
  - Opiates
  - Antidepressants
  - Antihistamines
  - Agents for BPH (finasteride/Proscar, dutasteride/Avodart)

*Including β-blockers, diuretics, α-adrenergic antagonists, central α-adrenergic agonists, spironolactone, guanethidine, methyldopa.

problems; and smoking[86,139,151] (Box 19-4). Being overweight or underweight is a risk factor; physical activity can reduce the risk of ED, but only in men who are obese.[32] Treatment for prostate cancer such as prostatectomy, external radiation therapy, and brachytherapy can contribute to the development of ED.

Etiologic Factors

The underlying causes of erectile dysfunction are commonly classified as *neurogenic, arteriogenic, venogenic,* or *psychogenic.* Approximately 50% to 80% of men seeking treatment for sexual dysfunction have an organic lesion. The ratio of organic to psychogenic lesions is directly proportional to age. In 70% of men younger than age 35 years, the cause is psychogenic. The psychogenic factors include anxiety, fear, depression, stress, fatigue, and so on.

In 85% of men older than age 50 years, the cause is organic. Conditions that can impede blood flow (e.g., atherosclerosis or medications) or impair nerve transmission (e.g., diabetes or surgery) are the most common organic causes.[93,98] Neurogenic or neurovascular ED can result from surgical or traumatic injury to the autonomic or somatic penile innervation or neurovascular mechanisms that initiate erections.

Autonomic denervation of the pudendal nerve and pelvic or perineal trauma from radical pelvic surgeries (e.g., for colon or prostate cancer) result in poor smooth muscle relaxation, arterial insufficiency, and venous inadequacy, thus preventing adequate erection.[90]

Both surgery and radiation therapy can cause this type of autonomic dysfunction. Radiation may also produce ED by accelerating microvascular angiopathy, causing cavernosal fibrosis or stenosis of the pelvic arteries, and by accelerating existing arteriosclerosis, leading to vascular impotence.[150]

Another possible neurologic mechanism is microscopic neuropathy with breakdown of cholinergic, adrenergic, noncholinergic, or nonadrenergic neurotransmission. Individuals with diabetes mellitus experience change in the ultrastructure of the cavernous nerves arising from the S2 to S4 spinal nerves. These changes include diffuse thickening of the Schwann cells and perineural basement membranes.

ED can be a hemodynamic event and can warn of ischemic heart disease in some men. Conditions resulting in arterial insufficiency can also result in local penile changes. Researchers refer to ED as *penis angina*[21] and a *penile stress test* that can be as predictive as a treadmill exercise stress test for atherosclerosis and subsequent peripheral vascular disease.[118]

Medications can also cause erectile dysfunction. Medications known to cause ED include antihypertensive agents, thiazide diuretics, antidepressants, anticholinergic agents, and opiates such as heroin and methadone.

Pathogenesis

Despite great strides in research into ED, knowledge and understanding of the pathophysiologic mechanisms responsible for ED are still not entirely clear. Numerous factors and structures can influence the process of sexual function and dysfunction. Coordinated interaction between regulatory centers in the diencephalon, brainstem, and spinal cord are required for sexual function. Penile erection is a neurovascular event modulated by neurotransmitters and hormonal status.

The penis is innervated by autonomic and somatic nerves. In the pelvis, the sympathetic and parasympathetic nerves merge to form the cavernous nerves, which enter the corpora cavernosa to regulate blood flow during erection and ejaculation. The corpus cavernosum is one of two chambers in the penis that run lengthwise and are surrounded by a membrane called tunica albuginea. A spongy tissue filling the chambers contains smooth muscles, fibrous tissues, spaces, veins, and arteries. The urethra along the underside of the corpus cavernosum is surrounded by the corpus spongiosum.[150]

The parasympathetic visceral efferent fibers arise from sacral roots 2 to 4 to supply the pelvic plexus located on the lateral wall of the rectum. The cavernous nerves leave the pelvic plexus and travel in the lateral pelvic fascia on the posterolateral surface of the prostate gland to supply the corpora cavernosa of the penis. The somatic component, the pudendal nerve, is responsible for penile sensation.[150]

During sexual stimulation, impulses from the brain and local nerves trigger the arteries in the penis to widen and the smooth muscle to relax. Blood moves into the spongy smooth muscle while the penile veins constrict to keep the penis engorged and rigid. The tunica albuginea helps trap the blood in the corpus cavernosum, sustaining the erection.[165]

Clinical Manifestations

Manifestations of erectile dysfunction include the following: need for more physical stimulation to induce an erection, less firm erections, longer time to reach orgasm, decreased force of ejaculation, increased time needed to get an erection after orgasm, fewer spontaneous erections, and erections that are lost during sexual intercourse. Most men (and their partners) experience significant feelings of emotional distress and/or depression associated with sexual dysfunction, especially when ED results in subsequent infertility for the couple. Quality-of-life issues are an important aspect of this disorder.

MEDICAL MANAGEMENT

PREVENTION. Without a better understanding of the pathophysiology behind ED, treatment rather than prevention is the main focus. Preventing coronary artery disease and diabetes mellitus may aid in preventing this condition. Anyone with ED should be counseled to avoid recreational drugs and excessive alcohol. Hypertension should be treated, and for anyone with diabetes, glucose levels must be monitored carefully and kept under control.

Regular exercise, keeping cholesterol levels below recommended levels, maintaining an ideal body weight, and quitting smoking are all healthy lifestyle choices that may help prevent ED.

DIAGNOSIS. Because of the sheer number of possible etiologic factors, a definitive diagnosis related to ED can be difficult. Differentiating between an organic versus psychogenic cause is the initial challenge. The nocturnal penile tumescence test, which monitors the incidence of nocturnal erections, helps with this distinction. Men with psychogenic ED/impotence will have nocturnal erections, whereas those with an organic lesion will not.

Physical examination includes an abdominal and genital inspection and palpation, assessment of peripheral pulses and blood pressure, and DRE to evaluate prostate size. Laboratory values, including serum chemistries, complete blood cell count, fasting lipid levels, thyroid function tests, and hormone levels may help rule out systemic diseases.

As a potential marker of cardiovascular risk, ED is no longer considered a benign result of aging. Its documented association with many chronic diseases and high-risk situations extends the significance of ED beyond the purely sexual domain, providing insight into general and cardiovascular health.[21] Arteriography is the standard test for vascular diagnostic testing, but ultrasonography is also used to assess the vascular integrity of the genital area.

TREATMENT. The goals of treatment for ED are to improve self-esteem, confidence, and overall sexual and relationship satisfaction. Management of ED can help restore men to their full erectile potential. Optimal treatment improves erection hardness and is designed to improve outcomes in overall sexual experience.[107]

Medical treatment for ED varies, depending on the cause. Pharmacologic treatment with phosphodiesterase type 5 (PDE-5) inhibitors, such as sildenafil (Viagra), vardenafil (Levitra), and tadalafil (Cialis), to increase blood flow to the penis by inhibiting a particular enzyme has become the new first-line treatment for anyone without heart disease. PDE-5 inhibitors can be used cautiously with α-blockers but are contraindicated in men who take any form of nitrate or nitrite medications because these drug combinations can cause serious hypotension.[165]

Other products are available for select individuals. For example, alprostadil (applied as a topical gel to the head of the penis or used as a suppository inserted into the urethra), previously only available as an injection into the penile tissue, can be used by anyone who is not hypersensitive to the drug, who does not have a history of venous thrombosis, or who does not have sickle cell anemia or sickle cell trait, thrombocytopenia, polycythemia, or multiple myeloma. An erection occurs within 10 minutes and will last for 30 to 60 minutes.

Testosterone injections are an option for men with documented androgen deficiency. Injection of vasoactive substances directly into the penis may also be used. These drugs relax the arterioles and smooth muscle of the corpus cavernosum and increase cavernous arterial blood flow, causing an erection. Penile prosthetic devices can be implanted surgically, and men with arterial and venous deficiencies are candidates for vascular reconstruction procedures. Constricting bands placed around the penis are helpful for men whose ED is associated with venous leakage Erections can be achieved mechanically with a vacuum pump device. It is important to encourage men to address the erectile function in a timely manner when symptoms first appear. Lack of erections over time can lead to fibrosis and cause further erectile difficulties.

Anyone with arteriogenic ED should be counseled regarding risk-factor modification, including lifestyle interventions such as exercise[68] and weight loss and pharmacologic management of hypertension and hyperlipidemia.[130] Psychologic counseling and/or behavioral therapy is indicated for those with a psychogenic basis for the sexual dysfunction. Counseling or behavioral therapy may be helpful for anyone who would like assistance coping with this dysfunction.

Other strategies can include engaging in sexual activity when rested, relaxed, and pain-free. Anyone with erectile dysfunction should be advised to use pillows or other props to create the most comfortable position possible when having sexual intercourse. Open communication with the sexual partner is of paramount importance in having a satisfying sexual experience.

PROGNOSIS. ED occurs immediately after radical prostatectomy, with variable return of function. Preservation of sexual function can be difficult even among men who have been treated with nerve-sparing surgery. Preservation of the nerves responsible for erection may depend on experience of the surgeon and preoperative potency. Younger, healthier men also may have better outcomes after surgery. In the case of radiation-induced ED, years may elapse before clinically significant ED develops.[150]

SPECIAL IMPLICATIONS FOR THE THERAPIST   19-7

Erectile Dysfunction

Many men are reluctant or uncomfortable discussing sexual function or dysfunction. Questions about sexual health must be culturally, ethnically, and spiritually sensitive; suggested questions for the physical therapist to ask are available.[62] To decrease the individual's discomfort, the therapist may want to explain that these questions are routinely asked of all clients.

Therapists usually ask clients with back pain about the presence of sexual dysfunction as part of the screening for cauda equina syndrome. Many people who answer yes to these questions may have a preexisting condition that accounts for the ED/impotence. Sexual dysfunction may be a postoperative complication related to some of the procedures described earlier in this chapter. If the person notes a sudden change in sexual function, communication with a physician is warranted.

The male pelvic floor muscles are active during sexual intercourse The perineal muscles, specifically the ischiocavernosus and bulbospongiosus, play a major role in gaining and maintaining penile erection *and preventing postmicturition urinary dribble.*

Weakness in the pelvic floor muscles may contribute to sexual dysfunction. Focused pelvic floor muscle exercises should be offered all men with intact nerve innervation and vascular supply as the first line of treatment for ED.[21,129,130] There is a limited amount of studies in this area, but results consistently show that pelvic floor reeducation and rehabilitation including biofeedback and electrical stimulation have an important role in restoring normal sexual, urologic, and erectile function.[13,43-46,158,159]

SEXUAL ABUSE IN MEN

Sexual abuse can be defined as nonconsensual sexual contact that includes but is not limited to touching, sexual assault, battery, rape, sodomy, coerced nudity, and sexually explicit photography.[38] Heterosexual men comprise 25% to 50% of all intimate partner violence (IPV) victims in a given year. Studies of male victims of sexual abuse suggest that 97% experience feelings of depression and 92% report anxiety.[40,162]

Much of the data on men is very similar (if not redundant) to what has been written about women. There does not seem to be a great deal of variation in how the abuse presents or the long-term effects of abuse between men and women. For these reasons, rather than write an extensive section on sexual abuse in men here, we refer the reader to "Domestic Violence" in Chapter 2.

REFERENCES

To enhance this text and add value for the reader, all references are included on the companion Evolve site that accompanies this textbook. The reader can view the reference source and access it online whenever possible.

CHAPTER 20

The Female Genital/Reproductive System

BETH SHELLY • VALERIE WANG • HOLLY TANNER • PATRICIA M. KING

The female genital or reproductive system is made up of the breasts, ovaries, fallopian tubes, uterus, vagina, and external genitalia (Fig. 20-1). The primary functions of this system are related to preparing the woman for conception and gestation (pregnancy) and for gestation itself. The female breast and hormonal systems, including the ovarian hormones, estrogen and progesterone, play a key role in these functions. Malfunctioning of this system can result in a multitude of local disorders, some benign and others life-threatening, as well as widespread systemic changes via the hormonal influences.

The diseases discussed in this chapter have several implications for therapists. Some conditions, for example, pelvic organ prolapse or postsurgical rehabilitation after mastectomy, may be the primary reason the woman is seeing the therapist. Other conditions, such as endometriosis, may be manifested solely by pain, and the woman presents to the therapist with back or pelvic pain of unknown cause.

The incidence of some of the disorders discussed in this chapter is quite high. For example, endometriosis is present in approximately 50% of women receiving treatment for infertility and in 10% to 15% of all premenopausal women. Breast cancer accounts for approximately one-third of all female cancers. Therapists frequently encounter disorders of this system.

The presence of some of these conditions places the woman at higher risk for developing other diseases. For example, a history of endometriosis increases the risk of ectopic pregnancy, a potentially life-threatening disorder. Menopause is known to contribute to disorders of aging, such as osteoporosis, cardiovascular diseases, and cancer.

Therapists are now involved in the field of urogynecology with specific evaluation and assessment tools, treatment modalities, and therapeutic interventions. Increasingly, therapists are involved in the management of conditions such as vaginismus, dyspareunia, vulvodynia, sexual dysfunction, pelvic pain, levator ani syndrome, endometriosis, pelvic organ prolapse, and incontinence. An online summary of discussions related to these topics throughout the text is available to gain a broad overview as well as a more complete understanding of how these conditions affect multiple systems and how other systems integrate with the pelvic floor.

Therapists' participation in women's health issues reflects the medical profession's changing view of women.

The traditional allopathic emphasis on women's breasts and reproductive system (the "bikini view") is shifting focus to a more holistic view of women as unique individuals during their reproductive years and beyond, both in health and in disease. In addition, many reproductive diseases are related to abnormal menstruation. It is helpful for physical therapists to know what is considered "normal" versus "abnormal" (Box 20-1).

AGING AND THE FEMALE REPRODUCTIVE SYSTEM

Patricia (Trish) M. King, PT, PhD, OCS, MTC

Menopause

Menopause is a normal consequence of aging that marks the end of a woman's reproductive years. Menopause is defined as the permanent cessation of menses specifically occurring when a woman has experienced 1 full year without menstruation.[287] Menopause is the end result of a progressive reduction of estrogen production by the ovaries that usually occurs gradually over a period of several years. Although the primary event of menopause, cessation of menses, is not a pathologic occurrence in aging females, the risk for certain pathologic conditions is increased by the anatomic and physiologic changes associated with menopause. A variety of physical, functional, and psychologic changes occur as a result of the estrogen deficiency associated with menopause and the transition to menopause.

Physiologic Changes of Menopause

During the reproductive years the primordial ovarian follicles, from which ova are expelled, steadily decrease in number. By middle age, the ovaries, which each held about 300,000 eggs at puberty, have resorbed or shed nearly all of them.[534] Ovarian production of estrogen and progesterone decreases significantly when the number of these follicles approaches zero. The reduced level of hormones results in a cascade of events altering the physiology of multiple systems leading to reproductive senescence.[181] Estrogens regulate growth hormone secretion and modulate the tissue responsiveness to growth hormone.[208a] After the menopause, and during aging, a decline in growth hormone secretion (referred to as somatopause) is physiologically observed. Estrogen has effects on various target organs in the body—not just the

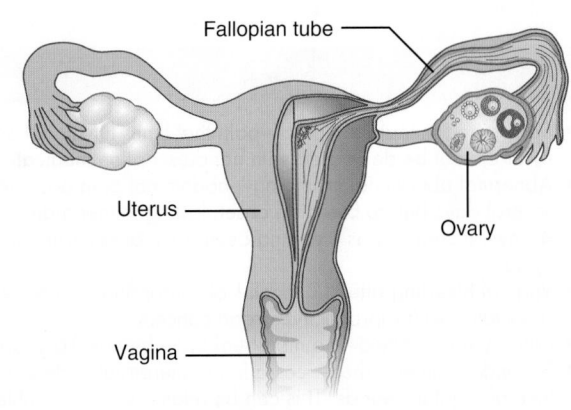

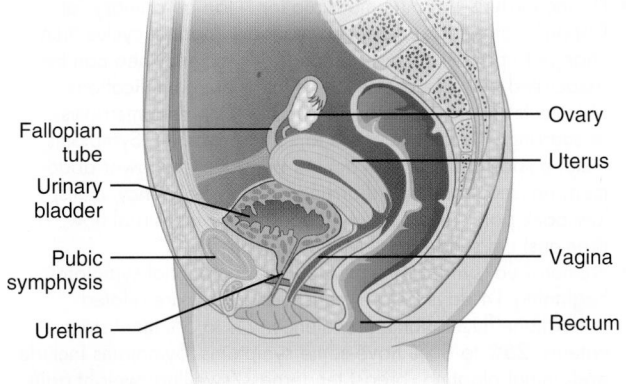

Figure 20-1

Female reproductive organs. See Figures 27-1 and 27-2 for visual representation of the pelvic floor muscles.

organs of reproduction. In fact, estrogen receptor sites are found throughout the body and in all organs of the body, including skin, blood vessels, bone, brain, heart, intestinal tract, and urinary bladder. Physiologic changes associated with declining estrogen include endometrial, vaginal, and breast atrophy; decreased thyroid function; hyperparathyroidism as well as decreased renal function, insulin release, and response to catecholamines.

Terminology

As mentioned, *menopause* is the permanent cessation of menses occurring when a woman has experienced 1 full year without menstruation. *Menopause transition* refers to the time period between when a woman experiences the initial reduction in ovarian function and when she reaches menopause. The term *menopause transition* was identified as the preferred terminology to *perimenopause* and *climacteric* following the STRAW meetings in 2003.[573,574] The term *perimenopause* continues to be commonly used; however, the recommendation is to limit its use when addressing patients/clients rather than in professional and scientific communication because of the imprecise definitions of perimenopause and climacteric. *Postmenopause* refers to the years in a woman's life following menopause. *Premature ovarian failure* refers to cessation of menses before age 40 years and is associated with an elevated follicle-stimulating hormone level). Premenopausal women who have a hysterectomy experience *surgical menopause*.

Age

The average reported age for menopause is 51.5 years[287]; however, age at menopause varies with the transition to menopause beginning as early as the late 30s for some women. Most women experience near-complete loss of production of estrogen by their mid-50s. Approximately 70 million women in the United States are beyond 50 years of age, with 2500 to 3500 women having their 50th birthdays each day. During the most recent U.S. census, close to 42 million women were age 55 years and older.[389,618] With the number of women in the 55-plus age group continuing to increase in the coming years, it is important for physical therapists to understand the impact of menopause.

Menopause Transition (Perimenopause)

Menopause transition (MT) is often referred to among women as "the change before the change." For some women, MT can begin as early as 10 years before the complete cessation of the menstrual cycle. For others, it can occur just a few months before menopause. Most women report a 3- or 4-year period of time when symptoms gradually escalate. MT is the physiologic reverse of puberty. Levels of reproductive hormones start to decline gradually with sudden fluctuations on a day-to-day basis as opposed to the gradual increase that occurs during puberty.

The intermittent variations in hormone levels account for the variations in the patterns of common symptoms women often experience during this time period. MT is further described as having two stages, early and late. Early MT is characterized by menstrual periods that continue to occur at regular intervals but with increasing distance between periods. During early MT ovulation continues but may alternate with anovulatory periods (menstrual cycles during which the ovaries do not release an oocyte [egg]). Increasing irregularity of the menstrual cycle occurs in late MT.

Premature Menopause

Approximately 1% of women experience *premature ovarian failure*, sometimes referred to as premature *menopause*. Smoking advances aging and may move the onset of menopause forward by approximately 2 years,[242] sometimes a factor in premature menopause. Premature menopause affects reproductive status and may affect sexual identity, sexual function, and sexual relationships. Factors modulating the individual's sexual outcome after premature menopause include associated medical, psychologic, and social and sexual comorbidities. Survivors of childhood and adolescent cancers also have increased risk for negative sexual outcomes following premature menopause. The biologic basis of desire, arousal, orgasm, and vaginal receptivity are impacted by premature menopause and combine with psychosocial factors to determine a woman's response to the changes in her reproductive status and the physical changes that impact sexual function.

Postmenopause

As life expectancy continues to increase, most women can now expect to live at least one-third of their lives

Box 20-1

COMPARISON OF NORMAL TO ABNORMAL MENSTRUAL CYCLE*

Many reproductive diseases are related to abnormal menstruation. It is helpful for physical therapists to know what is considered "normal" versus "abnormal."

Normal Menstrual Cycle

- Menarche—first menstrual cycle: 11 to 15 years old.
- Length of cycle—20 to 45 days; average 28 days (day 1 is the first day of bleeding).
- It is common to have several years of irregular bleeding when menstruation starts.
- Ovulation occurs around day 14 and may be associated with a small amount of transient lower abdominal pain.
- Normal menstrual bleeding lasts about 5 days.
- Menstrual pain—abdominal cramping begins shortly before bleeding begins, peaks within 24 hours of beginning of bleeding, decreases gradually, and is gone usually within 2 days (often before bleeding ends). Normal menstrual pain does not significantly limit most functional activities.

Abnormal Menstrual Cycle

- Infrequent menstrual cycle—longer than 31 to 35 days apart.
- Frequent menstrual cycle—less than 2 weeks from day 1 of your period to day 1 of your next period. Both infrequent and frequent cycles can indicate the onset of menopause but should be evaluated if the woman is not of the expected menopause age (48-52 years old) or if there are other symptoms present, such as severe pain or heavy bleeding.
- Heavy bleeding—fills a tampon or sanitary pad after 1 or 2 hours.
- Extended bleeding—bleeding lasting longer than 7 days.

- Severe abdominal cramping—pain that limits functional activity or cannot be decreased with nonprescription medications.
- Abnormal abdominal cramping—abdominal pain occurring several days before bleeding onset, lasting longer than 3 or 4 days, increasing as bleeding decreases, or occurring mid cycle.
- Vaginal bleeding after 12 months of menopause—may be associated with reproductive organ cancers.
- Primary amenorrhea—no menstrual cycle by age 16 years.
- Secondary amenorrhea—cessation of menstrual cycle after a time of regular periods. This can be related to female athlete triad and is indicative of pathology.
- Dysmenorrhea—painful menstruation. Can be primary (at first onset of menstruation) or secondary (normal cycles then change to painful cycles). Secondary dysmenorrhea can be associated with diseases such as infection, complications of intrauterine contraceptive device (IUCD), endometriosis, or scarring. Prevalence: 10% to 15% of women. Symptoms include spasmodic or dull aching pain over the lower abdomen, nausea, vomiting, diarrhea, urinary frequency, chills, low back pain, dizziness, syncope, heavy menstrual flow, premenstrual syndrome (PMS) symptoms.
- Premenstrual syndrome—physical and emotional symptoms beginning 14 days before menstruation that are related to hormone fluctuations. Prevalence: 2% to 5% meet strict criteria, 25% to 85% have some symptoms. Symptoms include abdominal bloating, breast tenderness/swelling, weight gain, fatigue, depression, irritability, headache, constipation, acne, rhinitis, edema, sleep problems, mood swings, poor concentration, noise sensitivity, and decreased motor skills.

*Information compiled from many sources.

after menopause. The physical, psychologic, and social changes associated with menopause are increasingly important for all health care practitioners to understand. The hormonal fluctuations of MT are expected to stabilize postmenopause, although hormonal and symptom variations may continue during this portion of the life cycle. Details of the changes that become the "new normal" for women in the postmenopausal years are outlined in this section using a body systems approach.

Surgical Menopause

Oophorectomy, or surgical removal of the ovaries, creates surgical menopause. Hysterectomy is the surgical removal of the uterus, which may or may not include the cervix and supporting ligaments. The ovaries and fallopian tubes are not removed during hysterectomy and so may continue to release reproductive hormones. In some cases, the remaining ovaries will stop functioning very soon after hysterectomy; in other cases, they may continue to function for several years more. Estrogen levels decline much more suddenly and symptoms are often more severe with surgical menopause than with natural menopause. Surgical menopause increases the risk for (and severity of) several common complaints associated with menopause, including thermoregulatory variations, vasomotor changes (hot flashes), vaginal atrophy, and cognitive decline.[212]

Clinical Manifestations

The signs and symptoms experienced during menopause vary among individuals and even cross-culturally; however, common patterns are reported.[625] Although most women experience spontaneous relief of symptoms within 5 years of onset, a substantial portion continue to experience symptoms beyond 5 years. In the reproductive system, temporal changes occur in the menstrual cycle in terms of both the length and frequency of the cycle. The intensity of menstrual bleeding and associated discomfort vary from a woman's previously typical patterns. Anovulation is most common in the later stages of MT, leading to skipped menstrual cycles.

Vaginal dryness and vaginal discomfort frequently occur and may lead to painful sexual intercourse (dyspareunia); vaginal dryness and painful intercourse are more common in the late stages of MT. The frequency of vaginal and bladder infections increases among women experiencing menopause, explained in part by vaginal pH changes, with a more alkaline environment resulting from the estrogen decline as well as the dehydration of the vaginal and urethral tissues.

Thermoregulatory and vasomotor changes during menopause are associated with "hot flashes" or "hot flushes" and "night sweats." Vasomotor complaints are the most well-known and most commonly reported complaints of women experiencing menopause also usually

Box 20-2

COMMON SYMPTOMS FROM PERIMENOPAUSE THROUGH POSTMENOPAUSE

- Hot flashes, flushing, sweats
- Vulvar or vaginal atrophy (dryness, burning, itching, dyspareunia)
- Anxiety, panic attacks, depression, mood swings, irritability
- Fatigue
- Urinary incontinence
- Insomnia, sleep disturbances
- Headache
- Decreased libido
- Prolonged bleeding, heavy bleeding, irregular menses, cessation of menses
- Heart palpitations, heart racing or pounding
- Short-term memory loss, difficulty concentration (brain fog)
- Changes in body composition: muscle loss, weight gain, central adiposity

reported as the most distressing of all menopausal symptoms. *Night sweats* are hot flashes combined with profuse perspiration, predominately reported to occur at night by menopausal women. Night sweats may negatively impact both the quality of sleep and mood. Dizziness and palpitations are also common during the MT. The vasomotor changes of menopause are often the most difficult for women to tolerate and reported to be positively correlated with anxiety among menopausal women.[108] Interesting cross-cultural variations in vasomotor symptoms are reported,[52,572] indicating that beliefs and attitudes attenuate both the manifestation and perception of menopausal symptoms.[336,572]

Fatigue, anxiety, sleeps disturbances, difficulty with memory and concentration, reduced libido, mood swings, and irritability are all commonly reported by menopausal women[108,440,604] (Box 20-2). Pain complaints also increase during the MT including headache, breast discomfort and enlargement as well as peripheral and spinal joint pain.[287] Additional signs and symptoms may occur in conjunction with the physiologic changes of menopause in the musculoskeletal, urologic, neurologic, cardiovascular, endocrine, gastrointestinal, integumentary, and psychosocial systems. Physical changes and pathologic correlates of menopause are presented in the following section.

Pathologic Correlates of Menopause

Although menopause is initiated in the reproductive system, pathologic conditions, symptoms, impairments, and functional changes occur across all body systems as a result of the complex physiologic interactions caused by the menopausal changes in estrogen levels. A body systems approach is used in this section to outline the pathologic consequences of menopause.

Reproductive System. A variety of changes occur in the reproductive organs as estrogen levels decrease. The myometrium, endometrium, cervix, vagina, and labia all become atrophic to some degree. Women who suffer from endometriosis may experience relief as the endometrium volume diminishes in the postmenopausal period. Pelvic ligamentous laxity contributes to the development of cystocele, rectocele, and uterine prolapse. Menstrual bleeding continues during the MT becoming irregular in timing with variations in flow and associated pain.

Vaginal Bleeding. Although *vaginal bleeding* should stop with menopause, 80% of all gynecologic or reproductive system problems in women older than age 60 years are related to postmenopausal bleeding (vaginal bleeding that occurs 1 year or more after the last period). Such bleeding can be a symptom of a life-threatening problem (e.g., cancer) or a benign condition (e.g., polyps) but always requires a medical evaluation. Women receiving continuous combined hormone replacement therapy, which is estrogen in combination with progestin taken without a break, are likely to experience irregular spotting until the endometrium (vaginal lining) atrophies, which takes about 6 months. A medical evaluation is required only if bleeding persists or suddenly appears after 6 months. Those women taking sequential hormone replacement therapy (HRT) (estrogen taken daily for 25 days each month with progestin taken for 10 or 12 days) normally bleed lightly each time the progestin is temporarily stopped.

Vaginal Atrophy. Vaginal atrophy, as well as flattening of the rugae (vaginal rugae are transverse epithelial ridges most commonly seen on the outer third of the female vagina), occurs during menopause. As a result of the surface epithelium thinning, the vaginal surface is friable and bleeding is common with minimal trauma. The blood vessels in the vaginal walls narrow, and over time, the vagina itself contracts and loses flexibility.

External Genitalia. External genitalia also experiences gradual changes to size and integrity during menopause. The vulvar epithelium atrophies and secretions from sebaceous glands diminish. Subcutaneous fat in the labia majora is lost and leads to shrinkage and retraction of clitoral prepuce and the urethra, to fusion of the labia minora, and to introital narrowing and then stenosis.[417] As a result of these changes, the clinical symptoms associated with vulvovaginal atrophy include vaginal dryness, itching, irritation, dyspareunia, and recurrent urinary tract infections.[373,585]

Pelvic Floor Dysfunction and Pelvic Organ Prolapse. Pelvic floor dysfunction and pelvic organ prolapse are both common during all stages of menopause. The development of pelvic organ prolapse and urinary incontinence is multifactorial. Estrogen receptors are found throughout the lower urinary and reproductive tracts, reduction of estrogen is associated with collagen changes and diminished vascularity of contributing to dysfunctions in the pelvic floor and support mechanisms for the pelvic organs. See further discussion of these conditions in Chapter 27.

Pelvic Pain. Pelvic pain encompasses a variety of conditions and pain patterns, some of which are more common during the menopausal years. Pelvic pain patterns are broadly categorized as cyclic, noncyclic and dyspareunia (painful sexual intercourse).[357] Dyspareunia is more common among older than younger women, with MT or perimenopause considered a risk factor (Table 20-1).[357] Hysterectomy, the second most common surgery among women in the United States and common in the medical history of menopausal women, is a risk factor for noncyclic pelvic pain.

Table 20-1	Pelvic Pain Risk: Positive and Negative Correlates

	Cyclic Pelvic Pain	**Noncyclic Pelvic Pain**	**Dyspareunia***
Positive correlates (increased risk)	Sex abuse	Child sex abuse	Child sex abuse
	Sex assault	Sex assault	Sex assault
	Stranger assault	PID	Spouse assault
	Physical threat	Depression	PID
	Pelvic inflammatory disease (PID)	Anxiety	Depression
	Age younger than 30 years	Miscarriage	Anxiety
	Early menarche	Long menstrual flow	Menopause transition
	Thin (body mass index <20)	Endometriosis	(perimenopause)
	Irregular flow	C-Section	Female genital mutilation/cutting
	Longer flow	Pelvic adhesions	
	Premenstrual syndrome	Hysterectomy	
	African American	Somatization	
Negative correlates (decreased risk)	Married	No abuse history	Younger age
	Fish intake		Premenopausal
	Physical exercise		
	High parity		

*Note to Reader: Dyspareunia (painful sexual intercourse) can occur in conjunction with cyclic or noncyclic pelvic pain or it can be the only type of pelvic pain a woman experiences. Dyspareunia increases when menopause stages start, which can be at least partly explained by the physical changes of menopause. Women may have other types of pelvic pain or no pelvic pain and then develop dyspareunia related to menopause transition (MT).

Sources: Golding JM: Sexual assault history and physical health in randomly selected Los Angeles women, *Health Psychol* 13:130, 1994; Golding JM: Sexual assault history and women's reproductive and sexual health, *Psychol Women Q* 20:101–121, 1996; Latthe P: Factors predisposing women to chronic pelvic pain: systematic review, *BMJ* 332(7544):749–755, 2006.

Courtesy of Baker, P (2008). *Biocultural correlates of chronic pelvic pain in women.* Unpublished doctoral dissertation/master's thesis, University of Florida, Gainesville.

Women experiencing pelvic pain prior to menopause may experience a worsening of the symptoms during menopause depending on the etiology of their pelvic pain. Some of the conditions and impairments that contribute to pelvic pain are worsened by the physical as well as psychosocial changes of menopause.[425] Women experiencing pelvic pain of musculoskeletal etiology prior to menopause may experience a worsening of symptoms during menopause as the support systems of the pelvis are weakened with the changes in muscle mass, bone and connective tissue strength, and atrophy of the pelvic organs associated with menopause.

In addition, there is indication that vulvar pain may increase during menopause for some women.[240] Pelvic pain associated with fibroids (which have estrogen receptors) may worsen in response to the naturally occurring hormone fluctuations of MT; theoretically, fibroid associated pelvic pain may also increase with HRT as a result of the estrogen stimulation although there are no studies to support the theory.

Vaginal Infections. *Vaginal infections* are increasingly common during menopause. The vaginal pH increases or becomes more alkaline during the MT and menopause. Elevated vaginal pH is a strong clinical indicator that menopause has occurred and may be used clinically to diagnosis menopause.[117,437] An alkaline pH is inhospitable to lactobacilli, the normal flora of the vagina; a decline in lactobacilli, increases the susceptibility to infection from urogenital and fecal pathogens.

Bacterial vaginosis is the most common cause of vaginitis in all women, both vaginosis and vaginitis are increasingly problematic for post-menopausal women. Symptoms of Bacterial vaginosis include vaginal itching, dysuria, and vaginal discharge with a fishy smell. Differential diagnosis considerations include yeast infection, urinary tract infection (UTI), and normal tissue irritation from the changes of menopause (tissue thinning, decreased blood flow and dehydration).[293] The fishy smell associated with Bacterial vaginosis does not accompany yeast infections and discharge should not accompany the normal changes of menopause nor should dysuria.[30]

Sexual Function. *Sexual function* is impacted by both biologic and psychosocial variables that occur during the stages of menopause. Dyspareunia is more common among women in the MT and postmenopause age groups than in women of other age groups. The biologic effects of menopause on vaginal tone and lubrication considered primary etiologic factor contributing to dyspareunia among menopausal women. Blood flow to the genitalia is reduced during menopause and vasocongestion, which is painful, is common with sexual activity. Reduced levels of testosterone and androgen as well as the declines in estrogen contribute to genital atrophy.

Diminishing libido is expected during postmenopause as the result of waning hormones, and is often reported; however, a sizeable study on sexuality and menopause found sexual intercourse, desire, arousal, or physical or emotional satisfaction were not significantly associated with age at MT.[50-52] Older age was associated with painful intercourse among the women who participated in that study. Relationship issues, as well as biologic factors, appear to explain more of the variance in diminished desire as well as sexual pain among older women.[2,50] Higher perceived stress, hot flashes, fatigue, depressed mood, anxiety, difficulty getting to sleep, early morning awakening, and awakening during the night are reported to significantly lower sexual desire. Better perceived health reported, exercise, and alcohol intake are reported to increase sexual desire and at least one study reports having a partner was associated with lower sexual desire among menopausal women.[656]

There is a significant volume of literature available on sexual symptoms and sexual functioning in menopausal women cross-culturally.[186,255,368,384,558,559] Sexual dysfunction was found less likely among African American than non-Hispanic white women and Asian women in a 2006 population-based study from Kaiser-Permanente.[2] Sexual dysfunction was more likely in postmenopausal women with higher educational levels, women who reported poorer overall health, women with urinary incontinence, and women in significant relationships (i.e., defined as married or in long-term relationship). Women in significant relationships were more likely to participate in regular sexual activity than women not in relationships, and they found that African American women were more likely to be satisfied with the sexual relationships; their study included 2109 women of whom 47.6% were white, 18.2% were African American, 16.4% were Asian, 16.6% were Hispanic, and 1.3% were Native American/other.

Lower body mass index (BMI) and better mental health scores were also associated with increased sexual satisfaction in the Addis study.[2] Avis and colleagues reported on a cohort of 3167 non-Hispanic white, African American, Hispanic, Chinese, and Japanese women from the Study of Women's Health across the Nation (SWAN) who were not using hormone replacement.[50] After controlling for a variety of variables, ethnic differences were significant for sexual arousal, pain, desire, and frequency of sexual intercourse. African American women reported higher frequency of sexual intercourse than white women; Hispanic women reported lower physical pleasure and arousal. Chinese women reported more pain and less desire and arousal than the white women, as did the Japanese women, although the only significant difference was for arousal.

Fertility. Although *fertility* ends when a woman reaches menopause, many women perceive themselves as infertile when the MT begins. Despite irregular menstrual bleeding and periods of anovulation, ovulation and conception can occur during the MT transition. Contraception choices are complicated during the MT transition as some commonly prescribed contraceptives can increase undesirable consequences of the MT such as reduced bone mineral density (BMD). As women age, they are more likely to acquire other medical conditions; comorbidities must be considered when contraceptives are prescribed by the appropriate health care practitioner. Guidelines are available from the Centers for Disease Control (CDC) that aim to assist clinicians with decision making when prescribing contraception.[132]

Infertility. *Infertility* is also a concern for women during the MT, as more women choose to delay marriage and childbearing until older ages. Sometimes desired pregnancy requires reproductive technologic assistance and other times it may occur spontaneously. Spontaneous pregnancies during the MT sometimes surprise women not using contraceptives because of their perception that infertility is a part of the MT. Pregnancies during the MT have increased risk for miscarriage, chromosomal abnormalities, cesarean delivery, gestational diabetes, pregnancy-induced hypertension, and stillbirth.[545]

Breast Tissue. *Breast tissue* volume diminishes during menopause in response to reductions in estrogen and progesterone. Estrogen and progesterone have proliferative effects on ductal and glandular structures in the breast. During menopause the volume and percentage of dense breast tissue is reduced and replaced with adipose tissue.[287]

Urologic System. Pelvic support mechanisms (pelvic floor muscles as well as ligamentous and other connective tissues) weaken during menopause in response to estrogen and other age-related changes in the musculoskeletal system. Risk is increased for urinary incontinence, cystocele (bladder prolapse), and urinary tract infections, and although the risk is clear, the exact role of menopause is complex and continues to be examined.[625]

Loss of collagen from around the urethra and within the trigone of the bladder may contribute to the development of urinary dysfunction. Women with preexisting urinary problems may experience increasing difficulty controlling urination as the decline in estrogen results in atrophic changes of the lower urinary tract, widening the urethra and decreasing resistance to the flow of urine. Women with detrusor muscle instability or neurogenic bladder who previously could manage their bladder control may suddenly find themselves with an unexpected loss (or worsening of incontinence).[646] Urinary incontinence (when combined with even minor skin changes associated with menopause) can create major problems for women confined to a wheelchair. Attention to dry skin, hydration, strategies to manage incontinence, and pressure ulcer prevention are very important.

Physical therapists must watch out for (and teach the client how to self-assess for) signs and symptoms of urinary tract infection, kidney and bladder stones, incontinence, and other changes associated with changes in kidney or bladder function.[646] See further discussion in Chapter 18.

Gastrointestinal System. Bowel discomfort, abdominal pain, bloating, nausea, changes in bowel patterns (including constipation and diarrhea), and the appearance or exacerbation of inflammatory bowel disease are associated with MT and menopause.[481] Similar patterns are reported during premenses and menses. Associations between menses, premenses, and gastrointestinal (GI) symptoms provide clinical support for argument that an effect association exists between GI symptoms and ovarian hormones.[278] Diet, hydration, exercise, and stress management may also impact the severity of the menopause associated GI symptoms as well as the presence of comorbidities such as Crohn disease or irritable bowel disease.

Integumentary System. Age-related skin changes enhanced by the hormonal changes of menopause include thinning, reduced elasticity, hyperpigmentation (age spots), wrinkles, and itching.[79,651] Collagen volume and collagen fiber strength are reduced and peripheral blood supply diminished during menopause. The changes in collagen integrity combine with a hormone related reduction in subcutaneous skin volume to give skin a looser appearance. Subcutaneous fat volume also decreases, usually most obvious in the face than other parts of the body as the facial muscles attach to the skin's undersurface creating facial lines. Many factors besides those directly attributable to menopause contribute to the rate and degree of the signs of skin aging, including genetics and health habits. Individuals with thin, dry, fair skin usually manifest the signs of skin aging earlier.

Other factors associated with earlier skin aging include overexposure to sunlight, tobacco use and alcohol use. Studies indicate that estrogen therapy may increase dermis thickness and skin collagen fibers with an overall beneficial effect on the skin of menopausal women.[539] Selective estrogen receptor modulators (SERMs) are being examined for effectiveness and safety in management of the skin changes that are associated with the estrogen decline of menopause.[555,584] The risk-to-benefit ratio of HRT specifically for skin changes is determined following clinical guidelines that continue to emerge as evidence is generated.[471]

Endocrine System. Even though estrogen levels decline as women age, the ovaries continue to produce significant amounts of testosterone and androstenedione after menopause. As a result, levels of testosterone may not decline sharply at menopause for women whose ovaries are intact. Testosterone is a natural means of preserving bone and muscle mass and of alleviating menopausal symptoms, particularly the loss of libido.[287] Androgen insufficiency can occur during menopause and is associated with fatigue, sexual function changes, diminished sense of well-being, as well as reduced levels of serum testosterone, which can impact tissue changes as well as libido.

Diabetes. Women with type 1 diabetes frequently go through menopause at an earlier age than women who do not have diabetes. Premature or early menopause may occur as a complication of type 1 diabetes.[191] As the woman with diabetes approaches menopause, changes in estrogen and progesterone affect how cells respond to insulin and, therefore, affect blood glucose levels. Menopause symptoms can mimic low blood glucose levels (e.g., moodiness or short-term memory loss). Sleep disturbance and weight gain associated with menopause make it harder to control blood glucose levels.

There is an increased risk of urinary tract infection, especially for the menopausal/postmenopausal woman on insulin and/or who has had diabetes for 10 or more years.[102] During the postmenopausal years when female hormone levels remain low, insulin sensitivity may increase with a drop in the expected blood glucose levels.[514] The benefits of HRT for postmenopausal women who have type 2 diabetes mellitus are not certain with the question of whether HRT improves glycemic control or worsens insulin sensitivity remaining unclear. Diabetes is a risk factor for several other conditions frequently occurring among menopausal women including carpal tunnel syndrome, rotator cuff impingement, biceps tendon impingement, osteoporosis and fractures.

Metabolic Changes. Body composition and fat distribution are altered during the stages of menopause, including loss of lean mass, increases in fat mass, and redistribution of fat from the periphery to the center.[582] Weight gain is common. Metabolism slows and caloric requirements decrease; if the balance of caloric intake and exercise is not modified in response to these changes, weight gain usually results. Studies support the theory that increases in physical activity as women age reduces weight gain; more weight gain occurs during the MT than postmenopause.[145] The evidence-supported relationship between physical activity and managing weight gain is an important consideration as physical therapists develop plans of care and/or educational programs for women who are approaching or beyond MT with weight gain as an identified health risk. Weight gain associated with menopause usually involves patterns of fat distribution such that fat deposition in the abdomen is increased. Abdominal fat is associated with increased risk for heart disease as well as for insulin resistance and type 2 diabetes mellitus.[172] Some women report weight gain with HRT; however, clinical trials do not support a positive association between weight gain and HRT.[216]

Vitamin D deficiency is high in the aging population, particularly among postmenopausal women, although the etiology of the deficiency is not well understood. Vitamin D deficiency is defined as a serum level of 25-hydroxyvitamin D below 10 ng/mL, whereas vitamin D "insufficiency" is characterized as a serum level of 25-hydroxyvitamin D of 10 to 30 ng/mL. The metabolite 25-hydroxyvitamin D is considered to be the best clinical measure of vitamin D stores.[152] Keep in mind that deficiency of vitamin D is associated with reduction in calcium absorption, hyperparathyroidism, muscle weakness, as well as increased bone turnover, increased rates of bone loss, and compromised mineralization of bone. The complications of vitamin D deficiency combine to increase fall risk. The daily recommended intake of vitamin D is 600 IU daily for the postmenopausal woman who is not at high risk for fractures or falls and 800 IU daily for the postmenopausal woman who is at high risk of osteoporosis or older than age 70 years.[653]

Cardiovascular System.[383]

Cardiac Events. Female gender has a cardioprotective effect for premenopausal women in large part due to estrogen's enhancement of levels of high-density lipoprotein, the beneficial cholesterol. Cardiac risk increases exponentially when women enter postmenopause with the risk increase predominately related to estrogen decline. The risk for mortality associated with menopause and subsequent coronary heart disease (CHD) is significant in this age group. CHD is the cause of death for 25% of all women across age groups, and is the number one killer of women (and men) in the United States.[462] The association between cardiovascular disease (CVD) and CHD risk and menopause was first noted in the Framingham studies,[321] which included the observation that increased CVD risk occurred among women in MT (regardless of the age of onset of menopause), indicating estrogen withdrawal to be more significant than other age-related factors in CVD risk for women. By the time women reach their 70s, the risk for cardiac events is identical to that of a comparably aged male.[287] Symptoms associated with cardiac disease vary among women by ethnic group and other sociodemographic variables, most notable, education, increasing the burden on practitioners to be alert to and aware of cross-cultural implications, as well as gender and age, when assessing risk for cardiac events.[255,547]

Vasomotor Changes. Vasomotor changes occur during MT and menopause and are usually reported as the most troublesome menopause symptoms by women experiencing MT. *Hot flashes* or *hot flushes* are a manifestation of central thermoregulation changes associated with the hormonal changes of MT. During hot flushes/flashes heart rate and blood pressure increase (in sleep and wakeful states), body temperature increases then declines; sweating begins in the chest and upper body. Risk factors for hot flashes include surgical menopause, early menopause, race/ethnicity, body mass, sedentary lifestyle, smoking, low circulating levels of estradiol, and use of SERMs. Surgical menopause is associated with a 90% probability of hot flashes during the first year after oophorectomy (removal of ovaries), and symptoms can be more abrupt and severe than those associated with natural menopause. Racial and ethnic variations exist but are not well understood. Hot flashes are more common among African American than Euro-American women and more common among Euro-Americans than Asians.[243] Ambient temperature seems to be a factor in hot flashes with more frequent and severe hot flashes reported by women in warmer climates.[502]

Central Adiposity. Central adiposity (truncal obesity) is a common pattern of weight gain among menopausal women. Central adiposity increases the risk for CHD and is strongly correlated with other cardiac risk factors, such as lipid and lipoprotein changes, blood pressure, and insulin level. The relationship between obesity and fat distribution on hot flashes is not clear with conflicting reports as to whether thinner or heavier women experience more frequent hot flashes.

Musculoskeletal System. Bone, muscle, and connective tissues are all affected by the physiologic changes of menopause increasing the risk for several musculoskeletal conditions and impairments for women beginning with MT. Increased risk for muscle injuries as well as slower rates of repair are noted among postmenopausal women that appear to be linked to lower levels of estrogen.[606,607] Muscle mass is positively correlated with estrogen levels[128] and declines with menopause, at least in part, in response to the decline in estrogen.

Inflammatory arthritis risk is higher in all stages of life for women compared to men. This risk increases with age, partly as a result of estrogen's suppressive effect on inflammatory responses, which begins to disappear during MT. Fibromyalgia[482] may either appear for the first time or worsen if already present for women entering the MT. On the other hand, the signs and symptoms of systemic lupus erythematosus (SLE) often diminish with menopause as do migraine headaches. In women with SLE, calcineurin (a molecule that initiates an increased inflammatory response) is induced by estrogen; in women without SLE calcineurin levels remain unchanged by the effects of estrogen. Reductions in estrogen during menopause appear to explain the reduced symptoms often occurring among women with SLE once they reach the menopausal years.[279]

Osteoporosis. Osteoporosis (decreased bone mass; statistically defined as BMD 2.5 standard deviations below the average for the healthy, young female) and *osteopenia* (BMD lower than normal peak BMD but above diagnostic level for osteoporosis) are both associated with MT, menopause, and postmenopause. Estrogen benefits bone integrity by limiting osteoclast formation and bone resorption. During MT BMD and periosteal bone size begin to diminish, partly from reductions in estrogen. Estrogen's effects on bone strength are not all positive; higher estrogen levels limit periosteal bone growth. As women progress through MT to menopause and postmenopause, periosteal apposition[6,595] (increase in periosteal diameter) rates increase, which may contribute to exogenous bone growth associated with the osteoarthritic changes that occur postmenopause.

Theoretically, acceleration in periosteal apposition during menopause could counteract the resorption of bone that occurs in response to decline in estrogen levels that would potentially protect bone integrity as BMD decreases; however, studies do not support that theory. Rates of periosteal apposition among older women are not adequate to counteract the rates of endocortical resorption. The natural variations in bone size differences that exist between women and men seem to contribute to the increased risk for diminished bone integrity among women despite the increase in apposition that occurs with menopause. Apposition rates needed to maintain stiffness over time for slender diaphyses are reported to be as high as 10 times that required by larger diameter bones.[358]

Interventions that stimulate periosteal apposition are recommended to gain balance between endocortical resorption and periosteal apposition for the treatment or prevention of osteoporosis. In addition to menopause and aging, race, ethnicity genetics, and lifestyle are factors in osteoporosis risk. Risk for osteoporosis is highest among Euro-American and Asian women; heredity appears to account for 50% to 80% of BMD variability.[287,499,500] Smoking, physical activity, exercise, and diet are also factors. See Chapter 24 for more information on osteoporosis and bone health.

Fracture Risk. Fracture risk increases with aging and is accelerated among aging women as BMD decreases. Two-thirds of the risk for all osteoporotic fractures in postmenopausal women is reportedly related to premenopausal peak bone mass.[209] The probability of a fracture of the forearm, humerus, spine, or hip increases as much as eightfold between ages 45 and 85 years for women.[319,320] Although osteoporosis is the dominant risk factor, fracture risk is also associated with prior fractures and family history of fractures. Ethnic differences also exist in fracture risk as they do for osteoporosis, although the mechanisms are not fully understood.[13] Models are available that predict fracture risk by combining a variety of clinical factors with BMD assessment[640] (see "Fractures" in Chapter 27).

Fracture location is also a factor with certain fractures predicting likelihood of fracture in other specific locations. For example, a vertebral fracture increases the risk of a second vertebral fracture as well as risk for fractures elsewhere; wrist fractures are predictive of vertebral and hip fractures. Although Colles fractures of the distal radius are more common among women of all ages, with risk increasing with menopause, low BMD is correlated with Colles fractures among premenopausal women.[292,322]

Fracture risk is closely tied to fall risk; factors related to both fracture and fall risk include age, gender/sex, balance, vision, as well as strength, activity and exercise.[164,560] Fracture risk (and thus risk for falls) also increases in the presence of rheumatoid arthritis[653] and other types of inflammatory arthritis, which are increased among women as they age.

Joint Mobility and Spinal Function. Spinal mobility and function are significantly reduced after women experience osteoporotic fractures of the spine. Limits to mobility and function may also occur among postmenopausal women without vertebral fracture. In one study of spine mobility and function among postmenopausal women, spinal range of motion and velocity were significantly reduced among women with osteoporosis compared with women with osteopenia,[611] underscoring the functional importance of preventive measures for osteoporosis among menopausal women.

Spinal Postural Deformity–Kyphosis/Hyperkyphosis. Kyphotic posture of the thoracic spine gradually increases in many women as vertebral height decreases in response to bone volume decrease and/or vertebral fractures during the menopausal years. Kyphotic posture can alter normal biomechanical and anatomical relationships in the shoulder girdle, cervical spine, and lumbopelvic girdle resulting in impairments to balance reaction and gait patterns that may increase fall risk.[291,562]

Adhesive Capsulitis, Rotator Cuff Impingements, and Biceps Tendon Impingement. Adhesive capsulitis, rotator cuff impingements, and biceps tendon impingement are common soft-tissue impairments among aging women and associated with or complicated by kyphotic posture. Kyphotic posture alters the position of the scapula and acromion, which may contribute to reduction in the size of the subacromial space and impingement, a relevant factor in the design of physical therapy programs for impingement syndrome.[375] Additional risk factors for impingements include degenerative processes at the acromioclavicular joint and structural abnormalities of the acromion that result in decreased subacromial space.[412]

Inflammation and fibrosis of the synovium and subsynovium occur with adhesive capsulitis; physical therapy is commonly utilized to treat adhesive capsulitis and is reported to have preventive value for postsurgical cases[616] of adhesive capsulitis. Risk factors for adhesive capsulitis, a condition characterized by sudden and painful loss of shoulder range of motion, include age greater than 40 years,[268] trauma,[512] diabetes,[45] prolonged immobilization,[257] thyroid disease,[654]stroke or myocardial infarction,[257] and the comorbidity of autoimmune disease (all more common among menopausal women).[112,375,616]

Oral Bone and Teeth. The beneficial effects of estrogen on skeletal bone mass impact oral bone and teeth with strong correlations reported between osteoporosis and tooth loss. Other factors, of course, impact dental health and tooth loss including strong negative correlations between cigarette smoking and good dental health.[287]

Tooth loss increases risk for craniomandibular dysfunction and related head, neck, and facial pain.

Osteoarthritis. After age 50 years more women than men are affected by osteoarthritis (OA), particularly of the hand, foot and knee.[653] Prior to age 50 years, OA is more prevalent among men than women. Estrogen is suggested as a factor in the increase in OA that occurs among women of menopausal age, however, findings are, inconsistent and inconclusive with varying explanations for the association. OA of the basilar joint of the thumb is of particularly high risk in menopausal women. occurring 10 to 20 times more often among women compared to men.[487]

Nervous System. Estrogen and progesterone both play key roles in neurologic health, with pathologic consequences possible as these hormones decline with menopause. Estradiol is a known neuroprotective factor; its effects promote attenuation of cell death, and proliferation of new neurons in the face of injury and disease. Progesterone modulates well-being and cognitive and memory processes in the central nervous system both in normal physiology and in pathology.[494]

The declines in estrogen and progesterone that begin during MT are occurring simultaneously with other age-related changes in the nervous system, contributing to a cascade of neurophysiologic changes that manifest later in life as a variety of impairments and functional changes. Estrogen deficiency is, in fact, suggested as the initial step in the chain of causality that increase risk for impairments to affective state, cognitive function, dementia, movement disorders as well as hot flashes and sleep disturbances.

Earlier onset menopause as well as surgical menopause is associated with increased risk for cognitive impairments, dementia and Parkinson disease, implying that timing of withdrawal of sex steroids is significant in the manifestation of neurologic pathology associated with menopause. Changes to memory, reasoning, affect and motor performance are all demonstrated to improve with HRT, reversing the sex steroid deficiency of menopause.[494]

Carpal Tunnel Syndrome. *Carpal tunnel syndrome* (CTS) is correlated with the presence of basilar joint OA in women and other risk factors associated with menopause. Additional correlates of carpal tunnel syndrome include a prior Colles fracture, inflammatory arthritis, hypothyroidism, diabetes mellitus, and use of corticosteroids and estrogens, all of which are common among women during the MT and in the postmenopausal years.[231,324,452,453] Further discussion on carpal tunnel syndrome is presented in Chapter 39.

Postpolio. Late menopause is associated with an increase in the severity of postpolio symptoms. Women in late menopause who were also postpolio reported more sleep disturbances,[317,394] and more difficulty with activities of daily living when compared to postpolio men of the same age. Symptoms of sensory loss and sleep disturbance typical of late polio are not easily differentiated from similar symptoms associated with menopause. Attention is needed during health care encounters to the psychologic and physical impact of menopause on women with postpolio as differentiated from the effects of postpolio.[318] Hysterectomy rates have been reported to be higher among postpolio menopausal women (35%) compared to the average rate for U.S. women (21%), although the explanation for the variation is not clear.

Psychosocial. Risk for *depression* is significantly increased for women during premenopause[93] and menopause.[325] The psychologic distress caused by the symptoms of menopause as well as a woman's reaction to aging and loss of fertility may contribute in the development of depression.[59] Grief over loss of childbearing status may be more likely among women with surgical menopause who are still of natural childbearing age. Loss of self-esteem as well as grief can encompass women emotionally and psychologically posthysterectomy.

Socially, menopause often occurs at a time when family structures and dynamics change with women either accepting increased responsibilities of extended families and care giving, or dealing with the increasing social isolation that occurs when children leave home and/or mid-life divorce or spousal death occurs. Multiple role strain is a factor in the development of depression, chronic pain, and other chronic illnesses among women.[58,576] Women in perimenopausal and menopausal years are particularly at risk for the multiple role strain as they manage relationships and responsibilities at work, at home as parents, spouses, and within their extended family and community. Midlife women may feel socially unsupported as they carry out multiple social roles with limited support from family members and others in their social network, further increasing the risk for development of depression.

The hormonal changes of menopause which are gradual in natural menopause are sudden and more severe with surgical menopause, magnifying the effects the hormonal changes of menopause on mood and emotion. Women who are depressed are more likely to have comorbid anxiety, substance abuse, cardiac disease, and an increased risk for suicide. A comorbidity of anxiety and CVD is associated with an increased risk for sudden death from cardiac events at an early age as well as in aging women, a fact heightening the importance of comprehensive multisystem screening during health care encounters.[391,527] A comorbidity of anxiety and CVD is associated with an increased risk for sudden death from cardiac events at an early age as well as in aging women, a fact heightening the importance of comprehensive multi-system screening during health care encounters.[391,527]

Estrogen and progesterone both have significant influence on neural mechanisms that impact mood and behavior. Progesterone in the central nervous system modulates well-being as well as cognition and memory. Declines in estrogen trigger reductions in serotonin; serotonin and other monoamine neurotransmitters (norepinephrine and dopamine) regulate mood disorders, sleep, and vasomotor functions. As serotonin levels drop, the likelihood of hot flashes, anxiety and sleep disturbance emerge; episodes of anxiety may include feelings of irritability and tension as well palpitations, chest discomfort, and other physiologic changes such as elevated blood pressure.[494] The shared neurotransmitter effects on vasomotor function and mood manifest as a twofold increase risk for depression among women who experience hot flashes during MT. In the later reproductive years, anxiety is found to predict the occurrence of hot flashes.[220]

Behaviors associated with depression include fatigue, inactivity, anhedonia (lack of enjoyment of activities that are usually enjoyable), and social isolation.[35] As women age, changes in energy level and activity may be perceived as normal by affected individuals and their health care practitioners, a perspective that can lend difficulty in diagnosing depression. Inactivity and reduced physical mobility further increase the risk for depression. Many aging women with incontinence choose to minimize social activities as a way of managing the risk or public accidents; social isolation is a behavior exhibited by depressed individuals as well as a behavior that can increase risk for depression.[432]

Loss of libido is an expected outcome of both surgical and natural menopause. Loss of sexual desire can negatively impact personal relationships negatively and increase risk for depression; women referred for *hypoactive sexual desire disorder* may benefit from screening for comorbid depression and anxiety by therapists and other health care practitioners. Relationship variables, attitudes toward sex and aging, vaginal dryness, and cultural background all impact sexual function during all stages of menopause.[50] Dyspareunia is more common in the MT, pointing to the biologic contributions of menopause; however, social factors are significant, more so for some women than the physical changes of menopause.[50]

Culture and ethnic differences are reported in women's attitudes toward menopause as well as in the physical signs and symptoms of menopause. African American and Euro-American women often welcome the cessation of menses, whereas the changes of menopause are reportedly more often regretted by Hispanic, Chinese American, and Japanese American women.[52,53,353,572] Hot flashes are usually perceived as solely determined by biology, however, the frequency and intensity of hot flashes are reported to vary among women by ethnic background. Hot flashes are not reported among traditional Japanese women but are reported by Japanese American women. There appears to be an emotional component to the frequency and severity of hot flashes that can vary by cultural beliefs and ethnicity. Hot flashes were found by Thurston and colleagues[604] to occur in response to both positive and negative emotions, with true physiologic hot flashes being associated with positive emotions, and perceived but nonphysiologic hot flashes associated with negative emotions.

Risk for all types of *violence and abuse* (physical, emotional, sexual) is higher for women than men throughout the life span.[490,605] A history of sexual violence and abuse in childhood is associated with more intense vasomotor symptoms during menopause; history of any type of violence or abuse is associated with delayed onset of menopause. Allsworth et al[12] found women reporting childhood or adolescent abuse entered perimenopause approximately 35% slower than women who reported no abuse with similar findings among women who reported first experiencing abuse during adulthood with the findings persisting when the cohort was restricted to nondepressed women. Violence and abuse are also associated with pelvic pain, dyspareunia, substance abuse and suicide risk,[357] all significant to practitioners during examination and screening.

MEDICAL MANAGEMENT

Medical management of menopausal signs, symptoms and associated conditions includes education, pharmacologic intervention, surgery and referrals to other medical practitioners or to practitioners or services outside of medicine. Medical treatment for abnormal uterine bleeding during the MT often includes low dose combination oral contraceptives, estrogens and progesterones, as well as progestin-containing intrauterine devices (IUDs). The treatment of women during the menopausal transition should be based primarily on the frequency and severity of symptoms. Androgen replacement has been used for hypoactive sexual desire disorder but is controversial. The benefits of androgens include enhancement of muscle mass, bone formation, and reducing hot flash frequency as well as the effects on libido. Long-term side effects are a concern and include male pattern baldness, voice deepening, clitoral hypertrophy, and adverse effects on lipid profile and cardiovascular risk.[287]

HORMONE REPLACEMENT THERAPY. Decisions about HRT for menopause related symptoms and conditions are based on a thorough medical understanding of the risks and benefits of HRT and how that understanding applies to each woman based on her individual symptoms, conditions, and risks. Table 20-2 presents the advantages and disadvantages of HRT. HRT is primarily used now in the short-term to manage vasomotor symptoms, vaginal atrophy, and/or for osteoporosis prevention or treatment. Reevaluation of need for HRT is recommended at

6- to 12-month intervals. Older women may choose to manage mood, sleep disturbances, and cognitive impairments (memory, concentration, decision making) through a more long-term use of HRT.

Bone-specific agents are usually considered more appropriate for long-term osteoporosis prevention or treatment (readers are referred to the discussion on osteoporosis in Chapter 24). If estrogen treatment is elected for isolated vaginal symptoms, low-dose local estrogen therapy is advised and safe for extended treatment. The lowest effective dose for the shortest period of time is recommended for all hormone therapies by the American College of Obstetricians and Gynecologists (ACOG). The North American Menopause Society provides guidelines to assist women in understanding the treatment choices related to HRT and menopause.[471]

Findings from the Women's Health Initiative (WHI) resulted in a halt to the routine use of estrogen and progestin in combination (medroxyprogesterone [Prempro]) in 2002 and estrogen alone (Premarin) in 2004. The initially perceived benefits to of HRT were determined to have stronger associations with lifestyle choices with women most likely to take hormone replacement being more health conscious in general than women who did not take HRT. Comparison to a placebo group in the WHI clarified those associations and revealed that hormone users were experiencing more breast cancer, heart disease, stroke, and blood clots. Estrogen replacement showed some benefit, but it was not enough to outweigh the risks.[655] HRT is now known to be associated with an

---

Table 20-2	Advantages and Disadvantages of Hormone Replacement Therapy (HRT)
Risks and Disadvantages	**Benefits**
Increased risk of heart attack in healthy women in the first year	Treats menopausal symptoms (e.g., hot flashes, night sweats, sleep disturbances, memory loss, fatigue, atrophic changes of vagina or urinary tract)
Increased risk of stroke in healthy women after 1 year	Maintains skin thickness and elasticity, prevents fine wrinkles
Increased risk of endometrial cancer (estrogen alone without progestin)	Prevents accelerated bone loss; maintains bone density; reduces risk of fractures by 50%
Increased risk of breast cancer with prolonged (>4 yr) use of HRT	Reduces risk of colon cancer and stroke
Side effects (e.g., vaginal bleeding, fluid retention, weight gain, bloating, breast swelling and tenderness, headaches, mood swings, depression, skin irritation, constipation, loss of libido*)	May improve blood pressure
Increased risk of gallstones, blood clots	Prevention or delay of Alzheimer disease (preliminary data)
Increased breast density and reduced specificity and sensitivity of mammography	Improves pain tolerance
Slight increased risk of dementia and Alzheimer disease in women older than 65 years	Increases production or prolongs action of serotonin
Contraindications/precautions:	
• History of blood clots	
• Pancreatic or liver disease	
• Hormone-sensitive breast or uterine cancer	
• Migraine headaches that are aggravated by estrogen	
Hypertension	
• Recent heart attack	
• History of uterine fibroids	
• Endometriosis	
• History of stroke or transient ischemic attacks	
• Benign breast disease	
• Current breast or endometrial cancer	

*Some side effects can be managed with a reduced dose, different schedule, or changing brands. Any woman experiencing intolerable side effects should see the prescribing physician for evaluation.

increased risk of CHD, stroke, venous thromboembolism, and cholecystitis. Breast cancer and ovarian cancer risk are also shown to increase. No longer considered a first choice for reducing CVD or preserving cognitive function, HRT is prescribed most often for short-term relief of menopausal-related symptoms such as hot flashes and vaginal.[211,287,471]

Whatever decision a woman makes should be in conjunction with her health care provider, keeping in mind that any decision made must be individualized for each women and can be changed as new information becomes available.[48] For the woman who cannot or prefers not to take long-term HRT, there are alternatives for preventing osteoporosis and heart disease and for modifying the transient and temporary symptoms of menopause.

SERMs are being tested to determine their effects in preventing bone loss, improving serum lipids, and reducing breast cancer risk. Tamoxifen is the most widely used SERM in the treatment and prevention of breast cancer; raloxifene is currently used in the prevention and treatment of osteoporosis in postmenopausal women. These pharmaceuticals stimulate estrogen receptors in some tissues but not in others. SERMs have no effect on symptoms associated with menopause. Alternately, antidepressants can help some women with severe hot flashes. The importance of lifestyle measures, such as exercising; maintaining a low-fat, calcium-rich diet; and not smoking, has been clearly demonstrated.

ALTERNATIVE AND COMPLEMENTARY THERAPIES. Alternative and complementary therapies to reduce the symptoms of menopause are sought by one-third or more of women.[492] Evidence supporting nonhormonal approaches to treatment (e.g., homeopathy,[603] phytoestrogens such as red clover isoflavones, black cohosh, dong quai, rose hips, soy products, flaxseed, and ginseng) are limited. The safety and efficacy of using herbal medicinal products in conjunction with other alternative approaches (e.g., yoga, meditation, and acupuncture) is also under investigation.[3,68,163,262,263,313,483,492]

SPECIAL IMPLICATIONS FOR THE THERAPIST | **20-1**

Menopause
Implications for Examination, Evaluation, Diagnosis, and Prognosis
History and Interview

Inquiring about menopause during the physical therapy examination of female patients and clients who are 40 years of age or older is consistent with the expanding role of therapists in primary care.[32,94] Appropriate topics to cover include date of onset of MT, signs and symptoms being experienced, any medical or nontraditional therapies, medications or behavioral strategies being utilized to manage the symptoms, as well as the woman's attitude about the changes of menopause.

The potential pathologic correlates of menopause are important to include in the *screening and risk assessment* components of the history and interview. Obesity, osteoporosis, heart disease, diabetes mellitus, incontinence, urinary tract infections, GI disturbances, sleep disturbance, memory impairment, depression, anxiety, falls, fractures, tooth loss, shoulder impingement, carpal tunnel syndrome, and inflammatory arthritis exacerbations are specific conditions to cover during screening.

The physical therapist may wish to develop a menopause-specific questionnaire or use published checklists for the body[94] systems and conditions most commonly associated with menopause. Utilization of a screening tool such as the Beck Depression Index (BDI) 35 or Zung36[71,552] to identify depression may reveal more cases of depression than self-report through an intake questionnaire.[637] Validated questionnaires may also be utilized to assess memory and cognition if answers to screening questions raise concern. Assessing attitudes about menopause are relevant as they may increase risk for depression, anxiety, and/or body image images. Individuals at increased risk for these effects may benefit from referral or informed of physical therapy approaches to care. Medical history should address prescription medications, supplements, and other interventions the patient or client is using to manage menopause signs and symptoms.

Physical Examination

The physical examination should be expanded beyond the requirements of the specific purpose of the therapy visit to screen for physical changes associated with menopause and aging. Height, weight, and BMI are not routinely recorded during therapy examination, however, since loss of height and weight gain are effects of aging and menopause, it is sensible to record those measurements and utilize the information in development of the plan of care.

Attention to spinal posture is indicated, particularly the presence of excessive kyphotic curve, a potential sign of reduced BMD and risk factor for compression fracture and painful musculoskeletal conditions such as shoulder girdle (adhesive capsulitis; rotator cuff impingement; biceps tendonitis). Early arthritis of the hip can be identified through assessment of hip rotation range of motion.[148,149] If fracture is suspected, tuning forks may be used to provoke symptoms from the suspected fracture site[94]; in the case of suspected femoral fractures,[97,98,261,601] the patella-pubic percussion test can be applied. Tests of balance and sensation are indicated, as well as visual and palpation examination of the skin integrity and signs of neurologic or cardiovascular compromise.

Assessment of weight distribution and waist circumference may identify those with truncal obesity, which increases risks for comorbidities such as heart disease and diabetes. Blood pressure should be assessed because CVD and hypertension are common among menopausal women and frequently undiagnosed. Muscle mass declines as the stages of menopause progresses, observation of overall muscle size and tone with follow-up questions and examination for strength and performance are appropriate. Counseling women about physical exercise, weight management, bone health and posture may be indicated.

Evaluation, Diagnosis, Prognosis

Identifying signs, symptoms, and risks associated with menopause informs the evaluation process so that the plan of care addresses a woman's health needs comprehensively. The woman's needs for education, consultation and/or referral for menopause-related changes may be discovered by expanding the examination to include attention to the known correlates of MT and menopause. Menopause associated physical impairments, functional limitations, conditions and/or indications or contraindications for planned interventions may be discovered during the expanded exam, which will also inform the therapist's evaluation and potentially lead to modifications in the plan of care, human movement diagnoses, and/or prognosis.

Implications for Intervention

Physical Activity and Exercise

Physical activity and exercise have a variety of effects that can be used therapeutically to address or prevent the changes and conditions associated with menopause. Assessment of current levels of physical activity and exercise beyond those related to the specific reason for the therapy visit is appropriate. Therapists may recommend modifications to type (mode), duration, intensity, and frequency of current activities or prescribe new activities or exercises tailored to the woman's specific symptoms, health and risks. By including physical activity prescription in the therapy plan of care, therapists can proactively assist women respond to and/or minimize the effects of aging and estrogen deficiency.

Regular physical activity may be prescribed to reduce the risk for weight gain, body composition and fat distribution (central adiposity) that accompany aging and the MT. *Moderate-intensity activities* are recommended to reduce many of the effects of menopause and aging, including osteoporosis, cardiovascular disease, and sleep disturbance.[8,614] *Vigorous intensity activity* may facilitate maintenance of or return to an optimal body composition, as well as provide additional health benefits.[74,583]

Endurance exercise training has positive effects on blood pressure and oxygen uptake regardless of menstrual status or hormone replacement.[159] Although cardiovascular activities, such as walking, are beneficial to maintaining condition and body weight and probably do prevent mobility disability, they do not substantially address the decline in musculoskeletal health of the older adult.[599]

Strenuous exercise may be more effective with somatic and psychological symptoms associated with menopause, including depression and anxiety.[428] Conversely, MT and menopause may impact a woman's physical exercise capacity and tolerance. Changes in peripheral vascular circulation associated with menopause in otherwise healthy women may limit exercise performance. Impaired exercise capacity or exercise intolerance may be helped by postmenopausal HRT.[421] Physical activity may also effect hormone levels by influencing protein carriers and receptors.

As muscle mass declines with aging and menopause exercise is important to the maintenance of muscle size and strength.[398] *Resistance training* and protein intake reduce the risk of sarcopenia and the loss of muscle. Nutrition, hormone replacement, and vitamin D consumption may also assist with enhancing muscle mass and are appropriate topics for discussion with women as they enter and progress through the stages of menopause.

Many of the musculoskeletal disorders that increase with aging are associated with patterns of muscle imbalance and weakness (i.e., shoulder impingement). Muscle strength is important among women with osteopenia or osteoporosis to provide protection to bones and joint during activities and trauma. Training specificity in the design of strength programs that focuses on potential problems known to face menopausal women as well any current problems is appropriate when physical therapists approach their role from a primary care and wellness perspective. For example, rotator cuff muscles are implicated in shoulder impingement that increases in prevalence for women during mid and late life supporting the use of specific exercises for rotator cuff strengthening in a general exercise regimen designed for older women who are patients or clients.

Pelvic Floor Muscle Rehabilitation

Pelvic floor muscle (PFM) rehabilitation is often a component of the physical therapist's plan of care for women in any of the stages of menopause. Incontinence and pelvic pain are the most common conditions associated with menopause that are indications for PFM rehabilitation. PFM rehabilitation may also be included as part of core stability exercise programs for women with a variety of musculoskeletal complaints and conditions associated with the low back and pelvic girdle and well as shoulder girdle. Detailed information on pelvic floor dysfunction is presented in Chapter 27.

Postsurgical Rehabilitation (Abdominal and Pelvic Surgeries)

Gynecologic and obstetric events often compromise abdominal and pelvic musculature with immediate and long-term effects. Rehabilitation focusing on abdominal and pelvic muscles injured during gynecologic surgery is usually warranted.[479,589] Restorative and preventive rehabilitation efforts after surgery focus on restoring normal neurophysiologic and biomechanical function to the muscles of the lower abdomen and pelvis.[205]

Hysterectomy (surgical menopause) was reported to increase the risk of moderate low back pain in women in one component of the Women's Health and Aging Study (WHAS).[205] Less muscle trauma occurs with laparoscopic procedures, which are increasingly utilized in common surgeries. However, stretching or ischemic injury during surgical retraction or compression in the abdominal wall may also lead to biomechanical dysfunction warranting inclusion of physical therapy in the postsurgical plan of care. Postsurgical physical therapy is often indicated to address problems with core stabilizing force production, secondary muscle deconditioning, and pain[205,248,285,330]

Manual Therapy

Manual therapy[501] is a safe and effective physical therapy intervention for many painful musculoskeletal conditions including those that have an increased risk among women as they enter the stages of menopause.[613] Thoracic spine dysfunction and pain, rotator cuff pathology, shoulder impingement, low back pain, and osteoarthritis of the hip and the knee are all musculoskeletal conditions of concern for menopausal women that are reported to respond favorably to physical therapy treatment that includes manual therapy.[42,78,109,189,199,224,480]

Manual therapy is demonstrated to be superior to exercise alone in the management of hip[286] OA and to have significant effects on symptoms when added to management of OA[189] of the knee. Manual therapy encompasses a variety of techniques using a continuum of forces with lower-grade techniques selected for use when conditions such as osteoporosis or osteopenia are present.[477] In addition to its use in the management of painful musculoskeletal conditions, manual therapy may also be effective in the management of other symptoms and conditions associated with menopause. For example, the manual technique myofascial release is reported to be effective in the managing pain and enhancing circulation in the treatment of venous insufficiency in postmenopausal women.[501]

Education and Consultation

As women enter the stages of menopause they need up-to-date, evidence-based information[153] about the physiologic processes of menopause, the signs and symptoms[59] they should expect, available treatment options (medical, surgical, pharmacologic, physical therapy, complementary), as well as recommended strategies for self-care. Therapists may include education as a component of the physical therapy plan of care and/or reach out to consulting or referral sources to address the information needs of women.

A woman's knowledge about the pathologic risks associated with menopause should be assessed along with an individualized risk assessment. Information about the risks and preventive measures for cardiovascular disease, osteoporosis, arthritis, incontinence, urinary tract infections, sexual problems, prolapse, depression, falls, and fractures are appropriate to share with all women entering MT as well as those already at menopause or postmenopausal. The younger the individual at the time of the encounter, the more likely the focus of the education will be on prevention rather than management or maintenance.

Information about diet, exercise, alcohol, and smoking cessation are important as applicable on a case-by-case basis. If sexual dysfunction is a problem, information about the multifactorial nature of sexual changes during menopause as well as treatment options and self-management strategies will need to be addressed by the physical therapist. Referrals to sex therapists may be indicated in some cases and/or it may be of benefit to include a patient or client's partner in educational sessions. Likewise, referrals to psychologists, counselors, psychiatrists, and massage therapists and other practitioners or community resources may be indicated based on risk assessment and the woman's interest and goals.

Menopause and Disability[318]

With advances in health care, women with physical disabilities are living longer than previous generations and making the transition through menopause in greater numbers than ever before. For the 16 million women older than 50 years of age with disabilities, there can be unique and challenging health concerns in clinical care. Because so little is known about menopause in women with physical disabilities, they are put in the position of having to educate both themselves and their health care providers about how they may experience menopause differently.[192]

Women with disabilities often experience menopause at an earlier age than their able-bodied peers, therefore the therapist may need to assess for early menopause.[626] The woman with a disability may have poorer general health and be at greater risk for comorbid disease. Estrogen loss compromises collagen content and vascular profusion of the skin, putting women who are wheelchair users or immobile at greater risk of skin breakdown and pressure ulcers.[192] Menopausal symptoms are similar for women with disabilities compared to the general population, but the effect of HRT and the potential interaction between HRT and other medications used to manage disabilities remains unknown.[72]

Particular attention to the musculoskeletal system, cardiovascular system, and the integumentary system is recommended for the physical therapy examination of women with disabilities nearing or in the MT or menopause. Cardiovascular health and fitness may be impacted by the limited mobility associated with disabilities. The risk of thrombosis related to hypercoagulation states associated with immobility may be made worse with exposure to hormone therapy, making this treatment option less likely for menopausal women with cerebral palsy, spina bifida, spinal cord injured, stroke, or other neurologic impairments.[170]

Bone loss associated with perimenopause and on through the transition to menopause may be more pronounced in women with mobility impairments.[192] Whereas the able-bodied woman usually reaches peak bone mass by age 35 years, the woman with a disability may never reach that peak. The risk of bone fracture and related impairments is higher in women with disabilities, especially for those who take medications that may further impair bone health (e.g., corticosteroids, tricyclic antidepressants, or anticonvulsants). Physical therapists can be instrumental in helping women with disabilities develop creative exercise strategies, taking into account their reduced mobility and weight-bearing status. Stretching to counterbalance repeated positions and motions is as important as resistance training in this population group. Studies are needed to determine the most effective means of preserving bone in women with disabilities.

A THERAPIST'S THOUGHTS*
MENOPAUSE

The number of women who seek care from physical therapists while also navigating the stages of menopause is and will continue to expand rapidly as the population ages. All women of menopausal age who enter physical therapy clinics are affected in some way by the changes associated with menopause. Even if the particular reason they are in physical therapy is not directly related to menopause, that woman is affected by menopause physically, socially, emotionally, or psychologically, or is at risk for an effect in the future. Physical therapists have a great deal to offer menopausal women that will benefit them both short-term and long-term—often beyond the initial reason the patient or client sought care or consultation from the therapist. Taking this broader approach to clinical interactions with women going through the stages of menopause is consistent with the expectations for primary care physical therapy practice, and one that will be rewarding for physical therapists who choose to take advantage of the opportunity.

Most of the changes associated with menopause that create difficulty and distress in women's lives are positively affected by exercise and physical activity; manual therapy is also helpful for many menopause-related complaints. Education about menopause is of benefit to all women no matter their age or stage of menopause. Physical therapists can use evidence regarding the benefits of exercise to support recommendations or prescriptions for physical activity to address osteoporosis, depression, cardiac disease, and many other conditions associated with menopause.

Providing physical therapy care for menopausal women from a primary care approach involves intentionally and comprehensively addressing menopause and its ramifications on overall health in addition to focusing on the particular health concern that initiated the physical therapy encounter. Taking the comprehensive, primary care approach requires some adjustment in approach to patient/client personal and family health history, interview, and physical examination to balance completeness with efficiency. A variety of resources, forms, and tools are available to assist physical therapists in setting up efficient examination procedures. By taking such a broad approach to examination, evaluation, and treatment planning, physical therapists have the opportunity to facilitate longstanding and far reaching effects on the overall health and quality of life of menopausal women in their care.

As women age, health declines and health related decisions for both patients/clients and practitioners increase in complexity. Patient/client education, consultation, and referrals are key strategies physical therapists can use to maximize the information and services available to inform and support women to move with good health through the stages of menopause.

Many of the issues that arise during menopause are of an intimate or potentially embarrassing nature requiring the physical therapist to assess the therapist's own comfort and competence addressing functional issues and impairments including sexual, intestinal, and urologic functions.

Referrals to other physical therapists or other types of practitioners are often warranted, so development of a network of colleagues for consultation and referral is often a necessary step. Therapists also have the opportunity to create consulting roles for themselves to serve as resources to other practices or to reach women in the community for non–clinic-based education and consultation about menopause, quality of life, physical functioning, and the benefits and services offered by physical therapy. Therapists have an excellent opportunity to provide women both information and care that can enhance a woman's overall health as she ages; hopefully many of us will choose to provide this type of primary and secondary intervention.

*Patricia (Trish) M. King, PT, PhD, OCS, MTC

DISORDER OF THE FEMALE UPPER GENITAL TRACT

Pelvic Inflammatory Disease

Overview and Incidence

Pelvic inflammatory disease (PID), the infection and inflammation of the female upper genital tract, is made up of a variety of conditions (i.e., it is not a single entity), including endometritis, salpingitis, tuboovarian abscess, and pelvic peritonitis. Any inflammatory condition affecting the female reproductive organs (uterus, fallopian tubes, ovaries, and cervix) may come under the diagnostic label of PID. It is a common cause of infertility, chronic pain, and ectopic pregnancy.[265]Approximately 1 million women are affected each year; 75% occur in women younger than age 25 years and 100,000 become infertile.[131]

Etiology and Risk Factors

PID occurs as a result of multimicrobial bacteria, such as *Neisseria gonorrhoeae, Chlamydia trachomatis,* and anaerobic and mycoplasmal bacteria. Either gonorrhea or chlamydia (two common sexually transmitted infections [STIs]) acquired through vaginal, oral, or anal intercourse is the most likely cause. Infection can occur when the uterus is traumatized. Infection can be introduced from the skin, vagina, or GI tract. It can be an acute, one-time episode or chronic with multiple recurrences.

PID is often associated with STIs/sexually transmitted diseases (STDs) or develops after birth or after a surgical procedure involving the reproductive tract such as an abortion or a dilation and curettage (D&C). D&C is a procedure to scrape and collect the tissue (endometrium) from inside the uterus. Dilation is a widening of the cervix to allow instruments into the uterus. Curettage is the scraping of the contents of the uterus.

Early age at first vaginal intercourse (higher prevalence for age younger than 15 years) and number of male sex partners are two major risk factors for PID.[135] The more partners the woman has, the greater the risk of PID. PID occurs if chlamydia is not treated and even if treated, some damage to the pelvic cavity cannot be reversed. Other risk factors include sexual activity without a condom, a sexual partner who reports symptoms or has a known history of chlamydia or gonorrhea, and previous pelvic infection(s).

Clinical Manifestations

Signs and symptoms of PID vary widely, making the medical diagnosis difficult. It is often asymptomatic but can present with vaginal bleeding and discharge and burning during urination. Constitutional symptoms associated with infection, such as fever or chills, and sometimes nausea and vomiting may be reported.

Painful intercourse (dyspareunia), painful menstruation, and back or pelvic pain are commonly reported. Pelvic pain does not occur until chlamydia leads to PID. Moderate (dull aching) to severe back, abdominal, and/or pelvic pain are possible. If the condition progresses to PID, scarring in the pelvic organs, including the ovaries, fallopian tubes, bowel and bladder, can cause chronic pain. The women can be left infertile because of damage and scarring to the fallopian tubes.

After one episode of PID, a woman's risk of ectopic pregnancy increases sevenfold compared with the risk for women who have no history of PID.[129,131] Ectopic pregnancy can occur when a partially blocked or slightly damaged fallopian tube causes an egg to get stuck in the fallopian tube where it is then fertilized.

MEDICAL MANAGEMENT

PREVENTION. PID can be prevented by making safer choices to avoid STDs (e.g., always using barrier methods during intercourse, limiting number of sexual partners and with frequent testing for treatment of STDs, choosing a partner who does not have a current or previous history of STD, and abstaining from sexual activity until infected partner has completed treatment). All medication prescribed must be taken to prevent reinfection.

DIAGNOSIS, TREATMENT, AND PROGNOSIS. PID is diagnosed on the basis of clinical presentation, a physical and pelvic examination, and laboratory tests. A vaginal swab or urine sample will be taken and sent to the laboratory. Ultrasound may be used to visualize the fallopian tubes or screen for pelvic abscess. Laparoscopic examination (thin, flexible tube with a light at the end is inserted through a small incision in the lower abdomen) allows the surgeon to view the internal organs and take tissue samples for diagnostic purposes.

PID is curable with antibiotics; prompt treatment does not reverse any damage already done. PID may require hospitalization and can be life-threatening. Complications of PID include chronic pelvic pain, infertility (inability or difficulty getting pregnant), and ectopic or tubal pregnancy.

The CDC recommends that all sexually active teens and young adult women be screened annually for STIs. Any woman who has had a new sexual partner (male or female) and those with multiple sexual partners should be screened regularly. Signs of infection or recurrence of infection should be investigated immediately and treated appropriately.[129,131]

DISORDERS OF THE UTERUS AND FALLOPIAN TUBES

Holly Tanner, PT, MA, OCS, WCS, LMP, BCB-PMD, CCI

Endometriosis

Overview

Endometriosis is an estrogen-dependent disorder defined by the presence of endometrial tissue (lining of the uterus) outside of the uterus. The disorder becomes apparent in the early teen years after menses have begun, and its symptoms continue until menopause. Each month as the woman's body prepares for a fertilized egg, the uterus becomes engorged with blood, providing a fertile place for the egg to attach and begin growing. If and when the unfertilized egg passes out of the body, the uterus sloughs off the lining of blood and the woman has a flow of menstrual blood for about 3 to 5 days.

Endometriosis occurs when the uterus sheds this blood up into the body, rather than down and out through the vagina. Endometrial tissue found outside of the uterus on other organs or structures within the pelvic cavity and the body responds each month the same way as the endometrium during the menstrual cycle. The misplaced tissue engorges with blood just as it would when lining the uterus. The blood cannot drain out of the body and the result is lesions, or "chocolate cysts," wherever the endometrial tissue is located with subsequent swelling, "bleeding," and scarring.[184]

The use of the word "bleeding" to describe the process may be a misnomer as the events are more likely that the pockets break down into blood and tissue, which can be deposited anywhere in the body. The most common sites of ectopic implantation include the ovaries, fallopian tubes, broad ligaments, pouch of Douglas, bladder, pelvic musculature, perineum, vulva, vagina, or intestines (Fig. 20-2). Deep endometriosis, referred to as adenomyosis externa, presents as a single nodule (larger than 1 cm in diameter) either in the vesicouterine fold or the lower 20 cm of the bowel.[343]

Although less common, endometrial tissue can also be found in the abdominal cavity, implanted on the kidneys, small bowel, appendix, diaphragm, pleura, bony elements of the spine,[210,215] and even on the surface of the skin. Whereas it was once thought that the blood just reached the pelvic and abdominal cavities, coating the viscera contained within, it is clear now that endometrial tissue migrates throughout the body. It has been recovered from bone, lungs, and even the brain.[236] Rarely, ectopic tissue has been found in joints, the nose, and the lungs.[631]

Wherever this tissue migrates, it is biochemically and endocrine active, behaving as if it were still under

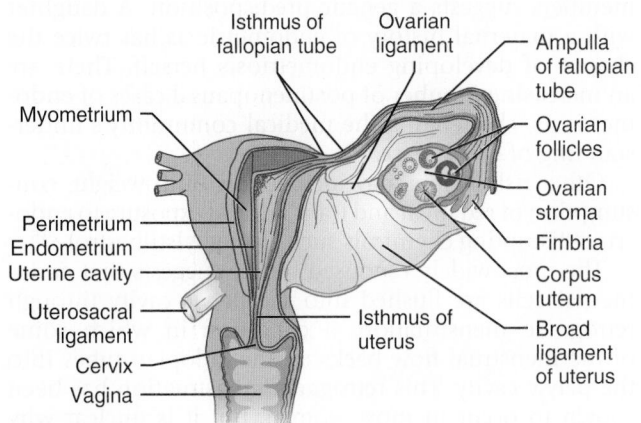

Figure 20-2

Potential sites of endometrial implantation.

the control of the hormonal system. Every month during the menses, a woman with endometriosis develops a host of symptoms that depend on where the uterine tissue resides. During menstruation, the dislocated tissue is responding just as the uterine lining, but since it cannot shed as the endometrium does, it remains where it is, eventually forming scar tissue and irritating the affected area. During menstruation, the dislocated tissue responds to the same hormonal influences as the uterine lining, yet the breakdown of the lesions creates chemical irritation, inflammation, and scarring rather than being shed by the body.

The American Society of Reproductive Medicine has classified endometriosis as I (minimal), II (mild), III (moderate), IV (severe), or V (extensive). Despite this classification system, a woman can have severe disease without symptoms or severe symptoms with minimal disease. This is most likely determined by the type of endometriosis and how biochemically active are the implants. Endometriosis is the most common diagnosis among women who have pelvic pain. In addition to severe pain, endometriosis negatively affects a woman's ability to work, her family relationships, and her self-esteem.[294]

Incidence

The incidence of endometriosis has increased in the past 40 to 50 years in Western countries. Reports of incidence vary from as low as 7% to as high as 60% of all women. In the general population, incidence of the disease is conservatively estimated at 11%. Endometriosis[111] is found in up to 50% of all infertile women. In young women who present with pelvic pain, the retrospective incidence of endometriosis is as high as 98%. Endometriosis[478] affects women of all ethnic origins, socioeconomic backgrounds, and geographic locations.[631]

Etiologic and Risk Factors

Any woman of childbearing age is at risk of developing endometriosis, but it is more common in those who have postponed pregnancy. In addition, other risk factors include early menarche; regular menstruation but 27-day or shorter cycles; and menstrual periods lasting 7 days or longer. The cause of endometriosis is unknown, although the high prevalence among family members suggests a genetic predisposition. A daughter with a maternal history of endometriosis has twice the chance of developing endometriosis herself. There are an increasing number of postmenopausal cases of endometriosis, challenging the medical community's understanding of the disease.[76]

Other risk factors may include low birth weight, consumption of red meat and trans fat, and exposure to endocrine-disrupting chemicals such as diethylstilbestrol.[235]

The most widely espoused theory suggests that endometrial cells are flushed into the pelvic cavity through retrograde menstruation, a condition in which some of the menstrual flow backs up the fallopian tubes into the pelvic cavity. This retrograde menstruation has been shown to occur in most women, but it is unclear why endometrial cells implant in some women and not in others. Because the fimbrial openings of the fallopian tubes are in the posterior aspect of the pelvis, more of the endometrial implants are found on posterior structures, sometimes giving rise to low back pain.

Another strongly held hypothesis is a dysregulation or dysfunction of the immune system that allows these cells to locate and survive where they do not belong. The cells from the uterine lining are resistant to the body's normal defense mechanisms and are not readily cleared away when they happen to stray outside the organ.

Other theories include the (1) dissemination of endometrial cells through the lymphatics or vascular system (explains presence of tissue in lungs); (2) metaplasia of the mesothelium (Meyer's theory), that is, endometrial cells change from one type of cell to another, whereby the endothelium undergoes transformation able to produce the same reproductive hormones (explains presence of tissue in joints); (3) intraoperative implantation associated with procedures such as hysterectomy and episiotomy; and (4) abnormal differentiation of precursor epithelial cells during early embryology, whereby these cells are seeded before birth. A significant positive association with endometriosis has been found with γ-hexachlorocyclohexane and β-hexachlorocyclohexane, used as insecticides and pharmaceuticals in lice and scabies treatments.[110]

Pathogenesis

Once endometrial cells migrate to other parts of the body, they can form pockets of tissue referred to as implants. These implants swell in response to the cyclic surge of estrogen and progesterone-forming cysts on the underlying organs that contain a dark, syrupy fluid composed of old blood and menstrual debris called *chocolate cysts*.

There are three primary pathologic types of endometriosis: (1) red or petechial implants are the most active with the greatest capacity to produce prostaglandins (inflammatory mediators) and also capable of producing endometrial protein and hormones; (2) brown or intermediate implants are moderately active and precursors to powder burns; and (3) black or brown powder-burn implants are inactive with little cellular material but associated with adhesions that stretch organs and cause direct nerve damage through devitalization and ischemia. The powder-burn implants adhere structures together, contributing to infertility, and are sometimes referred to as a *frozen pelvis*. The severity of the disease depends on which one of these three types is present.

Clinical Manifestations

The symptoms and signs associated with endometriosis depend on the location of the implants, but pain and infertility are the two major symptoms. Abdominal pain, fatigue, and mood changes are common beginning 1 or 2 days before the onset of the menstrual flow and continuing for the duration. The therapist may hear reports of intermittent, cyclical, or constant pelvic and/or low back pain (unilateral or bilateral). Deep endometriosis is associated with very severe pain and may involve the ureter causing hydronephrosis.[343]

Dysmenorrhea (painful menstruation) will be the chief complaint if the implants are on the uterosacral ligaments. These lesions swell immediately before or during menstruation, resulting in pelvic pain. Dyspareunia (painful intercourse) is also associated with this condition because penile penetration during intercourse can aggravate the local adhesions.

Pain during defecation can occur when there are adhesions on the large bowel. The fecal material moves through the intestine, stretching and aggravating the scar tissue. Surprisingly, the extent of the disease does not always correlate with the intensity of the symptoms. A woman with widespread lesions may be asymptomatic, whereas a woman with few implants may have considerable pain.

Other symptoms can include low-grade fever; diarrhea; constipation; rectal bleeding; and referred pain to the low back/sacral, groin, posterior leg, upper abdomen, or lower abdominal/suprapubic areas. Bleeding from anywhere else (e.g., nose bleeds, coughing up blood, or blood in urine or stools) is less common but still possible. Chronic abdominal pain can result in altered posture and body mechanics particularly maintaining trunk flexion. This, in turn, may contribute to other musculoskeletal disorders, which add another layer to the pain syndrome.

MEDICAL MANAGEMENT

DIAGNOSIS. Although the classic triad of cyclical dysmenorrhea, dyspareunia, and infertility strongly suggests the presence of endometriosis, accurate diagnosis requires direct visual examination by laparoscopy or laparotomy. One advantage of laparoscopy is that the technique is also therapeutic in that lesions can be removed immediately. Ultrasound and magnetic resonance imaging (MRI) are generally used to examine the pelvis, but MRI is more sensitive in detecting the implants. Researchers are trying to develop a radioimmune assay to measure endocrine protein associated or present with this disease toward the eventual development of a blood test.

TREATMENT. There is no cure for endometriosis; the goals of medical treatment are preservation of fertility (if fertility is an issue) and pain relief. Pregnancy does appear to suppress the disease, and in animal studies, the implants disappear during pregnancy.[631] Assisted reproduction may be recommended to stimulate ovulation and perform in vitro fertilization with transplantation of the embryo into the uterus.

Nonsteroidal antiinflammatory drugs may sufficiently relieve the pain, or other analgesics can be administered before or during menstruation. Other medications are used to inhibit ovulation and lower hormone levels to prevent the cyclic stimulation of the endometrial implants. Eventually, the implants will decrease in size. These medications include danazol, a combination estrogen-progesterone acetate; leuprolide (Lupron), which is injectable once per month into the muscle; goserelin, which is injectable under the skin, and nafarelin nasal spray, a gonadotropin-releasing hormone (GnRH) (these analogues act on the hypothalamus-to-pituitary interface to shut down the ovaries by blocking the ability to produce gonadotropins such as follicle-stimulating hormone and luteinizing hormone [LH]).

Danazol is a synthetic male hormone that inhibits the monthly surge of LH, reduces estrogen production, and influences the way estrogen affects endometriosis.

Primary adverse side effects include weight gain, edema, decreased breast size, acne, oily skin, headache, muscle cramps, and deepening of the voice. It can also adversely affect lipid metabolism and raise blood pressure.

Birth control pills may be used to reduce painful symptoms and inhibit menstrual periods, which stop the growth of endometriotic implants, but these do not cause complete regression of implants already present. Once the woman goes off the pill, these implants become active once again, sometimes with a rebound effect (symptoms are much worse).

Surgical intervention is another approach that is used less commonly than even 10 years ago because the etiology remains unchanged and regrowth occurs rather quickly. If the endometriosis is mild without extensive adhesions, laparoscopic cauterization or laser surgery may be indicated. If the woman is older than 35 years of age, disabled by the pain, and childbearing is completed, a total hysterectomy, bilateral salpingo-oophorectomy (removal of ovaries and fallopian tubes), and implant removal are considered. Surgical excision of deep endometriosis provides pain relief and may improve the woman's chances of conceiving.[343]

Nontraditional therapies, such as yoga, aromatherapy, reflexology, acupuncture,[641] naturopathic medicine,[525] and homeopathy, may be useful adjuncts to allopathic medicine. Many women are using this type of alternative/complementary intervention combined with diet and nutrition to self-treat without medications. Numerous resources are now available in this area.[61,182,203,426]

The future treatment of endometriosis may be based on the development of remodeling enzymes that work to remodel tissue at the cellular level. Understanding the mechanisms of growth factors for the growth and development of epithelial cells, the immune system, and implant physiology will help researchers develop more specific intervention techniques.

PROGNOSIS. As mentioned, there is no cure for endometriosis, although pregnancy and menopause appear to arrest its continued development with alterations in reproductive hormones.[664]

Endometriosis has been linked with reproductive cancers and melanoma.[115,233] The link between endometriosis and these diseases remains unclear, although a genetic predisposition or shared exposures to environmental toxins (especially dioxins) have been suggested, but the findings are inconsistent and inconclusive.[546,664]

SPECIAL IMPLICATIONS FOR THE THERAPIST 20-2

Endometriosis

As common as this disease is, therapists often encounter endometriosis as a primary diagnosis, as a comorbidity, or as an undiagnosed condition. Many women note that their back or pelvic pain is cyclic. Therapists often justify this observation with an explanation that the hormonal changes associated with menstruation can result in ligamentous laxity, thereby stressing the joints of the pelvis. This is only one possible scenario.

Therapists need to consider all possibilities, including pelvic disease. Dyspareunia is a common complaint associated with sacroiliac, lumbar, or hip dysfunction. If the painful intercourse is related to endometriosis, the pain will be present regardless of position. If the pain is related to joint dysfunction, typically certain intercourse positions will be comfortable and others painful. In addition painful penetration related to endometriosis is usually felt deep in the pelvis or abdomen with deep thrusting.

Endometriosis may account for false-positive findings during the therapist's physical examination. For example, if there are endometrial implants on the psoas major muscle, local palpation and length or strength testing of the psoas may be provocative. The therapist may be led to believe the psoas is the origin of the pain complaints. Endometrial implants on pelvic floor muscles and ligaments, sacroiliac ligaments, and abdominal wall muscle may lead to similar false-positive findings.

The medications commonly given to treat endometriosis can result in a variety of side effects that can account for a woman's symptoms. GI system complaints (dyspepsia, nausea, and so on) may be related to the pain or the antiinflammatory medication being taken. The GnRH medications can result in hot flashes and vaginal dryness. Danazol can cause weight gain, acne, decreased breast size, and hirsutism.

Physical therapists can help women with known endometriosis pain in several ways. General pain management would include: generalized regular exercise to release endorphins and maintain overall health, pain relieving modalities such as transcutaneous electrical nerve stimulator and heat, stress management training, and education on posture and body mechanics and pain physiology. Physical therapists can also offer evaluation and treatment for coexisting musculoskeletal disorders thus decreasing pain from other structures such as cramped muscles and strained joints. The abdominal muscle should also be evaluated for trigger points and treatment offered accordingly. In all cases, patients/clients should have a complete home management program for further flares and progression of symptoms.

Uterine Fibroids

Holly Tanner, PT, MA, OCS, WCS, LMP, BCB-PMD, CCI

Overview

Uterine fibroids (benign tumors of the uterus) forming on the outer surface of the uterus or within the walls or lining of the uterus are common, presenting in up to 50% of all premenopausal women[393] age 35 years or older. Risk factors include age, nulliparity, obesity, smoking, polycystic ovarian syndrome, diabetes, and hypertension; incidence is higher in African American than in white women.[207] These fibroids constitute the primary reason women have hysterectomies.[577]

Clinical Manifestations

Usually, uterine fibroids are asymptomatic, but pain, urinary or bowel discomfort, and abnormally heavy vaginal bleeding during or between menstrual periods can occur. Symptomatic women often become anemic, experiencing fatigue and weakness that contribute to an impaired lifestyle. In addition to pain and heavy bleeding, pelvic pressure, infertility, miscarriage and preterm labor are also associated with fibroids.[528]

Fibroids, also known as uterine leiomyomas, can and often do grow to the size of a grapefruit or larger. Growth is related to estrogen and progesterone; fibroids often regress after menopause, and may grow again if hormone replacement is initiated. Fibroids can place pressure on the bladder resulting in constipation, urinary frequency and urgency, and nocturia. Pressure on spinal nerves can also cause low back pain (Fig. 20-3).

MEDICAL MANAGEMENT

DIAGNOSIS. Diagnosis is made on the basis of history, clinical presentation, and clinical examination; uterine fibroids are frequently found incidentally during a routine pelvic exam (irregular shape of the uterus). Transvaginal ultrasonography or hysteroscopy (scope placed through the cervix into the uterus) may be used when diagnostic confirmation is needed.

TREATMENT. Pharmacotherapy to control fibroid-related symptoms may include nonsteroidal antiinflammatory drugs for pain control, oral contraceptives, or other hormonal agents to decrease bleeding. Other options may include surgical removal through a procedure called

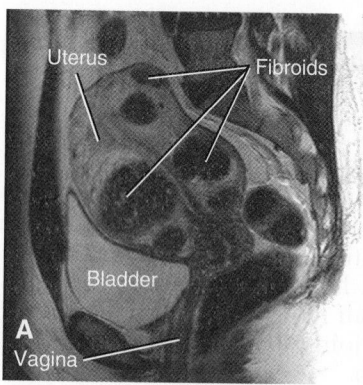
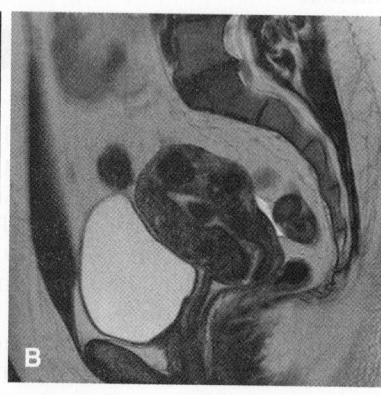

Figure 20-3

Uterine fibroids. A, MRI image of uterine fibroids. Note the position in relation to the sacrum, bladder, and pubic bone. Pressure on nerves and soft tissue in this area can cause painful pelvic, abdominal, low back, and sacral pain. **B,** MRI image of fibroids after uterine fibroid embolization (same individual). (Courtesy Robert L. Vogelzang, MD, Chicago.)

myomectomy. One way to perform this operation is to pass a fiberoptic scope through the vagina into the uterus (called *hysteroscopic myomectomy*) to remove the tumors. Fibroids embedded in the uterine wall usually require a laparoscopy or more invasive open abdominal surgery. Hysterectomy (removal of the entire uterus) may be needed.

A less-invasive technique and alternative to hysterectomy, called *uterine fibroid embolization* or *uterine artery embolization*, may be possible for select individuals. This procedure is performed with the woman under local anesthesia and mild sedation and involves the radiologist inserting a catheter into the femoral artery through a small incision in the groin and then using fluoroscopy to guide the catheter into the uterus. Tiny bead-like or small sponge particles (polyvinyl alcohol) are injected; they block off the blood supply to the smaller arteries supplying the fibroids, causing them to shrink and die.

Another alternative to hysterectomy is endometrial (or balloon) ablation in which the uterine lining is destroyed (but not the uterus) through electrical energy or heat from a balloon-tipped catheter inserted into the vagina, through the cervix, into the uterus. The balloon is then filled with a sterile solution until it conforms to the shape of the uterus and heated until the heat destroys the endometrial tissue. A conservative alternative, known as *magnetic resonance-guided focused ultrasound*, preserves the uterus and is safe and effective.[393]

Eliminating red meat and ham from the diet and eating green vegetables, fruit, and fish appear to have a protective effect. Presumably, diet influences levels of the estrogen hormone, which is known to affect fibroid growth.[143]

SPECIAL IMPLICATIONS FOR THE THERAPIST   20-3

Uterine Fibroids

Recovery after uterine fibroid embolization may require a few weeks before the woman feels "back to normal." Fatigue may persist and occur rapidly without warning for the first month after the procedure. Subjectively, some women report an immediate sense of relief from pain and congestion with gradual decrease in abdominal distention.

The therapist may address this problem in a similar way as for the treatment of endometriosis by addressing compensatory postures and gait for those individuals who had pain long enough to cause such changes. Assess for abnormalities and asymmetries in muscle strength and function throughout the abdomen, trunk, pelvis, and hips. If hysterectomy is warranted, postsurgical recovery may be more extensive.

Endometrial Carcinoma (Uterine Cancer)

Overview and Incidence

Endometrial carcinoma is commonly known as uterine cancer, but technically the term *uterine cancer* refers to all cancers found in the uterus body and the cervix. Cancer of the lining of the uterus (endometrium) is the fourth most common cancer in women and the most common cancer of the female reproductive organs, accounting for approximately 52,630 new cases and 8590 deaths in 2014 in the United States.[557] There is no apparent genetic component to endometrial cancer, but rather, environmental, social, and lifestyle factors are the most important.[600]

Risk Factors

Endometrial carcinoma is most common in women who are older (average age 60 years), white, affluent, obese (abdominal fat), sedentary, and of low parity. In fact, 75% of cases occur in postmenopausal women who have no other known risk factors; the remaining 25% occur in premenopausal women, including 5% in women younger than age 40 years. Hypertension, diabetes mellitus, and uterine fibroids[523] are also predisposing factors.

Any condition that increases exposure to estrogen unopposed by progesterone is a risk factor for uterine cancer. For example, obesity, polycystic ovary syndrome (PCOS), estrogen therapy, and some hormonal contraceptive formulations increase a woman's exposure to unopposed[213] estrogen and therefore increase the risk of endometrial cancer.

Tamoxifen (Nolvadex) therapy, estrogen replacement therapy without progestin, and the presence of estrogen-secreting tumors are also risk factors. Although tamoxifen is used as an antiestrogen treatment for breast cancer, in postmenopausal women with an intact uterus, it can enhance rather than suppress the action of estrogen. This action causes endometrial overgrowth, resulting in an increased incidence of uterine cancer in this population.

A great deal of attention has been paid to the possible induction of endometrial cancer by the antiestrogen tamoxifen, which has led to the development of new SERMs. The National Cancer Institute's Study of Tamoxifen and Raloxifene (STAR) trials to compare these two drugs and their side effects are ongoing. The current data on raloxifene after 10 years continue to show a preventive benefit for breast cancer with less risk of uterine cancer compared to tamoxifen.

Cigarette smoking, physical activity and exercise, and the use of hormonal contraceptives appear to decrease the risk. In fact, women who exercise are 80% less likely to develop endometrial cancer than women who do not exercise at all.[600] There is a strong link between obesity and endometrial cancer. Risk factors vary based on premenopausal versus postmenopausal status.

Pathogenesis

Epidemiologic and clinicopathologic evidence points to three separate types of endometrial cancer: endometrioid, serous, and clear cell. Each histotype has a distinct genetic etiology, presentation, and natural history.[474] Type I (low-grade endometrioid carcinoma) is the most common type and has the most favorable prognosis.[474] It is hormonally related and associated with hyperplasia. Most of the risk factors listed refer to type I endometrial carcinoma.[15] This type of endometrial cancer arises through a series of changes at the cellular level accompanied by specific alterations in gene expression and activity.[409,624]

Type II endometrial cancers (high-grade nonendometrioid carcinoma) account for approximately 10% of all uterine cancer. These are clinically aggressive tumors that are not hormonally related. They are associated with endometrial atrophy, with a worse prognosis, and disproportionate number of endometrial cancer deaths.[474]

There is some evidence that PCOS and insulin sensitivity may play a role in the pathogenesis of endometrial cancer, possibly through hormone disruption. The role of the tumor-suppressor gene *PTEN* in the development of endometrial cancers has also been reported. Loss of PTEN activity is frequently observed in endometrial cancers, although the exact mechanisms for initiation and progression remain unclear.[624,657]

Clinical Manifestations

Unlike ovarian cancer, endometrial cancer has a major identifiable symptom in its early stages: abnormal bleeding (present in 80% of all cases). Irregular bleeding is a normal consequence of menopause, but the woman who is at least 12 months past menopause (cessation of menses) and now presenting with abnormal vaginal bleeding is the most typical presentation of endometrial cancer. Metastases to the lymphatic system can result in abdominal or lower extremity swelling.

MEDICAL MANAGEMENT

PREVENTION AND SCREENING. At the present time, the best prevention plan is to maintain a healthy weight through diet and regular physical activity. A plant-based diet rich in vegetables, whole grains, and beans is advised.[350] Researchers at Johns Hopkins are investigating a new test as a broad screening tool for endometrial (and ovarian) cancer called the PapGene test; early studies with a small number of women showed the PapGene test accurately detected 100% of endometrial (and 41% of all ovarian) cancers.[335]

DIAGNOSIS. Abnormal bleeding in any woman of any age must be medically evaluated. Women with increased risk and those with postmenopausal bleeding or vaginal discharge should be screened for endometrial cancer. When metastatic spread occurs, the most common sites are lymph nodes, lung, or liver. More rarely, bone metastases with isolated lesions to the femur, tibia, fibula, and calcaneus may occur.[395]

Endometrial sampling is currently the most accurate and widely used screening technique, but ultrasonographic measurement of endometrial thickness and hysteroscopy have also been used. Staging to provide uniform terminology for better communication among health professionals and to provide appropriate treatment and inform patients of prognosis has changed significantly over the last 25 years. It is now determined surgically using the International Federation of Gynecology and Obstetrics (FIGO) classification. For complete TNM (tumor, node, metastasis) and FIGO staging, see the National Comprehensive Cancer Network (NCCN) Clinical Practice Guidelines in Oncology: Uterine Cancer, available at http://www.nccn.org/professionals/physician_gls/PDF/uterine.pdf.

Other less-invasive methods of staging are under consideration such as laparoscopic-assisted vaginal hysterectomy with lymphadenectomy.[63] Contrast-enhanced MRI may help decrease the number of unnecessary lymph node dissections.[221]

TREATMENT. Endometrial cancer is usually treated surgically with total laparoscopic or abdominal hysterectomy and bilateral salpingo-oophorectomy,[227] although fertility-sparing treatment is possible for some women.[228] Progestin therapy may be used in those women who decline surgical intervention,[122] and hormonal therapy (including progestin and antiestrogen tamoxifen for some women) has been used with recurrent disease. Most of these cancers are detected at an early stage when they are highly curable.

Advances in radiologic technology have brought about important changes in the standard of care for uterine cancer. External beam radiotherapy (EBRT) and 3D MRI-guided vaginal intracavity brachytherapy (VBT)[158] are available for stage 1 endometrial cancer following hysterectomy[342] but remain under investigation.[259]

Women with advanced stages of endometrial cancer may not be candidates for operative intervention in the presence of tumor fixation or deeply invasive cancer. Intense chemotherapy regimens for women with advanced or recurrent endometrial cancer are being studied.[622] Medically inoperable cases may be treated with radiotherapy alone (EBRT or VBT). Radiation may be used when the tumor spreads outside the uterus or in the case of advanced or recurrent disease after failed hormonal therapy. Cytotoxic combination chemotherapy also has been used with varying results.

The current and future focus of treatment lies with an understanding of the pathogenesis of endometrial cancer at the molecular level. There are efforts to identify biomarkers that can be used in targeted therapies.[409,532,566] Chemopreventive agents in the form of diet (foods that contain chemicals with anticancer properties, antioxidants, and plant-based phytochemicals) also show promising but sometimes conflicting results.[90,168,530,615]

PROGNOSIS. Most endometrial carcinomas are diagnosed at an early stage.[532] Early detection makes this disease curable, but recurrences occur in 15 to 20% of cases[532] and are associated with a poor prognosis.[622] Most recurrences occur within the first 3 years after surgery. Endometrial lining involvement of less than 50% is associated with 100% survival, but this drops precipitously when tumor growth involves more than half of the endometrium, especially with local or distant metastases.[229] Sexual dysfunction (or diminished sexual function) is prevalent following treatment for endometrial cancer; risk factors include postmenopausal status, lack of vaginal lubricant use, higher BMI, and laparotomy (open surgical approach).[173,341]

SPECIAL IMPLICATIONS FOR THE THERAPIST   20-4

Endometrial Carcinoma (Uterine Cancer)

Physical activity and exercise are known to decrease the risk of endometrial cancer. This is yet another area of preventive medicine in which the therapist can be very instrumental in conducting a screening examination consisting of a few questions and prescribing an appropriate exercise program.

Questions may include past personal or family history of endometrial (or other) cancer, presence of menses or menopause, use of HRT or nutraceutical supplements (e.g., rose hips, dong quai, or soy), presence of osteoporosis or bone density testing results, and current exercise/physical activity levels. Any time a woman who is at least 12 months after menopause, not taking hormone replacements, and reports vaginal bleeding, a medical evaluation is required.

For the woman who has been treated for endometrial cancer with lymphadenectomy and/or radiation, posttreatment lymphedema and other potential side effects (see Chapter 5 and Table 9-7) may require physical therapy intervention.

Cervical Cancer

Overview and Incidence

The cervix is the interface between the uterus and the vagina. It is made up of two layers of epithelial cells: the endocervix, which extends into the uterus, and the ectocervix, the portion visible when the cervix is viewed from the vaginal canal. There are two main types of cervical cancer, squamous cell carcinoma (80%-90%) and adenocarcinoma (20%).[535]

Every year in the United States, approximately 12,340 women are diagnosed with cervical cancer (half of those women have never been screened) and 4030 women die of this disease (288,000 worldwide deaths).[557] Mortality has declined by more than 50% in the last 30 years as a result of widespread screening with cervical cytology testing (Papanicolaou [Pap] screen).[466] It is now largely a preventable disease with preventive sexual practices, regular screening, and intervention at the precancerous stage. Twenty-five percent of new cases of cervical cancer develop in women 65 years and older, but the prevalence appears to be increasing disproportionately in young women.

Etiologic and Risk Factors

Clinical studies confirm that the transfer of human papilloma virus (HPV), also known as papillomas or genital warts, during unprotected sexual intercourse is the primary risk factor for squamous cell cervical cancer. HPV is the most common STD in the United States, affecting more than 50% of sexually active adults. The CDC estimates that 7.5 million Americans become infected with genital HPV each year. A new study suggests HPV infection rates are higher than previously thought, and perhaps as many as one-third of all American women are infected.[195]

More than 100 types of HPV have been identified; 23 of these infect the cervix, and 13 types are associated with cancer. All types can interfere with host-cell mechanisms that prevent cells from growing and replicating excessively. Infection with one of these viruses does not necessarily predict cancer, but the risk of cancer is increased significantly, and a link between HPV infection and female cervical cancer and male anal cancer has been demonstrated.[280]

Other risk factors include maternal use of diethylstilbestrol (DES, a synthetic estrogen [adenocarcinoma type]), smoking (even passive smoking), hormonal contraceptive use, high parity (number of births), low socioeconomic status, ethnic background (black women experience a 72% higher incidence compared with whites),[510] young age at first intercourse (17 years or younger), multiple sexual partners (more than three in a lifetime),[134] and the presence of other STDs.[304]

Alcohol and other drugs are additional risky behaviors that may play a role in young age of first sexual intercourse and more than five sexual partners. Impaired judgment from alcohol and other drug use can lead to unsafe sexual practices and with risky partners (partners more likely to have STIs) contributing to HPV infection.[314]

Greater understanding of the behavioral and biologic mechanisms accounting for early age of first sexual intercourse and subsequent HPV infection in adolescents may help direct primary prevention of HPV infection and HPV-related disease. In addition to the risky behaviors discussed previously, it is now known that the cervix is particularly vulnerable to HPV during adolescence and especially early puberty.[314] There are a number of potential reasons for increased vulnerability of the cervix. Cervical immaturity in the young girl and adolescent female is marked by inadequate cervical mucus, which acts as a protective barrier against infectious agents. Two other examples include cervical ectopy, which is characterized by rapid physiologic changes in the cervical epithelium, or immature immune response to HPV infection.[314]

Cervical ectopy refers to the condition in which a small ring of cells extend beyond the normal border of the endometrium (the inner wall of the uterus) to the cervical os (the neck of the uterus). Cervical ectopy is a normal physiologic phenomenon in women under hormonal influence, such as during puberty, but may increase cervical susceptibility to infection with STIs, including HPV.

The development of a protective cervical mucus is progressive through adolescence to full maturity. Until cervical maturity is reached, the woman remains at increased risk for HPV infection (and other STIs). Cervical immaturity is a risk factor for women who engage in sexual intercourse at a young age, including those who are sexually abused.[314] Other factors that determine whether an HPV infection will persist include cigarette smoking, a compromised immune system, and HIV infection.[466]

Pathogenesis

The common unifying oncogenic feature of the vast majority of cervical cancers is the presence of HPV. More than 99% of cervical cancers contain at least one high-risk HPV type (16, 18, 31, 45); approximately 70% contain HPV types 16 or 18.[315,535] The molecular basis for oncogenesis in cervical carcinoma can be explained to a large degree by the regulation and function of the two viral oncogenes E6 and E7 (see discussion of oncogenes in Chapter 9). The ability of HPV to target the function of tumor suppressors is typical of DNA tumor viruses. The E6 gene product binds to the p53 tumor-suppressor gene and induces p53 degradation. E7 targets another tumor suppressor that functions like *p53* in cell cycle control and inactivates it.[300]

As a result of these molecular disruptions, dysplastic changes occur in the thin layer of cells known as the *epithelium* that covers the cervix. The cells found covering the outer surface of the cervix are squamous (flat and scaly), whereas the cells lining the endocervical canal are columnar (column-like). Cervical cancer precursors identified with a Pap smear are known as cervical intraepithelial neoplasia or dysplasia. The degree of dysplasia is based on the depth of squamous epithelium replaced by atypical cells and the severity of the abnormality.

Clinical Manifestations

Most people never know they have had HPV because there are no symptoms and a healthy immune system clears the body of infection. When it persists, HPV can cause lesions in the cervix, vagina, or vulva. Left untreated, these lesions can progress to cancer. Early-stage cervical cancer, especially in the preinvasive stage, is usually asymptomatic. Often women have advanced disease before abnormal bleeding occurs. This can present as spotting between menstrual periods, longer and heavier periods, bleeding after menopause, or bleeding after sexual intercourse. Pelvic or low back pain can occur, but this is uncommon.

More advanced stages of cervical cancer may cause bowel and bladder problems because of pressure on the rectum or bladder or sexual difficulties because of the growth in the upper vagina, causing discomfort. Ureter blockage can lead to death because of uremia (the inability of the body to excrete waste), which causes uremic poisoning. The progression to this type of advanced cancer is relatively rare in developed countries.

The physical effects of cervical cancer after treatment are actually more significant. Women who have the conization procedure or loop electrosurgical excision procedure may experience cramping, bleeding, or a watery discharge. Hysterectomy, radiation therapy, surgery alone or combined with radiation, and/or chemotherapy may all cause significant side effects, which should improve over time with proper intervention.

The emotional effects of cervical cancer are often significant as well. Women treated with radiation almost always lose the benefits of estrogen because the ovaries are extremely sensitive to radiation. HRT is usually prescribed, and without this intervention, the emotional effects of cervical cancer can be compounded by hypoestrogenism and its emotional side effects.

Sexuality after hysterectomy or other interventions for this cancer can be impaired; women may experience depression from no longer being able to have children; and some women may feel guilt and shame associated with feeling "unclean" because of genital tract disease.

MEDICAL MANAGEMENT

PREVENTION. Risk of HPV and HPV-related cases of cervical cancer can be reduced and/or prevented using barrier contraceptives, engaging in monogamous sex with a likewise monogamous partner, or practicing sexual abstinence (see "Sexually Transmitted Disease" in Chapter 8).[204]

Although not preventive, studies show that consistent condom use can speed the regression of the HPV-related lesions on the cervix and on the penis and shorten the time it takes to clear HPV infections.[92,288] Women with five or fewer lifetime sexual partners have higher regression rates compared with women who have had more than five partners.[134]

The possibility of HPV infection among women who have sex with women has been reported based on limited data.[402,403] STDs can be spread between female sex partners, probably through the exchange of cervicovaginal fluid and direct mucosal contact.[404]

Fruits and vegetables and carotenoids (including high intake of carrots), along with vitamins C and E, may be protective against cervical cancer.[657] Although once considered a potential risk factor for cervical cancer, the use of IUDs may have a protective effect against cervical cancer among women who have not been infected with HPV.[127] IUDs do not protect against HPV; further study is needed to confirm and understand the association between IUD use and cervical cancer.

EARLY DETECTION AND SCREENING. Early detection is the key to a 100% cure rate for cervical cancer. Current recommendations[535] are age appropriate and suggest delaying the start of cervical cancer screening until age 21 years and then screening women ages 21 to 29 years every 3 years. For women 30 to 65 years old, screening with cytology tests (Pap smear and HPV) is recommended every 3 years. No screening is necessary after hysterectomy or after age 65 years if there have been previous negative test results. Women with known HIV infection, HPV, or other STDs must especially be screened for cervical cancer.[200] Women who have a history of cervical cancer or in utero exposure to DES should continue screening after age 30 years using the same protocol as for women before age 30 years.[569] For details of current screening recommendations, see Saslow[535]: http://onlinelibrary.wiley.com/doi/10.3322/caac.21139/pdf.

Women who have sex with women should receive Pap smear screening according to the current guidelines. It should not be assumed that testing is not needed for those who use condoms consistently or for women who have not been in a sexual relationship with men.[402,403] Women who have sex with women should be educated about preventive measures including washing hands, using rubber gloves, and cleaning sex toys or using a protective barrier, such as a condom, especially when partners share such devices.[404]

VACCINE. Two cervical cancer vaccines are now available (Gardasil, Cervarix) to protect females against four types of HPV that cause most cervical cancers. Ongoing studies are investigating the effectiveness of Gardasil in boys and men ages 16 to 26 years and in mid-adult women ages 24 to 45 years.

Currently, the vaccine is administered intramuscularly in a series over 6 months and costs between $300 and $400, which may make its use prohibitive as a routine vaccination. The vaccination is advised for females before becoming sexually active, but sexually active females can also benefit. Even if the woman is already infected with one or more of the four HPV strains covered by the vaccine, the vaccine will help protect her from the remaining strains.[270] The vaccine can be given to females between ages 9 and 26 years.[458]

The Advisory Committee on Immunization Practices (ACIP), which is part of the CDC, has issued its first summary statement about recommendations for HPV vaccination.[401] The interested reader can read the full summary at http://www.cdc.gov/mmwr/preview/mmw rhtml/rr56e312a1.htm?s_cid=rr56e312a1_e. The ACIP recommends routine immunization of girls age 11 to 12 years. This is a controversial social issue because safe sex practices can prevent HPV and its associated complications, making universal vaccination unnecessary. Both the ACIP and the National Women's Health Network advise that the vaccine should not replace routine cervical screening or education regarding sexual practices.[11] Guidelines from the American Cancer Society (ACS) suggest routine vaccination for females age 11 to 12 years, although girls as young as 9 years may receive the HPV vaccination. Universal vaccination for females age 19 to 26 years is not advised.[536]

Each woman should make an individual decision regarding HPV vaccination based on her own risk and the potential benefit from the vaccination. Ideally, the vaccine should be administered before exposure to genital HPV through sexual intercourse because the potential benefit is likely to diminish with an increasing number of sexual partners.[536] Vaccination is more imperative for women who do not have access to cervical cancer screening services. The protective effect of vaccination that is successfully provided to adolescent and young women who are unlikely to undergo regular Pap screening will yield greater positive outcomes than vaccination provided to women who will seek regular screening regardless.[536]

Note to Reader: Vaccination for males remains under investigation and is not universally recommended.[446,407] The HPV-related diseases that affect males are anogenital warts and cancers of the penis, anus and oropharynx. The quadrivalent vaccine against HPV has proved to be effective in preventing external genital lesions in males aged 16 to 26 years in 90.4% of cases.[370] Studies show that vaccination to both genders can be more efficacious. Recommendations have been made based on the scientific evidence for vaccination of 11- to 26 year-old males against HPV in order to guarantee protection to everyone.[307,360,370]

DIAGNOSIS. Information is gathered from examinations and diagnostic tests to determine the size of the tumor, how deeply the tumor has invaded tissues within and around the cervix, and the metastases to lymph nodes or distant organs. Staging to find out how far the cancer has spread is an important process and the key factor in selecting the right treatment plan.

Cervical cancer is detected using a Pap test, and the Pap test is credited with reducing the incidence of this cancer in the United States by 75% over the past 50 years. This test is used to detect changes in the cells of the cervix that may indicate a precancerous or cancerous condition. However, Pap tests have a 15% to 25% false-negative rate for detecting cervical dysplasia[554] and can be inconclusive, requiring further testing, including HPV testing, colposcopy (microscopic examination of the lower genital tract), conization (cone-shaped biopsy), or loop electrosurgical excision procedure.

New automated screening systems (PAPNET or AutoNet) have been approved by the U.S. Food and Drug Administration (FDA) for computer review of negative Pap smears and for primary screening. These systems have the ability to reduce human error, but their cost-effectiveness is under intense scrutiny. Numerous other cervical biomarkers are under investigation for possible diagnostic use.[300]

A new laparoscopic assessment of the sentinel lymph node in early-stage cervical cancer is under investigation with excellent preliminary results.[337,399] Computed tomography (CT) scanning may be used in women who are not candidates for surgical treatment.

STAGING. There are four stages of cervical cancer with intermediate steps within each stage. A comparison of TNM and FIGO classifications for cervical cancer can be found online at http://emedicine.medscape.com/article/2006486-overview[96]; FIGO staging is available at the National Cancer Institute website: http://www.cancer.gov/cancertopics/pdq/treatment/cervical/HealthProfessional/page3#Reference3.2. Staging of cervical cancer is based on clinical staging rather than surgical staging. This means that the extent of disease is evaluated by the physician's physical examination and in some cases, a few other tests that are done such as cystoscopy and proctoscopy. Surgery may determine that the cancer has spread more than initially assessed. This new information may change the treatment plan, but it does not change the woman's FIGO stage.

Stage 0 is the precancerous stage, and there are no gross lesions; carcinoma is limited to the mucosa and is referred to as carcinoma in situ or cervical intraepithelial neoplasia grade 1, grade 2, or grade 3. For premalignant dysplastic changes, the cervical intraepithelial neoplasia grading is used for stage 0. Grade 1 is most likely to regress naturally and does not require treatment; grade 3 is most likely to advance to cancer. Grades 2 and 3 both require treatment.

Stage I is strictly confined to the cervix, and lesions are measured as less than or greater than 4 cm in size. In stage *II*, the cancer extends beyond the cervix but has not extended to the pelvic wall. The vagina is minimally involved, and there may or may not be parametrial involvement.

In *stage III* the carcinoma has extended to the pelvic wall and involves the lower one-third of the vagina and there may be kidney involvement (spread via the ureters). *Stage IV* is characterized by carcinoma that has extended beyond the true pelvis or has infiltrated adjacent organs (e.g., mucosa of the bladder or rectum). There may be metastatic spread of the growth to distant organs.

TREATMENT. Advances in radiologic technology have brought about important changes in the standard of care for cervical cancer. EBRT is being replaced by 3D MRI-guided

VBT[158] for stage 1 cervical cancer following hysterectomy; this shift is somewhat controversial and comparisons of EBRT and VBT remain under investigation.[158]

Concurrent cisplatin-based chemotherapy and radiation have shown significant survival improvement for women with locally advanced cervical cancer. The use of hypoxic cell radiosensitizers and monoclonal antibodies that inhibit cell growth increase numbers of malignant cells killed.[518] More advanced cases are managed by surgery (i.e., hysterectomy) followed by radiation or chemoradiation therapy for high-risk or advanced stages.[300] In addition to a vaccine and chemopreventive agents, biologic response modifiers are under investigation for future treatment options.

Fertility-preserving radical trachelectomy (removal of the cervix and pelvic lymph nodes but preserving the uterus) is possible for the treatment of early-stage cervical cancer for select individuals. The procedure has been successful with conception and full-term births (C-section delivery) 6 months after surgery in 66% of cases studied.[333]

PROGNOSIS. Cervical cancer is a slow-growing neoplasm with a good response rate to intervention. Almost all women with preinvasive cancer are cured. Reconstructive surgery and ovary preservation may be able to preserve childbearing status in younger women. The majority of treated women who develop recurrences do so in the first 2 years after primary therapy. Women with more advanced-stage disease or with lymph node involvement have a significantly less favorable prognosis.

SPECIAL IMPLICATIONS FOR THE THERAPIST **20-5**

Cervical Cancer

The physical therapist can continue to function in the role of educator and prevention specialist when conducting a personal/family history that includes questions about the consistency of Pap testing and presence of STDs (e.g., HPV or genital warts), as these relate to cervical cancer for women of all ages.

Although new, more sensitive testing is available, the majority of medical specialists agree that being screened for cervical cancer on a regular basis is more important than the availability of the latest technology. Any woman with a previous history of cervical cancer who presents with suspicious supraclavicular (or other) unusual lymph node presentation must be referred to her physician for medical evaluation. Reported symptoms of vaginal bleeding and GI or genitourinary dysfunction must also be promptly investigated before initiating pelvic rehabilitation.

Ectopic Pregnancy

Holly Tanner, PT, MA, OCS, WCS, LMP, BCB-PMD, CCI

Overview

Ectopic pregnancy, also known as *tubal pregnancy,* is marked by the implantation of a fertilized ovum outside the uterine cavity (Fig. 20-4). The fallopian tube is the

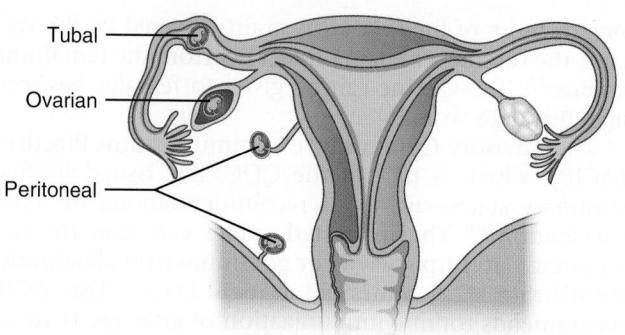

Figure 20-4

Ectopic pregnancy (outside the uterus) with implantation inside the fallopian tube (tubal pregnancy), abdomen (peritoneal or abdominal), or ovary. The majority of ectopic pregnancies (98%) are implanted inside the fallopian tube. (From Goodman CC, Snyder TE: *Differential diagnosis for the physical therapist: screening for referral,* ed 4, Philadelphia, 2007, WB Saunders.)

most common site of ectopic pregnancy, with approximately 95% implanting there, but extrauterine pregnancies can occur anywhere outside the uterus (e.g., ovary, abdomen, or pelvic peritoneum). Ectopic pregnancy is a true gynecologic emergency, as a ruptured ectopic pregnancy is the cause of 10% to 15% of all maternal deaths in the United States.[5]

Incidence and Risk Factors

The incidence of ectopic pregnancy is increasing in the United States and worldwide with approximately 19 to 26 per 10,000 ectopic pregnancies each year. This increased rate is accompanied by decreased rates of inpatient diagnosis as well as decreased surgical treatment.[610]

The reasons for this rise are unclear, although several risk factors have been identified, such as any condition that causes damage to the fallopian tubes that could impair transport of the ovum or impede the migration of the fertilized ovum to the uterus. For example, there could be a mechanical altering of the tube (e.g., narrowing or bending) and/or decreased motility of the ovum through the tube as a result of infection or inflammation.

Three risk factors that have been traditionally associated with an increased risk of ectopic pregnancy are STDs (especially chlamydia and gonorrhea), prior tubal or ovarian surgery, and current IUD. Other risk factors include ruptured appendix, endometriosis, smoking, PID or other pelvic infections, douching,[327] and previous ectopic pregnancy.[609] Adhesions related to some of these conditions can compress the fallopian tube or distort it in such a way that passage of the ovum is impaired. In addition, a history of infertility and the use of clomiphene citrate to induce ovulation or in vitro fertilization procedures are associated with an increased risk of this condition.

Etiologic Factors and Pathogenesis

Ectopic pregnancy is caused by delayed ovum transport secondary to decreased fallopian tube motility or distorted tubule anatomy. Advancements in diagnostic technology have revealed a number of etiologic factors, the most common being salpingitis. Salpingitis is an infection and inflammation of the fallopian tubes.

Three to 4 days are typically required for the ovum to travel through the fallopian tube to the uterus. The ovum is rapidly dividing and growing throughout the journey. During ectopic pregnancy, fertilization does not occur in the uterus. The sperm fertilizes the ovum soon after the ovum enters the ampulla of the fallopian tube. If the journey is slowed sufficiently (tubule motility), the ovum becomes too large to complete the passage through the tubule. If the tubule anatomy has been affected by recurrent infection or endometriosis, the same problem occurs. The trophoblasts that cover the surface of the ovum easily penetrate the mucosa and wall of the tubule, and implantation occurs.

Bleeding occurs during implantation with leakage into the pelvis and abdominal cavity. Vaginal bleeding that may be perceived as menstruation may occur. The pregnancy will typically outgrow its blood supply, terminating the pregnancy. If the pregnancy does not terminate, the thin-walled tubule will no longer support the growing fetus, and rupture can occur by the twelfth week of gestation. Tubal rupture is life-threatening because rapid intraabdominal hemorrhage can occur.

Clinical Manifestations

The classic presentation of ectopic pregnancy is marked by amenorrhea or irregular bleeding and spotting, non-specific lower abdominal quadrant or back pain, and a pelvic mass. The woman may believe she had a menstrual period but when questioned will report the period was atypical for her.

The pain reported can be diffuse and aching or localized and will progress to a sharper, lancinating acute type of pain. The pain can be sudden in onset and intermittent and may be accompanied by hemorrhage. The pain is thought to be primarily a result of the leakage of blood into the pelvic and abdominal cavity. Pain referred to the shoulder area can occur if the blood comes in contact with the kidney or diaphragm. Other symptoms include dizziness, fainting, paleness, and shock (if ectopic pregnancy bursts and causes significant bleeding).[609] Because the woman is pregnant, signs and symptoms associated with normal pregnancy may also be present. These findings include fatigue, nausea, breast tenderness, and urinary frequency.

MEDICAL MANAGEMENT

DIAGNOSIS. Physical examination reveals a pelvic mass in approximately 50% of the cases. Pelvic ultrasound studies can reliably reveal a gestational sac by 5 to 6 weeks into the pregnancy. An empty uterine cavity with elevated (slight) human chorionic gonadotropin-beta subunit (hCG-β) and symptoms strongly implies an extrauterine pregnancy. Blood studies may show anemia, and serum pregnancy tests (hCG-β hormonal levels) will be positive but show levels lower than expected in the presence of a normal pregnancy (lack of doubling over 2 days). Definitive diagnosis requires laparoscopy.

TREATMENT. Surgical intervention consisting of a noninvasive laparoscopic salpingostomy to remove the ectopic pregnancy is performed if the fallopian tube has not ruptured. Laparotomy is indicated if there is internal bleeding or if the ectopic site cannot be adequately visualized with the laparoscope.

A chemotherapeutic agent, methotrexate, can be administered to remove residual ectopic tissue after laparoscopy. This drug is also used when the pregnancy is intact and surgery is contraindicated or the diagnosis is made early enough that the condition is not life-threatening and preserving fertility is desirable.

SPECIAL IMPLICATIONS FOR THE THERAPIST   **20-6**

Ectopic Pregnancy

(See also Evolve Box 20-1 on the book's Evolve website for a list of other obstetrical conditions the physical therapist should know about.)

An awareness of this potentially life-threatening condition is important for the therapist. This awareness should include knowledge of the preexisting conditions that increase the risk of ectopic pregnancy and of the symptoms associated with pregnancy. If a woman of childbearing age complains of an onset of lower abdominal, ipsilateral shoulder, or back pain, the therapist should ask questions regarding her menstrual cycle and if any of the symptoms of pregnancy are present.

Anytime a sexually active woman of childbearing age presents with shoulder, back, pelvic, and/or abdominal pain with vaginal bleeding, medical referral is required. In general, if the therapist suspects ectopic pregnancy, an immediate telephone call to the physician or medical referral is warranted.

If follow-up care occurs, the therapist should be aware that perinatal loss can be a profound experience for the woman (and her family). A sensitive presence and validation of the loss may be helpful. Cultural responses to perinatal loss vary; the therapist should remain alert to any intervention needed.[118] Women who suffer an ectopic pregnancy may also have increased difficulty conceiving.[89]

DISORDERS OF THE OVARIES

Ovarian Cystic Disease

Overview

Ovarian cysts, most of which are benign, are the most common form of ovarian tumor. The different types of cysts include functional cysts (follicular cysts and luteal cysts), endometrial cysts, neoplastic cysts, and cysts that result from PCOS.

The follicle and corpus luteum are the source of most symptomatic ovarian cysts in premenopausal women. These cysts are called *functional cysts* and rarely produce symptoms (unless they rupture or hemorrhage) because they develop in the course of normal ovarian activity. A *follicular cyst* develops when an egg matures but does not erupt from the follicle but rather continues to swell as it fills with fluid. A *luteal cyst* develops from a corpus luteum when the tissue that is left after the egg has been expelled fills with blood or other fluid.

Endometrial cysts develop when endometrial tissue migrates to the ovaries, forming blood-filled cysts called *endometriomas*, or *chocolate cysts*, because of the dark-brown color of the contents. Endometrial cysts can grow large enough to impair ovulation and cause pain and cramping during menstrual periods.

Neoplastic cysts are "new growths" considered benign in the majority of cases; only a small percentage of neoplastic cysts are cancerous or have the capacity to invade neighboring tissues and metastasize to distant sites. Cyst-adenomas are the most common type of neoplastic cyst.

A disorder marked by the presence of multiple cysts is called *PCOS*. This polycystic disorder is a hormonal disorder affecting premenopausal women and one of the most common causes of infertility. The disease gets its name from the many small cysts that build up inside the ovaries, although there has been a recommendation that the name should be changed. The recommendation comes as a result of evidence in the literature that this condition is possibly made up of specific phenotypes with separate conditions (androgen excess, ovulatory dysfunction, and polycystic ovaries).[467]

Incidence and Etiologic and Risk Factors

Ovarian cysts are one of the most common endocrine disorders in women, affecting 3% to 7% of women of childbearing age. The exact etiology of ovarian cysts remains unknown, but intrinsic ovarian defect combined with factors outside the ovaries is suspected.

In the case of PCOS, a series of central and peripheral mechanisms related to insulin resistance occurs that is determined genetically and inherited[467]; PCOS is now considered a systemic metabolic disease.[64,194,344] Prevalence for PCOS ranges between 6% and 15% of women in the United States; more than half are obese. Among those women who seek treatment for infertility, more than 75% have some degree of PCOS.

Pathogenesis

Two types of ovarian cysts (the follicle and corpus luteum) are a normal part of the reproductive cycle. At least one follicle (a sac containing an egg and fluid) matures in an ovary during each cycle. During ovulation, the follicle ruptures to release the egg. The follicular remnant, or corpus luteum, is a smaller sac containing a viscous yellow liquid. The corpus luteum releases progesterone, which promotes the development of the uterine lining in preparation for the implantation of a fertilized egg.

Ovarian cysts develop when excess circulating androgens are converted to estrone in the peripheral adipose tissue. The elevated levels of circulating estrogens stimulate the release of GnRH by the hypothalamus and inhibit the secretion of follicle-stimulating hormone by the pituitary. GnRH stimulates the pituitary, which produces LH. The increased secretion of LH stimulates the ovary to produce and secrete more androgens. This self-perpetuating cycle results in abnormal maturation of the ovarian follicles, the development of multiple follicular cysts, and a persistent anovulatory state.

Several genes are implicated in the pathogenesis of PCOS. Researchers have discovered that many women are resistant to their own insulin. To counter this resistance, the pancreas makes extra insulin; over many years this may exhaust the pancreas' ability to make insulin and thus lead to diabetes and subsequent cardiovascular complications. In addition, high insulin levels boost the production of androgens that may induce muscular changes, leading to reduced insulin-mediated glucose uptake creating a repeated cycle and worsening condition.[289]

Clinical Manifestations

The likelihood of symptoms developing often has more to do with the size and location than the type of ovarian cyst. As cysts grow, their weight often pulls the ovary out of its customary position, sometimes cutting off the blood supply to the ovary. Pressure from the ovary in its new position against the uterus, bladder, intestine, or vagina may result in a variety of symptoms such as abdominal pressure; pain; abdominal bloating; or discomfort during urination, bowel movements, or sexual intercourse. Large cysts can impair ovarian function reducing ovulation and causing irregular periods or infertility in premenopausal women.

Depending on the type of cyst, if a cyst ruptures, the contents of the sac are usually absorbed by the body. When endometriomas rupture, the contents may be distributed on the uterus, bladder, and intestines. As the immune system moves in to clean up the debris, scar tissue develops, forming adhesions with resultant chronic pelvic pain. In the case of neoplastic cyst rupture, the more toxic contents can result in peritonitis.

Pain can be a manifestation of cysts. A dull, aching sensation experienced in the lower abdominal, groin, low back, or buttock areas can occur. The sensation may also be described as a heaviness. This pain is associated with bleeding into the cyst or with quick enlargement of the cyst. Sudden or sharp pain can indicate a cyst rupturing or hemorrhaging or a torsion occurring.

PCOS manifests in many different ways and is characterized by physical and metabolic changes. The affected girl or woman may present with one or more of the following manifestations: weight gain and obesity, prominent facial or body hair, severe acne, thinning scalp hair, infertility, and menstrual problems. They may seek medical care with a variety of different physicians depending on the primary presenting symptom (e.g., dermatologist for the skin involvement, internist for weight gain and elevated blood glucose, gynecologist for irregular periods and/or inability to get pregnant).

Fifty percent of these women have amenorrhea, and another 30% have abnormal uterine bleeding. PCOS is associated with endometrial cancer because high levels of androgen interfere with ovulation so women with PCOS do not regularly shed the endometrium. Impaired glucose tolerance is present in 40% of women with PCOS, and the subsequent risk for insulin resistance, type 2 diabetes, and heart disease have been documented.[163,467]

Other symptoms or conditions associated with PCOS include obstructive sleep apnea and daytime sleepiness[632] and benign breast disease (formerly fibrocystic breast disease).[174] There is a twofold increased risk for venous thrombosis embolism among women with PCOS who are taking combined oral contraceptives and a 1.5-fold increased risk for those women with PCOS who are not taking oral contraceptives.[64]

MEDICAL MANAGEMENT

DIAGNOSIS AND TREATMENT. The history and pelvic examination lead to suspicion of cystic disease. Confirmation is made by ultrasonography or laparoscopy. Ultrasound may be transvaginal (inserting a tampon-sized transducer into the vagina) or abdominal (moving a transducer across the lower abdomen) and can help identify the type of cyst and whether a cyst contains solid or liquid material. Laboratory tests include a complete blood count to identify infection or anemia (heavy bleeding) and a carcinoembryonic antigen-125 (CA-125) test for ovarian cancer. All women with PCOS should be screened for glucose intolerance.[365]

The treatment of ovarian cysts depends on the results of the diagnostic tests and the age of the woman (preserving childbearing status). In premenopausal women, the decision whether to drain or remove the cyst depends on the problems the cyst is causing (e.g., follicular or luteal cysts resolve without treatment, and endometriomas and neoplastic cysts may be removed surgically).

The treatment of PCOS is primarily hormonal with the goal being an interruption of the persistent elevated levels of androgens. Pharmaceuticals (e.g., metformin, clomiphene citrate) may be used to induce ovulation.[429,430] If medication is not effective, laser surgery can be instituted to puncture the multiple follicles.

It is now known that the application of diabetes management techniques aimed at reducing insulin resistance and hyperinsulinemia (e.g., weight reduction, oral hypoglycemic agents, and exercise) can reverse testosterone and LH abnormalities and infertility, as well as improve glucose, insulin, and lipid profiles.

SPECIAL IMPLICATIONS FOR THE THERAPIST   20-7

Ovarian Cystic Disease

Depending on the clinical presentation, therapists may ask women if menstrual dysfunction is present. A history of ovarian cystic disease could account for a woman's low back or sacral pain, but usually there is some indication in the menstrual history to suggest a gynecologic link.

In women with known PCOS, impaired glucose tolerance, or insulin resistance, elevated androgens with the associated muscular changes that further reduce glucose uptake and elevated cholesterol warrant the use of exercise and increased physical activity before the onset of macrovascular and microvascular symptoms.[289,344] See also "Diabetes Mellitus" in Chapter 11.

Considering how common PCOS is, therapists need to be aware of the potential side effects of clomiphene citrate. These include insomnia, blurred vision, nausea, vomiting, urinary frequency, and polyuria. The onset of any of these symptoms warrants communication with the physician.

Ovarian Cancer

Overview

Ovarian cancer is estimated to be the second most common female urogenital cancer and the most lethal of these cancers largely as a result of the advanced stage at diagnosis in most women.[303] Many different types of ovarian cancers can occur but the majority (85%-90%) are carcinomas. The classification of ovarian tumors is based on the tissue of origin.[49] The most common tumors (90%) have always been thought to arise from the surface epithelium or lining/covering of the ovary. Epithelial ovarian cancer is further classified as serous (most common), endometrioid, clear cell, mucinous, transitional cell (Brenner tumors), mixed, and poorly differentiated. However, recent studies suggest that histologically similar cancers can arise from the fimbriae (finger-like projections at the ends of fallopian tubes that brush the ovaries) and from deposits of endometriosis.[519] The origin and pathogenesis of ovarian cancer[49] (whether epithelial or fimbrial) is an area of current ongoing debate and controversy.

The term *extraovarian primary peritoneal carcinoma* (EOPPC) is sometimes used interchangeably with the term *ovarian cancer*. This is a relatively newly defined disease that develops only in women, accounting for approximately 10% of cases with a presumed diagnosis of ovarian cancer. Characterized by abdominal carcinomatosis, uninvolved or minimally involved ovaries, and no identifiable primary form of cancer, EOPPC has been reported after bilateral oophorectomy performed for benign disease or prophylactically for ovarian cancer.[201] The occurrence of EOPPC may be explained by the common origin of the peritoneum and the ovaries from the coelomic epithelium. The various histologic differences of ovarian and peritoneal lesions are under investigation.

Incidence

An estimated 22,800 women in the United States developed ovarian cancer in 2012 with 15,500 deaths from ovarian cancer.[557] The poor outcome is based on the difficulty of diagnosing the disease, which results in 60% to 70% of the women having metastatic disease at the time of diagnosis. Although there are a number of types of ovarian cancers, epithelial tumors make up approximately 90% of the cases and are the leading cause of death from gynecologic cancer in the United States. The incidence of epithelial tumors peaks in women during their 50s and 60s; it is rare before puberty.

In the United States, white and Hawaiian women have the highest incidence of ovarian cancer, whereas Native American and black women have the lowest incidence.

Etiologic and Risk Factors and Pathogenesis

The etiology of ovarian cancer is not well understood. No single cause of ovarian cancer has been discovered, but hormonal, environmental, and genetic factors appear to influence the development of the disease (Box 20-3). None is as important as a family history of ovarian or breast cancer. Loss of two tumor-suppressor genes (*p53* and *BRCA1*) occurs early in ovarian carcinogenesis in women who are *BRCA1* mutation carriers.[648] Overall,

RISK AND PROTECTIVE FACTORS FOR OVARIAN CANCER

Risk Factors

- Presence of *BRCA1* or *BRCA2* mutation*
- Lynch syndrome (hereditary nonpolyposis colorectal cancer)*
- Family history (mother or father's side) of breast, ovarian, or colon cancer
- Personal history of endometrial or breast cancer
- Increasing age (older than 40 years, most occur in women 55-75 years)
- Nulliparity (never given birth)
- Giving birth for the first time after age 35 years
- Never breastfed
- White race
- History of endometriosis
- Perineal use of talc (powder); exposure to asbestos (risk factor under investigation)[119,587]
- Living in an industrialized Western nation
- Obesity
- High dietary fat intake
- Prolonged exposure to estrogen (early onset of menarche/before age 12 years, menopause after age 50 years, postmenopausal estrogen-only replacement therapy)
- Infertility
- Fertility drugs (under investigation; not yet confirmed)
- Tobacco and alcohol use (mucinous ovarian cancer)

Protective Factors

- Suppression of ovulation
  - Increasing numbers of full-term pregnancies
  - Longer duration of lactation (breastfeeding)
  - Oral contraceptive use
  - Tubal ligation
  - Hysterectomy

*Women with either of these factors have the highest risk of developing ovarian cancer but account for only approximately 10% of those with the disease.

Data from Jelovac D. Recent progress in the diagnosis and treatment of ovarian cancer. *CA Cancer J Clin* 61(3):183–203, 2011.

more than 90% of all cases occur sporadically; only 10% of all women with ovarian cancer have a hereditary predisposition. However, genetic variants in the transforming growth factor β signaling pathway has also been shown to be a risk factor for the development of ovarian cancer.[661]

The average woman has less than a 2% chance of developing ovarian cancer in her lifetime (1 in 57 vs. 1 in 8 for breast cancer), whereas a woman with first-degree relatives with ovarian cancer or who has the *BRCA1* (*BRCA* stands for BReast CAncer) mutation has about a 45% lifetime chance, and for *BRCA2*, the risk is approximately 25%.[524]

The risk of ovarian cancer is inversely proportional to the number of lifetime ovulations[303] (incessant-ovulation theory).[630] For example, nulliparous women (never given birth) are at increased risk of developing ovarian cancer. Every time an egg is released, it ruptures the surface of one of the ovaries. Cells have to replicate to repair the damage, and the more times they do this, the greater the chances that a cancer-causing mutation will occur. Because epithelial tumors make up approximately 90%

of ovarian cancers, many of the risk factors in Box 20-3 relate to this entity.

Following ovulation, the mutated cells may become trapped within the connective tissue around the ovary. This can lead to the formation of cysts subjecting epithelial cells to a proinflammatory microenvironment (inflammation theory), which may increase the rate of DNA damage. This is why anything that interferes with ovulation (e.g., pregnancy, breastfeeding, or hormonal contraceptives) diminishes the risk of developing ovarian cancer.

A history of breastfeeding also is important, because women who breast feed are at decreased risk of developing this condition compared to nulliparous women and parous women who have not breastfed. At the present time, there are no established nutritional risk factors for ovarian cancer. The association of milk/dairy products or calcium consumption with ovarian cancer has not been proved. Moderate alcohol consumption may reduce the risk; the role of obesity and physical activity in this cancer is unclear.[350]

Oral contraceptives and tubal ligation substantially reduce the risk of serous, endometrioid, and clear cell subgroups, but have no apparent effect on mucinous tumors, which likely follow a different oncogenic pathway.[630] Once present, ovarian cancer spreads to the pelvis, abdominal cavity, and bladder, whereas lymphatic metastasis carries the disease to the paraaortic lymph nodes and to a lesser extent the inguinal or external iliac lymph nodes. Hematogenous spread of the cancer can result in liver and lung involvement.

Clinical Manifestations

In the past, most ovarian cancers were considered asymptomatic or "silent," presenting with symptoms so vague that the disease is advanced in many cases by the time the woman seeks care. But new evidence shows that up to 89% of women with early-stage disease seek medical care for symptoms including abdominal bloating, early satiety (difficulty eating/feeling full), flatulence, fatigue and malaise, gastritis, or general abdominal discomfort. Local pelvic pain is often an early symptom (1-6 months prior to diagnosis).[241] Abnormal vaginal bleeding, leg pain, pelvic mass, and low back pain are less common but still reported symptoms.

Symptoms associated with metastatic spread of the disease include unexplained weight loss, weakness, pleurisy, ascites, and cachexia (general feebleness and wasting). Ascites is an accumulation of fluid within the peritoneal cavity. This can occur when there is marked increased pressure within the liver sinusoids or portal hypertension that results in serum exuding through the superficial capillaries into the peritoneal cavity (see Fig. 17-5).

Paraneoplastic cerebellar degeneration is a type of paraneoplastic syndrome that primarily affects women with gynecologic cancers. It is associated with, but not directly caused by, the cancer or its metastases. Although rare, paraneoplastic cerebellar degeneration can occur years before any discernible symptoms of malignancy, especially ovarian cancer. Paraneoplastic cerebellar degeneration can also develop following the detection and treatment of ovarian cancer. Symptoms typically include ataxic gait, truncal and appendicular ataxia, nystagmus, peripheral neuropathy and speech impairment (dysarthria).[244] The syndrome can be debilitating with limited treatment options.

MEDICAL MANAGEMENT

SCREENING AND PREVENTION. Screening all women for ovarian cancer is not considered practical or cost-effective. However, women at high risk for ovarian cancer (e.g., those with a family history of ovarian cancer in a mother, sister, or daughter) and any woman with a personal history of breast, colon, or uterine cancer should receive annual screening with a combination of the CA-125 blood test, physical examination, and transvaginal ultrasound.

There is no reliable screening test to detect ovarian cancer in its early, most curable stages. Two diagnostic tests are used but both lack sensitivity and specificity. The CA-125 blood test (carcinoembryonic antigen, a biologic marker produced by ovarian cancer cells) is elevated in about half the women with early-stage disease and approximately 80% of those with advanced disease. This test is not adequate as a screening tool because it does not detect the disease early in women who are asymptomatic, results vary depending on menopausal status, and it can be elevated in other conditions, such as pelvic infections, fibroids, or endometriosis, and even during ovulation.[563]

Researchers are continuing to evaluate CA-125 as a screening tool (e.g., rapidly rising CA-125 may be more predictive than elevation on a single test) and also investigating other substances, such as lysophosphatidic acid, a growth factor for ovarian cancer cells measured in the blood.[513] Researchers at Johns Hopkins are investigating a new test as a broad screening tool for ovarian (and endometrial) cancer called the PapGene test; early studies with a small number of women showed the PapGene test accurately detected 41% of all ovarian (and 100% of endometrial) cancers.[335]

Some studies suggest that serous ovarian cancers detected at an early stage generally have a favorable underlying biology. Genetic-profiling of cancers detected at an early stage predict a favorable outcome. But this may be because slow-growing tumors are more likely to be detected before they spread. Conversely, most late-stage ovarian cancers seem to have a more virulent biology. This insight suggests that if screening approaches are to succeed it will be necessary to develop approaches that are able to detect virulent cancers at an early stage.[80]

Researchers at the University of Washington School of Medicine in Seattle have been able to accurately predict ovarian cancer based on the duration and frequency of key signs and symptoms, including pelvic/abdominal pain, urinary urgency or frequency, increased abdominal size and bloating, and difficulty eating/feeling full (early satiety). This symptom index is considered positive for ovarian cancer if any of these signs and symptoms occur more than 12 times a month for less than 12 months.[40]

Routine ultrasound imaging is also under investigation as an effective screening tool when used to identify enlarged ovaries.[538] Transvaginal ultrasonography helps determine whether an existing ovarian growth is benign or cancerous. Because the early-stage symptoms are quite nonspecific, most women do not seek medical attention until the disease is advanced.

Some women with a positive immediate family history of ovarian cancer choose to have prophylactic oophorectomies after completing childbearing to prevent the development of this disease. This intervention is not 100% protective because the lining of the peritoneal cavity comprises the same cells as the lining of the ovaries and development of primary peritoneal cancer after prophylactic oophorectomy can occur.[524]

A history of one or more full-term pregnancies, a history of breastfeeding, and the use of hormonal contraceptives reduce the risk of ovarian cancer. Hormonal contraceptives (whether in pill form, injectable, or patch form) are recommended as cancer prevention for women with a family history of ovarian cancer, especially if the *BRCA* mutation is present. The mechanism of protection is unclear, but it is probably a result of the inhibition of ovulation; there is a potential increased risk of cervical cancer with this treatment.[451,524]

As a result of analgesics reducing the risk for colorectal cancer, studies of the effect of similar pharmacologic effects on ovarian cancer have been conducted. Regular use of acetaminophen (but not aspirin) may be associated with lower risk of ovarian cancer.[446]

DIAGNOSIS AND STAGING. Despite the reputation of ovarian cancer as a silent killer, more than 90% of women with ovarian cancer (whether early or advanced) reported experiencing symptoms long before diagnosis.[273] However, these are often nonspecific and vague and frequently are misdiagnosed as indigestion or irritable bowel syndrome or some other nongynecologic condition including mechanical low back pain. Imaging, menopausal status, and biomarkers can aid in distinguishing malignant from benign pelvic masses. A cervical smear may reveal malignant cells, and a biopsy will reveal whether the mass is benign or cancerous.[67]

No one biomarker specific to ovarian cancer has been identified yet; researchers are investigating a panel of biomarkers to aid in earlier diagnosis.[663] Diagnostic tools currently in use and under investigation include serum CA-125,[563] serum human epididymal protein 4 (HE4),[147,434,435,436] risk of malignancy index (used to differentiate ovarian cancer from other pelvic masses), and the risk of ovarian cancer algorithm or the risk of ovarian malignancy algorithm[323,433,491,564] (based on age and fluctuations in CA-125 blood levels).[67] Current screening strategies (ultrasound, biomarker evaluation) may lower the stage at diagnosis but have not been shown to improve survival.[303]

FIGO staging of the disease is as follows: stage I—disease limited to one or both ovaries; stage II—extension to other pelvic organs; stage III—intraperitoneal metastasis (spread to other abdominal organs but not the liver); and stage IV—distant metastasis (spread to the liver or organs outside the abdominal cavity). The cancer is considered advanced at stages II to IV. For a more comprehensive breakdown of the American Joint Committee on Cancer (AJCC) TNM and FIGO staging systems for ovarian cancer, see the NCCN Clinical Practice Guidelines.

TREATMENT. Treatment of ovarian cancer depends on the specific tumor type but usually consists of cytoreductive surgery that includes total abdominal hysterectomy, bilateral salpingo-oophorectomy, omentectomy (removal of supportive tissue attached to organs in the abdominal cavity), and lymphadenectomy followed by adjuvant combination chemotherapy.[369]

Fertility-sparing surgery and comprehensive staging is done for any woman who desires to maintain her fertility.[460] Anyone (men and women) interested in more information about preserving fertility after cancer should talk to their physicians about future fertility. The ACS and NCCN offer excellent reviews of this topic.[27]

Giving intraperitoneal chemotherapy along with intravenous (IV) chemotherapy may improve survival of women with stage III ovarian cancer. Intraperitoneal chemotherapy allows higher doses and more frequent administration of drugs and appears more effective at killing cancer cells in the peritoneal cavity where ovarian cancer is likely to spread or recur first. Successful surgery to remove the bulk of the tumor is required first.[46,647]

New cancer drugs are being developed to treat resistant or recurrent disease. Ovarian growth is angiogenesis dependent, causing researchers to investigate the use of antiangiogenic treatment (e.g., angiostatin or endostatin) to inhibit tumor growth in this type of cancer.[662] Other new interventions and approaches under investigation include the use of molecular targeted therapy (laboratory-produced substances that find and bind to cancer cells, delivering tumor-killing agents without harming normal cells), genetic techniques (e.g., gene therapy to supply a working copy of the tumor-suppressing gene *p53*), vaccines to boost a woman's immune response to ovarian tumor cells that emerge after treatment, and new combinations and sequences of currently used drug interventions.[62,592]

PROGNOSIS. Ovarian cancer has a very poor prognosis because it is difficult to detect early and usually presents with advanced metastases (70% present in an advanced stage). The cancer is generally responsive to treatment if found early, with a 90% 5-year survival rate. In most cases, clinical response to treatment is approximately 80%, but tumor recurrence within 3 years after treatment occurs in most women.[201] Return of the tumor within 6 months after achieving complete remission is referred to as *drug resistant;* cancer that does not respond to initial therapy at all is labeled *drug refractory.* Either of these scenarios can have a poor prognosis; recurrent ovarian cancer is highly treatable but not curable. Salvage therapy (chemotherapy to help manage symptoms and prolong survival) may be recommended if a cancer cure is not possible but quality of life may be impaired by further aggressive therapy. Five-year survival without recurrence is a good prognostic indicator.

SPECIAL IMPLICATIONS FOR THE THERAPIST **20-8**

Ovarian Cancer

Therapists treating women with a history of ovarian cancer need to be cognizant of the moderate-to-high risk of recurrence of the disease. Gait disturbance may be the first sign of a paraneoplastic syndrome associated with gynecologic cancer. Other symptoms associated with metastases may include thoracic or shoulder girdle pain secondary to lymphadenopathy, symptoms associated with lung (dyspnea, see Chapter 15) or liver (see Chapter 17) disease, and weight loss and fatigue. Onset of any of these complaints warrants communication with the physician. Lymphedema associated with ovarian cancer can develop in the lower quadrant(s) requiring ongoing surveillance for early signs and lymphedema management.

Oophorectomy induces menopause in women. Therefore an onset of the symptoms described in the beginning of this chapter may occur in addition to headaches, depression, and insomnia. Ovary removal before age 65 years is also a risk factor for heart disease, hip fractures, dementia, and movement disorders (e.g., Parkinson disease), and even premature death.[517]

Side effects from cancer treatment are often present. Chemotherapy-induced peripheral neuropathy is a common problem after treatment with Taxol. Symptoms may or may not resolve. Removal of the ovaries and chemotherapy can result in vaginal atrophy, dryness, and resulting soft-tissue tightness (e.g., vaginal inlet stenosis) or soft-tissue tenderness or restriction (e.g., pelvic floor). These effects of treatment can create physical and emotional distress affecting quality of life that can be addressed by physical therapy.

Online educational resources of interest to the therapist and clients include: National Ovarian Cancer Coalition (www.ovarian.org), American Cancer Society (www.cancer.org/Cancer/OvarianCancer), and the National Cancer Institute (www.cancer.gov/cancertopics/types/ovarian).

Ovarian Varices

Incompetent and dilated ovarian veins (as well as other uterine and pelvic veins) are a known cause of abdominal and pelvic pain and contribute to pelvic congestion syndrome (Fig. 20-5). This is only one of many possible causes of chronic pelvic pain and pelvic congestion syndrome.[568] Ovarian varices may occur unilaterally or bilaterally, most often in women who have had children but occasionally in nonparous women.[214]

Reported symptoms include pain that worsens toward the end of the day or after standing for a long time, pain that occurs premenstrually and after intercourse, sensations of heaviness in the pelvis, and prominent varicose veins elsewhere on the body. This type of pelvic pain arises when blood pools in a distended ovarian vein rather than flowing back toward the heart and is more common among women with low blood pressure. This distention and pooling form a varicocele, a term traditionally

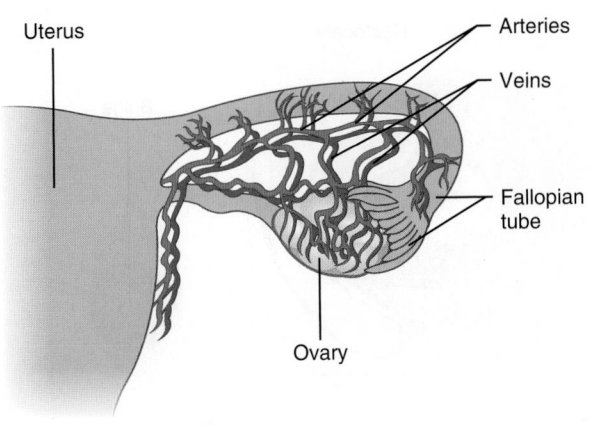

Figure 20-5

Varicose veins (varicosities) of the ovary. Ovarian varicosities associated with pelvic congestion syndrome are the cause of chronic pelvic pain for women. This form of venous insufficiency is often accompanied by prominent varicose veins elsewhere in the lower quadrant (buttocks, thighs, calves). Men may have similar varicosities of the scrotum (not shown). (From Goodman CC, Snyder TE: *Differential diagnosis for the physical therapist: screening for referral*, ed 5, Philadelphia, 2013, WB Saunders.)

applied to men to describe varicose veins in the testicles, but varicoceles can also occur in the female counterparts of those organs. In fact, 10% of men experience pelvic varices of the gonadal veins presenting as varicoceles similar to uteroovarian varices seen in women.[123]

Ovarian vein incompetence may be suspected from the presence of vulvar varicosities and can be diagnostically visualized with computed tomographic venography, contrast enhanced MRIs, or transvaginal ultrasound. If observed during pregnancy, these may disappear after delivery but become more prominent with subsequent pregnancies.

Treatment with embolization of the pelvic and ovarian veins (see discussion of this technique in "Uterine Fibroids" above) is relatively new but reportedly safe and effective in alleviating pain and symptoms, improving sexual functioning, and reducing anxiety and depression with subsequent improved quality of life reported.[331,568]

PELVIC FLOOR DISORDERS

Pelvic floor disorder is a general label given to a group of conditions involving the pelvic structures: organs, muscles, ligaments, joints. It is important for all physical therapists to have a basic knowledge of these conditions, symptoms and treatments (see the book's Evolve website for an expanded list of this information in Evolve Box 20-1; also see "A Therapist's Thoughts: Organizing Your Thoughts" below).

In the literature, the term "pelvic floor disorder" usually refers to conditions in which the muscles and ligaments of the pelvic floor become weakened and lose their ability to close and support. The most common pelvic floor disorders are pelvic organ prolapse (discussed here), urinary incontinence (see Chapter 18), and fecal incontinence (see Chapter 16).

Causes of pelvic floor disorders vary among the different conditions. However all pelvic floor disorders can be related to pelvic floor muscle (PFM) dysfunction. Pelvic floor muscle dysfunction refers specifically to a condition of the skeletal muscle layer of the pelvic floor (see Chapter 27 for a complete discussion of PFM dysfunction).

A cross-sectional survey of almost 2000 adult U.S. females reported an overall prevalence of 23.7% for at least one pelvic floor disorder. Prevalence increased with age from 9.7% in women 20 to 39 years old to 49.7% in those older than 80 years. A statistically significant increase in prevalence was also seen, with increasing parity from 12.8% among women without children to 32.4% in women with three or more deliveries. Weight differences also reached statistical significance with obese women reporting pelvic floor disorders[473] at a prevalence of 30.4% and normal weight women at 15.1%.

A THERAPIST'S THOUGHTS*
ORGANIZING YOUR THOUGHTS

Signs and symptoms in the pelvis and abdomen can originate from many structures including organs, joints, and skeletal muscles. It is helpful to categorize conditions:

- Organ based/medical (primarily treated by medical practitioners such as urinary tract infection and PID)
- Musculoskeletal conditions treated by most physical therapists (lumbar and sacroiliac dysfunction)
- Musculoskeletal conditions treated by specialized physical therapists (PFM dysfunction, painful bladder syndrome and others)

This helps the therapist determine his or her roles in the treatment of the individual (i.e., refer to a medical practitioner, self-treat, or refer to a specialist physical therapist).

*Beth Shelly, PT, DPT, WCS, BCB-PMD

Pelvic Organ Prolapse—Cystocele, Rectocele, and Uterine Prolapse

Overview

The three types of pelvic organ prolapse (POP) discussed here are cystocele, rectocele, and uterine prolapse. A *cystocele* or prolapsed bladder is the loss of support of the bladder and urethra resulting in falling of the urinary bladder and a bulging of the anterior vaginal wall into the vagina (Fig. 20-6, A and B). A *rectocele* is the loss of support of the rectum resulting in falling of the rectum and a bulging of the posterior vaginal wall into the vagina (Fig. 20-6, C and D). A *uterine prolapse* is the fall of the uterus into the vagina (Fig. 20-7).

Other types of pelvic floor prolapse may include cystourethrocele (bladder and urethra prolapse into the vagina), urethrocele (just the urethra prolapses into the vagina), enterocele (part of the intestine prolapses into the space between the vaginal and the rectum), rectal prolapse (the anal and rectal canal folds over and falls out the rectum) and vaginal vault prolapse (the apex of the vagina prolapses, occurring sometimes after a hysterectomy).

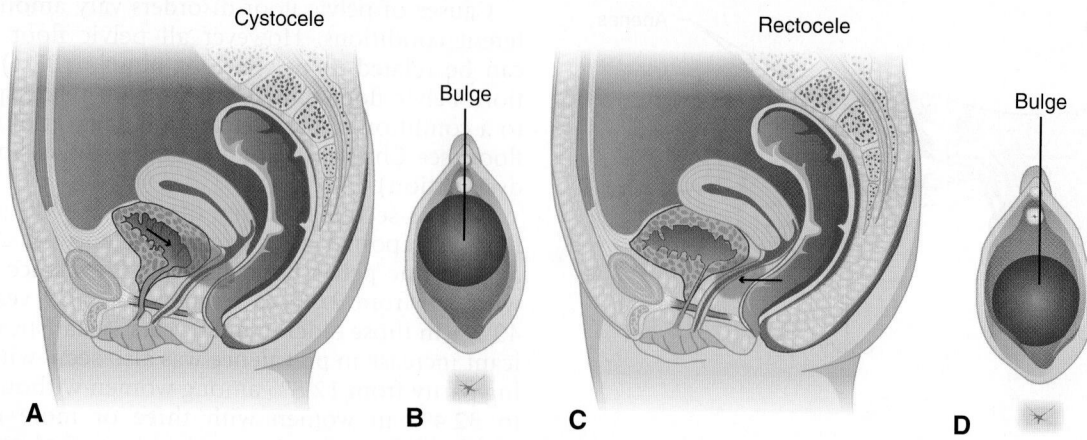

Figure 20-6

A, Cystocele (sagittal view). Note the bulging of the anterior vaginal wall. The urinary bladder is displaced downward. **B,** Lithotomy view: the bladder pushes the anterior vaginal wall downward into the vagina. **C,** Rectocele (sagittal view). **D,** Note the bulging of the posterior vaginal wall associated with rectocele (lithotomy view).

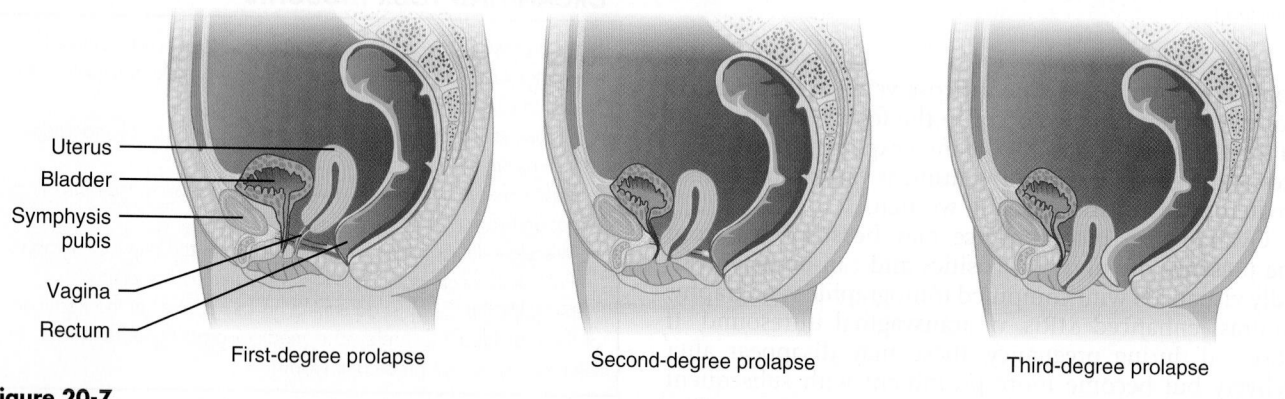

Figure 20-7

Stages of uterine prolapse. Herniation of the uterus through the pelvic floor resulting in protrusion into the vagina. *First-degree:* the cervix remains in the vagina. *Second-degree:* the cervix appears at the perineum or protrudes on straining. *Third-degree:* the entire uterus protrudes outside the body, and there is total inversion of the vagina.

Etiologic and Risk Factors

Cystocele, rectocele, and uterine prolapse are a result of loss of support of the PFM, fascial, and ligamentous structures of the pelvic organs. Multiple pregnancies (in particular the third vaginal delivery) increase the risk of these disorders developing. There is some disagreement as to whether there are identifiable labor or delivery parameters which contribute more to POP. Some professionals feel prolonged labor, bearing down before full dilation, and forceful delivery of the placenta are possible causes of prolapse. Trauma to the pudendal or sacral nerves during birth and delivery is an additional risk factor. Genetics may play a role as family history of prolapse increases the individual risk of prolapse.[424] Decreased tissue support because of aging, complications of pelvic surgery, a history of heavy lifting, obesity, prolonged coughing, or excessive straining during bowel movements may also result in prolapse of some or all of these structures.

Pathogenesis

The uterus and other pelvic structures are maintained in their proper position by three mechanisms: suspension by intact endopelvic fascia and ligaments such as the uterosacral, and cardinal ligaments, constriction by the PFM specifically the levator ani layer, and the structural geometry of the flap value mechanism.[643]

Overstretching, genetic weakness, partial or full avulsion of the endopelvic fascia can result in POP. The location of the weakening determines the type of prolapsed; anterior endopelvic fascia weakness results in cystocele, posterior endopelvic fascia weakness results in rectocele. The pelvic floor musculature forms a sling-like structure that supports the uterus, vagina, urinary bladder, urethra, and rectum (see Figs. 27-1 and 27-2).[185]

Multiple studies have documented the important role of the PFM in avoiding or improving POP.[284] Similar to loss of support in the noncontractile tissue, overstretching, weakness, partial or full avulsion of the PFM can contribute to downward movement of the pelvic organ on POP. As the organs move downward the canals straighten and the flap value mechanism is lost. Etiologic and risk factors listed above contribute to this loss of support.

Clinical Manifestations

The symptoms of POP vary greatly and are not related to type or severity, with some individuals having severe POP and no symptoms while others have a very small decedent of the organ and significant symptoms. The most common symptom is a sense of heaviness or pressure in the perineum, which is often worse after long periods of standing or upright weight-bearing postures, decreased with lying down, and may be felt by some people to be painful.

Often the woman notices a "lump" in the vaginal area and seeks medical advice to determine the cause. All POP can have these two symptoms. Many women have more than one type of POP and thus may have many of the symptoms below.

The symptoms associated with a cystocele may include urinary frequency and urgency, difficulty in emptying the bladder, and urinary incontinence. The symptoms associated with a rectocele include a feeling of incomplete rectal emptying, constipation, and aching or pressure after a bowel movement. If the rectocele becomes large enough to trap feces, manual pressure applied to the vaginal wall may be necessary in order to complete a bowel movement without excessive straining (a practice called *splinting*, or *stenting*, which is usually an indication of the need for corrective surgery).

Primary symptoms resulting from uterine prolapse are backache, and irritation and excoriation of the exposed mucous membranes of the cervix and vagina, especially from sexual intercourse and from wiping after toileting.

MEDICAL MANAGEMENT

DIAGNOSIS. The diagnosis of these disorders is primarily derived from observation and the pelvic examination. The two most common grading systems are the Baden-Walker[31] (Box 20-4) and POPQ.[597] The POPQ involves a complex set of measurements to map the shape of the vaginal walls. The Baden-Walker is simpler and used by most gynecologists. In this system, the organ position grade depends on how far the organ

---

Box 20-4
BADEN-WALKER SYSTEM FOR THE EVALUATION OF POP

Grade

0 Normal position
1 Descent halfway to the hymen
2 Descent to the hymen
3 Descent halfway past the hymen
4 Maximum possible descent

Data from ACOG Practice Bulletin No. 85: Pelvic organ prolapse, *Obstet Gynecol* 110(3):717–729, 2007.

---

protrudes through the introitus (entrance to the vagina). A *first-degree* uterine prolapse is marked by some descent, but the cervix has not reached the introitus. A *second-degree* uterine prolapse is marked by the cervix as part of the uterus having descended through the introitus. A *third-degree* prolapse is manifested by the entire uterus protruding through the vaginal opening (see Fig. 20-7).

TREATMENT. Treatment decisions are based on intensity of symptoms (i.e., how bothersome they are to the individual) and can include surgical, mechanical, or conservative options.

Surgical procedures that can be used to correct POP include colposuspension, colporrhaphy, sacrocolpopexy, and paravaginal repair. Many women have concomitant bladder suspension or hysterectomy. There are complications with surgery and approximately 30% require another surgery for reoccurrence.[137]

Mechanical treatments involve fitting of a pessary (a device inserted into the vagina to hold the organ(s) in place). Some women can remove their own pessary, others must report to the nurse every 3 months to have the device removed, washed, and replaced. Pessaries should always be worn during recreational activities or strengthening exercises.

Conservative options are becoming more popular with new research documenting its success. Rehabilitation[590] includes PFM strengthening exercises and muscle reeducation, postural education, self-care and possibly biofeedback, or electrical stimulation. Strengthening of the PFMs should be incorporated into the preoperative and postoperative rehabilitation program as well.[301]

Managing constipation with lifestyle changes, such as adequate hydration, fiber intake, developing regular bowel habits, and regular exercise, are often effective for rectocele.

SPECIAL IMPLICATIONS FOR THE THERAPIST   20-9

Cystocele, Rectocele, and Uterine Prolapse

As with urinary incontinence, physical therapists can have a primary role in the treatment of POP through treatment of pelvic floor muscle dysfunction (see Chapter 27). Therapists will also see people with pelvic floor disorders as a comorbidity. In these cases, therapists must be vigilant to avoid increased intraabdominal pressure, such as holding the breath or bearing down in any way similar to performing a Valsalva maneuver, as these could exacerbate the pelvic floor condition.

Some "core exercises" may also exacerbate POP symptoms. Slowly adding exercises, asking patients/clients to monitor and report change in POP symptoms, and educating women against bearing down during exercise can avoid complications. Women should also be educated in proper body mechanics and avoidance of lifting in a trunk flexed position which can exacerbate symptoms.

In addition, a woman with a second- or third-degree uterine prolapse may have difficulty tolerating extended periods of weight-bearing activities. Alternative positions for sexual intercourse should be discussed (e.g., pillow under the hips or avoiding being above the partner), and alternative positions for exercise will need to be incorporated into the rehabilitation program (include more sitting or reclined exercise and consider pool therapy if possible).

BREAST DISEASE

Valerie Wang, PT

Breast disease falls into two categories: *benign breast conditions* and *breast cancer*. Most breast lumps are benign or noncancerous. These include cysts and fibroadenomas, and a number of other conditions that are characterized by lumpy and sometimes painful breasts. Because cancerous tumors of the breast cannot be distinguished from benign lesions, persistent lumps, as well as breast pain, should always be medically evaluated.

Benign Breast Conditions

Overview

Benign breast conditions or *benign breast changes* (also referred to as *benign breast disease*) are the preferred terms for describing a number of breast irregularities. Use of the term *fibrocystic breast disease* is now considered an erroneous "wastebasket" designation. Some degree of tissue nodularity (sometimes referred to as "lumpiness") is normal in most younger women; tissue changes do not necessarily constitute true disease. Fibrocystic changes can only be confirmed by histologic examination. Other terms used to describe tissue nodularity include *diffuse cystic mastopathy* or *mammary dysplasia*. Diagnosis of *benign breast conditions* is based on symptoms and physical findings, which may include:
- Cyclical swelling, discomfort, tenderness
- Cysts
- Mastalgia (severe breast pain; may be cyclical or not)
- Nodularity (significant lumpiness; may be cyclical or not)
- Nipple discharge
- Infections and inflammations (mastitis, Mondor disease, abscess)

Cysts are fluid-filled lumps that may fluctuate in size. They may be microscopic or large enough to palpate. Their onset may be gradual or sudden (overnight). Less common than cysts, but also prevalent, are *fibroadenomas*. They are a solid tumor comprised of glandular and fibrous connective tissue in the elements that arise from the terminal duct lobular unit. Lumps may be easily moveable under the skin, firm, painless and rubbery with well-defined borders. They usually occur in single lumps, but in 10% to 15% of women they are multifocal and can be bilateral.

Incidence and Risk Factors

Benign breast changes, cysts, and fibroadenomas make up the majority of benign breast conditions. These changes are most often observed in women age 20 to 50 years; breast changes associated with the menstrual cycle are estimated to occur in half of all women. Peak incidence for benign breast changes is between the ages of 40 and 44 years. It is not known if risk factors for developing breast cancer also apply to the development of benign breast disease. Fibroadenomas occur most commonly in premenopausal women with peak incidence before the age of 30 years. Cysts present more often in women age 30 to 50 years, and especially preceding menopause. Assessment of benign breast conditions to rule out breast cancer currently accounts for more than half of all surgical procedures on the female breast.

Etiologic Factors and Pathogenesis

Because benign breast conditions are not one disease entity, etiology is not clearly known. Variations from the normal changes associated with breast development and reproductive life (pregnancy, lactation, involution) form the basis for most benign breast conditions. Nonproliferative tissue nodularity can be generalized, occurring in multiple areas of both breasts. Fibroadenomas are estrogen-sensitive and may be stimulated by pregnancy, lactation, and perimenopause. Cystic changes can be minimal without producing a discrete mass or can produce cysts up to 5 cm.

Hormonal factors, such as the use of postmenopausal hormones or a family history of breast cancer, can increase the risk of benign breast conditions.[85,169] The timing of certain lifestyle factors may be important in the development of benign breast conditions. Although alcohol use in adulthood does not appear to impact risk of benign breast conditions, regular alcohol consumption (7 drinks per week) during adolescence likely increases risk.[83]

Some types of benign breast conditions are linked to higher breast cancer risk, while others are not (Box 20-5). Benign breast conditions can be divided into three general groups, based on whether the cells are multiplying (proliferative) and whether there are abnormal cells or patterns of cells (atypia):
- *Nonproliferative lesions* do not seem to affect cancer risk
- *Proliferative lesions without atypia* slightly increase cancer risk
- *Proliferative lesions with atypia* raise the risk of cancer

Clinical Manifestations

Nodularity usually presents bilaterally as regular, firm nodules that are mobile and may be described as bubble wrap, small gravel, or small water balloons. Masses associated with nodularity may or may not be painful. Pain, tenderness, or discomfort may occur in association with fluid retention and/or accompany hormonal changes associated with the menstrual cycle such as during the premenstrual phase. Cysts can fluctuate in size with rapid appearance or disappearance. Fibroadenomas are typically solitary lesions around 2 to 4 cm in size when first detected. A typical fibroadenoma is nontender and easily moveable under the skin with well-defined borders.

MEDICAL MANAGEMENT

DIAGNOSIS AND TREATMENT. Detection of these benign lesions is based on physical examination, and imaging

Box 20-5

BENIGN BREAST CHANGES AND RISK FOR DEVELOPING BREAST CANCER

Nonproliferative Lesions

These conditions are not linked with the overgrowth of breast tissue. They do not seem to affect breast cancer risk, or if they do, the effect is very small.

- Fibrosis
- Cysts
- Mild hyperplasia of the usual type
- Adenosis (nonsclerosing)
- Phyllodes tumor (rare; usually benign)
- A single (solitary) papilloma
- Granular cell tumor
- Fat necrosis
- Mastitis
- Duct ectasia
- Benign lumps or tumors (lipoma, hamartoma, hemangioma, hematoma, neurofibroma, adenomyoepithelioma)
- Squamous and apocrine metaplasia
- Epithelial-related calcifications

Proliferative Lesions Without Atypia

These conditions are linked with the growth of cells in the ducts or lobules of the breast tissue. They seem to raise a woman's risk of breast cancer slightly (1.5-2 times the usual risk).

- Moderate or florid ductal hyperplasia of the usual type (without atypia)
- Fibroadenoma
- Sclerosing adenosis
- Multiple papillomas or papillomatosis
- Radial scar

Proliferative Lesions with Atypia

These conditions are linked with the excess growth of cells in the ducts or lobules of the breast tissue, and the cells no longer look normal. They can raise breast cancer risk about 3.5 to 5 times higher than normal.

- Atypical ductal hyperplasia
- Atypical lobular hyperplasia

Lobular Carcinoma in Situ

This condition raises breast cancer risk 7 to 11 times that of normal.

Data from American Cancer Society: How noncancerous breast conditions affect breast cancer risk. Available online at http://www.cancer.org/healthy/findcancerearly/womenshealth/non-cancerousbreast-conditions/non-cancerous-breast-conditions-benign-br-cond-and-br-cancer-risk. Accessed July 22, 2014.

such as mammography, ultrasound, and MRI. Because benign breast conditions are often indistinguishable from carcinomas, biopsy is often used to confirm the diagnosis. Breast ultrasound helps to differentiate cystic fluid-filled masses from solid masses. The presence of nodularity does not predispose a woman to cancer but may make diagnosis of cancerous lumps more difficult.

Treatment for benign breast conditions often takes a back seat to ruling out cancer. Palliative treatments may include aspirin, mild analgesics, and local heat or cold. Dietary changes may be recommended, including salt restriction (especially during the second half of the menstrual cycle), low fat or Mediterranean diet, and avoiding caffeine and other stimulants containing methylxanthines, which are found in coffee, chocolate, tea, and many soft drinks and energy drinks. Current research has not shown that the use of stimulants have a significant impact on symptoms.[26]

Other recommendations with anecdotal support include evening primrose oil, use of diuretics, and vitamin and mineral supplementation (vitamins A, B_6, D, E, calcium, and magnesium). The use of hormones, including oral contraceptives, tamoxifen, and androgens, as well as pain medication such as Danocrine (danazol) and Parlodel (bromocriptine) may be prescribed for women with severe symptoms. Women are encouraged to wear a supportive brassiere or to use fabrics that do not irritate the breast skin. In some cases, painful cysts have been aspirated with relief of symptoms.[386,416,427,623]

Breast Cancer

Overview

Breast cancer is the most common malignancy in females in the United States after nonmelanoma skin cancer, and accounts for one-third of all cancers diagnosed in American women. Breasts are made up of glandular milk-producing tissue (ducts and lobules) and stromal or connective tissue. Most breast cancers are adenocarcinomas (glandular) originating in the single layer of epithelial cells that line the ductal and lobular systems of all milk ducts (Fig. 20-8).

Major histopathologic categories of breast cancer (based on morphologic features of the tumor) include *ductal carcinoma in situ* (DCIS); *invasive (infiltrating) ductal carcinoma* (IDC); *invasive (infiltrating) lobular carcinoma* (ILC); *inflammatory breast cancer* (IBC); and *Paget disease of the breast*. Less-common subtypes of IDC include *medullary, tubular, mucinous, papillary*, and *cribriform cancers* of the breast. *Lobular carcinoma in situ* (LCIS) is not considered a true cancer but a precancerous condition with increased risk of developing into cancer. LCIS usually occurs in more than one lobule. *Phyllodes tumor* is usually benign; in rare instances it is a cancer of the breast arising in the stromal tissue. *Sarcomas* are rare cancers that start in connective tissues such as muscle tissue, fat tissue, or blood vessels.

DCIS is the most common type of in situ cancer, and is found in approximately 20% of newly diagnosed breast cancer cases. It develops at several points along a duct and appears as a cluster of microcalcifications or white flecks on a mammogram. DCIS is made up of small areas of atypical cells in an abnormal arrangement confined to the duct of the breast. For this reason, many pathologists do not consider DCIS to be true cancer. DCIS is represented by a broad continuum from slow-growing cells with little potential to be transformed into cancer to cells with more aggressive potential that may invade the duct wall and grow beyond it. It is considered to be stage 0 disease. Diagnosis and treatment of DCIS remains one of the most controversial areas in breast health medicine involving debate about potentially overly aggressive treatment.

IDC is the most common of the invasive breast cancers, originating in a duct, breaking through the duct

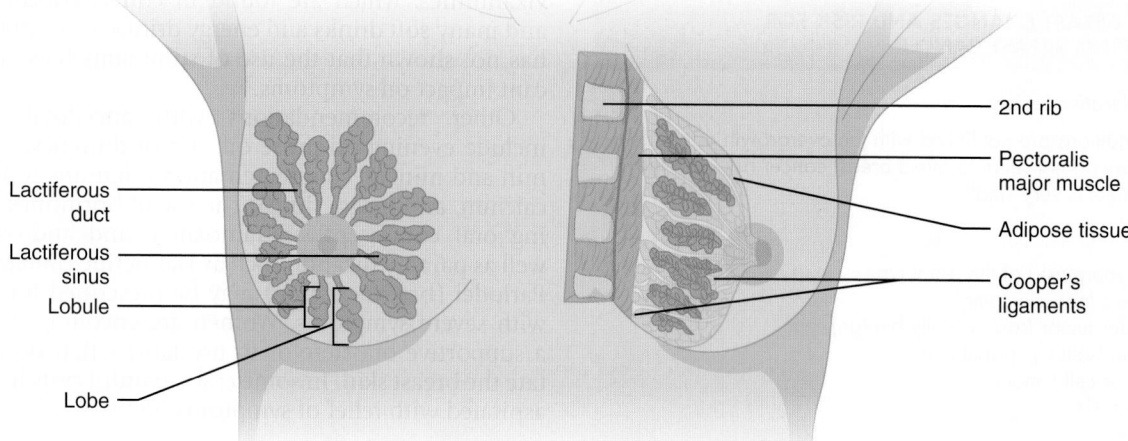

Figure 20-8

Breast anatomy. The breast is made up of glandular tissue, fibrous tissue, including suspensory ligaments, and adipose tissue. Glandular tissue contains 15–20 lobes radiating from the nipple and made up of lobules. Within each lobe are clusters of alveoli that produce milk. Each lobe is embedded in adipose tissue and empties into a lactiferous duct. There are 15–20 lactiferous ducts that form a collecting duct system converging toward the nipple. These ducts form ampullae or lactiferous sinuses behind the nipple, which are reservoirs for storing milk. The lobules and ducts are surrounded by fatty and connective tissue, nerves, blood vessels, and lymphatic vessels. The suspensory ligaments (Cooper ligaments) are fibrous bands extending vertically from the surface attaching to the chest wall muscle. These support the breast tissue and become contracted in cancer of the breast, producing pits or dimples in the overlying skin. (From Jarvis C: *Physical examination and health assessment,* ed 4, Philadelphia, 2004, WB Saunders.)

wall, and invading the stromal tissue of the breast with further possible metastasis via the lymphatic and/or circulatory systems. IDC is usually detected by mammogram or as a palpable lump during a breast examination. IDC represents 70% or more of all invasive breast cancer cases in women and 80% to 90% of all breast cancer cases in men.[386]

ILC is the second most common type of invasive breast cancer making up 5% to 15% of invasive cancers.[406] This type of breast cancer grows through the wall of the lobule and may spread via the lymphatic or circulatory system. ILC cells invade the stroma of the breast in a "single-file" pattern forming a diffuse pattern that can be difficult to detect. ILC has more of a tendency to be multifocal (discontinuous) than IDC, and some studies show that it is slightly more likely to affect both breasts (bilateral cancer).[362] Because of the single-file growth pattern, ILC often is poorly imaged on mammography with the tumor being larger than appears on mammogram or breast ultrasound.[634] Invasive lobular cancers are not typically felt as a lump; instead they may feel like an area of increased thickening or nothing palpated at all.

Medullary, tubular, mucinous, papillary, and cribriform carcinomas are less-common types of ductal carcinoma, together accounting for around 10% of breast cancers. These and other breast cancer variants present clinical challenges; because of their small numbers, treatment algorithms have relied largely on case studies and small series rather than large or randomized trials.[659] Medullary, tubular, and mucinous carcinomas are invasive but tend to have better outcomes than invasive ductal or invasive lobular carcinomas. Papillary and cribriform carcinomas are rare and are usually associated with DCIS.

IBC is a rare (1%-5%)[456] and very aggressive, rapidly progressive form of invasive breast cancer that is not

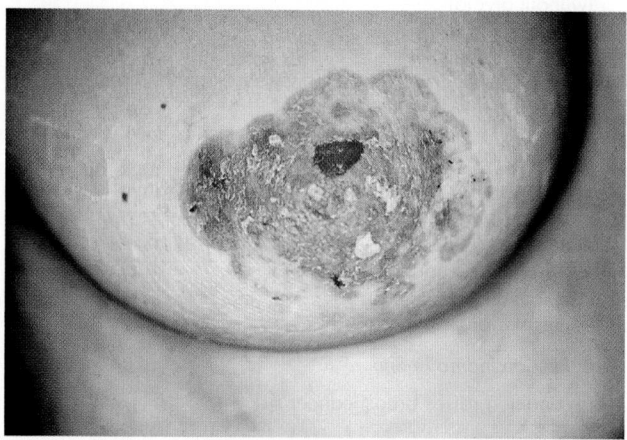

Figure 20-9

Paget disease of the breast. An erythematous plaque surrounds the nipple. (From Bolognia JL: *Dermatology,* St. Louis, 2003, Mosby.)

a true inflammatory process and is not usually associated with fever. In IBC, cancer cells obstruct lymphatic vessels in the breast, causing erythema and edema. IBC presents much like mastitis or cellulitis (see "Clinical Manifestations" below). The lymphatic blockage results in a rapid increase in breast size.[515] Because of its rarity, IBC is often misdiagnosed as mastitis or generalized dermatitis.[515]

Paget disease of the breast is a rare form of ductal carcinoma (1%-3%) that is located beneath the nipple, with itching, tingling, pain, and eczema-like rash; it can progress to crusting, ulceration, and weeping (Fig. 20-9).[272] It is usually unilateral and may involve the areola. Paget disease of the breast often occurs in conjunction with DCIS or invasive cancer. It may be dismissed at first because early symptoms are similar to those caused by some benign skin conditions.

Phyllodes tumors are rare and arise in the stroma as well as the glandular tissue of the breast. They are usually benign, but in rare cases can be malignant.[26]

In some cases, a single breast tumor can be a combination of these types or a mixture of invasive and in situ cancer. Rarely other kinds of cancers can occur in the breast: lymphoma, liposarcoma, angiosarcoma, and melanoma.

Male Breast Cancer. Male breast cancer is a uncommon disease comprising less than 1% of all breast cancers. Breast cancer was previously thought to be biologically similar in both genders, but new studies suggest differences despite the development of the same *types* of breast cancers that are found in women. Studies on men have been limited until recently; early results of a large ongoing study show that the risk of genetic variations is different for men and women.[22] Lobular carcinoma is rare in men because of the absence of lobules in the male breast. Most breast cancers in men are ductal carcinomas, most commonly IDC. Involvement of the skin or chest wall is more common in male breast cancers, possibly because of the relatively small amount of breast tissue.

Newer Classification Systems. It is clear that not all breast cancers are the same; breast cancer is not one disease but many. Different characteristics in clinical biomarkers and gene expression result in a multiplicity of clinical behaviors. More recent classification systems are based on gene profiling assays and immunohistochemical characterization of breast cancers. Assessment includes hormone receptor status, oncogene overexpression (see the discussion of oncogenes in Chapter 9), proliferative capacity, and other features. Currently there are four to five designations for primary molecular subtypes of different breast cancers: luminal A tumors, luminal B tumors, HER2/neu overexpressing tumors, basal-like tumors, and a normal breast-like group.[266,495,633]

Incidence

Breast cancer statistics for detection, mortality, and morbidity continue to improve with significant health focus, and screening and treatment advances. Even so, breast carcinomas still account for approximately 30% of all cancers affecting women in the United States. Additionally, breast cancer is the second largest cause of female cancer deaths in the United States, second only to lung cancer.

There are an estimated 235,030 new cases of breast cancer in women and 2360 in men for 2014. Projections for cancer deaths in 2014 were 40,030 deaths for women and 430 for men.[557] Rates appear to have stabilized with a decrease in newly diagnosed cases from 1999 to 2005 at 2% per year for women age 50 and older.

Etiologic Factors

As in every other cancer, breast cancer begins when something, an *initiator*, causes a gene to mutate. If the cell with the mutated gene survives to divide, it passes on the mutated gene to daughter cells, which, in turn, divide. Because they are abnormal, these cells are more vulnerable than normal cells to further mutations and may eventually become abnormal enough to be considered cancer. The immune system may recognize these cells to be abnormal and destroy them long before this happens.

The development of invasive breast cancer begins with epithelial hyperplasia, premalignant change, and in situ carcinoma, which, in turn, leads to invasive carcinoma. In approximately 80% of breast cancers, estrogen is believed to be a key factor in promoting (rather than initiating) cancer. It may not trigger the series of genetic changes that are required to transform normal breast cells into malignant ones, but it may spur the proliferation of altered cells, increasing the likelihood that they will develop into cancer. See further discussion below in "Diagnosis and Staging: Biomarkers."

In the case of families with a strong history of breast (and often ovarian) cancer in several members with cancer at young ages, the culprit is often one of two mutated genes, altered *BRCA1 or BRCA2* (BReast CAncer) genes. Other genes contribute and researchers are searching for more. *BRCA1* and *BRCA2* are tumor-suppressor genes present in all humans. When working properly, they produce proteins that repair DNA and monitor cell growth. Thus mutations can render these genes inactive, making DNA vulnerable to many kinds of damage such as aging and environmental factors (such as both environmental and medical radiation), that may increase the risk for developing breast, ovarian, and other cancers. Either of these mutated genes can pass at conception from a mother or father to a daughter or son. One abnormal gene confers significant risk of breast cancer for women with the mutation. The onset of breast cancer is at a much earlier age for these individuals as well. Approximately 57% of women with altered *BRCA1* develop breast cancer as do approximately 49% of women with altered *BRCA2*.[138]

Most breast cancers (90%-95%) are not linked to identifiable hereditary factors. Mutations in oncogenes and tumor-suppressor genes involved in cellular growth can be caused by external factors such as radiation, toxins, and other factors yet to be identified.

Risk Factors

Female gender, age, ethnicity, family history (including genetic risk factors) medical history, menstrual history, childbearing history, and environment are all factors linked to breast cancer (Box 20-6). Major risk factors for IBC include young age, high BMI (30 or higher), and white race.[515]

Gender and Hormone Exposure. Being female is the most significant risk factor associated with this disease. Although women have many more breast cells than men, the primary reason they develop breast cancer more often is thought to be related to exposure to the growth-promoting effects of the female hormones estrogen and progesterone. The average lifetime risk for a woman in the United States to develop breast cancer is 12%.[19] Fewer than 1% of breast cancers occur in males. (See discussion under "Risk Factors for Breast Cancer in Males" below).

Endogenous estrogen exposure throughout life, including in utero, may have an effect on breast cancer risk. The length of a woman's total number of reproductive years, including an early onset of menstruation (before age 12 years), and later cessation (menopause; after age 55 years) may affect breast cancer risk. Results from the Collaborative Group on Hormonal Factors in Breast Cancer

Box 20-6

FACTORS THAT INCREASE THE RELATIVE RISK OF BREAST CANCER IN WOMEN*

Relative Risk Factor; R > 4.0

- Age (65+ years vs. younger than 65 years, although risk increases across all ages until age 80 years)
- Biopsy-confirmed atypical hyperplasia or lobular carcinoma in situ
- Certain inherited genetic mutations for breast cancer (*BRCA1* and/or *BRCA2*)
- Dense breasts (as seen on mammography)
- Personal history of breast cancer

Relative Risk Factor; R = 2.1–4.0

- High endogenous estrogen or testosterone levels
- High bone density (postmenopausal)
- High-dose radiation to chest (younger than age 30 years, including treatment for Hodgkin lymphoma)
- Two first-degree relatives with breast cancer (mother, sister, daughter)

Relative Risk Factor; R = 1.1–2.0

- Alcohol consumption
- Ashkenazi Jewish heritage
- Early menarche (younger than 12 years)
- Height (tall)
- High socioeconomic status
- Late age at first full-term pregnancy (older than 30 years)
- Late menopause (older than 55 years)
- Never breastfed a child
- No full-term pregnancies (nulliparity)
- Obesity (postmenopausal) or adult weight gain
- One first-degree relative with breast cancer
- Personal history of endometrium, ovary, or colon cancer
- Recent and long-term use of menopausal hormone therapy containing estrogen and progestin
- Recent oral contraceptive use

*See also Box 20-5: Benign Breast Changes and Risk for Developing Breast Cancer.

See also the *Breast Cancer Risk Assessment Tool* (http://www.cancer.gov/bcrisktool/), an interactive tool developed by the National Cancer Institute (NCI) and the National Surgical Adjuvant Breast and Bowel Project (NSABP) for health professionals to assess a woman's risk of developing invasive breast cancer. The tool has been updated to include African American, Asian American, and Pacific Islander American women based on the Contraceptive and Reproductive Experiences Study (CARE) and the Asian American Breast Cancer Study (AABC).

Data from American Cancer Society. Breast Cancer Facts and Figures, 2011-2012. Available online at http://www.cancer.org/acs/groups/content/@epidemiologysurveillance/documents/document/acspc-030975.pdf. Accessed July 25, 2014.

suggest the effects of menarche and menopause may be increased by other risk factors such as obesity, with lobular cancers appearing to be more affected than ductal cancers by endogenous ovarian hormones.[157]

Eighty percent of all women diagnosed with breast cancer will have estrogen receptor–positive *(ER-positive)* biometrics. Tumors that are ER-positive have ERs and are stimulated to grow by estrogen. Estrogen attaches to the receptor molecule and activates genes that promote cell growth. Tumors that do not have ERs are called *ER-negative* and are not influenced by the hormone.

Previous history of first-generation hormonal contraceptive use (higher dose formulations before 1975) and more recent prolonged use of combined HRT (estrogen-progestin) have been linked with increased risk of breast cancer, often found at a more advanced stage. According to the National Institute of Cancer, there is solid evidence, that combination HRT is associated with an increased risk of developing breast cancer. In the WHI trial, there was a 26% increase in incidence of invasive breast cancer associated with combined HRT. For estrogen-only therapy, the evidence for association with breast cancer incidence is mixed.[139,454]

The role of estrogen in the development and progression of some breast cancers directs investigation into potential contributions from chemicals in the environment with estrogenic activity that can enter the human breast. A range of organochlorine pesticides and polychlorinated biphenyls possess estrogen-mimicking properties that have been measured in human breast adipose tissue and in human milk. These may enter the breast from contamination of food, water, and air. The role of these chemicals in promoting breast cancer is not yet definitively known.[178,179,608]

Age. Age is the second most significant risk factor for the development of breast cancer; incidence increases with advancing age. The cumulative lifetime risk of developing breast cancer for women in the United States is 1 in 8 (or 12%-13%) based on an 80-year life span. At age 25 years the risk of developing breast cancer is quite low: 1 in 1681, with increasing risk as a woman ages. From age 30 to 39 years, the absolute risk is 1:227, or 0.44%; from age 40 to 49 years the absolute risk is 1:67, or 1.5%; from age 50 to 59 years the risk is 1:36, or 2.8%; and from age 60 to 69 years the risk is 1:26, or 3.8%. Ninety-five percent of all new cases of breast cancer occur in women age 40 years and older; approximately 2 of 3 (of all) breast cancers occur in women older than age 55 years. The median age at which a woman in the United States is diagnosed with breast cancer is 61 years.[21] There are currently an estimated 2.75 million breast cancer survivors in the United States.

Women older than age 75 years are the most rapidly growing demographic of newly diagnosed breast cancers.[567] Further research is needed to improve outcomes for women in this age group. The number of complicating comorbidities will likely be a factor in the diagnosis and treatment in this age group.[448]

Diet, Weight Gain, and Obesity. Plant-rich diets versus consuming animal products may lower breast cancer risk, specifically for ER-negative breast cancers. Women whose diets most resembled the DASH diet (Dietary Approaches to Stop Hypertension), which emphasizes vegetables, fruits, fiber-rich grains, legumes, nuts, low-fat dairy, and low in refined carbohydrates, found a significant decrease in risk for developing ER-negative breast cancers.[225]

BMI, a known breast cancer risk factor, could influence breast risk through pathways related to sex hormones, insulin resistance, chronic inflammation, and altered levels of adipose-derived hormones. Current evidence shows the relationship between excess body weight and breast cancer risk to be somewhat mixed. A slightly lower risk of breast cancer has been found in overweight premenopausal women. However postmenopausal weight gain in is considered to be a significant risk factor.[505,593] Estrogen manufactured in adipose tissue may make the hormone available even when ovarian production stops at menopause. There is evidence to suggest that fat cells in different parts of the body metabolize differently. For example, central obesity (excess fat in the waist area) may affect risk more than the same amount of fat in the hips and thighs. Elevated serum insulin levels have been linked to some cancers, including breast cancer.[232] Individuals with lifelong obesity (from childhood) seem to have less risk for developing breast cancer.[17,354]

Personal History, Family History, and Heredity. A personal history of breast cancer in one breast increases a woman's risk of developing a new cancer in the other breast or in another part of the same breast three- to fourfold.[17] This is not the same as a cancer recurrence of the first cancer; it is a new cancer. Additionally, women with a personal history of uterine and ovarian cancer or a family history of breast cancer among first-degree relatives have a significantly increased risk of developing breast cancer. Benign breast disease when accompanied by proliferative changes, increases the risk of cancer (see Box 20-5).

Some breast cancers may be caused by inherited gene mutations. Hereditary breast cancers account for approximately 5% to 10% of all breast cancers,[17] with most of those related to altered *BRCA1* or *BRCA2* gene. Normally, these genes suppress cancer by making proteins that prevent cells from growing abnormally. Inheriting either mutated gene from a parent results in a significantly increased risk of breast cancer for members of some families with *BRCA* mutations.[422] Cancer in this population tends to develop at an earlier age and with a higher rate of bilateral disease than do non-*BRCA* carriers. They also have an increased risk for developing ovarian and pancreatic cancer.[422] Specific mutations of *BRCA1* and *BRCA2* are more common in women of Ashkenazi Jewish ancestry. Male carriers of *BRCA2* mutations are also at increased risk for breast cancer.[484] Other genes under investigation include growth factor receptor genes and oncogene overexpression (e.g., *ATM*, *TP53*, *CHEK2*, *PTEN*, *CDH1*, and *STK11*).

Although only a small percentage of breast cancer cases are hereditary, approximately 15% of women with breast cancer have a close blood relative with this disease. Conversely, most women (more than 85%) who are diagnosed with breast cancer do not have a family history of this disease.[17] Having one first-degree relative (mother, sister, or daughter) with breast cancer doubles a woman's risk; breast cancer in two or more first-degree relatives (mother, sister, daughter) increases the risk about threefold. Although the exact risk is not known, women with a family history of breast cancer in a father or brother also have an increased risk of breast cancer.[17]

Race/Ethnicity. Racial disparities in the United States exist between groups of women developing and dying from breast cancer.[649] White women have a higher rate of developing breast cancer than any other racial or ethnic group except for African American women younger than age 40 years. During 1999–2006, breast cancer incidence rates among white and Asian American/Pacific Islander women declined slightly, while the rates among African American, Hispanic/Latina, and American Indian/Alaska Native women remained stable. According to the latest statistics, African American women and Hispanic/Latina women are more likely to be diagnosed with large tumors than are white women. African American women have the highest cancer mortality rate, with a 5-year survival rate of 79%. The 5-year survival rate for white women and Asian women was 91%; rate for Hispanic/Latina and Pacific Islander it was 86%, and among American Indian/Alaska Native the rate was 84%.[20,23,24] Black men are at almost twice the risk dying from breast cancer than white men.

Genetic mutations among specific people groups have been studied extensively among Ashkenazi Jews and other people groups. These studies have helped to identify both genetic and environmental contributors to the development of breast cancer.

Radiation Exposure. Exposure to ionizing radiation is a risk factor for the development of cancer. In 2004, the National Toxicology Program classified x-rays and gamma rays as known human carcinogens. X-rays, gamma rays, and materials and processes that emit x-rays and gamma rays are used in the nuclear power industry, the military, medicine, scientific research, and in a variety of consumer products. Biologic damage by ionizing radiation is related to dose and dose rate.[310,463] Previous radiation therapy to the chest area as treatment for another cancer (such as Hodgkin disease or non-Hodgkin lymphoma) has been shown to be a significant risk for breast cancer in women. The risk varies with the individual's age when she had the radiation, the dose received, and the size of the radiation field. The risk of developing breast cancer from chest radiation is highest if the radiation was given during adolescence (during the time of breast development). There seems to be evidence of lowering secondary cancer risk with the addition of chemotherapy at the time of radiation therapy. Radiation treatment after age 40 years does not seem to increase breast cancer risk.[28] The secondary cancer risk to females seems to increase 10 years after the initial diagnosis and treatment of Hodgkin disease; it is recommended that these individuals be followed for 40 years or longer.[282,295,444,596]

Alcohol. The use of alcohol is linked to an increased risk of developing breast cancer,[155,329,376,423] particularly in hormonally sensitive cancers (ER-positive) and invasive lobular carcinoma. The risk increases with the amount of alcohol consumed; there appears to be a dose–response relationship over time.[140] Compared with nondrinkers, women who consume three to six alcoholic drinks a week over a long period of time have an increased risk for invasive breast cancer by a small but statistically significant amount. Breast cancer risk increases with as few as three drinks per week and each daily drink increases breast cancer risk by approximately 12%. Thus, compared to a woman who does not drink, a woman who has one drink a day has an increased breast cancer risk of approximately 12%.[106,140,449] Heavy alcohol consumption (three or more drinks per day) is associated with a 40% to 50% increased relative risk compared with not drinking at all.[140,377]

Several mechanisms have been proposed. Alcohol consumption is shown to increase levels of endogenous estrogens. This hypothesis is further supported by data showing that the alcohol–breast cancer association is limited to women with ER-positive tumors. Elevated blood concentration of acetaldehyde (a reactive metabolite of alcohol) is known to be toxic and hypothesized to cause DNA modifications that lead to cancer.[160] The effects of alcohol may be mediated through the production of prostaglandins, lipid peroxidation, and the generation of free radicals influencing hormone levels and ERs. Alcohol also acts as a solvent, enhancing penetration of carcinogens into cells.

Other Environmental Factors and Factors in Question. There is strong evidence that exposure to tobacco smoke increases breast cancer risk.[308,507] Exposure to acrylamide in food (high levels found in potato chips, French fries, and other food products produced by high temperature cooking) and its association with breast cancer is currently under investigation.[355,381] Other topics of research include work at night,[420,509] lack of sleep, DES daughters,[290] exposure to agricultural pesticides and herbicides,[95] radiofrequency fields,[269] and radiation exposure from accidents at nuclear power plants.[267] Scientific research thus far has been unable to establish a direct link between breast cancer and electromagnetic fields; silicone breast implants; abortion or miscarriage[281,305]; or chemicals in antiperspirants, deodorants, cosmetics or hair dyes.

Risk Factors for Breast Cancer in Males

Age and heredity are the most common risk factors for breast cancer in males, with a mean age of 67 years at the time of detection.[206] Men who inherit altered *BRCA1* or *BRCA2* genes have an increased risk for male breast cancer at a rate that is 80 times greater than those without these genetic abnormalities. An altered *BRCA2* gene is found in 40% of all male breast cancers. Because of this strong association, first-degree relatives (siblings, parents, and children) of a man diagnosed with breast cancer may desire genetic testing for *BRCA1* and *BRCA2*.

Men diagnosed with early-stage breast cancer have a lower 5-year survival rate than women diagnosed with early-stage disease, with a mean survival rate of 6 years. In a 2012 analysis of 13,000 male breast cancer cases, a higher percentage of individuals were African American than other ethnicities and they were diagnosed at an older age than were females. Males had larger tumors, higher grade tumors, and were more likely to have lymph node metastasis, including distant metastasis. They were less likely to have lobular carcinoma but more likely to have cancers that were ER-positive and progesterone receptor (PR)–positive. Males and females with advanced breast cancer at diagnosis were found to have an equivalent survival rate.[256]

Other established risk factors for male breast cancer include high estrogen exposure,[22] Klinefelter syndrome, and chest radiation before age 30 years (≥20 Gy). Men can have high estrogen levels because of taking hormonal medications, treatment with immunosuppressant medications after organ transplantation, obesity, estrogen exposure in the environment[540] (military service, estrogen-fed beef, or dichlorodiphenyltrichloroethane [DDT]

exposure), heavy alcohol use and liver disease. Nevertheless, when a man discovers a breast lump, it is usually unilateral gynecomastia, which can occur at any age and can be associated with medication for heart disease, hypertension, or with cannabis use. Men do not develop cysts or fibroademomas.[386]

Protective Factors

Factors that are considered protective against acquiring breast cancer include strenuous exercise more than 4 hours a week,[454] younger age at first livebirth, multiparity (more than 2 births), and breastfeeding[114,156] longer than 5 months.[161,628] (The relative rate of breast cancer decrease has been cited at 4.3% for every 12 months of breastfeeding, in addition to 7%-11% for each birth.)[612] See "Prevention" below.

Pathogenesis

Understanding the pathogenesis of cancer in general and breast cancer specifically is an evolving discipline (see "Cancer Pathogenesis" in Chapter 9). Gene mutations are the proximate cause of cancer, but according to ongoing inquiry mutations alone are not enough to explain the development of breast cancer. Most carcinomas develop in the glandular epithelium of the terminal duct lobular unit. In the normal breast, the milk ducts and lobules are neatly lined with epithelial cells. In the complex, multistep process that leads to the development of cancer, an overproduction (*hyperplasia*) of normal-looking cells progresses to abnormal-looking cells (*atypical ductal hyperplasia or atypical lobular hyperplasia*). When premalignant change or "cancer" cells multiply but remain contained within the duct, the condition is termed DCIS. IDC occurs when cancer cells break through the duct wall and enter other tissues. ILC occurs when cancer cells in the lobules break through to invade the stroma.

Clinical Manifestations

Eighty percent to 90% of breast masses that are large enough to palpate are discovered by the woman herself. In males, the lump is usually centrally located behind the areola; in women, the typical presentation is central behind the areola or in the upper, outer quadrant, although neoplasm can occur anywhere in the breast tissue (Fig. 20-10). Because of the single file development of lobular cancers, areas of increased tissue density may be felt rather than a lump.

Palpable masses tend to be firm and irregular and painless if it is a carcinoma versus smooth and rubbery if it is benign. Fixation of the breast to the underlying pectoral muscles and chest wall can cause significant asymmetry (Fig. 20-11). Other manifestations include a change in breast contour or texture, nipple discharge and retraction or inversion, local skin dimpling (Fig. 20-12), erythema, and/or a local rash or ulceration. Lymphadenopathy may also be the initial presentation of this disease.

IBC is characterized by unilateral breast enlargement, but bilateral involvement is possible. Warmth, redness of the skin with sensation of heat, sudden swelling, itching, pain, skin dimpling called *peau d'orange* (orange peel), and nipple changes (e.g., retraction, flattening, crusting, blistering) are typical. Some women describe the

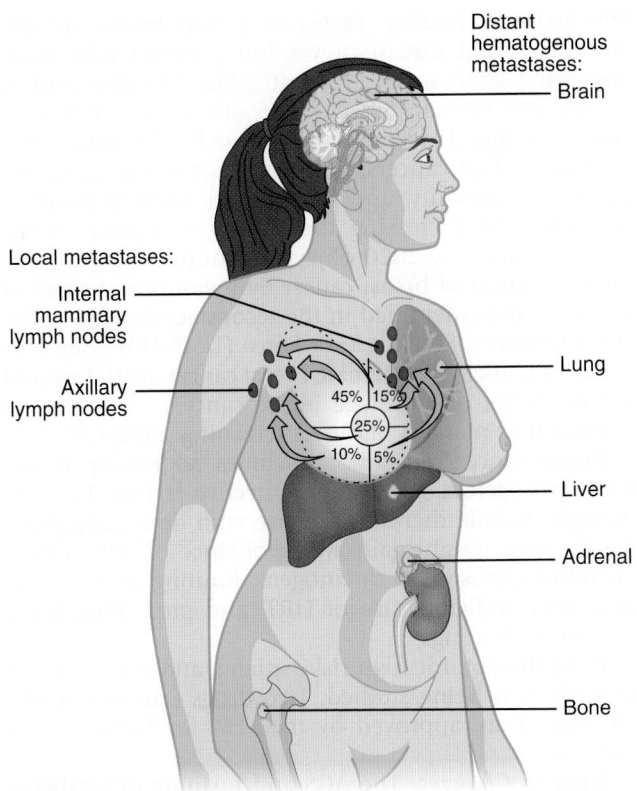

Figure 20-10

The distribution of breast carcinoma and the pathway of lymphatic metastases. Most tumors in women are found in the upper lateral quadrant and behind the nipple (areola) and for men, behind the nipple. (From Damjanov I: *Pathology for the health-related professions*, ed 3, Philadelphia, 2006, WB Saunders.)

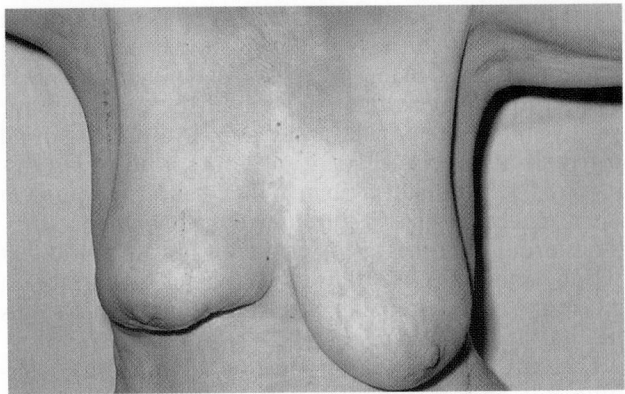

Figure 20-11

Fixation. Asymmetry, distortion, or decreased motility is observed in the woman's right breast as she lifts her arms. As cancer becomes invasive, fibrosis can fix the breast to the underlying pectoral muscle. Although at first glance, it looks as if the woman's left breast is enlarged compared to the right, in fact, the woman's right breast is held against the chest wall. (From Mansel R: *Color atlas of breast diseases*, London, 1995, Mosby.)

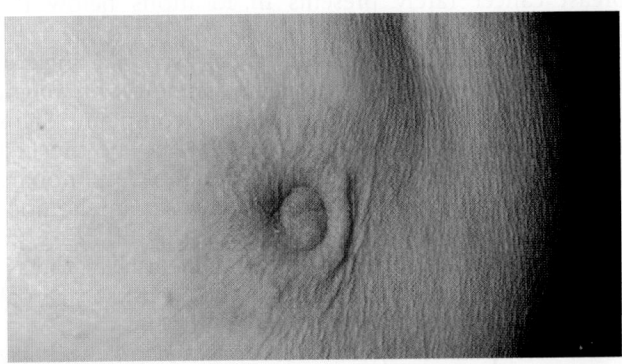

Figure 20-12

Dimpling. The shallow dimple above and slightly to the right of the nipple as viewed in this photograph shows signs of skin retraction or skin tethering. Cancer causes fibrosis, which contracts the suspensory ligaments of the breast, resulting in this clinical change in the breast tissue. The dimpling may be visible at rest, with compression, or with lifting of the arms. The fibrosis can also pull the nipple as seen by the distortion of the areola here. (From Evans AJ: *Atlas of breast disease management: 50 illustrative cases*, Philadelphia, 1998, WB Saunders.)

presentation as a bug bite or as a bruise on the breast that does not go away. Breast color ranges from pink to red to purple, and breasts can feel heavy, thick, and congested. Symptoms can intensify over hours and days. If such symptoms persist beyond the initiation of antibiotic treatment for a breast "infection," then a biopsy is strongly recommended as true mastitis almost always responds to antibiotic therapy. Although a palpable tumor may not be present, lymph node involvement (metastases) to the axillary or supraclavicular lymph nodes is present in 55% to 85% of women at the time of presentation.[515] For an excellent full review of IBC, see reference 675.

Cancer Recurrence. *Local recurrence* means that the cancer has returned to the previously diseased breast in the case of breast conservation, or along the incisional scar in the case of mastectomy. Local recurrence can present in the area of the lumpectomy excision or in an unrelated area of the breast. Recurrence in the scar of a mastectomy usually occurs in the skin and adipose tissue of the removed breast; it rarely includes muscle. As breast cancers continue to be differentiated by molecular subtyping, recurrence rates can be reported more specifically. (See "Biomarkers" below.)

Regional recurrence means that the cancer has now been found in the axillary, supraclavicular or internal mammary lymph nodes. Many studies investigate *locoregional recurrences*. Primary cancer involvement of the lymph nodes may predict those individuals who may be at greater risk of regional recurrence, but women without nodal metastases are still at some risk of cancer recurrence.

When comparing mastectomy alone with breast-conservation therapy (lumpectomy plus radiation therapy) for early stage disease, there is a slight benefit with mastectomy for local control. However, the overall survival rates for individuals who have undergone either procedure are equivalent.[382,561,594]

As breast cancers continue to be differentiated by molecular subtyping, recurrence rates can be reported with more specificity (see "Biomarkers" below). For example, in a 2012 analysis of 15 studies involving more than 12,000 women, those with luminal A subtype (ER+/PR+) tumors exhibited the lowest rates of local recurrence. Individuals with triple-negative and HER2/neu+

breast tumors exhibited a greater risk of local recurrence following breast-conserving therapy or mastectomy.[388]

Metastases. *Distant recurrence* is defined as cancer cells transported elsewhere in the body by the lymphatic system and/or the circulatory system. If cancer is found in lymph nodes elsewhere, it suggests spread of the disease by the lymphatic system. When cancer is found in other organs, it suggests spread by the circulatory system. Metastases from breast neoplasm typically are found first in bone and lungs. With disease progression, liver, brain and spinal cord, adrenal glands, and skin and GI systems may be also involved (see Table 9-2).

The type of breast cancer must be identified to determine not only treatment but to differentiate between cancer recurrence and a new cancer. Local metastases by direct extension of the primary disease site may involve the chest wall, ribs, pleura, pulmonary parenchyma, or bronchi. Erosion of the first and second ribs and associated vertebrae can also occur.[414] Individuals with IBC commonly present with metastases to the axillary or supraclavicular lymph nodes, and in 1 in 3 individuals there is distant metastases.[103] Metastatic spread from breast cancer rarely presents in locations below the elbows and knees.

Symptoms associated with metastases can include upper extremity edema, bone pain, jaundice, or weight loss. These findings are rarely the initial complaint. Signs and symptoms of the affected system may be the first clinical indication of a problem. For example, pulmonary lesions may present as vague, aching chest pain, hemoptysis, or unexplained dyspnea. Bone pain and fracture are the most common symptoms of bone metastases. Metastases to the liver may present as fatigue, jaundice, carpal tunnel syndrome, or skin changes.

Paraneoplastic Syndrome. *Paraneoplastic syndrome* (or *stiff person syndrome*) is a rare syndrome associated with breast cancer (as well as lung, ovarian, and lymphatic cancers). It is believed to be hormonally mediated and caused by tumor cell or immune response to the presence of cancer in the body, but not by the local presence of cancer cells. Sometimes the symptoms of paraneoplastic syndromes are present before the diagnosis of a malignancy. In paraneoplastic neurologic disorders, the central and/or peripheral nervous system may be affected.[180] Symptoms may include progressive symptoms of neuropathy or myelopathy with altered muscle tone. Additional symptoms may include gait ataxia, dizziness, nystagmus, difficulty swallowing, fine motor incoordination, slurred speech, visual disturbances, memory loss and dementia, and seizures.[504] For further discussion, see "Paraneoplastic Syndrome" in Chapter 9.

MEDICAL MANAGEMENT

Health care policy and scientific research on the detection, diagnosis, and treatment of breast cancer is rapidly expanding and changing with monthly and even weekly updates. The information presented here is based on current evidence. The reader is encouraged to keep abreast of new information through helpful internet websites provided for both the consumer and the therapist. A list of these websites is presented in Evolve Box 20-2 on the book's Evolve website.

PREVENTION. *Healthy People* is a nationwide health-promotion and disease-prevention program with comprehensive goals set by the United States Department of Health and Human Services.[4] *Healthy People 2020* supports continued advances in research, detection, and treatment of all cancers; it also reviews trends in cancer incidence, mortality, and survival that identify progress made toward decreasing the impact of cancer in the United States. The 2020 objectives continue to promote early detection of breast cancer by measuring the use of screening tests identified in the recommendations of the U.S. Preventive Services Task Force (USPSTF). They also focus on reducing the female breast cancer death rate and the incidence of late-stage breast cancers,[277] which are intermediate markers of cancer screening success.[457]

Breast cancer prevention includes addressing modifiable risk factors, as well as protective factors. Lifestyle changes include diet and exercise with decreasing postmenopausal weight gain and avoidance of risk factors, including exposure to carcinogens, limiting alcohol consumption, judicious use of HRT, and promoting long-term breastfeeding.

Drug therapy for high-risk patients and precancerous conditions is being studied. Two drugs (tamoxifen and raloxifene) are approved by the FDA for breast cancer prevention.

Lifestyle Changes. The ACS and Institute of Medicine summary of public health recommendations based on prevention of modifiable lifestyle factors includes:

- Avoid unnecessary medical radiation, especially at younger ages.
- Avoid combination menopausal hormone therapy.
- Avoid smoking (especially before first pregnancy).
- Avoid passive smoke.
- Limit alcohol consumption.
- Increase physical activity
- Maintain healthy weight; reduce obesity.
- Limit or eliminate workplace and consumer exposure to chemicals that are plausible contributors to breast cancer risk.
- If at high risk for breast cancer, consider chemoprevention.

Physical Activity and Exercise. Observational epidemiologic evidence consistently suggests that exercise and physical activity have an established effect on breast cancer prevention with an inverse dose–response effect in which risk decreases with increased activity level.[579,617] Studies support an average risk reduction for breast cancer of 25% to 30% in physically active individuals when an "optimum" level of moderate-intensity exercise is achieved for 30 to 60 minutes for 5 days per week.[60,223] Moderate-intensity activity is recommended as opposed to low-intensity activity[251] and activity can be cumulative throughout the day in 10-minute increments.

The National Cancer Institute recommends strenuous exercise for more than 4 hours per week for reducing breast cancer risk. The ACS publishes 5-year guidelines for cancer prevention. The 2010 recommendations for physical activity for cancer prevention in adults include 150 minutes or more of moderate-intensity or 75 minutes of vigorous-intensity activity each week, or an equivalent combination, preferably spread throughout the week.[347]

Examples of strenuous-exercise activity include swimming laps, aerobics/calisthenics, running, and jogging. Examples of moderate activity include brisk walking, golf, and volleyball.[171]

Research shows that in *premenopausal* women, physical activity among the most active women reduces risk by as much as 23%.[580] Possible biologic mechanisms include changes in metabolic and sex hormones, growth factors, adiposity, and immune function. *Postmenopausal* women who maintain a regular moderate-to-vigorous exercise program can reduce their risk for cancer by 20% to 40%.[175,222] In the WHI study of postmenopausal women, 1.25 to 2.0 hours per week of brisk walking was correlated with an 18% risk reduction compared with inactive women; 10 or more hours of exercise activity per week reduced the risk even more.[418] The RENEW (Reach Out to Enhance Wellness) study and the NEW (Nutrition and Exercise for Women) trial reported on the impact of different lifestyle interventions (diet and exercise interventions) on biomarkers that have been linked to breast cancer risk and prognosis.[188,378,379] Postmenopausal, sedentary, overweight women enrolled in the NEW study were randomly assigned to one of four groups: dietary weight loss, exercise alone, dietary weight loss plus exercise, or control.

The primary outcome in early phases of the study[379] was change in levels of sex steroid hormones, which have been linked to breast cancer risk and prognosis. Women randomly assigned to the weight-loss groups experienced significant favorable changes in estrogen, testosterone, sex hormone–binding globulin, insulin, c-peptide, leptin, and adiponectin levels, compared with controls. Individuals randomly assigned to exercise alone experienced smaller but significant changes in estrogen, testosterone, and leptin levels, but not other hormones. Additionally, biomarker change was significantly smaller in the exercise alone group versus the dietary weight loss plus exercise group. However, the degree of weight loss was related to the magnitude of biomarker change in the dietary weight loss alone group, but not in the diet plus exercise group, suggesting that modest weight loss was able to effect the same change in biomarkers as more significant weight loss, when the modest weight loss was combined with exercise.

Diet and Nutrition. There is emerging evidence that healthy dietary patterns may have a role in breast cancer risk reduction. Diets characterized by high intake of fruits and salad are shown to be associated with a slightly lower risk of breast cancer and for hormone receptive-negative breast cancer in particular.[56] There have been conflicting evidence from randomized controlled trials that common dietary recommendations (such as low-fat diets, foods low in glycemic index, and high in dietary fiber, antioxidants, micronutrients, and calcium) have an effect on breast cancer prevention other than limiting weight gain in adulthood and limiting alcohol intake (see below).[75,190,423]

Controlling weight (especially after menopause) is associated with preventing breast cancer, the recurrence of breast cancer, and death from breast cancer. It is known that metabolic syndrome (which is associated with weight gain, central adiposity, elevated serum insulin and glucose levels, and insulin resistance) increases the risk of breast cancer recurrence in postmenopausal women.[120,232] Weight gain after treatment for breast cancer may increase the recurrence rate for breast cancer.[250,378,408,497]

Increased health promotion seeks to address diabetes, prediabetes, and chronic inflammation in reducing breast cancer risk. Because androgens and estrogen are elevated in obesity and are risk factors for postmenopausal breast cancer risk, weight loss may help decrease breast cancer risk in hormonally sensitive cancers by decreasing levels of serum estrogen and free testosterone.[120,250,378,408,497]

Despite conflicting or null findings of dietary interventions in numerous randomized controlled trials, results do not necessarily indicate a lack of effect of dietary factors on breast cancer risk. A combination of dietary factors (rather than single components acting in isolation) may yet show benefit. Current recommendations include approaches that are low in some kinds of fats (such as the Mediterranean diet), high in fruits, vegetables, and whole grain carbohydrates, and low in sugar, alcohol, processed foods and hormone-treated milk, eggs, beef and chicken (or no animal products, strictly a plant-based diet). Many studies are investigating the role of reducing some kinds of dietary fat intake and cholesterol.[359,410] The data seems to support reduced breast cancer risk only when weight loss accompanies a low fat diet. Calcium, vitamin D, dietary fiber, and nut intake in adolescence is another research focus in the development of proliferative benign breast conditions and breast cancer.[591]

There are mixed results from research showing a relationship between high intakes of meat, red meat, processed meat, and meat cooked at high temperatures with increased breast cancer risk. Chemical byproducts (heterocyclic amines and polycyclic aromatic hydrocarbons) occur in or on the surface of well-cooked meat or in smoke, which is produced when fat burns or drips on hot coals. Heterocyclic amines and polycyclic aromatic hydrocarbons are carcinogenic. As a result, recommendations include the reduction of consumption of grilled and smoked meats cooked at high temperatures.[578]

Alcohol. There is good evidence that *restricting* alcohol consumption reduces breast cancer risk.[423] Recommendations regarding acceptable levels of alcohol intake vary from no alcohol at all to less than one drink a day. (One drink equals 12 ounces of beer, 5 ounces of wine, or 1.5 ounces of hard liquor.) There may a difference between consumption of red wine and white wine. Data suggests that red wine acts as a nutritional aromatase inhibitor[556]; this finding may explain why red wine does not appear to increase the risk of breast cancer. More study is needed as this seems to be an area of ongoing debate.[104,352]

Although only a few studies address the effect of drinking alcohol and the risk of recurrence, a 2010 study of women with previously diagnosed early-stage breast cancer, found that drinking even a few alcoholic beverages per week (three to four drinks) increased the risk of breast cancer recurrence. Antioxidant intake, folate, and B_{12}, specifically, may reduce alcohol-associated breast cancer risk.[55,69,299] Consumption of alcohol in adolescence is associated with an increased risk of proliferative benign breast conditions in a dose–response relationship.[104,352]

Childbearing and Breastfeeding. Reproductive factors such as late age at first birth (older than 34 years) and nulliparity are established risk factors for breast cancer. Earlier childbearing, multiple births, and breastfeeding have a protective effect on developing breast cancer. Delayed childbearing, low parity, and no or short duration breastfeeding are increasing social trends in developed countries that are associated with the high incidence of breast cancer in these countries. Parity, early age at first full-term pregnancy, and breastfeeding have been long believed to influence the risk of breast cancer predominantly through hormonal mechanisms that involve estrogen and progesterone. Studies confirm risk reduction for ER+/PR+ (luminal) cancers of 11% per birth.[144,450] This protective effect has also been observed in lobular cancers that are often positive for hormone receptors. Women younger than 20 years of age at first birth demonstrate a 27% lower risk than those in the "oldest age at first birth" category, when adjusted for parity. Reduced risk of ER– PR– cancers has not been correlated with parity or age at first birth. Both ER+PR+ and ER–PR– cancers have shown decreased risk associated with breastfeeding and late age at menarche. Duration of breastfeeding has shown a cumulative effect.[338,392,612]

Hormone Replacement Therapy. The use of HRT should be thoroughly analyzed by individual women and their physicians. The WHI trial of combined estrogen plus progestin HRT was stopped early when health risks, which included invasive breast cancer, outweighed benefits. Not only did researchers find an increased incidence of breast cancers among those women who received relatively short-term combined HRT, but these cancers were diagnosed at a more advanced stage than those who received placebo medication. HRT also increases the percentage of women with abnormal mammograms. These results suggest estrogen plus progestin may stimulate breast cancer growth and hinder breast cancer diagnosis.[144,450]

Chemoprevention. In 2009, the American Society of Clinical Oncology updated its guidelines concerning the use of chemotherapeutic agents for reducing breast cancer risk.[635] It includes specifics on the use of SERM drugs such as tamoxifen, raloxifene, and aromatase inhibitors (AIs). For women at *high risk* of developing breast cancer, treatment with tamoxifen reduces breast cancer by 30% to 50%.[361] Treatment with raloxifene has a similar effect on reduction of invasive breast cancer, but appears to be less effective for prevention of noninvasive tumors. Clinical tools and resources reviewing risks and benefits of breast cancer chemoprevention and summarizing recommendations are available online at http://www.asco.org/guidelines/bcrr.

Other Preventive Measures. The influence of many types of environmental exposures on breast cancer risk requires continued scrutiny. Preventive recommendations with the strongest evidence include avoiding radiation exposure (especially the use of computerized tomography in medical testing), avoiding combined postmenopausal hormone therapy, and avoiding active smoking. Other recommendations may include limiting exposure to passive smoking and other environmental carcinogens in certain consumer products (i.e., bisphenol A, phthalates), industrial chemicals (i.e., benzene, ethylene oxide), and pesticides (i.e., DDT/DDE [dichlorodiphenyldichloroethylene]). More research is needed to establish a conclusive link of these exposures to breast cancer.[308,309,571] Increased vitamin D intake by food or supplementation as well as exposure to the sun (needed by the skin to manufacture vitamin D) may be recommended. Epidemiologic studies suggest an association between vitamin D and calcium intake and breast cancer. Current research reveals a high prevalence of vitamin D deficiency and osteoporosis in individuals with breast cancer.[77]

Disturbed sleep–wake cycle with its disruption of the human circadian cycle and reduced sleep quality has been proposed as contributing to an increased risk of cancer in general and breast cancer specifically. Women in night-time jobs or doing rotating shift work with repeated disruption of the circadian system may be at increased risk of breast cancer.[275] Achieving the recommended 7 to 8 hours of sleep per night is advocated; a recent study found an association of aggressive breast cancers in postmenopausal women who routinely sleep fewer hours.[602]

Prophylactic mastectomy (also referred to as risk-reduction mastectomy) for women with a *BRCA1* or *BRCA2* mutation and positive family history has proved to be extremely effective. However, testing and managing hereditary cancer risk is a complex decision-making process. A decision support tool designed for joint use by women with *BRCA* mutations and their health care providers is available from the Stanford Medicine Cancer Institute online at http://brcatool.stanford.edu/.

SCREENING AND EARLY DETECTION. Discovery of identifiable masses on mammography and ultrasound *before* a palpable lump or nodule is found is the goal of screening technologies. For decades, early detection has been considered the hallmark of effective intervention in cases of breast cancer, with the goal of finding any breast cancer when it is as small as possible. Current evidence indicates that the biology of the individual cancer is also very important. A tiny, very aggressive breast cancer may be able to spread to distant sites before it is large enough to be detected, while a much larger, but slow-growing cancer may present a minimal problem even if it is never detected.[415]

In the past, women were advised to use a combination of three tools: monthly breast self-examination (BSE), clinical breast examination by a qualified health professional, and regular mammography. Routine screening mammograms for women in their 40s and the use of BSE has been challenged in the last few years. Differing guidelines currently exist in the medical community. Box 20-7 presents a summary of the ACS screening recommendations (current as of the writing of this text); the reader is encouraged to look for any updates published over time.

Mammography. Mammography is an x-ray of the breast and is an essential tool for the detection of a lesion before the mass (cancerous or benign) is large enough to be palpable. It can detect very small lesions of 0.5 cm. The term *screening mammography* implies the mammogram is done when there is no palpable lump or any other breast findings that lead to a suspicion of cancer. The role of mammography in reducing breast cancer mortality has been demonstrated in multiple randomized clinical trials.[553] There is good evidence from case-controlled studies and incidence-based mortality studies that screening

Box 20-7

AMERICAN CANCER SOCIETY RECOMMENDATIONS FOR EARLY BREAST CANCER DETECTION IN WOMEN WITHOUT BREAST SYMPTOMS

The ACS recommendations for breast cancer screening for women without breast symptoms are presented below in abbreviated form. Readers should refer to the original full text guideline document to see the complete recommendations, along with the rationale and summary of the evidence (http://www.cancer.org/Cancer/BreastCancer/MoreInformation/BreastCancerEarlyDetection/breast-cancer-early-detection-acs-recs).

Mammography

- Mammography should be done annually beginning at age 40 years. When clinical breast examination (CBE) is done along with mammograms it provides opportunity for women and their health care provider to discuss changes in their breasts, early detection testing, and factors in the woman's history that might make her more likely to have breast cancer.
- Women should be educated about the benefits, limitations, and potential harms associated with regular mammography.
- Mammograms should be continued regardless of a woman's age, as long as she does not have serious, chronic health problems, such as congestive heart failure, end-stage renal disease, chronic obstructive pulmonary disease, and moderate to severe dementia. Age alone should not be the reason to stop having regular mammograms. Women with serious health problems or short life expectancies should discuss with their doctors whether to continue having mammograms.

Clinical Breast Examination

- Beginning at age 20 years, CBE and counseling to raise awareness of breast symptoms; for women ages 20 to 39 years, CBE every 3 years; after age 40 years, CBE and mammogram yearly for asymptomatic women
- CBE should be performed by a qualified medical professional. There is increasing evidence that primary care providers and gynecologists have a need to improve their CBE skills instead of just relying on imaging studies.[249]

Additional screening (e.g., starting annual mammography at a younger age and/or at closer intervals, or adding magnetic resonance imaging or ultrasound examination to mammography screening) may be recommended for women with any of the following:

- Previous personal history of breast cancer
- History of chest wall radiation between the ages of 10 and 30 years
- Documented genetic mutation (*BRCA1* or *BRCA2*)
- Strong positive family history with first-degree relative (parent, brother, sister, or child) with *BRCA1* or *BRCA2* gene mutation and not having had genetic testing themselves
- High-risk benign pathology (ductal carcinoma in situ, lobular carcinoma in situ or atypical ductal hyperplasia, or atypical lobular hyperplasia
- Very dense breast tissue on mammography

Breast Self-Examination

Current recommendations regarding BSE are somewhat controversial (see text discussion). BSE is an option for women starting in their 20s. Women should be told about the benefits and limitations of BSE. Women should report any breast changes to their health professional right away. Women who choose to use a step-by-step approach to BSE should have their BSE technique reviewed during their physical exam by a health professional

Summary of New ACS Guidelines

- CBE every 3 years for women ages 20 to 39 years
- Annual CBE every year for asymptomatic women ages 40 years and older
- BSE occasionally or not at all; women ages 20 years and older should be educated about the benefits and limitations of the BSE
- Mammogram annually from age 40 years

Data from American Cancer Society (2011): Breast Cancer: Early Detection. Available online with further discussion at: http://www.cancer.org/Cancer/BreastCancer/MoreInformation/BreastCancerEarlyDetection/breast-cancer-early-detection-acs-recs

---

mammography in women age 50 to 75 years decreases breast cancer mortality by 38% to 70%.[498] For women age 39 to 49 years, the risk can be reduced by 15%.[465] For women older than age 70, there is less robust evidence. A recent U.S. study found that 84 women between the ages of 40 and 84 years need to be screened annually to save 1 life from breast cancer and 5.3 need to be screened annually to gain 1 life-year from breast cancer.[283]

The value of routine screening mammography was questioned in 2009 when the USPSTF recommended that routine screening mammograms for women with an average risk of breast cancer should start at age 50 years instead of age 40 years. The recommended changes were very controversial and amended. The guidelines are available online at http://www.annals.org/content/151/10/716.full. Since the USPSTF recommendations, studies are finding that screening mammography rates for women ages 40 to 49 years have declined by almost 6% (when comparing mammogram rates before and after the USPSTF recommendations on a sample size of nearly 8 million women ages 40-64 years).[1,10]

For women between the ages of 40 and 50 years, screening should be based on a shared discussion between women and their health care providers, taking into account personal circumstances and preferences. Many groups recommend that screening mammography for women at average risk of breast cancer should start at age 40 years. Among these groups are the American Medical Association, the American College of Obstetricians and Gynecologists, the American College of Radiology, the ACS, the National Cancer Institute, the National Comprehensive Cancer Network, the Mayo Clinic, the National Breast Cancer Foundation, and Susan G. Komen for the Cure. Cancers found in this age group are more commonly found at earlier stages and with less lymph node involvement. Excluding women in this age group could also impact early diagnosis of more aggressive cancers which may found disproportionately in nonwhite populations (African Americans, Latina/Hispanic, Asian/Pacific Islanders).[43,405]

For younger women who are at *high risk* for developing breast cancer the ACS recommends yearly mammograms and ultrasound or MRI (see "Imaging Technology" below). In these cases, addressing the biology of the cancer is paramount. For most of these women, screening should begin at age 30 years and continue for as long as the woman is in good health.[18,82] For *all* high-risk women, earlier initiation of screening, screening at shorter intervals, and screening with additional modalities, such as ultrasound and MRI, may be advised.[82]

The cost-effectiveness and efficacy of screening mammography in women ages 75 years and older also have come under scrutiny. It has been suggested that the small gain in life expectancy is a variable that should be considered. Decisions should be based on the overall health status of each individual woman.

There are limitations in the use of mammography in women with dense breast tissue. Radiologists have long known that there is decreased sensitivity of mammography in women with dense breasts and an increased risk of developing breast cancer in women with dense breasts. This information has not been routinely communicated to women in a mammography report.[234] Slightly more than 50% of women undergoing screening mammography can be classified as having dense breasts. A 2010 survey concluded that 95% of women older than age 40 years did not know their breast density, and almost 90% were unaware that increased breast density increases their risk of breast cancer.[271,298] Notification requirements of breast density (currently enacted in some states and proposed at the federal level) present implementation challenges. These include concerns about variation in the use of additional imaging technologies (usually ultrasound) and lack of uniform standards in the interpretation of breast densities, which may result in unnecessary surgical procedures with emotional, physical, and financial implications. Consumer advocacy for more reporting information may result in earlier detection of breast cancer in women with dense breasts.[44,296]

When a lump or other breast complaint is investigated or a mammogram is read as positive, then the study requested is a *diagnostic mammogram* (as opposed to a screening mammogram). It is a problem-solving mammogram, which may involve additional views of the breast. Suspicious findings are usually followed by evaluation with high-frequency ultrasound and/or stereotactic biopsy.

For women with breast implants, additional mammography screening, called an *implant displacement view* may be requested.

Clinical Breast Examination. See Box 20-7.

Breast Self-Examination. Although mammography has been the main focus of breast cancer detection, almost half of breast cancers found in women ages 50 to 69 years are found by the women themselves or their clinicians.[522] But because current research shows that a formal BSE plays a small role in finding breast cancer, the ACS no longer recommends that all women conduct regular BSEs (see Box 20-7). Breast cancer detection is more commonly associated with an incidental discovery of a breast lump or increased awareness of what is "normal" for an individual. Such discovery may be just as effective as a formal regimen.[91] The ACS has chosen to advise women that BSE is an "optional" screening tool. However, many experts still advocate monthly BSEs performed 1 week after menstrual bleeding begins, or in postmenopausal women, consistently on the same day each month.

The American College of Obstetricians and Gynecologists (ACOG) advocates performing BSE as one way to increase a woman's breast cancer awareness. Most breast cancer advocacy groups (e.g., The Mayo Clinic, the American Medical Association, the ACOG, the American College of Radiology, the ACS, the National Cancer Institute, and the National Comprehensive Cancer Network) recommend that women become familiar with their breasts by *any method* beginning at late puberty or in their 20s. If a woman chooses to perform BSE, she should learn the correct procedure from a qualified health care professional (including physical therapists)[246,247] who can evaluate her technique. Instruction in breast awareness/self-examination is available online at www.Komen.org, www.breastcancer.org, and www.cancer.org.

Genetic Testing. Genetic testing is recommended for selected individuals; it is not advisable for everyone with a breast cancer diagnosis. Inherited mutations of *BRCA1* or *BRCA2* increase the lifetime risk of breast (and ovarian) cancer; however, having an inherited gene mutation does not mean breast cancer is inevitable, even though first mutation has occurred by conception. Women who have a positive family history of breast cancer before the age of 40 years may want to seek genetic counseling. Testing may be advised for anyone with a family history described previously in "Risk Factors" above.

Genetic testing which results in a negative test for a mutation may be difficult to interpret if the family history is unknown. Coping with the results if they are positive and weighing all the options can be challenging.[146] Although most states have genetic privacy laws to prevent discrimination by health insurers, the guidelines do not always apply to life or disability insurance. Testing is done by a simple blood test, but the test may be expensive and is not always covered by health insurance.

Imaging Technology. Imaging has become increasingly important in the process of diagnosis of all breast problems; even biopsies are often image-directed. The use of imaging technology for screening versus diagnosis must be distinguished. Diagnosis requires a biopsy analysis. As described previously, mammography is an essential technology for detecting lesions that are too small to palpate and in aiding analysis of suspect lesions.

Studies have shown that the addition of screening ultrasound or MRI to mammography in women at increased risk of breast cancer results in a higher yield of cancer detection.[16,82] The false-negative rate of mammography alone ranges from 25% to 59%.[384a] *High risk* is defined as a 20% or higher chance of developing breast cancer over the course of a lifetime (as opposed to the average lifetime risk for a woman in the United States of 12%-13%.) Persons in the high-risk group include women who have received radiation treatment to the chest between ages 10 and 30 years (e.g., for Hodgkin disease); women who are prone to breast cancer because of the presence of genetic mutations, such as *BRCA1* or *BRCA2*; and those whose mothers, fathers, sisters, brothers, daughters, or sons carry those mutations. Other groups that may meet the definition of high risk include a personal history of breast cancer, previous atypical biopsy, dense breasts (more than 50%) and those with elevated risk by criteria of the Gail or Claus models (see also the Breast Cancer Risk Assessment Tool [http://www.cancer.gov/bcrisktool/]).[81,82,101,371]

Digital Mammography. Digital mammography has a number of advantages over conventional film-screen mammography and most radiology departments in Western countries are making the conversion. Benefits of digital mammography include the ability to electronically store and digitally enhance images. Images can also be electronically transmitted to specialists elsewhere for consultation. Studies show that digital mammography is equal or slightly superior to film-screen mammography in detecting and describing abnormalities.[274,297]

Ultrasound. Ultrasonography is primarily used to differentiate a cyst from a solid lesion. It is used to help interpret a mammogram and aids in the detection of cancers that may not show on mammography (mammography-occult). Ultrasound is being used more frequently to image dense breast tissue. Breast tissue density refers to the fibroglandular composition (as opposed to fatty tissue) of the breast. High density of breast tissue is a significant and independent risk factor for breast cancer and also reduces the sensitivity of mammography, as glandular tissue masks cancer on the mammogram. It is estimated that in women with dense breasts, as high as 35% of breast cancers go undetected by mammogram. The National Cancer Institute estimates that approximately 40% of women undergoing screening mammography have dense breasts (67% of premenopausal women and 25% of postmenopausal women).[101] These women have an increased risk of breast cancer, with detection usually at a more advanced stage. However, a recent study showed that those individuals with breast cancer and dense breasts did not have increased risk of death.[234] The FDA approved the first ultrasound imaging system for women with dense breast tissue in 2012. The somo-v Automated Breast Ultrasound System (ABUS) is intended for use in combination with standard mammography in women with dense breast tissue who have a negative mammogram and no symptoms of breast cancer.[621]

Magnetic Resonance Imaging. MRI is an imaging technology that uses powerful magnetic field and radio waves to create images of the breast. Breast MRI has been approved the FDA since 1991 as a supplement to mammography in detecting and staging breast cancer. MRI is a highly sensitive test for breast cancer and may reveal cancers missed by both mammography and ultrasound screening. However, because the cost associated with MRI is high (10 times the cost of a mammogram), MRI is not used for women at average risk for breast cancer for routine screening. Sensitivity is good, detecting 94% to 95% of invasive cancers when used in conjunction with mammogram, but specificity varies widely (30%-90%) with frequent false positives. MRIs are used more specifically for women with a high risk of breast cancer. They are also useful in determining the extent of disease or presence of multifocal (or multicentric) tumors, and in detecting the presence of contralateral disease.[366] MRIs may be employed for individuals with a proven history of breast cancer and in cases where conventional imaging presents difficulties, such as those with invasive lobular

carcinoma, or when dense breast tissue[37] precludes an accurate mammographic and physical assessment.

Breast cancer can remain dormant for years before becoming clinically apparent, so long-term follow-up is mandatory for all women, especially anyone with a previous history of breast cancer.[113] Improvement in breast cancer screening technology such as 3D mammography is a current research focus. Other investigators seek a more precise, noninvasive screening technique that does not involve the use of radiation. The use of minimally invasive tests that seek out biologic markers in blood, urine, and other fluids before a tumor develops is needed.

Ductal Lavage. *Ductal lavage* is one such method of collecting breast epithelial cells from breast duct fluid for cytologic examination. Ductoscopy (or endoscopy) has been found to be a useful diagnostic adjunct for individuals with pathologic nipple discharge. Its role in the early detection or management of breast cancer requires further investigation.

Elastography. *Elastography* is a noninvasive method in which soft-tissue stiffness or strain images are used to detect or classify tumors. Elastography is currently being used with ultrasound, but some research studies are using magnetic resonance elastography and CT. Use of ultrasound elastography may reduce unnecessary biopsies.[332,537]

Thermography. *Thermography* is a tool that records the temperature of the breasts by measuring infrared radiation emitted. Theoretically, cancerous tissue has a higher temperature than normal tissue as a result of increased vascularity and a higher metabolic rate of the cancerous cells. Although thermography is commercially available as a screening tool for detecting breast cancer, in 2011 the FDA warned against the use of breast thermography as a substitute for mammography. Currently, there is insufficient evidence to support the use of thermography in breast cancer screening, or as an adjunct to mammography. Additionally, there is a high incidence of false positives and lack of rigorous study makes its clinical benefit questionable at this time.[218]

Other Imaging Methods. A number of other imaging methods are available for detecting breast cancer and are used mainly in research studies or to obtain more information about a tumor found by another method. They have not been found reliable enough for routine use. *Scintigraphy* (also called *scintimammography* and *molecular breast imaging*), is used to image cellular absorption of a radioactive tracing agent. *PEM (positron emission mammography)* measures glucose metabolism with a radioactive tracer with increased metabolism indicating the possible presence of a tumor. PEM is an advanced application of positron emission tomography that produces sharp, detailed images of breast lesions as small as 1.5 mm. PEM may be used instead of breast MRI when obesity or metal implants preclude the use of an MRI machine. It can be helpful in individuals with breast implants and may be considered an effective tool in the evaluation of DCIS because of higher sensitivity.[316] *Breast-specific gamma imaging* (BSGI or *sestamibi nuclear breast imaging*) involves an injected radioactive substance (technetium sestamibi) with another agent that make the sestamibi collect in the breast. BSGI has a high rate of false-positive findings as well false negatives. BSGI cannot image extensions through the pectoralis muscle, making MRI a better choice for individuals with very large tumors (compared to breast size) and for anyone with aggressive cancers near the chest wall.

DIAGNOSIS AND STAGING. Detection of a breast abnormality happens through physical examination or imaging studies (see section above on "Screening and Early Detection" including Imaging Studies). Diagnosis, on the other hand, determines with certainty what the abnormality is, thus requiring biopsy and pathology examination. If the diagnosis is cancer, then the physician seeks additional information about how extensive the cancer is (*staging*) and how it appears and behaves (*grading*), so that effective treatment can be initiated.

Techniques utilized in the diagnosis of breast cancer include core biopsy, needle biopsy, incisional biopsy, and excisional biopsy (see further discussion in Chapter 9 "Diagnosis: Tissue Biopsy"). Sentinel lymph node (SLN) mapping is used to identify metastases in invasive cancers. *Sentinel lymph node biopsy* (SLNB) consists of the removal of one to three nodes; it is now standard practice to identify and remove only the first node or nodes that cancer cells may have reached after leaving the breast. This eliminates unnecessary axillary lymph node dissection (ALND), in which more than three nodes are removed. With SLNB, radioactive blue dye is injected preoperatively to identify the first (sentinel) node of drainage from the region of the breast where the cancer is present.

SLN biopsy (see discussion of technique in Chapter 9) has replaced ALND for the staging of *clinically* node-negative individuals with breast cancer, demonstrating equivalent survival to ALND for women with lymph node–negative status while resulting in reduced morbidity. For the majority of women with *pathologically* positive SLNs, completion of ALND is recommended by the ASCO Guidelines and the NCCN. However, recent data from the American College of Surgeons Oncology Group trial suggest that ALND may be omitted in selected individuals (those who have had lumpectomy and radiation) with one or more positive SLNs.[36,237,238,345,459] The data does not address those women who opted for mastectomy and did not receive radiation.

Biomarkers. Breast cancers are biologically heterogeneous. Current classification of subtypes of breast cancer is based on biomarkers and gene expression profiling. Commonly measured tumor markers are hormone receptors for estrogen and progesterone. These hormone receptors are proteins that signal cell proliferation. Breast cancers are labeled ER+ if they have receptors for estrogen and PR+ if they have PRs. Thus cancer cells (like normal breast cells) may receive signals from estrogen and progesterone that could promote growth. Hormone positive (ER+ or PR+) cancers represent up to 80% of all breast cancers.[239] Cancers that are ER+/PR+ have receptors for both hormones that could be supporting cancer growth; 60% to 65% of all breast cancers are ER+/PR+. ER−/PR− cancers represent up to 25% of breast cancers.[464] Hormone receptor testing determines a status that is used to identify whether the cancer is likely to respond to hormonal therapy or other treatments. Hormonal therapy

includes medications that either lower the amount of available estrogen or block estrogen from supporting the growth and function of breast cells. More research is needed to help understand cancers that are PR+.

Another biomarker that is analyzed at the time of biopsy is Her-2/neu (also called c-erbB2 or more often ErbB2). Her-2/neu stands for human epidermal growth factor; it is an oncogene that when overexpressed leads to cell proliferation.[136,485] Her-2/neu–positive cancers account for approximately 15% to 20% of invasive cancers. Cancers that are identified as Her-2/neu+ can benefit from targeted drug therapy with Herceptin (trastuzumab). Triple negative breast cancers (TN: ER−/PR−/HER2/neu−) represent 15% to 20% of invasive breast cancers and are considered to be more aggressive cancers with poorer prognosis.[105] The largest proportion of breast cancers (60%-70%) are ER+/HER2/neu−. Within these cancers there is a wide heterogeneity, with some cancers having a much better prognosis than others.

Gene expression studies have identified five common subtypes of breast cancer: *luminal A tumors, luminal B tumors,* HER2/neu overexpressing tumors, *basal-like/TN tumors,* and *normal breast-like tumors.*[469] Ongoing research shows variations in the occurrence of breast cancer subtypes by demographics (e.g., age, race, and ethnicity), screening detection, estimating risk of development of a second primary breast cancer in the contralateral breast, recurrence risk, and treatment and prognosis indicators (see "Grading and Staging" below for additional information). Discoveries of additional subtypes are expected as research advances.

Commercial tests available for identifying different types of tumors and customizing therapies include *Oncotype DX, MammaPrint,* and *Mammostrat.* Oncotype DX samples 21 genetic markers that are used for prognosis and prediction. In women with ER+, node-negative cancers, the test has been used to predict risk of recurrence as well as benefit from employing adjuvant chemotherapy *in addition* to the use of estrogen-inhibiting drugs such as tamoxifen. A low recurrence score (18 or lower) along with other favorable factors suggests that the person can decline chemotherapy but still benefit from hormonal therapy. A high recurrence score (31 and above) suggests significant benefit from adjuvant chemotherapy. Intermediate scores of 19 to 30 require a discussion between the patient and oncologist for decision making.[461]

Oncotype DX has been used to predict the risk of DCIS recurrence or the development of a new invasive cancer in the same breast. Data is being used to make recommendations regarding the benefit of radiation therapy after breast-conserving surgery for DCIS. The use of Oncotype DX test was been included in treatment guidelines for early-stage breast cancer by the American Society for Clinical Oncology and the NCCN.

The *MammaPrint* test is a microarray assay that is more commonly used in Europe. It analyzes the biology of the tumor through the activity of 70 genes and estimates the risk of recurrence for early-stage breast cancer (both hormone receptor–positive and –negative). The test provides a calculation of risk (low or high) for cancer recurrence that can be used to determine whether chemotherapy may reduce recurrence risk. *Mammostrat* is a newer test that analyzes five immunohistochemical markers that help to identify postmenopausal individuals with early-stage hormone positive cancers who may benefit from adjuvant chemotherapy.[66]

Grading and Staging. Once the diagnosis of cancer is established, pathologists have a number of ways of analyzing cancer cells and how they may behave. *Grading* refers to the study of cell appearance looking at differentiation as well as mitotic rate, nuclear grade, tubular formation and other features. A *well-differentiated* cancer tends to look more like normal cells and is considered less aggressive, while poorly differentiated cancers are the opposite. A commonly used scoring system that combines these observations is the Nottingham (or Bloom Richardson) histologic score. A grade of 1 to 3 is assigned, with 3 being the most aggressive. For further discussion, see "Grading and Staging" in Chapter 9.

The clinical *stage* of the tumor is ascertained in order to determine optimal management, including selection of candidates for adjuvant systemic therapies. A staging system is a standardized way to summarize information about how far a cancer has spread. Therapeutic decisions are formulated in part according to staging categories but primarily according to tumor size, histologic and nuclear grade of the primary tumor, proliferative capacity of the tumor, lymph node status, hormonal status (ERs and PRs), HER2/neu status, menopausal status, and the general health of the individual.[455] Box 20-8 summarizes the staging criteria for breast cancer.

TREATMENT. Breast cancer is commonly treated by various combinations of surgery, radiation therapy, and systemic therapy (chemotherapy, targeted therapy, and endocrine therapy). The timing and sequencing of these interventions varies according to each individual case. Prognosis and selection of therapy may be influenced by the aforementioned clinical and pathology features. The NCCN publishes an annual update of its original 1996 NCCN Breast Cancer Treatment Guidelines.[459] The Guidelines (http://www.nccn.org/professionals/physician_gls/f_guidelines.asp) are available online for professionals with a section for patients as well. They are an important resource for keeping abreast of constant changes and recommendations regarding treatment of all stages of breast cancer. Details of treatment for IBC can be found online.[515]

Surgery. Surgery is a part of every person's treatment who has breast cancer. Surgery may be employed in the initial biopsy and any additional biopsies, for local control (lumpectomy or mastectomy), accessing and analyzing the status of axillary lymph nodes, and in breast reconstruction options. Prior to the 1970s, *radical mastectomy* was the most commonly employed procedure for surgical treatment of breast cancer. This procedure included removal of the entire breast, pectoral muscles (pectoralis major and pectoralis minor), all axillary lymph nodes, and some additional skin. Postsurgical problems included lymphedema, restricted shoulder mobility, impaired muscle function, and paresthesia. In today's era, radical mastectomy is rarely performed. The goal of the breast surgeon is local control by removing the tumor with "negative" or "clean" margins (see discussion below). Surgical options include *modified*

Box 20-8

TNM STAGING SYSTEM FOR BREAST CANCER

Cancers are classified based on their T (tumor), N (node), and M (metastasis) stages:

- The letter T followed by a number from 0 to 4 describes the tumor's size and spread to the skin or to the chest wall under the breast. Higher T numbers mean a larger tumor and/or wider spread to tissues near the breast.
- The letter N followed by a number from 0 to 3 indicates whether the cancer has spread to lymph nodes near the breast and, if so, how many lymph nodes are affected.
- The letter M followed by a 0 or 1 indicates whether the cancer has spread to distant organs—for example, the lungs or bones.

Primary tumor (T) categories:

TX: Primary tumor cannot be assessed.

T0: No evidence of primary tumor.

Tis: Carcinoma in situ (DCIS, LCIS, or Paget disease of the nipple with no associated tumor mass)

T1 (includes T1a, T1b, and T1c): Tumor is 2 cm or less in diameter.

T2: Tumor is larger than 2 cm but not more than 5 cm in diameter.

T3: Tumor is larger than 5 cm in diameter.

T4: Tumor of any size growing into the chest wall or skin. This includes inflammatory breast cancer.

Nearby lymph nodes (N) (based on looking at them under a microscope):

NX: Nearby lymph nodes cannot be assessed (e.g., removed previously).

N0: Cancer has not spread to nearby lymph nodes.

N1: Cancer has spread to 1 to 3 axillary (underarm) lymph node(s), and/or tiny amounts of cancer are found in internal mammary lymph nodes (those near the breast bone) on sentinel lymph node biopsy.

- **N1mi:** Micrometastases (tiny areas of cancer spread) in 1 to 3 lymph nodes under the arm. The areas of cancer spread in the lymph nodes are 2 mm or less.
- **N1a:** Cancer has spread to 1 to 3 axillary lymph nodes with at least one area of cancer spread greater than 2 mm across.

N2: Cancer has spread to 4 to 9 lymph nodes axillary lymph nodes.

N3: Cancer has spread to 10 or more axillary lymph nodes, or growth of tumor in other lymph nodes around the breast (internal mammary, supraclavicular).

Metastasis (M):

MX: Presence of distant spread (metastasis) cannot be assessed.

M0: No distant spread is found on x-rays (or other imaging procedures) or by physical exam.

M1: Spread to distant organs is present. (The most common sites are bone, lung, brain, and liver.)

Data from American Cancer Society. *How is breast cancer staged?*. Available with further discussion online at: http://www.cancer.org/Cancer/BreastCancer/DetailedGuide/breast-cancer-staging; and National Comprehensive Canter Network. NCCN Guidelines for Patients: Breast Cancer. Version 2014.

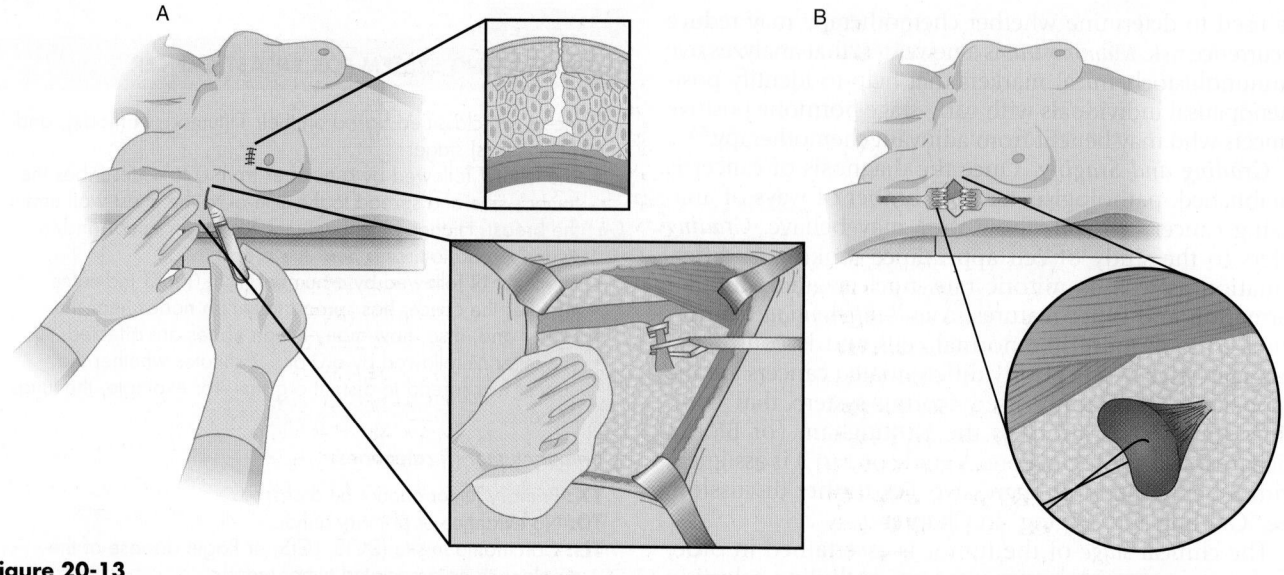

Figure 20-13

Breast-conserving therapy. A, Incisions to remove malignant tumors are made directly over the tumor without tunneling. A transverse incision in the low axilla is used for either the sentinel node biopsy or the axillary dissection. The *inset* shows the excision cavity of the lumpectomy; no attempt is made to approximate the sides of the cavity, which will fill with serous fluid and gradually shrink. **B,** In the sentinel node biopsy, a similar transverse incision is made and extended through the clavipectoral fascia and the true axilla entered. The sentinel node is located by virtue of its staining with dye or radioactivity, or both, and dissected free as a single specimen. (From Townsend CM: *Sabiston textbook of surgery,* ed 17, Philadelphia, 2004, WB Saunders.)

radical mastectomy, simple mastectomy (also known as total mastectomy) or *breast-conserving therapy* (BCT).

Breast-Conserving Therapy. Treatment recommendations for women with stage I or II breast cancer often include BCT, also known as *breast conserving surgery* or *lumpectomy.* Over half the women in the United States with early-stage breast cancer receive BCT and postsurgical radiation therapy (Fig. 20-13). Breast-conserving surgery followed by radiation therapy gives the same survival benefit as mastectomy for women with localized tumors. Lumpectomy may also be an option for women with larger tumors who receive neoadjuvant chemotherapy (before surgery) to shrink the tumor.

In BCT, only the tumor is removed along with a rim of normal breast tissue, thus preserving the remaining breast. The breast cavity fills with serous fluid over time and the breast itself is conserved. The removed cancer and surrounding tissues are submitted to the pathologist. A report of "negative," "clean," or clear" margins indicates that as far as can be determined, all the cancer has been successfully removed. A report of "positive" or "dirty" margins means that there are cancer cells at the edge of the removed tissue. Additional surgery is recommended when positive margins remain; however, this varies widely by surgeon and location. Studies show that 20% to 38% of women who have undergone BCT require reexcision surgery. Most of the women who require reexcision need only one additional surgery; approximately 10% need two or more surgeries, and 8% to 10% of women eventually have a mastectomy.[302,411,439] Risk factors for reoperation because of close or positive margins are multifocal tumors and tumors located in the outer upper quadrant of the breast.[230]

Although there is some concern that reoperation may be associated with increased rates of local and distant recurrence, evidence from recent studies supports the practice

of multiple reexcisions to obtain clear margins as a safe alternative to mastectomy for women with invasive breast cancer or DCIS. Consensus as to what constitutes tumor-free or "clean" margins in breast-conservation surgery has improved. Defining adequate surgical tumor clearance is an important area of research in the elimination of residual disease.[202] An emerging technology, the MarginProbe system was approved by the FDA for use in 2013. The MarginProbe uses electromagnetic waves to identify possible cancerous tissue. The benefit of using this system is that the surgeon can determine intraoperatively whether more tissue needs to be removed (as opposed to waiting for pathologic analysis of the removed lumpectomy tissue). MarginProbe can be used during lumpectomy for both DCIS and invasive breast cancer. Initial reports from use in Europe show that surgeons who used MarginProbe during lumpectomy were 56% less likely to perform a reexcision lumpectomy.[511]

The choice between breast-conserving surgery and mastectomy depends on balancing the need to achieve complete excision of the tumor with the woman's preferences with respect to cosmetic appearance and preserving sexual sensitivity of the breast. Clinical factors that influence this choice include the type, location, and spread of the tumor, multifocal disease, the ratio of tumor size to breast size, and the use of neoadjuvant systemic treatment. In many cases, a woman chooses mastectomy for greater peace of mind, to avoid radiation therapy, and for reconstruction options. On the other hand, if a surgeon recommends only mastectomy, then second and third opinions may be considered as surgeons gain expertise in newer oncoplastic techniques. Despite recommendations for BCT, there remains concern that mastectomy (and contralateral prophylactic mastectomy) may be overused.[54]

Mastectomy. Mastectomy is usually reserved for women with more extensive disease; although mastectomy may be desirable for some women with early breast cancer as noted above. Mastectomy is the total removal of the breast. It can be a *simple* (or *total mastectomy*), a *modified radical mastectomy*, or *partial mastectomy* (larger than a lumpectomy). In cases where immediate reconstruction is planned at the time of the mastectomy, it is possible to retain much of the woman's natural skin over the breast. This procedure is called a *skin-sparing mastectomy*; the surgeon removes only the skin of the nipple, areola, and the original biopsy scar. If no immediate breast reconstruction is planned, the surgeon removes as much skin as is required to make the scar and chest surface flat. Nipple-sparing procedures are gaining some acceptance as well.

Women who have a mastectomy as part of their breast cancer treatment have options. Many choose to use a breast prosthesis; others choose to go "breast-free." Breast reconstruction (see further discussion below) of one or both breasts by a plastic surgeon is increasingly chosen by women in the United States who have undergone mastectomy. Surgical reconstruction may be immediate (at the time of the mastectomy) or delayed (any time after the mastectomy, including many years later). The rate of reconstruction varies by geography, socioeconomic status (including insurance coverage), hospital type, age, and ethnicity.[346] Nationwide, 20% to 25% of individuals having a mastectomy also have immediate breast reconstruction.[142] The Women's Health and Cancer Rights Act of 1998 requires all health insurance providers and health maintenance organizations that pay for mastectomy to also pay for reconstruction of the breast removed by mastectomy, surgery and reconstruction of the opposite breast to achieve symmetry, the use of a breast prosthesis, and treatment for any complications of surgery including lymphedema.[29,619] An excellent website for supporting women making these decisions is www.breastfree.org.

Lymph Node Surgery. Surgery that addresses the lymph nodes and the possibility of regional metastases[476] has seen a change in the last decade. For early stage breast cancer, SLN biopsy has replaced ALND as the standard of care for the staging of clinically node-negative individuals with breast cancer (see discussion of technique in Chapter 9). SLN biopsy has demonstrated equivalent survival to ALND for individuals who were lymph node–negative while resulting in reduced morbidity.

For the majority of people with pathologically positive SLNs with suspicion of regional metastases, complete ALND is recommended by the American Society of Clinical Oncology Guidelines and the NCCN. During a traditional ALND, five to 30 lymph nodes may be removed; more recent practice for SLNB is to remove one to three nodes.[36,459,237,238,642,345] Recent data from the American College of Surgeons Oncology Group Z0011 trial and a 2011 position paper from the American Society of Breast Surgeons suggest that ALND may be omitted in *selected* individuals with one or two positive SLNs. Another approach under investigation is called reverse axillary mapping, which involves injecting the tracer dye under the skin of the upper arm.[468]

Breast Reconstruction. Breast reconstruction is a surgical solution to anatomic defects caused by breast cancer. Breast reconstruction can be implant-based or autologous using transplanted tissue from the woman's own abdomen, back, or buttocks, which is then used to create a breast mound. Of the more than 96,000 reconstruction surgeries performed in 2011 in the United States, 79% were implant-based with either a silicone or saline implant.[38] Reconstruction with an implant alone usually requires tissue expansion. This is a two-stage surgical process: first, a tissue expander is placed under the chest wall muscles (pectoralis major, serratus anterior, anterior rectus fascia). Then the woman returns to the office of the plastic surgeon over a period of 4 to 6 months for saline injections ("fills") through an internal valve, which gradually stretches the muscles and soft tissues. A second surgical procedure replaces the expander with the implant.

Breast Implants. Although silicone implants were once banned, their use has been reinstated. In 2011, the FDA released long-term results to date of the silicone implant monitoring program and concluded that there is no evidence that silicone implants increase the risk of breast cancer or autoimmune diseases.[620] However, recent studies suggest an increase in large cell lymphoma with the use of prosthetic implants.[486] See also "Breast Implantation" in Chapter 25.

Silicone implants have the advantage of feeling more natural than saline implants, but some surgeons prefer to use saline because of their long-term safety record. All breast implants (regardless of their intended use for augmentation or for reconstruction) have a tendency to become encapsulated in connective tissue over time. The result may be a firm breast that no longer matches the opposite breast.[475] In these cases, additional surgery over a woman's lifetime may be required to address the capsular contraction. Other complications that may require surgical intervention include infection,[639] implant rupture or leaks, deflation, or pain. Outcomes assessment of breast reconstruction is complex, but revision surgery within 5 to 10 years is common.[526]

Autologous Reconstruction. Breast reconstruction with autologous transplanted tissues uses the woman's own adipose tissue, muscle and skin that can be harvested from a number of sites to either form a breast or create a pocket for an implant. In 2011, nearly 20,000 women in the United States had autologous reconstruction surgeries with transverse rectus abdominal muscle (TRAM) flap and deep inferior epigastric perforator (DIEP) flap surgeries occurring in almost equal amounts, slightly ahead of latissimus dorsi flap reconstructions.[39] The benefits of using abdominal and lower extremity donor sites include the absence of a foreign implant with a natural-looking result. Additionally, the breast mound ages with the woman and responds to weight loss or weight gain.[493]

The most popular of these muscle flap procedures are the *latissimus dorsi* (*back*) *flap* and the *TRAM flap* (Fig. 20-14). A latissimus dorsi flap (or "lat flap") procedure utilizes a section of skin, fat, and latissimus dorsi muscle that is detached from the back region and then tunneled under the skin to the breast area (Fig. 20-15). The tissue may be shaped into a natural-looking breast and sewn into place; more commonly the latissimus muscle is used to form the base of a pocket to receive an implant in order to create a breast of moderate size. In these cases, the latissimus flap is a combination of autologous and implant-based reconstructive surgeries.

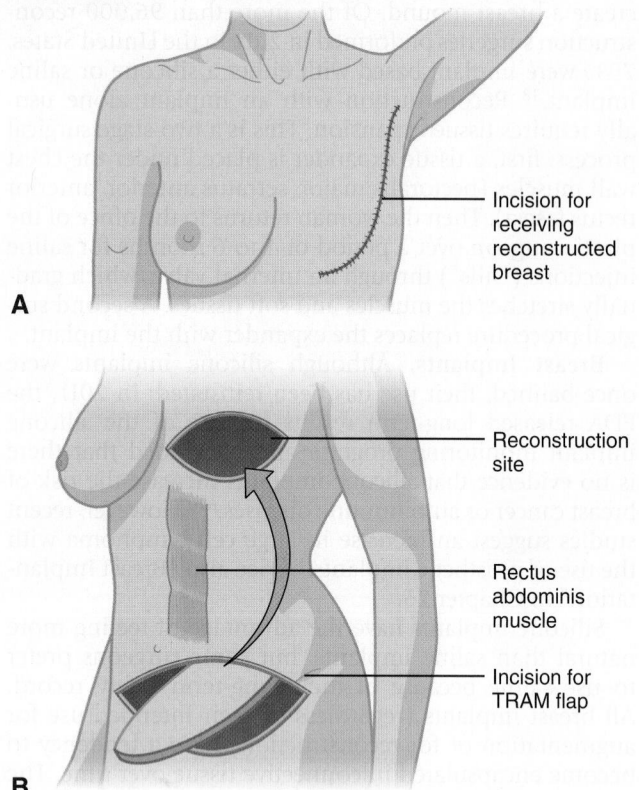

A

B

Figure 20-14

Transverse rectus abdominis myocutaneous (TRAM) flap. A, After mastectomy of the involved breast, **(B)** a breast is reconstructed using the lower abdominal skin and fatty tissue. In a *pedicled* TRAM, the tissue's own blood supply remains attached and the lower abdominal tissue is rotated into position on the chest. The tissue is tunneled under the skin to the chest area, where it is brought through the mastectomy incision. The reconstructed tissue is shaped to form a matching breast and placed in the mastectomy skin pocket. A *free* TRAM flap refers to using skin and tissue that are completely disconnected from their own blood supply, moved from the abdomen to the new site, and then reconnected to different blood vessels. A nipple and areola can be tattooed on later after healing has taken place.

Labels in figure:
- Incision for receiving reconstructed breast
- Reconstruction site
- Rectus abdominis muscle
- Incision for TRAM flap

The TRAM flap procedure can be either a pedicle flap or a free flap. In the *pedicle flap*, the tissue removed remains attached to its blood supply and is tunneled under the woman's skin into the mastectomy wound. In the case of free flaps, a plastic surgeon trained in microvascular technique is required. The donor tissue (adipose and vascular supply) is removed from the abdomen and anastomosed to the internal mammary blood supply. In the *free* TRAM procedure, muscle, fat and skin are harvested along with inferior epigastric vessels. This flap is separated from the abdomen and brought to the chest defect where it is anastomosed to either the thoracodorsal or internal mammary vessels.

Over the years, the TRAM procedure has evolved so that only a very small portion of the muscle around the necessary blood vessels is removed, a procedure now referred to as a *muscle-sparing TRAM*. If the blood vessels supplying the abdominal tissue are exceptionally good, then no muscle tissue is needed. The muscle is split rather than cut. This procedure is referred to as a *perforator flap* surgery

or *DIEP* flap. Contraindications for perforator flap surgeries include a history of heavy smoking (with unfavorable vascular conditions), significant cardiopulmonary disease, history of blood clots (deep venous thrombosis or pulmonary embolus), previous surgery of the vascular territories, and allergy to anticoagulants.

Muscle-sparing free TRAM or DIEP perforator reconstructions involve a significant surgery time (4 or more hours per breast) and 3- to 5-day hospital stay because of the microvascular techniques and tissue monitoring that are required. The donor defect is repaired by abdominoplasty ("tummy tuck"); mesh may or may not be used. The lower abdominal incision is made laterally from hip to hip (iliac crest) with removal of vascular supply, adipose tissue, and skin. The umbilicus is related.[548]

The goal of the plastic surgeon is to remove as little abdominal muscle tissue as possible while still transplanting a viable flap of lower abdominal fat and overlying skin. Dissection of nerve supply is an additional area of investigation by surgeons trained in DIEP flap reconstruction. If significant rectus abdominal muscle has been removed, synthetic mesh or acellular dermal matrix may be used to repair the defect to decrease the risk of herniation.

Other perforator flaps used less commonly include those from the buttocks: either the *superior* or *inferior gluteal artery perforator* flap, either of which has minimal donor-site morbidity. Like the DIEP, the superficial inferior epigastric artery flap transfers the same tissue from the abdomen to the chest for breast reconstruction as the TRAM flap without sacrificing the rectus muscle or fascia (Fig. 20-16).[252,253] The *transverse upper gracilis flap* harvests muscle and tissue from the inner thigh.

All of these autologous procedures are more complicated than implant surgery, requiring microvascular surgery and a longer hospital stay but with a result that is usually a softer, more natural appearing breast. The woman often has an additional surgery (3-6 months later) to create a new areola and nipple on the reconstructed breast with modification of the opposite breast if necessary to match the reconstructed breast. Tattooing or repigmentation of the nipple–areola complex is an option as well.

After surgery, the treatment plan may include radiation therapy and systemic therapies such as chemotherapy, hormone therapy, and targeted therapy or any combination of these approaches. The primary objective of these treatments is to reduce the odds of occult metastases from developing into disease.

Radiation Therapy. Most women receive radiation therapy after a lumpectomy to eradicate any residual cancer cells in the affected breast or adjacent lymph nodes. Postmastectomy radiation is an increasing trend in certain groups because of the concern of local recurrence in the scar after mastectomy. These include women with large tumors, those with lymphatic vascular invasion, a tumor close to the rib cage or chest wall, or four or more positive axillary lymph nodes. Usually whole-breast radiation is delivered once a day, 5 days a week, for 5 to 6 weeks using a linear accelerator machine (Fig. 20-17). This delivery system is termed EBRT. A later "boost" may be added by use of an external electron beam.

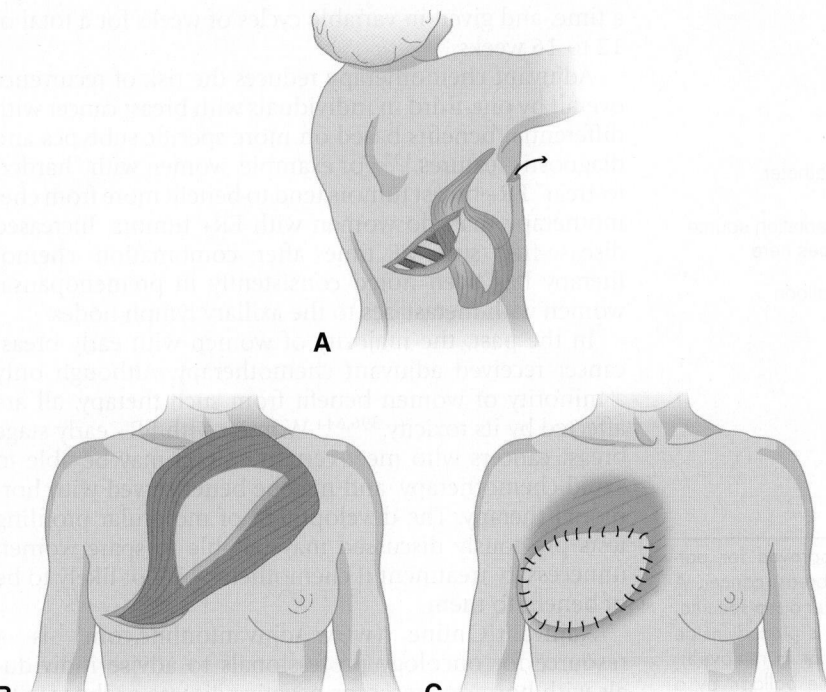

Figure 20-15

Latissimus dorsi flap. Schematic representation of latissimus dorsi flap. **A,** Flap elevation. **B,** Flap transposition. **C,** Flap inset. (From Townsend CM: *Sabiston textbook of surgery*, ed 19, Philadelphia, 2012, WB Saunders.)

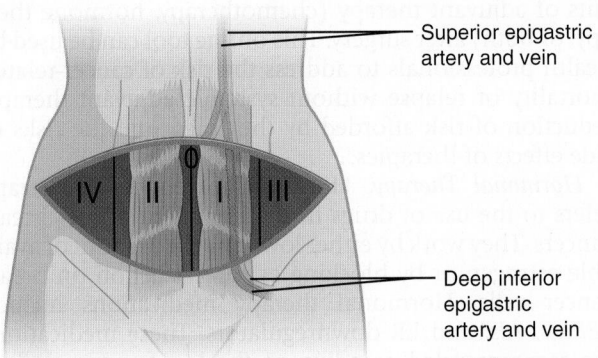

Superior epigastric artery and vein

Deep inferior epigastric artery and vein

Figure 20-16

Vascular territories of the abdominal wall provided by unilateral transverse rectus abdominis myocutaneous (TRAM) flap. Studies show that the most reliable cutaneous portion is directly overlying muscle zone I, followed by zones III, II, and IV, respectively. A deep inferior epigastric perforator flap (DIEP) is an alternative procedure to the TRAM. A small portion of the rectus abdominis muscle is dissected to harvest the blood vessels, but the muscle is preserved because no muscle or overlying muscle fascia is used. The DIEP flap relies on blood vessels that perforate the rectus abdominis muscle (e.g., deep inferior epigastric artery and vein). (From Townsend CM: *Sabiston textbook of surgery*, ed 17, Philadelphia, 2004, WB Saunders.)

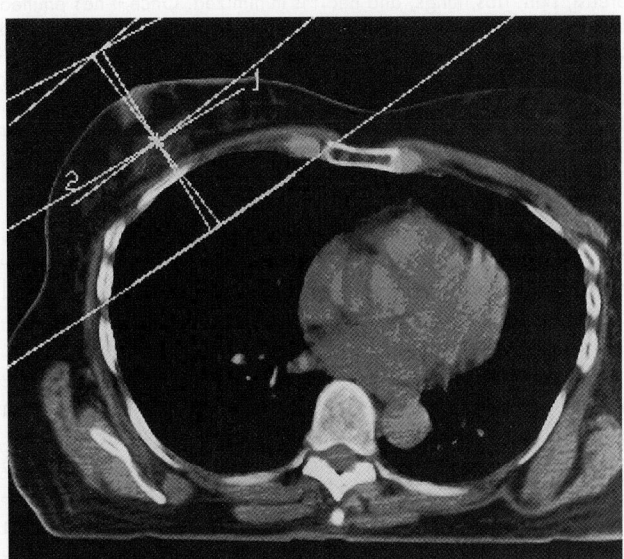

Figure 20-17

The standard radiation field configuration for breast cancer. Two tangentially directed fields encompass the breast with a minimal amount of underlying lung tissue. The contralateral breast and all of the critical structures are avoided. (From Abeloff MD: *Clinical oncology*, ed 3, Philadelphia, 2004, Churchill Livingstone.)

An alternative to whole-breast radiation is *internal radiation* or *accelerated partial-breast irradiation*. Varieties of accelerated partial-breast irradiation gain local control in less time. The radiation is directed to the tissue immediately around the tumor where cancer is most likely to recur. The two most commonly used forms of partial-breast radiation in the United States are balloon-delivered *intracavitary brachytherapy* (Fig. 20-18; MammoSite) and multicatheter internal radiation or *interstitial*

brachytherapy, both of which use radioactive "seeds." Studies are under way to determine optimum candidate selection and protocols. Initial results utilizing multicatheter internal radiation are comparable to conventional radiation therapy.[442,445]

Two other experimental approaches to radiation therapy are: (1) 3D *conformal* or *intensity-modulated partial-breast radiation therapy*, which uses a linear accelerator

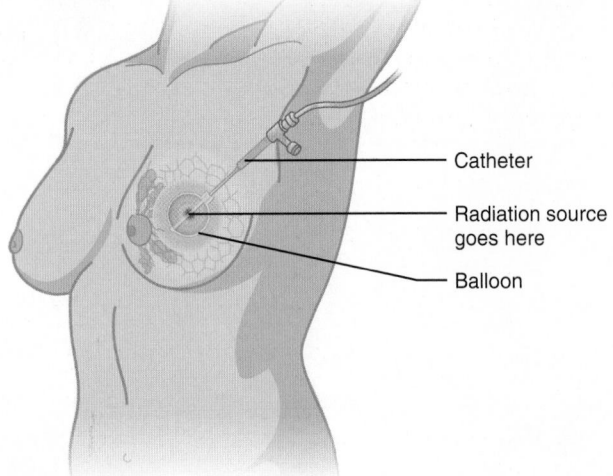

Catheter

Radiation source goes here

Balloon

Figure 20-18

Balloon brachytherapy. The MammoSite device approved for partial breast radiation in the treatment of early-stage breast cancer. A single-balloon catheter is inserted in the breast to deliver a site-specific, prescribed dose of radiation. The deflated balloon is placed inside the lumpectomy cavity (the space left after the tumor is removed). A tiny radioactive source (seed) is placed within the balloon by a computer-controlled machine. Because the radiation source is inside the balloon, radiation is delivered to the area of the breast where cancer is most likely to recur. Radiation exposure to the rest of the breast, skin, ribs, lungs, and heart is minimized. Once it has emitted the prescribed dose of radiation, the source is removed. When used as primary therapy (i.e., the only form of radiation after a lumpectomy), treatments are twice a day for up to 5 days. The applicator shaft, a tube connected to the balloon, remains outside the breast. After 10 sessions in 5 days, the balloon is deflated and the catheter is then removed.

machine to treat multiple or difficult-to-reach tumors, and (2) *intraoperative radiation therapy* (Axxent brachytherapy), which delivers a single dose of highly concentrated radiation directly to the tumor bed immediately following early-stage tumor removal.

Chemotherapy. Chemotherapy is used to treat the whole body via the vascular system and is employed with women with suspected or confirmed metastatic disease. *Adjuvant chemotherapy* is the term used for chemotherapy given at the time of breast cancer diagnosis, whereas *systemic therapy* is the term used for individuals with known metastases. *Neoadjuvant chemotherapy* refers to chemotherapy given prior to surgical excision with the intent of shrinking the tumor size.

Chemotherapy works by interfering with cell division thus causing cell death (for further discussion, see Chapter 9). There are many drugs commonly administered as adjuvant chemotherapy for breast cancer (see Table 9-6): cyclophosphamide (Cytoxan), methotrexate (amethopterin, Mexate, Folex), 5-fluorouracil (Adrucil), doxorubicin (Adriamycin), epirubicin (Ellence); and paclitaxel (Taxol or Abraxane) or docetaxel (Taxotere). Additional drugs are used chemotherapeutically for more advanced breast cancers. The drugs are delivered via a vascular access device, including Hickman, Groshong, and portacath devices. Treatments protocols developed by the oncologist and patient vary in the combination of drugs used and method of delivery, usually 10 minutes to 4 hours at

a time, and given in variable cycles of weeks for a total of 12 to 16 weeks.

Adjuvant chemotherapy reduces the risk of recurrence overall by one-third in individuals with breast cancer with differential benefits based on more specific subtypes and diagnostic features.[197] For example, women with "harder-to-treat" ER– breast tumors tend to benefit more from chemotherapy than do women with ER+ tumors. Increased disease-free survival time after combination chemotherapy has been noted consistently in premenopausal women with metastases to the axillary lymph nodes.

In the past, the majority of women with early breast cancer received adjuvant chemotherapy. Although only a minority of women benefit from such therapy, all are affected by its toxicity.[396,644] Women with ER+ early stage breast cancers who meet certain criteria may be able to avoid chemotherapy, and may be better served with hormonal therapy. The development of molecular profiling tests previously discussed may be able to spare women unnecessary treatment if chemotherapy is not likely to be of benefit to them.

Adjuvant!Online (www.Adjuvantonline.com) is a resource for oncology professionals to advise individuals with hormone receptor-negative disease or those with positive lymph nodes with either positive or negative hormone receptors. It is currently being updated to include HER-2/neu status. The tool evaluates the risks and benefits of adjuvant therapy (chemotherapy, hormone therapy, or both) after surgery. This online tool can be used by health professionals to address the risk of cancer-related mortality or relapse without systemic adjuvant therapy, reduction of risk afforded by therapies, and the risks of side effects of therapies.

Hormonal Therapy. Hormonal or endocrine therapy refers to the use of drugs in the treatment of ER+ breast cancers. They work by either lowering the amount of available estrogen or by blocking estrogen's action on breast cancer cells. Hormonal therapy medications include *SERMs, AIs,* and ER downregulators. These medications are recommended as adjuvant therapy for a period of 5 or more years to decrease risk of cancer recurrence or cancer in the contralateral breast. They are also used neoadjuvantly, to reduce tumor size, or for chemoprevention in individuals at high risk of breast cancer. Hormonal therapy is also used to arrest the growth of advanced hormone receptor–positive breast disease in both pre- and postmenopausal women.

SERMs work by blocking the effects of estrogen in the breast tissue by competing with estrogen at the cellular level in breast tissue. SERMs reduce the risk of cancer recurrence as well as development of a new cancer in the contralateral breast by approximately 50%. They also decrease the risk of cancer mortality.[25,311] Tamoxifen (Nolvadex) is the best-known and most widely used SERM and has been in use for more than 30 years. When tamoxifen is taken for 5 years, studies show a lowered recurrence rate of 45% to 50% in ER+ cancers in years 0 to 4. Clinical trials continue to explore the use of tamoxifen beyond 5 years. Recent studies may support recommendation of continuing hormonal medications for 10 years.[196]

Tamoxifen's selective estrogen activation effects may produce some serious, although rare, side effects, including blood clots, stroke, and endometrial cancer. Other side effects that have been reported include hot flashes, fatigue, weight gain, premature menopause, leg cramps, urogynecologic symptoms (including urinary incontinence), and cataracts.[636]

Raloxifene is another SERM that is less likely to promote thromboembolic events, endometrial cancer and benign uterine conditions, and cataracts. Its use is limited to chemoprevention in postmenopausal women. Currently, it is not approved for use in premenopausal women or as adjuvant treatment after breast cancer diagnosis.[636]

SERMs offer other health benefits unrelated to treating cancer. Even though SERMs block estrogen's action on breast cells, they activate the effect of estrogen in bone and liver cells. This results in reduced osteoporosis and increased heart protection by lowered cholesterol levels (higher high-density lipoprotein and lower low-density lipoprotein levels). The ongoing Co-STAR (Cognition in the Study of Tamoxifen and Raloxifene) trial is investigating effects of both medications on mood and cognitive performance.[176]

AIs work differently than SERMs. They interfere with the production of estrogen in postmenopausal women by blocking the enzyme aromatase, which converts the hormone androgen into small amounts of estrogen in the body. This results in reduced availability of estrogen to stimulate the growth of ER+ breast cancer cells. AIs are recommended as the drug of first-choice in postmenopausal women; there are more benefits and fewer serious side effects than with tamoxifen. However, AIs may cause more cardiac problems, osteoporosis, and joint pain than tamoxifen. Studies show that switching to an AI after taking tamoxifen for 2 to 3 years (for a total of 5 or more years of hormonal therapy) is superior to 5 years of tamoxifen alone. Data also show that taking an AI for 5 years after taking tamoxifen for 5 years continues to reduce the risk of the cancer recurrence, compared to no treatment after 5 years of tamoxifen.[57,193,431]

ER downregulators are another class of drugs that work by blocking estrogen in postmenopausal women with advanced ER+ breast cancer that has stopped responding to other hormonal therapy medicines.

Targeted (or Biologic) Therapy. Trastuzumab (Herceptin) is a highly effective drug used to treat breast tumors that are HER2/neu positive. HER2+ breast cancers are more aggressive and less likely to respond to conventional therapies. A defective growth-promoting oncogene, known as HER2/neu is found in 15% to 20% of women with invasive breast cancer. Trastuzumab may slow or stop the growth of breast cancer in individuals who have tumors with too many copies of the HER2/neu gene or too many HER2/neu receptors by *targeting* HER2/neu proteins. In addition to blocking HER2/neu receptors, trastuzumab may facilitate the immune system in the destruction of cancer cells. It is considered an immune-targeted therapy and thus an antibody that attacks cancer at its genetic roots.

Trastuzumab is approved by the FDA for individuals with metastatic HER2-positive disease and individuals with earlier stages of HER2/neu+ disease as adjuvant treatment either alone or as part of a regimen with chemotherapy.[233,489,565] The drug is given by infusion; on average, once every 3 weeks for early breast cancers and once a week for more advanced cancers. Side effects from the use of trastuzumab include an increase in cardiovascular events, including left ventricular dysfunction and congestive heart disease. A large number of individuals report flu-like symptoms. Less-common serious side effects (<1%) are pulmonary allergic reactions and pulmonary toxicity.

Bevacizumab (Avastin) is a targeted monoclonal antibody approved by the FDA in 2008; it is an antiangiogenic agent that works by decreasing blood supply to the cancer. Generally used along with chemotherapy in women with advanced disease, it has a number of severe risks and side effects, including hypertension, cardiovascular dysfunction, and thromboembolism.[165] In 2011, the FDA announced that it had removed the breast cancer indication from Avastin because the drug has not been shown to be safe and effective for that use. The medicine itself was not removed from the market. Studies are ongoing to identify a subset of individuals with breast cancer who may benefit from its use and combining its use with other drugs.

Ovarian Ablation. Removing estrogens from premenopausal women by surgically removing the ovaries or using drugs to suppress ovarian function is another way of treating ER-positive breast cancer.[258]

PROGNOSIS. Cancer prognosis is dependent on the age and menopausal status of the woman, the stage of the disease, type/subtype of cancer, histologic and nuclear grade of the primary tumor, biomarkers such as ER and PR status of the tumor, HER2/neu status, proliferative capacity of the tumor, and status of the axillary lymph nodes. A tumor's biology (hormone status, molecular subtype, histopathology) is more important than size and how much the cancer has spread. These factors hold for both men and women, although recent data shows that men are diagnosed with later stage disease than women, with larger tumors, and with a greater likelihood of lymph node involvement and distant metastases.

When cancer characteristics (age of the individual, tumor stage, grade, nodal status, ER/PR/HER2/neu status) are matched, survival rates for men with breast cancer are equivalent to those of females.[219] Other factors that influence prognosis include race/ethnicity (African Americans and Hispanic/Latinas are often diagnosed at later stages), activity level (sedentary individuals have poorer prognosis), and BMI (risk increased when BMI is greater than 30).

Breast tumors that lack estrogen responsiveness tend to have a poorer prognosis because of the cancer's limited response to current antiestrogen treatments available.[351] Individuals with TN disease (ER–/PR–/HER2/neu–) represent a particular therapeutic challenge because of the lack of molecular targets. However, for these individuals, advances in conventional IV chemotherapy have resulted in improved survival rates.[84]

Further understanding of less-common types of breast cancer and ongoing developments in molecular subtyping help to determine prognosis. For example, IBC constitutes only 2% of all breast cancers in the United States, but it represents a large percentage of locally advanced disease (this could be a consequence of late diagnosis with metastases already present rather than because of subtype). It is an extremely variable disease with poor prognosis despite recent therapies; the survival rate for all women with IBC is 35% to 40% and with local recurrence rates as high as 50% and survival time of less than 4 years even with multimodal treatment.[41,515] (See www.ibcsupport.org and www.ibcresearch.org for updated information.)

If detected early before metastases, most breast cancers are curable. There has been a reduction in mortality of 1% to 2% annually in the United States and other industrialized countries, possibly related to changes in lifestyle (e.g., diet, exercise, and reproductive behavior), early diagnosis, and improved success of treatment.[187] Up to 85% of all cases reported are diagnosed as stage 0 or I disease.[464]

Five-year survival statistics (reported in a study that compiled pooled data of four prospective cohort studies of 18,000 breast cancer survivors) are: 95.5% to 98.7% for stage I disease; 91.4% to 96.7% for stage II disease; and 67.0% to 89.7% for stage III disease.[464] Although stage IV disease is no longer considered curable, some women live a considerable amount of years with metastatic disease. However the reported median survival of stage IV disease is 18 to 24 months.[183] Negative prognostic indicators for bone and/or brain metastases include aggressive nature of primary lesion (e.g., tumor stage–high nuclear grade; poor histologic grade), TN cancers, size of the tumor, and lymph node involvement. Approximately 10% to 15% of individuals with breast cancer develop distant metastases within 2 years of diagnosis (early metastases) with a poor 5-year survival rate of 21%.[171,521]

Advancements in technology make early detection possible as well as new treatments available with an improving survival rate; even so, approximately 40,000 women died from this disease each year. Many women experience secondary complications of the disease and its treatments, including decreased quality of life, weight gain, sleep disturbances, poor body image, fatigue, increased risk for osteoporosis, CVD, premature menopause, peripheral neuropathy, cognitive changes, lymphedema, and the development of other cancers.

Recurrence. Local recurrence refers to cancer that occurs in the same breast that has been treated with BCT or in the scar of a mastectomy. The incidence of ipsilateral breast tumor relapse in individuals who were previously treated for early stage breast cancer by breast-conserving surgery and radiation therapy or by mastectomy is estimated to be 6%.[151] Differentiation between a true recurrence and a new primary tumor is necessary.[167,260] Local recurrences that occur more than 5 years after initial treatment have a better prognosis, as do those that occur in older women with smaller lesions.

Although the 5-year local recurrence rate for all breast cancers after BCT is low (less than 10% at 5 years for all subtypes) there is variation based on lymph node involvement and subtypes. If lymph nodes are positive, the 5-year recurrence rate is 11% for the individual with BCT. For women who have had a mastectomy with one to three positive lymph nodes, the 5-year local recurrence rates for BCT is approximately 16%; for four or more positive nodes, it is 26%. Radiation therapy to the chest wall

may be employed on those breast cancers with lymph node involvement. The use of systemic therapies can also further lower these risks.[245] Local recurrence is noted to be particularly low for the luminal A subtype (ER+/PR+/HER2/neu−). Recurrence rates are higher for breast cancers with higher grade, hormone-negative, TN cancers and HER2/neu+ cancers.[388] As described previously, the Oncotype DX test and others assign a recurrence score for hormone-positive, node-negative cancers treated with either tamoxifen alone or tamoxifen with chemotherapy.

Regional recurrence refers to cancer that is found in the axillary, supraclavicular, or (less commonly) internal mammary lymph nodes; this may occur after an ALND or SLNB. Risk of regional recurrence correlates with the pathologic detection of higher number of positive lymph nodes. Although SLNB is highly accurate in predicting the status of axillary nodes in individuals with breast cancer, the procedure is associated with a low rate (up to 10%) of false-negative results. Applying mapping and operative techniques to new anatomic findings of sentinel lymphatic channels and drainage patterns may improve this statistic.[638] Recurrence in lymph nodes other than ipsilateral lymph nodes suggests metastasis.

Distant recurrence denotes disease spread to other organs; it is metastatic disease. Common sites for breast cancer metastases are bone, lungs, liver, and brain. Women with advanced breast cancer (stage IV disease) may live a considerable amount of years with good quality of life. With the further identification of molecular subtypes of breast cancer there is anticipated progress in the treatment of metastatic breast cancer. Matching treatment to subtypes may improve outcomes. For example, in a 2012 analysis of 15 studies involving more than 12,000 women, individuals with luminal subtype (ER+/PR+) tumors exhibited the lowest rates of local recurrence. Women with TN and HER2/neu+ breast tumors were analyzed for local recurrence and predictive factors for prognosis following BCT versus mastectomy and treatment.[150,326,348] When BCT was chosen, HER2/neu+ cancers showed higher recurrence rates than did TN cancers. When mastectomy was chosen, there was no difference in recurrence rates reported between HER2-neu and TN cancers.

Contralateral Breast Cancer. Contralateral second primary breast cancers are estimated to occur in 3% to 15% of female breast cancer survivors who have not been identified as having a genetic component for breast cancer risk.[472,531] This is a 60% higher risk as compared to an individual's risk of developing a first primary breast cancer. It is well-known that the risk is significantly higher for those individuals who carry *BRCA1* or *BRCA2* mutations.[397,531]

Study is ongoing as to how the expression of tumor markers in primary breast cancers influences the risk of contralateral breast cancer. Studies demonstrate increased risk of developing another ER– cancer in the opposite breast in those individuals whose primary tumor was ER–[86,349] as well as elevated risk in cancers that are TN or HER2/neu+ (as opposed to those that were ER+/HER2/neu−). It is presumed that this is true for breast cancers that are considered aggressive cancers (such as IBC).[531]

Young age at time of primary breast cancer diagnosis coupled with a first-degree family history of breast cancer shows increased risk.[531,533] LCIS rarely develops into invasive breast cancer, but it is known that discovery in one breast increases the risk of developing cancer in the other breast. The development of a contralateral breast cancer is associated with an increased risk of distant cancer recurrence.

Prophylactic approaches to reduce the risk of a second breast cancer include pharmacologic, radiotherapeutic, and surgical approaches in addition to lifestyle changes (diet, weight reduction, and exercise). Because the risk of developing other primary malignancies in breast cancer survivors may be greater than the general population, it is recommended that in addition to screening for contralateral breast cancer and recurrences, breast cancer survivors should undergo screening for other malignancies.[660]

SPECIAL IMPLICATIONS FOR THE THERAPIST   20-10

Breast Cancer

There are many considerations for the therapist working with men and women who report upper quadrant symptoms of unknown origin or who have been diagnosed with breast cancer, both before and after treatment. Therapists who specialize in oncology rehabilitation are increasingly active in research and developing protocols for best practices. The therapist should have knowledge of diagnostic categories, surgical procedures, postoperative restrictions and recommendations, expected/adverse outcomes of surgery, chemotherapy, radiation therapy, hormonal therapy, and targeted therapies (see discussion in Chapter 9).

The therapist must be knowledgeable of time-related restrictions for performing soft-tissue mobilization, risk factors for the development of lymphedema (see discussion in Chapter 13), and recommendations regarding lifestyle changes and complementary treatments. The use of alternative treatments, which take the place of medical treatments, can also be an area in which the therapist can provide valuable input for the individual with breast cancer. And, finally, outcome measures are an increasingly important part of clinical practice. The reader is referred to the special issue of *Rehabilitation Oncology* (Vol. 31. No. 1, 2013) that highlights the American Physical Therapy Association Oncology Section's Task Force on Breast Cancer Outcomes recommendations on measures that can or should be used for individuals treated for breast cancer.[34] Campbell et al also published a prospective model of care for breast cancer rehabilitation with a rationale for the integration of measures of function to aid physical therapists in providing better rehabilitation care for breast cancer survivors that may further assist physical therapists.[121]

Screening for Disease and Cancer Recurrence

When treating a woman with a history of breast cancer, an awareness of the symptoms and signs associated with breast cancer is important. Therapists should be alert to signs and symptoms that may point to local, regional, and distant metastases. Additionally, breast cancer survivors are at increased risk of developing a second primary breast cancer; it is not a recurrence but a new cancer unrelated to the first. This may occur in either breast for the individual who has undergone BCT or mastectomy (rare ipsilaterally). Around 5% of breast cancer survivors are diagnosed with a second breast cancer within 8 years of their initial diagnosis.

A local recurrence or second primary breast cancer will present most commonly as a new lump or mass. Masses that are painless, hard, and with irregular edges should be considered suspicious and should be evaluated. Palpation of a lump or mass in these areas or new onset of edema or swelling in the upper quadrant should raise concern for the therapist and lead to further questioning regarding the clinical findings.

Therapists examining the shoulder and shoulder girdle region need to be aware of the soft tissue structures (including breast tissue and regional lymph nodes) located in these areas. The upper, outer quadrant of the breast can extend up toward the glenohumeral joint; more cancerous masses occur in this area of the breast than in any other part of the breast. Approximately 35% to 50% of women with breast cancer will have metastasis to the axillary lymph nodes at the time of breast cancer diagnosis.[364] Breast tumor metastases to lymph nodes can involve the axillary, supraclavicular, infraclavicular, and internal mammary lymph nodes. Disease spread to these lymph nodes groups may cause compression of adjacent structures, resulting in referred pain to the shoulder, upper extremity, and/or chest wall.[254,414]

If the mass lies within the pectoralis major muscle, the mass should change during palpation during active muscle contraction. Metastases to the thorax are common in breast cancer, and pulmonary symptoms can be very similar to pulmonary abnormalities that occur after radiotherapy. If the therapist is in doubt regarding any reported or observed manifestations, the client should be medically evaluated (see "Lymphedema" in Chapter 13).

Bone metastases occur in up to 70% of women with advanced breast cancer.[520,581] The most common sites for boney metastases are the humerus in the upper extremity and the femur the lower extremity. Any report of new onset or increased bone pain, especially at night and/or with weight-bearing activities, should be carefully assessed; pathologic fracture is a possibility. Positive nodal status, large tumor size, ER+ status, and age younger than 35 years are significant risk factors for bone metastases in this population. Individuals who use tobacco, have a poor diet and nutrition, report decreased physical activity, and engage in alcohol abuse are much more likely to develop metastases.

Preoperative Considerations

Preoperative evaluation of the upper quarter by the therapist is recommended for all women undergoing surgical intervention for breast cancer whether the intervention is SLNB, ALND, lumpectomy, or mastectomy of any kind. Also recommended is evaluation prior to breast reconstruction surgery (immediate or delayed). Therapists are working to provide evidence-based research supporting the role of the oncology rehabilitation therapist in preoperative assessment and education. Educating breast surgeons, radiation oncologists, medical oncologists, and plastic surgeons regarding the benefits of preoperative assessment and postoperative therapeutic interventions is needed, as referral to a physical therapist may be delayed by months or years until the individual requests help with longstanding impairments.

Preoperative Assessment

Preoperative assessment of the person with breast cancer includes taking a thorough history and recording baseline measurements of both upper extremities so that any postoperative changes can be more easily detected. Radiation changes and previous surgeries are risk factors for postural compromises that contribute to movement impairments of the shoulder. The prevalence of shoulder-related dysfunction has been cited at 7% to 36% in the general population.[650]

Assessment of the individual's current physical activity level includes activities of daily living, work and leisure activities, and fitness and exercise habits and preferences. Upper quadrant motion (including biomechanics and scapulohumeral timing), posture, joint range of motion (including accessory motions), flexibility, and soft-tissue conditions should be assessed. Arthrokinematic changes of the shoulder joint and other preexisting shoulder problems present prior to breast cancer diagnosis and treatment may contribute to less than optimal postoperative recovery of glenohumeral and scapular motion. The therapist can address these problems before surgery or during neoadjuvant treatment, facilitating postoperative functional recovery.

Education

The therapist is a key educator and care provider who may be involved prior to breast cancer diagnosis, throughout the treatment and recovery process, in the transition from breast cancer "patient" to breast cancer "survivor," and/or helping those living with end-stage disease. If BCT or reconstruction has not been discussed with the woman, the therapist may want to encourage the woman to discuss this with her surgeon before the scheduled procedure. Studies show that only approximately 25% to 35% of breast surgeons discuss reconstruction or refer clients for a reconstructive surgery consultation with a plastic surgeon at the time of treatment planning.[9,493,496] Therapists should provide support for the woman who chooses to use a breast prosthesis, or no prosthesis at all. A helpful website for making these decisions is www.breastfree.org. Meeting with the medical oncologist prior to breast surgery is also recommended. Breast health navigators (often nurses or social workers) are patient advocates and may help coordinate the multidisciplinary team, which includes clinicians in many different specialties, such as the breast surgeon, plastic surgeon, radiation oncologist, medical oncologist, physical therapist, imaging technologist, radiologist, pathologist, and other support members.

Preoperative education should be specific to the individual's surgery, teaching postoperative precautions and safe movement (such as log rolling), avoidance of overactivity, and recommended exercises in the early postoperative phase prior to outpatient therapy.[575] For women who plan to undergo breast reconstruction, information about postoperative drain care, lifting and activity restriction, abdominal and chest protection, lymphedema prevention, and return to activity guidelines may be presented at this time.

Therapists can provide education and exercise interventions to decrease risk of vertebral fracture associated with osteoporosis especially for those individuals experiencing treatment effects on bone. Instructions may include avoiding spinal flexion and rotational movements, use of appropriate body mechanics, and adaptive equipment. Strengthening of spinal extensors, neutral core, and lower extremities may be employed along with balance training (and vestibular rehabilitation if indicated) to reduce fall risk and risk of fracture (hip, upper extremity, ribs) or other injury.

Side Effects of Treatment

(For a more complete discussion, see Chapters 5 and 9.)

Individuals receiving neoadjuvant or adjuvant therapy (chemotherapy, radiation therapy, hormonal therapy, or targeted therapy) may experience numerous side effects that may impact rehabilitation (see Chapters 5 and 9). Potential side effects of therapy are listed in Table 9-8; see also Tables 5-7 and 5-8.

Chemotherapy

The vast majority of individuals receiving chemotherapy experience fatigue and experience flulike symptoms.[400] This has been minimized to some extent with erythropoietin used to treat anemia by stimulating bone marrow production of red blood cells. Other common side effects include nausea, hair loss, mouth sores, neutropenia, and neuropathy (especially with taxanes). Less-common side effects that are serious include sepsis, cardiac damage, and secondary leukemia.[650] Cognitive difficulties can be pronounced during treatment, but long-term cognitive deficits after chemotherapy for breast cancer are reportedly small in magnitude, most often affecting verbal ability (word finding) and visuospatial ability (getting lost more easily in unfamiliar locations).[306]

For the individual with low nadir (lowest point of blood cell production after neutrophil and platelet count have been depressed by chemotherapy) and/or anemia, the timing of scheduled therapy visits is important to maximize productivity during the session. Exercises and functional activities may need to be paced or therapy visits adjusted to accommodate the person's energy level. Conditioning exercise can address the need for increased endurance for activities of daily living, family responsibilities and occupational demands.

Radiotherapy

Radiation therapy uses high-energy beams to destroy cells; both cancer and native cells are affected.

Immediate radiation risks include skin redness, blistering, fatigue, and breast tenderness. Long-term effects include tissue scarring, poor wound healing, lymphedema, ischemic heart disease,[177] increased breast firmness, loss of breast volume, and permanent skin changes (e.g., telangiectasias and hyperpigmentation). Surgeons typically wait 6 months after radiotherapy to assess tissue quality for surgical options including reconstruction.[650]

Radiotherapy to the left breast is associated with higher rates of chest pain, coronary artery disease, and myocardial infarction. Cardiotoxic drugs such as doxorubicin (Adriamycin) and trastuzumab (Herceptin) may compound the problem. The therapist can screen women treated for breast cancer for cardiac symptoms and risk factors such as blood pressure and smoking. Regular cardiac surveillance is important for all breast cancer survivors regardless of whether they had radiation therapy because of the increased risk of cardiac disease with aging.[208,544]

Hormonal Therapy

Although SERMs have a protective effect on bone mineral density, the majority of AIs have been linked with a decrease in bone density and increased fracture risk. Further research is needed to address prevention and management of osteoporosis with the use of AIs and quality of life after breast cancer.[73] Baseline and follow-up bone density studies are recommended for individuals on AIs; drug therapy may include bisphosphonates and other medications (e.g., monoclonal antibody therapy). Education should include adequate calcium and vitamin D supplementation and modifying risk factors such as alcohol intake, tobacco use, and lack of exercise.[390]

There has been an increased frequency of lower-extremity arthralgias reported with the use of hormonal therapy, specifically with the use of AIs and, to a lesser degree, tamoxifen. Adverse effects can include complaints of joint and muscle pain and stiffness, carpal tunnel syndrome, and trigger finger. AI-induced musculoskeletal syndrome is associated tendon-sheath thickening and intraarticular fluid retention with loss of grip strength.[380,438] The effect of estrogen deprivation and arthralgias is under investigation. It is hypothesized that both systemic and local effects of estrogen deficiency may impair cartilage maintenance. The role of vitamin D is the subject of ongoing research. Symptoms of arthralgias are reported in 25% to 40% of individuals on AIs, with the intensity of symptoms being a factor in the 20% of individuals who choose to discontinue use of this medication.[226,419,516] Switching to another AI may significantly improve symptoms such that the individual is able to maintain therapeutic benefit for hormonal adjuvant therapy benefit.[107]

A variety of interventions for joint pain have been studied, including physical therapy, movement therapies such as tai chi or yoga, acupuncture, heat, massage, diuretics, acetaminophen, nonsteroidal antiinflammatory drugs, cyclooxygenase-2 inhibitors, magnesium, vitamin D, and glucosamine chondroitin sulfate (taken with the AI). Some of these treatment approaches are effective for some women, but it is not clear yet if there is one optimal treatment or combination of interventions that is optimal for everyone.

Other complications of hormonal therapy include vasomotor symptoms, mood disorders, sexual dysfunction, venous thrombosis, endometrial pathology, and cataract formation. Therapists should be alert to signs and symptoms of these conditions.

Postoperative Considerations

Recovery after individual surgical procedures may vary. Many centers have postoperative protocols for each procedure available for review. For further discussion, see "Breast Reconstruction," later in this section. Potential complications after all types of breast cancer surgery (BCT, mastectomy, and reconstruction) may include pain, sensory changes (dysesthesias and numbness), infection (cellulitis), tissue necrosis, seroma development, hematoma, and local tissue swelling. Despite the adoption of more conservative surgical approaches, pain and functional compromise after surgery remain significant clinical challenges.

Breast surgery and surgical assessment of axillary lymph nodes (either by SLNB or ALND) are commonly associated with pain, decreased shoulder range of motion, weakness, movement impairment, swelling, neuropathy, fatigue, axillary web syndrome (or cording), and lymphedema of the upper extremity and trunk. Between 10% and 64% of women report upper-body symptoms between 6 months and 3 years after breast cancer.[276] Functional impairments with upper-extremity tasks such as household chores, lifting, and carrying have been reported in 35% or more women at 1 year postsurgery.[374]

Therapeutic interventions employed by the oncology rehabilitation therapist address soft-tissue fibrosis, deficits in muscle strength and flexibility, lymphatic insufficiency, muscle hypertonicity, and neural hypersensitivity. Proactive and preventative approaches should be employed rather than delaying treatment until problems persist. It is well-known that functional impairments can persist many years after the completion of breast cancer treatment. Prospective surveillance models have been proposed as a model of ongoing evaluation of physical functioning as opposed to a traditional model of impairment-based care.[588] This surveillance model uses physical therapists as experts in movement dysfunction to provide preoperative examination, education, ongoing clinical monitoring, early identification, and intervention for common conditions result from breast cancer treatment. These include upper-extremity dysfunction, pain, weakness, fatigue, arthralgias, lymphedema, neuropathy, weight gain, cardiovascular changes, and osteoporosis and fracture risk reduction.[141,544a,588]

Medical caregivers as well as therapists can review simple range of motion exercises that can be done postoperatively once the drains are removed prior to any outpatient therapy.[141] Restricting shoulder abduction in the first week after mastectomy (or drains out plus 5 days) is recommended to allow lymphatic collecting vessels to regenerate and reconnect. This is facilitated by promoting close proximity of severed vessels to one another. Restricting shoulder abduction during this time period has been observed to decrease the risk of seroma development.[387,588]

The therapist must assess the biomechanics of shoulder motion after radiation therapy and surgery and employ interventions that address dysfunction of the upper quarter. Scapular and genohumeral movement along with cervical and thoracic spine are likely to be compromised. Anterior chest muscle tightness and hypertonicity secondary to pain is common. Postural changes may result from efforts to protect the surgical site, which efforts promote further muscle and soft-tissue shortening. Radiation fibrosis of the pectoral tendons and muscle sheaths may exacerbate tissue tightness. When the pectoralis major muscle is incorporated into the muscular pouch which houses breast implants, muscle tension markedly increases resulting in scapular protraction. Myofascial pain in the scapular retractors is common.[141] The therapist may employ manual therapy, modalities, and therapeutic exercises, which include stretching and strengthening for endurance and proper sequencing of motor recruitment.[198]

Ongoing education and support are significant aspect of the therapist–client relationship. Therapists working with oncology clients require a specialized skillset to assist individuals who are coping with the emotional challenges of living with a life-threatening and body-altering disease. They are integral to the healing and recovery process as empathetic companions throughout the treatment continuum: surgeries, radiotherapy, chemotherapy, and targeted and hormonal therapies. They assist the client with emotional and physical adjustments to body image, sexuality, stress management, potential changes in vocational and family-life roles, and end-of-life issues.

Barriers to individuals receiving physical therapy treatment after surgery for breast cancer include a lack of evidence-based protocols and research challenges to acquiring such evidence, which include the multi-factorial nature of rehabilitation. Other barriers include the limited number of clinicians who specialize in oncology rehabilitation and lack of traditionally established relationships between the therapist and breast surgeons, oncologist, radiation oncologists, and plastic surgeons. Logistical barriers may include the person's distance to clinic, as well as financial and insurance limitations. Individuals with cancer may be treated with simplistic algorithms that may afford little benefit and may in fact be harmful.[141]

Breast-Conserving Therapy

BCT usually does not affect the pectoralis major muscle or overlying fascia, but the therapist should request the operative report for more details; lobular breast cancer can progress to the chest wall requiring deep resection. The therapist should be aware that tissue destruction caused by radiation therapy may include muscle damage.

A THERAPIST'S THOUGHTS*
BREAST-CONSERVING SURGERY

Although women who have breast-conserving surgery may not have as much trauma to the chest muscles, they can still benefit from the services of a physical therapist. These women can benefit from preoperative education about precautions and movement of the upper extremity, and they may need physical therapy because of the side effects of radiation therapy. This is a group of women who are often neglected after their surgery.

*Margaret Rinehart-Ayres, PT, PhD

Mastectomy

Mastectomy without reconstruction has different rehabilitation considerations from mastectomy with reconstruction (immediate or delayed). Women who have undergone mastectomy should be instructed postoperatively and assisted with breathing and splinted coughing techniques to prevent pulmonary complications. Lower extremity exercises may be employed to prevent thromboemboli. Management of postoperative drains and activity modification, as well as when to begin active shoulder range of motion (not too early; not too late), are important functions of the oncology rehabilitation therapist. (See "Shoulder/Upper Extremity" later in this section.)

A significant number of women (reported to be between 20% and 65%) undergoing mastectomy or levels 1 and 2 lymph node removal experience a neuropathic pain phenomenon called *postmastectomy pain syndrome* (PMPS) or *post–breast therapy pain syndrome* (PBTPS).[14,340] PMPS/PBTPS is an imprecise term used to describe any pain persisting beyond the period of "normal" healing (usually defined as 3 months) after a mastectomy.[14,340] It is thought to arise from neural injury during surgery, specifically the intercostobrachial nerve, a peripheral nerve with tributaries that branch into the axilla and upper arm. Neuroma formation, intercostals brachial nerve sacrifice, fibrotic entrapment, and intraoperative compromise of cutaneous innervations have been implicated. It is now recognized that similar presentations occur after BCT and axillary surgeries.[141] The pain occurs at the incision site, axilla, arm, or shoulder and may be experienced as burning, numbness, tingling, pins and needles, lancinating or shock like.[570] Severity ranges from mild to extremely distressing; onset and frequency are highly variable (immediate to 3 months postoperatively and experienced as continuous or episodic: daily, weekly, and monthly).

Because PMPS/PBTPS seems to be increasingly reported, it is important for the clinician to inquire about postmastectomy pain. Prognostic risk factors that predispose an individual to PMPS/PBTPS are unknown, with the possible exception of age (more common in women younger than 30 years).[126,570] An oncology rehabilitation program to promote flexibility and prevent adhesive capsulitis, and restore strength, range of motion, and normal neuromuscular recruitment patterns should be employed with a focus on functional mobility, instrumental activities of daily living and vocational capacity. Use of desensitization techniques (deep pressure, light touch, sharp or vibratory stimulation), nerve gliding techniques, transcutaneous electrical nerve stimulation and topical cold have been anecdotally employed.[141]

Pharmaceutical and interventional pain techniques are increasingly offered. These include medications for neuropathic pain. Nonsteroidal antiinflammatory drugs work by desensitizing central nervous system effects. Opioid trials may be warranted for intense or refractory pain. Interventional techniques include intercostal or paravertebral nerve blocks.

Breast Reconstruction

Autologous Reconstruction

The therapist should be aware that in the pedicled TRAM flap and the free TRAM there is a risk of sacrifice of the entire rectus muscle and risk of abdominal weakness, hernia, and fat necrosis. The lower abdominal hernia rate for TRAM surgeries is 1% to 15%.[650] The free TRAM procedure has less of a risk of fat necrosis because of a better blood supply. A mesh patch may or may not be utilized in the rectus area. Altered kinesthesia and musculoskeletal mechanics (e.g., altered tension of the thoracolumbar fascia and resulting back pain, substitution by the abdominal oblique muscles, and compensation of the contralateral rectus muscle) require intervention. Gradual advancement to assure correct muscle recruitment is advised. A TRAM protocol–therapist's guide, courtesy of Nicole L. Stout, PT, MPT, CLT-LANA, is available on the Evolve website in Evolve Table 20-1.[650]

Perforator flap surgeries dissect the blood vessels out from the muscle which minimizes donor site morbidity. The DIEP perforator flap surgery has a lower abdominal hernia rate of less than 1% with preservation of 70% of the rectus abdominis muscle function.[650]

Postoperative protocols vary. Typically, room temperature is kept warm and supplemental oxygen is provided with close tissue monitoring, including tissue oximetry, employed to minimize risk of flap necrosis. The patient is kept in flexion (head of bed elevated, hips and knees flexed) and on bedrest for 1 to 2 days to facilitate wound healing. Precautions in the first 2 days include no pressure on the central chest, no rolling, no covering of incisions or flap, and no bathing.[650]

The acute care therapist instructs the patient in use of incentive spirometry, splinted coughing techniques, and bed mobility with good technique for getting out of bed with minimal use of upper extremities. After the person has tolerated out of bed in a chair, ambulation is initiated. Activities of daily living training includes drain care, showering protocols, and intensive education on avoiding central chest pressure, return to home environment with precautions, and graded exercises to the upper quadrant and abdominal muscles. The woman should not wear a bra for approximately 30 days or use any hot or cold on the breast mound as it is insensate. Driving and lifting is restricted. Limited activity is enforced for 2 weeks and monitored exercise (e.g., avoiding abdominal "crunches") is employed after 6 or more weeks (depending on the surgeon's protocol).[650] The outpatient therapist should request an operative report to ascertain whether any synthetic or acellular mesh has been used in the surgical reconstruction.

Complications and Problems

Donor-site morbidity is more pronounced with autologous procedures that involve muscle transfer. Post-TRAM flap complications have received the most attention.[141] Isokinetic testing reveals weakness of the truncal flexors following TRAM flap harvesting. Trunk flexion deficits up to 23% have been reported in subjects with pedicled-TRAM flap procedures and trunk extension deficits up to 14%. For the free-TRAM procedure, trunk flexion deficits up to 18% have been reported, with no deficits in trunk extension.[47] Further research is needed to support reports of even fewer deficits in patient's after DIEP and other perforator flap surgeries.

Eventual recovery has been noted by some authors,[217] but imbalance between truncal flexors and extensors may persist. TRAM-associated functional deficits related to proprioceptive denervation include impaired balance and interference of truncal "righting" reflexes, and increased risk of low back pain. A graded postoperative abdominal muscle reeducation and strengthening program is essential to prevent further spine-related musculoskeletal complications and associated postural compromise.

Lymph vessel damage may occur during the separation of the rectus sheath from the overlying dermis resulting in truncal lymphostasis. Truncal edema is common and can last for up to a year; it generally responds to lymph clearing techniques. Trauma may also produce fibrosis and tethering of the dermis to underlying tissue. This fibrosis limits truncal extension and may result in neural entrapment producing chronic pain. Although uncommon (occurring in 1%-5% of cases), the most serious complication of the flap procedure is a loss of blood circulation to the transferred tissue, leading to necrosis and the loss of all or part of the reconstructed breast. Despite the potential for functional morbidity, a significant majority of women recommended TRAM reconstruction and report enhanced health-related quality of life following the procedure.[627]

Breast Implants

Women who receive breast implants for reconstruction after mastectomies undergo a much less extensive operation than autologous reconstructions. Acellular dermal matrix (such as AlloDerm) may be used to help define the natural breast landmark at the inframammary fold and lateral breast curve.[650] There is a much shorter recovery time and no loss of other tissues with minimal scarring. There are however multiple office visits during the "fill" phase of tissue expansion prior to the placement of the permanent implant. Postoperative restrictions may include limiting shoulder range of motion to 90 degrees or less for 2 weeks.

Complications associated with implant reconstruction surgery include those caused by tissue damage from the cancer surgery and adjuvant chemotherapy and radiation to the surrounding tissue. The most common complication of implant reconstruction is *capsular contraction* in which scar tissue formation around the implant deforms or hardens the implant. Capsular contraction occurs in up to 30% of breast implant reconstructions with surgical intervention usually required.[645] For women who have radiation therapy following breast reconstruction, the risk of scar tissue and hardening around the breast implant increases to as high as 50%. Other risks include implant rupture or leakage and less often bruising, infection, and chronic pain.

As noted previously there may be musculoskeletal impairments because the tissue expander and implant is placed under the pectoralis major, serratus anterior, and anterior rectus sheaths. These include pectoral muscle spasm, splinting and guarding, chest wall tightness, scarring, and decreased shoulder range of motion and function. Pectoral tightness may affect scapular retractor muscles with postural compromise. This is manifest in stretch weakness and irritability resulting in periscapular pain and subsequent myofascial dysfunction in the back and neck muscles. Mobilization, manual therapy, and myofascial release techniques may be helpful.

Latissimus Dorsi Myocutaneous Flap

The latissimus dorsi myocutaneous flap (or "lat flap") is another common surgery chosen particularly for *bilateral* reconstruction. It is a pedicled procedure in most cases and may be performed without an implant, with an immediate implant, or more commonly with use of a tissue expander (with implant exchanged at a second surgery.) Thus the "lat flap" may be considered to be a combination of autologous and implant reconstructive surgeries. High rates of capsular contraction have been cited, but in recent studies, more acceptable rates of 7% to 10.5% (requiring capsulectomy) have been achieved by some clinics.[629] Patient satisfaction is high with acceptable functional upper extremity use in daily activities.[385,488] More information is needed on function-related donor-site morbidity following latissimus dorsi harvesting. There are reported risks of shoulder morbidity with diminished range of motion (47%) and strength (33%)[154] with physical activity limitations; the latissimus dorsi is an important shoulder adductor, internal rotator, and depressor. Therapy should address abnormal motion at the scapula–thoracic joint, as well as scapular stabilization for upper-extremity activities.

Axillary Node Dissection

A number of dysesthesias have been reported after lymph node surgery. Sensations have been described as tender, sore, pulling, aching, painful, twinge, tight, stiff, pricking, throbbing, shooting, tingling, numb, burning, hard, sharp, nagging, and deep or penetrating.[65] Numbness under the arm (axillary and medial upper arm area) is often a clue that axillary node dissection was performed. Frequently, the individual does not know how many nodes were removed. The therapist should request the pathology report to determine the number of nodes removed and to help educate the individual on risk for lymphedema and other complications. See www.lymphedemarisk.com. Postoperative deficits following axillary lymph node dissection can become chronic conditions for many breast cancer survivors.[264] Many of these problems develop within 3 months of surgery, whereas others can develop many years later independent of shoulder problems.[413,575]

Axillary Web Syndrome

Axillary web syndrome (AWS), also known as axillary cording or lymphatic cording, is a condition associated with surgery to the axilla. It is not uncommon and can occur with ALND or SLNB. Lymphatic cording is described as a visible and palpable web or fibrous cord of subcutaneous tissue that may be confined to the axilla or extend distally along the anterior, medial aspect of the arm as far as the palm (Fig. 20-19). Proximal cording into the torso and breast tissue have also been described.[356]

The cords are most visible in the axilla when the shoulder is abducted or in the antecubital space when the elbow is extended (Fig. 20-20). Radiating pain down the arm during shoulder abduction and limitation of shoulder abduction and/or elbow extension are the most common symptoms. Usually there are two or three palpable cords under the skin that are hard and painful, but not erythematous. Typically, the affected individual has a normal postoperative course but with delayed complaints of intense pain along with limited range of motion, especially shoulder abduction (less than 90 degrees in 74% of cases).[443,508] The incidence of AWS and predisposing patient and surgical

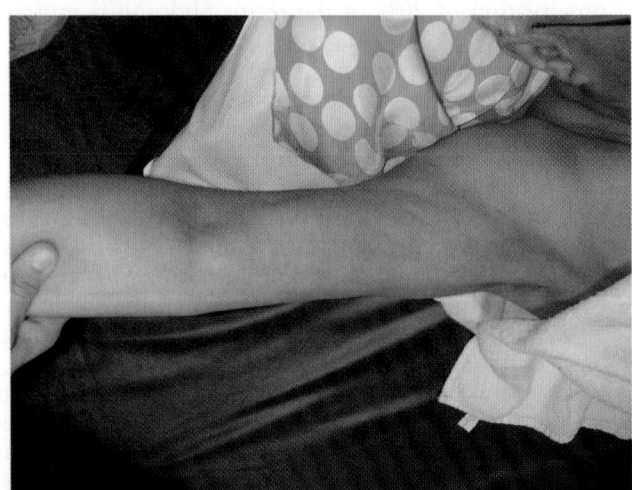

Figure 20-19

Axillary web syndrome 2 weeks after initiation of physical therapy intervention. The cording is less prominent but still visible as the skin is pulled back by the cord. This effect can make the arm look swollen as if there is some swelling from lymphedema. Edema can also accompany cording. (Courtesy Jane Kepics, MS, PT, CLT-LANA, Phoenixville Hospital, Phoenixville, PA.)

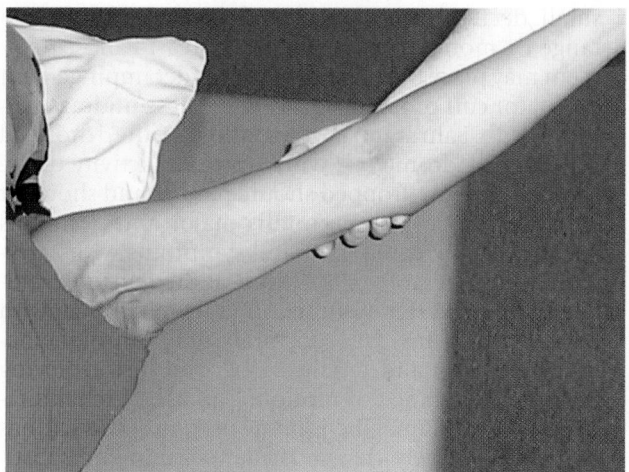

Figure 20-20

Photo shows a pretreatment axillary cord that limits shoulder abduction. This client had a biopsy of a swollen axillary lymph node. The biopsy was benign, but the woman had pain and limited range of motion for about 6 weeks. (Courtesy Jane Kepics, MS, PT, CLT-LANA, Phoenixville Hospital, Phoenixville, PA.)

characteristics are poorly defined. Reports range from 6% to 72% of women who develop AWS after lymph node surgery (ALND or SLNB). Symptoms typically present between weeks 1 and 5 postoperatively.[367,443] The condition may be self-limiting, resolving within 3 months' time.[503] However, some women do report persistent discomfort (even severe pain) in the chest wall or axilla for longer periods. Treatment may improve movement and reduce pain sooner than without treatment.[312,339,658]

The physical therapist may be very instrumental in discovering unreported or unresolved AWS. Physical therapy intervention may have a role in reducing the length of time clients suffer from this condition, especially for women for whom the condition persists beyond the expected time due to concurrent cancer care.[658] Early recognition of symptoms (e.g., arm pain and decreased shoulder motion) and intervention may help prevent postural changes, movement dysfunction, and restriction of activities of daily living.[650]

Clinicians report good success with gentle and slow manual therapy techniques including myofascial release, soft-tissue mobilization, skin traction, cord bending, and scar massage directly to the cords and to the surrounding tissues. The therapist must avoid being too aggressive with this approach. Even with gentle techniques, palpable and audible "releases" of the cord can be felt and heard by the therapist and the client with sudden increase in arm movement.[356] Length of therapy treatment has been reported in the literature to be 4 to 18 weeks, with range of motion typically regained within 2 months of initiating physical therapy. Patient/client education includes frequent and gentle active range of motion with self-stretching and cautious use of local heat and careful monitoring (because of compromised sensation from intercostal brachial nerve damage and increased risk of lymphedema).[650]

This condition may occur from lymphatic disruption after breast or axillary surgery or possibly disruption of fascial planes during the surgery. The exact mechanism is unknown. It may be attributed to lymphovenous injury (e.g., lymph vein rupture, superficially dilated veins with thrombi inside [superficial lymphatic thrombosis], or lymphatic outflow obstruction) from prolonged positioning during surgery, or lymphovenous stasis from removal of nodes in the axilla. The cords may represent thrombosed lymphatics after an inflammatory phase with thickening of the vessels, temporary shortening, and tightening, which later remits.[328,367,443]

It is important to differentiate articular or postoperative muscular shortening, as well as the fear-avoidance behavior (i.e., fear of pain from movement) from AWS.

A THERAPIST'S THOUGHTS*
AXILLARY WEB SYNDROME

Although the literature reports axillary web syndrome (AWS) occurs in the early weeks after surgery, clinical physical therapists note scarring can continue and this syndrome can develop even a year after surgery. There is some debate about the effect of early exercise and stretching on the development of AWS. The question of whether early exercise and stretching can trigger versus prevent AWS (some surgeons seem to think this type of protocol can serve to prevent or reduce AWS) remains unanswered. The definition of "early" also remains unclear. Waiting 5 to 8 days after the drain(s) is (are) removed before addressing lost shoulder/elbow range of motion may allow for regeneration of the deeper vessels.[506]

Oncology therapists report anecdotal observations that women who rest adequately in the early days following surgery have their drains removed sooner and do not require aspiration as often (or at all) compared with women who have a difficult time following the guidelines to rest and avoid exercise/overuse of the involved extremity. In other words, women who are more active seem to be the ones who develop AWS, especially the more aggressive cases. Rest may promote anastomotic development of the lymphatic collecting vessels.

My theory is that when they overuse an area that has been traumatized and still easily creating increased inflammation due to the lack of adequate fibroblastic regeneration protection, then the lymphatic fluid and inflammatory cascade of chemicals drips down distally while resting. Rest allows for adequate healing and fibroblastic activity to complete the repair process without developing cording.

To aid in limiting range of motion early on (especially shoulder abduction) it has been suggested the woman use a safety pin or cloth restraint attached to clothing to remind the individual of the recommended motion restrictions. The therapist can aid in restoring motion through the *careful* use of moist heat (this is an area of controversy; see further discussion of physical agents, Chapter 9), especially in any areas with sensation changes secondary to treatment followed by myofascial release, gentle stretching, and ice. Patients are instructed in a home program of self-stretching, nerve gliding exercises, contract-relax techniques, and encouraged to maintain motion through light daily activities.

*Loraine Lovejoy-Evans, MPT, DPT, CLT-Földi

Shoulder/Upper Extremity

Upper quarter impairments with activity and participation limitations are commonly reported in individuals receiving treatment for breast cancer. The most common complaints are pain and weakness in the involved extremity; approximately 80% of women with these complaints indicate that the impairments limit them on daily basis.[598] Most women present with more than one symptom such as arm and breast edema, shoulder stiffness, weakness, movement impairment, axillary and/or chest wall pain, and sensory changes.

Shoulder girdle movement is affected by surgery and/or radiation. Limited shoulder abduction and external rotation is commonly reported after surgery with women reporting more shoulder restrictions and impairments after mastectomy than with breast-conserving surgery. Altered movement patterns of the scapula (with associated pain and dysfunction) on the side of the cancer have been demonstrated with mastectomy.[550] Altered kinematics may be the physical manifestation of pain pathways or may induce pain. Loss of motor activity may alter force couple produced by muscles of the rotator cuff, increasing upward rotation of the scapula, which has been implicated in movement dysfunctions currently labeled impingement syndrome and glenohumeral instability. It has been proposed that loss of lateral shoulder rotation contributes to increased posterior tilt of the scapula as a compensatory movement.[550] The incidence of shoulder morbidity is also higher in those who have undergone postsurgical radiation therapy.[166]

In the breast cancer population, 40% of patients have metastasis in the axillary lymph nodes. For those who undergo ALND, 73% report restricted shoulder mobility, tightness, edema, pain and numbness and limitations in activities of daily living.[598] Limited shoulder range of motion is common following surgery and especially ALND. Efficacy of physical therapy following ALND has been demonstrated with improved shoulder mobility, lessened pain, enhanced psychosocial adjustment, and improved quality of life.[87,100,133,363] The pathophysiology of adhesive capsulitis after breast cancer surgery is presumably the same as the development of this condition in other situations with decreased mobility.[174] Reports conflict whether there is a lowered incidence of adhesive capsulitis with SLNB versus ALND.

Radiation-induced changes of the pectoralis major muscle and decreased size of pectoralis major and minor muscles have also been reported.[166,372,551] However, surgery itself can create fibrotic changes with healing. Fibrosis in the pectoralis major and minor muscles increases the risk of shoulder impingement with greater scapular anterior tipping, decreased upward rotation and increased scapular medial rotation under load conditions. Individuals with a clinically determined shortened pectoralis minor muscle demonstrate scapular kinematics similar to those found for subjects with shoulder impingement.[99] Even small decreases in shoulder abduction and flexion range of motion in women after breast cancer treatment may place them at risk for shoulder impingement or rotator cuff problems over time. These findings correlate with Sahrmann's designation of the "dropped shoulder syndrome,"[529] with decreased activity of the upper trapezius, dropped shoulder, neck and shoulder pain, atrophy of the pectoralis major and pectoralis minor, and increased pain and symptoms with carrying objects. The role of the physical therapist in evaluating upper quarter dysfunction in the individual with breast cancer involves postural and arthrokinematic assessment, and retraining beyond just achieving postoperative range of motion. The use of rehabilitative ultrasound imaging is being used in some settings to more effectively view muscular recruitment, substitution, inhibition, and overactivity.[650]

Restricting activity of the involved arm following surgery until all the drains are removed has shown to decrease wound complications including seromas.[549] Limiting shoulder abduction to 90 degrees for an additional 5 days after drains are removed has been advised by expert therapists. A proactive multidisciplinary approach is advocated. Some surgeons restrict movement for up to 6 weeks after surgery so as to decrease the risk of seroma formation; there is much controversy over this and little evidence regarding the optimum timeline for inactivity and resuming activity.

Excessive limiting of motion can result in stiffness and loss of mobility throughout the entire upper quadrant on the affected side. Scarring with facial tightness complicates the therapist's treatment intervention. Early rehabilitation that respects the need for adequate healing yet allows for graded movement and tissue stress will result in minimized stiffness. For the therapist and the patient/client, this includes manual stretching, gentle aerobic conditioning, low-intensity resistance training, and postural modifications.[650]

Current evidence suggests that upper-extremity impairments from treatment for breast cancer can extend beyond the acute stages of recovery and may be considered a component of chronic illness. The most common impairments 6 months after surgery are breast and axillary scar tightness, axillary edema, altered scapular kinematics, and neck and shoulder pain. Older women with depressive symptoms at 2 months after diagnosis have been shown to have reduced range of motion 12 months postdiagnosis and posttreatment.[116] Risk factors for chronic pain include acute postoperative pain, radiation therapy, and more invasive treatment.

Functional assessment tools currently in use by therapists include the DASH (Disability of Arm, Shoulder and Hand), SPADI (Shoulder Pain and Disability Index), and the Penn Shoulder Scale. Functional scales that have been adapted for the individual with breast cancer include the visual analogue scale (VAS) and Scale for Breast Cancer Patients (based on the Oswestry Low Back Pain Disability Questionnaire), and Functional Assessment of Cancer Therapy for Breast Cancer

(FACT-B). Notable limitations in lifting, carrying and reaching have been highlighted by these tools.[550]

Lymphedema

Education about the incidence and prevention of lymphedema including lifetime precautions is a primary task of the oncology rehabilitation therapist (see Table 13-2). Physical therapists have demonstrated how early diagnosis and treatment of breast cancer-related lymphedema can reduce costs and the need for intensive rehabilitation.[586] As previously mentioned, a surveillance model to identify impairment at the earliest onset has been proposed as a standard of care for breast cancer treatment. A preoperative exam to establish a baseline level of function with follow-up examinations postoperatively at 1-month and then 3-month intervals for up to 1 year are advised instead of the traditional model of treating lymphedema once it has progressed with its concomitant functional limitations.[33,586]

A nomogram for predicting lymphedema risk for individuals who have had ALND is available online at: www.lymphedemarisk.com. Factors contributing to risk include age, body mass index (>30), number of chemotherapy cycles in ipsilateral arm, location of the radiation field, and the development of postoperative seroma, infection, or early edema.[88] Studies show the risk of lymphedema to be least, but not nonexistent, among those individuals who have had SLNB. More study between the association of cancer treatment and lymphedema is needed.[470]

Secondary lymphedema of the upper quarter remains a chronic and distressing condition for some women after breast cancer treatment. It is most commonly seen in the ipsilateral arm, but can also affect the trunk, abdomen, and breast. Conservative therapies, such as complete decongestive therapy, compression bandaging and garments, and exercise, have proved effective in reducing fluid volume and improving subjective arm symptoms and quality of life.[441] Lymphedema and its treatment are presented in depth in Chapter 13.

Low-level laser treatment has been approved by the FDA since 2007 for the treatment of postmastectomy lymphedema. The laser-beam pulses produce photochemical reactions at the cellular level, thereby influencing the course of metabolic processes and reducing the volume of the affected arm, extracellular fluid, and tissue hardness.[124] In a double-blinded, randomized, controlled trial, laser treatment was found to be effective in reducing the limb volume, increasing shoulder mobility, and improving hand grip strength in approximately 93% of patients with postmastectomy lymphedema.[7]

Exercise and Breast Cancer

Exercise During Treatment

Decline in physical activity is common during treatment for breast cancer. Chemotherapy for breast cancer may cause unfavorable changes in physical functioning, body composition, psychosocial functioning, and quality of life. Studies of aerobic or

A THERAPIST'S THOUGHTS*

LASER FOR BREAST CANCER-RELATED LYMPHEDEMA (BCRL)

In the double-blinded, randomized, controlled trial study on laser referenced above,[7] the laser group had 29% reduction compared to 22% in the control group. Each group did some exercise and wore compression garments of 40 to 60 mm Hg compression (which in my opinion is too high for the upper extremity). They report improved shoulder range of motion of 10 degrees more in the study group compared with the control group.

The results are not statistically significant enough to support laser treatment as a successful treatment modality to be encouraged. In our clinic, we have used the Rhian corporation laser but our women with breast cancer-related lymphedema have not had significant volume reductions from the laser treatment. The laser treatment was given after women had undergone complete decongestive therapy and their limbs were stabilized for several months/years wearing compression garments. The hope was that further reduction would be achieved through the laser treatment. This did not occur. We have observed some good results with pain and scar softening in secondary arm and leg lymphedema, and fibrosis softening in primary lymphedema but no significant volume reductions. We have also used it trying to reduce significant hand edema/fibrosis secondary to breast cancer-related lymphedema with limited success.

As the subtitle of this section suggests, this is just my opinion; but for me, the evidence from the study is not very convincing. Readers must be very objective when reviewing papers encouraging us to see something as significant that may not be so on closer inspection. Carati's[125] report of 200-mL reductions in limb volume may seem significant, but upon closer examination, this is not a significant amount of decrease in lymphedema. Moreover, only 26 of 37 subjects who received the "active laser treatments" (27 were in the placebo group; there was no control group) were available for limited follow-up in 2 to 3 months. Data was missing on one-third of the experimental group—this is not highlighted in the abstract but is something that as critical readers of research we need to look for.

If one theory of how laser works in this patient population is that it stimulates the mitochondria to release more growth hormone, would that not perhaps encourage cancer cell growth, particularly if the laser is applied in the axilla as in the Carati study? The manufacturer and literature have so far not answered that question. I advise caution when using this modality for breast cancer–related lymphedema.

See also comments regarding the use of modalities with all cancer patients in Chapter 9.

*Bonnie Lasinski, MA, PT, CSCI, CLT-LANA

resistive exercise during adjuvant treatment for breast cancer have shown benefit in areas of self-esteem, physical fitness, body composition, and chemotherapy completion rate.[162] The impact of all types of aerobic exercise is significant in maintaining functional ability and reducing fatigue in women with breast cancer who are receiving chemotherapy or radiation therapy. Moderate-intensity (40%-70% of predicted maximum heart rate) aerobic exercise is effective during adjuvant therapy for breast cancer to increase peak VO_2 and, therefore, aerobic capacity reserves. Improved physical

Note to Reader: Throughout this text, the benefits of exercise and lifestyle changes in relation to various diseases, disorders, and conditions have been discussed, including (pertinent to the diagnosis of breast cancer) exercise and immunology (see Chapter 7), exercise and cancer from a variety of viewpoints (see Chapter 9), exercise and the cardiovascular system (see Chapter 12), and exercise and the lymphatic system (see Chapter 13). The reader is encouraged to read all of those sections in order to gain a perspective that takes into consideration all aspects of care for individuals with breast cancer throughout their lives.

For a full discussion of the influence of exercise and cancer and more evidence-based specifics regarding mode, intensity, frequency, and duration, see Chapter 9. See also previous Prevention section for guidelines related to exercise and breast cancer and a review of the most recent literature. This is an area of ongoing research and the reader is advised to continue keeping up with current published studies.

function, decreased fatigue, and improved psychologic factors are the final outcomes.[334]

Exercise After Treatment

Survivors of breast cancer are at increased risk of breast cancer recurrence, second primary breast cancers and early mortality. Physical activity guidelines (2008) for 2.5 hours (10 MET-hours) of moderate intensity activity per week have been reviewed as they apply to breast cancer survivors. Engaging in at least 10 MET-hours/week of physical activity has is associated with a 27% reduction in all-cause mortality and a 25% reduction in breast cancer mortality. Meeting the physical activity guidelines has not yet been proven to be associated with reducing risk of breast cancer recurrence.[70]

Physical activity at any time after completion of primary breast cancer treatment is associated with reduced rates of mortality,[223] improved immune function, improved health-related quality of life, improved bone density, increased muscle strength, and decreased fatigue.[652] Most research studies have been of home-based or supervised exercise. While exercise for sedentary individuals requires behavior change, group physical activity programs can foster social support and feelings of connectedness.[447]

Exercise for Cancer-Related Fatigue

See "Exercise for Cancer-Related Fatigue" in Chapter 9.

Exercise and Breast Cancer-Related Lymphedema

(See also "Exercise and Lymphedema" in Chapter 9.)

Exercise restrictions for women with or at risk for breast cancer–related lymphedema have changed as a result of updated research. Previous recommendations to avoid vigorous, repetitive or strenuous upper-body exercise (believing that such types of exercise might induce lymphedema) have been overturned. Studies of upper-extremity resistance training in women after surgery for breast cancer have included teams of dragon boat racers and weight lifting. In randomized controlled trials of women at risk for lymphedema and for those with stable lymphedema after breast cancer surgery, a slowly progressive weight-lifting program has shown no significant effect on developing lymphedema or exacerbating limb swelling. Benefits of exercise have been shown to reduce overall symptoms and result in increased strength.[541,542,543]

REFERENCES

To enhance this text and add value for the reader, all references are included on the companion Evolve site that accompanies this textbook. The reader can view the reference source and access it online whenever possible.

CHAPTER 21

Transplantation

CHRIS L. WELLS • COURTNEY FRANKEL • EVA GOLD •
G. STEPHEN MORRIS

Transplantation for the treatment of end-stage organ failure has been one of the major medical advances of the last 40 years. The success of this form of treatment has improved dramatically with improved surgical procedures, better understanding and management of the rejection process, and more options in immunosuppressant medications.

Advances have been made in the prevention and management of bacterial, viral, and fungal infections so that recipients of transplanted organs or cells live longer. A number of people have survived for well over 25 years. Unadjusted adult survival rates at 5 years range from 80% for recipients of living related kidney transplants to 40% for the small number of heart-lung recipients, with the 5-year survival rate averaging 70%.[281,407]

The first successful live-donor kidney transplantation was completed in 1954 by Dr. Murray and Dr. Harrison. They performed a living-donor kidney transplantation between identical twins with the recipient living 8 years at that time with no immunosuppressant medication. In 1990, Dr. Murray was awarded the Noble Prize in Physiology or Medicine for his contribution in the advancement of transplantation.[289]

By the end of the 1960s, the great advances in surgical techniques combined with immunologic and pharmacologic discoveries led to further successful organ transplantation, including the first heart, liver, and pancreas. With the commercial introduction of cyclosporine in 1983, the world of transplantation has made remarkable strides in becoming an acceptable medical intervention in the treatment of various end-stage organ diseases, including lung transplantation.[296]

In the past 3 decades we have seen great advances in the preservation of donor organs and surgical techniques to transplant multiple organs. There also have been advances in the preservation of donor organs, expansion of living related and deceased donor organs, detection of early rejection; further advances in immunotherapy and management of infections have made treatment even more successful. More than 535,500 lives have been saved or enhanced by transplantation.[312,411]

A case study about a transplantation patient is presented in Evolve Box 21-1 on the book's Evolve site.

INCIDENCE

Transplantation remains limited by an acute worldwide shortage of available and suitable human organs. Early in 2012 there were more than 113,000 people waiting for transplants. In 2011, more than 6500 people died while waiting for a suitable organ. It is estimated that every 10 minutes an individual is listed on United Network for Organ Sharing (UNOS) waiting list for an organ transplantation and that 18 people die each day while waiting on the UNOS transplantation list. This number has not changed significantly despite more people being aware of transplantation. In 2008, an estimated 12,000 deaths in the United States had the potential to yield suitable organs, yet less than half of these deceased individuals donated organs.[297] This leads to a large disparity between the need for organ transplantation and the availability of organ donations.[411]

Each cadaveric donor can donate up to 25 organs and tissues to help as many as 50 recipients. This means up to 500,000 organs should be available for transplantation each year, but only approximately 25,000 transplantations are performed (Table 21-1).[410] One positive highlight in the incidence of transplantation has come from the increase in living related organ donation.[412] In 2001, the number of live-donor organs recovered was more than the number of deceased- or cadaver-donor organs. In 2001, almost 6000 individuals donated a kidney or a portion of their liver, lung, or pancreas to provide an opportunity for another to survive an end-stage organ disease.[312,411]

TYPES OF TRANSPLANTATION

Many types of tissues and organs can be donated and therefore transplanted, including the heart, lungs, liver, pancreas, kidneys, intestines, skin, bone and bone marrow, umbilical cord blood, veins, soft tissues, heart valves, corneas, and eyes.

Many different terms are used to describe types of transplantations (Box 21-1). *Allograft* (homograft) transplantations are between individuals of the same species (e.g., human being to human being). *Autologous* transplantations are within the same individual (e.g., skin graft from leg to hand; blood or bone marrow for own use later).

| Table 21-1 | National Waiting List for Organ Transplantation | | | |

Organ	2014	2008	2004	2001
	YEAR			
Kidney	100,958	100,597	61,020	47,574
Liver	15,739	76,089	16,858	17,889
Heart	3,996	2711	3164	3864
Lung	1,605	2016	3816	3671
Heart-lung	not reported	91	169	207
Kidney-pancreas	2,053	2334	2362	3367
Pancreas (including PAK)	1,188	1437	1522	1051
Intestine	263	212	191	164
Total (candidates)	123,101	100,597	85,170	76,787

PAK, pancreas after kidney.
From U.S. Department of Health and Human Services. Health Resources and Services Administration. Organ Procurement and Transplantation Network. *2014 National Report* http://optn.transplant.hrsa.gov/data/. Accessed July 27, 2014. Figures related to active waiting list candidates are updated online daily.

Box 21-1
TYPES OF TRANSPLANTS

- *Allogeneic:* between individuals of the same species but of different genetic constitution (e.g., human to human)
- *Allograft* (homograft; homologous; autologous): between individuals of the same species (e.g., human to human)
- *Autologous:* within the same individual (e.g., transfer of skin from one site to another on the same body; donation of blood or bone marrow for own use later)
- *Heterologous* (heterograft; xenogeneic): between individuals of different species (e.g., pig to human)
- *Heterotopic* (autograft): transfer of organ or tissue from one part of a body of a donor to another area of the body of a recipient
- *Homologous* (homogenous): corresponding or similar in structure, position, origin (e.g., pig heart, human heart)
- *Orthotopic:* tissue transplant grafted into its normal anatomic position
- *Syngeneic* (isograft): between genetically identical members of the same species (identical twins)
- *Xenogeneic* (heterograft): between individuals of different species (e.g., pig to human)

Xenogeneic (heterograft) transplantations are between individuals of different species (e.g., pig to human being). *Allogeneic* transplantation is one in which the source comes from a human leukocytic antigen (HLA; see Chapter 7)–matched donor (usually a sibling). *Syngeneic* transplants are between genetically identical members of the same species (identical twins); the syngeneic transplant is also called an isograft.

Orthotopic homologous transplantation refers to the surgical placement (grafting) of the donor organ into the normal anatomic site. In the *heterotopic homologous* transplantation, the recipient's diseased organ is left intact and the donor organ is placed in parallel with anastomoses between the two organs.

Box 21-2
COMBINED ORGAN TRANSPLANTS

- Kidney-heart
- Kidney-heart-lung
- Liver-kidney-pancreas
- Kidney-intestine
- Liver-kidney-pancreas-intestine
- Liver-pancreas-lung
- Liver-lung
- Kidney-lung
- Liver-lung-heart
- Liver-heart
- Liver-pancreas
- Liver-intestine
- Liver-pancreas-intestine
- Liver-kidney
- Pancreas-intestine
- Liver-kidney-heart

From U.S. Department of Health and Human Services. Health Resources and Services Administration. Organ Procurement and Transplantation Network. *2014 National Report.* A total of 8,543 multiple organ transplants were performed in 2014 (compared with 578 in 2011). Comparisons by year, age, gender, ethnicity, region, and center, are available online at: http://optn.transplant.hrsa.gov/latestData/step2asp?.

Combined-Organ Transplantation

Combined-organ transplantations from a single donor are uncommon relative to single-organ transplantations (Box 21-2). Research to date generally suggests that there has been a continued increase in combined-organ transplantation, although the total numbers are low. Organ rejection is lower in cases of combined-organ transplantation compared with single-organ transplantation. Despite the increase in surgical risk and complex posttransplant medical care, the short-term survival in combined-organ transplantation seems to be acceptable, but long-term recipient and graft survival remains unknown at this time. No single center has accumulated a significant experience, and as a result long-term results in the current era are unknown.[28]

Organ Retransplantation

Retransplantation is necessary because of acute graft failure, chronic graft rejection or injection, or the recurrence of the primary disease as in the case liver or heart and lung transplantation. When the body mounts a defense against the transplanted organ, a clinical picture of chronic rejection presents itself. This form of rejection leads to a destruction of the donor organ over time. As improvements in survival rates for all transplantation occur, the need for retransplantation will also increase; for example, since the year 2000, there has been a 4% increase in heart retransplantation.[412] There is concern in dedicating more organs for retransplantation because these recipients have lower survival rates.

In many cases, the immunosuppressive medication is no longer able to suppress the immune response and rejection persists, which will eventually cause organ failure. One option is for the recipient to undergo another transplantation procedure. Transplant recipients in need of a retransplantation once again become organ candidates and must meet certain criteria for transplantation of that specific organ.

There is typically an increased risk of morbidity and/or mortality for these candidates when compared with outcomes of first-time transplantation procedures. For most organs, the 3- and 5-year survival is not as high for recipients who have undergone retransplantation.[205,206,411]

Ethical issues centered on the availability (i.e., shortage) of organs are always a consideration with retransplantation. Graft survival after retransplantation is less than for primary transplants, both for immunologic (e.g., rejection) and nonimmunologic (e.g., donor age, donor size, cadaver vs. live donor) reasons, and requires more aggressive monitoring for rejection.

Pediatric Transplantation

Solid-organ transplantation has become accepted therapy for the treatment of end-stage organ dysfunction in children. As with adult organ transplantation, the supply of cadaver pediatric organ transplants is limited. And, like adult organ transplantation, living related donation is on the rise in pediatrics. Close tissue match of the related donor allows a higher compatibility rate and transplantation scheduling before the child is in critical condition and improves overall outcomes.

Children can receive adult organs; in the case of the liver, only a portion of the adult donor liver is needed. Preoperative and postoperative assessment and care are very similar to adult care. Management may be complicated by infections such as hepatitis B and cytomegalovirus. Morbidity and mortality are often attributed to the consequences of long-term immunosuppression and include graft failure, increased incidence of cancer,[138] hypertension, and renal failure or diabetes from overimmunosuppression.

There are known age-related differences in all phases of pharmacokinetics (absorption, distribution, metabolism, elimination); information specifically related to age and differences in the pharmacokinetics of immunosuppressants is very limited at this time. Biologic and psychologic changes common during the transition from childhood to adolescence and adolescence to adulthood present some unique challenges.[200] Children receiving orthotopic liver transplantation are at risk for endocrine complications such as growth failure, hepatic osteodystrophy, pubertal delay, adrenal insufficiency, and drug-induced diabetes.

Parent training and education are essential components in the transplantation process. The care team pays special attention to the psychosocial and emotional needs of the child and family. Noncompliance and nonadherence are common behaviors among all age groups but especially among adolescents. The consequences of this behavior include increased rejection, late graft loss, and death. Despite the best 1-year graft survival of any age group, the long-term transplantation outcomes in this age group are not as optimal.[127,311,340]

ORGAN PROCUREMENT AND ALLOCATION

Organ Distribution

With the passage of the National Organ Transplant Act in 1984, the U.S. government began the process of establishing a comprehensive framework for the development and administration of a national transplant system.[408] The Organ Procurement and Transplant Network (http://optn.transplant.hrsa.gov/) was created to maintain a national registry to track the process and outcomes related to organ donation and transplantation. Since 1998, more than 530,000 people have received organ transplants at 250 U.S. transplantation centers, and the national waiting list now exceeds 113,000 people who are waiting for a suitable organ.[410,411]

In 2004, the Organ Donation and Recovery Improvement Act (Public Law 108-216) was signed with a legislative provision to establish a federal grant program to provide assistance to living donors for travel and other expenses. This act focused on strengthening efforts to increase donation rates, including ways to make live donation an easier and more appealing option. Removing financial barriers from living organ donations may help expand access to transplantation for members of lower socioeconomic groups who may not be able to consider living donation.[182]

In 2006, the revision of the Uniform Anatomical Gift Act allowed individual states to develop their own donor registration process and strengthen the wishes of the deceased to donate. This allowed the organ procurement organizations (OPOs) to proceed with the donation process and prevents others from overriding donor wishes. The result of this effort was an increase by 24% in donor registration in many states and more than nine states exceed a 50% increase in registration.[437]

This legislation also grants money to states for organ donor awareness, public education, and outreach activities designed to increase the number of organ donors, establish programs coordinating organ donation activities, and conduct studies of long-term effects associated with living organ donation.[441]

Further work in improving the procurement process, including care for the donor to allow organs to be recovered from the associated trauma has also led to an increase in available organs. Surgeons are able to accept organs from donors who do not match the general criteria, from an extended donor pool, and from more marginally suited organs. Preliminary work shows that these once discarded donor organs have equal outcomes regarding hyperacute rejection, and short-term survival of graft and recipient. Unfortunately, with these advancements there are additional stresses placed upon hospital centers to report outcomes related to length of stay and cost. These are new barriers to efforts to increase available donors. For example, because of increased required reporting procedures, transplantation centers are less likely to use organs from an extended donor pool, from donation after cardiac death, or to accept high-risk transplantation candidates.[437]

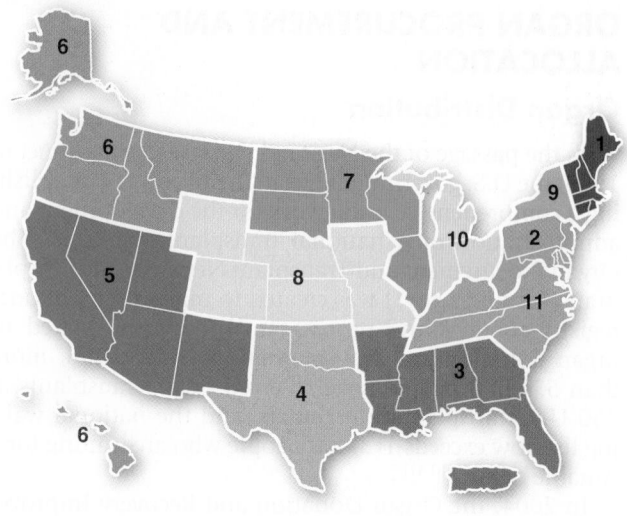

Figure 21-1

The United Network for Organ Sharing (UNOS) is divided into 11 geographic regions. (Courtesy United Network for Organ Sharing, Richmond, VA.)

United Network for Organ Sharing

To establish a means to procure and distribute donor organs in an appropriate and ethical manner, the United States was divided into 58 local procurement areas, ranging in population from 1 million to 12 million, and those areas were then divided into 11 regions (Fig. 21-1). Each local area has a designated OPO responsible for recovering and transporting organs to transplantation hospitals in their territories. At present there are 246 transplantation centers across the United States. The local OPO also provides a wealth of medical and public education about organ transplantation and the promotion of donation.

On the national level the UNOS (www.unos.org) is a private, nonprofit organization that provides critical services in the area of organ transplantation. UNOS administers the national organ waiting list, coordinates the matching and distribution of donor organs via the local OPO throughout the United States, tracks outcomes, establishes physician training for the medical and surgical management of transplant recipients, and provides public education.[407]

UNOS is composed of every transplantation center, tissue-matching laboratory, and OPO within the United States, which are required to report a massive amount of data to UNOS. The Organ Procurement and Transplant Network analyzes all data provided regarding transplantation candidates, recipients, and living and decreased donors.

Great detail in the process to match candidates with a donor organ(s) has been developed to ensure equity based on medical need. There are two large processes occurring simultaneously to match and allocate organs. One side involves the identification and management of the potential transplantation candidate (someone waiting for an organ) through the transplantation center; on the other side is the identification and procurement of viable organs for donation.

After a thorough evaluation the transplantation center reports vital medical information about each candidate to UNOS. When a possible deceased organ donor has been identified, the local OPO will obtain and report valuable medical information about the donor to UNOS. The UNOS computer system will search for a suitable match between the donor and candidate.

A list of potential candidates will be provided in a priority order, and the organ is offered to the candidate who has the highest medical need as well as the greatest likelihood of a successful outcome based on the analysis of prior transplantation.

This allocation begins with the transplantation center being contacted at the local level, but if a local candidate does not match the donor organ or has a lower medical need, the organ will be offered to a candidate in the region where the donor organ was procured and then to adjacent regions and then finally nationally, with the goal to utilize every suitable organ.[408]

Allocation Policy. UNOS has developed a status coding or allocation system to prioritize the candidates waiting for transplantation when a donor organ has been recovered. The goal of this allocation system is to promote an equitable system that saves as many lives as possible. The creation of these new allocation systems have been critical to making the system more equitable for candidates who suffer from an aggressive or highly progressive disease, like many forms of pulmonary fibrosis. Each waiting list and the prioritization of possible candidates vary from organ to organ.

The allocation of deceased donor organs has significantly changed over the years, with the goal to ensure that people who have the most urgent medical need will be given priority despite the amount of waiting time a person has on the UNOS list.[410] The change in allocation policy is known as *transplant benefit*.

In response to a perceived unfairness in organ allocation, Congress issued a "Final Rule" in 1998. The rule called for a more objective ranking of potential recipients on a waiting list and more equality in disease severity among transplant recipients across OPOs.

The policy is intended to balance anticipated duration of survival on the transplantation list with length of benefit from receiving a transplant. Priority for transplanted organs will go to those candidates most urgently needing a transplant and expected to receive the most survival benefit from the transplant. Waiting time is used to decide allocation if there is more than one potential candidate with equal medical urgency scores.

This distribution system is also designed to decrease the disadvantage some people have because of the progressive nature of their disease or the uneven distribution of transplantation centers within the United States. The new policy considers the waiting list urgency and transplantation benefit of each candidate based on individual clinical diagnostic factors. The improved computerized organ-matching system has made these important changes possible.

For example, it is known that an individual who has a cardiac index of less than 1.8 L/min/m^2 and who is on a high dose of one or more inotropic medications (drugs that affect the force of heart muscular contractions) has a shorter life expectancy than someone who is only on oral medication with compensated heart failure. In this scenario, the first person would be assigned a status 1A, listed higher on the transplantation listing, and offered an organ before the second person (see Box 21-8).

Organ Donation

Deceased organ donation continues to be the primary source for available organs, either when complete and irreversible loss of all brain and brainstem activity occurs or when the heart stops in the case of cardiac death. The Organ Donation Breakthrough Collaborative is an effort by the U.S. Department of Health and Human Services and the Health Resources and Services Administration to unite the various agencies involved in transplantation and to define their roles and efforts to increase the identification of potential organs.

The transplantation center, donor hospitals, and the local OPO work together to procure organs to save and enhance the lives of people who are dying from end-stage organ disease. The other source of donated organs is living donation. This collaborative effort between 2003 and 2006 resulted in a 22.5% increase in donation which is a fourfold increase from the precollaborative period.[363] However, in 2011 there were just over 6000 living donors, a decrease from the high of 7000 in 2004.[407]

Source of Organ Donations

The characteristics of what constitutes an acceptable donor, both deceased and living, have been changed over the years in an attempt to maximize the number of potential donor organs as organ shortage is still a limiting factor. The effect of these changes on the outcome for recipients is not fully known. Early on it was typical that the deceased donor was a young individual who was declared brain dead from a traumatic brain injury. Today, more deceased donations are from the older person, individuals with certain comorbidities, or individuals who have suffered a fatal cerebral vascular injury from stroke or aneurysm.[407,437]

There is also an increased use of organs harvested from non–heart-beating deceased donors, especially in kidney transplantation. Most transplantation centers are still reluctant to transplant other organs from the non–heart-beating donor because of the risk of ischemic injury to the organs,[113] but recent studies show acceptable and encouraging results.[194]

There has been some preliminary research that has used extracorporeal membrane oxygenation (ECMO) to support the donor and improve organ perfusion. Using ECMO for the organ recipient in the early posttransplant period is another way to support a marginal donor organ.[240] Currently, researchers are using an ex vivo lung perfusion device in animal models (pigs) to improve normal lung physiology in the hopes that this effort can improve lung function and thus increase the amount of available organs.[105]

There has also been increased utilization of organs from an "extended" or "high-risk" donor pool. These are deceased donors who fall outside the general criteria to be an acceptable donor, such as older individuals,

individuals with diabetes, those with some forms of cancer, and individuals who are positive for the hepatitis B or C virus. There are reports of promising results when organs from this extended donor pool have been used with no increase in primary organ failure and equivalent early survival rates.[437] More time will be needed to examine long-term organ and recipient survivals.

Individuals previously considered unacceptable transplantation candidates may be offered a donor organ from this extended donor pool. Seropositive hepatitis B or C candidates can now receive a transplant from a positive donor. In the past, these individuals were not considered acceptable candidates for transplantation.[63] Successful kidney transplantations have been completed from deceased donors who have a medical history of diabetes.[4]

Many so called "marginal" or "suboptimal" organs have been discarded by centers even though people die each day while on the waiting list. Marginal organs can provide a viable solution to organ shortage. Studies have been performed to use aggressive methods to improve the suitability of organs which were once thought to be suboptimal.[103,324] When used with appropriate surgical techniques and immunosuppression protocols, suboptimal organs can increase the supply of donor organs by 25% to 30%.[2]

The source of organ donation is also changing in regard to the living donation. In previous years living donation was conducted primarily between relatives referred to as a *directed donation*. Directed donation also can be between nonrelated individuals, spouse, or friend.[312] The living donation can occur indirectly (a nondirected donation); that is, the living donor is placed on a national living donor list and the donor's gift is anonymous to the recipient. Living donors can donate a kidney, portion of a lung, liver, intestine, and pancreas.[409]

Living donors need to make a fully informed consent because of the risk to their health and life. Reports of long-term effects of living donation are limited at this time. There are some studies of psychosocial and socioeconomic issues facing living kidney donors.[118] UNOS is aware of 11 donors who donated between 1998 and 2008 (out of approximately 64,000) and were subsequently listed for kidney or liver transplantation as a consequence of complications from their donation. This report is limited to only the individuals who have registered on UNOS. There is a poor understanding of long-term morbidity and mortality complications for living donors who never initiate transplant procedures for themselves.[118,409]

Guidelines for Donor Candidates

There are general guidelines that are used when determining the acceptability of a donor; criteria vary slightly depending on organ type. These guidelines have been expanded as procedures to procure organs improve and as transplantation centers become more effective at surgical procedures and medical management of transplant recipients.

Most donors are younger than 50 years of age, although this is not exclusive because of the high need for donors and advances in postoperative management. Smoking history must be less than 30 pack-years with acceptable oxygenation measured as a PO_2 greater than 300 mm Hg.

Other criteria for donors vary according to the organ being harvested. For example, a living related lung donor must not have a history of lung disease, previous thoracic surgeries, or be larger in size than the recipient (weight, height, chest size); the latter requirement is required because only two lung lobes will support the recipient's full pulmonary function.

For all organ donations, there must be no evidence of malignancy, human immunodeficiency virus (HIV), hepatitis B, or sepsis. Although rare, HIV transmission from a living organ donor has been documented.[41,136] To reduce the risk for transmission of HIV through living-donor organ transplantation, transplantation centers are advised to screen living donors for HIV as close to the time of organ recovery and transplantation as possible. Transplant candidates should be informed of the potential risks for disease transmission. Potential donors must be cautioned to avoid behaviors that would put them at risk for acquiring HIV before organ donation.[41]

Hepatitis C present in the donor is considered a precaution but not a contraindication. If the candidate already has hepatitis C or is critically ill, the risk of developing hepatitis C is not considered a contraindication in the decision to progress with the procedure.

Body weight must be within 20% of the ideal (using the body mass index for heart and lung organ donation; see the discussion of body mass index in Chapter 2) because of the ischemia–perfusion injury associated with obesity.[227] Biologically related donors with clear and altruistic motivation (as opposed to coerced by the family or guilt driven) are preferred.

Testing is performed to assess the function of each donor organ considered for procurement. For potential renal donors, urinalysis, creatinine, blood urea nitrogen, and liver function are tested. For the heart, an echocardiogram, 12-lead electrocardiogram, serial arterial blood gas measurements, and possibly a right- and left-heart catheterization are ordered. Pancreatic function is assessed with amylase and lipase studies. Serial arterial blood gases, sputum Gram stain, and bronchoscopy to inspect the airways are used to assess the function of the lungs.[311,403,408]

Organ Recovery

Hearts and lungs can be preserved for up to 6 hours, livers up to 24 hours, and kidneys up to 72 hours. Lungs cannot be preserved outside the body for any extended period of time, although the effects of ex vivo lung perfusion on lung function posttransplant is being explored in an animal model[240] and in clinical trials with small numbers of humans.[8] This length of allowable ischemic time helps determine allowable distances between centers.

Efforts are being made to improve organ harvest and preservation techniques and the number of organs harvested. For example, eliminating medical failures before donation through aggressive resuscitation, coagulopathy control, invasive monitoring, and dedicated intensive care unit (ICU) management while implementing a rapid brain death determination protocol has been documented as successfully increasing the number of donor organs available.[139,265,437] Since the year 2000, there has been a slight increase in *donation after cardiac death.*

Although liver transplantation does not appear to be a viable option postdeath, kidney recipients show similar long-term outcomes when a candidate receives a donation-after-cardiac-death kidney organ. Results of other organs and tissues are still under investigation.[437]

Technology to improve organ recovery, maintain organ perfusion, and recover normal cell metabolism is under investigation using a kidney transporter, a portable organ preservation device. The ability to maintain and monitor organ viability over an extended period of time may allow live donors to avoid traveling to the recipient's location for explant surgery. Eventually, this type of technology may be extended to include transport devices for all other organs.

Efforts to obtain consent for donation continue to improve as part of the Organ Donation Breakthrough Collaborative's efforts. Public education now includes National Donor Awareness Week and the choice to indicate organ donation on a driver's license. According to Health Care Financing Administration regulations, hospitals are now required to report every death and impending death to their local OPO in order to continue receiving Medicare benefits.[141]

Early referral of all imminent deaths to OPOs results in the OPO conferring with the medical team regarding the best medical plan of care for the recipient, including specific needs of the family, as well as procedures necessary for the donor, once consent is obtained. These steps help ensure that care of potential organ donors continues without premature termination.[362]

A new approach to obtaining family consent is being utilized. Instead of informing the family of the individual's death and at a later time discussing organ donation (referred to as *decoupling*), now most families are approached about organ donation at the time when they are making end-of-life decisions. Policies and laws have strengthened the wishes of the donor, making it easier for the OPO to begin the process of donation while discussing with the family the process and positive benefits of organ donation.[437] The discussion about organ donation has become a team approach between the OPO staff, physicians, nurses, and clergy. In 2005, 57% of families approached about donation consented, which is up 17% from 2001.[407]

During this critical period of time assessing a potential donor, personnel from the OPO request medical evaluation from various specialists (e.g., cardiologist, pulmonologist, nephrologist, gastroenterologist, and surgeon) to determine the viability of the organs that were consented for harvesting and to provide instructions for continued medical care to ensure adequate organ function until the procurement process begins.

Criteria for Organ Candidates

People waiting for transplants (candidates) are listed at one or more of the transplantation centers where they plan to have surgery. A national, computerized waiting list of potential transplantation candidates in the United States is maintained by UNOS with active input from treatment centers. UNOS maintains a 24-hour telephone service to aid in matching donor organs with people on the waiting list and to coordinate efforts with transplantation centers.

Each possible transplantation candidate undergoes various testing, and many of these test results, such as organ(s) needed, blood type, body size, various organ functions, walking ability, life support need, virology, and other pertinent comorbidities, are reported to UNOS.

There are criteria for most organs to classify candidates into levels of medical urgency or status based on the medical workup. When a donor becomes available, UNOS is notified and a list of potential organ candidates for that region is identified. UNOS notifies the OPO, which, in turn, notifies the transplantation center to verify that the candidate is currently medically appropriate and has consented to the transplantation process. Arrangements are then made to transport the donor organ and candidate to the transplantation center and proceed with the surgery.

Several factors are taken into consideration in identifying the best-matched candidate or candidates. In general, preference is given to candidates with the most critical status from the same geographic area as the donor because timing is a critical element in the organ procurement process. Waiting for combined-organ transplantation is much more complicated. The candidate must be listed on each organ waiting list. Once the potential candidate reaches the top of the one organ list and is offered an organ, the other organs from the same donor would be offered as long as there is not a higher status candidate ahead of this candidate. For example, if an individual is listed for heart-lung transplantation and has the highest lung allocation score (LAS) for the region and matches the other necessary characteristics for the organ, then this candidate would be offered the heart (as long as there is not another candidate who is a status 1 in that named region and who also matches the donor). This process makes multiple-organ transplantation difficult.

The transplantation team bears the responsibility to conserve scarce resources for those who can benefit, requiring careful screening of potential candidates. Transplantation centers follow UNOS guidelines, but criteria may vary from center to center. Some centers require a medical evaluation for the acceptance of applicants for transplantation.

Many centers have medical and nonmedical criteria, with exclusion criteria for people with severely problematic behavior or other psychosocial risk factors (Box 21-3). There has been a recent trend toward recognizing the importance of nonmedical issues, such as psychologic stability, family support, functional status, and history of compliance or adherence to medical care, when evaluating applicants, because of the impact of these issues on outcomes.[117,348,349,350]

A history of problematic behavior, such as lack of adherence to treatment and the presence of psychiatric instability, leads to higher posttransplant mortality and morbidity.[120,246,367] Compliance issues associated with substance abuse usually include personality disorders, living arrangements, and/or global psychosocial factors. A history of substance abuse requires documentation of abstinence; ongoing drug and/or alcohol abuse can potentially impair the success of the transplantation and requires referral for treatment before placement on a transplantation waiting list.

Box 21-3

GENERAL CRITERIA FOR ORGAN CANDIDATE

NOTE: This is a *general* list of criteria for potential organ recipients; considerations will vary from organ to organ, and transplantation center as well.

Medical Considerations

- Matched blood type required
- Body weight (morbid obesity more than 20% of ideal body weight contraindicated; severe malnutrition less than 70% of ideal body weight contraindicated)
- Presence of other illness or disease contraindicated
  - Other end-stage organ disease
    - Irreversible renal insufficiency
    - Irreversible hepatic insufficiency
    - Severe pulmonary disease: FVC 50%, FEV$_1$ 60%
    - Fixed pulmonary hypertension
- At risk for cardiac problems (death, myocardial infarction, coronary angioplasty, bypass surgery, unstable angina)
- Uncontrolled infection or acute sepsis
- HIV
- Malignancy with metastases
- Malignancy with an expected 5-year survival of 75%
- Irreversible neuromuscular or neurologic disorder
  - Severe peripheral vascular disease or cerebrovascular disease
  - Abdominal aneurysm
  - Peripheral ischemic ulceration
  - Carotid disease
- Decrease in chest wall mobility
- Nonambulatory with poor rehabilitation potential

Nonmedical Considerations

- History of noncompliance with medical therapy (last 5 years)
- History of ongoing alcohol or drug dependence
- Active or recent (within last 6 months) cigarette smoking (lung transplant)
- History of psychologic instability
- Financial resources available
- Family and community support available

FEV$_1$, forced expiratory volume in 1 second; FVC, forced vital capacity.

In the case of live-donor transplantation, psychosocial risk to donors must be taken into consideration. Most published reports have indicated an improved sense of well-being and a boost in self-esteem for living donors, but there have been some reports of depression and disrupted family relationships after donation, and even suicide after a recipient's death.[111,214]

Medical compatibility of the donor and candidate or candidates is determined based on characteristics such as blood type, weight, and age. Illness in the recipient that cannot be treated or that will prevent transplantation success must be evaluated carefully. For example, in the case of someone with heart failure who is being considered for heart transplantation, pulmonary arterial pressure will be evaluated. If the pulmonary artery pressure is high and unresponsive to medication, the pressure is considered refractory, or fixed. If a new heart is placed in this system, the donor heart, particularly the right ventricle, will not be able to pump against the high pulmonary pressure and will result in right-sided heart failure. This candidate would more likely benefit from a ventricular assist device (VAD) to support cardiac function; it has been clearly documented that pulmonary arterial pressure does decrease with VAD, which may then allow the individual to qualify for transplantation.[69]

Transplantation is usually not recommended if another illness is predicted to rapidly cause graft failure or impact survival in other deleterious ways after transplant. In addition, a previous history of cancer or osteoporosis is considered carefully as postoperative medications can greatly advance these diseases.

Pretransplantation Evaluation

Extensive medical testing is required before someone is placed on the transplantation waiting list (Table 21-2). Blood and tissue typing, including Rh factor analysis for histocompatibility, are used as some of the first eligibility criteria for donor-candidate matching. The process of determining histocompatibility, that is, finding compatible donors and candidates, is called *tissue typing*. Before transplantation, testing in the laboratory is carried out to determine whether antibodies incompatible with the donor have been formed by the candidate (a positive crossmatch). If the crossmatch is positive, the transplant will fail; a negative test result is necessary for a successful transplant.

Predictor values for acute and chronic rejection are evaluated, such as panel reactive antibodies (a measure of the amount of antibodies circulating in the system), and offer some predictive value of hyperacute rejection. In some cases, treatment will be performed to lower the panel reactive antibodies in a recipient to help increase the donor pool for that individual.

Other serology testing determines exposure to cytomegalovirus (CMV), Epstein-Barr virus (EBV), herpes simplex viruses, and hepatitis because complications can arise related to individual exposure to viral loading (i.e., the greater the viral replication, the higher the incidence of active infection).

CMV infection may contribute to an increased incidence of chronic rejection and result in CMV syndrome (e.g., viremia: spread of virus throughout the body with fever and malaise) or organ-specific tissue-invasive disease.[377] Herpes simplex virus is associated with an increased incidence of necrotizing pneumonitis and cervical cancer; and EBV is associated with an increase in posttransplantation lymphoproliferative diseases. (See further discussion of these infectious diseases in Chapter 8.) Transplant recipients are placed on appropriate medications to reduce the risk of infection and undergo repeated serologic testing if clinical signs and symptoms suggest infection or infectious disease (see Box 8-1).

Fasting lipids, liver function studies, prostate-specific antigen levels to determine prostate function, and tests specific to the potential organ transplant are carried out. Other tests will be completed to rule out other organ dysfunction. Functional testing and dual-energy x-ray absorptiometry (DEXA) scans are commonly included to determine activity tolerance and bone health, respectively.

A person with isolated end-stage organ failure with no other complications has a better chance for selection than someone with other complicating factors. In addition to all the testing procedures, the organ candidate meets with a large team of professionals (listed in Table 21-2), including, in some centers, rehabilitation staff, such as physical and occupational therapists.

ADVANCES AND RESEARCH IN TRANSPLANTATION

Advances in Medications

Tremendous advancement has been made in the pharmacologic management of transplant recipients. Medications are used with transplant recipients to prevent rejection and treat rejection or infection. Research is ongoing to find ways to reduce or eliminate the long-term use and adverse effects of medications, especially immunosuppressants. New discoveries in cellular immunology have led to a greater understanding of the immune system and its implications for tissue transplantation. Immunosuppressive

Table 21-2	Referral to Transplant Center			
Blood Work	**Testing***		**Consultations***	**Other**
ABO blood type	Multigated acquisition		Surgeon	Urinalysis
Panel reactive antibodies	Echocardiogram		Pulmonologist	Sputum cultures
Serology	Transesophageal echocardiography or		Cardiologist	Creatinine clearance
Liver function tests	transthoracic echocardiogram		Nephrologist	Purified protein
Fasting lipids	Pulmonary function tests		Transplant coordinator	derivative
Prostate-specific antigen	6-Minute walk test		Social Service	Mammogram
Prothrombin time	V̇/Q̇ scan (ventilation-perfusion)		Credit analysis	Pap smear
Partial prothrombin time	Arterial blood gases		Neuropsychology	
Complete blood count	Diffusion capacity of carbon monoxide		Physical therapy	
Nicotine level	Organ catheterization (heart, kidney)		Rheumatologist	
Drug/toxicity screen	X-ray		Gynecologist	
	Electrocardiogram		Dentist	
	VO2max or VO2peak		Nutritionist	
	Glucose testing (diabetes mellitus)			
	Peripheral vascular disease			
	DEXA scan (osteoporosis)			

*Specific consultants and the special tests orders are determined by the type of organ transplantation planned.

regimens continue to improve, and newer immunomodulatory strategies are evolving. In particular, new immunosuppressive drugs may allow the recipient to overcome or reduce the early antibody-mediated rejections.[39]

Most transplant recipients are placed on a three-drug regimen to control the incidence of rejection and minimize the adverse effects that are common if any one drug is given in too high a dosage. This drug cocktail commonly consists of a calcineurin inhibitor, an antimetabolite, and a corticosteroid. New research continues to attempt to decrease the dosage and the number of immunosuppressive medications the transplant recipient is exposed to in order to promote long-term, effective graft function without the harmful side effects of these potent medications.

There has been a decline in the use of cyclosporine and Neoral for most organs. These drugs have been replaced with the administration of tacrolimus (Prograf). Cyclosporine and tacrolimus are classified as *calcineurin inhibitors*.[407] Calcineurin is an enzyme, protein phosphatase, that is responsible for activating the transcription of interleukin-2, which stimulates the growth and differentiation of T cells. Calcineurin is also linked to the differentiation of fiber types and hypertrophy of muscle fibers[130]

The mechanism of action for tacrolimus and cyclosporine is similar in that they both inhibit calcineurin, although tacrolimus is more selective in its action and may be one of the reasons its use has become more popular (Fig. 21-2). Both drugs bind to specific lymphoid tissues and block the production of interleukin-2, which is a critical substance in the growth and proliferation of activated T cells and other immune response cells, such as natural killer cells, macrophages, and lymphocytes.[95]

The second class of drugs is the antimetabolites including azathioprine (Imuran), mycophenolate mofetil (Cell-Cept), and cyclophosphamide (Cytoxan).[407] There has been an increased utilization of mycophenolate mofetil

over other drugs in this classification. Azathioprine works by suppressing the bone marrow (as exhibited by thrombocytopenia, leukopenia, and anemia), and mycophenolate mofetil inhibits the inflammatory response mediated by the immune system (Fig. 21-3).[251,252] Cyclophosphamide, which is typically thought of as an anticancer drug, has been used in transplant recipients. It inhibits the replication of DNA and RNA in the lymphocytes and other key cells involved in mounting an immune response against the transplanted organ.[95]

The third drug is prednisone, a corticosteroid with an effect at the level of the macrophages. Prednisone blocks the production of interleukin-2 in the presence of an antigen to stimulate a major histocompatible complex, thus stimulating both B-cell and T-cell response (Fig. 21-4).

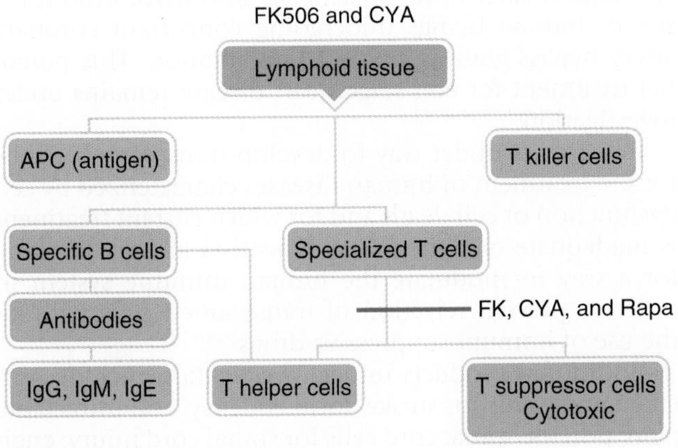

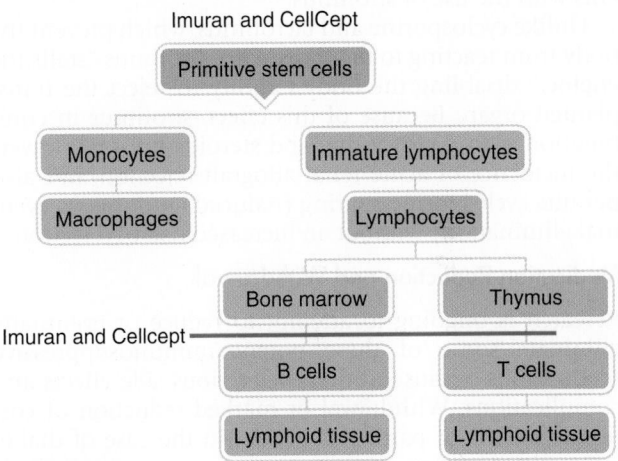

Figure 21-3

Azathioprine (Imuran) and mycophenolate mofetil (CellCept) are theorized to block lymphocytes from maturing into T cells. This inhibits the immune-mediated inflammatory response. (Courtesy Chris L. Wells, University of Maryland School of Medicine, James H. Dauber, University of Pittsburgh Medical Center-Health Systems, and Carla Peterman, University of Maryland Medical Center.)

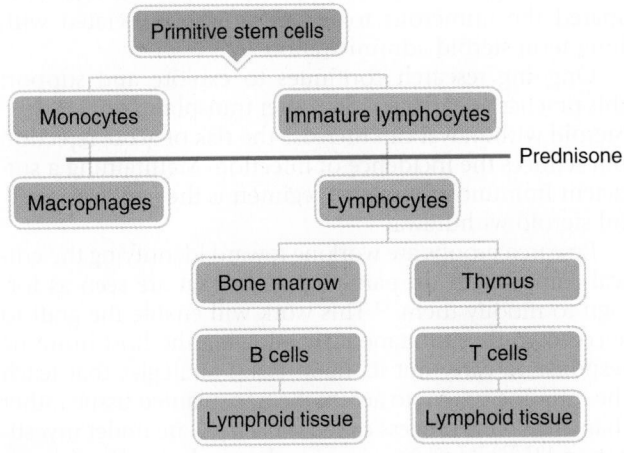

Figure 21-4

Prednisone works at the macrophage level and is theorized to block the production of interleukin-2, thus preventing the formation of major histocompatible complexes that normally stimulate both B- and T-cell response. (Courtesy Chris L. Wells, University of Maryland School of Medicine, and James H. Dauber, University of Pittsburgh Medical Center-Health Systems.)

Figure 21-2

Cyclosporin (CsA, CYA, Neoral, Sandimmune) and tacrolimus (Prograf) block the sensitization of T cells. Cyclosporin and tacrolimus inhibit calcineurin in lymphoid tissues and thus inhibit the production of immune mediators such as interleukin-2. In general, sirolimus (Rapamune) structure is similar to cyclosporin but its action is different. It does not interfere directly with the cytokine production but inhibits the growth and proliferation of T and B lymphocytes by inhibiting the lymphocytes from taking action in response to stimulatory signals from certain cytokines. (Courtesy Chris L. Wells, University of Maryland Medical Center, and James H. Dauber, University of Pittsburgh Medical Center-Health Systems.)

Research continues to attempt to decrease the exposure and utilization of corticosteroids because of the adverse effects of this medication, including diabetes, osteoporosis, muscle wasting (steroid myopathy), and fat deposition.

Sirolimus (rapamycin, Rapamune) is an immunosuppressant that inhibits cytokine-driven cell proliferation and maturation. It was approved for use with renal transplants and was introduced for use with other organ transplants in the late 1990s. Sirolimus is presently being used in a low percentage of transplant recipients. It may be used in combination with a calcineurin-inhibiting drug and mycophenolate mofetil. Some centers use sirolimus and mycophenolate mofetil alone, particularly with pancreas kidney recipients.[221,407] Some studies have reported a decrease in chronic rejection in heart transplant recipients with the use of sirolimus.[222]

Unlike cyclosporine and tacrolimus, which prevent the body from reacting to the transplant, sirolimus "stalls the engine," disabling the body's ability to reject the transplanted organ. Because of this effect, sirolimus in combination with cyclosporine and steroids not only lowers the incidence of acute renal allograft rejection, but also permits cyclosporine sparing (reduced amounts or eventual elimination) without an increased risk of rejection.

Medication Reduction and Withdrawal

Research is ongoing to attempt to reduce or eventually eliminate some of these potent immunosuppressive medications because of their deleterious side effects and complications. Withdrawal or marked reduction of corticosteroids is of particular benefit in the case of diabetes mellitus and in the presence of severe osteoporosis or aseptic necrosis of bone. Steroid withdrawal is possible in up to 70% of pancreas transplant candidates who are otherwise maintained on tacrolimus-based immunosuppression.[203,215]

Among individuals who initially received sirolimus in combination with cyclosporine and steroids, those who had steroid treatment stopped 1 month after transplantation had significantly fewer rejection episodes and were spared the numerous toxic side effects associated with long-term steroid administration.[193]

Ongoing research continues to explore and support this practice as early as 4 days after transplantation.[10,12,436] Steroid withdrawal can increase the risk of acute rejection but reduces the incidence of infection. Maintaining a sufficient immunosuppressive regimen is the key to successful steroid withdrawal.

Research groups are working toward identifying the critical components on particular grafts that are seen as foreign to modify them.[50] This work will enable the graft to succeed while simultaneously allowing the host immune response to carry out its main tasks. Strategies that teach the immune system to accept the transplanted tissue rather than attack it, a process called *chimerism*, are under investigation.[192,229,382] Chimerism involves inducing the donor's immune system onto the candidate's so that the candidate's immune system no longer rejects the organ or tissue. In bone marrow transplantation (BMT) chimerism is achieved when bone marrow and host cells exist compatibly without signs of graft-versus-host disease (GVHD).

A potential breakthrough may have been discovered in a recent study in which eight kidney transplant recipients were also given a mixture of stem cells from their organ donor. Five of the eight people were able to stop taking their immunosuppressant medications because the mixing of stem cells from the donor with the recipient helped make the recipients' immune system not view the donor's tissues as foreign.[248]

Researchers studying how the developing fetus avoids destruction may be able to identify protective biologic pathways and then use this model to develop drugs to interrupt the rejection process and promote tolerance of foreign tissue.[206,404]

Advances in Research

Advances in understanding of immunology and organ preservation, surgical technique, pharmacology, and postoperative care have permitted the rapid development of other organ transplantation procedures than just the heart and lung (e.g., liver, pancreas, intestine).

New transplantation is being developed for other organs, such as pancreatic islet cells for the treatment of diabetes and ovarian preservation for later use in cases of cancer requiring removal of the ovaries. The use of hepatic segments for transplantation (either from cadavers or from living related donors) has decreased the number of people (especially children) awaiting liver transplantation.

The first transplantation of skeletal muscle cells to test whether the cells can repair damaged heart muscle took place at Temple University's heart transplantation program in 2000. Muscle tissue taken from the individual's arm was transplanted into his own heart during a surgical procedure to implant an assistive device while waiting for a heart transplant.[134]

Since then, researchers have successfully injected autologous skeletal myoblast cells into myocardium tissue in human beings undergoing concurrent coronary artery bypass grafting or VAD implantation. This potential treatment for end-stage heart disease remains under investigation.[123,188]

Research is under way to develop transplantable cells for the treatment of human diseases characterized by cell dysfunction or cell death and for which current treatment is inadequate or nonexistent. Scientists are also looking for a way to modulate the human immune system in order to prevent rejection of transplanted cells without the use of immunosuppressive drugs.[300]

Additional products under investigation include porcine neural cells for stroke, focal epilepsy, and intractable pain; porcine spinal cord cells for spinal cord injury; engineered blood vessels for use as vascular grafts; neurologic cell transfer for Parkinson disease or Huntington chorea; human liver cells for cirrhosis; and porcine retinal pigment epithelial cells for macular degeneration.[15,300]

The diverse research directions being undertaken around the world will continue to change the field of transplantation in the years to come. Gene therapy (including in utero), xenotransplantation, tissue engineering, chimerism, and new fields of study developing daily can only be presented briefly in this text but help represent the overall picture of rapid change in treatment approaches.

Xenotransplantation

Allotransplantation remains the preferred treatment for human organ failure, but shortages of acceptable donor organs and the lack of success in developing suitable artificial organs have led researchers to investigate the use of organs from other species (xenotransplantation). Xenotransplantation is defined more fully as the interspecies transplantation of cells, tissues, and organs or ex vivo interspecies exchange between cells, tissues, and organs.[17]

Nonhuman primates are now considered an unethical and unsafe source of donor organs, so other species are being considered, in particular the pig. Baboon organs are too small to sustain human beings for long periods. The risk of transmitting deadly infectious agents from nonhuman primates is greater than from other animal species.

Physicians are already successfully using various pig components (e.g., heart valves, clotting factors, islet cells, brain cells) to treat human diseases. Researchers are now breeding genetically manipulated donor pigs whose cells, tissues, and organs could be permanently transplanted into human beings without being destroyed by the human immune system.[160] Concerns still exist about the potential for transfer of infectious agents from animals to humans and the introduction of diseases foreign to the human, leading to a possible epidemic. Scientists hope that, by using modern biotechnology, it may be possible to generate pigs free of threatening viruses in the future.[375]

Previously, hyperacute rejection or acute vascular rejection was the biggest disadvantage to xenotransplantation. Circulation of recipient blood through the transplanted organ caused graft failure within 24 hours. Scientific progress has eliminated this obstacle.[375] Considerable progress has been made in pig-to-primate organ xenotransplantation resulting in transplant functioning for days and weeks rather than minutes. Researchers have successfully implanted pig organs as a short-term bridge (up to 10 hours) until a human donor organ can be found and implanted.[249]

Other hurdles to xenotransplantation include anatomic, physiologic, and biochemical differences. The upright position of human beings is unique in nature. Gravity therefore exerts a different impact on the anatomic location of organs such as lung, heart, liver, and kidney. More pronounced are differences on the humoral and enzymatic basis.

Complex interactions existing in allografts are totally disturbed in xenogeneic situations. Regaining physiologic function of the graft in the foreign environment may be prevented by molecular incompatibilities between the donor and recipient. Experts say that before xenotransplantation can become an everyday reality, safeguards must be developed to ensure the minimization of risk to the recipient and to society. The decision to proceed with clinical application of this technique depends on ethical, regulatory, and legal frameworks established by consensus.[160]

Issues yet to be resolved include the recipient's right to privacy, selection of the first recipients of xenografts, concern that the socioeconomically disadvantaged will be used as test subjects for the first xenografts, and animal rights are just a few of the concerns expressed by various interest groups.[17,160,345]

Tissue Engineering and Regenerative Medicine

> **Note to Reader:** What we report to you in this short section is just the tip of the iceberg for the kinds of research under way in this area. Although in its infancy stages in some areas, tissue engineering and regenerative medicine is growing rapidly, with continued expansion of clinical applications expected.

Tissue engineering, the science of growing living human tissues for transplantation and other therapeutic applications, is a rapidly expanding industry—so much so that biomedical engineering and technology is a college-degree program, and in some areas a PhD program, designed to develop engineers able to bridge the gap between biology, medicine, and engineering. Tissue engineering applies the principles of biology and engineering toward the development of biologic substitutes that restore, maintain, or improve tissue function.

The science of tissue engineering has given birth to a new clinical discipline called *regenerative medicine* aimed at replacing or regenerating living tissues so as to restore the functions of damaged or defective tissues and organs. The reader is referred to a comprehensive review of the field, including stem cell types, in an excellent review article on the subject.[164] Aging, associated with a progressive failing of tissues and organs and the leading cause of many diseases, is also one of the primary forces behind a branch of regenerative medicine designed to "rejuvenate" the failing, aging body.[21,217]

In addition, the military has been a major force in advancing the field as a result of the numerous traumatic and burn injuries to thousands of soldiers during the wars in Iraq and Afghanistan. In 2008, the federal government invested $85 million to create the new Armed Forces Institute of Regenerative Medicine (AFIRM); research at more than 2 dozen institutions is being integrated to develop and provide cutting-edge technologies and treatments to wounded soldiers.[112] Total funding has now reached more than $300 million and includes support from the Department of Defense, state governments, universities, and private industry.

Tissue engineering, or the fabrication of functional living tissue, uses cells seeded on highly porous, synthetic, biodegradable, polymer scaffolds as a new approach toward the development of biologic substitutes that may replace lost tissue function. Over the past decade, the fabrication of a wide variety of tissues has been investigated, including both structural and visceral organs.

Bioengineered skin, bone, ligaments, tendons, and articular cartilage are already available in some clinical settings.[31] The use of muscle-derived stem cells to aid in muscle healing after muscle injury is a biologic treatment being investigated. The intention is to increase angiogenesis and decrease scar formation.[313] Platelet-rich plasma (a form of blood injection therapy) is being used and studied in promoting tendon healing by increasing the concentration of growth factors.[176]

In another direction, research efforts are also focusing on collagen synthesis, cell proliferation, and cartilage repair.[279] Collagen meniscus implants used to regenerate or regrow new meniscus-like tissue and stem cells are being tested for anterior cruciate ligament reconstruction,[278] with the goals of slowing down and preventing further degenerative joint disease, enhancing joint stability, providing pain relief, and returning people to activities at their desired level.

Autologous chondrocyte implantation and osteochondral autologous transplantation take plugs of cartilage or bone from one site, multiply the cells in culture, and place them into a lesion or hole in the native cartilage or bone, respectively. Repair tissue of high quality requires at least 2 years to regenerate and mature.[96]

Functional bone tissue with the necessary strength for load-bearing applications is still under development. Injectable hydrogels have resulted in materials with significantly enhanced compressive strength.[368] Several growth factors contained in demineralized bone matrix (e.g., bone morphogenetic protein) are now being used to stimulate bone healing. Tissue engineering for bone healing has great potential for many people who experience nonunion, slow-to-heal bone fractures, or traumatic bone loss associated with war injuries.[169]

Other research is under way to generate stronger bone substitutes either by increasing osteoblast differentiation and mineralization[109] or culturing the engineered tissue for a longer period of time before implantation to allow matrix maturation.[68] Learning to tailor the strength of tissue-engineered bone to the person's need requires further research.[114,242]

Other examples of current progress in the area of bioengineering include implants filled with islets for people with diabetes to replace insulin injections, a method to generate natural breast tissue to replace saline implants, heart valves, dental tissue (gums, teeth), skeletal muscle, tissue isolated from synthetic polymers, and formation of phalanges and small joints from bovine-cell sources. Tissue engineering models are being developed to treat different conditions with the urinary bladder, such as bladder cancer, acontractility, and inflammatory disease.[328]

Laboratory-grown organs are under investigation, with the hope for producing donor tissue and organs for transplantation on demand and developing living prosthetics (incorporating living tissue with electronics) for every organ system in the body.[244,415] Embryonic and adult stem cells, able to differentiate into all types of cells, remain the hope of many scientists in the treatment of systemic diseases and local tissue defects, as a vehicle for gene therapy, and to generate transplantable tissues and organs in tissue-engineering protocols.[37,217,307]

state-of-the-art science is directed at manipulating cell fate. However, the biomechanical environment of these cells is pivotal to their ultimate differentiation, health, and function. Given this notion, now is an ideal time for physical therapists to become involved. As a profession, we have the skills to integrate biology, biomechanics, and physiology in a way that allows the timing and intensity of physical interventions to be optimized for tissue regeneration and, ultimately, function.[14] We will be involved in designing and implementing regenerative rehabilitation aimed at maximizing function as the transplanted tissue replaces, repairs, or regenerates injured, aged, or diseased tissues.[13] The first annual symposium on regenerative rehabilitation was held in November 2011. The American Physical Therapy Association (APTA) Section on Research sponsors research and continuing education on regenerative medicine; see the APTA website (http://www.apta.org/) for more information (type in search window: regenerative medicine for podcasts and audio conferences).

BIOPSYCHOSOCIAL IMPLICATIONS

Many different ethical, social, moral, economic, and legal issues are associated with the procurement and allocation of living or bioengineered tissue. In addition, new information concerning the psychoneuroimmune responses (see "Psychoneuroimmunology" in Chapter 1) in healthy tissues and organs has added new dimensions to understanding the emotional adjustment for recipients of living organ and tissue transplants.

Legal and Ethical Considerations

Before alternate treatment methods can be fully implemented, scientific and medical communities and the general public will have to seriously consider and attempt to resolve legal and ethical issues. For example, federal law prohibits the sale of human organs in the United States, and violators are subject to fines and imprisonment. However, individuals have taken matters into their own hands and established donor-matching services on the Internet.

In some countries of continental Europe, organ donation is governed by "presumed consent" legislation. Unless legally designated otherwise, organ donation is presumed on the death of each individual. Consent legislation has had a proven and positive, sizeable effect on organ donation rates.[1]

Although Western opinion is almost universally against the practice of paid organ donation and the use of organs from judicially executed prisoners, similar laws are not in place worldwide. The ethics of both issues continue to be debated.

Bioethical Considerations

Another area of concern involves researchers growing human cells into tissues using stem cells derived from human embryos left over from attempts at artificial

---

SPECIAL IMPLICATIONS FOR THE THERAPIST 21-1

Regenerative Rehabilitation

Currently, biochemists, cell biologists, and developmental biologists dominate the field because the

fertilization or following abortions. Currently in the United States, embryonic stem cell lines are being made in the private sector and in private universities that use private funding. Federal funding for stem cell research (banned under the Bush administration) has been reinstated. This change occurred after a 2010 U.S. Court of Appeals ruling upheld President Obama's executive order (2009) to allow research funding by the National Institutes of Health and Department of Health and Human Services.[255,272]

Legislation in the United States to allow federal funding for research using stem cells derived from embryos originally created for fertility treatments and willingly donated by consenting adults has been introduced and remains a debated issue. For the most part, embryonic stem cells are only used in fundamental research. It is predicted that it will be at least 5 to 8 years before they can be put to use in clinical trials.

Many bioethicists and lawmakers still question the appropriateness of this research until the ethical issues and appropriate concerns can be voiced and resolved. Questions about the nature of human life and its protection, the safeguard of human dignity, and the use of genetic material have been raised. However, new discoveries in the rapidly developing field of stem cell research, such as the discovery of master stem cells (see "Hematopoietic Cell Transplantation" below) replacing the use of embryonic tissue, may bypass these bioethical concerns.

Other countries, such as Israel, England, and India, and in parts of Asia, have moved ahead in the area of stem cell research. Since January 2006, stem cell trials for the treatment of stroke, spinal cord injury, leg ischemia, and myocardial infarction have been conducted in India using bone marrow–derived stem cells.

Concerns related to animal-derived matrix proteins have also been raised. Some private bioengineering companies are proactively researching ways to develop human tissue with matrix proteins naturally secreted by the cells rather than developing tissue from animal-derived matrix proteins. In the area of animal organ transplantation (xenotransplantation), rules governing the welfare of animals bred for transplants are being formulated. For example, a ban on having children has been placed on all people receiving animal organ transplantation.

Psychoemotional Considerations

Pretransplantation

Transplant applicants face many challenges, including the obvious physical illness, complex assessment protocols, uncertainties about surgery and outcome, the possibility of relocation to obtain transplant services, and large expenses. Waiting for a transplant can be accompanied by a vast range of changing emotions, such as relief, despair, elation, depression, excitement, and apprehension.

No single attitude is common or expected; each person's reaction is a valid expression of his or her experience. Most candidates find waiting for surgery a stressful time and, of course, the longer the wait, the greater the stress. The evaluation process itself and the wait for the results after tests and procedures require complex coping strategies, especially if the person is denied for transplantation.

When death is a possibility, candidates may worry that negative thinking will harm their health. Others are distressed that someone else must die before an organ will be available for transplantation or that receiving an available organ deprives someone else of life. Candidates are encouraged to focus on the desired outcome without completely ignoring the alternatives for themselves and outcomes for others. Counseling and support groups are often recommended.

Anxiety and depression are common complications of medical illness of any kind and may interfere with the candidate's or recipient's participation in rehabilitation. Symptoms of posttraumatic stress disorder are not uncommon in the recipient or partner after organ implantation or mechanical assist device implantation followed by heart transplantation.[60,280]

Clinical symptoms of posttraumatic stress disorder, anxiety, or depression can be subtle and mimic the individual's health condition, requiring candidate or recipient self-awareness and careful screening by all members of the transplantation team to identify and treat early. The therapist can take an active role by administering simple evidence-based questionnaires to screen for the need for referral to an appropriate health provider (for example, social work or psychology). Attention to the supporting members of the recipient's family and partners is also advised.[60] In some centers, caregivers start their own support groups while they are relocated to help with their needs during the stressful process.

A condition severe enough to require organ transplantation can sometimes impair concentration, memory, judgment, or ability to process thoughts. In particular, approximately one-third of all liver transplant candidates have severe impairment of mental abilities (i.e., hepatic encephalopathy) and may be extremely confused or even delirious at the time of transplantation. Similar mental impairment can occur with heart, lung, and kidney candidates, although it is less common.

Posttransplantation

Postoperatively, recipients face a long recovery period, the potential for graft rejection, reintegration into family and work roles, and lifelong changes, such as the need for drug compliance and changes in diet. Adaptation after transplantation is a lifelong process and depends on several factors, such as the success of the transplantation, expectations before the transplantation and perceived outcomes, postoperative complications or side effects of the antirejection drugs, permanent physical changes or changes in appearance, as well as other individual considerations.

Identification of recipients most likely to have compliance and psychiatric problems early after transplantation is important in focusing interventions that maximize recipients' psychosocial status in these areas and thus improve long-term physical health outcomes.[120,391] Pretransplantation psychiatric disorders, female gender, longer hospitalization, more impaired physical function, and less social support from caregivers and family in the perioperative period are known risk factors for posttransplantation anxiety and depressive and psychologic disorders.[119]

Stress on the family and the need for family support and counseling also affect treatment outcomes. Health care staff may observe a deterioration of family relationships after transplantation (especially between husband and wife or between partners). Older children receiving organ transplantation may face the challenge of parents not allowing or unable to allow the child to grow into adulthood. Support groups can be extremely helpful in these types of situations and should be recommended early by the health care team.

POSTTRANSPLANTATION COMPLICATIONS

With advances in technology and immunology, transplantation of almost any tissue is feasible, but the clinical use of transplantation to remedy disease is still limited for many organ systems because of the rejection reaction and other posttransplant complications.

Complications following organ transplantation can be classified into three broad categories: (1) complications associated with the procurement and surgical procedure, (2) complications of the transplantation, and (3) complications as a result of the immunosuppressive agents used to prevent rejection. Each type of organ transplantation has its own accompanying surgical risks and complications (see discussion in each section).

Following surgery, two main complications of organ transplantation remain infection and organ rejection. The most serious posttransplantation complication is death, which can be caused by infection, organ toxicity, GVHD, relapse, and various other causes (Fig. 21-5). The overall incidence of infection is in the range of 10% to 15%,[98] occurring most often (60%) in kidney transplant recipients.[231]

Infection and organ rejection are common and treatable, but prevention is the first step. For this reason, pretransplantation serologic testing is done to determine histocompatibility and to avoid transmitting infectious agents (e.g., CMV, vancomycin-resistant enterococci, hepatitis B virus, hepatitis C virus) from donor to recipient. Herpes zoster infection can be a serious complication of organ transplantation, with postherpetic neuralgia occurring in almost half of the recipients affected. Heart and lung recipients have the highest incidence (15%), followed by renal (7.4%) and liver (5.7%) transplant recipients.[171]

As survival rates improve, other complications arise, such as the increased risk of other diseases (e.g., cancer, diabetes). Compared with the general population, recipients of a kidney, liver, heart, or lung transplant have an increased risk for diverse infection-related and unrelated cancers[138] (see further discussion in "Cancers in Solid-Organ Transplant Recipients" below).

Ischemic Reperfusion Injury

Ischemic injury occurs when normal blood and oxygen supply to the donor organ is stopped at the time of organ harvest, whereas *reperfusion injury* can occur when blood flow is returned to the organ after transplantation. The donated organ is very sensitive to the amount of time it is not being perfused or supplied with blood, which can

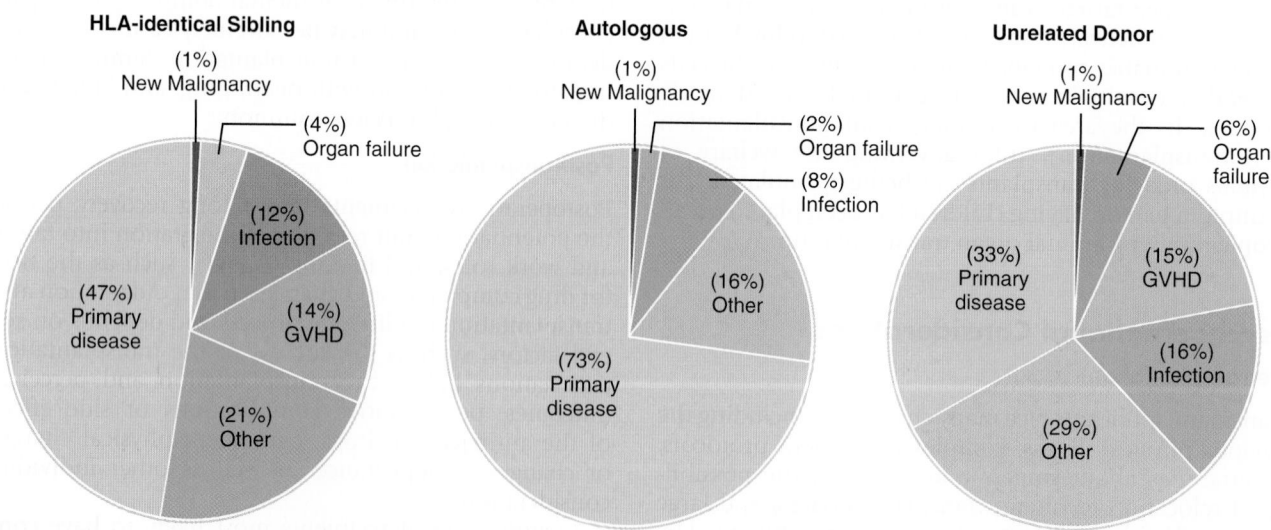

Figure 21-5

Causes of death after transplants performed in 2008–2009. The effect of disease stage is even more apparent for allogeneic transplants. Individuals receiving an HLA-identical sibling transplant for acute myelogenous leukemia in remission have a 100-day mortality rate of 7% to 9%, compared to 22% for recipients with active leukemia at the time of transplantation. Early mortality after an unrelated donor transplant is higher than after an HLA-identical sibling transplantation, but the rate also depends on the disease and disease stage. The causes of death in the first 100 days posttransplantation mainly relate to the primary disease, graft-versus-host disease, infection, and end-organ damage. After an autologous transplant, primary disease is the most commonly reported cause of death. Among allogeneic transplant recipients, unrelated donor transplants have fewer deaths related to the primary disease; however, organ failure and infections are higher after unrelated donor transplants. (Courtesy Center for International Blood & Marrow Transplant Research (CIBMTR). *CIBMTR Summary Slides–HCT Trends and Survival Data.* March 2012.)

lead to ischemia.[89] Ischemic reperfusion injury may occur with any organ transplantation; it results in the onset of the inflammatory response, which has both immediate and long-term effects on the donated organ.

After the organ has been surgically implanted, the clamps are removed to allow blood to once again perfuse the organ. It has been suggested that the abrupt return of blood to the donor organ (now transplanted into the recipient) may create further trauma to the epithelial lining of the blood vessels because the transplant recipient may be circulating blood at a higher pressure than the donor organ.

This phenomenon is especially common in heart or lung transplantation in the presence of comorbid pulmonary hypertension. This results in a reperfusion injury, which leads to leukocytes and platelet aggregation, which further causes endothelial permeability and inflammatory cell activation and adherence.

Mild ischemic reperfusion injury is common, and recovery usually occurs within 3 to 5 days. If the injury is significant, organ dysfunction and failure and possible death of the recipient are possible. More recently it has been shown that there is a significant relation between the presence of an ischemic reperfusion injury and development of chronic rejection via the activation of both the innate and adaptive immune responses and organ regeneration.[53] See "Graft Rejection" below.

Histocompatibility

In all cases of graft rejection, the cause is incompatibility of cell surface antigens. The rejection of foreign or transplanted tissue occurs because the recipient's immune system recognizes that the surface HLA proteins of the donor's tissue are different from the recipient's.

Certain antigens are more important than others for successful transplantation, including ABO and Rh antigens present on red blood cells and histocompatibility antigens, most importantly, the HLA. As expected, there is a better chance of graft acceptance with syngeneic or autologous transplants because the cell surface antigens are identical. For all categories of transplantation, minimizing HLA mismatches is associated with a significantly lower risk of graft loss.[81]

It has been shown that in a person with HLA antibodies, the antibodies are directed against the antigen of the donor kidney and will result in immediate graft failure. It also has been documented that the when specific HLA antibodies are directed against B cells, hyperacute rejection is produced, leading to graft dysfunction and possible failure.[396]

Rh antigen is more important in heart and kidney transplants than in lung transplantation. In renal transplants HLA crossmatches are routinely performed, whereas this is not commonly done in lungs (unless the candidate has a high panel reactive antibody count). Crossmatching policies may vary by institution.

Graft Rejection

Transplant rejection may occur for immunologic or nonimmunologic reasons. When the body recognizes the donor tissue as nonself and attempts to destroy the tissue shortly after transplantation, rejection occurs as an immunologic phenomenon. Transplant rejection is most often caused by histocompatibility.

Nonimmunologic factors can occur as a result of the draining reperfusion process necessary in organ harvest and transplantation. Ischemic reperfusion injury is associated with an increase in acute and chronic rejection.[53] See "Ischemic Reperfusion Injury" above.

As residual blood is drained from the transplanted organ into the host's general circulation, the body recognizes the transplanted tissue cells as foreign invaders (antigens) and immediately sets up an immune response by producing antibodies. These antibodies are capable of inhibiting metabolism of the cells within the transplanted organ and eventually actively causing their destruction.

Research to develop a reliable method to reduce the ischemic reperfusion injury is currently ongoing. Eliminating the occurrence of poor early graft function and consequently reducing the chances for rejection episodes are the primary goals of these investigations.[126,129]

Types of Graft Rejection

There are three types of transplant rejection—the *hyperacute* rejection, the *acute* or late acute rejection, and the *chronic* rejection—depending on the amount of time that passes between transplantation and rejection (Table 21-3).

Hyperacute Rejection. Hyperacute rejection (rare with antibody screening and tissue typing) is dominantly mediated by humoral responses of the immune system (natural antibodies, complement cascade) and the activation of coagulation factors. There is an immediate rejection after transplantation when the recipient has preformed antibodies to donor tissue.

This reaction necessitates prompt medical action, which may include surgical removal of the transplanted tissue or the use of life-support devises such as a temporary VAD or ECMO, in the case of a heart or lung transplantation. These devices can be used to support blood circulation and gas exchange while the individual undergoes such treatment as plasmapheresis and immunoglobulin therapy in an attempt to remove the reactive antibodies. Medical treatment may diminish the hyperacute rejection response and allow the donor organ to recover, or it may allow time for another donor organ to be implanted.[251]

Acute or Late Acute Rejection. The acute or late acute rejection can appear days to years after the transplantation. This type of rejection involves a combination of cellular and humoral reactions. Acute antibody-mediated rejection or vascular rejection typically occurs days to weeks posttransplantation. There is an interaction between the recipient's antibody and donor HLA or endothelial cell antigens that leads to graft vessel injury and thrombosis formation. Acute cellular rejection is most common in the first 3 to 6 months posttransplantation and involves the proliferation and infiltration of T lymphocytes and macrophages.[189,251] Despite the early pattern of acute rejection, both humoral and cellular rejection can occur at any time.

Clinically, there is sudden onset of organ-related symptoms, which may be associated with fever and graft

Table 21-3	Clinical Manifestations of Organ Rejection		
Hyperacute Rejection	**Acute (Late) Rejection**		**Chronic Rejections**

Immediate reaction
Severe graft dysfunction or failure, then death
Death
	Occurs days to years after transplantation
	May be asymptomatic in early stages
	Fever; constitutional symptoms (flu-like)
	Loss of appetite
	Graft tenderness
	Blood pressure changes
	Dyspnea
	Fatigue
	Peripheral edema, weight gain
	Inflamed skin lesions
	Reduced exercise capacity
	Organ related-symptoms
	• Kidney:
	  • Proteinuria
	  • Uremia
	  • Neurologic symptoms
	  • Nausea and vomiting
	• Liver:
	  • Palpable liver
	  • Jaundice
	  • Hematemesis (vomiting blood)
	  • Abdominal pain
	  • Ascites
	  • Neurologic symptoms (see Box 21-6)
	  • Elevated transaminase
	  • Elevated bilirubin
	• Heart:
	  • S3 gallop
	  • Arrhythmias
	  • Jugular vein distention
	• Lung:
	  • Changes in respiratory status; breathlessness; prolonged need for ventilatory support
	  • Fall in spirometric values (>10% change/reduction from baseline; <90% at rest)
	  • Decreased FEV_1 >10%
	  • Dry or productive cough
	  • Change in sputum (color amount)
	  • Decreased oxygen saturation
	  • Reduced vital capacity; decreased exercise capacity
	  • Radiographic changes
	• Pancreas:
	  • Nausea
	  • Vomiting
	  • Anorexia
	  • Other gastrointestinal symptoms
	  • Urologic symptoms
			Occurs 3 months to years after transplantation
			May be asymptomatic in early stages
			Organ-related symptoms
			Histologic changes
			Graft dysfunction
			Graft failure

FEV_1, forced expiratory volume in 1 second.

tenderness, fatigue, or decrease exertional tolerance, or the recipient may be totally asymptomatic. Graft rejection must be differentiated from immunosuppressive toxicity.

This form of rejection can be reliably graded using a system of categories of mild, moderate, and severe rejection. Acute rejection, if detected in its early stages, can be reversed with immunosuppressive therapy. With the advancement in immunosuppressive medications and management, there has been a decline in acute rejection, which has led to an increase in 1-year graft and recipient survival.[407]

Chronic Rejection. Chronic rejection can occur as early as 3 months posttransplantation, but it is usually months to years before the chronic rejection occurs. This type of rejection develops as a function of both cell-mediated and humoral-mediated reactions and is characterized by slow, progressive organ failure.

Growing evidence indicates that chronic rejection is the aggregate sum of irreversible immunologic and nonimmunologic injuries to the graft over time. Chronic rejection is associated with chronic vascular changes, such as arteriopathy or diffuse atherosclerosis with intimal proliferative changes, depending on the type of organ. In the presence of a chronic immune/inflammatory process within the donor organ, the intimal lining of the vascular tissue undergoes fibrosis and vascular remodeling. This leads to a decrease in the lumen size and ischemia of the distal tissue and perpetuates the inflammatory reaction.[116,169]

A history of acute rejection episodes, either asymptomatic or clinically apparent, and inadequate therapeutic level of the immunosuppressive medications or poor compliance are among the most recognizable immunologic risk factors for chronic rejection.[189]

Adherence to immunosuppressive therapy is a key factor contributing to transplant failures that occur within 2 years after surgery. Financial barriers, such as the lack of insurance coverage, are the most common reason for noncompliance or spreading out antirejection medications, taking them less often.[87] Chronic rejection results in irreversible cellular damage within the donor organ and leads to graft dysfunction and eventually failure.[185,251] Rarely is chronic rejection responsive to medical therapies.

Immunosuppression

That a primary role of the immune system is to distinguish between self and nonself (the immunologic response of the recipient to the donor's tissues) presents a major problem for the transplant recipient. In the person with an intact immune system (immunocompetence), the recipient's immune system recognizes the transplanted tissue or organ as foreign (nonself) and produces antibodies and sensitized lymphocytes against it.

The ultimate objective of immunosuppressive therapy (see "Advances in Medications" under "Advances and Research in Transplantation" above) is to block transplantation candidate reactivity to the donor's organ while sparing other responses. Because these drugs suppress immunologic reactions, infection is a leading cause of death, particularly within the first postoperative year.[253] However, increased understanding of rejection mechanisms has made it possible to suppress specific elements of the immune response and has led to a decrease in death-related infection and rejection.[47,407]

Although lower amounts of immunosuppressive drugs are now prescribed, these drugs usually must be taken for the life of the recipient and physical changes and other side effects remain a well-known problem (see Table 5-3).

Side Effects of Long-Term Immunosuppression

(See also Chapter 5.)

Long-term immunosuppression can have serious consequences for the recipient, such as diabetes and accelerated hyperlipidemia, with associated atherosclerosis and subsequent cardiovascular disease.

There is a high incidence of musculoskeletal effects that will concern the therapist, such as decreased bone density and osteoporosis. Half of all transplant recipients are diagnosed with osteoporosis and one-third have documented vertebral fractures,[257] steroid- and calcineurin inhibitor–induced myopathies, as well as avascular necrosis and musculoskeletal injuries.

Within the first 6 months after transplantation, the organ candidate can lose more bone density than any woman during the postmenopausal period. Osteoporosis

has become a silent contributor to mortality in organ transplantation.[380] Physical therapy intervention must address this concern.

Neurotoxic reactions are manifested by a fine tremor, paresthesias, and, occasionally, seizures. Sensorimotor demyelinating polyradiculoneuropathy has been reported as a rare side effect in liver transplant recipients receiving tacrolimus (Prograf).[260] Neuropathies and paresthesia, including foot drop (anterior tibialis weakness), can occur with this drug[430]; quadriplegia is a rare adverse event.

The individual may report difficulty completing fine motor activities of daily living, such as poor handwriting and difficulty eating. These changes may be significant enough to stop some people from going out publicly or dining out in restaurants. Reports of memory loss may not be secondary to actual alterations in memory, but rather a decrease in executive function.[102,388] Most of these events are dose related and reversible.

Cancers in Solid-Organ Transplant Recipients

Organ recipients have three times the incidence of various cancers, and some specific cancers are 100 times more frequent in the immunosuppressed population after transplantation than in the general population. Cancer incidence is proportional to immunosuppression drug levels and the risk increases each year after transplant.[113] It has been suggested that immunosuppressive agents may cause DNA damage and interfere with normal DNA repair mechanisms. Immune surveillance, which ordinarily prevents the growth and development of malignancies, may be impaired by certain immunosuppressive medications.

The most common tumors among transplant recipients (40%-50% incidence) are squamous cell cancers of the lips and skin owing to the enhanced photosensitivity. Squamous cell carcinoma is often more aggressive than in nonimmunosuppressed people, with multiple sites of presentation and frequent recurrence.[139] The incidence of basal cell carcinoma is 10% higher than the general population, and the incidence of squamous cell carcinoma has been reported to be 250 times greater in orthotopic homologous transplantation recipients.[208]

Organ recipients are also at increased risk for some malignancies such as Kaposi sarcoma, non-Hodgkin lymphomas and other posttransplant lymphoproliferative disorders, soft-tissue sarcomas, carcinomas of the vulva and perineum, carcinomas of the kidney, and hepatobiliary tumors.[116,138,402]

Solid organ cancer risk involving the lung, colon, pancreas, prostate, stomach, breast, and ovary is twofold higher in transplant recipients than in the general population, while kidney cancer risk is 15 times greater.[138,218] Malignant lymphomas occur 11.8 times more often in kidney transplant recipients compared with the general population. The majority of lymphomas occur after the first posttransplant year.[310] Exactly why kidney transplantation is more affected by these factors than other organs remains unknown.[216]

Cardiac transplant recipients have a higher incidence of cancer than do other transplant recipients, perhaps because of the higher levels of immunosuppression.

There have been studies that have reported an increase in lung cancer in heart transplant recipients who have a history of smoking. There is an increased incidence in posttransplant lymphoproliferative disease in heart transplant recipients who underwent OKT$_3$ induction therapy or use of antithymocyte globulin for rejection therapy.

Gastrointestinal Problems

Gastrointestinal complications of solid-organ transplantation have been well described in the literature. Disorders of the colon and rectum are a considerable source of morbidity, especially after heart and lung transplantation. Colorectal problems occur among 7% of lung transplant recipients, 6% of heart-lung transplant recipients, and 4% of heart transplant recipients. Major events include diverticulitis, perforation, and malignancy. More minor complications include polyps, pseudoobstruction, and benign anorectal disease.[168] Acute nausea, vomiting, weight loss, restrictions to diet and eating can be barriers to rehab; feeding tubes are often used to supplement nutrition in transplant recipients.

Wound Healing

Advances in surgical techniques and immunosuppression have led to an appreciable reduction in postoperative complications following transplantation. However, wound complications, as one of the most common types of posttransplantation surgical complications, can still limit these improved outcomes and result in prolonged hospitalization, hospital readmission, and reoperation.[273]

Chronic immunosuppressive drug therapy impairs and prolongs wound healing, especially common among those organ recipients with diabetic or neuropathic pedal ulcers. The two most important risk factors for wound complications are immunosuppression and obesity. Other risk factors include surgical and/or technical factors (e.g., type of incision, reoperation, surgeon's expertise), advancing age, diabetes mellitus, malnutrition, and uremia.[273]

Therapists should be involved in preventive management of wound complications; identifying and minimizing risk factors whenever possible is important. Therapists involved in wound therapy should inform their clients, members of the clients' families, employers of clients, and third-party payers to expect longer times in healing plantar ulcers because of long-term immunosuppressive therapy.[370]

Total-contact casting remains a highly effective and rapid method of healing neuropathic pedal ulcers in diabetic immunosuppressed clients and transplant recipients, although it may take several weeks longer than it would for those individuals who were not immunocompromised. Transplant recipients who are immunocompromised appear to be no more at risk for wound failure complications when using total-contact casting as a treatment modality than those individuals without these additional variables.[370]

Posttransplantation Pain Syndromes

Reports of chronic pain among solid-organ transplant recipients were first recorded in the late 1990s.[146] Since that time more understanding of posttransplantation pain syndromes has come to light. Pain associated with posttransplantation syndrome is described as burning, stabbing, or dull, and may be linked with depression; a correlation between pain intensity and organ rejection has been established.[146] Primary musculoskeletal pain can occur following solid-organ transplantation often (but not always) linked with immunosuppressive medications (e.g., cyclosporine). Individuals who experience partial sympathetic reinnervation following heart transplantation may experience chest discomfort and/or shoulder and arm pain.

ORGAN TRANSPLANTATION AND EXERCISE, ACTIVITY, AND SPORTS

Whereas some people will have a period of only a few days of physical inactivity before transplantation (e.g., toxic liver failure), the majority of organ candidates will live with their diseased organs for a prolonged period of time, often years. By the time of organ transplantation, candidates usually have experienced a period of long-term ill health leading to end-stage organ failure accompanied by severe deconditioning and exercise intolerance.

Complications of long-term immunosuppressive therapy and the kind of organ that has failed will determine some of the problems an individual may face in relation to exercise, activities, and sports. Most transplantation candidates experience an impaired physical performance level that not only interferes with the ability to perform leisure-time exercise, but also often limits the ability to perform even simple physical tasks, such as rising from a chair or climbing stairs.[226]

Weakness, dyspnea on exertion, and fatigue are often present, and there may be little motivation for exercise and sport. Finding an activity or exercise that the person can do successfully is the first step to initiating regular lifelong exercise.

Whether or not a potential candidate receives a transplant, therapy can be focused toward more function and improved quality of life. Exercise training increases work capacity as measured by increased oxygen consumption (VO$_2$), increases efficiency of oxygen utilization in the muscles, normalizes distribution of muscle fiber types, increases aerobic metabolism with delays in the onset of lactic acid buildup, and promotes modulation of the parasympathetic nervous system with more sensitive baroreceptors.[33,212] Exercise training also improves psychologic factors such as depression in pretransplant and posttransplant individuals.[76,232,323]

An assessment of transplant candidates must take into consideration daily life and daily activities, including potential return to work requirements. For example, a job that requires lifting requires assessment of cardiovascular compliance and hemodynamic stability during lifting, whereas someone at home must be safe in activities of daily living.

Pretransplantation Activity and Exercise

It has been proposed that peripheral skeletal and respiratory (in the case of thoracic involvement) muscle work capacity is reduced before transplantation and contributes to the limitations of exercise seen in the posttransplantation population.[422] Preservation of muscle strength before transplantation becomes difficult for some who are acutely ill. Muscular dysfunction attributable to detraining and deconditioning is common.[239]

While an individual waits on the transplant list, it is important that the candidate participate in an exercise program with the goal to promote functional mobility. Exercise programs should be individualized to focus on the needs of each person required to maintain function, self-control, and esteem.

Exercises should be functional, with an emphasis on strengthening the proximal muscles of the pelvis and the lower extremities, especially the gluteal and quadriceps muscles, as well as muscles of the shoulder girdle and trunk to support upper extremity function and accessory respiratory efficiency.

Weight training to maintain or increase muscular strength may help the candidate counteract the effects of steroids on muscle and the adverse effects of immobility and chronic inflammation.[93,308,323] It has been reported by transplantation centers around the United States that transplantation candidates who take part in an exercise program before surgery are likely to recover more rapidly following transplantation. Researchers are beginning to publish data on exercise performance before and after transplantation.[79,146,184,331,376]

Educational sessions can be extremely beneficial to both the organ recipient and the caregivers with regard to the transplant process and its aftercare. Preparing the potential recipient for complications such as weakness and osteoporosis before surgery and how to best treat issues when they arise can improve the individual's success in overcoming them after transplantation.

Posttransplantation Activity and Exercise

After organ transplantation, the underlying pathophysiologic process returns to normal if the donor organ is functioning appropriately. For example, exercise performance in individuals with heart transplants increases with respect to pretransplantation performance but remains subnormal and may not improve with time after surgery.[42] The extent of recovery depends on the function of the transplanted organ, which, in turn, is determined by the quality and function of the organ implanted, the presence of any rejection or infection, and the development of other comorbidities.

Despite the pretransplantation physical deconditioning and exercise limitations, transplant recipients can progressively return to a normal life with return to work and even safely participate in sporting activity and exercise.[226] National and International Transplant Games, a multidisciplinary sporting event started in 1978, illustrates the degree to which organ candidates can return to exercise and sports. At the 2006 National Kidney Foundation–sponsored games in Louisville, KY, transplant recipients from all 50 states, with the oldest recipient being 84 years of age, participated to celebrate the gift of life and experience competition.

Regular exercise enhances quality of life and lowers the risk of cardiovascular disease, hypertension, and diabetes. This is especially important in transplant recipients, because many immunosuppressive drugs can be atherogenic and diabetogenic.[110,149,278] It is recommended that physical therapy should begin on postoperative day 1, with the goal to mobilize out of bed as soon as medically stable. Progressive physical training should begin as soon as the recipient is up and walking.

Despite the restoration of system function that allows most recipients to return to an improved quality of life, including returning to work, having and caring for children, and participating in leisure recreational activities, transplant recipients often experience a persistent limitation in peak aerobic and anaerobic capacity when compared with health- and age-matched normal subjects.[274]

There is a decrease in maximal and peak VO_2, decrease in workload, earlier onset of anaerobic threshold, and lower VO_2 at the anaerobic threshold. Heart transplant recipients have lower exercise capacity than other transplant recipients.[274] There is evidence to suggest that recipients continue to have abnormalities in both central and peripheral chemoreflex mechanisms along with the adverse effects of the immunosuppressive medications that contribute to prolonged deficits of exercise capacity.[26,59]

Despite the inherent limitations caused by the posttransplantation state, exercise training after transplantation can increase exercise capacity, improve endurance, and increase muscle strength, contributing to higher quality of life after transplantation even in the presence of posttransplantation limitations.[152,193,204,209,274] Physical activity and exercise may reduce or attenuate side effects of immunosuppression. Transplant recipients tolerate progressive exercise training and can achieve near-normal and even normal levels of function.[210] There is evidence that rehabilitation can improve muscle function and exercise parameters compared with those who had a transplant and did not participate in rehabilitation.[271]

Various exercises have been prescribed for transplant recipients. Studies document various training programs, including aerobic programs of low-to-high intensities, muscle endurance, and resistive training. It is difficult to draw any specific conclusions about the optimal exercise program. The best recommendation that can be made is to prescribe a comprehensive exercise program that includes muscular strength and endurance training, restoring functional mobility and improving cardiopulmonary endurance.[27,175]

Gaining density in the lumbar spine is especially important because up to 35% of transplant recipients develop lumbar spine bone fractures.[58] Resistive training has been shown to restore bone density to pretransplantation levels compared with an additional 6% loss in subjects who did not participate in resistance training. Marked increase in muscle mass, strength, and exercise capacity was also observed.[386]

Guidelines for Activity and Exercise

Whether assessing aerobic, anaerobic ability, or activities of daily living (Table 21-4), measurements of vitals,

Table 21-4   Exercise Guidelines for Organ Candidates and Recipients*

Weight training has become an acceptable component of a comprehensive exercise program. It is recommended to begin strength training at low-to-moderate intensity levels along with a progressive aerobic and stretching program. It is important to assess blood pressure response during exercise and evaluate for signs and symptoms of right-sided heart failure in the presence of pulmonary hypertension. The recipients should also be monitored for hemoptysis, overuse injuries, poorly regulated glucose, electrolyte and nutritional imbalances and surgical precautions. Anyone with documented pulmonary hypertension may have the following associated signs and symptoms (light headedness, dizziness, angina-like pain, decreased cardiac output with exercise or development of abnormal heart sounds with exertion) needs to be supervised during low level interval exercises.

Once the person is medically stable and basic level of function is restored, the therapist can more accurately prescribe a supervised exercise program by completing a symptom-limited aerobic exercise test as well as a 1 or 3 RM (repetition maximum). As a reminder, a 1 RM is defined as the heaviest weight that can be lifted safely at the weakest position in the range of motion one time. The therapist must take into account any significant impairments present and the effects of long-term steroid use, especially muscle wasting, osteoporosis, and coagulopathy. Risk for injury is higher in this group when using 1 RM.

- Select an enjoyable activity or exercise and always have a goal! Some centers target a long-term goal by organizing an annual fun run/walk or join one already organized.
- Include adequate warm-up, stretching, and cool-down periods.
- Progress activity or exercise as described in text.
- Include interval training, aerobic activity, strength training, muscular endurance training, and flexibility.
- Combine activities and/or exercise program with energy conservation techniques (see Box 9-4).
- Maintain a normal breathing pattern; breath holding may contribute to excessive elevation in blood pressure and produce associated symptoms, such as dyspnea and light-headedness.
- Exercise 4-5 days a week; allow 24-48 hours recovery time after strenuous activity and 48 hours after moderate to vigorous resistance training for those involved muscles.
- Follow guidelines for neuropathy and myopathy.

Endurance Training: High Repetitions/30-90 Seconds High-Intensity Intervals/Low to Moderate Resistance

- Muscle endurance: 2-3 days per week
- Weights that are 50%-60% of 1 RM (to cause fatigue in 30-90 seconds of time)
- Perform 12-30 repetitions per set at 30- to 90-second intervals
- Perform 2-5 sets of each exercise per workout

Strength Training: Low Repetitions/3-8 Repetitions, Moderate to High Resistance

- Strength training 2-3 days per week
- Determine actual and predicted 1 RM
- Resistance is high with goal of 3-8 repetitions, 70%-85% of 1 RM
- Perform 3-5 sets of each exercise per workout
- Consider closed kinetic chain functional activities
- Perform each exercise through a full functional range of motion

Aerobic Training

- Aerobic training completed 5 days a week for minimal 30 minutes of moderate intensity or 20 minutes of vigorous intensity
- Activity should use large muscle in repetitious manner
- Intensity 40%-85% of maximal work capacity

Weight Training: Low Repetitions/More Resistance

- Use weights that are 40%-60% of the 1 RM.†
- Perform 3-8 repetitions per set.
- Perform 3-5 sets of each exercise per workout.
- Perform each exercise through a functional range of motion.

For the Therapist

Maintain or Monitor	Terminate Exercise If...
Observe client response to exercise: allow minimal to moderate dyspnea; respiratory rate should be <30 breaths/min with minimal rales heard on auscultation	Respiratory rate >40 breaths/min with increased rales
Allow only mild level of fatigue; use rate of perceived exertion (RPE, Borg scale; see Table 12-13)	(3/10 on Borg scale)
Maintain stable vital signs (heart rate [HR], blood pressure); maintain stable cardiac output (rate pressure product [RPP], pulse pressure [PP])	HR exceeds target zone; decrease in systolic blood pressure (SBP), pulse pressure (PP) narrows (SBP – diastolic blood pressure [DBP]), decrease in RPP (RPP = HR × SBP)
Maintain stable electrocardiogram (ECG)	Increased incidence of arrhythmias or perceived palpitations
Maintain central venous pressure (CVP)	Monitor in the presence of right-sided heart failure; maintain CVP 20 at mm Hg; terminate exercise relative to other symptoms

Table 21-4	Exercise Guidelines for Organ Candidates and Recipients*—cont'd	
Maintain or Monitor	**Terminate Exercise If...**	
Maintain pulmonary arterial pressure (PAP)	Rest is indicated if PAP rises 5 mm Hg; terminate exercise if PAP rises and persists after rest and/or in the presence of other symptoms	
Maintain oxygen saturation 90% (this is individually determined by each center according to each person's medical status)	Oxygen saturation less than 90% (or saturation below prescription)	
Monitor for signs of bleeding	(See Tables 40-8 and 40-9)	
Maintain or expect an increase in CVP	Change in mental status (e.g., level of confusion, hostility); onset of pallor or diaphoresis; client request	

*Guidelines for exercise are modified for the organ recipient but follow the *ACSM's Guidelines for Exercise Testing and Prescription*. These are only guidelines; each exercise program must be individually tailored to the organ recipient's condition and comorbidities. Progression must be according to tolerance.

†Intensities of 80% to 100% have been shown to produce the most rapid gain in muscle strength within the normal population. However, because of the possibility of overtraining or injury in the pretransplantation or posttransplantation population, caution must be used when overloading a muscle or muscle group.[4a]

including blood pressure, heart rate, oxygen saturation, respiratory rate, and rate pressure products (heart rate and systolic blood pressure), can provide valuable information and can be used as measurable outcomes of treatment intervention.

In general, as the intensity of activity increases, the heart rate and systolic blood pressure increase, with a concomitant return to baseline with cessation of activity (see Appendix B). The response the transplant recipient has to exercise will depend on the type of transplant, medications taken, and present level of fitness. For example, heart transplant recipients typically have a blunted heart rate response with exercise as a result of the denervated state of the heart.

Monitoring the recovery may be an objective measure of improvement in physical capacity. Consistent abnormal responses should be reported to the physician for further evaluation. Other considerations are determined according to the underlying pathologic condition (e.g., cardiomyopathy, congestive heart failure, renal failure, diabetes, cirrhosis) and pretransplantation treatment (e.g., VADs, medications, dialysis). See the "Special Implications for the Therapist" features for each specific diagnosis in this chapter.

For all transplant candidates and recipients, the duration of beginning aerobic exercise should be until fatigue begins; allow for a short recovery period and repeat in an interval manner until the duration is at least 20 minutes of continuous exercise. The goal is to perform at least 30 minutes of nonstop activity daily at a moderate exertional level before reducing exercise frequency to four to five times weekly. Individuals trying to control blood pressure or lose weight should work for a longer duration, 45 to 60 minutes, at a lower intensity (e.g., 50%-65% of predicted maximal heart rate).[144] The exercise program should consider the recipient's comorbidities and be individualized to the needs and goals of the transplant recipient.[71,226]

Limitations on Activity and Exercise

Transplant trauma is a theoretic possibility, so organ recipients are advised not to participate in contact sports. Except for this general broad precaution, limitations on sporting and exercise must be evaluated on a case-by-case basis and may be determined by the course of the illness. For example, the person who undergoes emergency liver transplantation for acute liver failure will have relatively little secondary damage. Therefore, vigorous exercise training for competition is not contraindicated for healthy transplant recipients. However, cardiorespiratory fitness and strength training should progress gradually before the client engages in more strenuous sports participation.

On the other hand, someone with chronic renal failure can develop renal osteodystrophy (see Fig. 18-7 and the section on chronic renal failure in Chapter 18), decreased bone density, osteoporosis, reduced peak cardiac output (because of the arteriovenous fistula required for vascular access), and irreversible neuropathies and myopathies. Anyone experiencing renal failure secondary to diabetes will have multiple other secondary complications (see "Diabetes" in Chapter 11).

Many other potential limitations on sporting and exercise must be recognized and evaluated, such as the condition of the recipient at the time of transplantation and the type of organ that has failed. For example, people with severe pulmonary disease necessitating heart-lung transplantation often experience malnutrition and muscle wasting before transplantation. Liver failure can cause abnormalities of lung function, including ventilation–perfusion mismatching, pulmonary hypertension, and loss of oxygen-diffusing capacity.

Denervation

Denervation of the transplanted heart, pancreas, liver, or kidneys results in a loss of sympathetic nerves to the organ (e.g., loss of vagal response in the heart, impaired insulin in the pancreas, and altered renin responses in the kidney) requiring some modifications in the exercise program. In contrast, surgical removal of sympathetic liver nerves does not inhibit hepatic glucose production during exercise, and denervation of the lungs does not impair the ability to increase ventilation during physical exertion.[226]

The denervated lung will experience reduced tidal volumes and decreased lung compliance. There is a delay in the bronchodilation response requiring an extended warm-up period in order to obtain the catecholamine response necessary for organ vasodilation and, thereby, increased tidal volume during exercise.[61,83]

There is evidence that reinnervation does occur to some extent for some recipients. For heart transplant recipients who have some degree of autonomic nervous system function restored, there is an increase in heart rate greater than 35 beats/min with peak exercise levels and also an immediate decrease in heart rate after exercise. This restoration results in an increase in exercise capacity that is closer to healthy age-matched control subjects.[333] Without a balance in parasympathetic–sympathetic responses, heart rate variability during and after exercise is impaired. In the absence of parasympathetic activity, an increase in blood pressure may occur during exercise. For the individual who does not experience parasympathetic recovery, exercises should be performed under supervision with close monitoring of pulse and blood pressure (and possibly electrocardiogram) during the first several exercise sessions. Arrhythmias during the acute recovery period may be an early sign of rejection.[309]

Medications

Besides the usual exercise-related risks anyone faces, recipients have additional medication-related risks associated with the long-term immunosuppressive therapy, including exaggerated hypertensive response, myopathies, neuropathies, osteoporosis, and fractures.

The adverse effects of the immunosuppressive medications on skeletal muscle, including the muscle-wasting effects of glucocorticoids, are well-known. It is documented that quadriceps strength of renal transplant candidates is only 70% of normal, although this side effect can be counteracted by resistance exercise training.[195,196,333] Also documented are decreased type 1 muscle fibers, decreased capillary density as a result of calcineurin-inhibitor medications[270] Other potential side effects[339] are listed in Tables 5-3 and 5-4; see also "Immunosuppression" under "Posttransplantation Complications" above.

Chronic Rejection

Finally, transplanted organs may be exposed to chronic rejection, limiting the function of the organ. With the decline in organ function, there is a decrease in exercise tolerance. For example, in heart transplant recipients, chronic rejection is associated with a decrease in cardiac output, onset of heart failure, and accelerated atherosclerosis.[416]

With lung transplantation, the recipient suffering from chronic rejection may present with an impairment in gas exchange, leading to desaturation and increased air trapping and work of breathing. However, despite all these variables, the benefits of exercise in maintaining a healthy lifestyle and sense of well-being are much greater than the risks (e.g., rejection, respiratory impairments) imposed by organ transplantation. Exercise should be reduced in duration and intensity but not necessarily discontinued during rejection episodes.[315]

Psychosocial Factors

Although it is assumed that transplant recipients will spontaneously increase their physical activity after transplantation, fear of harming the new organ or protective family members may discourage vigorous activity. As a member of the transplantation team, the therapist should encourage a program of regular activity immediately after transplantation and provide exercise guidelines (specifically aerobic, resistive, and core exercise) as a part of the long-term transplantation care plan.

Education

Education regarding the need for lifelong exercise to improve endurance, strength, and function specifically to counteract the deleterious effects of the immunosuppression regimen is essential to motivate the transplant recipient to succeed. It is recommended that the recipient be referred for supervised outpatient services because many studies have documented an increase in recovery with supervised exercise as opposed to a home exercise program.[386]

HEMATOPOIETIC CELL TRANSPLANTATION

HSCs is the abbreviation used to refer to hematopoietic stem cells. Several excellent sources for more information are suggested: Harvard Stem Cell Institute (HSCI) www.hsci.harvard.edu, Center for International Blood and Marrow Transplant Research (CIBMTR) www.cibmtr.org, and Be the Match, from the National Marrow Donor Program (http://bethematch.org/).

> **Note to Reader:** Hematopoietic cell transplantation (HCT) is the preferred term but you may still see this referred to as hematopoietic stem cell transplantation (HSCT). HSCs is the abbreviation used to refer to hematopoietic stem cells. Several excellent sources for more information are suggested: Harvard Stem Cell Institute (HSCI) www.hsci.harvard.edu, Center for International Blood and Marrow Transplant Research (CIBMTR) www.cibmtr.org, and Be the Match, from the National Marrow Donor Program (http://bethematch.org/).

Definition and Overview

The purpose of this section is to introduce the physical therapist to the process of hematopoietic cell transplantation (HCT) and the adverse outcomes that can accompany this procedure. Hematopoiesis is the process by which all mature, functioning blood cells develop. Central to this process are HSCs, which are undifferentiated cells that reside primarily in the bone marrow. HSCs are unique in that they are self-renewing and, in response to appropriate signals, able to differentiate into all types of mature, functional blood cells (Fig. 21-6). That is, the differentiation of HSCs gives rise to all approximately 10^{11} to 10^{12} new blood cells that are produced daily across all cell lineages.

Efforts to therapeutically replace or transplant the contents of the bone marrow and specifically provide new hematopoietic cells have been ongoing for more than a century. Early in the 20th century people with blood diseases were given bone marrow cells orally. Perhaps a more realistic starting point for hematopoietic stem cell transplantation (HCT) is a 1959 report of a person who received 18 mL of intravenous marrow from his brother as a treatment for aplastic anemia.

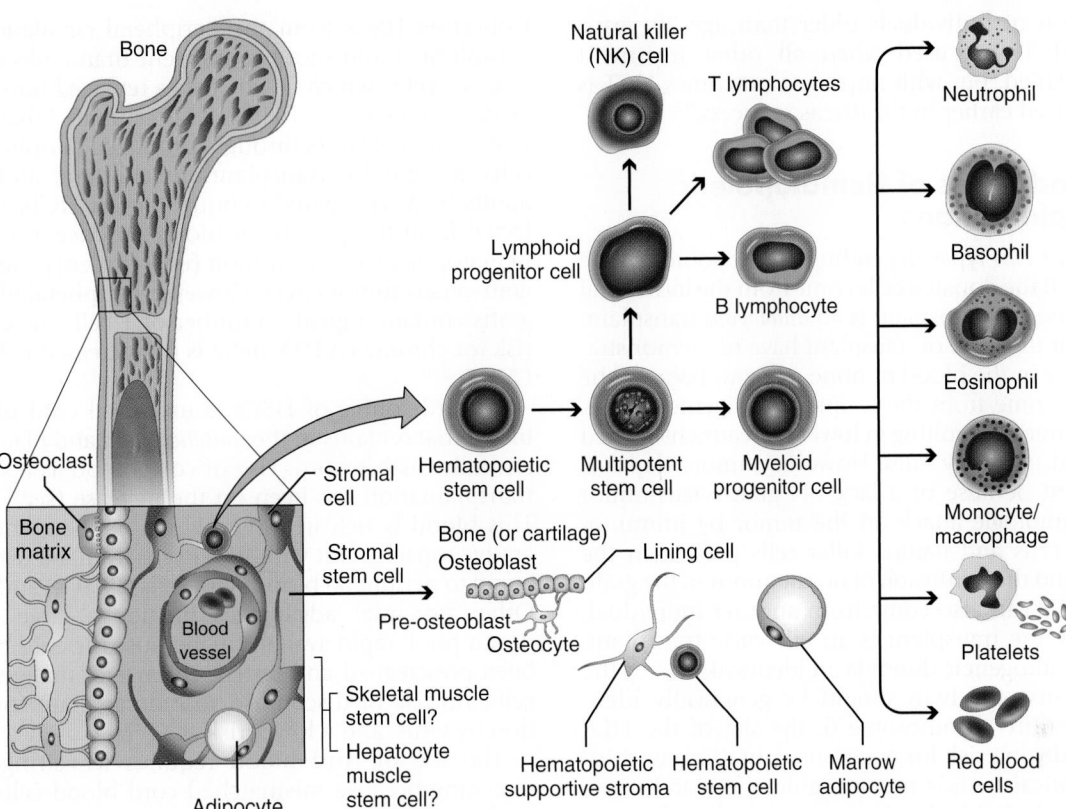

Figure 21-6

Adult stem cells. Adult stem cells can be multipotent and have the capacity to differentiate into a limited number of different cell types, often restricted to a given tissue or organ system, as in the case of adult hematopoietic or epidermal stem cells. Two stem cell types have been isolated from adult bone marrow—the hematopoietic stem cell and the mesenchymal stem cell. Adult mesenchymal stem cells of bone marrow origin, although their range of differentiation has been shown to be broader than that of any other adult stem cell type, do not reach pluripotency (able to develop into different cells). It is thought that in some organ systems, such as the gastrointestinal epithelium, a unipotent pool of progenitors exists for repopulating a rapid population turnover of only one type of cell—although it is difficult to be certain whether such progenitors can be distinguished from the overall population of fully differentiated cells in tissues with high cellular turnover. (From Goldman L, Schafer AI: *Goldman's Cecil medicine*, ed 24, Philadelphia, WB Saunders, 2012. Used with permission).

In the mid-1950s bone marrow was unsuccessfully transfused into several nuclear workers who had received excessive radiation exposure. In 1959, it was reported that an individual with end-stage leukemia survived for 3 months after first receiving a lethal dose of radiation followed by an infusion of bone marrow collected from the patient's identical twin.[398]

These early efforts at HCT failed because little was known about tissue rejection and immune suppression. The identification of and ability to type the major histocompatibility complex or HLA system in humans in the early 1960s made it possible to match donor with recipient, thus reducing graft rejection. This advance combined with the discovery of immune suppression compounds such as cyclosporine reduced tissue rejection and brought about the modern era of HCT.[97]

Today, HCT is widely used to treat a number of blood diseases. Worldwide, approximately 30,000 to 40,000 HCTs are performed annually, and the number continues to increase each year with 5-year survival rates exceeding 50% depending on the disease, age of the recipient, and source of donor material. There has been a dramatic increase of recipients older than 50 years in the last decade.[298]

Diseases Treated by Hematopoietic Cell Transplantation

A variety of hematologic cancers are treated by HCT including multiple myeloma, non-Hodgkin lymphoma, Hodgkin disease, acute and chronic myeloid leukemia, acute and chronic lymphocytic leukemia, and myelodysplastic syndromes. Multiple myeloma and lymphoma account for approximately 60% of all HCTs. Multiple myeloma continues to be the most common indication for autologous transplantation and acute myeloid leukemia for allogeneic transplantation.[320]

Noncancer blood diseases, including aplastic anemia, sickle cell anemia, severe combined immune deficiency, and thalassemia, may also be treated with HCT. Solid tumors, including medulloblastomas and germ cell tumors, have been treated with HCT. Age was once a limiting factor for receiving an HCT, but the introduction of less myeloablative induction regimens has allowed the transplantation of individuals older than age 70 years. Previously, HCT was used when all other treatment options had failed, but with improved outcomes HCT is increasingly used earlier in the disease process.[97]

Sources and Types of Hematopoietic Cell Transplantations

HCTs can be of two types depending on the source of the donated cells. If the donated cells come from the individual with the disease, the transplant is an *autologous* transplant. Candidates for this type of transplant have no demonstrable malignancy in the blood or bone marrow. Because the donated cells come from the recipient, antigenic incompatibility is reduced, resulting in lowered treatment-related morbidity and mortality rates. However, tumor relapse is more prevalent because of a lack of "graft-versus-tumor effect" (immunologic attack on the tumor by immunocompetent T cells and natural killer cells present in the donor graft) and the reinfusion of occult tumor in the graft.

Donor HCTs can also come from another individual, in which case the transplant is an *allogeneic* transplant. Preferably, an allogeneic donor is an identical twin of the recipient because the twin should be genetically identical for the entire chromosome 6, the site of the HLA genes thus reducing risk for posttransplantation morbidity. If an identical twin is not available, the search for a donor turns to individuals who are genetically related to the recipient—usually a sibling. While not perfect, such matched, related donors increase the likelihood of an optimal HLA match.

If no related donors are available, the search turns to a matched *unrelated donor*. Such donors are found through bone marrow registries. An optimal HLA match between the donor and recipient drives donor selection so as to reduce the risk of posttransplantation morbidities, including GVHD (see discussion under "Transplantation of Hematopoietic Stem Cells" below). The choice of performing a transplant using donor cells from an unrelated donor is generally determined by the urgency of the transplant.[97,163]

HSCs are collected from three different sites including the bone marrow, peripheral blood and umbilical cord blood (Fig. 21-7). In the past, HSCs collected from *bone marrow* aspirates have served as the traditional source of HCTs; today, this is no longer the primary source of HSCs, now accounting for only approximately 20% of HCTs.[299]

These cells are collected from the bone marrow of the donor's superior iliac crest and require the donor to be anesthetized; a needle is inserted into the bone marrow to collect its contents. Adverse effects are generally rare and include discomfort at the harvesting site that typically lasts 1 to 2 weeks. Priming the bone marrow with granulocyte colony-stimulating factor increases the production of HSCs into the blood, reducing the required number of aspirations. Infrequently, additional collection of marrow is required for graft failure, but this is the exception not the rule.

A second (and now primary) source of HCTs comes from those that circulate in the *peripheral blood*. Normally these cells are present in the blood in low numbers. Priming the bone marrow with granulocyte colony-stimulating factor increases their number in the circulating blood.

Collecting HSCs from the peripheral circulation is less complicated and more convenient than collecting bone marrow cells, which is why it has replaced bone marrow as the main source of HSCs. It is estimated that approximately 91% of HCTs through mobilized peripheral blood cells account for transplants in children, and 98% in adults.[320] As compared to bone marrow HCTs, those collected from the peripheral blood produce a more rapid hematopoietic reconstitution (engraftment) and a greater graft-versus-tumor effect. However, peripheral blood HSC grafts contain a greater number of T cells increasing the risk for chronic GVHD; there is no increased risk of acute GVHD.[299]

A third source of HSCs is umbilical cord blood, the blood that remains in the *umbilical cord* and placenta after an individual is born. Use of cord blood as a source for transplantation has been on the increase (see Fig. 21-7). This blood is rich in HSCs, which have superior proliferative capacity, but with fewer cells available when compared to peripheral blood stem cells (PBSCs) and marrow. Other potential advantages include a large potential donor pool, rapid availability because the cord blood has been prescreened and tested, absence of malignant stem cells, no risk or discomfort to a donor, rare contamination by virus, and a lower risk of GVHD.

The use of cord blood requires less-stringent HLA matching because mismatched cord blood cells are less likely to cause GVHD. Unfortunately, cord blood occurs in only small volumes, limiting the numbers HSCs that can be collected from individual donors. In addition, hematopoietic reconstitution is slower when cord

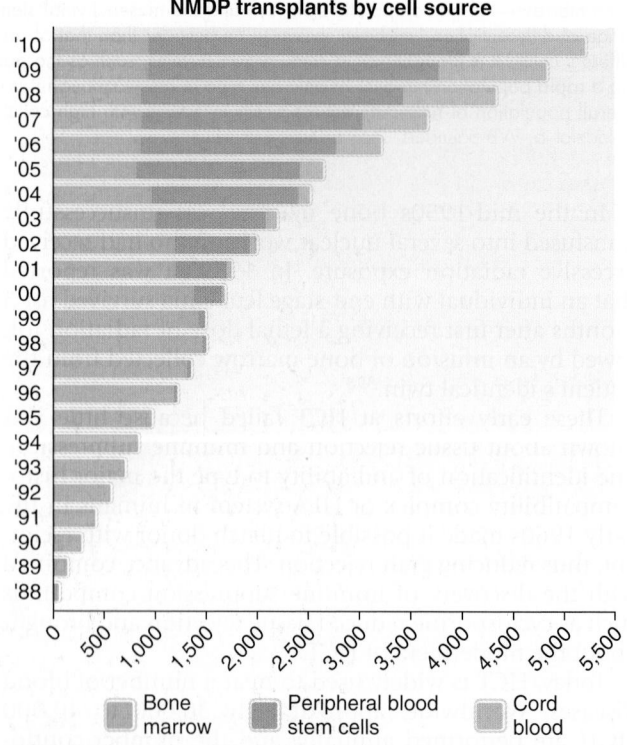

Figure 21-7

National Marrow Donor Program transplants by cell source, 2014. (Courtesy of the National Marrow Donor Program. Used with permission.)

blood is used, increasing the risk for posttransplantation infection.[97,163]

Transplantation of Hematopoietic Stem Cells

The transplantation of HSCs consists of several phases including conditioning, harvest, infusion, preengraftment and engraftment. *Conditioning* is a critical element in the HCT process. The primary purpose of the conditioning regimen is to render the recipient sufficiently immune suppressed to prevent rejection of the graft and to eradicate any remaining malignant cells. Myeloablative conditioning is achieved by delivering maximally tolerated dose of multiple chemotherapeutic agents with nonoverlapping toxicities, with or without radiation. This regimen is undertaken 7 to 10 days prior to transplantation, causes myelosuppression (myeloablative regimens), and has a number of potential adverse effects including mucositis, nausea, vomiting, alopecia, diarrhea, rash, peripheral neuropathies, and pulmonary and hepatic toxicity.

Nonmyeloablative preparative regimens are used in individuals with less aggressive tumors. These regimens use substantially lower doses of chemotherapy drugs and radiation than myeloablative regimens. These regimens are immunosuppressive but not myeloablative and rely on a graft-versus-tumor effect to kill tumor cells with donor T lymphocytes. They result in fewer adverse effects and are frequently used in individuals age 55 years or older, and in people with notable comorbidities. All conditioning regimens result in some myelosuppression, which continues after completion of the preparative regimen. The nadir or low point in cell numbers or blood values typically occurs 5 to 7 days posttransplant.

Harvesting involves the collection of HSCs and has been previously discussed. *Infusion* of the harvested cells is a relatively simple process that is performed at the bedside. HSCs are infused through a central vein over a period of several hours. The transplanted cells migrate to the bone marrow cavities by mechanisms that have not yet been fully elucidated. Once in the bone marrow, the goal is for the HSCs to begin repopulating the marrow with cells that will differentiate and mature into fully functioning blood cells.

The *preengraftment* period is the period when the transplanted cells migrate to the bone marrow and begin to populate this area. During this period the recipients face continued adverse effects of the induction strategies as white and red blood cell and platelet counts drop to their lowest value. With decline in circulating blood cell numbers, clinical manifestations can include nausea, vomiting, and hair loss, particularly if the individual has received ablative conditioning (side effects are not as likely for individuals receiving a reduced-intensity regimen).

During preengraftment, the recipient remains particularly vulnerable to infection. In fact, infection remains the primary cause of posttransplant, nonrelapse mortality. To help combat infection, some facilities keep patients in isolation rooms during this period, whereas others restrict these individuals to their units. All recipients receive antibacterial, antifungal, and antiviral prophylaxis during this period, as well as immune-suppression drugs such as tacrolimus. It is worth noting that these individuals have venous access devices in place, which further increases the risk for infection, thus requiring careful antisepsis on the part of all health care providers.

As the stem cells repopulate the bone marrow, hematopoiesis progressively improves and circulating levels of blood cells increase. When cell numbers reach specific threshold levels, *engraftment* is said to have occurred. The duration of time required for engraftment varies, but is generally 9 to 14 days from infusion (day 0) for PBSC, 12 to 18 days for marrow, and 25 to 56 days for cord blood transplants. Specifically, neutrophil engraftment has occurred in allogeneic transplant recipients when an absolute neutrophil count exceeds $1500/mm^3$ for 48 hours (normal values are 3000-$7000/mm^3$). This may take 3 to 4 weeks, but if complications occur (e.g., GVHD, infection, slow engraftment) the recipient may be hospitalized for months. A platelet count of 20,000 to 50,000 $cells/mm^3$ is a mark of platelet engraftment.

These measures suggest that the recipient now has some minimal inherent protection against infection and abnormal bleeding. Infection control prophylaxis and immune suppression continues after engraftment has occurred. At this point, recipients may be discharged from the hospital but at most transplantation centers, they are asked to remain within 1 to 2 hours distance from the hospital until they are approximately 100 days posttransplantation. During this outpatient period, they are carefully monitored and treated for abnormal blood counts, infection, and symptom control.[163]

Complications of Hematopoietic Cell Transplantation

Advances in transplantation techniques and supportive care strategies have resulted in significant improvement in survival for those who have undergone treatment. Subsequently, HCT survivors are at risk of developing a range of long-term complications. Two-thirds of HCT survivors develop at least one chronic health condition and one-fifth develop severe or life-threatening conditions. HCT recipients who have survived for at least 5 years posttransplantation are at a fourfold to ninefold increased risk of late mortality for as long as 30 years from HCT, producing an estimated 30% lower life expectancy compared with the general population.[45]

Some people entering transplantation may already have significant multisystem damage, including cardiopulmonary, nutritional, musculoskeletal, and neurologic impairments secondary to either the underlying disease or its treatment. Bone metastasis, steroid myopathy, polyneuropathies, depleted protein stores, and impaired skin integrity are common comorbidities present before HCT transplantation (Box 21-4). Virtually all HCT recipients rapidly lose all T and B lymphocytes during and after conditioning, losing immune memory accumulated through lifetime exposure to infectious agents, environmental antigens, and vaccines.

Although not very common, neurologic complications occur in accordance with the stage of HCT. For example, during conditioning, drug-related encephalopathies and seizures or complications secondary to medical

COMPLICATIONS ASSOCIATED WITH HEMATOPOIETIC CELL TRANSPLANTATION

Pretransplantation

- Effects of immune suppression (see Table 5-4)
  - Steroid myopathies, neuropathies
  - Immobility
  - Weakness
  - Renal failure
- Effects of chemotherapy and radiation therapy (see Tables 5-8 and 5-9)
  - Cognitive impairment
  - Neurologic impairment
  - Neutropenia
  - Thrombocytopenia
  - Hemorrhage
  - Anemia
  - Cardiopulmonary toxicity
    - Arrhythmias
    - Cardiomyopathy
    - Interstitial pneumonitis
    - Obstructive or restrictive disease
  - Nutritional deficits
  - Bone metastasis
  - Impaired skin integrity

Posttransplantation

- Infection
- Graft-versus-host disease (see Box 21-5)
- Recurrence of malignancy
- Sterility
- Cystitis
- Venoocclusive liver disease
- Fatigue
- Hearing loss (ototoxic antibiotics)
- Delayed effects of radiation
  - Visual loss (cataract formation)

procedures are possible. During bone marrow depletion, metabolic and drug-related encephalopathies and seizures, septic cerebral infarctions, and hemorrhages may occur. The risk of neurologic complications is modest with myeloablative regimens and minimal with nonmyeloablative regimens.

Chronic immunosuppression results in infections by viruses and opportunistic organisms, and late events such as central nervous system relapses of the original disease, neurologic complications of GVHD, and second primary malignancies.[234,378] Recurrence of malignancy is always a possibility. The frequency and type of neurologic complication depends on the type of HCT and the underlying disease.[355] Therapists should pay attention to altered level of consciousness, headaches, motor or sensory deficits, visual disturbances, involuntary movements, cranial nerve palsies, or seizures as these are clinical significant and may be a sign of neurologic complications.[228]

HCT recipients may be at an increased risk of developing hypertension, diabetes, congestive heart failure,[20] and dyslipidemia (referred to as cardiovascular risk factors); and these can potentially increase the risk of cardiovascular disease.[19] Recipients of allogenic transplants are more likely to report diabetes and hypertension than

control siblings, and are more likely to report hypertension than autologous recipients.[26] Cardiac or pulmonary toxicity also may occur as a result of the irradiation and immunosuppressive drugs used to prepare candidates for the transplantation. Arrhythmias may be the first sign that a chemotherapeutic agent is becoming cardiotoxic. Interstitial pneumonitis, an inflammation of the lungs, is a common complication, especially among allogeneic transplantations, which leaves the person susceptible to obstructive small airway disease.

Infections and hemorrhagic complications during the period of bone marrow aplasia, emerging immune competence, and GVHD are the most life-threatening complications following HCT, and they may be fatal. Infections include early bacterial infections or later opportunistic infections, especially CMV interstitial lung disease. EBV-associated lymphoproliferative disorders (posttransplantation lymphoproliferative disorders) are a significant problem after stem cell transplantation from unrelated donors or mismatched family members.[186]

Other long-term complications of HCT include sterility/infertility, osteoporosis, cystitis, thyroid problems, cataract formation, cardiomyopathy, and venoocclusive liver disease. Neuromuscular changes, such as peripheral neuropathies, muscle cramping, and steroid myopathies, may also develop.[97,163] A condition known as *posttransplant distal limb syndrome* has been reported with constant bilateral pain, bone marrow edema, and soft-tissue swelling in the lower legs and ankles.[369] Decreased bone mineral density, such as osteopenia, has been identified in childhood survivors of BMT, which places them at higher risk for fracture or osteoporosis.[352]

The complications of peripheral blood stem cell transplantation (PBSCT) are essentially the same as those of BMT, but hematologic recovery after PBSCT is much more rapid (typically 11 to 14 days, and as early as 9 days), thereby significantly shortening the period of postchemotherapy neutropenia (decreased neutrophils, a type of granular leukocyte used to fight infection) and thrombocytopenia (decreased platelets in peripheral blood). Faster engraftment makes PBSCT a preferred procedure over BMT. However, there is no difference in overall survival between marrow and PBSC as stem cell sources.[16]

Long-term psychologic effects of HCT on survivors are being reported as more information becomes available from studies conducted over a period of 10 or more years. Adverse psychologic outcomes reported include anxiety, depression, somatic distress, and thoughts of suicide.[393]

Prognosis

Enormous progress has been made in understanding the biology, therapy, and prophylaxis strategies of transplantation and in extending the range of potential stem cell donors to include unrelated people. Dramatic advances have occurred in the prevention of serious infection, including CMV infection, formerly a significant cause of mortality.

One-hundred-day mortality, defined as death before 100 days after transplant, is often used as a gauge of procedure-related toxicity. Relapse can occur in stem cell recipients as a result of the growth of residual cancer cells (e.g., leukemia) not killed by chemotherapy or radiation. Allogeneic transplants are associated with relatively high risks of GVHD, failure of engraftment, infections, and liver toxicity, resulting in high early mortality. Long-term survival rates are improved with HCT (compared with no HCT), but this type of transplantation does not confer a normal life span.[379,397]

Unfortunately, posttransplant toxicities with myeloablative regimens (not the case with reduced-intensity HCT), remain a major limitation to successful application of the procedure. Primary disease recurrence continues to account for the majority of deaths in autologous transplant recipients. New cancer, organ failure, and suicide are also cited as causes of death among long-term survivors after HCT. The incidence of suicide is infrequent but still higher among such survivors than among healthy subjects.[282,351]

Despite substantial morbidity and mortality after HCT in some cases, recipients who survive long term are likely to enjoy good health. For those who survive more than 5 years after HCT, 93% are in good health and 89% return to work or school full time. Eighty-eight percent of those who survive 10 years after HCT report that the benefits of transplantation outweigh the side effects.[82]

Although the success rates of transplantation have been improving over time, the prognosis still depends on the underlying disease, delays in transplantation, associated risk of relapse (e.g., leukemia) and current remission state, the development of acute GVHD based on the level of match between donor and recipient, and the age of the recipient. There is no effective therapy for severe acute GVHD, and people stricken with it rarely recover.

With understanding of the many issues facing the individual receiving an HCT, one may wonder why anyone would agree to undergo such a challenging treatment. It may be helpful to remember that most people facing an HCT expect either certain death or a high probability of death without it. This perspective may help health care professionals working with these individuals to understand why the procedure is performed.

SPECIAL IMPLICATIONS FOR THE THERAPIST   21-2

Hematopoietic Cell Transplantation

The therapist's subjective evaluation must include past medical and social history to assess other medical conditions, relevant past surgeries, living situation, and prior level of function/exercise/activities.

The recipient's goal(s) for therapy must be directly inquired and therapy aimed toward that goal if appropriate. Objective data may include assessment of strength, skin condition, general cognition, neuropathy and/or myopathy involvement, functional range of motion, and analysis of transfers, gait, and balance. The rate of perceived exertion (RPE) scale, oxygen saturation level, heart rate, and blood pressure in relation to activity level are also helpful tools to assess ability to function outside the hospital environment. Remember that each specific medical treatment regimen is associated with its own comorbidities.

The combination of these factors puts the person at risk for immobility and subsequent pneumonia, pressure ulcers, muscle weakness, and overall deconditioning. It

is important to remember that autologous transplant recipients may receive treatment as outpatients, but allogenic recipients may be hospitalized for 1 month or even considerably more, if complications occur.

Skin inspection and skin care are of primary importance to prevent pressure or shear injuries. Any skin opening is an invitation to an opportunistic infection. The therapist must evaluate the need for appropriate footwear, turning schedules, specialized mattress surfaces, and chair or wheelchair cushions. The client must be instructed in self-inspection, especially when splinting is used to treat neuropathic weakness and proprioceptive loss.

In addition, long-term side effects of chemotherapy include peripheral neuropathy, and the prolonged use of steroids can induce steroid myopathy and osteoporosis. Any of these conditions places the individual at risk for falls and associated injuries.

A THERAPIST'S THOUGHTS*

Falls Prevention

During transplant induction and in the acute posttransplantation phase, recipients must be encouraged to remain mobile and maintain activities of daily living despite the many unpleasant symptoms present. The loss of white blood cells exposes the individual to infection, while the depletion of red blood cells reduces energy, resulting in profound fatigue and increasing the risk for falls. Oral mucositis is a painful condition that may be present as a consequence of chemotherapy, and may make eating, and therefore available energy, deficient.

The increased risk of injury from falling with low platelet counts (e.g., subdural hemorrhage) makes activity and balance training and assessment during hospitalization increasingly critical as well. Cognitive impairment, including that due to medications such as pain medications and/or sedatives, also increases the risk of falls for these individuals.

At our facility, all our HCT patients are automatically on falls precautions. We are constantly working on trying to reduce falls with our patients. There seems to be a greater risk of falls at night with toileting, whether with bed-to-commode transfers or even use of a urinal at the edge of the bed.

*Eva Gold, PT

Exercise During and After Hematopoietic Cell Transplantation

Note to Reader: Although we report on results of studies examining the effects of physical activity and exercise on recipients during and after hematopoietic cell transplantation, these studies are not all equal. Some studies specifically evaluate people receiving bone marrow transplantation, whereas others focus on the broader hematopoietic cell transplantation (which includes peripheral blood, cord blood, and bone marrow). Comparing outcomes from these various studies is a bit like comparing apples to oranges if different sources of hematopoietic cells are used in the transplantation process. So we encourage you to continue your own literature research and review based on the treatment your patients are receiving and modify your programs accordingly as new evidence presents itself.

Very early involvement of the physical therapist in designing an individualized and structured self-directed exercise program for recipients is of great benefit to their well-being and sense of control. There is also evidence that aerobic exercise can be safely carried out immediately after HCT and can partially prevent loss of physical performance,[124] depending on the medical and physical condition both before transplantation and after transplantation and chemotherapy. See also "Organ Transplantation and Exercise, Activity, and Sports" above.

Exercise capacity in BMT recipients is much lower when transplantation is preceded by cardiotoxic chemotherapy or irradiation. Reduced exercise endurance, reduced maximal oxygen consumption, reduced rise in cardiac output during exercise, and reduced ventilatory anaerobic threshold are closely related to the potential effects of chemotherapy.[210]

Extremely abnormal responses require consultation with the physician before therapy is initiated or continued. These clients may need continuous monitoring over many therapy sessions rather than just using symptoms as a guide to exercise tolerance once a baseline is established.

Training studies of candidates before HCT to evaluate the impact of inactivity have not been performed. However, it has been demonstrated in individuals who have undergone BMT that a treadmill walking program started 18 to 42 days after transplantation results in significant improvement in maximal physical performance, walking distance, and lowered heart rate at a given workload.[128] Active exercise, muscle stretching, and treadmill walking have been shown to increase muscle strength after allogeneic BMT.[275]

Exercise in the form of 3 days/week aerobic exercise (20-40 minutes) plus 2 days/week of resistance training (bands or weights) performed 1 to 4 weeks prior to, during, and after transplantation, can also help improve cancer-related fatigue, physical capacity, overall physical function, anger/hostility, pain, and global distress.[181,432] In addition, the EXIST (Exercise Intervention after Stem Cell Transplant) Study is currently being performed to further evaluate the benefit and cost-effectiveness of a high-intensity strength and interval training program.[325]

Aerobic exercise improves the physical performance of peripheral stem cell recipients who have undergone high-dose chemotherapy. To reduce fatigue, this group of individuals should be counseled to increase physical activity rather than rest after treatment.[73] The therapist should be aware of potential side effects of cytokine growth factors used to mobilize peripheral stem cells including bone pain, myalgias, and flulike symptoms; some people may develop a low-grade fever.[294]

Pulmonary conditioning with inspiratory muscle training, muscular strengthening, and endurance exercises is important to help maintain mobility but must be balanced with pacing, prioritizing, and other energy conservation techniques (see Box 9-4) as an important part of treatment.

Range of motion, supervised or assisted ambulation, and resistive or endurance exercises can be utilized. Active assisted and passive range of motion is sometimes required for joint disuse and stiffness. Resistive exercises in the form of functional activities such as bridging, transfers, and walking are individually prescribed.[99] Resistance training may also help offset the decreased bone mineral density observed in childhood survivors of BMT by increasing fat-free mass and decreasing the fat mass index (kg of fat mass/height [m^2]).[352]

Interval activity training (see Appendix B) combined with energy-conservation techniques is an important component of therapy because the client's blood counts drop (including hemoglobin count, resulting in anemia), thereby reducing the body's capacity for exertion or aerobic activity.

Decreased platelet counts increase the person's susceptibility to bleeding from minor injuries. The amount of resistance and the use of equipment to provide resistance depend on platelet count. The therapist must monitor blood values to avoid causing joint hemorrhage (see Tables 40-8 and 40-9). Safety education is important, and assistive devices may be needed.

A THERAPIST'S THOUGHTS*

Physical Activity, Exercise, and Hematopoietic Cell Transplantation

From Eva Gold, PT

The discussion of "exercise" is often a challenge with these individuals. To most of them, it doesn't make sense to "exercise" when they are sicker than they ever have been and are fighting for their life! So at our hospital we refer to "activity" whenever possible, and we do as much activity as possible with all our HCT recipients, even though many are on experimental protocols and profoundly ill.

Our program ranges from supine exercises to treadmill and stationary biking (sometimes at very slow pace but often following Frank Dimeo's interval idea (http://frankdimeofitnesss.blogspot.com/2013/03/how-to-do-interval-training.html) although trying to encourage our hospitalized patients to exercise for 30 continuous minutes is typically challenging and probably inappropriate). We use the Borg Rating of Perceived Exertion. We encourage our patients to work out in the rate of perceived exertion range of 11 (fairly light) to 13 (somewhat hard). With aerobic (treadmill, bike, or even walking in the halls) intervals, we'll encourage them to build up during the warm-up to 11, then push it toward 13, then back to 11, and up to 13—back and forth as tolerated. We've even had some lower-level patients walk on the treadmill, then sit in a chair on the stopped treadmill, then start up again.

The functional and energy levels vary so widely between our patients and even with the same patient over time that we need to be quite creative and adjust with each treatment. Some of our patients who were very active prior to diagnosis may have a treadmill or bike in their room and use it frequently! It is important to ensure that these patients do not overdo their workouts.

From Cyd Dashkoff, PT-CSLT

During the recipient's stay in a hospital setting, the physical therapy and occupational therapy staff attempt to keep recipients active. We teach them how to follow the daily blood counts, monitor their heart rate, and adjust activities accordingly. They are instructed not to allow their heart rate to get above a target heart rate determined by the formula: 220 – recipient's age × 60%.

*Eva Gold, PT, and Cyd Dashkoff, PT-CSLT

Infection

Myelosuppression as a result of specific chemotherapeutic agents or drug combinations is the number one factor that predisposes the person to infection (see Box 8-1). Until bone marrow function returns, the HCT recipient is extremely susceptible to life-threatening infection, which requires all staff to practice interventions to minimize or prevent infection, such as good handwashing technique. Some facilities require "surgical scrubbing" and mask when going into a recipient's room.

Preventing infections among HCT recipients is preferable to treating infections. Any therapist working with this population is advised to obtain the guidelines for preventing opportunistic infections among HCT recipients available from the Centers for Disease Control and Prevention.[401] See also Chapter 8.

Therapists and nursing staff must work closely together to prevent infection, recognize early signs of infection or rejection, and reinforce the educational program, which is complex and is often taught in a short time under less-than-ideal conditions. Very early on, therapists instruct recipients on deep breathing exercises, ventilatory strategies, airway clearance including effective coughing technique as important ways of minimizing infections.

Monitoring Vital Signs

Vital signs must be monitored before, during, and after exercise to assess each HCT recipient for an abnormal response. Monitoring responses over time during the recovery process can alert the therapist to any developing cardiopulmonary compromise. RPE and heart rate can also be used to monitor patients during exercise and activity with a goal of keeping the RPE between 11 (fairly light) and 13 (somewhat hard) on the 6 to 20 scale. This scale correlates with expected heart rates, so adding a zero behind the RPE gives the likely heart rate at that level of exertion in healthy individuals.

The concept of routine monitoring applies to anyone who is seemingly healthy after transplant and may also provide helpful information about when to advance an exercise program. Knowledge of past medical history and preexisting conditions that could affect physical conditioning is essential. Preexisting conditions in the presence of extended periods of inactivity can contribute to further physical deconditioning.

Normal changes in vital signs include an increased heart rate and increased systolic blood pressure proportional to the workload, with minimal change in diastolic blood pressure (no more than 10 mm Hg). Hypertension or the use of antihypertensive medications (or other medications) can alter the normal response of blood pressure to exercise. Recipients may be deconditioned with a less than normal (sluggish) blood pressure response (see Appendix B).

Monitoring Laboratory Values

In addition to monitoring vital signs, the therapist must be aware of daily laboratory values for red blood cells, white blood cells, and platelets. Each facility will have its own guidelines for activity and exercise based on blood counts. For example, in some facilities, absolute neutrophil count must be more than $500/mm^3$ on 3 consecutive days for allogeneic HCT recipients before ambulating in the hallway while wearing a high-efficiency particulate air (HEPA) filter mask. Individuals with platelets less than 10,000 cells/mm^3 may require transfusion before activity and exercise can be resumed or progressed. Resistive bands are used only if platelets are 20,000 cells/mm^3 or more. Exercise tolerance is not based on white blood cell count unless elevated due to infection, and accompanying fever and elevated heart rate.[165]

Often symptomatology is used as the primary measure of acceptable activity. Neutropenia precautions may be in effect limiting activity outside the individual's room and requiring an N-95 (respirator and dust) mask whenever leaving the room. Platelet levels must be evaluated (thrombocytopenia) before chest percussion is performed. See also "Radiation Injuries" and "Chemotherapy" in Chapter 5.

GRAFT-VERSUS-HOST DISEASE
Overview

The use of HCT in bone marrow–depleted or immunodeficient people has resulted in the complication of GVHD. GVHD remains a major obstacle in the curative potential of allogeneic HCT.

GVHD does not occur with organ transplantation. In organ transplantation, it is host-versus-graft disease when the recipient recognizes the transplanted organ as foreign and rejects it because the recipient has a competent immune system. In individuals who receive HCT, there is no longer a competent immune system; it is the infusion of immune-competent cells that begin to recognize the recipient as foreign. In other words, GVHD occurs when immunocompetent T lymphocytes in the grafted material (donated stem cells) recognize foreign antigens in the recipient (person receiving cells), thus initiating an

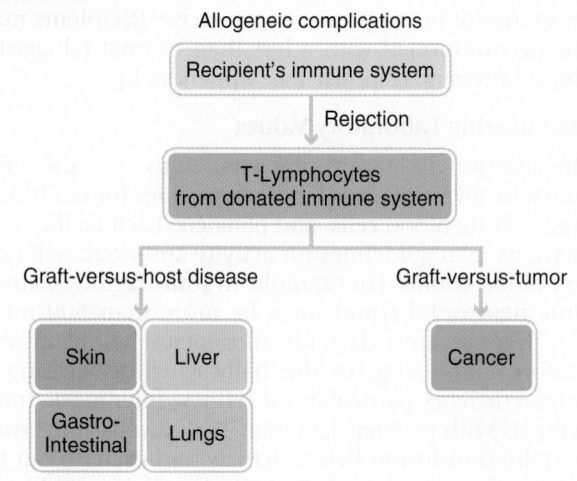

Allogeneic complications

Recipient's immune system

Rejection

T-Lymphocytes
from donated immune system

Graft-versus-host disease   Graft-versus-tumor

Skin   Liver   Cancer

Gastro-   Lungs
Intestinal

Figure 21-8

Several forces are at work inside a recipient's body when undergoing an allogeneic stem cell transplant. First, remnants of the recipient's own immune system may attack the donated immune system, which is called *rejection*. Factors that help prevent rejection include finding the best possible match, total-body irradiation, and chemotherapy conditioning. A second complication occurs when the donated immune system T cells attack the recipient's own body, which is defined as graft-versus-host disease. GVHD is not desirable in and of itself. However, if the donated immune system attacks the cancerous cells and destroys them, then there is less chance of relapse and better long-term survival; this is a desirable situation. This effect is called *graft-versus-tumor* (GVT). Researchers are looking for ways to promote the GVT effect without causing GVHD. (Courtesy Linda M. Tripp, PT, University of Minnesota Medical Center, Fairview–University Campus, Minneapolis, MN. Used with permission.)

immune response against the recipient's tissues and rejection of the host/recipient.

GVHD may be acute, typically occurring within the first 100 days after transplantation, or chronic, usually developing 3 to 6 months after transplantation.[86] Chronic GVHD is associated with a reduced risk of relapse, mediated by graft-versus-tumor effect (Fig. 21-8). Acute GVHD remains the most significant complication of the HCT process, with survival dependent on the response to therapy. To date, it has not been possible to dissociate detrimental chronic GVHD and beneficial graft versus disease effect.[30,35,101,433]

Risk Factors

Key risk factors for the development of GVHD include older age of donor or recipient, source of allogeneic stem cells (higher risk for chronic GVHD with PBSC than marrow, which is higher than cord blood), and degree of HLA disparity.[86] Donor/recipient sex mismatch increases the risk of GVHD; a female donor into a male recipient increases the risk over same-sex transplants.

Conditioning regimens containing total-body irradiation are associated with higher incidence and severity of GVHD compared with those involving only chemotherapy.[9] The disease state and the intensity of the conditioning regimen also influence the risk of developing GVHD. The fact that individuals prepared with low-dose conditioning regimens and transplanted with cells from HLA-identical siblings have an incidence of acute GVHD of 40% speaks to the biologic challenges of HCT.[35,101]

Clinical Manifestations

Acute Graft-Versus-Host Disease

Acute GVHD primarily involves the skin, with the liver and gastrointestinal tract being secondary sites. Diagnosis may be challenging and require tissue-based diagnosis because posttransplant infections, diarrhea, or other transplant-related toxicities could be the causative agent, rather than acute GVHD. Signs and symptoms of GVHD include fever, skin rash (first affecting the palms, soles of the feet, back of the neck and shoulders, but with eventual spread throughout the body possible), hepatitis, diarrhea, abdominal pain, ileus, vomiting, and weight loss. Ocular involvement may also occur.

If acute GVHD progresses, skin involvement may advance from 25% or less involvement of the integument to spread over the entire body. The skin rash may progress to skin blistering, desquamation, and erythema. The presence of a damaged integument increases the risk of infection with normal skin flora; for individuals with severe skin involvement, medical management resembles that used to care for severe burns.

Diagnosis of hepatic GVHD is graded primarily on serum bilirubin levels but in the absence of specific tests for liver involvement diagnosing hepatic GVHD may be questionable. Gastrointestinal GVHD may cause nausea, anorexia, pain and watery, secretory diarrhea. Endoscopy and mucosal biopsies are used to diagnosis gut GVHD. Fluid loss may be high in these patients making frequent monitoring of electrolytes and intake/output measurements essential.[35,101,433]

Low level (grades 1-2 acute GVHD) is not typically substantially quality-of-life impairing; what matters most is the rate of grades 3 to 4 acute GVHD, which carry with them a poorer prognosis.

Chronic Graft-Versus-Host Disease

Chronic GVHD affects upwards of 60% of recipients who survive 100 days beyond transplantation. Chronic GVHD presents similarly to an autoimmune disease. Common characteristics include scleroderma-like hardening of skin, muscle pain or weakness, and joint contractures that may severely decrease function.[321]

Gastrointestinal symptoms may include mucositis of the oral mucosa, progressing into the remainder of the gastrointestinal tract with esophageal narrowing and dysphagia, chronic diarrhea, and malabsorption. The patient may develop dyspnea and nonproductive cough (bronchiolitis obliterans). Hepatitis and cholestasis are also common symptoms (Box 21-5).

A generalized polyneuropathy coincident with the occurrence of GVHD has been reported. The neuropathy affects proximal and distal muscles and demonstrates hyporeflexia or areflexia. Electrophysiologic studies do not meet strict criteria for demyelination. The signs of neuropathy may improve after immunosuppressive treatment has been completed or simultaneously with the resolution of GVHD.

There is some evidence that individuals with cancer who undergo HCT are at risk for cognitive deficits. Cumulative clinical risk factors (e.g., length of hospital stay, history of cranial irradiation, intrathecal chemotherapy,

Box 21-5

SIGNS AND SYMPTOMS OF GRAFT-VERSUS-HOST DISEASE

Gastrointestinal

- Mucositis
- Esophageal inflammatory changes (esophageal narrowing, dysphagia)
- Abdominal cramping
- Nausea, vomiting
- Diarrhea, malabsorption
- Anorexia
- Ileus
- Hepatic injury (hepatitis, cholestasis)

Pulmonary

- Constrictive bronchiolitis (formerly bronchiolitis obliterans)
  - Wheezing
  - Rapid, shallow breathing
  - Nonproductive cough
  - Skin and soft-tissue retractions during respirations
  - Fever
  - Cyanosis
  - Dehydration
  - Respiratory failure
- Progressive dyspnea

Integument

- Hypopigmentation or hyperpigmentation of the skin
- Progressive maculopapular rash
- Sclerodermatous changes
- Pressure ulcer formation
- Alopecia
- Photosensitivity
- Keratoconjunctival sicca

Neuromusculoskeletal

- Generalized polyneuropathy
- Muscle wasting and weakness
- Distal joint pain and stiffness
- Joint contractures (chronic graft-versus-host disease)
- Changes in deep tendon reflexes (hyporeflexia or areflexia)
- Guillain-Barré syndrome (rare)
- Polymyositis (rare)

Other

- Hemorrhage
- Infection
- Vision changes (dry eyes, blurred or double vision)
- Severe headaches

allogeneic transplantation, unrelated donor, and post-HCT complications such as severity of mucositis and enteritis, GVHD) are more likely to demonstrate cognitive decline and less neuropsychologic recovery over time than recipients who have less risk. Individuals who have a complicated clinical course should be referred for evaluation and management of cognitive deficits.[213]

MEDICAL MANAGEMENT

PREVENTION AND TREATMENT. GVHD is a multisystem alloimmune disorder characterized by immune dysregulation, immunodeficiency, impaired organ function, and decreased survival. Virtually every organ and organ system in the body is adversely impacted by chronic GVHD, and management is focused largely on immune suppression therapies.[49]

Mitigating the risk of GVHD can be done by finding the best match possible for allogeneic cells, depleting T-lymphocytes in the donated stem cells, and using prophylactic immunosuppressives (e.g., cyclosporine or tacrolimus). Although antirejection drugs, such as tacrolimus and cyclosporine, are given prophylactically, some 40% to 90% of individuals receiving HCT still develop acute GVHD.[30,35,101,433] Untreated GVHD is often fatal as a result of hemorrhage and infection.

High-dose corticosteroids are the preferred treatment for acute GVHD. The dosages of steroids used to treat GVHD, as well as pulmonary hemorrhage and engraftment syndrome in patients post-HCT are significantly greater than those used in treating rejection in organ transplantation. Additionally, steroids have their own adverse effects (avascular necrosis, osteoporosis, steroid myopathy, diabetes, and glaucoma) further adding to the symptom burden of these patients.

Treatment with immunosuppressive therapy, including prednisone, cyclosporine, tacrolimus (Prograf), thalidomide, or a combination of these agents, has improved the long-term outlook for people with chronic GVHD. Even so, high-dose corticosteroids increase the risk of infection and myopathy and there is a high mortality rate. Chronic GVHD may resolve slowly (sometimes taking years) with gradual restoration of cell-mediated and humoral immunity function.

GVHD plays an important role on function and overall quality of life. Fatigue, dyspnea, gastrointestinal side effects, worries/anxieties, and skin problems can create severe impairments of quality of life in survivors of HCT suffering from GVHD. Taking into account that the prevalence of GVHD might be higher in patients after PBSCT compared with recipients after BMT, PBSCT may lead to more severe impairments of quality of life than BMT.[317,330]

FUTURE TRENDS. There are many other treatment strategies under investigation, such as donor lymphocyte infusion, tandem transplants, and the use of natural killer cells.

Donor lymphocyte infusion is an important therapeutic intervention for treating individuals who have relapsed or developed refractory disease following an allogeneic HCT. The procedure involves infusing peripheral lymphocytes collected from the original HCT donor with the goal of hastening or intensifying the graft-versus-disease (in the case of leukemia, graft-versus-leukemia) reaction.[293] Donor lymphocyte infusion has proven to be most effective against chronic myeloid leukemia but with some success against other leukemias, multiple myeloma, and lymphomas. Despite the utility of donor lymphocyte infusion, postinfusion development of GVHD remains a significant problem.[115]

Tandem transplants are used in clinical trials in an effort to increase survival in select individuals with multiple myeloma and other types of cancer. This process of tandem stem cell transplants involves receiving two autologous stem cell transplants weeks apart or an autologous transplant followed by reduced-intensity conditioning and an allogeneic stem cell transplant.[292,303]

Natural killer (NK) cells are components of the innate immune system, capable of recognizing targets without prior sensitization in order to recognize and attack malignant cells. They provide a first line of defense against malignant cells and virally infected cells. In an effort to make use of the anticancer properties, NK cells can be collected and infused to try to kill tumor cells. NK cells therapy can be used as a stand-alone treatment in individuals with lymphoma, breast, or ovarian cancer.

These cells may be infused prior to HCT to achieve remission in poor prognosis relapsed acute myelogenous leukemia or with umbilical cord transplant for relapsed leukemia. They may be infused after HCT in an effort to kill remaining tumor cells, prevent relapse, promote engraftment, and mediate control of infections without inducing GVHD.

Treatment precautions for individuals receiving NK cells are based on the protocol, the specific concerns of the physician for that person, and other factors. Precautions may vary from clinical site to site, but these individuals usually are permitted to ambulate in the halls, even though their absolute neutrophil count is below 500 cells/mm³, as long as they wear an N-95 mask. In other facilities, they may not be permitted to leave their rooms to walk in the hallways even with a mask.[145]

SPECIAL IMPLICATIONS FOR THE THERAPIST   21-3

Graft-Versus-Host Disease

Early symptoms of GVHD (see previous discussion in this chapter) usually appear within 10 to 30 days after transplantation and may include rash, dryness of eyes, blurred or double vision, severe headaches, distal joint pain and stiffness, hepatomegaly, persistent nausea and vomiting, stomach cramps, and diarrhea. For a video of an assessment protocol for chronic GVHD see: http://www.fhcrc.org/en/labs/clinical/projects/gvhd.html.[77]

Although some cardiopulmonary abnormalities can only be detected by echocardiography, early warning symptoms of cardiopulmonary complications, such as progressive dyspnea, sensation of heart palpitations, irregular heartbeats, chest pain or discomfort, or increasing fatigue, may be reported by the recipient or observed by the therapist. The physician must be notified of such changes and modifications made to the exercise program for mildly to moderately abnormal responses.

In most centers, there is no waiting period for exercising individuals undergoing HCT. Stationary bikes in isolation rooms can be provided. Strengthening exercises for large proximal muscle groups are prescribed. Manual therapy, exercise, and education are aimed at improving functional mobility and quality of life. Modification of activities, home safety, and ambulation devices when warranted are included. The therapist should watch for steroid myopathy (see discussion, Chapter 5). An extended period of time may be required before normal strength and function

return because of the combination of fatigue and steroid myopathy.

From the National Marrow Donor Program

The National Marrow Donor Program has resources that can be very useful for clinicians as well as recipients. To view their Allogeneic and Autologous Transplant Guidelines, visit https://bethematchclinical.org/Resources-and-Education/Materials-Catalog/HCT-Guidelines-for-Referral-Timing-and-Post-Transplant-Care/

These are available in a mobile app, online, and in print. Their posttransplant guidelines toolkit contains posttransplant care recommendations for late effects and screening for GVHD.

ORGAN TRANSPLANTATION

Kidney Transplantation

Overview

The first kidney transplantation was done in 1954 by Dr. Joseph Murray, and resulted in a successful graft and provided the recipient with an additional 8 years of life. It was the first organ transplantation of any kind ever performed, with the success credited to the live donor (adult twin brother). Kidney transplantation remains the most common type of solid-organ transplant (see Table 21-1).

As people older than age 65 years become the fastest growing segment of the population, the number of cases of end-stage renal disease (ESRD) requiring kidney transplantation will continue to increase. Diabetes is now the most common cause of ESRD. Almost half of adults undergoing transplantation already have diabetes.

Renal replacement remains the most successful form of treatment for ESRD and, in the case of diabetes, offers an opportunity to eliminate dependence on dialysis and exogenous insulin. Simultaneous kidney-pancreas transplantation has become a safe and effective method to treat advanced diabetic nephropathy and results in stable metabolic function, reduced cholesterol, and improved blood pressure control.[392]

Until recently, almost all candidates for renal transplantation had been treated for months or years with hemodialysis; now it is possible to plan a kidney transplant before the complete shutdown of the kidney or kidneys, avoiding dialysis completely. Studies show that when dialysis is used, peritoneal dialysis is associated with a lower incidence of delayed graft function and may be preferred over hemodialysis.[46,418]

Continuous ambulatory peritoneal dialysis is a maintenance system of dialysis in which an indwelling catheter permits fluid to drain into and out of the peritoneal cavity by gravity. The individual remains able to complete this type of dialysis three or four times per day while at home rather than coming to a hemodialysis clinic three or four times per week for 3 or 4 hours at a time while the blood is filtered through a dialysis machine.

Receiving a kidney transplant without a prior history of hemodialysis or peritoneal dialysis presents some problems in adjustment for those people who, never having experienced the intrusion of dialysis, must now learn to live with the side effects of antirejection drugs and potential complications of surgery. Whereas the person on dialysis may see transplantation as a welcome relief, recipients who have never been treated with dialysis may be more likely to view the surgery and recovery as an ordeal and therefore experience more difficulties in adjustment.

Indications and Incidence

As mentioned, the primary indication for renal transplantation is type 1 diabetes with ESRD, which occurs in more than one-third of all cases of type 1 diabetes.[174] Cardiac autonomic neuropathy develops as a result of uremia and diabetes with severe cardiac dysfunction when these conditions are present at the same time. Both kidney transplantation and kidney-pancreas transplantation result in improved cardiac autonomic function and modulation of heart rate.[55]

A more unusual indication for kidney transplantation would be polycystic kidney disease, especially when combined with polycystic liver disease. As of 2008, more than 80,000 people were waitlisted for kidney-alone transplant, while just over 16,000 transplants were performed (5966 of which were living donor).[24]

Transplantation Candidates

As discussed above, people with type 1 diabetes and ESRD can choose dialysis or transplantation for renal replacement therapy. Recent studies show a survival advantage with kidney transplant in elderly adults compared with those on dialysis therapy; inclusion of kidney transplant across different ages, including older adults is referred to as *expanded criteria donor*.[283]

Those individuals with type 1 diabetes younger than 45 years with little or no atherosclerotic vascular disease are ideal candidates for a combined kidney-pancreas transplantation. The addition of a pancreas transplant is associated with greater morbidity and may require higher levels of immunosuppression, but can result in stabilization of neuropathy and improved quality of life.[262]

Some renal transplant candidates are at high risk for cardiac events, sometimes fatal. Analysis of these clinical risk factors (including age at least 50 years, type 1 diabetes mellitus, and abnormal electrocardiogram) may assist in identifying candidates who may be at risk for cardiac death.[250] For those choosing transplantation, a kidney from a living related donor is associated with longer graft and individual survival.

Transplantation Procedure

Kidney grafts may be positioned intraperitoneally, anastomosed to the iliac vessels, and then drained into the bladder (Fig. 21-9); extraperitoneally in the iliac fossa through an oblique lower abdominal incision; or in small children, retroperitoneally with a midline abdominal incision. The diseased or damaged kidney may or may not be removed from the patient. The new kidney will usually start to work right away, but it may not start producing urine for 10 to 14 days.

More recently, a procedure called *laparoscopic nephrectomy* was introduced to remove the live-donor kidney. Four small incisions called ports are made in the abdomen. The ports allow the surgeon to insert the laparoscope

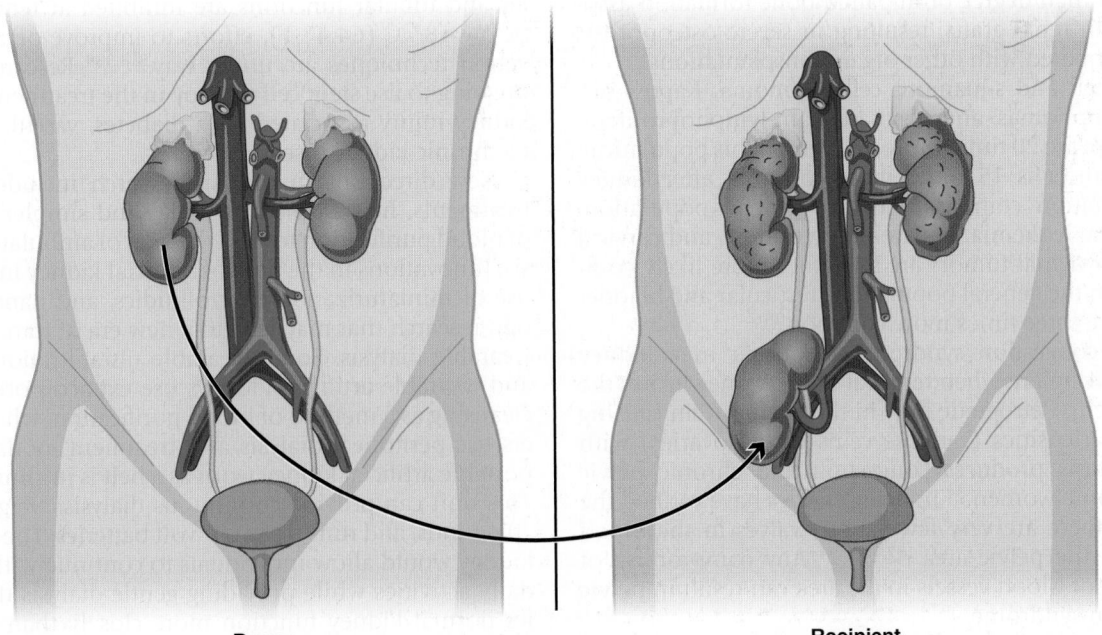

Donor   **Recipient**

Figure 21-9

In a minimally invasive live-donor kidney transplantation, surgeons remove the donor's kidney through a 3- to 4-inch incision below the donor's umbilicus. For the recipient, blood vessels of the donor kidney are attached to the major abdominal blood vessels. The ureter of the donor kidney is attached to the recipient's bladder. The donor kidney begins working immediately. The recipient's own malfunctioning kidney is not always removed.

and other instruments used in the procedure to clamp off arteries and the ureter and cut the kidney loose.

Complications

As with other solid-organ transplantation, renal recipients experience graft dysfunction, organ-related infection (nephrotoxicity), and graft rejection as the three most common complications. Surgical complications include renal artery thrombosis, urinary leak, and lymphocele, although chronic rejection accounts for most renal allograft losses after the first year following transplantation. Donor organ quality, delayed graft function, and other donor and recipient variables leading to reduced nephron mass are nonimmunologic factors that contribute to the progressive deterioration of renal graft function.[284]

Cardiovascular and cerebrovascular diseases are major causes of morbidity and mortality after kidney transplantation. Extensive carotid vascular wall abnormalities increase significantly despite kidney and pancreas transplantation in those individuals with type 1 diabetes mellitus and progressive uremia.

Although initiation of plaque development is related to systemic factors, progression of established plaque is largely influenced by local factors within the arterial wall and therefore unaffected by organ transplantation.[290] In fact, research shows an association between CMV infection and atherosclerotic plaque formation in coronary heart disease, a finding that also found in posttransplant cardiac complications in kidney recipients with CMV.[202]

Other complications may include renal dysfunction with prolonged use of cyclosporine, hypertension, lipid disorders, hepatitis, cancer, and osteopenia. Hypertension occurs in up to 80% of renal graft recipients; approximately 15% of graft recipients develop chronic hepatitis. There is a high degree of impaired bone formation associated with renal grafts, resulting in severe osteoporosis when compared with other organ transplantations.

Basal cell and squamous cell carcinoma, Kaposi sarcoma, lymphomas, and posttransplant lymphoproliferative disease are 20 times more frequent in this population. Kidney cancer is 15 times more common after kidney transplantation compare with the general population. Melanoma, leukemia, hepatobiliary tumors, and cervical and vulvovaginal tumors are five times more likely compared with the general population. Testicular and bladder cancers are three times more common.[216]

Pelvic congestion syndrome can occur in a kidney donor or recipient when removal of the kidney ligates the ovarian vein. Retrograde flow in the ovarian vein causing ovarian varicosities (varicose veins of the ovaries) with venous stasis produces congestion and chronic pelvic pain in some women.[34] Imaging studies have verified the fact that there are very few venous valves in the blood vessels of the pelvic area.[137,188,394] Any compromise of the valves or blood vessels in the area can result in pelvic congestion syndrome.

Prognosis

Long-term renal transplant survival has improved from 23% (graft) and 36% (recipient) for cadaveric donor in 1986, to 92% and 93%, respectively, in 1996.[269]

According to the United States Renal Data System annual report in 2012, the 10-year renal transplant survival rate remains high but depends in part on whether the recipient received a transplant from a deceased or living donor. The probability of returning to dialysis or being retransplanted is much less now for all donated sources.[413]

With the ability to accept a donor kidney from family members, closer tissue and blood matches may improve long-term results. For deceased donors, expanded criteria donor kidneys are not associated with increased mortality or transplant failure in recipients older than 70 years. For all types of donors, the persistent association between living donor kidneys and lower all-cause mortality across all ages suggests that, if possible, elderly recipients gain longevity from living donor kidney transplant.[283]

The National Kidney Foundation reports the national average for survival rates of kidney-pancreas transplants is 94.1% still functioning well 1 year after the operation, 90% after 2 years, and 87.1% at 3 years. The success rates are good for combined kidney-pancreas transplants from deceased donors, but the best results are usually achieved with a closely matched kidney from a living donor (usually from a sibling). The next best results are achieved with a kidney from a less closely matched living donor (such as a spouse or friend).[295]

Future Trends

The renal research community has made great strides in improving client outcomes on dialysis and following organ transplantation. However, only a small fraction of individuals with ESRD undergo transplantation because of a lack of donor organs, requiring continued research to find alternative methods of successful treatment. Alternately, preserving donor organs more effectively may ensure better graft survival rates. Because both glomerular and tubular functions are inhibited at temperatures below 18° C (64.4° F), efforts to improve organ preservation techniques are under way.[318,389] Research is also ongoing to use stem cell therapy in the treatment of acute kidney injury associated with diabetes, vascular disease, or chronic kidney disease.[400]

New directions in dialysis research include cheaper treatments, home-based therapies and simpler methods of blood purification toward the goal of ambulatory dialysis. Innovations in the field of artificial kidney include the use of miniaturization, microfluidics, and nanotechnology, research that may lead to a new era of transportable, wearable dialysis. Some wearable ultrafiltration systems and wearable artificial kidneys use extracorporeal blood cleansing as a method of blood purification, whereas others use peritoneal dialysis as a treatment modality.[343] A portable artificial kidney worn as a belt is in clinical trials. This unit can provide continuous dialysis, weighs about 10 pounds, and runs on two 9-volt batteries. The wearable kidney would allow individuals to continue with normal daily activities while providing gentle dialysis that mimics normal kidney function more closely than standard dialysis.[110,343]

A complete system for hemofiltration in neonates and infants (referred to as CA.R.PE.DI.E.M. [Cardio-Renal Pediatric Dialysis Emergency Machine]) has been developed. The miniaturization of a dialysis circuit for acute kidney injury in the pediatric population may help reduce the high mortality rate (more than 50%) for these children.[342]

Kidney Transplantation

As an increasing number of studies document the effectiveness of exercise in disease prevention and prevention of transplant complications, timely and effective rehabilitation programs will be implemented. Physical and occupational therapy can offer a great deal to aid renal rehabilitation, especially to increase endurance and physical strength and to improve function and independence (see "Organ Transplantation" and "Exercise, Activity, and Sports" in this chapter).

Given the high rate of malignancies in this population, the therapist should continue to work with the recipients in cancer education and prevention. Cancer screening is an important ongoing feature of any physical therapy examination and evaluation with this population. Skin protection and tobacco use cessation should be emphasized as part of patient education by all health care professionals, including physical therapists.

Acute Care Phase

Most kidney recipients are discharged about 5 days after surgery and are not seen by the therapist until later in the recovery process (or perhaps not at all) as an outpatient, approximately 1 month postoperatively. At that time, the recipient will most likely still be monitoring both blood pressure and blood glucose levels. The therapist should pay close attention to both measurements as the rehabilitation component is added.

Exercise

Kidney transplants have been performed longer than any other organ transplant, providing a greater number of retrospective studies to assess the influence of exercise on kidney transplantation. It has been shown that pretransplantation and posttransplantation exercise training improves lipid profile, increases hematocrit level, normalizes insulin sensitivity, and lowers the requirement for antihypertensive medication.[166,167]

Although a kidney transplant recipient may be normotensive at rest, there is an elevated blood pressure response to exercise, possibly caused by altered function of blood pressure control and by the effects of cyclosporine. This requires careful monitoring and documentation of vital signs in the exercise program planning and assessment.

Training effectively modifies factors known to be associated with atherogenesis and cardiac disease in hemodialysis clients. However, exercise training alone after renal transplantation is not enough to modify cardiovascular risk profile. Research to determine the effects of multiple risk interventions is needed.[316]

Before transplantation, clients with kidney disease, especially those receiving hemodialysis, are susceptible to bone loss as a result of altered vitamin D_3 function and its role in calcium absorption. Resistive exercises can help increase bone density (in the general population and in all organ transplantations) and should be initiated before transplantation or as early after transplantation as possible.[57,241,285]

Overuse tendon injuries occur at a high rate in kidney transplant recipients[5,288]; whether the mechanism for this is immunologic, metabolic, or medication induced remains unclear. The use of fluoroquinolones (potent oral antibiotics such as levofloxacin, ciprofloxacin, norfloxacin) has been linked as a responsible factor.[265,274,440] The Achilles is the most commonly reported tendon injury, but injury can occur in the upper extremities as well. For anyone taking fluoroquinolones, care should be taken to avoid overloading tendons as dramatic ruptures following even small trauma have been reported.[374]

The deep inferior epigastric artery, which feeds the lower rectus abdominis muscle, is usually transected in kidney transplantation. The physical therapist will have to take this into account when prescribing exercises and addressing core strength. Studies investigating whether preservation of the deep inferior epigastric artery can prevent lower rectus abdominis muscle atrophy show that this is possible.[209] The therapist will want to read the operative report to determine the status of the lower rectus abdominis muscle before beginning rehabilitative efforts.

Liver Transplantation

Overview

The first liver transplantation in a human being was performed in 1963. Since that time, the success of this procedure has improved so much that more than 6000 liver transplantations were completed in the United States in 2011.[410] In the following decade, a team of surgeons at the University of Chicago developed the living-related transplant that required only a lobe of a liver or small pieces taken from living donors, although today this still represents a fraction of total transplants per year (247 living-donor transplants in 2011). This technique has also been applied to cadaveric donor livers by splitting the liver to expand the donor pool.[62]

Indications

Orthotopic liver transplantation has become an established therapy for end-stage liver disease (e.g., cirrhosis caused by alcoholism, hepatitis C), acute liver failure, and primary biliary cirrhosis or primary sclerosing cholangitis, as well as for nonalcoholic cirrhosis and hepatic or biliary malignancy.

Biliary atresia (bile ducts not formed normally) is the most common indication for pediatric liver transplantation. Five hundred pediatric liver transplants are performed annually; more than half are for biliary atresia. Other indications include neonatal cholestasis (children born with liver failure for unknown reasons), metabolic error leading to liver failure, and acute liver failure for any reason (e.g., viral infection, drug overdose, tumor, cirrhosis).

Theoretically, anyone with advanced, irreversible liver disease with certain mortality may be considered for a liver transplant provided the disease can be corrected by liver transplantation (Table 21-5).

Hepatitis B is not eliminated by transplantation, but its recurrence and the damage it can cause may be substantially reduced by giving the client hepatitis B globulin. Hepatitis recurs in the transplanted liver in 80% to 90% of cases, but the damage to the new liver is slow, so many years of symptom-free living can occur.

With the exception of metastatic malignancy and hepatic lymphoma, there are few absolute contraindications to liver transplantation. Liver transplantation for large primary liver cancers is very limited; transplantation remains the best treatment for small tumors (less than 5 cm) in a liver that is already cirrhotic.[435]

People with metastatic disease that has spread to the liver are no longer treated with liver transplantation because of the poor outcome. The exception is a small group of people whose liver cancer is characterized by neuroendocrine tumors that are very slow growing. The results of transplantation in this group are not as good as for those individuals with benign disease but acceptable enough to qualify for transplantation.

Some metabolic disorders (e.g., familial hypercholesterolemia) that arise in the liver but produce damage elsewhere in the body can be cured if the liver is replaced with a liver from a normal individual. Many inborn errors of liver metabolism are benign and are not associated with end-stage liver disease. Acute fulminant liver failure secondary to severe hepatitis owing to a virus, toxin, or poison can be life threatening and requires liver transplantation to prevent death.

Transplantation Candidates

The decision to perform a liver transplantation may be determined by how long the procedure will extend the candidate's life. In general, people with nonmalignant, nonalcoholic liver disease between ages 2 and 60 years are considered most suitable. A definite age cutoff has not been determined; although many transplantation centers do not accept most people as candidates if they are older than 60 years, this limit is being expanded. Older people may be unable to survive the procedure, and clients with considerable damage to other major organs (e.g., heart, lungs) cannot handle the stress of the surgery. For technical reasons, with small birth weight infants surgeons may prefer to wait until significant growth has occurred.

The potential candidate with an end-stage liver disease that is correctable by a liver transplant must also be a good operative candidate. Many potential risk factors have been reported to increase the risk of transplantation (Table 21-6). Clients with alcoholic cirrhosis may be required to remain abstinent 6 months before the transplant, although it has been suggested that liver transplantation itself contributes to recovery from alcoholism.

The recidivism (relapse) rate following liver transplantation varies in reported studies from 4% to 32%, although the majority of studies report a recidivism rate in the 4% to 9% range.[301,314] The use of the biologic markers to screen for alcoholic relapse has been used in liver graft candidates but remains controversial.[40,207,359,383,425,427]

Transplantation Procedure

The liver from the cadaveric donor is removed through a midline incision from the jugular notch to the pubis including a median sternotomy, with particular care to

Table 21-5	Liver Transplantation
Indications	**Possible Contraindications**
Primary biliary cirrhosis	Sepsis
Neoplasm (selected cases)	Hepatic lymphoma
Acute fulminant liver failure	AIDS
Inborn errors of metabolism	Poor client understanding
Alcoholic cirrhosis after documented treatment and recovery	Alcoholic cirrhosis (documented continued abuse)
Drug-induced liver disease	Cirrhosis secondary to drug abuse
Chronic active hepatitis (see text)	Chronic active (type B) hepatitis
Neonatal cholestasis (bile suppression)	Advanced cardiopulmonary disease
Biliary atresia	Inability to follow up with treatment
Sclerosing cholangitis	
Budd-Chiari syndrome	
Congenital hepatic fibrosis	
Cystic fibrosis	

AIDS, Acquired immunodeficiency syndrome.

Table 21-6	Liver Transplant Risk Factors	
Low	**Intermediate**	**High**
Increasing age	Active extrahepatic infection	More than one other failing organ
Severity of liver dysfunction in otherwise stable person without encephalopathy	Hepatobiliary sepsis	Prolonged, severe coma
Preexisting thrombotic disorder	Hepatorenal syndrome	Preoperative hemodynamic instability
	Small-sized infant	Extrahepatic malignancy
	Short-duration coma	Immunosuppressive disorders
	Transplantation across ABO barrier	
	Previous portosystemic shunt	
	Portal vein thrombosis	
	Operative variable	

Data from Busuttil RW (ed). *Transplantation of the liver*, ed 2, Philadelphia, 2005, WB Saunders; and Chakravarty D. *Liver transplantation*, Maryland Heights, MO, 2010, Jaypee Brothers Medical Publishers.

avoid hepatic injury or portal vein transection. The iliac artery and vein are also harvested in the event that vascular reconstruction is required.

Living-related transplantation requires a much less extensive operative opening, and the reduced-size graft is usually taken from the donor's left lobe (Fig. 21-10). In some situations (e.g., presence of metabolic abnormalities), the autologous graft is placed in an anatomically altered site, thereby preserving the orthotopic position for future use in the case of graft failure; this technique is not possible with disorders leading to portal hypertension.

Successful engraftment of the donor organ requires a recipient hepatectomy to remove the diseased liver, a procedure that can be difficult when there is severe portal hypertension and excessive collateral formation. In many centers, the recipient is placed on heart-lung bypass to avoid congestion of the portal circulation and improve venous return to the heart during implantation, thus improving hemodynamic stability.

The implantation procedure begins with anastomoses, that is, surgical formation of a connection between the donor and the recipient's suprahepatic and then infrahepatic vena cava. Alternatively, the donor vena cava can be anastomosed side-to-side with the recipient vena cava if it is left in situ during the recipient hepatectomy (piggyback technique). The operation then proceeds to the portal anastomosis. After all venous connections are made, the liver is reperfused.

Complications

Transplantation of the liver differs from renal, lung, or heart transplantation because there is no intervening assistance from an artificial liver; the technical aspects of liver transplantation require precise connection of the hepatic artery, hepatic and portal veins, and the bile duct. In the case of a living donor, there is a risk of hemorrhage and death if an artery is accidentally severed.

Rejection is the most common cause of liver dysfunction after transplantation, most likely after the first week and during the first 3 postoperative months. As with all organ transplantation procedures, the chance of organ rejection requires the use of immunosuppressants with their associated complications, especially suppression of the body's natural defenses, making infections a common complication and cause of graft dysfunction.

Each person is also placed on prophylactic medications and preemptive therapy for a period of time to decrease the risk of opportunistic infection.[287] CMV, a common infectious process, can occur early after liver transplantation. CMV remains a major cause of morbidity but is no longer a major cause of mortality after liver transplantation.

Extrahepatic complications may include renal failure, neurologic disorders, and pulmonary involvement (e.g., pneumonia, atelectasis, respiratory distress syndrome, pleural effusion). Hepatocellular carcinoma, hepatitis B, and Budd-Chiari syndrome may recur in the transplanted liver, but other chronic liver diseases do not recur.

In Budd-Chiari syndrome, occlusion of the hepatic veins impairs blood flow out of the liver, producing massive ascites and hepatomegaly. It is associated with any condition that obstructs the hepatic vein (e.g., abdominal trauma, use of oral contraceptives, polycythemia vera, paroxysmal nocturnal hemoglobinuria, other hypercoagulable states, congenital webs of the vena cava).

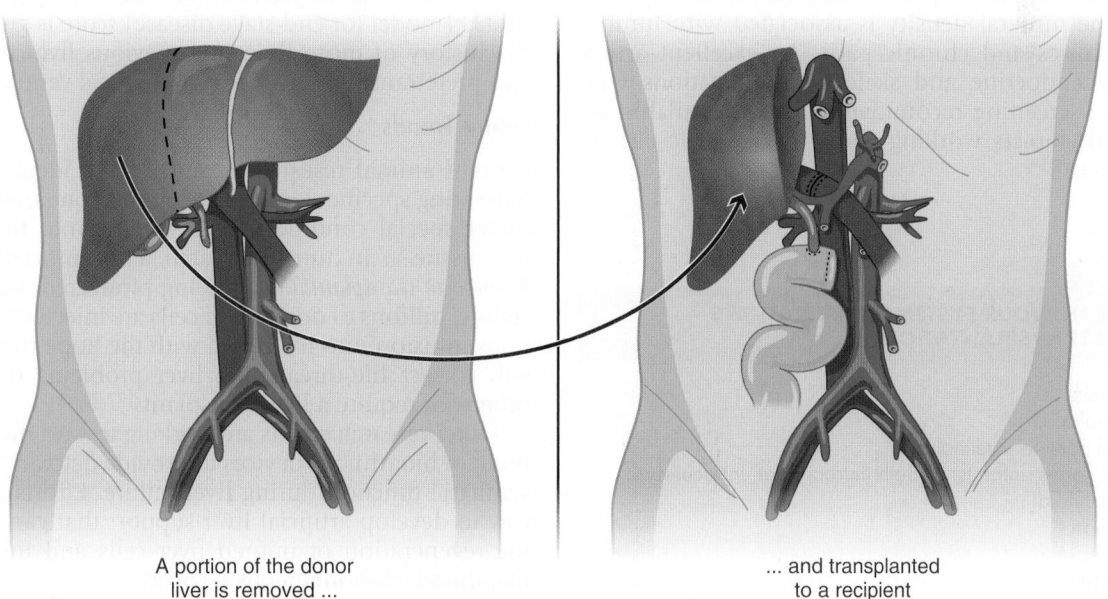

A portion of the donor liver is removed ...

... and transplanted to a recipient

Figure 21-10

In a minimally invasive live-donor liver transplant, an incision is made just under the donor's rib cage. A portion of the liver is removed; the donor's liver will grow back to a normal size within a few weeks. For the recipient, the diseased liver is removed through an incision in the upper abdomen. The donor liver is placed into the abdomen and blood vessels are reattached to the new liver. The bile duct of the donor liver is attached to the recipient's bile duct or to a segment of intestine so the bile can drain into the small intestine.

Mechanical postoperative complications include biliary strictures, nonfunction of the graft (i.e., the transplanted liver does not function), hemorrhage, and vascular thrombosis of the hepatic artery, portal vein, or hepatic veins. Mononeuropathy of the ulnar and peroneal nerves occurs in approximately 5% to 10% of orthotopic liver transplantation, primarily attributed to intraoperative compression (tilting of the surgical table) or postoperative trauma. Poor nutritional status, use of intermittent pneumatic compression devices, and body shape (tall and slender) are other potential contributing factors to peroneal neuropathy following liver transplantation.[372,439] Other upper-extremity mononeuropathies may occur as a result of vascular cannulations (flexible tube inserted to deliver medication or drain fluid).[75]

Other clinically significant neurologic events occur in a substantial percentage of adult liver transplant recipients. Central nervous system complications after liver transplantation may be a consequence of liver disease itself, may be caused by the adrenergic effects of immunosuppressants (e.g., tacrolimus, cyclosporine), or may result from a wide array of metabolic abnormalities or vascular insults occurring in the early postoperative period.

Box 21-6 lists the most common central nervous system complications. The therapist is likely to be familiar with most of these terms, with the possible exception of central pontine myelinosis, which is demyelination of the central pons that causes a locked-in syndrome characterized by paralysis of the limbs and lower cranial nerves with intact consciousness.

Children receiving orthotopic liver transplantation are at risk for endocrine complications such as growth failure, hepatic osteodystrophy, pubertal delay, adrenal insufficiency, and drug-induced diabetes. Other potential complications include bone fractures caused by malnutrition, malabsorption, and osteodystrophy. Low spine bone mineral density is associated with lumbar spine fractures and chronic pain. An excellent article reviewing endocrine and skeletal complications with preventive screening recommendations is available for physical therapists working with the pediatric patient population.[190]

Box 21-6

CENTRAL NERVOUS SYSTEM COMPLICATIONS OF LIVER TRANSPLANTATION

- Focal seizures
- Encephalopathy
- Central pontine myelinolysis
- Hemorrhages, infarcts, or both (intracranial, intracerebral, subarachnoid)
- Confusion
- Coma
- Psychosis
- Cortical blindness
- Quadriplegia
- Tremors
- Alzheimer type II astrocytosis
- Central nervous system aspergillosis (fungal infection)
- Cytomegalovirus (viral infection)

Prognosis

Factors determining survival include the underlying cause of liver failure (e.g., poorer prognosis for advanced cirrhosis), the person's ability to stop the intake of alcohol in the case of alcoholic cirrhosis, and the presence of complications or symptoms of hematemesis, jaundice, and ascites. Continued advances in the use of immunosuppressant-steroid combinations have increased survival rates through effective immunosuppression with minimal toxicity.

In the case of liver transplantation, survival rates correlate with the number of liver transplantation procedures performed in transplantation centers. Overall 1-year survival rates have improved from 70% 10 years ago to more than 85% in many high-volume centers.[131]

More than 50% survive 20 years and report improved quality of life compared with those who have liver disease.[373] Unadjusted deceased-donor transplant survival at 1, 5, and 10 years is now 85%, 69%, and 55%, respectively, while living-donor survival at the same intervals is 88%, 75%, and 60%, although far fewer living-donor transplants are performed.[311] Survival after emergency liver transplantation for acute liver failure is less because such clients are seriously ill at the time of the operation.

The expected 1-year survival rate after a second or subsequent liver transplantation is approximately 50%. Two groups of people qualify for liver retransplantation: those with serious postoperative complications because of mechanical failure or rejection and those who have a slow, progressive course of chronic hepatic dysfunction, usually caused by rejection or recurrence of primary disease.

Risk factors have been identified recently to help predict graft failure in retransplant. These include recipient is older than age 55 years, donor older than age 45 years, MELD (model for end-stage disease) score is greater than 27, history of more than one previous liver transplant, and preretransplant need for mechanical ventilation.[191]

Future Trends

Current animal research is centered on identifying and harvesting specific stem cells from the bone marrow that, under special conditions, will convert into functioning liver tissue.[327] In human research, a new procedure called *hepatocyte transplantation* is being pioneered. In this procedure, billions of donor liver cells are injected by intravenous infusion into the blood with the hope that the cells will correct life-threatening liver problems that would otherwise require a liver transplant.[177,201,341]

Other research efforts are working toward the development of bioartificial devices to provide detoxification and synthetic function during liver failure. Efforts are under way to develop artificial liver support that can stimulate the regeneration of injured liver cells and increase the likelihood of spontaneous recovery.[304]

Bioartificial liver devices are not purely mechanical devices but rather cell-based biologic devices; they create a flow of blood through an extracorporeal circuit lined with healthy hepatocytes.[243] An effective temporary extracorporeal liver support system could improve the chance of survival with or without transplantation as the final treatment.[161] Bioartificial liver systems have been tested in human beings with acute liver failure but are not available for general use yet. Although the device may serve as a bridge to transplantation, no mechanical devices have favorably impacted the outcome of acute liver failure.[304] No device has been developed that can perform all the necessary functions of a healthy liver; researchers are trying to develop liver cells that will perform as many of these tasks as possible.[78,84,304]

SPECIAL IMPLICATIONS FOR THE THERAPIST 21-5

Liver Transplantation

The majority of transplanted livers begin to function well within minutes to hours after the vascular clamps are released. The client must be closely monitored for signs of respiratory compromise, bleeding, infection, rejection, and fluid or electrolyte imbalance (see Chapter 5). Vital signs must be monitored as activities are slowly resumed with physician approval and according to the client's tolerance levels (see Appendix B).

Acute Care Phase

Postoperatively, the client will have multiple intravenous lines, drains, and a Foley catheter, as well as a painful abdomen with a large abdominal incision and a 4- to 5-inch left axillary incision (bypass procedure) restricted by staples and dressings. Standing postoperative orders are usually followed in the ICU.

The typical ICU stay is 24 to 48 hours, with ventilatory support for the first 24 hours. The patient must relax and let the machine breathe for him or her. The patient cannot talk and may be very anxious. The staff should make every effort to keep the patient informed about what is going on and help the patient communicate.

The large incisions are contraindications for resistive exercises; gradual low-resistance training can be introduced according to the physician's protocol. Physical therapy orders for nonspecific out of bed activity and mobility begin by postoperative day 1. The therapist can assess joint motion, observe for thrombosis or infection, begin thrombosis prevention, and take a look at potential discharge needs. Falls prevention is an important aspect of rehabilitation postoperatively. A multidisciplinary approach to mobility coordinated by the physical therapist may help with falls prevention as well as reduce length of stay and increase the rate of return home.[420]

Any signs or symptoms of infection should be reported immediately. This may include headache, fever, skin rash or red streaks, change in pulse rate, confusion, burning with urination, or other constitutional symptoms (see Box 8-1). Mild signs and symptoms of rejection are present during the first few days to weeks, but are controlled in most cases. The patient may report pain caused by the liver, fever, fatigue, and change in color of stool (gray) or urine (tea color). In terms of morbidity or mortality after liver transplantation, infection is usually a much greater concern than rejection.

Upper-extremity range-of-motion exercises and client education for prevention of adhesive capsulitis (i.e., frozen shoulder) are important concerns. Coughing and deep breathing with a pillow splint are taught early. These people do not want to cough, and respiratory infection is a hazard to avoid.

Often postoperative ascites is a significant problem, making functional training (e.g., bed mobility training, transfers) more difficult in the presence of an altered center of gravity. Hand, pedal and, in men, scrotal edema from dependent positioning frequently develops, requiring active-range-of-motion and bed mobility training as soon as possible.

Assisted ambulation should occur as soon as the client is stable in the upright position; placement of the gait belt can be problematic because the T-tube to drain bile is placed in the right lower abdomen and should be avoided. Try using the gait belt around the upper trunk instead.

Once the telemetry is removed, rehabilitation can progress rapidly. Ascites and associated edema usually resolve within 3 to 4 weeks, but if edema persists, comprehensive lymphedema therapy may be required (see discussion in Chapter 13).

Outpatient Phase

Outpatient therapy continues for approximately 8 weeks postoperatively. The liver transplant recipient with healthy heart and lungs can usually function well at home and resume independent activities of daily living. Rest and energy conservation balanced with nutrition, exercise, and correct, consistent, lifelong drug self-administration are all considered important features of the rehabilitation process.

Pretransplant hepatic encephalopathy usually resolves slowly in the posttransplant period if the donor organ is functioning well; client and therapist will see a reduction or cessation of associated signs and symptoms.

Common problems during the outpatient phase are centered around balance and coordination. Fatigue and reduced endurance add to the client's instability. Sleep disturbance may occur as a side effect of medications contributing to fatigue.

The therapist must be alert to any self-medicating or use of nonprescription drugs by the client; the client should be encouraged to check with the physician before continuing unmonitored drug use. Steroid usage in older women can cause posttransplant mental confusion; the woman may become uncooperative and disoriented to time and place and experience hallucinations.[371] Observe for steroid myopathy in all recipients (see Table 5-5).

The therapist should be aware of incisional precautions because of the abdominal incision. Often surgeons place weight-lifting restrictions for a period of time (usually 6-8 weeks if the incision is healing well).

The abdominal scar may result in a kyphotic posture and altered breathing. Some people continue to use an assistive device. The therapist may be able to assist in improving posture, strength, balance, coordination, and fatigue levels. Exercise is an extremely valuable part of the postoperative recovery phase.

Exercise

Extreme weakness and fatigue reducing clients' activity level are common in many liver transplant candidates with chronic liver disease. Low VO_2max is common in pretransplant liver candidates with primary biliary or alcoholic cirrhosis along with alcohol-induced myopathy contributing to exercise limitations.

Improvement in exercise capacity with training before transplantation has been demonstrated, and new studies confirm the same outcome after liver transplantation on physical fitness, muscle strength, and functional performance in candidates treated for chronic liver disease (see also "Organ Transplantation" and "Exercise, Activity, and Sports" presented earlier in this chapter).[43,44]

Compliance with a home program of exercise and activity may be a problem; fatigue and quality of life are cited most often for poor adherence. Education is the key as both of these symptoms can be improved with exercise.[233,266,344,373,417]

The liver plays an important role in providing glucose for oxidation and the maintenance of glucose homeostasis during physical exercise. Denervation of the liver does not alter the release of glucose during physical activity. Consequently, liver transplant candidates can perform quite heavy exercise and maintain acceptable glucose levels.

Heart Transplantation

Overview

In 1905, Drs. Carrel and Guthrie began to perform experimental procedures to prove heart transplantation was possible. In 1946, Dr. Demikhov performed the first heterotrophic heart transplantation in a dog. In 1960, Lower and Shumway developed the technique for heart transplantation that remains the basis of standard clinical surgical transplantation technique worldwide. The first human heart procedure was performed in South Africa by Dr. Christiaan Barnard (1967), followed shortly by the first U.S. transplant by Norman Shumway at Stanford in 1968.[156]

Incidence and Prevalence

Despite the various initiatives to increase the number of available donor hearts, there is a relatively constant number of heart transplants performed each year, ranging from 2050 to 2350. At present there are more than 52,000 individuals who have received a heart transplant and more than 20,000 alive today because of a heart transplantation procedure. In 2011, there were 2322 heart transplants done, with approximately 370 transplants being completed in pediatric recipients (age 17 years or younger).[411]

At any one time, there are approximately 3600 individuals waiting for a heart transplantation.[297] The average wait (median) for heart transplantation is 135 days in 2009 with a range of 1 to slightly longer than 12 months. Twenty-four percent of recipients in 2009 waited less than 30 days.[412] During this wait period the candidate is constantly monitored and medically managed to assure proper candidacy, accurate UNOS listing, and minimize the adverse effects of any further progression of the heart failure or the onset of new medical issues.

The decline in waiting candidates is a result of multiple factors, including improvement in the medical and surgical management of heart disease and heart failure, including VADs. The waiting list has also declined because there are fewer people who have been classified as a status 2 being activated in the UNOS list. This is partly a result of the advances in health care and the fact that the data do not support the efficacy of organ allocation to individuals with a status 2. This has resulted in an increase in allocation of available organs to candidates with more current medical needs. There has been almost a 30% decline in candidates with a status 2 listing in the past decade.[312]

There have been some other subtle changes in the characteristics in candidates waiting for a heart transplantation. There has been a 4% increase among African Americans and a 7% increase among the number of women awaiting transplantation. There has been an increase in the candidates with a primary diagnosis of congenital defects or valve disease. The largest change, slightly more than 7%, has been in the number of individuals listed for transplant surgery with the primary diagnosis of coronary artery disease.

Indications

Potential candidates of cardiac transplantation must have end-stage heart disease with severe or advanced heart failure (New York Heart Association class III or IV end-stage heart disease) with a life expectance of less than 1 year. The most common underlying cause of heart failure leading to cardiac transplantation is cardiomyopathy either because of end-stage ischemic coronary heart disease or nonischemic dilated cardiomyopathy.

Other, less-common cardiac diseases that may be treated with a heart transplantation include sarcoidosis, restrictive cardiomyopathy, hypertrophic cardiomyopathy, congenital heart disease, life-threatening arrhythmias and retransplantation.

One other criterion for heart transplant includes cases where further medical or surgical intervention would not extend the individual's life or improve physical capacity. The presence of other irreversible organ diseases such as liver or renal failure, stroke, peripheral arterial disease, and diabetes with organ disease are considered exclusion criteria for transplantation. Severe chronic obstructive pulmonary disease or irreversible pulmonary hypertension are also contraindications to heart transplantation.

Transplantation Candidates

The selection of candidates for heart transplantation involves the use of multiple prognostic variables (Box 21-7; see also Box 21-3) in conjunction with medical urgency criteria established through UNOS status listings (Box 21-8). People accepted as candidates for heart transplantation are expected to have a limited survival if they do not have surgery and to have exhausted other medical or surgical options that extend the individual's life or improve their physical capacity.

Box 21-7

INDICATIONS AND REQUIREMENTS FOR HEART TRANSPLANTATION

- Cardiogenic shock or low cardiac output state requiring mechanical support
- Low cardiac output or refractory heart failure requiring inotropic support
- ESHD with NYHA class III or IV not responding to medical intervention
- Intractable severe angina not amenable to intervention
- Life expectancy <50% of expected survival at 1 year that includes:
  - LVEF <20%
  - Maximal VO_2 <12 mL/kg/min
  - Peak VO_2 <10 mL/kg/min
  - Ventricular arrhythmias not responsive to medical therapy
  - Cardiac Index <2.0 L/min/m^2
  - Pulmonary capillary wedge pressure >16 mm Hg
- Age typically <65 years old
- No irreversible organ dysfunction
- No irreversible pulmonary hypertension
- Free of cancer (time of remission depends on type of cancer)
- Free from substance abuse (minimally >6 months)
- Diabetes mellitus with peripheral end-stage organ complications
- No active infections
- Good compliance
- HIV negative
- Psychologic stability
- Financial support
- Family Support

ESHD, end-stage heart disease; LVEF, left ventricular ejection fraction; NYHA, New York Heart Association.

The candidate needs stable social support and financial resources to cover medications and follow-up care. Ideally, the candidate should be younger than 65 years of age and have no other disease, such as cancer, that would shorten the life of the individual or limit the life expectance of the transplantation.[414] Age cutoff is also controversial and has increased since the year 2000; although the upper age limit for transplantation candidates is currently 65 years, an increasing number of centers will consider candidates who are in their 70s if there are no other contraindications.[261]

Pediatric listings differ slightly. Status 1A characterizes a child younger than 6 months of age with pulmonary arterial pressure greater than 50% of systolic pressure who is being supported by a mechanical circulatory device, balloon pump, or mechanical ventilator; or receives high doses of multiple inotropes (agents that alter the force of muscular contractions). Status 1B indicates growth failure in a child younger than 6 months of age with a pulmonary arterial pressure less than 50% of systolic pressure or low-dose inotropes. Status 2 includes all actively listed children who do not meet the criteria of Status 1. Status 7 includes any child who is actively waiting for transplant.[360]

Risk factors in the adult heart transplant candidate must be assessed to provide guidelines about the timing of placing a person on the UNOS waiting list and when to perform the transplantation. The measure of exercise VO_2

has become an indicator of prognosis in advanced heart failure and is currently being used as a major criterion in many centers for the selection of candidates for heart transplantation.

Individuals with a maximal VO_2 of less than 12 mL/min/kg have a lower survival rate unless treated successfully with transplantation. However, VO_2 can be affected by age, gender, muscle mass, and conditioning status. The multiple factors that affect exercise capacity may explain why some people with congestive heart failure and a peak VO_2 of less than 14 mL/kg/min have a favorable prognosis even when transplantation is deferred.[38,65,261,335]

Ejection fraction, cardiac index, and diabetes status are also used to assess risk. Anyone with an ejection fraction of less than 20% and a cardiac index of less than 2 L/min/m^2 is also considered a potential candidate for transplantation. Ejection fraction is the amount of blood the ventricle ejects; the normal ejection fraction is approximately 60% to 75%. A decreased ejection fraction is a hallmark finding of ventricular failure. Normal cardiac index ranges from 2.5 to 4 L/min/m^2.

Transplantation Procedure

Heart transplantation is a procedure using homologous (allograft) transplant procedure. Almost all heart transplantations done at this time are *orthotopic*; that is, the diseased heart is removed and the donor heart is grafted into the normal anatomic site. There are three surgical procedures that can be used to implant the heart: biatrial, bicaval, and total procedure. The biatrial procedure involves suturing the new heart on the native atrial wall. This procedure is not used as much anymore because of the increased incidence of arrhythmias and valvular dysfunction when compared with the other two procedures. The bicaval procedure is the most common at this time, and involves the anastomoses of the superior and inferior venae cavae. The total procedure includes the bicaval approach plus the anastomosis of the pulmonary veins.[170,347]

In the *heterotopic* cardiac transplantation, the recipient's diseased heart is left intact and the donor heart is placed in parallel with anastomoses between the two right atria, pulmonary arteries, left atria, and aorta. In the heterotopic transplantation, the donor heart assists the diseased heart. This type of procedure accounts for less than 1% of the transplantation population and may be performed in an individual with fixed pulmonary hypertension or someone who is physically very large, requiring a higher cardiac output than a donor heart from an average-size donor.

One of the effects when an orthotopic transplantation is performed is the recipient loses the connection between the donor heart and the autonomic nervous system because it is surgically disconnected to remove the diseased native heart. The autonomic nervous system is not reconnected at the time of the donor heart implantation. This leaves the transplant recipient with the loss of the fight-or-flight response. The heart relies on its own intrinsic properties for sufficient contractility and cardiac output at rest.

In general, the recipient will have an elevated heart rate at rest because of the loss of the parasympathetic input, a decrease in compliance (the heart's ability to relax to completely fill), and a blunted heart rate response with

Box 21-8

UNOS ORGAN ALLOCATION STATUS LIST

Heart

Status 1A:

- Individual admitted to listed treatment center with mechanical circulatory support (VAD, total artificial heart, intraaortic balloon pump, ECMO) for acute hemodynamic decompression. Status for 1A must be recertified every 14 days. An individual with total artificial heart discharge from hospital can be listed for 30 days
- Individual with mechanical circulatory support with complications including thromboemboli, device infection, ventricular arrhythmias
- Individual with mechanical ventilation support
- Individual with single high-dose inotropic medication or multiple low-dose inotropic medications with administration via a central venous line
- Exceptions are reviewed on an individual bases

Status 1B:

- Individuals with VAD support
- Individuals with continuous inotrope infusion
- Exceptions are reviewed on an individual basis

Status 2:

- An individual waiting for transplant but does not meet the criteria for Status 1A or 1B.

Status 7:

- An individual who is considered temporarily unsuitable to receive a transplant

Lung

Lung allocation system is a method to calculate the medical urgency of transplantation. A lung allocation score (LAS) is calculated for each individual based upon the following medical items:

- LAS medical score items: factors used to calculate the LAS
  - Lung diagnosis
  - Date of birth
  - Functional status
  - Assisted ventilation
  - Height and weight
  - Diabetes
  - Supplemental oxygen
  - Percent predicted forced vital capacity (FVC)
  - Six-minute walk distance
  - Serum creatinine
  - Pulmonary artery systolic pressure
  - Mean pulmonary artery pressure
  - Pulmonary capillary wedge mean
  - PCO_2
- Factors used to predict risk of death on the lung transplant waitlist
  1. FVC
  2. Pulmonary artery (PA) systolic pressure (groups A, C, and D)

  3. O_2 required at rest (groups A, C, and D)
  4. Age
  5. Body mass index (BMI)
  6. Diabetes
  7. Functional Status
  8. Six-minute walk distance
  9. Continuous mechanical ventilation
  10. Diagnosis
  11. $PaCO_2$
  12. Bilirubin (current bilirubin: all groups; change in bilirubin: Group B)
- Factors that predict survival after lung transplant
  1. FVC (Groups B and D)
  2. Pulmonary capillary wedge pressure ≥20 (Group D)
  3. Continuous mechanical ventilation
  4. Age
  5. Serum creatinine
  6. Functional status
  7. Diagnosis

  Group A: Includes candidates with obstructive lung disease, including without limitation, chronic obstructive pulmonary disease (COPD), α_1-antitrypsin deficiency, emphysema, lymphangioleiomyomatosis, bronchiectasis, and sarcoidosis with mean PA pressure ≤30 mm Hg.

  Group B: Includes candidates with pulmonary vascular disease, including without limitation, primary pulmonary hypertension, Eisenmenger syndrome, and other uncommon pulmonary vascular diseases.

  Group C: Includes, without limitation, candidates with cystic fibrosis and immunodeficiency disorders such as hypogammaglobulinemia.

  Group D: Includes candidates with restrictive lung diseases, including without limitation, idiopathic pulmonary fibrosis, pulmonary fibrosis (other causes), sarcoidosis with mean PA pressure >30 mm Hg, and obliterative bronchiolitis (non-retransplant).

Heart-Lung Transplantation

When the candidate is eligible to receive an available heart organ, the lung shall be allocated to the heart-lung candidate from the same donor. When the candidate is eligible to receive a lung organ, the heart shall be allocated to the heart-lung candidate from the same donor if no suitable Status 1A isolated heart candidates are eligible to receive the heart. Heart-lung candidates shall use the ABO matching requirements for both heart and lung.

Data from United Network for Organ Sharing (UNOS): *2011 Annual report of the U.S. Scientific Registry for Transplant Recipients and the Organ Procurement and Transplantation Network-transplant data*, Richmond, VA, 2012.

exertion because of the loss of the sympathetic nervous system. The heart relies on the release of catecholamines to increase rate and contractility, and there is a delay in recovery of this function following transplantation. The therapist should also expect a delay in recovery until the body processes the released hormones. In general, the recipient has an exercise capacity of 65% to 70% of predicted VO_2 capacity.[189,381] There is promising evidence,

however, that partial normalization of heart rate can be achieved by 6 to 12 months after transplant.[305] See further discussion of denervation in "Special Implications for the Therapist 21-6: Heart Transplantation" below.

Complications

One of the most common posttransplant complications is rejection. (see also "Posttransplantation Complications:

Graft Rejection" discussed above).With the increased understanding of the immune system there has been a decrease in hyperacute rejection to approximately 2%. This type of rejection occurs within minutes to hours postimplantation and involves a catastrophic immune response from the interaction between the recipient's circulating antibodies and donor antigens.[156,251]

Acute Rejection. Acute rejection can occur at any time after transplantation. Twenty-four percent of recipients will experience acute rejection within the first year. Recipients can present with signs and symptoms such as fever, malaise, heart rate alteration or arrhythmias, jugular vein distention, decreased exercise tolerance, or heart failure. Rejection can also be asymptomatic.[189,254]

Acute rejection can be an antibody-mediated response and or T-cell–mediated response. The antibody-mediated acute rejection occurs early in the postoperative period and is associated with capillary endothelial changes with macrophage and neutrophil infiltrations and interstitial edema.

T-cell–mediated rejection is associated with increased lymphocytes and macrophages, which lead to a complex immune response and the activation of cytotoxic T cells, B cells, and NK cells, resulting in the destruction of interstitial and vascular graft tissue.[189,251,254]

Cardiac Allograft Vasculopathy or Transplant Coronary Artery Disease. Chronic rejection is a medical issue that a recipient may face months to years after transplantation. This immune-mediated rejection is experienced by 8%, 32%, and 43% of recipients 1 year, 5 years, and 8 years posttransplantation, respectively, as diagnosed by angiography. In the heart transplant recipient, chronic rejection presents itself as cardiac allograft vasculopathy (CAV).[358]

Chronic rejection is thought to be mediated by indirect allorecognition and is associated with both humoral and cellular acute rejection and correlated with persistent inflammation. This leads to a diffuse proliferation of smooth muscle cells, concentric intimal narrowing, and accelerated diffuse obliterative atherosclerosis of both intramyocardial and epicardial arteries and veins (Figs. 21-11 and 21-12).[135,170,358]

Risk factors associated with CAV include hypertension history of the donor, older donor age, recipient's body mass index, recipient CMV infection, and treatment with antibiotics within the first 2 weeks posttransplantation for an infection. There is an increased risk of developing CAV within the first 3 years posttransplantation. Other risk factors include elevated C-reactive proteins and troponin I, and the use of cyclosporine and corticosteroids.[357]

Recipients who are suffering from CAV may initially be asymptomatic, but as the disease progresses the recipient will present with signs and symptoms of heart failure. These signs and symptoms include dyspnea, syncope, jugular vein distention, peripheral edema, malaise, low grade fever, general fatigue, and variable arrhythmias (most likely atrial tachycardiac arrhythmias).

With the denervation of the donor heart many recipients will not experience angina despite the atherosclerosis and decrease in myocardial perfusion. Symptoms of angina cannot be ignored because it is now recognized that a portion of recipients will obtain some degree of

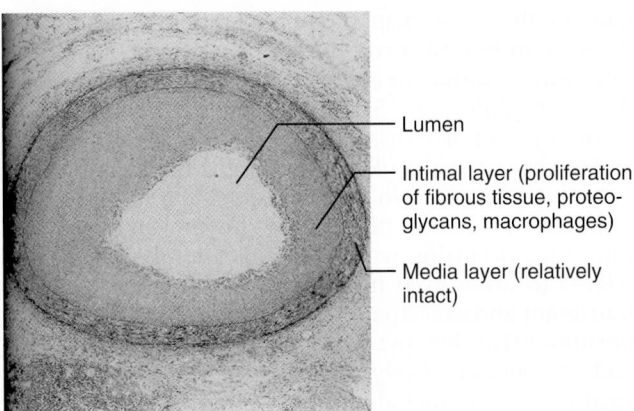

Figure 21-11

Transplant coronary artery disease. Proliferation of the intimal layer of the epicardial coronary artery from a 14-year-old cardiac transplant recipient 1 year after transplant. This condition produces a significant reduction in diameter of the arterial lumen that will compromise blood flow to the myocardium. (Reprinted from Gajarski RJ: Update on pediatric heart transplant: long-term complications, *Tex Heart Inst J* 24(4):260–268, 1997.)

Lumen

Intimal layer (proliferation of fibrous tissue, proteoglycans, macrophages)

Media layer (relatively intact)

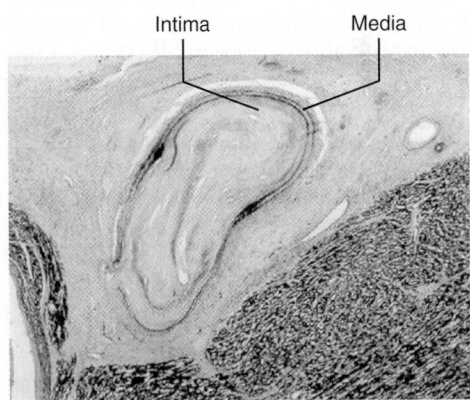

Intima   Media

Figure 21-12

Transplant coronary artery disease resulting in complete occlusion of epicardial coronary artery in an 11-year-old heart transplant recipient 4 years after transplantation. The lumen is obstructed with dense fibrous tissue with thinning and fibrosis of the media layer. (Reprinted from Gajarski RJ: Update on pediatric heart transplant: long-term complications, *Tex Heart Inst J* 24(4):260–268, 1997.)

sympathetic nervous reinnervation.[36,189,125] The classic angiogram diagnosis is not as useful for diagnostic purposes for CAV because CAV is more diffuse with small arterial disease initially. Dobutamine stress echocardiography is more effective in the diagnostic process. CT scan and intravascular ultrasound are particularly effective in diagnosing early CAV by assessing the entire cardiac arterial tree and assessing the hyperplasia of the intimal layer of the arteries.[357]

Infection. There has been a continuous decrease in the infection rates posttransplantation despite the higher-risk populations. This has come about from the improvement in immunosuppressive medications, less induction therapy, further development of antimicrobial medications, and improved prophylactic management.[178] Prophylactic management for CMV infection also results in a decrease in complications as well as a decrease in CAV development later in the posttransplantation period.[377] Despite the decrease in infection complications posttransplantation, infections continue to account for approximately 30% of deaths in adults and 15% in pediatric recipients between 1 and 3 years posttransplantation.[224,385]

The characteristics of infection in the transplant recipient can be classified in several ways. For example, infections can be classified in relation to the time of transplant. Infections occurring within the first month may be (1) related to unresolved infection of the recipient prior to transplant and exacerbated by the surgery and the immunosuppressive therapy; (2) transmitted from the donor; and (3) perioperatively related to the medical and surgical procedure, including line, wound, and pulmonary infections (most common).

The most common infectious pathogen that heart transplant recipients face is bacterial, primarily from the increase in antibiotic resistance. The recipient will be monitored and treated for other infectious pathogens (e.g., viral and fungal). Sources of bacterial infections are *Staphylococcus*, which continues to increase in incidence and *Pseudomonas aeruginosa*, which has decreased in incidence in the past decade.[178] The primary site of the infection is pulmonary with bacteremia and sternal wound accounting for the almost 70% of all bacterial infections.

Viral infections, CMV, herpes simplex virus, and EBV have also decreased as a result of prophylactic management but continue to need close monitoring and intervention. This is especially true for the recipient who was negative for viral exposure and mismatched with a donor who is seropositive.[178] Fungal infections such as *Aspergillus* and *Candida* are also a concern, but there has been a significant decrease in invasive *Aspergillus* infections in the past decade. These infections are most common between 1 and 6 months posttransplantation, usually related to a prior infection that has not resolved within the first 30 days, expanded donor pool, and the particular immunosuppressant medication used.

Acute Graft Failure. In the early postoperative phase, the donor heart may not sufficiently support the circulatory demand of the body and is associated with early morbidity and mortality. The dysfunction of the graft may be related to an ischemic injury sustained in the procurement process. There may be a reperfusion injury sustained at the time when the circulation is reestablished through the donor heart. Finally, graft dysfunction may be the result of acute right ventricular failure because the right ventricle is not accustomed to contracting against the elevated pulmonary arterial pressures within the recipient's pulmonary vascular resistance. Within the first 30 days posttransplantation, acute graft failure accounts for approximately 35% of deaths.[189,385]

Neuromuscular. Reports have also been made of generalized polyneuropathy accompanying solid-organ rejection of the heart and kidneys. The neuropathy affects proximal and distal muscles and demonstrates hyporeflexia or areflexia.

Musculoskeletal. There is a decrease in muscle mass and strength from the effects of immobility, chronic effects of the inflammatory response, and effects of immunosuppressive medications. Tacrolimus and cyclosporine inhibit and transform myosin heavy chain and oxidative enzymes from fast to slow muscle twitch. There

is also a decrease in skeletal muscle perfusion because of the increased sensitivity of peripheral chemoreceptors.[93]

Osteopenia and osteoporosis are significant complications for transplant recipients of all ages. Osteopenia has been reported to affect 20% to 49% of candidates waiting for transplantation and accounts for 14% of vertebral compression fractures.[237] Posttransplantation, the risk of bone disease increases with the use of immunosuppressive medications and renal dysfunction with the greatest degree of bone loss within the first year posttransplantation. Evidence of osteoporosis rates are 15% and 25% for the spine and hip, respectively, and up to 36% of vertebral compression fractures reported within the first year.[237]

The adverse effect on bone density is multifactorial. Corticosteroids inhibit bone formation proliferation, and function by decreasing the levels of type I collagen. Corticosteroids also reduce intestinal calcium stimulating an increase in osteoclastic activity and have adverse effects on skeletal muscles that further contribute to decreased bone density. Calcineurin inhibitors, cyclosporine A, and tacrolimus directly decrease bone density by increasing osteoclastic activity and indirectly decrease bone density by altering T-cell function and impairing renal function. Tacrolimus and cyclosporine also have adverse effects on skeletal muscles.[56,236,237,257]

Cancer. The incidence of cancer is proportional to the drug levels of the immunosuppressive medications and survival time posttransplantation; in general, average onset of malignancy is between 2.5 and 4 years posttransplantation in 10% of heart transplant recipients. By 15 years posttransplantation, almost 50% of recipients are diagnosed with some form of malignancy. Skin cancer is the most common form of cancer present, at a rate of 29% at 15 years posttransplantation (basal cell more often than squamous cell carcinoma).[385]

Heart transplant recipients have a higher incidence of lymphomas related to high drug levels and the use of OKT$_3$. Posttransplant lymphoproliferative disease is associated with EBV, which causes a proliferation of B cells. More recently, however, there appears to be an association with EBV and T-cell proliferative lymphomas. Posttransplant lymphoproliferative disease may begin in the donor organ or in extranodal sites such as the lung, gut, or central nervous system, or it can present as a disseminated disease.[253,322,334,385]

Other. Other complications occur as a result of longterm use of immunosuppressive medications and their adverse effects (see "Immunosuppressants" in Chapter 5). It has been reported that 50% to 95% of recipients are treated for hypertension because of medications and renal insufficiency, and that 60% to 80% of recipients develop hyperlipidemia. Approximately 35% to 40% develop diabetes.[385]

One-third of recipients have renal dysfunction, with approximately 5% to 8% progressing to ESRD and requiring hemodialysis or renal transplantation.[189,253] Cyclosporine- or tacrolimus-induced hyperuricemia, along with renal insufficiency and use of loop diuretics, can lead to an increase in gout. Gout is characterized by early symptoms, including arthralgias and monoarthritis affecting the first metatarsophalangeal joint, knees, ankles, heels, and insteps. Over time, upper-extremity joints become involved, progressing to polyarticular chronic arthritis. Treatment is as for primary gout (see Chapter 27).

Finally, 25% of recipients are treated for depression. There are reports that approximately 10% of recipients suffer from posttraumatic stress disorder.[152,170,253]

Prognosis

In general, people tolerate the transplantation procedure well, and the graft resumes normal function promptly. Recipients are often extubated and out of bed into a chair 1 to 2 days after surgery. Survival times were short 30 years ago, but new immunosuppressive drugs developed in the mid-1980s and improved in the 1990s have extended survival for more recipients.

UNOS reports continued improvement in the survival rates after cardiac transplantation. Survival rates are excellent, with a 3-month survival rate of 94% and 1-year, 5-year, and 10-year survival rates of 89%, 75%, and 56%, respectively. Whites have the highest survival rates, with African American recipients having an approximately 15% lower 5-year survival rate. Young adult recipients also have 5-year survival rates below 70%, and women have a 2% lower 5-year survival rate than men.[189,407]

More careful candidate selection, endomyocardial biopsy to allow for early rejection detection, and advanced medical-surgical techniques also have contributed greatly to improved longevity. Only a decade ago, infection and acute and/or chronic rejection were the major causes of death in heart transplant recipients. With improved longevity, chronic graft vasculopathy (accelerated atherosclerosis, transplant coronary artery disease) and malignancies are now the primary causes of death among heart transplant recipients. Infection, rejection, and sequelae of long-term immunosuppression (especially renal insufficiency or renal failure) remain the primary treatment issues.

A recent study found that heart transplant recipients older than age 65 years reported better quality of life, adherence to medical regimen, and better psychosocial adjustment 5 years after heart transplant than their younger counterparts.[364] One report shows completion of the Ironman Triathlon 22 years after heart transplant.[182,364]

The data for long-term success, including functional mobility and quality of life, is limited at this time. Few studies have addressed geriatric issues in transplant patient selection or management, or addressed the implications on health span and disability when recipients age into late life with their transplanted organ, thus making it difficult for health care providers to speculate on the transplant recipient's long-term needs.[2]

Current Trends

Ventricular Assist Devices. VADs have become an accepted surgical intervention for the management of heart failure. Since the early 1990s, VADs have been used as a *bridge to transplant* when an individual was not expected to survive the wait time for a heart transplant. In many cases, VAD implantation was the last resort; the patients were medically unstable, leading to complications, higher mortality rates, prolonged hospitalization, and complicated rehabilitation. More recently, the use of VADs as a bridge to transplant is done prior to irreversible dysfunction of other organs (e.g., renal or liver dysfunction and cardiac cachexia).[54]

In 2001, Rose reported that VAD recipients had lower mortality and depression and improved quality of life than did individuals receiving optimal medical therapy for heart failure. This report led to the FDA approving the HeartMate XVE VAD for implantation for individuals who were not heart transplant candidates. This is referred to as *destination* therapy.[247,346]

VADs have significantly changed in the last 2 decades. Many of the devices are smaller, and easier to operate now. This has allowed for longer VAD support, decrease in complications, and possible discharge home. VADs are most commonly implanted for left-heart failure. Currently, the most common implanted devices for left-heart failure are the HeartMate II (www.thoratec.com) (Fig. 21-13), HeartWare (www.heartware.com) (Fig. 21-14), and Jarvik 2000 (www.jarvikheart.com) (Fig. 21-15).

There is no VAD similar to the left ventricular assist device at this time that was designed for right heart failure, although the Thoratec pVAD can provide long-term right ventricle support. For biventricular failure, the most common long-term devices are the Thoratec pVAD (Fig. 21-16) and the CardioWest total artificial heart (SynCardia Systems, Inc., Tuscon, Ariz.; not shown). The CardioWest total article heart is a true replacement of the person's native ventricles. The diseased ventricles are excised and two mechanical ventricles are sewn to the native atria. Total artificial hearts are currently restricted to cases where medications and a left ventricular assist device are not enough to sustain life until a transplant can be done. The total artificial heart is a life-saving therapy for advanced stages of heart failure from a variety of underlying causes.

The VADs are designed to support heart function and can be described as pulsatile or nonpulsatile depending on how the device circulates blood. VADs can be classified as providing short- or long-term support. Pulsatile pumps like Thoratec pVAD or Abiomed mimic heart

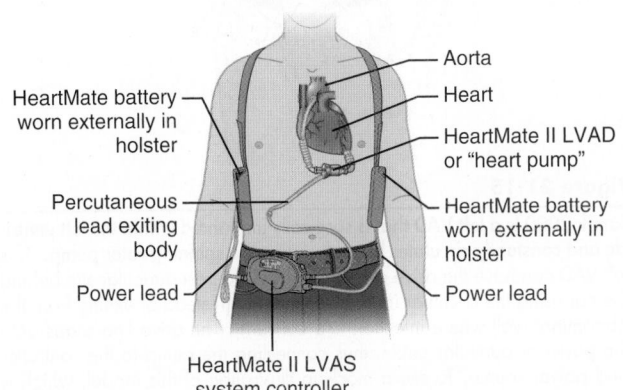

Figure 21-13

HeartMate II left ventricular assist system is a nonpulsatile left VAD that works in parallel with the native heart to support left ventricular function. HeartMate II provides sufficient continuous systemic circulation and allows for relatively free mobility so that the person can return home and actively participate in a comprehensive exercise program and other noncontact recreational activities. (Courtesy Thermo Cardiosystems, Inc., Woburn, MA.)

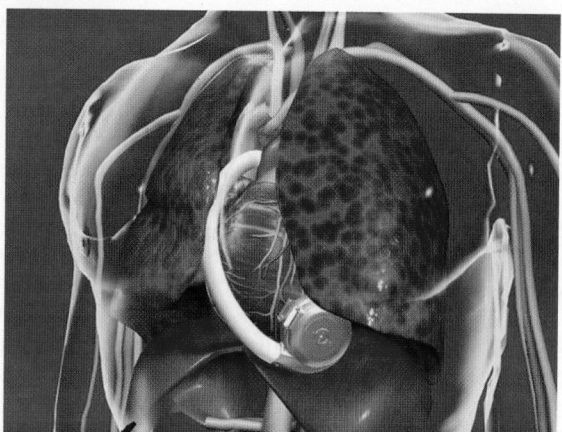

Figure 21-14

HeartWare is a centrifugal nonpulsatile left VAD that provides continuous systemic circulation. The components of the device include a pump which is implanted intrathoracic, a very short inflow conduit or cannula, and outflow conduit or cannula. Additional components not shown in the image are the percutaneous lead (driveline), controller, and power source. Blood circulates from the left ventricle through the inflow cannula into the pump that continuously delivers blood forward to the ascending aorta via the outflow cannula. (Courtesy HeartWare International Inc., Framingham, MA. Used with permission.)

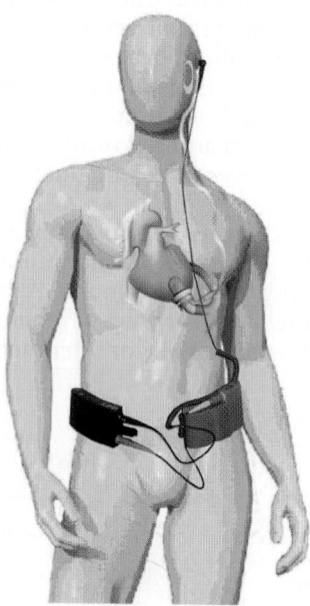

Figure 21-15

Jarvik 2000 is a left VAD that is surgically implanted within the left ventricle and constantly circulates blood by way of a spinning rotor pump. This left VAD can have the drive exit the body at the post auricular site behind the ear using the cochlear implant technology (instead of exiting from the abdominal wall where infection is a concern). The drive line snaps onto the posterior auricular cable, thus connecting the pump to the controller and power source. To see a mock-up illustration of this model, which is under clinical trials in the United States, go to http://www.jarvikheart.com/basic.asp?id=74. (Courtesy Robert Jarvik, MD, used with permission.)

function in that the atrium fills the VAD, which then pumps the blood out into systemic circulation. For the nonpulsatile pumps the VAD circulates blood continuously. The patient may or may not have a palpable pulse or ausculatory blood pressure depending on how fast the

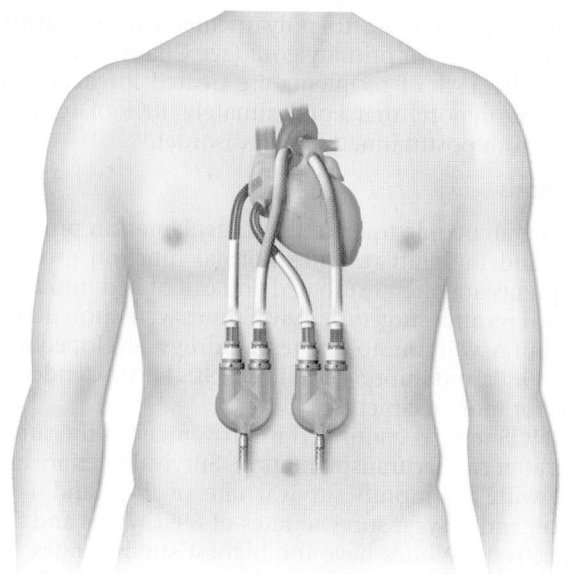

Figure 21-16

The Thoratec is a pneumatically driven VAD shown here with various cannulation options. It can support the right, left, or both ventricles. This device is used as a bridge to transplantation or in the case of possible recovery of the native heart function. The actual pump is external to the body, which allows this device is be used for people of smaller stature. Another special feature of this device is its ability to support a patient in biventricular or only right ventricular failure. (Courtesy Thoratec Laboratories, Pleasanton, CA. Courtesy Chris L. Wells, University of Maryland Medical Center, Baltimore, MD.)

VAD is spinning or rotating to circulate blood and providing sufficient cardiac output. The faster the VAD circulates blood, the less likely traditional methods for monitoring a patient's vitals will be possible.

Indications for Ventricular Assist Device. As mentioned, the use of VADs in the management of heart failure has significantly changed in the last decade. Forty percent of VADs are used as a *bridge to transplant*, and whose wait may be longer than they can be medically managed with optional care.[142] An equal number of VADs are used to determine the candidacy for heart transplantation or to qualify a patient for transplantation.[142] The implant of a VAD allows the transplant center and potential candidate to address medical or psychosocial issues to transform the VAD recipient into a more suitable heart transplant candidate. A small portion of individuals placed on VADs (approximately 5%) will be able to be weaned from the device once the native heart recovers from the cause of the acute dysfunction.[142]

Besides the use of VADs as a bridge to transplantation, this technology now allows selected people to receive long-term (permanent) support as a substitute for cardiac transplantation. This is referred to as *destination therapy*. The use of VAD as destination therapy and alternative to heart transplantation accounts for 15% of VAD implantation.[225,247]

The HeartMate II is the first second-generation device approved for use both as a bridge to transplant and as a destination therapy. (This is a link to a video that demonstrates its use: http://www.youtube.com/watch?v=PsHpKbwX1Yg.) A third-generation continuous flow device

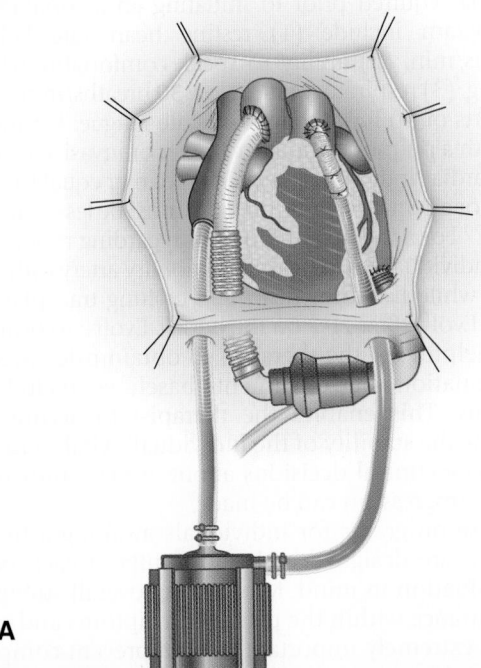

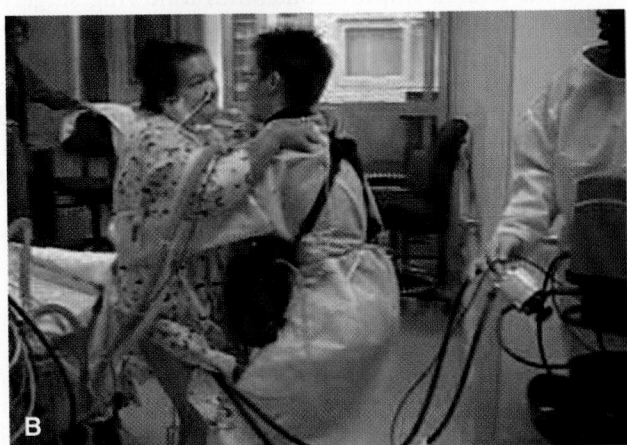

Figure 21-17

A, Thoratec CentriMag is a VAD that is designed to provide emergent and temporary (up to 14 days) right, left, or biventricular support with the goal to achieve hemodynamic stability. **B,** A patient is initiating gait training while being supported by a right VAD (CentriMag), another more long-term left VAD (VentrAssist), and mechanical ventilation. (A, Courtesy Thoratec CentriMag, LLC, Waltham, MA. B, Courtesy Chris L. Wells, University of Maryland Medical Center, Baltimore, MD.)

(HeartWare) is currently available and is approved by the FDA as a bridge to transplant (http://www.youtube.com/watch?v=HK8HSW3wZQg). A randomized, controlled trial (called ENHANCE) is under way comparing Heart-Ware as destination therapy against the HeartMate II.

Another study[235] comparing exercise tolerance and quality of life of a destination left ventricular assist device versus a heart transplant demonstrated that both groups increased exercise tolerance, although the heart transplant group showed greater improvement. Quality of life improved similarly in both groups. More research is needed to determine optimal modes of support and predictive factors for those individuals likely to recover.

Precautions and Considerations. There are several common components of all VADs that the physical therapist should understand (e.g., what they are, what their function is, and how to manage each component if an alarm is activated). There is a surgically implanted pump with cannulas (tubes) that circulate blood forward. The pump can be implanted internally or external to the body, and is connected to a controller that is external to the body via a drive line. The drive line typically exits the body at the right abdominal wall where it connects to the controller.

It is critical that the therapist makes sure the drive line is secured to the body with an adhesive anchor or abdominal binder. If the tissue around the drive line is disrupted, there is a significant likelihood that an infection could occur; it is very difficult to eradicate the infection once it contaminates the drive line. The controller is the computer that is programmed by the engineer to operate the pump. Finally, there is some type of power source. Most VADs can operate on AC power or portable batteries. For some VADs, there is a computer monitor or console that allows the therapist to monitor the function of the VAD. The VAD team can use the computer to make programming changes as indicated. See Figure 21-13 (HeartMate II) for an example of the common VAD components.

Besides the development of nonpulsatile pumps there has been the development of a short-term VAD. These pumps have become important because they can provide right, left, or biventricular support for days or weeks. These short-term devices have become extremely useful to temporarily support cardiac function for a transplanted heart that initially is not functioning properly. These VADs provide circulatory support while also supporting the donor heart with the goal for recovery. The most common devices for short-term support are the CentriMag (Fig. 21-17, A), Impella LP 5.0 (Fig. 21-18) (www.abiomed.com), and Tandem Heart (not shown; www.cardiacassist.com).

Future Trends

Current research centers on the role of stem cells in cardiac regeneration for use following myocardial infarction and as possible treatment for heart failure. Embryonic stem cells can differentiate into true cardiomyocytes, making them a potential source of transplantable cells for cardiac repair.[99]

SPECIAL IMPLICATIONS FOR THE THERAPIST   21-6

Heart Transplantation
Pretransplantation

The therapist's role in transplantation varies from region to region. In some areas, the therapist is only involved with the candidate pretransplantation if that person has been hospitalized. Some therapists will treat these clients in the outpatient setting to address muscle and endurance deficits. Goals are to improve function, strength, and exercise capacity, either to make them a stronger candidate for transplantation or to assist the transplantation team in determining timing for transplantation listing or timing for other medical or surgical interventions. Potential transplant

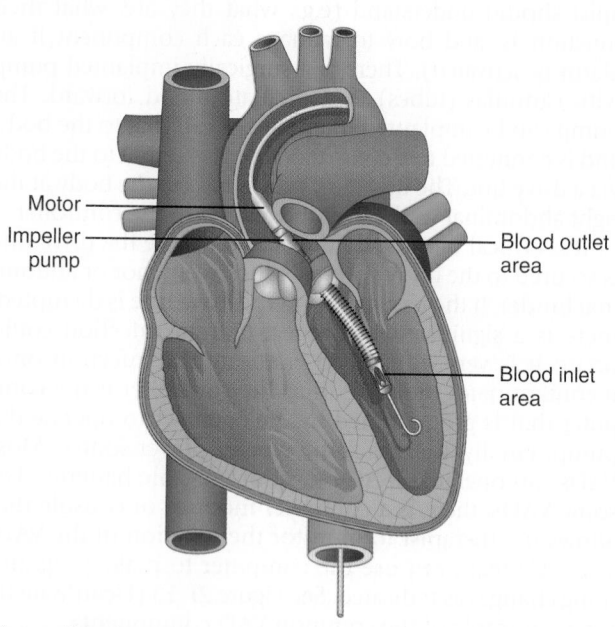

Motor
Impeller pump
Blood outlet area
Blood inlet area

Figure 21-18

Abiomed Impella LP 5.0. The Impella is the smallest VAD. This pump is positioned across the aortic valve, which allows continuous flow of blood from the left ventricle to the aorta. This pump can provide pump output up to 5 L/min. (Courtesy Abiomed Inc, Danvers, MA.)

recipients are educated on the role of physical therapy during the pretransplantation and posttransplantation periods.[173]

The outpatient pretransplantation physical therapy evaluation should include a general assessment of strength, functional mobility, range of motion, balance, and symptom inventory.[173] For all therapists working with individuals with heart disease, the 6-minute walk test provides a clinical assessment tool that is useful in developing an effective rehabilitation program and also offers the therapist some guidelines for recommending someone as a potential transplantation candidate.[74]

Other functional tests, such as gait speed, sit-to-stand test, short physical performance battery, and the physical performance tests, may be helpful in objectively assessing function and monitoring changes in capacity. This information may be very helpful to the medical and surgical management plan of care for the individual.

An individualized home exercise program is provided, including active and/or resistive upper- and lower-extremity exercises. These activities should be as functional as possible, as opposed to traditional open kinetic therapeutic exercises. Increasing the overall activity level is encouraged in any way possible (e.g., walking, stationary biking, swimming). Individuals with chronic heart failure tolerate exercise intervention only when they are well compensated with medications and/or close monitoring; consequently, the therapist should monitor the patient closely for signs and symptoms of heart failure and declines in activity tolerance.[173]

Criteria required prior to initiating an aerobic exercise program include (1) resting heart rate below 120 beats/min, (2) ability to speak comfortably while exercising, (3) respiratory rate below 30 breaths/min, and (4) reports of no more than moderate fatigue. For inpatients with a pulmonary artery catheter or invasive monitoring, cardiac index must be greater than or equal to 2 L/min/m² or a central venous pressure must be less than 12 mm Hg.[70] For a therapist's thoughts regarding mobilization of individuals who have a pulmonary artery catheter in place while listed for heart and/or lung transplantation, see Evolve Box 21-2 on the book's Evolve website.

It is helpful for the therapist to obtain prior medical information that documents baselines, including vital signs. This enables the therapist to accurately determine the stability of the individual's vital signs so appropriate clinical decisions about exercise prescription and progression can be made.

Exercise programs for individuals awaiting a heart transplant are designed with the results of each person's evaluation in mind. Maximizing overall strength and endurance within the person's symptoms and tolerance is extremely important to help prevent complications and to improve outcomes following surgery. Exercise intensity is largely based on ambulation time and the rate of perceived exertion.[173]

Side effects of medications contribute to the high incidence of musculoskeletal injuries (e.g., steroid myopathies and neuropathies, avascular necrosis, osteoporosis). Prevention is an important component of the pretransplantation habilitation (and posttransplantation rehabilitation) programs. See specific recommendations in "Osteoporosis" in Chapter 24.

Acute Care Phase

Postoperative

In the acute care setting, immediate postoperative considerations are important. Because most cardiac transplant candidates have experienced months of restricted activity before surgery, airway clearance and general strengthening are important aspects of early treatment.

The primary physical therapy goals in the early postoperative period are to focus on increasing functional mobility, restore balance, and fall prevention education, to prepare for discharge. The overall plan-of-care (Table 21-7) should include sternal precautions training (see Box 12-3), a plan for exercise progression, outpatient rehabilitation services, and a home exercise program. Client education is a key component of the posttransplantation program, and each member of the team must perform this role seriously. An excellent summary of acute care and outcomes for cardiac transplantation is available for acute care therapists.[72,381]

Physical and occupational therapy initiated in the ICU focuses on restoring mobility and functional skills, increasing strength, and improving balance and coordination; strengthening should be functional in nature and focus on muscles of the lower extremity, pelvic girdle, and trunk. Bed mobility, transfer training, and ambulation can begin as early as postoperative day 1 and progress as tolerated.

Table 21-7	Physical Therapy Management

Acute	Outpatient
Progress functional mobility	Exercise capacity testing and/
Sternal precaution training (see Box 12-3)	or functional field testing
Airway clearance techniques	Monitor vital signs
Monitor hemodynamics	Functional strengthening program and general stretching
Monitor anticoagulation/ antiplatelet levels	Re-entry into community (work, recreational, leisure activities)
Monitor for dysfunction	Monitor anticoagulation/antiplatelet levels
OHTx: infections and rejection	Monitor for dysfunction
VAD: pump dysfunction	OHTx: infections and rejection
Assess for neuromuscular changes, especially for patient with VAD support	VAD: pump dysfunction
Education:	Assess for neuromuscular changes, especially for patient with VAD support
• Side effects of medications	Education:
• Vital response to exercise	• Side effects of medications
Self-monitoring:	• Vital response to exercise
• Signs of infection/rejection/VAD alarms (see Table 21-3 and Box 8-1)	Self-monitoring:
• Home exercise program	• Signs of infection/rejection/VAD alarms
	• Home exercise program: osteoporosis care (weight-bearing activities, spine care, scar management)

OHTx, orthotopic heart transplantation; VAD, ventricular assist device.

Airway clearance and breathing exercises are essential to improve lung volume and prevent atelectasis. Frequent ambulation or cycling, along with slow, rhythmic reaching, turning, bending, and stretching of the trunk and all extremities many times throughout the day, help alleviate the surgical pain–tension cycle and facilitate pulmonary function.

Posttransplantation upper-extremity activities and restrictions may vary depending up the surgeon's preference and the individual's risk factors for sternal complications. Most activities can be completed within pain tolerance for each individual. For most individuals, upper extremities can be raised above 90 degrees in forward flexion or to tolerance; abduction may be limited to 90 degrees, but it is possible for the arms to complete abduction above 90 degrees with no increase in sternal wound complications.[73]

Postoperative reports of chest pain may be a result of the sternal incision and musculoskeletal manipulation during surgery. During the sternotomy, the costovertebral and costotransverse joint, thoracic spine as well as local musculature may be overstretched resulting in pain and dysfunction.[419] Sternal precautions are standard postoperative orders and must be reinforced; these vary from center to center[73] (see Box 12-3). It is important for the physical therapist to instruct the patient and caregivers in safe modifications for basic mobility while healing occurs. Precautions may need to be varied along with functional mobility modifications based upon individual patient risk factors.

Chest pain secondary to myocardial ischemia or coronary insufficiency does not occur in the early postoperative months because the heart has been denervated.[358] Any other symptoms that may be associated with ischemia (e.g., dyspnea, lightheadedness, faintness, or increase in perceived exertion) should be attended to and reported. Chest pain may also be associated with postoperative bleeding, pericarditis, and pleural effusion.

Progressive ambulation can be initiated as soon as the client can transfer. It is safe to use a cardiac or standard rolling walker. If the person has a dysfunctional lower extremity that requires an increase in upper-extremity weight bearing, the situation should be discussed with the surgeon. Upper-extremity weight bearing varies based on the surgeon's preference, quality of the bone, placement of the sternal wires, and comorbidities of the patient.

Ambulation and endurance training (e.g., use of a stationary bike or treadmill) should be progressed as tolerated (i.e., stable vital signs with electrocardiogram and good recovery without fatigue carrying over from day-to-day).

Heart recipients should be instructed in the use of the rate of perceived exertion scale or Borg scale as heart rate is no longer a viable means to indicate intensity. It is recommended to begin at a low intensity level (2-3 out of 10 on the modified rate of perceived exertion scale or 12-13 out of 20) and then progress to 16 out of 20 (equivalent to 75%-85% of predicted heart rate; see Table 12-13).[153,381] Intensity is always based on the individual's present medical condition and prior level of function.[52,153,381]

Once basic functional mobility has been restored, the use of a treadmill or bicycle or other aerobic activities can be introduced. The therapist should keep in mind the patient's goals and preferences, and assess for the presence of any musculoskeletal or neuromuscular deficits when prescribing an aerobic exercise program. The minimal goal is patient participation in at least 30 minutes of aerobic exercise at a moderate intensity level at least 5 days a week; this is the basic recommendation for all adults made by the American Heart Association.

Strength training should be a key portion of the posttransplantation rehabilitation to address the chronic decrease of muscular strength. For the upper extremities, resistive training will need to be consistent with sternal precautions and should be progressed once the surgeon has lifted the activity restrictions. Lower-extremity resistive training can be prescribed when the recipient is hemodynamically stable and should focus on functional activities such as closed-chain exercises, sit to stand, and step ups. Resistive training should be prescribed at 50% of 1 maximal repetition for 8 to 15 repetitions, 1 to 3 sets, and include 4 to 10 exercises that are repeated twice a week.[199,381]

Discharge Planning

There are many topics of clinical education that need to be disseminated to the recipient prior to discharge and continued in outpatient services. The therapist should educate the recipients on the adverse effects of the immunosuppressant medications on the neuromuscular and musculoskeletal system and how to minimize some of these effects with exercise and activities modifications.

The recipient also needs to know how to monitor heart rate, blood pressure, and use of the Borg Rate of Perceived Exertion Scale at rest and during exercise. The therapist should work with the medical team to reinforce healthy living behaviors and continue to reduce cardiac risk factors, including proper nutrition, healthy weight management, smoking cessation, medication adherence, and maintaining a routine exercise program. The recipient can even continue to exercise during bouts of rejection as long as there are no signs of unstable heart failure and vital signs are stable.[381]

By the time of discharge, the recipient and caregiver should be independent with monitoring vitals and proper hand washing techniques. They should demonstrate knowledge of signs and symptoms of infection and rejections and be able to articulate what action they to take when they suspect changes in health. This is an important topic for the therapist to assist the transplant team with, especially as these clinical health changes may be noticed first during exercise with a decrease in exercise tolerance, fatigue or an increase in fatigue, and abnormal changes in vital signs. Finally the recipient and caregiver should be independent with basic functional mobility and be able to comply with sternal precautions during mobility and activities.

Outpatient Rehabilitation

Rehabilitation should continue upon discharge with the focus on restoring functional independence, increasing muscle mass and strength, and increasing exercise capacity. If the patient has muscle atrophy, decrease in muscle strength and endurance, and is taking corticosteroids, it is advised for the recipient to be referred to outpatient physical therapy for comprehensive muscular strength and muscular endurance training, advance balance, coordination and community entry activities.[184]

Outpatient services should also continue to address osteoporosis rehabilitation and introduce scar management. After completion of outpatient physical therapy, the individual should be referred to outpatient cardiac rehabilitation to increase aerobic capacity. Typically cardiac rehabilitation programs focus on aerobic training and therefore it is important that the recipient see a physical therapist for a comprehensive exercise program to reach muscle mass, muscular endurance, and strength potential as described.

Although assessing work capacity is important, performing an assessment of transplant recipients must take into consideration daily life and daily activities first. Assessing potential for return-to-work and work requirements may occur as early as 3 to 4 months postop, depending on the recipient's occupation.

For more physical jobs (e.g., manual labor, any job that requires lifting, carrying, or repetitive load), work assessment typically does not occur until 6 to 12 months after transplantation. For example, a job that involves lifting requires assessment of cardiovascular compliance and hemodynamic stability during lifting. The team will assess hemodynamic status; the therapist will make objective assessments of the recipient's hemodynamic responses to activity and exercise.

Exercise

Individuals undergoing heart transplantation, like those undergoing coronary artery bypass surgery, are affected by preoperative inactivity, the adverse systemic effects of heart failure, postoperative deconditioning, and medication effects.

These individuals can benefit greatly from exercise rehabilitation (see also "Organ Transplantation" and "Exercise, Activity, and Sports" presented earlier in this chapter). Heart transplant recipients can experience significant improvements with exercise. Exercise can improve hemodynamics and assist in managing blood glucose level, hypertension, and weight management.[91]

There are many reasons why a heart transplant recipient demonstrates a decrease in exercise tolerance, but the appropriately prescribed exercise program and adherence can potentially minimize these adverse effects. Reasons for limitation include cardiac denervation, diastolic dysfunction, lack of pericardium, use of corticosteroids, and immunosuppressant medications, deconditioning and muscle atrophy, decrease in arteriovenous oxygen ($A\text{-}VO_2$) difference, and chronic stress effects of skeletal muscles related to heart failure.[184,199,381] With a comprehensive rehabilitation program, the heart transplant recipient can increase muscle mass and strength, increase VO_2, improved $A\text{-}VO_2$ difference, and improved quality of life, and experience a decrease in anxiety and depression.[91,199,381]

Effects of Denervation

Heart transplantation results in a denervated myocardium and an impaired ability by the autonomic nervous system to regulate cardiac function (Box 21-9). The resting heart rate after transplantation and denervation is higher than normal (usually in the range of 90-115 beats/min); an external pacemaker may be used if there is not an efficient heart rate to sustain cardiac output. Besides the effect of organ denervation on heart rate, most recipients are on antihypertensive medications that will further delay or blunt an increase in heart rate in response to exercise.

Persisting denervation and sympathetic vasoconstriction inducing functional vascular abnormalities prevent adequate increase in blood flow to exercising limbs and may contribute to decreased exercise performance.[42] Residual abnormalities of ventilatory and gas exchange responses to exercise following heart transplantation are also attributed to the chronotropic incompetence associated with denervation.[338] Chronotropic incompetence is a term used to describe the

Box 21-9

EFFECTS OF CARDIAC DENERVATION

- Heart rate
  - Elevated at rest
  - Blunted rise with exertion
- Stroke volume: blunted rise with exertion
- Cardiac output: 70%-75% of predicted
- VO_2: 70%-80% of predicted
- Pulmonary arterial pressure
  - Elevated at rest
  - Marked rise with exertion
- Anticipatory effect: lost
- Abnormal diffusion capacity
- Ventilation: increased response to exertion
- Loss of anginal pain as a warning sign of myocardial ischemia during early years of denervation

Clinical Meaning

- Need for extensive warm-up
- Decrease in exercise capacity
- Marked blood pressure response
- Rely on other data to detect ischemia

Modified from Braith RW: Exercise training in patients with congestive heart failure and heart transplant recipients, *Med Sci Sports Exerc* 30(10):S367–S378, 1998.

reduced heart rate response to exercise in heart transplant recipients.[33]

Decreased peripheral blood flow is only one variable to consider. Reduced oxygen extraction and utilization, differences in muscle fiber type, and decrease in oxidative enzymes may also contribute to reduced exercise tolerance.[80,381]

In addition to reduced cardiac and skeletal muscle performance, it is likely that the mood state of the individual; level of depression and anxiety; and decreases in cognitive function such as attention, concentration, and mental flexibility may affect the person's ability to participate in activity by affecting frequency, intensity, and duration of exercise.[80,102]

Over time some recipients may regain partial reinnervation, in which case the individual should be able to exercise at higher workloads, have fewer exertional symptoms related to cardiac limitation, and increase in heart rate may surpass 35 beats/min.[146] Partial reinnervation can be recognized when there is an increase in heart rate for each minute during a graded exercise test and when the heart rate decreases every minute during the recovery phase.[381] This phenomenon of reinnervation may begin months to years posttransplantation; the magnitude of reinnervation is variable.[381]

Studies show a functional significance during exercise in people with marked reinnervation, including a higher maximal heart rate, increased peak oxygen uptake, increased oxygen pulse, and earlier heart rate recovery after cessation of exercise (and falling more rapidly) than in the non-reinnervated cases.[219,220,395,406,431]

Importance of Warm Up and Cool Down

In the denervated myocardium, peak heart rate will (on average) only increase 15 to 25 beats/min from the resting level during moderate to high submaximal exercise. The therapist needs to remember that the recipient is catecholamine dependent, which means a minimal of 5 minutes is needed to warm up and allow the body to release catecholamines. Catecholamines will allow a minimal increase in heart rate and contractility, thus increasing cardiac output. Exercise should include large muscle groups to promote venous return, thereby maximizing filling of the ventricles.[51,277]

If the recipient does not warm up sufficiently, the feeling of fatigue and stress (similar to an athlete "hitting the wall") is experienced because of the inability to increase cardiac output to meet demands. The recipient is functioning in anaerobic metabolism.

The physiologic changes unique to heart transplant clients require a thorough warm-up before exercise to stimulate catecholamine release (epinephrine, norepinephrine) and to give the heart necessary time to prepare for peak activity. The warm-up period should be mild and long so as to prevent a large oxygen deficiency. Each step in the exercise protocol should be prolonged for up to 5 minutes to allow for a steady state of heart rate.[74]

Likewise, a cool-down period is essential after cessation of exercise to allow for the decrease in blood pressure and return to baseline. The recipient's heart rate can remain elevated for several minutes to an hour as a result of the loss of parasympathetic input and high levels of circulating catecholamines combined with an adrenergic hypersensitivity.

Individuals must be monitored for intensity and tolerance according to symptoms and by an rate of perceived exertion scale while working within an acceptable range for heart rate response. Remember that a rise in heart rate of more than 35 beats/min with a moderate to high level of exertion should not be observed during the early postop period. If this occurs, the person should be monitored closely for rejection.

Although denervation eliminates the sympathetic and parasympathetic nervous system input to the heart, the Bainbridge reflex, catecholamine response, and the Starling law allow for increased stroke volume. The Bainbridge reflex causes heart rate to increase as venous return to the heart stimulates volume receptors in the atria to trigger an increased heart rate. Release of catecholamines such as epinephrine and norepinephrine results in sympathetic stimulation to increase rate and force of muscular contraction of the heart. The net effect is to increase heart rate and stroke volume thus increasing cardiac output. At the same time, peripheral blood vessels constrict, resulting in elevated blood pressure.

The Starling law states that the greater the myocardial fiber length (or stretch), the greater will be its force of contraction. The more the left ventricle fills with blood, the greater will be the quantity of blood ejected into the aorta. This is like a rubber band: the more it is stretched, the stronger it recoils or snaps back. Thus a direct relation exists between the volume of blood in the heart at the end of diastole (the length of the muscle fibers) and the force of contraction during the next systole.

With the start of an activity there will be an increase in venous return associated with large muscle contraction that is responsible for early increases in heart rate; within 5 to 6 minutes after warm-up, catecholamines are activated and heart rate continues to increase. The heart rate may remain elevated after exercise secondary to remaining circulating catecholamines. Some recipients, particularly those with insufficient reinnervation, will achieve peak heart rate response postexercise rather than during exercise.[381]

A similar catecholamine response is not observed during isometric or isotonic contractions thus it is very important to incorporate a sufficient warm up or design an exercise program that includes evenly spaced short bouts of aerobic training (8 to 10 minutes), interspersed among the strength training component of the exercise program to allow the recipient's cardiovascular system to adjust to the new demands. The recipient may increase tolerance to strength, power, and muscle endurance training, which may improve compliance.[80,381]

With the loss of autonomic nervous system input over time, diastolic dysfunction occurs. The ventricles hypertrophy because of a loss of compliance and from working against elevated pulmonary and systemic pressures. These changes, combined with the reduced cardiac output, altered kidney function, and use of antihypertensive medications, lead to a reduction in cardiac reserve, or the ability to increase output from rest to exertion. This reduced reserve will be most evident during exercise, requiring close monitoring for exertional hypertension.

Importance of Monitoring Vital Signs

With the loss of vagal innervation, hypotension can be a problem, especially if there has not been an adequate warm-up or cool-down period. It is not uncommon to see a change in diastolic blood pressure (increase or decrease by 10-15 mm Hg) during exertion. Each transplantation center typically has guidelines for blood pressure parameters. In general, an increase or decrease in diastolic pressure greater than 20 mm Hg from baseline, a drop in systolic pressure greater than 10 mm Hg, or rise greater than 40 mm Hg above baseline or a peak pressure of 180 to 200 mm Hg warrants physician notification and adjustments to workload intensity or duration.

Following heart transplantation, there may be allograft vasculopathy, a manifestation of chronic rejection, which will cause increasing ischemia of the transplanted heart during increasing activity and exercise. This cardiac allograft vasculopathy can contribute to reduced oxygen uptake and a ventilation–perfusion mismatch, limiting exercise capacity.[361] With insufficient reinnervation, this ischemic condition may not be detected, except through the monitoring of vital signs and diagnostic testing.[183,357]

If the recipient has concomitant pulmonary involvement, abnormal diffusion capacities with altered ventilation responses may occur. These pulmonary components can cause a decrease in cardiac function with possible myocardial ischemia and possible mild desaturation.

Although there have been some documented cases of angina, most of these clients will not experience ischemia-induced angina as an early warning sign of cardiac impairment. This is another reason the therapist must follow appropriate exercise guidelines to stimulate a catecholamine response and monitor vital signs to assess cardiac function. The signs of decreasing activity tolerance should be reported to the transplant center because it may be associated with CAV.

Isometric Exercise

Isometric exercise, exercises that typically cause a breath hold, puts a volume stress rather than a pressure stress on the heart and cannot be graduated. This section is not considering such common exercises as quadriceps or gluteal muscle isometric contractions. In the acute care phase, the recipient's heart is very volume or preload dependent; consequently, aggressive isometric exercise will decrease preload and should be avoided at first.

This type of exercise should be initiated only with the physician's approval and performed with extreme caution only after considerable dynamic warm-up to raise the heart rate. Blood pressure response should be monitored closely during these stressful exercises. Once the client has moved past the acute care phase of rehabilitation and is function is restored, isometric exercise can be utilized if indicated and progressed as tolerated. The recipient should be instructed in breath control exercises to avoid a Valsalva effect.

Rehabilitation of Individuals with Ventricular Assist Device Support

Patients with acute decompensation as a consequence of myocardial ischemia and heart failure may be placed on an intraaortic balloon pump (see discussion in Chapter 12 and Fig. 12-14). This device improves myocardial perfusion and decreases left ventricular afterload. The catheter or balloon is typically inserted into the aorta via the femoral artery. If the patient is stable, low-level strengthening, range of motion, modified bed mobility, and airway clearance activities can be prescribed. The principal restriction is typically no hip flexion beyond 30 degrees. The therapist should monitor peripheral perfusion of the involved extremity and skin inspection for signs of limb ischemia or wound development. If the catheter is placed in the upper extremity, more functional mobility and reconditioning can be prescribed during time of support.

The key to the rehabilitation of patients being supported on a VAD is for the physical therapist to be competent on the operation and management of any alarms (see Fig. 21-15). With the nonpulsatile VADs, the therapist will need to modify how the patient is monitored because it is common for these individuals not to have a palpable pulse; the typical blood pressure method and use of pulse oximetry are commonly inaccurate or are unable to obtain the intended data. It is important that the patient fully understands how to use a subjective scale so the therapist can monitor the recipient's tolerance during the therapy sessions.

One of the benefits of VAD support is that the patient is no longer restricted in activity tolerance because of low cardiac output. This means that a comprehensive and aggressive rehabilitation program can be instituted including functional strengthening, functional mobility, and aerobic and anaerobic reconditioning. The therapist should monitor the patient and VAD function closely during exercise and report findings to the VAD team in case they need to make adjustments in the VAD setting to optimize VAD performance. Many of these patients can be discharged home within 2 to 3 weeks postimplant. Besides monitoring the VAD function, the rehabilitation goals and procedures are very common to what has been discussed earlier in this chapter for heart transplant recipients.

The therapist should monitor the patient for any VAD alarms and complications. The most common complications include bleeding in the early postoperative period, infections, thrombus formation, and stroke. It is advised that the therapist know and teach the patient what the normally functioning VAD units actually sound like. The sound of the VAD may change if there is pump dysfunction or thrombus.

The therapist should always follow the strict guidelines on drive line care to minimize the risk of drive line infection. If the pathogen gets seeded on the device the VAD may need to be explanted to address the infection and this typically leads to a high mortality rate. Finally, because stroke is still a major concern for patients being supported by a VAD, the therapist should conduct thorough neurologic screening, including cranial nerve, coordination, and functional testing. This is important to obtain a functional baseline for the individual in case a problem arises.

The prognosis for patients with VAD support is still under investigation and depends on the reason for the VAD implantation and medical status of the patient. In general the 1-year survival rate for destination therapy patients is 67% for all types of devices and 74% for nonpulsatile devices. The 2-year survival for all devices is only 46%.[225]

SPECIAL IMPLICATIONS FOR THE THERAPIST 21-7

Mechanical Circulatory Support

With an increasing number of centers nationwide routinely implanting these devices along with the increase in clinical trials to use VADs as a destination therapy, and patients allowed to be discharged home, it is likely that therapists in a variety of settings will be exposed to clients with these devices and become involved in the evaluation and treatment progression. For a therapist's thoughts regarding mobilizing individuals who have a pulmonary artery catheter in place while listed for heart and/or lung transplantation and mobilization of individuals on ECMO see Evolve Boxes 21-2 and 21-3, respectively, on the book's Evolve website.

Throughout the rehabilitation process, the therapist must monitor the international normalized ratio values for risk of bleeding (see "International Normalized Ratio" in Chapter 40), monitor drivelines during transfer training to avoid torsion or pulling, monitor VAD pump rate and pump output at rest and during exercise, observe for volume overload or dehydration (see "Fluid and Electrolyte Imbalances" in Chapter 5),

assess for neurologic and musculoskeletal complications, and observe for any signs of infection (see Box 8-1). In addition, there is a high incidence of orthostatic hypotension in this population, requiring monitoring of vital signs.

Lung Transplantation

Overview

The first lung transplant was performed in 1963 on a 58-year-old man with bronchogenic carcinoma; he survived for 18 days. Other lung transplantations were attempted without success because of lung rejection, anastomotic complications, or infection in the transplant recipients.

Long-term survival was achieved in 1965 with the discovery of chemical immunosuppression. The real breakthrough came in 1981, when the first successful human heart-lung transplantation was performed for the treatment of pulmonary vascular disease and again in 1983 with the first double-lung transplant.[347,426]

The lung is the most difficult organ to preserve its function during harvest and reimplantation. Upon the brain death of an individual there is a catecholamine storm that occurs, which leads to the disruption of the pulmonary capillary beds. The consequence is pulmonary edema and difficulty with ventilation and oxygenation.[143] There is also an increased risk of lung injury because of pulmonary contusion if the death of the donor was traumatic, as well as the risk of aspiration and ventilatory-related trauma and pneumonia.[347] Less than 15% of cadaveric donors have lungs suitable for harvest.[85] In 2011, the Organ Procurement and Transplant Network reported that only 1081 lungs were recovered while there were approximately 1700 candidates waiting for a suitable lung transplantation. Approximately 2300 individuals are registered for lung transplants annually.

With the shortage of available donor lungs, approximately 13% of people die while waiting on the transplantation list. The shortage has also led to the development of new preservation and organ improvement techniques, such as ex vivo lung perfusion.[103] The shortage has also led surgeons to accept more marginally functioning organs.

The original criteria for a suitable lung donor were very strict making lung transplantation a rare occurrence. The criteria included the age 55 years or younger, less than 20 pack-years (cigarette smoking), clear chest radiography, a PaO_2/FiO_2 ratio of 300 mm Hg or greater (partial pressure of oxygen in arterial blood/fraction of inspired oxygen), short period of mechanical ventilation support, absence of chest trauma, no evidence of aspiration/sepsis, absence of negative Gram stain organisms in sputum, and absence of purulent secretions.[48,158] The use of lungs from an extended donor pool has not significantly increased the number of procedures for many complex reasons.

Lungs are being accepted from older donors, with positive cultures for viral and negative Gram infections, and lower PaO_2/FiO_2 ratios. And organs are now being harvested from nonbeating heart-donor death; the decision to accept the organ lies with the transplantation center. In the past, it was common practice to perform more single-lung transplants as opposed to bilateral transplantations because of the insufficient number of suitable organs. More recently, surgeons are returning to bilateral transplantations, particularly for patients with pulmonary hypertension and even emphysema. The results indicate a decrease in chronic rejection complications, and slight improvement in median survival for bilateral transplants.

The surgeon can offer a living donor lung transplantation for the right candidate, but completion is rare. There was no living related lung transplantation reported in the United States for 2011. This reduction is attributed primarily due to the decrease of candidates with high acuity with the implementation of the Lung Allocation Scoring System. In 2011, 400 living donor lung transplantations were performed for all disease processes.[107]

Another advancement in improving and increasing the number of available organs and improving the transplant process has been in the clinical research of extracorporeal lung perfusion (ex vivo perfusion). The ex vivo perfusion and low-to-normal ventilation support as reported from the University of Toronto has allowed for the donor organ to be supported for up to 12 hours at normal temperatures of perfusion and ventilation that has permitted an active metabolic function for the lung.[105] In turn, this permits further time for medical treatment of such medical conditions as aspiration, pulmonary embolism, pneumonia, and pulmonary edema.

This procedure has allowed treatment for these conditions that typically would have rendered the lung unsuitable for transplant. This process may allow for more donor lungs to be treated, assessed, and used for transplantation. The authors[105] reported the ability to heal and use approximately 70% of the donor organs that were harvested and treated with ex vivo perfusion method in the preliminary research. With only 15% of multiorgan donors able to have their lungs harvested for transplant because of ICU management or related to brain dead event, this line of research shows promise. If normothermal conditions are maintained (instead of hypothermia) to allow for healing, more organs would become available for transplantation.

Indications

At present there are 65 active lung transplantation centers in the United States. Over the past 25 years there has been an expansion in the number of diseases that can be successfully treated by lung transplantation. In the past decade with the new LAS system, there has been a change in the distribution of recipients based upon their primary disease.

In 2001, 53.3% of lung recipients had chronic obstructive pulmonary disease (usually smoking-related emphysema, but also including emphysema caused by α_1-antitrypsin deficiency). In 2009, this percentage had been reduced to 29.2% with an increase in transplants occurring as a result of pulmonary fibrosis, from 16.2% to 33.6%. Other common indications include cystic fibrosis, idiopathic pulmonary hypertension, and secondary hypertension as a result of congenital diseases.[230,412]

Less frequent indications include lymphangioleiomyomatosis, eosinophilic granuloma, drug-induced and radiation-induced pulmonary fibrosis, and occupational-induced pulmonary diseases, such as silica farmer's lung, that lead to pneumonitis and pulmonary fibrosis. Pulmonary disease arising from an underlying collagen vascular disorder, such as scleroderma and lupus, can also lead to end-stage lung disease.

Although lung cancer has traditionally represented an absolute contraindication to transplantation, successful transplantation for bronchoalveolar carcinoma has been documented.[6,23,421]

Transplantation Candidates

There are many factors that are analyzed in the determination of a lung transplantation candidate because of the potential complications associated with these factors (see Box 21-3). Some of these variables include the presence of severe osteoporosis, the degree of systemic and pulmonary hypertension, diabetes mellitus, and coronary artery disease that may worsen after transplantation; severe gastroesophageal reflux disease (GERD), obesity, mechanical ventilation at the time of transplantation (higher mortality rate); underlying collagen vascular disease; presence of antibiotic-resistant infections, especially *Burkholderia cepacia* (a multiresistant bacterial respiratory infection associated with severe and often lethal postoperative infections); and previous thoracic surgery.[18]

It is both science and art to determine the best time to list a person for transplantation based on the disease process and its progression, blood type, other medical conditions, and even the activity level of the transplantation center. The important thing is to list a potential candidate for transplantation when the data suggest that the person can survive the expected waiting time for transplantation without developing other contraindications to transplantation.

Contraindications may include irreversible damage to other organs (unless a multiorgan transplant would be appropriate), certain types of infection, dependency on mechanical ventilation, cancer within at least 2 years from listing, chronic extrapulmonary infections from such viruses as HIV or hepatitis, untreatable psychiatric disorder, severe chest wall/spinal deformity, and documented poor adherence to medical care.[100,196] The candidate must be free of clinically significant cardiac, renal, or hepatic impairment. Some relative contraindications include severe functional limitations, mechanical ventilator support, obesity or severe osteoporosis.[158]

Until 2005 the allocation of donor lungs was primarily decided by the amount of waiting time a potential candidate had registered with UNOS. In 2005, the LAS was implemented with the goal to better identify candidates and utilize the very limited resources to achieve the best possible outcomes.

Lung Allocation System. The LAS is based on the previous 6 months of medical information. Box 21-10 presents the International Guidelines for selection criteria for transplant candidates. The LAS is the method to estimate for each candidate the risk of dying before transplantation, which is then mathematically combined with the probability of survival for the recipient after transplantation. The goal is to implant the most appropriate candidate at the most appropriate time to maximize outcomes

Box 21-10

INTERNATIONAL SELECTION CRITERIA FOR LUNG TRANSPLANTATION

General Criteria

- Must meet criteria listed in Box 21-3

Chronic Obstructive Pulmonary Disease

- BODE Index of 7-10 or at least 1 of the following:
  1. History of hospitalization for exacerbation with acute hypercapnia ($PaCO_2$ >50 mm Hg)
  2. Pulmonary hypertension or cor pulmonale or both
  3. FEV_1 <20% and either DLCO <20% or homogenous distribution of emphysema
- BODE: Index that includes body mass index, degree of airflow obstruction (FEV_1) degree of dyspnea (Modified Medical Research Council Scale), and exercise capacity (6MWT)

Cystic Fibrosis (and Other Bronchiectatic Diseases)

- FEV_1 <30%
- O_2-dependent respiratory failure
- Hypercapnia
- Pulmonary hypertension
- Other indicators of rapidly declining lung function (e.g., increasing numbers of hospitalizations, massive hemoptysis, increasing cachexia)

Idiopathic Pulmonary Fibrosis and Nonspecific Pulmonary Fibrosis

- DLCO <39% predicted

- 10% or greater decrement in FVC during 6-month follow-up
- Decrease in pulse oximeter <88% during 6MWT
- Honeycombing on high-resolution CT (fibrosis score >2)

Nonspecific

- DLCO <35% predicted
- 10% or greater decrement in FVC or decrease of 15% in DLCO in 6 months

Pulmonary Fibrosis Associated with Vascular Disease

- Persistent NYHA class III or IV on maximal medical therapy
- Low (<350 m) or declining 6MWT
- Failing therapy with intravenous epoprostenol (inhibits platelet activation and a vasodilator) or equivalent
- Cardiac index <2 L/min/m²
- Right atrial pressure >15 mm Hg

Pulmonary Arterial Hypertension

- Symptomatic, progressive disease (NYHA functional class III or IV with optimal treatment)
- Limited life expectancy (2-3 years)
- Hemodynamic parameters
- Cardiac index 2 L/min/m²
- Right atrial pressure 15 mm Hg
- Mean pulmonary artery pressure 55 mm Hg

6MWT, 6-minute walk test; DLCO, diffusing capacity for carbon monoxide (the extent to which oxygen passes from the air sacs of the lungs into the blood); FVC, forced vital capacity; NYHA, New York Heart Association.

Data from Orens JB, Estenne M, Arcasoy S, et al: International guidelines for the selection of lung transplant candidates: 2006 update—a consensus report from the Pulmonary Scientific Council of the International Society for Heart and Lung Transplantation, *J Heart Lung Transplant* 25(7):745–755, 2006.

---

and decrease the rate of deaths while waiting for a suitable organ to be found.

The LAS is calculated based upon the following measures: (1) expected number of days lived without a transplant during an additional year on the waitlist, (2) expected number of days lived during the first year post-transplantation, (3) the transplantation benefit measure which is calculated by posttransplantation survival minus the waitlist urgency measure. See Box 21-8 for the LAS formula and the variables that are factored in to calculate the waiting list urgency and the posttransplantation benefit.

General categories to cluster diseases have been made to allow the factors such as degree of pulmonary systolic pressure and amount of supplemental oxygen be more sensitive as a predictor in the LAS formula based upon the disease. Each candidate is assigned an LAS score; the procurement centers then allocate donor organs based on those LAS scores. The score is given as 0 to 100, and the higher the LAS score, the higher the probability of receiving an offer. The scores can be updated as the candidate's state of heath changes (see Box 21-8).

Allocation is based upon ABO compatibility and waiting time in descending order. Priority 1 includes patients who are suffering from respiratory failure. Respiratory failure is defined as need for mechanical ventilation, or using an FiO_2 greater than 50% to maintain oxygen saturation at greater than 90% or having a PaO_2 less than 50 mm Hg or a PCO_2 greater than 56 mm Hg. Priority 1 candidates

also include individuals with pulmonary hypertension because of pulmonary vein stenosis or hypertension with cardiac index less than 2 L/min/m². All other patients are classified as priority 2.

With the implementation of the LAS system there has been a decrease in the number of active patients waiting on the list, a decrease in waiting times, and an increase in the number of candidates transplanted, peaking in 2009 with a reported 3272 transplant procedures being completed worldwide.[92]

In 2009, 66% of the people actively waiting for transplantation were transplanted less than 12 months from listing. The mean wait time for a patient with a LAS score of 50 or greater has been less than 2 months. Since 2004 there has also been an increase in the number of older adults receiving a transplant, with older adults making up 22% of the total recipients.[92] There appears to be a trend of increasing mortality rates on the waiting list among patients with diseases such as pulmonary fibrosis, cystic fibrosis, and pulmonary hypertension, although still lower than the mortality rates prior to 2004. This trend and others are monitored and reassessed every 6 months by the Thoracic Organ transplant Committee to determine if changes need to occur to obtain the goals of the LAS.

The last reported death rate while waiting for a lung transplantation was 141 per 1000 patients, with potential candidates with idiopathic pulmonary fibrosis having the highest death risk, 261.8 per 1000 patients. Candidates who were 18 to 34 and 12 to 17 years of age had the highest death rate per 1000 deaths, with the death rate for candidates older than age 65 years declining since 2004.[412] With increased listing of older and sicker patients, including 9% of transplants needed by patients waiting in the ICU, the average mortality rate for candidates is approximately 13%.[158]

Transplantation Procedure

The four major surgical approaches to lung transplantation are single-lung transplantation, bilateral sequential transplantation, heart-lung transplantation, and transplantation of lobes from living donors. Since 2002, bilateral lung transplants have exceeded the number of single-lung transplants. Bilateral lung transplants accounted for 72% of the number of transplants completed in 2009.[92] This is attributable to the improved posttransplantation survival, and the possibly to the changes in the characteristics of waiting lists and LAS scores. Living-related procedures have markedly declined in frequency; heart-lung transplantation continues to consist of low numbers.[412]

Single-lung transplantation typically requires a posterolateral thoracotomy but some surgeons are using an anterior approach, whereas double-lung transplantations are typically done through bilateral anterior thoracotomies and a horizontal disruption of the sternum, referred to as a "clam shell." In this latter procedure, the rib cage and sternum are lifted anteriorly and superiorly as you would lift the hood of your car. This procedure allows good visibility of the mediastinum. The heart-lung procedure is still generally performed through a mediastinotomy.

In general, donor lungs should be the same size or just slightly larger than the recipient so that the donor lobes fill each hemithorax, avoiding persistent pleural space problems in the recipient. However, donor lungs must have a lung volume similar to (or less than) that of the intended recipient; larger lungs in single-lung transplantation can be placed on the left side, where the diaphragm has the potential to descend because of the absence of the liver under the left hemidiaphragm. In living-related donations, a lobe (generally the right or left lower lobe) is removed from each of the two donors and is used to replace the lungs of the recipient.

Denervation. The lung loses autonomic nervous system innervation below the bronchial anastomosis. This results in a loss of the cough reflex of the donor lung. There is a delay in bronchial dilation during exertion and impairment of ciliary function. These neurologic deficits increase the recipient's risk for sputum retention and pneumonia.

Complications

Postoperative complications of primary lung transplantation include infection; dysfunction of the bronchial and/or vascular anastomoses, including bronchial stricture or malacia, stenosis, or occlusion of the venous anastomoses; and acute or chronic rejection.

Primary Graft Dysfunction/Failure. Primary graft dysfunction (PGD), a severe form of ischemic–reperfusion injury after lung transplantation, affects as many as 25% of recipients and is associated with mortality rates as high as 50% within the first 30 days posttransplantation. Graft dysfunction or failure in lung recipients is similar to acute lung injury or adult respiratory distress syndrome and characterized by severe hypoxemia, lung edema, and parenchymal infiltrates with a low PaO_2/FiO_2 ratio (less than 300 mm Hg) and diffuse alveolar damage.[104]

In the immediate postoperative period, there is a change in ventilation and perfusion. This change may cause an injury to the pulmonary vascular system, depending on donor lung preservation, ischemic time, and primary pulmonary disease, particularly in the presence of pulmonary hypertension. These factors lead to epithelial ischemia and set up an increase in the inflammatory response, apoptosis, cellular necrosis, dysfunction of fibrinolytic and coagulation cascades, and alterations in the sodium–potassium adenosine triphosphatase pathway.[122]

There are donor- and recipient-related risk factors associated with PGD. Donor-related factors include age, African American ethnicity, female gender, history of smoking, prolonged mechanical ventilation, aspiration pneumonitis/pneumonia, trauma, and hemodynamic instability. Recipient-related risk factors include idiopathic pulmonary hypertension, use of cardiopulmonary bypass, and large blood transfusion.[48]

The leading causes of death for lung transplant recipients vary based upon the posttransplantation time. Causes of death within the first 30 days include non-CMV infections, which account for 20% of the deaths, and other complications, such as coagulopathy, disruption of one of the anastomoses, and ventilatory-induced injury.[92] In the case of acute PGD, ventilation needs may exceed the parameters of standard mechanical ventilation and ECMO may be required, in which case gas exchange takes place entirely, or in part, outside the body (see Fig. 21-19). See further discussion in "Future Trends" below.

The leading cause of death within the first year is from non-CMV infections (35.3%) followed by graft failure and other complications such as bronchial anastomosis dysfunction. After 3 years the primary cause of death is related to chronic rejection, which is referred to as bronchiolitis obliterans (25%), and there is an increasing rise in death associated with renal failure and cancer and complications of diabetes.[92,108,390,424]

Bone Density Loss. Glucocorticoid-induced changes in bone density are a significant medical complication after lung transplantation. In fact, unlike other transplant recipients who develop osteoporosis after surgery from antirejection drugs, lung recipients are more at risk for osteopenia or osteoporosis as a result of pretransplant decreased muscle mass, exposure to acute, high-dosage, or long-term use of corticosteroids, and lack of weight-bearing activities.

Besides the pretransplantation exposure to corticosteroids, lung transplant candidates commonly suffer from poor absorption of nutrients associated with the underlying disease process (e.g., cystic fibrosis, collagen vascular diseases). Malabsorption deficits and deficits of enzymes needed to utilize vitamin D further increase the risk for bone loss in individuals with these particular pathologies.

Immunosuppressive medications such as cyclosporine, mycophenolate mofetil, and azathioprine may be used in the pretransplantation period for the management of interstitial lung disease and autoimmune diseases such as scleroderma and lupus, which can result in further bone loss. The incidence of osteoporosis of the vertebral spine is 29% in pretransplant lung candidates; bone loss continues posttransplantation at a rate of 2% to 5% in the first year, with up to 20% of recipients having a significant progression of their disease. The incidence of fractures has been reported as high as 37% within the first year, primarily related to the adverse effects of immunosuppressive drugs on bone remodeling and bone quality.[56,88,236,375]

Lung transplant recipients are more likely to be exposed to higher immunosuppressive levels and longer exposure to corticosteroids than other organ transplant recipients as a result of the highly vascular and immunogenic nature of the lung, which further compromises the health of bone.[424,426] (See the section "Side Effects of Long-Term Immunosuppression" in this chapter, and see also Chapter 5.)

Gastrointestinal Disorders. Gastrointestinal problems are a considerable source of morbidity for lung transplant recipients, often because of the poor absorption patterns of nutrients previously mentioned in association with the underlying pathologies. The most common major complication is diverticulitis, requiring colectomy. Malignancy occurs slightly less often; minor problems such as polyps and benign anorectal disease have also been reported.[168]

Nutrition/Swallowing. Many recipients fail initial swallow studies after transplantation as a result of vocal cord injury or weakness. Many are also kept NPO (nothing by mouth) because of severe GERD requiring a gastrojejunostomy tube for nutrition during the NPO status. The therapist should be alert to the diet requirements of the individual, specifically whether the patient is cleared to take oral medications, liquids, solid foods, or whether the liquids need to be thickened to prevent aspiration. This is especially important if the individual has diabetes and requires quick increases of blood glucose but is unable to take juice or glucose tablets by mouth.

Diabetes Management. A large percentage of post–lung transplant recipients develop steroid-induced diabetes in the early postoperative phase. Lung recipients should be trained to check and manage their blood glucose; the therapist needs to be aware of the individual's glucose status before and during exercise. Patients should be encouraged to bring their glucometers to rehabilitation in case the need arises to check. The therapist should be aware of the facility guidelines and policies regarding blood glucose and exercise and be able to assist patients as needed to maintain blood glucose in an acceptable range for exercise.

Pulmonary Problems. The transplanted lung may have deficiencies in lymphatic drainage, especially in the early period after transplantation. Ventilation and ventilation–perfusion may be impaired if effusion is clinically significant. If effusion is persistent, affected by dietary intake, and cloudy in appearance, the patient should be evaluated for a chylothorax. Disruption of the lymphatic system appears to be restored 3 to 6 weeks after implantation, and mucociliary function may be depressed for up to 16 weeks.

Recipients frequently develop chronic bronchitis and may lack bronchus-associated lymphatic tissue as a result of chronic rejection. There is a delay in bronchodilation with the onset of exertion because of the denervated nature of the lung. Unlike the partial reinnervation of the autonomic nervous system in heart recipients, there is a long-term persistence of denervation in the donor lung.[390]

Other pulmonary complications include surgical trauma to the phrenic nerve, anastomosis dysfunction, pneumothorax, pulmonary embolus, and native lung hyperinflation. Although phrenic neuropathy is an infrequent complication of lung transplantation, the therapist may see evidence of it with subsequent diaphragmatic dysfunction. Clinical evidence of phrenic nerve damage may include atelectasis, pneumonia, elevated hemidiaphragm, and prolonged ventilatory support, and is reported in up to 30% of lung transplant recipients.

Narrowing of the bronchus can occur from the formation of granulation tissue or fibrosis or narrowing because of malacia. A stent can be placed within the airway to stabilize the lumen and allow for sufficient air flow.[7,158]

In individuals with an underlying obstructive disease (most commonly emphysema) who undergo a single-lung transplant, either acutely or chronically, the native lung can develop further hyperinflation because of increased lung compliance and the presence of bullous disease. The lung can displace the mediastinum away from the native lung; lead to a decrease in pulmonary function, dyspnea, tachycardia, and flattening of the diaphragm; and, if severe, can alter the flow of blood through the cardiac system.[7]

Increased attention is being paid to gastric reflux and dysphasia. One report indicates up to 70% of lung transplant recipients have an abnormal swallow on diagnosis testing. Dysphasia can lead to aspiration, pneumonitis, and an increased risk of pneumonia.[158] It is theorized that dysphasia is the result of intubation and use of the transesophageal echocardiogram probe placed during the surgery.

Rejection. The lung transplant recipient needs to be continuously monitored for rejection with 37% of all recipients suffering at least 1 episode of rejection within the first year.[92] Hyperacute rejection is predominantly an antibody-mediated response that results immediately after revascularization and leads to a massive immune response, thrombus formation, and destruction to the donor lung. Treatments may include plasmapheresis, intravenous immunoglobulin therapy, and augmented B lymphocytes-targeted therapy such as mycophenolate or azathioprine. The patients may be so critically ill, they require ECMO (see "The Medically Complex Patient: Critical Illness" in Chapter 5). There is a high mortality rate for individuals who suffer from hyperacute rejection.[302,426,434]

Acute rejection is generally a T-cell–mediated response. Class 1 HLA antigens located in all nucleated cells are recognized by CD8-recipient cells that mediate the immune response, whereas class 2 HLA antigens are found in endothelial cells that activate CD4 T lymphocytes. Both T-cell–mediated responses lead to the activation and proliferation of the recipient's immune response.[302,434]

Some people in acute rejection will be asymptomatic; but when a person in rejection is symptomatic, clinical manifestations may present as dyspnea, fatigue, fever and chills, oxygen desaturation, decreased exercise tolerance, and changes in x-ray findings (see Table 21-3). The recipient may suffer significant respiratory distress or even failure, requiring mechanical ventilator support.[158] Recipients should use a home spirometer daily to check for expiratory indices (e.g., FEV_1), and monitor exercise tolerance, which will show a decline as a consequence of acute rejection. Infection control should be heightened when any recipient is being treated for rejection. Careful handwashing and use of a surgical mask may be recommended.

Chronic rejection, referred to as bronchiolitis obliterans syndrome (BOS), accounts for 5% of deaths in the first-year posttransplantation. BOS is the fibrotic occlusion of small airways as a result of the adverse effects of rejection on the donor lung and is diagnosed by biopsy. It is a cluster of signs and symptoms of chronic rejection that has not been diagnosed as having cellular changes; BOS cannot be confirmed in up to 50% of recipients. BOS is defined as a decrease in FEV_1 greater than 20% that cannot be attributed to acute rejection or infection.[332,424] BOS is associated with the following risk factors: frequent and severe episodes of acute rejection, lymphatic bronchitis, viral infection, GERD, CMV, and prolonged ischemic times.[424]

BOS is also the leading cause of death in recipients 1 to 5 years posttransplantation at a rate of 25.4%; an additional 37% are diagnosed with BOS during this midterm time period.[92] The exact cause of late graft failure (more than 5 years posttransplantation) is difficult to determine, but death from graft failure is most likely a result of BOS and accounts for an additional late mortality rate of 16.4% to 19.3%.[92,158]

Infection. The absence of the cough reflex and diminished mucociliary function in the denervated lung leads to insufficient mucus clearance and contributes to the elevated frequency of pulmonary infection (at least three times more common than in heart transplant recipients). Pulmonary infection is also related to the increased level of immunosuppressive medications required posttransplantation, poor nutritional status, and the fact that the lung is exposed to environmental factors. Signs and symptoms of infection may be very difficult to distinguish from acute rejection (fever, tachycardia, tachypnea, fatigue, malaise, decrease in exercise tolerance, oxygen desaturation, and respiratory failure) except there is an increase in sputum production with a productive cough in most cases.

Infections are associated with a significant negative impact upon transplant outcomes. Non-CMV infections are associated with an 18% to 35% mortality rate across the posttransplantation continuum. Pulmonary bacterial infections accounts for a 25% mortality rate in patients confirmed with bacteremia.[92] Lung transplant recipients may develop a viral infection; these infections peak within the first 3 months posttransplantation and typically involve the CMV or Epstein-Barr virus. CMV infections account for 2.5% mortality within the first year.[92]

Much effort is taken to test the donor and recipient for viral infections so proper medications can be administered to decrease the risk of infection. Finally, the recipient may develop a fungal infection, commonly *Candida* or *Aspergillus*, although mortality and morbidity rates associated with fungal infections have decreased with the availability of new antifungal medications.

Other. Lung transplant recipients are at risk for other complications as previously discussed in other transplantation sections of this chapter. These complications significantly reduce quality of life, and increase mortality and morbidity rates. For example, cancer accounts for up to 12% of recipient deaths after 5 years posttransplantation. Renal dysfunction is present in almost 24% and 33% of lung transplant recipients at 1 and 5 years posttransplantation, respectively. There is a high prevalence of cardiac risk factors as well, with 57% of recipients having been diagnosed with hyperlipidemia, 39% develop diabetes, and almost 83% with systemic hypertension.[92] Slightly more than 9% of deaths after 10 years are related to cardiovascular disease.[92,158]

Prognosis

Survival rates for lung transplantation continue to improve as surgical techniques and postoperative care improve despite the fact that the recipients are older and there has been an expansion of the medical criteria for donor lungs. The 1-, 3-, and 5-year survival rates for single and bilateral transplants are 83.8%, 63%, and 47.5%, respectively. Lower survival rates are found for retransplantation, with a 27.9% survival at 5 years.[411] There are differences in survival rates based upon primary pulmonary diagnosed and by age. For example, individuals with congenital defects, pulmonary fibrosis and pulmonary hypertension and graft failure have approximately a 10% decrease in survival rates when compared with cystic fibrosis and chronic obstructive pulmonary disease.[411] Patients who are either 11 to 17 years old or older than 65 years of age have a lower survival rate when compared to other age groups.[411]

There are few heart-lung transplantations performed annually. The complexity of candidate medical status, the technical surgical issues, and the management of both heart and pulmonary function lead to a decrease in survival when compared with isolated lung transplantation. The 1-, 3-, and 5-year survival rates for combined heart-lung transplantation are approximately 67.5%, 49.6%, and 40.1%, respectively.[411]

Future Trends

With the increasing history of lung transplantation there is much research to be done in fully understanding and assessing the effects of transplantation. Research should continue in the assessment of survival rates based upon new advances in procurement and candidate selection and pretransplant management. But beyond these topics, research needs to expand in the area of post-operative management including further studies in dysphasia and dysfunction of other neuromotor structures such as the phrenic nerve and vagus nerve that may impact mortality and morbidity. Research is needed in the arena of quality of life, rehabilitation, and community reentrance for these recipients.

Extracorporeal Membrane Oxygenation. One of the most exciting areas of pretransplantation management is the use of ECMO as a bridge to transplantation (Fig. 21-19). Once thought of as an extreme medical intervention to salvage an individual for possible transplant, which was very controversial, ECMO is becoming more common in the management of individuals with refractory hypoxemia.

ECMO is a device that allows the gas exchange to occur outside the body to aid or replace the function of the lungs that no longer can properly regulate the body's pH by performing adequate gas exchange. ECMO could interface with the body via venous-to-venous or venous-to-arterial

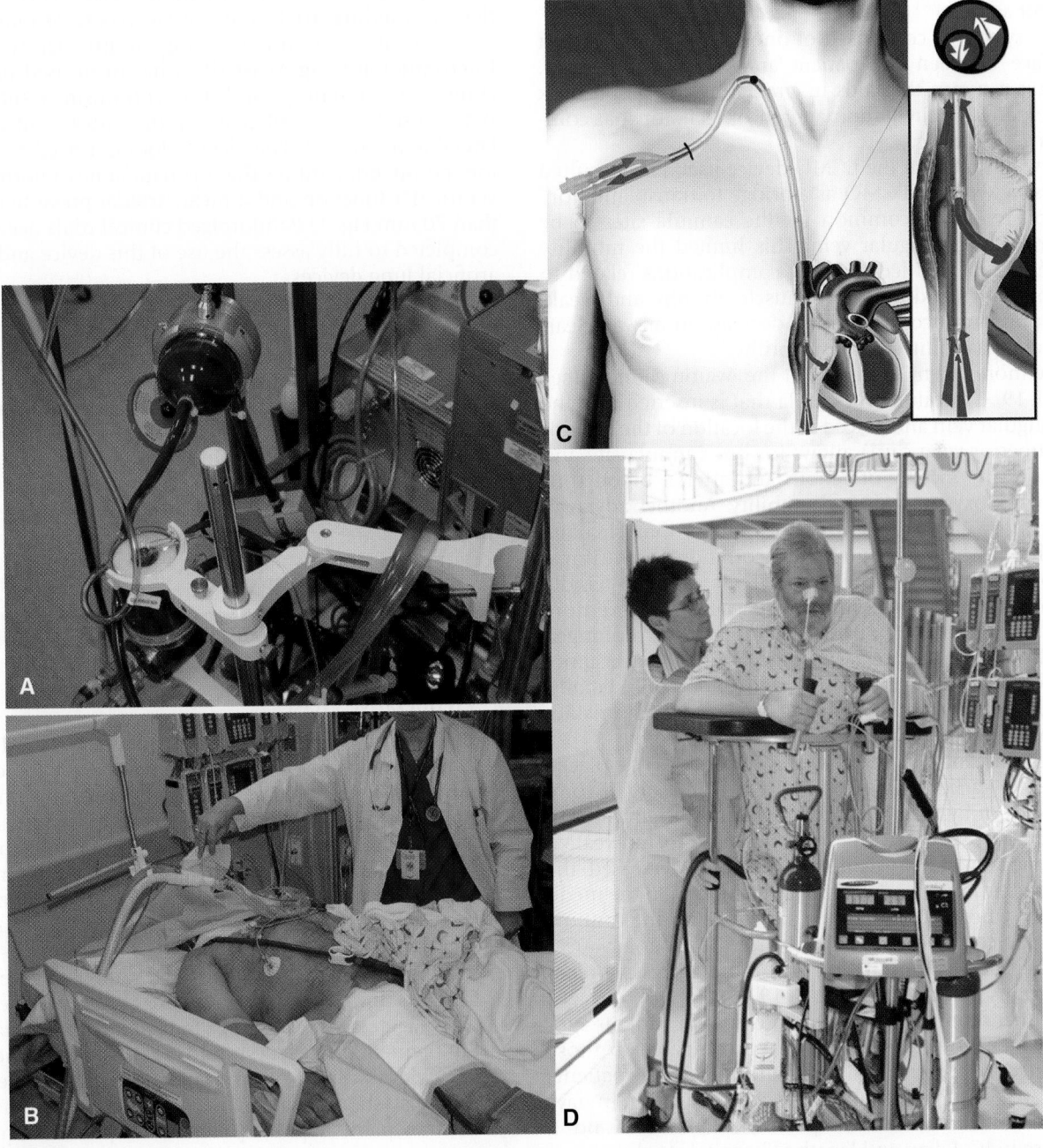

Figure 21-19

Extracorporeal membrane oxygenation (ECMO). A, ECMO is used to support the cardiopulmonary system by controlling gas exchange and assisting the heart in blood circulation. With ECMO, venous blood is circulated through a CO_2 scrubber and membrane oxygenator (white canister) and returned to the body via a centrifuge pump (red and silver machine) as oxygenated blood with a desired $PaCO_2$ and PaO_2. **B,** Depending on how the machine is cannulated to the patient, ECMO can assist or control cardiopulmonary function. The cannulation sites in this individual are the femoral vein and artery. In more critically ill patients the cannulas can be inserted in the inferior vena cava or right atrium and the aorta, primarily bypassing cardiopulmonary function. This photo illustrates the traditional nonambulatory ECMO. **C,** Work is currently being done to develop an ECMO system that would allow the patient to be mobilized out of bed and allow more aggressive rehabilitation to prevent adverse effects of immobility. With the new Avalon cannula (Avalon Laboratories, LLC, Rancho Dominguez, CA), the surgeon can connect the patient to ECMO via one site allowing more mobility. **D,** With a portable nonpulsatile pump (Thoratec CentriMag) and new oxygenator system, the physical therapist can now promote early mobility. (A, B, and D courtesy Chris L. Wells, University of Maryland Medical Center, Baltimore, MD. **C,** From Garcia JP: Ambulatory venovenous extracorporeal membrane oxygenation: innovation and pitfalls. *J Thoracic Cardiovasc Surg* 142(4):755–761, 2011. Used with permission.)

circulation. In venous-to-venous circulation, the common cannula sites are the femoral and jugular veins. Venous-to-arterial ECMO cannulas are typically femoral vein to femoral artery or right atria to pulmonary trunk or to left atria for cardiac support; this latter approach is only used when the chest has already been surgically open for another reason and the heart needs circulatory support as well.[264]

The system is comprised of one or two cannulas that interface between the patient and the ECMO device. There is a pump that aids in circulating the blood back to the patient's circulation and an oxygenator that completes gas exchange.

New advances in the ECMO device itself have resulted in this new use of ECMO as a bridge to transplantation. Previously, it was common for the cannula sites to be femoral vein to jugular vein. This limited the mobility of the patient and led to many complications related to immobility including severe muscle atrophy and weakness, pressure ulcers, delirium, decrease in airway clearance, and gastrointestinal dysmotility.[147]

The more recent invention of the Avalon cannula (see Fig. 21-19, *C*; a bilumen cannula that is inserted into the right jugular vein and placed in the location of the inferior and superior vena cava) allows for one cannula site and decreases the mixing of venous and arterial blood thus improving oxygenation and mobility. Another advancement is the improvement of the pumps that circulate the blood. The new pumps are commonly centrifugal pumps that have the ability to increase speed to handle the increase in cardiac output, especially with exertion. The oxygenators have also been designed for prolonged use. They have a smaller surface area and lower resistance therefore decreasing the trauma to the blood cells. Finally, heparin-coated circuits are being used to decrease risk of thrombus formation.[147]

These advances have allowed individuals to be placed on ECMO earlier to decrease the additional organ complications of hypoxemia and prolonged mechanical ventilation. In many cases patients are able to be weaned from mechanical ventilation, which has decreased the risk of pneumonia and decreased the burden to the medical team when mobilizing the patient. With the cannula site in the cervical region, along with the other advances described above, ambulation and more aggressive rehabilitation is possible (see Fig. 21-19, *D*).[154,155,405]

Fuehner reported significant outcomes in patients supported by venovenous ECMO when compared to those supported by mechanical ventilation.[151] These patients had a 30% reduction in mortality, 23% reduction in days on mechanical ventilation posttransplantation, and a decrease in ICU days and length of hospital stay by 21 and 29 days, respectively.[151]

The ECMO device is also being used more in the postoperative period for the management of PGD. Marasco[264] reported the increase success of using ECMO within the first 48 hours posttransplantation for PGD. His group reported success in supporting the patient and the new donor lungs through the initial period of PGD to allow for healing and medical intervention.[179,240,264] This allowed for a significant reduction in the patient requiring emergent retransplantation. In his study, Marasco also

reported that patient's outcomes were poor when ECMO was introduced after postoperative day 7 for reasons of graft failure that may have been infectious or rejection.[264]

Artificial Lung. Work continues in the areas of developing an artificial lung device that would further allow function and improve quality of life for the treatment of end stage lung disease. For example, oxyRVAD is a device that is in animal trials and the University of Pittsburgh continues its work in developing an artificial lung. The Interventional Lung Assist (iLA) has been used in 1500 clinical cases in Europe and shows promising results. The iLA is inserted into bilateral femoral artery and contralateral femoral vein. This device does not need a circulatory pump, but requires that the patient has a normal left ventricular function and a mean arterial pressure greater than 70 mm Hg.[286] Randomized clinical trials need to be completed to fully assess the use of this device and other artificial lung devices.

The potential benefits in utilizing either an artificial lung device or ambulatory ECMO device are significant and include a more effective way of oxygenating the individual while preventing the adverse effects of immobility. A study reported a case of a patient ambulating with a physical therapist while on ECMO to improve functional mobility and endurance prior to transplant.[256] It may even provide a means for long-term "respiratory dialysis."[258] Xenotransplantation is also under intense scrutiny, with some encouraging experimental results (see section on Xenotransplantation in this chapter).[256]

Lung Transplantation
Preoperative Phase

The therapist working with transplantation candidates is usually treating people who may have a life expectancy of less than 2 years. In the preoperative therapy program, functional goals are the primary focus, with attention directed toward increasing functional mobility, maintaining or improving strength and muscle endurance, improving breathing patterns whenever possible, and educating the recipient and the caregiver regarding the transplant process.

Many people with end-stage lung diseases are able to improve their aerobic capacity, especially with aggressive pre–lung transplant rehabilitation. Supplemental oxygen should be increased as needed to achieve a SpO_2 of at least 88% with exercise. The therapist should stay in close communication with the transplant team if a potential recipient is requiring more oxygen to complete the same level of exercise or if the person's performance declines significantly for several days in a row. Prompt assessment by the transplant pulmonologist is recommended if the individual is exhibiting signs and symptoms of exacerbation of the individual's disease.

The psychosocial elements of care, especially depression and anxiety, are an important aspect of intervention. Helping the recipient manage anxiety during rehabilitation in the preoperative phase is extremely important, and often requires referral to a psychologist, social worker, or psychiatrist. Often there is significant anxiety posttransplantation; the more the recipient is able to deal with it preoperatively, the better the recipient can manage it after surgery. This is especially true given that maximizing psychosocial status improves long-term physical health outcomes in the transplantation population.[117,349]

More recently, investigators are reporting the safe and successful rehabilitation of patients with pulmonary fibrosis and pulmonary arterial hypertension. The pulmonary rehabilitation studies have small numbers, but report promising results with improvements in 6-minute walk test, decreased dyspnea and anxiety, and improvement in various quality of life measures. These studies do have mixed results regarding improved oxygen capacity for patients with pulmonary fibrosis.[157] Currently, studies are under way that are examining the benefits of pulmonary rehabilitation for individuals with pulmonary hypertension. Fox et al reported an increase in 6-minute walk test and oxygen capacity and noted no medical events during rehabilitation.[148]

Acute Care Phase

Following the initial surgery, the ICU plan will focus on supporting respiratory function and initiating airway clearance techniques to minimize the risk of infections and resolve atelectasis, stabilize hemodynamics, and mobilize out of bed to begin functional training. During this acute phase the patient should be monitored closely for an ischemic and reperfusion injury and rejection.

It is important that the therapist monitor vital signs, including oxygen saturation and breathing patterns. A few centers place these patients on reverse isolation, but for most the medical staff will follow standard precautions. Therapy may be initiated on postoperative day 1 and may range from positioning for skin care and pulmonary management to beginning functional mobility.

Posttransplantation pulmonary blood flow and ventilation are variable and may be affected by the function of the graft, function of the native lung, presence of pulmonary hypertension, a change in cardiac output, or diaphragmatic function. For the patient who is having difficulty with ventilation and perfusion, the therapist will need to assess oxygenation and breathing patterns to determine the optimal position to maximize respiratory function.

Positioning

In some transplantation centers, it has been advised that single-lung transplant clients should be placed in the side-lying position with the transplanted side up and the native lung down. This was thought to help to decrease the edema and compression in the new lung and promote drainage, as well as decrease mediastinal shift toward the operative side, thus promoting optimal inflation. Other opinions favor placing the transplanted lung down to improve ventilation and perfusion matching. However, patient intolerance for lying on their transplanted side may not make this possible because of pain and discomfort from the thoracotomy incision and chest tubes.

In contrast, it has been advised that during an episode of acute rejection, when perfusion to the transplanted lung is severely diminished, the transplanted lung be positioned down with the native lung up to increase perfusion. Research in this area is needed; one study has shown that positioning needs to be evaluated on an individual basis and may change over the course of the postoperative period.[159]

Positioning may depend on the severity of an ischemic reperfusion injury and its state of healing, which can usually be determined within the first 10 days postoperatively. If the injury is severe, it may progress to diffuse alveolar disease. Other factors that may affect positioning tolerance include rejection, infection, cardiac output, renal function, and skin integrity.

The simple use of towel rolls or pillows can aid in optimal positioning of the chest and spine in any of the intervention or resting postures to help decrease the work of breathing. Careful attention must be given to the positioning of the upper extremity to aid in or discourage the recruitment of accessory muscles in conjunction with surgical incision precautions (see Box 12-3).

The client may be weaned from a ventilator within 24 to 48 hours if the organ is functioning well and patient is able to clear airway effectively, but some people may remain on a ventilator longer. Supplemental oxygen is usually no longer necessary by the time of hospital discharge. Client education, including various airway clearance techniques, handwashing skills, strength training, and breathing exercises, are initiated early in the recipient's recovery.

Airway Clearance and Breathing Techniques

The therapist will need to assess respiratory function along with a complete evaluation to determine the best airway clearance technique (ACT) and ventilatory strategies to maximize ventilation and oxygenation. Traditional chest physical therapy can be completed early in the postoperative period if the person is hemodynamically stable.

The therapist must consider the risk and benefits of completing percussion and vibration in Trendelenburg positions and should confer with the surgeon to determine whether the position is contraindicated. Along with the increase in reports of dysphasia in lung transplant recipients,[22] current research suggests there is an increase in silent aspiration resulting from gastroesophageal reflux that worsens pulmonary function.[66,67]

If the therapist does position the person in a Trendelenburg position, the therapist should not complete the treatment right after feeding. The postpyloric position of the feeding tube should be documented and feeding should be stopped a minimum of 30 minutes before treatment or wait at least 30 minutes until after the person has consumed food or beverages. Many transplant patients experience delayed gastric emptying and stomach contents remain for longer than normal. The therapist should also coordinate ACT with pain medications and ventilation weaning protocols.

Before and after every manual ACT, the therapist should inspect the chest tube sites to rule out air leak and subcutaneous emphysema. Care should be taken not to apply any ACT directly over the insertion site. The recipients will have a decrease in coughing and efficient breathing because the lung is denervated (Box 21-11). Pain, anxiety, and any decrease in mental alertness needs to be considered when selecting an ACT for the recipient

Conditioned breathlessness is a term that applies to the lung transplant recipient. These clients often need to relearn how to normalize the breathing pattern and to understand that the feeling of breathlessness does not necessarily indicate a lack of oxygen, infection, or rejection, but is instead a function of anxiety and muscle fatigue. Exertional dyspnea and tachypnea may be seen for several weeks to months postoperatively.

There are several techniques that can be used to improve the recipient's breathing pattern. Diaphragmatic breathing should be facilitated if the phrenic nerve is intact. Positioning in slight trunk and hip flexion will relax the abdominal wall to decrease the work of the diaphragm.

The therapist will need to examine the movement of the diaphragm in various positions (supine, sidelying, prone, sitting) to determine the best position for training. Segmental breathing exercises can be used to facilitate diaphragmatic breathing and chest wall expansion. Inspiratory hold, pursed-lipped breathing, and phonation exercises may also be effective tools to improve breath control.

Soft-tissue and joint mobilization to the thoracic spine, rib cage, and abdominal wall can be effective manual techniques to improve chest wall mobility and therefore decrease the work of breathing. Once the surgical incision is healed, scar management should begin in order to avoid soft tissue restriction, decreased rib mobility, and chronic pain.

Finally, upper-extremity muscle endurance exercises should focus on improving accessory respiratory function. Strengthening of scapula and thoracic spine musculature should be addressed to further improve the breathing pattern and decrease dyspnea.[32,267]

Box 21-11

EFFECTS OF LUNG DENERVATION

- Decreased tidal volume
- Decreased lung compliance
- Decreased chest wall compliance
- Delay in bronchodilation
- Impairment of mucociliary blanket
- No cough reflex
- Decreased breath holding
- Loss of Hering-Breuer reflex*
- Increased work of breathing (WOB)
- Increased dyspnea
- Exercise
  - Decreased tidal volume
  - Decreased minute ventilation
  - Increased respiratory rate

*Increased volume on inspiration will reflexively decrease respiratory rate with a period of apnea (cessation of breathing).

Anxiety control in clients with severe hypoxemia can help decrease respiratory rate and improve the breathing pattern. However, it is very difficult to decrease respiratory rate in people with lung disease, especially interstitial pulmonary fibrosis, even during nonanxious periods. Anxiety can be a barrier to rehabilitation and ventilation management if the person does not have a sufficient coping mechanism.[121]

Telling the client to "slow your breathing down" is not an effective instructional or biofeedback technique. Instructing the individual to use pursed-lip breathing with a pause at the top of inspiration, then an inspiratory hold before exhaling is an effective means of decreasing the respiratory rate and aid in gas diffusion. Biofeedback may be a useful technique with this population, but there are no studies available in this area. There are several excellent resources to guide the therapist in establishing specific therapeutic exercises to improve respiration and phonation.[150,187,268,269]

It is important for the therapist to monitor vitals and signs and symptoms of rejection and infections as well as the critical complications such as pulmonary embolus and pneumothorax. A decrease in tolerance to exercise and desaturation may be the first identified symptoms during exercise. Subtle desaturation may also be related to insufficient warm-up periods before exertion. Saturation levels should be normally above 93%; supplemental oxygen may be needed when saturation levels are at or below 90% (see Table 21-4).

It may be beneficial to use supplemental oxygen during therapy to maximize the rehabilitation potential. Any changes in exercise tolerance and vitals should be reported to the transplantation center for further investigation.

Rehabilitation in the early postoperative period should focus on airway clearance, functional strength, and functional mobility training. Once basic functional mobility is restored, therapy should focus on progressing aerobic exercise, muscular strength, and muscular endurance tolerance. Once rehabilitation goals are met, the recipient should begin to increase cardiovascular and pulmonary endurance and continue completing their muscular training. If pulmonary function is insufficient for extubation, functional mobility training and strengthening should progress as appropriate with proper mechanical ventilation support, including supplemental oxygen to help the person progress and contribute to the weaning process.

Outpatient Phase

Client education regarding the importance of consistently following an at-home or community-based program to increase and maintain metabolic equivalent level (multiples of resting oxygen consumption) with exercise is essential. There is some evidence that recipients with poorer caregiver relationships and greater psychologic distress may need additional support to perform the self-care behaviors expected after lung transplantation. Recognition of problems in this area may require consultation with the case worker or discussion with the transplant team to plan intervention prior to discharge.[117]

It is recommended that the recipient be referred to outpatient physical therapy immediately after hospital discharge for further strength and functional training, with the goal of improving muscular strength and endurance along with aerobic capacity so that the person can maximize the benefits from traditional pulmonary rehabilitation and participate easily in community-based activities without fatigue. The recipient should be able to self-monitor and progress through the exercise program independently by the time they are discharged from the supervised rehabilitation program.

A traditional pulmonary rehabilitation program is an effective therapy for recipients whose primary limitations are decreased aerobic capacity and muscle weakness and who would benefit from extensive client education and support. The majority of people should participate in a walking program to help minimize weight gain, muscle atrophy, osteoporosis, and edema (effect of cyclosporine on kidneys). In addition, resistance exercise especially for the lower extremities is essential to improving strength and function. The therapist should verify on a weekly basis that the recipient is compliant with self-monitoring of blood pressure, blood glucose, and spirometry volumes and report any changes to the physician's office.

The peak effect of transplantation on lung function is typically within 3 to 6 months, at which point the limiting effects of surgically related factors (e.g., postoperative pain, altered chest wall mechanics, respiratory muscle dysfunction, acute lung injury) have dissipated. After double-lung replacement, normal pulmonary function is usually achieved.

Communication with the transplant team, especially the transplant coordinator, is important during the outpatient phase of rehabilitation, particularly when complications arise. It is essential to keep the transplant team informed of the patient's progress with rehabilitation and any deficits that are noted.

Exercise

Before lung transplantation, candidates are characterized by very low exercise capacity (VO_2max 14 mL/kg/min) because of the restricted oxygen uptake caused by reduced ventilatory capacity, ventilation–perfusion mismatching, or decreased diffusion capacity and/or blood shunting.[263]

After transplantation, overall pulmonary function improves and exercise capacity increases because the lungs can now perform improved oxygen uptake and maintain oxygen saturation levels greater than 90% during submaximal exercise (see also "Organ Transplantation" and "Exercise, Activity, and Sports" discussed earlier in this chapter). An aerobic endurance training program improves submaximal and peak exercise performance significantly in lung transplant recipients.[387,390] Muscular endurance and strength training has shown improvements in strength or muscle function and improvements in bone density.[428]

By the end of the first year after transplantation, approximately 80% of recipients report no limitations in activity; exercise is not limited by ventilation despite a decrease in tidal volume and increased respiratory rate with exercise.[338] However, the recipients reach only 40% to 60% of predicted VO_2 capacity.[7,172,197,428] The therapist should continue to follow the guidelines outlined in Table 21-4.

Despite these improvements, cardiopulmonary exercise testing consistently shows that VO_2max in recipients of single- and double-lung transplants is still lower than sedentary, healthy, matched control subjects.[162,429] Maximal oxygen consumption is depressed despite the absence of clinically significant cardiac or ventilatory limitations on exercise. There is evidence that the continued decrease in exercise capacity is related to deficits in oxygen extraction, abnormal microcirculation oxygen delivery, anemia, and alterations in muscle fiber type and oxidative enzymes.[7,172,239,338] Evidence shows, however, that posttransplantation rehabilitation can improve aerobic capacity closer to predicted levels.[271]

A number of studies show that lower-limb skeletal muscle dysfunction may be a major factor in exercise limitation. Clients report lower-extremity fatigue rather than dyspnea as the main reason for exercise intolerance. There may be an intrinsic abnormality of the skeletal muscle in recipients of transplants. An in-depth summary of exercise limitations in this population is available.[428]

It is essential to emphasize to all lung transplant recipients the importance of lifelong exercise to improve and maintain function and well-being. In addition, the therapist should convey to the patient that it may take much longer to achieve optimal strengthening and endurance capabilities when compared with nontransplant patients as a consequence of the many factors discussed in this section.

Pancreas Transplantation

Overview

Pancreas transplantation has become an accepted therapeutic approach to treat type 1 diabetes, which is caused by the autoimmune destruction of pancreatic islet β cells, thereby successfully restoring normoglycemia. Pancreas transplantation is mainly performed for individuals with type 1 diabetes mellitus.

Although whole pancreas transplantation represents a physiologic approach to reverse diabetes mellitus, a new technique of pancreas islet β-cell transplantation is now available for carefully selected individuals with severe, unstable type 1 diabetes. Islet transplantation remains an experimental procedure in the United States and awaits formal results of ongoing phase III trials to justify biologic licensure and transition to standard of care. Transplanting insulin-secreting cells is a low-invasive procedure with the possibility of modulating graft immune response before transplantation, allowing reduced or minimized immunosuppressive medications.[423]

In June 2000, the *New England Journal of Medicine* prereleased the findings of a report (the Edmonton protocol) from researchers injecting pancreas cells near the liver in eight people with type 1 diabetes. The cells took up residence in the liver and began producing insulin.[366]

Since that time continued advancement has occurred through extensive collaboration between key centers.[238] For example, the Collaborative Islet Transplant Registry (CITR) reports continued improvement in efficacy and safety outcomes of islet transplantation with fewer islet infusions and adverse events per recipient.[29]

A current trial is ongoing by the Clinical Islet Transplantation (CIT) Consortium in which islet cells are transplanted into two groups: islet-alone treatment in individuals with type 1 diabetes with severe hypoglycemia unawareness, and islet after kidney transplant in patients with prior successful kidney transplant.[211]

There are still limitations with this approach, but newer pharmacotherapies and interventions designed to promote islet survival, prevent apoptosis, promote islet growth, and prevent immunologic injury are approaching clinical trial status.[276]

Indications

Unlike heart, lung, or liver transplantations, pancreas transplantations are not an immediately lifesaving procedure. Recipients have to be carefully selected in order to reduce morbidity and mortality; investigation of myocardial and cerebral vascularity is essential.

Even with these guidelines, pancreas transplantation has become a routine treatment for type 1 diabetes with uremia or for those who previously received a kidney transplant. Pancreas transplantation at the same time as a renal transplant is considered more often now, especially if the diabetes has been difficult to control.[354]

Although the recipient must remain on lifelong immunosuppressive medications, 80% to 90% 1-year survival rates are considered very acceptable given the alternatives of insulin therapy, dietary restrictions, hypoglycemic and hyperglycemic episodes, dialysis, and potential long-term complications associated with diabetes mellitus.[94] Recent research shows that pancreas transplants can provide excellent glucose control in recipients with type 2 diabetes as well.[291,356]

Diabetic nephropathy is the leading cause of kidney failure in people with type 1 diabetes. Successful pancreas transplantation leads to normal glycemic control in people with type 1 diabetes, but historically this type of transplantation has been limited to people with both kidney failure and diabetes. Pancreas transplantation does not reverse the advanced complications (e.g., diabetic retinopathy, vascular sclerosis) present with long-term diabetes. However, the effect of pancreas transplantation on reversing neuropathy (i.e., improved nerve action and potential amplitudes) is possible.[11]

Despite the difficulty of this surgical procedure and the many potential complications, pancreas transplantation before the development and progression of diabetic nephropathy is being suggested for this population group.[198,384] However, this is a controversial subject because others believe that, in the absence of end-stage renal failure, there is no justification for pancreas

transplants alone, except where diabetes itself poses a greater risk to life than the transplantation procedure.

Individuals with diabetes and renal involvement and individuals with unstable diabetes may be helped with an islet or pancreas transplant, but this approach is still considered experimental. Such transplantation may speed up the need for a kidney replacement. For individuals with well-controlled diabetes and intact function, pancreas or islet transplantation may not be advised given the risks of immunosuppression following transplantation.[354]

Simultaneous pancreas-kidney transplantation is an accepted treatment for carefully selected candidates with type 1 diabetes and ESRD and in a small group of individuals with uncontrolled severe metabolic problems.[365]

Transplant Candidates. Many centers consider pancreas transplantation contraindicated in people with cardiovascular disease, especially atherosclerotic vascular disease and congestive heart failure, because of the poor outcome after pancreas transplantation when either of these risk factors is present. Some centers may consider transplantation in cases of atherosclerotic vascular disease if coronary lesions are corrected before transplantation. Other risk factors include age older than 45 years, obesity, and hepatitis C.[262]

Transplantation Procedure. The donor pancreas is most often placed extraperitoneally on the right side using the recipient's (native) vessels. It is necessary to drain the pancreatic exocrine secretions by channeling them to the urinary bladder or into the stomach. This may be accomplished with a variety of surgical techniques.

In the case of pancreas islet cell transplantation, cells removed from a cadaver are injected into the blood vessel leading to the liver (portal vein). Because development of these procedures is in its infancy, they presently require the cells from two pancreases, matched for blood type, to produce an apparent cure. Better methods for extracting cells from the donated pancreas or a way to grow the cells in the laboratory are being investigated.

Complications. Surgical complications remain the primary source of morbidity after pancreas transplantation (especially when combined with a simultaneous kidney transplantation), affecting approximately 35% of studied cases.[337] This may change with continued advances in surgical techniques, but data are limited at this time. Specific complications include graft vascular thrombosis, pancreatic hemorrhage, intraabdominal bleeding or infection, allograft failure, and urologic problems associated with the bladder drainage surgical technique.

Other nonsurgical complications may include posttransplant pancreatitis possibly secondary to ischemia reperfusion microvascular injury and the more typical transplantation complications associated with other solid organs, such as infection and side effects of prolonged immunosuppression.

Complications of the pancreatic islet cell transplantation are minimal, but long-term safety and effectiveness of this technique remain to be proven. The recipients must take a combination of three immunosuppressive medications to prevent the body from rejecting the transplanted cells. The increased risk of cancer, infection, and other long-term side effects associated with these medications has been discussed.

Prognosis. Over the past 20 years there has been a progressive improvement in outcomes after pancreas transplant alone, simultaneous pancreas-kidney, and pancreas after kidney transplantation.[174] Vascular disease remains the major cause of both morbidity and mortality after transplantation in recipients who have diabetes and is correlated with the degree of vascular disease before transplantation. Graft and recipient survival rates in diabetic recipients are higher when the recipient receives simultaneous pancreas-kidney transplantation. These survival rates are even higher when the kidney donor is a living related donor.[336]

Compared with other abdominal transplantations, pancreas transplants have had the highest incidence of surgical complications. This trend may be reversing owing to identification of donor and candidate risk factors, better prophylaxis regimens, refinements in surgical technique, and improved immunosuppressive regimens.[223] Steroid withdrawal is possible in up to 70% of pancreas transplant recipients as long as the person is maintained on some form of immunosuppression (usually tacrolimus).[204,215]

Even with surgical complications, pancreas transplant recipients' survival rates are 96% to 98% at 1 year and 92% at 3 years.[24,174] Data on survival rates following islet transplantation are limited given the recent development of this technique and the scarcity of donor islet cells. Of those people who have received autotransplants worldwide following total or subtotal pancreatectomy, insulin independence has been achieved in 40%. Islet allotransplantations have demonstrated improved metabolic control in more than 50% of cases, and insulin independence in approximately 20%.[306]

Future Trends. More widespread application of pancreas transplantation is expected in the future, with earlier transplantation indicated in the course of diabetic disease.[130] Successful transplantation of human fetal pancreatic tissue into recipients who have type 1 diabetes is under investigation.[38] Strategies to reduce the metabolic consequences of hyperglycemia on nerves and to enhance axonal regeneration are being studied.[319,329,438]

As previously mentioned, pancreatic islet β-cell transplantation may replace whole-organ transplantation, or may be used in combination with kidney transplantation or after pancreas transplantation failure. Xenogeneic sources of cells, engineered islet cells with genes that induce immunoprotection, some form of β-cell replacement therapy, and sustaining populations of transplanted β cells are all part of current research.[132,133,353]

Research is under way to develop an artificial pancreas with the ability to automate insulin delivery based on continuous glucose monitoring data while taking into consideration exercise and meals.[180,245,259,399,442] Availability of preliminary systems is still sometime down the road, with estimates of Europe by 2016 and the United States in 2018.[326]

Skin Transplantation

Human cadaver allograft skin is widely used for covering excised burn wounds when limited available skin donor sites or the overall client condition does not permit immediate grafting with autologous skin. However, recurring problems are associated with human cadaver allograft skin, including limited supply, variable quality, ultimate immune rejection, and the potential for bacterial and viral disease transmission.

Several biotech companies are working on tissue-engineered skin substitutes that could revolutionize the treatment of severe burns as well as pressure ulcers and other serious wounds. Engineers can now mass produce postcard-size sheets of durable, uniform tissue that the body readily accepts. Cells can be grown on biodegradable lattices to produce the functional equivalent of dermis and epidermis.

The FDA has already approved products for use in burn cases requiring immediate closure of wounds but where there is not enough undamaged skin to be used as autografts. These products are also approved in Europe for plastic and reconstructive surgery and for the treatment of excisional wounds.

One type of patch is made up of two layers; the chemicals within the bottom layer help the new cells form a pattern similar to the normal dermis instead of the normally developing pattern of scar tissue. As dermis cells regenerate, blood vessels grow into this microscopic scaffolding over a 7- to 10-day period.

Within 3 weeks, the scaffolding dissolves as the new dermis grows in under the top layer of silicone. Acting as a pseudoepidermis, these patches close the burn injury to invading bacteria much like a normal skin graft would do.[64] Later, the top silicone layer can be pulled away easily for skin grafting.

Another type of newly developing artificial skin product is dermal fibroblast cells (connective tissue in the skin that produces collagen and elastic fibers) constructed from the foreskin of newborns and cultured onto a mesh that serves as the scaffolding. During the formation of tissue, the fibroblasts proliferate within the mesh, where they secrete human dermal collagen, matrix proteins, and growth factors.

One foreskin the size of a postage stamp can produce as many as 200,000 grafts. The separation process discards the immune stimulating cells and saves the fibroblasts (stimulate growth and regeneration of the dermis) and keratinocytes (provide protective epidermis). It takes approximately 6 days for the layer of dermis to grow, at which time the keratinocytes are added, forming the tough outer layer known as the *stratum corneum*, which is capable of resisting injury and infection. The complete process takes approximately 20 days.

In both types of artificial skin products, the patches act as a template or scaffolding on which new dermis cells can form, allowing early wound excision and immediate wound closure with control of fluid loss. Reduced cases of rejection and reduced risk of infection and disease transmission potentially allow for early ambulation, earlier rehabilitation, and faster recovery.

Recognizing wound infection after graft application can be challenging because the graft appears white or yellow after hydration with wound fluid. Any change from baseline at the wound site; in the amount or type of edema, erythema, drainage, odor, and warmth; unexplained fever; or pain should be reported to the physician.

Normal skin grafting is still necessary for burns, but the new developing dermis allows surgeons to place over the wound a thinner, smaller skin graft from donor sites that heal within 1 week. Temporary skin replacement for excised burn wounds before autografting has been attached as long as 74 days without rejection and without hypertrophic scarring.

The drawbacks to this procedure are the cost (approximately $1000 for one 4- to 10-inch sheet) and patch fragility, making the grafts difficult to work with and more easily dislodged than skin grafts. Researchers are continuing to explore the concept of an off-the-shelf full-thickness skin product that would be a permanent replacement for skin.

Stem cell-based therapy has been explored much over the last few years in the area of burns and wound healing. One study demonstrated improved closure by applying a topical treatment of mesenchymal stem cells to patients with chronic skin wounds.[25] In another study, patients treated with bone-marrow derived mesenchymal stem cells demonstrated improved healing and reduced pain of their chronic lower-extremity ulcers.[106] Mesenchymal stem cells have also been studied in an application of fibrin/thrombin spray, which accelerates wound closure.[140,164]

In addition to wound healing, burn wounds represent a major clinical challenge because of loss of large areas of skin, but stem cell therapy has not played a large clinical role to date. However, trials are ongoing using bioreactors, which serve to grow cells in a three-dimensional environment to isolate and grow skin stem cells from the patient and the apply them to burned areas of skin using a spray gun for maximal coverage and healing.[112]

REFERENCES

To enhance this text and add value for the reader, all references are included on the companion Evolve site that accompanies this text book. The reader can view the reference source and access it online whenever possible.

CHAPTER 22

Introduction to Pathology of the Musculoskeletal System

KEVIN HELGESON

The new century, characterized by increasing individual participation in high-speed travel, complex industry, and competitive and recreational sports, also is marked by significant increases in primary musculoskeletal system injury and conditions that have enormous impact on society.

The fact that the skeletal system with its associated soft tissues provides a protective covering for important structures such as the brain and heart and essentially makes up the limbs puts this system at risk for traumatic and repetitive insults and injuries (Box 22-1).

More than ever, the gap between science and clinical applications of therapeutic exercise has been narrowed. New diagnostic technology and the new branch of study called genomics are providing an increasing understanding of the molecular basis for disease and injury. This new knowledge is changing the approach for health care intervention in many areas, including the musculoskeletal system.[114]

The ability to document the influence and effects of exercise at the molecular and cellular levels has resulted in early functional rehabilitation, preventive exercise programs, and the use of exercise as a first-line intervention for many conditions. Maintaining good musculoskeletal health and recovering quickly from musculoskeletal injury or disease contribute to an individual's overall health, welfare, and quality of life.

Better technology has made it possible to measure what happens to muscle with age without painful and invasive muscle biopsies. For example, newer imaging methods are measuring fatty infiltration of skeletal muscle, a contributor to metabolic problems and muscle dysfunction with aging. Magnetic resonance spectroscopy (MRS) and computed tomography (CT) are being used to characterize this fatty infiltration. Scientists are looking for ways to reduce the risk of falls, fractures, and disability from changes in the supportive and protective skeletal muscle.[15] Intervention strategies including various kinds of exercise are under investigation.

Preclinical disability is a new concept observed in aging adults (65 years of age or older). It is defined as progressive and detectable but unrecognized decline in physical function.[52] Early signs of decline in physical function are observed in the ability to perform mobility tasks and activities of daily living needed to maintain an independent living status.[2,20]

Preclinical disability may be seen as an increased time to complete a task, modification of a task, or decrease in the frequency with which a task is performed. Individuals with preclinical disability are at increased risk for progression to more severe disability; early identification of decline in physical function is important if intervention to stop the decline is possible.[51,52]

More than 50% of injuries in the United States are to the musculoskeletal system; 28.6 million Americans incur musculoskeletal injuries each year. Fractures, sprains and strains, and dislocations account for nearly half of all musculoskeletal injuries.

Annually, an estimated 7 million Americans receive medical attention for sports-related injuries.[34] Children younger than age 15 years account for more than 3.8 million sports-related injuries in the United States each year.[26] Violence-related sports and recreational injuries (e.g., being pushed, hit) are increasing among children and adolescents.[33] See "Occupational Injuries and Diseases" in Chapter 4.

Severe cerebral palsy and other developmental disorders (see Chapters 23 and 35) are more common than ever before, because many infants with these complications at birth now survive and live into adulthood. The age span of humans has become progressively longer, with a variety of accompanying age-related conditions such as osteoporosis and degenerative joint or disc disease. Arthritis is the leading chronic condition reported by Americans age 65 years and older.[12]

In addition, the musculoskeletal system often is confronted with immobilization secondary to major illness or injury, bed rest, or casting or splinting of a specific

---

Box 22-1

COMMON MUSCULOSKELETAL DISORDERS

- Fracture
- Dislocation
- Subluxation
- Contusion
- Hematoma
- Repetitive overuse, microtrauma
- Strain, sprain
- Degenerative disease

body region. The musculoskeletal system reacts quickly to the lack of mechanical stress and normal loading (immobilization) in ways that may adversely affect recovery and rehabilitation.

The physical and physiologic responses of the musculoskeletal tissues and resultant deterioration occur within days but take many months to reverse. In fact, 3 weeks of bed rest has a more profound impact on physical work capacity than three decades of aging.[43,53] (See "Tissue Response to Immobilization" in Chapter 6; see Table 6-7.)

Like all other body systems, the musculoskeletal system does not function in isolation. Therefore, primary disease of the musculoskeletal system can significantly affect other body systems and vice versa. In addition, certain diseases are systemic, meaning that all body systems, including the musculoskeletal system, can be involved to some degree. The challenge to develop an effective rehabilitation program is heightened when one is faced with complex, multisystem disorders (see Chapter 5).

Many musculoskeletal disorders are drug induced or are side effects of treatment for conditions such as cancer. Drug-induced musculoskeletal disorders represent a broad clinical spectrum, from asymptomatic biologic abnormalities to severe and even life-threatening diseases. Myopathies, arthralgias, arthropathies, connective tissue diseases, and periarticular disorders (e.g., tendinopathy, enthesopathy, adhesive capsulitis) have been linked with medications. An increasing number of drugs have been implicated in inducing rheumatic symptoms and/or syndromes. All drug classes can induce musculoskeletal disorders, but the majority are caused by corticosteroids, vaccines, antibacterials, and lipid-lowering agents.[13]

The purpose of this section is to provide an overview of the musculoskeletal system, keeping in mind the biologic response to trauma discussed in Chapter 6 and examples of how primary diseases in other organs affect the musculoskeletal system, and vice versa, and to begin to examine the local (musculoskeletal) and systemic (e.g., immune system, endocrine system, gastrointestinal system) effects of exercise. An approach that assesses all the systems and considers underlying pathology is essential when identifying the source of impairments.

ADVANCES IN MUSCULOSKELETAL BIOTECHNOLOGY

Advances in molecular biology techniques have extended the potential for understanding musculoskeletal disorders from the microscopic (histologic) level down to the molecular level of gene expression within individual cells. These advances are initiating new avenues of research and, ultimately, novel clinical interventions.

Orthopedic surgery has been revolutionized by tissue engineering, including biologic manipulation for spinal fusion[41]; synthetic skeletal substitute materials[13]; preservation and restoration, transplantation, or fabrication of avascular tissue (e.g., meniscus, articular cartilage)[86,99]; and joint restoration instead of joint replacement.[62,108]

Other technologic advances are under scientific investigation, such as bone implants to stimulate bone development and prevent limb loss associated with cancer[17,112,124]; injectable degradable scaffolds as bone substitute for bone

defects, to strengthen osteoporotic vertebral bodies, or heal compression and nonunion fractures[39,41,66,77]; synthetic muscle regeneration; and new materials and plastics, making it possible to replace spinal discs or extend joint replacements by an additional 10 years or more.

In addition, the first nerve tubes for the repair and regeneration of peripheral nerves is now available for clinical use.[74] Biodegradable polymer scaffolds to support axonal regeneration in the transected spinal cord are being investigated in animal studies. Multichannel scaffolds are seeded with neural stem cells and Schwann cells needed to facilitate regeneration across the cord. The hope is to have such treatment available immediately for anyone with a spinal cord injury.[76]

The influence of biopsychosocial-spiritual stress on the physical body (an area of study referred to as psychoneuroimmunology) has become an acknowledged and accepted factor to consider in the healing process for each individual. Approximately 40% to 80% of adults in primary care report only their physical symptoms (including musculoskeletal manifestations), leaving a large portion of clients with significant psychologic distress undiagnosed.[64] Physical therapists often see clients demonstrating various somatoform disorders (see Chapter 3); recognizing this underlying component is important in understanding the biology (and pathology) of the musculoskeletal system and therefore planning appropriate intervention.

Gender discrepancies in rates of injuries and muscle mass response to strength training or deconditioning continue to be established in specific work and sports populations.[11,24,35] Differences in ligamentous laxity, muscle strength, endurance, muscle reaction time, and muscle recruitment time in males versus females and athletes versus nonathletes may provide additional important information for prevention and rehabilitation of musculoskeletal injuries.[36,71,107]

Women double their rate of injury during ovulation, when levels of estrogen are the highest. Training and conditioning differently during different times of the month may help protect women from injury.[29,37,60] The effectiveness of neuromuscular and proprioceptive training in preventing anterior cruciate ligament injuries in female athletes has been demonstrated.[78]

Men increase their muscle volume about twice as much in response to strength training compared with women; men also experience larger losses in response to detraining than women.[63,79]

The military has recognized that females undertaking strenuous exercise alongside males are at increased risk of injury. Equal opportunities legislation has been interpreted to require identical training for males and females, but some segregation of training may be necessary to reduce the excess risk of injury to females, provided the outcome of training is no less favorable to either gender.[16,97]

BIOLOGIC RESPONSE TO TRAUMA

An understanding of the biologic processes related to trauma is essential when considering the information in this chapter. The reader is encouraged to review Chapter 6 for a complete update on this topic when reading the next sections of this chapter.

AGING AND THE MUSCULOSKELETAL SYSTEM

Much has been written about the effects of aging on the musculoskeletal system, especially in light of exercise as an effective intervention for so many diseases and conditions. Participation in a regular exercise program is an effective intervention to reduce or prevent a number of functional declines associated with aging.

Endurance training can help maintain and improve various aspects of cardiovascular function (as measured by maximal VO_2, cardiac output, and arteriovenous oxygen difference) and enhance submaximal performance. Importantly, reductions in risk factors associated with disease states (e.g., heart disease, diabetes) improve health status and contribute to an increase in life expectancy.[8,10]

Strength training helps offset the loss in muscle mass and strength typically associated with normal aging. Additional benefits from regular exercise include improved bone health and therefore reduction in risk for osteoporosis; improved postural stability, thereby reducing the risk of falling and associated injuries and fractures; and increased flexibility and range of motion.[9]

Although not as abundant, evidence also suggests that involvement in regular exercise also can provide a number of psychologic benefits related to preserved cognitive function, alleviation of depressive symptoms and behavior, and an improved concept of personal control and self-determination.[8,10]

Sports-related injuries among people born between 1946 and 1964, now referred to as "boomeritis,"[93] are on the increase as older adults continue to participate actively in sports of all kinds. Physical therapists can provide valuable preventive education regarding the aging process as it relates to the musculoskeletal system and exercise. This presentation is a brief summary of the findings to date; more in-depth discussion is available.[58,72]

Muscle

Sarcopenia

Overview and Definition. Age-related loss in muscle mass, strength, and endurance accompanied by changes in the metabolic quality of skeletal muscle is termed *sarcopenia*. Sarcopenia involves both the reduction of muscle mass and/or function as well as the impairment of the muscle's capacity to regenerate.[40]

Muscle mass is lost at a rate of 4% to 6% per decade starting at age 40 in women and age 60 in men.[61] The greatest decline in both men and women occurs with inactivity, acute illness, and after age 70, at which time the mean loss of muscle mass has been measured as 1% per year.[117] At all ages, females appear to be more vulnerable to loss of lean tissue than males; however, in men and women, muscle strength can be maintained through exercise well into the eighth decade.[48,49,65]

Etiology. The etiology is multifactorial, involving changes in muscle metabolism, endocrine changes (e.g.,

low testosterone levels), nutritional factors, and mitochondrial and genetic factors.[84,89] It remains uncertain how much age-related loss of muscle function is an inevitable consequence of aging, nutritional status, or dysregulation of neurologic, hormonal, and/or immunologic homeostasis.

Likewise, it remains unknown how much sarcopenia reflects a decline in physical activity and exercise capacity, and as part of a broad cycle, whether this decline is a function of age, lack of motivation, decline in neuromuscular function from disuse or loss of motoneurons, age-associated decreases in metabolism, or other factors such as anemia or high levels of inflammatory markers.[1,27,30,118]

Pathogenesis. The identification of the molecular chain able to reverse sarcopenia is a major goal of studies on human aging. Animal studies suggest that myofiber regeneration in sarcopenic muscle is halted at the point where reinnervation is critical for the final differentiation into mature myofibers.

Combined evidence points to a decreased capacity among motoneurons to innervate regenerating fibers. There are also changes observed in the expression of several cytokines known to play important roles in establishing and maintaining neuromuscular connectivity during development and adulthood.[44]

The decline in muscle mass previously thought to be the result of proteins' breaking down faster than they were being created and restored may be linked instead to other potential reasons such as diet and nutrition, the body's ability to use protein from food, and hormonal changes.[116] For example, inadequate dietary intake of protein also results in loss of skeletal muscle mass; the current recommended daily allowance (RDA) may not be adequate to completely meet the metabolic and physiologic needs of virtually all older people.[25]

Loss of muscle function appears to be due to decreased total fibers, decreased muscle fiber size, impaired excitation-contraction coupling mechanism, or decreased high-threshold motor units. For example, at midthigh, muscle accounts for 90% of the cross-sectional area in young, active adults. However, this same measurement taken in older adults is only 30%.[53]

Additionally, selective loss of motor unit number or atrophy (particularly after 70 years) of fast twitch (type IIa) muscle fibers may occur.[22] Some researchers suggest that no preferential loss of type I or type II muscle fibers occurs with age, but rather, both types are equally affected and type II fiber cross-sectional area is reduced, which accounts for the significant decrease in muscle strength.[3]

Other studies have shown that type II fibers are preferentially affected by aging and that fiber II atrophy is associated with a decline in satellite cells (essential for skeletal muscle growth and repair).[116]

Other researchers hypothesize an extrinsic apoptotic pathway to explain how type II fiber–containing skeletal muscles may be more susceptible to muscle mass losses.[91] Several signaling pathways of skeletal muscle apoptosis are currently under intense investigation, with particular focus on the role played by mitochondria.[80] However it occurs, the clinical significance of this loss is that it leads to diminished strength and exercise capacity.[113]

Effects of Sarcopenia. From a clinical perspective, loss in muscle mass accounts for the age-associated decreases in basal metabolic rate contributing to metabolic disorders such as type 2 diabetes mellitus and osteoporosis and decreases in muscle strength and activity levels, which, in turn, are the cause of the decreased energy requirements of the aging adult.[46]

Loss of muscle mass (i.e., atrophy) and definition and loss of muscle function resulting in subsequent muscle weakness are implicated in difficulty accomplishing activities of daily living (e.g., rising from a chair, climbing stairs, carrying groceries), slow gait speed, impaired balance reactions, and increased risk of vertebral compression (and other) fractures. There does not appear to be a relationship between age-related sarcopenia and the bone mass loss also prevalent in the same age group.[31]

Aging workers notice increasing difficulty continuing a job they have previously performed without trouble. Slowing down of reflexes and coordination combined with loss of muscle mass and strength can make it difficult to remain in the same job or train for a new job.

By age 65, changes in the muscle mass, muscle weakness, and decreased levels of physical activity are evident in the increased numbers of falls and injuries. Injuries in an aging musculoskeletal system take longer to recover, contributing to further physical deconditioning, potentially creating additional comorbidities.

Exercise and Sarcopenia. (See also "Musculoskeletal System, Aging, and Exercise" below.) Appropriate exercise can alter, slow, or even partially reverse some of the age-related physiologic changes that occur in skeletal muscle, including sarcopenia. Skeletal muscle adaptations in response to strength training in older adults occur with progressive resistance training (PRT) or high-intensity training (e.g., two to six sets of eight repetitions at approximately 80% of the person's one-repetition maximum).[119]

Understanding muscle fiber types and the impact of physical therapy interventions on muscle fiber type conversions is becoming increasingly important in today's evidence-based practice. An excellent review of these concepts is available.[98] We know, for example, that age-related changes can be counteracted and physical function improved by increased physical activity of a resistive nature.[109] Mechanical load on muscle can increase the cross-sectional area of the remaining fibers but does not restore fiber numbers characteristic of young muscle.[3]

Strength training has been shown to improve insulin-stimulated glucose uptake both in healthy older adults and in individuals with diabetes. Strength training also improves muscle strength in healthy adults and in those who have chronic diseases. Increased strength leads to improved function and a decreased risk for falls, injuries, and fractures.[38] These results also promote increased independence and improved quality of life.[123]

Aging muscle may be resistant to insulin-like growth factor I (IGF-I); IGF-I promotes myoblast proliferation, differentiation, and protein assimilation in muscle through multiple signaling mechanisms. Exercise may be able to help aging muscle that is resistant to IGF-I by reversing this effect.[3]

High-resistance training exercise has been of significant benefit to sarcopenia.[84] In fact, after 6 months of exercise training, resistance exercise has been shown to reverse mitochondrial dysfunction for genes that are affected by both age and exercise.[83] Combinations of resistance exercise, aerobic exercise, and stretching have shown beneficial effects on sarcopenia, but the optimum regime for older adults remains unclear.[57,68,90]

Many older adults would like to be more physically active but do not have the experience or knowledge to develop and build up an exercise regimen without appropriate supervision such as the physical therapist can offer. Others have participated in athletics throughout adulthood and continue to train and remain in good health. The therapist can help educate older adults about the importance of maintaining strength training and endurance with the emphasis on strength, which decreases more rapidly than endurance.[54]

Joint and Connective Tissue

At the same time as changes in bone and muscle are taking place, a progressive loss of flexibility and changes in connective tissue starts contributing to an increased incidence of joint problems beginning in middle age and progressing through old age. Loss of flexibility also contributes to increased risk of falls and other injuries. Connective or periarticular tissue, including fascia, articular cartilage, ligaments, and tendons, becomes less extensible, with resultant decreased active and passive range of motion.

Increased Stiffness and Decreased Flexibility

Decreased flexibility occurs with a combination of biologic aging, inactivity, structural and biochemical changes, and degenerative diseases.[105] The extracellular matrix of skeletal muscle will undergo changes that increase the concentration of collagen, changes in the composition of elastic fibers, and increase the infiltration of fat within the matrix. These changes will have a significant effect on increasing muscle stiffness and limiting muscle force generation.[69]

Others have shown that aging collagen has increased cross-links between molecules, increasing the mechanical stability of collagen but also contributing to increased tissue stiffness.[94] Increased collagen content in the endomysium of animal intramuscular connective tissue has been shown to correlate with increased stiffness of the whole muscle.[6]

Another possible source of extracellular matrix changes is related to fibrinogen, produced in the liver and converted to fibrin, which constantly circulates throughout the body to serve as a clotting mechanism (with superglue-like effects) should an injury occur. Fibrinogen normally leaks out of the vasculature in small amounts into the intracellular space and then adheres to cellular structures, causing microfibrinous adhesions among the cells. Activity and movement normally break down these adhesions along with macrophagic activity to dissolve unused fibrinogen and fibrin. In the aging process, less fibrinogen and fewer (less efficient) macrophages are available. These factors, along with less physical activity and movement, allow these microadhesions to accumulate in muscle and fascia, resulting in an increased sense of overall stiffness.[70]

Regardless of the exact physiologic mechanism for the gradual increase in stiffness associated with aging, physical activity has an important influence in alleviating stiffness. Further research is needed to understand how and what kind of physical activity influences or possibly prevents stiffness.[18,121]

Changes in Articular Cartilage

Articular cartilage, which cushions the subchondral bone and provides a low-friction surface necessary for free movement, contains few cells, is aneural and avascular, and often starts to break down with increasing age.[75] The main proteoglycan in articular cartilage (aggrecan) binds with hyaluronan to form massive aggregates that expand the collagen matrix of the tissue to provide it with its compressive and tensile strength.

With age, proteoglycan aggregation is reduced and smaller proteoglycans are synthesized with an increase in keratin sulfate and reduced chondroitin sulfate content. The hydrophilic proteoglycans have been shown to become shorter in aged tissue and therefore lose their ability to hold water in the matrix.[23] Dehydrated articular cartilage may have a reduced ability to dissipate forces across the joint.[58]

Degeneration and thinning or damage of articular cartilage with loss of water content contribute to a significant increase in incidence of osteoarthritis with aging. By age 60, as much as 80% of the population shows evidence of such, although only about 15% present with symptoms.[105]

Knowledge of these changes has resulted in new interventions such as glucosamine-chondroitin supplementation, platelet-rich plasma therapy, hyaluronic acid, and other joint viscosupplementation for osteoarthritis (see Chapter 27).[28,50,87] With or without a symptomatic presentation, educating adults about the importance of joint protection is an important role of the physical therapist.

Tendons

Tendons exhibit a lower metabolic activity associated with aging that has implications for injury and healing in the aging population.[4,5] A reduction in the stiffness of tendon with aging will affect the contractile properties of a musculotendinous structure, reducing maximal force production and the slower transmission of forces. Also an age-related decrease occurs in the tensile strength of some tendons and ligament-bone interfaces, and loss of integrity of some joint capsules occurs.[85] For example, rotator cuff impairment with loss of joint function is common in older people. A gradual loss of connective tissue resistance to calcium crystal formation occurs in the older adult, leading to an increase in the incidence of crystal-related arthropathies (e.g., gout, pseudogout; see Chapter 27).[42]

Proprioception

Joint proprioception, described as sensations generated to increase awareness of joint orientation at rest and in motion, declines with age, especially in the knee and ankle.[55,88,100] Joint proprioception provides both a sense of joint position and sense of joint movement. Mechanoreceptors located in the joint capsules, ligaments, muscles, tendons, and skin provide the sensory information needed for a sense of joint position.

The presence of osteoarthritis seems to make joint proprioception even worse, though it is unclear whether impaired joint sense promotes arthritic change or whether arthritic change causes the sensory loss. There is some evidence that proprioception may be reduced before the development of joint degenerative change.[67]

Bone

The skeletal system serves numerous functions in the human body throughout the life span. Bone is the primary storage depot for calcium, phosphate, sodium, and magnesium. Bones are the hosts for the hemopoietic bone marrow (growth and development of elements of blood). Bones also serve important mechanical functions, such as protection of components of the nervous system and visceral organs; provision of rigid internal support for the trunk and extremities; and provision of attachment sites for numerous soft tissue structures.

Bone is remodeling constantly throughout life. While osteoclasts resorb the existing bone, new bone is being formed by osteoblasts. Three primary influences affect this remodeling process: (1) mechanical stresses; (2) calcium and phosphate levels in the extracellular fluid; and (3) hormonal levels of parathyroid hormone, calcitonin, vitamin D, cortisol, growth hormone, thyroid hormone, and sex hormones.

Aging adversely affects the "quality" of human bone material, both the stiffness and strength of bone and its "toughness." These effects are caused by factors such as architectural changes, compositional changes, physiochemical changes, changes at the micromechanical level, and the degree of prior in vivo microdamage.[125]

The bone density of the skeleton reaches its peak during an adult's twenties and remains stable for about two decades. Around the time of menopause for women, resorption, the process by which bone is broken down and calcium is released from the bone for use by the body, increases, while formation, the bone-rebuilding process, fails to keep pace. This imbalance, which is triggered by declining estrogen levels, leads to rapid bone loss during the first decade after menopause, with moderate bone loss thereafter. In women with low peak bone mass, it can result in osteoporosis with the increased potential for vertebral, hip, or other fracture.[95]

The same progressive decrease of calcium can occur in men, only at a reduced and slowed rate. In women, loss occurs at a rate of approximately 1% per year after age 35 with acceleration especially during the first 5 years after menopause. Men lose 10% to 15% by age 70 years and 20% by age 80.

In women the loss is greater, amounting to about 20% by age 65 and 30% by age 80.[7,104] In both genders, by age 65, bone loss generally has progressed to a point where the older adult is predisposed to fractures, especially when other comorbidities exist (e.g., diabetes, balance or vestibular impairment, renal impairment, immobilization).[120]

THE MUSCULOSKELETAL SYSTEM, AGING, AND EXERCISE

By the year 2030, 70 million people in the United States will be age 65 years or older; people 85 years and older will be the fastest-growing segment of the population. As more individuals live longer, the importance of exercise and physical activity to improve health, functional capacity, quality of life, and independence will increase in this country.[8,10]

Strength training is considered a promising intervention for reversing the loss of muscle function and the deterioration of muscle structure that is associated with advanced age. The capacity of older men and women to adapt to increased levels of physical activity is preserved, even in the most aged adult.[21,48,115]

For example, the relationship of exercise to insulin action is important because increased body fat (especially abdominal obesity) and decreased exercise is linked to the increased incidence of diabetes in the aging population.

Regularly performed exercise can affect nutritional needs and functional capacity in the older adult, contributing a preventive effect.[44] Combining knowledge of exercise principles with nutrition is important for all people but especially in the older adult population, disabled individuals, athletes, adolescents, and anyone with a medical condition, disease, or illness.[122]

Muscle

Human muscles contain two different types of muscle fibers based on speeds of shortening and morphologic differences. Type I muscle fibers, known also as *slow oxidative slow twitch fibers*, are the fatigue-resistant red fibers. The red color is the result of high amounts of myoglobin and a high capillary content. Greater myoglobin and capillary content contributes to the increased oxidative capacity of red muscles compared to white muscles (type II).[98]

Type II fibers, or fast twitch fibers, have two different characteristics. Type IIa, which are bigger and faster than type I, are also fatigue resistant and are referred to as *fast oxidative fibers*. Type IIb fibers are the classic white fibers, which lack aerobic enzymes and therefore fatigue rapidly. Each muscle contains type I and type II fibers in various proportions.

The basic distribution of fiber types is thought to be an inherited characteristic. Although distribution varies among individuals, the average ratio of fast to slow twitch fibers is 50 : 50. Individuals trained in endurance activities usually have a higher proportion of slow twitch fibers, and those trained for high-intensity, high-speed activities have more high twitch fibers. The oxidative capacity of both fibers can be increased greatly by endurance training, but the glycolic capacity and contractile properties are not modified.[101]

Muscle function can be described in terms of strength and endurance, which is also how we focus training of muscle. Strength can be defined in several ways depending on the specific method of measurement but is usually related to the diameter of the muscle fiber, which has been consistently shown to increase with strength training.

Endurance can be measured as the ability to work over time; local muscle endurance is distinguished from general body endurance as the ability of an isolated muscle group to continue a prescribed task rather than the ability to continue an activity such as running, swimming, or jogging for an extended period of time.[101]

As a result of specificity of training and the need for maintaining muscular strength and endurance, and flexibility of the major muscle groups, a well-rounded training program including aerobic and resistance (strength and endurance) training and flexibility exercises is recommended.

Strength Training

Strength training refers to exercise directed at improving the maximum force-generating capacity of muscle. There is evidence that strength training has a positive effect on aging skeletal muscle.[56,119]

Collectively, studies indicate that strength training in the older adult (1) produces substantial increases in the strength, mass, power, and quality of skeletal muscle; (2) can increase endurance performance; (3) normalizes blood pressure in those with high-normal values; (4) reduces insulin resistance; (5) decreases both total and intraabdominal fat; (6) increases resting metabolic rate in older men; (7) prevents the loss of bone mineral density with age; (8) reduces risk factors for falls; and (9) may reduce pain and improve function in those with osteoarthritis in the knee.[8,10]

Significant strength gains are possible in all populations, including older adults, when exposed to an adequate strength training program. Strength gains occur from enhanced neuromuscular activation over the initial 8 weeks and from increased fiber density and hypertrophy during subsequent weeks.[73]

Considerable evidence exists that sarcopenia can be prevented, reduced, and reversed with prescriptive strength training programs that emphasize gradual, progressive, high-intensity resistance exercises (e.g., high load/low repetition) for the upper and lower extremities.[14,96,98]

Resistance training significantly increases muscle size and increases energy requirements and insulin action in adults over age 65 years. A program of once- or twice-weekly resistance exercise (carried out at a level described as "reasonably difficult" or "difficult") achieves muscle strength gains similar to 3 days/wk training in older adults and is associated with improved neuromuscular performance.[111] The goal is to design a program for each individual to provide the proper amount of physical activity and exercise to attain maximal benefit at the lowest risk.

Strength training does not increase maximal oxygen uptake beyond normal (i.e., individuals attain the same maximal VO_2 before and after training).[81,82] In postmenopausal women, muscle performance, muscle mass, and muscle composition are improved by hormone replacement therapy. The beneficial effects of hormone replacement therapy combined with high-impact physical training appear to exceed those of hormone replacement therapy alone.[102,103,110] Long-term results remain under investigation.

Endurance Training

Endurance training refers to exercise directed at improving stamina (the duration that a person can maintain strenuous activity) and aerobic capacity (VO_{2max}). Endurance training places a high metabolic demand on the muscle and will increase the oxidative capacity of all muscle fiber types.[98]

Endurance exercise can reverse the decline in physical conditioning associated with aging. An endurance training program using relatively modest intensity of training can reverse 100% of the loss of cardiovascular capacity, returning some healthy older adults to levels of aerobic power present in young adulthood. Even an older person who has failed to maintain fitness over time can benefit from an exercise program.[81,82]

In middle-aged adults, the mechanism responsible for decline in cardiovascular capacity appears to be a reduced plasticity of heart muscle; improved aerobic power after training appears to be directly related to peripheral oxygen extraction (i.e., the muscles' ability to take up and use oxygen).

Aerobic exercise results in improvements in functional capacity and reduced risk of developing type 2 diabetes mellitus in the older adult. Aerobic endurance training for fewer than 2 days/wk at less than 40% to 50% VO_2 and for less than 10 minutes is generally not a sufficient stimulus for developing and maintaining cardiovascular fitness in healthy adults.

Joint

As discussed earlier, tendons, ligaments, and muscles around the joints have less water content, resulting in increased stiffness, with increasing age. Articular cartilage has less tensile strength and the biochemical composition changes, often leading to osteoarthritis.[92]

Joint changes with deterioration of subchondral bone and atrophy of the synovium also can occur. Well-regulated exercise does not produce or exacerbate joint symptoms and actually may improve symptoms.[32] This concept is discussed in greater detail in "Osteoarthritis" (see Chapter 27).

Bone

The relationship between bone mass and activity is well established. Complete immobilization and weightlessness result in rapid onset of accelerated bone resorption; bone mass recovers when activity resumes, but whether bone loss is completely reversible is unknown. Immobilization also leads to changes in collagen, ligaments, and the musculotendinous junction at the joint, causing reduced range of motion.

Osteopenia, osteomalacia, and osteoporosis affect the mineralization of bone matrix and can impact the bone health of the aging adult. Older adults are at greater risk for osteoporosis-related fractures, both age related for all adults and postmenopause related for women. Fractures are discussed in more detail in Chapter 27.

Specific Exercise Guidelines

Resistance training is an integral component in the comprehensive health program promoted by major health organizations such as the American Heart Association, American College of Sports Medicine, Surgeon General's office, and others. Population-specific guidelines have been published, and the current research indicates that for healthy people of all ages and many people with chronic diseases, single-set programs of up to 15 repetitions performed a minimum of two times per week are recommended.

Each workout session should consist of 8 to 10 different exercises that train the major muscle groups. Single-set programs are less time consuming and generally result in greater compliance. The goal of this type of program is to develop and maintain a significant amount of muscle mass, endurance, and strength to contribute to overall fitness and health.

Although age in itself is not a limiting factor to exercise training, a more gradual approach in applying prescriptive exercise at older ages may be necessary because exercise programs also can cause injury, especially in the presence of comorbidities such as arthritis, obesity, neurologic disease, postural instability, cardiovascular impairment, previous joint injuries, joint deformity, or other musculoskeletal complications, such as tendonitis or shoulder impingement syndrome. High-intensity resistance training (>60% of the one-repetition maximum) has been demonstrated to cause large increases in strength in the older adult (older than 65 years).[19,45]

People with chronic diseases may have to limit range of motion for some exercises and use lighter weights with more repetitions.[47,59] Otherwise, older adults do not have to "take it easy" when performing exercise. The presence of heart disease, diabetes, cancer, or other comorbidities may require some initial progression in the prescribed program.[119]

Overall, therapists should pay careful attention to finding exercise intensities that are optimally suited to induce the desired training effects. The skeletal muscle of older people is more easily damaged with the loading that occurs during training compared with the skeletal muscle of younger adults. Care should be taken to monitor soreness and prevent muscle injuries after exercise.[119]

Recommendations for the quantity and quality of exercise for developing and maintaining cardiorespiratory and muscular fitness and flexibility in healthy adults also have been published. A certain combination of *frequency* (3-5 days/wk), *intensity* (55%-90% of maximum heart rate or 40%-85% of VO_{2max}), and *duration* (20-60 minutes continuously or 10-minute bouts intermittently throughout the day) of exercise performed consistently over time has been found effective for producing a training effect.[8,10]

Fatigue, the inability to continue to maintain a given activity, may develop as a result of depletion of muscle and liver glycogen, decreases in blood glucose, dehydration, and increases in body temperature. In a strength training program for adults older than age 65 years, repeated maximum voluntary contractions resulting in fatigue may differ from those for younger populations. This may be relevant for designing optimal strength training programs for older adults specifically requiring closer supervision to ensure that each repetition is completed without substitution or incomplete range of motion and to adjust rest times between contractions. Alternatively, electrical stimulation may provide more consistent muscle activation during strength training in this age group.[106]

Exercise guidelines for the very old (age >85 years) also have been published by the American College of Sports Medicine as follows: *frequency* of at least 2 days/wk, preferably 3 days; *intensity* of 40% to 60% of heart rate reserve; *duration* of at least 20 minutes. Walking, leg/arm ergometry, seated stepping machines, and water exercises are recommended.

Additional recommendations for resistance training include two to three sets of 8 to 12 repetitions performed with good form and through the entire range of motion for each exercise performed on each training day (one set may be sufficient); some standing postures with free weights and balance training should be included.[8,10] When 12 repetitions can be completed without difficulty (observe for increased respiration, extremity tremors, facial grimacing), the weight can be increased by 5% with a lower number of repetitions to begin a new training cycle.

REFERENCES

To enhance this text and add value for the reader, all references are included on the companion Evolve site that accompanies this textbook. The reader can view the reference source and access it online whenever possible.

CHAPTER 23

Genetic and Developmental Disorders

ALLAN M. GLANZMAN

Pediatric diseases and disorders comprise a large number of conditions. Entire volumes have been devoted just to pediatric pathologies. Given the format of this book and space limitations, this chapter includes as many of the more commonly encountered genetic and developmental disorders as possible. Cerebral palsy is discussed separately as a neurologic condition in Chapter 35.

A brief discussion of several other rare but important diagnoses also is included. Because physical and occupational therapy intervention is not the focus here, the reader is referred to other, more appropriate resources for specific and thorough intervention guidelines for these conditions.[39,126,187,228,236]

DOWN SYNDROME

Definition and Incidence

Down syndrome was the first genetic disorder attributed to a chromosomal aberration and is referred to as trisomy 21. Down syndrome is characterized by muscle hypotonia, cognitive delay, dysmorphic facial features, and other distinctive physical abnormalities.

Down syndrome is the most common inherited chromosomal disorder, occurring once in every 700 livebirths. The incidence of Down syndrome rises with maternal age. Before maternal age 30 years the incidence is 1 in 2000 births; it is 1 in 50 for mothers age 35 to 39 years, and 1 in 20 for mothers older than 40 years. There is a 2% risk of recurrence for a couple who have had a child with Down syndrome. The prevalence has been increasing because of a number of factors and at birth is 11.8 per 10,000 infants.[222]

Etiologic Factors and Pathogenesis

The actual cause of the phenotype in Down syndrome is not yet known; however, some hints have begun to emerge as researchers continue to explore gene mapping and develop genetic models for Down syndrome.[11] Evidence from cytogenetic and epidemiologic studies supports multiple causality.

Chromosomal Abnormality

Trisomy 21 produces three copies of chromosome 21 instead of the normal two because of faulty meiosis (cell division by which reproductive cells are formed) of the ovum or, sometimes, the sperm. This results in a karyotype (chromosomal constitution of the cell nucleus) of 47 chromosomes instead of the normal 46.[128] The faulty cell division can also occur after fertilization, leading to only a portion of cells being affected, with a milder clinical picture. This situation is referred to as mosaicism. Because of the positive correlation between increasing age and Down syndrome, it is hypothesized that deterioration of the oocyte (immature ovum) or environmental factors such as radiation and viruses may cause a predisposition to mistakes in meiosis and the resulting chromosomal abnormality. In a small number of cases, Down syndrome occurs as a result of a translocation of chromosome 15, 21, or 22 (i.e., the long arm of the chromosome breaks off and attaches to another chromosome). Chromosomal translocation can be hereditary or associated with advanced parental age. Although Down syndrome usually is attributed to the aging woman, evidence suggests that in 5% to 10% of cases Down syndrome correlates with paternal age.[214,270]

The third copy of chromosome 21 is the cause of the phenotypic characteristics that are observed in people with Down syndrome. Some of the genes are dosage sensitive and contribute to the Down syndrome phenotype; however, this is complicated by the fact that there might be downstream effects in some cases that impact the expression of genes on other chromosomes. The 21st chromosome is the smallest and there are approximately 305 coding genes that are present in triplicate in individuals with Down syndrome. Another possible explanation for some features of the phenotype might be caused by not only elevated expression of specific genes, but by the elevated expression of groups of genes and a resulting lack of genetic stability.[180] Only a few specific genes have been identified as causative of specific pathology in Down syndrome and the specific causative factors that contribute to the Down syndrome phenotype are still being considered. It is likely that there will emerge a more comprehensive model of phenotypic causation in the future.

Alzheimer Disease

Alzheimer disease is also more common in people with Down syndrome, occurring at an earlier age than that of the Alzheimer population in general. By the age of 40 years, symptoms of Alzheimer disease can be seen in almost everyone with Down syndrome. The increased rate of Alzheimer disease in individuals with Down syndrome is a result of abnormally high production of β-amyloid that makes up the extracellular plaques seen in individuals with Down syndrome. This results from the increased expression of amyloid precursor protein gene, which not only increases β-amyloid but also impairs mitochondrial function in Down syndrome. This effect of amyloid precursor protein gene expression is also found in familial Alzheimer disease.[208]

Amyloid precursor protein is processed through a variety of enzymatically driven steps, with the ultimate aggregate being pathogenic. This is a direct result of the amyloid precursor protein genes location on the 21st chromosome found in triplicate in children with Down syndrome.[103] In addition to the extracellular plaques, intracellular tangles and striated neurophil threads are found within the cell, which result from a hyperphosphorylation of protein tau, is a protein that contributes to the cytoskeleton of the cell and acts to stabilize the microtubule infrastructure of the cell.

Role of Free Radicals

Amyloid precursor protein gene expression also has an impact on energy metabolism in the mitochondria. This phenomenon, and the fact that the gene for superoxide dismutase (an important free radical defense) is also found on the long arm of chromosome 21, suggests a role in the neuropathology of Down syndrome through the action of free radical-induced damage. Although superoxide dismutase shows normal expression in the fetus of individuals with Down syndrome, it is over expressed in the brains of adults with Down syndrome and declines as symptoms of dementia appear. There is also an imbalance between superoxide dismutase and glutathione peroxidase activity and this imbalance is related to the presence of free radicals in the brain. This suggests that the imbalance may play a role in the developmental brain abnormalities found in people with Down syndrome. However, this imbalance is likely a result of chronic oxidative injury as opposed to an underlying primary cause of the developmental disability.[169, 178,180]

Growth Factors

Astrocyte-derived neurotrophic factor (S100β), an astroglial-derived Ca^{2+} binding protein, is also coded for on the 21st chromosome. In Down syndrome this growth factor is overexpressed prior to birth in the brains of those with Down syndrome. This overexpression increases as the person ages, and in the second decade can be correlated with the degree of β-amyloid found in the brain. In addition, astrocyte-derived neurotrophic factor may also play a role in neuronal injury via calcium toxicity and it may have a role in initiating gliosis through its proinflammatory action, by facilitating the release of nitric oxide and cytokines.[169,180]

The resulting gross pathology observed in the brains of people with Down syndrome is an overall reduction in brain weight with a reduced size of the cerebral and cerebellar hemispheres, the hippocampus, the pons, and the mammillary bodies. Additional abnormal findings may include smaller convolutions within the brain, structural abnormalities in the dendritic spines of the pyramidal neurons of the motor cortex, and abnormalities of the pyramidal system as a whole, including decreased pyramidal neurons in the hippocampus. This last finding and the decreased size of the amygdala in people with Down syndrome who develop dementia have particular significance as these factors are associated with the increased incidence of Alzheimer's symptoms in older adults with Down syndrome.[6]

Clinical Manifestations

Children with Down syndrome are readily identified by their flattened nasal bridges, up slanting palpebral fissures, epicanthic folds, short broad hands, transverse palm crease, and mild to moderate hypotonia. Table 23-1 lists the most frequently observed clinical characteristics.

Many other associated clinical manifestations may also be present. For example, people with Down syndrome tend to exhibit increased susceptibility to infections[191] such as respiratory infection and otitis media (ear infection). They are more likely to contract hepatitis B if exposed and there is a decreased antibody response to immunization. There is an increased incidence of ophthalmologic disorders (35%), thyroid dysfunction (8%), and gastrointestinal anomalies and associated constipation (13%).

Both acute lymphoblastic and myeloid leukemia[144] occur at between 10 and 20 times the rate found in the typically developing population with a 1 in 300 risk (0.3%) as compared to a risk in the general population of a tenth of that level. Congenital cardiac anomalies (50%),[254] such as atrioventricular and ventricular septal defects, represent a larger proportion of defects in this population, and a relative underrepresentation of disorders of the vessels, such as transposition of the great vessels or aortic coarctation,[254] is seen. All of these conditions, however,

Table 23-1	Down Syndrome: Clinical Characteristics	
Most Frequently Observed Manifestations	**Associated Manifestations**
Flattened nasal bridge (90%)	Other congenital anomalies
Almond eye shape	• Absence of kidney
Flat occiput	• Duodenal atresia
Muscle hypotonia and joint hyperextensibility	• Tracheoesophageal fistula
Congenital heart disease	Feeding difficulties
Language and cognitive delay	Atlantoaxial instability
Short limbs, short broad hands and feet	Sensory impairment
Epicanthal folds	• Hearing loss (conductive)
High arched palate; protruding, fissured tongue	• Visual impairment
Delayed acquisition of gross motor skills	• Strabismus
Simian line (transverse palmar crease)	• Myopia
	• Nystagmus
	• Cataracts
	• Conjunctivitis
	Delayed growth and sexual development
	Obesity
	Diabetes mellitus

are present at rates that are greater than those found in the population as a whole.[186]

Children with Down syndrome frequently present with a variety of musculoskeletal or orthopedic problems[157] thought to be acquired secondary to soft-tissue laxity and muscle hypotonia. Some of the more common findings include recurrent patellar dislocation, excessive foot pronation, scoliosis, slipped capital femoral epiphyses, and late hip dislocation (after 2 years).

Atlantoaxial or occipitocervical instability of the cervical spine is a found in 10% to 15% of children[157] with Down syndrome. This instability is thought to be secondary to ligamentous laxity, odontoid maldevelopment, or defect in the formation of the posterior arch. Atlantoaxial displacement can be identified on plane radiographs with anterior–posterior, lateral, mouth open and flexion–extension views. Occipitocervical instability is harder to identify on plain radiographs because of overlap of the boney structures at the base of the skull; an MRI with supervised flexion and extension might be needed. Anyone with instability should be educated on symptomatology to watch for and instructed in activity modification. For example, they should avoid contact sports, gymnastics, and diving, and should be followed closely by a medical team.[157] The majority of cases are asymptomatic; however, clinical changes indicative of symptomatic spinal compression include hyperreflexia, clonus, positive Babinski sign, torticollis, progressive weakness, changes in sensation, loss of established bladder and bowel control, and a decrease in motor skills.

Children with Down syndrome often present with feeding difficulties and delayed acquisition of motor skills. These skills, however, improve with age. Because of the hypotonia, midline upper-extremity movement is difficult and emerges later in development than would be expected. Gait[47] usually is characterized by a smaller step length, decreased knee flexion at heel contact, and knee hyperextension in stance. There is also a decreased single-limb support time, and a decreased push off at terminal stance. These children present with slower reaction times and postural reactions. Movement patterns are typically characterized by increased variability, which is often magnified[227] with advancing age. Secondary disorders often develop after age 30 or 35 years, including obesity, diabetes mellitus, and cardiovascular disease. Other significant problems can include osteoarthritic degeneration of the spine and osteoporosis,[93] in addition to vertebral or long bone fractures.

MEDICAL MANAGEMENT[252]

DIAGNOSIS. Measurement of α-fetoprotein (AFP), human chorionic gonadotropin, and unconjugated estrogen in maternal serum (triple screen) allows detection of an estimated 60% to 70% of fetuses with Down syndrome. Using this screening test, prenatal diagnosis may be made during the second trimester (between 15.5 and 20 weeks' gestation).

Nuchal translucency ultrasound at 10 to 14 weeks' gestation provides a good way to identify the fetus with Down syndrome. Ultrasound carries a 6% false-positive rate and will identify only 77% of affected fetuses.[143]

Postnatal diagnosis usually begins with suspected physical findings at birth. Genetic studies showing the chromosomal abnormality can confirm the diagnosis. Specific diagnostic testing for the secondary problems discussed earlier varies depending on the involved organ systems suspected of dysfunction.

TREATMENT. Because no known cure exists for Down syndrome, treatment is directed toward specific medical problems (e.g., antibiotics for infection, cardiac surgery, monitoring of thyroid function, and monitoring for development of Alzheimer disease). Larger medical centers are pursuing plastic surgery to eliminate the hypoplastic facial features based on the premise that this type of surgery has a positive influence on rehabilitation. The overall goal of treatment intervention is to help affected children develop to their full potential. This involves a team of experts, including therapists.

PROGNOSIS. The improved life expectancy of people with Down syndrome as a result of the greater availability of surgery and advances in medical care has been documented, but life expectancy still remains lower than that for the general population.[135]

The presence of congenital malformations, especially of the heart and gastrointestinal tract, can result in high mortality rates in the affected population[80]; lack of mobility and poor eating skills are also predictors of early death.[69] Respiratory tract infections are very common and contribute significantly to morbidity and mortality.[99]

Significant health problems contributing to mortality have been reported in the adult population with Down syndrome, including untreated congenital heart anomalies, acquired cardiac disease, pulmonary hypertension, recurrent respiratory infections and aspiration leading to chronic interstitial lung disease, and complications from Alzheimer disease.

Over the last 40 years the life span of those with Down syndrome has increased significantly. In 1968, the average age of death was 2 years of age; by 1997, it had increased to 50 years of age. Unfortunately, this degree of improvement has not occurred for everyone with Down syndrome. There is a significant disparity that exists based on race, with whites with Down syndrome enjoying a significantly longer life span than nonwhites.[41]

SPECIAL IMPLICATIONS FOR THE THERAPIST 23-1

Down Syndrome
Precautions

Because atlantoaxial instability is a potential problem, activities that could result in a direct downward, traction, or translational force on the cervical area require caution and may be contraindicated (e.g., surgery, especially head and neck surgery; manual therapy; tumbling; diving; horseback riding, football, soccer, gymnastics, trampoline). Transportation in a car or bus or on a bicycle alone or with an adult may be considered a potentially risky activity requiring specific support. Likewise, riding carnival-type rides such as fast-moving carousels, roller coasters, and so on should be discussed with the family.

Some disagreement exists on the degree of screening and restriction that is required. The Committee on Sports Medicine and Fitness of the American Academy of Pediatrics has published a position paper on atlantoaxial instability in children with Down syndrome that disfavors screening of this population.[34] Plain radiographs do not predict which children are at increased risk and cannot assure that children will not develop problems in the future; other sources favor radiologic examinations of the cervical spine of children with Down syndrome.[190] The therapist is an important source of information for increasing family and community awareness regarding the potential precautions and contraindications associated with atlantoaxial instability. Symptomatic children should have radiographs taken in the neutral position with further evaluation based on the initial result and referral as needed for further evaluation.

Decreased muscle tone compromises respiratory expansion. In addition, the underdeveloped nasal bone causes a chronic problem of inadequate drainage of mucus. The constant stuffy nose forces the child to breathe by mouth, and dries the oropharyngeal membranes. These anatomical differences, as well as immunologic factors, increase the individual's susceptibility to upper respiratory tract infections and ear infections.

Low oral motor tone and a protruding tongue can interfere with feeding, especially solid foods. Because the child breathes by mouth, sucking for any length of time is difficult. When eating solids, the child may gag on food because of mucus in the oropharynx.

The parents should be instructed in taking measures to lessen these problems, such as clearing the nose with a bulb-type syringe, especially before each feeding; providing frequent feedings with opportunities for rest; rinsing the mouth with water after feedings; changing the child's position frequently; practicing good hand washing; and performing postural drainage and percussion if necessary.

Gross and Fine Motor Development

The therapist concerned with motor development as well as other clinical, educational, psychosocial, or vocational issues relevant to people with Down syndrome is referred to other more intervention-oriented resources.[30,100,263]

Physical Activity and Exercise

Developing an active lifestyle early in childhood is important given the risk factors for the development of obesity, diabetes mellitus, and cardiovascular disease in this group. The presence of cardiac defects may affect the client's overall level of activity, fitness, and endurance training, especially in the school setting.

Some evidence suggests that individuals with Down syndrome physiologically work harder when engaged in physical activity or exercise (e.g., higher heart rate, greater oxygen consumption, and minute ventilation) compared to peers who are without impairment or who are developmentally delayed but do not have Down syndrome.[71]

Anyone with Down syndrome interested in participating in the Special Olympics must work closely with the therapist, support staff, and physician to establish guidelines for safety. These individuals can benefit from aerobic conditioning, but the frequency, intensity, and duration must be modified from the general recommendations of the American College of Sports Medicine (ACSM).

Lower peak heart rate and lower VO_2 in this population require a lower level of aerobic conditioning. Vital signs should be monitored throughout the exercise program as a means of determining workload levels and progressing the activity or exercise.[96]

SCOLIOSIS

Definition

Scoliosis is an abnormal lateral curvature of the spine. The curvature may be toward the right (more common in thoracic curves) or the left (more common in lumbar curves). Rotation of the vertebral column around its axis occurs and causes an associated rib cage deformity. Scoliosis is often associated with kyphosis and lordosis.

Overview and Incidence

Scoliosis is classified as idiopathic (unknown cause; 60% of all cases[201]), osteopathic (as a result of spinal disease or bony abnormality), myopathic (as a result of muscle weakness), or neuropathic (as a result of a central nervous system [CNS] disorder), with the latter two often being combined and denoted as a neuromuscular scoliosis.

Age of onset can vary from birth onward and is referred to as infantile (0-3 years), juvenile (ages 3-10 years), adolescent (age 10 until bone maturity at between 18 and 20 years of age), or adult (after skeletal maturation). Between 0.4% and 5.5% of children may present with some type of scoliosis,[232] with one in four of those requiring some type of treatment intervention. The incidence is increased with associated neuromuscular impairments such as cerebral palsy, spina bifida, neurofibromatosis, and muscular dystrophy, with one-third of all cases of scoliosis occurring in the context of a primary neuromuscular disorder.[201]

As a whole the overwhelming majority of cases of progressive idiopathic scoliosis are found in the adolescent age group when the growth velocity of the spine increases after relatively slow growth period between the ages of 5 and 11 years for girls and up to age 13 years for boys.[43]

Infantile idiopathic scoliosis (rare in the United States) accounts for 1% of cases.[201] It is characterized by curvatures that are most often thoracic and toward the left, and most commonly affects males. Juvenile idiopathic scoliosis is characterized most often by a right thoracic curvature and can be rapidly progressive. This type of scoliosis has a much more variable natural history and can lead to significant deformity if left untreated.[129] Adolescent idiopathic scoliosis of greater than 30 degrees is seen most often in females without any neurologic impairments in a 10:1 female-to-male ratio.[260] In its milder forms (10-degree curve or less), scoliosis affects boys and girls equally, but girls are more likely to develop more severe curvatures requiring intervention.

Adult scoliosis (curves greater than 30 degrees) affects approximately 500,000 people in the United States and the prevalence of scoliosis in adults older than age 50 years is reportedly between 6% and 10% (based on routine radiographs).[25]

Etiologic Factors

Scoliosis may be functional or structural. Functional or postural scoliosis may be caused by factors other than vertebral involvement, such as pain, poor posture, leg-length discrepancy, or muscle spasm induced by a herniated disk or spondylolisthesis. These curves disappear when the cause is remedied. Functional scoliosis can become structural if untreated.

Structural scoliosis is a fixed curvature of the spine associated with vertebral rotation and asymmetry of the ligamentous supporting structures. It can be caused by deformity of the vertebral bodies and may be congenital (e.g., wedge vertebrae, fused ribs or vertebrae, hemivertebrae), musculoskeletal (e.g., osteoporosis, spinal tuberculosis, rheumatoid arthritis), neuromuscular (e.g., cerebral palsy, polio, myelomeningocele, muscular dystrophy), or, most commonly, idiopathic.

At the present time, despite extensive study, the cause of idiopathic scoliosis remains unknown. Researchers hypothesize that this type of scoliosis relates to the maturation disturbances of the CNS, including neurohormonal transmitters or neuromodulators secondary to genetic defect.[142]

Multiple areas of research including abnormalities of connective tissue, neuromotor mechanisms, neurohormonal imbalances (e.g., melatonin, calmodulin), and biomechanics (e.g., the importance of the erect posture) have been explored for a potential relationship to the cause of idiopathic scoliosis. However, no clear evidence supports any one area as an etiologic factor of this disorder; rather, it appears to be multifactorial.[138] Genetic studies have identified a genetic predisposition to some types of scoliosis[265]; and polymorphisms that contribute to susceptibility are actively being investigated.[115,231]

Pathogenesis

The pathogenesis of scoliosis remains unclear but may be better understood in relation to the underlying cause. Abnormal embryonic formation and segmentation of the spinal column are possible pathologic pathways in congenital scoliosis. Neuromuscular scoliosis is often the result of an imbalance or asymmetry of muscle activity through the trunk and spine.

The earliest pathologic changes associated with idiopathic scoliosis occur in the soft tissues as the muscles, ligaments, and other tissues become shortened on the concave side of the curve. Some hypothesize[232] that scoliosis sets up abnormal forces across the spine as a consequence of the differences in length–tension relationships,

with the muscles on the convexity being in a lengthened position and those on the concavity positioned in a relatively shortened state, and as a result a muscle imbalance is present.

Evidence establishes the existence of hypertrophy of the muscles on the side of the convexity[134]; however, the muscles on the concavity still are at a mechanical advantage and facilitate the progression of a curve once it is established. In time, bone deformities occur, as compression forces on one side of the vertebral bodies apply asymmetric forces to the epiphyseal ossification center, resulting in increased bone density on that side. The compressive force is greatest on the vertebrae in the apex of the concavity, so the apical vertebrae become most deformed (Fig. 23-1).

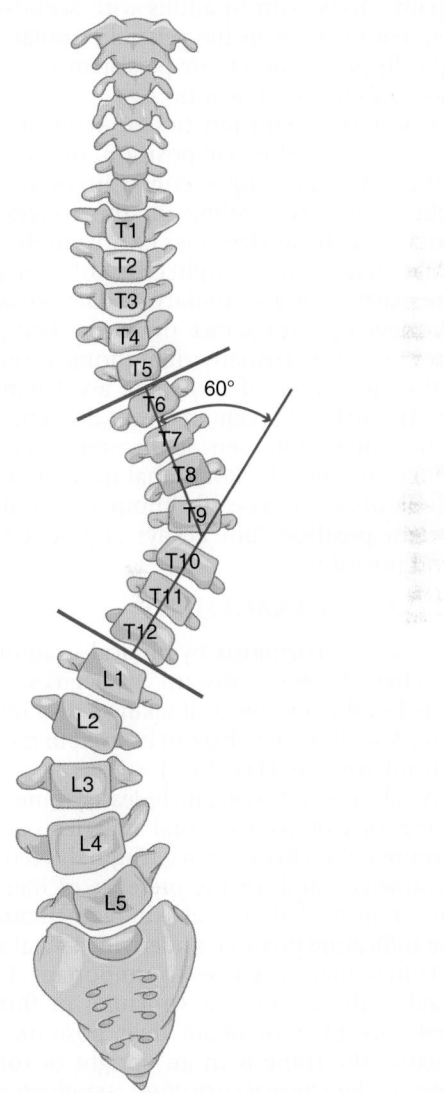

Figure 23-1

The Cobb method of measuring scoliosis. The top vertebra used in the measurement is identified as the uppermost vertebra whose upper surface tilts toward the curvature's concave side (the superior surface of the vertebra that is most tilted). The bottom vertebra is the lowest vertebra whose inferior surface tilts most toward the curvature's concave side. A line is drawn parallel to each of these vertebrae. The angle formed by the two perpendicular lines drawn to each of these lines creates the angle of the curvature.

Clinical Manifestations

Curvatures of less than 20 degrees (mild scoliosis) rarely cause significant problems. Severe untreated scoliosis (curvatures greater than 60 degrees) may produce pulmonary insufficiency and reduced lung capacity, back pain, degenerative spinal arthritis, disk disease, vertebral subluxation, or sciatica.

Back pain is not typical in children or adolescents with mild scoliosis[52] and should be evaluated by a physician who can rule out spondylolisthesis, tumor, infection, or occult trauma. Back pain may be associated with curve progression after institution of brace treatment for idiopathic scoliosis.[193] The adult with scoliosis often presents with back pain that is considered multifactorial, arising from muscle fatigue, trunk imbalance, facet arthropathy, spinal stenosis, degenerative disk disease, and radiculopathy. Back pain in adults with scoliosis occurs more frequently[52] than in the general population; the pain is typically greater and more persistent,[25] affecting function and disability level measures.[52]

Common characteristics of scoliosis are asymmetric shoulder and pelvic position, often identified when clothes do not hang evenly. Curves are designated as right or left, depending on the convexity (e.g., right thoracic scoliosis describes a curve in the thoracic spine with convexity to the right). Usually one primary curvature exists with a secondary or compensatory curvature that develops to balance the body. Two primary curvatures may exist (usually right thoracic and left lumbar). If the curvatures of the spine are balanced (compensated), the head is centered over the center of the pelvis; if the spinal alignment is uncompensated, the head is shifted to one side. Rotational deformity on the convex side is observed as a rib hump sometimes seen in the upright position, but always apparent in the forward bend position.

MEDICAL MANAGEMENT

DIAGNOSIS. Diagnosis by clinical examination requires the client to bend forward 90 degrees with the hands joined in the midline as if taking a dive into a swimming pool. A scoliometer also can be used to measure the angle of trunk rotation (Fig. 23-2).

An abnormal finding includes asymmetry of the height of the ribs or paravertebral muscles on one side. The examiner also checks for leg length discrepancy and other asymmetries and for the presence of hair patches, nevi, pits, or areas of abnormal skin pigmentation in the midline indicating possible underlying spinal abnormality.

Differential diagnosis is important in determining whether the scoliosis is structural or functional. Structural curvatures maintain their position irrespective of whether the spine is in an upright or forward bending position. Functional curvatures straighten when placed in a forward bend position. The physician also performs a neurologic examination to rule out an underlying neurologic disorder, especially in the presence of left thoracic curvature.

Full-length radiographs of the spine, using posteroanterior views instead of anteroposterior views can minimize breast radiation dosage[59] by 20 times. The radiographs are evaluated using the Cobb method (see Fig. 23-1) to measure the degree of curvatures. A curve must be larger than 10 degrees to be considered scoliotic.

The Risser sign is also determined from the film as an indication of maturation and is used as a prognostic predictor of progression.[181] Typically, the iliac crest ossifies from anterior to posterior. Risser divided the crest into four quarters according to ossification, grading the ossification from 1 to 4, with a grade 5 indicating that the whole apophysis has ossified and is fused to the iliac crest.

Neuroimaging beyond plain films may be necessary. For example, bone scan may be used to rule out neoplasms, infections, spondylolysis, or compression fractures as the underlying cause. Magnetic resonance

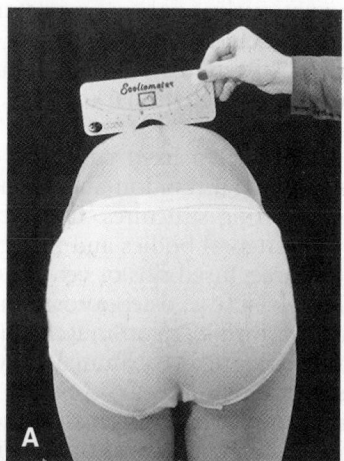

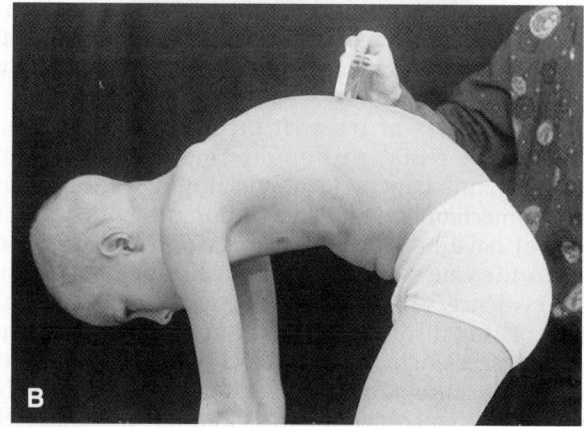

Figure 23-2

The scoliometer. This device can be used by any health care worker trained to screen for scoliosis. Some medical personnel also use this device to monitor curvatures over time, thereby avoiding unnecessary radiographs. Ask the client to bend forward slowly (the Adam position), stopping when the shoulders are level with the hips. View the client from both the front and back, keeping your eyes at the same level as the back. Before measuring with the scoliometer, adjust the height of the person's bending position to the level where the deformity of the spine is most pronounced. This position varies from one person to another depending upon the location of the curvature (e.g., a low lumbar curvature requires further bending than an upper thoracic curvature). Lay the scoliometer across the deformity with the 0 mark over the top of the spinous process. A measurement of 5 degrees or more in the screening test is considered positive and requires medical follow-up. Visually observe for asymmetry of the ribs or paravertebral muscles. In this child, hamstring tightness (greater on the left) accounts for the positional shift to the left. The scoliometer reading was zero. (Courtesy Todd Goodrich, University of Montana, Missoula.)

imaging (MRI) is used to differentiate cord lesions, disk herniations, neoplasms, infections, spondylolysis, spinal stenosis, and compression fractures.

TREATMENT. Prevention of postural or idiopathic structural scoliosis is the key to management of the majority of scoliosis cases. Early detection allows for early treatment without surgical intervention and with good long-term results. Overall goals of management are to prevent severe and progressive deformities that might lead to decreased cardiorespiratory function.

Conservative care in the past has included exercise and electrical stimulation; however, this has not been shown to be efficacious.[172] Observation and monitoring every 4 to 6 months for curvatures less than 25 degrees, spinal orthoses for curvatures 25 to 45 degrees (Table 23-2), and surgery for curvatures greater than 45 degrees is recommended.[160,198] The goal of using spinal orthoses is to serve as a passive restraint system to maintain curvatures within 5 degrees of the curve measurement at the time of initial application. This is accomplished successfully in 85% to 88% of cases.[262] Curves with an apex between T8 and L2 and compensated thoracolumbar curves respond the most favorably to bracing,[181] whereas curves with an apex at T6 or above have the poorest outcome.

Researchers continue to explore improved dynamic orthotics and holistic treatment approaches as well as aerobic training.[10] Exercise has not traditionally been viewed as effective for scoliosis; however, there is some renewed interest in its potential effect on the flexibility of an existing scoliotic curve.[102] For many years, exercise has been dismissed as an ineffective treatment for adolescent scoliosis.

Orthotic regimens have varied for late-onset idiopathic scoliosis, but typically bracing is indicated for curves greater than 20 degrees in the skeletally immature individual, or earlier if progression has been noted.[25]

Interventions in the adult with scoliosis should follow a conservative nonoperative course of physical therapy to improve aerobic capacity, strengthen muscles, and improve flexibility and joint motion. In addition, nonnarcotic analgesics, nutritional counseling, smoking (or tobacco-use) cessation, nerve root blocks, facet injections, and epidural steroid injections should be considered to address the problem of pain before surgery (if pain is the primary concern). Bracing has never been shown to have an effect on the natural history of adult scoliosis, but may be used symptomatically for certain people who are not operation candidates.[25]

Table 23-2	Scoliosis: Bracing Options
Brace	**Use**
Milwaukee (cervicothoracolumbosacral orthosis)	Best with curvature at T8 or above
Boston (thoracolumbosacral orthosis)	Best with curvature apex lower than T9 or T10
Lyon	For idiopathic scoliosis with thoracic hypokyphosis
Charleston	For idiopathic curves fabricated in maximum side-bend correction

Surgical intervention (e.g., fusion with posterior segmental spinal instrumentation) may be necessary for curvatures greater than 45 degrees, in the presence of chronic pain, or when the curvature appears to be causing neurologic changes. Surgical goals are to halt progression of the curvature, improve alignment, decrease deformity, prevent pulmonary problems, and eliminate pain. The surgical options include a variety of segmental instrumentation systems. These are combined with a posterior fusion and, in more severe cases, anterior fusion. In children and adolescents who are not skeletally mature, instrumented fusion is not possible and either growing rods or a vertical expandable prosthetic titanium rib is considered. These methods of instrumentation allow the spine and thoracic cavity to continue to grow while providing internal stabilization for the scoliosis until a final spine fusion can be completed.[192,268]

Minimally invasive surgery can be used in the population who need an anterior release along with a spinal fusion to decrease the morbidity associated with open thoracotomy. This procedure is designed to maximize the stability of the spine. This technique is still evolving and long-term data is needed but it may result in faster recovery, fewer complications, and less pain along with adequate alignment.[184,213]

PROGNOSIS. Postural curvatures resolve as the primary problem is treated. Structural curvatures are not eliminated but rather increase during periods of rapid skeletal growth. If the curvature is less than 40 degrees at skeletal maturity, the risk of progression is small. In curvatures greater than 50 degrees, the spine is biomechanically unstable, and the curvature will likely continue to progress at a rate of 1 degree/yr throughout life.[25]

Poor seating can contribute to this progression.[125] In severe kyphoscoliosis, pain and the inability to achieve comfortable positioning can complicate care, and ultimately pulmonary compromise can lead to death.

SPECIAL IMPLICATIONS FOR THE THERAPIST 23-2

Scoliosis
Intervention

Key roles of the therapist are screening for scoliosis and the education of the public about scoliosis. Consumer education must include recommendations for adequate calcium intake and participation in weight-bearing activities. This is especially important for girls since studies show a higher risk of developing osteoporosis in women.[45]

Traditional exercise programs of stretching and general strengthening continue to be employed but have not been found to halt or improve scoliosis even when used in conjunction with orthoses. When utilized, the focus of strengthening programs is on trunk extensors, abdominals, and gluteal muscles (especially hip extensors).

Postoperative

During the hospital stay after surgery the therapy and nursing staff must check sensation, color, and blood supply in all extremities to document neurovascular status. A serious complication following spinal surgery that is monitored for intraoperatively is neurovascular compromise.

Initially, the person should be log-rolled and deep-breathing exercises encouraged to prevent the development of pulmonary complications. For those who are ambulatory, mobilization can begin within 24 to 48 hours, depending on the surgeon's protocol. Adults are treated with antiembolic stockings and sequential compression devices until they are ambulatory, and most patients (depending on the instrumentation used) are fitted soon after surgery with a custom-molded lightweight plastic thoracolumbosacral orthosis. The brace is to be worn full-time when out of bed; in some cases, a progressive tolerance schedule may be required initially to achieve this. A vigilant preventive skin care program is also important.

Activities of daily living (brushing the hair or teeth) and active range of motion exercises of the extremities help maintain circulation and muscle strength. Clients should be instructed in quadriceps setting, ankle pumps, and other range of motion exercises. These should be performed frequently on their own throughout the day.

Cast syndrome (superior mesenteric artery syndrome) is a rare but serious complication that can follow spinal surgery and application of a body cast that is infrequently used for immobilization. It is characterized by nausea, abdominal pressure, vomiting, and vague abdominal pain; cast syndrome probably results from hyperextension of the spine. This hyperextension accentuates lumbar lordosis with compression of a portion of the duodenum between the superior mesenteric artery and the aorta and vertebral column posteriorly. The therapist encountering anyone in a body jacket, localizer cast, or high hip spica cast must be aware of this condition, because it can develop as late as several weeks to months after application of the cast. Medical treatment is necessary for this condition.

The incidence of other postsurgical complications is low but may include infection at the surgical site, dislodgment or fracture of instrumentation, failure of fusion, and urinary tract infection, among other common postoperative complications. Osteophytes and foraminal narrowing in the concavity of the lumbar curvature may develop in older clients, causing nerve root impingement and radicular pain. Recovery in the adult may take 6 to 12 months with improvement continuing for up to 2 years.[25]

Precautions

Precautions after spinal fusion depend on the type of fusion, segmental stabilization versus Harrington rod, and physician preference. Segmental stabilization provides some advantages over the traditional Harrington rod, including the ability to get out of bed on the first or second day after surgery and home from the hospital a few days after surgery. The more rigid segmental stabilization may make osteoporosis more likely to occur; however, the rate of pseudarthrosis is lower.[118]

Segmental instrumentation provides a better correction of the scoliosis, and postoperative casting or bracing often is not required. Precautions generally include avoiding excessive bending, trunk rotation, or hyperextension. Lifting limitations are often imposed depending on type of fusion. These precautions are to help prevent breaking or dislodging of the hardware while promoting bony union in the corrected position.

Functional mobility is severely limited for the first 4 weeks after surgery. After 3 months any type of noncontact sport is acceptable, including aerobic exercise such as walking or stationary bicycling; swimming especially is encouraged and can be started once the incision is healed after some types of fusions; however, diving is contraindicated. Vigorous activities and contact sports usually are avoided unless the client is directed otherwise by the physician. Restrictions can vary from one physician to another and with various types of fixation devices.

Skin care and prevention of breakdown are essential for anyone wearing a cast or spinal orthosis or brace. The client should be taught good skin care and how to recognize signs of irritation that can lead to lesions. For individuals with neuromuscular scoliosis who are not ambulatory, it is important to be aware of the degree of residual pelvic obliquity and accommodate this in wheelchair seating systems while monitoring skin tolerance.

KYPHOSCOLIOSIS

Overview and Etiologic Factors

Scheuermann disease (juvenile kyphosis, vertebral epiphysitis) is a structural deformity classically characterized by anterior wedging of 5 degrees or more of three adjacent thoracic bodies affecting adolescents between the ages of 12 and 16 years. Scheuermann disease is the most common cause of structural kyphosis in adolescence with an incidence of between 4% and 8%.[243] The mode of inheritance is likely autosomal dominant, but the etiologic factors and pathogenesis of this excessive kyphosis remain unknown.

Scheuermann originally proposed that a vascular disturbance of the vertebral epiphyses during periods of rapid growth was the underlying cause; however, this has not been subsequently supported. Scheuermann disease also has been associated with increased levels of growth hormone, and individuals with this disease are frequently taller than average.

In the aging population, kyphoscoliosis (adult round back) is more likely to develop as a result of poor posture, degeneration of the intervertebral disks, vertebral compression fractures or osteoporotic collapse of the vertebrae. In addition, endocrine disorders (e.g., hyperparathyroidism, Cushing disease), arthritis, Paget disease, metastatic tumor, or tuberculosis can also result in Kyphosis.

Clinical Manifestations

Adolescent kyphosis is usually asymptomatic despite the prominent vertebral spinous processes. Some adolescents experience mild pain at the apex of the curvature in addition to fatigue, and tenderness or stiffness in the involved area or along the entire spine. The pectoral, hamstring, and hip flexor muscles are often tight, producing a crouched posture with anterior pelvic tilt and lumbar lordosis. Signs and symptoms associated with adult kyphosis are similar to those of the adolescent form, but rarely produce local tenderness, unless caused by vertebral compression fractures.

In both adolescent kyphoscoliosis (Scheuermann disease) and adult kyphosis, the vertebrae are wedged anteriorly and disk lesions called Schmorl nodes develop. Schmorl nodes are localized extrusions of the nuclear material through the cartilage plates and into the spongy bone of the vertebral bodies. The cancellous bone reacts by encapsulating the herniated tissue within a wall of fibrous tissue and bone, producing the Schmorl node.

MEDICAL MANAGEMENT

DIAGNOSIS. Adolescents may be referred for medical evaluation as a result of school screening, or they may present because of concerns over posture and appearance. Adults more commonly present because of increased pain. Diagnosis is based on clinical examination and confirmed by radiographic findings, including Schmorl nodes, endplate narrowing, and irregular endplates.

TREATMENT. Indications for treatment remain controversial, because the true natural history of this disease has not been clearly defined. Presently, the choice of treatment in Scheuermann kyphosis is based on the severity and progression of the curve, the age of the individual, and the symptomatology present.

Bracing appears to be very effective if the diagnosis is made early in adolescents who have not reached skeletal maturity and have curves of less than 50 to 65 degrees, where a correction of more than 15 degrees can be achieved in the brace.[137,243] Surgical management is warranted in those with more severe curves and in adults who continue to show progression of the curve or who have progressive neurologic symptoms or unmanageable pain.

| SPECIAL IMPLICATIONS FOR THE THERAPIST | 23-3 |

Kyphoscoliosis

Scheuermann kyphosis usually responds to physical therapy intervention combined with anti-inflammatory medications and behavioral modifications.[241] Exercises (e.g., postural exercises, hamstring stretching, and core stability exercises) are helpful to maintain flexibility and improve strength in the thoracic musculature.

Precautions and implications for postoperative care are discussed in the previous section (see "Special Implications for the Therapist 23-2: Scoliosis" above). Physical load capacity after extensive surgical correction and spinal fusion for Scheuermann kyphosis is unknown; an individualized decision must be made in each case.

SPINA BIFIDA OCCULTA, MENINGOCELE, MYELOMENINGOCELE

Definition

Congenital neural tube defects (NTDs) encompass a variety of abnormalities. The term *spina bifida* is the one most often used to describe the more common congenital defects of neural tube closure. Normally, the spinal cord and cauda equina are encased in a protective sheath of bone and meninges (Fig. 23-3). Failure of neural tube closure during development produces defects that may involve the entire length of the neural tube or may be restricted to a small area.

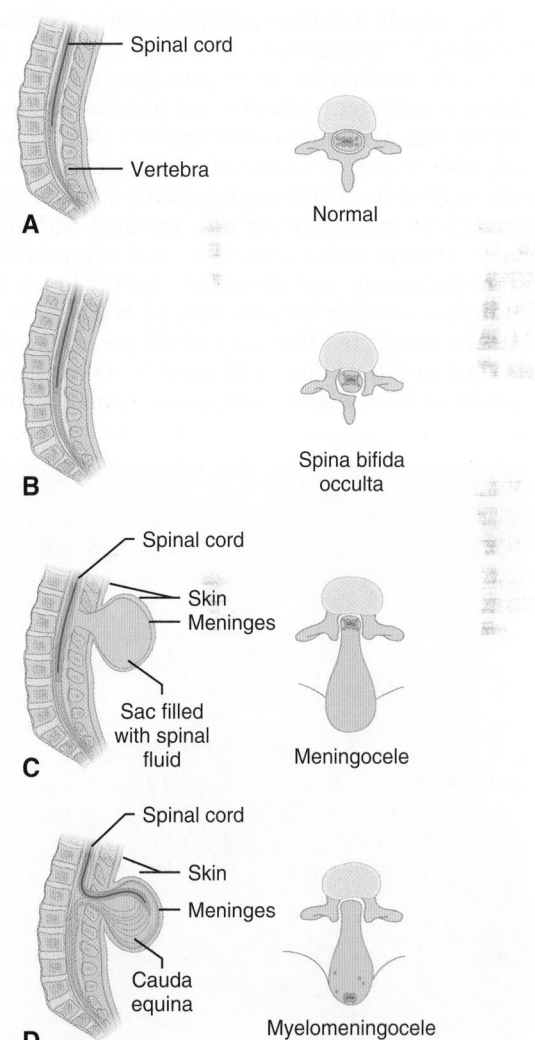

Figure 23-3

Various degrees of spina bifida. A, Normal anatomic structure. **B,** Spina bifida occulta results in only a bony defect, with the spinal cord, meninges, and spinal fluid intact. **C,** Meningocele involves the bifid vertebra, with only a cerebrospinal fluid (CSF)–filled sac protruding; the spinal cord or cauda equina (depending on the level of the lesion) remains intact. **D,** Myelomeningocele is the most severe form because the spine is open and the protruding sac contains CSF, the meninges, and the spinal cord or cauda equina.

The three most common NTDs—spina bifida occulta (incomplete fusion of the posterior vertebral arch), meningocele (external protrusion of the meninges), and myelomeningocele (protrusion of the meninges and spinal cord)—are presented here. Generally, these defects occur in the lumbosacral area but also may be found in the sacral, thoracic, and cervical areas (Fig. 23-4).

Incidence and Etiologic Factors

The incidence of NTDs varies by ethnic background, geographic area, and socioeconomic status. And is estimated at 3.4 per 10,000 livebirths.[24,176] Regional variations are significant. For example, in Scandinavia the rate can be as low as 2 per 10,000, whereas in China it can be as high as 100 per 10,000.[220]

The overall incidence of spina bifida appears to be declining.[269] Termination of pregnancies as a result of the wider availability of maternal serum screening in addition to better nutrition and prenatal vitamins containing folic acid have contributed to this decline. Folic acid, also known as vitamin B_9, is found chiefly in green leafy vegetables, legumes, egg yolks, baker's yeast, and bread products, which are now fortified with folic acid. Multivitamins containing folic acid taken when planning a pregnancy and during at least the first 6 weeks of pregnancy prevent 50% to 70% of NTDs.[40,161] Women must be cautioned that half of all pregnancies are not planned and that folic acid must be taken before conception to be effective. Taking supplements containing folic acid is the safest and most effective way of preventing NTDs.[158]

Evidence supports the hypothesis that the etiology of NTDs is multifactorial and related to the interaction of a genetic predisposition, teratogenic exposure (i.e., substances or agents that can interfere with normal embryonic development), and an essential folic acid deficiency or folic acid metabolic disorder. Genetic factors are considered important in the pathogenesis of spina bifida. Couples who have had one child with spina bifida have a recurrence rate of 3% to 8%. Several individual genes have been identified in the folate–homocysteine metabolism pathway and have been linked to elevated risk.[159] There is interest in developing genetic risk profiles based on alterations in different metabolic pathways that have been proposed as underlying factors in the alteration of risk in different groups with similar ethnic backgrounds. In the Hispanic population, it has been proposed that alterations in the groups of genes that govern various steps in purine biosynthesis may be at the root of an elevation of basil risk level, while in the non-Hispanic white population genes that govern homocysteine metabolism may underlie alterations in risk.[149] Increased rates of spina bifida are found in individuals with trisomies 13 and 18 and in the case of triploid (having three times the number of normal chromosomes in the cell nucleus),[57] and in chromosome 13q deletion syndrome.[136,219]

Teratogenic exposure and epigenetic influences also are associated with an increased incidence of NTDs. Exposure to vitamin A, valproic acid, solvents, lead, herbicides, glycol ether, clomiphene, carbamazepine, aminopterin, and alcohol is linked to increased rates of NTDs. A number of occupations have also been linked to NTDs, presumably because of teratogenic exposure. Finally, insulin-dependent diabetes is associated with increased risk of NTDs in addition to maternal obesity, weight gain, and elevation of glycemic index in nondiabetic women.[96,202]

Pathogenesis

Normally, about 20 days after conception, the embryo develops a neural groove in the dorsal ectoderm. The neural groove deepens as the two edges fuse to form the neural tube. By about day 23 this tube is completely closed except for an opening at each end. The upper end closes on day 25 and continues to fold and develop, forming the brain, whereas the bottom end closes on day 27 and forms the spinal cord.

The neural groove is formed by both cell proliferation and the production of a hyaluronic acid extracellular matrix. The first opportunity for failure of vertebral architecture to develop and close normally is through abnormalities in the hyaluronic acid matrix or the actin microfilaments that support elevation of the neural crest. A second opportunity for failed closure is slightly later in development when an abnormal overgrowth at the caudal end may develop, causing closure to fail. Just before closure of the neural tube surface glycoproteins are produced by the ectoderm and act as the glue that holds the cells together. A third opportunity for failed closure is abnormal production of these glycoproteins, leading to failure of the neural tube to close. A final possible genesis of myelomeningocele is the rupture of the neural tube

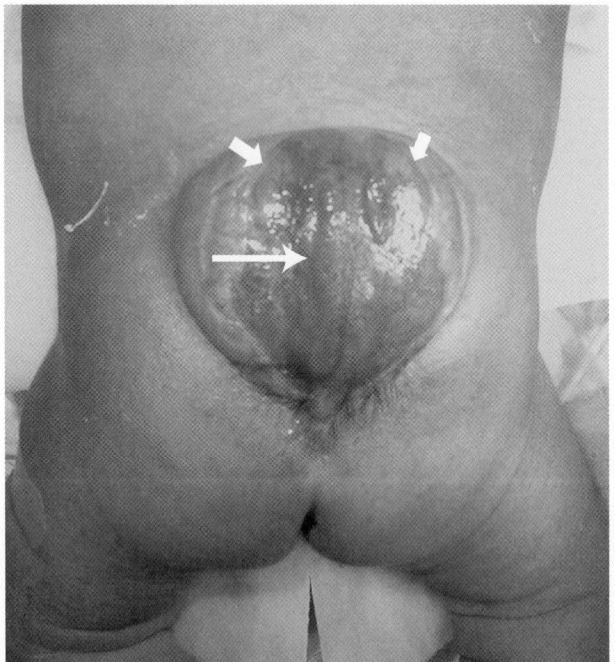

Figure 23-4

Myelomeningocele in a newborn. The neural placode is visible at the surface *(long arrow)* in this lumbosacral myelomeningocele. A placode is an area of thickening in the embryonic epithelial layer where the spinal cord develops later. Abnormal epithelium lines the edges of the cerebrospinal fluid–filled cyst *(short arrows)*. (From Burg FD, Ingelfinger JR, Polin RA, et al: *Current pediatric therapy*, ed 18, Philadelphia, WB Saunders, 2006.)

after its closure as a result of cerebral spinal fluid (CSF) pressure. In this case development of Chiari II malformation occurs, in which the cerebellar tonsils develop below the foramen magnum or are forced through the foramen magnum because of pressure leading to increased CSF pressure and forcing the neural tube open. The defect in myelomeningocele can be identified by the eighth week of gestation and is complete by the 12th week.[8]

Some animal models support the presence of a defect in homocysteine metabolism in the pathogenesis of NTD, which correlates with an increased risk of NTD in some populations.[147] Plasma homocysteine levels and folic acid levels show an inverse relationship, and current research is focusing on the metabolism of folic acid and its genetic determinants,[161] in addition to the importance of these genetic defects in spina bifida. It appears that the genetics of NTDs are multifactorial.

Clinical Manifestations

NTDs are typically divided into two groups: occulta (hidden) and aperta (visible). Approximately 75% of vertebral defects are located in the lumbosacral region, most commonly at the L5 to S1 level. Motor dysfunction depends on the level of involvement and sparing of sensory and motor innervation (Fig. 23-5 and Table 23-3).

The loss of motor function is not evenly distributed over the limbs and spine, resulting in muscle imbalance contributing to the development of scoliosis and various musculoskeletal deformities and contractures that are related to the specific denervated muscles and the resulting imbalance across the joint. Table 23-4 lists the clinical features and other associated characteristics of NTD.

Spina Bifida Occulta

Spina bifida occulta does not protrude visibly but is often accompanied by a depression or dimple in the skin, a tuft of dark hair, soft fatty deposits (subcutaneous lipomas or dermoid cyst), port-wine nevi, or a combination of these abnormalities on the skin at the level of the underlying lesion. Spina bifida occulta usually does not cause neurologic dysfunction, but occasionally bowel and bladder disturbances or foot weakness occurs.

Spina Bifida Aperta

In spina bifida aperta (meningocele and myelomeningocele), a sac-like cyst protrudes outside the spine. Like spina bifida occulta, a meningocele rarely causes neurologic deficits, whereas myelomeningocele is associated with permanent neurologic impairment the severity of which is correlated with the level of involvement.

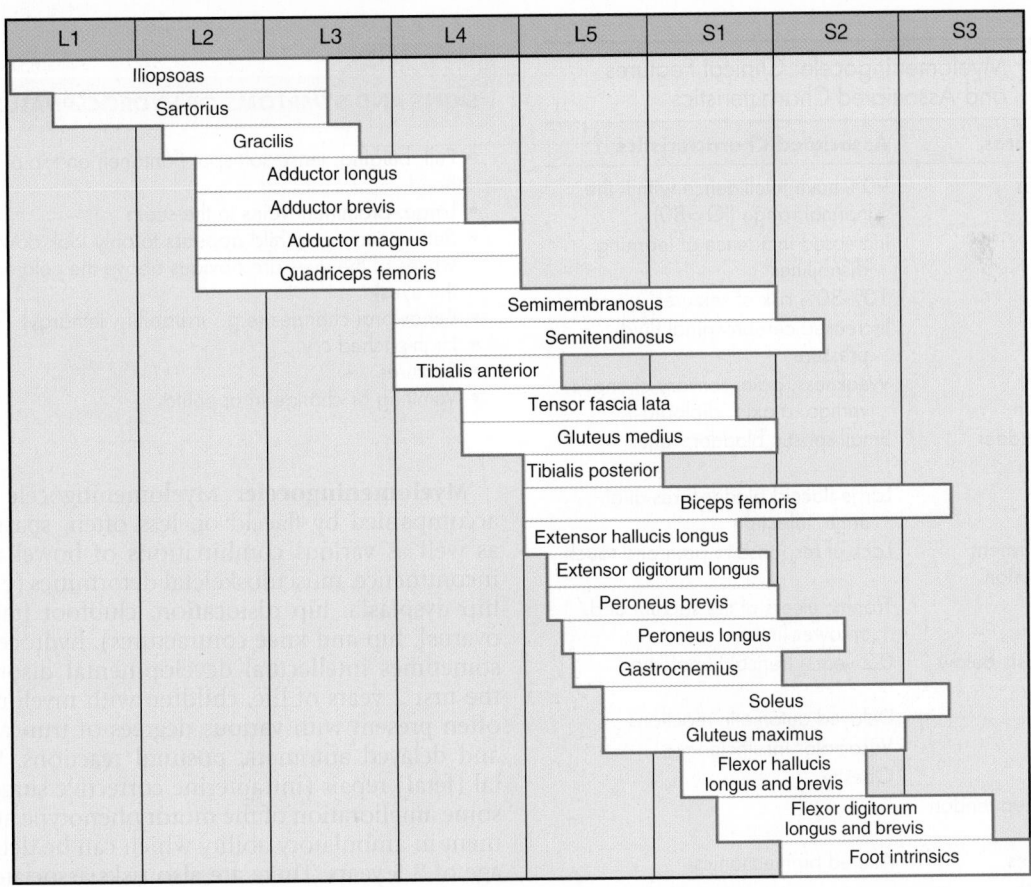

Figure 23-5

Normal lumbar and sacral segmental innervation. For the child with myelomeningocele, once the level of the lesion has been identified, the therapist can begin to assess muscle involvement above and below that level. (From Sharrard VVJ: The segmental innervation of the lower limb muscles in man, *Ann R Coll Surg Engl* 35:106–122, 1964.)

Table 23-3	Myelomeningocele: Functional Mobility		
Motor Level Spinal Cord Segment	**Critical Motor Function Present**	**Bracing/External Support For Ambulation**	**Typical Functional Activity**
≤T10	No LE movement	Standing brace or equipment	Supported sitting*
T12	Strong trunk	HKAFOs	Sliding board transfers
	No LE movement	Sometimes with thoracic corset	Good sitting balance*
			Therapeutic ambulation
			Independent wheelchair mobility
L1-L2	Unopposed hip flexion, some adduction	Standing brace or equipment	Household ambulation*
		HKAPOs, KAFOs, or RGOs	May community ambulate if motivated
		Crutches once ambulating with walker	
L3-L4	Quadriceps†	KAFOs	Household and short community ambulation*
	Medial hamstrings	Crutches	
	Anterior tibialis	Floor reaction	Wheelchair for long distances
		AFOs/twister cables	
L5	Weak toe activity	KAFOs	Household and short community ambulation*
		Crutches (yes and no)	
		Floor reaction	Community ambulation‡
		AFOs (yes and no)	
S1	Lateral hamstring	Usually no AFOs or upper limb support	Community ambulation
	Peroneals		
S2-S3	Mild intrinsic foot weakness	Possible crutch or cane with increased age	Community ambulation

AFO, ankle-foot orthosis; HKAFO, hip-knee-ankle-foot orthosis; KAFO, knee-ankle-foot orthosis; LE, lower extremity; RGO, reciprocating gait orthosis;
*Do not usually walk as adults.
†Approximately 50% probability of long-distance ambulation with muscle grades 4/5.
‡Able to use ambulation as the primary means of locomotion outside the home.

Table 23-4	Myelomeningocele: Clinical Features and Associated Characteristics
Clinical Features	**Associated Characteristics**
Hydrocephalus	90% have intelligence within the normal range (IQ >80)
	Increased incidence of learning disabilities
	10%-30% risk of seizures
	Increased cerebrospinal fluid pressure
Arnold-Chiari malformation	Weakness, pain, sensory changes, vertigo, ataxia, diplopia
Bowel and bladder incontinence	Small spastic bladder: reflux
	Large flaccid bladder: residual urine, infection
Sensory impairment below the lesion	Lack of response to pain and touch
	Trophic ulcers of the sacrum and/or lower limbs
Flaccid paralysis below the lesion	0-2 years: truncal hypotonia
	Delayed automatic reactions
	Vasomotor insufficiency
	Obesity
Absence of deep tendon reflexes	
Clubfoot (talipes equinovarus)	Altered biomechanics
Hip subluxation/dislocation	30% demonstrate decreased ambulation status by age 12 years
Scoliosis	Late childhood and early adolescence: kyphoscoliosis

Box 23-1

SIGNS AND SYMPTOMS OF HYDROCEPHALUS

- Full, bulging, tense soft spot (fontanel) on top of the child's head
- Large, prominent veins in the scalp
- Setting sun sign (child appears to only look downward; the whites of the eyes are obvious above the colored portion of the eyes)
- Behavioral changes (e.g., irritability, lethargy)
- High-pitched cry
- Seizures
- Vomiting or change in appetite

Myelomeningocele. Myelomeningocele is typically accompanied by flaccid or, less often, spastic paralysis, as well as various combinations of bowel and bladder incontinence, musculoskeletal deformities (e.g., scoliosis, hip dysplasia, hip dislocation, clubfoot [talipes equinovarus], hip and knee contractures), hydrocephalus, and sometimes intellectual developmental disorder. During the first 2 years of life, children with myelomeningocele often present with various degrees of truncal hypotonia and delayed automatic postural reactions. With prenatal (fetal) repair (intrauterine corrective surgery) there is some amelioration of the motor phenotype and improvement in ambulatory ability which can be detected by the age of 2.5 years. There are also risks associated with prenatal repair including inducement of premature labor and uterine rupture.

Between 83% and 90% of children born with this condition have an associated hydrocephalus if closure is completed after birth (Box 23-1). Between 40% and

54% of those who have an in utero closure of the myelomeningocele have hydrocephalus.[2,29] Hydrocephalus accompanying myelomeningocele usually occurs in the presence of a type I or type II Arnold-Chiari malformation; that is, the cerebellar tonsils are displaced through the foramen magnum (Fig. 23-6), resulting in obstruction of CSF flow and increased CSF pressure and hydrocephalus.

Generally speaking, most children with myelomeningocele have some degree of type II Arnold-Chiari malformation, regardless of the presence of hydrocephalus. This picture has been altered by the advent of fetal repair, and the Arnold-Chiari malformation may be reversed after repair and lower rates of hydrocephalus are noted after fetal closure.[1,28,159,246] Even though an Arnold-Chiari malformation may be present radiographically, it may not be symptomatic.

Tethered cord syndrome is also a common comorbidity following surgical closure of the primary lesion and can occur at any time during growth. As the child grows, the spinal cord can become tethered or bound down, resulting in progressive neurologic compromise. The presenting features are consistent with neurologic compromise and include incontinence, progressive weakness, and back pain. Tethered cord syndrome occurs in 3% to 5% of children with spina bifida.[117]

Syringomyelia

Syringomyelia, a cavity or syrinx, present within the spinal cord or medulla also can be present. This can progress, with increased pressure impinging on the surrounding tissue. Severe Arnold-Chiari malformations and syrinxes are rare, but can lead to potentially fatal consequences. Because of the location of the respiratory centers of the brainstem, central apnea can be serious and necessitate the use of mechanical ventilation and can potentially result in death. Sleep problems, including hypersomnolence, sleep fragmentation, choking, snoring, and morning headaches, are all potential clinical findings.[23] Cranial nerve involvement with resulting feeding difficulties, choking, pooling of secretions, aspiration, and stridor is also a common finding. Vertigo, ataxia, or spasticity, as well as pain, progressive weakness, or diplopia, can also be presenting findings in the older child.

Integumentary

Sensory disturbances usually parallel motor dysfunction. Pressure ulcers at the sacrum, ischial tuberosities, knees, and the dorsum of the feet can be a significant comorbidity. Box 23-2 lists the factors that contribute to pressure ulcers in this population. Many of these same risk factors are present in other conditions prone to pressure ulcers (e.g., diabetic neuropathy; see also Box 10-13 and Figure 10-32).

Urologic

Bladder (and bowel) problems are present in virtually all children with myelomeningocele because these functions are controlled at the S2 to S4 levels. Even children with sacral lesions and normal leg movement often have bowel and bladder problems.

Problems with urinary incontinence and infection can occur if the bladder is small and spastic (bladder holds little urine) or large and hypotonic (incomplete emptying of the bladder and ureteral reflux). Bladder dyssynergy occurs with either a flaccid or spastic sphincter. Normally, when the bladder contracts, the sphincter relaxes, allowing urine to flow. In a dyssynergistic state, the bladder and sphincter contract together, predisposing the child to urethral reflux.

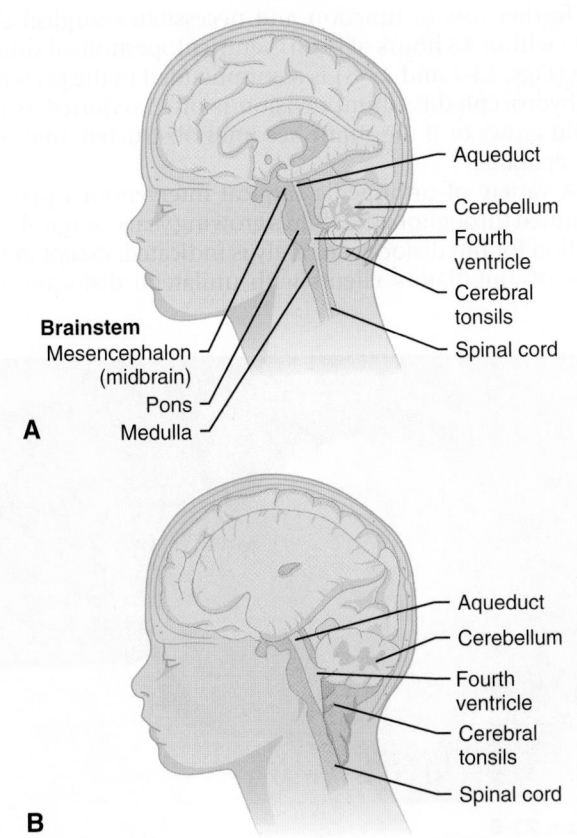

Aqueduct
Cerebellum
Fourth ventricle
Cerebral tonsils
Spinal cord

Brainstem
Mesencephalon (midbrain)
Pons
A Medulla

Aqueduct
Cerebellum
Fourth ventricle
Cerebral tonsils
Spinal cord

B

Figure 23-6

Arnold-Chiari malformation. A, Normal brain with patent cerebrospinal fluid (CSF) circulation. **B,** Arnold-Chiari type II malformation with enlarged ventricles, which predisposes a child with myelomeningocele to hydrocephalus. The brainstem, fourth ventricle, part of the cerebellum, and the cerebral tonsils are displaced downward through the foramen magnum, leading to blockage of CSF flow. Additionally, pressure on the brainstem housing the cranial nerves may result in nerve palsies.

Box 23-2

FACTORS CONTRIBUTING TO PRESSURE ULCERS IN MYELOMENINGOCELE

- Ammonia from urine burns
- Friction burns (feet and knees of young active children)
- Pressure from casts or splints
- Bony prominences
- Vascular problems
- Poor transfer skills
- Obesity
- Asymmetric weight bearing or posture (scoliosis, orthopedic deformities)

MEDICAL MANAGEMENT

DIAGNOSIS. Frequently, NTDs are detected prenatally with ultrasonic scanning and serum AFP testing. Elevated AFP usually occurs by 14 weeks' gestation in the presence of NTDs. This type of screening will not detect skin-covered (closed) neural defects such as spina bifida occulta. The potential for false-positive results with this test may result in unnecessary intervention.

Additionally, as the incidence of this condition continues to decrease, the less reliable the test becomes, because the positive predictive value of the AFP test is dependent on the prevalence of the disease in a population. The less prevalent the disease, the less accurate laboratory results may be. See Chapter 40 for further explanation of the limitations of laboratory tests.

Amniocentesis can detect only open NTDs and is recommended for pregnant women who have previously had children with NTDs or in the case of a large lesion noted with ultrasonic scanning. The need for more accurate, noninvasive imaging of the CNS is recognized, and fetal MRI is an effective, noninvasive means of assessing fetal CNS anatomy with superior ability to resolve posterior fossa anatomy over ultrasonography. However, to date fetal MRI has not surpassed ultrasonography in evaluating hydrocephalus and the level and nature of the spinal lesion.[33,146]

Postnatally, meningocele and myelomeningocele are obvious on examination. Transillumination of the protruding sac usually can distinguish between these two conditions. In meningocele, the sac with its CSF contents is transilluminated (light shines through the sac); in myelomeningocele, the light does not shine through the neural bundle that is present. Spinal films can be used to boney detect defects, and the computerized tomographic scan or MRI demonstrates the presence of hydrocephalus. Other laboratory tests may include urinalysis, urine cultures, and tests for renal function.

TREATMENT. Timing of the closure is important. Prenatal diagnosis has made planned cesarean sections, fetal repair,[12] and therapeutic abortion possible. A cesarean section is the preferred method of birth to avoid trauma to the neural sac that occurs during vaginal delivery. Prenatal closure is now available by fetal surgery and has been found to decrease the incidence of shunt-dependent hydrocephalus and Arnold-Chiari malformation from above 90% in each case to 59% and 38%, respectively.[28,246] By interrupting the flow of CSF during gestation, intrauterine repair enables the cerebellum and brainstem to resume a normal (or nearly normal) configuration.

Prospective parents should be cautioned not to expect improvement in leg function as a result of this surgery. The potential benefits of surgery must be weighed carefully against the potential risks of preterm labor and delivery, potential infection, and blood loss.[245] If postnatal closure is chosen, infection and drying of the nerve roots can lead to further loss of function and necessitates surgical closure within 48 hours of birth. Ventriculoperitoneal shunting (Figs. 23-7 and 23-8) is recommended in the presence of hydrocephalus; shunt revision is often required as the child grows or if the shunt becomes obstructed, infected, or separated.

A variety of orthopedic surgical interventions may be required throughout the child's growing years. Surgical correction for hip dislocation rarely is indicated, except in the case of ambulatory clients with unilateral dislocation.[78]

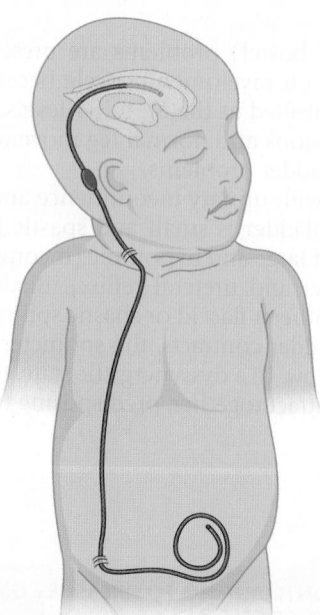

Figure 23-7

Ventriculoperitoneal shunt. This shunt provides primary drainage of cerebrospinal fluid from the ventricles to an extracranial compartment (usually either the heart [ventriculoatrial] or the abdominal or peritoneal [ventriculoperitoneal] cavity, as shown here). Extra tubing is left in the extracranial site to uncoil as the child grows. A unidirectional valve designed to open at a predetermined intraventricular pressure and close when the pressure falls below that level prevents backflow of fluid.

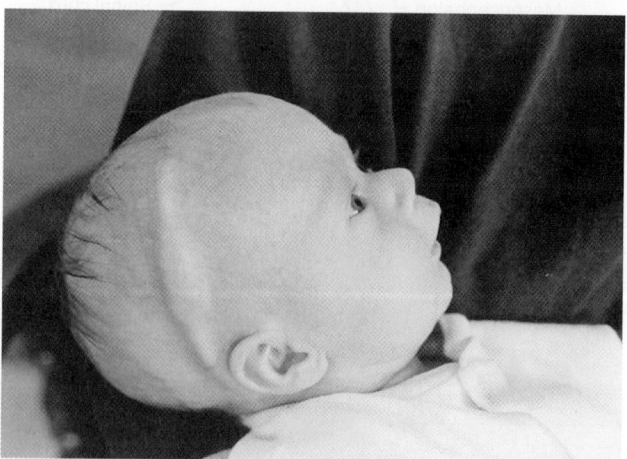

Figure 23-8

Placement of the shunt. The shunt is placed very superficially, necessitating caution when handling the infant. The therapist must be careful to avoid placing pressure over the shunt, stretching the neck, or placing the child in the head-down position. Parents may be distressed initially by the cosmetic appearance of the shunt, but as the child grows, and with hair growth, the shunt is no longer visible. See Fig. 23-10 of this same child with no obvious signs of a shunt. (Courtesy Todd Goodrich, University of Montana, Missoula.)

Investigation shows that a level pelvis and good range of motion of the hips are more important for ambulation than is reduction of bilateral hip dislocation.[104]

Spinal fusion for kyphotic deformity of the spine has had mixed results and frequent complications. Hip flexion and knee flexion contractures often are addressed with muscle releases, and foot deformity correction often is achieved with soft-tissue procedures and in more-severe cases with bony procedures (Figs. 23-9 through 23-11).

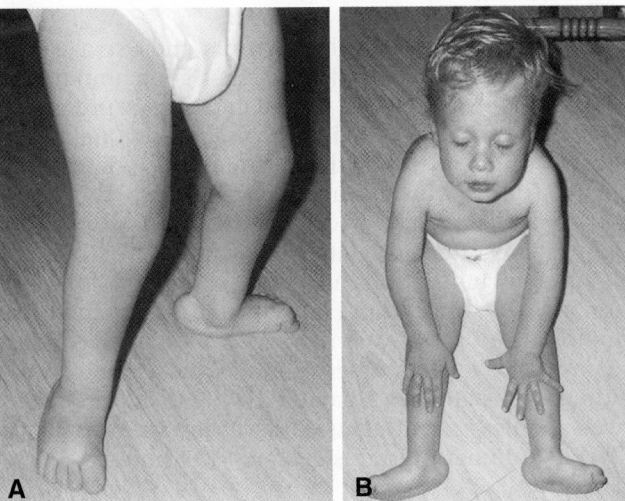

Figure 23-9

Orthopedic involvement. A, Three-year-old boy with bilateral congenital vertical talus resulting in rocker-bottom foot deformities caused by an L4 to L5 myelomeningocele. Note the compensatory knee flexion and genu valgus along with developing toe flexion contractures (the latter from loss of motor control). **B,** Rocker-bottom foot deformity seen more clearly in the non–weight-bearing position. (Courtesy Zane and Dianna Kuhnhenn, Missoula, MT.)

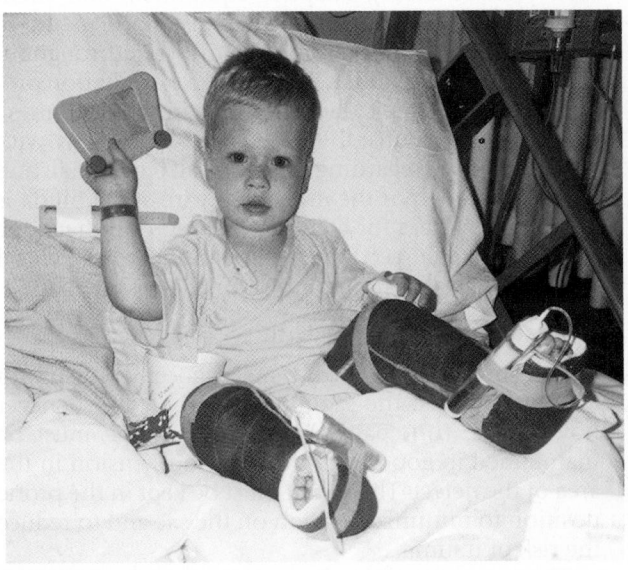

Figure 23-10

Postoperative inpatient after orthopedic reconstructive surgery for congenital vertical talus deformity. Drainage tubes directly from the incision sites were used for 12 hours. (Courtesy Zane and Dianna Kuhnhenn, Missoula, MT.)

Medical management of the bowel and bladder dysfunction is of critical importance from both a medical and social standpoint. The muscles of the bladder can show either spasticity or flaccidity, leading to either a condition where the bladder is small and under high pressure from urine or large and stretched out and under low pressure. However, during early childhood neurologic status is not always stable and can be volatile in the context of a tethered cord and subsequent release. As a result, urologic function should be monitored serially with urodynamic and upper tract evaluations.[167]

In children with spastic bladders under high pressure, vesicoureteral reflux and decreased bladder volume and compliance are critical factors. These factors together contribute to damage to the upper urinary tract and kidneys if not managed effectively.

Children with hypotonic bladders often have more residual urine and are more prone to infection. Infection is treated prophylactically in most children with spina bifida, with antibiotics and high fluid intake as a critical part of an overall management program. Kidney damage is unusual in children with hypotonic bladders because bladder urine is under low pressure and reflux is less of a problem.

Complete bladder emptying using clean intermittent catheterization provides a means to manage urine flow and avoid elevated pressures; in addition, the use of anticholinergic medication can also help avoid elevated

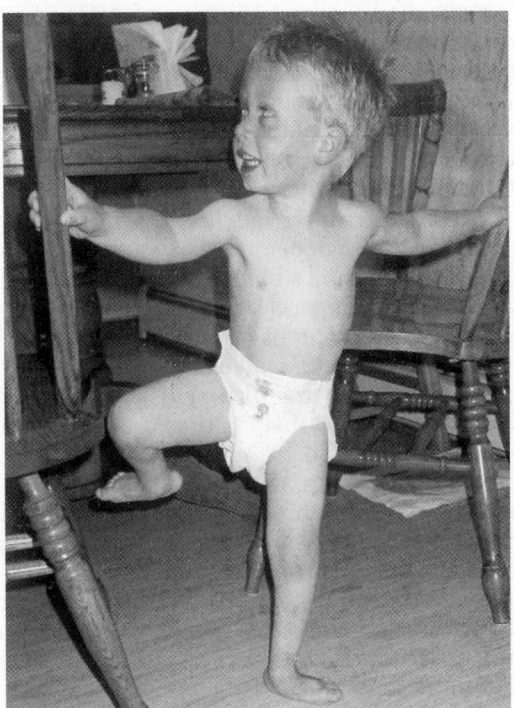

Figure 23-11

Postoperative result. Risk for skin breakdown is reduced around the great toe (no longer contracted into flexion), and base of support is improved for ambulation and allows the child to stand on one leg with support (note the more neutral alignment of lower extremity, especially the knee). The child wears ankle-foot orthoses to maintain proper alignment; there may be some regression of alignment in time because of the continued lack of motor control. (Courtesy Zane and Dianna Kuhnhenn, Missoula, MT.)

pressures by increasing bladder capacity. Manual pressure on the bladder (the Credé method) is used less often because of its tendency to cause reflux. Implantation of an artificial urinary sphincter has been used in the older child or adolescent,[183] and bladder augmentation or urinary diversion are options for the child with high pressures and insufficient volume.

Artificial urinary sphincters can also be implanted to accomplish the opening and closing of the bladder outlet by use of a cuff placed around the outlet. The cuff can be constricted to close the outlet or relaxed to open the outlet and allow urine to flow however these devices come with a relatively high complication rate.[167] Intravesical electrical stimulation remains controversial; however, it has been employed at some centers, with the benefits of increased bladder compliance and increased bladder volume being the most common positive outcomes.[119] Renal function can lead to significant morbidity or mortality in this population and should be monitored regularly.[199]

Stool incontinence is managed most commonly by a program to regulate bowel movements using diet, timed enemas, or suppositories. In some centers, the Malone antegrade continence enema procedure is being used to aid in bowel control. This procedure places a cecostomy, bringing the cecum to the abdominal wall in a procedure similar to the placement of a percutaneous endoscopic gastrostomy tube. Antegrade enemas are then used to control bowel function.[56]

PROGNOSIS. Early, aggressive care of NTDs has now improved the overall prognosis associated with this condition. Prognosis varies with the degree of accompanying neurologic deficit. At present, prognosis is poorest for those children who have total paralysis below the lesion, kyphoscoliosis, hydrocephalus, and progressive loss of renal function secondary to chronic infection and reflux.

At present, survival to adulthood is approximately 85%; most deaths occur before age 4 years. Overall adjustment of the parents and siblings to having a family member with myelomeningocele can be stressful and should not be overlooked in terms of its impact of the affected individual or family as a whole. Often either depression or anxiety, in addition to impairments in social functioning, can be challenges that children with myelomeningocele face and should be addressed with psychologic support.[110]

Approximately two-thirds of children with myelomeningocele and shunted hydrocephalus have intelligence that falls in the normal range. The remaining one-third fall into the range for intellectual developmental disorder, usually mild. Irrespective of IQ, children with spina bifida still have difficulties in perceptual and organizational abilities, attention, speed of motor response, memory, and hand function, in addition to mental flexibility, efficiency of processing, conceptualization, and problem solving. Overall cognitive delays occur less often as a result of improved medical treatment for these children.

Adult outcome data are incomplete and evolving[199] as individuals cared for in different time periods age. Most adults older than 50 years of age survived the preshunt era of the 1950s and are without hydrocephalus, whereas adults now in their 30s include people with more severe disabilities who benefited from the advances in medical and surgical management.

Adults with myelomeningocele continue to need therapy and medical management secondary to joint and spinal deformities, joint pain, pressure ulcers, neurologic deterioration, depression, and poor social interaction and adjustment.

Prognosis for Motor Function. The child's motor abilities vary according to the level of the lesion, but delay in achieving ambulation can be expected in all children with spina bifida, including those with low neurosegment-level lesions.

A child's ability to walk outdoors and use a wheelchair by age 7 years usually suggests a good ambulation prognosis.[61] If functional ambulation is not present by 7 to 9 years of age, it is unlikely to occur subsequently.[5,74] A third of all people with myelomeningocele demonstrate a decline in ambulatory status with increasing age, usually around age 12 years. These losses in ambulatory status often correlate with a variety of adolescent changes, including increasing body size and composition, loss of upper- and lower-extremity strength, or immobilization for varied periods of time secondary to musculoskeletal surgery or fracture healing. Adult ambulatory status in spina bifida is highly influenced by two variables, including motor level and sitting balance. Overall ambulation status declines over time.

SPECIAL IMPLICATIONS FOR THE THERAPIST ▷ 23-4

Spina Bifida Occulta, Meningocele, Myelomeningocele

Throughout the life span of an individual with any of these conditions, the therapist participates actively in providing direct intervention, preventive care that can reduce complications and morbidity (and the associated costs of these), adaptive equipment, and client and family education. The therapist participates in both preoperative and postoperative care throughout the life of the individual. Functional rehabilitation provided by the therapist facilitates functional outcomes.

A helpful resource to the therapist and family with practical advice regarding the physical, emotional, and cognitive growth of the individual with spina bifida is available.[140] Areas for consideration beyond the scope of this text are also covered in this resource (e.g., legal issues, financial planning, vocational assessment).

Neonatal Intensive Care Unit

Before surgery to repair the meningocele, pressure of any kind against the sac must be avoided. Whenever holding the (unrepaired) infant, the spine must be maintained in good alignment without tension in the area of the defect. The infant must be kept in the prone position to minimize tension on the sac and to reduce the risk of trauma.

The prone position allows for optimal positioning of the legs, especially in cases of associated hip dysplasia. The infant is placed flat with the hips slightly flexed to reduce tension on the defect. The legs are maintained in abduction with a pad (a folded diaper or towel) between the knees, and a small diaper roll is placed under the ankles to maintain a neutral foot position.

The prone position is maintained after operative closure, although many neurosurgeons allow a side-lying or partial side-lying position unless it aggravates a coexisting hip dysplasia (see "Developmental Dysplasia of the Hip" above) or permits undesirable hip flexion. The side-lying positioning offers an opportunity for position changes, which reduces the risk of pressure sores and facilitates feeding.

In all handling procedures, care must be taken to avoid pressure on the sac preoperatively or on the operative site postoperatively. If permitted, the infant can be held upright against the body. For the infant with hydrocephalus, until the shunt is in place and draining well, activities that position the head above the body tend to decrease intracranial pressure. Activities that position the head below the body increase intracranial pressure; as a result, care should be taken with handling. In the older child, positional headaches may be indicative of shunt malfunction.

Skin Care

Areas of sensory and motor impairment are subject to skin breakdown and require close attention. The loss of skin sensation accompanied by lack of pain can lead to injury and pressure ulcers. Inadequate circulation increases the problem, because wounds do not heal properly.

Placing the infant on a soft foam or fleece pad reduces pressure on the knees and ankles. Periodic cleansing, application of lotion, and gentle massage can aid circulation, which often is compromised. Bath water must be tested prior to submerging the child to protect against burns because the child cannot feel the water temperature. The family should be advised to use sunscreen to prevent sunburn and to assure that shoes and braces fit appropriately, as these can also be a source of pressure resulting in skin breakdown. The skin should be checked daily for red areas that do not disappear readily when the pressure is removed.

Early and Ongoing Intervention
Precautions

Passive range of motion exercises must be performed slowly and cautiously given the tendency toward fracture in this population. When the hip joints are unstable, stretching into hip flexion or adduction may aggravate a tendency toward subluxation. For this reason the prone hip extension test for measuring hip extension is the method of choice over the traditional Thomas test.[107] An early role of the therapist in assessment is to assist in establishing baseline information regarding the level of initially available muscle function and sensation. Information regarding strength assessment specific to this population is available.[107]

Ongoing assessment includes an awareness of signs and symptoms associated with changes resulting from increased CSF pressure in the presence of hydrocephalus with or without a shunt (Box 23-3). A shunting

---

Box 23-3

SIGNS AND SYMPTOMS OF SHUNT MALFUNCTION

- Congestion of scalp veins
- Firm or tense soft spot on cranium (fontanel)
- Listlessness, drowsiness, irritability
- Vomiting, change in appetite
- Marked depression of the anterior fontanel (overdrainage)
- Disturbance in urinary and bowel patterns
- Increasing head circumference
- Swelling along the shunt
- Seizures
- Nuchal (nape of the neck) rigidity
- Additional symptoms for older children and adults:
  - Gradual personality change
  - Headaches
  - Blurring vision
  - Memory loss
  - Progressive coordination problems
  - Declining school or work performance
  - Decrease in sensory or motor functions

Box 23-4

SIGNS AND SYMPTOMS OF TETHERED CORD SYNDROME

- Changes in bowel and bladder function
- Scoliosis
- Increased spasticity
- Increased asymmetric postures or movement
- Altered gait pattern
- Decreased upper extremity coordination
- Changes in muscle strength (at or below the lesion)
- Back pain

---

mechanism is used for hydrocephalus associated with a variety of conditions other than myelomeningocele. Depending on the underlying condition, shunts can become obstructed or stop functioning for many reasons (e.g., occlusion resulting from blood clots or brain fragments, tumor cell aggregates, bacterial colonization, or other debris; the tube itself can become kinked or blocked at the tip; or growth of the infant or child or physical activities can result in disconnection of the shunt components or withdrawal of a distal catheter from its intended drainage site). Shunt systems also may fail because of mechanical malfunction, including fracture of the catheters, leading to underdrainage or overdrainage.

Infants do not show typical signs of increased intracranial pressure, because skull suture lines are not fully closed. In this age group, a bulging fontanelle is the most obvious sign of pathology. Once the skull bones have fused and the anterior fontanelle is no longer palpable (9-16 months of age), pressure can build inside the closed space, resulting in a variety of symptoms, including headache, vomiting, and irritability.

Tethering of the spinal cord may develop with myelodysplasia. The cord becomes caught or tethered from scar tissue and is stretched as the vertebral canal continues to elongate (Box 23-4). Other causes of a tethered cord include meningomyelocele repair, obstructed CSF shunt, syringomyelia, benign tumor, and spinal cord hypoplasia (i.e., the cord is progressively shorter than the canal and pulled as a result).

Likewise, children with spina bifida have been identified as having the greatest risk of becoming allergic to latex[95] (see "Latex Rubber Allergy" in Chapter 4). Typical symptoms include watery eyes, wheezing, hives, rash, swelling, and, in severe cases, anaphylaxis, a life-threatening reaction. These responses occur when items containing latex touch the skin, mucous membranes (mouth, genitals, bladder, or rectum), or open areas.

The therapist must avoid using toys, feeding utensils, or other items made of latex that the infant or child might put in the mouth. Parents must be advised to read all labels and avoid products, especially toys and utensils, containing latex. If latex content is not indicated, the manufacturer should be contacted for verification before purchase or use of the item. More information on this topic is available for parents (American Latex Allergy Association, http://www.latexallergyresources.org; http:/www.latexallergy help.com).

Controversies

The timing of the operative repair of the lesion remains under heavy debate. Some centers are repairing the defect before birth and are having good results. In most centers, early closure (within the first 24-48 hours) after birth is the standard, and care is taken to prevent local infection, avoid trauma to the exposed tissues, and avoid stretching of other nerve roots, with the goal of preventing further motor impairment.

Other experts contend that surgical repair is best delayed until after further assessment of neurologic function, intellectual potential, and extent of complications. This delay increases the infant's ability to tolerate the surgical procedure, allows for better epithelialization of the sac (thereby reducing the risk of infection), and permits easier mobilization of skin for closure.

A variety of plastic surgical procedures can be used for skin closure. The goal is to place the sac and its contents back in the body with good skin coverage of the lesion and careful closure. Excision of the membranous covering or removal of any portion of the sac may damage functioning neural tissue and is avoided. Although this corrective procedure may prevent an infection of the spinal cord or brain, the goal of surgery is not an improvement in neurologic function.

Philosophic differences exist regarding the necessary characteristics of management programs for children with myelomeningocele. Children whose programs emphasize upright activities and ambulation show better outcomes in terms of, bone density, lower-extremity fracture risk, pressure ulcer risk, transfer skills (even after they have stopped ambulating) compared with children whose programs focus primarily on wheelchair mobility.[152] High-level lesions do not preclude ambulation; however, this may be a relatively energy-intensive activity as compared with wheeled mobility and may have a negative impact on some aspects of school performance. This needs to be balanced with the long-term benefits noted above related to an emphasis on ambulation in the early years.[77]

Controversy also exists regarding the best choice of lower extremity bracing and ambulation method. One area of contention involves the hip-knee-ankle-foot orthosis (HKAFO) for swing-through gait only versus the reciprocating gait orthosis (RGO), which allows the individual options of a swing-to, swing-through, or reciprocating gait. Precautions when considering HKAFO or RGO include severe spinal deformity, spasticity, decreased upper-extremity strength, moderate obesity, knee flexion or plantar flexion contractures greater than 15 to 20 degrees, and hip flexion contracture greater than 35 degrees.

Another area of bracing controversy is whether to brace high and provide a more normal- appearing pattern and protect against progressive orthopedic deformity or to brace low and allow more freedom of movement. Given the many improvements and number of bracing options available, the key to maintaining ambulatory status is good lower-extremity range of motion and a level pelvis. The choice of bracing depends on a careful evaluation of the individual's range of motion, strength, and gait pattern.

DEVELOPMENTAL DYSPLASIA OF THE HIP

Overview

Developmental dysplasia of the hip (DDH), previously known as congenital hip dysplasia or dislocation, is a common hip disorder affecting infants and children. The change in name reflects the fact that DDH is a developmental process occurring dynamically in utero and during the first year of life; this condition is not necessarily present at birth as the word *congenital* implies.

DDH can be unilateral or bilateral and occurs in three forms of varying severity: (1) unstable hip dysplasia, in which the hip is positioned normally but can be dislocated by manipulation; (2) subluxation or incomplete dislocation, in which the femoral head remains in contact with the acetabulum but the head of the femur is partially displaced or uncovered; and (3) complete dislocation, in which the femoral head is totally outside the acetabulum.

Incidence and Risk Factors

The incidence of DDH is between 8.6 and 11.5 per 1000 livebirths.[133] Approximately 85% of affected infants are females. The risk of hip dysplasia increases dramatically in the presence of certain obstetric conditions (e.g., breech delivery, large neonate, twin or multiple births) and other conditions such as idiopathic scoliosis, myelomeningocele (spina bifida), arthrogryposis, and cerebral palsy. The presence of other musculoskeletal deformities such as torticollis,[255] metatarsus adductus, and calcaneal valgus deformity should alert the medical practitioner to the need for further evaluation. Other risk factors include family history, first pregnancies, multiple fetuses, and oligohydramnios (deficient volume of amniotic fluid limiting fetal movement). Certain ethnic groups (Eastern Europeans, Lapps, and Native Americans) also have an increased risk of DDH. One-fourth of all cases involve both hips; when only one hip is involved, the left hip is affected three times more often than the right.

Etiologic Factors

The cause varies depending on the associated condition but is usually the result of mechanical, physiologic, or environmental factors. Hormonally derived (maternal hormone relaxin may affect the child in utero and during the neonatal period) or hereditary laxity of the ligaments about the joint and positioning are possible etiologic factors.

Infant positioning, both prenatally and postnatally, may affect the formation of the acetabular cup and hip stability because the acetabulum is formed as a result of contact with the femoral head, and this is thought to be one possible cause of DDH.[60]

Cultural customs of how babies are carried affect rates of DDH; those cultures that swaddle infants with the hips in extension and adduction are at greater risk of DDH. Conversely, carrying the infant or young child with hips and lower extremities abducted, flexed, and externally rotated may increase stability of the femoral head in relation to the acetabulum.

Pathogenesis

DDH can affect the acetabulum, the femoral head, and the relationship of the femoral head to the acetabulum. The femur, acetabulum, and hip joint capsule usually are well developed by approximately 10 weeks' gestation but continue to enlarge throughout gestation and develop through contact between the femoral head and acetabulum. Most dislocations result in a progressive deformation of the femoral head and acetabulum during gestation.[60]

The subluxated hip maintains contact with the acetabulum but is not well seated within the hip joint. Often this occurs because the acetabulum is shallow, with the roof of the acetabulum sloping at an increased angle in people with DDH, rather than showing a normal cup shape. The dislocated hip has no contact between the femoral head and the acetabulum, the femoral head sits on the iliac wing and the ligamentum teres is elongated and taut (Fig. 23-12).

If the dislocation is not diagnosed and treated early, secondary changes in both soft tissues and bony structures occur. The longer the dislocation has been present, the greater the secondary changes that occur. These changes include stretching of the hip capsule, contracture and shortening of the structures of the hip joint, changes in the blood supply to the hip, flattening of the femoral head, and acetabular dysplasia, sometimes with development of a false acetabulum.

Clinical Manifestations

Clinical manifestations of DDH vary with age. In the newborn and nonambulatory period up to 12 months of age, one or more positive signs may be present (Fig. 23-13). Any observed physical asymmetries in range of motion (even as little as 10 degrees is considered significant, especially as a limitation of hip abduction), asymmetry in the buttock or gluteal fold (higher on the affected side), extra thigh skin folds, or leg-length discrepancy requires medical evaluation.

In the ambulating child, uncorrected bilateral dysplasia may cause a characteristic gait pattern known as a compensated Trendelenburg gait. As the child sways the torso from side to side to compensate for an ineffective gluteus medius, the child assumes a waddling gait pattern.

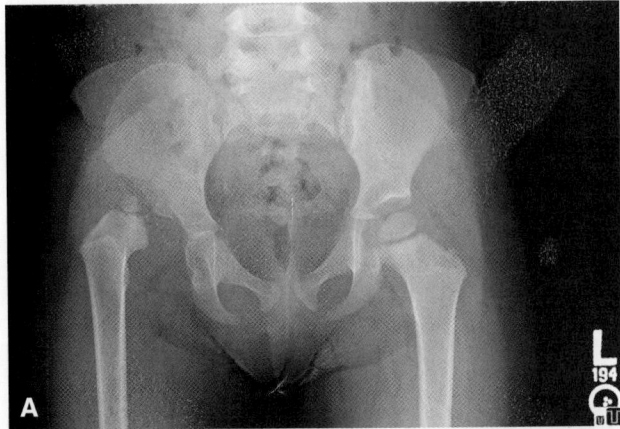

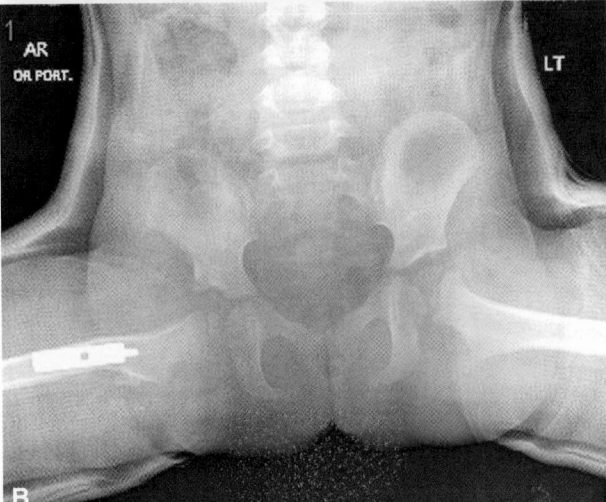

Figure 23-12

Developmental dysplasia of the hip. Three-year-old child with unilateral developmentally dysplastic hip. **A,** Note the head of the femur sitting lateral to the acetabulum. The roof of the acetabulum appears dysplastic and the proximal femur somewhat valgus. **B,** Postoperative: the femur has been relocated in the acetabulum and a varus derotation osteotomy performed. A wedge is cut from the femoral shaft, then internally rotated and positioned in varus to correct the femoral anteversion and valgus. It is also common when there is acetabular insufficiency for portion of the iliac crest to be removed and used as a wedge above the acetabulum to deepen the acetabulum. (Courtesy Allan Glanzman, The Children's Hospital of Philadelphia, PA.)

Unilateral dysplasia usually is characterized by a limp with a positive Trendelenburg sign during the stance phase of gait on the involved side (Fig. 23-14). A flexion contracture on the involved side(s) develops as a result of posterior displacement of the hips, which then contributes to marked lumbar lordosis.

MEDICAL MANAGEMENT

DIAGNOSIS. In the newborn period, clinical examination is the most important diagnostic tool and continues to be the standard screening tool. A positive Ortolani or Barlow click confirms DDH in the first month of life, with a specificity of greater than 99% but a sensitivity of only 60% (see Fig. 23-13).[221] These tests are considered significantly less diagnostic past 2 to 4 weeks.[90] As ligamentous structures become stronger or if the joints become stretched and worn, it is more difficult to elicit the characteristic popping in and out described.

In some cases, dislocation is not diagnosed by these standard tests, and the disorder may not be apparent at birth. Because a normal neonatal examination cannot guarantee that a hip will not become dysplastic, serial examination throughout infancy is essential. Well-baby checkups should include hip examination until the child begins to walk with a normal gait pattern.

The Galeazzi sign becomes positive in the older infant once shortening of the thigh becomes apparent. Radiographic examination is unreliable in the infant and is used more commonly in older infants and children. Plain radiographs are not able to image the hip adequately until the head is ossified and may not confirm the diagnosis if the unstable hip is in the reduced position at the time the film is taken.

For this reason, ultrasonography is suggested in cases of suspected but unconfirmed DDH. Ultrasonography by the Graf method allows visualization of the bony acetabular roof and rim and the cartilaginous roof of the acetabulum, with a score of 1 to 4 assigned. A dynamic assessment to assess stability of the hip involves a Barlow maneuver under ultrasound guidance and is graded as normal, subluxed, or dislocated.[221] It is especially accurate during the first 4.5 to 6 months of life; however, its use as a screening tool remains controversial.[90,223]

TREATMENT. The goal of treatment for DDH is to ensure stability of the femoral head in the acetabulum, thereby encouraging the development of a normally shaped socket and femoral head. This is accomplished by replacing the head of the femur into the acetabulum with no intervening soft tissue. The proper position then must be maintained for a period of time sufficient for the bony and cartilaginous structures to develop sufficient stability

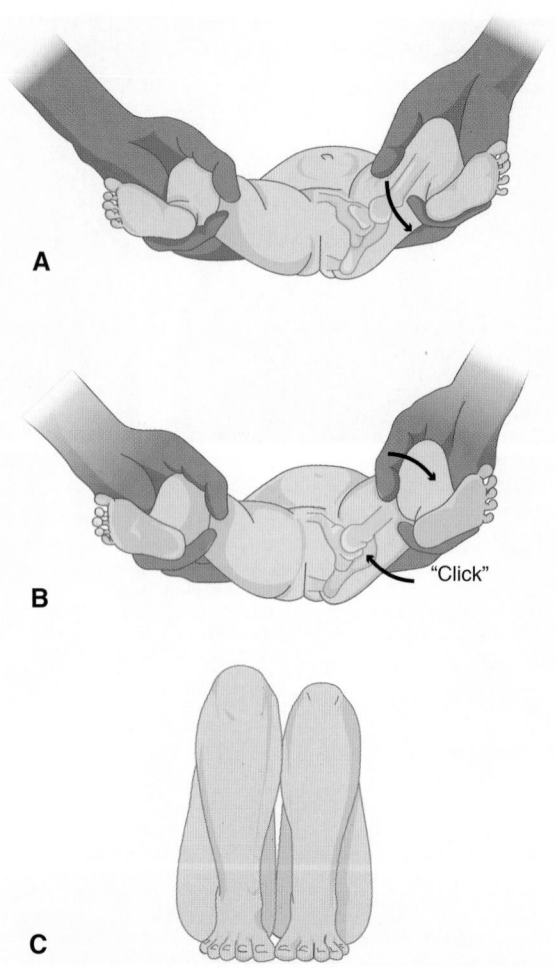

Figure 23-13

Signs of hip dislocation. **A,** Ortolani maneuver No. 1 (also the second part of the Barlow test): hip flexion and adduction with downward pressure dislocates the hip. **B,** Ortolani maneuver No. 2: gentle hip flexion, abduction, and slight traction reduce the hip with a discernible click or clunk, and increased hip abduction is possible in a positive test. This test is valid only for the first few weeks after birth. **C,** Galeazzi test (the Allis sign): in the supine position, with hips and knees flexed and feet flat on the floor, the knee is lower on the dislocated side, indicating that the head of the femur is positioned posterior or superior to the rim of the acetabulum. This test is used to assess unilateral hip dislocation and can be used in older children (from 3 months on).

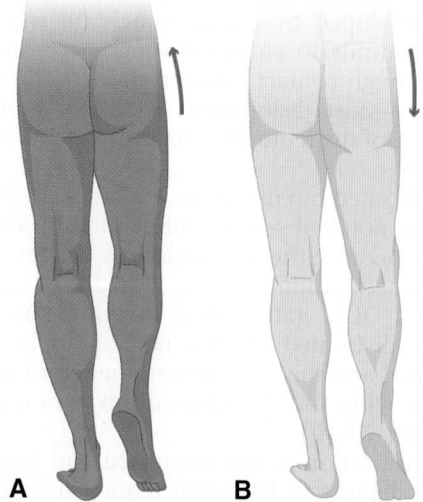

Figure 23-14

Trendelenburg sign. **A,** Negative: with the weight on one leg, the pelvis on the opposite side is slightly elevated (observed from behind the client). **B,** Positive: with weight on one leg, the pelvis drops on the opposite side because of muscle weakness or pain in the hip joint on the stance side. The Trendelenburg sign measures weakness of the hip abductor muscles, especially the gluteus medius.

so that the hip does not subluxate or dislocate with normal movement. Lack of contact of the femoral head in the acetabulum will allow the persistence of acetabular dysplasia. Treatment depends on the age of the child and the severity and duration of the dysplasia.

The most common treatment in the infant is placement of the hip in a position of 100 to 110 degrees flexion and 40 to 60 degrees abduction until the joint capsule tightens and the acetabulum is molded to assume a cup shape. This can be accomplished through the use of a hip harness such as the Pavlik harness (Fig. 23-15). The former standard of treatment with triple diapering is no longer recommended, because proper positioning cannot be ensured and the treatment results in an unacceptable incidence of avascular necrosis of the femoral head. Although the current standard improves this risk there are still reports of avascular necrosis that range between 0 and 28% in the literature, with a higher risk found when there is delay in the onset of treatment and with increased severity of the underlying hip dysplasia.[221] The infant must wear the apparatus continuously for 3 to 9 months to stabilize the hip in the correct alignment. The infant is gradually weaned from the harness so it's used at nighttime only before its final discharge. Criteria for discontinuation of the harness are not standard. Some physicians advocate complete removal of the harness 6 weeks after the hip can no longer be moved in and out of the acetabulum. Others recommend discontinuation when radiographic findings confirm hip stabilization.

In the child treated between ages 6 months and 2 years, a closed reduction is used, often with an adductor release and psoas tenotomy. An arthrogram is used to confirm the reduction followed by 3 to 5 months in a hip spica cast. Treatment after the age of 18 months requires surgical reduction, often with both femoral varus derotational osteotomy and pelvic osteotomies to augment the acetabulum in addition to tenotomy of contracted muscles (see Fig. 23-12, *B*) depending on the clinical presentation. Traction is used before closed reduction by some in an attempt to aid in reducing the dislocation by applying a distractive force to the joint to loosen the surrounding tissue before the closed reduction.

PROGNOSIS. Outcome is directly related to the child's age at initiation of treatment. If the dislocation is corrected in the first few weeks of life, the dysplasia is completely reversible and a normal hip can develop, with rates of success as high as 95%.[145] If surgical reduction is required, 86% have a satisfactory outcome with rates of long-term osteoarthritis of 25% in those individuals who required a closed reduction and 49% in those needing an open reduction.[221] When the condition is untreated, long-term problems can include degenerative joint disease, hip pain, antalgic gait, scoliosis, back pain, or the need for total hip replacement.

| SPECIAL IMPLICATIONS FOR THE THERAPIST | 23-5 |

Developmental Dysplasia of the Hip

Often therapists are involved early and regularly in managing a child's program for some condition other than hip dysplasia and may be the first health care workers to observe signs of hip pathology. An awareness of quick screening strategies for hip dysplasia is critical (Box 23-5).

Physical therapy preoperatively and postoperatively is often a vital part of the rehabilitation process.

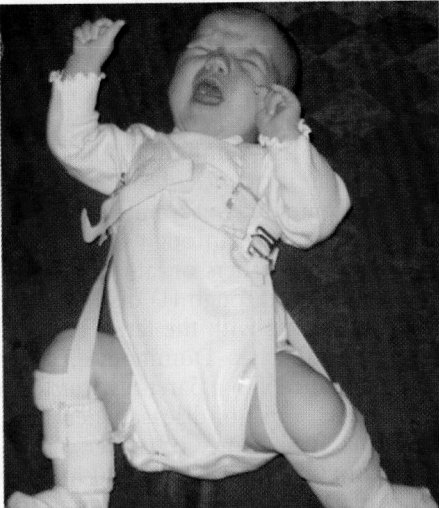

Figure 23-15

Pavlik harness. A 7-month-old with developmental hip dysplasia wearing a Pavlik harness that holds her legs in flexion and abduction. The harness is worn 23 hours a day, removed only for bathing and diaper changes. The goal of treatment is to keep the femoral head in good contact with the acetabulum. A stable hip encourages the development of a normally shaped socket and rounded head of the femur. The proper hip position must be maintained for enough time to stabilize the joint. The hip should be flexed to 95 degrees and abducted (apart) at least 90 degrees. This position keeps the femoral head in the best position and allows the ligaments and joint capsule to tighten up. (Courtesy Allan Glanzman, The Children's Hospital of Philadelphia, PA.)

Box 23-5

HIP DYSPLASIA: QUICK SCREEN

History
- Breech delivery
- Family history
- Female

Lower-extremity examination
- Foot alignment
- Hip range of motion (asymmetry, limited abduction)
- Asymmetric skin folds (thigh, gluteal)
- Buttocks appear flattened
- Leg-length discrepancy

Hip stability (only one positive test required)
- Ortolani sign
- Barlow sign
- Galeazzi sign

Gait (if ambulating)
- Abnormal (waddling gait, limp)
- Positive Trendelenburg sign
- Pain

Typical posture
- Lower-extremity hip flexion, adduction, internal rotation
- Asymmetric head and neck alignment when associated with torticollis

Preoperative intervention may include lower extremity and trunk strengthening and parent/caregiver education. Positioning and handling techniques are an important aspect of the child's care both before and after surgery. Postoperatively, the therapist reviews cast care (or traction/orthotic care) with the child's family/caregivers.

Precautions

Positioning and splinting strategies focus on hip abduction and external rotation. Care must be taken not to set the harness in too much flexion (more than 120 degrees) or abduction (more than 70 degrees) secondary to the potential for impingement on the vascular supply to the femoral head. Force should not be used in flexing and abducting the hip as the excessive pressure can cause avascular necrosis. The ideal "safe zone" for the hip in the harness should be 100 to 110 degrees of flexion and 40 to 60 degrees of abduction.[261]

Positions to avoid include lower-extremity adduction and flexion as occurs in the side-lying position, especially with one lower extremity drifting across the midline.[39] Tests for hip subluxation or dislocation (see Fig. 23-13) should not be repeated too often, because they can result in persistent laxity, articular damage to the head of the femur, and dislocation.

When transferring a child immediately after casting, make sure the casts are dry, plaster casts typically need 1 to 2 hours to completely air dry, whereas fiberglass will cure faster. Use the palms to avoid making dents in the cast as indentations in the cast can predispose the child to pressure ulcers. Check capillary refill, color, sensation, and motion of the child's legs and feet periodically while the cast is in place and notify the physician immediately of delayed capillary refill, or dusky, cool, or numb toes is noted.

Motor Development

The widely abducted position of the lower extremities limits opportunities to initiate or continue development of low back and hip extension, especially in the absence of the prone position. Likewise, the widely abducted base of support in sitting decreases opportunities for the use of trunk rotation necessary for transitioning in and out of positions such as sitting and lying prone. The therapist must closely monitor overall progression of motor development during this time and provide as many opportunities as possible for the development of these important skills.

NEUROMUSCULAR DISORDERS

Neuromuscular disorders, including the muscular dystrophies, congenital myopathies, and spinal muscular atrophy, are presented in this chapter. Other neuromuscular disorders, such as Charcot-Marie-Tooth disease, amyotrophic lateral sclerosis, Guillain-Barré polyneuritis, and chronic inflammatory demyelinating polyneuropathy, are discussed in other chapters in this text.

The Muscular Dystrophies

Definition and Overview

The muscular dystrophies (MDs) comprise the largest and most common group of inherited progressive neuromuscular disorders of childhood. They affect all population types, even animals. Signs of MD can occur at any point in the life span. These disorders, in general, have a genetic origin and are characterized by ongoing, typically symmetric, muscle wasting with increasing deformity and disability. Paradoxically, in some forms (e.g., Duchenne, Becker) wasted muscles tend to hypertrophy because of connective tissue and fat deposits, giving the visual appearance of muscle strength. Six major types of MD are included in this text discussion: (1) Duchenne muscular dystrophy (DMD), (2) Becker muscular dystrophy (BMD), (3) facioscapulohumeral (Landouzy-Dejerine) dystrophy (FSHD), (4) limb-girdle dystrophy (LGMD), (5) myotonic dystrophy, and (6) congenital muscular dystrophy (CMD), also known as muscular dystrophy congenita. These forms of MD involve a primary degeneration of muscle with a gradual loss of strength, but each type differs as to which muscle groups are affected, age of onset, and rapidity of progression (Fig. 23-16).

Incidence and Etiologic Factors

The incidence of DMD is approximately 1 in 3500 livebirths. Rates of occurrence for each type are listed in Table 23-5. DMD and BMD are X-linked recessive disorders caused by mutations in the dystrophin gene *Xp21* that codes for the muscle membrane protein dystrophin. The affected gene on the short arm of the X chromosome *(Xp21)* is one of the largest genes in the human genome. In these two forms of MD, males are affected clinically and females are typically carriers. Male offspring have a 50% chance of being affected and females have a 50% chance of being carriers.

FSHD is an autosomal dominant disorder with onset in adolescence. The son or daughter of a person affected with FSHD is at 50% risk of inheriting the defective gene. FSHD occurs with an incidence of 5 in 100,000 births.

LGMD may be inherited in several ways depending on the type. LGMD type 2 (A through O, Q) disorders are autosomal recessive disorders of late childhood or adolescence and type 1 (A through H) disorders are autosomal dominant disorders with the latter only accounting for 10% to 14% of all cases. Dominant disorders have a 50% risk of inheritance if one parent is affected; recessive disorders carry a 25% risk of disease when both parents are carriers and a 50% chance of carrier status. Overall, the prevalence of LGMD is 1 in 100,000 individuals and the prevalence of various types is often dependent on ethnic background.[200] The incidence of the sarcoglycanopathies can be quite variable by population.[124]

Myotonic dystrophy has an incidence that varies between 1 in 5000 and 1 in 50,000 births, with rates in some populations that approach 1 in 550 because of local founder effects.[271] A founder effect occurs when there is a loss of genetic variation in a population. For example, when the population is isolated or reduced in size because of environmental or social factors the genes of the "founders" of the smaller population are disproportionately frequent. Myotonic dystrophy demonstrates an autosomal dominant inheritance pattern, with each generation

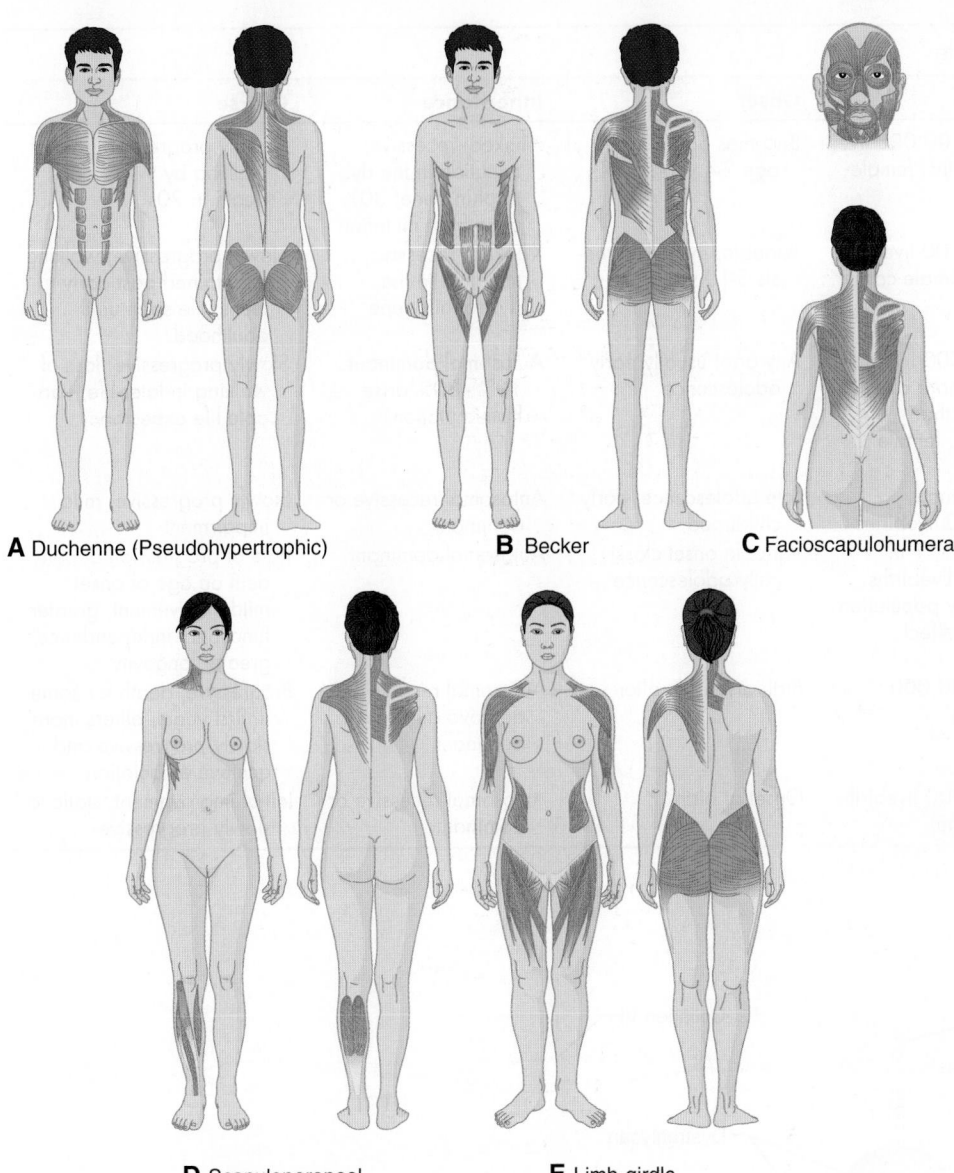

A Duchenne (Pseudohypertrophic)   **B** Becker   **C** Fascioscapulohumeral

D Scapuloperoneal   **E** Limb-girdle

Figure 23-16

Muscle groups involved in muscular dystrophies. These are presented in relative terms; that is, unlike spinal cord injury with definitive muscle involvement, in muscular dystrophy, proximal or distal muscle groups are affected in varying ways with individual differences noted. For example, in the facioscapulohumeral form, the lower erector spinae is featured here but may be spared, and in limb-girdle dystrophy, the lower abdominal muscles may be involved but are not shown in this illustration. **A,** Duchenne: shoulder girdle (trapezius, levator scapulae, rhomboids, serratus anterior), pectoral muscles, deltoid, rectus abdominis, gluteals, hamstrings, calf muscles. **B,** Becker: neck, trunk, pelvic and shoulder girdle. **C,** Facioscapulohumeral: muscles of the face and shoulder girdle. **D,** Scapuloperoneal: muscles of the legs below the knees (first), shoulder girdle (later). **E,** Limb-girdle: upper arm (biceps and deltoid) and pelvic girdle.

being somewhat more severely affected than the last. This increase in the phenotypic severity of the disease state with succeeding generations is referred to as anticipation and can be correlated with an expansion in the size of the triple-repeat genetic enlargement that is the causative factor in this disease.[131]

CMD represents a group of recessively inherited disorders that can be divided into two groups based on the presence of brain involvement. Only the most common forms are included here. The overall incidence has been placed at 4.65 per 100,000 in the Italian population.[165] In Japan, however, Fukuyama MD, one form of CMD, is as common as DMD.

A number of classification schemes have been proposed for the CMDs. For our purposes we will use a biochemical classification that divides the disorders based on the location of the abnormality in the muscle. In this way, CMDs can be divided into (1) those that are the result of protein deficits found in the extracellular matrix including merosin negative (Laminin alpha 2-LAMA2) and Ullrich (collagen VI) CMD; (2) defects in the endoplasmic reticulum

including Selenoprotein 1 (SEPN1); and (3) defects of glycosylation of dystroglycan including Walker-Warburg syndrome (WWS), muscle-eye-brain disease (MEB), Fukutin and Fukutin-related protein defects (FKRP), and like-glycosyltransferase (LARGE) defects making up the final group.[171]

Pathogenesis

Knowledge of the MDs and an understanding of their complexities has escalated dramatically since the late 1980s, when the protein dystrophin was identified as the causative factor in DMD and BMD. Subsequently, other members of the dystrophin glycoprotein transmembrane complex have been identified as causative factors in many other forms of MD.

In addition to transmembrane proteins of the dystrophin glycoprotein complex, there have been proteins in the extracellular matrix, sarcomere, and nuclear membrane identified as causative factors in MD (Fig. 23-17). Recently, it has become apparent that

Table 23-5	Disorders of Muscle			
Type	**Incidence**	**Onset**	**Inheritance**	**Course**
Duchenne (DMD) (pseudohypertrophic)	20-30 in 100,000 live male births; female carrier	Becomes apparent at age 2-4 years	X-linked; recessive; mutation in the dystrophin gene; 30% arise from mutation	Rapidly progressive; loss of walking by 9-10 years; death in 20s
Becker (BMD)	5 in 100,000 live-births; female carrier	Variable, initial diagnosis 5-10 years	X-linked; recessive; mutation in the dystrophin gene	Slowly progressive; walking maintained past early teens; life span until adulthood
Facioscapulohumeral (FSHD)	5 in 100,000 livebirths (males more often affected than females); female carrier	Any age: usually early adolescence	Autosomal dominant; 10% - 30% arise from mutation	Slowly progressive; loss of walking in later life; variable life expectancy
Limb-girdle (LGMD)	1 in more than 100,000 livebirths	Late adolescence: early childhood	Autosomal recessive or dominant	Slowly progressive; mild impairment
Myotonic dystrophy	1 in 5000 to 1 in 50,000 livebirths Variable by population founder effect	Variable onset classically adolescence	Autosomal dominant	Rate of progression dependent on age of onset; mild involvement, greater functional independence, greater longevity
Congenital muscular dystrophy	4.65 in 100,000 livebirths	Birth or shortly after	Autosomal recessive or de novo autosomal dominant	Progressive; death for some in first years, others more slowly progressive and achieve ambulation
Congenital myopathies	2 in 100,000 livebirths (Nemaline)	Onset at birth	Autosomal recessive or dominant	Initial improvement, static to slowly progressive

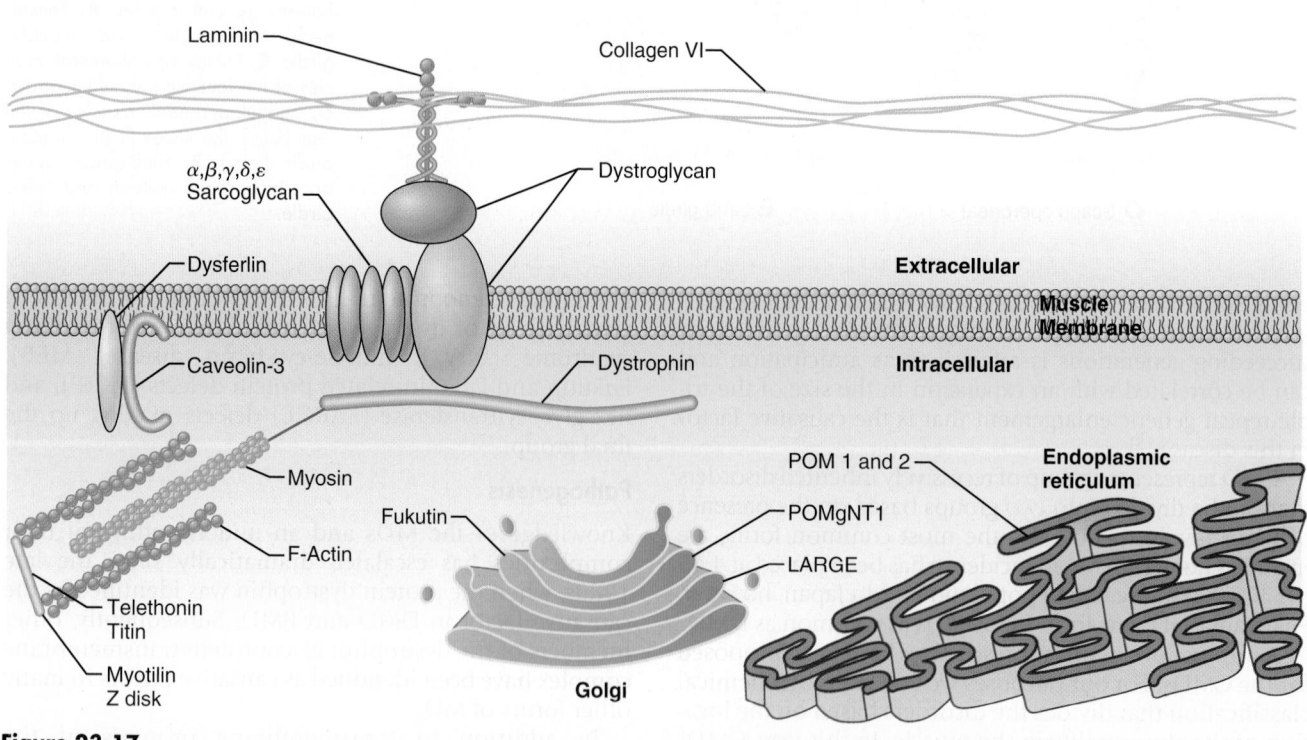

Figure 23-17

Diagram showing the most common muscle protein defects that lead to muscle disease. The dystroglycan complex spans the muscle membrane and connects dystrophin and the myosin/F-actin contractile mechanism to the extracellular matrix. The Golgi complex and endoplasmic reticulum are also displayed with the causative factors related to glycosylation defects. (*Courtesy Allan Glanzman, The Children's Hospital of Philadelphia, PA.*)

in addition to structural proteins, enzymatic defects in glycosylation (the posttranscriptional modification of proteins by the addition of sugars) can also create MD. These discoveries, along with advances in genetic testing, have brought new information on the molecular pathogenesis of these disorders, including the genetic and molecular characterization of many forms of MD.

Duchenne and Becker Muscular Dystrophies. The affected gene in DMD/BMD encodes for the protein dystrophin, which, along with its binding partners, is needed for incorporation of the dystroglycan complex in the muscle membrane and the resulting membrane stability that it conveys. Muscle membrane lesions play a fundamental role in the pathogenesis of DMD/BMD, involving skeletal, cardiac, and smooth muscle membranes.

Dystrophin is the protein that links the muscle membrane (sarcolemma) with the contractile muscle protein (actin). Lack of normal dystrophin makes the sarcolemma susceptible to damage during contraction–relaxation cycles. Disruption of the muscle membrane and muscle fiber necrosis are initiated by muscle contraction, especially eccentric contraction.[182] In addition the dystroglycan complex, which is dependent on the proximal attachment with dystrophin to integrate properly in the membrane, is important not only for structural stability of the membrane but also for its role in cell signaling. Cell signaling is accomplished through the detection of mechanical strain and its regulation of satellite cell recruitment, modulation of protein turnover, and control of blood flow to the muscle.[130] The underlying biochemical defect in all types of MD does not necessarily disrupt the integration of dystrophin in the membrane. While the absence of some sarcoglycan molecules in LGMD (see "Limb-Girdle Muscular Dystrophy" below) can lead to susceptibility to mechanical trauma, the absence of other muscle-based proteins does not.[91]

The absence of dystrophin acts to destabilize the membrane and allow the uncontrolled influx of Ca^{2+}. This action triggers the destruction of the cell from the inside through the activation of calpain, a calcium-activated proteinase.[177] This process is accompanied by inflammation and oxidative stress, which may play a role in the pathogenesis of muscle damage.[130] The inflammatory state following the initial mechanical damage initiates necrosis and apoptosis. These actions may impact the persistence of satellite cells and muscle cell nuclei,[130] impairing the muscles ability to regenerate and possibly altering the differentiation of satellite cells to favor fibroblasts or adipocytes. Muscle cells are replaced by fatty and connective tissues, and contractures develop. Fat cells then continue to accumulate between damaged muscle fibers as a response to the ongoing muscle atrophy. Disorganization of tendinous insertions also is associated with fat accumulation.

Males with undetectable levels of dystrophin typically have DMD, whereas those with dystrophin of an abnormal size or structure or with lower levels of dystrophin typically have BMD. The division between BMD and DMD, however, is determined by the age that ambulation is lost. Those who lose ambulation prior to 13 years of age fall into the DMD group, and those who walk past age 16 years fall into the BMD group, with the middle group defined as intermediate.

Limb-Girdle Muscular Dystrophy. LGMD represents a collection of genetically heterogeneous disorders that can be broadly divided on a genetic basis into two groups. LGMD type 1 (LGMD1A through 1H) are all inherited dominantly, and LGMD type 2 (LGMD2A through 2Q) are inherited recessively. Some of the forms of LGMD are the result of proteins that are part of the sarcoglycan transmembrane complex. Often, in these cases, not only the primary protein will be absent but many of the proteins binding partners will not integrate properly into the membrane and be diminished as well. Although there is little data on the impact of exercise in children with LGMD, an understanding of the protein structure allows one to be more conservative with those forms of LGMD that might limit the full integration of the transmembrane glycoprotein complex where contraction induced muscle cell damage has been demonstrated in animal models.

LGMD type 1A (5q31) is the result of the absence of myotilin and is very rare. Myotilin is a thin filament protein associated with the Z disk and involved in assembly of the contractile mechanism of the cell.[206]

LGMD1B (Lamin A/C or LMNA) (1q21) results from the absence of lamin A and lamin C. Lamins A and C are both produced from the same gene, which is spliced in different ways to produce these two similar proteins that function in the nuclear membrane and are involved in nuclear membrane stability and cell differentiation.[92]

LGMD1C results from the absence of Caveolin 3 (3p25). Caveolin 3 is found as part of the muscle membrane and acts in cell signaling.

LGMD1D is caused by mutations in the *DNAJB6* gene (7q36), which codes for one of a class of proteins called "J" proteins that act as modulatory proteins or cochaperones. The mutations found in *DNAJB6* result in an impairment of inhibition of toxic protein aggregation and protein turnover within the cell.

LGMD1E is related to an abnormality in the gene for DESMIN (2q35) and is located on chromosome 2q35.[89] Desmin, a filament protein is needed for organization of the cytoskeleton within the cell acting as both a transport system within the cell and providing physical stability to the cell to keep it from collapsing. This is especially important in muscle cells where physical demands are significant. In addition, the connections are important for signaling between the nucleus, the sarcolemma, and the actin and myosin of the cell. Additionally connections with the extracellular matrix aid the overall structural composition and alignment of the z disks within the muscle cell. Finally, there is an interaction with mitochondria to facilitate its localization adjacent to the contractile mechanism of the muscle so that sufficient energy is available. This interruption in the Desmin filamentous network of the cell is also seen in other disorders of cardiac or skeletal muscle and comprises a group of disorders sometimes referred to as Desmin-related myopathies or myofibrillar myopathies.[152]

LGMD1F (chromosome 7q32.1), G (chromosome 4q21), and H (chromosome 3p25.1-p23) have been identified in single families and are not discussed in detail here. The reader is referred to the primary descriptions.[19,179]

The second group of LGMDs (2A through 2O and 2Q) are more common than the dominant forms and are inherited recessively. LGMD2A is one of the most common with an estimated carrier frequency of 1 in 103.[185] The underlying defect in LGMD2A is that of a cellular regulatory enzyme P94, calpain 3 (*CAPN3*) gene (15q15.1), one of the calpain family of molecules (calcium-activated protein enzymes). The function of calpain 3 is not well understood, but it appears to play a role in the organization of the muscle cell as it forms during the regenerative process and is likely involved in sarcomere remodeling following exercise.[101,177] *CAPN3* is attached to the structural protein titin, as well as possibly to parts of the sarcomere, and becomes activated with exercise over a certain threshold when it interacts with myosin light chain 1. In addition, *CAPN3* is involved in the muscle membrane repair[101] and some have suggested that *CAPN3* is necessary to protect against exercise-induced muscle damage. This theory is based on animal models of LGMD2A that show exercise-induced muscle damage and abnormal adaptation of the muscle architecture following the stress of exercise.[175]

LGMD2B is caused by an absence of dysferlin (2p13). This is also the protein defect found in Miyoshi myopathy. Miyoshi myopathy presents with a distal dystrophic phenotype in contrast to the proximal LGMD2B proximal phenotype.[259] Dysferlin acts as a membrane repair molecule and interacts with other molecules[38] (Mitsugumin 53, annexin, and calpain) at the muscle membrane to execute membrane repair by a process of intracellular vesicle aggregation at the site of membrane damage and subsequent vesicle fusion with the sarcolemma. In addition, the pathology associated with this form of LGMD is accompanied by a significant inflammatory response in the muscle secondary to the primary protein defect.[97]

The absent genes in LGMD2C (13q12.12), 2D (17q21.33), 2E (14q12), and 2F (5q33.3) all code for a specific proteins in the sarcoglycan–glycoprotein complex and as a group can be referred to as sarcoglycanopathies. This portion of the glycoprotein complex consists of six proteins, the absence of four of which (γ, α, β, and δ) represent the four sarcoglycanopathies (ε and ζ abnormalities have not been found to cause pathology). These proteins are found in close association with dystrophin in the muscle membrane and act to stabilize the membrane. Sarcoglycan-deficient muscle is sensitive to eccentric, contraction-induced disruption of the plasma membrane. δ-Sarcoglycan is strongly associated with β-sarcoglycan and β-dystroglycan,[124] and forms the core of this group of proteins. In the absence of these core proteins, none of the members of this group of proteins integrate properly. Reduced levels of other sarcoglycans (e.g., γ, α, β) also appear to be involved with the stability at the muscle membrane but do not as significantly account for contraction-induced muscle injury as those in the core of the complex.[242]

LGMD2G is the result of a genetic defect on the seventeenth chromosome (17q12), which codes for the protein Telethonin. Telethonin is a protein that acts together with titin (discussed later) in the formation of the muscle cell sarcomere. In the adult muscle, it is found at the Z disk in the sarcomere.[163] Telethonin also plays a role in interactions between the contractile apparatus of the muscle cell and the membrane in sensing the degree of stretch that the sarcomere is experiencing.

LGMD2H results from the absence of the tripartite-motif–containing (*TRIM 32*) gene (9q33), which belongs to a family of similar proteins. *TRIM 32* is not well understood, but acts in conjunction with other enzymes in the muscle and is found to be upregulated in situations where muscle remodeling is occurring, as is the case when changes in weight bearing occur. In addition, it is found in increased levels when muscle cells are differentiating and is expressed in animal models of myogenic stem cells. It impacts differentiation through the modulation of c-Myc, a regulator gene that modulates transcription.[174] *TRIM 32* is also found associated with the thick myosin filaments of the sarcomere.[127]

LGMD2I is a common form of LGMD caused by a mutation in the FKRP gene (19q13.3). FKRP encodes for an enzyme that is involved in glycosylation of α-dystroglycan and can be referred to along with the other LGMDs and CMDs that involve proteins that impair glycosylation as dystroglycanopathies.[240] Glycosylation is a process by which a protein is modified after it is transcribed by the addition of a carbohydrate to a portion of the protein. In this case both α- and β-dystroglycan are produced by the same gene and function differently because of alternative patterns of glycosylation. α-Dystroglycan (and β) is a component of the dystrophin glycoprotein complex and is thought (along with β-dystroglycan) to be an important component of the dystrophin-associated glycoprotein complex that spans the cell membrane, providing both structural and signaling functions. The glycosylation process provides the structure of the extracellular binding site with Laminin, an important extracellular protein that provides extracellular input, as well as a structural connection to the extracellular matrix, that is transferred through the cell membrane by the dystroglycan complex for signaling purposes.[162]

LGMD2J results from a mutation at 2q24.3 in the Titin gene. Titin is a large intracellular protein that is responsible for elasticity and stability of the sarcomere as well as playing a signaling roll related to sensing mechanical stress.[211] In addition it plays a role in the assembly of the sarcomere in the developing muscle cell. Titin extends from the M line and connects the thick-filament myosin to the Z line, where it forms an elastic connection.[141] Clinically titinopathies can present as the LGMD2J when there is homozygous mutation (mutations on both alleles) and in this case there is also a secondary absence of calpain-3. When there is a heterozygous mutation (only one allele affected) the phenotype is milder and presents as tibial MD.[247]

LGMD2K (POMT1) (9q34) represents the LGMD form of one of the disorders of glycosylation and can also present in a more severe form as a CMD (see discussion below).

The exact role of LGMD 2L Anoctamin 5 (*ANO5*) (11p14) is not known, but it is thought that it might code for a segment of a calcium-activated chloride channel. Recessive mutations result in this LGMD phenotype, whereas dominant mutations result in gnathodiaphyseal dysplasia, a sclerotic disorder of bone.[106]

LGMD 2M is the designation for another one of the dystroglycanopathies that results from abnormalities in

Fukutin (9q31). This LGMD form is a milder presentation for what was originally identified as a Fukuyama CMD (see below) and later found to present also in this milder form. In the Japanese population this is one of the more common neuromuscular disorders.[108]

LGMD 2N POMT2 (14q24) is an uncommon, mild presentation of this dystroglycanopathy (see below for discussion).

LGMD 2O POMGnT1 (1p32) is an uncommon LGMD presentation of one of the dystroglycanopathies that typically presents as a CMD (see below).

LGMD 2Q Plectin 1f (8q24) results in an abnormality in the connection between the sarcomere and muscle cell membrane with additional abnormalities noted in overall sarcomeric structure.[94]

Congenital Muscular Dystrophy. The first group of CMDs are disorders of glycosylation that present to varying degrees with muscle, brain, and eye involvement. Glycosylation is the addition of sugars or chains of sugars (glycans) to proteins and can be grouped in to N-glycans and O-glycans based on their binding characteristics. This process takes place in the endoplasmic reticulum and Golgi complex and is regulated by a series of enzymes that control the addition of glycans. Glycan chains are thought to be important in signaling between cells and intracellular signaling as well as the establishment of the proper folded structure of the proteins.[66]

O-mannose glycans develop into very complicated structures and are carried by α-dystroglycan, which is closely associated with β-dystroglycan and is an integral part of the dystrophin-associated protein complex and important in both muscle and brain development. The dystroglycan complex also spans the muscle membrane and binds to both actin, inside the cell, and laminin 2, in the extracellular matrix and glycosylation has been identified as necessary for the binding of laminin 2 to dystroglycan in the extracellular matrix.

Five of the CMDs are linked to mutations in the process of glycosylation. Different mutations in this gene can produce a wide range of phenotypic severity, which in some cases results from the varied amounts of residual enzyme activity.

WWS (POMT1) is the most severe CMD and is the result of defects in the first step in the glycosylation process where O-mannose is added to α-dystroglycan caused by the absence of O-mannosyltransferase 1 that facilitates this reaction. The gene that is responsible is the POMT1 gene. WWS is a phenotypic diagnosis and POMT1 is only responsible for approximately 20% of the cases. An additional 10% of cases may also be contributed by abnormalities in ISPD (7p21.2) whose absence affects O-mannosylation. Mutations in POMT2 and the enzyme O-mannosyltransferase 2 is also a cause of WWS, and the combination of these two genes in the endoplasmic reticulum modulates transferase activity.[258]

MEB can be caused by mutations in the *POMGnT1* gene (1p34.1) that encodes for the transferase in the next step in the O-mannosyl glycosylation pathway. Clinically MEB represents a spectrum of phenotypic expression from mild (those who will live into adulthood) to a severe MEB; in general, MEB presents a phenotype that is less severe than WWS. Because of this variability, other factors are presumed to affect the severity of the presenting phenotype. One such factor might be overexpression of LARGE.

Fukuyama CMD is caused by a mutation in the fukutin gene (9q31.2); the products are expressed in muscle in the same location as dystroglycan. Fukutin is found in the *cis*-Golgi, but beyond that its function has not been established although it is thought to participate in glycosylation of α-dystroglycan. The pathology of the CNS that is seen is that of a cobblestone lissencephaly where the layering of the cerebrum is disrupted as the result of abnormal neuronal migration. Fukutin is likely involved in both neuronal migration and synapse function in addition to formation of the basement membrane, the glia limitans, which separates the cerebral cortex and the pia mater of the meninges.[267]

CMD resulting from a mutation in LARGE can present phenotypically as MEB, WWS, or more mildly with Intellectual disability and only mild weakness. LARGE is found in the Golgi complex and is the rate-limiting step in the glycosylation of α-dystroglycan. When it is overexpressed, α-dystroglycan is hyperglycosylated in animal models. Despite this knowledge, its exact function still remains unclear. The potent effect of LARGE makes it an ideal target for drug development as its overexpression can rescue both in vitro and in vivo models of a variety of glycosylation-based MDs.[79]

Merosin-negative CMD results from a mutation in the laminin alpha-2 *(LAMA2)* gene (6q22-23) and in deficiency or absence of merosin (also known as laminin) the protein effected in merosin-negative CMD.[123] The underlying pathophysiology is not well understood, but the function of laminin 2 is primarily one of cell-adhesion. It is found as a three-chained structure composed of three subunits: $α_2$, $β_1$, and $γ_1$. It binds to dystroglycan (as well as integrin) and provides structural support for the basement membrane protecting the cell from contraction induced damage.[83]

Ullrich CMD (and Bethlem myopathy; see below) is one of the more common CMDs and is the result of a defect in the extracellular matrix protein collagen type VI. Collagen type VI is made up of three strands, COL6; A1, A2, and A3, These three strands are coded for on 21q22.3 or 2q37.3 and form a triple helix, which then associates into a dimeric structure consisting of two associated subunits that are aligned in an antiparallel "head-to-toe fashion." Finally two of these dimeric proteins become aligned in a parallel fashion creating a tetrameric four-protein complex, which is then the final product and is transported out of the cell and becomes a component of the extracellular matrix. It is found both near the basement membrane and within tendons surrounding fibroblasts, which is the cell of origin of COL6. The underlying structural defect that leads to poor force transmission might relate to interaction with the muscle cell membrane and biglycan, which might provide an intermediate connection to the membrane because it binds with both COL6 and the dystrophin-associated transmembrane protein complex, but the exact function still remains unclear.[22]

Facioscapulohumeral Dystrophy. The genetic defect has been found at 4q35 in 90% to 95% of individuals with FSHD.[36,250] FSHD occurs as the result of a decrease in the typical number of tandem repeats on chromosome 4q35; however, the pathogenesis of this is impacted by other genetic factors possibly ones found both proximal and distal to the gene on the fourth chromosome.[215] The assumed impact of other genetic factors is the result of observations that not all individuals with a decreased number or D4Z4 repeats demonstrate phenotypic characteristics of FSHD. Seventy percent of affected individuals have between four and eight repeats, but this range is also found in 3% of the normal population, suggesting the presence of other factors that impact phenotypic expression. The presence of a reduced number of repeats along with these other factors causes production of a protein called double home box protein 4 (DUX4), which is normally not produced in healthy subjects. The presence of DUX4 causes the symptomatology associated with FSHD. This is in contrast to most other genetic disorders where the absence of a protein is the disease causing factor. Here the presence of a previously silent gene, which has been turned on, now produces a protein which causes phenotypic expression.[215]

Myotonic Dystrophy. There are three forms of myotonic dystrophy. The major form of myotonic dystrophy, also known as Steinert type or MD11 myotonic dystrophy with protein kinase *(DMPK)* gene (9q13.3) being the identified abnormality and it represents 98% of the cases. A second type of myotonic dystrophy has been identified, myotonic dystrophy type 2 (MD2) zinc finger protein (ZNF9) (3q21.3).[154] In MD1, the underlying defect of the gene is a trinucleotide repeat in which cytosine, thymine, and guanine are repeated an abnormally large number of times (see Fig. 1-4). With succeeding generations this defect expands, a condition known as anticipation, also seen in other triple-repeat disorders. In diseases that demonstrate anticipation, each succeeding generation is more affected than the last.[131]

The precise pathophysiology remains poorly understood, but the triple repeat results in abnormal splicing of RNA. There are two similar RNA binding proteins CUG-BP and MBNL-1 that mediate a subset of splicing events that are impaired in MD1. This results in abnormalities involving the creation of abnormal RNA transcript processing and alterations in other genes, some of which code for the chloride channel,[17] the insulin receptor, and microtubule-associated protein tau, each related to a portion of the underlying phenotype (myotonia, risk of diabetes mellitus, and cognitive delay).[18] In myotonic dystrophy muscle fibers demonstrate altered resting muscle membrane potentials, possibly resulting from a dysregulation of ion channel function.[14]

Clinical Manifestations

Duchenne Muscular Dystrophy. DMD is usually identified when the child has difficulty getting up off the floor (the Gowers sign; Fig. 23-18), falls frequently, has difficulty climbing stairs, and starts to walk with a waddling gait (proximal muscle weakness) and an increased lumbar lordosis (compensation for abdominal and hip extensor weakness). At the same time, the child begins to walk on the toes because of contracture of the posterior calf musculature and weakness of the anterior tibial, peroneal, and proximal muscles.

Hip abductor weakness produces a positive Trendelenburg sign (see Fig. 23-14), which eventually changes to a compensated Trendelenburg emblematic of the gluteus

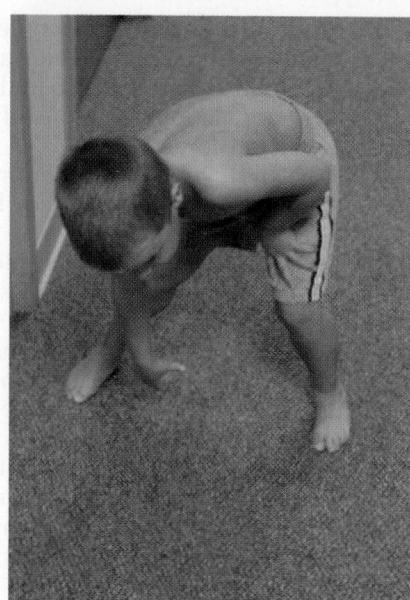

Figure 23-18

The Gowers sign. This boy adopts the typical movement seen with proximal weakness, such as myopathies, when arising from the floor, a chair, or even when climbing stairs. During the Gowers maneuver, the client places the hands on the thighs and walks up the legs with the hands until the weight of the trunk can be placed posterior to the hip joint. This sign is characteristic of weakness of the lumbar and gluteal muscles. (Courtesy Allan Glanzman, The Children's Hospital of Philadelphia, PA.)

medius weakness. Classically ambulation continues to deteriorate up to the age of 7 to 12 years, at which time the majority of people with DMD lose the ability to walk.[26,229] However, treatment with prednisone or deflazacort may delay the cessation of ambulation for 2 to 5 years, allowing children to continue to walk until an older age.[168]

The shoulder girdle becomes involved, with excessive scapular winging, which is made more prominent by the presence of an excessive lumbar lordosis (Fig. 23-19). Shoulder girdle weakness and the need to maintain the weight line posterior to the hips and anterior to the knees to enhance stability at those joints often prevents the use of crutches or a walker to support the body weight.

Weakness of the shoulder girdle also causes difficulty in performing overhead activities related to hygiene and work. Biceps tendinitis, subacromial bursitis or other impingement disorders at the shoulder occur as the children get older as the result of weakness and the repeated manual lifts that become necessary for transfers. Muscle imbalances create biomechanical dysfunction, and weakness impairs the ability to stabilize the shoulder girdle, contributing to shoulder problems.

With the progression of weakness, scoliosis occurs at a rate of 80% to 90% in individuals who are untreated with corticosteroids and usually progresses more rapidly after the person is wheelchair bound. Spinal fusion is usually considered when the spinal curve approaches 40 degrees. Early fusion, when a good correction and level pelvis can be obtained, and when the individual's respiratory status is relatively more intact, produces the best result. The rate of scoliosis is significantly reduced by the use of corticosteroids.

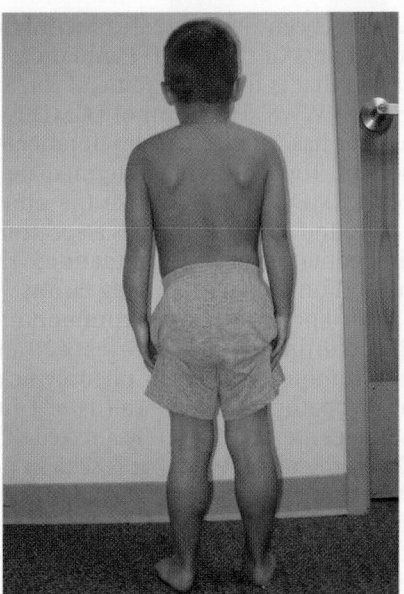

Figure 23-19

Duchenne muscular dystrophy with pseudohypertrophy of calves and lordotic posture that places the weight of the trunk behind the hip joint. Even though weakness occurs symmetrically, habitual standing postures may create asymmetries in flexibility in some cases. (Courtesy Allan Glanzman, The Children's Hospital of Philadelphia, PA.)

Common comorbidities associated with DMD include cognitive, respiratory, cardiac, and gastrointestinal dysfunction. The average IQ of individuals with DMD is 1 standard deviation below the mean, with specific reading disorders noted irrespective of IQ. Even so, many children with DMD have normal or above-normal intelligence.

Children with DMD develop a progressive restrictive respiratory impairment secondary to weakness and contracture of the respiratory muscles. Respiratory problems become more of a problem after the children become wheelchair bound. Nocturnal hypoventilation is one of the earlier manifestations of respiratory involvement and is usually accompanied by morning headaches, sleep disturbance, or nightmares. Chest muscle deterioration combined with joint contractures and spinal scoliosis results in diminished ventilation and ability to produce pressure to cough up secretions, leading to upper respiratory infections or pneumonia.

Dilated cardiac myopathy and, less frequently, conduction abnormalities can be life-threatening and with the improvements in pulmonary care this has often become the life-limiting impairment.

Gastrointestinal problems are common, and constipation, pseudoobstruction and gastric dilation can result from the smooth muscle deterioration.

Becker Muscular Dystrophy. Signs and symptoms of BMD resemble those of DMD but with a slower progression and longer life expectancy. Ambulation is preserved into midadolescence or later, but often is marked by the toe walking with bilateral calf muscle hypertrophy and contracture.

Proximal muscles tend to be affected to a greater degree and before the involvement of the distal musculature, with primary effects observed in the neck (relatively preserved in BMD versus DMD), trunk, pelvis, and shoulder girdle. Muscle cramps are a common complaint in late childhood and early adolescence. Scoliosis and contractures (elbow flexors, forearm pronators, and wrist flexors in the upper extremity and plantar flexors, knee flexors, and hip abductors in the lower extremity) and other comorbidities also found in DMD are common; however, these occur less frequently and with less severity in the BMD type.

Limb-Girdle Muscular Dystrophy. LGMD affects proximal more than distal muscles and follows a steady progressive course, although the course can vary widely even in a given family in some forms. Early symptoms develop as a result of muscle weakness in the pelvic and shoulder girdle muscles, usually the first symptoms are noticed in adolescence or early adulthood. Winging of the scapulae, lumbar lordosis, abdominal protrusion, waddling gait, poor balance, and inability to raise the arms may also develop.

LGMD1A (myotilin) also known as myofibrillar myopathy has a typical age of onset in adulthood as late as the seventh decade of life. Some individuals have cardiac involvement and there is an associated neuropathy that is axonal in character associated with LGMD1A. As a result, some people with this type will have prominent distal weakness superimposed on the proximal LGMD phenotype.[218]

LGMD1B (Lamin A/C or LMNA) has a wide variability in phenotype depending on mutation type. This ranges from severe Emery-Dreifuss muscular dystrophy to a somewhat less-aggressive LGMD-type phenotype. Cardiac conduction defects are common and need to be aggressively managed. In addition, the development of dilated cardiomyopathy is also seen in this population.[44] The contracture pattern in this population includes the development of elbow flexion and ankle plantar flexion contractures, along with trunk and cervical extension contractures, with relative sparing of the quadriceps muscle strength in most cases.[170]

LGMD1C (caveolin 3) is one of a number of ways that abnormalities in Caveolin 3 can present. In this form, first symptoms are typically seen in the first decade with proximal weakness and the Gowers sign. In addition, calf hypertrophy similar to DMD and postexercise soreness is common. Caveolin 3 can also present with isolated elevated creatine kinase without weakness, rippling muscle disease (percussion-induced muscle contraction), or as an isolated hypertrophic cardiomyopathy.[32]

LGMD 1D (DNAJB6) onset is typically between the third and sixth decade of life and ambulation is typically preserved with functional deficits characterized by problems climbing steps and running. Contracture is not a prominent feature in LGMD1D. The distribution of weakness of the legs is characterized by proximal weakness in addition to posterior compartment (hamstring more than quadriceps) weakness with inconsistent involvement of the arms.[209,212]

LGMD1E (Desmin) presentation is typically between the second and sixth decade of life, with the distribution of weakness in a typical LGMD distribution or more distally in a scapuloperoneal pattern. Affected individuals can develop respiratory, as well as oral, motor dysfunction. Cardiac findings are common in this population.[217]

Clinical manifestations of LGMD2A Calpain-3 (p94 protein) (CAPN3) include phenotypic variability from first decade of life onset and rapid progression to onset later onset and slower progression. Approximately 70% of affected individuals present between ages 6 and 18 years.[173] The typical pattern of involvement is that of a classic limb-girdle pattern, with the gluteal and adductor muscles most affected. The average age of ambulation loss varies considerably (5-39 years) and is related to age of onset. The underlying genetics seems to be related to the phenotypic severity. Individuals with two null mutations are much more homogeneous, with an average age of presentation of 15 years.[197]

The phenotypic presentation of LGMD2B (Dysferlin) can be that of classic LGMD or, alternatively, either a Miyoshi myopathy phenotype, which presents with gastroc-soleus involvement as the defining factor, or as a more rapidly progressive wasting of the anterior tibialis.[98]

The typical presentation of LGMD2C-F Sarcoglycan (gamma 13q12.12, alpha 12q21.33, beta 4q12, delta 5q33.3) is in the later first decade of life with proximal weakness similar to that of DMD. However, there is significantly more variability and some individuals present later in the second decade of life or even in adulthood. Cardiomyopathy is most common in individuals with β and δ sarcoglycanopathies. Respiratory failure is also a concern in a pattern similar to that found in DMD, although with somewhat more variability in onset. The contracture pattern[124] associated with this form includes plantarflexion contractures.

LGMD2G (Telethonin) presents primarily as an LGMD pattern of skeletal muscle weakness; however, there are some reports of congenital presentation or hypertrophic cardiomyopathic presentation.[72]

LGMD2H (TRIM32) presents with significant variability between groups of individuals and with typically proximal weakness that ranges from nonprogressive to slowly progressive.[239]

LGMD2I (FKRP) is one of the dystroglycanopathies. Its clinical presentation is widely distributed, ranging from mild, late-onset disease as is found in the LGMD2I phenotype to a severe form of CMD with brain and eye abnormalities in addition to severe weakness at birth.[21] The severity of the phenotype is dependent on the efficacy of the underlying protein that is produced in the glycosylation of dystroglycan. Many of the genes implicated have both more-severe and less-severe forms, depending on the specific mutation characteristics and how severely the final protein is effected in terms of its function in the glycosylation process.[162]

LGMD2J (Titin) can present in two phenotypic varieties. In the case where there is a mutation on one allele, the phenotype is one of a tibial muscular dystrophy, with anterior tibialis and long toe extensor weakness as the first symptoms which may progress to proximal weakness in old age. When there is a mutation to the gene on both alleles, the phenotypic picture is one of LGMD2J and dilated cardiac myopathy, sometimes without skeletal muscle involvement owing to different splicing in the two different tissues.[247]

LGMD2K has been designated to identify the milder phenotypic variants of the POMT1 mutation. This is the same mutation that is found in some of the more severe CMD cases with WWS. This form of LGMD is one of the only forms that has intellectual developmental disorder as a component. There are some intermediate forms that fall between LGMD and WWS. Like the other glycosylation defects found in FKRP, there is a spectrum of severity found in people with POMT1 mutations. This is likely the result of still unknown modifying factors.[51]

Proximal weakness is the most common presentation of LGMD2L, occurring between the ages of 20 and 50 years, with a less-common form that is phenotypically similar to Miyoshi myopathy where the calf is first involved. In both cases, males are more severely affected.[106]

LGMD2M is the phenotype that is seen in people with the LGMD form of Fukuyama congenital muscular dystrophy, which has a very broad spectrum of phenotype ranging from the severe CMD presentation to that of isolated hypercalcemia all resulting from the same FKTN gene.[256]

LGMD2N is a rare LGMD presentation of Walker-Warberg CMD.

LGMD2O is the LGMD milder presentation of MEB.

LGMD2Q presents with early onset of weakness and delayed motor skills in the first years of life followed by a plateau with a continuation of ambulation until the third decade (ages 20-30 years).[94]

A THERAPIST'S THOUGHTS*
Clinical Phenotypes

The details of clinical phenotyping as described in these sections may be easy to skip over but this information is important for the physical therapist when establishing a plan of care in the absence of a known natural history. Therapists need to provide anticipatory guidance and treatment in the context of progression that is expected.

To expand on this point further, remember that clinical features are often dependent on the specific underlying LGMD type and even then the severity of presentation can be quite variable between individuals, making this type of MD more difficult to diagnose. Identification of the specific type of LGMD should be pursued to provide the best guidance for the client and to allow the therapist and physician to treat the person proactively with full knowledge of the natural history of the specific disorder rather than approaching the case reactively. For example, an understanding of the natural history of the specific form of LGMD will aid in anticipating the pattern of potential contracture and weakness in addition to the anticipated functional course and typical timing of functional decline.

*Allan Glanzman, PT, DPT, PCS

Congenital Muscular Dystrophy. CMD represents a spectrum of disease states that most commonly present at the more severe end of the spectrum in infancy, with rapidly progressive muscle strength loss and progressive respiratory symptoms. The first group includes those with disorders of glycosylation. Affected individuals demonstrate a mixed central and peripheral picture with involvement of both the brain and muscle in addition to involvement of the visual system.

WWS is the most severe of the CMDs and presents at birth with a rapidly progressive course, with death most commonly occurring prior to 1 year of age. Ocular impairments include retinal abnormalities, microphthalmia glaucoma, cataracts, and anterior chamber abnormalities. The CNS complications include a cobblestone lissencephaly[58] with polymicrogyria. Cerebellar abnormalities are also present and include hypoplasia in addition to fourth ventricular dilation. MEB has similar clinical findings as WWS but a wider range of phenotypic presentations.

Fukuyama MD can also present as a CMD but is more often found in its milder LGMD form. Common phenotypic presentation includes onset at or shortly after birth with weakness and delayed gross motor skills with progressive contractures and weakness, with very few individuals achieving ambulation and a typical loss of ambulation by the age of 10 years. Cognitive impairment is common and often severe, with MRI findings somewhat similar to those found in WWS.

Ullrich CMD can present along a spectrum of severity, with its milder form, Bethlem myopathy, representing the mildest presentation. In its more severe forms, children have significant weakness that either prevents ambulation or allows them to walk only for a short time prior to adolescence.[156] The most prominent feature of the phenotype is the distal laxity mixed with proximal contractures, particularly of the knee and the elbow, with prominent shoulder protraction resulting from contracture of the pectoral muscles. The distal laxity in the Achilles tendon can contribute to a crouched gait pattern or the gastrocsoleus and posterior tibialis can present with contracture and a plano varus foot position in standing.

Merosin-negative CMD typically presents with weakness at birth. However, most infants attain the ability to sit and a spectrum of severity exists, including an LGMD phenotype that has been reported with the milder phenotypes include the ability to ambulate in childhood in those patients with partial merosin deficiency.[123] Contracture pattern includes limitation in neck flexion and early development of hip flexion contractures. Muscle strength of the quadriceps is typically relatively spared. Respiratory insufficiency develops, typically in the first decade.

Facioscapulohumeral Dystrophy. FSHD is a mild form of MD beginning with weakness and atrophy of the facial muscles and shoulder girdle, usually presenting in the second decade of life. Phenotypic expression is more common in males than in females (95% vs. 69%), with more females being carriers. Inability to close the eyes may be the earliest sign; facial expressions are limited even when laughing or crying, forward shoulders and scapular winging is a prominent feature, as is difficulty raising the arms overhead (Fig. 23-20).

Other changes in the face include diffuse facial flattening, a pouting lower lip, and inability to pucker the mouth to whistle. Progression is descending, with subsequent involvement of either the distal anterior leg (quadriceps and anterior tibialis) or hip girdle muscles.[235] Weakness of the lower extremities may be delayed for many years. Contractures, skeletal deformities, and hypertrophy of the muscles are uncommon.

There is wide variability in age at onset, disease severity, and side-to-side symmetry, even within affected members of

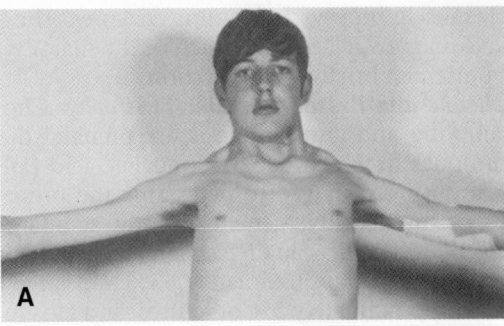
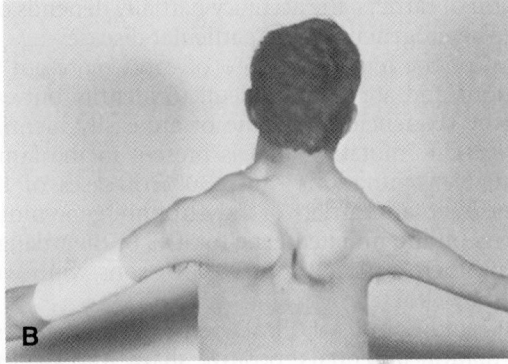

Figure 23-20

Facioscapulohumeral dystrophy. Weakness of subscapular musculature makes it difficult to perform overhead activities; wasting also causes the clavicles to jut forward and the shoulders to have a drooping appearance. During humeral movement, the scapulae wing and ride up over the thorax. (From Morgan-Hughes JA: Diseases of striated muscle. In Asbury AK, McKhann GM, McDonald WI, editors: *Diseases of the nervous system: clinical neurobiology*, ed 2, Philadelphia, 1992, WB Saunders, p. 170.)

the same family. Associated non–skeletal muscle manifestations include high-frequency hearing loss and retinal telangiectasias, both of which are usually asymptomatic.[235,250]

Myotonic Dystrophy. The clinical presentation of myotonic dystrophy represents a spectrum of disease severity that is based on the size of the genetic triple repeat. Three phenotypes have been identified. The most severe is congenital myotonic dystrophy with weakness and myotonia at birth. The classic form is characterized by weakness and some degree of disability, with mild myotonia and cataracts.

The clinical symptomatology of myotonic dystrophy includes muscle weakness and wasting with a delayed relaxation of the muscle and increased excitability. Ocular cataracts are also a defining feature; cardiac conduction defects represent a serious comorbidity. A wide variety of other symptoms, including sensorineural hearing loss, hypersomnia, testicular atrophy (and sterility), and endocrine dysfunction, are also found in myotonic dystrophy.[14] People with myotonic dystrophy have muscular weakness, wasting, and hypotonia.

MEDICAL MANAGEMENT

DIAGNOSIS. Researchers continue to develop noninvasive imaging procedures for evaluating the localization, extent, subtype, and mechanisms of skeletal muscle damage in MD. Diagnosis is currently based on clinical presentation, family history, and diagnostic testing such as muscle ultrasound or MRI, genetic testing, electromyography

(EMG), muscle biopsy, and serum enzymes. The use of these five diagnostic tests with each of the major types of MD is presented briefly in this section.

Duchenne and Becker Muscular Dystrophy. Chorionic villi sampling and amniocentesis are prenatal diagnostic techniques in which deoxyribonucleic acid (DNA) is removed during gestation to determine the presence or absence of the defective gene. Currently, standard laboratory genetic testing can detect large deletions of the dystrophin gene in approximately 65% and large duplications in approximately 5% of fetuses, and aids in identification of carriers; the accuracy partially depends on the genetic heterogeneity of the particular disease.

Most of the remaining 35% of cases represent point mutations and are more difficult to identify but can be found by sequencing the gene or are easily identifiable if the specific mutation that is present in the family is known. New mutations cause 30% of cases of DMD. Mothers who are carriers of a dystrophin gene mutation will pass on the mutated gene to 50% of their daughters (making them carriers) and 50% of sons, who will be affected by DMD.

EMG studies in DMD/BMD demonstrate the presence of fibrillation potentials, positive sharp waves (more in DMD), and long-duration polyphasic motor unit action potentials (MUAPs) (more in BMD) with full recruitment at low force. Nerve conduction velocities are normal in both DMD and BMD.[62] A muscle biopsy specimen shows variation in the size of muscle fibers; central nuclei, inflammatory cells, and fat and connective tissue deposits are prominent characteristics of the biopsy specimen. In DMD, the muscle stains negative for dystrophin antibodies, whereas in BMD, levels of dystrophin vary.

Serum enzyme levels are used to identify the presence of active muscle breakdown. Levels are extremely high in the first years of life before the onset of clinical weakness and persist as symptoms develop. Eventually, after replacement of muscle substance has become chronic and extensive, the creatinine kinase (CK) level may be either normal or only mildly elevated (less than five times normal). The CK may be increased in DMD, especially in the earlier phase of the illness. Approximately 50% to 60% of female carriers of DMD/BMD have elevated CK. Males affected by DMD/BMD present with CK levels that are approximately 2 to 10 times normal, reflecting active muscle damage (see "Serum Enzymes" in Chapter 40; see Table 40-15).

Limb-Girdle Muscular Dystrophy. LGMD presents with markedly increased levels of CK, however, often not to the same magnitude seen in DMD. EMG and muscle biopsy results demonstrate myopathic changes. EMG findings reveal positive sharp waves, and fibrillation potentials are absent in some individuals and increased in others. Short-duration, small-amplitude MUAPs and an increased number of MUAPs are characteristic of LGMD.[62]

Muscle biopsy specimens present with variable fiber size and atrophy alternating with hypertrophy; in the later stages connective tissue is increased. Muscle in LGMD can be stained for a variety of components of the sarcoglycan complex as well as many other known protein defects. In the context of a suspected sarcoglycanopathy, this often does not provide a specific diagnosis, because defects

in one sarcoglycan can affect incorporation of the others; however, the clues provided can lead to appropriate genetic testing to confirm the diagnosis.[242]

Congenital Muscular Dystrophy. A good clinical examination will provide insight into the basis of an infant's hypotonia and determine if it is thought to be central in origin (based on soft neurologic signs) or peripheral. However, most of the disorders of glycosylation show a mixed central and peripheral picture, which can complicate the interpretation of the examination. Initial CK will be increased in CMD, and a muscle biopsy specimen will present as an active dystrophic process with a variation in fiber size, fiber splitting some increase in central nuclei, degenerating fibers, and basophilic staining of regenerating fibers. Combined MUAPs will be diminished, and in merosin-deficient CMD, a mixed picture may be noted, including demyelination.

Facioscapulohumeral Dystrophy. In FSHD, serum CK is elevated in 75% of affected individuals. Electrodiagnostic testing demonstrates a myopathic pattern, with positive sharp waves and fibrillation potentials often noted; however, these are less prominent than in DMD. The most striking characteristic in FSHD is short-duration, small-amplitude, polyphasic MUAPs.[62]

Muscle biopsy findings are somewhat dependent on which muscle is biopsied with variable fiber size and necrotic and regenerating fibers being common; central nuclei, and inflammatory infiltrates can also be noted. Analysis for the underlying genetic defect 4q35 can be used to confirm the diagnosis.

Myotonic Dystrophy. In myotonic dystrophy microscopic evaluation of muscle and nerve demonstrates alterations. In the muscle selective atrophy of the type I fibers is noted, with central nuclei and hypertrophic fibers and increased connective tissue present. Nerve biopsy results show a variable degree of demyelination, particularly in large fibers, in addition to regenerating fibers characteristic of axonal neuropathy.[257] EMG is used to document myotonia, with the unmistakable "dive bomber" sound produced by a myotonic discharge.

TREATMENT. At present no known treatment halts the progression of MD. Despite recent advances in our understanding of the MDs, current therapy for these disorders remains primarily supportive. Research in the area of molecular biology that has brought specific information about the molecular pathogenesis involved may one day lead to effective treatment.

Presently, treatment intervention is directed toward maintaining function in unaffected muscle groups for as long as possible, utilizing supportive measures such as physical and occupational therapy, orthopedic appliances, orthopedic surgery, and pharmaceuticals (corticosteroids for DMD). Children who remain active as long as possible avoid complications (e.g., contractures, pressure ulcers, infections) and deconditioning that are common once they are wheelchair bound.

It is important to remember that there is an active muscle degeneration underlying some of the MDs. Strengthening, especially eccentric exercise, is not helpful and may cause increased weakness, particularly in DMD and other disorders that impact the muscle membrane. Contracture management is the focus of treatment for the therapist and is important in maintaining function in those with MD. Splinting, stretching, serial casting, and assistive technology are mainstays of treatment in this group and should be considered when approaching these clients.

Glucocorticoid therapy (e.g., prednisone and deflazacort) has been used to slow the progression of DMD and BMD. The use of glucocorticoids has become the mainstay of treatment for many individuals with these forms of dystrophy. The use of glucocorticoids has been demonstrated to increase myogenic differentiation, myoblast fusion, and laminin expression in animal models[4] and has been shown to improve muscle force and function in children with DMD.[48] The functional advantage of this medical treatment is the child's ability to maintain independent ambulation, respiratory function, and spinal alignment for longer periods of time.

Stem cell and gene therapy for MD are currently under investigation. Investigators are exploring a variety of ways to exogenously deliver healthy copies of the dystrophin gene to dystrophic muscles[132,153] or to pharmacologically treat the effects of this disease.[42] Experiments in the MDX mouse have investigated gene therapy techniques through the use of viruses to implant a miniversion of the dystrophin gene into dystrophin-deficient muscles to delay or stop muscle degeneration. The main obstacle has been immunologic; however, human trials are on the horizon.

In other research models, attempts have been made to inject skeletal muscles with donor cells, a gene transfer method referred to as myoblast transfer therapy. These myoblasts fuse with diseased muscle fibers and provide the missing gene to replace dystrophin. However, this has not produced a viable treatment approach for clinical application to date.[166,230,253]

There are also treatments on the horizon for specific genetic defects. DMD is the end result of a variety of different genetic mutations in the dystrophin gene. Most people with DMD have large mutations; others have point mutations, duplications, or early stop codon mutations. There is the potential that some of these may be amenable to drug treatments, either to reestablish the reading frame or to facilitate read through in the case of a premature stop codon.

In a small portion of people (up to 15%) with DMD and other genetic disorders, the underlying genetic defect is a premature stop codon or nonsense mutation (a stop codon normally Ribosome stop reading at the appropriate time).The inability to read the genetic material and produce dystrophin in these individuals potentially can be suppressed by compounds that induce read through. This has been investigated in animal models and in cell culture as well as in human trials.[9,15]

People with point mutations might be amenable to a treatment with antisense oligonucleotides designed to induce exon skipping. Genes are read in sets of three base pairs. When someone has a point mutation, if it is an out-of-frame mutation, everything after the mutation is shifted and the groups of three base pairs do not produce the appropriate amino acids. These drugs cause RNA to skip over the exon where the point mutation is present during the transcription process when the introns are removed and the messenger RNA is formed. In this way, the effected exon is removed and the gene is allowed to continue reading in sets of three base pairs with the remaining exons being assembled appropriately. If these drugs are effective in clinical trials, the hope is that this strategy could induce production of increased levels of dystrophin and result in an effective treatment for people with DMD.[76]

PROGNOSIS. Prognosis varies with the type of MD present. As a general rule, the earlier the clinical signs appear the more rapid, progressive, and disabling the dystrophy, with puberty and the onset of middle age often creating the tipping points for functional decline. DMD generally occurs during early childhood with rapid progression of symptoms and results in death, often in the third decade of life. Pulmonary complications, resulting from respiratory muscle dysfunction, and cardiac dysfunction in the form of conduction defects or myopathy are the common sources of morbidity and mortality. People with BMD usually live into the fifth decade (their forties) or beyond; mortality most often related to cardiac dysfunction. Those with FSHD involvement may appear almost stable over a period of years; variable progression occurs among those with LGMD. People with both FSHD and LGMD have a relatively normal life span.

SPECIAL IMPLICATIONS FOR THE THERAPIST 23-6

Muscular Dystrophy
Precautions

When people with MD become ill or injured and are on bed rest (at home or in the hospital) even for a few days, they may lose many of their functional abilities. For example, a child who falls and breaks a leg and is on bed rest or otherwise immobilized will lose muscle strength and may never regain the ability to ambulate. These children should be encouraged to be as mobile as possible, and, if possible, ambulate for even a few minutes every day during the course of any illness.

Although activity helps individuals maintain functional abilities, strenuous exercise may facilitate the breakdown of muscle fibers, so that exercise must be approached cautiously. Low-repetition maximum weightlifting, especially eccentric strengthening, is not recommended. Exercise is best done in the pool, where exercise is concentric. Any exercise program should produce only minimal fatigue with no postexercise soreness, because the amount of damage to the muscle membrane with exercise is related directly to the magnitude of the stress placed on it during contraction.[182]

Respiratory involvement requires careful monitoring of breathing techniques, respiratory movements, and oxygen saturation levels. Monitoring oxygen during exercise and activity is recommended. See Appendix B. The client should be instructed in diaphragmatic, deep-breathing exercises. Airway clearance techniques, including the use of percussion and postural drainage and mechanical insufflator–exsufflator for assisted cough, are especially useful during illness.[7]

Investigators have shown that the inspiratory muscles can be trained for both force and endurance in this population. These training-related improvements in inspiratory muscle performance are more likely to occur in those who are less-severely affected by the disease. In those clients who have disease to the extent that they are already retaining carbon dioxide, little change occurs in respiratory muscle force or endurance with training.[151]

In the later stages of respiratory compromise nighttime mechanical ventilation (e.g., continuous positive airway pressure or bilevel positive airway pressure delivered by face mask) is an intervention used to rest the respiratory muscles. A major priority for these children is to avoid or delay the need for intubation and full-time mechanical ventilation; these noninvasive methods can aid in this goal.[54]

Therapy Interventions

For individuals with the more disabling forms of MD such as DMD, the therapist can provide anticipatory guidance about the course of the disease and valuable information regarding the use of various types of adaptive equipment. Initially, grab bars provide for safety, but eventually a rolling commode or combination commode and bath chair is needed. As DMD progresses, a power wheelchair provides functional mobility once ambulation is no longer possible.

Eventually, adapted controls (mini-joystick, touch pad, or fiberoptic switches) may be required for the power chair to accommodate the severe weakness and contracture that develop in the later stages of DMD. Power Tilt-In-Space wheelchair systems allow for pressure relief where air or gel cushions are no longer sufficient.

In the individual who no longer has access to a computer for school or work secondary to severe weakness, environmental control systems allow computer access by inferred link and mouse emulation to allow control of the mouse from the wheelchair control or completely hands-free control through the use of voice recognition software.

Overhead slings and mobile arm supports are helpful with feeding and other upper-extremity activities, especially after spinal surgery, when axial flexibility is removed and greater active range of motion is required for these functional tasks.

Splinting and night positioning in addition to active and passive range of motion exercises will aid in delaying the onset of contractures and reducing the associated morbidity. Once the formation of contractures has occurred serial casting can be considered if ambulation has not progressed to end stage and the person is still able to rise from the floor independently.[86] Home environmental assessment and careful family and client interviews are important in planning out the appropriate adaptive equipment and home modifications.

Both children and adults can benefit from ambulation and pool therapy programs aimed at improving endurance. For a more in-depth discussion of the direct intervention protocols for this condition, the reader is referred to other resources.[39,55,188]

Congenital Myopathy

Definition and Overview

Congenital myopathy describes a group of disorders with somewhat similar phenotypic course, including central core disease, nemaline myopathy, multicore-minicore disease, and myotubular myopathy/centronuclear myopathy. A full appreciation of the specifics of each disease is necessary for treatment planning. As a group they are characterized by weakness at birth or shortly thereafter, with a course that is relatively stable or slowly progressive. Often there are developmental gains made early in the course of the disease while the natural developmental progression of the child is in full force. Later the child might lose skills, as muscle strength does not keep up with the gain in body size or contractures interfere with function.

Incidence

Nemaline myopathy is the most common of these diseases and occurs at a rate of 2 per 100,000 live births.[31] The remaining types each account for a smaller incidence but greater total number of cases (prevalence).

Pathogenesis

Nemaline myopathy is a heterogeneous disease with a number of genetic loci identified. The genes, loci, and protein products responsible for the resulting pathology include α-tropomyosin slow (1q22-23, TPM3), β-tropomyosin (p13.2, TPM2), troponin 1 (19q13.4, TNNT1), nebulin (2q21-22, NEB), and α-actin (1q42.1, ACTA1). These genes can have either autosomal dominant or recessive inheritance.

Central core disease is the result of a mutation in the ryanodine receptor protein (RYR1) gene (19q13.1) with a defect in the ryanodine receptor and can be inherited both as a recessive or dominant gene. RYR1 functions as part of a calcium release channel. It sits between the T-tubule and the sarcoplasmic reticulum and is integral to the process of excitation-contraction coupling through its regulation of cytosolic calcium homeostasis.

Multicore-minicore disease can be the result of a mutation in Selenoprotein N1 *(SEPN1)* gene (1p36), which is inherited recessively, or it can have the same mutation as central core disease (RYR1). Both central core and multicore-minicore disease are named because of the characteristics of the muscle biopsy findings. In multicore-minicore disease there are several intracellular collections within the muscle cell. In central core, there is one larger collection. These cores occur in type I fibers and lack oxidative enzyme activity. Early in the course of a ryanodine receptor defect, the muscle biopsy specimen can present with multiple intracellular cores. As the disease progresses it may be that these cores coalesce and form one central core, which accounts for the overlap in the genetics of these two diseases.

Myotubular (centronuclear) myopathy is X-linked and caused by a mutation in the myotubularin gene *(MTM1)* located on Xq28.[31]

Clinical Manifestations

Nemaline Myopathy. Nemaline myopathy presents in a phenotypically heterogeneous way with five different types identified. Type 1 is the severe congenital form, type 2 the intermediate form, type 3 the most typical, and types 4 and 5 present in childhood or adulthood, respectively.

The typical form presents in infancy and is characterized by hypotonia throughout the body, including the face. Feeding difficulties, including aspiration and respiratory insufficiency, initially present at night and are common comorbidities. Contractures and spinal rigidity are also common; there is both weakness of the extremities and a lack of flexibility of the trunk, especially in flexion. Rigid spine presentation is typical in individuals who have selenoprotein defects.

Central Core Disease. Central core disease typically presents in infancy but can also present later. CK levels are usually normal or only mildly elevated. Common comorbidities include congenital hip dislocation, scoliosis, and talipes equinovarus. Because there is often variable penetrance, members of the same family can have varied phenotypic presentations. Anyone with central core disease is at risk for malignant hyperthermia, a severe and life-threatening reaction to certain anesthetics.

Multicore-Minicore Disease. Four groups of multicore-minicore disease have been identified. The classic form is characterized by proximal weakness and scoliosis, as well as pulmonary insufficiency. Distal joint laxity is a common finding. Myopia is a common visual finding. Individuals with group II have ophthalmoplegia and severe facial weakness in addition to more global weakness. Individuals classified as having group III disease also have arthrogryposis and early onset.

Myotubular (Centronuclear) Myopathy. Myotubular myopathy is very phenotypically variable, with a range of presentations possible. The severe neonatal form is the most common type and can lead to death in the first year of life. Despite the fact that many have life-threatening pulmonary involvement, those who receive intensive ventilatory support can survive past the first year, gain strength, and show improvement in their respiratory status as they progress past the first year. Even so, upper respiratory infections remain significant challenges for many affected individuals. A less-common form presents with a milder course and survival into adulthood.[31,234]

MEDICAL MANAGEMENT

DIAGNOSIS. Diagnosis of congenital myopathy is made first by clinical examination. The differentiation of central versus peripheral causes of the hypotonia will help guide the physician's workup. These factors include deep tendon reflexes, upper motor neuron signs, and cognitive status.

If a peripheral process is suspected, an EMG can differentiate a neurogenic versus myogenic process and then a muscle biopsy can be performed to evaluate the pathologic characteristics. Special stains or electron microscopy can be ordered to further narrow the possible diagnoses. Finally, genetic testing can be ordered to confirm the diagnosis.

TREATMENT. Treatment is primarily symptomatic. Management of contractures is important in maintaining function, and supportive pulmonary care is important, especially in those clients who develop nocturnal hypoventilation. Cardiac monitoring is important for those with a propensity toward cardiac symptoms.

Spinal Muscular Atrophy

Overview and Incidence

Spinal muscular atrophy (SMA) is a neuromuscular disease characterized by progressive weakness and wasting of skeletal muscles resulting from anterior horn cell degeneration. SMA is the second most common fatal autosomal recessive disorder after cystic fibrosis. The overall incidence is 1 in 6000 to 1 in 10,000 live births, and 1 in 40 to 1 in 60 individuals carry the genetic defect (Table 23-6).[50,155]

Childhood SMA is divided into SMA type I, SMA type II, and SMA type III. SMA type I, the more severe or acute form, is referred to as Werdnig-Hoffmann disease and causes respiratory failure and early death, typically in the first few years of life, if respiratory support is not provided. Kugelberg-Welander disease, or type III SMA, is the mildest form. These individuals learn to walk without assistance; a relatively slow progression is noted in type III. SMA type II represents an intermediate form; affected individuals demonstrate the ability to sit independently at some point, but significant functional impairment and reliance on power mobility is typical (see Table 23-6). Despite the classification system which divides SMA into three types based on the maximal independent motor skill achieved, SMA really represents a continuous spectrum of severity.

Etiologic Factors and Pathogenesis

The basis of this recessively inherited motor neuron disease is a genetic mutation in the *SMN1* gene found on the long arm of chromosome 5 (5q13.1).[84] The *SMN1* gene is defective in 99% of all cases of SMA and is the cause of SMA. The *NAIP* gene is defective in 45% of the more severely involved type I individuals, and it has been proposed that an NAIP deletion can increase SMA severity.[116,164] The *SMN1* gene has a homologous gene, *SMN2*, that can compensate for the absence of SMN1 by producing survival motor neuron (SMN) protein, although in reduced quantities. SMN2 can be present in multiple copies; the more copies of SMN2 present, the more SMN protein is produced, and the milder the phenotype becomes.

Progressive degeneration of anterior horn cells of the spinal cord is noted in SMA, with selected motor nuclei of the brainstem being variably affected. In the remaining axons, sprouting occurs, resulting in enlarged motor units. The underlying pathogenesis of anterior horn cell loss appears to be the persistence of programmed cell death in the anterior horn cells.[225]

The *SMN1* gene mutation decreases intracellular levels of SMN protein[84] present in the cytoplasm and nucleus of all cells. SMN protein function is not fully understood but it is involved in all cells and functions as part of the splicing mechanism during protein production as well as

Table 23-6   Spinal Muscular Atrophy

Type	Incidence	Onset	Inheritance	Features	Course
SMA type I (Werdnig-Hoffmann; acute or severe form)	Overall incidence for all types of SMA is 1 in 6000-10,000 livebirths[179a,179b]	0–3 mo	Autosomal recessive	LEs flexed, abducted, and externally rotated (frog position) UEs abducted, externally rotated, unable to move to midline against gravity Poor head control Significantly decreased muscle tone/weakness Decreased newborn movements, decreased diaphragmatic movements High risk of scoliosis Proximal muscle weakness greater than distal weakness Weak cry and cough Normal sensation and intellect	Rapidly progressive Severe hypotonia 65% survive 4th year[177a] but only 28% of those with less than 16 hours of ventilation 50% survive 10 years but only 16% of those with less than 16 hours of ventilation[177a]
SMA type II (intermediate form)	27% of SMA Dx is type II	Before 18 months	Autosomal recessive	LEs flexed, abducted, and externally rotated Limited trunk control Weakness Increased risk of scoliosis Normal sensation and intellect	Progressive but stabilizes Moderate to severe hypotonia Shortened life span,[161] although a 100% survival has been reported to 10 years of age[146a] Attain the ability to sit at some point Reliance on power mobility
SMA type III (Kugelberg-Welander; mild form)	13% of SMA Dx is type III	Present after 18 months	Autosomal recessive	Proximal weakness (greatest with trunk, hip, knee extension) Trendelenburg gait, especially with running Slow continued development progression; sits independently Walks independently (lumbar lordosis, waddling gait, genu recurvatum, protuberant abdomen) Wheelchair bound early adulthood (dependent on age of onset) Good UE strength	Slowly progressive Attain the ability to ambulate at some point Wheelchair dependence determined by age of onset: with onset prior to 2 years of age, 50% lose ambulation ability by 12 years of age; with onset after 2 years of age, 50% lose ambulation by 44 years of age[204]

LE, Lower extremity; UE, upper extremity.

preventing motor neuron cell death.[122] The variability of phenotype in SMA is related to the presence of multiple copies of the *SMN2* gene. SMN2 is an almost identical copy of SMN1. Because of a difference in exon 7, which then is spliced differently at the pre–messenger RNA stage, SMN2 is less effective at producing the gene product SMN with each SMN2 copy. Only 10% of the protein that SMN1 produces occurs as a result of the altered splicing.[70] This results in various intracellular levels of SMN that is dependent on how many copies of the SMN2 gene are present.

From the many animal models of SMA that have been produced, it is known that SMN is found in the nucleus and cytoplasm of all cells and is needed functionally for all cells. SMN functions as part of the spliceosome in the nucleus where it is initially produced. However, it is first trafficked out of the nucleus where it binds with Unrip and seven Gemin proteins. This complex facilitates the formation of small nuclear ribonucleoproteins that are important in the structure of the spliceosome once the complex is transported back into the nucleus. The spliceosome functions in the removal of the introns and assembly of the exons in preparation for formation of amino acids by the ribosome.[70]

The spinal motor neurons are specifically sensitive to low levels of SMN and the result is a reduced pool of anterior horn cells. In addition, in the remaining anterior horn cell pool there is an alteration of the structure and function of the existing motor neurons such that acetylcholine distribution is altered in the presynaptic terminal and, ultimately, acetylcholine release into the neuromuscular junction is impaired. Recently, it was suggested that SMN may have a roll in axon formation beyond its function as part of the spliceosome.[70]

Clinical Manifestations

Progressive atrophy of skeletal muscles is noted by the partial denervation, with a variable degree of weakness, and fatigue reported as the primary phenotypic characteristics of SMA. Often restrictive lung disease is present and this is a major source of mortality. Initial weakness and loss of motor strength is noted around the time of presentation but muscle strength can remain stable over long periods of time. There is a slowly progressive loss of motor function that is detectable only over years. Explanations for this loss of function remains undetermined, but decrease in motor function could be caused by factors such as increased body size.[113]

Children with SMA type I present with features of this disorder within the first days or few months of life. Hypotonia and severe generalized weakness is characteristic and is infants with SMA type I are unable to sit unsupported. Children with type II present before age 18 months with chronic weakness and attain independent sitting but never walk without assistance. Individuals with type III SMA are able to ambulate independently at some point in their lives, although they often require the use of a wheelchair by puberty or middle age, with the rate of progression dependent on the age of the onset of symptoms. Clinical problems associated with the muscle weakness seen in SMA include feeding and nutrition, respiratory, and orthopedic including scoliosis.

MEDICAL MANAGEMENT

DIAGNOSIS. The diagnosis is suspected on the basis of clinical manifestations, muscle biopsy, or EMG in which a neuropathic pattern is found. Nerve conduction velocities should be normal; combined motor action potentials are decreased in magnitude.

Clinically, the first symptom that is noted is the presence of weakness that should be evaluated in the context of the rapidity of onset and the child's age. Deep tendon reflexes are decreased or absent, suggesting a disorder of the peripheral nerve and sensation will be intact including vibratory sense. Fasciculations may also be noted in the tongue and more reliably will be seen on muscle ultrasound.

On needle EMG, fibrillations and sharp waves (hyperexcitability caused by denervation) are usually present and action potentials are high amplitude (showing large motor units) with polyphasic morphology (indicating denervation/reinnervation).[233] Muscle biopsy specimens show groups of small atrophic fibers alternating with large hypertrophic fibers, representing those without anterior horn cells and those with anterior horn cells, respectively. Genetic testing for SMA also confirms the diagnosis.

TREATMENT. Treatment is symptomatic and preventive, primarily preventing pulmonary infection and treating or preventing orthopedic problems, including contracture and scoliosis. Feeding problems are common, especially in cases with bulbar muscle weakness; gastrostomy tube feedings are often necessary to optimally manage nutrition.

Respiratory problems (involvement of the intercostals) are common, and percussion and postural drainage and treatments with an in-exsufflator (also known as coughalator, a machine that helps in the removal of bronchial secretions from the respiratory tract) can aid in airway clearance, especially during intercurrent illness and will maintain flexibility of the chest wall with chronic use. Positive-pressure ventilatory support, typically by bilevel positive airway pressure (initially at night), can extend the life span in these individuals.

The majority of people with SMA type I or II develop some degree of scoliosis; individuals with SMA type III who become nonambulatory are also at risk for the development of scoliosis. Bracing has not been found to delay the progression of scoliosis but might help with sitting balance (Fig. 23-21). Care should be taken to allow good diaphragmatic movement and not create increased respiratory effort if a soft spinal orthosis is chosen to manage sitting posture.

Spinal fusion is the primary means of management for scoliosis. Although fusion is often necessary, there is some consequence to function. Many will not return completely to their prior functional level.[81] In addition, the thorax no longer grows once a fusion is complete and as a result vital capacity is diminished. Two types of spinal instrumentation (growing rods and vertical expandable prosthetic titanium rib) allow the thorax to continue to grow when scoliosis in noted at a young age so a spinal fusion can be delayed till the majority of growth is complete at 12 years of age. Individuals with type II SMA can also develop hip subluxation or dislocation, but this is not typically painful, and the literature on surgical correction is not supportive.

Individuals with type II SMA should participate in a standing program (Fig. 23-22). Knee-ankle-foot orthoses

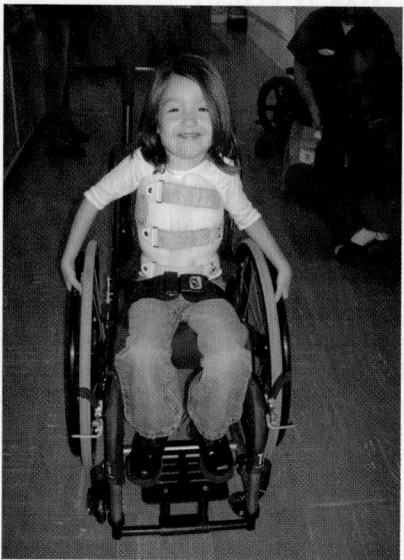

Figure 23-21

Spinal muscular atrophy (SMA). This 4-year-old child with SMA type II is fitted with a one-piece body jacket or thoracolumbosacral orthosis (TLSO). The TLSO offers support and control of the trunk and lower spine for improved sitting posture, balance, and greater stability. Full body jackets of this type may increase the work of breathing; an abdominal cutout (not present in this body jacket) to allow diaphragmatic excursion is typically provided for individuals with SMA who rely on diaphragmatic respiration due to the pattern of muscular weakness. The chair is a titanium ultralight wheelchair, which this child can propel for independent mobility. (Courtesy Tamara Kittelson-Aldred, Access Therapy Services, Missoula, MT. Used with permission.)

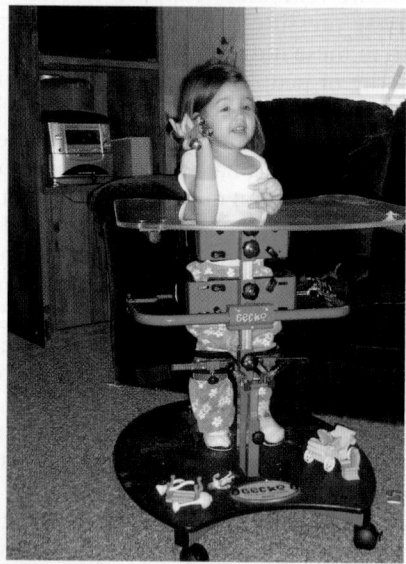

Figure 23-22

Static vertical standing frame provides support and stability in the upright position for the child with spinal muscular atrophy. Ankle-foot orthoses provide support for weight bearing through the lower extremities. (Courtesy Tamara Kittelson-Aldred, Access Therapy Services, Missoula, MT. Used with permission.)

(KAFOs) with ischial weight bearing or parapodiums are ideal for this in the younger age group and standers for older children may be best. However, as contractures develop, standing will become more difficult despite the most aggressive splinting, range of motion, and serial casting program. SMA type III clients initially ambulate, although about half of this group loses ambulatory skills in childhood or adolescence.

PROGNOSIS. Prognosis varies according to age of onset or type of SMA (see Table 23-6). The earlier the disease occurs, the faster the progression of muscle weakness and the poorer the prognosis. The presence of respiratory distress also contributes to a poorer prognosis.

SMA type I is the most severe with death likely in the first years of life as a result of respiratory insufficiency or infection. Most children with this form of SMA do not survive past 3 years without the aid of mechanical ventilation. Clients with type III (with onset after 2 years of age) typically remain independently ambulatory into adult life; if onset is before 2 years, loss of ambulatory ability at an average age of 12 years is typical.[204]

| SPECIAL IMPLICATIONS FOR THE THERAPIST | 23-7 |

Spinal Muscular Atrophy

A variety of opinions exist regarding the usefulness or effectiveness of an active developmental program for children with SMA. However, children with SMA type I or II often outlive predictions, and therapy intervention is helpful in improving function and preventing musculoskeletal problems.

Precautions

The infant or child with SMA who lacks independent mobility requires frequent changes of position to prevent skin problems and other complications, especially pneumonia. The pharynx may require suctioning to remove secretions in the more severe cases, and feeding must be carried out slowly and carefully with good positioning to prevent aspiration in those individuals with oral motor involvement. The involvement of a therapist with specialization in feeding (usually an occupational therapist or speech-language pathologist) is essential for these children.

Respiratory weakness or diminished head control may prevent the child from benefiting from prone positioning. This is especially problematic when the child cannot lift the head to clear the airway. The use of prone positioning must be evaluated and monitored carefully by the therapist because children with SMA breath primarily with the diaphragm and prone position restricts abdominal expansion; vertical positions (sitting and standing) tend to be the most functional primarily for biomechanical reasons because the head is balanced above the trunk and the strength required is less than in prone or quadruped.

Monitoring oxygen saturation levels may be necessary in evaluating programming effectiveness especially in the person with type I SMA. Observe how much work is required to breathe, and whenever possible use a pulse oximeter (see Fig. B-1, Appendix B) to measure oxygen saturation noninvasively. Pulse oximetry can provide an outcome measure for documentation (see Appendix B).

Therapy Intervention

Specific treatment protocols for this condition are beyond the scope of this book. The therapist is referred to a more appropriate resource.[39,236] An overall management program should include positioning to encourage head and trunk control and to promote functional strengthening, in addition to splinting to maintain range of motion. Assistive technology can provide the maximum possible independence for children with SMA.

Power mobility for the child with SMA who has no independent mobility is essential and should be considered in the child as young as 18 months to 2 years of age (Fig. 23-23).[237] Low-technology solutions, such as "slings and springs" or mobile arm supports, also may be very liberating for the child who has limited antigravity upper extremity movement by providing a wide variety of exploratory opportunities.

Facilitation and active assistive work toward standing and ambulation can be effective in increasing strength through closed chain exercise and standing can help reduce the incidence of contracture. More severely involved clients may benefit from positioning in a standing frame or KAFOs.

Inspiratory muscle training also has been found to be effective in neuromuscular disorders in improving maximal voluntary ventilation, maximal inspiratory mouth pressure, as well as respiratory load perception[88,264] and should be considered in this population.

Aquatic therapy can be a valuable adjunct to traditional intervention strategies for people at all levels of the SMA continuum. By using the physical properties of water such as buoyancy, hydrostatic pressure, viscosity, and turbulence, the therapist provides additional tools for intervention, especially in the case of extreme weakness characteristic of this disorder.[73]

TORTICOLLIS

Definition and Overview

Torticollis (congenital muscular torticollis [CMT]; wry neck) means twisted neck and is a contracted state of the sternocleidomastoid muscle (SCM), producing head tilt to the affected side with rotation of the chin to the opposite side (Fig. 23-24). Four types of muscle abnormalities have been identified on ultrasonography: 15% have a fibrotic mass in the SCM (type 1), 77% have diffuse fibrosis mixed with normal muscle (type II), 5% have fibrotic tissue without normal muscle (type III), and the last group (type IV) present with a fibrotic cord and represent only 3% of the population.

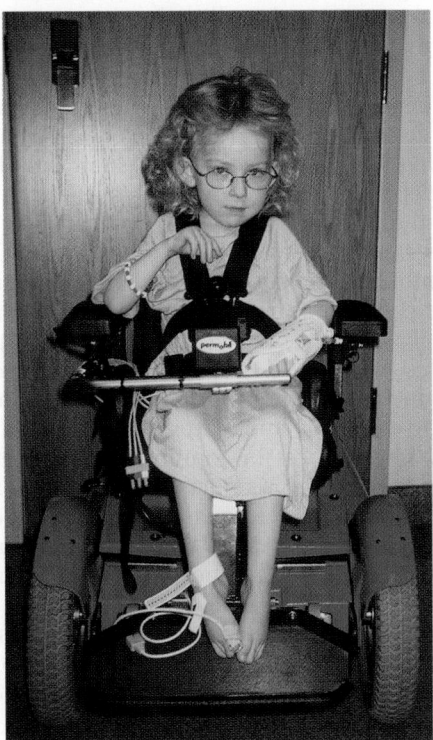

Figure 23-23

Spinal muscular atrophy (SMA). Three-year-old with SMA in her power wheelchair, which allows her to adjust the seat height so that she can be on the floor to aid with transfers or at eye level with her peers. The adjustable seat allows the child to participate in activities at elevated surfaces (e.g., counter or table heights), retrieve objects from a shelf, or help decorate the tree at Christmas. (Courtesy Allan Glanzman, The Children's Hospital of Philadelphia, PA.)

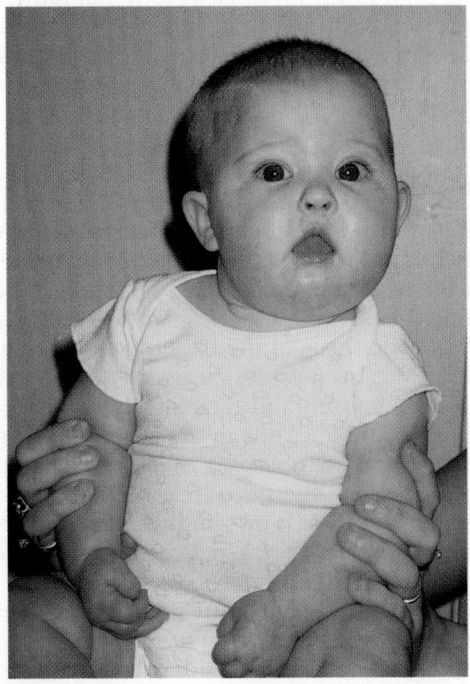

Figure 23-24

Torticollis. Five-month-old with torticollis (head tilt toward the involved side and rotation away from the involved side). (Courtesy Allan Glanzman, The Children's Hospital of Philadelphia, PA.)

Torticollis often is confused with a separate disorder known as cervical dystonia (also referred to as acquired torticollis or spasmodic torticollis). These are two separate entities and are presented separately in this text. CMT as it is presented in this section is a musculoskeletal phenomenon, whereas cervical dystonia is a movement disorder with an underlying CNS pathology (see "Dystonia" in Chapter 31).

Incidence and Etiologic Factors

Reports of the overall incidence of CMT vary significantly from 0.6 to 400 per 100,000 livebirths, but this condition is not considered uncommon.[109] A variety of possible causes of CMT exist, but the etiology remains unknown.

Initially it was thought that the fibrosis was related to birth trauma, because incidence is increased in breech (19%) and forceps (6%) delivery, vacuum extraction (30.5%), and cesarean section (17.9%).[46] Predisposing factors can include a restrictive intrauterine environment, poor muscle tone, or cervical–vertebral abnormalities. A genetic contribution also has been proposed in a portion of cases of CMT.[68]

Pathogenesis

The possible pathogenesis of the muscular fibrosis seen in CMT has been explored experimentally in animal models and has been produced through venous occlusion, and this, in addition to arterial occlusion, has been proposed as the possible pathogenesis.[109]

One theory postulates that the malposition of the head potentially leads to a compartment syndrome. In this scenario, the SCM is not stretched or torn, but rather kinked or compressed. With the head and neck in a position of forward flexion, lateral bend, and rotation, the ipsilateral SCM kinks, causing an ischemic injury and subsequent edema.[53]

Clinical Manifestations

The first sign of CMT identified in only a portion of affected children is a firm, nontender, palpable enlargement of the SCM often referred to as a sternocleidomastoid tumor of infancy. A portion of cases demonstrate bulbous fibrotic tissue at the base or midportion of the involved SCM. This local lesion usually reaches its maximal size by 1 month and then slowly regresses within 4 to 8 months and does not always result in torticollis.[244] The typical position observed of lateral head tilt and rotation to the opposite side predominates regardless of whether a fibrotic mass is present (estimated in 15%-66% of cases[109,112]) or no mass is palpated and the muscle is uniformly fibrotic and shortened.

If the torticollis is left untreated the deformity can become severe, the infant's face, ear, and head flatten from resting on the affected side, a condition referred to as plagiocephaly ("oblique head"); this cranial asymmetry gradually worsens. The infant's chin turns away from the side of the shortened muscle, the head tilts to the shortened side, and the shoulder is elevated on the affected side, further limiting cervical movement. Plagiocephaly (best observed by looking down on the head from above) is usually marked by the side of the flattened forehead, which is accompanied by the contralateral occipital flattening. When torticollis and plagiocephaly occur together, this condition is referred to as plagiocephaly–torticollis deformation sequence (Fig. 23-25).

The incidence of other deformities such as hip dislocation and clubfoot is elevated in cases of CMT.[46] Subluxation or bony anomalies of the cervical spine can also be associated with CMT and should be ruled out by cervical spine radiographs.[109,226]

MEDICAL MANAGEMENT

DIAGNOSIS. Clinical examination combined with the history forms the basis of the initial diagnostic process. Medical evaluation including radiographic studies of the spine is always indicated to rule out congenital deformities of the cervical spine, ocular disorders, and, less frequently, tumors or other CNS pathology in children with presumed torticollis.

TREATMENT. Initial management involves a period of physical therapy to correct the contracture in present in the SCM is the mainstay of treatment for CMT. Interventions include twice-daily passive range of motion to stretch the shortened muscle; stabilization of the proximal attachment of the SCM and trapezius is important during range of motion. Positioning is also important to encourage erect and midline head posture. Strengthening activities should include both active and active assistive exercises in addition to the incorporation of postural reactions in treatment when these reactions begin to develop.[120]

Splinting has been advocated by some for older children (older than 4 months) who continue to demonstrate head tilt.[114] A cervical collar or tubular orthosis for torticollis can be helpful in providing tactile cueing for movement in the direction opposite the lateral tilt. Usually these collars are the most effective at a time that is compatible with active head control (Fig. 23-26).

In cases of delayed treatment or where craniofacial asymmetry persists, nonsurgical remodeling of the skull using externally applied pressure can be used (Fig. 23-27). With advances in computer software and technology (e.g., pressure scanners), researchers are determining the pressure per square inch (psi) that applies the appropriate force needed to achieve the remodeling process for each individual head diameter, volume, and topography.[248,249]

Surgical intervention is rare (e.g., SCM tenotomy, plastic surgery for craniofacial asymmetry) and is considered only if the individual continues to demonstrate significant motion restrictions of 30 degrees after 6 months of age or the deformity persists past 12 months of age. Increased thickening of the SCM or increased deformity are also indications to consider surgical intervention.[120]

PROGNOSIS. CMT usually resolves with conservative treatment. Complete recovery, including full passive range of motion, can be expected to take approximately 3 to 12 months; however, recurrence with growth is

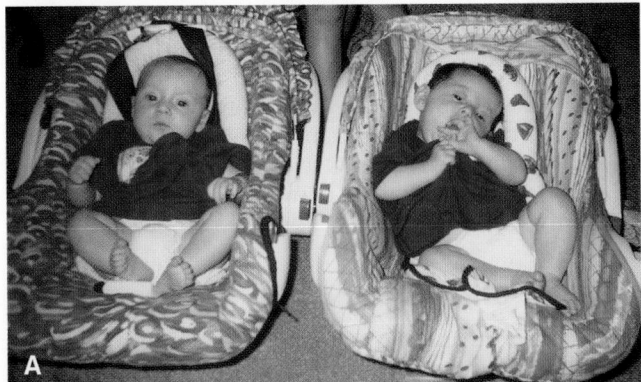

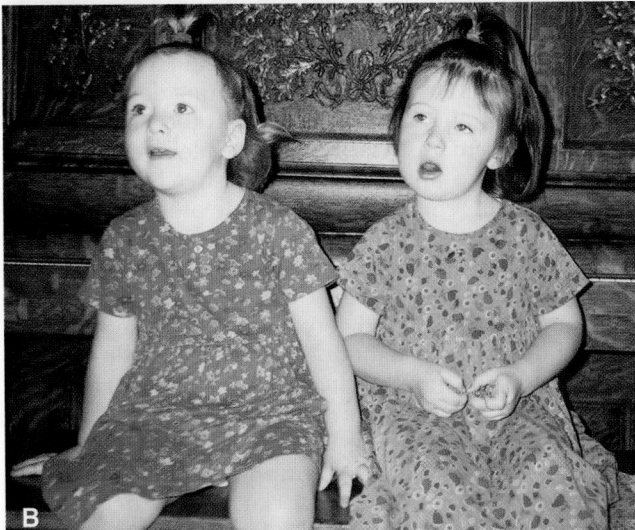

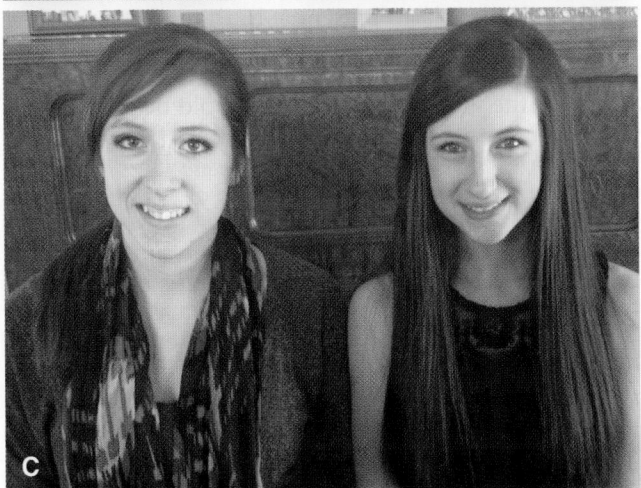

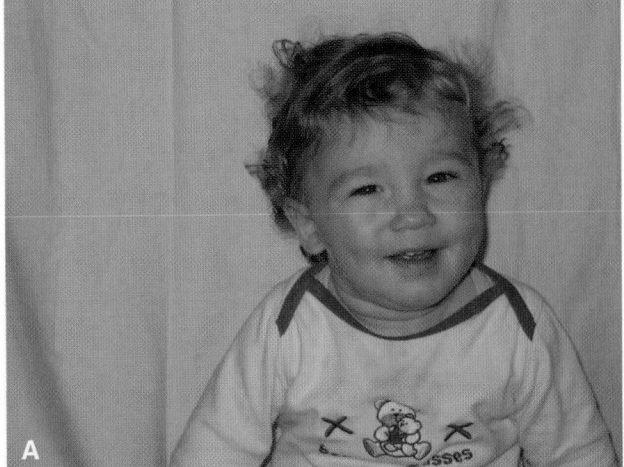

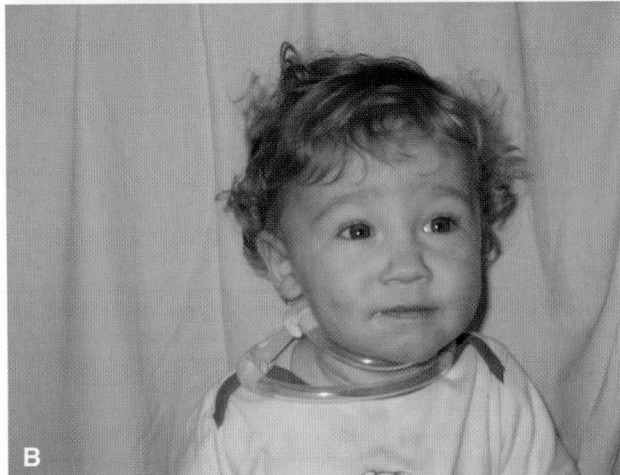

Figure 23-26

Congenital torticollis. A, Note the head tilt in this toddler with right-sided congenital torticollis. Despite his full range of motion, he has an occasional residual head tilt to the right and turn to the left. **B,** The same child wearing a TOT Collar (tubular orthosis for torticollis) to encourage a more vertical head position. (Courtesy Allan Glanzman, The Children's Hospital of Philadelphia, PA.)

sometimes seen and a period of follow up after resolution is warranted. Fewer than 16% of children presenting in the first year ultimately requiring surgery.[64] Left untreated or poorly managed, chronic, unresolved torticollis can result in persistent deformity and asymmetry of the head shape and position.

Figure 23-25

Plagiocephaly–torticollis deformation. A, Four-month-old fraternal twins: the child on the right has marked untreated congenital muscular torticollis (CMT) with plagiocephaly. Note the positional pelvic asymmetry from placement in a car seat. **B,** The same twins (2 years old) after physical therapy (PT) intervention at age 6 months for the child on the right. PT intervention over a 3-month period of time included passive range of motion, facilitated active range of motion, positioning, and a cervical collar. A home exercise program was prescribed with periodic rechecks. Eventually the use of a helmet was instituted to remodel craniofacial asymmetry (see Fig. 23-27). Some craniofacial asymmetry persists, although full active and passive range of motion are present. **C,** The same twins as teenagers in high school. (Courtesy Laurie Matteson, Great Falls, MT. Used with permission.)

SPECIAL IMPLICATIONS FOR THE THERAPIST   23-8

Torticollis

The prognostic information provided makes it possible for therapists to better predict treatment duration at the time of initial assessment. When parents are provided with more precise information about the length of treatment, parents may be more willing to adhere to the exercise program.[65] Torticollis that does not respond to physical therapy may have a nonmuscular cause, such as bony anomaly or ocular disorders, and may require further medical evaluation and should be referred for reevaluation if a child does not respond to therapy.

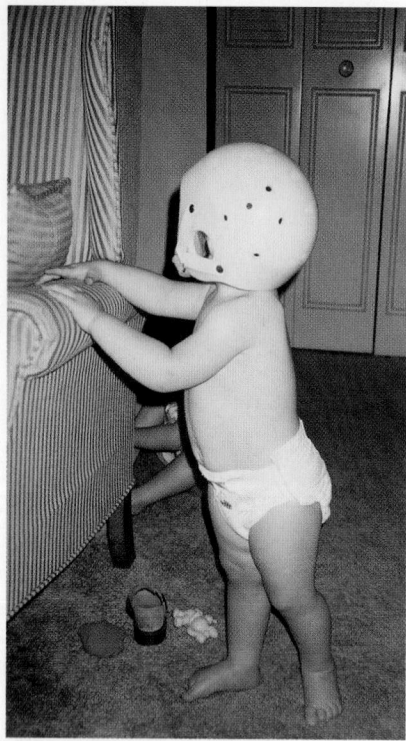

Figure 23-27

Fourteen-month-old girl wearing a polypropylene helmet lined with durometer foam. This helmet placed remodeling pressure on the cranium to reshape unresolved craniofacial asymmetry that persisted as a result of delayed medical intervention and inconsistent use of a cervical collar. The helmet was accepted readily by the child and worn at all times (except for bathing) for approximately 4 months. Pressure was applied to the right posterior occiput to bring the head and neck into midline alignment while space was created where the skull was flattened in the left posterior occipital area to allow for bony growth in that area. See Fig. 23-25, *B*, for intervention outcome. (Courtesy Laurie Matteson, Great Falls, MT. Used with permission.)

Postoperative

After surgery for this condition, postoperative bracing to position the lengthened muscle on stretch has been advocated to allow the muscle to heal in the lengthened position.[114] Standard postoperative monitoring of vital signs and skin condition is recommended.

BRACHIAL PLEXUS BIRTH PALSY

Definition and Overview

Brachial plexus injury at birth can be divided into a number of categories. Erb palsy is a paralysis of the upper limb typically resulting from a traction injury to the brachial plexus at birth. Erb palsy actually is made up of three distinct types of brachial plexus palsies: (1) Erb-Duchenne palsy affecting the C5 to C6 nerve roots (95%-99% of all cases), (2) whole-arm palsy affecting C5 to T1, and (3) Klumpke palsy affecting the C8 and T1 (lower plexus) nerve roots.

Incidence

The incidence of brachial plexus injuries has decreased secondary to improved obstetric management of difficult labors. Traction injuries are most common in newborns, occurring in 0.1% of spontaneous, 1.2% of breech, and 1.3% of forceps deliveries. Overall, the incidence of birth-related traction injuries is between 0.5 and 2 per 1000 live births.

Etiologic and Risk Factors

The major contributing factor to these injuries has been attributed to stretching of the brachial plexus, that is, a pulling away of the shoulder from the head secondary to a traction maneuver during the birth process.

The lower plexus injury resulting in Klumpke palsy usually is caused by manipulation during delivery resulting from hyperabduction of the arm at the shoulder; that is, the trunk remains relatively immobile in the mother's pelvis while the upper extremity is stretched. However, some question remains about the role of the obstetrician as compared with the position of the infant and the forces encountered in the canal before birth. Evidence suggests that the propulsive nature of the birth process when stretching of the involved nerves occurs is something over which the birth attendant does not have full control.[210]

Obstetric history associated with Erb palsy is characterized by high birth weight or vertex delivery with shoulder dystocia (i.e., during delivery the baby's shoulder impinges on the mother's symphysis pubis). Klumpke palsy more commonly is associated with heavy sedation, difficult breech delivery, and brow or face presentation. Rarely, neoplasm present at birth results in brachial plexus palsy. The absence of signs of a traumatic injury accompanied by the onset of weakness and progressive course in the first few days of life should be investigated by MRI.[3]

Pathogenesis

Plexus injury during birth is usually the result of a stretch or avulsion of the plexus. A mild lesion is characterized by stretching of the nerve fibers, whereas a moderate injury involves some nerve fibers being stretched and others actually torn. A more severe injury is characterized by a complete rupture of the plexus trunks with avulsion of the roots from the spinal cord. The degree of disability depends on the site and severity of injury. Diaphragmatic and serratus anterior paralysis suggests an avulsion injury as indicated by the location of the nerves with respect to the plexus. Persisting disability in neonatal brachial plexus palsy is partly a result of impaired motor unit activation. This impairment may be a form of developmental apraxia caused by defective motor programming in early infancy.[27]

Clinical Manifestations

Children with brachial plexus injuries are unlikely to demonstrate postural or placing responses with the involved upper extremity when tested. In Erb palsy the arm is maintained in adduction and internal rotation at

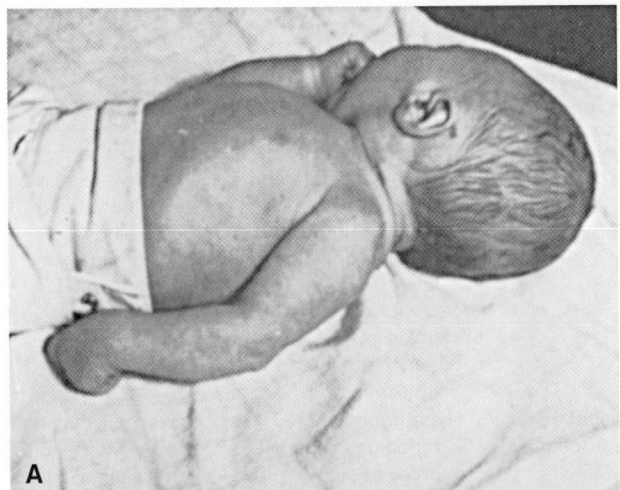

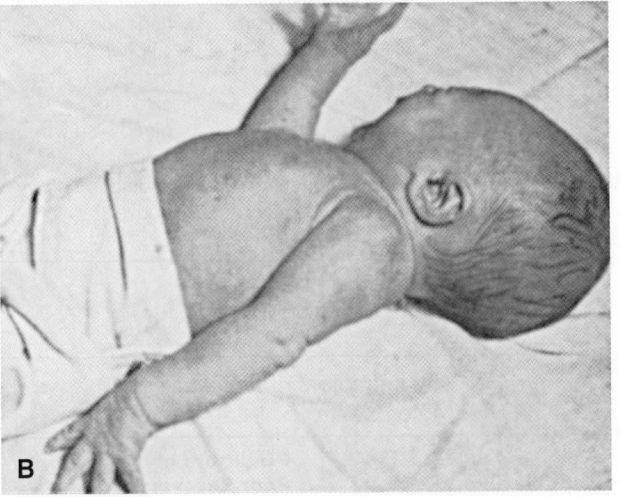

Figure 23-28

Erb palsy. **A,** In this infant with Erb palsy, the arm is maintained in a position of adduction and internal rotation at the shoulder with the lower arm pronated and fingers flexed. **B,** Same infant demonstrating an asymmetric Moro reflex with opening of the left hand but still in the "waiter's tip" position. (From Behrman RE, Kliegman RM, Jenson HB: *Nelson textbook of pediatrics,* ed 17, Philadelphia, 2004, WB Saunders.)

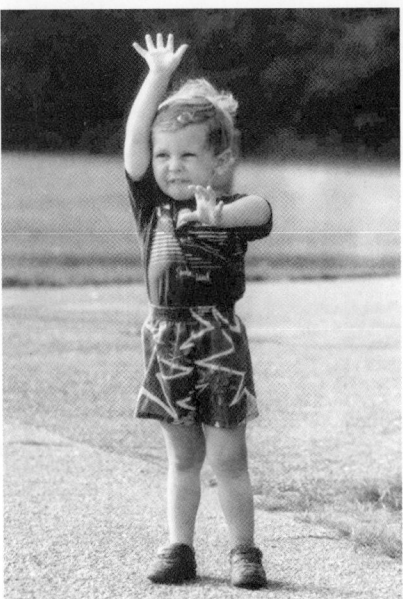

Figure 23-29

Brachial plexus palsy. Child with limited shoulder external rotation and abduction of the left arm associated with whole-arm palsy. Full motion of the upper extremity is demonstrated on the right side. (From Green DP, Hotchkiss RN, Pederson WC: *Green's operative hand surgery,* ed 5, London, 2005, Churchill Livingstone.)

MEDICAL MANAGEMENT

DIAGNOSIS. Some injuries are recognizable readily at or soon after birth. Radiographs may be taken to rule out associated fractures of the clavicle. Imaging of the brachial plexus using MRI is not invasive and can demonstrate proximal and distal lesions.

MRI can be used to detect nerve root avulsions, nerve ruptures, brachial plexus scarring, posttraumatic neuroma, brachial plexus edema, spinal cord damage, abnormalities of the shoulder joint, trauma, neoplasms, and infection. This type of imaging allows diagnosis and careful preoperative evaluation of children with brachial plexus injuries.[16]

EMG can be used to delineate the extent of injury and aid in the prognosis and assist the surgeon in identifying appropriate surgical procedures. EMG usually is delayed until 4 to 6 weeks after birth and may be followed serially over time to track recovery. Conduction studies can aid in separating actual axonal loss from conduction block. Needle EMG can help determine the portion of the plexus damaged as well as the severity of the damage.[62]

TREATMENT. Treatment is often delivered as part of a multidisciplinary team that includes a neurologist, surgeon, and therapist. The therapy approach is typically one that follows the strategies outlined in Table 23-7. Microneurosurgical intervention at an early stage can improve the outcome in some cases, especially in more severe cases where acceptable recovery is not anticipated (C5-T1 global injury without some recovery by 8-10 weeks of age). For example, some children have no chance of recovery unless they undergo early aggressive surgical reconstruction of the injured brachial plexus. In children with global or total paralysis, surgery is performed by

the shoulder with the lower arm pronated and fingers flexed, assuming the waiter's tip position (Fig. 23-28). Children with this type have difficulty with activities such as hand-to-mouth, hand-to-head, and hand–to–back of neck movements but usually have control of the wrist and fingers.

In Klumpke palsy, paralysis of the small muscles of the hand and wrist flexors causes a claw hand appearance. Proximal shoulder control is good, but voluntary wrist and hand control is difficult. In severe forms of brachial palsy (whole-arm palsy), the whole plexus can be affected but to a varying degree (Fig. 23-29). In this case careful examination is necessary to identify affected muscles. In all three cases (Erb, Klumpke, and whole-arm palsy) normal sensation is diminished; however, gross pain sensation may not be decreased to the same degree as movement.

Table 23-7 summarizes the clinical characteristics of brachial plexus injury.

Table 23-7 Brachial Plexus Injury: Clinical Characteristics

Type	Typical Posture	Strength Losses	Sensory Losses	Skeletal Changes	Treatment Strategies
Erb palsy (C5-C6)	Shoulder IR, adduction, finger flexion (difficulty with hand to mouth, hand to head, and hand to back of neck)	Deltoid, supraspinatus, infraspinatus, teres minor, biceps, brachialis, brachioradialis, supinator	C5-C6 deficits	Flattening of glenoid fossa/humeral head Elongating deformity of coracoid process hooking down and lateral Scapular winging potential Posterior shoulder dislocation	Active/active assistive exercise: shoulder abduction; elbow flexion; forearm supination and shoulder ER
Klumpke (C8-T1)	Pronation, elbow flexion contractures; no grasp reflex	Wrist flexors, long finger flexors; hand intrinsics	Diminished sensation	Hypertrophy of olecranon and coronoid process: elbow flexion contracture; posterior dislocation of radial head (25%)	Active/active assistive exercise: forearm supination, elbow extension, finger flexion Positional splint to assist with elbow extension; combined with UE weight bearing
Total plexus injury (whole arm)	Combinations of above	Combination of Erb and Klumpke types	Moderate losses	Posterior glenohumeral dislocation	Combination of above

ER, external rotation; IR, Internal rotation; UE, upper extremity.

3 to 4 months to maximize ultimate extremity function and minimize disability.[91,238]

Options for surgical care include tendon transfers considered after a plateau in recovery has occurred or microneurosurgery. The latter procedure is best considered between the ages of 6 months and 12 months for optimal functional results.[205] The role of surgery in those individuals affected at the C5-6 and C5-7 levels is less clear. There are a number of predictive models that can be used at 3 months to anticipate the degree of recovery that can be expected and aid in treatment planning. In many cases, referral for microsurgical intervention is initiated too late for primary nerve surgery, which has the best outcomes when surgery is performed at the proper stage in development. Secondary reconstructive procedures at a later date can still improve the outcome in many cases.[121]

PROGNOSIS. In most instances full recovery can be expected, with 53% recovering normal or near-normal function and an additional 39% achieving good functional recovery. Erb palsy has the best rate of recovery, with up to 90% of cases demonstrating spontaneous recovery. If C7 is involved in an Erb palsy, poor outcome is more likely, with the lower plexus palsies having the poorest prognosis.[203] Some children do have long-term disability as an outcome and require careful follow-up to prevent the development of contractures and to facilitate active motor control.

The first muscles to return are the elbow, wrist, and finger extensors, followed by the deltoid and biceps and later the external rotators. The timely recovery of these muscles (beginning at 6 weeks and continuing through 3 months) is prognostic of good functional recovery with

Table 23-8 Key Indicators of Recovery of Motor Control*

Predictors of Good Recovery	Predictors of Poor Recovery
Return of biceps function by 3 months of age C5-6 involvement only	Minimal bicep and deltoid function at age 6 months C7 involvement with lack of improvement between ages 3 and 6 months Global palsy or lower plexus involvement

Data from Ruchelsman DE, Pettrone S, Price AE, Grossman JA. Brachial plexus birth palsy: an overview of early treatment considerations, *Bull NYU Hosp Jt Dis* 67(1):83–89, 2009.

the lack of antigravity elbow flexion at 3 months predicting poor recovery.[62]

The long-term prognosis for recovery of motor control is poor beyond 18 months (Table 23-8), and probably 15% of infants experience significant disability, with reports showing a wide range of long-term impairments.[205]

SPECIAL IMPLICATIONS FOR THE THERAPIST 23-9

Brachial Plexus Birth Palsy

An integrated team approach to congenital brachial plexus injuries is imperative. Each child must be carefully evaluated, therapy interventions maximized, and the surgical approach (when required) individualized to obtain the best outcome.

An aggressive and integrated physical and occupational therapy program is essential in the treatment of these injuries. The therapist uses a problem-solving approach and adjusts the interventions based on each child's unique needs. The maintenance of full passive range of motion during the period of neurologic recovery is essential for normal joint development and optimal long-term recovery.

Early surgical correction of shoulder contractures and subluxations reduces permanent disability. Postoperative rehabilitative therapy can preserve and build on gains made possible by medical or surgical interventions.[189,194]

Treatment should focus on activities that encourage active and active assistive movement and that maintain the normal joint kinematics. The shoulder requires particular attention to maintain the normal scapulohumeral and scapulothoracic relationships in addition to maintaining the normal "roll and glide" of the glenohumeral joint and preventing subluxation.

Some strategies used to maintain functional upper extremity range of motion, prevent subluxation, and improve active movement include neuromuscular electrical stimulation, biofeedback, joint mobilization, and positioning using splints. Scapulothoracic stabilization for winging of the scapula using taping may be helpful if there is scapulothoracic weakness.

Passive range-of-motion exercises should be performed day in the direction of limited movement to help prevent the development of contractures, and a well-thought-out home program is an integral part of the therapy program with the intensity of the program determined by the clinical course. When splints are used, careful follow-up and family education by the therapist is necessary, especially if sensory impairment is present.

OSTEOGENESIS IMPERFECTA

Overview and Incidence

Osteogenesis imperfecta (OI), sometimes referred to as brittle bones, is a rare congenital disorder of collagen synthesis affecting bones and connective tissue. Four primary types of OI[224] were identified by Silence in 1979; however, with the ongoing identification of the genetics of OI, several expansions have been recommended.[37,195,251] Individuals with OI present with varying degrees of severity and clinical phenotypes (Table 23-9). Clinical features

Table 23-9	Sillence Classification of Osteogenesis Imperfecta (OI)*	
Type	**Severity**	**Description**
I (most common form)	Mildest form of OI	Dominantly inherited with blue sclerae
		Mild to moderate fragility without deformity Most fractures occur before puberty
		Associated with blue sclerae, triangular face, hearing loss (beginning in 20s or 30s); easy bruising
II	Most severe form (perinatal lethal)	Stillbirth or death during infancy or early childhood
		Extreme fragility of connective tissue
		Multiple in utero fractures
		Usually intrauterine growth retardation
		Severe bone deformity
		Soft, large cranium
		Micromelia: long bones crumpled and bowed; ribs beaded
III	Moderately severe	Progressive deformities
		Scoliosis
		Triangular-shaped face, large skull
		Severe osteoporosis
		Severe fragility of bones; usually in utero fractures
		Fractures heal with deformity and bowing
		Normal sclerae
		Extreme short stature
		Usually wheelchair bound by teenage years
IV	Variable but usually milder course; normal or near-normal life span	Mild to moderate skeletal fragility and osteoporosis (more severe than type I); dominant inheritance
		Associated with bowing of long bones
		Barrel-shape rib cage
		Bone fracture easily before puberty; some children improve at puberty
		Light or normal sclerae; may or may not have moderate short stature and joint hyperextensibility

Note: As mentioned in the text, classifications of OI are currently under expansion and/or revision. For this edition, the original Sillence classification, as presented here, was not replaced with one of the emerging classifications that have been proposed as no consensus has been reached regarding updated changes. The reader is advised to seek additional information regarding any future proposed (or actual) changes made.

From Sillence DO, Senn A, Danks DM: Genetic heterogeneity in osteogenesis imperfecta. *J Med Genet* 16(2):101–116, 1979.

vary widely between types, within types, and even within the same family. Experts estimate that between 30,000 and 50,000 people have OI in the United States (prevalence), or about 1 in 20,000 (incidence).[160a]

Etiologic Factors and Pathogenesis

Most children with OI inherit the disorder from a parent (autosomal dominant inheritance). Genetic counseling requires recognition that the parent can be a carrier of the dominant gene by parental mosaicism (i.e., the parent carries the mutation in a portion of the parent's germ cells).

Approximately 25% of children with OI, however, are born into a family with no history of the disorder. In these cases, the genetic defect occurred as a spontaneous mutation. Because the genetic defect is usually dominant (whether inherited from a parent or resulting from a spontaneous mutation), affected people have a 50% chance of passing on the disorder to each of their children.

Many different mutations have been identified in association with OI. There are two general groups of mutations that result in autosomal dominant OI. The first group tends to have milder phenotypic presentation. This group is composed of either nonsense mutation (premature stop codon) or frame-shift mutation (an alteration of the three base pair sequence) both resulting in haploinsufficiency where one allele does not produce functional protein and the other allele produces insufficient quantity for the biologic demands. The second group of mutations produce proteins with structural abnormalities. The most typical are mutations that alter glycine in the triple helical structure of collagen and alter its function with respect to both its stability and communication with the extracellular matrix. These mutations tend to have more severe phenotypes.[13] Type I collagen (see "Collagen" in Chapter 6 and Fig. 6-23) is found in the extracellular matrix of bone, skin, and tendon and is the major structural protein (scaffolding) of these tissues.

In endochondral and intramembranous bone formation the final structure of bone is similar, despite different mechanics of formation. Collagen is produced by osteoblasts that, in normal bone, become surrounded by a collagen matrix. Once the matrix is formed, calcium is laid down, trabeculae develop, and cancellous bone is formed. As the trabeculae become thicker and the density increases, a cortex of compact bone is formed.

Bone modeling in OI appears to be defective, with a smaller cross-sectional area observed and thinner cortex noted in the long bones, leading to diminished strength. The overall mass of cancellous bone also is decreased in OI as a result of a smaller number of trabeculae, possibly resulting from decreased production in endochondral ossification.

In individuals with OI cancellous bone volume does not increase with age as it does in children who do not have OI. This is related primarily to decreased rates of trabecular thickening in people with OI. In type I OI the annual rate of trabecular thickening is decreased, and in type III and type IV no trabecular thickening is noted over time.

The rate at which matrix is laid down in these three types of OI is slowed when compared with the normal rate. Because this slowing is uniform across types I, III, and IV of OI, severity probably is not related to the decreased rate of matrix production.[196]

The underlying causes of the bony abnormalities seen in people with OI are not entirely understood but probably result from one or a combination of factors. These factors have a potential role in the ultimate phenotypic expression in OI and include the unique structural characteristics of the abnormal collagen created by the mutation; the absence of other connective tissue proteins that impact the assembly of the extracellular matrix; and the degree to which the collagen is incorporated into that matrix.[63,148]

Clinical Manifestations

This disease has a wide range of clinical presentations ranging from a normal appearance with occasional fractures to severe involvement with growth retardation and long bone and spinal deformities (Fig 23-30; see Table 23-9). In its severe forms, OI is evident at birth because of the fractures and deformity that have occurred in utero.

The less-severe forms may not become evident until the child begins to walk and fractures develop. The tendency to fracture declines after puberty when cortical bone density increases despite trabecular density remaining low. The fracture rate in women increases after menopause. Some children with OI can be mistaken for abused children until the diagnosis is made.

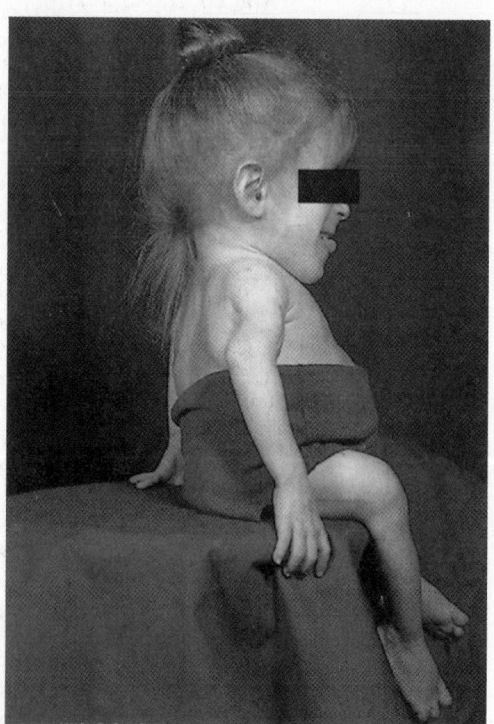

Figure 23-30

Child with osteogenesis imperfecta type III. This shows defect of all four limbs and increased anteroposterior diameter of the chest. Note the spinal deformity. (From Bullough PG: *Bullough and Vigorita's orthopaedic pathology*, ed 3, St Louis, 1997, Mosby, p. 133.)

Shortened stature is common in children with OI. This is partly caused by the abnormal development of epiphyseal growth plates, deformity after fractures, osteoporosis, and vertebral collapse, which contribute to loss of height with increasing age. Lower extremities tend to be more involved than upper extremities. These children often bruise easily, and ligaments tend to show increased laxity.

Additional clinical features may include thin skin, joint hypermobility, deformity of bony auditory structures with subsequent hearing impairment, scoliosis, pectus deformity, deformed teeth, a tendency toward recurrent epistaxis, excess diaphoresis, cardiovascular complications (e.g., aortic and mitral valve insufficiency, aortic dissection), and metabolic defects (e.g., elevated serum pyrophosphate, decreased platelet aggregation). Children with type III or IV OI are born with a triangular face, a feature that makes them easily identifiable.

Blue or tinted (purple, gray) sclerae are present. The sclerae are blue or tinted because they are abnormally translucent like thin skin, and consequently they filter the red color of the underlying choroid plexus of blood vessels, just as a bruise or a subcutaneous hematoma appears blue through thin translucent skin.[207]

Developmental motor skills often are delayed because of poorly developed muscles (atrophy), hypermobility of joints, and multiple fractures requiring immobilization. The majority of children with type I OI ambulate either as functional or household ambulators, and approximately 50% walk without any type of assistive device as community ambulators.

Almost half of children with type III OI are dependent on power mobility, with only 27% becoming household ambulators. Of those children with type IV disease, 26% are community ambulators and 57% household ambulators. The best predictors of ambulatory status are disease type and the ability to sit by 9 or 10 months of age.[49,67]

MEDICAL MANAGEMENT

DIAGNOSIS. Diagnosis of OI is based on clinical manifestations and skin biopsy that looks at collagen. The collagen defect is used to determine what type of OI the person has according to the Sillence classification. Bone scans and x-ray films show evidence of multiple old fractures and skeletal deformities. Skull radiographs show wide sutures with small, irregularly shaped islands of bone called wormian bones.

TREATMENT. Orthopedic management is central to the overall care of symptomatic OI. Fracture prevention and control are the primary focus; careful positioning and handling are required to prevent fractures in the neonate. Lightweight hip-knee-ankle-foot orthoses and splints also may be used to help support the limbs, prevent fractures, and aid in ambulation. Hip-knee-ankle-foot orthoses are used more often than KAFOs because KAFOs have a longer lever arm for rotational force, resulting in greater risk for proximal femur fractures.[85]

Fracture immobilization is as minimal as possible to prevent disuse atrophy. A repeated cycle of fractures-immobilization of the same bone can inhibit progress in mobility and the development of strength (Fig. 23-31).

The use of intramedullary rods is one way of managing recurring fractures (Fig. 23-32). Indications for this procedure include more than two fractures in the same long bone within a 6-month period, lower-extremity bone angles greater than 40 degrees, or very unstable lower extremities in a child who appears ready to walk. Telescoping intramedullary rods are used to stabilize the bones, elongating as the bone grows, although this procedure is not without risk.

The reoperation rate is significant, with complications related to osteopenia that occurs around the rods (greater

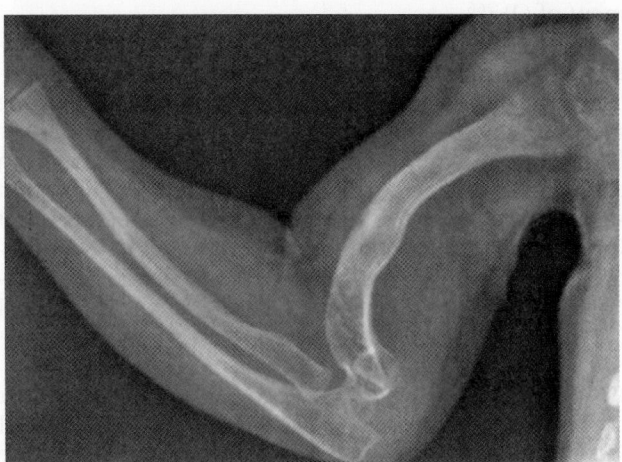

Figure 23-31

Radiograph of upper extremity in a person with osteogenesis imperfecta. This radiograph shows severe osteoporosis, slender bones, and multiple healed fractures. (From Bullough PG: *Bullough and Vigorita's orthopaedic pathology,* ed 3, St Louis, 1997, Mosby, p. 134.)

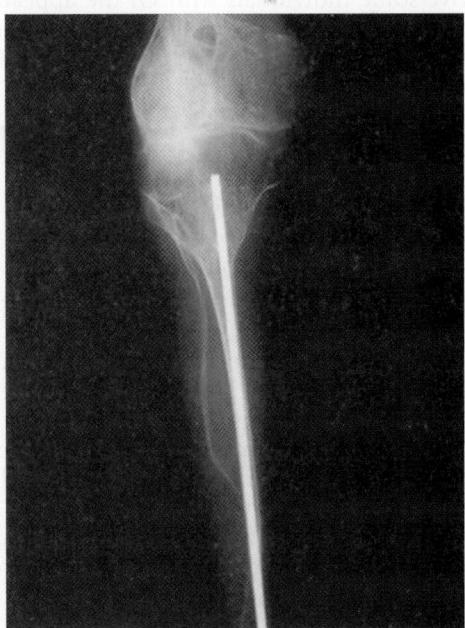

Figure 23-32

Radiograph of the leg of an individual with severe clinical osteogenesis imperfecta that has been treated by rodding of the tibia. The extreme ribbon-like quality of the bones is apparent in the fibula. (From Bullough PG: *Bullough and Vigorita's orthopaedic pathology,* ed 3, St Louis, 1997, Mosby, p. 135.)

around thicker rods), rod migration, and bony growth even beyond the available expansion. Osteotomies also are performed to help control rotational deformities, with appropriate bracing to prolong the time period between potential surgeries.

Medical management has included the use of bisphosphonates, a class of medications (including pamidronate) that inhibit osteoclast function, improve bone mineral density, and decrease the incidence of fractures. Some data exist on the use of growth hormone in OI, but reports of an increased rate of fractures have prevented the use of growth hormone as a first-line drug in the treatment of OI.[266]

Initial reports of allogeneic bone marrow transplantation of mesenchymal cells (progenitors of osteoblasts) have been promising, with increased bone mineral content and histologic evidence of new bone formation 3 months after engraftment.[111] Studies in cell cultures and in mice have raised the possibility that several additional strategies may be developed to treat OI through the use of gene therapy; a review of current gene therapy strategies under investigation is available.[75] At present, no effective treatment exists for type II (perinatal lethal) OI.

PROGNOSIS. People with OI types I and IV have a milder course and live a relatively normal life span. In type III OI, mortality can be related to cardiorespiratory failure stemming from kyphoscoliotic deformity. A significant risk also exists of basilar invagination of the skull and intracranial bleeding.[150]

Incomplete and relatively painless fractures after birth that receive no treatment can produce deformities from bones healing in poor alignment. Short stature and deformities give some individuals with OI the appearance of having achondroplasia. Milder forms of this condition have fewer clinical problems, and these children survive into adulthood.

SPECIAL IMPLICATIONS FOR THE THERAPIST `23-10`

Osteogenesis Imperfecta
Precautions

Infants and children with this disorder require careful handling to prevent fractures. They must be supported when they are being turned, positioned, moved, burped, and cuddled or held. Diaper changing must be carried out gently, never lifting the legs by the ankles but rather by gently lifting the buttocks.

With the older child, passive range-of-motion exercises (especially to obtain hip extension) can be used with caution and are considered safe if used in moderation. Rotational forces are contraindicated, but gentle stretching in straight planes and myofascial stretching are acceptable if done carefully and with the client's participation.

The child must be encouraged to use full active range of motion without force. Strengthening activities should avoid placing weight near joint lines, and if manual resistance is applied, long lever arms should be avoided.

Family Education

Educational material and information can be obtained from the Osteogenesis Imperfecta Foundation (www.oif.org). The family must be instructed in handling and positioning techniques. Precautions should be given to avoid lifting the child under the arms or by the hands. The young child should not be tossed into the air or be involved in roughhouse play.

At the same time, families should be encouraged to hold and play with their child appropriately and to help the child develop interests that do not require strenuous physical activity. Fine motor skills are encouraged, and activities of daily living modifications for personal hygiene may be necessary.

Swimming frequently is recommended, but the child must be monitored carefully to avoid falls in the shower and pool area. Nonskid aquatic shoes can be worn (by the child or by the caregiver carrying a nonambulatory child in the aquatic area) to assist with this precaution.

Family members must also be instructed to assess for fractures daily. The child may bruise easily, but it is common for a child to have no bruises around the fracture site. Symptoms to look for include limited use of an extremity, malposition of an extremity, focal swelling or tenderness, or crying when a body part is moved or when the child attempts to move.

In the case of diagnosed OI involving child abuse allegations, the parents are encouraged to carry a letter from the primary care physician documenting the diagnosis. Even so, any suspicion of actual abuse in the case of a child with OI requires careful documentation and appropriate referral.

Therapy Intervention

Therapy helps to prevent disuse weakness or loss of bone stock and strengthens muscles and builds bone density. Light resistance to exercise or movement can be used; aquatic programs are especially helpful in allowing exercise with light resistance.

Strengthening programs emphasize hip extension, hip abduction, trunk extension, and abdominal muscles. A hip extension, hip abduction, and spinal muscular strengthening program complemented by a swimming program two times per week correlates with an increased ability to assume and maintain an upright position and subsequent ambulation.[20]

Positioning is a significant part of the overall management program for these children. Positioning emphasizes a neutral position of the head, trunk, and lower extremities; neutral hip rotation; and hip extension. In fragile cases, the prone position should be avoided except when fully supported or while being supported in the swimming pool.

The ability to stand is important and should be implemented at approximately 10 to 14 months' chronologic age. Standing can be initiated in a standing frame for 30 minutes twice daily. Special care must be taken to avoid fractures when placing and securing the child in the stander. Aquatic therapy also can be used as a medium for initiating standing activities in more-severe cases. Throughout any standing activity the therapist must continue to monitor for lower extremity bowing secondary to bone instability.

Mobility

The therapist may have to use a significant amount of creativity to adapt ambulating devices and to accommodate for various musculoskeletal deficiencies while fostering the skills necessary for independent mobility. If ambulation is unlikely, the therapist should not hesitate to move quickly toward a wheelchair as the child's primary means of mobility.

When upper extremities are not involved (or minimally affected), manual propulsion chairs offer a functional means of strengthening. Wheelchair fit is extremely important, as bones can bow around supporting surfaces such as armrests. Although children as young as 2 years old cognitively can use and benefit from powered mobility,[237] whenever possible, powered mobility is delayed in this population until the child is older (e.g., 5 or 6 years).

ARTHROGRYPOSIS MULTIPLEX CONGENITA

Definition and Overview

Arthrogryposis multiplex congenita (AMC) is the presence at birth of multiple congenital contractures resulting from decreased fetal movement in an intact skeleton. Contracture can result from any number of underlying pathologies. Contractures may occur either in flexion or extension, and the muscles may be nothing more than fibrous bands.

Three different types of AMC exist: (1) contracture syndromes, (2) amyoplasia (lack of muscle formation or development), and (3) distal arthrogryposis, primarily affecting the hands and feet. Occasionally, the child presents with associated abnormalities such as cleft palate, cardiac lesions, urinary tract malformations, and cryptorchidism (failure of testes to descend into the scrotum); however, their presence or absence depends on the underlying cause of the arthrogryposis.

Incidence and Etiologic Factors

AMC affects 1 in 4300 individuals[139] and can result from any condition that limits fetal movement. Various investigations have attributed the basic defect to an abnormality of muscle, CNS, lower motor neuron, or fetal environment. Hereditary factors have been identified in a number of isolated cases of AMC, with autosomal dominant, recessive, X-linked recessive, and mitochondrial inheritance patterns being identified.[87] AMC also is associated with a variety of CNS disorders, including migrational brain disorders and neurodegenerative disorders. CMD also is associated with a smaller percentage of cases of AMC. Other possible causes are prenatal viral infection, drugs, maternal hyperthermia, vascular compromise between mother and fetus, and decreased amniotic fluid

in utero (oligohydramnios) limiting fetal movement. The joint deformities present in AMC appear to be secondary to the lack of active motion during intrauterine development and the presence of joint contractures and abnormal weight bearing across the joint.

Pathogenesis

The underlying cause of AMC is unknown and the contracture phenotype is the result of potentially many different causes; however, the underlying condition in all cases results in decreased fetal movement.[35]

Clinical Manifestations

The dominant features of AMC include joint contracture, articular rigidity, muscle weakness, and in some cases replacement of the muscle with fibrous and fatty tissue. Arthrogryposis can affect all joints of the body but tends to have a preference for the feet, hips, wrists, knees, elbows, and shoulders (in order of decreasing frequency). Box 23-6 outlines a typical clinical picture of a child with arthrogryposis.

Because many of these children demonstrate average or above-average intelligence, they are able to accommodate for loss of motion with a variety of alternative mobility patterns, such as seat-scooting or rolling. Typical postures include hip flexion with knee extension or a "jackknife" posture, which affects the child's ability to attain certain developmental postures, including quadruped, short sit, and ring sit, because of the contractures. Those children with knee flexion and hip external rotation or a "frogleg posture" are typically slower to roll but quicker to sit and

---

Box 23-6

ARTHROGRYPOSIS: CLINICAL PICTURE

- Speech, cognition usually within average limits
- Facial asymmetry
- Oral-motor: hypotonia, congenitally absent muscles, jaw stiffness contribute to oral-motor difficulties
- Trunk: thoracolumbar scoliosis (20%), rigid movement, slow responses, minimal rotation, all affecting equilibrium and balance
- Lower extremity jackknife posture (55%)
  - Flexed dislocated hips with extended knees
  - Clubfeet (talipes equinovarus)
- Lower extremity frog posture (45%)
  - Abducted, externally rotated hips
  - Knee flexion
  - Clubfeet (talipes equinovarus)
- Upper extremity posture
  - Shoulder adduction and internal rotation
  - Extended elbow, wrist ulnar deviation
  - Flexed wrists with stiff straight fingers; poor thumb control
- Functional reach impaired requiring multiple muscle substitution, co-contraction of flexors and extensors, use of opposite arm or hand to assist
- Delayed motor development
  - Sitting independently: approximately 15 months
  - Ambulation: approximately 2 to 3 years if musculoskeletal limitations allow

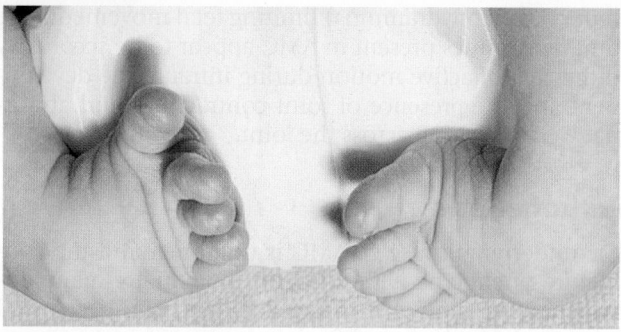

Figure 23-33

Clubfoot deformity, talipes equinovarus (bilateral deviation). This 4-month-old child was diagnosed with spina bifida, hemivertebrae, and clubfoot. Early intervention can include serial casting to provide stretch to the contracted structures and to provide a more normal plantigrade foot position. Clubfoot is a common morbidity found in children with spina bifida. The casts are typically changed every 1 to 2 weeks and followed by the use of a molded ankle-foot orthosis to maintain the corrected position. Often, as the child grows, surgical releases and osteotomies also are required to provide an optimal correction. (From Zitelli BJ, Davis HW: *Atlas of pediatric physical diagnosis,* ed 4, St Louis, 2002, Mosby.)

scoot. Many of the children are unable to make the transition from sitting to standing and can't maintain a standing position once placed upright, often because of hip extension weakness and hip flexion contractures.

As adults, arthritis is a common comorbidity in a variety of different joints as a result of overuse and the abnormal stresses that are placed across the joints. Many affected individuals will benefit from some type of wheeled or powered mobility for long distances, either because of the wear and tear on malaligned joints and the amount of energy required to move in a malaligned position or to improve functional mobility.

MEDICAL MANAGEMENT

DIAGNOSIS. Prenatal diagnosis may be made by ultrasonic examination based on diminished fetal movement and detection of joint contractures. These findings usually do not become evident until 16 to 18 weeks' gestation.[216] A definitive diagnosis is made by neonatal examination and, if needed, radiographs. However, congenital joint contractures may be secondary to many conditions, requiring differential diagnosis.

TREATMENT AND PROGNOSIS. Physical therapy and occupational therapy are the mainstays of early treatment, with passive mobilization of the joints, positioning, strengthening, and enhancement of functional adaptation skills (e.g., prevention of falls, mobility training, movement up and down stairs or on uneven terrain).

Orthopedic surgery often is used to address the many musculoskeletal limitations associated with AMC and often is combined with serial casting. Some of the more common surgical procedures include posterior spinal fusion for thoracolumbar scoliosis; quadriceps lengthening to increase knee flexion for functional movement; and posterior capsulotomies, hamstring lengthening, and wedge osteotomies to allow for increased functional knee extension.

Clubfoot deformity (Fig. 23-33) often is treated with a heel cord lengthening and capsulotomy, in addition to a talar procedure if needed to achieve a good correction. Hip procedures are associated with a fairly high risk of failed reduction; in addition, there is a risk of avascular necrosis if the hip is not able to be reduced and is splinted in abduction.

Other less-common procedures are being attempted, such as the successful use of the latissimus dorsi muscle to restore elbow flexion.[82] A variety of opinions exist regarding the place for the various soft tissue and bony procedures available, with some advocating nontreatment.

| SPECIAL IMPLICATIONS FOR THE THERAPIST | 23-11 |

Arthrogryposis Multiplex Congenita
Therapeutic Intervention

The child benefits maximally from therapy from 0 to 2 years of age and during periodic growth spurts, with functional goals related to optimal functional mobility and activities of daily living. Strengthening programs focus on weak muscles or movement in opposition to typical resting postures.

Removable splints, such as ankle-foot orthoses, are recommended for positioning and to maintain muscle length. These should be worn a minimum of 6 to 8 hours per day and preferably up to 22 hours per day if they don't interrupt sleep. In children who are nonambulatory, power mobility should be considered as early as 2 years of age if the underlying weakness or contractures make manual wheelchair mobility impractical. A variety of adaptive equipment (including powered feeding devices)[105] are available to aid in the completion of activities of daily living.

REFERENCES
To enhance this text and add value for the reader, all references are included on the companion Evolve site that accompanies this textbook. The reader can view the reference source and access it online whenever possible.

CHAPTER 24

Metabolic Disorders

KEVIN HELGESON

Metabolic disorders can affect numerous body tissues, including bony structures. Primary metabolic diseases and their implications for the therapist are discussed in Chapter 11. Metabolic disorders primarily affecting the skeletal system are the focus of this chapter.

The skeleton is a metabolically active organ that undergoes continuous remodeling throughout life with an annual turnover of cortical and trabecular bone of about 10% of the adult skeleton.[125] This remodeling is necessary both to maintain the structural integrity of the skeleton and to serve a metabolic function as a storehouse of calcium and phosphorus. These dual functions can come into conflict under conditions of changing mechanical forces or metabolic and nutritional stress.[116]

Clinical disorders in which bone resorption is increased are common and include Paget disease of bone, osteoporosis, and the bone changes secondary to cancer such as occur in myeloma and metastases from breast or prostate cancer. Clinical disorders of reduced bone resorption are less common and have a genetic basis (e.g., osteopetrosis).

Metabolic bone disease is typically manifested by diffuse loss of bone density and bone strength, but increased bone density and decreased bone strength can occur such as with Paget disease. Significant disability, marked by bone pain, postural deformity, and fracture, can occur secondary to these bony changes. The commonly observed accentuated thoracic spine kyphosis in clients with vertebral collapse secondary to osteoporosis can compromise cardiopulmonary function, affecting the person's ability to participate in a rehabilitation program.

The most serious, potentially life-threatening and costly complication of metabolic bone disease is fracture (see "Fractures" in Chapter 27). Osteoporosis alone is estimated to be responsible for more than 1.5 million fractures annually and this is expected to double in the next 15 years with the aging of the baby boomers in the United States (currently 700,000 vertebral fractures, 300,000 hip fractures, 250,000 wrist fractures, and 250,000 other fractures); 1 in 3 women older than 50 years of age experience a fracture in their lifetime.[98] The monetary cost of these fractures is estimated at $10 billion to $15 billion annually in the United States. This estimate does not include the indirect costs of lost wages or productivity of either the individual or the caregiver.

Therapists have an important role in the primary prevention of disability secondary to the complications associated with metabolic bone disease. Client education regarding posture, body mechanics, and proper exercise is an important component of any prevention program. Physical therapy intervention is also a vital part of the rehabilitation of clients disabled by the resultant pain or postural deformities that can accompany these diseases. Therapists also treat many clients who have experienced traumatic injury precipitated by the presence of metabolic bone disease or, conversely, people who are experiencing the metabolic consequences of trauma.

The regulation of all metabolic functions requires proper fluid and electrolyte balance, which in turn relies on a finely tuned integration between the endocrine system and the nervous system. The effects of metabolic disorders on muscle and muscle performance are discussed more completely in Chapter 5. Finally, therapists treat many people with a primary diagnosis of low back, knee, or shoulder conditions with osteoporosis as a secondary diagnosis. The presence of such a secondary diagnosis may influence the therapist's choice of evaluation and intervention. A thorough understanding of this group of diseases will enable the therapist to treat clients safely and effectively.

OSTEOPOROSIS

Definition and Overview

Osteoporosis is a chronic, progressive disease characterized by low bone mass, impaired bone quality, decreased bone strength, and enhanced risk of fractures.[98] Osteoporosis can be classified as primary or secondary, depending on the underlying etiology. *Primary osteoporosis*, the most common, can occur in both genders at all ages but often follows menopause in women, and occurs later in life in men. Osteoporosis associated with medications, other conditions, or diseases is referred to as *secondary osteoporosis* (Box 24-1).

Incidence

Osteoporosis is by far the most common metabolic bone disease, affecting more than 10 million people living in

Box 24-1

RISK FACTORS AND CONDITIONS ASSOCIATED WITH OSTEOPOROSIS

Risk Factors

Nonmodifiable

- Age 50 years and older
- Caucasian/Asian
- Northern European ancestry
- Menopausal (occurs early in those <45 years and can be surgically induced through bilateral oophorectomy)
- Family history of osteoporosis; personal history of fragility fracture; fragility fracture in first-degree relative
- Long periods of inactivity, immobilization, long-term care
- Depression
- Lactose intolerance
- Femoral neck BMD

Risk Factors for Which Intervention Might Reduce Incidence of Osteoporosis and Fractures

- Inactivity or sedentary lifestyle
- Excess intake of:
  - Alcohol (>2 drinks/d)
  - Tobacco (active or passive)
  - Caffeine* (equivalent to >3 cups caffeinated coffee/d)
- Amenorrhea (abnormal absence of menses)
- Estrogen deficiency (women)/testosterone deficiency (men)
- Medications (>6 months)
  - Corticosteroids/steroids
  - Immunosuppressants
  - Anticoagulants (Heparin; Coumadin)
  - Nonthiazide diuretics (furosemide)†
  - Methotrexate (MTX)
  - Cisplatin (chemotherapy)
  - Aromatase inhibiters (breast cancer treatment)
  - Antacids (containing aluminum)
  - Laxatives
  - Anticonvulsants
  - Benzodiazepines (Valium, Librium, Xanax)
  - Some antibiotics (e.g., tetracycline derivatives)
  - Buffered aspirin
  - Excessive thyroid hormones
  - Lithium
  - Androgen deprivation (prostate cancer)
  - Depo-Provera (contraceptive)
  - Gonadotropin-releasing hormone agonists

- Low body weight and body mass index (see Table 2-3), thin, small body frame
- Diet and nutrition
  - Calcium and magnesium deficiency
  - Vitamin D deficiency
  - Vitamin C deficiency (helps with calcium absorption)
  - High ratio of animal to vegetable protein intake
  - High-fat diet (reduces calcium absorption in the gut)
  - Excessive sugar (depletes phosphorus)
  - High intake of low-calcium beverages such as coffee and carbonated soft drinks
  - Eating disorders (bulimia, anorexia nervosa, binge eating)
  - Repeated crash dieting or "yo-yo" dieting

Associated Diseases and Disorders

- Endocrine disorders
  - Hyperthyroidism
  - Hyperparathyroidism
  - Type 2 diabetes mellitus
  - Cushing disease
  - Male hypogonadism (testosterone deficiency)
- Malabsorption
  - Celiac disease
  - GI disease; gastric surgery
  - Hepatic disease
- Medication related
- Organ transplantation
  - Chronic pulmonary disease
  - Rheumatic diseases, including juvenile idiopathic arthritis
- Chronic renal failure
- Osteogenesis imperfecta
- Sickle cell disease
- Cancer and cancer treatment (children and adults), skeletal metastasis
- Eating disorders
- Spinal cord injury
- Cerebrovascular accident or stroke
- Acid-balance imbalance (metabolic acidosis)
- Depression
- Erectile dysfunction
- Hypogonadal states
- HIV/AIDS

GI, Gastrointestinal; *HIV/AIDS,* human immunodeficiency virus/acquired immunodeficiency syndrome.
*Caffeine from any source in excess of 300 mg/d should be avoided.
†Some diuretics such as the nonthiazide diuretics have calcium-retaining properties with reduced incidence of hip fracture with long-term use.

the United States. An additional 34 million Americans already have low bone mass (osteopenia) that places them at increased risk of osteoporosis. With the aging of America, osteoporosis is expected to increase in prevalence.[16]

The disease is much more common in women, especially postmenopausal women who are estrogen deficient. However, osteoporosis in men represents a major public health problem, which until recently has received little recognition. Approximately 2 million men are affected by osteoporosis and another 12 million are at risk as a result of low bone mass. This condition in men remains underdiagnosed, undertreated, and underreported.[34,36,100]

One in every 2 women older than 50 years of age will experience fragility fractures secondary to osteoporosis.[44] One in 4 men will experience an osteoporosis-related

fragility fracture during their lifetime, usually later (because of greater bone mass than women) at approximately age 70 years. When affected, men have a higher morbidity and mortality than that of women (30% versus 9%).[12,147] This is because men are older at the time they sustain a fracture and are more likely to have comorbid disease, malnutrition, and complicated hospitalizations.[149]

Etiologic Factors

The cause of *primary osteoporosis* is unknown, but many contributory factors exist such as mild but prolonged negative calcium balance, declining gonadal and adrenal function, relative or progressive estrogen deficiency, or sedentary lifestyle. *Secondary osteoporosis* may be caused by prolonged therapy with corticosteroids, heparin, anticonvulsants, and other medications; alcoholism, malnutrition, malabsorption, or lactose intolerance; endocrine disorders; or other conditions or diseases (see Box 24-1).

Risk Factors

Between the ages of 25 and 35 years, bone mass peaks, and the rate of bone resorption begins to exceed the rate of bone formation. This physiologic mismatch can progress to a point at which osteopenia (Box 24-2) may be noted radiographically and a progression of osteoporosis is suspected. Box 24-1 lists the many risk factors and conditions or diseases associated with osteoporosis. Chronic diseases, or medications used to treat these diseases, may have side effects that can damage bone or interfere with bone formation, leading to osteoporosis.

A difference is certainly evident between risk factors for osteoporosis and risk factors for fractures (see Box 27-16). Estrogen status, heredity, and ethnicity are important risk factors for osteoporosis in women; alcoholism, cigarette smoking, steroid therapy, and hypogonadism or androgen withdrawal therapy for prostate cancer are the most common factors for men,[171] although in 50% of cases, a cause is unknown.[147] Age is a risk factor for both men and women; the 10-year fracture risk at age 50 years quadruples by age 80 years; although women are affected earlier in the decades compared to men, the associated mortality and morbidity is much greater for men.[1]

Hormonal Status

Postmenopausal women are at higher risk to develop the disease. Diagnosis of primary postmenopausal osteoporosis occurs with increasing frequency from age 51 to 75 years. The increased risk of osteoporosis related to menopause is due primarily to the decreased production of estrogen. Estrogen deficiency is linked mostly to the loss of cortical bone, which is linked to the increased risk for fractures.[71] Decreased intestinal calcium absorption, increased bone resorption to compensate for low calcium levels, and impaired osteoblastic activity have all been associated with estrogen deficiency.

Women lose bone at the usual rate of 1% per year after peak bone density has been achieved; however, bone loss accelerates to a varying degree (depending on such factors as calcium intake and absorption, hormonal balance, and activity level) for about 5 to 8 years after menopause, increasing the risk of fracture. Researchers report a wide range from 2% to 11% loss for the 10 years after menopause, slowing after that to about 0.5% to 1% of bone mass per year.

Men experience a gradual slowing of testosterone production with age, and below-normal testosterone levels have been associated with loss of bone mineral mass. The outward signs of this phenomenon (e.g., loss of muscle strength, fatigue, and a decreased interest in sex) are often attributed to aging without considering the accompanying osteoporosis that ensues. Other risk factors include androgen-deprivation treatment for prostate cancer and hypogonadism associated with erectile dysfunction.[15] Low serum testosterone levels have also been documented

Box 24-2

TERMINOLOGY OF METABOLIC BONE DISEASE

Osteomalacia: Softening of the bones
Osteopenia: Low bone mass
Osteopetrosis: Increased bone density
Osteoporosis: Decreased bone density (strength)

Osteoporosis is contrasted from osteopenia (low bone mass) by its characterization as "low bone mass, microarchitectural deterioration of bone tissue and decreased bone strength with bone fragility and consequent increase in fracture risk" [as defined by the National Osteoporosis Foundation].

in men treated with corticosteroids for chronic inflammatory conditions such as sarcoidosis.[2]

Heredity/Genetics

Peak bone mass is partly genetically determined as evidenced by the varying prevalence of osteoporosis among different ethnic groups, but other variables also exist such as differences in bone geometry and rate of bone loss. Individual differences among people of the same ethnic background can occur, possibly in part because of inheriting specific genes that affect bone mass and turnover.[128]

Eight genes have been linked to bone density with a strong connection to the receptor for parathyroid hormone (PTHR1). This hormone plays a crucial role in determining the level of calcium in the blood. Genetic differences in the levels of receptors for PTH in the blood may determine bone density. The results of some research suggest that gender specificity as to how these genes are expressed plays a key role (i.e., men and women may inherit these genes differently).[35]

Body build is related to bone fragility. Older women who weigh less than 127 pounds tend to have less cortical bone and are therefore at greater risk of fractures. Obesity, by increasing the mechanical strain on bone, may result in increased peak bone mass, reducing bone fragility. In addition, obesity increases the amount of biologically available estrogen, protecting against fracture. Women with a family history of osteoporosis are at high risk of developing osteoporotic fractures.[130]

Ethnicity

Ethnicity is also considered a risk factor because bone mass correlates positively with skin pigmentation. Whites have the least amount of bone mass, whereas blacks have the greatest amount. Men have wider long bones than women, and blacks have wider long bones than whites. Therefore black men are at lowest risk of developing osteoporosis.[135] Because white women generally have lower peak bone mass, the complications of the bone loss associated with aging can affect them earlier in life.

Limited information available suggests that Native American women have lower bone densities than white non-Hispanic women, and Mexican American women have bone densities intermediate between those of white non-Hispanic women and black women.[91] On the other hand, skin pigmentation also correlates with vitamin D synthesis, with more heavily pigmented people requiring greater amounts of sunshine to synthesize vitamin D needed for bone strength. Early reports indicate that osteoporosis may be more prevalent in Hispanic, Native American, Asian, and black women than once thought.

Physical Inactivity

Inactivity and immobilization have been associated with decreased bone formation. The prolonged inactivity results in reduced gravitational and muscular forces acting on the skeletal system. The decreased mechanical stress on bony structures alters bone physiology, resulting in decreased bone mass.

Disuse osteopenia, which can be caused by immobilization (e.g., cast, bed rest, long-term care, or neurologic impairment), results from a change in cellular function or an increase in the recruitment of osteoclasts. The difference in the quality of bone produced is in the decreased number of trabeculae and in increased osteoclastic performance. Residents in nursing home or long-term care facilities have a 5- to 10-fold greater fracture risk than community dwellers.[37]

Tobacco

Cigarette smoking is associated with a reduction of bone mass and is a well-known risk factor for spinal and hip fractures. The effects of smokeless tobacco and second-hand smoke have not been evaluated as risk factors but may be important considerations. Some evidence suggests that cigarette smoke may affect bone progenitor cells by directly contributing to the development of osteoporosis.[32,77,145]

Alcohol

More than two "units" of alcohol per day is a risk factor for osteoporosis.[66] A unit is defined as one 12-oz beer, one 5-oz glass of wine, or 1.5 oz of hard liquor. Excessive alcohol intake alters osteoblast gene expression and matrix synthesis, thereby reducing the number of effective cells.[168] Chronic alcohol use can impair intestinal absorption and increase renal excretion of calcium, contribute to poorer overall nutrition, and increase the likelihood of a fall.

In men, consuming large amounts of alcohol is a major independent risk factor for hip fractures[55]; combined alcohol and corticosteroid use has a significant impact on the development of osteoporosis.[90] (See "Tobacco" and "Depressants" in Chapter 2.)

Medications

Long-term use of medications, including corticosteroids, has been associated with the presence of osteoporosis. People with a wide range of medical conditions (e.g., asthma, chronic obstructive pulmonary disease [COPD], organ transplantation, renal impairment, arthritis, systemic lupus erythematosus [SLE], Crohn disease or regional enteritis, sarcoidosis, and others) may be taking corticosteroids.

Most bone loss occurs during the first 6 months of systemic corticosteroid therapy. Loss of 10% to 15% of spinal trabecular bone mass is possible; after that, bone loss averages 1% to 2% annually. Corticosteroids impair osteoblastic activity and the maturation of preosteoblastic cells to osteoblasts, increase osteoclastic activity, and

impair vitamin D–dependent intestinal calcium absorption, which can result in secondary hyperparathyroidism. The hyperparathyroidism increases bone resorption and decreases renal resorption of calcium, thereby increasing the amount of calcium excretion.

Other medications have also been implicated (see Box 24-1). Selective serotonin reuptake inhibitors (SSRIs) are not on this list, but there is some preliminary evidence that links the use of SSRIs to the increased risk of fracture for those older than age 50 years.[124,132] More research is needed to identify if depression itself is the source of endocrine changes that can damage bone.[52]

Depression

Depression is now recognized as a risk factor for osteoporosis.[133,174] Individuals with a history of a major depressive disorder are more likely to have lower bone densities and higher levels of cortisol than people without depression, regardless of physical activity levels. Major depressive disorders are thought to cause bone loss primarily due to immune and endocrine mechanisms. Depressive disorders are also associated with poor lifestyle habits that are potential contributory factors to bone loss.[21] Depression may be a risk factor in other ways. A study of bone loss in premenopausal women with and without major depression showed that those who were depressed had unfavorable levels of cytokines that specifically affect bone mass.[20,21] Cytokines act as chemical messengers between the immune, nervous, and endocrine systems.[20,86]

Diet and Nutrition

Different sources of dietary protein may have different effects on bone metabolism. Women age 65 and older with a high dietary ratio of animal-to-vegetable protein intake have more rapid femoral neck bone loss and a greater risk of hip fracture than do those with a low ratio.

Animal foods provide predominantly acid precursors, whereas protein in vegetable foods is accompanied by base precursors not found in animal foods. Imbalance between dietary acid and base precursors leads to a chronic net dietary acid load that may have adverse consequences on bone.[134,136] Excess acid is excreted in the urine, but with aging, the kidneys are less capable of excreting acid.

Bone density is decreased in anorexic and bulimic women and is possibly the result of estrogen deficiency, low intake of nutrients, low body weight, early onset and long duration of amenorrhea, low calcium intake, reduced physical activity, and hypercortisolism. This type of reduced bone density is associated with a significantly increased risk of fracture even at a young age.[46] The female athlete triad describes the combination of disordered eating, amenorrhea, and osteoporosis, which is a situation that often goes unrecognized and untreated.[101,154]

A significant number of people with osteoporosis also have celiac disease, a gastrointestinal (GI) disorder that impairs the absorption of calcium, various nutrients, and vitamin D needed for maintaining healthy bones. Identification and effective dietary therapy for celiac disease can lead to improved absorption of vital nutrients and potentially reverse the decline in bone mineral density (BMD). Celiac disease increases the long-term risk of fracture, especially hip fracture.[54,80]

New information about the role of cholesterol in bone health has come to light. High cholesterol associated with a high-fat diet may decrease overall bone production through the process of oxidation. Oxidative stress modulates differentiation of vascular and bone cells oppositely so that a parallel buildup and loss of calcification occur in vascular calcification and osteoporosis, respectively.[94] Preliminary studies in animals suggest that an atherogenic diet inhibits bone formation by blocking differentiation of osteoblast progenitor cells.[111,112]

Pathogenesis

Bone is composed of a meshwork of collagen fibers inlaid with calcium and phosphate. These minerals are mixed with water to form a hard, cement-like substance called *hydroxyapatite*. Sodium, magnesium, and potassium are also present in smaller amounts. The human skeleton is composed of two main bone types: trabecular and cortical. Bone strength is made up of two components: bone density and bone quality. Bone density refers to how many bone cells are present in a square inch. That measure also reflects how close together the bone cells are. But density isn't the only component of bone strength. There is also bone quality. Bone quality reflects the health of the bone cells present. Quality of the collagen cells that make up bone, thickness of the bone, and architecture of the bone all make up this entity we call bone quality. Bone quality reflects the condition of the supportive structure of bone.

BMD increases during growth and development, and the peak bone mass is achieved in the third decade of life. This is the bone bank for the rest of a person's life.[19] An individual with a high peak bone mass who starts to lose bone later in life and loses it slowly is unlikely to sustain osteoporotic fractures, whereas someone with suboptimal peak bone mass who starts to lose bone earlier in life or loses bone rapidly is more likely to develop osteoporosis with fractures.

Osteoporosis develops when new bone formation falls behind resorption, possibly related to impaired new bone formation due to declining osteoblast function (Fig 24-1, Fig. 24-2). The onset of bone loss is likely to be genetically predetermined, and the subsequent rate of bone loss may also be influenced by genetic factors.

Bone loss increases at the time of menopause as a result of the marked reduction in the circulating concentrations of estradiol and progesterone (Fig. 24-3).[41] Other causes of age-related bone loss have been discussed previously in this chapter. Each one of those contributing factors has its own pathologic process. Only the general pathogenic concepts are discussed here.

Small defects in formation remaining at the completion of a normal remodeling cycle accumulate and also contribute to age-related losses in bone mass. Thus the bone that experiences the greatest number of remodeling cycles is at the highest risk for age-related losses in mass. New information about metabolic bone diseases has revealed that maintenance of adult skeletal mass is controlled not only by changes in the production of osteoclasts and osteoblasts but also by altering the duration of their respective life spans through regulated apoptosis (programmed cell death). During bone remodeling,

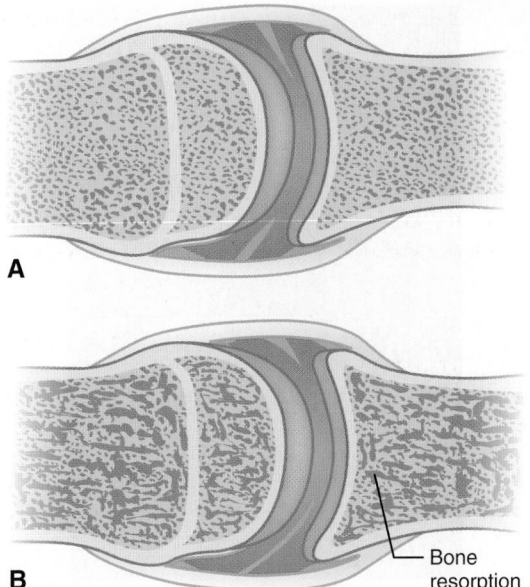

Figure 24-1

Osteoporosis. A, Normal bone and joint. **B,** Osteoporotic changes shown with bone resorption greater than bone formation resulting in weakened trabeculae and increasing risk for fracture. (From Jarvis C: *Physical examination and health assessment,* ed 6, Philadelphia, 2012, WB Saunders.)

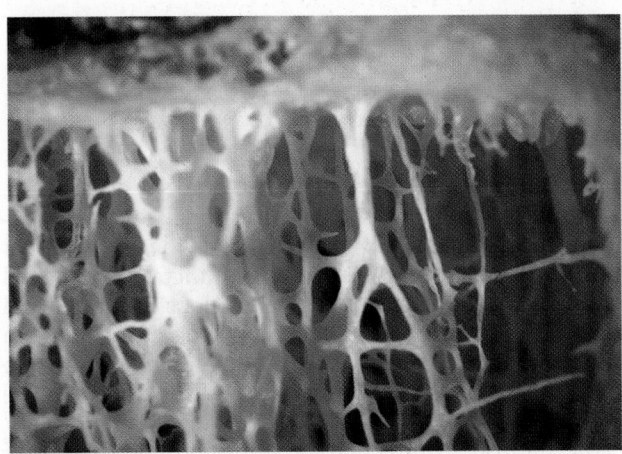

Figure 24-2

Osteoporosis of the lumbar vertebra with generalized loss of bone. The vertical plates have become perforated and the number of horizontal cross-braces are decreased markedly in proportion to the vertical plates. (From McPherson RA: *Henry's clinical diagnosis and management by laboratory methods,* ed 21, Philadelphia, 2006, WB Saunders.)

disruption of the rate of supply of new osteoblasts and osteoclasts and the timing of this supply by apoptosis may be an important mechanism behind the deranged bone turnover found in most metabolic disorders of the adult skeleton.[63,166]

Defects in a protein called *alphaV beta3 integrin* appear to play a role in the development of osteoporosis. The effects of this protein can be reversed by enhancing another protein, macrophage colony-stimulating factor (M-CSF). The interaction between M-CSF and alphaV beta3 integrin is under investigation. These proteins may have a role in bone cell differentiation and the signaling

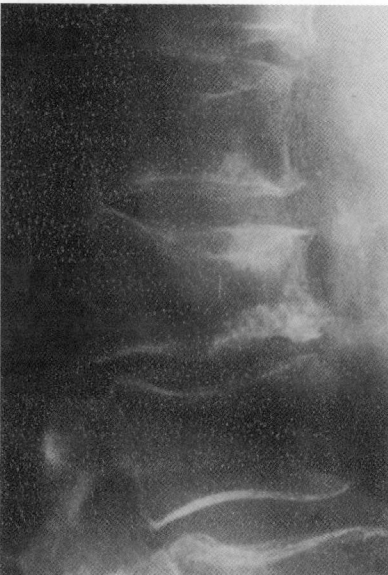

Figure 24-3

Postmenopausal osteoporosis in a 59-year-old woman. Lateral view of the thoracolumbar spine sows protrusion of disc material through a weakened end plate (Schmorl's node). Note also the biconcave appearance of several vertebral bodies. (From Grainger: RG: *Grainger & Allison's diagnostic radiology: a textbook of medical imaging*, ed 4, Philadelphia, 2001, Churchill Livingstone.)

pathway that causes a change in osteoclast and osteoblast balance.[151,152,175]

Bone Demineralization

Bone demineralization, which can lead to osteopenia, takes place when a deficit in hormonal levels, inadequate physical activity (mechanical load), or poor nutrition occurs. Bone strength is a function of skeletal load—that is, bone responds to alterations in mechanical forces. Although the exact physiologic mechanism causing bone to sense and respond to alterations in mechanical loads is unclear, adaptations appear to be site specific.

Mechanical stimuli may be the only type of stimuli capable of inducing modeling in mature bone; young bone responds more favorably to mechanical loading than old bone, again emphasizing the importance of physical activity and exercise in the adolescent and young adult.[163] Physical activity transmits mechanical loads to the skeleton through gravitational forces and muscular pull at sites of attachment. In the absence of mechanical forces (space flight or prolonged bed rest), urinary calcium excretion increases and bone density decreases. BMD changes induced by loading are not maintained long-term, which is why regular site-specific and weight-bearing exercises must be done routinely to prevent osteoporosis and reduce bone fracture risk.[163] Subsequently, hormonal levels, physical activity, and nutrition are the key factors that facilitate bone growth because they regulate the osteoblastic and osteoclastic remodeling cycles, initiate a natural cycle of microscopic bone damage and subsequent repair, and foster solid bone architecture.[113]

Gender Differences

Studies of normal age-related changes in human bone have been investigated by using a combination of different techniques. Men show an age-related compensatory increase in bone size (cross-sectional area of the vertebral bodies), which cannot be found in women. Women have a higher tendency, after age 50 years, to demonstrate disconnection of the trabecular network that can be positively affected by physiologic loading such as occurs during exercise.[95]

Clinical Manifestations

Loss of height, postural changes, back pain, and fracture are the most common presenting features of osteoporosis. Postural changes may include lax abdominal musculature, protuberant abdomen, forward head, kyphosis, dowager's hump, loss of lumbar lordosis, posterior pelvic tilt, knee hyperextension, shoulder internal rotation, scapular forward rotation, palms facing backward, and other deviations in alignment observed when assessed by a physical therapist. Marked thoracic spine kyphosis and loss of overall body height are common findings, especially after a vertebral compression fracture.[68] Similarly, bone loss in the mandible can contribute to changes in facial appearance.

Muscular pain and spasm can occur in the lower back paravertebral muscles, as can burning pain in the midthoracic region lateral to the spine because of excess stretch placed on the rhomboid muscles from the compensatory forward rotation of the scapulae. Trigger points secondary to kyphoscoliosis, rhomboid imbalance, and paravertebral muscle spasm are common. Similar muscle imbalance and muscular symptoms are observed or reported in the lower quadrant with involvement of the lumbosacral and sacroiliac joints and surrounding musculature.[64]

Fractures

The vertebral bodies, hip, ribs, radius, and femur are the most common fracture sites (in that order) although any bone in the body can be affected. A first fracture is a risk factor for a second fracture, which, in turn, increases the risk of death.[11] Fractures are often "silent" compression fractures of vertebral bodies, sacral insufficiency fractures, or complete fractures of the spine or femoral neck. Metatarsal insufficiency fracture in both men and women maybe an unrecognized early sign of osteoporosis.[155]

Vertebral compression fractures (VCFs) are the most common osteoporosis-related spinal fractures presenting with clinical symptoms of back pain, posture change, loss of height, functional impairment, disability, and diminished quality of life (Fig. 24-4). These can occur without injury or fall when the bone becomes so porous or weak and it begins to compress (see "Fractures" in Chapter 27). By age 90 years, the force required to produce failure of the L3 vertebrae is approximately one-fourth the compressive failure force at age 30 years.[69]

The prevalence of vertebral fractures increases steadily with age, ranging between 20% for 50-year-old postmenopausal women and 64% for older women. The majority of vertebral fractures are not connected with severe trauma,

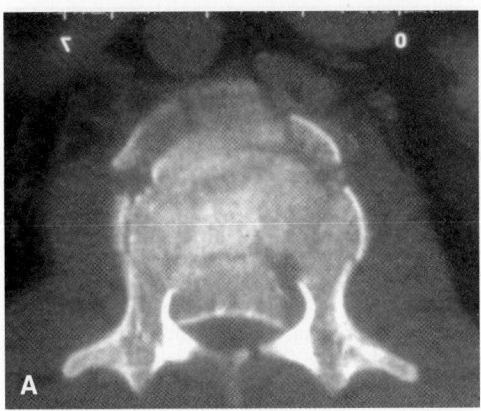

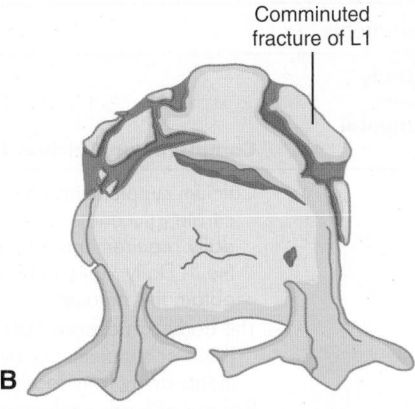

Comminuted
fracture of L1

Figure 24-4

Computed tomography of unstable comminuted vertebral compression (burst) fracture of the lumbar vertebra (L1). (From Marx JA: *Rosen's emergency medicine: concepts and clinical practice,* ed 6, St Louis, 2006, Mosby.)

Box 24-3

MANAGEMENT OF OSTEOPOROSIS

Prevention

Client education
Optimize calcium and magnesium intake (see Table 24-1)
Exposure to sunlight; vitamin D therapy
Regular physical activity (weight bearing) and prescriptive exercise
Other lifestyle changes (e.g., reduce or eliminate alcohol and tobacco)
Maintenance of menstrual cycles from youth through adulthood
Minimize intake of carbonated soft drinks and caffeine
Minimize use of medication(s) known to cause bone loss
Recognize and treat any medical conditions that can affect bone health
Adequate nutrition and calories; avoid chronic dieting or "yo-yo" dieting
Reduce animal sources of protein; increase vegetable sources of protein
Phytoestrogens (under investigation)
Psychosocial support

Management

Same as for Prevention
Pharmacotherapy (single or combination)
• Bisphosphonates
  • Intravenous: pamidronate (Aredia); zoledronate (Zometa)
  • Oral: risedronate (Actonel); ibandronate (Boniva); etidronate (Didronel); alendronate (Fosamax sodium); tiludronate (Skelid)
  • Oral/IV: clodronic acid
• Hormonal therapy (ERT/HRT for women, testosterone for men)
• SERMs (Raloxifene/Evista)
• Calcitonin (nasal or injection):
  • Miacalcin
  • Calcimar
• Parathyroid hormone (PTH; rhPTH: teriparatide/Forteo)
• Osteoprotegerin (OPG)
Osteoporosis education, balance assessment, and falls prevention
Psychosocial support
Falls and fracture prevention (see Chapter 27)

IV, Intravenous; *ERT,* estrogen replacement therapy; *HRT,* hormone replacement therapy; *SERMs,* selective estrogen receptor modulators; *PTH,* parathyroid hormone; *rhPTH,* recombinant human PTH; *OPG,* osteoprotegerin.

---

and only one in three is diagnosed clinically. Almost 20% of women will experience another fracture within 1 year after a vertebral fracture.[48]

Pain associated with VCFs is usually severe and localized to the site of fracture, typically midthoracic, lower thoracic, and lumbar spine. Tenderness to palpation over the fracture is common in both symptomatic and otherwise asymptomatic cases. Pain may radiate to the abdomen or flanks and is aggravated by prolonged sitting or standing, bending, or performing a Valsalva maneuver. Side lying with hips and knees flexed may alleviate the pain. Generalized bone pain is more suggestive of metastatic carcinoma or osteomalacia. Neurologic symptoms may not occur immediately but rather develop insidiously over days to months.[103]

MEDICAL MANAGEMENT

PREVENTION. Since no cure is available for osteoporosis, prevention and, more effectively, early intervention is essential for everyone (men, women, young, and old) but especially for those at risk (Box 24-3). By minimizing modifiable risk factors, people at high risk for developing osteoporosis may be able to achieve higher peak bone mass in the hope of delaying or preventing the onset of osteoporosis.[98] Because peak adult bone density depends on factors during growth and development, preventing osteoporosis in the aging adult begins by providing necessary dietary calcium intake during bone development and calcification in childhood and adolescence (Table 24-1).

A recent longitudinal study has determined that maternal consumption of magnesium, fat, and milk during the third trimester of pregnancy will greatly influence an adolescent's bone mineral density. This study suggests that a child's in utero diet will affect the programming of bone responses.[173] Other studies to assess the influence of maternal milk and soft drink consumption on children's consumption show that parents play a powerful role in children's eating behavior. They influence children's developing preferences and eating behaviors by making

Table 24-1	Daily Calcium Requirements	
Age Group	**Minimum Daily Requirements (mg of elemental calcium)**	**Comments on Calcium Administration**
Birth to 6 mo	200 mg	Calcium supplements come in several preparations (e.g., acetate, carbonate, citrate, gluconate, glucarate, glubionate, lactate, phosphate). Recommended daily requirements refer to elemental or actual calcium. Check the label in the % Daily Value and note how many tablets or capsules are required to obtain this amount.
6 mo to 1 y	260 mg	The body can absorb 500 mg of calcium at a time. Spread calcium intake (food or supplements) over the course of a day. Separate calcium supplements away from foods high in calcium or vitamins with calcium added.
1-3 y	700 mg	Beware of foods containing wheat bran or oxalic acid (e.g., chocolate, cauliflower, rhubarb, beet greens, brussels sprouts) that interfere with calcium absorption. Take calcium supplements away from these foods.
4-8 y	1000 mg	Calcium can interfere with the effectiveness of a variety of tetracycline antibiotics and fluoroquinolones such as Cipro, Floxin, Levaquin, Avelox, Factive, Vibramycin, and Minocin. Avoid consuming calcium (food or supplements) within 2-4 hours of taking these drugs.
9-18 y	1300 mg	Calcium, especially in antacids, may interfere with certain calcium channel- and beta-blockers and thyroid medication (Thyroxine). Check with prescribing physician about how to take calcium.
19-50 y	1000 mg	Calcium can interfere with bisphosphonate absorption. If taking bisphosphonates, delay consuming calcium (food or supplements) at least 30 minutes. Spend at least 10 minutes daily in the sun (longer if using sunscreen) to obtain vitamin D necessary for calcium absorption and bone formation.
51-70 y	1000 mg for males 1200 mg for females	For every ounce over 4 oz of animal protein, an additional 100 mg of calcium is required to stay even.
>70 y	1200 mg	Take calcium supplements with a meal rather than on an empty stomach, unless the foods contain significant amounts of calcium.
Pregnant or lactating females	1000-1300 mg	Extra-strength antacid made with calcium-carbonate in tablet form (e.g., Tums) is used by some people to obtain calcium. Beware of this antacid; decreased stomach acid alters calcium and absorption. For the individual with reduced stomach acid and especially the older adult, this may not be a good choice.

For anyone with osteoporosis (or trying to prevent osteoporosis), the RDA of calcium is as stated for his or her age group in the table above.
Data from National Women's Health Information Center, Department of Health and Human Services, 2000; Swan KG et al. Osteoporosis in men: a serious but under-recognized problem, *J Musculoskelet Med* 18(6):310-316, 2001; Institute of Medicine of the National Academies. Dietary reference intakes (DRIs): recommended dietary allowances and adequate intakes, elements. In: Ross CA, Taylor CL, Yaktine AL, Del Valle HB, editors. DRI: Dietary Reference Intakes. Calcium, Vitamin D. Washington (DC): The National Academies Press: 2011;1108; DiPiro JT, Talbert RL, Yee GC, Matzke GR, Wells BG, Posey LM, editors. *Pharmacotherapy. A Pathophysiologic Approach.* 8th ed. New York (NY): McGraw Hill; 2011.

some foods available rather than others, and by acting as models of eating behavior.[40,129]

Serum screening for celiac disease in anyone with osteopenia or osteoporosis is advised because dietary changes can restore normal absorption of dietary nutrients in this group, including calcium and vitamin D, contributing to a reversal in the decline of BMD associated with osteoporosis.[146]

Calcium. Peak bone mass is attained around age 30 years, at which time the pattern of bone building and bone loss is reversed, with more calcium loss than deposit. Regular exercise and physical activity, combined with adequate calcium, is considered both a prophylactic and treatment measure for osteoporosis from childhood through the adult years. The risk of fractures can be reduced by 50% if vitamin and nutrient requirements are met in the first 2 to 3 decades of life.[53] Low-fat dairy and other calcium- and magnesium-rich foods (e.g., broccoli or kale, sardines or salmon with the bones, fresh or dried apricots, figs, turnip greens, oranges or calcium-enriched orange juice, or tofu) and calcium supplements are the primary means of achieving an adequate calcium intake.[18]

Vitamin D. Vitamin D helps the body absorb, synthesize, and transport calcium within the body, therefore necessitating adequate sunshine each day. Vitamin D requirements vary by geographic location and age. In northern areas (above the 42-degree latitude parallel; in the United States, imagine a line stretching from the California–Oregon border to Boston), the sunlight in winter angles too obliquely to produce the ultraviolet light needed for adequate vitamin D production. Additional vitamin D (food or supplementation) is recommended; many calcium supplements contain vitamin D.

Diet. Dietary considerations, such as reducing animal sources of protein, increasing vegetable sources,[134,136] and increasing whole soy foods,[131] may result in reduced risk for both cardiovascular disease and osteoporosis. Soybeans and foods made from soy are high in phytoestrogens, which are plant chemicals classified as isoflavones that display estrogen-like activity because of their structural similarity to human estrogens. These substances exhibit high affinity binding for the estrogen receptor and may have a beneficial influence in the prevention of osteoporosis, cardiovascular disease, and endocrine-controlled cancer (e.g., breast, prostate). This claim remains highly controversial.[22]

According to some reports, the lipid-lowering oral statins (HMG-CoA reductase inhibitors; see Table 12-5) increase BMD by enhancing bone morphogenetic protein-2 (BMP-2), a powerful stimulator of osteoblast differentiation and osteoblastic expression, thereby promoting mineralization while reducing the risk of fractures. However, further testing is necessary before more specific recommendations can be made.[62,148]

Individuals with high risk for developing osteoporosis should consider a combination of dietary modifications and supplements. For women, baseline BMD tests performed at the time of menopause (cessation of menstrual flow) or even earlier (during the perimenopausal phase) can provide a baseline assessment for future reference. Falls prevention (as a means of fracture prevention) is a separate component of osteoporosis management but not necessarily osteoporosis prevention (see "Falls Preventions" in Chapter 27).

SCREENING. Whereas osteoporosis was once called a "silent disease" because it was not recognized until a fracture signaled its presence, the widespread availability of technology to measure bone density has made it possible to identify people at risk for osteoporosis before fractures are imminent. The NOF recommends that all men and postmenopausal women age 50 and older should be assessed for their risk of osteoporosis and relater fractures. A BMD test is recommended or women at age 65 and older and men age 70 and older. For men and women ages 50 to 69, a BMD test is recommended for those with high risk factors or who have had a recent fracture.[98]

Until evidence supports the cost-effectiveness of routine screening or the efficacy of early initiation of preventive drugs, an individualized approach has been recommended.[115] However, even given this guideline, appropriate screening is not taking place. According to at least one study of Medicare recipients, bone density testing was the lowest for women in the highest fracture risk group based on age. This may occur because physicians do not realize the benefit of screening and intervention in fracture prevention for older adults.[102] There is accumulating evidence that more and more younger adults are developing osteoporosis at an earlier age (ages 50-70), suggesting that baseline screening should begin even earlier. Therapists treating anyone with fragility fractures, vertebral compression fractures, or fractures anywhere in a postmenopausal woman should advise these individuals to ask their physician about medical screening for osteoporosis, including dual energy x-ray absorptiometry (previously DEXA, now DXA) scans and blood tests for metabolic bone markers (e.g., vitamin D, calcium, parathyroid hormone).[33]

Screening is particularly important for men at risk because fragility fractures are more likely to lead to fatal consequences than in women. Without a diagnosis of osteoporosis, treatment interventions that can prevent fractures are not initiated.[2]

DIAGNOSIS. Careful assessment of the osteoporotic person is essential in developing a comprehensive plan that reduces fracture risk and improves quality of life. Assessment of the individual with osteoporosis includes history and physical examination, laboratory testing, and imaging studies. Information gathered during this assessment assists clinicians in targeting strategies to prevent fractures. Diagnosis and intervention are based on bone density and risk assessment[140]; in the case of secondary osteoporosis, the specific underlying cause must be determined through the diagnostic process before intervention can be initiated.

History. The medical history should contain the personal and family history of fractures, lifestyle, intake of substances such as vitamin D, calcium, corticosteroids, and other medications. Clinicians should be aware of problems with vitamin D measurement, including seasonal variation, variability among laboratories, and the desirable therapeutic range. The physical examination can reveal relevant information such as height loss and risk of falls.[75]

Bone Mineral Density Testing. A BMD test is the simplest way to assess for osteoporosis. Without this test, most people are unaware they have osteoporosis until a fracture occurs, although some fractures can be painless or the pain may be mistaken for arthritis, delaying diagnosis. BMD is a measurement of the mineral content of bone in grams per square centimeter (g/cm^2) for the area of the body that has been scanned. A person's BMD measurement is compared to norm values of those of the same age and sex (called a Z score) or can be compared to young adults of the same sex (T score). A decrease in BMD will be reported in the absolute measure of bone in grams per square centimeter or in standard deviations below the average bone mass density. The WHO has developed a diagnostic classification system for postmenopausal women based on their BMD compared to the mean bone density of a young adult. A "normal" level is a BMD within one standard deviation of young adult (T score at 1.0 or above), the "osteopenia" level is a BMD between 1.0 and 2.5 standard deviations below a young adult, and "osteoporosis" being a BMD is 2.5 standard deviations or more below a young adult. For premenopausal women and men under age 50, a Z score adjusted for ethnicity of 2.0 standard deviations below the mean along with an assessment of their risk factors are used to make the diagnosis of osteoporosis.[98,108]

Multiple imaging modalities can be used to evaluate BMD and diagnose osteoporosis, including DXA, which measures spine, hip, or total body density; peripheral DXA (pDXA), which measures wrist, heel, or finger density only; quantitative ultrasound (QUS), in which sound waves are used to measure calcaneal, tibial, or patellar density; peripheral computed tomography (pCT); or radiographic absorptiometry (RA), which is a radiograph of the hand. These methods are not interchangeable and do not provide equivalent information.

DXA is the preferred procedure because it measures bone density at the femoral neck and lumbar vertebral

Table 24-2	WHO Classification for Bone Mineral Density
T Score	**Significance**
–1.0 or higher	Normal; low risk for fracture
–1.0 to –2.5*	Osteopenia (low bone mass)
–2.5 or lower†	Osteoporosis

*Half of fragility fractures occur in this group.
†The National Osteoporosis Foundation (NOF) suggests that anyone with a T score of –2.0 or less or –1.5 or less with at least 1 risk factor should be treated to reduce fracture risk.
From World Health Organization Study Group: Assessment of fracture risk and its application to screening for postmenopausal osteoporosis, Tech Rep Series, No 843, Geneva 1994, The Organization.

bodies where bone loss occurs more rapidly (Table 24-2). DXA has the highest sensitivity and specificity but sensitivity may not be adequate. The World Health Organization (WHO) recommends combining BMD to predict fracture risk with clinical risk factors.[140] DXA best predicts fracture risk in adults without previous fracture. BMD testing is most efficient in women over 65 years of age but is also helpful for men and women with risk factors. Serial BMD tests can identify individuals losing bone mass, but clinicians should be aware of what constitutes a significant change.[75]

Predicting Fracture Risk. The World Health Organization has developed a computerized tool called the *Fracture Risk Assessment* or FRAX to calculate the 10-year risk of sustaining a fracture.[98,170] It is based on individual patient models that integrate the risks associated with clinical risk factors as well as BMD at the femoral neck. Medication treatment is recommended for postmenopausal women and men age 50 or older who have a 3% to 10% risk of a hip fracture or 20% risk of major fracture elsewhere in the body (e.g., wrist, spine, upper arm) according to the test.

Radiographs. Fractures are usually diagnosed by radiograph examination (x-ray) that demonstrates the fracture (Fig. 24-5) and also reveals the signs of osteopenia leading to the diagnosis of osteoporosis. Once osteopenia is noted, other causes of metabolic bone disease must be ruled out, including hyperthyroidism, hyperparathyroidism, osteomalacia, testicular failure, malignancies, and so on. Histologically, a thinning of cortical bone and a reduction in the number and size of the trabeculae of cancellous bone occurs (see Fig. 24-1). Thirty percent or greater bone density loss must occur before such abnormalities can be noted on a radiographic film.

Laboratory Testing. Laboratory testing can detect other risk factors and can provide clues to etiology. Selection of laboratory tests should be individualized because there is no consensus regarding which tests are optimal. Biochemical markers of bone turnover (e.g., alkaline phosphatase, osteocalcin, urinary hydroxyproline, urinary deoxypyridinoline, urinary N-telopeptide, and others) reflect the rate of bone remodeling and may be helpful in assessing for fracture risk and for effectiveness of the treatment regimen but are not widely used at present.[75] Levels of serum total testosterone may be obtained for men.[108]

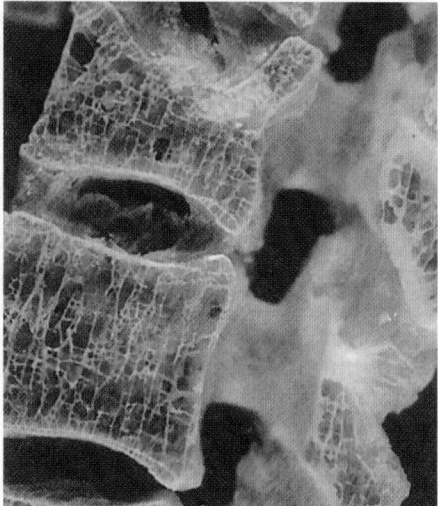

Figure 24-5

Decreased bone density of vertebrae with compression fracture. (From Schiller AL: Bones and joints. In Rubin E, Farber JL, eds: *Pathology*, ed 2, Philadelphia, 1994, JB Lippincott.)

TREATMENT. Osteoporosis is not curable, but intervention can stop the progression of bone loss and prevent further morbidity. Secondary osteoporosis intervention begins with treatment of the underlying cause. Management of primary and secondary osteoporosis in the adult should include lifestyle measures to reduce bone loss such as a high calcium intake, smoking cessation, reducing alcohol intake, and physical activity and exercise. Besides eliminating factors, such as chronic alcohol abuse and cigarette smoking, a key to prevention is developing as great a peak bone mass as possible through adequate calcium intake and regular exercise. Calcium is required for bone mineralization and also suppresses bone turnover, slowing the remodeling process. Fall prevention is an important intervention for anyone with low bone mass and high risk factors.

Reports suggest that premenopausal women need more than 1000 mg of calcium daily, and postmenopausal women need more than 1500 mg daily (see Table 24-1). The average calcium intake of postmenopausal women is 400 to 500 mg/d, well below the recommended levels. Vitamin D (800 units/d) is advocated to assist in maximal absorption of dietary calcium.[105]

Medications. Pharmacotherapy to reduce fracture risk in women with reduced BMD is initiated when the T score is below 2.0 in the absence of risk factors or below 1.5 if other risk factors are present.[98,105] A T score is not the only measure of fracture risk. A 70-year-old woman with a T score of 2 is at greater immediate risk of fracture than a woman 50 years of age with the same T score because of other variables common in the older-age population that can increase fracture risk (e.g., poor eyesight, reduced muscle mass, balance problems, or medications).

Paying attention to individuals who are osteopenic (low bone mass but without the microarchitectural bone changes seen in osteoporosis) is important because there are increasing numbers of people who are osteopenic and who do experience bone fracture.[140] Despite the availability and favorable safety profile of bisphosphonates, many people are not receiving therapy, including men who have low BMD or who are at risk of fracture from osteoporosis.[13,15]

Postmenopausal women need estrogen replacement with selective estrogen receptor modulators (SERMs), which maximize the beneficial effect of estrogen on bone and minimize or antagonize the deleterious effects on the breast and endometrium, or antiresorptive agents, such as bisphosphonate, to help prevent bone loss. Although calcitonin is not approved for prevention, it is approved for treatment because it acts directly on osteoclasts, suppressing activity.[105]

Bisphosphonates are a family of drugs that inhibit bone resorption and actually reverse bone loss. These drugs are currently being used in various bone conditions involving increased levels of bone resorption such as osteoporosis from a variety of clinical causes, glucocorticoid-induced bone loss, hypercalcemia of cancer, and Paget disease of bone. The use of bisphosphonates in reducing bone pain associated with cancer is described in Chapter 26.

Researchers are evaluating two long-term effects of various treatment interventions: (1) the effect of each agent on BMD and (2) the effect of each agent on fracture development. For women in a state of estrogen deficiency, exercise or estrogen supplementation alone does not prevent bone loss, but exercise combined with estrogen causes a synergistic effect.[106] Criticism of studies using exercise alone includes the nonspecificity of the exercise to the targeted area being measured. For example, walking and lifting weights are not enough of a stimulus for the forearm. Further research is needed to clarify the role of specific loading exercises in exercise prescription for postmenopausal women.[6,104]

Estrogen and estrogen plus progestogen supplementation has been found to reduce the risk of fractures, but once discontinued, within 1 year fracture risk resumes at a level similar to that in women who have not received such therapy.[105] For this reason, the labeling of estrogens has been modified to state that they may be used to "manage" osteoporosis. The lack of efficacy of calcitonin to prevent bone loss during the first 5 years after menopause and the lack of prospective fracture reduction data for estrogen have resulted in these labeling restrictions. SERMs and bisphosphonates have been shown to increase BMD and decrease fracture risk.[105] For men, the addition of testosterone therapy for those individuals with normal gonadal function is inconclusive, but may be beneficial in improving bone mineral density for those with lowered testosterone levels.[7,87,158]

Raloxifene (Evista) is the only SERM approved by the Food and Drug Administration (FDA) for the treatment and prevention of osteoporosis. It is the first compound with selective estrogen agonist activity in bone but with estrogen antagonist activity or no activity in reproductive tissues and breast.

Other second-generation SERMs, bazedoxifene, lasofoxifene (Oporia) and strontium ranelate (Protelos), remain under investigation. Raloxifene reduces the risk of positive estrogen-receptor breast cancer, decreases total cholesterol and low-density lipoprotein (LDL) cholesterol, and increases high-density lipoprotein (HDL) cholesterol but does not increase the risk of endometrial cancer or cause spotting and bleeding.[45,105] After 4 years of treatment, raloxifene reduces the risk of first vertebral fracture by 50% with sustained efficacy in the continued reduction of fracture reduction in the fourth year.[84] Raloxifene treatment does not change the physiologic structure of bone quality and does not cause fibrosis, osteomalacia, or other toxic effects.[121]

All resorptive agents currently approved for treatment of osteoporosis (e.g., bisphosphonates, SERMs, or nasal calcitonin) decrease bone resorption but cannot induce new bone formation. Consequently, their effects are limited. The use of agents that stimulate new bone formation, such as recombinant human PTH (rhPTH [teriparatide]), is recognized as a single agent and in combination with antiresorptive agents.[98,105]

A once-a-year pharmacologic treatment with zoledronic acid (Zometa) has been reported from the HORIZON Pivotal Fracture trials involving multiple investigators from several countries. Postmenopausal women with osteoporosis treated with a single infusion of intravenous zoledronic acid had a 70% reduced risk of vertebral fracture during a 3-year period and a 41% reduced risk of hip fracture. This treatment is most effective in preventing vertebral fractures in younger women with lower risk factors. The advantage of this drug is the increased compliance rate because of the convenience of a once-yearly infusion as opposed to a weekly or monthly dose regimen. It should be noted that higher rates of serious atrial fibrillation occurred in the zoledronic acid group.[10,14,61]

Combined administration of hormone replacement therapy (HRT) and bisphosphonates appears to have a more pronounced effect in the appendicular skeleton than the axial skeleton with greater increases of bone mass at the lumbar spine and hip than for either of the therapies alone.[51]

The use of an ultra-low-dose estrogen patch has been shown to improve bone density in animal and human trials. The skin patch contains a very small amount of estrogen with no progestin and has been used to increase bone density without harmful side effects in small groups of women. There is some evidence that the protective effects of ultra-low-dose estrogen therapy depends on a woman's endogenous estrogen levels before treatment. The optimal dose levels for this therapy have not yet been defined.[38,58,70]

An important research finding has been the discovery of osteoprotegerin (OPG), a protein belonging to the tumor necrosis factor receptor family. OPG occurs naturally in the body and plays a key role in the physiologic regulation of osteoclastic bone resorption. Animal studies have shown that OPG increases bone mass by reducing osteoclast production. Limited data suggest that OPG and PTH work together synergistically to improve bone mass and strength beyond what either can accomplish alone. The discovery of OPG has opened a new era in bone research by increasing the molecular knowledge available and providing new therapeutic targets in bone disease.[43,73,78]

Exercise. Exactly how much benefit can be gained from given levels or types of exercise remains unclear, but the consensus is that regular exercise has a positive effect on bone mass levels. Weight-bearing exercises (against gravity), such as walking and jogging, stress the skeletal system and are associated with greater changes in bone remodeling and result in larger bone mass, although the effects on bone mass differ in premenopausal versus postmenopausal women.

Exercises combined with bracing or other rehabilitative measures aimed at reducing the anterior translation of the cervicothoracic spine and thoracic hyperkyphosis may be beneficial in reducing the risk or occurrence of osteoporotic fractures.[69]

Vibration. *Whole body vibration,* also known as *oscillating plate therapy,* is a new method of treatment being tested as a tool for the prevention and treatment of osteopenia, osteoporosis, and bone fractures. Vibrating plates that the size and shape of a bathroom scale have shown effectiveness in increasing BMD (and balance). Vibratory exercise may be more effective than walking to improve both these measures. Researchers continue to investigate the physiologic mechanisms involved and to identify the most appropriate parameters to use that are both safe and effective.[3,17,47,59,172]

Surgery. Because of the challenges of reconstruction of osteoporotic bone, open surgical management is reserved only for those rare cases that involve neurologic deficits or an unstable spine.[138] New minimally invasive procedures for management of acute vertebral fractures, vertebroplasty, and kyphoplasty, which involve the injection of bone cement into the fractured vertebra, are discussed in Chapter 27.

PROGNOSIS. Osteoporosis, once thought to be a natural part of aging among women, is no longer considered age- or gender-dependent. Although osteoporosis is one of the greatest deterrents to women's health and accounts for significant morbidity and mortality, it is largely preventable because of the remarkable progress in the scientific understanding of its causes, diagnosis, and treatment. Even so, at the present time, 24% of women over the age of 50 years die from complications (e.g., pneumonia, infections, and fracture emboli) in the first year after an osteoporotic-associated hip fracture.[98] As mentioned, a first fracture has a 2- to 4-fold increased risk of a second fracture with associated morbidity and mortality. The exact mechanism for increased fracture-associated mortality is unclear. It could be secondary to the underlying (poor) health of the affected individual (e.g., poor nutrition, dementia, weakness, deconditioning, low bone density).[11]

Medical treatment for osteoporosis has been shown to decrease the incidence of vertebral fractures by 40% to 60% after just 1 year of treatment. The occurrence of a single vertebral fracture substantially increases the likelihood of future fractures and progressive kyphotic deformity.[105] Even so, only 50% of women with vertebral compression fractures diagnosed incidentally with chest radiographs are started on any pharmacologic treatment. Only 40% of patients admitted with an osteoporotic hip fracture are referred for osteoporosis treatment and only 6.2% receive osteoporosis treatment at the time of discharge.[60,93] Vertebral fractures are accompanied by increased mortality,

with the relative risk of death after such a fracture being almost nine times higher than the person without osteoporosis-associated vertebral fracture.[48,153] Low bone density at the hip is a strong and independent predictor of all-cause and cardiovascular mortality in older men age 65 years and older.[159]

Adverse side effects of long-term use of bisphosphonates have been reported that affect the GI system and include esophagitis, heartburn, abdominal pain, and diarrhea. Intravenous bisphosphonates can cause transient acute phase reactions with fever, myalgia, and flu-like symptoms. Osteonecrosis of the jaw has also been raised as a possible concern, most often with intravenous administration of bisphosphonates used to manage hypercalcemia associated with metastatic disease.

Adherence to osteoporosis medications is relatively poor, with up to 30% of individuals suspending their treatment within 6 to 12 months of initiating therapy. Poor adherence is usually attributed to drug-induced adverse effects and results in increased risk of fracture and hospitalization.[110] Some women have discontinued pharmacologic treatment early because of bothersome side effects or from a misinterpretation of their BMD test results.[156]

SPECIAL IMPLICATIONS FOR THE THERAPIST   24-1

Osteoporosis

Physical therapists may initially see someone with osteoporosis for problems that are secondary to this condition. Medical diagnoses and impairments can include cervical and thoracic pain from hyperkyphotic postures, vertebral fractures and degenerative disc disease, and falls from balance disorders. There may be additional activity limitations as well. All older adults need to be asked about their history of bone health and for known results of prior tests for bone mineral densities such as with a DEXA scan. These individuals may have been given their DEXA scan T scores but may not have been assessed for risk of fracture using the newer FRAX assessments. Therapists should keep in mind that the diagnosis of osteoporosis has implications for the quality of movement, independence with daily activities, and risk for other disease conditions.

Treatment programs for osteoporosis and osteoporosis-related conditions should be designed to address the common impairments found with these individuals and to prevent problems associated with falls and vertebral fractures. The goals for a treatment program need to be set at 3 to 6 months in length in order to see key changes in impairments and activities limitations. The treatment program should be designed to be continued by the patient/client independently for up to a year before a reevaluation will be needed.

Plan of Care and Interventions

Intervention begins with the identification of people at risk or who have been identified as osteoporotic but who have not received any education, training, or rehabilitation. Management of fractures and special implications for the therapist regarding fractures are discussed in Chapter 27. Many questions, issues, and concerns about future intervention and exercise parameters for osteoporosis remain unsolved at this time. Therapists should be aware of the various aspects of the osteoporosis and the overall medical and rehabilitation management of this condition. The connection between osteoporosis, postural changes (see "Postural Assessment" below), and movement must be appreciated by the therapist when formulating a plan of care.

The role of the physical therapist in maximizing these goals is an important key to the success of these individuals. Clients must be educated about the importance of each aspect of the intervention program. For example, calcium alone, without exercise and adequate vitamin D, cannot prevent osteoporosis regardless of how much calcium is taken. Since we do not store up calcium as adults, supplementation only provides necessary calcium for as long as the supplements are taken.

Importance of Compliance

When evaluating the effect of medical treatment or rehabilitation intervention, the outcome is only as good as the individual's compliance. A long-term commitment to any program is required. No immediate benefit may be perceived, especially when the individual is asymptomatic and has an overall lack of appreciation of the seriousness of the problem. Older adults experiencing cognitive decline and forgetfulness are also at risk for noncompliance. Management goals are centered on stabilizing or increasing bone mass, preventing fractures, maximizing physical performance and function, improving quality of life, and managing symptoms, especially in the presence of pain from fractures and deformity.[68,99]

Screening Assessment

The clinical implications of osteoporosis are varied, numerous, and significant. Considering the prevalence of primary osteoporosis and the diseases and medications with which osteoporosis can be associated, therapists will encounter this disease often. Anyone who has had a first osteoporotic-induced or low-trauma fracture should be screened for weakness (especially quadriceps muscle weakness) and level of (decreased) physical activity—both are risk factors for death following this type of fracture.[11] The Osteoporosis Assessment Questionnaire and the health-related quality of life (HR-QOL) can be used to assess the functional levels of individuals with osteoporosis.[76,117,157]

Postural Assessment

Older adults should be routinely assessed for postural changes secondary to osteoporosis. The assessment of posture in supine and prone position may reveal problems not seen in standing including tightness in pectoral and hip flexor muscles and weaknesses in the extensor muscles of the trunk and hips. A hyperkyphotic posture may be associated with movement dysfunction in the lower and upper extremities as well as limiting pulmonary function. Older individuals with hyperkyphosis may choose to limit their walking patterns and activities to prevent falling episodes and may not report this as problem or concern. The assessment

of balance, functional activities, and walking speed may show deficits compared to age-matched norms.

Therapists should be aware of the symptoms and signs associated with osteoporosis, since they may be in a position to refer a client to a physician for examination based on a change in the person's status, especially in the presence of significant risk factors. For example, a 65-year-old woman being treated for a rotator cuff disorder may report the onset of sharp midthoracic pain associated with sneezing since her last visit, but she now notes a constant, dull ache in the area. In addition, the client and therapist note an increase in the thoracic kyphosis. Communication with a physician regarding these clinical changes is warranted because of the concern about a possible fracture.

The therapist should also be aware of the potential side effects common to osteoporosis medications. For example, calcium can cause constipation, calcitonin may be accompanied by nausea and flushing, raloxifene may cause leg cramps, and the bisphosphonates are associated with GI intolerance and/or esophagitis. Side effects of estrogen replacement therapy are listed in Box 24-4.

Numerous medications (e.g., antihypertensives, sedatives, psychotropics, diuretics, narcotics, antidepressants, and antipsychotics) can contribute to a loss of balance and falls. A balance and fall assessment and falls prevention program is essential for anyone at risk for osteoporosis, anyone with diagnosed osteoporosis, or anyone with a past history of fragility fractures associated with osteoporosis.

Exercise and Osteoporosis

Therapists have an important role in the promotion of exercise as a preventive measure for osteoporosis. As mentioned, exercise is considered to have an important role in maintaining and possibly increasing peak bone mass. Exercise should be started early in life to increase peak bone mass and should be maintained across the life span to minimize the risks of osteoporosis. Exercise not only improves musculoskeletal health but also reduces the chronic pain syndrome and decreases depression associated with osteoporosis.[4,143]

Box 24-4

SIDE EFFECTS OF ESTROGENS

- Sudden onset of or change in headache, coordination, vision, breathing, speech, or extremity strength or sensation*
- Chest pain*
- Groin or calf pain*
- Change in vaginal bleeding
- Urinary incontinence
- Increased blood pressure
- Breast discharge or lumps
- Skin rash
- Extremity edema
- Jaundice
- Abdominal pain
- Tremors

*The above side effects warrant communication with a physician. Those marked with an asterisk call for *immediate* communication.

The American College of Sports Medicine has published a position stand on physical activity and bone health, including suggestions for exercise prescription for children and adolescents and for adults (Table 24-3).[72] Some evidence that exercise-induced gains in bone mass in children are maintained into adulthood suggests that physical activity habits during childhood may have long-lasting benefits on bone health. Quantitative dose-response studies are still lacking in this area so the guidelines offered are suggestions based on best evidence.

Exercise For Adults

The results of numerous studies of exercise and bone health as they are presented here represent four different exercise-related issues: (1) building bone mass, (2) slowing the decline of BMD, (3) preventing fracture, and (4) maintaining muscle mass and strength. An excellent summary of many studies of specific types of exercise in differing populations is available.[104]

Although the effect of exercise on slowing the decline of BMD later in life is modest, studies have shown that the factors associated with falls such as balance, strength, and mobility are improved with moderate-level exercise program.[57,65] The level of exercise must be maintained because the benefits are lost if exercise is discontinued. A physical therapist understands the musculoskeletal system and the underlying pathologies and comorbidities and can implement an effective intervention plan that takes these variables into consideration.

Weighted exercise combined with calcium citrate supplementation has been shown in the Bone Estrogen Strength Training (BEST) study to increase bone density even in women who did not take HRT. Exercises, such as leg presses, seated rows, wall squats, and back extensions and latissimus pull downs, improve bone in the wrist, hip, and spine by 1% to 2% even in women who did not take a hormone replacement.[24]

Type of Exercise

Exercises to build bone density must be directed at the muscles supporting or attached to the affected bone. Both aerobic and resistance training exercise can provide weight-bearing stimulus to bone, but research indicates that resistance training has a more profound site-specific effect (directed at the areas that demonstrate bone loss) than aerobic exercise.[89,104,143]

Many cross-sectional and longitudinal studies have shown a direct, positive relationship between the effects of resistance training and bone density.[67,85,104,169] On the other hand, aerobics, yoga, Pilates, and tai chi chuan are more likely to increase muscle strength and help maintain coordination and balance, which help prevent loss of balance and provide protection during loss of balance or falls.[9,82,114,149]

More studies are available now regarding the effects of tai chi on BMD, especially in postmenopausal women. Limited evidence suggests that tai chi may be an effective, safe, and practical intervention for maintaining BMD in postmenopausal women.[97,164,165]

For the more active adult with osteoporosis, activity assessment is also important. For those with vertebral osteoporosis or previous history of vertebral fractures, activities, such as golfing, bowling, biking, rowing, sit-ups, or other exercise, with a major component of spinal flexion, side bending, or spinal rotation should be excluded. Swimming is an excellent physical activity, especially for those individuals with arthritis or other joint involvement, but without a weight-bearing component, it is not beneficial to offset the complications of osteoporosis nor does it build bone density.

Intervention modalities may include therapeutic exercise, resistance bands, foam rolls or balance balls,

Table 24-3	ACSM Position Stand: Physical Activity and Bone Health	
Parameter	**Children and Adolescents**	**Adults**
Mode	Impact activities • Gymnastics • Plyometrics • Jumping Resistance training (moderate intensity) Participation in aerobic sports (involving running and jumping)	Weight-bearing endurance activities • Tennis • Stair-climbing • Walking/Jogging Jumping • Basketball • Jump rope • Volleyball Resistance exercise (weight training)
Intensity	High intensity required for bone loading Resistance training: less than 60% of 1 repetition maximum (1-RM) advised for this population (safety considerations)	Moderate to high intensity required for bone loading
Frequency	At least 3 times/wk 5-7 times/wk preferred	Weight-bearing endurance activities: at least 3-5 times/wk; 5-7 preferred Resistance exercise: at least 2 times/wk
Duration	At least 10 minutes/session Two sessions per day preferred when time is limited to 10-20 minutes/session	30-60 minutes of combined weight-bearing endurance activities, jumping, and resistance training that targets all major muscle groups

Data from Kohrt WM: Physical activity and bone health. American College of Sports Medicine Position Stand. *Med Sci Sports Exerc* 36(11): 1985-1996, 2004.

electrotherapy modalities, spinal orthoses or corsets, soft tissue mobilization, and so on. During an acute symptomatic episode, local modalities are often used to control pain and improve movement and function. Using the osteoporosis disability index can help document improvements and positive outcomes.[109]

Exercise Prescription

Similar to muscle strengthening, the intensity of the challenge to the bone must be gradually increased (principle of overload) and must exceed the level of challenge to which the bone has already adapted. The program must be continued or these changes will reverse.

Overall, it appears that high-load, short-duration stimulus causes a minimal effective strain that induces bone growth. The remodeling process seems to respond best to changes in the distribution of strain, suggesting that exercise should be diverse, involve different loading situations, and involve strains imposed at fast rates, with few repetitions needed to obtain the maximal osteogenic effect.[104]

Site-specific extensor isometric stabilization exercises are key to the prescriptive exercise program but must be augmented by a total program of reducing risks; implementing postural correction and scapular stabilization; and improving weight-bearing patterns, strength, balance, and flexibility. The parameters of duration, frequency, and intensity (dosage) and other concepts of prescriptive exercise (Box 24-5) need to be better defined and further investigated with randomized controlled studies. Therapists may find comprehensive information provided for our profession in regards to safety in movement for persons with low bone mass (osteopenia) and skeletal fragility (osteoporosis) through the materials and seminars offered by Sara Meeks, PT (see www.sarameekspt.com).

To minimize the risk of development of musculoskeletal repetitive overuse syndromes, education regarding the proper use of exercise equipment, proper body mechanics, variety in the exercise program, and awareness of warning signs of overuse injuries is essential. Exercising excessively can have detrimental effects. For example, women who exercise to the point of amenorrhea may lose bone rapidly, enhancing the risk of developing osteoporosis.[28,39,167]

Aquatic Therapy

(See also general guidelines for aquatic physical therapy, Appendix B.)

Although swimmers have been shown to have higher mineral densities than those of control groups, the protective effect of swimming as an effective exercise against osteoporosis and subsequent fractures has not been demonstrated. Activities with substantial muscular involvement but without gravitational forces are associated with lower BMD than those with a weight-bearing component.[26,150]

Although swimming and aquatic therapy are not weight-bearing activities and therefore are not preventive, they still help maintain range of motion, build strength, and increase cardiovascular fitness with minimal stress on bones and joints. Walking in the water against the resistive force of the water is a better alternative for those individuals participating in an aquatic exercise program.

One study done to assess the effects of a water-based exercise and self-management program on balance, fear of falling, and quality of life in community-dwelling women 65 years of age or older with a diagnosis of osteopenia or osteoporosis indicated that water-based therapy improves dynamic standing balance.[29] There was significant improvement in the physical functioning, vitality, social functioning, and mental health for the intervention group. The improvements in these psychosocial domains could have resulted from the benefits of increased activity, effects of the water, or the group interaction and socialization.[29]

Fracture Prevention

Therapists also have a role in the prevention of the most serious complication associated with osteoporosis: fracture. A prescriptive exercise program designed to improve flexibility, balance, and strength may help prevent osteoporosis, fractures, and falls. Based on our understanding now that there is a link between depression and osteoporosis, the therapist's intervention for people who are experiencing major depression should include fracture prevention.[133,174] (See "Depression" in Chapter 3.)

A physical therapist can design an exercise program that can help increase bone density with proper strengthening and weight-bearing exercises; lessen

---

Box 24-5

EXERCISE PRESCRIPTION GUIDELINES

The following guidelines are used in providing prescriptive exercise:

- **Specificity:** Activities selected for osteogenic effects should stress those skeletal sites at risk for osteoporotic fractures.
- **Overload:** Progressive increase in the intensity of the exercise for continued improvement must be evident, but applied skeletal loads must be within the structural capacity of the bone to sustain the given stress.
- **Initial Values:** Those with the lowest bone mass and weakest muscles will have the greatest improvement; those with average or above average bone mass and muscle strength will have the least.
- **Diminishing Returns:** A biologic ceiling for exercise-induced improvement in the functioning of any physiologic system is evident. As this ceiling is approached, more effort is required to attain smaller gains.
- **Maintenance:** Exercise to maintain healthy bone and muscle is a lifelong endeavor; once peak bone mass has been reached, regular physical activity, aerobic exercise, and site-specific exercise is required to maintain strength.
- **Reversibility:** The positive effect of exercise on bone and muscle will be lost if the exercise program is discontinued. It takes longer to build bone than to lose it.

Data from National Osteoporosis Foundation (NOF): Clinicians Guide to Prevention and Treatment of Osteoporosis (2009) stress on bones through improved balance, posture, and body mechanics; and identify potential hazards in the home or workplace environment that could lead to fractures in those with osteoporosis. Choosing the appropriate gait-assistive device and teaching the person how to use the walker, cane, and other aids properly could also prevent injury. Educating the individual and family regarding home ambulatory hazards, such as throw rugs, faulty footwear, is important for fall prevention. (See extensive discussion of this topic in "Fracture" in Chapter 27.)

Quality of Life

Because of the costs involved in treating osteoporosis and the potential benefits offered by exercise, a need exists to expand the evaluation of exercise programs to include other relevant endpoints, such as quality of life and general fitness and well-being. Among older women who have exceeded average life expectancy, quality of life is profoundly threatened by falls and hip fractures. Any loss of ability to live independently in the community has a considerable detrimental effect on their quality of life. In a landmark study, the majority of women 75 years and older reported being willing to trade almost their entire life expectancy to avoid a hip fracture that would result in being admitted to a long-term-care facility. In short, 80% said they would rather be dead.[126]

The Female Athlete and Osteoporosis

(See further discussion in "Female Athlete Triad," Chapter 3.)

The therapist working with female athletes must be aware of the documented decrease in bone density despite normal calcium intakes and regular exercise. A unique challenge exists with this population: the need to reduce bone stress while maintaining adequate muscular and aerobic conditioning in female athletes who are amenorrheic.[101] The therapist can offer important client education, since many athletes do not realize the long-term orthopedic consequences of menstruation cessation. In the presence of bone density decline, the therapist should identify and initiate alternative training regimes. Non–weight-bearing and minimal weight-bearing activities, such as aquatic therapy and cycling, will significantly decrease the forces acting on the bone while still maintaining the training effect. Pool running is a viable activity for maintenance of cardiovascular and muscular training that closely simulates the sport itself.[154]

Most athletes do not seek physical therapy intervention until pain has developed after the occurrence of a stress reaction or fracture. The main objective of intervention at this point is to use physical agents for pain reduction combined with alternative non–weight-bearing therapies. A slow, careful progression back to normal training intensity and duration of weight bearing should be instituted. Education of the client throughout the entire process for prevention of fracture recurrence is of utmost importance.[120]

Precautions and Considerations

In people with known osteoporosis or those at high risk of having the disease, caution should be taken with examination and treatment techniques. For example, using a posteroanterior pressure technique at the thorax for provocation and mobility assessment with the client positioned prone will place significant stress on the rib cage, possibly resulting in a fracture.

Thoracic spine mobilizations using gentle mobilizations in a seated position has been used as part of successful rehabilitation program to attenuate thoracic kyphosis in elderly women with osteoporosis. Although it is important that provocation and mobility information be collected and joint dysfunction be treated to improve functional abilities, precautions must be taken, including using other techniques or altering the person's position (e.g., side lying or sitting) so that the anterior thorax is not stabilized.[160]

As with other metabolic bone diseases, delayed healing and poor retention of internal fixation devices after fracture can occur in clients with osteoporosis. Postoperatively, the response to rehabilitation may be slowed, and adjustments may have to be made in the program to protect the injured area as recovery takes place. Close communication with the physician is called for to ensure safety.

BMD of the spine is correlated with the strength of spine extensors, so maintaining muscular strength of the spine muscles is important.[56] Reduction of back extension strength is correlated with increasing age and body mass index in both men and women, although men have a greater loss than women with increasing age. In both genders, more loss of back extension strength than appendicular muscle strength occurs.[142]

Flexion exercises are clearly contraindicated for anyone with osteoporosis. Anterior compressive forces associated with forward flexion of the spine can contribute to vertebral compression fractures. Posterior pelvic tilt and partial sit-ups (minimal abdominal crunches, lifting the head and upper torso only to the level of T6) do not appear to cause any anterior compressive force.[141]

The inflammatory nature of rheumatic diseases may predispose people to osteoporosis as it interferes with normal bone metabolism; this is compounded by the inactivity related to pain, joint inflammation and discomfort, muscle weakness, fatigue, and functional impairment. Weight-bearing exercise (sometimes even that performed during normal daily activities) helps maintain bone mass, but these clients often have limited ability to exercise or even walk. In such cases, aquatic therapy may be the only viable alternative despite the limitations mentioned.

The medical interventions for the prevention or management of osteoporosis also have implications for the therapist. Medication side effects may occur at any time and may warrant communication with the physician. Box 24-4 lists the side effects of estrogens. Estrogen therapy has been associated with blood clots, heart attack, stroke, and breast and endometrial cancer. To reduce the risk of endometrial carcinoma, estrogen is taken with a progestin.

Clients with a history of these conditions are at greater risk of developing side effects. Nevertheless, HRT has an important role in reducing the rate of bone mass loss, although its role in reducing the risk of developing cardiovascular disease has come under question (see "Menopause and Hormone Replacement Therapy" in Chapter 20). A side effect of calcium supplements that warrants immediate communication with a physician is urinary dysfunction. Mild diarrhea or constipation or a chalky taste that does not resolve should be brought to a physician's attention.

OSTEOMALACIA

Definition

In contrast to osteoporosis, which results in a loss of bone mass and brittle bones, osteomalacia is a progressive disease in which lack of mineralization of the bone matrix results in a softening of bone without loss of the present bone matrix. Osteomalacia is a generalized bone condition in which insufficient mineralization of the bone matrix results from deficiency of calcium, vitamin D, and/or phosphate. The disease is sometimes referred to as the adult form of *rickets*, with the absence of epiphyseal plates in adults precluding the epiphyseal plate changes seen in rickets.

Etiologic Factors

The two primary causes of osteomalacia are insufficient intestinal calcium absorption and increased renal phosphorus losses. The insufficient calcium absorption occurs because of either a lack of calcium or a resistance to the action of vitamin D. Excessive levels of the fibroblast growth factor-23 will inhibit reabsorption of phosphate in the renal tubules.[42] Increased renal phosphorus losses can also occur associated with renal osteodystrophy (see "Chronic Renal Failure" in Chapter 18 and Fig. 18-7) and renal tubular insufficiency. In addition, the long-term use of antacids, which contain aluminum hydroxide that bind with dietary forms of phosphate to prevent GI absorption, and the presence of long-standing hyperparathyroidism can lead to phosphate deficiencies, contributing to the development of osteomalacia.

The dietary deficiency type of osteomalacia has been eradicated in the United States for the most part by the widespread supplementation of dairy products with vitamin D. However, osteomalacia does occur in the malnourished aging adult who may not receive adequate nutrition or enough exposure to sunlight.[127]

Incidence and Risk Factors

Osteomalacia is essentially a histologic diagnosis, so little information on its overall prevalence in the adult population is available. Diseases of the small intestine, cholestatic disorders of the liver, biliary obstruction, and chronic pancreatic insufficiency increase the risk of developing osteomalacia. These conditions adversely affect the absorption of calcium and the action of vitamin D. The incidence of osteomalacia is greater in the world's colder regions, which is related to decreased exposure to sunlight, affecting vitamin D levels.

Osteomalacia is seen with greater frequency in cultures where the population has increased skin pigmentation and the diet is deficient in vitamin D (e.g., northern China, Japan, and northern India).[31] Osteomalacia is common in the aged adult because of calcium- and vitamin D–deficient diets and decreased sunlight exposure. Housebound and institutionalized individuals are especially at risk; thus the prevalence of osteomalacia is expected to increase with the aging of the American population.[31] This situation is worsened by the intestinal malabsorption problems associated with aging or the presence of SLE that usually requires avoidance of sunlight to prevent ultraviolet-induced flare-ups.[128]

Long-term use of commonly prescribed medications also increases the risk of developing osteomalacia. Anticonvulsant medications, such as phenobarbital and phenytoin, accelerate breakdown of the active forms of vitamin D by inducing hepatic hydroxylases. As mentioned, antacids can cause phosphate deficiency. Box 24-6 summarizes the risk factors associated with osteomalacia.

Pathogenesis

Osteomalacia develops from the lack of calcium salts depositing in the boney matrix resulting in an increase in the extent of the uncalcified or osteoid matrix. The structure of the bone is unchanged, but is greatly weakened from the lack of mineralized content.

The radiographic appearance of the osteomalacia is found in the textural changes of osteoid seams. The decalcification results in an exaggeration of the osteoid seams seen adjacent to the relatively sparse areas of calcified bone (Fig. 24-6). These exaggerated seams occur because of the excessive time lag between collagen deposition and the appearance of the calcium salt. As the osteoid accumulates, bone strength declines. Areas of abundant osteoid

---

Box 24-6

RISK FACTORS ASSOCIATED WITH OSTEOMALACIA

- Old age
- Residence in cold geographic area
- Vitamin D deficiency
- Gastrectomy
- Intestinal malabsorption associated with:
  - Diseases of the small intestine
  - Cholangiolitic disorders of the liver
  - Biliary obstruction
  - Chronic pancreatic insufficiency
- Long-term use of:
  - Anticonvulsants
  - Barbiturates
  - Antacids, especially those containing aluminum
  - Lithium
  - Etidronate
  - Sodium fluoride
  - Acetazolamide
- History of:
  - Hyperparathyroidism
  - Chronic renal failure
  - Renal tubular defects (decreased reabsorption of phosphate)

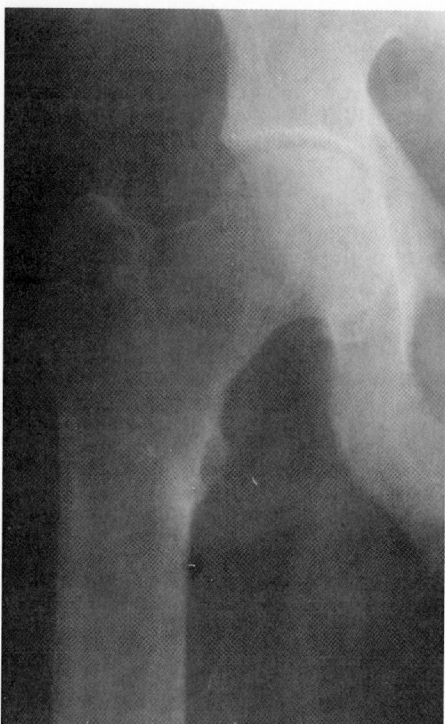

Figure 24-6

Osteomalacia of the femur. Note the loss of the sharp interface between cortical bone and cancellous bone caused by demineralization of the cortex. (From Richardson JK, Iglarsh ZA: *Clinical orthopaedic physical therapy*, Philadelphia, 1994, WB Saunders.)

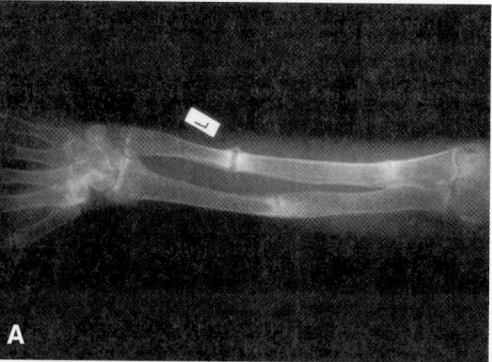

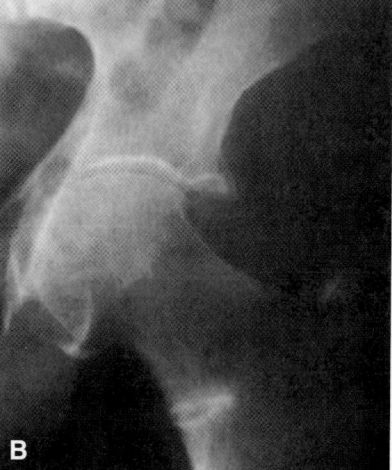

Figure 24-7

Osteomalacia. A, Forearm and **B,** femoral neck. Looser zones are seen as translucent zones with sclerotic margins. Usual sites include the medial femoral neck, pubic rami, lateral borders of the scapulae, and ribs. Complete fractures can extend through Looser zones; these will heal with appropriate treatment. (From Bullough P: *Orthopaedic pathology*, ed 3, London, 1997, Mosby-Wolfe.)

appear as radiolucent stripes. These stripes are known as *Looser zones or pseudofractures* and occur most commonly on the concave side of long bones, the ischial and pubic rami, and the ribs and scapula (Fig. 24-7). Pseudofractures also develop from the healing of multiple microstress fractures in the moderately severe form of osteomalacia sometimes referred to as *Milkman's syndrome.*[127]

Clinical Manifestations

The diagnosis of osteomalacia is difficult and often delayed because many people present initially with diffuse, generalized aching and fatigue in the presence of anorexia and weight loss. Proximal myopathy and sensory polyneuropathy may also be present, resulting in a confusing clinical presentation. Bone pain and periarticular tenderness can occur in the spine, ribs, pelvis, and proximal extremities.

The combination of muscle weakness and softening of bone contributes to postural deformities, including increased thoracic kyphosis, a heart-shaped pelvis, and marked bowing of the femurs and tibias. The muscular weakness (proximal myopathy) may lead to a waddling gait and difficulties with transitional movements such as rising from sitting to standing, climbing stairs, or moving into and out of bed. Occasionally, the hypocalcemia associated with osteomalacia leads to latent tetany, with paresthesias of the hands and around the mouth, muscle cramps, and positive Chvostek and Trousseau signs (see Figs. 5-8 and 5-9).

MEDICAL MANAGEMENT

DIAGNOSIS. Osteomalacia may present with a variety of clinical and radiographic signs mimicking other musculoskeletal disorders (e.g., fibromyalgia or polymyalgia rheumatica). For this reason, numerous methods are used to diagnose osteomalacia, including radiographs, bone scan, bone biopsy, and a laboratory workup. Blood serum levels of calcium, albumin, phosphate, alkaline phosphatase, and PTH are obtained and urine is collected to assess calcium and phosphate excretion rates.[122]

Radiographically, osteomalacia, like osteoporosis, may appear as osteopenia. A bone biopsy at the site of osteopenia will evaluate the calcification levels of the bone matrix. Besides osteopenia, radiolucent bands in the bone cortex (Looser zones) may be revealed radiographically (see Fig. 24-7).

Although not occurring nearly as often as in osteoporosis, acute fracture may be what leads to the diagnosis of osteomalacia. The radius, femur, vertebral bodies, ribs, and pubic ramus are common sites of fracture.

TREATMENT. The treatment of osteomalacia depends primarily on the cause. If inadequate nutrition is the problem, strengthening the dietary regimen with calcium and vitamin D is necessary. This step may be sufficient to improve the calcification of the organic matrix and thereby result in healing of the pseudofractures and strengthening the bones in general.

If osteomalacia is a result of intestinal malabsorption, treatment is directed to correct the primary disease. Phosphate supplementation can be prescribed in the presence of renal phosphate wasting. If used, vitamin D must be given to enhance calcium absorption impaired by the phosphate.

SPECIAL IMPLICATIONS FOR THE THERAPIST   **24-2**

Osteomalacia

See "Special Implications for the Therapist 24-1: Osteoporosis" above.

Considerable overlap occurs between osteomalacia and osteoporosis regarding implications for the therapist. The reader is directed to the section associated with osteoporosis for the discussion of client injury during examination and intervention, recognition of possible fracture, postoperative care, and side effects of calcium agents. See Chapter 27 for a discussion of prevention of fracture.

PAGET DISEASE

Definition

Paget disease (also known as *osteitis deformans*) is the second most common metabolic bone disease after osteoporosis. The disease is a progressive disorder of the adult skeletal system, characterized by increased bone resorption by osteoclasts and excessive, unorganized new bone formation by osteoblasts. Eventually, the normal bone marrow is replaced by vascular and fibrous tissue. Although Paget disease is a state of high bone turnover, the excess bone that is formed lacks the structural stability of normal bone (enlarged bone but weakened), leading to complications such as deformity, fracture, arthritis, and pain. The disease may involve one or more sites.

Incidence and Prevalence

Paget disease is a common disease of the aging adult population, rarely presenting before age 35 years with increasing prevalence among adults over age 50 years. Approximately 3% of the population over age 50 years and 10% of those over age 70 years may be affected, with the prevalence decreasing over the past 50 years.[5,92]

Although still unclear, both prevalence and severity of Paget disease seem to be declining. Current prevalence is only approximately 50% of that in 1983.[23] Men and women are both affected, although a slight increased prevalence is evident among men. The disease is often familial and has an unusual geographic distribution. Populations of the British Isles and countries where migration from Britain occurred (the United States, Australia, New Zealand, and Canada) have a greater incidence. The disease is almost nonexistent in Asia and in the native African and South American populations.[118]

Etiologic Factors

The cause of Paget disease is unknown. Sir James Paget, who described the disease more than a century ago, thought it was likely a bone infection. Paget disease is often inherited in an autosomal dominant pattern, but the genetic basis of the condition is not well understood.[25,79]

Family studies have localized gene susceptibility to Paget disease at three different chromosomal regions, although these defects do not appear to account for the majority of cases. The results of a number of studies suggest that variations in the protein p62 affect the function of osteoclasts and that the production of p62 is directed by the sequestosome 1 gene.[119] Genomic studies of human sequestosome 1 gene containing a Paget disease mutation are ongoing. Because of the late age of onset of this disease, finding large families with a number of generations with the disease has been difficult and has hindered progress in research.

Environmental factors, specifically slow viruses that take years to progress to a point where symptoms become evident, may play a role in the development of Paget disease[74]; the hereditary factor may be the reason family members are susceptible to the suspected virus.[92,137] Exactly how the viruses affect osteoclasts remains unknown. Paget disease has become less prevalent and people are presenting even later and with less severe disease than before; thus, environmental factors may be an important etiologic factor in this disease.[23]

Pathogenesis

Traditionally, Paget disease has been considered a disorder of the osteoclasts (bone-resorbing cells) rather than the osteoblasts (bone-forming cells). However, osteoblasts are major regulators of osteoclast development and function, and a tightly coupled pathway of communication and collaboration is evident between these two groups of cells. The exact mechanism by which these two cell types contribute to the formation of Paget disease is under investigation.

An initial resorptive stage where abnormal osteoclasts proliferate unrestrained is evident. The bone resorption is so rapid that osteoblastic activity cannot keep up and fibrous tissue replaces bone. Radiographically, the resultant lytic areas are sharply defined and appear as flame- or wedge-shaped. The initial resorption stage is followed by abnormal regeneration called the *osteoblastic sclerotic phase*.

In the sclerotic phase, the normal cancellous architecture is replaced by coarse, thickened struts of trabecular bone, and the cortical bone is irregularly thickened, rough, and pitted. The abnormal arrangement of the lamellar bone, separated by so-called cement lines, gives the bone the look of a mosaic. Although heavily calcified, the bone is now enlarged but weakened with a chaotic woven pattern, rather than the well-organized lamellar structure seen in normal bone.

Involvement of the vertebral bodies presents with a picture-frame appearance radiographically as the cortical shell and endplates become greatly exaggerated in comparison to the coarse, cancellous bone portion of the vertebral body (Fig. 24-8). The final stage of the disease is characterized by little cellular activity.[27]

Clinical Manifestations

Paget disease begins insidiously and progresses slowly. In mild cases, a person may have a few symptoms or may be symptom free over a very long period, eventually presenting with bone pain and skeletal deformities. When Paget disease is active in several bones, overactive osteoclasts can release enough calcium in the blood to cause hypercalcemia resulting in fatigue, weakness, loss of appetite, abdominal pain, and constipation.[5]

Musculoskeletal

The progressive deossification that weakens the bony structure primarily affects the axial skeleton. The lesions occur at multiple sites, particularly the skull, spine, pelvis, femurs, and tibias. Pathologic fractures can occur in any bone (Fig. 24-9), especially in the proximal femurs, pelvis, and lumbar spine.

Affected bones change in size, shape, and alignment, resulting in bone pain, deformities, fractures, and arthritis (Box 24-7). The most common presenting symptom is pain, which may be of a headache, radicular, osteoarthritic, muscular, or other skeletal origin. Pain from periosteal irritation of involved bones is deep and boring, worse at night, and reduced but not eliminated with activity. In some people, this pain may be referred to nearby muscles and joints.[161]

Clients may also experience fatigue, lightheadedness, and general stiffness. New onset of pain may be related to pathologic fracture of the vertebral bodies, pelvis, or long bones. Damage to the cartilage of joints adjacent to the affected bone and distortion of the normal joint alignment from bony changes may lead to osteoarthritis. The osteoarthritis is often more disabling than the Paget disease itself and will not respond to treatment of the underlying bone disease.[41]

Clinical findings also include postural deformities such as increased thoracic kyphosis and bowing of the femurs and tibias (Fig. 24-10). Bony softening of the femoral neck can cause coxa vara (reduced angle of the femoral neck) and may result in a waddling gait. These changes may produce increased local mechanical stresses resulting in pain.

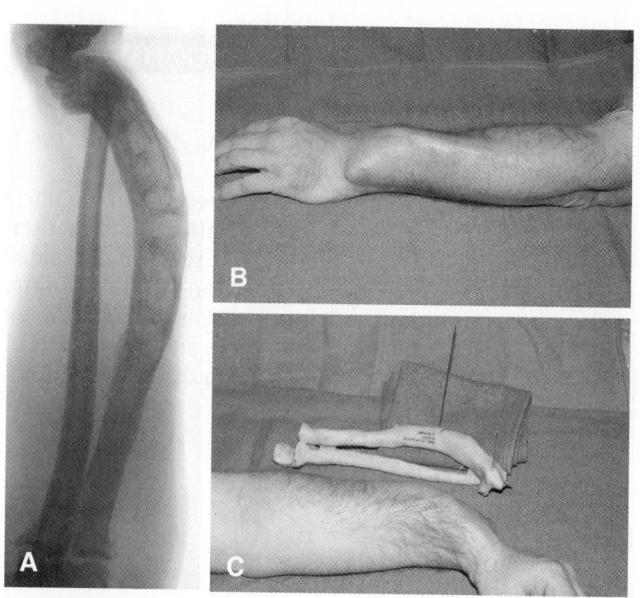

Figure 24-9

Paget disease. A complex malunion of the radius in a 62-year-old man after several fractures. **A,** The presenting lateral radiograph of the severe deformity. **B,** The clinical appearance. **C,** A bone model made from computed tomographic scans and used for preoperative planning for correction of the deformity. (From Browner BD: *Skeletal trauma: basic science, management, and reconstruction*, ed 3, Philadelphia, 2003, WB Saunders.)

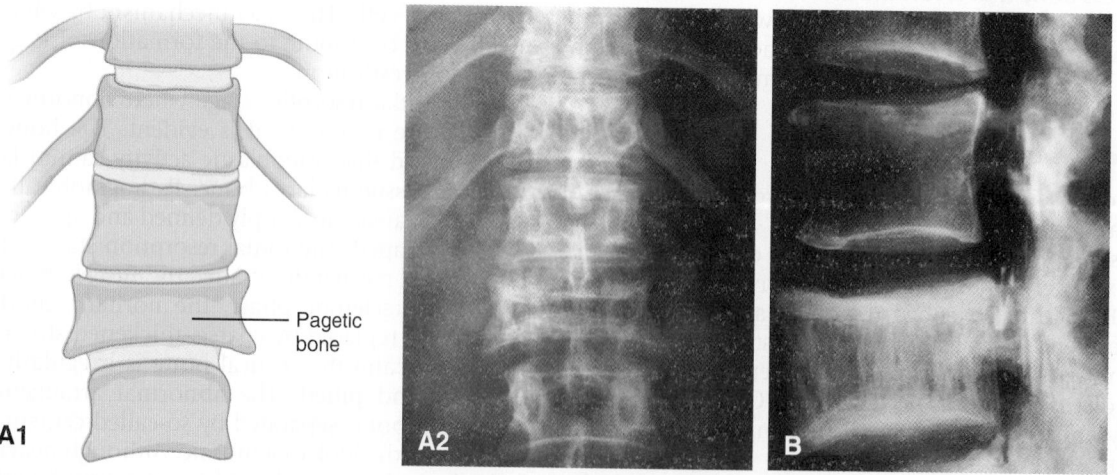

Pagetic bone

A1   **A2**   **B**

Figure 24-8

A, Clinical radiograph of the spine shows a solitary focus of pagetic bone. A loss of height of the vertebra (compression), some increases in the width of the vertebra, and a typical "picture frame" appearance are evident. **B,** Radiograph of the lumbar spine in a 66-year-old male shows enlargement of L4 with coarsening of the trabecular pattern and a margin sclerosis, the so-called picture-framing characteristic of Paget disease. (From Bullough P: *Orthopaedic pathology*, ed 3, London, 1997, Mosby-Wolfe; B, Courtesy Dr. Alex Norman.)

Neurologic

Paget disease of the skull and spinal column can produce neurologic complications as a result of either direct impingement (myelopathy) or ischemia related to a *pagetic steal syndrome* (hypervascular pagetic bone "steals" blood from the neural tissue).[161]

Affected individuals also report tinnitus, vertigo, and hearing loss. Typical neurologic deficits include eighth cranial nerve involvement with hearing loss related to involvement of the ossicles or bony foraminal encroachment. Headaches may occur if the skull is involved, and the forehead may enlarge as the amount of bone in the skull expands and the foramen for the cranial nerves becomes smaller (Fig. 24-11).

Other nerve or spinal cord compression syndromes may occur as enlarged pagetic bones put pressure on various nerve structures. Findings may include myelopathy, spinal stenosis, radiculoneuropathy, cauda equina syndrome, peripheral nerve entrapment, carpal and tarsal

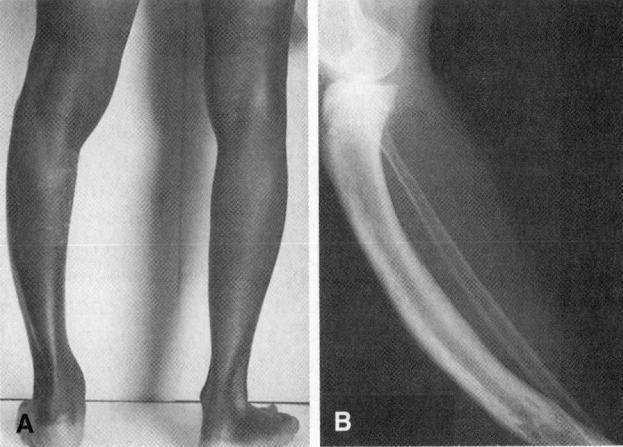

Figure 24-10

A, Bowing of the leg is often seen in Paget disease. **B,** Radiograph of a person with Paget disease affecting the tibia (but not the fibula). Overgrowth has resulted in an increase in length of the tibia, associated with bowing. Irregularity of both the periosteal and endosteal surfaces is shown. (From Bullough P: *Orthopaedic pathology,* ed 3, London, 1997, Mosby-Wolfe.)

Box 24-7

CLINICAL MANIFESTATIONS OF PAGET DISEASE

Pain

- Headache
- Muscular
- Osteoarthritis
- Radicular
- Skeletal

Skeletal

- Pain (bone pain that may be referred to nearby joints and muscles)
- Deformities
  - Kyphoscoliosis
  - Bone thickening or enlargement (including skull)
  - Bowing (outward bowed femur, forward bowed tibia)
  - Coxa varus (waddling gait); acetabular protrusion
  - Vertebral compression or collapse
- Fractures
- Osteoarthritis

Muscular

- Pain (myalgia)
- Stiffness

Neurologic

- Nerve compression syndromes (including cranial, spinal, and peripheral nerves)
- Mental confusion, deterioration in cognitive function
- Sensorineural hearing loss

Cardiovascular

- Increased cardiac output
- Increased vascularity (increased skin temperature over involved bone)
- Heart failure

Miscellaneous

- Fatigue
- Tinnitus
- Lightheadedness, dizziness, vertigo

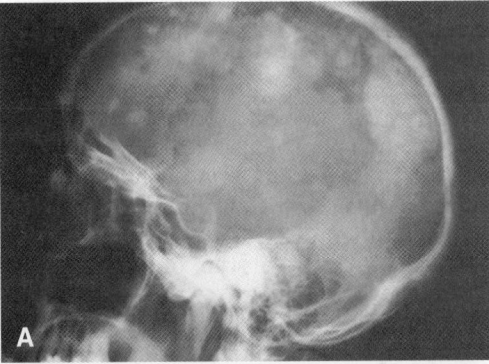
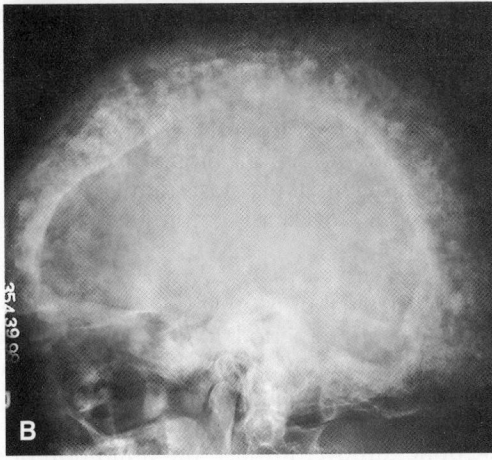

Figure 24-11

Clinical radiographs of the skull in later stages of Paget disease. **A,** Marked patchy sclerosis appears in the bone, the organized architecture is lost, and the bone becomes extremely thick, on occasion several times thicker than normal. **B,** Advanced involvement of the skull with marked thickening of the entire vault, areas of osteolysis, and patchy new bone formation resulting in a "cotton-wool" appearance called *osteoporosis circumscripta cranii.* This person experienced progressive hearing loss. (A from Bullough P: *Orthopaedic pathology,* ed 3, London, 1997, Mosby-Wolfe; B from Goldman L: *Cecil textbook of medicine,* ed 22, Philadelphia, 2004, WB Saunders.)

tunnel syndromes, and any of the effects of cranial nerve compression.[161]

Cardiovascular

Other findings may include mental deterioration (Paget disease causes reduced blood flow to the brain) and cardiovascular disease (rare). The cardiovascular disease is due to vasodilation of blood vessels in the bones and skin and subcutaneous tissues overlying the affected bones. When one-third to one-half of the skeleton is involved, an increase in cardiac output may be severe enough to cause heart failure. This is the most common cause of death in people with advanced Paget disease.[161]

MEDICAL MANAGEMENT

DIAGNOSIS. Because Paget disease progresses slowly and the severity of the disease varies considerably among individuals, it may be many years before a diagnosis is made or the person may be misdiagnosed with arthritis or other disorders. In fact, the diagnosis is often made incidentally on the basis of radiographs or laboratory tests done for other conditions.

A screening test that measures alkaline phosphate blood levels can be used to detect those at risk of Paget disease. Alkaline phosphatase is an enzyme that is produced by bone cells and overproduced by pagetic bone. Siblings and children of those with Paget disease may have a standard alkaline phosphatase blood test every 2 or 3 years. Alkaline phosphatase levels can also be used to diagnose Paget disease and to monitor response to therapy (see Table 40-5). If the alkaline phosphatase level is above normal, other tests, such as the bone-specific alkaline phosphatase test, bone scan, or radiographic examination, can be performed.

The diagnosis is usually based on the characteristic bone deformities and radiologic bony changes. Bone scans are positive only if the disease is active and marked by rapid bone turnover but provide information that helps determine the extent and activity of the condition. Bone scans must be confirmed by radiographic examination as other conditions are also accompanied by a metabolically active lesion. A bone biopsy may be performed for a medical differential diagnosis to rule out hyperparathyroidism, bone metastasis, multiple myeloma, and fibrous dysplasia.

TREATMENT. The goal of treatment is to normalize bone health for a prolonged period. Inhibitors of bone resorption, nitrogen-containing bisphosphonates such as oral alendronate or risedronate, are the first line of treatment.[119] These pharmacologic agents (see Box 24-3) decrease bone turnover through the inhibition of osteoclastic activity to improve bone density, and reduce fracture incidence. These pharmacologic agents have a long lasting effect on biochemical processes and provide long-lasting remissions in the majority of people.[55]

Treatment response is assessed by the extent of reduction of the biochemical markers of bone turnover, especially plasma total alkaline phosphatase. The goal of treatment is to induce full remission, through normal levels of alkaline phosphatase and prevention of complications of the disease.[107] Some experts in the field are recommending treatment of asymptomatic people who have active disease at sites where complications are likely to develop, although no data are available at this time to prove that complications can be prevented by pharmacologic intervention.[119]

Individuals under long-term oral bisphosphonate use are treated with caution because of the potential side effects, especially osteonecrosis of the jaw (ONJ).[96] Well-controlled, prospective clinical trials on the effect of oral bisphosphonates on bone are needed to determine which individuals may be at risk for such complications.[123,162]

Management of Paget disease depends on the degree of pain and extent of the pathologic changes. Nonsteroidal and other antiinflammatory agents are used to control the pain. Surgical intervention may include fracture repairs, occipital craniectomy to relieve basilar and nerve compression, tibial osteotomy if the deformity is severe, and joint replacement(s) if severe degenerative joint disease is present (Fig. 24-12).

PROGNOSIS. The course of Paget disease varies widely from stable and asymptomatic, to rapid progressions of signs and symptoms. The outlook is generally good, particularly if treatment is given before major changes have occurred. Biochemical remission with bisphosphonates is achievable in a majority of individuals.[144]

Paget disease is accompanied by osteogenic sarcoma in less than 1% of all cases; but represents an increase in risk that is several thousand-fold higher than the general population.[49,50,88] There may be a link between the putative gene for Paget disease and the tumor suppressor gene for osteosarcoma on chromosome 18q.[8,88]

Peak incidence of the associated sarcoma occurs in the seventh and eighth decades. Tumors tend to be high grade and found in areas commonly affected by Paget disease, especially in the pelvis, femur, humerus, and skull. Metastases have often already occurred at the time of discovery.

Prognosis for individuals with Paget sarcoma is poor and is unrelated to the site or stage of presentation.[30]

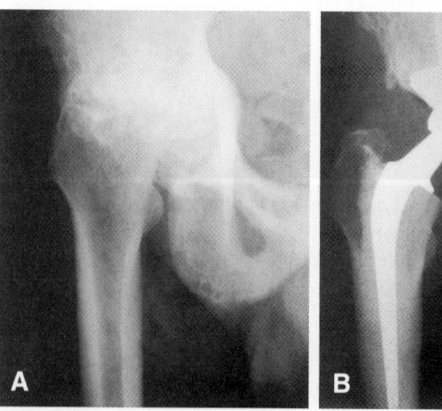

Figure 24-12

Extensive Paget disease of the acetabulum and femur in an 82-year-old man. **A,** Protrusion deformity and varus femoral neck are seen. **B,** After total hip replacement. Acetabulum required autogenous bone graft from femoral head. Cementless acetabular component appears bone ingrown 5 years after surgery. (From Canale ST: *Campbell's operative orthopaedics,* ed 10, St Louis, 2003, Mosby.)

Little progress has occurred in the treatment of Paget sarcoma over the years despite improvement in the treatment of standard osteosarcoma.[83] See Chapter 26 for an overview of osteogenic sarcoma.

SPECIAL IMPLICATIONS FOR THE THERAPIST   24-3

Paget Disease

Although Paget disease and osteoporosis can occur in the same person, these are completely different disorders, with different causes. However, despite their marked differences, considerable overlap is evident between Paget disease and osteoporosis regarding interventions and implications for the therapist (see "Osteoporosis" above). The overlap includes the discussion of client injury during examination and treatment, recognition of possible fracture, and postoperative care. For a discussion of fractures, and fracture prevention, see Chapter 27.

Screening Assessment

Other important considerations exist for the therapist. If working with an aging adult population, therapists need to be aware of the symptoms and signs of Paget disease. Because pain is often the initial symptom and is usually a vague diffuse ache, difficulty in distinguishing this disease from degenerative joint disease of the lumbar spine, hips, or knees can be evident.

Clients with diffuse headaches may present to the therapist with undiagnosed Paget disease. These clients may report hearing loss, tinnitus, incontinence, diplopia, or swallowing difficulties. Slurring of speech or the onset of signs or symptoms associated with heart disease is evident. The presentation of any of the above clinical manifestations warrants communication with a physician. Awareness of the side effects of antiinflammatory medications is also important. These side effects include indigestion, nausea, vomiting, melena, tinnitus, hearing loss, vertigo, and hyperapnea. Again, if any of these signs or symptoms are reported to the therapist, communication with a physician is warranted.

Exercise and Paget Disease

Exercise is very important in maintaining skeletal health and is recommended for people with Paget disease. Joints adjacent to involved bone may function at a mechanical disadvantage, causing muscular pain that can be reduced with exercise. Strengthening muscles can also help minimize skeletal complications of Paget disease with its mechanical stresses and resultant structural abnormalities of bone.[97,161]

The pain associated with Paget disease often leads to less physical activity in daily life. Loss of muscle strength, joint motion, and cardiovascular endurance occur, leading to functional limitations such as slower walking and shorter distances.[81] Exercise helps with weight control, improving cardiovascular function and cardiac output, and maintains muscular strength and joint motion.[139]

Severity of Paget disease will determine the exercise program. Stretching, strengthening, endurance, aerobics, balance, and coordination exercises are all important. Some types of exercise should be avoided such as jogging, running, jumping, and if the spine is affected, forward bending and twisting exercises.[139]

Complications of orthopedic surgery on pagetic bone include hemorrhage, infection, pathologic fracture, delayed union or nonunion, and aseptic loosening of the hardware. The therapist may be involved in management of extremity deformities requiring management with orthotics.

REFERENCES

To enhance this text and add value for the reader, all references are included on the companion Evolve site that accompanies this textbook. The reader can view the reference source and access it online whenever possible.

CHAPTER 25

Infectious Diseases of the Musculoskeletal System

KEVIN HELGESON

Understanding the epidemiology, pathogenesis, and treatment of musculoskeletal infections will allow the clinician to play an active role in all phases of diagnosis and intervention. From early detection of signs and symptoms that identify those clients who are at risk and need of further medical evaluation to the rehabilitation of those clients who undergo surgical intervention for musculoskeletal infections, the role of therapists and their impact on the outcome of treatment cannot be underestimated.

The use of temporary and permanent implants and prosthetic materials, including bioprosthetic implants, is now commonplace. Therapists often treat clients with biomaterial implants. Joint replacements, heart valves, vascular prostheses, artificial disk replacements, shunts, dental implants, baclofen/insulin/pain pumps, sutures, catheters, and allografts are a few of the devices that can harbor infections. Musculoskeletal infections can require drastic measures to treat and prevent morbidity. For example, infection after total joint replacement often requires removal of the hardware, and joint sepsis may require extensive surgical debridement.

Only the most common infectious diseases seen in a therapy practice are included in this chapter (e.g., osteomyelitis, diskitis, infectious arthritis, and tuberculosis [TB]). Necrotizing fasciitis, streptococcal myositis, and soft tissue infection leading to gangrene are discussed in Chapter 8; cellulitis is discussed in Chapters 8 and 10.

OSTEOMYELITIS

Overview

Osteomyelitis is an inflammation of bone caused by an infectious organism such as bacteria, but fungi, parasites, and viruses can also cause skeletal infections (see Chapter 8). Areas affected most often include the spine, pelvis, and arms or legs.[69] The pathophysiology of osteomyelitis is complex and poorly understood. Key factors include the virulence of the infecting organism; the individual's immune status; any comorbidities; and the type, location, and vascularity of the involved bone.

Acute osteomyelitis is the clinical term for a new infection in bone that can develop into a chronic reaction when intervention is delayed or inadequate. It is a rapidly destructive pyogenic infection often seen in children, older adults, and intravenous (IV) drug abusers. The infectious agent enters the body through an open wound or the GI tract. The infection has the capability to spread quickly through the bloodstream, resulting in septicemia or a septic infectious joint.

In adults, osteomyelitis is usually a subacute or chronic infection that develops secondary to an open injury to bone and surrounding soft tissue. *Chronic osteomyelitis* is often the result of a persistent bone infection or acute disease remaining undiagnosed.

Incidence

Acute osteomyelitis is a relatively uncommon but potentially serious disease occurring more often in children than adults and affecting boys more often than girls. Acute hematogenous osteomyelitis is the most common type and is usually seen in children. Chronic osteomyelitis is more common in adults and immunocompromised people. The incidence of osteomyelitis was expected to decline with more widespread availability of antibiotics. However, with the presence of drug-resistant organisms, the number of IV drug abusers, and the increased use of implantable prosthetic devices, osteomyelitis is actually becoming more common.[8,63]

Etiologic Factors

Staphylococcus aureus is the usual causative agent of acute osteomyelitis.[101] It has the ability to bind to cartilage, produce a protective glycocalyx, and stimulate the release of endotoxins. Glycocalyx is the glycoprotein and polysaccharide covering that surrounds many cells; in bacterial cells, the glycocalyx forms masses of fibers that extend from the bacterial cell and are the means by which the bacteria adhere to surfaces.

Other organisms such as group B streptococcus, pneumococcus, *Pseudomonas aeruginosa*, *Haemophilus influenzae*, and *Escherichia coli* also produce bone infections.[30,53,63] Among people with sickle cell anemia, *Salmonella* infection is associated with osteomyelitis. Osteomyelitis can be acquired from exogenous or hematogenous sources.

Exogenous osteomyelitis is acquired by invasion of the bone by direct extension from the outside as a result of inoculation into the bone by a penetrating or puncture wound, extension from an overlying abscess or burn, or other trauma such as an open fracture.[12] Surgical procedures, open fractures, and implanted orthopedic devices are common sources of acute osteomyelitis infection. These examples of osteomyelitis secondary to a contiguous area of infection are common in immunocompromised people and in those with diabetes or severe vascular insufficiency.[109]

Hematogenous osteomyelitis is acquired from spread of organisms from preexisting infections such as occurs in impetigo; furunculosis (persistent boils); infected lesions of varicella (chickenpox); and sinus, ear, dental, soft tissue, respiratory (through alveoli when an upper respiratory infection is present), and genitourinary infections. Vaginal, uterine, ovarian, bladder, and intestinal infections can lead to iliac or sacral osteomyelitis.[56]

Osteomyelitis of the arm and hand bones may occur in drug abusers, and vertebral osteomyelitis is seen in adults from hematogenous spread from pelvic or urinary tract infections. The lumbar spine is the most commonly involved area. In children, the infection is spread hematogenously and usually develops in the metaphyseal regions of the long bones, adjacent to the growth plates (e.g., distal femur, proximal tibia, humerus, and radius).[63]

Risk Factors

In general, anyone who is chronically ill (e.g., diabetes or alcoholism) or who receives large doses of steroids or immunosuppressive drugs is particularly susceptible to osteomyelitis (Box 25-1). Infection with methicillin-resistant *S. aureus* increases the risk of developing osteomyelitis.[10]

Risk factors for osteomyelitis of the foot in individuals with diabetes include ulceration, sausage toe, or visible or palpable bone. Infected or nonhealing ulcers following several weeks of appropriate care and off-loading pressure increases the risk of osteomyelitis. An ulcer area deeper than 3 mm, over boney prominences, or larger than 2 cm^2 are additional risk factors.[10]

Older adults with additional preexisting medical conditions, such as malignancy, malnutrition, and renal or hepatic failure, are also at a greater risk.[72] Individuals with spinal cord injury with complete motor and sensory paralysis at the paraplegic level appear to be at risk for vertebral osteomyelitis.[42]

Nutritional status is an often overlooked variable in acute and chronic illness. Anyone who is at risk for malnutrition or is compromised by a poor nutritional status is at risk for infection, slowed tissue healing, and an increased incidence of postsurgical complications.

Infection is the second most common cause of prosthetic joint failure, after mechanical loosening. Some cases of prosthetic joint infection may be misclassified as aseptic loosening. The incidences of prosthetic joint infection is higher after a revision.[97]

Pathogenesis

The pathophysiology of osteomyelitis is complex and poorly understood. Key factors include the virulence of the infecting organism; the person's immune status; any underlying disease; and the type, location, and vascularity of the involved bone. Regardless of the source of the pathogen, the pathogenesis of bone infection initially involves an inflammatory response. Acute osteomyelitis may develop in the metaphysis of long bones because of the decreased amount of phagocytosis and/or slower rate of blood flow in the terminal arterioles. The vascular loop in growing bone is a common site of bacterial seeding because the arterioles form a loop and then drain into the medullary cavity without establishing a capillary bed (Fig. 25-1). Trauma, including microtrauma, may also increase susceptibility to infection by slowing the blood flow.[22]

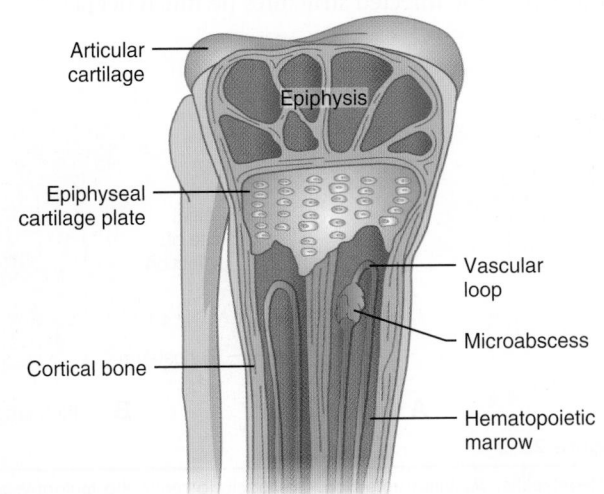

Figure 25-1

The vascular loop in growing bone is a common initial site of bacterial seeding.

The metaphysis of long bones is very porous, allowing exudate from the infection to spread easily. As the organisms grow and form pus within the bone, tension builds within the rigid medullary cavity, forcing pus through the haversian canals. Haversian canals contain blood, lymph vessels, and nerves. Once bacteria gain access to these channels, they are able to proliferate unimpeded, forming a subperiosteal abscess that deprives the bone of its blood supply and eventually may cause necrosis. Necrotic cells then become a fertile bed for the organisms to multiply. Because sensory nerve endings are absent in cancellous bone, this process can progress without pain. Necrosis then stimulates the periosteum to create new bone.

A sheath of new bone, called an *involucrum*, forms around the *sequestrum* of necrotic tissue that has become separated from the surrounding bone (Fig. 25-2). By the time the sequestrum forms, the osteomyelitis is considered to be chronic. In adults, this complication is rare because the periosteum is firmly attached to the cortex and resists displacement. Instead, infection disrupts and weakens the cortex, which predisposes the bone to pathologic fracture.

In vertebral osteomyelitis, the infection is first found in the metaphysis or cartilaginous endplates and quickly spreads to the intervertebral disk. Abscess formation is common through direct extension of the infection to adjacent tissues. The abscesses can advance posteriorly to involve the epidural area or anteriorly to produce a paravertebral abscess that can extend to the psoas muscle, producing hip pain.[107]

Clinical Manifestations

The primary manifestations of osteomyelitis vary between adults and children. Back pain is typically the chief complaint in adults, but once the infection becomes systemic (as opposed to an abscess) a low-grade fever may be present. Children are more likely to present with acute, severe complaints, such as high fever and intense pain, but in some cases, local manifestations will predominate such as edema, erythema, and tenderness. These signs are easier to detect in the extremities, unlike vertebral osteomyelitis where the infected structures lie much deeper.[56]

In the initial phases of the infection, pain may not be a factor because of the lack of pain fibers in cancellous bone. This makes diagnosis and intervention difficult because of the potential rapid spread of the infectious agent, which is facilitated by the delay in the administration of appropriate antibiotics. When the infection extends into the periosteum, increased joint pain; diminished function; and systemic signs, such as fever, swelling, and malaise may rapidly develop.

The pain will likely be described as deep and constant, increasing with weight bearing when the infection is anywhere in the lower extremity. Clients presenting with chronic osteomyelitis complain of local pain and swelling and may limp but otherwise are often asymptomatic. The clinical sign of "sausage toe" has been used to detect underlying pedal osteomyelitis. This clinical sign has been demonstrated to have good sensitivity and specificity in clients with diabetes.[92]

Once present, spinal osteomyelitis can produce intermittent or constant back pain. The pain can be aggravated by motion but is also present regardless of activity level in some individuals and throbbing at rest. It may radiate in a radicular distribution and is commonly accompanied by spinal tenderness and rigidity; accessory motions of the spine are often difficult to perform. As mentioned, pyogenic vertebral osteomyelitis may result in a psoas abscess causing painful hip extension and/or an antalgic limp. Cervical abscess formation may lead to torticollis or dysphagia.[107,108]

Radiculopathy, myelopathy, or even complete paralysis can occur with neural compression as a result of abscess, instability, or spinal deformity associated with vertebral osteomyelitis. Direct spread of the infection into the epidural space can cause meningitis.[108]

Sacroiliac osteomyelitis is usually characterized by severe, local pain with tenderness and an antalgic gait. The pain may radiate to the buttocks or abdomen. The history will be a recent onset of localized pain. Besides pain, other symptoms may include fever, local tenderness, and swelling. Any unexplained cellulitis should be considered a sign of osteomyelitis in children, even if no other contributing signs or symptoms are evident.

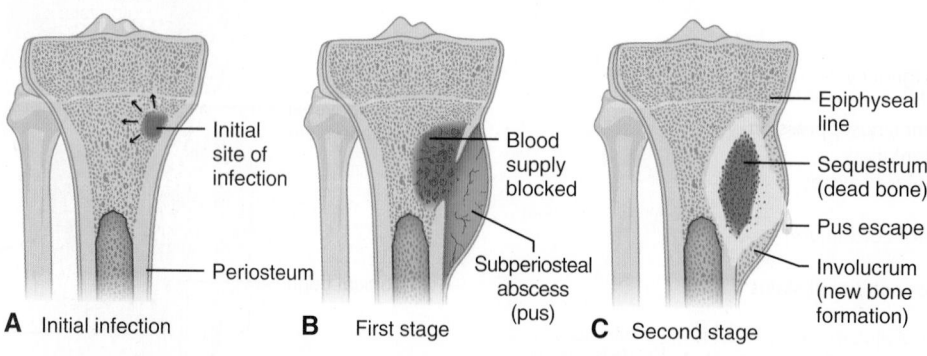

Figure 25-2

Osteomyelitis. A, Initial infection. The bacteria reach the metaphysis through the nutrient artery. **B,** First stage: bacterial growth results in bone destruction and formation of an abscess. **C,** Second stage: from the abscess cavity, the pus spreads between the trabeculae into the medulla, through the cartilage into the joint, or through the haversian canals of the compact bones to the outside. These sinuses traversing the bone persist for a long time and heal slowly. The pus destroys the bone and sequesters part of it in the abscess cavity. Reactive new bone is formed around the focus of inflammation. (From Damjanov I: *Pathology for the health-related professions*, ed 3, Philadelphia, 2006, W.B. Saunders.)

MEDICAL MANAGEMENT

PREVENTION. Because chronic osteomyelitis is also recognized as a complication of treatment of open fractures, prevention of infection is important. The risks can be minimized if the wound is thoroughly debrided, irrigated, and left open for delayed primary closure. Delayed primary closure allows the wound bed to be inspected, and further debridement can be carried out if necessary.

Clients with any of the conditions listed in Box 25-1 or with any additional risk factors should be taught proper preventive measures and be aware of early warning signs. As mentioned, nutritional status plays a critical role in the prevention of infection and the body's ability to combat infection once it occurs. Anyone with biomaterial implants will have an increased risk of infection, especially in the immediate postoperative period. Although rare, late infections occurring 1 year postoperatively have been reported.[102]

SCREENING. Although diagnosing infectious diseases is outside the scope of the therapist's practice, screening is still appropriate, using a thorough history and a review of systems to help identify pathologies that require further medical evaluation. For screening purposes, the presence of a fever, unexplained weight loss, history of cancer, and failure to respond to adequate treatment are good indicators of more serious pathology.[51]

Disturbances in the sleep pattern, such as awakening with pain, requiring sleep medications, or inability to fall asleep, along with symptoms that increase with walking, have been found to be associated with serious back problems.[93] In other areas of the body, localized pain in the presence of other risk factors may raise suspicion.

DIAGNOSIS. Medical diagnosis is often delayed because of the lack of specific signs and symptoms, especially in chronic osteomyelitis. Signs and symptoms that are generally associated with infection may be masked by (or mistaken for) normal postoperative changes. Laboratory values and radiographs are often negative in the early stages. Positive cultures are obtained in only half of the cases; however, this is improving because of advancements in molecular techniques.[25,101] Any unexplained cellulitis in children is suggested to be considered as a possible indicator of underlying osteomyelitis.[10]

Radiographs may not detect bony abnormality in infections of less than 10 days' duration. Lytic lesions may be demonstrable on radiographs within 2 weeks of onset of the disease (Fig. 25-3). A periosteal reaction develops later (Fig. 25-4). Magnetic resonance imaging (MRI) and isotope bone scans are the procedures of choice in delineating the disease's anatomic extent. Imaging tests are often used to localize or confirm the presence of infection. MRI is sensitive and provides valuable detail of septic arthritis, spinal osteomyelitis, and diabetic foot infections.[86] Radionuclide bone scan can detect early-stage disease and is helpful in detection and identifying multiple sites of involvement.[20] This procedure may be used as an alternative when MRI cannot be performed or as an adjunct diagnostic tool in people with an uncertain diagnosis.

Nuclear medicine imaging techniques, such as fluorine-18-fluorodeoxyglucose positron emission tomography scans, provide accurate localization of infection and/or source of fever of undetermined origin, thereby guiding additional testing. Fluorine-18-fluorodeoxyglucose positron emission tomography helps diagnose spinal osteomyelitis and can be useful in measuring the extent of disease and monitoring response to treatment.[71,85,115]

Identification of the infectious pathogen is of utmost importance because the type of medication used often depends on the infecting microorganism. Specimens are obtained for culture or stains by aspiration, needle biopsy, or swab. Accurate identification is often difficult because of the technical problems of obtaining an acceptable sample. Image-enhanced needle biopsy can improve the specimen quality.

Early acute postoperative prosthetic joint infection in most cases occurs in the first 3 months after surgery.

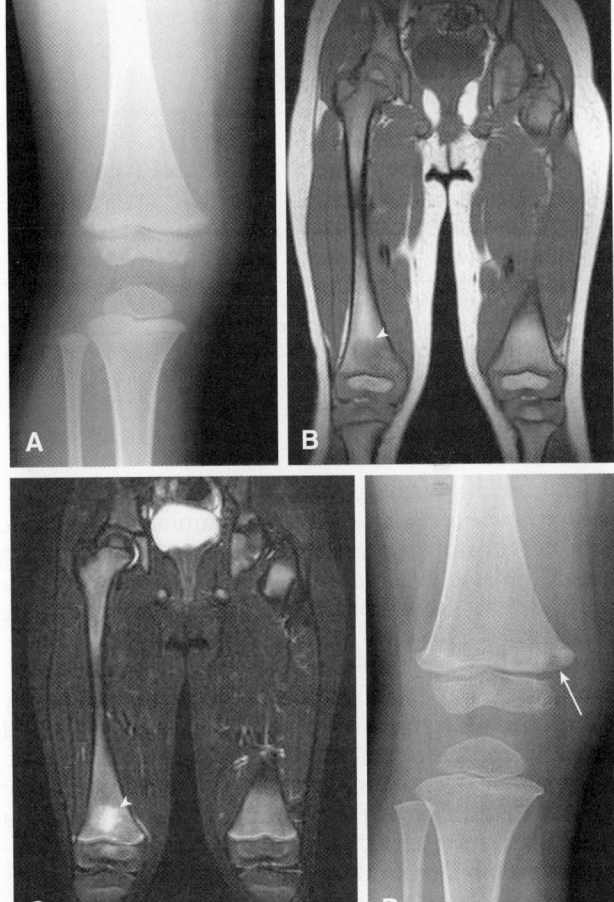

Figure 25-3

Acute osteomyelitis in a child. A, Frontal radiograph of the knee. This 3-year-old child presented with knee pain and a limp. The film is normal. **B,** T1 coronal image of the thighs. There is a rounded focus of abnormal, low signal intensity in the distal right femoral metaphysis *(arrowhead)*. **C,** Coronal STIR image of the thighs. The lesion shows strikingly increased signal at this site of acute osteomyelitis. **D,** Frontal radiograph of the knee. This film, obtained 3 weeks after the first radiograph, now shows a small metaphyseal lucency abutting the medial aspect of the physis at the site of infection *(arrow)*. (From Helms CA. Helms: *Musculoskeletal MRI*, ed 2, Philadelphia, 2008, W.B. Saunders.)

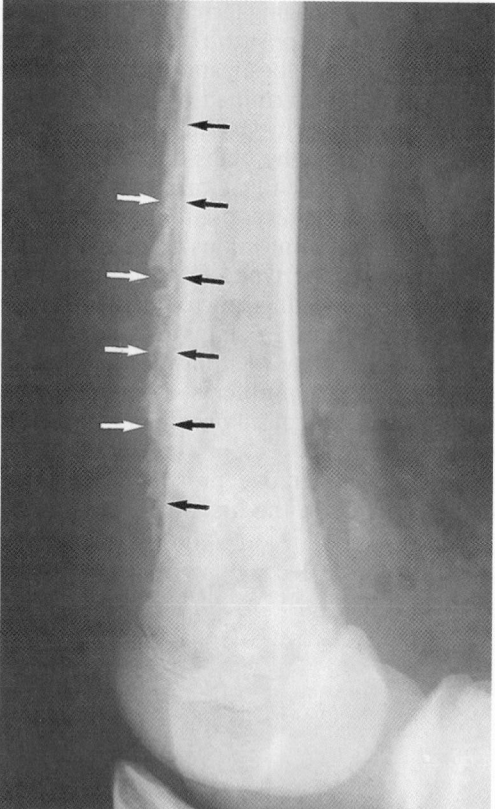

Figure 25-4

Chronic osteomyelitis. A lateral view of the knee shows the periosteal reaction *(arrows)* suggestive of chronic osteomyelitis. The bone of the distal femur has a mottled appearance as a result of the infection. (From Mettler FA: *Essentials of radiology,* ed 2, Philadelphia, 2005, W.B. Saunders.)

Chronic, postoperative prosthetic joint infection is characterized by more subtle signs of inflammation, chronic persistent postoperative pain, and/or early loosening of the implant. Differentiating late postoperative prosthetic joint infection from aseptic implant failure can be challenging.

TREATMENT. Immediate treatment is called for, especially in acute osteomyelitis. The successful use of sequential IV and high-dose antibiotic therapy is now an accepted modality and has lessened the role of surgery in these infections. The choice of antibiotics is based primarily on the culture results as well as the client's age and health status, site of infection, and previous antimicrobial therapy.

Antibiotics are delivered intravenously to hasten their effect when faced with serious infection that can progress rapidly. Evaluation of response to treatment by monitoring C-reactive protein levels has decreased the average duration of therapy to 3 to 4 weeks with few relapses.[65,101]

Surgery is indicated if the infection has spread to the joints as this is considered an orthopedic emergency. Articular cartilage can be damaged in a matter of hours. The goal of surgery is to drain exudate or pus from the bone or joint. Often, extensive debridement of both bone and surrounding soft tissue is required. Various reconstructive procedures may be considered once the infection

is eliminated. These include soft tissue procedures to provide well-vascularized soft tissue coverage of defects and revascularized bone for stabilization of the affected area. In adults, both surgery and antibiotics are often required.

The goals for treatment of chronic osteomyelitis are to eliminate the infection by use of antibiotics if possible or by surgically removing infected tissue. If surgery is indicated, then the current trend is toward more radical surgery rather than serial debridements. In general, chronic osteomyelitis is more difficult to treat than the acute type because it is difficult to eradicate completely. Exacerbations may respond well to treatment with rest and antibiotics, only to flare up again months later.

In the spine, surgery may be necessary to treat the infection and to address spinal deformity. Deformity of the spine from the infection or subsequent surgery may lead to pain or neurologic compromise. If surgery is not indicated, the person may be treated with short-term bed rest or the use of a brace for immobilization.

The use of appropriate antibiotics prophylactically is standard for some procedures, such as total joint replacements, and in open wounds that are contaminated. Antibiotic bead chains can be implanted in the infected area to achieve concentrated levels of antibiotics in the local tissue without raising serum levels to toxic ranges. These bead chains can be an effective method of prophylaxis and treatment of established infections.[31,66]

PROGNOSIS. There is a small risk of death for the majority of individuals with acute osteomyelitis, but treatment remains a challenge. With early medical interventions, an infection arrest rate of 70% to 90% can be expected, even in chronic cases.[88,109] If the process is unattended for a week to 10 days, a permanent loss of bone structure and changes to the surrounding soft tissues almost always occurs. When osteomyelitis is diagnosed in the early clinical stages and treated with antibiotics, the prognosis is excellent. For skeletally immature children and adolescents, there is a greater possibility of an infection, resulting in a growth abnormality in the affected bony structures.

When osteomyelitis persists for a long period of time, infected necrotic bone serves as an isolated reservoir for infection that will not respond well to systemic antibiotics. Reduced blood flow will facilitate the likelihood that an infection will be established and the pharmacologic agent will be prevented from reaching the locus of infection. The comorbidities of diabetes and peripheral vascular disease increase the risk of a recurring infection.[109] The emergence of antibiotic resistance, particularly resistance to methicillin and vancomycin by *S. aureus* organisms, contributes to long-term sequelae and morbidity.[101]

Chronic osteomyelitis has a poor prognosis, even when treated surgically. People with chronic osteomyelitis are often in great pain, require prolonged medical care, and may, although rarely, require amputation of an extremity. In the older adult population, the reoccurrence of chronic osteomyelitis ranges from 3% to 40% and the mortality rate is reported as being less than 5%.[72,109] The bottom line is that the best way to minimize the mortality and morbidity observed in osteomyelitis is to practice preventive measures and reduce the time between the onset of the infection and the initiation of an appropriate intervention.

Osteomyelitis
SURGERY

If surgery is indicated, current resection and debridement techniques may result in soft tissue and bony defects that require secondary microsurgical reconstruction with split-thickness skin grafting, muscle flaps, or bone grafting. If the infection has affected the articular cartilage, controlling weight-bearing and compressive forces with exercise should be a priority.[34,114] For example, weight bearing on the affected leg may be restricted, and crutches may not be advised when arm(s) and leg(s) are affected simultaneously until sufficient healing occurs to avoid pathologic fractures. The physician must make this determination.

Often, surgery and initial management are performed without adequate consideration for adjacent joints. Prolonged immobilization or limited mobility and weight bearing with external fixators may lead to significant impairment of previously uninvolved joints and muscles. Attention must not be focused on the infection site to the exclusion of the rest of the limb. Important elements of a successful rehabilitation include minimizing the original effects of the trauma or disease process and preventing as many complications as possible.

Preventing Complications

Preventing complications is best done by beginning rehabilitation early. Therapists should first recognize the possible side effects of medical intervention that may lead to complications such as contractures, atrophy, impaired joint mechanics, and loss of function. Treatment of osteomyelitis is complex, and rehabilitation is sometimes perplexing under the best of circumstances.

Sequelae of hip joint sepsis can include joint destruction, avascular necrosis, and fracture. When complications such as these arise, a full recovery is jeopardized. In addition to the musculoskeletal problems, the therapist should consider other involved organ systems, such as the cardiovascular system, and what impact the comorbidities may have on healing, rehabilitation, and return to a high level of function.

Strict aseptic technique must be used when changing dressings and performing wound care. Reconstructive surgery to cover bone or soft tissue defects requires careful monitoring, dressing changes, and protection. If the client is in skeletal traction for fractures, the insertion points of pin tracks should be covered with small, dry dressings.

Pins used in external fixators also deserve close inspection. Therapist and client must avoid touching the skin around the pins and wires. Assess vital signs, wound appearance, and any new pain daily for signs of secondary infection. During the acute phase of this illness, any movement of the affected limb will cause discomfort or pain. The affected limb should be firmly supported and kept level with the body.

Active, active assisted, and passive range of motion (ROM) exercises of adjacent joints are essential. Good skin care is essential with proper positioning; frequent (but careful and gentle) position changes (at least every 2 hours); and skin assessment for any signs of developing pressure ulcers. Massage or any technique that can possibly spread the infection through mechanical means is to be avoided.

INFECTIONS OF PROSTHESES AND IMPLANTS

Overview

Over the past decades, joint replacement surgery has become commonplace, which is largely attributed to the success of these procedures in restoring function to people with disabling arthritis. Implant infection remains the primary cause of prosthetic failure, occurring either acutely within the first month postoperatively or months to years after the joint replacement.[6] Nearly 80% of these infections are caused by staphylococcus organisms, which enter by perioperative, hematogenous, or contiguous means. Perioperative infections occur around the time of surgery and are probably caused by contaminated instruments at the surgical site. Hematogenous infections occur as a result of a primary infection somewhere else in the body. Contiguous infections occur secondary to a nearby infection.[112]

Other types of prostheses or implants susceptible to infection include internal fixation of the spine, breast implants, penile implants, dental implants, cardiac implants, other orthopedic devices and hardware, shunts, and even contact lenses (external to epithelial surfaces that can give rise to serious life-threatening infections).

Incidence

The successful development of synthetic materials and the introduction of artificial devices into nearly all body systems have been accompanied by the adaptation of microorganisms to the opportunities these devices provide for eluding defenses and invading the host. With improvements in surgical procedures and prophylactic antibiotics, the incidence of infection has been reduced to less than 1.5%. The incidence of infection does increase with longer procedures and revisions.[87] However, as the number of people undergoing replacements has grown, reoperations have become increasingly common. Bioprostheses, implanted in large numbers in the early 1980s, have now gone into the second or third decade of life since implantation, a time when biodegradation becomes more common. Multiple reoperations carry a higher risk of infection. Likewise, as the population ages, an increasing number of total hip, knee, shoulder, elbow, wrist, and finger arthroplasties are coming up for revision.

Infection of a prosthetic joint causes loosening of the prosthesis and sepsis with significant mortality and morbidity. Two-thirds of prosthetic joint infections occur within 1 year of surgery and are the result of intraoperative inoculations of bacteria into the new joint or postoperative bacteremias. Early infections have been substantially reduced by preoperative use of antibiotics, the use of laminar flow in operating rooms, and improved surgical technique.[87]

Risk Factors

Certain groups have been identified as predisposed toward infection of their prosthetic joints, including those with prior surgery at the site of the prosthesis, rheumatoid arthritis, corticosteroid therapy, diabetes mellitus, poor nutritional status, low albumin, obesity, and extremely advanced age.[18]

Any factor that delays or impairs wound healing increases the risk of infection. Psoriasis, steroids, diabetes mellitus, and immunodeficiency increase the risk of prosthetic infection. Immunodeficiency can be either local (e.g., wear debris from the implant) or systemic (e.g., *Candida albicans*, rheumatoid arthritis, or immunosuppressive medications). Risk factors for infection of spinal instrumentation may include IV drug use, paraplegia with neurogenic bladder, and pyelonephritis secondary to renal calculi.

Certain factors or events can enhance the ability of bacteria to multiply rapidly and increase the risk of infection (e.g., wound hematomas, seromas, hemarthroses, fresh operative wounds, ischemic wounds, and tissues in diabetic and steroid-treated people). In the early postimplantation period, the fascial layers have not yet healed, and the deep, periprosthetic tissue is not protected by the usual physical barriers. Any superficial infection that develops, such as an infected wound hematoma, wound infection, or suture abscess, can become a preceding event for joint prosthesis infection.

Joint replacement has been shown to be responsible for reactivation of quiescent infections that occurred earlier in a person's life. Evaluation of a client for history of osteomyelitis, tuberculosis, human immunodeficiency virus (HIV), or other infection caused by bacteria with latent capabilities is important before joint replacement surgery.[35]

Etiologic Factors and Pathogenesis

Locally introduced forms of infection account for about 70% of all prosthetic joint infections and occur as a result of wound infection next to the prosthesis, or to operative contamination.[70] Operative contamination may be a result of direct implantation at the time of the operation by the operating team, from environmental sources, or from contaminated implant materials. Holes in the implants (e.g., press-fit acetabular cups) are potential pathways through which debris can gain access to the implant–bone interface, resulting in infection, creating periprosthetic bone loss, and potentially initiating loosening.[84] In general, these infections are caused by a single pathogen, but polymicrobial sepsis can occur.[79]

Staphylococci (coagulase-negative staphylococci and *S. aureus*) are the principal causative agents of joint prosthesis infection (approximately 40% and 20%, respectively), aerobic streptococci and gram-negative bacilli are each responsible for 10% and 5% of cases, mixed flora constitutes 10%, and anaerobes are involved in about 5% of these infections. No organism is found in about 10% of cases.[119] Rarely, latent foci of chronic, nonactive osteomyelitis are reactivated by the disruption of tissue associated with prosthetic surgery. Previous *S. aureus* and *Mycobacterium tuberculosis* infections can recur postoperatively.[18]

Bacteria adhere tightly to the implant surface by adhesins, which recognize specific host proteins absorbed on the material surface. They also use biofilms, a type of slime that protects bacterial colonies from destruction by phagocytes. Multiple layers of biofilm allow staphylococci to cling to the surface of the implant and avoid both immune system defenses and antibiotic diffusion. The slimes can even alter the host's immune capability and increase antibiotic resistance. Bacteria can lie dormant on the prosthetic device for years until the person becomes immunocompromised from aging or other health issues.[6,7]

Prostheses that are cemented into place with polymethyl methacrylate can develop infection at the bone–cement interface, whereas cementless prostheses are more likely to develop sepsis in the bone contiguous with the metallic alloy. As foreign bodies, these prostheses facilitate local sepsis by decreasing the quantity of bacteria necessary to establish infection and by permitting pathogens to persist on their avascular surface, sequestered from circulating immunologic defenses (leukocytes, antibodies, and complement) and from systemic antibiotics.[18]

In the presence of prosthetic or implantable devices, many bacteria form a fibrous material called *glycocalyx*. Organisms can reproduce within this matrix and form a thick biofilm that is protected in part from host defense mechanisms. Biofilms are an important issue for surgery involving prosthetic or implantable devices. For example, only 32% of infections caused by slime-producing staphylococci resolved with antibiotics compared with 100% recovery in non–slime-producing strains.[89]

The implant and its adherent biofilm must be removed for the infection to resolve because recurrent, acute infections or disseminated, persistent infection may develop if these reservoirs are allowed to continue. Meticulous protocols for sterilization of implants should be followed, because biofilms may be an important mechanism of antibiotic resistance.[89]

Clinical Manifestations

Persistent joint pain may be the only symptom with no clinical signs of infection at all. Staphylococcus infections are usually characterized by symptoms similar to wound infection such as edema, hematoma, fever, and local pain. Late-onset or delayed infection usually presents as increasing joint pain followed by rapid onset of systemic symptoms.[111]

Prosthetic joint infections can be divided into the following three categories: early (infection that develops less than 3 months after surgery), delayed (3 to 24 months after surgery), and late (more than 24 months).[95]

Early infections typically present with acute symptoms such as fever, joint pain, warmth, and redness. These individuals may form a sinus tract from the prosthesis to the skin with purulent drainage. Virulent organisms, such as *S. aureus* or gram-negative bacilli, are usually responsible for early infections.

People who present with delayed infections often lack systemic symptoms, making diagnosis difficult. These individuals display joint pain and/or joint loosening. Organisms responsible for these infections are less virulent such as coagulase-negative staphylococci (particularly *S. epidermidis*) and *Propionibacterium acnes*. Early and delayed infections are typically acquired at the time of surgery, whereas late infections develop from hematogenous seeding. In one study of 63 infected hip prosthesis, 29% were early infections, 41% delayed, and 30% were late infections.[48]

When a bloodborne infection arises in a prosthetic joint several months or years after implantation surgery, the fully healed connective tissue often is capable of restricting the septic process to a relatively small focus at the bone–cement interface. Joint pain is the principal symptom of deep tissue infection, irrespective of mode of presentation, and suggests either acute inflammation of the periarticular tissue or loosening of the prosthesis caused by subacute erosion of bone at the bone–cement interface.

MEDICAL MANAGEMENT

PREVENTION. Sterilization and attention to infection control guidelines reduces the risk of infection.[6] Proper handwashing remains the key to reducing the transmission of pathogens to others and the spread of antimicrobial resistance. Despite this well-known fact, adherence by surgeons and other important health care workers remains low.[110] Researchers are working to design self-sterilizing materials and more effective infection-resistant materials. New coatings with an antiadhesive or biocide capabilities are the next step.[98]

DIAGNOSIS. Clinical manifestations of joint pain, swelling, erythema, and warmth all reflect an underlying inflammatory process in the surrounding tissues but are not specific for infection. When a painful prosthesis is accompanied by fever or purulent drainage from overlying cutaneous sinuses, infection is likely. The physician must differentiate infection from aseptic and mechanical problems (e.g., hemarthrosis, mechanical loosening, or dislocation). Constant joint pain is suggestive of infection, whereas mechanical loosening commonly causes pain only with motion or weight bearing.

The diagnosis of joint prosthesis infection is dependent on isolation of the pathogen by aspiration of joint fluid or by obtaining tissue at arthrotomy. Gram stain and culture will typically identify the responsible organism in 65% to 94% of cases.[119] Special media may be required if fungus or atypical organisms are suspected. Culture of sinus tract drainage or overlying skin should be avoided. Elevated serum leukocyte count, erythrocyte sedimentation rate, and C-reactive protein level are suggestive but not diagnostic of joint infection. Ultrasound-guided (ultrasonography) aspiration in suspected sepsis of arthroplasty has been developed to facilitate this process.

Radiologic abnormalities may be helpful when changes are noted over serial radiographs, but some changes can lag behind symptoms by 3 to 6 months. When both the distal and proximal components of a prosthetic joint demonstrate pathology on radiography, infection is more likely than simple mechanical loosening. However, such radiographic changes are not specific for infection and may also be seen with aseptic processes.

The use of CT and MRI scans is limited because of the artifacts created by the prosthesis. A bone scan will demonstrate increased uptake in areas of bone with enhanced blood supply or increased metabolic activity (a normal finding during the first 6 months postimplantation). Positive scans at 6 months after implantation are abnormal but do not differentiate among inflammation, possible loosening, and infection. The best method for determining an infected prosthetic joint is the use of scintigraphy with radioisotope-labeled leucocyte and bone marrow.[46]

A series of tests before, during, and after surgery are needed for early detection of implant infection. Periimplant infection does not respond well to oral antibiotic therapy because of antibiotic resistance from widespread clinical use of broad-spectrum antibiotics. The biofilm-forming strains of staphylococcus seem to have an even higher degree of resistance to antibiotics. The person is at risk for implant failure and possible death.[6,98]

Successful treatment requires a combination of surgical intervention (usually removal and replacement of the entire implant) and long-term antimicrobial therapy.[111,112] A temporary implant coated with antibiotics may be put in place while the person is treated with IV antibiotics. When there are no further signs of infection, a permanent replacement prosthesis can be implanted.

TREATMENT. Prosthesis removal accompanied by extensive and meticulous surgical debridement of surrounding tissue and effective antimicrobial therapy are usually necessary to treat deep infections, especially infections involving the interface between prosthesis and bone. Surgical debridement with retention of the prosthesis followed by a course of antibiotics may be appropriate for a limited and select group or people.[75]

For more predictably effective treatment of prosthetic joint replacement sepsis, complete removal of all foreign materials (metallic prosthesis, cement, and any accompanying biofilm) is essential. This can be done in a one- or two-stage exchange. The most successful protocol incorporates standardized antimicrobial therapy with a two-stage surgical procedure: (1) removal of prosthesis and cement and placement of an antibiotic impregnated cement spacer, followed by a 6-week course of bactericidal antibiotic therapy and (2) reimplantation of a new prosthesis using cement impregnated with an antibiotic at the conclusion of the 6-week antibiotic course.[98] Cementless two-stage hip procedures may result in infection rates similar to total hip arthroplasties done with cemented components.[67,113]

Sometimes, surgical intervention is not possible because of a medical or surgical condition or refusal on the part of the affected individual. In such cases, lifelong oral antibiotic treatment may be required to suppress the infection and retain function of the joint. Serial radiographs are needed to monitor progressive bone resorption at the bone–cement interface. In such cases, the localized septic process may still extend into adjacent tissue compartments or become a systemic infection, or the person may develop side effects of chronic antibiotic administration.

PROGNOSIS. Infection associated with prostheses and implants can produce significant morbidity and occasionally death. Early recognition and prompt therapy for infection in any location is critical to reducing the risk of seeding the joint implant hematogenously. Situations likely to cause bacteremia should be avoided.[18]

The American Academy of Orthopedic Surgeons currently recommends routine use of microbial prophylaxis for anyone undergoing joint replacements, while the American Dental Association advises that a single dose of prophylactic antibiotic be given to selected individuals undergoing dental procedures associated with significant bleeding and potential hematologic bacterial contamination.[98] The selected populations include people with inflammatory arthropathies, immunosuppression, diabetes mellitus, malnutrition, hemophilia, or previous prosthetic joint infection and anyone undergoing these dental procedures within 2 years after joint replacement.

Perioperative antibiotic prophylaxis has been shown to reduce deep wound infection effectively in total joint replacement surgery. Cephalosporins continue to be the antibiotic of choice for orthopedic surgeons because of the broad spectrum of activity against the most common pathogens. The antibiotic is given within 60 minutes before the incision is made (120 minutes if vancomycin or a fluoroquinolone is added), and if the procedure is long, another dose is administered during surgery. The medication is then continued for less than 24 hours after surgery.[17] Although only 2% to 3% of prostheses become infected within 10 years after implantation, there is considerable risk of morbidity (e.g., hospitalization, amputation, or disability) and even death.[4]

| SPECIAL IMPLICATIONS FOR THE THERAPIST | 25-2 |

Infections of Prostheses and Implants

Many cases of infection after instrumentation or prosthetic implantation occur months to years after the surgery. In most cases, a distant cause of infection can be identified, but usually no preceding breakdown of the overlying skin occurs to help identify the presence of underlying infection. The therapist may not be aware of existing hardware and must include questions in the interview to elicit this information. A recent history of infection from dental caries, pulmonary or upper respiratory tract, GI tract, or genitourinary tract in such a person requires medical evaluation. Any spontaneous drainage from previous scars or sites of surgery may be a sign of infection and must also be evaluated by a physician.

Anyone with implants of any kind with onset of increasing musculoskeletal symptoms (especially in the area of the surgery) must be screened for the possibility of infection. Normal radiographs and negative needle aspirates can delay medical diagnosis of infection. Knowing the risk factors for developing an antibiotic-resistant infection (e.g., multiple surgical procedures, previous S. aureus infection, or multiple antibiotics) and recognizing red flag symptoms of infection can help the therapist in recognizing the need for persistence in obtaining follow-up medical care.

Breast Implantation
(See also "Breast Reconstruction," Chapter 20.)

Silicone breast implants are medical devices implanted subcutaneously or subpectorally for cosmetic breast augmentation or reconstruction after mastectomy. Postoperative infection can occur in up to 35% of postmastectomy reconstructions and in up to 2.5% of breast augmentation procedures.[116] Factors that increase the risk for infection have not been well studied, but surgical technique and underlying disease appear to be the principal reasons.

Women who undergo reconstruction with placement of implant after mastectomy for cancer are up to 10 times more likely to develop an infection than women receiving cosmetic augmentation. This is often the result of the side effects of chemotherapy and radiation therapy required with surgery.[90,96,116] Two-thirds of infections occur during the acute postsurgical period, whereas one-third appear months to years later. Infections that develop months to years later most likely result from organisms seeded from a distant location.[90,96]

Other complications of breast implants include hematomas, seromas, visible wrinkles or folds, scarring, asymmetry or displacement of the implant, capsular contracture, implant leak or rupture, silicone gel bleed, or prolonged pain of the breast. Implants may interfere with mammography, causing some women to discover breast cancer at later stages. Some studies have shown that silicone devices can prolong wound healing and delay formation of granulation tissue.[90,96]

Although complication with silicone gel–filled implants have been widely discussed, most women with silicone gel–filled breast implants do not experience serious problems; some women have reported symptoms otherwise associated with connective tissue and immune-related disorders.[100] Such symptoms may include joint pain and swelling; skin tightness, redness, or swelling; swollen lymph nodes; unusual and unexplained fatigue; swollen hands and feet; and unusual hair loss.

SPONDYLODISKITIS
Overview and Incidence

Spondylodiskitis is a range of conditions from a self-limiting inflammatory process to a pyogenic infection. The intervertebral disk is the most common site for a spinal infection, with the infection affecting the annulus, nucleus, or the vertebral endplates.

Etiologic and Risk Factors

A bacterial origin is usually the cause of the infection. *S. aureus* is commonly found, but in some cases, no organism can be isolated. *M. tuberculosis* is also detected in disk infections. Children as young as 2 years old can develop diskitis, which may be confused with vertebral osteomyelitis. The origin of the infection in children may be traumatic, but the source of infection is more likely to be the hematogenous spread of a bacterial infection preceding the diskitis, such as in the upper respiratory or urinary tract. Fungal or yeast infections can also lead to spondylodiskitis.[28]

A spondylodiskitis is the most common complication after a diskectomy. The infection may involve the adjacent vertebrae and spread to the disk through the cartilaginous endplates. Other procedures capable of directly inoculating the disk, such as diskography, also carry the risk of infection. Direct inoculation is the only method by which an infection can arise from within the disk. As with children, urinary tract infections as the result of catheterization or cystoscopy may also be the underlying source of disk space infections.

Pathogenesis

If the infection arises within the disk itself, formation of a peridural abscess is not common. However, an infection extending to the disk from the cartilaginous plate can spread to cause an epidural abscess posteriorly or a paravertebral abscess anteriorly.[50] The pathogenesis of infection formation is described in this chapter (see "Pathogenesis" under "Infectious Arthritis" below).

Clinical Manifestations

Diskitis presents in different ways at different ages, but fever and spinal pain are classic symptoms in children. In the very young child, back pain or a refusal to walk and pain with hip extension may be the first symptoms and must be taken seriously. Abdominal pain and weight loss may occur, and the child may not be able to flex the lower back.[19] In children presenting with diskitis the concern is whether the diagnosis is actually vertebral osteomyelitis. Clinically, either condition will result in children refusing to walk, limping, or complaining of back pain. However, those with vertebral osteomyelitis often appear more ill and febrile.[27,41]

In adults, disk infection after spinal procedures usually is noted within a few days, whereas those developing from an infection at a distant site may not be evident for months. Spinal pain will be common and sometimes severe with radiation of the pain into the lower extremities. The lower extremity pain is not usually radicular; instead, it may involve multiple nerve levels. People may present with unusual posture and movement patterns that could be erroneously labeled pain of psychogenic origin. In both children and adults the back pain may range from mild to severe. The client will often report that the pain is made worse with activity and that rest does not relieve the pain.

MEDICAL MANAGEMENT

DIAGNOSIS. Inflammatory markers may be elevated, but often laboratory tests are inconclusive and cultures of blood and disk tissue are negative. Plain radiographs should be taken for anyone suspected of having spinal infection. Disk space narrowing, endplate irregularity, and a loss of lumbar lordosis may be visualized. Bone scans are also used for initial evaluation.[27] However, MRI is essential in providing the differential diagnosis when vertebral osteomyelitis is a possibility; MRI reduces diagnostic delay and may help avoid the requirement for a biopsy.[19,28,41]

In adults, the use of MRI in conjunction with bone scans using gadolinium enhancement has been found to be useful in differentiating normal postoperative disk space changes from those caused by infection. MRI is most useful in determining the extent of the infection and the required duration of oral antibiotic therapy after initial IV antibiotics but less valuable in demonstrating the type of infection (e.g., pyogenic vs. tuberculous). The sclerosis present later in the disease course may be confused with a benign degenerative process or even with metastatic disease. MRI and biopsy may be used to differentiate chronic cases.

TREATMENT. Treatment for the younger person may consist of bed rest, hip spica casting, and bracing. Antibiotics are used but do not appear to radically alter the natural course of the infection in children.[19] In adults, a removable body jacket can be used along with specific or empiric antibiotic therapy. The use of antibiotics prophylactically is common after spinal surgery in adults to prevent this condition from developing. Antifungal agents may first be tried for Candida diskitis. Surgery will be necessary in 10% to 20% of all cases.[28,27]

PROGNOSIS. In both adults and children the prognosis is good, although pain may persist for several months up to several years. In children, long-term follow-up care has shown a resolution of the pain in spite of persistent radiographic changes.[27]

Late radiographic changes in adults include vertebral collapse, kyphosis, and eventually, bony ankylosis, which can take up to 2 years to run its course. Adults can expect similar spontaneous healing to occur, especially in those individuals with a strong immune response.

Complications can arise when the infection spreads or when an abscess forms. An epidural abscess can result in paralysis and is noted in older people, in those who have involvement of the cervical region, and in those with associated medical problems, such as diabetes.

SPECIAL IMPLICATIONS FOR THE THERAPIST   25-3

Diskitis

Because very young children can be affected, diskitis must be considered a possible cause of spinal pain or refusal to bear weight or walk. Because the pain is usually related to activity and increases with weight bearing, it is easy to mistakenly attribute the symptoms to musculoskeletal origins. The presence of hip or back pain of unknown cause, especially after spinal surgery or recent infection, must be evaluated by a physician.

Box 25-2

CAUSATIVE AGENTS OF INFECTIOUS (SEPTIC) ARTHRITIS

Bacterial

- Gonococcal
- Infectious endocarditis
- Lyme disease
- Syphilis
- Tuberculosis

Fungal

- Candida

Viral

- Epstein-Barr virus
- Hepatitis
- Human immunodeficiency virus
- Mumps
- Rubella

Reactive

- Acute rheumatic fever
- Chlamydial infection
- Enteric infection
- Reiter syndrome

Box 25-3

PREDISPOSING FACTORS IN ADULT SEPTIC ARTHRITIS*

- Immunosuppression/immunodeficiency
  - Systemic corticosteroid use
  - Chemotherapy
  - Radiation therapy
  - Human immunodeficiency virus (HIV)
- Preexisting arthritis
- Arthrocentesis
- Diabetes mellitus (poorly controlled)
- Sickle cell disease
- Alcohol or drug abuse
- Trauma
- Other infectious diseases
- Chronic renal failure
- Unknown or none

*More than one factor may exist.
From Esterhai J, Gelb I: Adult septic arthritis, *Orthop Clin North Am* 22:504, 1991.

Box 25-4

INTRODUCTION OF BACTERIAL ARTHRITIS

- Hematogenous spread (via bloodstream)
- Direct inoculation and penetrating injury
  - Penetrating or puncture wound; fracture; human bite
  - Surgery
  - Arthrocentesis
  - Arthroscopy
  - Total joint arthroplasty
- Direct extension
  - Periarticular osteomyelitis
  - Contiguous soft tissue infection, abscess, cellulitis

From Esterhai J, Gelb I: Adult septic arthritis, *Orthop Clin North Am* 22(3):504, 1991.

INFECTIOUS ARTHRITIS

Overview and Incidence

Infectious causes of fever and arthritis can be divided into four groups by causative agent (Box 25-2). This section is confined to the discussion of bacterial arthritis (also called *septic* or *infectious arthritis*), which differs from reactive arthritis (see Chapter 27) in several ways. *Bacterial arthritis* may be a local response with joint destruction and sepsis, whereas *reactive arthritis* is defined as the occurrence of an acute, *aseptic*, and inflammatory arthropathy arising after an infectious process but at a site remote from the primary infection. Some of the other infectious causes of arthritis are discussed in other chapters (see Chapter 8 for Lyme disease and Epstein-Barr virus [EBV], Chapter 12 for rheumatic fever, and see Chapter 7 for HIV).

Etiologic and Risk Factors

Bacteria, viruses, and fungi are all capable of infecting a joint, by invading and inflaming the synovial membrane.[62] *S. aureus, streptococcus pneumoniae, Kingella kingae,* and *Neisseria gonorrhoeae* are the most common organisms responsible for infectious arthritis.[54] Predisposing factors for development of septic arthritis are listed in Box 25-3. Microorganisms can be introduced into the joint by direct inoculation, direct extension, or by hematogenous (through the bloodstream) spread, which is the most common route (Box 25-4). In addition, direct penetrating trauma, joint arthroplasty, and chronic joint damage as seen in diseases, such as rheumatoid arthritis, are also considered to put a joint at risk.[40,43]

The primary risk factor for septic arthritis is a preexisting abnormal joint from rheumatoid or degenerative conditions. A history of alcohol abuse, IV drug abuse, HIV infection, or other infectious disease increases the likelihood of having an infectious joint that becomes septic. Although nongonococcal infectious arthritis can affect individuals across the life span, infants, children, and older adults are at greatest risk.[13] Risk factors for poor outcomes after septic arthritis include delayed diagnosis, onset earlier than 3 months, osteomyelitis, and methicillin-resistive *S. aureus* as the underlying organism.[15]

Pathogenesis

After being directly inoculated into the joint cavity, bacteria rapidly multiply in the liquid culture medium of the synovial fluid and are phagocytosed by synovial lining cells. Bacteria are either killed by the synovial cells or form microabscesses within the synovial membrane. Organisms that reach the synovium through the bloodstream multiply in enlarging microabscesses of the synovium until they break into the articular cavity.

Bacterial products, such as endotoxins and cell wall fragments, stimulate synovial cells to release tumor necrosis factor and interleukin 1. These cytokines up-regulate expression of adhesion ligands in synovial membrane vessel endothelial cells, resulting in leukocyte attachment and migration into synovial fluid and articular tissues. Bacterial fragments form antigen–antibody complexes that activate the classic pathway of complement, and bacterial toxins activate the alternative complement pathway to produce proinflammatory products C3a and C5a (see Chapter 6).

The phagocytosis of bacteria also results in autolysis of neutrophils with release of lysosomal enzymes into the joint, which causes synovial, ligament, and cartilage damage. Cellular immune mechanisms also appear to play a role in acute joint infection. After 48 hours of synovial infection, T lymphocytes infiltrate the synovium, interleukin 6 levels are increased, and B-cell activation results in immunoglobulin G antibody production.

Bacterial toxins also activate the coagulation system, causing intravascular thrombosis in the subsynovial vessels and fibrin deposition on the surface of the synovium and articular cartilage. This layer of fibrin provides a gelatinous nidus for bacterial replication. Microvascular obstruction leads to ischemia and necrosis, further permitting abscess formation, destroying the cartilage matrix.

Finally, after the acute necrotic inflammatory synovitis, the synovial membrane proliferates, forming an inflammatory exudate called *pannus* that erodes articular cartilage of the joint capsule and subchondral bone. All of this can take place in 17 days, quickly destroying a joint in the process. This underscores the need for urgency in detection and intervention in septic arthritis.

A chronic inflammatory synovitis may persist even after antibiotics have eradicated the infection. The threshold for starting empiric therapy with antibiotics for those individuals with acute joint pain and swelling should therefore be low.[36]

Clinical Manifestations

People with infectious arthritis can be any age and can present with an acute onset of joint pain, swelling, tenderness, and loss of motion. Fever, chills, and other systemic symptoms depend on the stage of the illness. Physical examination may reveal the classic signs of infection such as increased temperature of the joint, swelling, redness, and loss of function. Pus may drain outside through a sinus formed from the joint to the outside. Only the severity and the nature of these signs will differentiate the septic joint from more mundane causes such as tendinitis and other noninfectious inflammatory diseases.

A child with a septic joint will often refuse to bear weight on the affected leg or use the affected arm; there may be extreme tenderness to palpation at the joint and along the metaphysis. Destruction of the joints can proceed rapidly and have long-lasting effects with pathologic fracture, growth arrest in children, deformity, and joint dislocation.[21] In addition to the infection, the WBCs that enter the joint to combat the infection release enzymes that have a deleterious effect on articular cartilage. In more severe cases, septic shock, multiorgan disease, pericarditis, or pyelonephritis can develop, especially if diagnosis and treatment have been delayed. Long-term complications of septic arthritis in children include joint instabilities and lower extremity deformities.[105]

In adults, *S. aureus* produces a monarticular sepsis, usually at the hip or knee. In children, the ankle and elbow are also common sites.[54] Although not as common, shoulder septic arthritis and polyarticular involvement have been reported.[15] *Gonococcus* affects mostly women and may produce skin lesions, tenosynovitis, and polyarthralgias, in addition to systemic symptoms. Prosthetic joints are also sites of infection, which is probably introduced at the time of surgery. *S. epidermidis* is often the cause.

In general, the coexistence of fever and the signs and symptoms of an acute exacerbation of arthritis must arouse suspicions of a septic joint and be managed as a medical emergency until proved otherwise.[40,61,64]

MEDICAL MANAGEMENT

DIAGNOSIS. Besides a detailed history and physical examination, the confirmation of the diagnosis is made by analysis of the joint fluid obtained by aspiration. The decision to aspirate the joint, however, is made on the basis of history and physical examination. The method to obtain a sample of the aspirate depends on the joint that is involved. Needle aspiration when possible is often considered the method of choice. Aspiration of the sacroiliac and hip joints is difficult, and may be aided by the use of fluoroscopy (real-time X-ray). Imaging studies such as X-rays, contrast MRI (arthrograms), and ultrasonography may be done before joint aspiration. Decisions on treatment and appropriate antibiotics are aided by the results of cultures, stains, and laboratory studies such as the WBC count, C-reactive protein, and erythrocyte sedimentation rate.[78]

With the development of advanced deoxyribonucleic acid (DNA) analysis techniques, identification of traces of bacterial genomes may eventually make it possible to develop specific vaccines or pharmacologic agents to prevent or treat septic arthritis.

TREATMENT. As already mentioned, any joint infection is considered a medical emergency. Admission to the hospital for treatment with specific IV antibiotics is required. Continued treatment with oral medication for an additional 2 to 3 weeks is standard. The combined use of antibiotics along with corticosteroid medications such as dexamethasone has been shown to produce a chondroprotective response, speed recovery, and reduced hospitalization time.[54,64] Aspiration of the joint is critical. Besides needle aspiration, more aggressive techniques of tidal irrigation, arthroscopy, or arthrotomy may be used depending on the situation.[64] Surgical drainage may be indicated for hip or shoulder joint infections. In prosthetic joints, the infection may require removal of the hardware and cement, along with a more prolonged course of antibiotics.

Early in the course of intervention, the joint should be rested. This may be accomplished by splinting, traction, or casting. Care in application of the splint will preserve function, and the splint should be removed periodically for ROM exercise. The importance of these simple ROM exercises cannot be overlooked because the risk for joint contracture as a complication of immobilization is a concern, especially in the older adult. More vigorous types of exercise and aggressive mobilization activities are performed when signs of infection have resolved.[62]

The aggressiveness of intervention is dictated by the specific organism, the joint involved, duration of symptoms, and the health of the individual. Surgical drainage is often required to preserve function and prevent complications. In some cases, joint instability (e.g., chronic or repeated hip subluxation) may require more extensive surgical intervention.

PROGNOSIS. As for other infectious diseases, prompt treatment is the key to a successful outcome. If treatment is initiated within 5 to 7 days of onset, a good or excellent long-term result can be expected.[72,106] Currently, the mortality rate has dropped considerably for infections caused by nongonococcal agents; however, sequelae in the form of destructive changes in the bone or joint can result in significant functional limitations.

Mortality is higher in the older adult (increases after age 65 years) even with quick and correct interventions.[72] Overall mortality from septic arthritis ranges from 10% to 25%, and permanent joint disability occurs in 25% to 50% of survivors. Septic arthritis of the knee is associated with better outcomes than that of the hip or shoulder.[15,36] The more common complications include osteomyelitis, abscess formation, and permanent loss of joint motion and joint instability. If the infection is not controlled, toxemia and septicemia can cause death. The risk of morbidity and mortality are increased when there are multiple sites of infection and when the individual has multiple comorbidities.

SPECIAL IMPLICATIONS FOR THE THERAPIST 25-4

Infectious Arthritis

Immediate referral of a client with a suspected septic joint to a specialist may save the joint from unnecessary destruction. Being aware of client history, potential risk factors, and assessing for signs and symptoms of infection are essential. Including joint infection in the differential diagnosis of some clients with joint pain may expedite early intervention. This is important because the prognosis is related to the time between onset of symptoms and definitive treatment.

Treatment of hip infections within 4 days of symptomatic presentation can result in preservation of the joint and complete resolution of the infection. However, delayed intervention can result in serious complications leading to total hip replacement.[10] Unfortunately, even with prompt and appropriate intervention, the chance of some degree of joint dysfunction is likely.[21,64]

The age of the client and the previous condition of the joint are also important factors. The older adult, who often has additional joint pathology, such as degenerative joint disease, rheumatoid arthritis, or complications from diabetes, may not recover full function of the joint. The presence of associated joint pathology also tends to confound the diagnosis of sepsis, which further diminishes the chances of a favorable outcome and may result in a significant amount of residual impairment (e.g., contractures or fibrous ankylosis), especially among the aging.[72]

INFECTIOUS (INFLAMMATORY) MUSCLE DISEASE

Myositis

Overview

Myositis is a general term used to describe inflammation of the muscles that can be an autoimmune condition or directly caused by viral, bacterial, and parasitic agents. Infection-induced myositis is most often caused by *S. aureus* and parasites such as trichinella and the tapeworm larva *Taenia solium*.

When affecting skeletal muscle, these infectious agents result in inflammatory changes with sequela, ranging from significant functional losses to a minor self-limiting condition. Autoimmune conditions can be activated or aggravated by infections, which may explain the link between myositis, infections, and autoimmune processes.

The most common forms are dermatomyositis (DM), polymyositis (PM), and inclusion body myositis (IBM) (Box 25-5). DM appears to occur more often in children and older adults. Inflammatory myopathies are discussed further in Chapter 27; PM and DM are included in Chapter 10.

Incidence

IBM is the most common acquired muscle disease in adults over 50 years and often misdiagnosed. Myositis is diagnosed in 1 in 100,000 people a year, although some experts suspect that many cases may go unidentified because it is so often mistaken for the symptoms of aging or in women, depression.[44]

Etiology and Pathogenesis

The primary pathology is from intra–muscle fiber degeneration that leads to muscle fiber destruction and severe weakness.[9] This form is often progressive and debilitating and often does not respond to available treatments.[9,16,39] Inflammation is a major cause of the muscle damage. Numerous drugs may induce myopathies, including cholesterol-lowering statins. Lipid-lowering drugs associated with myotoxicity can cause symptoms ranging in severity from myalgias to rhabdomyolysis, resulting in renal failure and death (discussed in Chapter 27).[11,29,74,80] Myositis caused by parasites is considered a relatively uncommon condition; however, the parasitic infection trichinosis is reported to affect up to 4% of the population.[37]

Myositis can be the first sign of a malignancy. Some experts theorize that the autoimmune rheumatic diseases that occur in people over age 40 years may reflect an anticancer immune response in a large number of people.

Box 25-5

TYPES OF MYOSITIS

- Dermatomyositis (see Chapter 10)
- Polymyositis
- Inclusion body myositis
- Myositis ossificans (see Chapter 27)
- Idiopathic inflammatory myopathies (see Chapter 27)
- Rhabdomyolysis (see Chapter 27)
- Pyomyositis

Studies have quantified the risk, finding that people with DM face a threefold risk of cancer, whereas those individuals with PM face a 40% increase in risk.[47,70] In effect, these people may be cancer survivors without knowing it because the muscle cells are accidentally harmed during the immune system's assault on a tumor.[23,70]

The antigens that produce the immune response are present in normal muscle tissue but at low levels. They are much more prevalent in myositis cells of individuals with autoimmune myositis and in muscle cells that are regenerating such as those that occur after an injury. It is hypothesized that a feed-forward loop occurs when damaged muscle cells start to repair themselves. These cells express higher amounts of the antigens, causing the immune system to respond; the immune response causes further damage to the muscle, which in turn repairs itself, its regenerating cells expressing even more antigens, and continuing the feed-forward cycle.[24]

The IBM form of myositis appears to be autoimmune-mediated by cytotoxic T cells and deposits of amyloid-related proteins. There is a strong association of IBM with human leukocyte antigens (HLA) I and II. IBM tends to develop in individuals with other autoimmune disorders or immunodeficiency.[33,83] A small number of IBM cases may be hereditary (h-IBM) but most are "sporadic" (s-IBM), meaning there is not a direct genetic link.[44]

Clinical Manifestations

The commonly observed symptoms of this family of conditions are as would be expected for any inflammatory process. These nonspecific symptoms include malaise, fever, muscle swelling, pain, tenderness, and lethargy. Specifically, the inflammatory response found in PM and DM is in connective tissue and muscle fibers.

Other than the symptoms associated with these infections, there is a risk of tissue necrosis and extensive muscle tissue damage with atrophy and weakness, especially if left untreated. Other clinical features of myositis are dysphagia, decreased esophageal motility, vasculitis, Raynaud phenomenon, cardiomyopathy, and interstitial pulmonary fibrosis. A purple skin rash and eyelid edema are often associated with DM. The distribution of the rash includes the eyelids, face, chest, and extensor surfaces of the extremities. In adults, subcutaneous calcium deposits are a sign of severe long-term DM.[2]

In most cases, IBM progresses slowly over months or years and is characterized by frequent falling episodes, trouble climbing stairs or standing from a seated position. Drop foot and subsequent tripping may be reported. Weak grip, difficulty swallowing, and muscle atrophy and weakness are often accompanied by functional decline and pain or discomfort secondary to weakness.

MEDICAL MANAGEMENT

DIAGNOSIS. In addition to careful and thorough history, a muscle biopsy is the primary diagnostic tool. Muscle aches and pains associated with a bout of influenza often may actually be a subacute viral myopathy. A differential diagnosis requires muscle biopsy, electromyography, and laboratory values.

The muscle biopsy will make the differentiation between PM, DM, and IBM and exclude other myotonic disease. Electromyography will demonstrate muscle irritability and myopathic changes. Because of the associated release of creatine kinase (CK) into the blood with skeletal muscle damage, this enzyme can be a useful measure of the extent of the infection (see Table 40-13). CK levels are 5 to 10 times higher than normal in PM, but only mildly increased in IBM.[16,81]

TREATMENT AND PROGNOSIS. Aggressive early treatment of any of these conditions will lead to an improved prognosis. Trichinosis can be very successfully treated with pharmacologic agents. The treatment of PM and DM often includes immunosuppressive therapy and corticosteroids. There is no established treatment that improves, arrests, or slows the progression of IBM; it is resistant to treatment with antiinflammatory, immunosuppressant, or immunomodulating agents.[52] Because of the resulting muscle weakness and possible extensive skeletal muscle damage associated with myositis, the client must be prepared for an aggressive and prolonged rehabilitative process.

The role of the physical and occupational therapist should not be underestimated in the attainment of a successful outcome. Submaximal exercise has been shown to be effective, although eccentric or intense exercise is not recommended.[16,58,81]

Other clinical trials are testing new drugs to add to the arsenal of corticosteroids, immunosuppressants, and IV immunoglobulin, a plasma product. Scientists are conducting trials of rituximab, an artificial antibody used to treat certain types of cancer; infliximab, which blocks the effect of tumor necrosis factor, which is a protein associated with inflammation; and etanercept, which blocks tumor necrosis factor alpha, also involved in inflammation.[2]

For people with PM and DM, existing medications work well, although many of the drugs have serious side effects and may cease being effective over time.

SPECIAL IMPLICATIONS FOR THE THERAPIST 25-5

Myositis

Muscle pain and weakness in anyone at risk for myositis and especially for individuals taking lipid-lowering statins should be a red flag for the therapist. Underlying neuromuscular diseases may become clinically apparent during statin therapy and may predispose the individual to myotoxicity.[11] Exercise may be an additional risk factor for the symptomatic presentation of myotoxicity.[5] The alert therapist will recognize this potential condition and make an appropriate medical referral sooner rather than later.

Infections of Bursae and Tendons

Overview and Incidence

Acute infections affecting the bursae and tendons are uncommon and must be treated appropriately to avoid complications. The hand is very susceptible to scratches, bites, and subsequent infections. Hand infection can range from cellulitis to tenosynovitis. Because of the superficial nature of these tissues and the potential for dysfunction, hand infections are given special attention in this section.

Etiologic and Risk Factors

The bursae and tendons that lie close to the skin surface are most susceptible to infection from direct contact with microorganisms. Trauma to the elbow and knee is common, especially in sports such as wrestling. Anaerobic bacteria are more commonly seen in wounds from bites and in people with diabetes. The bacteria enter the body by direct inoculation through a local skin abrasion or with common procedures such as a cortisone injection into the inflamed bursae. *S. aureus* is the most common organism isolated and may cause up to 80% of infections.

Hand infections often develop from untreated injuries. Up to 60% of hand infections are related to trauma, 25% are caused by human bites, and 10% are a result of animal bites.[73] As with all infections, people with diabetes or who are immunocompromised have a greater risk of developing an infection in the hand. In addition, the risk of osteomyelitis is also of concern because of the proximity of bone.[68]

Pathogenesis

Infection in the hand can spread along synovial sheaths, fascial planes, and via lymphatic channels. Bursae are lined with a membrane similar to synovium and are therefore subject to the same pathologic processes, namely, inflammatory conditions caused by acute or chronic infections. (See "Pathogenesis" under "Infectious Arthritis" below.)

Clinical Manifestations

The olecranon and prepatellar bursae can be sites of localized infection. An olecranon bursal infection will cause pain, loss of function, and swelling, which may be accompanied by cellulitis. Infections of other bursae, such as the prepatellar and subdeltoid bursae, have similar presentations.[117]

Tendon sheaths of the extremities can also become infected. As mentioned earlier, the hand is a common site because of its susceptibility to minor trauma. The anatomy of the hand determines the nature and presentation of the infection. For example, the tendon sheaths of the thumb and small finger extend proximally to the wrist, whereas the sheaths of the index, long, and ring fingers stop at the proximal pulley.

An infection of the flexor tendon of the thumb could rapidly spread to the small finger. Common signs associated with an infectious tenosynovitis include a finger maintained in slight flexion; fusiform (spindle-shaped) swelling; pain on extension (passive or active); and tenderness along the tendon sheath into the palm.

MEDICAL MANAGEMENT

DIAGNOSIS,TREATMENT, AND PROGNOSIS. In most joints, examination will identify a localized swelling, not a joint effusion. Aspiration of fluid for laboratory analysis is performed before treatment. The use of antibiotics is often adequate, but surgical incision and drainage are

sometimes required; occasionally, bursectomy is required. Prompt treatment with drainage, irrigation, and antibiotics is crucial.

Appropriate treatment of hand infections is based on an accurate identification by culture of the organism causing the infection. In addition to the appropriate antibiotic, the hand is immobilized and elevated, and often, surgical drainage is necessary. Necrotic tissue is cautiously debrided, and the wound is left open to drain.[77]

Early and aggressive rehabilitation is essential, especially for a structure as complicated and integrated as the hand. Both physical and occupational therapists may play a role in this process. Given the potential complications of surgery and immobilization and the potential for tissue loss, a comprehensive rehabilitation program is necessary to maximize function.

SPECIAL IMPLICATIONS FOR THE THERAPIST 25-6

Infections of Bursae and Tendons

Treatment of hand injuries has developed into a subspecialty, and rightfully so, not only for the orthopedic surgeon but also for the therapist. Clients recovering from infection and surgery must be monitored carefully, and their treatment should be adjusted often. Splinting of the hand is an important feature throughout the course of treatment.

Early immobilization must be done with eventual recovery and function in mind. The wrist should be placed in 30 to 50 degrees of extension, the metacarpophalangeal joints in 75 to 90 degrees of flexion, and the interphalangeal joints in full extension. Active ROM exercise is initiated early, as soon as the infection begins to subside and treatment appears to be successful, which is often within 48 hours.

Prognosis depends on the extent of the infection and how soon treatment was initiated. Delayed intervention usually requires more extensive surgical debridement, an increased chance of scar tissue formation, the need for possible skin grafts, and a prolonged rehabilitation to maximize function.

EXTRAPULMONARY TUBERCULOSIS

TB is an acute or chronic infection caused by *M. tuberculosis* that can affect multiple organ systems via lymphatic and hematogenous spread during the initial pulmonary infection (see Chapter 15). Disseminated or miliary TB involves not only the lungs but also most other organ systems. Systems involved may include the pulmonary, genitourinary, musculoskeletal, and lymphatic. Of these, the lymphatic system is most commonly involved in immunocompromised hosts such as those with HIV.

Extrapulmonary TB is more difficult to diagnose and treat than pulmonary TB. This is due in part to clinicians' lack of familiarity with the condition. In addition, extrapulmonary TB is often in inaccessible areas, which makes aspiration or biopsy, and therefore diagnosis, more difficult. Also, smaller numbers of bacilli can cause extensive damage to joints but are harder to detect. TB involving the bone is usually transferred hematogenously from some other organ, usually the lung. Only one-fourth of people with skeletal TB have a known history of TB.[103]

Skeletal Tuberculosis

Overview and Incidence

Because skeletal TB is relatively uncommon, delays in diagnosis are frequent. After a 40-year decline, the incidence of TB has increased over the past several decades. The World Health Organization (WHO) estimates that more than 8 million new cases of TB occur annually and approximately 3 million individuals die from TB and associated complications every year.[3] More than 15 million people in the United States are estimated to be infected with TB. This increase is due in part to the presence of acquired immune deficiency syndrome (AIDS). The causes for this change in number of active cases of TB are discussed at length in Chapter 15. Although TB is found in all 50 states, New York, California, and Hawaii have had the highest incidence. Skeletal TB is uncommon, but infection rates have held constant over the years. From 10% to 15% of TB is extrapulmonary, and only 10% of extrapulmonary TB is skeletal.

Pathogenesis and Clinical Manifestations

Extrapulmonary TB is spread hematogenously from other organs. In adults, the onset of skeletal TB is insidious, developing 2 to 3 years after the primary infection. Early signs and symptoms include pain and stiffness; the pain may be localized or referred. The lower thoracic and lumbar spine is commonly involved (Pott disease), but other sites (e.g., weight-bearing joints or elbows) have been reported.[32] Systemic signs, such as fever, chills, weight loss, and fatigue, are not common in the early phase. Joint effusion often occurs with TB arthritis and has been shown to affect muscles and nerves around the joint.[118]

In the case of spine involvement (occurring 5% in the cervical spine, 25% in the thoracic spine, and 20% in the lumbar and lumbosacral spine), infection begins in the cancellous bone of the vertebral body and eventually spreads to the intervertebral disk and adjacent vertebrae. As the disease progresses, nerve root irritation, pressure from abscess, and collapse of the vertebral body will cause a progressive increase in pain and protective spasm with cord compression and possible paraplegia.[82,97] The abscess may extend from the lumbar region to the psoas muscle, producing hip pain (see Figs. 16-13 and 16-14).

MEDICAL MANAGEMENT

DIAGNOSIS. Early diagnosis is very helpful in preserving articular cartilage and the joint space but is often delayed for several months to years after the initial presentation because there are no symptoms pathognomonic of extrapulmonary TB. Treatment may be delayed because symptoms are consistent with chronic sciatica, when the true cause of the radiating pain is tuberculous sacroiliitis with an anterior synovial cyst.[26]

Conventional radiographs and bone scans are important in the initial detection, and computed tomography (CT) and MRI can assist in further evaluation.

Confirmation of skeletal TB requires microbiologic assessment with smear and culture. In the spine, this confirmation can be accomplished with fine-needle aspiration. Tissue biopsy is more often required for extrapulmonary disease.[76]

TREATMENT AND PROGNOSIS. Treatment does not differ for pulmonary and extrapulmonary TB. Although surgical debridement is sometimes necessary, usually pharmacologic treatment is sufficient. (See Chapter 15 for discussion of medical management of TB.) Chemotherapy is the mainstay in the management of TB spondylitis, but decompressive surgery may be required in the presence of Pott paraplegia.[60,82]

Rehabilitation after surgery for TB of the spine or extremities follows standard orthopedic principles. Medical intervention and subsequent rehabilitation are individualized based on the extent of the infection. Surgical treatment of joint infection may include arthrotomy, synovectomy, and treatment of articular erosions.

Extraarticular infections can sometimes be treated with curettage and bone grafting. For more advanced infections, resection of bones and joints, arthrodesis, and limb salvage or amputation may be indicated. Factors to be considered include the affected bone, extent of surgical excision, and involvement of soft tissue, articular cartilage, or bone. Weight bearing is often limited, but active movement is often encouraged.

In the spine, surgery is more often needed to address nerve compression or deformity secondary to collapse of the vertebral body rather than the infection. The resultant deformity often includes a marked kyphotic curve with a gibbus formation (Fig. 25-5). Paralysis can be a serious complication of vertebral TB and can be a result of the disease process or a secondary spinal deformity. Paralysis persisting longer than 6 months is unlikely to improve, and late paralysis with inactive disease and significant kyphosis is much less responsive to treatment.[82]

In the joint, if TB is diagnosed early when the infection is confined to the synovium, rest, medication, and joint protection may be adequate. In advanced disease with caseation, fibrosis, and scarring, the vascularity is reduced (Fig. 25-6), which makes medications less effective. Surgical excision or curettage of the affected areas may be necessary. In joints, the granulomatous tissue acts to separate the articular cartilage from the underlying bone.

SPECIAL IMPLICATIONS FOR THE THERAPIST 25-7

Extrapulmonary and Skeletal Tuberculosis

Extrapulmonary (skeletal) TB is not often seen in a physical therapy practice but can present as arthritis or other musculoskeletal manifestations of unknown cause. Anyone with this type of clinical presentation with a compromised immune system, especially HIV/AIDS; past or recent release from incarceration; a history of immigration to the United States from an area where TB is endemic; or any other risk factor for TB listed in Chapter 15 should be screened for medical disease.

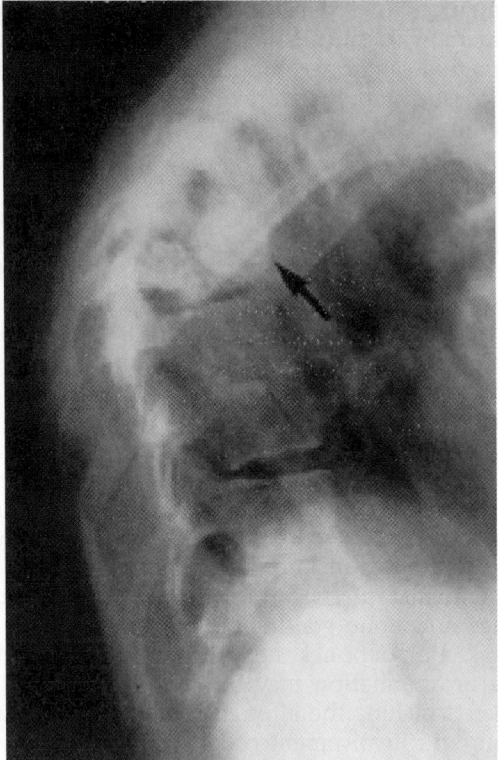

Figure 25-5

Tuberculous spondylitis. Involvement at multiple levels. Gibbus deformity is seen in the upper thoracic region *(arrow)*. (From Yao D, Sartoris D: Musculoskeletal tuberculosis, *Radiol Clin North Am* 33:681, 1995.)

Therapists may provide treatment to clients with pulmonary TB that involves postural drainage and percussion to remove secretions from the lung. Care must be taken with clients' sputum. All health care professionals must be aware of the risk to themselves of contracting or spreading to others the infection when working with people who have TB. This is equally important for extrapulmonary TB. (See Box 15-4 and "Pulmonary Tuberculosis" in Chapter 15, including "Special Implications for the Therapist 15-5: Pulmonary Tuberculosis.") Although it is thought that once the client is started on appropriate medical therapy the risk of transmission decreases in as little as 2 weeks, there are types of drug-resistant TB that may be infectious for longer periods.

In addition to the obvious orthopedic concerns that will evolve during the treatment of skeletal TB, therapists should be aware of psychosocial issues that may develop. Clients undergoing long-term treatment for infectious diseases will undoubtedly have some difficulties in managing their disease.

Chronic pain, repeated hospitalizations, frequent setbacks, fear of long-term disability, and loss of independence may all contribute to a number of abnormal, but expected, illness behaviors. A multidisciplinary team that includes physical and occupational therapists, psychologists, community health nurses, and others will be useful in achieving functional goals.

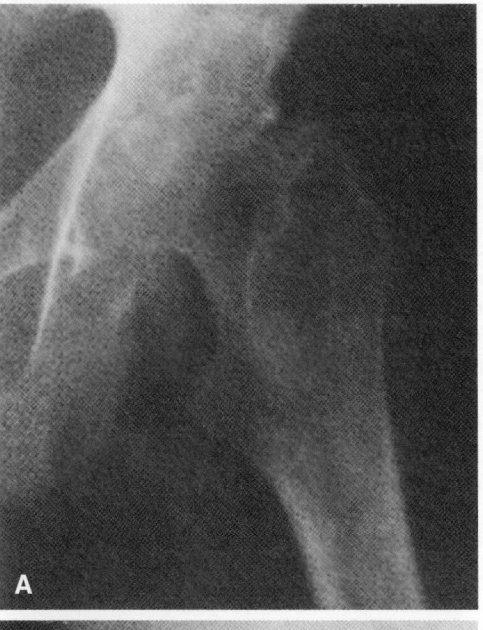

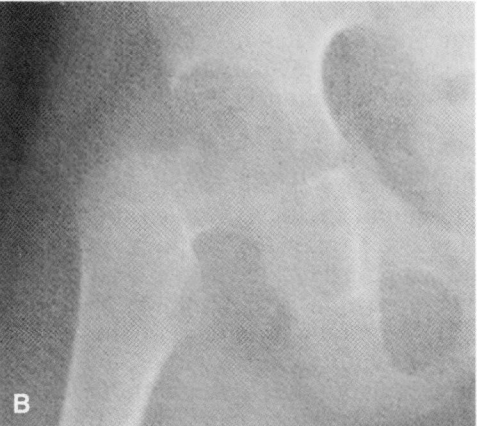

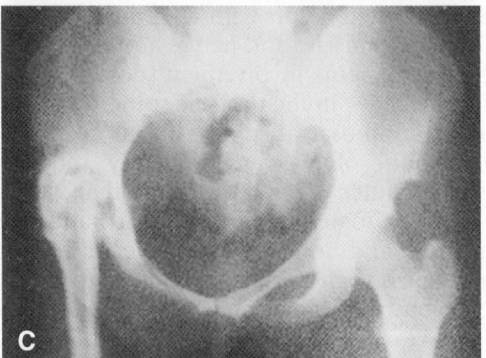

Figure 25-6

Tuberculous arthritis. A, Bony erosion of acetabulum and femoral head with joint space loss. There also is evidence of periarticular osteopenia. **B,** Similar findings to **A** but with further destruction of the femoral head and acetabulum. **C,** Advanced TB of the hip with superior displacement and ankylosis of the right hip joint. (From Yao D, Sartoris D: Musculoskeletal tuberculosis, *Radiol Clin North Am* 33:687, 1995.)

SUMMARY OF SPECIAL IMPLICATIONS FOR THE THERAPIST

Rehabilitation after medical interventions for infectious diseases must proceed in a comprehensive and coordinated fashion. The pathology of each type of infectious disease process and the medical decisions made for treatment will have some bearing on the rehabilitation plan. The patient's goals and expectations, general health and potential for repair of the affected bone and structures must be considered in the rehabilitation plan.

The hip joint is commonly affected and has been alluded to in several chapters as a site of infectious processes of many origins and will be used here again to illustrate some factors that should be considered in planning rehabilitation. The client and therapist may be anxious for an exercise program to begin, but this must be done in concert with medical treatment and consideration of the stage of recovery.

Early in the course of intervention, rest and protection of healing tissues will be the primary objective. All health care providers must be made aware of the potentially adverse effects of apparently simple movements. For example, using a bedpan and performing isometric exercises produce acetabular contact pressure close to that of walking.[59] Therefore, clinicians should not assume that a client who is on bed rest is not producing elevated joint compressive forces. Clients must be instructed in proper methods of moving, transferring, and positioning themselves.

Active ROM exercise is often the first type of supervised exercise permitted. These movements must be done while noting limits set by pain, spasm, or apprehension. Active hip flexion has been found to increase acetabular contact pressure similar to that of full weight bearing.[104] However, passive ROM exercise has been found to have a beneficial effect on healing joints.[45,94] Restoring full ROM may not be as realistic or as necessary as obtaining the ROM required to restore function.

Continuous passive ROM is a means of early mobilization in a postoperative rehabilitation regimen that may improve early motion and decrease postoperative pain. Continuous passive ROM has not been found to have no long-term benefit for regaining function compared with daily standardized exercises and has not been shown to prevent deep vein thrombosis.[14,55,57]

Once the client is ambulatory, his or her weight-bearing status must be determined and monitored. This will depend on the type of infection, surgical procedure, stage of recovery, and extent of joint destruction. Articular cartilage heals very slowly, and the cartilage on weight-bearing surfaces should be protected from undue compressive or shear forces. In addition, immobilization has deleterious effects on articular cartilage and other periarticular tissue[1] (see "Cartilage Injury and Healing" in Chapter 6 and Table 6-7).

Exercise after prolonged immobilization should take these factors into consideration. Often, a non–weight-bearing status is used with the intention of minimally loading the joint. In fact, the compressive forces may actually increase when compared with those of a touch-down, weight-bearing gait pattern.[91] Other factors, such as the weight of the limb and muscular contraction, must be considered. Long-term use of an ambulatory aid may be indicated for as long as a 2- to 3-year period.[49] The use of a cane in the contralateral hand can reduce weight-bearing forces by up to 15%.[38,99]

REFERENCES

To enhance this text and add value for the reader, all references are included on the companion Evolve site that accompanies this textbook. The reader can view the reference source and access it online whenever possible.

CHAPTER 26

Musculoskeletal Neoplasms

KEVIN HELGESON

Neoplasm is defined as a new or abnormal growth of cells and is often used interchangeably with *tumor*, which means any swelling or mass. Neoplasms are divided into two broad categories: benign and malignant. Benign neoplasms show no tendency to metastasize, are noninvasive, and are usually slow growing. A malignant neoplasm is one that can be invasive or can metastasize (see further discussion, Chapter 9).

Although neoplasms represent a small portion of the spectrum of pathology seen in clinics, their severity and potential for serious consequences necessitate an understanding of their detection and treatment.

The purpose of this chapter is to review the characteristics of primary and secondary musculoskeletal neoplasms. Those that may be encountered by therapists are highlighted. It is hoped that by increasing awareness of the clinical manifestations, earlier detection will be possible.

PRIMARY TUMORS

Overview

Description

Primary musculoskeletal tumors are those that have developed from or within tissue in a localized area. Primary musculoskeletal neoplasms can be benign or malignant, soft tissue or bone. A soft tissue tumor may originate from muscle, cartilage, nerve, collagen, adipose, lymph or blood vessel, or skin (see Table 9-1). Common sites in the body and location within the bone vary depending on the type of tumor (Table 26-1; Fig. 26-1).

Modern classification of soft tissue tumors recognizes more than 200 benign and approximately 70 malignant (sarcomatous) lesions with a ratio of benign tumors to malignant sarcomas of 100 : 1. The focus of this chapter will remain on the most common bone and soft tissue tumors encountered in the physical therapist's practice.

Other soft or connective tissue tumors (e.g., skin, heart, myeloma, lymphatic, hematologic, neurologic) are discussed elsewhere in this text. An excellent comparison of soft tissue sarcomas in adults and children, including rehabilitation, is available elsewhere.[4,71] A review of solid bone cancers occurring during adulthood and the implications for physical therapy is also available.[51]

Benign Neoplasm

Benign tumors are well differentiated, resemble normal tissue, rarely invade locally, and have low potential for autonomous growth. However, benign does not necessarily mean innocuous. For example, osteoblastomas in the spine may produce serious neurologic problems requiring resection, with additional complications possible from the surgical procedure.

Some benign bone tumors pose difficult evaluation and management decisions and can result in a significant level of impairment. For example, large fibrous defects in weight-bearing bones can cause pathologic fractures. A *pathologic fracture* refers to bone that has been weakened by local destruction (osteoclastic resorption) from any cause; bone with this type of impairment is more readily fractured than normal bone. This complication is referred to as a *pathologic fracture* because it occurs through an area of abnormal or pathologic bone.

Although rare, some benign lesions can develop into a malignancy. Benign lesions usually do not cause the constant, severe pain that is commonly associated with progressive malignant disease, but benign tumors can impair blood supply or compress nerve tissue.

Malignant Neoplasm

Malignant primary tumors of bone by definition have the capacity to spread to other sites and often do so aggressively by invading locally and destroying adjacent tissues and by metastasizing to distant sites. Skeletal neoplasms often metastasize to the lungs through the bloodstream.

Fortunately, malignant tumors are not as common as benign lesions; however, this rarity has made it difficult to standardize treatment interventions and management. For this reason, most individuals with malignant primary tumors are referred to regional centers, where valuable experience concerning evaluation and treatment can be gained and then applied to future cases.

Incidence

Primary tumors of the musculoskeletal system are uncommon, although the incidence is difficult to determine because these lesions often escape diagnosis (Table 26-2). Excluding myeloma and skin cancer, as few as 2400 new cases of primary bone tumors and 9200 cases of soft

Table 26-1	Classification of Soft Tissue and Bone Tumors

Tissue of Origin	Benign Tumor	Malignant Tumor
Connective Tissue		
Fibrous	Fibroma	Fibrosarcoma
		Malignant fibrous histiocytoma
Cartilage	Chondroma	Chondrosarcoma
	Enchondroma	
	Chondroblastoma	
	Osteochondroma	
Bone (osteogenic)	Osteoma; osteoblastoma (giant osteoid osteoma)	Osteosarcoma (osteogenic sarcoma)
Bone marrow (myelogenic)		Leukemia
		Multiple myeloma
		Ewing sarcoma
		Hodgkin lymphoma of bone
Adipose (fat)	Lipoma	Liposarcoma
Synovium	Ganglion, giant cell of tendon sheath	Synovial sarcoma
Muscle		
Smooth muscle	Leiomyoma	Leiomyosarcoma (uterus, gastrointestinal system)
Striated muscle	Rhabdomyoma	Rhabdomyosarcoma (can occur anywhere)
Endothelium (Vascular/Lymphatic)		
Lymph vessels	Lymphangioma	Lymphangiosarcoma
		Kaposi sarcoma
		Lymphosarcoma (lymphoma)
Blood vessels (angiogenic)	Angioma	Angiosarcoma
	Hemangioma	Hemangiosarcoma
Neural Tissue		
Nerve fibers and sheaths	Neurofibroma	Neurofibrosarcoma
	Neuroma	Neurogenic sarcoma (also known as neurosarcoma or schwannoma)
	Neurinoma (neurilemmoma)	
Glial tissue	Gliosis	Glioma
Epithelium		
Skin and mucous membrane	Papilloma	Squamous cell carcinoma
	Polyp	Basal cell carcinoma
Glandular epithelium	Adenoma	Adenocarcinoma

tissue sarcomas are detected annually in the United States with a 3 : 1 ratio of men to women affected.[149] This does not mean that they are unimportant. A great deal of time is devoted to research, reporting, and educating physicians in the proper management of people with primary tumors. These efforts are indicative of the serious nature of the problem rather than the frequency.

Risk Factors

Little progress has been made in our knowledge of the risk factors involved in the etiopathogenesis of malignant bone tumors. Although bone tumors may have a predilection for certain sites, age groups, and gender, most causes of osteosarcoma are unknown. The main factors implicated are Paget disease, Li-Fraumeni syndrome, antineoplastic drugs, ionizing radiation, and hereditary retinoblastoma.[54]

Exposure to alkylating chemotherapeutic agents such as cyclophosphamide, used in the treatment of acute lymphocytic leukemia, has been associated with subsequent development of osteosarcoma in a small percentage of cases.

Several genetic conditions are related to the development of soft tissue sarcoma (e.g., neurofibromatosis, tuberous sclerosis, basal cell nevus syndrome), but this is only a small number of cases.[174] Soft tissue tumors also may be associated with high doses of radiation or exposure to toxic chemicals in the workplace (herbicides, dioxin, preservatives, and so on).

A very small number of periprosthetic malignancies have been reported, most commonly malignant fibrous histiocytoma associated with joint replacements. Increases in sarcomas have been observed in animals presumably linked with metallic ions (debris) from metal implant materials such as cobalt, chromium, titanium, and nickel. A causal relationship between metal joint implants and carcinogenicity in humans remains under investigation.[49]

Etiologic Factors and Pathogenesis

The histogenesis of tumors is generally poorly understood, although significant progress has been made toward understanding tumor development as a biologic phenomenon. For a detailed description of the

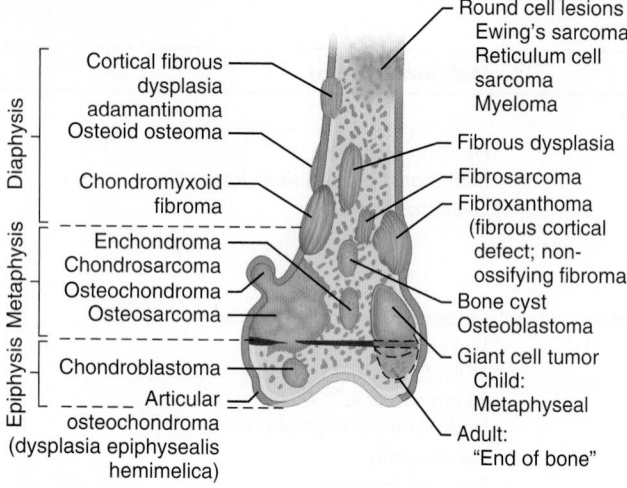

Figure 26-1

Composite diagram illustrating frequent sites of bone tumors. The diagram depicts the end of a long bone that has been divided into the epiphysis, metaphysis, and diaphysis. The *epiphysis* refers to the articular end of the long bones, which is primarily cartilaginous in the growing child. The *metaphysis* is the wider part of the shaft of the long bone. The *diaphysis* refers to the shaft itself. The typical sites of common primary bone tumors are labeled. (From Madewell JE, Ragsdale BD, Sweet DE: Radiologic and pathologic analysis of solitary bone lesions: I. Internal margins, *Radiol Clin North Am* 19:715, 1981.)

Table 26-2	Relative Frequency of Primary Bone Tumors*
Benign	
Osteochondroma	35% of benign tumors; 10% of all bone tumors
Osteoid osteoma	10%–12% of benign bone tumors
Enchondroma	10% of benign bone tumors; some report as high as 24%
Osteoblastoma	1%–2% of benign bone tumors
Chondroblastoma	<1% of all bone tumors
Hemangioma	<1% of all bone tumors
Malignant	
Metastatic neoplasm	Most common form of bone malignancy; *secondary* neoplasm of bone
Multiple myeloma	Most common *primary* neoplasm of bone; plasma cell malignancy (bone marrow)
Osteosarcoma	Most common form of primary bone tumor; 35% of all malignant bone tumors; 15%–20% of primary sarcomas (excluding multiple myeloma)
Chondrosarcoma	25% of malignant bone tumors (excluding multiple myeloma)
Ewing sarcoma	16% of malignant bone tumors; second most common in children; fourth overall *primary* bone tumor for adults and children (after myeloma)
Malignant fibrous histiocytoma	2%–5% of malignant bone tumors (excluding multiple myeloma)
Chordoma	1%–4% of all malignant tumors; slow-growing but locally aggressive
Angiosarcoma	14% of malignant bone tumors (excluding multiple myeloma)

*Listed by decreasing order of frequency; with the exception of metastatic neoplasm listed, these statistics refer to primary bone tumors. Primary neoplasms of the skeleton are rare, amounting to only 0.2% of the overall primary bone tumors.
Data from:
Dorfman HD, Czerniak B: Bone cancers, *Cancer* 75:203–10, 1995.
Zhang PJ: *Essentials in bone and soft tissue pathology,* New York, 2010, Springer.
Sundaresan N: Primary malignant tumors of the spine, *Orthop Clin North Am* 40(1): 21-36, 2009.
Fletcher C: *Pathology and genetics of tumours of soft tissue and bone,* ed 4, Geneva, 2013, World Health Organization.
International Association [IARC]/World Health Organization [WHO]: WHO Classification of Bone Tumours (2006). Available online at http://www.iarc.fr/en/publications/pdfs-online/pat-gen/bb5/bb5-classifbone.pdf [Accessed October 8, 2012].

molecular biology of bone formation, apoptosis and its role in bone cancer, and molecular and oncogenetic concepts of bone neoplasia, the reader is referred to other sources.[87,176]

Bone Tumors. To grasp the concepts of tumor formation, one must understand that bone metabolism is a balancing act of bone formation and resorption. The coupling of these two processes usually results in a balance of bone resorption and formation. When metabolic bone disease and neoplastic formations occur, this balance is upset.

Under normal circumstances, bone remodeling involves a fine balance between osteoblast activity, which promotes new bone synthesis, and osteoclasts, which stimulate bone resorption. This balance is disrupted by the presence of malignant cells, resulting in uncoupling of the process of remodeling.

Bone remodeling is a structured process governed by highly specialized cells. Osteoblasts are derived from mesenchymal fibroblast-like cells and are responsible for bone formation. Bone formation is accomplished by synthesizing various collagens, alkaline phosphatase, and other chemicals. A variety of paracrine factors, including tumor necrosis factor alpha, tumor necrosis factor beta, interleukin-1, and prostaglandins are released during the remodeling process and may ultimately contribute to growth of the metastatic cells.[81]

Cortical bone is most abundant in the outer walls of the shafts of long bones and is quite dense. The haversian canal system, which refers to the concentric rings of lamellae, is found in cortical bone. Cortical bone surrounds the trabecular or cancellous bone, which is the honeycomb-like bone found in the ends of long bones. Trabeculae are aligned with applied stresses in the bone. The metabolic activity is higher in cancellous bone than cortical bone, which accounts for why many disorders that create disturbances in metabolic activity are first noted in cancellous bone.

Bone tumors are considered to be either osteoblastic or osteolytic, although most have characteristics of both processes. The osteoblastic process can be preceded by tumor cells or by normal cells in the host bone reacting to the tumor. Because the host bone continues with the normal process of resorption and bone formation, there will likely be a variety of cell types within the lesion. This makes histologic interpretation difficult.

Neoplastic cells do not themselves destroy bone, but their presence incites local osteoclastic resorption of bone. The cells of certain neoplasms also incite local osteoblastic deposition of normal bone, referred to as reactive bone. The neoplastic cells of the osteogenic group of neoplasms are capable of producing osteoid (young bone that has not undergone calcification) and bone, which are then referred to as tumor bone or neoplastic bone. The radiographic appearance of lesions affecting bone reflects varying proportions of bone resorption (osteolysis) and bone deposition (osteosclerosis)—some of the latter being reactive bone, and some being neoplastic bone.[87]

Soft Tissue Tumors. Four types of genetic disorders underlying soft tissue sarcomas have been identified: translocations, gene amplifications, mutations, and complex genetic imbalances. Detection of these molecular changes can guide treatment and may predict response to treatment. Techniques used to detect translocations are very sensitive and in some cases may be used to detect microscopic metastasis.[21]

Soft tissue sarcomas have a predictable growth pattern, beginning as small masses and often growing in a centripetal pattern. The leading edge of the tumor (reactive zone) contains edema, fibrous tissue, inflammatory cells, and tumor cells. Uncontrolled growth often causes loss of blood supply at the center of the tumor.

Benign soft tissue tumors also have a centripetal growth pattern, but the expansion is more controlled and much slower. Benign lesions tend to be more superficially located compared with malignant lesions, which often grow within tissues under the deep fascia.[68,159] Soft tissue tumors found in the abdomen tend to be larger in size and result in poorer outcomes than those in the extremities.[27]

Clinical Manifestations

The clinical features must be well understood to ensure that the diagnostic evaluation proceeds expeditiously. Unfortunately, many tumors are not diagnosed on their initial presentation. This is due to the ambiguous presentation of most tumors in their early stages; rarely does one actually find the case that is described as typical for a given lesion. This may be true regarding benign or malignant tumors, the initial presentation, and the appearance of the lesion.

Pain. Pain is a hallmark of tumor development, especially with malignant lesions. With bone tumors, intense pain is more likely to occur with rapidly growing lesions caused by pressure or tension on the sensitive periosteum and endosteum. Constant pain that is not dependent on position or activity and is increased with weight-bearing activities is a red flag symptom. The presence of night pain is considered an additional important finding. When the client reports night pain, further questioning is required.

The therapist should ensure that the client is reporting true night pain, which awakens the person from sleep, rather than a pain that makes it difficult to fall asleep. Ask the individual if rolling onto the involved side or painful area awakens him or her. Ascertain whether the pain subsides with movement and change in position, possibly indicating mechanical ischemia or positioning as the cause of the night pain. Determine the effects of eating on pain, as this may be an indicator of gastrointestinal (GI) involvement.

It is also important to remember the common referral patterns for pain. These may give important clues to the origin of symptoms. The varied pain pattern is a result of the nature, site, and rate of growth of the tumor.

Because pain is the overriding symptom in many people who seek treatment, a great deal of information should be obtained concerning the pain. The onset, progression, nature, quality, intensity, and aggravating factors are just some of the factors that may be important in identifying a tumor in the early stages.[147]

Keep in mind that with cancer, pain is not always a measure of disease progression. Some tumors can progress to advanced stages without causing significant pain. Soft tissue tumors can occur in any anatomic region, although most develop in the extremities, usually the legs. These tumors may progress with relatively little pain because the soft tissue allows the growth to occur without putting undue pressure on nerve endings. Any swelling present is often attributed to a minor injury, delaying medical examination.

In fact, clients often report a recent history of trauma, although no scientific evidence directly connects such injury to the inception of soft tissue or bone sarcomas. Instead, such traumatic episodes are thought to call attention to a specific body part or location, thereby increasing the likelihood of detecting an otherwise painless and often innocuous soft tissue mass or bone lesion.[174]

Fractures. Pathologic fractures are rare in primary neoplasms, but if the lytic process affects a significant portion of the cortex (over 50%) or occupies 60% of the bone diameter, the risk of fracture increases. A relatively small lytic lesion in the femoral neck that destroys the inferior cortex of the femoral neck also places the client at increased risk. In benign lesions, no other symptoms may warn of the impending fracture.

A history of sudden onset of severe pain may be an indication of a pathologic fracture. Solitary bone cysts, fibrous dysplasia, nonossifying fibroma, and enchondromas may only be detected after presentation with a pathologic fracture. In addition to the tumor itself, other factors such as disuse, treatment (biopsy, radiation), and other health problems (osteoporosis) may increase the risk of pathologic fracture.[175]

Miscellaneous. Other signs and symptoms often encountered include swelling, fever, and the presence of a mass. Other factors that are useful in screening for serious pathology include unexplained weight loss, failure of rest to provide relief of pain, age, and history of cancer. The history will often give more meaningful information regarding the possibility of skeletal neoplasms than the physical examination.

Swelling. Swelling surrounding a tumor may not be detectable in a bone tumor, but with soft tissue tumors close to the skin surface, swelling may be one of the first presenting signs. The nature of swelling, including the location, amount, temperature, and tenderness, is somewhat dependent on the vascularity of the lesion.

Mass. A careful physical examination may reveal a mass or other signs of an inflammatory process. The presence of a mass should raise questions concerning the location, mobility, tenderness, dimensions, and recent changes in any of these factors. As with pain, the size of the mass is not indicative of the severity of the lesion but is one factor to consider. Any change in size, appearance, or other characteristics of a lump, local swelling, or lesion of any kind within the previous 6 weeks to 6 months should be reported to the physician.

Metastases. Sarcomas spread by hematogenous routes rather than through the lymphatics. The most common site of metastases for individuals with extremity sarcomas is the lung, followed by liver and other bone sites. Anyone diagnosed with soft tissue sarcoma has an approximately 50% chance of local recurrence, because these tumors spread along tissue planes and involve adjacent tissue. Lymph node involvement is uncommon and is often associated with poor prognosis.[85,166]

MEDICAL MANAGEMENT

DIAGNOSIS. Physical examination, imaging studies (e.g., x-rays, computed tomography [CT], magnetic resonance imaging [MRI]), and biopsy are the primary diagnostic tools.

Physical Examination. Many tumors cannot be observed or palpated during the physical examination, but if a mass is present its characteristics must be noted. The presence of café au lait spots (associated with neurofibromatosis), skin ulceration, or neurologic findings (e.g., footdrop, calf pain) may be significant.

Because synovial sarcoma, rhabdomyosarcoma, and epithelioid sarcoma can metastasize via the lymphatics, examination of the lymph nodes is essential.[89] A tumor overlying bone and muscle can be evaluated by contracting the muscle and checking for movement or change in consistency of the tumor.

Radiographic Examination. Radiographs also help differentiate between bone and soft tissue involvement. Plain radiographs are a mainstay in the detection and evaluation of many skeletal tumors.[17] In many cases, skeletal tumors are found incidentally on routine radiographs for associated injuries. The radiograph provides unique information concerning skeletal tumors. MRI has emerged as the most useful imaging tool for evaluating soft tissue tumors, although biopsy is essential for a definitive histologic diagnosis.

The location of the tumor will give many clues to the type of lesion (see Fig. 26-1). Some tumors develop exclusively in the epiphysis, whereas others develop in the diaphysis of long bones. Bone tumors tend to predominate in those ends of long bones that undergo the greatest growth and remodeling and hence have the greatest number of cells and amount of cell activity (shoulder and knee regions).

When small tumors, presumably detected early, are analyzed, preferential sites of tumor origin become apparent within each bone, as shown in Fig. 26-1. This suggests a relationship between the type of tumor and the anatomic site affected. In general, a tumor of a given cell type arises in the field in which the homologous normal cells are most active. These regional variations

suggest that the composition of the tumor is affected or may be determined by the metabolic field in which it arises.

The effect that the tumor has on bone is described as destructive or lytic if the normal bone pattern is disrupted (Fig. 26-2). Approximately 50% of the bone must be destroyed before the lesion can be detected. This may be evident by an irregular, erosive border surrounding the lesion; loss of trabeculae; or disruption of the cortex.[110]

The response of surrounding bone to the tumor is another important feature to note on plain radiographs. Sclerotic borders give an indication of the growth characteristics of the tumor. A well-defined border with definite sclerotic margins is seen with a slow-growing lesion.

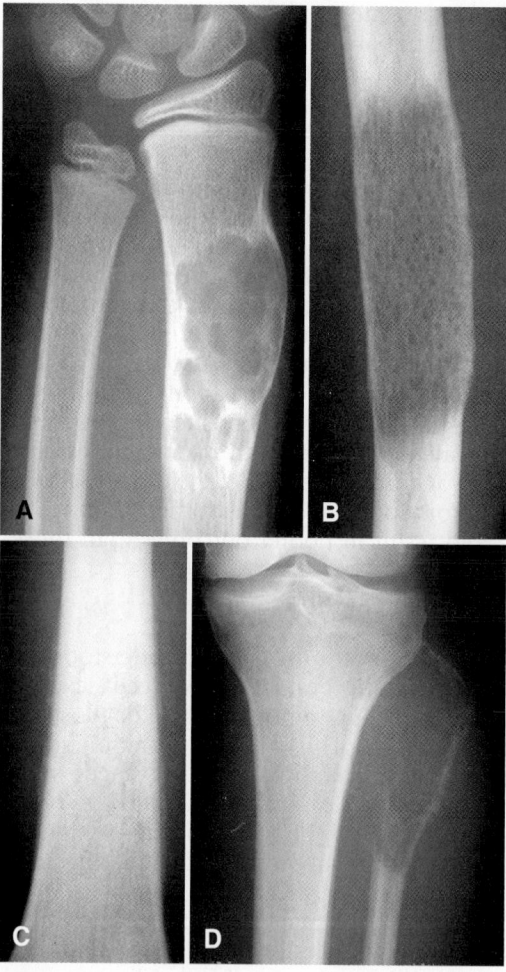

Figure 26-2

Patterns of bone destruction. A, AP radiograph of the distal radius in a patient with nonossifying fibroma (NOF), demonstrating the sharp, "geographic" margin indicating slow growth. Endosteal scalloping and bone expansion with an intact overlying cortex are additional features of slow growth. **B,** AP radiograph of the humerus showing a "motheaten" appearance caused by the coalescence of multiple small lytic areas in a patient with renal carcinoma metastasis. **C,** AP radiograph of the distal femur showing a "permeative" pattern of bone destruction in a patient with primary bone lymphoma. **D,** AP radiograph of the fibula showing a lytic lesion with expansion and destruction of the cortex indicating an aggressive growth pattern. *AP,* anteroposterior. (From Adam A: *Grainger & Allison's diagnostic radiology,* Philadelphia, 2008, Churchill Livingstone.)

A tumor with a permeated or moth-eaten appearance (i.e., an area with multiple holes with irregular edges randomly distributed) with an expansive cortical shell indicates an aggressive malignant lesion. Codman's triangle, a triangular-shaped area of reactive bone, is formed when the neoplasm has eroded the cortex, elevating the periosteum and producing reactive bone in the angle where it is still attached (Fig. 26-3).

The tumor's location, its effect on bone, and the local bone response to the lesion are just some of the radiographic features to be noted and will help in planning the rest of the evaluation.

Imaging. Radionuclide bone scan (scintigraphy), CT, MRI, angiography, and ultrasonography all have a place in the evaluation of bone lesions. *Bone scans* help locate skip metastases and the presence of bone metastases as well as metastatic bone lesions, and they assess tumor activity by the amount of radioisotope uptake in and around the tumor. Greater uptake indicates a more aggressive and malignant tumor. *CT scans* will allow for good visualization of the tumor's location, matrix and the surrounding tissues responses to the tumor. CT is also good for detecting pulmonary metastases. *MRI* is more valuable for determining the extent of the marrow involvement and soft tissue masses outside the bone.[1,50] The surgical team uses the information provided by an MRI to help visualize the involvement of the tumor and to plan limb salvage techniques.

Angiography plays an important role when limb-sparing surgery is being considered by providing information regarding the neovascularity of the tumor and mapping the vascular anatomy. *Ultrasonography* is a noninvasive imaging method that can be used to determine the size and consistency of a soft tissue mass and the need for other imaging studies. It may be used to establish intraarterial access for subsequent chemotherapy.[84]

Biopsy. A biopsy is the definitive diagnostic procedure in both bone and soft tissue tumors and is usually performed after physical examination and imaging. This procedure can take many forms. The decision to do an open or incisional, core needle or fine-needle biopsy, or excisional biopsy is based on the location and type of tumor.

Laboratory Tests. Various laboratory studies are used to detect, diagnose, and differentiate musculoskeletal neoplasms. Laboratory tests that may be of value include the complete blood count, urinalysis, erythrocyte sedimentation rate (elevated in Ewing sarcoma), serum calcium (elevated in metastatic bone disease), phosphorus (decreased with "brown tumors" associated with hyperthyroidism), alkaline phosphatase (elevated in osteosarcoma and Paget disease), and serum protein electrophoresis (abnormal in metastatic bone disease).

Serum levels of alkaline phosphatase and calcium are often elevated with metastatic disease. Elevated alkaline phosphatase and lactic dehydrogenase also occur with osteosarcoma (see Table 40-5).

STAGING AND GRADING. The purpose of much of the extensive workup once a tumor is identified is to determine the grade and stage of the tumor. Grading determines the histologic characteristics, such as the extent of anaplasia or differentiation of the cells from grade I, indicating cells that are very differentiated, to grade IV, those that are undifferentiated.

Staging of a tumor is concerned with the extent of its growth, both local and distant. The tumor-node-metastasis staging system (see Box 9-1) reflects the degree of local extension at the primary tumor site, involvement of local nodes, and presence of metastasis. This classification group is strongly correlated with survival.

The relative rarity of soft-tissue sarcomas, the anatomic heterogeneity of these lesions, and the presence of more than 30 recognized histologic subtypes of variable grade have made it difficult to establish a functional system that can accurately stage all forms of this disease.[172] The staging system of the AJCC and the UICC, now in its seventh edition (2010), is the most widely employed staging classification for soft-tissue sarcomas.[131] Staging helps in planning and standardizing the intervention strategy for these rare lesions. Outcomes do not always correspond

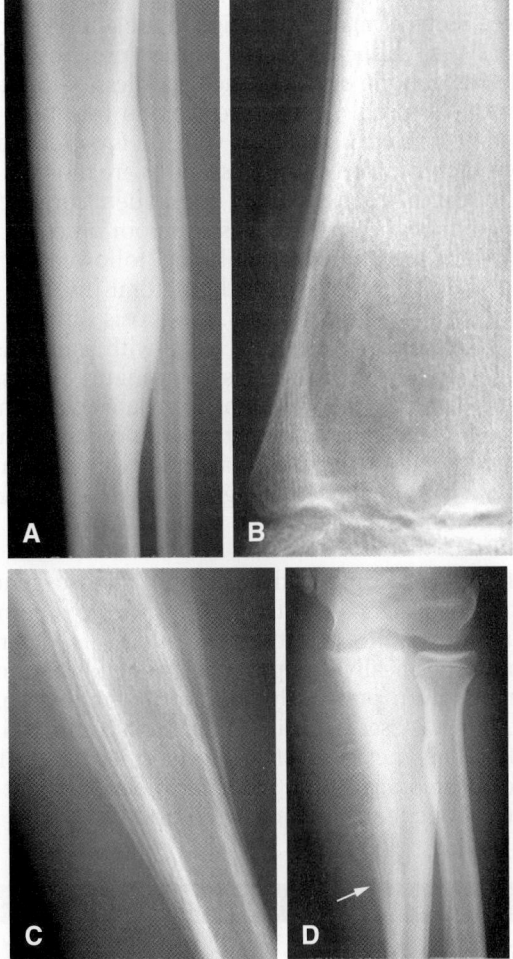

Figure 26-3

Patterns of periosteal reaction. A, Lateral radiograph of the tibia showing a solid periosteal reaction due to osteoid osteoma. **B,** AP radiograph of the distal tibia showing a single, laminated periosteal reaction associated with a Brodie abscess. **C,** AP radiograph of the humerus showing a multilaminated periosteal reaction associated with Ewing sarcoma. **D,** AP radiograph of the proximal ulna showing a "hair-on-end" type vertical periosteal reaction associated with Ewing sarcoma. Note also the Codman triangle *(arrow)*. (From Adam A: *Grainger & Allison's diagnostic radiology*, Philadelphia, 2008, Churchill Livingstone.)

to grades, and some tumors are "ungradable." Diagnosis and grading are increasingly based on tissue obtained by core needle biopsy, which presents its own challenges.[44]

TREATMENT. Once a tumor has been identified and staged, decisions about management and intervention can be considered. Treatment ranges from *observation* in the case of some benign bone tumors to *surgical intervention*. Principles of treatment are similar for some of the malignant bone tumors such as Ewing sarcoma and osteosarcoma. Chemotherapy or surgery alone cures few people. Multimodal measures are needed for a long-term successful response.[6]

Complete tumor resection is the best surgical strategy and is attempted whenever possible. A marginal excision removes the tumor at its border, resulting in some of the tumor remaining. A wide excision (sometimes referred to as an en bloc incision) removes some of the normal surrounding tissue, leaving none of the tumor. Soft tissue sarcomas often require wide excision to reduce the recurrence rate. Radical resection may be required in which the entire involved bone and all the tissue compartments adjacent to the tumor are removed.

The spine, sacrum, pelvis, ankle, hand, mediastinum, and chest wall are just a few examples of bone cancer locations that make surgery difficult. When local excision has positive margins (not all the cancer was removed), local control may be increased with radiation and chemotherapy regimens. Immunotherapy and biotherapy are additional treatment methods used to prevent cancer recurrence.[6]

Limb salvage or limb-sparing procedures have largely replaced amputation as the principal method to eradicate primary sarcomas. The three phases to any limb-sparing procedure are (1) resection of the tumor, (2) reconstruction of the skeletal area involved, and (3) soft tissue and muscle transfer to complete the reconstruction.

Obtaining a wide surgical margin while preserving limb viability and function remains the challenge to the medical team, requiring close coordination of surgical, medical, and oncologic staff. Often, soft tissue reconstruction is necessary to provide wound coverage after tumor removal.

The use of *radiation* is recommended for some tumors such as Ewing sarcoma and myeloma, but many malignant tumors are not affected by radiation. For some soft tissue tumors, adjunctive radiation is used in an attempt to limit the degree of surgical excision needed. In general, radiation is not recommended for benign conditions. Irradiation creates a suboptimal tissue bed susceptible to wound breakdown, seroma, and hematoma formation and infection, which may complicate the success of soft tissue reconstruction.[174]

Because hematogenous spread occurs early in musculoskeletal tumors, *chemotherapy* is also used to help eradicate malignant tumors. For example, combination chemotherapy has resulted in increased survival rates in clients with Ewing sarcoma and rhabdomyosarcoma as well. When chemotherapy is combined with other modalities such as surgery and radiation, less toxic doses can be used.[117]

Future improvements in treatment may come about as a clearer understanding of cellular and molecular pathways of pathogenesis is elucidated. The development of less toxic, more specific therapies remains an important challenge. Newer strategies under investigation include stem cell transplantation, gene therapy, biotherapy such as biologic response modifiers, antibody targeting of immunotoxins to tumor cells, and vaccines designed to elicit T-cell immunity with specificity for tumor peptides.

As discussed in Chapter 9, modern clinical oncology is moving toward tailored therapy according to genetic profiling. Treatment can be stratified with different intensities prescribed based on the genetic characteristics of the individual cancer. Individuals with a poor prognosis may do better with aggressive therapies such as stem cell transplantation for an improved cure rate. Gene silencing techniques may make it possible for the development of specific drugs that will target malignant cells without causing damage to normal tissue.[11]

PROGNOSIS. The prognosis is based in part on the type of tumor and whether it is benign or malignant. Survival is influenced by the grade of malignancy, tumor stage, and achieved surgical margins. A high grade and evidence of metastasis are associated with a poor prognosis for all neoplasms of bone or soft tissue regardless of the staging system that is used.[129] Tumor extension into both anterior and posterior columns of a vertebra is correlated with a poor outcome. Incomplete resections are more likely to result in tumor recurrence with subsequent surgeries and increased risk for complications and poor outcome.[178]

Slow-growing tumors should be followed for prolonged periods, to determine the natural history and to identify the ultimate prognosis. Prognosis can vary from 3- to 5-year survival rates for clients with sarcomas and myeloma, to tumors that are asymptomatic. Successfully treated individuals may develop severe late effects, including second cancers (e.g., radiation-induced sarcomas or treatment-related leukemia), particularly after high-dose therapy with an alkylating agent, and chemotherapy-induced cardiomyopathy.[9]

RECURRENCE. People with recurrent disease generally have a poor prognosis but need to undergo a complete reevaluation of the extent of the disease to determine this more specifically. The prognosis depends on the type of therapy given previously, duration of remission, and extent of metastases. The lung is the most common initial site of distant metastases for the majority of soft tissue and bone sarcomas. Other sites may include distant osseous sites, bone marrow, and lymph nodes.

SPECIAL IMPLICATIONS FOR THE THERAPIST 26-1

Primary Tumors

Screening Assessment

A therapist's involvement with clients with musculoskeletal neoplasms should begin with increased efforts directed toward early detection and education. Although many musculoskeletal tumors produce symptoms that are also present with more mundane conditions, careful examination and monitoring of a client's response to intervention may lead to earlier detection and treatment.

Assessing for past history of cancer, family history, and risk factors may alert the therapist to the need to screen further for medical disease. This is especially true in the case of musculoskeletal symptoms of unknown cause or when the individual does not respond to physical therapy intervention as expected for a musculoskeletal problem.

The presence of suspicious lymph nodes or aberrant soft tissue masses can be identified by the therapist but must be further evaluated by a physician. By including the possibility of a primary musculoskeletal tumor in the differential diagnosis of clients who have continued pain despite appropriate rest and treatment, further medical evaluation may be recommended, which may help reveal other pathology.

Rehabilitation

An achievable goal for the majority of people with soft tissue and bone sarcomas is freedom from disease with long-term resumption of nearly normal function. Therapists are key to the successful attainment of this goal for individuals who are undergoing treatment for primary musculoskeletal neoplasms. A comprehensive approach should be used to ensure that both psychosocial-spiritual aspects and physical problems are addressed.[66] Occupational status, family structure, and age are all important factors.[71]

Communication among the team members such as social workers, rehabilitation counselors, physicians, nurses, and therapists cannot be overemphasized. Communication is essential to coordination and follow-through in the treatment and rehabilitation program. A detailed approach to evaluation and treatment of clients with cancer should be formulated.[66]

Therapists must understand the pathology of the tumor to understand the entire management plan. Specific interventions and goals can be developed with a thorough understanding of the pathology and the medical treatment being undertaken.

Early postoperative mobilization is essential to prevent complications such as pressure ulcers, deep venous thrombosis, lymphedema, pneumonia, muscle wasting, and generalized weakness associated with prolonged bed rest. Surgical procedures will have an effect on multiple organ systems, as will chemotherapy and radiation therapy. A detailed assessment and description of pain is always indicated, as described in Chapter 9, because pain control is a critical component in successful acute rehabilitation.

Many other factors to consider before implementing a treatment plan following orthopedic procedures include controlling compressive forces and weight bearing. Wolf's law demonstrates bone strength to increase in response to imposed mechanical stress, such as the pulling force of muscles and the pressures of weight bearing. When bone resorption exceeds bone formation, osteopenia develops.

After excision of cancerous bone (sometimes accompanied by muscle resection), mechanical weakening and resultant bone instability may limit or contraindicate weight bearing and use of the involved extremity.[51] Remaining muscles should be strengthened and

substitution patterns of muscle control implemented and encouraged where necessary.[71]

Other considerations in the rehabilitative process may include rehabilitation for the amputee, evaluation of adaptive equipment needs, ambulation devices, use of orthoses to support involved extremities, wound care management, environmental adaptations (e.g., access ramps, accessible doorways, bathroom grab bars), work site modifications, and quality-of-life issues. Client education is essential regarding proper body mechanics, energy conservation, side effects of treatment (see Chapter 9), and prevention and recognition of complications such as infection (see Box 8-1), deep vein thrombosis (see Chapter 12), skin breakdown (see Chapter 10), lymphedema (see Chapter 13), scar formation, and the loss of flexibility, strength, balance, or endurance.

Prescriptive Exercise

As discussed, treatment of tumors can result in amputation (sometimes as extensive as a hemipelvectomy[19]), prolonged immobilization, bone or muscle resection, or extensive surgical reconstruction, all of which require consideration of postoperative complications (e.g., ischemia, infection) and the involvement of many different types of rehabilitation.

An individualized program of exercise that takes into account the diagnosis, underlying pathology, physical condition of the individual, effects of various interventions, strength deficits, structural instability, and so on is essential. Toward this end, the therapist should be aware that studies are underway concerning the long-term effects of prosthetic knee replacement after wide resection, risk factors for prosthetic failure, and the most effective rehabilitative strategies after limb salvage procedures for bone tumors. Limb-sparing techniques (instead of amputation and/or disarticulation) such as the endoprosthetic replacement (distal femoral replacement with rotating hinge device; expandable for pediatric population) continue to undergo modification and refinement. Surgeons are attempting to minimize muscle resection, maintain mechanical function, and successfully reattach the muscles to the endoprostheses or to surrounding soft tissue structures, thereby reducing functional impairment.[59,78]

Rehabilitation techniques for these clients remain conjectural. Despite loss of range of motion (ROM) and muscle power, most clients report good limb function (depending on their definition of "good"). Early gait training and weight bearing with active assisted range are indicated, and isometric exercises about the joint are recommended.[71]

General principles regarding energy conservation (see Box 9-4) and exercise for the person with cancer, especially following chemotherapy or radiotherapy, are discussed in Chapter 9. Additionally, the therapist must keep in mind safety guidelines for the use of laboratory values as discussed in Chapter 40 (see Tables 40-8 and 40-9) and "Special Implications for the Therapist 26-9: Metastatic Tumors" below.

PRIMARY BENIGN BONE TUMORS

Bone Island

Overview and Incidence

Bone islands also known as enostoses (singular: enostosis) are oval, usually small, sclerotic lesions of bone. They are one of the most common benign bone lesions. Bone islands have been observed in all bones and may present as solitary or multiple lesions. The lesion is well defined and made up of cortical bone with a well-developed haversian canal system.[133] The borders blend in with the surrounding bone. The presence of spicules of cortical bone extending from the margins to the surrounding trabeculae is characteristic.

True frequency of these lesions remains unknown, but the estimated prevalence of bone islands of the pelvic bone is about 1%. In the spine, enostoses may be apparent in 1% to 14% of persons.[134] Bone islands are seen in both men and women and in all age groups, with perhaps a lower frequency in children. Any osseous site can be affected, but the lesions have a predilection for the pelvis, proximal femur, and ribs.[135]

Clinical Manifestations

Bone islands do not usually cause any symptoms although there have been isolated reports of mild arthralgias and/or skin lesions.[133] They are seen on radiographs as incidental findings.

MEDICAL MANAGEMENT

When the bone islands are small (less than 1 cm), diagnosis with plain radiographs is adequate. They are usually oblong and align themselves with the axis of the bone. A bone scan is usually normal, confirming the absence of malignancy.[69] The emphasis is not on intervention but on the judicious use of diagnostic tools. Biopsies should be avoided, as they are usually unnecessary. Although some bone islands can enlarge, they do not transform into malignant lesions.

| SPECIAL IMPLICATIONS FOR THE THERAPIST | 26-2 |

Bone Islands

Bone islands are seen in radiographs of clients with a variety of musculoskeletal traumas. If clients are aware of these lesions, they should be reassured that they pose no significant health concern. Many physicians do not inform clients that bone islands are present. Care must be taken not to alarm the client. The word *tumor* is foreboding and should be used sparingly.

Osteoid Osteoma

Overview, Incidence, and Etiologic Factors

Osteoid osteoma is a rare benign vascular osteoblastic lesion. The lesion usually presents as a osteoid nidus within loose vascular tissues found in the cortex of long bones such as the femur and tibia. Spine and pelvis may also be affected but osteoid osteomas can occur in

almost any bone except the skull. The tumors occur near the end of the diaphysis (Fig. 26-4). Tumors in the hip acetabulum have been reported but are rare.[143] Osteoid osteoma accounts for about 10% to 12% of benign bone tumors.[94,135] Most of these lesions are found in men under the age of 25. The cause of osteoid osteoma remains unknown.

Pathogenesis

Pathologic study shows areas of immature bone surrounded by prominent osteoblasts and osteoclasts. The lesion is vascular, but no cartilage is present. Osteoid osteoma is probably a "reactive" bone-forming lesion rather than a true neoplasm, consisting of a small, round nidus (nest) of osteoid tissue surrounded by reactive bone sclerosis. Soft tissue and bone changes are caused by local secretion of prostaglandins by the tumor.

The zone of sclerosis is not an integral part of the tumor and represents a secondary reversible change that

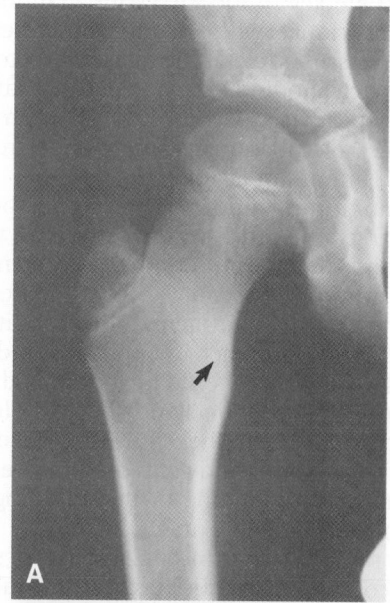

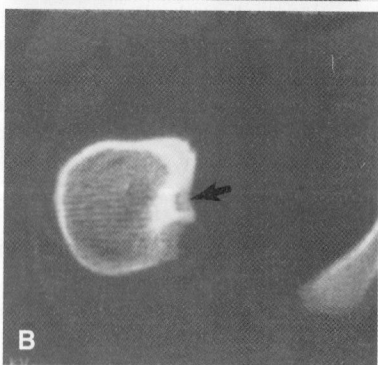

Figure 26-4

Osteoid osteoma. A, Bony sclerosis with cortical thickening is seen in this person with pain in the proximal femur. A faint lucency *(arrow)* can be seen in the area of sclerosis, which is the nidus of an osteoid osteoma. **B,** A computed tomographic (CT) scan through the nidus shows it to lie just dorsal to the lesser trochanter *(arrow)*. This is a characteristic appearance of an osteoid osteoma with CT. (From Helms C: *Fundamentals of skeletal radiology: benign cystic lesions,* Philadelphia, 1989, WB Saunders.)

gradually disappears after the removal of the nidus. Osteoid osteomas are not progressive and rarely grow larger than 1 cm in diameter. They are uncalcified and therefore radiolucent.

Clinical Manifestations

Gradually increasing and persistent local pain in the area of the tumor, described as a dull ache progressing to intense pain, is the primary complaint. The pain is often worse during rest and at night and is characteristically relieved by aspirin and other nonsteroidal anti-inflammatory drugs (NSAIDs). Pain relief may be due to the inhibitory effect on prostaglandins produced by osteoid osteomas. Systemic symptoms are uncommon with normal blood and chemistry tests. Left untreated, an osteoid osteoma can be symptomatic over a 2- to 3-year period, followed by a recovery period lasting 3 to 7 years needed for ossification of the osteoid nidus.[94]

When the lesion is located near a joint, synovial effusion may develop and interfere with joint function, with local muscle atrophy developing.[92] A significant leg length discrepancy can occur, caused by the increased growth rate of affected bone in young individuals with open growth plates.

Though they occur rarely in the spine, if present, they are found in the lower thoracic or lumbar spine located in the posterior vertebral arch. The tumor can lead to joint pain and dysfunction, often delaying the diagnosis by masquerading as a more common problem such as an overuse syndrome.[124]

Spine involvement may result in an unexplained backache or painful type of scoliosis with unilateral spasticity of spinal muscles. Some people with vertebral lesions may have clinical symptoms suggestive of a neurologic disorder, lumbar disc disease, or both.[45] In the case of spine involvement, neurologic deficits can be caused by extradural compression.[124]

MEDICAL MANAGEMENT

DIAGNOSIS. Radiographs can be diagnostic for osteoid osteoma, although these are often normal early in the course. Later, a small (less than 1 cm) translucency or nidus forms, surrounded by sclerotic bone. Lesions in the cortex of the bone may appear with a reactive sclerosis that will make visualization of the lucent nidus difficult.[94] When the tumor is not easily identified on radiographs (e.g., vertebral nidus), further testing is required, such as a bone scan (scintigraphy), which will show a focal uptake of the radiotracer. Plain films may not be adequate when the tumor is intraarticular; in such cases, CT or MRI can be used to accurately locate the nidus. The use of percutaneous needle biopsy will confirm only half of the cases.

TREATMENT AND PROGNOSIS. Initial treatment of this condition is to control symptoms with use of aspirin or NSAIDs with most people having some relief of symptoms. Follow-up radiographs at 3 to 6 month intervals will determine if the nidus is growing or starting to show signs of recovery. Osteoid osteomas have no potential for malignant transformation.[177]

Because this condition is primarily found in young men wanting active lifestyles, most will choose a surgical excision of the nidus. Surgical excisions can be performed with an en bloc resection if the lesion is found in a long bone; otherwise, an unroofing and curettage method will be used in order to preserve the bone tissue surrounding the nidus. A surgical excision is usually a curative treatment for an osteoid osteoma, with the incidence of a recurrence being rare. Lesions that are found in the spine or near joint surfaces can be treated with use of percutaneous needle excisions guided with use of a CT scan or radionuclides. Radiofrequency or laser ablation can also be used for difficult to localize lesions. These treatments have a one-third rate of incomplete resection and greater potential for persistent symptoms and recurrence of the osteoma.[94]

SPECIAL IMPLICATIONS FOR THE THERAPIST | 26-3

Osteoid Osteoma

The size and extent of the resection may mandate some activity restrictions or weight-bearing limitations if the risk of fracture exists. Monitoring bone healing with serial radiographs may help guide the weight-bearing progression. Intraarticular lesions certainly require more extensive rehabilitation for restoration of normal function.

Osteoblastoma

Overview

Osteoblastoma is another reactive but benign bone lesion similar to osteoid osteoma, only larger, with a tendency to expand. Some aggressive forms of osteoblastoma have been recognized. Unlike osteoid osteoma, osteoblastomas are often found in the spine, sacrum, and flat bones. Osteoblastomas involve the spine in approximately 35% of affected individuals, with the cervical spine affected in up to 39% of those people (Fig. 26-5).[25]

Those found in the long bones are usually in the diaphysis, although as with most tumors, they can be seen elsewhere (Fig. 26-6). The histologic makeup of osteoblastoma is very similar to that of an osteoid osteoma. In fact, sometimes it is size alone that differentiates the two, with osteoblastoma being the larger. The lesions are osteolytic and have a sclerotic border.

Incidence

Osteoblastoma occurs most often in men less than 30 years old, but cases have been reported in children as young as 2 years old and adults in their seventies.[177] Osteoblastoma is a rare osteoblastic tumor that makes up only 1% to 2% of all benign bone tumors.

Clinical Manifestations

A dull aching pain that is poorly localized is a common presentation for an osteoblastoma.[145] In general, the pain of osteoblastoma is not as severe as with osteoid osteoma, and will not be relieved with nonsteroidal antiinflammatory drugs. Larger tumors will become tender to palpation and symptoms will be more localized to the diaphysis of the bone or pedicles of the spine. Spinal tumors may result in a functional scoliosis and produce neurologic deficits due to nerve compressions. Metastases and even death have been reported with the aggressive variant, which can behave in a fashion similar to that of osteosarcoma.

MEDICAL MANAGEMENT

DIAGNOSIS. Osteoblastoma is seen on plain radiographs, but when it is located in the spine, other imaging techniques are also useful.[12] The lesion can have variations in its appearance. Often it looks like a large osteoid osteoma with a well-defined radiolucency in the central portion and a thin, sclerotic border. It also can be similar to an aneurysmal bone cyst that is expansile, lytic, and has a soap bubble appearance (see Fig. 26-3). CT and MRI are valuable in localizing the tumor and determining the extent of tissue involved. An aggressive lesion can expand beyond the cortex and involve soft tissue.

TREATMENT. In the long bones, curettage (scraping to remove the contents of the bone cavity) is often adequate. A wider excision is sometimes recommended because of the unpredictable nature of osteoblastoma and high recurrence rate (up to 15%). Recurrence is often attributed to incomplete resection.

Extramarginal excisions can result in the need to perform reconstructive procedures using autografts or allografts and internal fixation when the tumor is located in the diaphysis of long bones. If the joint is affected, implants may be needed. In the spine, removal of the tumor may lead to instability, which may require fusion and internal fixation.

In the cervical spine, their presence so close to neurovascular structures (e.g., vital blood vessels and the spinal cord) makes treatment of this problem very complex. Embolization (either partial or complete) may be done first before surgery. Embolization is a nonsurgical, minimally invasive procedure using metal sponges or other devices to purposefully block blood flow. Surgery to remove the tumor is then done within 24 hours of the embolization. When necessary, bone defect filling and instrumented fusion may be done.[41]

PROGNOSIS. Ninety percent to 95% of osteoblastomas are cured by the initial treatment,[10] but even with careful removal of the tumors, they recur in about 10% to 20% of affected individuals.[16] There is a risk of malignant transformation into an osteosarcoma, which can sometimes be determined early. Appropriate intervention with adjunctive chemotherapy or radiation is the current standard of care. Embolization before marginal resection may reduce the rate of recurrence.[41]

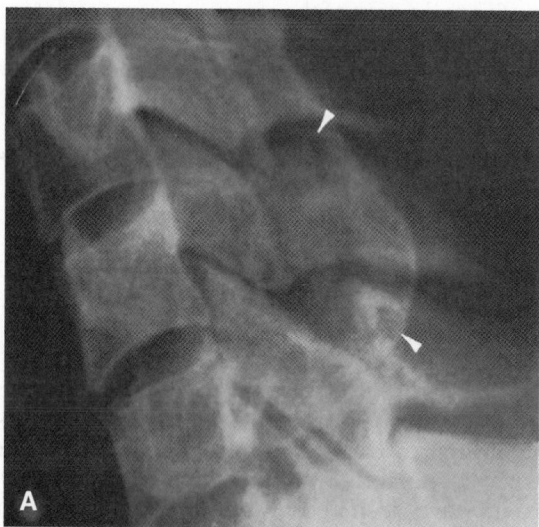

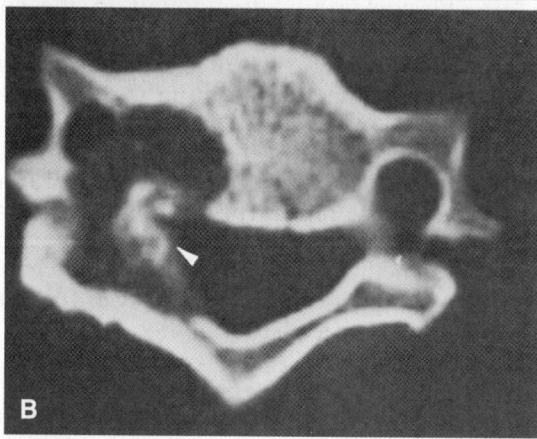

Figure 26-5

Osteoblastoma: spine. Two different examples are shown. **A,** An expansile lesion *(arrowheads)* in the lamina of the fifth cervical vertebra is evident. **B,** Note an osteolytic lesion containing calcification or ossification *(arrowhead)* affecting the body, transverse and costal elements, and lamina of a cervical vertebra as depicted on a transaxial CT scan. (From Resnick D: *Bone and joint imaging,* ed 3, Philadelphia, 2005, Saunders.)

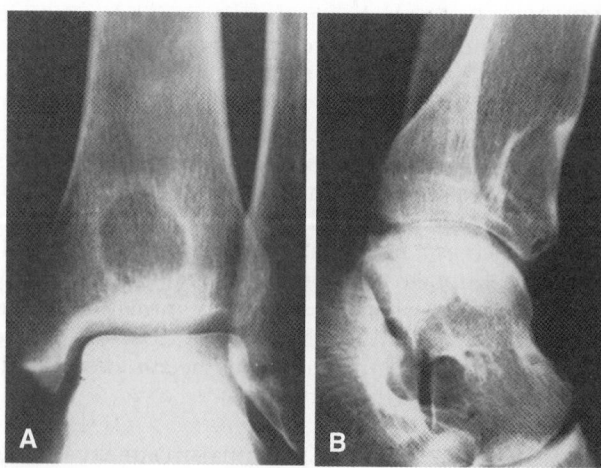

Figure 26-6

Genuine (conventional) osteoblastoma of the tibia in a 24-year-old woman. Anteroposterior **(A)** and lateral **(B)** radiographs show a round radiolucent lesion with slightly sclerotic borders at the lower and anterior aspect of the tibia. (From Gitelis S, Schajowicz F: Osteoid osteoma and osteoblastoma, *Orthop Clin* 20:320, 1989.)

Osteoblastoma

Surgical excision may be extensive. In the long bones, the risk of pathologic fracture is often present. The use of external fixation, allografts, immobilization, and limited weight bearing is common.

PRIMARY MALIGNANT BONE TUMORS

Primary malignant bone tumors are relatively rare, representing about 6% to 7% of all pediatric neoplasms. They can be broadly categorized into low-grade (chordoma, chondrosarcoma) and high-grade tumors (osteosarcoma, Ewing sarcoma).[156] Osteosarcomas are the most frequent type, followed by chondrosarcoma and then Ewing sarcoma. Osteosarcomas make up more than half of all malignant bone tumors; Ewing sarcomas account for one-third of all primary malignant bone tumors (Table 26-3).[54]

Osteosarcoma

Overview

Osteosarcoma, also known as *osteogenic sarcoma*, is an extremely malignant tumor with destructive lesions and abundant sclerosis, both from the tumor itself and from reactive bone formation. Most deaths associated with osteosarcomas are from metastatic pulmonary diseases. A characteristic of osteosarcoma is the production of osteoid by malignant, neoplastic cells. This is seen on photomicrographs and is one of the features used to help differentiate this tumor. Resected specimens usually show that the cortex has been broken by the destructive tumor. Although various types of osteosarcoma exist, including parosteal, periosteal, telangiectatic, and small cell, only the most common, conventional or classic intramedullary osteosarcoma, is discussed here.

Incidence

Osteosarcoma is the second most frequent malignant condition of bone, accounting for 15% to 20% of all primary bone tumors; only myeloma is seen more often. It is still fairly rare, with about 560 new cases diagnosed each year in the United States.[107,144] Osteosarcoma occurs most often in male children, adolescents, and young adults under the age of 30, with a peak frequency during the adolescent growth spurt when there is rapid bone turnover and another smaller peak in people older than 50 years.[45]

Osteosarcoma can develop in many bones but is more common in long bones, the site of the most active epiphyseal growth. The distal femur (knee) is the most common site, followed by the proximal tibia and proximal fibula (50% are located in the knee region), proximal humerus, pelvis, and occasionally the mandible, vertebrae, or scapula.

Etiologic and Risk Factors

Osteosarcomas can be primary or secondary. Certain genetic or acquired conditions increase the risk of osteosarcoma (e.g., retinoblastoma, Paget disease of bone, enchondromatosis, ionizing radiation). Alterations of multiple chromosomes and their extra copies have been demonstrated but only in distinct clinical subsets of osteosarcoma. Secondary osteosarcomas are those that develop from other lesions such as Paget disease, chronic osteomyelitis, osteoblastoma, or giant cell tumor.

Pathogenesis

The mechanisms involved in the development of osteosarcomas are still obscure. Osteosarcoma originates from primitive (poorly differentiated) cells from the osteoblasts of the mesenchyme. This suggests that early osteoprogenitor cells with the ability for chondroblastic differentiation are affected in the development of osteosarcoma. Approximately 70% of osteosarcoma tumor specimens demonstrate a chromosomal abnormality. Genetic predisposition commonly involves mutations in tumor-suppressor genes or as DNA helicases unwind for replication. Tumor-suppressor genes regulate the cell cycle; mutations will result in uncontrolled cell proliferation.[107]

Osteosarcoma grows rapidly and is locally destructive. It may be osteosclerotic (producing considerable neoplastic or tumor bone), or it may arise from more primitive cells and remain predominantly osteolytic, eroding the cortex of the metaphyseal region and resulting in pathologic fracture. As it continues to grow beyond the confines of the bone, the tumor lifts the periosteum, resulting in the formation of reactive bone in the angle between elevated periosteum and bone called *Codman's triangle* (see Fig. 26-3).

Table 26-3	Malignant Bone Tumors*				

Tumor	Age (y)	Sex Ratio (M : F)	Common Sites	Location
Osteosarcoma	10-25	2 : 1	Long bones of extremities (knee joint), jaw	Metaphysis
Ewing sarcoma	10-20	2 : 1	Long bones; multiple sites	No predilection for specific part of the bone; diaphysis most common
Chondrosarcoma	50+	2 : 1	Pelvis, ribs, vertebrae, long bones (proximal)	Diaphysis or metaphysis
Chordoma	65+	1 : 1	Skull, sacrum, spine (cervical, lumbar)	Axial skeleton, medullary canal
Giant cell tumor	20-40	1 : 1	Long bones (knee joint)	Epiphyses

*In order of descending frequency.
Adapted from Damjanov I: *Pathology for the health professions*, ed 4, Philadelphia, 2011, Saunders.

Clinical Manifestations

Osteosarcoma seems to appear in bones undergoing an active growth phase and appears at the epiphyseal plate of rapidly growing bone in adolescents. The long bones such as the distal femur, proximal humerus, and proximal tibia have a relatively more active growth period than other bones, which makes them more vulnerable (Fig. 26-7).

Pain that has continued for several weeks to months is the presenting complaint. The tumor is often located in the metaphysis but does not cross the physis. Even so, joint pain and tenderness can be present as the lesion penetrates the cortex and invades the joint capsule, also spreading to other nearby structures (e.g., tendons, fat, muscles).

Because osteosarcoma can be a rapidly destructive tumor, the pain increases, and swelling may develop in just a few weeks, accompanied by some limitation of motion. Systemic symptoms are rare, although occasional fever may occur. This aggressive neoplasm is very vascular, and the overlying skin is usually warm. Metastases appear in the lungs early in 90% of cases and occur in 20% to 25% of cases at the time of presentation.[107]

MEDICAL MANAGEMENT

DIAGNOSIS. Reports of dull, aching pain and night pain that persist over many months' duration that become more severe are common presentations that lead to the suspicion of a tumor. Adolescents may delay receiving care as lower extremity pain at night may be interpreted to be normal growing pains. There may also be localized swelling, tenderness, and limited joint motion present. Plain radiographs will demonstrate dramatic changes and obvious tumor formation.

CT scans and especially MRI are used to evaluate the extent of disease. In Fig. 26-8 plain films of a pelvis demonstrate minimal changes that could easily be dismissed as insignificant. The CT scan, however, reveals a large osteosarcoma involving the ilium. More commonly, radiographs show a rapidly growing lesion with poorly defined margins, and a permeated or moth-eaten appearance in the lytic area. PET-CT scan is used to monitor treatment response and conduct surveillance to detect recurrence.[79]

A biopsy is performed to determine the histologic makeup of the lesion. The level of vascular endothelial growth factor at the time of diagnosis may be prognostic for the risk of metastasis and the 5-year survival rate for individuals with osteosarcomas.[132] Serum alkaline phosphatase level is often elevated, but this is not diagnostic.

TREATMENT. Many factors such as age, remaining growth, expected functional outcome, and prognosis

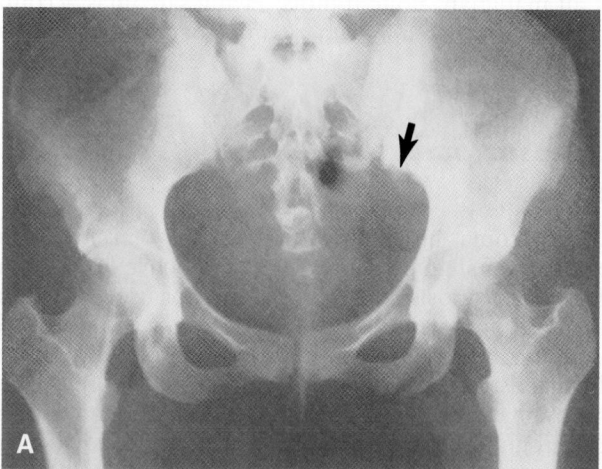

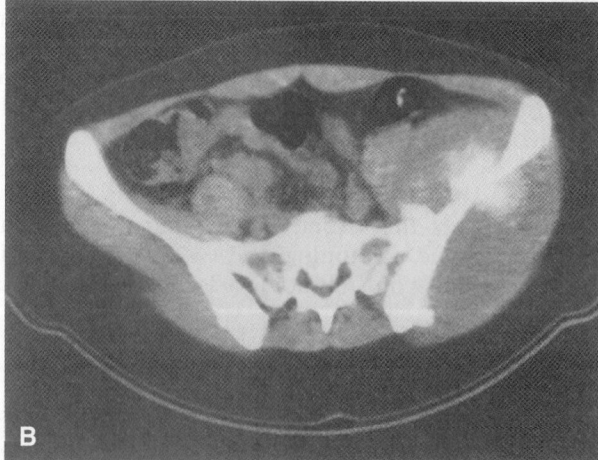

Figure 26-8

Osteosarcoma. A, A subtle sclerotic lesion is seen in the left ilium adjacent to the sacroiliac joint that was initially diagnosed as osteitis condensans ilii, a benign entity. Because of persistent pain, the person returned for a follow-up visit, and a small amount of cortical destruction on the pelvic brim was noted *(arrow)*. **B,** A computed tomographic scan was performed, which showed a large tissue mass and new bone tumor around the ilium, which is characteristic of an osteogenic sarcoma. (From Helms C: *Fundamentals of skeletal radiology: benign cystic lesions,* Philadelphia, 1989, WB Saunders.)

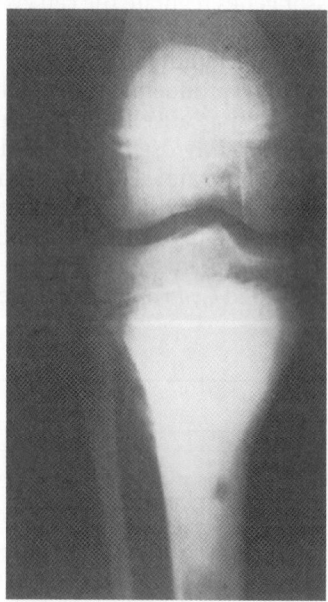

Figure 26-7

Osteosarcoma. An extremely sclerotic lesion in the proximal tibia of a child is noted, which is characteristic of an osteogenic sarcoma. (From Helms C: *Fundamentals of skeletal radiology: benign cystic lesions,* Philadelphia, 1989, WB Saunders.)

are considered in making the best treatment choices for osteosarcoma. Preoperative and chemotherapy often precedes surgery. Chemotherapy may also help lessen the chance of skip lesions and treats presumed micrometastases or multiple foci of tumor that can cause recurrence of the tumor after surgery. Postoperative chemotherapy may still benefit people who do not respond with more than 90% tumor necrosis at the time of surgery. New discoveries about the molecular genetics of osteosarcoma eventually may lead to effective targeted therapy for osteosarcoma.

Surgical Excision and Salvage. Surgical removal of the tumor with wide margins is the definitive treatment for an osteosarcoma, with chemotherapy used in the preoperative and postoperative care of the individual. Preoperative chemotherapy is used to stimulate tumor necrosis to allow for better tumor resections and to begin treatment of any metastasis. Some osteosarcomas result in limb amputation, but most are treated using limb salvage techniques to insure complete tumor removal and will lead to reconstruction of a functional extremity.[120,170]

Expandable Prosthesis. The use of a noninvasive expandable prosthesis for skeletally immature children and adolescents following limb salvage for malignant tumors in the leg is becoming more popular (Fig. 26-9). Prostheses allow better local tumor control and improved cosmesis, with the potential for equal limb length at skeletal maturity[120]; however, more revisions may be required over time[63] with this approach. An expandable metal rod prosthesis for pediatric osteosarcoma can be used to replace the bone and does not require repeated procedures to lengthen as the child's other leg grows. Painless electromagnetic rays are used to expand the rod slowly without compromise to the surrounding skin and muscle.[67]

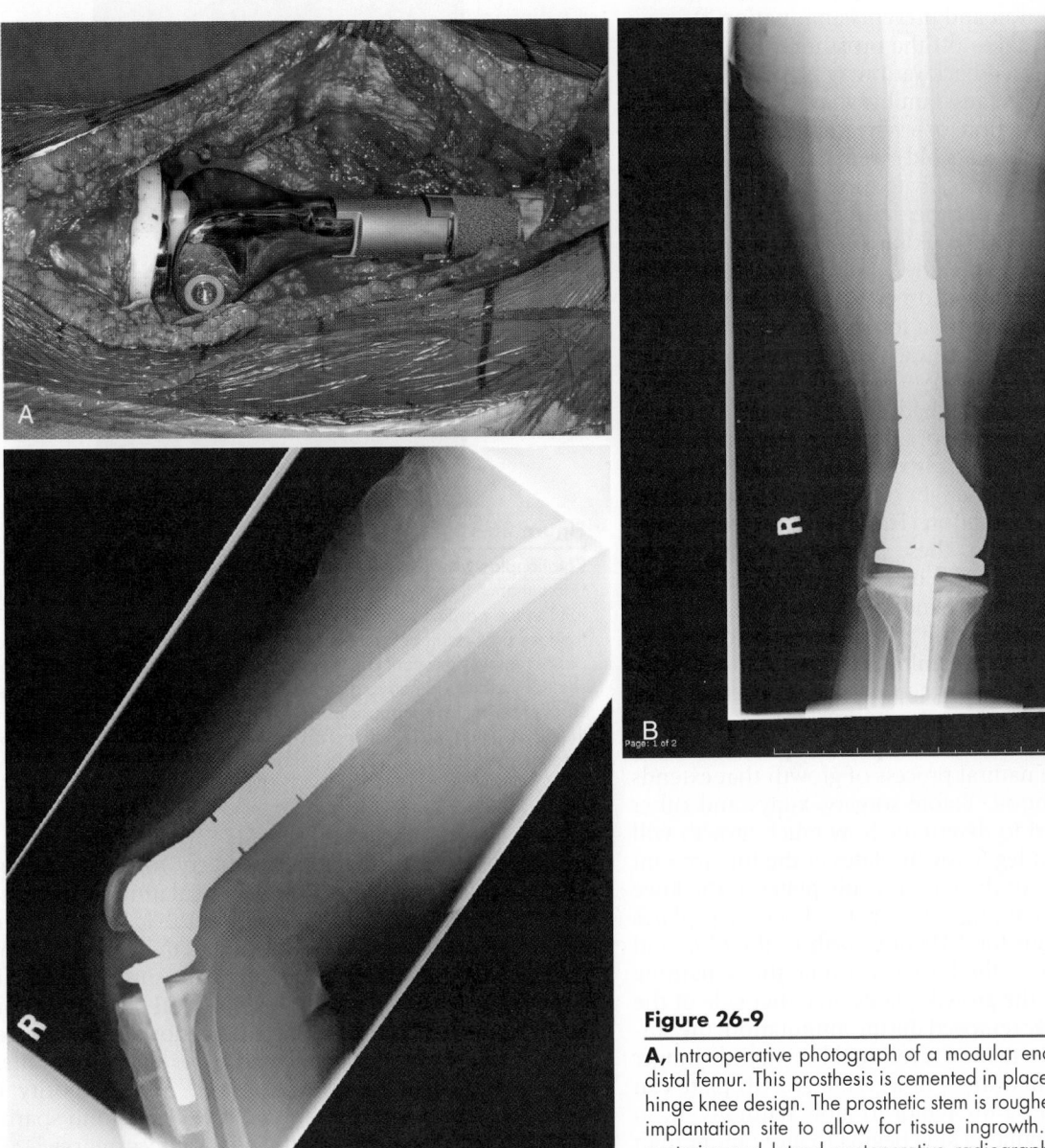

Figure 26-9

A, Intraoperative photograph of a modular endoprosthesis for the distal femur. This prosthesis is cemented in place and has a rotating hinge knee design. The prosthetic stem is roughened near the femur implantation site to allow for tissue ingrowth. **B** and **C,** Anteroposterior and lateral postoperative radiographs of the prosthesis shown above. (From Abeloff MD: *Abeloff's clinical oncology,* ed 4, Philadelphia, 2008, Churchill Livingstone.)

Review of current literature demonstrates that this procedure has generally good reported outcomes but has a high complication rate. Aseptic loosening and mechanical dysfunction are common modes of failure and often necessitate one or more large revision surgeries. Further improvement in implant design and biomaterials may decrease the incidence of these complications, and promising work in these areas is ongoing.[120]

Rotationplasty. Another creative procedure called *rotationplasty* removes the cancerous portion of the bone below the knee, then uses the remaining bottom segment of the leg and ankle joint as a new knee. The surgeon removes the affected bone, rotates the lower portion of the leg 180 degrees so the foot faces the opposite direction, and reattaches it to the upper femoral area. Nerves, muscles, and blood supply are preserved. The posterior-facing ankle now functions as a weight-bearing knee joint in a specially fitted prosthesis (Fig. 26-10). Although the outcome is visually unusual, such a procedure improves gait and knee function and prevents amputation.[95]

When the child takes off the prosthesis, the cosmesis of seeing a foot turned backward may not be acceptable. In such cases, children and families may still prefer endoprosthetic reconstruction or even amputation. Younger children (less than 10 years old) seem better able to adapt psychologically and physically to the rotationplasty.[58,102]

The tibia turn-up is another important procedure that is an option in cases of osteosarcoma (Fig. 26-11). The leg is amputated above the knee, and the tibia bone from the lower leg is inverted, or turned up, making it possible for the ankle end of the tibia to be fused to the bottom of the femur. The muscles are then sutured back onto the tibia.[28,29]

Tibia turn-up is an alternative that people may consider when the appearance of a rotationplasty seems too extreme. Tibia turn-up is also an option when cancer occurs in the thigh that might otherwise require a high-level above-knee amputation (Fig. 26-12). By having the tibia fused to the femur, these individuals now have a long residual limb that will be easier to fit with a prosthesis, providing them with increased function. Although these individuals will wear an above-knee prosthesis with a mechanical knee, their comfort and mobility will usually exceed that of above-knee prosthesis users with a short residual limb.[28]

Rotationplasty and tibia turn-up techniques both make allowances for the natural process of growth that extends into young adulthood. Before surgery, x-rays and other tests are performed to determine how much growth will occur in the sound leg. Growth plates at the hip account for 30% of growth in the femur, while plates at the knee contribute the remaining 70%. In the lower leg, plates at the ankle account for 40% of growth in the tibia and fibula, while those at the knee contribute the remaining 60%. Therefore, if the growth plates on either side of the knee are completely removed during amputation, the surgeon may choose to make the residual limb a little longer to compensate. Oftentimes, however, a growth plate can be salvaged, enabling the femur to grow naturally. If, in the future, the amputated side begins to grow more than desired, the surgeon can stop the growth by suturing the growth plate.[28]

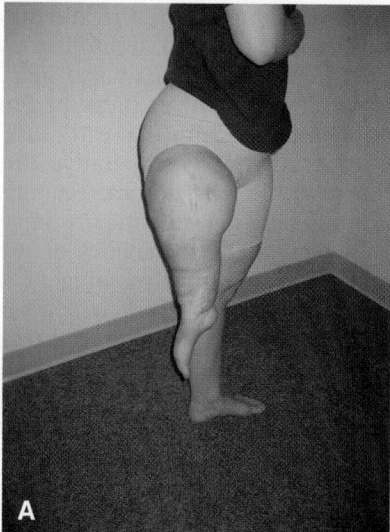

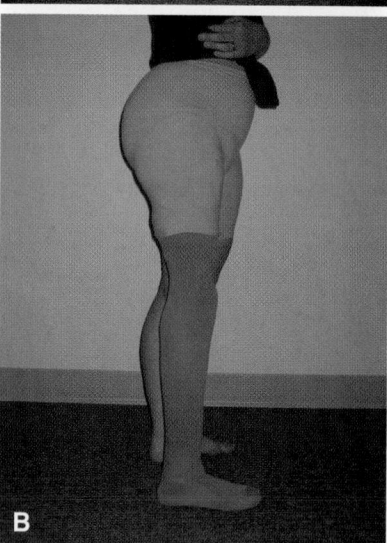

Figure 26-10

Rotationplasty for osteosarcoma. The primary reason for rotationplasty is to enhance the person's mobility as a prosthesis user. Placing the ankle joint in the position of the knee creates a functional, natural knee, and the toes provide important sensory feedback to the brain. **A,** Rotationplasty removes the cancerous portion of the femur (proximal to the mid-shaft of the femur), then rotates the lower portion of the leg 180 degrees so the foot faces the opposite direction. The proximal tibia is fused to the distal femur; the remaining bottom segment of the leg and ankle joint function as a new knee. **B,** Standing on the prosthesis with the cover on it. (Courtesy Kevin Carroll, Hanger Prosthetics and Orthotics, Orlando, FL.)

PROGNOSIS. Until the 1970s, surgery for osteosarcoma consisted of amputation or disarticulation. The 5-year survival rate at that time was about 20%, with frequent pulmonary micrometastasis.[38] Today the use of adjunctive (preoperative) chemotherapy with surgery results in 5-year cure rates of 70% to 80% for local disease without known metastases at the time of diagnosis. The expected 10-year survival rate is only 20% to 30% when there is clinically detectable metastases.[107] The majority of affected individuals (more than 90%) have limb-sparing surgery or rotationplasty with few local recurrences.[153,168] Individuals who do develop lung metastases have a 20% to 30% 5-year survival rate.

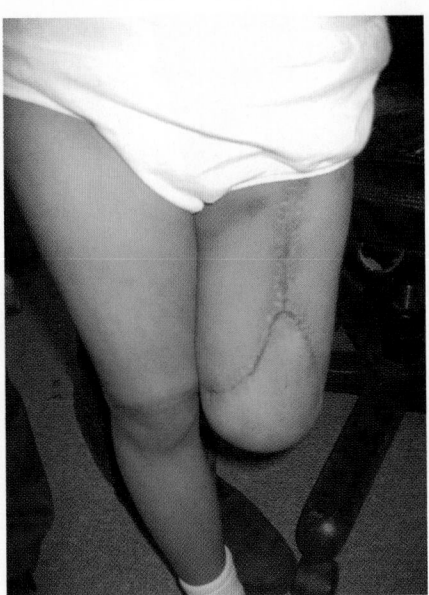

Figure 26-11

Tibia turn-up procedure. Sarcoma just below lesser trochanter in a 7-year-old girl. There were three surgical options for this client: (1) transtrochanteric amputation (major loss of limb), (2) tibia turn-up procedure (shown here), or (3) rotationplasty (see Fig. 26-10). The tibia turn-up procedure was chosen for cosmetic reasons with excellent functional outcomes with the use of a prosthesis. The tibia turn-up procedure avoids high-level transfemoral amputation and provides an outcome similar to that of a knee disarticulation amputation. (Courtesy Kevin Carroll, Hanger Prosthetics and Orthotics, Orlando, FL.)

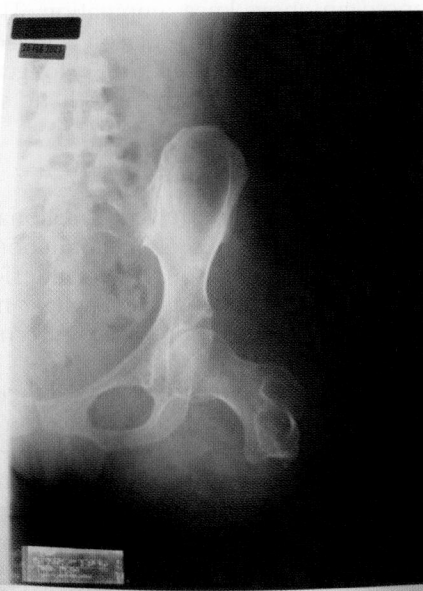

Figure 26-12

Rotationplasty or tibia turn-up can be a good alternative to high-level above-knee amputations such as this. (Courtesy Kevin Carroll, Hanger Prosthetics and Orthotic, Orlando, FL.)

The outcome is dependent on the stage at diagnosis and the ability of the surgeon to achieve a tumor-free margin. Osteosarcoma survivors have received significant chemotherapy and have undergone substantial surgeries, which can have an impact on very long-term outcomes.[113]

Local recurrence occurs in up to 40% of individuals with osteosarcoma within 3 years of treatment and is a poor prognostic sign.[107] Local recurrence of craniofacial lesions after treatment is 50% for mandibular tumors and even higher for maxillary and skull lesions (80% and 75%, respectively); metastases occur in about one-third of craniofacial osteosarcomas.[5] In older people, osteosarcoma may develop as a complication of Paget disease, in which case the prognosis is extremely grave.

Childhood osteosarcoma survivors reportedly do relatively well, considering their extensive treatment, but are at risk of experiencing chronic medical conditions, activity limitations, and adverse health status. Survivors warrant life-long follow-up.[113]

SPECIAL IMPLICATIONS FOR THE THERAPIST	26-5

Osteosarcoma

See previous discussion and "Special Implications for the Therapist 26-1: Primary Tumors" above.

Many survivors of cancer experience lasting, adverse effects caused by either their disease or its treatment. Physical therapy interventions can reverse or ameliorate the impairments (body function and structure) found in these individuals, improving their ability to carry out daily tasks and actions (activity), and to participate in life situations (participation). Measuring the efficacy of physical therapy interventions in each of these dimensions is challenging but essential for developing and delivering optimal care. An ICF framework for the physical therapist's assessment in oncology rehabilitation is available.[66]

Malignant neoplasms usually necessitate aggressive intervention, and therefore rehabilitation is more intensive, prolonged, and individualized. Extensive surgery, such as limb-sparing techniques, has provided therapists with an opportunity to assist these clients in maximizing their function (Fig. 26-13).[117] When musculoskeletal structures are involved, it is important to be aware of reduced tensile strength of malignant tissue as compared with uninvolved bone tissue. Studies also show that ROM correlates with functional mobility and quality of life in individuals with lower-extremity sarcoma after limb-sparing surgery. ROM exercises are important component of a physical therapy program for children and adolescents with this condition.[104]

Preoperative Assessment[28]

People who have been diagnosed with cancer and are faced with the impending amputation of a leg find themselves in a state of shock and grief. Parents of children who are born with a lower limb difference experience similar emotions. Under these circumstances, it is difficult to talk openly with a surgeon about amputation and to meet with a prosthetist to discuss future prosthetic needs. The fact that the majority of these clients are children, teenagers, and young adults only increases the level of anxiety. Yet beneath the surface of these painful conversations are seeds of hope: amputation can save a person's life, preoperative consultations

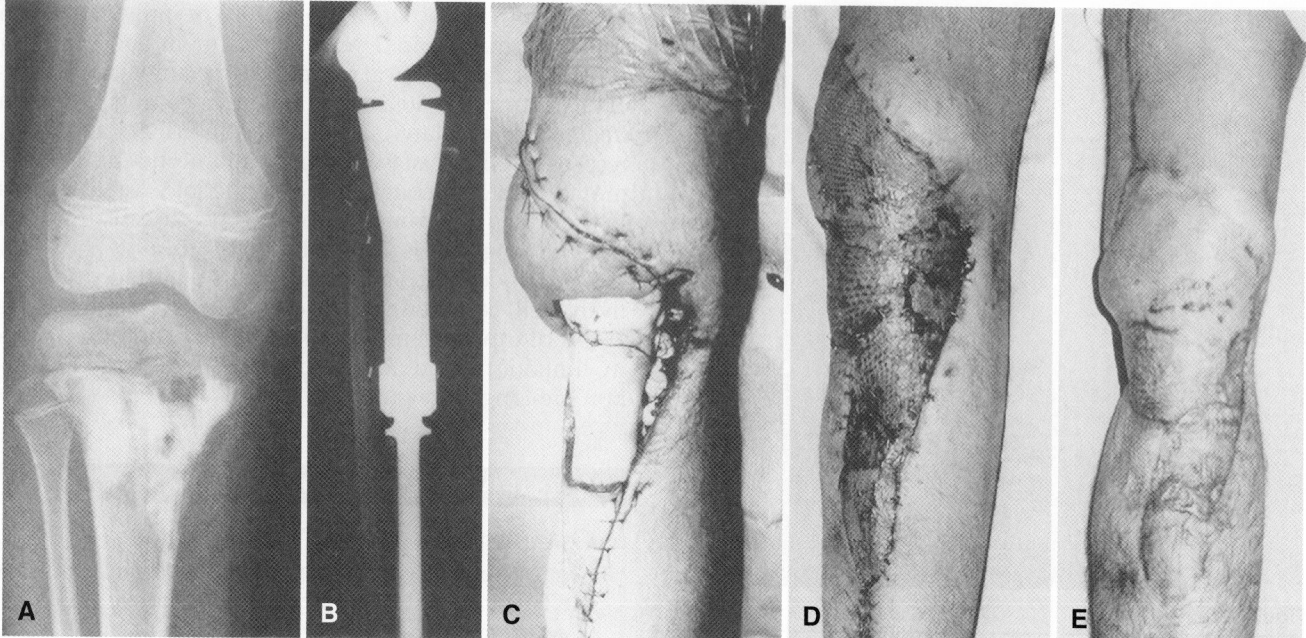

Figure 26-13

Use of a free muscle transfer to salvage an infected massive prosthesis. A, Preoperative radiograph of a 9-year-old boy with an osteosarcoma. **B,** After radical resection, an expandable prosthesis was inserted. **C,** When infection occurred, with subsequent breakdown of the wound, the prosthesis was removed, and the area was widely debrided. A spacer of antibiotic-impregnated methacrylate was inserted. **D,** Infection was controlled, and the knee was reconstructed with another prosthesis and a free latissimus transfer. **E,** A satisfactory result was obtained, sparing the leg. (From Hausman M: Microvascular applications in limb-sparing tumor surgery, *Orthop Clin* 20:434, 1989.)

can help people make better decisions, and children who are fitted early with a prosthesis can lead very active lives.[28]

Knowing what the options are before surgery can enable individuals and their families to make the best choice for each specific situation. Limb-sparing procedures, some of which involve bone replacement with human or laboratory-grown bone, or prosthetic implants are used much more often now compared with even 10 years ago. Conservative recommendation for a standard above-knee amputation at a point significantly higher than the site of the cancer is no longer considered the standard of care for each individual. Treatment of these conditions requires highly specialized physicians and medical facilities.[28]

The therapist can be instrumental in discussing a rotationplasty and tibia turn-up, two surgical procedures that may increase client mobility as prosthesis users. At first glance, both procedures appear somewhat extreme and are difficult for people to visualize. As mentioned earlier, younger individuals (up to age 24) may have more emotional and relational difficulty, which may be overcome in adulthood. According to one study, emotional and physical scars may decrease self-reported quality of life.[58] However, the long-term positive results experienced by most people are impressive.

Ideally, rotationplasty gives the affected individual a level of function that may be equivalent to that of a below-knee prosthesis user, even though he or she has

experienced an above-knee amputation. The goal of tibia turn-up is to provide the person who faces a high-level, above-knee amputation with a longer, stronger residual limb onto which the prosthetic socket can lock.[28]

Postoperative Rehabilitation

Because these tumors are treated at regional medical centers, the initial phases of rehabilitation may be implemented by therapists with a great deal of experience working with clients with malignant neoplasms and those who have undergone various reconstructive surgical procedures.

When the client returns home, a local therapist may be called on to continue the rehabilitation program. Communication with the therapist at the regional medical center to confirm initial management plan, progression, and prognosis is recommended.

The Functional Mobility Assessment with reference values has been examined in clients with lower extremity sarcoma. Functional Mobility Assessment requires the individual to physically perform functional mobility tasks and provides a reliable and valid measure of objective functional outcome and may help therapists guide children and adolescents in returning to daily activities.[102,103]

As might be expected, rehabilitation following limb-sparing surgery or rotationplasty focuses on retraining muscles and increasing weight bearing and balance, ROM, and strength.

Chondrosarcoma

Overview and Incidence

Chondrosarcoma is usually a relatively slow-growing malignant neoplasm that arises either spontaneously in previously normal bone or as the result of malignant change in a preexisting nonmalignant lesion, such as an osteochondroma or an enchondroma. The pelvic and shoulder girdles are common sites of tumor and related pain, as are the proximal and distal femur, proximal humerus, and ribs.

Chondrosarcoma is the second most common solid malignant tumor of bone in adults (after osteosarcoma, third after myeloma). Primary chondrosarcomas are more common, but their origin is idiopathic. Secondary tumors are those that arise from previously benign cartilaginous tumors or from a preexisting condition such as Paget disease.

Men in their forties to sixties are most likely to be affected by primary chondrosarcoma.

Pathogenesis

In general, chondrosarcomas develop from cells committed to cartilaginous differentiation. The neoplastic cartilaginous cells produce cartilage rather than the osteoid seen with osteosarcoma. Alterations of programmed cell death (apoptosis) may play a significant role in the pathogenesis of low- to intermediate-grade chondrosarcomas, whereas high-grade lesions most likely develop by means of a multistep mechanism involving multiple transforming genes and tumor suppressor genes.[32,151]

Chondrosarcoma is classified by location of the lesion: central, peripheral, or juxtacortical. With *central chondrosarcoma*, the neoplastic tissue is compressed inside the bone, and areas of necrosis, cystic change, and hemorrhage are common. *Peripheral chondrosarcoma* arises outside the bone and then invades the bone. The *juxtacortical chondrosarcoma* is thought to be periosteal (affecting the periosteum) or parosteal (affecting the outer surface of the periosteum) in origin. Chondrosarcomas can be graded based on their microscopic appearance. The presence of a chondroid matrix, extent of necrosis, and type of cells are some of the grading standards used.

Clinical Manifestations

Pain is the most common presenting complaint, although this is a slow-growing tumor, so in some cases the tumor can exist for years without symptoms. The lesion can range from a slow-growing lesion to an aggressive malignancy capable of metastasizing to other organs. The metastatic potential of chondrosarcoma is less than for osteosarcoma. The majority of chondrosarcomas are grade I or II, which rarely metastasize. When metastasis occurs, it is via the hematogenous route to the lungs, others bones, or organs.[32]

MEDICAL MANAGEMENT

DIAGNOSIS. On radiograph, the tumor often shows an expansile lesion in the diaphysis of long bones with cortical thickening and destruction of the medullary bone (Fig. 26-14). The appearance is somewhat variable depending on the rate of growth and the host bone response. Biopsy

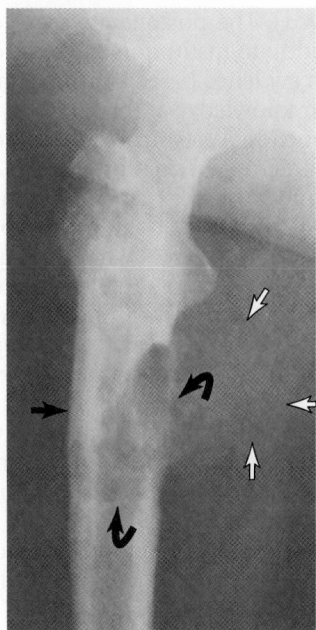

Figure 26-14

Characteristic radiographic features of chondrosarcoma include thickening of the cortex *(black arrow)*; destruction of the medullary and cortical bone *(curved arrows)*; and soft tissue mass *(white arrows)*. Note the characteristic punctate calcifications in the proximal part of the tumor. (From Greenspan A: Tumors of cartilage origin, *Orthop Clin* 20:359, 1989.)

is important not only for accurate diagnosis but also for guiding treatment. Chondrosarcoma can develop on the surface of bone or present as multicentric, involving several bones.

TREATMENT. Treatment of chondrosarcoma is surgical, with complete tumor removal. Wide resections or limb-sparing procedures are often required, and internal fixation after tumor removal to prevent fracture may be recommended. As with osteosarcoma, radiation therapy is ineffective. Because of the slow-growing nature of this malignancy, chemotherapy is limited in its effectiveness.[151]

PROGNOSIS. The prognosis is dependent on the aggressiveness and stage of the lesion. For example, a grade I lesion is unlikely to metastasize, and if it is completely resected, a good prognosis follows, with 75% to 80% chance of cure.[39] A grade III lesion is much more likely to metastasize. Undifferentiated lesions found in the pelvis or any bone where complete resection is difficult have a poorer prognosis. Secondary chondrosarcomas are usually of a low-grade malignancy and have a good prognosis with adequate intervention; metastasis is rare.[32]

SPECIAL IMPLICATIONS FOR THE THERAPIST   26-6

Chondrosarcoma

Recovery and restrictions may vary depending on the size and location of the tumor and postoperative condition (once the tumor and surrounding bone have been removed). The postoperative protocol may vary from institution to institution and surgeon to surgeon. There are no evidence-based treatment guidelines published to our knowledge at this time.

Some functional restrictions reported across the country include no driving for 6 weeks, no lifting for 3 months, and no work (depending on type of occupation) for 3 months. Shoulder motion is restricted at first to below 90 degrees when the upper extremity is affected. Use of the hand below the elbow may be allowed for writing and other functional activities in the first few days to week. Food and meal preparation is not allowed until the arm can be moved above 90 degrees.

Again, the progression of movement and activities is dependent on the size and location of the tumor and subsequent treatment. For example, tumors confined to the periosteum can be excised without resecting the bone. Postoperative rehabilitation will resemble protocols used for proximal humeral fractures. The time frame may be slightly extended depending on healing response. Factors affecting wound and bone healing include age, presence of comorbidities, general health, and nutrition.

More complex chondrosarcomas with wide surgical excision may require longer recovery time because of reconstruction, allografts, hardware, or prosthetic implants. Rehabilitation may be further compromised by adjunct therapy such as chemotherapy and/or radiotherapy. The therapist is advised to read the surgical report and consult with the surgeon when formulating a specific plan of care for each individual.

Ewing Sarcoma

Overview and Incidence

Ewing sarcoma is a malignant nonosteogenic primary tumor that can arise in bone or soft tissue.[91] It is the third most common primary malignant bone tumor of children, adolescents, and young adults and the fourth most common overall, although it only accounts for approximately 3% of all pediatric malignancies.[100] Most tumors of this type (80%) occur in young people under the age of 20; approximately 225 new cases are diagnosed each year in the United States.[15] Ewing sarcoma has been reported in children as young as 5 months, but can occur at any age. The median age is 15 with more than half of all tumors presenting in adolescents. The Ewing sarcoma family of tumors rarely occurs in the black population.[114]

Although this type of bone tumor was noted as early as 1866, it was not until 1921 that James Ewing described his experience with the lesion. The pelvis and lower extremity are the most common sites. Unlike with many tumors, no predilection for a certain part of the bone is evident.

Risk Factors, Etiologic Factors, and Pathogenesis

Based on different levels of scientific evidence, the main risk factors related to Ewing sarcoma include Caucasian race, parental occupation (exposure to pesticides, herbicides, fertilizers), and parental smoking.[54]

Cytogenetic studies show that 95% of these tumors are derived from a specific genetic translocation between chromosomes 11 and 22, although the molecular oncogenesis remains unknown. The formation of the EWS-FLI1 fusion protein from the chromosomal translocation contributes to the pathogenesis of Ewing sarcoma by modulating the expression of target genes.

Ewing sarcoma is composed of islands of small, uniformly round cells of neural origin characterized by strong membrane expression of CD99.[15,42] It is the least differentiated tumor in a group of neuroectodermally derived lesions in bone and soft tissue. These morphologic features are characteristic enough to serve as useful diagnostic markers.[86] The most common sites for a primary tumor are the lower extremities and the pelvis with extraosseous tumors primarily starting in the trunk and extremities.[114]

The tumor is soft, sometimes viscous, with hemorrhagic necrosis caused by the rapid tumor growth outpacing its blood supply. The cortical bone is affected through the haversian canals. The medullary cavity is affected, and infiltration of the bone marrow can progress extensively without radiographic evidence of bone destruction. When the tumor perforates the cortex of the bone shaft and elevates the periosteum, the consequent reactive bone formation causes layered calcification referred to as an "onion-skin" appearance seen radiographically (Fig. 26-15).

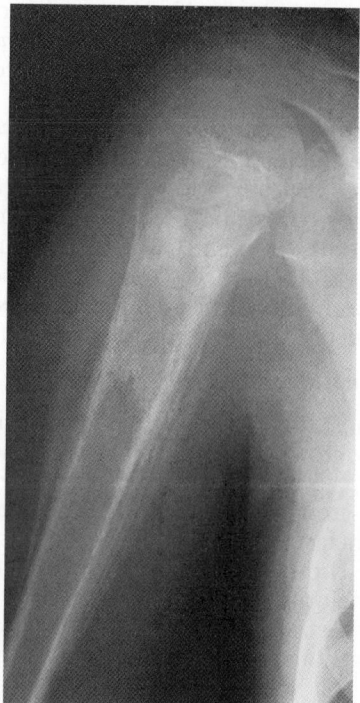

Figure 26-15

Ewing sarcoma of the humerus. Bone destruction is seen in the proximal metadiaphysis. The cortex is infiltrated and a multilaminar periosteal reaction with an onion-skin appearance is present medially; Codman triangles are present on the lateral aspect. (From Grainger RG, Allison D: *Grainger and Allison's diagnostic radiology: a textbook of medical imaging*, ed 4, Philadelphia, 2001, Churchill Livingstone.)

Clinical Manifestations

As with other malignant bone tumors, local bone pain is the most common presenting symptom after an injury (e.g., sports-related injury), a factor that sometimes delays diagnosis. Ewing sarcoma presents most often in the long (tubular) bones (e.g., femur, tibia, fibula, humerus) and the pelvis. Less often, the ribs, scapula, vertebrae, feet, and craniofacial bones are involved.

Swelling occurs in approximately 70% of all cases, and both pain and swelling are usually progressive. The pain may be intermittent, which also delays diagnosis. There may be a palpable or observable mass. Pathologic fractures occur at the site of the tumor in long bones but only in 5% to 10% of cases. In young children, flu-like symptoms, including a low-grade fever, may be present, which may lead to the mistaken diagnosis of osteomyelitis.[91]

Ewing sarcoma frequently metastasizes to other bones, especially late in the course of the disease. When the cervical or lumbar spine is involved, neurologic deficit may lead to a mistaken diagnosis of disc disease.[70]

MEDICAL MANAGEMENT

DIAGNOSIS. Anyone suspected of having Ewing sarcoma is staged for both local and metastatic disease. Radiographs show an obvious lytic process with a moth-eaten appearance involving a diffuse area of bone and soft tissue extension (Fig. 26-16). As mentioned, an onion-skin formation may be seen, which is due to layers of reactive bone (see Fig. 26-15). On radiographs, the appearance may not differentiate this lesion from osteomyelitis or osteosarcoma.[155]

An elevated erythrocyte sedimentation rate may be noted but is not diagnostic. CT, MRI, and bone scans can help diagnose and define the extent of the tumor. MRI is more sensitive than CT scan in assessing soft tissue involvement and bone marrow spread.[95] The MRI or CT scan is repeated after several cycles of chemotherapy to better assess the response to chemotherapy and help plan further treatment of the local site with radiation or surgery.

Metastatic disease is evaluated at the time of presentation with chest x-ray or chest CT scan looking for pulmonary metastases. Bone scan to detect bone metastases, bone marrow aspirate at a site far from the local tumor site, and tumor biopsy are used to assess the spread of the disease and help with staging and treatment planning.

TREATMENT. Significant progress has been made in the management of Ewing sarcoma in the past 25 years. Cure requires intensive therapy to control both local and distant disease. The treatment plan is individualized based on the stage and respectability of the primary tumor. Multimodal treatment can include multiagent chemotherapy, radiotherapy, immunotherapy or biotherapy, embolization, and surgery.[7,15,18] Local tumors are very responsive to high-dose radiation. In some cases, radiation is associated with the additional morbidities of second malignancy and a significant adverse impact on both cardiac and pulmonary function.[148]

Effective repeated cycles of combination chemotherapy over a period of 6 months to a year have been developed to eradicate distant metastases. Presurgical chemotherapy can result in a minimally sized tumor that will result in a less invasive surgical procedure and a better chance of survival.[114]

Selective surgery in the treatment of primary Ewing sarcoma can result in amputation, but the development of limb-sparing techniques has reduced amputations considerably. There is no ideal method of reconstruction in limb salvage surgery. The choice of method is individualized based on many factors, including age; location and extent of the tumor; preferences of the client or, in the case of a child, the family; the availability of surgical facilities and expertise; and cost of the procedure.[115,164]

Targeted therapies using drugs against the insulin-like growth factor receptor I (IGF-IR or CD99) are under clinical investigation. CD99 is a cell surface transmembrane protein that is highly expressed in Ewing sarcoma. Neutralizing IGR-IR functions has been shown in animal studies to significantly affect tumor cells by causing massive apoptosis of Ewing sarcoma cells, thus reducing their malignant potential.[146] Studies incorporating intensive therapy followed by stem cell infusion show no clear benefit.[15,47]

PROGNOSIS. Although Ewing sarcoma is extremely malignant with a high frequency of both metastatic spread and local recurrence, the prognosis for clients with this tumor is improving steadily with improved treatment.[18] Just a few decades ago, only about 5% to 10% of clients with Ewing sarcoma lived longer than 5 years after detection. The 5-year survival rate is as high as 80% if metastasis has not occurred at the time of diagnosis and treatment.[77] Delay between symptom onset and diagnosis is common and a negative prognostic factor.[100]

Long-term survival is determined by the presence or absence of metastasis and the site and extent of the local tumor.[86] As many as 35% of clients will have metastatic disease at the time of diagnosis, usually to the lung. More than four metastatic nodules is a poor prognostic

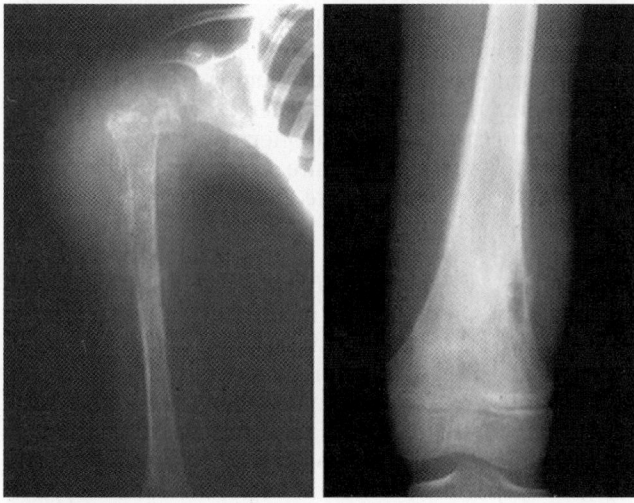

Figure 26-16

Ewing sarcoma. Radiographs of the left humerus *(left)* and right distal femur *(right)* show destructive permeative lesions with soft tissue extension. (From Weidner N: *Modern surgical pathology*, ed 2, Philadelphia, 2009, Saunders.)

indicator; recurrent or progressive disease is a poor prognostic factor. Long-term survival rates for metastatic Ewing sarcoma remain below 20%.[90]

People with Ewing sarcoma of distal sites such as the bones of the hands and feet have a much better prognosis than people with lesions in central sites such as the pelvis and sacrum. Tumors larger than 8 to 10 cm have a significantly poorer outcome than smaller tumors.[163] The presence of uncommon sites of metastasis confers a worse prognosis.[128]

Many individuals without metastasis are remaining continuously disease free at 5 and 10 years. A good response to chemotherapy (e.g., decrease in the size of the tumor mass, greater than 95% tumor kill) is a favorable prognostic sign.[171] Positive surgical margins (i.e., not getting clear margins) after resection is a negative prognostic risk factor for local recurrence and survival.[100]

There is much debate about the role of age at diagnosis. Some studies show older age to be associated with poorer outcome; others show no association between age and survival. It may be that younger children with small, well-defined, distal lesions have the best prognosis.[142] With the increase in long-term survival rates following improved treatment intervention, the problems of late local recurrence, late functional impairment secondary to complications of radiation therapy, and radiation-induced sarcomas are on the rise.[98,163]

SPECIAL IMPLICATIONS FOR THE THERAPIST 26-7

Ewing Sarcoma

As with osteosarcoma, initial intervention is aggressive, involving extensive surgical resection, limb salvage, and sometimes amputation. Saving the person's life is the first priority. After that, rehabilitation becomes the focus, including recovery of function, social reintegration, and return to work.

Analysis of rehabilitation suggests that clients with cemented modular oncologic endoprostheses recover faster than individuals treated using other techniques. The level of functional performance may be different depending on the treatment plan chosen. For example, sparing the extremity may lead to greater functional impairment compared to some people undergoing amputation who are provided with a modern prosthesis.

Some of the newer amputation surgeries and reconstructive techniques provide greater function but possibly less cosmetically acceptable results for some people. Some clients complete the entire course of rehabilitation but eventually decide that an amputation will provide greater functionality.

Chordoma

Overview and Incidence

Chordomas develop from the remnants of the primitive notochord along the vertebral column and primarily begin in the sacrococcygeal or sphenooccipital regions. Chordomas are usually slow-growing but locally aggressive malignant neoplasms and account for 1% to 4% of all malignant bone tumors, primarily affecting older adults.[20,121,178]

Chordomas do not have a capsule and tend to infiltrate into neighboring soft tissues. Metastases can occur to the liver, lungs, lymph nodes, peritoneum, skin, heart, brain, and distant regions of the spine but often remain asymptomatic and are discovered only on postmortem examination. Metastases occur most often when there is local recurrence of the primary tumor.[106]

Clinical Manifestations

Most chordomas arise in the midline of the body, involving the clivus (central skull base) in half the cases. One-third of all chordomas occur in the sacrum and account for half of all sacral tumors,[145] with the remaining found in the cervical and lumbar spine. The high cervical region, especially C2, is affected most often.[178] Clival chordomas are frequently midline lesions whose posterior growth may breach the dura and invaginate the brainstem.

Clinical manifestations based on the biologic behavior of chordoma appear to differ from person to person. The most common presenting symptom is pain; generally, symptoms depend on the location of the tumor. For example, clival chondromas may cause headaches, visual disturbances, dysphagia, muscle weakness, and even hemiparesis.[76] Sacral tumor often present with nonspecific symptoms such as low-back pain, sacrococcygeal pain, or referred buttock or leg (sciatica) pain.[145]

Night pain or pain at rest that is not relieved by analgesics is a red flag finding. Other symptoms can include bowel and/or bladder dysfunction, gait disturbances, and motor impairment.

MEDICAL MANAGEMENT

TREATMENT. The mainstay of treatment for chordoma is aggressive surgical resection preceded by chemotherapy to stabilize the tumor.[121] Complete resection of the tumor is not always possible, especially when it is located in the high cervical region. Adjuvant therapy (radiation and/or chemotherapy) may be administered before and/or after surgery.[165] Recurrence is seen, often requiring subsequent treatment. Metastases require resection and chemotherapy unless metastases are too extensive for systemic treatment.[106]

PROGNOSIS. Although chordoma is a relatively slow-growing tumor, it has a high incidence of local recurrence and poor long-term prognosis.[165,178] Tumor seeding (transfer of a small number of cancer cells) can occur during biopsy or incomplete debulking procedures. The result is an increased risk of local recurrence and metastasis. The biopsy tract must be excised en bloc along with the tumor specimen.[14] Cancer recurrence often necessitates repeat surgical procedures with risk for complications. The 5-year survival rate for a chordoma tumor has been estimated to be 50%.[121]

Metastases are becoming more common as people with chordomas live longer as a result of more aggressive surgical and adjuvant treatments. Researchers hope to identify markers that will help predict which tumors will behave aggressively in order to direct treatment toward early diagnosis and intervention for people with aggressive tumors.[106]

Giant Cell Tumor

Overview and Incidence

Giant cell tumor of bone (also known as giant cell myeloma) is a distinct, locally aggressive neoplasm that accounts for approximately 5% of all primary bone tumors.[144] Although classically considered benign, these tumors are now considered a low-grade (malignant) sarcoma because of their high rate of recurrence and potential for malignant transformation with metastases to the lungs.[43,72]

The tumor most frequently involves the epiphyseal ends of long tubular bones in skeletally mature adults between the ages of 20 and 55 years of age, with a peak age incidence in the third decade of life. Giant cell tumor occurs more often in Chinese people (up to 20% of the population are affected) compared to Caucasians in Western countries.

Sixty percent occur around the knee; 10% to 12% involve the distal radius. The bones of the hand and wrist are rarely affected.[80] Giant cell tumors are the second most frequent primary bone-involved tumor in the sacrum[72]; this type of tumor is extremely rare in the vertebrae.

Etiology and Pathogenesis

The etiology of giant cell tumor is unknown. The tumor cells have been reported to produce chemoattractants that can attract osteoclasts and osteoclast precursors.[152]

Pathologic examination of the neoplasm reveals a tumor that is soft, friable (easily breaks apart), fleshy, and red-brown with yellow areas. The tumor usually extends to but not into the articular cartilage. Destruction of the bone cortex with expansion into soft tissue can occur (Fig. 26-17). Hemorrhage, cyst formation, and necrosis can be seen on gross pathology. Hemorrhage and necrosis (often accompanied by pathologic fracture) occur often in the weight-bearing bones. The tumors can be locally invasive (into bone and soft tissue) with extensive bone destruction and cortical expansion.

Clinical Manifestations

Symptoms depend on the location but pain on weight bearing with pathologic fracture may be the presenting clinical feature when tumors occur in the weight-bearing bones. Sacral tumors may present with localized pain in the low back radiating to one or both of the legs. Abdominal discomfort and bowel and bladder symptoms may be present.[72]

Pulmonary metastases referred to as benign pulmonary implants occur in 1% of cases. The nodules grow slowly and can be excised effectively. They are usually asymptomatic and discovered when a routine chest x-ray is taken. Multiple lung lesions or progressive spread can result in death.

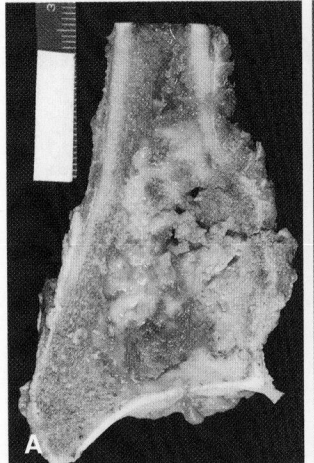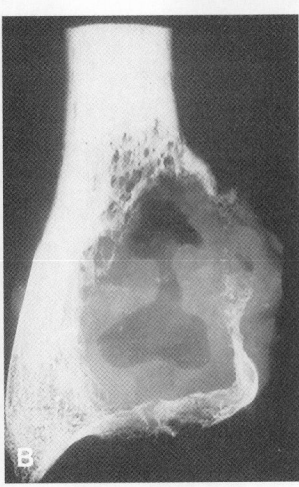

Figure 26-17

Giant cell tumor. Gross morphologic features of giant cell tumor. **A,** Bisected distal end of radius with well-demarcated tumor mass expanding bone contour. Tumor tissue is red-brown with yellow septations. **B,** Radiographic presentation of tumor showing focal destruction of cortex. (From Dorfman HD, Czerniak B: *Bone tumors,* St. Louis, 1998, Mosby.)

MEDICAL MANAGEMENT

Diagnosis is by radiographs and confirmed by histologic assessment with findings typical of this particular type of tumor observed. Treatment is with surgical excision; bone grafting to fill the cavity and further reconstruction may be needed.[160]

Recurrence is usually confined to the bone and does not extend to the soft tissue. Recurrence after excision occurs in up to half of clients. Recurrence usually occurs within 3 years of the index removal but can occur many years (even decades) later. Some experts suggest this is because of bleeding into the surgical site when the tumor is removed. Any tumor cells that spill into the open area can reseed the area and/or be carried away by the blood to the lungs. Improved surgical technique with effective control of intraoperative bleeding may reduce the rate of recurrence.[72]

Limiting bleeding makes it possible for the surgeon to see the outline of the tumor and remove it without contaminating the surgical site. Surgical sponges can be packed around the outside of the tumor to keep any cells from spilling into the area. In the case of sacral giant cell tumors, improved intraoperative control of hemorrhage has made it possible to preserve bowel and bladder function by sparing the S3 sacral nerves.[72] Filling the resected areas with polymethylmethacrylate during surgery have also been used to prevent the recurrence of these tumors.[88]

Radiation is not a mainstay of treatment but may be utilized in cases of surgically inaccessible or incompletely resectable lesions.[108] The use of adjuvant treatment such as chemotherapy and radiotherapy is debated. Studies using radiofrequency ablation, bone substitutes, and liquid nitrogen and phenol as alternative therapies are under way.[65]

MULTIPLE MYELOMA

Multiple myeloma is a hematopoietic neoplasm involving bone marrow. It is a primary bone cancer with plasma

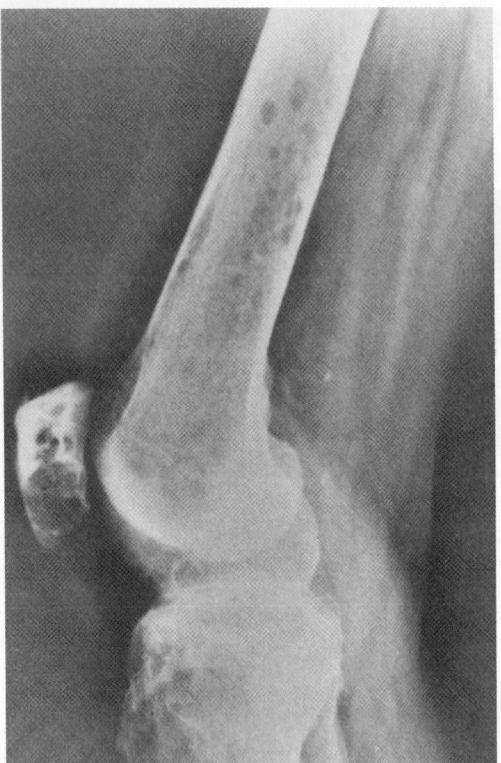

Figure 26-18

Multiple myeloma. Small lucencies in the distal femur, proximal tibia, and patella. (From Ghelman B: Radiology of bone tumors, *Orthop Clin* 20:307, 1989.)

cell proliferation and is one of a group of disorders called *plasma cell dyscrasias* (see Chapter 14 for a detailed description of this condition).

Skeletal involvement is most common in the spine, pelvis, and skull, because bone marrow is found in high concentrations in these structures. Deep bone pain is often present clinically, and radiographs may demonstrate osteopenia and punched-out areas of bone with sclerotic borders (in flat bones) (Fig. 26-18).

The prognosis is generally poor, with the 5-year survival rate of 33 percent, and the median survival length of 33 months.[118]

PRIMARY SOFT TISSUE TUMORS

Benign Soft Tissue Tumors

Common benign soft tissue tumors include lipoma, ganglia, popliteal cyst (Baker cyst), nerve sheath tumor (neurofibroma and schwannoma), and desmoid tumors.

Lipoma is the most common soft tissue tumor, generally occurring during middle age and late adulthood and composed of mature fat cells. These tumors are usually superficially located in the subcutaneous tissue and remain asymptomatic. Occasionally a lipoma of the breast will grow large enough to cause tenderness and block lymphatic drainage, requiring removal. Even without surgical excision, lipomas are unlikely to ever undergo malignant transformation, but recurrence is possible if the lesion, including microscopic cells, is not completely removed.

Ganglia arise from a joint capsule or tendon sheath, usually on the dorsal aspect of the wrist but sometimes on the volar aspect of the wrist or on the lower extremity. Pain or tenderness may or may not be present; pressure on a nerve can cause focal neurologic symptoms.

Popliteal cyst, more commonly referred to as a *Baker cyst*, is a subtype of ganglion that often communicates with a joint space. A Baker cyst is most often palpated behind the knee in older adults with osteoarthritis. Rupture of the cyst or hemorrhage from the joint into the cyst causes episodes of severe pain.[140] Swelling distal to the lesion (calf and foot) may also occur.

Nerve sheath tumor is a tumor of the nerve sheath arising in a peripheral nerve and growing concentrically from the center of the nerve. Neurofibromas infiltrate the nerve and splay apart the individual nerve fibers. They are usually superficially located, painless, and benign but can sometimes degenerate into cancer.

Neurofibromas can occur as a single lesion or in greater numbers as part of a collection of symptoms in association with von Recklinghausen disease (neurofibromatosis) and schwannomas. Neurofibromas contain cells and features of Schwann cells but also contain fibroblasts and perineural cells. Both neurofibromas and schwannomas are benign, grow slowly, and can be cured surgically.[2,93]

Schwannomas and neurofibromas arise from the coverings of peripheral and cranial nerves. Schwannomas arise from Schwann cells as the name suggests. Schwannoma is a rare tumor of the sheath or lining around the peripheral nerves. It starts in the Schwann cells, which is how it gets its name. Schwann cells help form the cover around the nerves called the myelin sheath. Schwannomas can be benign or malignant. The malignant type is called *neurosarcoma* or *neurogenic sarcoma*.

In the benign form, growth is slow and painless. The tumor stays on the outside of the nerve. The benign form does not spread to other areas and is not likely to cause death. But if it grows large enough to put pressure on the nerve, then pain, numbness, and even paralysis can occur.

Schwannomas can arise from Schwann cells covering the vestibular portion of cranial nerve VIII, causing benign acoustic neurinomas. Although the tumors grow slowly and are considered benign, they can compress the eighth cranial nerve, resulting in hearing loss and tinnitus. Vestibular function is lost but slowly enough that the body compensates; for this reason, vertigo is uncommon with acoustic neuromas. Large tumors can compress the cerebellum and brainstem, resulting in ataxia and hydrocephalus. The affected individual may also experience facial paralysis if the trigeminal nerve is compressed.[93]

Schwannomas can also occur as intradural extramedullary tumors, most often in individuals with neurofibromatosis. Multiple schwannomas in this population group are common. The tumors often extend through the intervertebral foramen into the abdomen or thoracic cavity. Compression causes local or radicular pain and may progress to include symptoms of spinal cord compression (e.g., motor weakness, sensory disturbances, autonomic changes). As with all benign schwannomas, surgical resection is curative.

Table 26-4	Soft Tissue Sarcoma		
Tumor	**Age**	**Sex Ratio**	**Common Sites**
Malignant fibrous histiocytoma	50-70 y	3 : 1(M/W)	Leg, thigh, retroperitoneum; extremities (lower > upper)
Liposarcoma	40-60 y	1 : 1	Any site of adipose tissue; extremity, trunk, retro-peritoneum, breast
Rhabdomyosarcoma	Children <15 y; 2 peaks: 2-6 y and 15-19 y	1.4 : 1(M/W)	Any site; four main areas: head and neck, genitourinary (bladder, prostate, testes), extremities, trunk
Leiomyosarcoma	50-70 y	Women > men	Skin, deep soft tissues of the extremities, retro-peritoneum, uterus
Malignant schwannoma	20-50 y; can occur at any age	Men > women	Peripheral nerves, any site; flexor surface extremities
Synovial sarcoma	Young adult, 15-40 y	Men > women	Extremity, knee (popliteal area), feet, hands, forearm
Epithelioid sarcoma (rare)	Young adult	Men > woman	Extensor surface of the extremities, tendon sheath, joint capsule (shoulder), hands, feet
Clear cell sarcoma (rare)	Young adult	Women > men	Deep to dermis; tendon, aponeuroses; spinal nerve root (rare)
Fibrosarcoma (rare)	35-55 y	Men > women	Fibrous connective tissue (thigh, posterior knee); scars, subcutaneous fibrous tissue, deep connective tissue, around tendons or nerve sheaths, ligaments, muscle fascia; can occur as bone tumors (periosteum)

Data from:

Pisters PWT: Soft-tissue sarcomas, *Cancer management*, ed 14, CancerNetwork, 2011. Available online at: http://www.cancernetwork.com/cancer-management/soft-tissue-sarcomas/article/10165/1802713.

Zhang PJ: *Essentials in bone and soft tissue pathology*, New York, 2010, Springer.

Fletcher C: *Pathology and genetics of tumours of soft tissue and bone*, ed 4, Geneva, 2013, World Health Organization.

*Listed in approximate descending order of prevalence. Most soft tissue sarcomas are rare; some (as labeled) are extremely rare.

Malignant Soft Tissue Tumors

Overview and Incidence

Soft tissue sarcomas are a heterogeneous group of rare tumors that arise predominantly from the embryonic mesoderm and present most often as an asymptomatic mass. They can occur anywhere in the body, but most originate in the extremities (59%), trunk (19%), retro-peritoneum (15%), or head and neck (9%).[22] Sarcomas account for 1% of all newly diagnosed adult cancers. The incidence is much higher in children, constituting 15% of annual pediatric malignancies.[149]

Types of Soft Tissue Sarcomas. Currently there are more than 50 histologic types of soft tissue sarcoma that have been identified. The most common are malignant fibrous histiocytoma, leiomyosarcoma, liposarcoma, synovial sarcoma, and malignant peripheral nerve sheath tumors. Rhabdomyosarcoma is the most common soft tissue sarcoma of childhood (Table 26-4).[35]

Malignant schwannoma, also known as *neurosarcoma* or *neurogenic sarcoma*, is a rare nerve sheath tumor of the peripheral nerves arising from Schwann cells or within existing neurofibromas. They can occur anywhere in the body but are often located on the flexor surface of the extremities. They are usually slow growing and painless, often present for years.[159] When pressure is placed on the involved nerve, then pain, paresthesia, and paralysis may occur.

Rhabdomyosarcomas constitute more than half of all soft tissue sarcomas in children under 15 years of age. Occurrence in adults is possible but relatively rare.[125] Eighty percent of the affected individuals are white. Boys are affected slightly more than girls; approximately 250 children in the United States are diagnosed each year with rhabdomyosarcoma.[40]

Rhabdomyosarcoma is a malignancy of striated muscle but can occur sporadically at any site in the body (e.g., bladder, prostate, head and neck, limbs, testes, muscle) and is of unknown cause. Symptoms are site dependent, but the tumor presents as a painless mass in the soft tissues. About one-third of all people with rhabdomyosarcoma have readily resectable tumors, half do not, and in about half of all cases, regional lymphatic spread at diagnosis is evident, with a much less favorable prognosis.[119] Diagnosis is often delayed as lesions are frequently attributed to sports-related trauma.

Other sites of metastases include the lungs, bone, and bone marrow. Tumors are aggressive and must be excised whenever possible. If tumors are too large to remove surgically, preoperative chemotherapy is used first to shrink the tumor. This allows for the possibility of complete resection and possibly a lower dose of radiation to achieve local control. Reduced exposure to radiation may decrease the late effects of radiation.[40]

Other common soft tissue sarcomas include malignant fibrous histiocytoma, liposarcoma, synovial sarcoma, epithelioid sarcoma, and clear cell sarcoma. *Malignant fibrous histiocytoma* is now recognized as the most common (although still occurring rarely) soft tissue sarcoma in adults, primarily affecting men 50 to 70 years old. Malignant fibrous histiocytoma occurs as a deep-seated mass that typically enlarges to 5 cm or more by the time of diagnosis and is usually located on the leg, especially the thigh.

Liposarcoma is a soft tissue malignancy with a peak incidence between ages 40 and 60 years. These are slow-growing lesions that can achieve a large size (10-15 cm), usually located in the thigh but occasionally retroperitoneally, causing pain and weight loss. *Synovial sarcoma* occurs most often in a young adult as a slow-growing mass of the extremities, often located near the knee. These lesions are painful and tender to palpation and often present similarly to a Baker cyst or ganglion. Reclassification of this sarcoma will eventually reflect the fact that the synovium is not involved in this type of sarcoma.

Epithelioid sarcoma, a small, firm, slow-growing mass, typically occurs in young adults on the extensor surface of an extremity but can also occur on the shoulder. These can develop deep enough to be undetectable on physical examination. Epithelioid sarcoma can look like a rheumatoid nodule, ganglion, or draining abscess and is often confused with a benign lesion.[8]

Clear cell sarcoma arises deep to the dermis, has a uniform growth pattern, and is often located on tendons or aponeuroses. In rare cases, this type of tumor can also originate in the spinal nerve roots with dissemination to the vertebral bodies, resulting in cauda equina. In approximately 20% of individuals, the tumor has a dark appearance resulting from production of melanin, and it is often confused with benign soft tissue tumors.[159]

Etiology and Risk Factors

Most soft tissue sarcomas will develop without an identifiable cause.[150] Specific inherited genetic alterations are primarily associated with an increased risk of soft tissue sarcomas. Distinct chromosomal translocations that code for oncoproteins are associated with certain histologic subtypes of soft tissue sarcomas. Oncogenes identified in the development of soft tissue sarcomas include *MDM2*, *N-myc*, *c-erbB2*, and members of the *ras* family.[35] Ras proteins regulate cell proliferation, survival, and differentiation and are activated by mutations in many cancers.

Risk factors for soft tissue sarcomas include radiation therapy for cancer of the breast, cervix, testes, or lymphatic system with a mean latency period of approximately 10 years. Other risk factors include occupational exposure to chemicals, including herbicides and wood preservatives. Chronic lymphedema following axillary dissection is an additional risk factor for the development of lymphangiosarcoma.[35]

Pathogenesis

All sarcomas share a mesodermal cellular origin, but research has not been able to completely identify the pathogenesis involved. Sarcomas probably do not originate from normal tissue but arise from aberrant differentiated and proliferative malignant mesenchymal cell formations. There are some genetic origins that have been specifically identified for individual sarcoma types. Many sarcoma-linked oncogenes appear to be triggered by viruses; sequencing of these viruses may eventually allow for the development of specific antibodies against oncogenic activation.[161]

Clinical Manifestations

Soft tissue sarcomas present most often as painless, asymptomatic masses. They can grow quite large before being observed but do not usually produce pain when compressing surrounding structures. Metastasis occurs primarily hematogenously, with lymph node dissemination in rare cases.[150]

MEDICAL MANAGEMENT

DIAGNOSIS. Diagnostic imaging, fine-needle aspiration, biopsy, and clinical studies are the mainstay of diagnosis. X-rays are used to look for lung metastases; CT scans and contrast-enhanced techniques provide details of high-grade lesions and large tumors, and assess the extent of tumor burden and proximity to vital structures. MRI is the preferred imaging modality for sarcomas of the extremities.[74,150]

Staging of soft tissue sarcomas follows the AJCC method of staging based on anatomic location (depth), grade, size of the tumor, and presence of distant or nodal metastases (nodal status). Metastases occur to the lungs first, but also to the bone, brain, and liver. Intracompartmental or extracompartmental extension of extremity sarcomas is important for surgical decision making and planning.[116]

TREATMENT. Treatment depends on the type of tumor, stage, and location. For example, a multidisciplinary approach is taken for people with soft tissue sarcomas of the extremities. Surgical excision with clear margins combined with radiation yields good local control, but metastasis and death remain significant problems, especially for those individuals who have sarcomas at sites other than the extremities.

Systemic therapy (i.e., cytotoxic chemotherapy) is effective only for certain histologic subtypes; the adverse toxic side effects in individuals who do not respond to chemotherapy negate the routine use of this form of treatment. Many studies with randomized controlled trials have now shown that chemotherapy does not improve disease-free and overall survival in people with soft tissue sarcomas.[62,130,150]

Likewise, there are few supportive data to show that the use of preoperative chemotherapy can improve survival rates. Studies are under way to combine systemic chemotherapy with radiosensitizers and concurrent external beam radiation in hopes of treating microscopic disease, thus producing favorable local as well as systemic results.

There has been a gradual change in the local treatment of soft tissue sarcomas from amputation to a more conservative, limb-sparing, function-preserving approach combined with radiation.[55,130] Amputation may be required for high-grade extremity sarcomas in about 5% of people whose tumor cannot be removed, while still preserving function using limb-sparing techniques.[35] See previous discussion in "Primary Tumors" above.

PROGNOSIS. The overall 5-year survival rate for soft tissue sarcomas of all stages remains about 60% to 80%.[114] Death from recurrence and metastatic complications occurs within 2 to 3 years of the initial diagnosis in 80% of cases.[115] Despite improvements in local control rates, individuals with high-risk soft tissue sarcomas have poor long-term results. There is some evidence that individuals who had limb sparing surgery display superior functional outcomes over those who have amputations. Pain and perceiving that the cancer negatively influenced opportunities has been associated with poor outcomes.[157]

Advanced, metastatic sarcomas are always incurable; management is palliative. Factors associated with a poorer prognosis include age older than 60, tumors larger than 5 cm, and high-grade histology.[116] Individuals with leiomyosarcomas, clear cell sarcomas, and malignant fibrous histiocytomas may have a poorer survival rate compared with those individuals who have fibrosarcomas, liposarcomas, and neurofibrosarcomas.[101]

Rhabdomyosarcoma. Current 5-year survival in rhabdomyosarcoma reaches 60% to 70% in nonmetastatic cases and remains below 20% in metastatic situations.[47] Children with relapsed, recurrent, or metastatic sarcomas represent a complex challenge for the pediatric oncologist.[37,73] Over the last 30 years, the prognosis for children with rhabdomyosarcoma has improved dramatically with the use of multiagent chemotherapy, aggressive surgery for local disease, and more precise delivery of radiation therapy. Prognosis depends on the type of gross residual tumor (histology), location of the tumor, and the presence and number of metastases at the time of diagnosis. Age and completeness of resection are additional prognostic factors.[136]

Cartilaginous Tumors

Many tumors of cartilaginous origin can occur. Three of the more common tumors of a cartilaginous origin are the enchondroma, osteochondroma, and chondrosarcoma. Cartilage tumors involving some parts of the skeleton (e.g., small bones of the hands and feet) are almost always benign, whereas cartilaginous lesions of the ribs, sternum, and flat bones such as the pelvis and scapula are more likely to be aggressive.[30]

Determining the aggressiveness of cartilaginous tumors is especially difficult, and even the histologic differentiation is troublesome. Sometimes the presence of pain or the development of pain in a previously diagnosed benign cartilaginous tumor such as an enchondroma is all that raises suspicion of a malignant process or transformation.

Benign Cartilaginous Tumors

ENCHONDROMA.

Overview and Incidence. Enchondroma is a common, benign tumor arising from residual islands of cartilage in the metaphysis of bones (Fig. 26-19). The tubular bones of the hands and feet (phalanges, metacarpals, metatarsals) are common sites, although the long tubular bones (femur, humerus) can be affected. They are rarely seen in sites most commonly affected by chondrosarcoma (trunk bones).[57] Enchondromas account for approximately 10% of benign skeletal tumors. They are seen in people between the ages of 20 and 40 but can occur at any age in both men and women.

Pathogenesis and Clinical Manifestations. Cartilaginous tumors are lesions in which cartilage is produced, rather than osteoid as in the osteosarcomas. These lesions are classified as chondromas. Enchondral ossification is the process by which most bones in the skeleton are formed—that is, bone is slowly absorbed from the inner cortex while periosteal reactive bone is deposited on the outer surface. A cartilaginous model exists as a precursor to mature bone. A tumor may then develop from cartilage islands displaced from the growth plate during

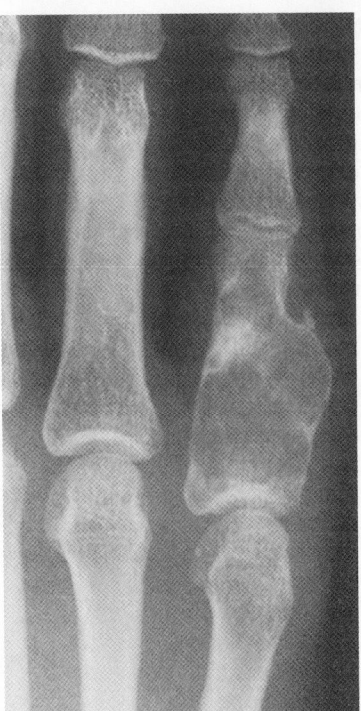

Figure 26-19

Enchondroma of the proximal phalanx of the small finger in a 27-year-old woman. Note radiolucent, expansile lesion that resulted in attenuation and thinning of the cortex. (From Greenspan A: Tumors of cartilage origin, *Orthop Clin* 20:351, 1989.)

development. This is thought to occur perhaps secondary to trauma or to an abnormality in the growth plate.

Histologically, enchondroma consists of hyaline cartilage appearing as lobules rimmed with a narrow band of reactive bone. These may be difficult to differentiate from a slow-growing chondrosarcoma, and in a small percentage of cases, a single enchondroma (usually in a large, long bone) does undergo malignant change to become a chondrosarcoma.[122]

Enchondromas may be asymptomatic. In some cases, some swelling may occur. When present in the hands, pain may be a symptom of pathologic stress fracture.

MEDICAL MANAGEMENT

DIAGNOSIS. In those cases where no symptoms are present, plain radiographs or bone scans performed for other reasons reveal the tumor as an incidental finding. Once detected, differentiating the lesion from a chondrosarcoma is crucial. The radiograph and clinical history, not the histologic makeup, are the most informative. Radiographs of enchondromas do not show cortical destruction. Pain without evidence of a fracture is also suspicious of malignancy rather than enchondroma.

TREATMENT AND PROGNOSIS. Curettage is a common form of treatment, with or without spongy bone grafting, depending on the size and location of the lesion. Clients with enchondromas in the hand may develop stress fractures, which often respond to splinting. Recurrence of enchondromas after curettage is less than 5%, and malignant transformation occurs in 2% of all cases (usually adults).[56]

OSTEOCHONDROMA.

Overview and Incidence. Osteochondroma is the most common primary benign neoplasm of bone, accounting for 90% of all benign bone tumors.[64] A continuous osseous outgrowth of bone with a cartilaginous cap is characteristic (Fig. 26-20). The outgrowth arises from the metaphysis of long bones and extends away from the nearest epiphysis. The metaphyses of long bones, especially the distal femur, proximal humerus, and proximal tibia, are common sites. The flat bones of the ilium and scapula can also be involved.[64]

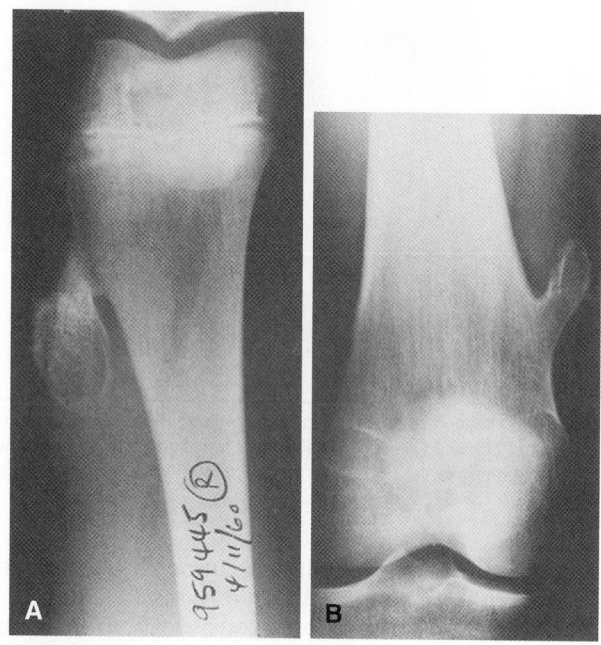

Figure 26-20

Osteochondroma. Two radiographs (**A** and **B**) showing mature osteochondroma: stalked lesion pointing toward the diaphysis and away from the growth plate. (From Bogumill G, Schwamm H: *Orthopaedic pathology*, Philadelphia, 1984, WB Saunders.)

The incidence of osteochondroma is unknown. Some reports indicate that men are affected more often, but this may be due to the fact that it is often an incidental finding, and men may be more likely to have a radiograph taken during the second decade of life when the lesion is usually seen.

Pathogenesis. Osteochondromas appear to result from aberrant epiphyseal development. They are an extension of normal bone capped by cartilage that forms a prominent "tumor" (lump, swelling), sometimes referred to as *osteocartilaginous exostosis.* The younger the individual, the larger is the cartilage cap, because during the growing years, an osteochondroma has its own epiphyseal plate from which it grows.[105]

The lesion will usually cease growing when the individual reaches skeletal maturity. The central portion of the lesion is normal medullary bone. The lesion may begin as a displaced fragment of epiphyseal cartilage that penetrates a cortical defect and continues to grow.

Osteochondroma in older adults is rare but cases involving the spine have been reported. Because this type of tumor develops during skeletal growth, pathological accelerating bone turnover such as occurs with psoriatic arthritis may be the underlying mechanism in the elderly.[173]

Clinical Manifestations. In some people, a hard mass will be detected, sometimes present for many years. When the tumor is palpable it may, owing to the cartilaginous cap, feel much larger than is apparent on radiographs.

Osteochondromas are not painful lesions in themselves, but they may interfere with the function of surrounding soft tissues such as tendons, nerves, or bursae. Blood vessels can also be compromised by the tumors (Fig. 26-21), and if tumors are sufficiently large, they may even limit joint motion.[105]

Synovial osteochondromatosis can occur secondary to benign proliferation of the synovium and presents as multiple loose bodies within a joint.

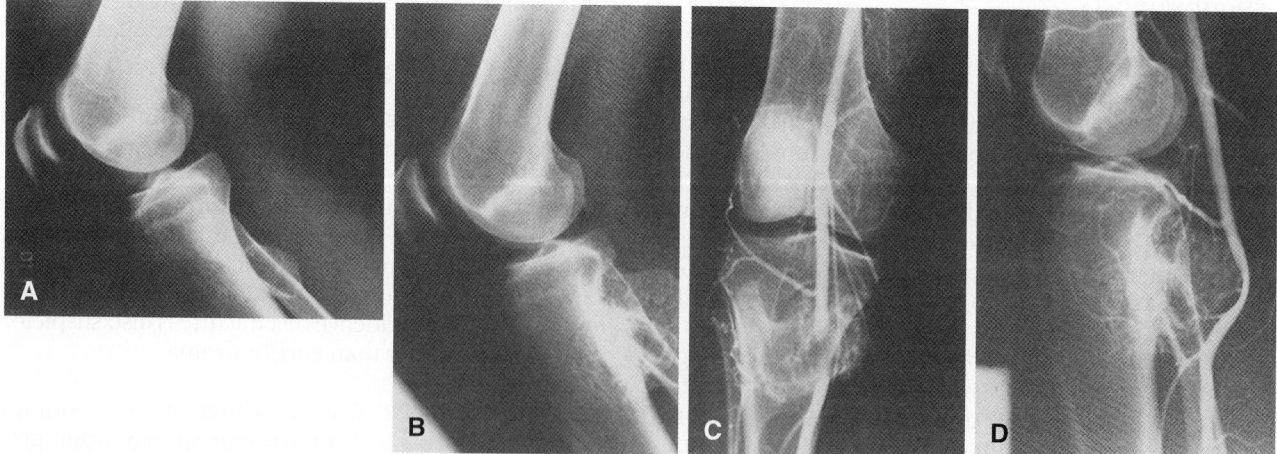

Figure 26-21

Osteochondroma of the proximal fibula in a young man. **A,** Lateral radiograph of the right knee obtained when the patient was 17 years old demonstrates an exophytic lesion arising from the proximal fibula. **B,** Lateral radiograph obtained 8 years later shows considerable interim growth of the osteochondroma, although a smooth outline is maintained. **C,** Anteroposterior and **D,** lateral angiograms demonstrate displacement and marked narrowing of the distal popliteal artery by the tumor. (From Guidici M, Moser R, Kransdorf M: Cartilaginous bone tumors, *Radiol Clin North Am* 31:247, 1993.)

MEDICAL MANAGEMENT

DIAGNOSIS. Plain radiographs may show a slender stalk of bone directed away from the nearest growth plate. This is referred to as a *pedunculated osteochondroma*. A sessile osteochondroma has a broad base of attachment (Fig. 26-22). In both types, the most important feature to note is the continuity of the cortex between the host bone and the tumor.

CT and MRI are not commonly used in the diagnostic workup of benign lesions, but if atypical clinical manifestations or recent changes in the appearance of the lesion on plain radiographs are evident, MRI may be indicated. For example, MRI can demonstrate the continuity of the marrow between the tumor and the host bone, thereby ruling out a periosteal osteosarcoma.

TREATMENT AND PROGNOSIS. Because osteochondromas usually cease their growth at skeletal maturity, no intervention is needed unless they are symptomatic or interfering with normal limb function. Removal of the lesion is sometimes required when symptoms such as vascular compromise, chronic bursitis, or pain develop secondarily.[105] Rarely, an osteochondroma can transform into a chondrosarcoma. Those symptomatic lesions that are removed have a very low recurrence rate.

Malignant Cartilaginous Tumors

Chondrosarcoma. *Chondrosarcoma* is defined as a malignant tumor of cartilage in which the matrix formed is uniformly or entirely chondroid in nature.[57] These tumors are classified as malignant bone tumors and therefore are discussed in "Primary Malignant Bone Tumors" below.

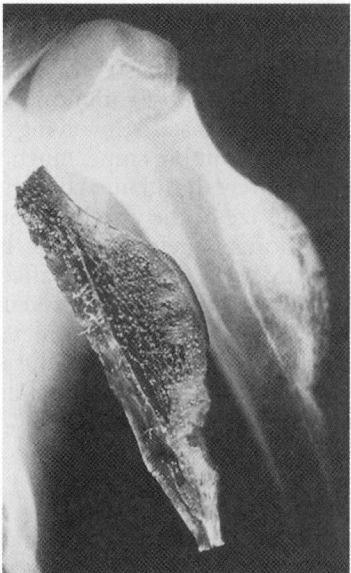

Figure 26-22

Osteochondroma. Radiograph and gross specimen of the sessile osteochondroma. Note the cartilaginous component causing the radiographic defect in the distal portion. Note also incorporation of hematopoietic tissue into the base of the osteochondroma. (From Bogumill G, Schwamm H: *Orthopaedic pathology*, Philadelphia, 1984, WB Saunders.)

Fibrous Lesions

Overview

Fibrous (fibroosseous) lesions (also referred to as fibrous dysplasia) within bone are a common osseous anomaly of mesenchymal tissue. They are usually solitary lesions found in the femur, skull, humerus, and tibia. Adolescents and young adults are affected. These lesions vary from small, fibrous cortical defects to larger fibrous dysplasias. Although most are benign, fibrosarcoma has many of the features of osteosarcoma. Many children have defects in the metaphysis, but most resolve spontaneously. Those that persist are seen in young adult men. The distal femur and tibia are common sites.

Pathogenesis and Clinical Manifestations

The hallmark of this disease is the inability of bone-forming tissue to produce mature bone. The process is arrested at the level of woven bone; even if a large amount of osteoid tissue is produced, it cannot or does not mature to lamellar bone. The pathogenesis is unknown, but it appears the underlying molecular mechanism involves the fundamental cell differentiation process.[99]

Although the defect occurs in the metaphysis, during normal bone growth the defect may be displaced into the diaphysis. Microscopic examination reveals disorganized, haphazard deposits characteristic of woven bone, sometimes accompanied by local hemorrhage and serous fluid accumulation. Growth of lesions is often stabilized during puberty.

Most fibrous defects are asymptomatic. Some individuals experience mild to moderate pain with swelling or deformity of the affected site. The more extensive the disease, the earlier the onset of symptoms. Pathologic fractures may be the initial symptom and occur where large lesions exist. Depending on the specific form of dysplasia, affected bones include ribs; craniofacial bones; long, tubular bones; and pelvis.

There may be associated extraskeletal symptoms such as hyperpigmentation of the skin (café au lait spots corresponding to the site of musculoskeletal involvement) or endocrine dysfunction (e.g., early menarche in females, acromegaly, hyperthyroidism, hyperparathyroidism, Cushing syndrome).

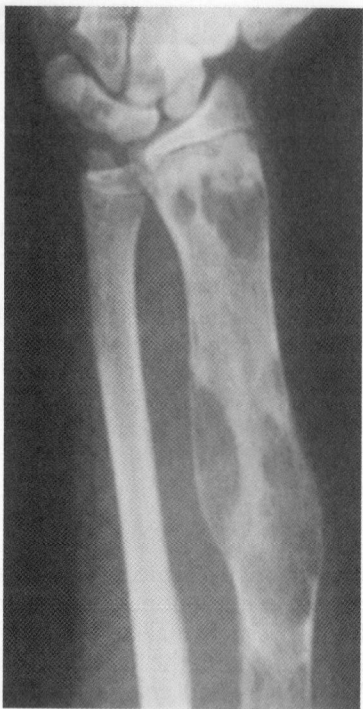

Figure 26-23

Fibrous dysplasia. A predominantly lytic lesion with some sclerosis and expansion is seen in the distal half of the radius in a child. Expansion and bone deformity are commonly seen in fibrous dysplasia. The sclerotic areas are described as having a ground-glass appearance. (From Helms C: *Fundamentals of skeletal radiology: benign cystic lesions,* Philadelphia, 1989, WB Saunders.)

MEDICAL MANAGEMENT

Plain radiographs are usually diagnostic and are usually found as an incidental finding on radiographs. The appearance of the lesion is dependent on the amount of mineralized and fibrous tissues, with most lesions having an irregular shape with a thin sclerotic border (Fig. 26-23). Most fibrous lesions will be treated with observation, but will not resolve spontaneously. Even though this is a benign lesion, treatment sometimes requires surgery. When the dysplasia thins the cortex of a weight-bearing bone or occupies more than half of the diameter of the bone, the risk of pathologic fracture increases. Benign fibrous defects generally have a good prognosis.[53] Implications for the therapist are similar to those with other benign bone tumors.

METASTATIC TUMORS

Overview

Cancer commonly metastasizes to bone; skeletal involvement represents the third most common site of metastatic spread (after lung and liver).[154] *Secondary* or *metastatic neoplasms* refer to those lesions that originate in other organs of the body.

All malignant tumors have the capability to spread to bone; the skeleton is the third most common site of metastatic carcinoma, exceeded only by lung and liver. Malignant tumors that have metastasized to the bone are the most common neoplasm of the bone.

Although all of the factors that affect the timing and location of metastasis are not known, bone tissue contains a number of growth factors that can stimulate the proliferation of tumor cells that may metastasize to these sites.[89] Cancer metastases (both carcinomas and sarcomas) to bone are a common clinical problem, because the cancers that cause them are prevalent and often metastasize.[23] Primary cancers responsible for 75% of all bone metastases include prostate, breast, lung, kidney, GI, and melanoma.[137]

Common sites for *breast* cancer to metastasize include the pelvis, ribs, vertebrae, and proximal femur. *Lung* cancer can metastasize to the bone early in the disease, remaining asymptomatic until widespread dissemination has taken place; therefore, treatment is often not successful. Neoplasms in the *kidney* metastasize to the vertebrae, pelvis, and proximal femur in about 40% of the cases. The *prostate* is the most common source of skeletal metastases in men.[175]

Early detection is important for successful intervention. Therapists should be aware of this possible cause of lumbar spine and hip pain, especially in men older than age 50. Cancer of the thyroid is uncommon but does metastasize to bone. Women are affected by bone metastases from the thyroid three times more often than men. Therapists should remember that the development of metastasis may be delayed and may even occur after removal of a cancerous thyroid. For discussions of specific primary cancers, see the relevant chapters.

Incidence and Etiology

Metastatic bone neoplasms are much more common than primary bone lesions; about half of all individuals with cancer (except skin cancer) will develop bone metastases at some point. Incidence increases to 80% of individuals with advanced cancer. The incidence of bone metastasis is expected to increase with the prolonged survival associated with improved antineoplastic therapies now available. The spine is the site most commonly affected, with more than 50% of the metastases involving the spine[158]— usually the thoracic or lumbar spine, much less often the cervical spine, and rarely the atlantoaxial region.[3]

In the spine, the size of the vertebral body may influence the distribution of metastases. The larger lumbar vertebral bodies are more commonly affected than the smaller thoracic or cervical vertebrae. Neurologic compromise is more likely to occur when metastatic lesions affect the thoracic spine because of the smaller ratio between the diameter of the spinal canal and the spinal cord within the thoracic spine.[167]

Risk Factors

Risk factors are those related to the primary cancer. For some cancers, the risk factors are well documented, and efforts to educate individuals on health risks should be stressed. Adequate exercise, proper diet and nutrition, and avoidance of tobacco use are the primary preventive measures. It is likely that the increase in incidence of spinal (and other) metastases can be attributed to the improving survival of clients with cancer.[167]

Pathogenesis

The pathophysiology of metastasis is not completely understood, but new information on the biology of tumor metastases derived from advanced techniques in molecular pathology is contributing new insight daily (see "Invasion and Metastases" in Chapter 9). The development of metastatic disease, regardless of the eventual target organ, usually follows a common pathway.

Cancer can spread through the bloodstream, lymphatic system, or by direct extension into adjacent tissue. Hematogenous spread of the cancer is most common, and therefore skeletal metastases are found in areas of bones with a good blood supply. These include the vertebrae, ribs, skull, and proximal femur and humerus.

The skeletal vasculature represents a significant proportion of the body's total vasculature. At the same time, the vertebral plexus of veins has no valves, so that the retrograde venous pressure is often increased in the abdominal and chest regions. This enables the retrograde blood flow to bypass the caval system, reaching the bones of the vertebral column instead via the extradural Batson venous plexus.[13,45] Batson plexus may be the route by which breast cancer cells metastasize directly to the thoracic spine.[167]

The unique vasculature of the spine contributes to the high rate of spinal involvement in metastatic disease. The vertebral venous system is a valveless channel that extends from the sacrum to the skull. Venous connections to this system exist from the breasts, lungs, thyroid gland, kidneys, and prostate gland. Cells from the primary tumor mass enter the circulation by traversing either the walls of small blood vessels in normal tissue or those of vessels induced by the tumor itself.[111] Once having gained access to the vertebral vein system, tumor cells can travel to distant organ sites. There are also direct connections to the vertebrae, ribs, pelvis, skull, and the shoulder and pelvic girdles.[51]

From a biologic point of view, it is very unlikely that the abundance of the vascular network within the bone is the only factor that predisposes to metastasis, because metastases rarely develop in other tissues that have an equally rich vascular supply. It is proposed that the biologic conditions of bone tissue must be important factors in promoting the growth of tumor cells that reach the marrow through the venous and arterial blood network.[45,89]

The development of skeletal metastasis involves a series of events that begins when a tumor cell separates from the primary site, enters the blood system, and then extravasates from the blood vessel to the secondary site.[167] Adhesion molecules control separation and clustering of cancerous cells. The presence or absence of certain molecules controls the ability of cells to metastasize. Various types of adhesion molecules have been implicated. Cadherins, integrins, and selectins each have distinct properties that can regulate the propensity for a primary lesion to metastasize to a specific organ.

Metastasis to bone often results in osteolysis, because cancer cells secrete a number of paracrine factors that stimulate osteoclast function. The cancer tries to destroy the bone (lytic process), and in response, the bone attempts to grow new bone (blastic process) to surround the cancer. If the cancer overwhelms the bone, it becomes weak and fractures easily. Bone metastases may be lytic (most common), blastic, or mixed. Lesions originating from the breast, lung, kidney, and thyroid are usually lytic. Blastic metastases are commonly associated with advanced carcinomas of the prostate and sometimes the breast.[112,175]

Clinical Manifestations

Although as many as 50% of people with breast or prostate metastasis have no bone pain, pain remains the most common presenting symptom, often characterized as sharp, severe, worse at night, transient or intermittent in the early course but eventually constant in more advanced cancer, and mechanical (see "Cancer Pain" in Chapter 9).

Bone pain of a mechanical nature associated with skeletal metastases occurs as a result of significant bone destruction, joint instability, mechanical insufficiency, and fracture. It is often incapacitating and persistent despite local and systemic therapies. Long bone or vertebral fractures with or without spinal cord compression may be the first indication of advanced disease. Spinal cord compression, the most serious complication of bone metastasis, occurs secondary to increased pressure on the spinal cord or as a result of vertebral collapse. Classic signs and symptoms of cord compression include pain, numbness, and/or paralysis.[51]

Pain may also arise from a biologic origin for a number of reasons. It may occur as a result of rapid growth of the tumor stretching the periosteum. Increased blood flow or angiogenesis (sometimes giving a throbbing or pulsatile sensation) and the release of cytokines at the site of the metastases gives rise to bone pain. And neuropeptides elaborated by or acting on bone-associated nerves in the endosteum can result in bone pain.[46,109] Because the skeleton provides both form and support, growing tumors that deform the cortical bone contribute to activity-associated pain. This type of pain is often intermittent and related to weight bearing and movement.[109,162]

Bone often functions as a metastatic conduit for peripheral nerves, as bone metastases travel hematogenously from distal body parts to the central nervous system. Therefore, bone tumor growth and invasion into surrounding tissues can result in neuritic pain syndromes, plexopathies, and spinal cord compression.

These pain syndromes contribute to increasing loss of mobility and bed rest, the effects of which are increasing generalized weakness, risk of thromboembolism, hypercalcemia, atelectasis, and pneumonia. The latter occur particularly in anyone with painful rib metastases. Mechanical failure or pathologic bone fracture may occur as a result of prolonged immobilization (osteoporosis). As with primary tumors, pathologic fractures can occur directly from the tumor itself or from the secondary effects of intervention.[109]

Metabolic changes can also occur as a result of the disease or the treatment, increasing the risk of fracture. In people with multiple metastases, the resultant hypercalcemia may cause anorexia, nausea, vomiting, general weakness, and depression. Unexplained weight loss is typically a late sign of metastatic disease.

Left untreated, hypercalcemia may lead to diffuse osteoporosis, renal insufficiency, and dehydration (see

Chapter 5). These symptoms may be relieved (and possibly prevented)[127] by the use of bisphosphonates (e.g., intravenous pamidronate [Aredia] and clodronate; oral ibandronate and clodronate), small molecules that inhibit osteoclast-induced bone resorption. The reactive bone formation stimulated by these lesions accounts for the elevation of serum alkaline phosphatase.[139]

MEDICAL MANAGEMENT

DIAGNOSIS. A history of malignancy raises the suspicion of recurrent disease or a metastatic lesion. The evaluation of an individual with a previous history of cancer or a current malignancy and bone pain begins with a physical examination and basic radiographic studies.[110] Because much of the bone matrix must be destroyed before the lytic process is noted on radiographs, plain films are not useful in early detection but are more important in staging and treatment planning. Spinal metastasis may be evident by the loss of the pedicle as seen in the anteroposterior view of a standard spinal radiograph or with a pathologic fracture of a long bone.

Whole-body bone scans are much more sensitive for early detection of skeletal metastasis but are not useful in predicting fractures. Approximately one-third of those with skeletal metastatic disease have positive bone scan findings yet negative radiographic results. Scans are also used to determine the extent of dissemination.

CT and MRI also have roles in delineating various types of metastasis and assessing the size and extent of the lesion. More advanced technology using single-photon emission tomography allows for better determination of anatomic location of the areas of radioisotope uptake.[141,167] Biopsy is sometimes necessary to confirm a diagnosis when the primary source is not known. CT-guided biopsy is used to assess spinal lesions; diagnostic accuracy is greater for lytic lesions (93%) compared to sclerotic lesions (76%).[97]

Other diagnostic tests may include serum chemistries, urinalysis, serum protein electrophoresis, and prostate-specific antigen determination (for men). Biochemical markers of bone turnover such as N-telopeptide and pyridinium cross-links (pyridinoline and deoxypyridinoline) may provide information on bone dynamics that reflect diseases activity in bone.

Several studies have shown bone turnover markers to be correlated with the extent of metastatic disease and the number of skeletal sites involved. Rises in such markers may be the first indication of bone involvement and possibly a useful early diagnostic sign of progression. Markers of bone turnover may be helpful in identifying those individuals likely to respond to bisphosphonate treatment and as a means of monitoring the effectiveness of bisphosphonate therapy in the management of bone metastases.[82,96]

TREATMENT. Therapeutic interventions may depend, in part, on the extent of involvement. The person with localized disease may be offered potentially curative therapy, whereas the individual with extensive skeletal and visceral involvement may only benefit from palliative treatment.[81,123,175]

Treatment of bone metastasis is problematic, costly, and primarily palliative. Prolonging survival is not always possible, so improving function with pain relief, local control of disease, and bone stability is often the primary goal. This is becoming more important as treatment for primary cancers improves. Individuals may die from the primary tumor or from the metastasis (e.g., breast cancer). When survival rates and longevity increase, the likelihood of skeletal metastasis increases.

Intervention for skeletal neoplasms requires a multidisciplinary approach to optimize therapy options and coordinate their sequencing.[48] Intervention modalities may include endocrine therapy (for breast and prostate cancer), chemotherapy, biotherapy (immunotherapy), use of bone-seeking radioisotopes (a therapy that has analgesic and antitumor effects), and bisphosphonates to suppress bone resorption. These are often combined with other localized interventions such as surgery and site-directed radiation therapy.[52,138]

Surgery is rarely curative but can be an effective therapy to decompress neural tissue for resolution of symptoms and/or restoration of function (especially ambulation), reduce anxiety, improve mobility and function, facilitate nursing care, preempt fracture (i.e., repair bony lesions before they fracture), and control local tumor when nonsurgical therapies fail.[112,174]

Pathologic fractures that occur in the femur and humerus often require surgical stabilization. Intramedullary fixation with interlocking devices to limit motion at the fracture site is indicated in many instances. The desire to restore normal anatomy must be weighed against the reality that the individual may have a terminal disease. An estimated life expectancy of at least 6 months is desirable before extensive joint reconstructive procedures are carried out.[75]

Where the risk of fracture is great, as when more than 50% of the cortex is destroyed, prophylactic nailing of the femur may be indicated (Fig. 26-24). See the discussion of fractures and fracture treatment, including newly developing fracture treatment procedures, in Chapter 27.

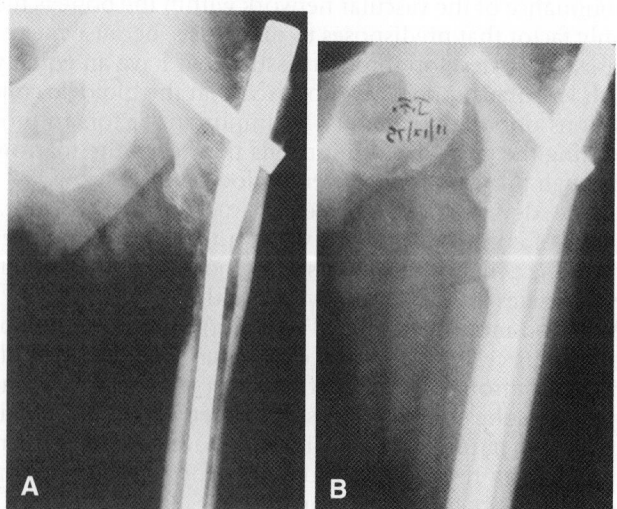

Figure 26-24

A, Prophylactic fixation in a 63-year-old woman with an impending fracture secondary to breast metastasis treated by Zickel nailing. **B,** Complete healing of this subtrochanteric lesion 5 months after radiation and chemotherapy. (From Habermann E, Lopez R: Metastatic disease of bone and treatment of pathologic fracture, *Orthop Clin* 20:475, 1989.)

Spinal metastases can cause severe pain, instability, and spinal cord compression with neurologic compromise. Management of metastatic spinal cord compression is challenging as affected individuals have widely different symptoms, comorbidities, adjuvant therapies, and tumor prognosis. For example, people with metastatic breast cancer often survive longer than those with metastatic spinal disease from lung cancer; aggressive surgical options may be pursued depending on the type of primary cancer.[31,169]

Pathologic fractures of the spine can be immobilized in an appropriate spinal brace, but a progressive neurologic deficit is an indication for surgical intervention. Surgery can take the form of decompression, posterior stabilization, excision, and reconstruction or prosthetic replacement.[126] Vertebroplasty or kyphoplasty may be considered for the person with a vertebral compression fracture and minimal bone deformity.[60] The decision to pursue surgery to prolong ambulation is an individual one and must take into consideration the person's health status, individual prognosis, attitudes, and expectations.[31]

PROGNOSIS. Although management of the skeletal metastasis may be successful in terms of restoring stability to a pathologic fracture, the prognosis for the primary cancer is still guarded. Only rarely is the skeletal metastasis actually the cause of death. Skeletal morbidity includes bone pain, hypercalcemia, pathologic fracture, spinal cord or nerve root compression, and immobility, all of which can impact mortality rates.[34]

The median survival for people with tumors that have metastasized to the bone is determined by the type of tumor (e.g., prostate: 29 months; breast: 23 months; kidney: 12 months; lung: less than 4 months). The overall median survival after detection of bone metastases is approximately 19 months; this significant amount of time allows for interventions that can dramatically improve a person's quality of life and functional independence.[46] Metastases to the vertebrae with epidural spinal cord compression can increase morbidity and hasten mortality. Loss of function, poor quality of life, and poor survival rates accompany spinal metastases.[31]

Favorable prognostic factors include indolent nature of the primary lesion (e.g., prostate cancer); well-differentiated tumor on histologic examination; a long recurrence-free survival (greater than 3 years); sclerotic lesion on radiograph as opposed to a lytic lesion, especially after treatment; a single bone lesion; a single system involved with metastatic disease; low tumor markers; no vital organ involvement; and general good condition of the individual. Unfavorable prognostic factors include the following[46]:

- Aggressive nature of the primary lesion (e.g., lung cancer)
- Poorly differentiated tumor on histology
- Short recurrence-free survival (less than 1 year)
- Lytic lesion
- No sclerosis on radiograph following treatment
- Multiple bone lesions
- Multiple system metastases
- High tumor markers
- Vital organ involvement
- General poor condition of the individual

The risk of pathologic fracture is greater in osteolytic lesions of the long bones. A direct relationship exists between the degree of cortical destruction and the risk of pathologic fracture. When cortical destruction is less than 25% to 35%, the risk for fracture is low. Destruction greater than 50% correlates with a much higher risk for pathologic fracture. The presence of pain with weight-bearing activities indicates compromised structural integrity and therefore also places the individual at greater risk of fracture.[51,61]

SPECIAL IMPLICATIONS FOR THE THERAPIST 26-9

Metastatic Tumors
Early Detection

Metastases to the skeleton are important to the therapist because the presence of musculoskeletal pain may be the initial symptom of an undetected primary carcinoma elsewhere. Early detection is essential for effective intervention. A thorough history and a high index of suspicion can lead to the timely communication with a physician. In people with a history of cancer, the clinician should be vigilant regarding the likelihood and common sites of metastasis. Autopsy-based analyses of the distributions of bone metastases demonstrate that the most favored sites are the vertebrae, pelvis, femur, and bones of the upper extremity. Metastases distal to the elbow or knee are rare; when they do occur, the kidney is most likely the site of the primary tumor.[112]

Preoperative Intervention

Exercise is recommended for individuals with bone metastases before and after surgery, focusing on increasing muscle strength and endurance while maintaining bone protection. Exercise programs directed at strengthening and stretching are often needed; high-impact and high-torsion activities should be avoided.[46]

An understanding of common postoperative impairments helps in treatment planning, preventing or minimizing length of hospitalization, and fostering an early return to independence. Chemotherapy for some cancers includes the use of steroids that can lead to muscle atrophy, especially of the type II fibers (see Chapter 5). Isometric exercises may prevent marked atrophy. Radiation therapy can lead to contracture of soft tissues, and clients should be taught to stretch and self-mobilize the soft tissues of susceptible areas before treatment.

Instruction in fall prevention strategies, including optimal body mechanics and exercises to maintain strength and balance, is essential before and after surgery.[46] This is especially true for anyone taking pain medication that causes drowsiness and decreased coordination.[51]

Rehabilitation

People who have had a pathologic fracture stabilized are often referred for rehabilitation. Hypercalcemia is common in the acute or subacute phase[24] and occurs when bone resorption is greater than new bone formation. The osteolysis that occurs with bone metastasis is one cause of hypercalcemia.

Treatment of the primary cancer with chemotherapy and/or radiation therapy often provides additional challenges, such as fatigue and increased risk of infection. For a client with lung cancer, baseline pulmonary status should be established and proper breathing techniques taught. Management of clients with metastatic disease is challenging, because in addition to these complications, clients often need extensive rehabilitation after the medical treatment.[36]

Management of skeletal metastasis, including fracture, is aimed at improving or restoring function, especially maintaining ambulatory function to preserve quality of life and prevent the negative sequelae of immobility (see Table 6-8).[66] If the bone has been compromised or fractures have occurred, surgical intervention will attempt to stabilize the defect.

After the surgery, early mobilization, including gait training, bed mobility, and transfers, is essential. Maximizing functional independence is the driving force behind all rehabilitation efforts. Safety and bone protection are important during mobility and strengthening activities. Evaluation of upper extremity function and coexisting upper extremity metastases before allowing weight bearing through the arms is important.[46]

There is a reluctance to ambulate clients who are at risk of pathologic fracture because a measure of risk has not been developed, but in fact an active rehabilitation program may not place a client at increased risk of fracture.[25] The risk of producing pathologic fractures in clients with cancer by increasing mobility and function is low.[26] Many individuals with skeletal metastases and pathologic fracture have been shown to be good candidates for intensive rehabilitation programs if they do not have hypercalcemia caused by lytic metastases or pain severe enough to require parenteral narcotics.[22]

Because many of the people with metastatic disease are at risk for pathologic fractures, the risk of falling must be considered when planning for ambulation training, especially among older adults. Assessments of mental status, balance, strength, ROM, endurance, vision, ambulation history, and symptoms of dizziness are all important and will help plan ambulation training. Even with the most critical analysis of the risks and benefits, therapists who work with individuals who have serious medical conditions such as metastatic lesions and pathologic fractures must be prepared for setbacks and unexpected events to occur when attempting to preserve or maximize function.

Rehabilitative decision making in this area requires collaboration between the therapist and the medical staff (e.g., oncologist, surgeon) and takes into primary consideration the degree of cortical involvement. It is very helpful if the therapist has access to imaging studies with accurate information about the extent of involvement, specific levels affected, and knowledge of stability (or instability) of spinal segments to assist in treatment planning. The following guidelines are just that: a guide to be used as a template to begin with but modified by individual differences and interests, postoperative protocols, physician input, and so on.

For clients with less than 25% of the cortex invaded, submaximal isometrics and gentle aerobics (e.g., bicycling at low resistance, aquatics if approved by the physician for those with wounds or fractures that are healing) are generally permitted, and the involved limb most typically is cleared for weight bearing as tolerated.

When cortical involvement increases to 25% to 50%, restrictions tighten and allow for gentle ROM without pressure into the end ROM and limb offloading to partial weight bearing. Finally, with greater than 50% cortical involvement, exercise may need to be deferred and the limb maintained non–weight bearing.[33,51] See Chapter 9 for other exercise guidelines for the individual with cancer and "Special Implications for the Therapist 26-1: Primary Tumors" above.

REFERENCES

To enhance this text and add value for the reader, all references are included on the companion Evolve site that accompanies this textbook. The reader can view the reference source and access it online whenever possible.

CHAPTER 27

Soft-Tissue, Joint, and Bone Disorders

KEVIN HELGESON

People presenting with muscle, joint, and bone disorders make up a significant percentage of the therapist's practice. These conditions are primarily manifested by pain, deformity, and loss of mobility and function. Many of the people seen by therapists have these conditions secondary to trauma or repetitive overuse; these conditions are local in terms of the involved tissues and nonprogressive in nature.

Therapists may treat impairment in other regions of the body to reduce the mechanical stresses on the involved region, but the disorder itself (i.e., degenerative joint disease, bursitis, tendinitis) does not spread to other body regions. This is in contrast to rheumatic diseases and systemic disorders, which can be manifested not only by local joint or muscle pain and impairments but also by additional complaints associated with other body systems.

Although this book is primarily a compilation of diseases and conditions of all systems, this chapter contains both orthopedic and systemic conditions that affect the bones, joint, or muscles that may not fall into any other category. Because the focus of this text is not orthopedics, many orthopedic conditions have not been included. For the most part, those conditions with a more generalized effect or accompanied by a systemic component are included here. The concepts presented in Chapter 22 are especially important to the discussion of this chapter and should be reviewed or read along with this chapter.

This chapter is divided into three distinct anatomic areas (soft tissue, joint, and bone) with conditions and diseases placed in the area most notably affected. Frequently there is overlap, and one condition affecting more than one area is found in a single section. As always, the reader is encouraged to keep a broad perspective whenever studying an isolated condition or anatomic area.

SOFT TISSUE

Soft-Tissue Injuries

Soft-tissue injuries, such as strains and sprains, lacerations, tendon ruptures, muscle injuries, myofascial compartment syndromes, dislocations, and subluxations, are described briefly in this section. For a more detailed description of these conditions, the reader is referred to Chapter 6 of this text and the more comprehensive text by Magee, Zachazewski, and Quillen (2007): *Scientific Foundations and Principles of Practice in Musculoskeletal Rehabilitation*.

Strains refer to stretching or tearing of the musculotendinous unit; they may be partial or full tears. The musculotendinous junction is a region of highly folded basement membranes between the end of the muscle fiber and the tendon. These involutions maximize surface area for force transmission but contain a transition zone where the compliant muscle fibers become relatively noncompliant tendon, placing this junction at increased risk for injury.[112] The sarcolemma of the muscle fiber is the usually site for the initial injury from an excessive stretching force.

Strains can be classified as mild, moderate, or severe (complete) tears or as injuries of first, second, or third degree depending on the severity of tissue damage. Stretching or minor tearing of a few fibers without loss of integrity is classified as *first degree* (mild), with only minor swelling and discomfort accompanied by no or only minimal loss of strength and restriction of movement.[422]

Second-degree (moderate) strain refers to partial tearing of muscle tissue with clear loss in function (ability to contract). Pain, moderate disabilities, point tenderness, swelling, localized hemorrhaging, and slightly-to-moderately abnormal motion are typical.

A *third-degree* (severe) strain refers to complete loss of structural or biomechanical integrity extending across the entire cross section of the muscle and usually requires surgical repair. An alternate classification scheme uses three grades of injury (I, II, III). Common sites for this type of injury include the ankle, knee, and fingers.

The tendon is most vulnerable to injury (*tendinitis, tendon rupture*) when it is tense or the attached muscle is maximally contracted or stressed and tension is applied quickly or obliquely. Tendon injuries can also be created by extrinsic forces that excessively cause compression or a frictioning on the tendon. Tendinosis or tendinopathy reflects more of a chronic condition with minimal or no inflammatory process detected histologically. Changes have been documented at the cellular level with expansion of local cells and thinner collagen fibrils resulting in what is now referred to as a "failed healing response."[688]

Tendinitis and spontaneous tendon ruptures have been reported to occur as a potential side effect of antibiotic treatment, especially with the use of fluoroquinolone antibiotics (e.g., drugs ending in "floxacin," such as ofloxacin, norfloxacin, levofloxacin). Reports suggest that fluoroquinolone-associated tendon disorders are more common in people older than 60 years of age, especially those who are also taking oral corticosteroids.[848] Fluoroquinolone-related tendon injuries also occur at a higher rate in heart, lung, and kidney transplant recipients. In such cases, care should be taken to avoid overloading tendons, because dramatic ruptures following even small trauma have been reported.[57,773] Therapists should monitor for tendon injuries for people with previous history of tendinopathy, magnesium deficiency, hyperparathyroidism, diuretic use, peripheral vascular disease, rheumatoid arthritis (RA), diabetes mellitus, or after participation in strenuous sports activities.[57,300,737]

Muscle contusion (bruising with intact skin) is common in contact sports and incites an inflammatory response, sometimes involving hematoma formation. The clinical manifestations of this soft-tissue injury are local pain, edema, increased local tissue temperature, ecchymosis, hypermobility or instability, and loss of function.

Myofascial compartment syndromes develop when increased interstitial pressure within a closed myofascial compartment compromises the functions of the nerves, muscles, and vessels within the compartment. Compartment syndromes may be acute or chronic and are most likely to occur within the "envelopes" of the lower leg, forearm, thigh, and foot where the fascia cannot give or expand.

Many clinical conditions predispose to the development of compartment syndromes, including fractures, severe contusions, crush injuries, excessive skeletal traction, and reperfusion injuries and trauma. Other risk factors may include burns, circumferential wraps or restrictive dressings, or a cast or other unyielding immobilizer. Ischemia and irreversible muscle loss can occur, resulting in functional disability (and even potential loss of limb) if the condition is left untreated.[283]

The earliest clinical symptom of impending acute compartment ischemia is pain disproportionate to that expected from the injury. The pain is described as deep, throbbing pressure. There may be sensory deficit or paresthesia within the region distal to the area of involvement. In severe compartment syndromes, objective signs are visible, such as a swollen extremity with smooth, shiny, or red skin. The extremity is tense on palpation, and passive stretch increases the pain.[567] Prompt surgical decompression is the standard intervention.

Injury to the *growth cartilage* can occur in skeletally immature children and adolescents. During adolescent growth spurts, the cartilage cells of the physis not only become more active but apparently become more prone to injury. Hypertrophy and weakening of the hypertrophic zone of cartilage are thought to be the cause.[268]

The three areas of growing cartilage in a skeletally immature individual include the physis (growth plate), articular cartilage of joint surfaces, and major bone–tendon attachments (apophyses). These sites account for a large number of sports injuries in young athletes, including osteochondritis dissecans (articular surface) and Osgood-Schlatter disease (apophysis); both conditions are discussed later in this chapter.

The terms *subluxation* and *dislocation* relate to joint integrity. Subluxation is partial disruption of the anatomic relationship within a joint. Mobile joints are at risk of subluxation. These include the glenohumeral, acromioclavicular, sacroiliac, and atlantoaxial joints. Once the joint condition has stabilized, rehabilitation should address local muscle imbalances and adjacent joint hypomobility, which could increase mechanical stresses at the joint.

Dislocation implies complete loss of joint integrity with loss of anatomic relationships. Often significant ligamentous damage occurs with this type of injury. Dislocations most often occur at the glenohumeral joint. Congenital dislocations are most frequently seen at the hip joints (see "Developmental Dysplasia" in Chapter 23).

Joint dislocation can also be a late manifestation of chronic disease, such as RA, paralysis, and neuromuscular disease. In the presence of a joint dislocation, the integrity of nerve and vascular tissue must be assessed. If compromise is suspected, timely reduction is essential to prevent serious complications.

SPECIAL IMPLICATIONS FOR THE THERAPIST 27-1

Soft-Tissue Injuries

Immediate immobilization is required with soft-tissue lesions to avoid excessive scar formation and prevent rerupture at the injury site. Both further retraction of the ruptured muscle stumps and hematoma size can be minimized by placing the injured extremity to rest.[421] Immobilization appears to provide the new granulation tissue with the needed tensile strength to withstand the forces created by muscle contractions. Immobilization should not extend beyond the first few days following the injury.[422]

Early mobilization for the treatment of acute soft-tissue injuries has proven effective, especially in treating injured athletes. Early mobilization induces rapid and intensive capillary ingrowth into the injured area, with better repair of muscle fibers and more parallel orientation of the regenerating myofibers in comparison to immobilization. Early mobilization has the added benefit in muscle of improved biomechanical strength, which returns to the level of uninjured muscle more rapidly using active mobilization.[422]

The therapist can guide the injured individual in following a recovery protocol to enhance healing. Crutches may be advised with severe lower extremity muscle injuries, especially injuries where adequate early immobilization is difficult to achieve (e.g., groin area).[472] Movement during the first 3 to 7 days should be with care to avoid stretching the injured muscle.

Preventing the Effects of Immobilization

The therapist can be very helpful in treating soft-tissue injuries by preventing the detrimental effects of immobilization (see Table 6-7), by promoting tissue flexibility and strength, by minimizing inflammation, and by enhancing tissue healing.

Between days 7 and 10 after an injury, the therapist can gradually progress the individual in using the injured muscle more actively, using pain and tolerance as a guide to setting limits. All rehabilitation activities should begin with a warm-up of the injured muscle, as warming up reduces muscle viscosity and relaxes muscles neurally.[627] Stimulated, warm muscles absorb more energy than unstimulated muscles and can better withstand loading. Combining a warm-up with stretching can improve the elasticity of injured muscle.[714]

Isometric training should be started first and progressed to isotonic training; isotonic strengthening begins without a resisting load–counterload, then one is progressively added. All exercises should be done within the limits of the client's pain. When the individual can complete isometric and isotonic exercises without pain, then isokinetic training with minimal load can begin.[422]

The effects of loading on the musculotendinous unit during rehabilitative exercise are increased tendon size, tensile strength, and enhanced collagen fiber organization of newly formed collagen. Restoring kinesthetic and proprioceptive awareness at the site of injury and restoring mobility and strength are also important elements of the rehabilitation program. A protocol of eccentric contraction is advocated for chronic tendinopathies, especially for the Achilles tendon.[688]

Creatine Supplementation in Athletes

The therapist working with athletes at all levels (high school, collegiate, recreational, amateur, professional) and of all ages should be aware that performance-enhancing supplements can cause muscle damage despite their intended use to build muscle mass so as to increase strength or power.[83]

One example of this type of supplement is creatine used to increase lean body mass in conjunction with a resistance training program. Potential side effects of creatine supplementation include muscle cramping, diarrhea and other gastrointestinal symptoms, and dehydration.[680]

Fluoroquinolones

Any time athletes are taking fluoroquinolones, the therapist should guide them in reducing intensity and volume of training routines until the antibiotic has been completed. Gradual return to full level of physical activity, exercise, training, and competitive play must be delayed until the full antibiotic course is completed. All athletic activity should be stopped if any adverse reactions are experienced. Monitoring for any complication (e.g., cardiac arrhythmia, photosensitivity, rashes, tendinopathies, central nervous system disorders, and hepatic and renal dysfunction) is advised for a full month after cessation of the antibiotic.[331]

Injury Prevention

Overuse injuries from repetitive stresses and microtrauma are common among children and adults, especially young athletes participating in organized sports. The therapist working with athletes from any sport can emphasize injury prevention by educating both the athletes and their parents and encouraging coaches to emphasize injury prevention.

Prevention begins with conditioning, especially at the beginning of the season for one-sport athletes who do not play year round. Training errors, variable skeletal and muscle growth rates, anatomic malalignment, and faulty equipment are just a few of the key factors that contribute to injury. For those individuals involved in multiple sports, volume and intensity of athletic involvement combined with inadequate time for recovery after injuries of any kind are key issues.[136,664]

Learning and practicing the basic skills (e.g., sliding into bases correctly, making a tackle in football, learning how to head-butt the ball in soccer) and understanding the fundamentals for each sport activity is essential. Many more injuries occur during practice than during actual competitive play, since this is where more time is spent. Early participation in organized sports at younger ages often results in overuse injuries, likely because of strength and flexibility imbalances.[664]

The therapist can help identify and correct such risk factors before they translate into injury. Early detection of risk factors and injuries can help minimize the severity of injury and reduce long-term consequences of soft-tissue damage. Everyone should be encouraged to think about injury prevention during practices as well as during competitions.

Heterotopic Ossification

Overview and Definition

Heterotopic ossification (HO) is defined as bone formation in nonosseous tissues (usually muscles and other soft-tissue areas). It is considered a benign condition of abnormal bone formation in soft tissue that occurs most commonly after trauma such as fractures, surgical procedures (especially total hip replacements), spinal cord and traumatic brain injuries, burns, and amputations. HO is the most common complication of total hip arthroplasty.[147] Classification of HO is based on the anatomic location and effect on functional motion (Box 27-1).

There is an increased incidence of HO among military personnel with blast injuries. The extreme force destroys bone, muscles, and tendons, resulting in amputation. Bone growth associated with HO in the residual limb does not follow a predictable pattern, and bone may grow into long spikes or develop more like cobwebs.

In addition to acquired forms of HO, there are forms resulting from hereditary causes such as fibrodysplasia ossificans progressiva, progressive osseous heteroplasia, and Albright hereditary osteodystrophy. These conditions are extremely rare but do provide helpful information on the pathophysiology of the condition.[845]

HO and *myositis ossificans* are terms often used interchangeably. Both conditions represent the deposition of mature lamellar bone and share radiographic and histologic characteristics, but the locations in which they occur are different. HO develops in nonosseous tissues, whereas myositis ossificans forms in bruised, damaged, or inflamed muscle.[139]

HO in people with spinal cord injuries is often referred to as *neurogenic HO*. Neurogenic HO appears to be related more to the degree of completeness of spinal cord injury than the level involved; individuals with complete transverse spinal cord injuries are more likely to develop HO compared to those with incomplete spinal cord injuries.[45,139]

Risk Factors

Risk factors for HO include a serious traumatic injury, previous history of HO, hypertrophic osteoarthritis, ankylosing spondylitis (AS), and diffuse idiopathic skeletal hyperostosis (DISH). Men seem to be at higher risk for HO than women. Other risk factors may include Paget disease, RA, posttraumatic arthritis, neural axis and thermal injuries, and osteonecrosis.[139,147]

Surgery-related factors may contribute to the formation of HO. Surgeries of the hip region may pose additional risk for the development of HO.[855] Individuals who have undergone multiple surgical interventions over a short period of time are at increased risk of HO. This may be attributed to the extensive damage to soft tissues, presence of disseminated bone dust, or formation of hematoma. Length of time in surgery also has been implicated.[68]

HO occurs in 1% to 3% of the burn population. It appears to be related more to the degree of thermal injury than to the location of the burn. Individuals with third-degree burns affecting more than 20% of the total body surface are at greatest risk for the development of HO. Systemic physiologic factors in conjunction with local factors are the likely underlying etiology.[230,396]

Etiology and Pathogenesis

The cause of HO remains unknown. Direct trauma is the most common cause of heterotopic bone formation in the elbow. It appears that there is a link between the severity of injury and the amount of ectopic bone formation that develops. Someone who sustains a massive traumatic injury is very likely to develop HO; HO is five times more likely if there is both fracture and dislocation of the elbow.[139]

It is most likely that pluripotent mesenchymal (stem) cells that could differentiate into cartilage, bone, or tendon/ligament become osteoblasts instead. Differentiation begins early after surgery and peaks at 32 hours, possibly induced by a bone-inducing substances such as bone morphogenetic protein. The stimulus and mechanism that causes this to happen in soft tissues after trauma has not been determined. There may be local factors, such as mechanical stress (e.g., articular disruption, muscle damage), and/or systemic factors.[425,517]

Individuals with traumatic brain injury are predisposed to HO, most likely because of osteoinductive factors released at the site of the brain injury, although little is known about this process.[274] In the case of bone fracture or reaming of the bone during joint replacements, bone marrow, which is capable of forming bone, may spread into well-vascularized muscle tissue. Bone marrow combined with growth factors from traumatized tissues may set off a series of steps leading to bone development and HO.[52,147]

Histologically, in the acute phase, the inflammatory process results in edema and degeneration of muscle tissue. After a few weeks, the inflamed tissue is replaced with cartilage and bone, and the bone undergoes intensive turnover. Histologically, this process cannot be distinguished from the formation of bone callus in fractures.[800]

There are histologic differences between normal bone and the ectopic (displaced) bone formed in HO. In normal bone, the periosteal layer covering the external surface of the bone has an inner vascular cambium layer surrounded by an outer fibrosis layer. In HO, the ectopic bone is not enveloped by periosteum. Instead there are three zones: the center is made up of dense cells and is surrounded by a layer of osteoid. The outermost layer consists of highly organized bone, although ectopic bone has twice the number of osteoclasts compared with normal bone and a higher number of osteoblasts as well.[895]

Clinical Manifestations

Muscle pain and loss of motion are the most common presenting symptoms, often within 2 weeks of the precipitating trauma, surgery, burn, or neurologic insult. Swelling, warmth, erythema, and tenderness mimic a low-grade infection or, in the case of surgery, the normal postoperative inflammation that is often present. The hallmark sign of HO is a progressive loss of range of motion at a time when posttraumatic inflammation should be resolving.

As the ectopic ossification advances, the acute symptoms described may subside, but motion continues to decrease, even with intervention such as dynamic and/or static progressive splinting. Over the next 3 to 6 months, the HO matures and the individual develops a rigid or abrupt end feel with pain at the end range of motion. Delayed nerve palsy is common when the elbow is affected.[139]

Areas of calcification and bone spurs may progress to ankylosis. Sites affected most often include the hip, elbow, knee, shoulder, and temporomandibular joints. The elbow is the most common site of HO in burn patients; of the 1% to 3% of individuals affected, the elbow is involved more than 90% of the time.[396] Typically, a bridge of ectopic bone forms across the posterolateral aspect of the elbow, possibly filling in the olecranon fossa.[68] Pressure from the bone formation can result in pressure ulcers and interfere with skin grafts. Loss of motion can have serious consequences for daily function, especially for those individuals who are already neurologically compromised.

Different classification schemes are used depending on the site affected. Most grade the condition based on a scale from 0 to 3 or 0 to 4. Grade 0 is no islands of bone visible on x-ray. The final grade is bony ankylosis, with progressive involvement between the lowest and highest grade (e.g., bone spurs, periarticular bone formation).[830]

MEDICAL MANAGEMENT

PREVENTION. Measures can be taken to prevent HO, such as radiation treatment and pharmaceuticals (e.g., nonsteroidal antiinflammatory drugs [NSAIDs], diphosphonates).[855] Diphosphonates inhibit osteoid cells from calcifying, thereby preventing HO. The effect lasts only as long as the drug is taken. Gastrointestinal disturbance and osteomalacia are adverse side effects of this treatment, making it less than optimal.

NSAIDs, such as indomethacin and rofecoxib, are effective in reducing the frequency and magnitude of ectopic bone formation in some areas (e.g., hip). Used during the first 3 weeks postoperatively, NSAIDs inhibit precursor (undifferentiated) cells from developing into osteoblasts.[45]

Low-dose external-beam radiation is another effective preventive measure. Fractionated radiation of the pluripotent mesenchymal cells has been shown to be effective in preventing HO from developing when delivered within 72 hours after surgery.[506] It can be used alone or in combination with NSAIDs. Prevention is recommended for individuals at high risk of ectopic ossification, including those with neurologic injury, burns, past history of HO, and/or a previous history of other conditions previously mentioned.

The best prevention for HO is to avoid soft-tissue trauma, especially among high-risk individuals undergoing surgery of any kind. Complete wound lavage and the removal of all bone debris and reamings may help prevent HO.[147]

DIAGNOSIS. A bone scan is the best method for early detection of a heterotrophic ossification. Radiographic evidence with mineralization may be observed 4 to 6 weeks after the trauma (sometimes as early as 2 weeks after the incident event). Radiographs show the location, extent, and maturity of pathologic bone. HO must be differentiated from metastatic calcification, most often associated with hypercalcemia, and from dystrophic calcifications in tumors. History and radiographic examination usually provide the tools needed to diagnose this condition. Ultrasound may prove useful in diagnosing HO around the hip or elbow and distinguishing HO from a deep vein thrombosis in someone with a spinal cord injury.[596]

A computed tomographic (CT) scan may be best to show the exact location and involvement of the articular surfaces. Laboratory tests to measure the level of serum alkaline phosphatase are used by some, but they are not consistently accurate.

TREATMENT AND PROGNOSIS. Radiation applied to the damaged limb site within a few days after the injury may respond but there is always the risk of impaired healing for those with bone fractures. The use of bisphosphonate drugs may be useful in the prevention or early stages of ossification.[45] Surgical resection is delayed until the bone matures and develops a distinct fibrous capsule so as to minimize trauma to the tissues and reduce the risk of recurrence and may only be done in cases where activities of daily living (ADLs) are compromised by loss of motion.[396]

Indication for surgery may not be just the presence of HO but rather the severity of functional restriction when loss of motion prevents the individual from using the affected extremity. A comprehensive rehabilitation program is needed to maximize motion, restore function, and reduce the risk of developing ankylosis. Once surgical removal is done, radiation and NSAIDs are continued to prevent recurrence.

SPECIAL IMPLICATIONS FOR THE THERAPIST 27-2

Heterotopic Ossification

The therapist's management of HO has evolved based on knowledge of the condition. Traditional thinking that passive range of motion is contraindicated with HO has been abandoned. There was concern that passive range of motion could lead to further bone growth, but this has not proven accurate. Forcible muscle stretching can lead to muscle tears and ossification within the muscle and is contraindicated but should not be confused with passive range-of-motion exercises, which can be effective in preventing loss of motion and ankylosis.[139]

A specific program of physical therapy intervention can be planned based on the timing of the referral. During the acute and edematous phase (first 1-2 weeks postoperatively), proper measures are taken to reduce swelling, minimize scar formation, and provide pain management to allow for maximum participation in the program. Range-of-motion exercises (passive and active) can begin but must take into account the type and extent of injury present (e.g., fracture, joint instability).

Phase 2 occurs during the inflammatory stage approximately 2 to 6 weeks after the injury or incident event. Unorganized scar tissue forms during this phase but remains soft and deformable so that range-of-motion gains can be made. The soft tissues still respond to various modalities, and self-passive stretching with weighted stretches and/or dynamic or static progressive splinting is most likely to recapture lost motion. Specific recommendations for HO affecting the elbow are available.[139]

The therapist should continue to encourage functional use of affected areas, including strengthening when appropriate, and emphasize motion throughout all motions, even if x-rays show HO developing around weeks 4 to 6 in this phase. By week 6, bone fractures are typically healed, allowing for more aggressive splinting. Scar tissue is fully formed but still malleable during this third (fibrotic) phase from 6 to 12 weeks. Splinting and resistive exercises can continue to maximize gains in motion.

Finally, during the last phase, 3 to 6 months after injury or surgery, scar tissue is organized and fibrotic. The individual may continue to make small gains, but often motion has reached a plateau and splints are discontinued gradually. Clients should be encouraged to continue a home strengthening program for at least another 6 months.[139]

Connective Tissue Disease

Overview and Incidence

Sometimes people have features of more than one rheumatic disease. This has been called the overlap syndrome or mixed connective tissue disease (MCTD). This category includes people who have overlapping features of systemic lupus erythematosus (SLE), scleroderma, or polymyositis. The incidence of this disease is unknown, but adults, particularly women, are predominantly affected.[637]

Initially, MCTD was considered a distinct entity defined by a specific autoantibody to ribonuclear protein (RNP). In the late 1980s, this concept of MCTD was considered flawed, because with time, in many of the affected people, the manifestations evolve to one predominant disease, and because many people with autoantibodies to RNP have clear-cut SLE. Consequently, the designation *overlap connective tissue disease (OCTD)* became the preferred name for the disorder in people having features of different rheumatic diseases.[406]

There is also a condition called undifferentiated connective tissue syndrome in which the systemic rheumatic diseases present have several properties shared to a variable extent by RA, SLE, polymyositis, dermatomyositis, and Sjögren syndrome, which makes a specific diagnosis for a recognizable connective tissue disease difficult.[10]

More advanced technology has brought about immunogenetic and serologic studies that demonstrate once again that MCTD is quite distinctive from other disorders, especially SLE and systemic sclerosis. There is now good evidence that the clinical and serologic features of MCTD are not just a haphazard association but represent a distinctive subset of connective tissue disease in which specific autoimmune response is relevant to clinical expression and to understanding the underlying pathogenesis.[132,526]

Etiologic and Risk Factors and Pathogenesis

The cause of connective tissue disease is unknown, but hypotheses implicating modified self-antigens or infectious agents in the pathogenesis of MCTD have been advanced.[380] Persons with this condition often have hypergammaglobulinemia and test positive for rheumatoid factor, suggesting an immune injury.

There is also a high titer of antibody to RNP (anti-RNP), but as previously mentioned, this feature is also present in SLE. The cause for the formation and maintenance of the high titer of anti-RNP antibody is unclear. There is no direct evidence that these antibodies induce the characteristic involvement of the various organ systems.

There is considerable controversy over the possible connection between silicone breast implants (and other silicone-containing devices, such as shunts and catheters) and the risk of connective tissue diseases. To date, there is no convincing evidence of an association between breast implants in general, or silicone gel–filled breast implants specifically, and any of the individual connective tissue diseases or other autoimmune or rheumatic conditions.

From a health perspective, breast implants appear to have a minimal effect on the number of women in whom connective tissue diseases develop; the elimination of implants would not be likely to reduce the incidence of connective tissue diseases.[419,477] See also "Infections with Prostheses and Implants" in Chapter 25.

Likewise, efforts to prove an association between organic solvents and connective tissue disease have not been consistently replicated; which solvents convey risk remains unknown.[272]

Clinical Manifestations

OCTD/MCTD combines features of SLE (rash, Raynaud phenomenon, arthritis, arthralgia), scleroderma (swollen hands, esophageal hypomotility, pulmonary interstitial disease), polymyositis (inflammatory myositis), and, in most people, polyarthralgias; 75% have RA. Proximal muscle weakness with or without tenderness is common.

Pulmonary, cardiac, and renal involvement, as well as such findings as Sjögren syndrome, Hashimoto thyroiditis, fever, lymphadenopathy, splenomegaly, hepatomegaly, intestinal involvement, and persistent hoarseness, may occur. Neurologic abnormalities, including organic mental syndrome, aseptic meningitis, seizures, multiple peripheral neuropathies, and cerebral infarction or hemorrhage, occur in approximately 10% of people affected by this disorder. A trigeminal sensory neuropathy appears to be seen much more frequently in MCTD/OCTD than in other rheumatic diseases.[637]

MEDICAL MANAGEMENT

DIAGNOSIS, TREATMENT, AND PROGNOSIS. The diagnosis is considered when additional overlapping features are present in persons appearing to have SLE, scleroderma, polymyositis, RA, juvenile idiopathic arthritis, Sjögren syndrome, vasculitis, idiopathic thrombocytopenic purpura, or lymphoma. High titers of serum antibodies to U1-RNP are a characteristic serologic finding seen much more often with OCTD/MCTD than with any other rheumatic disease.

General medical management and drug therapy are similar to the approach used in SLE. Most persons are responsive to immunosuppression with corticosteroids, especially if administered early in the course of the disease. Mild disease often is controlled by salicylates, other NSAIDs, antimalarials, or very low doses of corticosteroids. High doses of steroids may be used in combination with cytotoxic drugs when the disease is progressive and widespread. People with this condition should be encouraged to develop regular exercise habits and participate in an active lifestyle.[379]

The overall mortality has been reported as 13%, with the mean disease duration varying from 6 to 12 years. Individuals who respond well to steroid therapy have a good prognosis. Pulmonary and cardiac complications (e.g., pulmonary hypertension) are the most common cause of death in MCTD.[345] Sustained remissions for several years in some people receiving little or no maintenance corticosteroid therapy have been observed.

Polymyalgia Rheumatica

Overview

Polymyalgia rheumatica (PMR; literally "pain in many muscles") is a disorder marked by diffuse pain and stiffness that primarily affects the shoulder and pelvic girdle musculature. This condition is significant in that diagnosis is difficult and often delayed; severe disability can occur unless proper intervention is initiated. PMR may be the first manifestation of a condition called giant cell arteritis, an endocrine disorder, malignancy, or an infection.[782]

The initial symptoms associated with PMR are often subtle and of gradual onset, resulting in a delay in the person's seeking care. The complaints also may be localized to one shoulder, leading to an initial diagnosis of bursitis. As the disease progresses, carrying out ADLs becomes increasingly difficult. Bed mobility and sit-to-stand transfers are among the functional activities affected.

Finally, a significant number (15%-20%) of those with PMR also develop giant cell arteritis, a condition characterized by inflammation in the arteries of the head and neck (see further discussion in Chapter 12). The risk related to the arteritis is blindness secondary to obstruction of the ciliary and ophthalmic arteries from inflammation-associated swelling.[449]

Incidence and Risk Factors

Female gender, age, and race are the three primary risk factors associated with PMR. Women are affected twice as often as men, and the disease is rare before the age of 50 years; most cases occur after age 70 years. White women are more commonly affected than are women of other ethnicities. PMR is a relatively common condition, with incidence estimated at 1 in 200 for the general population.[718]

Etiologic Factors and Pathogenesis

The cause of PMR is unknown, but experts suspect that genetic factors, infection, or an autoimmune malfunction may play a role. There is a genetic predisposition for PMR; the immune system gene human leukocyte antigen (HLA) DR4 (see Table 40-21) has been linked to this condition. Besides associations with HLA, tumor necrosis factor (TNF) appears to influence susceptibility to both PMR and giant cell arteritis. Additional studies are under way to clarify the genetic influence on susceptibility to these conditions.[306]

Despite complaints of pain and stiffness in the muscles, PMR is not associated with any histologic abnormalities. Serum creatinine kinase levels, electromyograms, and muscle biopsy results are negative in this population.

Rather, the aching and stiffness typical of this condition are caused by joint inflammation.[852]

A number of imaging studies can be used to image the effects of this condition, with ultrasound and scintigraphy the most promising techniques. Magnetic resonance imaging (MRI) studies show that subacromial and subdeltoid bursitis of the shoulders, iliopectineal bursitis, and hip synovitis are the predominant and most frequently observed lesions in active PMR.[125] The inflammation of the bursa associated with glenohumeral synovitis, bicipital tenosynovitis, and hip synovitis may explain the diffuse discomfort and morning stiffness.

Clinical Manifestations

PMR may begin gradually, taking days or weeks for symptoms to become fully evident, but more often it develops suddenly, and the person wakes up one morning feeling stiff and sore for no apparent reason. Getting out of bed in the morning can be the biggest challenge for individuals with PMR before initiating drug therapy.

Even though the initial muscle pain and stiffness may occur unilaterally, the symptoms are often bilateral and symmetric, affecting the neck, sternoclavicular joints, shoulders, hips, low back, and buttocks. Painful stiffness lasts more than 1 hour in the morning upon arising and is a hallmark feature of this disorder. Flu-like symptoms, such as fever, malaise, and weight loss, are not uncommon.[852]

Peripheral manifestations (e.g., wrists or metacarpophalangeal joints) are present in approximately 50% of all cases of PMR and include joint synovitis, diffuse swelling of the distal extremities with or without pitting edema, tenosynovitis, and carpal tunnel syndrome.[719] Many people are misdiagnosed with fibromyalgia, myositis, tendonitis, thyroid problems, or depression and spend months searching for answers and help before the correct diagnosis is made.

Despite the complaints of difficulties with bed mobility, sit-to-stand maneuvers, and accomplishing ADLs such as combing the hair or brushing the teeth, muscle weakness is not the problem. Pain and stiffness are the primary issues. Local tenderness of the involved muscles is noted with palpation. In addition, fever, malaise, unexplained weight loss, and depression may occur.

For those individuals with concomitant giant cell arteritis, additional symptoms of headache, jaw pain, scalp tenderness, fever, fatigue, weight loss, anemia, or blurred or double vision can occur.

MEDICAL MANAGEMENT

DIAGNOSIS. Because there are no definitive tests to identify PMR, the diagnosis is often based on the presence of a constellation of findings and the person's rapid response to a trial of prednisone. Besides the complaints noted under "Clinical Manifestations" above, the person may be anemic and present with an elevated erythrocyte sedimentation rate (ESR; measure of viscosity); lowered hemoglobin and elevated platelet count (indicators of inflammation); and elevated C-reactive protein (indicator of current disease activity).[188,577]

The current diagnostic criteria include as a requirement an ESR higher than 30 or 40 mm/hr. However, several reports indicate that a large number of people with PMR (7%-22%) have a normal or slightly increased ESR at the time of diagnosis, supporting the notion that an increased ESR should not be an absolute requirement for the diagnosis of PMR. This subset is characterized by younger age, less marked predominance of females, lower frequency of constitutional symptoms (e.g., weight loss, fever), and a longer diagnostic delay.[544]

The lack of rheumatoid factor, the presence of antinuclear antibodies, and the lack of histologic changes in the muscles contribute to the diagnosis by excluding other conditions. MRI or ultrasonography of the joint or joints may facilitate diagnosis in anyone with typical proximal symptoms of PMR who also has normal ESR values.[130]

TREATMENT AND PROGNOSIS. Untreated, PMR can result in significant disability. It is imperative that the individual be checked for giant cell arteritis, a frequently concurrent condition that can cause irreversible blindness.[843]

Treatment is with corticosteroids (e.g., prednisone); the response is dramatic. In fact, if dramatic improvement is not noted within 1 week of starting the prednisone, the diagnosis of PMR is questioned and the person must be reevaluated.[577]

Two to 4 weeks after these symptoms are controlled, the slow tapering begins, the rate of which is based on clinical symptoms and some laboratory parameters. Most people require a maintenance dosage of prednisone for 6 months to 3 years that is gradually tapered to the lowest effective dose required to control symptoms. Treatment may take up to 5 years or longer before complete clinical remission occurs.[843] Methotrexate is not as effective as steroids but may be used for or in combination with corticosteroids for individuals who develop a dependency on corticosteroids in order to decrease the corticosteroid load.[437]

PMR is not life-threatening but it can limit daily activities, decrease restful sleep with nighttime awakenings and difficulty turning in bed, and decrease a sense of well-being and quality of life. With proper treatment, the prognosis is good, as the disease is self-limiting in many people with resolution within a period of 1.5 to 2 years; however, recurrence can be as high as 30% in people who received treatment for 1 to 2 years. Those individuals with temporal arteritis are at increased risk for stroke or blindness.[843]

SPECIAL IMPLICATIONS FOR THE THERAPIST 27-3

Polymyalgia Rheumatica
When treating someone with a history of PMR, the therapist must be aware of the potential risk of giant cell or temporal arteritis. An adult older than age 65 years with sudden onset of temporal headaches, exquisite tenderness over the temporal artery, scalp sensitivity, or visual complaints should be seen by his or her physician immediately as this vasculitis is associated with stroke and blindness.[449]

Increased complaints of muscle pain and stiffness should direct the therapist to ask if the client is still taking the prednisone as directed. Because of the dramatic

relief obtained with prednisone, clients may quit taking it prematurely. Careful monitoring of the dosage level is necessary for proper tapering of the medication. Communication with the primary physician is warranted in the presence of this scenario.

Potential side effects of prednisone include weight gain, mood swings, cataracts, glaucoma, diabetes, easy bruising, rounding of the face, difficulty sleeping, and hypertension (see further discussion in Chapter 5).

Side effects are less likely to occur at low doses; any of these side effects must be evaluated by the physician. Accelerated bone loss and compression fractures are important concerns.[852] The therapist can be very instrumental in client education about preserving bone strength through the use of calcium, vitamin D, and exercise (see "Osteopenia and Osteoporosis" in Chapter 24).

Because PMR is an inflammatory response involving bursitis and tenosynovitis, therapy intervention can begin with this pathogenesis in mind. For example, the use of ultrasound as a deep heating agent in the presence of inflammation should be reconsidered when approaching this type of problem.

Rhabdomyolysis

Overview and Definition

Rhabdomyolysis is the rapid breakdown of skeletal muscle tissue as a consequence of mechanical, physical, or chemical traumatic injury (Box 27-2). The principal result is a large release of the creatine phosphokinase enzymes and other cell by-products into the blood system. Accumulation of muscle breakdown products can lead to acute renal failure.

Box 27-2

CAUSES OF RHABDOMYOLYSIS

Physical
- Prolonged high fever; hyperthermia
- Electric current (electrical and lightning injuries)
- Excessive physical exertion (pushups, cycling, marathon running)

Mechanical
- Crush injury
- Burns (including electrical injuries)
- Compression (e.g., tourniquet left on too long)
- Compartment syndrome

Chemical
- Medications (e.g., antibiotics, statins, first-generation H_1-receptor antagonists)
- Herbal supplements containing ephedra (rare)
- Excessive alcohol use
- Electrolyte abnormalities
- Infections
- Endocrine disorders
- Heritable muscle enzyme deficiencies
- Mushroom poisoning (rare)

Etiology and Risk Factors

Of particular note is the potential rhabdomyolysis from high-dose statins (cholesterol-lowering medications).[190] Less than 5% of the adult population who take statins develop this problem. However, with more than 15 million Americans taking these drugs, the prevalence is on the rise.[735,829]

Underlying neuromuscular diseases may become clinically apparent during statin therapy and may predispose to myotoxicity.[48,170] Rhabdomyolysis also has been reported in performance athletes taking herbal supplements containing ephedra; there are similar reports of rhabdomyolysis in individuals using weight-loss herbal supplements.[539,790]

Strenuous exercise, including marathon running, biking, and exercises such as push-ups, sit-ups, or pull-ups can result in damage to skeletal muscle cells, a process known as exertional rhabdomyolysis.[178]

Pathogenesis and Clinical Manifestations

The individual may report muscle pain (myalgia) and weakness ranging from mild to severe.

The exact mechanism for statin-induced rhabdomyolysis remains unknown. There may be a drug influence on deoxyribonucleic acid (DNA), an enzyme deficiency, or autoimmune reaction triggered by the drug.[170] Regardless of the cause, the effect of the process is well known; specifically, when muscle proteins are released into the blood, one of these proteins (myoglobin) can precipitate in the kidneys and spill into the urine. The client may report a change in color of the urine, most often tea colored or the color of cola soft drinks.

The therapist is most likely to see this with military recruits or marathon runners who have been exercising in hot and humid weather, or who have taken analgesics, had a viral or bacterial infection, and/or have a preexisting condition.[178] Acute excessive consumption of alcohol exacerbated by a hot environment and dehydration can also predispose individuals competing in athletic events to exercise-induced rhabdomyolysis.

Massive skeletal muscle necrosis can also occur, further complicating the situation with reduced plasma volumes leading to shock and reduced blood flow to the kidneys resulting in acute renal failure. As the injured muscle leaks potassium, hyperkalemia may cause fatal disruptions in heart rhythm.

MEDICAL MANAGEMENT

DIAGNOSIS, TREATMENT, AND PROGNOSIS. The diagnosis is typically made by history and clinical presentation and confirmed by laboratory studies when an abnormal renal function and elevated creatine phosphokinase are observed. To distinguish the causes, a careful medication history is considered useful. Often the diagnosis is suspected when a urine dipstick test is positive for blood, but no cells are seen on microscopic analysis. This suggests myoglobinuria, and usually prompts a measurement of the serum creatine phosphokinase, which confirms the diagnosis.[646]

Treatment is directed toward rehydration and correction of electrolyte imbalances by administering intravenous fluids, and in the case of renal failure, dialysis may be necessary. In most cases of rhabdomyolysis, especially in the case of exertional rhabdomyolysis, damage to skeletal muscle cells resolves without consequence. Clinically significant rhabdomyolysis is uncommon but, when present, can be life-threatening.[735]

SPECIAL IMPLICATIONS FOR THE THERAPIST 27-4

Rhabdomyolysis

Recovery from statin-induced rhabdomyolysis occurs with cessation of the medication, but there may be some evidence that muscle training can speed up the recovery process.[149] The presence of peripheral rhabdomyolysis should prompt the therapist to assess the individual for impaired muscle performance, especially proximal muscle weakness, including the inspiratory muscles. Changes in cardiorespiratory function in individuals taking statins and presenting with muscle weakness anywhere in the body should be investigated more closely.[149]

The natural history of skeletal muscle recovery after statin-induced rhabdomyolysis has not been investigated. One case report has shown the potential benefit of intense muscle training following statin-induced muscle damage. Research is needed to answer the questions of whether exercise aids, inhibits, or exacerbates muscle weakness in affected individuals. If, indeed, exercise is beneficial, then exercise parameters (type, frequency, intensity, duration) must also be investigated. With the increasing number of adults taking cholesterol-lowering statins, therapists may expect to see a concomitant increase in adverse events such as rhabdomyolysis.

Myopathy

Definition and Overview

Myopathy is a term used to describe nonspecific muscle weakness secondary to an identifiable disease or condition. The term *myositis* is also used to describe idiopathic inflammatory myopathies.

Many metabolic and hormonal diseases and autoimmune diseases can cause muscle weakness. Myopathies are usually classified as either hereditary or acquired (Box 27-3; see also Table 39-3) Myopathy associated with polymyositis or dermatomyositis is discussed in Chapters 5 and 10.

A new disorder called *critical illness myopathy (CIM)* has also been introduced (see "The Medically Complex Patient: Critical Illness" in Chapter 5). Disorders associated with prolonged stays in intensive care units (ICUs; e.g., acute respiratory illness, septic inflammatory response syndrome, acute respiratory distress syndrome) often result in excessive and prolonged weakness. CIM is a nonnecrotizing myopathy accompanied by fiber atrophy, fatty degeneration of muscle fibers, and fibrosis. As improvements in medical technology and medical management of individuals with severe illness continue to improve, the incidence of CIM is expected to rise.[235,700,676]

CLASSIFICATION OF MYOPATHIES*

Hereditary

- Muscular dystrophy
- Congenital myopathy
- Myotonia
- Metabolic myopathy
- Mitochondrial myopathy (e.g., zidovudine [AZT] myopathy [rare])
- Neurologic (e.g., Charcot-Marie-Tooth disease)

Acquired

- Inflammatory myopathy
  - Idiopathic
  - Dermatomyositis, polymyositis
  - Rheumatoid arthritis
  - Autoimmune diseases
  - Human immunodeficiency virus (HIV)–associated myopathy
- Endocrine myopathy
  - Diabetes mellitus
  - Thyroid disease
- Myopathy associated with systemic illness
  - Renal impairment
  - Cancer
  - Acute lung injury
  - Acute respiratory distress syndrome
  - Septic inflammatory response syndrome
- Drug-induced or toxic myopathy
  - Corticosteroids
  - Alcohol
  - Statins (cholesterol-lowering drugs)

*See Table 39-3.
Data from Goldman L, Schafer AI. *Goldman's Cecil medicine, expert consult premium edition*, ed 24, Philadelphia, 2011, WB Saunders; and McDonald CM: Myopathic disorders. In Braddom R, editor: *Physical medicine and rehabilitation*, ed 4, St Louis, 2012, Elsevier.

Myopathy (myositis) associated with infectious causes is mentioned briefly in Chapter 25. Information about other sources of muscle pain not discussed in this chapter and their neurophysiologic bases is also available.[571]

Etiologic Factors and Pathogenesis

The idiopathic inflammatory myopathies are thought to be immune-mediated processes that are triggered by environmental factors in genetically susceptible individuals. The pathogenesis of acquired myopathies and their course are highly variable and depend on the underlying cause. For example, in thyrotoxicosis, the high metabolic rate reduces the muscle stores of nutrients, whereas in hypothyroidism, the entire metabolism, including the energy-generating metabolism of muscles, is slowed down. Myopathy associated with RA is caused by the rheumatic joint disease.

Expression of proinflammatory cytokines such as interleukin (IL)-1 on endothelial cells and expression of major histocompatibility complex class I antigens on muscle fibers are associated with muscle weakness in individuals with active and chronic disease.[7]

Diabetes is associated with myopathy of three origins: vascular, neurogenic, and metabolic. Diabetes affects the small blood vessels and is associated with chronic hypoperfusion of muscles with blood. Diabetes also affects the peripheral nerves and causes neurogenic muscle atrophy and weakness. The disturbances of carbohydrate and lipid metabolism caused by insulin deficiency or insulin resistance adversely affect muscle function.

Acquired myopathy can also occur as part of a paraneoplastic syndrome (see discussion in Chapter 9). Tumors may produce muscle weakness with or without inflammation. Human immunodeficiency virus (HIV)–associated myopathies are less common now with improved medical intervention, but may still be encountered by the therapist.

Medications such as the cholesterol-lowering statins are associated with tendinitis and muscle abnormalities. Use of systemic corticosteroids combined with prolonged exposure to neuromuscular blocking (paralytic) agents during the treatment of various critical illnesses in the ICU mentioned above may be the key risk factor for this type of acute myopathy. Septic inflammatory response syndrome may be another risk factor.[700]

Clinical Manifestations

Myopathy is characterized by progressive proximal muscle weakness with varying degrees of pain and tenderness. Distal involvement is possible but is more common in myositis. During the early stages of disease, the muscles may be acutely inflamed and painful to move and touch. Muscle weakness and easy fatigability eventually compromise aerobic capacity and affect the person's endurance, ability to work, socialize, and complete ADLs.[368] Other symptoms of systemic illness may be present, including fever, fatigue, morning stiffness, and anorexia. Statin-induced myopathy can produce respiratory myopathy with impaired inspiratory muscle performance characterized by fatigue, muscle pain, and weakness.[149]

MEDICAL MANAGEMENT

DIAGNOSIS. The management of myopathy is determined by the underlying cause. Muscle biopsy, electromyography, and laboratory findings (measurement of muscle enzymes) are essential to ensure diagnostic accuracy, especially in the case of idiopathic myopathy. Electromyography can allow differentiation between myopathy and neuropathy and can localize the site of the neuropathic condition. The typical laboratory profile reveals mild to marked elevations in muscle enzymes, including creatine kinase and aldolase.

Some imaging techniques of muscles, such as MRI and magnetic resonance spectroscopy, can assess changes in local inflammatory activity. Changes in protein and gene expression patterns in repeated biopsy specimens provide molecular information that may lead to a more precise disease classification scheme and improved treatment, but these are research tools at this time.[516]

TREATMENT AND PROGNOSIS. Inflammatory myopathies may respond to pharmacologic treatment, especially corticosteroids, but also immunosuppressives and antimalarial agents. Oral creatine supplements combined with exercise have proven effective for improving muscle function without adverse effects in adults with inflammatory myopathies.[172]

Effective therapy for noninflammatory myopathies remains lacking; antiinflammatory agents do not appear to be helpful in these cases. Presently there is no known pharmacologic treatment or prevention for CIM. Medical management to minimize the risks is suggested.[700]

Prognosis is variable, with some people responding well to medical therapy and rehabilitation and others continuing to decline. Longstanding disability is not uncommon despite aggressive immunosuppressive treatment; the reasons for the persisting disability remain unknown.[7] Additionally, corticosteroid-related complications can have a significant impact.

Factors associated with poor survival include onset after age 45 years, delayed diagnosis and intervention, severe weakness and pharyngeal dysphagia, malignancy, myocardial involvement, and interstitial lung disease. CIM is reversible, but there is often considerable morbidity (e.g., persistent pain and weakness, HO with frozen joints).[476] ICU-acquired myopathy prolongs hospitalization because of the need for extensive rehabilitation. Even with rehabilitation, many affected individuals remain heavily dependent upon others for personal care and ADLs.[542]

SPECIAL IMPLICATIONS FOR THE THERAPIST   27-5

Myopathy

See also "Special Implications for the Therapist 10-14: Dermatomyositis and Polymyositis" in Chapter 10 and "Corticosteroids" and "Immunosuppressive Agents" in Chapter 5.

Reduced muscle strength, endurance, and coordination accompanied by fatigue are commonly reported with myopathies. Myalgia occurs at rest and with exercise in half or more of all affected individuals in all stages of the disease. Left untreated, most cases of muscle weakness associated with inflammatory myopathies progress slowly over months and result in further decline of muscle strength and endurance.[13]

Baseline measurement of muscle function using manual muscle testing assesses strength but not endurance, an important feature with this condition. A functional index to specifically test muscle impairment is under investigation but has not been finalized. For now, outcome measures are limited to activity limitation and participation restriction.[13]

Acute Care

Physical therapists in the acute care setting frequently see the effects of bed rest, even without associated injury and after only as little as 1 week as disuse atrophy causes decrease in muscle mass. Often this occurs in the older adult population who have already experienced significant decline in muscle mass.

The effects of ICU-acquired myopathy are even more pronounced in the person who is both on bed rest and

critically ill. CIM is also often accompanied by critical illness polyneuropathy, a disorder of the peripheral nerves triggered by the same events as CIM.[700] For further discussion, see "The Medically Complex Patient: Critical Illness" in Chapter 5.

Patients with the combination of these two conditions have difficulty weaning from the ventilator. Once the individual is alert and less sedated, weakness and atrophy of the limbs becomes more readily apparent. Severe flaccid tetraparesis may even be observed. Muscles innervated by the cranial nerves appear to be spared. Whereas critical illness polyneuropathy can affect all limbs and muscle groups, distal weakness and sensory changes are more common. CIM typically affects larger, more proximal muscle groups; sensation is not impaired.[700]

Recovery can be delayed by weeks to months. Further details regarding intervention and prognosis are available in Chapter 5. The therapist is a key member of the rehabilitation team, recognizing the need for psychologic and emotional support to the patient and the family. Understanding that the patient is not just deconditioned and has a complex pathologic condition can help facilitate appropriate referrals to other disciplines (e.g., occupational therapy, psychology, social work, physiatry, speech pathology).[700]

Exercise and Myopathy

Early rehabilitation is important in the course of myopathy, with careful application of rest and exercise (rest during the active inflammatory phase; rebuilding of muscle strength during remission). During periods of severe inflammation, bed rest and passive range of motion are recommended; active range of motion exercises are contraindicated.[198]

It is important to design a rehabilitation program according to the type, stage, and severity of myopathy. Muscle assessment and functional evaluation are prerequisites to determining an appropriate intervention program. In extremely acute cases, a tilt-table may be necessary to reacclimatize the cardiovascular system and assist with balance training for the individual who has been on bed rest.

The exercise program begins in the acute phase with stretching and passive range of motion and progresses throughout the recovery process according to the person's tolerance to include isometric, isotonic, and low-intensity aerobic activities. Moist heat applied before stretching inflamed or sore muscles may be helpful. Performing exercises in a gravity-eliminated environment (aquatic program) or gravity-eliminated position may be necessary in the beginning.[368] Attention to the muscles of respiration and breathing assessment are also important, and anyone with cardiac involvement must be evaluated before initiating an aerobic program.

Concern about stressing the already inflamed muscles with a resultant increase in creatine phosphokinase level has traditionally prevented the use of strengthening exercises for anyone with inflammatory myopathies. But exercise itself can cause elevated serum creatine kinase levels in healthy individuals,[535] and studies have shown that people with stable active disease can perform isometric exercise without causing a sustained rise in creatine phosphokinase level.

The effects of exercise training on inflammatory myopathies have determined the potential role of exercise as method for lowering systemic inflammation markers.[369,370,611] Studies show improvement in adults with stable myopathies after a 12-week 20-minute home exercise program combined with a 15-minute walking program 5 days per week. Improvement was measured as reduced impairment and reduced activity limitation/participation restriction.[14,16]

Similar results have been reported for individuals with active myopathies performing an intensive resistive exercise program.[12,15] People in a variety of exercise programs, including stair climbing, stationary cycling, strength training, group exercise in a pool or at a gym, and outdoor walking using a wide range of frequency, intensity, and duration, have all shown improvement in fatigue and aerobic fitness while serum creatine kinase levels remain unchanged.[13] Experts advise a general recommendation of daily physical activity for 30 minutes 5 to 7 days each week. Supervised continuous aquatic exercise adapted to the individual's disease level and disability is also recommended.[13]

A home program including heat modalities, prescriptive exercise, and assistive devices assists the individual to manage with functional disability. Upper-extremity splinting and lower-extremity bracing may be necessary to prevent contractures, prolong mobility, and enhance functional skills. A weak quadriceps mechanism combined with foot drop or a shuffling gait can contribute to increased falls, necessitating an assessment of muscle strength and balance, and risk for falls with necessary intervention.

Client education about this condition is important and should include energy conservation (see Box 9-4) and joint protection education. Serious side effects can accompany high-dose corticosteroid therapy, compounding the functional difficulties already present with the myopathy (see further discussion in Chapter 5).

Myofascial Pain Syndrome

Jan Dommerholt, PT, DPT, MPS

Overview

Myofascial pain syndrome and trigger points (TrPs) have been described for centuries, but continue to be overlooked and often ignored in general clinical practice.[358,762] Pain management specialists are more likely to recognize the importance of TrPs[255,340] and often realize that TrPs are one of the most common primary musculoskeletal pain conditions.[144] Frequently, TrPs are concomitant with other pain diagnoses, such as migraines and tension-type headaches,[121,246,252,293] epicondylalgia,[256,251] carpal tunnel syndrome,[678,774] arthritis,[50,51] shoulder problems, including impingement syndromes,[371,107] pelvic pain conditions,[30,208,420,886,907] fibromyalgia,[3,276,278] and whiplash injuries,[210,211,266] among others.

Janet Travell and David Simons are credited for bringing TrPs and their referred pain patterns back to the foreground.[767,835] Long before she described TrPs, Travell was intrigued by Kellgren's studies of experimentally induced referred pain published in the late 1930s.[445,446] As a cardiologist, Travell wondered about the implications of Kellgren's work for the field of cardiology.[760] Soon after she started exploring muscle referred pain, she realized that skeletal muscles harbor TrPs and that these feature typical referred pain patterns. In just a few years, she shifted her attention from cardiology to muscle pain and dysfunction,[832,834] although she continued to publish in the field of cardiology.[313,696] In 1952, she published the typical referred pain patterns for 32 muscles and their TrPs.[833]

Definition and Classification

The most broadly accepted definition of a TrP states that a TrP is a hyperirritable spot in a taut band of a skeletal muscle that is painful on compression, stretch, overload or contraction of the tissue, which usually responds with a referred pain that is perceived distant from the spot.[767]

TrPs are classified as *active*, when they cause spontaneous local and referred pain, and as *latent*, when they only cause pain upon stimulation. Active TrPs are more sensitized,[249] feature more endplate noise,[471] involve a greater area of a muscle,[833] have a significantly altered chemical milieu,[740,741] and significantly lower pain thresholds with electrical stimulation in the muscle, the overlying cutaneous, and the subcutaneous tissues than latent TrPs and non-TrP muscle tissue.[857,858]

Nevertheless, recent research confirms that latent TrPs also provide nociceptive input into the dorsal horn even though they are not spontaneously painful.[275,277,279,497,882,899,909] Whether a TrP is considered active or latent depends at least partially on the degree of sensitization. It is often assumed that TrPs represent strictly local muscle phenomena, but it is now known that TrPs are peripheral sources of persistent nociceptive input, leading to peripheral and central sensitization.[121,248,251,293]

Both active and latent TrPs can cause allodynia and primary and secondary hyperalgesia, which suggests that afferent fibers from TrP nociceptors make new effective connections with dorsal horn neurons that normally only process information from remote body regions.[569,570] Secondary hyperalgesia is usually referred to as referred pain.

Etiologic and Risk Factors

Trigger points have been reported in all age groups, except infants.[17,174,436,856,905] There is evolving evidence that they develop following various forms of muscle overload, including unaccustomed eccentric and concentric loading,[288,412] but also with low-load repetitive tasks and sustained postures.[386,836]

In addition to mechanical overload, TrPs may also develop in association with visceral pain and dysfunction,[420,254,292,859] such as endometriosis, interstitial cystitis, irritable bowel syndrome, and prostadynia, with psychologic or emotional conditions,[55,763] or even with respiratory stress, such as overbreathing.[145,418]

In other words, any sustained or repetitive activity may contribute to TrPs. Mechanical and structural factors, including anatomical variations such as forward head posture, significant leg-length deficiencies or scoliosis, that affect or overload muscles must be identified, resolved, or alleviated.[247,715] Medical and psychologic problems that affect muscle function must also be identified and corrected where possible.[287]

Pathogenesis

At the sarcomere level, TrPs are linked to a possibly damaged or at least dysfunctional sarcomere assembly, leading to shortened sarcomeres, fiber degeneration and inflammatory responses within the muscle fiber.[286,312,555,612,766,878] Damage to the muscle filaments may breakdown the barrier formed by the actin and titin, with the filaments becoming stuck in this barrier at the Z-line of the sarcomere.[626,879] TrP formation is linked to motor endplate changes, including an excessive release of acetylcholine, an inhibition of acetylcholine esterase, and an upregulation of nicotinic acetylcholine receptors,[287,764] that causes the muscle to become hypertonic. Human and animal studies have shown that the excessive acetylcholine release correlates with the occurrence of endplate noise that does not require an electrical activation of the α-motor neuron.[114,146,152,153,183,521,677,761,765]

The "integrated TrP hypothesis" was developed by Simons, Travell, and Simons and has been updated based on new evidence about TrPs.[288,562,764,765,767] The integrated TrP hypothesis describes how the sensory, motor, and autonomic systems all contribute to the developing and sustaining a TrP. The sustained contractures create a local hypoxia, which triggers an immediate drop in the tissue pH. A lowered pH will inhibit acetylcholine esterase, but stimulate release of adenosine triphosphate, bradykinin and other proinflammatory mediators that will maintain contraction of the muscle fiber, initiate hyperalgesia and central sensitization, and affect the sympathetic nervous system. Muscle nociceptors will respond to the local chemical changes from a TrP by inducing neuroplastic changes in the dorsal horn of the spinal cord that is partially responsible for the referred pain phenomena associated with TrPs.

Clinical Manifestation

TrPs are usually very painful to touch and often palpation results in verbalizations, body movements, and recognition by the patient of the familiar pain complaint. TrPs can restrict range of motion,[243,250,314,531] alter movement activation patterns,[513,514] cause local and referred pain, and cause weakness without signs of atrophy,[212] which need to be assessed.

Referred pain phenomena may be a feature in the clinical presentation. The term "referred pain" should

be interpreted broadly as the term encompasses not just pain, but also other paresthesia, such as tingling, burning, and numbness. The presence of referred pain can be rather confusing for clinicians and patients, as the location of the pain complaint usually does not match the source of the pain.[291] For example, pain in the medial aspect of the patella and knee may be caused by TrPs in the adductor longus muscle, and retroorbital headaches may originate in TrPs in the sternocleidomastoid or trapezius muscle.[246] Knowledge of typical referred pain patterns is necessary to link the history to clinically relevant TrPs.

MEDICAL MANAGEMENT

DIAGNOSIS. Although myofascial pain is recognized as a legitimate clinical entity, there are no uniformly accepted diagnostic criteria.[515,608,831] Lucas and colleagues noted that the reliability of locating active TrPs in symptomatic individuals has not been examined and concluded that high-quality studies are needed.[515] There is, however, some level of consensus among expert clinicians and researchers.[108,285,387,609]

The most relevant criteria for the identification of TrPs include the presence of a taut band in a relevant muscle, the presence of a TrP in that band, and reproduction of the familiar pain complaint.[285,831] The medical diagnosis is made based on history and physical examination. The problem may be confined to just a few muscles or may be more widespread, regional or generalized. Although taut bands and TrPs can be visualized with magnetic resonance and sonoelastography, these tests have no clinical utility at this point in time.[154,155,758] TrPs can be located and treated with shockwave technology, but because of the high costs of these units, few clinicians use shockwave therapy in the diagnosis and management of myofascial pain.[67,68,603,604]

Physicians should evaluate patients for any possible underlying causes or contributing factors, such as structural or mechanical perpetuating factors, including scoliosis, leg-length discrepancies, localized or widespread joint hypermobility, and nutritional, metabolic, or systemic perpetuating factors, including vitamin insufficiencies or hormonal imbalances. Physical therapists also need to be familiar with the most common perpetuating factors and communicate with patients' physicians when they suspect any underlying problems.

Although there is a lack of randomized, controlled, double-blind studies or even epidemiologic correlational studies verifying the clinical observations that certain metabolic and nutritional factors are relevant in the treatment of individuals with myofascial pain, clinical observations are part of the accepted hierarchy of evidence-based medicine and should be considered. The most common metabolic factors in myofascial pain are hypothyroidism, iron, vitamin B_{12} and vitamin D insufficiencies or deficiencies.[213] Possible side effects of medications (e.g., statins) may include widespread myalgias.[759,771]

TREATMENT. Medical management must address any contributing and perpetuating factors and possible comorbidities based on common differential diagnostic considerations. Pain, depression, anxiety, and poor sleep hygiene must be addressed using contemporary approaches, including pharmacologic interventions. As many people with persistent pain have poor sleep hygiene, sleep studies may be needed. Referral to other health care providers may be indicated, including physical therapy and cognitive behavioral psychology or clinical social work.

PROGNOSIS. The prognosis of myofascial pain is directly related to the awareness of clinicians with the current scientific literature and their training and experience. Well-trained health care providers are able to provide effective treatments, inactivate TrPs, and return patients to full functional status. However, few medical and physical therapy schools include myofascial pain and TrPs in their curriculum.

SPECIAL IMPLICATIONS FOR THE THERAPIST 27-6

Myofascial Pain Syndrome

Clinically, a detailed history and physical examination are required. The clinician needs to explore the occurrence of any precipitating event, habit, or activity that may have caused muscle overload. The history taking should consider the presence of muscle pain and TrPs secondary to visceral pathology. The physical therapist's examination needs to include a biomechanical assessment with appreciation of which muscles could potentially be subjected to repetitive or sustained overload and an assessment of any compensatory movement strategies.

Unusual asymmetries and abnormal breathing patterns should be noted.[145] Range of motion of clinically relevant joints must be assessed before and after TrP inactivation. It is common to see an immediate improvement in range of motion, muscle strength, movement coordination, and pain levels. Palpation of relevant muscles is the last step in the process and starts with the identification of the taut bands. The taut band is further assessed for the presence of TrPs. When properly identified, TrPs can be treated very effectively with manual techniques, dry needling, and injections as part of a comprehensive management strategy.[3,50,151,153,167,243,388,389,495,513,514,677] Perpetuating factors must be addressed. There is some evidence that laser,[19,135] high-power ultrasound,[531] and some electromodalities[703] may be useful, but not all studies support this.[695] Conventional ultrasound has only a temporary antinociceptive effect.[788,789] Many people with myofascial pain syndrome present with inadequate posture, including forward head posture, which must be addressed through education and proprioceptive training.[267]

Physical therapy intervention can also contribute to improved sleep patterns. Once pain levels are reduced and TrPs have been inactivated, physical therapy should include common treatment interventions, such as strengthening, flexibility, and cardiovascular conditioning, among others.

A THERAPIST'S THOUGHTS*
Myofascial Pain Syndrome

Although the textbooks by Simons, Travell, and Simons are among the best-sold medical texts in the world, with translations in many languages, it is striking that awareness of the existence and implications of TrPs is not widely integrated in the thought process of health care providers. An increasing number of schools of physical therapy are including the assessment and treatment of TrPs in their curriculum, as new scientific evidence about TrPs emerges.

The growing interest in dry needling is bringing the problem of TrPs to the foreground, but it seems that the intrigue is more focused on the "new modality" than on the evidence-informed utilization of helping reducing or eliminating pain and improving function. There is still strong opposition to TrP concepts by some physical therapy groups even though, from my observations in exchanges on websites and blogs, it appears that most opponents of TrP concepts are not familiar with the surge in scientific studies and do not really have a basis for their concerns.

Some argue that "pain is produced by the brain" and therefore a focus on muscle pain would be counterproductive. Yet, as persistent sources of peripheral nociceptive input, TrPs should be considered within the context of contemporary pain sciences. It is my hope that in the near future, there will be universal understanding and education to explore the current scientific knowledge base and incorporate TrP concepts throughout physical therapy curricula. In the end, patients and society at large will benefit from this change in direction and focus.

*Jan Dommerholt, PT, DPT, MPS

Pelvic Floor Muscle (PFM) Dysfunction

Beth Shelly, PT, DPT, WCS, BCB-PMD

Overview

The pelvic floor muscles (PFMs) are a collection of voluntary, skeletal, internal muscles stretching like a sling from the pubic bone to the coccyx and surrounding the vagina, urethra, and rectum (Fig. 27-1). They work together to support the internal pelvic organs and close off the urethra and rectum to maintain continence (Fig. 27-2). These muscles also participate in sexual arousal and orgasm. The nomenclature of the skeletal muscles in this area is not consistent throughout the literature. In this text "pelvic floor muscles" includes all the skeletal muscles of the pelvic floor.

Pelvic floor muscle dysfunction is the specific dysfunction of the skeletal muscle layer in the pelvic floor (Table 27-1). Physical therapists who have expertise in skeletal muscle dysfunction have a great deal to offer individuals with these dysfunctions.

Etiologic Factors

Many diagnoses and symptoms that result in dysfunction of the pelvic floor musculature or chronic pelvic pain are included under the heading of PFM dysfunction (Box 27-4). Only general concepts related to the multitude of causes and symptoms can be covered in this text. For more specific information related to each of these conditions, the reader is referred elsewhere.[86,349]

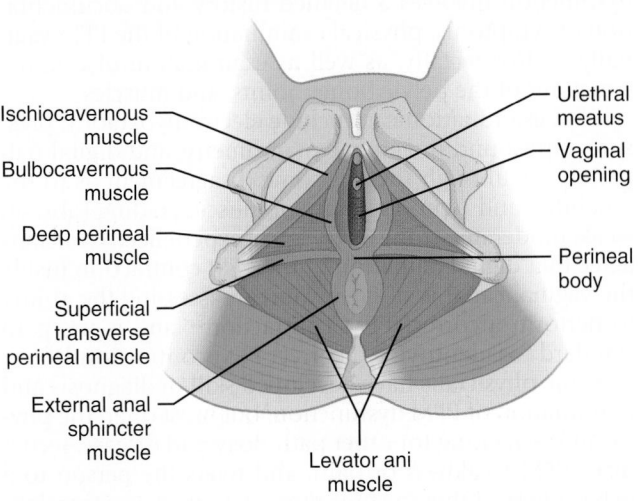

Figure 27-1

Pelvic floor muscles. There are three layers of the pelvic floor muscles (PFMs) from superficial to deep; the most superficial layer of the PFMs include the external anal sphincter for control of gas and feces, the sexual muscle (bulbocavernous and ischiocavernous), and the superficial transverse perineal muscles. The second layer, sometimes referred to as the *urogenital diaphragm*, includes the sphincter urethra and urethrovaginal sphincter and participates in urinary continence. (From Myers RS: *Saunders manual of physical therapy*, Philadelphia, 1995, WB Saunders.)

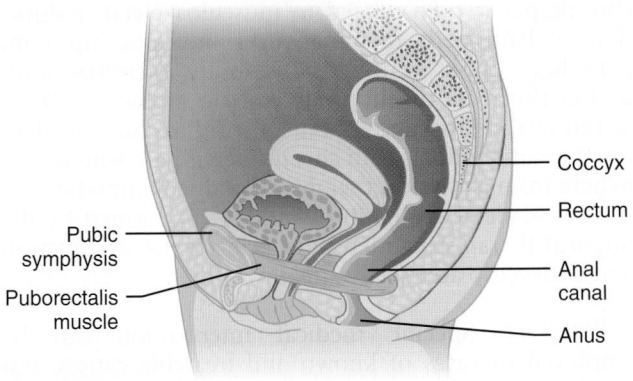

Figure 27-2

Pelvic floor muscles. The deepest layer is collectively known as the levator ani muscles. The levator ani muscle is made up of four muscles: the puborectalis, pubococcygeus, coccygeus, and ischiococcygeus muscles (not shown) and supports the pelvic viscera in both the male and female. (From Myers RS: *Saunders manual of physical therapy*, Philadelphia, 1995, WB Saunders.)

Prevalence

The prevalence of PFM dysfunction remains unknown, but it is considered a common problem among women of reproductive age, many of whom have never been diagnosed. Prevalence is available for the pathologies of PFM dysfunction such as urinary and fecal incontinence and pelvic organ prolapse (see discussion in Chapter 20). The lack of a consensus on the definition of chronic pelvic pain and lack of a classification scheme hinder epidemiologic studies. One large U.S. study[546] reported 15% of females age 18 to 50 years describe symptoms of chronic pelvic pain. A similar study in the United Kingdom showed a prevalence of chronic pelvic pain of 24%.[546,911] Although the majority of these conditions affect women, men can also be affected.

Pathogenesis

Underactive PFM is defined as "a situation in which the PFM cannot voluntarily contract when it is appropriate."[352] This is reflected in decreased strength and endurance, and poor PFM coordination during increased intraabdominal pressure such as coughing and sneezing. Underactive PFM is associated with urinary incontinence and pelvic organ prolapse. Pathogenesis of underactive PFM and pelvic floor disorders such as urinary incontinence, fecal incontinence, and pelvic organ prolapse, is investigated in several recent studies.[42,140,204] PFM avulsion, over stretching of the muscle and connective tissue and damage to the pudendal nerve are all implicated as possible causes of pelvic floor disorders and muscle dysfunction. Forceps, episiotomy, long pushing stage and large fetal head appear to contribute to the trauma.[204]

Overactive PFM is defined as "a situation in which the PFMs do not relax, or may even contract when relaxation is functionally needed."[352] Overactive PFM is characterized by an increase in PFM tension, active spasm, or incoordination causing musculoskeletal pain or dysfunction of the urogenital and/or colorectal system.

The pathogenesis of overactive PFM and chronic pelvic pain remains poorly understood, and laparoscopic investigation often reveals no obvious cause for pain.[460] Injury to the pudendal nerve as a result of pelvic surgery, childbirth, ruptured disk, injury to the coccyx, or the herpes zoster virus may account for some cases of chronic pelvic pain. Origin of dysfunction can be categorized as tissue based/nociceptive or neuropathic/central sensitization.[372]

Table 27-1	Pelvic Floor Muscle (PFM) Disorders		
Name of Condition	**Description**	**Symptoms/Diagnosis**	**Signs/Impairments**
Normal PFM	PFM is able to contract and relax on command and in response to increased intraabdominal pressure as appropriate	Normal urinary, bowel and sexual functioning	Normal voluntary and involuntary contraction and relaxation of the PFM
Underactive PFM	PFM is unable to contract when needed	Urinary or fecal incontinence, pelvic organ prolapse	Absent or weak voluntary PFM contraction; noncontracting PFM
Overactive PFM	PFM is unable to relax and may contract during functions such as defecation or micturition	Obstructive voiding or defecation, dyspareunia, pelvic pain	Absent or incomplete voluntary PFM relaxation; nonrelaxing PFM

Based on data from Haylen BT: An International Urogynecological Association (IUGA)/International Continence Society (ICS) joint report on the terminology for female pelvic floor dysfunction, *Int Urogynecol J* 21(1):5–26, 2010.

CAUSES OF PELVIC FLOOR MUSCLE DYSFUNCTION

Underactive PFM

- Pregnancy alone and/or birth-related trauma
- Abdominal or pelvic surgery
- Chronic increased intraabdominal pressure: obesity, chronic constipation, chronic coughing, poor exercise and lifting techniques
- Psychogenic origin
- Spinal cord injury or other neurologic condition (e.g., stroke, Parkinson disease, multiple sclerosis)

Overactive PFM

Research has been unable to clearly identify causation. This represents conditions that appear with or precede overactive PFM:

- Musculoskeletal injury or trauma (back, sacrum, sacroiliac area, hip, pelvis)
- Habitual postural dysfunction
- Fibromyalgia, chronic fatigue syndrome
- Nerve entrapment or injury, nerve root irritation
- Myofascial pain syndrome, trigger points
- Abdominal or pelvic surgery
- Childbirth trauma and episiotomy
- Pain related to rectal hemorrhoids, rectal fissures
- Psychogenic origin
- Sexual assault, sexual abuse, or negative sexual experiences
- Bowel and bladder disorders, including endometriosis, interstitial cystitis, diverticulitis, constipation, irritable bowel syndrome, regional enteritis (Crohn disease)
- Unknown cause

Current evidence points to the occurrence of central sensitization as the primary origin of pain in some conditions of chronic pelvic pain.[372] In these cases, there will be little tissue impairments and treatments would be directed at the hypersensitive nervous system.

Clinical Manifestations

Clinical manifestations of PFM dysfunctions are determined by the underlying etiologic factors and pathologic findings. For example, the primary presentation of someone with *underactive* PFM can vary from urinary incontinence to perineal pressure of pelvic organ prolapse.

Clinical presentation of individuals with *overactive* PFM is a pain, pressure, or ache, usually poorly localized in the perivaginal, perirectal, and lower abdominal quadrants and pelvis (suprapubic or coccyx regions) and sometimes radiating down the posterior aspect of the thigh. Symptoms of overactive PFM are often reproduced by manual palpation and examination of the PFMs. Other symptoms of overactive PFM dysfunction may include low back pain that is intermittent and unpredictable, changes location often, and is difficult to reproduce; sharp, fleeting rectal pain; painful intercourse or inability to penetrate; extreme rectal pressure; and pubic bone pain or tenderness. See website resource for more on overactive PFM.

MEDICAL MANAGEMENT

DIAGNOSIS. Diagnosis and diagnostic testing depends on history and clinical presentation. Evaluation of PFM dysfunction involves a detailed history and documentation of symptoms, physical examination of the PFM vaginally and/or rectally, as well as examination of external structures of the pelvic bones, joints, and muscles.

PFM examination can include electromyography, pressure, ultrasound imaging, dynamometry, and digital palpation.[87] Although there is some disagreement as to the reliability and reproducibility of muscle grading (absent, weak, moderate, strong),[85,572] most experienced clinicians agree that digital palpation of the PFM contraction inside the vaginal canal is of great value in assessing the ability to perform a correct PFM contraction[86] and is the gold standard for identifying a correct PFM contraction.[484]

Some physicians have developed skill in diagnosis and examination of PFM dysfunction, but most often the physician is screening for other pathology and disease, recognizes PFM weakness or pain, and refers the person to a pelvic physical therapist for more definitive examination.

Examination for Overactive Pelvic Floor Muscle. According to Neville et al,[620] ultrasonography and MRI are being used more often to image the PFM now that the technology has advanced. Previously, laparoscopic examination was used with poor results in more than half of all pelvic pain cases.

PFM tenderness and a positive Patrick or FABER (flexion, abduction, external rotation) test with overpressure results in 100% specificity in identifying women with chronic pelvic pain related to musculoskeletal dysfunction.[620] Pain with this maneuver indicates hip joint pathology, pubic symphysis instability, sacroiliac joint dysfunction, or an iliopsoas muscle spasm.[232] These screening tests are suggested in an effort to correctly identify those individuals with chronic pelvic pain who would benefit from a physical therapy referral. A comprehensive musculoskeletal evaluation would be performed by the physical therapist to identify specific tissue dysfunction and to develop an effective treatment plan.

TREATMENT. Specific medical intervention can be employed in cases of known and treatable causes, but more often, medical management has been limited to treatment of symptoms using pharmacologic and hormonal agents and surgical intervention with variable results.

Physical therapy intervention is quickly becoming the first-line therapy of choice for many causes of PFM dysfunction. Working with a counselor or other skilled professional is recommended when treating someone with a past (or current) history of abuse.

Proper instruction in PFM exercise is an important part of prevention and treatment. PFM exercises, also called *Kegel* exercises, were named for Dr. Arnold Kegel who did research using the exercise in the mid-1900s.[444] Although the lay public refers to them as "Kegel" exercises, the preferred term is *PFM* exercises. Brief verbal or written instruction in performing a PFM contraction is not adequate preparation as measured in more than 50% of cases investigated.[53,117] A properly performed PFM exercise should result in a significant increase in the force of the urethral closure without an appreciable Valsalva effort. Improperly done, the PFM exercise technique can potentially promote incontinence.

The best time to explain a PFM contraction is during a pelvic examination. The medical practitioner can describe the exercise and verify that it is done correctly during digital palpation of the muscle inside the vagina or rectum. A trained practitioner, such as a physical therapist, can also provide follow-up assessment and training with necessary biofeedback to ensure the success of a properly performed exercise program. This may be particularly helpful in older adults, who often have a difficult time localizing pelvic muscles.

SPECIAL IMPLICATIONS FOR THE THERAPIST 27-7

Pelvic Floor Muscle Dysfunction
Prevention and Education

It is imperative that women (including adolescent females) receive education about the functions and dysfunctions of the pelvic floor complex to promote preventive exercises rather than waiting for the need of restorative pelvic floor exercise. Exercises for the pelvic floor should be part of every woman's fitness regimen, either as prevention or specific to the type of pelvic floor muscle dysfunction and its causes.

Therapists need to routinely ask women questions about pelvic floor function (e.g., presence of urinary incontinence, pain with sexual intercourse or other sexual dysfunction, presence of known reproductive organ or pelvic floor dysfunction, and past history; see questions in "Special Implications for the Therapist 18-8: Urinary Incontinence" in Chapter 18) and provide education and exercise programs for these muscles, making a medical referral when appropriate.

Physical Therapist Intervention

Intervention must be determined based on examination, including external assessment and, in the case of those therapists with additional training, internal pelvic floor muscle examination. Patients may be instructed to visualize the perineal area in a mirror or palpate lightly to sense an inward movement of the area during PFM contraction. Internal vaginal assessment by a skilled physical therapist would be recommended if there is outward movement, no movement, or the person is unsure of the proper technique. Remember, more than 50% of individuals tested could not perform PFM exercises correctly with verbal instructions alone and over 20% were performing them in a way that might increase leakage.[117]

Any unspoken behaviors or indication of discomfort on the part of the client should prompt the physical therapist to stop and communicate with the client before continuing or discontinuing. Issues of childhood incest or sexual assault or adult sexual issues may be a significant contributing factor, requiring combined pelvic muscle rehabilitation and psychotherapy or sexual abuse counseling. Special considerations include cultural differences in modesty, the possibility of current substance use or abuse, and past (or present) sexual abuse or sexual dysfunction.

Pelvic Floor Muscle Training

(See Evolve Site for more information.)

To date, many systematic reviews, Cochrane reviews, and meta-analyses have documented the benefits of PFM exercises for female stress urinary incontinence. Comparing PFM training to no treatment,[216] women with stress urinary incontinence who were treated were 17 times more likely to report cure or improvement and were 5 to 16 times more likely to be continent on pad test. Dumoulin[216] concludes that it is "no longer a question of whether PFM training programs work but what components and combinations thereof are most effective."

Men, children, older adults, and individuals with neurological dysfunction can also benefit from specialized PFM training and conservative management provided by a pelvic physical therapist.[128,347,365,373] PFM training should be tailored to the needs of the individual and may include increasing PFM force and endurance, decreasing PFM resting tone, and coordinating the PFM to contract and relax when needed.

Therapists are encouraged to provide instructions and monitor results. The patient should be referred to a specialized physical therapist if expected improvements are not reported.[216] A skilled evaluation is needed to fully identify each person's needs and is beyond the scope of this text; however, a brief review of PFM strengthening is included here.

Exercise Prescription

PFM exercises can be prescribed in several modes: active assistive, active, and resistive.

Active Assistive Pelvic Floor Muscle Exercises

Active assistive PFM exercises would include exercises with overflow facilitation. The adductors, gluteals and external rotators are thought to assist in strengthening the PFMs.[88,216,394] Contraction of overflow muscles, such as squeezing a ball between the knees or pushing the knees apart against elastic band resistance, can decrease urinary incontinence symptoms, especially in the elderly and pediatric populations.[216] However, these are not a substitution for the individually instructed, isolated, active PFM exercises that have been shown in high-level research to be effective.[166,216,353]

Active Pelvic Floor Muscle Exercises

Active PFM exercises form the bulk of training and have been studied and reported most often. These exercises can be combined with several forms of biofeedback (pressure or electromyography). Despite expert opinion, multiple randomized controlled trials have failed to show a statistically significant difference between outcomes with and without electromyography training as long as the exposure to individual PFM training is the same.[76,297,363,601]

Individualized PFM training includes attention to several factors (more specific information about PFM training is available on the Evolve website). Components of PFM training program would include determining the *number of seconds* the PFM contraction is held and amount of rest between contractions. *Number of repetitions* performed and the *number of times the set is repeated* during the day would also be determined.

Exercise prescription would also include choosing the *position* (supine, sitting, or standing) used for static exercises. Likewise, consideration is given when selecting positions used during PFM training for dynamic activities (such as lifting and bending) and PFM training in combination with abdominal muscle contraction.[431] "The Knack" is a technique in which the individual practices squeezing the PFM before sneezing and coughing and can result in 98% decrease in urinary incontinence.[583] Attention is also given to breathing phase to restore normal intraabdominal pressure and avoid bearing down.[376,431]

Resistive Pelvic Floor Muscle Exercises

Resistive PFM exercises would include insertion of a vaginal weight or changing to upright position for exercises. Some practitioners believe that exercises done in an upright position (sitting or standing) provide gravity resistance and are more difficult. However at least one randomized study comparing supine-only PFM exercises to supine and upright PFM exercises showed no significant difference in decreasing urinary incontinence.[95] Still most physical therapists start exercises in the supine position and add upright exercises as needed. Vaginal weights can result in decreased urinary incontinence,[362] but comparison studies do not show a significant advantage over PFM exercises alone.[89]

There is some research to show optimum *frequency* of supervised PFM training. Dumoulin (2011) reports training carried out under supervision more than two times per month to be the most effective.[216] *Individual versus group training* is another decision that must be made when planning prescriptive training exercise for PFMs. In a study comparing individual PFM training to group PFM training,[655] participants undergoing individual training were dryer on pad test but otherwise both groups had improvement in strength, quality of life, and personal satisfaction (86% in both groups). Group PFM exercises are significantly better than no treatment.[655]

Studies on long-term effects of PFM training found that adherence was a significant predictor of success both during the period of therapy and thereafter.[11] Meta-analysis of PFM training shows the program must last for at least 6 weeks (*duration*).[166] There is no standard agreement on maintenance; this aspect of the plan of care should be individualized for each person.

Underactive Pelvic Floor Muscle

In addition to the PFM exercise training discussed above, intervention for underactive PFM may focus on postural education to place the pelvic floor in the most optimal position for strengthening and function and motor learning techniques (e.g., use of a Swiss ball), and behavioral training (see Evolve site for urge suppression techniques). Principles of motor learning guide the therapist in incorporating pelvic muscle function with breathing (work of the diaphragm muscle), the abdominal muscles, and low back muscles. This is an important step in creating sensory awareness of the pelvic floor that takes time and repetition.

Restoring normal pelvic floor strength and bladder control is essential before resuming vigorous physical activity or exercise.

The therapist is very instrumental in teaching contraction of the appropriate muscles without muscle contraction of the gluteal muscles and with complete relaxation of the pelvic muscles between contractions. With verbal and manual cues, or biofeedback (auditory, visual, or electronic), the client can be taught to contract the pelvic floor muscles while maintaining decreased activity in other hip and trunk muscles. Patients are also taught to maintain pelvic floor muscle tone while avoiding a Valsalva maneuver.

Overactive Pelvic Floor Muscle

Intervention for overactive PFM may focus on postural education to place the pelvic the pelvic floor in the most optimal position for relaxation and function and aerobic exercise to mobilize the pelvis; behavioral training; joint alignment; soft-tissue, scar, and/or visceral mobilization; myofascial release therapy; trigger point therapy; strain–counterstrain; and stretching for the adductors, iliopsoas, piriformis, internal obturator, abdominals, and other muscles as determined by the assessment. Biofeedback and relaxation training can enhance normalization of overactive tone and dilators may be used to stretch the vaginal tissues and train relaxation during intercourse. Education on the physiology of pain and cognitive behavioral therapy may also contribute to success in individuals with chronic pelvic pain syndromes.

A THERAPIST'S THOUGHTS*

Advanced Training

There are several certificate course series specifically for physical therapists interested in treating urinary incontinence and other pelvic dysfunctions. Postgraduate training is necessary to fully treat PFM dysfunction. For an internal pelvic floor assessment or treatment therapists should be fully educated in consent-to-treat and issues of third person in the room. Further resources are available on the Evolve website.

*Beth Shelly, PT, DPT, WCS, BCB-PMD

Coccygodynia

Beth Shelly, PT, DPT, WCS, BCB-PMD

Overview and Etiology

Coccygodynia (also coccydynia) was first used by Dr. Thiele in his description of pain related to the coccyx and the muscles attached to the coccyx in the 1930s.[818] Causes are often unclear, but fall into several categories: musculoskeletal, direct trauma related to childbirth or direct fall, inflammation related to trauma or sacrococcygeal calcium deposits,[670,694] infections,[650, 818] referred pain from visceral sources in the pelvis,[650] neoplasm (sacral chordoma), or centralized pain syndrome.

Musculoskeletal causes include poor sitting posture, pelvic asymmetry/malalignment, PFM spasm, sacrococcygeal luxation or hypermobility, coccygeal spicule (hook on end of coccyx), lumbosacral disk degeneration.[296] (Note: Luxation is a translation type slippage of the joint—not in a physiologic direction. Hypermobility refers to the excessive movement in a physiologic movement like flexion and extension.)

Sacral chordoma is a rare, slow growing tumor that should be considered in the medical differential diagnosis, especially when there are neurologic symptoms present.[424] Overactivity of the ganglion impar (cluster of nerve cells in front of the sacrum or coccyx joint where the sympathetic trunks of the two sides unite) can also cause chronic coccyx pain.

Clinical Manifestations

Symptoms are primarily related to pain with sitting; however, pain on transfer from sit-to-stand is often related to the musculoskeletal causes of coccyx pain. In individuals with coccygodynia, movement of the coccyx may be painful. In addition, palpation of the PFMs rectally may identify TrPs, overactive PFM, and decreased ability to relax the PFM.

MEDICAL MANAGEMENT

Medical examination includes radiography in standing and lateral sitting positions,[296,694] which could reveal posterior luxation, hypermobility in flexion, coccygeal spicule, and/or crystal deposits in the sacrococcygeal or intercoccygeal joints.

Medical treatments include medications (e.g., oral analgesics and NSAIDs) as a first-line treatment.[650,694] A short course of oral corticosteroids for calcific deposits may be recommended.[694] Corticosteroid injection (with or without anesthesia) can result in 60% to 65% improvement in some musculoskeletal cases.[529,650] Local anesthetic injections to block ganglion impar (ganglion impar is the location where two pelvic sympathetic trunks converge ending in a ganglion at the front of the coccyx) often produces 50% to 75% relief of coccyx pain.[120,650] A study by Foye and colleagues[264] reported that some individuals can receive 100% relief from just one injection of this type when performed under fluoroscopic guidance.

Partial or total coccygectomy is not recommended based on a review in the pain literature,[650] while the same procedure is recommended by a systematic review published in the orthopedic literature.[437] Studies supporting the use of this type of surgical intervention are levels 3 and 4 and report 54% to 96% success with overall complication rate of 11% related to infections.[437] Removal of the distal segment of a nonunion coccyx fracture appears to provide some surgical success. Chordoma and other sacral tumors are curable with surgery and early diagnosis may lead to preservation of bladder, bowel, motor and sexual function.

SPECIAL IMPLICATIONS FOR THE THERAPIST   27-8

Coccygodynia

Physical therapy treatments include manipulations of the coccyx, massage to levator ani muscles, and manual treatment of pelvic joint malalignment. The therapist assesses and treats muscle imbalances and prescribes exercises to address biomechanical dysfunction of the PFMs. The therapist will also provide patient/client education on sitting posture, use of appropriate cushions, and avoidance of aggravating factors such as lifting and constipation.[530,694]

JOINT
Chondrolysis
Overview

Chondrolysis is a process of progressive cartilage degeneration resulting in narrowing of the joint space and loss of motion. It is seen most often as a complication of slipped capital femoral epiphysis, but can occur in association with infection, trauma, and prolonged immobilization for any reason. Trauma can also include orthopedic procedures such as arthroscopic meniscectomy, shoulder arthroscopy, anterior cruciate ligament reconstruction, and thermal capsulorrhaphy.[148,338,492,660]

The hip is the most likely location for chondrolysis to occur, but cases have been reported affecting the knee, shoulder, and ankle. Spontaneous chondrolysis without known risk factors occurs occasionally, most commonly in adolescent girls. In fact chondrolysis occurs five times more often in females than in males; adolescence is the most common period of onset.[675,892]

Etiology and Pathogenesis

The etiology is unknown; many theories have been proposed, including nutritional abnormalities, mechanical injury, ischemia, abnormal chondrocyte metabolism, ischemia, and abnormal intracapsular pressure. There may be some evidence to support an autoimmune mechanism responsible for the cartilage destruction.[675]

Various studies have implicated IL-1, which has chondrolytic action by stimulating the release of inflammatory mediators, enhancing the breakdown of cartilage proteoglycans. Clearly, some disruption of the cartilage extracellular matrix occurs leading to chondrolysis, but the key to the process has not been discovered.

Clinical Manifestations

Regardless of the underlying cause of this condition, the affected individual presents with progressive joint stiffness with progressive loss of motion and pain. Chondrolysis of the hip causes anterior hip and/or groin pain accompanied by an antalgic gait. Soft-tissue contracture can result in an apparent leg-length discrepancy and pelvic obliquity with muscle atrophy. Painful ankylosis may develop in some individuals, whereas others experience an improvement in pain and range of motion.[902]

MEDICAL MANAGEMENT

DIAGNOSIS, TREATMENT, AND PROGNOSIS. Imaging studies are used to make the diagnosis. Plain radiographs may exhibit signs of joint narrowing, erosions of subchondral bone or even signs of osteopenia. For advanced cases, the definitive diagnosis may be made on the basis of scintigraphy and/or MRI.

Treatment is with NSAIDs to control synovial inflammation. Protected weight bearing and maintenance of joint motion are important components of the treatment plan. Surgery may be indicated (e.g., capsulectomy, tendon release of the adductor and iliopsoas), but the best course of operative treatment is unknown.[902]

Osteoarthritis

Overview

Osteoarthritis (OA), or degenerative joint disease, is a slowly evolving articular disease that appears to originate in the cartilage and affects the underlying bone, soft tissues, and synovial fluid.

OA is divided into two classifications: primary and secondary. Primary OA is a disorder of unknown cause, and the cascade of joint degeneration events associated with it is thought to be related to a defect in the articular cartilage. Secondary OA has a known cause, which may be trauma, infection, hemarthrosis, osteonecrosis, or some other condition.

OA is present worldwide as a heterogeneous group of conditions that lead to slow, progressive degeneration of joint structures with defective integrity of articular cartilage in addition to related changes in the underlying bone at the joint margins. OA can lead to loss of mobility, chronic pain, deformity, and loss of function.

Incidence

OA is the single most common joint disease, with an estimated prevalence of 60% in men and 70% in women after age 65 years, affecting an estimated 27 million people in the United States.[483] In fact, it is the most common musculoskeletal disorder worldwide affecting the hands and large weight-bearing joints such as the hip and knee and causing disability.[289] And the overall prevalence is expected to increase dramatically over the next 20 years as the population ages.

Before age 50 years, the prevalence of OA in most joints is higher in men than in women, but this pattern changes after age 65 years. In the United States, OA is second only to ischemic heart disease as a cause of work disability in men older than 50 years.[84]

In the United States, approximately 6% of adults older than 30 years of age have OA of the knee and 3% have OA of the hip; incidence rises with increasing age. Both incidence and prevalence are expected to rise in the coming decades as a result of the aging of America combined with more extreme sports and activities (see "Etiologic and Risk Factors" below). OA is the most common indication for total joint replacements.[483]

Etiologic and Risk Factors

The etiology of OA is multifactorial, including many components of biomechanics and biochemistry. Evidence is growing for the role of systemic factors such as genetics, nutrition and weight control, estrogen deficiency (menopause), bone density, immune system response, and local biomechanical factors (e.g., muscle weakness, obesity, femoral dysmorphia, soft-tissue laxity, mechanical properties of the cartilage and labrum, and loads and positions imposed on the joint by functional activities).[242,547]

Serious injury and an inherited predisposition account for half of all cases of OA in the hands and hips and knees.[241,280,704] Smokers with knee OA sustain greater cartilage loss and have more severe knee pain than those who do not smoke, suggesting a role for tobacco in cartilage degeneration.[27]

There is low or no additional risk of OA from regular, moderate running, but sports that involve high-intensity, acute, direct joint impact from contact with other players do carry an increased risk of OA, especially when repetitive joint impact and twisting are combined. Football players, soccer players, hockey players, and baseball pitchers are especially at increased risk. Anterior cruciate ligament injury may predispose athletes to knee OA, especially when accompanied by meniscectomy.[179,580] Labral tears and femoroacetabular impingement are risk factors for the development of hip OA. Labral tears can also disrupt the synovial seal that contains the synovial fluid within the joint. The resulting increase in joint friction can further damage the joint and contribute to the development of osteoarthritic changes.[547]

Although the theory is as yet unproven, some experts warn that extreme sports, such as snowboarding, mountain biking, and aggressive in-line skating, with the increased incidence of repeated impact or injury, may be risk factors for OA developing earlier in life. Much of the OA in men is attributable to occupational activities, particularly kneeling or squatting, along with heavy lifting and repetitive use of heavy machinery.[6,241,242]

Generalized ligamentous laxity appears to be a predisposing factor; this may be related to the presence of estrogen receptors on the ligaments. Postmenopausal women appear to be at increased risk.[817] Some women have a condition called *hypermobility joint syndrome* (or *hypermobility syndrome*), with loose, unstable joints resulting from a dominant inherited connective tissue disorder.[325,896]

Hypermobility syndrome is characterized by excessive laxity of multiple joints, a condition that is separate from the generalized hypermobility associated with disorders such as Ehlers-Danlos syndrome, RA, SLE, or Marfan syndrome. Hypermobility syndrome appears to be a systemic collagen abnormality with a decreased ratio of type I to type III collagen (see Table 6-2).[712]

Women with this syndrome may develop OA earlier than the norm. Muscle weakness in anyone can also cause joint changes leading to OA, such as occurs with prolonged immobilization, polymyositis, multiple sclerosis, or any of the myopathies listed in Box 27-3.

Some studies show a link between patellar alignment and patellofemoral OA manifested by a loss of cartilage thickness and knee pain and disability.[399] Other studies suggest that malalignment is not a risk factor for OA, but rather a marker of disease severity and its progression.[398] Additional studies are needed to establish the normal and abnormal ranges of patellar alignment indices and their relationship to patellofemoral OA.[433]

Pathogenesis

The pathophysiologic events associated with OA are beginning to be understood more definitively. It is quite clear now that OA is a disorder of the whole synovial joint organ, not just "wear and tear" on the cartilage. In fact, it may be that damage to the articular cartilage is the by-product of a disease process that is centered in subchondral bone in particular.[576]

In recent years, the view of OA has shifted to that of both a local and systemic condition in which inflammation plays an important part in determining the symptoms and disease progression.[239,536] The former wear-and-tear concept has been replaced by the idea that OA is an active disease process with joint tissue destruction and aberrant repair as a result of alterations in cellular function.[240]

Although joint cartilage is the final target of the pathologic processes, the underlying subchondral bone may be the primary etiologic agent. Treatment focused on modifying changes in the bone may alter the pathologic processes observed in the adjacent cartilage.[2] The use of new, potent bone antiresorptive agents in clinical use will help test this hypothesis.[501,781]

Tissue changes in OA are the result of active joint remodeling processes involving an imbalance between catabolic and anabolic repair activity. People with OA may have a general tendency toward increased bone metabolic activity, especially in response to biomechanical or other stimuli such as occurs with obesity and injury.[2]

As OA develops, loss of cartilage, hypertrophic changes in neighboring bone and joint capsule, mild synovial inflammation, and degenerative changes in the menisci, ligaments, and tendons all contribute to pain and loss of joint function, resulting in joint failure.[743] These changes lead to a mechanopathology where abnormal loading of joint structures leads to excessive loading of joint structures that allows for further damage and dysfunctional movements.[240]

It has been discovered that essential inflammatory cytokines, such as IL-1β and TNF-α, initiate this cycle of catabolic and degradative events in the cartilage, mediated by metalloproteinases, enzymes that degrade cartilage extracellular matrix as part of the normal turnover in all tissues. These enzymes are upregulated after joint injury.[2]

The role of inflammation in the pathophysiology and progression of early OA is supported further by the observation that C-reactive protein levels are raised in women with early knee OA and higher levels predict those whose disease will progress. The synovium from OA joints stains positive for IL-1β and TNF-α. Nitric oxide, which exerts pro-inflammatory effects, is released during inflammation. In experimental OA, nitric oxide induces chondrocyte apoptosis, thus contributing to cartilage degradation. Hence, unregulated nitric oxide production in humans plays a part in the pathophysiology of the disease.[159,730]

Articular cartilage has an important role in joint physiology by providing a smooth, relatively friction-free surface between the bony ends making up the joint. In addition, the cartilage attenuates the mechanical load transmitted through the joint. With progressive loss of cartilage, inflammation develops, with resultant bony overgrowth, ligament laxity, and progressive muscle weakness and atrophy accompanied by joint pain. The finding of estrogen receptors on chondrocytes suggests that estrogen deficiency so common in the postmenopausal woman who is not on hormone replacement plays a role in the health of the articular surface.[813]

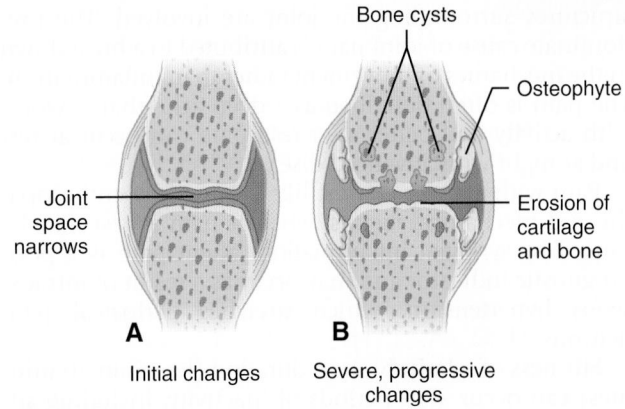

Figure 27-3

A, Early degenerative changes associated with osteoarthritis include joint space narrowing and articular cartilage erosion. **B,** Late degenerative changes associated with osteoarthritis include osteophyte formation and articular cartilage fissuring and eburnation.

Once the cartilage begins to break down, excessive mechanical stress begins to fall on other joint structures. Eventually, fissuring and eburnation of the cartilage (thinning and loss of the articular cartilage resulting in exposure of the subchondral bone, which becomes denser with the surface becoming worn and polished) can occur.

The joint space narrows as the cartilage thins, and sclerosis of the subchondral bone occurs as new bone is formed in response to the now excessive mechanical load. New bone also forms at the joint margins (osteophytes) (Fig. 27-3) with the end result being mechanical joint failure and varying degrees of loss of joint function.

Immobilization is another factor that can result in articular cartilage degeneration. Secondary to the lack of vascular supply, articular cartilage depends on repetitive mechanical loading and unloading for the nutritional elements to reach the chondrocytes and the cellular waste products to return to the synovial fluid and eventually to the bloodstream.[80] This nutritional mechanism of articular cartilage is interrupted by immobilization. If the nutritional cycle is interrupted long enough, structural changes will occur.

Clinical Manifestations

The most common symptoms of OA include bony enlargement, limited range of motion, crepitus on motion, tenderness on pressure, joint effusion, malalignment, and joint deformity. Inflammation is a prominent sign that plays a role in symptom generation. Soft-tissue inflammation and edema are observed during acute exacerbations.[239] The most commonly involved joints associated with this disorder are the weight-bearing joints, especially the hip and knee but also the shoulder, lumbar and cervical spine and the first carpometacarpal and metatarsophalangeal joints.[348]

The onset of symptoms related to OA can occur insidiously or suddenly. Only a portion of people who have radiographic evidence of OA have associated pain.[656] For most people, however, the pain complaints progress slowly and gradually. Because the cartilage is not innervated, pain is not perceived until the bone or other structures surrounding the joint are involved. The predominate cause of joint pain is attributed to a breakdown in the mechanics of movement rather than inflammation. The pain is often described as a deep ache that is worse with activity and better after rest; pain can occur at rest and at night with advanced disease.[259,428]

Pain with activity is most likely caused by enthesopathy and mechanical factors, whereas pain at rest may be caused by synovial inflammation. Night pain is a poor prognostic indicator and may occur as a result of intraosseous hypertension, which stretches periosteal pain neurons.[301]

Stiffness of relatively short duration (less than 30 minutes) can occur after periods of inactivity, including sitting and sleeping. Morning stiffness usually only lasts 5 to 10 minutes after awakening. Movement and activity dissipate this stiffness until the individual sits or rests for a long period of time. This differs from RA, in which the morning stiffness or gelling can last until noon or even midafternoon. Swelling, if present, is mild and localized to the joint. Loss of flexibility is usually associated with significant disease and can occur secondary to soft-tissue contractures, intraarticular loose bodies, large osteophytes, and loss of joint surface congruity.

Crepitus (audible crackling or grating sensation produced when roughened articular or extraarticular surfaces rub together during movement) may be noted on physical examination, and enlarged joint surfaces, including osteophytes, may be palpable. Although many people have physical and radiographic findings of OA, they may not have symptoms, whereas others with minimal changes observed develop significant symptoms. The reasons for this remain unknown.

For many women, OA typically develops within a few years of menopause and is often associated with mild inflammation for the first year or two that a particular joint is involved.[348] The joints may intermittently be warm and tender. The disease is strikingly symmetric, although the degree of involvement may vary somewhat.

OA of the hands affecting the distal interphalangeal and proximal interphalangeal joints occurs most often in this group of women.[817] The gradual loss of joint motion can assume major significance, with the person finding it difficult to grasp small objects.

After 1 or 2 years of inflammation, the joints enlarge with osteophyte (spur) formation, referred to as Heberden nodes (affecting the distal interphalangeal joints) and Bouchard nodes (affecting the proximal interphalangeal joints) (Fig. 27-4) and become unsightly. Pain may also be noted with loss of joint articular cartilage. Lateral deformities of the joints are common, with stretching of the collateral ligaments and bone resorption. This leads to overlapping of the fingers and considerable loss of functional ability.

Some individuals experience OA of the carpometacarpal joint. With advanced disease, individuals with carpometacarpal involvement may develop joint subluxation as the metacarpal flexes and adducts, leaving the metacarpal base prominent. Axial loading (e.g., pinching) and rotation characteristically reproduce symptoms and cause crepitus.[817]

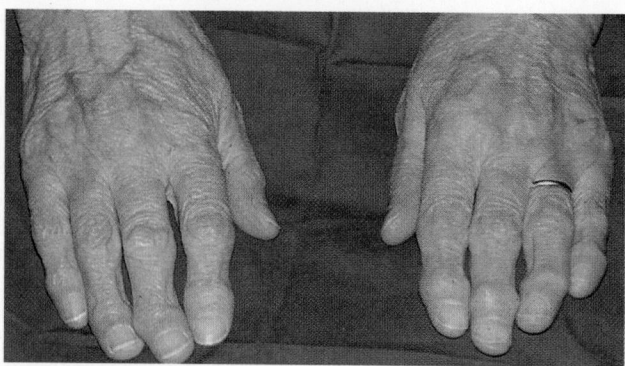

Figure 27-4

Typical hand deformities in osteoarthritis. Heberden nodes are seen on the distal interphalangeal joints, and Bouchard nodes are at the proximal interphalangeal joints. (From Forbes CD, Jackson WF: *Color atlas and text of clinical medicine*, ed 3, London, 2003, Mosby.)

MEDICAL MANAGEMENT

PREVENTION. Arthritis (including OA and rheumatic conditions) is the leading cause of disability in the United States, affecting more than 50 million people, with an estimated prevalence of nearly 67 million by the year 2030.[158] The Arthritis Foundation, Centers for Disease Control and Prevention (CDC), and *Healthy People 2020* are working together to implement the National Arthritis Action Plan to address the public health challenges of arthritis.[35,355]

Arthritis research is providing a growing body of knowledge about prevention as well as slowing the disease's progression and new, more effective combinations of drug and behavioral interventions. Education is a cornerstone of prevention and management for this condition. A healthy lifestyle helps prevent OA, and exercise can lessen disability if OA has developed. Moderate exercise has been shown to improve the knee cartilage glycosaminoglycan content in individuals at high risk of developing OA.[705] Strengthening the quadriceps muscle and maintaining an appropriate body weight for height reduce risk of OA at the knee by 30%.[240-242]

Sports officials and athletes need to work with athletic trainers, exercise physiologists, and physical therapists to evaluate and modify rules, equipment, and playing surfaces while providing adequate training to help reduce injuries. Early diagnosis and intervention with complete rehabilitation of joint injuries can decrease the risk of subsequent OA.[241,242] In the future, biomarkers found in joint fluid, blood, or urine that indicate changes in bone or cartilage may help identify people at risk for OA, allowing for prevention of disease progression and early intervention.

High intakes of vitamin C are associated with lower rates of OA on radiograph examination and less knee pain from OA. High levels of vitamin D protect against new and progressive OA.[241,361]

DIAGNOSIS. OA is diagnosed by correlation of history, physical examination, radiologic findings (Figs. 27-5 and 27-6), and laboratory tests, which rule out rheumatic

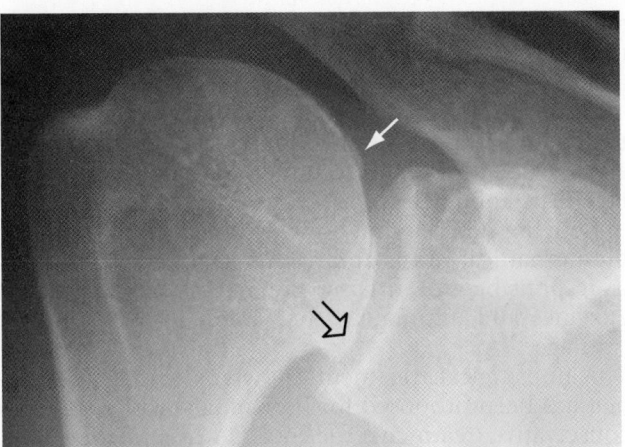

Figure 27-5

Osteoarthritis of the shoulder. There is osteophytic lipping *(open arrow)* from the humeral head, including new bone formation deep to the cartilage *(closed arrow)*. (From Harris ED: *Kelley's textbook of rheumatology,* ed 7, Philadelphia, 2005, WB Saunders.)

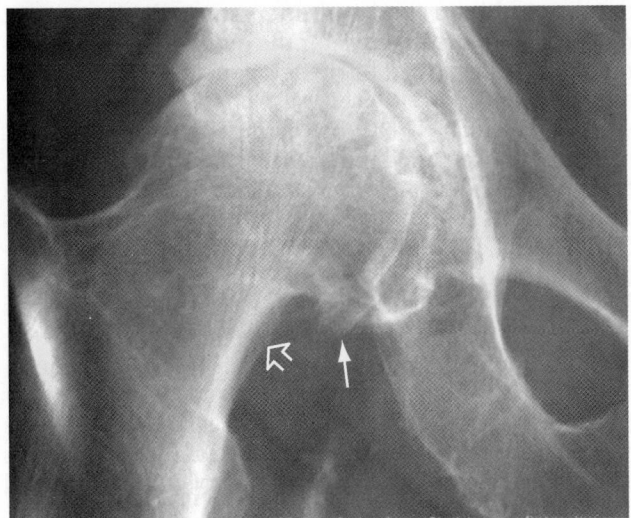

Figure 27-6

Osteoarthritis of the hip. The anteroposterior view of the hip shows complete cartilage space loss superiorly. There is osteophytic lipping from the femoral head, especially medially *(arrow)*, and buttressing bone *(open arrow)* is present along the femoral neck. (From Harris ED: *Kelley's textbook of rheumatology,* ed 7, Philadelphia, 2005, WB Saunders.)

Box 27-5

OSTEOARTHRITIS: RADIOGRAPHIC FINDINGS*

- Joint space widening (early evidence)
- Subchondral bone sclerosis
- Subchondral bone cysts
- Osteophytes
- Joint space narrowing

*Listed in order of progression.

Box 27-6

KELLGREN AND LAWRENCE GRADING SYSTEM FOR THE KNEE

Grade	Radiographic Findings
1	Possible osteophytes; no joint space narrowing
2	Definite osteophytes; possible narrowing of joint space
3	Moderate multiple osteophytes; definite joint space narrowing; some sclerosis and possible deformity of bone ends
4	Large osteophytes; marked joint space narrowing; severe sclerosis and definite deformity of bone ends

Data from Kellgren J, Lawrence J: Radiologic assessment of osteoarthritis, *Ann Rheum Dis* 16(4):494–501, 1957.

---

the signs of OA of the hand are typically seen first in the more distal interphalangeal joints.[21]

The physician also relies on findings from the physical examination, such as joint line or bony tenderness, joint effusion (not always present), joint giving way sensations, quadriceps muscle atrophy, unsteadiness on uneven surfaces or stairs, varus or valgus deformity (knee), and any abnormalities such as Heberden nodes, a classic osteoarthritic change observed in the distal interphalangeal joints of the hands (see Fig. 27-4). Laboratory evaluation may include ESR and rheumatoid factor, but generally these tests are not needed.[20]

OA is classified based on clinical information and radiologic evidence. The classification system proposed by Kellgren and Lawrence is used to classify stages of OA and to determine progressions of the disease. The classification is based on grades of 0 to 4, using the criteria of joint space narrowing and changes to bony structures (Box 27-6).[224,447] Grade 4 changes include large osteophytes, severe joint space narrowing, bony sclerosis, and bone exposure (Fig. 27-7).

MRI is becoming increasingly helpful in determining OA pathology because of its ability to show the condition of cartilage and the surrounding soft tissues. MRI is used to identify the presence of bone marrow lesions, synovitis, and periarticular inflammation that can the source of chronic pain for patients with OA.[240]

A goal of current research is to develop laboratory tests (i.e., serum, synovial, or urine biomarkers) that would help identify people who are predisposed to OA, detect the disease in its earliest stages, and assess the response to therapy.

TREATMENT. OA is managed on an individual basis, and treatment consists of a combination of nonsurgical and surgical options.[908] Treatment is modified based

---

disease. Box 27-5 lists radiographic changes associated with OA. The history of location of symptoms, symptom duration, functional limitations, trauma, medical comorbidities, and family history helps guide the physician in making the diagnosis.

The American College of Rheumatology's guidelines for the clinical diagnosis of knee OA were published in 1986 and continue to include knee pain with at least three of the following: older than age 50 years, morning stiffness lasting less than 30 minutes, or crepitus on motion, bony tenderness, bony enlargement, and no palpable warmth over the knee joint. These clinical findings along with radiographic signs of degeneration are most commonly used to make the diagnosis of knee OA. Guidelines for the diagnosis of hip OA are similar, while

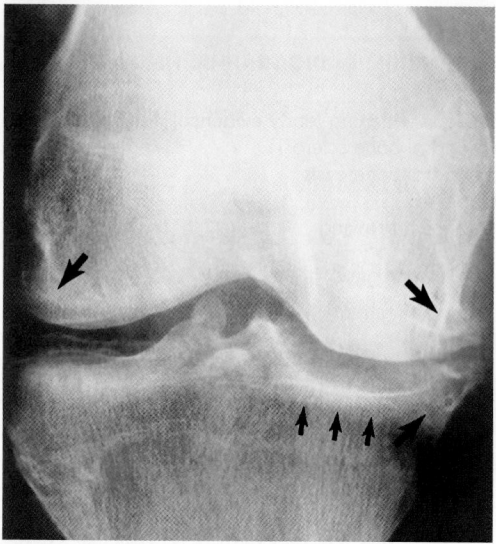

Figure 27-7

Osteoarthritis of the knee. Proliferative marginal osteophytes *(larger arrows)*, narrowing of the medial weight-bearing joint space, and eburnation (exposure of the subchondral bone, surface becomes smooth and polished as it wears down) *(smaller arrows)*. (From Noble J: *Textbook of primary care medicine*, ed 3, St Louis, 2001, Mosby.)

on response and should begin with conservative care, including education, weight loss, exercise, orthotics and/or braces, medications, and complementary approaches.

The combination of modest weight loss and moderate exercise provides better overall improvements in function, pain, and mobility in older adults who are overweight or obese with knee OA.[573,858,869] Greater improvements in function have been observed in older obese adults with the most weight loss.[581] Surgery is avoided and considered only when debilitating pain and major limitation of functions interfere with walking and daily activities or impair ability to sleep or work.[401]

Pharmacotherapy. Acetaminophen is recommended as a first line of treatment. Topical capsaicin and glucosamine/chondroitin should also be considered. NSAIDs and cyclooxygenase (COX)-2 inhibitors should be tried if acetaminophen is ineffective. Current recommendations for NSAID use include utilizing the lowest effective dose for the shortest possible period in order to reduce pain and preserve mobility.[662,692] Newly discovered information about the pathophysiology of OA is paving the way for researchers to design medical therapy that targets specific sites of pathophysiologic pathways involved in the pathogenesis of OA. Medical attention has shifted from easing the pain of OA to slowing the disorder's progression and actually preventing it.

Other medications that can be considered include COX-2 inhibitors, nitric oxide synthesis inhibitors, and antioxidants; chondrocyte and bone growth promoters; metalloproteinase and cytokine inhibitors; and gene therapy.[156] Inhibitors of eicosanoids (signaling molecules in inflammatory and immune responses) and nerve growth factors inhibitors are other considerations for future therapeutic options.

Research on cytokines, growth factors, and signaling pathways that was started in the 1990s is now producing new concepts for disease-modifying OA drugs, much like the disease-modifying drugs developed and now available for RA.[400,729,844]

Antiresorptive drugs aimed at altering the increased metabolic states of the subchondral bone may have an effect in altering damage done to the overlying cartilage. This approach is based on the hypothesis that the underlying subchondral bone, either indirectly through biomechanical effects or directly via release of cytokines, is responsible for driving the release of degradative enzymes and, ultimately, the destruction of overlying cartilage.[439]

A nonsurgical treatment known as *viscosupplementation* has been proposed for individuals whose standard conservative treatments for knee OA (e.g., medications, physical therapy, and behavioral therapy) have been inadequate or ineffective. This intervention involves direct injections into the knee of substances derived from sodium hyaluronate a principal component of natural synovial fluid. These injections were proposed to help restore some of the viscosity and elasticity of the diseased joint fluid and offer pain relief for 6 to 12 months.[74] Recent analyses for the outcomes of this treatment have questioned the benefits versus risk for serious adverse events.[713]

Education. The CDC has launched a major public health initiative, called the National Arthritis Action Plan, to identify and change behaviors that may cause OA, calling for a significant change in the way this disease is treated. Medical interventions involving expensive medications, joint injections, and surgery are now suggested for use in the 10% to 30% of cases in which OA will progress to severe joint damage.[35]

Multimodal treatment should include client education and self-management. Two excellent websites for consumer education and self-management of OA are available from the Arthritis Foundation[35] and Arthritis Self-Management.[40] Behavioral interventions directed toward enhancing self-management are important, including prevention (see previous discussion), diet and weight control, and low-impact exercise. More attention to psychosocial problems (e.g., isolation, depression) that may influence the person's perception of pain, and to exercise is recommended. The value of a well-designed exercise program including training for strength and endurance also has been recognized.[870,908] Aquatic therapy is especially helpful as a form of moist heat and gravity-eliminated resistive exercise.[60]

Complementary, Alternative, and Integrative Therapy. An area of medicine called complementary and integrative medicine has developed as more health care professionals, including medical doctors, have started incorporating these treatment methods into their overall management plans. The Arthritis Foundation has published an excellent resource on alternative therapies[34]; some experts advise people not to think of these therapies as "alternative" but rather as synergistic measures that can be integrated into a total care plan. Best available evidence suggests that acupuncture, several herbal preparations (e.g., devil's claw root, white willow bark, frankincense), and capsaicin cream may be beneficial.[199,228]

Evidence is weak or contradictory but shows promise for some alternative therapies (e.g., homeopathy, magnet therapy, tai chi, leech therapy, Reiki, music therapy, yoga,[218,321,647,840] imagery, and therapeutic touch).[173,227,647] The use of acupuncture for pain has been shown to be helpful for some, but not all, types of pain.[485] Results from several systematic reviews conclude "there is not sufficient evidence to recommend many of the practitioner-based complementary therapies for the management of OA, but neither is there sufficient evidence to conclude that they are not effective or efficacious."[229,434,519]

Nutraceuticals are foods or food products having potential benefits as a treatment or preventative for a disease process.[361] Glucosamine and chondroitin sulfate are components of articular cartilage. Glucosamine is derived from the shells of lobster, shrimp, and crabs; chondroitin sulfate is derived from cow cartilage. These can be taken orally with potential effects of decreasing joint inflammation, inhibiting proteolytic enzymes that breakdown cartilage and stimulating the synthesis of proteoglycans and hyaluronic acid.

Long-term use of these agents may provide combined structure-modifying and symptom-modifying effects, making these potentially disease-modifying agents for OA. For those taking glucosamine and chondroitin, most take 1500 mg of glucosamine and 1200 mg of chondroitin daily; anyone weighing more than 200 lb should increase the dosage to 2000 mg of glucosamine and 1600 mg of chondroitin sulfate.[366]

The symptomatic benefit of glucosamine and chondroitin has been more promising, but few well controlled studies exist to establish a consistent effect for patient symptoms and function.[584,690] The Glucosamine/Chondroitin Arthritis Intervention Trial (GAIT) studied the efficacy of glucosamine sulfate, glucosamine hydrochloride, and chondroitin sulfate for the treatment of OA using a rigorous study design to elicit the cause and effects of these agents. The authors concluded that after 24 months of use these nutraceuticals had minimal effects on pain and function for older adults with knee OA.[725] Investigators in various trials report a range of results with this treatment, making conclusions difficult. Differences in studies are too great to make comparisons or draw meta-analysis conclusions. Different glucosamine preparations add to the complexity of comparative studies.[689,874] The safety of this product used over a long period of time has also been questioned.[511]

Surgery. Surgical intervention is considered when pain and loss of function are severe. Arthroscopic management, including lavage and debridement, abrasion arthroplasty, subchondral penetration procedures such as drilling and microfracture, and laser/thermal chondroplasty, may benefit some individuals, potentially delaying reconstructive procedures (e.g., osteotomy, joint arthrodesis or fusion, total joint replacement). Each of these procedures is under investigation for efficacy and long-term results.[397,908]

To help joint replacements last longer, research is focusing on wear- and corrosion-resistant materials as well as investigating how the tissue around the replacement

responds. Replacement of damaged cartilage using one of three types of cartilage is also under investigation: one's own cartilage, donor cartilage, and cartilage produced by tissue engineering of progenitor cells (see "Tissue Engineering" in Chapter 21). Medications that stimulate human cartilage matrix formation without stimulating the chondroresorption processes are also under investigation.[360, 614]

PROGNOSIS. OA is a major contributor to functional limitations and reduced independence in adults older than 65 years of age. It is a chronic condition with unpredictable symptoms that often cause fluctuations in pain and function.[5]

Mobility disability, defined as needing help walking or climbing stairs, is common for those with hip and/or knee OA. The social burden in terms of personal suffering and use of health resources is expected to increase with the increasing prevalence of obesity and the aging of the American population.[401]

Although there is no known cure for OA, by following the guidelines for lifestyle changes, pain management, and self-management incorporating exercise and weight loss, affected individuals can substantially decrease the pain and dysfunction associated with OA.

SPECIAL IMPLICATIONS FOR THE THERAPIST 27-9

Osteoarthritis

Therapists need to be aware of the potential poor correlation between the extent of radiographic degenerative changes and the presence of symptoms. The assumption that a person with significant, extensive joint degeneration will not improve should not be made until a thorough rehabilitation program has been attempted.

Conversely, it should not be assumed that someone with minor radiographic degenerative changes cannot be experiencing severe, intense pain. Therapists should rely primarily on the clinical examination findings for direction regarding the development of prognosis (including plan of care) and intervention.

Medications and Nutraceuticals

The medications commonly prescribed for OA have significant potential side effects. The NSAIDs have ulcerogenic potential, especially when taken with nonprescription drugs. Gastric irritation can result from inhibition of prostaglandin production, which can reduce mucus and bicarbonate production and decrease local blood flow.

Peptic ulcer disease can be manifested by a multitude of complaints, including indigestion, nausea, vomiting, thoracic pain, and melena (black tarry stools). The onset of any of these complaints calls for communication with a physician.

Nutraceuticals, such as chondroitin, can also cause problems in some individuals. Chondroitin is chemically similar to blood-thinning drugs, such as heparin, warfarin (Coumadin), and even aspirin, and could cause excessive bleeding. Anyone taking these supplements with unexplained back or shoulder pain or excessive bruising or bleeding from any part of the body (nose, gums, vagina, urine, and rectum) must be evaluated by a physician. Anyone taking these supplements who also has diabetes should be aware that some studies in animals show that glucosamine increases blood glucose levels. Studies in humans have not found any long-term associations for increased risk of hyperglycemia.[594,736]

Joint Protection

People with symptoms associated with OA must understand their role in minimizing the mechanical stresses on the involved joint or joints. The diseased joints need to be protected from excessive mechanical forces. Educating the client on how to reduce the daily wear and tear on the joint is essential. This may include the use of postural supports or a cervical collar or an exercise program to vary the stresses with which the involved joints are dealing.

Proper posture and avoidance of prolonged stressful postures, use of supports, varying of physical activities to vary the stresses (i.e., alternating biking with swimming or walking), and following through with a flexibility and strengthening exercise program are all components under the affected individual's control.

Wearing shoes that fit properly and are appropriate for the activity may help avoid injury. Good alignment of the joints is important, especially in the knee. Evaluating the need for an assistive ambulatory device, a shock-absorbent shoe insert or heel wedge, brace, or other orthotic devices is important to unload the pressure on affected joints. A simple lateral wedge insole of 5 or 10 degrees directly reduces the knee varus torque in individuals with medial knee OA and can interrupt the OA cycle, slowing the progression of the disease and disability.[236,450]

Exercise and Osteoarthritis

Since the realization that structured exercise programs can improve function without exacerbating symptoms, exercise and joint protection techniques have become mainstays of treatment. In fact, attempts to alleviate pain through pharmacologic or physical modalities may not improve symptoms unless accompanied by some form of physical conditioning.[537, 880]

The plan of care for someone with OA is dictated by the extent of the disease and the joints involved, but everyone with OA should be encouraged to continue exercising, including strength training and low-intensity aerobic components.

General Concepts

Physical therapy has been shown effective in OA of the knee to reduce pain; improve physical function; increase isometric muscle strength, gait speed, and stride length; and improve quality of life.

A combination of manual physical therapy and supervised exercise provides beneficial effects still present 1 year later and delays or prevents the need for surgical intervention, with fewer joint replacements reported.[202,265] Such supervised exercise/manual therapy programs have been shown to increase improvement and provide greater symptomatic relief compared with a similar unsupervised home exercise program.[201,518,780]

Optimizing existing and potential joint function by improving flexibility and strength is important. In fact, exercise combined with self-management appears to have a similar effect to drug treatments and is generally safer.[231] Low-intensity, controlled movements that do not increase pain can help individuals regain or maintain motion and flexibility.[241,242]

The therapist can use the same guidelines for all individuals when establishing frequency, intensity, and duration by following well-known general concepts (e.g., establish *intensity* by calculating heart rate at 60% of the heart rate maximum, begin at the individual's level of *duration* from 1 to 2 minutes and build up to 30 minutes, work toward a *frequency* of five to seven times per week). Clients should be taught how to monitor and progress frequency, intensity, and duration; use good biomechanics; and avoid exacerbating musculoskeletal symptoms.

In the presence of mild joint swelling, the client should be taught to use ice before exercise and to incorporate a program of submaximal exercise to warm up before beginning the prescribed exercise program.[561] If there is joint effusion, the surrounding muscles cannot contract maximally because of reflex inhibition caused by joint distention. Submaximal exercise for 3 or 4 minutes on a swollen joint decreases this inhibition mechanism, allowing for continued strength training. Moderate to severe joint effusion may require additional physical therapy intervention, such as electrical stimulation.

Resistance and low-intensity aerobic exercise may reduce the incidence of disability related to ADLs and prolong autonomy in adults older than 60 years of age, specifically those with knee OA. The lowest ADL disability risks were found for participants with the highest compliance to the exercise program.[653] Long-term weight training and aerobic walking programs significantly improve postural sway in older adults with OA, thereby improving static postural stability.[574]

In the case of the frail older adult, progressive resistive exercises have been shown to be safe and effective following an acute illness when monitored carefully (e.g., measuring vital signs, observing for signs of physiologic distress).[801] Other specific exercise recommendations and safety considerations are available,[24,202,587,591] but the optimal type of exercise and duration for the prevention and treatment of OA remain under investigation.

Successful management of degenerative joint disease may require evaluating and treating dysfunction of other body regions. For example, someone with OA of the knee and pain on ambulation may have significant foot or ankle dysfunction. Treating joint and soft-tissue hypomobility and muscle imbalances and fabricating orthoses may considerably alter the mechanical stresses on the arthritic knee.

For those individuals who do not seem to respond, progress, or improve with physical therapy intervention, a number of factors should be considered. Mode of treatment delivery is not the only parameter. Treatment compliance, mechanical characteristics (e.g., joint laxity, malalignment), and radiographic severity should be carefully considered. Research is needed to focus on predictive factors and outcomes for individual characteristics and type of exercise protocols prescribed.[253]

In clinical trials of older adults, exercise at moderate levels of training has been shown to be effective in improving generalized and localized pain and functional status. There is no evidence that one type of exercise is better than others.[880] The exercise prescription must be individualized to the needs and preferences of each person.

Clients should be encouraged to exercise to the extent that they are capable. Many older adults are more likely to adhere to a program that is short and sweet (i.e., short, frequent episodes of exercise) rather than long, once-a-day programs. Educating, motivating, and providing prescriptive exercise are important roles the therapist plays to help maximize function and prevent significant recurrence of symptoms.

The therapist should take into account psychosocial factors, especially self-efficacy, which is an important variable in the rehabilitation process predictive of physical function.[257,346] Self-efficacy is defined as a person's belief about the person's ability to successfully complete a task or activity.[54] See further discussion of self-efficacy in Chapter 2.

Sometimes increasing physical activity does cause increased pain, but studies show this is short-lived. The therapist can help clients get over the "pain hump" by assuring them that this response is normal and temporary.[258] Older adults may become more motivated to exercise if they understand the benefits. Teach them the overall health benefits of exercise in preventing chronic conditions such as diabetes, heart disease, osteoporosis, and cancer.

The therapist can help educate them about how exercise can help reduce their risk factors for OA as well as decrease risk for falls with a program of balance and gait training.[822] Use the information in this chapter on falls prevention to personalize the message and remind the client that people who exercise have a lower incidence of falls, fractures, hospitalizations, and premature death.[575]

Specific Exercise Training

Muscles have been shown repeatedly to be the major shock-absorbing mechanism of joints, especially the knee. Eccentric muscle performance serves this shock-absorbing function, supporting the idea that rehabilitation programs should include activities to enhance eccentric function, especially of the quadriceps muscle.[870]

The quadriceps muscle group must absorb the force and decelerate the increasing load as the weight-bearing limb stabilizes under the load. Overloading the bones' capacity to accept force may be what leads to osteoarthritic changes and/or pain in the knee.[319]

Studies show that quadriceps weakness might be from muscle dysfunction and not necessarily muscle atrophy.[75,839] Quadriceps weakness may be present in people who have OA but do not have knee pain or muscle atrophy. Pain may be a consequence of the changes in muscle activity rather than the other way around. More study is needed to identify the level of motor units' activation and contractile properties of the muscle in OA during concentric and eccentric contractions.[776,777]

The strength of the quadriceps can be enhanced with a variety of clinical and home exercise methods.[209] Open chain quadriceps-strengthening exercises can cause exercise-induced arthralgias in this population and generally should be avoided. Closed chain kinetic strengthening exercises (e.g., leg press, wall slide) can be effective for quadriceps strengthening and are usually well tolerated when performed correctly.[659] Hamstring strengthening should be included when weakness is present. Research on strengthening exercises for people with hip OA is not as abundant as that for people with knee OA, but the evidence supports a similar approach.[795]

It is likely that the loss of joint proprioception associated with OA may contribute to gait alterations, muscle imbalances, repetitive microtrauma, loss of coordination, and, ultimately, excessive joint loading.[127,491] Functional ability is also limited in individuals with OA who have poor proprioception combined with muscle weakness.[847] Exercises to facilitate proprioception and closed kinetic chain exercises for knee OA have both been shown to improve functional score, walking speed, and muscle strength.[499]

Aquatic Physical Therapy

Aquatic physical therapy is used often in the management of individuals with hip and knee OA. Studies with short-term follow-up, have found aquatic exercises did not make the joint condition worse or result in injury.[374,881] Studies to confirm the efficacy of this treatment and the long-term outcomes yield inconsistent results, but have found reduced disability levels, but no significant effects on pain relief.[880]

Degenerative Intervertebral Disk Disease

Overview and Definition

The degenerative joint process described in the previous section applies to any synovial joint, including the facet joints of the spinal column. Degenerative joint changes are not limited to synovial joints, however, and in the spine (particularly the low lumbar segments) they commonly occur at the intervertebral disk articulations as well. Currently, there is no consensus on what "disk degeneration" actually is or how it should be defined or distinguished from the physiologic processes of growth, aging, healing, and adaptive remodeling. The following working definition has been proposed as a starting point: *The process of disk degeneration is an aberrant, cell-mediated response to progressive structural failure.*[1]

Lumbar disk degeneration begins early in life with macroscopic changes being visible from the age of 30 years onward. It is estimated that half of all Americans older than age 40 years are affected by degenerative disk disease (DDD).[582]

Disk degeneration follows a predictable pattern. First, the nucleus in the center of the disk begins to lose its ability to absorb water. The disk becomes dehydrated. Then the nucleus becomes thick and fibrous, so that it looks much the same as the annulus. As a result, the nucleus isn't able to absorb shock as well. Routine stress and strain begin to take a toll on the structures of the spine. Tears form around the annulus. The disk weakens. It starts to collapse, and the bones of the spine compress.[575] This process is discussed in greater detail later in the "Etiology and Pathogenesis" section.

Incidence

Lumbar DDD is a common musculoskeletal disease estimated to affect up to 5% of all adults. This disease and resulting condition can occur before age 20 years, usually in a familiar pattern or in elite athletes who have been exposed to repetitive physical loading of the spine from frequent trunk rotations, frequent kicking or jumping, or repeated spinal flexion and extension.[335] In the general population, it tends to peak in the fourth and fifth decades of life and declines after that. It has been reported that men suffer from sciatica due to disk herniation approximately 1.5 to 3 times more often than women, but it is not clear if this is a true difference in prevalence of DDD or can be attributed to anatomic and mechanical factors that contribute to nerve root compression.[9]

Risk Factors

The greatest risk factor for disk degeneration is familial aggregation including genetic inheritance,[64,66] which accounts for approximately 50% to 70% of the variability in disk degeneration between identical twins. Individual genes associated with disk degeneration have been identified (e.g., aggrecan, collagen type IX, matrix metalloproteinase-3, vitamin D receptor).[1,63,720] Age and body weight also appear to be two other significant risk factors for DDD.[734]

Twin and family studies show that the risk of developing a lumbar disk herniation is approximately five times greater in people who have a positive family history. Mutations that alter collagen I structure (the major component of the outer annulus) may contribute to annular tears and disk ruptures. Sequence variations in the genes for collagen IX may also be linked with DDD.[9]

There has been a prevailing view that DDD occurs as a result of excessive forces, particularly from the cumulative effects of repeated loading from occupational physical demands, such as manual material handling. Results of research to confirm or refute this hypothesis have been mixed; some studies find a correlation between disk degeneration and physical demands, while other do not.[65,868] Results of the Finnish Twin Cohort suggest that routine (daily) physical loading of the spine may actually have a training (rather than detrimental) effect. Occupational lifting or repeated loading of the spine from physical activity may in fact benefit the disks[868] as cyclic

mechanical stresses may increase the growth rate and collagen fibers of the nucleus pulposus.[548]

Body height has been suggested but not consistently found to be a risk factor in all studies; the link between DDD and obesity and smoking also remains controversial. The role of psychosocial factors has also been investigated, and they have been found to have a positive link as risk factors for disk herniation, which can lead to further DDD. Atherosclerosis is another potential risk factor. Obstruction in the abdominal aorta, lumbar, and middle arteries can lead to ischemia in the lumbar spine, resulting in hypoxia and tissue dysfunction with eventual disk degeneration.[442]

Etiology and Pathogenesis

The intervertebral disk undergoes marked changes with age, although genetic inheritance, inadequate metabolite transport, and loading history combined with age contribute significantly to structural failure that can occur during ADLs.[1]

The most significant alterations occur in the nucleus pulposus. The number of cells and the concentration of proteoglycans and water decrease. In addition, there is fragmentation of proteoglycans, which contributes to water loss. As the nucleus breaks down, the fibrocartilaginous inner annulus expands. Fissures and clefts may form within the disk, and the height of the disk decreases. This loss of disk height can contribute to the age-related condition of spinal stenosis.[31,69]

A number of events can contribute to the three stages of age-related disk degeneration (Box 27-7).[458] The most important event appears to be the decreased cellular function and concentration. The progressive decline in arterial supply to the periphery of the disk and the impairment of nutrient delivery across the cartilaginous endplate contribute to the reduced nutritional supply to the cells, affecting cellular function. In addition, the impaired cartilaginous endplate diffusion results in reduced cellular waste product removal and an increased lactic acid concentration. The resultant decreased pH level compromises cellular metabolism and biosynthesis and can lead to cell death. The reduced biosynthesis can adversely affect the biomechanical properties of the matrix over an extended period of time.

Besides the internal events affecting the general health of the intervertebral disk, repetitive external mechanical loading on the structure can lead to fatigue failure of the matrix. When enough structural breakdown occurs, what once were normal mechanical loads acting on a normal disk are now excessive loads on a compromised disk. At this point the degenerative process is accelerated.[113,322]

Collapse of the inner annulus into the nucleus is a common feature in the disks of older adults, with the anterior annulus being affected more than the posterior (Fig. 27-8). This could be caused by nucleus decompression following endplate fracture. In many older disks, the cartilage endplate becomes detached from the underlying bone, presumably because the high internal pressure that presses it against the bone in young disks has been lost.[1,323]

The results of the Videman[868] and Twin Spine[64] studies go against the traditional view that physical loading and repetitive spinal movements are responsible for

Box 27-7

DISK DEGENERATION

Three Stages of Disk Degeneration[239]

- Dysfunction
  - Circumferential and radial tears in the disk annulus
  - Localized synovitis and hypermobility of the facet joints
- Instability
  - Internal disruption of the disk
  - Progressive disk resorption
  - Degeneration of the facet joints with capsular laxity
  - Subluxation
  - Erosion
- Stabilization
  - Osteophytosis (bone spur formation)
  - Spinal stenosis

Events Leading to Disk Degeneration

- Impaired cellular nutrition
- Reduced cellular viability
- Cellular senescence
- Accumulation of degraded matrix macromolecules
- Fatigue failure of the matrix

Risk Factors for Disk Degeneration

- Age
- Body mass index
- Heredity
- Physical loading*
- Occupational (repetitive) lifting*

*New evidence suggests that these factors may not be as strongly linked with degenerative disk disease as previously thought. Regular physical activity may benefit the disks. Age, body weight, and hereditary factors may be the greatest risk factors for degenerative disk disease.[4,493]
Data from Schoenfeld AJ, Nelson JH, Burks R, Belmont PJ Jr: Incidence and risk factors for lumbar degenerative disc disease in the United States military 1999–2008, *Mil Med* 176(11):1320–1324, 2011; and Beattie PF: Current understanding of lumbar intervertebral disc degeneration: a review with emphasis upon etiology, pathophysiology, and lumbar magnetic resonance imaging findings, *J Orthop Sports Phys Ther* 38(6):329–340, 2008.

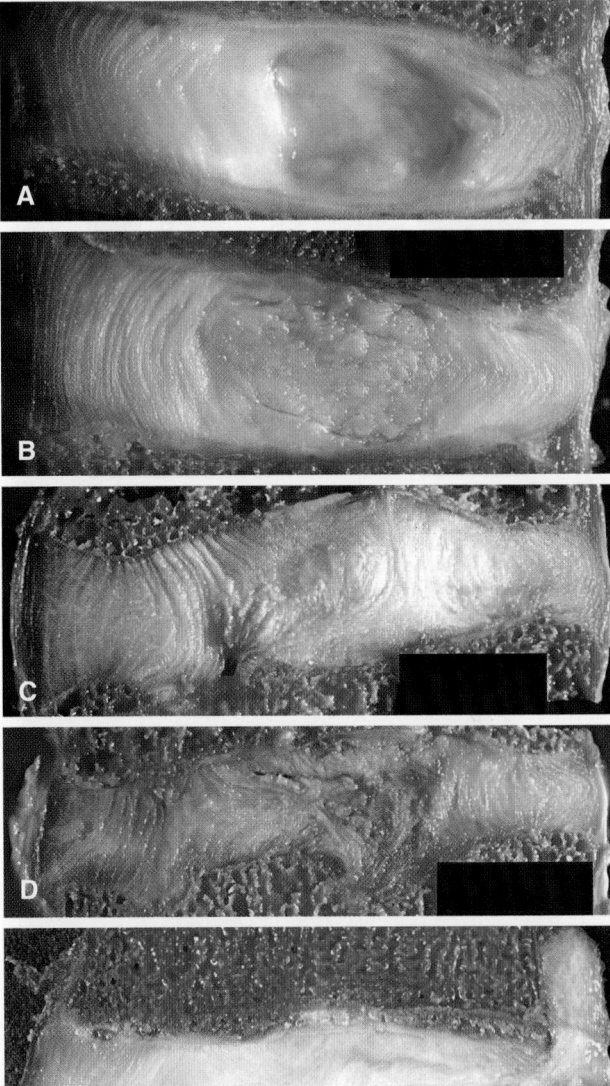

Figure 27-8

Lumbar intervertebral disks (midsagittal section; anterior on the *left*). **A,** Young disk in a male, 35 years old. **B,** Mature disk in a male, 47 years old. **C,** Disrupted disk in a male, 31 years old. Note the endplate and inward collapse of the inner anulus. **D,** Severely disrupted disk in male, 31 years old. Note the collapse of disk height. **E,** Disk induced to prolapse in cadaver male, 40 years old. Some nucleus pulposus has herniated through a radial fissure in the posterior anulus *(right)*. (From Adams MA: *The biomechanics of back pain,* Edinburgh, 2002, Churchill Livingstone.)

mechanical "wear and tear" on the disk. The authors suggest that loading from daily physical activity and higher body weight may actually help offset the effects of aging.[866] Forces across the lumbar spine vary with body weight and lifting strength; this may explain why some disks degenerate more than others. The authors also suggest that smaller disks hold up better because it is easier for nutrients to reach each cell. The results of the Twin Spine study also support the idea that disk degeneration appears to be determined in great part by genetic influences. Although environmental factors also play a role, it is not primarily through routine physical loading exposures (e.g., heavy vs. light physical demands) as once suspected.[64]

Associated with intervertebral disk degeneration are spinal stenosis and degenerative spondylolisthesis, two common conditions in the adult older than age 65 years. As the intervertebral disk loses height, the annulus may bulge circumferentially and the ligamentum flavum can buckle. Both encroach on the spinal canal, subarticular (facet) recesses, and lateral intervertebral foramina. With

a loss of disk height, compressive force increases on the neural arch,[666] causing OA of the facet (apophyseal) joints and osteophytes around the margins of the vertebral bodies (Fig. 27-9).[867] In addition, concurrent osteophyte formation on the vertebral bodies or articular processes may occur, compounding the stenosis.

Degenerative spondylolisthesis as a result of disk degeneration and degenerative changes of the posterior facet joint is marked by anterior slippage of one vertebra over another with an intact posterior neural arch. The

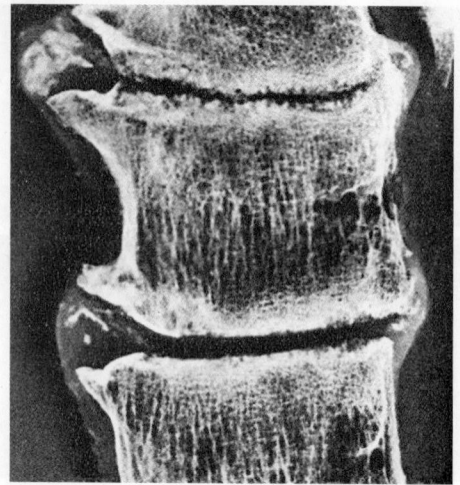

Figure 27-9

Radiograph of a lumbar spine (anterior on *left*) with severe disk narrowing, vertebral osteophytes, sclerosis of the endplates, and selective loss of horizontal trabeculae from the vertebral body. (From Adams MA: *The biomechanics of back pain*, Edinburgh, UK, 2002, Churchill Livingstone.)

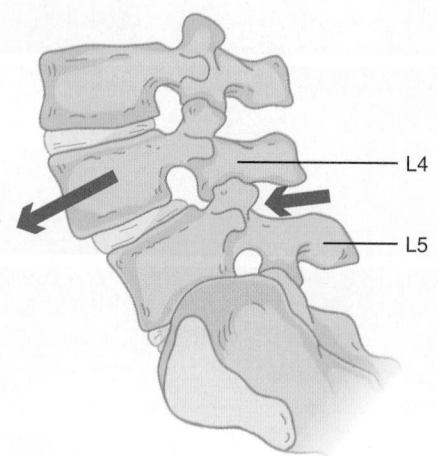

Figure 27-10

Degenerative spondylolisthesis at L4-L5. (From DeRosa C, Porterfield JA: Lumbar spine and pelvis. In Richardson JK, Iglarsh ZA, editors: *Clinical orthopaedic physical therapy*, Philadelphia, 1994, WB Saunders, p. 144.)

L4-L5 spinal segment is the most common site for this to occur (Fig. 27-10). Lytic or isthmic spondylolisthesis (a separate etiology from degenerative spondylolisthesis and more common in younger groups) is marked by anterior slippage of one vertebra over another with a defective posterior neural arch (Fig. 27-11). The L5-S1 spinal segment is the most common site for lytic spondylolisthesis to occur. The loss of disk height associated with degeneration allows for a buckling of the annulus and ligamentum flavum, slackening them somewhat. This allows the vertebrae to migrate anteriorly in response to the shear forces inherent to the lumbar lordosis.[364]

In contrast to the L5-S1 segment, the facet joint orientation at the L4-L5 segment tends to be more in the sagittal plane, so there is no structural bar to anterior slippage. The facet joint orientation at L5-S1 tends to be more in the frontal plane, making anterior migration of L5 difficult unless there is a structural defect in the posterior

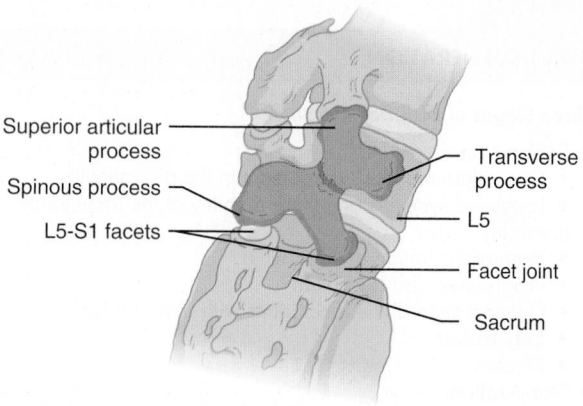

Figure 27-11

Spondylolysis or posterior arch defect, which can lead to a lytic spondylolisthesis. The Scottie dog with a collar, which is visible on the radiograph (posterior oblique view), is outlined. (From Magee D: *Orthopedic physical assessment*, ed 5, Philadelphia, 2008, WB Saunders.)

neural arch. Stenosis can be caused by the displacement of one vertebra over another as well as by the concurrent buckling of the annulus and ligamentum flavum.

Clinical Manifestations

Disk degeneration is most likely to affect the lower lumbar spine but can affect the upper lumbar spine and cervical spine as well. Low back pain is often the first symptom, but DDD is asymptomatic in up to one-third of all affected individuals.[91,423]

DDD is one of the most common causes of low back pain with radiculopathy. The intervertebral disk changes include alterations in volume, shape, structure, and composition. Although there is not a 100% correlation between the presence of DDD and pain complaints, the structural alterations will decrease motion and alter the mechanical properties of the spine.[113]

Most people with DDD have a gradual onset of increasingly severe midline lower back pain. At first, symptoms only last a few days. This type of back pain is often intermittent but recurring over the years. Each time it occurs, the pain may seem worse than the time before. Eventually the pain may spread into the buttocks or thighs, and it may take longer to subside.[168]

When pain is present, it tends to get worse after heavy physical activity or after a prolonged time in one position. The back may also begin to feel stiff. Resting the back eases pain. Aching of the buttock(s) and posterior thigh(s) with ambulation is common.

The symptoms of DDD should not be confused with disk herniation, which may occur as part of the process of disk degeneration but is not a constant feature and is a separate entity from DDD. Clinical presentation of disk protrusion and herniation can vary widely but can occur as a result of tears of the annulus fibrosus, causing acute back or neck pain or radicular pain if there is herniation of the nucleus pulposus.

In the lumbar spine, radiculopathy causing sciatic pain and restricted straight-leg raise may occur as the sheath of the nerve root is compressed,[803] or as a result of inflammatory irritation from chemicals released by the damaged disk.

Centralization of radiating pain is characteristic of sciatica from disk protrusion or herniation. Specifically, leg pain routinely reduces or "retreats" to the lumbar midline before the disappearance of back pain. This distinctive pain pattern was first described by McKenzie.[559]

Other signs of disk herniation include ankle dorsiflexion weakness; great toe extensor weakness; impaired ankle reflexes; loss of light touch sensation in the medial, dorsal, and lateral aspects of the foot; and positive ipsilateral or crossed straight leg raise test. These six neurologic tests allow detection of most clinically significant nerve root compromises resulting from L4-L5 or L5-S1 disk herniations.[332,894]

Gait abnormality, muscle weakness, sensory changes such as numbness and tingling, and bowel or bladder dysfunction can occur as a result of myelopathy associated with either disk herniation or degeneration. In the case of cervical disk involvement, difficulty swallowing, hand numbness, the Lhermitte sign, and hoarseness or voice difficulties may occur. MRI observations of disk degeneration and herniation are poorly correlated with clinical signs and symptoms. For example, a large, extruded disk may be clinically tolerable if the spinal canal is large and the spinal nerve roots are not compressed. On the other hand, a focal, contained subligamentous herniation may produce severe symptoms if it occurs in the foramen adjacent to the dorsal root ganglion of the affected nerve.[560]

Degeneration of the intervertebral disks in the lumbar spine may create enough instability or a Spondylolisthesis. There is not a clear consensus that low back pain is associated with spondylolisthesis. In the case of disk degeneration associated with stenosis and spondylolisthesis, the person can be asymptomatic, even when moderate to severe changes are observed on imaging studies. Conversely, early or mild changes can be accompanied by severe pain and neurologic symptoms.[432]

MEDICAL MANAGEMENT

DIAGNOSIS. The diagnosis of degenerative disk disease is made from the history of a person's condition, physical examination and imaging studies. Standard radiographs of the lumbar spine can demonstrate disk space narrowing and the presence of spondylophytes along the margins of the vertebral bodies, which are common signs of degenerating vertebral disk. MRI is the best choice for the visualization and grading of the degenerating disk material. MRI will also allow for the assessment of the surrounding soft tissues, adjacent facet joints, and the possible effects on the spinal nerves. CT scans may be a better tool for the assessment of spondylolysis and spondylolisthesis.[432,532]

TREATMENT. Conservative care, including NSAIDs, mild analgesics for short-term pain control, physical therapy, cognitive behavioral therapy, lifestyle changes (e.g., smoking cessation, weight loss, fitness program), and aerobic conditioning are the first line of treatment for painful DDD.[438,560] The goal is to reduce painful symptoms and enable the person to get back to normal activities as soon as possible. Bed rest is no longer the standard of care.

Surgery. Surgery to remove the disk or disk fragments (diskectomy), laminectomy, and/or spinal fusion may be considered if conservative care has been unsuccessful and/or neurologic symptoms persist. The use of surgical procedures for the treatment of lumbar spine conditions continues to be controversial as long-term outcomes have not proven to significantly better than conservative management approaches.[438] Surgical procedures can be appropriately used to avoid permanent nerve damage and foot drop.

A number of procedures have been proposed to address the effects of a degenerating vertebral disk. Injection of steroid, denervating and anesthetic agents into the disk or adjacent facet joints have been used to diminish local inflammation and decrease nociceptor activity. The use of electrothermal and radiofrequency energy have been used to induce a shrinkage of disk material or to destroy pain receptors surrounding the disk. Many of these methods have provided short-term relief of pain associated with degenerative disk disease, but have not demonstrated enough consistent long-term benefits.[168]

For some individuals, artificial disk replacement (ADR) is an alternative to spinal fusion. After removing what is left of the damaged or worn-out disk, the ADR device is inserted in the space between two lumbar vertebrae. The goal is to replace the diseased disk while keeping the normal spinal motion. ADR devices are not designed at this time for the treatment of herniated disks but for one or two levels of DDD. Cervical arthroplasty is also available now, with primary indications for the treatment of radiculopathy and myelopathy at one or two levels.[438]

The advantages of this treatment over spinal fusion are maintenance of spinal movement, disk height, and neural foramina, thus simulating a more normal spinal alignment, angulation, and mechanics. Immobilization is avoided with ADR, and early return of function is possible. There is the additional advantage of preventing adjacent-segment deterioration that can occur after spinal fusion.

There are also risks and disadvantages (e.g., infection; ossification; neurologic impairment; implant failure; and fracture, migration, or subsidence or sinking down into the bone).[222] Although short-term and medium-term results are favorable, long-term results are not yet available.[416,455,837]

For individuals with classic symptoms of spinal stenosis from a herniated disk, the use of an interspinous process spacer (e.g., X-STOP) helps prevent spinal extension without removing bone. By placing this metal device between the interspinous processes, the spine is blocked from moving backward into extension. The X-STOP is best suited for those people who have stenosis at one or two levels of the lumbar spine. Anyone who has more severe symptoms with muscle weakness and/or sensory loss is not likely to be helped by this procedure.[904]

Gene Therapy. Researchers are investigating the use of gene therapy to slow, prevent, or reverse the biochemical changes associated with disk degeneration. Alternatively, if the correct gene could be identified, it might be possible to manage an annular tear by direct repair or regeneration.[20] In other areas of study, autologous chondrocyte transplantation may become a future treatment for DDD. Animal studies show that chondrocytes removed from damaged cartilaginous tissues maintain a capacity to proliferate and reproduce tissue similar to normal intervertebral disk material.[566]

PROGNOSIS. Disk structural failure is irreversible, always progresses by physical and biologic mechanisms, and is closely associated with mechanical dysfunction and pain.[1] The potential for recovery varies based on the size of the protrusion, the size of the canal, the person's age and activity level, the extent of disk disruption, and similar parameters related to spondylolisthesis and stenosis.[134] Levels of disability during episodes of back pain, maladaptive coping behaviors and genetic factors have also been identified as important for the recovery and return to function for DDD.[438]

SPECIAL IMPLICATIONS FOR THE THERAPIST 27-10

Degenerative Intervertebral Disk Disease

Degenerative changes of the spine affecting the intervertebral disks often occur concomitantly with other spinal degenerative and osteoarthritic changes such as spinal stenosis and with the effects of vascular occlusion from atherosclerosis. There are two additional conditions associated with spinal stenosis: cauda equina syndrome and vascular/neurogenic claudication.

Cauda equina syndrome is characterized by pain in the upper sacrum, with paresthesias of the buttocks and genitalia possibly resulting in bowel or bladder incontinence or sexual dysfunction (difficulty achieving orgasm or inability to achieve or maintain an erection). Numerous conditions may lead to these manifestations, including spinal canal stenosis. Therapists working with anyone with back or neck pain should ask about these symptoms, and if any are present, immediate communication with a physician is recommended.[192]

Even with the local degenerative changes in the spine, stenosis may be marked primarily by lower-extremity symptoms (neurogenic claudication) as opposed to back pain. The symptoms may include pain, altered sensation, or muscle weakness.

The symptoms are typically brought on by walking and are relieved by prolonged rest (sitting or lying down) or by flexion of the spine. When a person is upright and walking, the lumbar spine is in a relatively backward-bent position, which further reduces the size of the foramina and subarticular recesses. When the spine is flexed, the foramina are opened, relieving pressure on the nerves. Similar symptoms are noted with vascular claudication (tissue ischemia secondary to vascular insufficiency), except that vascular symptoms are not dependent on the position of the spine but rather on the level of activity.

Functionally, people with neurogenic claudication lack the backward-bending range of motion to tolerate walking. If the therapist can improve overall backward-bending range of motion by mobilizing the thoracic and upper lumbar regions and by stretching the hip flexors, the affected individual may be able to assume an upright posture without reaching the end range of motion at the involved segments where the nerve compression is occurring. If this can be accomplished, walking tolerance should improve.

Exercise and Degenerative Disk Disease

Chronic low back pain from DDD is difficult to treat.[69] Nonsurgical care is the first line of treatment, often involving the physical therapist. Each individual must be assessed carefully and the plan of care provided based on presenting features. Back extension exercises, abdominal strengthening, postural training, and flexibility exercises for the spine and hamstrings may be helpful.

There is some evidence supporting the efficacy of exercise therapy.[351,538,854] At least one study shows stability exercises are effective for the treatment of DDD. When compared with mobilization treatment, stabilization exercises improved pain and function significantly more than mobilization.[498]

More studies are needed to identify the exact type of exercise along with frequency, duration, and intensity. Predictive factors for outcome need to be identified along with identification of candidates most likely to improve with exercise therapy (or type of exercise needed for each person).[853]

Aerobic conditioning is an important feature of the exercise program, especially to address the vascular component of this condition. Walking, swimming and/or water aerobics, and stationary bicycle are some possible choices. Each individual's lifestyle and overall physical condition will dictate the most likely course of action to prescribe or suggest.

Rheumatic Diseases

Rheumatic disorders are systemic diseases encompassing more than 100 different diseases divided into 10 classification categories. The pathogenesis and progression of these disorders can affect any and all body systems. The onset of joint pain and loss of function may be accompanied by fever, rash, diarrhea, scleritis, or neuritis symptoms that are not typically associated with joint or muscle conditions normally brought on by repetitive overuse or trauma.

Rheumatic disorders are also often marked by periods of exacerbation and remission. During a period of exacerbation the therapist will often need to modify the treatment approach considerably. In addition, aggressive medical intervention (i.e., medications) may need to be initiated to prevent or minimize the tissue destruction that can occur with these disorders. Many of the rheumatic conditions are chronic and progressive, requiring long-term rehabilitation and ongoing adjustment of functional goals.

Therapists must be able to differentiate between degenerative joint disease (OA) and rheumatic joint conditions (Table 27-2). If there is any suspicion of the presence of a rheumatic disorder, immediate referral to a physician is warranted. When someone with RA presents with systemic symptoms or if existing complaints worsen, communication with a physician is advised. An understanding of the diseases discussed in this chapter will assist the therapist regarding this clinical decision-making process.

Table 27-2	Osteoarthritis and Rheumatoid Arthritis	
	Osteoarthritis	**Rheumatoid Arthritis**
Onset	Usually begins at age 40 yr Gradual onset over many years; affects majority of adults older than age 65 yr	Initially develops between ages 25 and 50 yr Onset may be sudden over several weeks to months, intermittent exacerbation and remission
Incidence[70]	12% of U.S. adults; 21 million people	1%-2% of U.S. adults; 600,000 men, and 1.5 million women; estimated prevalence rate of juvenile RA in children younger than 16 yr is between 30,000 and 50,000
Gender	Most common in men before age 45 yr; after age 45 yr more common among women	Affects women 3 times as often compared with men, but more disabling and severe when present in men
Etiology	Etiology remains unknown; immunologic reaction with massive inflammatory response; possible genetic and environmental triggers	Multifactorial; local biomechanical factors, biochemistry, previous injury, inherited predisposition
Manifestations	Usually begins in joints on one side of the body Primarily affects hips, knees, spine, hands, feet	Symmetric simultaneous joint distribution Can affect any joint (large or small) predilection for upper extremities
	Inflammation with redness, warmth, and swelling in 10% of cases	Inflammation almost always present
	Brief morning stiffness that is decreased by physical activity movement	Prolonged morning stiffness lasting 1 hour or more
Associated signs and symptoms	No systemic symptoms; possible associated trigger points	Systemic presentation with constitutional symptoms (e.g., fatigue, malaise, weight loss, fever)
Laboratory values	Effusions infrequently, synovial fluid has low WBC and high viscosity	Synovial fluid has high WBC, and low viscosity
	ESR may be mildly to moderately increased	ESR markedly increased in the presence of an inflammatory process but not specifically diagnostic for RA
	Rheumatoid factor absent	Rheumatoid factor usually present but is not specific or diagnostic for RA (can be elevated C-reactive protein)
	New biomarkers under investigation (e.g., C-telopeptide, CTX, C-reactive protein YKL-40)	C-reactive protein, a true indicator of systemic inflammation, strong predictor of disease outcome (RA progresses more rapidly in the presence of elevated C-reactive protein) Other biomarkers are under investigation (e.g., vascular endothelial growth factor,* matrix metalloproteinase 3)

ESR, Erythrocyte sedimentation rate; RA, rheumatoid arthritis; WBC, white blood cell count.
*Vascular endothelial growth factor is an angiogenic cytokine. Its presence supports the theory that expansion of the synovial vasculature is important for the development of joint destruction in RA.

Rheumatoid Arthritis

Overview. RA is a chronic systemic inflammatory disease presenting with a wide range of articular and extraarticular findings. Chronic polyarthritis, which perpetuates a gradual destruction of joint tissues, can result in severe deformity and disability. Systems that may be involved include the cardiovascular, pulmonary, and gastrointestinal systems. Eye lesions, infection, and osteoporosis are other potential extraarticular manifestations.[38]

RA is a major subclassification within the category of diffuse connective tissue diseases that also includes juvenile arthritis, SLE, progressive systemic sclerosis (scleroderma), polymyositis, and dermatomyositis.[317]

Incidence and Risk Factors. RA has a worldwide distribution and affects all races. Approximately 1% to 2% of the U.S. adult population (1.3 million people) has RA, which is the second most prevalent form of arthritis after OA.

Age and female gender are the two primary risk factors associated with RA. Although the onset of the disorder can occur at any age, the peak onset is usually between 30 and 60 years; with the aging of America, the prevalence of RA is expected to rise. Women are affected nearly three times more frequently than men; although it is less common, children can also develop the disorder (see "Juvenile Idiopathic Arthritis" below). The cause of RA is unknown, but is most likely from a combination of genetic and environmental factors. Some genetic markers have been identified for the disease, but not all persons with RA have these genes.[39] Pregnancy and oral contraceptives appear to influence the incidence and severity of the disease. The incidence of RA in women who have borne a child is lower, and oral contraceptives diminish the incidence of severe arthritis.[98,731]

Prophylactic administration of recombinant hepatitis B vaccine may trigger the development of RA in those with a genetic predisposition, such as the major histocompatibility complex class II molecules, but it is a safe and effective vaccine for individuals with RA.[220,668] An association between autoimmune thyroid diseases and rheumatic diseases has been established, although its precise mechanism is unclear. For example, RA often occurs in association with Graves disease and Hashimoto thyroiditis. In these individuals, there is a significant presence of antithyroid autoantibodies.[545]

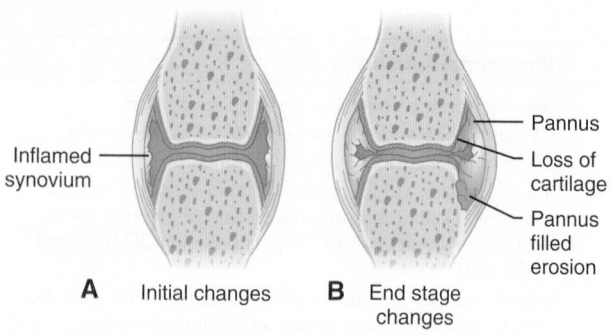

A, Early synovial changes associated with rheumatoid arthritis. **B,** Late joint changes associated with rheumatoid arthritis, including pannus formation and articular cartilage eburnation.

Figure 27-12

Drinking decaffeinated coffee (4 or more cups per day) may be an independent risk factor among older women, especially in the presence of seropositive disease. The mechanism for this to occur remains unknown.[579]

Etiologic Factors. Little is known about the exact causes of RA, except that joint inflammation is a consequence of massive infiltration of immune cells, especially T lymphocytes, into the synovial fluid. Genetic predisposition and environmental triggers, such as a bacteria (e.g., *Mycoplasma fermentans*), are both considered possible etiologic factors in the stimulation of T cells.[169,237,384]

Pathogenesis. RA is considered an autoimmune disease, with inflammation and destruction targeted at the joint capsule (articular) and elsewhere throughout the body (extraarticular). Approximately 80% of people with RA are rheumatoid factor positive.[344]

Rheumatoid factors are autoantibodies that react with immunoglobulin antibodies found in the blood. Rheumatoid factor has also been found in the synovial fluid and synovial membranes of those with the disease. It is hypothesized that the interaction between rheumatoid factor and the immunoglobulin triggers events that initiate an inflammatory reaction.

RA begins attacking the joint in the synovium. The normal synovial membrane consists of loose connective tissue that contains blood vessels and is covered by a layer of synovial lining consisting of macrophages and synoviocytes and is only minimally infiltrated by lymphocytes. In RA, the cells of the synovial lining multiply, there is an influx of leukocytes from the peripheral circulation, and the synovium becomes edematous. The synovial lining thickens, resulting in the clinical synovitis seen so often.

These changes can result in the development of thickened synovium, a destructive vascular granulation tissue called *pannus.* The inflammatory cells found within the pannus are destructive, preventing the synovium from performing its two primary functions: lubricating the joint and providing nutrients to the avascular articular cartilage. As this tissue proliferates, encroaching on the joint space at the margins where the hyaline cartilage and synovial lining do not adequately cover the bone, it dissolves collagen, cartilage, subchondral bone, and other periarticular tissues in its path (Fig. 27-12).

Although the cause of RA remains unknown, recent advances in molecular techniques have allowed for identification of distinct cell subtypes, surface markers, and products that may initiate and propagate the inflammatory and destructive components of the disease. Cytokines, TNF-α, IL-1, and IL-6, found in abundance in the rheumatoid synovium, appear to play a major role in the pathophysiologic process of RA.[605]

The interaction of cytokines, immune and nonimmune cells (e.g., synovial fibroblasts and osteoclasts) prompts a massive inflammatory response. As the attracted leukocytes, monocytes, and lymphocytes phagocytize the immune complexes, these cytokines stimulate the secretion of matrix metalloproteinases (protein-degrading enzymes that lyse the cartilage and destroy the joint), leading to articular cartilage destruction and synovial hyperplasia with local tenderness, swelling, and intense joint pain. Elevated cytokines also inhibit bone formation and induce bone resorption by directly or indirectly activating osteoclasts. Elevated levels of IL-6 contribute to anemia and fatigue associated with RA by disrupting iron homeostasis and stimulating the hypothalamic–pituitary–adrenal axis, respectively.

The result of the synovial changes that occur in RA can be irreversible joint instability, joint deformity, or ankylosis (adhesions and fibrous or bony fusion of the joint). Joint destruction eventually leads to laxity of the tendons and ligaments, which contributes to the altered biomechanics and deformities frequently observed.[221] The wide range of extraarticular problems is also probably a result of local inflammatory injury induced by the immune complexes traveling through the circulatory system.

Clinical Manifestations. RA is a systemic disease typically manifested by articular and extraarticular complaints (Box 27-8). The symptoms usually begin insidiously and progress slowly as the disease process moves from cartilage degradation to ligamentous laxity and, finally, synovial expansion with erosion. Complaints of fatigue, weight loss, weakness, and general, diffuse musculoskeletal pain are often the initial presentation. Deconditioning and depression are common complications of this disease.[191]

The course of RA can vary considerably from mild to severely disabling and is difficult to predict, but it appears that adults with RA today have less-severe symptoms and less functional disability than even a decade ago. This positive trend and more favorable course of disease may be attributed to earlier diagnosis with a shorter duration of symptoms at the time of diagnosis and more aggressive use of drug therapy.[887]

Joint. The musculoskeletal symptoms gradually localize to specific joints. Multiple joints are usually involved, with symmetric, bilateral presentation. The most frequently involved joints are the wrist, knee, and joints of the fingers, hands, and feet, although RA can affect any joint, including the temporomandibular joints. The metacarpophalangeal and proximal interphalangeal joints of the hand are involved early. The involved joints can be edematous, warm, painful, and stiff. After periods of rest (e.g., prolonged sitting, sleeping), intense joint pain and stiffness may last 30 minutes to several hours as activity is initiated.

As the disease progresses, joint deformity can occur, including subluxation. Deformities in the fingers are

Box 27-8

ARTICULAR AND EXTRAARTICULAR MANIFESTATIONS OF RHEUMATOID ARTHRITIS

Cardiac

- Conduction defects (usually asymptomatic)
- Pericarditis
- Interstitial myocarditis
- Coronary arteritis
- Vasculitis
- Aortitis

Hematologic

- Anemia of chronic disease
- Felty syndrome (splenomegaly, neutropenia)
- Lymphoma, leukemia

Musculoskeletal

- Osteopenia, osteoporosis (associated fractures)
- Joint pain (reflects severity of synovitis; may not be present at rest)
- Joint stiffness (present in most cases, especially after inactivity; duration reflects degree of synovial inflammation; improves with physical activity)
- Joint contracture (extension of involved joints most commonly affected)
- Swelling (synovial tissue)
- Muscle atrophy (hands, feet; occurs rapidly in severe disease)
- Muscle weakness; often out of proportion to the degree of muscular atrophy
- Tenosynovitis, tendonitis, tendon triggering, tendon rupture
- Joint deformity

Neurologic

- Compression neuropathies; nerve entrapment syndromes (e.g., carpal tunnel syndrome, tarsal tunnel syndrome)
- Polyneuropathy
- Peripheral neuropathy (mononeuritis multiplex, stocking-glove peripheral neuropathy)
- Myelopathy; subluxation or instability of C1-C2
- Lhermitte sign (upper-extremity paresthesias that increase with neck flexion)

Integumentary

- Nodulosis (see Fig. 27-15; subcutaneous nodules, especially over olecranon and proximal ulna, extensor surfaces of fingers, Achilles tendon ["pump bumps"])

- Nodules can occur in tendon, bone, sclerae, over pinna or ear, and in visceral organs, especially lung
- Palmar erythema (identical to changes found in liver disease and pregnancy; persists even in remission)
- Sweet syndrome
- Vasculitis

Ocular

- Episcleritis (inflammation of the superficial sclera and conjunctiva)
- Scleritis (inflammation of the sclera)
- Sicca syndrome (dry eyes)

Psychologic

- Depression (common); other mood disorders

Pulmonary

- Effusions
- Interstitial pneumonia
- Interstitial fibrosis
- Nodules (rheumatoid nodulosis)
- Pleurisy, pleuritis
- Empyema
- Pulmonary hypertension

Renal

- Interstitial nephritis, nephritic syndrome
- Vasculitis

Vascular

- Skin changes (rash, ulcers, purpura, bullae)
- Infarctions (brain, viscera, nail folds; see Fig. 27-16)
- Digital gangrene
- Medium-vessel arteritis
- Small-vessel vasculitis

Other

- Unexplained weight loss, anorexia
- Malaise, fatigue
- Lymphadenopathy (lymph node enlargement; more common in men)
- Colon cancer

Data from: McInnes IB, O'Dell JR. State-of-the-art: rheumatoid arthritis. *Ann Rheum Dis* 69(11):1898–1906, 2010; and Arthritis Foundation. *Who gets rheumatoid arthritis*. Available at: http://www.arthritis.org/who-gets-rheumatoid-arthritis.php. Accessed on November 19, 2012.

common, including ulnar deviation, swan-neck deformity, and boutonnière deformity. The ulnar deviation occurs as the extensor tendons slip to the ulnar aspect of the metacarpal head. Hyperextension of the proximal interphalangeal joint and partial flexion of the distal interphalangeal joint make up the swan-neck deformity (Fig. 27-13). The boutonnière deformity is marked by flexion of the proximal interphalangeal joint and hyperextension of the distal interphalangeal joint (Fig. 27-14).

Soft Tissue. Soft-tissue manifestations of RA can include synovitis, bursitis, tendinitis, fasciitis, neuritis, and vasculitis. These problems are often overlooked but can be very debilitating. Soft-tissue imbalance combined with joint involvement can result in significant deformity, especially in the hands and feet.

Spine. Early involvement of the spinal column is common and typically limited to the cervical spine, with deep, aching neck pain radiating into the occipital, retroorbital, or temporal areas reported in 40% to 88% of persons.[90,456,693] Neck movement precipitates or aggravates neck pain; facial and ear pain and occipital headaches occur frequently with active disease from irritation of the C2 nerve root supply to the spinal trigeminal tract, greater auricular nerve, or greater occipital nerve.[456]

There is a potential for atlantoaxial subluxation (usually anterior) and brainstem or spinal cord compression. The upper cervical spine is affected most commonly because the occiput-C1 and the C1-C2 articulations are purely synovial and are thus primary targets for rheumatoid involvement. In addition, because the C1 and C2 facets are oriented in the axial plane, there is no bony interlocking to prevent subluxation in the face of ligamentous destruction.[693]

The natural history of cervical instability in people with RA is variable, and only some develop neurologic deficits.[215,631] Symptoms of C1-C2 subluxation include a sensation of the head falling forward with neck flexion, loss of consciousness or syncope, dysphagia, vertigo, seizures,

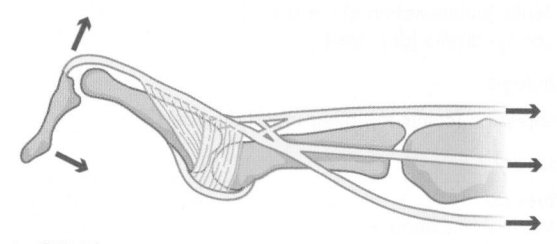

Figure 27-13

Swan-neck deformity. (From Jacobs JL: Hand and wrist. In Richardson JK, Iglarsh ZA, editors: *Clinical orthopaedic physical therapy*, Philadelphia, 1994, WB Saunders, p. 309.)

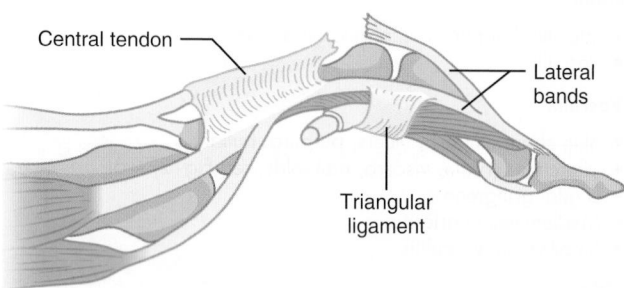

Central tendon —

Lateral bands

Triangular ligament

Figure 27-14

Boutonnière deformity. (From Jacobs JL: Hand and wrist. In Richardson JK, Iglarsh ZA, editors: *Clinical orthopaedic physical therapy*, Philadelphia, 1994, WB Saunders, p. 664.)

hemiplegia, dysarthria, nystagmus, peripheral paresthesias, and loss of dexterity of the hands.[96] Urinary retention and later incontinence are symptoms of more severe involvement. Sleep apnea may be caused by brainstem compression associated with atlantoaxial impaction.[654]

There may be a positive Lhermitte sign with shock-like sensations of the torso or extremities with neck flexion. Atlantoaxial instability may result in vertebrobasilar insufficiency with visual disturbances, loss of equilibrium, vertigo, tinnitus, and dysphagia. These symptoms can also be caused by mechanical compression of the cervicomedullary junction or brainstem.[693] Asymmetrical destruction of the lateral atlantoaxial joints may result in a clinical presentation of head tilt down and to one side. When the neck is flexed, the spinous process of the axis may be prominent.

Pain associated with RA in the subaxial segments of the cervical spine is located in the lateral aspects of the neck and clavicles (C3-C4) and over the shoulders (C5-C6). Neurologic symptoms include burning paresthesias and numbness, which may be attributed to carpal tunnel syndrome, delaying the diagnosis of cervical myelopathy.

Cutaneous. The visible rheumatoid nodule is a characteristic skin finding in RA, occurring in approximately 25% of all cases. These granulomatous lesions usually occur in areas of repeated mechanical pressure, such as over the extensor surface of the elbow, Achilles tendon, and extensor surface of the fingers (Fig. 27-15). Nodules are usually asymptomatic, but they can become tender or cause skin breakdown and become infected. Nodules that cannot be seen visibly can also occur in the heart, lungs, and gastrointestinal tract, causing serious problems such as heart arrhythmias and respiratory failure.

Neurologic. One third of adults with RA have cervical spine involvement leading to compressive cervical myelopathy presented as neck pain and stiffness, the Lhermitte sign, weakness of the upper or lower extremities, hyperactive distal tendon reflexes, and presence of the Babinski sign. In severe cases, urinary and fecal incontinence and paralysis can occur.[270]

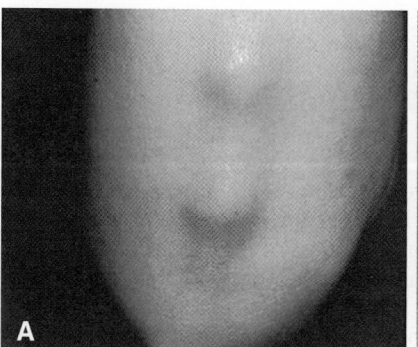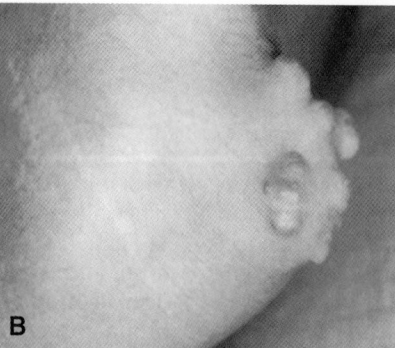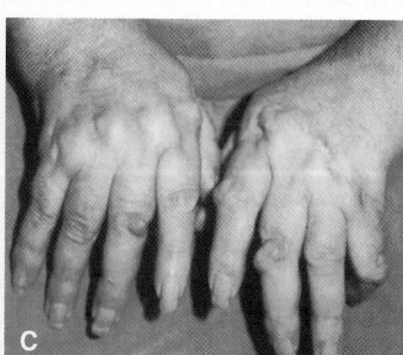

Figure 27-15

A, Rheumatoid nodules may be firm, raised, nontender bumps over which the skin slides easily. Common sites are in the olecranon bursa (elbow), along the extensor surface of the forearm, and behind the heel (calcaneus). **B,** These nodules are also associated with rheumatoid arthritis and are firm, nontender, and freely moveable. These are most common in people with severe arthritis, high-titer rheumatoid factor, or rheumatoid vasculitis. **C,** Multiple rheumatoid nodules of the digits with typical ulnar deviation deformity from longstanding rheumatoid arthritis. Histologically identical lesions have been found in the sclera (eye), larynx, heart, lungs, and abdominal wall. The lesions develop insidiously and may regress spontaneously but usually persist. (**A,** from Callen JP, Greer KE, Hood AF: *Color atlas of dermatology*, Philadelphia, 1993, WB Saunders, p. 130. **B** and **C,** from Callen JP, Jorizzo J, Greer KE: *Dermatological signs of internal disease*, Philadelphia, 1988, WB Saunders, pp. 41, 42.)

Chronic inflammation of the atlantoaxial joint can lead to laxity of the transverse ligament, which normally keeps the dens closely abutted against the anterior arch of the atlas. With loss of integrity of the ligament, the dens moves backward and presses against the spinal cord during forward neck flexion. The individual experiences a shock like sensation and numbness down the arms with forward flexion of the neck (the Lhermitte sign, previously mentioned). Arthritic changes with erosive involvement of the lower cervical spine facet (zygapophyseal) joints can also lead to compressive myelopathy or radiculopathy.

Peripheral neuropathies are common as the nerves become compressed by inflamed synovia in tight compartments. Pain, dysesthesias, motor loss, and muscle atrophy can occur, leading to dysfunction and disability. Rheumatoid vasculitis involving medium-sized arteries to the muscles can lead to mononeuritis multiplex, while small-vessel vasculitis causes stocking-glove peripheral neuropathy.[270]

Extraarticular. The extraarticular manifestations are numerous and affect men and women equally (see Box 27-8 and Fig. 27-16). Many of these manifestations impair cardiopulmonary function, restrict activity, decrease endurance, and are disabling; some are life-threatening. They could easily hamper rehabilitation efforts, delaying or preventing progress. See Chapters 12 and 15 for descriptions of the cardiovascular and pulmonary manifestations, respectively.

Sjögren syndrome (discussed below) is marked by lymphocytic and plasma cell infiltration of the lacrimal and parotid glands. This can result in diminished salivary and lacrimal secretions. Felty syndrome is marked by splenomegaly and leukopenia. Mood disorders, especially depression, are common (see "Depression" in Chapter 3).[18,876]

Individuals with RA are also at increased risk for severe infection, including tuberculosis, requiring hospitalization.[59,133,214] There is also a greater risk of cardiovascular and cerebrovascular morbidity and mortality among adults with RA compared to adults with OA.

The increased risk of myocardial infarction, congestive heart failure, and cerebrovascular accident is not explained by traditional cardiovascular risk factors, but the mechanism for this association is unknown at this time. Altered immunologic function may possibly explain the increased association, but other factors, such as the

new biotherapies for RA (e.g., TNF-α blockers), may be at work as well.[214,625,897]

MEDICAL MANAGEMENT

PREVENTION. As mentioned in "Osteoarthritis" above, there is a need to implement interventions such as supervised exercise programs, weight loss, and self-education courses such as found at the Arthritis Foundation's website, which have been shown to reduce pain and physician visits.[41,508]

DIAGNOSIS. In the early stages of RA, the diagnosis can be difficult because of the gradual, subtle onset of the complaints. The symptoms may wax and wane, delaying the visit to a physician's office. Early diagnosis can help prevent or reduce erosive and irreversible joint damage, as well as reduce morbidity and mortality associated with this chronic disease. The diagnosis is ultimately based on a combination of history, physical examination, imaging studies, and laboratory tests, with careful exclusion of other disorders.[191]

Table 27-3 lists the diagnostic criteria for RA as recently modified by the American College of Rheumatology.[23]

Table 27-3	2010 American College of Rheumatology (ACR)-European League Against Rheumatism (EULAR) Classification Criteria for Rheumatoid Arthritis

Target population (Who should be tested?): Individuals who
1. have at least 1 joint with definite clinical synovitis (swelling)
2. with the synovitis not better explained by another disease
Classification criteria for RA (score-based algorithm: add score of categories A–D; a score of ≥6/10 is needed for classification of a person as having definite RA)‡

	Score
A. Joint involvement	
1 large joint	0
2-10 large joints	1
1-3 small joints (with or without involvement of large joints)	2
4-10 small joints (with or without involvement of large joints)	3
>10 joints (at least 1 small joint)	5
B. Serology (at least 1 test result is needed for classification)	
Negative RF and negative ACPA	0
Low-positive RF or low-positive ACPA	2
High-positive RF or high-positive ACPA	3
C. Acute-phase reactants (at least 1 test result is needed for classification)	
Normal CRP and normal ESR	0
Abnormal CRP or abnormal ESR	1
D. Duration of symptoms	
<6 weeks	0
≥6 weeks	1

ACPA, Anticytoplasmic antibody; CRP, C-reactive protein; ESR, erythrocyte sedimentation rate; RF, rheumatoid factor
From Aletaha D, Neogi T, Silman AJ, et al: 2010 Rheumatoid arthritis classification criteria: an American College of Rheumatology/European League Against Rheumatism collaborative initiative, *Arthritis Rheum* 62(9):2569-2581, 2010.

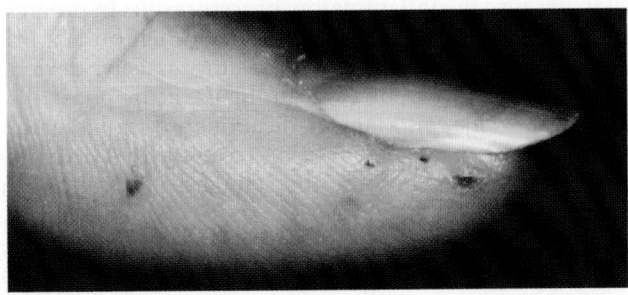

Figure 27-16

Vasculitis splinter infarction around the finger of a person with systemic vasculitis associated with rheumatoid arthritis (extraarticular manifestation). Clinical features are diverse, because virtually any blood vessel anywhere in the body can be affected. (From Moots RJ, Bacon PA: Extraarticular manifestations of rheumatoid arthritis, *J Musculoskelet Med* 11:10-23, 1994.)

The classification is based on the presence of synovitis in at least one joint that cannot be accounted for by an alternative diagnosis, with a score of 6 or higher in 4 individual score domains of the ACR criteria.[191] The presence of serum rheumatoid factor supports the diagnosis but can also be found in healthy persons. Synovial fluid analysis will reveal an elevated white blood cell count, protein content, and protein antibodies. Also, a decrease in synovial fluid volume and poor viscosity and an increased turbidity may be noted (see Table 27-2). C-reactive protein, an acute-phase reactant, may be helpful when obtained in a series over time to predict those individuals who are at increased risk for joint deterioration and as a measure of response to treatment. Persistent elevation in C-reactive protein is a predictive factor for cervical spine subluxation.[269,645]

Most individuals will be symptomatic for a long period before seeing a physician. At least half of all adults with RA are not referred for rheumatologic consultation until they have had their disease for at least 6 months (sometimes more than 1 year).[599]

Conventional radiography, ultrasonography, and MRI studies allow more accurate diagnosis of RA.[811] The earliest joint changes (periarticular swelling and cortical thinning with erosion at the margins of the articular cartilage and joint space narrowing) are seen on plain radiographs (Fig. 27-17). Screening cervical spine radiographs should be considered for all individuals with RA, but especially for those with advanced peripheral joint disease.[456]

MRI is more sensitive than conventional radiography for detecting early RA and can show lesions of the synovium and cartilage, and joint effusions.[221] MRI has the ability to visualize synovitis and detect bone edema, which is emerging as a predictor of future erosive bone changes.[104] Ultrasonography enables the visualization of small superficial structures and can reveal synovial inflammation and tenosynovitis as well as effusions and bone erosions.[811]

TREATMENT. The primary goal for the treatment of RA is a state of remission, with an absence of or having minimal signs and symptoms for the disease process. A process described as "treating to target" is used to customize the use of pharmacologic agents and other therapeutic measures to reach this goal for each person with RA.[779] Early treatment of RA is critical to improving long-term outcomes, as clinical evidence clearly shows that joint destruction in RA begins early in the disease.[669] The treatment goals for someone with RA are to reduce pain, maintain mobility, and minimize stiffness, edema, and joint destruction. Aggressive combination drug therapy (Box 27-9) in conjunction with other management techniques, including physical therapy, is the mainstay of treatment.[180]

The management approach is individualized, especially in the presence of extraarticular manifestation. The physician has a challenging task trying to optimize the pharmacologic management when there is no way to identify which people will need aggressive therapy. The physician must balance the need for conservative care without being too conservative to avoid unchecked inflammation and joint damage, while at the same time avoiding being too aggressive, leading to exposure to potentially toxic medications when less expensive, safer drugs would have been as effective.[104, 779]

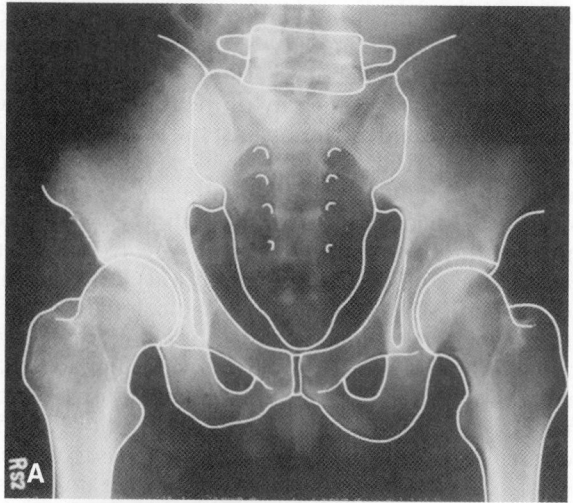

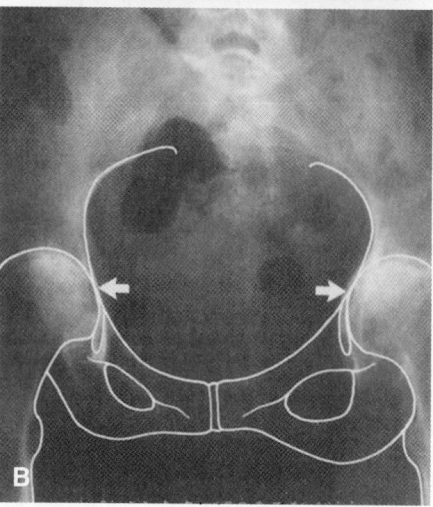

Figure 27-17

A, Radiograph of normal hips and pelvis. **B,** Radiograph of rheumatoid arthritis of the hips. Note the narrowed joint space (loss of articular cartilage) and periarticular bone density changes. (From McKinnis LN: *Fundamentals of radiology for physical therapists.* In Richardson JK, Iglarsh ZA, editors: *Clinical orthopaedic physical therapy,* Philadelphia, 1994, WB Saunders, p. 673.)

The chronic nature of the disease makes client education and continual adherence to the treatment program vital. Because the inflammatory process results in progressive joint destruction, controlling inflammation is a primary goal. Medications, rest, ambulatory assistive devices, orthoses, and ice can be used during the acute phase.

Pharmacotherapy. Many medications are available now to help in the management of RA (see Box 27-9). Methotrexate (MTX) has become the standard medication for those with newly diagnosed RA, and is the most widely used immunosuppressant for RA management because of its long-term efficacy.[191] Although its exact mechanism remains unknown, it allows for rapid remission of joint pain and stiffness found in the early stages of the disease process. Effects tend to plateau after 3 to 6 months, and side effects can be numerous; regular serum monitoring of liver and renal function is required.

Disease-modifying antirheumatic drugs (DMARDs; also known as biologic DMARDs), are examples of newer

Box 27-9

PHARMACOTHERAPY FOR RHEUMATOID ARTHRITIS

Analgesics

- Various nonprescription and prescription drugs, including acetaminophen (Tylenol), tramadol (Ultram), and codeine

Nonsteroidal Antiinflammatory Drugs (NSAIDs)

- Nonprescription and prescription formulas, including aspirin, ibuprofen (Advil, Motrin), naproxen (Aleve, Anaprox, Naprelan, Naprosyn), ketoprofen (Orudis, Oruvail), diclofenac (Voltaren), diflunisal (Dolobid), indomethacin (Indocin)

Corticosteroids

- Oral or injection formulas, including prednisone (Cortan, Deltasone, Meticorten), methylprednisolone (Medrol)

Disease-Modifying Antirheumatic Drugs (DMARDs)

- Antimalarials (hydroxychloroquine [Plaquenil])
- Non–antibiotics sulfonamides (sulfasalazine [Azulfidine], minocycline [Minocin, Dynacin])
- Injectable and oral gold (Ridaura)
- D-penicillamine (Depen, Cuprimine)
- Methotrexate (Amethopterin, Rheumatrex)

- Immunosuppressants (azathioprine [Imuran], cyclophosphamide [Cytoxan], cyclosporine [Neoral, Sandimmune], Leflunomide [Arava])

Cytokine Inhibitors*

- Tumor necrosis factor (TNF) inhibitors† (etanercept [Enbrel], infliximab [Remicade], adalimumab [Humira])
- Interleukin-1 inhibitor (anakinra [Kineret])
- Golimumab (Simponi; human monoclonal antibody to TNF-α)
- Certolizumab (Cimzia; human monoclonal antibody to TNF-α)

Lymphocyte Inhibitors

- Rituximab (Rituxan; antibody originally developed for the treatment of B-cell lymphoma)
- Abatacept (Orencia; interrupts the activation of T cells, leading to T-cell anergy and apoptosis)
- Belimumab (Benlysta; inhibits B-cell growth and survival)

Investigational Drugs (in Clinical Trials)

- HuMax-CD20 (antibody that targets B cells)
- Atacicept (inhibits B-cell growth and survival)
- Tocilizumab (Actemra; anti–interleukin-6 receptor monoclonal antibody)

*Pegylation is a new way to deliver anti–TNF-α agents that are site specific. Polyethylene glycol is added to enhance the pharmacokinetic properties of a molecule, decreasing its volume of distribution and clearance and increasing its half-life.
†May also be referred to as TNF-α antagonists.
Data from Yazici Y, Abramson SB: Bright Future for RA Therapies, *J Musculoskelet Med Suppl* S32-S35, 2006; and McInnes IB, O'Dell JR: State-of-the-art: rheumatoid arthritis. *Ann Rheum Dis* 69(11):1898–1906, 2010.

types of drugs used in combination with analgesics, antiinflammatories, and steroids to alter the course and clinical presentation of RA. Some DMARDs block the activity of a protein (TNF) that triggers and prolongs the inflammatory process, leading to joint destruction. Others block IL-1, a protein present in excess in people with RA, thus inhibiting inflammation and cartilage damage.

DMARDs, often used in combination, are started as early as possible to reduce or prevent joint damage. These drugs take weeks to months to begin working and must be monitored carefully for adverse side effects. DMARDs are often given along with a steroid, which quiets inflammation and improves symptoms while the individual is waiting for the DMARD to take effect. Then the steroid is withdrawn slowly.

Analgesics are used to help relieve pain. NSAIDs reduce pain, swelling, and inflammation. Corticosteroids help reduce inflammation and pain and can slow joint damage. Biotechnology has made new pharmacologic agents possible with genetically engineered products that can relieve symptoms and slow the progression of this disease. These new agents can "reset the inflammatory thermostat" and avoid joint damage.[644]

NSAIDs are effective for pain and swelling associated with inflamed joints caused by RA, but these pharmacologic agents do not affect disease progression. Corticosteroids may be prescribed in addition to DMARDs and NSAIDs to relieve pain, and in clients with unremitting disease with extraarticular manifestations. Intraarticular injections can provide relief of acute inflammation. Administration of these drugs for periods of 3 to 6 months is often necessary for benefit to be noted.

The development of cytokine inhibitors has had an important role in treating individuals with RA. Targeting TNF-α, an important proinflammatory cytokine present in the rheumatoid synovium, has been a great help in treating this disease. IL-1 has several actions that overlap those of TNF-α; TNF-α appears to be more important in early inflammation, while IL-1 may be more important in erosive arthritis. Cytokine targets such as IL-6, IL-12, and IL-18 remain under investigation.[461,558]

Biologic response modifiers were developed to target the interaction sites in the pathologic pathway blocking the action of TNF-α, which initiates the inflammatory response, thereby suppressing inflammation more effectively. Etanercept (Enbrel) is a genetically engineered (recombinant) version of a receptor for TNF that helps bind and inactivate excess TNF, thereby reducing the inflammatory response (cytokine inhibitor). When used in combination with MTX, results are superior to those of MTX alone.[600,885]

Fortunately, a new member of the tumor necrosis family has been identified: osteoprotegerin (OPG). This protein plays a key role in the physiologic regulation of osteoclastic bone resorption, counteracting the destruction and bone degradation caused by the cytokine-induced inflammatory process. OPG might represent an effective therapeutic option for diseases, such as RA, that are associated with excessive osteoclastic activity.[814] Other drugs under investigation block protein signals that cause inflammation. Reducing the number of these proteins or blocking the receptors that receive their signals might help control RA.

Drugs that stop B cells from causing inflammation, such as rituximab, intercept B cells and stop them from completing their tasks. Several other approaches to stopping B cells are under investigation. One drug that was investigational but now available is belimumab (Benlysta); this medication blocks signals that drive B cells.

The additional use of bone-active agents can reduce the rate of bone loss (e.g., OPG, a regulator of osteoclast formation, may prevent bone erosion without inhibiting the inflammatory process necessary in other parts of the body).[309] Minocycline, an antibiotic, is another effective DMARD that can be used in people with early seropositive RA, making it possible to reduce the amount of corticosteroids used.[633]

Surgery. Surgery may be indicated if conservative care is insufficient in achieving acceptable pain control and level of function. Synovectomy to reduce pain and joint damage is the primary operation for the wrist. Total joint replacement procedures are performed at the shoulder, hip, knee, wrist, and fingers. The most common soft-tissue procedure is tenosynovectomy of the hand. Studies support prophylactic stabilization of the rheumatoid cervical spine to prevent paralysis in high-risk individuals.[177,615]

Complementary and Alternative Medicine/Complementary and Integrative Medicine. Some complementary approaches, such as acupuncture and autogenic training, have been advocated by some in the treatment of RA, but have not shown adequate efficacy for the management of RA.[520] Nutraceuticals, such as fish and plant oils; vitamin, mineral, and other supplements (e.g., S-adenosylmethionine [SAMe]) have also been advocated for individuals with RA. Safety and effectiveness are not yet proven in long-term studies. Physical therapists may be more involved in studying the effects of movement therapies such as tai chi, qi gong, and yoga (see text discussion).

PROGNOSIS. There is no known cure for RA at this time, and joint changes are usually irreversible. Restrictions in the ability to perform specific actions and difficulty in performing ADLs can result in functional limitations and disability. It is now established that the longer a person has RA, the greater the likelihood of having cervical spine disease.[632]

More specific predictors of neurologic recovery from brainstem or spinal cord compression include location of the disease (basilar invagination has a poorer prognosis than isolated atlantoaxial or subaxial instability), degree of preoperative neurologic deficit, and spinal canal diameter.[693]

Knowledge of the natural history of RA affecting the cervical spine is limited. Studies are small in size and limited in scope. Transition from reducible subluxation to irreducible subluxation often accompanies atlantoaxial impaction an average of 6 years after atlantoaxial subluxation. Up to 80% of individuals with rheumatoid subluxations demonstrate radiologic progression but may not experience corresponding clinical symptoms.[456]

There is a high rate of sudden death linked with untreated myelopathy. The presence of myelopathy increases the risk of mortality dramatically; without surgery, most people die within 1 year. Even with surgery to stabilize the spine, death from cord compression does occur.[619]

Quality-of-life issues are central to this disease when people who expected to be active and productive are severely capacitated in early adulthood. The natural history of RA varies considerably, but people who present at an early stage and receive early intervention continue to do well years later, with reduced joint pain and inflammation and preservation of function.[805]

Mortality in adults with extraarticular manifestations of RA is significantly greater than in those whose disease is limited to the joints; in many people, the extraarticular manifestations are more debilitating than the arthritis itself.[270] Death from complications associated with RA and its treatment can occur. These complications include subluxation of the upper cervical spine; infections; gastrointestinal hemorrhage and perforation; and renal, heart, and lung disease. The same factors that contribute to joint inflammation also accelerate atherosclerosis and heart disease; early death resulting from coronary artery disease will be the focus of future treatment efforts.[193]

As the complex pathogenesis is better understood, new drugs that can interrupt tissue and joint destruction without interfering with host defense mechanisms or causing other adverse effects may be developed to stop the progression of this disease.

SPECIAL IMPLICATIONS FOR THE THERAPIST 27-11

Rheumatoid Arthritis
Medical Screening of Joint Pain

Therapists see many people with joint pain. Most of these people have joint pain secondary to degenerative OA as opposed to rheumatic joint disease, but the therapist must be aware of the symptoms and signs associated with RA. The therapist can ask a series of questions to help identify the cause of joint pain.[307] An abbreviated version of this list includes the following:

- *Are you stiff in the morning?* If yes, *how long does this stiffness last?*
- *Does your stiffness increase after sitting?*
- *Where do you think the pain is coming from?*
- *If joints, which ones are involved?*
- *Do you ever notice any joint swelling or other changes?*
- *Does anyone else in your family have RA or other kinds of arthritis?*
- *Does aspirin or ibuprofen help you feel better?*

Being aware of the clinical signs and symptoms of RA will help the therapist make an early referral. The distribution of joint involvement is an important clue. RA usually affects the small joints of the feet and hands symmetrically; generalized pain ("I hurt all over") is not characteristic of RA.

Quick, aggressive medical treatment is necessary to minimize joint destruction. Unexplained joint pain for 1 month or more, especially accompanied by systemic complaints, skin rash, or extensor nodules, no matter how mild, should raise concern on the therapist's part. Cervical pain with reports of urinary retention or incontinence warrants immediate medical evaluation. Also, insidious onset of polyarthritis or joint pain within 6 weeks of taking a medication should raise suspicion regarding the nature of the pain complaints.

Any of these red flags suggests the need for a medical referral if a physician has not recently evaluated the affected individual.

Anyone with known RA should be instructed in recognizing the signs and symptoms of progression of disease (e.g., increased duration of morning stiffness, increased number of tender and painful joints, increased intensity of joint pain, increased fatigue, increased gait disturbances, worsening of visible deformities) so that the intervention plan can be modified to meet the individual's needs.

When distinguishing articular pain from periarticular involvement, remember that true arthritis produces pain and limitation during both active and passive range of motion, while limitation from tendinitis is much worse during active than during passive motion. Inflammatory joint involvement typically produces warmth, erythema, and tenderness. Frequently, there is bogginess related to underlying synovitis or effusion. These indicators are not present with joint pain of a mechanical cause.

Patient/Client Education

Helping individuals affected by RA understand the disease, disease process, treatment, possible outcomes, and role of exercise and self-care is a major part of the therapist's task. Self-management includes learning pacing, joint protection, and energy conservation; monitoring symptoms; and maintaining or progressing an exercise program.[41]

Each person must be taught ways to minimize trauma to inflamed joints by unloading joints and reducing mechanical joint stresses. This can be done through modification of activities such as using assistive devices to open doors and jars, and avoiding excessive weight bearing on inflamed joints by reducing movements such as bending and stooping. Energy conservation (see Box 9-4) should become a way of life for anyone with acute or subacute disease. The systemic nature of this disease produces global fatigue; the demand for energy to move joints may increase if biomechanics are altered.[414]

The need for frequent rest breaks, change in level of activity, and change in positions throughout the day should be taught and their use encouraged, but they should be balanced by the need to avoid muscle wasting and weakness from immobilization. Range of motion, stretching, and isometric exercises must be taught, monitored, and reinforced for as long as the therapist follows the individual, always teaching the client how to modify the program during periods of active inflammation.

Cervical Spine Involvement

Cervical collars may be used for comfort but do not protect against progressive subluxation or neurologic compromise. Rigid cervical collars can partially limit anterior atlantoaxial subluxation, but they also prevent reduction of the deformity in extension.[440,441] Rigid orthoses are also poorly tolerated in these individuals because of skin sensitivity and temporomandibular joint involvement. Anyone with cervical spine involvement should be taught to avoid cervical flexion. The therapist can focus on isometric strengthening of neck muscles and overall postural training.

In the case of conservative intervention with nonsurgical management, the therapist must observe for (and teach the client to observe for) gradual deterioration in function that may indicate the development of subtle myelopathy (see "Clinical Manifestations" below). Radiographic evaluation is important in observing for impending neurologic compromise.[693,884]

Rehabilitation

RA is a chronic, progressive disease requiring an interdisciplinary team approach that is individual to the client and comprehensive, with long-range planning that extends beyond the initial acute phase. The role of the physical therapist in the management of RA is well established,[115,496,503,622] especially with the renewed focus on outcome-based intervention.

The American College of Rheumatology developed criteria for classification of functional status for individuals with RA that may help guide the therapist in designing and monitoring the results of an appropriate plan of care (Box 27-10).

The Ottawa Panel identified nine goals in the rehabilitation of individuals with RA, including decreasing pain, effusion (swelling), and stiffness; correcting or preventing joint deformity; increasing motion and muscle force (decreasing weakness); improving mobility and walking; increasing physical fitness; reducing fatigue; and increasing functional status.[640]

Before initiating any rehabilitation program for this group of individuals, a thorough limb and joint examination must be done to provide an objective way to assess and document disease activity and progression or, conversely, remission and improved function. Numerous resources are available to assist the clinician in carrying out a thorough clinical assessment of the individual with RA, including a helpful joint-by-joint guide (describing where and how to palpate).[592,717,755,756,791] Physical therapy examination should also include observation of activity limitations, impairments, and a systems review as outlined in the *Guide to Physical Therapist Practice*.[25]

Box 27-10

CLASSIFICATION OF GLOBAL FUNCTIONAL STATUS IN RHEUMATOID ARTHRITIS

Class I: Completely able to perform usual activities of daily living (self-care, vocational, avocational)

Class II: Able to perform usual self-care and vocational activities, but limited in avocational activities

Class III: Able to perform usual self-care activities, but limited in vocational and avocational activities

Class IV: Limited in ability to perform usual self-care,* vocational, and avocational activities

*Usual self-care activities include dressing, feeding, bathing, grooming, and toileting. Avocational (recreational and/or leisure) and vocational (work, school, homemaking) activities are patient-desired and age- and sex-specific.

From American College of Rheumatology. Available at: http://www.rheumatology.org/practice/clinical/classification/ra/raclass.asp. Accessed August 10, 2014.

Complete bed rest is rarely indicated and is saved for those with severe, uncontrolled inflammation. For many people, a rest period of up to 2 hours during the day is important for dealing with general body fatigue and protection of involved joints. Splints can be applied to rest involved joints, prevent excessive movement, and reduce mechanical stresses. Crutches, canes, or walkers can be used to reduce weight-bearing stresses and enhance balance.

Adaptations may be necessary (e.g., platform crutches) because of upper-extremity involvement. A home program of self-management will include instruction in proper body mechanics, positioning, joint protection, and energy conservation (see Box 9-4). Adaptive equipment designed to make tasks easier may include large key handle attachments allowing the person to use the whole palm to turn a key, spring-open scissors with big loops for anyone with hand involvement, jar openers and electric can openers, clip-on bottle openers, and ergonomic kitchen utensils with large handles and ergonomically angled handles.[554]

Instability at any joint, particularly at the atlantoaxial segment, requires caution on the therapist's part. Such a joint may present with a marked reduction in range of motion, such as the shoulder or neck feeling stuck or caught with a certain movement. A history of periods of significant loss of range of motion alternating with full range of motion suggests joint hypermobility. Restoration of mobility is an important goal, but choosing techniques that are gentle or applying traction while stretching is necessary.

The extraarticular problems may affect the rehabilitation program. For example, if fatigue is present, the therapist may have to allow periods of rest during the treatment session. During periods of symptom exacerbation there is a fine line between overextending the client and maximizing activity. There are times when active exercise may have to be curtailed, but passive stretching remains important to prevent contractures.

Splenomegaly may account for tenderness on palpation and fullness or increased resistance of the left upper abdominal quadrant. Deep soft-tissue techniques are contraindicated in this area. Percussion techniques may help the therapist delineate the caudal boundaries of the spleen.

Remission

The primary goal for the treatments of RA is to attain and maintain a long period of remission. Physical therapists should regularly assess a patient's functional abilities and joint mobility as assessment for the remission of the inflammatory process. The complete absence of tender or swollen joints is the most important sign of remission.[636]

An absence of joint symptoms for 2 consecutive months is needed to determine a remission, but a definitive time line has not been established. Some people with longstanding disease may achieve remission, although this is not possible for everyone. After remission, researchers hope to be able to affect a curative approach.

Postoperative Care

Surgical treatment of RA is often complicated by the client's generalized debilitated condition. People with RA tend to have poor skin condition, poorly healing wounds, and osteopenic bone. Generalized bone loss occurs early in the course of RA and correlates with disease activity.[541] This condition is further affected by the use of corticosteroids.

Poor nutritional status has been associated with higher complication rates following surgery, including infection. Following standard precautions with adequate hand washing is important. Likewise, promoting respiration with good breathing techniques is an important component of the therapist's postoperative intervention.

Anyone with RA should be taught early on that, if surgery is ever indicated, a program of isometric and range-of-motion exercises before surgery is advised. Review dislocation precautions and restrictions prior to the surgical procedure. After arthroplasty, correction of deformity and relief of pain are typical, but recurrence of deformity can occur even with appropriate rehabilitation. Many clients are still very satisfied with the improved cosmesis, reduced pain, and improved function. Maximum benefit from arthroplasty may not occur for up to 1 year after surgery.[150]

The postoperative rehabilitation regimen must be tailored to the specific needs of each individual. The surgeon's intraoperative assessment of the quality of tissues, component stability, and any associated repairs is critical to the rehabilitation protocol selected. Specific motion limitations vary depending on intraoperative repairs made, complications, and adverse events (e.g., infection, wound dehiscence, dislocation, implant fracture or failure, nerve damage).

Exercise and Rheumatoid Arthritis

Therapeutic exercises, including specific functional strengthening and whole-body functional strengthening, are a beneficial intervention for individuals with RA. The benefit may vary depending on the stage of disease (acute, subacute, inactive) but includes reduced pain, improved overall function, and decreased number of sick leaves.[403,415,641]

Whereas rest has often been the treatment of choice, a balance must be attained between rest required during acute flare-ups and activity necessary to prevent the deconditioning effects of prolonged rest, immobilization, and inactivity. Education as to the efficacy of exercise and its proper use in self-management of RA has been shown effective in reducing stiffness and improving function in as little as 4 hours of a community-based physical therapy intervention delivered over a period of 6 weeks.[73]

To date, there is no evidence that active exercise beneficially affects the inflammatory processes associated with adult RA, but it has been shown that a short-term intensive exercise program in active RA is more effective in improving muscle strength than a conservative exercise program and does not have deleterious effects on disease activity.[403,846]

Individual studies of long-term intensive exercise have not shown an increase in joint swelling or pain with such a regimen. In fact, those who exercise rigorously at least twice a week for an hour show more improvement in physical abilities, such as stair climbing, and reduced psychologic distress compared to those who received standard care.[195]

The beneficial effect of exercise in lowering cytokine levels and increasing antiinflammatory compounds in plasma has been demonstrated in children with juvenile RA.[860] Other effects of exercise on the immune system are discussed in "Exercise Immunology" in Chapter 7.

General Concepts

Exercises to prevent contractures, improve strength and flexibility, and enhance cardiorespiratory or aerobic conditioning are important components of the rehabilitation program.[342,462,622] Joint pain leads to a reflex inhibition of muscle surrounding the joints, causing disuse atrophy of these muscles. Use of corticosteroids may lead to an additional decrease in strength and function.[622]

The feet are often overlooked in people with RA, but foot involvement occurs frequently, can impair gait, and can prevent safe participation in an exercise program. Foot involvement resembles that of the hand, with one important difference being that alterations in biomechanics may cause excessive stress to proximal lower extremity joints and to the spine areas forced to compensate for the altered gait.

Careful assessment of the feet may reveal uneven or pathologic weight-bearing patterns. Gait analysis and assessment of shoe wear can provide additional significant information regarding altered biomechanics.[47] Providing assistive devices or orthotics before initiating an exercise program may be essential.[359,717,755,756]

Range-of-motion exercises should begin with low repetitions several times throughout the day. Isometric exercises with short holds (4-6 seconds) have been suggested, again using low repetitions (start with one or two and build up gradually to four to six).[414]

Range-of-motion exercises can be increased up to eight to 10 repetitions in subacute cases, with the addition of dynamic strengthening exercises. Stable, quiescent, or inactive disease makes it possible to add an aerobic component such as walking, aquatics, or biking for at least 15 minutes each day, three times a week. Range of motion and strengthening can be continued and monitored.[414]

During active exercise programs the therapist should monitor fatigue levels and should avoid overtraining. For the individual with active (acute) disease, adequate sleep is essential for controlling mood, fatigue and pain levels. Encourage 8 to 10 hours of rest each night.[410,842]

Exercise Prescription

A helpful guide in establishing the level of acceptable exercise intensity is as follows: acute pain during exercise indicates a need to modify the program; if joint pain persists for more than 1 hour after exercise is completed, the exercise was probably excessive.[284]

Engaging in moderate-level exercise for 30 minutes per day 4 or 5 days per week appears to substantially increase physical fitness, even for older adults.[804] Exercise spaced out over the course of the day can help loosen up stiff, achy joints while still providing cardiovascular benefits.[588]

The Arthritis Foundation website describes the benefits and types of exercises, how to start, and how to keep going. This website educates people about the possible effects of not exercising (e.g., increased joint stiffness, muscle weakness, muscle atrophy, increased risk of fracture and deformity). The foundation also provides valuable exercise tips for before, during, and after exercise.[37]

Currently the National Arthritis Foundation offers the largest standardized exercise program to individuals with arthritis through two community-based programs: an on-land exercise program called Arthritis Foundation Exercise Program (AFEP)[37] and an aquatic exercise program called the Arthritis Foundation Aquatic Program (AFAP).[36] The AFEP program is led by a certified instructor using a variety exercises to improve motion, strength, endurance, balance, coordination, posture, and body mechanics. Other recommendations and guidelines for including conditioning exercise in a comprehensive management program for RA are available.[24,36,590]

Strength Training

Dynamic strengthening (gradually increasing resistance) through the full available range of motion helps stabilize joints, reducing erosive wear and tear on the structures. Regular, dynamic strength training combined with endurance-type physical activities improves muscle strength and physical function, but not bone mineral density, in adults with early and longstanding RA, without causing detrimental effects on disease activity.[49,327,328]

Low-load resistive muscle training has been shown to increase functional capacity and is a clinically safe form of exercise in mild to moderate RA.[462] Other studies report that moderate- or high-intensity strength training programs have better training effects on muscle strength in RA. It is essential to maintain the training routine to obtain long-term benefits.[326]

Strengthening in some cases of RA can be difficult, because exercise may lead to increased joint swelling and subsequent joint destruction, persons with RA may be hesitant to participate in a regular exercise program.[863] Before initiating a strengthening program, the physical therapist must be sure that pain is controlled, range of motion is optimized, and contractures are minimized.[622] Paying attention to biomechanics, deformities, and muscle imbalances is important. Exercising misaligned joints without properly distributing the load can place too much pressure on vulnerable joints.[745]

Aerobic Exercise

Aerobic exercise in this population is necessary to help reduce weight and improve cardiovascular fitness without increasing pain.[568,728] Aerobic exercises are safe to perform during the subacute and inactive stages of RA. Aerobic capacity can be estimated using a single-stage submaximal treadmill test.[589] Training programs begin at 50% (and work toward 80%) of maximal oxygen uptake based on the baseline test results. Without baseline testing, the therapist can rely upon (and teach the client to use) the Borg scale for rate of perceived exertion (see Table 12-13). Heart rate monitors are also helpful in enabling clients to track their cardiovascular responses.[414]

Screening for unknown coronary artery disease is recommended before initiating resistance or aerobic exercise. RA can also affect the bony structures of the rib cage and cause a decrease in chest expansion. The usual precautions for cardiopulmonary screening still apply based on the individual's age, risk factors, and health history (especially heart health history).

People with RA may have normal pulmonary function tests but reduced respiratory muscle strength and endurance with reduced aerobic capacity compared to adults without RA.[175] Assessment of respiration and intervention to improve breathing patterns are important components of the rehabilitation program.

Aquatic Therapy

Aquatic therapy may be beneficial for conditioning, strengthening, and flexibility while reducing mechanical stress on the joints. Water exercise provides the means by which people with RA can reach needed training levels in a comfortable environment. The AFAP program consists of 72 exercises similar to the PACE (personalized aerobics for cardiovascular enhancement) program that can be done in water with decreased joint loading, a reduced effect of gravity, increased buoyancy, and increased circulation.[36]

Modalities and Rheumatoid Arthritis

Various modalities provide temporary pain relief and may be used in effectively and safely controlling symptoms of the acute inflammatory phase of RA. Information on the rationale for use and effectiveness of the various physical modalities is available.[126,578,591]

Although cold may be more suitable in acute inflammation, people with RA usually prefer heat. Superficial heat (e.g., paraffin baths, moist hot packs, hydrotherapy or aquatic therapy) is recommended for palliative treatments of acute flare-ups. Caution must be used with prolonged or deep heat because it may increase intraarticular temperature, leading to increased collagenase activity, possibly contributing to joint destruction.[701]

Electrotherapeutic modalities and thermotherapy physical agents are often used as part of a rehabilitation program mainly for pain relief, to control inflammation, and to reduce joint stiffness.

The Ottawa Panel recommends the use of low-level laser therapy, therapeutic ultrasound, thermotherapy, electrical stimulation, and transcutaneous electrical nerve stimulation for the management of RA.[640] This recommendation is based on the analysis of systematic and literature reviews. Specifics of studies reviewed and a summary of the findings have been published.[111,402]

Box 27-11

SUBCATEGORIES OF JUVENILE IDIOPATHIC ARTHRITIS (JIA)

- Pauciarticular JIA (PaJIA; oligoarthritis)
- Polyarthritis JIA (PoJIA RF+)
- Polyarthritis JIA (PoJIA RF−)
- Systemic-onset JIA (SoJIA)
- Psoriatic JIA
- Enthesitis-related arthritis
- Other (undefined)

RF+, Rheumatoid factor positive; RF−, rheumatoid factor negative.
Data from Petty RE: ILAR classification of JIA: second revision, Edmonton 2001, *J Rheumatol* 31(2):390, 2004.

Medications

Because of the long-term nature of RA, intervention is usually an ongoing process. Aspirin and NSAIDs are potentially ulcerogenic, and prolonged use of corticosteroids can lead to osteoporosis.

The analgesics and slow-acting antirheumatic drugs, such as gold and penicillamine, can impair renal function. Periodic screening of each of the body systems is imperative when working with this population; anyone taking DMARDs but still having joint pain and swelling should be reevaluated by the rheumatologist.

Numerous other side effects can occur with any of the pharmacologic agents used in the management of RA. The therapist should be aware of the potential side effects with any of the medications each client is taking.

For the individual with Felty syndrome (RA in combination with low white blood cell count or leukopenia and an enlarged spleen), there is an increased risk of infection, even when treatment with DMARDs raises the white blood count. Careful hand washing and standard precautions are always warranted, but especially in the case of this syndrome.

Juvenile Idiopathic Arthritis

Overview and Incidence. Although the term *juvenile idiopathic arthritis* (JIA; formerly juvenile RA) brings to mind a single disease similar to adult RA, it is actually an umbrella term for a heterogeneous group of arthritides (Box 27-11) of unknown cause that begin before 16 years of age and occur in all races. Each subtype has a different presentation, genetic background, and prognosis.[94,308,686]

Many other forms of arthritis (e.g., SLE, dermatomyositis, scleroderma) that affect adults occur less frequently in children. Approximately 30,000 to 50,000 children in the United States are affected by one of the subtypes discussed here (Fig. 27-18). The general classification of JIA is based on the number of involved joints and the presence of systemic signs and symptoms.[308]

Pauciarticular JIA (also known as oligoarthritis or oligoarticular JIA), meaning "few joints," generally affects four or fewer joints during the first 6 months of disease, usually in an asymmetric pattern, and most commonly involves the knees, elbows, wrists, and ankles. Girls are

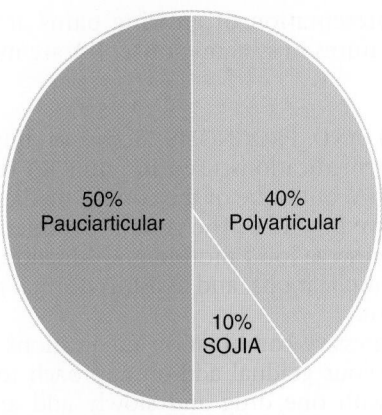

Figure 27-18

Breakdown in types of juvenile idiopathic arthritis.

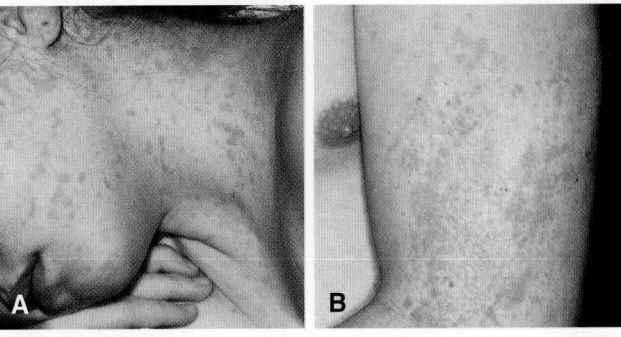

Figure 27-19

A and **B**, Skin rash associated with juvenile idiopathic arthritis. (A, from Paller AS, Mancini AJ: *Hurwitz clinical pediatric dermatology: a textbook of skin disorders of childhood adolescence*, ed 3, Philadelphia, 2006, WB Saunders. B, from James WD, Berger T, Elston D: *Andrews' diseases of the skin: clinical dermatology*, ed 10, Philadelphia, 2006, WB Saunders.)

affected more often than boys and usually between the ages of 1 and 5 years. This type of JIA is relatively mild with few extraarticular features. Parents may notice a swollen joint and limp or abnormal gait, usually early after the child wakes up in the morning. Leg-length discrepancy is common. Pain is not a central feature at first, and the disease rarely manifests any constitutional symptoms.[597]

Pauciarticular JIA is the most common type of JIA, comprising half of all JIA cases; it has three subtypes. The first is characterized by the presence of antinuclear antibodies and a high risk of uveitis, a potentially dangerous inflammation of the eye resulting in irreversible damage and blindness. The second subtype affects the spine as well as other joints, although spinal involvement may not occur until the child reaches late adolescence. Children with this subtype may test positive for the HLA-B27 gene (see Table 40-21), which is common in adults with AS (this subtype is sometimes referred to as juvenile AS). In the third subtype, joint involvement is the extent of the disease. Usually pauciarticular JIA runs a benign course; recurrences occur in up to 20% of children, most often during the first year but possibly delayed by as much as 5 years after the initial diagnosis. There are some children who develop persistent joint disease, referred to as extended oligoarthritis.[597]

Polyarticular JIA affects five or more joints, most commonly including the large and small joints (wrists, cervical spine, temporomandibular joint, small joints of the hands and feet, as well as the knees, ankles, and hips). Joint involvement is usually symmetric and is most like that of adult RA, with the potential for severe, destructive arthropathy.

Polyarticular JIA comprises 40% of all cases of JIA and affects girls more often than boys. There are two subtypes depending on whether children are rheumatoid factor positive or negative. The rheumatoid factor–positive subtype is characterized by the presence of rheumatoid factor (a type of autoantibody found in the blood of adults with RA) and the *DR4* genetic type, also common in adults with RA. Subcutaneous nodules, cervical spine fusion, chronic uveitis, and destructive hip disease can occur in this type of polyarticular JIA.[597]

The second subtype is characterized only by joint involvement, usually less severe. Children with this subtype

do not test positive for rheumatoid factor.[217] Morning stiffness and fatigue with possible low-grade fever are common clinical manifestations of this type of JIA.

Systemic-onset JIA (also called Still disease; sometimes also affecting adults, although rare) affects boys and girls equally with involvement of any number of joints. This subtype has the most severe extraarticular manifestations, affecting many body systems, and comprises 10% of all cases of JIA.

It often begins with a high-spiking fever and chills that appear intermittently for weeks and may be accompanied by a rash on the thighs and chest that often goes away within a few hours (Fig. 27-19). The fever pattern is marked by spikes exceeding 39° C (102° F) and periods between the spikes during which the child feels much better.

Inflammatory arthritis typically develops at some point, and 95% of the children have joint complaints within 1 year of the initial presenting symptoms. Approximately half of the children who have systemic-onset JIA recover almost entirely; unfortunately, one-third of the children remain ill, with persistent inflammation manifesting as fever, rash, and chronic destructive arthritis.[597]

In addition to inflamed joints, the child may experience enlargement of the spleen (hepatosplenomegaly) and lymph nodes (lymphadenopathy); inflammation of the liver, heart, and surrounding tissues; and anemia.[90] Box 27-12 lists clinical manifestations associated with Still disease.

Psoriatic JIA is more common in girls, presents with psoriasis, arthritis, and at least two of the following: dactylitis, nail abnormalities, and a family history of psoriasis. Diagnosis may be delayed because joint symptoms precede skin manifestations by years. Treatment with aggressive immunosuppressives may be required; uveitis is a feature in some cases.

Enthesitis-related arthritis presents as inflammation of the tendon attachments to the bone, especially along the spine and Achilles tendon, along with arthritis and any two of the following: sacroiliac joint tenderness, inflammatory spinal pain, the presence of HLA-B27, positive family history, acute uveitis, and pauciarticular or polyarticular arthritis in boys older than 8 years.

Box 27-12

CLINICAL MANIFESTATIONS ASSOCIATED WITH STILL DISEASE

Systemic

- Fever
- Rash
- Lymphadenopathy
- Polyarthritis
- Pericarditis
- Pleuritis
- Peptic ulcer disease
- Hepatitis
- Anemia
- Anorexia
- Weight loss

Musculoskeletal

- Polyarthritis, polyarthralgias
- Myalgia, myositis
- Tenosynovitis
- Skeletal growth disturbances (short stature, failure to thrive)

Data from Bagnari V, Colina M, Ciancio G, Govoni M, Trotta F. Adult-onset Still's disease. *Rheumatol Int* 30(7):855–862, 2010.

Etiologic and Risk Factors and Pathogenesis. The cause is still poorly understood, but JIA may be triggered by environmental factors and infection (viral or bacterial) in children with a genetic predisposition. Genomic studies hope to identify genetic traits that will predict disease risk and other characteristics such as disease course, age of onset, and disease severity. Eventually, researchers may be able to identify molecular biomarkers to help diagnose and treat this group of arthritides.[308,661]

JIA can occur in boys or girls of any age (girls more often than boys) and most commonly begins during the toddler or early adolescent period. The pathogenesis is similar to that of adult RA, with immune cells mistakenly attacking the joints and organs, causing inflammation, destruction, fatigue, and other local and systemic effects.

TNF and the interleukins (IL-1 and IL-6) seem to be the primary cytokines responsible for many systemic features. These cytokines increase collagenase activity, osteoclast activation, body temperature, and muscle and fat breakdown, as well as acute-phase reactants.

MEDICAL MANAGEMENT

DIAGNOSIS. Early disease recognition is needed to help improve the clinical outcome, but symptoms of rheumatic disease are often mistaken for "growing pains," delaying diagnosis by many months. Diagnosis involves a medical history, physical examination, and laboratory tests, including serum evaluation to measure inflammation and to detect antinuclear antibodies, rheumatoid factor, or sometimes HLA-B27.[378]

For a diagnosis of JIA, objective arthritis must be seen in one or more joints for at least 6 weeks in children younger than 16 years; it may take up to 6 months to determine which subtype is present. Pain is often dull and aching and less severe, but presents in the morning and early during the day rather than the more common presentation of growing pains at night. The systemic features in systemic-onset JIA are more readily diagnosed.

TREATMENT AND PROGNOSIS. Some of the immuno-modulatory medications used in adult RA can be used in cases of JIA, but none of the current medications used has a curative potential. The goal of treatment is to control pain, preserve joint motion and function, minimize systemic complications, and assist in normal growth and development.

Early aggressive combination medications are replacing the previous gradual add-on approach to treatment (i.e., start with one drug and slowly add another and another to gain the desired effects without too many side effects).[877] Medications are administered to control the systemic and articular complaints and, in some cases, halt the progression of the disease.

These agents may include immunosuppressives, DMARDs (e.g., MTX), and biologic agents such as TNF inhibitors (etanercept [Enbrel], infliximab [Remicade]).[308,320] MTX is the most common medication for the person with JIA. The medication is administered either orally or with subcutaneous injections and may need 6 to 12 months for full therapeutic effect to be maintained.[308]

Adverse effects from taking anti-TNF agents (e.g., neurologic disorders, weight gain, severe infection, hemorrhagic diarrhea) have been reported and should be monitored for carefully. In systemic JIA, approximately 50% respond to anti-TNF agents, but in many children, the response is not sustained.[275] Corticosteroids are indicated if severe anemia, unrelenting fever, or vasculitis is present. Bone marrow transplantation may be used in cases of JIA that are resistant to standard medical management.[802]

The prognosis has greatly improved as a result of substantial progress in disease management, especially the use of anticytokine agents in children who are resistant to conventional antirheumatic agents. Early-onset, progressive forms of JIA have a guarded prognosis. Between 25% and 70% of children with JIA will still have active arthritis 10 years after disease onset; more than 40% enter adulthood with active arthritis.[510]

The mortality risk for children with JIA is estimated to be three to five times higher than in the general population.[820] Morbidity and mortality may be improved (including increased rates of disease remission) with the changes in treatment approaches, but this has not yet been documented.[510]

Autologous stem cell transplantation is used for some individuals whose disease is refractory to MTX and other DMARDs. Complete remission is possible for up to half of the individuals receiving autologous stem cell transplantation, with improvement reported in those individuals who are not resistant. Infection is a common morbidity associated with this treatment, observed in up to 71% of cases, in addition to an associated death rate of 15%.[196]

As the immune mechanisms and inflammatory processes are better understood, new drugs able to inhibit single molecules or pathways will be developed.[686] Investigations continue to study biologic therapies that block IL-1 and IL-6 in systemic JIA.[510]

Juvenile Idiopathic Arthritis

Children with JIA may have no disability, especially if they have the oligoarticular form of the disease. Severe disability is seen most often in cases of rheumatoid factor–positive polyarticular and systemic disease, followed by rheumatoid factor–negative polyarthritis, enthesitis-related arthritis, and psoriatic arthritis. Physical therapy is an important adjunctive therapy for JIA.[94,308]

Efforts have been made to identify early predictive clinical, laboratory, demographic, genetic, or treatment-related factors for functional disability. It appears that there are complex interactions between disease subtypes but with specific predictors of outcome for each disease subtype. More study is needed to completely define predictive factors.

Physical therapy and occupational therapy are utilized for pain control, facilitation of mobility, and function. Equally important is the role of exercise in improving strength, endurance, and aerobic capacity.[316,770] In children with JIA, resistive exercise produces a change in the immune response, with significantly lower levels of cytokines and higher levels of antiinflammatory compounds compared with those who did not exercise.[860]

With respect to joint impairment, loss of joint motion is the strongest indicator of functional disability in children with systemic JIA, and loss of joint motion has a greater effect on lower limb function than on upper limb function.[72] By the time children become adults, only 20% of them have moderate to severe limitations.

The role of the therapist in preventing joint loss should not be underestimated. Cervical spine involvement can occur in polyarthritis JIA and systemic JIA, with cervical stiffness as the most common finding. Neck pain is uncommon, and neurologic complications are less likely to develop in JIA than in adult RA.

The therapist should keep in mind the significant impact JIA has on the children and their families. The cost of this disease can be staggering, with pharmacotherapy, hospitalizations, medical visits, and other professional services, including physical and occupational therapy.

Psychosocial-spiritual and quality-of-life issues should also be addressed.[308] Appearance and body image are affected directly by JIA (e.g., generalized growth failure, local growth anomalies such as micrognathia), side effects of drug therapy, surgical scars, and severity of pain and fatigue. The therapist may be the first to recognize overall problems with adjustment, as reflected by anxiety, depression, and/or social withdrawal.[94]

For those children with JIA who reach adulthood, significant problems can result from arthritis and uveitis, medication morbidity, and lifelong disability.[586] Young women may face the issue of pregnancy and childbirth with fears of transmitting JIA to the offspring, and possible reduced ability to conceive along with increased rates of miscarriages have been reported by some.[638]

If the therapist is seeing a young child with joint pain who has not been diagnosed, sensitivity to soft tissue manipulation despite improved or restored joint range of motion warrants further medical investigation. For children with a known diagnosis, the use of physical modalities may be appropriate but must be used with caution as children are not always able to perceive and/or report discomfort.

Exercise and Juvenile Idiopathic Arthritis

Very few studies have been done to determine the safety and efficacy of exercise for children with JIA. A study with nine children suggested that bicycle and treadmill exercise is safe and feasible for children who do not have severe hip disease.[433] Aquatic physical therapy is an excellent way to complete exercises while providing joint protection and engaging the child in a fun activity. One study engaged 54 children with JIA, ages 5 to 13 years, in a supervised aquatic training program 1 hour per week for 20 weeks. Measures of functional ability, health-related quality of life, joint status, and physical fitness showed no improvement, but there were also no signs of worse health status, suggesting that swimming is a safe exercise program.[807] More studies are needed to determine at what frequency, level, intensity, and duration a swimming training program would make a significant difference (improvement) in the areas tested and measured.

Strengthening programs for children with rheumatic disease can be part of the exercise program, even for children younger than 6 years of age. Twice-daily sessions of 15 to 20 minutes are advised.[697] A strengthening program using jump roping and lower extremity weightbearing exercises has been shown to be well tolerated and resulted in improved muscle strength in a study of children and adolescents with JIA.[721a]

Active exercise is not advised during flare-ups when joints are inflamed, but most children usually self-limit their physical activity according to symptoms. Passive stretching and modified aquatic physical therapy are better choices during exacerbations. Parents and children should be educated on the importance of avoiding forced or deep flexion of inflamed joints. Some activities may need to be modified or avoided.

Children with quiescent JIA can participate in some sports activities. With improved medical therapies, children with JIA are able to lead a more active lifestyle than similar children were able to do even 10 years ago.[489] The therapist can be helpful in assessing each child for abnormal biomechanics that can place the child at increased risk for injury or future articular damage. Neuromuscular training may be needed to improve neuromuscular function and biomechanics. Proper technical performance during athletics may allow children with JIA to use joint-loading techniques (e.g., during jumping and landing) in a safe and controlled manner.[610]

Low bone mineral density is a common secondary condition associated with JIA. Weight-bearing exercise programs to reduce the risk of low bone mineral density are safe and effective for children with JIA who are healthy and should be included in the plan of care.

More research is needed to determine the amount, duration, and frequency of weight-bearing activity needed to reduce the risk for low bone mineral density in this population.[271]

The role of physical activity and an active lifestyle in cardiorespiratory fitness has been documented, but long-term follow-up is still needed to show if such a program protects from loss of aerobic fitness in this population group.[808] The 6-minute walk test has been shown to be a good test for measuring functional exercise capacity in a small study of children (boys and girls) with JIA ages 7 to 17 years.[643] This might be a good place to begin baseline studies and evaluate response to the aerobic component of the plan of care for individuals with JIA.

Spondyloarthropathies

Spondyloarthropathies (SpAs), a group of disorders formerly considered variants of RA, are in fact distinct entities with similar features affecting the spine (Box 27-13). SpAs are characterized by inflammation of the joints of the spine and include several distinct entities: AS, Sjögren syndrome, psoriatic arthritis, and reactive arthritis, including arthritides that accompany inflammatory bowel disease (known as enteric arthritides), and Reiter syndrome. Inflammatory eye disease (e.g., uveitis, conjunctivitis, iritis) occurs in approximately 25% of clients.

Enteropathic arthritis (arthritis associated with inflammatory bowel disease) occurs in approximately 20% of clients who have inflammatory bowel disease (e.g., Crohn disease, ulcerative colitis) and is discussed further in Chapter 16. Arthritic symptoms flare with inflammatory bowel disease and usually affect the lower extremities in an asymmetric pattern. Vasculitis, clubbing of the fingers, and skin changes may be present.

New biomarkers for SpAs have been reported. Changes in synovial tissue may be good biomarkers to assess the effectiveness of treatment. Specific changes in the cells of the synovial tissue correspond to treatment with TNF blockers. Biopsy specimens of synovial tissue taken after treatment, showing changes in synovial macrophages,

polymorphonuclear leukocyte levels, and expression of matrix metalloproteinase-3, which are thought to play a role in the degradation of collagen, may lead scientists to use these same biomarkers for early identification and treatment of RA.[470]

Ankylosing Spondylitis

Overview and Incidence. AS, sometimes referred to as Marie-Strümpell disease, is an inflammatory arthropathy of the axial skeleton, including the sacroiliac joints, apophyseal joints, costovertebral joints, and intervertebral disk articulations.

Approximately one-third of those with AS have asymmetric involvement of the large peripheral joints, including the hip, knee, and shoulder. Figure 27-20 shows the most commonly involved joints. The disorder can ultimately lead to fibrosis, calcification, and ossification with fusion of the involved joints. The pain, resultant postural deformities, and complications associated with this disease can be disabling.

Prevalence of AS is 0.1% to 0.2% in the U.S. general population. Nearly 2 million people in the United States have this condition, making it almost as common as RA. It is higher in whites and some Native Americans than in African Americans, Asians, or other nonwhite groups.[7]

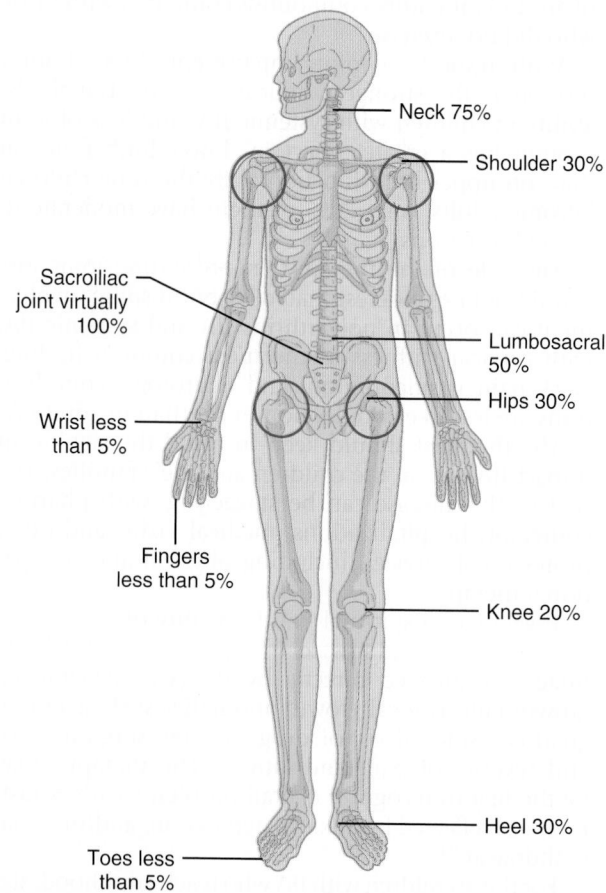

Figure 27-20

Joints most commonly involved in ankylosing spondylitis and incidence of involvement. Not shown: jaw 15%, eye 20%, ribs 20%, and costovertebral junction 70%. (From Ramanujan T, Schumacher HR: Ankylosing spondylitis: early recognition and management, *J Musculoskelet Med* 1[1]:75–91, 1992.)

AS typically affects young people, beginning between the ages of 15 and 30 years (rarely after age 40 years). This differs from back pain of mechanical origin, which is much more likely to develop between 30 and 65 years of age. Men are affected two to three times more often than women, although this disorder may be just as prevalent in women but diagnosed less often because of a milder disease course with fewer spinal problems and more involvement of joints such as the knees and ankles.[849,900] Overall sibling risk is approximately 5.9%.[494]

Etiologic and Risk Factors. Although the molecular basis of AS remains unclear, evidence points to a genetic or environmental link. Approximately 90% of those with AS are HLA-B27–positive, but of all of the people with this antigen only 1% to 2% develop AS. However, in individuals with inflammatory back pain and the HLA-B27 gene, the risk of AS increases to 59%.[333,540]

Proof that this disorder is an autoimmune disease attributable to cross-reactivity between bacteria and HLA-B27 is still lacking.[408] However, approximately 20% of people who develop AS have a first-degree relative who is HLA-B27–positive.

Gender, age, race, and family history are all important factors related to the risk of developing AS. Although it is more prevalent in males, there is significantly less disparity in incidence between the genders than was once thought. The belief is that the disorder has been grossly underdiagnosed in women because the disease tends to be milder and peripheral joint involvement is more common, confusing the clinical picture.

No direct linkage of the X chromosome with susceptibility to AS has been found, but the influence of female gender is greater than that of male gender in determining increased susceptibility to AS in children. The striking maternal effect is greatest for women with young age at onset, which is not seen in men.[124] It has been hypothesized that women tend to have a milder form of AS because they have the susceptibility genes, which they pass on to their children, whereas men have the severity genes.[110]

Studies under way using the results of the Human Genome Project are searching for other genes that, in combination with HLA-B27, constitute risk for AS. The results of the first genome scan show areas where there appear to be some other genes that have been implicated in Crohn disease and psoriasis, suggesting a shared genetic basis in these conditions. The identification of new genes responsible for AS will alter the current view of AS pathogenesis with earlier diagnosis and intervention.[333]

Other researchers have demonstrated that environmental factors, such as infectious microbes, are essential for the development of AS, in particular, normal bacteria in the bowel.[33,405,494]

Pathogenesis. The pathogenesis of AS is poorly understood, but the fundamental lesion appears to be chronic inflammation at sites of attachment of cartilage, tendons, ligaments, and synovium to the bone.[672] AS is marked by a chronic nongranulomatous inflammation at the area where the ligaments attach to the vertebrae (an area called the enthesis), initially in the lumbar spine and then in the sacroiliac joint.

Disruption of this ligamentous–osseous junction results, and reactive bone formation occurs as part of the repair process. Cartilage of the sacroiliac joints may also be involved (Fig. 27-21). The replacement of inflamed cartilaginous structures by bone contributes to progressive ossification with bony growth between the vertebrae, leading to a fused, rigid, or bamboo spine, characteristic of end-stage disease (see Fig. 27-22).

Clinical Manifestations. Insidious onset of low back, buttock, or hip pain and stiffness lasting for at least 3 months are often the initial presenting complaints. Early onset of back pain, stiffness, and fatigue during childhood often goes unrecognized for what it is. Onset of symptoms leading to a diagnosis occurs most often during early adulthood.[672]

At first the pain is described as a dull ache that is poorly localized, but it can be intermittently sharp. Over time, pain can become severe and constant, increased by prolonged rest or immobility and decreased by active movement. Coughing, sneezing, and twisting may worsen the pain.[494]

Pain may radiate to the thighs but does not usually go below the knee.[7] Buttock pain is often unilateral but may alternate from side to side. Significant morning stiffness, lasting more than 1 hour, is often present. There may be tenderness over the spinous processes and sacroiliac areas with associated paraspinal spasms.

Enthesitis (inflammation of the tendons, ligaments, and capsular attachments to bone) may produce tenderness, pain and/or stiffness, and restricted mobility in the costosternal, costovertebral, and manubriosternal joints, iliac crest, ischial tuberosities, greater trochanters, spinous processes, or ligamentous attachments at the calcaneus.

Other clinical features include early loss of normal lumbar lordosis with accompanying increased kyphosis of the thoracic spine, painful limitation of cervical joint motion, and loss of spine mobility (flexibility) in all planes of motion.

In some cases the initial complaints may occur in the extremities (e.g., hips or knees), with back symptoms appearing on average 3 years after onset of the peripheral involvement. Shoulder symptoms and loss of shoulder mobility are common but are rarely disabling. Involvement of the shoulder joint in AS correlates with involvement of other peripheral joints as well as the extent of radiographic change on shoulder films.[893]

Hip flexion contractures are often present bilaterally and can be assessed using the Thomas test (in the supine position, ask the individual to maximally flex the contralateral hip joint; observe for loss of lumbar lordosis and flexion of the opposite leg, signaling a positive Thomas test result for the presence of a hip flexion contracture; repeat on the other side). Loss of hip mobility can result in reduced functional ability.

Loss of chest wall excursion is an indicator of decreased axial skeleton mobility because of involvement of the thoracic spine and the costovertebral and costosternal joints. If the ligaments that attach the ribs to the spine (costovertebral junction) become ossified, the chest may be unable to expand, compromising breathing. Circumferential measurements taken at the fourth intercostal space (or just below the breasts in women) before and at

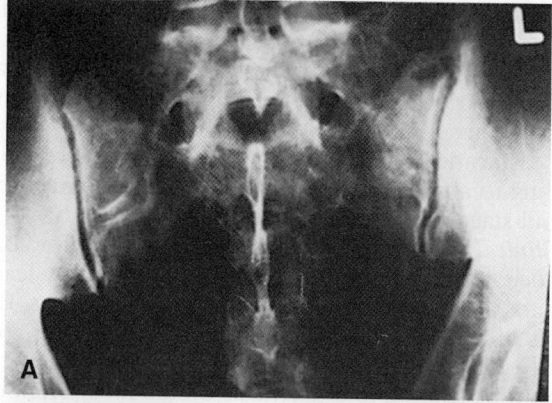

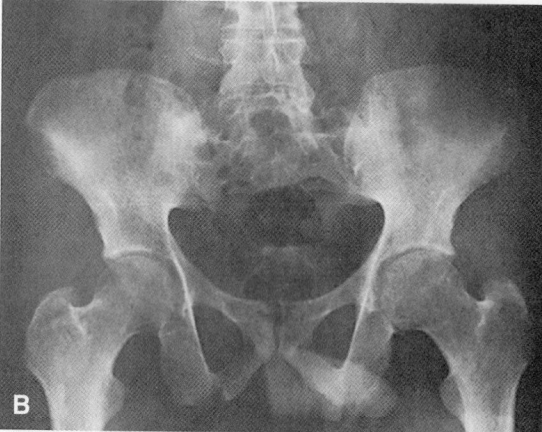

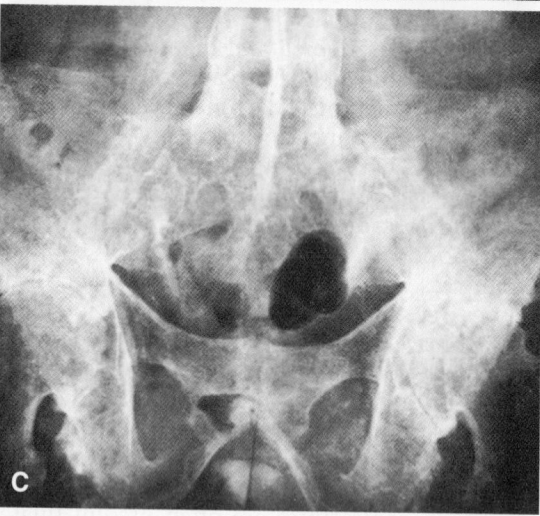

Figure 27-21

Progression of ankylosing spondylitis of the sacroiliac joints. A, Normal sacroiliac joints. **B,** Fusion of sacroiliac joint spaces; the sclerosis has resorbed, and there is slight narrowing of the left hip joint. **C,** Advanced ankylosing spondylitis with generalized osteoporosis and fusion of the spinous process, intervertebral disks, sacroiliac joints, and symphysis pubis. The entire skeletal unit has been transformed into one continuous osseous mass. (A, from Magee D: *Orthopedic physical assessment*, ed 2, Philadelphia, 1992, WB Saunders, p. 329. B, from Rothman RH, Simeone FA: *The spine*, Philadelphia, 1982, WB Saunders, p. 921. C, from Bullough PG: *Orthopaedic pathology*, ed 3, London, 1997, Mosby-Wolfe, p. 300.)

the end of inspiration should reveal an excursion of 4 to 5 cm. Excursion less than 4 cm, and especially anything less than 2.5 cm, is a suspicious finding.

Complications. Longstanding disease is associated with multiple complications. Skeletal complications

include osteoporosis, fracture, atlantoaxial subluxation, and spinal stenosis. In the most severe cases, the spine becomes so completely fused that the person may become locked in a rigid upright or stooped position, unable to move the neck or back in any direction. Flexion contractures, rigid gait, and flexing at the knees in order to maintain an upright position are not uncommon findings.

The stiff and osteoporotic spinal column is prone to fracture from even a minor insult; a significant proportion of individuals with AS experience vertebral fracture during the course of the disease.[850] Fracture sites range from T7 to S1.[187,238] In fact, the incidence of thoracolumbar fractures in AS is four times higher than in the general population.[182,375,888]

Fractures can also occur in the cervical spine from the effect of osteoporosis, spinal stiffness and cervical kyphotic deformity. These fractures result is significant loss of functional mobility and may be unstable enough to result in neurologic changes in the spinal cord and cervical nerve roots. These fractures may result in surgical fixations and correction of the kyphotic deformity.[732]

The atlantoaxial segment is among the last areas of the axial skeleton to fuse. Because of the inherent mobility of C1 and C2 and the immobility of the remainder of the cervical spine secondary to the disease, attempts to move the head could result in subluxation. Spinal stenosis can result from the proliferation of bony tissue from the spinal ligaments and facet joints. Stenosis may cause neurogenic claudication and cauda equina syndrome.

AS is a systemic disease with widespread effects. In addition to arthritis in the spine, arthritis in other joints may be accompanied by inflammatory bowel syndrome with fever, fatigue, loss of appetite, weight loss, and other extraarticular complications. These clinical features distinguish AS from mechanical pain.

The most common extraarticular manifestation is uveitis, occurring in 20% to 30% of affected individuals. Cardiomegaly, pericarditis, aortic regurgitation or insufficiency, amyloidosis (rare), and pulmonary complications may also occur. Pulmonary problems include upper lobe fibrosis and decreased total lung capacity and vital capacity (late stages of AS).[543]

MEDICAL MANAGEMENT

DIAGNOSIS. AS is not easily detectable in the early stages without an MRI and only then with specialized MRIs, which are not routinely ordered. Early, accurate diagnosis allows treatment to start before the onset of permanent rigidity and deformity.

Intraarticular inflammation, early cartilage changes, and underlying bone marrow edema and otitis can be seen with a specific MRI technique called short tau inversion recovery sequences.[672] Diagnosis is usually based on identification of the clinical manifestations and radiographic findings.[7] History, physical examination, radiography, and laboratory tests are all used in the diagnosis.

In the physical examination, range-of-motion tests provide important information. The Schober test, chest expansion (measured at the fourth intercostal space or

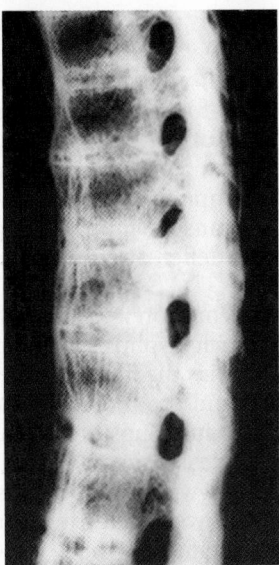

Figure 27-22

Radiograph of a sagittal vertebral column in a person with ankylosing spondylitis. There is complete fusion of the spine, accentuated kyphosis, and loss of lumbar and cervical lordosis. There is also complete fusion of the intervertebral disk spaces. (From Bullough PG: *Orthopaedic pathology,* ed 3, London, 1997, Mosby-Wolfe, p. 301.)

just below the breasts in women on inspiration after forced maximal expiration), and military stand against the wall are the clinical tests used most often. A distance of less than 15 cm for the Schober test and less than 2.5 cm for chest expansion on inspiration are suspicious findings.

Clinical manifestations alone are not diagnostic, but when taken along with the history and radiographic results, they become significant for the diagnosis. Radiographs may be negative in the early stages of the disease (for up to 10 years); MRI enables the examiner to identify sacroiliitis earlier than plain radiography.

Radiographic findings of symmetric, bilateral sacroiliitis include blurring of joint margins, juxtaarticular sclerosis, erosions, and joint space narrowing. The replacement of ligamentous tissue by bone at the site where the annulus fibrosus of the intervertebral disk inserts into the vertebral body results in a characteristic square-shaped vertebral body. In addition, as bony tissue bridges the vertebral bodies and posterior arches, the thoracic and lumbar spine takes on the appearance of a bamboo spine on radiographs (Fig. 27-22).

No laboratory test is diagnostic of AS; laboratory tests assist primarily by ruling out other diseases. The presence of the HLA-B27 antigen is a useful adjunct to the diagnosis but is not diagnostic itself, as so many people with other causes of back pain also are HLA-B27–positive. ESR and C-reactive protein are elevated in 75% of affected individuals and may correlate with disease activity in some people, but these levels can be normal even in individuals with active disease.[672,757]

There are several classification schemes used in the diagnosis of AS. Calin's criteria for classification of inflammatory back pain lists age at onset younger than 40 years, back pain for more than 3 months, insidious onset, morning stiffness, and improvement with exercise

as diagnostic.[123] Rudwaleit and colleagues suggest morning stiffness lasting more than 30 minutes, improvement of back pain with exercise but not with rest, awakening with back pain during the second half of the night, and alternating buttock pain.[710]

The New York Criteria for classification of AS and the modified New York Criteria add decreased chest expansion and radiographic findings to their classification schemes. Armor's criteria for classification of SpA as a broader diagnostic scheme assigns 1 to 3 points to each of more than a dozen criteria. If the criteria points add up to at least 6, the person will be considered to have spondyloarthritis.[32] And finally, the European Spondyloarthropathy Study group criteria for the classification of SpA lists inflammatory back pain or synovitis in the lower extremities accompanied by at least one of seven key features including history, pain patterns, and accompanying systemic symptoms such as uveitis, psoriasis, ulcerative colitis, urethritis, and so on (again, this is a broader diagnostic scheme for arthropathies including but not exclusive to AS).

TREATMENT. The primary focus of intervention is to maximize health-related quality of life through the control of inflammation and stiffness in the joints, maintaining mobility and proper postural alignment of the spine to prevent structural damage, while providing pain relief.[100] Effective education is essential, because much of the management requires lifestyle adjustments and cooperation, especially compliance with the exercise program.[494]

Joint involvement can be managed with NSAIDs (including COX-2–specific inhibitors), but in some cases DMARDs, such as MTX or sulfasalazine, may be used for peripheral disease.[100]

Persistent symptoms of spinal involvement, peripheral arthritis, or enthesitis unresponsive to NSAIDs or DMARDs can be managed with biologic agents such as TNF-α antagonists (e.g., etanercept, infliximab, adalimumab). These agents are effective in preventing the progression of disease by reducing disease activity, decreasing inflammation, and improving spinal mobility.[7,101]

Other targeted therapies may be needed to treat specific organ involvement, such as eye inflammation. To avoid long-term complications associated with severe postural deformities, a lifetime commitment to exercise is important.

Surgery has a limited role in the management of AS and is most appropriate for individuals with a severe deformity that impedes vision, walking, eating, abdominal expansion, or respiratory function. Spondylodiskitis or spinal fracture may require surgical intervention.[96] Spinal fusion may be needed but is not routinely recommended. The most valuable surgical intervention is total joint arthroplasty, especially a total hip replacement.[494] It is expected that with the new biologic therapies, the need for surgical intervention will become a rare event.[96]

PROGNOSIS. The extent of disability in persons with AS varies considerably, but fewer than 1% experience complete remission and more than 80% who are ill for longer than 20 years still have daily pain.[102,900] Periods of exacerbation and remission are common during the course of the disease.

The severity of symptoms during the first decade indicates the long-term severity and disabling nature of the disorder. Severe disease is usually marked by peripheral joint and extraarticular manifestations. The onset of hip disease in anyone with AS at any stage of the disease is a major prognostic marker for long-term severe disease and is more common in people with onset at a young age.[110]

Individuals with AS have an increased mortality rate. The impact of this disease can be seen in various aspects of workforce participation, such as needing more assistance, withdrawal from the workforce, and reduced quality of life. Early diagnosis and management will likely help prevent functional disability and improve outcomes.[93]

SPECIAL IMPLICATIONS FOR THE THERAPIST | 27-13

Ankylosing Spondylitis

Whenever someone presents with new onset of back, sacroiliac, or hip pain in the absence of trauma or overuse that is accompanied by associated signs and symptoms of systemic disease (e.g., fever, fatigue, respiratory compromise) the therapist must recognize that these are not symptoms typically associated with mechanical causes of back pain. If present, these features are considered red flags that should raise concern regarding the underlying cause of the complaints.

The therapist can assess for limitation of spinal mobility, most evident as a decrease in forward flexion of the spine, using the Schober test. In the standing position, place a mark at the lumbosacral junction, which is represented by the intersection of a line joining the dimples at the posterosuperior iliac spines. Place a second mark 5 cm below and 10 cm above the lumbosacral junction. The client is then asked to bend forward and attempt to touch the toes.

Now remeasure the distance between the upper and lower marks. The distraction between these two marks has been found to correlate very closely with anterior flexion measured radiologically. The distance increases more than 5 cm in the absence of AS and less than 5 cm when AS is present.

Alternatively, measure the horizontal distance between the posteroinferior iliac spine in both the prone and sitting positions, observing for a change in the distance with a change in position. Expect to see the posteroinferior iliac spine a half inch closer in the prone position compared to sitting in the normal young adult and suspect AS if there is no change.

Treating a client with a diagnosis of AS requires that the therapist entertain different considerations. If the client complains of sharp pain associated with a fall, sneeze, or lifting a moderately heavy object, one must consider the possibility of a fracture.[642] With osteoporosis being a potential complication, technique modification is warranted. See "Special Implications for the

Therapist 24-1" and "Osteoporosis" in Chapter 24 for further discussion.

Management should follow guidelines similar to those outlined for fibromyalgia (see Chapter 7). With the fragility of the spine in AS and the risk of fractures from even a minor injury or fall, falls prevention is also important. This is an area for careful attention, because a number of people with AS suffer neurologic deficit after injury, especially spinal fracture.[375]

Trunk range-of-motion and strengthening exercises to minimize thoracic kyphosis are essential. The more severe the kyphosis, the more hindered pulmonary function will be and the more pronounced the compensatory forward head posture. Postural deformities contribute to cervical pain and headaches and may also affect balance. Avoiding obesity is recommended to reduce stress on weight-bearing joints and the cardiopulmonary system.

Finally, smoking should be discouraged because of its adverse effects on the cardiopulmonary system. The therapist can also monitor clients taking NSAIDs for early signs of gastrointestinal bleeding or other adverse side effects (see Chapter 6).

For individuals receiving TNF-α blockers, slowing the progress of AS is possible in the majority of cases. They are used to treat arthritis of the joints as well as the spinal arthritis associated with AS. One drawback with these drugs that the therapist should be aware of is an increased risk of infections. Any sign of infection (even a sore throat) should be reported to the physician as the drug therapy may have to be suspended because of the involved immunosuppression.[100]

Exercise and Ankylosing Spondylitis

Therapists play a potentially important role in the rehabilitation of this population.[222] Although more studies are available now than ever before in this area, there still is not sufficient evidence to base recommendations for or against specific physical therapy interventions. Continued research is needed to address those modalities and applications commonly used in practice.[187] A summary of the available scientific evidence on the effectiveness of physical therapy interventions in the management of AS is presented here and elsewhere.[849]

General Concepts

Although exercise is a commonly recommended intervention for AS, little is known about the effectiveness of unsupervised recreational and back exercises. Findings from one study[841] suggest that exercise improves pain, stiffness, and function when performed at least 30 minutes per day and back exercises at least 5 days per week, although these effects vary with the duration of the AS. There may be an optimal duration for exercise performed independently over a weekly period, but consistency rather than quantity appears to be a much more significant variable. Although there is no difference in disease activity with a regular program of exercise, improved function has been demonstrated.[722]

Interpreting the results of some studies can be difficult. For example, one study showed that younger individuals with AS who had a shorter duration of disease and were less disabled also exercised less compared to older, more disabled adults who exercised more often. Without careful analysis and understanding of the results, the conclusion could be made that those people who exercised more frequently were more disabled, when in fact, affected individuals did not get serious about exercising consistently until the disease had progressed.[234]

Exercise Prescription

The question of what type of exercise is best for this condition has not been adequately answered. Persons with AS have been found to have lower cardiorespiratory fitness levels compared to age-matched controls, which fitness tends to worsen as their disease progresses.[334] Exercising does benefit people with AS, but, again, consistency, not quantity, seems to be the key factor in influencing posture, strength, motion, balance, mobility, fitness, and overall health.[667,722] Both home programs and group programs are beneficial for individuals with AS.[186,245]

A multimodal physical therapy program including aerobic, stretching, and pulmonary exercises along with routine medical management has been shown to yield greater improvements in spinal mobility, work capacity, and chest expansion compared with medical care alone. After 3 months, individuals in a 50-minute, three-times-a-week multimodal exercise program were significantly improved in chest expansion, chin-to-chest distance, occiput-to-wall distance, and the modified Schober flexion test.[407]

Functional and breathing capacity, as well as balance, should be assessed and developed. Stretching of the shortened muscles and chest expansion exercises should be encouraged. Improving and/or maintaining cardiovascular fitness is important.

Strengthening of the trunk extensors is equally important, so that if and when spinal fusion occurs, the spine is aligned in the most functional position possible. This requires a coordinated effort among all team members, including the affected individual and family.

High-impact and flexion exercises should be avoided, whereas low-impact, aerobic exercise with extension and rotational components can be emphasized. Each individual will need to identify personal limitations and safe levels of participation.

In general, contact sports and high-risk activities, such as downhill skiing, horseback riding, boxing, football, soccer, and water skiing, should be avoided; aquatic therapy is an excellent option for most people, provided extension principles are emphasized. In the presence of spinal fusion and osteoporosis, other activities requiring high levels of balance, agility, and coordination (e.g., bicycling, ice skating, rollerblading) can result in falls and fractures.

Overexercising can be potentially harmful and can exacerbate the inflammatory process; principles of relaxation, proper body mechanics, and energy conservation should be a part of the education program offered (see Box 9-4), including assessment of ADLs and providing necessary aids or devices such as long-handled reaching tools, adaptations for the car, special garden tools, or elastic shoelaces. Learning and using proper breathing techniques throughout all activities will help maintain chest expansion, improve oxygenation, and minimize muscle fatigue.

At present, aggressive but careful stretching to address the areas of hypomobility and the muscle imbalances is purported to help maintain as optimal a posture as possible.[892] An exercise program focusing on specific strengthening and flexibility exercises of the shortened muscle chains offers promising short- and long-term results in the management of this condition.[55,244,892]

Outcome Measurements

Mobility tests to establish a baseline and measure the effectiveness of short-term intensive physical therapy and exercise on spinal, hip, and shoulder motion have been evaluated.

Finger-to-floor distance, thoracolumbar rotation, and thoracolumbar lateral flexion are the most sensitive tests to detect improvements (or progression) in short-term clinical trials, whereas the Schober test, thoracolumbar flexion, and occiput-to-wall distance are insensitive measures of improvement. Hip internal rotation, shoulder flexion, and abduction measurements are also sensitive, although more suitable for individuals with articular symptoms. Thoracolumbar rotation and hip rotation are the only measurements that correlate with disease duration, but not with age.[356]

The Bath Ankylosing Spondylitis Functional Index (BASFI), along with the Dougados Functional Index score, Bath Ankylosing Spondylitis Metrology Index, and Bath Ankylosing Spondylitis Disease Activity Index (BASDAI), and miniBASDAI are self-assessment tools that can be used both by the therapist and by the client to establish a baseline and document improvement or decline.[62,122,329,616]

The therapist must be vigilant for an exacerbation of the inflammatory process. Assess (and periodically reassess) the spine and peripheral joints for mobility, range of motion, and strength. Modalities such as ultrasound, heat and cold, and electrotherapy may be effective during the acute phase if used judiciously.

Aggressive stretching must be avoided during these phases; teaching the individual a progressive relaxation program may be helpful. Communication with the physician is necessary for the development of a proper medication regimen.

Positioning

The affected individual may need help modifying home or work situations. Appropriate footwear advice should be provided; some people benefit from functional foot orthoses. Resting in the prone position is advised to help avoid hip and spine flexion contractures. The Spondylitis Association of America[787] recommends a firm, supportive sleeping surface to maintain good spinal alignment. Soft mattresses or waterbeds can contribute to excessive flexion and stooped postures.

The therapist can provide additional recommendations for the use of pillows or towel rolls for proper alignment in the various positions. The person may not stay positioned all night, but with time and training, changing positions and realigning props can be incorporated into the sleep cycle at least part of the time.

Proper lifting techniques can be demonstrated, with return demonstration provided by the client. The therapist should assess the work area or instruct the individual in appropriate ergonomics given the diagnosis of AS.

Diffuse Idiopathic Skeletal Hyperostosis

Overview and Definition. DISH is a disease entity considered to be an idiopathic variant of OA. The condition was first described by Forestier and Rotes-Querol, and has been called Forestier disease.[160,260,708]

The condition results in ossification of ligaments, especially the longitudinal ligaments of the spine causing stiffness and back pain. The ossification of the anterior longitudinal ligament leads to the development of a lengthy and complex, paravertebral mass along the anterior aspect of the vertebral column (Fig. 27-23). The condition more commonly affects men than women (2:1), presenting between the ages of 50 and 70 years.

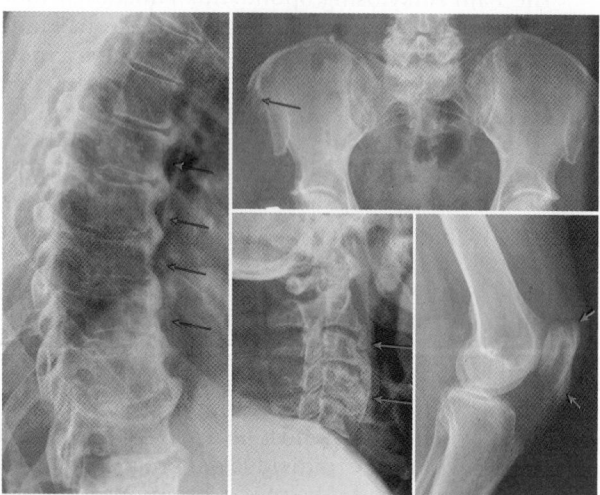

Figure 27-23

Diffuse idiopathic skeletal hyperostosis (DISH). DISH is seen in older individuals, predominantly involving the thoracic spine with flowing anterior ossification (at least four levels); associated with enthesophytes elsewhere (especially pelvis). Patients are at increased risk for heterotopic bone formation after joint replacement. DISH is differentiated from ankylosing spondylitis by age (older), location (C, T spine > L spine, no sacroiliac involvement), and morphology (loosely flowing ossification on lateral view). (From Morrison WM, Sanders TG: *Problem solving in musculoskeletal imaging*, St Louis, 2008, Mosby.)

The thoracic spine is most commonly affected by the ossification of the anterior longitudinal ligament. Radiographically, the condition is identified with the appearance that can be described as "candle wax" dripping down the spine. Ossification of ligaments in the lumbar and the lower cervical spine are usually found with ossification extending into the thoracic spine. Unlike OA, the condition does not directly result in degeneration of vertebral facet joints, joint space narrowing, or spondylophytes (lipping of vertebral bodies); instead, it presents with syndesmophytes (bony outgrowths attached to ligaments), resulting in decreased mobility of the spine, especially for the lumbar spine. The condition can aggravate the effects of OA and other degenerative conditions of the spine.[160]

Extraspinal forms of this condition have been identified for the large synovial joints of the upper and lower extremities.[524] Efforts are underway to develop a new classification criteria that will more accurately reflect what is known and has been observed about this condition. At present there is no agreement about the inclusion of extraspinal, constitutional, and metabolic manifestations in a new classification of DISH.[523]

Risk Factors. Diseases that produce endothelial cell damage, causing aggregation of platelet-derived growth factor, will stimulate osteoblast production that may be the genesis of the hyperostosis. The disease processes associated with hypertension, coronary artery disease, diabetes mellitus, AS, and metabolic diseases such as Paget and hyperparathyroidism have been hypothesized to be precursors to the development of DISH.

DISH has been found in individuals with high levels of uric acid, type II diabetes, severe atherosclerotic cardiovascular diseases, and high body mass index levels.[525,738,910] People who have undergone surgical procedures using periosteal stripping or who have experienced blunt trauma to the spine and peripheral joints have subsequently developed DISH.

Environmental exposure to excessive levels of fluoride or fluorine vapors can result in thickening of the periosteum and may be a factor for the development of ligament calcifications. Genetic influences have been investigated, such as with other seronegative SpAs, but no specific genetic factors have been identified.[160]

Etiology and Pathogenesis. DISH is characterized by ossifications starting at the insertion of ligaments, tendons, and joint capsule insertion points (entheses) to bone. The ossification usually starts along the body of a vertebra, extending along the longitudinal ligaments. The ossification process is separate from the subjacent vertebral body and any sclerotic changes occurring along the vertebral disk. Fusion of cortical bone of the vertebrae with the ossification of ligament has been observed only with advanced cases of the disease.[261]

The etiology of DISH has not yet been identified. A number of disease processes, genetic, environmental, and anatomical causes have been investigated without a clear cause for why the ossification process develops in some individuals. The presence of elevated endogenous insulin, the serum matrix Gls protein, and other growth factors have been identified as possible stimuli to ossification. AS is a similar condition resulting in proliferation of bony growths in the spine that has been linked to the presence of the HLA-B27 antigen (Fig. 27-24). No definitive relationship has been established between those individuals with DISH and the presence of this antigen.[635]

Clinical Manifestations. This condition begins and develops asymptomatically and is usually identified inadvertently from radiographs taken for other conditions. Individuals with this condition will have spinal and joint mobility that is normal for their age and may not find any limitations in their daily functions or recreational activities during the early stages of the disease.

Symptoms are usually complaints of dull pain and stiffness in the spine following prolonged periods of rest/sleep (e.g., upon waking in the morning) or with activities that require spinal bending or twisting motions. The symptoms will usually subside with rest and the use of NSAIDs.[708] Patient with extensive hyperostosis formations along the anterior surface of the cervical spine may present with symptoms of hoarseness, stridor/snoring, or difficulties swallowing (dysphagia).[118,262,862] As the condition progresses to more extensive calcifications along the spine or peripheral joints, an individual will experience more persistent symptoms, limitations in joint mobility, and abnormal spinal posture.

Individuals with advanced cases of DISH are more susceptible to suffering vertebral fractures of the cervical and thoracic spine[203] that can lead to neurologic complications.[99] In some cases, extra bone growth around the spinal cord can also cause loss of sensation and even paralysis.[888]

MEDICAL MANAGEMENT

DIAGNOSIS. DISH is most commonly identified from radiographic findings of a "flowing" ossification along the anterolateral margins of the vertebral column (see Figs. 27-23 and 27-24). The ossification along at least four contiguous vertebral bodies, preservation of disk height, and absence of facet joint ankyloses are the criteria for the diagnosis of DISH of the spine.[809] For extraspinal cases of the condition, calcification is found along the attachment sites for ligaments and tendons of the joint.[524]

Further evaluation for the extent and effects of the ossifications can be made using CT and MR images. Upon radiographic findings of DISH, further work-up of other rheumatologic conditions, especially AS is performed. Anyone with signs of cardiovascular and metabolic syndrome associated with DISH should be evaluated and treated for these conditions.[910]

The use of imaging will determine the extent of the ligamentous ossifications and risks for spinal fractures. The presence of hyperostosis along peripheral joints can be well visualized with radiographic views. CT images can provide accurate visualization of spinal ossifications with sagittal and coronal views with good resolutions to assess the facet apophyseal joints.

The lower segments of the *cervical spine* are more commonly involved, with ossifications extending to the atlantoaxial joint and occiput. Progression of hyperostosis along the cervical spine can restrict function of the larynx and pharynx that may require swallowing studies. For the *thoracic spine*, there is usually more ossification along the right lateral aspect of the spine with advanced cases having hyperostosis extending to the posterior aspect of the ribs. Involvement of the *lumbar spine* will usually affect the upper segments, with advanced conditions extending to the posterior ligaments of the spine.

Individuals who have suffered a vertebral fracture secondary to having DISH will need extensive imaging studies to determine the extent of the fracture and to plan surgical procedures to treat the fracture and possibly remove the ossifications along the spinal column.[613,809]

TREATMENT. For individuals identified in the early stages of DISH, a conservative approach that treats symptoms of pain and stiffness using pharmaceuticals, such as NSAIDs, and exercise is warranted. Ongoing evaluation of the hyperostosis is also advised. Many of these people are at risk for coronary artery disease, type 2 diabetes, and other metabolic diseases, and will need further medical evaluation and preventive measures for these conditions.[522]

Individuals with cervical hyperostosis that affects swallowing or breathing function will need imaging and a fiberoptic laryngoscopy to assess the extent of the ossifications. A rehabilitation approach may be possible using modifications to diet and compensations to improve swallowing function to allow for satisfactory management of this problem.[262] For advanced cases, surgical procedures to remove the ossifications from the cervical spine allows for a return to normal breathing and swallowing functions.[673]

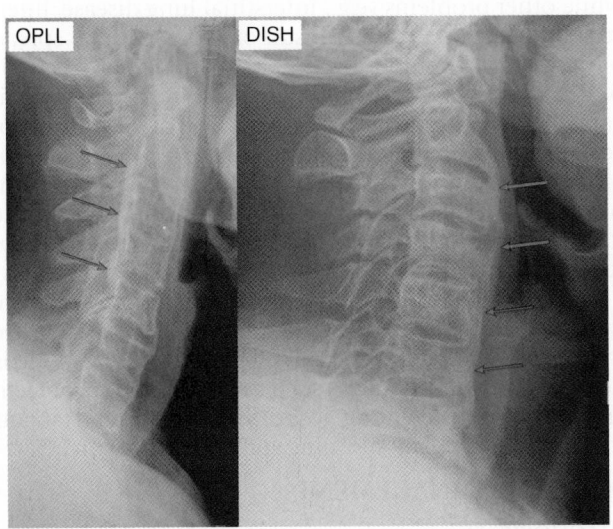

Figure 27-24

Contrast findings of ankylosing spondylitis with ossification of the posterior longitudinal ligament (ossification of the posterior longitudinal ligament; note linear ossification along the posterior vertebral bodies) and diffuse idiopathic skeletal hyperostosis (diffuse idiopathic skeletal hyperostosis; note undulating anterior ossification). Occasionally, there is overlap of these disorders. (From Morrison WM, Sanders TG: *Problem solving in musculoskeletal imaging*, St Louis, 2008, Mosby.)

SPECIAL IMPLICATIONS FOR THE THERAPIST 27-14

Diffuse Idiopathic Skeletal Hyperostosis

Therapeutic exercise programs for this condition have been employed with the goals of diminishing back pain, improving spinal range of motion, and decreasing disability. Al-Herz reported on the use of a daily program of trunk and hip stabilization exercises, active trunk range of motion, and stretching for the hamstrings and lumbar spine.[8] After 6 months, participants demonstrated improvements in trunk mobility, but had inconsistent improvements in symptoms and disability levels.[8]

Therapists should develop an individualized plan to address mobility and symptoms for individuals with DISH. A multimodal approach of modalities, spinal mobility and stretching, postural exercises, and aerobic exercises should be considered to best address symptoms and activity limitations.[838]

Sjögren Syndrome

Overview. Sjögren syndrome is a chronic arthritis-related disease that can affect several organs, most commonly the moisture-producing glands (e.g., mouth, eyes) but also joints, lungs, kidneys, or liver. Sjögren syndrome is an autoimmune disease, sometimes also considered as a connective tissue disease that is characterized by the body's inability to distinguish healthy cells from foreign substances.[682]

In Sjögren syndrome, the immune system mistakenly attacks its own moisture-producing glands and other organs. It may be a primary condition occurring alone or secondary to other autoimmune diseases, such as RA or lupus.[176]

Incidence and Risk Factors. Sjögren syndrome is the second most common autoimmune rheumatic disease, affecting an estimated 2–4 million Americans, developing most often in postmenopausal women. It can occur in children and men or women of any age; women are affected nine times more often than men.[263]

Information from rheumatology clinics suggests that primary Sjögren syndrome is as common as SLE and that approximately 30% of people with RA or systemic sclerosis have histologic evidence of Sjögren syndrome. Other risk factors include having another autoimmune disease or having a family member with Sjögren syndrome.

Etiologic Factors and Pathogenesis. The primary symptoms of Sjögren syndrome are the result of exocrine gland (mainly salivary and lacrimal gland) destruction by focal T-lymphocytic infiltrates. The infiltrating T and B cells interfere with glandular function at several points.[273] Additional potential contributing factors are B-cell hyperreactivity (these locally produce immunoglobulins having autoantibody reactivity) and long-term immune system stimulation.[772]

Evidence supports a genetic component in its etiology, but there is no strong evidence for a specific candidate gene.[29] Neurogenic regulation of the salivary gland is impaired, with structural abnormalities of the secretory acinar apparatus. The acinar basement membrane is abnormal, as it lacks the laminin α_1 chain; this loss may impair its ability to induce stem cells to differentiate into acinar cells.[464]

Organ-specific autoantibodies are present, but the role of the autoantibodies in the disease process is not clear, and it is unknown whether they contribute to tissue dysfunction before tissue inflammation is observed.[699] Researchers suspect that a common immunologic mechanism (e.g., infiltration by activated T cells and expression of HLA-class molecules on epithelial cells) is involved in the development of autoimmune disorders, especially autoimmune thyroid diseases and Sjögren syndrome, but the details remain unknown.

The interactions between the neuroendocrine and immune systems as these relate to autoimmune diseases such as Sjögren syndrome are the topic of numerous research studies.[427] Significantly lower basal adrenocorticotrophic hormone and cortisol levels have been found in individuals with Sjögren syndrome, associated with a blunted pituitary and adrenal response to ovine corticotropin-releasing factor compared to normal controls. Research findings suggest adrenal axis hypoactivity as well as adrenal and thyroid axes dysfunction.[426]

Clinical Manifestations. Clinical manifestations vary according to the systemic problems present from integumentary, respiratory, renal, hepatic, neurologic, and vascular involvement. Associated symptoms may include extremely dry throat, esophagitis, gastritis, and dental cavities from a lack of saliva; vaginal dryness with painful sexual intercourse; fatigue; joint and muscle pain; joint and muscle stiffness; swelling; rashes (vasculitis); numbness (peripheral neuropathy as a consequence of small-vessel vasculitis); Raynaud phenomenon; B-cell lymphoma; and inflammation of the lungs, kidneys, or liver.

The hallmark symptoms of Sjögren syndrome are dry eyes and dry mouth. This syndrome may also cause dryness in other areas, such as the kidneys, gastrointestinal tract, blood vessels, sinuses, respiratory tract, liver, pancreas, and central nervous system.

Some of the problems (e.g., recurrent bronchitis or sinusitis) arise from exocrine dysfunction in other organs, while other problems (e.g., interstitial lung disease, interstitial nephritis) occur as a result of extraglandular spread of lymphocytic infiltration discussed in the pathogenesis of this disease.[873] Primary Sjögren syndrome causes salivary gland swelling and tenderness. The dry eyes (keratoconjunctivitis sicca) are described as the feeling of sand or a burning sensation in the eyes with decreased secretion of tears. Dry mouth (xerostomia) and dry cough make it difficult for affected individuals to chew and swallow food or speak continuously.

Depression, anxiety, thyroiditis, and fibromyalgia are frequent comorbid illnesses requiring a comprehensive management approach to this condition. Quality of life is decreased by complications such as sleep loss, loss of teeth and poorly fitting dentures, loss of vision, profound fatigue, musculoskeletal pain, morning stiffness, and so on.[623]

MEDICAL MANAGEMENT

DIAGNOSIS. Many conditions present similarly to Sjögren syndrome with dry eyes and dry mouth, such as lupus, vasculitis, thyroid disease, and scleroderma; side effects of some medications (e.g., tricyclic antidepressants, antihistamines, radiation treatments of the head and neck) can mimic Sjögren syndrome. Sjögren syndrome is a systemic disease with the potential to affect almost every organ system in the body, so the proper diagnosis is important.

Diagnosis is based on a complete physical examination; medical history; and specific tests such as a slit-lamp test to detect damage to the surface of the eye by using a dye that exposes eroded areas of the conjunctiva (the membrane that covers the eye and lines the inside of the eyelids), Schirmer test to assess degree of dryness in the eyes, lip biopsy to show inflammation of the salivary glands, and blood tests to detect antibodies (e.g., rheumatoid factor, antinuclear antibody, anti–Sjögren syndrome A antibody, and anti–Sjögren syndrome B antibody) that are associated with primary Sjögren syndrome.[750]

Many serum and salivary biomarkers for Sjögren syndrome have been proposed, but none has been specific enough for diagnostic purposes or correlated with disease activity measures. Modern genomic investigation is looking for candidate biomarkers and possible etiopathologic mechanisms underlying this disorder.[263]

TREATMENT. There is no cure for Sjögren syndrome, but it can be managed effectively. Ocular involvement is managed with local and systemic stimulators of tear secretion. Treatment of oral manifestations includes intense oral hygiene and prevention and treatment of oral infections. The use of saliva stimulants and mouth lubricants can help with the dryness.[551] Avoiding situations and activities that contribute to dryness, and moisturizing other areas of dryness, such as the skin and vagina (women), are advised.

Intervention typically involves medications (e.g., corticosteroids such as prednisone, NSAIDs, or hydroxychloroquine [Plaquenil]) to help reduce joint pain and stiffness and ease fatigue and muscle pain, as well as other palliative measures for symptomatic relief. Exercise and proper nutrition may help with the fatigue and joint symptoms.[683]

Mild cases of peripheral neuropathy can remit spontaneously, but usually symptomatic treatment (e.g., gabapentin) is needed. More severe involvement affecting ambulation may require the use of steroids, azathioprine, or intravenous gammaglobulin or cyclophosphamide.[873] Anti–B-cell therapy is a new potential therapy for glandular and extraglandular manifestations such as glomerulonephritis or vasculitis. Gene transfer has been attempted in animal models with promising results.[551] The use of green tea polyphenols, which have both antiinflammatory and antiapoptotic properties, is also under investigation based on the knowledge that the incidence of Sjögren syndrome is much lower in China and Japan, two leading green tea–consuming countries. Animal studies show that green tea polyphenols could provide protective effects against autoimmune reactions in skin and salivary glands.[391]

PROGNOSIS. Sjögren syndrome progresses slowly, with the interval between first symptoms and diagnosis ranging from 2 to 8 years. Left untreated, dryness of the eyes can lead to eye infections and may result in damage to the cornea and visual loss.

Sjögren syndrome is a benign disease that affects quality of life. When extraoral and extraocular exocrine gland dysfunction or lymphocyte-mediated tissue destruction involves other organs, significant morbidity and mortality can occur. There is a high risk of malignant transformation that requires close follow-up.

SPECIAL IMPLICATIONS FOR THE THERAPIST 27-15

Sjögren Syndrome

Special implications and preferred practice patterns are determined by the presenting clinical features but follow the general guidelines for RA. See "Special Implications for the Therapist 27-11: Rheumatoid Arthritis" above.

Physical capacity is reduced in Sjögren syndrome, and fatigue is a dominating and disabling symptom.[797] Evidence-based studies on the effect of exercise in Sjögren syndrome are limited, with small sample sizes. The available studies indicate that clients with Sjögren syndrome can benefit from moderate- to high-intensity levels of exercise, with positive effects on aerobic capacity, fatigue, physical function, and depression (mood).[798]

Further research is needed to evaluate the effect of exercise on groups with varying degree of disease severity and to document the long-term impact on the disease.[798]

Psoriatic Arthritis

Overview and Incidence. Psoriatic arthritis is a seronegative inflammatory joint disease afflicting a small percentage of people who have psoriasis. This joint disorder is associated with radiographic evidence of periarticular bone erosions and occasional significant joint destruction. Psoriatic arthritis tends to progress slowly, and for most of those affected, it is more a nuisance than a disabling condition.[303]

Approximately 1% of the population of the United States has psoriasis. Psoriatic arthritis occurs in approximately 20% of persons with psoriasis, and more often in those with severe psoriasis. Uncomplicated psoriasis typically presents during the second and third decades of life, with the onset of the arthritis occurring up to 20 years later. The disease can occur in children, with onset typically between the ages of 9 and 12 years. Psoriatic arthritis does not appear to have a strong predilection for one gender.

Etiologic and Risk Factors. A strong familial association has been noted with this disease. Although specific marker genes have not been discovered, there is general agreement that a genetic predisposition exists for psoriatic arthritis. There is approximately an 80% to 90% chance of contracting psoriatic arthritis if one has a first-degree relative with the disorder.[343]

Pathogenesis. An inflammatory synovitis results in the joint changes associated with psoriatic arthritis. Lymphocyte infiltration into the synovium occurs. Initially, the synovium is pale, with edematous granulation tissue extending along the contiguous bone. The synovium later becomes thickened with villous hypertrophy. Eroded articular margins begin to appear at this time. In severe cases, the joint space tends to be filled in with dense fibrous tissue.[563]

Clinical Manifestations. The arthritis can be oligoarticular or polyarticular. There is a predilection for the distal interphalangeal joints of the hands. Other joints of the digits may be involved. The joint changes may

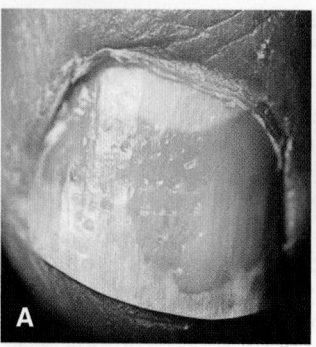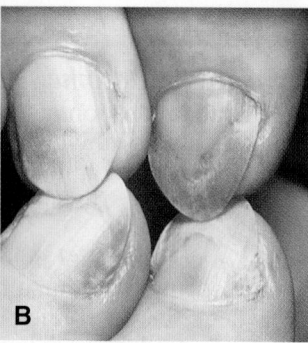

Figure 27-25

Nail changes associated with various forms of arthritis. A, Pitting of the nail beds associated with psoriasis. **B,** Onycholysis associated with reactive arthritis, a separation of the nail plate from the nail bed beginning at the free margin and progressing inward. (A, from James WD, Berger T, Elston D: *Andrews' diseases of the skin: clinical dermatology,* ed 10, Philadelphia, 2006, WB Saunders. B, from Arndt KA: *Primary care dermatology,* Philadelphia, 1997, WB Saunders.)

lead to significant hand deformities, including claw deformity. The digital joint changes and associated flexor tenosynovitis can result in an edematous, thickened digit.[556]

Joints of the axial skeleton can also be affected but typically become involved several years after the onset of the peripheral joint disease. The sacroiliitis is usually unilateral, unlike that in AS. Sacroiliitis can occur in 20% to 40% of clients.

Although not as common as in RA or Reiter syndrome, extraarticular manifestations can occur with psoriatic arthritis. Inflammatory eye disease, including conjunctivitis and iritis, renal disease, mitral valve prolapse, and aortic regurgitation are associated with this disorder. Pitting of the nails and onycholysis (Fig. 27-25) are also commonly associated with psoriatic arthritis.

There are some differences in the manifestations of this disease between children and adults. A slight predilection for females is noted in children. In addition, the arthritis may appear before the skin manifestations in a number of children. Compared with adults, the onset of the arthritis tends to be more acute in children, with the involvement of multiple asymmetric joints. The hip joint is much more commonly involved in children.

MEDICAL MANAGEMENT

DIAGNOSIS. The diagnosis of psoriatic arthritis is usually easily made because of the onset of inflammatory arthritis in the presence of obvious psoriasis. Differential diagnosis can be difficult, however, if the psoriasis is absent or equivocal. Laboratory tests do not help except to rule out RA. Box 27-14 lists common radiographic findings in psoriatic arthritis.[28]

TREATMENT AND PROGNOSIS. There is currently no cure for psoriasis or psoriatic arthritis. People with mild arthritis are treated symptomatically with NSAIDs. If there is an acute flare of only one or two joints, local corticosteroid injections may help. Anyone with more aggressive disease may benefit from DMARD therapy with MTX, sulfasalazine, and the TNF-α antagonists.[563]

Box 27-14

RADIOGRAPHIC FEATURES OF PSORIATIC ARTHRITIS

- Asymmetric oligoarticular distribution of disease
- Relative absence of osteopenia
- Involvement of distal interphalangeal joints
- Involvement of sacroiliac joint (unilateral)

Data from Amrami KK: Imaging of the seronegative spondyloarthropathies, *Radiol Clin North Am* 50(4):841–854, 2012.

Because of the association between severe skin involvement and severe arthritis, treatment of the psoriasis is emphasized with the hope of reducing the arthritis. Multiple medications have been used in an attempt to control progressive psoriatic arthritis but with equivocal results. As noted earlier, for most persons with psoriatic arthritis, the disease is mild, not destructive.

SPECIAL IMPLICATIONS FOR THE THERAPIST 27-16

Psoriatic Arthritis

See "Special Implications for the Therapist 27-11: Rheumatoid Arthritis" above.

The goals for therapy are to prevent the development of joint degeneration while increasing functional abilities and improving quality of life. With the goal of early remission of the disease, a team approach of working with a rheumatologist, dermatologist, occupational therapist, and psychologist, will provide the best outcome for these people. Because a person with this disease can present with a variety of inflammatory conditions in the axial skeleton and the extremities, the therapist will need to develop a treatment plan that is specific to each individual.[303] If a flare-up of the skin condition is noted, encourage the client to see the client's physician. If the joint inflammation worsens, prompt communication with the physician should occur so the client can be placed on an appropriate medication regimen.

Reactive Arthritis

Overview. This section is confined to the discussion of reactive arthritis, which differs from bacterial arthritis (discussed in Chapter 25) in several ways. Reactive arthritis is defined as the occurrence of an acute, *aseptic,* inflammatory arthropathy arising after an infectious process but at a site remote from the primary infection, whereas bacterial arthritis may be a local response with joint destruction and sepsis.

The borderline between reactive arthritis and true septic arthritis may be obscure, as several organisms can cause both, with overlapping symptoms and laboratory features. Other infectious causes of arthritis are discussed in other chapters (e.g., HIV in Chapter 7; Lyme disease and Epstein-Barr virus in Chapter 8; rheumatic fever in Chapter 12).

Etiologic and Risk Factors and Pathogenesis. Reactive arthritis is a recognized sequela of infection with a number of enteric pathogens, such as *Campylobacter jejuni* (gastrointestinal tract), *Salmonella typhimurium*, *Shigella* (dysentery), *Chlamydia trachomatis* (genitourinary tract), *Chlamydia pneumoniae* (respiratory tract), *Yersinia, M. fermentans,*[384] and *Clostridium difficile* (colitis associated with antibiotic therapy; with chlamydiae the most common cause of reactive arthritis.[137,138]

The overall prevalence of reactive arthritis has declined, although an increase has been seen in a small population group composed of intravenous drug users with acquired immunodeficiency syndrome. Reactive arthritis is most common in young, sexually active adults, especially men who have been infected with *C. trachomatis.* However, children and older adults of both genders are affected by the postenteric form. Reactive arthritis following urogenital infection is underdiagnosed in women. The tendency for chlamydial infection to be subclinical or asymptomatic and the relative infrequency of pelvic examinations are contributing factors.[607]

A particular major histocompatibility complex class I antigen, HLA-B27, is well recognized as a genetic marker of susceptibility to reactive arthritis (see Table 40-21). Bacteria in the joint may stimulate the immune system to produce antibodies and protein factors (cytokines), several of which produce local inflammation and tissue damage, leading to an arthritic joint.[337]

Clinical Manifestations. The arthritis first manifests 1 to 4 weeks after the infectious insult and is usually asymmetric affecting more than one joint, typically the large and medium joints of the lower extremities. Sacroiliac joint involvement occurs in approximately 10% of acute cases and 30% of chronic cases. The clinical picture varies from mild arthralgia and arthritis to incapacitating illness that may result in bed rest for several weeks. Joint pain may be minimal with no signs of inflammation, but stiffness, pain, tenderness, and loss of motion are often present.[137,607]

Associated findings may include uveitis, enthesitis (inflammation involving the sites of bony insertion of tendons and ligaments), sacroiliitis, urethritis, and conjunctivitis. Reactive arthritis encompasses a subgroup that demonstrates the classic clinical triad of arthritis, urethritis, and conjunctivitis, which is called Reiter syndrome (see further discussion in the next section). Reactive arthritis is a broader category that includes some but not all of the more restrictive features associated with Reiter syndrome. The distinction between these two conditions is somewhat arbitrary.[443]

Extraarticular manifestations of reactive arthritis may include onycholysis of the fingernails or toenails, dactylitis (sausage like swelling of the toes and fingers because of joint and tenosynovium inflammation), painless mucosal ulcers in the mouth, discharge from the vagina or penis, urologic symptoms (urgency, frequency, difficulty starting or continuing a flow of urine), or various types of skin lesions. Rarely, neurologic or cardiac involvement occurs secondary to inflammatory and fibrotic lesions.

MEDICAL MANAGEMENT

DIAGNOSIS. There is considerable clinical overlap among the various types of inflammatory arthritides. Usually, a careful clinical and family history and physical examination will lead to the diagnosis. Laboratory evaluation, synovial fluid aspiration, cultures for bacteria, antibody testing, measurement of serum immunoglobulin, and imaging studies contribute to the differential diagnosis.[137]

TREATMENT AND PROGNOSIS. NSAIDs and disease-modifying drugs are the basis of medical management. A short course of corticosteroids may be necessary in some cases, and antirheumatic agents may be beneficial in chronic reactive arthritis. Antibiotics are recommended if the infection is identified.

The overall prognosis for reactive arthritis is good even in severe cases, but full recovery does not always occur. Many people will experience some form of persisting symptoms, with degeneration of lower extremity joints that can lead to chronic disability.

Recurrence is possible, and a chronic form of this condition can develop, characterized by recurring arthritis that is accompanied by tendinitis or tenosynovitis. Sacroiliitis and spondylitis may not resolve but may persist, with ongoing pain and stiffness of the neck and back.[607]

SPECIAL IMPLICATIONS FOR THE THERAPIST 27-17

Reactive Arthritis

See "Special Implications for the Therapist 27-11: Rheumatoid Arthritis" above.

The relationship of infections of the gastrointestinal or genitourinary system to the joint is well documented (see "Arthritis and Inflammatory Intestinal Diseases" in Chapter 16), so that anyone with new onset of joint involvement must be medically evaluated for an underlying bacterial or infectious cause.

Past medical history may reveal a recent infectious process, use of antibiotics, presence of a sexually transmitted disease, or bowel disease to alert the physician. The presence of joint involvement accompanied by (or alternating with) gastrointestinal signs and symptoms such as diarrhea, abdominal pain or bloating, constitutional symptoms (e.g., fever, night sweats), or positive iliopsoas or obturator sign (see Figs. 16-13 and 16-14) must be reported to the physician.

Anyone taking NSAIDs for reactive arthritis must take them as prescribed and not just for analgesia or on occasion. The therapist can help educate affected individuals that a stoic attitude of enduring the pain and restricted mobility with a refusal to "take pills" will result in less optimal and delayed recovery.

Physical therapy intervention is very valuable during convalescence to regain full motion, strength, and function. Temporary splinting may be advised in the most painful cases, but muscle atrophy can be rapid, and therefore immobilization should be minimized.[607]

If new symptoms develop or the person does not respond to therapy, medical evaluation is advised; modification of medications may be needed.

Reiter Syndrome

Overview. Reiter syndrome is one of the most common examples of reactive arthritis. Reiter syndrome usually follows venereal disease or an episode of bacillary dysentery (enteric infection) and is associated with typical extraarticular manifestations.

The prevalence and incidence of Reiter syndrome are difficult to establish because of (1) the lack of consensus regarding diagnostic criteria, (2) the nomadic nature of the young target population, (3) the underreporting of venereal disease, and (4) the asymptomatic or milder course in affected women.

Etiologic and Risk Factors. The most common microbial pathogens are *Shigella, Salmonella, Yersinia, Campylobacter,* and *Chlamydia* species. Age, gender, and medical history are important risk factors associated with Reiter syndrome. The peak onset of this disorder occurs during the third decade of life, although children and older adults can also develop this disease. Individuals with the HLA-B27 antigen have been found to have more severe symptoms.[512]

Males are more commonly affected than females but not to the extent once thought. The incidence in women is potentially underestimated because their clinical manifestations are less severe than men's and women are more prone to occult genitourinary disease, leading to misdiagnosis.

A history of infection, especially venereal or dysenteric, is associated with increased risk of developing this condition. Men and women are equally affected by enteric infections. Reiter syndrome is the most common form of reactive arthritis observed in HIV-infected adults and appears to be more strongly associated with male homosexuality than with injection-drug use or other risky behaviors.[739]

Pathogenesis. Reiter syndrome is believed from a combination of immune and infectious causes and is primarily marked by inflammatory synovitis and inflammatory erosion at the insertion sites of ligaments and tendons (enthesitis). Heterotopic bone formation can occur at these sites. Synovial findings include edema, cellular invasion (lymphocytes, neutrophils, plasma cells), and vascular changes. Extensive pannus formation is rare, unlike in RA.[898]

Clinical Manifestations. The triad of symptoms classically associated with Reiter syndrome includes urethritis, conjunctivitis, and arthritis. The urethritis and conjunctivitis often occur early in the disease. Other ocular manifestations include uveitis and keratitis (fungal infection of the cornea).

Three musculoskeletal manifestations are acute inflammatory arthritis, inflammatory back pain, and enthesitis. Only about one-third of individuals affected by Reiter syndrome have all three. Low back pain is found in 50% of the people with the syndrome, with signs of decreased lumbar flexion. As discussed in the previous section, the arthritis is usually asymmetric, is often acute, and typically involves joints of the lower extremity, including the knees, ankles, and first metatarsophalangeal joint. Isolated hand joints can be involved. Although most of the symptoms and signs disappear within days or weeks, the arthritis may last for months or years.[512]

Extraarticular manifestations are as previously mentioned for reactive arthritis. The skin lesions may be indistinguishable from those of psoriasis. Low back pain is also a common complaint. The arthritis can progress and spread to the spine and even to the upper extremities.

MEDICAL MANAGEMENT

DIAGNOSIS. The diagnosis of Reiter syndrome may require months to establish, because the various manifestations can occur at different times. The combination of peripheral arthritis with urethritis lasting longer than 1 month is necessary before the diagnosis can be confirmed.

Laboratory tests typically reveal an aggressive inflammatory process. Elevated ESR and C-reactive protein are detected, and thrombocytosis and leukocytosis are common findings. Urine samples, genital swabs, and stool cultures are useful laboratory tests for identifying the triggering infection.[898]

Up to 70% of those with established Reiter syndrome may have radiographic abnormalities, including (1) asymmetric involvement of the lower-extremity diarthroses, amphiarthroses, symphyses, and entheses; (2) ill-defined bony erosions with adjacent bony proliferation; and (3) paravertebral ossification.

TREATMENT AND PROGNOSIS. Although Reiter syndrome is precipitated by an infection, there is no evidence that antibiotic therapy changes the course of the disorder. Treatment in general is largely symptomatic, with NSAIDs being the primary intervention.

If the arthritis persists, joint protection and maintenance of function become important. Immobilization and inactivity are usually discouraged, whereas range-of-motion and stretching exercises are emphasized. TNF-α antagonists may improve the outcome, but no controlled trials have been performed. Typically the arthritis resolves in 3 to 12 months, but can reoccur. Chronic articular or spinal disease affects 30% of the population affected; severe disability occurs in less than 15% of those individuals afflicted.[7]

SPECIAL IMPLICATIONS FOR THE THERAPIST 27-18

Reiter Syndrome

See "Special Implications for the Therapist 27-11: Rheumatoid Arthritis" above.

Questions related to the presence and treatment of infection, current and past, should be asked during the history taking. Also inquire into the person's general health, both current and before the onset of the presenting pain complaints. Typically, the onset of joint pain associated with concurrent systemic complaints would raise suspicion.

New-onset inflammatory joint disease with a history of recent enteric or venereal infection or new sexual contact strongly suggests a systemic origin of symptoms. Reiter syndrome is one condition in which past medical history and general health status may provide the most important information.

If the client is undiagnosed or has not yet been seen by a physician, medical evaluation is required. See also "Reactive Arthritis" above, including the "Special Implications for the Therapist 27-17: Reactive Arthritis."

Gout

Overview. Gout represents a heterogeneous group of metabolic disorders marked by an elevated level of serum uric acid and the deposition of urate crystals in the joints, soft tissues, and kidneys. Gout is the most common crystalopathy (crystal-induced arthritis) in the United States.

Hyperuricemia and gout are generally classified into one of three groups. *Primary hyperuricemia* is an inherited disorder of uric acid metabolism. *Secondary hyperuricemia* occurs as a result of some other metabolic problem, such as glucose-6-phosphatase dehydrogenase deficiency, reduced renal function (from any number of causes), certain medications that block uric acid excretion, or neoplasms. The third category, *idiopathic hyperuricemia*, encompasses conditions that do not fit into either of the other categories.

Although gout is a metabolic disorder and could be presented in Chapter 24 as such, it is so predominantly viewed as a form of arthritis because of its clinical presentation (gout can be manifested as a joint disorder characterized by acute or chronic arthritis) that it is included here instead. Crystals other than uric acid crystals can also form inside joints, such as occurs in a condition called *pseudogout* when calcium pyrophosphate dihydrate (CPPD) crystals are present.

The presence of CPPD crystals in the synovial fluid can cause symptoms identical to those of acute gout. Unlike gout, however, CPPD most often affects the knees of older women and may have polyarticular involvement. Pseudogout, also known as chondrocalcinosis, is associated with a number of metabolic disorders, such as hypothyroidism, hemochromatosis, hyperparathyroidism, and diabetes mellitus.

Incidence. Primary gout is predominantly associated with middle-aged men, with a peak incidence during the fifth decade of life. It is the most common inflammatory disease in men older than 30 years, generally becoming symptomatic after a period of hyperuricemia lasting 10 to 20 years.[593] New cases of gout have doubled in the last few decades.[474,483]

Gout is rare in children, and less than 10% of the cases occur in women. Most women with gout are 15 years or more postmenopausal (later for women taking hormone replacement therapy; a few years of estrogen deficiency are necessary before gout becomes evident in this population).[324,395]

Etiologic and Risk Factors. A family history of gout increases the risk of developing the disorder. The prevalence of gout increases with increasing serum urate concentration and age; with the aging of the American population, decreased renal function is becoming more prevalent, accompanied by a rise in the number of cases of gout.

Secondary hyperuricemia (gout) can be a result of urate overproduction or decreased urinary excretion of uric acid. People at risk for urate overproduction are those with a history of leukemia, lymphoma, psoriasis, or hemolytic disorders and those receiving chemotherapy for cancer.

Heavy alcohol consumption (especially beer), obesity, fasting, medications (e.g., thiazide diuretics, levodopa, and salicylates), renal insufficiency, hypertension, hypothyroidism, and hyperparathyroidism can all lead to decreased excretion of uric acid. Among the associated factors, age, duration of hyperuricemia, genetic predisposition, heavy alcohol consumption, obesity, thiazide drugs, and lead toxicity contribute the most to the conversion from asymptomatic hyperuricemia to acute gouty arthritis.[161,783]

A diet rich in purines (nitrogen-containing compounds found in foods such as shellfish, trout, sardines, anchovies, meat [especially organ meats], asparagus, beans, peas, spinach) can increase the risk of gout or make gout attacks more severe. Ingestion of fructose-sweetened foods and beverages has also been implicated with an increased risk of hyperuricemia and gout. Fructose is the only sugar known to elevate serum uric acid levels.[163,164] Conversely, there is a lower prevalence of gout in vegetarians and with supplemental vitamin C intake.[165,395]

In many cases of primary gout, the specific biochemical defect responsible for the hyperuricemia is unknown. A majority of cases probably result from an unexplained impairment in uric acid excretion by the kidneys. This impairment could result from decreased renal filtration, increased reabsorption, or decreased urate excretion by the renal tubules.

Pathogenesis. Uric acid is a substance that normally forms when the body breaks down cellular waste products called *purines*. In healthy people, uric acid dissolves in the blood, passes through the kidneys, and is then excreted through the urine. If the body produces more uric acid than the kidneys can process or if the kidneys are unable to handle normal levels of uric acid, then the acid level in the blood rises.

When the uric acid in the blood reaches high levels, it may precipitate out and accumulate in body tissues, forming supersaturated body fluids, including in the joints and kidneys. These crystals frequently collect on articular cartilage, epiphyseal bone, and periarticular structures. The crystal aggregates trigger an inflammatory response, resulting in local tissue necrosis and a proliferation of fibrous tissue secondary to an inflammatory foreign-body reaction. The genetics of gout are under investigation; there is some evidence that genetic variants of urate transporters that aid in the excretion of urate may contribute to altered serum uric acid levels.[162]

Clinical Manifestations. The disease occurs in four stages: asymptomatic hyperuricemia (defined as serum urate of more than 7 mg/dL), acute gouty arthritis, intercritical gout, and chronic tophaceous gout.[595] Many people with elevated uric acid levels for prolonged period of time never develop signs or symptoms.

The most common clinical presentation is the acute, monoarticular, inflammatory arthritis manifested by exquisite joint pain, occurring suddenly at night. Although the first metatarsophalangeal joint (i.e., the big toe) is a common site of pain, the ankle, instep, knee, wrist, elbow (olecranon bursa), and fingers can all be the site of the initial attack (Fig. 27-26). Besides local, intense pain of quick onset, erythema, warmth, and extreme tenderness and hypersensitivity are typically present. Chills, fever, and tachycardia may accompany the joint complaints.[711]

After recovering from the initial episode the person enters an asymptomatic phase called the *intercritical period*. This period can last months or years despite persistent hyperuricemia and synovial fluid that contains monosodium urate crystals.[595]

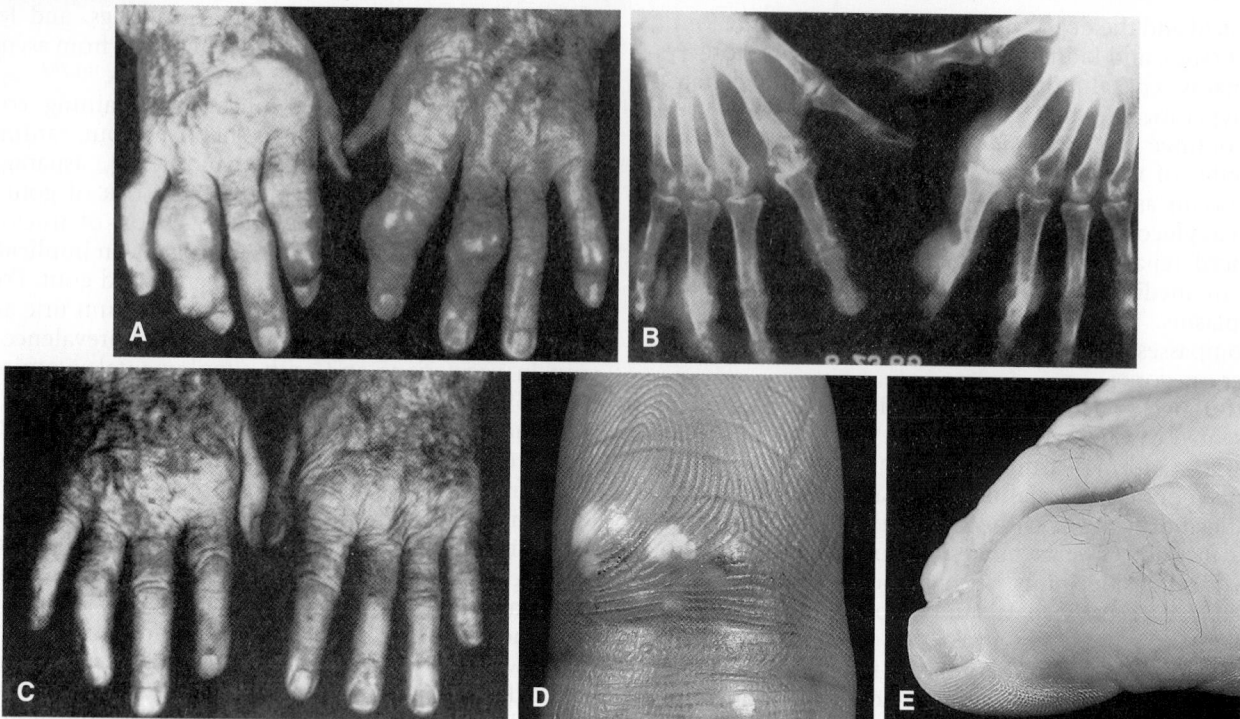

Figure 27-26

Tophaceous gout. A to **C,** Chronic gouty arthritis with tophaceous destruction of bone and joints. **D,** Tophaceous deposits in the digital pad of a 28-year-old man with systemic lupus erythematosus. **E,** Tophaceous enlargement of the great toe in a 44-year-old man with a 4-year history of recurrent gouty arthritis. (From Goldman L: *Cecil textbook of medicine,* ed 22, Philadelphia, 2004, WB Saunders.)

The gouty attacks return suddenly with increasing frequency and severity and often in different joints. These attacks may be precipitated by trauma, surgery, alcohol consumption, or overindulgence in foods with high purine content. The arthritis can enter the chronic phase up to a decade after the initial attack, characterized by joint damage, functional loss, and disability. Deposits of monosodium urate crystals in soft tissue (tophi) and bone abnormalities are the hallmarks of chronic disease (Fig. 27-27).[783] Tophi can be located in tendons, ligaments, cartilage, subchondral bone, bursa, synovium, and subcutaneous tissue around the joints. Common sites of these hard, sometimes ulcerated masses that extrude chalky material include the helix of the ear, forearm, knee, and foot.[595]

MEDICAL MANAGEMENT

DIAGNOSIS. Often termed "the great imitator," gout may masquerade as septic arthritis, RA, or neoplasm. The diagnosis can be delayed for weeks or months. A definitive diagnosis of gout is made when monosodium urate crystals (tophi) are found in synovial fluid, connective tissue, or articular cartilage.

Serum uric acid levels are elevated in approximately 10% of the affected population (more than mg/dL); the presence of hyperuricemia alone does not equal a diagnosis of gout, nor does a normal serum level exclude its presence. The diagnosis is made most often on the basis of the triad of acute monoarticular arthritis, hyperuricemia, and prompt response to drug therapy.[595,711]

Bone abnormalities seen on imaging studies (e.g., calcification, overhanging edges of bone erosions with sclerotic margins but with normal bone density) may be

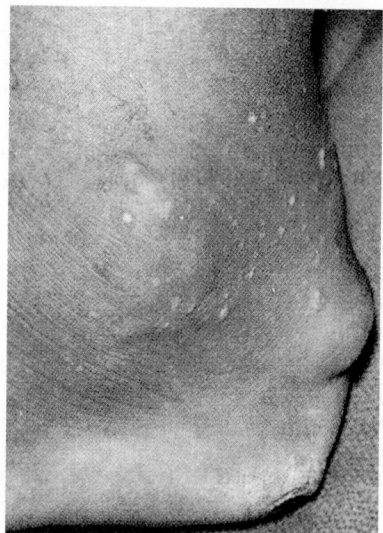

Figure 27-27

Tophus, a chalky deposit of sodium urate present in the Achilles tendon and foot, occurs in cardiac transplant recipients who have an associated history of gout. These tophi form most often around the joints in cartilage, bone, bursa, and subcutaneous tissue, producing a chronic foreign-body inflammatory response. Tophi are not clinically significant for the therapist, but indicate an underlying condition that requires medical attention. (From Howe S, Edwards NL: Controlling hyperuricemia and gout in cardiac transplant recipients, *J Musculoskelet Med* 12:15–24, 1995.)

present in a small number of affected individuals. These are usually late findings in the disease process, occurring most often in the chronic phase.

Musculoskeletal ultrasonography is another imaging method used to evaluate gouty joints. This noninvasive technique shows where the crystals have been deposited in the joint. Ultrasound pictures show the hyaline cartilage—the cartilage that coats the ends of the bones to protect them.

Ultrasonography can also show the *double contour sign*. This sign looks like a top covering or extra coating of the joint surface when crystals are deposited in the hyaline cartilage. Ultrasound studies do not replace fluid removal and examination under a microscope because ultrasound does not confirm infection.[474]

TREATMENT AND PROGNOSIS. The goals of intervention are twofold: (1) to end acute attacks and prevent recurrent attacks and (2) to correct the hyperuricemia. The American College of Rheumatology have established treatment guidelines for pharmacological and nonpharmacologic treatments. The guidelines are based on the acute and chronic presentation of this disease.[452]

The first line of pharmacologic treatments is the use of an xanthine oxidase inhibitor (e.g., allopurinol) to lower the level of urate in the bloodstream. These agents should lessen the level of symptoms and can prevent or lessen future gout attacks by slowing the rate at which the body makes uric acid in cases of excess uric acid production.

NSAIDs are effective in treating the pain and inflammation of an acute attack. Occasionally intraarticular injection of corticosteroids is used to manage acute attacks. These pharmacologic agents must be taken on a continuous basis to maintain a lower concentration of uric acid in the blood. Colchicine with its antiinflammatory effects is another medication given during the acute phase but is less commonly used now because of its narrow therapeutic range and numerous side effects. Involved joints should also be rested, elevated, and protected (e.g., crutches, foot cradle, assistive devices, orthotics, proper shoe wear).

Once the acute attack has been relieved, the hyperuricemia may be treated, especially in the case of recurrent attacks of acute gouty arthritis or chronic gout. This requires lifelong management, and compliance is absolutely necessary. Dietary changes, weight loss, and moderation of alcohol intake are all important. Controlling the hyperuricemia is the key to preventing this disease from becoming chronic and disabling.[223]

New understanding of the exact mechanisms behind gout has led to the development of new agents for individuals with *refractory* gout. Refractory means the symptoms are not resolved with standard treatment and the condition has become chronic and unmanageable.

These new treatments, called *uricase therapy*, are not available yet for use in the general public. They are just in the experimental stages. Drug companies are looking to find ways to use enzymes that convert uric acid into an acid that will be readily absorbed and passed out of the body. One of these enzymes is uricase. Humans don't have this enzyme naturally but other animals do. The use of pig and baboon uricase (called *pegloticase therapy*) is under investigation and pending FDA approval.[474]

Some researchers are using medications off-label (i.e., drugs already on the market but used for other problems).

One drug in particular (rasburicase) is used to reduce subsequent elevation of plasma uric acid released as a result of tumor lysis after cancerous tumors have been treated. It seems to work, but it is very expensive ($8000) per dose so its use may not be feasible if it turns out that long-term use is required.[474]

Right now uricase (biologic) therapy is an induction therapy, which means it is administered intravenously. Infusion reactions are holding things back a bit. At least 10% of the people receiving induction therapy experience severe adverse reactions, including flushing, hives, low blood pressure, chest pain, and muscle cramping. It may be possible eventually to start with an intravenous dose, get the symptoms under control, and then switch to a pill form of the same medication to maintain results.

The future looks promising for gout sufferers. It seems certain that better understanding of purine metabolism will come to light in the very near future. Experts feel sure that it's only a matter of time before scientists hit upon a pharmaceutical "cure" for cases of gout that can't be managed otherwise with diet and exercise.

SPECIAL IMPLICATIONS FOR THE THERAPIST 27-19

Gout

Education on the causes and risk factors for gout will be the keystone treatment for gout. Those individuals who are obese will need a well-monitored exercise program to improve physical health and to promote weight loss.[452] The onset of severe joint pain with a swollen, hot joint should always concern the therapist. Gout, infection, and hemarthrosis are all conditions that could account for this clinical scenario. Gout may be associated with fever and malaise, making it difficult to distinguish clinically from a septic joint.

People with long-term gout often develop numerous complications, including orthopedic conditions of the foot and lower extremities, diabetes, and cardiovascular diseases. These individuals report difficulties with their quality of life that include physical and mental health issues. The therapist's plan of care should include interventions to address these comorbidities and to address quality-of-life issues.[487]

A septic joint is an orthopedic emergency so anytime a red, hot painful joint is observed without prior medical diagnosis, immediate medical evaluation is necessary. Quick diagnosis and initiation of intervention are necessary to control or prevent damage to the joint structures.

Sometimes individuals with gout experience a flare-up after taking urate-lowering agents. This reaction can come as a surprise, as the expectation is that the pain and swelling will get better. Flares of this kind occur when old deposits of crystals stored in the tissues are being released. The increase in symptoms is not a sign that new crystals are forming. The affected individual should not stop taking prescribed medications without first checking with the medical doctor. Getting rid of the old crystals can help protect the joint from further damage.[474]

Neuroarthropathy

Neuroarthropathy, or neuropathic arthropathy, is an articular abnormality related to neurologic deficits, regardless of the nature of the primary disease. Other terms applied to this disorder are Charcot joint, neurotropic or neuropathic joint disease, and neuropathic osteoarthropathy. Many underlying diseases or conditions can cause neuropathy, such as syphilis, syringomyelia, meningomyelocele, injury or trauma, multiple sclerosis, congenital vascular anomalies, diabetes mellitus, alcoholism, amyloidosis, infection (e.g., tuberculosis, leprosy), pernicious anemia, and intraarticular or systemic administration of corticosteroids.[304] See the individual discussions of each condition.

Early joint changes as seen on imaging studies may look very similar to those of OA. When present, advanced neuroarthropathy is more clearly defined, with enlarging and persistent effusion and minimal subluxation, fracture, or fragmentation. Microfractures can progress quickly into gross fragmentation, and the joint may appear to deteriorate quickly over a period of days to weeks.

Malalignment with angular deformity, subluxation, or dislocation leads to increased stress on the articular bone, contributing to sclerosis and fractures. Fracture lines can originate in the subchondral region and extend in an extraarticular direction. Management with arthrodesis or arthroplasty is often unsuccessful. More specific intervention approaches are discussed with each individual underlying condition.

BONE

Fracture

Overview

A fracture is any defect in the continuity of a bone, ranging from a small crack to a complex fracture with multiple segments. Fractures can be classified into four general categories: (1) fracture by sudden impact (traumatic), (2) stress or fatigue fracture, (3) insufficiency fracture, and (4) pathologic fracture.

A *stress* or *fatigue* fracture, sometimes referred to as a stress reaction or bone stress injury, is defined as a partial break (reaction) or complete break (fracture) in the bone caused by the bone's inability to withstand stress applied in a rhythmic, repeated, microtraumatic fashion. More simply stated, a fatigue fracture occurs if normal bone is exposed to repeated abnormal stress, and an insufficiency fracture occurs if normal stress is applied to abnormal bone.

These types of overuse stress or fatigue fractures are most common in track and field athletes, distance runners, and soldiers in training. Most occur in the lower extremity and affect the tibial shaft and metatarsal bones, but they can also occur at the pubic ramus, femoral neck, or fibula; an increasing number of stress fractures have been reported in the knee (tibial plateau, proximal tibial shaft, femoral condyles).[707,733]

The two kinds of stress fractures are compressive and distractive. Compressive stress fractures occur as a result of forceful heel strike during prolonged marching or running. Distractive stress reactions occur as a result of muscle pull and can become more serious if displacement occurs.

Insufficiency fractures (sometimes referred to as insufficiency stress fractures) result from a normal stress or force acting on bone that has deficient elastic resistance or has been weakened by decreased mineralization. Reduced bone integrity can result from many factors but occurs most commonly from the effects of radiation, postmenopausal or corticosteroid-induced osteoporosis, or other underlying metabolic bone disease (e.g., hyperparathyroidism, osteomalacia, rickets, and osteodystrophy). Insufficiency fractures arise insidiously or as a result of minor trauma. It has been proposed that weight bearing alone can be enough "trauma" to transmit a traumatic force to the compromised spine.[490]

Pathologic fracture is a term used to describe a fracture that occurs in bone rendered abnormally fragile by neoplastic or other disease conditions. Insufficiency fractures can be thought of as a subset of pathologic fractures, occurring in bones with structural alterations due to osteopenia, osteoporosis, or disorders of calcium metabolism. A complete fracture extends through the entire bone; a greenstick fracture does not. A greenstick fracture often has to be completed before effective healing occurs. Other incomplete fractures may be called torus (or buckle), crack, or hairline fractures.

Fractures can be described for the orientation of the fracture line through the bone. Transverse, oblique, and spiral fracture lines are commonly found from traumatic causes of bone fractures. Comminution describes a fracture with multiple fragments at the fracture site and can be associated with different fracture lines. Fractures can also be described by the orientation of the fracture fragment ends and the long axis of the bones to describe if they are in a position and alignment that will allow for normal healing of the fracture. Figures 27-28 and 27-29 show the different types of fractures (Box 27-15). Displaced, open fractures are more likely to be unstable. Compressive or shear forces can cause stable fractures to shift, becoming unstable. Unstable fractures are more likely to require surgery to stabilize them.

An *epiphyseal* fracture occurs in the growth centers of children and adolescents, located in the long bones. Growth can be arrested or altered in this type of fracture, and immediate intervention is required. An *articular* fracture occurs on or near a joint and is described by the course of the fracture line (e.g., T- or Y-shaped, transcondylar, supracondylar, intercondylar).

Pelvic and *sacral* fractures were traditionally classified according to stability, but with improvements in orthopedic procedures, these types of fractures are more often classified based on causative force vectors; this system is more appropriate as they direct surgical fixation.[775,903] The mechanisms of force vectors from the injury include anteroposterior compression, lateral compression, vertical shear, and combined/mixed mechanisms.

Pelvic and sacral fractures may include a single pubic or ischial ramus, ipsilateral pubic and ischial rami, pelvic wing of the ilium (Duverney fracture), or fracture of the sacrum or coccyx. If the injury only results in a slight widening of the symphysis pubis or the anterior sacroiliac

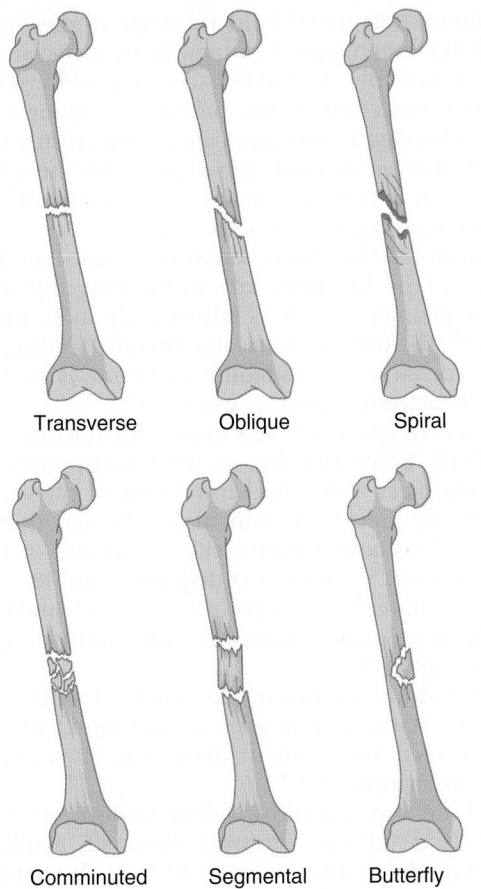

Figure 27-28

Classification of fractures. In a transverse fracture, the fracture line is at a right angle to the long axis of the bone; this fracture is usually produced by shearing force. An oblique or spiral fracture occurs following a twisting or torsional force; fragments displace easily in the oblique fracture, whereas nonunion rarely occurs in a spiral fracture because of the wide area of surface contact. A fracture is comminuted if the bone is broken into more than two fragments and segmental if a fragment of the free bone is present between the main fragments. The separation of a wedge-shaped piece of bone is called a butterfly fracture. See Box 27-15 for other types of fractures and their definitions.

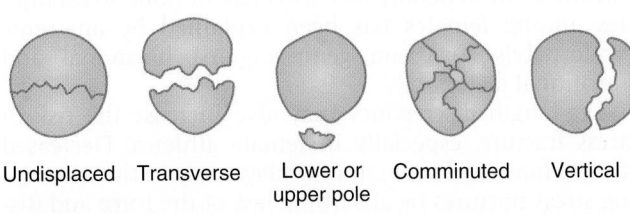

Figure 27-29

Types of patella fracture. Patella fractures are classified as transverse, stellate, or vertical. These three categories can be further divided into displaced and undisplaced. The arterial blood supply to the patella is derived from two systems of vessels from branches of the geniculate arteries. These two systems supply the middle third and apex of the patella. In cases of displaced transverse fractures, the proximal blood supply may be compromised, leading to avascular necrosis of the proximal segment. (From Shankman G: Fundamental orthopedic management for the physical therapist assistant, St Louis, 1997, Mosby.)

joint and the pelvic ligaments are intact, the fracture is considered stable. Unstable pelvic fractures can cause rotational instability, vertical instability, or both.

Vertically unstable pelvic fractures occur when a vertical force is exerted on the pelvis such as occurs when an individual falls from a height onto extended legs or is struck from above by a falling object. Disruption of the ligaments (posterior sacroiliac, sacrospinous, and sacrotuberous) is usually complete, and the hemipelvis is displaced anteriorly and posteriorly through the symphysis pubis.

Sacral fractures occur from stress transmitted through the pelvic ring to the sacrum. Lateral compression fractures are seen most often in motor vehicle accidents. Direct stress to the sacrum from a high fall onto the buttocks occurs less often and produces a transverse, rather than vertical fracture.[457]

Vertebral compression fracture (VCF) is one of the most common osteoporosis-related fragility fractures. VCFs often occur with only minor trauma. Only 20% to 25% of people who sustain a VCF develop symptoms severe enough to seek medical attention.[502,709] VCFs are classified as wedge, crush, or biconcave according to their morphologic appearance.[411] The greater prevalence of wedge fractures may be related to DDD, a condition that causes normal intradiscal pressure to shift and concentrate load to the peripheral aspects of the vertebral body.[475]

Etiology

Bone mass is known to reach its maximum size and density (peak bone mass) by the time an adult reaches age 30 years. Women have a tendency to lose bone mass sooner than men, often beginning in their late 30s during the perimenopausal years. Bone loss is accelerated for women during and after menopause; men are more likely to experience bone loss in their mid to late 60s.

Cancellous bones have a greater percentage of trabecular bone (e.g., spine, ribs, jaw, wrist) and are more porous with a greater surface area and are therefore more susceptible to bone loss and fractures. But low bone mass does not always result in fractures. Scientists are actively studying the differences between bones that fracture and those that do not, especially among people of different ethnic backgrounds. It appears that differences in bone structure and repair capability are two major factors to explain differences in fracture rates.

Risk Factors and Incidence

By far the most common traumatic fractures are those associated with sudden impact, such as occurs with assault, abuse, traumatic falls, or motor vehicle accidents.

Motor vehicle accidents involve fractures of the skull, nasal bone, and mandible most often; high-velocity injuries including automobile or motorcycle accidents often result in open fractures of the lower extremity. In the general population, radius and/or ulna fractures comprise the largest proportion of upper-extremity fractures. The most affected age group is children ages 5 to 14 years as a result of accidental falls at home.[171]

Age is an important risk factor for fractures. The rate of hip fracture increases at age 50 years, doubling every 5 to 6 years. Increasing age and low bone mineral density (BMD) are the two most important independent risk factors for an initial vertebral or nonvertebral fracture.[92]

Decreased BMD associated with osteoporosis accounts for the largest number of fractures among the older adult population (see "Osteoporosis" in Chapter 24). In fact, a fracture may be the first sign of an underlying diagnosis of osteoporosis, and a serious fracture is a risk factor itself for future fractures in high-risk groups. There are an estimated 1.5 million osteoporosis-related fragility fractures in the United States each year.

VCFs are the most common osteoporosis-related fractures, accounting for approximately 700,000 injuries. The incidence increases with age and with decreasing bone density. Factors that increase the risk of a first vertebral fracture include previous non–spine fracture, low BMD at all sites, low body mass index, current smoking, low milk consumption during pregnancy, low levels of daily physical activity, previous fall(s), and regular use of aluminum-containing antacids.[621]

One in every two women older than 50 years of age will experience fragility fractures secondary to osteoporosis.[302] Data collected from the U.S. Medicare population older than age 65 years revealed a pattern of rapidly rising rates with age for fractures of the pelvis, hip, and other parts of the femur among women.

Fractures at the hip were most common, accounting for 38% of the fractures identified. The proximal humerus, distal radius/ulna, and ankle also were common fracture sites. Fractures distal to the elbow or knee had only small increases in incidence with age older than 65 years. Women have higher fracture rates than men of the same race, and whites generally have higher rates than blacks of the same gender.[58,82]

Men are less likely to develop osteoporosis and subsequent fracture, but they are not immune to this condition and are frequently undertreated for osteoporosis even after a fracture.[453] Epidemiologic studies have confirmed that osteoporosis in men is an increasing health problem, possibly attributable to increased longevity and increased awareness of the problem.[282] Bone loss as a result of hypogonadism associated with erectile dysfunction, or induced by androgen-deprivation therapy in the treatment of prostate cancer, increases the risk of osteoporosis and thus fracture for some men.

Fracture risk has been consistently associated with a history of falls, including falls to the side, and attributes of bone geometry, such as tallness, hip axis, and femur length.[617] The way a person falls, laterally landing directly on the trochanter versus falling backward, is an independent risk factor for hip fractures.[82,311,648]

Box 27-16 lists other risk factors for fracture; see also Box 27-18. Some risk factors for fracture, such as age, low body mass index, and low levels of physical activity, probably affect fracture incidence through their effects on bone density and propensity to fall and inability to absorb impact.[617] Vitamin D deficiency and its link with generalized muscle weakness leading to falls and fractures is likely more prevalent among older adults than previously thought.[290,861]

Low vitamin D status has been linked with decreased functional status and progress during inpatient rehabilitation in men and women (mean age: 70 years) with a variety of diagnoses.[454]

The long-term use of high-dose proton pump inhibitors, such as Prilosec, Protonix, Prevacid, Aciphex, and Nexium used to reduce stomach acid has also been linked with hip fractures. The presumed mechanism is reduced bone density via interference with calcium absorption. A certain amount of acid is needed to absorb most forms of calcium. Proton pump inhibitors may also inhibit another proton pump important in bone remodeling. Until further information is known about this effect, individuals at risk for fractures who are also taking proton pump inhibitors should talk with their physicians about fracture prevention.[624,901]

Stress Fractures. In the case of stress reactions and fractures, an abrupt increase in the intensity or duration of training (i.e., military trainees, athletes preparing for marathons) is often an additional risk factor.[733] Female recruits are at increased risk for pelvic and sacral stress fractures. The generally increased risk of bone stress injuries among females has been explained by anatomic (wide pelvis, coxa vara, genu valgum), hormonal, and nutritional factors.[549]

Leg-length discrepancy may also increase the risk of stress fracture, especially in female athletes. Decreased muscle mass and strength may play a role in the developing stress fractures by absorbing less of the force and distributing or exerting more load to the bone. Good muscle strength may decrease the strain on bone and delay muscle fatigue. Muscle fatigue may cause alterations in running mechanics that could increase ground reaction forces exerted on the bone.[448,549]

Pathogenesis

The repair or regeneration of bone involves a complex sequence of cellular activities, beginning with acute hematoma formation and early inflammatory response

Box 27-16

RISK FACTORS FOR FRACTURES

- Trauma
  - Motor vehicle accidents
  - Industrial or work-related accidents
  - Assault
  - History of falls; risk factors for falls (see also Boxes 27-18 and 27-19)
  - Overuse (marathon runners, military); sudden changes in training (duration, intensity)
  - Participation in sports, including dance (recreational or competitive)
- Advanced age
- Women: postmenopausal osteoporosis; military: stress fractures
- Men: hypogonadism (erectile dysfunction, prostate cancer)
- Any insufficiency* or fragility fractures, especially vertebral fractures
- Residence in a long-term care facility
- Poor self-rated health
- Low physical function
  - Slow gait speed; gait disorders or movement dysfunction; low levels of physical activity
  - Difficulty in turning while walking; inability to pivot
  - Use of a walking aid (cane, walker)
  - Decreased quadriceps strength (e.g., inability to rise from chair without using arms)
  - Increased postural (body) sway†[425,698]
  - Impaired cognition, dementia
- Physical attributes
  - Low physical fitness
  - Decreased bone mineral density
  - Bone geometry (see text description)
  - Leg-length discrepancy
  - Height
  - Low body mass index; low muscle mass
  - Poor nutrition; eating disorder; vitamin D deficiency
- Alcohol and/or substance use
- Other diseases or conditions
  - Osteoporosis; failure to treat or undertreatment of osteoporosis
  - Osteogenesis imperfecta
  - Osteonecrosis
  - Neoplasm; skeletal metastases; surgical resection for tumor
- Radiation treatment
- High-dose, long-term use of proton pump inhibitors

*Fracture in bones with nontumorous disease (e.g., rheumatoid arthritis, osteoporosis, following radiation) at normal load.[256]

†Postural sway is a corrective mechanism associated with staying upright and can be used as a measure of balance. Postural sway increases with age (reflecting decreased balance) and with the use of benzodiazepines.[698]

and followed by granulation tissue infiltration, recruitment, proliferation, and differentiation of osteogenic and often chondrogenic cells; matrix formation and mineralization; and eventual remodeling.[305]

The process is orchestrated and guided by a series of biologic and mechanical signals. Molecular signaling cascades and nutrition are key factors in the success of bone repair or regeneration. Bone response to injury and the phases of the reparative process are discussed in greater detail in Chapter 6 (see also Fig. 6-26).

When a bone is fractured, its normal blood supply is disrupted. Osteocytes (bone cells) will die from the trauma and the resulting ischemia. Bone macrophages will remove the dead bone cells and the damaged bone. A precursor fibrocartilaginous growth of tissue occurs before the laying down of primary bone, eventually followed by the laying down and remodeling of normal adult bone.

This complex process of fracture healing can be broken down into five stages: (1) hematoma formation, (2) cellular proliferation, (3) callous formation, (4) ossification, and (5) consolidation and remodeling. Some resources describe the phases of bone healing more succinctly as inflammatory, reparative, and remodeling.[382]

During the initial 48 to 72 hours after fracture, hematoma formation occurs as clotting factors from the blood initiate the formation of a fibrin meshwork. This meshwork is the framework for the ingrowth of fibroblasts and capillary buds around and between the bony ends.

During the cellular proliferation phase, osteogenic cells proliferate and eventually form a fibrocartilage collar around the fracture site. Eventually the collars and the ends of the bones unite. The cartilage is eventually replaced by bone as osteoblasts continue to move into the site (callous formation and ossification). Finally, the excessive bony callus is resorbed and the bone remodels in response to the mechanical stresses placed on it.

Clinical Manifestations

The primary manifestations of fracture include pain and tenderness, increased pain on weight bearing, edema, ecchymosis, loss of mobility, and loss of function of the involved body part. Point tenderness over the site of the fracture is usually present, but not all fractures are equally painful. Insufficiency fractures of the spine, pelvis, or sacrum often present with nonspecific low back, groin, or pelvic pain, mimicking other clinical conditions such as local tumor or metastatic disease or disk disease.

With many fractures, attempts to move the injured limb will provoke severe pain, but in the presence of a fatigue fracture (stress reaction) active movement is typically painless. Resistive motions or repetitive weight bearing will cause pain, and the area will be exquisitely tender to local palpation. There may be edema observed in the area of the fracture. Clinical manifestations are most severe when the fracture is unstable.

VCFs are often painless but are associated with height loss and respiratory dysfunction. When painful, the initial pain may be sharp and severe, but after a few days it may become dull and achy. The pain may be reproducible on examination with pressure over the spinous process of the involved level. Pain associated with VCFs tends to be postural (i.e., worse with spinal extension or even standing up straight); it can be debilitating enough to confine some older adults to a wheelchair or bed.

Complications

The deformity associated with an extremity fracture is often obvious, but the deformity of a spinal fracture is not always so. For example, a compression fracture of a thoracic vertebral body may result in an anterior wedging of the body but only a mildly accentuated thoracic kyphosis. When thoracic kyphosis does occur, decreased trunk strength and decreased pulmonary function are possible.[488]

Older adults with VCF are two to three times more likely to die secondary to pulmonary causes (e.g., congestive heart failure, pneumonia) and have an increased risk for hospitalization and mortality.[225] Urinary retention and gastrointestinal symptoms are also common manifestations in people with VCFs. Neurologic deficits can also occur, but these symptoms usually resolve; less than 5% of affected individuals need surgical decompression.[746]

Occasionally, in an adolescent or young adult who has not achieved mature bone growth, a persistent but painless prominence may occur 1 to 3 months after a minimally displaced fracture. It is located on the compression side of the fracture within the newly formed subperiosteal bone (intracortical) as a result of encapsulation or calcification of a hematoma. This transient postfracture cyst is benign, but must be medically diagnosed as such, as it cannot be distinguished clinically from infection or tumors.[810]

The healing of a fracture can be abnormal in one of several ways. The fracture may heal in the expected amount of time but in an unsatisfactory position with residual bony deformity called *malunion*. The fracture may heal, but this may take considerably longer than the expected time (*delayed union*); or the fracture may fail to heal (*nonunion*) with resultant formation of either a fibrous union or a false joint (*pseudoarthrosis*).

Loss of blood supply to the fracture fragments may impede healing by preventing adequate revascularization. Motion at the fracture site or an excessively wide gap can also contribute to nonunion. Individuals with nonunion often have pain, heat, and tenderness at the fracture site.

Other complications may include associated soft-tissue injury, complications secondary to treatment, infection, skin ulceration, growth disturbances, posttraumatic degenerative arthritis, soft tissue or connective tissue adhesions, arthrodesis, myositis ossificans, osteomyelitis, refracture, nerve injury and neurologic complications, and vascular compromise.[716]

MEDICAL MANAGEMENT

PREVENTION. Therapists have a key role in the prevention of falls. Education and risk evaluation are two important variables in preventing fractures from occurring (Box 27-17). Combining BMD with fracture assessment (e.g., use of dual x-ray absorptiometry to assess vertebral fractures) has a positive impact on lowering repeat fractures.[281, 617]

Studies are under way to determine the most cost-effective strategy for fracture prevention. In the case of hormone replacement therapy, treating those people with low BMD levels (secondary prevention) seems to be more cost-effective than general treatment (primary prevention).

High-risk groups can be identified (e.g., long-term care residents) and treated with low-cost interventions (e.g., calcium plus vitamin D or external padded hip protectors). Use of hip protectors (padded, convex plastic shields worn inside specially designed undergarments) to prevent hip fracture for those people at risk has met with mixed results.[81,295,435,727] Problems such as insufficient supply, discomfort while sleeping, difficulty toileting,

---

Box 27-17

PREVENTION OF FALLS

- Wear low-heeled, closed footwear with rubber soles or good gripping ability; avoid smooth-bottomed shoes or boots. This applies to slippers; wear slippers or shoes when getting out of bed at night.
- Provide adequate lighting for hallways, stairways, bathrooms; use a flashlight outdoors. Wear glasses at night when getting out of bed for any reason.
- Conduct a home safety evaluation. Remove loose cords, slippery throw rugs; repair uneven stairs, steps, sidewalks.
- Avoid oversedation; carefully monitor medications (especially sleep medications, antidepressants) and drink alcohol in moderation (never drink alcohol if taking medications without your physician's approval).
- Provide sturdy handrails on both sides of stairways.
- Provide grab bars on bathroom walls and nonskid strips on mats in tub or shower and beside tub or shower.
- Avoid going outdoors when it is wet, icy, or slippery; wear footwear with good traction or clip-on ice grippers; avoid walking on wet leaves or garden or yard clippings or debris.
- Carry items close to the body and leave one hand free to grasp railings or for balance.
- Know the location of pets before walking through a room or area of the house or apartment; maintain floors free of clutter and small objects.
- Put aside pride and use an appropriate assistive device as recommended by the therapist (e.g., cane, walking stick, walker); walkers equipped with a seat work well for people with limited endurance.
- Encourage a program of physical activity and exercise that is attainable.
- Avoid changing position quickly, such as when getting out of a chair or bed. Stand for a moment to see if you are dizzy so that you can sit down again if necessary. See discussion of postural hypotension for prevention strategies (see Chapter 12).
- Keep items on shelves in the kitchen and elsewhere within reach. Do not stand on a chair or stepladder to reach items. Consider the consequences of a fall and broken hip if you are tempted and if you are thinking, "Nothing will happen, I will be fine."

---

correct positioning of the shield, and ease of application for anyone who is overweight or obese and/or has arthritis has made the use of hip protectors less than optimal. Instead of relying on hip protectors, older adults should be encouraged to increase bone mass through nutrition and physical activity and take extra care with medications that cause dizziness. The use of hip protectors has been advocated for institutionalized individuals. Cognitive impairment is actually helpful in terms of compliance and positive results.[634,726]

Fall prevention is important in adults older than 60 years of age (see Box 27-17). Further studies comparing different preventive regimens are needed.[864] Fracture prevention in the athlete begins with assessment of the athlete's past history, training variables, biomechanical factors, and shoe wear. In the military population, most bone stress injuries occur during the 8-week basic training period; injury-prevention programs to target this group are advised.[549] The reader is referred to other sources for more specific assessment techniques.[24,105,106,553]

DIAGNOSIS. Fractures are often diagnosed by visual inspection and confirmed by plain radiographs. Many VCFs are detected incidentally on chest radiographs. Fractures can often involve surrounding soft tissue, vascular, and neurologic structures, requiring careful assessment at the time of injury.

In the case of stress reactions (stress fractures), conventional radiographic studies (x-rays) are usually inadequate; often the lag time between manifestation of symptoms and detection of positive radiographic findings ranges from 1 week to several months. Up to 35% of sacral fractures are undetected on plain radiographs; cross-sectional imaging such as CT or MRI may be needed to identify and confirm sacral fractures. MRI is the gold standard for identifying bone stress injuries of the lower extremities, especially during the early stages of developing injury. CT is the imaging technique of choice to identify pathologic fractures.[504,549,890]

Radionuclide bone scanning (scintigraphy) has become a useful imaging study because it can demonstrate subtle changes in bone metabolism long before conventional radiography. MRI is also sensitive for detecting pathophysiologic changes associated with stress injuries but is more expensive and is reserved for cases in which other imaging findings are indeterminate.[310, 598]

TREATMENT. The medical approach to management of fractures is based on the location of the fracture, assessment of fracture type, need for reduction, presence of instability after reduction, and functional requirements of the affected individual. For example, stress fractures are usually uncomplicated and can be managed by rest and restriction from activity, whereas an unstable fracture of any bone may require immediate surgical intervention.[504]

Individual factors such as age, activity level, the person's general health and overall condition, and the presence of any other injuries must also be taken into consideration. The goal of treatment is to promote hemostasis, hemodynamic stability, comfort, and early mobilization to prevent potential complications from immobility (e.g., constipation, deep vein thrombosis, pulmonary embolism, pneumonia). In the case of stress fractures, the initial period of rest is followed by a gradual return to activity. The progression of return to sports is based on symptomatic response to increasing activity.

The presence of osteoporosis complicates the need for immobilization or spinal fusion. Nonoperative treatment for VCFs includes activity modification, bracing, assistive devices, pharmacology (e.g., narcotic analgesics, calcitonin), and physical therapy. Hospital admission and bed rest is required for up to 20% of the population for whom conservative care is not possible or adequate.

The debilitating effects of immobilization and keeping older adults bed bound is well recognized, with increased risks for developing pulmonary complications, pressure ulcers, deep vein thrombosis, and urinary tract infections. And BMD is further reduced by immobility and bed rest, thereby increasing the risk of additional VCFs and other fragility fractures.[746]

Surgery. Surgical intervention may be required for VCFs, including bone grafts or bone graft substitutes, internal fixation (e.g., metal plating, wiring, screws),

traction, or reduction and casting or immobilization. VCFs also may be treated by surgical decompression and fusion, vertebroplasty, and kyphoplasty.[413] Analgesic therapy is effective for most people with VCFs from bone metastases.[665]

Minimally invasive procedures for the management of acute vertebral fracture have been developed. Injection of FDA-approved polymethylmethacrylate bone cement into the fractured vertebra is being used around the United States in procedures known as *vertebroplasty* or *kyphoplasty.*[702]

In kyphoplasty, using a fluoroscope, the surgeon locates the spinal fracture, inserts a needle into that vertebra, and inflates a tiny balloon at the tip of the needle, pushing the vertebral body as close to its normal position as possible and leaving a defined cavity that can be filled. Once the collapsed portion of the vertebra has been raised, the balloon is deflated and removed and bone cement is injected through the same needle into the vertebral body. The cement hardens, quickly sealing the fracture. No postsurgery bracing is required. Reports of acute pain relief have been documented, but the long-term effect of one or more reinforced rigid vertebrae on the risk of fracture of adjacent vertebrae remains unknown at this time.

A similar technique is being developed for the treatment of a fractured distal radius with calcium phosphate bone cement injected into the trabecular defect of the fracture site. Using a gene transfer vector, this remodelable bone cement allows for earlier removal (at 2 weeks instead of 6 weeks or more) of the cast or splint and early mobilization.

Results have been very encouraging, with better clinical and radiologic results than with conventional treatment.[721] In the United States, other researchers are experimenting with the use of this cement on other bones, such as the calcaneus, and for use in cranial reconstruction.[4,185,459,494]

Rehabilitation and Fractures. With or without surgical intervention, following bone fracture there is usually a period of immobilization (casting or splinting, fracture brace) to remove longitudinal stress. This period allows for the phagocytic removal of necrotic bone tissue and the initial deposition of the fibrocartilaginous callus.

For any type of fracture, management during the perifracture period is directed toward blood clot prevention (mechanical and/or pharmacologic), the avoidance of substances that inhibit fracture repair (e.g., nicotine, corticosteroids), and the possible need for supplemental caloric intake. Treatment should be initiated for anyone with osteoporosis, including calcium and vitamin D supplements, oral bisphosphonates, selective estrogen receptor modulators, calcitonin, and teriparatide (see discussion of treatment of osteoporosis in Chapter 24).

Gradually progressive stress will be applied to stimulate fracture callus formation and healing. In the case of pelvic or lower extremity fractures, the timing and extent of mobilization depend on the type of fixation used. For example, if an external fixation is applied for fracture stabilization, mobilization can occur within tolerance of the person's symptoms almost immediately.

Modalities and Fractures. Many studies carried out on the effect of ultrasound waves on fracture healing show that bone heals faster when it responds to applied pressure. Low-intensity (0.1 W/cm^2) pulsed ultrasound (2-msec bursts of sine waves of 1.0 MHz [frequency]; duration of 20 minutes daily) is an established therapy for fracture repair.[61,883]

In both animal and human trials, such ultrasound has been shown to facilitate fresh fracture repair and initiate healing in fractures with repair defects. However, the mechanism by which ultrasound achieves these outcomes is not clear. One possible mechanism is the direct stimulation of bone formation. Ultrasound has a direct effect on blood flow distribution around a fracture site, resulting in greater callous formation. This increased circulation serves as a principal factor facilitating the acceleration of fracture healing by ultrasound.[46,806,883]

Bone Grafting. Bone grafting to enhance bone repair can be applied during the repair stage of bone formation. Autogenous bone grafting takes bone from another part of the body and implants it in the bony defect that requires healing. The graft is most often taken from the iliac crest or fibula and contains all the components needed for bone healing. Donor site pain is a common complaint and the primary reason why some people prefer to use allogenic bone graft material from a donor (bone bank).

Tissue engineering of bone has emerged as a new treatment alternative in bone repair and regeneration.[205] The use of biodegradable plastics has been developed to provide scaffolding for the regrowth of tissue with the potential for healing fractures and repairing bone lost to tumors, osteoporosis, trauma, and other disorders. The use of osteoconductive scaffolds, growth factors and osteoprogenitor cells have been proposed as methods for inducing bone formation when blood supply and osteoporotic conditions are present.

Commercially available demineralized bone matrix can be used to enhance bone healing, especially in people with nonunions or after the removal of bone cysts or fibrous lesions. Demineralized bone matrix still retains some of the original trabecular structure, which can function as a scaffold for osteoconduction.[336]

The addition to this scaffolding of growth hormones or other bioactive molecules that enhance bone repair to create a "smart matrix" has the potential of speeding up the healing of fractures and repair of more serious crush injuries or nonunion of bone. Further development of the concept includes gene transfer as a cellular vehicle for delivery of bone morphogenetic protein to promote bone formation.[22,479]

Gene Therapy. Gene therapy involves the introduction of DNA into cells (exogenous or endogenous) in an effort to direct them to overexpress a selected biofactor and thus promote bone repair. Gene transfer may be accomplished in one of several different ways. Cells may be grown in culture and reimplanted into the wound. DNA may be mixed into bone marrow during surgery and then implanted. Or DNA may be injected directly into the wound site. Gene-based strategies are still in the laboratory phase. Introduction into the clinic is expected in the next decade.[205,305]

PROGNOSIS. In general, fractures in children heal in 4 to 6 weeks, in adolescents in 6 to 8 weeks, and in adults in 10 to 18 weeks. This process from fracture to full restoration of the bone will take weeks to months, depending on the type of fracture, location, vascular supply, health, and age of the individual. Nonunion or delayed union is more likely to occur in adults and occurs in up to 10% of all fractures (affecting nearly 500,000 people each year in the United States).[671]

Older adults who have suffered a hip fracture have the highest rate of nonunion complications (15%-30%). These individuals are almost four times more likely to die in the first year after fracture compared with those without fracture. Delay until surgery after hip fracture increases mortality and risk for complications of pneumonia and pressure ulcers significantly.[557, 768] Older women (older than 65 years) who survive the first year after a hip fracture may be at increased risk of death up to 5 years after the injury.[392,528]

Many people are at high risk for premature death or loss of independence following fracture; mortality after fracture is higher among men than among women.[79,92] Less than 50% of older adults with a hip fracture will regain their prior level of function, with approximately half experiencing at least one fall in the year after their fracture.[505,753] The inability to stand up, sit down, or walk 2 weeks after surgery is the strongest predictor for mortality among older adults with surgically repaired hip fractures.[357,812]

A person's condition before fracture (especially that of older adults with hip fractures) has important prognostic implications. Older adults who fall within 6 months following a hip fracture are more likely to demonstrate poorer balance, slower gait speed, and greater decline in ADL from the prefracture level than those who do not fall.[753]

Healthy functional status contributes to faster recovery time with fewer complications and reduced medical expenses.[181] Negative predictors for healing include medications, such as calcium channel blockers and NSAIDs, renal or vascular insufficiency, smoking, alcoholism, and diabetes mellitus. Treatment can also affect healing via inadequate reduction, poor stabilization and fixation, distraction damage to blood supply, and postoperative infection.

Associated complications, such as nerve injury, can occur, and it can take up to 18 months before reinnervation of the motor endplate is complete. Return of function is dependent upon this factor. If there are no signs of improvement by 7 months, spontaneous recovery is unlikely.[890] Exploratory surgery may be indicated at that time.

SPECIAL IMPLICATIONS FOR THE THERAPIST   27-20

Fracture

There are excellent resources regarding fractures available for the therapist managing fractures, including special considerations, orthopedic intervention, rehabilitation considerations, precautions, goals, and therapeutic exercise with expected time frames for healing and rehabilitation.[119,219,382, 466,716]

For the older adult, there are many potential consequences of fractures. These include biomechanical, functional, and psychologic effects that can limit function and result in considerable disability. Biomechanical consequences can include anorexia and weight loss, compression of abdominal contents and decreased lung function from kyphotic posture, and the risk of more fractures.

Chronic, debilitating pain and increased dependence on family and friends occur as part of the functional consequences. Often there is a significant decrease in the individual's ability to perform ADLs because of impaired physical function. These factors, combined with depression and anxiety (and for some people, sleep disorders), result in psychologic consequences.[665] The therapist must remain alert to all of these potential consequences when evaluating each client and planning the best approach to clinical management.

Tobacco use, especially cigarette smoking (both the nicotine and the smoke itself), exposes individuals to toxins that can delay bone healing considerably. Nicotine occupies receptor sites on the stem cells' surface that are intended for acetylcholine, a chemical that helps nerve cells communicate. Normally, stem cells turn into cartilage-forming cells needed to create the scaffold for callus development over the break.[778]

Nicotine's effect on stem cells is to cause them to produce too much cartilage while at the same time blocking nerve transmission and delaying or preventing bone healing. Therapists should review the hazards of smoking with clients who have fractures and encourage smoking cessation or reduction. Using nicotine patches or gum immediately after bone injury may have the same negative effect as continuing to smoke.

Fall (Fracture) Prevention

Physical therapists can have a major impact on fall prevention, contributing to the savings of high costs to the health care industry by assessing for risk factors and preventing falls that lead to fractures (see Boxes 27-17 and 27-18).

Given the risk for fracture and other complications and associated emotional and monetary costs, falls are of significant concern for older adults, their families, and the health care system. Complications caused by falls are the leading cause of death from injury in men and women older than 65 years[724]; a cluster of falls has been observed in older individuals during the months preceding death.[315]

Incidence

Half of all older adults who fall die as a direct or indirect result of that fall; men are more likely to die after a fall than women. The fall rates and mortality rates from falls are on the rise in the United States.[141,651] Other important statistics include the following:

- In 2010, an estimated 21,700 older adults died from fall injuries in the United States.
- At least one out of every four adults age 65 years and older will fall at least once during the next year; it is likely that older adults are falling even more often than is generally reported.[97]

- Some sources say that one out of every three adults 65 years of age and older fall each year.[350,294,383]
- Of adults who fall, 14% return to the hospital within 2 weeks.
- Falls are the second leading cause of traumatic brain injury among persons age 65 years and older.[142,184]
- Older adults who fall often sustain more severe head injuries than their younger counterparts.
- Falls are a major cause of intracranial lesions among older persons because of their greater susceptibility to subdural hematoma.[184]
- Even among older adults who do not sustain an injury during a fall, half cannot get up off the floor; this is a predictive factor for functional decline and/or death.[823,827]
- The complaint of dizziness is one of the most common reasons older adults visit the doctor; the incidence of dizziness doubles, triples, and quadruples decade by decade from 60 to 80 years of age.[891]
- Of these dizziness cases, 45% are caused by vestibular problems.

Risk Factors and Red Flags

Complex layers of skill are required to maintain balance in the upright position. Strength, coordination, endurance, flexibility, vision, vestibular control, and hearing are just a few of the skills involved.

At the same time, there are more than 400 risk factors identified for falls. It may be best to focus on the most common risk factors that are modifiable. Age is certainly a primary risk factor, and although age itself is not modifiable, we must be very aware of which adults are at risk requiring screening and intervention (Box 27-18). The rates of falls and fall injuries increase with age; adults 85 years and older are four to five times more likely to injure themselves in a fall than are adults age 65 to 74 years; the risk of being seriously injured in a fall increases with age.[794]

Movement impairments, cognitive deficits, errors in judgment, and an unsafe environment are common hazards for the aging adult. Gait changes such as an increase in base of support or stride width increases the risk of falls.[468] The use of an assistive device such as a cane or walker is a risk factor, especially when learning to use it for the first time. Incontinence (including functional incontinence) is a risk factor by itself, but when combined with any of these other risk factors raises the risk even more.[354]

Gait or balance instability combined with muscle weakness is among the highest risk factors.[233] Combine any one of these with side effects of medication, the use of alcohol or other drugs (especially when combined with medications), and multiple comorbidities and the risk for falls increases disproportionately.

Many gait disturbances really are a reflection of underlying red flag histories and risk factors. For example, visual impairments can cause increased sway and increased stride width. A past history of falls is a predictor of fear of falling, and a fear of falling will lead to changes in gait such as shorter stride length and slower speed.

Box 27-18

RISK FACTORS FOR FALLS

Age Changes

- Muscle weakness; loss of joint motion (especially lower extremities)
- Abnormal gait
- Impaired or abnormal balance
- Impaired proprioception or sensation
- Delayed muscle response/increased reaction time
- ↓ Systolic blood pressure (<140 mm Hg in adults older than age 65 years)
- Stooped or forward bent posture
- Hearing loss[500]

Environmental/Living Conditions

- Living alone
- Poor lighting
- Throw rugs, loose carpet complex carpet designs, pets underfoot
- Cluster of electric wires or cords
- Stairs without handrails
- Bathroom without grab bars
- Slippery floors (water, urine, floor surface, ice); icy sidewalks, stairs, or streets
- Restraints
- Use of alcohol or other drugs
- Footwear, especially slippers

Pathologic Conditions

- Vestibular disorders; episodes of dizziness or vertigo from any cause
- Orthostatic hypotension (especially before breakfast)
- Chronic pain condition
- Neuropathies
- Cervical myelopathy
- Osteoarthritis; rheumatoid arthritis
- Visual or hearing impairment; multifocal eyeglasses; change in perception of color; loss of depth perception; decreased contrast sensitivity

- Cardiovascular disease
- Urinary incontinence
- Central nervous system disorders (e.g., stroke, Parkinson disease, multiple sclerosis)
- Motor disturbance
- Osteopenia, osteoporosis
- Pathologic fractures
- Any mobility impairments (e.g., amputation, neuropathy, deformity)
- Cognitive impairment; dementia; depression

Medications

- Antianxiety; benzodiazepines
- Anticonvulsants
- Antidepressants
- Antihypertensives
- Antipsychotics
- Diuretics
- Narcotics
- Sedative-hypnotics
- Phenothiazines
- Use of more than four medications (polypharmacy/hyperpharmacotherapy)

Other

- History of falls
- Female sex; postmenopausal status
- Elder abuse/assault
- Nonambulatory status (requiring transfers)
- Gait changes (decreased stride length or speed)
- Postural instability; reduced postural control
- Fear of falling; history of falls[473]
- Dehydration from any cause
- Recent surgery (general anesthesia, epidural)
- Sleep disorder/disturbance; sleep deprivation; daytime drowsiness; brief disorientation after waking up from a nap[796]

From Goodman CC, Snyder TE: *Differential diagnosis for physical therapists: screening for referral*, ed 5, Philadelphia, 2012, WB Saunders. Used with permission.

Past history of joint replacement (knee) increases the risk of tripping, which increases the risk of falling and injury.[550] Painful feet from bunions, corns, overgrown or ingrown toenails, and other podiatric conditions are reported by 50% of older adults when asked. Loss of protective sensation in the feet occurs with diabetes or other peripheral neuropathies.

Neuromusculoskeletal impairments such as muscular weakness, loss of motion, and balance instability, especially when combined with comorbidities such as arthritis, Parkinson disease, multiple sclerosis, stroke, and so on, can result in positive Trendelenburg sign, uneven stride length, limping, uneven weight bearing, and many other changes in gait pattern. Sleep deprivation can lead to slowing in motor reaction time, thus increasing the risk of falls.[226,785]

Comorbidities, such as osteoporosis, arthritis, and other orthopedic problems, limb amputation, diabetes, dementia, chronic lung disease, stroke, and heart disease, are actually more important than polypharmacy

(use of four or more medications of any kind) as risk factors for falls, although polypharmacy is still an important risk factor.[482]

Many of the risk factors fall under the category of red flag histories, too. A past history of falls is one of the most important red flag histories. Obtaining an accurate history can be very challenging. Older adults may forget or deny problems with balance, coordination, and falls (or near falls). They may have lost self-confidence or experience postfall anxiety. Often they modify their behavior and activity level to avoid anything that might cause a fall, so they can honestly answer that they are not having any trouble with falls and have not fallen in the last weeks to months.

Meanwhile, their hygiene is poor because they are afraid to get in and out of the tub or shower. They may restrict and even eliminate community activities for fear of falling. Fear of falling (and especially the fear of not being able to get up) leads to self-imposed functional limitations such as prolonged sitting and all of the natural sequelae that come with an increasingly sedentary lifestyle. Predictors of fear of falling include the following:

- Past history of falls
- Use of assistive device
- Balance or gait instability
- Depression or anxiety

Gait and Movement Characteristics Associated with Falls

In the older adult, gait disturbances and gait changes are often an outward manifestation of an inward or other problem. The therapist should not seek to change the gait pattern *until* the underlying cause of the problem is known. Consider the following gait characteristics associated with falls and assess carefully[56]:

- Decreased gait speed and stride length (linked with weak hip extensors and ankle plantar flexors, reduced push-off phase, reduced ability to propel the body forward during gait)
- Increased stride frequency (linked with muscle weakness and impaired balance requiring increased duration of double support)
- Increased (wider) stance (neurologic changes in diabetes or other conditions, muscle weakness)
- Unsteady gait (speed changes abruptly when unintended and/or person cannot adopt new movement patterns when the task requires it; alcohol or other drug use, dizziness, side effect of medication, decreased ankle/knee proprioception)
- Grabbing for support or stumbling
- Decreased medial–lateral sway (gluteus medius weakness)
- Unsafe or incomplete transfers
- Poor sitting balance; difficulty sitting or unsafe sitting down
- Difficulty rising from a seated position

Visual Impairment

Bifocal or multifocal eyeglasses combined with decreased contrast sensitivity and decreased depth perception lead to bending the head up and down to see the edge of a step. Decreased peripheral vision results in increased postural sway necessary to find center; with decreased reaction times, client cannot regain lost balance, resulting in an injurious fall.

Blindness and visual impairment are among the 10 most common causes of disability in the United States, associated with shorter life expectancy and lower quality of life.[143] Visual impairment (especially combined with cognitive deficits) can lead to errors in judgment such as climbing up on counters, overreaching, and the use of step stools, resulting in falls.

The therapist can assist in identifying possible untreated visual impairment by asking a few simple visual screening questions and making an appropriate referral when indicated:

- *How much difficulty would you have recognizing a friend across the street? [Choose one.]*
  No difficulty

  Some difficulty

  Moderate difficulty

  Extreme difficulty

- *How much difficulty do you have watching television? [Choose one.]*
  No difficulty

  Some difficulty

  Moderate difficulty

  Extreme difficulty

- *When was the last time you had an eye examination in which the pupils were dilated (you had to wear the wraparound sunglasses after the examination)?*

Screening Questions to Identify History of Falls

It may be best to avoid asking the question, Do you have a fear of falling? It is less threatening to ask about the *degree of confidence* in performing an activity, especially for people who view admitting fear as a sign of weakness.[533,826] It may be better to ask questions with answers on a continuum from "no confidence" to "complete (100%) confidence." For example:

- *How confident are you when walking on sidewalks, grass, or uneven surfaces? [Choose one.]*
  Not confident at all

  Slightly confident

  Moderately confident

  Completely confident

- *How confident are you when getting in and out of a car? [Choose one.]*
  Not confident at all

  Slightly confident

  Moderately confident

  Completely confident

- *How confident are you when using a public restroom? [Choose one.]*
  Not confident at all

  Slightly confident

  Moderately confident

  Completely confident

  Follow-up questions may include the following:

- *In the past month, have you had any falls?*
- *In the last month, have you slipped or tripped or lost your balance and almost fallen?*
- *In the last month, have you hit against furniture and bruised yourself?*
- *In the past month, have you landed on the floor? If yes, were you able to get up by yourself or without help?*

Testing

Tests and measures are important in identifying individuals at risk for falls and finding ways to reduce risk factors and prevent falls. The therapist should collect baseline data using validated, reliable tests, keeping in mind that many tests do not identify why the individual is at risk or what intervention strategies would be most effective.[256]

Advances in technology are beginning to provide computerized assessments of sensory integration and motor control that can objectively identify and differentiate balance system disorders (e.g., NeuroCom, Biodex). Since these are not yet available in all facilities, other test measures must be relied upon. For example, the Semmes-Weinstein monofilament test (see Fig. 11-15) can be used to check the protective level of sensation in the feet; impairment of this peripheral system could be the primary risk factor for falls and subsequent fracture.

Decreased sensation in the feet associated with diabetic neuropathy can affect both the timing and quality of gait, requiring retraining of the somatosensory and vestibular systems to help compensate for the somatosensory deficit.[657,658,891] A neurologic miscue can create foot drop and the toe hitting the ground can cause a fall, easily leading to a hip fracture or broken arm.

A loss of protective sensation and diminished information being received by the brain about how much muscle to use at corresponding sequences of toe-offs during gait can occur. Gait and strength training are important in the management of large-fiber neuropathies when impaired vibration, depressed tendon reflexes, and shortening of the Achilles tendon occur.[871]

At the same time, keep in mind that diabetes gait may occur independent of sensory impairment. The increased joint movement, wider stance, and slower pace demonstrated in some individuals with type 2 diabetes may be neurologic in origin and not related to muscle weakness or loss of sensation in the feet.[657,658]

Test for ankle and knee proprioception. Determine the lowest threshold for detecting joint movement, determine the accuracy of joint position sense by comparing or matching each joint to the contralateral joint, and perform the joint repositioning test (test limb segment repositioning without the aid of vision).

Dizziness can be a result of benign paroxysmal positional vertigo caused by particles containing calcium collected in a semicircular canal provoking episodes of spinning vertigo when the head is moved into certain positions. A canalith repositioning procedure (e.g., Epley maneuver, canalith repositioning treatment, liberatory maneuver) "cures" this problem by repositioning the person (from sitting to side-lying or supine) to move particles out of the canal into the utricle, where they can be reabsorbed.

Test for benign paroxysmal positional vertigo by performing the Dix-Hallpike maneuver: assist the person from sitting to supine with the head extended over the edge of the treatment table and rotated 45 degrees to the side of the suspected ear. A positive test result is present when nystagmus is induced after a delay of about 10 seconds. See further discussion in Chapter 38.

Test Functional Limitations

The therapist should use a standardized fall assessment tool and use it consistently.

Tests for functional limitations are useful but do not necessarily identify the cause(s) of balance dysfunction. Many tests are available; the therapist should choose one that best matches the individual's current level of functioning.[197] Some examples include the following:

- Berg Balance Scale: 14-item test measures balance on a continuum from sitting to standing. Valid and reliable measure of balance in older adults; predictive of individuals at risk; helps goal setting and directs intervention; use with lower-functioning patients.
- Timed Up-and-Go Test: used to screen individuals at risk for falls. The client must be able to follow directions. Score of 13.5 seconds indicates that the individual is at risk for falls.[819]
- One-Legged Stance Test: measures postural stability needed to make turns, climb stairs, get dressed, get in a car, step into a bathtub, or step up onto a curb. Risk of falls increases two times if test score is less than 5 seconds; client is at risk if response is 12 seconds or less; marginal risk if response is 13 to 20 seconds; 20+ is considered "safe"; the individual must not sway more than 45 degrees to remain in the "safe" category.
- Sit-to-Stand: must be able to rise from a chair 10 times without using the arms in less than 20 seconds.
- Four Square Step Test: reliable, valid, easy to administer and score; timed test to assess the rapid change in direction while stepping over low objects and movement in four directions; requires higher level of cognitive function and ability to shift weight from one foot to the other while changing direction. Consider using with adults who report falls or near loss of balance as a result of hurrying. Correlates with functional reach test and timed up-and-go test; this means the tests measure similar constructs, so only one of the tests needs to be administered.[206]

Predictive fall risk information can also be obtained and can be useful when putting together the plan of care; fall risk assessment for use with the acute care inpatient population and assessing fear of falling may be appropriate (Box 27-19). No one scale best predicts falls risk in older adults. The activities-specific balance confidence scale and falls efficacy scale are highly correlated with each other. These two tests are moderately correlated with Survey of Activities and Fear of Falling in the Elderly (SAFE).[385]

The therapist should adopt a task- or function-oriented approach. This requires analysis of all the systems involved in the required movement. Rather than focus on individual exercise movements, identify the systems involved in the task and direct intervention to each of those systems.

For example, suppose the person's goal is to be able to pick up objects from the floor. Physical therapy goals are to improve reactive responses to external challenge during stance and ambulation activities as measured by the following: Goal 1—Increase Berg Balance Scale score from 34/56 to 50/56 in 6 weeks; Goal 2—Increase Tinetti's Performance-Oriented Mobility Assessment score from to 19/28 to 24/28.

The intervention should be customized for each individual, targeting the specific underlying impairments, which may include the following:

- Task-specific activities in sitting, standing, and walking (including reaching; weight shifting; progressing from flat surfaces to rocker board, curbs)

PREDICTIVE FALL RISK ASSESSMENT

- Functional reach test: must be able to reach 6 or more inches
- Tinetti's Performance-Oriented Mobility Assessment/Tinetti's Balance Index: objectify gait and balance; predict risk of falls; can be used with people who have an assistive device; does not detect small changes in gait deviation—Gait Abnormality Rating Scale is better for assessing early, minute gait deviations
- Dynamic Gait Index: provides predictive fall-risk information
- Gait Abnormality Rating Scale—Modified: used to assess risk of falling in community-dwelling, frail older adults based on several gait variables
- Physiologic Profile Assessment: series of simple tests of vision, peripheral sensation, muscle force, reaction time, and postural sway that are easy to administer quickly with minimal equipment[507]
- Measurement of vital signs and assessment for postural hypotension: these are important assessment tools in predicting falls

For Use with Acute Care Inpatient Population—Fall Risk Assessment

- STRATIFY: St. Thomas's Risk Assessment Tool in Falling Elderly Inpatients
- Hendrich II Fall Risk Model (http://consultgerirn.org/uploads/File/trythis/try_this_8.pdf)

Fear of Falling

- Falls Efficacy Scale: good for adults who are frail
- Survey of Activities and Fear of Falling in the Elderly (SAFE): assesses 11 activities of daily living
- Activities-Specific Balance Confidence Scale: measure of balance confidence; good with higher functioning older adults; used in studies of amputee populations

---

- Functional strengthening of the ankle, hip, and trunk muscles
- Range of motion in the trunk, hip, lower extremity (especially ankle)
- Static and dynamic balance activities with lateral sway, reach, grasp, manipulation of arms
- Treadmill training

Keep in mind that general strengthening is not enough. Specific muscle groups must be targeted and given enough resistance to build strength. The ankle is considered the most important joint governing balance.[505] Older folks often have reduced ankle motion and strength; these deficits are linked with reduced balance.[564,784] Check for loss of ankle motion; mobilize the calcaneus before stretching. Resistive exercises that produce overload of the hip extensors or ankle dorsiflexors are more effective in improving balance and reducing falls than general low-resistance exercises for the lower extremities.[189]

Exercise and Fall Prevention

Three types of exercise that can help prevent falls and fractures are balance training (prevents falls), strength training (builds bone and muscle), and aerobic training (builds muscle and endurance).

Walking while performing an additional attention-demanding cognitive task is a means to measure whether the client is able to walk automatically. The therapist can assess for dual-task interference, which is the worsening of performance of the main task (e.g., walking) as a result of simultaneously performing an attention-demanding cognitive task (e.g., counting backward).

Automaticity of the main task is reflected by a low or absent dual-task interference effect. Nonautomaticity can have an impact on daily living; gait changes caused by performing an additional cognitive task while walking are associated with increased risk of falling among older adults.[70,851]

Steps to Take

Almost all hip fractures in adults older than age 65 years are caused by falls, and very few are spontaneous, answering the question of whether falls are the result of fractures or vice versa.[630] Hip fractures among older adults occur mainly in well-known environments, during everyday activities, and without overwhelming hazards, emphasizing again the importance of fall prevention/fracture reduction programs for all adults older than age 65 years.

The CDC has recommended community-based falls prevention programs as an effective strategy based on research identifying interventions that can reduce falls.[141] The therapist can be very instrumental in falls prevention by reviewing each of these with all clients age 65 years and older. Four key fall prevention strategies are the following:

- Review of medications to reduce side effects and interactions
- Annual eye examination
- Regular exercise
- Reduction of fall hazards in every room of the home or facility

Modifying the environment is important; it may not prevent falls but it may reduce the severity of injury. The therapist should have the client and/or family complete an environmental safety check. Some studies show that this step is more effective when people are provided with a checklist and encouraged to make the changes themselves. An excellent checklist is available.

Fall-proofing homes; fall prevention education; osteoporosis and fall assessment; osteoporosis prevention (see Chapter 24); and exercise programs to improve balance, coordination, flexibility, strength, endurance, breathing, and posture are all important components of fall prevention and subsequent fracture prevention. Exercise to address all these components is key in fall prevention.[754] For example, lower-extremity weakness or loss of motion, particularly at the ankle and knee, is significantly associated with recurrent falls in the older adult population.[564,784,889]

Specific intervention programs,[752,825] exercise suggestions,[317,330,706] and educational materials[26,404] are available (Box 27-20). Sometimes even the simple step of teaching clients adequate hydration can improve their muscle strength, coordination, and balance, reducing risk for falls (see "Dehydration" in Chapter 5).

Box 27-20

RESOURCES FOR FALLS ASSESSMENT AND PREVENTION

1. American Geriatrics Society, British Geriatrics Society, and American Academy of Orthopaedic Surgeons Panel on Falls Prevention: Guidance for prevention of falls in older persons, *Ann Longterm Care* 9:42–47, 2001. Available online at http://www.healthinaging.org/aging-and-health-a-to-z/topic:falls/. Accessed August 10, 2014.
   Falls: General information
   Medical Evaluation of Falls
   Choosing a Cane or Walker
   Choosing and Starting an Exercise Program
   Improve Your Balance in 10 Minutes/Day
   Decrease Your Risk of Falling
   Tips for Patients with Low Vision
2. Department of Health and Human Services (HHS), Bureau of Primary Health Care: Lower extremity amputation prevention (LEAP) program. Available online at www.hrsa.gov/leap. Accessed December 4, 2012.
3. Rose D. *Fallproof—a comprehensive balance and mobility training program,* ed 2, Champaign, IL, 2009, Human Kinetics.
4. Fall risk assessment for older adults: The Hendrich II model. Available online at http://consultgerirn.org/uploads/File/trythis/try_this_8.pdf. Accessed December 4, 2012.
5. Centers for Disease Control and Prevention. Preventing falls among older adults. Available online at: http://www.cdc.gov/Features/OlderAmericans/. Accessed on November 30, 2012.
6. National Safety Council: Falls. Available online at http://www.nsc.org/safety_home/HomeandRecreationalSafety/Falls/Pages/Falls.aspx. Accessed December 4, 2012.
7. National Council on Aging (NCAA). Falls prevention. Available online at http://www.ncoa.org/improve-health/falls-prevention/. Accessed Jan. 16, 2013.

Computerized assessments of sensory integration and motor control can objectively identify and differentiate balance system disorders. Through advances in technology, therapists are now better able to identify the underlying impairments that may increase a person's risk for falling.[618,865] In addition, clinical risk factors predictive of fracture (e.g., age, gender, height, weight, use of walking aid, current smoking) have been identified. The presence of five or more of these factors increases the rate of fracture (tested in white women).[875] These models have not been validated in other population groups.

Instituting and following a fall protocol in an extended or acute care facility may be able to reduce the incidence of repeated falls. The therapist can help staff set up a study to find out what time of day most falls occur and establish well-supervised small group activities during those times, especially for residents with dementia who are more likely to be put by themselves, get bored, and attempt to get up without assistance and fall. Residents of long-term care facilities may require individualized exercise interventions that can be adapted to their changing needs in reducing falls.[629]

Current use of physical restraints with acute care clients or residents of long-term care facilities is based largely on the assumption that these devices prevent falls and fall-related injuries. Numerous studies have reported a significant incidence of falls and injuries in restrained older adults rather than a lower risk of falls and injuries. With growing acceptance of restraint-free care as a standard of practice, therapists can be instrumental in educating personnel in these facilities of these findings when instituting a program.[131,465,828]

A THERAPIST'S THOUGHTS*
Falls and Fall Prevention

The vestibular system controls head, neck, and eye movements and is certainly an important component of balance and falls prevention. The three semicircular canals positioned in each spatial plane accurately sense head position and rapidly send signals to the eyes to keep our vision stable. After the age of 40 years, the number and size of vestibular neurons decrease. In individuals older than age 70 years, 40% of the vestibular sensory cells are gone.[77,786]

Vestibular impairment or dysfunction is certainly a possible cause of falls, and the therapist should test for this and intervene appropriately, but often the underlying etiologies are impairments of the peripheral systems feeding into the vestibular system. The vestibular system may react too little or inappropriately because external stimuli are deficient. Keep in mind that there may be other causes of vestibular system failure, which may not be failure at all but merely compensation for impairment or failure of other systems.

Take into consideration motor, visual, and especially oculomotor, vestibulomotor, and oculovestibular reflexes; it is not a single-system issue. The *visual* or *ocular system* determines movement and position in space and provides visual reference points. And the *proprioceptive* or *somatosensory* system consisting of pressure sensors in muscles, tendons, and joints (especially in the lower extremities) senses gravity and joint position. Any change in these systems can result in dizziness, fear of falling, and limited activity, leading to increased postural instability and contributing to further weakness and imbalance in a downward declining spiral of events.

Consider the effects of macular degeneration, loss of peripheral vision, and the loss of visual cueing mechanisms from these systems.[786] A person may be able to compensate with one problem or system dysfunction, but when all three systems are impacted, it is much more difficult. The person starts to experience dizziness as the vestibular system tries to increase input. The person's natural tendency is to sit more to avoid dizziness and falls.

Sometimes use of a simple cane to increase peripheral messages can make a big difference. But what is the typical response to this? "That will make me look old." "I'd rather fall than use that thing." Issues of pride enter in; the individual is unwilling to use a cane to help increase proprioceptive cues to make up for a loss of vestibular, visual, or motor input. You may need to have an honest, frank discussion with that person. Try to reframe the client's view of the situation into something more acceptable; for example, help the individual see this as a short-term situation or even consider using a more direct approach. For instance, convey the following information to your patient/client:

Studies show that 50% of the people older than 65 years who fall fracture their hip and do not return home from the hospital. They often end up in a nursing home or extended care facility. Fifty percent of those people die within 1 year. Are you going to let a simple cane keep you from going home? If you do not want to use a cane, then how about getting a walking stick and letting me help you learn how to use it to your best advantage?

The therapist can also help older adults determine their own problem list and solutions in order to effect successful changes in behavior by asking the following questions[481]:

- What do you think is the problem?
- What can be done to change your situation? Alternatively: What do you think will help?
- What needs to happen for you to be able to _____ (repeat what the person just told you)?
- Can you do it? Can you _____ (repeat back what the person said needs to happen).
- Will you do it?

If the patient/client hesitates, you can ask, "What is one thing you *can* do to improve matters?"

The therapist can also make some changes in how the therapist practices in regards to screening individuals for falls risk, reducing or modifying risk factors, and preventing falls leading to fractures. If implementing a falls screening and prevention program for your facility seems too overwhelming, then at least choose one test and perform it consistently for 6 months or 1 year. Consider providing and/or participating in health fairs offering balance and posture screening.

Put together a task force with the express purpose of developing a screening checklist to fit your population base. Complete the checklist for every patient/client and conduct appropriate test measures. Make an appropriate referral sooner rather than later.

*Kevin Helgeson, DHSc, PT

Stress Reaction/Fracture

In the case of individuals reporting isolated or pinpoint pain of the lower extremity associated with overuse in the presence of negative radiographic examination (x-ray), the therapist may need to assess further for the possibility of a stress fracture. This is also true for the client who shows minimal improvement (or a worsening of symptoms) following therapy intervention.

Applying a translational, rotational, or impact stress to the bone often reproduces the symptoms when the stressed bone lies deep within the tissue. Testing may start by applying a striking (percussive/compressive) force through the heel as the client lies supine and observing for any associated increase in painful symptoms, especially at the hip or groin. Pull the leg into a position of internal rotation and resist as the person tries to externally rotate the leg; then move the leg into external rotation as the person tries to internally rotate the leg. For a differentiation of stress reactions of the femoral neck versus the pubic ramus, see Box 27-21.

Any suspicion of stress reaction/fracture warrants communication with the physician. Further imaging studies may be necessary.[733] Any woman with a stress fracture should be evaluated for the female athlete triad (amenorrhea, eating disorder, osteoporosis). Treatment of the underlying factors that contribute to the injury is important, including these three factors.[906]

Rehabilitation will vary depending on the age, condition, and goals of the affected individual. For

---

Box 27-21

DIFFERENTIATION OF STRESS REACTION/FRACTURE

Pubic Ramus

- Adductor muscles may be in spasm (adductor avulsion from stress fracture at the inferior ramus); limited abduction
- Negative heel strike/percussion test result
- Pain with activity that is relieved with rest, usually no pain at night
- Pain with resistance to the muscles of adduction and external rotation; positive Patrick or FABER (hip and knee flexion, hip abduction, hip external rotation) test (e.g., pain is reproduced as the person tries to internally rotate from a position of external rotation)
- Gait may be normal or antalgic depending on the fracture location

Femoral Neck

- Vague, nonspecific description and onset of pain; unrelieved by rest; aggravated at night by rolling onto that side
- Positive Trendelenburg sign (see Fig. 23-16) with compensated gait pattern
- Positive heel strike/percussion test; symptoms reproduced with hopping
- Positive test of femoral neck integrity (pain as person tries to externally rotate from an internally rotated position; may be unable to even assume test position in passive internal or medial rotation)*
- Noncapsular pattern (capsular pattern of the hip is defined as gross limitation of flexion, abduction, and medial rotation and slight limitation of extension with little or no limitation of lateral rotation)
- Localized tenderness at the greater trochanter unrelieved by treatment intervention for bursitis; pain may occur in the buttocks and/or groin

Tibia

- Painful pinpointed symptoms reproducible on palpation, frequently bilateral (one side more symptomatic than the other side); must be differentiated from shin splints
- Increased pain on weight bearing and walking (person assumes a wide-based waddling gait)
- May have a positive reaction to painful heel strike (more common in a hip fracture); symptoms reproduced with hopping

*This may be differentiated from trochanteric bursitis, which is characterized by painful hip abduction and lateral rotation (but not medial rotation).

Data from Ozburn MS, Nichols JW: Pubic ramus and adductor insertion stress fractures in female basic trainees, *Mil Med* 146(5):332–334, 1981; and Schneiders AG; The ability of clinical tests to diagnose stress fractures: a systematic review and meta-analysis, *J Orthop Sports Phys Ther* 42(9):760–771, 2012.

---

example, rehabilitation for military personnel will differ greatly from that prescribed for a postmenopausal woman. Specifics of progressing an exercise program are available.[553,707]

Acute Care and Complications

Complications of fractures require vigilance on the therapist's part and possibly quick action. Significant swelling can occur around the fracture site, and if the swelling is contained within a closed soft-tissue compartment, compartmental syndrome may occur (see "Soft-Tissue Injuries" above). Because of the progressively increased intracompartmental pressure, nerve and circulatory compromise can occur. This condition may be acute or chronic. The compartment becomes exquisitely painful.

A thorough sensory and motor examination may be warranted. If the therapist notes skin changes, decreased motor function, burning, paresthesia, or diminished reflexes, physician contact is necessary. Permanent damage and loss of function may result if this condition is not treated. The therapist's examination may be helpful in establishing the extent of the injury and baseline function.[194]

Another complication associated with fractures is fat embolism, a potentially fatal event.[742] The risk of developing this condition is related to fracture of long bones and the bony pelvis, which contain the most marrow. The fat globules from the bone marrow (or from the subcutaneous tissue at the fracture site) migrate to the lung parenchyma and can block pulmonary vessels, decreasing alveolar diffusion of oxygen.

The initial symptoms typically appear 1 to 3 days after injury, but this complication can occur up to a week later. Subtle changes in behavior and orientation occur if there are emboli in the cerebral circulation. There may also be complaints of dyspnea and chest pain, diaphoresis, pallor, or cyanosis. A rash on the anterior chest wall, neck, axillae, and shoulders may develop. The onset of any of these symptoms warrants immediate physician contact.

Individuals with acute VCFs (see Fig. 24-5) can be difficult to treat, because pain and fear can be severe. Even when extra care is taken with logrolling techniques, transitional movements can be exquisitely painful, with the client crying and begging the therapist to stop.

Arranging for premedication 45 to 60 minutes before treatment is advised, followed by modalities to modulate the pain and promote relaxation before attempting movement or exercise. Adaptive equipment, from wheelchair modifications to spinal orthotics to assistive devices (e.g., reachers/grabbers, stocking aids, raised toilet seats, bed grab bars), helps to improve posture, function, mobility, confidence, and independence.

The therapist must be alert to other complications that can occur following fracture, such as breakage of wires, displacement of screws, loss of fixation, refracture, delayed union and malunion, and infection.[744] Anyone on bed rest is at risk for complications from immobility, including constipation, deep vein thrombosis, pulmonary embolism, and pneumonia.

Fracture Rehabilitation

Like medical treatment, fracture rehabilitation is shaped by fracture type, need for reduction, presence of instability after reduction, and functional requirements of the affected individual. Postoperative rehabilitation can begin immediately to within 1 week after surgery depending on the physician's protocol.

There are some widely accepted guidelines and rehabilitation protocols for various types of fractures. The American Academy of Orthopaedic Surgeons offers guidelines for the rehabilitation of many different types of fractures. Several publications with fracture rehabilitation protocols are available specifically for the physical therapist.[109,552,639,824]

Many older adults never return to the same level of function after a hip fracture and most will need 6 months of recovery to regain the prefracture level of function.[78] Mortality rates following hip fractures in older adults may be improved by a more intensive rehabilitation program immediately after the operation. The best predictor of mortality immediately after hip fracture up to 1 year after fracture is the inability to stand up, an indicator of frailty.[357]

Older adults admitted for care of a fall-related hip fracture should be evaluated early in their hospital stay to determine risk for falls following discharge. Indicators may include a previous history of falls and prefracture use of an assistive device for ambulation. The plan of care should include balance and mobility training to prevent future falls. A previous history of falls is a risk factor for future falls; poor balance, slow gait speed, and decline in ADLs have been identified in older adults who fall within 6 months following a hip fracture.[753]

Early mobilization accompanied by transfer training, and maintaining strength and range of motion after fracture surgery are essential to reduce the risk of deep vein thromboembolism, pulmonary or infectious complications, skin breakdown, and decline in mental status.

Following a fracture in the lower extremity (including the hip), some orthopedic surgeons advocate unrestricted weight bearing, advising the client to decide himself or herself how much weight to put on the leg. Stable fractures can usually tolerate weight bearing. Rotationally stable but potentially long unstable femur fractures may be allowed toe-touch weight bearing. Clients with vertically and rotationally unstable femoral fractures may be restricted to non–weight-bearing status, using a wheelchair or electric scooter (if not in a spica hip cast).[685]

Although immediate weight bearing may cause initial bone loss, the long-term success of achieving bone growth remains unchanged,[748] and the short-term benefits of functional recovery and quicker return to independent living that accompany unrestricted weight bearing are important.[463,649]

Again, depending on the type of fracture, some movements may be restricted to allow for proper fracture consolidation. Most importantly, a non–weight-bearing status can actually place greater forces on the hip as a result of the biomechanics involved in maintaining correct positioning of the lower extremity.[393,606] In the case of femoral neck or intertrochanteric fractures, there is little biomechanical justification for restricted weight bearing; indeed, there is far greater pressure generated from performing a hip bridge while using a bedpan (almost equivalent to the effect of unsupported ambulation).[628]

Partial weight bearing is usually considered 30% to 50% of body weight. Touch or touchdown weight bearing is 10% of body weight, but this is a subjective decision that is not easily determined. Allowing for unrestricted weight bearing according to the client's tolerance is less restrictive, but the therapist must assess for intact cognition and decision-making abilities, intact sensation, upper body strength, vestibular function and balance, and proprioception before allowing unsupervised weight-bearing as tolerated.

Early fracture repair and physical therapy reduce hospital stays, increase chances of returning home (rather than being discharged to a nursing facility or rehabilitation facility), reduce complications, and improve functional mobility and independence at discharge,[44,318] and are associated with higher rates of 6-month survival.[181,377] Although the evidence has not clearly supported specific recommendations for an exercise program after hip fracture, there are a number of smaller studies show benefits of an exercise program to improve function.[747] Therapists are encouraged to share the results of studies such as these with hospital administrators when developing fall and fracture prevention programs.

The literature supports recommending follow-up for strength and functional assessment 7 to 9 months after fracture.[723,748] Muscle strength around the hip remains weak after hip fracture, with joint arthroplasty requiring an exercise program for strengthening for 1 year or longer.[207,751] Short-term intervention with a therapist can be very cost-effective in reducing refracture rates.[748,749]

Older adults who receive physical therapy while still in the hospital following hip replacement for hip fracture are more likely to be discharged directly home rather than to a rehabilitation or assisted living facility.[339] People with hip fractures who receive additional home health visits are less likely to be hospitalized and more likely to need fewer medical visits, which usually translates into lower Medicare costs.[409]

For clients with VCFs, the plan of care should include trunk extension strengthening and a cognitive-behavioral component to improve coping, especially for older adults. Improvements have been retained for at least 6 months in one randomized, controlled trial.[299]

Osteochondroses

A number of clinical disorders of ossification centers (epiphyses) in growing children share the common denominator of avascular necrosis and its sequelae. These disorders are grouped together and referred to as the *osteochondroses*,[43] with multiple synonyms (epiphysitis, osteochondritis, aseptic necrosis, ischemic epiphyseal necrosis). There are additional eponyms based on the name of the person or persons who described the disorder as well, such as Kohler disease (tarsal-navicular bone disease), Osgood-Schlatter disease, and Legg-Calvé-Perthes disease.

The underlying etiologic factors and pathogenesis are similar in all these entities, and the clinical manifestations are determined by the stresses and strains present. Most susceptible areas are the epiphyses, which are entirely covered by articular cartilage and therefore poorly vascularized.

Osteochondritis Dissecans

Osteochondritis dissecans is a disorder of one or more ossification sites with localized subchondral necrosis followed by recalcification. This condition affects the subchondral bone and the adjacent layer of articular cartilage; a piece of articular cartilage and fragment of bone separate and pull away from the underlying bone. These fragments can become loose bodies in the joint; the most common sites of involvement are the concave surfaces of synovial joint, such as the medial femoral condyle, talar head and capitellum of the humerus.

Osteochondritis dissecans is caused by repetitive microtrauma resulting in ischemia and disruption of the subchondral growth. The articular cartilage softens, and fragment separation leads to cartilage injury that can progress to form a crater. Activity-related pain, swelling, and giving way are common symptoms. Pain is increased with passive knee extension and tibial internal rotation and relieved with tibial external rotation (Wilson sign).[200]

Signs of an osteochondritis dissecans can be seen on a plain radiographs with MR images used to determine if the lesion is stable or unstable.[679] Management varies with the person's age and the severity of the lesion and includes nonoperative management for stable lesions (activity modification, protected weight bearing, immobilization for 4-6 weeks). Arthroscopic procedures can be used to fixate the lesion, debride tissues from the defect, and implant tissues to stimulate healing.[200]

Osteonecrosis

Overview and Incidence

The term *osteonecrosis* refers to the death of bone and bone marrow cellular components as a result of loss of blood supply in the absence of infection. *Avascular necrosis* and *aseptic necrosis* are synonyms for this condition.

The femoral head is the most common site of this disorder (sometimes called Chandler disease), but other sites can include the scaphoid, talus, proximal humerus, tibial plateau, and small bones of the wrist and foot. Avascular necrosis is the underlying cause for approximately 10% of total hip replacement surgeries and overall affects approximately 20,000 people annually, often between the second and fifth decades of life.[480]

Etiologic and Risk Factors

Osteocytic necrosis results from tissue ischemia brought on by the impairment of blood-conducting vessels. A minimum of 2 hours of complete ischemia and anoxia is necessary for permanent loss of bone tissue.[417] The bony ischemia may be secondary to trauma disrupting the arterial supply or to thrombosis disrupting the microcirculation.

Bones or portions of bones that have limited collateral circulation and few vascular foramina are susceptible to avascular necrosis. Box 27-22 lists conditions associated with osteonecrosis. A number of these conditions are linked to osteonecrosis by the development of fat emboli (caused by altered fat metabolism) in the vascular tree of the involved bone.

The conditions associated with the development of fat emboli include alcoholism, obesity, pregnancy, pancreatitis, medications (e.g., oral contraceptives, corticosteroids), and unrelated fractures. Many cases of femoral head osteonecrosis are idiopathic (i.e., no known cause or risk factor can be identified).

Osteonecrosis has also been recognized as a complication in HIV-positive individuals; in fact, individuals who are HIV-positive have a 100-fold greater risk of developing osteonecrosis than the general population.[602] The exact mechanism for this remains unknown. It may be caused by hyperlipidemia secondary to the use of protease inhibitors; however, avascular necrosis was reported before the era of highly active antiretroviral therapy.[687] It does not appear to be related to the degree of immunodeficiency.

More recently, the use of bisphosphonates has been linked with osteonecrosis of the jaw (sometimes referred to as "dead jaw syndrome"), especially after trauma to the teeth or bones of the jaw such as occurs with dental surgery (e.g., tooth extraction). The reason this happens is not entirely clear. Scientists hypothesize that because the jaw has a high rate of bone renewal in response to stress via generation of an inflammatory response by the gums and teeth, bisphosphonates keep osteoclasts from reabsorbing damaged bone cells in the jaw. The damaged bone builds up and eventually results in osteonecrosis.[692]

This phenomenon is most likely to occur in individuals treated for bone cancer with intravenous bisphosphonates. The dosage of intravenous bisphosphonates can be as much as 12 times more than the oral bisphosphonate dosage prescribed for osteoporosis. Individuals with cancer treated this way also undergo other bone-weakening treatments (e.g., chemotherapy, radiation therapy).[652]

Pathogenesis

Certain bones are more vulnerable to osteonecrosis than others. These bones are covered extensively by cartilage, have few vascular foramina, and have limited collateral circulation. The femoral head is a prime example of a bone at risk. The superolateral two-thirds of the femoral head receives its blood supply almost entirely from the lateral epiphyseal branches of the medial femoral circumflex artery (Fig. 27-30).

The only other source of blood for the femoral head is the medial epiphyseal artery (contained within the ligamentum teres), which has limited anastomoses with the lateral epiphyseal vessels. Hip dislocation or fracture of the neck of the femur can compromise the precarious vascular supply to the head of the femur. The talus, scaphoid, and proximal humerus are also susceptible to osteonecrosis.[534]

As the ischemia progresses, repair processes occur but are not capable of preventing necrosis and deformation of the bone, such as flattening and collapse of the femoral head. The articular cartilage and acetabulum are usually spared until late in the disease process, but the articular cartilage may be lifted off the underlying bone, resulting in irreparable damage to the joint.[191] The entire process extends over many years, and unlike in osteochondrosis of immature bone (e.g., Legg-Calvé-Perthes disease), spontaneous healing never occurs.

Clinical Manifestations

Often no symptoms are observed during the initial development of osteonecrosis even though an ischemic condition of the bone exists.[381] Hip pain is the usual initial presenting complaint, with a gradual onset, sometimes of many weeks' duration, before diagnosis. The pain may be

---

Box 27-22

CONDITIONS ASSOCIATED WITH OSTEONECROSIS

- Idiopathic
- Trauma (e.g., fall)
- Systemic lupus erythematosus
- Pancreatitis
- Diabetes mellitus
- Hyperlipidemia
- Cushing disease
- Gout
- Sickle cell disease
- Alcoholism
- Obesity
- Pregnancy
- Medications
  - Oral contraceptives
  - Corticosteroids
  - Bisphosphonates (under investigation)
- Organ transplantation (medication related)
- Human immunodeficiency virus (HIV) infection
- Radiation therapy (less common)
- Dysbaric disease (deep sea diving; rare)

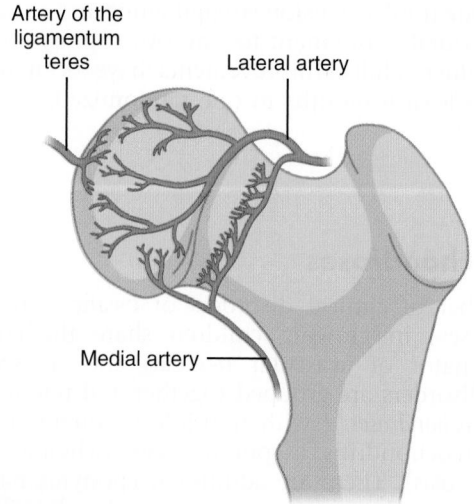

Figure 27-30

Blood supply to the femoral head in a child. (From Bullough PG: *Orthopaedic pathology,* ed 3, London, 1997, Mosby-Wolfe, p. 263.)

mild and intermittent initially but will progress to become severe, especially during weight-bearing activities.

If the femur is involved, the pain may be noted in the groin, thigh, or medial knee area. An antalgic gait is noted, and pain provocation occurs with weight-bearing activities and hip range-of-motion exercises, especially internal rotation and flexion and adduction. The affected individual will report a slowly progressive stiffening of the joint. When fracture occurs, it is usually at the junction between necrotic bone and reparative bone, possibly extending down through the reparative interface to the healthy inferior cortex of the femoral neck.[585]

Eventually degenerative joint changes and osteoarthrosis occur at the involved hip joint; the pathologic process is often relentless, with collapse of the femoral head imminent in spite of medical intervention.[381]

Osteonecrosis of the jaw is characterized by exposed bone in the mouth, numbness or heaviness in the jaw, pain, swelling, infection, and loose teeth. Delayed or poor wound healing after dental surgery may be the first indication of a problem. Crepitus as the jaw opens and closes may be present and is often described as like the sound of someone walking on ice.[691]

MEDICAL MANAGEMENT

DIAGNOSIS. Plain films may be normal initially. Bone scan, MRI, and CT scans are much more sensitive procedures and detect subtle bony changes.

TREATMENT. The choice between conservative and surgical intervention depends on the size of the lesion, how early the diagnosis is made, and whether bony collapse has occurred. If surgery is not indicated, protected weight bearing is essential to prevent collapse of the lesion.[742]

Surgical intervention may consist of core decompression for small lesions without evidence of structural collapse (most common procedure in early diagnosis) to relieve pain and delay or prevent structural collapse, hemiarthroplasty, or total joint replacement.[509] Core decompression removes a core of bone from the femoral head and neck in an attempt to relieve intermedullary pressure, thereby promoting revascularization. This may be accompanied by bone grafting.[792]

Joint replacement may be required if femoral head collapse occurs or in order to prevent this complication. However, this procedure is limited by young age and high activity level as well as the limited life expectancy of the prosthesis.[681]

New techniques for bone stimulation may be used, such as replacing the dead bone with living bone from the individual's fibula to give added strength to the damaged area and possibly prevent or postpone joint arthroplasty in young individuals; see also "Fracture: Treatment" above.[681]

An osteotomy may be performed to shift the site to where maximal weight bearing occurs on a particular joint surface. Analgesics and NSAIDs are used for symptomatic relief of pain.

PROGNOSIS. The prognosis depends on the extent of damage that has occurred before diagnosis in the case of nontraumatic disease. Unfortunately, many cases are diagnosed in an advanced stage of disease, when minimally invasive surgical procedures are no longer helpful.[480] Early intervention (both surgical and nonsurgical) has definitely improved the outcome, but many people with femoral head osteonecrosis experience irreversible damage to the joint and will need total arthroplasty.

SPECIAL IMPLICATIONS FOR THE THERAPIST   27-21

Osteonecrosis

Therapists are always advised to obtain a thorough and complete history from clients, especially in the presence of musculoskeletal manifestations of apparently unknown cause. Because osteonecrosis is difficult to identify early, knowledge of causative factors (see Box 27-22) is important. Differential diagnosis of lumbar, hip, thigh, groin, or knee pain is essential, because osteonecrosis may present referred pain and symptoms as if coming from any one of these.

When treating people at risk for osteonecrosis, therapists must consider the possibility of fracture if there is a sudden worsening of pain complaints followed by a sudden, dramatic loss in range of motion. Once the diagnosis is made, close communication with the physician is important for safe progression of weight bearing and exercise.

Following surgical intervention, the usual postoperative precautions and indications apply for minimization of complications (e.g., deep vein thrombosis), early mobilization, assessment for gait-assistive devices, gait training, demonstration of motion restrictions, and pain management.

In the case of microvascular bone transplantation, some physicians caution clients to avoid high-impact activities such as jumping, skiing, competitive tennis, and carrying more than 100 lb, although long-term studies of these stresses on repaired or reconstructed bones have not been carried out.

Legg-Calvé-Perthes Disease

Definition and Overview

Legg-Calvé-Perthes disease, also known as *coxa plana* (flat hip) and *osteochondritis deformans juvenilis*, is epiphyseal aseptic necrosis (or avascular necrosis) of the proximal end of the femur. It is a self-limiting disorder characterized by avascular necrosis of the capital femoral epiphysis (the center of ossification of the femoral head). Complete revascularization of the avascular epiphysis occurs over a period of time without any treatment.

This condition occurs in approximately 1 in 1200 children, primarily boys (5:1 ratio of boys-to-girls) between the ages of 3 and 12 years, making it the most common of the osteochondroses. Legg-Calvé-Perthes disease occurs 10 times more often in whites than in blacks.

Deformation of the epiphysis with changes in the shape of the femoral head and the acetabulum occur during the process of revascularization in a significant portion of affected individuals. This may lead to degenerative arthritis in young adult life.[429] Stulberg's classification used five classes to describe the shape and size of the femoral head, configuration of the acetabulum, and congruency of the joint surfaces. Individuals with classes I and II have retained a spherical femoral head. Class III is an ovoid femoral head. Classes IV and V have a flattened or irregular femoral head.[430,799]

Etiologic Factors

The direct cause is a reduction in blood flow to the joint, although what causes this is unknown. It may be that the artery of the ligamentum teres femoris closes too early, not allowing time for the circumflex femoral artery to take over. Genetic coagulopathy has been suggested,[793] possibly triggered by exposure to cigarette smoke in utero and during childhood.[298]

Delay in bone age relative to the child's chronologic age suggests a possible general disorder of skeletal growth with focal expression in the hip. Mechanisms proposed to explain the delay in bone maturation include genetic, endocrine, nutritional, and socioeconomic factors.[486]

Pathogenesis

The disease process consists of four stages lasting from 2 to 5 years (Table 27-4 and Fig. 27-31). Because the growth plate of the femoral head lies above the insertion of the capsule of the hip joint in children and because the epiphyseal plate acts as a firm barrier to blood flow between the metaphysis and epiphysis, the femoral head depends on vessels that track along the surface of the neck of the femur to enter the epiphysis above the growth plate.[527]

Injection studies have demonstrated that the most important vessels supplying the epiphysis are the lateral epiphyseal vessels. These vessels are vulnerable to interruption of blood flow by trauma or by increased intraarticular pressure. It is possible that in Legg-Calvé-Perthes disease the ischemic events are episodic in nature and result from increased intraarticular pressure.[116]

Delays in bone maturation observed with this disease are correlated with the stage of the disease. The decrease in bone age delay in the later stages of the disease indicates that as the disease progresses, bone maturation accelerates and tries to catch up with the chronologic age. This phenomenon is referred to as *bone maturation acceleration*. This process occurs earlier in the epiphyses of the lower ends of the radius and ulna and short bones of the hands compared to the carpal bones.[486]

Clinical Manifestations

The Legg-Calvé-Perthes condition is characterized by insidious onset, initially presenting as the intermittent appearance of a limp on the involved side with hip pain described as soreness or aching with accompanying stiffness. The pain may be present in the groin and along the entire length of the thigh following the path of the obturator nerve or referred pain just in the area of the knee. There is usually pinpoint tenderness over the hip capsule.

Painful symptoms are aggravated by activity and fatigue and relieved somewhat by rest. Mild Legg-Calvé-Perthes

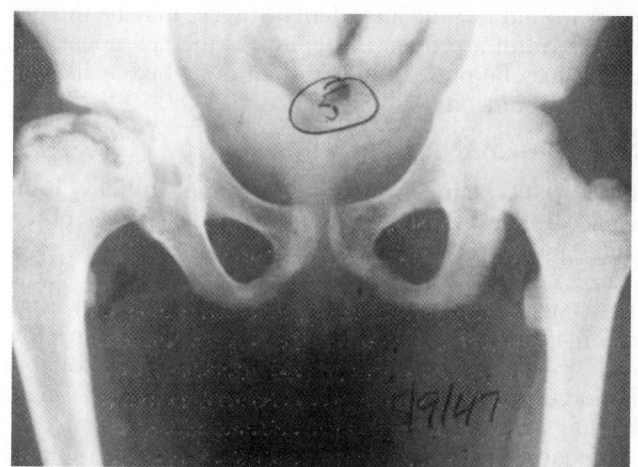

Figure 27-31

Radiograph of lower pelvis in Legg-Calvé-Perthes disease after revascularization of the necrotic femoral head shows enlargement of the right femoral head, with the original necrotic ossification center seen as a "head within a head." (From Bullough PG: *Orthopaedic pathology*, ed 3, London, 1997, Mosby-Wolfe, p. 263.)

Table 27-4	Stages of Legg-Calvé-Perthes Disease	
Stage	**Time Period**	**Pathogenesis**
Avascular (stage 1)	1-2 weeks	Quiet phase: spontaneous vascular interruption to the epiphysis causes necrosis of the femoral head with degenerative changes, hip synovium and joint capsule are swollen, edematous, and hyperemic; joint space widens; cells of the epiphysis die, but bone remains unchanged
Revascularization (stage II; fragmentation stage)	6-12 months	Vascular reaction: new blood supply causes bone resorption and deposition of new bone cells; deformity from pressure on weakened area occurs; the entire or anterior one half of the epiphysis of the femoral head is necrotic; increased blood supply and decalcification of bone cause softening at the junction of the femoral neck and the capital epiphyseal plate; granulation tissue and blood vessels invade the dead bone now detectable on radiographic examination
Reparative (stage III; residual stage)	2-3 years	New bone replaces necrotic bone; the necrotic: femoral head is placed or surrounds by new bone (sometimes giving it an appearance of a head inside a head; see Fig 27-31), flattening of the femoral head causes the femoral neck to become short and wide with subluxation, progressive deformity; and even fracture possible
Regenerative (intravascular)	Final months	Completion of healing or regeneration gradually reforms the head of the femur into live spongy bone; restoration of the femoral head to a normal shape is more likely in younger children and only if the anterior epiphysis was involved; residual deformity may exist in some cases that can lead to the gradual development of joint disease (osteoarthritis)

disease is characterized by partial femoral head collapse, retention of a full range of hip abduction and rotation, and lack of subluxation on radiographic examination.

Delay in bone maturation is a common feature of this condition. Skeletal development is unevenly timed in the growing bones, with the maximum delay occurring in the distal limb segments. As the condition progresses, there are decreases in active and passive range of motion, as well as limited physiologic (accessory) motion affecting walking and running.

Severe Legg-Calvé-Perthes disease begins later and involves collapse of the whole femoral head, stiffness, and subluxation. Atrophy of the thigh musculature and restriction of hip abduction and rotation may develop. Short stature may develop as a result of epiphyseal dysplasia, and in those individuals who are left untreated, a flat femoral head will develop that is prone to degenerative joint disease.[684]

Late complications in adults with a childhood history of Legg-Calvé-Perthes include early OA of the hip and acetabular labral tears. Hip, groin, or back pain may be the first symptom in affected adults. Postural asymmetry, leg length discrepancy, decreased range of motion, and decreased strength may be accompanied by an abnormal gait pattern.[71]

MEDICAL MANAGEMENT

DIAGNOSIS. Physical examination, clinical history, and radiographic examination (Fig. 27-32) confirm the diagnosis. MRI is widely accepted as the imaging method of choice, allowing early diagnosis and providing staging information necessary for adequate management.[451]

There are several different classifications used to determine severity of disease and prognosis. The Catterall classification specifies four different groups defined by radiographic appearance during the period of greatest bone loss.

The Salter-Thomson classification simplifies the Catterall classification by reducing it down to two groups: group A (Catterall I, II), in which less than 50% of the ball is involved, and group B (Catterall III, IV), in which more than 50% of the ball is involved. Both classifications share the view that if less than 50% of the ball is involved, the prognosis is good, while more than 50% involvement indicates a potentially poor prognosis.

The Herring classification studies the integrity of the lateral pillar of the ball. In lateral pillar group A, there is no loss of height in the lateral third of the head and little density change. In lateral pillar group B there is a lucency and loss of height of less than 50% of the lateral height. Sometimes the ball is beginning to extrude the socket. In lateral pillar group C, there is more than 50% loss of lateral height.[527,674]

Many doctors utilize these classifications as they provide an accurate method of determining prognosis and help in determining the appropriate form of treatment.

TREATMENT. The goal of treatment is to limit deformity and preserve the integrity of the femoral head. Mild disease may not require intervention, but careful follow-up with radiographic examination every 3 months is

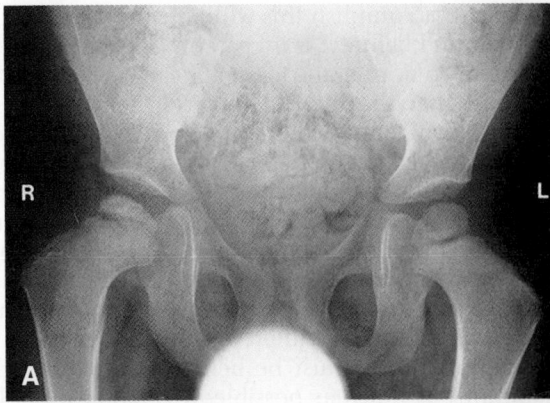
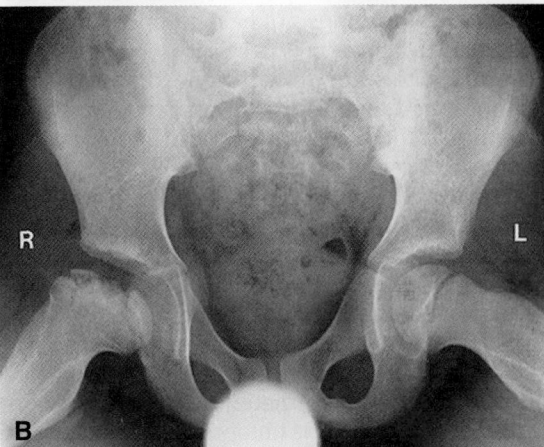
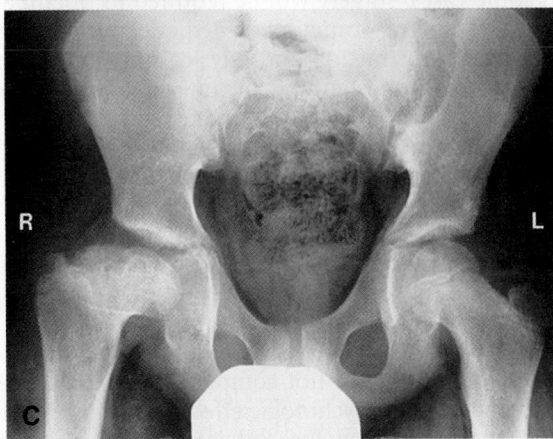

Figure 27-32

Legg-Calvé-Perthes disease. **A,** Anterior view of the pelvis demonstrates fragmentation and sclerosis of the right femoral epiphysis *(arrow)* in a 6-year-old male. **B,** Follow-up film obtained 8 years later shows continuing deformity resulting from osteonecrosis. **C,** The child developed significant degenerative arthritis by age 12 years. (From Mettler FA: *Primary care radiology*, Philadelphia, 2000, WB Saunders.)

needed to observe for deterioration and progression of the disease.[565]

Current methods of treatment attempt to prevent deformation of the femoral head and restore the spherical and congruent femoral head contour of the acetabulum. This is done by ensuring that the vulnerable anterolateral part of the avascular capital femoral epiphysis is contained within the acetabulum, a process called *containment*. The femoral head can be molded to a normal shape as it heals.

The idea is to accomplish this while the bone is biologically plastic and before it is irreparably deformed.[429]

The closer to normal the femoral head is when growth stops, the better the hip will function in later life.[390] The way that surgeons achieve this goal is through containment. In the past, weight bearing was minimized, but more recently, therapy allows the child to continue weight bearing with the femur in an abducted and internally rotated position. Keeping the head of the femur well seated in the acetabulum decreases focal areas of increased load and minimizes distortion, thereby maintaining range of motion and preventing deformity.

The femoral head must be held in the joint socket (acetabulum) as much as possible. It is better if the hip is allowed to move and is not held completely still in the joint socket. Joint motion is necessary for nutrition of the cartilage and for healthy growth of the joint. All treatment options for Legg-Calvé-Perthes disease try to position and hold the hip in the acetabulum as much as possible. This healing process can take several years.[478]

Conservative care is usually continued for 2 to 4 years. A variety of splints, braces, and positional devices may be used to maintain the proper position.[341] When lack of motion has become a problem, the child may be admitted to the hospital and placed in traction. Traction is used to quiet the inflammation. Antiinflammatory medications may be prescribed. Physical therapy is used to restore the hip motion as the inflammation comes under control. Home traction may also be an option.

In some cases, surgery will be required to obtain adequate containment. Sometimes, adequate motion cannot be regained with traction and physical therapy alone. If the condition is longstanding, the muscles may have contracted or shrunk and cannot be stretched back out.

To help restore motion, the surgeon may recommend a *tenotomy* of the contracted muscles. When a tenotomy is performed, the tendon of the muscle that is overly tight is cut and lengthened. This is a simple procedure that requires only a small incision. The tendon eventually scars down in the lengthened position, and no functional loss is noticeable.

Surgical treatment for containment may be best in older children who are not compliant with brace treatment or where the psychologic effects of wearing braces may outweigh the benefits. Surgical containment does not require long-term use of braces or casts. Once the procedure has been performed and the bones have healed, the child can pursue normal activities as tolerated.

Surgical treatment for containment usually consists of procedures that realign either the femur (thighbone), the acetabulum (hip socket), or both. Realignment of the femur is called a *femoral osteotomy*. This procedure changes the angle of the femoral neck so that the femoral head points more toward the socket.[816]

To perform this procedure, an incision is made in the side of the thigh. The bone of the femur is cut and realigned in a new position. A large metal plate and screws are then inserted to hold the bones in the new position until the bone has healed. The plate and screws may need to be removed once the bone has healed.

Realignment of the acetabulum is called a *pelvic osteotomy*. This procedure changes the angle of the acetabulum (socket) so that it covers or contains more of the femoral head. To perform this procedure, an incision is made in the side of the buttock. The bone of the pelvis is cut and realigned in a new position. Large metal pins or screws are then inserted to hold the bones in the new position until the bone has healed. The pins usually must be removed once the bone has healed.[821]

If there is a serious structural change in the anatomy of the hip, there may need to be further surgery to restore the alignment closer to normal. This is usually not considered until growth stops. As a child grows, there will be some remodeling that occurs in the hip joint. This may improve the situation such that further surgery is unnecessary.

In severe cases, both femoral osteotomy and pelvic osteotomy may be combined to obtain even more containment.

PROGNOSIS. Legg-Calvé-Perthes disease may vary in severity from a mild self-healing problem with no sequelae to a condition that will destroy the hip unless serious action is taken. Early on, it may be difficult to determine which course the disease will follow.[157]

Even though the disease is self-limiting, the prognosis varies according to the age of onset (better prognosis in children whose onset is before age 5 years). Children older than age 8 years at the time of onset have a better outcome with surgical treatment than with nonoperative care.[367] There is some evidence to suggest that early delay in bone age (stage I of the disease) is linked with more severe disease.[486]

Older age, complete involvement of the femoral head, and noncompliance with treatment contribute to a poorer prognosis. Although girls are less likely to develop Legg-Calvé-Perthes disease compared to boys, they often have a poorer prognosis. The reason for this difference is unknown.

A delay in bone age maturation of more than 2 years in stage I of the disease has been linked with greater severity of the disease. However, children with Legg-Calvé-Perthes disease have a normal onset of puberty, and by the time they are 12 to 15 years old, their stature and bone age are the same as those of their peers.[469]

SPECIAL IMPLICATIONS FOR THE THERAPIST 27-22

Legg-Calvé-Perthes Disease

Therapists may be involved in gait training, aquatic therapy, and range of motion exercises during this period.[103] It should be emphasized to the child and family that Legg-Calvé-Perthes disease is a long-term problem with treatment aimed at minimizing damage while the disease runs its course. Performing exercises daily is essential during the healing process to ensure that the femur and hip socket have a perfectly smooth interface. This will minimize the long-term effects of the disease. As sufferers age, problems in the knee and back can arise as a result of the abnormal posture and stride adopted to protect the affected joint.

Surgery may be performed to contain the femoral head in the acetabulum, especially in children older than 6 years with serious involvement of the femoral head. Hip replacements are relatively common during the sixth decade as the already damaged hip suffers routine wear; this varies from individual to individual.

See also "Special Implications for the Therapist 23-5: Developmental Dysplasia of the Hip" in Chapter 23. For specific intervention guidelines, the reader is referred to a more appropriate text.[129,815]

Osgood-Schlatter Disease

Overview

Osgood-Schlatter disease (osteochondrosis) results from fibers of the patellar tendon pulling small bits of immature bone from the tibial tuberosity. In the past, Osgood-Schlatter was considered a form of osteochondritis (inflammation of bone and cartilage), but more recent thinking suggests that the process is one part of the spectrum of mechanical problems related to the extensor mechanism. Rather than being an actual degenerative "disease," Osgood-Schlatter is considered a form of tendinitis of the patellar tendon.[289]

It is most commonly seen in active adolescent boys ages 10 to 15 years, but can also affect girls ages 8 to 13 years. The ratio of boys to girls affected by Osgood-Schlatter disease is 3:1. It is estimated that 20% of adolescents actively involved in sports have some symptoms of Osgood-Schlatter disease with an equal number among military recruits affecting kneeling and squatting during military training.[473, 663]

Etiologic Factors and Pathogenesis

Osgood-Schlatter disease is probably the result of indirect trauma (force produced by the sudden, powerful contraction of the quadriceps muscle during an activity) or repetitive stress (repeated knee flexion against a tight quadriceps muscle) before complete fusion of the epiphysis to the main bone has occurred. It is further aggravated by the longitudinal traction associated with bone growth in adolescents and the presence of external tibial torsion. Longstanding tension on the patella and patellar tendons during rapid growth spurts sets up an imbalance between the femur and the anterior structures of the knee. The result can be Osgood-Schlatter disease.[872]

Another possible cause of Osgood-Schlatter lesions is abnormal alignment in the legs. Children who are knock-kneed or flat-footed seem to be most prone to the condition. These postures put a sharper angle between the quadriceps muscle and the patellar tendon. This angle is called the *Q angle*. A large Q angle puts more tension on the bone growth plate of the tibial tuberosity, increasing the chances for an Osgood-Schlatter lesion to develop. A high-riding patella, called *patella alta*, is also thought to contribute to development of Osgood-Schlatter lesions.[289]

In young athletes, the tendon is attached to prebone, which is weaker than normal adult bone. With excessive stresses on the tendon from running and jumping, the structure becomes irritated and a tendinitis begins. Often fragments representing cartilage or bone formations are

found on the surface of the patellar tendon and are a potential cause of pain. These patellar tendon fibers can actually pull fragments away from the tibial epiphysis. This process is described as avulsion of the secondary ossification center of the tibial tuberosity (Fig. 27-33).[289]

Clinical Manifestations

Clinically, clients report constant aching and pain at the site of the tibial tubercle (just below the kneecap), which is often enlarged on visual examination. Symptoms are aggravated by any activity that causes forceful contraction of the patellar tendon against the tubercle, such as active knee extension or resisted knee flexion (e.g., going up or down stairs, running, jumping, biking, hiking, kneeling, squatting).

Besides the obvious soft-tissue swelling, there may be localized heat and tenderness, the latter elicited with direct pressure over the anterior aspect of the proximal tibial tubercle. Many children with this condition also have significant tightness in the hamstrings, iliotibial band, triceps surae (bellies of the gastrocnemius and soleus), and quadriceps muscles. Tightness in these areas can potentially increase the flexion moment and subsequent stresses at the tibial tubercle.

MEDICAL MANAGEMENT

DIAGNOSIS. On physical examination, the examiner is able to palpate tenderness at the tibial tubercle; later there will be a bony bump at that site that distinguishes this problem from other conditions affecting the knee.

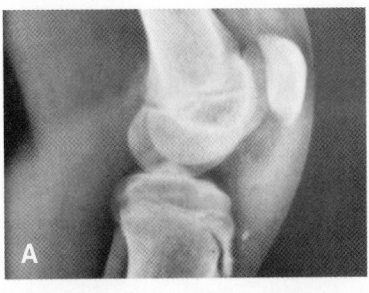

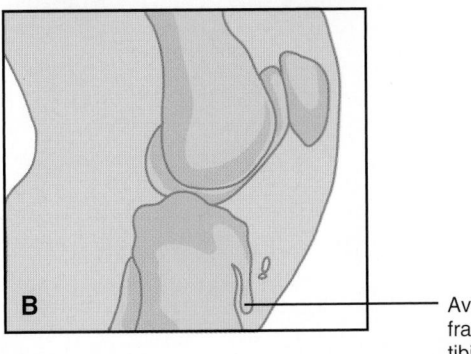

Avulsed and fragmented tibial tubercle

Figure 27-33

Clinical radiograph of the knee in a 12-year-old child shows fragmentation and avulsion of the tibial tubercle. Swelling below the knee and an enlarged tibial tuberosity may be observed clinically. This condition, known as Osgood-Schlatter disease, is probably posttraumatic. (From Bullough PG: *Orthopaedic pathology*, ed 3, London, 1997, Mosby-Wolfe, p. 98.)

Clinical diagnosis may be confirmed by radiograph (or ultrasonography to avoid exposure to x-ray), as many conditions are very similar (e.g., patellar tendinitis, chondromalacia patella, synovial plica). Although the films may be normal, epiphyseal separation, soft-tissue swelling, and bone fragmentation can be visualized in many cases.

TREATMENT AND PROGNOSIS. Immobilization is no longer advocated with this condition, although rest from aggravating activities and/or activity modification/restriction is recommended until symptoms have subsided. This time frame ranges from 2 to 3 weeks in some individuals to 2 to 3 months or longer in others. Enough time must be allowed for revascularization, healing, and ossification of the tibial tubercle before resumption of unrestricted athletic participation. NSAIDs and ice are used regularly.[289]

Treatment should include exercises to address the mechanical inefficiencies of the extensor mechanism, stretching for any areas of inflexibility, and strengthening areas of weakness (e.g., ankle dorsiflexion, pain-free quadriceps strengthening).

Balance and coordination should be assessed and rehabilitation provided as appropriate. Support may be provided through the use of a knee sleeve, brace, or narrow strap around the leg placing pressure over the tibial tubercle. This latter device is used to reduce the pulling stresses of the patellar tendon on the tubercle and subsequently reduce pain.

Approximately 90% of children with this condition respond well to nonoperative treatment. Complete recovery is expected with closure of the tibial growth plate but in fact, 60% of affected individuals report discomfort with kneeling long after skeletal maturity.[467] Conservative measures are usually sufficient to provide pain relief and resolution of local swelling.

When conservative care fails to resolve painful symptoms, full-extension immobilization of the leg through reinforced elastic knee support, cast, or splint may be prescribed for 6 to 8 weeks. In chronic, unresolved cases (rare), surgery may be necessary to remove the prominent tibial tubercle and any epiphyseal ossicles that have formed in the tendon. Sometimes ossicle removal without tibial tubercle excision is performed. In extreme cases, the epiphysis may actually be removed or holes drilled into the tibial tubercle to facilitate revascularization of the area. Response to surgical treatment for symptomatic unresolved disease in skeletally mature adults is reportedly good to excellent with resolution of pain and return to daily activities including unrestricted sports participation. Pain on kneeling remains a persistent problem.[663]

REFERENCES
To enhance this text and add value for the reader, all references are included on the companion Evolve site that accompanies this textbook. The reader can view the reference source and access it online whenever possible.

Introduction to Central Nervous System Disorders

KENDA S. FULLER

OVERVIEW

The central nervous system (CNS) controls and regulates all mental and physical functions. The nervous system is unparalleled among organ systems in terms of diversity of cellular constituents. It is composed of a network of neural tissue that includes both receptors and transmitters. There is a complex interaction among the areas that control both thought and movement, dysfunction in one area will cause changes in the other. Disease or trauma of the CNS may affect the nervous system through damage to several types of tissues in a local area, such as in stroke, or it may cause dysfunction in one type of tissue throughout many areas of the CNS such as in multiple sclerosis. Dysfunction of the neurons in particular areas of the brain can disrupt the complex organization of firing, resulting in abnormal perception of the environment, uncoordinated movement, loss of force production, and decreases in cognition.

Behavior is shaped by the interplay between genes and the environment. There are genes that control entry into the cell cycle where cells synthesize DNA and undergo mitosis. Proliferation can be triggered by internal signals or in response to external growth factor stimulation. There is a complex spectrum of alterations produced by aging, disease, and neoplastic transformation. Mutations of genes cause changes in cell growth, differentiation, and death. A set of genes appear to inhibit cellular proliferation; these genes are the "brakes" of the cell cycle, and loss of these genes may lead to neoplastic, tumor growth.[27]

Inherited patterns of DNA expression appear to cause a predisposition for neurologic disease and affect the ability to repair damage from an insult in the nervous system. Genetic information is stored in the chromosomes within each individual cell in the body; about 80,000 genes are represented and arranged in a precise order. More than one-third of the genes are expressed as messenger ribonucleic acid (RNA) in the brain, more than in any other part of the body. An anomaly or alternative gene version is referred to as an *allele*. Single-gene mutations or alleles have been identified and can be associated with degenerative neurologic disease such as Huntington disease. However, for most chronic disorders, there appear to be multiple abnormalities, and it is clear that environmental conditions have an effect on how the abnormality is manifested.[2] Pathologic derangements of normal cellular processes are a way of looking at possible causes of disease.

The following chapters describe typical neurologic disorders, and the differential diagnosis to identify each. The incidence, risk, and etiologic factors are described in each chapter. As more understanding evolves, it is clear that there is overlap in the pathologic processes. Symptoms can be both similar and distinguishing. Treatment for one disorder may have the some of the same components as another with neurotransmitter substances the main target. In general, science is discovering the value of nutrition, exercise and mindfulness as contributing to what is termed "neuroprotection."

PATHOGENESIS

Cellular Dysfunction

Neuronal cell death is a hallmark of many disorders of the nervous system through the processes of necrosis and apoptosis. The intensity of cellular injury determines whether the cell dies or is able to survive. Very severe injury leads to the passive process of necrosis, less severe but irreparable injury leads to the active process of apoptosis, and survivable injury leads to reactive changes such as gliosis or scarring.

Apoptosis is programmed cell death, or a type of cellular suicide, but apoptosis does not cause inflammatory responses. It is a more organized process with fragmentation of the cells and degradation of the DNA. It is common during the development of cells to eliminate the overproduction of one cell type. The biochemical pathway is present in all cells of the body and is used normally in the maturation and regulation of the nervous system with systematic removal of neurons from the brain. In apoptosis, the cell is removed by macrophages and leaves no residual damage to other components of the CNS. If the cell sustains genetic damage through neurodegenerative disease or injury and cannot be repaired by the system, the cell dies. Damage to the CNS can cause excessive apoptosis through the process of trophic factor withdrawal, oxidative insults, metabolic compromise, overactivation of glutamate receptors, and exposure to bacterial toxins.[60] Both necrosis and apoptosis underlie diseases as diverse as stroke, trauma, demyelinating disorders, infections, and neurodegenerative disorders.

When cell death is caused by necrosis, there is cellular swelling, fragmentation, and cell disintegration. Necrosis causes the internal structure of the cell to swell as water enters the cell through osmosis and cell membranes to rupture. Lymphocytes and polynuclear cells can cause inflammatory cells to surround the necrotic debris, resulting in release of cytotoxic compounds and destruction of neighboring cells. Excitotoxicity results from the inappropriate activation of excitatory amino acid receptors leading to the entry of calcium ions into the cell. The calcium activates intracellular function. Damaged cells release excitotoxins that cause further destruction within surrounding cells.[27]

Free radical formation is a by-product of excitotoxicity. Free radicals are capable of destroying cellular components and triggering apoptosis. Free radicals are molecules with an odd number of electrons. The odd, or unpaired, electron is highly reactive as it seeks to pair with another free electron. Free radicals are generated during oxidative metabolism and energy production in the body. Free radicals are related to normal metabolism but can be the cause of oxidative stress in brain injury and disease. Oxidative stress refers to cells and tissues that have been altered by exposure to oxidants. Oxidation of lipids, proteins, and DNA leads to tissue injury. Nitrogen monoxide (nitric oxide [NO]) is a free radical generated by NO synthase. This enzyme modulates physiologic responses, such as vasodilation or signaling, in the brain. Oxidative stress, rather than being the primary cause, appears to be a secondary complication in many progressive disorders, such as Alzheimer disease, Parkinson disease, and amyotrophic lateral sclerosis (ALS), as well as disorders of mental status. An enhanced antioxidant status is associated with reduced risk of several diseases.[75]

The extracellular environment is critical to the function of the neurons and is managed by a variety of methods. The blood-brain barrier is made from endothelial cells and its tight junctions that block diffusion, so that substances can pass only through the cell and not in between cells. This process is regulatory in nature and not completely protective. Entry into the CNS is determined by lipid solubility. Glucose and amino acid cross the endothelial cell barrier via protein transporters.[83]

The ependymal cells line the ventricles and spinal canal and regulate metabolism between the channels of the extracellular space and the ventricles. The ependyma forms the basis of the cerebral spinal fluid barrier. There is movement of molecules through the extracellular space with the possibility of long-range and relatively diffuse actions of neurotransmitters released into the extracellular space. This type of signaling is known as *volume transmission* and may have a major role in setting large-scale neuronal excitability or inhibition.[27]

Dysfunction within the nervous system can affect either or both of the two main classes of cells: the glial cells and the neurons. Stem cells create new glia and new neurons. The region immediately beneath the ependymal cell layer produces new cells at a very low rate in the adult compared to the amount created during neurogenesis in early development. They migrate widely through the brain and conform phenotypically to the regions where they end up.

Glial Cells

Aside from neurons, macroglia and microglia are the two primary cell types located throughout the CNS. The macroglia are derived from a nerve cell lineage and are classified into three distinct subtypes: astrocytes, oligodendrocytes, and Schwann cells. These macroglia are the most populous cells of the CNS and support and maintain neuronal plasticity throughout the CNS. Glial cells are often implicated in the disease process that affects brain tissue.[46]

Microglia are the resident immune cells of the brain. Microglia are interspersed throughout the brain and represent approximately 10% of the CNS population of cells. Microglia differ from the macroglia because they are derived from a monocyte cell lineage. Microglia respond to CNS insult by diffuse proliferation and infiltration of CNS tissue. Microglia are pivotal in innate immune activation and function to modulate neuroinflammatory signals throughout the brain. In the absence of a stimulus indicating inflammation, microglia are dormant. Inflammatory cytokines produced within the CNS target neuronal substrates, triggering a response of fever, increased sleep, reduced appetite, and lethargy. Collectively, these behavioral symptoms of sickness are evolutionarily conserved and function to increase the metabolic demand for clearance of pathogens via the microglia.[33] Active microglia show macrophage-like activities, including scavenging, phagocytosis, antigen presentation, and inflammatory cytokine production. Activated microglia and monocytes coming in from the bloodstream can assume the form of macrophages. Microglia recruit and activate astrocytes to propagate these inflammatory signals further. Normally, these neuroinflammatory changes are transient and beneficial, with microglia returning to the dormant state after the resolution of the immune challenge. However, nearby neurons may be damaged by toxins released from activated macrophages and microglia. Aging provides a brain environment in which microglia activation is not resolved, leading to a heightened sensitivity to immune activation; this lack of resolution may also contribute to the pathogenesis of neurologic disease.[91]

Astrocytes, another type of glial cell, are named because they look like star cells. They are the most numerous cells in the brain and outnumber neurons 10 to 1. Figure 28-1 shows the relationship of the glial cell to the neuron. The glial cells provide support and structure for the CNS and play the role that connective tissue performs in other parts of the body. The neurons communicate information to one another in order to process sensory information, program motor and emotional responses, and store information through memory. In addition to their support function, the cells serve a nutritive function, since they connect to the capillary wall and to the nerve cell. Astrocytes are permeable to potassium and therefore are involved in maintaining the correct potassium balance in the extracellular space. Astroglia have the ability to monitor and remove extracellular glutamate and other residual neuronal debris after brain injury and can seal off damaged brain tissue.[46,85]

When the astroglial cells become dysfunctional as part of an injury or degenerative process, it may reinforce

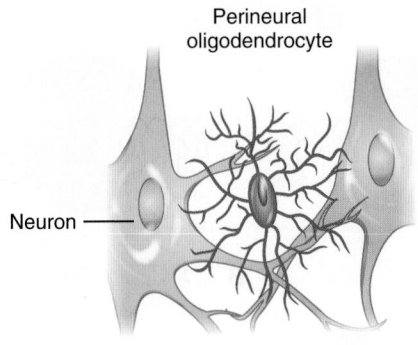

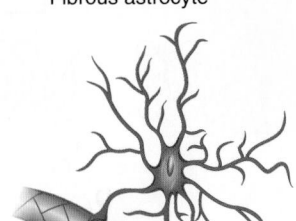

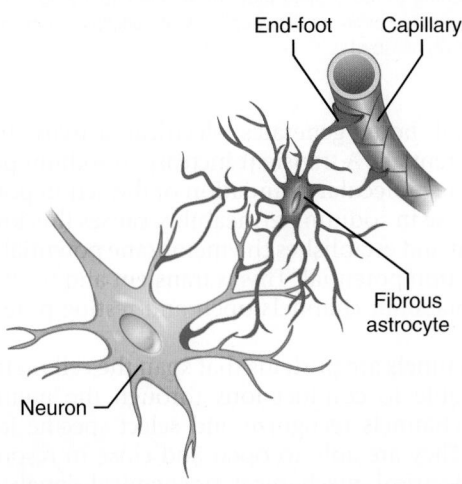

Figure 28-1

The relationship of the glial cells (astrocytes, oligodendrocytes) to the neurons and capillaries. (From Kandel ER, Schwartz JH: *Principles of neural science*, ed 2, New York, 1985, Elsevier.)

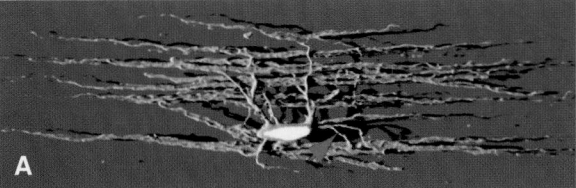

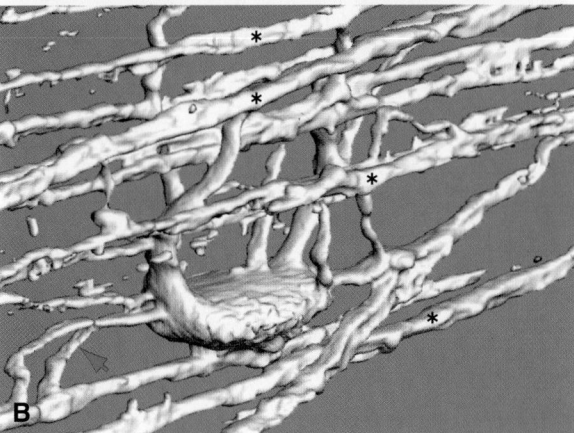

Figure 28-2

A, Single oligodendrocyte from a rat. **B,** More magnified view showing the process as they emerge from the cell body. (From Nolte J: *The human brain: an introduction to its functional anatomy*, ed 5, St Louis, 2002, Mosby. Courtesy Dr. Peter S. Eggli, Institute of Anatomy, University of Bern, Bern, Switzerland.)

neuronal damage. Astroglial changes are widely recognized to be one of the earliest and most remarkable cellular responses to CNS injury via both hypertrophy and regeneration.[70] Astrocyte swelling is a common pathologic finding and is often seen at the interface with the vascular system. Astrocytes are in involved in creating glial scarring, or fibrillary gliosis.[69] Astrocytes may alter their gene expression in response to brain injury. Astroglial cell tissue can also be the site of neoplastic disorders that disrupt nerve cell function by compressing the neurons and blood supply in the surrounding area (see Chapter 30).

Pain was classically viewed as being mediated solely by neurons, as are other sensory phenomena. It is clear now that spinal cord glia amplify pain and are activated by certain sensory signals arriving from the periphery. These glia express characteristics in common with immune cells in that they respond to viruses and bacteria, releasing proinflammatory cytokines, which create pathologic pain. (See Chapter 7 for more information about interactions between the immune system and the CNS.) An apparently discrete CNS lesion may lead to glia activation throughout the pain neuraxis, and systemic rather than localized treatment may be required to effectively treat neuropathic pain. Modulation of glia activity is the goal; as a total block leads to anesthesia and adverse neurologic side effects.[36]

The two other glial cell types, the oligodendrocyte, a part of the CNS, and the Schwann cell found in the peripheral nervous system, are responsible for the production of the myelin sheath, which surrounds the axon. (See Chapter 39 for information on the peripheral disorders that are associated.) Demyelinating disorders that target the CNS, such as multiple sclerosis, are often the result of disrupted function of the oligodendrocyte.[1] This process is further described in "Multiple Sclerosis" in Chapter 31. Figures 28-2 and 28-3 show the oligodendrocyte and describe the process of myelination.[70]

Nerve Cells

Communication between nerve cells is related to the structure and function of each cell type. The location in the nervous system, the input cells, and the target cells will determine how a cell communicates. The cell body size as well as the shape and configuration of dendrites and axons will also affect the method of communication. However, almost all neurons will typically fire through a

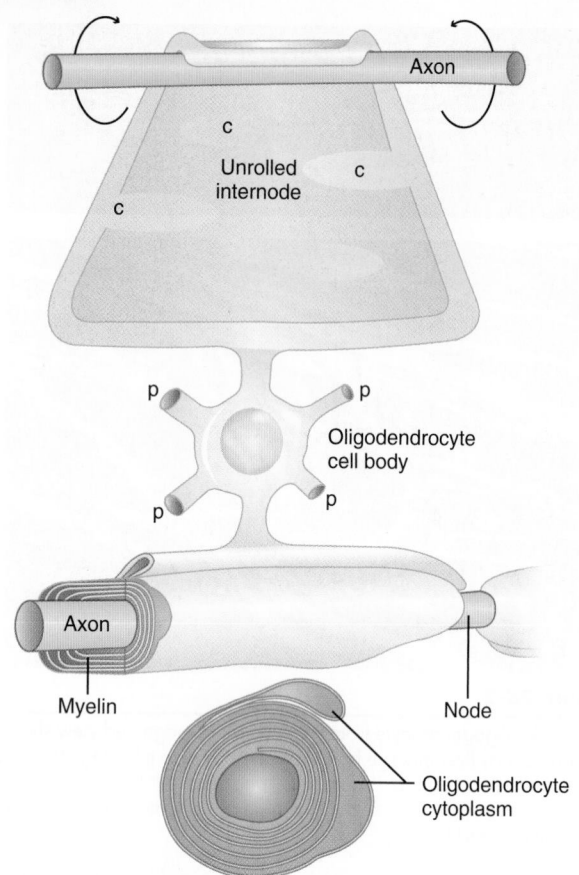

Figure 28-3

Schematic diagram of the formation of myelin in the central nervous system (CNS). (From Nolte J: *The human brain: an introduction to its functional anatomy*, ed 5, St Louis, 2002, Mosby. Redrawn from Krstić RV: *Illustrated encyclopedia of human histology*, Berlin, 1984, Springer-Verlag.)

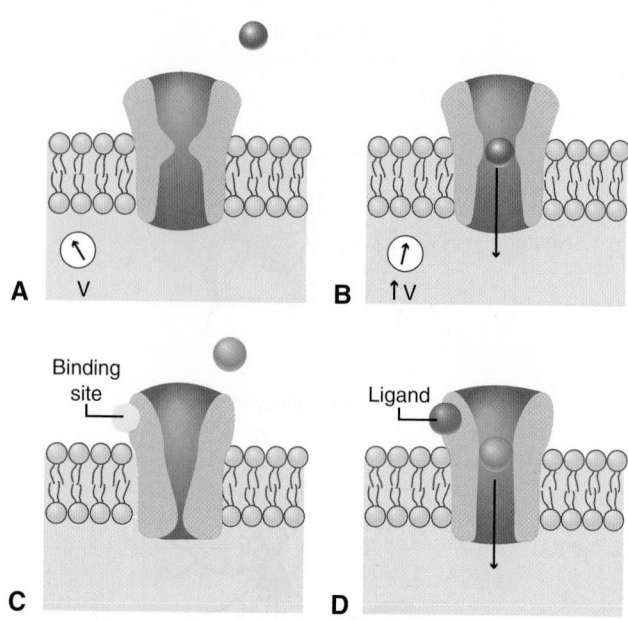

Figure 28-4

Ion channels respond to the changes in voltage. A represents the closed state, and **B** represents the open state that allows neurotransmitters to gain entry into the cell. **C** and **D** represent the opening based on the ligand attaching to the protein that causes the channel to open. (From Nolte J: *The human brain: an introduction to its functional anatomy*, ed 5, St Louis, 2002, Mosby.)

manner that can be described schematically. Essentially, the chemical information encoded by a gene within one nerve cell is delivered to the appropriate postsynaptic genome through a series of molecular reactions.[92] Information is transferred via electrical signals that travel along the neuron and is carried to the next neuron through a series of biochemical events that will influence the behavior of the second-order neuron.

The cell body of the neuron is the metabolic center of the neuron and includes the nucleus where the genetic material is located. The gene expressed in a cell directs the manufacture of proteins that determine the structure, function, and regulation of the neural circuits. Mutation, or changes in the structure of the DNA, can lead to the production of abnormal proteins that can be associated with vulnerability to neurologic disease. Abnormalities within the gene structure leading to predisposition for mutations can be inherited. Toxicity or abuse of drugs can also affect the ability of the DNA to replicate in a normal manner and can cause long-term dysfunction of the nervous system. Cell body inclusions are growths that occur within the cell body as a part of aging, such as Lewy bodies, but can also be a part of the disease process and can cause loss of function of the cell as a result of the obliteration of the nucleus of the cell.[75]

The cell body generates electrical activity through action potentials. A transient increase in sodium permeability is the molecular foundation of the action potential. The increase in sodium permeability causes this ion to be dominant and establishes the membrane potential as +40 mV, or action potential. This is transient and soon closed as the potassium channels open and resting potential is restored.

Ion channels are proteins that span the cell membrane and are able to conduct ions through the membrane. The ion channels recognize and select specific ions for transfer. They are able to open and close in response to specific electrical, mechanical, or chemical signals. Figure 28-4 describes the gating properties.[69] Sodium channel blockers bind the outer axonal surface of the channel and prevent the flux of sodium. The nerve cells sequentially generate four different signals at different sites within the cell: an input signal, a trigger signal, a conducting signal, and an output signal. The input signal depolarizes the cell membrane. Dendrites are typically the site for receiving incoming signals from other neurons. It is in the trigger zone on the initial segment of the axon that the receptor signals are summed, and the neuron then fires an action potential through the length of the axon. The intensity of the conducting signals is determined by the frequency of individual action potentials. As the action potential reaches the neuron's terminal, it stimulates the release of a chemical neurotransmitter cell through the presynaptic terminals.[46] Figure 28-5 shows the processes related to transmitter release.[69] Excitatory synapses are distributed distally in the dendritic receptive field, and inhibitory synapses exist in the proximal dendritic field or on

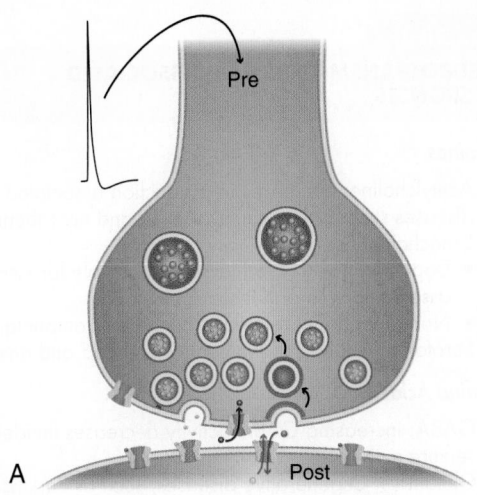
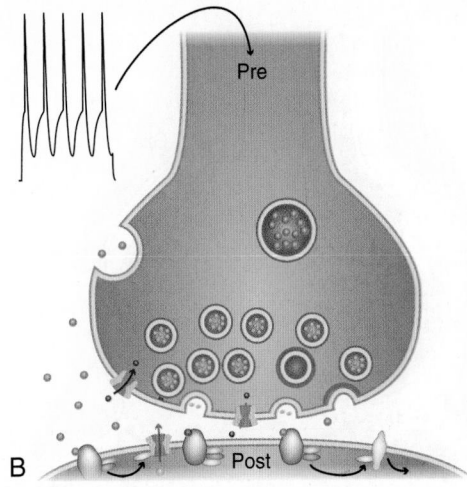

Figure 28-5

A, Depolarization of the terminal causes sodium influx and opening of the channels in the postsynaptic neuron. **B,** Release of transmitters from large and small vesicles, the status of the postsynaptic proteins will affect the binding capability. (From Nolte J: *The human brain: an introduction to its functional anatomy,* ed 5, St Louis, 2002, Mosby.)

the cell body. The combined firing creates modulation of input.

The axon serves as the entry route of a number of pathogens and toxins and presents a large target as a result of its large volume. The axon of the nerve can selectively be damaged, without destruction of the cell body, causing a decrease or loss of presynaptic activity. The stretch damage to the axon is responsible for the abnormal or delayed firing associated with damage to the brainstem in head trauma. Axonal spheroid formation is a reaction to injury resulting in formation of axon retraction balls and can be seen in radiation necrosis and traumatic brain injury. It is clear now that axon degeneration plays a part in secondary and primary progressive multiple sclerosis.[27]

Neurotransmission

By means of its axonal terminals, one neuron contacts and transmits information to the receptive surface of another neuron. The release of neurotransmitter from the presynaptic terminal and the uptake of that substance in the postsynaptic receptor are known as a synapse. A simplified diagram is shown in Figure 28-6. Virtually all communication between neurons occurs via chemicals. The chemical communication involved in this process is universally known as either neurotransmission or neuromodulation.[47] Changes in neurotransmitter substances in the space surrounding the neurons have been implicated in many nervous system disease processes.

Neurotransmitters are synthesized within each neuron, stored in presynaptic vesicles, and released from depolarized nerve terminals. They bind specifically to presynaptic or postsynaptic receptors, which recognize the neurotransmitter's chemical conformation. A single neuron can release several different neurotransmitter substances, and a single neuron can be selectively receptive to different types of neurotransmitters because of the differences in ion channels.[93] Activation of a receptor in response to neurotransmitter can cause changes in a variety of molecules. Modification, or modulation, of the

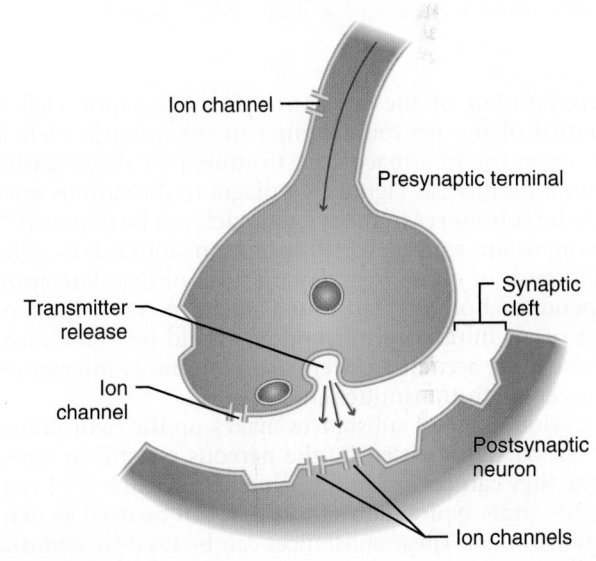

Figure 28-6

Schematic representation of the postsynaptic neuron and the presynaptic terminal. Transmitter substances are synthesized in presynaptic terminals, released into the synaptic cleft, and occupied in the postsynaptic terminal.

system can take place presynaptically, postsynaptically, or within the cell body.

Changes in the target cell can cause abnormal responses to normal levels of transmitters. The amount of neurotransmitter released in the synaptic cleft is determined by the neuronal firing rate, the quantity of transmitter in the nerve terminal, and the cumulative regulatory actions of excitatory and inhibitory neurotransmitters. These biochemical actions alter the electrical activity of the postsynaptic neurons. One aspect of chemical transmission that is extremely important in signaling is the time course of transmitter in the synaptic cleft. The breakdown of a transmitter is an important variable and can change the

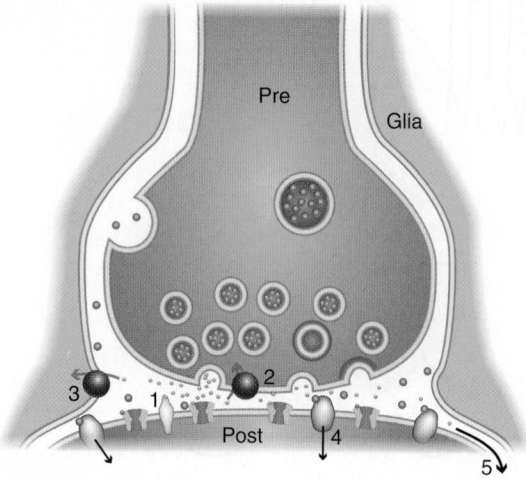

Figure 28-7

The transmitter substances can be removed by (1) enzymatic inactivation of neurotransmitter, (2) reuptake of the neurotransmitter by the presynaptic terminal, (3) removal by the nearby glial cells, (4) uptake by the postsynaptic terminal, or (5) it may just move out of the synaptic space into adjoining spaces. (From Nolte J: *The human brain: an introduction to its functional anatomy*, ed 5, St Louis, 2002, Mosby.)

Box 28-1

NEUROTRANSMITTERS AND ASSOCIATED RESPONSES

Amines

- Acetylcholine: decreases in production associated with diseases such as Alzheimer disease and myasthenia gravis
- Catecholamines
  - Dopamine: decreased levels responsible for symptoms associated with parkinsonism
  - Norepinephrine: related to cocaine or amphetamine
- Serotonin: involved in the control of mood and anxiety

Amino Acids

- GABA: increasing GABA activity decreases incidence of seizure activity
- Glutamate: degenerative diseases, such as Parkinson, ALS, or Alzheimer, may be related to increases in glutamate; increased levels contribute to the secondary damage associated with stroke and spinal cord injury
- Glycine: more active in the spinal cord than CNS

*Neuroactive Peptides**

- Enkephalins and β-endorphins: pain control achieved by use of drugs (opiates) that bind to endorphin and enkephalin receptors
- Substance P: involved in pain pathways

GABA, γ-Aminobutyric acid; *ALS*, amyotrophic lateral sclerosis; *CNS*, central nervous system.
*More than 50 neuroactive peptides have been identified, these are most typical.

concentration of the substance in the synaptic cleft.[37] Control of the neurotransmitter in the synaptic cleft is the basis for pharmacologic treatment in degenerative neurologic disease. Figure 28-7 diagrams the various ways that the substances in the synaptic cleft can be removed.[69] An important concept for all neurotransmitters is that the final result of either hyperpolarization or depolarization depends on both the transmitter and its receptor. The concept of an inhibitory transmitter should be abandoned for the more accurate concept of an inhibitory interaction between neurotransmitter and receptor.

A wide range of substances makes up the neurotransmitter substances used by the nervous system. In some cases, they can coexist in the same neuron. Box 28-1 represents some typical substances that can be used as neurotransmitters. These substances can be used by neurons in different ways, according to the function of the specific neuron. To be used as a neurotransmitter, these substances are packaged in vesicles within the neuron and respond to the particular enzymes that are specific to that neuron.[93]

Amino Acids. One of the small-molecule neurotransmitters, glutamate, is an excitatory amino acid transmitter used throughout the brain and spinal column. It is an intermediate transmitter in cellular metabolism, so the presence of glutamate in a cell does not necessarily suggest neurologic activity. Glutamate functions with its receptors in an excitatory or depolarizing system at primary afferent nerve endings, the granule cells of the cerebellum, the dentate gyrus, and the corticostriatal and subthalamopallidal pathways important to basal ganglia function. When the levels of glutamate rise above normal, it can become neurotoxic and cause cell death. Glutamate opens ion channels to bring calcium into the cell. In the case of excess glutamate, too much calcium is allowed into the cell, and the calcium eventually destroys the cell.

Excess glutamate can be an effect of neuronal injury, as in stroke, and brain or spinal cord injury. It appears that the genes in the nerve cell body may trigger this excitotoxic mechanism, resulting in release of excess glutamate that may lead to the degenerative processes associated with diseases such as ALS, Alzheimer, Huntington, and Parkinson.[72] Part of the activation of seizure is due to glutamate receptors. Toxins or drug abuse can also trigger an excitotoxic level of glutamate.[92]

γ-Aminobutyric acid (GABA) is a tiny amino acid that serves both as a neurotransmitter and as an intermediate metabolite in the normal function of cells. GABA is synthesized from glutamate by way of the vitamin B_6–dependent enzyme, glutamate decarboxylase. GABA is the major transmitter for brief inhibitory synapses. GABAergic cells have a dense representation within the basal ganglia.[34] Loss of GABAergic neurons that inhibit glutamate results in increased excitation. Glycine is another amino acid neurotransmitter that is the transmitter at some inhibitory CNS synapses. The distributions of GABA and glycine synapses overlap, but glycine is more prominent in the spinal cord.[69]

The N-methyl-D-aspartate (NMDA) receptor has a complex process using glutamate and glycine activation at the same time but also requiring membrane polarization to remove magnesium from inside the cell, so that the cell can allow sodium to be active within the cell. NMDA receptors are widely distributed throughout the neocortex, hippocampus, and anterior horn motor neurons. The NMDA response thus works when the membrane bearing the receptor has already been depolarized by another stimulus, so it prolongs or augments the initial depolarization. This activity supports the activities of learning and memorization. During cellular energy failure induced by ischemia, there is collapse of membrane potentials (depolarization) and uncontrolled synaptic and transmembrane release of excitatory amino acids into the extracellular space. NMDA receptors will open and allow calcium into the intracellular space causing damage to the mitochondria, limiting the production of adenosine triphosphate (ATP). Drugs that are NMDA receptor antagonists include ketamine and eliprodil. Antiepileptic drugs, such as felbamate and lamotrigine, block the glutamate and glycine activity at the NMDA receptors.[27]

Amines. Cholinergic neurons play two different roles in the nervous system. Acetylcholine was the first neurotransmitter discovered and has primary activity at the level of the peripheral nervous system. It is the transmitter released by the motor neurons at neuromuscular junctions and within the autonomic nervous system. Disorders related to acetylcholine are discussed in Chapter 39. The role of the cholinergic neurons in the CNS is quite different because it is involved with the regulation of the general level of activity. Cholinergic systems can be mapped to the medial cortex and to the areas responsible for information flow to the hypothalamus and amygdala through the reticular formation. They also constitute a major element of the autonomic nervous system as preganglionic neurons of sympathetic ganglia and postganglionic parasympathetic neurons. The cholinergic and biogenic amine systems appear to establish the activity set point of the cortex and basal ganglia rather than point-to-point neural firing.[27] Biogenic amines are synthesized from amino acid precursors, dopamine, serotonin, and norepinephrine. Two transmitters known as catecholamines are dopamine and norepinephrine.

Dopamine is synthesized in four major CNS pathways. The most important and most widely understood involves the nigrostriatal pathway of the basal ganglia. Dopaminergic function is decreased in individuals with Parkinson disease and attention disorders affecting the frontal lobe. The synthetic pathway for dopamine is tyrosine to dopa to dopamine. It is possible that biomarkers α-synuclein aggregation can be detected in gastrointestinal tract neurons in Parkinson disease.[86]

Norepinephrine is a neurotransmitter found in the hypothalamus and the locus ceruleus in the brainstem. It is synthesized from dopamine and therefore shares the same enzymes, including the rate-limiting tyrosine hydroxylase. Like dopamine, norepinephrine is removed from the synapse by active reuptake into the presynaptic cell and then is metabolized by two enzymes, monoamine oxidase (MAO) and catechol-O-methyltransferase (COMT).[34] Dopamine and norepinephrine are the primary neurotransmitters associated with the task of attending. Both need to be enhanced to achieve sustained clinical benefit.

The catecholamines appear to have an important role in working memory. The cholinergic system appears to be critical for the acquisition of long-term declarative memories. Cholinergic function decreases somewhat with age and greatly in individuals with Alzheimer disease, and these changes may contribute importantly to corresponding reductions in declarative memory ability. Centrally acting cholinesterase inhibitors are marketed for improvement of memory.

Serotonin has its main cell bodies in the dorsal raphe nucleus of the brainstem as well as the spinal cord, hippocampus, and cerebellum. In parallel to dopamine, it is synthesized by a two-step process, first with a rate-limiting enzyme and then a general enzyme. The first step takes tryptophan to 5-hydroxytryptophan (5-HTP) with the rate-limiting enzyme, tryptophan hydroxylase. The second step takes this intermediate to serotonin (5-hydroxytryptamine [5-HT]) by aromatic amino acid decarboxylase, which is the same enzyme involved in dopamine synthesis. There are several types of serotonin receptors spread throughout the brain. Serotonin is metabolized like the catecholamines by active reuptake into the presynaptic cell and then metabolism by MAO. Serotonin is removed from the synaptic cleft by reuptake pumps rather than by degradation. Antidepressant medications work by inhibiting this reuptake.[27]

Neuropeptides. Neurons can secrete hormones, or neuropeptides, and most or all of them can function as neurotransmitters. Neuropeptides are metabolically difficult for cells to make and transport, and can be effective at very low concentrations. Synthesis of neuropeptides begins in the nucleus of the cell, where the gene is transcribed into RNA. Five genes related to control of emotion have been identified: COMT, serotonin transporter (SLC6A4), neuropeptide Y (NPY), a glucocorticoid receptor-regulating co-chaperone of stress proteins (FKBP5), and pituitary adenylate cyclase–activating polypeptide receptor (ADCYAP1R1). The effects of genes on emotion, as well as the variety of mechanisms and factors (such as stress) that modify these effects, are being studied.[9]

Gaseous Neurotransmitters and Others. NO and carbon monoxide are gases that can diffuse easily through neuronal membranes and can influence subsequent transmitter release. Astrocytes may be the target, mediating cell-to-cell communication between vessel endothelium and smooth muscle and are critical in vasomotor control, inflammation, and neuronal communication. NO sets the functional state of adjacent cells and has a short half-life. NO released from endothelial cells acts on vascular smooth muscle causing vasodilation. NO released from inflammatory cells occurs in high concentrations and kills cells. NO may play a role in neurodegeneration, and acute elevations may contribute to damage in ischemia and trauma. NO synthesis is augmented by NMDA receptor activation by glutamate; therefore, NO may synergize excitotoxity.[47]

Neurotrophic factors are essential to maintenance and survival of neurons and their terminals but are produced by the body in a limited supply. Four major neurotrophins have been identified in humans: nerve growth factor, brain-derived neurotrophic factor, neurotrophin 3, and neurotrophin 4/5. Neurotrophins interact with receptor cells to prolong the life of the neuron. Although this class of substances is also not fully understood, it is clear that it plays a role in the development of the nervous system.

It appears to work by suppressing the pathway that leads to apoptosis.[46]

CLINICAL MANIFESTATIONS

Sensory Disturbances

The skin, muscles, and joints contain a variety of receptors that create electrical activity as described previously[12,90] (see Chapter 39). The electrical input is carried to the CNS through the *afferent axons* via the spinal cord. The cell bodies rest in the ganglion of the dorsal root that lies adjacent to the spinal cord. The afferent fibers are arranged somatotopically in the spinal column and ascend to the brainstem and the sensory cortex. Figure 28-8 shows the simplified synapse.[69] A characteristic of the fibers that run in the dorsal column of the spinal cord is that they synapse at the level of the brainstem nuclei, where they cross over to the contralateral (opposite) hemisphere of the brain. This phenomenon is illustrated in Figure 28-9.[69] When there is a disorder of the brain that affects the afferent system above the level of the brainstem, symptoms occur on the side contralateral to the lesion.[46,69]

The brainstem receives information from specialized senses. For example, vestibular information is received via cranial nerve VIII and integrated through the brainstem nuclei, contributing to postural control and locomotion. Disorders of the afferent nerve, dorsal columns of the spinal cord, and brainstem result in changes in the sensory input available. This can manifest as lack of cutaneous sensation, numbness, tingling, paresthesias, or dysesthesias in the distribution of the nerves affected. Sensory input from the joints and muscles is known as *proprioception*. When this sensory function is lost or disturbed, the person will have difficulty maintaining the body in the appropriate position for the voluntary and involuntary movements necessary for most functional activities, especially those required for postural control. Movements become ataxic or uncoordinated because of the loss of feedback on position from the joints.[3]

The nervous system has several pain-control pathways available, some of which suppress and some of

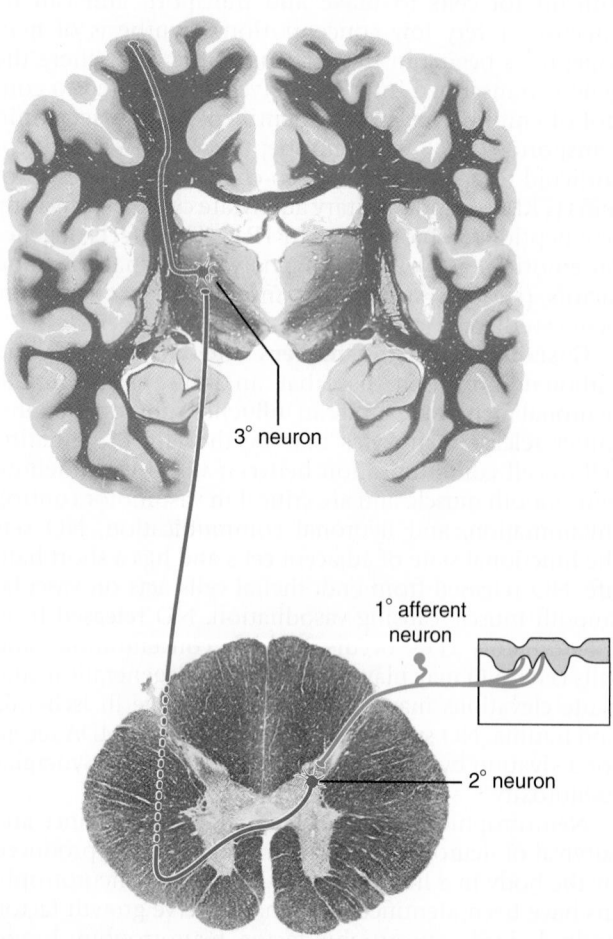

Figure 28-8

The minimum sensory pathway from the periphery to the cerebral cortex.
(From Nolte J: *The human brain: an introduction to its functional anatomy*, ed 5, St Louis, 2002, Mosby.)

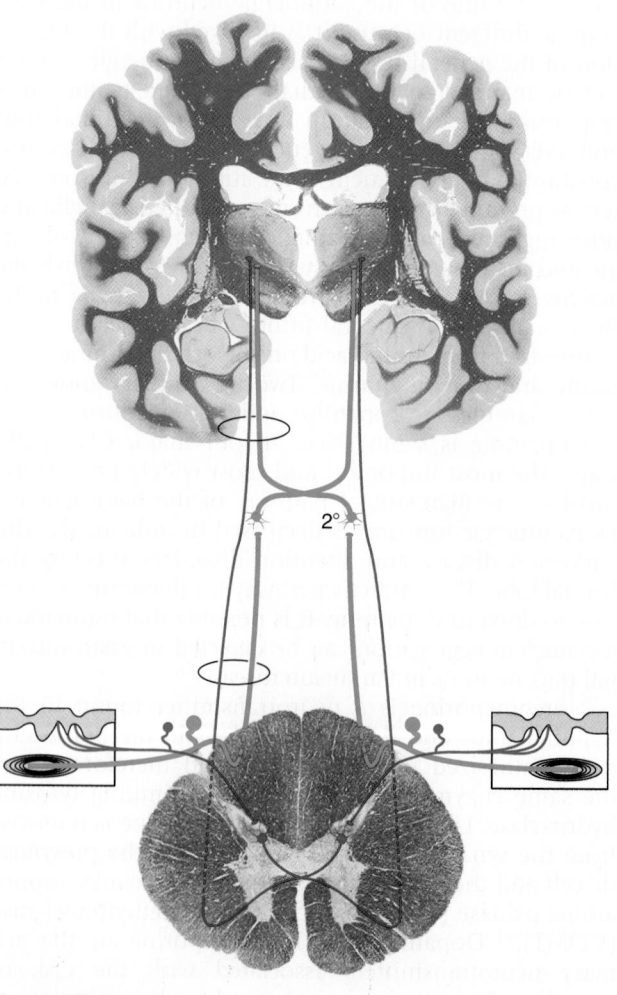

Figure 28-9

A, In the spinal cord, a lesion would result in decreased touch on the same side of the lesion and decreased pain sensation on the contralateral side. **B,** A lesion above the medulla would cause decreased touch and pain on the contralateral side. (From Nolte J: *The human brain: an introduction to its functional anatomy*, ed 5, St Louis, 2002, Mosby.)

which facilitate the experience of pain. Modulation of noxious stimuli is directed by the reticular formation. Noxious stimuli can be experienced as more or less painful, depending on the individual's circumstances. If an individual is focused on a task during an injury, such as a soldier or athlete, the pain of the injury may be suppressed until the task is completed. When a lesion affects the midbrain areas that modulate and interpret sensory input, such as the thalamus, the result can cause exaggeration of sensory stimuli.

Disruption of the sensory input provided by the optic nerve is evident in some disorders of the brain and will result in loss of vision in some or all of a field of view. Visual-field cuts are common with stroke (see Chapter 32). Visual hallucinations can also be part of a CNS disorder when the optic radiations or occipital lobe is disrupted, which may also be caused by stroke or a degenerative disease such as multiple sclerosis.

Our survival instincts are related to smell, taste, vision, hearing, and vestibular balance. They are the first signal for the "fight, flight or freeze" behavior for survival. The sensation of vertigo, from inner ear injury, causes more concern for the individual than pain does.

Movement Disorders

Control of movement is accomplished by the cooperative effort of many brain structures.[12,90] Abnormal movement patterns in neurologic disorders can result from lesions of the CNS at many levels. A simplified representation of the typical synaptic flow of neurons and interneurons is seen in Figure 28-10. It is important to recognize that there are many synapses not represented here in the levels of the brainstem and central modulation centers of the basal ganglia and limbic. Activity initiated in the cerebral cortex triggers interneurons that regulate interaction of the lower motor neurons. The parietal and premotor areas of the cerebral cortex are involved in identifying targets in space, determining a course of action, and creating the motor program. The cortex determines strategies for movement. The brainstem and spinal cord are responsible for the execution of the task. The same signal may be processed simultaneously by many different brain structures for different purposes, showing parallel distributed processing.

Various areas of the brain, such as the cerebellum and basal ganglia, interact to establish a motor program that modifies the hierarchic information going from the cortex to the spinal cord. For example, parietal and premotor regions, together with basal ganglia–sustained activation underlie the special skill of handwriting with the dominant hand.[42] The reticulospinal and corticospinal pathways work in parallel to generate a large repertoire of diverse, coordinated movement in the hand. The reticulospinal pathway may likely become a therapeutic target when the corticospinal tract is absent or injured.[41] During motor adaptation, goal locations and movement vectors are differentially remapped, and separate motor plans based on these features are effectively averaged during motor execution.[105]

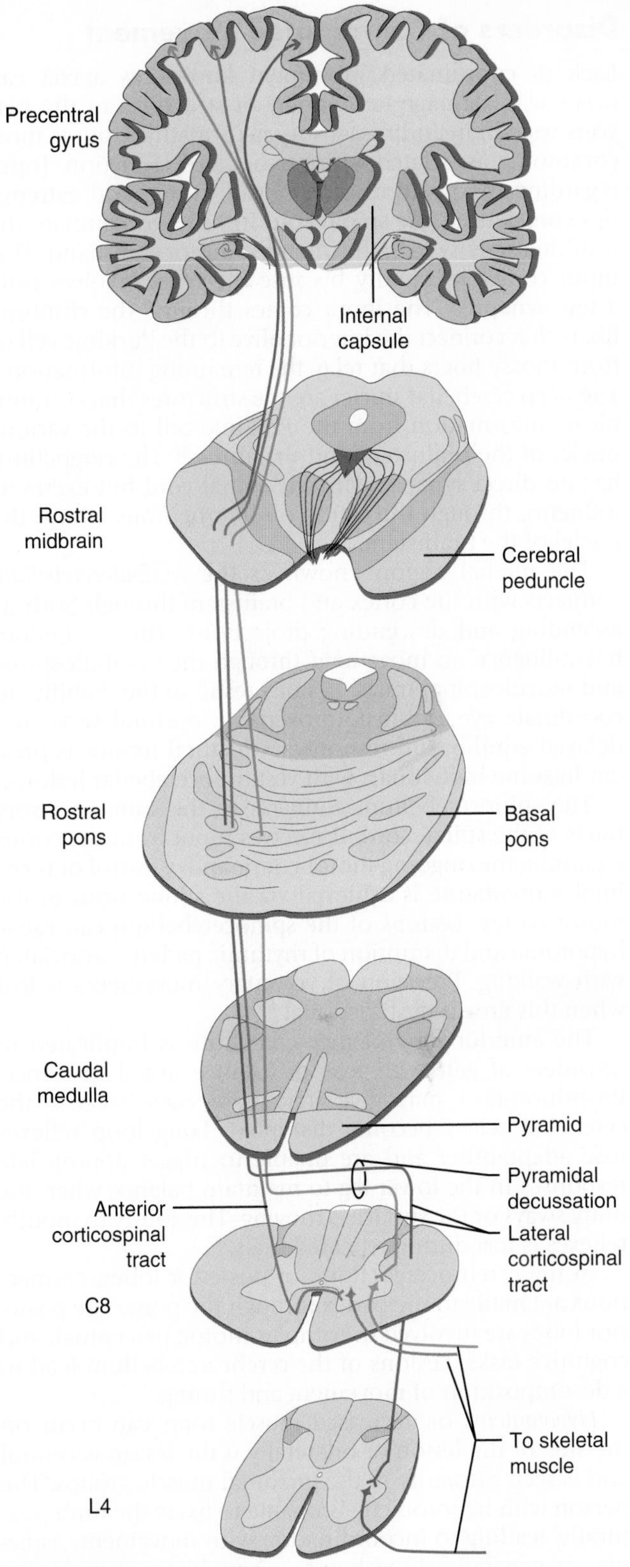

Figure 28-10

Pathway of the motor system from the cortex to the skeletal muscle as it courses through the brainstem structures and spinal cord. (From Nolte J: *The human brain: an introduction to its functional anatomy,* ed 5, St Louis, 2002, Mosby.)

Disorders of Coordinated Movement

Lack of coordinated movement known as ataxia can occur with damage to a variety of structures of the nervous system, including sensory neuropathies, but is most commonly associated with cerebellar dysfunction. Input regarding the position of the head, trunk, and extremities comes from the spinal cord in order to compare the resulting activity with the intended motor command. This input comes in rapidly because the relay involves only a few synapses. The input comes through the climbing fibers that connect the inferior olive to the Purkinje cell or from mossy fibers that relay the remaining information.[5] The deep cerebellar nuclei are the structures that communicate information from the Purkinje cell to the various nuclei of the brainstem and thalamus.[46] The cerebellum has no direct synapse with the spinal cord but exerts its influence through the action on interneurons within the nuclei of the brainstem.

The medial region known as the *vestibulocerebellum* connects with the cortex and brainstem through both its ascending and descending projections. The cerebellum has influence on movement through the vestibulospinal and reticulospinal tracts. Lesions result in the inability to coordinate eye and head movement, postural sway, and delayed equilibrium responses.[5] Postural tremor is present in some individuals with vestibulocerebellar lesions.

The spinocerebellum connects to the somatosensory tracts of the spinal cord. It receives input from the cortex regarding the ongoing motor command. Control of proximal musculature is achieved via the connections to the motor cortex. Lesions of the spinocerebellum can cause hypotonia and disruption of rhythmic patterns associated with walking. Precision of voluntary movements is lost when this area is dysfunctional.[63]

The anterior lobe of the cerebellum is implicated in disorders of gait with loss of balance noted in stance. Proprioception may give inaccurate cues because the cerebellar relays become disrupted. Long loop reflexes lose adaptability and are unable to trigger appropriate responses in the lower leg to maintain balance when the body sways or the surface is moving. The ability to modify reflexes is lost during repeated trials.[97]

In the cerebrocerebellum, or posterior lobes, connections are made to the cortex through the pons. The posterior lobes are involved in complex motor, perceptual, and cognitive tasks. Lesions of the cerebrocerebellum lead to a decomposition of movement and timing.

Hypotonicity, or decreased muscle tone, can occur on the side of the lesion or bilaterally if the lesion is central and is seen primarily in the proximal muscle groups. The person with hypotonicity is unable to fixate the limb posturally, leading to incoordination with movement. *Asthenia*, or generalized weakness, is sometimes seen in the person with cerebellar lesions. Hypotonicity and asthenia, however, do not always occur together. It is believed that both disorders represent loss of input from the cerebellum to the cerebral cortex, but they may represent loss of input to different areas of the cortex.

Dysmetria, the underestimation or overestimation of a necessary movement toward a target, is commonly seen with cerebellar disorders. There is an error in the production of force necessary to perform an intended movement. The initiation of movement is prolonged compared to normal, and the ability to change directions rapidly is impaired. The resulting overshoot and undershoot during movement are known as an *intention tremor*. *Dysdiadochokinesia*, the inability to perform rapidly alternating movements, is related to the inability to stop ongoing movement. The movement becomes slow, without rhythm or consistency.

Decomposition of movement, termed dyssynergia, is seen in persons with cerebellar dysfunction. Instead of performing a movement in one smooth motion, the person will move in distinct sequences to accomplish the motion. Multijoint movements are more affected than single-joint movements. Disruption in force and extent of movement will result in difficulty with grip control and maintaining static hold against resistance. When the resistance is removed, for example, the extremity will oscillate because of lack of feedback regarding position and force needed to maintain static hold.

Scanning speech is a component of cerebellar dysfunction representing complexity of the motor activity. Word selection is not affected, but the words are pronounced slowly and without melody, tone, or rhythm. This reflects the incoordination or hypotonicity of the muscles of the larynx in controlling the voice.

Eye movements are disrupted in the person with cerebellar dysfunction, in both a static head and eye position and with movement of the head. *Gaze-evoked nystagmus*, or nonvoluntary rhythmic oscillation of the eye, occurs when the cerebellum is unable to hold the gaze on an object, especially in a lateral position. When looking at a lateral target, the eyes drift back toward midline and then immediately back to the target. Eyes flickering on and off the target, eyes fluttering around the target, or spastic bursts of eye oscillations may be present when there is brainstem or midline cerebellar lesions.

Ocular dysmetria is similar to the dysmetria seen in the extremities. This dysmetria is seen in cerebellar lesions when the eyes are moving from one target to another (known as *saccadic movement*) or when attempting to follow a target (known as *smooth pursuit*).

Vestibuloocular function is disrupted in medial lesions, and the ability to maintain eye stability during head movement is affected. See "Vestibular Dysfunction" in Chapter 38 for more information on vestibuloocular dysfunction.

Gait disturbance is another disorder related to dysfunction of the cerebellum. The gait becomes wide based and staggering without typical arm swing. The step length is uneven, the step widths are inconsistent, and the feet are often lifted higher than necessary. Stance and swing become irregular, and there is loss of adaptation to changes in terrain. It becomes difficult to perform heel-to-toe walking or walking a straight line, which is the standard sobriety test. In some persons, there is a surprising ability to avoid a fall, although the standing balance is abnormal.[32] Impedance control, the ability to adjust the mechanical behavior of limbs to account for instability, allows adaptation to environmental disturbances. The ability to selectively modulate the endpoint stiffness of the arms, adjusting for varying directions of environmental disturbances is affected in cerebellar injury.[31]

The cerebellum plays a major role in motor learning. The cerebellum is vital in anticipatory, or feed-forward, activity and modification of response.[52] The cerebellum learns or memorizes small movements that are integrated into complex activity. During the acquisition phase of motor learning, the cerebellum is active.[39] Increased activity has also been noted during mental imagery or mental rehearsal of a motor program.[80] The cerebellum is active during cognitive and emotional processes, and lesions can cause difficulty in shifting attention from one sensory or thought domain to another.

Deficits of Higher Brain Function

The cortex has a great deal to do with the abilities and activities that are a part of the highest development in humans, including language and abstract thinking. Perception, movement, and adaptive response to the outside world depends on an intact cerebral cortex. Crystallized intelligence refers to the knowledge and skills that are accumulated over a lifetime. This type of intelligence tends to increase with age. Crystallized intelligence involves learning, knowledge, and skills, whereas fluid intelligence involves our ability to reason and make sense of abstract information. Both can be compromised as a result of damage to the processes of the cortex and deeper components of the brain. The cortex is subdivided for ease of understanding the separate functions, although the structure and function is full of overlap. Figure 28-11 represents some of the functional specialization of the brain. Figure 28-12 describes the lobar relationship to the cerebellum and brainstem.

The *frontal lobe* is the largest single area of the brain, constituting nearly one-third of the brain's cortical surface. It is phylogenetically the youngest area of the brain and has major connections with all other areas of the brain. The frontal lobe is responsible for the highest levels of cognitive processing, control of emotion, and behavior. An individual's personality is established as a frontal lobe function, and one of the most disturbing deficits seen with lesions affecting the frontal lobe is change from the person's premorbid personality. A person's character and temperament are changed by damage to the frontal lobe. Slow processing of information, lack of judgment based on known consequences, withdrawal, and irritability can be the result of an insult to the frontal lobe. Lack of inhibition and apathy are common clinical problems related to frontal lobe damage. The person with a frontal lobe disorder may lack insight into the deficits, and therefore behavior can be difficult to control.

The *right hemisphere syndrome* represents the inability to orient the body within external space and generate the appropriate motor responses. Hemineglect is one of the most common deficits seen with right hemisphere lesions. The individual does not respond to sensory stimuli on the left side of the body and does not respond to the environment surrounding the left side. Hemineglect is evident in the involved extremities and trunk during mobility and self-care activities. The ability to draw in two and three dimensions is lost along with other drawing skills, such as perspective and accurate copying. Spatial disorientation can result, with the person losing familiarity with the environment and becoming lost in areas that should be familiar. Inability to read and follow a map can be an indication of right hemisphere deficit.[24]

Disorders of emotional adjustment often follow a lesion in the right hemisphere. These disorders are primarily in the affective domain of interpersonal relationships and socialization. Cortical control of the limbic system is believed to be responsible, but the exact mechanism of control of more complex emotional behavior is not completely understood at this time. There appears to be hemispheric lateralization of emotions with suggestions that the right hemisphere is the dominant hemisphere in controlling emotions.

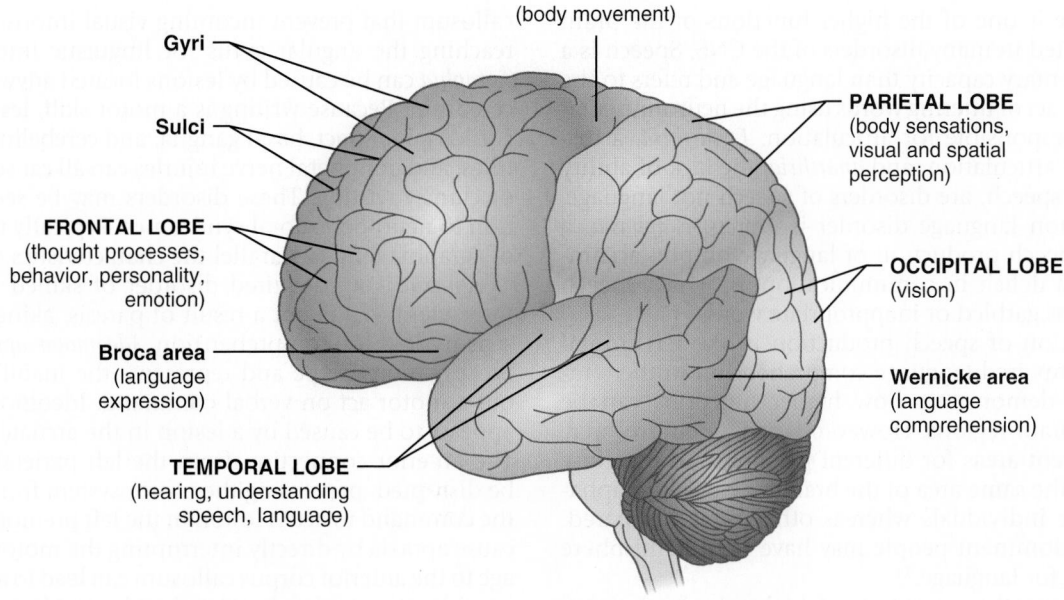

Figure 28-11

Schematic representation of functional specialization in the cortex. (From Chabner DE: *The language of medicine*, ed 8, Philadelphia, 2007, Saunders.)

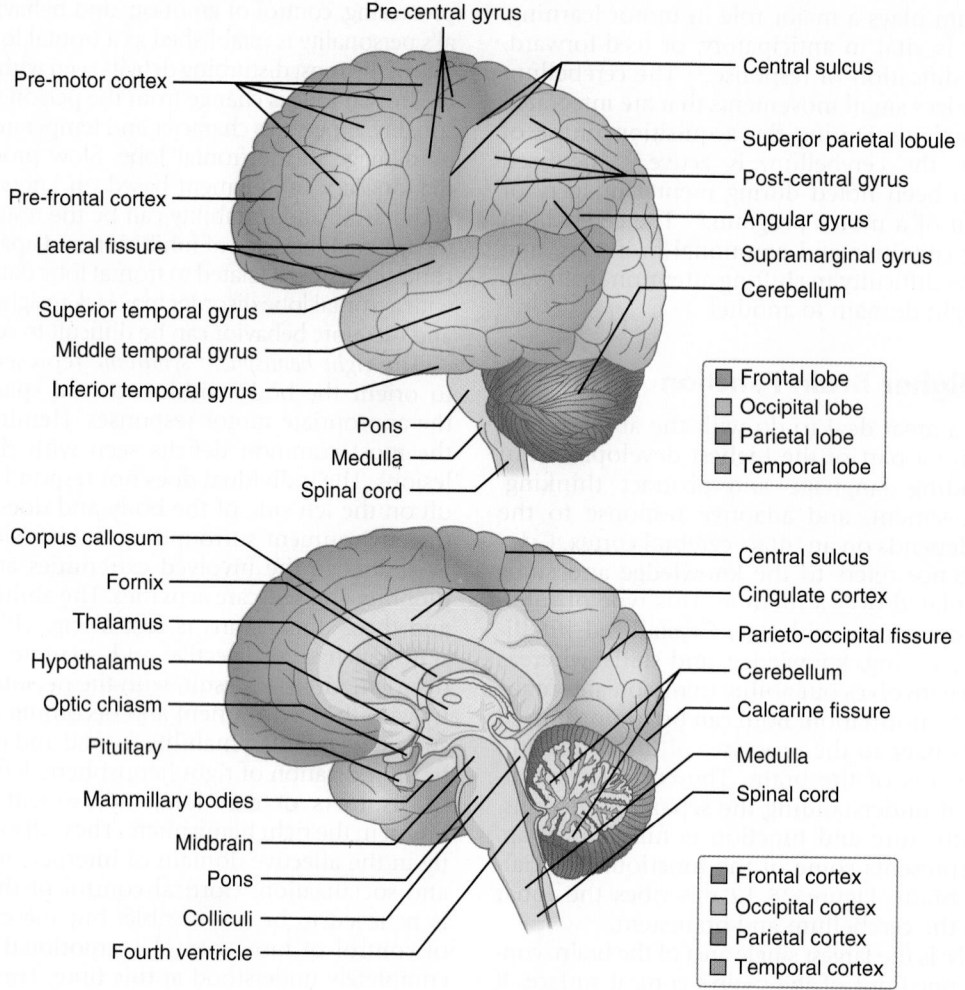

Pre-central gyrus
Pre-motor cortex
Pre-frontal cortex
Lateral fissure
Superior temporal gyrus
Middle temporal gyrus
Inferior temporal gyrus
Pons
Medulla
Spinal cord

Central sulcus
Superior parietal lobule
Post-central gyrus
Angular gyrus
Supramarginal gyrus
Cerebellum

☐ Frontal lobe
☐ Occipital lobe
☐ Parietal lobe
☐ Temporal lobe

Corpus callosum
Fornix
Thalamus
Hypothalamus
Optic chiasm
Pituitary
Mammillary bodies
Midbrain
Pons
Colliculi
Fourth ventricle

Central sulcus
Cingulate cortex
Parieto-occipital fissure
Cerebellum
Calcarine fissure
Medulla
Spinal cord

☐ Frontal cortex
☐ Occipital cortex
☐ Parietal cortex
☐ Temporal cortex

Figure 28-12

The lobes of the cortex and their relationship to the cerebellum, midbrain, and brainstem. (From Farber SD: *Neurorehabilitation: a multisensory approach,* Philadelphia, 1982, WB Saunders.)

Language is one of the higher functions of the brain that is affected in many disorders of the CNS. Speech is a more elementary capacity than language and refers to the mechanical act of uttering words using the neuromuscular structures responsible for articulation. *Dysarthria*, a disturbance in articulation, and *anarthria*, the lack of ability to produce speech, are disorders of speech not language. One common language disorder is *expressive aphasia*, a deficit in speech production or language output, accompanied by a deficit in communication, in which speech comes out as garbled or inappropriate words.

Localization of speech production in the left frontal lobe and impaired language comprehension in the temporal lobe demonstrate how higher functions can be related to brain regions. However, language control may be in different areas for different persons, and therefore damage to the same area of the brain may produce aphasia in some individuals whereas others may be spared. Left hand–dominant people may have right hemisphere dominance for language.[54]

Alexia is another symptom of higher brain dysfunction. It is the acquired inability to read. Alexia is typically caused by lesions in the left occipital lobe and the corpus callosum that prevent incoming visual information from reaching the angular gyrus for linguistic interpretation. *Agraphia* can be caused by lesions located anywhere in the cerebrum. Because writing is a motor skill, lesions of the corticospinal tract, basal ganglia, and cerebellum; myopathies; and peripheral nerve injuries can all cause abnormal or clumsy writing. These disorders may be seen in addition to neurobehavioral syndromes. Typically the features of agraphia tend to parallel the characteristics of aphasia.

Apraxia is an acquired disorder of skilled purposeful movement that is not a result of paresis, akinesia, ataxia, sensory loss, or comprehension. *Ideomotor apraxia* is the most common type and represents the inability to carry out a motor act on verbal command. Ideomotor apraxia appears to be caused by a lesion in the arcuate fasciculus. The anterior connection from the left parietal lobe may be disrupted, preventing the motor system from receiving the command to act. A lesion in the left premotor area can cause apraxia by directly interrupting the motor act. Damage to the anterior corpus callosum can lead to apraxia that is evident in the left hand only. *Ideational apraxia* is failure to perform a sequential act even though each part of the act can be performed individually. The lesion causing

Table 28-1	Characteristics of Comas	
Manifestations	**Metabolic and Drug-Induced**	**From Space-Occupying Lesions**
Onset	Behavioral changes, decreased attention and arousal	Usually severe headache, focal seizures
Pain response	Present and equal	May be different on each side
Reflexes	Intact deep tendon reflexes equal responses,	Deep tendon reflexes may be unequal; positive Babinski sign (UMN lesion)
Pupillary reaction	Bilateral normal response	May be unequal
Size of pupil	May be at midpoint with anticholinergics; pinpoint from opiates; dilated from anoxia	Midbrain lesion—midpoint Pons lesion—pinpoint Herniation to brainstem—large
Corneal reflex	Bilateral, intact	Unequal, may be absent
Eye movement	Spontaneous movement without intention; no reaction to VOR	May have paresis of lateral gaze with CN III compression
Decorticate or decerebrate posturing	Absent; movement is normal	Posturing may be present depending on level of lesion
Extremity movement	Equal movement on both sides	Paresis may be unilateral

UMN, Upper motor neuron; VOR, vestibuloocular reflex; CN III, third cranial (oculomotor) nerve.

ideational apraxia appears to be in the left parietal lobe, as in hemiparesis, or in the frontal lobe, as in Alzheimer disease. The syndrome is seen as well with diffuse cortical damage associated with degenerative dementia.

Agnosia is the inability to recognize an object; the previously acquired meaning of an object is no longer attached to it. Agnosia is associated with lesions of the sensory cortices involved with seeing, hearing, and feeling and with the loss of one sensory modality. It is difficult to assess because the person is often easily able to compensate. Although the ability to recognize an object by vision is gone, the ability to recognize that same object by hearing or feeling is retained.

Altered States of Consciousness

Alteration of consciousness is not considered an independent disease entity but a reflection of some underlying disease or abnormal state of brain function. The human brain possesses a mechanism that allows a waking and sleeping state (arousal), as well as a separate ability to focus awareness on relevant environmental stimuli (attention).[24,62] To achieve a state of consciousness the cerebral cortex must be activated by the ascending reticular formation fibers in the brainstem. The fibers extend to the thalamus, limbic system, and cortex. The upper part of this system acts as an on/off switch for consciousness and controls the sleep-wake cycle. The lower part controls respiration.

Disturbances of arousal and attention can range from coma after brainstem injury to confusional states caused by drug intoxication. Metabolic or systemic disorders generally cause depressed consciousness without focal neurologic findings.[96] CNS disorders may or may not have concomitant focal signs. Table 28-1 compares metabolic and drug-induced coma with coma caused by space-occupying lesions.

Clinical disorders of arousal may result in hyperaroused states and can appear as restlessness, agitation, or delirium. This is presumably a result of the loss of hemispheric inhibition of brainstem function. Hypoarousal can be described on a spectrum ranging from drowsiness to stupor and coma. Stupor is a state of unresponsiveness that requires vigorous stimulation to bring about arousal. Coma is a state of unarousable unresponsiveness. Small and restricted lesions of the brainstem can result in stupor and coma. Massive bilateral hemispheric lesions are necessary to cause coma. Table 28-2 identifies the brainstem reflexes in coma.

Damage to the cerebral cortex can be caused by loss of blood flow, subarachnoid hemorrhage, anesthetic toxicity, hypoglycemia, hypothermia, or status epilepticus (see "Epilepsy" in Chapter 36). If the link to the brainstem is destroyed, the person will remain in a persistent vegetative state (PVS). Although the person may make random movements and the eyes may open, mentation remains absent. Akinetic mutism, similar to PVS, reflects damage to the mediofrontal lobe and results in lack of motivation to perform any motor or mental activity (abulia). In the *locked-in syndrome*, there is damage to the pons resulting most often from thrombosis of the basilar artery. This is a remarkable impairment, involving no mental deficit at all but resulting in inability to move anything but the eyes. It is in essence the opposite of PVS.

Supratentorial lesions that cause increased pressure, such as hemorrhage, cerebral edema, or neoplasm, can cause coma by producing tentorial herniation and subsequent compression of the brainstem. There is usually a hemiparesis with a dilated pupil on the side of the lesion because of central compression involving the third cranial nerve by the herniation.

In infratentorial lesions, brainstem damage can be related to drugs, hemorrhage, infarction, or compression from the posterior fossa. Disruption of ocular movements is an early sign of brainstem involvement.[102] There is loss of the pupillary reaction to light while the corneal reflex remains intact.

Brain death relates to destruction of both the upper and lower parts of the reticular formation in the brainstem, which will eventually lead to death. Cortical electrical activity and spinal reflexes may be preserved, but these are of no consequence because they are unable to be used for thought or movement.

Table 28-2	Brainstem Reflexes in the Comatose Patient				
	Examination Technique	**Normal Response**	**Afferent Pathway**	**Brainstem**	**Efferent Pathway**
Pupils	Response to light	Direct and consensual pupillary constriction	Retina, optic nerve, chiasm, optic tract	Edinger-Westphal nucleus (midbrain)	Oculomotor nerve, sympathetic fibers
Oculocephalic	Turn head from side to side	Eyes move conjugately in direction opposite to head	Semicircular canals, vestibular nerve	Vestibular nucleus. Medial longitudinal fasciculus. Parapontine reticular formation (pons)	Oculomotor and abducens nerves
Vestibulo oculocephalic	Irrigate external auditory canal with cold water	Nystagmus with fast component beating away from stimulus	Semicircular canals, vestibular nerve	Vestibular nucleus. Medial longitudinal fasciculus. Parapontine reticular formation (pons)	Oculomotor and abducens nerves
Corneal reflex	Stimulation of cornea	Eyelid closure	Trigeminal nerve	Trigeminal and facial nuclei (pons)	Facial nerve
Cough reflex	Stimulation of carina	Cough	Glossopharyngeal and vagus nerves	Medullary "cough center"	Glossopharyngeal and vagus nerves
Gag reflex	Stimulation of soft palate	Symmetric elevation of soft palate	Glossopharyngeal and vagus nerves	Medulla	Glossopharyngeal and vagus nerves

Attention is more difficult to relate to specific brain structure than arousal. However, the acute confusional state is one of the most common neurologic disorders encountered. Although there is not a clear understanding of the mechanism of attention from the neuroanatomic perspective, there appears to be a major role played by the parietal and frontal lobes. Frontal and prefrontal areas of the brain are responsible for mental control, concentration, vigilance, and performance of meaningful activity. Cognition and emotional control are established by extensive white matter connections between the frontal lobes and the remainder of the cerebrum.[89] Diseases that affect the white matter, such as multiple sclerosis, can affect the level of attention without decreasing arousal. Psychiatric disease has an effect on both arousal and attention.[62] The acute confusional state may be the result of a number of causes. Intoxicants, metabolic disorders, infections, epilepsy, blood flow disorders, traumatic injuries, and neoplasms can all be responsible for the change in orientation or attention.

Emotional Instability

The orbital prefrontal region is especially expanded in the right cortex and is dominant for selectively attending to facial expressions. It has extensive connections with limbic and subcortical regions, important in regulation of emotional information and mediation of pleasure and pain. Muscles of the head and neck represent a unique relationship to the primary senses. Humans have more facial muscles than any other species, and the connections to the limbic lobe reflect emotion. Maternal-infant connection and bonding and social-emotional connection between individuals depend on facial expression. Primitive emotions that serve fundamental motivational and social communication functions and nonverbal affects are spontaneously expressed on the face. Psychic systems process unconscious information. Empathetic cognition and the perception of the emotional states of other human beings are developed within the first 3 years of life. Control of vital functions enable the individual to cope actively with stress and environmental challenge. Self-regulation functions are learned through this region.[87]

The thalamus is a two-lobed medial structure that that sits just above the brainstem and is bounded on its dorsal surfaces by the lateral ventricles. The thalamus consists of multiple nuclei receiving input from sensory receptors and brainstem arousal systems and then relays this information to the frontal cortex, the cingulate gyrus, the amygdala, and the hippocampus. With the exception of olfaction, all sensory input goes through thalamic nuclei before being sent onto the cortex. The thalamus affects the quantity and quality of sensory processing. The fact that basic sensory information and arousal signals converge in the thalamus explains why even basic sensory signals can be distorted under conditions of high arousal. Although moderate arousal may facilitate transmission, conditions of high stress likely will distort or hinder transmissions to target structures throughout the brain.

Although the limbic system defies exact definition, it is recognized as the area of control of human behavior and is widely studied in behavioral neurology. The limbic system, sometimes referred to as the limbic lobe, is generally considered to encompass part of the cortical, diencephalon, and brainstem structures. This system includes the orbitofrontal cortex, hippocampus, parahippocampal gyrus, cingulate gyrus, dentate gyrus, amygdala, septal area, hypothalamus, and portions of the thalamus. The limbic lobe structures are seen in Figure 28-13.[69] Working together, these structures provide the essential, need-directed motor activity necessary for survival. This is the area that integrates the motivation and intentional drive to trigger a motor act. Both the automatic and somatic systems are influenced by the limbic system.[99] Limbic syndromes involve the primary emotions, which are those associated with pain, pleasure, anger, and fear. The processing of the

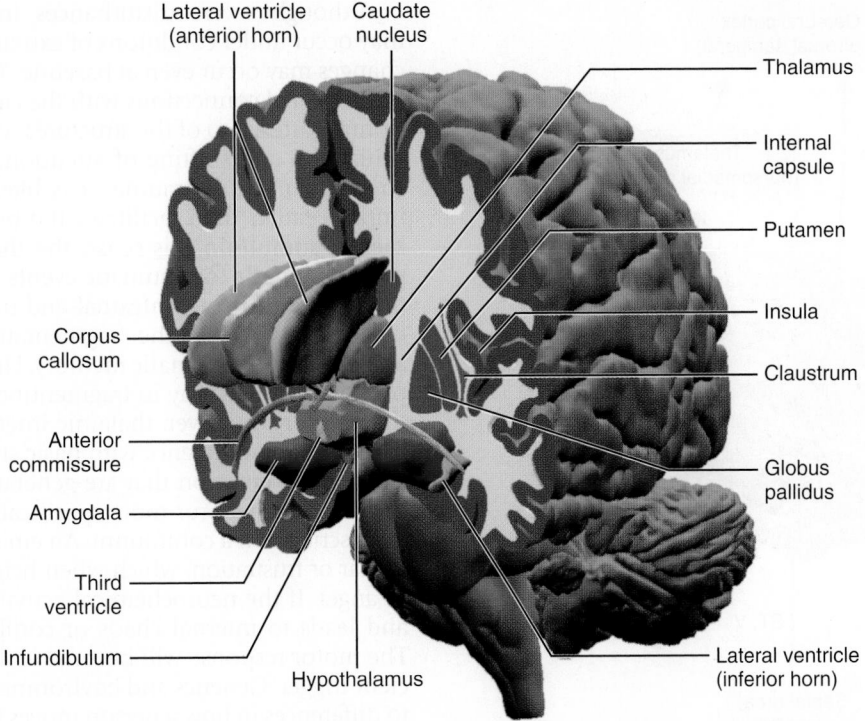

Figure 28-13

Three-dimensional representation of the structures of, and those surrounding, the limbic lobe. (From Nolte J: *The human brain: an introduction to its functional anatomy*, ed 5, St Louis, 2002, Mosby.)

limbic system is responsible for the fact that emotionally charged experiences will be more easily remembered than those with less emotional stimulation.[24] In lower animals, the limbic system is concerned primarily with the sense of smell, and it is a common observation that smells can trigger a strong emotional response in humans.

The amygdala are nuclei located in the medial temporal lobe anterior to the hippocampus as illustrated in Figure 28-14. The amygdala is involved in sensory processing and determining the value of the information received. The patterns of emotional memories are formed here, and this is the area that establishes the anxiety and panic or the pleasure that is unconsciously related to an experience that may or may not be remembered.[3] The amygdala is richly connected with the prefrontal cortex, the thalamus, hypothalamus, and brainstem as seen in Figure 28-15.[69] Not represented here is the influence that the prefrontal cortex has on the amygdala, which is thought to be inhibitory. The amygdala is the central structure associated with the learning of fear, fearful responding, and associated autonomic and behavior responses.

Kindling is a term originally used to describe how subthreshold seizure activity becomes increasingly active and severe with successive seizures. Partial kindling also can occur in the amygdala, and it appears related to increased defensive responses and anxiety-like behavior in animals. In humans, the amygdala is involved in integrating emotional and contextual information that are parts of the human stress response. Amygdaloidal lesions result in hampered fear conditioning, whereas amygdaloidal stimulation results in classic fear responses such as defensive and aggressive behavior and autonomic reactivity. It

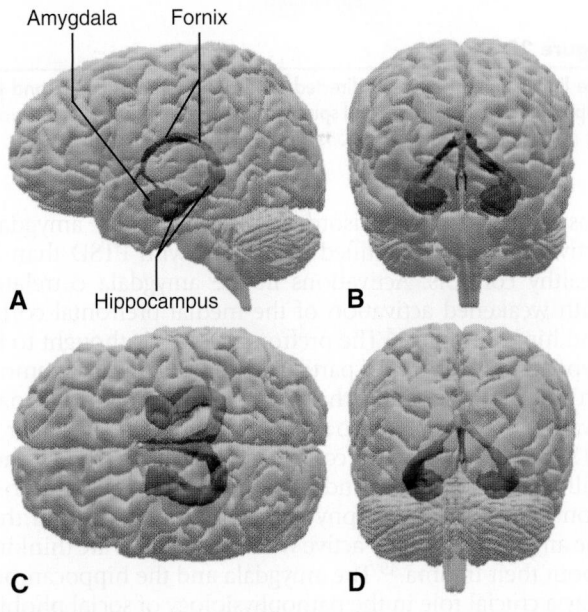

Figure 28-14

Placement of the main structures of the limbic lobe as seen from left (A), back (B), above (C), and behind (D). (From Nolte J: *The human brain: an introduction to its functional anatomy*, ed 5, St Louis, 2002, Mosby.)

has been demonstrated that the amygdala plays a role in conditioned fear responding in general and the startle response in particular.

Perhaps the best example of an anxiety disorder that seems to follow the classic fear-conditioning model is

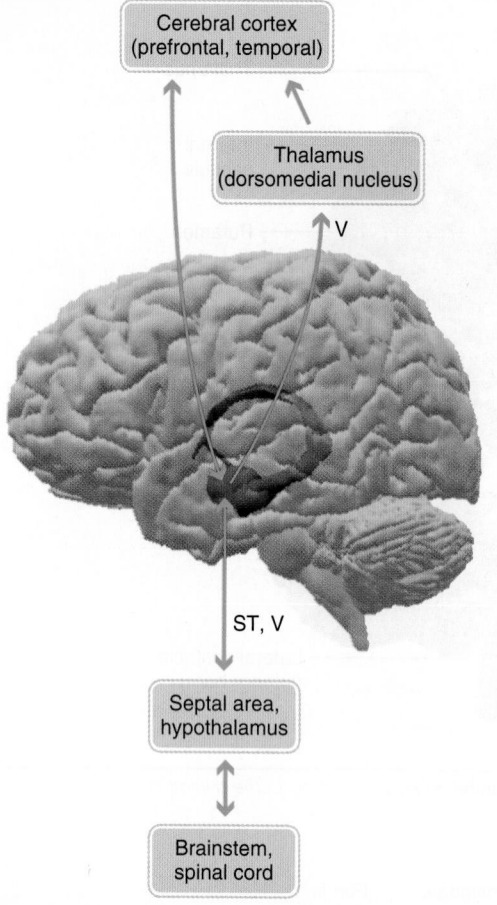

Figure 28-15

The limbic lobe gives input directed toward the cerebral cortex and the hypothalamus, brainstem, and spinal cord. (From Nolte J: *The human brain: an introduction to its functional anatomy*, ed 5, St Louis, 2002, Mosby.)

posttraumatic stress disorder (PTSD). Greater amygdala activations were identified in persons with PTSD than in healthy controls. Activations in the amygdala correlated with weakened activation of the medial prefrontal cortex and hippocampus.[65] The prefrontal cortex is thought to be hypoactivated in PTSD, particularly during trauma memory activation. It is possible that such prefrontal cortex hypoactivation may be related to startle responses that are larger in PTSD when exposed to contexts in which they know they will be exposed to reminders of their trauma. Recent positron emission tomography (PET) studies have found that the amygdala is clearly active when individuals are thinking about their trauma.[49] The amygdala and the hippocampus play a crucial role in the pathophysiology of social phobia.

Dissociative symptoms are common among survivors of trauma, and maladaptive levels of dissociation can develop alongside other pathologic responses to trauma. Dissociation is defined as a disruption in the usually integrated functions of consciousness, memory, identity, or perception of the environment, and the term *dissociative symptoms* in the literature has been used to capture a range of symptoms that can include changes in time perception, altered sensory perception, flashbacks, psychogenic amnesia, reduction in awareness, affective blunting, feelings of detachment, depersonalization, multiple identities, and derealization.[26,49]

Although severe disturbances in sensory processing may occur under conditions of extreme stress, more subtle changes may occur even at baseline. The thalamus has rich bidirectional connections with the cingulate gyrus and the frontal cortex, two of the structures responsible for the prioritization and shifting of attention. During the extreme stress of an actual trauma, it is likely that the thalamus impairs rather than facilitates the processing of environmental stimuli. In this sense, the thalamus has a role to play in amnesia for traumatic events. For example, disruption in the relay of contextual and traumatic information could contribute to the fragmentation and inaccuracies associated with traumatic memory. Unlike the role the hippocampus might play in fragmenting sensory elements of the memory, however, thalamic interference would result in an initial interference with basic stimulus encoding.[49]

Levels of emotion that are generated and advanced by the limbic system, or more specifically the amygdala, can be described on a continuum. An emotion can be triggered as fear or frustration, which when heightened can manifest as anger. If the neurochemical activity continues to build and leads to internal chaos or conflict, it becomes rage. The motor response will become violent if there is a sufficient trigger. Genetics and environmental history will lead to differences in how a person moves from fear to violence. When there is damage to the area of the limbic lobe that results from injury or disease, there can be an increase in rage and easy progression to violence. The diffuse axonal damage of head injury can cause a tendency to become easily frustrated or to have unsubstantiated fears.[101] Fear conditioning is a fast process, with a long-lasting effect, but repeated exposure to the conditioned stimulus in the absence of the unconditioned stimulus can lead to extinction. Extinction reduces the likelihood that the conditioned stimulus will elicit the fear response. The medial prefrontal and anterior cingulate cortices have been implicated in extinction learning. Understanding how learned fears are diminished and how extinction learning is changed in individuals who have anxiety disorders might be an important step in translating neurobiologic research to diagnosis and treatment of these individuals.

Functional (psychogenic) movement disorders are part of the spectrum of functional neurologic disorders, some of the most prevalent disorders seen in neurologic practice. In common with other functional disorders, there is an absence of appropriate health-service provision and research interest for functional movement disorder, despite their prevalence. These disorders occupy a grey area between neurology and psychiatry. The key clinical feature that separates patients with functional movement disorder from those with organic movement disorders is that the movements have features that one would usually associate with voluntary movement (distractibility, resolution with placebo, and presence of pre-movement potentials), but patients report them as being involuntary and not under their control. There seem to be just two logical explanations for this feature: either movements are deliberately feigned or there must be a brain mechanism that allows voluntary movement to occur but to be experienced subjectively as involuntary. Understanding this mechanism would seem to be key to understanding the development of symptoms and their treatment. Table 28-3 presents terms used to describe the various psychogenic disorders.[22]

Table 28-3	Terms Commonly Used to Describe Psychogenic Disorders and Their Implications

Psychogenic Disorder	Implication
Psychogenic	Suggests psychological causation
Conversion disorder	Operationalized within DSM: requires an identified psychological triggering factor for diagnosis
Somatization disorder	Operationalized within DSM: requires presence of multiple physical symptoms including one conversion neurologic symptom
Medically unexplained symptoms	Suggests that a medical explanation might one day be apparent
	Could refer to many medical symptoms that are not thought to be psychogenic, but still are not of a known cause
Functional	Broad term suggesting a functional rather than a structural deficit, which could apply to several neurologic disorders not regarded as psychogenic but where structural pathology is absent (e.g., migraine)
Hysteria	Historical term that carries substantial stigma in society and implies a link between symptoms and the uterus
Nonorganic	Defines the condition by what it is not; the term organic is itself not well defined

DSM, Diagnostic and Statistical Manual of Mental Disorders, 4th Edition, American Psychiatric Association.

Some terms, such as psychogenic, conversion, or somatization, directly suggest that the cause of physical symptoms is psychologically mediated. Conversion and somatization are operationalized diagnoses that specifically need the presence of a psychological triggering factor and exclusion of feigning. However, for most movement disorder clinicians, the presence of a psychological triggering factor is not a requirement for diagnosing a patient with FMD, and the difficulties of routinely excluding feigning in clinical practice are complex.

From Edwards MJ: Functional (psychogenic) movement disorders: merging mind and brain, *Lancet Neurol* 11(3):250–260, 2012.

The different symptom dimensions of obsessive compulsive disorder and other anxiety disorders are likely to share common neural substrates dedicated to general threat detection and emotional arousal because these reactions are adaptive and useful to deal with different kinds of threat. Research suggests that syndrome-specific neural substrates may have evolved to deal with specific threats. In evolutionary terms, general anxiety, which is common to individuals who have obsessive compulsive disorder and other anxiety disorders, may have evolved to deal with nonspecific threats; for example, cleanliness is important for protection against infections. Harming obsessions and checking rituals keep people safe, and hoarding helps people survive periods of scarcity; however, it can be manifested outside of the physical threat. The neuroimaging findings, showing increased activation of limbic and ventral frontal-striatal regions in obsessive compulsive disorder, could reflect exaggerations of normal emotional responses to biologically relevant stimuli rather than fundamentally abnormal neuronal responses.[59]

Borderline personality disorder, including affective dysregulation, identity disturbance, and self-mutilating behaviors, were originally thought to involve a disorder of character. In recent studies, it appears that borderline personality disorder individuals are compromised significantly in executive skill and/or other frontal lobe functions, visuomotor speed, attention, and verbal memory. These fairly consistent neuropsychologic findings in adults are supported by developmental studies of children with borderline features. These children appear to have greater difficulty with executive skills, including planning, organizing, and sequencing; perceptual motor functioning; and memory proficiency.[65]

Memory Problems

Memory is associated with various areas of the brain, and a particular area may be responsible for different aspects of memory. The hippocampus, the thalamus, and the basal forebrain are critical to the performance of recent memory (Table 28-4). Figure 28-16 shows the relationship of learning strategies and brain regions. For immediate auditory memory, left and right temporal-parietal cortices mediate auditory verbal and nonverbal material. Neurogenesis has been observed in the dentate gyrus of the hippocampus throughout the lives of many species, including humans. Not all newly generated hippocampal neurons survive, but hippocampal-dependent memory tasks can enhance the survival of these neurons.[34] Inflammatory cytokines reduce hippocampal neurogenesis and impair the ability to maintain long-term potentiation in the hippocampus, which is a critical physiologic process involved in memory consolidation.[33]

Working memory, the ability to hold information in short-term storage while permitting other cognitive operations to take place, appears to depend on the prefrontal cortex. Keeping a spatial location in mind may involve a right frontal area that directs the maintenance of that information in a right parietal area, whereas keeping a word in mind may involve a left frontal area that directs the maintenance of that information in a left temporal or parietal area. Specific basal ganglia and cerebellar areas appear to support the working memory capacity of particular frontal regions. It appears that the brain performs problem solving based on working memory that is found and lost in the course of a task. This fluid memory, related to reasoning, can be trained and needs to be reestablished with constant mental workout. Essentially the goal is to expand the work space of the brain. This is the area that is being explored in relation to "brain training," and it is critical to the rehabilitation process.

Disorders of recent memory, known as *amnesia*, are a significant neurobehavioral phenomenon and common in persons after traumatic brain injury. *Declarative memory* is retention of facts and events of a prior experience or the memory of what has occurred and is related to explicit learning. *Procedural memory* describes the learning of skills and habits, or how something is done. Implicit learning is based on procedural memory. The relationship to memory and relearning motor skills is discussed in "Special Implications for the Physical Therapist 28-1: Motor Learning Strategies" below.

Anterograde amnesia is the failure of new learning or formation of new memory. *Retrograde amnesia* is the loss of

Table 28-4	Correlation of Anatomic Site to Disorders of Memory and Other Neurologic Findings	
Anatomic Site of Damage	**Memory Finding**	**Other Neurologic and Medical Findings**
Frontal lobe	Lateralized deficit in working memory. Right spatial defects, left verbal defects, impaired recall with spared recognition	Personality change Perseveration Chorea, dystonia Bradykinesia, tremor, rigidity
Basal forebrain	Declarative memory deficit	
Ventromedial cortex	Frontal lobe–type declarative memory deficit	Upper visual field defects
Hippocampus and parahippocampal cortex	Bilateral lesions yield global amnesia, unilateral lesions show lateralization of deficit Left: verbal deficit; right: spatial deficit	Myoclonus Depressed level of consciousness Cortical blindness Autonomations
Fornix	Global amnesia	
Mammillary bodies	Declarative memory deficit	Confabulation, ataxia, nystagmus, signs of alcohol withdrawal
Dorsal and medial dorsal nucleus thalamus	Declarative memory deficit	Confabulation
Anterior thalamus	Declarative memory deficit	
Lateral temporal cortex	Deficit in autobiographic memory	

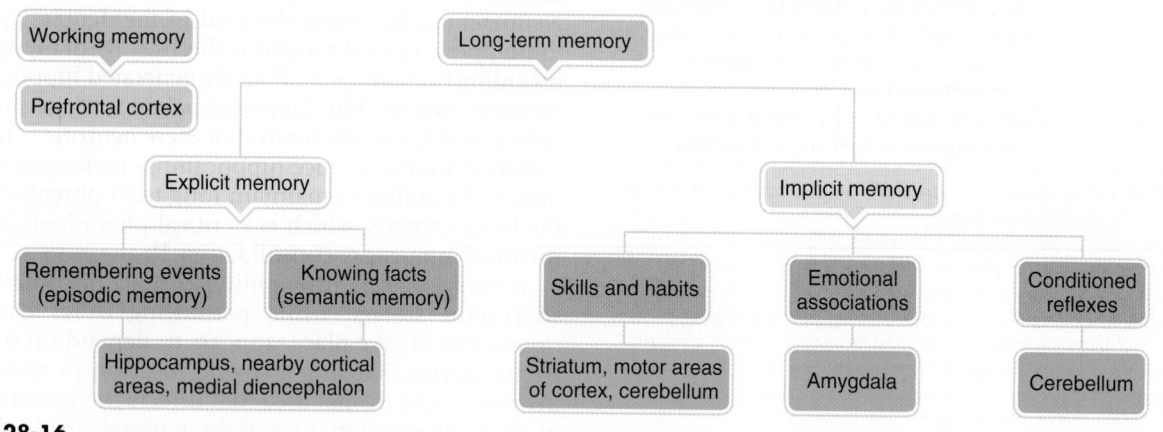

Figure 28-16

Anatomic correlates for explicit and implicit learning. (From Nolte J: *The human brain: an introduction to its functional anatomy,* ed 5, St Louis, 2002, Mosby.)

ability to recall events. The inability to acquire new learning is often accompanied by *confabulation,* the fabrication of information in response to questioning. *Traumatic amnesia* refers to an individual's inability to recall significant aspects of their traumatic experience. Traumatic memories are reported to be fragmented, compartmentalized, and disintegrated, suggesting that the hippocampus still may have a role to play in the phenomenon of traumatic amnesia. Dysregulation in the hippocampal system has the potential to generate narratives of traumatic events that are spotty and unreliable.

Neuromodulators, such as norepinephrine, have the potential to affect hippocampal functioning in a more dynamic fashion. The locus ceruleus, located in the brainstem, for example, projects directly to the hippocampus and modulates its functioning through norepinephrine release. The effects of such a network are unclear, although the implications are that stress-related memory alterations might occur on a split-second basis and deficient or extreme locus ceruleus input may disrupt normal hippocampal processing severely. Given that the hippocampus

plays a role in integrating input from diverse sources when encoding memory, disruptions in its functioning may lead to memories that seem fragmented and nonlinear. Over time, fragments of the memory may become consolidated, vivid, and easily recalled, while other fragments rarely are accessed.[49]

The role of stress in neurologic disease often is overlooked. Several chronic neurologic disease states, such as Alzheimer disease, are associated with elevated secretion of stress hormones, in particular cortisol, which results from overactivity of the hypothalamic-pituitary-adrenal axis. The stress or perceived threat activates the hypothalamus, triggering release of hormones that cause increased adrenal output of cortisol.[82] Stress also can trigger or exacerbate symptom onset and perhaps progression of chronic illness such as Parkinson disease. Stress hormones also can mitigate the impact of acute neurotrauma; for example, there is a positive correlation between cortisol levels and mortality after head injury. Thus neurologic disease states can occur within a context of elevated glucocorticoids, which may have profound influences on recovery and neuroplasticity. In addition, abnormal regulation of glucocorticoid release is associated with many affective disorders, such as depression and PTSD, that are overrepresented in populations with neurologic disease; Parkinson disease is a prime example. Acute and sustained glucocorticoid release also can precipitate changes in peripheral and central immune signaling, resulting in cytokine profiles that may be deleterious for functional recovery in the face of neurologic challenge.[38] General adaptation syndrome, described in Chapter 2, has been identified as a continuum of alarm, resistance, and exhaustion and has been implicated in the stress response.

Accumulation of risk is another concept that plays a pivotal role in the life-course model of chronic diseases. Allostasis is defined as the ability to achieve stability through change. The price of this accommodation to stress has been defined as the allostatic load. It follows that acute stress (the "fight, flight, or freeze" response) and chronic stress resulting from the cumulative load of minor day-to-day stresses can add to the allostatic load and have long-term consequences. Subacute stress is defined as an accumulation of stressful life events over a duration of months and includes emotional factors, such as hostility and anger, as well as affective disorders such as major depression and anxiety disorders. Chronic stressors include factors such as low social support, work stress, marital stress, and caregiver strain and present as feelings of fatigue, lack of energy, irritability, and demoralization.

The link between chronic psychologic distress and adverse behavior, such as overeating, may be centrally mediated. Normally, glucocorticoids help end acute stress responses by exerting negative feedback on the hypothalamic-pituitary-adrenal axis. The combination of chronic stress and high glucocorticoid levels seems to stimulate a preferential desire to ingest sweet and fatty foods, presumably by affecting dopaminergic transmission in areas of the brain associated with motivation and reward.[29]

Brain areas associated with reward are linked with those that sense physical pain. Chronic pain can cause depression, and depression can increase pain. Most individuals who have depression also present with physical symptoms. Studies using functional magnetic resonance imaging (fMRI) have shown that social rejection lights up brain areas that are also key regions in the response to physical pain. The area of the anterior cingulate cortex that is activated by visceral pain also is activated in cases of social rejection.

Disturbances of neurologic function can result in behavioral disturbances that mimic disturbances of mental function in psychiatric disorders. *Delusions*, or fixed false beliefs, have been reported in a great variety of neurologic conditions and appear to be associated with the limbic system. Paranoid delusions are common in disorders of the medial temporal lobe or a combination of the frontal and right parietal lobes. *Hallucinations* are sensory experiences without external stimulation. Visual hallucinations generally suggest neurologic involvement; auditory hallucinations imply psychiatric disease. Midbrain lesions in the cerebral peduncles can cause hallucinations involving animals. Temporal lesions can cause recurrent auditory experiences.[24]

Box 28-2

RAPID EYE MOVEMENT SLEEP BEHAVIOR DISORDER AND RELATED BRAINSTEM STRUCTURES

- Substantia nigra (midbrain-dopaminergic)
- Locus coeruleus (brainstem-noradrenergic)
- Pedunculopontine nucleus (pons-cerebellum)
- Dorsal vagus nucleus
- Dorsal raphe nucleus (involved in serotonin pathways)
- Gigantocellular reticular nucleus (control of arousal)

Modified from Gagnon JF: Rapid-eye-movement sleep behaviour disorder and neurodegenerative diseases. *Neurology* 5:424–432, 2006.

Rapid eye movement sleep behavior disorder is characterized by loss of muscular atonia and prominent motor behaviors during rapid eye movement sleep. Sleep behavior disorder can cause sleep disruption. The disorder is strongly associated with neurodegenerative diseases such as multiple-system atrophy, Parkinson disease, dementia with Lewy bodies, and progressive supranuclear palsy. The symptoms of sleep behavior disorder precede other symptoms of these neurodegenerative disorders by several years. Furthermore, several recent studies have shown that sleep behavior disorder is associated with abnormalities of electroencephalographic (EEG) activity; cerebral blood flow; and cognitive, perceptual, and autonomic functions. Sleep behavior disorder might be a stage in the development of neurodegenerative disorder. Box 28-2 lists the areas of the brain that play a role in sleep behavior.[28]

Lesions of the hemispheres or lobes may cause loss of the functions that each hemisphere controls. Because diseases and damage caused by trauma will often affect one area of the brain, the associated syndromes for the main areas of the brain are described.[56]

Brainstem Dysfunction

The brainstem contains the lower motor neurons for the muscles of the head and does the initial processing of general afferent information concerning the head. The cranial nerves enter the system at the brainstem through the respective nuclei and provide sensation and motor control of the head and neck.[69] The sensory and motor functions of the cranial nerves are outlined in Table 28-5. A working knowledge of the attributes of the cranial nerves assists in the understanding of the level and impact of lesions within the CNS.

Distinctive brainstem functions include a conduit for spinal cord activity in both ascending sensory tracts and descending motor tracts. The nuclei in the brainstem provide relay functions to divert the information to the appropriate higher level structures for further modification.

The brainstem has been divided into three major subdivisions related to a characteristic set of features. The medulla, attached directly to the spinal cord, houses the inferior olivary nucleus that has direct output connections to the cerebellum and gets direct input from the spinal cord and cerebellum. The pons extends from the medulla and is attached to the cerebellum through both the middle and superior cerebellar peduncles receiving major outflow from the cerebellum. Vestibular nuclei sit within the pons, making it the center for integration of vestibular input.

The third level of the brainstem, the midbrain, contains the red nucleus with fibers that connect the cerebellum to the thalamus. The substantia nigra found here connects to the basal ganglia structures and shares the dopamine pathway related to the initiation and control of movement. It is also connected to the cortex through the cerebral peduncle containing descending fibers.

The reticular formation is a diffuse network of neurons, extending through the brainstem to higher levels, and is important in influencing movement. The reticular regions are closely related to the cerebellum, basal ganglia, vestibular nuclei, and substantia nigra and involved with complex movement patterns. It is through the reticular formation that there is inhibition of flexor reflexes, so that only noxious stimulus can evoke the flexor response such as the reflexive pulling a hand away from a hot stove.

This is a brief reflection of the complexity of the brainstem and is not intended to be comprehensive.

However, it is clear that advanced knowledge of the interface and connections of the brainstem helps the therapist understand the functions that are described throughout this text.

Autonomic Nervous System Dysfunction

The term *autonomic nervous system* was introduced to describe the system of nerves that controls the unstriated tissue, the cardiac muscle, and the glandular tissue of mammals involved in the control of autonomic function. The autonomic CNS neurons are located at many levels from the cerebral cortex to the spinal cord. Efferent autonomic pathways are organized in two major outflows: the sympathetic and parasympathetic. Finally, the enteric nervous system, which is considered a separate and independent division of the autonomic nervous system, is located in the walls of the gut. The schematic diagram of the autonomic nervous system is seen in Figure 28-17.

Table 28-5	The Cranial Nerves and Their Functions		
Cranial Nerve	**Component**	**Function**	
I—Olfactory	S	Olfaction	
II—Optic	S	Vision	
III—Oculomotor	M	Innervation of inferior oblique muscle and medial, inferior, and superior rectus muscles of eye	
	A	Innervation of ciliary ganglion, which regulates papillary constriction (papillary constrictor muscle) and accommodation to near vision (ciliary muscle)	
IV—Trochlear	M	Innervation of superior oblique muscle of eye	
V—Trigeminal	S	Sensation (epicritic, protopathic) from face, nose, mouth, nasal and oral mucosa, anterior two-thirds of tongue, and meningeal sensation, through all three divisions (ophthalmic, maxillary, mandibular)	
	M	Innervation of muscles of mastication and tensor tympani muscle (through mandibular division only)	
VI—Abducens	M	Innervation of lateral rectus muscle of eye	
VII—Facial	S	Taste from anterior two-thirds of tongue	
	M	Innervation of muscles of facial expression and stapedius muscle	
	A	Innervation of pterygopalatine ganglion, which innervates lacrimal and nasal mucosal glands, and submandibular ganglion, which innervates submandibular and sublingual salivary glands	
VIII—Vestibulocochlear	S	Hearing (cochlear division); linear and angular acceleration, or head position in space (vestibular division)	
IX—Glossopharyngeal	S	Taste and general sensation from posterior one-third tongue; sensation (epicritic, protopathic) from pharynx, soft palate, tonsils; chemoreception from carotid body and baroreception from carotid sinus (unconscious reflex sensory information)	
	M	Innervation of pharyngeal muscles	
	A	Innervation of otic ganglion, which supplies parotid gland	
X—Vagus	S	Visceral sensation (excluding pain) from heart, bronchi, trachea, larynx, pharynx, gastrointestinal tract to level of descending colon; general sensation of external ear; taste from epiglottis	
X—Vagus	S	Visceral sensation (excluding pain) from heart, bronchi, trachea, larynx, pharynx, gastrointestinal tract to level of descending colon; general sensation of external ear; taste from epiglottis	
	M	Innervation of pharyngeal and laryngeal muscles and muscles at base of tongue	
	A	Innervation of local visceral ganglia, which supply smooth muscles in respiratory, cardiovascular, and GI tract to level of descending colon	
XI—Spinal accessory	M	Innervation of trapezius and sternocleidomastoid muscles	
XII—Hypoglossal	M	Innervation of muscles of tongue	

S, Sensory nervous system; M, motor nervous system; A, autonomic nervous system; GI, gastrointestinal.
From Felten DL, Felten SY: A regional and systemic overview of functional neuroanatomy. In Farber SD: *Neurorehabilitation: a multisensory approach,* Philadelphia, 1982, Saunders, pp 53-54.

Neurons in the cerebral cortex, basal forebrain, hypothalamus, midbrain, pons, and medulla participate in autonomic control. The central autonomic network integrates visceral, humoral, and environmental information to produce coordinated autonomic, neuroendocrine, and behavioral responses to external or internal stimuli. A coordinated response is generated through interconnections among the amygdala and the neocortex, forebrain, hypothalamus, and autonomic and somatic motor nuclei of the brainstem. The insular and medial prefrontal cortices (paralimbic areas) and nuclei of the amygdala are the higher centers involved in the processing of visceral information and the initiation of integrated autonomic responses. The central nucleus of the amygdala projects to the hypothalamus, periaqueductal gray (PAG), and autonomic nuclei of the brainstem to integrate autonomic, endocrine, and motor responses to emotionally relevant stimuli.

The hypothalamus integrates the autonomic and endocrine responses that are critical for homeostasis. The PAG matter of the midbrain is the site of integrated autonomic, behavioral, and antinociceptive stress responses. It is organized into separate columns that control specific patterns of response to stress. The lateral PAG mediates sympathoexcitation, opioid-independent analgesia, and motor responses consistent with the fight-or-flight reaction. The ventrolateral PAG produces sympathoinhibition, opioid-dependent analgesia, and motor inhibition.

Neurons in the medulla are critical for the control of cardiovascular, respiratory, and gastrointestinal functions. The medullary nucleus of the solitary tract is the first relay station for the arterial baroreceptors and chemoreceptors, as well as cardiopulmonary and gastrointestinal afferents.

Preganglionic sympathetic neurons are organized into different functional units that control blood flow to the skin and muscles, secretion of sweat glands, skin hair follicles, systemic blood flow, as well as the function of viscera. Selectivity is refined by the release of different neurotransmitters. Acetylcholine is the neurotransmitter of the sympathetic and parasympathetic preganglionic neurons. The main postganglionic sympathetic neurotransmitter is norepinephrine.

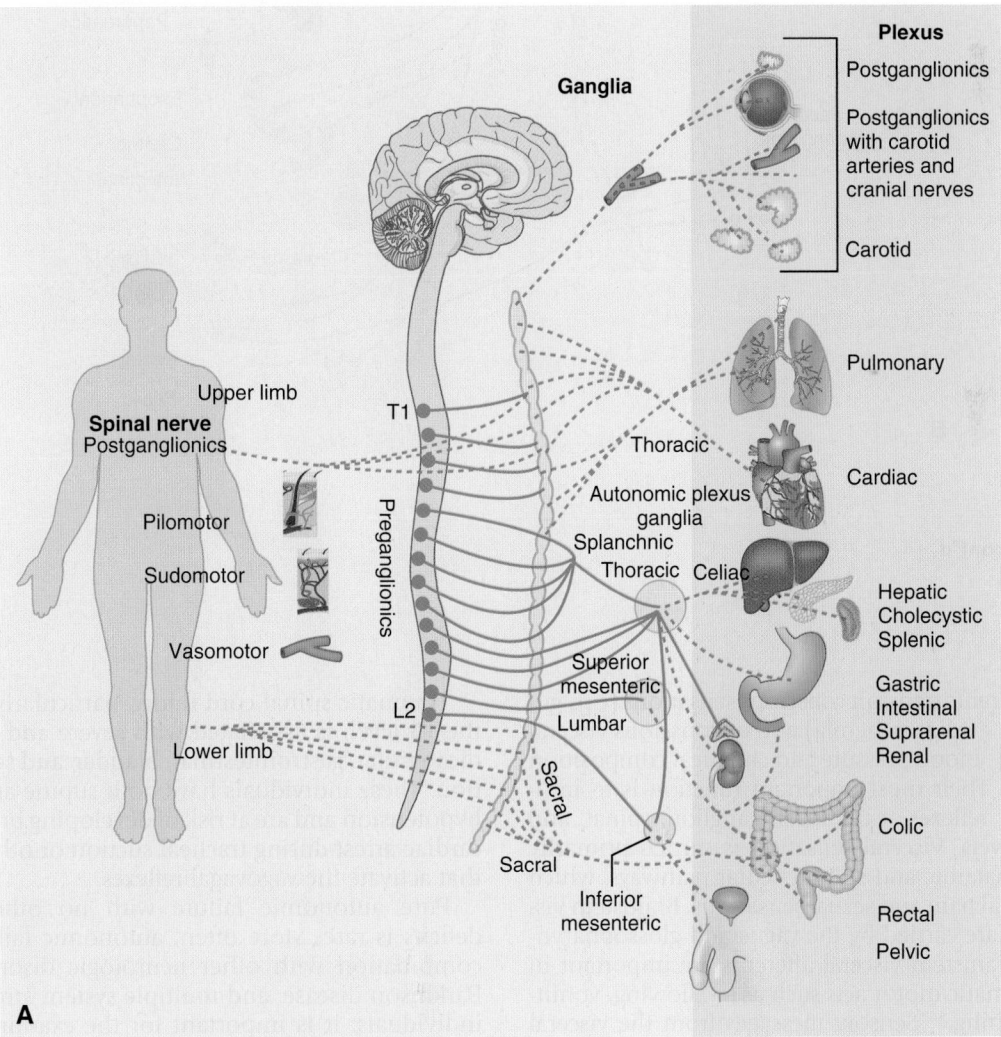

Figure 28-17

Sympathetic (**A**) and parasympathetic (**B**) divisions of the autonomic nervous system: efferent systems. (From Levy MN, Koeppen BM: *Berne and Levy principles of physiology*, ed 4, St. Louis, 2006, Mosby.)

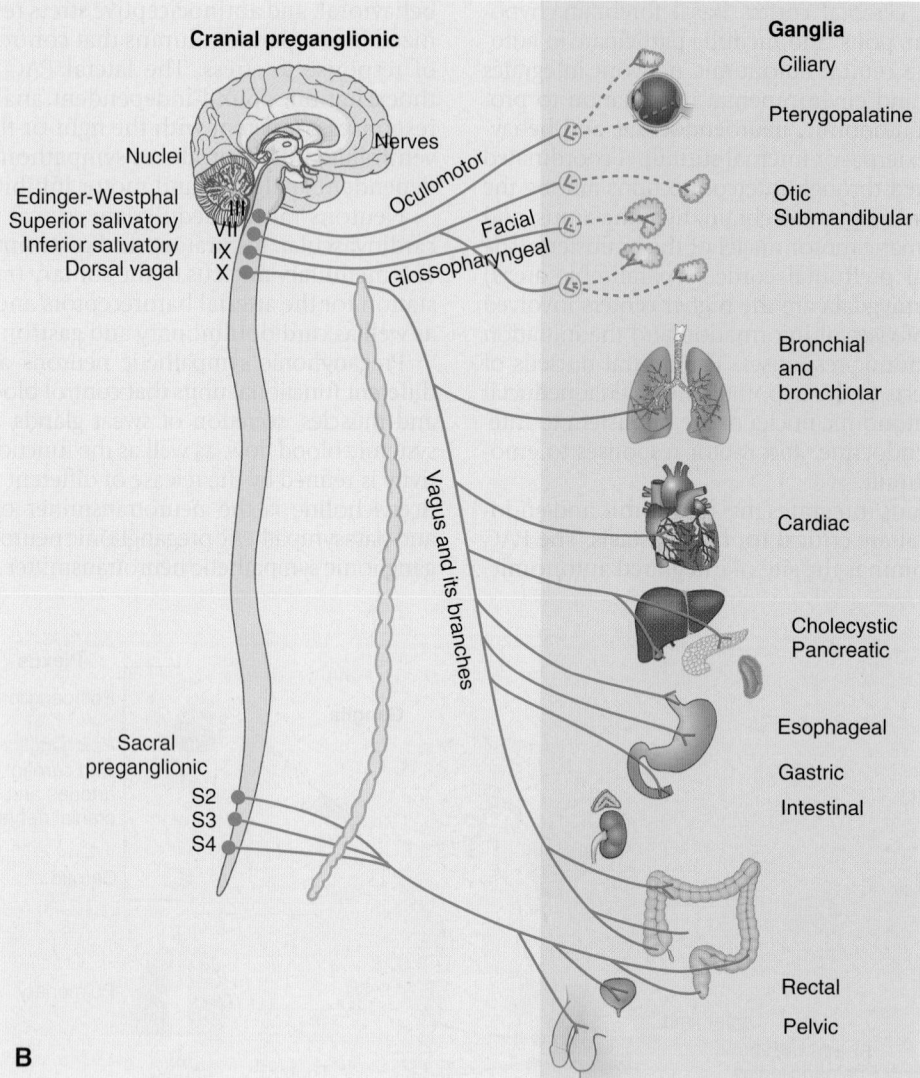

Figure 28-17, cont'd

Visceral afferents transmit conscious sensations (e.g., gut distention and cardiac ischemia) and unconscious visceral sensations (e.g., blood pressure and chemical composition of the blood). Their most important function is to initiate autonomic reflexes at the local, ganglion, spinal, and supraspinal levels. Visceral sensation is carried primarily by the spinothalamic and spinoreticular pathways, which transmit visceral pain and sexual sensations. Brainstem visceral afferents are carried by the vagus and glossopharyngeal nerves. Brainstem visceral afferents are important in complex automatic motor acts such as swallowing, vomiting, and coughing.[34] Sensory messages from the visceral organs travel back to the medulla and the limbic lobe. This may be the explanation for the term "gut feeling." The walls of the intestinal organs contain independent nerve sell clusters that operate independently from the vagus nerve, and use the same neurotransmitters as the brain.[81]

Traumatic spinal cord injury, particularly injury above the T5 level, is associated with severe and disabling cardiovascular, gastrointestinal, bladder, and sexual dysfunction. These individuals have both supine and orthostatic hypotension and are at risk of developing bradycardia and cardiac arrest during tracheal suction or other maneuvers that activate the vagovagal reflexes.

Pure autonomic failure with no other neurologic deficits is rare. More often, autonomic failure occurs in combination with other neurologic disorders, such as Parkinson disease, and multiple system atrophy. In these individuals, it is important for the examiner to inquire about abnormalities in gait, changes in facial expression, the presence of dysarthria, difficulty in swallowing, and balance problems. Autonomic failure also occurs in individuals with some peripheral neuropathies such as those associated with diabetes. Because autonomic failure may be caused by lesions at different levels of the nervous system, a history of secondary trauma, cerebrovascular disease, tumors, infections, or demyelinating diseases should be established. Additionally, because the most frequent type of autonomic dysfunction encountered in medical practice is pharmacologic, there should be a thorough review of medication use, especially antihypertensive and psychotropic drugs.

Some conditions may be confused with autonomic failure, including neurally mediated syncope, which is referred to as vasovagal, vasodepressor, or reflex syncope. This condition is caused by a paroxysmal reversal of the normal pattern of autonomic activation that maintains blood pressure in the standing position; these individuals do not have autonomic failure. A detailed history is important to differentiate this disorder. In contrast to individuals with chronic autonomic failure in whom syncope appears as a gradual fading of vision and loss of awareness, individuals with neurally mediated syncope often have signs and symptoms of autonomic overactivity such as diaphoresis and nausea before the event. This distinction and the episodic nature of neurally mediated syncope should be part of a thorough clinical history.

The complexity of the nervous system cannot be overstated. The information provided in this overview of the components of the CNS is meant to illuminate the many facets of the system that can be affected by pathologic processes. Figure 28-18 shows the relationship of the areas that have been described here.[41] Familiarity with this relationship is the basis of attempting to understand the pathologies that will be considered in the next chapters. To understand pathology, one must have a good working knowledge of brain structure and function. The Whole Brain Atlas web site provides dynamic images of the brain integrating imaging techniques that link anatomy and pathology.[103]

Aging and the Central Nervous System

Senescence, or aging, results from changes in DNA, RNA, and proteins. Errors in the duplication of DNA increase with age because of random damage over time. There may be a specific genetic program for senescence. Fibroblasts from an older individual double fewer times than those of an embryo.

Age-related reduction in adult brain weight represents loss of brain tissue. There is highly selective atrophy of brain tissue in the aging CNS. It is not clear how much of the change represents actual loss of nerve cells, since the changes in vascular tissue and glial cells may represent some of the loss. Simple loss of cells is common. Nerve cell shrinking, causing possible changes in functional efficiency, may be a more important effect of old age than cell loss. Nerve conduction velocity decreases with age in both the motor and sensory systems. By the eighth decade, there is an average loss of 15% of the velocity in the myelinated fibers.[55]

The inner structure of the nerve cell changes with aging. The presence of lipofuscin, or wear and tear pigment, a pigmented lipid found in the cytoplasm, may interfere with normal cell function via pressure on the cell nucleus. The pigmented nuclei of the brainstem

catecholaminergic neurotransmitter accumulate with age. Damage to an axon close to the neuronal cell body results in changes in the area of the cell body and is referred to as an axonal reaction. The mechanism and relationship to dysfunction are still not clearly understood. The deposition of amyloid-β protein creating plaques in the cerebral cortex is found in many but not all older people. Neuritic, or senile, plaques are found outside the neuron filled with degenerating axons, dendrites, astrocytes, and amyloid. They represent damage to brain tissue. The neuritic plaques are thought to occur most often in the cortex and hippocampus and have been associated with dementia and Alzheimer disease.[25]

Neurofibrillary tangles, or abnormal neurologic fibers that displace and distort the cell body, are found in higher concentrations in the older brain. Neurofibrillary tangles and amyloid are also found in higher concentrations in people with Alzheimer disease (see Chapter 31).

The blood supply also diminishes during aging, with a net reduction of 10% to 15%. The relationship of cerebral blood flow, the resultant decrease in the glucose supply to the brain, and decreased metabolism are not well established as to cause and effect. All three are noted in the aging brain.[75]

Morphologic changes in the aging brain are accompanied by neurochemical changes. Aging has a more deleterious effect on myelinated primary afferents than their unmyelinated counterparts. Neuronal atrophy, axonal lesions, loss of peripheral nerve endings, receptor organs and centrally projecting nerve terminals represent large myelinated primary afferent neurons. An inability to maintain appropriate neuronal function in senescence may result from a disturbance in the trophic signaling between neurons and their target cell. There is a decreased capacity of peripheral target tissues such as skeletal muscle and skin to synthesize neurotrophic factors of the nerve growth factor family of neurotrophins. Neurotrophins have been shown to regulate the expression of neurofilaments, which affect neural plasticity. Neurotrophins also influence the capacity of neurons to withstand the damaging effects of free radicals. Decreased neurotrophin signaling may be related to abnormal neuropeptide and other neurotransmitter substances that influence important functional aspects of primary sensory neurons process as it affects sensory neurons.[21] Changes in these neurotransmitters may be reflected in decreased control over visceral functions, emotions, and attention. Serotonin, involved in central regulatory activities of respiration, thermoregulation, sleep, and memory, appears to be reduced in the older brain. Depression in the older adult may be related to increased production of MAO, which breaks down catecholamines and results in a loss of the feeling of well-being.[47]

Other changes in the brain related to neurotransmission, such as Parkinson and Alzheimer disease, are described in the chapters that follow. Mood and depressive symptoms also are common in elderly individuals who are ill and are associated with increased morbidity and mortality. A growing body of data suggests that hyperactivation of the immune system has been implicated in the pathophysiology of major depressive disorder. Several proinflammatory cytokines, such as tumor necrosis

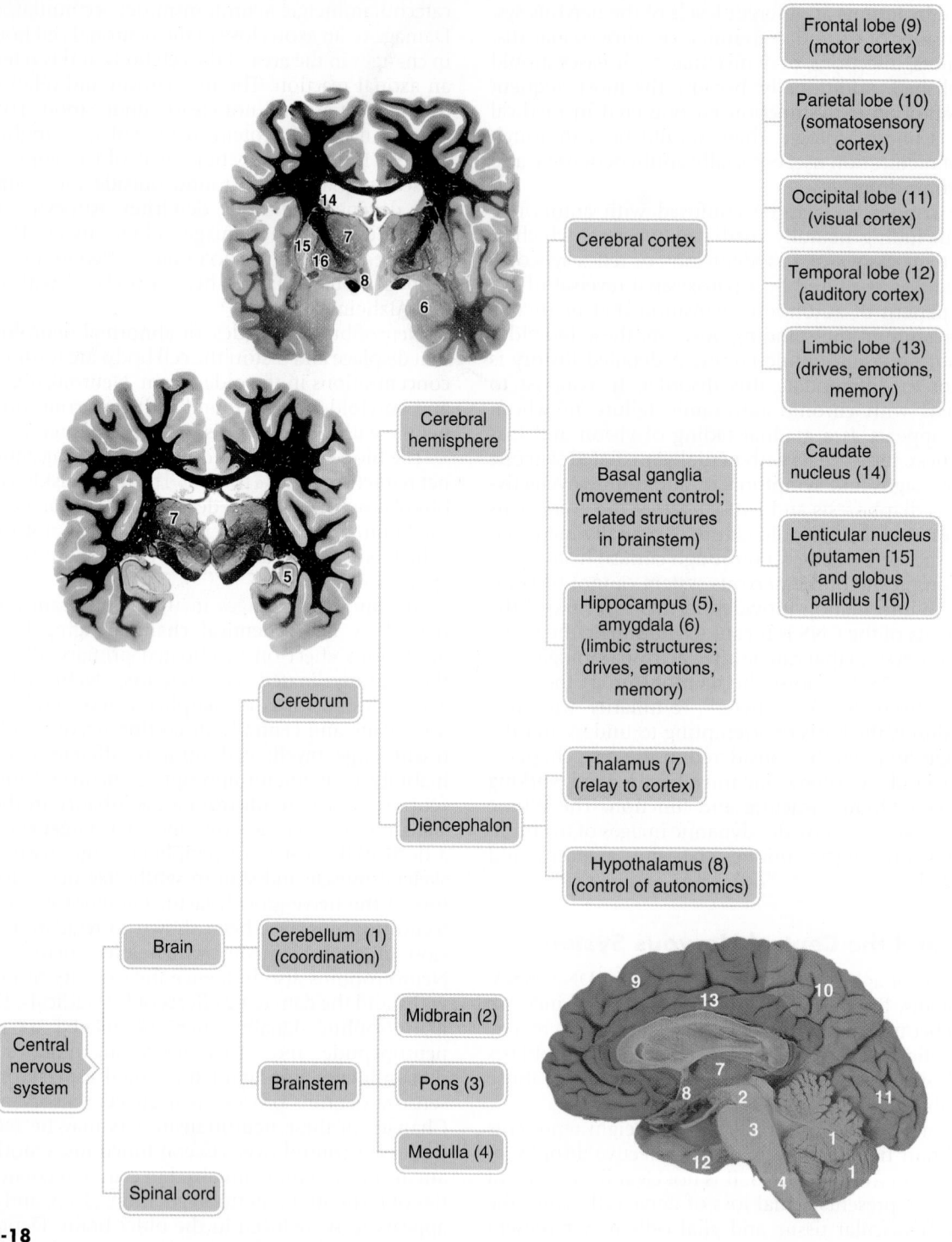

Figure 28-18

Overview of the subdivisions of the central nervous system (CNS). (From Nolte J: *The human brain: an introduction to its functional anatomy,* ed 5, St Louis, 2002, Mosby.)

factor-alpha and interleukin-1, have been found to be significantly increased in patients with major depressive disorder.[48] Age-associated alterations in immunity are apparent in the innate immune cells of the brain. There is an elevated inflammatory profile in the aging brain consisting of an increased population of reactive glia. A potential consequence of a reactive glial cell population in the brain is an exaggerated inflammatory response to innate immune activation. Even in the absence of detectable disease, the glia population undergoes an age-related transformation that creates a more sensitive brain environment.

An amplified and prolonged inflammatory response in the aged brain promotes protracted behavioral and cognitive impairments, and the behavioral consequences of illness and infection in the elderly, if prolonged, can have deleterious effects on mental health. There is an increased prevalence of delirium in elderly individuals who present to the emergency department as a result of infections unrelated to the CNS. Viral or bacterial pneumonia in the aged frequently presents clinically as delirium, even in the absence of classic pneumonia symptoms.[33]

Both neurophysiological and neuropsychological investigations support the general concept that the speed of central processing is reduced with advancing age.[71] The central mechanisms that are involved in the control of balance do not appear to change excessively with age but are more likely to be affected by degenerative neurologic diseases such as Parkinson or Alzheimer. Age-related changes in the peripheral vestibular system include hair cell receptors that begin to decrease at the age of 30 years, and by 55 to 60 years, there is a loss of the vestibular receptor ganglion cells. The myelinated nerve cells of the vestibular system show up to a 40% loss. Partial loss of vestibular function in the older population can lead to complaints of dizziness, with less ability of the nervous system to accommodate the loss compared with younger persons.

In addition to vestibular losses, there is concomitant loss of other sensory inputs relating to balance and mobility: vision and somatosensation. Maintaining equilibrium, or balance, requires a multimodal system integrating vestibular, visual, and somatosensory signals. The integration of these signals in the CNS coordinates multiple output responses: eye movement, postural correction, motor skill, and conscious awareness of spatial orientation. There are longer response latencies and delayed reaction times. Vision changes include loss of acuity, decreased peripheral fields, and loss of depth perception. The loss of input from this combination is slow, with compensation developing through the years.[16] Eventually, a loss of functional reserve, or redundant function, that is normally present in virtually all physiologic systems is seen with aging. There is an apparent decrease in the ability to integrate conflicting sensory information to determine appropriate postural responses. Changes occur as well in motor output that may contribute to the loss of balance and mobility.[14] Although the response patterns are the same in young and old people, with responses being activated in the stretched ankle muscle and radiating up to the thigh, in some older people, this response is disrupted, with the proximal muscles being activated before the distal muscles. In the older person, there appears to be more cocontraction of muscles around the ankle as a result of perturbation.[88]

There are data showing alterations in peripheral and central autonomic nerve activity, and decreases in neurotransmitter receptor action that lead to diminished autonomic reactivity with decreased control of blood pressure and cerebral blood flow regulation and poorly coordinated autonomic discharge such as bladder function. Strategies for autonomic function improvement and increasing cortical blood flow include walking and somatic afferent stimulation through activities including stroking skin or acupuncture to increase sympathetic, parasympathetic, and central cholinergic activity.[43]

Neurologic disease is more prevalent in older persons, as is the risk of neurologic sequelae as a result of intracranial hemorrhage, subdural hematoma, and neoplasms. Awareness of the signs and symptoms of these disorders is essential. The therapist may be the person able to identify a disease or the potential for a disorder that may manifest during a treatment session.

DIAGNOSIS

Clinical Localization

Clinical localization is the first step to differential diagnosis for an individual with neurologic disease. Coupling the time course of the illness with the clinical localization is the essence of neurology. The history of the onset and nature of the symptoms is critical to establish the diagnosis related to the neurologic disorder. In many cases, based on the history and symptoms, the clinician is able to generate a hypothesis regarding the site in the nervous system that has been affected and the nature of the lesion. A complete history of the nature of the symptoms is also critical to determining which diagnostic tools will provide the most accurate differential diagnosis and best determine the cause.

The examination of the client with neurologic dysfunction often begins with mental status changes. Alterations of consciousness and disturbances of higher brain function give the clinician clues about the nature of the disease process and the location of damage within the brain[96] (Table 28-6).

Motor and sensory changes will also reflect the type, level, and extent of damage to the system in the case of both disease and trauma. Understanding the typical motor and sensory changes associated with a particular disease or disorder leads the evaluation. For example, knowing that ALS involves both upper and lower motor signs may help the clinician when this otherwise perplexing condition presents in the clinic. Understanding the functional deficits related to each condition can also lead the clinician to a diagnosis. Gait disorders are often representative of the level or location of damage within the nervous system.

The diagnosis of neurologic disorders remains a clinical specialty, although the use of sophisticated imaging and measurement of neural function have provided insight into the pathologic state of the nervous system. With the development imaging such as fMRI and noninvasive brain stimulation techniques there is hope for new strategies focused on enhancing neurologic recovery and functional ability, even in the chronic phase.[10] The following are examples of diagnostic test currently performed.

Computed Tomography

CT scans allow a snapshot of the CNS, and damage within tissue can be identified. Disorders affecting blood flow, multiple sclerosis, neoplasm, and infection can be identified with these scans. CT is an excellent study to evaluate for acute intracranial hemorrhage, particularly in the subarachnoid space. Active bleeding may be detected in either epidural or subdural hemorrhages as a relative lucency, which is commonly referred to as the "swirl sign."

Table 28-6 Useful Studies in the Evaluation of Disorder of Level of Consciousness

Syndrome	Neuroimaging	Electrophysiology	Fluid and Tissue Analysis	Neuropsychological Tests
Bilateral cortical dysfunction; confusion and delirium	Usually normal; may show atrophy; rarely bilateral chronic subdural hematoma or evidence of herpes simplex encephalitis; dural enhancement in meningitis, especially neoplastic meningitides	Diffuse slowing; often, frontally predominant intermittent rhythmic delta activity (FIRDA); in herpes simplex encephalitis, periodic lateralized epileptiform activity (PLEDS)	Blood or urine analyses may reveal etiology; CSF may show evidence of infection or neoplastic cells	In mild cases, difficulty with attention (e.g., trailmaking tests); in more severe cases, formal testing is not possible
Diencephalic dysfunction	Lesion(s) in or displacement of diencephalon; also displays mass displacing the diencephalon	Usually, diffuse slowing; rarely, FIRDA; in displacement syndromes, effect of the mass producing displacement (e.g., focal delta activity, loss of faster rhythms)	Usually not helpful	Usually not obtained
Midbrain dysfunction	Lesion(s) in the midbrain or displacing it	Usually, diffuse slowing; alpha coma; evoked response testing may demonstrate failure of conduction above the lesion	Rarely, platelet or coagulation abnormalities	Usually not performed
Pontine dysfunction	Lesion(s) producing syndrome; thrombosis of basilar artery	EEG: usually normal; evoked responses usually normal	Rarely, platelet or coagulation abnormalities	Usually not performed
Medullary dysfunction	Lesion(s) producing dysfunction	EEG: normal; brainstem auditory and somatosensory evoked responses may show conduction abnormalities	Rarely, platelet or coagulation abnormalities	Usually not performed
Herniation syndromes	Lesion(s) producing herniation; appearance of perimesencephalic cistern	Findings related to etiology	Findings related to etiology	Usually not performed
Locked-in syndrome	Infarction of basis pontis	EEG and evoked potential studies: normal	Findings related to etiology	Usually not performed
Death by brain criteria	Absence of intracranial blood flow above the foramen magnum	EEG: electrocerebral silence; evoked potential studies may show peripheral components (e.g., wave I of brainstem auditory evoked response) but no central conduction	Absence of hypnosedative drugs	Not done
Psychogenic unresponsiveness	Normal	Normal	Normal	Helpful after patient "awakens"

CSF, Cerebrospinal fluid; *EEG,* electroencephalogram; *FIRDA,* frontally predominant intermittent rhythmic delta activity; *PLEDS,* periodic lateralized epileptiform activity.

From Koenigsberg RA, Faro SH, Hershey BL et al.: Neuroimaging, Chapter 23, in Goetz: *Textbook of Clinical Neurology,* ed 2, Philadelphia, 2003, Saunders.

Edema from excitotoxic damage associated with infarct or diffuse anoxia can be seen representing intracellular fluid, and vasogenic edema is the abnormal accumulation of extracellular fluid in the white matter that looks like fingers following the white matter tracts. Evaluation of ventricular size can be done by CT. Enlargement of the temporal horns out of proportion to the lateral ventricular bodies is helpful in recognizing early hydrocephalus. CT can be helpful to follow ventricular size after shunting.

CT is very useful for detecting intracranial calcifications such as those seen in congenital infections, vascular lesions, and metabolic disease. The location and distribution of calcifications is helpful in differentiating these various causes. The identification of calcification in a neoplasm aids in differential diagnosis.[34]

Magnetic Resonance Imaging

MRI signal patterns are recognizable with common diseases such as cerebral edema, neoplasm, abscess, infarcts, or demyelinating processes. MRI is the study of choice to evaluate all lesions in the brain and spine. CT, however, is more sensitive than MRI for the evaluation of calcifications, subtle fractures, and remains pivotal in the diagnosis of acute subarachnoid hemorrhage. Additionally, MRI cannot be performed in individuals who have intraorbital foreign bodies, pacemakers, or non-MRI-compatible implants, such as artificial heart valves, vascular clips, cochlear implants, or ventilators. The use of MRI is the modality of choice for detecting congenital malformations. Infection of the spine is better evaluated by MRI.

Functional Magnetic Resonance Imaging

fMRI is based on blood oxygenation level–dependent imaging of the brain and provides functional data of cerebral activation during any given task (e.g., motor, visual, or cognitive). fMRI shows both neuroanatomy and functions of the brain and is a brain-mapping tool for clinicians, researchers, and basic scientists. A noninvasive procedure with no known risks, fMRI is used for presurgical mapping of motor, language, and memory functions and allows neurosurgeons to be aware of, and to navigate, the precise location of cortices and structural anomalies from a space occupying lesions.[40]

Positron Emission Tomography

PET and single-photon emission CT scanning can show cellular activity via regional blood flow in the brain and are now used to monitor changes in the brain with functional activity. Both techniques can be used to depict the regional density of a number of neurotransmitters, allowing researchers to better understand the role of different parts of the brain during activity. PET and combined PET/CT provide powerful metabolic and anatomic information together in a single exam.[64]

DaTSCAN

Routine clinical studies with single-photon emission CT markers of the presynaptic dopamine transporter system (DaT) are now a reality. Two radiopharmaceuticals, both cocaine analogs labeled with iodine-123, are commercially available under the name of DaTSCAN and demonstrates excellent ability to separate patients with Parkinson disease from normal controls and other patients with nonparkinsonian tremor, particularly benign essential tremor. The DaT radiotracers show specific uptake in the striatum within the caudate nucleus and putamen with almost homogeneous distribution. Patients with benign essential tremor demonstrate similar findings, whereas in idiopathic Parkinson disease there is marked reduction of the tracer uptake in the putamen contralateral to the most affected side (Fig. 28-19). In patients with dopa-responsive dystonia, the striatal uptake of DaT ligands is clearly normal and distinct from patients with early-onset Parkinson disease.

Diffusion Tensor Imaging

Diffusion tensor imaging is capable of quantifying anisotropy of diffusion in white matter. Diffusion is *isotropic* when it occurs with the same intensity in all directions. It is *anisotropic* when it occurs preferentially in one direction, as along the longitudinal axis of axons. For this reason, DTI finds its greatest current application in

MRI examinations of the white matter. In normal white matter, diffusion anisotropy is high because diffusion is greatest parallel to the course of the nerve fiber tracts. These images can also be color coded, allowing for more spectacular visualization of nerve fiber tracts (Fig. 28-20).

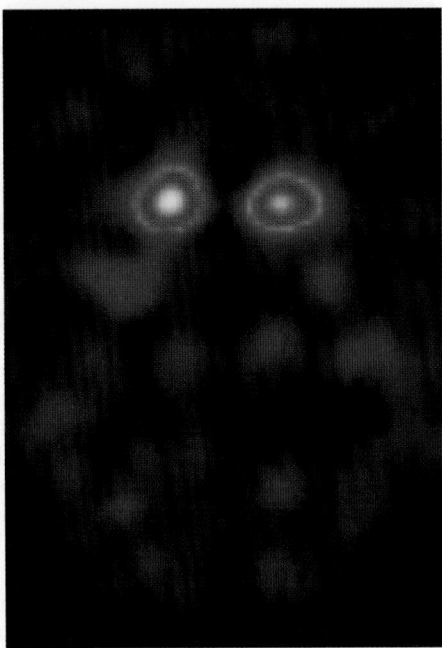

Figure 28-19

Transverse slice from a single-photon emission CT study with β-FP-CIT in a 61-year-old patient with idiopathic Parkinson disease. There is marked reduction of the tracer uptake in the putamen, worse on the left hemisphere contralateral to the more affected body side. (From Ell PJ, Gambhir S: *Nuclear medicine in clinical diagnosis and treatment*, ed 3, London, 2004, Churchill Livingstone.)

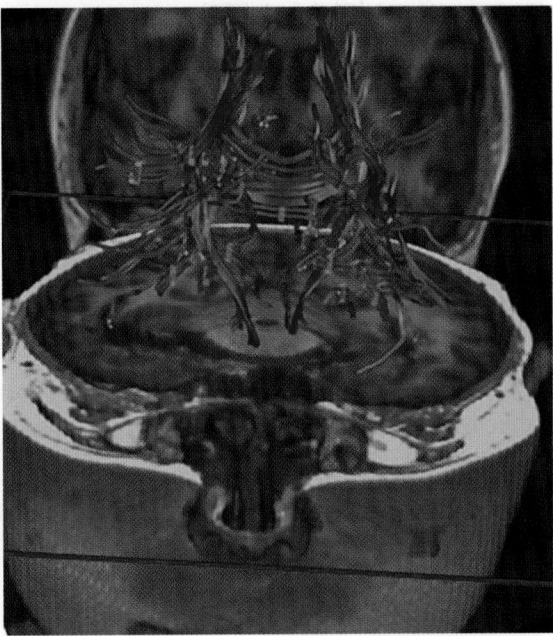

Figure 28-20

Diffusion tensor image (DTI) obtained with a 3-Tesla scanner. (From Daroff RB: *Bradley's neurology in clinical practice*, ed 6, Philadelphia, 2012 Saunders.)

Any disruption of a given nerve fiber tract (e.g., MS, trauma, gliosis) will reduce anisotropy, and the disruption of the white matter tract can be visualized.

Electroencephalography

Cerebral ischemia produces neuronal dysfunction, leading to slowing of frequencies or reduced amplitude in the EEG tracing. These changes may be generalized (global ischemia) or regional (focal ischemia). The depth of ischemia is associated with the severity of EEG changes. EEG cannot assess the whole cerebral cortex, however, and is less reliable at assessing subcortical structures. Chapter 36, "Epilepsy," further describes the uses of EEG in recording brain activity.

Brainstem Auditory Evoked Potentials

Potentials generated in the auditory nerve and in different regions of the auditory pathways in the brainstem can be recorded. The attention of the subject is not required. Because the brainstem auditory evoked potential (BAEP) is of very low voltage, between 1000 and 2000 responses are generally recorded so that the BAEP can be extracted by averaging from the background noise. Wave III probably arises in the region of the superior olive, whereas waves IV and V arise in the midbrain and inferior colliculus. Waves VI and VII are of uncertain origin and little clinical utility because of their inconsistency in normal subjects. The most consistent components are waves I, III, and V, and it is to these that attention is directed when BAEPs are evaluated for clinical purposes.

The BAEP is an important means of evaluating function of the cranial nerve VIII and the central auditory pathways in the brainstem. In infants, young children, and adults who are unable to cooperate for behavioral testing, BAEPs can be used to evaluate hearing. The wave V component of the response is generated by auditory stimuli that are too weak to generate other components. The BAEP is also useful in assessing the integrity of the brainstem. The presence of normal BAEPs in comatose individuals suggests either that the coma is due to bihemispheric disease or that it relates to metabolic or toxic factors; abnormal BAEPs in this context imply brainstem pathology and a poorer prognosis than otherwise. When coma is due to brainstem pathology, the BAEP findings help in localizing the lesion.

BAEPs have been used to detect subclinical brainstem pathology in individuals with suspected multiple sclerosis. However, the yield in this circumstance is less than with the visual or somatosensory evoked potentials, possibly because the auditory pathway is relatively short or is more likely to be spared. Cerebral ischemia results in delay in the arrival of or reduction in amplitude of evoked responses.[34]

Transcranial Doppler Ultrasonography

Transcranial Doppler ultrasonography uniquely measures local blood flow velocity in the proximal portions of large intracranial arteries. Hemodynamic compromise is inferred when there is reduction in mean flow velocities or when there is slow flow acceleration. In addition, transcranial Doppler ultrasonography can detect cerebral microembolic signals, reflecting the presence of gaseous or particulate matter in the cerebral artery. Solid, fat, gas, or air materials in flowing blood are larger and of different composition and, thus, have different acoustic impedance than surrounding red blood cells. Thus, the Doppler ultrasound beam is both reflected and scattered at the interface between the embolus and blood, resulting in an increased intensity of the received Doppler signal. A completely accurate and reliable characterization of embolus size and composition, however, is not yet possible with current technology.

Near-Infrared Spectroscopy

In brain tissue, the venous oxygen saturation predominates (70%-80%), and cerebral oximetry relies on this fact. Near-infrared spectroscopy uses light optical spectroscopy in the near-infrared range to evaluate brain oxygen saturation by measuring regional cerebral venous oxygen saturation. Table 28-7 describes the use of various imaging techniques correlated to anatomic site.

Transcranial Magnetic Stimulation

Transcranial magnetic stimulation (TMS) is a brain stimulation technique that allows study of the physiology of the CNS, identifying the functional role of specific brain structures and, more recently, exploring large-scale network dynamics. TMS has diagnostic value as well as therapeutic potential for several neuropsychiatric disorders. The stimulation involves restricted cortical and subcortical regions and, when used in combination with a visually guided technique, results in improved accuracy to target specific areas including functional maps of the motor and visual cortex. New combinations of these techniques, in conjunction with neuroimaging, will further advance the utility of their application.[18,79]

TREATMENT

Treatment is based on an understanding of the level and type of neuronal dysfunction. Treatment of neurologic disorders has been a frustrating science in the past, but with better understanding of the cellular processes and changes related to disease, treatment holds more promise.

Methods to Control Central Nervous System Damage

Damage or disease of the nervous system often results in changes in the production and uptake of neurotransmitters. Many important drugs that alter nervous system function act by selective interaction with neurotransmitter receptors. Drugs that act at synapses either enhance or block the action of these neurotransmitters. Most neurotransmitters with a prominent role in brain function produce very brief receptor-mediated actions at specific groups of synapses. A few neurotransmitters are more prolonged and act more widely throughout the extracellular space. The combined action of both a briefly acting and a

Table 28-7   Neuroimaging Applications in Diagnosis and Therapy

Technique	Diffuse or Multifocal Cerebral	Focal Cerebral	Subcortical	Brainstem	Spinal Cord
Plain film	Neoplasm Metabolic Congenital	Neoplasm	Not useful	Not useful	Trauma Neoplasm Degenerative
CT	Hemorrhage Calcification Infarct Neoplasm Inflammation Vascular	Hemorrhage Calcification Infarct Neoplasm Inflammation Vascular	Hemorrhage Calcification Infarct Neoplasm Inflammation Vascular	Hemorrhage Calcification Infarct Neoplasm Inflammation Vascular	Hemorrhage Calcification Neoplasm Inflammation
MR	Neoplasm Inflammation Hemorrhage Vascular White matter disease Congenital Infarct	Neoplasm Inflammation Hemorrhage Vascular White matter disease Congenital Infarct	Neoplasm Inflammation Hemorrhage Vascular White matter disease Infarct	Neoplasm Inflammatory Hemorrhage Vascular White matter disease Infarct	Neoplasm Inflammatory Hemorrhage Vascular White matter disease Infarct
Myelography	Not useful	Not useful	Not useful	Not useful	Degenerative Neoplasm Hematoma Inflammatory Vascular Congenital
Angiography	Mass effect Vasculopathy Atherosclerosis	AVM tumor Aneurysm Atherosclerosis	AVM tumor Aneurysm Atherosclerosis	AVM tumor Aneurysm Atherosclerosis	AVM
Ultrasonography	Hemorrhage (Neonatal) Congenital Neoplasm Infection Vascular	Hemorrhage (Neonatal) Congenital Neoplasm Infection Vascular	Hemorrhage (Neonatal) Congenital Neoplasm	Congenital Neoplasm	Congenital Neoplasm
PET-SPECT	Vascular Neoplasm Infection Degenerative Trauma	Vascular Neoplasm Infection Degenerative Trauma	Vascular Neoplasm Infection Degenerative Trauma	Not useful	Not useful

AVM, Arteriovenous malformation; *PET-SPECT*, positron emission tomography–single-photon emission CT.

more enduring neurotransmitter produces a modulation of postsynaptic neuronal activity. Pharmacologic strategies are aimed at modulation of neurotransmitter synthesis, release, reuptake, and degradation.[45] Some drugs mediate inhibition of neurotransmitter release by acting at presynaptic receptors. Opiates are one group of drugs that act by the inhibition of neurotransmitter release. Drugs used to control excessive tone in specific muscle groups often work by inhibiting neurotransmitter release. Anesthetic drugs modify the actions of neurotransmitter receptors by changing the membranes of cells on or within which the receptors are located.[19]

Drug therapy can stimulate neurotransmitter release. Drugs aimed at maintaining neurotransmitter activity in the synaptic cleft can be useful in neuromuscular junction diseases. Another way to regulate the level of neurotransmitters is to influence the rate of chemical degradation.

Drugs can inhibit the breakdown of certain elements that may be broken down by natural processes such as oxidation. One action of these drugs is to prolong the efficacy of released neurotransmitters by inhibiting their degradation.[98] An example of this process is the regulation dopamine. Dopamine activity can be increased by four mechanisms:

• Increased synthesis
• Increased release
• Prolongation of neurotransmitter activity
• Direct receptor stimulation

Synthesis of the neurotransmitter can be increased by giving dopa because it is the product beyond the rate-limiting enzyme and there is ordinarily an abundant amount of aromatic amino acid decarboxylase in the CNS. When dopa is combined with a peripherally active decarboxylase inhibitor, more dopa is delivered across the blood-brain barrier and can be used to synthesize central dopamine. Drugs such as cocaine, amphetamine, and methylphenidate can increase release.

The normal metabolism of dopamine involves reuptake of dopamine into the presynaptic cell, with subsequent metabolism by two enzymes, MAO and COMT. Prolongation of dopamine activity can be effected by blocking reuptake or altering enzyme activity. Amantadine and possibly some tricyclic antidepressant medications operate on the dopaminergic system through blockade of reuptake. MAO inhibitors and COMT inhibitors for human use also increase dopaminergic activity. Finally, direct activation of the dopamine receptors on the striatal cell can be induced by agonists like bromocriptine, pergolide, and other drugs. Importantly, orally administered dopamine itself has no place in altering the CNS dopamine levels, because, being a positively charged molecule, it cannot cross the blood-brain barrier.[34]

Other drugs protect the cell membrane in the presence of toxins that act on the membrane, such as the toxic effects of the free radicals produced in brain tissue after hypoxia, ischemia, and seizures. Damage to the neuron occurs when the free radical is allowed to penetrate the membrane.[76]

The best defense is to prevent penetrance. Antioxidant therapies are being examined for a variety of neurodegenerative disorders and the sequelae of stroke and spinal cord injury. Oxidative stress has been consistently linked to ageing-related neurodegenerative diseases. Among the cellular pathways conferring protection against oxidative stress, a key role is played by vitagenes, which include Hsp70, heme oxygenase-1, thioredoxin and sirtuins. Cellular signaling pathways and molecular mechanisms that mediate hermetic responses typically involve antioxidant enzymes and transcription factors such as Nrf-2 and NFÎ°B. Vita genes, either individually or by acting in concert, contribute to counteract the radical oxygen species–mediated damage.[30] As oxidative stress invariably contributes to various forms of cell death, a better understanding of how antioxidant defenses are maintained in particular brain cells will probably help to develop protective strategies in degenerative insults specifically affecting these cells.[35] Optimal functioning of the central and peripheral nervous system is dependent on a constant supply of appropriate nutrients.[51] Ongoing studies are looking at the natural substances noted above as well as manufactured substances that will provide antioxidant or free radical scavenging. There is great hope that substances that will slow down the destruction related to oxidative stress will prove to be curative for progressive diseases of the CNS, as well as other degenerative processes associated with connective tissue, neoplasm, and aging.[8] There are similar cellular mechanisms underlying neuronal loss, neurodegeneration and disease which share common mechanisms such as protein aggregation, oxidative injury, inflammation, apoptosis, and mitochondrial injury. Although cerebrovascular disease has different causes from the neurodegenerative disorders, many of the same common disease mechanisms come into play following a stroke. Novel therapies that target each of these mechanisms may be effective in decreasing the risk of disease, abating symptoms, or slowing down

their progression. Although most of these therapies are experimental, and require further investigation, a few seem to offer promise.[94] Brain training, specialized exercises designed to keep the brain functioning at the highest levels possible, is gaining momentum in controlling the effects of aging and has potential to impact the training to maximize brain activity after injury or in relationship to progressive disease.

Stem cells are unspecialized living cells that have the capacity to renew themselves for long periods of time through cell division. Under certain physiologic or experimental conditions, they can be induced to become cells with special functions such as the beating cells of the heart muscle or the insulin-producing cells of the pancreas. *Embryonic stem cells* are derived from embryos that develop from eggs that have been fertilized in vitro and then donated for research purposes with the informed consent of the donors. The embryos from which human embryonic stem cells are derived are typically 4 or 5 days old and consist of a hollow microscopic collection of cells called the *blastocyst*. An *adult stem cell* is an undifferentiated cell found among differentiated cells in a tissue or organ. The primary roles of adult stem cells in a living organism are to maintain and repair the tissue in which they are found. Some researchers now use the term *somatic stem cell* instead of adult stem cell. Unlike embryonic stem cells, which are defined by their origin, the origin of adult stem cells in mature tissues is unknown. A single adult stem cell could have the ability to generate a line of genetically identical cells, or *clones*.[2]

There is evidence for the impact of immune system dysfunction in these diseases despite the blood-brain barrier protection of the CNS from the direct effects of autoimmune responses. Identification of immune system elements is leading researchers toward an understanding of the role of the immune system in diseases such as multiple sclerosis, ALS, Parkinson disease, and Alzheimer disease.

Use of catheters to deliver drugs directly into the cerebrospinal fluid or brain tissue has enhanced the ability to deliver drugs that act directly on the neuron. Although the catheters have been made more sophisticated and can deliver the drugs in measured doses, complications of administration and uneven levels of absorption continue to be limiting factors.

Treatment of Nonneural Dysfunction

Many drugs used to treat neurologic disorders influence nonneural tissue, including cerebral blood vessels and glia. Cerebral edema can increase the permeability of the blood-brain barrier, causing an increase in fluid within the brain. The resulting compression of brain tissue can be life-threatening. Drugs, such as mannitol, that control cerebral edema, or drugs that provide diuresis can help preserve neuronal function. In demyelinating disease, antiinflammatory and immunosuppressive drugs are used to preserve the function of the glial cells that produce the myelin sheath.

For some of the viruses that invade the CNS, there is replication of cells in nonneural tissue. Use of drugs that inhibit RNA or DNA synthesis can prevent viral replication without disrupting neuronal integrity. Acyclovir, used in the treatment of herpes encephalitis, is an example of this type of drug.

In infants and children, there is an altered drug metabolism that should be considered whenever administering drugs that act on the nervous system. Concomitant illness and fever will further alter drug metabolism. An immature blood-brain barrier can also affect the absorption of drugs into brain tissue. When anticonvulsants are administered, close monitoring of blood levels is necessary.

PROGNOSIS

Prognosis is the keystone to management of neurologic disorders because it links diagnosis to outcomes and identifies need for treatment. Prognostic studies can also identify if available treatment is ineffective. In addition, these studies can indicate which diseases have an important impact on function or disability.[57]

Disability resulting from neurologic disease and trauma can be extensive, and care of these clients often requires use of limited resources: time and money. With the tremendous advances made in the emergent medical care of trauma victims and people with significant neurologic disease, the number of people living with neurologic disorder is increasing at a steady rate.[6]

Permanent or progressive impairments can be demoralizing to clients and their families. Clients must reorganize their perspectives in order to learn alternative ways of regaining as much control as possible over life activities. Success builds a sense of efficacy, and failure undermines self-worth. Tackling challenges in successive attainable steps will lead to further competencies in associated tasks. When individuals see others with similar disabilities perform successfully, they may have increased confidence in their own abilities. The persuasion of health care providers and caregivers can boost effort but must be realistic. Perceived self-efficacy can influence the course of health outcomes and functional status. The prognosis for an individual should consider both the social and cognitive status of the individual in relationship to the diagnosis.[4]

The economic evaluation of health care reflects the complexity of the disease treatment process and the value of health effects. Policy makers are demanding information about the economic outcomes of diseases and their treatments. Research methodologies oriented toward cost-of-illness and cost-benefit analysis have emerged. Clinicians should be involved in this analysis to maintain perspective, especially in catastrophic and degenerative processes.[52]

As noted above, several chronic neurologic disease states, such as Alzheimer disease, are associated with elevated secretion of stress hormones such as cortisol. Stress also can trigger or exacerbate symptom onset and perhaps progression of chronic illness such as Parkinson disease. Stress hormones also can mitigate the impact of acute neurotrauma; for example, there is a positive correlation between cortisol levels and mortality after head injury. Thus, neurologic disease states can occur within a context of elevated glucocorticoids, which may have profound influences on recovery and neuroplasticity. In addition, abnormal regulation of glucocorticoid release is associated with many affective disorders, such as depression and PTSD, that are overrepresented in populations with neurologic disease. Release of glucocorticoids, however, also can occur in anticipation of adverse events. Anticipatory release of glucocorticoids occurs in the absence of a frank physical stimulus, keyed by memories or instinctual predispositions.[81]

Measures of health-related quality of life address the impact of health on physical, social, and psychologic aspects of life. The particular scale may address issues related to a specific population or may be sensitive to a clinical intervention. The therapist should be familiar with the measurement tools typically used during intervention for a condition or disease. As much as possible, these tools are described in the appropriate chapter in this section.[6]

Physiologic Basis for the Recovery of Function

After injury to the nervous system, there are changes in the structure and function of the neurons. In some instances, the changes can lead to further damage, whereas other changes facilitate recovery.

Diaschisis, or neural shock, occurs when there is injury to a nerve and disruption of the neural pathway that extends a distance from the site of injury. When the neurons distal to the injury regain function, which may be soon after the injury, partial function may return.

Injury may be secondary to either swelling of the axon or edema in the surrounding tissue that blocks *synaptic activity* in the injured neurons, as well as that in the surrounding area. With reduction of the edema, function may return. This is the reason that medications that reduce edema are often given in the context of diffuse brain swelling.

When there is a loss of presynaptic function in one area, the postsynaptic target cells for that area may become more sensitive to neurotransmitters that are now produced in lower concentrations. The compensatory mechanism is known as *denervation supersensitivity*. *Regenerative synaptogenesis* occurs when injured axons begin sprouting. *Collateral sprouting* is the process of neighboring axons sprouting to connect with sites that were previously innervated by the injured axon.

Suppression of a response to a stimulus is considered habituation, whereas sensitization is an increased response to a stimulus, usually related to noxious stimuli or pain. Adaptation is the ability to modify a motor response based on changes in the sensory environment or input received.

Long-term potentiation occurs when a weak input and a strong input arrive at a dendrite at the same time. The weak stimulus is enhanced by the strong stimulus. With repeated activation of combined stimuli, there is an increase in the presynaptic transmitter associated with the stimulus. After the long-term potentiation has been established, the weak input will elicit a stronger response than it had initially.[54]

The characteristics of a lesion will have a profound effect on recovery from a brain injury. Small lesions of the brainstem may in fact be as devastating as large lesions of the cerebral cortex. Cerebellar damage can affect both learning and memory of movements. Lesions that occur gradually appear to cause less disruption of function than lesions that occur all at once, such as with strokes. Advanced age will adversely affect the return of function. Studies show that a person's prior level of activity and environment will affect the rate and extent of recovery. An enriched environment will positively affect recovery when it is available, either before the insult or during the recovery period.

Redistribution of cortical mapping is seen after a lesion in the brain.[13] These changes may involve unmasking of previously nonfunctional synaptic connections from adjacent areas, or the ability of the neighboring inputs may take over. It is clear that both sensory and motor maps in the cortex are constantly changing according to input from the environment. In addition, the brain appears to increase use of ipsilateral pathways after a lesion that affects one side.[77]

Neural modifiability or adaptation may be seen as a change in the organization of connections among neurons and is often referred to as plasticity.[88] The elements described above are active in this process, including genetic coding, neuronal networks, individual synapses, and neurotransmitters. Physiologic studies suggest that motor relearning and recovery of function may be accomplished through the same neural mechanisms and reflect the plasticity of the brain. Learning alters our capability to perform the appropriate motor act by changing both the effectiveness of the neural pathways used and the anatomic connections.

Learning involves storage of memory and can occur in all parts of the brain with both parallel and hierarchic processing. The area of representation within the brain becomes specialized for both inputs and outputs. Areas of the brain used during the early phase of learning movement are different from those used once a skill is learned. Initially, more areas of the brain are active, since skill develops both the number of neurons firing and location of activity change. The use of sensory input is increased in the early stages of learning. The prefrontal areas are also more active in the learning phase and become less active during automatic movements.[13] The stimuli repeatedly excite cortical neuron populations, and the neurons progressively grow in numbers. Repetition will lead to greater specificity, and the responses become stronger. With skill acquisition, sensory feedback appears to be less critical.

Control of learning comes from many areas of the CNS working together. The area involved may depend on a number of variables associated with the type of learning taking place and is influenced by the environment. The cortex is involved in learning through sensorimotor integration. It is postulated that there are widely distributed groups of neurons acting as a cortical engram, composed of multiple functional groupings. Thus, when an activity is repeated and stored in memory, the engrams are available to trigger groups of cells that fire synchronously during movement. The engrams appear to influence the precision, speed, and accuracy of movement.[54]

The limbic system is critical to the learning phase because it generates need-directed motor activity and communicates the intent to the rest of the brain. The limbic system is a critical part of the neural representation necessary for memory that includes the cortex and thalamus.

The cerebellum is active during procedural learning. A possible mechanism is through the influence of the climbing fibers on the mossy fibers with eventual change in the output fibers, the Purkinje fibers.[95] The lateral cerebellum affects cognition through its relationship to the frontal areas active during cognitive processes.[66,80]

The basal ganglia appear to be highly involved in the cognitive aspects of motor behavior although the level of contribution remains unclear. Habit formation appears to be associated with functions of the basal ganglia, and the control of internally generated movement here appears to be a part of the motor learning continuum.[54]

SPECIAL IMPLICATIONS FOR THE THERAPIST | 28-1

Motor Learning Strategies: Neuroplasticity

Comorbid impairments should always be considered, as well as the individual's prior health status, age, motivation, and established life practices. In every case, it is important to remember the focus of intervention should not be so much on the disease that the person has as it should be on the person that has the disease. For maximal effectiveness, CNS injury should be treated as soon as possible beyond the initial injury phase, when the chance of exacerbating the cellular damage is past. The location of the injury should drive the intervention. The interaction between the client with neurologic dysfunction and the therapist is critical for optimal motor learning to take place. To elicit the highest level of function within the motor system and allow insight regarding the program, goal-directed activities must be included.[100,104]

During the examination and evaluation of disability the therapist should recognize the impairments that contribute to abnormal motor control.[17,68,84,88] Force production, speed of motion, coordination of movement, and cognition are often affected in neurologic disorders. Identification and modification of environments that can alter responses should be made early in the management process. Difficulty with bowel and bladder control can affect progress with recovery and should be managed with either physical or medical means. Treatment of nonneural tissue changes secondary to weakness or changes in tone should be addressed in the intervention. Substitution devices, assistive devices, and environmental changes should be considered when it is clear that the client will not recover from specific impairments. Reintegration into social and personal roles is of prime importance to the client with neurologic dysfunction. Functional status is the critical outcome marker, and physical therapists are able to positively influence outcomes in this area. Determining the correlation between impairment and functional limitation, disability or participation is paramount in the rehabilitation process and is the basis of studies relating task specificity to levels of impairment.[53]

The recovery of function after CNS injury involves the reacquisition of complex tasks. Inherent in the recovery of function that has been lost secondary to a neurologic insult is the process of motor relearning, which can be defined as the process of acquisition or modification of movement.[16,88] Motor learning is a modification of behavior by experience and includes perceiving, remembering, thinking, and acting. Behaviorally important inputs are trained through specialization. Interaction and integration of critical systems can facilitate improvement in movement despite anatomic or physiologic deficits in the CNS. Learning-based activities drives reorganization, stimulates neurons from adjacent areas, create new synapses, and activates neurons in the uninjured areas of the brain. Changes in the cortical synaptic structure and function, with increases in dendritic activity, as the result of learning are seen both in the course of child development and after behavioral training in the adult.

Memory is the retention of these modifications; therefore, memory plays a critical role in motor learning.[54] Memory for motor behaviors is developed through different forms of learning and involves different brain regions. Memory associated with fear or other emotional stimuli is thought to involve the amygdala. Memory established through operant conditioning requires the striatum and cerebellum. Memory acquired through classical conditioning and habituation involves changes in the sensory and motor systems included in the learning. Input to the brain is processed into short-term working memory before it is transformed into a more permanent long-term storage.[34]

Motor learning, or the precision of movement, takes place as the client determines the optimal strategy of movement to perform a motor task. There are several models that incorporate defined stages of motor learning involved in skill acquisition. The Fitts and Posner Model includes the *cognitive stage* as the first stage, which requires a great deal of thought, experimentation, and intervention. Performance is variable, as is seen in the first attempts to walk after brain injury. In the cognitive stage, the treatment environment is highly structured to allow clients to think and focus on a task. Feedback is given more frequently and may involve more sensory systems. Problem solving is focused on the movement strategies necessary to complete the task. The task may be broken down at this time to work on component parts of the total movement and practiced with repetition.[82,84]

The second stage of skill acquisition is the *associative stage*, represented by refining of the skill. Fewer errors of performance are experienced, and the motor programs elicited are more consistent and efficient. Feedback can be given in a summary format, often after a few trials. The individual will use trial and error to fine-tune the movement. The final stage is the *autonomous stage*, in which the movement is efficient and the need for attention to the activity is decreased. The motor program has been integrated by the basal ganglia, and each component is initiated with little thought. This activity can now be performed in conjunction with another activity.

The need for feedback during each stage is different. The therapist can enhance treatment by providing the correct amount of feedback for the client attempting to perform a task. For a skill to be acquired, learning principles that promote associative and automatic phases need to be incorporated in the intervention. This appears to be related to the practice conditions. It is clear that repetition is required in every stage. Initially blocked or serial practice is used until the learner understands the dynamics of the task. When cognition is limited, it may be better to keep to a blocked practice schedule longer. For a skill to become learned or transferred to other activities, random practice is more effective. Part-task training can be beneficial if the task can naturally be broken down into component parts that create the whole movement when put back together. Differences in input sources, including afferent activity from different components of sensory systems may create different representational activities within the thalamic nuclei and associated cortical areas. Representation changes can occur as a result of environmental interaction and purposeful behavioral practice.[44,78] Motor learning is reflected in changes to the brain's functional organization as a result of experience, and motor learning also changes sensory systems.[67] Integrated motor imagery practice has been shown to improve function in many areas and shows functional carryover.[20] Use of imagery can be effective throughout the rehabilitation process.

Neuroprotection

Aging and neurodegenerative conditions such as Alzheimer and Parkinson diseases are characterized by tissue and mitochondrial changes that compromise brain function. Alterations can include increased reactive oxygen species production and impaired antioxidant capacity with a consequent increase in oxidative damage, mitochondrial dysfunction that compromises brain ATP production, and ultimately increases apoptotic signaling and neuronal death. Among several nonpharmacologic strategies to prevent brain degeneration, physical exercise is an effective strategy, which antagonizes brain tissue and mitochondrial dysfunction.[58] Forced exercise appears to increase cerebral glycolysis even more than voluntary exercise via increased cerebral metabolism.[50,73]

Animal studies have shown efficacy in neuroprotection related to hippocampal cell survival and further maturation and neurogenesis.[7,11,23] Exercise interventions in individuals with Parkinson disease incorporate goal-based motor skill training to engage cognitive circuitry important in motor learning. With this exercise approach, physical therapy helps with learning through instruction and feedback (reinforcement) and encouragement to perform beyond self-perceived capability.[15,61,74]

The general idea is that exercise that incorporates goal-based motor skill learning improves motor skill performance and can be enhanced through cognitive engagement. Studies suggest that with combined goal-based and aerobic training, the possibility for improving automatic cognitive motor control may be possible,

Experience-dependent neuroplasticity

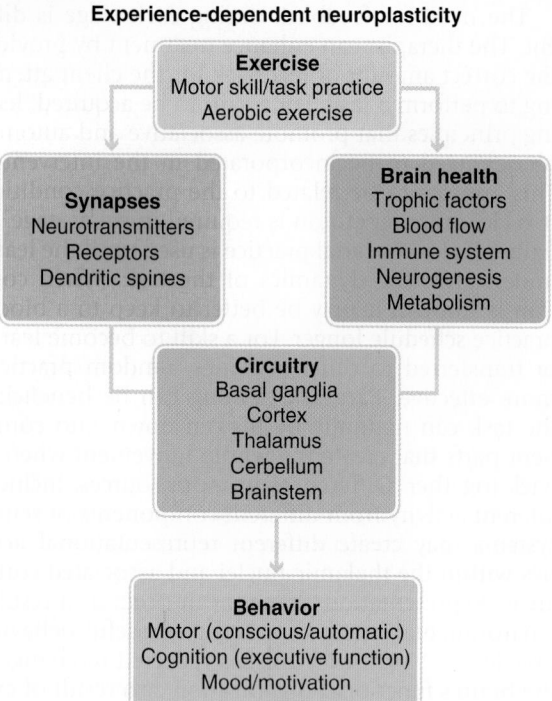

Figure 28-21

Exercise and neuroplasticity in Parkinson disease. Clinical and basic research studies support the effects of exercise on neuroplasticity in Parkinson disease. Neuroplasticity is a process by which the brain encodes experiences and learns new behaviors and is defined as the modification of existing neural networks by adding or modifying synapses. Evidence is accumulating that both goal-directed and aerobic exercise may strengthen and improve motor circuitry through mechanisms that include but are not limited to alterations in dopamine and glutamate neurotransmission, as well as structural modifications of synapses. In addition, exercise may promote neuroprotection of substantia nigra neurons and their existing connections. Finally, exercise-induced alterations in blood flow and general brain health may promote conditions for neuroplasticity important for facilitating motor skill learning, including cognitive and automatic motor control and overall behavioral performance. Although more studies are clearly needed, taken together these findings are supportive of a disease-modifying effect of exercise in Parkinson disease. (Adapted from Petzinger GM, Fisher BE, McEwen S, et al.: Exercise-enhanced neuroplasticity targeting motor and cognitive circuitry in Parkinson's disease. *Lancet Neurol* 12:716–726, 2013.

reducing the attention demands of walking. Aerobic exercise may contribute to more general improvement in brain health and repair, through the recruitment of the immune system and/or increasing blood flow and trophic factor signaling. These aerobic exercise benefits are likely to impact connectivity through *priming* the brain environment conducive for promoting synaptic neuroplasticity leading to altered circuitry. Exercise can restore important circuits in motor behavior by modulating glutamate neurotransmission as well as influencing general brain health. Figure 28-21 shows the process that is considered to explain the concept of neuroprotection with exercise.

REFERENCES

To enhance this text and add value for the reader, all references are included on the companion Evolve site that accompanies this textbook. The reader can view the reference source and access it online whenever possible.

CHAPTER 29

Infectious Disorders of the Central Nervous System

KENDA S. FULLER

OVERVIEW

Infection of the central nervous system (CNS) remains relatively rare in that many protective responses limit the access of harmful organisms to the nervous tissue. However, neurologic infections are a major cause of mortality and morbidity worldwide. Bacterial infections can be serious and life-threatening. Biologic adaptations of infectious agents and altered modes of transmission present new challenges. Drug-resistant strains create new threats, and travel has increased the exposure to both viruses and the bacteria that can cause infection of the nervous system.[18,40]

Despite protective mechanisms, once there is access to the brain, viruses produce a large range of neuropathologic conditions including oncogenic states, producing astrocytomas.[59] CNS infections can affect the brain's parenchyma, directly causing abscess. Remote infectious processes, such as bacterial endocarditis, resulting in infected emboli, can cause infectious intracranial aneurysms.[46] Sepsis can cause diffuse, multifactorial involvement of the CNS, including invasion of the meninges with resulting meningitis.[58] The cerebrospinal fluid (CSF) can be contaminated when an object penetrates the meninges. This is often a result of trauma or a neurosurgical procedure.[10] Trauma to the front of the face that causes damage or fracture of nasal structures or the cribriform plate can lead to infection in the CSF. Infection of the inner ear can spread to the brain via the CSF.[48]

MENINGITIS

Definition

In meningitis, the meninges of the brain and spinal cord become inflamed. The three layers of the meningeal membranes (dura mater, arachnoid, and pia mater) can be involved. The relationship of the meninges to the brain tissue is shown in Figure 29-1. The pia mater and arachnoid become congested and opaque. The inflammation extends into the first and second layers of the cortex and spinal cord and can produce thrombosis of the cortical veins. There is an increased chance of infarction, and the scar tissue can restrict the flow of CSF, especially around the base of the brain. This block of CSF can result in hydrocephalus or a subarachnoid cyst. Stretch or pressure on the meninges will cause the cardinal sign of headache.[2]

Incidence

The estimated incidence of meningitis is 2 to 6 per 100,000 adults per year in developed countries and is up to 10 times higher in less-developed countries. The incidence of bacterial meningitis is highest among children younger than 1 year of age. Extremely high rates are found in Native Americans, Alaskan Natives, and Australian aboriginals, suggesting that genetic factors play a role in susceptibility. Other risk factors include acquired or congenital immunodeficiencies, hemoglobinopathies such as sickle cell disease, functional or anatomic asplenia, and crowding such as occurs in some households, day care centers, or college and military dormitories. A CSF leak resulting from congenital anomaly or following a basilar skull fracture increases the risk of meningitis, especially that caused by *Streptococcus pneumoniae*.

Enteroviruses cause meningitis with peaks during summer and fall. These infections are more prevalent among low-socioeconomic-status groups, young children, and immunocompromised persons. The prevalence of arboviral meningitis is determined by geographic distribution and seasonal activity of the arthropod (mosquito) vectors. In the United States, most arboviral infections occur during the summer and fall.[39]

Etiologic and Risk Factors

Vaccines developed in the past 15 years to protect against the development of meningitis, primarily against *Haemophilus influenzae* type B (Hib) infection, have dramatically decreased the incidence in the countries where there is access to the vaccine. There appears to be a second period of increased susceptibility during late adolescence. In adulthood, bacterial meningitis is mostly associated with conditions that affect the defense mechanisms of the host.[18] Individuals with compromised immune function related to other conditions, such as HIV, remain at high risk to develop meningitis.[40] When there is damage or removal of the spleen, a person becomes more susceptible to pneumococcal disease.

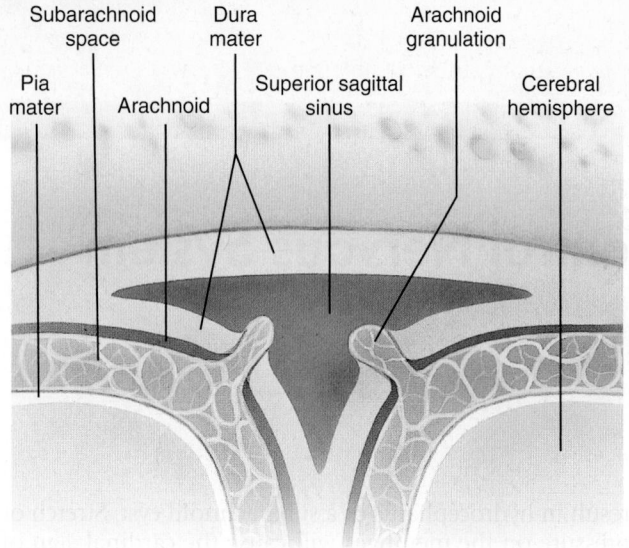

Figure 29-1

The meninges, showing the relationship of the dura, arachnoid, subarachnoid space, pia, and brain tissue. (From Lundy-Ekman L: *Neuroscience: fundamentals for rehabilitation*, ed 3, Philadelphia, 2007, Saunders.)

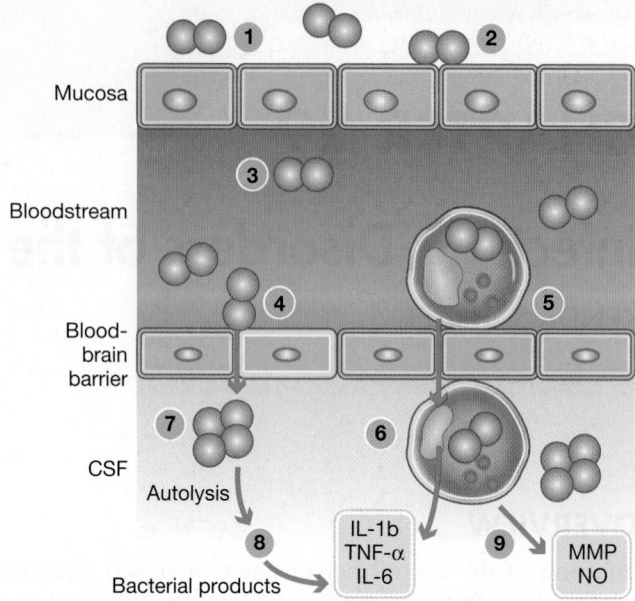

Figure 29-2

Pathogenesis of bacterial meningitis. (1) Adherence and colonization of mucosa; **(2)** invasion of bloodstream; **(3)** multiplication in bloodstream; **(4)** increased permeability of the blood-brain barrier and bacteria cross the blood-brain barrier; **(5)** infiltration of CSF by white cells; **(6)** release of proinflammatory cytokines; **(7)** uncontrolled replication of bacteria in sanctuary site, CSF; **(8)** bacterial products stimulate inflammatory cascade; **(9)** activated leukocytes lead to production of matrix metalloproteinase (MMP) and oxidants. (From Magill AJ, Ryan ET, Hill D, et al: *Hunter's tropical medicine and emerging infectious disease*, ed 9, Philadelphia, 2012, Saunders.)

Otitis, mastoiditis, and sinusitis are common predisposing conditions that may need specialized treatment. Neoplastic meningitis is a complication that occurs infrequently but is characterized by neurologic signs and symptoms and has a poor outcome.[19] Meningitis associated with cutaneous anthrax became an urgent health concern with the 2001 bioterrorism threat. Although there is meningeal involvement in only 5% of persons exposed, studies of experimental inhalation anthrax in monkeys have demonstrated meningeal involvement in 40% to 50% of cases.

Pathogenesis

The most common bacteria causing acute bacterial meningitis (*S. pneumoniae, N. meningitidis,* and *H. influenzae*) have neurotropic potential, which allows them to invade the host mucosal epithelium, multiply in the bloodstream and cross the blood-brain barrier into the CSF.[58] Figure 29-2 shows the process that allows access into the CNS. Young children mount inadequate immune responses to bacterial capsular polysaccharides, rendering them particularly vulnerable to these infections.[38]

Once there is penetration of the blood-brain barrier and infectious agents move into the CSF and parenchyma of the brain, there is less immune protection than in the rest of the body. The CSF has about 1/200 the amount of antibody as blood, and the number of white blood cells is very low compared with the blood. The brain lacks a lymphatic system to fight infection despite the fact that the level of leukocytes in the brain increases.[17] Cytokines, chemokines, macrophages, and microglia respond to viral and bacterial infections. The polymorphonuclear cells recruited to the infection cause damage to the surrounding brain tissue by the release of cytotoxic free radicals and excitatory amino acids such as glutamate. Neuronal cell death occurs mainly in the hippocampus,

through apoptosis, and in the cortex, through necrosis. White matter injury also occurs, secondary to small-vessel vasculitis, focal ischemia, or venous thrombosis. Oxidative stress may be responsible for apoptosis in the hippocampus. Vasculitis can lead to infarction and decreases in cerebral blood flow, causing a drop in the glucose level of the CSF. Responses to inflammation in the brain can block CSF, resulting in hydrocephalus, edema, and increased intracranial pressure.[9,52]

Aseptic (Viral) Meningitis

Viral infection is the most common cause of inflammation of the CNS. Viral meningitis is an acute febrile illness with signs and symptoms of meningeal irritation, usually with a lymphocytic pleocytosis of the CSF and negative CSF bacterial stains and cultures. Aseptic meningitis most often is caused by enteroviruses, which are the major cause of meningitis in 40% of those 30 to 60 years old.[24] The second most common cause of meningitis is herpes simplex virus 2, which is detected in approximately 20% of individuals with meningitis. Epstein-Barr virus can also be responsible and is more often seen in late adolescence and early adulthood. Systemic lupus erythematosus, a disorder of connective tissue, can cause aseptic meningitis. Sarcoid tumors and other intracranial tumors or cysts can lead to aseptic meningitis through rupture.[4] Often the meningitis occurs days or weeks after the exposure. Recurrent aseptic meningitis is two or more episodes with a disease-free interval between. This must be distinguished

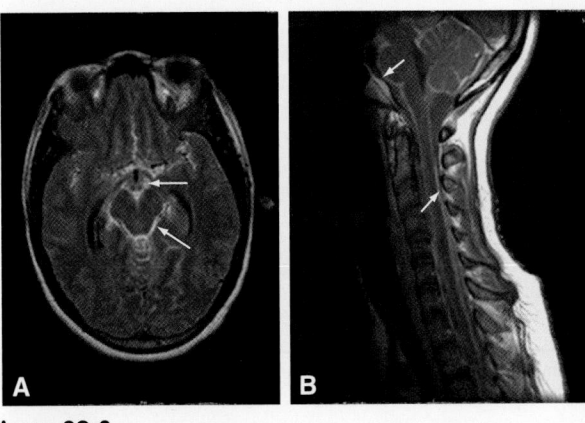

Figure 29-3

Tuberculous meningitis. A, T1-weighted transverse MRI of the brain. **B,** Sagittal MRI of base of brain and spinal cord in patient with tuberculous meningitis. Note enhanced meninges *(arrows)* in basilar regions of brain, brainstem, and spinal cord. (From Vincent J, Abraham E, Kochanek P, et al: *Textbook of critical care,* ed 6, Philadelphia, 2011, Saunders.)

from the waxing and waning of chronic meningitis.[19] Certain drugs or chemicals can cause aseptic meningitis. The drugs most commonly involved are the nonsteroidal antiinflammatory medications. Chemicals can cause direct meningeal irritation and are often related to surgical procedures that expose the chemical.

Tuberculous Meningitis

Tuberculous meningitis is a severe form of extrapulmonary tuberculosis and is rare (0.5%-1%) but is associated with high mortality and disability among survivors.[32] Tuberculous meningitis is an infection by *Mycobacterium tuberculosis*, which enters the body by inhalation.[18,62] CNS involvement includes abscess or spinal cord disease. The hallmark pathologic processes are meningeal inflammation, basal exudates, vasculitis and hydrocephalus. Diagnosis is based on the characteristic clinical picture, neuroimaging abnormalities, and CSF changes (increased protein, low glucose, and mononuclear cell pleocytosis). CSF smear examination, mycobacterial culture, or polymerase chain reaction is mandatory for bacteriologic confirmation. Prompt diagnosis and early treatment are crucial. Decision to start antituberculous treatment is often empirical. WHO guidelines recommend a 6-month course of antituberculous treatment; however, other guidelines recommend a prolonged treatment extended to 9 or 12 months. Corticosteroids reduce the number of deaths. Resistance to antituberculous drugs is associated with a high mortality. Patients with hydrocephalus may need ventriculoperitoneal shunting. Bacillus Calmette-Guérin vaccination protects to some degree against tuberculous meningitis in children.[26]

Tuberculous brain abscesses may produce mass effect and edema. CSF may demonstrate formation of multiple cysts with lymphocytes and an elevated protein. Infected bacilli enter the subarachnoid space to cause diffuse meningitis.[43] A CT image of a tuberculoma is seen in Figure 29-3.[42]

Bacterial Meningitis

The organisms generally responsible for bacterial meningitis are those found in mucosal surfaces in the upper respiratory tract. Bacteria in the birth canal can be transferred from the mother to the infant during birth. Group B streptococcus, *Escherichia coli*, and *Listeria monocytogenes* are bacteria that can cause infection in the neonate, although antibodies are passed through the placenta. As these antibodies decline, the susceptibility to Hib, pneumococcus, and meningococcus increases, especially in the second half of the first year of life. On the other end of the spectrum, *S. pneumoniae* and *Neisseria meningitis* are the most common bacteria causing infection in the adult and geriatric populations.[45,52]

In bacterial meningitis, inflammation initially is confined to the subarachnoid space, then spreads to the adjacent brain parenchyma. Vasculitis starts in the small subarachnoid vessels. Thrombotic obstruction of vessels and decreased cerebral perfusion pressure can lead to focal ischemic lesions. Veins are more frequently affected than arteries, probably because of their thinner vessel walls and the slower blood flow. Damage to the cell bodies causes the production of amyloid-β precursor protein that is carried through the axon and accumulates within terminal axonal swellings, or spheroids. This axonal pathology contributes to neurologic sequelae seen after bacterial meningitis.

Anthrax Meningitis

Bacillus anthracis is a gram-positive spore-forming bacterium that causes anthrax disease in humans and animals. It is a systemic infection that causes septicemia, toxemia, and meningitis, the latter associated with high mortality. Acute infection with *B. anthracis* Sterne and the Î"LF mutant results in disruption of human brain microvascular endothelial cell integrity.[22]

Clinical Manifestations

Headache, vomiting, meningeal signs, focal deficits, vision loss, cranial nerve palsies, and raised intracranial pressure are dominant clinical features in tuberculous meningitis. Adults with acute bacterial meningitis usually present with features of fever, neck stiffness, and altered mental status. More advanced disease may include opisthotonus, focal neurologic deficit, seizures, and a reduced level of consciousness. Pain in the lumbar area and the posterior aspects of the thigh identified as Kernig sign, or pain with combined hip flexion and knee extension. As the inflammation progresses, flexion of the neck will produce flexion of the hips and knees. This is known as a positive Brudzinski sign.[53] The positions for Kernig and Brudzinski tests are shown in Figure 29-4. If the infection remains undetected or untreated, the brainstem centers may be affected. The individual may then experience seizures and coma, vomiting, and papilledema. Focal neurologic signs, including cranial nerve palsies and deafness, can also be seen when the brainstem is affected.

MEDICAL MANAGEMENT

DIAGNOSIS. Early symptoms of meningitis and septicemia often resemble viral illnesses such as influenza, making the condition difficult to diagnose. Classic symptoms such as a nonblanching rash and a stiff neck are often late symptoms of the disease, and neck stiffness is rarer in

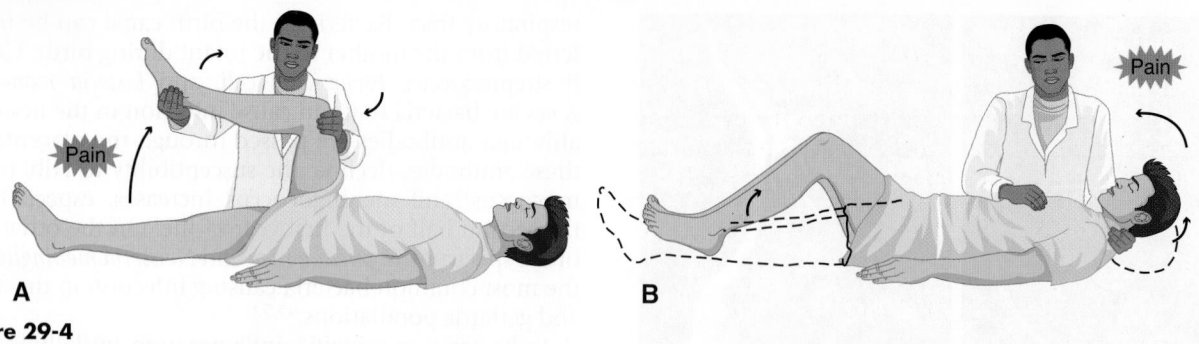

Figure 29-4

Assessing a client with meningeal irritation. A, Kernig sign. **B,** Brudzinski sign. (From Black JM: *Medical-surgical nursing: clinical management for positive outcomes,* ed 7, Philadelphia, 2004, WB Saunders.)

infants and young children. The presence of ear or upper respiratory tract infections does not necessarily exclude a diagnosis of meningitis. The emphasis should therefore be on regular, close monitoring of an ill child and assessment of the vital signs. Awareness of the recognized "red flag" symptoms of septicemia—cold hands and feet, limb pain, and pale or mottled skin—could also aid earlier diagnosis and hence potentially improve prognosis.[33]

Lumbar puncture is the only absolute means of substantiating a diagnosis of meningitis. The viruses causing viral meningitis can be isolated in CSF and include enteroviruses, lymphocytic choriomeningitis, and herpes simplex virus. Lumbar puncture reveals mononuclear cells in the hundreds, a normal glucose level, a mild increase in protein, and absence of bacterial organisms (see "Laboratory Values" in Chapter 40). Radiographs are taken to rule out fracture, sinusitis, and mastoiditis. A CT scan or MRI will reveal evidence of brain abscess or infarction that may be responsible for the symptoms. Figure 29-3 shows evidence of abnormal MRI with tuberculous meningitis.

Viral infection is the most common cause of inflammation of the CNS in children. Differentiation from bacterial infection of the CNS is made on the basis of signs and symptoms and CSF changes. Clinical symptoms consistent with meningeal involvement are milder but overlap with those of bacterial infection.[45]

Prompt diagnosis is critical in bacterial meningitis because death can occur without antibiotic treatment. Because determining the bacterial etiology can take up to 48 hours with CSF cultures, an alternative diagnostic test should be considered. Gram stain examination of CSF is recommended when meningitis is suspected. It is fast, inexpensive, and accurate up to 90% of the time. Polymerase chain reaction is useful for excluding a diagnosis of bacterial meningitis and may eventually, with further refinement, be used for determining etiology.[17]

When CSF findings suggest bacterial meningitis, but Gram stain and culture results are negative, a combination of laboratory tests is necessary to distinguish bacterial from viral meningitis. In bacterial meningitis, the opening pressure generally is between 200 and 500 mm H_2O (lower in children), white blood cell count and protein concentration are elevated, glucose concentration may be low, and there may be a neutrophil or lymphocyte predominance.[59]

When there is a neoplasm or brain tumor, the infection may be the result of pleomorphic manifestations

of neoplastic meningitis and co-occurrence of disease at other sites. Useful tests to establish diagnosis and guide treatment include MRI of the brain and spine, CSF cytology, and radioisotope CSF flow studies. Assessment of the extent of disease of the CNS is valuable because large-volume subarachnoid disease or CSF flow obstruction is prognostically significant.[29]

Anthrax meningitis produces CSF that is marked by polymorphonuclear pleocytosis and hemorrhage. Characteristic gram-positive rods abundantly found in the smear of the CSF, blood, etc. make diagnosis certain in most of the cases. Resistance to penicillin, the drug of choice, is now being occasionally reported. Other antibiotics that are found to be very effective are doxycycline and ciprofloxacin. Fear of use of anthrax spores as a biological weapon has also given a new dimension to the problem.[21] CSF protein elevation is generally present, and CSF glucose concentrations are generally decreased, as is seen with causes of other bacterial meningitis.[55]

The time course after onset of the disease indicates the type of organism involved. Viral meningitis is hyperacute, with symptoms developing within hours. Acute pyogenic bacterial meningitis can also develop in 4 to 24 hours. Individuals with fungal meningitis or tuberculous meningitis develop symptoms over days to weeks. In tuberculous meningitis, there is a predominance of mononuclear cells, the glucose level is decreased, and protein is increased. It is difficult to identify the tuberculosis bacterium, so clinical signs are important to follow.[15]

TREATMENT. Guidelines for the diagnosis and treatment of bacterial meningitis from the Infectious Diseases Society of America are updated on a regular basis. Prompt treatment of bacterial meningitis with an appropriate antibiotic is essential. Optimal antimicrobial treatment of bacterial meningitis requires bactericidal agents able to penetrate the blood-brain barrier, with efficacy in CSF. Several new antibiotics have been introduced for the treatment of meningitis caused by resistant bacteria, but their use in human studies has been limited. More complete understanding of the microbial and host interactions that are involved in the pathogenesis of bacterial meningitis and associated neurologic sequelae is likely to help in developing new strategies for the prevention and therapy of bacterial meningitis.[57]

When acute bacterial meningitis is suspected, antimicrobial therapy should begin as soon as possible.

Bacterial meningitis is a neurologic emergency; progression to more severe disease reduces the likelihood of a full recovery. Targeted antimicrobial therapy can begin in adults following a positive CSF Gram stain result. Antibiotic therapy should not be delayed pending the results of Gram stain or other diagnostic tests. Antimicrobial therapy should be modified as soon as the pathogen has been isolated. Duration of therapy depends on individual responses.[59]

Suspected bacterial meningitis in a child or infant is considered a medical emergency. The general picture involves fever, decreased feeding, vomiting, bulging fontanel (in infants), seizures, and a high-pitched cry. In neonates with meningitis caused by gram-negative bacilli, the duration of therapy should be determined in part by repeated lumbar punctures documenting CSF sterilization. If there is no response after 48 hours of appropriate therapy, repeated CSF analysis may be necessary. Because any complications of bacterial meningitis usually occur within the first 2 or 3 days of treatment, outpatient management requires close follow-up. Criteria for outpatient therapy are inpatient antimicrobial therapy for 6 or more days; no fever for at least 24 to 48 hours; no significant neurologic dysfunction, focal findings, or seizure activity; stable or improving condition; and ability to take fluids by mouth. There should be an established plan for physician and nurse visits, laboratory monitoring, and emergencies. Seizures can be controlled with antiseizure medications. As the infection is controlled, the seizures are resolved, so a short course is all that is usually necessary.[59]

The addition of dexamethasone can reduce the subarachnoid space inflammatory response that is related to morbidity and mortality and may therefore alleviate many of the pathologic consequences of bacterial meningitis related to cerebral edema or cerebral vasculitis. Change in cerebral blood flow, increase in intracranial pressure, and neuronal injury can be controlled by judicious steroid use.

Radiologic treatment is effective with neoplastic meningitis. Because neoplastic meningitis affects the entire neuraxis, chemotherapy treatment can include intra-CSF fluid. Neoplastic meningitis is often a part of a progressive systemic disease, and consequently treatment is palliative.[29]

Usual treatment for viral meningitis is symptomatic. Medication is given for the headache and nausea. The prognosis in viral meningitis is excellent, and most individuals recover within 1 to 2 weeks. Treatment of acute episodes of herpes meningitis with acyclovir has been shown to decrease the duration and severity of symptoms. It may work as well for prophylactic control of episodes. Tuberculous meningitis is managed with drugs given to treat the tuberculosus. In addition, adjunctive therapy with corticosteroids may reduce mortality and decrease neurologic sequelae in severe meningitis. Drugs that scavenge for free radicals and the use of N-methyl-D-aspartate (NMDA) receptor blockers can help reduce tissue injury.[59]

PROGNOSIS. Mortality ranges from 5% to 25% depending on the infecting bacteria and the health and age of the person infected. At least one neurologic complication, such as impairment of consciousness, seizures, or focal neurologic abnormalities, typically develops in 75% of individuals with bacterial meningitis. Systemic complications, cardiorespiratory failure, or sepsis are also common and found about 40% of the time. Hyponatremia occurs about 30% of the time, with an average duration of 3 days, well managed by fluid restriction.

Cranial nerve palsies occur about 30% of the time, with hearing impairment during hospitalization a common complaint, but more than half have full return of hearing. The severity of hearing loss was graded as mild one-third of the time, moderate one-third, and profound in another third. When there is hearing loss, it is more likely to be bilateral than unilateral.[65]

In children, long-term neurologic consequences of bacterial meningitis include developmental impairment, hearing loss, blindness, hydrocephalus, hypothalamic dysfunction, hemiparesis, and tetraparesis. There is a 30% mortality rate, with increasing death with individuals over 60 years. Most death occurs within 2 weeks, as a result of both systemic and neurologic complications. Aseptic or viral meningitis is usually self-limiting, and there is not the same degree of neurologic sequelae involved. Mortality rates for tuberculous meningitis range from 20% to 50%, and survivors may be left with neurologic sequelae similar to those seen in acute bacterial meningitis.[35,36] With better understanding of the role of cytokines, therapies targeting these processes are under study and show promise. These therapies may help to further control damage to the nervous system during the infectious or inflammatory process.[9] Poor outcome is significantly associated with the severe consciousness disturbance, and the presence of intracranial brain swelling, seizure, cerebral hemorrhage or pneumonia.[56]

ENCEPHALITIS

Definition

Encephalitis is an acute inflammatory disease of the parenchyma, or tissue of the brain, caused by direct viral invasion or hypersensitivity initiated by a virus. Encephalitis is characterized by inflammation primarily in the gray matter of the CNS. Neuronal death can result in cerebral edema. There can also be damage to the vascular system and inflammation of the arachnoid and pia mater.[3] Viruses carried by mosquitoes or ticks are responsible for most of the worldwide known cases of primary CNS infection. In many cases, such as West Nile virus and herpes simplex virus, the individual can develop either encephalitis or meningitis. This is reflected in the different levels of impairment that may be experienced after exposure.

Incidence. Before 1994, outbreaks of West Nile virus were sporadic and occurred primarily in the Mediterranean region, Africa, and Eastern Europe. Since 1994, outbreaks have occurred with a higher incidence of severe human disease, particularly affecting the nervous system. By 2002, incidence was 4 to 14 per 100,000 population in the Midwest. West Nile virus is now endemic throughout the contiguous United States, with 17,000 human neuroinvasive disease cases and more than 1500 deaths

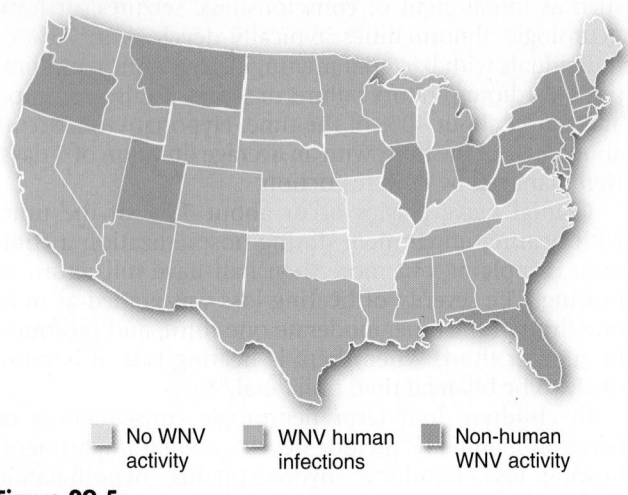

No WNV activity

WNV human infections

Non-human WNV activity

Figure 29-5

West Nile virus activity by state—United States, 2013. (From CDC ArboNET, www.cdc.gov./westnile, accessed July 2013.)

reported since 1999. More than 780,000 illnesses have likely occurred. Figure 29-5 illustrates the spread of the virus through the United States. Incidence is highest in the Midwest from mid-July to early September. West Nile fever develops in approximately 25% of those infected, varies greatly in clinical severity, and symptoms may be prolonged. The virus has caused meningitis, encephalitis, and poliomyelitis.[27] Up to 20% of infected people suffer permanent neurologic damage, and less than 2% die.[8,47]

Etiologic and Risk Factors

West Nile virus is a flavivirus that was originally isolated in 1937 from the blood of a febrile woman in the West Nile province of Uganda. The virus is widely distributed in Africa, Europe, Australia, and Asia, and since 1999, it has spread rapidly throughout the Western Hemisphere, including the United States, Canada, Mexico, and the Caribbean and into parts of Central and South America.

Since the first detection of West Nile virus in the Western Hemisphere in 1999, the virus has spread rapidly across the North American continent and as far south as Argentina. An unprecedented pattern of large annual epidemics of human neuroinvasive disease continues in North America, resulting in considerable public health impact. The high infection incidence in humans has resulted in non-mosquito transmission modes, such as through transfused blood and transplanted organs. West Nile virus incursion into Latin America and the Caribbean Islands has resulted in surprisingly low human, avian, and equine morbidity and mortality despite evidence that West Nile virus strains circulating in those regions are similar to those in North America.

Acute viral encephalitides, such as Eastern and Western equine encephalitis, St Louis encephalitis, and California virus encephalitis, and the most recent outbreak of West Nile virus depend on mosquitos for transmission and tend to occur in the mid- to late summer. The Eastern variety is the least common but most deadly. It occurs in outbreaks along the entire east coast of the United States.

It is rapidly progressive, with lesions in the basal ganglia. It carries high mortality and morbidity rates. The Western version has a much lower mortality but appears to be particularly severe in infants and children.[14]

West Nile virus is transmitted primarily between avian hosts and mosquitos. Figure 29-6 shows the cycle of transmission. Mosquitoes of the genus *Culex* carry the virus, and it is maintained during the dormant period of the adult mosquito and reintroduction of the virus by migratory birds from their winter breeding grounds or from locations where the virus may be transmitted all year round.[13] Norwegian scientists have reported that an unexpectedly large number of dogs in the Arendal area of southern Norway have antibodies to tick-borne encephalitis virus caused by flavivirus passed on by forest-living, blood-sucking ticks. Human beings, dogs, sheep, cows, and other mammals become infected when fed on by a tick, although the virus also spreads through the consumption of raw milk from infected animals, and it can cross the placenta from mother to fetus.[1]

Pathogenesis

Encephalitis produces an inflammatory response and pathologic changes in the brain. Ballooning of infected cells and degeneration of the cellular nuclei can lead to cell death. Plasma membranes are destroyed, and cells form multinucleated giant cells. There is perivascular cuffing causing damage to the lining of a vessel and hemorrhagic necrosis. The oligodendrocytes are affected, creating gliosis, or scarring. Widespread destruction of white matter can occur through inflammation and thrombosis of perforating vessels. Focal damage can hit discrete areas such as the optic nerve.[28]

West Nile virus is thought to initially replicate in dendritic cells after the host has been bitten by an infected mosquito. The infection then spreads to regional lymph nodes and into the bloodstream. The way in which the virus invades the nervous system is still unknown; retrograde transport along peripheral nerve axons has been proposed. Histologic CNS findings of West Nile virus infection are usually characterized by perivascular lymphoplasmacytic infiltration, microglia, astrocytes, necrosis, and neuronal loss with predilection to structures like the thalamus, brainstem, and cerebellar Purkinje cells. These variable anatomic involvements explain different clinical presentations.[34]

Herpes simplex virus is found in neonatal infants and appears to arise from maternal genital infection with the virus. It is acquired as the baby passes through the birth canal. Fifty percent of those who contract herpes simplex virus will develop CNS disease, whereas others may only develop skin, eye, and mouth disease. Herpes simplex encephalitis is found after the age of 3 months and is often a latent infection found in the gray matter of the temporal lobe and surrounding structures of the limbic system and the frontal lobe. It is the most common cause of sporadic nonepidemic encephalitis in the United States. Possible genetic factors are undergoing study, and in animal studies, there appears to be a connection to the $\gamma_1 34.5$ gene.[2]

Encephalomyelitis can result from viral infections such as measles, mumps, rubella, or varicella. Mumps is usually benign and self-limited, but it can trigger encephalitis and

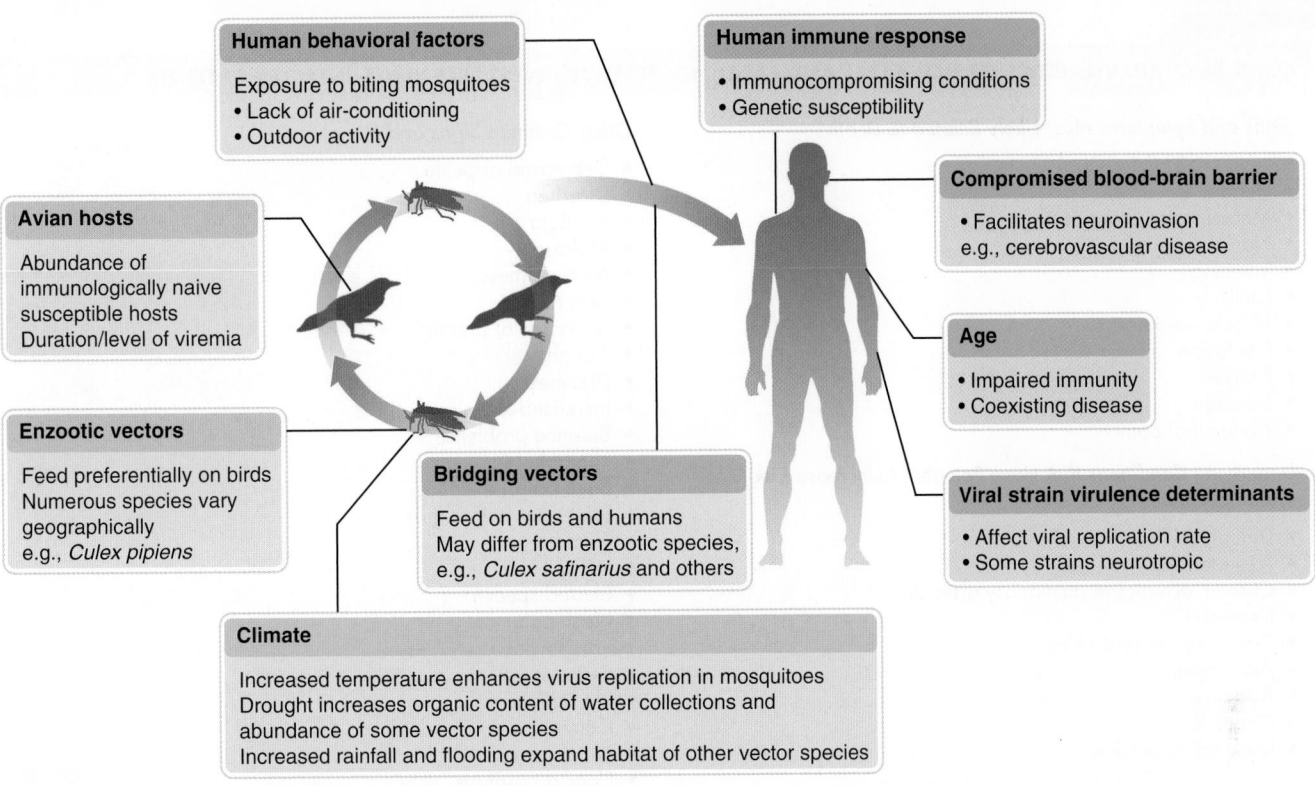

Figure 29-6

West Nile virus transmission cycle and examples of modifying climatologic, vertebrate, mosquito, and human factors on infection and illness. (From Tsai TF, Vaughn DW, Solomon T: Flaviviruses. In Mandell GL, Bennett JE, Dolin R, eds: *Principles and practice of infectious diseases*, ed 6, New York, 2005, Churchill Livingstone.)

other CNS complications such as acute, hydrocephalus, ataxia, transverse myelitis, and deafness.[60] Vaccines that contain neuronal antigens have been known to precede these infections, particularly for rabies or smallpox. When there is an illness at the time of vaccination, the risk of developing infection increases. Neurologic problems typically occur within 3 weeks of the illness or vaccination.[4]

Epstein-Barr virus and hepatitis A have been associated with CNS disorders of an infectious nature. Acute toxic encephalitis occurs during the course of a system infection with a common virus. Parasites, bacteria, and toxic drug reactions can lead to infection of the brain and cause encephalitis or encephalopathy.

Clinical Manifestations

Signs and symptoms of encephalitis depend on the etiologic agent, but in general, headache, nausea, and vomiting are followed by altered consciousness. If the person becomes comatose, the coma may persist for days or weeks. Agitation can be associated with the degree of infection and may be associated with abnormal sensory processing. Depending on the area of the brain involved, there may be focal neurologic signs, with hemiparesis, aphasia, ataxia, or disorders of limb movement. There can be symptoms of meningeal irritation with stiffness of the back and neck. With herpes simplex encephalitis, there can be repeated seizure activity, hallucinations, and disturbance of memory, reflecting involvement of the temporal lobe.[48]

Although many individuals infected with West Nile virus are asymptomatic, symptoms develop in 20% to 40% of people with West Nile virus infection. The incubation period is 2 to 14 days before symptom onset. Most complaints are of flu-like symptoms. West Nile virus is characterized by fever, headache, malaise, myalgia, fatigue, skin rash, lymphadenopathy, vomiting, and diarrhea. Kernig and Brudzinski signs may be found on physical examination. Less than 1% of infected individuals develop severe neuroinvasive diseases. West Nile meningitis usually presents with fever and signs of meningeal irritation such as headache, stiff neck, nuchal rigidity, and photophobia. Box 29-1 lists the findings that are most critical to watch for to determine potential for high level of disability or death. In addition, West Nile virus can present as acute flaccid paralysis. Figure 29-7 shows the pattern of weakness found in some individuals with this form of West Nile virus infection. The lesion of spinal anterior horns results in a paralysis similar to polio and reaches a plateau within hours. Deep tendon reflex can be diminished in severely paralyzed limbs. Reports of substantial muscle ache in the lower back and bowel and bladder functions are common. There is minimal or no sensory disturbance.[34,63]

Encephalitic lesions appear to alter sleep patterns as sequelae of brain-immune interactions. Responses of the immune system to invading pathogens are detected by the CNS, which responds by orchestrating complex changes in behavior and physiology. Sleep is one of the behaviors altered in response to immune challenge. Cytokines may play an active role in infectious challenge by regulating sleep.[44]

Box 29-1

CLINICAL CHARACTERISTICS OF NONFATAL AND FATAL HOSPITALIZED WEST NILE VIRUS–INFECTED PATIENTS

Signs and Symptoms Most Likely Related to Death

- Fever >38° C (>100.4° F)
- Headache
- Mental status changes
- Nausea
- Vomiting
- Chills
- Muscle weakness
- Confusion
- Fatigue
- Lethargy
- Abdominal pain

Underlying Conditions that Have Potential to Increase Risk of Complications

- Diabetes
- Hypertension
- Chronic obstructive pulmonary disease
- Dementia
- Coronary artery disease
- Alcoholism
- Asthma
- Cancer
- Immunosuppression

Other Common Signs and Symptoms

- Decreased appetite
- Diarrhea
- Myalgia
- Malaise
- Neck stiffness
- Skin rash
- Shortness of breath
- Cough
- Dizziness
- Increased sleepiness
- Balance problems
- Photophobia
- Back pain
- Joint pain (arthralgia)
- Tremor
- Weight loss
- Slurred speech
- Neck pain
- Sore throat
- Seizures
- Blurred vision
- Coma
- Numbness
- Flaccid paralysis
- Lymphadenopathy
- Paresthesias

From Mazurek JM: The epidemiology and early clinical features of West Nile virus infection. *Am J Emerg Med* 23:536-543, 2005.

MEDICAL MANAGEMENT

DIAGNOSIS. Diagnosis usually rests on detection of IgM antibody in serum or CSF. Differential diagnosis of the types of infections of the brain has improved with the use of MRI and polymerase chain reaction to diagnose herpes simplex encephalitis. The electroencephalogram (EEG) will show seizure activity in the temporal lobe in herpes simplex. In general, lumbar puncture is abnormal, with increased proteins. The glucose level, however, may be normal or moderately increased. CT scans do not show much until the damage is extensive. MRI shows cerebral edema and vascular damage earlier in the process and leads to earlier detection.[2] In West Nile virus, lesions can sometimes be seen in the white matter, pons, substantia nigra, and thalamus. An important MRI finding is the focal abnormal signal intensity within the anterior horns; the level of abnormal spinal MRI findings corresponds to the paralysis. Change can be seen in the spinal roots, possibly a result of axonal degeneration secondary to spinal motor neuron loss or Wallerian degeneration in the spinal roots. Figure 29-8 shows the imaging studies of individuals with West Nile virus.

West Nile virus infection begins with nonspecific symptoms, making early clinical diagnosis challenging. Immunoglobulin M (IgM) antibodies against the virus (usually by enzyme-linked immunoassay [ELISA]) are generally indicative of a recent West Nile virus infection. Blood samples that are collected between the 8th and 21st day after onset are likely to give the best yield. IgM antibodies are only detectable 8 days after symptom onset. There may be a negative result from a blood sample obtained before the 8th day after symptom onset. After the 21st day, the titer of IgM could decline. The lymphocyte count, particularly the degree of relative lymphopenia, is a readily available test; the degree of relative lymphopenia (≥10%) appears to have prognostic importance in West Nile encephalitis. Clinicians should maintain a high index of suspicion for West Nile virus infection during the epidemic season, particularly when evaluating the elderly with neurologic or gastrointestinal symptoms.[15,41]

West Nile meningitis and encephalitis have similar degrees of pleocytosis, or multiple cystic lesions. However, West Nile encephalitis tends to create higher concentrations of total protein in the CSF and leads to a more severe outcome. Electrophysiologic studies are helpful for the diagnosis of paralysis induced by West Nile virus. Motor nerve conduction studies may reveal severely reduced amplitudes of compound muscle action potentials in symptomatic limbs. However, if the nerve conduction study is done in the early phase of the illness, compound muscle action potentials can be normal because Wallerian degeneration can take 7 to 10 days to complete. Nerve conduction velocities are usually preserved, and sensory nerve conduction is typically normal. Needle electromyography shows severe denervation in muscles of weak limbs and its corresponding paraspinal muscles. Taken together, these abnormalities in the paralyzed limbs localize the lesions to the anterior horn

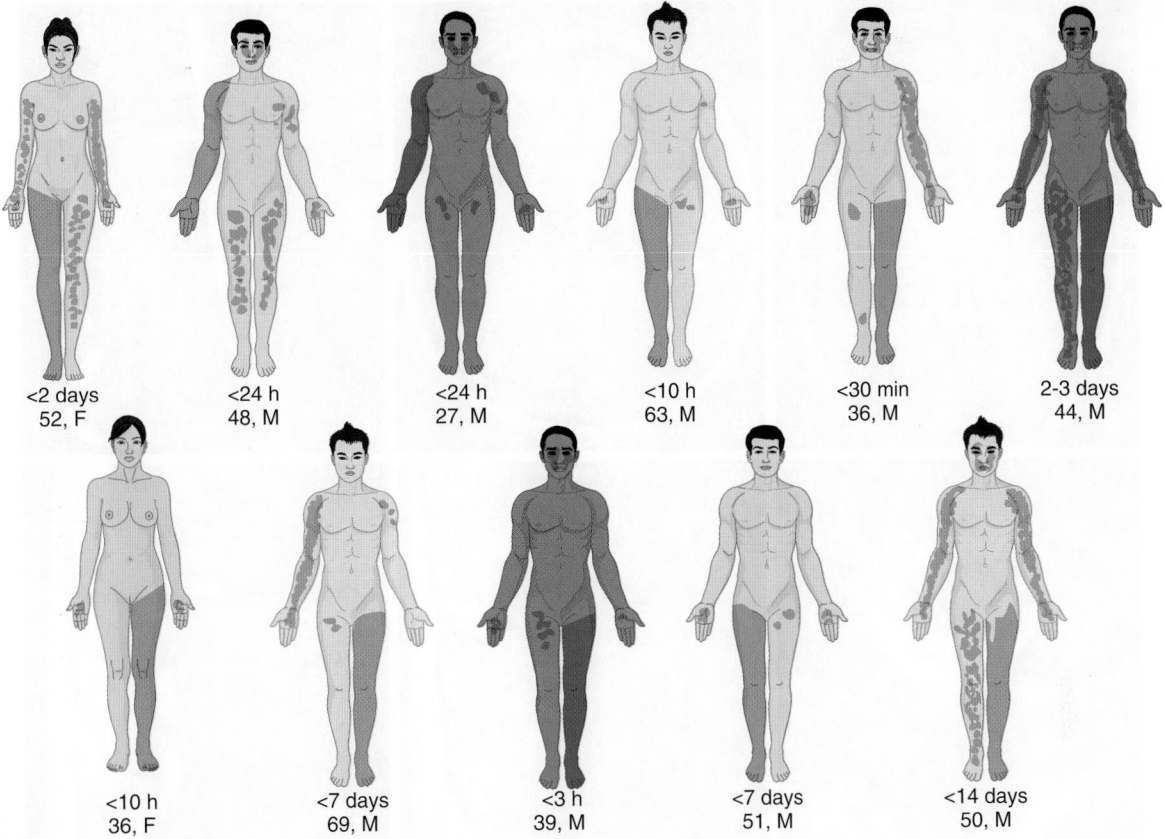

Figure 29-7

Clinical features induced by West Nile virus paralysis in 11 representative individuals. Weak limbs at the peak of paralysis are darkened. Degree of darkness corresponds to the severity of weakness. Duration of weakness, age and sex are noted. (From Kramer LD: West Nile virus, *Lancet Neurol* 6:171-181, 2007.)

motor neurons or their ventral nerve roots. The localization is typically consistent with the MRI findings. Individuals presenting with an otherwise unexplained facial palsy during the summer should be tested not only for neuroborreliosis but also for West Nile virus. West Nile encephalitis may present with cranial nerve abnormalities involving the cranial nerves VI or VII.[16,34]

TREATMENT. Treatment varies with the infectious agent. No antiviral treatment is available for encephalitis except for that caused by the herpes simplex virus. Acyclovir appears to improve the outcome in herpes simplex encephalitis. Close monitoring of the symptoms is critical, especially with the complication of cerebral edema, which may require surgical decompression, hyperventilation, or administration of mannitol. The use of corticosteroids is controversial because of the potential suppression of antibody protection within the CNS. Human vaccines for flavivirus infections are currently available only for yellow fever, Japanese encephalitis, and tick-borne encephalitis.[14] For West Nile virus, treatment is supportive; no licensed human vaccine exists. Prevention uses an integrated pest management approach, which focuses on surveillance, elimination of mosquito breeding sites, and larval and adult mosquito management using pesticides to keep mosquito populations low. During outbreaks or impending outbreaks, emphasis

shifts to aggressive adult mosquito control to reduce the abundance of infected, biting mosquitoes. Pesticide exposure and adverse human health events following adult mosquito control operations for West Nile virus appear negligible.

PROGNOSIS. The prognosis depends on the infectious agent. The rate of recovery can range from 10% to 50% even in individuals who may have been very ill at the onset. Individuals with mumps meningoencephalitis and Venezuelan equine encephalitis have an excellent prognosis. Other encephalitides, such as western equine, St Louis, and California encephalitis and West Nile virus, have a moderate to good rate of survival. Although, with the use of medication, herpes simplex encephalitis has a moderately good outcome (20% mortality), neurologic sequelae are common in 50% of persons.[3,14] Recovery for paralysis is remarkably variable. The variation may be caused by different degrees of motor neuron or motor unit loss.[34]

Some recovery is complete within weeks, but outcome is highly variable. The severity of the original illness does not always predict the final outcome. Prediction of post–West Nile virus poliomyelitis syndrome similar to post-polio syndrome is not yet possible. Permanent cerebral problems are more likely to occur in infants. Young children will take longer to recover than adults with similar

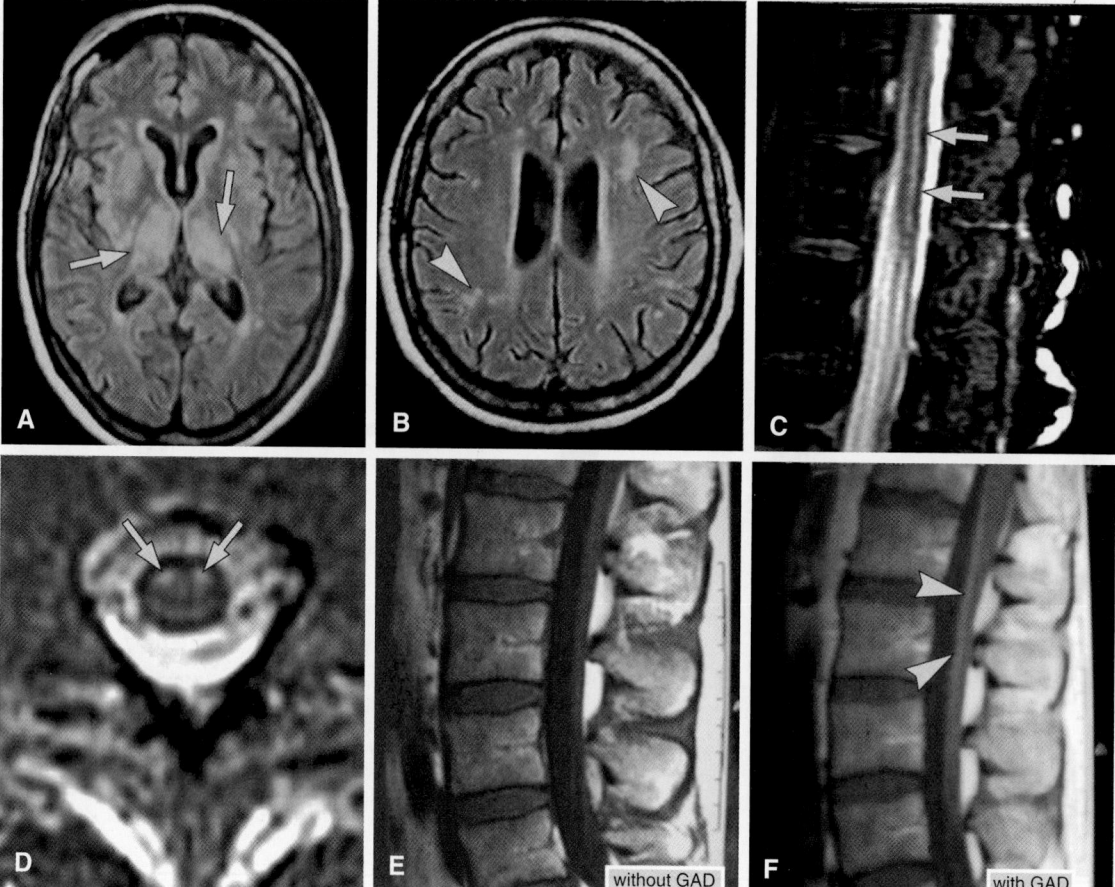

Figure 29-8

Abnormal MRI findings in patients with West Nile virus. A, Image of the brain from a 57-year-old woman with encephalitis shows abnormal signals in bilateral thalamus and weighted MRI in other areas of basal ganglion. **B,** Focal white matter lesions are also seen. **C,** Sagittal T2-weighted MRI of the lumbar spinal cord shows abnormal signal intensity *(arrows)* conspicuous within the cord. **D,** Transverse view of the cord at the midlumbar level; abnormal signal intensity *(arrows)* is confined to the anterior horns. **E,** T1-weighted lumbar spine MRI from a patient with both meningitis and acute flaccid paralysis shows no discernible abnormality; however, after giving gadolinium contrast, spinal roots are significantly enhanced **(F).** (From Kramer LD: West Nile virus, *Lancet Neurol* 6:171-181, 2007; C and D from Li J, Loeb JA, Shy ME, et al: Asymmetric flaccid paralysis: a neuromuscular presentation of West Nile virus infection, *Ann Neurol* 53:703-710, 2003.)

infections. Anti–West Nile virus IgM can persist for 1 year or longer.

Development of West Nile virus vaccines have been explored, including immunization of animals with recombinant viral proteins, inactivated West Nile virus, deoxyribonucleic acid (DNA) that expresses viral antigens, or attenuated West Nile virus isolates.[34]

BRAIN ABSCESS

Definition

Brain abscess is an uncommon disorder accounting for only 2% of intracranial mass lesions. CNS abscesses are circumscribed, enlarging, focal infections that produce symptoms and findings similar to those of other space-occupying lesions such as brain tumors. Brain abscesses, however, often progress more rapidly than tumors and more frequently affect meningeal structures. Brain abscesses occur when microorganisms reach the brain and cause a local infection. There may be only one area of abscess, or many areas may be infected because of spread

by blood-borne pathogens. Although the site and size of the abscess influence the initial symptoms, evidence of increased intracranial pressure is common.[58]

Risk Factors and Pathogenesis

Persons with a compromised immune system receiving steroids, immunosuppressants, or cytotoxic chemotherapy or persons with a systemic illness, such as HIV infection, have an increased risk of developing a brain abscess. Whereas viruses tend to cause diffuse brain infections as described previously, most bacteria, fungi, and other parasites cause localized brain disease. Brain abscesses may develop from other infections in the cranium such as sinusitis or mastoiditis.

Infections leading to brain abscess can come from extracerebral locations; blood-borne metastases; infection from lung or heart; or infections within the cranium such as otitis, cranial osteomyelitis, and sinusitis. Recent or remote head trauma or neurosurgical procedures may be the cause. Blood-borne infections seed the brain and spread and produce abscesses in brain regions in proportion to the blood flow; accordingly, parietal lobe abscesses predominate. Extension of infection from otitis and mastoiditis involves contiguous brain regions of the temporal lobe and cerebellum, whereas abscesses resulting from sinusitis affect the frontal and temporal lobes. Neurologic complications develop in nearly one-third of patients with infective endocarditis, and neurologic manifestations can be the initial symptom. Infective endocarditis should always be considered in a patient with a fever and stroke.[23]

Subdural empyema is an infection in the space between the dura and the arachnoid. It usually results from infected paranasal sinuses and rarely from infected mastoid sinuses by extension of thrombophlebitis from the sinuses into the subdural space. The infection is most commonly unilateral because bilateral spread is prevented by the falx. The empyema may evolve to cause cortical vein thrombosis, cerebral abscesses, or purulent meningitis.

Most brain abscesses evolve over a number of stages, with involvement of the cerebrum occurring during the first 1 to 3 days. Inflammatory infiltrates of polymorphonuclear cells, lymphocytes, and plasma cells follow within 24 hours. By 3 days, the surrounding area shows an increase in perivascular inflammation. The late cerebritis phase develops approximately 4 to 9 days after infection, during which time the center becomes necrotic, containing a mixture of debris and inflammatory cells Early reactive astrocytes surround the zone of infection and proceed to early capsule formation between approximately 10 and 13 days. At this time, the necrotic center shrinks slightly, and a well-developed peripheral fibroblast layer evolves. The late capsule stage continues to evolve between 14 days and 5 weeks, with continual shrinking of the necrotic center and a relative decrease in the inflammatory cells. The capsule thickens with astrocyte scarring.[58]

If the infection is carried in the blood from another site in the body, the abscess will usually develop at the junction of the gray and white matter. Anaerobic bacteria are found in more than one-half of brain abscesses. The infection usually begins as local encephalitis with necrosis and inflammation of the neurons and glial cells. As the process continues, a capsule wall is formed by the proliferation of fibroblasts. There is usually an area of cerebral edema around the abscess. Bacterial and fungal abscesses will continue to grow until they become lethal. Abscesses caused by other parasites are usually self-limiting.[48]

Clinical Manifestations

Normal body temperature is common, and white cell counts are not always high. Neck stiffness is rare in the absence of increased intracranial pressure. Otherwise, the presenting features resemble those of any expanding intracranial mass, like a slow-growing neoplasm, or it may be rapid and progress to possible herniation and brainstem compression, causing death. A headache of recent onset is the most common symptom, representing distortion or irritation of pain-sensitive structures within the cranial vault, especially those of the great venous sinuses

Table 29-1	Manifestations of Brain Abscess
Headache	55%
Disturbed consciousness	48%
Fever	58%
Nuchal rigidity	29%
Nausea, vomiting	32%
Seizures	19%
Visual disturbance	15%
Dysarthria	20%
Hemiparesis	48%
Sepsis	17%

Data from Lu CH, Chang WN, Lin YC, et al: Bacterial brain abscess: microbiological features, epidemiological trends and therapeutic outcomes. Q J Med 2002;95:501-509.

and the dura mater about the base of the brain. If the process continues untreated, isolated headache increases in severity and becomes accompanied by focal signs, such as hemiparesis or aphasia, followed by obtundation and coma. The period of evolution may be as brief as hours or as long as many days to weeks with more indolent organisms. Seizures may occur with abscesses that involve the cortical gray matter.[58] Lethargy and confusion progress with the increased intracranial pressure present with the growing mass. Focal signs reflect the area of the brain that is affected, with paresis resulting from frontal and parietal lesions and visual disturbances noted with occipital lobe dysfunction.[48] Table 29-1 lists typical manifestations of brain abscess.

The most common symptoms of subdural empyema are headache, fever, a neurologic deficit, and a stiff neck. However, subdural empyema may progress and cause signs of raised intracranial pressure, such as vomiting, altered level of consciousness, seizures, and papilledema. A high degree of suspicion is needed to establish the diagnosis early in the course of the illness. In patients with sinusitis, the symptoms of subdural empyema may be incorrectly attributed to the sinusitis.

MEDICAL MANAGEMENT

DIAGNOSIS. A history of infection or immunosuppression will lead to suspicion of abscess rather than neoplasm. Imaging plays an important role in the diagnosis and treatment of brain abscess, pyogenic infection, and encephalitis. MRI can detect early changes, such as brain edema, and is preferable to CT. The area of cerebritis that is seen initially as a low-signal-intensity, ill-defined area later progresses to a central cavity with slightly higher signal intensity than CSF, surrounded by edema that is slightly hypointense in comparison to brain parenchyma. Later stages of infection show central necrosis and formation of a rim of slightly high signal intensity on T1-weighted imaging.[51] Gadolinium administration shows a ring-enhancing lesion. Diffusion-weighted imaging helps differentiate abscesses from brain tumors; an abscess cavity demonstrates high signal with decreased apparent diffusion coefficient values, whereas necrotic tumor cavities demonstrate the opposite.[30] When combined with CSF, serologic studies, and patient history, imaging findings can suggest the cause of encephalitis.[5]

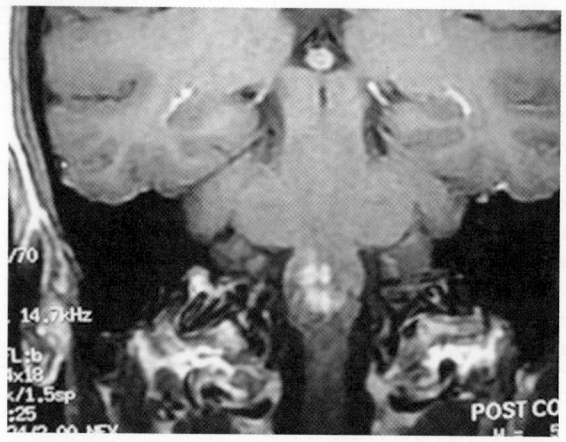

Figure 29-9

Brain stem abscess. MRI with gadolinium shows an enhancing lesion in the brain stem caused by *Listeria* species infection. (From Goldman L, Schafer AI: *Goldman's Cecil medicine*, ed 24, St. Louis, 2011, Saunders.)

Figure 29-9 shows the effect seen on MRI. Although the early signs are similar to those of meningitis, the focal signs of compression in one area of the brain distinguish the abscess over time. The EEG is often abnormal.[28]

TREATMENT. Appropriate and timely antibiotic protocol and surgical drainage is required to reduce the mass effect. Careful clinical observation is necessary with multiple abscesses, and CT scans should be repeated often to determine if the abscess continues to expand. Initially, corticosteroids may be used to control the cerebral edema caused by the abscess, but these are used for a short time only because of their interference with capsule formation and immunosuppressive action in the brain. Treatment of patients with infective endocarditis and cerebral emboli requires prevention of embolization with appropriate antibiotic therapy and sometimes cardiac surgery Anticoagulation is contraindicated in patients with cerebral infarcts and septic emboli because of the high risk for complications from intracerebral bleeding.

Medical treatment alone is not generally advocated, although it may be considered if a patient is too sick to undergo surgical therapy. Medical therapy alone is more likely to be successful if treatment is begun in the cerebritis stage before a capsule forms (generally within 10 days of symptom onset), if the lesions are small (<3 mm), and if patients show definite clinical improvement in the first week. If the location is surgically inaccessible or if the surgical approach would traverse eloquent tissue or the ventricular system; if there is concomitant meningitis or ependymitis; or if the patient has hydrocephalus requiring a shunt that could become infected during the operative procedure, surgery should be avoided. Surgical excision of an abscess can be done only if the abscess is encapsulated (usually after 10 days of symptom onset) but can dramatically reduce the length of antibiotic therapy, down to as short as 2 weeks. If an abscess is larger than 3 cm or if a patient is deteriorating clinically, surgical therapy should be initiated. Two surgical options currently in

use are aspiration and excision. Stereotactic aspiration can be done under local anesthesia if necessary. Because of the limited space in the posterior fossa and the mild clinical deficits associated with removal of cerebellar tissue, cerebellar abscesses should be managed surgically unless the patient cannot tolerate surgery because of excessive bleeding risk. Figure 29-10 shows the process of determining care that might be followed to decide the best clinical action to take.

For supportive therapy, patients need to be hospitalized to initiate IV antibiotics, and a neurosurgeon should be involved in the patient's care. The hemodynamic and respiratory status of the patient may need to be supported. Steroids can be considered in patients who have clinical deterioration due to vasogenic edema surrounding the abscess. The use of steroids is not advocated in all patients because it may reduce the penetration of antibiotics into the abscess, and they may increase the risk of rupture into the ventricle. The use of steroids can slow the reduction of capsule formation and may reduce the amount of contrast enhancement on CT, so when these patients are followed up with CT, it is important to not consider the lessening degree of contrast enhancement as a sign of improvement. Serial CTs (once every week or two) should show decrease in the size of the abscess. If the patient develops seizures, an antiepileptic medication should be started. The role of prophylactic anticonvulsant therapy is controversial, but such therapy is likely not to be of benefit in cerebellar or deep cerebral abscesses.[67]

PROGNOSIS. Mortality from brain abscess can be lowered from 65% to 30% with control of the infection with antibiotics and surgery. Nearly one-half of the clients are left with some neurologic sequelae, which may include focal signs and seizure activity.[58]

Mortality rates in patients with infective endocarditis and cerebral emboli range from 30% to 80%. Mortality is high if there is hemorrhagic transformation of the infarct. Mortality in patients with ruptured mycotic aneurysms is 80%, and even patients with unruptured aneurysms have a mortality rate of 30%.

PRION DISEASE

Definition

Rare forms of encephalopathies include the prion diseases of Creutzfeldt-Jakob disease (CJD), kuru, and bovine spongiform encephalopathy (BSE), also known as mad cow disease. The incubation period is slow and can be up to 5 to 8 years.[13] Classic CJD is a rare, fatal, and degenerative neurologic disease with a long asymptomatic latent period that was first described in 1920. The causative agent of CJD is thought by most experts to be a prion protein (PrPsc), an abnormal conformation of a normal cellular protein (PrPc) that can recruit additional PrPc to PrPsc, resulting in deposition of insoluble precipitates in neural tissue. CJD is one of a variety of prion diseases of humans that occur spontaneously at a rate of approximately 1 per million throughout the world and can be transmitted vertically in familial conditions, such

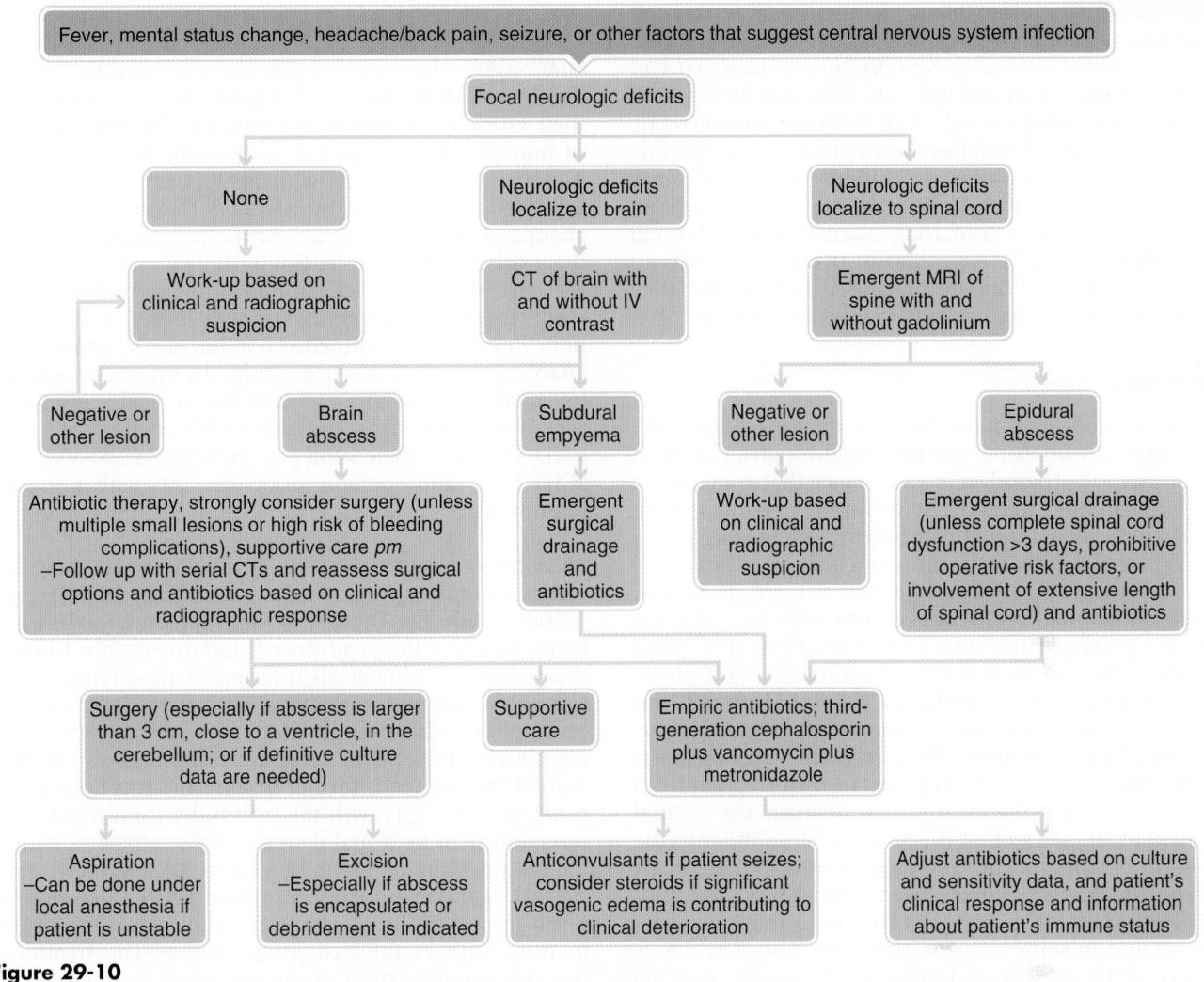

Figure 29-10

Approach to the patient with possible brain abscess or parameningeal infection. (From Brain Abscess and Parameningeal Infection in Johnson: *Current therapy in neurologic disease*, ed 7, St. Louis, 2008, Mosby.)

as Gerstmann-Sträussler-Scheinker syndrome, or through ritualistic cannibalism (kuru).[49]

Like classic CJD, variant CJD (vCJD) is a fatal, degenerative neurologic disease, although it occurs in younger persons and has distinctive clinical, histopathologic, and biochemical features, including the presence of readily detectable prion protein in non–CNS lymphoreticular tissues such as appendix, spleen, tonsil, and lymph nodes. In contrast to classical CJD, vCJD disease is new, first reported in the United Kingdom in 1996. The causative agent of vCJD, a prion, is the same agent that causes BSE. A massive epidemic of BSE occurred in Great Britain in the 1980s and early 1990s as a result of the recycling and processing of material from dead sheep and cattle into food meal for cattle. Although this practice was stopped in the mid-1990s after appreciation of the BSE epidemic, an estimated 250,000 cattle had already been infected with BSE. Transmission of the BSE prions to humans occurred by oral consumption of beef and other cattle products containing reticular endothelial or neural tissue, resulting in a delayed outbreak of vCJD in the United Kingdom.[25]

Incidence and Etiologic and Risk Factors

The annual incidence of all human prion diseases is generally reported to be about 1 case per million individuals. The incidence peaks at nearly 6 cases per million between the ages of 65 and 74 years, and prion disease accounted for about 1 in 8500 deaths in the United States between 1999 and 2008.[12]

The classic forms, sCJD MM1 or sCJD MV1, are by far the most common, accounting for 55% to 70% of sporadic prion diseases. In Italy, the incidence of genetic transmissible spongiform encephalopathy diseases is the second highest among European countries.[24] Infection with BSE-derived or vCJD-derived prions depends on the host's genetic makeup, which means that there could be a substantial number of symptom-free human carriers of these infectious agents. There is now evidence that vCJD prions can be transmitted through blood transfusion and other iatrogenic routes.[6,7]

Iatrogenic transmission has occurred via corneal and dural transplants and depth cerebral electrodes. Hormone therapy using human pituitary products can be a cause.

Transmission of prion disease is also possible through ingesting nervous system products that contain infected material. Eating nervous system products of beef that had been fed rendered protein led to the increased incidence in the United Kingdom in the 1990s.[54] Skeletal muscle tissue from CWD-infected deer has shown prion infectivity, however, the implications of these findings for human beings are unclear. Studies are looking at the role of the PrP encoding gene (PRNP) in conferring susceptibility to human prion diseases.[31] It is very difficult, if not impossible, to predict how prions from one species will behave when they transit species barriers; however, studies are ongoing.[50,61]

Pathogenesis

In the prion formation mechanism, a pathogenic protein is generated from its normal isoform through a change in conformation. The prion is a substance that contains no nucleic acid but can replicate within the nervous system. Prions and other alternatively folded proteins might also be involved in normal cell function, including the formation of biochemical memory at the synapse. Therefore, the term *prion* currently applies not only to a disease-specific pathogen but also to a mechanism that could have a wide and crucial role in pathologic and physiological processes.[49] Similar to oncogenes, mutations of the normal cellular prion protein gene cause disease. Abnormal prion protein differs from oncogene products in that the prion protein programs its own creation from normal cellular proteins and then instructs the normal protein to change so that it is functionally similar to the abnormal protein. The microscopic alterations consist of spongy change in neuropil, neuronal loss, and gliosis. The spongiform change is similar to that seen after anoxia and in some cases of Alzheimer disorders. There appears to be accelerated death of Purkinje cells, resulting in the ataxia that is commonly seen.[20]

Clinical Manifestations

Prion disease occurs most commonly between 50 and 70 years and shows rapidly progressive multidomain cognitive impairment and confusion, occasionally accompanied by cortical visual disturbances, ataxia, and spontaneous or induced myoclonus. It is common to see a gaze that expresses apprehension or fear and shows heightened reactivity to external stimuli. This syndrome is frequently preceded by mild psychiatric symptoms such as malaise, anxiety, mood changes, and diminished ability to concentrate. Extrapyramidal and cerebellar signs occasionally occur at onset, but the neurologic examination can also be unremarkable. Less common presentations include a prominent ataxia eclipsing the cognitive impairment, concomitant epilepsy, and visual deficits such as field defects, distortion, and cortical blindness. Neurologic signs can be unilateral.

Movement progressively becomes abnormal, with dementia that also worsens over time. Sleep-wake symptoms develop with severe sleep EEG abnormalities with loss of sleep spindles, very low sleep efficiency, and virtual absence of rapid eye movement (REM) sleep.[37] Akinetic mutism will eventually develop with overriding myoclonic jerks.

MEDICAL MANAGEMENT

DIAGNOSIS. Human prion diseases present a formidable diagnostic challenge to clinicians, mainly because of their rarity and varied manifestations. The heterogeneity of human prion diseases is attributable not only to the presence of three forms with distinct causes—sporadic, inherited, and acquired by infection. Detection of spongy change alone is not sufficient for the neuropathologic diagnosis of prion disease but must be corroborated with Western blot testing. If familial prion proteinopathy is suspected, molecular genetic analysis of DNA from lymphocytes can be performed.[20] For the practical purpose of enabling a prompt diagnosis, sporadic prion diseases can be separated into three groups: the cognitive subtypes, including sCJD MM1 and sCJD MV1, sCJD MM2, and sCJD VV1; the ataxic subtypes, including sCJD VV2 and sCJD MV2; and sporadic prion diseases with non-CJD phenotypes.[49]

TREATMENT AND PROGNOSIS. Once diagnosed, these disorders are rapidly progressive and eventually fatal. The key barrier to effective therapy is that they present clinically when neuronal loss is advanced, and irreversible. Current treatments are almost all directed at modifying symptoms; few address underlying pathogenic mechanisms and are inevitably delivered too late to rescue dying neurons. A new therapeutic target for prion disease, effective animal studies, lends further insight into mechanisms of prion neurotoxicity with the possibility for a window of reversibility in neuronal damage characterized as neuronal rescue. Using lentivirally mediated RNA interference (RNAi) against native prion protein (PrP) interventions result in prevention of symptoms and increased survival in mice with established prion disease. The treatment prevents the formation of the neurotoxic prion agent at a point when diseased neurons can still be saved from death; however, the target and the timing of the intervention appears to be critical.[27,64,66]

SPECIAL IMPLICATIONS FOR THE THERAPIST 29-1

Infectious Disorders of the Central Nervous System

The therapist must understand and observe all isolation procedures. Often the treatment of these clients begins in the intensive care unit. Monitoring vital signs throughout the treatment session may be necessary when the client is in the acute stage. The client may demonstrate symptoms that are similar to many noninfectious brain disorders. The clinical picture may represent the diffuse disorders typical of brain trauma, or there may be only focal neurologic symptoms that may appear similar to stroke or neoplasm.[53]

Initially, when the inflammatory response is greatest, there may be a profound alteration of consciousness. The therapist should be familiar with the scales used to monitor levels of consciousness such as the Glasgow Coma Scale. The client may be agitated, with difficulty in processing sensory input resulting in increased sensitivity to sound and light. Cognitive and perceptual disorders with memory deficits probably represent the involvement of the brain in the area of the ventricles.[48] It is essential that the therapist understand the behavioral changes that accompany diffuse brain disorders. See Chapter 33 for further details.

Sensory dysfunction should be thoroughly evaluated. If the client has a history of instability of heart rate, blood pressure, or respiration, these should be monitored during the evaluation of sensation, because sensory input may aggravate responses in some individuals. Cutaneous sensation may be affected in different distributions, depending on whether the damage is diffuse or deep in one area of the brain. Distorted or absent sensory input can affect mobility and functional status in a dramatic way. For further description of sensory and motor deficits related to specific areas of damage, see Chapter 32.

Movement disorders also reflect the nature and depth of the insult to the brain. Abnormal posturing of the client in the acute phase may be noted, and abnormal postural reflexes may be present. Decorticate posturing and decerebrate posturing are often seen in the early stages of these brain disorders.[11] Positioning and range-of-motion exercises are critical in the early phases because the stiffness of the back and neck can exacerbate the pain. Often, maintaining a darkened environment during treatment will decrease the complaints of headache. Understanding motor learning strategies is important, because movement often must be relearned in the context of residual damage or agitated behaviors (see "Special Implications for the Therapist 28-1: Motor Learning Strategies" in Chapter 28).

When interacting with the client and family, it is important to be familiar with the acute, subacute, and chronic prognosis related to the type of infection causing the brain injury. Knowing there may be a good outcome will be encouraging during the acute and devastating onset of the infections. Neurologic recovery will continue for many years if the brain remains stimulated as a course of appropriate physical rehabilitation.[48]

During the late summer season, the therapist should be aware of the manifestations of mosquito-or tick-borne illnesses. Changes in clients that are consistent with infections should be monitored and a referral made to the appropriate health care provider when necessary.

A THERAPIST'S THOUGHTS*

"Until the therapist determines that the vital functions, such as rate of respiration, heart rate, and blood pressure vary appropriately with the demands of the intervention; these factors should be monitored."

*Judith A. Dewane, PT, Dsc, NCS

REFERENCES

To enhance this text and add value for the reader, all references are included on the companion Evolve site that accompanies this textbook. The reader can view the reference source and access it online whenever possible.

CHAPTER 30

Central Nervous System Neoplasms

STEPHEN A. GUDAS

INTRODUCTION

Several categories of neoplasia affect the central nervous system (CNS). *Primary* tumors, which may be either benign or malignant, may develop in the brain, spinal cord, or surrounding structures. Secondary, or *metastatic,* tumors may spread to the CNS from another site, such as the lung or breast. *Paraneoplastic syndromes* may occur because of remote or indirect effects on the CNS from cancer elsewhere in the body. Additionally, and less commonly, *leptomeningeal carcinomatosis* may occur, in which carcinoma metastasizes to the pia mater and arachnoid with multiple lesions to the meninges and cerebrospinal fluid (CSF) pathways of the brain and/or spinal cord.

The presence of any CNS tumor is cause for concern because of the vital functions of the brain and spinal cord. The critical areas and confined spaces in the CNS make it vulnerable to a space-occupying lesion. Most primary malignant CNS tumors are locally invasive and cause significant morbidity and mortality.[88]

The early effects of a CNS tumor are related to mechanical displacement of brain or spinal cord tissue, or a mild block in CSF circulation, causing increased intracranial pressure (ICP). As a tumor grows, compression or destruction of local brain or nerve tissue may occur, resulting in specific neurologic deficits. Symptoms of brain tumors may range from minimal, such as mild lethargy, to marked, such as seizures, blindness, and paralysis, as the tumor progresses. Likewise, symptoms of spinal cord tumors may range from mild to severe and include pain, sensory impairments, weakness, and paralysis. Although primary CNS tumors typically do not metastasize outside the CNS because of the lack of a CNS lymphatic system to transport cancer cells, some tumors, such as medulloblastoma may infrequently travel through the CSF to the spinal cord as "drop metastasis" and cause spinal cord complications. Hematogenous dissemination of a primary brain tumor to a site outside the skull does not usually occur.

The diagnosis of a CNS tumor with its threat of significant loss of neurologic and cognitive function is devastating to the client and family. A CNS tumor robs a person of independence and dignity, and is viewed as a humiliating and inextricably fatal process.[80] Difficult decisions about treatment options and quality-of-life issues add stress for the client and family. In children with brain tumors, the diagnosis creates parental fear and emotional upheaval, and requires adjusting and decision making for the different needs at varying stages of the illness.[45] Caregiving and financial struggles frequently are encountered with both brain and spinal cord tumors.

Despite the inescapable realities of these difficult issues, the situation is improving, with dramatic new advances in radiologic imaging, neurosurgery, and adjuvant therapy. At present, including those with both benign and malignant tumors, approximately 50% of patients with CNS tumors can be successfully treated and have an excellent long-term prognosis.[143] A knowledge and awareness of current treatment advances provide the health professional with the information and skills to care for the client and family in a sensitive, compassionate, and hopeful but realistic manner.

Classification

The major purpose of tumor classification is to facilitate communication about tumor behavior and treatment, and to design studies to learn more about the tumors.[160] Primary brain tumors are classified by light microscopy according to their predominant cell type.[148] The World Health Organization (WHO) classification system, which incorporates the Ringerz system for astrocytomas, is becoming the most commonly accepted system, making it easier for clinicians to accurately compare the effects of treatment.[17,33,101,148] It is a three-tiered system, based on neuroembryonal origin, that is, naming a tumor by the most likely cell of origin, and adding qualifying phrases to describe its behavior.[160]

Table 30-1 provides the WHO classification of primary tumors. The grading, from I to IV, indicates the aggressiveness of the tumor, with grade IV being the most aggressive. The St. Anne–Mayo (Daumas-Duport)[116] system is another classification system in use. It is four tiered, based on the presence or absence of four major criteria (nuclear atypia, mitoses [cells in a state of division], endothelial proliferation, and necrosis), with grade I having none of these features, grade II having one, etc. Various other systems exist, based on a number of distinguishing criteria: neuroembryonal origin, primary versus secondary, benign versus malignant, histologic grade, anatomic

Table 30-1	World Health Organization Classification of Primary Brain Tumors According to Histology*	
Most Common Tumors		**Grade (WHO)**
Astrocytic Tumors		
Pilocytic		I
Astrocytoma (diffuse, infiltrative, fibrillary)		II
Anaplastic		III
Glioblastoma multiforme		IV
Oligodendroglial Tumors and Mixed Gliomas		
Oligodendroglioma, well differentiated		II
Anaplastic oligodendroglioma		III
Mixed oligodendroglioma/astrocytoma*		II
Mixed anaplastic oligodendroglioma/anaplastic astrocytoma*		III
Ependymal Tumors		
Myxopapillary ependymoma		I
Ependymoma		II
Anaplastic		III
Choroid Plexus Tumors		
Choroid plexus papilloma		I
Choroid plexus carcinoma		III
Neuronal and Mixed Neuronal-Glial Tumors		
Ganglioglioma		I-II
Central neurocytoma		II
Filum terminale paraganglioma		I
Dysembryoplastic neuroepithelial tumor (DNET)		I
Pineal Parenchymal Tumors		
Pineocytoma		II
Pineoblastoma		IV
Embryonal Tumors		
Medulloblastoma		IV
Supratentorial primitive neuroectodermal tumor (PNET)		IV
Atypical teratoid/rhabdoid tumor		IV
Meningeal Tumors		
Meningioma		I
Atypical, clear cell, choroid		II
Rhabdoid, papillary, or anaplastic (malignant)		III
Pituitary Tumors		
Adenomas		I
Carcinomas		II
Tumors of Cranial and Spinal Nerves		
Neurinomas (schwannomas) (acoustic neuromas)		I-II

*Mixed tumors that consist of oligodendroglioma/anaplastic astrocytoma or anaplastic oligodendroglioma/astrocytoma are usually graded according to the highest grade component, although there is no consensus from the WHO on the issue.

Adapted from UpToDate, Schiff D, Batchelor T. Classification of brain tumors. Available at http://uptodateonline.com. Accessed September 25, 2006; and Kleihues P, Cavenee, WK, editors: *Data from pathology and genetics—tumors of the nervous system*, Lyon, France, 2000, International Agency for Research on Cancer.

location, and childhood versus adult tumors. The multiplicity of grading systems has been confusing, making it difficult for clinicians to accurately compare the effects of treatment,[116] so the acceptance of one system will be beneficial.

Primary brain tumors originate from the various cells and structures normally found within the brain. Secondary or metastatic brain tumors originate from structures outside the brain, most often from primary tumors of the lungs, breast, gastrointestinal tract, or genitourinary tract,[58] or from melanoma.[153]

Primary CNS tumors also may be subdivided into *malignant* tumors, such as astrocytomas, and so-called *benign tumors*, such as meningiomas, neurinomas, and hemangioblastomas. A histologically benign tumor has a slow growth rate and is relatively noninvasive. However, because of space-occupying properties in vital tissue with a resultant high threat of functional limitation, the use of the term *benign* is somewhat misleading. Some authors insist that because of location even a very slow-growing CNS tumor should be considered basically malignant.[44,148] The histologically benign tumor may be surgically inaccessible or located in a vital area, such as the pons or medulla, and will continue to grow, thereby causing an increase in ICP, neurologic deficits, herniation syndromes, and, finally, death.

Malignant CNS tumors typically have a high growth rate and are invasive and infiltrative. They are capable of modulating the surrounding extracellular matrix by secretion of substances that allow for invasion of surrounding tissue by the tumor cells.[116] Tumors also have the ability to create new blood vessels to sustain the tumor, a process called *angiogenesis*.

Anatomic brain tumor location refers to the location of the lesion in reference to the tentorium or cerebral tissue. Knowing the anatomic location helps to predict probable deficits based on the function of that particular area in the brain. Box 30-1 lists the anatomic location of the most common CNS tumors.

There are other typically recognized subdivisions. There are two main groups of primary tumors in the brain: *gliomas*, the most common type, which includes astrocytomas and glioblastomas, and tumors arising from supporting structures, such as meningiomas, neurinomas, and pituitary adenomas. A third group arising from embryonal undifferentiated nerve cells has been termed *primitive neuroectodermal tumors (PNETs)*[53] and arise more frequently in children. Examples of primary tumors in the spinal cord include the more common neurinomas (schwannomas or neurilemomas) and the less frequent gliomas and meningiomas.

Further subgroups of gliomas have been established based on cellular atypism, the presence of mitotic figures, the incidence of endothelial hyperplasia, and the presence of necrotic areas. It is hoped that newer techniques of molecular biology, such as the ability to identify growth factors and inhibitors necessary for cell growth and differentiation, may lead to a more sophisticated subclassification. Molecular and genetic signatures may predict brain tumor behavior and may soon guide not only tumor classification and diagnosis but also tumor-specific treatment strategies.[40]

ANATOMICAL SITES OF THE MOST COMMON CENTRAL NERVOUS SYSTEM TUMORS

Supratentorial Tumors
- Cerebral hemispheres
  - Metastases
  - Meningiomas
  - Gliomas (malignant gliomas: anaplastic astrocytoma and glioblastoma multiforme, astrocytoma, oligodendroglioma)

Midline Tumors
- Pituitary adenomas
- Pineal tumors
- Craniopharyngiomas

Infratentorial Tumors
- Adults
  - Acoustic schwannomas (neurinomas, neurilemomas)
  - Metastases
  - Meningiomas
  - Hemangioblastomas
- Children
  - Cerebellar astrocytomas
  - Medulloblastomas
  - Ependymomas
  - Brainstem gliomas

Spinal Cord Tumors
- Extradural
  - Metastases
- Intradural
  - Extramedullary
  Meningiomas
  Schwannomas, neurofibromas
  - Intramedullary
  Ependymomas
  Astrocytomas

Adapted from Weiss HD: Neoplasms. In Samuels MA, editor: *Manual of neurologic therapeutics*, ed 5, Boston, 1995, Little, Brown, p. 225.

Because the clinical presentation, treatment, and prognosis are heavily dependent on the location of involvement and whether the tumor is primary or metastatic, this discussion is divided into four parts: (1) primary brain tumors, (2) primary intraspinal tumors, (3) metastatic tumors, and (4) childhood brain tumors.

PRIMARY BRAIN TUMORS

Incidence and Prevalence

Tumors of the CNS are not uncommon. The National Cancer Institute projected that 24,620 new *malignant primary* tumors of the brain and nervous system would be diagnosed in 2013 in the United States.[3] The National Cancer Institute Surveillance, Epidemiology, and End Results (SEER) data indicate that in 2010 there were approximately 141,553 people alive who had had a history of CNS cancer. The mean age at diagnosis of brain and nervous system cancer is 57 years of age. The overall 5-year relative survival rate for 2003–2009 was reported to be 33.5%. Estimates are that 23,130 new cases (12,770 men and 10,360 women) of brain and nervous system cancer would occur and that 14,080 men and women would die from these cancers in 2013.[2,149]

Benign primary brain tumors add to the total incidence. The American Brain Tumor Association reported a combined estimate of 69,720 new primary malignant and benign brain tumors in 2013, the most recent estimate available,[3,4] or 14 per 100,000 U.S. population. The number of people living with either a benign or malignant brain tumor (prevalence) in the United States in 2013 was estimated to be approximately 350,000 to 400,000.[3] Of brain tumor survivors, approximately 75% have a diagnosis of benign tumors, approximately 23% have malignant tumors, and 2% have tumors of uncertain behavior.

Although malignant brain tumors accounted for a small percentage of the approximately 1.5 million new cases of *all* types of cancer, brain tumors kill more Americans each year than multiple sclerosis and Hodgkin disease combined.[133] For all the intracranial diseases, death from intracranial neoplasms is second only to stroke.[53] Approximately 12,820 deaths each year in the United States are caused by primary brain and nervous system tumors.[4] The incidence of primary brain and nervous system tumors peaks in the pediatric population, then increases by approximately 1.2% per year until it plateaus in the population older than 70 years of age.[116] Primary brain tumors are the second most common form of cancer in children,[11,97] and primary CNS tumors are the second leading cause of death from cancer in children. Gliomas account for approximately 50% of CNS tumors. The average age of onset for all primary brain tumors is 53 years.[115] Table 30-2 summarizes the frequency of primary CNS tumors.

More than 60% of tumors in adults are supratentorial, or located in the cerebral hemispheres, above the tentorium. The tentorium is a flap of meninges separating the cerebral hemispheres from the posterior fossa structures. The majority of pediatric tumors are infratentorial, involving primarily the cerebellum and brainstem.[29] Certain tumor types have a predilection for specific areas of the brain, although they may arise elsewhere in the brain. Figure 30-1 illustrates the topologic distribution and preferred sites of primary CNS tumors.

Pathogenesis

Brain tumors affect the brain through compression of cerebral tissue, including brain substance and cranial nerves; invasion or infiltration of cerebral tissue; and sometimes erosion of bone.[58] These mechanisms precipitate pathophysiologic changes such as cerebral edema and increased ICP.

In most brain tumors, vasogenic edema develops in the surrounding tissue of the tumor because of compression and obstruction of CSF pathways, moving CSF across ventricular walls.[53] Substances released from tumor cells altering the blood-brain barrier also may cause rapid cerebral edema. Increased permeability of the capillary endothelial cells of the white matter impairs cellular activity and causes electrochemical instability, resulting in seizures. As the edema continues to develop, signs and symptoms of increased ICP become more apparent.

Table 30-2 | Frequency of Primary Central Nervous System Tumors

CHILDREN (AGE 0–14 YEARS)		ADULTS (AGE ≥15 YEARS)	
Type	**Percentage**	**Type**	**Percentage**
Glioblastoma	20	Glioblastoma	50
Astrocytoma	21	Astrocytoma	10
Ependymoma	7	Ependymoma	2
Oligodendroglioma	1	Oligodendroglioma	3
Medulloblastoma	24	Medulloblastoma	2
Neuroblastoma	3	Pituitary adenoma	4
Neurinoma	1	Neurinoma	2
Craniopharyngioma	5	Craniopharyngioma	1
Meningioma	5	Meningioma	17
Teratoma	2		
Pinealoma	2	Pinealoma	1
Hemangioma	3	Hemangioma	2
Sarcoma	1	Sarcoma	1
Others	5	Others	5
Total	100	Total	100

Adapted from Janus TJ, Yung WKA: Primary neurological tumors, In Goetz C, editor: *Textbook of clinical neurology*, ed 2, Philadelphia, 2003, WB Saunders.

Initially, the brain may have a surprising tolerance to the compressive and infiltrative effects of brain tumors, particularly with slow growing tumors, and early symptoms may be few. Compensatory mechanisms to accommodate the edema and maintain normal ICP are limited. When the brain can no longer compensate, the resultant increase in ICP leads to more evident signs and symptoms. Intracranial herniation and herniation through the foramen magnum are potential results of serious ICP elevation. Figure 30-2 illustrates intracranial herniation syndromes evoked by supratentorial masses.

Clinical Manifestations

The particular clinical presentation of a brain tumor depends on the compression or infiltration of specific cerebral tissue, the related cerebral edema, and the development of increased ICP.[58] Cerebral edema surrounding the tumor results from the inflammatory response of tissues to the tumor and contributes to the increase in ICP. Box 30-2 lists common signs and symptoms of brain tumors.

The initial clinical signs of an intracranial tumor are related to the generalized effect of an increase in ICP. Headache is commonly present (in one-third to one-half of cases), is typically generalized or retroorbital, and is typically worse in the morning and better later in the day. The headache is intensified or precipitated by any activity that tends to raise the ICP, such as stooping, straining, coughing, or exercising. Irritation, compression, or traction of pain-sensitive structures such as the dura mater and blood vessels causes the headache.[119] Although tension-type headache is more common, migraine-type and other types may be exhibited.[154] The sixth cranial nerve (abducens) is highly susceptible to elevated ICP because of its local anatomic relationships as the basis pontis slips caudally during transtentorial herniation, not,

Box 30-2

SIGNS AND SYMPTOMS OF BRAIN TUMORS

- Headache
- Visual changes (double vision, blurred vision)
- Nausea
- Vomiting
- Cognitive changes—impairment of memory, judgment, personality
- Lethargy
- Behavioral changes
- Seizures
- Syncope
- Weakness
- Hemiparesis, hemiplegia
- Apraxia
- Cortical sensory deficits (graphesthesia, stereognosis difficulties)
- Sensory impairments (tingling, spatial orientation changes)
- Cranial nerve palsies
- Aphasia
- Facial numbness
- Hearing disturbances
- Anosmia
- Swallowing difficulties
- Paralysis of outward gaze (sixth cranial nerve)
- Papilledema
- Incoordination
- Ataxia
- In children, diastases of cranial sutures and enlarging head size

as previously believed, because of its long intracranial path.[55] This causes weakness in the lateral rectus muscle and diplopia. Nausea and vomiting are common, often caused by increased ICP. In glioblastoma multiforme (GBM), about one third of patients suffer nausea and vomiting. Box 30-3 lists signs and symptoms of intracranial hypertension.

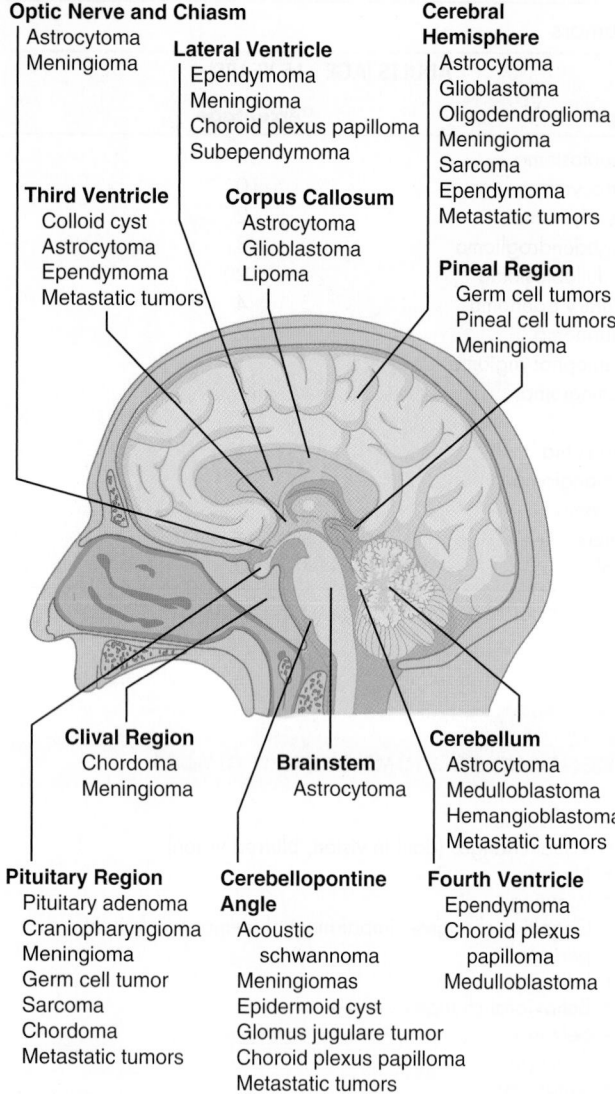

Optic Nerve and Chiasm
Astrocytoma
Meningioma

Lateral Ventricle
Ependymoma
Meningioma
Choroid plexus papilloma
Subependymoma

Cerebral Hemisphere
Astrocytoma
Glioblastoma
Oligodendroglioma
Meningioma
Sarcoma
Ependymoma
Metastatic tumors

Third Ventricle
Colloid cyst
Astrocytoma
Ependymoma
Metastatic tumors

Corpus Callosum
Astrocytoma
Glioblastoma
Lipoma

Pineal Region
Germ cell tumors
Pineal cell tumors
Meningioma

Clival Region
Chordoma
Meningioma

Brainstem
Astrocytoma

Cerebellum
Astrocytoma
Medulloblastoma
Hemangioblastoma
Metastatic tumors

Pituitary Region
Pituitary adenoma
Craniopharyngioma
Meningioma
Germ cell tumor
Sarcoma
Chordoma
Metastatic tumors

Cerebellopontine Angle
Acoustic schwannoma
Meningiomas
Epidermoid cyst
Glomus jugulare tumor
Choroid plexus papilloma
Metastatic tumors

Fourth Ventricle
Ependymoma
Choroid plexus papilloma
Medulloblastoma

Figure 30-1

Topologic distribution and preferred sites of primary central nervous system tumors. (Adapted from Burger PC, Schneithauer BW, Vogel FS: *Surgical pathology of the nervous system and its coverings*, ed 3, New York, 1991, Churchill Livingstone.)

Other common initial signs are mental clouding, lethargy, alterations in consciousness and cognition, syncope (fainting), and easy fatigability. Behavioral changes may include irritability, flat affect, emotional lability, and lack of initiative and spontaneity. Increasing intracranial CSF pressure may precipitate an increase in perioptic pressure, which, in turn, impedes venous drainage from the optic head area and retina, causing papilledema, or edema of the optic disc. Papilledema, present in approximately 70% to 75% of patients with brain tumors, is associated with visual changes, such as decreased visual acuity, an enlarged blind spot, diplopia, and deficits in the visual fields. Often deterioration in vision may be the precipitating factor in the patient's seeking an appointment with an optometrist or ophthalmologist. A dilated ophthalmologic examination showing papilledema is fairly crucial to the diagnosis when it is not straightforward.

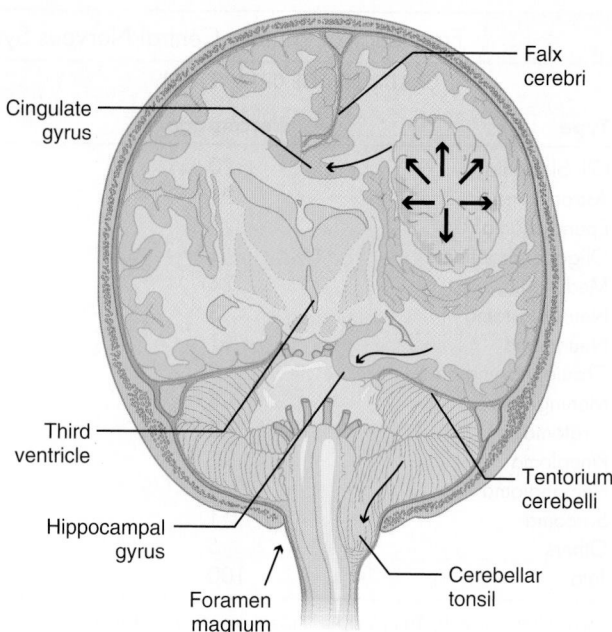

Cingulate gyrus

Falx cerebri

Third ventricle

Hippocampal gyrus

Foramen magnum

Tentorium cerebelli

Cerebellar tonsil

Figure 30-2

Intracranial herniation syndromes evoked by supratentorial masses. The tumor and its edema *(arrows)* have produced the following *(curved arrows)*: cingulated gyrus herniation under the falx cerebri; diencephalic herniation across the midline compressing the ipsilateral ventricle and producing hydrocephalus in the contralateral ventricle; hippocampal gyrus herniation through the tentorial notch compressing the posterior cerebral artery and brainstem; and herniation of the cerebellar tonsils through the foramen magnum. (From Abeloff MD, Armitage JO, Niederhuber JE, et al: *Clinical oncology*, ed 3, Philadelphia, 2004, Churchill Livingstone; and adapted from Plum F, Posner JB: *The diagnosis of stupor and coma*, ed 2, Philadelphia, 1980, FA Davis.)

Approximately 20% to 50% of adults with brain tumors develop seizure activity.[24] The cerebral edema causes hyperactive cells, which produce abnormal, paroxysmal discharges or seizure activity.[121] Seizures may be the first presenting sign of a tumor. In patients presenting with seizures, detection of low-grade gliomas is becoming increasingly frequent with magnetic resonance imaging (MRI). Figure 30-3 is an MRI scan of a low-grade glioma presenting with a seizure. In the later stages of illness, seizure activity is present in 70% of patients.[107] A common feature of a tumor-related seizure is its repetitive nature, with seizures being very stereotypical in a given patient.[154]

As the tumor grows, causing progressive destruction or dysfunction of tissue, locally referable signs may occur (hemiparesis, specific cranial nerve dysfunction, aphasia, visual symptoms, ataxia), which may help to localize the tumor site. Table 30-3 provides a list of signs associated with localized brain lesions.

SPECIFIC PRIMARY BRAIN TUMORS

A wide variety of specific types of primary brain tumor exist, with similarities in medical management and implications for physical therapy. Therefore, the specific tumors are first presented individually, followed by a discussion of diagnosis, medical management, and therapy implications for all primary brain tumors.

Box 30-3

SIGN AND SYMPTOMS OF INTRACRANIAL HYPERTENSION

Common

- Headache
- Tinnitus
- Vomiting (with or without nausea)
- Visual obscurations, visual loss, photopsias
- Papilledema
- Diplopia
- Lethargy and increased sleep
- Psychomotor retardation
- Pain on eye movement

Less Common

- Hearing distortion or loss
- Vertigo
- Facial weakness
- Shoulder or arm pain
- Neck pain or rigidity
- Ataxia
- Paresthesias of extremities
- Anosmia
- Trigeminal neuralgia

Adapted from DeAngelis LM: Tumors of the central nervous system. In Goldman LM, Ausiello D, eds: *Cecil textbook of medicine,* ed 22, Philadelphia, 2004, WB Saunders.

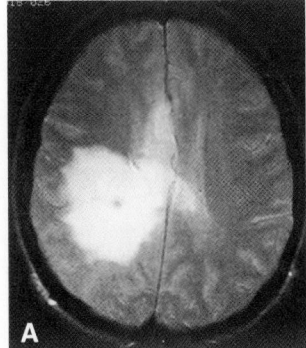 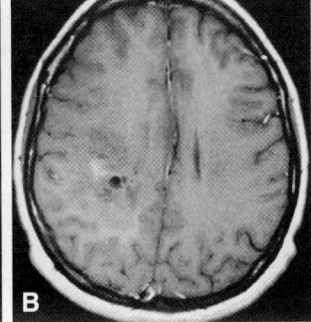

Figure 30-3

MRI of a low-grade glioma. A, T2-weighted image. **B,** T1-weighted image, gadolinium contrast with minimum enhancement. The images are typical of this tumor, which is being detected with increasing frequency by MRI in seizure patients. Many are invisible on computed tomographic scans. (From Goldman LM, Ausiello D, eds: *Cecil textbook of medicine,* ed 22, Philadelphia, 2004, WB Saunders.)

Gliomas

Overview and Incidence

Gliomas are the most common of the primary brain tumors, accounting for 30% to 40% of all brain tumors, with men more frequently affected than women in a 3:2 ratio.[3] Gliomas are divided into *benign* or *low-grade gliomas,* such as the low-grade astrocytomas, and *malignant gliomas,* such as anaplastic astrocytomas and GBMs. Other gliomas are oligodendrogliomas, ependymomas, and medulloblastomas. Terms such as *brainstem glioma* and *optic nerve glioma* refer to the location of these tumors. Only a tissue sample will give the specific diagnosis.

Low-grade astrocytomas account for 7% to 10% of primary brain tumors[1,3] and are the most common type of intracranial tumor in children. Malignant astrocytomas (anaplastic astrocytoma and GBM) are much more common in adults than low-grade astrocytomas, making up 20% to 30% of primary brain tumors. Oligodendrogliomas and ependymomas make up another 5% to 7%. Medulloblastomas, sometimes termed *embryonal tumors* or *PNETs,* make up approximately 1% of primary brain tumors. Brainstem gliomas often affect children between 5 and 10 years of age but can also be found in adults between 30 and 40 years of age. Most optic gliomas occur in children younger than age 10 years. Table 30-4 lists the types of primary brain tumors, the cell of origin, and the distribution of primary CNS tumors by histologic type. The age of peak incidence is 45 to 55 years in adults, and 2 to 10 years in children.[157]

Gliomas are tumors of the glial cells, the group of cells that support, insulate, and metabolically assist the neurons. Glial cells are derived from glioblasts. It is of interest to note that neurons, despite their prevalence in the CNS (100 billion in the adult brain, according to some authors), are rarely the cellular basis of neoplastic transformation.

Glial cells, which numerically exceed the number of neurons, are subdivided into astrocytes (star-shaped cells, sometimes termed *long arms*), which provide nutrition for neurons; oligodendrocytes (glial cells with few processes, sometimes termed *short arms*), which produce the myelin sheath of the axonal projections of neurons; and ependymal cells, which line the ventricles and produce cerebral spinal fluid.[58] Gliomas are subdivided into *astrocytomas, oligodendrogliomas,* and *ependymomas,* named for the cell of origin of the tumor. A combination glial cell tumor may occur as well, such as an oligoastrocytoma. *Medulloblastomas* are tumors of the vermis of the cerebellum and are classified by some authors as gliomas and by some as PNETs or embryonal tumors. Medulloblastoma is grouped with the PNETs because of common features, but some pathologists and clinicians prefer to distinguish these two; currently the debate continues.[115]

Astrocytomas are given histologic grades of I through IV to indicate the rate of cell division (mitosis), nuclear atypia, endothelial proliferation, and necrosis. Grades I and II astrocytomas are the slowest-growing, and grades III and IV astrocytomas are progressively faster growing with higher rates of mitosis.[111] Astrocytomas are capable at any time of converting to a higher grade.[104] Refer to Table 30-1. (See "Grading of Tumors" in Chapter 9.)

Etiologic and Risk Factors

Relatively little is known about the cause of gliomas. They are characterized by a significant genetic heterogeneity, which makes the basic biology of glial neoplasms difficult to understand. A relationship may exist with chromosome abnormalities. Advances in the fields of molecular biology have allowed identification of mutated genes that increase the cell's susceptibility to the development of certain cancers.[104] These mutated genes that lead to the development of cancer are known as *oncogenes* (see Chapter 9).[116] Another type of chromosome abnormality leads to deletion of the cell's defense mechanism or its normal

Table 30-3 Signs Associated with Localized Brain Lesions

Location of Lesion	Associated Signs
Prefrontal area	Loss of judgment, failure of memory, inappropriate behavior, apathy, poor attention span, easily distracted, release phenomena
Frontal eye fields	Failure to sustain gaze to opposite side, saccadic eye movements, impersistence, seizures with forced deviation of the eyes to the opposite side
Precentral gyrus	Partial motor seizures, jacksonian seizures, generalized seizures, hemiparesis
Superficial parietal lobe	Partial sensory seizures, loss of cortical sensation including two–point discrimination, tactile localization, stereognosis and graphism
Angular gyrus	Agraphia, acalculia, finger agnosia, allochiria (right–left confusion) (Gerstmann syndrome)
Broca area	Motor dysphasia
Superior temporal gyrus	Receptive dysphasia
Midbrain	Early hydrocephalus; loss of upward gaze; pupillary abnormalities; 3rd nerve involvement–ptosis, external strabismus, diplopia; ipsilateral cerebellar signs; contralateral hemiparesis; parkinsonism; akinetic mutism
Cerebellar hemisphere	Ipsilateral cerebellar ataxia with hypotonia, dysmetria, intention tremor, nystagmus to side of lesion
Pons	Sixth nerve involvement–diplopia, internal strabismus; seventh nerve involvement–ipsilateral facial paralysis; contralateral hemiparesis; contralateral hemisensory loss; ipsilateral cerebellar ataxia; locked-in syndrome
Medial surface of frontal lobe	Apraxia of gait, urinary incontinence
Corpus callosum	Left-hand apraxia and agraphia, generalized tonic–clonic seizures
Thalamus	Contralateral thalamic pain, contralateral hemisensory loss
Temporal lobe	Partial complex seizures, contralateral homonymous upper quadrantanopsia
Paracentral lobule	Progressive spastic paraparesis, urgency of micturition, incontinence
Deep parietal lobe	Autotopagnosia, anosognosia, contralateral homonymous lower quadrantanopsia
Third ventricle	Paroxysmal headache, hydrocephalus
Fourth ventricle	Hydrocephalus, progressive cerebellar ataxia, progressive spastic hemiparesis or quadriparesis
Cerebellopontine angle	Hearing loss, tinnitus, cerebellar ataxia, facial pain, facial weakness, dysphagia, dysarthria
Olfactory groove	Ipsilateral anosmia, ipsilateral optic atrophy, contralateral papilledema (Foster–Kennedy syndrome)
Optic chiasm	Incongruous bitemporal field defects, bitemporal hemianopsia, optic atrophy
Orbital surface frontal lobe	Partial complex seizures, paroxysmal atrial tachycardia
Optic nerve	Visual failure of one eye, optic atrophy
Uncus	Partial complex seizures with olfactory hallucinations (uncinate fits)
Basal ganglia	Contralateral choreoathetosis, contralateral dystonia
Internal capsule	Contralateral hemiplegia, hemisensory loss, and homonymous hemianopsia
Pineal gland	Loss of upward gaze (Parinaud syndrome), early hydrocephalus, lid retraction, pupillary abnormalities
Occipital lobe	Partial seizures with elementary visual phenomena, homonymous hemianopsia with macular sparing
Hypothalamus, pituitary	Precocious puberty (children), impotence, amenorrhea, galactorrhea, hypothyroidism, hypopituitarism, diabetes insipidus, cachexia, diencephalic autonomic seizures

From Gilroy J: *Basic neurology*, ed 2, Elmsford, NY, 1990, Pergamon Press, pp. 228–229.

tumor-suppressing activity. This tumor suppressor gene, when altered, is unable to inhibit or limited in its normal ability to inhibit cellular proliferation.[116] The presence of an oncogene and/or the absence of a tumor-suppressor gene may be only one step toward tumor formation. Tumorigenesis is thought to be a multistep process, with other contributing factors in addition to chromosome abnormalities.[23]

Certain specific chromosome abnormalities have been linked to specific brain tumor types.[133] The oncogene *c-sis* has been identified with GBM. The oncogene *C-erb*B has been identified in 30% of malignant gliomas and is associated with the transforming growth factor receptor. Chromosome 17 abnormalities are present in all grades of astrocytomas.[133] Oncogenes may have some bearing on other genetic disorders associated with brain tumors. Neurofibromatosis, or von Recklinghausen disease (a familial condition involving the nervous system, muscles, bones, and skin and characterized by multiple soft tumors over the entire body associated with areas of pigmentation), is associated with spinal neuromas, acoustic neuromas, meningiomas, and gliomas. Tuberous sclerosis is associated with astrocytomas.[43] Von Hippel-Lindau disease, a hereditary condition characterized by angiomatosis of the retina and cerebellum, is associated with hemangioblastomas.[157] The best-described tumor suppressor genes are Rb and p53, associated with retinoblastoma and Li-Fraumeni syndrome, a familial breast cancer associated with soft-tissue sarcomas and other tumors.

No risk factors have been identified for the development of brain tumors, other than exposure to ionizing radiation.[118,125,160] The effects of carcinogenic viruses or agents are unclear. Associations have been made between certain viruses and brain tumors, such as the Epstein-Barr virus and primary CNS lymphoma, but they are insufficient to constitute direct cause-and-effect relationships.

Table 30-4 Cell of Origin and Distribution of Primary CNS Tumors by Histologic Type

Tumor	Cell of Origin	Frequency (%)
Meningioma	Arachnoidal fibroblast	27.4
Glioblastoma	Astrocyte	23.0
Astrocytoma	Astrocyte	11.3
Ependymoma	Ependymal cell	2.2
Oligodendroglioma	Oligodendrocyte	4.0
Embryonal, including primary neuroectodermal tumor (PNET)/medulloblastoma	Unknown*	1.9
Pituitary adenoma	Pituitary	6.6
Craniopharyngioma	Cells from Rathke pouch	0.8
Nerve sheath	Schwann cell	7.5
Lymphoma	Lymphocyte	2.7
All others		12.6
Choroid plexus papilloma or carcinoma	Choroid epithelial cell	
Hemangioblastoma	Endothelial cell	
Germ cell tumor	Primitive germ cell	
Pineocytoma	Pineal parenchymal cell	
Chordoma	Notochordal remnant	

Gliomas (glioblastomas, astrocytomas, oligodendrogliomas, and ependymomas) and neuroepithelial tumors account for 44.4% of all tumors.
Data from Central Brain Tumor Registry of the U.S., Statistical Report 2002–2003, analysis of data collected from 1995 to 1999 (n = 37,788); and Abeloff MD, Niederhuber JE, McKenna WG, editors: *Clinical oncology: a clinical perspective balanced with relevant basic science*, ed 3, 2004, Churchill Livingstone, Philadelphia.

Sustained exposure to certain pesticides, vinyl chloride, nitrosoureas, and polycyclic hydrocarbons has been implicated in astrocytic tumors, but epidemiologic surveys of workers in the farming, petrochemical, and rubber industries have produced conflicting results.[143] Certain industries, such as synthetic rubber processing, vinyl chloride production, and petrochemical and oil refining do show increased risk.[115,136] Infection, trauma, and immunosuppression are other suspected triggers. Radiation treatment for scalp ringworm in children is associated with an increased rate of developing brain tumors late in life.[50] A history of frequent exposure to full-mouth dental x-rays, particularly at an early age, also is associated with certain brain tumors.[23] Most of the extensive research in the area of nonionizing radiation exposure such as that from cellular phones, household appliances, and high-voltage electrical lines does not support an association with cancer.[5] Although some of the studies may show an association with exposure to electromagnetic fields, either many other confounding variables, such as exposure to other carcinogens, may account for the association[23] or a direct causal relationship cannot be proven (see Chapter 4).[115] An increased risk of childhood tumors is also associated with maternal diet, including consumption of cured meats containing nitrites during pregnancy.[23,115]

Low-Grade Astrocytoma—Grades I and II

Incidence. Low-grade astrocytomas make up 10% to 12% of primary brain tumors in adults.

Pathogenesis. Low-grade astrocytomas include grades I and II. Grade I includes pilocytic astrocytoma (composed of fiber-shaped cells), sometimes termed juvenile astrocytoma, and is considered benign by some and malignant by others.[83,150] Grade I astrocytoma grows slowly and often becomes cystic. It is composed of astrocytes with densely staining nuclei and scanty cytoplasm and is usually relatively acellular. The cells are uniform and closely resemble mature resting or reactive nonanaplastic astrocytes (well differentiated). Mitoses are absent or very rare.[67,83] Although these are slow-growing tumors, they may become large.[4] Figure 30-4 is a photograph of a well-differentiated astrocytoma. Grade II astrocytomas may be diffuse, infiltrative, and/or fibrillary, and have more anaplastic features. *Fibrillary* refers to the neuroglial fibrils. Other types are protoplasmic (cells that consist largely of protoplasm) and gemistocytic (large, densely packed cells with a globoid appearance).[150] There is moderate cell density. Figure 30-5 shows the appearance of computed tomographic (CT) and MRI astrocytoma scans with and without the use of contrast. The contrast agent, such as gadolinium, distinguishes the edema from the actual tumor. The larger the extent of the edema after administration of an intravenous contrast agent, the more malignant the lesion is likely to be.[97] Cerebral astrocytoma presents as a solid, gray mass with indistinct boundaries. Differentiation falls somewhere within a spectrum from well-differentiated (grade I) tumors to more anaplastic (grade II) tumors.[50] Astrocytomas in the cerebellum are often cystic and well circumscribed.

Clinical Manifestations. In adults, astrocytomas typically occur in the third and fourth decades of life and are usually located in the cerebrum, most commonly in the frontal lobes, but also may be found in the temporal lobes, parietal lobes, basal ganglia, and occipital lobes. Astrocytomas usually appear in the cerebellum in children.

In adults, typical initial symptoms are unilateral or focal headaches that become generalized as ICP increases. Frontal lobe tumors may produce personality disorders with changes in behavior and emotional state. Parietal and temporal lobe tumors may cause seizures

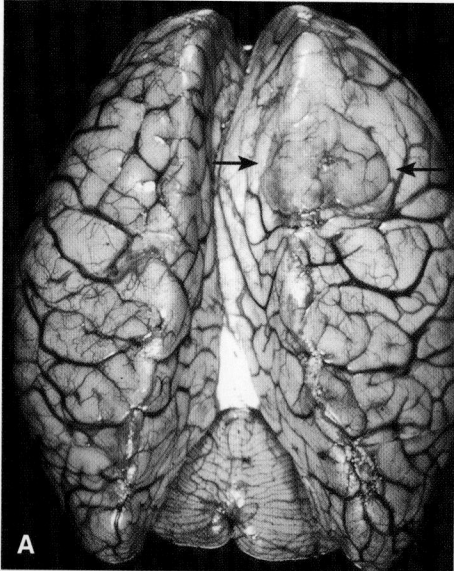

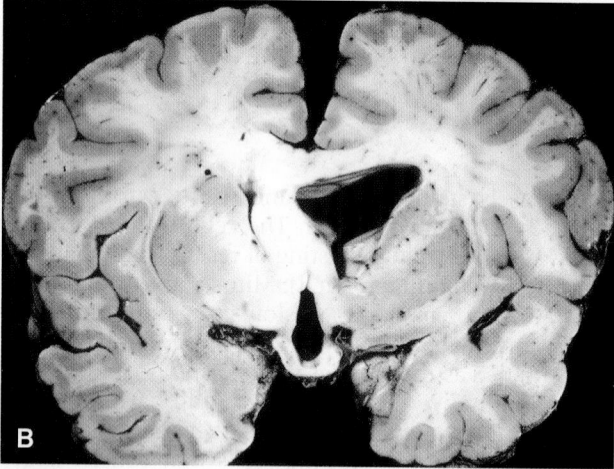

Figure 30-4

A well-differentiated astrocytoma. A, The right frontal tumor has expanded gyri, which led to flattening *(arrows)*. **B,** Expanded white matter of the left cerebral hemisphere and thickened corpus callosum and fornices. (From Kumar V, Abbas, AK, Fausto N, eds: *Robbins and Cotran pathologic basis of disease,* ed 7, Philadelphia, 2005, WB Saunders.)

on one side of the body. Occipital lobe tumors produce visual changes. Involvement of the optic apparatus or optic pathways also may produce visual changes. Refer to Table 30-3 for more details of signs associated with tumor location. In time, astrocytomas, like other gliomas, tend to become more malignant. In children, cerebellar astrocytomas lead to symptoms of unilateral cerebellar ataxia involving the limbs and trunk followed by signs of increased ICP.

Prognosis. Individuals with low-grade astrocytomas treated optimally have 5- to 10-year survival rates of 100% for completely excised lesions, and a 60% 5-year survival and 35% 10-year survival for partially excised lesions with radiation therapy. For many there will be a period of relative clinical stability that averages 5 to 7 years.[113,150] Untreated low-grade astrocytomas have a 5-year survival rate of 32% and a 10-year survival rate of 11%.[143] Despite the benign categorization, it must be understood that astrocytomas are nearly always infiltrative lesions and

generally progressive. Conversion of a low-grade astrocytoma to a higher-grade lesion over the years is a common phenomenon.[96]

High-Grade Astrocytoma—Grades III and IV

Incidence. High-grade malignant astrocytomas, grades III and IV, are much more common in adults than are low-grade astrocytomas. Grade III is often termed anaplastic astrocytoma and grade IV is termed GBM, although both are highly anaplastic. Grades III and IV astrocytomas make up 20% to 35% of primary brain tumors.

Pathogenesis. Anaplastic astrocytomas, grades III and IV, are diffusely infiltrative tumors that invade into the cerebral parenchyma. They typically involve the white matter of the cerebral hemispheres.[146] They often contain a mix of cells and cell grades, but are graded by the highest-grade cell seen in the tumor. GBM is a particularly rapidly growing, aggressive, infiltrative tumor that tends to invade both cerebral hemispheres via the corpus callosum. Figure 30-6 provides MRI and intraoperative pictures of a GBM. A GBM is a pinkish-gray or multicolored, well-demarcated mass with scattered areas of grossly visible hemorrhage. The blood vessels show endothelial proliferation: it is a highly vascular tumor, with vascular endothelial growth factor implicated, suggesting that the malignant progression from low-grade astrocytoma to GBM includes an "angiogenic switch."[146] The histologic distinction of an anaplastic astrocytoma from a glioblastoma is based largely on the absence or presence of tumor necrosis[157] and microvascular proliferation.[146] Microscopically, the tumor is pleomorphic (having various distinct forms) and hypercellular, with the cells showing hyperchromatic nuclei. There are many mitoses, giant cells, and young glial forms.

Of interest is the advance in molecular genetics in astrocytoma. Two moderately common genetic alterations are found to occur: inactivation of the TP53 tumor-suppressor gene and loss of chromosome 22q.[81] Further inactivation of tumor-suppressor genes on chromosomes 9p, 13q, and 19q leads to anaplastic astrocytomas.[81] The EphA receptor is overexpressed in GBM, and is a functional, targetable receptor that can be altered for treatment.[34] Many further mutations occur, and an understanding of the complexity of these mutations is beginning to suggest methods to intervene therapeutically. Also, understanding tumor stem cells that are responsible for populating and repopulating the tumors may also have therapeutic implications, as therapies that do not ablate the tumor stem cells will be ineffective in eradicating the tumor.[46,84,85,146]

Clinical Manifestations. Anaplastic astrocytoma and GBM most frequently arise in the frontal and temporal lobes, with the cerebellum, brainstem, and spinal cord being rare sites for adults. They most frequently occur in the fifth and sixth decades of life. Signs and symptoms progress rapidly, with grade IV GBM being particularly aggressive. The presentation may be of unilateral headache that is followed by generalized headache, indicating an increase in ICP. The development of seizures is not unusual. Lethargy, memory loss, motor weakness, and personality changes may occur.

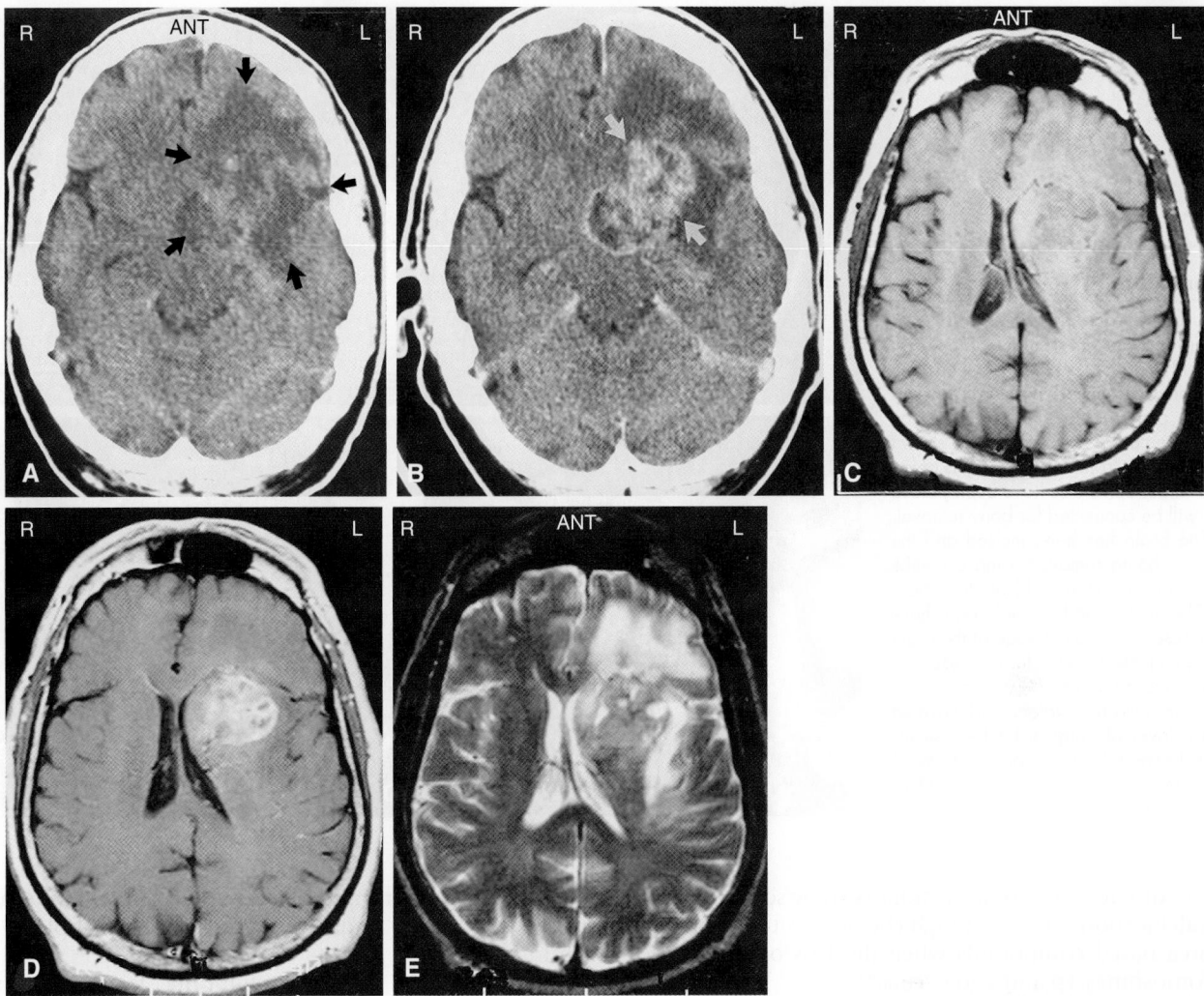

Figure 30-5

Astrocytoma. These contrasted and noncontrasted CT and MRI scans were obtained in the same patient and demonstrate a left astrocytoma with a large amount of surrounding edema. **A,** The noncontrasted CT scan shows only a large area of low density that represents the tumor and edema *(arrows)*. **B,** A contrasted CT scan shows enhancement of the tumor *(arrows)* surrounded by the dark or low-density area of edema. **C,** A noncontrasted T1-weighted MRI scan clearly shows a mass effect caused by impression of the tumor on the left lateral ventricle and some midline shift. **D,** A gadolinium-enhanced T1-weighted MRI scan clearly outlines the tumor, but the edema is difficult to see. **E,** A T2-weighted MRI scan shows the tumor rather poorly, but the surrounding edema is easily seen as an area of increased signal *(white)*. (From Mettler FA Jr: *Essentials of radiology*, ed 2, Philadelphia, 2005, WB Saunders.)

Prognosis. All malignant astrocytomas will eventually recur. With optimal treatment (excision, radiation therapy), clients with anaplastic astrocytoma (grade III) have a 70% 1-year survival rate, a 40% 2-year survival rate, and a 10% to 20% 5-year survival rate. GBM (grade IV) has a grimmer prognosis with a 50% 1-year survival rate, a less than 15% 2-year survival rate, and rare long-term survival.[143] The relationship between genetic alterations and prognosis is complex and may be age dependent.[61,146] For patients younger than 50 years, the most significant prognostic factor is histology, with median survival for anaplastic astrocytoma of 49.4 months and for GBM of 13.7 months. For patients older than 50 years, the most significant prognostic factor is the performance status. Patients with an anaplastic astrocytoma or a GBM with a high performance status live a median of 10.3 months, compared with 5.3 months for those with a lower performance status.[103,115]

Oligodendroglioma

Incidence. Oligodendrogliomas make up 2% to 3% of gliomas.[3] It is not uncommon to have a combination of cell types, such as astrocytes, creating a mixed oligodendroglioma/astrocytoma, or oligoastrocytoma. Oligodendrogliomas occur most frequently in young and middle-aged adults, but can also be found in children.

Pathogenesis. Oligodendroglioma is a slow-growing, solid, calcified tumor arising from oligodendrocytes, the myelin-producing cells of the CNS. It stains for myelin basic protein. It can be either low-grade (II) or high-grade (III). It is a gray-pink to red cystic area in the brain and has a honeycomb appearance at low microscopic power because of the presence of a fibrovascular stroma. On higher power the cells have a uniform appearance, with a central nucleus surrounded by a clear cytoplasm, or a fried egg appearance. Mitotic figures are infrequent.

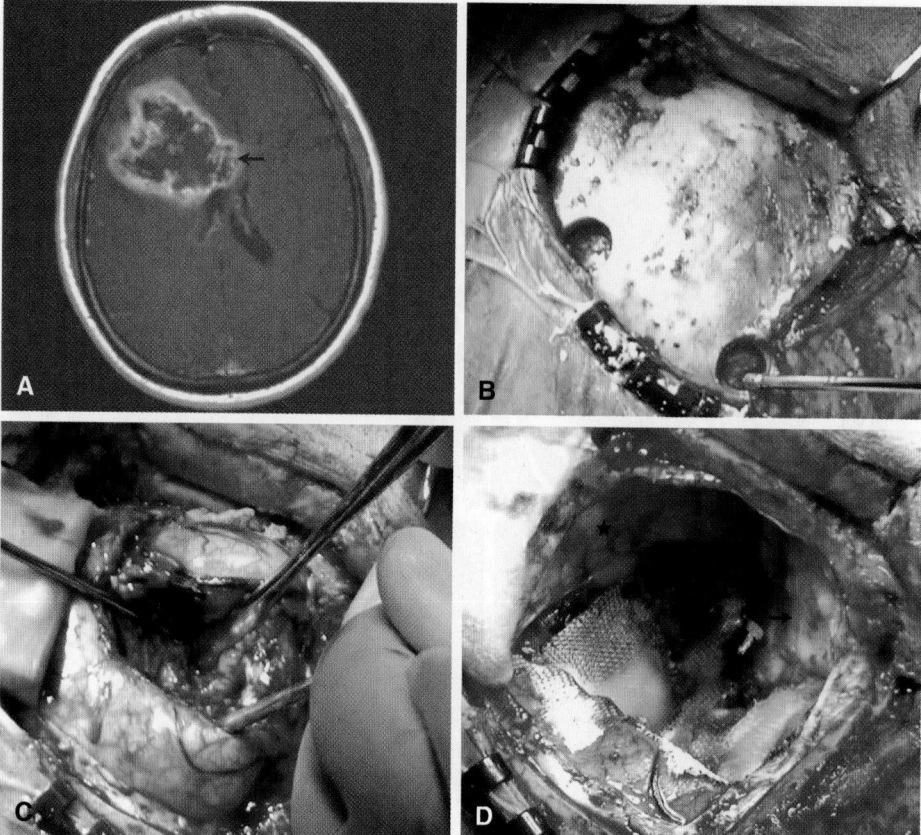

Figure 30-6

MRI and intraoperative pictures of a patient with a right frontal GBM. **A,** An axial T1-weighted MRI scan. The enhancing lesion demonstrates central necrosis and is causing mass effect. Infiltration along the corpus callosum is also shown (arrow). **B,** A frontal craniotomy is being performed. Burr holes have been placed and will be connected for bony removal. **C,** The brain has been incised and the tumor is being removed using a combination of suction and blunt dissection. **D,** The tumor and frontal lobe have been resected. The cut edge of the brain is seen at the lower left. The resection cavity has been lined with carmustine polymer (Gliadel) wafers and covered with a layer of Surgicel for hemostasis. (From Townsend CM Jr: *Sabiston textbook of surgery*, ed 17, Philadelphia, 2004, WB Saunders.)

Approximately 70% of these tumors show some evidence of calcification. There is a high chemosensitivity to nitrosourea based compounds when the loss or deletion of chromosomes 1p and 19q occurs.[65]

Clinical Manifestations. Oligodendrogliomas are located predominantly in the cerebral hemispheres, often in the frontal lobes. They expand toward the cortex and may spread through it and eventually attach to the dura.[50] A history of partial or generalized seizures, usually of long duration and sometimes with chronic headache, is the typical presentation pattern of oligodendrogliomas. They tend to bleed spontaneously and may present with a stroke-like syndrome.[133] The hallmark of this tumor radiologically is calcification, which can be identified in the vast majority of people by CT. It is usually nonenhancing with gadolinium, meaning that the surrounding edema is limited.[150] If an oligodendroglioma contains astrocytoma cells, it is graded at the highest level of anaplasia present.

Prognosis. With optimal treatment, 5- and 10-year survival rates are 80% to 100% and 45% to 55%, respectively. The median overall survival is 17 years.[106] Radiotherapy alone is no longer considered the primary treatment choice.[95] Although a long interval of quiescence may occur after treatment, oligodendrogliomas eventually reoccur, often as a more aggressive tumor with progressing symptoms.[143]

Ependymoma

Incidence. Ependymomas have a low incidence, comprising only approximately 2% of gliomas.[3] Ependymoma is much more prevalent in children than adults and is the third most frequent posterior fossa neoplasm of children.

Pathogenesis. An ependymoma is a neoplasm derived from the ependymal cell lining of the ventricular system and the central canal of the spinal cord. It is graded I to IV, depending on the degree of anaplasia. It is usually reddish, lobulated, and well-circumscribed, resembling a cauliflower in shape. Pseudorosette formation, in which the cells are arranged about a clear space or a blood vessel, may occur, and blepharoplasts (small round or rod-shaped intracytoplasmic bodies) may be seen.

Clinical Manifestations. Ependymoma is more common in the fourth ventricle and is likely to be detected early because of the signs and symptoms of increased ICP in the posterior fossa (e.g., headache, nausea, vomiting, and papilledema). Many of the symptoms and eventually survival depend on the grade and location of the tumor. In a recent series, 69% were supratentorial, and 31% were infratentorial.[28] Greatest mortality for ependymoma is in those patients receiving subtotal resection, regardless of whether or not radiation therapy is employed post surgically. Radiation therapy can be avoided even in anaplastic tumors if total resection is achieved.[156] However, supratentorial ependymomas often grow large before detection. Figure 30-7 depicts an ependymoma of the fourth ventricle.

Prognosis. The prognosis for ependymomas is improving: 5-year survival rates exceed 80% and 10-year survival rates are 40% to 60%.[143]

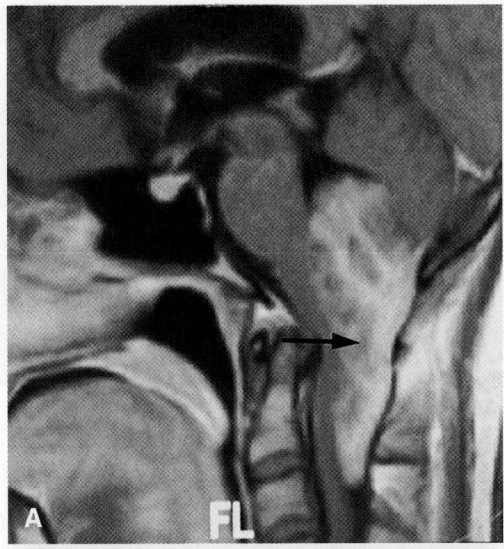

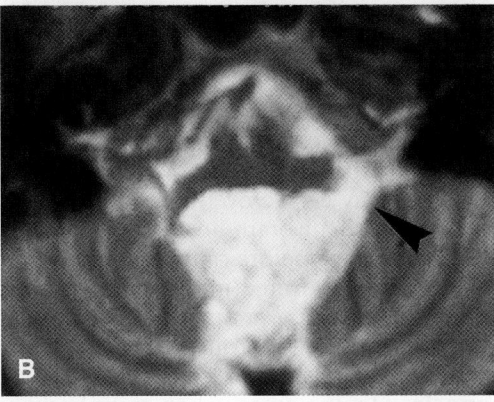

Figure 30-7

Ependymoma of the fourth ventricle. Sagittal gadolinium-enhanced T1-weighted **(A)** and axial T2-weighted **(B)** magnetic resonance images. A heterogeneously enhanced mass *(arrow)* fills the lower half of the fourth ventricle and extends through the foramina of Luschka *(arrowhead)* and Magendie to lie posterior to the medulla oblongata and upper cervical spinal cord, which are compressed from behind. There is obstructive hydrocephalus. (From Grainger RG, Allison DJ, Adam A, Dixon AK, eds: *Grainger and Allison's diagnostic radiology: a textbook of medical imaging,* ed 4, Philadelphia, 2001, Churchill Livingstone.)

Medulloblastoma

Incidence. Medulloblastomas make up less than 2% of primary brain tumors.[3] The age of peak incidence is 45 to 55 years in adults. In children, the tumor occurs mainly between the ages of 2 and 10 years. Medulloblastoma is the most common malignant primary CNS tumor in children and the second most common posterior fossa tumor in children.

Pathogenesis. Medulloblastoma is a typically a rapidly growing malignant tumor. The cell of origin is unknown, but it is presumed to arise from the embryonal external granular layer of the cerebellum. It is considered to belong to a group of tumors known as PNETs. It has a tendency to metastasize to the surface of the remaining CNS via the subarachnoid spaces. Grossly it is red and soft and is composed of many closely packed cells, with oval nuclei and many mitoses. Pseudorosette formations are common. It is highly vascular, containing numerous small blood vessels.[143] Four separate types of medulloblastoma can be classified: classic, large cell (anaplastic), desmoplastic, and nodular.[161]

Clinical Manifestations. Medulloblastoma often develops in the cerebellar vermis and is very aggressive in younger children. Because of its proximity to the fourth ventricle, early development of hydrocephalus is common, along with other signs of cerebellar dysfunction, such as ataxia. Medulloblastomas tend to metastasize through CSF pathways, more predominantly into the spine but also into the supratentorial compartment. Drop metastases to the spinal subarachnoid space, causing cord compression and possible paraplegia, are a common enough complication that close monitoring is warranted.

Prognosis. Early in the century medulloblastomas were uniformly fatal tumors. Improvement in therapeutic strategies during the past 30 years has dramatically improved the prognosis.[140] Favorable prognostic factors include age greater than 2 years, undisseminated local disease, and greater than 75% tumor resection. In these clients, the 5-year disease-free survival rate exceeds 60% to 70% in most studies.[57,143] In poorer-risk cases, the 5-year disease-free survival rate is approximately 45%.[143] After recurrence, the survival rate at 1 year is 22%, but 0% at 3 years.[90]

Tumors Arising from Supporting Structures in the Brain

Meningioma

Overview. Meningiomas are slow-growing, usually benign lesions that occur most commonly along the dural folds and cerebral convexities, although they may occur in the spinal cord as well. The WHO classification recognizes three groups, grade I or benign, grade II or atypical, and grade III or malignant (anaplastic).[42,143] Although 90% of meningiomas are grade I, making their prognosis favorable in many cases, complete resection is only possible in fewer than 50% of patients.[42]

Incidence. Meningiomas represent up to 34% of all intracranial neoplasms and are the second most common primary intracranial tumor in adults and the most common of benign brain neoplasms.[4] Ninety percent are considered benign and approximately 5% are grade III. Most are single lesions, but multiple meningiomas also occur. They are most common between the ages of 40 and 70 years, and are two to three times more prevalent in females than in males.[143] They are increased in neurofibromatosis, in women who use postmenopausal hormone replacement therapy, and in patients who have had breast cancer.

Pathogenesis. Meningiomas originate in the arachnoid layer of the meninges and are believed to be derived from the cells and vascular elements of the meninges. Cytogenetic analysis demonstrates multiple deletions on chromosome 22 in most people with meningioma. Gene downregulation is observed in recurrent and advanced cases, and this gene repression may be caused by gene promotion hypermethylation, suggesting that this type of epigenetic event may play an important role in meningioma progression or recurrence.[110] Tumors are most often

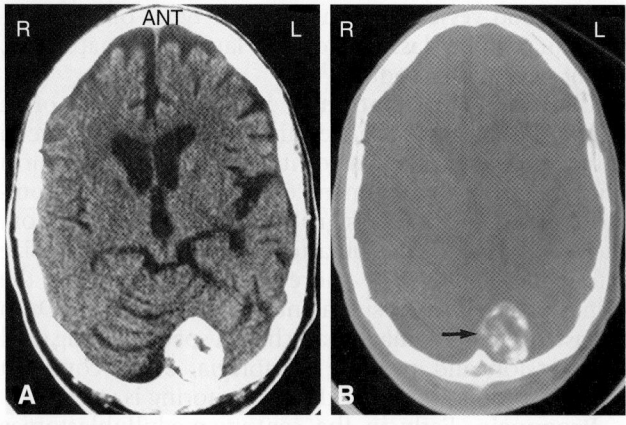

Figure 30-8

Meningioma. A, A noncontrasted CT scan shows a very dense, peripherally based lesion in the left cerebellar area. **B,** A bone window image obtained at the same level shows that the density is caused by calcification within this lesion. (From Mettler FA Jr: *Essentials of radiology*, ed 2, Philadelphia, 2005, WB Saunders.)

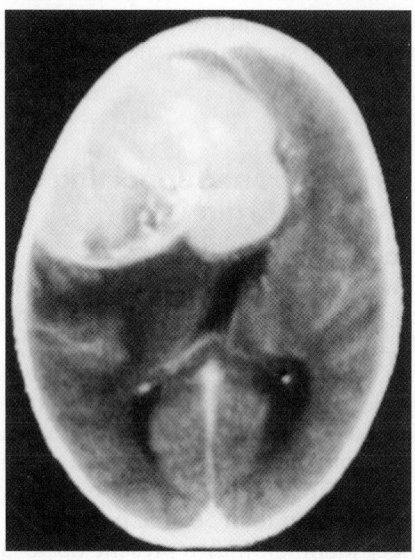

Figure 30-9

CT scan with contrast of a meningioma in a patient who presented with mild cognitive deficits, illustrative of the size a slow-growing tumor can attain in the brain. The tumor was completely resected. (From Goldman LM, Ausiello D, eds: *Cecil textbook of medicine*, ed 22, Philadelphia, 2004, WB Saunders.

located between or over the cerebral hemispheres, at the skull base, or in the posterior fossa. Meningiomas are typically well-circumscribed globular masses. Interestingly, they may infiltrate the dura, the dural sinuses, or bone, but generally do not invade the underlying brain parenchyma. Figures 30-8 and 30-9 are CT scans of meningiomas. Most meningiomas grow as well-encapsulated tumors, but others develop in relatively thin sheets along the dura.

Meningiomas, because of their proximity to or invasion of the bone, are known to provoke a local osteoblastic response termed *hyperostosis*. This may cause a profuse local thickening of the skull. Figure 30-10 shows diffuse reactive hyperostosis, as well as facial distortion from the growing meningioma.

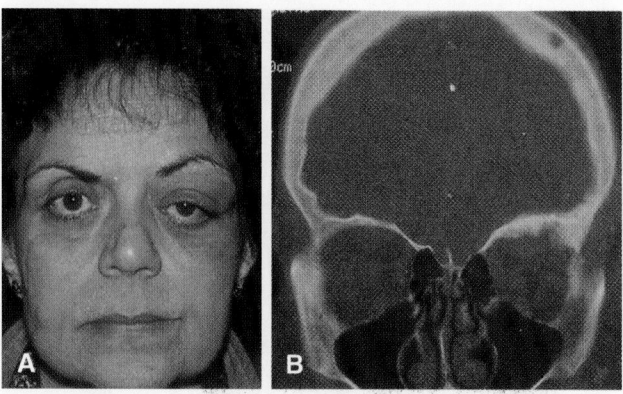

Figure 30-10

A, Upper eyelid edema, mild proptosis, and downward displacement of the eye as a result of en plaque sphenoid wing meningioma. **B,** CT scan of the same patient demonstrating lytic bone lesions and diffuse reactive hyperostosis as a result of bone infiltration by meningioma. (From Abeloff MD, Armitage JO, Niederhuber JE, et al: *Clinical oncology*, ed 3, Philadelphia, 2004, Churchill Livingstone.)

Clinical Manifestations. Meningiomas are more common in the later years of life and are more frequent in women. Because they are slow growing, abnormal signs and symptoms may evolve over a period of many years. When located in silent brain areas, some meningiomas can become very large before causing clinical symptoms. Also, they can be discovered incidentally as masses that show little or no growth over time. Neurologic abnormalities depend on the location of the tumor; seizures are a common finding with skull-based lesions.

Prognosis. Meningiomas, when completely resected (surgical accessibility determines excision capabilities), have excellent prospects of long-term cure. Patients with completely excised lesions experience a 10-year survival rate of 80% to 90%. Partially resected meningiomas have a 50% to 70% 10-year progression-free survival. Malignant meningiomas, approximately 1% to 10% of meningiomas, have a shorter disease-free interval[143] and a tendency to recur.

Pituitary Adenoma

Overview. Pituitary adenomas are benign tumors derived from cells of the anterior portion of the pituitary gland. The pituitary gland, located at the base of the brain, sits in the sella turcica, the saddle-shaped transverse depression on the superior surface of the body of the sphenoid bone. Figure 30-11 gives the anatomic relations of the pituitary gland, optic chiasm, and surrounding parasellar structures. Although pituitary adenomas are the most common of the pituitary tumors, infrequently other types of pituitary tumors may occur in the location of the pituitary gland and may be primary or metastatic. See also "Pituitary Gland" in Chapter 11.

Incidence. Pituitary adenomas are common lesions, accounting for approximately 13% of all intracranial tumors, making them the third most common primary brain tumor in adults after meningiomas and the gliomas.[101] They are usually found in middle-aged or older people. Women are more affected more often than men, particularly during childbearing years. Almost 70% are

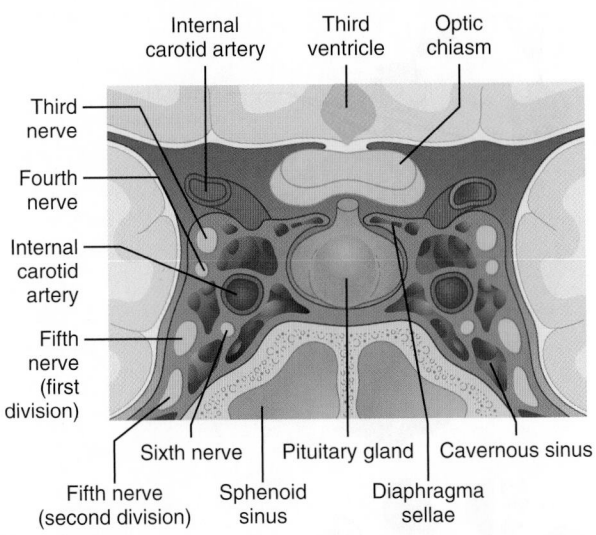

Figure 30-11

Anatomic relations of pituitary gland and surrounding parasellar structures. (Adapted from Warwick R: *The orbital vessels.* In Warwick L ed: Eugene Wolff's anatomy of the eye and orbit, ed 7, Philadelphia, WB Saunders, 1976.)

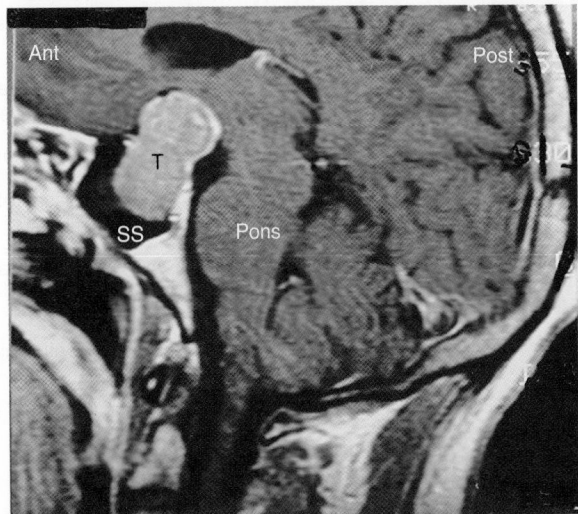

Figure 30-12

Pituitary adenoma. A sagittal view of the base of the brain on a T1-weighted magnetic resonance image shows the pituitary tumor *(T)* and its extension down into the sphenoid sinus *(SS).* (From Mettler FA Jr: *Essentials of radiology,* ed 2, Philadelphia, 2005, WB Saunders.)

functional, or secreting, tumors, and these tend to occur in younger adults. Nonfunctioning tumors (nonsecreting), also called nonfunctioning adenomas, tend to occur in older adults.

Pathogenesis. With recent advances in molecular techniques, genetic abnormalities associated with pituitary tumors are becoming clearer. The great majority of pituitary adenomas are monoclonal in origin, suggesting that most arise from a single somatic cell. Additional molecular abnormalities present in aggressive pituitary adenomas and include mutations of the RAS oncogene and overexpression of the c-MYC oncogene, which suggests that these genetic events are linked to disease progression. Small lesions of the pituitary gland, called *microadenomas,* are less than 10 mm in diameter and may be asymptomatic. Most grow in the front two-thirds of the pituitary gland. Larger tumors, or macroadenomas, may compress the adjacent normal pituitary gland. Figure 30-12 shows a pituitary tumor extension down into the sphenoid sinus. Extension of the tumor above the sella turcica compresses the optic chiasm.

Clinical Manifestations. In the majority of pituitary tumors, the release of excess pituitary hormones or pituitary insufficiency results in dramatic and unique clinical syndromes. Galactorrhea and amenorrhea, gigantism and acromegaly, and the symptoms of Cushing disease (hypertension, facial and truncal obesity, osteoporosis, muscle weakness, menstrual abnormalities, and female hirsutism) are among the hormonal symptoms. Pituitary insufficiency, or hypopituitarism, can lead to symptoms such as fatigue, weakness, and hypogonadism. A second pattern of presentation consists of regression of secondary sexual characteristics and hypothyroidism. The third pattern of presentation is one of neurologic findings, including headache, bitemporal visual loss, and ocular palsy. Figure 30-13 localizes masses such as a pituitary tumor

Localization and identification of masses by pattern of field loss

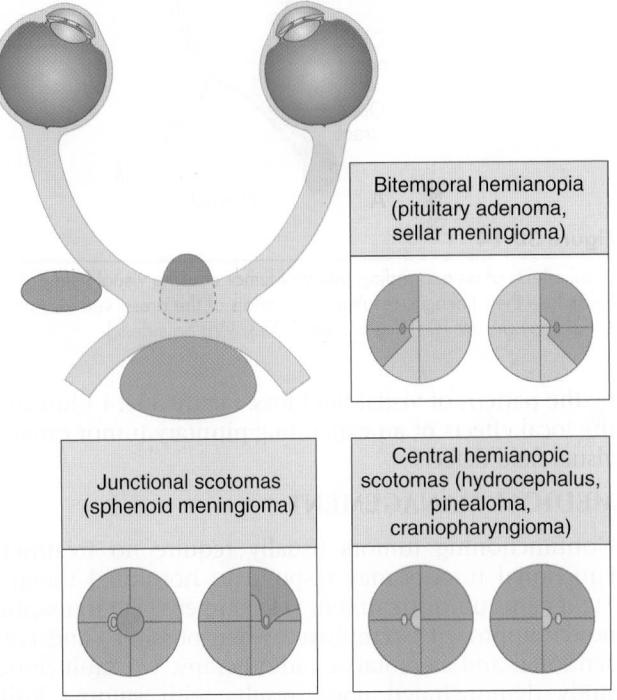

Figure 30-13

Localization and probable identification of masses by pattern of field loss. Junctional scotomas occur with compression of the anterior angle of the chiasm (sphenoid meningioma). Bitemporal hemianopia results from compression of the body of the chiasm from below (e.g., because of pituitary adenoma, sellar meningioma). Compression of the posterior chiasm and its decussating nasal fibers may cause central bitemporal hemianopic scotomas (e.g., because of hydrocephalus, pinealoma, craniopharyngioma). (From Yanoff M, Duker JS, Augsburger JJ, et al., eds: *Ophthalmology,* ed 2, St Louis, 2004, Mosby.)

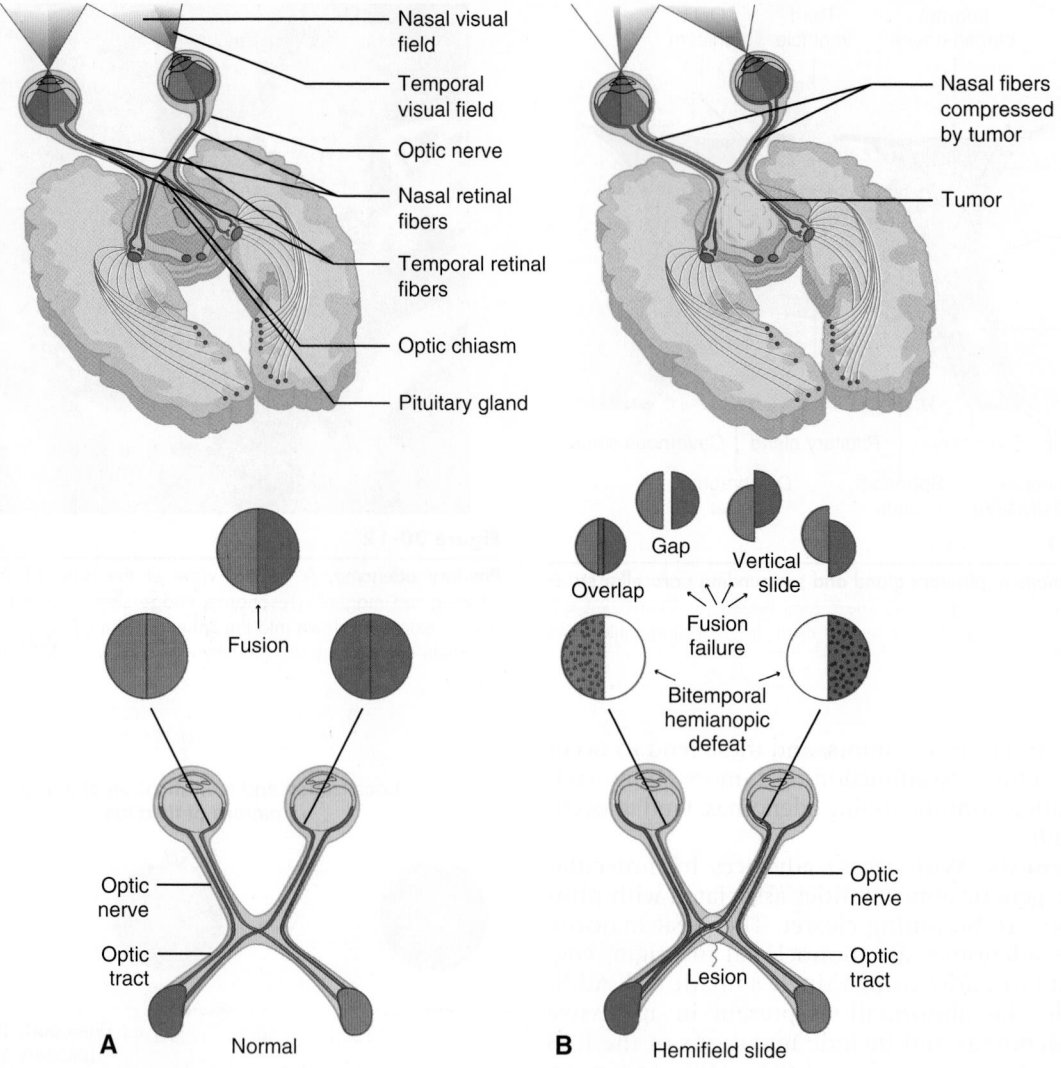

Figure 30-14

Local effects of an expanding pituitary tumor causing visual field defects: **(A)** normal vision and **(B)** bitemporal hemianopsia. The nasal and temporal fields lose their linkage, resulting in overlap of the preserved visual field. (From Larsen PR, Kronenberg HM, Melmed S, et al, eds: *Williams textbook of endocrinology*, ed 10, Philadelphia, 2003, WB Saunders.)

by the pattern of visual field loss. Figure 30-14 illustrates the local effects of an expanding pituitary tumor causing visual field defects.

MEDICAL MANAGEMENT

Nonfunctioning tumors usually require no treatment Functional tumors may respond to hormonal therapy. Malignant tumor treatment is by surgery (the transsphenoidal approach is employed when possible) and conventional and stereotactic radiotherapy.[72] A multicenter study demonstrated good results with gamma knife radiosurgery for the management of nonfunctioning pituitary adenomas.[131]

PROGNOSIS. Tumors of the pituitary are very treatable, with the majority of people enjoying long-term survival or cure. Because visual compromise is a complicating feature of many pituitary tumors, serial recording of visual field deficits can document disease progression in addition to responses to treatment.

Neurinoma, Neuroma

Overview and Incidence. Neurinomas are slow-growing, benign tumors originating from Schwann cells. In the brain, they most commonly develop on the vestibular component of the eighth cranial nerve and are also called *acoustic neurinomas*, *acoustic neuromas*, or *schwannomas*. Acoustic neurinomas account for 3% to 10% of all brain tumors.[101] They occur mainly in the fourth to sixth decades of life, with a 2:1 female-to-male occurrence ratio. Approximately 5% occur in the context of neurofibromatosis. It is of note that bilateral lesions are most likely to occur in neurofibromatosis.

Pathogenesis. Acoustic neurinomas typically originate in the internal auditory canal in the transition zone of the oligodendroglial cells and peripheral nervous system Schwann cells. Neurinomas also may be found attached to other cranial nerves, such as the trigeminal nerve. The tumor grows into the cerebellopontine angle, eventually compressing the facial nerve, and encroaches

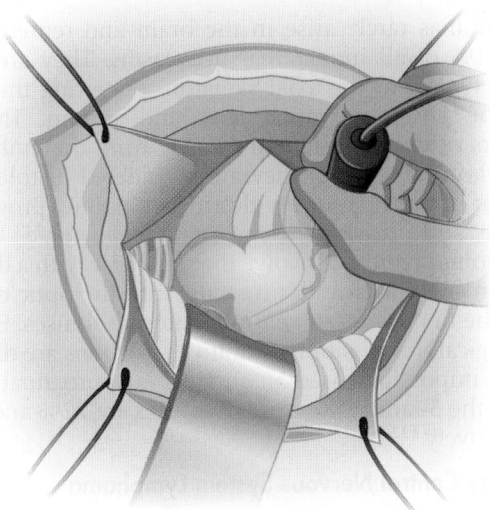

Figure 30-15

Surgical view of a large acoustic neuroma (retrosigmoid approach) showing use of a flexible-tipped probe to locate the facial nerve on the medial surface of the tumor out of direct view. Early identification of the facial nerve "around the corner" on the ventral surface of the tumor helps speed the procedure by allowing rapid removal of the remaining capsule. Tumor is drawn as if transparent to show details of anatomy on the hidden surface. (From Yingling CD, Gardi JN: Intraoperative monitoring of facial and cochlear nerves during acoustic neuroma surgery, *Otolaryngol Clin North Am* 25(2):413–448, 1992.)

on the brainstem. Some lesions may remain relatively quiescent for long periods of time, but the majority are slow-growing, progressive lesions. The tumor is thickly encapsulated, often highly vascular, and microscopically consists of spindle-shaped cells with rod-shaped nuclei often lying in parallel rows.

Clinical Manifestations. Acoustic neurinomas typically present with progressive unilateral sensorineural hearing loss. Other symptoms include tinnitus, vertigo, and unsteadiness. Facial numbness, difficulty swallowing, impaired eye movement, and taste disturbances may occur. Weakness of the facial muscles is generally a late feature. Deformity and obstruction of the fourth ventricle leads to hydrocephalus with headache, vomiting, and other symptoms of increased ICP. Figure 30-15 provides a surgical view of a large acoustic neuroma.

Prognosis. In the majority of cases, cure is achieved with surgical resection. Stereotactic radiotherapy may be possible, reducing surgical side effects.[6] As acoustic neurinomas are slow growing, and surgery often accelerates hearing loss, the decision to delay surgery until necessary may be made. However, because the likelihood of hearing retention is greatest when the tumor is small, surgery may be done as soon as possible.

Choroid Plexus Papilloma

Choroid plexus papilloma is a low-grade neoplasm of the choroid plexus, the vascular coat along the ventricles carrying blood vessels within the pia mater to each ventricle. It is relatively rare and usually is found in children. It often is associated with overproduction of CSF and hydrocephalus. Complete removal of the tumor usually results in

an excellent prognosis and resolution of the hydrocephalus. The prognosis for choroid plexus carcinoma, another variation of a choroid plexus tumor, is dismal.

Pinealoma

Overview and Incidence. Pineal region (posterior to the third ventricle) tumors are rare (1% of all intracranial tumors), more common in children, and more common in males than females. They tend to occur in adults between 20 and 40 years of age. These are a heterogeneous group of tumors. Germ cell pinealomas have an embryonal basis, and although some are very radiosensitive, others are aggressive, highly malignant, and generally incurable. Germinomatous tumors have a survival rate of 98%; nongerminomatous tumors do not fare as well and are less radiosensitive.[98] Pineal parenchymal tumors have a tendency to disseminate craniospinally.

Clinical Manifestations and Prognosis. Pineal region tumors typically result in obstructive hydrocephalus because of the proximity of the pineal gland to the ventricular system. Symptoms include headache, nausea, vomiting, and ocular abnormalities. Management is by shunting the hydrocephalus, if present; radiation therapy; and/or surgical excision. Individuals with responsive tumors have a 5-year survival rate of 70%.[143] Those with nonresponsive tumors have a 1-year survival rate of only 33%.

Craniopharyngiomas

Overview. Craniopharyngiomas are histologically benign congenital tumors and occur most commonly in the suprasellar region in the pituitary stalk adjacent to the optic chiasm.

Incidence. Craniopharyngiomas are rare and account for 1% to 3% of all intracranial tumors.[26] They are the third most common intracranial tumor in children, accounting for 10% of all intracranial tumors in this age group.

Pathogenesis. Craniopharyngiomas presumably arise from embryonic remnants of Rathke pouch and grow slowly from birth. They vary in size from small, solid, well-circumscribed masses to huge multilocular cysts that invade the sella turcica, reaching a large size before they are diagnosed. They often involve the pituitary gland, optic nerve, and third ventricle. Two basic histologic subtypes have been described: adamantinomatous and papillary.[147] Sixty percent to 80% of tumors are calcified.

Clinical Manifestations. Based on the location, craniopharyngiomas can compromise a number of important intracranial structures and produce multiple signs and symptoms. The most common presentations are pituitary hypofunction, visual difficulties, and severe headaches. Other signs are increased ICP, neuroendocrine disorders, hypothalamus involvement, cranial nerve palsies, hydrocephalus, and progressive dementia. Sexual dysfunction is the most common endocrine problem in adults, with 90% of men complaining of erectile dysfunction and most women having amenorrhea. Depression may occur, presumably because of extension of the tumor into the frontal lobes, striocapsulothalamic areas, or limbic system.[151]

Prognosis. Optimal treatment is controversial, but radiation and/or surgical resection are used. Intracavitary radiation is used in select tumors. With complete resections or resections followed by radiation therapy, 10-year survival rates of 78% have been reported. Recurrence rates are higher in patients receiving less than 54 Gy of radiation. The tumors do have a tendency to recur, and even though histologically they are benign, they may be better thought of as low-grade malignancies.

Epidermoid and Dermoid Tumors (Cysts)

Incidence. Epidermoid and dermoid tumors are rare benign tumors that arise from imperfect embryogenesis of the CNS and account for 2% of intracranial tumors. The most common cysts in the brain are epidermoid, arachnoid, colloid, and dermoid.

Pathogenesis. Cysts are fluid-filled spheres composed of desquamated epidermal cellular debris, keratin, and cholesterol. During embryologic development, groups of cells are diverted from the areas of the face or skin to the neural tube. They grow in basal regions of the brain and tend to enlarge along CSF pathways. Most cysts are benign and grow slowly, and may not cause symptoms for many years.

The epidermoid cyst often contains remnants of skin cells or tiny pieces of cartilage and occurs near the cerebellopontine angle or the pituitary gland. The arachnoid cyst is found in the subarachnoid space, often in the Sylvian fissure, the cerebellopontine angle, the cisterna magna, or the suprasellar region of the brain, and may cause increased ICP. The colloid cyst is most frequently found in the third ventricle and may block CSF, causing headache, seizures and increased ICP. The dermoid tumor has epidermal cellular debris, but it is mixed with additional dermal elements such as hair, hair follicles, sweat glands, and sebaceous glands. Dermoid cysts are usually located in the posterior fossa or the adjacent meninges, or in the lower spine.

Prognosis. In most cases, complete surgical excision of the tumor capsule and contents is curative.[143] If the tumor is unable to be totally removed, it may recur, although growth is slow.[2]

Hemangioblastoma

Incidence. Hemangiomas make up 2% of all intracranial tumors, are the most common adult intraaxial tumor of the posterior fossa, and occur more frequently in males. They most commonly occur in people about 40 years old.

Pathogenesis. Hemangiomas are benign, slow-growing tumors typically arising in the posterior fossa, primarily in the cerebellar vermis or pons, as solitary lesions with clearly indicated borders. The origin is thought to be cells in the blood vessel lining. Hemangioblastomas are a vascular conglomerate of endothelial cells, pericytes (found wrapped about precapillary arterioles), and stromal cells. These highly vascular tumors attached to the wall of a surrounding cyst are often associated with von Hippel-Lindau syndrome.[120]

Clinical Manifestation and Prognosis. Blockage of the CSF results in ICP and hydrocephalus. Common symptoms include headache, nausea and vomiting, balance and gait disturbances, and poor coordination. Complete surgical excision for tumors arising in the cerebellum is curative.

Chordoma

Chordomas rarely arise in the brain and represent less than 1% of all intracranial neoplasms. They are much more typical in the axial skeleton, preferring the clivus (in the posterior cranial fossa)and sacrum. They are tumors of bone, presumed to arise from the embryonal notochord remnants. They are considered histologically benign but have a locally destructive nature, progressive course, and occasionally metastatic behavior.[143] Cranial chordomas typically involve the skull base with a destructive process that invades rostrally into the optic chiasm, into the brainstem, or ventrally into the sinuses. Because of surgical inaccessibility, curative resections are difficult, if not impossible. Median survival is approximately 7.7 years; the 5- and 10-year survival rates are 72% and 45%, respectively.[132]

Primary Central Nervous System Lymphoma

Overview and Incidence. Primary CNS lymphoma (PCNSL) is a non-Hodgkin lymphoma and occurs in the absence of systemic lymphoma. It is also called an extranodal lymphoma. This tumor was formerly quite rare, but between 1973 and 1985, it tripled in frequency in immunocompetent patients and also increased in the immunosuppressed population—that is, in clients with acquired immunodeficiency syndrome (AIDS) and collagen vascular disorders, organ transplant recipients, and the congenitally immunodeficient.[4,157] There was a decrease in incidence in young men and patients with AIDS between 1995 and 1998, which was explained by the introduction of highly active antiretroviral therapy for patients with human immunodeficiency virus (HIV) infection.[158] PCNSL in the patient with AIDS continues to decrease in incidence with the advent of highly active antiretroviral therapy.[51] It currently accounts for 4% to 7% of all primary brain tumors.[1,26,28,56,87]

Pathogenesis. The pathophysiologic basis for development of these tumors is unclear, particularly in immunocompetent patients. PCNSL most commonly originates from B lymphocytes and is associated with cytokines. In immunosuppressed patients, it is almost always associated with latent infection of neoplastic B cells by Epstein-Barr virus.[56] The lymphoma cells typically assume a periventricular pattern, involving the deep white matter, basal ganglia, corpus callosum, and thalamus. PCNSL may also involve the CSF, the eyes, or the spinal cord. Lesions may be multiple. Lesions in immunocompetent patients more often may be a single brain lesion, in a supratentorial location, and with frontoparietal lobe involvement. The diagnostic procedure of choice is a stereotactic (x-ray–guided) biopsy, as patients derive little clinical benefit from surgical resection.[66]

Clinical Manifestations. Symptoms and signs generally evolve over several months, including personality and behavioral changes, confusion, generalized seizures, and symptoms associated with increased ICP (headaches, nausea and vomiting). The most frequent presenting symptom in 30% to 40% of patients is impaired cognition.[35] Focal neurologic signs, such as hemiparesis or blurred or double vision, may occur. The appearance on MRI or CT of multiple deep cerebral and periventricular lesions, along with an immunodeficient state, suggests the diagnosis.[77]

Differential diagnosis includes infections, other tumors, and inflammatory disorders.

Prognosis. The prognosis is generally poor, with median survival of 10 to 14 months, although adding systemic chemotherapy (methotrexate and cytosine arabinoside) to radiation has improved median survival to 32 to 60 months.[66,143] Age affects prognosis significantly; younger patients have better outcomes.

Other Miscellaneous Brain Tumor Types

Other infrequent brain tumors bearing mention are as follows:

- **Chondromas** tend to arise at the base of the skull, are slow growing, and are composed of cartilage-like cells often attached to the dura mater.
- **Chondrosarcomas** are the malignant variant of chondromas.
- **Atypical teratoid rhabdoid tumors** are high-grade tumors occurring most commonly in the cerebellum in children and are aggressive with frequent metastasis through the CNS.
- **Dysembryoplastic neuroepithelial tumors** are slow-growing, benign, grade I tumors, often containing a mix of neurons and glial cells, and typically found in the temporal or frontal lobe.
- **Gangliocytomas** and **gangliogliomas** arise from ganglia-type cells (groups of neurons), and are most commonly located in the temporal lobe and third ventricle.
- **Germ cell tumors** include the germinoma, teratoma, embryonal carcinoma and yolk sac tumor, and choriocarcinoma. These tend to arise in the pineal or suprasellar regions and occur primarily in children and young adults. Teratomas are composed of various tissue types within the tumor, often containing calcium, cysts, fat, and other soft tissues.

More details on these CNS tumors, as well as further information on the numerous other infrequent CNS tumors, are available in various references.[1,5,18,67,78,88]

Diagnosis of Primary Brain Tumors

When a brain tumor is suspected on clinical evaluation, a thorough neurologic examination as well as brain imaging studies are done to confirm its presence and exact location.

MRI has evolved as the most informative brain imaging study because of its superior imaging capabilities and lack of artifact from the temporal bones. With the addition of gadolinium contrast enhancement, which distinguishes tumor from surrounding edema, MRI detects tumors even a few millimeters in size. MRI also defines critical anatomic relationships between the tumor and surrounding neurovascular structures. The multiplanar capability of MRI allows optimal visualization of the anatomy. MRI is particularly useful in visualizing the brainstem and other posterior fossa structures.[157] New MRI techniques are being developed to investigate the biochemical basis of tumors, such as the proton magnetic resonance spectroscopy, which measures the signals from nuclei other than water.[115]

Although MRI has many advantages over CT, CT scanning is widely accessible, convenient, and effective in revealing most brain tumors if they are large enough. The increased vessel formation or neovascularization accounts for the enhancement of these tumors and allows them to be visualized. Although its brain imaging capabilities are inferior to those of MRI, CT can identify cerebral edema, midline shift, and ventricular compression of obstructive hydrocephalus. In intraventricular masses, CT is highly sensitive in detecting calcification. CT also is better than MRI for demonstrating bone destruction. CT imaging may be needed when a patient has precautions for a magnetic study (e.g., pacemaker or other metallic implants). Intravenous contrast greatly increases the sensitivity of CT scan for brain tumors.

Once a tumor has been detected with MRI or CT, other particular parameters may help to characterize it further. For example, establishing the location of an intracranial neoplasm in either the extraaxial or intraaxial compartment is valuable in differential diagnosis.[157] For example, astrocytomas are intraaxial and meningiomas are extraaxial. The MRI or CT may detect a cleft between the brain parenchyma and the tumor, which indicates a possible extraaxial mass such as a meningioma. Resting functional MRI and connectivity mapping, a relatively new technique, demonstrate the connections between motor, premotor, and somatosensory cortex, and can be utilized in the presurgical evaluation of patients.[87] There are numerous new techniques to image tumors. Single-photon emission CT imaging uses preoperative thallium-201 emission CT in which the maximum uptake area of the brain tumor distinguishes benign from malignant tumors and localizes the area for biopsy. Iodine-123-α-methyl-L-tyrosine single-photon emission tomography imaging uses a radioisotope to distinguish glioma recurrence from benign posttherapeutic change. The positron emission tomography (PET) scan is able to localize the areas of maximum glucose utilization within a tumor, guiding the neurosurgeon to perform biopsy of locations with the most aggressive biologic behavior and differentiating viable tumor from necrosis.[29,53,115] The PET scan also maps functional areas of the brain prior to surgery or radiation so as to minimize injury to eloquent areas.[157] Fluorodeoxyglucose PET measures glucose utilization and helps to differentiate recurrent tumor from radiation necrosis. It also is not influenced by corticosteroid therapy. Echo planar MRI is a new technique of functional MRI imaging that provides maps of tumor blood flow and may allow better resolution of tumor versus surrounding edema at the tumor borders. Magnetic resonance spectroscopy may show pathologic spectra outside the area of contrast enhancement, suggesting infiltrative lesions.[105,121] More recent imaging developments include the use of diffusion tensor imaging, functional MRI, and magnetic resonance spectroscopy imaging.[76] Additional tests may be indicated to further delineate the tumor and identify possible surgical hazards. Cerebral angiography delineates the vascularity within the brain and can help determine the best surgical approach. Visual field and funduscopic examination identifies visual defects that are specific to a particular area. Audiometric studies determine hearing loss. Chest films help to rule out lung cancer with metastatic lesions to the brain, and other studies are used to rule out a primary lesion outside the brain when a metastatic lesion is suspected. Endocrine studies are done when a pituitary adenoma or craniopharyngioma is suspected.[58,102] A needle biopsy using CT-guided stereotactic (x-ray–guided) technique through a burr hole in the cranium may be performed to identify the specific tumor type and grade. A needle biopsy may not be possible, however, with vascular tumors or tumors near vital centers for fear of precipitating bleeding or respiratory distress. As tumors may have variation in grading throughout the tumor, a needle biopsy may potentially miss the higher-graded area, limiting the accuracy of the diagnosis.

MEDICAL MANAGEMENT

Surgery, radiation therapy, chemotherapy, and immunotherapy are the treatment options for brain tumors. Management of symptoms and side effects is a major component of medical management.

TREATMENT

Surgery. Surgical excision is the most important form of initial therapy, because it provides histologic confirmation of the tumor and a basis for determining the treatment and prognosis. The new stereotactic neurosurgical techniques have had a profound impact on neurosurgery efficacy and safety. Intraoperative magnification and the operating microscope have allowed stereoscopic visualization of otherwise inaccessible tissues and have reduced the morbidity and mortality of brain surgery.[115] MRI scanning combined with computer-aided navigation tools helps the neurosurgeon map the exact tumor location and track its removal during the procedure. Surgery reduces tumor load and quickly relieves the ICP and mass effect, thereby reducing symptoms and improving neurologic function. The surgical cytoreduction also enhances the effectiveness of adjuvant therapy (e.g., radiation therapy).

A traditional operative technique is the *craniotomy*, a resection of the skull overlying the tumor, removal of the tumor, and replacement of the bone flap (Fig. 30-16). *Stereotactic biopsy* of the lesion without craniotomy is used when deep mass lesions are surgically unresectable or when the risk of craniotomy outweighs the benefits. Stereotactic procedures involve creating a burr hole in the brain at an exact location using a computer, radiologic equipment, and a special head-fixation device.

The technologic and conceptual advances in neurosurgery (e.g., intraoperative magnification, ultrasonic aspirators, microinstrumentation, computer-based stereotactic resection procedures) have allowed safer and more precise approaches to previously inaccessible tumors.[134,143] Awake cortical mapping before and during surgery identifies critical areas of brain functioning to avoid and/or reduce damage to these areas.[20,41,87] Endoscopic surgery for pituitary adenomas, tumors of the orbit, vestibular (acoustic) neuromas, meningiomas, and other skull-based tumors, uses endoscopes attached to an endocamera and a video monitor system.[135] Transsphenoidal resections are possible through the nose (transnasal), which avoid an external craniotomy (Fig. 30-17). Actual short videos of endoscopic brain surgeries are available for viewing on the Internet.[71] As Figure 30-18 shows, facial craniotomy

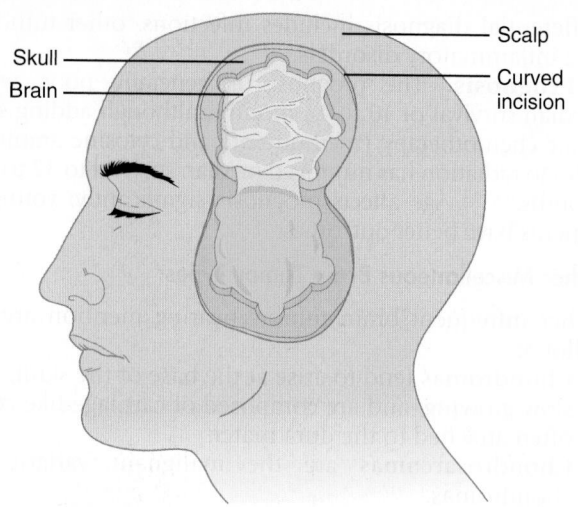

Figure 30-16

Craniotomy with osteoplastic bone flap. (From Schnell SS: Nursing care of clients with cerebral disorders. In Black JM, Matassarin-Jacobs E, eds: *Luckmann and Sorensen's medical-surgical nursing*, ed 4, Philadelphia, 1993, WB Saunders, p. 734.)

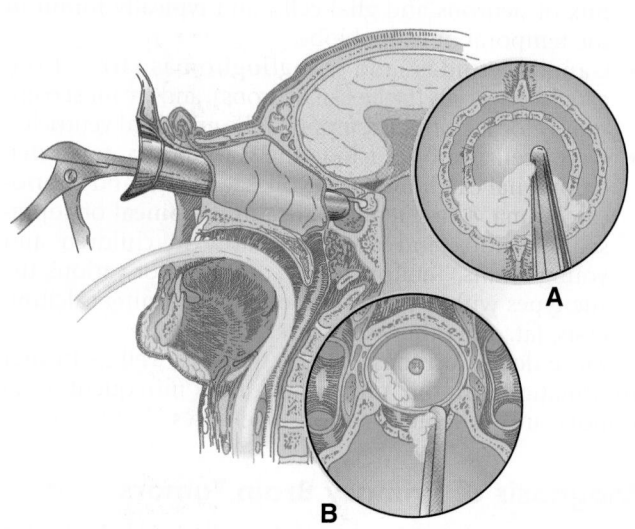

Figure 30-17

Endonasal transsphenoidal resection of the pituitary tumor. A, Removal of the sella floor with small rongeurs. **B,** Exposed inferior aspect of a pituitary adenoma. (From Tindall GT, Barrow DL: *Disorders of the pituitary,* St Louis, 1986, Mosby.)

or endoscopy utilizes incisions positioned between facial cosmetic subunits.

The goal of surgery is total excision, while minimizing trauma to vital neural structures. The survival rates of patients undergoing total resections for brain tumors are significantly higher than those of patients undergoing partial resections.[103] In infiltrative intraaxial lesions, in which total excision is not possible, the goal is to provide a measure of temporary control by reducing mass effect and ICP. If the preoperative neurologic deficit is caused by destruction of brain tissue by tumor, surgical resection will not improve the situation. In the case of many benign extraaxial tumors (e.g., meningiomas, schwannomas, pituitary adenomas), cure can be achieved.

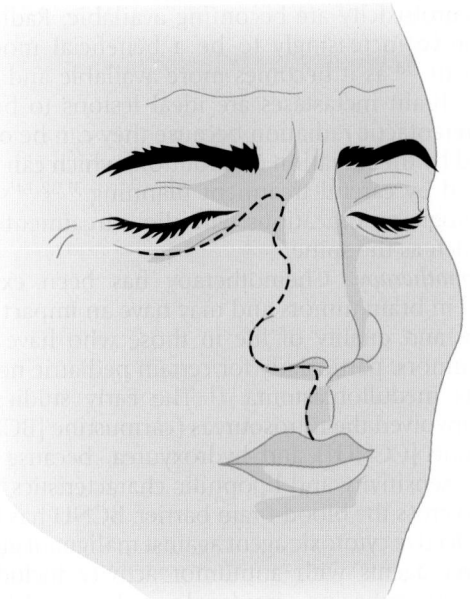

Figure 30-18

Illustration of standard location for facial incisions, with craniofacial resection completed using traditional methods. These incisions are positioned between facial cosmetic subunits *(dashed lines)*. (From Cummings CW Jr, Haughey BH, Thomas JR, et al, eds: *Cummings otolaryngology—head and neck surgery,* ed 4, Philadelphia, 2005, Mosby.)

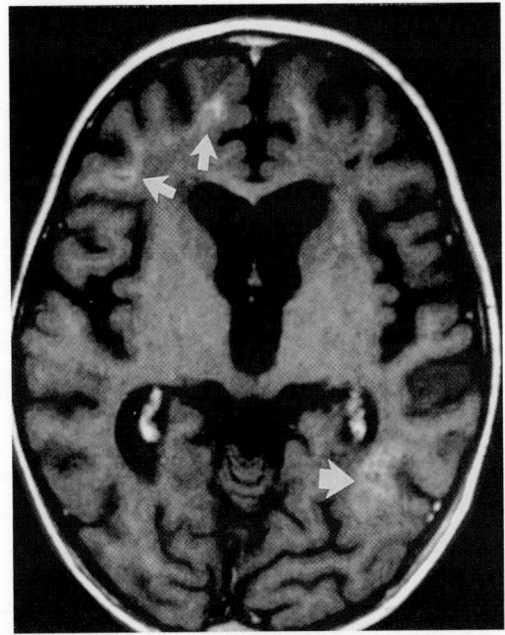

Figure 30-19

Generalized brain changes after radiotherapy. T1-weighted magnetic resonance image of a child shows both central and cortical atrophy, as well as high-signal areas *(arrows)*, owing to mineralizing microangiopathy. (From Behrman RE, Kliegman M, Jenson HB, eds: *Nelson textbook of pediatrics,* ed 17, Philadelphia, 2004, WB Saunders.)

Operative complications include hemorrhage, infection, seizures, hydrocephalus resulting from an impairment of CSF absorption, and neuroendocrine disturbances, especially if surgery is in the region of the pituitary. Brain edema, usually present before surgery, may be severely aggravated during surgery. Corticosteroids usually are given for several days before craniotomy to reduce preoperative edema. Improved surgical techniques have reduced the complications of hemorrhage, infection, and permanent neurologic injury to less than 10% of cases.[143] Postoperative survival is prolonged but complication risks increase in patients who undergo multiple cranial surgeries for brain tumors.[60]

Radiation Therapy. Radiation therapy following surgical resection is of proven effectiveness for most malignant brain tumors.[36,74] Various brain tumors have different susceptibilities to radiation therapy, but the survival advantage is unquestionable. A greater degree of tumor anaplasia and a younger age may result in a better response to radiation.[13] Unresectable or incompletely resected tumors in particular are candidates for radiation therapy. Established radiation doses that avoid exceeding thresholds of CNS tolerance are in the range of 40 to 60 Gy (4000-6000 rad). Radiation using a linear accelerator is typically given in fractionated doses five times a week over 34 to 36 weeks.

Radiation is delivered to a localized area of the brain to minimize the volume of tissue irradiated. Acute reactions to radiation are a result of acute brain swelling, occur during or immediately after radiation, and manifest as an increase in neurologic deficit or increased ICP. Steroid therapy is given to reduce this effect during radiation therapy. A similar delayed postirradiation syndrome 1 to 3 months after radiation also can be controlled by steroids. A third brain reaction known as *radiation necrosis* may occur months to years after irradiation and is severe and irreversible.[75,139] It is presumed to be the result of direct toxic effects on the brain and its microvasculature (Fig. 30-19). There is progressive deterioration, dementia, and focal neurologic signs.

As survival time increases, other long-term complications of irradiation are of concern. Hypopituitarism, radiation-induced occlusive disease of cerebral vessels, radiation-induced oncogenesis, leukoencephalopathy, and myelopathies from spinal axis irradiation are included in these complications (Fig. 30-20). White matter injuries correlate significantly with radiation dose in long-term survivors (longer than 18 months). These changes correlate with functional neurologic status,[33] including altered mental status, speech impairments, motor deficit, cranial nerve deficit, personality changes, altered memory, and other neurologic signs.[7]

Advances in radiation therapy have led to newer methods of radiation delivery. Interstitial radiation therapy, or *brachytherapy,* involves the placing of the radiation source, such as radium seeds, within the tumor for a period of several days. Brachytherapy has shown promise in treating GBM and other primary brain tumors.

Stereotactic radiosurgery is a technique to deliver a large single fraction of highly focal radiation to a brain tumor.[82] It originally was used to treat functional disorders (e.g., pain and movement disorders) but is now being used in the treatment of primary and metastatic brain tumors.[130] There are several methods: The linear accelerator–based systems, which are the most widely available, deliver high-energy photon beams using converging arcs, which intersect at the target site. Various modifications in the linear accelerator

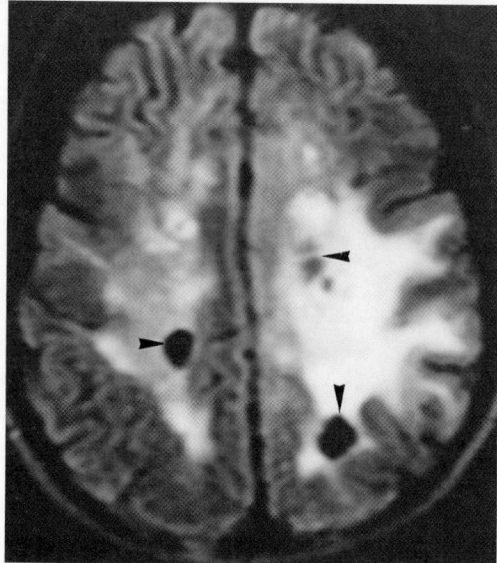

Figure 30-20

Postradiotherapy encephalopathy. Axial fluid-attenuated inversion recovery magnetic resonance image. Extensive high signal in the white matter of both cerebral hemispheres is caused by radiation-induced leukoencephalopathy. There are also areas of cystic necrosis in this case *(arrowheads)*. (From Adam A, Dixon AK, Grainger RG, et al, eds: *Grainger and Allison's diagnostic radiology: a textbook of medical imaging*, ed 4, Philadelphia, 2001, Churchill Livingstone.)

are available. Three-dimensional conformal radiation therapy allows shaping of the radiation beams to match the tumor's contours. Intensity-modulated radiation therapy is a refinement of three-dimensional conformal radiation therapy; it ensures that maximum intensity is directed at a specific site, reducing the dose to the surrounding tissues. Gamma knife radiotherapy uses high-energy photon beams from cobalt-201 sources, each directed at a specific isocenter. A halo device is attached to the skull, and the patient's head is positioned into a collimator that delivers focused gamma beams to the targeted tumor.

Synchrocyclotron proton beam therapy delivers heavy charged particle beams through a small number of portals in the skull.[143] The *CyberKnife* is a frameless robotic radiosurgical device with increased fractionation flexibility and the ability to treat extracranial lesions. It is capable of changing the target of the beam delivery instantaneously.[122,130]

In some specific primary and metastatic brain cancers, radiosurgery, instead of surgery, may be the first line of treatment. The advantages of radiosurgery compared to surgery are avoiding the risk of hemorrhage, infection, and tumor seeding; linking treatment directly to three-dimensional visualization, which reduces the chances of a marginal miss; and requiring minimal hospitalization.[63,130] The use of pegylated gold nanoparticles in animals increases survival, increases tumor cell radiosensitization, and preferentially targets tumor-associated vasculature that may be of future benefit.[69] Although gamma knife, proton beam, and CyberKnife equipment are expensive, and treatment requires collaboration between radiation oncologists and neurosurgeons, the use of these modalities is rapidly increasing, and data on their effectiveness

and neurotoxicity are becoming available. Radiotherapy may prove increasingly to be a beneficial modality of client care[108] as it becomes more available and easier to deliver. Brain metastases are ideal lesions to be treated with stereotactic radiation because they can be optimally covered by the radiation distribution, which can be easily designed by careful treatment planning.[31,32,145] In time, technologic modifications will allow treatment at other sites, such as the spine.

Chemotherapy. Chemotherapy has been extensively studied in brain tumors and may have an impact on both survival and quality of life in those who have primary brain tumors, particularly for certain pediatric neoplasms such as medulloblastoma.[143] The early studies in the 1960s involved the nitrosoureas (carmustine [BCNU] and lomustine [CCNU]) and hydroxyurea, because of their in vitro sensitivity and lipophilic characteristics allowing them to cross the blood-brain barrier. BCNU has been the most effective cytotoxic agent against malignant glioma.[157]

Newer agents with antitumor activity include diaziquone, procarbazine, imidazole carboxamide (DTIC), vincristine, cisplatin, carboplatin, tamoxifen, CPT-11 (irinotecan or Camptosar), and temozolomide (Temodar or TMZ).[115,157] TMZ is emerging as the chemotherapy drug of choice for high-grade gliomas in the adjuvant setting; it is associated with significant improvements in median progression-free survival.[9,64,137,138,142] It is thought that TMZ may be especially useful for elderly patients with glioblastomas as an alternative to radiation therapy to maintain a reasonable performance status.[22] A three-drug regimen of procarbazine, lomustine, and vincristine also benefits patients with anaplastic glioma, but offers no survival benefit for those with GBM.[115] Current clinical trials are investigating paclitaxel (Taxol), phenylacetic acid, and other novel techniques such as the thymidine-kinase gene, continuous infusion chemotherapy, and the use of antiangiogenesis drugs such as thalidomide. Trials of intracavitary placement of carmustine polymer wafers (Gliadel) are demonstrating prolonged survival without the systemic side effects of chemotherapy.[157] Targeting vascular endothelial cell growth factor with agents such as bevacizumab has demonstrated promising results.[120] To bypass the blood-brain barrier, intrathecal delivery (through an Ommaya reservoir surgically placed in the scalp with its tube inserted into the lateral ventricle) can be done. Another technique is an intraarterial (intracarotid) delivery allowing much higher concentration of drugs such as methotrexate, vincristine, or cisplatin than intravenous injection allows, which overcomes molecular resistance. Intrathecal chemotherapy may be given when leptomeningeal involvement occurs with tumor or to increase the CSF concentration. Addition of chemotherapy to surgery and irradiation for malignant gliomas does provide some increases in 24-month survival, up to 23.4% from 15.9%.[143]

Hormonal Therapy. Hormonal therapy is often used to treat functioning pituitary tumors. Dopamine agonists are used to control the production of prolactin. Somatostatin analogues are used to reduce growth hormone levels and relieve the associated symptoms. If satisfactory results are achieved, surgery and/or radiation may not be necessary.

Immunotherapy. Immunotherapy or biotherapy is the most infrequently used and least-proven therapy for brain

Table 30-5	Emergency Treatment of Elevated Intracranial Pressure in Acutely Decompensating Patients		
Therapy	**Treatment**	**Onset (Duration of Action)**	**Other**
Hyperventilation	Lower $PaCO_2$ to 25-30 mm Hg	Seconds (minutes)	Usually requires intubation and mechanical ventilation
Osmotherapy	Mannitol 0.5-2 g/kg IV, repeat as necessary	Minutes (hours)	Brisk diuresis Requires Foley catheter Strict attention to electrolytes
Corticosteroids	Dexamethasone 50-100 mg IV, followed by 50-100 mg/day in divided doses	Hours (days)	Most effective on vasogenic edema (tumors, abscesses) Less effective on cytotoxic edema (stroke)

IV, Intravenous; $PaCO_2$, arterial partial pressure of carbon dioxide.
From DeAngelis, LM, Tumors of the central nervous system. In Goldman LM, Ausiello D, eds: *Cecil textbook of medicine*, ed 22, Philadelphia, 2004, WB Saunders.

tumors. Immunotherapy, originally the use of donor serum containing preformed antibodies, now includes the use of interferons and interleukin-2 (see "Interferons" in Chapter 7 and "Immunotherapy" in Chapter 9) to boost immune function.[58] The depressed immunocompetence of clients with malignant glioma gives at least a theoretical basis for the potential roles of biologic response modifiers in the treatment of these tumors. Preliminary studies show some promise.[143] Many advances have occurred in immunotherapy and hold promise as advances in surgery, radiation therapy, and chemotherapy have been modest.[10]

Symptom Management. Brain tumors lead to edema of tissue surrounding the tumor, and brain swelling can be massive and extend the neurologic deficits caused by the tumor alone. Antiinflammatory drugs (corticosteroids, such as dexamethasone [Decadron], prednisone, hydrocortisone) are used to provide prompt and effective reduction in peritumoral edema. Improvement in symptoms of ICP and in focal neurologic signs begins within 24 to 48 hours after steroid initiation, and by the fourth and fifth day the maximum degree of improvement is obtained.[157]

Corticosteroids generally are used perioperatively and are tapered gradually after tumor resection, because long-term high-dose corticosteroids precipitate undesirable side effects. Corticosteroids also may be used periirradiation because radiation also precipitates edema. Upon tumor recurrence or progression, corticosteroids may again be instituted to temporarily maximize residual neurologic function.

It is possible for a brain tumor to cause an acute increase in ICP that may be life-threatening because of imminent cerebral herniation. Emergency treatment is required if ICP reaches 20 mm Hg or more. Quick-acting agents are needed to lower the pressure. Mannitol is used as a temporary agent to quickly reduce brain water and relieve the pressure. Steroids are used in conjunction with mannitol to decrease edema. Table 30-5 lists emergency treatments for elevated ICP in acutely decompensating patients.

Anticonvulsants also may be needed to prevent or control seizure activity. These drugs also are used before and after surgery to control symptoms and are continued as long as they are indicated.[29] One of the most common anticonvulsant therapies used today in the brain tumor population is phenytoin (Dilantin).[107]

Brain tumors also cause a variety of motor, speech, hearing, visual, and other neurologic signs and symptoms. Although control of the tumor and edema through medical management is the first priority, residual neurologic problems can significantly lower the quality of life. Timely referral to rehabilitation specialists for management of these functional deficits can improve performance status and quality of life. Strengthening, motor and balance evaluation and training, splinting, bracing, fatigue and pain management, incontinence training, home adaptation, activities of daily living retraining, speech therapy, hearing adaptations, auditory retraining, and vision programs are available to improve and alleviate these functional deficits.

Other specialists are also part of the rehabilitation team. Pharmacists provide assistance with pain management; the oncology nurse provides symptom management, psychosocial support, and education; the nutritionist provides diet and nutrition counseling; the social worker assists with community resources and placement in settings for necessary further care; and clergy provide assistance with personal and spiritual issues.

The psychosocial implications of brain tumors are enormous. Referral to psychooncology specialists for alleviation of psychologic distress and family disruption, and promotion of role reorganization and adaptation are often of great value. Brain tumor support groups, psychotropic medications, oncology educational classes for the client and family, and enrollment in one-on-one support programs can be very helpful. Survivors of childhood tumors may experience neurocognitive effects that may manifest after many years; surveillance for these problems is paramount.[25]

SPECIAL IMPLICATIONS FOR THE THERAPIST 30-1

Primary Brain Tumors
Rehabilitation Referrals

Therapists will undoubtedly encounter clients with brain tumors in any practice arena because of the significant neuromuscular and cardiopulmonary impairments. Neurologic or orthopedic practices may see patients with brain tumors presenting with gait and balance instability or cervical pain. When the signs and symptoms of a yet undiagnosed brain tumor bring the person to therapy (e.g., unsteady gait and poor balance, weakness), differential diagnosis skills are needed by the therapist to determine a cluster of signs and symptoms indicating a possible tumor, such as headache, nausea and vomiting, lethargy, and so on (refer to Boxes 30-2 and 30-3 and Table 30-3) or a progression of symptoms despite physical therapy intervention requiring referral to the physician.

Knowledge Needed for Rehabilitation

Brain tumor studies are beginning to demonstrate rehabilitation effectiveness.[16,52] As the survival of those with brain tumors increases, rehabilitation needs become more prominent.[16] A general knowledge of primary brain tumor and medical treatment is needed to provide the therapist with skills for differential diagnosis, examination and evaluation, treatment planning, and goal setting. Knowledge of malignant versus benign status, disease progression, expectations, complications, prognosis, and precautions such as seizures and deep vein thromboses (DVTs) are needed to plan intervention and establish goals. The therapist should also be aware of expected focal symptoms in relation to tumor location to anticipate functional changes that may require treatment modifications, as well as possible paraneoplastic syndromes that may complicate rehabilitation. In geriatric populations, managing the patient with brain cancer may require comprehensive geriatric assessment to identify comorbidities.[11,12]

It is important to be able to distinguish between a meningioma (a benign, potentially curable tumor) and a malignant glioma (a rapidly growing fatal tumor) in order to set goals, to interact with the family, and to provide appropriate intervention. The advancements in brain tumor medical management (e.g., the promising effectiveness of TMZ for malignant gliomas) and the developing preciseness of radiation therapy brings longer survival and opportunities for better quality of life.[137] The therapist must be aware, prepared, and hopeful that, as the demand for rehabilitation grows, the rehabilitation outcomes will improve.

In addition, knowledge of medical treatment complications from surgery, radiation, chemotherapy, and other interventions will give the therapist the ability to adjust the rehabilitation program as needed, to accommodate, for example, myelosuppression from chemotherapy or fatigue from radiation therapy. Overall, the fact that there are no randomized or controlled clinical trials existing for best evidence to support multidisciplinary rehabilitation after treatment of brain tumors highlights the challenge of design, rigor, and outcome measurements in this population.[73]

Acute Postoperative Management

When a referral is received for acute postoperative rehabilitation therapy, awareness of general postoperative complications, including atelectasis, pneumonia, cardiac arrhythmias, fluid and electrolyte imbalances, infection, meningitis, intracranial hemorrhage, and renal and gastrointestinal disorders, is important. Potential symptoms after brain surgery include confusion, pain, weakness, and headache. Observing the client closely during therapy intervention for any significant signs and symptoms, and making appropriate adaptations during therapy, are part of the role of the therapist.[127]

Postoperative Complications of Intracranial Surgery

Potential complications of intracranial surgery may be very serious, even fatal, because of the significant functions performed by the structures involved. Some postoperative complications may improve; others may be permanent.

Increased ICP (resulting from cerebral edema or bleeding) is the major complication of intracranial surgery. Findings may include decreased level of consciousness with headaches, visual and speech disturbances, muscle weakness or paralysis, pupil changes, seizures, vomiting, and respiratory changes (see Box 30-3). Approximately 50% of primary pediatric brain tumors will present with hydrocephalus; shunting is often necessary during surgical resection.[159]

In at-risk patients, there are several methods that can be used to continuously measure ICP, including intraventricular catheters, subarachnoid or subdural screws or bolts, epidural sensors, and intraparenchymal catheters. Other monitored parameters include mixed venous oxygen saturation (SvO_2) and jugular oxygen saturation (SjO_2), which reflects oxygen saturation of the blood returning from the brain. Normal ICP ranges from 0 to 15 mm Hg, with a midrange of 8 mm Hg and fluctuations occurring with active movement of the extremities and trunk, coughing, suctioning, noxious touch, and other physical stress maneuvers. Use of pleasant sensations, such as music and therapeutic touch, to reduce ICP are being investigated. Sustained ICP above 20 mm Hg requires emergency treatment. A therapist noting a rise in ICP above 15 mm Hg should contact the nurse or physician.

Because of increased ICP, further surgical intervention may be needed to release excess fluid. A catheter may be inserted to drain excess fluid from a ventricle or other fluid-filled space, called a shunt, or a Jackson-Pratt suction drain may be needed. CSF postoperative leaks are evidenced by saturation of the surgical head dressing or leaking of a clear, thin fluid from the ear or nose that dries in concentric circles.

Management of the postoperative client with increased ICP typically includes, among other things, elevation of the head to about 20 to 30 degrees is often prescribed. The client should be protected from any position that allows stasis of the CSF drainage and should be taught to observe the drainage and to be aware of signs of infection. The client also should be instructed against coughing, sneezing, or blowing the nose. An erratic body temperature may occur after intracranial surgery. Either hypothermia or hyperthermia may be present. The therapist should check with the nursing staff before beginning therapy if concern exists regarding abnormal temperature.

DVT occurs in one-third of patients who have surgery. Seizures,[59] CSF leakage, and wound infection are also risks. Periocular edema is common, as are temporary visual field deficits. Patients may have other temporary deficits resulting from cerebral edema, such as communication, motor, and sensory deficits; diminished gag and swallowing reflexes; diplopia; loss of corneal reflex; and personality changes.[58] *Pneumocystis carinii* pneumonia (PCP) is a life-threatening opportunistic infection that occurs in immunocompromised hosts, such as with corticosteroid used. Signs of PCP are fever and dyspnea with or without a prominent dry cough, though the onset may be subtle. The risk of PCP is increased while steroids are being tapered.[107,126]

Meningitis also may occur, caused by irritation of the meninges by infection or blood in the subarachnoid space. If it develops, meningitis typically appears 2 or 3 days after surgery. Chills, fever, nuchal rigidity, headache, irritability, increased sensitivity to light, and decreased level of consciousness are signs of meningitis. Other signs to be aware of include ecchymosis, stress ulcer, swallowing difficulties and aspiration, and impaired airway. Respiratory changes should be monitored carefully. An abnormal respiratory rate and depth may indicate rising ICP. By carefully observing the client during therapy, protecting the client from harm, and alerting medical staff of seizure activity or other adverse signs and symptoms, the therapist can provide a valuable adjunct to postoperative care.

Positioning in the Acute Postoperative Phase

If there is any question about positioning of a client during therapy, the therapist should communicate with the nursing staff. Incorrect positioning may have serious, possibly fatal, consequences. In the acute phase after surgery above the tentorium, orders may be given to avoid lowering the head, to avoid extreme flexion of the legs, and to keep the neck in a neutral position. After surgery below the tentorium, the client may be kept flat and turned every 2 hours or have orders for elevation of the head of the bed. It is recommended that the neck not be angulated anteriorly or laterally, but there are usually no restrictions placed on turning. For infratentorial tumors that may cause dizziness on arising, elevating the head of bed gradually while concurrently monitoring vital signs is recommended. The dizziness is caused by transient edema in the area of the eighth cranial nerve. For posterior fossa surgery, the client is typically positioned on the side with a pillow under the head. This protects the operative site from pressure and minimizes tension on the suture line.[58]

If a bone flap was removed for decompression, the orders may be to place the client only on the nonoperated side or the back. This facilitates brain expansion. If a large tumor has been removed from a cerebral hemisphere, there may be an order to avoid positioning on the operative site to prevent shifting of the cranial contents because of gravity.

If a client is neurologically unstable, and with ICP in a critical range (more than 20 mm Hg), therapy procedures that require a flat position (e.g., lowering the head of the bed for range-of-motion exercises) should be avoided. Placing a pillow under the head facilitates good venous outflow. When the client is side lying, protecting the hips from sharp flexion avoids an increase in intrathoracic pressure, which can in turn increase cerebral ICP.

Intervention Preparation

Before physical therapy intervention, examination should include a review of the medical chart. If indicated, physicians should be contacted for pertinent information and guidelines. Hematologic values may be of critical importance for exercise training plans. Anemia causes fatigue, leukopenia increases infection susceptibility, and thrombocytopenia increases bleeding susceptibility and is of particular concern because it may lead to intracranial hemorrhage.[105,107]

Familiarity with cancer terminology and the behavior of the particular tumor aids communication with others on the team. For example, knowledge of tumor staging and grading, the prognosis, the medical management such as the surgical procedure, presence of an Ommaya reservoir, and the various types of central lines and monitoring devices facilitate interdisciplinary care planning and intervention. Knowledge of the Karnofsky scale (Table 30-6), a functional performance scale used by many oncologists to indicate the client's activity level in the hospital, home, or community, is helpful. It can facilitate communication among the team on issues such as a client's candidacy for home discharge with home health assistance or need for more supervised care. The ECOG (Eastern Cooperative Oncology Group) 1 to 4 scale is another tool that may be used to identify functional performance.

Initial outcomes expected for clients with brain surgery include full range of motion, active where possible, of all extremities and optimal functioning of respiratory, cardiovascular, and other systems within the precautions indicated. When the client's condition is stable, functional outcomes include independent bed mobility and transfers, ambulation, and self-care skills (activities of daily living).

Rehabilitation Examination for Postoperative Care

During the acute postoperative phase, a thorough examination within the constraints of the precautions, including strength, joint range of motion, sensory and perceptual status, neurologic signs, pain patterns, presence of fatigue, and mobility, helps to identify treatable impairments that affect function.[91] During examination and intervention, the therapist should avoid any Valsalva maneuver that would increase intrathoracic pressure, thus increasing ICP.

Rehabilitation Intervention

After intracranial surgery bed rest precautions may initiated, usually for 24 hours, and should be observed by the therapist. If the client is stable, passive range of motion exercises may begin.

Table 30-6	Karnofsky Performance Status Scale	
Condition	**Percentage**	**Comments**
Able to carry on normal activity and to work. No special care is needed.	100	Normal; no complaints; no evidence of disease
	90	Able to carry on normal activity; minor signs or symptoms of disease
	80	Normal activity with effort; some signs or symptoms of disease
Unable to work. Able to live at home, care for most of personal needs. A varying degree of assistance is needed.	70	Cares for self; unable to carry on normal activity or to do active work
	60	Requires occasional assistance but is able to care for most needs
	50	Requires considerable assistance and frequent medical care
Unable to care for self. Requires equivalent of institutional or hospital care. Disease may be progressing rapidly.	40	Disabled; requires special care and assistance
	30	Severely disabled; hospitalization is indicated, although death is not imminent
	20	Hospitalization is necessary; very sick; active supportive treatment necessary
	10	Moribund; fatal processes progressing rapidly
	1	Unconscious
	0	Dead

From Baird SB, McCorkle R, Grant M: *Cancer nursing: a comprehensive textbook*, Philadelphia, Saunders, 1991.

Position changes are important, and use of a draw sheet and adequate help ensure that the patient will not strain with position change and increase ICP. When movement to the bedside chair is safe but ICP precautions preclude active supine to sitting movements, lifting the client to a reclining chair by a draw sheet with the help of several caregivers and then gradually raising the client's back and head in the chair protects him or her from straining. Bedside sit-and-dangle exercises also may be requested. Blood pressure checks for postural hypotension, close assessment for dizziness and faintness, and monitoring of respiratory rate, heart rate, and ICP during activities are essential. General conditioning activities early in the recovery are valuable to address the fatigue cycle typical of cancer.

Subacute and Ambulatory Rehabilitation

As the patient becomes more stable and is moved into lower levels of acuity, including inpatient and ambulatory care, continued monitoring is imperative. The therapist must monitor vital signs and observe for any neurologic change; any adverse indications such as seizures, bleeding at the operative site, or signs of a DVT; or sudden changes in mental status.

Medical treatment modalities and side effects have a pronounced effect on the client's participation in therapy. Chemotherapeutic and radiation side effects, such as myelosuppression, nausea, and fatigue, may temporarily lower energy levels, requiring adjustment of the therapy program. Irradiated areas should be protected against skin injury. No heat or cold or topical agents should be used in the irradiated area during the treatment series or for several weeks after the treatment series until the skin damage has cleared. The radiation oncologist will determine the topical agent(s) to be used. If persistent trophic change occurs to the skin with obvious circulatory impairment, heat or cold should not be applied over the site because of poor dissipation effects.

Examination and intervention are based on the impairments and disabilities identified. Safety in mobility, gait and balance training, protection from falls, strengthening, equipment decisions, functional training and aerobic capacity training are important rehabilitation interventions.[155] Written educational materials are increasingly requested.

The efficacy of increasing the activity level has been demonstrated, and functional training, gait training, and exercise are well-accepted postoperative interventions.[117] Long-term management may include family training and education and more advanced treatment aimed at self-care and safety, return to family roles, and work and leisure activity.

More attention is being paid at the present time to cancer-related fatigue, identifying possible causes such as myelosuppression, anorexia, pain, sleep deprivation, and somnolence. Treatment modalities including surgery, radiation therapy, and chemotherapy are associated with fatigue. Understanding fatigue and the ameliorating factors is increasingly becoming the subject of studies. In a recent glioblastoma study, fatigue was associated with decreases in almost all aspects of quality of life.[86] Addressing fatigue with a structured progressive exercise program has some efficacy.[38,39,99,128] Although there is no consensus on the ideal type of exercise, frequency, intensity, duration, or mode, there is good cardiopulmonary response to interval training at 50% to 70% of heart rate reserve or working at an exertion level of 11 to 14 on the 6 to 20 rate of perceived exertion scale. While treatment is being given, most studies recommend decreasing the intensity to the lower end of the heart rate range.[30] Some studies suggest careful monitoring to avoid overstressing the immune system.[109] Other problems associated with fatigue should be addressed as they occur.[123] Throughout the rehabilitation process, activities that increase ICP, such as vigorous resistive exercises or isometrics, should be avoided.

Studies support the benefits of comprehensive and interdisciplinary rehabilitation for patients with primary and metastatic brain tumors.[62,100,107] Outcomes of physical therapy intervention may be measured by standardized tools, such as the Karnofsky scale, the European Organization for Research and Treatment of Cancer Quality of Life Questionnaire 30 (EORTCQ-30), the Psychosocial Adjustment to Illness Scale, the Functional Living Index—Cancer (FLIC) Scale, the Functional Assessment of Cancer Therapy—Brain (FACT) tool,[48,89] and the Functional Assessment of Chronic Illness Therapy (FACIT) Scale. Fatigue measures include the 1 to 10 analogue scale, the Brief Fatigue Inventory (BFI),[21] the Piper Fatigue Scale, and numerous other new fatigue measures. Some studies have used the Functional Independence Measure (FIM) to evaluate changes in function with inpatient rehabilitation[62,89,100,105] and have demonstrated improvements. Considerations of quality of life are increasingly part of medical oncologic studies.

Steroid Effects

Corticosteroids are prescribed during surgery and again during radiation to reduce cerebral edema. Long-term effects include many adverse problems, including proximal weakness, behavioral changes, osteoporosis, increased appetite, bloating, hypertension, and many more. Long-term steroid use is avoided, and the drugs are typically discontinued after the acute surgical or radiation management is completed. However, with steroid tapering and discontinuation, there may be a possible increase in cerebral edema and a recurrence of symptoms previously present before surgery or radiation. For example, a person receiving brain radiation taking dexamethasone during the radiation series may demonstrate improved hemiparesis as a result of the steroid. However, when radiation therapy is completed and steroid therapy is tapered and discontinued, the hemiparesis may worsen. The therapist needs to be aware of decreasing function related to steroid tapering during this time and report it to the physician. The decision may be made to continue the steroid at a low dose. If corticosteroids are tapered too rapidly after surgery or radiation therapy, causing peritumoral edema, a bolus dose of dexamethasone followed by a more gradual weaning schedule may alleviate the symptoms.[49] Edema fluctuations from the tumor effect itself may cause a puzzling improvement and regression in neurologic status. Mobility issues and goals should be planned with the client and family, keeping in mind this potential of variable symptoms from edema fluctuations. The therapist must avoid creating either false hope or pessimism when patient performance varies because of edema fluctuations.

Psychosocial Impact

The impact of the diagnosis may be difficult for the client to comprehend. The client who does comprehend may demonstrate extreme behavioral responses or a profound sense of hopelessness. The client should be encouraged to ask questions and express his or her feelings about the situation. Depression is difficult to distinguish from apathy caused by the brain tumor,[68] but a differential diagnosis, if possible, through depression testing, is important to help the therapist to advocate for improved management of depression. Managing cognitive effects of radiation therapy is difficult for the client and family.[27,123] The caregiver's support, realistic reassurance, and inclusion of the client and family in the decision-making process will have a positive impact on the quality of life.[58]

Because the diagnosis of a brain tumor is so devastating to the client and family, causing fear and uncertainty, the therapist must have sufficient maturity and psychosocial skills to be supportive and understanding. The challenge is not necessarily to provide solutions to these psychosocial problems but to provide support and validation and to facilitate referrals to appropriate professionals while addressing the physical problem for which the person was referred.

The Rehabilitation Team

The therapist involved in rehabilitation of the person with a brain tumor is part of a rehabilitation team of professionals. The team may include representatives from nursing, nutrition, respiratory therapy, speech therapy, social work, psychology, the chaplain's office, durable medical equipment suppliers, hospice staff, and the physician office staff. An interdisciplinary approach allows access to needed resources.

The therapist must understand that the term *cancer rehabilitation* is used by many specialists and community programs that provide services for the person with cancer and may mean different things in different contexts. Oncology nurses are increasingly supportive of cancer rehabilitation and an interdisciplinary approach,[92] and include symptom control and psychosocial issues in their definition of rehabilitation. Many local groups, such as church and synagogue support groups, provide another aspect of rehabilitation. The National Cancer Institute has identified four objectives for cancer rehabilitation: psychologic support, optimal physical functioning, vocational counseling, and optimal social functioning.[94] Financial issues, nutrition, spousal relationships, sexual counseling, vocational rehabilitation, employment opportunities, physician–patient communication, patient education, and coping skills are broader aspects of rehabilitation.

In some acute care and outpatient settings, the therapist may be fortunate enough to be part of a more formalized cancer rehabilitation program that includes these facets of rehabilitation. The advantages for the client with access to such a program include early and appropriate referrals to skilled professionals and resources, coordination of care and information, and a smooth transition across the continuum of care. Other benefits include enhancement of program

Intraspinal location and relative incidence of spinal tumors

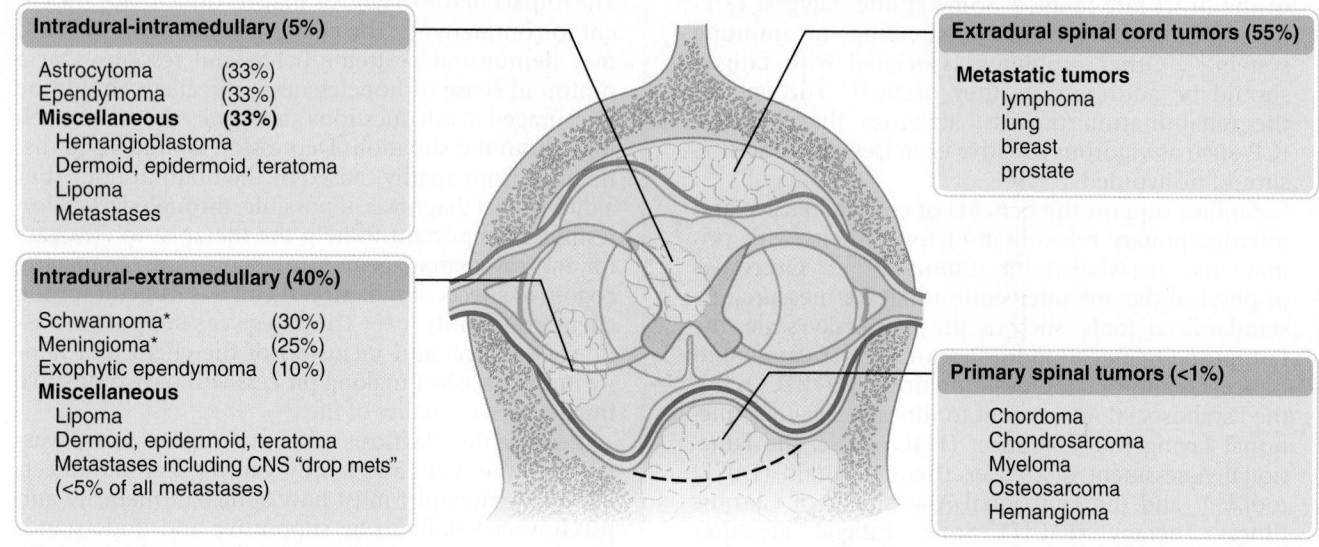

Intradural-intramedullary (5%)	
Astrocytoma	(33%)
Ependymoma	(33%)
Miscellaneous	**(33%)**
Hemangioblastoma	
Dermoid, epidermoid, teratoma	
Lipoma	
Metastases	

Extradural spinal cord tumors (55%)
Metastatic tumors
lymphoma
lung
breast
prostate

Intradural-extramedullary (40%)	
Schwannoma*	(30%)
Meningioma*	(25%)
Exophytic ependymoma	(10%)
Miscellaneous	
Lipoma	
Dermoid, epidermoid, teratoma	
Metastases including CNS "drop mets" (<5% of all metastases)	

Primary spinal tumors (<1%)
Chordoma
Chondrosarcoma
Myeloma
Osteosarcoma
Hemangioma

*Can be partially or wholly extradural

Figure 30-21

Primary and metastatic tumors of the spine and spinal cord. (Adapted from Poirier J, Gray F, Escourelle R: *Manual of basic neuropathology*, ed 2, Philadelphia, 1990, WB Saunders.)

development resulting from collaboration of professionals, outcome studies that will improve the quality of care, and the potential for rehabilitation research.

PRIMARY INTRASPINAL TUMORS

Primary spinal cord tumors are about one-sixth as common as primary brain tumors. The histologic types of tumor cells in the spinal cord are the same as those found in the brain, although the prevalence of certain types may differ. The most common tumor in the spinal cord is the schwannoma or neurinoma, followed by the meningioma and glioma.[97]

A convenient anatomic classification system of spinal cord tumors is based on the relationship of the tumor to the spinal cord and dura. Figure 30-21 diagrams the location and relative incidence of spinal tumors. Intradural–intramedullary tumors arise within the spinal cord substance. Intradural–extramedullary tumors arise outside the spinal cord but within the dura. Extradural spinal cord tumors arise outside the spinal cord and the dura (Fig. 30-22).[143] The specific spinal cord tumor types and their incidence are discussed first, followed by the clinical presentation and medical management.

Intradural–Intramedullary Tumors

Incidence

Intradural–intramedullary (within the dura, within the cord) tumors are the least-common type of primary intraspinal tumors in adults, but the most common type in children. These tumors account for 5% to 10% of intraspinal tumors. The dominant tumor types are astrocytomas and ependymomas.[152]

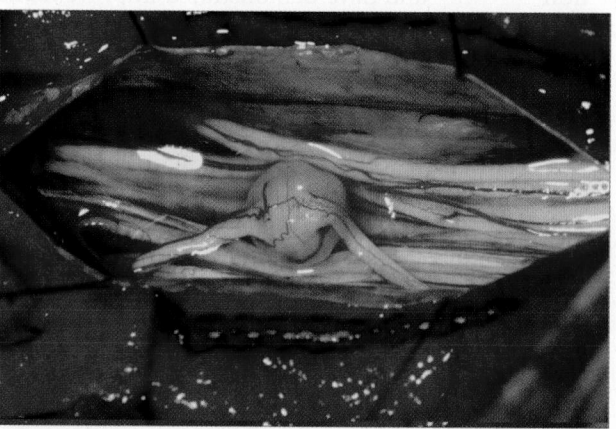

Figure 30-22

Spinal-cord neoplasms are extradural or intradural tumors according to their relation to the thecal sac. (From *Lancet Oncol* 8[1], 2007.)

Pathogenesis

Because they are located within the cord itself, intradural–intramedullary tumors generally are derived from the cellular substrate of the spinal cord, such as the astrocytes and ependymal cells, or from the primitive embryonal cells. Astrocytomas may occur anywhere along the spinal cord and may span several cord segments longitudinally. In children they may run the entire length of the cord.

Although all astrocytomas are infiltrative, most are low grade and slow growing in the spinal cord. Ependymomas are generally slow growing as well and less infiltrative, and therefore more amenable to surgical excision. Other less-frequent types of intradural–intramedullary tumors are hemangiomas, epidermoid and dermoid cysts, teratomas, lipomas, and neuroenteric cysts. Of interest to therapists is chemical meningitis with its significant chronic pain that can occur when epidermoid or dermoid cysts leak debris into the CSF. Very infrequently, a primary intramedullary spinal lymphoma (PCNSL) may occur.[15,144]

Intradural–Extramedullary Tumors

Incidence

Intradural–extramedullary (within the dura, outside the cord) tumors are the most-common type of primary intraspinal tumor in adults, and they account for approximately 45% of all spinal tumors. Neurinomas (schwannomas) and meningiomas are the dominant tumors in this group. Meningiomas are 10 times more common in women than in men and occur in middle age.[152]

Pathogenesis

Intradural–extramedullary tumors are primarily derived from the supporting elements of the CNS, including the meninges and nerve sheath. Occasionally, tumors in this compartment are carried down as drop metastases by the CSF from malignant brain tumors (medulloblastomas, less commonly ependymomas and PNETs). Figure 30-23 shows a PNET in the brain and spinal cord surfaces. Intradural-extramedullary tumors cause compression of the spinal cord, rather than invasion of the cord. Neurinomas are soft, globular masses that arise at the sensory or dorsal nerve root. Occasionally they may straddle the intervertebral foramen and extend outside the foramen, in the so-called *dumbbell configuration*. Spinal meningiomas are benign, slow-growing globular tumors that often grow in the thoracic, cervical, and foramen magnum regions. They may be present for many years before symptoms occur.

Extradural–Extramedullary Tumors

Incidence

Extradural–extramedullary tumors are most often metastatic tumors and are addressed in "Metastatic Tumors" below. Extradural–extramedullary tumors represent approximately 45% of all spinal cord tumors. An occasional meningioma, neurinoma (schwannoma), or spinal chordoma arises extradurally. Spinal chordomas represent less than 1% of spinal cord tumors.[152]

Pathogenesis

Spinal chordomas are primary tumors that arise from the vertebral bodies, usually in the cervical or sacral regions of the axial skeleton. They are prone to metastasize outside the spinal column. Lesions are characterized by expansive destruction of the bone, for example, the sacrum, or by varying degrees of vertebral collapse. Box 30-4 summarizes the type and location of spinal tumors.

Clinical Manifestations of Primary Intraspinal Tumors

Spontaneous pain caused by nerve root irritation is a common clinical feature of primary spinal tumors and is usually worse at night. Intramedullary tumors give rise to a poorly localized, deep, burning type of pain in the spinal region. Extramedullary tumors produce a knife-like radicular type of pain typically radiating to the periphery

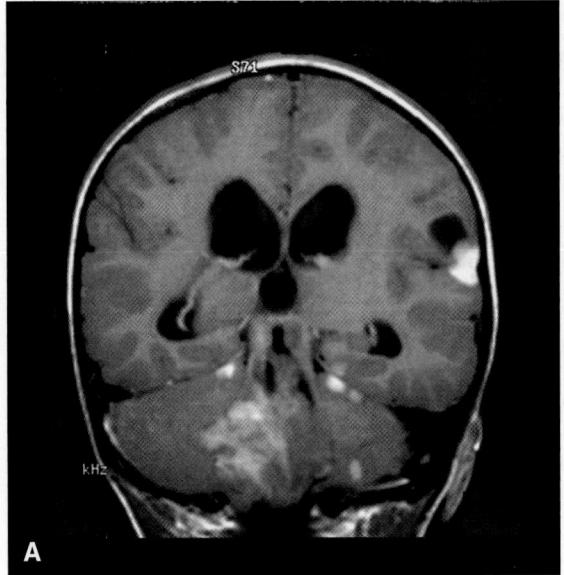

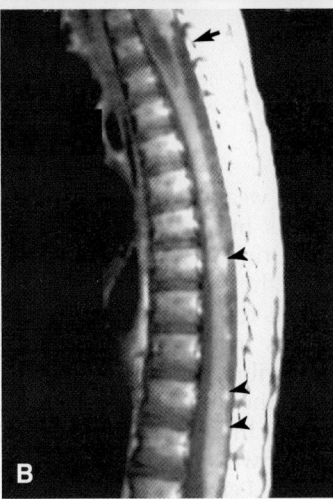

Figure 30-23

Primitive neuroectodermal tumor (PNET). A, T1-weighted coronal MRI scan after injection of contrast medium in a 5-year-old boy. There is a large multifocal tumor in the posterior fossa causing hydrocephalus. There are multiple smaller, contrast-enhancing, tumors along the surface of cerebellum and in the cerebrum. **B,** A T1-weighted sagittal postcontrast MRI scan of the spinal canal shows a large mass *(arrow)* in the junction of the cervical and thoracic spine with a syrinx and multiple small enhancing nodules *(arrowheads)* over the surface of the spinal cord. (From Adam A, Dixon AK, Grainger RG, et al, eds: *Grainger and Allison's diagnostic radiology: a textbook of medical imaging,* ed 4, Philadelphia, 2001, Churchill Livingstone.)

of the nerve, often aggravated by coughing, sneezing, or straining. The association of asymmetry of reflexes with nerve root pain and an insidious onset is strongly suggestive of a spinal cord tumor.

Nerve root pain may be followed by motor weakness of muscles supplied by the nerve. The motor changes of intramedullary tumors include lower motor neuron changes at the level of the lesion and may also include upper motor neuron changes at lower levels. The motor changes of extramedullary lesions begin with segmental weakness at the lesion site and may progress to a Brown-Séquard syndrome or later to a transverse cord

Box 30-4

SPINAL TUMORS

Extradural

- Metastasis
- Primary bone tumors arising in the spine

Intradural and Extramedullary

- Meningiomas
- Neurofibromas
- Neurinomas (schwannomas)
- Lipomas
- Arachnoid cysts
- Epidermoid cysts
- Metastasis

Intramedullary

- Ependymoma
- Glioma
- Hemangioblastoma
- Lipoma
- Metastasis

From DeAngelis LM: Tumors of the central nervous system. In Goldman LM, Ausiello D, eds: *Cecil textbook of medicine*, ed 22, Philadelphia, 2004, WB Saunders.

Box 30-5

SIGNS AND SYMPTOMS OF SPINAL CORD TUMORS

- Pain
- Weakness
- Sensory changes
- Urinary frequency
- Urinary urgency
- Sphincter disturbances
- Syringomyelia-like symptoms
- Brown-Séquard syndrome–like symptoms
- Hydrocephalus
- Increased intracranial pressure
- Papilledema
- Atrophy
- Hyporeflexia
- Spasticity
- Hyperreflexia
- Gait disturbances
- Sexual dysfunction

syndrome.[143] The weakness is characterized by upper motor neuron signs, including spasticity. Sphincter weakness, increasing urinary frequency, and urgency may develop. In men, the development of sphincter disturbances frequently is followed by impotence.

Sensory changes in extramedullary tumors are usually along the distribution of the involved nerve roots. Intramedullary tumors result in dissociated sensory disturbances in the limbs below the level of the lesion because of their growth pattern of crossing fibers of the spinothalamic tract. People often report a feeling of temperature change, particularly a feeling of cold below the level of the lesion. Pain and temperature sensation are compromised, but proprioception and light touch may be preserved.

Syringomyelia-like symptoms of loss of pain and temperature sensation below the level of the lesion on one or both sides of the body may occur from damage to the decussating lateral spinothalamic fibers. This often is accompanied by progressive spastic paraparesis caused by pressure on the descending corticospinal tracts. Anterior growth of the tumor produces anterior horn signs, such as muscle weakness, wasting, and fasciculations in the muscles supplied by the anterior horn cells.

Other symptoms of intramedullary cord tumors are papilledema, hydrocephalus, and elevations in ICP. The reason for development of papilledema is unclear, but it is more common with tumors of the thoracic and lumbosacral regions. Box 30-5 lists signs and symptoms of spinal cord tumors.

MEDICAL MANAGEMENT

DIAGNOSIS. After a history and neurologic examination, MRI is the method of choice for the identification of spinal cord tumors. Gadolinium-enhanced MRI is helpful to differentiate between edema and tumor. Occasionally

plain films may be helpful in treatment planning. Lumbar puncture and CSF examination are no longer used as diagnostic tools.

TREATMENT AND PROGNOSIS. Surgery is the principal treatment for all primary intraspinal tumors. Complete and curative resection is the objective. Radiation therapy is not required when lesions are completely excised. Intraspinal astrocytomas have a lower rate of cure, although surgery and radiation may prolong the disease-free survival. Childhood astrocytomas, however, have a more favorable prognosis, with a 5-year survival rate of 90%.

SPECIAL IMPLICATIONS FOR THE THERAPIST 30-2

Primary Intraspinal Tumors
Alertness to Signs and Symptoms

As specialists in motor function, therapists may be involved even before a diagnosis of cancer has been made in observing and identifying the signs of spinal cord tumors. Clients referred to physical therapy because of back pain symptoms who have intractable pain that worsens with recumbency and is not relieved by physical therapy should raise the suspicion of an intraspinal tumor. Progressive neurologic signs should alert the therapist to the need for medical referral and an MRI or computerized axial tomography scan to elicit the diagnosis. A thorough initial examination and evaluation of any person with back pain, including symptoms, pain patterns, strength assessment, and other neurologic signs such as impaired bowel and bladder function, changes in deep tendon reflexes, and signs of spasticity, should be the standard of practice to rule out tumors and other systemic disorders.

Rehabilitation Referrals

Neurologic deficits from primary spinal cord tumors may result in impairments such as spinal pain, weakness in the extremities and trunk, sensory loss, bowel and bladder dysfunction, spinal instability, and impaired aerobic capacity. Bed mobility limitations, difficulties with transfers in and out of bed, knowledge deficit regarding spinal safety, ambulation limitations, decreased self-care, equipment issues, and difficulties in returning to work, community activities, and leisure activities all require rehabilitation therapy. Because of a favorable prognosis with completely excised primary tumors, the approach of the therapist should be toward achieving maximal function and support of the client and family toward long-term goals. Many patients will survive their tumors but residual deficits and functional limitations are common. Medical management, including surgery (resections, kyphoplasty, fusions), chemotherapy, and radiation therapy, causes complications over a prolonged time period that require rehabilitation intervention at numerous time points during recovery.

Knowledge Needed for Rehabilitation

As with primary brain tumors, therapists should know the medical management plan, the prognostic expectations, the side effects of treatment, and precautions to prepare for the rehabilitative approach to a client with an intraspinal tumor. Knowledge of the most common intraspinal tumors, their patterns of growth, and neurologic changes assists the therapist in assessing the patient accurately, setting goals, and providing intervention.

Rehabilitation Evaluation

A thorough examination of the neurologic and musculoskeletal systems is very important to identify impairments that affect function. For example, an anterior tibialis muscle weakness or a lower extremity paraparesis may be the impairment that limits mobility and transfers and may be amenable to therapy. The therapist should review medical records, laboratory and radiologic reports, and other studies. If the treatment is provided on an outpatient basis, blood value determinations should be requested to assist the therapist in planning exercise programs. Communicating with the oncologist, the surgeon, and nurse; keeping abreast of imaging reports and other diagnostic tests; and being alert to other medical management, such as the effect of steroids and chemotherapy, allow the therapist to be more effective in treatment. Postoperative precautions may include protection from spinal torsion and use of an external support. Protection of irradiated skin follows the same guidelines as given under "Primary Brain Tumors" above.

METASTATIC TUMORS

The extended survival in all types of cancer has allowed time for metastasis to occur from primary tumors elsewhere in the body. Metastatic complications are an escalating problem. Metastases to the brain and spinal cord are among the most serious complications of metastatic cancer.[17,143]

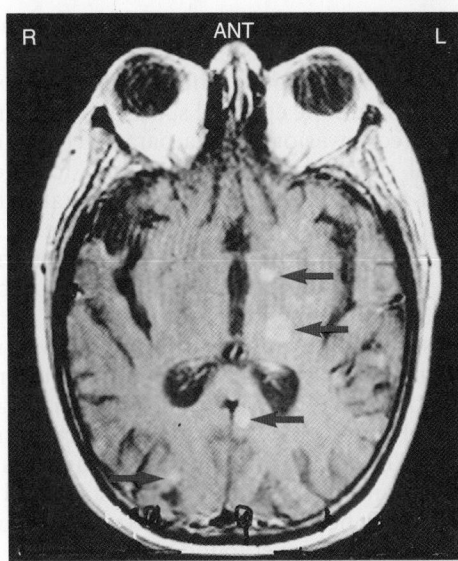

Figure 30-24

Metastatic disease in the brain. A gadolinium-enhanced T1-weighted magnetic resonance image shows multiple metastases as areas of increased signal *(arrows)*. (From Mettler FA Jr: *Essentials of radiology*, ed 2, Philadelphia, 2005, WB Saunders.)

Incidence

The incidence of metastatic CNS tumors is estimated to be 150,000 to 180,000 per year, although exact figures are difficult to ascertain.[3] The number of metastatic brain tumors is estimated to be 150,000 per year, and the number of metastatic spinal cord tumors is estimated to be approximately 80,000 per year.[3] These tumors are the most common intracranial tumor in adults.[152] The incidence of metastatic CNS tumors is on the rise as a result of improved life expectancies from advances in cancer treatment. Here they find a safe haven behind the blood-brain barrier through which many chemotherapeutic agents for the primary cancer cannot pass. The blood-brain barrier restricts passage of high-molecular-weight compounds through its tight capillary endothelial junctions.[116] The brain is a metastatic site in approximately 20% of people with primary cancer elsewhere, and the spinal cord is a metastatic site for 10% of primary cancers.[143]

Pathogenesis[8]

Metastatic tumors reach the brain generally through the arterial blood system. A smaller number arise by direct extension from extracranial sites such as the neck or paranasal sinuses. The cascade of events for formation of a metastasis includes tumor cells at the primary site reaching a critical volume in proximity to a blood vessel, dislodging from the primary tumor and entering blood vessels, embolizing, traveling, extravasating from the blood vessel, and growing in parenchyma of another organs.[44,17] Most metastatic tumors arise in the distribution area of the middle cerebral artery to the cerebral hemispheres, with most lesions located in the parietal or frontal lobes. Approximately 20% are found in the posterior fossa, primarily the cerebellum. About half of cases include multiple metastatic lesions in the brain (Fig. 30-24).

Metastatic tumors reach the spine and spinal cord through direct arterial dissemination to the vertebral body, by retrograde spread via the vertebral venous plexus as it perforates into the epidural space and vertebral bodies, or by direct invasion from a paravertebral tumor to the epidural space via the intervertebral foramen. The majority of spinal metastases are extradural–extramedullary, although in less than 5% of cases the location is intramedullary. The thoracic spine is the most frequent site of metastasis (70%), followed by the lumbosacral spine (20%) and the cervical area (10%).[143]

The most common cancers resulting in brain metastases are lung cancers, especially small cell carcinoma; cancers of the breast, kidney, and gastrointestinal tract; and melanoma. Figure 30-25 shows dural metastasis from breast cancer. The most common cancers metastasizing to the spinal column are lung, breast, prostate, and kidney cancers and lymphomas. In approximately 10% of cases, the primary tumor is never found.

Clinical Manifestations of Brain Metastasis

Metastatic brain tumors present with headache, seizures, elevated ICP, and similar signs of primary tumors. Table 30-7 provides a more complete listing. However, symptoms may progress much more rapidly, often in days to weeks, as a result of the significant edema that accompanies a metastasis. Cerebellar metastases may cause obstructive hydrocephalus and abrupt deterioration.

MEDICAL MANAGEMENT

DIAGNOSIS, TREATMENT, AND PROGNOSIS. MRI is the diagnostic procedure of choice because it is the most sensitive in revealing multiple small lesions. A review of the chest film is often enough to give a presumptive

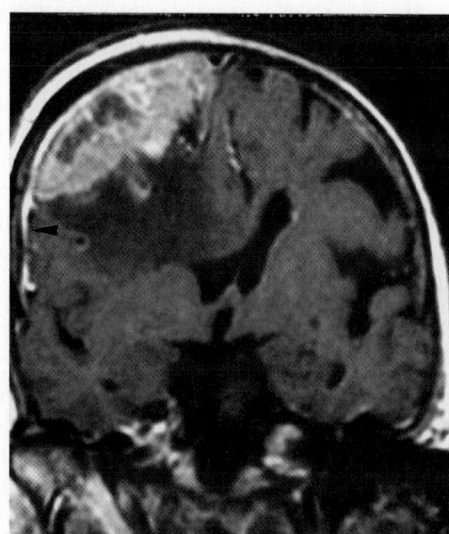

Figure 30-25

Dural metastasis from breast carcinoma. Coronal T1-weighted postcontrast magnetic resonance image. There is a heterogeneously enhancing mass with an irregular surface that arises from the dura over the right cerebral convexity. It displaces the underlying brain and causes considerable low-signal edema within it. There is a dural "tail" extending away from the tumor (arrowhead). (From Adam A, Dixon AK, Grainger RG, et al, eds: Grainger and Allison's diagnostic radiology: a textbook of medical imaging, ed 4, Philadelphia, 2001, Churchill Livingstone.)

diagnosis of lung cancer. With a history of cancer elsewhere in the body, a solitary brain lesion has approximately a 90% certainty of being a metastatic deposit.[143] Because meningiomas have a high prevalence in people with breast cancer, metastatic breast lesions in the brain must be differentiated pathologically from meningiomas for optimal treatment.

Medical management includes corticosteroids, surgical excision when solitary or small numbers of metastases are accessible, and irradiation in almost all cases. Of solitary brain metastases associated with non–small cell lung cancer, up to one-third may be cured with surgery followed by radiation therapy. Steroids have a dramatic effect in relieving symptoms caused by the significant peritumoral swelling. Radiotherapy provides adequate palliation for many people, because death occurs from the primary cancer, not the brain metastasis.[70] Brain metastases from breast cancer are increasing in incidence.[141] The treatment of brain metastases with gamma knife radiosurgery, stereotactically, gives an average survival time of 8 months.[129] In general, the prognosis for people with brain metastasis is poor, because the metastasis indicates that the primary cancer has already escaped control.

Clinical Manifestations of Spinal Metastasis

Back pain is the most common and prominent symptom of metastasis to the spinal column and cord, and is present in 95% of cases. Anyone with a known cancer history who presents with new-onset back pain of unknown etiology should be considered to have spinal metastasis until proven otherwise.[119] Pain is caused by stretching of the periosteum, tension or traction on the spinal nerve roots and cord, or compression of the cord and meninges. It is usually a dull ache, worse at night in the recumbent position, and may be local in the spine or may be a radicular pain. Intradural–intramedullary metastases are less common than primary tumors in this location, and overall their occurrence is rare.[152]

Without treatment, pain progresses in weeks or months (sometimes days) to weakness, sensory loss, and bowel and bladder sphincter disturbance. These tumors characteristically progress quickly after onset of weakness to cause paraplegia and permanent loss of sphincter control.

Table 30-7	Presenting Symptoms and Signs of Brain Metastasis	
Symptom	**Common Signs**
Headache	Focal weakness or unexplained falls
Mental status change	Focal sensory deficits
Altered level of consciousness	Speech difficulty
Seizures occurring when older than 35 years of age	Aphasia, focal weakness
Papilledema or visual obscurations	Ataxia
Visual complaints or unexplained motor vehicle accidents	Visual field defect

From Goetz: Textbook of clinical neurology, ed 2, Chap 47, Philadelphia, 2003, WB Saunders, 1991.

Diagnosing and treating the metastasis early is important, because people treated while still ambulatory are likely to remain so, but those who have reached the stage of paraplegia and sphincter loss do not typically regain function.

MEDICAL MANAGEMENT

DIAGNOSIS. A careful neurologic examination, followed by plain films of the spine, is an important first approach and results in a diagnosis in the majority of cases. The most common findings are pedicular erosion, vertebral collapse, pathologic fracture-dislocation, and a soft-tissue shadow suggestive of a paraspinal mass.[143] Bone scans are the next test of choice. If results of any of these tests are positive, MRI or CT is then done for more definitive imaging of the lesion. This will also determine whether the tumor is intramedullary and can be performed in the absence of vertebral disease. Figure 30-26 is an MRI showing focal spine metastases.

TREATMENT. Radiotherapy is typically the treatment of choice for spinal metastasis to reduce pain, reduce tumor compression, and restore neurologic function. Radiotherapy and/or chemotherapy is also helpful in preserving spinal stability. For those tumors that are chemotherapy sensitive, urgent management with chemotherapy is indicated to preserve spinal integrity.

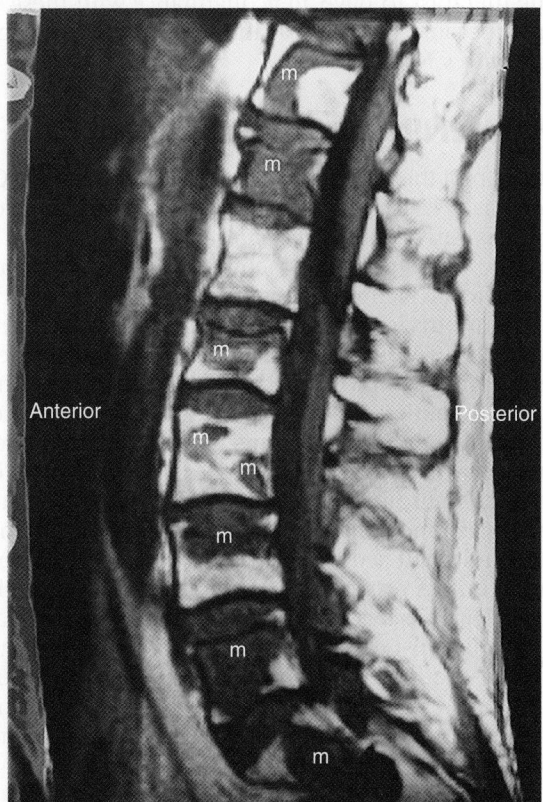

Figure 30-26

Focal spine metastases. A sagittal or lateral T1-weighted magnetic resonance image of the lumbar spine shows the normal white or high signal in fat within the bone marrow. In many of the vertebral bodies, the high signal of normal marrow has been replaced by dark areas of metastatic deposits *(m)*. (From Mettler FA Jr: *Essentials of radiology*, ed 2, Philadelphia, 2005, WB Saunders.)

Surgery is reserved for people with a worsening neurologic deficit during radiation therapy, for those with a spinal instability causing cord compression, for tumors known to be radioresistant, and for individuals who already have received the maximum radiation.

It should be noted that past attempts at surgical decompression with laminectomy have proved to be disappointing, with neurologic improvement occurring in only 30% of cases.[143] Surgical access via laminectomy to the typically anterior tumors compressing the cord from a ventral direction is technically difficult. Evidence exists that very high doses of corticosteroids relieve local spinal edema. Current practice is to begin very large doses of corticosteroids as soon as a spinal cord compression from metastatic tumor is diagnosed. This dose is continued for several days, then reduced, allowing time for decisions to be made for radiation or surgery.[157]

PROGNOSIS. Prognosis for return of neurologic function is based on the degree of loss before radiotherapy. With radiotherapy, 80% of clients who are ambulatory at the time of treatment remain so, and 30% who are nonambulatory regain gait.[143] Pain and neurologic function improve in the majority of people. Because the metastasis indicates loss of containment of the primary tumor, cure is beyond expectation. However, early diagnosis and treatment lead to the optimal result, the prevention of paraplegia.

Radiation to the spinal cord may cause complications of myelopathy. Although radiation has no acute effects on the cord, an early delayed radiation myelopathy after irradiation of the neck is common. The Lhermitte sign (a sudden electric shock sensation radiating down the back and lower extremities brought on by neck flexion), the hallmark of this radiation myelopathy, is present for several months and then abates. It is not a predictor of late delayed radiation spinal cord injury.[37] A late effect of radiation to the cord, occurring between 6 and 36 months after radiation, is a chronic progressive myelopathy that begins as a Brown-Séquard syndrome and progresses over weeks or months to a spastic paresis. No effective medical treatment exists, but the therapist can provide mobility management, skin precautions, and safety education for these clients.

SPECIAL IMPLICATIONS FOR THE THERAPIST 30-3

Primary Intraspinal Tumors
Rehabilitation Referrals

Neurologic deficits resulting from metastatic CNS tumors in the brain or spinal cord often require physical and occupational therapy. The neurologic impairments from either intracranial or intraspinal tumors may include weakness, paralysis, decreased sensation, and pain leading to loss of mobility and self-care skills. Paraplegia from spinal metastasis requires much rehabilitative intervention. The incidence of metastatic CNS tumors is increasing.

Prediagnosis Alertness to Signs and Symptoms

Because therapists are often in a position to observe the mobility and neurologic status of clients before a diagnosis of a CNS metastasis is made, being alert to abnormal neurologic signs in anyone with a cancer history is vital. In someone with a cancer history, any signs of intracranial metastasis, such as visual symptoms or mental status changes, should be reported immediately to the physician. Knowing the signs and symptoms of an intraspinal metastasis and immediate referral to the physician cannot be overemphasized. Spinal cord compression can progress in a matter of hours or days to paraplegia. Spinal pain complaints, particularly in the thoracic spine, and/or progressive strength changes, sensory changes, and/or bowel or bladder function changes in a patient with a cancer history are red flags. A therapist who refers the patient to the physician in time may prevent irreversible paraplegia and sphincter function loss.

Knowledge Needed for Rehabilitation

As with primary CNS tumors, therapists need to know the medical management plan, the prognostic expectations, and the hematologic guidelines for exercise. Goal setting needs to be realistic for noncurable disease, yet not without hope for good management.[19] Families and caregivers may need to have an even greater role in goal setting and training. As with primary brain tumors, the psychosocial implications have a profound impact on the client and family, and the therapist can provide support, as well as be a sounding board for decision making. It is helpful to realize that in some cases, paraplegia from a metastatic spinal cord tumor may respond to irradiation and improve enough for some return of function, such as limited ambulation. The physical therapist must be alert to any neurologic improvement.

Rehabilitation Precautions

As with primary CNS tumors, clients and their families must have an awareness of the side effects of the various treatment modalities. Postoperative acute care precautions are discussed under "Primary Brain Tumors" above. A general knowledge of metastatic spread and behavior is helpful.[8,93] Myelosuppression, fatigue, nausea, and precautions need to be understood. Avoiding modalities such as heat or cold or any topical agents over skin being irradiated is important for skin protection, because poor circulation inhibits normal heat and cold dissipation. Once the irradiation sessions are completed and the skin has healed, and depending on skin integrity and adequate circulation, modalities such as heat or cold or transcutaneous nerve stimulation may be used. Although ultrasound is not usually recommended for pain management because of concerns about tumor growth, its use for palliation of pain in end-stage disease may be allowed.

PARANEOPLASTIC SYNDROMES

Cancer may cause effects on the nervous system that are not directly related to the primary tumor mass or a metastasis. These so-called remote effects, or paraneoplastic

syndromes (see Chapter 9), include such problems as paraneoplastic cerebellar degeneration, brainstem encephalitis, myelitis of the spinal cord, and motor neuron disease.[47] Paraneoplastic syndromes are also termed paraneoplastic neurologic disorders. The cause of most paraneoplastic syndromes is unknown, although an immune mechanism is the most likely hypothesis. The response of the immune system to the antigen may be misdirected and cause neurologic dysfunction. Paraneoplastic syndromes may be the first sign of the presence of cancer.[14,114,124]

Although paraneoplastic syndromes involving the CNS are rare, they are often severe, associated with an inflammatory CSF, and leave the person with severe neurologic disability. Treatment effectiveness has been limited. Some syndromes are associated with particular tumors, such as paraneoplastic cerebellar degeneration with lung cancer. In this syndrome, the early symptoms are a slight incoordination in walking, with progressive gait ataxia; incoordination of arms, legs, and trunk; dysarthria; and often nystagmus. After a few months the illness reaches its peak and stabilizes. By this time, most clients must have assistance to walk, handwriting is impossible, many cannot sit unsupported, and speech is with great effort.

It is not within the scope of this chapter to elaborate on CNS paraneoplastic syndromes. However, it is helpful for the therapist to have an acquaintance with these syndromes, because they appear in the practice of caring for people with CNS neoplasms.[17]

LEPTOMENINGEAL CARCINOMATOSIS

Infiltration of the meninges and CSF pathways of the CNS by neoplastic cells is a less-common complication of cancer and is known as *leptomeningeal carcinomatosis*. This metastatic seeding of the meninges can be widespread and multifocal. Neurologic signs will depend on location. Brain symptoms may include headache, change in mental status, seizures, double vision, abducens palsy, and hemiparesis; spinal symptoms include radicular pain, numbness, and weakness.[115] Meningeal carcinomatosis occurs in approximately 5% of patients with cancer, but is being diagnosed with increasing frequency as patients live longer and as neuroimaging studies improve.[54,114] Cancers of the breast and lung, non-Hodgkin lymphoma, melanomas, and adult acute leukemias are the most common primary tumors responsible for leptomeningeal carcinomatosis. Diagnosis is by CSF studies, which show malignant cells in most cases. MRI is also done to assess bulky disease in the brain or spine. Current therapy includes radiotherapy to symptomatic sites, with concurrent intrathecal chemotherapy.[143] Survival is measured in months from treatment.

PEDIATRIC TUMORS

Incidence and Pathogenesis

Approximately 4300 primary brain tumors were diagnosed in children and adolescents in 2013.[3,79] The incidence of primary brain and nervous system tumors peaks

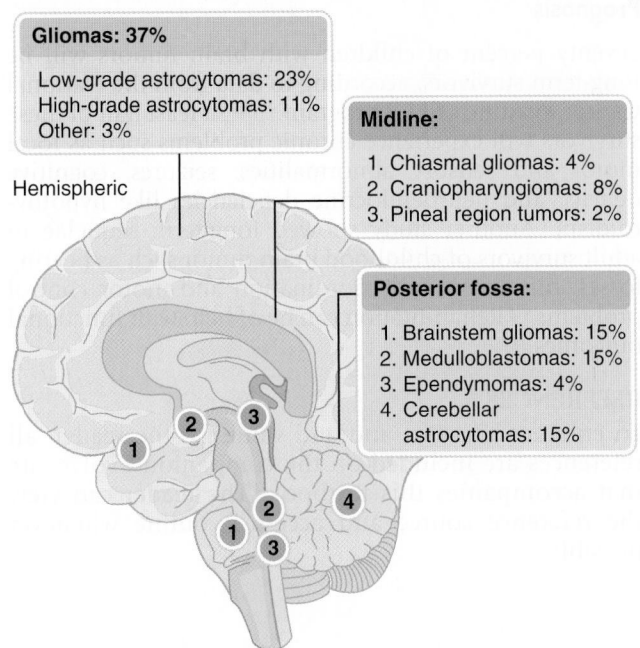

Gliomas: 37%

Low-grade astrocytomas: 23%
High-grade astrocytomas: 11%
Other: 3%

Hemispheric

Midline:

1. Chiasmal gliomas: 4%
2. Craniopharyngiomas: 8%
3. Pineal region tumors: 2%

Posterior fossa:

1. Brainstem gliomas: 15%
2. Medulloblastomas: 15%
3. Ependymomas: 4%
4. Cerebellar astrocytomas: 15%

Figure 30-27

Childhood brain tumors occur at any location within the central nervous system. The relative frequency of brain tumor histologic types and the anatomic distribution are shown. (From Kliegman RM, Behrmann RE: *Nelson textbook of pediatrics*, ed 18, Philadelphia, 2007, WB Saunders.)

in the pediatric population from age 0 to 6 years, drops at age 7 to 10 years, remains steady until age 18 years, then drops. In infants and young children, intracranial tumors are the second most common form of cancer, after leukemia.[143] The peak incidence of these tumors occurs between birth and age 6 years. Brain tumors are the second leading cause of cancer-related deaths in children younger than age 15 years. Table 30-2 compares the frequency of childhood tumors with the frequency of adult tumors.

The etiology of pediatric brain tumors is little understood. Cranial exposure to radiation and possible evidence of a heritable syndrome are causes. Other factors being studied include maternal diet and intake of vitamins during pregnancy.

The most frequently encountered types of intracranial tumors in children are the astrocytoma, medulloblastoma, ependymoma, and brainstem glioma.[43] Brain tumors in children are typically located infratentorially, primarily in the cerebellum and brainstem, although they may occur at any location. Figure 30-27 shows the relative frequency and location of brain tumors.

Astrocytomas are the most common type of pediatric intracranial tumor, accounting for approximately 47% of all brain tumors in children. They are usually well-differentiated grade I tumors. About half of them occur supratentorially, most commonly in the frontal lobes, but also in the temporal and parietal lobes. The cerebellum is the most common infratentorial site of the astrocytoma in children. Cerebellar astrocytoma is more common in males and usually occurs in the first two decades of life, with the median incidence at age 18 years. Children with grade I astrocytomas have a 10-year postoperative survival rate of 85%.[50] Infrequently, high-grade astrocytomas occur, with a poorer prognosis.

Medulloblastomas account for 20% to 25% of childhood brain tumors and are the most common malignant tumor in children. These aggressive tumors are more common in males than females and have a peak incidence at age 5 years in children. Evolution of therapeutic strategies including multimodal chemotherapy followed by surgery has dramatically improved the outlook for children with medulloblastomas.[143] Medulloblastomas belong to the group of tumors known as *PNETs* and arise in the fourth ventricle. Medulloblastomas have a predilection for meningeal seeding. The 5-year survival rate is approximately 50%.

Ependymomas usually arise in children from the floor of the fourth ventricle and make up 9% to 20% of childhood tumors. The 5-year survival is 85% when complete resection is possible and approximately 45% overall.

Brainstem gliomas may be of several tumor types; the most common is astrocytoma, but they also may be glioblastomas or ependymomas. The overall prognosis for brainstem tumors is relatively poor, but occasionally gratifying treatment results are obtained.[143]

Clinical Manifestations

Clinical manifestations of CNS neoplasms in children are more difficult to evaluate because children are less able to relate and report symptoms. Parents, teachers, and caretakers may notice problems before the child is aware of a change. Most supratentorial astrocytomas present initially with seizures. Cerebellar astrocytomas produce typical cerebellar findings such as ataxia, and many produce symptoms of increased ICP. Tumors of the cerebral aqueduct or the fourth ventricle, such as an ependymoma or medulloblastoma, typically present at an early stage with headache, nausea, and cranial nerve palsies, but also may produce long-tract signs such as hemiparesis. Hydrocephalus is a complication in patients with ependymoma and medulloblastoma, and a late manifestation of brainstem gliomas.[50]

Diagnosis and Treatment

Diagnosis is by MRI or CT scan, although the CT scan may not be adequate to detect the early stages of brainstem or fourth ventricle tumors. Early treatment includes high-dose dexamethasone, emergency ventricular drainage in the case of hydrocephalus, and surgical resection. Radiation is the principal form of treatment for brainstem gliomas. Postoperative radiation is indicated for medulloblastomas and may be helpful for ependymomas and gliomas. Chemotherapy, although generally not beneficial, has been helpful for medulloblastomas.

The risks of brain radiation therapy in children are of great concern. These may include learning disabilities, hypopituitarism, occlusive disease of cerebral vessels, and radiation-induced secondary tumors. Because myelinization of the CNS is not generally complete until 2 to 3 years of age, radiation therapy performed before this age can be especially devastating and is not usually done.[143] Long-term effects from childhood tumors and treatment have been reported by R. J. Packer.[73,108]

Spinal cord tumors rarely occur in children. Spinal ependymoma is the most prominent primary intraspinal tumor and has a predilection for the lumbosacral spine. It is treated with resection and radiation therapy. The risks of radiation therapy in children include myelopathy and spinal deformities.

Metastatic spinal cord tumors in children arise most commonly from sarcomas and less often from neuroblastomas, lymphomas, and leukemias. Metastatic tumors in children occur principally by direct extension from an adjacent primary cancer[143] and can be the presenting feature of the primary cancer. This is in contrast to adult spinal tumors, in which access is by a vascular route and usually occurs in the setting of an advanced malignancy.

Because pediatric metastatic spinal cord tumors usually are not associated with extensive vertebral column destruction, they generally can be removed through a simple laminectomy. An aggressive approach to metastatic spinal tumors in children results in a more favorable outcome in children than in adults.[143] Approximately 96% of children have improvement or stabilization of neurologic deficits, and 60% of nonambulatory children regain the ability to walk after treatment.

Prognosis

Seventy percent of children with brain tumors will be long-term survivors, according to data from the National Cancer Institute's SEER program.[79,83] At least half of these survivors will experience chronic problems such as focal motor and sensory abnormalities, seizures, cognitive deficits, and neuroendocrine deficiencies like hypothyroidism. Another study showed long-term sequelae in adult survivors of childhood brain tumor such as hearing losses, blindness, and coordination and motor control problems.[79] Rehabilitation can be of help with functional outcomes.[112]

REFERENCES

To enhance this text and add value for the reader, all references are included on the companion Evolve site that accompanies this textbook. The reader can view the reference source and access it online whenever possible.

CHAPTER 31

Degenerative Diseases of the Central Nervous System

KENDA S. FULLER • ERICA DEMARCH • PATRICIA A. WINKLER

Degenerative diseases of the central nervous system (CNS) can affect gray matter, white matter, or both. The neurodegenerative disorders are characterized by loss of functionally related groups of neurons. The pattern of neuronal loss is selective, affecting one or more groups of neurons while leaving others intact. The cause of the neuronal loss is unknown but is clearly multifactorial. The diseases appear to arise without any clear inciting event in individuals without previous neurologic deficits. The clinical symptoms produced depend on which neuronal populations are lost. Degenerative changes in gray matter diseases interfere with the function of the neuronal cell bodies and synapses. The diseases can affect the cortex, the gray matter of the spinal cord, or both. The most common factor in this group of diseases is the slow deterioration of body functions controlled by the brain and spinal cord.

The neuropathologic findings observed in the degenerative diseases reflect changes in different components. In some disorders there are intracellular abnormalities, such as Lewy bodies and neurofibrillary tangles, whereas in others there is primary loss of neurons.[35] Some degenerative diseases have prominent involvement of the cerebral cortex, such as Alzheimer disease; others are more restricted to subcortical areas and may present with movement disorders such as tremors and dyskinesias, such as Parkinson disease. Demyelination has the major impact on other disorders such as multiple sclerosis. Through genetic and molecular studies of these diseases it is becoming clearer that there are many shared features across the disorders.

Cellular stress is a major component of neurodegenerative disease. When the cell is stressed, the proteins that form filaments and microtubules creating the cytoskeleton can collapse and form perinuclear bundles or clumps of protein aggregates. If the stress experienced by the cell is not lethal, the cell adapts and manufactures several proteins that may restore functional activity of partially denatured proteins. If the proteins cannot be restored, then a process begins to destroy the proteins. If the proteins do not fully degrade, they become clumped together to form intracellular inclusions. The inclusions in neurodegenerative disorders are examples of such aggregates. The aggregated proteins are generally cytotoxic, but the mechanisms by which protein aggregation is linked to cell death may be different in these various diseases. The histologic characteristics of the inclusions often form the diagnostic hallmarks of these different diseases.

Disorders of movement associated with gray matter destruction are reflected in functional loss and decreased fractionation of movement. Dementia can be present and always represents a pathologic process; dementia, despite popular belief, is not part of normal aging. The majority of the degenerative diseases that affect the basal ganglia are associated with involuntary movements. Disruption of smooth coordination of muscles can be seen in diseases affecting the cerebellum and brainstem. Many of the disorders appear later in life and mimic the normal deterioration of the nervous system that comes with aging.

The cost of care for people with degenerative neurologic disease is significant as a consequence of the protracted time of disability before death and the extent of the disability. Although medical science has made tremendous progress in the past few years, degenerative disorders continue to be a challenge to health care providers and a scourge to modern society.

AMYOTROPHIC LATERAL SCLEROSIS
Overview and Definition

Amyotrophic lateral sclerosis (ALS) is a disorder that is generally recognized as an adult-onset progressive motor neuron disease, but is also a complex disease process underlying a multisystem illness. The first detailed description was by Jean Martin Charcot in 1869, in which he discussed the clinical and pathologic characteristics of "la sclérose latérale amyotrophique," a disorder of muscle wasting (amyotrophy) and gliotic hardening (sclerosis) of the anterior and lateral corticospinal tracts involving both upper and lower motor neurons. It is the most physically devastating of the neurodegenerative diseases. Peripheral nerve changes result in muscle fiber atrophy or amyotrophy. The resulting weakness causes profound limitation of movement.[169] Executive dysfunction, characterized by deficiencies in attention, language comprehension, planning, and abstract reasoning, represents cortical involvement.

Incidence and Etiologic and Risk Factors

The incidence of ALS is approximately 2 per 100,000 adults and seems to be consistent around the world with the exception of the Western Pacific where the incidence increases to 14 to 55 per 100,000 adults.[144]

Approximately 90% of cases of ALS occur sporadically and are clinically manifest in the fifth decade or later. The cause is still unknown. Clusters of ALS have been noted, where there have been three or four individuals living or working in close proximity or individuals participating in the same sport; military service appears to hold a possible risk for ALS. Chronic intoxication with heavy metals, such as lead or mercury, has been suggested as an etiologic agent, but there still does not seem to be a clear cause. ALS occurs predominantly in men, although bulbar onset occurs more often in women. There may be an increased incidence in white males, with a lower rate reported in Mexico, Poland, and Italy.[33,169]

Familial ALS (FALS) is an inherited autosomal trait. It occurs in 5% to 10% of all ALS cases. The identification of at least one additional family member with ALS in successive generations is essential for the diagnosis of FALS. Most FALS is inherited in an autosomal dominant pattern and is characterized by an early onset. Family linkage may be missed if there was a death of a family member before the usual age of onset. Copper and zinc superoxide dismutase (SOD1) gene mutation may account for approximately 15% of cases of FALS. SOD1 genetic testing can be used for genetic counseling in families in which SOD1 mutations are already established.

Pathogenesis

The pathologic hallmarks of ALS are the degeneration and loss of motor neurons, with astrocytic gliosis and microglial proliferation in the presence of intraneuronal inclusions in degenerating neurons and glial cells. Upper motor neuron cell loss occurs in the motor cortex, with loss of Betz cells from Brodmann area 4, frontotemporal cortex, hippocampus, thalamus, and substantia nigra. Astrocytic gliosis with axonal loss occurs in corticospinal tracts. There is loss of lower motor neuron axons in the brainstem and spinal cord, spinocerebellar tracts, and dorsal columns.

Eighty percent of FALS cases have degeneration of the spinocerebellar tract. Dementia may be a result of changes in the frontotemporal cortices or in the substantia nigra (basal ganglia). Some histologic changes seen in ALS are consistent with those in other lower motor neuron diseases. Destruction of large motor neurons of the anterior horn cells is greatest in the cervical and lumbar regions of the cord and between the internal capsule and the bulbar pyramids. Critical neurons are sparse, and the dendrites are shortened, fragmented, and disorganized. Microscopic examination demonstrates a reduction in the number of anterior horn neurons throughout the length of the spinal cord, with associated reactive gliosis and loss of anterior root myelinated fibers. There are similar findings in the cranial nerve nuclei in bulbar manifestations. Diffuse and patchy loss of myelin appears in all areas of the spinal cord except the posterior columns, allowing for preservation of sensation.[175]

Ribonucleic acid (RNA) content is reduced in the damaged cells. An evolving theory in ALS pathogenesis is that mutations in such proteins as TDP43, FUS/TLS, senataxin, peripherin, SMN1, SOD1, and angiogenin may result in aberrant interactions in RNA metabolism. Excessive accumulation of the pigmented lipid (lipofuscin) develops that normally is not seen until advanced age. The production of free radicals may be responsible for the changes in the lipid molecules, eventually causing cell death.[21] Spheroids, the axonal swelling containing packed neurofilaments found in the dendrites and axons distant from the cell body, are found more frequently in the early cases with shorter clinical courses. Spheroids are not found in FALS. The spheroids may represent the slowing of transport in the axon and the abnormal processing of neurofilaments. The aggregation of protein into inclusion bodies in cells has been described in many other neurodegenerative disorders including Parkinson disease, Huntington disease, and Alzheimer disease. It is still unclear whether protein aggregation is directly toxic to cells or is a defense mechanism to reduce intracellular aggregation of toxic proteins.[59]

Immune processes are active in the pathogenesis, if not the initiation, of ALS. Immune complexes have been identified in gut and renal tissue from patients with ALS. Antibodies have been found in some cases of ALS that may indicate involvement of hormones in the immune process; however, there appears to be a poor response to immunologic treatment.[19]

Glutamate, the principal excitatory neurotransmitter in the human motor system, can cause excitotoxic damage when the extracellular glutamate concentration increases. Plasma glutamate levels in individuals with motor neuron disease can be twice that of normal. This may be related to a defect in the transport and breakdown of excitatory amino acids predisposing the person to neurotoxicity. Astrocytic glutamate transporter, termed *GLT1* or *EAAT2*, is markedly reduced in the motor cortex and anterior horn cells of patients with ALS resulting in significantly raised levels of glutamate in cerebrospinal fluid (CSF) in ALS. Environmental toxins may act as excitotoxins.[28,207]

Oxidative damage appears to play a role in the damage to nerve cells in ALS. Calcium-mediated excitotoxicity can generate free radicals. In FALS, the mutated SOD1 appears to cause increased reactivity to hydrogen peroxide and lead to an increase in free radicals. Copper ions in a reduced state will cause this process to become harmful to the neuron. Oxidative damage and glutamate toxicity may interact or potentiate each other. They may also contribute to other mechanisms of motor neuron degeneration, including axon transport abnormalities and apoptosis.[169]

The death of the peripheral motor neuron in the brainstem and spinal cord leads to denervation and atrophy of the corresponding muscle fibers. In the early phases of the illness, denervated muscle may be reinnervated by sprouting of preserved nearby distal motor axon terminals, although reinnervation in this disease is less extensive than in other chronic neurologic disorders.[33]

There is remarkable selectivity of neuronal cell death, involving motor neurons of the brainstem and spinal cord with relative sparing of the oculomotor nuclei. There is eventual spread into the prefrontal, parietal, and temporal areas, as well as into the subthalamic nuclei and reticular formation. In persons kept breathing with ventilatory support, there may eventually be sensory system changes.

Clinical Manifestations

Cognitive impairments are noted in up to 50% of individuals with ALS. With careful assessment, these deficiencies can be noted early on. Executive function deficits can be found in visual attention, working memory, cognitive flexibility, problem solving, and visual-perceptual skills. Verbal fluency declines before dysarthria develops. The cognitive deficits are a result of changes in frontal lobe function and may be related to frontotemporal dementia. Bulbar onset is more predictive of cognitive impairment than limb onset. Pseudobulbar affect, resulting in emotional lability, emotional outbursts, and pathologic laughing or crying, is not related to a psychologic or psychiatric condition and is not a part of the frontotemporal dementia.

The motor control manifestations of ALS vary depending on whether upper or lower motor neurons are predominantly involved. With lower motor neuron cell death and early denervation, the first evidence of the disease typically is insidiously developing asymmetric weakness, usually of the distal aspect of one limb progressing to weakness of the contiguous muscles. Extensor muscles become weaker than flexor muscles, especially in the hands. Cervical extensor weakness develops and can lead to drooping of the head and pain associated with overstretched muscles. Increased lumbar lordosis occurs as part of the compensatory strategy to attempt to right the head and bring the eyes level.

The neurons innervating muscles controlling articulation, chewing, and swallowing originate in the medulla, or the "bulb," and any weaknesses in the muscles are considered bulbar signs. In the lower motor or flaccid component, facial muscles are affected. Inability to hold the eye closed against pressure is a standard test. Weakness around the mouth develops, and air leaks out. The movement of the tongue is decreased, and atrophy is present. Fasciculations in the tongue are present with lower motor neuron dysfunction. Dysarthria associated with lower motor neuron involvement is reflected by inability to shout or sing, a hoarse or whispering quality of the voice, and nasal tone. Manipulating food inside the mouth becomes difficult. Eventually, weak swallowing may trigger reflex coughing.

Individuals with ALS complain of drooling because of the absence of automatic swallowing, which is made worse by the forward head position. Breathing becomes difficult, and accessory breathing replaces diaphragmatic breathing. Respiratory distress can occur when sleeping, especially on the back.

Deformities of the extremities are common, especially since weakness causes shortening of the extensor muscles. Clawhand develops as the weakness of lumbricals and interossei hinders metacarpal flexion and tenodesis flexes the distal joints. Figure 31-1 shows the hands of an individual with ALS.

Weakness caused by denervation is associated with progressive wasting and atrophy of muscles. Cramping

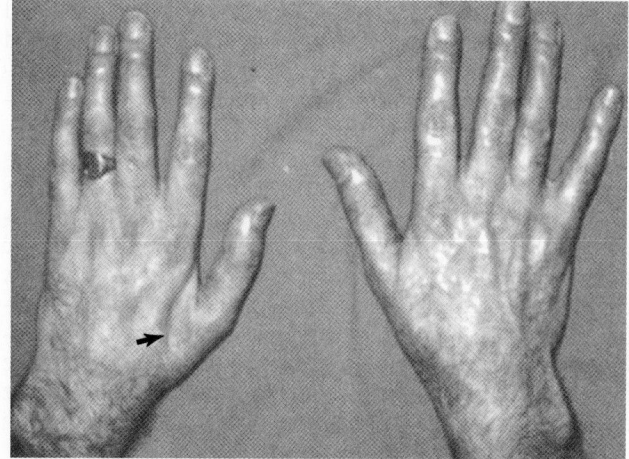
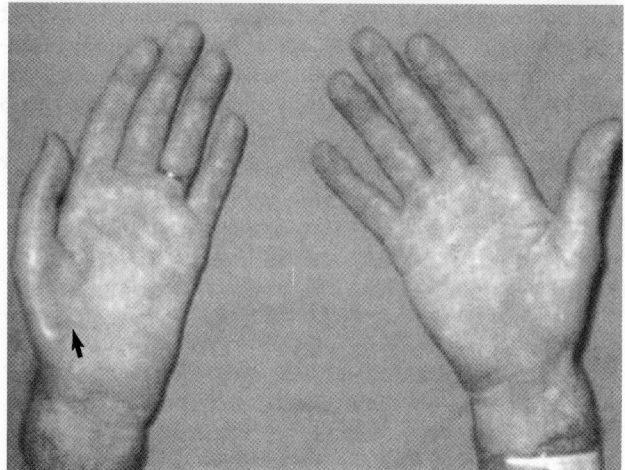

Figure 31-1

Wasting of hand muscles in amyotrophic lateral sclerosis. (From Parsons M: *Color atlas of clinical neurology*, London, 1993, Wolfe.)

with volitional movement in the early morning is often reported, with complaints of stiffness. Muscle cramps indicate lower motor neuron dysfunction. It may be related to hyperexcitability of distal motor axons. Early in the disease there are fasciculations, or spontaneous twitching of muscle fibers. Fasciculations are the result of spontaneous contractions of a group of muscle fibers belonging to a single motor unit. The impulse for the fasciculation appears to arise from hyperexcitable distal motor axons. This is random in time and in muscles affected. It should be noted that both muscle cramping and fasciculations are found in healthy adults and should never be taken alone as a concern for the development of ALS.

Upper motor neuron symptoms are characterized by loss of inhibition and the resulting lack of dexterity and spasticity. Muscle strength is decreased along an upper motor neuron pattern. Extensor muscles of the upper extremity and flexor muscles of the lower extremity are weakened, as spasticity develops as the result of loss of brainstem control of the vestibulospinal and reticular formation control. As in other upper motor lesions, spasticity can limit the ability to accurately assess muscle strength.

Spastic bulbar palsy occurs when upper motor neurons and the corticobulbar fibers controlling speech, mastication, and swallowing are affected. This is termed *pseudobulbar palsy* and differs from the palsy associated with lower motor neuron loss in the brainstem. Pseudobulbar affect may manifest as inappropriate laughter, irritability, anger, and tearfulness.

The tendon, or muscle stretch, reflexes become hyperactive based on the loss of the Ia inhibitory reflex. This also extends to the development of clonus, in which manual quick stretch of a muscle induces repeated rhythmic muscle contraction. The Babinski response is positive, characterized by extension of the great toe, often accompanied by fanning of the other toes in response to stroking the outer edge of the ipsilateral sole upward from the heel with a blunt object. If there is enough wasting of the dorsiflexors, the response may appear to be flexor despite upper motor neuron involvement.

It is characteristic of ALS that, regardless of whether the initial disease involves upper or lower motor neurons, both categories are eventually implicated. In most persons with ALS, the Babinski and Hoffmann signs are present or the tendon jerks are disproportionately active.[139] Throughout the course of the disease, eye movements and sensory, bowel, and bladder functions are preserved.

ALS is characterized by differing areas of CNS involvement and has been categorized in terms of four major groups of symptoms listed below.[97,150] Figure 31-2 shows the levels of dysfunction associated with the terms that describe them.

1. *Pseudobulbar palsy* reflects damage in the corticobulbar tract.
2. *Progressive bulbar palsy* is a result of cranial nerve nuclei involvement. There is weakness of the muscles involved in swallowing, chewing, and facial gestures. Fasciculations of the tongue are usually prominent. With early bulbar involvement, there can be difficulty with respiration before weakness of the limbs. Dysarthria and exaggeration of the expression of emotion, or pseudobulbar affect, indicate involvement of the corticobulbar tract. The oculomotor system is usually not involved, and eye movement remains normal.
3. *Primary lateral sclerosis* results in neuronal loss in the cortex. Signs of corticospinal tract involvement include hyperactivity of tendon reflexes with spasticity causing difficulty with active movement. Weakness and spasticity of specific muscles represent the level and progression of the disease along the corticospinal tracts. There is no muscle atrophy, and fasciculations are not present. This form of ALS is rare.

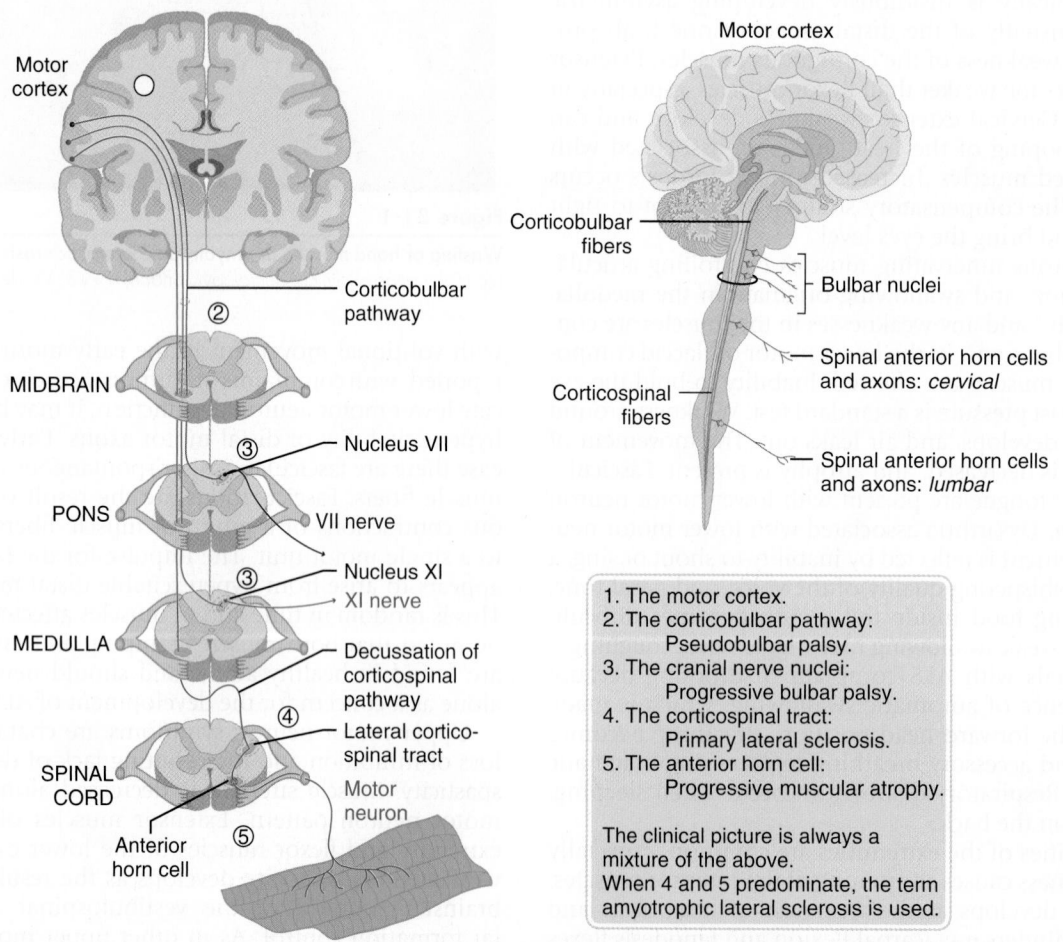

Figure 31-2

Areas of damage in the central and peripheral nervous system as a result of amyotrophic lateral sclerosis. (From Lindsay KW, Bone I, Callander R: *Neurology and neurosurgery illustrated*, New York, 1986, Churchill Livingstone. Insert from Noble J: *Textbook of primary care medicine*, ed 3, Copyright 2001, Mosby, Inc., and borrowed from Pryse-Phillips WM, Murray TJ: *Essentials of neurology: a concise textbook*, New York, 1992, Medical Examination Publisher, p. 660.)

4. In *progressive spinal muscular atrophy* there is progressive loss of motor neurons in the anterior horns of the spinal cord, often beginning in the cervical area. There is progressive weakness, wasting, and fasciculations involving the small muscles of the hands. Other levels of the spinal cord can be the site of the initial disease process, with symptoms reflecting the level involved. These areas of weakness can be present without evidence of higher-level corticospinal involvement, such as spasticity.

ALS with probable upper motor neuron signs is a condition in which there are no overt upper motor neuron signs, but involvement of the corticospinal tracts is indicated by the incongruous presence of active tendon reflexes in limbs with weak, wasted, and twitching muscles. Upper and lower limbs are usually affected first, with progression to facial symptoms and respiratory failure.

MEDICAL MANAGEMENT

DIAGNOSIS. Diagnosis is predominantly made by the combination of clinical presentation and electromyogram (EMG). The time to diagnosis differs, typically according to the first presenting symptoms. With upper limb onset the time to diagnosis is approximately 15 months, with lower extremity onset it is 21 months, and with bulbar involvement as the first sign it is approximately 17 months.[32] Box 31-1 describes diagnostic criteria.

The symptoms are generally first reported to a primary care physician, and it appears that there is a greater delay in reaching the diagnosis in such cases than when the initial symptoms are reported to a neurologist. Often in the early cases and those that are progressing slowly, there may be minimal abnormality on the first EMG, and the changes that lead to diagnosis may not appear for 6 to 12 months. In electrodiagnosis, rapidly progressive ALS shows different changes on the EMG compared with slowly progressive ALS. It is thought that some of these differences comes from the adaptation and sprouting that occur early in the process. This adaptation cannot be sustained as the disease progresses.[142]

EMG studies include the muscles of the extremities and trunk, and are selected based on the propensity for weakness in ALS. EMG criteria for the diagnosis of ALS include the presence of fibrillations, positive waveforms, fasciculations, and motor unit potential changes in multiple nerve root distributions in at least three limbs and the paraspinal muscles. These changes occur without change in sensory response.[170]

In 1990 the World Federation of Neurology El Escorial criteria for the diagnosis of ALS were established, and four categories of ALS were outlined (Box 31-2). Suspected ALS is characterized by lower motor neuron signs alone in two or more regions, to which might be added upper motor neuron signs on the basis of the clinical examination. Possible ALS is defined as upper and/or lower motor neuron signs in only one region, possibly with a grouping of upper or lower motor neuron signs in other regions. Exclusion of structural lesions would be attempted. Probable ALS is considered if there are upper and lower motor neuron signs in two regions, and the upper motor neuron signs are above the lower motor neuron signs. Structural lesions must definitely be ruled out by neuronal imaging studies. Definite ALS requires lower motor neuron signs to be present in addition to upper motor neuron signs in three CNS regions concomitantly with upper or lower motor neuron signs in other regions with structural lesions excluded. Definite EMG signs of lower motor neuron degeneration require the presence of evidence of acute denervation with fibrillations or positive sharp waves and

---

Box 31-1

ABNORMAL DIAGNOSTIC FINDINGS IN AMYOTROPHIC LATERAL SCLEROSIS

- Clinical features of weakness, atrophy, and fatigue
- EMG: shows fibrillations and fasciculations
- Unstable motor units (in rapidly progressing ALS)
- Increased duration/amplitudes (in slowly progressing ALS)
- Low-amplitude polyphasic motor unit potentials
- Muscle biopsy: shows denervation atrophy
- Muscle enzymes, such as creatine phosphokinase, elevated
- CSF normal
- No changes on myelogram

Box 31-2

WORLD FEDERATION OF NEUROLOGY EL ESCORIAL CRITERIA FOR DIAGNOSIS OF AMYOTROPHIC LATERAL SCLEROSIS (ALS)

WEAKNESS/ATROPHY/HYPERREFLEXIA/PLASTICITY EMG/NCV/NEUROIMAGING			
Suspected ALS	**Possible ALS**	**Probable ALS**	**Definite ALS**
LMN signs in more than two regions	UMN + LMN signs in one region	UMN + LMN signs in two regions	UMN + LMN signs in three regions
UMN signs in more than one region	UMN + LMN signs in more than two regions	UMN + LMN signs in more than two regions	UMN + LMN signs in more than three regions
	Add LMN signs to UMN regions	Add LMN signs to UMN regions	(Discern from ALS plus, ALS LAUS, ALS mimics)
	Add UMN signs to LMN regions	Add LMN signs to UMN regions	
	Exclude structural lesions	Exclude structural lesions	Exclude structural lesions
	(Exclude other causes)	(Exclude other causes)	(Exclude other causes)

( ), Proposal to add this category to diagnostic criteria for ALS, WFN El Escorial Revisited; EMG, electromyography; LAUS, laboratory abnormalities of uncertain significance; LMN, lower motor neuron; NCV, nerve conduction velocity; UMN, upper motor neuron.
Data from Brooks BR: Introduction: defining optimal management in ALS: from first symptoms to announcement, *Neurology* 53(Suppl 5):S1–S3, 1999.

Box 31-3

DISORDERS THAT CAN MIMIC AMYOTROPHIC LATERAL SCLEROSIS

- Myasthenia gravis
- Cervical myelopathy
- Multifocal motor neuropathy
- Hypoparathyroidism
- Inclusion body myositis
- Bulbospinal neuronopathy
- Lymphoma
- Radiation-induced effects

chronic denervation represented by large-amplitude and long-duration motor unit potentials, as well as reduced recruitment in each muscle.[32]

There are several disorders that resemble ALS that are treatable. ALS must be differentiated from other conditions that produce a combination of upper and lower motor neuron lesions. Lymphoma and Lyme disease can cause diffuse lower motor axonal neuropathy. Disorders of the cervical cord, such as skull base deformities, syringomyelia, cord tumors, and cervical spondylosis, must be ruled out.[19] Box 31-3 describes disorders that can mimic ALS.

In such cases, however, there should not be any evidence of anterior horn cell involvement in the legs or trunk, but only in the upper limbs. Cervical myelopathy can look like ALS if cord compression is combined with root involvement. The lower motor neuron findings are only in the arms, an important diagnostic feature, and this situation can be confirmed by imaging of the cervical cord and use of EMG to determine if there are fasciculations in the legs. Any signs of disease caused by a lesion above the foramen magnum, such as bulbar signs or cranial nerve V or VII involvement, would rule out a cervical cause. Lower motor neuron lesions may be predominant with spinal arachnoiditis (usually syphilitic) and radiculitis, cervical ribs, and peripheral nerve lesions, including the postpolio syndrome. Weakness and wasting are typical of all forms of hereditary motor neuropathy, some of which occur first in adult life, and in hereditary motor and sensory neuropathy. The same findings, although without fasciculations, are also seen in primary muscle disease, rheumatoid arthritis, and myotonic dystrophy. If there is doubt about evidence of anterior horn cell disease in the trunk or legs, EMG should be able to demonstrate that which cannot be seen clinically.

Weight loss may suggest carcinoma, and investigations should be undertaken to rule out underlying malignancy if there is any atypical feature on examination or investigation, such as marked slowing of motor nerve conduction velocities. Most other mimics can be excluded by history, such as hereditary neuropathy, prior gastrectomy, polio, or electrical injury. Dyspnea may suggest chronic obstructive pulmonary disease or heart failure. Thorough examination will reveal hyperthyroidism or acromegaly. Laboratory tests will reveal lead or other metal poisoning. ALS symptoms may mimic nonneurologic diseases, and neurologic signs may be missed.[16] Involvement of the sensory system or conduction block with evoked potential testing may indicate other neurodegenerative disease processes.

TREATMENT. Riluzole remains the only Food and Drug Administration (FDA)–approved drug for ALS. Riluzole has a broad range of pharmacologic effects, including inhibition of glutamate release, postsynaptic glutamate receptor activation, and voltage-sensitive sodium channel inactivation. Riluzole appears to be neuroprotective and slows the disease course by approximately 10% to 15%, but it is not curative. There is controversy over the best time to begin therapy with riluzole.[102] Neuroprotective effects would be more extensive when there are more motor units intact to preserve, and this argument supports early treatment.[45] Asthenia and gastrointestinal side effects are common, and the long-term neurotoxic effects are unknown.

Although neuroinflammation occurs in the brainstem and spinal cord of individuals with ALS, suggesting that antiinflammatory agents may be effective in treating this disease, use of medications directed toward inflammation has not proved to change the course of ALS.

Myotrophin (insulin-like growth factor I) appears to affect motor dysfunction by promoting the survival of motor neurons and regeneration of motor nerves.[113]

The high metabolic load of motor neurons and the consequent dependence of these cells on oxidative phosphorylation may make them particularly vulnerable to the loss of mitochondrial function. Coenzyme Q10 is an antioxidant and an essential mitochondrial cofactor facilitating electron transfer in the respiratory chain. Studies have not proven significant changes when given after diagnosis is made. Use of vitamin E as an antioxidant early in the course has been advocated, but studies show limited effect. The impetus for studying and treating individuals with antioxidant therapy is its role in protecting against motor neuron injury.[225]

Oxidative stress appears to put people at risk for ALS comparable to that found in those with Alzheimer disease. People at risk for ALS might be identified by use of bioassays showing increased oxidative damage comparable to that in individuals with diagnosed disease. These assays could lead to early intervention and primary prevention. A ketogenic diet similar to the one employed to control epilepsy may be of some effect as ketones have the ability to alter mitochondrial function and have a positive effect in ALS based on animal studies.[227]

Although no medication can stop the disease, much can be done in the form of symptomatic therapy. Health care providers should emphasize the value of maintaining the highest level of function throughout the course of the disease, providing education and support to prepare for the rapid decline in function. Symptomatic measures may include the use of anticholinergic drugs to control drooling and baclofen or diazepam to control spasticity. Dextromethorphan-quinidine, commonly used for coughs, shows benefit in the treatment of pseudobulbar emotional lability.[229] Table 31-1 lists medications used for symptomatic control.

Maintenance of nutrition is a significant problem because of the difficulty chewing and swallowing. Weakness of jaw movement, loss of tongue mobility, and difficulty in lip closure, in addition to impairment of the swallowing reflex, are common. This may lead to respiratory complications from aspiration. By modifying the consistency and texture of food and fluids, the risk of

Table 31-1 | Symptomatic Treatment in Amyotrophic Lateral Sclerosis

Symptoms	Pharmacotherapy	Other Therapy
Fatigue	Pyridostigmine bromide Antidepressants Methylphenidate Amantadine Modafinil	Energy conservation, work modification Sleep study: BiPAP if abnormal
Spasticity	Baclofen Tizanidine Dantrolene sodium Diazepam	Movement to inhibit tone, Botox injections
Jaw clenching	Benzodiazepines	Botulinum toxin injections into masseters
Cramps	Quinine sulfate Baclofen Vitamin E Clonazepam	Massage Physical therapy
Fasciculations	Carbamazepine	Assurance
Sialorrhea	Hyoscyamine sulphate Diphenhydramine Scopolamine patch Glycopyrrolate Atropine TCAs	Suction machine Botox injection into salivary glands Parotid gland radiation therapy Steam inhalation Nebulization Dark grape juice
Pseudobulbar laughing or crying	TCAs SSRIs Levodopa/carbidopa Lithium Mirtazapine Venlafaxine Quinidine/dextromethorphan	
Thick phlegm	Guaifenesin Nebulized N-acetylcysteine Nebulized saline Propranolol	Insufflation–exsufflation High-flow chest wall oscillation therapy Cool mist humidifier Rehydration Pineapple or papaya juice Reduced intake of dairy products, caffeine, alcohol
Aspiration	Cisapride	Modified food consistency, tracheostomy, modified laryngectomy and tracheal diversion
Joint pains	Antiinflammatory drugs Analgesics	Range-of-motion exercise, warmth-generating modalities
Depression	TCAs SSRIs, venlafaxine, mirtazapine, bupropion	Counseling Support group meetings, psychiatry
Insomnia	Zolpidem tartrate Lorazepam Opioids TCAs	Pressure air pad/gel mattress Noninvasive positive pressure ventilation where appropriate
Laryngospasm	Sublingual lorazepam	
Respiratory failure	Bronchodilators Morphine sulfate	Hospital bed Nocturnal noninvasive ventilator IPPB
Constipation	Increase oral liquid Metamucil Dulcolax suppositories Lactulose and other laxative	Exercise "power pudding": prune juice, prunes, applesauce, bran

BiPAP, Bilevel positive airway pressure; IPPB, intermittent positive-pressure breathing; SSRI, selective serotonin reuptake inhibitor; TCA, tricyclic antidepressant.

From Daroff RB, Fenichel GM, Jankovic J, Mazziotta JC: *Bradley's neurology in clinical practice*, 6th ed, Philadelphia, 2012, WB Saunders, Table 74.4.

aspiration is reduced.[11] Percutaneous endoscopic gastrostomy is used to provide nutrition when eating is no longer an option.

Noninvasive ventilation should be considered to treat respiratory insufficiency in order to lengthen survival and to slow the decline of forced vital capacity. Noninvasive ventilation may be considered to improve quality of life. Early initiation of noninvasive ventilation may increase compliance and insufflation–exsufflation may be considered to help clear secretions.[166]

Multidisciplinary ALS clinics provide coordinated care. Survival has been found to be longer for individuals with bulbar symptoms, the use of aids and appliances was greater, and the mental quality of life was better for the individuals with ALS who were treated at the multidisciplinary clinics than for individuals who did not receive specialty clinic care. With focused care, up to 80% of individuals with ALS can die at home.[70]

PROGNOSIS. The course of ALS is relentlessly progressive. It appears that earlier onset (younger than 50 years of age) has a longer course. Death from the adult-onset sporadic type usually occurs within 2 to 5 years, resulting mainly from pneumonia caused by respiratory compromise. In general, those with bulbar palsy have a more rapid course than those with primary lateral sclerosis, in whom the prognosis is markedly better. Respiratory failure and inability to eat are part of the final stages of ALS. Nasogastric tube feeding and use of a respirator may be options to prolong the life of the client. Individual and family wishes concerning these procedures should be discussed as early as possible in the course of the disease, as some clients may experience a rapid decline in function at any time.

SPECIAL IMPLICATIONS FOR THE THERAPIST   31-1

Amyotrophic Lateral Sclerosis

The ALS-Specific Quality of Life Instrument (ALSSQOL) is based on the McGill Quality of Life Questionnaire (MQOL), modified by changes in format and by adding questions on religiousness and spirituality. A 59-item tool with a completion time averaging 15 minutes, it is a practical tool for the assessment of overall quality of life in individuals with ALS and appears to be valid and useful across large samples. Validation studies of a shortened version are now under way.[223]

The ALS Functional Rating Scale (ALSFRS-R), which can be found at and downloaded from http://www.alsconnection.com/ALSFRS.asp, is a functional scale that can be used to follow the progression of ALS. Six months are needed to detect changes in the ALSFRS-R score because of variability, due principally to differing rates of progression among patients.[95]

The relationship between verbal associative fluency, verbal abstract reasoning, and judgment in ALS can be evaluated using a 20-minute screening evaluation. Deficiencies in these measures were found in 20% to 35% of patients with limb-onset ALS and in 37% to 60% of patients with bulbar-onset ALS. This simple screen identifies deficits that affect discussions of treatment interventions and end-of-life issues.

Muscle strength declines in an overall linear progression throughout the course of the disease. Staging of ALS helps the therapist to determine the most effective intervention based on the current functional status and on the predicted progression of the disease. Table 31-2 describes interventions associated with the various stages of the disease. Moderate exercise programs can be safely adapted to abilities, interests, specific response to exercise, accessibility, and family support.[155]

The rate of loss is stable within a broad range after the first year, but during the first year there is fluctuation of strength that may be a result of the potential for adaptation within the CNS. At this point, the goal of therapy is to maintain general physical activity and muscular tone. Regular exercise in moderation can help alleviate fatigue and have a beneficial effect on the client's general well-being.[25] Complaints of diffuse pain will start in the early stages, related to joint stiffness and decreases in muscle control in the limbs or trunk.

Spasticity contributes to complaints of weakness. Consistent slow stretching that decreases tone may be of benefit. The Ashworth scale can be used to measure the degree of spasticity. Cramps, which can be a source of pain, also respond to a daily stretching routine.

Changes in gait are significant, and gait analysis is necessary to assess the need for assistive devices. Falls caused by weakness are a major problem. Ankle dorsiflexion is lost before loss of strength in plantar flexion. Hamstring strength appears to correlate with walking, and the decrease parallels the loss of walking ability. Isometric muscle strength as a percentage of normal shows a dramatic decrease late in the course of the disease when fewer muscle fibers are available. This is when the greatest functional losses are noted. A surprisingly small amount of muscle activity is necessary across the joints to allow normal function of a joint. Some movement and joint stability are maintained until the degeneration causes atrophy of muscle activity to less than 20% of normal. The weakness and wasting often produce painful subluxation of the scapulohumeral joint, and the arm should be supported.[2] Contractures should be routinely stretched, taking care to support the joints, since there is minimal control of muscle activity in the late stages. Complaints of pain may begin when the client is unable to shift weight in bed or in sitting. Changing the reclining angle of the bed or wheelchair or the position of the legs will give some relief. Caregivers need to be educated in this aspect of care.

Braces, other assistive devices, and motorized scooters or wheelchairs help to maintain mobility and freedom. Many upper-extremity devices are available to maintain joint alignment at rest, to make daily activities easier to perform, and to support mobility when it is lost. Braces for the lower extremity can extend the time of upright walking, and braces for the back and neck can assist with head and trunk control. Pain is often a complaint brought to the therapist. Thermal modalities and transcutaneous electrical nerve stimulation can help the pain associated with muscle shortening, joint stiffness, and muscle cramping.

Evaluation of the home environment, providing rails, hoists, or supports; eliminating stairs where possible; and advising on helpful devices for feeding, shaving, dressing is essential as the individual becomes limited to household mobility. Posture for activities of daily living may be improved with a collar, a brace, or spring-loaded splints. Special beds can be leased or borrowed. Family and friends may organize a roster of people to sleep over, sparing the spouse from waking

Table 31-2	Exercise and Rehabilitation Programs for Clients with Amyotrophic Lateral Sclerosis
Stage	**Treatment**

Phase I (Independent)

Stage I:

Patient characteristics
- Mild weakness
- Clumsiness
- Ambulatory
- Independent in ADL

- Continue normal activities or increase activities if sedentary to prevent disuse atrophy
- Begin program of ROM exercises (stretching, yoga, tai chi)
- Add strengthening program of gentle resistance exercises to all musculature with caution not to cause overwork fatigue
- Provide psychologic support as needed

Stage II:

Patient characteristics
- Moderate, selective weakness
- Slightly decreased independence in ADL
- Difficulty climbing stairs
- Difficulty raising arms
- Difficulty buttoning clothing
- Ambulatory

- Continue stretching to avoid contractures
- Continue cautious strengthening of muscles with MMT grades above F+ (3+); monitor for overwork fatigue
- Consider orthotic support (i.e., AFOs, wrist, thumb splints)
- Use adaptive equipment to facilitate ADL

Stage III:

Patient characteristics

- Continue stage II program as tolerated; caution not to fatigue to point of decreasing patient's ADL independence
- Keep patient physically independent as long as possible through pleasurable activities, walking
- Encourage deep-breathing exercises, chest stretching, postural drainage if needed
- Prescribe standard or motorized wheelchair with modifications to allow eventual reclining back with head rest, elevating legs

Phase II (Practically Independent)

Stage IV:

Patient characteristics

- Active assisted passive ROM exercises to the weakly supported joint— caution to support, rotate shoulder during abduction and joint accessory motions
- Encourage isometric contractions of all musculature to tolerance
- Try arm slings, overhead slings, or wheelchair arm supports
- Motorize chair if patient wants to be independently mobile; adapt controls as needed

Stage V:

Patient characteristics
- Severe lower-extremity weakness
- Moderate to severe upper-extremity weakness
- Wheelchair-dependent
- Increasingly dependent in ADL
- Possible skin breakdown secondary to poor mobility

- Encourage family to learn proper transfer, positioning principles, turning techniques
- Encourage modifications at home to aid patient's mobility and independence
- Electric hospital bed with antipressure mattress
- If patient elects HMV, adapt chair to hold respiratory unit

Phase III (Dependent)

Stage VI:

Patient characteristics
- Bedridden
- Completely dependent in ADL

- For dysphagia: soft diet, long spoons, tube feeding, percutaneous gastrostomy
- To decrease flow of accumulated saliva: medication, suction, surgery
- For dysarthria: palatal lifts, electronic speech amplification, eye pointing
- For breathing difficulty: clear airway, tracheostomy, respiratory if HMV elected
- Medications to decrease impact of dyspnea

ADL, Activities of daily living; *AFOs*, ankle-foot orthoses; *HMV*, home mechanical ventilation; *MMT*, manual muscle test; *ROM*, range of motion.
Modified from Sinaki M: Exercise and rehabilitation measures in amyotrophic lateral sclerosis. In Yase Y, Tsubaki T: *Amyotrophic lateral sclerosis: recent advances in research and treatment:* Amsterdam, 1988, Elsevier.

every 3 hours to turn the patient. The legs should be elevated and elastic stockings used if leg swelling is a problem. Avoid using diuretics for leg swelling.

Frustration and boredom are common. Family and volunteers can be mobilized from neighborhood groups, such as church or social groups, to visit to talk, listen, play cards, turn pages or read, or just to be there for a while.

Sexual frustration is common and is not often discussed. The clinician should do so freely and without embarrassment with both the patient and spouse; the problems are mainly matters of method. The partner may need counseling to understand that he or she needs to take the active role and to learn effective techniques that overcome weakness and muscle spasms.

Respiratory changes cause the most disability and eventually lead to death. Respiratory distress is a mechanical problem because of lack of muscle support. From the earliest stages of care of the client with ALS, prevention of respiratory complications should be emphasized. Box 31-4 lists the symptoms and signs of potential respiratory impairment.

Early evidence of respiratory involvement may be shortness of breath, poor cough reflex, and headache. Some clients can be taught to use their abdominal muscles to increase inspiration and expiration when the muscles of the diaphragm and intercostal muscles become weak. Swallowing becomes difficult and should be evaluated by a speech pathologist. Pseudobulbar affect causing uncontrolled laughing or crying decreases the capacity to regulate breathing

and increases risk of shortness of breath. Aspiration is common, and techniques to control this can be taught. Mechanical ventilation is an option to prolong the ability to breathe. Individuals with a relatively slow disease progression, and those with spinal onset, might benefit more from treatment with noninvasive ventilation than patients with rapid disease progression or bulbar onset. Noninvasive positive-pressure ventilation improves the patient's quality of life, despite progression of ALS, and without increasing the caregiver burden or stress.[109] In addition, suction, intermittent positive pressure breathing, and postural drainage appear to be useful in maintaining bronchial hygiene. Only 5% of individuals choose long-term, invasive ventilation because of the restriction of activity, caregiver involvement, and overall cost.[141] Communication becomes limited, again because of loss of oral muscle control and breath support. Communication strategies can be taught, and augmentative equipment is available. In all cases, the individual becomes dependent over time. In the terminal stages, the comfort of the patient is the therapeutic goal.

As patients with ALS weaken, the decisions facing the patient progress from issues of morbidity to mortality. Traditionally, the neurologist and other therapeutic support staff have deferred to the wishes of the patient and family members in determining level of support in response to progressive physical decline. Impairments in judgment have potentially significant clinical implications that should be considered by health care providers and caregivers when discussing treatment interventions and end-of-life issues with patients.[81]

All patients with ALS and their families have to come to grips with the many end-of-life decisions that confront them. These include the need to get the many events in life in order, come to terms with relationships, and decide how forthcoming disabilities will be handled. Decisions regarding care at home versus in a nursing facility should be made as early as possible. Information about advance directives, living wills, and power of attorney should be available. Patients may raise the question of suicide or assisted suicide, and the caregivers should be comfortable not only talking about these issues but also calling on others who may have more expertise and experience in discussing these issues. It makes things more difficult for the patient and family if the caregivers avoid these sensitive areas and talk only about the disease and medical management. Psychologic and emotional support for the individual and the family is critical. A direct and informative approach is appreciated; giving false hope should be avoided.

Box 31-4

SYMPTOMS AND SIGNS OF POTENTIAL RESPIRATORY IMPAIRMENT

Symptoms

Breathlessness
Orthopnea
Recurrent chest infections
Disturbed sleep
Nonrefreshing sleep
Nightmares
Daytime sleepiness
Poor concentration and/or memory
Confusion
Hallucinations
Morning headaches
Fatigue
Poor appetite

Signs

Increased respiratory rate
Shallow breathing
Weak cough
Weak sniff
Abdominal paradox (inward movement of the abdomen during inspiration)
Use of accessory muscles of respiration
Reduced chest expansion on maximal inspiration

From NICE Clinical Guideline 105. Available at: http://nice.org.uk/guidance/CG105/chapter/1-guidance. Accessed July 31, 2014.

ALZHEIMER DISEASE AND VARIANTS
Overview and Definition

In 1907, Alois Alzheimer described the case of a 51-year-old woman who presented with a relatively rapidly deteriorating memory along with psychiatric disturbances resulting in death 4 years later. Alzheimer disease (AD), as it is now labeled, is described by the hallmark pathology of neurofibrillary tangle and continues with relentless neurologic deterioration.

Dementia is a term for a decline in intellectual functioning severe enough to interfere with a person's relationships and ability to carry out daily activities. A significant decline in memory is a hallmark of dementia, but is not the only characteristic. Age-associated memory impairment, or benign senescent forgetfulness, is a decline in short-term memory that does not progress to other mental or intellectual impairments. Other causes of dementia must be carefully ruled out, and there are syndromes that mimic AD in relationship to the dementia but have different neurologic causes.

AD is the most common cause of dementia overall. It is one of the principal causes of disability and decreased quality of life among older adults.[2] Progress in clinical knowledge of AD has led to more reliable diagnostic criteria and accuracy; the earliest manifestations and even the presymptomatic phases of the disease may soon be identifiable. Table 31-3 lists definitions related to dementia.

Incidence and Etiologic and Risk Factors

There are approximately 25 million people with AD worldwide, 5 million in the United States. The prevalence of AD rises with each decade of age. The known prevalence is 6% in people older than 65 years of age, 20% in people older than 80 years of age, and more than 95% in those older than 95 years of age.[256]

Data from Alzheimer's Disease International forecast that the prevalence of AD worldwide will double every 20 years, to 65.7 million by 2030 and 115.4 million by 2050, with higher proportions in developed versus undeveloped countries.[193] Because life expectancy continues to rise, so does the potential for more individuals to be afflicted. It is thought that many individuals with the symptoms go undiagnosed and untreated. The cause of AD remains unknown, but there appears to be a relationship among genetic predisposition; the abnormal processing of a normal cellular substance, amyloid; and advanced age.[124] Lifetime risk of developing AD is estimated to be between 12% and 17%. Twin studies show evidence that in identical twins, one may develop AD while the other remains dementia free. People with a family history of the disease are at higher than average risk for AD.

The apolipoprotein E (*APOE*) gene, on chromosome 19, is the major genetic source of the common forms of late-onset AD. The APOE2 allele may be protective, and the APOE4 allele is associated with increased risk. Individuals inherit a copy of one type of allele from each parent, but AD is not inevitable, even in people with two copies of the APOE4 allele. People without APOE4 have an estimated risk of between 9% and 20% for developing AD by age 85 years. In people with one copy of the gene, the risk is between 25% and 60%. In people with two copies, the risk ranges from 50% to 90%. But only 2% of the population carries two copies of the APOE4 allele. No evidence exists that these mutations play a role in the more common, sporadic, nonfamilial form of late-onset AD. However, there is a subtype of early-onset AD seen in families with histories of late-onset disease. The exact genetic abnormality and transmission are still unclear. *APOE4* accounts for only part of the genetic risk for Alzheimer disease. A family history of dementia, regardless of *APOE4* status, can also increase the risk of developing the disorder. Specifically, persons with a first-degree relative with dementia have a 10% to 30% increased risk of developing AD.

The underlying mechanism through which *APOE* influences AD risk has not yet been determined. Scientists have explored several possibilities, including the idea that *APOE* may play a role in cholesterol transport, neuronal integrity, and amyloid deposition.[127]

The amyloid precursor protein (APP) gene is located on chromosome 21. Studies report the greatest deposits of β-amyloid in people with APOE4. It appears that the APOE protein removes β-amyloid but that the APOE4 variant does so less efficiently than other APOE types. Genetic mutations in the genes that control APP are also being targeted as causes of early-onset AD. In the genetic disease Down syndrome, for example, β-APP, the source of β-amyloid, is overproduced, which almost always leads to early AD.

Mutations in genes known as presenilin 1 and presenilin 2 account for most cases of early-onset inherited AD. The defective genes appear to accelerate β-amyloid plaque formation and apoptosis, a natural process by which cells self-destruct.

Mutations of these and other genes have been identified and provide strong support for the "amyloid cascade hypothesis" of AD (Fig. 31-3). Although the amyloid cascade is currently considered by many researchers as a key contributor to the pathogenesis of AD, some researchers have challenged this assertion and have proposed that β-amyloid occurs secondary to neuron stress and functions as a protective adaptation to the disease rather than causing cell death.

The same genes may have different effects depending on the ethnic population. Dietary and other cultural factors that increase the risk for hypertension and unhealthy cholesterol levels may also play a role. For example,

Table 31-3	Key Definitions Related to Dementia
Term	**Definition**
CIND	A clinical syndrome with deficits in memory or other cognitive abilities that have minimal impact on day-to-day functioning and does not meet criteria for dementia
MCI	A clinical subsyndrome of CIND. Amnestic or nonamnestic
Dementia	A clinical syndrome consisting of global cognitive decline, memory deficits plus 1 other area of cognition, and significant effect on day-to-day functioning. Not delirium
Alzheimer dementia	A dementia syndrome that has gradual onset and slow progression and is best explained as caused by Alzheimer disease
Alzheimer disease	A brain disease characterized by plaques, tangles, and neuronal loss

CIND, Cognitive impairment not dementia; MCI, mild cognitive impairment.

From Nowrangi MA, Rao V, Lyketsos CG: Epidemiology, assessment, and treatment of dementia. *Psychiatr Clin North Am* 34(2):275–294, 2011, Table 1.

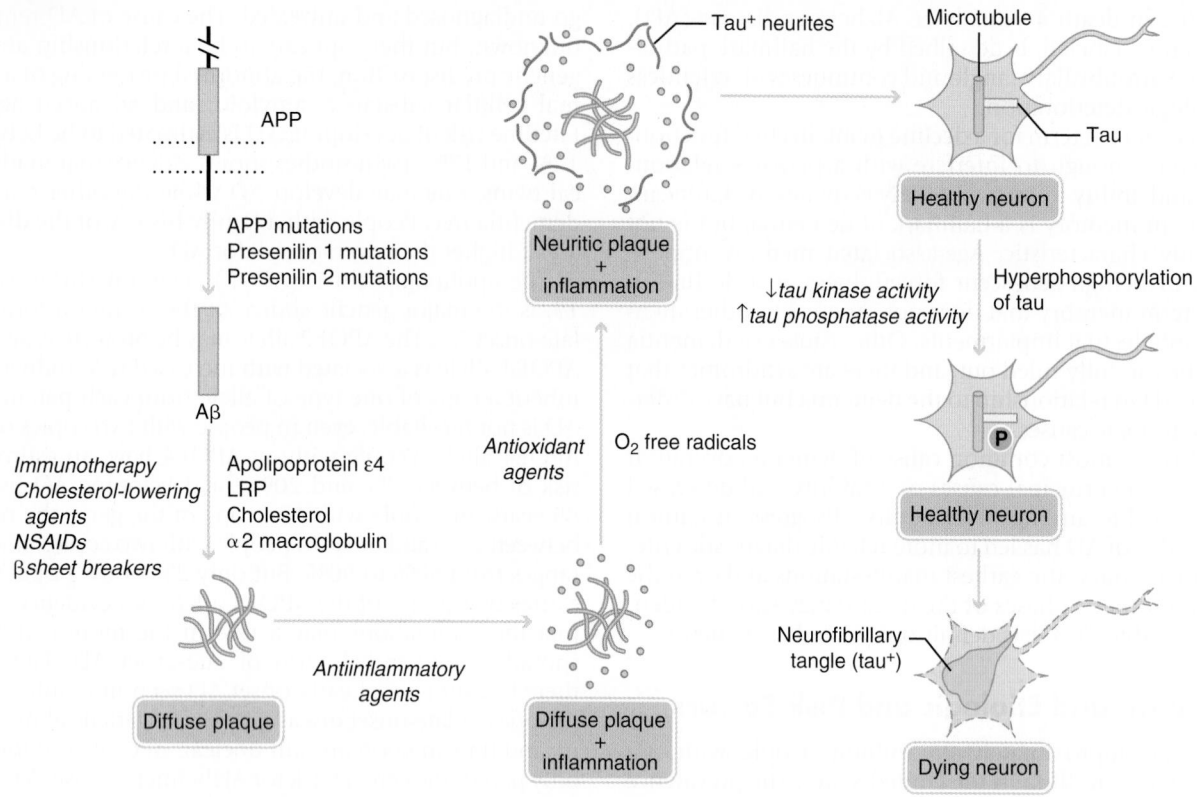

Figure 31-3

The amyloid cascade hypothesis of Alzheimer disease pathogenesis and potential therapeutic targets. (From Goetz CG: *Textbook of clinical neurology,* ed 3, Philadelphia, 2007, WB Saunders.)

a study of Japanese men showed that their risk increased if they emigrated to America. And the disease is much less common in West Africa than in African Americans, whose risk is the same as or higher than that of white Americans.

Some studies have reported an association between AD and systolic hypertension. Furthermore, some studies report a lower risk for AD in individuals whose blood pressure was reduced. Nevertheless, although hypertension is strongly linked to memory and mental difficulties, stronger evidence is needed to prove any causal relationship between hypertension and AD.

Vascular risk factors increase the risk for AD, including hypertension, diabetes, and hyperlipidemia. There has been research suggesting an association between high cholesterol levels and AD in some people. A number of recent studies support the link between AD and cholesterol by suggesting that certain cholesterol-lowing drugs known as statins may be protective against AD. The APOE genotype is linked with both atherosclerosis and AD. The APOE4 genotype reflects abnormal cholesterol transport.[252] Level of education may be a marker for some other risk factor.

Highly educated (or highly intelligent) people may have a higher cognitive reserve, allowing longer and more effective adaptation to declining brain function. People with less education (often less wealthy), may be at higher risk because of exposure to malnutrition and noxious substances early in life. Some studies suggest that depression is a risk factor for dementia Additional studies revealing the true mechanism could eventually lead to more specific treatments for AD. Indeed, studies

---

Box 31-5

KEY RISK FACTORS AND PROTECTIVE FACTORS FOR ALZHEIMER DISEASE

- Primary risk factors: age; family history; genetic markers such as apolipoprotein E ε4 gene; trisomy 21; mutations in presenilins 1 and 2; female gender after 80 years of age; cardiovascular risk factors such as hypertension, diabetes, obesity, and hypercholesterolemia
- Possible risk factors: head injury; depression; progression of Parkinson-like signs in older adults; lower thyroid-stimulating hormone level within the normal range; hyperhomocysteinemia; folate deficiency; hyperinsulinemia; low educational attainment
- Possible protective factors: apolipoprotein E ε2 gene; regular fish consumption; regular consumption of omega-3 fatty acids; high educational level; regular exercise; nonsteroidal antiinflammatory drug therapy; moderate alcohol intake; adequate intake of vitamins C, E, B$_6$, and B$_{12}$, and folate

From Desai AK: Diagnosis and treatment of Alzheimer's disease, *Neurology* 64(12 Suppl 3):S34–S39, 2005.

---

of asymptomatic *APOE4* carriers show that these persons are more likely to display subtle abnormalities on brain scans, such as positron emission tomography (PET) or magnetic resonance imaging (MRI) scans. Combining information on *APOE4* carrier status with other informative biologic marker data is a promising research strategy for detecting individuals who might be candidates for AD prevention strategies.[266] Box 31-5 outlines some of the key risk factors as well as possible protective factors related to AD.

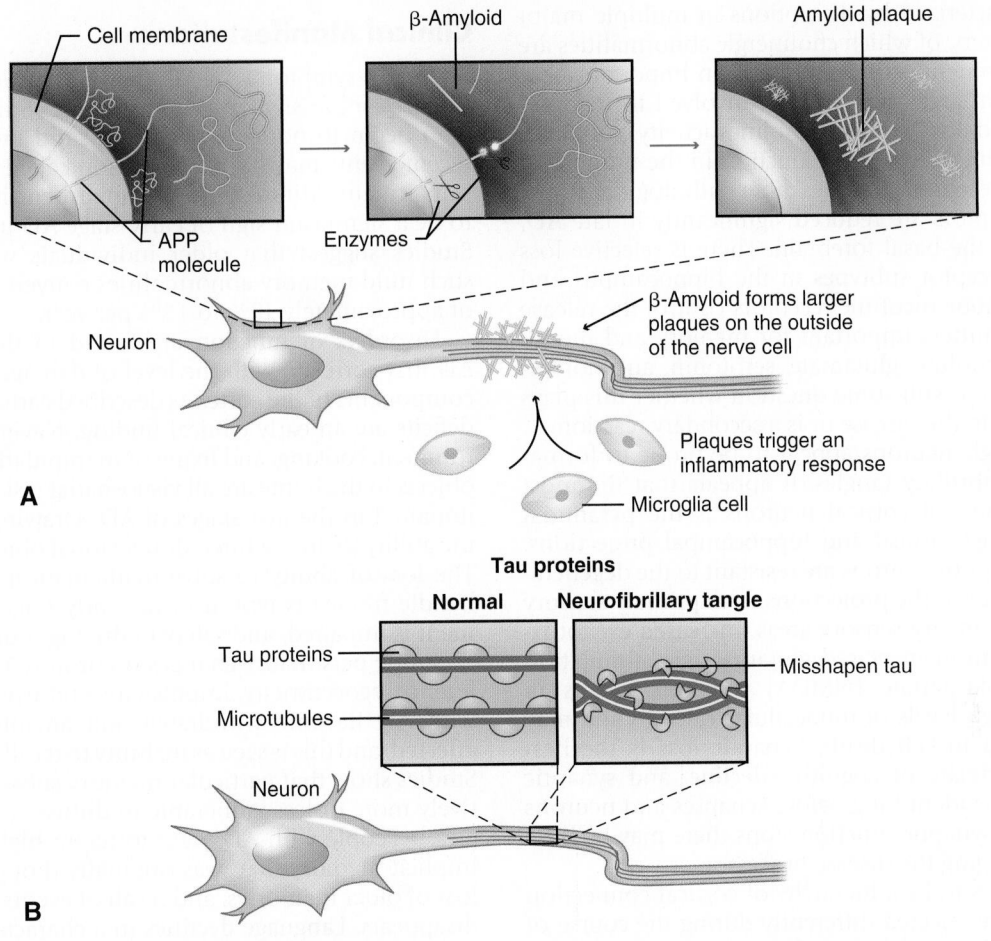

Figure 31-4

Current etiologic theories for the development of Alzheimer disease. A, Abnormal amounts of β-amyloid are cleaved from the amyloid precursor protein (APP) and released into the circulation. The β-amyloid fragments come together in clumps to form plaques that attach to the neuron. Microglia react to the plaque, and an inflammatory response results. **B,** Tau proteins provide structural support for the neuron microtubules. Chemical changes in the neuron produce structural changes in tau proteins. This results in twisting and tangling (neurofibrillary tangles). (From Lewis SM: *Medical-surgical nursing: assessment and management of clinical problems,* ed 8, St. Louis, 2011, Mosby.)

Pathogenesis

Like other degenerative conditions, AD has no single identified cause. The loss of neurons is thought to be a consequence of the breakdown of several processes necessary for sustaining brain cells. There are several neuropathologic hallmarks of AD. There is progressive accumulation of insoluble fibrous material, amyloid. Senile plaques consisting of extracellular amyloid are found in higher concentrations in the brains of individuals with AD than in normal aging brains. The amyloid deposition appears to have a relationship to β-amyloid protein, a natural substance that is required to maintain fibroblasts and cell function. Components of this protein occur typically as a by-product of neuron function. Normally, the β-amyloid dissolves and is reabsorbed by the brain tissue. When it remains in the fluid surrounding the neurons, the β-amyloid protein may deform its shape by folding in on itself. This abnormal protein then sticks together with other β-amyloid material, forming a sheet of connected proteins; the result is a plaque. The amyloid plaque also includes fragmented axons, altered glial cells, and cellular debris. This plaque triggers an inflammatory response, resulting in increased free radicals that cause damage to the nervous system.

APP is a large nerve-protecting protein that is the source of β-amyloid. In AD, certain enzymes, particularly those called γ-secretases, snip APP into β-amyloid pieces. This process is controlled by presenilin proteins. An additional protein in the areas of the brain affected by AD is endoplasmic reticulum–associated binding protein, and it appears to combine with β-amyloid, which in turn attracts new β-amyloid from outside the cells. High amounts of endoplasmic reticulum–associated binding protein may also enhance the toxicity of β-amyloid. It appears that the amyloid plaque, when it comes in contact with a neuron, causes chemical changes that may lead to the destruction and destabilization of microtubules, the structural components of the neural cells. A protein molecule called tau normally responsible for holding the microtubules together detaches and causes the microtubule to disintegrate. This process may be caused by an enzyme that escapes its normal restraints and breaks down the tau. As the microtubule disintegrates, neurofibrillary tangles form and remain in the system. The overall effects are decreased cell division and loss of axonal transport of neurotransmitters. Figure 31-4 shows a typical neuritic plaque and neurofibrillary tangle.

AD is characterized by disruptions in multiple major neurotransmitters, of which cholinergic abnormalities are the most prominent. Acetylcholine is an important neurotransmitter in areas of the brain involved in memory formation, and loss of acetylcholine activity correlates with the severity of AD. The reduction in the number of acetylcholine receptors precedes other pathologic changes, and these receptors are reduced significantly in late AD, particularly in the basal forebrain. There is selective loss of nicotinic receptor subtypes in the hippocampus and cortex. Presynaptic nicotinic receptors control the release of neurotransmitters important for memory and mood, such as acetylcholine, glutamate, serotonin, and norepinephrine. There is still some question whether this plays a primary role in the disease or is a secondary reaction.

Glutaminergic neurons appear to be prone to formation of neurofibrillary tangles. It appears that the most vulnerable group of cortical neurons is the pyramidal cells with corticocortical and hippocampal projections. Other subgroups of neurons are resistant to the degenerative process, such as the projections from primary sensory to adjacent secondary sensory areas. Increased excitotoxicity resulting from increased glutamatergic stimulation of N-methyl-D-aspartate (NMDA) receptors results in abnormally high levels of intracellular calcium and may ultimately lead to cell death. Synaptic loss is the best pathologic correlate of cognitive decline, and synaptic dysfunction is evident long before synapses and neurons are lost. Once synaptic function stops there may be little chance of changing the disease process.

There appears to be a hierarchy of cortical connection systems that are affected differently during the course of AD. A progression of the neurofibrillary tangles seems to move from the entorhinal cortex and hippocampus to the limbic system to the cortex, including the frontal, temporal parietal, and occipital cortices. One study suggests that the effect of AD on hippocampal volume equals the effect of roughly 17 years of aging.[249] This may correlate with the changes seen in memory, behavior, and motor skills as the disease progresses. The distribution of the lesions in the cerebral cortex may be different in AD compared with that in other disease processes that cause dementia.

Cerebral amyloid angiopathy may predispose an individual to develop AD. Cerebral amyloid angiopathy is an important feature of senile dementia and AD along with senile plaques, neurofibrillary tangles, neutrophil threads, and synapse loss. Amyloid gradually causes atrophy of the medial smooth muscle cells of the arteries of the brain that weakens them, causing predisposition to hemorrhage.[181] There appears to be a relationship between strokes and AD (see Chapter 32). Abnormalities have been reported in fibroblasts, red and white blood cells, and platelets. Alterations in blood proteins have been observed.[147]

Protein kinase R (PKR) is a kinase that has been shown to play a role in recognizing and signaling viral infection is altered in several neurologic disorders in which it negatively modulates memory and can become toxic. PKR accumulates in the brain of patients with AD and can indirectly induce the phosphorylation of tau can induce the death of neurons. PKR levels in the CSF and the activity of PKR in the brain are highly elevated in patients with AD.[116,266]

Clinical Manifestations

The early symptoms of AD may be overlooked because they resemble signs of natural aging. Still, older adults who begin to notice a persistent mild memory loss for recent events may have a condition called mild cognitive impairment. Mild cognitive impairment is now thought to be a significant sign of early-stage AD in older people. Studies suggest that older individuals who experience such mild memory abnormalities convert to AD at a rate of approximately 10% to 15% per year.

Disorders of function are found in the person with AD that correlate with the level of damage in the various components of the cortex as described earlier. Visuospatial deficits are an early clinical finding. Navigating the environment, cooking, and fixing or manipulating mechanical objects in the home are all visuospatial tasks that often are impaired in the first stages of AD. Drawing is abnormal; the ability to draw a three-dimensional object is often lost. The loss of ability to solve mathematical problems and handle money is typical in the early stages of AD. Judgment is impaired, and safety in driving is diminished.

Subtle personality changes occur in AD, such as indifference, egocentricity, impulsivity, and irritability. People with AD become withdrawn and anxious. Memory is affected, and this is seen as inability to recall current events. Studies show that particular memory subsystems are relatively more or less vulnerable to diffuse cortical pathologies.[36] People with AD seem to retain higher capacity in implicit memory than was originally thought. AD causes loss of older memories, and recall of events from early life disappears. Language declines in a characteristic progression. Word-finding difficulty is first, followed by inability to remember names (anomia), and finally diminished comprehension. Social situations become difficult, and mood swings are common.[162] Between 40% and 60% of individuals with late-onset AD suffer from psychotic symptoms, which may include hallucinations, delusions, and dramatic verbal, emotional, or physical outbursts. This is a severe form of AD, with a genetic basis, that has a more rapid and aggressive course. Table 31-4 describes the difference between normal aging and AD.

Major depression is uncommon, but many persons with AD have periods of depressed mood associated with feelings of inadequacy and hopelessness. AD-associated depression is often more modifiable by environmental manipulation than depressions not associated with AD. As AD progresses, delusions, agitation, and even violence may occur.

Abnormal motor signs are common, related to the area of the brain that is involved, and perhaps caused by the type of neurotransmitter dysfunction. A relationship between the motor impairments and levels of function can be seen. Presence of tremor appears to be associated with increased risk for cognitive decline, presence of bradykinesia with increased risk for functional decline, and presence of postural-gait impairments with increased risk for institutionalization and death. Disorders of sleep, eating, and sexual behavior are common. The electroencephalogram shows more awake time in bed, longer latencies to rapid eye movement sleep, and losses in slow-wave sleep.[164]

Table 31-4	Differences Between Normal Signs of Aging and Dementia

Early Signs of Alzheimer Disease
Memory and Concentration

Normal	Dementia
• Periodic minor memory lapses or forgetfulness of part of an experience. • Occasional lapses in attention or lapses in attention or concentration.	• Misplacement of important items. • Confusion about how to perform simple tasks. • Trouble with simple arithmetic problems. • Difficulty making routine decisions. • Confusion about month or season.

Mood and Behavior

• Temporary sadness or anxiety based on appropriate and specific cause. • Changing interests. • Increasingly cautious behavior.	• Unpredictable mood changes. • Increasing loss of outside interests. • Depression, anger, or confusion in response to change. • Denial of symptoms.

Later Signs of Alzheimer Disease
Language and Speech

• Unimpaired language skills.	• Difficulty completing sentences or finding the right words. • Inability to understand the meaning of words. • Reduced and/or irrelevant conversation.

Movement/Coordination

• Increasing caution in movement. • Slower reaction times.	• Visibly impaired movement or coordination, including slowing of movements, halting gait, and reduced sense of balance.

Other Symptoms

• Normal sense of smell. No abnormal weight changes in either men or women.	• Impaired sense of smell. Severe weight loss, particularly in female patients.

Data from *Alzheimer's disease: early warning signs and diagnostic resources.* The Junior League of NYC, Inc. 1988.

MEDICAL MANAGEMENT

DIAGNOSIS. The most important diagnostic step in evaluating dementias is to determine whether a chronic encephalopathy results from a potentially reversible cause. Interaction of multiple medications can also trigger dementia and should be assessed.

A decline from previous levels of functioning and impairment in multiple cognitive domains beyond memory are critical in establishing dementia. Determining the rate of change is useful, since abrupt changes are not consistent with AD.[26] The progression is usually continuous and does not fluctuate or improve. Box 31-6 shows the Global Deterioration Scale. Information obtained from family members or caregivers can provide data when there seems to be lack of insight from the client. The Functional Activities Questionnaire is a useful informant-based measure.

Clinical screening tests, such as the Short Test of Mental Status, the Mini-Mental State Examination, and Mattis Dementia Rating Scale, provide a baseline for monitoring the course of cognitive impairment over time and document multiple cognitive impairments.[2]

A clock drawing test is also a good test for AD. The individual is given a piece of paper with a circle on it and is first asked to write the numbers in the face of a clock and then to show "10 minutes after 11." The score is based on spacing between the numbers and the positions of the hands.

Neuropsychologic tests can accurately predict the probability of conversion to incident AD after 5 or 10 years.[72,236] Clues on physical examination include a variety of findings that may be common in elderly individuals but are not part of the typical picture of AD, such as ataxia, hyperreflexia, and tremulousness. Depression can be difficult to distinguish from dementia, and it can coexist with dementia.

Ruling out a partially or completely reversible dementia by performing a blood count, chest radiography, and general neurologic examination is critical in the diagnostic evaluation of a person with suspected AD. Autoimmune and paraneoplastic serologic studies may be helpful in such individuals as well.

Forming a complete differential diagnosis requires ruling out other potential causes of disease. The American Academy of Neurology recommends serum analyses that include thyroid function tests, hepatic panels, metabolic panel, complete blood count, vitamin B_{12} levels, and folate levels. In addition, heavy metal screens, syphilis serology, urine or serum toxicology, electrocardiogram, and chest radiograph may be considered. Brain imaging may include either noncontrast head computed tomography, brain MRI, and PET based on clinical findings. Other biomarkers, such as CSF tau, β-amyloid levels, and genetic screening for APOE4, continue to be used in research but may soon be used in the clinical setting.

Use of neuroimaging can be beneficial in the diagnosis of AD. Both MRI and computed tomography (CT) can identify the changes in brain size that are associated with AD. Diagnostic criteria are based on the measurement of medial temporal lobe atrophy or on the volumetric measurement of the entorhinal cortex and hippocampus.[23] The brain demonstrates atrophy with normal aging, so this is not the only diagnostic test.[160]

Single-photon emission computed tomography (SPECT) can be used to determine brain activity, especially in areas where information is processed for memory functions. This may be used in the future to predict potential for development of AD. Fluorodeoxyglucose PET imaging reveals a patient's pathology, and provides a marker of clinical status and disease progression.

Hippocampal atrophy, decreased CSF amyloid, and decreased brain glucose metabolism when present together in a patient appear to lead on to development of AD.[92]

Box 31-6

GLOBAL DETERIORATION SCALE

Stage 1

NO COGNITIVE DECLINE: During the first of the dementia stages, there is no subjective complaints of memory deficit. No memory deficit evident on clinical interview.

Stage 2

VERY MILD COGNITIVE DECLINE (Age Associated Memory Impairment): Subjective complaints of memory deficit, most frequently in following areas: (a) forgetting where one has placed familiar objects; (b) forgetting names one formerly knew well. No objective evidence of memory deficit on clinical interview. No objective deficits in employment or social situations. Appropriate concern with respect to symptomatology.

Stage 3

MILD COGNITIVE DECLINE (Mild Cognitive Impairment): During this stage of the **dementia stages,** one might observe clear-cut deficits. Manifestations in more than one of the following areas: (a) patient may have gotten lost when traveling to an unfamiliar location; (b) coworkers become aware of patient's relatively poor performance; (c) word and name finding deficit becomes evident to intimates; (d) patient may read a passage or a book and retain relatively little material; (e) patient may demonstrate decreased facility in remembering names upon introduction to new people; (f) patient may have lost or misplaced an object of value; (g) concentration deficit may be evident on clinical testing. Objective evidence of memory deficit obtained only with an intensive interview. Decreased performance in demanding employment and social settings. Denial begins to become manifest in patient. Mild to moderate anxiety accompanies symptoms.

Stage 4

MODERATE COGNITIVE DECLINE (Mild Dementia): Clear-cut deficit on careful clinical interview. Deficit manifest in following areas: (a) decreased knowledge of current and recent events; (b) may exhibit some deficit in memory of one's personal history; (c) concentration deficit elicited on serial subtractions; (d) decreased ability to travel, handle finances, etc. **Frequently no deficit in following areas:** (a) orientation to time and place; (b) recognition of familiar persons and faces; (c) ability to travel to familiar locations. Inability to perform complex tasks. Denial is dominant defense mechanism. Flattening of affect and withdrawal from challenging situations frequently occur.

Stage 5

MODERATELY SEVERE COGNITIVE DECLINE (Moderate Dementia): Patient can no longer survive without some assistance. Patient is unable during interview to recall a major relevant aspect of their current lives, for example, an address or telephone number of many years, the names of close family members (such as grandchildren), the name of the high school or college from which they graduated. Frequently some disorientation to time (date, day of week, season, etc.) or to place. An educated person may have difficulty counting back from 40 by 4s or from 20 by 2s. Persons at this stage retain knowledge of many major facts regarding themselves and others. They invariably know their own names and generally know their spouses' and children's names. They require no assistance with toileting and eating, but may have some difficulty choosing the proper clothing to wear.

Stage 6

SEVERE COGNITIVE DECLINE (Moderately Severe Dementia): May occasionally forget the name of the spouse upon whom they are entirely dependent for survival. Will be largely unaware of all recent events and experiences. Retain some knowledge of their past, but this is very sketchy. Generally unaware of their surroundings, the year, the season, etc. May have difficulty counting from 10, both backward and, sometimes, forward. Will require some assistance with activities of daily living, for example, may become incontinent, will require travel assistance but occasionally will be able to travel to familiar locations. Diurnal rhythm frequently disturbed. Almost always recall their own name. Frequently continue to be able to distinguish familiar from unfamiliar persons in their environment. Personality and emotional changes occur. These are quite variable and include: (a) delusional behavior, for example, patients may accuse their spouse of being an impostor, may talk to imaginary figures in the environment, or to their own reflection in the mirror; (b) obsessive symptoms, for example, person may continually repeat simple cleaning activities; (c) anxiety symptoms, agitation, and even previously nonexistent violent behavior may occur; (d) cognitive abulia, that is, loss of willpower, because an individual cannot carry a thought long enough to determine a purposeful course of action.

Stage 7

VERY SEVERE COGNITIVE DECLINE (Severe Dementia): Here in the last stage of the **dementia stages** all verbal abilities are lost over the course of this stage. Frequently there is no speech at all—only unintelligible utterances and rare emergence of seemingly forgotten words and phrases. Incontinent of urine, requires assistance toileting and feeding. Basic psychomotor skills, for example, ability to walk, are lost with the progression of this stage. The brain appears to no longer be able to tell the body what to do. Generalized rigidity and developmental neurologic reflexes are frequently present.

From http://www.7dementiastages.com/dementia-stages. Accessed on June 10, 2013.

Researchers are looking at different components of the human brain cell to identify molecular changes in deoxyribonucleic acid (DNA) and RNA seen in individuals with dementia and AD. Approaches are widespread, as it is clear that the disease is multifactorial. Patients with AD typically have a selective reduction in CSF β-amyloid 42, the brain effectively acting as a "sink" for the molecule. Conversely, tau and phosphorylated-tau are excessively *released* from the brain and into the CSF in patients with AD, with an increase in total tau representing neuronal damage and increased phosphorylated-tau reflecting neurofibrillary tangle formation.

Disease states that can mimic AD include Pick disease, Lewy body dementia, and frontotemporal dementia.

Pick Disease. Much less common and sometimes clinically indistinguishable from AD, Pick disease is characterized by cortical atrophy involving predominantly the frontal and temporal regions with sparing of the posterior two thirds. Loss of frontal inhibition of socially unacceptable and previously suppressed behavior emerges early in the disease, often overshadowing the memory disturbance. The inclusions are known as Pick bodies. The neurons balloon in the area of involved tissue, but there are not the plaques or tangles seen in AD.

Lewy Body Dementia. This disorder exhibits highly variable clinical and neuropathologic overlap with AD and Parkinson disease. It is characterized by initial parkinsonism unresponsive to standard medications, progressing to deterioration of cognition. Cellular changes include presence of the Lewy bodies found in Parkinson disease and neurofibrillary tangles, senile plaques, and granulovacuolar degeneration similar to those in AD.

Corticobasal ganglionic degeneration is characterized by striking asymmetrical gait and speed apraxia, "alien hand" syndrome, rigidity, myoclonus, and cortical sensory loss. Dementia is usually a late manifestation of the disease. Affected patients generally present with dementia preceding motor signs, particularly with visual hallucinations and episodes of reduced responsiveness.

Frontotemporal Dementia. Frontotemporal dementia is used to describe the various progressive disorders that have a predilection for the frontal lobes. The cellular neuropathology is variable, and in some cases it seems to be the frontal lobe manifestations of AD, Pick disease, and Lewy body dementia.

TREATMENT. There is currently no cure for AD. Current treatment focuses on establishing an early accurate clinical diagnosis, early institution of cholinesterase inhibitors, and/or NMDA receptor–targeted therapy. Treating medical comorbidities and dementia-related complications, ensuring that appropriate services are provided, addressing the long-term well-being of caregivers, and treating behavioral and psychologic symptoms with appropriate nonpharmacologic and pharmacologic interventions also are important.[148] Individuals who are genetically predisposed to AD are advised to closely control their blood pressure as hypertension was recently shown to interact with *APOE* ε4 genotype to increase amyloid deposition in cognitively healthy middle-aged and older adults.

The importance of defining factors that may delay the onset, slow the progression, or even prevent AD and cognitive decline cannot be overestimated. With the aging of world populations, the burden of individuals with all degrees of cognitive impairment on societies will be enormous. A great deal of research has been conducted concerning these factors over the past decades. Although it is true that there are no definitive interventions that have been defined to prevent or slow the cognitive decline in aging, there are very strong trends in the literature. The available evidence suggests that physical activity, intellectual activity, and social engagement are the most helpful factors at reducing AD and cognitive decline. These same factors are helpful for enhancing quality of life. There is optimism in the field with respect to possible disease-modifying effects that can be achieved through a variety of nutritional, pharmacologic, and lifestyle modifications. Box 31-7 outlines the medications currently in use.

Treatment oriented at preventing the breakdown of tau, or the formation of plaques, is being tested now and shows promise. The treatment of those persons identified as at high risk may someday be protective gene therapy.[157]

Box 31-7

COMMON MEDICATIONS USED IN ALZHEIMER DISEASE

- **Donepezil** (Aricept) has only modest benefits, but it does help slow loss of function and reduce caregiver burden. It works equally in patients with and without *APOE* ε4. It may even have some advantage for patients with moderate to severe AD.
- **Rivastigmine** (Exelon) targets two enzymes (the major one, acetylcholinesterase, and butyrylcholinesterase). This agent may be particularly beneficial for patients with rapidly progressing disease. This drug has slowed or slightly improved disease status even in patients with advanced disease. (Rivastigmine may cause significantly more side effects than donepezil, including nausea, vomiting, and headache.)
- **Galantamine** (Reminyl). Galantamine not only protects the cholinergic system but also acts on nicotine receptors, which are also depleted in AD. It improves daily living, behavior, and mental functioning, including in patients with mild to advanced-moderate AD and those with a mix of AD and vascular dementia. Some studies have suggested that the effects of galantamine may persist for a year or longer and even strengthen over time.
- **Tacrine** (Cognex) has only modest benefits and has no benefits for patients who carry the *APOE* ε4 gene. In high dosages, it can also injure the liver. In general, newer cholinergic-protective drugs that do not pose as great a risk for the liver are now used for AD.
- **Memantine** (Namenda), targeted at the NMDA receptor, is used for moderate to severe AD.
- **Selegiline** (Eldepryl) is used for treatment of Parkinson disease, and it appears to increase the time before advancement to the next stage of disability.

Combining information on *APOE4* carrier status with other informative biologic marker data is a promising research strategy for detecting individuals who might be candidates for AD prevention strategies.[115]

A management model for AD that incorporates a diagnostic protocol to identify and assess people with possible dementia and care management addressing individual function, caregiver support, medical treatment, psychosocial needs, nutritional needs, and advance directives planning is critical. To improve end-of-life care for people with AD, any treatment model should also incorporate patient-centered care and palliative care from the initial diagnosis of AD through its terminal stages. Short-term intensive counseling can significantly reduce the long-term risk for depression among those who care for spouses or partners with AD.[64]

Management of the client with AD is a challenge to health providers and to the family who become caregivers. Manipulation of the environment can be effective. It is difficult to manage aggressive behavior in the home, and long-term care in a facility with a special Alzheimer unit is often the most appropriate place for that client. In many individuals with AD, treating comorbid conditions such as depression, hearing or vision impairment, congestive heart failure, symptomatic urinary tract infection, or hypothyroidism may produce a greater benefit than focusing treatment only on AD. Cardiovascular disease may influence the expression and clinical manifestations of the disease.

There is compelling evidence for the important role of regular physical activity.[157] Exercise training combined with behavioral management techniques can improve physical health and depression in individuals with AD. Leisure-time physical activity at midlife is associated with a decreased risk of dementia and AD later in life. Regular physical activity may reduce the risk or delay the onset of dementia and AD, especially among genetically susceptible individuals.[61,209]

Diet in midlife shows potential for neuroprotection, and findings can be generalized to a combination of the following: consumption of a diet low in fat, high in omega-3 oils, and high in dark vegetables and fruits; use of soy (for women only); supplementation with vitamin C, coenzyme Q10, and folate; and moderate alcohol intake. It appears that no single item creates the protection, but the foods and supplements may work together to lower risk.

There is growing evidence indicating that oxidative damage caused by the β-amyloid peptide in the pathogenesis of AD may be hydrogen peroxide (H_2O_2) mediated. Polyphenols from apple and citrus juices, such as quercetin, are able to cross the blood-brain barrier and show neuroprotection against H_2O_2. The effect of polyphenols from citrus is similar to that of vitamin C, but quercetin from apple juice gives stronger neuroprotection than vitamin C. In addition to their antioxidant properties, many polyphenols, such as quercetin, have potent antiinflammatory properties. In addition to antioxidant vitamins and polyphenols, fruit and vegetable juices also may possess other protective components, such as folate and minerals.[58]

The mutations in APP, presenilin 1, and presenilin 2 allow genetic screening to be used in suspected cases of familial AD with early onset and for appropriate genetic counseling and support. Although preimplantation genetic diagnosis of the embryo, prenatal diagnosis, preimplantation embryo selection, and presymptomatic testing have been offered to families of individuals who have early-onset familial AD, complex legal and ethical issues surrounding these interventions must be addressed before these interventions can be routinely recommended.

PROGNOSIS. AD is the fourth leading cause of death in adults. The period from onset to death typically is 7 to 11 years. Initially, deficits in higher cortical function are the most noticeable. Motor signs may reflect higher burden or different type or more biologically detrimental localization of neuropathology. The association of different aspects of motor signs with different outcomes may reflect varying underlying neurotransmitter systems being affected. For example, in Parkinson disease, tremor and bradykinesia are viewed as representing more purely dopaminergic manifestations, whereas posture, balance, and gait disorders may be mediated by other neurotransmitter systems in addition to dopamine. Changes caused by the dementia may advance relentlessly over many years, creating not only deep emotional and psychologic distress, but also practical problems related to caregiving that can overwhelm affected families. During the middle stages of the disease, the client often develops behavioral and motor problems. Finally, the client becomes mute and unable to comprehend. Death is often secondary to dehydration or infection.

SPECIAL IMPLICATIONS FOR THE THERAPIST | 31-2

Alzheimer Disease

Dementia syndromes almost always affect ability to independently perform activities of daily living such as grooming, toileting, and eating. Instrumental activities of daily living include complex activities such as meal preparation, banking, driving, and decision making.

Cognitive decline consistent with the diagnosis of primary degenerative dementia is a unique clinical syndrome with characteristic phenomena and progression. The Global Deterioration Scale (see Box 31-6) can be used for the assessment of primary degenerative dementia and delineation of its stages.[200,201]

Use of a comprehensive cognitive stimulation program in AD patients enhances neuroplasticity, reduces cognitive loss, and helps the patient to stretch functional independence through better cognitive performance. Remarkable effects have been observed also in the areas of mood and behavior. Behavioral disturbances influence caregiver burden and institutionalization as well as being associated with patient and caregiver distress. Increase in social attention and interaction improves mood and behavior in demented elderly. Important mood benefits are reported from stimulation programs predominantly aimed at cognition.[182] Changes in functional abilities correlate with cognitive deficits and prognosticate clinical course because they significantly affect caregiver burden and rates of institutionalization. Tools to be used are the Functional Activities Questionnaire and the Assessment of Motor and Processing Skills.

Cognitive rehabilitation programs can minimize demands on executive control systems in favor of structured tasks that are designed to exploit implicit memory. Appropriate feedback is critical, as there is increased agitation and anxiety when mistakes are recognized. Nonverbal cues can be helpful when language is the source of confusion. Moving through parts of a task with guidance can facilitate understanding and promote confidence to proceed. When the experience is more pleasurable, the response is improved, as the stress of the task may be reduced.

The client with AD has generalized weakness and abnormality of movement. Movements become more stereotyped and rigid. Postural reflexes are diminished, and the incidence of falls increases. Falls occur in approximately 30% of clients with AD, which may be attributable to their lack of perception of where their bodies are in space and their inability to move adequately around objects. Having the client move in a space that has few obstacles appears to decrease the number of falls. The use of increased lighting, especially in the early evening, will decrease the agitation often referred to as *sundowning*.[260]

The therapist often sees a client with AD in a structured living environment, since many people become difficult to maintain at home. Movement and exercise can provide the client with an activity that the client can succeed in, as well as maintain mobility, good breathing patterns, and endurance. Restlessness and wandering are typical of the client with AD, and a structured exercise program appears to decrease restlessness. Daytime exercise can also help control nighttime pacing and the resulting daytime drowsiness. Some residential programs have set up areas that the client can access without wandering out of the facility. The use of these areas may decrease agitation and allow individuals to pace safely.[27]

Group therapy with simple exercises that use images rather than commands is most effective. Storytelling integrated into the exercise program helps to stimulate thinking as well as movement. Clients need to be able to attend to an activity for at least 5 minutes, and the group therapy session must not provide more stimulation than clients are able to tolerate. Exercises should be short and simple and done in the same order each day. Repetition and reassurance can help keep clients engaged. The exercise program should include group interaction with physical touching, such as holding hands or working in pairs. Use of exercise bands, balls to kick and throw, and light weights works well.[24,151] Community-dwelling individuals with Alzheimer disease and sleep problems can benefit from walking and increased light exposure, alone or in combination, but these interventions must be implemented with caregiver assistance.[159]

Top of Form

Word fluency scores appear to improve with community based walking.[156] A multimodal exercise program is associated with a reduction in the neuropsychiatric symptoms of patients with AD and contributes to the attenuation of the impairment in the performance of instrumental activities of daily living in elderly women with AD.[177] The Preventing Loss of Independence through Exercise (PLIÉ) program combines elements of Eastern and Western exercise traditions, including yoga, tai chi, Feldenkrais, physical therapy, occupational therapy, mindfulness, and dance movement therapy. PLIÉ instructors have patients sit in a circle, which promotes group movement and social interaction. Conversations tend to build and become more complex in this setting.[13]

In working with the individual with AD, knowing something about the individual might enable the therapist to use words and terms that are more familiar to the individual. Approach to the person should be slow and from the front. Always identify yourself and use the person's name before intervention begins. Identifying pain during activity is important, because pain may be involved in aggressive behavior. Use of modalities to decrease the client's pain may result in improved behavior. The Alzheimer's discomfort rating scale is useful.[118]

Intervention should be based on the individual's stage of progression. In the early stages, work on high-level balance and gait activities will help to maintain mobility and balance. Strength gains have been reported to be significant in older persons in a strengthening program, and strength is an important component of balance. Maintaining range of motion, especially in the trunk and distal extremities, will help to maintain function. Caregiver training is important for consistent follow-through with activities and provision of appropriate cues. When assistance is needed for mobility, caregiver training on transfers, contracture management, and assistance with gait is included in the intervention.

Choosing the appropriate orthotic, assistive device, and wheelchair can be a challenge as dementia develops. Walkers have been designed for the AD client to use on flat surfaces with appropriate support and safety.

The therapist should be familiar with the warning signs of AD. Because the disease mimics other signs of old age, the symptoms may go unreported. It is often the spouse who asks questions regarding the possibility of the client's developing AD. Information regarding the types of symptoms related to the disease can be helpful to the family in deciding whether more evaluation is needed. Box 31-8 lists the Alzheimer's Association's 10 warning signs of AD.

Box 31-8

10 WARNING SIGNS OF ALZHEIMER DISEASE

1. Memory loss that disrupts daily life
   One of the most common signs of AD is memory loss, especially forgetting recently learned information. Others include forgetting important dates or events; asking for the same information repeatedly; increasingly needing to rely on memory aids (e.g., reminder notes or electronic devices) or family members for things they used to handle on their own.

2. Challenges in planning or solving problems
   Some people may experience changes in their ability to develop and follow a plan or work with numbers. They may have trouble following a familiar recipe or keeping track of monthly bills. They may have difficulty concentrating and take much longer to do things than they did before.

3. Difficulty completing familiar tasks at home, at work or at leisure
   People with AD often find it hard to complete daily tasks. Sometimes, people may have trouble driving to a familiar location, managing a budget at work, or remembering the rules of a favorite game.

4. Confusion with time or place
   People with AD can lose track of dates, seasons and the passage of time. They may have trouble understanding something if it is not happening immediately. Sometimes they may forget where they are or how they got there.

5. Trouble understanding visual images and spatial relationships
   For some people, having vision problems is a sign of AD. They may have difficulty reading, judging distance and determining color or contrast, which may cause problems with driving.

6. New problems with words in speaking or writing
   People with AD may have trouble following or joining a conversation. They may stop in the middle of a conversation and have no idea how to continue or they may repeat themselves. They may struggle with vocabulary, have problems finding the right word or call things by the wrong name (e.g., calling a "watch" a "hand-clock").

Continued

10 WARNING SIGNS OF ALZHEIMER DISEASE—cont'd

7. Misplacing things and losing the ability to retrace steps
   A person with AD may put things in unusual places. They may lose things and be unable to go back over their steps to find them again. Sometimes, they may accuse others of stealing. This may occur more frequently over time.
8. Decreased or poor judgment
   People with AD may experience changes in judgment or decision making. For example, they may use poor judgment when dealing with money, giving large amounts to telemarketers. They may pay less attention to grooming or keeping themselves clean.

9. Withdrawal from work or social activities
   A person with AD may start to remove themselves from hobbies, social activities, work projects, or sports. They may have trouble keeping up with a favorite sports team or remembering how to complete a favorite hobby. They may also avoid being social because of the changes they have experienced.
10. Changes in mood and personality
   The mood and personalities of people with AD can change. They can become confused, suspicious, depressed, fearful, or anxious. They may be easily upset at home, at work, with friends, or in places where they are out of their comfort zone.

From Alzheimer's Association: 10 Early Signs and Symptoms of Alzheimer's. Available at: http://www.alz.org/alzheimers_disease_10_signs_of_alzheimers.asp. Accessed June 11, 2013.

CAUSES OF DYSTONIA RELATED TO CAUSES THAT ARE NONGENETIC

- Drugs, including neuroleptics, dopamine agonists, anticonvulsants, antimalarial drugs
- Intramedullary lesions of the cervical cord
- After hemiplegia: often a delayed reaction to stroke
- Focal brain lesions: vascular malformation, tumor, abscess
- Demyelinating lesions, such as with multiple sclerosis
- Traumatic brain injury with lesion to contralateral basal ganglia or thalamus
- Encephalitis
- Environmental toxins: manganese, carbon monoxide, methanol
- Hypoparathyroidism
- Degenerative disease: Parkinson disease, Huntington disease, Wilson disease, progressive supranuclear palsy, multiple system atrophy
- Cerebral palsy

DYSTONIA

Definition and Overview

Dystonia is a movement disorder characterized by sustained or intermittent muscle contractions causing abnormal, often repetitive, movements, postures, or both. Dystonic movements are typically patterned, twisting, and may be tremulous. Dystonia is often initiated or worsened by voluntary action and associated with overflow muscle activation.[3]

Testing of people with dystonia has identified many central and peripheral abnormalities. Nerve conduction velocity studies have shown a failure of neural activities preparing for movement. Defective retrieval of specific motor programs in response to sensory stimuli results in cocontraction of both agonist and antagonist muscles around a joint.[208,247] In focal dystonia of the hand, there are somatosensory degradations in the involved hand, with graphesthesia and astereognosis.[40]

Currently, according to the American Dystonia Society (ADS), three characteristics are used to classify the different types of dystonia; age at onset, area of body affected, and the underlying cause.[8] The consensus update by the International Consensus Committee of the European Federation of Neurologic Societies was established to clarify terminology to improve clinician diagnosis, prognosis, and treatment. It published its final recommendations in May 2013.[3] Its recommendations include two divisions to classify dystonia: clinical characteristics and etiology. This better reflects current genetic findings and assists in diagnosis. This section is based on its recommendations, with older terminology defined, when appropriate, to facilitate communication among health care providers.

Clinical characteristics include the following four subcategories.

1. **Age of onset** (ADS uses two categories: early onset from birth to 28 years and older than 28 years)
   - Infancy (birth to 2 years)
   - Childhood (3-12 years)
   - Adolescence (13-20 years)
   - Early adulthood (21-40 years)
   - Late adulthood (>40 years)

   These age groups were recommended to provide consistency with terminology in other neurological disorders.

   Dystonia that begins in the first year of life is often an inherited metabolic disorder that suggests a poor prognosis. Dystonia manifesting between 2 and 6 years of age often is consistent with dystonic cerebral palsy. Dopa-responsive dystonias tend to manifest between 6 and 14 years of age. Focal dystonia usually occur after 50 years of age.[3]
2. Body distribution of symptoms
   - Focal. Limited to one body segment. Examples are cervical dystonia, writer's cramp, and blepharospasm.
   - Segmental. Affects adjacent body parts. An example is cranial dystonia, which involves blepharospasm with jaw involvement.
   - Multifocal. Involves two more noncontiguous body regions. An example is the right arm and left leg.
   - Generalized. Affects the trunk and at least two other body parts.
   - Hemidystonia. Mainly affects one side of the body. These labels are consistent with ADS terminology.
3. **Temporal pattern** describes the disease course which can be static, progressive, variable, persistent, action-specific, diurnal, or paroxysmal. There is no current category equivalent.
4. **Associated features**
   - Isolated
   - Combined with other movement disorders

The ADS currently uses four classifications by cause. (1) Primary dystonia (now isolated) ruled out secondary causes. (2) Secondary resulted from environmental causes such as exposure to carbon monoxide, cyanide, manganese, and methanol, or underlying disease such as brain tumors, cerebral palsy, Parkinson disease, stroke, multiple sclerosis, hypoparathyroidism, vascular malformation, CNS injuries, infections of the brain, and some antipsychotic medications. (3) Dystonia-plus are dystonias that are from nondegenerative neurochemical disorders associated with other neurologic conditions. For example, myoclonus-dystonia and dopa-responsive dystonia. (4) The final category, heredodegenerative, includes neurodegenerative disorders that are heredity based. These include X-linked dystonia-parkinsonism, Huntington disease, Wilson disease, and Parkinson disease. See Box 32-9 for causes of dystonia that are not genetic.

The second major classification of dystonia is based on its etiology. It is as follows.
1. Nervous System Pathology
   - Evidence of degeneration
   - Evidence of structural lesions
   - No evidence of degeneration or structural lesions
This category covers the secondary and dystonia-plus conditions of the ADS.
2. Inherited or Acquired
   Inherited
   - Autosomal dominant
   - Autosomal recessive
   - X-linked recessive
   - Mitochondrial
This category covers primary and heredodegenerative dystonia categories in the ADS. There have been many types of dystonia of proven genetic origin including DYT1, -5, -6, -11, and -12, which are autosomal dominant.
   Acquired
   - Perinatal brain injury
   - Infection
   - Drug/toxic
   - Vascular
   - Neoplastic
   - Brain injury
   - Psychogenic
There is an ongoing discussion about dystonia that may have a psychogenic basis.[57] Posttraumatic dystonia, a controversial diagnosis, has been the focus of whether dystonia seen after injury is mainly psychogenic. Evidence is divided.[106,250]
   Idiopathic
   - Sporadic
   - Familial
These two categories cover secondary conditions in the ADS categories.

Nonmotor features of dystonia have been delineated. They vary depending on the type of dystonia, but include cognitive decline and psychiatric symptoms in some of the degenerative categories. Finally, *cervical dystonia, sometimes confused with spasmodic torticollis,* a neurologically based movement disorder affecting the head and neck, which is a separate entity from spasmodic torticollis. Torticollis is a musculoskeletal phenomenon treated as an orthopedic condition (see discussion of torticollis in Chapter 23).

Incidence

An estimated 250,000 persons are afflicted with dystonia in North America. About 1.1 in 100,000 persons per year develop dystonia, with a female-to-male ratio of 1.6:1.[69] The Mayo Clinic in Rochester found 3.4 cases of primary generalized dystonia and 29.5 cases of focal dystonia per 100,000 persons.[180] Focal dystonia is estimated to be six times more common than other well-known neuromuscular disorders such as muscular dystrophy, Huntington disease, and ALS.

The average age of onset of primary or genetic dystonia is 12 years old. For focal dystonias, the age of onset is between 30 and 50 years.[8]

Etiologic and Risk Factors

Genetic-based dystonia, previously considered primary dystonia, is the most common diagnosis, accounting for two-thirds of all cases. There are multiple genetic forms of dystonia. The DYT1 and DYT6 genes have been recognized as genetic forms of dystonia for several decades.[74] The DYT1 dystonia typically begins in one extremity and progresses to increased involvement in other limbs/trunk. The cranial and cervical muscles are rarely involved. DYT6 has early involvement of the cervical area and oromandibular, laryngeal, and speech are commonly involved. It appears that persons with generalized dystonia carry a different gene than those with focal dystonias.[73] Another inherited dystonia is dopa-responsive dystonia, or Segawa dystonia.[5]

Focal dystonias, sometimes called writer's cramp, involving hand function, are particularly common among those in certain occupational groups, such as keyboard operators and musicians. Focal dystonia related to occupational cramps may be a result of abnormal or repetitive biomechanics. Focal dystonia involving the hand may also occur as part of a peripheral nerve disorder. Although generally listed as idiopathic, recent evidence supports a genetic basis, at least in some cases of focal dystonia.[215]

Drug-induced extrapyramidal symptoms may include dystonia as a common side effect associated with antipsychotic drugs (neuroleptics). This results in various acute and chronic manifestations of neuroleptic-induced dystonia (e.g., blepharospasm [difficulty in opening the eyelids], torticollis, or retrocollis [involuntary extension of the neck]).[120] The fact that β-blocking agents are effective in reducing symptoms in these cases points to the possibility that neuroleptic drugs increase the activity of β-adrenergic transmitters.

Pathogenesis

Three neurophysiologic deficits underlie the clinical manifestations of dystonia: deficient inhibition at the cortex, brainstem, and spinal cord levels; abnormal plasticity; and sensory processing dysfunction. However, how one uses their motor system appears linked to the manifestation, in many cases, of dystonia.

Chemical dysfunction or scarring within the striatum (caudate nucleus and putamen) is the probable mechanism for deficient inhibition.[100] Overactivity of the direct pathway within the basal ganglia loop (cortex–striatum–internal globus pallidus–thalamus–premotor/motor cortex) is speculated to result in an overflow of motor cortex activity, thus creating the dystonic movements. A defect in the body's ability to locally process inhibitory neurotransmitters such as γ-aminobutyric acid (GABA), dopamine, acetylcholine, norepinephrine, and serotonin may contribute to poor inhibition of motor control. Dysfunction of the lenticulothalamic neuronal circuit seems to be related to the development of dystonia following head trauma.[149,231] The striatum also has strong thalamocortical somatosensory connections, with potential to disrupt normal sensory processing.

The striatum is strongly associated with neuroplasticity. Abnormal neuroplasticity is present in many dystonias and especially in focal dystonias.[259] An in-depth review of research and discussion of striatal basis for dystonia is available.[188]

Patterns and types of motor use may be the final key in developing dystonia. Clinical symptoms (penetrance) of dystonia are only present in 30% of those with the DYT1 gene and in 60% of those with the DYT6 gene. Because several types of dystonia do not appear to have a genetic basis, an environmental "use-dependent" factor is also proposed (with or without a genetic basis) for many dystonias, particularly focal dystonias.[5,38,198,213] Use-dependent environmental factors like peripheral injury or repetitive movement training, may trigger dystonic movement development in people with abnormal neuroplasticity. Research suggests that the somatosensory cortex may function abnormally, contributing to the altered motor output.[39,100,128,129,237] Both somatosensory cortex and somatotopic representation at the thalamus degrade in individuals with dystonia.[151] Studies of musicians and writers with dystonia in the hand show a less differentiated or smeared corticosensory cortex.

MEDICAL MANAGEMENT

DIAGNOSIS. Dystonia is a clinical diagnosis except for those cases that have a genetic basis. Testing for genetic forms of dystonia is now recommended. Tests to rule out other neurologic diseases are important. Otherwise, there is no definitive test for dystonia, and the diagnosis of idiopathic dystonia is often delayed 1 year or more. The clinical presentation of dystonic movements, such as head deviation or neck pain, may be the first diagnostic sign. The person usually has a normal perinatal and developmental history. EMG studies show sustained simultaneous contractions of agonists and antagonists.

Five features of dystonia that guide diagnosis are:

1. Dystonic postures—a body part is flexed or twisted along its longitudinal axis and sensation of rigidity and traction is present.
2. Dystonic movements—movement is a twisting nature or a pull in a preferred direction, repetitive and patterned attitude (consistent and predictable).
3. Geste antagoniste (sensory trick)—alleviation of dystonia occurs during the geste movement, which may or may not last through the entire movement. The geste movement is natural and never forceful so it does not push or pull the affected body part, but is a sensory input. (A common geste is a light touch to the chin for people with cervical dystonia.)

4. Mirror dystonia—mirror movements are observed in the opposite body side.
5. Overflow dystonia—dystonic movement or postures extend beyond the commonly involved body region. Observed at peak of dystonic movement. Determining that there is no evidence for other neurologic disorders, or secondary dystonia is essential in the diagnosis of idiopathic dystonia.[4]

TREATMENT. Treatment remains symptomatic and includes drug therapy, including botulinum toxin type A and type B injections, physical and occupational therapy, and sometimes surgery. Deep brain stimulation of the globus pallidus internus has also been successful in some patients, especially in children and people with genetic-based generalized dystonia.[10,186] It is less effective for patients with dystonia as part of other neurologic disease processes. Anticholinergics such as trihexyphenidyl (Artane) have been the most widely used medications to decrease acetylcholine and correct a cholinergic imbalance in the basal ganglia. Side effects of these drugs vary, with blurred vision, dry mouth, confusion, voiding, sleeping difficulties, and personality changes observed, but the medication is effective. Baclofen and other muscle relaxants are used occasionally for relief.

Botulinum toxin types A and B, injected intramuscularly, have emerged as a safe and effective symptomatic treatment for a number of conditions associated with excessive muscle activity, particularly focal dystonias involving a limited number of muscles. These injections are effective in improving postural deviation and pain in approximately 80% to 90% of people with cervical dystonias.[122,123] Injection directly into the actively contracting muscles blocks the neuromuscular junction by acting presynaptically to reduce the release of acetylcholine, producing a chemical denervation. Muscle weakness can result from this treatment. Response occurs in 3 to 7 days and lasts 3 to 4 months. Dysphagia is the most serious side effect, but can be decreased in incidence and severity by injecting lower doses, particularly into the sternocleidomastoid. The need to continue indefinitely with repeat injections approximately every 3 months is a major drawback.[187]

Surgery may be considered only when other treatments are no longer effective, although surgical intervention may also lose its effect over time, providing only temporary symptomatic relief. Surgeries to interrupt the pathways or foci responsible for the abnormal movements can be effective. Thalamotomy is the destruction of a portion of the thalamus. Pallidotomy is a destructive operation on the globus pallidus. Pallidus stimulation is achieved by placing an electric stimulator in the globus pallidus. Rhizotomy involves the surgical resection of the anterior cervical spinal nerve roots and is used along with selective peripheral denervation, or removal of the nerves at the point where they enter the contracting muscles.

PROGNOSIS. Age of onset is the best predictor of prognosis. If dystonia starts at or near birth and affects other members of the family, it tends to get progressively worse over the years. If the condition starts in childhood and is secondary to cerebral palsy or other brain injury close to the time of birth, the dystonia tends to remain static for many years. In one-third of cases of adult-onset focal dystonia there is progression to segmental dystonia, although there is less than a 20% chance that the disease will progress to generalized dystonia.

Spontaneous remission occurs in some cases within the first year, but the majority of clients show steady progression of their focal dystonia, with maximal disability occurring after 5 years. Neck pain, occurring in 70% to 80% of clients, contributes significantly to disability. Cervical dystonia has important psychosocial consequences, since many people with this condition withdraw from their jobs and social activities.[251]

SPECIAL IMPLICATIONS FOR THE THERAPIST 31-3

Dystonia

Testing

The Toronto Western Spasmodic Torticollis Rating Scale (TWSTRS)[53] and the Tsui are two commonly used impairment and disability scales for rating the severity of cervical dystonia. The TWSTRS is more involved but has good reliability and validity.[243,244,245] The Barry-Albright Dystonia Scale[14] is used for dystonia associated with other neurologic diseases. Range of motion, pain, and descriptions of active motion, as well as limitations in functional activities, are also useful measurements. Outcomes can be measured with life satisfaction scales, such as the SF-36 (Short Form-36 General Health Survey).[29]

Intervention

There is little high-quality research to guide the therapist in intervention, so interventions are often based on the basic pathophysiology of dystonia in areas where there is no research.

The therapist should address all aspects of functional ability with the client who has been affected by dystonia, including stress and pain management, energy conservation, adaptive equipment, mobility, and selective splinting, which can improve or deteriorate symptoms depending on the type of dystonia.[37,96]

Sensory processing abnormalities, as discussed under pathogenesis, may be involved in the abnormal movements of dystonia and can provide some direction for intervention. In owl monkeys that developed dystonic movements of the hand and particularly the fingers in response to a high number of repetitive movements of the forearm and hand,[40] the sensory cortex reorganized by decreasing the representation (dedifferentiation) of the hand and fingers. The cortical thalamic reorganization occurred after the monkeys began experiencing dystonia of the hand secondary to overuse. Later research by the same laboratory demonstrated recovery of the cortical representation and redifferentiation using sensory stimulation therapy rather than motor retraining. These studies suggest that treatment approaches should focus on sensory retraining, and particularly active interpretation of sensory stimuli. A case series using sensory retraining demonstrated success with this method in humans who had writer's cramp, a focal dystonia.[41] A recent literature review[31] of effective therapies for focal hand dystonia reported support for sensory retraining, motor sensory retuning, and limb immobilization however, it appears important not to do repetitive stereotyped movements during retraining.[264,265]

Other sensory approaches, such as EMG biofeedback, have the potential to improve dystonia also. Theoretically, visual input provides an alternate, functional route for sensory input to reach the motor output system through the surface EMG visual feedback.[139] The primary motor cortex, which is responsible for initiating motor tasks, receives highly processed visual information from cortical areas other than the somatosensory cortex (i.e., parietal lobe, basal ganglia). These pathways may be able to override the malfunctioning input systems.[139] Surface EMG feedback is effective in reducing symptoms in persons with focal hand dystonia.[41,139] Trials using surface EMG for hand dystonia demonstrated results in as few as five sessions although long term retention was questionable.[60] Several studies using a series of cases demonstrate EMG biofeedback is effective for treatment of patients with cervical dystonia.[138] Other studies of EMG biofeedback do not appear to be as effective, especially studies using EMG as a relaxation training technique.[71]

There is weak support for modalities, stretching, and strengthening alone. However, Tassorelli et al[232] reported success using physical therapy of stretching, strengthening, postural control and balance exercises along with surface EMG biofeedback in a study comparing outcomes of two groups, one receiving Botox (BTX) only and the other receiving BTX and physical therapy. The group given physical therapy and BTX showed significantly better outcomes than the BTX-only group.

Task-oriented treatment, rather than more traditional strengthening and stretching exercises, has a better potential for improving function. Having clients do highly skilled tasks in treatment that are challenging and stimulating will improve learning. A combination of treatments often is most effective. For example, a client with right lower-extremity dystonia of 8 years' duration used a combination of surface EMG feedback on the anterior tibialis and gastrocnemius during stepping to targets and using the foot to identify and manipulate small objects in order to normalize motion. BTX type A injections into the hip flexor and gastrocnemius were done later to assist in reducing the abnormal hip flexor component of walking. The outcome was a normal gait pattern.

In some cases of dystonia, splinting has been effective for improving function. In cases in which the foot or feet turn in, insoles placed in the shoes to build up the outer border of the foot may help to put the foot in a neutral position and produce a more normal gait pattern. The use of a cervical collar has been tried by some with good results, but it may be that the sensory information to the skin accounts for this success rather than the mechanical support provided. If the collar minimizes pain or provides a more functional midline position, there may be some merit in its use. Otherwise, if it only works as a sensory trick, a piece of cloth wrapped around the neck may accomplish the same effect. The person who uses a cervical collar should be taught to do task-oriented exercises outside the collar to minimize weakness in the noninvolved muscles; for example, reading letters placed on the side opposite head rotation while the body stays facing forward.

When the jaw, tongue, or lips are involved, gentle pressure on the lips or teeth may lessen spasm. Exerting slight pressure against the jaw on the side to which the head is rotated may decrease or inhibit muscle spasm, although this is an immediate and short-term reaction. Guidelines for chewing and swallowing may be helpful for the client with oromandibular dystonia.

Swimming therapy can be especially helpful in reducing discomfort and facilitating movement.

Aggressive strengthening and range-of-motion treatments may increase the symptoms of dystonia; any treatment should be carried out within the client's tolerance and without increasing the manifestations of the dystonia. Because dystonia originates in the CNS, passive techniques such as massage provide only temporary relief from symptoms and do not affect the underlying movement disorder. Likewise, focal dystonia does not respond to facilitatory or inhibitory techniques used for modulating spasticity. When relief of spasm allows the client to assume a more normal or correct posture, underlying tight soft tissues may benefit from short-term use of physical therapy modalities and soft-tissue mobilization to restore full range of motion.[37,232]

HUNTINGTON DISEASE
Overview and Definition

Huntington disease (HD) is a progressive hereditary disorder characterized by abnormalities of movement, personality disturbances, and dementia. Known also as Huntington chorea, it is most often associated with choreic movement that is brief, purposeless, involuntary, and random. However, the disease course involves more than just a movement disorder, and hence the name HD. HD is a disorder of the CNS and is classified as a neurologic disorder, but because it is a condition with effects that are complex, management requires a multidisciplinary approach.[102,262]

Incidence and Etiologic and Risk Factors

The prevalence of HD in North America ranges from 4 to 8 per 100,000 persons. It is estimated that there are 25,000 cases in the United States. HD may begin at any time after infancy but usually starts in middle age. Twenty-five percent of persons with HD have disease of late onset, which is defined as onset of motor symptoms after age 50 years. There is almost always a history of an affected parent. There is a 50% risk in each child of an affected adult.[11] Transmission of the juvenile form of HD (onset before age 20 years) appears to be primarily from the father. With adult onset there is more equal transmission from both parents.[80]

HD is an autosomal dominant disease with the IT15 or HD genetic marker found on the tip of chromosome 4. In a subset of cases, the junctophilin-3 gene is responsible for the HD genotype. All the people who inherit the gene will develop symptoms of the disease if they do not die prematurely. Because there is no cure for HD, there is an ethical dilemma associated with testing. Studies are underway to determine the psychiatric and social problems that may result from the knowledge that one will develop HD.[83]

Pathogenesis

Although the cause remains unknown, pathologic findings show a consistent pattern of tissue changes in the brain. The ventricles are enlarged as a result of atrophy of the adjacent basal ganglia, specifically the caudate nucleus and putamen (collectively the striatum) (Fig. 31-5). This is a result of extensive loss of small and medium-sized neurons. The volume of the brain can decrease by as much as 20%. Caudate atrophy correlates with a measured decline

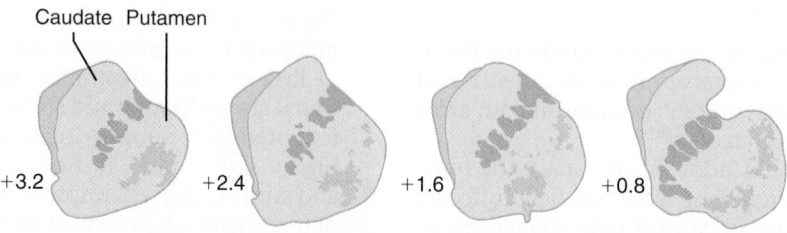

Caudate   Putamen

+3.2   +2.4   +1.6   +0.8

Figure 31-5

Atrophy seen in the caudate and putamen in a person with Huntington disease. As the disease progresses there is a change in the caudate at the interface with the ventricle. The outline becomes more and more concave, representing the progressive atrophy.

in Mini-Mental State Examination scores, but not with the severity or duration of neurologic symptoms. It is the atrophy of the putamen that correlates with neurologic symptoms. The atrophy of the cortices appears to occur at the same rate as that of the striatum. White matter degeneration in the frontal cortex appears to be associated with the course of the disease. Slower disease progression appears to be correlated with more white matter changes. The more aggressive progressive disease is related to less white matter and more striatal damage. Other subtle changes occur in the cortex and cerebellum, including both loss of neurons and production of glial cells that inhibit neural transmission.[101]

As with other progressive diseases, there is selective vulnerability of neurons in a particular region with preservation of others. In the early and middle stages of HD, neurons projecting from the striatum to the substantia nigra are depleted. This reduces the amount of neurotransmitters, including GABA, acetylcholine, and metenkephalin. This leaves relatively higher concentrations of other neurotransmitters, such as dopamine and norepinephrine. The normal balance of inhibition and excitation responses in the complex organization of the basal ganglia and thalamus that allows for smooth, controlled movement is disrupted. The result is an excess of dopamine and excessive excitation of the thalamocortical pathway. This may explain the excessive abnormal involuntary movements described as chorea.[16,197,262]

In the later stages of HD, there is a loss of the direct inhibitory substance that causes more inhibition of the thalamocortical output with resultant rigidity and bradykinesia, or slowness of movement. By the late stages of HD, virtually all the caudate nucleus projection neurons are affected. The mechanism of neuronal loss is not known. One hypothesis is that an excitotoxin causes the cell death noted in the basal ganglia.[196]

Clinical Manifestations

Movement Disorders

Many individuals with suspected early HD will show almost no neurologic abnormality on routine examination other than minor choreic movements. The movements may be suppressed during the examination as they can often be integrated into a purposeful movement, such as raising the hand to the head as if to smooth the hair. Early in the course the involuntary movements may appear to be no more than an exaggeration of normal restlessness, usually involving the upper limbs and face. The chorea is increased by mental concentration, emotional stimuli, performance of complex motor tasks, and walking. Problems with voluntary movement may be detected by asking for rapid tongue movements or finger-to-thumb tapping, or testing for dysdiadochokinesia, the inability to make rapid alternating movements.

Assessment of muscle strength will usually be normal in early cases but may be affected by any significant bradykinesia or general motor disturbance. Tone will usually be normal initially, but rigidity will become part of the clinical picture in many cases as the disease progresses. The tendon reflexes are usually normal.

Abnormalities in eye movement are common in HD. The ability to execute a saccade, a rapid movement of the eyes from one target to another in order to move the visual focus rapidly to different objects, is disturbed. There is often a decrease in the velocity of eye movement, an undershooting of the target, or latency in initiation of movement. Gaze fixation abnormalities have been noted; that is, inability to fix on a light source without the intrusion of small saccadic movements. Smooth pursuit, or tracking of the eye to follow a moving object, is interrupted by the same small, jerky saccadic movements. There is often an inability to suppress reflex saccades to a visual stimulus, which leads to visual distractibility.

The term *chorea* is derived from the Greek word for dance, and gait abnormalities are common in HD. When chorea is a predominant sign, persons walk with a wide-based, staggering gait. Those persons with bradykinesia and hypertonicity may walk with a slow, stiff, unsteady gait.

Dysarthria, reflected as a decrease in the rate and rhythm of speech, may be mild in the early course with an increase to the point where speech may be unintelligible. In addition to the mechanical problems, neuron loss disrupts linguistic abilities, resulting in reduced vocabulary and syntactic errors. Some persons become mute at a stage before motor disability is severe.

Abnormalities of swallowing, or dysphagia, can cause choking and asphyxia. Dysphagia may involve multiple abnormalities of ingestion, including inappropriate food choices, abnormal rate of eating, poor bolus formation, and inadequate respiratory control.

Cachexia, or the wasting of muscle with weight loss, is found despite an adequate diet. This appears to be independent of the hyperkinesia and is found in persons with rigidity as well.

Sleep disorders become a progressive problem throughout the course of HD. An increased latent period before sleep and increased periods of wakefulness are common in moderately affected persons. Sleep reversal—daytime somnolence and nighttime restlessness—is seen in severely affected persons and is probably related to the dementia. Choreic movements are reduced during the deepest part of sleep.

Urinary incontinence is often a problem. This could be related to dementia, depression, decreased mobility, or hyperreflexia of the muscles that control urine output. There can be a concomitant increase in the incidence of urinary tract infections.

Memory. Individuals with HD are often reported to be unaware of their neurologic, cognitive, and behavioral symptoms; however, it is not the case for memory deficits at an early stage. Loss of awareness of memory deficits in HD is associated with the severity of the disease in terms of CAG repeats, functional decline, motor dysfunction, and cognitive impairment, including memory deficits and executive dysfunction.[49]

Neuropsychologic and Psychiatric Disorders

Early mental disturbances in persons with HD include personality and behavioral changes, such as irritability, apathy, depression, decreased work performance, violence,

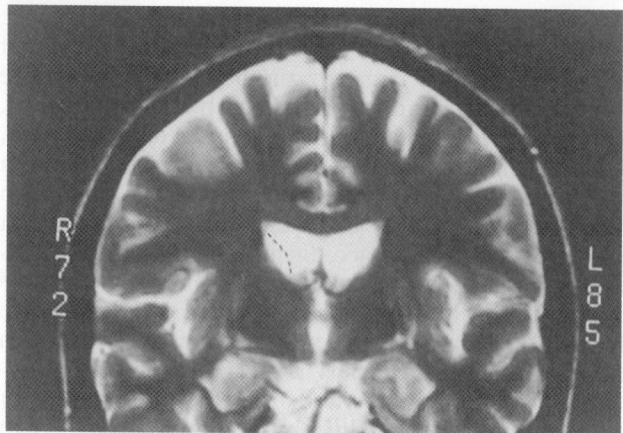

Figure 31-6

Magnetic resonance scan showing the degeneration of the caudate in a person with Huntington disease (HD). The *dotted lines* show where the tissue would be in a person without HD. (From Ramsey R: *Neuroradiology,* Philadelphia, 1994, WB Saunders.)

impulsivity, and emotional lability.[173] Intellectual decline usually follows the personality changes. The neuropsychologic profile characteristically includes a type of memory disturbance that suggests an impairment of information retrieval. Individuals often have difficulty recalling information on command, but are able to give the correct answer in a multiple-choice format. There is difficulty with organization, planning, and sequencing, even when all the information is provided. Other prominent abnormalities include visuospatial deficits, impaired judgment, and ideomotor apraxia, the inability to perform previously learned tasks despite intact elementary motor function.

More than one-third of persons with HD will develop an affective disorder. Depression is the most common psychiatric condition and does not appear to be simply a reaction to a fatal illness. Evidence for this is the fact that mood disorders are not randomly distributed but occur in subsets of families with HD.[83]

MEDICAL MANAGEMENT

DIAGNOSIS. The clinical diagnosis of HD depends on recognition of patterns of symptoms given in the client's history and clinical signs, and the family history. Difficulties in diagnosis arise when the family history appears negative. Some families deny the presence of cognitive or psychiatric disease. Understanding of the clinical signs must take into account the fact that signs change during the course of the illness. Different patterns may be observed depending on the age of onset.[102] PREDICT-HD found cognitive changes decades before the expected date of motor diagnosis.[153]

MRI demonstrates atrophy of the striatum that is most easily appreciated as enlargement of the frontal horn of the lateral ventricles. Figure 31-6 shows this change in brain structure. This is not of great diagnostic value unless it is very pronounced, given the normal reduction in brain mass with age and the occurrence of atrophy in other disorders that might be confused with HD. PET will also show atrophy, but its value as a diagnostic tool has the same limitations as MRI.

In addition to genetic linkage analysis, which requires testing of family members, it is now possible to evaluate the DNA of an individual to identify specific components that are diagnostic for HD. This eliminates the need to compare DNA of affected family members, but there are still problems with this method, because there is a small percentage of affected individuals who do not display the characteristics on the specific gene and there are nonaffected individuals who carry the gene. Identification of easily obtainable, reliable, and robust biomarkers of HD progression will be important for the development and evaluation of disease-modifying treatments.[258]

Recognition of HD in older persons is critical to establish the genetic link for future generations. Often the diagnosis is overlooked in favor of the label of senile chorea, because there are minimal changes in behavior and cognition. The differential diagnosis of HD in the older population includes various degenerative, systemic, and drug-related conditions. An individual treated with neuroleptics for a psychiatric presentation of HD, for example, may go on to develop movement disorders, and these may be confused with the typical side effects of the medication.[174]

TREATMENT. Management of HD requires a team approach, including medical and social services. Education of clients and their families about the implications of the disease is important. Genetic, psychologic, and social counseling are started as soon as the diagnosis is confirmed. Organizations designed to help families with HD are often of great help. Nabilone shows some promise to change motor behaviors but larger and longer randomized studies are needed.[56] Dopaminergic stabilizer pridopidine, shows some effect on voluntary motor function with most effect related to eye movements, hand coordination, dystonia, gait, and balance problems.[67,79]

Medical treatment, at this time, primarily is symptomatic. The most useful drugs for the symptomatic relief of chorea are anticonvulsants or antipsychotic agents that block dopamine neurotransmission. They can also help with the emotional outbursts, paranoia, psychosis, and irritability seen in HD. Drug therapy for chorea should be held in reserve if the abnormal movements are slight. There is a high incidence of side effects with the drugs, including acute dystonias, pseudoparkinsonism, and akathisia, which is characterized by uncontrollable physical restlessness. The most serious effect is chronic tardive dyskinesia resulting in involuntary movement of the face, tongue, and lips. Another adverse reaction is neuroleptic malignant hyperpyrexic syndrome, characterized by fever and rigidity.

Tetrabenazine (TBZ), now available in the United States, was recently approved by the FDA for the treatment of chorea associated with HD. It is a reversible inhibitor of the vesicle monoamine transporter type 2. It inhibits primarily dopamine and to a lesser degree serotonin and norepinephrine. Side effects include parkinsonism and depression.

Surgical procedures to remove the medial globus pallidus, thought to be overexcited by neuronal loss in the striatum, have been tried with mixed results. Implantation of adrenal medullary grafts has not been encouraging;

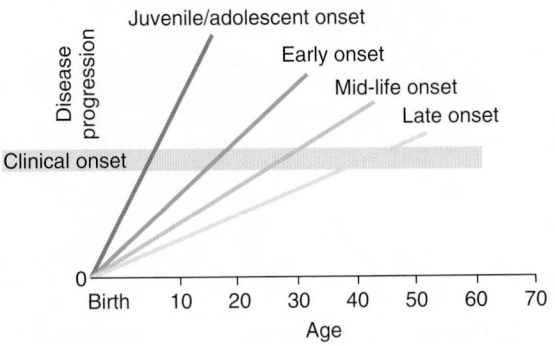

Figure 31-7

Progression of HD related to age at onset. (From Fahn: *Principles and practice of movement disorders*, ed 2, Philadelphia, 2011, WB Saunders.)

the improvement appears to be transient. Several patients with HD have been treated with fetal cell implantation in the striatum. Despite a few positive reports, in most cases no improvement has been observed. Autopsy studies have shown that the grafts survive but do not integrate with host striatum.[88]

PROGNOSIS. It is characteristic of the disease that younger people, with onset of symptoms at age 15 to 40 years, will experience a more severe form of the disease than older people, with onset in their 50s and 60s. The advance of the disease is slow, with death occurring on average 15 to 20 years after onset. Survival into the 80s is not uncommon, and persons living to past 90 years old have been recorded. Age at onset and age at death frequently show a familial correlation. Clinicopathologic studies demonstrate a strong inverse correlation between the age at onset and the severity of striatal degeneration.[117] Figure 31-7 shows the relationship of time of onset to progression of disease.

Increasing disability from involuntary movements and mental changes often results in death from intercurrent infection. Suicide accounts for approximately 6% of deaths, and 25% of persons with HD attempt suicide at least once.

SPECIAL IMPLICATIONS FOR THE THERAPIST   31-4

Huntington Disease

Education of the client and family about movement disorders, including gait and safety in mobility, is the basis for therapeutic intervention. *Apraxia*, the inability to perform skilled or purposeful movements, may become severe. This impairment may lead to significant disability in performance of activities of daily living. The client may lose the ability to dress and do self-care activities, such as grooming, regardless of cues provided by caregivers. Positioning to prevent soft-tissue deformities and safety in transfers should be taught according to the current movement disorder identified. Both the therapist and the family should understand that these techniques may need to be changed as the movement disorder progresses. The therapist should be aware that it is possible that chorea and bradykinesia

are manifested in the patient at the same time owing to the progressive neuronal loss in the basal ganglia described earlier. In clients whose bradykinesia is predominant, there is a propensity to freeze, especially in confined spaces, and this may precipitate falls.

Clients with HD do fall, but it is surprising that mobility is maintained despite the seemingly precarious arrangements of the limbs and trunk. As the disease progresses, postural stability becomes impaired and axial chorea may throw the client off balance. Lower scores on the Tinetti mobility test and younger age were significant predictors of falls.[136] Use of a metronome to drive modulation of gait may have a training effect to increase gait speed.[235] Intensive rehabilitation treatments may positively influence the maintenance of functional and motor performance in patients with HD and may last as long as 3 years.[267]

The ability to intervene with neurotherapeutic techniques, including motor learning, may be limited in the face of the concomitant decline in mental function as the motor system impairments progress. Participation in typical activities declines.[65] Role changes, sense of isolation and concerns for children are commonly described by individuals with HD and therefore should be addressed.[261]

MULTIPLE SCLEROSIS

Overview and Definition

Multiple sclerosis (MS) is a major cause of disability in young adults. The name is descriptive of the sclerotic plaques disseminated throughout the CNS that are the hallmark of the disease. There are multiple lesions found throughout the brain and spinal cord. These lesions slow or block neural transmission, resulting in weakness, sensory loss, visual dysfunction, and other symptoms. The course of MS is highly variable. Complications of MS may affect multiple body systems and require profound adjustments in lifestyle and expectations for clients and their families; therefore, a multidisciplinary approach is necessary to optimize clinical care.

MS is a chronic illness that may be manifested in multiple forms and courses. There are four generally recognized subtypes. Relapsing-remitting MS is characterized by relapses or attacks, which are periods of neurologic dysfunction lasting days to months and followed by full or partial recovery. By convention, new symptoms must last at least 24 hours and be separated from other symptoms by at least 30 days to qualify as a new attack. The hallmark is that there is a stable course between relapses. This is the most common pattern, seen in approximately 85% of newly diagnosed individuals. After presenting with a pattern of relapsing-remitting MS early in the disease course, many patients go on to develop fewer acute relapses and over time develop a more insidious progression of neurologic decline. This stage is referred to as secondary progressive MS, and approximately 60% of patients progress to this stage within 2 decades from onset of disease. Primary progressive MS is a steady decline in neurologic function from the outset with episodes of minimal recovery. The most common clinical presentation of primary progressive MS is myelopathy, a gradual, progressive weakening and wasting of muscles, which is typically seen in persons with onset after the age of 40 years. Typically, these patients present with insidious onset of asymmetric leg weakness or gait imbalance Progressive-relapsing MS is progressive disease from the onset with clear exacerbations. This is considered the rarest form of MS.

The term *clinically isolated syndrome* has emerged to define the first demyelinating attack that is suggestive of MS, typically optic neuritis, transverse myelitis, or a brainstem syndrome. For some patients, this is an isolated event, but many others go on to have subsequent attacks and develop relapsing-remitting MS. Studies show that for patients with an initial demyelinating event that have even one lesion characteristic of MS on brain MRI, the risk of having a second attack, and thereby meeting diagnostic criteria for MS, is 88%. To date, only the first-line injectable therapies have been studied for intervention.

Incidence

Marked differences in the prevalence of MS exist among different populations and ethnic groups. MS is a disease of temperate climates. Highest known prevalence occurs in the Orkney Islands, off Scotland. MS is also common in Scandinavia and elsewhere in northern Europe. There are more than 2 million persons affected worldwide; the incidence is 12 per 100,000 persons. In the United States, it is estimated that 450,000 people are affected, with about 10,000 new cases per year. Whites of north European descent have significantly higher rates of the disease than do other racial groups. MS is extremely rare in Japan and virtually unknown in black Africa, but Japanese Americans and African Americans show an increased prevalence.[204] African Americans with MS have a greater likelihood of developing opticospinal MS and transverse myelitis and have a more aggressive disease course than white Americans.[107] Figure 31-8 shows the incidence rates worldwide.

MS rarely manifests before adolescence; it rises steadily in incidence from the teens to age 35 years and declines gradually thereafter. Similar to many other autoimmune diseases, MS has a predilection for women, with a female-to-male ratio of 2.5:1. Men have a slightly later age of onset and more severe clinical outcomes than women. Men with MS transmit the disease to their children (independently of the child's sex) more often than do women who have MS.[46] Relapse rates may decline 70% in the third trimester of pregnancy, most likely from circulating levels of estriol. These facts suggest a complex hormonal modulation of the immune system.

Etiologic and Risk Factors

There is a clear genetic component in the risk of developing MS.[37] When one parent is affected, and especially if that parent developed MS before 20 years of age, a child has a fivefold higher risk of developing MS.[212] Absence

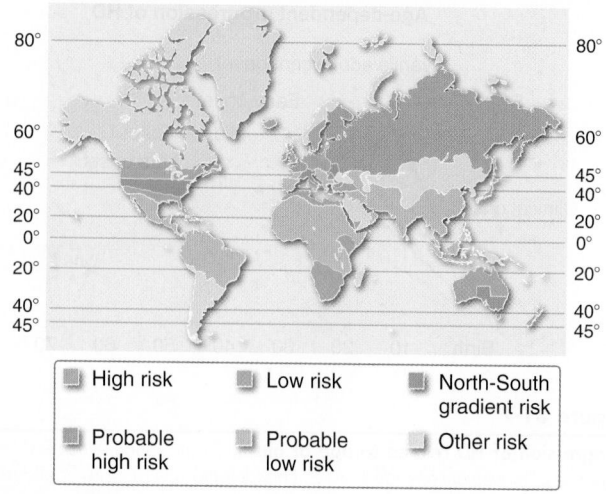

Figure 31-8

World map showing the relative incidence of multiple sclerosis. Areas of greatest risk are in the northern latitudes. (Adapted from National Institute of Neurological and Communicative Disorders and Stroke: *Multiple sclerosis: hope through research.* Publication no. 79-75, Washington, DC, 1981, National Institutes of Health. In Umphred DA: *Neurological rehabilitation,* ed 5, St Louis, 2007, Mosby.)

of the inhibitory *KIR2DL3* gene is associated with the development of MS. There does not seem to be any association between the presence or absence of *KIR* genes with clinical disease parameters.[123] The human leukocyte antigen (HLA) region on chromosome contributes a small fraction to the genetic basis of MS.[53] The linkages are complex and may involve multiple weak links that are difficult to identify using current research methods. In Scotland, where risk of developing MS is high, there is an increase in the incidence of the HLA-DR2 allele in the population, which has a proven correlation to MS. The presence of HLA-DR2 is associated with a nearly twofold increase in the likelihood of having a second attack of MS within 5 years. A variety of genes have been associated with the disease, including interleukin-1b receptor, interleukin-1 receptor antagonist, and immunoglobulin Fc receptor.

Coexisting autoimmune disorders are seen in a majority of individuals, such as Hashimoto thyroiditis, psoriasis, inflammatory bowel disease, and rheumatoid arthritis. Families with a history of MS have autoimmune disorders in greater than 65% of first-degree relatives. Hashimoto thyroiditis, psoriasis, and inflammatory bowel disease are the most common disorders also occurring in family members. The presence of various immune disorders in families with several members with MS suggests that the disease might arise on a background of a generalized susceptibility to autoimmune disorders. Viral infection often precipitates an attack of MS. In fact, it is the only natural event that has been shown unequivocally to increase the risk of a new attack of MS. Less than 10% of infections are followed by relapses, but more than one-third of the relapses are proceeded by infection.[53] The possibility that infections, especially viral infections, actually may cause MS has been investigated for many years. Numerous candidate viruses and a smaller number of bacteria have been proposed and then rejected.

Pathogenesis

MS is the classic example of a primary demyelinating disorder, but demyelination alone does not account for the persistent functional disturbances that characterize the disease as it progresses. After myelin is damaged, nerve conduction properties, initially abnormal, can recover, in part related to redistribution of sodium channels. Myelin loss occurs initially around the small veins and venules in brain and spinal cord. There are focal abnormalities referred to as plaques disseminated throughout the cerebral hemispheres in the white matter, especially in the white matter surrounding the ventricles, the optic nerves, and the brainstem. The corpus callosum is usually involved in MS because this structure receives a unique double blood supply. Spinal cord pathology has been hypothesized to be an important factor in disease progression in primary progressive MS but is not always predictive.[220]

The pathologic conditions that occur in MS include inflammation, demyelination, and axon loss. MS is predominantly a T-cell–mediated inflammatory disorder with overproduction of proinflammatory cytokines. Demyelination can result from either direct damage to neuronal myelin by inflammatory cells or indirectly because of the extracellular environment. This demyelination can cause neurons to be more susceptible to apoptosis. Although demyelination may produce the relapses that occur during the disease, long-term disability is primarily caused by irreversible axon loss and cell death.[86]

The initial event in MS may be priming of autoreactive, peripheral T cells against myelin antigens by an infectious agent. It is thought that preexisting autoreactive T cells are activated outside the CNS by foreign microbes, self-proteins, or microbial superantigens. Activated T cells cross the blood-brain barrier through a multistep process. In this trafficking process, lymphocytes attached to endothelial cells proceed to pass through the endothelial cell cytoplasm. Chemokines, like cytokines, are secreted polypeptides that can induce increased production of integrin molecules by lymphocytes and switch these integrin molecules into a higher affinity state that allows them to transmigrate more effectively across CNS endothelium. The activated T cells secrete cytokines that stimulate microglial cells and astrocytes, recruit additional inflammatory cells, and induce antibody production by plasma cells. Antimyelin antibodies, activated macrophages or microglial cells, and tumor necrosis factor are thought to cooperate in producing demyelination. In the neurodegenerative phase of the disease, excessive amounts of glutamate are released by lymphocytes, microglia, and macrophages. The glutamate activates various glutamate receptors, causing the influx of calcium through ion channels associated with toxic damage to oligodendrocytes and axons. The oligodendrocyte is a nonneural component of the CNS that is directly related to the cell body or axon. The oligodendrocyte produces the myelin that wraps around the axon of the nerve cell. The myelin sheath increases the speed of the action potential and is critical for smooth and rapid movement.

Both necrosis and apoptosis play a role in the progression of MS. When necrosis occurs in MS lesions, it produces enhancing lesions caused by the substantial breakdown of the blood-brain barrier. In MS lesions, apoptosis occurs in neurons, oligodendrocytes, and leukocytes. Apoptosis occurs pathologically in MS, in part because the loss of myelin causes neurons to be much more susceptible to binding of agents that induce apoptosis rather than necrosis. Apoptosis is probably at least partially responsible for the progression that leads to permanent disability and explains why lesion activity on MRI scans can be quiescent at a time when the disability of the individual continues to increase. Apoptosis of oligodendrocytes may represent a very early stage in the evolution of lesions that underlie acute relapses of MS. Therefore, myelin destruction in MS lesions may be caused by processes other than those mediated by macrophages.

Brain atrophy is a clinically relevant component in MS and begins early in the disease course. The caudate (part of the basal ganglia) can be smaller in volume and also have changes in shape. The demyelinated cortex contains apoptotic neurons. Cortical demyelination may influence dendrite and axon function and decrease neuronal viability, which may further activate disease progression. Axonotmesis as a result of inflammation in MS lesions can lead to retrograde neuronal degeneration and apoptosis.[190] In chronic lesions, demyelinated axons undergo a slow, disseminating wallerian degeneration along neural tracts away from the initial site of injury, contributing to long-term disability.

New lesions frequently appear at sites of previous activity or within or at the edges of previously stable lesions. New lesions can form within or overlap shadow plaques (areas of thin remyelination) and may contribute to failed remyelination or the conversion of shadow plaques into classic demyelinated plaques.[194] Thus some lesions may appear to be quite large.

The plaques may be acute or chronic lesions. The acute plaques are small, circumscribed areas of hypocellularity, demyelination, and axonal loss. Astrogliosis, resulting in scar tissue formation, is more severe in MS lesions than in most other neuropathologic conditions. Periventricular infiltrates consisting of macrophages, T cells, immunoglobulins, and microglia fill the plaque.[248] Axons passing through may be spared, but there seems to be more and more evidence of axon loss within the plaques. New active plaques are pink with faint borders that exhibit an intense inflammatory response. Old inactive plaques are gray and firm, with sharp edges with a gliotic background crossed by axons but lacking oligodendrocytes.[179] Abnormal immune function in the blood and CSF is a common finding.[112]

A variety of pathogenic mechanisms may be involved in the development of MS plaques, which occur as a result of diversity in the sequence of events that causes the condition to arise. The features of the lesions, including the amount and nature of T-cell–, macrophage-, and immunoglobulin-related damage, seem to vary from individual to individual, but there is much less variation among the active lesions within an individual. For example, the survival of oligodendrocytes varies among individuals.[40] In some individuals, it appears that oligodendrocyte dystrophy and apoptosis are the primary cause of demyelination. In others, the presence of immunoglobulins suggests that demyelinating antibodies have a pathogenic role.[145,154] As with demyelination, axonal destruction could result from direct immunologic attack or inflammatory mediators or from secondary effects of chronic demyelination.[240] As in other chronic inflammatory diseases of the CNS, vascular pathology is profound in the brains of patients with MS, seen both within the lesions and in normal-appearing white matter. Inflammatory changes occur in the perivascular space. Dysfunction of the blood-brain barrier is shown by changes in endothelial tight junctions. In chronic lesions, vascular fibrosis is common. The relation between inflammation, blood-brain barrier damage, and structural vascular pathology is complex. Serum protein leakage from vessels is seen early stages of the disease and seems to decrease with progression. Widespread hypoperfusion in normal-appearing white matter and in cortical and deep gray matter has been recorded in patients with relapsing-remitting MS and progressive MS. Neurophysiologically, fatigue in MS is associated with more anteriorly widespread event-related desynchronization during a movement (indicating hyperactivity during movement execution), and lower postmovement contralateral event-related synchronization (indicating failure of the inhibitory mechanisms intervening after movement termination) compared with normal individuals and patients with MS without fatigue. This finding is consistent with central dysfunction and a central origin of fatigue in MS.

Clinical Manifestations

In most individuals, MS is characterized by progressive disability over time, but the amount of accumulated disability varies widely. A benign course may affect up to 20% of individuals and is characterized by an abrupt onset with one or a few relapses followed by complete or nearly complete remitting periods. These individuals experience little or no permanent disability and remain relatively symptom free. This is a designation that can only be made with certainty in retrospect, since there are no perfect prognostic markers. More recent MRI scan data suggest that even in individuals with benign MS there is likely significant progression of lesions.

Each individual's CNS appears to have a different threshold for producing symptoms and signs reflecting the affected regions of the CNS. This threshold, or the capacity of the individual's brain to adapt to the lesions, will determine the severity of the clinical manifestations.[161]

Optic neuritis is often the first manifestation of MS. The optic nerve is an extension of the cerebral cortex, virtually a tract of the CNS, and is therefore subject to the effects of demyelination with the syndrome of optic neuritis. Optic neuritis typically presents as a unilateral, painful decrease or loss of vision. It is commonly associated with visual field defects, decreased color vision, and reduced clarity of vision.[87] Individuals with optic neuritis must be carefully evaluated for an ocular mobility abnormality to determine the possibility of a second anatomically distinct lesion, because the symptoms of blurring may be caused by an eye movement disorder.[131]

Sensory changes are also common initial complaints. This is often a paresthesia or dysesthesia noted in one extremity or in the head and face. Visual blurring, diplopia, weakness, and balance problems also may be early signs. Often these symptoms are transient and not even reported. It is usually when there is a pattern or the symptoms are unchanging that the person seeks medical attention. Dorsal column symptoms include paresthesias (tingling, pricking) and hypoesthesia (diminished sensitivity). These may begin in an extremity and ascend over hours or several days to include the rest of the leg or arm, the perineum, the trunk, and perhaps other extremities. Other sensory complaints include a feeling of swelling, of wetness, or that the body part is tightly wrapped. Involvement of a cord level is diagnostically helpful in distinguishing this attack from a peripheral neuropathologic incident. Other positive dorsal column signs are loss of vibration, position, and two-point discrimination. Sensory complaints are often not substantiated by objective findings, especially if the symptoms are mild or the remission has already begun before the individual is examined. For example, the feeling of numbness may not result in a loss of response to pinprick.

The single most common and most disabling symptom of MS is fatigue.[89] Many patients recall that fatigue often preceded diagnosis or the occurrence of identifiable neurologic lesions by several years. Fatigue is typically present in midafternoon and may take the form of increased motor weakness with effort, mental fatigue, and sleepiness. MS-related fatigue presents as an overwhelming feeling of tiredness in those who have not exerted themselves and are not depressed. Neuromuscular or short-circuiting fatigue is common. The demyelinated nerve fires again and again until it shorts when it is called upon to do a repetitive task. Thus, progressive resistive exercises often result in a feeling of increased fatigue and weakness rather than a feeling of increased strength. Short breaks with energy conservation can make this fatigue less prominent.

Sleep dysfunction is related to fatigue in MS. Excessive limb movements, nocturia, and pain are the main symptoms resulting in fragmented sleep and poor sleep efficiency in MS. Insomnia is a common complaint, with pain and discomfort being linked to sleep initiation insomnia, and nocturia being linked to sleep maintenance insomnia.[22]

Spasticity, velocity-dependent stiffness about a joint, is an extremely common problem with MS, occurring in 90% of all cases caused by abnormal firing of the ascending and descending excitatory and inhibitory pathways in the brain and spinal cord. It can vary from nonexistent to severe, even in the same person, and from moment to moment, making its management challenging. GABA and other neurotransmitters are involved. Often those who have significant spasticity use their spasticity to walk, transfer, and manage their daily living. Treatment becomes an issue only if the spasticity is causing discomfort, pain, or problems with daily living. Pain, either from an injury or from a bladder infection, exacerbates spasticity. Thus, the management of spasticity begins with the removal of noxious stimuli. In some individuals, spasticity can be intractable. The high doses of medications necessitated by this circumstance sedate and cause disability on their own. Spasms may accompany the spasticity and usually are more severe and frequent at night. They often interrupt the sleep cycle, even in those who do not recognize their awakenings. This may lead to severe fatigue the next day; thus, minimizing nocturnal spasms is important. Associated signs of upper motor neuron syndrome may include clonus, spontaneous extensor or flexor spasms, positive Babinski sign, and loss of precise autonomic control.[158,167,218]

Weakness in MS usually is a result of decreased neuromuscular impulses secondary to demyelination and axonal loss. As discussed previously, progressive resistive exercises may contribute to fatigue and give the appearance of increasing weakness. Signs of muscle weakness secondary to damage of the motor cortex and tracts reflect the loss of orderly recruitment and rate modulation of motor neurons. Muscle activation patterns and agonist–antagonist relationships are disturbed. Heat, either from increased ambient temperature or from fever, often increases weakness. This may be the result of a conduction block. Cooling often allows more efficient conduction and improved strength if there is appropriate innervation.

Involvement at the level of the brainstem reflects lesions of cranial nerves III through XII at the root, nuclear, or bulbar level. Trigeminal neuralgia (also called tic douloureux) is a shock-like pain in the face. Although not a common finding, it is highly characteristic of MS in a young person. Spasm or weakness of facial muscles can also be seen. Dysarthria, abnormal speech resulting from poor control of the muscles of speech, and dysphagia, including signs of gurgling, coughing, weight loss, pneumonia, choking, or a weak voice, can present in brainstem involvement.

There can also be gaze palsies, the loss of active control of eye movement, and nystagmus, involuntary rhythmic tremor of the eye. Intranuclear ophthalmoplegia is the most common gaze palsy, resulting in lateral gaze paralysis, and is caused by demyelination of the pontine medial longitudinal fasciculus, an area of the brain's white matter involved in the control of eye movement. Other lesions in the brainstem and reticular formation can cause other palsies, resulting in difficulty with conjugate gaze and ipsilateral gaze palsy. Idiopathic nystagmus that improves over time also can be caused by lesions in the vestibular nuclei or cerebellum.

Other abnormalities of ocular mobility, such as instability of fixation or inability to suppress the vestibuloocular response, are related to lesions involving brainstem nuclei and tracts. Vertigo, the sensation of spinning, may appear suddenly and in dramatic fashion with gait unsteadiness and vomiting. In MS, this reflects a brainstem rather than end-organ vestibular disorder; a careful look at associated brainstem symptoms will help to distinguish the cause (see Chapter 38).

Coordination (ataxia) problems often accompany tremor and are among the most difficult symptoms to manage. Compensatory techniques taught via exercises can be helpful but rarely enough to satisfy. Cerebellar syndrome deficits may be symmetric, with all four limbs involved, or asymmetric, with only one side affected. Manifestations include ataxia, hypotonia, and truncal weakness, causing postural and movement disorders. Dysarthria of cerebellar origin (scanning speech, producing

abnormalities in the rhythm of speech) is common. Cerebellar signs are often associated with the progressive phases of the illness.[239]

Pain is surprisingly common in MS, occurring in 50% of individuals. The pain usually is a burning neuropathic type. It may be disturbing, and pain medicine offers little if any relief. The distribution of the pain may not follow any recognizable neurologic distribution. It can be paroxysmal in nature but often is fairly constant, with nocturnal worsening when the body is at rest in bed. Another clinical symptom is the Lhermitte sign, a momentary electricity-like sensation evoked by neck flexion or cough.

Depression is a primary symptom of MS occurring because of actual changes in the brain and its chemistry. Depression can occur as a direct result of the MS plaques or as a reaction to the diagnosis or disability. Depression may lead to greater disability than that caused by the level of neurologic impairment. Medication use for other symptoms may contribute to the cognitive problems with sedation and confusion; thus, these must be reviewed regularly in those who have dulled cognition. Depression may be an additive culprit and is treatable if recognized. There is no question that reactive (exogenous) depression occurs frequently in MS and is amenable to counseling and other nonpharmacologic techniques, but the brain disease seen in MS clearly leads to chemical (endogenous) depression in many. Cognitive decline is of significance in up to 50% of persons with MS.[219] Memory loss is the most common cognitive problem, and there commonly are a variety of slowed response types. The suicide rate for MS seems greater than that for many other neurologic diseases, some of which have a worse perceived prognosis.

Bladder and bowel symptoms are common and usually occur when the spinal cord is involved. Bladder urgency, frequency, and incontinence associated with an overactive bladder are often seen early in the disease and generally precede incontinence. Bladder issues are prominent in those who have MS. The bladder can present itself with frequency, urgency, hesitancy, and incontinence with differing mechanisms. Most frequent is the small, failure-to-store bladder characterized by a low postvoid residual. This can be measured by catheterization or ultrasound. It often has uncontrollable contractions.

More problematic from a management point of view is the large, failure-to-empty bladder. It overfills with residuals from 200–900 mL and presents with the same symptomatology despite looking different anatomically and physiologically. Frequently, there is a dyssynergia between the bladder and the urinary sphincter, causing similar symptoms from yet another mechanism. Residual urine after emptying, with subsequent overflow incontinence and heightened risk of urinary tract infections, is a problem for 50% of persons with MS, especially later in the course of the disease. This may require intermittent or chronic catheterization, or use of the Credé method (manual pressure on the bladder to express urine).[21] Neurogenic disorders may also impair bowel function, resulting in incontinence or constipation.

Bowel function is affected less than bladder function but can be problematic. Irritable bowel is a common associated problem, and regulating the bowel often means changing treatments, depending on the circumstances. It is better to be slightly constipated than slightly loose.[218]

Sexual expression may require special attention in MS. Relationships remain of utmost importance and need to be stressed, without diminishing the importance of the actual sexual performance in the face of disability. In men, erectile dysfunction is frequent. Occasionally, penile prostheses may be placed. This is less common today because of alternative treatment options. Female sexual expression may be diminished by vaginal dryness or decreased or altered sensation in the vaginal area.

Unique symptoms in MS are called paroxysmal because they come in bouts. Sometimes they are sensory in nature and may be painful. Trigeminal neuralgia is a common example of this type of painful, paroxysmal symptom. This lancinating, electrical sensation along the distribution of a branch of the trigeminal nerve can be terribly disabling. It may be a standalone problem in some individuals, but also is a symptom associated with MS. Periodic electrical sensation down the spine with the bending of the neck is called the Lhermitte sign, another paroxysmal sensory symptom. These types of sensations occasionally may be felt in other parts of the body. Often the paroxysmal symptoms are motor in nature. They may be twitching of an eyelid or myokymia in the facial muscles. They may manifest as a true spasm of an arm in an extended or, occasionally, flexed position lasting for seconds. They can occur frequently, several times an hour. The spasm may occur with speech, a paroxysmal dysarthria or speech arrest. All of these can be disconcerting to the individual and the clinician.

The aggressive use of immune-modulating agents to slow down the actual disease process has contributed to the development of a whole new set of symptoms that the clinician must recognize and manage. Interferon initiation often brings about a fever reaction, which may be disabling to the person who has MS. It often is recommended that interferon be administered in the evening before going to bed. This allows for the impact of the fever during the night, when it may be less disabling to activities of living. Antipyretic medications (ibuprofen or acetaminophen) may be administered 4 hours before the injection, at the time of injection, and then, if necessary, 4 hours after the injection.

Subcutaneous injections can lead to immune reactions within the skin, with inflammation, redness, and significant irritation. Good injection technique is essential. This may involve icing the area before injecting. A common error is injecting too shallowly. Injection devices use improved techniques and have decreased many of these side effects but may contribute to the problem if they are set to deliver the medication too shallowly within the skin rather than beneath it. It is important to allow the air bubble in the syringe to remain to push the medication through the skin and it is recommended that the needle be free of lingering medication as it pierces the skin. Rotation of the injection sites is an absolute necessity to preserve as much skin area as possible and allow healing between injections. For some individuals, the addition of a cortisone cream or a local anesthetic cream may be helpful. With some treatments, pain can linger after the injection. Applying cooling can offer symptomatic relief. Understanding the issues often is helpful in the development of compensatory strategies.

MEDICAL MANAGEMENT

DIAGNOSIS. The McDonald Criteria of the International Panel on Diagnosis of MS, updated in 2010, is widely used diagnostic criteria (Table 31-5). The presence of both gadolinium-enhancing and nonenhancing lesions on the baseline MRI can substitute for a follow-up scan to confirm dimension in time, as long as it can be reliably determined that the gadolinium-enhancing lesion is not due to non-MS pathology.[191] Box 31-11 show some examples of differential diseases for which screening should be done.

Gray matter lesions are different from white matter lesions showing little T-cell inflammation or disruption of the blood-brain barrier but with leakage of plasma proteins. Cortical demyelination might be primarily related to meningeal inflammation. Within the white matter; glutamate excitotoxicity and mitochondrial dysfunction have the potential to cause axonal damage with secondary effects in the cortex.

Early-onset MS is associated with lesions within the spinal cord. The spinal cord may be abnormal when the brain MRI is normal. However, an abnormal spinal cord is found more than half the time when there are nine or more brain lesions. Approximately 80% to 85% of individuals present with a relapsing-remitting course, with symptoms and signs evolving over days and typically improving over weeks.[224]

The whole spinal cord can be imaged with high resolution and phased-array coils, showing abnormalities in 80% to 90% of individuals with MS, usually without accompanying neurologic symptoms or signs. Hypoxic–ischemic disease does not present with spinal cord abnormalities. Incidental spinal cord lesions do not occur with aging and are rarely reported in other immune-mediated disorders. Most individuals with early MS have lesions within the spinal cord. But imaging may not be performed, so they may not be isolated. Spinal cord lesions tend to increase as the number of brain lesions rises; this is associated with higher risk for a second attack and a diagnosis of clinical MS. Ultimately, abnormal brain MRI scans are present in more than 90% of individuals with clinically definite MS. Normal brain MRI scans may represent disease that is relatively restricted to the spinal cord. Reductions in nerve fiber density are seen in the spinal cord, including in otherwise normal-appearing tissue, and are likely related to permanent disability. Axonal loss can be profound in later stages of disease.

Figure 31-9 shows the plaques seen on MRI. The lesions do not always correlate with the clinical signs, and there can be evidence of focal lesions in the absence of disease. In fact, the vast majority of enhancing lesions are considered to be asymptomatic when they first appear on the brain scan. However, there is a correlation between periods of clinical worsening of the disease and increases in the total number of lesions, the number of new lesions, and the total area of enhancement on MRI.[30] Thus, a single brain MRI scan after a first event is highly prognostic of development of clinically definite MS.[183] Figure 31-10 shows an example of aggressive MS over 2 years revealed in MRI imaging.

Table 31-5	The 2010 McDonald Criteria for Diagnosis of MS Clinical Presentation and Additional Data Needed for MS Diagnosis

Clinical Presentation	Additional Data Needed for MS Diagnosis
≥2 Attacks*; objective clinical evidence of ≥2 lesions or objective clinical evidence of 1 lesion with reasonable historical evidence of a prior attack[†]	None[‡]
≥2 Attacks*; objective clinical evidence of 1 lesion	Dissemination in space, shown by ≥1 T2 lesions in at least 2 of 4 MS-typical regions of the CNS (periventricular, juxtacortical, infratentorial, or spinal cord)[§]; or await a further clinical attack* implicating a different CNS site
1 Attack*; objective clinical evidence of ≥2 lesions	Dissemination in time, shown by simultaneous presence of asymptomatic gadolinium-enhancing and nonenhancing lesions at any time; or A new T2 and/or gadolinium-enhancing lesion(s) on follow-up MRI, irrespective of its timing relative to a baseline scan; or Await a second clinical attack*

1 Attack*; objective clinical evidence of 1 lesion (clinically isolated syndrome)	Dissemination in space and time, shown by:
	For DIS:
	  ≥1 T2 lesion in at least 2 of 4 MS-typical regions of the CNS (periventricular, juxtacortical, infratentorial, or spinal cord)[§]; or await a second clinical attack* implicating a different CNS site;
	For DIT:
	  Simultaneous presence of asymptomatic gadolinium-enhancing and nonenhancing lesions at any time; or
	  A new T2 and/or gadolinium-enhancing lesion(s) on follow-up MRI, irrespective of its timing relative to a baseline scan; or
	  Await a second clinical attack*

Insidious neurologic progression suggesting MS (primary progressive MS)	1 yr of disease progression (retrospectively or prospectively determined) plus 2 of 3 of the following criteria[§]: 1. Evidence for DIS in the brain based on ≥1 T2 lesions in the MS-characteristic (periventricular, juxtacortical, or infratentorial) regions 2. Evidence for DIS in the spinal cord based on ≥2 T2 lesions in the cord 3. Positive CSF (isoelectric focusing evidence of oligoclonal bands and/or increased IgG index)

DIS, Dissemination in space; DIT, dissemination in time; IgG, immunoglobulin G.

If the criteria are fulfilled and there is no better explanation for the clinical presentation, the diagnosis is MS; if suspicious, but the criteria are not completely met, the diagnosis is possible MS; if another diagnosis arises during the evaluation that better explains the clinical presentation, then the diagnosis is not MS.

*An attack (relapse; exacerbation) is defined as patient-reported or objectively observed events typical of an acute inflammatory demyelinating event in the CNS, current or historical, with duration of at least 24 hours, in the absence of fever or infection. It should be documented by contemporaneous neurologic examination, but some historical events with symptoms and evolution characteristic for MS, but for which no objective neurologic findings are documented, can provide reasonable evidence of a prior demyelinating event. However, reports of paroxysmal symptoms (historical or current) should consist of multiple episodes occurring over not less than 24 hours. Before a definite diagnosis of MS can be made, at least one attack must be corroborated by findings on neurologic examination, visual evoked potential response in patients reporting prior visual disturbance, or MRI consistent with demyelination in the area of the CNS implicated in the historical report of neurologic symptoms.

[†]Clinical diagnosis based on objective clinical findings for two attacks is most secure. Reasonable historical evidence for one past attack, in the absence of documented objective neurologic findings, can include historical events with symptoms and evolution characteristics for a prior inflammatory demyelinating event; however, at least one attack must be supported by objective findings.

[‡]No additional tests are required. However, it is desirable that any diagnosis of MS be made with access to imaging based on these criteria. If imaging or other tests (for instance, CSF) are undertaken and are negative, extreme caution needs to be taken before making a diagnosis of MS, and alternative diagnoses must be considered. There must be no better explanation for the clinical presentation, and objective evidence must be present to support a diagnosis of MS.

[§]Gadolinium-enhancing lesions are not required; symptomatic lesions are excluded from consideration in patients with brainstem or spinal cord syndromes.

From Sheremata W, Tornes L: Multiple sclerosis and the spinal cord, *Neurol Clin* 31(1):55–77, 2013.

Contrast enhancement in CT and MRI suggests inflammation but is more accurately a measure of leakage of moderate-size molecules across the damaged tight junctions of the CNS endothelium. The enhancement pattern (size, shape, solid versus ring) may be variable within and more so between individuals, which reflects a heterogeneous pathology. Ring enhancement, for example, may suggest a more severe pathology. Figure 31-11 demonstrates the development of a T2-weighted hyperintense lesion by serial MRI. Monitoring serial MRI studies with enhancement helps to identify agents that may be active against the early inflammatory stage of MS.[228] Figure 31-12 shows changes related to progressive forms of MS. Functional MRI maps the brain areas activated using a task paradigm. Functional disturbances have been the basis for hypotheses suggesting that compensatory mechanisms develop in early MS, which initially may mask injury and delay the appearance of dysfunction. Functional

Box 31-11

DIFFERENTIAL DIAGNOSIS OF MULTIPLE SCLEROSIS

Other Inflammatory Demyelinating Central Nervous System Conditions

- Acute disseminated encephalomyelitis
- Neuromyelitis optica

Systemic or Organ-Specific Inflammatory Diseases

- Systemic lupus erythematosus
- Sjögren syndrome

Inflammatory Bowel Disease

- Vasculitis
- Periarteritis nodosa
- Primary central nervous system angiitis
- Susac syndrome
- Eales disease
- Granulomatous diseases
- Sarcoidosis

Infectious Disorders

- Lyme neuroborreliosis
- Syphilis
- Viral myelitis
- Progressive multifocal leukoencephalitis
- Subacute sclerosing panencephalitis

Cerebrovascular Disorders

- Multiple emboli
- Hypercoagulable states

- Sneddon's syndrome
- Neoplasms
- Metastasis
- Lymphoma
- Paraneoplastic syndromes

Metabolic Disorders

- Vitamin B_{12} deficiency
- Vitamin E deficiency
- Central (or extra) pontine myelinolysis
- Leukodystrophies (especially adrenomyeloneuropathy)
- Leber hereditary optic neuropathy

Structural Lesions

- Spinal cord compression
- Chiari malformation
- Syringomyelia/syringobulbia
- Foramen magnum lesions
- Spinal arteriovenous malformation/dural fistula

Degenerative Diseases

- Hereditary spastic paraparesis
- Spinocerebellar degeneration
- Olivopontocerebellar atrophy

Psychiatric Disorders

- Conversion reactions
- Malingering

From Goetz CG: *Textbook of clinical neurology,* ed 2, Philadelphia, 2003, WB Saunders.

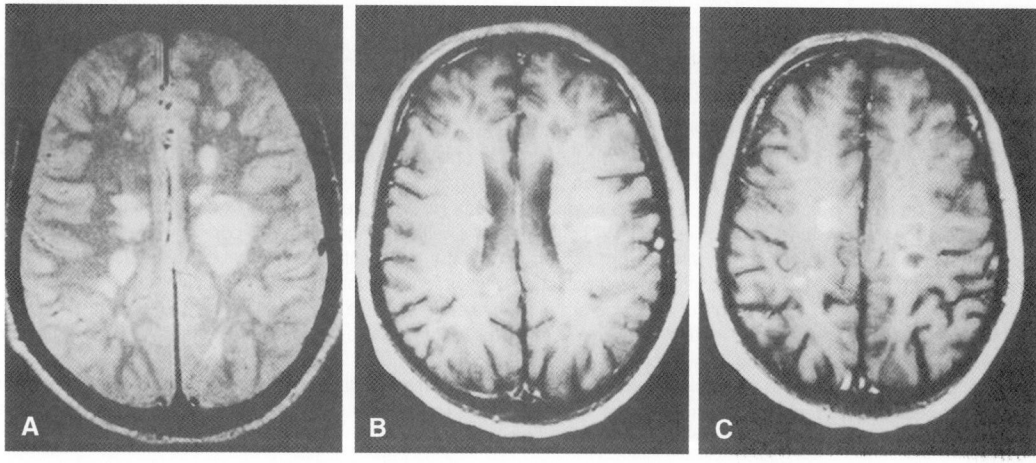

Figure 31-9

A, Typical scattered, variably sized plaques in the brain associated with the diagnosis of multiple sclerosis (MS). **B,** Contrast-enhanced magnetic resonance imaging reveals scattered area of solid and ring-shaped enhancement. **C,** Note the atrophy, greater than would be expected for the person's age, a common finding in MS. (From Ramsey R: *Neuroradiology,* Philadelphia, 1994, WB Saunders.)

disturbance may only become apparent after exhaustion of these adaptive mechanisms. Fatigue severity is correlated with the reduction in thalamic and cerebellar activation. Although abnormal functional MRI patterns may be observed in given individuals with MS, their interpretation may not be straightforward. Functional MRI findings reflect functional adaptation, they do not necessarily serve as direct evidence for gray matter pathology.

Functional MRI appears to identify sensorimotor and cognitive disturbances in MS. The most consistent finding by functional MRI studies in populations of individuals with MS is impairment in sensorimotor activation indicated by abnormally increased contralateral blood oxygenation level and ipsilateral supplementary motor activation. Sensorimotor functional MRI is sensitive even in the early stages of disease.

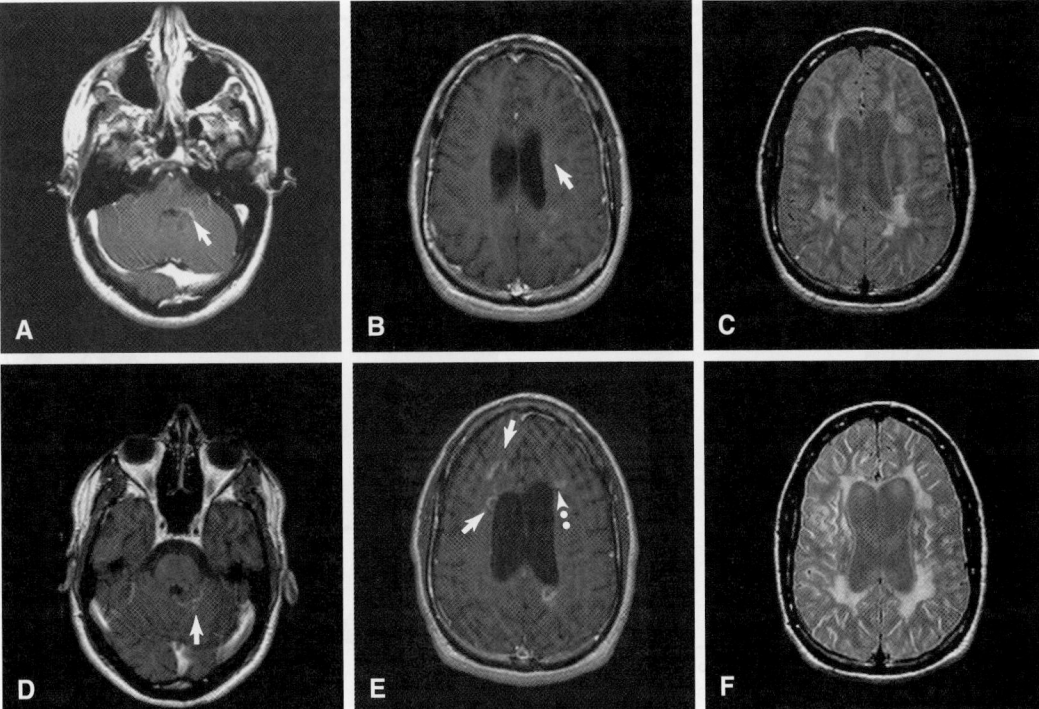

Figure 31-10

Aggressive multiple sclerosis over 2 years. Disease was initially relapsing-remitting but converted relatively quickly to secondary progressive MS. *Top row:* Contrast-enhanced left pons **(A)** and left frontal-parietal white matter **(B)**, both showing a relatively rare edge enhancement pattern *(arrows)*. Typical confluent T2 hyperintensities and mild-moderate volume loss based on lateral ventricle size **(C)**. *Bottom row:* Two years later magnetic resonance image shows different edge-enhancing lesions *(arrows)* in posterior fossa **(D)** and both edge enhancement *(arrows)* and ring enhancement *(dotted arrow)* in deep white matter along the lateral ventricles **(E)**. Progressive volume loss based on moderately large lateral ventricles and more extensive confluent T2 hyperintensity is seen in **(F)**. (From *Radiol Clin North Am*, 44 [1]:____, 2006.)

Measures of regional brain atrophy are useful to determine neuropsychologic dysfunction. Imaging data suggest that neuropsychologic impairment in MS is related, in part, to atrophy of gray matter regions and in the juxtacortical areas. Gray matter atrophy is associated with impairments in verbal memory, euphoria, and disinhibition.

Whole-brain atrophy reflects the destructive aspects of the disease. The data linking brain atrophy to clinical impairments suggest that irreversible tissue destruction is a major determinant of disease progression, whereas white matter lesion activity has less correlation. The strongest correlations between MRI measures and disability may be those provided by atrophy measures. Confounding factors must be considered when assessing whether loss of brain volume directly indicates tissue atrophy. Secondary progressive disease causes significantly more atrophy of both white matter and gray matter and a significantly higher lesion load than relapsing-remitting disease.[233] Primary progressive disorders show decreased numbers and volume of enhancing lesions, related to the less intense inflammation. Cellular imaging based on superparamagnetic iron oxide–tagged cells is a more specific probe of the migration occurring at the level of the blood-brain barrier basic to the inflammatory process.

PET scans, and functional MRI show widespread cerebral hypometabolism, as well as selective hypometabolism in the bifrontal and basal ganglial regions in MS. The regional analysis of deep and cortical gray matter atrophy suggests an association between the neurodegenerative process taking place in the striatum–thalamus–frontal cortex pathway and the development of fatigue in relapsing-remitting MS. The inclusion of the posterior parietal cortex as one of the best predictors of the modified fatigue impact scale cognitive domain suggests the major role of the posterior attentional system in determining cognitive fatigue in relapsing-remitting MS.[41]

CSF analysis often shows increased mononuclear cell pleocytosis, an elevation in total immunoglobulins, and the presence of oligoclonal bands. These responses suggest an inflammatory response in the CNS. In 85% to 95% of individuals with clinically definite MS, these values are abnormal. In people with suspected MS, the number is much lower. Abnormal values, including oligoclonal bands, also may be seen in a smaller percentage of those with a variety of disorders, especially other inflammatory or infectious disorders that may affect the CNS. Metabolites from the breakdown of myelin may also be detected in CSF but are very nonspecific. Measurement of these myelin basic proteins in CSF is more useful as a predictor of response to steroids used during acute exacerbations than as a diagnostic tool.

Evoked potential response testing may detect slowed or abnormal conduction in visual, auditory, somatosensory, or motor pathways. These tests employ computer averaging techniques to record the electrical response evoked in the nervous system following repetitive sensory or motor stimuli. Evoked potentials are abnormal in up to 90% of

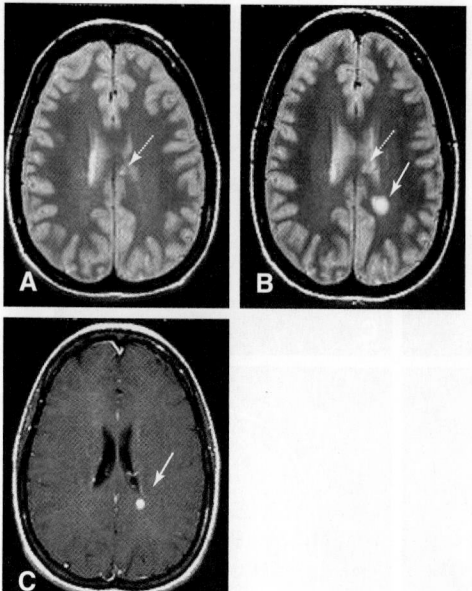

Figure 31-11

Development of a T2 hyperintense lesion by serial magnetic resonance imaging. A, Case of relapsing multiple sclerosis with low T2 hyperintense lesion burden, including chronic lesions in the corpus callosum *(arrow)*. **B,** One month later, a new T2 hyperintense lesion develops in the left parietal-occipital white matter *(solid arrow)*, whereas the corpus callosum lesions remain stable *(dotted arrow)*. **C,** Corresponding enhancement in acute lesion *(arrow)* from blood-brain barrier breakdown and concurrent inflammation. **D,** Exploded view of the new lesion showing the complex structure, centrally hyperintense, most likely from mixed pathology including demyelination, matrix including glial change, and, importantly, axonal degeneration. The intermediate black ring may be a zone of macrophage infiltration, and the outer ring is likely from edema. (From *Radiol Clin North Am*, 44[1], 2006.)

individuals who have clinically definite MS. Testing can provide evidence of a second lesion in an individual with a single clinically apparent lesion, or it can demonstrate an objective abnormality in an individual with subjective complaints and a normal examination.

Myelography and CT are both insensitive to the pathologic changes in MS and should not be used where the diagnosis of MS is a possibility. Both may still be used to rule out other disorders that mimic MS symptoms.

TREATMENT. Keeping an activated immune system from getting to the central myelinated fibers slows the process of demyelination in MS. Therefore, the principle of treatment in MS today revolves around immune modulation. Different steps of the pathologic cascade in MS may eventually be targeted therapeutically for optimal treatment of MS. Understanding the inflammatory process in MS is important because inflammation includes destructive components that should be targeted for inactivation and potentially beneficial mechanisms that should be enhanced or not disturbed by treatment. Despite earnest research efforts, there is no cure for or immunization against MS.

Disease-modifying drugs significantly decrease new cortical lesions development and cortical atrophy progression and can reduce relapse rates, disability progression and transition to secondary progressive MS without long-term safety issues.[42]

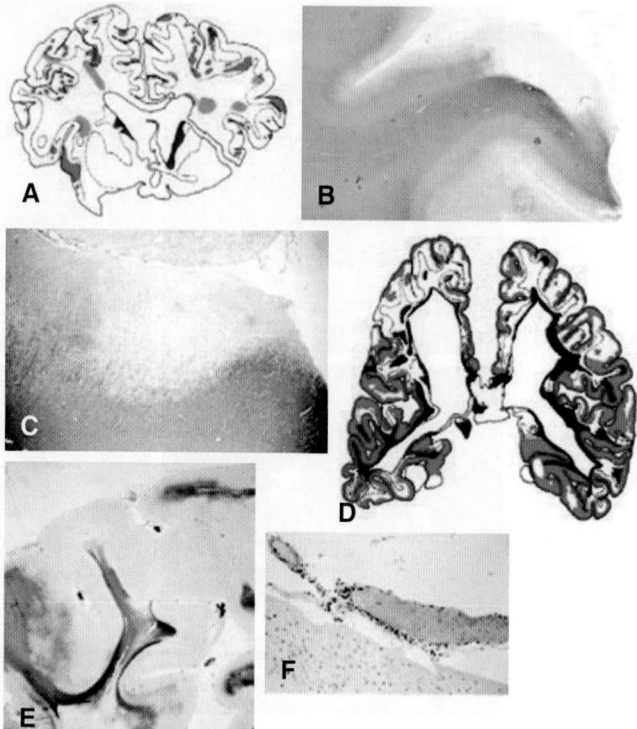

Figure 31-12

Cortical plaques in progressive forms of multiple sclerosis (MS). Cortical demyelination and diffuse white matter inflammation are hallmarks of primary progressive MS (PPMS) and secondary progressive MS (SPMS). **A** and **D,** Schematic lesion maps based on whole hemispheric sections from two archival cases of progressive MS. Case A (PPMS): A 37-year-old man with a history of gradually progressive hemiparesis (left greater than right), sphincter dysfunction, and dysarthria, requiring use of a wheelchair within 6 years of disease onset. Patient died at age 72 of aspiration pneumonia and acute myocardial infarction. Case D (SPMS): A 33-year-old woman initially presenting with diplopia and hemiataxia that partially resolved following short course of corticosteroids. Subsequent course characterized by gradually progressive dysarthria, dysphagia, ophthalmoplegia, and limb and gait ataxia, requiring use of a wheelchair within 7 years of disease onset. She also developed a focal seizure disorder 4 years prior to death and died at age 46 of aspiration pneumonia. **B** and **C,** Subpial cortical demyelination is demonstrated in case A at low **(B)** and high **(C)** magnification. **E,** Extensive subpial demyelination involving multiple gyri is illustrated in case D at low magnification. **F,** Meningeal inflammation may be prominent, often in close proximity to areas with subpial cortical demyelination. Proteolipid protein immunocytochemistry; *green* = focal demyelinated plaques in the white matter; *orange* = cortical demyelination; *blue* = demyelinated lesions in the deep gray matter. (From Pirko I: Gray matter involvement in multiple sclerosis, *Neurology* 68[9]:634–642, 2007.)

First-generation injectable disease-modifying therapies, including interferon (IFN)-β-1b, IFN-β-1a, and glatiramer acetate, have more similarities than differences. All these agents reduce the number of exacerbations by approximately 30%. In addition, these medications reduce the risk of new MRI activity. IFN-β-1a IM/SC was also shown to reduce the risk of sustained disability progression. In general, the injectable disease-modifying therapies are safe and well tolerated. Because of the risk of hematologic abnormalities and hepatotoxicity, a blood count and liver function tests should be monitored with the IFN therapies.[97]

The drugs have become known as "ABC." A is for IFN-β-1a (Avonex, Biogen Idec), and B is for IFN-β-1b (Betaseron, Berlex Laboratories). The higher the dose of interferon, the more potent is the response. Rebif, another INF-β-1a drug, is used in higher doses. Rebif is given subcutaneously at a 46% higher dose three times weekly, for a total of 4.4 times as much drug as Avonex. The potent antiinflammatory effects of interferons have a dramatic effect on the MRI scans, with a decrease in contrast-enhancing lesions.[143,146] INF-β-1a also has been shown in relapsing individuals to slow progression of disability, brain atrophy, and cognitive dysfunction.[125] The treatment effect can be delayed by at least several months. This delay might indicate the fact that the atrophy occurring in the first months is the culmination of a cascade of events that began before the onset of therapy. Alternatively, the ongoing loss of brain volume might be the result of "pseudoatrophy," such as that caused by treatment-related resolution of brain edema and inflammation. Proposed mechanisms by which interferon might limit brain atrophy include increasing nerve growth factors, limiting immune-mediated destructive inflammation, and limiting toxic mechanisms such as pathologic iron deposition.[165] Thus, the question remains as to whether controlling acute relapses and inflammation will ultimately be adequate. Other factors may have an influence on demyelination and axon injury.[179]

The C drug, glatiramer acetate (Copaxone, Teva Pharmaceutical Industries), is a polypeptide that appears to fool the immune system. It seems to decrease the attack by blocking immune cells headed toward myelin and thereby preventing damage. The principal effect may be a shift from a proinflammatory cell bias to an antiinflammatory cell bias. It also has a partial and delayed but significant effect of limiting the rate of brain atrophy in relapsing-remitting MS and there is less occurrence of the flulike symptoms that are associated with the interferons.[85] Glatiramer acetate is effective in treating MS-related fatigue. Glatiramer acetate occasionally induces a systemic reaction. This rare, but real, symptom complex presents with a feeling of panic, chest discomfort, shortness of breath, and a feeling of doom and gloom. It usually lasts for 20 minutes and then clears rapidly, but if panic sets in and an emergency is called, the issue may be magnified and complicated. The treatment is to realize that the problem is associated with the medication and requires resting for the duration of the symptoms to allow them to abate on their own. This usually is not a recurrent problem but occasionally can repeat.[163]

Mitoxantrone (Novantrone, Immunex) is used to modify relapsing and secondary progressive MS. Mitoxantrone is the only drug approved for treatment of secondary progressive MS. It presumably works by depression of T-cell counts and removal of activated T cells from the immune repertoire. Because of potential side effects, its use is being limited at present to individuals whose MS is clearly advancing in spite of aggressive ABC therapy or who already are in a secondary progressive phase. The ABC drugs have not yet been found conclusively to be helpful in secondary progressive disease, and no drugs have been found effective in primary progressive disease.[226]

Natalizumab (Tysabri) is a monoclonal antibody that prevents immune cells from moving from the blood to the CNS. It was originally approved by the FDA based on a dramatic lowering of relapse rate and a 50% reduction in the development of a sustained increase in disability. This treatment is a once-monthly intravenous infusion.[189]

Fingolimod is an oral immunomodulating agent. Its final effect is also to reduce the normal circulation and trafficking of leukocytes. It also nears the 50% mark for decreasing the mean cumulative number of lesions also reduced the risk of disability progression.[130]

Dalfampridine (Ampyra) is a broad-spectrum potassium channel blocker, and is thought to enhance signal conduction in the nerves by blocking potassium leaks. Studies show increased walking speed in persons with MS after taking dalfampridine. History of seizure or kidney disease are both contraindications for this medication.[94]

Despite the time and effort given to slow the disease, the bulk of current intervention is devoted to symptomatic management. Improvement in the ability to control symptoms through therapy and medications can enhance quality of life in the individual with MS. Amantadine, pemoline, modafinil, and other medicines can reduce fatigue. Depression and sleep disorders may contribute to fatigue and must be recognized and treated appropriately. Centrally acting and peripherally acting muscle relaxants, such as baclofen (Lioresal), tizanidine, and dantrolene, decrease hypertonicity and leg spasms. Anticonvulsants and antidepressant medicines are used to treat pain. Intrathecal baclofen pumps reduce severe spasticity. Oxybutynin and tolterodine diminish bladder hyperactivity. Focal injections of Botox can be helpful in decreasing muscle spasticity.[1] Repetitive transcranial magnetic stimulation may improve spasticity in MS. The antiepileptic agents and antidepressant treatments often are effective in modulating the painful symptoms. Gabapentin in relatively high doses often is necessary for the desired effect. Spasms occurring during the day usually are handled best by the addition of the antiepileptic medications, including gabapentin and topiramate.

Amitriptyline is helpful, especially at night as it can sedate and provide pain relief. Clonazepam, given at bedtime, can aid in sleep initiation and decrease spasms with minimum side effects. Diazepam has a similar effect. Dose escalation should be avoided. Dopamine agonists and dopamine itself also decrease nocturnal spasms reasonably effectively at low dosages. All of these treatments require adjustment from time to time to maintain some relief. All medications currently available to control symptoms of MS have potential side effects and therefore must be used judiciously.[211]

Treatment of fatigue in MS has proved to be challenging. Modafinil is a popular and relatively safe drug, with the most common side effect being headache, and is considered first line for MS-related fatigue. Amantadine produced small but statistically significant improvements in fatigue related to energy level, concentration, problem solving, and sense of well-being. Given the strong coexistence of depression and fatigue in MS, treatment with antidepressants, such as selective serotonin reuptake inhibitors, monoamine oxidase inhibitors, tricyclic antidepressants, selective serotonin-norepinephrine reuptake inhibitors, and dopamine-norepinephrine reuptake inhibitors, is considered, although there are few systematic studies assessing their efficacy in MS-related fatigue as a separate symptom. Corticosteroids remain the first-line treatment of acute exacerbations. There is no consensus regarding optimal dosing; however, a regimen of 1000 mg intravenous (IV) methylprednisolone daily for 3 to 5 days is considered standard. It is typically thought that oral corticosteroids are equal in efficacy, but the key is that one must use high-dose steroids. There is now a consensus statement from the American Academy of Neurology regarding treatment of acute optic neuritis with methylprednisolone. Corticosteroids can alter almost every aspect of the immune system. Corticosteroid-induced restoration of the blood-brain barrier, which becomes less effective during active demyelination or plaque formation, has an antiedema benefit and may prevent circulating toxins, viruses, or immunoactive cells from entering the CNS. Decreased activity of the macrophages and lymphocytes results in less damage to the myelin in response to steroid therapy.[54] Individuals with severe demyelination who do not respond to corticosteroids may improve with plasma exchange.[132,257] Activated leukocyte cell adhesion molecule is involved in leukocyte migration across the blood-brain barrier, which is a key stage in MS pathogenesis. Observations suggest protective role against MS for both rs11559013GA and rs34926152GT genotypes in HLA-DRB1*1501–positive individuals.[254] Estriol treatment prevents neuropathologic alterations that occur in the hippocampus with the possibility of prevention of deficits in synaptic function and hippocampal neuropathology. The rationale for combination therapy in MS seems strong. Data from many preliminary studies lend support to the safety, tolerability, and efficacy of several combination regimens.[54] There are no FDA-approved therapies for primary progressive MS, and to date no study has shown clear benefit of disease-modifying therapies for this group of patients.[97]

PROGNOSIS. The average frequency of attacks of MS is approximately 1 per year. The attacks vary in severity; therefore close observation is required to reliably track the attack frequency. Attacks tend to be most common in the early years of MS and become less frequent in later years, regardless of the disability. The risk for rapid development of moderate disability may be greater in persons in whom the frequency of attacks is higher than average.

Multiple factors may predict a severe course, such as motor and cerebellar symptoms, disability after the first attack, and short time interval between attacks. Numerous relapses within the first year negatively influence the clinical course. Conversely, sensory symptoms, infrequent attacks, full neurologic recovery after a relapse, and a low level of disability after 5 to 7 years may be associated with an improved prognosis.

Burden of disease on MRI scans may be the strongest predictor of clinical outcomes. Over 14 years, there was no significant disability accrued in individuals with normal MRI findings at the time of diagnosis, whereas MRI scans with greater than 10 lesions predicted that individuals would require a cane for walking within that same time frame. A change in lesion load within the first year also is a negative predictor of outcome. Late-onset MS is not necessarily associated with a worse outcome.

Progression of primary progressive and relapsing MS differed little between late-onset and early adult-onset disease. The individuals with late-onset disease were older when reaching an Expanded Disability Status Scale score of 6.[241]

Because disability is often significant in individuals with MS, lifestyle changes are frequently necessary. Movement impairment is frequently associated with MS, and difficulty in walking is a major disability. If MS is untreated, 15 years after diagnosis 50% of individuals with MS will require the use of an assistive device to walk, and at 20 years 50% will be wheelchair bound. About one-fourth of persons with MS will require human assistance with activities of daily living.[131]

It is the coexistence of physical and cognitive impairments together with emotional and social issues in a disease with an uncertain course that makes MS rehabilitation unique and challenging. Individual rehabilitation improves functional independence but has only limited success in improving the level of neurologic impairment. Severely disabled people derive as much as or more benefit than those who are less disabled, but cognitive problems and ataxia tend to be refractory. Cost and utility are significantly correlated with functional capacity.[137] There is now good evidence that exercise can improve fitness and function for those with mild MS and helps to maintain function for those with moderate to severe disability. Several different forms of exercise have been investigated. For most individuals, aerobic exercise that incorporates a degree of balance training and socialization is most effective. Time constraints, access, impairment level, personal preferences, motivations, and funding sources influence the prescription for exercise and other components of rehabilitation. Just as immunomodulatory drugs must be taken on a continual basis and be adjusted as the disease progresses, so should rehabilitation be viewed as an ongoing process to maintain and restore maximum function and quality of life.[34]

Life expectancy is reduced by a modest amount in MS; the risk of dying of MS is strongly associated with severe disability. The death rate in persons who are unable to stand or walk is more than four times that in persons the same age without MS. In mildly disabled individuals, the death rate is approximately 1.5 times that of the age-matched population. Persons with more frequent initial episodes with rapidly developing disability have a poorer long-term outcome. Individuals with primary progressive disease also have decreased life expectancy. Suicide is more than seven times more common than in age-matched controls, and depression must be treated aggressively.

SPECIAL IMPLICATIONS FOR THE THERAPIST 31-5

Multiple Sclerosis

Because MS is typically progressive, it is expected that individuals will need to access the medical community with greater needs over time. Maintaining function in the household and community is a typical rehabilitation goal. Although people with MS are advised to be as active as possible in all ways of life, there is no consensus on the best method to attain that goal. Activity carried out in accordance with individual strength and abilities, avoiding exhaustion, will help to prevent or diminish the complications leading to disability. Skin breakdown following sensory loss and immobility is a common problem that can be controlled by appropriate skin care and positioning.

Fatigue and weakness are the complaints most often taken to a therapist. The Modified Fatigue Index is a self-report scale to monitor changes in the level of fatigue. This can be helpful for therapists to measure changes associated with interventions or to describe changes in function following a relapse.

The replacement of oral spasticity medications with intrathecal baclofen has become more routine, and the therapist should be involved in the dosing and management. Any spasticity the individual is using for activities of daily living may be altered. Thus, transferring techniques may require a different approach. The perception of strength that may be given by stiffness may disappear, giving the perception of weakness. Determining the appropriate muscle for use of Botox should also be done with the therapist who is most familiar with the individual's movement disorder and functional status.

In establishing a training program for endurance and strengthening, careful consideration of the neurologic changes is critical.[109] Careful monitoring of exercise appears to be necessary because of impaired cardiopulmonary systems. Individuals with MS have poor exercise tolerance as a result of respiratory muscle dysfunction.[78] Repetitive submaximal strength training appears to be of benefit to most people, with an increase in both peak torque generated and a decrease in the reported perception of fatigue.[153] Changes achieved in strength and endurance are probably the result of the normal physiologic changes that are associated with this type of training. Clients demonstrating increased reflex activity with exertion will need a longer time to recover after fatigue and may notice increased extensor tone and difficulty with flexion. Use of cooling vests to lower core temperature during exercise can be beneficial to those who have heat intolerance. It is important to realize that for most people with MS, fatigue will exacerbate symptoms.[45,161]

Nonpharmacologic measures for managing fatigue are more consistently beneficial in patients with MS-related fatigue. The cumulative evidence supports the theory that exercise training is associated with a small improvement in quality of life among individuals with MS.[22,107]

Understanding movement disorders common to lesions in specific brain regions and the spinal column is essential for the therapist. Analysis of movement is the most critical skill necessary to determine sensory and motor deficits that may be contributing to loss of postural control and mobility. The therapist must be able to identify the specific impairments to establish the appropriate stretching and strengthening exercises. A successful exercise program depends on a number of factors essential to motor learning, including practice, adequate feedback, and knowledge of results. The client with MS is often restricted in practice by neurologic fatigue and by impairments that disrupt sensory feedback, attention, memory, and motivation. The therapist will need to carefully identify the client's resources and abilities and capitalize on them to minimize the level of disability.[184,253] Establishing individually designed fitness programs is an important role of the physical therapist. Models for such programs can lead the therapist in the appropriate direction and provide protocols taking into consideration the common concerns associated with MS.[135,108]

The day-to-day variation in MS makes determination of an appropriate training program challenging. Use of both impairment and disability scales will assist in monitoring changes. The scales show the relative improvement after intervention or overall decline regardless of intervention. The scales are useful in tracking the disease process for both the client and the health care provider. Therapists making decisions regarding the need for adaptive equipment can use the scales to establish trends in the course of the disease. A common disability scale used by rehabilitation professionals and researchers working with patients with MS is the Kurtzke Expanded Disability Status Scale (Box 31-12). It is used to monitor changes in disability levels and has value in determining prognosis. Therapists working with this patient population should become adept at using this tool.[105] Anther scale in use is the Multiple Sclerosis Functional Composite (MSFC) a measure of disability progression which correlates with the Kurtzke Expanded Disability Status Scale, relapse rates, and SF-36 PCS; and is capable of demonstrating therapeutic effects in randomized, controlled clinical studies.[210]

Box 31-12

KURTZKE EXPANDED DISABILITY STATUS SCALE

0.0	Normal neurologic examination
1.0	No disability, minimal symptoms
1.5	No disability, minimal signs in more than one functional level
2.0	Slightly greater disability in one functional system
2.5	Slightly greater disability in two functional systems
3.0	Moderate disability in one functional system; fully ambulatory
3.5	Fully ambulatory but with moderate disability in one functional system and more than minimal disability in several others
4.0	Fully ambulatory without aid, self-sufficient, up and about 12 hr/day despite relatively severe disability; able to walk about 500 m without aid or rest

Continued

Box 31-12

KURTZKE EXPANDED DISABILITY STATUS SCALE—cont'd

4.5	Fully ambulatory without aid, up and about much of the day, able to work a full day; may otherwise have some limitation of full activity or require minimal assistance; characterized by relatively severe disability; able to walk about 300 m without aid or rest
5.0	Ambulatory for about 200 m without aid or rest; disability severe enough to impair full daily activities (e.g., to work a full day without special provisions)
5.5	Ambulatory for about 100 m without aid or rest; disability severe enough to preclude full daily activities
6.0	Intermittent or unilateral constant assistance (cane, crutch, brace) required to walk about 100 m with or without resting
6.5	Constant bilateral assistance (canes, crutches, braces) required to walk about 20 m without resting
7.0	Unable to walk beyond approximately 5 m with aid; essentially restricted to a wheelchair; wheels self in standard wheelchair and transfers alone; up and about in wheelchair 12 hr/day
7.5	Unable to take more than a few steps; restricted to wheelchair; may need aid in transfer; wheels self but cannot carry on in standard wheelchair a full day; may require motorized wheelchair
8.0	Essentially restricted to bed or chair or perambulated in wheelchair but may be out of bed itself much of the day; retains many self-care functions; generally has effective use of arms
8.5	Essentially restricted to bed much of the day; has some effective use of arm or arms; retains some self-care functions
9.0	Helpless bed patient; can communicate and eat
9.5	Totally helpless bed patient; unable to communicate effectively, eat, or swallow
10.0	Death from multiple sclerosis

Modified from Kurtzke J: Rating neurological impairment in multiple sclerosis: an expanded disability status scale (EDSS), *Neurology* 33:1444, 1983.

PARKINSONISM AND PARKINSON DISEASE

Overview and Definition

Atrophy of the brain leading to degeneration of neurons in the basal ganglia can be caused by a variety of disorders that are not well understood. These include multiple system atrophy, progressive supranuclear palsy, corticobasal ganglionic degeneration, and diffuse Lewy body disease. Parkinsonian features can be manifested as a part of other diseases affecting the CNS, such as atherosclerosis, ALS, and HD.[255]

Parkinson disease (PD), or idiopathic parkinsonism, is a chronic progressive disease of the of the CNS, characterized by rigidity, tremor, and bradykinesia and postural instability. The disease is thought to result from a complex interaction between multiple predisposing genes and environmental effects, although these interactions are still poorly understood. PD is still regarded as a sporadic neurodegenerative disorder, characterized by the loss of midbrain dopamine neurons and presence of Lewy body inclusions.

Incidence

PD, following AD, is the second-most common neurodegenerative disorder in the United States. Parkinsonism, including PD, affects more than 800,000 adults in the United States, with prevalence rates of 350 per 100,000 adults. Approximately 42% of parkinsonism is related to PD. The lifetime risk of developing parkinsonism is 7.5% according to a Mayo study. There appears to be a higher rate among white Americans and Europeans compared with black Africans. Black persons in America and Chinese in Taiwan have higher rates of the disease than their counterparts in West Africa or China.[20] PD becomes increasingly common with advancing age, affecting more than 1 person in every 100 older than age 75 years. A possible explanation of the correlation between age and prevalence may be the age-related neuronal vulnerability. Because of the increase in life expectancy, the aging of the baby boomers, and the precision of diagnosis, the incidence of PD is expected to rise. It is estimated that approximately 630,000 people in the United States were diagnosed with PD in 2010, with diagnosed prevalence likely to double by 2040. The national economic burden of PD exceeds $14.4 billion in 2010 (approximately $22,800 per patient).[140] The majority of cases begin between the ages of 50 and 79 years. Approximately 10% will develop initial symptoms before the age of 40 years.[145]

Etiologic and Risk Factors

An increasing number of chromosomal features linked to familial parkinsonism have been found, notably PARK1 to PARK11. Among these, seven genes have been identified, four causing autosomal dominant parkinsonism (*synuclein, UCHL1, NURR1, LRRK2*), which means one copy of an altered gene in each cell is sufficient to cause the disorder. In most cases, an affected person has one parent who has both the condition and three altered genes that cause autosomal recessive disease (*DJ1, PINK1, parkin*). This type of inheritance means that two copies of the gene in each cell are altered. Most often, the parents of an individual with autosomal recessive PD each carry one copy of the altered gene but do not show signs and symptoms of the disorder.[93] These provide insights into the molecular pathogenesis of the disease, but genetic testing for these mutations is of little clinical relevance. The chance of identifying parkin mutations is less than 5% in sporadic cases with onset at younger than 45 years. The probability is much greater in those with onset at younger than 30 years of age and in those with an affected sibling. Confirmation of this recessive form of disease might be helpful in genetic counseling, because it renders transmission to the subsequent generation very unlikely.[63] Given the late onset of typical PD, it is likely that by the time individuals become symptomatic, many first-degree relatives are deceased from other causes. Parkinson Progression Marker Initiative started in 2010 as a 5-year observational, international, multicenter study designed to identify PD progression biomarkers both to improve understanding of disease etiology and course and to provide crucial tools to enhance the likelihood of success of PD disease-modifying therapeutic trials.

Many potential exposures have been cited as possible risk factors for PD. Three major groups include toxic exposures, infection exposures, and a heterogenic group of miscellaneous exposures. Some toxic agents, such as carbon monoxide, manganese, cyanide, and methanol, can damage the basal ganglia and produce parkinsonian symptoms. A rapidly developing Parkinson-like disease has been linked to the use of MPTP (1-methyl-4-phenyl-1,2,3,6-tetrahydropyridine), a synthetic narcotic related to heroin. Some neuroleptics can produce a parkinsonian syndrome. In drug-induced parkinsonism, the symptoms can usually be reversed by withdrawal of the drug.

The link to infection exposure remains unresolved, despite years of study. There may still be a possibility that infection plays a role, based on observations of serum antibody titers for measles virus, rubella virus, herpes simplex virus types 1 and 2, and cytomegalovirus in persons with PD. Pesticides and herbicides may be environmental causes and are likely to produce between 2% and 25% increased risk. If some individuals are determined to be particularly susceptible to low environmental exposure, then pesticides may pose a more serious risk. In every age group, men are more likely than women to develop parkinsonism. This finding is not completely understood, but perhaps hormones may protect women, whereas men may be exposed to more environmental toxins according to their occupational choices. Long-term exposure to either manganese or copper has been linked to an increased incidence of parkinsonism.

More years of formal education appear to increase the risk of PD. Physicians are at significantly increased risk of PD when occupational data are used. By contrast, four occupational groups show a significantly decreased risk of PD according to one source: construction and extractive workers (miners, oil well drillers), production workers (machine operators, fabricators), metalworkers, and engineers.[91]

There is a relatively well-established relationship between PD and a history of smoking. Individuals with a history of smoking seem to have a lower risk of developing PD.

High levels of physical exercise may lower PD risk. The risk of PD appears to be lower among women who report strenuous exercise during early adulthood. Physical exercise can promote secretion of growth factors in the CNS that in turn may contribute to the survival and neuroplasticity of dopaminergic neurons. Moreover, exercise decreases the ratio between dopamine transporter and vesicular monoamine transporter; a decrease in this ratio may lower the susceptibility of dopaminergic neurons to neurotoxins and reduce dopamine oxidation. Finally, physical exercise may activate the dopaminergic system and increase dopamine availability in the striatum. Any of these or other mechanisms may be responsible for the beneficial effects of forced exercise in animal experiments. In the rat model of PD, forced exercise prior to chemically induced parkinsonism caused a significant increase of glial-derived neurotrophic factor that has neuroprotective effects for dopaminergic neurons.[47] Studies to determine if results found in animal studies are relevant to neuroprotective effects of physical exercise in human PD pathogenesis are ongoing.

Pathogenesis

Parkinsonian symptoms come primarily from dysfunction within the subcortical gray matter in the basal ganglia. Physiologic studies have shown the basal ganglia to be actively involved in almost all types of movement, including postural responses, alternating movements, and spontaneously occurring movements. The basal ganglia are active prior to recorded EMG activity in the muscles involved in a movement. Lesions do not produce paralysis or weakness, but rather change the character of movement, leading to loss of adaptive control, slowing of movement, and poor coordination. The motor loop that determines the initiation and scaling of motor activity derives its input from the premotor, motor, and somatosensory cortices. This is the process of preparation for forthcoming movement, and when disrupted it can cause a reduction in size and speed of the movement.

Basal ganglia–cerebral cortex interactions are disrupted by the abnormal function of the basal ganglia. This reflects a delay in motor programming related to the unconscious initiation of motor preparation, or lack of "response set" or readiness to move. The complex loop that includes the basal ganglia is involved in motivation and in planning global aspects of behavior.[143] The basal ganglia interact with the frontal cortex and with the limbic system, including the hippocampus and amygdala, and therefore have a role in cognitive and emotional function. The basal ganglia, in association with the frontal lobe, appear to play an important role in the integration of sensory information. It is now recognized that diffuse neuronal loss in the cerebral cortex may also contribute to changes observed in PD.

The basal ganglia are large subcortical structures that are interconnected and functionally interposed between the cortex and the thalamus. They also have direct connections to the limbic lobe, frontal cortex, and brainstem. It is likely that the fundamental principles that will be described here in relationship to the cortex–basal ganglia–thalamus–cortex system can also explain the disorders related to the connections between the basal ganglia and the frontal cortex, limbic lobe, and brainstem. The failure to facilitate desired behaviors and simultaneously inhibit unwanted behaviors may be responsible for the cognitive, emotional, and memory problems that coexist with movement disorders.

The signs and symptoms of parkinsonism are neurochemical in origin. The pathologic hallmark is the degeneration of a nucleus that is part of the basal ganglia, the substantia nigra. It loses its ability to produce dopamine, a neurotransmitter necessary to normal function of basal ganglia neurons. A depletion of 70% to 80% of the dopamine is estimated to occur before clinical signs of the disease are noted.[46,121] Initially, the system adapts, and there is increased efficiency in the pathways that depend on dopamine, but over time, as the dopamine depletion continues, function declines.

Abnormal protein breakdown, which may occur spontaneously or in relationship to a gene mutation, contributes to the neurodegeneration of PD. It appears that there are many possible triggers for the programmed cell death that results in mitochondrial dysfunction and oxidative stress. Despite significant research in this area, many observations are correlative in nature, and a precise process has not been identified. The inherited, early-onset forms of the disease may have a mutation that causes degradation of protein that may mimic the changes found in those individuals with sporadic, later-onset disorder. The changes in neurochemistry and protein are both consistent with aging. There is some overlap of degeneration that is similar to the processes seen in the dementias, including AD.

Free radical or oxidative stress appears to also have a role in the dysfunction of the basal ganglia.[24] Compared to the rest of the brain, the substantia nigra is exposed to higher levels of oxidative stress. Evidence of inflammation is typically found in the area of the substantia nigra pars compacta in conjunction with programmed cell death. It is proposed that neuroinflammation does not initiate PD but can promote progression and add to the worsening of symptoms. Recent animal study findings appear to support the "dying back" hypothesis of PD, which proposes that the tyrosine-hydroxylase-positive terminal loss in the striatum is the first neurodegenerative event in PD, which later induces neuronal degeneration in the substantia nigra.

Shedding Light on Early Parkinson's Disease Pathology

The motor pattern generators, thoughts and behaviors, and processes for memory are all initiated through the cerebral cortex. The parietal-occipital-temporal lobes, prefrontal areas, thalamic nuclei, limbic lobe, amygdala, and hippocampus use glutamate projections into the striatum (caudate and putamen). The input into the striatum comes in a topographic organization that is maintained to some degree throughout the basal ganglia.

Dopamine is produced in the substantia nigra pars compacta. Dopamine has more than one configuration, and the D_1 configuration either increases the efficiency or decreases the effect of cortical input to the striatum depending on the context of the desired movement. D_2 primarily decreases the effect of cortical input to the striatum. The striatum (caudate and putamen) has medium spiny neurons that project outside of the striatum. Dopamine input to the striatum terminates largely on the shafts of these dendritic spines and is able to modulate transmission from the cerebral cortex to the striatum. Cholinergic interneurons and GABA interneurons also synapse on these dendrites. Although there are fewer GABA interneurons, they have a powerful inhibitory effect. Through long-term potentiation and long-term depression, dopamine may be involved in the neural mechanism of habit learning. Depletion of dopamine in the striatum impairs the learning of new movement sequences.

D_1 dopamine goes from the striatum primarily to the internal globus pallidus and substantia nigra pars reticulata. (These two groups of neurons are functionally related and often grouped together.) The second population contains GABA and enkephalin and expresses D_2 dopamine receptors. These neurons project to the external globus pallidus. The external globus pallidus sends inhibitory input via GABA receptors to the internal globus pallidus.

The primary basal ganglia output comes from the internal globus pallidus, representing the body below the neck, and the substantia nigra pars reticulata, representing the head and eyes. The output is to the thalamus and, via several additional pathways, eventually to the brainstem and spinal cord. The output to the brainstem and spinal cord is through GABA neurotransmitters and is inhibitory.

There is another parallel circuit via the subthalamic nucleus. Excitatory input using glutamate via the hyperdirect pathway comes from the frontal lobe and motor areas and goes directly to the subthalamic nucleus, forming a somatotopic organization. There also appears to be a topographic separation of motor and cognitive inputs to the subthalamic nucleus. The output of the subthalamic nucleus is excitatory, using glutamate, and facilitates the external globus pallidus and the substantia nigra pars reticulata, producing a GABA inhibition to the thalamus.

The subthalamic nucleus also participates in a third or indirect pathway. This pathway involves signaling from the striatum (caudate and putamen) to the external globus pallidus to the subthalamic nucleus to the basal ganglia outputs.

The basal ganglia intrinsic circuitry is complex, with the direct pathway through the striatum (caudate and putamen) and a hyperdirect pathway through the subthalamic nucleus to the basal ganglia outputs. The hyperdirect pathway through the subthalamic nucleus is excitatory and fast, and the direct pathway through the striatum (caudate and putamen) is slower and inhibitory but more powerful.[168]

The cumulative inhibitory output of the basal ganglia acts as a brake on the motor pattern generators in the cerebral cortex and brainstem. The interaction among these pathways allows for a planned movement to be executed while competing movements are prevented, thereby increasing the precision of the movement without losing the power necessary to perform an activity. This is thought also to allow one part of a movement sequence to be activated in order for another sequence to begin. Through these mechanisms, movement and thought can be adapted quickly when the environment requires a different response.

When dopamine stimulation is decreased or withdrawn from the cycle, the overall effect is increased inhibition of input into the thalamus. The final effect of increased inhibition of the thalamus decreases the ability of the thalamus to send excitatory input back to the frontal cortex. So the ultimate outcome is less activity in the cortex, resulting in slowed movement and less power generated through the musculoskeletal system (Fig. 31-13).

These abnormal responses also influence the pathways to the brainstem that travel through the superior colliculus to the nucleus raphe magnus resulting in abnormal facial expression, blinking, and eye and eyelid movements. Although less clearly understood, abnormal firing or sequencing to the pedunculopontine tegmental nucleus can influence locomotion, sleep cycle regulation, attention, arousal, and startle.

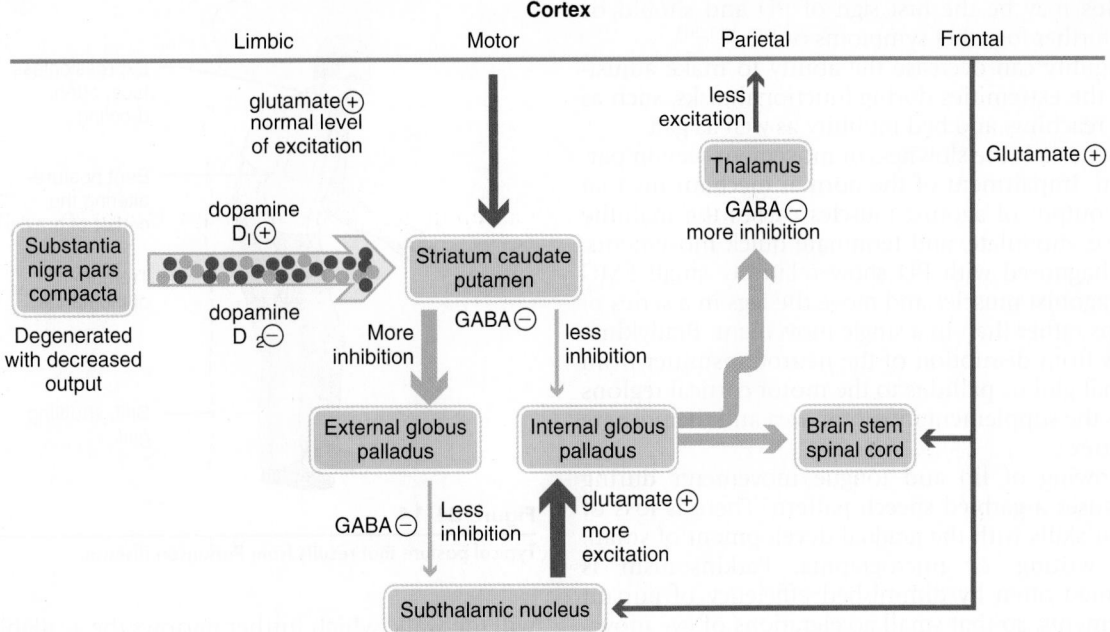

Figure 31-13

How the loss of dopamine production in the substantia nigra causes the eventual decrease in excitation of the cortex in the motor loop that involves the basal ganglia. Glutamate (positive transmission) is *red* and GABA (negative transmission) is *blue*. The decreased dopamine causes less than normal inhibition of the striatum (caudate/putamen), so there is more output to the internal globus pallidus. This output is inhibitory, so the cycle of inhibition is already started. Because the internal globus pallidus has been inhibited, there is less output, resulting in less inhibition of the subthalamic nucleus. This results in increased output of the subthalamic nucleus, this time causing more facilitation of the external globus pallidus. The increased output of the external globus pallidus, because it is inhibitory, causes greater inhibition of the thalamus, and the final end result is decreased excitation of the frontal or motor cortex. So the movement coming out of the cortex is less forceful than intended.

Note the other available pathway from the frontal cortex directly to the subthalamic nucleus. The subthalamic nucleus then facilitates the external globus pallidus, and the output of the external globus pallidus is inhibitory to the internal globus pallidus. The output of the internal globus pallidus is inhibitory to the thalamus as well as the brainstem and spinal cord. In this case, because of the double inhibition (sometimes referred to as disinhibition) the final output is excitatory. This pathway is not dependent on dopamine, but because it sends signals to the same nuclei that have already been affected by the decreases in dopamine, the system gets out of balance and the result is loss of normal modulation. Note also the pathway out of the basal ganglia to the brainstem and spinal cord.

Although the relationship of the substantia nigra and the striatum (caudate and putamen) are foremost in the disorder of parkinsonism, neuropathologic findings can be found in many other dopaminergic and nondopaminergic cell groups. The pathway responsible for postural stability may be affected outside of the basal ganglia.

Clinical Manifestations

Movement disorder is the hallmark of parkinsonism, although other symptoms are evident and may actually precede the impairment of movement. The ability to move is not lost, but there is a problem with movement activation and loss of reflexive or automatic movement. Movement becomes reliant on cortical control. The ability to perform known tasks, such as walking, changing direction, writing, and basic activities of daily living, is diminished. The considerable variation among individuals in the clinical manifestations and the level of deterioration in movement over time can be explained by the complex mechanism of dysfunction defined in "Pathogenesis" above.[68]

The tremor of PD, the most common initial manifestation, often appears unilaterally and may be confined to one upper limb for months or even years. It is first seen as a rhythmic, back-and-forth motion of the thumb and finger, referred to as the pill-rolling tremor. It is most obvious when the arm is at rest or during stressful periods. The tremor starts unilaterally but can eventually spread to all four limbs as well as neck and facial muscles. Tension or exertion will cause the tremor to increase, and it will disappear during sleep. Tremor does not usually impact the functioning of the individual.

Rigidity is an increased response to muscle stretch that appears in both antagonist and agonist muscle groups. Rigidity, like tremor, usually appears unilaterally and proximally in an upper limb and then spreads to the other extremities and trunk. One of the earliest signs of rigidity is the loss of associated movements of the arms when walking. Rigidity is identified when another person is trying to passively move the extremity and there is a jerky response (tremor under rigidity), known as cogwheel rigidity, or a slow and sustained resistance, known as lead-pipe rigidity. Rigidity does not appear to have a direct effect on volitional movement. Axial rigidity usually limits rotation and extension of the trunk and spine. Reduced variability and less adaptation of movement between thoracic rotation and pelvic motion appears early in the onset of PD. One of the most common musculoskeletal complaints is shoulder stiffness, sometimes diagnosed with frozen shoulder;

in fact, this may be the first sign of PD and should be screened further for other symptoms of PD.[133,203]

This rigidity can decrease the ability to make adjustments of the extremities during functional tasks, such as transfers, reaching, and bed mobility as well as gait.

Bradykinesia is the slowness of movement seen in parkinsonism. Impairment of the normal mechanisms that scale the output of agonist muscles causes the inability to produce, modulate, and terminate quick movements. Persons diagnosed with PD show relatively small EMG bursts in agonist muscles and move the legs in a series of small steps rather than in a single movement. Bradykinesia results from disruption of the neurotransmitter from the internal globus pallidus to the motor cortical regions known as the supplementary motor area and the primary motor cortex.

The slowing of lip and tongue movements during talking causes a garbled speech pattern. There is loss of fine motor skills with the gradual development of small, cramped writing, or micrographia. Parkinsonism is accompanied often by diminished efficiency of pursuit eye movements, so that small accelerations of eye movement (saccades) are required to catch up with a moving target, which causes smooth pursuit eye movements to be jerky instead of smooth. Eye movement in the vertical plane may be reduced.

Akinesia is a disorder of movement initiation and is seen in parkinsonism as a paucity of natural and automatic movements, such as crossing the legs or folding the arms. Hypokinesia refers to decreasing range and size of movement. Small gestures associated with expression are reduced. The face is mask-like, with infrequent blinking and lack of expression. Freezing, or gait akinesia, is the sudden cessation of movement in the middle of an action sequence, as if the foot is stuck to the floor. Sometimes it is the environment that seems to trigger freezing, such as when the individual walks through a doorway or over a change in surface like stepping from a carpet to a hard floor. Freezing most often affects walking turning, and dual-task performance is a common trigger.[221] It can also affect speech, arm movements, and blinking. Freezing is uncommon in the early phase but increases over time.[77,171] Research shows "reduced connectivity of the pedunculopontine nucleus with the cerebellum, thalamus and multiple regions of the frontal cortex. These results support the notion that freezing of gait is strongly related to structural deficits in the right hemisphere's locomotor network involving prefrontal cortical areas involved in executive inhibition function."[15,82]

The gait pattern in parkinsonism is highly stereotyped and characterized by impoverished movement with distinctive features of stooped posture, short shuffling steps, foot drags or "catches," arms swing less, difficulty initiating walking or turning and slowness. Range of motion in the joints of the lower extremity is often limited. Trunk, pelvic, and hip movements are diminished, resulting in a decreased step length and reciprocal arm swing. Increased left/right gait asymmetry and diminished bilateral coordination occurs with a loss of ability to produce a steady gait rhythm.[104]

The gait is narrow based and shuffling and the speed is decreased. Persons with plantar flexion contractures

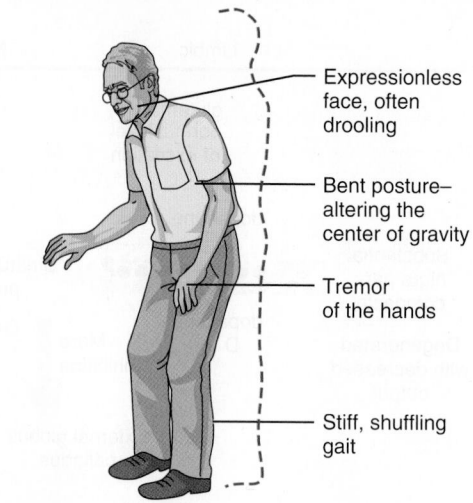

Figure 31-14

Typical posture that results from Parkinson disease.

will toe-walk, which further narrows the available base of support. In gait, there is a loss of heel strike, reduced toe elevation, reduced movement at the knee joints, loss of dynamic vertical force, reversal of ankle flexion–extension movement, and loss of backward-directed shear force.[199] Festination is common when attempting to stop or change direction; the stride becomes smaller but more rapid, and instead of stopping, the individual actually increases speed and is usually stopped by running into something or by falling. Preparatory postural responses to move from a bipedal to single-limb stance are frequently absent for induced steps, which may increase instability during first step.[205] There is reduced ability to adapt to changes of environments or to perform new tasks. Difficulty with "ambulation" is a "clinical red flag" that marks emerging disability.[178,222]

The posture in PD is characterized by flexion of the neck trunk, hips, and knees with elbows bent and arms adducted (Fig. 31-14). Other postural abnormalities include extreme neck flexion (antecoli), increased lateral flexion of the trunk (Pisa syndrome), or abnormal posture of the trunk in the anteroposterior plane with marked flexion of the thoracolumbar spine. Kyphosis, or extensive flexion of the spine, is the most common postural deformity. Scoliosis, an abnormal lateral curvature of the spine, can result from the unequal distribution of rigidity in posture.

Postural instability in people with PD is a result of impairments of multiple systems. Musculoskeletal constraints of persistent posturing of a forward head and trunk, decreased joint mobility, narrow foot stance, and axial rigidity tend to pull the center of gravity forward and reduce functional limits of stability especially in the backward direction. Central motor drive is impaired causing bradykinetic movements, poorly timed and scaled anticipatory postural adjustments. Feedforward control to stabilize posture before and during voluntary movements is compromised. Abnormal patterns of postural responses, including excessive antagonist activity, results in coactivation of distal and proximal muscles. Adapting to changing support conditions is less efficient in individuals with PD.[172] The ability to sequence motor activity appears to have an impact on postural correction. During posterior perturbations, lack of stability appears to be the result of lack of appropriate knee flexion.

Most people with PD experience weakness and fatigue once the disease becomes generalized. The person has difficulty sustaining activity and experiences increasing weakness and lethargy as the day progresses. Repetitive motor acts may start out strong but decrease in strength as the activity progresses. This compounds bradykinesia and increases immobility. Performing dual tasks causes more slowing in individuals who have parkinsonism. Smooth performance of sequential motor tasks is broken down into distinct components. The functions of the basal ganglia incorporate motor program selection and adaptation, which involves maintenance of coordination between body parts, task-specific adjustments of movement and quick shifts from one task to the next. Changing the "set" for an activity is more difficult for the individual with parkinsonism when the context or environment requires a sudden change in activity.

Nonmotor symptoms, such as those related to autonomic dysfunction, are common and potentially disabling manifestations of the disease. Loss of neurons in the sympathetic ganglia may cause autonomic dysfunction. This results in excessive sweating, excessive salivation, incontinence, and disabling orthostatic hypotension.[66] There is a greasy appearance to the skin of the face and occasional drooling because of loss of the swallowing movements that normally dispose of saliva. Olfactory dysfunction is an early sign of PD in most individuals, and overlaps with multiple system atrophy and progressive supranuclear palsy.

Rapid eye movement sleep behavior disorders result in lack of the normal muscle atonia and jerking of body and limbs causing disrupted sleep. Restless leg syndrome appears to be associated, mostly because of the similarities in treatment response. Abnormal sleep patterns may also contribute to the daily fatigue.

Fatigue is related to other nonmotor features such as depression and excessive daytime sleepiness. In more than half of the individuals, mental fatigue is persistent and seems to be an independent symptom that develops parallel to the progressive neurodegenerative disorder of PD.[7]

Dysfunction of the basal ganglia also influences sensory integration. The inability to distinguish self-movement from movement in the environment can contribute to abnormal balance reactions.[31] There is an increased dependence on visual information for motor control. There is strong visual dependency for balance, resulting in the inability to choose a balance strategy based on vestibular information even when the visual surround is unavailable for visual stability.[27] Box 31-13 outlines some of the contributions to imbalance seen in individuals with parkinsonism. Olfactory function is diminished, along with impaired color vision and visual perception.[246] Spatial organization is often disturbed, resulting in difficulty with orientation to the environment.

Pain syndromes and discomfort in PD usually arise from one of five causes: (1) a musculoskeletal problem related to poor posture, awkward mechanical function, or physical wear and tear; (2) nerve or root pain, often related to neck or back arthritis; (3) pain from dystonia,

---

Box 31-13

CAUSES OF BALANCE IMPAIRMENT IN PARKINSON DISEASE

- Loss of postural reflexes
- Visuospatial deficits
- Retropulsion
- Start hesitation
- Freezing
- Festinating gait
- Orthostatic hypotension
- True vertigo

---

the sustained twisting or posturing of a muscle group or body part; (4) discomfort caused by extreme restlessness; and (5) a rare pain syndrome known as "primary" or "central" pain, arising from the brain.[84]

Dementia and intellectual changes occur in almost 50% of persons with PD. Development of dementia is associated with more rapid progression of disability and potential for need for assisted living. Bradyphrenia, a slowing of thought processes, with lack of concentration and attention may also occur. Coexisting AD, organic brain disease, and vascular compromise may also contribute to the dementia.[192]

Depression is common and is probably related to the dopamine depletion. Loss of serotonin in the brainstem and limbic lobes has been found using PET studies. Behavioral changes, such as apathy, lack of ambition, indecisiveness, and anhedonia, are common and may be related to depression. Depressive episodes or panic attacks can precede onset of motor symptoms.

Although reduced motor activity by itself would not seem to be a functional disorder, many of the small automatic muscular adjustments are important for successfully carrying out functional activities. For example, in attempting to rise from a chair a person may fail to make the small initial adjustments of legs that are crucial to standing up and fail to be able to get from sitting to standing without assist.

The person with PD typically becomes deconditioned. Rapid heart rate and difficulty breathing are common. Vital capacity is reduced as the kyphosis increases and the intercostal muscles develop rigidity.[195] Respiratory complications are the leading cause of death. The Hoehn and Yahr classification (Table 31-6) is a common scale used to define the level of disability associated with PD.

MEDICAL MANAGEMENT

DIAGNOSIS. There is no single blood or imaging test that can definitively diagnose PD. In most cases, the diagnosis is made on the basis of the classic triad of signs (tremor, rigidity, and akinesia), a typical medical history, and characteristic findings on physical examination.[238] The combination of asymmetry of symptoms and signs, the presence of a resting tremor, and a good response to levodopa best differentiates PD from parkinsonism as a result of other causes. Diagnostic problems may occur in mild cases. Other movement disorders that do not fall under the category of parkinsonism need to be

Table 31-6	Hoehn and Yahr Classification of Disability

Stage	Character of Disability
I	Minimal or absent; unilateral if present
II	Minimal bilateral or midline involvement; balance not impaired
III	Impaired righting reflexes; unsteadiness when turning or rising from chair; some activities restricted but patient can live independently and continue some forms of employment
IV	All symptoms present and severe; standing and walking possible only with assistance
V	Confined to bed or wheelchair

Modified from Hoehn MM, Yahr MD: Parkinsonism: onset, progression and mortality, *Neurology* 17:427, 1967.

recognized by clinicians to establish a differential diagnosis. Box 31-14 lists features of parkinsonism as a result of causes other than PD.

Depression, with its associated expressionless face, poorly modulated voice, and reduction in voluntary activity, may be difficult to distinguish from mild parkinsonism. Olfaction is frequently impaired in PD, suggesting that deficiencies in smell may be a potentially useful test to distinguish PD from related disorders.

CT or MRI is not helpful in diagnosis of PD but can identify other causes of symptoms, such as Wilson disease, or mass effects causing disruption of the basal ganglia function, such as stroke or hydrocephalus. In 2011, the United States Food and Drug Administration approved the use of DaTSCAN for detecting images of the level of dopamine transporters in the brains of people with suspected parkinsonian syndromes. DaTSCAN binds to the presynaptic dopamine active transporter (DAT) on neurons that communicate with areas controlling movement, including the striatum. The DaTSCAN SPECT is most helpful in differentiating between PD and essential tremor, drug-induced parkinsonism, and psychogenic parkinsonism. It is not able to differentiate between PD, progressive supranuclear palsy, multiple systems atrophy and other neurodegenerative diseases affecting the dopamine neurons in the brain. For the classic motor symptoms of PD to be present, typically 50% or more of these neurons must be lost. DaTSCAN is able to detect this decreased activity early in the course of PD, when the diagnosis may still be uncertain. Neither DaTSCAN nor a doctor's examination is a perfect (gold standard) method for diagnosing PD. Both methods will occasionally miss actual cases of PD, while misdiagnosing other diseases that resemble PD.[62] Only an autopsy can conclusively determine whether a person's brain exhibits PD pathology.

Functional imaging through PET is highly sensitive to regional changes in brain metabolism and receptor binding associated with movement disorders. SPECT shows differences in the posterior putamen, contralateral to the predominantly affected limb. Asymmetric scan findings have been observed in individuals with mild, newly recognized symptoms. Unilateral disease produces a significant difference in striatal uptake between the ipsilateral and contralateral sides in both the caudate and putamen

Box 31-14
PARKINSONISM VERSUS PARKINSON DISEASE

Multisystem Atrophy: Striatonigral Degeneration, Sporadic Olivopontocerebellar Atrophy, Shy-Drager Syndrome

- Orthostatic hypotension, sexual impotence, bladder dysfunction
- Cerebellar dysfunction
- Myoclonus of face and hands
- Neck flexion
- Mottled, cold hands
- Dysarthria
- Good response to levodopa initially for a small percentage; dyskinesia and cranial dystonia associated with use of levodopa

Progressive Supranuclear Palsy

- Vertical ophthalmoplegia
- Oculomotor dysfunction
- Axial rigidity greater than limb rigidity
- Early falls
- Speech and swallowing disturbances
- Cognitive or behavioral changes
- Hypertension
- Poor response to levodopa

Corticobasal Degeneration

- Apraxia, cortical sensory changes, alien limb phenomenon
- Asymmetric rigidity
- Limb dystonia
- Myoclonus
- Negligible response to levodopa

Vascular Parkinsonism

- Dysfunction in lower extremities
- Gait disturbances
- Additional focal signs of midbrain lesion
- Poor response to levodopa

Dementia with Lewy Bodies

- Early dementia
- Rigidity more prominent than bradykinesia or tremor
- Hallucination
- Fluctuating cognitive status
- Falls
- Motor features may respond to levodopa but with psychiatric side effects

Modified from Lang AE, Lozano AM: Parkinson's disease, *N Engl J Med* 339(15):1044–1053, 1998.

nuclei. One explanation is that there is a preceding unequal functional reactivity of the basal ganglia, which results in an asymmetrical clinical response.

Altropane (a close cousin of cocaine), a component of radioactive technetium-99m, is a compound that can measure the concentration of dopamine transporters imaged by SPECT. This may lead to diagnosis of PD based on identifying decreasing levels in the brains of persons when only mild symptoms appear.

Assessing progression of PD using clinical rating scales such as the United Parkinson's Disease Rating Scale is a common way to track progression. However, the progression may be masked by medication, and because of the multitude of symptoms that may change at different rates, it is hard to determine a change in the course of the disease.

TREATMENT. Overall, the treatment is to preserve a patient's independence and quality of life. The current therapeutic approach to PD is symptomatic; major studies to determine possible therapeutic neuroprotection are still being researched, but no single intervention has proven to be disease modifying. Drug therapy is adapted to the person's needs, which may vary with the stage of the disease and the predominant manifestations.[9] When mobility becomes affected to the degree that walking and self-care activities become difficult, medications improve the control of movement. As the disease progresses over time, the effectiveness of medication changes, leaving the individual with a shorter "on" time during which symptoms are reduced and more rigidity during "off" times when symptoms are active. Long-term use of medication can also increase the dyskinesia or chorea-like movement resulting from the change in activity in the basal ganglia. Side effects can become more problematic as the dosages needed to control symptoms are increased. The management of these medications becomes the focus of intervention.[78]

Levodopa (L-dopa), which is taken up by remaining dopaminergic neurons in the basal ganglia and converted to dopamine, improves most of the major features of parkinsonism, including tremor, rigidity, bradykinesia and walking problems. Initially it leads to nearly complete reversal of symptoms, with effects lasting up to 2 weeks, known as long-duration levodopa response. As the disease progresses, the length of the effect becomes shorter, it takes longer for the effect to be noticed after dosing, and symptoms increase during the end of the dose period. Eventually there is dose failure or lack of any effect at all. Levodopa can cause dyskinesias that produce chorea, athetosis, dystonia, tics, and myoclonus. Predictable fluctuations include a wearing-off effect and early-morning akinesia. The duration of effect of each dose becomes shorter and will often match the drug's half-life of less than 2 hours. Although levodopa is the most effective drug for PD, the time to start taking it is controversial. Early use may contribute to greater activity levels and employability but cause more disability at later stages when the effect fluctuates and ultimately decreases. Protein in food uses the same mechanism as levodopa for crossing the blood-brain barrier. When levodopa is given with protein, the protein blocks the ability of the levodopa to cross the blood-brain barrier. This is usually managed by having the individual eat most of the daily protein in the evening, when immobility will cause the least inconvenience. Caffeine administered before levodopa may improve its pharmacokinetics in some individuals with parkinsonian symptoms.[44] Infusion of levodopa directly into the intestines gives a more stable response but is expensive and invasive. Levodopa should be avoided in persons with malignant melanoma and in persons with active peptic ulcers, which may bleed.

Carbidopa (Sinemet) inhibits the breakdown of levodopa and is often used in combination with levodopa. Carbidopa reduces the amount of levodopa required daily for beneficial effects and is often combined with levodopa in a single preparation (Sinemet).

Catechol-O-methyl transferase (COMT) inhibitors slow the breakdown of dopamine in the body. Of these, entacapone (Comtan) and tolcapone (Tasmar) reduce the off time, and allow for decreased dosing of levodopa.[185] Liver function must be monitored regularly with the use of tolcapone. Tolcapone must be used with levodopa but can decrease the amount of levodopa needed. A combination pill called Stalevo combines carbidopa/levodopa and entacapone.

Dopamine agonists act directly on dopamine receptors. Bromocriptine (Parlodel) seems to be the best tolerated, and its use in parkinsonism is associated with a lower incidence of response fluctuations. It is often given in combination with levodopa and carbidopa. Pramipexole (Mirapex) or ropinirole (Requip) can be used either to delay starting levodopa or to decrease the amount needed. Transdermal application of dopamine agonists can be provided with rotigotine (Neupro Patch) and lisuride. Apomorphine (Apokyn) is injected under the skin to provide quick action, typically 20 minutes, and is used for rescue treatment when wearing off is abrupt or unpredictable. One possible adverse effect of dopamine agonists is sedation, sleep attacks and the occurrence of drug-induced compulsive behaviors (shopping, gambling, eating, hypersexuality).

Monoamine oxidase type B (MAO-B) inhibitors (Selegiline (Eldepryl) and rasagiline (Azilect)) block the effect of the enzyme MAO-B that naturally breaks down several chemicals in our brain, including dopamine allowing more dopamine to be available. These inhibitors are usually used early in treatment when symptoms are mild and can be added when problems with wearing off occur and symptoms return between medication doses. Research has shown the neuroprotective functions of rasagiline and selegiline with an increase in glial-derived neurotrophic factor and brain-derived neurotrophic factor.[48,176]

Persons with mild symptoms but no disability may be helped by amantadine. Amantadine (Symmetrel) is the only medication that can reduce dyskinesia that develops later in the course of the disease. Coadministration of levodopa and amantadine controls dyskinesia without disrupting the effect of levodopa.

In the striatum the low level of dopamine is accompanied by increased cholinergic transmission. Anticholinergic drugs help reduce rest tremor only and are not used to treat other motor symptoms. The side effects of the anticholinergic medications, including sedation, confusion, and psychosis, limit their usefulness, especially with advancing age. MAO-B inhibitors have replaced the use of anticholinergics in treatment of PD.[43]

Antioxidants have been studied for neuroprotection, such as coenzyme Q10, which helps stabilize mitochondria and appears to decrease the worsening of symptoms. Trophic factors, antiinflammatories, antiapoptotics, and antioxidants have been identified by the National Institutes of Health for further study for control of neuronal death.

Deep brain stimulation uses a pacemaker-like device surgically implanted with electrodes in the nuclei of choice and a pulse generator implanted in the chest. The generator is controlled externally through a magnetic field. Stimulation through the electrodes can be applied to the internal globus pallidus and the subthalamic nucleus or thalamus. Thalamic stimulation is most effective for tremor, with less effect on dyskinesia and rigidity. Electrode implantation in the globus pallidus appears to have good initial effect; however, there is a chance of psychosis and punding activity over time. Most centers are now stimulating the subthalamic nucleus bilaterally, but the individual's profile leads the decision. Although the picture is not yet clear on the issue of target choice, the subthalamic nucleus does seem to provide more medication reduction, whereas globus pallidus may be slightly safer for language and cognition. Preoperative response to levodopa predicts better outcome after deep brain stimulation of the subthalamic nucleus. Stimulation can increase on time and decrease off time, as well as the severity of the off periods. Dyskinesia typically improves over time, either as a result in medication reduction or as an effect of stimulation. The ability to perform activities of daily living is improved, and there is typically improved sleep time. Apathy and abulia can occur over time; this may be related to withdrawal of levodopa. There can be an increase in sadness or the opposite response with excessive hilarity that may be related to stimulation of the surrounding area or change in subthalamic limbic activity. Edema around the electrode may contribute to the psychotropic effects. The implant is thought to last approximately 5 years and can be removed if another more effective type of treatment is found.[14] Bilateral subthalamic stimulation, alone or in combination with levodopa, causes improvement in axial signs for posture and postural stability.

Although there is little evidence for drug effect on postural stability and gait disorders, researchers in motor control are making progress in identifying the nature of the abnormal responses both inside and outside of the basal ganglia.[217] See "Special Implications for the Therapist 31-6: Parkinson's Disease" below. Based on the strong evidence that relates prior exercise and activity status to risk of PD, and the recent knowledge gained about neuroplasticity in the brain, it is likely that changes in postural control may come through interventions that drive neuroplastic changes.

Although orthostatic hypotension affects less than 20% of individuals with parkinsonism, it can limit activity. Use of midodrine (Proamatine), fludrocortisone (Florinef), and pyridostigmine (Mestinon) can be helpful in maintaining normal blood pressure. Supine hypertension may result and must be monitored. Urinary dysfunction is treated via antimuscarinic agents or α-agonists. Anticholinergics or scopolamine patches may be helpful for drooling, and use of intraparotid injection of botulinum toxin-A can help. Constipation is common and may precede the motor symptoms in PD; it is usually managed by fluids, fiber, stool softeners and exercise.

Depression is found in more than 40% of individuals with PD. Medication interactions must be looked at carefully. Use of serotonin uptake inhibitors may interact with selegiline. Tricyclics can be useful, but the central effects must be monitored more carefully than in the healthy younger population.

Respiratory complications, which are the leading cause of death, can be prevented to some extent with an early aggressive aerobic exercise program, followed by regular moderate activity as the disease progresses. Control of breathing can be facilitated using verbal and tactile stimuli and should be integrated into any intervention.

Behavioral abnormalities can be associated with high doses of dopaminergic replacement therapy, including the phenomenon of punding, characterized by fascination with technical equipment and excessive sorting of objects, grooming, hoarding, or use of a computer. This may be related to the impaired frontal lobe function and a result of psychomotor stimulation. Other abnormalities in reward-seeking behavior related to dopamine are hypersexuality and excessive gambling. Reducing the level of medication is helpful, and some neuroleptics such as clozapine will lessen symptoms of psychosis.

Experimental therapeutics targeted at improving dopaminergic drugs to increase selectivity for various receptor subtypes and at controlling the uptake of dopamine are currently under study. Improved plasma stability is achieved through transdermal application, which bypasses the fluctuations in gastric release. Studies are aimed at potential substances that evoke antiparkinsonism through neurotransmitter systems outside of dopamine.[2] Pharmacologic manipulation of glutamate and GABA neurotransmission includes the drug istradefylline, which completed phase III trials. In Japan, istradefylline is approved to use in the adjunctive treatment of PD, but is still not an FDA approved drug in United States.[206] Opiate, serotonin, and histamine receptors are possible sites for intervention. A more careful look at the cholinergic system may help to manage the issues of dementia and find possibilities for reducing the apparent dysfunction at the level of the brainstem that affects sleep wake cycles and orthostasis. Clinical study of the drug droxidopa in patients with neurogenic orthostatic hypotension is in phase 3. Droxidopa augments norepinephrine levels, which should lead to improved cerebral perfusion following orthostatic challenge thereby reducing rapid drop in blood pressure and symptoms of dizziness, fainting and falls.[50,216]

Tozadenant as an adjunct to levodopa experienced significant reductions in off-time without worsening dyskinesia, compared with those on placebo. Tozadenant is an oral, selective adenosine 2α receptor antagonist. It is currently in phase 2 studies.

Cell transplantation of grafted dopaminergic neurons in PD continues to hold promise. The striatum (caudate and putamen) are primary targets for the implants.[103,242]

PROGNOSIS. In general, all the clinical manifestations in PD worsen progressively, although not to the same extent. Tremor as a presenting symptom may be used to predict a more benign course and longer therapeutic benefit to levodopa. In individuals with newly diagnosed PD, older age at onset and rigidity/hypokinesia as an initial symptom can be used to predict more rapid rate of motor progression.[230]

The presence of associated comorbidities, stroke, auditory deficits, and visual impairments as well as male sex may be used to predict faster rate of motor progression. Older age at onset and initial hypokinesia/rigidity may be used to predict earlier development of cognitive decline and dementia. Older age at onset, dementia, and decreased dopamine responsiveness may be used to predict earlier nursing home placement as well as decreased survival. Lack of mobility, loss of balance reactions, and weakness result in more falls than in an age-matched normal population. Osteoporosis can result from prolonged inactivity and may be present secondary to advanced age at onset. Falls more often lead to fractures owing to the prevalence of osteoporosis. Fracture healing may be delayed. Posture and gait abnormalities are the most difficult to control in advanced cases.

PD does not significantly reduce life span in most persons who develop the generalized form between 50 and 60 years of age. However, because there is progressive neuronal loss despite the response to treatment, deterioration continues until death occurs, often from infection or other conditions associated with debilitation.

As the onset of disease is typically in the fifth or sixth decade of life and is progressive despite medication, the economic cost of the disease can be quite high because of loss of income, cost of drugs, assistive devices, and assisted living. Pain, fatigue, and depression also adversely affect the quality of life compared with that of age-matched normal subjects.[214]

| SPECIAL IMPLICATIONS FOR THE THERAPIST | 31-6 |

Parkinson Disease

There are clearly various and separate components of the movement disorders related to parkinsonism, especially in PD. As we become better able to identify the relationship between specific impairment and the resulting function, intervention by the therapist will have more impact on ability to participate in typical activities. Each individual's needs and goals must be addressed and programs modified as the movement disorders change as the disease progresses.[34,60,64,202] Skills are learned most effectively when they are practiced repeatedly in relation to meaningful goals. The benefits of exercise are well established for people with PD, but long-term compliance is limited. Research is now studying how to promote increased activity/exercise/walking in the community. The use of community-based wellness exercise classes, a virtual exercise coach, pedometers, and tandem bikes are all being explored.[76]

Of course we understand the benefits of exercise "use it or lose it" theory, but educating and improving our patient's confidence is important for them to adhere to a program and make life long changes in exercise and physical activity habits. Low outcome expectation from exercise, lack of time to exercise, and fear of falling appear to be important perceived barriers to engaging in exercise in people who have PD, are ambulatory, and dwell in the community. These may be important issues for physical therapists to target in people who have PD and do not exercise regularly.[75]

Following the World Health Organization in the International Classification of Functioning, Disability,

and Health (ICF) model intervention should address all of the ICF categories: body structure and function (directly related to PD: tremor, bradykinesia, rigidity, akinesia, postural instability; indirectly related to PD: decreased flexibility decreased endurance), activity (gait, transfers, bed mobility) and participation (ability to work, interact socially self-care, recreational sports, quality of life). Environmental factors (home and community settings) and personal factors (resources, personal attitudes, self-efficacy, emotions and feelings) all need to be considered. In addition understanding the timing and effects of their medication and collaborating with the multidisciplinary team will optimize the benefits of your treatment plan. The elements of repetition, intensity, and challenge together with skilled training will lead to improved goal directed motor skill learning.

Exercises to Address Rigidity

Spinal flexibility or axial mobility contributes to function. It can impact ability to perform many of the components of tasks, including functional reach, movement in bed and turning while walking. Exercises should minimize co-contraction, promote axial rotation, lengthen the flexor muscles, strengthen the extensor muscles, promote erect posture and teach relaxation strategies.[18,214]

Exercises to Address Bradykinesia

Bradykinesia is associated with slow and weak postural responses to perturbations and anticipatory adjustments. Slowed rate of muscle activation patterns occurs. "Because bradykinesia is due to impaired central neural drive, rehabilitation to reduce bradykinesia should focus on teaching patients to increase speed, amplitude and temporal pacing of their self-initiated and reactive limb and body center of mass movements.[134]

Exercises to Improve Balance/Postural Stability

More research is now looking at how balance control relies on the interaction of several physiological systems (the musculoskeletal, neuromuscular, cognitive, sensory systems) with environmental factors and the performed task. Exercises need to improve sensory integration of the vestibular and somatosensory system and decrease visual dependency, improve timing and amplitude, and task specific adaptation. Whole-body coordination, the ability to shift between different tasks and control center of mass and base of support to increase functional limits of stability should be a part of the exercise regimen in those with fall risk. Each component of balance needs to be progressed in difficulty and complexity.[52] Tai Chi, tango dancing, and boxing have all shown improvements in postural stability.[51,55,98,99,152]

Exercises to Improve Gait

The use of external cues is effective in replacing the absent internal control that disturbs automatic and repetitive movements and allow movement to be directly controlled by cortical control. The use of rhythmic auditory stimulation in persons with PD leads to an increase in gait velocity, cadence, and stride length associated with an increase in the EMG activity around the ankle.[234] Complexity of task appears to be related to gait. Individuals with moderate disability associated with PD experience considerable difficulty when they are required to walk while attending to complex visuomotor tasks involving the upper limbs.[26] Visual cueing for improved gait appears to have the most effect on stride length and decreases time spent in double stance during walking. Walking speed, arm swing amplitude, and step length can be increased by verbal instructional sets, using cognitive strategies.[12] Many studies support the benefits of treadmill training to improve gait speed, stride length, walking distance and quality of life. Treadmill training offers opportunity for a lot of practice, high number of reps may facilitate retention, external cue to provide rhythmic and somatosensory feedback, used with external cues (auditory) paired with attentional strategy maximizes benefits.[44,90,110,111]

Gait training strategies and goals will vary according the progression of the disease.[171]

Managing the home environment is critical, as most falls occur at home. The training of a caregiver to give the appropriate verbal and visual cues can be beneficial.[119] Use of grab bars can be valuable, especially if there is a bathtub, since stepping over the edge requires significant weight shift. Recognizing areas that may induce freezing (doorways, narrow spaces) may decrease the fall risk in those areas. Keeping a diary of falls can be helpful. Strategies mentioned earlier can work by means of bypassing the basal ganglia and making use of the supplementary motor area. External feedback can be effective in improving movement when it cannot be controlled from internal organization. Use of virtual reality has been shown to be effective in persons with parkinsonism. Until the time that it is readily available, techniques employed by persons with PD to trigger movement or to "unfreeze" are used by most individuals with PD. Parkinsonian syndromes studies are limited but are starting to be researched more than case studies. Findings support the use of balance and eye movement exercises to improve gaze control in progressive supranuclear palsy.[263]

Nonmotor symptoms may have an effect on therapy. Anxiety, apathy and/or depression can cause low energy, fear, poor motivation, poor compliance. Cognitive impairment may impact the ability of individuals with PD to learn new motor skills and/or answer questions.[17,114] Pathways leading to and from the frontal cortex, limbic lobe, and hippocampus are affected in PD. Learning strategies and environments that best eliminate stress need to be identified. Decreased attention (shifting or selecting and decreased concentration (increased distractibility) may need a quiet environment, redirection, simple commands and repetition. Decreased executive functioning may decrease problem solving, poor self-analysis and self-correction. Decreased organizational ability may need lists, reminders, timers, simplification. Decreased multi- or dual-tasking may need to

begin with one task at a time before adding increased cognitive and motor loads. Sleep disturbances may cause fatigue and/or low energy. Bladder urgency and frequency may shift focus from task at hand. Orthostatic hypotension may cause dizziness, unsteadiness and/or falls. Pain or paresthesia may limit activity level, and cause fear. Dyskinesia may increase instability and safety and compensatory techniques may need to be taught. Medication side effects may impact the client's ability to participate in therapy, modifications may be necessary if the medication level drops during the session. Caregivers can be trained to assist in mobility during "off" periods.

Intervention strategies have been established and can be used to establish programs. Clinical trials with randomized approaches are under way to provide evidence of interventions addressing the movement disorders discussed here. This will assist therapists the most when the components studied can be extrapolated into functional tasks.

Disease-modifying aspects of exercise shows strong promise. Future research may look at the complexity of the motor skills and degree of protection. With evidence for exercise benefit within this population, it should also be recognized by the therapist that submaximal responses to exercise testing occur in PD, with higher heart rate and increased oxygen consumption.[126]

Secondary Parkinson Syndrome

Parkinsonian syndromes, also called *atypical parkinsonism* or *Parkinson plus syndromes*, are a family of neurodegenerative disorders that result from neuronal loss in different components of the basal ganglia, the brain system of which the dopaminergic midbrain neurons affected in PD are a part. All of these disorders can be difficult to differentiate from PD early in the course of the illness. These disorders have distinctive clinical features, which may emerge only after the onset of parkinsonism. Important clinical clues that one of these disorders is present are symmetric onset of parkinsonism, absence of typical resting tremor, early autonomic dysfunction, prominent dystonia, significant early cognitive impairment, and prominent early falls.[6]

Iatrogenic parkinsonism or drug-induced parkinsonism results from the use of pharmacologic agents that block dopamine effects or interfere with dopamine metabolism. The most common causes of drug-induced parkinsonism are dopamine antagonist antipsychotic medications. The risk of drug-induced parkinsonism is reduced significantly with newer atypical antipsychotic agents. Another group of drugs that can cause drug-induced parkinsonism is older (non–serotonin antagonist) dopamine antagonist antiemetics. Agents interfering with dopamine production or synaptic vesicular storage can cause drug-induced parkinsonism. These include methyl-para-tyrosine, methyldopa, and reserpine. Flunarizine and cinnarizine, when they are used as vestibular suppressants or cerebral vasodilators, can cause parkinsonism. Sodium valproate may cause tremor that can progress to parkinsonism. Features of iatrogenic parkinsonism are bilateral onset and predominant bradykinesia with increased involvement in the arm compared to the legs in the younger population, but more consistent with PD in older individuals. If drug-induced parkinsonism is suspected, the suspected offending agent is withdrawn, and the individual should improve. With dopamine antagonists or reserpine, improvements can occur within days to weeks after medication withdrawal, but there is sometimes a prolonged latency of months before marked improvement occurs.

Vascular parkinsonism involves primarily the lower extremities. It is associated with lacunar infarcts (see Chapter 32) and probably represents small infarcts in the basal ganglia or corticobasilar pathways. A stroke in the region of the striatum (caudate and putamen) and hemiparesis of the arm is common. Systemic lupus erythematosus may also cause cerebral vasculitis. Vascular parkinsonism presents typically with start hesitation, a broad-based shuffling gait (rather than the narrow-based gait associated with PD), and frequent falls. Depending on the level of damage and the cause, the response to levodopa will vary.

Infectious causes of parkinsonism are suspected when the symptoms develop during the acute or recovery phase of an illness with fever. Cases of parkinsonism have been reported as a result of West Nile virus infection and have historically been associated with encephalitis. Human immunodeficiency virus (HIV) infection can cause parkinsonism via the viral damage in encephalopathy or opportunistic infections.

Toxicity, often related to manganese accumulation in the substantia nigra, can cause parkinsonism and dystonia, seen in miners, factory workers making dry cell batteries, and those exposed to some fungicides.

Disorders with Parkinsonian Characteristics

Benign Essential Tremor

Benign essential tremor is not associated with any underlying cause, is common after the age of 50 years, and is usually hereditary. This tremor is of a different character, and there is a lack of other neurologic signs.

Progressive Supranuclear Palsy

Progressive supranuclear palsy has symptoms of bradykinesia, rigidity, and postural instability similar to those of PD and is frequently misdiagnosed as PD. Neurofibrillary tangles are the main pathology in progressive supranuclear palsy; oligodendrocytes are also affected. Postural instability is the most pronounced symptom, with early falls that are not associated with obstacles or change in surface. Motor recklessness may occur, getting abruptly out of a chair. There is usually lack of tremor, progressive onset of symmetric symptoms, gait freezing and apraxia. Dysarthria and dysphagia are on a continuum, with dysphagia typically occurring later than 2 years after onset. Loss of upward gaze, saccades, and smooth pursuit eye tracking progresses over time. Inhibition of eyelid opening and closure, or blepharospasm, can cause functional blindness. Inability to perform vestibuloocular reflex cancellation is lost. Apathy, intellectual slowing, and impairment of executive function progress, and there can be pseudobulbar features (emotional lability, dysarthria, dysphagia). The autonomic nervous system maintains near-normal function.

Levodopa and deep brain stimulation are effective for the movement disorder, and Botox can help to improve blepharospasm.

Multiple System Atrophy

There is extreme clinical variability within the multiple system atrophy group of disorders that is primarily familial but can be sporadic. Neuronal atrophy is seen to a variable degree in the brainstem, cerebellum, spinal cord, and peripheral nerves. The differential pathology is associated with gliosis and cytoplasmic inclusion in the glia. Multiple system atrophy (MSA) typically has its onset in the fifth to seventh decade, and parkinsonism is the primary condition; however, there is more evidence of cerebellar involvement, and autonomic dysfunction is greater and more disabling than that found in PD. Levodopa is used in the treatment, but with less success than when it is used in PD. Cerebellar and autonomic nervous system dysfunction respond poorly to anticholinergics. Large European studies are underway to examine pathogenesis and intervention strategies. There are different types of MSA. MSA-A, sometimes called Shy-Drager syndrome, is characterized by akinetic rigid parkinsonism with early onset severe postural hypotension not related to drugs. Autonomic abnormalities are predominant and include bowel and bladder dysfunction, impotence, upper airway obstruction, cardiac arrhythmia, disturbances of sweating and temperature regulation and pilary changes. MSA with predominant parkinsonism (MSA-P) MSA-P is defined as MSA where extrapyramidal features predominate. The term striatonigral degeneration, parkinsonian variant, is sometimes used for this category of MSA. MSA-C is defined as MSA where cerebellar ataxia predominates. It is sometimes termed sporadic olivopontocerebellar atrophy.

Olivopontocerebellar atrophy is one of the most common and variable of the non-PD parkinsonian conditions. Neuronal loss with gross atrophy is concentrated in the pons, medullary olives, and cerebellum. Ataxia, rigidity, spasticity, and oculomotor movement disturbances are present in variable degrees and combinations. The intracytoplasmic inclusions are predominantly oligodendrocytic, and there is modest tau and synuclein immunoreactivity.

Wilson Disease

Wilson disease, or progressive hepatolenticular degeneration, is rare but also represents degeneration of the basal ganglia and is related to excess deposition of copper. Cysts or cavities form in the basal ganglia with necrosis. The lateral ventricles can be enlarged with associated brain atrophy. This can be imaged using MRI, PET, or SPECT studies. Cerebellar and brainstem damage is common, and there can be spheroid bodies in the cerebral cortex. The symptoms of Wilson disease go far beyond movement disorder mimicking PD and include

A THERAPIST'S THOUGHTS*

Parkinson Disease

Every patient with PD should be educated on neuroprotection and neuroplasticity, and the earlier they are educated, the better. In treating those diagnosed with a progressive disorder, you want to empower them on how they can change their brain and maximize the benefits of their exercise program. The intensity, difficulty, complexity and specificity of exercises need to be explained and incorporated in their exercise routine. Although they may consider themselves "active," their intensity may not be at a sufficient level to promote the most benefits. An easy way to assess the intensity of their walking is to count their steps per minute and use a metronome or music to maintain their speed and/or increase it (100 steps/min would be considered moderate intensity). Your role as a therapist is to increase the intensity level of practice beyond their self-selected energy expenditure. Many of my patients report therapists do not work them hard enough and give in to their complaints. Make sure you always try to motivate and work your patient to their fullest ability; help them understand they are capable of moving more than they think.

Besides the intensity of exercise, the quality of movement maintained during repetitive movements is very important. One of the main movement problems due to basal ganglia disorder is the failure to automatically maintain an appropriate amplitude and timing of sequential movements. Training should include the awareness of complete muscle activation, attention to effort and amplitude of movement. Use of auditory cues (music or metronome while walking on a treadmill), visual or tactile cues (touching a target to maintain range of motion during calf raises) will immediately enhance the size and timing of their movement and therefore maximize overall performance.

You should become aware of your patient's goals and interests (i.e., sports, hiking, dancing) and incorporate task specific exercises to help improve outcomes and compliance. For example if your patient plays tennis, incorporate the racket in your session during reaching and stepping exercises.

*Erica DeMarch, PT, MS

profound affective disorders. Ophthalmologic signs of brownish or greenish rings in the periphery of the cornea are a hallmark sign. The disorder is treated via copper chelating.

Restless Leg Syndrome

Restless leg syndrome is reported as the desire to move the extremities associated with paresthesia, motor restlessness with worsening of symptoms at rest (typically at night), and relief with activity or sensory stimulation. It is familial in 60% of cases, and the effect is related to reduced iron stores in the substantia nigra. There is no loss of dopaminergic neurons as is seen in PD, but the dysfunction lies within the presynaptic and postsynaptic junction of dopaminergic neurons. Levodopa is the traditional treatment, and it is effective when movement is the most problematic symptom. Opioids such as methadone can help when dopamine agents are not effective. For the individual with pain or dysesthesia, neuroleptics can be of benefit.

REFERENCES

To enhance this text and add value for the reader, all references are included on the companion Evolve site that accompanies this textbook. The reader can view the reference source and access it online whenever possible.

CHAPTER 32

Stroke

KENDA S. FULLER

STROKE

Overview and Definition

Stroke often occurs in well-appearing adults as a sudden, devastating focal vascular event that results in destruction of surrounding brain tissue. Stroke is primarily a consequence of changes in both the function of the heart and in the integrity of the vessels providing blood to the brain. See Chapter 12 for cardiac structure and function and related pathogenesis.

Transient ischemic attack has been the term used for focal neurologic symptoms that completely resolve within 24 hours. However, the etiology is the same as stroke, and it is becoming more common for the symptoms to be regarded and named as such, resulting in hospitalization, closer observation, and early use of imaging to determine level of brain damage.

Although stroke deaths have declined, and have dropped to the fourth leading cause of death after being the third leading cause for many years, it is still a leading cause of serious long-term disability. The direct and indirect cost determined by stroke is estimated at $70 billion per year. Most survivors return home and rely on spouses or children for support; four out of five families are affected by stroke. Two-thirds of strokes occur in low-income and middle-income countries, where the average age of stroke onset is 15 years below that in high-income countries. Therefore, stroke has a substantial impact on worldwide society, affecting workplace productivity, not only of the survivors, but also of their caregivers. Work is often interrupted or abandoned based on the need to provide care for a family member.[131] Attempts to decrease the stroke burden related to intrinsic damage at onset, and control of recurrence, underlie most current studies. Effective rehabilitation strategies are also at the forefront of research.

Incidence

Stroke is a major global health problem that will continue to increase over the next 20 years as the population ages. Of the 16 million people worldwide who suffer a first-time stroke each year, more than 10 million survive and the prevalence of stroke survivors is estimated to reach 77 million by the year 2030.[6,112] The average incidence rate of first strokes is 114 per 100,000 persons, which accounts for approximately 800,000 new or recurrent strokes that occur each year in the United States. First strokes account for about 75% of acute events, and recurrent strokes account for about 25%.

Men of Latin and African descent living in the United States have a 50% higher chance of having a stroke than do Caucasian men; this is associated with large artery–occlusive disease, which is most pronounced in strokes at earlier ages.[41] Sickle cell disease is increased in the African population and leads to a higher incidence of stroke.[75] Incidence of stroke is increased with a family history of stroke, with both paternal and maternal influence.[63] Strokes occur more often in the spring.[85] There are several stroke types with different etiology and risk factors; therefore, management is driven by the stroke subtype. Figure 32-1 shows the prevalence of stroke types.

Risk Factors

Cerebrovascular disease, the primary cause of stroke, is caused by one of several pathologic processes involving the blood vessels of the brain. The damage may be intrinsic to the vessel, or the damage may originate remotely, such as when an embolus from the heart or extracranial circulation lodges in an intracranial vessel. The stroke may result from the rupture of a vessel in the subarachnoid space or intracerebral tissue. Figure 32-2 shows the effects of different types of stroke on brain tissue.[116]

Risk factors for stroke can be divided into those that are potentially modifiable and those that are not. Among the nonmodifiable risk factors (age, race, and sex), age constitutes the greatest risk. The incidence of stroke doubles with every decade after age 55 years. Approximately 5% of men aged 65 to 69 years have had stroke compared with the 10% of men aged 80 to 84 years. Women have a 20% less chance of stroke than men, but age increases the risk just as with men.

Stroke is a heterogeneous multifactorial disorder, but epidemiologic data provide substantial evidence for a genetic component. Genetic variants appear to be most related to specific stroke subtype. This has implications on both prevention and treatment related to stroke.

There is an association between two gene regions (*PITX2* and *ZFHX3*) and cardioembolic stroke, including atrial fibrillation. Two additional genes, *HDAC9* and *9p21*, are associated with large vessel stroke.[121]

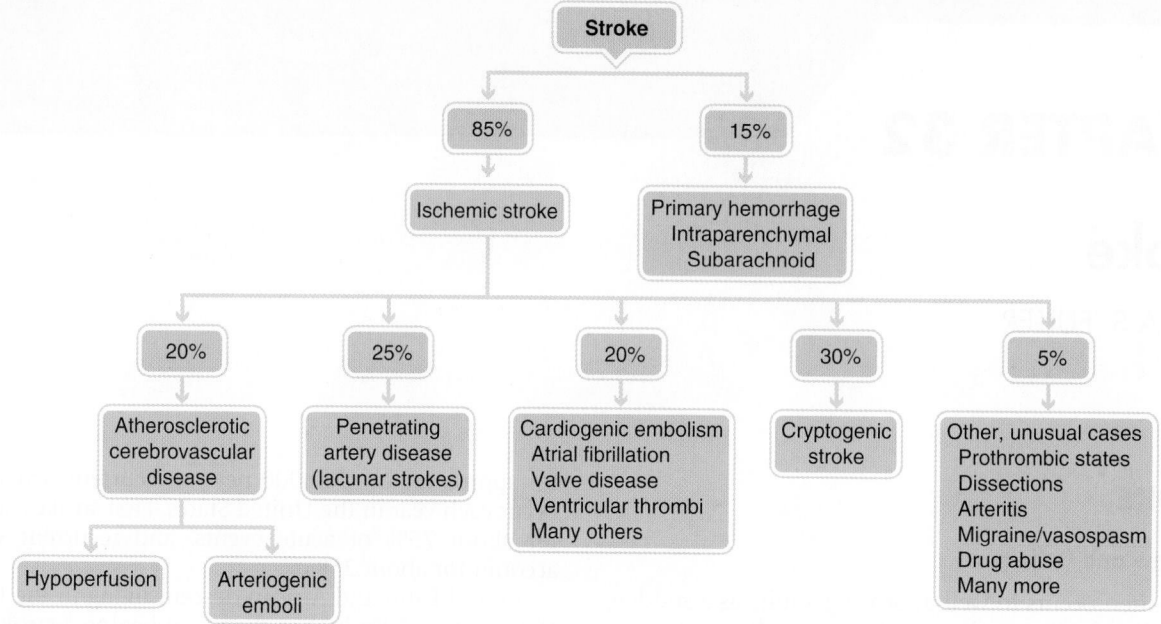

Figure 32-1

Percentage of strokes caused by different etiologies. (Reprinted from Townsend CM: *Sabiston textbook of surgery*, ed 17, Philadelphia, 2004, Saunders.)

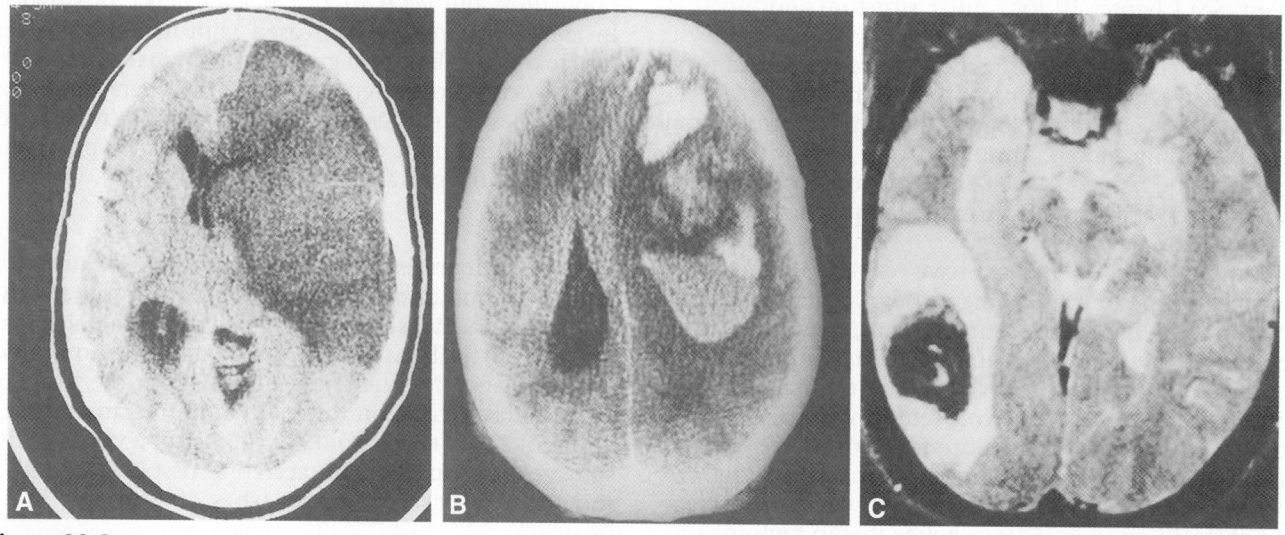

Figure 32-2

Radiographic images of the brain after stroke. A, An acute infarct with mass effect and compression of the ventricle. **B,** An acute intracerebral hemorrhage in the hemisphere. **C,** Amyloid angiopathy with acute hemorrhage; the edema surrounding the area results in a slight mass effect on the midbrain. (Reprinted from Ramsey R: *Neuroradiology*, Philadelphia, 1994, WB Saunders.)

The identification of *NOTCH3* mutations has been found in individuals with cerebral autosomal-dominant arteriopathy with subcortical infarcts and leukoencephalopathy. Studies of sickle cell disease have drawn attention to the importance of modifier genes and of gene-gene interactions in determining stroke risk. There are probably many alleles with small effect sizes associated with multifactorial stroke. Genetic association studies on a wide range of candidate pathways are currently underway. Figure 32-3 shows the interaction of genetics, disease, and environment.[20]

Hypertension (blood pressure above 160/95 mm Hg) is the most prevalent and modifiable risk factor for stroke. Decreasing diastolic blood pressure by 5 to 6 mm Hg

decreases risk of stroke by up to 40%.[26] Prehypertension describes blood pressure at the upper end of normal range (between 120/80 and 129/89 mm Hg), which in combination with other risk factors as described below may increase the risk of cardiovascular disease and stroke.

Various cardiac diseases have been shown to increase risk of stroke, including coronary heart disease, left ventricular hypertrophy, and cardiac failure. The stroke risk increases with the degree of stenosis. Death is more often from fatal coronary artery disease than stroke. The risk of stroke after myocardial infarction (MI) is 30% in the first month.[116] If cerebral microembolism occurs after stroke, there is increased risk of an embolic event.[81] Development

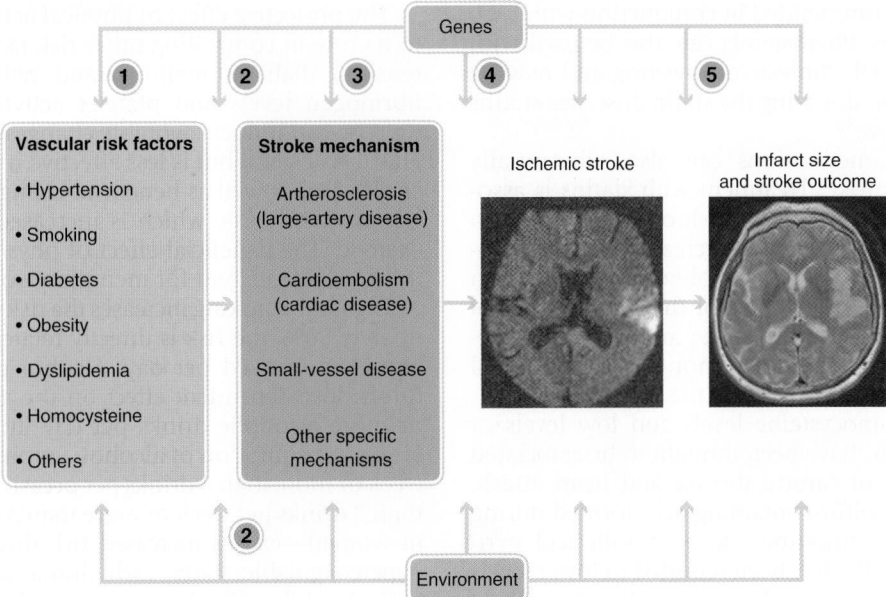

Figure 32-3

Genetic factors and ischemic stroke. Genetic factors may affect stroke risk at various levels. They could act through conventional risk factors (1), interact with conventional and environmental risk factors (2), or contribute directly to an established stroke mechanism such as atherosclerosis or small vessel disease (3). Genetic factors could further affect the latency to stroke (4) or infarct size and stroke outcome (5). Similarly, environmental factors and interactions between genes and the environment could occur at various levels. (Reprinted from Dichgans M: Genetics of ischaemic stroke, *Lancet Neurol* 6:149–161, 2007.)

of neurologic deficits preceded by brief symptoms of focal symptoms in the same vascular territory usually suggests atherothrombosis as the vascular mechanism. Cardiac valve abnormalities such as mitral stenosis and mitral annular calcification are moderate risk factors. Structural abnormalities of the heart, such as patent foramen ovale and atrial septal aneurysm increase risk. Atrial fibrillation is an important risk factor for stroke.[98] It increases the stroke risk by a factor of six, and 8% of individuals over the age of 80 years have atrial fibrillation.[136]

Fibrinogen is a coagulation factor that has been demonstrated to be associated with increased stroke risk. Fibrinogen plays a crucial role in platelet aggregation. Platelets initiate thrombosis by attracting fibrin and other clot-forming substances. Conditions associated with increased fibrin deposition or increased blood viscosity are rheumatic heart disease, endocarditis, atherosclerosis, polycythemia, and thrombocytosis.

Leukemia is complicated occasionally by brain hemorrhages and microinfarcts. When the white blood cell count is very high (increased leukocrit), the white blood cells can pack capillaries, leading to microinfarcts and vascular rupture with small hemorrhages in the brain. Larger intraparenchymatous hemorrhages and subarachnoid hemorrhages (SAHs) are most often related to thrombocytopenia because of replacement of the bone marrow with leukocyte precursors.[35]

Diabetes mellitus, a common endocrine disorder, has long been established as a risk factor for stroke. Diabetes is known to cause large artery atherosclerosis, increased cholesterol levels, and plaque formation. The ability of the cerebral arterioles to dilate is reduced in long-standing type 2 diabetes.[57]

Lifestyle choices have a significant effect on several of the risk factors for stroke, and there is a large body of research focused on making recommendations regarding diet and exercise. For example, level of cholesterol has long been considered a part of the stroke risk profile; however, the relation between raised lipid level and stroke remains unclear.[110] High total cholesterol levels create increased risk of ischemic stroke. These include the large artery and lacunar subtypes that have atherosclerotic pathogeneses. Younger individuals and those with low high-density lipoprotein (HDL) levels are at greater risk; higher levels of HDL cholesterol are associated with decreased risk of ischemic stroke. Low-density lipoprotein (LDL) cholesterol levels currently are thought to be biochemical predictors of coronary artery disease associated with carotid athrerosclerosis.[119]

Dietary factors that increase LDL cholesterol include saturated fatty acids, *trans*-fatty acids, and dietary cholesterol. Soluble fiber as is present in foods such as beans, oats, barley, and some fruits and vegetables reduces LDL cholesterol through decreased absorption of cholesterol and bile acids. The potential for soy protein to decrease serum cholesterol levels has been studied extensively, with recent meta-analyses demonstrating that 30 to 50 g per day of soy protein can reduce LDL cholesterol by 3% to 5%.

Phytosterols are cholesterol-like compounds that are found mostly in vegetable oils, nuts, and legumes. When included in the diet, they inhibit cholesterol absorption by displacing cholesterol from mixed micelles, as opposed to statin drugs, which inhibit cholesterol synthesis. Phytosterols create additional lipid lowering when combined with a heart-healthy diet using other LDL-lowering strategies. Carotenoids in carrots, pumpkin, apricots, spinach, and broccoli are recommended in conjunction with consuming phytosterols. Phytosterols can also be used with statins for greater LDL cholesterol lowering and may be more preferable than doubling the statin dose. See statins in "Treatment" below.[58]

Lipid-modifying medications can also substantially reduce the risk of stroke. Treatment with statins is associated with the reduction in the risk of a first stroke in various populations of patients at increased risk of cardiovascular events. National Cholesterol Education Program III guidelines recommend statins for the management of patients who have not had a stroke and who have elevated total cholesterol or elevated non–HDL cholesterol in the presence of hypertriglyceridemia.

High plasma homocysteine levels and low levels of folate and vitamin B_6 have been thought to be associated with increased risk of carotid disease and heart attack. Homocysteine is a sulfur-containing acid formed during the metabolism of methionine. The use of folic acid, pyridoxine, and vitamin B_{12} has been reported to lower levels of homocysteine in the blood. However, the strength of association of homocysteine with risk of cardiovascular disease showed a weak correlation in meta-analysis.[71] Cardioprotective benefits have been found with consumption of even modest amounts of omega-3 fatty acids provided by an average intake of 1 to 2 oz of fish daily.[93]

There are many countries in the Mediterranean region that have distinct dietary patterns with an overlap of similar characteristics. The Mediterranean diet is associated with a low incidence of cardiovascular disease, which is attributed in part to a high consumption of olive oil and low consumption of saturated fat. Box 32-1 outlines the common characteristics of the diet.

Significant obesity, particularly abdominal adiposity, worsens the prognosis of individuals with coronary disease. Weight loss provides approximately 10% effect on lipid lowering, improves glycemic control, blood pressure, inflammation, and fibrinolysis. In addition, sustained weight loss also may increase life expectancy.

Box 32-1

THE MEDITERRANEAN DIET

The International Conference on the Diet of the Mediterranean summarized the key dietary components in 1993. They are:
1. An abundance of plant foods (e.g., fruits, vegetables, potatoes, breads, grains, beans, nuts, and seeds)
2. Minimally processed and, whenever possible, seasonally fresh foods
3. Fresh fruits as the typical daily dessert
4. Olive oil as the principal source of dietary fat
5. Dairy, poultry, and fish in low to moderate amounts
6. Fewer than five eggs per week
7. Red meat in low frequency and amounts
8. Wine in low to moderate amounts (one to two glasses per day for men and one glass per day for women)
   The Mediterranean diet, being largely plant based, also includes a high intake of fiber and phytosterols (~400 mg per day).

From: Katcher HI: Lifestyle approaches and dietary strategies to lower LDL-cholesterol and triglycerides and raise HDL-cholesterol. *Endocrinol Metab Clin North Am* 38:45–78, 2009.

The protective effect of physical activity may be related to its role in controlling other risk factors such as hypertension, diabetes mellitus, and reductions in plasma fibrinogen levels and platelet activity. Regular aerobic exercise can induce favorable changes in triglycerides and HDL cholesterol but is less effective in lowering total LDL cholesterol as well as beneficial changes in the activity of lipoprotein lipase, which is increased following aerobic exercise. The beneficial effect of physical activity appears to be more apparent for men than women.

Cigarette smoking increases the risk of stroke by approximately 50%; the risk is directly related to the number of cigarettes smoked per day. Alcohol consumption has a direct dose-dependent effect on the risk of stroke. Three or more alcoholic drinks per day increase risk by 45%. Heavy consumption of alcohol—more than 14 drinks per week or more than 4 drinks per occasion in men and more than 7 drinks per week or more than 3 drinks per occasion in women—causes increased risk through hypertension, hypercoagulable states, arrhythmia, and decreased cerebral blood flow. Evidence suggests that light to moderate drinking may have beneficial effects by increasing HDL cholesterol levels and decreasing platelet aggregation and fibrinogen levels, with a 32% decrease in risk.

Cocaine use is associated with hemorrhagic stroke by increased risk related to focal arterial vasoconstriction and occasionally to inflammatory vasculitis. Although the evidence remains inconclusive, other recreational drugs such as lysergic acid diethylamide (LSD) and marijuana are thought to increase the risk. Some concern exists regarding the use of over-the-counter cold medications, diet pills, ephedrine, and pseudoephedrine.

Young women have a low absolute risk of stroke, and use of oral contraceptives seems to be insignificant. However, the absolute risk of stroke is much greater in postmenopausal women simply because they are older. In older women, a modest relative increase in stroke risk when using oral contraceptives may produce a much larger absolute increase in risk of stroke. Thus, differences in prescribing estrogen-containing compounds to premenopausal versus postmenopausal women appears to be justified. Women with hypertension or a history of smoking have a higher absolute risk. Individuals who have had an ischemic stroke are at risk of a second stroke. Thus, oral contraceptive use should be discouraged in women with prior stroke and should certainly be stopped in women who have had a stroke while taking oral contraceptives.

Recognition of the multiple risk factors that can interact to increase the probability of stroke is important. Use of risk profiles can assist in the ability to predict stroke in a single individual, such as the one established as a part of the Framingham study.[135] The percentage of individuals with "no known risk factors" is declining, and the prevalence of high blood pressure, type 2 diabetes, and obesity is increasing.

Pathogenesis

Energy failure following a reduction in blood flow induces a region of cell death known as the *infarct* and a surrounding area of damaged tissue called the *penumbra*. Inflammatory processes in the penumbra exacerbate the infarct. Endothelial and glial cells become activated, releasing free radicals, cytokines, and chemokines, in addition to increasing the production of enzymes causing neuronal cell death and changes in the blood-brain barrier, leading to leukocyte infiltration. Inflammatory processes are further activated by the C-reactive protein and cytokine-induced functions. Cytokines also signal the CNS, thereby initiating brain-mediated defenses such as fever. Uncontrolled or excessive inflammatory responses to injury can have devastating results in the CNS, where tissues lack the capacity to regenerate (Fig. 32-4). Damage related to the different stroke subtypes varies and is discussed further in each section.

Clinical Manifestations

The first indication of the onset of stroke may be transient with focal symptoms, but it is the first warning that a stroke is about to occur. Early warning signs are listed in Box 32-2. Although the risk factors and early warning signs have been well publicized, individuals at highest risk do not appear to be aware of warning signs and may not consult a physician when the symptoms occur. Clinical manifestations are related to the type of stroke that occurs and are addressed later in the chapter in the individual stroke subtypes.

Treatment

The chain of events favoring good functional outcome from an acute ischemic stroke begins with the recognition of stroke when it occurs. The public's knowledge of stroke warning signs remains poor. Fewer than half of 9-1-1 calls for stroke events were made within 1 hour of symptom onset, and fewer than half of those callers thought stroke was the cause of their symptoms.

Although the routine use of supplemental oxygen remains unproven, supplemental oxygen to maintain oxygen saturations >94% is recommended after cardiac arrest and is reasonable for patients with suspected stroke. Antihypertensive medications are considered in extreme hypertension with systolic blood pressure ≥220 mm Hg. Hypoglycemia, with levels <60 mg/dL, is frequently found in patients with stroke-like symptoms; thus, prehospital glucose testing is critical.[55]

Stroke is the major cause of disability in the Western world and is the third greatest cause of death, but there are no widely effective treatments to prevent the devastating effects of stroke. Extensive and growing evidence implicates inflammatory and immune processes in the occurrence of stroke and particularly in the subsequent injury. Several inflammatory mediators have been identified in the pathogenesis of stroke, including specific cytokines, adhesion molecules, matrix metalloproteinases, and eicosanoids. An early clinical trial suggests that inhibiting interleukin-1 may be of benefit in the treatment of acute stroke.

Prognosis

The University of Oxford ABCD scale can be used to determine the chance of progression to a stroke with greater

Box 32-2

WARNING SIGNS OF STROKE

- Sudden weakness or numbness of the face, arm, or leg
- Sudden dimness or loss of vision, particularly in one eye
- Sudden difficulty speaking or understanding speech
- Sudden severe headache with no known cause
- Unexplained dizziness, unsteadiness, or sudden falls

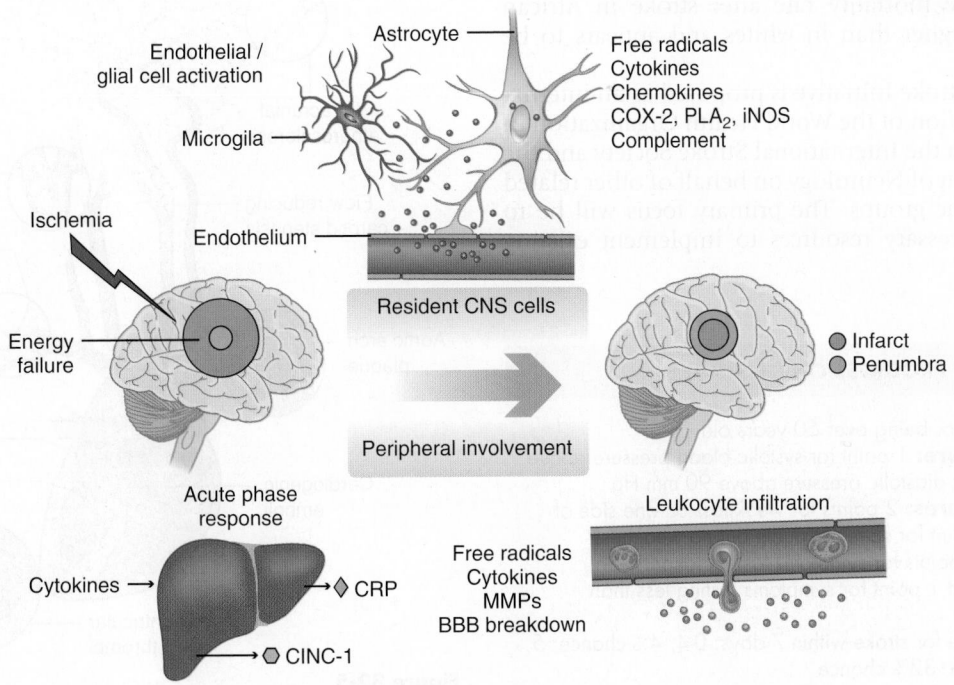

Figure 32-4

Immune/inflammatory responses and their contribution to ischemic injury after stroke. (From Skinner R, Georgiou R, Thornton P, Rothwell N: Psychoneuroimmunology of stroke. *Immunol Allergy Clin North Am* 29[2]:359–379, 2009.)

consequences (Box 32-3). Risk of second stroke varies between 3% and 5% in 5 years and is related to the concomitant cardiac and vascular disorders. The recurrence rate of stroke is highest in the first 30 days after the first stroke and remains higher for 1 year. The presence of atherosclerosis increases the chance of another thrombotic event. Men have 30% to 80% higher rates of recurrence than do women.[99]

Living with stroke can be a challenge, with the onset of impairments causing difficulty eating, urinary incontinence, and difficulty speaking or understanding language. Hemiparesis remains a long-term consequence in almost half of stroke survivors. Cognitive changes, anxiety, and confusion can be very disturbing for the individual and add to caregiver stress. Quality of life often is reported as poor.

Concomitant diseases of aging such as arthritis, diabetes, osteoporosis, and decreased plasticity of the nervous system associated with aging often make the recovery from stroke a challenge. Medical complications occur in up to 85% of stroke survivors and present potential barriers to optimal recovery. Infections occur in almost 25% of stroke survivors, primarily in the urinary tract and chest. Incidence of deep vein thrombosis and pulmonary emboli is increased. Falls resulting from impaired mobility are also prevalent, with serious injury reported in 5% of the reported falls. Approximately 75% of stroke survivors will have a fall within the first 6 months after stroke. Pain and depression are reported in more than 30% of stroke survivors.[70] Urinary incontinence after stroke is a bad prognostic feature, both for survival and functional recovery.

Mortality associated with stroke has decreased in the past 20 years in all age groups. However, stroke still remains the number one cause of disability in the adult population. The mortality rate after stroke in African Americans is higher than in whites and appears to be increasing.[37]

The Global Stroke Initiative is proposed as an international collaboration of the World Health Organization in partnership with the International Stroke Society and the World Federation of Neurology on behalf of other related professional civic groups. The primary focus will be to harness the necessary resources to implement existing knowledge and strategies for stroke prevention, especially in low-income and middle-income countries and in disadvantaged populations in high-income countries.[7]

Ischemic Stroke

Pathogenesis

Occlusion of Major Arteries. Thrombosis and embolic occlusion of a major vessel are the most common causes of ischemic stroke. The heart is the most common source of embolic material as a result of damage to heart tissue from atherothrombotic disease. Atrial fibrillation is thought to cause thrombus formation in the fibrillating atrium. Left ventricular MI can be a source of emboli, especially in the first few weeks following the event when thrombus formation is most prevalent.[102] Mitral valve prolapse or congenital septal defects are also sources of emboli. Formation of emboli during or after coronary artery surgery or intracardiac surgery is a well-recognized complication.

Artery-to-artery embolism, usually arising from an atherothrombotic lesion in the carotid or vertebrobasilar system, may lead to stroke. The emboli from this lesion may travel along the course of circulation and may cause occlusion in the smaller branches. The proximal internal carotid artery is the most common site of atherosclerosis and atherothrombosis leading to stroke. Other causes of emboli may be thrombus in the pulmonary vein, fat emboli in the blood, and tumor emboli from a neoplastic process.[31] Sources of emboli are shown in Figure 32-5.

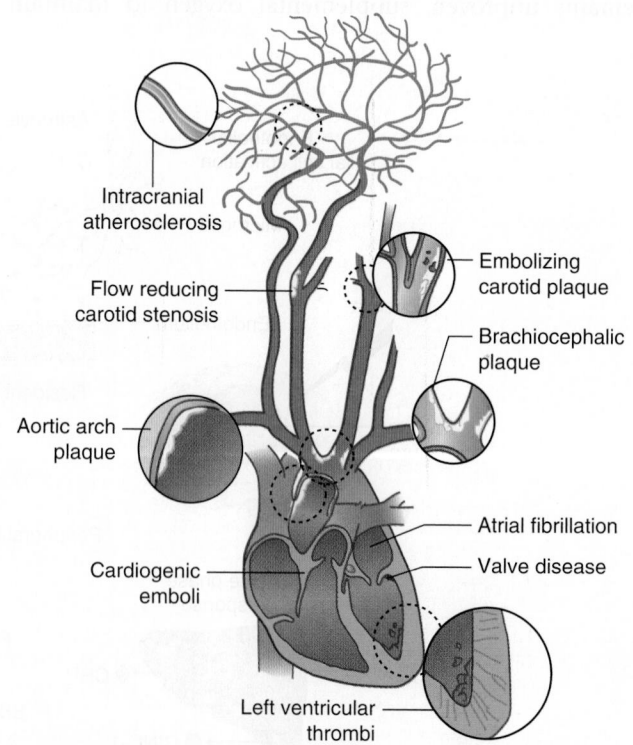

Intracranial atherosclerosis

Flow reducing carotid stenosis

Aortic arch plaque

Cardiogenic emboli

Embolizing carotid plaque

Brachiocephalic plaque

Atrial fibrillation

Valve disease

Left ventricular thrombi

Figure 32-5

Cardiogenic and arterial atherosclerotic sources for stroke. (Reprinted from Townsend CM: *Sabiston textbook of surgery,* ed 17, Philadelphia, 2004, Saunders.)

Box 32-3

ABCD PREDICTS PROGRESSION OF STROKE

- **Age:** 1 point for being over 60 years old
- **Blood pressure:** 1 point for systolic blood pressure above 140 mm Hg or diastolic pressure above 90 mm Hg
- **Clinical features:** 2 points for weakness on one side of the body; 1 point for speech trouble but no weakness
- **Duration:** 2 points for symptoms lasting longer than 60 minutes and 1 point for symptoms lasting less than 60 minutes
- Predictive value for stroke within 7 days: 0-4, 4% chance; 5, 12% chance; 6, 32% chance

Modified from Rothwell PM: A simple score (ABCD) to identify individuals at high early risk of stroke after transient ischaemic attack. *Lancet* 366:29–36, 2005.

Changes in the collateral pathways of the circle of Willis are apparent in response to internal carotid artery obstruction that may provide some protection against neurologic damage associated with occlusion. The anterior circle of Willis and the posterior communicating artery show increased diameter in some individuals when the internal carotid artery is blocked.[48] Figure 32-6 shows the distribution of the circle of Willis.

Secondary Vascular Responses. When a cerebral artery is occluded, the formation of thromboemboli probably begins in the distal vessels of that artery. These presumed microvascular occlusions progressively increase in number and continue to impair blood flow in the brain. Cell death surrounding the area of blocked blood flow may be due to the squeezing effects of microvessels by the swelling of the *astrocyte*, one of the cellular support structures of the nervous system. Astroglial swelling is one of the earliest cell changes induced by single-artery occlusion. The formation of fibrin in the grey matter surrounding the occluded vessel also may contribute to the lack of reperfusion of microvessels. Other factors include bleeding into the parenchyma, increased platelet aggregation, endothelial cells swelling in the walls of the vessels, and vasospasm.[40,86]

Secondary Neuronal Damage. The tissue of the brain, or the *parenchyma*, is highly vulnerable to an interruption in its blood supply. When the cerebral blood flow falls below 20 mL/100 mg of tissue per minute, neuronal functioning is impaired. Neuronal death, or infarction, occurs when the brain receives less than 8 to 10 mL/100 mg/min. Frequently, in an acute infarction, a portion of the affected brain receives no blood, while a surrounding area receives sufficient blood from collateral circulation to maintain viability but not to sustain function. This territory has been termed the *ischemic penumbra*.[122] The major injury to the neurons in the brain is the hypoxia-ischemia related to the occlusion of the artery causing cell death near the core. Further damage to the brain tissue and neurons occurs as a secondary response. There is decreased perfusion relative to the necessary oxygen requirements causing decreased metabolism in the infarcted area. If blood flow to this ischemic area is restored before irreversible damage occurs, then the tissue will likely recover and resume normal function.

After an ischemic event, the cells that normally clear excess glutamate are compromised, and excess glutamate is found in the extracellular space. Depolarization of the postsynaptic cell occurs in response to this increase in glutamate. Excess glutamate allows abnormally high entry of calcium ions into the cells. Excessive numbers of calcium ions begin the process that causes cell death. Catabolic enzymes are activated by the release of calcium ions and can cause damage of the proteins that support neurons, the glial cells. It appears that other mechanisms cause excess calcium during the ischemic process in addition to glutamate, including the dysfunction of the electrochemical gradient in the damaged membrane.

Apoptosis, or programmed cell death occurs in response to the hypoxic damage.[76] The changes in the perfusion pressure associated with hypoxia can also cause the endothelial cells to trigger the release of neurotoxic substances such as free radicals. Oxygen free radicals can initiate many destructive processes in the brain tissue. The overall result of the hypoxic event is a chain of reactions, some that occur simultaneously, extending the damage and death of brain tissue beyond the area of vascular supply. Figure 32-7 shows the cascade of destruction after ischemia. See Chapter 28 for further information on apoptosis and free radicals.

Distant from the ischemic and stroke sites are regions that also show alterations in metabolism despite being normal on anatomic imaging studies such as CT or MRI. There appears to be an uncoupling of oxygen consumption and glucose use that may reflect a change in brain metabolism caused by deafferentation while other areas are hypometabolic after a cortical infarct. This decline in oxygen metabolism in the unaffected hemisphere from the acute to the subacute stage suggests a delayed effect. Neurologic recovery appears to be influenced by prefrontal metabolism, possibly because this region is part of a network that has an important compensatory role in motor recovery.[82]

Clinical Manifestations

Syndromes. Syndromes reflect the dysfunction associated with disruption of blood flow in specific areas of the brain.[62,73] The syndromes are named according to the arteries that feed the specific areas. The syndrome can be

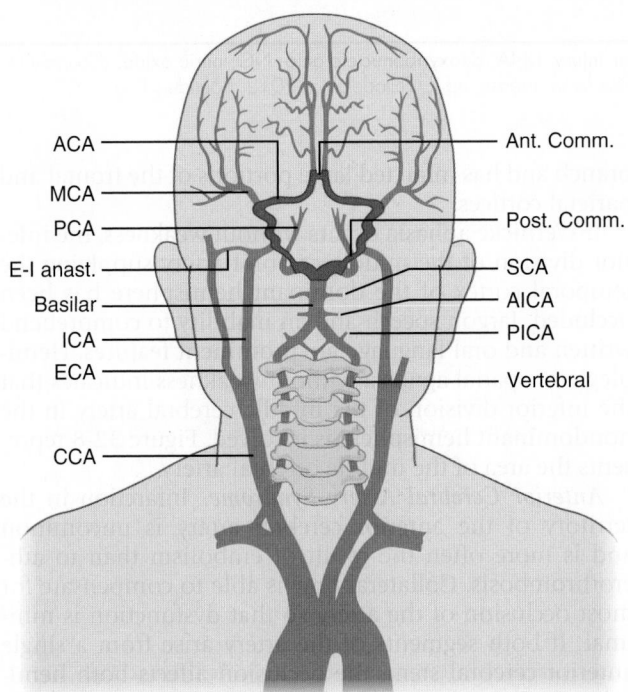

Figure 32-6

Extracranial and intracranial arterial supply to the brain. Vessels forming the circle of Willis are highlighted. *ACA*, Anterior cerebral artery; *AICA*, anterior inferior cerebellar artery; *Ant. Comm.*, anterior communicating artery; *CCA*, common carotid artery; *ECA*, external carotid artery; *E-I anast.*, extracranial-intracranial anastomosis; *ICA*, internal carotid artery; *MCA*, middle cerebral artery; *PCA*, posterior cerebral artery; *PICA*, posterior inferior cerebellar artery; *Post. Comm.*, posterior communicating artery; *SCA*, superior cerebellar artery. (Modified from Lord R: *Surgery of occlusive cerebrovascular disease*, St Louis, 1986, C.V. Mosby.)

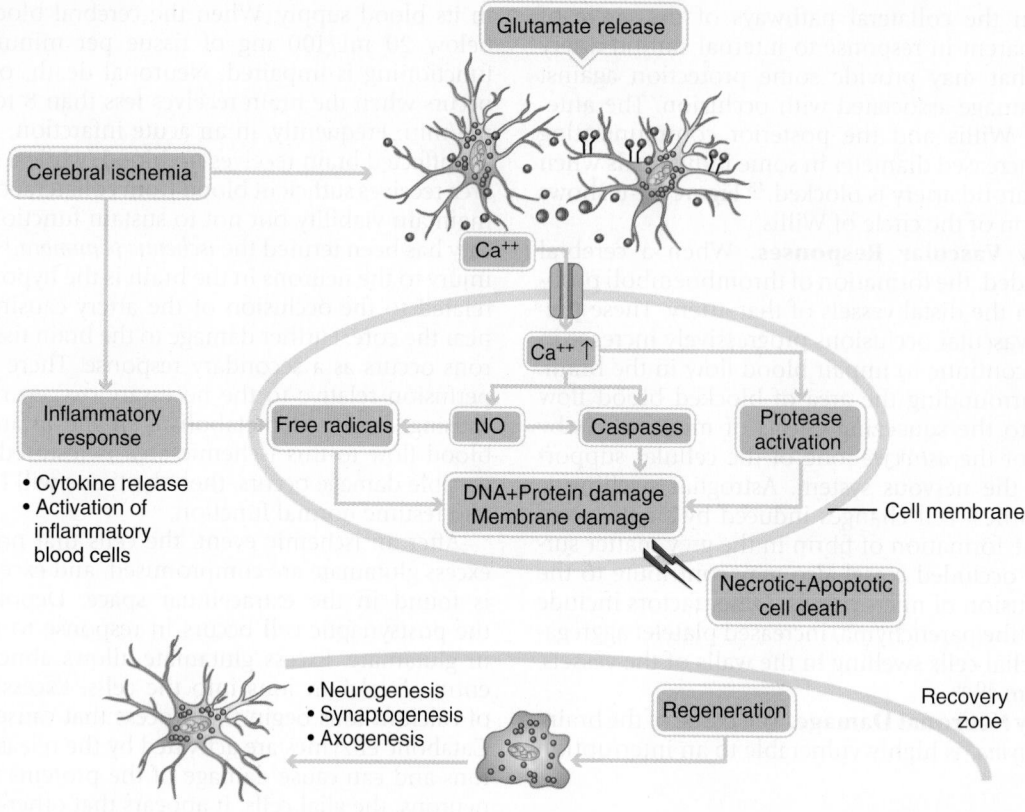

Figure 32-7

Depiction of the major events that encompass the ischemic cascade of cellular injury. DNA, deoxyribonucleic acid; NO, nitric oxide. (Courtesy Dr. Wolf-Rudiger Schaebitz. Creager: *Vascular medicine: a companion to Braunwald's heart disease*, ed 2, Philadelphia, 2012, Saunders.)

partial or complete. When the blockage is in the more proximal component of the artery, the resulting area of hypoxia is greater than if the clot is lodged in a more distal part of the artery. Because of the collateral circulation provided by the circle of Willis, some areas of the brain are supplied by more than one artery. When one artery is blocked, circulation is provided to the tissues through the blood supply of other arteries. In this case, the clinical syndromes are not as extensive. The actual configuration of arteries is different in each individual, so the syndromes described here are not to be considered all encompassing. This is an overview of the types of symptoms that might be encountered when a particular artery is blocked.

Middle Cerebral Artery Syndrome. If the entire middle cerebral artery is occluded at its stem, blocking both the penetrating and cortical branches, the clinical findings are contralateral *hemiplegia* and *hemianesthesia*, or the loss of movement and sensation on one-half of the body. If the dominant hemisphere is affected, *global aphasia*, or the loss of fluency, ability to name objects, comprehend auditory information, and repeat language, is the result. (See "Parietal Lobe Syndromes" in Chapter 28.)

Partial syndromes resulting from embolic occlusion of a single branch include brachial syndrome, or weakness of the upper extremity, and frontal opercular syndrome, or facial weakness with motor aphasia with or without arm weakness. A combination of sensory disturbance, motor weakness, and motor aphasia suggests that an embolus has occluded the proximal superior division

branch and has infarcted large portions of the frontal and parietal cortices.

If Wernicke aphasia occurs without weakness, the inferior division of the middle cerebral artery supplying the temporal cortex of the dominant hemisphere has been occluded. Jargon speech and an inability to comprehend written and oral language are prominent features. Hemiplegia or spatial agnosia without weakness indicates that the inferior division of the middle cerebral artery in the nondominant hemisphere is involved. Figure 32-8 represents the area of the middle cerebral artery.

Anterior Cerebral Artery Syndrome. Infarction in the territory of the anterior cerebral artery is uncommon and is more often the result of embolism than to atherothrombosis. Collateral flow is able to compensate for most occlusion of the artery so that dysfunction is minimal. If both segments of the artery arise from a single anterior cerebral stem, the occlusion affects both hemispheres. Contralateral hemiparesis and sensory loss are usually seen with the lower extremity more involved. Profound *abulia*, a delay in verbal and motor response, is common. Akinetic mutism also can result in significant disability. Figure 32-9 represents the area of blood flow of the anterior cerebral artery.

Internal Carotid Artery Syndrome. The clinical picture of internal carotid occlusion varies depending on whether the cause of ischemia is thrombus, embolus, or low flow. The cortex supplied by the middle cerebral territory is affected most often. Occasionally, the origins of both the anterior

Middle cerebral artery

Anatomy

Lateral surface of cerebral hemisphere.

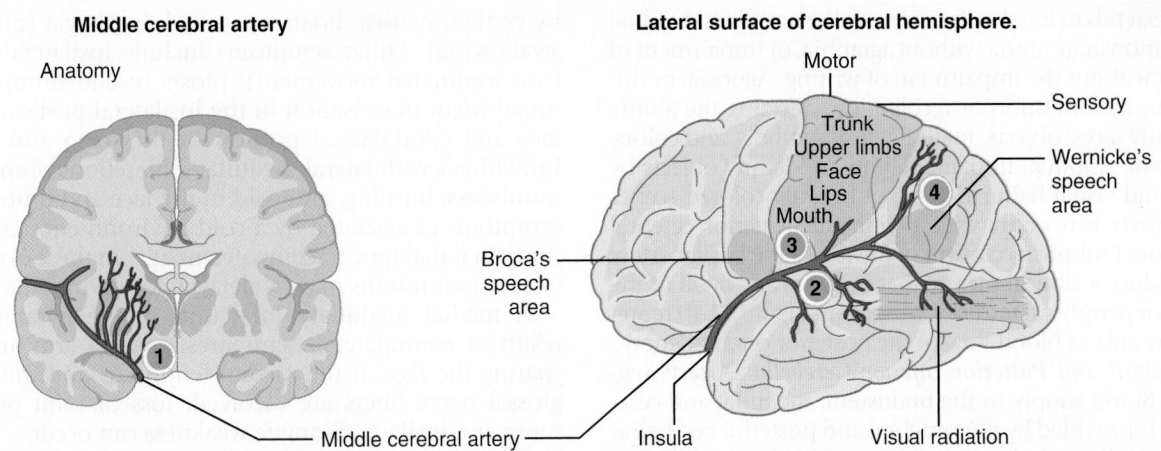

Figure 32-8

The middle cerebral artery is the largest branch of the internal carotid artery and the most common site of emboli. Its deep branches feed the internal capsule and basal ganglia. On the lateral surface, the branches feed areas of the parietal, frontal, and temporal lobes. (Reprinted from Lindsay KW, Bone I, Callander R: *Neurology and neurosurgery illustrated*, New York, 1986, Churchill Livingstone.)

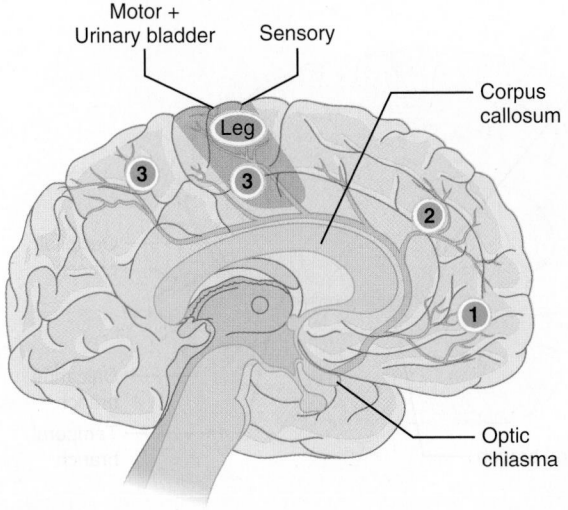

Figure 32-9

The anterior cerebral artery branches from the internal carotid. Deep branches supply the internal capsule and basal ganglia. Superficial branches supply the frontal and parietal lobes. (Reprinted from Lindsay KW, Bone I, Callander R: *Neurology and neurosurgery illustrated*, New York, 1986, Churchill Livingstone.)

and middle cerebral arteries are occluded at the top of the carotid artery. Symptoms consistent with both syndromes result. With a competent circle of Willis producing adequate collateral circulation, the occlusion can be asymptomatic.

Posterior Cerebral Artery Syndrome. If the proximal posterior cerebral artery is occluded, including penetrating branches, the areas of the brain that are affected are the subthalamus, medial thalamus, and ipsilateral (same side) cerebral peduncle and midbrain. Signs include thalamic syndrome, including abnormal sensation of pain, temperature, proprioception, and touch. Sensations may be exaggerated and light pressure may be interpreted as painful stimuli. This may develop into intractable, searing pain, which can be incapacitating. The anterior pattern consists mainly of perseverations and superimposition

of unrelated information, apathy, and amnesia. After paramedian infarct, the most frequent features are disinhibition syndromes with personality changes, loss of self-activation, amnesia and, in the case of extensive lesions, thalamic dementia; this pattern may often be difficult to distinguish from primary psychiatric disorders, especially when neurologic dysfunction is lacking. After inferolateral lesion, executive dysfunction may develop but is often overlooked, although it may occasionally lead to severe long-term disability. After posterior lesion, cognitive dysfunction with neglect and aphasia are well known.[15]

If the posterior cerebral artery is completely occluded at its origin, hemiplegia results from infarction of the cerebral peduncle. Involvement of the red nucleus or dentatorubrothalamic tract can produce contralateral ataxia. When palsy of cranial nerve III occurs with contralateral ataxia, it is known as Claude syndrome. Third nerve palsy occurring with contralateral hemiplegia is known as Weber syndrome. Hemiballismus, or flailing of the extremity, usually results from a deep penetrating vessel causing infarct in the contralateral subthalamic nucleus. Paresis of upward gaze, drowsiness, and abulia (the lack of interest in movement) can be attributed to occlusion of the artery of Percheron. If the posterior cerebral stem is occluded, there can be infarction of the subthalamus; coma and decerebrate rigidity may result.

Peripheral supply of the posterior cerebral artery includes the temporal and occipital lobes. Occlusion of this component of the artery often affects the occipital lobe with homonymous hemianopsia, in which the visual field defect is on the side opposite to the lesion. Cortical blindness, the inability of the brain to record an image although the optic nerve is intact, is one of the visual disturbances that is seen with infarcts in this region.

Medial temporal lobe involvement (including the hippocampus) can cause an acute disturbance in memory, particularly if it occurs in the dominant hemisphere. This typically resolves because memory has dual representation. Memory is represented on both sides of the brain; if one area is affected the intact side can compensate to a considerable extent. If the dominant hemisphere is affected and the infarct extends to involve the corpus callosum, the individual may demonstrate alexia without agraphia, or impairment of reading without the impairment of writing. Agnosia, or difficulty in identification or recognition, affecting the ability to identify faces, objects, mathematical symbols, and colors, may occur. Anomia, impaired ability to identify objects by name, and visual hallucinations of brightly colored scenes and objects can occur with peripheral posterior cerebral infarction. Embolic occlusion of the top of the basilar artery can produce a clinical picture that includes any or all of the central or peripheral territory symptoms. Figure 32-10 represents the area of blood flow of the posterior cerebral artery.

Vertebral and Posterior Inferior Cerebellar Artery Syndrome. Blood supply to the brainstem, medulla, and cerebellum is provided by the vertebral and posterior cerebellar arteries. Collateral circulation is provided by the bilateral component of the vertebral artery so that ischemia often is not manifested in the presence of atherothrombosis.

Wallenberg syndrome is related to the lateral medulla and the posteroinferior cerebellum and is characterized by vertigo, nausea, hoarseness, and dysphagia (difficulty swallowing). Other symptoms include ipsilateral ataxia (uncoordinated movement), ptosis (eyelid droop), and impairment of sensation in the ipsilateral portion of the face and contralateral portion of the torso and limbs. Individuals with lateral medullary infarction complain of numbness, burning, and cold in the face and limbs, with symptoms exaggerated by a cold environment, reflecting the spinal thalamic tract involvement.[61] In these cases, the onset of symptoms may be delayed for up to 6 months.[51]

A medial medullary infarction of the pyramid can result in contralateral hemiparesis of the arm and leg, sparing the face. If the medial lemniscus and the hypoglossal nerve fibers are involved, loss of joint position sense and ipsilateral tongue weakness can occur.

The edema associated with cerebellar infarction can cause sudden respiratory arrest from raised intracranial pressure (ICP) in the posterior fossa. Gait unsteadiness, dizziness, nausea, and vomiting may be the only early symptoms. Figure 32-11 shows the area of distribution of

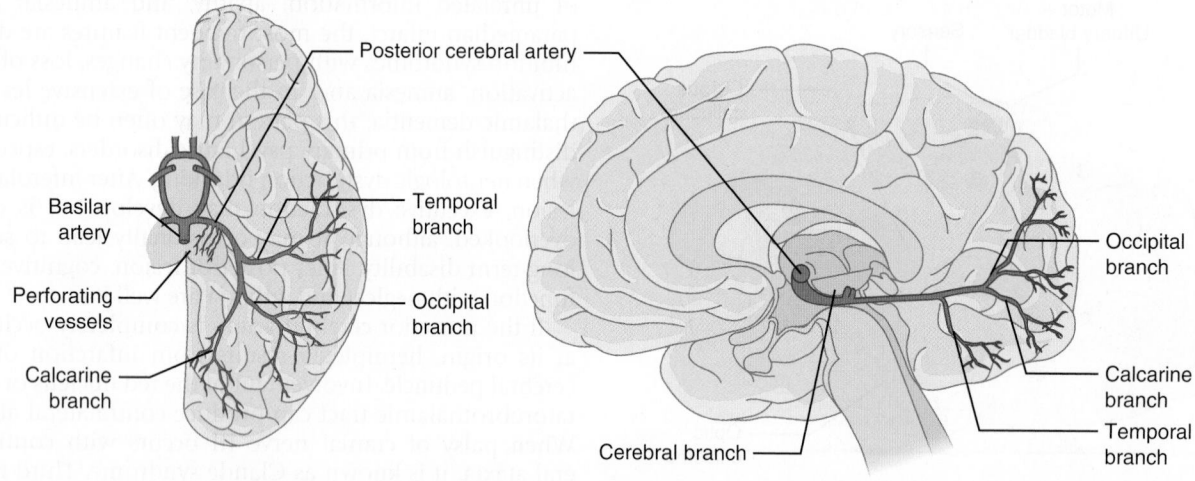

Figure 32-10

The posterior cerebral arteries branch from the basilar artery. The small perforating branches supply the midbrain structures and posterior thalamus. The temporal branch supplies the temporal lobe, and the occipital and calcarine supply the occipital lobe, including the visual cortex. (Reprinted from Lindsay KW, Bone I, Callander R: *Neurology and neurosurgery illustrated*, New York, 1986, Churchill Livingstone.)

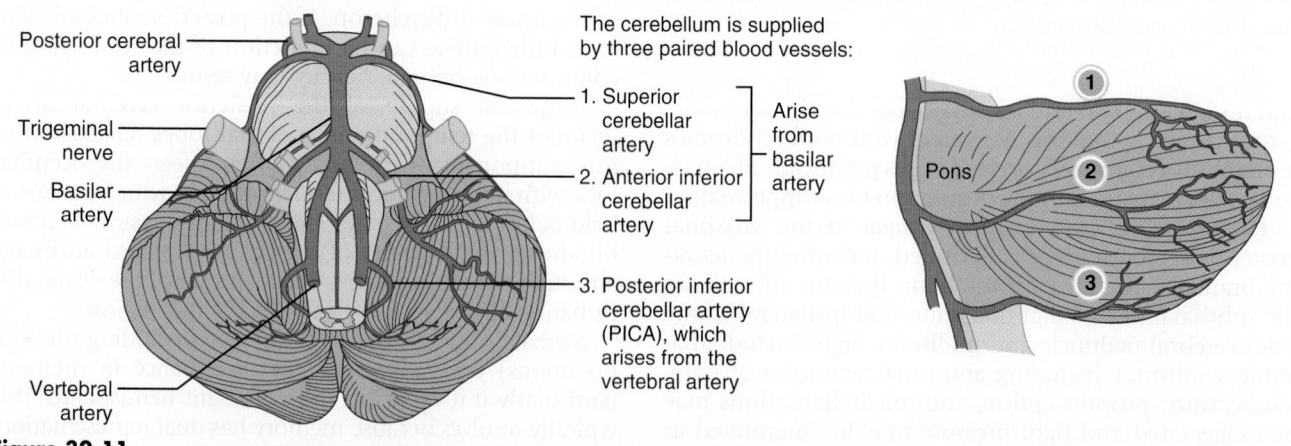

Figure 32-11

A lesion in the cerebellar territory will produce both cerebellar and brainstem signs and symptoms. (Reprinted from Lindsay KW, Bone I, Callander R: *Neurology and neurosurgery illustrated*, New York, 1986, Churchill Livingstone.)

the superior cerebellar, anterior inferior cerebellar, and posterior inferior cerebellar arteries.

Basilar Artery Syndrome. Atheromatous lesions can occur anywhere along the basilar trunk, but they occur most often in the proximal basilar and distal vertebral area. Ischemia as a result of occlusion of the basilar artery can affect the brainstem, including the corticospinal tracts, corticobulbar tracts, medial and superior cerebellar peduncles, spinothalamic tracts, and cranial nerve nuclei.

If the basilar artery is occluded, the brainstem symptoms are bilateral. When a branch of the basilar artery is occluded, the symptoms are unilateral, involving the sensory and motor aspects of the cranial nerves.

Superior Cerebellar Artery Syndrome. Occlusion of the superior cerebellar artery results in severe ipsilateral cerebellar ataxia, nausea and vomiting, and dysarthria, or slurring of speech. Scanning speech, a drawn-out and monotone speech pattern, reflects damage to the cerebellum. Loss of pain and temperature in the contralateral extremities, torso, and face occurs. Dysmetria, characterized by the inability to place the extremity at a precise point in space, is common, affecting the ipsilateral upper extremity.

Anterior Inferior Cerebellar Artery Syndrome. Principal symptoms include ipsilateral deafness, facial weakness, vertigo, nausea and vomiting, *nystagmus* (rhythmic oscillations of the eye), and ataxia. *Horner syndrome* ptosis, miosis (constriction of the pupil), and loss of sweating over the ipsilateral side of the face may occur. A paresis of lateral gaze may be seen. Pain and temperature sensation are lost on the contralateral side of the body.

Lacunar Syndrome. Lacunar infarcts are small infarcts of the end arteries typically found in the basal ganglia, internal capsule and pons. The lacunar infarcts have the characteristics of ischemic necrosis and the cysts are surrounded by astrocytic gliosis, or scarring of the support structures of the brain.[52] These small cystic spaces resulting from healed ischemic infarcts are common in individuals with hypertension or diabetes. A large majority are asymptomatic, but in about 20% of cases a stroke syndrome occurs with a slowly progressive (over 24-36 hours) dysfunction of the cells in the area of the lacune.[78] The lacunar syndrome is representative of the area of infarct in which the lacunae are predominant in the deep structures of the brain and have their effect often on white matter. If the posterior limb of the internal capsule is affected, a pure motor deficit may result; in the anterior limb of the internal capsule, weakness of the face and dysarthria may occur. If the posterolateral thalamus is affected, there is a pure sensory stroke. When the lacunae occur predominantly in the pons, ataxia, clumsiness, and weakness may be seen. Parkinsonism can manifest due to involvement of the basal ganglia, as can subcortical dementia. Figure 32-12 shows the areas of predilection for lacunae to develop.

MEDICAL MANAGEMENT

DIAGNOSIS. History of the neurologic event should be obtained, including timing, pattern of onset, and course. An embolic stroke occurs rapidly, with no warning. A more progressive and uneven onset is typical with thrombosis. The presenting symptoms will help to determine the location of the lesion. Information about the nature and severity of the ischemic insult may be just as important as the

"time" of the ischemic event for predicting outcome and making therapeutic judgments. Neuroimaging of the brain has become a standard procedure in the diagnosis of stroke. In the acute stroke setting, there is a trade-off between the increased information provided by perfusion imaging and the increased time needed to acquire additional imaging sequences. The performance of these additional imaging sequences should not unduly delay treatment with intravenous recombinant tissue plasminogen activator (rt-PA) in the ≤4.5-hour window in appropriate patients. Non–contrast-enhanced computed tomography (NECT) remains sufficient for identification of contraindications to fibrinolysis and allows patients with ischemic stroke to receive timely intravenous fibrinolytic therapy, but it should be obtained within 25 minutes of the patient's arrival.

CT scan is the fastest, most convenient and widely available test to use for the diagnosis and early treatment of acute stroke. CT scans may be normal in the acute stage of an embolic stroke. CT can rule out other pathologies and help determine the extent of the lesion. It can also determine where there is bleeding, which would prevent the use of clot-busting drugs. Figure 32-13 shows

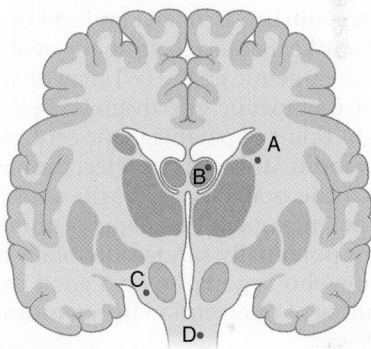

Figure 32-12

Usual sites of lacunar infarcts in the deep white matter. A, Internal capsule/putamen. **B,** Thalamus. **C,** Mesencephalon. **D,** Pons. (Reprinted from Pryse-Phillips W, Murray TJ: *Essential neurology: a concise textbook,* ed 4, New York, 1992, Medical Examination Publishing.)

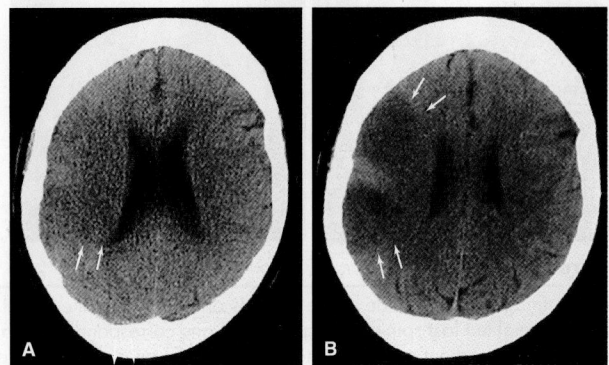

Figure 32-13

A, CT scan taken 2 hours 50 minutes after large right middle cerebral artery occlusion. There are subtle, ultra-early ischemic changes, including loss of the gray-white interface *(arrows)* and subtle evidence of sulcal effacement. **B,** CT scan of same patient approximately 8 hours after symptom onset shows acute hypodensity *(arrows)* and more prominent sulcal effacement. (Reprinted from Marx JA: *Rosen's emergency medicine: concepts and clinical practice,* ed 6, St Louis, 2006, Mosby.)

how an acute stroke looks on CT. Displacement of brain structures, such as the ventricles, by edema sometimes can be seen early in a large infarct. In ischemic stroke, CT scans reveal the area of decreased density and loss of grey/white matter differentiation resulting from edema. Cortical lesions appear wedge shaped and deeper lesions appear to be round or oval. Potential for hemorrhagic transformation of the ischemic infarct can often be seen on CT.[90] Lacunar infarcts are sometimes visible on CT scans as small, punched-out, hypodense areas. Images of lacunae can be seen in Figure 32-14. Identification of the penumbra and infarct core on hyperacute noncontrast and perfusion-weighted CT may lead to potentially more aggressive treatments related to reperfusion and to arrest progression of stroke damage in the early part of the stroke.[89] Figure 32-15 demonstrates how the use of new imaging techniques may assist in this goal.

MRI allows for the identification of an ischemic event within 2 to 6 hours of onset. The soft tissue contrast and multiplanar imaging capability offered by MRI have led to its wide acceptance as the method of choice for high-resolution brain imaging. Diffusion-weighted MRI (DWI) provides an indication of the brain tissue's physiologic response to ischemia and can document the evolution of stroke. Because halting the evolution of the stroke is the therapeutic goal, DWI may be useful in the evaluation of therapeutic effectiveness. Perfusion imaging uses a tight bolus of paramagnetic contrast agent and a sequence of rapid MRI scans to detect the passage of the agent through the brain tissue.[28] MRI stroke sequences can be used as a measure of ischemic penumbra and can help pinpoint potentially salvageable brain tissue, helping to identify who is going to be a good candidate for the later window of intervention using thrombolysis and who is not.[101]

Positron emission tomographic (PET) imaging has been of great benefit in advancing the understanding of the pathophysiology of cerebrovascular disorders. PET imaging allows for the detection of stroke earlier and with higher sensitivity than anatomic imaging with either MRI or CT. Furthermore, PET imaging has been useful in evaluating the extent of the functional damage because areas not immediately affected by the infarct may show hypometabolism or decreased blood flow. Initial stroke severity has been shown to correlate with the initially affected volume as determined by PET, whereas neurologic deterioration during the first week after stroke correlates with the proportion of the initially affected volume that infarcted, and functional outcome correlates with

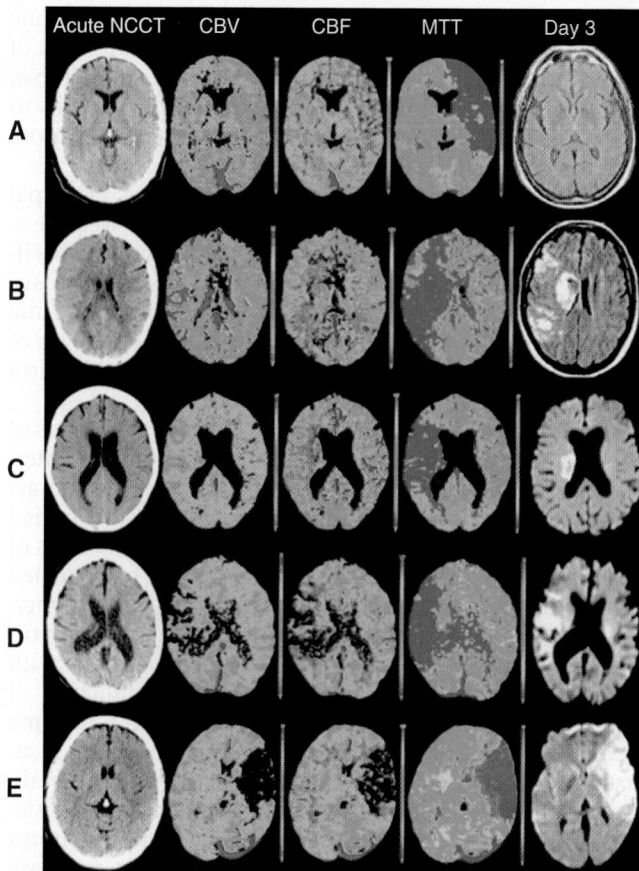

Figure 32-15

Patient A: Isolated focal swelling (IFS) on noncontrast CT (NCCT), hypoperfusion on mean transit time (MTT), and increased cerebral blood volume (CBV) on acute CT perfusion (CTP) maps, and no progression to infarction with subsequent major reperfusion. *Patient B:* IFS on NCCT, hypoperfusion on MTT, and increased CBV on acute CTP maps, but progression to infarction occurred without major reperfusion. *Patient C:* Hypoperfusion on MTT and increased CBV on acute CTP maps without any change apparent on acute NCCT. No infarction in cortical regions on follow-up with major reperfusion. *Patient D:* Hypoperfusion on MTT and decreased CBV on acute CTP maps without any apparent change on NCCT. Subsequent infarction present in reduced CBV regions on follow-up MRI. *Patient E:* Profound decrease in CBV and CBF on acute CTP maps with associated parenchymal hypoattenuation on NCCT. Extensive infarction on follow-up MRI. (Reprinted from Parsons M, Pepper EM, Bateman GA, et al: Identification of the penumbra and infarct core on hyperacute noncontrast and perfusion CT. *Neurology* 68:730–736, 2007.)

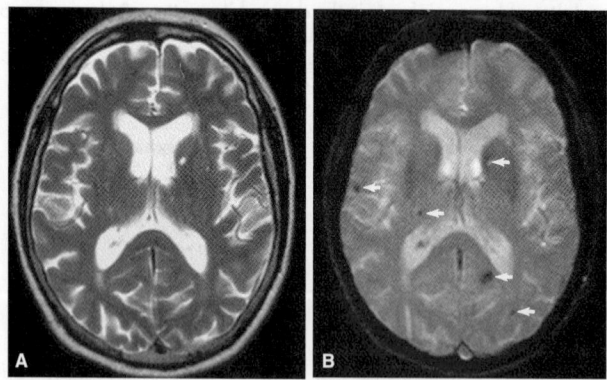

Figure 32-14

In these images, the left side of the brain is on the right of the panel. Axial T2-weighted fast spin-echo sequence (**A**) and corresponding axial T2*-weighted gradient echo sequence (**B**) from a 57-year-old man who presented with a left lacunar syndrome; his risk factors included hypertension and smoking. The T2-weighted fast spin-echo sequence shows several hyperintense foci in the cerebral white matter and basal ganglia but no microbleeds. The T2*-weighted gradient echo image shows several areas of focal signal loss consistent with microbleeds *(arrows)* in the right frontal lobe, right thalamus, left parietal lobe, and left caudate nucleus. (Reprinted from Werring DJ, Coward LJ, Losseff NA, et al: Cerebral microbleeds are common in ischemic stroke but rare in TIA, *Neurology* 65(12):1914–1918, 2005.)

the final infarct volume. Crossed cerebellar diaschisis is seen as hypometabolism and hypoperfusion in the cerebellar cortex contralateral to the site of the infarct and usually occurs during the first 2 months after infarction (Fig. 32-16).[82]

Cerebral angiography can be used in the absence of CT or MRI but is an invasive procedure and used only when other forms of imaging are not appropriate.

Studies of the carotid artery and vertebral arteries are performed using ultrasound evaluation. Doppler ultrasound looks at the flow velocity of the blood through the artery. Plaque accumulation and ulceration can be identified by Doppler. Doppler studies are used to determine the need for carotid endarterectomy.[44]

All acute stroke patients should undergo cardiovascular evaluation, both for determination of the cause of the stroke and to optimize immediate and long-term management. This cardiac assessment should not delay reperfusion strategies. Atrial fibrillation may be seen on an admission electrocardiogram; however, its absence does not exclude the possibility of atrial fibrillation as the cause of the event. Thus, ongoing monitoring of cardiac rhythm on telemetry or by Holter monitoring is indicated in some patients.

TREATMENT. The American Stroke Association recommends that blood pressure be kept less than 180/105 mm Hg after infusion of IV rt-PA and permissive hypertension up to a systolic blood pressure of 220 mm Hg and diastolic blood pressure of 120 mm Hg for those who do not receive thrombolysis unless there is a compelling indication otherwise.[1] An excessive rise in blood pressure may cause an increase in edema. When clinically stable, individuals with blood pressure greater than 140/90 mm Hg should be given medication to lower blood pressure. Unless contraindicated, use of diuretics and β-blockers should be the medication of choice. Angiotensin-converting enzyme inhibitors have been used with diabetes mellitus, heart failure, and MI.[83]

Emboli that lodge in the artery stem can cause edema. If not controlled, the edema can spread and create pressure in the area of the cerebellum and brainstem. Even a small amount of edema in the cerebellum can cause respiratory arrest from compression of the brainstem and lead to coma and death. It is the most common fatal complication. Water restriction and agents that raise the serum osmolarity should be considered with the onset of significant edema.

Thrombolytic and antithrombotic agents form the cornerstone of ischemic stroke treatment and prevention[3]: rt-PA is used for the emergent care of embolic stroke; t-PA activates plasminogen to form plasmin, which actively digests fibrin strands, and is effective in dissolving the thrombosis or blood clot responsible for the blockage.[4,128]

By promoting early recanalization of occluded vessels and early reperfusion of ischemic fields, there is potential to salvage penumbral neuronal tissue. If it is received within 4.5 hours after the initial stroke, the person is significantly more likely to recover function.[46] Recently, IV rt-PA has been used for up to 6 hours after the onset of symptoms.[32] The risk of brain hemorrhage with IV t-PA is about 5% in stroke patients and the inappropriate use in a stroke that is hemorrhagic will increase that risk. It must be determined on CT that the stroke is purely embolic; guidelines are established by the National Institute of Neurological Disorders and Stroke study.[35] With the use of DWI imaging and further understanding of the status of the ischemic penumbra, the window of opportunity may become larger and therapies more effective. Thrombolysis reduces the overall risk of dependency in the long term, although the incidence of fatal intracranial hemorrhage is increased.[127]

Several prognostic factors must be considered for selecting candidates for intravenous thrombolysis. Younger age, absence of cardiac disease or diabetes, lower blood pressure on admission, lower neurologic score, absence of early ischemic parenchymal changes, large artery thrombus visible on baseline brain CT, and a developed collateral circulation are all factors associated with a more favorable outcome. Risk factors for developing brain hemorrhage include time to treatment, dose of thrombolytics, blood pressure level, severity of neurologic deficit, and severity of ischemia.

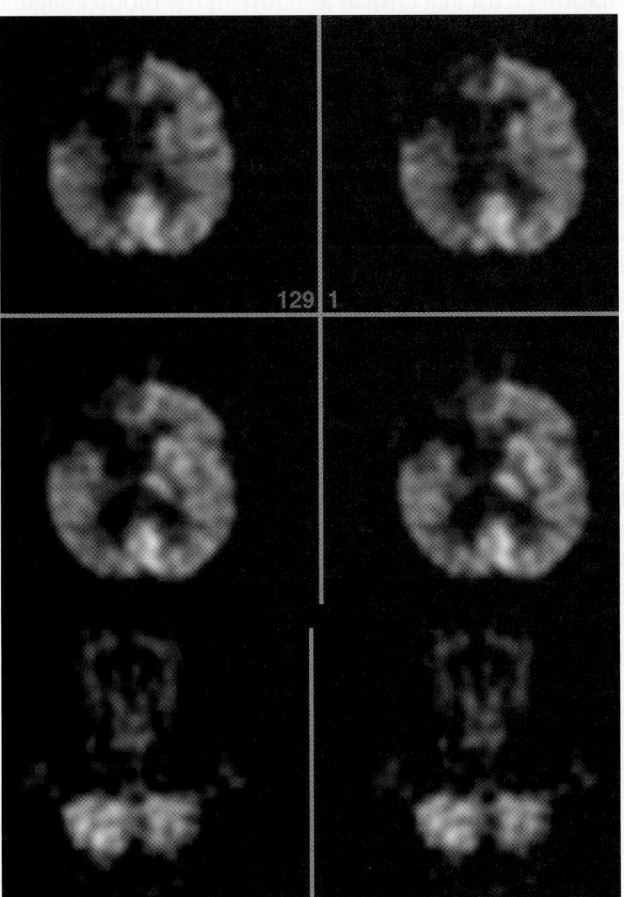

Figure 32-16

Fluorodeoxyglucose PET scan of a patient after embolic stroke in the distribution of the right anterior cerebral artery. There is severely decreased metabolism in the right frontal lobe extending to the midline. There is also crossed cerebellar diaschisis with decreased metabolism in the left cerebellum. (Reprinted from Newburg AB, Alavi A: The role of PET imaging in the management of patients with central nervous system disorders. *Radiol Clin North Am* 43:49–65, 2005.)

Besides hemorrhage, potential complications of thrombolysis include reperfusion injury, arterial reocclusion, and secondary embolization due to thrombus fragmentation. Thus, adequate hospital facilities and personnel are required for administration of thrombolytic therapy as well as for monitoring and managing potential complications. Following t-PA administration, blood pressure should be closely monitored and kept at less than 180/105 mm Hg and antithrombotic agents should be avoided for 24 hours.

Intracranial clot retrieval is now possible with endovascular thrombectomy. Endovascular thromboaspiration, sonothrombolysis, angioplasty, or stent placement can be performed. Most stroke centers are now offering these options, with trials done up to 8 hours after symptom onset when used with very large clots.[106] Mechanical interventions have seemed to be of the most benefit to patients who are either ineligible for thrombolysis or with large artery occlusions unlikely to resolve with thrombolysis by itself.[103]

Acute ischemic stroke is recognized as the third leading cause of death in the United States; improved treatments for management are important to reduce disability and death. The standard of care of acute stroke therapy has been reperfusion/recanalization of the occluded vessels using pharmacologic management, endovascular management, or a combination approach. Significant improvements have been made in the management with the use of endovascular therapy.

Prophylaxis

Anticoagulation. Anticoagulation therapy has played a prominent role in the prevention of acute infarction for several decades, and current research supports its use in high-risk individuals. The prevention of cardioembolic stroke is best accomplished with oral anticoagulation, barring any contraindications. Antiplatelets such as aspirin are used to decrease risk of second MI and may reduce the chance of stroke after MI.

Aspirin has become the antiplatelet standard for individuals with acute ischemic stroke who are not receiving thrombolysis. Several other antiplatelet agents such as ticlopidine, clopidogrel, and aspirin-dipyridamole have been shown to be more effective. The American Heart Association/American Stroke Association evidence-based guidelines for patients with noncardioembolic ischemic stroke recommend treatment with an antiplatelet agent, including aspirin, plus extended-release dipyridamole, and clopidogrel.[39]

Clopidogrel, a platelet adenosine diphosphate receptor antagonist, appears to be an effective antiplatelet drug that has rare interactions with other medication, although it should be used with caution in conjunction with heparin or warfarin or nonsteroidal antiinflammatory drugs.[25] Clopidogrel is deemed a reasonable alternative for patients allergic to aspirin.

Anticoagulation should not be used with high blood pressure or other risk factors of hemorrhagic stroke. Studies are underway to determine use in acute poststroke management.[56] Heparin can be used prophylactically against deep venous thrombosis and pulmonary embolism.

Warfarin sodium (Coumadin, Panwarfin) appears to be about twice as effective as aspirin in the prevention of stroke in individuals with atrial fibrillation. Use of warfarin after MI has shown reduced stroke risk overall but increases the chance for hemorrhagic stroke. Persons older than 75 years have the highest risk of stroke and can benefit from anticoagulation. The risk of bleeding increases with age, and the ability to determine the risk/benefit ratio is complex. These medications are probably currently underutilized in the older individuals at risk for stroke.[88] When there are contraindications to warfarin, aspirin is an alternative therapy.

Patients with atrial fibrillation (AF) at risk of stroke are not always anticoagulated with vitamin K antagonists (VKAs) despite lack of contraindication. Dabigatran, an oral direct thrombin inhibitor, is a new option with proven safety and effectiveness in these patients. Dabigatran is superior to warfarin for stroke prevention in patients with atrial fibrillation, with similar rates of major bleeding. Because it does not require laboratory monitoring, dabigatran therapy is less complicated than warfarin therapy, but it costs significantly more.[13]

Rivaroxaban is a direct inhibitor of factor Xa, a coagulation factor at a critical juncture in the blood coagulation pathway leading to thrombin generation and clot formation without significant rates of major bleeding, showing there is a favorable benefit-to-risk profile.[91] The high bioavailability and pharmacokinetic predictability of once- or twice-daily oral rivaroxaban is advantageous for extended prophylaxis and for treatment. Rivaroxiban is cleared by both renal and hepatic routes, but is contraindicated in cases of severe renal or hepatic dysfunction. There are also potential drug interactions with azole compounds or human immunodeficiency virus–protease inhibitors. The FDA has approved the anticoagulant apixaban (Eliquis) for a selective active site inhibitor of factor Xa to reduce the risk of stroke and systemic embolism in patients with nonvalvular atrial fibrillation. Apixaban is well absorbed after oral administration and is cleared by renal routes and other metabolic pathways. The most common and most serious adverse reactions observed in clinical trials were related to bleeding. If anticoagulation with Eliquis must be discontinued for a reason other than pathologic bleeding, coverage with another anticoagulant should be strongly considered.[80]

Lipid-Lowering Agents. Cholesterol-lowering agents such as statins decrease the risk of stroke after MI. Studies show that the anti-stroke effects may be separate from the lipid-lowering properties through changes in the endothelium, inflammatory response, plaque stabilization, and thrombus formation. Several organizations have endorsed the use of statins for stroke prevention. The FDA has added ischemic stroke as an indication for statin therapy. The use of statins, in accordance with National Cholesterol Education Program Adult Treatment Panel III guidelines, is endorsed by the American Heart Association and American Academy of Neurology for both primary and secondary prevention of stroke.[105]

Despite the success of the statins, a second class of agents, cholesterol absorption transport inhibitors, also has been developed and approved in the past decade for LDL cholesterol lowering, although only ezetimibe is currently available. It provides excellent tolerability and safety along with moderate reductions in LDL cholesterol of approximately 18%. There is the possibility of achieving LDL cholesterol reductions of up to 65% with combination therapy.[107]

PET studies have been used to monitor the success of various treatment regimens. PET has been used to evaluate the effects of thrombolytic therapy in acute stroke and has found that critically hypoperfused tissue can be preserved by early reperfusion and that large infarcts can be prevented by early reperfusion to viable tissue. In the future, functional imaging modalities that could eventually include tracers for neuronal integrity might be used to help in the selection of individuals for thrombolytic therapy, possibly permitting the extension of the critical time period for inclusion of individuals to aggressive stroke management strategies.[82]

Neuroprotection. Medications aimed at creating neuroprotection to decrease the amount of cell death secondary to excitotoxicity are being developed, and clinical studies are underway; however, results continue to be limited, and few studies have progressed to phase III.[33]

Excitotoxicity has been a widely investigated area in stroke. Ischemic neuronal injury in vitro depends on synaptic release of excitatory amino acids (EAAs) and resultant elevation of intracellular free calcium. Even transient exposure to excess excitatory amino acids is toxic to cultured neurons, and alterations in neuronal energy balance increases the vulnerability of neurons to excitotoxic damage even in the presence of physiologic concentrations of EAAs.[63] Evidence that this process progresses for several hours after the ischemic insult highlights a potential role for neuroprotective strategies administered during the critical window before irreversible loss, although the exact duration of this window in humans remains unknown. The action of glutamate on N-methyl-D-aspartate receptors seems to play an important role in glutamate-mediated toxicity. Compounds that decrease glutamate levels or interfere with its binding to this receptor have been the focus of many studies.[117]

Magnesium ion, which electrophysiologically behaves as a noncompetitive N-methyl-D-aspartate antagonist, has demonstrated efficacy as a neuroprotective agent in focal and global models of cerebral ischemia prompting current phase III trials.

Approaches directed at presynaptic reduction of pathologic glutamate release may control the damage caused by excess extracellular glutamate. Reducing the amplification of excitotoxic calcium ion release also may help control cell death. Neuroprotection is evident for the presynaptic glutamate release inhibitors 619C89 and lubeluzole when administered within 6 hours of induced ischemia. Both drugs are currently in phase II trials in stroke. A tetracycline derivative, minocycline, reduces inflammation and appears to protect against focal cerebral ischemia after stroke. It is most effective when started before ischemia develops but can be effective after the onset of ischemia. It has no therapeutic effect on astrogliosis or

spreading depression but may provide some protection from glutamate toxicity.[139]

Timing is critical in the administration of these drugs. The window of opportunity may be 2 to 6 hours after infarction. These antiexcitotoxic therapies may be suitable for either hemorrhagic or ischemic stroke and someday may be given by paramedics before full neurologic evaluation.[125]

Nerve Growth Factor. Animal studies providing treatment with bone marrow stromal cells ameliorates neurological functional deficits after stroke. Nerve growth factor is a neurotrophic factor that supports the survival and growth of neural cells. Noggin, an antagonist of bone morphogenetic protein, promotes the differentiation of stem cells into neurons. Treatment of stroke with a combination of transfection of nerve growth factor and Noggin in bone marrow stromal cells induced a synergistic effect on improved neurologic functional outcome.[21]

Surgical Intervention. Carotid endarterectomy is the treatment of choice for low-flow or embolic transient ischemic attack in individuals younger than 80 years old.[5] If stenosis is greater than 70% in a sclerotic lesion at the origin of the internal carotid artery, endarterectomy is indicated. Because women have arteries that are 10% smaller than men to begin with, the absolute size of the artery becomes significantly smaller with 70% occlusion. Therefore this equation may need to be looked at differently in women.

Careful selection of candidates for surgery is essential, as it takes an experienced team of surgeons and other health care providers to manage the postoperative course. Controversy surrounds the role of prophylactic endarterectomy in persons with asymptomatic extracranial carotic stenosis.[29]

Control of Symptoms. Pharmacotherapy of spasticity in stroke is controversial. Weakness of the extremities can result, and if the spasticity is contributing to stability, that may be lost with use of medications. Baclofen and benzodiazepines work at the level of the spinal cord; dantrolene works on the muscle fibers.

Treatment to decrease the firing of specific muscles with incobotulinumtoxinA (Botox) gives more discrete control of the choice of muscle to be injected and shows significant improvements in muscle tone and disability in patients with poststroke upper limb spasticity. It is also in common use for lower extremities; however, the studies to support this are not as evident as those on the upper extremities. Choosing the appropriate muscle or group of muscles is critical in a successful outcome. The effects of botulinum toxin usually last for approximately 3 to 6 months, so it is a temporary solution.[114]

Urinary incontinence can be a disabling sequela of stroke. Urge incontinence is treated with behavioral therapy and anticholinergics. An areflexic bladder can be managed with self-catheterization or use of a Foley catheter.

Depression after stroke is common and does not appear to be related to the area of lesion. Depression after stroke responds to treatment and should be guided by the other concomitant medical conditions and the side effects of the particular medication. Use of tricyclic antidepressants shows improvement within 3 to 6 weeks and should be continued for a minimum of 6 months.[47]

PROGNOSIS. The prognosis for survival after cerebral infarction is better than after intracerebral infarct or SAH. Loss of consciousness after an ischemic stroke implies a poorer prognosis than remaining conscious. Individuals with ischemic stroke are at risk for other strokes or MIs. The risk factors and type of damage related to the stroke syndrome relate to degree of disability and mortality.

Neurobiochemical markers of brain damage are being studied to determine a relation with outcome after stroke. Two such markers, protein S-100B and neuron-specific enolase, show a relation between the blood level 2 to 4 days after stroke and functional impairment and discharge from acute level of care.[138]

Recovery from stroke is the fastest in the first few weeks after onset, with the most measurable neurologic recovery (approximately 90%) in the first 3 months.[87] However, movement patterns can continue to be influenced by intervention with goal-directed activities, and repetition of movement appears to improve the speed and control of the movement in the individual up to 5 or more years after stroke. (See "Special Implications for the Therapist 32-1: Stroke Rehabilitation" below.)

Intracerebral Hemorrhage

Overview and Definition

Intracerebral hemorrhage (ICH) is bleeding from an arterial source into brain parenchyma (often referred to as an *intraparenchymal hemorrhage*) and is regarded as the most deadly of stroke subtypes. Primary ICH describes spontaneous bleeding in the absence of a readily identifiable precipitant and is usually attributable to microvascular disease associated with hypertension or aging. Secondary ICH occurs most often in association with trauma, impaired coagulation, toxin exposure, or an anatomic lesion. Chronic hypertension causes fibrinoid necrosis in the penetrating and subcortical arteries, weakening of the arterial walls, and formation of small aneurysmal outpouchings, or microaneurysms, that predispose to spontaneous ICH. Bleeding usually arises from the deep penetrating arteries of the circle of Willis, including the lenticulostriate, thalamogeniculate, and thalamoperforating arteries and perforators of the basilar artery. Acute rises in blood pressure and blood flow can also precipitate ICH even in the absence of preexisting severe hypertension. A ruptured vascular malformation is the second most common cause of ICH.

Bleeding is limited by the resistance of tissue pressure in the surrounding brain structures. If a hematoma is large, distortion of structures and increased ICP cause headache, vomiting, and decreased alertness. Because the cranial cavity is a closed system, enlargement of a hematoma or development of severe edema may shift brain tissues into another compartment, or herniate, and cause deterioration in the clinical condition.

Supratentorial ICH, so named because it occurs above the cerebellar tentorium, is classified as being lobar (i.e., involving the hemispheres of the cerebrum) or deep (i.e., implying involvement of structures of the midbrain, such as the thalamus, putamen, or caudate nucleus). Infratentorial, below the tentorium, refers to involvement of either the brainstem, usually the pons, or cerebellum.[100]

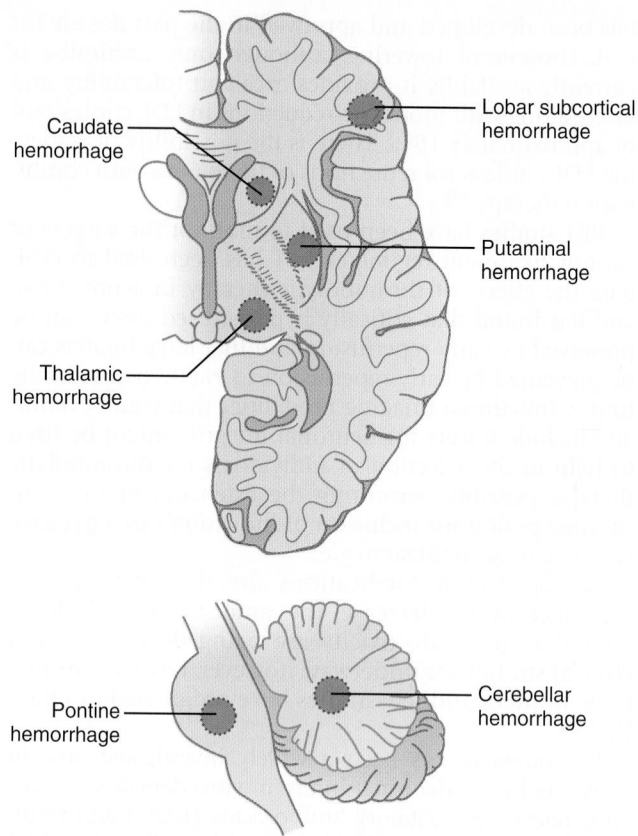

Figure 32-17

Horizontal cerebral section *(top)* and sagittal brainstem section *(bottom)* showing most common sites of ICH. (Modified from Caplan LR: *Caplan's stroke: a clinical approach*, ed 3, Boston, 2000, Butterworth-Heinemann.)

Incidence

The incidence of ICH is low among persons younger than 45 years, and it increases dramatically after the age of 65 years. In one study, the incidence of ICH doubled with each advancing decade until age 80 years, after which the incidence became 25 times higher.[99] ICH tends to occur more frequently in men. In the United States, African Americans are more likely to have an ICH than are whites. Worldwide rates are higher in Asian populations than in Western populations. ICH is a major cause of morbidity and death and accounts for 10% to 15% of all strokes in whites and about 30% of strokes in African Americans and individuals of Asian origin. Locations of hypertensive ICHs are the putamen (40%), lobar (22%), thalamus (15%), pons (8%), cerebellum (8%), and caudate (7%). Figures 32-17 and 32-18 represent the areas most likely to be involved in ICH and occurrences.

Spontaneous ICH can also occur in association with the prescription of anticoagulants, primary or metastatic brain tumors or granulomas, and use of sympathomimetic drugs. Aneurysms rarely bleed only into the brain, but when they do, they cause a local hematoma near the brain surface.

Etiologic and Risk Factors

Spontaneous ICH in the parenchyma of the brain usually is from an anomaly of the vessel structure or changes brought on by hypertension. Hypertension represents

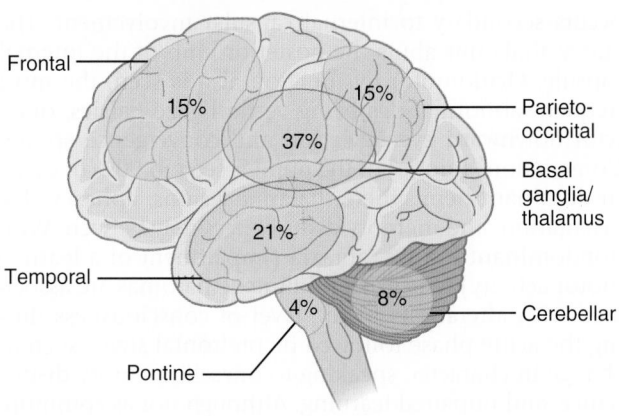

Figure 32-18

Sites of predilection of ICH. (Modified from Lindsay KW, Bone I, Callander R: *Neurology and neurosurgery illustrated*, New York, 1986, Churchill Livingstone.)

the single most important modifiable risk factor for ICH. Cerebral amyloid angiopathy (CAA) causing abnormal changes in the vessels of the brain accounts for approximately 10% of ICHs. CAA is recognized as an important cause of ICH in elderly persons.[37]

Excessive use of alcohol has been associated with massive spontaneous ICH. Alcohol has a number of acute and chronic effects that may contribute to hemorrhagic stroke, such as direct effects on cerebral vessels, hypertension, and impaired coagulation. Cocaine and amphetamine use is an important cause of ICH.

ICH is the most important adverse effect of thrombolytic therapy. Hemorrhage from fibrinolytic agents can occur within 12 to 24 hours and are typically lobar, occurring in the cortex and subcortical white matter.[104] Long-term anticoagulant therapy is associated with an increased risk for ICH. Many individuals with anticoagulant-associated ICH are also hypertensive, so that the extent of increased risk is difficult to clearly identify independently.[98]

Use of other medications in conjunction with thrombolytic therapy may place individuals at risk for ICH. A number of drugs, such as nonsteroidal antiinflammatory agents, nitrates, and propranolol, may affect platelet function and contribute to bleeding.[140]

Other possible risk factors include liver disease, prior ischemic stroke, and cigarette smoking. Obesity, sickle cell anemia, mitral valve prolapse, patent foramen ovale, and polycythemia have been identified as possible risk factors. More research in this area is ongoing and will provide more insight into the relation of chronic disease and lifestyle to ICH. Pregnancy may increase the risk of ICH. Eclampsia accounts for more than 40% of ICHs in pregnancy.

Pathogenesis

Histopathologic changes in the cerebral microvasculature of hypertensive individuals include processes that affect both the contents and the walls of the blood vessels of the brain. These changes are seen in small cerebral arteries and arterioles where they branch, and they are more severe in the small penetrating vessels in the deep white matter than in cortical vessels of similar size. Changes are more severe

distally than proximally. Smooth muscle cells are progressively replaced by collagen (hyalinization). Altered permeability of the vessel wall leads to fibrinoid changes in the vessel wall. This results in accumulation of proteinaceous material and fat deposits on the subintimal wall. The vessel wall becomes prone to leakage or rupture.[133]

Those with hypertension have a substantial reduction in the percentage of smooth muscle in the vessel wall. This decreased smooth muscle mass most likely represents structural weakening, resulting in rupture and hemorrhage. Necrosis of the endothelium may be a result of vessel ischemia. The changes in smooth muscle and the thickening of the intimal wall increase the metabolic requirements and impede the flow of oxygen to the outermost part of the vessel wall.

CAA is characterized by protein fibrils in the arterioles and small cerebral arteries and is formed by aberrant protein synthesis. Amyloid replaces smooth muscle in the media separating the elastic membranes. Lymphocytic infiltrates, hyaline arteriole degeneration, and fibrinoid necrosis are characteristic changes in the vessel wall. The parenchymal changes seen in CAA reflect the consequences of the vascular pathology and direct deposition of amyloid in the brain tissue. Brains with evidence of CAA frequently demonstrate periventricular demyelination, thought to be caused by ischemia from amyloid deposition in the vessels supplying the deep white matter.[38,47]

In drug-related ICH, some underlying vascular pathologic lesion may be present, such as an arteriovenous malformation (AVM) or chronic vasculitis. The ICH occurs as a result of a sudden increase in blood pressure triggered by the drug. The proposed mechanism for the increased incidence of ICH in the individual with increased alcohol ingestion is decreased circulating levels of clotting factors produced by the liver. Thrombocytopenia, which is often associated with alcoholism, may underlie or potentiate hemorrhage.[42]

Hemorrhagic transformation, or conversion of an ischemic cerebral infarction, refers to secondary bleeding thought to occur either with early reperfusion into a damaged vascular bed with impaired autoregulation or as a result of development of collateral circulation into the same vascular bed.

When hemorrhage occurs, it spreads along a path of least resistance, primarily following the fiber tracts of the white matter. Grey matter, with its dense cell structure, is more resistant to the shearing forces of the growing hematoma and is more likely than white matter to be compressed rather than infiltrated by the spreading hematoma. Edema forms in the parenchyma surrounding the hematoma. Blood is reabsorbed by macrophages at the periphery of the hemorrhage, leaving a cavity surrounded by necrotic tissue. This process usually takes weeks to months.[132]

Clinical Manifestations

Neurologic symptoms occur gradually in most cases, representing the expansion of the hematoma. In some cases (approximately 30%) onset is sudden, which is also characteristic of an ischemic stroke. The earliest signs relate to blood issuing into parenchymatous structures. For example, a hematoma in the left putamen and internal capsule would first cause weakness of the right limbs; a cerebellar hematoma would cause gait ataxia. As the hematomas enlarge, the focal symptoms increase. If the hematoma becomes large enough to raise ICP, headache, vomiting, and decreased alertness develop. Some hematomas remain small and the only symptoms relate to the focal collection of blood. Once the condition is stabilized, the symptoms improve in parallel with the resorption of the hematoma.

Although headache is an important symptom of ICH, it is present in severe form in only 30% to 40% of cases. Headache is most common as a sign of superficial and large hemorrhages.

The incidence of seizure correlates with the location of the hemorrhage. Cerebral cortex hemorrhage causes the most prevalent seizure activity. Two-thirds of the seizures are generalized and one-third are focal. Focal seizures affect the body on the contralateral side (see Chapter 36). The level of consciousness at onset is unrelated to the occurrence of seizure.

Syndromes. Syndromes associated with ICH are representative of the area of bleed and reflect brain activity of the particular site.[9] Table 32-1 gives typical signs in individuals with ICHs at various sites.

Putamen. Approximately 50% to 80% of hemorrhages occur in the putamen. The result is contralateral sensorimotor deficit resulting from its proximity to the internal capsule. Small putamen hemorrhages may mimic lacunar syndromes, such as pure motor weakness. A type of aphasia may be present that mimics Broca aphasia when the lesion is in the midputamen. Wernicke aphasia is seen with a posterior putamen lesion. Pupillary abnormalities, visual field loss, and oculomotor deficits are common. Conjugate gaze deviation toward the side of the lesion may be present. Abulia and motor impersistence are seen when the anterior putamen is affected. Headache and vomiting also occur in about 25% of cases.

Thalamus. Sensory losses, or dysesthesias, are common with thalamic hemorrhage, and some motor deficit

occurs secondary to internal capsular involvement. The lateral thalamus abuts the posterior limb of the internal capsule. Oculomotor dysfunction also is seen, the most frequent abnormalities being vertical gaze palsies, often with downward eye deviation and convergence spasm. Constriction (miosis) of the pupil is seen in 50% of cases. In dominant hemisphere thalamic lesions, aphasia, disorientation, and memory disturbances may be seen. With nondominant lesions, apraxia (impairment of a learned motor activity) may exist. Midline hematomas are associated with alterations in the level of consciousness during the acute phase followed by prefrontal signs, such as change in character, speaking to oneself, memory disturbance, and impaired learning. Although not as common, the individual may experience symptoms such as headache, nausea, and vomiting to the same degree as with putamen hemorrhage.

Cerebellum. A hallmark of cerebellar hemorrhages is ataxia. Additional symptoms may be nausea and vomiting, and dizziness with nystagmus and vertigo often is present. The individual may be dysarthric. Brainstem signs, such as facial paresis, can be present with a hemorrhage that extends to the brainstem. The signs of cerebellar hemorrhage should be carefully monitored, as the progression to compression of vital structures in the region of the fourth ventricle and medulla can be rapid and can produce life-threatening changes.

Pons. Brainstem hemorrhages commonly arise in the midline of the pons, leading to coma, quadriparesis, and nonreactive pupils with absent horizontal eye movement. Lateral pontine hemorrhage can result in extraocular paresis with deviation away from the side of the lesion. Quick, downward jerks of the eye occur with a slow, upward drift. Pupils are small but reactive. Contralateral sensory and motor symptoms and ipsilateral cerebellar signs also are seen.

Table 32-1	Signs in Patients with Intracerebral Hemorrhages at Various Sites			
Location	**Motor/Sensory**	**Eye Movements**	**Pupils**	**Other Signs**
Putamen or internal capsule	Contralateral hemiparesis and hemisensory loss	Ipsilateral conjugate deviation	Normal	Left: aphasia Right: left-sided neglect
Thalamus	Contralateral hemisensory loss	Down and in upgaze palsy	Small; react poorly	Somnolence, decreased alertness; left: aphasia
Lobar				
Frontal	Contralateral limb weakness	Ipsilateral conjugate gaze	Normal	Abulia
Temporal	None	None		Hemianopia Left: aphasia
Occipital	None	None		Hemianopia
Parietal	Slight contralateral hemiparesis and hemisensory loss			Hemianopia; left: aphasia; right: left neglect; poor drawing and copying
Caudate	None or slight contralateral hemiparesis	None	Normal	Abulia, agitation, poor memory
Pons	Quadriparesis	Bilateral horizontal gaze paresis, ocular bobbing	Small; reactive	Coma
Cerebellar	Gait ataxia, ipsilateral limb hypotonia	Ipsilateral gaze or cranial nerve VI paresis	Small	Vomiting, inability to walk, tilt when sitting

Caudate. Caudate hemorrhages can rupture into the ventricles and therefore have a presentation like that of an SAH. Headache, vomiting, and loss of consciousness may occur. The internal capsule may be involved, causing sensorimotor involvement.

Internal Capsule. Internal capsule hemorrhages often result in a pure motor, pure sensory, or sensorimotor stroke with ataxia. The internal capsule is a white matter tract that is situated lateral to the basal ganglia as it connects to the cerebral cortex.

Lobar. Lobar hematomas are centered in the immediate subcortical white matter. Symptoms are lobe-specific (see "Clinical Manifestations" in "Ischemic Stroke" above and "Higher Brain Disorders" in Chapter 28). Seizures are more common with lobar hemorrhages than with deeper bleeds.

MEDICAL MANAGEMENT

DIAGNOSIS. The availability of CT allows for prompt diagnosis of ICH. The specific area of damage can be imaged and the amount of blood identified. CT also has documented acute clot retraction progression of hypertensive ICH and early hemorrhagic infarction. It accurately documents the size and location of the hematoma, the presence and extent of any mass effect, and the presence of hydrocephalus and intraventricular hemorrhage. CT scans should be performed immediately in individuals suspected of having an ICH. Follow-up CT scans are utilized when there is a change in clinical signs or state of alertness in order to monitor changes in the size of the lesion and ventricular system and to detect important pressure shifts. If the clinical syndrome and CT findings are typical of hypertensive hemorrhage in the basal ganglia, caudate nucleus, thalamus, pons, or cerebellum, angiography is usually not necessary. If the hemorrhage is in an atypical location, and the individual is young and not hypertensive, angiography is indicated to exclude an AVM, aneurysm, vasculitis, or tumor. Individuals who have ICH after cocaine use have a high likelihood of vascular malformations and aneurysms and need angiography. Particular attention should be directed to the presence of a coagulopathy. A drug screen should be obtained to evaluate use of sympathomimetics if substance abuse is suspected. Increased sympathetic outflow due to the hemorrhage may lead to an increase in dysrhythmias. Dysrhythmias also may signal impending brainstem compression from an expanding hemorrhage.

MRI can provide multiplanar views and can discriminate subtle tissue changes and rapidly flowing blood. However, it is of limited usefulness in the first 24 hours after ICH. MRI has the capability to detect previous hemorrhage, and it can image the posterior fossa more clearly than can CT.

Prothrombin time, partial thromboplastin time, and platelet count should be performed in all individuals to rule out a bleeding disorder. Coagulation factor deficiencies can be detected by evaluation of liver enzymes. Bleeding time, platelet aggregation studies, and fibrinogen assay also can be indicators of disorders related to possible repeat hemorrhage.

The differential diagnosis for ICH is similar to that of ischemic stroke and includes migraine, seizure, tumor, abscess, hypertensive encephalopathy, and trauma. Hypertensive encephalopathy and migraine also can present with headache, nausea, and vomiting. Although focal neurologic signs are uncommon, they may occur with these entities. With hypertensive encephalopathy, individuals usually have marked elevation in blood pressure and other evidence of end-organ injury, including proteinuria, cardiomegaly, papilledema, and malignant hypertensive retinopathy. These individuals usually improve significantly with treatment of hypertension. Migraines often are associated with an aura, and the individual often has a history of similar headaches.

The difference between ICH and labyrinthitis can be especially difficult to determine in the elderly. The abrupt onset of vertigo, vomiting, and nystagmus can represent a peripheral process, such as labyrinthitis, or a central process, such as cerebellar or brainstem infarct or hemorrhage. Age older than 40 years and a history of hypertension or other risk factors for ICH increase the possibility of a cerebellar hemorrhage. Findings specifically referable to the brainstem must be sought; these include hiccups, diplopia, facial numbness, dysphagia, and ataxia. Vertiginous individuals often have a strong desire to remain immobile with their eyes closed, but this must not preclude a thorough cranial nerve and cerebellar examination, including gait. Gross ataxia is present with cerebellar stroke and absent with labyrinthine disease. A head CT scan should be strongly considered in individuals older than age 40 years to assist in differentiating labyrinthitis and cerebellar hemorrhage.

A screen for toxic substances in the blood should be performed, especially in the younger population. Acquired immunodeficiency syndrome should be considered as a possible cause of ICH. Biopsy of brain tissue can be diagnostic of CAA, cerebral vasculitis, and neoplasm. Evaluation of cerebrospinal fluid may indicate levels of toxicity; however, individuals with increased ICP are at risk during the procedure for possible herniation causing compression of the brainstem.

TREATMENT. The acute reduction of elevated blood pressure is advisable and is most readily accomplished with rapid-acting, potent antihypertensive medication along with effective control of increased ICP, which exacerbates blood pressure elevation.[60] A major issue in the management of ICH is control of edema (see "Treatment" under "Ischemic Stroke" above). Anticonvulsant therapy should be considered with lobar hemorrhage.

The frequency of ICH may increase with the use of long-term anticoagulation therapy. Treatment with vitamin K is useful to correct an elevated prothrombin time; however, this takes 12 to 24 hours. Fresh-frozen plasma immediately restores diminished clotting factors. Protamine sulfate is the treatment of choice for reversal of the heparin effect. Thrombocytopenia responds to plasma infusion and plasma exchange.

An individual with a potential ICH requires rapid assessment and transport to a facility that has CT scanning capability and intensive care management. The prehospital management is similar to that for ischemic stroke. The circumstances surrounding the event and other concomitant medical conditions also should be ascertained. An evaluation of the initial level of consciousness, Glasgow Coma Scale, any gross focal deficits, difficulty with speech, clumsiness, gait disturbance, or facial asymmetry should be noted.

Supportive care involving attention to airway management and perfusion is of the highest priority. Individuals with hemorrhagic stroke are more likely to have an altered level of consciousness that may progress rapidly to unresponsiveness, requiring emergent endotracheal intubation. Intravenous access and cardiac monitoring should be initiated. Evaluation of blood glucose and appropriate dextrose and naloxone administration should be considered in any patient with altered mental status.

There is disagreement regarding optimal blood pressure management in an individual with ICH. Hypertension may cause deterioration by increasing ICP and potentiating further bleeding from small arteries or arterioles. Hypotension may decrease cerebral blood flow, worsening brain injury. In general, recommendations for treatment of hypertension in individuals with ICH are more aggressive than those for individuals with ischemic stroke. The current consensus for ICH is to recommend antihypertensive treatment with parenteral agents for systolic pressures greater than 160 to 180 mm Hg or diastolic pressures greater than 105 mm Hg. Treatment for lower blood pressures is controversial. Disadvantages include the need for careful monitoring (ideally with an indwelling arterial catheter) and the theoretical risk of worsening the hemorrhage secondary to the vasodilatory effects of nitroprusside on cerebral vessels. Labetalol is another therapeutic option.

Hyperventilation and diuretics such as mannitol move fluid from the intracranial compartment, thereby reducing cerebral edema. These interventions should not be used prophylactically. Although this effect may be temporarily helpful in the acute setting, because the brain tissue reequilibrates, rebound swelling can occur and worsen the individual's clinical status. These agents also can cause dehydration and lead to hypotension. The use of steroids in cerebral hemorrhage, previously a common practice, may be harmful and is not recommended. Other experimental modalities include barbiturate coma and hypothermia. Seizure activity can cause neuronal injury, elevations in ICP, and destabilization of an already critically ill individual. In addition, nonconvulsive seizure may contribute to coma. Seizure prophylaxis (18 mg/kg phenytoin) should be considered for individuals with ICH, especially individuals with lobar hemorrhage.

Selected individuals with sizable lobar hemorrhage and progressive neurologic deterioration may benefit from surgical drainage. Surgery is more efficacious in individuals with cerebellar hemorrhage. The clinical course in cerebellar hemorrhage is notoriously unpredictable. Individuals with minimal findings may deteriorate suddenly to coma and death with little warning. For this reason, most neurosurgeons consider emergent surgery for individuals with cerebellar hemorrhage within 48 hours of onset.

PROGNOSIS. Although the overall mortality from ICH is high, functional recovery among survivors is also high. The most important predictor of mortality is hemorrhage size. The individuals who are comatose at onset or who have a wide spectrum of neurologic deficits tend to do poorly compared with those who remain alert and have focal neurologic symptoms. Survival depends on the location, size, and rapidity of development of the hematoma. ICHs are at first soft and dissect along white matter fiber tracts. If the individual survives the initial changes in ICP, blood is absorbed and a cavity or slit forms that may disconnect

brain pathways. Individuals with small hematomas located deep and near midline structures often develop secondary herniation and mass effect and have a high mortality rate. Survivors invariably have severe neurologic deficits. In individuals with medium-sized hematomas, the deficit varies with the location and size of the hematomas. Most individuals survive with some residual neurologic signs. Survival for individuals with hemorrhage in the posterior fossa is more dependent on location of hemorrhage than size. Midline pontine hemorrhage is often fatal, whereas lateral hemorrhages carry a better prognosis.

Subarachnoid Hemorrhage

Overview and Definition

SAH can begin with the sudden onset of a "thunderclap" with searing pain; sometimes the headache begins with exertion. SAH results in frank blood in the subarachnoid space between the arachnoid and the pia, which are contiguous membranes that surround the brain tissue. SAH can be spontaneous, is often seen in normotensive persons, and results in a sudden, severe headache. One percent to 4% of all individuals presenting to the emergency department with a headache have an SAH.

Etiologic and Risk Factors

Aneurysm and vascular malformations are responsible for most SAHs. SAH can be the result of trauma, developmental defects, neoplasm, or infections that cause rupture into the subarachnoid space. Hypertension may be seen in 32% and fever in 5%. Vascular malformations are responsible for approximately 6% of hemorrhages into the subarachnoid space. Included in vascular malformations are venous malformation, AVM, and cavernous malformation. The highest incidence of SAH is in women over the age of 70 years. Risk factors for SAH include smoking, excessive alcohol consumption, and hypertension. Genetic associations are being studied. A total of nine suggestive linkage regions have been identified with 2 that have appeared in several populations: the 7q11.2, also known as the intracranial berry aneurysm-1 (ANIB1) and the region at chromosome 19q13.3.[79]

First-degree relatives of persons who have experienced an SAH have a threefold to sevenfold increased risk of an SAH. If transmitted genetically, the effect will most likely be on the connective tissue. Aneurysms are also more common among individuals with hereditary connective tissue disorders. Individuals with hemorrhage resulting from an aneurysm tend to be younger than those with hemorrhage secondary to hypertension.

Individuals with fibromuscular dysplasia, polycystic kidney disease, or connective tissue diseases have a higher incidence of aneurysms. Embolization, often from endocarditis, can cause mycotic aneurysms. Fungi or tumor tissue can travel to the brain. About one-fifth of individuals with aneurysms have more than one vascular anomaly or other aneurysms.

Types of Subarachnoid Hemorrhage

Berry aneurysm is a congenital abnormal distention of a local vessel that occurs at a bifurcation, where the medial layer of the vessel is the weakest. About 90% of SAHs are due to berry aneurysms. Aneurysms are probably caused by a combination of congenital defects in the vascular wall and degenerative changes. Aneurysms usually occur at branching sites on the large arteries of the circle of Willis at the base of the brain. When an aneurysm ruptures, blood is released under arterial pressure into the subarachnoid space and quickly spreads through the cerebrospinal fluid around the brain and spinal cord. Aneurysms are less often caused by arterial dissection through the adventitia of arterial walls, embolism of infected material of distal cerebral arteries (mycotic aneurysms), and degenerative elongation and tortuosity of arteries (dolichoectasia). Figure 32-19 shows the typical formations of berry aneurysms.

Venous malformations are composed entirely of veins, which are usually thickened and hyalinized, with minimal elastic tissue or smooth muscle. The veins converge on a draining vein. Normal brain parenchyma is interspersed among the vessels. Venous malformation is the most common form of vascular malformation, constituting approximately 50% of malformations. The risk of hemorrhage from venous malformation has been estimated at 20% per year. Individuals with a cerebellar malformation have the greatest risk of hemorrhage. Occasionally, seizures may be associated with venous malformations. Headaches and focal neurologic deficits are manifested according to the area of the brain that is disrupted.

Arteriovenous malformation is characterized by direct artery-to-vein communication without an intervening capillary bed. The blood vessel contains elastin and smooth muscle cells. Brain parenchyma is found within the AVM, and it is usually gliotic and nonfunctional. AVMs are the result of abnormal fetal development at approximately 3 weeks' gestation. More than 90% of AVMs occur in the cerebral hemispheres. Most AVMs are sporadic, but familial AVMs occur; these appear to have an autosomal-dominant inheritance with incomplete penetrance.

The annual risk of bleeding from an AVM is 1% to 4%. AVMs result in an SAH more than 50% of the time. Seizures, headache, or an audible bruit may precede a hemorrhage. Progressive focal neurologic deficits develop in some individuals, and cognitive decline may also precede a hemorrhage. AVM-associated hemorrhages occur predominantly in the third and fourth decades of life.

Malformations less than 3 cm in diameter are more likely to bleed than are larger AVMs because arterial pressure is higher in the smaller vessels. A single draining vein, obstructed drainage, or a periventricular or intraventricular location increases the risk of hemorrhage.

Angiography is the definitive diagnostic procedure for an AVM. CT scanning is diagnostic for a dense lesion in the brain. Suspicion of an AVM arises when an area of decreased density is seen around the hematoma and heterogeneous densities appear within the hematoma. MRI is not useful in the diagnosis; however, AVM can be suspected based on MRI with evidence of intravascular moving blood. An AVM should be suspected as a cause of hemorrhage in persons younger than 40 years, especially if they are normotensive. Figures 32-20 and 32-21 represent the vascular disorder and its appearance on imaging.[94]

Approximately 10% of individuals die from an AVM hemorrhage. In the first year following the hemorrhage,

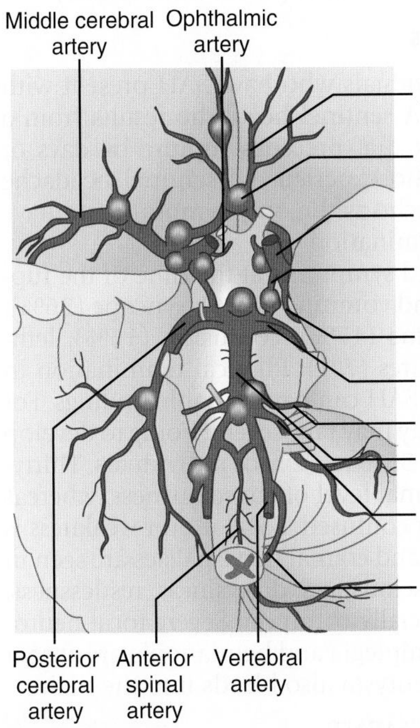

Middle cerebral artery

Ophthalmic artery

Anterior cerebral artery

Anterior communicating artery

Internal carotid artery

Posterior communicating artery

Anterior choroidal artery

Superior cerebellar artery

Internal auditory artery

Basilar artery

Anterior inferior cerebellar artery

Posterior inferior cerebellar artery

Posterior cerebral artery

Anterior spinal artery

Vertebral artery

Figure 32-19

Berry aneurysms typically develop at the bifurcations of arteries on the undersurface of the brain. (Reprinted from Goldman L: *Cecil textbook of medicine,* ed 22, Philadelphia, 2004, WB Saunders.)

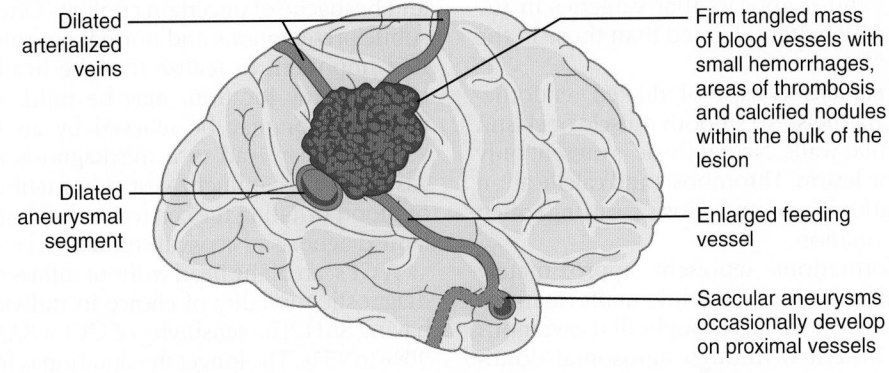

Dilated arterialized veins

Dilated aneurysmal segment

Firm tangled mass of blood vessels with small hemorrhages, areas of thrombosis and calcified nodules within the bulk of the lesion

Enlarged feeding vessel

Saccular aneurysms occasionally develop on proximal vessels

Figure 32-20

Typical deformation of blood vessels and brain tissue in relation to an AVM. (Reprinted from Lindsay KW, Bone I, Callander R: *Neurology and neurosurgery illustrated,* New York, 1986, Churchill Livingstone.)

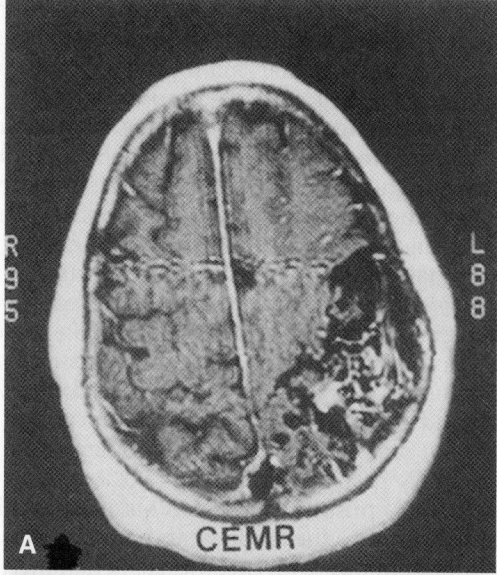
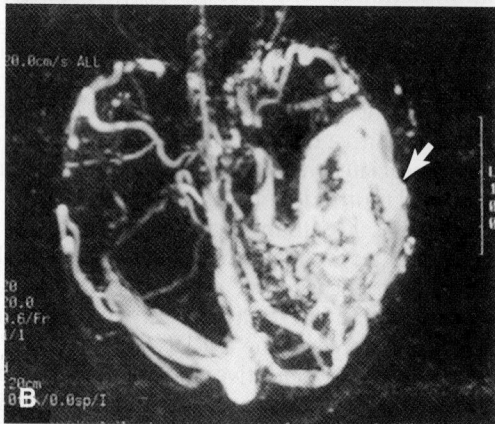

Figure 32-21

The AVM as seen with MRI (**A**) and MR angiography (**B**). *Arrow* points to enlarged vessel in periphery of AVM. (Reprinted from Ramsey R: *Neuroradiology*, Philadelphia, 1994, WB Saunders.)

the chance of recurrence is 6%. A concomitant aneurysm increases the chance of recurrent bleeding to 7%.[8]

Neuroradiologic embolization, stereotactic radiotherapy, and surgery are the current treatments for AVM. These techniques are used alone or in combination depending on the size and site of the lesion. Vasospasm after surgery is a side effect, and it appears that surgeries in the posterior circulation are better tolerated than those in the anterior circulation.[67]

Cavernous malformations consist of dilated, endothelium-lined, fibrous channels. No smooth muscle or elastin is present in the vascular walls. Neural tissue is present only at the periphery of the lesion. Thrombosis and calcification within the malformation occur, and gliosis (scarring) often surrounds the malformation.

Cavernous malformations represent approximately 10% of vascular malformations. Multiple malformations can occur in the same person. It is thought that cavernous malformations are inherited through autosomal dominance, with close to 100% penetration. Hispanics are at particular risk for the familial disorder. No apparent relation exists between malformation size and age and the

likelihood of hemorrhage. Women tend to be more susceptible to hemorrhage than men. Subclinical bleeding frequently occurs around the malformation.

MRI is the imaging procedure of choice for visualizing cavernous malformations. The malformation appears as a well-defined region with a central area of mixed signal intensity surrounded by a rim of hypointensity.

The majority of individuals recover from a cavernous malformation hemorrhage, and the risk of repeat bleeding is low. Spontaneous rupture of a venous malformation is not common, and the resulting hemorrhage is often not of great consequence. Surgery is the treatment of choice for malformations that have hemorrhaged and are in an accessible part of the brain. The majority of individuals recover from a cavernous malformation hemorrhage, and the risk of recurrence is low.

Syndromes are associated with the location of the hemorrhage, as they are in ICH. (See section above.)

Clinical Manifestations

Forty percent of individuals who have SAH present with a sentinel headache. A sentinel headache results from a minor aneurysm leak that precedes rupture by days or weeks. Individuals who experience a sentinel headache typically report headache as the only symptom and have a normal physical examination

Common associated symptoms at the time of the rupture include nausea and vomiting (75%), syncope (36%), neck pain (24%), coma (17%), confusion (16%), lethargy (12%), and seizures (7%). Physical examination in individuals who have SAH can have variable findings. For example, nuchal rigidity may take several hours to develop and is present in only 35% to 52% of individuals. Thirty-six percent have a normal level of consciousness, whereas 28% are somnolent or confused. Focal motor weakness is detected in only 10%, and cranial nerve palsies are seen in 9%. Alteration of consciousness, drowsiness, restlessness, and agitation are especially common. Severe focal neurologic signs such as hemiplegia and hemianopia are absent at onset unless the aneurysm also bleeds into the brain.

MEDICAL MANAGEMENT

DIAGNOSIS. Up to 38% of individuals who have an SAH are misdiagnosed initially. Misdiagnosis of SAH is associated with increased morbidity and mortality. The most common misdiagnoses for SAH are viral meningitis, migraine, and headache of uncertain etiology. Often individuals have subtle presentations and normal neurologic examinations. It is important to realize that the headache of SAH may occur in any location, may be mild, may resolve spontaneously, or may be relieved by analgesics. Prominent vomiting may lead to a misdiagnosis of viral syndrome, gastroenteritis, influenza, or viral meningitis. The presence of blood irritating the cervical or lumbar theca may lead to a misdiagnosis of cervical strain or sciatica.

A CT scan of the head without intravenous contrast is the diagnostic modality of choice in individuals suspected of having SAH. The sensitivity of CT for SAH is approximately 90% to 95%. The longer the duration is from onset of symptoms, the lower is the sensitivity of CT for SAH. Therefore, a lumbar puncture should be performed in all individuals suspected of having an SAH when the CT scan is negative or inadequate. The hematoma caused by an aneurysm tends to be of a different character than that caused by hypertension. The location of hemorrhage is also a clue to the diagnosis of aneurysm. Primary sites for hematoma resulting from aneurysms are in the area of the corpus callosum and anterior horns, the frontal lobe, and the temporal lobes. Angiography is required to establish that an intracerebral hematoma has been caused by a ruptured aneurysm.

TREATMENT. Once the diagnosis of SAH is made, a neurosurgical consultation and arrangement for transport to the closest emergency department is critical. The treatment of individuals with SAH involves the prevention and management of the relatively common secondary complications of SAH: rebleeding, vasospasm, hydrocephalus, hyponatremia, and seizures. About one-half of individuals with SAH have vasospasm, and this problem may resolve or progress to cerebral infarction. Fifteen percent to 20% of individuals with vasospasm die despite maximal therapy. Angiographic vasospasm has a typical temporal course: onset between 3 and 5 days after hemorrhage, maximal narrowing at 5 to 14 days, and gradual resolution over 2 to 4 weeks. Decreasing the risk of delayed cerebral ischemia involves fluids, avoidance of antihypertensive drugs, and administration of the calcium antagonist nimodipine.[120]

The International Subarachnoid Aneurysm Trial confirmed endovascular treatment as the treatment of choice for intracranial berry aneurysms. Isolating the aneurysm or rupture site from the circulation is the primary goal of treatment via coiling or clipping. Spontaneous rupture of a venous malformation is not common, and the resulting bleed is often not of great consequence. Surgical resection of the hematoma may be necessary if it is significantly extensive. With evacuation of the hematoma, the malformation is left intact in most cases.

PROGNOSIS. Mortality rate from SAH is high in elderly persons. Functional outcomes are poor, and few individuals 75 years or older are able to live independently at discharge. Early aggressive surgical treatment of elderly individuals admitted in good condition may lead to better outcomes. Seizure-like episodes occur in 25% of individuals after SAH.

If the resulting hematoma is less than 3 cm, the prognosis is good. Evacuation of hematomas that are larger should include resection of the causative aneurysm. Prompt removal may result in dramatic and early improvement of neurologic function. Repeat hemorrhage is more likely to occur if the hematoma is evacuated without treatment of the ruptured aneurysm.[88,108]

Subdural Hemorrhage

A subdural hemorrhage, or hematoma, is most often the result of tearing of the bridging veins between the brain surface and dural sinus. It results in accumulation of blood in the dural space. If it is a small amount, the body can reabsorb the fluid; if the blood is of great enough volume, as can occur with trauma, it becomes a space-occupying lesion. The lesion is reflected in the area of the hemorrhage and the result can be herniation of the cortex into the adjoining spaces. Figure 32-22 illustrates the

actual spaces and potential spaces in the cranial meninges. Compression of the brain tissue can result in both localized lesions and general decrease in the level of consciousness. Figure 32-23 represents the pressures on the brain that accompany a subdural hemorrhage. Chronic subdural hematoma (CSH) is defined as a subdural hemorrhage that is more than 20 days old. The peak incidence for CSH occurs in the sixth and seventh decades, with up to 80% occurring in elderly men. In elderly persons, CSH often is caused by minor trauma, especially falls. In the majority of cases, there is no underlying brain injury. Fragility of the bridging veins and cerebral atrophy allow increased movement of the brain within the skull, thereby predisposing elderly individuals to CSH.

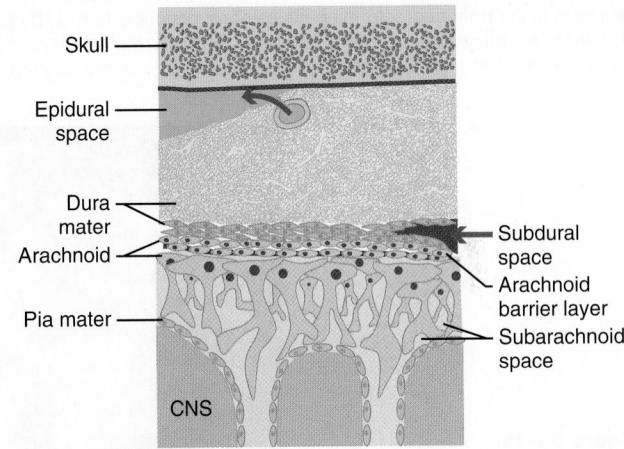

Figure 32-22

Actual spaces and potential spaces in the cranial meninges. Epidural space between dura and skull can be opened up by blood from a ruptured meningeal artery. Subdural space may be opened up by blood from a vein that tears as it cross the arachnoid to enter a dural sinus. (Reprinted from Nolte J: *The human brain*, St Louis, 2002, Mosby.)

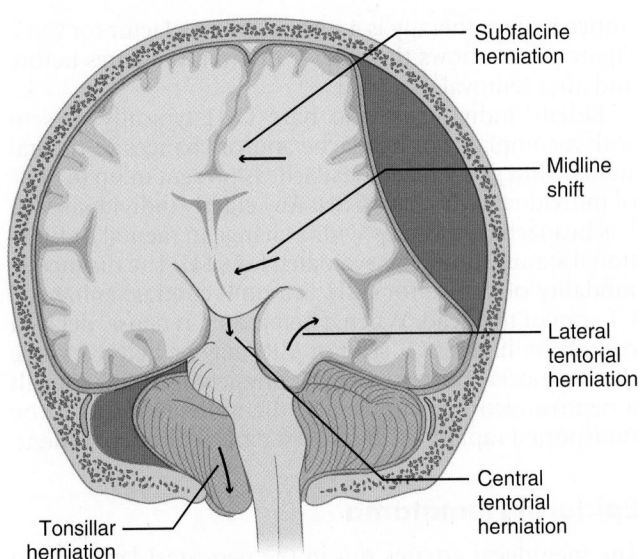

Figure 32-23

Compression of brain tissue with herniation into adjacent structures produced by the subdural hemorrhage. (Reprinted from Lindsay KW, Bone I, Callander R: *Neurology and neurosurgery illustrated*, New York, 1986, Churchill Livingstone.)

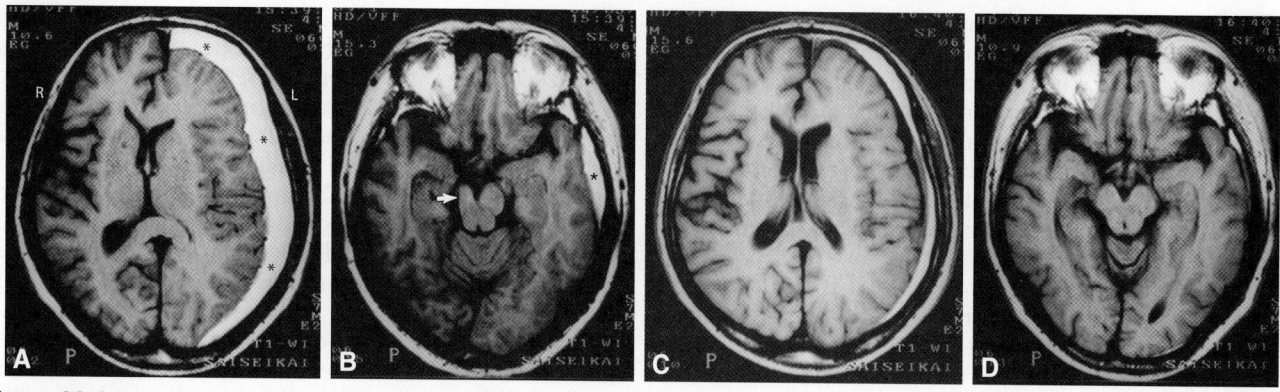

Figure 32-24

A, CSH *(asterisk)* over the surface of the left cerebral hemisphere, compressing its subarachnoid spaces and lateral ventricle. **B,** Shifting midline structures to the right and deforming the cerebral peduncle *(arrow)* by pressing it against the tentorium cerebelli, causing left-sided weakness. **C** and **D,** Return to midline of structures and release of pressure after surgical evacuation. (Reprinted from Itoyama Y, Fujioka S, Ushio Y: Kernohan's notch in chronic subdural hematoma: findings on magnetic resonance imaging: case report. *J Neurosurg* 82:645–646, 1995.)

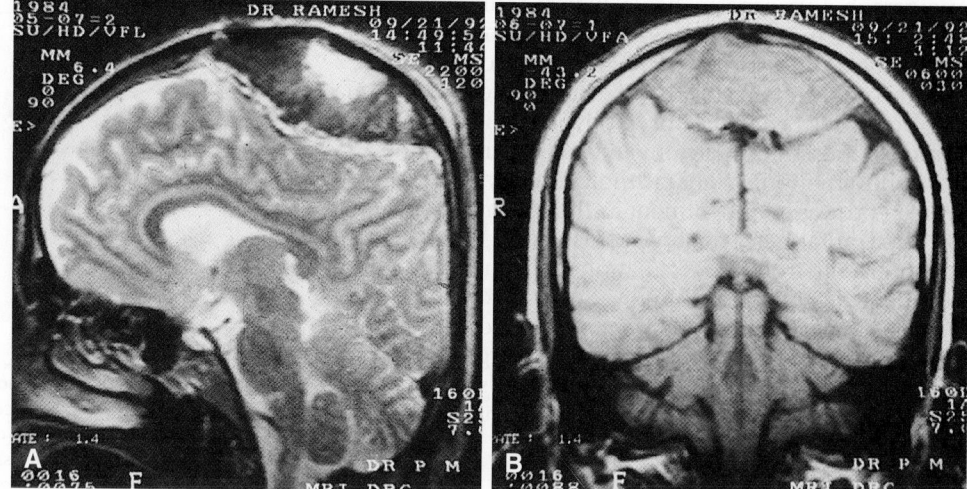

Figure 32-25

Epidural hematoma seen on MRI. A, Sagittal view. **B,** Coronal view. (Reprinted from Ramesh VG, Sivakumar S: Extradural hematoma at the vertex: a case report. *Surg Neurol* 43:138, 1995.)

Anticoagulant therapy is a recognized risk factor for CSH. Figure 32-24 shows the change in brain pressures before and after removal of a CSH.[126]

Elderly individuals who have CSH typically present with a complaint of headache and/or changes in mental status. Mild generalized headache is present in up to 90% of individuals who have CSH. Any elderly individual who has headache, especially with a change in mental or functional status, should be evaluated for CSH. The diagnostic modality of choice for CSH is a non–contrast-enhanced CT scan of the head. When a hematoma is dense, delayed contrast-enhanced CT scan or MRI may be helpful. Once the diagnosis is confirmed, the physician should consult a neurosurgeon promptly, and the individual should be transported rapidly to the closest emergency department.

Epidural Hematoma

The meningeal arteries run in the periosteal layer of the dura. They can be torn during a traumatic skull injury, and bleeding occurs between the periosteum and the skull, resulting in an epidural hematoma. The damage comes from compression of the brain. Because there is potential for extensive pooling of blood, this is considered a medical emergency and should be evacuated immediately to prevent compression on the posterior structures, which may cause death. Figure 32-25 presents an MRI showing an epidural hematoma.

VASCULAR DISORDERS OF THE SPINAL CORD

Vascular disorders of the spinal cord are rare; however, vascular disorders of the brain and spinal cord have many common factors. Because of anatomic differences, some special issues must be considered in vascular disorders of the spinal cord. Infarctions in the spinal cord can be a result of any of the same causes as those in the brain; however, some of the symptoms appear to affect the lower motor neuron at the site of the anterior horn, and the result may be more flaccid extremities and muscle atrophy.

An AVM in the spine can cause pain and burning below the level of the lesion with progressive spastic paraparesis, with or without lower motor neuron lesion. Bowel and bladder dysfunction are seen when the AVM occurs in the lumbar region.

Transverse myelitis, the dysfunction of both halves of the spinal cord in a transverse section, can be related to vascular disorders. In addition to congenital vascular malformation, transverse myelitis can be caused by viral infection, multiple sclerosis, and degenerative disorders. Necrosis of the spinal cord often occurs at several levels, resulting in sensory and motor loss and pain. The lesion may involve nerve roots or just the central structures. The majority of individuals with transverse myelitis experience some degree of recovery (see also Chapter 34).

SPECIAL IMPLICATIONS FOR THE THERAPIST 32-1

Stroke Rehabilitation

The disability resulting from stroke is a major problem for the stroke survivor, the family, and health care providers. A team of professionals is necessary to address the multitude of problems present after stroke. Therapists play a key role in this team, and there is now stronger evidence relating therapeutic intervention to decreased levels of disability. Stroke is highly heterogeneous in its effects, and each individual must be managed according to the particular impairment and disability that remains after the onset of stroke.[16]

The organization of movement changes after stroke. Mobility can be limited by a number of impairments. These changes reflect damage in specific areas of the brain. Basic reflex patterns can change and limit the ability to rely on automatic postural control mechanism for balance. A lack of normal inhibition of the H-reflex in the soleus during activation of tibialis anterior during balance activity has been noted in individuals after stroke. The increased H-reflex activity disrupts the normal on-off cycle in the muscles of the distal extremity and can cause an abnormal balance strategy.[66,72] Transmitter depletion at the synapse of group Ia afferents is known as homosynaptic depression. When group Ia afferents are activated repetitively at low frequencies the release of excitatory transmitter at the synapse on the motoneuron is depressed. When they occur in reflex pathways, the resulting changes in transmitter release will contribute to the "habituation" of reflexes that are elicited too rapidly, which is associated with the degree of spasticity.[11] Box 32-4 gives examples of typical motor impairments after stroke.

Poststroke fatigue differs from the normal fatigue caused by exertion that resolves with rest. Rather it is described as pervasive, abnormal, persistent, and excessive weariness not consistent with the amount of energy expended. Physical activity has been linked with the IL-6 system, and through this system regular activity influences mood, performance, and cognitive function. The IL-6 processing, related to inflammatory responses, is one of the mechanisms that become abnormal after stroke. Stroke is also associated with increased mental fatigue resulting in poor concentration, memory difficulties, irritability, and emotional lability. Poststroke fatigue results in decreased functional independence, institutionalization, and mortality even after adjustment for age.

Examination

Identification of which impairments may be causing an inability to perform functional activities and cause

Box 32-4

MOVEMENT PROBLEMS ASSOCIATED WITH STROKE

- Decreased force production
- Sensory impairments
- Abnormal synergistic organization of movement
- Altered temporal sequencing of muscle contractions
- Impaired regulation of force control
- Delayed responses
- Abnormal muscle tone
- Loss of range of motion
- Altered biomechanical alignment

disability is critical. There is a degree of spontaneous recovery after stroke, but typically, some impairment persists over time. A good understanding of the characteristics of the different stroke syndromes is critical to establishing the appropriate strategies for intervention. Figure 32-26 represents areas of brain damage and associated clinical signs.

Qualitative as well as quantitative measures should show sensitivity to change over time and identify relevant issues for the stroke survivor, including quality of life.[130] Many measures are currently used and there are efforts to benchmark levels of function that can help determine rehabilitation potential as early in the process as possible.[24,53,109]

Predicting upper limb recovery after stroke appears to be related to the early ability to shoulder shrug and perform at least synergistic hand movement.[59] Measurement of movement with a computer-assisted reach can quantify constraint forces and range of motion of the upper extremity. This may lead to more precise monitoring of movement and ability to determine recovery.[95]

The focus of measurement tools has traditionally been directed toward the contralateral side; however, the degree of impairment and disability of the ipsilateral side always has been questioned.[14] Unilateral tapping speed of the ipsilateral fingers may point toward ability to determine if the unaffected side has maintained functional integrity.[92] MRI demonstrates ipsilateral activation in the primary sensory cortex during contralateral tasks performed in an individual after stroke.[45]

Discrete differences exist according to the side of hemispheric lesion, with a right hemisphere lesion causing impairment of pacing, transporting, and coordinating two body parts and left hemisphere lesions resulting in impairment in calibrating movements. Despite these differences, there does not appear to be an overall difference in functional level as measured by instrumental activities of daily living between individuals according to which hemisphere the stroke affected.[12]

Intervention

Brain reorganization after neural injury is of great interest to therapists, as understanding the relation between alterations in neural structure and functional recovery are critical to the interventions chosen for each individual. It appears that the nature of the infarct may drive the plasticity related to recovery, and while a recovery after a small infarct may result in

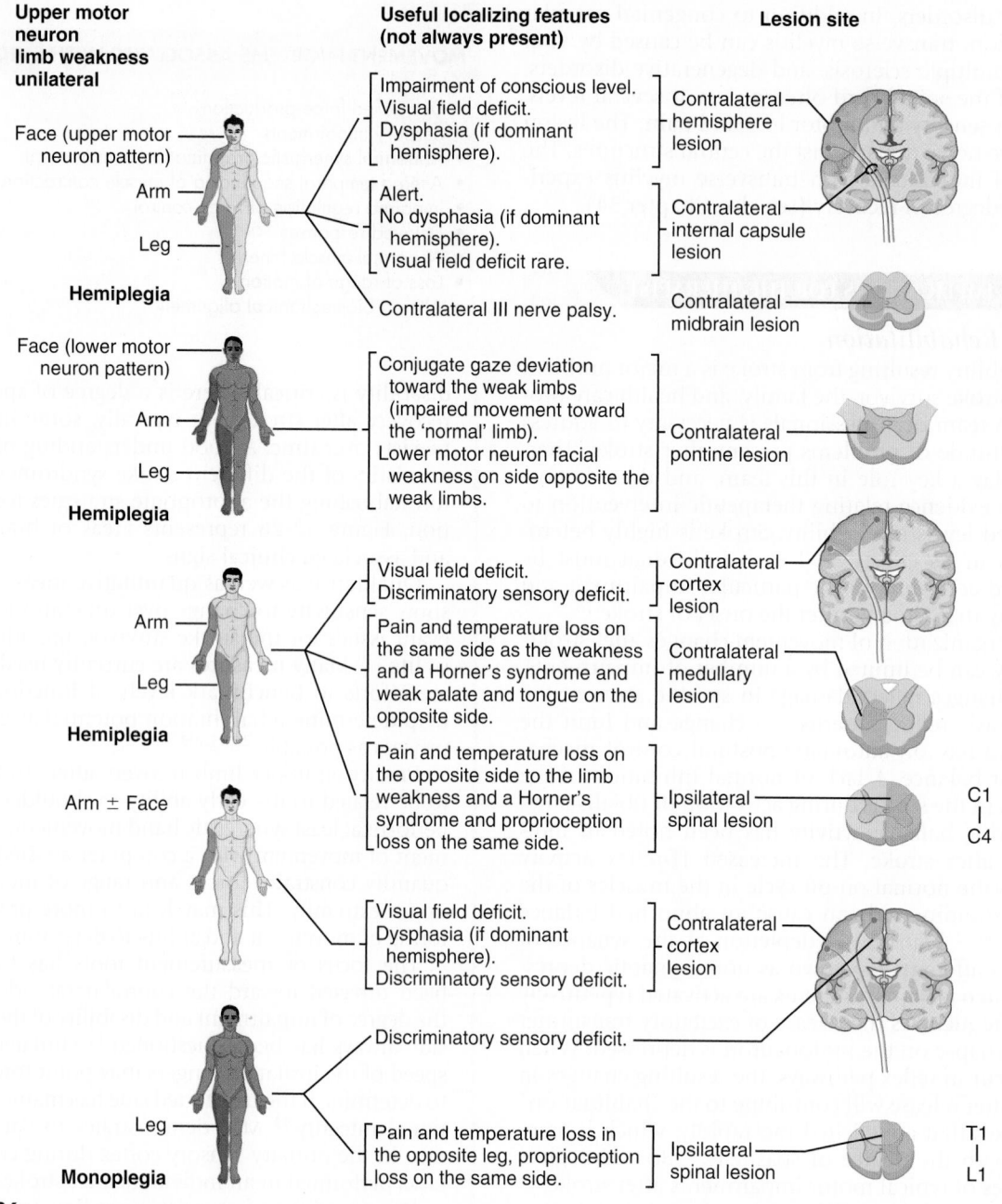

Figure 32-26

Localizing features of damage to specific areas of the brain and spinal cord. (Reprinted from Lindsay KW, Bone I, Callander R: *Neurology and neurosurgery illustrated*, New York, 1986, Churchill Livingstone.).

reorganization around the area of the infarct, a large lesion may require more extensive changes in remote metabolism, blood flow, neurotransmitter function, and axonal sprouting that may not follow the same pattern of plasticity. Inherent in the processes of rehabilitation-dependent motor recovery are restoration and reorganization of motor maps within the cortex surrounding the lesion.[34,84,111]

Skill acquisition for recovery of function is the main goal in movement retraining. Increased knowledge of neural plasticity will lead to more precision in determining the optimal task practice for motor learning. Problem solving is critical for improving skill,

but impairments of motor control such as decreased force production, increased tone, and poor control of degrees of freedom in movement must be adequately addressed. Implicit motor learning also depends on a neural network that can be affected in the pathogenesis of stroke.[8,64]

Many interventions are based on the manipulation of the environment to both guide and induce adaptive changes in the brain function. In some cases, the therapy sets out to trick the brain into activity. For example, there is evidence for the effectiveness of mirror therapy for improving upper extremity motor function, activities of daily living and decreasing pain, at least as an adjunct to normal rehabilitation for patients after stroke.[118] Significant gains in voluntary strength and muscle activation on the untrained, more-affected side after stroke can be invoked through training the opposite limb. Residual plasticity existing many years after stroke requires the clinical application of the cross-education effect where training the more-affected limb is not initially possible.[22] Bilateral arm training allows for greater force generated at movement initiation. Distributed constraint-induced therapy (dCIT) leads to higher functional ability and better performance in the amount and quality of use of the affected arm.[137] The specifics of training, including problem solving and manipulating the spatial and temporal aspects of the performance, appear to be inherent in the successful outcomes.[123] Movement of the upper extremity facilitated with electromyography-triggered stimulus and use of electrical stimulation orthoses continues to be studied with positive effects on movement and functional use of the upper extremity.[36,129]

Obtaining functional and normal-looking gait has long been the goal of therapists and stroke survivors.[78,115] Treadmill training with partial body weight support shows functional changes over typical terrain, with more normal movement of the affected limb during both stance and swing.[51,124] Computer-assisted gait training results in increased stride length and speed of walking.[113,115] There has been a rapid increase in available robotic devices that allow augmentation to hands-on therapy.[2,30] Wearable robots that assist three-dimensional movement show success because they mimic the trajectories of human movement.[69] Active subject participation in robot-driven gait therapy is vital to many of the potential recovery pathways and is therefore an important feature of gait training. Higher levels of participation and activity may be achieved when designs allow sufficient degrees of freedom to facilitate other aspects of gait such as balance.[139] A Virtual Model Controller for supporting one of these subtasks, namely the foot clearance, provides virtual support at the ankle, to increase foot clearance. This enables the therapist to focus the support on the subtasks that are impaired, and leave the other subtasks up to the patient, encouraging him to participate more actively in the training. Additionally, the speed-dependent reference patterns provide the therapist with the tools to easily adapt the treadmill speed to the capabilities and progress of the patient.[65]

Virtual reality applications are being developed with a focus on attention, executive function, memory, and spatial ability. Functional training for activities such as crossing the street, driving, preparing meals, and navigating by wheelchair are possible with virtual reality.[18,96]

Brain stimulation techniques designed to augment traditional neurorehabilitation hold promise for reducing the burden of stroke-related disability. Repetitive transcranial magnetic stimulation (rTMS), transcranial direct current stimulation, and epidural cortical stimulation can enhance neural plasticity in the motor cortex post-stroke.[27] rTMS has shown to have a positive effect on motor recovery in patients with stroke, especially for those with subcortical stroke. Low-frequency rTMS over the unaffected hemisphere may be more beneficial than high-frequency rTMS over the affected hemisphere.[54]

Control of spasticity and contractures by antispastic pattern positioning, range-of-motion exercise, stretching, and splinting has long been a part of the rehabilitation process. Maintaining soft tissue mobility in the distal extremities is a critical link to the performance of a motor activity. Traditionally it was thought that the activity of the spastic muscle should be limited to prevent further increase in tone; however, it has been shown that increased workload in a spastic muscle can be performed without increasing the spasticity.[10]

Fall prevention is always a primary goal for the individual sustaining a stroke. Falls are frequent, and in more than 5% of cases result in significant injury. Falls are common during the transition from sit to stand, and the kinematics of this activity has been studied. Evidence shows that people who fall take more time to rise and to sit down and demonstrate increased center of pressure sway in mediolateral directions. Weight on the nonparetic leg is significantly increased during the activity.[17,49] Balance retraining with center of pressure feedback provides more even distribution and control of center of gravity.[102]

Although a therapeutic goal is often to move clients out of assistive devices, studies show that for some parameters of gait the orthosis or assistive device still provides control over some of the critical components of gait. Rigid ankle braces resulted in longer relative single-stance duration, improved swing symmetry, and ankle excursions. The decreased activity in the anterior tibialis continues to be a drawback.[50] Use of a cane improves weight shift to prepare for the next step and results in decreased circumduction. Joint angles were more normal during the swing phase.[68]

Cardiovascular endurance training is indicated for the stroke survivor; programs incorporating such activities should be part of rehabilitation programs. Treadmill training has been shown to reduce the energy expenditure and cardiovascular demands of gait within the stroke population.[77] Submaximal all-extremity exercise shows potential in the rehabilitation programs for stroke.[74] Research is ongoing to establish the parameters of cardiovascular training within the limits created by neurologic deficits.

Based on the theory of motor learning, the ability to learn a new motor program or a different way of moving does not follow a specific time frame following brain damage.[6] It appears that the stroke-related sensorimotor deficits affect the processes underlying the control execution of motor skills but not the learning of those skills. Potential for adaptation based on learning goes beyond the time frame of spontaneous recovery.[134]

Failure to maintain functional gains after the course of therapy is a concern for all individuals involved in the management of poststroke rehabilitation. Functional exercise done on a regular basis has been shown to have a positive impact on recovery.[23] Early and consistent involvement of the family or primary caretakers is paramount, as is the follow-through of a home management program of activity and exercise. Compliance of stroke survivors and caregivers continues to be low despite efforts toward better education.[97] The functional consequence of fatigue in physical, professional, and social activities should be considered.[43]

The clinician and family should watch for symptoms related to angina, peripheral vascular disease, and deep vein thrombosis that may arise after stroke.

Osteoporotic bone loss has been demonstrated with immobility of the upper extremity, especially in women, and should be addressed as a part of a standard protocol.[19]

REFERENCES

To enhance this text and add value for the reader, all references are included on the companion Evolve site that accompanies this text. The reader can view the reference source and access it online whenever possible.

CHAPTER 33

Traumatic Brain Injury

KAREN L. McCULLOCH • KENDA S. FULLER

TRAUMATIC BRAIN INJURY

Overview and Definition

Traumatic brain injury (TBI) is damage that impairs brain function resulting from external physical force. The severity of brain injury varies widely, with the majority of injuries in the mild category. Concussion is a subset of mild traumatic brain injury (mTBI) that is generally self-limited and at the less-severe end of the brain injury spectrum but still involves a complex pathophysiological process. Moderate to severe injuries have a significantly worse outcome. Regardless of the severity of injury, there is a diminished or altered state of consciousness, at least initially. Impairment of cognition and physical function are common and may be temporary or permanent. Changes may be seen in behavior and emotional control. Functional disability or psychological maladjustment can be persistent and can have a devastating impact on lifestyle. Differences in recovery are seen in people who appear to have similar injuries.

Incidence and Risk Factors

It is estimated that as many as 3.8 million concussions occur in the United States per year during competitive sports and recreational activities; however, as many as 50% of the concussions may go unreported. Concussions occur in all sports, with the highest incidence in football, hockey, rugby, soccer, and basketball. The reported incidence of concussion is higher in female athletes than in male athletes despite similar playing rules in most sports. Certain sports, positions, and individual playing styles have a greater risk of concussion. Younger age and level of play is a risk factor for prolonged recovery. Preinjury mood disorders, learning disorders, attention-deficit disorders, and migraine headaches complicate diagnosis and management of a concussion.[30] Early posttraumatic headache, history of headaches fatigue/fogginess, amnesia, alteration in mental status, or disorientation lead to prolonged symptoms.[33] Concussion may occur in sports and situations not typically thought to put the athlete at risk and not necessarily during games, and often without a loss of consciousness, rather with an alteration in mental status, such as feeling disoriented or confused. A single concussion does not necessarily lead to cognitive impairment, but individuals who have had previous concussion are more likely to have future concussions with longer recovery times. In fact, a history of concussion is a highly probable risk factor for recurrent concussion. It is also highly likely that there is an increased risk for repeat concussion in the first 10 days after an initial concussion according to pathophysiologic studies.[32]

TBI peaks at three different age levels. The first peak occurs in early childhood at age 1 to 2 years and is related most often to child abuse. The second occurs in late adolescence and early adulthood between ages 15 and 24 years and may be related to risk-taking behaviors. Sports concussion is becoming more common in this age group. Between 2001 and 2009, the number of sports and recreation–related emergency department visits for TBI among persons aged ≤19 years increased 62%. Injury occurs most often during football, soccer, and playground activities. One of the most widespread causes of head injury among young people is bicycling. Wearing an appropriate helmet reduces the risk of severe head injury by 88%.[2]

The third peak in TBI occurs in the elderly population and is related most often to falls. This group is the most likely to be hospitalized, and approximately 7% will die while hospitalized. Although elderly individuals account for less than 15% of trauma admissions due to falls, they account for half of deaths due to falls. There is more susceptibility with age to tearing of the bridging vessels over the surface of the brain. In addition, there seems to be a significant, age-related decline in cerebrovascular autoregulation that may partially explain the worse outcomes seen in elderly individuals with TBI.[1]

Of those who sustain severe brain injury, approximately 60% of adults and 92% of children are injured in a motor vehicle accident. The increasing mandate for seatbelt use and availability of air bags appear to be reducing injuries. Pedestrians injured by automobiles represent some of the most seriously injured individuals after trauma. The elderly are at particular risk for being struck as pedestrians and make up a significant percentage of pedestrians who have been struck by a motor vehicle. Slow ambulation, impaired reflexes, misjudgment, and visual, auditory, and gait impairment contribute, as elderly individuals are frequently struck within marked crosswalks or walk directly into the path of an oncoming vehicle. In the elderly, there are significantly increased mortality rates, with a majority of deaths occurring at the scene or at the emergency department.[1] The incidence of penetrating TBI from gunshot wounds is increasing, and in some urban communities it is now the most common type of injury seen.[18] Brain injury due to firearms is associated most often with attempted suicide.[35] Alcohol use and abuse are frequently associated with brain trauma. Fifty percent of people admitted into hospitals with head trauma are intoxicated at the time. Brain injury may be two to four times higher in alcoholics than in the general population.[24]

The past 2 decades have witnessed a significant decline in overall TBI mortality from the mid-30% range in the 1970s to less than 20% in the 1990s, affected by improved preventive measures such as speed limits, seatbelt laws, airbag protection, helmet use, etc. This decline in mortality has paralleled an understanding of the secondary injury process and an appreciation that all neurologic damage does not occur at the moment of insult but evolves over the ensuing hours and days from various biochemical and molecular derangements, so that acute medical management can address these issues more effectively. Despite the recent advances in safety, TBI contributes to a third of all injury-related deaths in the United States. Those who survive TBI often experience persistent morbidity, driving the need for long-term rehabilitation. Appropriate management of the brain injury results in improved outcome from trauma.[29]

Etiologic Factors

TBIs can come from open or closed head injury. With an open head injury, the meninges have been breached, leaving the brain exposed. Penetrating missile injuries create localized, focal lesions that, when not fatal, cause limited damage to the brain. It is not the size of a missile but its velocity that generally determines the extent of damage. Penetrating injury also causes vascular injury, including disruption or the formation of aneurysms or pseudoaneurysms.[38] Figure 33-1 shows the kind of damage that can occur from a gunshot wound.

A closed head injury occurs when there is no skull fracture or laceration of the brain, but the soft tissue of the brain is forced into contact with the hard, bony, outer covering of the brain, the skull. The initial blow occurs under the point of impact (termed the "coup" injury); then, as the brain decelerates against the contralateral skull, injury occurs to tissue on the opposite side (the "contre-coup"). Such contre-coup injury is frequently worse than the injury underlying the impact.

Actual loss of consciousness does not always occur, although an altered state of consciousness is a hallmark of brain injury. Mild closed head injuries can occur after a severe neck injury without the head actually striking any surface. The symptoms are worse when there is a rotational component to the head injury in addition to the back-and-forth jarring.[17] Subdural and subarachnoid hemorrhage can occur in the presence of diffuse injury and rupture of veins bridging the brain to the venous sinuses. Rotational forces are the most likely forces to cause diffuse axonal injury (DAI), including damage to brainstem structures, such as the reticular activating system.

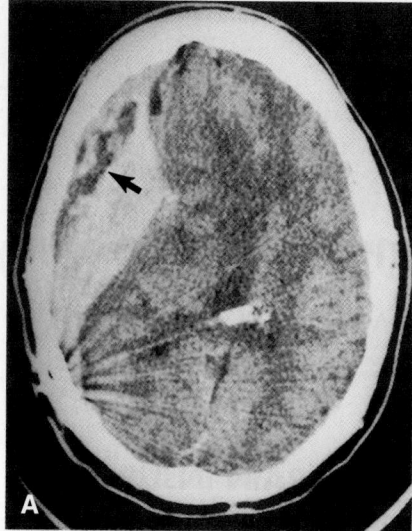

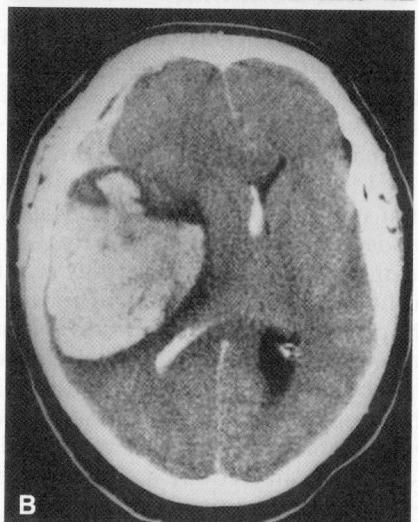

Figure 33-1

Gunshot wound resulting in both intracerebral and epidural hemorrhage. A, The bullet is shown on CT scan resting in a midline position with streaking effect of fragments also seen. The *arrow* points to area of decreased density thought to be epidural bleeding. **B,** Large intracerebral hemorrhage is noted with blood present in the ventricle. (Reprinted from Ramsey R: *Neuroradiology,* Philadelphia, 1994, WB Saunders, p 407.)

Severe head injury may cause significant bruising and bleeding within the brain. Approximately 25% of people with a normal initial computed tomographic (CT) scan will develop late hemorrhages. Contusions are usually more severe in persons with skull fracture than in those without fracture. Although contusion is the hallmark of TBI, severe or even fatal damage to the brain can occur without contusion.[4]

Pathogenesis

Primary injury is the result of forces exerted on the brain at impact. Secondary injury refers to changes compromising brain function that result from the brain's reaction to trauma or other system failure, such as brain swelling and impaired cerebral perfusion (Fig. 33-2).

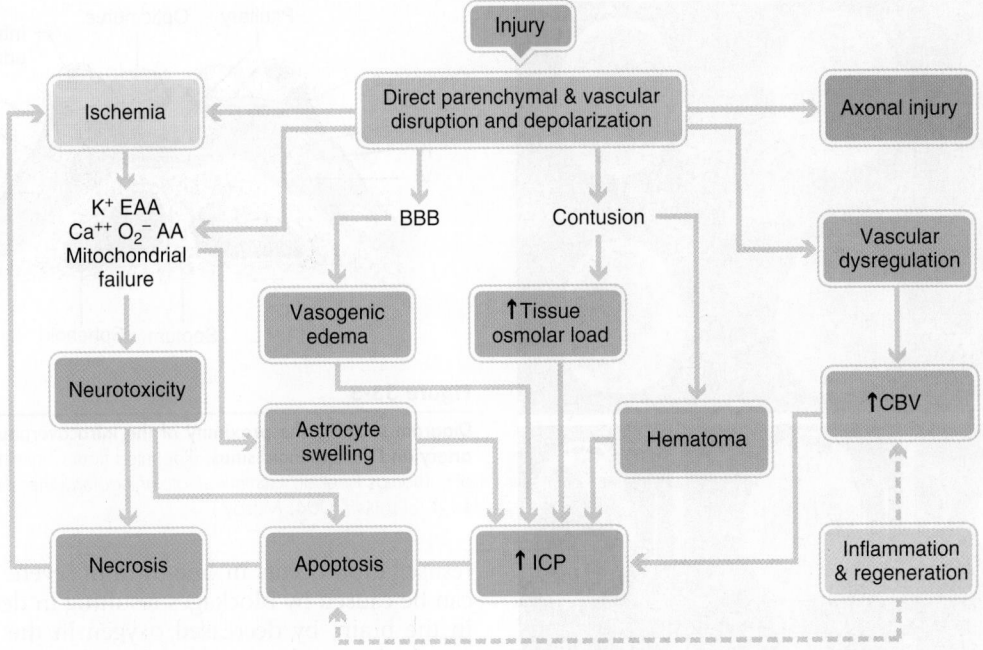

Figure 33-2

Categories of mechanisms proposed to be involved in the evolution of secondary damage after severe TBI *from* biochemical and molecular substrates of the secondary injury cascade. (From Kochanek PM, Clark RSB, Jenkins LW: Pathobiology of secondary brain injury. In Salaman M, ed: *Current techniques in neurosurgery*, ed 2, Philadelphia, 1993, Current Medicine.)

Vascular Changes

Internal or extremity injuries caused by trauma can cause excessive bleeding and decreased blood pressure, which if persistent can cause hypoperfusion to the brain, accentuating secondary injury. Vascular damage can lead to infarction within the cortical gray matter. Typically, contusions occur at the poles and on the inferior surfaces of the frontal and temporal lobes. Occipital blows are more likely to produce contusions than are frontal or lateral blows. Areas where the cranial vault is irregular, such as on the anterior poles, undersurface of the temporal lobes, and undersurface of the frontal lobes are commonly injured. With fracture of the cranial vault, there may be damage to the superficial epidural vessels and, particularly in the case of falls, there can be rupture of the bridging vessels between hemispheres.[49] Figure 33-3 shows CT scan images of changes seen after TBI with the presence of epidural and subdural hematomas.

TBI can be associated with other forms of vascular change. Gliding contusions, or hemorrhagic lesions in the cortex, may be the result of movement of the cortical grey matter in relation to the underlying white matter, causing shear strains to damage the penetrating vessels found at the grey and white matter interface.[63] Figure 33-4 shows the effects of shearing injury as seen on CT scan. Subarachnoid hemorrhage is common because of the rupture of pial vessels within the subarachnoid space. This may trigger vasospasm that can lead to reduced regional blood flow. Injury to the vessels within the white matter can also cause significant neurologic consequences, especially if it is in the area of the basal ganglia.[27]

An increase in cranial blood volume is considered to be the most important cause of increased intracranial pressure (ICP) after trauma. There can be bleeding into

the epidural compartment, creating a mass effect that can displace the brain and increase ICP. The shear and tensile forces of traumatic injury can also create a subdural hematoma by disruption of the bridging veins. Acute hydrocephalus occurs when blood accumulates in the ventricular system, expanding the size of the ventricles and causing increased pressure on brain tissue being compressed between the skull and the fluid-filled ventricles.[16] Vascular volume can increase if venous outflow is blocked or increased cerebral blood flow (CBF) increases passively because of loss of autoregulation. Cerebrospinal fluid volume increases may be the result of blockage of outflow pathways or interference with reabsorption. When the volume of one compartment changes slowly, compensatory decreases in the volume of other compartments may prevent a rise in ICP. When the volume change is rapid or the compensatory mechanisms are exhausted or dysfunctional, the ICP goes up.[10]

The overall result of these vascular changes is the decreased ability of the cerebral vessels to maintain necessary homeostasis in the face of changing blood pressure or blood gas composition. Initially, within the first few hours after severe injury, there is decreased CBF both globally and at the impact site, which can induce ischemia. Within 24 hours, the blood flow can be at normal or above-normal levels.[27] The management of brain perfusion can conflict with therapeutic goals focusing on problems with infection, ventilation, renal function, or even systemic circulation. For this reason, integration of brain and systemic care is critical on all levels, from understanding the pathophysiologic principles to treatment through interdisciplinary communication.[10]

Hypoxia. Hypotension (systolic blood pressure less than 90 mm Hg) occurring between injury and

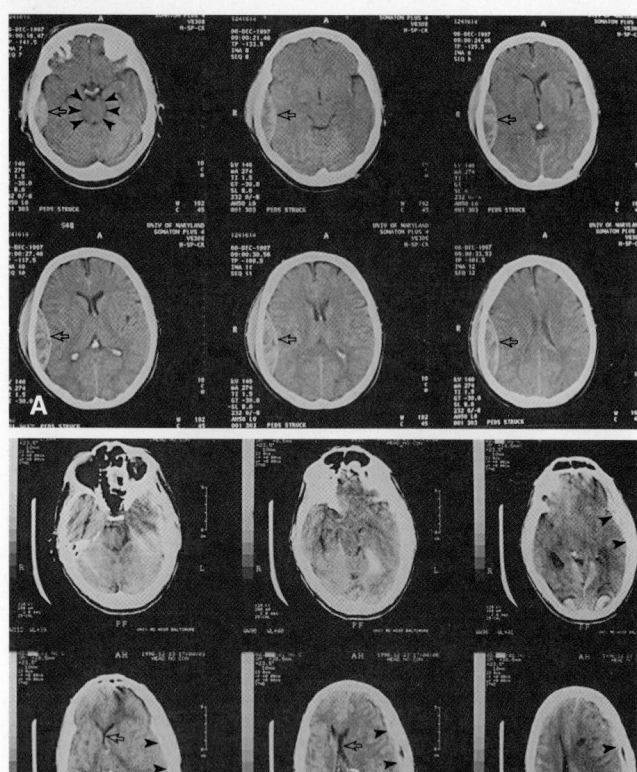

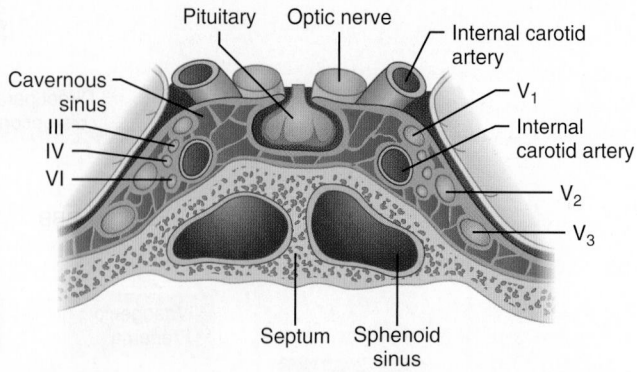

Figure 33-5

Diagram showing the proximity of the intracavernous internal carotid artery and the sphenoid sinus. (Reprinted from Cummings CW, Haughey BH, Thomas R, et al: *Cummings otolaryngology: head and neck surgery*, ed 4, St Louis, 2004, Mosby.)

Figure 33-3

CT scans of two patients with brain injury. **A,** This patient has a right temporal epidural hematoma *(arrows)*. The mesencephalic cisterns are patent in the top left, indicating a lack of brainstem compression despite mass *(arrowheads)*. **B,** This patient has suffered an acute left subdural hematoma *(arrowheads)* with midline shift *(arrows)*. (Reprinted from Townsend CM: *Sabiston textbook of surgery*, ed 17, Philadelphia, 2004, Saunders.)

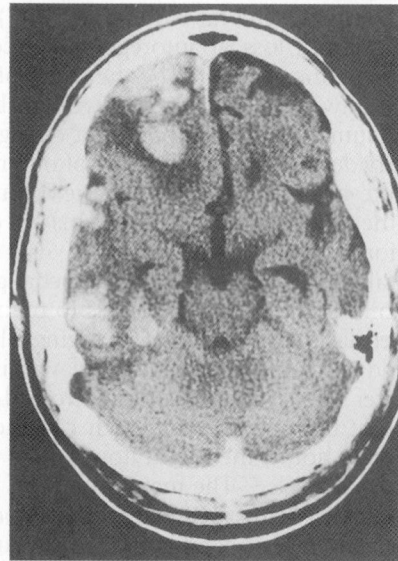

Figure 33-4

Contusion with shearing injury. CT scan shows multiple rounded areas of blood density with surrounding edema. Many of these areas are at the junction of grey and white matter consistent with shear injury. (Reprinted from Ramsey R: *Neuroradiology*, Philadelphia, 1994, WB Saunders, p 409.)

resuscitation occurs in one-third of severe TBI victims. It can be caused by blockages resulting in decreased blood in the brain, by decreased oxygen in the blood due to concomitant pulmonary insult, or by internal or extremity injuries that cause excessive blood loss. It is associated with doubling of mortality rate and a significant increase in morbidity. Early hypotension is also a strong predictor of poor outcome.[51]

Hypertension. Intracranial hypertension can interfere with perfusion by lowering the cerebral perfusion pressure (CPP). Under normal circumstances, cerebral pressure autoregulation maintains CBF constant over a CPP range of approximately 50 to 150 mm Hg. Following trauma, this relationship may be partially or totally disrupted.

Impaired vascular responsiveness of blood gas changes after brain injury results in abnormal arteriolar vasoconstriction in the presence of carbon dioxide. Vascular volume in the skull can increase if venous outflow is blocked or increased CBF is recruited for metabolic reasons (e.g., seizures, pyrexia) or increases passively because of loss of autoregulation.

Posttraumatic aneurysms of the intracavernous internal carotid artery can be associated with delayed and sometimes lethal massive epistaxis. This can be a result of basal skull fractures in the region of the carotid canal or cavernous sinus and/or orbital fractures and compromise of the optical nerves. Knowledge of these risk factors and early diagnosis can minimize the high mortality risk. Figure 33-5 demonstrates the proximity of these structures. It can take from days to years for the artery weakening to develop, with an average time of 3 weeks. Because of the close anatomic relationship of the intracavernous portion of the internal cerebral artery to the oculomotor, optic, abducens, trochlear, and trigeminal nerves, these structures may also be damaged during the aneurysm development, resulting in effects such as blindness, facial numbness, and/or oculomotor palsy.[19]

There appears to be a change in the endothelium, or walls, of the blood vessels following brain injury. In the normal brain, neurotransmitters such as acetylcholine induce dilation of the vessels through the release of endothelium-derived releasing factor, causing relaxation of the smooth muscle in the vessel wall. In the injured brain this reaction can be missing, resulting in abnormal vasoconstriction.[15] Additional changes at the level of the endothelium result in a disturbed blood-brain barrier in the injured brain. This results in leakage of serum proteins and neurotransmitters into the parenchyma, causing edema. The effects of edema in the brain are described in Chapters 28 and 32.

Parenchymal Changes

Axonal injury is a consistent feature of the traumatic event. Shear and tensile forces disrupt the axolemma. The distal axon segment can detach and trigger wallerian degeneration. These reactive axonal swellings, or retraction balls, full of axon material develop and can be detected in the injured brain within 12 hours of injury in animal models. The myelin sheath pulls away from the axon. The axonal changes are seen throughout the brain regardless of site of impact. The damage is different from that of stroke or tumor, which produces a more complete but local deafferentation. Typically, with DAI, there remain intact axons interspersed with the damaged axons.

This primary injury triggers a metabolic cascade that can add to secondary injury through excitotoxicity and free radical formation. Secondary cell death by necrosis of the cellular membrane can be a result of edema. Apoptosis, or programmed cell death from within the cell through changes in the DNA, can result in cell loss that occurs days, weeks, or months after injury.[50] There is evidence of the potential for recovery of function based on the possible sprouting of undamaged axons to reoccupy the areas left vacant by degenerating axons.

Excitotoxicity is a common occurrence with diffuse brain injury and results in an increase in extracellular neurotransmitters and increased potassium, causing a massive depolarization of the injured brain. The excitatory neurotransmitter glutamate rises to abnormal amounts following brain injury. Glutamate is neurotoxic when concentrations increase. A complex interaction of the various amino acids and neurotransmitters, may affect postsynaptic functions, resulting in secondary injury of the neural mechanisms of the brain. Inhibition function of the synaptic receptors can be altered, and may relate to both functional and behavioral changes. See Chapter 28 for information on the damage to the nervous system associated with glutamate.

Free radicals are generated by TBI. Extensive membrane depolarization, induced by trauma, allows for a nonselective opening of the voltage-sensitive calcium channels and an abnormal accumulation of calcium within neurons and glia. Such calcium shifts are associated with activation of lipolytic and proteolytic enzymes, protein kinases, protein phosphatases, dissolution of microtubules, and altered gene expression.[18]

Compressive Damage

Intracranial hypertension and mass bleeding inside the skull can produce herniation, causing a shift from its normal symmetric position. The most common herniation occurs at the lateral tentorial membrane separating the cerebral hemispheres from the posterior fossa. This shift may cause compression of the brainstem, the pituitary, or other delicate brain structures. Because the brainstem

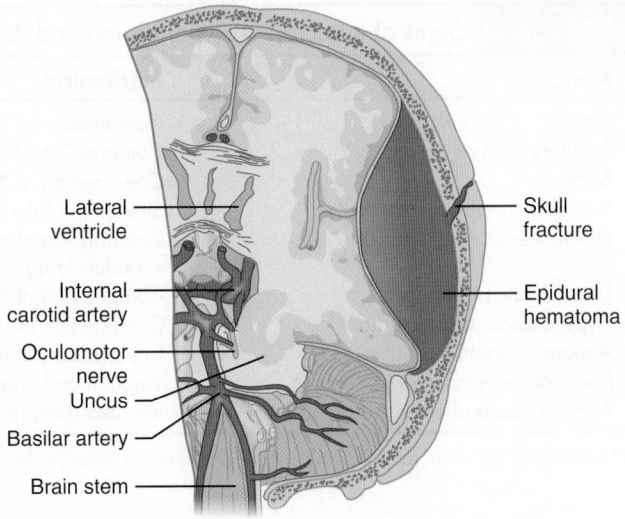

Figure 33-6

Anterior view of transtentorial herniation caused by large epidural hematoma. Skull fracture overlies hematoma. (Reprinted from Rockswold GL: Head injury. In Tintinalli JE et al, eds: *Emergency medicine*, New York, 2004, ed 6, McGraw-Hill, p 915.)

controls the body's major visceral functions, brainstem involvement may result in paralysis or death. In less severe situations, autonomic nervous system changes may include changes in pulse and respiratory rates and regularity, temperature elevations, blood pressure changes, excessive sweating, salivation, tearing, and sebum secretion. Because the adult brain is surrounded by the rigid skull, swelling of the brain or pooling of blood pushes tissue through openings in the base of the skull, resulting in herniation through the foramen magnum. Figures 33-6 and 32-23 show the herniation possible with epidural bleeding. Table 33-1 lists the possible signs of intracranial hypertension and associated herniation syndromes.

Clinical Manifestations

Signs and Symptoms

Acute clinical symptoms of concussion largely reflect a functional disturbance rather than a structural injury; with rapid onset of short-lived impairment of neurologic function that resolves spontaneously. Symptoms usually associated with concussion are headache, disorientation, dizziness, and nausea. The client may be irritable or distractible and have difficulty with reading and memory. These symptoms typically resolve in 7 to 10 days. A single concussion does not typically result in long-term neuropsychologic or cognitive complications. However, prediction of which individuals will experience persistent postconcussive symptoms is difficult. Factors that may increase recovery time include loss of consciousness for more than 1 minute, significance of cognitive symptoms, younger age, female gender, and depression. Nonspecific psychological symptoms such as personality change and depression are reported by more than one-half of individuals within 3 months of mild TBI. Fatigue and disruption of sleep patterns are also often reported. Ongoing

Table 33-1	Signs of Intracranial Hypertension and Associated Herniation Syndromes	

Sign	Mechanism	Type of Herniation
Coma	Compression of midbrain tegmentum	Uncal, central
Pupillary dilation	Compression of ipsilateral third nerve	Uncal
Miosis	Compression of the midbrain	Central
Lateral gaze palsy	Stretching of the sixth nerves	Central
Hemiparesis*	Compression of contralateral cerebral peduncle against tentorium	Uncal
Decerebrate posturing	Compression of the midbrain	Central, uncal
Hypertension, bradycardia	Compression of the medulla	Central, uncal, cerebellar (tonsillar)
Abnormal breathing patterns	Compression of the pons or medulla	Central, uncal, cerebellar (tonsillar)
Posterior cerebral artery infarction	Vascular compression	Uncal
Anterior cerebral artery infarction	Vascular compression	Subfalcine (cingulate)

*Hemiparesis will occur ipsilateral to the hemispheric lesion (false localizing sign).

clinical symptoms associated with persistent neurocognitive impairments can be demonstrated on objective testing. Animal and human studies support the concept of postconcussive vulnerability, showing that a second blow before the brain has recovered results in worsening metabolic changes within the cell. Experimental evidence suggests the concussed brain is less responsive to usual neural activation, and when premature cognitive or physical activity occurs before complete recovery, the brain may be vulnerable to prolonged dysfunction.[39]

Second impact syndrome has been described as a rare but catastrophic reaction to a second concussion that occurs before recovery from a previous concussion. The existence of this condition is controversial—having been documented in case reports—and its actual incidence is unclear. The theory is that the second injury causes rapid and severe lack of cerebral autoregulation, loss of consciousness, and rapid progression to severe disability or death if not identified and treated emergently. Second impact syndrome has been suspected primarily in the sport-related deaths of adolescents, underscoring the importance of identifying every concussion in middle or high school sports to reduce risk of this catastrophic condition.[41]

Current research suggests that damage may occur from multiple concussive blows over a lifetime may be associated with chronic traumatic encephalopathy (CTE), even though the incidence and cause(s) of CTE is unclear. This condition was first identified in boxers who have sustained many blows to the head during sport. CTE is a progressive degenerative condition marked by deterioration in cognition (memory loss, impaired judgment) and behavior (impulse control, aggressiveness, depression) that eventually results in dementia.[6,21,42]

Postmortem analysis of brain tissue reveals evidence of degenerative brain changes and the deposition of an abnormal protein, tau. CTE has been documented in well-publicized cases of college and professional athletes who have a history of repetitive exposure to concussive and subconcussive forces during sport, mostly who were retired, but one athlete as young as 18. Unfortunately, repeated concussion has been implicated by the media as the cause of CTE, when the full clinical history of these individuals has not been examined in detail. Factors such as chronic steroid use, substance abuse, psychiatric response to chronic pain, chronic health conditions, and genetic predisposition to dementia could contribute to signs and symptoms associated with CTE. Careful study of athletes who exhibit cognitive and behavioral changes is necessary to clarify the role of repeated concussion to long-term cognitive deficits. Parents and athletes should manage recovery from concussion carefully after an injury, and follow medical advice in deciding to continue in a sport with high concussion risk after one or more injuries has occurred.[21]

Brain injury during military conflict is increasingly a result of blast exposure. The injuries that result from proximity to an explosion include damage to fluid- and air-filled cavities from the pressure wave, injury from projectiles or being thrown by the force of the blast, and the potential for toxic exposure to fumes that could affect tissue oxygenation. Polytrauma may occur that affects systemic blood supply and adds to potential ischemia in the brain. If the injury is severe, the need for state-of-the-art field medicine and immediate transport for ongoing care is clear. Mild injury is more difficult to detect. A service member may underreport symptoms in the face of more seriously injured colleagues. Injury in a combat situation is very different from that on the playing field, as the risk to life is clear. Acute stress reactions and longer term posttraumatic stress co-occurs with TBI and share common symptoms. Careful assessment by a multidisciplinary team accustomed to working with service members is necessary to determine what symptoms may be the result of TBI versus other behavioral health conditions, so that appropriate treatment can be chosen.

Headache is the most common complaint following mTBI. Migraine headaches with and without aura can develop in the hours to weeks after a concussion. Immediately after mild TBI in sports such as soccer, football, rugby, and boxing, children, adolescents, and young adults may have a first-time migraine with aura. This syndrome may be triggered multiple times after additional mild TBI and has been termed *footballer's migraine*. Cluster headaches can develop after mild TBI. Subdural hematomas can result in headaches that are nonspecific and that can be mild to severe, paroxysmal or constant, and bilateral or unilateral.[18] Refer to Chapter 37, "Headache."

Moderate TBI often involves structural injury such as hemorrhage or contusion. Epidural hematomas frequently result from skull fractures with subsequent laceration of the middle meningeal artery. Classically, epidural hematoma leads to an initial loss of consciousness, which is followed by recovery of consciousness and a lucid period. The athlete then progressively deteriorates neurologically, with development of headache, a decline in mental status, and focal neurologic findings such as contralateral weakness or numbness, pupillary reflex abnormalities, or facial asymmetry. This injury resulting from rapid accumulation of pressure from arterial blood, if not recognized and treated, can result in death. Severe TBI generally results in some form of cognitive and/or physical disability or in death, especially with very low Glasgow Coma Scale (GCS) scores.[18]

Disorders of Consciousness. Altered level of consciousness is a state that can occur with diffuse or focal head injury, or when there is a combination of the two types of injury. This can be a result of diffuse bilateral cerebral hemispheric damage or a smaller lesion that affects the brainstem. In moderate or severe head injury, unconsciousness can be prolonged or persistent. Arousal that is associated with wakefulness depends on an intact reticular formation and upper brainstem.

Coma is regarded as the lowest level of consciousness and is characterized as not obeying commands, not uttering words, not opening the eyes, or a state of unresponsiveness. This indicates advanced brain failure, with bilateral cerebral hemispheric or direct involvement of the brainstem. Coma rarely lasts longer than 4 weeks. The GCS is the most widely used instrument for determining level of consciousness; it is used in the acute setting to determine current status and potential for improvement (Box 33-1). In rehabilitation contexts, individuals with disorders of consciousness are best examined using the Coma Recovery Scale–Revised, as it allows for more detailed assessment of responses to various sensory stimuli and basic functions that are observed when emerging from coma.[9]

Some individuals may continue to exhibit a reduced level of consciousness, a condition that has been referred to as postcomatose unawareness, characterized by a wakeful, reduced responsiveness with no evident cerebral cortical function. This includes eye opening with resumption of sleep-wake cycles and respiration, controlled at a subcortical level. Eyes may open spontaneously, but do not track or fix gaze. There is no purposeful movement or communication, although startle reactions, sounds made especially with tight muscle stretch, and facial expressions unrelated to the environmental context may be observed, and result from diffuse cerebral hypoxia or from severe, diffuse white matter impact damage, but the brainstem is usually relatively intact. The use of the term *vegetative state* is considered derogatory by some, with "wakeful unconsciousness" suggested as a more respectful term. Vegetative state may be defined as persistent if present for more than 4 weeks.

The minimally conscious state is a progression from wakeful unconsciousness but has some similarities. Individuals in the minimally conscious state demonstrate eye-opening, sleep-wake cycles, and often will track

Box 33-1	
GLASGOW COMA SCALE	

Eye Opening	**E**
spontaneous	4
to speech	3
to pain	2
no response	1

Best Motor Response	**M**
To Verbal Command:	
obeys	6
To Painful Stimulus:	
localizes pain	5
flexion-withdrawal	4
flexion-abnormal	3
extension	2
no response	1

Best Verbal Response	**V**
oriented and converses	5
disoriented and converses	4
inappropriate words	3
incomprehensible sounds	2
no response	1

E+M+V = 3 to 15

- 90% less than or equal to 8 are in coma
- Greater than or equal to 9 not in coma
- 8 is the critical score
- Less than or equal to 8 at 6 hours—50% die
- 9–11 = moderate severity
- Greater than or equal to 12 = minor injury

Coma is defined as (1) not opening eyes, (2) not obeying commands, and (3) not uttering understandable words.

Adapted from Teasdale G, Jennett B: Assessment of coma and impaired consciousness: A Practical Scale, *Lancet* 304(7872):81-84, 1974.

objects visually. The hallmark of the minimally conscious state is an inconsistent but clearly observable ability to sometimes follow simple commands, communicate (yes or no, by talking or gesture), show appropriate emotion, or to reach for or hold an object appropriately. Because the ability to do these tasks is inconsistent, differentiating between wakeful unconsciousness and minimally conscious state can be difficult. Once an individual can consistently communicate, follow instructions, or use an object (e.g., brush or pen), they are no longer in a minimally conscious state.

As a patient progresses in consciousness, they may emerge into a confused state marked by disorientation, severe cognitive deficits (memory, attention, e.g.), inconsistent arousal from drowsy to restlessness, sleep disturbances, and delusions or hallucinations. A confused state may be further characterized by exhibiting signs of appropriate or inappropriate behavior or communication. Fatigue during the course of a day may cause someone to display aspects of appropriate and inappropriate behavior at different times or as they emerge from being more or less confused about their environment and surroundings.

A rare but alternative form of injury associated with injury to the ventral pons is "locked-in syndrome" that involves quadriplegia but preserved awareness and arousal.[18] Locked in syndrome typically spares vertical eye movements, so these movements can be used to communicate. Disordered breathing patterns associated with injury to brainstem respiratory centers are also common.

Respiratory abnormalities associated with brain injury include *Cheyne-Stokes breathing*, a rhythmic pattern of alternating rapid breathing and momentary stopping of breathing, associated with hemispheric lesions that are bilateral or diencephalon; *hyperventilation*, with pontine or midbrain lesions; *apneustic breathing*, characterized by a prolonged pause at the end of inspiration, associated with lesions of the mid- and caudal portions of the pons; and *ataxic breathing*, irregular in both rate and tidal volume, seen with damage to the medulla.

Cognitive and Behavioral Impairments. Residual cognitive and behavioral deficits often remain despite a return to full consciousness including problems with attention, memory, and executive function. Disorders of learning, memory, information processing, abstract thinking, and complex problem solving reflect the prefrontal cortex pathology associated with TBI.

Loss of executive functions that regulate, control, and coordinate cognitive processes (planning, problem solving, inhibition, mental flexibility, task switching, initiation, and monitoring of actions) are observed when the dorsolateral prefrontal cortex is damaged.

When the damage is in the orbitofrontal area, behavior may be excessive and disinhibited. Inappropriate social and interpersonal behaviors, including inappropriate sexual behavior, occur with lesions in this area. Mood disturbances may include depression and anxiety. Septal area lesions result in irritability and rage. Pseudobulbar injuries can result in emotional liability, including euphoria, involuntary laughing, or crying that is not associated with negative emotions.

Cognitive deficits are not always directly observable, but observation of behavior provides information regarding the ability to integrate cognitive processes and adjust to the environment. Typical behaviors include erratic wandering; motor, sensory, and verbal perseveration; imitation of gestures; restlessness; refusal to cooperate; and striking out in response to stimulus or in random fashion. Often the individual will attempt to run away from the institution or home. Impulsivity, hyperactivity, and difficulty sustaining attention. Behavioral changes can be present without cognitive or physical deficits.[56] Table 33-2 includes some of the behavioral disturbances and their manifestations in people with TBI.

Memory function is dispersed throughout the brain (see Chapter 28), and there appears to be a lack of ability to use semantic organizational strategies to remember something by associating it with relevant cues. Complaints of memory problems are associated with poor performance on tests of speed, reaction time, attention tasks, and complex perceptual-motor abilities. Language deficits are often seen as word- and name-finding problems. However, recovery of language function appears to surpass that of memory in individuals with minor head injury.[14]

Impairment of memory common with head injury includes retrograde amnesia, the partial or total loss of ability to recall events that have occurred during the period immediately preceding head injury. Posttraumatic amnesia is the time lapse between the injury and the point at which functional memory returns.[7] During this time, there may be improvement in automatic activities, but a lack of carryover of tasks requiring memory or learning. The duration of posttraumatic amnesia is an indicator of the severity of the injury.[43] Anterograde memory is the ability to form new memory. Loss of anterograde memory is common and manifests as decreased attention or inaccurate perception. The capacity for anterograde memory is frequently the last function to return following recovery from loss of consciousness.

TBI is associated with several neuropsychiatric disturbances that can range from subtle deficits to severe disturbances, including cognitive deficits, mood disorders including depression, anxiety disorders, psychosis, and behavioral problems. More than 50% of individuals with TBI develop psychiatric sequelae.[47]

Pain. Pain is a common complaint after brain injury with complex interaction of physical and neuropsychological function. Even with a mild concussion, there is some level of trauma associated. Head and neck pain is common with whiplash, and there is an increased incidence of physical trauma associated with the severity of head injury. Pain can cause a persistent distraction that pulls the individual's attention away from activity and can decrease the ability to concentrate. It can affect the ability to sleep, which leads to daytime lethargy, and it contributes to emotional reactions such as anxiety and depression.[52]

Neuropathic pain can result from the aberrant somatosensory processing in the peripheral or central nervous system, most commonly with damage in the area of the thalamus. Myofascial pain is common with trigger points, stiffness, and weakness. A deep, burning pain followed by persistent, involuntary, and irregular movements of the toes and feet, termed *painful legs and moving toes*, can be associated with minor foot and ankle injuries. Fibromyalgia can develop, as it is related to sleep disturbances, anxiety, and depression. Another component of pain is suffering, in which the intensity is dependent on the person's mood, life experience, and level of social support. The result can often be that the cycle of pain and limitation of central processing can lead to a condition that mimics chronic pain syndrome. Chronic pain can have an impact on the neuropsychological function as part of a vicious cycle. Managing this syndrome in the individual with head injury can be challenging and warrants good decisions regarding both the pharmacologic and neuropsychological approaches.[14]

Cranial Nerve Damage. Focal damage in the brainstem can be reflected in the loss of cranial nerve function. The following are signs of specific cranial nerve deficits.[22,53] Examination of the eyes may yield valuable information about the level of brainstem disease causing coma, given the proximity of centers governing eye movement, pupillary function, and elements of the reticular activating system. Completely normal pupillary function and eye movements suggest that the lesion causing coma is rostral to the midbrain.

Table 33-2	A Typology of Behavioral Disturbances After Traumatic Brain Injury

Symptom	Description
Behavioral Excesses	
Inappropriate abrupt physical action	Responds to a situation too quickly without thinking about the adequacy or consequences of the behavior: doing before thinking. Does not include verbal interruptions
Tangential verbal output	Expresses one thought after another in disconnected or unrelated sequences: rambling speech, unable to get to the point
Excessive verbal output	Provides too much information; content may be overly detailed or redundant; may be unaware of conversational turn exchange signals or unable to terminate conversation.
Verbal interruptions	Inserts comments that disrupt the flow of conversation or the task at hand; may force other person to relinquish conversational turn before completing the thought.
Inappropriate topic selection	Poor discrimination of appropriate topics for the social context. Revealing statements about personal matters, relationships, feelings that are inappropriate for the social context or level of relationship: excessive self-disclosure.
Inappropriate word choice	Use of profanity or emotionally charged words that are inappropriate for the social context. Overly explicit descriptions and explanations.
Physical proximity violation	Positions body within a spatial proximity of another person that is inappropriate for the level of relationship or social context: violating personal space
Sexual inappropriateness	Acts with intent to develop intimate or sexual contacts or relationships inappropriate for the level of relationship or in violation of social mores (e.g., with adolescent minors); conversation contains sexual innuendos or lewd comments. May misinterpret others' expression of friendship as sexual advances, and responds as above.
Poor social judgment	Unaware of or does not apply rules governing social behavior; does not consider personal safety or safety of others in social context: rude, immature, coarse, tactless. Violates rules of etiquette.
Irritability	Feelings of annoyance or impatience; may accompany restlessness; easily provoked but generally does not escalate into an anger outburst. Tends to be a constant state, usually neither improving nor worsening by a significant degree.
Lability of affect	Magnitude of affect displayed is disproportionate to the antecedent event or social context and does not necessarily reflect the true nature or extent of feelings.
Anxious affect and rumination	Feelings of worry, tenseness, fearfulness, uncertainty about the future. Complains or verbalizes concern over trivia.
Angry transition—verbal	An escalation of verbal output, where pitch, volume, or speaking rate increases, dysfluency occurs, aggressive content is delivered. Still within the realm of appropriate. A building-up phase before an outburst.
Angry transition—behavioral	Facial flush; posture threatening; personal space may be violated, body positions exaggerated; agitation behavior is evident such as hair pulling, wringing of hands, clutching the fist.
Anger outburst—verbal	Explosive speech, screaming, abusive language, forceful or harmful content, self-deprecating content, or threats toward another person.
Anger outburst—behavioral	Hitting objects, striking out, exaggerated motions, forceful actions.
Behavioral Deficits	
Absence of or decrease in self-directed action	Decrease in spontaneous behaviors, requires prompts for behavioral action.
Depressed mood	Downcast facial expression, tearfulness, verbalizations of sadness, hopelessness, helplessness, low self-esteem; paucity of interest in pleasant events.
Restricted affect	Display of affect less than proportional to the event; face expressionless; voice monotonous; movement fails to reflect stated feelings.

Modified from Vomoto JM: Neuropsychological assessment and rehabilitation after brain injury. In Berrol S, editor: *Physical medicine and rehabilitation clinics of North America. Traumatic brain injury*, Philadelphia, 1992, WB Saunders, p 307.

The olfactory nerve (CN I) is well protected in the cribriform plate, but shearing of the fibers to the extent of damage occurs in about 7% of head injuries. In about 50% of those cases, this is a temporary condition.

The optic nerve (CN II) is not a true cranial nerve but rather a direct extension of the brain. The most vulnerable component of the optic nerve in people with head injury is the portion of the nerve located within the optic canal. Damage to this portion can result in monocular blindness, a dilated pupil with an absent direct pupillary response, and a brisk consensual response to light. Partial visual defects may take the form of scotomata, sector defects, and upper or lower hemianopia.

The oculomotor nerve (CN III) works in conjunction with the trochlear and abducens nerves to move the eyeball in the orbit to maintain gaze stability and scanning. Damage is often due to direct insult to the musculature, but it can also be due to cerebral herniation. This nerve is damaged in less than 3% of people with head injury. In some cases, there is development of misdirection of regeneration, resulting in constriction of the pupil when any one of the extraocular muscles supplied by the third nerve is activated. Also, because of misdirection of the growing axons, the levator muscle of the lid may receive fibers destined for other muscles. When the person affected attempts to look down, instead of the globe moving down, the lid becomes elevated.

It is important to understand the difference between peripheral damage to the oculomotor system and the abnormal movement that represents damage of a central nature that affects eye movements. Conjugate lateral deviation of the eyes is a sign either of an ipsilateral hemisphere lesion, a contralateral hemisphere seizure focus, or damage involving the contralateral pontine horizontal gaze center. Lateral gaze palsy may signal central herniation with compression of bilateral sixth nerves. Tonic downward deviation of gaze is suggestive of injury or compression involving the thalamus or dorsal midbrain, such as may occur with acute obstructive hydrocephalus or midline thalamic hemorrhage. Tonic upward gaze has been associated with bilateral hemispheric damage. Ocular bobbing, a rapid downward jerk followed by a slow return to mid-position, is indicative of pontine lesions. Rapid intermittent horizontal eye movements suggest seizure activity.[18]

The fourth cranial nerve is the least frequently injured oculomotor nerve (CN IV). Damage is usually in the form of contusion or stretching. With severe frontal blows, there can be direct damage to the fourth nerve or hemorrhage of the tentorial incisura. There can be a vertical diplopia mimicking a third nerve palsy. The prognosis for recovery in fourth nerve palsy is poor because the nerve is so slender that it is often avulsed by the trauma.

The most common form of trigeminal nerve (CN V) injury after head trauma involves the supraorbital and supratrochlear nerves as they emerge from the orbit. Damage results in anesthesia of a portion of the nose, eyebrow, and forehead. Facial trauma may extend the sensory deficits to the cheek, upper lip, gums, teeth, and hard palate. In deep coma, the eyelids can be opened easily, and the corneal reflex (indicating fifth nerve palsy) is often absent.

The abducens nerve (CN VI) is often injured when the head is crushed in an anteroposterior plane with resultant lateral expansion and distortion of the skull. It can also be damaged in fractures of the petrous bone. Vertical movement of the brainstem may severely stretch the sixth nerve as it leaves the pons. There can also be damage in relation to the third and fourth nerves in the orbital fissure. There is failure of the eye to abduct when the head is passively turned away from the side of the lesion. Abnormal wandering movements are present in midbrain lesions, and they usually disappear when the person regains consciousness.

Trauma to the facial nerve (CN VII) is common in head injury. With injury to the temporal bone or swelling of the nerve, external compression caused by hematoma symptoms of facial nerve palsy may occur. Loss of tear production, saliva secretion, and taste in the anterior two-thirds of the tongue and loss of stapedius muscle function may be noted. Muscles controlling facial expressions become weak.

Hearing and vestibular dysfunction occur in head injuries. Transverse fractures of the temporal bone may cause disruption of the auditory and vestibular end organs or result in transient eighth nerve dysfunction (vestibulocochlear nerve, CN VIII). A blow to the head creates a pressure wave that is transmitted through the petrous bone to the cochlea, resulting in hair cell damage and degeneration of cochlear nerves. For further information on dizziness and vertigo, see Chapter 38.

The glossopharyngeal (CN IX), vagus (CN X), spinal accessory (CN XI), and hypoglossal (CN XII) cranial nerves pass through the jugular foramen at the base of the skull. The twelfth nerve passes through the hypoglossal foramen nearby. Injury is most often from a missile wound, but fractures of the occipital condyle can also produce lower cranial nerve palsies. Symptoms include cardiac irregularities, excessive salivation, loss of sensation and gag reflex of the palate, loss of taste on the posterior third of the tongue, hoarse voice, dysphagia, and deviation of the tongue to the side of the lesion.

Motor Deficits. Abnormalities of movement are dependent on the area of the brain injured, with more focal lesions resulting in involvement of a single limb or hemiplegia with abnormal reflexes. The specific manifestations of hemiparesis may include loss of selective motor control, abnormal balance reactions, and sensory loss. Cerebellar damage may result in ataxia and may be on one side of the body or more global in presentation. Basal ganglia dysfunction can result in tremor or bradykinesia. See Chapter 32 for further information regarding focal damage to the brain associated with specific areas of infarct.

Often there is *flaccidity*, the absence of motor responses, at the onset, which is gradually replaced by increased tone, spasticity, and rigidity. *Decorticate posturing*, or hyperactive flexor reflexes in the upper extremities and hyperactive extensor response in the lower extremities, is common initially and reflects the loss of cortical control with motor patterns similar to those seen in a cortical stroke. *Decerebrate posturing*, or hyperactive extensor reflexes in both the upper and lower extremities, reflects injury at the superior border of the pons resulting in the loss of inhibitory control of the cortex and basal ganglia.[2,37] The progression from decorticate to decerebrate posturing in the acute phase of care is seen as a negative sign, as lower levels of the brain are affected.

Direct trauma to subcortical and substantia nigral neurons can result in movement disorders occurring shortly after an injury. Movement disorders occurring months following the injury have been hypothesized to be related to sprouting, remyelination, inflammatory changes, oxidative reactions, and central synaptic reorganization. Peripheral trauma that precedes the development of a movement disorder may alter sensory input, leading to central cortical and subcortical reorganization.

Postural and kinetic tremor can be due to direct traumatic lesions of the dentatothalamic circuit. Postural-kinetic tremors of the arms, legs, or head may occur within weeks of mild TBI even without loss of consciousness. Peripheral trauma can induce tremor, which can occur along with complex regional pain syndrome, dystonia, and myoclonus. Myoclonus, dystonia, and athetosis may be present in individuals with posttraumatic tremors.

Contralateral dystonia can be due to a lesion in the striatum, particularly the putamen. The onset of dystonia may have a latency period from 1 month to 9 years. Spastic dystonia due to pyramidal and extrapyramidal injury and paroxysmal nocturnal dystonia are variants of posttraumatic dystonia. Individuals may develop posttraumatic dystonia as a delayed sequela of severe TBI, initially characterized by coma and quadriplegia. After the individual awakens and the movement improves, severe action dystonia develops.[18]

Heterotopic Ossification. Another complication associated with head injury is the formation of *heterotopic ossification* (HO), or abnormal bone growth in the periarticular tissue. The cause and pathogenesis of HO is unknown, but is associated with trauma around a joint, immobility, and increased tone. Bone scans show evidence of increased uptake reflecting osteogenic activity with elevation of alkaline phosphatase.

The onset of HO is usually 4 to 12 weeks after the head injury, and it is first detected with a loss of range of motion. Local tenderness and a palpable mass eventually can be detected, and there can be erythema, swelling, and pain with movement. HO in the hip area can mimic deep vein thrombosis. Peripheral nerve compression will sometimes develop, especially if the HO is in the elbow. HO can also result in vascular compression and possible lymphedema.[59]

Medical Complications. Multiple medical complications can also occur after TBI. Cardiovascular effects of TBI include neurogenic hypertension and cardiac dysrhythmias. Respiratory complications such as neurogenic pulmonary edema, aspiration pneumonia, and pulmonary emboli usually caused by deep venous thrombosis are common. Other complications include disseminated intravascular coagulation, hyponatremia, diabetes insipidus, and stress gastritis. Iatrogenic infections are common.

MEDICAL MANAGEMENT

DIAGNOSIS. Concussion remains a clinical diagnosis ideally made by a health care provider familiar with the athlete and knowledgeable in the recognition and evaluation of concussion. Every concussive event should be reported and maintained as part of an individual's medical record. Recognition and initial assessment of a concussion should be guided by a symptoms checklist, cognitive evaluation (including orientation, past and immediate memory, new learning and concentration), balance tests, and further neurologic physical examination.

Graded symptom checklists provide an objective tool for assessing a variety of symptoms related to concussions, while also tracking the severity of those symptoms over serial evaluations. Standardized assessment tools provide a helpful structure for the evaluation of concussion. Although limited validation of these assessment tools is available, it is important to remember that the sensitivity, specificity, validity, and reliability of these tests differ among age and cultural groups. Balance disturbance is a specific indicator of a concussion, but not very sensitive. There should be no same-day return to play for an athlete with possible concussion because he or she should be monitored for changes in physical or mental status. Sideline assessment using the Sport Concussion Assessment

Tool SCAT-3 developed at the 3rd International Consensus on Concussion in Sport is becoming standard regulation to monitor cognitive status and symptom complaints in some states and countries.[28]

Neuropsychological tests are an objective measure of brain-behavior relationships and are more sensitive for subtle cognitive impairment than clinical exam. The evaluation consists of a series of cognitive challenges given to the individual, including assessment of sensorimotor status, attention span, memory, language, sequencing, problem solving, and verbal and spatial integration tasks. An example of testing protocol is seen in Figure 33-7. Comparisons of healthy controls and persons with brain injury have been well documented, but the results must be interpreted with recognition of the reliable change index, baseline variability, and false-positive and false-negative rates within the different components of the exam, and never used in isolation of other indications of severity. Previous tests of intellectual function, including IQ tests and achievement tests, can be helpful for comparison, especially in clients with mild brain injury. Cognitive impairment is the primary contributor to disability with moderate to severe brain injury.[31]

Athletes should undergo neuropsychological evaluation when injury is suspected because this may unmask subtle continued deficits if baseline testing is available for

Sample Clinical Report

ImPACT™Clinical Report

Sample Student

Exam Type	Baseline	Post-Injury 1	Post-Injury 2		
Date Tested	07/14/2009	08/25/2010	08/31/2010		
Last Concussion		08/23/2010	08/23/2010		
Exam Language	English	English	English		
Test Version	2.0	2.0	2.0		

Composite Scores							
Memory composite (verbal)	90	80%	72	17%	94	88%	
Memory composite (visual)	79	69%	55	8%	71	39%	
Visual motor speed composite	29.08	33%	19.65	<1%	33.17	34%	
Reaction time composite	0.55	93%	0.79	4%	0.59	56%	
Impulse control composite	8		13		13		
Total Symptom Score	0		31		0		

Scores in **bold RED** type exceed the Reliable Change Index (RCI) when compared to the baseline score. However, scores that do not exceed to RCI index may still be clinically significant. Percentile scores if available are listed in small type.

Figure 33-7

Baseline and postinjury neurocognitive tests (From The ImPACT Test, ImPACT Applications, Inc., Pittsburgh, Pennsylvania [http://www.impacttest.com/about/?The-ImPACT-Test-4])

comparison. The use of computerized testing has become more commonplace to provide a preinjury baseline. Analysis of these test results is ideally offered by a neuropsychologist. Postural stability testing may also be undertaken for adjunctive data in determination of concussion severity with the use of computerized balance testing systems or more simple clinical tests in standing (Balance Evaluation Scoring System) or Sensory Organization Testing. Collegiate and some high school athletic programs have preseason testing programs that allow comparison of cognitive and balance scores to postinjury results when a concussion occurs. This is ideal, but not always possible because a concussion can happen to anyone and are not always as a result of sports activity.

Cognitive and behavioral dysfunctions caused by brain injury are similar to posttraumatic stress syndrome, conversion or hysterical reactions, malingering, depression, and anxiety. Therefore careful evaluation of each individual should be performed to determine cause of symptoms. The trauma occurring at the time of the injury may trigger posttraumatic stress reactions or other psychoses in susceptible individuals with history of prior trauma.

When a person sustains a severe head injury, the GCS is used to assess level of consciousness. Using this scale, three aspects of response are observed independently: eye opening, best motor response, and verbal response. A score of 3 to 8 indicates a severe brain injury. Reflex responses tested by applying a noxious stimulus, such as pressure on a nail bed, fall into three categories: appropriate, inappropriate, or absent.

There is some controversy over including motor responses to describe the depth of coma because neural structures regulating consciousness differ from and are more anatomically distant from those regulating motor function.[48]

Oculomotor and pupillary signs are valuable in assisting with the diagnosis, localizing brainstem damage, and determining the depth of coma. Pupillary examination should document size and reactivity to light. Greater than 1 mm difference in size or asymmetry should be considered abnormal. Once the baseline neurologic status has been determined, repeated evaluations are critical to monitor improvement, provide prognostic data, or detect deterioration, which should be addressed immediately. Symptoms of focal neurologic deficits, lethargy, or skull fractures should be monitored. A mental status examination is important for all individuals with brain injury. Subtle abnormalities may be indicators of significant intracranial injury.

Higher GCS scores are associated with greater than normal cardiac index responses and better tissue oxygenation. Poor outcomes are related to low GCS, hypertension, mild tachycardia, normal pulmonary function, and reduced tissue oxygenation.[45]

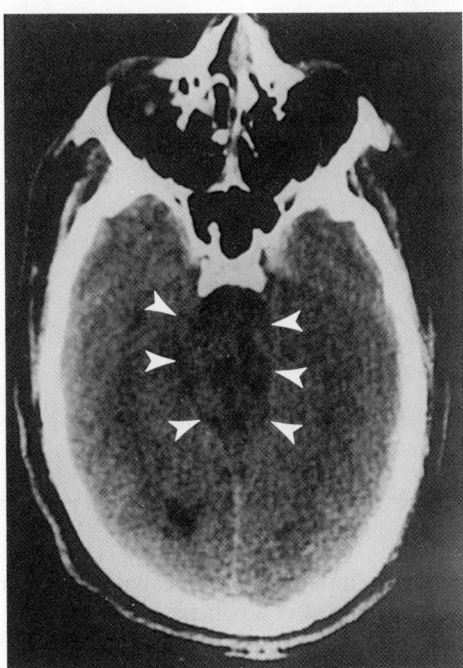

Figure 33-8

CT scan of the head in a patient with a closed head injury. Severe compression of mesencephalic cisterns is seen, indicating midbrain compression. (Reprinted from Townsend CM: *Sabiston textbook of surgery*, ed 17, Philadelphia, 2004, Saunders.)

Diagnostic imaging can provide significant information, which can guide the intervention and allow a more accurate prognosis. CT is the primary imaging modality for the initial diagnosis and management of the person with brain injury. CT scanning of the head reveals the presence of hemorrhage, swelling, or infarction rapidly and less expensively to rule out the need for surgical intervention. In individuals with traumatic coma, patterns on CT that have been associated with worse neurologic outcome include lesions in the brainstem, encroachment of the basal cisterns, and DAI (Fig. 33-8).[57]

DAI is a frequent CT and pathologic correlate of severe TBI, accounting for about 50% of primary brain injuries. DAI is usually associated with a poor outcome. Severe DAI is identifiable on CT as multiple punctate hemorrhages, typically in the deep white matter and corpus callosum and occasionally in the brainstem. DAI may also occur as a result of mild TBI and may culminate in subtle types of cognitive deficits. Approximately 10% to 15% of individuals with clinically severe TBI have a normal CT scan. In such situations, the possibility of extracranial or intracranial vascular disruptions may exist, and angiography should be considered.[18]

Current imaging with CT or magnetic resonance imaging (MRI) does not permit quantification of neural injury that occurs after a concussion. Proton magnetic resonance spectroscopy can be used to assess the neurochemical damage derived from a cerebral concussion by monitoring N-acetyl-L-aspartate levels over time. Current research indicates that N-acetyl-L-aspartate diminution appears to be linked to a general mitochondrial dysfunction, and therefore N-acetyl-L-aspartate restoration may be a surrogate marker of metabolic recovery. Other imaging approaches that show promise for demonstrating damage as a result of concussion include functional MRI, positron emission tomography, diffusion tensor imaging, and functional connectivity techniques; however, these are not routinely used in practice. The combination of metabolic data, physiologic data, and clinical observations may address the complete recovery from concussion.[39]

In severe TBI, a CT is routine because of the likelihood that some intracranial bleeding could be underway. If arterial bleeding occurs, an epidural hematoma can progress very rapidly and cause herniation. Warning signs that may portend need for urgent intervention include any vomiting, restlessness, any GCS score decrease, severe headache, and confusion, and focal temporal blow.[12] Vomiting may also be associated with individuals with migraine familial characteristics, so this should also be considered.[13]

MRI is complementary to CT and is used in conjunction with, not as a replacement for, CT. The multiplanar capabilities of MRI are important to better demonstrate extra-axial hemorrhage located subfrontally, subtemporally, or along the tentorium. Lesions in the posterior fossa, as well as shear injury, are better demonstrated on MRI than on CT. MRI can also detect small hemorrhages in the corpus callosum, intraventricular hemorrhages, or effacement of basal cisternal structures in the absence of brain shift or mass lesions.[26] Positron emission tomography can be used to identify both structural and functional consequences and is valuable for identifying activation patterns after mild head injury, but it is primarily used in a research context. Prediction of outcome should not be based on imaging in isolation from other physical markers.[23]

Electrophysiologic tests that have been used for predicting coma outcomes include somatosensory evoked potentials, transcranial motor evoked potentials, brainstem auditory evoked potentials, and event-related potentials. Visual, auditory, and somatosensory evoked potentials test the integrity of sensory circuits relaying information to the brain and can be used to document changes in a lesion, and therefore may aid in prognosis, but they are not routinely used in isolation.

Approximately 5% to 10% of individuals with severe TBI have an associated spine and/or spinal cord injury. Initial head injury evaluation and management thus require simultaneous evaluation and management for potential spinal injuries. The majority of individuals with severe TBI have multisystem injury. Possibility of other significant and potentially life-threatening injuries should be evaluated and the proper treatment priorities accordingly established.

TREATMENT. Treatment of TBI requires coordinated care and service from the onset of injury through the person's lifetime. The Brain Trauma Foundation provides clinical practice guidelines updated in 2012.[4,7]

Mild TBI or concussion is a topic of significant interest as a result of media attention on sports-related injury and the frequency of brain injury during the recent military conflicts in Iraq and Afghanistan. The American Academy of Neurology and the 4th Zurich Consensus Conference

Table 33-3	Zurich Consensus Guidelines for Progressive Return to Activity after Concussion, 2013[50]	
GRADUATED RETURN TO PLAY PROTOCOL		
Rehabilitation Stage	**Functional Exercise at Each Stage of Rehabilitation**	**Objective of Each Stage**
1. No activity	Symptom-limited physical and cognitive rest	Recovery
2. Light aerobic exercise	Walking, swimming, or stationary cycling, keeping intensity <70% of maximum permitted heart rate. No resistance training	Increase HR
3. Sport-specific exercise	Skating drills in ice hockey, running drills in soccer. No head-impact activities	Add movement
4. Noncontact training drills	Progression to more complex training drills, e.g., passing drills in football and ice hockey. May start progressive resistance training	Exercise, coordination, and cognitive load
5. Full-contact practice	Following medical clearance, participate in normal training activities	Restore confidence and assess functional skills by coaching staff
6. Return to play	Normal game-play	

on Concussion in Sport[50] provide guidance for management of concussion in the sports context. Although 80% to 90% of those who sustain sports concussion will recover fully in 7 to 10 days, this timeline for recovery may be longer for younger athletes. Identification and management of symptoms following concussion is critical, because education and an expectation for recovery is an important part of treatment. Rest is recommended on a short-term basis following injury with a stepwise approach to return to activity, school, or work, and eventually return to play.

Individuals with suspected concussion should be removed immediately from play and not be allowed to return to play on the same day. The Zurich guidelines for progression of return to activity after injury has not been well studied, but conventional practice encourages absent symptom complaints before activities are resumed. For school-aged athletes, the return to school is recommended first, with resumption of typical routine while monitoring responses to the cognitive and activity demands of a usual day. If well tolerated, a graded return to sport activity is recommended as described in the Zurich guidelines[50] (Table 33-3). Components of the concept are as follows: RETURN TO CLASS: Students will require cognitive rest and may require academic accommodations such as reduced workload and extended time for tests while recovering from a concussion. RETURN TO PLAY (RTP): Concussion symptoms should be resolved before returning to exercise. Symptoms of dizziness is one of the significant factors for more prolonged time before RTP. An RTP progression involves a gradual, stepwise increase in physical demands, sports-specific activities, and ongoing assessment to determine readiness for contact drills and eventually full participation. If symptoms occur with activity, the progression should be halted and restarted at the preceding symptom-free step. RTP after concussion should occur only with medical clearance from a licensed health care provider trained in the evaluation and management of concussions. The primary concern with early RTP is decreased reaction time with increased risk of a repeat concussion or other injury and exacerbation or prolongation of symptoms. DISQUALIFICATION FROM SPORT: There are no

evidence-based guidelines for disqualifying/retiring an athlete from a sport after a concussion. Each case should be carefully deliberated and an individualized approach to determining disqualification taken. EDUCATION: Greater efforts are needed to educate involved parties, including athletes, parents, coaches, officials, school administrators, and health care providers to improve concussion recognition, management, and prevention.[39] Figure 33-9 presents the Symptom Wheel, in which symptoms guide progression of activity in classroom and field of play.

Prehospital management of the person with severe TBI includes rapid triage, resuscitation, and efficient transport. Survival and medical management with the goal of stabilization and prevention of secondary complications are the primary medical focus. In the face of hypoxia determining if the upper airway is obstructed, and clearing the airway, is the first treatment administered. Intubation and ventilation are critical procedures, with positive-pressure breathing techniques supplemented by 100% oxygen and early intervention.[26] Hypotension (systolic blood pressure less than 90 mm Hg) and hypoxia (PaO_2 less than 60 mm Hg or oxygen saturation of less than 90%) should be avoided if possible and corrected if present.

Emergency department treatment includes determination of head injury severity, identification of persons at risk of deterioration, and control of hypoxia and hypotension. Prevention of secondary brain damage caused by edema, increased ICP, or bleeding should be addressed. Treatment of the medical complications of the trauma are paramount but not discussed here; the focus of this chapter is on the control and treatment of neurologic sequelae. Close clinical observation remains the best tool for neurologic monitoring in the early stages of brain injury.

Surgical intervention is critical in the presence of hemorrhage to prevent neurologic compromise and can improve both short- and long-term outcomes. Uncal, transtentorial, or tonsillar herniation can occur with hematomas. In some cases, the individual may be lucid after the injury and, then, in the presence of undetected hematoma, lapse into coma and die.

Injury to the dural sinus can occur with a depressed fracture over a major sinus and requires evacuation. Decompression of the skull, often using burr holes, is

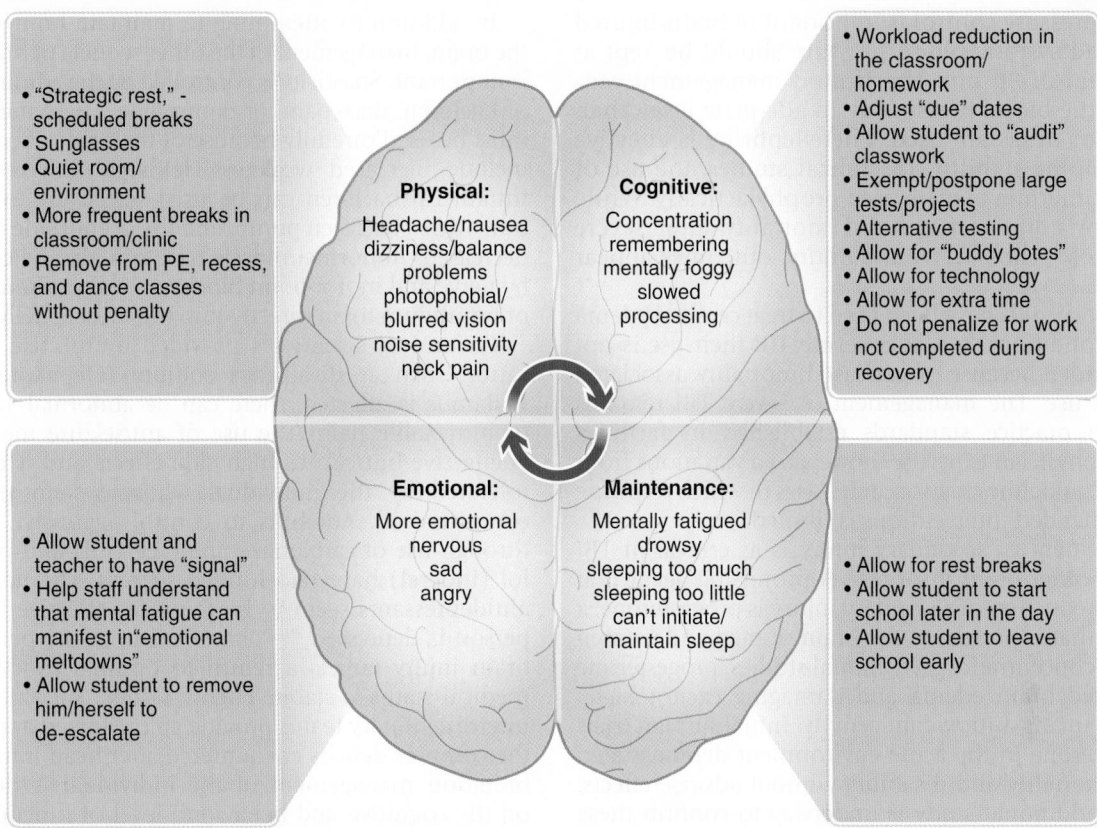

Figure 33-9

Symptom wheel. Certain symptoms lend themselves to certain interventions. The *Symptom Wheel* helps educators align concerns with solutions. (From Colorado Department of Education, Concussion Management Guidelines 2012; http://www.cde.state.co.us/HealthAndWellness/BrainInjury. htm, accessed July 15, 2013.)

warranted in the presence of significant cerebral edema or subdural hematoma. Decompressive craniectomy for intractable brain swelling is an older treatment that has recently received renewed attention to counter the effects of intractable increased ICP. This intervention may be used in particular with younger patients (Brain Trauma Foundation guidelines).

ICP monitoring is recommended for adults with severe TBI (GCS score 3-8) and an abnormal CT scan. Additional consideration or ICP monitoring include individuals whose neurologic status cannot be assessed because of administration of sedative drugs or neuromuscular blocking agents, age greater than 40 years, presence of limb posturing, and systolic BP <90 mm Hg (Brain Trauma Foundation). Indications for ICP monitoring in children are less clearly defined. CPP is monitored to characterize blood supply to the brain. CPP is derived by subtracting ICP from mean arterial pressure. If ICP increases, the level of systemic arterial pressure can be increased to maintain healthy levels of CPP. Sometimes mean arterial pressure is increased in order to increase CPP. Medications can be used to increase mean arterial pressure to counteract increased ICP and drive CPP to acceptable levels. There are guidelines from the Brain Trauma Foundation that suggest what levels of ICP are recommended and what range of CPP is desired.

For adults, the recommended range of CPP is 50 to 70 mm Hg. Higher CPP carries with it the risk of respiratory distress syndrome, whereas lower CPP is associated with brain ischemia. Recommended values for children are 40 to 50 mm Hg, with variation in acceptable values for infants and adolescents. Surgery can be performed to relieve increased ICP unilaterally or bilaterally depending on the presentation. Elevation of ICP more than 20 mm Hg is a significant predictor of a poor outcome. Monitoring of ICP can be accomplished in a number of ways. The ventriculostomy catheter allows monitoring and drainage of cerebrospinal fluid but it is the most invasive method and is associated with risk of infection. The epidural catheter, hollow subarachnoid bolt, and subarachnoid fiberoptic catheter are other options. All must be surgically placed. The noninvasive Doppler waveform can also provide information regarding ICP. If an ICP monitor is in place, the drainage of cerebrospinal fluid may have significant therapeutic benefits.

Cerebral fluid volume can be reduced pharmacologically. Mannitol is used to reduce blood viscosity and thereby improve circulation to brain tissue. Hyperventilation has been used as mechanism for controlling cerebral blood volume by increases in $PaCO_2$, resulting in vasoconstriction of the central vessels and reduced CBF. This must be considered a short-term procedure to be used judiciously because the cerebral vasoconstriction induced may produce ischemia; therefore, it is not recommended in the first 24 to 48 hours after injury and then only used on a short-term basis to reduce ICP.

Blood pressure control is important in brain-injured clients, and systolic blood pressure should be kept at a minimum of 90 mm Hg. If fluid management cannot keep the blood pressure at an adequate level, then vasopressor drugs are used. Phenylephrine is effective at maintaining stability. In clinical studies, the use of mild hypothermia may be used prophylactically. While hypothermia has not reduced mortality after severe TBI, in those who survive the injury, outcomes appear to benefit.

Glucocorticoids have been used to treat cerebral edema in other conditions, but after severe TBI their use is not recommended because of increased mortality associated with their use. The management of severe TBI remains subject to practice standards established in facilities based on physician expertise, however, so variations from published guidelines may occur in cases in which response to recommended interventions is limited.

Management of secondary injury is as critical in TBI as it is in other brain disorders. A promising agent that may offer reduction of secondary injury is progesterone, a hormone that is present in the brain of men and women in similar concentrations. In animal studies, progesterone has reduced brain edema and damaging excitotoxicity while enhancing antioxidant activity. Initial human trials of progesterone in the acute environment demonstrated reduced mortality and disability without adverse effects; however, additional study is underway to confirm these results in a larger sample to guide future practice.[40] Study of various neurotrophic and antioxidant agents show benefits in animals, but the transfer of these benefits to humans has been limited.

An active area of TBI research is the area of molecular genetics. It has been noted that certain genes are upregulated, whereas others are downregulated, after both trauma and ischemia. Particular attention has been focused on the apolipoprotein E gene (ApoE) and its various alleles. This gene is associated with susceptibility for late-onset and familial Alzheimer disease and also has been linked to greater risk of CTE in boxers. Certain alleles have been associated with an increased susceptibility and severity of brain injury, and others have been linked to improved recoveries after TBI.

Because of the intense sympathetic stimulation seen with head injury, hypertension and tachycardia are prevalent. Cushing phenomenon, or a rise in blood pressure in the presence of an acute rise in ICP (most often caused by brainstem compression), may be present. Moderate increases in blood pressure can be tolerated, but extreme hypertension should be treated because it could lead to increased blood volume.[26]

In the military context, past history of mild TBI and current symptoms influence the duration of rest that is recommended after exposure to blast or injury where concussion is suspected. Guidelines have been developed through collaboration of Defense and Veterans Brain Injury Center and Defense Centers of Excellence for Psychological Health and Traumatic Brain Injury to direct military physicians and therapists in best practice to manage concussion complaints and maintain health of service members with brain injury (see http://dcoe.health.mil/TraumaticBrainInjury.aspx).

In addition to attempting to maintain homeostasis in the brain, management of the other sequela of brain injury is important. Spasticity is controlled by the administration of baclofen, diazepam, or dantrolene. These medications must be used carefully because of their side effects, which include increased weakness, lethargy, and drowsiness. Intrathecal baclofen can be used selectively to decrease tone with a baclofen pump, and the overall side effects are decreased. Abnormal muscle tone can also be controlled by nerve and motor point blocks or by the administration of botulinum toxin directly into the muscle belly.[26]

Control of seizures is provided by the use of medication such as divalproex sodium (Depakote). If the thalamus is affected, there can be abnormal sensations or intractable pain. The use of antiseizure medications is effective but carries high side effects and is often not tolerated by the individual whose system is already compromised. Attempts to control aggressive behavior through use of carbamazepine (Tegretol) and propranolol (Inderal) have had limited success. The nontricyclic antidepressants seem to be the most effective when the person is depressed.[20] Rehabilitation of the person with brain injury targets a return to optimal function once medical status is stable. Highly skilled, specially trained interdisciplinary teams provide an organized approach to the complex deficits encountered after head injury. Rehabilitation management of the individual is dependent on the cognitive and behavioral level of function of the individual. A useful tool to assess behaviors as a function of cognitive recovery is the Rancho Los Amigos Levels of Cognitive Function Scale (Table 33-4). This scale was developed in the late 1970s, so some of the terminology currently in use in clinical practice is not included. The Braintree Neurologic Stages of Recovery from Diffuse TBI (Box 33-2) scale provides more contemporary terminology and corresponding Rancho stages. The Rancho Motor abilities are also critical in dictating the focus in rehabilitation. Cognitive and motor abilities may progress at different rates, such that some patients may be close to preinjury level in one area and remain very impaired in another, with diverse presentations.

Restoration of mobility, self-care, employment, and recreational activities are important goals, each depending on the level of sensorimotor impairment as well as cognitive status. See "Special Implications for the Therapist 33-1: Traumatic Brain Injury," below. Psychotherapy is critical in posttraumatic stress disorder and can be helpful to establish coping mechanisms to address the cognitive deficits and problem solving in relationship to daily activity.

Community-based programs for the person with brain injury that enhance the transition from rehabilitation unit to independent living have become less available. However, therapists still play a significant role addressing the need for intervention as the individual transitions to community living. In order to return to a lifestyle that may include work or school, the person with TBI needs to learn how to cope with the multiple demands on his or her attention that are part of that lifestyle. The person with TBI will have difficulty with executive functions such as organizing time and information, self-monitoring, and self-correcting. Self-motivation is often lacking,

Table 33-4	Rancho Los Amigos Scale for Levels of Cognitive Functioning
Level	**Behaviors Typically Demonstrated**
I.	No response: Client appears to be in a deep sleep and is completely unresponsive to any stimuli.
II.	Generalized response: Client reacts inconsistently and nonpurposefully to stimuli in a nonspecific manner. Responses are limited and are often the same regardless of stimulus presented. Responses may be physiologic changes, gross body movements, or vocalization.
III.	Localized response: Client reacts specifically but inconsistently to stimuli. Responses are directly related to the type of stimulus presented. May follow simple commands in an inconsistent, delayed manner, such as closing eyes or squeezing hand.
IV.	Confused–agitated: Client is in heightened state of activity. Behavior is bizarre and nonpurposeful relative to immediate environment. Does not discriminate among persons or objects; is unable to cooperate directly with treatment efforts. Verbalizations frequently are incoherent or inappropriate to the environment; confabulation may be present. Gross attention to environment is very brief; selective attention is often nonexistent. Client lacks short-term and long-term recall.
V.	Confused–inappropriate: Client is able to respond to simple commands fairly consistently. However, with increased complexity of commands or lack of any external structure, responses are nonpurposeful, random, or fragmented. Demonstrates gross attention to the environment, but is highly distractible and lacks ability to focus attention on a specific task. With structure, may be able to converse on a social-automatic level for short periods of time. Verbalization is often inappropriate and confabulatory. Memory is severely impaired, often shows inappropriate use of objects; may perform previously learned tasks with structure but is unable to learn new information.
VI.	Confused–appropriate: Client shows goal-directed behavior but is dependent on external input for direction. Follows simple directions consistently and shows carryover for relearned tasks with little or no carryover for new tasks. Responses may be incorrect because of memory problems but appropriate to the situation; past memories show more depth and detail than recent memory.
VII.	Automatic–appropriate: Client appears appropriate and oriented within hospital and home settings; goes through daily routine automatically, but frequently robot-like with minimal-to-absent confusion; has shallow recall of activities. Shows carryover for new learning, but at a decreased rate. With structure is able to initiate social or recreational activities; judgment remains impaired.
VIII.	Purposeful–appropriate: Client is able to recall and integrate past and recent events and is aware of and responsive to environment. Shows carryover for new learning and needs no supervision once activities are learned. May continue to show a decreased ability relative to premorbid abilities, abstract reasoning, tolerance for stress, and judgment in emergencies or unusual circumstances.

Modified from Hagen C, Malkmus D, Durham P: Levels of cognitive functioning. In *Rehabilitation of the head injured adult: comprehensive physical management,* Downey, Calif, 1979, Professional Staff Association of Rancho Los Amigos Hospital, pp 87–88.

and structure is necessary to ensure follow-through on assigned activities. Use of checklists, devices that provide reminders, and environmental cues are helpful when attempting to reintegrate the client into the community.

Individuals with high-level physical skills and moderate- or low-level cognition skills are often the most difficult to reintegrate into the family and society. Family and coworker expectations are high because physical function appears at the preinjury level, but cognitive and behavioral deficits can severely limit safety and the ability to participate in life roles. In general, it is cognitive function that makes one more successful in society. Aggressive counseling should start as soon as the behavioral and cognitive impairments are identified. Neuropsychologists and counselors can suggest interventions that help with cognitive functions, especially techniques to deal with memory loss, decreased attention span, and inappropriate behavior.

Significant deficits in motor skills but higher levels of cognitive skills generally lead to a higher quality of life. There are numerous upper and lower extremity adaptive devices to help perform activities of daily living. Electric wheelchairs controlled by the head, mouth, or hand and electric lifts for vans as well as hand controls for driving can assist with mobility. Computerized communications systems can improve interactions when speech is disrupted and cognition is still present.

The lack of motivation associated with TBI becomes a challenge for the therapist. Lack of internal initiation and decreased ability to learn may persist despite cues from the external environment. Setting goals that are meaningful to the client, even though they may seem to be unrealistic, is the first step in motivating the individual.

Alterations in attention span can be detrimental to progress in therapy. Reducing distracting stimuli can be helpful initially; distractions can be reintroduced as the ability to manage multiple inputs improves. In most cases, the family of the survivor needs help understanding their family member's social and behavioral changes.[55]

PROGNOSIS. TBI accounts for a disproportionate share of morbidity and mortality across the life span. Of these, 3% (approximately 52,000) die, 16% (275,000) are hospitalized; and 81% (1.365 million) are seen in the emergency room and then released. The incidence of severe long-term disability is small.[18]

Factors that affect outcome can be categorized in three major areas: injury severity, preinjury factors, and postinjury factors.[5,46] Injury severity is the area that has been most studied. The depth of impaired responsiveness and the duration of altered consciousness is related to outcome.[33] In addition, the duration of posttraumatic amnesia has been used as a predictor of severity of the brain injury. Other aspects of neurologic functioning

BRAINTREE NEUROLOGIC STAGES OF RECOVERY FROM DIFFUSE TBI AND CORRESPONDING RANCHO LOS AMIGOS SCALE LEVELS

1. *Coma*: unresponsive, eyes closed, no sign of wakefulness (Rancho Level I) (emergency medical services; acute inpatient hospital)
2. *Vegetative state (VS)/wakeful unconsciousness*: no cognitive awareness; transition marked by beginning spontaneous eye opening and sleep-wake cycles (Rancho Level II) (acute hospital)
3. *Minimally conscious state (MCS)*: Inconsistent, simply purposeful behavior, inconsistent response to commands begin; transition can be documented using Coma Recovery Scale–Revised (CRS-R) subscale criteria for minimally conscious state (47); often mute (Rancho Level III) (acute hospital; acute inpatient rehabilitation; subacute rehabilitation)
4. *Confusional state*: Interactive communication and appropriate object use begin; transition can be documented using CRS-R subscale criteria for emergence from minimally conscious state (47); amnesic (PTA), severe basic attentional deficits, hypokinetic or agitated, labile behavior; later more appropriate goal-directed behavior with continuing anterograde amnesia (Rancho Levels IV, V, and partly VI) (acute inpatient rehabilitation; acute hospital)
5. *Postconfusional/emerging independence*: marked by resolution of PTA; transition can be marked using scales such as the Galveston Orientation and Amnesia Test (GOAT) (4B); cognitive impairments in higher level attention, memory retrieval, and executive functioning; deficits in self-awareness, social awareness, behavioral, and emotional regulation; achieving functional independence in daily self-care; improving social interaction; developing independence at home (Rancho Level VI and partly VII) (acute inpatient rehabilitation, subacute inpatient rehabilitation, outpatient rehabilitation, residential treatment, outpatient day hospital, and community reentry)
6. *Social competence/community reentry*: marked by resumption of basic household independence and ability to be left home unsupervised for the better part of a day; developing independence in community, household management skills, and later returning to academic or vocational pursuits; recovering higher level cognitive abilities (divided attention, cognitive speed, executive functioning), self-awareness, and social skills; developing effective adaptation and compensation for residual problems (Rancho Levels VII and VIII) (outpatient community reentry programs, community-based services—vocational, special education, supported living services, mental health services)

Katz DI, Zasler NC, Zafonte RD: Clinical continuum of care and natural history. In Zasler ND, Katz DI, Zafonte RD (eds): *Brain Injury Medicine: Principles and Practice*, ed 2, New York, Demos Medical, 2013.

that indicate injury severity are also correlated with outcome.

Loss of pupillary light reflexes reflects significant damage to the brainstem and portends a poor prognosis. Oculomotor deficits often signal concomitant cerebral damage, resulting in severe cognitive deficits. The degree of hypoxemia and hypotension encountered in the early stages can also have an effect on the long-term prognosis.[54]

CT has increased the ability to predict outcome when there are lesions of the brain parenchyma, intercranial hematoma, subdural hematoma, or massive hemispheric swelling. Acute hemispheric swelling with an extracerebral hematoma is associated with the worst prognosis. Unilateral brain contusion and DAI also carry a poor prognosis. A midline shift of brain structures, absent or compressed basal cisterns (indicating rising ICP), and subarachnoid hemorrhage will increase the risk of death or remaining in a vegetative state.[57]

With severe injury, the possibility of cognitive and behavioral deficits increases. Cognitive deficits that affect motivation, attention, emotion, memory, or learning will limit recovery. A lack of awareness of deficits and lack of social skills reduces the ability to reintegrate into the community.[58]

Epilepsy occurring within 7 days is often related to severe injury, depressed fracture, penetrating injury, or intracranial hemorrhage. Posttraumatic epilepsy may emerge months or years following brain trauma and is more common after severe brain injury. Late epilepsy occurs most often as grand mal seizures or temporal lobe seizures.[24] Further information on seizures is available in Chapter 36.

Many studies of outcome relate injury severity to mortality as an important indicator. Once a person survives an injury, factors that affect outcome are complex but include preinjury characteristics and postinjury factors. Neuropsychologic dysfunction appears greater in people who sustain injury over the age of 30 years and those with less education. History of substance abuse, low educational level, prior brain injury, and psychiatric disorders can also limit success. Social and family problems are common and can cause isolation and poor quality of life.[36]

Postinjury factors such as access to appropriate care and adequate supports are critical to optimize recovery. A multidisciplinary rehabilitation team is effective in facilitating TBI recovery. However, it is important that the individual is able to be active in the rehabilitation process to take full advantage of the benefits. If an individual is in a vegetative state for a period of time after injury, more intense rehabilitation may be more effective once emergence from the vegetative state occurs. Family and social supports are key factors in recovery. Families require education and support in order to understand how to best help their family member. Often it becomes difficult to sustain relationships that were stable before the injury. Working with professionals who recognize these deficits and are trained to treat them will improve the chances of increasing quality of life after brain injury. Because change in functional abilities is common with moderate and severe injury, supports that will allow for community-based treatment and living are important, but are not always available.

Measures that address global functioning/outcome are the Glasgow Outcome Scale–Extended and the Disability Rating Scale (http://tbims.org/combi/drs/index.html). These scales measure function from coma to community reintegration, so they capture gross abilities. As a result, they are not very sensitive to small changes in function or for those with milder injuries. The Mayo-Portland Adaptability Inventory may be more useful for considering common obstacles to community reintegration, including physical, cognitive, emotional, behavioral, and social factors (http://tbims.org/combi/mpai/index.html). For specific recommendations of outcome measures for use in physical therapy practice across a range of clinical practice settings, refer to the TBIEDGE recommendations developed by a task force from the APTA Neurology Section. These recommendations are available on the neuropt.org site and are also shared on the rehabmeasures.org site.[60]

TRAUMATIC BRAIN INJURY IN CHILDREN

TBI is one of the leading causes of death and disability in children of all ages.[44] Nonaccidental injury is a common cause of brain injury in infants and toddlers and is often the result of the battered child or shaken baby syndrome. Injury is caused by shaking or striking the child.

Although the pathology of the brain injury in the child reflects damage similar to that in the adult, there are differences. Infants typically have tears in the white matter of the temporal and orbitofrontal lobes. The infant will more often sustain a subdural or epidural hemorrhage than an older child but is less likely to have skull fracture because of the pliancy of the skull.

Drowning is the third leading cause of death in children aged 1 to 4 years. Peak incidences occur in 1- to 4-year-olds and in adolescent boys. Boys are three times more likely to be injured. Rapid resuscitation leads to better outcomes, with poor outcome associated with near-drowning. As in adults, the motor activity return and pupillary light response are prognosticators of outcome (see Chapter 15).

A children's coma scale has been developed for use in children younger than age 3 years (Box 33-3). The highest level of ocular response is eye tracking. The verbal response is rated highest by crying, then by spontaneous respirations, with the lowest score given for apneic breathing. The highest motor response score is for flexing and extending the extremities.

Early management of the infant or child with TBI is similar to that of the adult, with some difference in the child's ability to tolerate the medications used. Late seizures are less common with children than with adults, so the need to be maintained on seizure medication is less.[34]

Rehabilitation goals for the child are similar to those of the adult, although play is used during therapy. Orthotic and assistive devices are used frequently but for a shorter time than for adults. Agitation is common and is often difficult for the parents and siblings to handle. Aggression, decreased attention span, hyperactivity, and socially inappropriate behavior are seen. These children often require a great deal of behavior modification.

Community reintegration can be as difficult for the child as it is for the adult. Schools are better prepared to handle cognitive delays than abnormal behaviors. Cognitive status may return in one area and remain defective in another. Attention and memory deficits may produce the greatest obstacles to learning.

SPECIAL IMPLICATIONS FOR THE THERAPIST   33-1

Traumatic Brain Injury

Rehabilitation of the brain-injured person involves the therapist at many different levels and in different settings. Typical progression through the system of care is illustrated in Figure 33-10. Understanding the deficits common in acute injury and the natural recovery patterns of the brain dependent on the site and type of injury is paramount for the therapist treating brain injury. The therapist working with individuals with brain injury must understand the interaction between the deficits related to cognitive and social behaviors and the ability to learn to move.[61] Cognitive rehabilitation and physical rehabilitation are closely related. Functional outcomes are limited by the cognitive status, and the understanding of the techniques that foster behavioral modification and learning should be used by the therapist during motor skill acquisition.[56] Occupational therapists assess individuals with brain injury in functional contexts to observe for the ability to integrate motor, sensory, and cognitive function in common activities of daily life. In some settings, occupational therapists may test components of cognitive and perceptual abilities. Language and cognitive problems are examined as well by speech pathologists and can include naming tests, aphasia examinations, as well as tests of auditory comprehension and speed of comprehension. Speech-language pathologists also assess for oral-motor control difficulties such as dysphagia (difficulty swallowing) and dysarthria (difficulty with articulation for speech).

Often the therapist will be involved in a dedicated brain injury unit or in a community reentry program. Even in a more general setting, the therapist is often responsible for intervention with individuals sustaining brain injury, often acutely, or when an individual has been through a rehabilitation setting and is referred for follow-up based on residual deficits. Provision of therapy in the long-term care setting involves care for

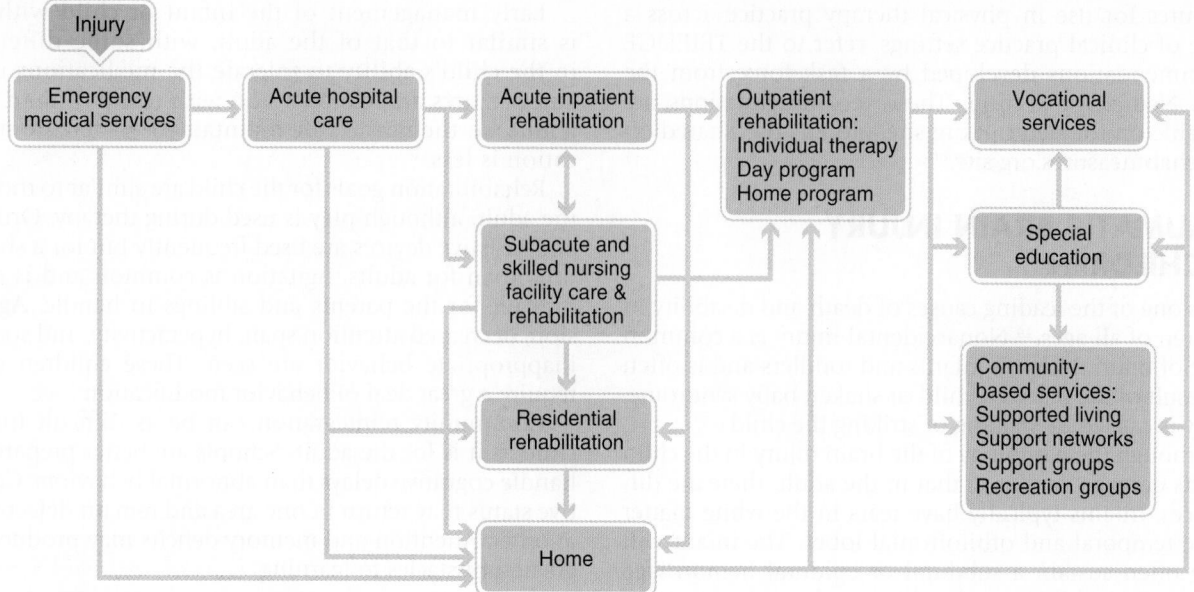

Figure 33-10

Typical flow of patients through the continuum of care. (From Zasler ND, Katz DI, Zafonte RD: Brain injury medicine: principles and practice, ed 2, New York, Demos Medical, 2013.)

individuals in the minimally conscious state, or with behavioral deficits precluding independent living.[8]

In the acute care setting, the therapist is responsible for the evaluation of neurologic function in conjunction with physicians and nurses. One role may be consistent monitoring of cranial nerve function. In addition, the therapist is involved in monitoring reflexive and voluntary motor behaviors. The treatment plan often includes pulmonary care, positioning, range-of-motion exercises, and relaxation techniques. Movement facilitation begins early in the treatment and continues throughout rehabilitation in many cases. Because treatment starts while the individual is still in the intensive care unit, a discussion of life-sustaining equipment follows.

Chest tubes are common with a pneumothorax or hemothorax. The drainage tube should be kept below the level of the chest at all times. Upper extremity movement should be monitored so as not to interfere with the tube. Nasogastric tube feeding is also common initially, and when a tube is in place, the head of the bed should be placed at 30 degrees to avoid aspiration. It is important that cerebral venous blood volume be controlled in head injury. Maintaining the head in a neutral nonrotated position and at a 20- to 40-degree tilt will usually provide adequate drainage. However, compression of venous drainage from tracheal ties and collars and extreme neck flexion or extension can occur if precautions are not followed. Lines such as central venous pressure catheters, pulmonary or arterial lines, and ICP monitors can be compromised during movement, and often the movement will trigger an alarm that can be upsetting for the client and family. Close communication with the nursing staff will give the therapist confidence in moving the person in the intensive care setting.

Pulmonary management is another critical area. Techniques such as percussion, vibration, and suctioning are used to keep the airway clear but must be done with caution and may be contraindicated in the presence of increased ICP. Monitoring blood gases and oxygen saturation is critical in some clients, because movement may alter these values. Weaning from the ventilator is an individual endeavor. Some clients are able to continue to incorporate activity during weaning, but for others it may mean a decrease in tolerance to movement.[25]

Management of decreased range of motion from spasticity or HO is another intervention provided by therapists. Joint contractures are a secondary problem produced by inability of the muscle to return to its normal resting length. Serial casting and dynamic splinting are used to maintain joint motion in the presence of spasticity, rigidity, or HO.[4] Managing excessive muscle and reflex activity through movement and positioning begins in the acute phase and often must still be addressed in the rehabilitative phase.

Similar concepts apply to decisions for wheelchair seating and positioning in the nonambulatory individual. Prevention of secondary joint disorders, pain, and disfigurement is facilitated by provision of support in the anatomically proper position. Materials and equipment that are lightweight and provide total contact provide the most comfortable support.[11]

Swallowing deficits and related problems with respiration or coughing occur in approximately one-third of persons with head injury. Head, neck, and trunk control affect the ability to swallow. Intervention based on lack of strength and mobility of the perioral structures often starts in the acute phase. Sensation, dentition, tongue control, and laryngeal control are assessed to determine the level of impairment relating to disability of speech and swallowing.[62]

Hemiplegia often persists and is seen in more than 50% of individuals with brain injury 6 months after onset. Diffuse damage to the central white matter tracts and midbrain with loss of integration of reflexes can have a devastating effect on function. See Chapter 32 for further information on hemiplegia.

Because somatosensory, visual, and vestibular inputs can be disrupted after TBI, dizziness and imbalance is common. A thorough evaluation of sensory integration function is necessary in order to design intervention. Therapists must be knowledgeable about the effects of brain injury so as to intervene without overstimulating, and attend to cognitive and behavioral aspects of the brain injury to ensure adherence to therapy. Visual stimulation may be disorienting so the client prefers to maintain an environment without peripheral visual stimuli, has difficulty reading, and avoids situations with fluorescent lighting. The individual may be hypervigilant in regard to the vestibular input and is already overstimulated by the time he or she reaches the therapist. Often there is a sensation of moving when at rest that is uncovered by sitting with the eyes closed. This can be an indication of maladaptation of the vestibular system. Settling techniques, such as putting weights on the shoulders, or pressing down on the top of the head can increase somatosensory input. Sensitivity to vestibular input can be decreased with activities that gradually increase exposure to vestibular challenges.

The individual with TBI will have complex movement disorders related to force production, timing, reaction time, and fatigue, and movements may be too slow for function. Sensory disturbances are significant, and the therapist should be adequately trained to evaluate and understand the sensory contributions to function. Learning new tasks is difficult, as described above in relation to central dysfunction, and cognitive deficits can limit progress. However, there are many opportunities to work with patients on high levels of balance and mobility function. The High-level Mobility Assessment Test (HiMAT) is an outcome measure developed specifically to monitor progress in people with brain injury who are interested in returning to running (http://tbims.org/comb i/himat/index.html).

The therapist should understand that with repetition of appropriate activities, these individuals can make significant gains. Although recovery may be rapid closer to the time of injury, small incremental changes can continue over months and years post injury. The use of appropriate environmental supports may be necessary to compensate for abilities that are lost, but quality of life can be restored. There are excellent resources available to assist the therapist in treatment. Many therapists have special expertise, and institutions are focused on management of the individual with brain injury.

Thank you to Nicole Miranda for her review and contributions to the information regarding concussion.

REFERENCES

To enhance this text and add value for the reader, all references are included on the companion Evolve site that accompanies this text book. The reader can view the reference source and access it online whenever possible.

CHAPTER 34

Traumatic Spinal Cord Injury

CANDY TEFERTILLER • LAURA S. WEHRLI • KENDA S. FULLER

SPINAL CORD INJURY

Spinal cord injury (SCI) is a catastrophic event of low incidence and high cost. It is most often highly active persons who incur the types of accidents that cause severe SCI. Within a matter of seconds, the person sustaining a traumatic SCI will become dependent on others or on assistive devices to perform even the most basic activities of self-care. SCI rarely occurs in isolation, and more than 75% of these individuals have some other systemic injury. In 10% to 15%, there is an associated head injury. This concern has led to the widely quoted clinical maxim that all traumatized patients or any patient with a severe head injury should be presumed to have a spine injury or SCI until proven otherwise.[42]

Incidence and Risk Factors

Males account for more than 80% of all cases of traumatic SCI. Most of the injured have traditionally been young people, but the mean age of SCI increased in the 1990s and is now recorded as the early forties. There is now a higher survival rate in the older population; in addition, the mean age of the general population also has increased. It is estimated that there are approximately 30 to 40 cases per 1 million persons on an annual basis, with an additional 6 to 8 deaths (per 1 million) occurring before hospitalization; however, the number of deaths occurring before hospitalization is decreasing. The number of individuals living with SCI is approximately 270,000, with 12,000 new cases each year.[76]

The primary cause of SCI is motor vehicle accidents, accounting for nearly 40% of SCIs. Falls are the second most common cause at 28%. Approximately 15% of SCIs are caused by violence; these include job-related injuries to security guards, policemen, workers shot during robberies, victims of violent crimes, and others. The likelihood of SCI from a gunshot wound appears to be higher among those who have had previous gunshot wounds (30%) or who have had prior involvement in the criminal justice system (52%). Unlike sports injuries, which peak nationwide during the summer months, the incidence of penetrating wounds of the spine remains the same throughout the year, and 40% of them occur on a Saturday or Sunday.[35]

Sports-related injuries account for less than 7% of the total. Accidents resulting in SCI are most prevalent in the contact sports of football and wrestling, high-speed sports such as snow skiing and surfing, and sports in which injuries can involve a fall from a height, such as a trampoline or a horse. Figure 34-1 shows a breakdown of the typical incidence of injury types.

Approximately 43% of all persons with SCIs have paraplegia, and 57% have tetraplegia. Twenty-one percent of all thoracic and lumbar cord injuries are complete lesions, as are 16% of cervical injuries. For penetrating wounds of the spine, however, a significantly greater proportion are complete, and there is a much greater shift toward thoracic spinal injuries as compared with injuries of the neck or lumbar spine.[75,99]

Definition and Etiologic Factors

Traumatic spinal cord injury is classified as concussion, contusion, or laceration. A *concussion* is an injury caused by a blow or violent shaking and results in temporary loss of function, similar to the cerebral concussion associated with head injury. In *contusion* injury, the glial tissue and spinal cord surface remain intact. There may be a loss of central grey and white matter, which creates a cavity that is surrounded by a rim of intact white matter at the periphery of the spinal cord. *Laceration* or *maceration* of the cord occurs with more severe injuries in which the glia is disrupted and the spinal cord tissue may be torn. Occasionally, this can result in complete transection of the cord. Gunshot wounds, knife wounds, and puncture injuries fall into this category.

Hemorrhages into the dura are common, although they rarely become large enough to compromise the spinal cord. Subarachnoid hemorrhages, caused by contusion and laceration of the cord, are frequent and can cause further compression of the cord.

The mechanism of injury influences the type and degree of the spinal cord lesion. Figure 34-2 shows the flexion damage that is referred to as the hangman's fracture, related to excessive flexion. Approximately 50% of injuries come from excessive flexion of the spinal column that results in a severe neurologic disorder.[21] Figure 34-3 shows how extension can cause SCI in the elderly

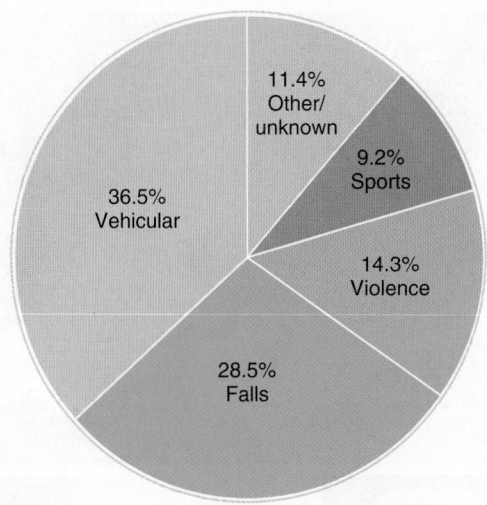

Figure 34-1

Approximate causes of traumatic spinal cord injury in 2010. (From National Spinal Cord Injury Statistical Center (NSCISC). Available at www.uab.edu/nscisc. Accessed June 3, 2013.)

population. Figure 34-4 shows vascular changes that may result from displacement of spinal components. The spinal cord is often violently displaced or compressed momentarily during an injury with forceful flexion, extension, and rotation of the spine. The vertebral body can burst and cause pressure or scatter bone fragments into the spinal cord. Figure 34-5 illustrates this phenomenon. Complete spinal cord lesions occur in about one third of flexion injuries. With crush fractures of the vertebrae, there is a 75% chance of a complete spinal cord lesion.

The majority of spinal cord–injured patients have at least one other system injury. Occasionally these injuries take precedence in evaluation and treatment. If one level of bony injury has been identified, it is necessary to survey the entire spine, because there is a 10% to 15% incidence of spinal injury at other levels.[42]

The difference between a complete and an incomplete spinal cord lesion may depend on the survival of a small fraction of the axons in the spinal cord. Evidence of axonal conduction across the lesion site has been found in individuals with clinical neurologic diagnoses of complete SCI at that level. The surviving axons may be injured and therefore have a decreased response to stimuli. The injured axon conducts slowly and fatigues rapidly.[106]

Pathogenesis

The development of the spinal lesion occurs over time and in a neuroanatomic distribution. In the first 18 hours, there is necrotic death of axons that were directly disrupted by the trauma. In the following weeks, there is further progression of tissue injury in both directions from the lesion. The immune system probably plays a major role during this phase. It appears that immune cells, such as monocytes and macrophages, emit chemical signals, such as cytokines and chemokines, that trigger apoptosis, or programmed cell death. This breakdown of cell function can occur away from the lesion site, often by as far away as four spinal segments.[19]

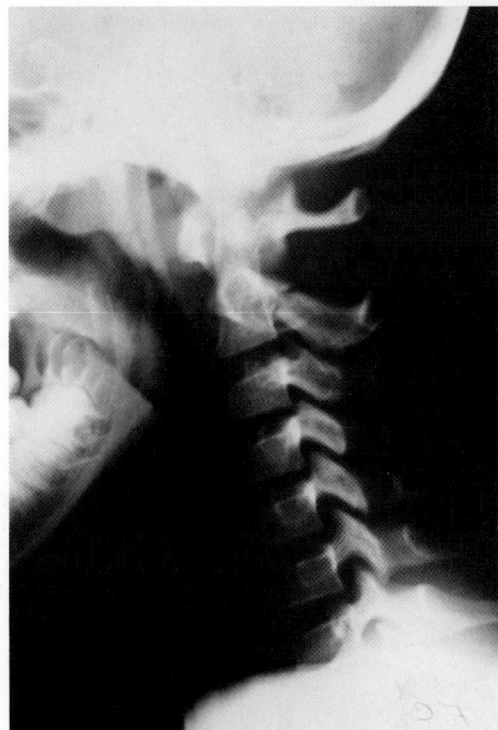

Figure 34-2

Fracture of C2 (hangman's fracture). (From Green NB, Swiontkowski MF, eds: *Skeletal trauma in children*, ed 3, Philadelphia, 2003, Saunders.)

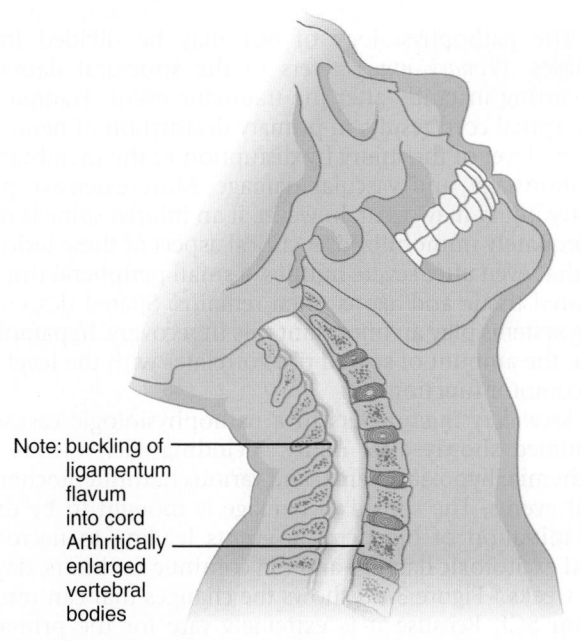

Note: buckling of ligamentum flavum into cord
Arthritically enlarged vertebral bodies

Figure 34-3

Elderly patients subjected to extension forces can sustain cervical spinal cord injury as a result of compression of the spinal cord between the posterior hypertrophic ligamentum flavum and the arthritically enlarged anterior vertebral bodies. (From Marx JA, ed: *Rosen's emergency medicine: concepts and clinical practice*, ed 6, Philadelphia, 2006, Mosby.)

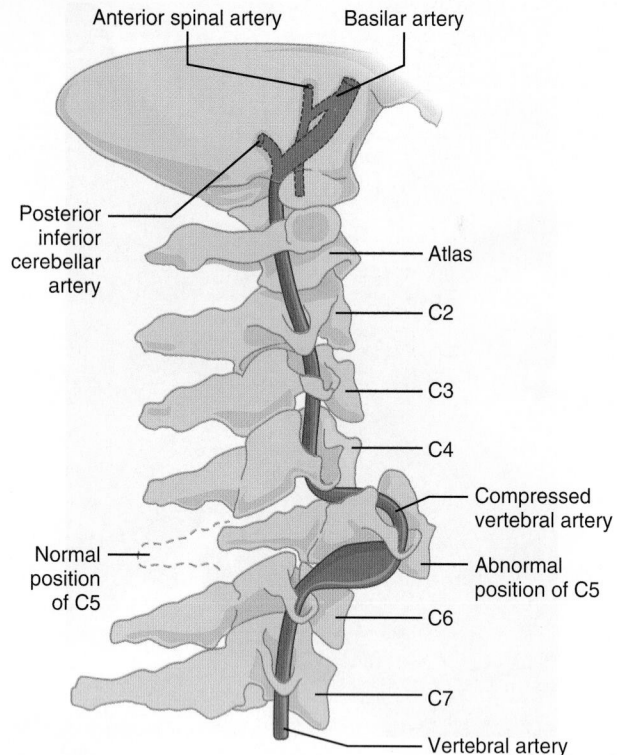

Figure 34-4

Mechanism of vascular injury of the spinal cord resulting from cervical vertebral injury. (From Marx JA, ed: *Rosen's emergency medicine: concepts and clinical practice*, ed 6, Philadelphia, 2006, Mosby.)

The pathophysiology of SCI may be divided into phases. *Primary injury* refers to the structural damage occurring instantly after the traumatic event. Trauma to the spinal cord results in primary destruction of neurons at the level of the injury by disruption of the membrane, hemorrhage, and vascular damage. More extensive primary injury may occur, however, if an injured spine is not adequately immobilized. A critical aspect of these lesions is that even after severe injuries, a small peripheral rim of spared tissue and axons often remains. Spared descending systems play an important role in recovery. In paraplegia, the amount of spared rim correlates with the level of locomotor function.[7,98]

Secondary injury refers to a pathophysiologic cascade initiated shortly after injury, including such insults as ischemia, hypoxia, edema, and various harmful biochemical events. The spread of damage is thought to be due to initiation of biochemical events leading to necrosis and excitotoxic damage and can continue for hours, days, or weeks.[4] Figure 34-6 shows the changes that can result from SCI. Because it is extremely rare for the primary injury to cause transection of the spinal cord, and it has been shown that less than 10% of the cross-sectional area of the spinal cord supports locomotion, it is very important to focus clinical attention on the secondary injury process.

Electrolyte disturbances following SCI include increased intracellular calcium level, increased extracellular potassium level, and increased sodium permeability. The route of calcium entry rather than the amount may

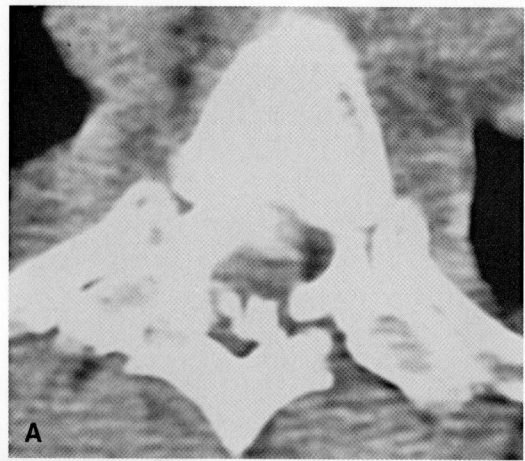

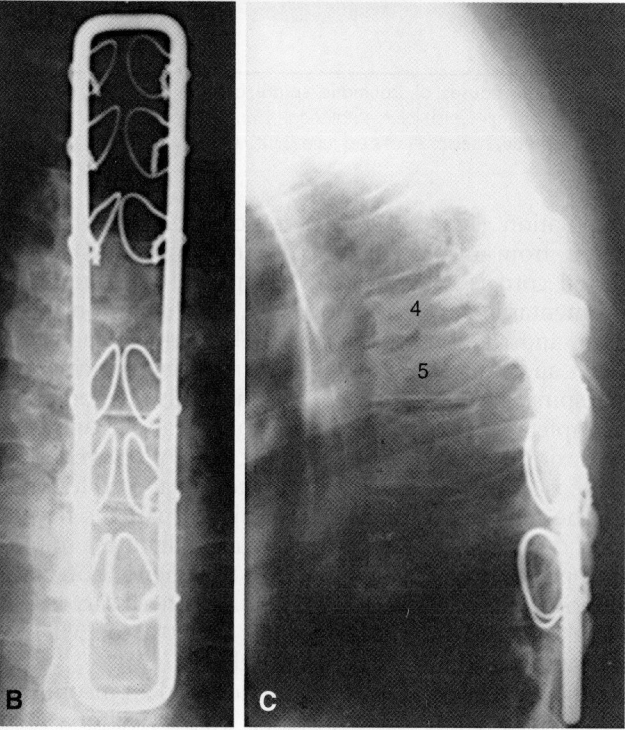

Figure 34-5

A T4-T5 fracture-dislocation resulted in a complete spinal cord injury in a 30-year-old man. **A,** A computed tomographic scan through the injured level demonstrates marked displacement and comminution at T4-T5, with multiple bone fragments within the canal. **B,** A postoperative anteroposterior radiograph shows stabilization with a Luque rectangle and sublaminar wires. This instrumentation provided rigid fixation and allowed early mobilization with minimal external support. The strength of fixation could have been improved with the use of double wires around the lamina bilaterally. **C,** Postoperative lateral radiograph. (From Browner BD, Jupiter JB, Levine AM, et al: *Skeletal trauma: basic science, management, and reconstruction*, ed 3, Philadelphia, 2003, Saunders.)

be the critical component. The influx of calcium ions in the neuronal cell can then lead to activation of various secondary processes, resulting in cellular death. Excitatory neurotransmitter accumulation, arachidonic acid release, endogenous opiate activation, and prostaglandin production can cause damage as part of the postinjury cascade. Free radical production and lipid oxidation play a central role in this process. See Chapter 28 for information regarding the effects of these disturbances. This results in

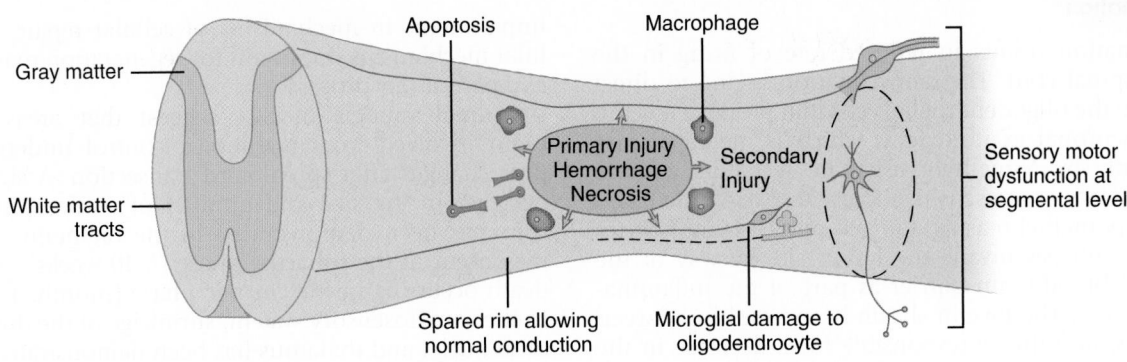

Figure 34-6

Spinal cord contusion lesions are characterized by a primary area created by hemorrhage of blood vessels causing necrosis of cells. This area eventually spreads because of secondary injury associated with apoptosis (programmed cell death), macrophages acting as immune mediators, and microglia causing damage to oligodendrocytes. The secondary damage may continue for days to weeks and move along the segmental levels, causing sensory and motor dysfunction. The spared rim may allow normal processing and preservation of function.

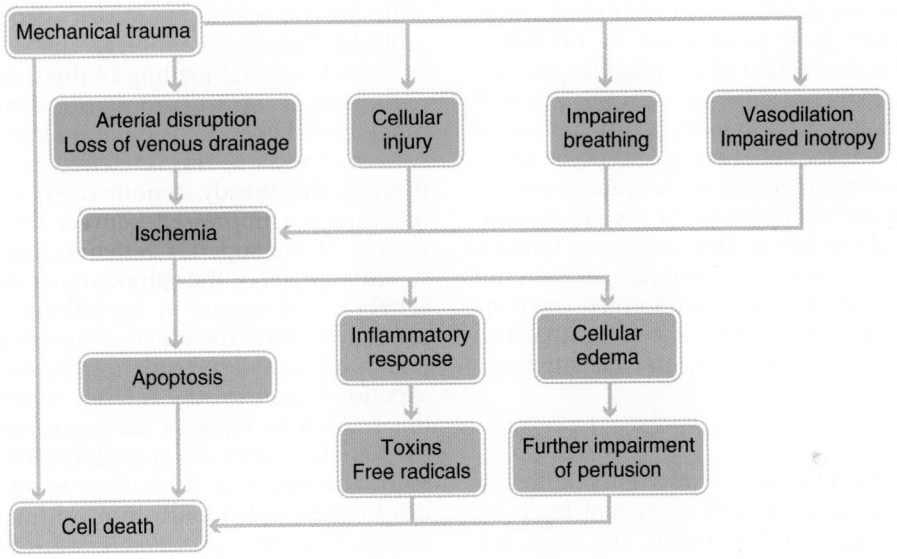

Figure 34-7

Mechanisms of spinal cord injury. Mechanical trauma to the spinal cord is exacerbated by systemic hypoperfusion or hypoxia. (From Miller RD, ed: *Miller's anesthesia*, ed 6, New York, 2005, Churchill Livingstone. Redrawn from Dutton RP: Spinal cord injury, *Int Anesthesiol Clin* 40:109, 2002.)

ischemia, edema formation, membrane destruction, cell death, and eventually permanent neurologic deficits.[42] The relationship of mechanisms of damage leading to cell death is shown in Figure 34-7.

Blood Flow Changes

Ischemia related to reduced blood flow is a very prominent feature of post-SCI events. Damage to blood vessels, microhemorrhage in the central grey matter, spreads radially and axially. The resulting hypoxic and ischemic events deprive grey and white matter of oxygen and nutrients necessary for neural cell survival and function. Ischemia in the area of injury may be due to the presence of norepinephrine, serotonin, histamine, and prostaglandins, all of which cause vasoconstriction. This ischemia may be compounded by loss of the normal autoregulatory response of the spinal cord vasculature.

Autoregulation of circulation is disabled at the injury site. Systemic pressure changes may be responsible for changes in spinal blood flow, which may cause nervous tissue damage by direct effects. The changes in blood flow may reflect rather than cause secondary injury.[46]

After several hours, there appear to be gross hemorrhages present, preceded by endothelial breakdown and pathologic coagulation products in the blood vessels. Macrophages enter the lesion and begin to digest the necrotic debris, converting the complex myelin lipids to neutral fat. Axonal swelling and increased permeability of blood vessels result in a visibly swollen spinal cord. Glial cells become active after about 6 days, and astrocytic fibers form scar-like tissue that lines the cavities created by the necrosis.

Edema

Edema is another feature of the secondary injury process. Edema develops first at the injury site and subsequently spreads into adjacent and sometimes distant segments of the cord. The relationship between this edema and worsening of neurologic function is not well understood

Demyelination

Demyelination results in reduced rate of firing in the injured spinal cord. The demyelination is due to direct trauma to the oligodendroglial cells that produce myelin. Unlike neuronal excitotoxicity, which is mediated predominantly by *N*-methyl-D-aspartate receptors, mature oligodendrocytes are sensitive to excitotoxicity mediated by non-*N*-methyl-D-aspartate receptors. Lymphocytes and macrophages invade the lesion site by way of the disrupted blood-brain barrier as part of the inflammatory response. The myelin sheath becomes thin between the nodes, and this is responsible for a decrease in the peak currents along the axon. Loss of a single segment of myelin renders an axon dysfunctional; therefore, a large subset of axons crossing the lesion eventually become nonfunctional despite the axons remaining physically intact.

Changes in white matter begin with Wallerian degeneration in the ascending posterior columns above the level of the lesion and in the descending corticospinal tracts. Wallerian degeneration may be triggered by microglial activation and by the destruction of the oligodendrocytes via the release of cytokines or other neurotropic factors.[56] The immune system appears also to trigger the release of nerve growth factor, which can be neuroprotective to some cells while being toxic to other cells in the spinal cord.

A prominent feature of subchronic SCI is the maturation of a scar around the lesion. This scar tissue forms a cellular and molecular barrier to axonal regeneration. By the chronic injury phase, the scar is well formed and consists of several cell types, such as the reactive astrocytes, fibroblasts, Schwann cells, microglia, and macrophages that have invaded the scar.

Grey Matter

Typically, the loss of central grey matter is confined to between one and one and one-half segmental levels of the spinal cord, causing central cavitation. The result is a fluid-filled cyst or syrinx (see later), or the cord collapses around the loss of tissue in an hourglass shape, with the minimal diameter located at the spinal segment of the original injury.

Dural Scarring

Scarring of the dura can cause a permanent connection of the cord to the overlying dura. Because the cord is normally freely mobile within the spinal canal, restricted motion attributable to dural scarring produces unusual forces on the cord when the neck is bent or with normal breathing or the cardiac cycle. These forces can produce microscopic injury, which may limit optimal regeneration and recovery.

Neural Function

Neural activity below the injury level is related to passive and active limb movements and sensory stimuli from the moving limbs. Substantial reduction of neural activity limits the body's ability to maintain the cellular functions of the spinal cord circuitry. Slow progressive loss of function is normal in chronic SCI. It is thought that the injured central nervous system (CNS) undergoes accelerated aging, with abnormal cell production and impairments in mechanisms of cellular repair. The cellular mechanisms important for regeneration may be lost as a part of this process.

Animal models of SCI suggest that areas of the brain involved in sensorimotor control undergo atrophic changes after spinal cord transection. A significant decrease in the size and number of corticospinal neurons has been demonstrated in the rat brain. Atrophy may occur in the subacute phase (5-10 weeks), with cell death occurring in the chronic phase (months to years). In the somatosensory system, shrinkage of the dorsal column nuclei and thalamus has been demonstrated in primates following upper limb deafferentation. Thus, both the somatosensory and motor systems are susceptible to atrophy after nervous system damage.[55]

Neurapraxia

The syndrome of neurapraxia is of special concern after athletic injury. Affected individuals experience dramatic, although transient, neurologic deficits, including tetraplegia. Transient tetraplegia most commonly occurs as a result of axial loading of the spine. In athletes with narrowing of the anteroposterior diameter of the spinal canal, both hyperextension and hyperflexion can lead to cord compression. This is referred to as the pincer mechanism. In the already stenotic canal, with hyperextension the cord is compressed between the posterior inferior margin of the superior vertebral body and the anterior superior aspect of the spinolaminar line of the subjacent vertebra. Conversely, in hyperflexion the cord is compressed between the anterior superior aspect of the spinolaminar line of the superior vertebra and the posterior superior margin of the inferior vertebra. In both cases, this sudden decrease in the anteroposterior diameter of the spinal canal results in compression of the spinal cord. Many attempts have been made to quantitate the level of risk to these individuals from continued athletic participation; however, considerable controversy still exists.[36]

Syringomyelia

One type of pathologic condition that can appear over time in the spinal cord related to trauma is syringomyelia. It is a clinical syndrome that results from cystic cavitation and gliosis of the spinal cord. This is reported to occur in close to 2% of persons with paraplegia and in 0.2% of quadriplegic individuals. In the chronic spinal cord lesion, the cysts may continue to develop, become tubular in shape, like that of a syrinx, and extend over several spinal levels (Fig. 34-8). Posttraumatic syringomyelia can develop up to 30 years after the initial lesion, but most commonly occurs within 4 to 9 years after trauma. One mechanism of syrinx formation is an initial hematomyelia followed by resorption and formation of a cyst cavity.[42]

In some cases, there are multiple cavities. The cavity may occupy almost the entire cross-sectional area of the cord, compressing the posterior columns. As the cyst develops, usually below the level of the initial lesion, there can be significant pain as a result of the compromise of the central spinal cord structures, such as the substantia gelatinosa and the posterior root entry zone.[100] The spinothalamic tracts are involved, which can result

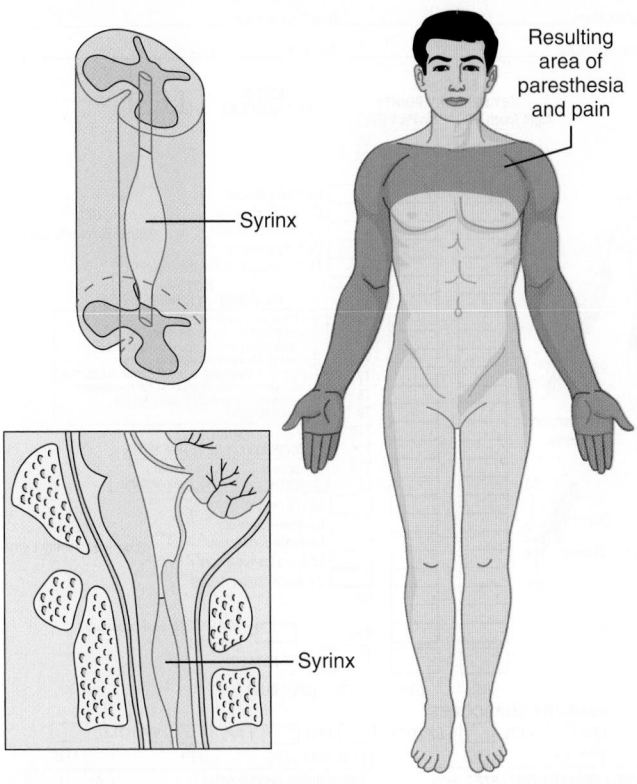

Figure 34-8

The syrinx formed in the late stages of spinal cord injury as a part of syringomyelia.

in the sharp pain that is often the first presenting symptom. There can be lower motor neuron dysfunction, causing weakness, atrophy, and loss of reflex activity. Sensory loss is common, and the sympathetic nervous system can become involved, resulting in syndromes such as Horner syndrome.[65]

The thoracic area of the spine is the most common site for the syrinx to develop, with descending and ascending fibers running in the walls of the cavitated lesions. The size and extent of the syrinx are represented by the symptoms, but because of location below the site of the lesion, changes are not easily recognized. The syringomyelia may be responsible for the spasms, phantom sensations, reflex changes, and autonomic visceral phenomena that may occur. Scoliosis can result from the loss of input to the paraspinals.[56] Anything that blocks the free flow of cerebrospinal fluid (CSF) can keep this fluid from moving normally in and out of the head. Pressure can build up in the syrinx, causing expansion and possible rupture, damaging normal spinal cord tissue and injuring nerve cells. Many people with posttraumatic syringomyelia do not develop any symptoms until midlife or later.[44]

Syringomyelia can be a very disabling condition. Spasms, phantom sensations, and autonomic visceral (organ) changes can occur. Sexual dysfunction, muscle spasticity, and loss of bowel or bladder control can develop. The first symptom may be sharp pain. Muscle atrophy, stiffness, and weakness of the neck, back, shoulders, arms, or legs, along with loss of reflexes, are common. Symptoms may be distributed like a cape over the shoulders and back. Headaches and loss of sensation

(pinprick and temperature) in the hands may be reported. The symptoms may only occur on one side of the body, depending on where the syrinx develops.

Clinical Manifestations

Level of Injury

SCIs are named according to the level of neurologic impairment. Differences may exist in the motor versus sensory levels identified. International Standards for Neurological Classification of SCI is widely used for assessment and classification (Fig. 34-9). The ASIA Impairment Scale (AIS) is a multidimensional approach to categorize motor and sensory impairment in individuals with SCI (ASIA 2002). Currently in its sixth edition, it identifies sensory and motor levels indicative of the most rostral spinal levels demonstrating "unimpaired" function. Twenty-eight dermatomes are assessed bilaterally using pinprick and light touch sensation and 10 key muscles are assessed bilaterally with manual muscle testing. The results are summed to produce overall sensory and motor scores and are used in combination with evaluation of anal sensory and motor function as a basis for the determination of AIS classification.

A clinical examination is conducted to test whether sensation is 0 = absent; 1 = impaired; or 2 = normal. Muscle function is rated from 0 = total paralysis to 5 = normal (active movement, full range of motion [ROM] against significant resistance). The presence of anal sensation and voluntary anal contraction are assessed as a yes/no. Bilateral motor and sensory levels and the AIS are based on the results of these examinations. The AIS (5 point ordinal scale)[51a] classifies individuals from "A" (complete SCI) to "E" (normal sensory and motor function). Preservation of function in the sacral segments (S4-S5) is key for determining the AIS. The AIS scores are clearly defined and understood by most clinicians working with individuals with SCI.[92]

Lesions are reported as *complete* when there is complete loss of sensory and motor function below the level of the lesion. Complete lesions are a result of spinal cord transection, severe compression or contusion, or extensive vascular dysfunction.

Incomplete lesions are the partial loss of sensory and motor function below the level of the injury. Incomplete lesions often occur when there is contusion produced by bony fragments, soft tissue, or edema within the spinal canal. The resulting motor or sensory function is called *sparing*.

Spinal Cord Injury Syndromes

Within the category of incomplete spinal cord lesions are the recognizable syndromes that have been identified. Several syndromes are illustrated in Figure 34-10.

Brown-Séquard syndrome is characterized by damage to one side of the spinal cord. The most common causes are stab and gunshot wounds. Loss of the entire hemisection of the spinal cord is rare; the natural lesion is always irregular. There is weakness ipsilateral to the lesion. Lateral column damage results in abnormal reflexes, including a positive Babinski sign, and clonus. Often there is ipsilateral spasticity in the muscles innervated below the lesion. As a result of dorsal column damage, there is loss

ASIA | INTERNATIONAL STANDARDS FOR NEUROLOGICAL CLASSIFICATION OF SPINAL CORD INJURY (ISNCSCI) | **ISCOS**

Patient Name _____ Date/Time of Exam _____

Examiner Name _____ Signature _____

RIGHT MOTOR KEY MUSCLES

SENSORY KEY SENSORY POINTS
Light Touch (LTR) Pin Prick (PPR)

C2
C3
C4

UER (Upper Extremity Right)

Elbow flexors C5
Wrist extensors C6
Elbow extensors C7
Finger flexors C8
Finger abductors (little finger) T1

Comments (Non-key Muscle? Reason for NT? Pain?):

T2
T3
T4
T5
T6
T7
T8
T9
T10
T11
T12
L1

LER (Lower Extremity Right)

Hip flexors L2
Knee extensors L3
Ankle dorsiflexors L4
Long toe extensors L5
Ankle plantar flexors S1

S2
S3
S4-5

(VAC) Voluntary anal contraction (Yes/No)

RIGHT TOTALS

(MAXIMUM) (50) (56) (56)

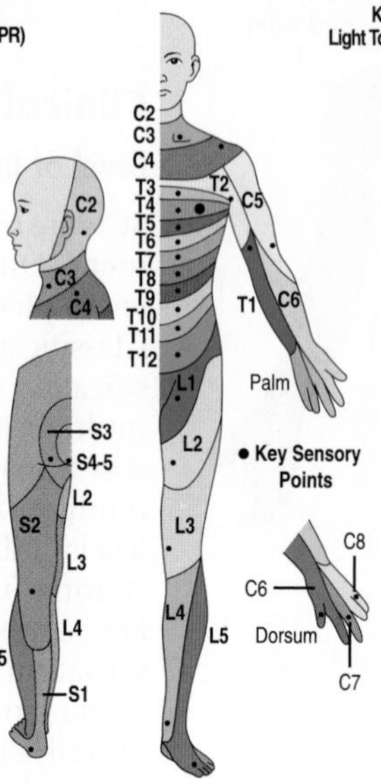

SENSORY KEY SENSORY POINTS
Light Touch (LTL) Pin Prick (PPL)

C2
C3
C4

● Key Sensory Points

Palm

Dorsum

LEFT MOTOR KEY MUSCLES

C5 Elbow flexors
C6 Wrist extensors
C7 Elbow extensors
C8 Finger flexors
T1 Finger abductors (little finger)

UEL (Upper Extremity Left)

T2
T3
T4
T5
T6
T7
T8
T9
T10
T11
T12
L1

MOTOR (SCORING ON REVERSE SIDE)
0 = total paralysis
1 = palpable or visible contraction
2 = active movement, gravity eliminated
3 = active movement, against gravity
4 = active movement, against some resistance
5 = active movement, against full resistance
5* = normal corrected for pain/disuse
NT = not testable

SENSORY (SCORING ON REVERSE SIDE)
0 = absent   2 = normal
1 = altered   NT = not testable

L2 Hip flexors
L3 Knee extensors
L4 Ankle dorsiflexors
L5 Long toe extensors
S1 Ankle plantar flexors

LEL (Lower Extremity Left)

S2
S3
S4-5

(DAP) Deep anal pressure (Yes/No)

LEFT TOTALS

(56) (56) (50) (MAXIMUM)

MOTOR SUBSCORES
UER ___ + UEL ___ = UEMS TOTAL ___ LER ___ + LEL ___ = LEMS TOTAL ___
MAX (25) (25) (50) MAX (25) (25) (50)

SENSORY SUBSCORES
LTR ___ + LTL ___ = LT TOTAL ___ PPR ___ + PPL ___ = PP TOTAL ___
MAX (56) (56) (112) MAX (56) (56) (112)

NEUROLOGICAL LEVELS Steps 1-5 for classification as on reverse	R L	3. NEUROLOGICAL LEVEL OF INJURY (NLI)	4. COMPLETE OR INCOMPLETE? Incomplete = Any sensory or motor function in S4-5	(In complete injuries only) ZONE OF PARTIAL PRESERVATION Most caudal level with any innervation	R L
	1. SENSORY			SENSORY	
	2. MOTOR		5. ASIA IMPAIRMENT SCALE (AIS)	MOTOR	

This form may be copied freely but should not be altered without permission from the American Spinal Injury Association. REV 02/13

Muscle Function Grading

0 = total paralysis

1 = palpable or visible contraction

2 = active movement, full range of motion (ROM) with gravity eliminated

3 = active movement, full ROM against gravity

4 = active movement, full ROM against gravity and moderate resistance in a muscle specific position

5 = (normal) active movement, full ROM against gravity and full resistance in a functional muscle position expected from an otherwise unimpaired person

5* = (normal) active movement, full ROM against gravity and sufficient resistance to be considered normal if identified inhibiting factors (i.e. pain, disuse) were not present

NT = not testable (i.e. due to immobilization, severe pain such that the patient cannot be graded, amputation of limb, or contracture of > 50% of the normal range of motion)

Sensory Grading

0 = Absent

1 = Altered, either decreased/impaired sensation or hypersensitivity

2 = Normal

NT = Not testable

Non Key Muscle Functions (optional)

May be used to assign a motor level to differentiate AIS B vs. C

Movement	Root level
Shoulder: Flexion, extension, abduction, adduction, internal and external rotation **Elbow:** Supination	C5
Elbow: Pronation **Wrist:** Flexion	C6
Finger: Flexion at proximal joint, extension. **Thumb:** Flexion, extension and abduction in plane of thumb	C7
Finger: Flexion at MCP joint **Thumb:** Opposition, adduction and abduction perpendicular to palm	C8
Finger: Abduction of the index finger	T1
Hip: Adduction	L2
Hip: External rotation	L3
Hip: Extension, abduction, internal rotation **Knee:** Flexion **Ankle:** Inversion and eversion **Toe:** MP and IP extension	L4
Hallux and Toe: DIP and PIP flexion and abduction	L5
Hallux: Adduction	S1

ASIA Impairment Scale (AIS)

A = Complete. No sensory or motor function is preserved in the sacral segments S4-5.

B = Sensory Incomplete. Sensory but not motor function is preserved below the neurological level and includes the sacral segments S4-5 (light touch or pin prick at S4-5 or deep anal pressure) AND no motor function is preserved more than three levels below the motor level on either side of the body.

C = Motor Incomplete. Motor function is preserved below the neurological level**, and more than half of key muscle functions below the neurological level of injury (NLI) have a muscle grade less than 3 (Grades 0-2).

D = Motor Incomplete. Motor function is preserved below the neurological level**, and at least half (half or more) of key muscle functions below the NLI have a muscle grade ≥ 3.

E = Normal. If sensation and motor function as tested with the ISNCSCI are graded as normal in all segments, and the patient had prior deficits, then the AIS grade is E. Someone without an initial SCI does not receive an AIS grade.

** For an individual to receive a grade of C or D, i.e. motor incomplete status, they must have either (1) voluntary anal sphincter contraction or (2) sacral sensory sparing with sparing of motor function more than three levels below the motor level for that side of the body. The International Standards at this time allows even non-key muscle function more than 3 levels below the motor level to be used in determining motor incomplete status (AIS B versus C).

NOTE: When assessing the extent of motor sparing below the level for distinguishing between AIS B and C, the **motor level** on each side is used; whereas to differentiate between AIS C and D (based on proportion of key muscle functions with strength grade 3 or greater) the **neurological level of injury** is used.

ASIA AMERICAN SPINAL INJURY ASSOCIATION

INTERNATIONAL STANDARDS FOR NEUROLOGICAL CLASSIFICATION OF SPINAL CORD INJURY

ISCOS INTERNATIONAL SPINAL CORD SOCIETY

Steps in Classification

The following order is recommended for determining the classification of individuals with SCI.

1. Determine sensory levels for right and left sides.
The sensory level is the most caudal, intact dermatome for both pin prick and light touch sensation.

2. Determine motor levels for right and left sides.
Defined by the lowest key muscle function that has a grade of at least 3 (on supine testing), providing the key muscle functions represented by segments above that level are judged to be intact (graded as a 5).
Note: in regions where there is no myotome to test, the motor level is presumed to be the same as the sensory level, if testable motor function above that level is also normal.

3. Determine the neurological level of injury (NLI)
This refers to the most caudal segment of the cord with intact sensation and antigravity (3 or more) muscle function strength, provided that there is normal (intact) sensory and motor function rostrally respectively.
The NLI is the most cephalad of the sensory and motor levels determined in steps 1 and 2.

4. Determine whether the injury is Complete or Incomplete.
(i.e. absence or presence of sacral sparing)
If voluntary anal contraction = **No** AND all S4-5 sensory scores = **0** AND deep anal pressure = **No**, then injury is **Complete**.
Otherwise, injury is **Incomplete**.

5. Determine ASIA Impairment Scale (AIS) Grade:

Is injury **Complete**? If YES, AIS=**A** and can record ZPP (lowest dermatome or myotome on each side with some preservation)

NO ↓

Is injury Motor Complete? If YES, AIS=**B**

NO ↓ (No=voluntary anal contraction OR motor function more than three levels below the motor level on a given side, if the patient has sensory incomplete classification)

Are at least half (half or more) of the key muscles below the neurological level of injury graded 3 or better?

NO ↓ → AIS=**C**   YES ↓ → AIS=**D**

If sensation and motor function is normal in all segments, AIS=**E**
Note: AIS E is used in follow-up testing when an individual with a documented SCI has recovered normal function. If at initial testing no deficits are found, the individual is neurologically intact; the ASIA Impairment Scale does not apply.

Figure 34-9

American Spinal Injury Association (ASIA) Motor Assessment Form. (Courtesy American Spinal Injury Association International, Atlanta.)

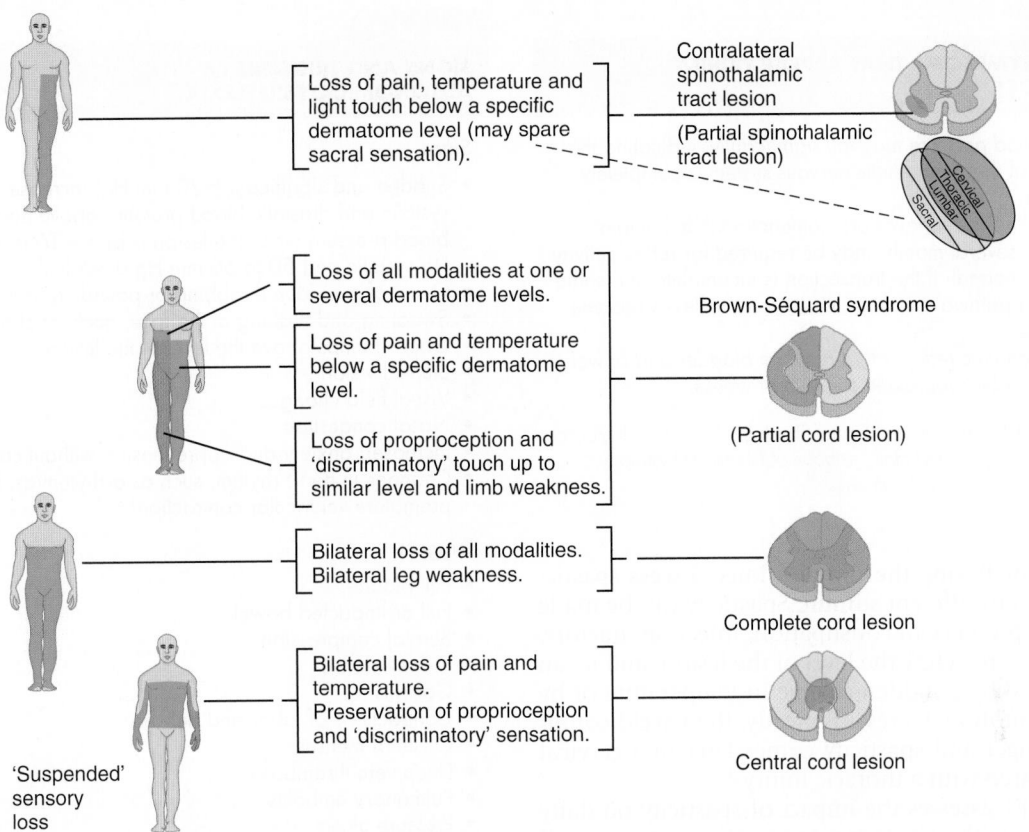

Figure 34-10

Spinal cord syndromes. Patterns of sensory loss and weakness. (From Lindsey KW, Bone I, Callander R: *Neurology and neurosurgery illustrated*, New York, 1986, Churchill Livingstone, p. 188.)

of proprioception, kinesthesia, and vibratory sense. On the contralateral (opposite) side, there is pain and temperature loss starting a few levels below the lesion. The lateral spinothalamic tract ascends on the same side for several segments before crossing, giving rise to the discrepancy between the level and contralateral signs.

Anterior cord syndrome is frequently associated with flexion injuries and is often the result of loss of supply from the anterior spinal artery. Damage to the anterior and anterolateral aspect of the cord results in bilateral loss of motor function and pain and temperature sensation because of interruption of the anterior and lateral spinothalamic tracts and corticospinal tract.

Central cord syndrome is a result of damage to the central aspect of the spinal cord, often caused by hyperextension injuries in the cervical region. There is characteristically more severe neurologic involvement in the upper extremities than in the lower extremities. Peripherally located fibers may not be as severely affected, and therefore function may be retained or recovered in the thoracic, lumbar, and sacral regions, including the bowel, bladder, and genitalia.

Posterior cord syndrome is extremely rare, with preservation of motor function, pain, and light touch sensation. There is loss of proprioception below the level of the lesion, leading to a severe gait deviations.

Conus medullaris syndrome and *cauda equina syndrome* reflect damage at the base of the spinal cord and generally result in flaccid lower limb paralysis, flaccid bowel and bladder sphincters, resulting in difficulty with bowel

accidents and bladder leakage as well as lack of penile erection in males.

The site of spinal cord damage determines the extent of the physical impairments. Injury of the cord in the cervical region creates tetraplegia, or paralysis of all four limbs. In addition to the limbs, the trunk and muscles of respiration are involved. Damage in the thoracic or lumbar region will result in paraplegia or paraparesis involving only the lower extremities and generally the lower trunk.

Changes in Muscle Tone

When the spinal cord is transected, all cord functions below the transection become substantially depressed; this is referred to as *spinal shock*. Spinal shock involves the loss of deep tendon reflexes and voluntary control as well as flaccidity below the level of the lesion. The condition may persist for a few hours, days, or weeks. It is thought to represent a period during which the excitability of spinal neurons is dramatically reduced owing to the loss of all descending projections. Autonomic symptoms, including sweating and reflex incontinence of bladder and rectum follow. As is the case in other areas of the nervous system, the affected neurons gradually regain their excitability as they reorganize and adapt to the new levels of reduced synaptic input.[45] Box 34-1 outlines the common physiologic events related to spinal shock.

Spasticity is an inevitable consequence of spinal cord lesions. There is an essential or basic spasticity, which may be of some benefit to the individual when emptying

COMMON SYMPTOMS THAT APPEAR DURING SPINAL SHOCK

- *Arterial blood pressure may fall significantly*, indicating that the output of the *sympathetic* nervous system is completely interrupted.
- *All skeletal muscle reflexes are nonfunctional.* In humans, 2 weeks to several months may be required for reflex activity to return to normal. If the transection is incomplete and some descending pathways remain intact, some reflexes become hyperactive.
- *Sacral autonomic reflexes that regulate bladder and bowel function may be suppressed for several weeks.*

From Spinal Cord Transection and Spinal Shock (p. 665) in Hall: *Pocket Companion to Guyton and Hall Textbook of Medical Physiology*, 12th ed., St. Louis, 2011, Saunders.

SIGNS AND TRIGGERS OF AUTONOMIC DYSREFLEXIA

Signs

- Sudden and significant (>20 mm Hg) increase in both systolic and diastolic blood pressure above normal (Normal blood pressure when the lesion is above T6 is 90 to 110 mm Hg systolic and 50 to 60 mm Hg diastolic.)
- Onset of a sudden throbbing or pounding headache
- Sweating and flushing of the face, neck, or shoulders
- Goose bumps above the level of the lesion
- Blurred vision
- Visual field changes
- Nasal congestion
- Increased anxiety and apprehension without cause
- Changes in heart rhythm, such as arrhythmias, fibrillation, premature ventricular contractions

Triggers

- Full bladder
- Full or impacted bowel
- Scrotal compression
- Kidney stones
- Gastritis
- Contractions of labor and delivery
- Onset of menses
- Deep vein thrombosis
- Pulmonary embolus
- Pressure ulcers
- Insect bites
- Bruises caused by sharp objects
- Tight and constrictive clothing or apparatus
- Changes in temperature
- Pain or irritation below the level of the lesion

Adapted from Zabel RJ, Forest BH: Autonomic dysreflexia: an acute care emergency, *Acute Care Perspect* 7(3):9–14, 1999.

the bladder or flexing the hip and knee. Excess spasticity is triggered by afferent stimuli. Spasticity can be made worse by the presence of constipation, infection, fracture, or a pressure sore below the level of the lesion, and it can be exacerbated by a sudden change in temperature or by physical or emotional stress. Typically, the flaccid condition lasts longer and spasticity comes later in a cervical injury compared with a thoracic injury.[51,57]

The SCI-SET assesses the impact of spasticity on daily life in people with SCI. It requires participants to recall their past 7 days when rating spasticity on a 7-point scale ranging from –3 (extremely problematic) to +3 (extremely helpful). The SCI-SET assesses the impact of spasticity on daily life in people with SCI.[1] The PSFS is a self-report measure of the frequency of reported muscle spasms that is commonly used to quantify spasticity The PSFS is a 2-component self-report scale developed to augment clinical ratings of spasticity and provide a more comprehensive understanding of an individual's spasticity status. The first component is a 5-point scale assessing the frequency with which spasms occur, ranging from 0 = no spasms to 4 = spontaneous spasms occurring more than ten times per hour. The second component is a 3-point scale assessing the severity of spasms, ranging from 1 = mild to 3 = severe. The second component is not answered if the person indicates they have no spasms in part 1.[80]

The SCATS is a physiologically based measure for spastic reflexes for use in individuals with SCI. It was developed in response to the demand for a standardized, simple clinical measure that encompasses the primary spastic reaction in the SCI population. The SCATS is split into three subscales, each addressing a separate spasm: clonus, flexor spasms, and extensor spasms. For each subscale, the spasm is triggered and then rated with a score ranging from 0 to 3.[11]

Autonomic Nervous System Changes

Autonomic dysreflexia (AD) can occur with a lesion above T6 and is the result of impaired function of the autonomic nervous system (ANS) caused by simultaneous sympathetic and parasympathetic activity. The ANS regulates body functions such as heart rate, blood pressure, and gland activity. Noxious stimuli, such as overextended bladder or bowel, pain, or other visceral stimuli will typically elicit a sympathetic response, resulting in vasoconstriction below the level of injury, which leads to an increase in blood pressure. In the non–spinal cord injured individual, the descending parasympathetic output compensates for this increase in blood pressure by causing vasodilation to bring blood pressure to a more normal level. Following SCI, sensory nerves below the level of the injury continue to transmit excitatory impulses, causing similar vasoconstriction and increased blood pressure. With the lack of inhibition of sympathetic output below the lesion, however, the blood pressure keeps rising unchecked. Secretions of neurotransmitters, such as norepinephrine, epinephrine, and dopamine, support this sympathetic response leading to parasympathetic stimulation to slow the heart rate (bradycardia) through stimulation of the vagus nerve. This response is not strong enough to overcome the extreme vasoconstriction. Vasodilation occurs above the level of the lesion and results in profuse sweating and skin flushing. A severe pounding headache may follow, with sweating and chills without fever. The increase in blood pressure makes the person susceptible to subarachnoid hemorrhage, renal or retinal hemorrhage, and seizure or myocardial infarction. AD should be handled as a medical emergency.[2,37] Box 34-2 lists signs and triggers of AD.[108]

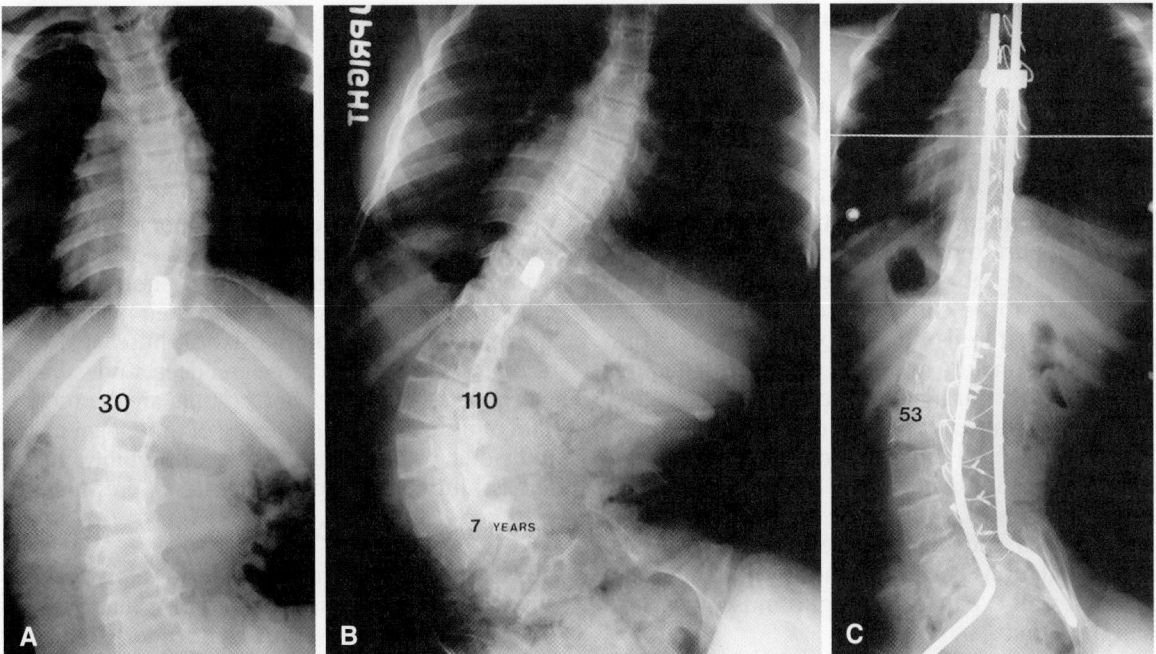

Figure 34-11

Progressive paralytic scoliosis after gunshot wound. **A,** Initial curve of 30 degrees. **B,** Seven years later, curve is 110 degrees. **C,** After fusion and segmental instrumentation, correction to 53 degrees. (From Canale ST, ed: *Campbell's operative orthopaedics,* ed 10, St. Louis, 2003, Mosby.)

Loss of thermoregulation below the level of the spinal cord lesion is a result of the disruption of the autonomic pathways from the hypothalamus, resulting in subnormal body temperature in a normal ambient environment. Vasoconstriction and the ability to sweat are lost. The body temperature, then, is greatly influenced by the external environment, and sensory feedback from the head and neck must be used to assist in regulating body temperature. The higher the lesion, the more severe the problem becomes.

Skeletal Changes

Joint ankylosis caused by heterotopic ossification (HO) or ectopic bone formation in the soft tissue, such as the tendons and connective tissue, can limit ROM, cause pain, and impair seating and posture. It often develops near the large joints, such as the anterior area of the hip, knee, shoulder, and elbow. It is always found below the level of the lesion, and it begins to develop within the first year after injury. The initial symptoms are soft tissue swelling, pain, redness, and increased temperature in the affected area. Asymmetric loss of ROM at the affected joint is a common sign of HO. Changes in bony alignment can develop secondary to muscle imbalances caused by unopposed contractions. Scoliosis can develop over time due to lack of paraspinal support, as is evidenced in Figure 34-11.

Pain

Individuals with SCI must deal with a number of secondary complications in addition to any disability caused by the injury itself. Pain, weakness, and fatigue appear to be most common and most closely linked to individual social and mental health functioning.[53] The number of reported pain sites increases with time, regardless of level or completeness of injury. While physical independence, mobility, and social integration remained relatively stable

despite increasing numbers of pain sites, increases in depressive symptoms are associated with increased pain. Smokers with SCI report more pain sites than their non-smoking counterparts.[84]

Pain caused by irritation of the nerve root is common, especially in cauda equina injury. Dysesthesia, impairment of sensation usually perceived as pain, can occur in areas with sensory loss and is often described as burning, pins and needles, or tingling. Disturbances of proprioception are related, and the person feels that a limb is in a different position than it is.

Musculoskeletal pain can result from faulty posture and overuse of limbs. Joint, ligament, and tendon deterioration is common, and secondary injury from muscle imbalances are related to significant dependence on upper extremities for all activities of daily living (ADLs) and functional mobility—frequent use of anterior shoulder muscles for wheelchair propulsion, for example, without equal use of shoulder extensors. Proper strength training can reduce these injuries and lead to more independence.

Fatigue

Complaints of fatigue, noted to be higher than in the general population, may be associated with changes in several systems. ANS changes with inadequate sweating and thermoregulation can cause activity intolerance. Psychologic well-being is associated with fatigue; depression and decreased community mobility can be predicted by increasing complaints of fatigue. The amount of effort it takes to accomplish even small tasks such as getting out of bed, showering, and dressing after an SCI may also contribute to increase in levels of fatigue.

Respiratory Complications

Respiratory complications associated with spinal cord lesions can be life-threatening. Paralysis of inspiratory muscles, thoracic injuries, and pain can reduce vital capacity.

Lesions above C4 result in paralysis of the diaphragm and generally require artificial ventilation because of loss of the phrenic nerve innervation. Pulmonary complications with lesions at C5 through T12 arise as a result of loss of innervation of the abdominal and intercostal muscles. Without the presence of abdominal muscles to provide anterior support to the abdominal cavity, the organs tend to sag forward and inferiorly, causing the position of the diaphragm to be compromised. In addition, the abdominal musculature is unable to exert pressure during forced expiration impairing the ability to cough or create force necessary during loud vocalization or singing. Paralysis of the external oblique muscles also inhibits the person's ability to cough and expel secretions.

An altered breathing pattern, the paradoxical breathing pattern, develops in conjunction with the loss of the intercostal muscles and dependence solely on the diaphragm for inhalation. The upper chest wall flattens and the abdominal wall expands, leading to musculoskeletal changes in the trunk.

Aspiration and pneumonia occur frequently in individuals with SCI and is usually associated with high-level injuries and complete lesions and advanced age. Pneumonia is the most common cause of death, especially in the period immediately after the injury. With no other complications, proper rehabilitation, and stable respiration, the death rate from pneumonia matches that in the general population.[82]

Impaired autonomic nervous system control affects the cardiovascular system and includes altered hormonal effects on the cardiovascular system, loss of the muscle pump causing decreased venous return, muscle weakness, and atrophy. Decreasing size of cardiac chamber along with greater use of type II over type I muscle fibers and a sedentary lifestyle affect cardiac status.[79]

Deep vein thrombosis and pulmonary embolism are associated with SCI because of increased coagulability of blood and decreased venous return. This may be associated with sympathetic dysfunction and unopposed vagal action. Risk of cardiovascular involvement comes from a greater prevalence of obesity, lipid disorders, metabolic syndrome, and diabetes. Daily energy expenditure is significantly lower in individuals with SCI, not only because of a lack of motor function but also because of a lack of accessibility and fewer opportunities to engage in physical activity.[73]

Metabolic Conditions

Persons with SCI are prone to abnormal carbohydrate metabolism and are found to develop hyperinsulinemia and insulin resistance. During the acute phase of SCI, there is significant weight loss, especially with tetraplegia, associated with increased metabolic demands, muscle atrophy, and a negative nitrogen and calcium balance. Hypoproteinemia can be caused by pressure ulcers. Over time, there is usually an increase in body fat in proportion to lean tissue in the person with chronic SCI. A more sedentary lifestyle as a result of SCI may predispose a person to some of these conditions.

Soon after SCI, bones start losing minerals and become less dense. This may be due to alteration of the ANS and circulatory system. Inactivity and lack of weight bearing also foster the development of osteoporosis. It is thought that individuals with SCI may have an earlier onset and a greater extent of osteoporosis with higher risk of fracture.

Pressure Ulcers

Pressure ulcers are a frequent complication of SCI. They arise primarily because of persistent pressure in the area of a bony prominence. Moisture, poor nutrition, complete lesions, acute illness, and cigarette smoking predispose the skin to breakdown. Persons who do not follow through on self-care requirements because of their own choice, depression, lack of motivation, substance abuse, or alcoholism are also prone to develop more and deeper pressure ulcers. Initially, the sacrum, heel, and scapula are the most common sites of ulcer formation because of time spent in bed. As the individual begins to use a chair for mobility, the trochanter and ischium become common sites of pressure ulcers.[105]

Bowel and Bladder Control

Bowel and bladder control is always affected in the person with SCI. The spinal center for urination is the conus medullaris. Primary reflex control originates from the sacral segment. During the stage of spinal shock, the urinary bladder is flaccid. All muscle tone and bladder reflexes are absent. Lesions above the conus medullaris, called upper motor neuron lesions, will cause a reflex neurogenic bladder, reflected by spasticity, voiding difficulties, detrusor muscle hypertrophy, and urethral reflux. Lesions at the conus medullaris cause nonreflex bladders, resulting in flaccidity and decreased tone of the perineal muscles and urethral sphincter. These are called lower motor neuron lesions. Bowel patterns mimic bladder responses in their response to spinal shock; reflex bowel occurs in upper motor neuron lesions above the conus medullaris, and nonreflex bowel is caused by lower motor neuron damage to the conus and cauda equina.[62] Figure 34-12 shows bladder reflex pathways.

Urinary tract infection is the most frequent secondary medical complication seen in persons with SCI. This persists despite improved catheter materials and design and use of antibiotics. In concert with this is the increased concentration of calcium in the urinary system, which leads to formation of kidney stones. Calculi in the kidney are a complication found more frequently in individuals using an indwelling catheter.[16]

Sexuality

Sexual response is directly related to the level and completeness of injury. Sexual function relies on nervous pathways similar to those of the bladder and bowel and is altered as described earlier. There are two types of responses: reflexogenic, or a response to external stimulation seen in persons with upper motor neuron lesions, and psychogenic, a response that occurs through cognitive activity such as fantasy, associated with lower motor neuron lesions. Men with higher-level lesions can often achieve a reflexive erection but typically do not ejaculate. With cauda equina lesions, erection and ejaculation are not usually possible. The primary reason for pursuing sexual activity is for intimacy needs, not fertility. Bladder and bowel concerns during sexual activity are not strong enough to deter the majority of the population

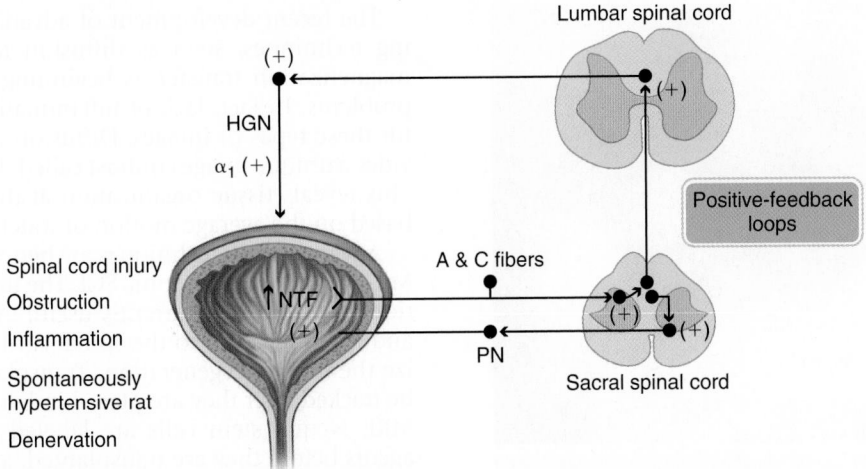

Figure 34-12

Possible mechanisms underlying spasticity in bladder reflex pathways induced by various pathologic conditions. Bladders from rats with chronic spinal cord injury exhibit increased level of neurotrophic factors (NTFs), such as nerve growth factor. NTFs can increase the excitability of C-fiber bladder afferent neurons and alter reflex mechanisms in parasympathetic excitatory pathways in the pelvic nerve (PN) as well as in sympathetic pathways in the hypogastric nerve (HGN). These reflex circuits are organized in the spinal cord as positive-feedback loops that induce involuntary bladder activity. (From Wein AJ, Kavoussi LR, Novick AC, et al: *Campbell-Walsh urology*, ed 9, Philadelphia, 2007, Saunders.)

from engaging in sexual activity. In addition, the occurrence of AD during typical bladder or bowel care is a significant variable predicting the occurrence and distress of AD during sexual activity.[3] Menses are typically interrupted for approximately 3 to 6 months after SCI; when restored, they can be another cause of AD. Fertility and pregnancy are uninterrupted by SCI, but the pregnancy must be observed closely, especially in the last trimester. Labor may begin without the woman's knowing it because of loss of sensation, and labor may initiate AD.[88]

Sleep Disorders

The prevalence of obstructive sleep apnea–hypopnea syndrome (OSAHS) is high after cervical cord injury. OSAHS is characterized by repeated oxygen desaturation. OSAHS should be suspected especially in individuals with daytime sleepiness, obesity, and frequent awakenings during sleep.[66] The changes in heart rhythm associated with OSAHS include sinusal arrhythmia, severe bradycardia, and ventricular and supraventricular tachycardia. The risk of sudden death, particularly of cardiovascular cause, is well known.[18]

MEDICAL MANAGEMENT

DIAGNOSIS. Delayed recognition of SCI is a significant problem in emergent care of traumatic injuries, occurring in more than 20% of cases.

Lateral film studies with plain radiographs are a rapid and effective way of evaluating cervical SCI, with the ability to detect approximately 85% of such injuries. When the open-mouth odontoid view and supine anteroposterior view are added, the accuracy rises to almost 100%. Any area that is inadequately demonstrated in the three-view spinal series is examined by computed tomography (CT). Flexion-extension studies are used primarily to evaluate instability caused by occult ligamentous injury and should not be done if there is any neurologic, bony, or soft tissue injury. The sensitivity of CT scanning is much

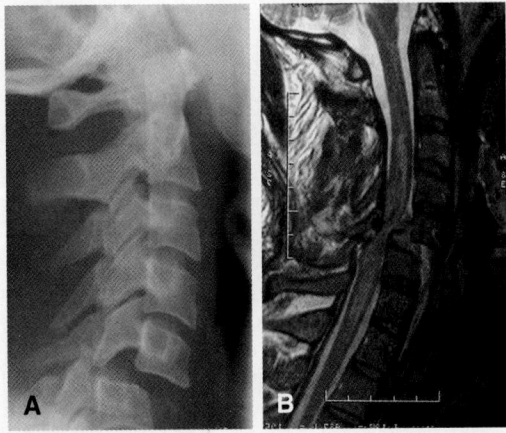

Figure 34-13

A, Plain lateral x-ray of the cervical spine showing a C5/6 dislocation. **B,** T2-weighted MRI of the same patient as in showing severe spinal cord damage. (From Bersten AD, Soni N: *Oh's intensive care manual*, ed 6, Oxford, 2008, Butterworth-Heinemann.)

greater than plain x-rays in the detection of spinal injuries especially with the newer multidetector CT machines. CT is superior to other diagnostic procedures in demonstrating impingement on the neuronal canal.[27]

MRI can show the extent of soft tissue damage when x-ray may not show the full extent (Fig. 34-13). Figure 34-14 shows a Jefferson fracture seen on x-ray and magnetic resonance imaging (MRI) scan. Figure 34-15 compares fractures at time of injury and after stabilization. Myelography is indicated for optimal visualization of compression of the spinal cord after trauma. Myelography alone is rarely indicated, and it is used in conjunction with CT in cases where MRI is not available.

In acute SCI, MRI is sometimes problematic because of its limited use around ferromagnetic objects such as respirators, oxygen tanks, and traction devices. When these

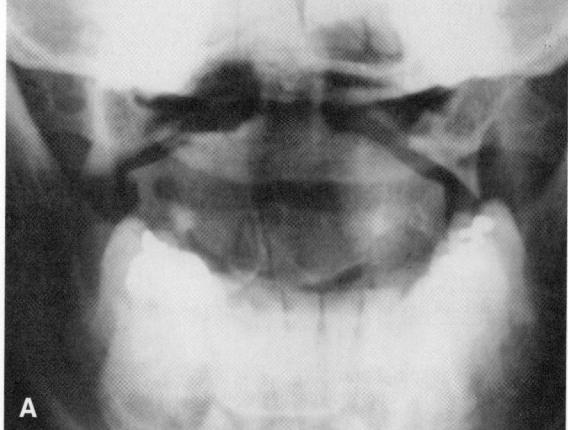

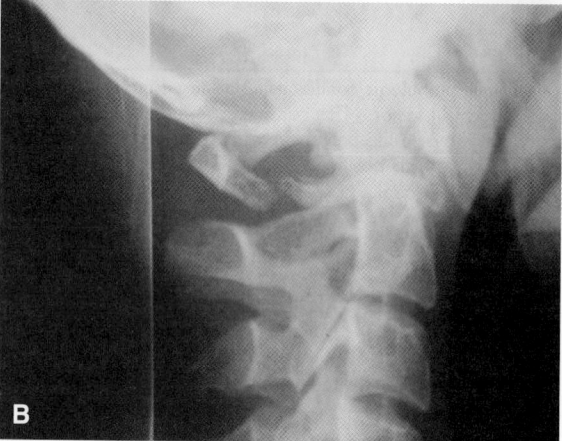

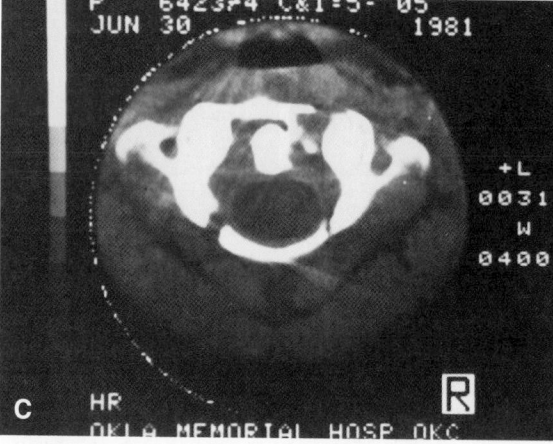

Figure 34-14

Fracture of C1 (Jefferson fracture). A, Anteroposterior view showing lateral displacement of the lateral mass and articulating facets of C1 on C2. **B,** Oblique view illustrating disruption of the posterior aspect of the ring of C1. **C,** Computed tomographic scan revealing the true extent of the injury. (From Green NE, Swiotkowski MF, eds: *Skeletal trauma in children,* ed 3, Philadelphia, 2003, Saunders. Courtesy Dr. Teresa Stacy.)

obstacles do not exist, the extent of spinal cord damage and the possibility of disk herniation can be more readily assessed by MRI. The presence of intradural or extradural hematoma can often be demonstrated on MRI. MRI is useful in excluding spinal cord contusion or hemorrhage in persons with neurologic deficits and normal CT scans and plain films.[30]

The recent development of advanced structural imaging techniques, such as diffusion tensor imaging and magnetization transfer, is beginning to overcome these problems. In fact, lack of inflammation is advantageous for these types of images. Diffusion tensor imaging provides a unique image contrast called diffusion anisotropy. This reveals tissue organization at the microscopic level based on the average motion of water molecules.[7,72]

Advanced MRI techniques are better than conventional MRI in visualizing chronic SCI. The development of functional MRI (fMRI), currently useful in imaging the brain, and its application to the spinal cord should revolutionize the field of regeneration. Transplanted cells can now be tracked after they are placed in living organisms using MRI. Neural stem cells are labeled with paramagnetic agents before they are transplanted, and MRI tracks their distribution and migration after they are placed in the damaged spinal cord.

In spinal trauma with severe neural malfunction, neurophysiologic studies help in determining which neural elements are involved; which spinal segment is responsible for mechanical or other irritation; and whether the lesion is chronic, acute progressing, or resolving. Neurophysiologic studies allow intraoperative monitoring and include somatosensory evoked potentials, motor evoked potentials, neurography, F-wave and H-reflex electromyography, and sympathetic skin response. Somatosensory evoked potentials and motor evoked potentials are useful in the investigation of the CNS. Electromyography, neurography, and F-wave and H-reflex studies are used for evaluation of the peripheral component of spinal injury.[106]

A unique SCI syndrome, burning hands syndrome, was first described in sports injury. This syndrome appears to be a variation of central cord syndrome associated with severe burning paresthesias and dysesthesias in the hands and/or the feet. Other signs of neurologic dysfunction are minimal or absent. More than 50% of the time there is an underlying spinal fracture-dislocation. It is important to differentiate this syndrome from the much more common and usually innocuous "burning" or "stinging" of brachial plexus origin. Box 34-3 outlines the combined evaluation of head and neck injuries that should be performed beginning at the sideline.[42]

Diagnosis of syringomyelia may be delayed because the early symptoms are so similar to those of other, more common neurologic disorders. The accident that caused the initial damage may have been months to years previous to the onset of symptoms. MRI is the best imaging study for diagnosing this disorder in the beginning stages. MRI will show the syrinx number, size, and location, and any other abnormalities of the spine and spinal cord. Functional MRI allows the surgeon to see the spinal fluid pulsating within the syrinx.

TREATMENT. Interventions at several levels are required to improve mortality, morbidity, and quality of life.

Emergent Care. The emergent phase of care is crucial for the person with traumatic SCI. It can make the difference between living the rest of life with a disability or recovering with only temporary neurologic deficits. An incomplete injury can be made worse by mishandling and can be made better by prompt attention to critical

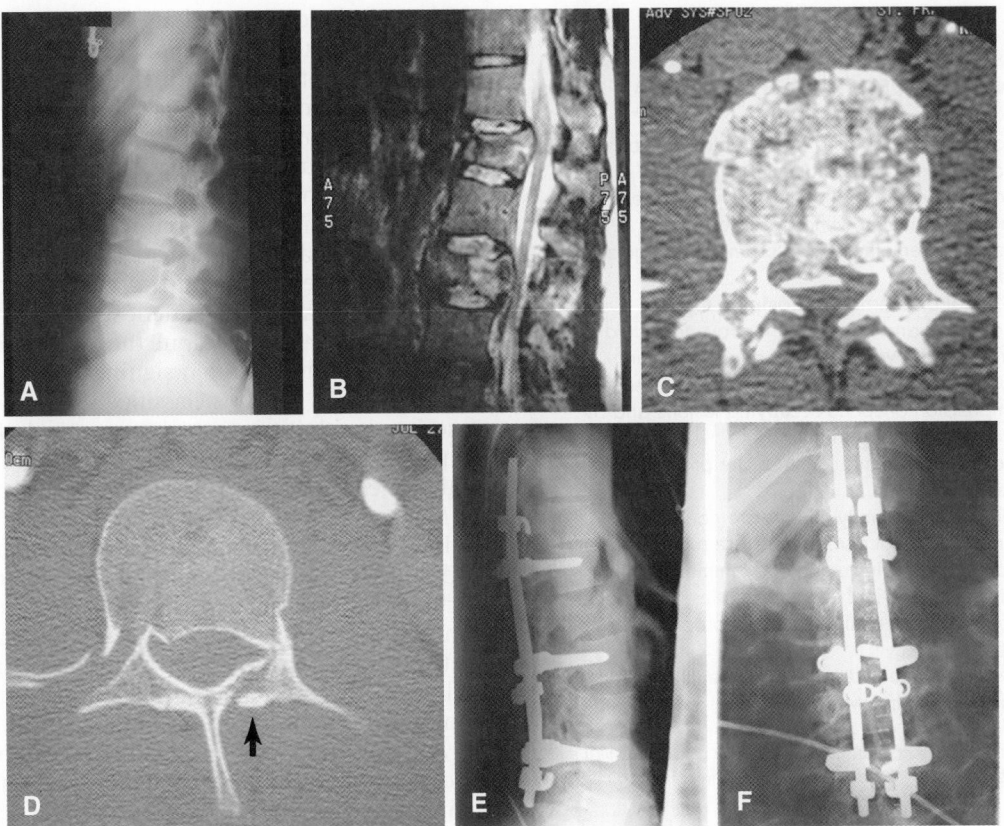

Figure 34-15

A 21-year-old man involved in a motor vehicle accident sustained a burst fracture of L1 and L3. The patient had an incomplete spinal cord injury. **A,** A preoperative lateral view shows loss of height predominately at L1. **B,** A sagittal-cut magnetic resonance image shows compression at both L1 and L3. **C,** An axial-cut computed tomographic (CT) scan at L3 shows a retropulsed fragment filling half the canal. **D,** An axial CT scan at L1 shows a fracture of the lamina and retropulsion of a fragment into canal. **E,** This injury was stabilized with Isola instrumentation combining both pedicle screws and laminar hooks. Sagittal alignment was maintained. **F,** Postoperative anteroposterior radiograph showing a cross-connection added for additional stability. (From Browner BD, Jipiter JB, Levine AM, et al: *Skeletal trauma: basic science, management, and reconstruction*, ed 3, Philadelphia, 2003, Saunders.)

Box 34-3

COMBINED EVALUATION OF HEAD AND NECK INJURIES

- Note exact time of injury. Management decisions are based on duration of symptoms.
- Assess loss of consciousness. Management of unresponsive athletes should follow the ABCs of trauma care (i.e., check airway, breathing, and circulation).
- Assess peripheral strength and sensation without moving the athlete's head or neck.
- Palpate the neck for asymmetric spasm or tenderness at the spine.
- Assess isometric neck strength without moving the athlete's head or neck.
- Assess active range of motion at the neck.
- Perform axial compression and Spurling test; if negative, athlete may be moved.
- Assess recent memory and postural instability.
- Inquire about symptoms such as headache, nausea, dizziness, or blurred vision.

From Whiteside JW: Management of head and neck injuries by the sideline physician, *Am Fam Physician* 74(8):1357–1362, 2006.

procedures. Box 34-4 includes the guidelines endorsed by the International Association for Trauma Surgery and Intensive Care.

Assessment of the likelihood of SCI includes understanding the mechanics of the trauma and obtaining vital signs. In the case of a cervical injury, paradoxic respiration or abdominal breathing may be present, and immediate immobilization should be instituted. Use of a rigid collar and spinal board can help to prevent movement of the spinal column. Oxygen and medication should be given to control the hyperperfusion and swelling of the spinal cord.

Monitoring in the critical care phase includes cardiac and neurologic status. Orthopedic management may begin at this phase and includes closed and open reduction of the vertebrae and decompression of the spinal cord. Surgery, including fusion and internal fixation, is the most common procedure performed prior to use of an orthosis for 8 to 12 weeks. The goal is to restore spinal alignment, establish spinal stability, and prevent further neurologic deterioration, enhancing recovery. The tetracycline antibiotic minocycline and the immunosuppressants FK-506 and cyclosporine are under investigation. In animal models of contusive SCI, preliminary results with minocycline suggest a promising reduction in apoptotic

Box 34-4

ESSENTIAL TRAUMA CARE SERVICES ENDORSED BY THE IATSIC AS THE "RIGHTS OF THE INJURED"

- Obstructed airways are opened and maintained before hypoxia leads to death or permanent disability.
- Impaired breathing is supported until the injured person is able to breathe adequately without assistance.
- Pneumothorax and hemothorax are promptly recognized and relieved.
- Bleeding (external or internal) is promptly stopped.
- Shock is recognized and treated with intravenous fluid replacement before irreversible consequences occur.
- The consequences of traumatic brain injury are lessened by timely decompression of space-occupying lesions and by prevention of secondary brain injury.
- Intestinal and other abdominal injuries are promptly recognized and repaired.
- Potentially disabling extremity injuries are corrected.
- Potentially unstable spinal cord injuries are recognized and managed appropriately, including early immobilization.
- The consequences to the individual of injuries that result in physical impairment are minimized by appropriate rehabilitative services.
- Medications for these services and for the minimization of pain are readily available when needed.

From Mock C, Lormand JD, Goosen J, et al: *Guidelines for essential trauma care*, Geneva, 2004, World Health Organization; with permission.
IATSIC, International Association for Trauma Surgery and Intensive Care.

death at the injury site and improved locomotor function. Cyclosporine acts at the mitochondrial membrane to impede apoptosis and has been shown to promote tissue sparing and inhibit lipid peroxidation in models of brain injury and **SCI** in experimental models.[86,107]

CNS/AANS guidelines discourage steroids in spinal injury which is in contrast to the old guidelines. The current recommendation is that methylprednisolone not be used for the treatment of acute SCI within the first 24 to 48 hours. The standard was revised because of the lack of medical evidence supporting the benefits of these drugs in the clinical setting. In fact, the report includes strong evidence that high-dose steroids are associated with harmful adverse effects.[83] Loss of ANS control affects the function of the cardiovascular system. Acute management of blood pressure is critical. The autonomic lesion predisposes persons with high spinal cord lesions to abnormal cardiovascular responses to vasoactive agents.

Management of Complications. Management of complications of SCI is critical. High cervical injuries require immediate placement of ventilation equipment and maintenance of pulmonary hygiene. Therapy consists of intermittent positive-pressure breathing, bronchodilators, and mucolytics. Prevention of pulmonary infection is critical in SCI.

Bilateral diaphragmatic pacing can be considered as an alternative method of ventilatory support in a select group of patients who have high SCI and preserved function of the phrenic nerve–diaphragm unit. The most suitable candidates for pacing are considered to be those patients with a preserved response to peripheral phrenic

nerve stimulation but lacking a response to transcranial stimulation of the diaphragm motor area.[93]

Treatment of spasticity includes use of muscle relaxants and spasmolytic agents.[87] Peripheral nerve blocks, such as botulinum toxin (Botox) and phenol, provide a temporary reduction of spasticity. Therefore, spasticity-related interventions need to be aimed at what matters most to the individual. It is critical for clinicians to understand individuals' experiences to make accurate assessments, effectively evaluate treatment interventions, and select appropriate management strategies.[67,68]

Pain Management. Despite the fact that SCI causes loss of sensation, there is often significant pain that develops over time. Pain in SCI is classified in many different ways associated with intrinsic or neurogenic dysfunction, such as pain associated with syringomyelia and musculoskeletal or mechanical pain.

Management of neurogenic pain in SCI is by systemic or local drug therapy and by neuroaugmentative and neurodestructive intervention. The pharmacologic approach includes nonsteroidal analgesics, opioids, antidepressants, and anticonvulsants.[50] Pregabalin (Lyrica) is associated with relief of central neuropathic pain and with reduction in pain-related sleep interference and significant improvement in sleep problems. Action on centrally located calcium channels may be important in the effectiveness of pregabalin in managing central neuropathic pain.

Neurodestructive procedures include both chemical and surgical destruction of nervous structures. Procedures may include deafferentation, interruption of ascending pain systems, or destruction of cells in the dorsal horn.

Decompressive surgery is performed in individuals with spinal cord syringomyelia, depending on which area is affected. Surgery to create a pseudomeningomyelocele, an artificial CSF reservoir, performed to normalize the CSF flow, has been shown to be effective. By draining the cyst, it is possible to prevent the cyst from reexpanding. Draining the fluid can relieve pain, headache, and a sensation of tightness in the head or neck. In a dural graft procedure, the space around the spinal cord is enlarged to allow free flow of fluid and reduce pressure.

Strategies for Future Consideration. Transplantation of stem cells is being studied extensively in relation to the treatment of SCI. Processes include producing regenerative growth factors, expressing substances capable of breaking down scar tissue and modulating the immune system's response to injury. It appears that there will be potential for reprogramming the host microenvironment; for example, embryonic stem cell transplantation reduces macrophage influx by more than 50%.

Critical components of optimal care following SCI are protection of neural tissue and limitation of secondary damage, facilitation of axonal regrowth, and control of factors that inhibit intrinsic neural repair. Because the consequences of SCI are complex, it is most likely that a hierarchy of intervention strategies will be needed to restore suprasegmental control leading to the recovery of function in the spinal cord.[10,48] The phases of injury and the neurophysiologic events will create both limitations and advantages related to potential treatments administered during the different phases of injury. Based on the premise that the relative inability of the CNS to regenerate can be largely attributed to the insufficient recruitment and activation of macrophages within the immune-privileged injured CNS, preclinical studies using transplantation of activated autologous macrophages after experimental SCI have been performed. Studies from several laboratories have demonstrated the ability for peripheral macrophages to synthesize nerve growth factor as well as the capability of these cells to phagocytose myelin, providing additional rationale for using hematogenous macrophages to repair the injured spinal cord. Human studies are under way; however, issues of cost and timing of application have limited outcomes.

Embryonic stem cells are true stem cells that show unlimited capacity for self-renewal. In contrast, adult stem cells are progenitor cells or cells that are immature or undifferentiated. Numerous preclinical studies suggest that embryonic and adult stem cells, along with their lineage-specific progenitors, may improve the outcome after experimental SCI. Transplanted stem cells may potentially act through several proposed mechanisms, which include providing trophic support to promote the survival and regrowth of host tissue, acting as a cellular scaffold to permit axonal elongation through the site of injury, and the replacement of lost or damaged cells. The demyelination of intact axons is a prominent feature of SCI and contributes to loss of function after injury, leading to potential therapeutic strategies which involve the replacement of myelin-producing cells through the transplantation of embryonic stem cells.[12]

Upon tissue damage or injury, progenitor cells can be activated by growth factors or cytokines, leading to increased cell division important for the repair process. Progenitor cells participate in the normal maintenance of the CNS. These mechanisms include production and replacement of cells lost to normal aging and cell turnover. Human embryonic stem cells (hESCs) may offer a renewable source of a wide range of cell types for use in research and cell-based therapies to treat disease. Researchers have successfully differentiated hESCs along the oligodendrocyte lineage, obtaining highly purified oligodendrocyte progenitor cells (OPCs). The transplantation of hESC-derived OPCs into adult rat spinal cord injuries has been shown to enhance remyelination and promote improvement of motor function. There may be feasibility of predifferentiating hESCs into functional OPCs and with potential therapeutic potential. However, it remains unclear whether the improved functional recovery that has been seen in preclinical studies is due to enhanced remyelination, to the secretion of trophic factors by OPCs, or to other neuroprotective effects of OPC transplantation that have yet to be identified.[12]

Progenitor cells transplanted during the acute injury phase are vulnerable to the same set of cell death mechanisms predominant during the secondary phase of acute injury. Understanding the function of growth-inhibiting factors within the adult CNS may lead to control of the neural destruction after SCI.[14]

Astrocytes can express molecules that are both growth permissive and growth inhibitory at the same time. Reactive astrocytes appear to create an inhibitory environment within the injured spinal cord and form an astroglial scar

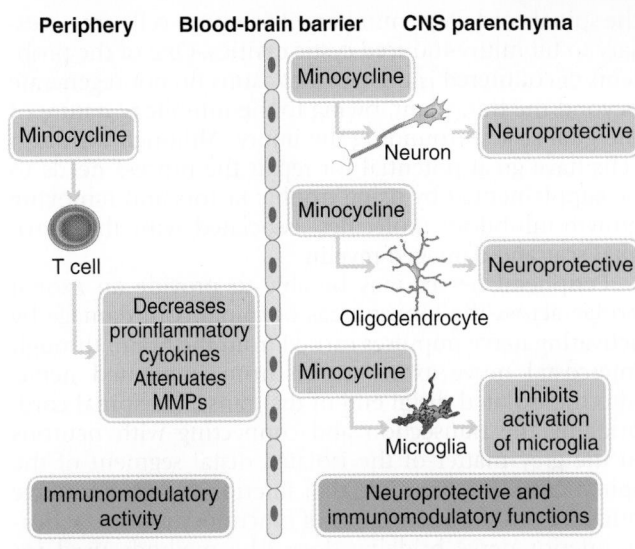

Figure 34-16

Peripheral and central functions of minocycline. Minocycline has immunomodulatory activity in the periphery and both immunomodulatory and neuroprotective capacity within the central nervous system. (From *The Lancet Neurology*, vol 3, issue 12, 2004, Fig. 3, Elsevier.)

that acts as a physical and chemical barrier to axonal regeneration. Maintaining an environment to support the growth of axons may involve the selective removal of astrocytes from the site of injury.[28,94] In contrast, glial restricted precursor–derived astrocytes may promote axonal regeneration via suppression of astrogliosis, realignment of host tissues, and delaying of expression of inhibitory proteoglycans. The glia, not the neurons, are the critical elements in preventing growth and in restoring it. Neurons retain the power to grow, and their sprouts only await the provision of a suitable glial pathway to be able to advance across the lesion. Several studies have suggested that an established, but not necessarily ongoing, glial scar is largely responsible for the failure of remyelination.

Inflammatory reactions in the CNS have a dual nature; they may be neuroprotective as well as neurotoxic. Studies illustrate that the nervous and immune systems have overlapping rules of organization and intercellular communication. Schwann cells have been used to facilitate a permissive environment for the injured spinal cord to regenerate. The Schwann cell is one of the most widely studied cell types for repair of the spinal cord. These cells play a crucial role in endogenous repair of peripheral nerves because of their ability to dedifferentiate, migrate, proliferate, and express growth-promoting factors and extracellular matrix molecules and myelinate regenerating axons. Following SCI, Schwann cells migrate from the periphery into the injury site, where they participate in endogenous repair process. Previous experiments have shown compressive mechanical stress to be important in stimulating the regenerative behavior of Schwann cells. Transplantation of highly permissive Schwann cell–enriched peripheral nerve grafts may enhance regeneration in SCI.[31] Figure 34-16 demonstrates the neuroprotective processes that may be integral within the immunomodulation. For transplantation into the spinal cord, large numbers of Schwann cells are necessary to fill injury-induced cystic cavities. One of the problems encountered is the fact that axons do not regenerate beyond the transplant, owing to the inhibitory nature of the glial scar surrounding the injury. Although Schwann cells have great potential for repair the process needs to be supplemented by using trophic factors and removing growth-inhibitory molecules associated with the astroglial scar and damaged myelin.

Peripheral nerves may be able to provide an axonal bridge across the longer areas of spinal cord damage by activating nerve impulses carried from the brain, through intercostal nerve axons grown from implanted nerve, into the isolated distal end of the transected spinal cord, bridging the transection and connecting with neurons in the grey matter of the isolated distal segment of the spinal cord. It is possible that inferior-to-superior nerve bridging can produce return of function, just as superior-to-inferior nerve bridging does. The methods used for peripheral nerve grafting continue to be explored and refined. Peripheral nerve grafting techniques have been developed using segments of sciatic nerve placed either directly between the damaged rostral and caudal ends of the injury site or used to form a bridge across the lesion to restore functional connectivity across the lesion site.[12]

PROGNOSIS. Prognosis related to ambulation is a concern to most persons who have sustained spinal cord injuries. The prognosis for recovery depends on the level of the injury, muscle strength, and ASIA Impairment scale at the initial injury.[58] The age of the individual also seems to contribute to recovery, with the best potential related to a younger age.[102]

Most motor recovery occurs during the first 6 months, and strength may continue to increase with appropriate facilitation. The muscles graded 1 to 3 in the zone of partial preservation have potential to recover motor function; however, less than 50% of the most cephalad muscle graded 0/5 at initial testing regained strength at 1 year. Overall, more than one-half of the SCI population will have return of some neurologic function. Compression fractures have the most favorable prognosis for return of function, with crush fractures having the least chance for return of function.[56] Preservation of axonal integrity and regrowth of neural tissue is anticipated to have a significant effect on the recovery of mobility after SCI. Turning this nervous system recovery into improved functional status is part of current and ongoing research in the rehabilitation field.

Morbidity and mortality during the first year following SCI are significantly higher than those following the first year. Those with Asia Impairment Scores (AIS) of D at any level have higher life expectancy rates as compared to those with AIS A–C. Clients with paraplegic injuries live longer than those with low cervical and high cervical injuries. Clients who depend on ventilators have the lowest life expectancy. Long-term urinary tract infection continues to be a cause of death, but control of sepsis has improved markedly since 1970.[75]

This is thought to be primarily a result of improvement in bladder training, antibiotic treatment, control of fluid intake, and surgery for obstruction of the lower urinary tract. Another common cause of death is respiratory disease, specifically atelectasis and pneumonia, and this is the leading cause of death among high cervical injury clients.[26]

Pneumonia continues at a rate higher than in the general population, with pulmonary edema associated with injuries above T6. Heart disease is common, including myocardial infarction, cardiac arrest, myocarditis, and pulmonary embolism. However, the mortality rate is not much higher than that in the general population and is improving with increased pharmacologic control and improved medical knowledge of the cardiovascular changes accompanying SCI.

People with SCI experience significant problems in a number of areas of life, resulting in ongoing stress related to pain, lack of income and financial problems, spasticity, stress, and difficulty in their sex lives. These problems do not appear to be highly correlated with aging, suggesting that they will not necessarily become more problematic, nor are they likely to self-remediate.[59]

Age, employment status, motor level and completeness of injury, and ambulatory mode (use of hand-propelled or motorized wheelchair, use of crutches or canes, or walking independently) are independently associated with health-related quality-of-life scores. Chronic cough, chronic phlegm, persistent wheeze, dyspnea with ADLs, and lower forced expiratory volume and forced vital capacity are each associated with a lower health-related quality of life.[17,52,90] A recent study reported that 58% of visits to family physicians by individuals with SCI were the result of complications that accompany immobility, including bowel and bladder dysfunction, pathologic fractures, skin breakdown, pain, AD, and spasticity. Therefore, exercise, prevention of secondary complications, injury prevention, good nutrition, and education are important components of health and wellness programs for individuals with spinal cord injuries.[26,58,75,102]

SPECIAL IMPLICATIONS FOR THE THERAPIST | 34-1

Traumatic Spinal Cord Injury

Rehabilitation to enhance the function and lifestyle of SCI clients has traditionally been aimed at helping clients to achieve the ability to perform ADLs and mobility-related ADLs.[91]

This approach attempts to facilitate maximal independence with most daily tasks and allows clients to return to desired activities, both occupational and recreational. Rehabilitation strategies address functional mobility skills, health maintenance, and vocational adjustments. Although the ideal goal is to reach the point where the disability is no longer the major focus of clients' lives, the client often has to perform their desired activities in a different way than prior to their injury. Psychosocial adjustment can be a primary focus of rehabilitation as clients experience a mix of emotions and reactions to their injury. They may be thankful for their own survival yet grieving the loss of body function and their ability to fill their previous roles and social responsibilities. Clients should be involved in all aspects of rehabilitation and be provided the information and environment to foster independence. Most importantly, clinicians should "respect expressions of

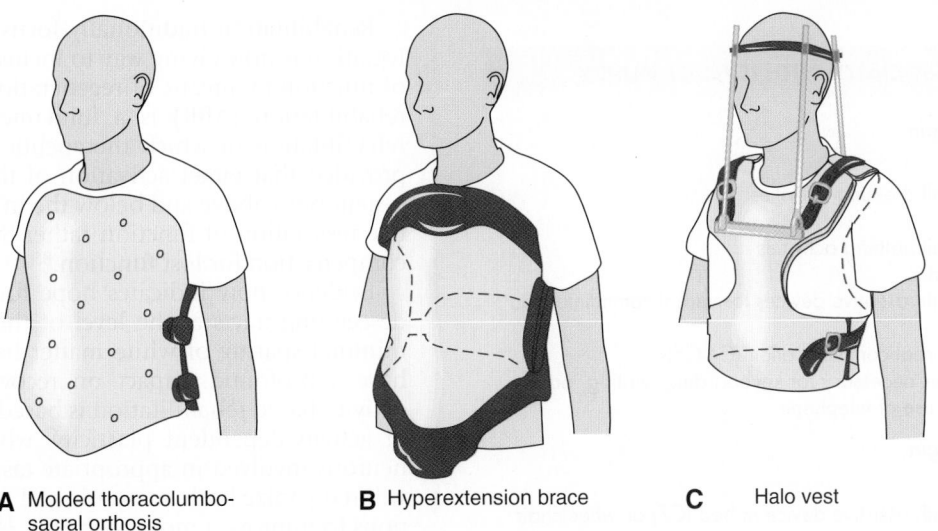

A Molded thoracolumbo-sacral orthosis **B** Hyperextension brace **C** Halo vest

Figure 34-17

A, Molded thoracolumbosacral orthosis, designed to control extension and rotary movements. **B,** Hyperextension brace, which restricts flexion in the thoracic area. **C,** Halo vest, which restricts upper thoracic and cervical motion.

hope" and incorporate the client's goals into the rehabilitation plan.[23]

It is critical throughout the rehabilitation process that the therapist be prepared for secondary medical complications that could be life-threatening, such as orthostatic hypotension, AD, deep vein thrombosis, and pulmonary emboli. Guidelines for management of these conditions can be found in the clinical practice guidelines published by the Consortium for Spinal Cord Medicine.[22,24,25,70]

At minimum, in initial stages of rehabilitation, clinicians should monitor blood pressure, oxygen saturation, and pulse rate and be familiar with the signs and symptoms of these complications. In cases of AD, identification and elimination of the causal factor and notification of the occurrence to other team members are critical.[67] AD and pulmonary emboli require emergent medical attention. Refer to Box 34-2 for symptoms and triggers of AD.[15,22]

In intensive care, physical therapists are concerned with preparation for and mobilization of the client. Emphasis here is on respiratory management, increasing ROM, and prevention of pressure ulcers. Postural drainage and assisted coughing should be initiated for secretion clearance.[26,40,101]

Monitoring blood pressure and oxygen saturation at rest and during activity is critical. Use of an abdominal binder during upright activity has been found to assist with maintenance of blood pressure as well as promotion of optimal diaphragm efficiency.[13]

Maintaining or increasing ROM, the beginning of a strength and endurance program, and education of both the client and family are key components for preventing secondary complications of SCI and promoting optimal functional potential.[77] When possible, the client and/or family should be taught to maintain ROM of the extremities independently. Adequate hamstring length and shoulder flexibility is critical for performance of transfers, bed mobility, and independent dressing during later stages of rehabilitation.[91]

Proper padding and positioning both in bed as well as while seated in a wheelchair are imperative for maintenance of skin integrity. A pressure-relieving cushion (usually filled with air or gel), which is engineered to disperse the pressure under the weight-bearing surface, should be used when sitting. Weight shifts or pressure reliefs should be performed every 15 to 30 minutes for 2 to 3 minutes at a time. A pressure relief offloads the weight-bearing tissue, allowing blood flow to return to that area and preventing ischemia in the tissues. Ischemia leads to skin breakdown and pressure ulcers.[24,69,89]

Orthotic management of the unstable and postoperative spinal column is often necessary, and the therapist should be familiar with the types of orthotic devices used. Figure 34-17 illustrates several orthoses used with different levels of spinal cord lesions.[81,82]

As the client progresses through acute rehabilitation and into outpatient treatment phases, physical therapy focuses on achieving optimal functional independence. As Box 34-5 demonstrates, the level of the lesion will determine the degree to which independence can be expected in certain activities.[25] For those with motor complete injuries, the therapeutic program must work toward developing the necessary ROM, strength, as well as the appropriate mechanics and strategies for efficient performance of transfers and bed mobility using only the innervated muscles. Clients with thoracic and lumbar levels of injury will attain independence with bed mobility, transfers, and wheelchair mobility barring any significant medical complications or comorbidities such as obesity, significant ROM restrictions, and persistent pain. Wheelchair mobility skills include propelling the manual or power wheelchair on indoor and outdoor surfaces, management of the wheelchair components, and, most important, weight shifts in the chair to prevent skin breakdown. Skills needed for mobility without assistive devices and adaptive equipment may be different from skills needed for mobility with equipment. In some cases, transfers into and out

DISABILITIES ASSOCIATED WITH LEVEL OF INJURY

C1-C5 Quadriplegia

- Dressing
  Dependent in all dressing activities
- Bathing
  Dependent in all bathing activities
- Communication
  Independent with assistive devices for verbal communication (C1-C3)
  Independent verbal communication (C4-C5)
  Assistive devices necessary for keyboarding, writing, page turning, and use of telephone

C6-C8 Quadriplegia

- Dressing
  Independent with assistive device in bed (C7) or wheelchair (C8)
  Minimal assistance with lower body dressing in bed
  Moderate assistance undressing lower body in bed
  Able to dress and undress in wheelchair with assistive devices (C8)
- Bathing
  Minimal assistance for upper body bathing and drying
  Moderate assistance for lower body drying (C6)
  Independent with assistive devices (C7-C8)
  Assistive devices (tub chair necessary for tub or shower)
- Communication
  Independent in verbal communication
  Assistive devices necessary for keyboarding, writing, and use of telephone
  Setup required (C6)

T1 and Below Paraplegia

- Dressing
  Independent with use of assistive device
- Bathing
  Independent with use of assistive device (tub bench or cushion on bottom of tub)
- Communication
  Independent

Modified from Altrice MB et al: Traumatic spinal cord injury. In Umphred DA, ed: *Neurological rehabilitation*, St. Louis, 1995, Mosby–Year Book, pp. 502–506.

of bed can only be done with special equipment, such as a transfer board or loop ladder.[60,91] Adaptations within the environment may be necessary for the client with weak upper extremities or poor hand control.

Depending on the motor level of the spinal cord injury, a client may require a significant amount of physical assistance after discharge from acute rehabilitation. More than 87% of persons admitted to an acute care hospital for treatment of SCI are ultimately discharged home. Among young adults, 50% of people with traumatic SCI are unmarried at the time of the incident.[75] Available caregiver support tends to be more limited, and external support systems will need to be established. For those with higher levels of injury, long-term care may be indicated if adequate caregiver support is not available. For older individuals sustaining SCI, there are more preexisting medical conditions, more secondary medical complications, and more need for long-term care.[42]

Rehabilitation traditionally focused on social reintegration is now giving way to inclusion of restoration of function by means of regeneration.[8] Activity-based rehabilitation (ABR) is a fundamental approach to rehabilitation in which therapeutic interventions are provided that target activation of the neuromuscular system both above and below the injury level to facilitate restoration of function rather than teaching pure compensation for lost function.[85]

Evidence now indicates hope for more sparing of descending tracts at the level of the lesion and even minimal sparing of white matter has been shown to have a profound impact on recovery of function.[6] Activity-based rehabilitation is based on the principles of activity-dependent plasticity, which assumes that neurons involved in appropriate task-specific training will reorganize both anatomic and functional connections to improve a motor behavior.[34]

Activity-based rehabilitation generally involves using intense practice and repetition of task-specific mobility training to promote neural recovery and elicit lasting changes in spinal cord function. Intensive therapy programs focused on recovery often utilize specialized rehabilitation interventions including but not limited to the following: locomotor training with body weight support (BWS) utilizing robotic and manual assistance, functional electrical stimulation (FES) cycling, FES neuroprosthetics designed to augment walking function, and whole body vibration (WBV).

The recovery of walking is typically a priority for individuals who have sustained a spinal cord injury. Locomotor training utilizing a treadmill with BWS is an activity-based therapy intervention that has gained popularity in recent years in the rehabilitation community. There is a growing body of evidence depicting that this type of intensive repetition of the walking pattern may be beneficial for individuals with incomplete SCIs to improve overground walking speed, endurance, and independence.[9,38,47,103,104] Locomotor training with BWS and manual assistance generally requires three to four therapists/trainers to deploy the intervention and can be very labor intensive for staff. Locomotor training devices utilizing a robotic orthosis have been developed and are also being used to train walking function after individuals have sustained an incomplete SCI and require fewer staff members while also causing less physical stress on staff. Although evidence supports that locomotor training with BWS may be beneficial for improving walking function in individuals with motor incomplete SCI, there is insufficient evidence at this time to demonstrate that one locomotor training strategy is superior over another.[32,38,64,71,78]

Robotic exoskeleton devices are an emerging technology that has recently become available for use in select rehabilitation centers. Many clinicians and consumers who have experience with these first robotic exoskeleton prototypes agree that these devices need to be smaller and more adaptable to be considered community mobility devices utilized by a significant number of individuals with SCIs. Currently, there are no commercially available devices that have been approved by the FDA to be sold for individual home/community use, but they offer exciting possibilities into the future for individuals who have sustained both motor complete and motor incomplete SCIs.[95]

ABR may also include the use of numerous forms of electrical stimulation for individuals with spinal cord injury. Augmenting the force production of specific muscle groups of the trunk, upper and lower extremities, lower extremity FES cycling, upper extremity FES cycling, FES-assisted standing, and FES-assisted ambulation are commons ways that FES is utilized in spinal cord rehabilitation. The goals of utilizing FES in the clinic may include the following: strengthening of impaired or paralyzed muscle groups, as a neuroprosthesis for the upper and lower extremities, and to assist in the prevention of the secondary complications associated with immobility. When utilizing FES in the clinic, it's important to remember that there are differences in the response of the neuromuscular system to electrical stimulation versus voluntary activation of a muscle group. During voluntary activation of a muscle group, the order of recruitment is generally from the smallest-diameter fibers to the larger-diameter fibers based on the muscle's load requirements, whereas electrically stimulating a muscle group often leads to a reversed pattern of recruitment. This reversed pattern of recruitment is not as efficient as voluntary activation and may lead to premature fatigue of the muscle group. Attempts to minimize fatigue related to FES have led to use of units that are fired by feedback on voluntary muscle activity.

Lower extremity neuroprosthesis designed to address foot drop as well as knee control are commercially available to augment walking in individuals with incomplete SCIs. Stimulation of the common peroneal nerve can facilitate swing phase activity, and stimulation of the hamstrings and quadriceps can support stance phase control and may assist with correction of knee hyperextension (genu recurvatum).[18] Improvements in gait speed, endurance, kinematics, and the physiologic cost of walking have been reported with the use of these FES-assisted ambulation in individuals who have sustained incomplete SCIs.[5,63,64,96,97]

Neuroprostheses via surgically implanted FES devices are rehabilitative tools with the potential to increase independence. Currently, there are studies under way assessing the efficacy and safety of implanted FES systems for standing and walking, but there are no commercially available implantable systems at this time. Therefore, even though implanted FES systems may be a promising hope for the future of spinal cord injury rehabilitation, they currently do not offer a possible alternative to wheelchair use.

Cycling in combination with FES is an intervention often considered to be an activity-based rehabilitation strategy. During FES cycling, software is used to stimulate lower extremity muscle groups including the quadriceps, hamstrings, gluteals, tibialis anterior, and gastroc/soleus at the appropriate intervals to allow an individual with little or no voluntary motor control to turn an ergometer utilizing their own power. Improved cardiorespiratory fitness, improved lower extremity function, increased lower extremity circulation, muscle hypertrophy, decreased spasticity, decreased blood glucose and insulin levels, as well as improvements in bone mineral density have been reported by some authors.[20,29,33,39,54,61]

Deficits in upper extremity function in individuals with tetraplegia can significantly limit their functional independence. An intensive training intervention may induce both functional and neurophysiologic changes by driving cortical reorganization.[49] FES-assisted hand movement can enable clients with tetraplegia to perform many of their simple ADLs. Upper extremity FES cycling is also an available intervention for individuals with spinal cord injury. Multiple muscle groups of the arms and scapula may be stimulated to augment upper extremity ergometry with the goals of increasing upper extremity strength, limiting atrophy, and improving cardiovascular fitness. However, clinicians should be cautious when using this intervention with high cervical injuries as shoulder subluxation and instability are concerns.

Exercise is critical to the individual with SCI to maintain cardiac fitness levels. There are numerous reports of strategies for exercises.[4] Circuit resistance exercise (CRT) improves muscle strength, endurance, and anaerobic power in individuals with paraplegia while significantly reducing their shoulder pain.[74] Skeletal muscle atrophy is associated with accumulation of greater intramuscular fat in thigh muscle groups in SCI and continues to increase over time in incomplete SCI.[43] There is a link between adiposity (accumulation of fat in adipose tissue) and defining characteristics of metabolic syndrome. Adiposity is related to dyslipidemia, vascular inflammation, hypertension, and insulin resistance.[41] There is persistent adaptive capability within chronically paralyzed muscles. Preventing musculoskeletal adaptations after SCI may be more effective than reversing changes in the chronic condition.

Recent evidence supports that activity-based rehabilitation may be beneficial for individuals who have sustained SCIs, promoting restoration of function, maximizing health and wellness, as well as limiting the impact of the secondary complications associated with immobility. Although this evidence is encouraging, compensatory strategies and ABR approaches must be utilized in parallel for individuals who have sustained SCIs to maximize functional independence while at the same time promoting recovery of the injured nervous system. Further research needs to be completed in this area of rehabilitation to determine who benefits most from ABR approaches and at what phase of the recovery process these interventions can be most beneficial. As new modalities of treatment are becoming available for individuals with SCIs, it is important that they are critically evaluated for their efficacy and utilized appropriately within the context of evidence-based practice.

REFERENCES

To enhance this text and add value for the reader, all references are included on the companion Evolve site that accompanies this textbook. The reader can view the reference source and access it online whenever possible.

CHAPTER 35

Cerebral Palsy

ALLAN M. GLANZMAN

CEREBRAL PALSY

Overview

Cerebral palsy (CP) is a nonprogressive lesion of the brain occurring prior to 2 years of age resulting in a disorder of posture and movement. CP may be accompanied by impairment of the skeletal system, including hip dislocation and scoliosis; oral motor and gastrointestinal (GI) function, including speech, feeding, and GI motility; as well as sensory disturbances, including vision, visual perception, and hearing. Common comorbidities include visual and hearing deficits, seizure disorders, scoliosis, hip dislocation, and mental retardation.

Classification

CP is often classified by the type of muscle tone, distribution of limb involvement, or functional skills. The types of muscle tone include hypotonia (low tone); hypertonia (high tone, spasticity); ataxia; and choreoathetosis, rigidity, or dystonia.[52]

Dystonia is characterized by involuntary sustained or intermittent muscle contraction resulting in sustained end-range posture, with some including twisted postures and repetitive movements.[58] *Choreoathetosis* is characterized by involuntary distal writhing movements (athetosis) and poorly graded proximal voluntary movement (chorea). *Rigidity* is characterized by a lead-pipe quality of resistance to passive movement which is independent of movement speed. *Spasticity* is characterized by a velocity-dependent resistance to passive stretch and is graded most commonly by using the modified Ashworth scale or by using Tardau's R1 and R2.[10] *Ataxia* is characterized by incoordination of voluntary movement patterns characterized by poor accuracy, targeting, and grading of movement. The patterns of motor involvement and distribution are described in Table 35-1.

Spastic CP, particularly quadriplegia and spastic diplegia, accounts for the majority of cases, with hemiplegia and triplegia being less common. The overwhelming majority of children have tone that is characterized by spasticity with ataxia, dystonia, and choreoathetosis affecting a minority of children[26] affect a relatively smaller number of children. New cases of choreoathetoid CP have become rare in the United States and Canada as a result of improved prenatal care in the prevention of Rh incompatibility and hyperbilirubinemia. The disorder remains a problem in developing countries.

Functional skills can also be used to classify individuals with CP. The Gross Motor Function Classification System provides a five-level system to classify motor involvement of children with CP on the basis of their functional status and their need for assistive technology and wheeled mobility (Box 35-1). The Gross Motor Function Classification System provides a means of grading age-related developmental skill.[42,43]

Level I includes children with neuromotor impairments whose functional limitations are less than what is typically associated with CP. It also includes children who have traditionally been diagnosed as having "minimal brain dysfunction" or "cerebral palsy of minimal severity." The distinctions between levels I and II therefore are not as pronounced as the distinctions between the other levels, particularly for infants less than 2 years of age.[42,43]

The descriptions of the five levels are broad and not intended to describe all aspects of the function of individual children. The focus is on determining which level best represents the child's present abilities and limitations in motor function. Emphasis is on the child's usual performance in home, school, and community settings (not best performance).[43]

The levels are described on a time line in categories as follows: before second birthday, between second and fourth birthdays, between fourth and sixth birthdays, between sixth and twelfth birthdays, and the expanded version now contains a category for children between their 12th and 18th birthday which is available at http://canchild.ca/en/measures/gmfcs_expanded_revised.asp. Distinctions between adjacent levels are outlined in Box 35-1.

Incidence and Etiologic and Risk Factors

The reported prevalence of CP ranges from 2.05 to 2.45 cases per 1000 births in most developed countries that have been surveyed.[27] Advances in perinatal care have improved the chances for survival of infants of extremely low birth weight and immature gestational age but it appears that the prevalence of Children with CP has increased as well.[26,29,32]

Despite the increased use of fertility drugs, survival of infants in multiple births, and survival of

Table 35-1	Classification of Cerebral Palsy	
	Category	**Description**
Topography	Monoplegia	Only one limb affected
	Diplegia	Involves trunk and lower extremities; upper extremities to a lesser degree
	Hemiplegia	Primarily one total side involved; upper extremity usually more than the lower extremity
	Quadriplegia (tetraplegia)	Involvement of all four limbs, head, and trunk usually lower extremity more than upper extremity, but upper extremity with limitation of function.
Type of tone abnormality	Ataxia	Irregularity of muscular action manifested by dysmetria; may be pure or combined with other forms
	Dyskinesia (dystonic or choreoathetosis)	Presence of involuntary movement; poor control of proximal movement (chorea) alternating with repetitive, involuntary, slow, distal writhing movements (athetosis); or stereotypic sustained, intermittent involuntary muscle contractions resulting in end range posture (dystonic); movements increase with emotional stress and around adolescence
	Hypotonia	Abnormally reduced muscle tone characterized by decreased consistency of the muscle belly or decreased ability of the muscle to generate force as the result of diminished central drive. This is often associated ligamentous laxity.
	Rigidity	Lead-pipe quality to the resistance to passive stretch
	Spasticity	Velocity-dependent resistance to stretch

Box 35-1

GROSS MOTOR FUNCTION CLASSIFICATION SYSTEM, EXPANDED AND REVISED, FOR CEREBRAL PALSY (GMFCS-E&R)

Before 2nd Birthday

LEVEL I: Infants move in and out of sitting and floor sit with both hands free to manipulate objects. Infants crawl on hands and knees, pull to stand and take steps holding on to furniture. Infants walk between 18 months and 2 years of age without the need for any assistive mobility device.

LEVEL II: Infants maintain floor sitting but may need to use their hands for support to maintain balance. Infants creep on their stomach or crawl on hands and knees. Infants may pull to stand and take steps holding on to furniture.

LEVEL III: Infants maintain floor sitting when the low back is supported. Infants roll and creep forward on their stomachs.

LEVEL IV: Infants have head control but trunk support is required for floor sitting. Infants can roll to supine and may roll to prone.

LEVEL V: Physical impairments limit voluntary control of movement. Infants are unable to maintain antigravity head and trunk postures in prone and sitting. Infants require adult assistance to roll.

Between 2nd and 4th Birthdays

LEVEL I: Children floor sit with both hands free to manipulate objects. Movements in and out of floor sitting and standing are performed without adult assistance. Children walk as the preferred method of mobility without the need for any assistive mobility device.

LEVEL II: Children floor sit but may have difficulty with balance when both hands are free to manipulate objects. Movements in and out of sitting are performed without adult assistance. Children pull to stand on a stable surface. Children crawl on hands and knees with a reciprocal pattern, cruise holding onto furniture and walk using an assistive mobility device as preferred methods of mobility.

LEVEL III: Children maintain floor sitting often by "W-sitting" (sitting between flexed and internally rotated hips and knees) and may require adult assistance to assume sitting. Children creep on their stomach or crawl on hands and knees (often without reciprocal leg movements) as their primary methods of self-mobility. Children may pull to stand on a stable surface and cruise short distances. Children may walk short distances indoors using a hand-held mobility device (walker) and adult assistance for steering and turning.

LEVEL IV: Children floor sit when placed, but are unable to maintain alignment and balance without use of their hands for support. Children frequently require adaptive equipment for sitting and standing. Self-mobility for short distances (within a room) is achieved through rolling, creeping on stomach, or crawling on hands and knees without reciprocal leg movement.

LEVEL V: Physical impairments restrict voluntary control of movement and the ability to maintain antigravity head and trunk postures. All areas of motor function are limited. Functional limitations in sitting and standing are not fully compensated for through the use of adaptive equipment and assistive technology. At Level V, children have no means of independent movement and are transported. Some children achieve self-mobility using a powered wheelchair with extensive adaptations.

Between 4th and 6th Birthdays

LEVEL I: Children get into and out of, and sit in, a chair without the need for hand support. Children move from the floor and from chair sitting to standing without the need for objects for support. Children walk indoors and outdoors, and climb stairs. Emerging ability to run and jump.

LEVEL II: Children sit in a chair with both hands free to manipulate objects. Children move from the floor to standing and from chair sitting to standing but often require a stable surface to push or pull up on with their arms. Children walk without the need for a handheld mobility device indoors and for short distances on level surfaces outdoors. Children climb stairs holding onto a railing but are unable to run or jump.

Continued

Box 35-1

GROSS MOTOR FUNCTION CLASSIFICATION SYSTEM, EXPANDED AND REVISED, FOR CEREBRAL PALSY (GMFCS-E&R)—cont'd

LEVEL III: Children sit on a regular chair but may require pelvic or trunk support to maximize hand function. Children move in and out of chair sitting using a stable surface to push on or pull up with their arms. Children walk with a hand-held mobility device on level surfaces and climb stairs with assistance from an adult. Children frequently are transported when traveling for long distances or outdoors on uneven terrain.

LEVEL IV: Children sit on a chair but need adaptive seating for trunk control and to maximize hand function. Children move in and out of chair sitting with assistance from an adult or a stable surface to push or pull up on with their arms. Children may at best walk short distances with a walker and adult supervision but have difficulty turning and maintaining balance on uneven surfaces. Children are transported in the community. Children may achieve self-mobility using a powered wheelchair.

LEVEL V: Physical impairments restrict voluntary control of movement and the ability to maintain antigravity head and trunk postures. All areas of motor function are limited. Functional limitations in sitting and standing are not fully compensated for through the use of adaptive equipment and assistive technology. At Level V, children have no means of independent movement and are transported. Some children achieve self-mobility using a powered wheelchair with extensive adaptations

Between 6th and 12th Birthdays

Level I: Children walk at home, school, outdoors, and in the community. Children are able to walk up and down curbs without physical assistance and stairs without the use of a railing. Children perform gross motor skills such as running and jumping but speed, balance, and coordination are limited. Children may participate in physical activities and sports depending on personal choices and environmental factors.

Level II: Children walk in most settings. Children may experience difficulty walking long distances and balancing on uneven terrain, inclines, in crowded areas, confined spaces or when carrying objects. Children walk up and down stairs holding onto a railing or with physical assistance if there is no railing. Outdoors and in the community, children may walk with physical assistance, a hand-held mobility device, or use wheeled mobility when traveling long distances. Children have at best only minimal ability to perform gross motor skills such as running and jumping. Limitations in performance of gross motor skills may necessitate adaptations to enable participation in physical activities and sports.

Level III: Children walk using a hand-held mobility device in most indoor settings. When seated, children may require a seat belt for pelvic alignment and balance. Sit-to-stand and floor-to-stand transfers require physical assistance of a person or support surface. When traveling long distances, children use some form of wheeled mobility. Children may walk up and down stairs holding onto a railing with supervision or physical assistance. Limitations in walking may necessitate adaptations to enable participation in physical activities and sports including self-propelling a manual wheelchair or powered mobility.

Level IV: Children use methods of mobility that require physical assistance or powered mobility in most settings. Children require adaptive seating for trunk and pelvic control and physical assistance for most transfers. At home, children use floor mobility (roll, creep, or crawl), walk short distances with physical assistance, or use powered mobility. When positioned, children may use a body support walker at home or

school. At school, outdoors, and in the community, children are transported in a manual wheelchair or use powered mobility. Limitations in mobility necessitate adaptations to enable participation in physical activities and sports, including physical assistance and/or powered mobility.

Level V: Children are transported in a manual wheelchair in all settings. Children are limited in their ability to maintain antigravity head and trunk postures and control arm and leg movements. Assistive technology is used to improve head alignment, seating, standing, and and/or mobility but limitations are not fully compensated by equipment. Transfers require complete physical assistance of an adult. At home, children may move short distances on the floor or may be carried by an adult. Children may achieve self-mobility using powered mobility with extensive adaptations for seating and control access. Limitations in mobility necessitate adaptations to enable participation in physical activities and sports including physical assistance and using powered mobility.

Between 12th and 18th Birthdays

Level I: Youth walk at home, school, outdoors, and in the community. Youth are able to walk up and down curbs without physical assistance and stairs without the use of a railing. Youth perform gross motor skills such as running and jumping but speed, balance, and coordination are limited. Youth may participate in physical activities and sports depending on personal choices and environmental factors.

Level II: Youth walk in most settings. Environmental factors (such as uneven terrain, inclines, long distances, time demands, weather, and peer acceptability) and personal preference influence mobility choices. At school or work, youth may walk using a handheld mobility device for safety. Outdoors and in the community, youth may use wheeled mobility when traveling long distances. Youth walk up and down stairs holding a railing or with physical assistance if there is no railing. Limitations in performance of gross motor skills may necessitate adaptations to enable participation in physical activities and sports.

Level III: Youth are capable of walking using a hand-held mobility device. Compared to individuals in other levels, youth in Level III demonstrate more variability in methods of mobility depending on physical ability and environmental and personal factors. When seated, youth may require a seat belt for pelvic alignment and balance. Sit-to-stand and floor-to-stand transfers require physical assistance from a person or support surface. At school, youth may self-propel a manual wheelchair or use powered mobility. Outdoors and in the community, youth are transported in a wheelchair or use powered mobility. Youth may walk up and down stairs holding onto a railing with supervision or physical assistance. Limitations in walking may necessitate adaptations to enable participation in physical activities and sports including self-propelling a manual wheelchair or powered mobility.

Level IV: Youth use wheeled mobility in most settings. Youth require adaptive seating for pelvic and trunk control. Physical assistance from one or two persons is required for transfers. Youth may support weight with their legs to assist with standing transfers. Indoors, youth may walk short distances with physical assistance, use wheeled mobility, or, when positioned, use a body support walker. Youth are physically capable of operating a powered wheelchair. When a powered wheelchair is not feasible or available, youth are transported

GROSS MOTOR FUNCTION CLASSIFICATION SYSTEM, EXPANDED AND REVISED, FOR CEREBRAL PALSY (GMFCS-E&R)—cont'd

in a manual wheelchair. Limitations in mobility necessitate adaptations to enable participation in physical activities and sports, including physical assistance and/or powered mobility.

Level V: Youth are transported in a manual wheelchair in all settings. Youth are limited in their ability to maintain antigravity head and trunk postures and control arm and leg movements. Assistive technology is used to improve head alignment, seating, standing, and mobility but limitations are not fully compensated by equipment. Physical assistance from one or two persons or a mechanical lift is required for transfers. Youth may achieve self-mobility using powered mobility with extensive adaptations for seating and control access. Limitations in mobility necessitate adaptations to enable participation in physical activities and sports including physical assistance and using powered mobility.

Distinctions Between Levels I and II

Compared with children and youth in Level I, children and youth in Level II have limitations walking long distances and balancing; may need a hand-held mobility device when first learning to walk; may use wheeled mobility when traveling long distances outdoors and in the community; require the use of a railing to walk up and down stairs; and are not as capable of running and jumping.

Distinctions Between Levels II and III

Children and youth in Level II are capable of walking without a hand-held mobility device after age 4 (although they may choose to use one at times). Children and youth in Level III need a hand-held mobility device to walk indoors and use wheeled mobility outdoors and in the community.

Distinctions Between Levels III and IV

Children and youth in Level III sit on their own or require at most limited external support to sit, are more independent in standing transfers, and walk with a hand-held mobility device. Children and youth in Level IV function in sitting (usually supported) but self-mobility is limited. Children and youth in Level IV are more likely to be transported in a manual wheelchair or use powered mobility.

Distinctions Between Levels IV and V

Children and youth in Level V have severe limitations in head and trunk control and require extensive assisted technology and physical assistance. Self-mobility is achieved only if the child/youth can learn how to operate a powered wheelchair.

From Palisano R, Rosenbaum, P, and Bartlett D. *The Gross Motor Function Classification System (GMFCS), Expanded and Revised (E &R)* (2007). CanChild Centre for Childhood Disability Research, Institute for Applied Health Sciences, McMaster University, Hamilton, Ontario, Canada. User instructions and more information are available online at http://motorgrowth.canchild.ca/en/GMFCS/resources/GMFCS-ER.pdf. Used with permission.

Table 35-2   Risk Factors for Cerebral Palsy

Prenatal	Perinatal	Postnatal
Maternal infection	Prematurity	Neonatal infection (meningitis, encephalitis)
• Rubella	Obstetric complications	Environmental toxins
• Cytomegalovirus	• Mechanical birth trauma	Trauma
• Herpes simplex	• Breech delivery	Kernicterus
• Toxoplasmosis	• Forceps delivery	Brain tumor
Maternal diabetes	• Twin or multiple births	Anoxia (e.g., near-drowning, assault)
Rh incompatibility	Prolapsed umbilical cord or umbilical	Cerebrovascular accident
Toxemia (undiagnosed or untreated)	cord flow abnormalities	Neonatal hypoglycemia
Maternal malnutrition	Low birth weight (<1750 g)	Acidosis
Maternal thyroid disorders	Small for gestational age (SGA)	
Maternal seizures	Low Apgar scores (≤4 at 5 min)	
Maternal radiation	Placenta previa (intrauterine bleeding)	
Abnormal placental attachment	Abruptio placentae	
Congenital anomalies of the brain		
Coagulation abnormalities		
Antiphospholipid antibodies		

---

extremely-low-birth-weight infants, the incidence (number of cases occurring over a certain period) of neurodisabilities, including CP, has remained constant among surviving premature infants.[35,44] In fact, incidence may have begun to show some recent decline,[28] although the prevalence (overall number of cases present at a specified time) has increased because of the improved survival rates.

The cause of CP may be unknown and is often multifactorial. In children of normal birth weight who have disabilities associated with CP, 80% of the disabilities are a result of factors occurring before birth and 10% to 28%

are attributed to factors occurring around the birth in term or near-term infants.[19]

In children of low birth weight who develop disabilities associated with CP (approximately 0.7 per 1000 live births), often uncertainty remains as to when the brain damage occurred (i.e., during fetal development or during or after birth). Any prenatal, perinatal, or postnatal condition that results in damage to the motor control systems of the brain can cause CP (Table 35-2). CP is the second most common neurologic impairment in childhood (mental retardation is the first).[69]

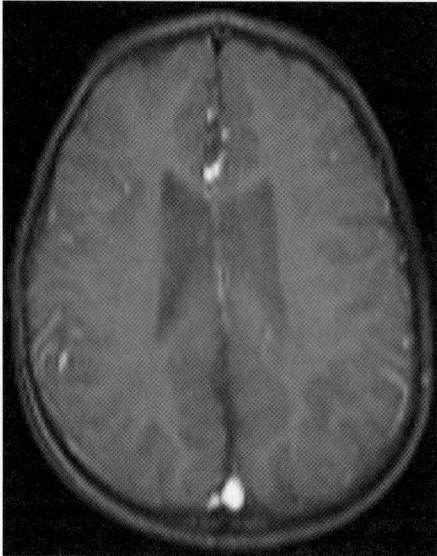

Figure 35-1

Magnetic resonance image of an interventricular hemorrhage with expansion of the lateral ventricles. This child was born at 26 weeks' gestation and diagnosed with diplegic cerebral palsy. (Courtesy Allan Glanzman, Children's Seashore House of the Children's Hospital of Philadelphia, PA.)

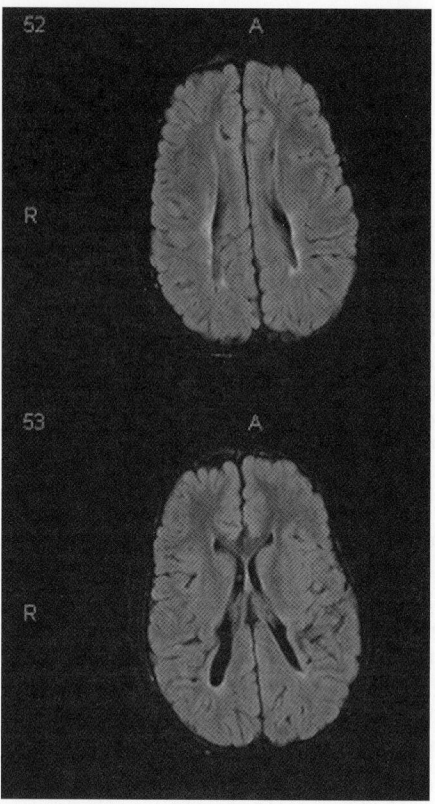

Figure 35-2

Magnetic resonance image of a periventricular leukomalacia with cystic formation extending into the parenchyma in a child with quadriplegic cerebral palsy. Top and bottom are serial sections in the same brain. In this child, the ventricles are a normal size. The abnormal finding is in the bottom slice where the cystic changes (black) extend into the brain tissue. (Courtesy Allan Glanzman, Children's Seashore House of the Children's Hospital of Philadelphia, PA.)

Pathogenesis

No consistent or uniform pathology is associated with CP. Several types of neuropathic lesions have been identified on the basis of autopsy: (1) hemorrhage below the lining of the ventricles (subependymal or interventricular), (2) hypoxia causing encephalopathy, and (3) malformations of the central nervous system (CNS).[76]

Until recently, interventricular hemorrhage was the most common form of brain injury in the premature infant (Fig. 35-1). In recent years, the incidence of interventricular hemorrhage has declined from an incidence of 49% in very-low-birth-weight infants to 20% in the same population.[54] As a result, periventricular white matter injury has become the more common cause of long-lasting brain injury in this population.

Periventricular lesions can be either cystic, as in periventricular leukomalacia (PVL), or more diffuse and result in abnormal myelination (Fig. 35-2). Diffuse periventricular myelination abnormalities can be found in up to 65% of premature infants when they reach full term (9 months from conception). The incidence of PVL has declined somewhat, but when the mildest forms of PVL are included it can be seen in more than 20% of preterm infants. During the preterm period, infants are at heightened risk for ischemia in the periventricular areas. The heightened risk is the result of passive-pressure circulation in the premature infant. The autoregulation of CNS blood flow normally present in full-term infants is absent, and the CNS blood pressure is more dependent on peripheral pressure. The premature infant between 23 and 32 weeks' gestation is at the highest risk of periventricular injury. As the periventricular white matter begins to myelinate and the vasculature matures, the risk of hypoxic injury declines.[18]

Hypoxic injury can also occur in the full-term infant; however, this represents only a small portion of infants with CP. It often occurs in the presence of bradycardia, intrauterine growth retardation, and preeclampsia and may also be facilitated by the presence of infection.[5]

Hypoxic-ischemic injury can be the result of three possible underlying causes: (1) decreased perfusion resulting from systemic hypotension and poor autoregulation of cerebral blood flow; (2) emboli, which block distal perfusion, and thrombosis; or (3) clot formation from polycythemia or a hypercoagulable state.[53] Hypoxic-ischemic injury is known to disrupt the normal metabolic processes, starving the cells of oxygen because of poor perfusion and poor oxygen delivery to the cells, resulting in a reliance on the cells' limited ability to maintain homeostasis through anaerobic energy metabolism.

Eventually, insufficient energy is all that is available for powering the sodium-potassium pump in the cell membrane, and the ionic gradients across the cell membranes break down. The resulting influx of calcium begins a cascade that, along with the osmotic pressure gradient that has developed, ends in cell death. The second phase of cell damage occurs with reperfusion when vasodilation allows increased blood flow and oxygen free radicals (see Fig. 6-3) are released that trigger programmed cell death or apoptosis. The severity and topography of the damage depends on the gestational age at the time of the injury and the degree of injury sustained.[7,18]

The primary hypoxic-ischemic lesion found in the premature infant is PVL (bilateral necrosis of the white matter of the brain adjacent to the lateral ventricles), present in 42% of term and 87% of preterm infants with CP.[34,74] A portion of premature infants demonstrate impaired autoregulation of cerebral circulation and also demonstrate a passive-pressure cerebral circulation (i.e., blood pressure in the CNS is not able to remain constant with fluctuations in the peripheral circulation, placing them at risk of cerebral injury when fluctuations in peripheral pressure occur). The periventricular arterial border zones are at particular risk for hypoxic-ischemic injury in these children.[74]

Focal injury to the brain can also result from hemorrhage and ischemia, with the resulting collection of blood creating injury from direct mechanical pressure on the tissue and secondary ischemia. In the premature infant, hemorrhage of the germinal matrix (the cells from which the nervous system arises; in the adult, these cells, called ependymal cells, lie adjacent to the ventricular system) into the lateral ventricle (see Fig. 35-1) is a common cause of CP and can result in venous infarction of the periventricular area with a resulting cystic lesion in that portion of the brain.[74]

Hypoxic-ischemic injury in the mature neonate most commonly results from either selective neuronal cell damage or parasagittal brain damage. These hypoxic-ischemic insults affect the border zones of the major cerebral arteries, either in the cerebral cortex, cerebellum, or the parietal or occipital regions. Focal or multifocal brain damage can result from either arterial embolism or venous thrombosis and is more common in the more mature neonate. The incidence of this mechanism of injury increases with gestational age greater than 28 weeks and typically presents as a unilateral injury.[7]

Children who develop CP fail to demonstrate normal CNS maturation after a CNS injury. Persistence of immature layers of the primary motor cortex is often present, and many of the other layers demonstrate abnormalities, particularly those with projections to the pyramidal tract.[2]

Clinical Manifestations

Although the neurologic manifestations of CP are nonprogressive, the motor impairments change with growth and maturation and may become more apparent as the affected child grows. Clinical manifestations of motor impairments associated with CP may include alterations of muscle tone, delayed postural reactions, persistence of primitive reflexes (Fig. 35-3), delayed motor development, and abnormal motor performance (e.g., delay in movement onset, poor timing of force generation, poor force production, inability to maintain antigravity postural control, decreased speed of movement, and increased cocontraction).[15]

Persistence of primitive reflexes and impaired motor function can affect the head, neck, trunk, and extremities and impair sucking and swallowing, as well as delayed GI motility and gastroesophageal reflux, resulting in feeding difficulties (Fig. 35-4).[61]

Associated disabilities may include cognitive impairments (e.g., mental retardation, learning disabilities,

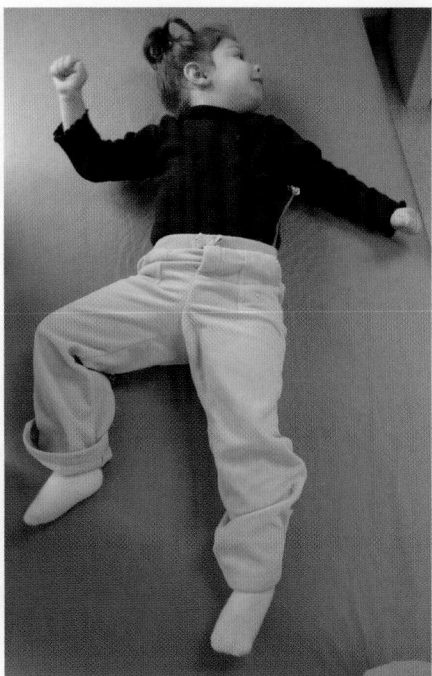

Figure 35-3

Asymmetric tonic neck reflex. Four-year-old with quadriplegic cerebral palsy demonstrating the asymmetric tonic neck reflex. This primitive reflex contributes to an obligatory change in body posture resulting from a change in head position. With head turning to one side, the arm and leg on the same side extend while the arm and leg on the opposite side flex. This posture resembles a fencing position and prevents the child from bringing the left hand to her mouth for exploration and self-feeding. (*Courtesy Allan Glanzman, Children's Seashore House of the Children's Hospital of Philadelphia, PA.*)

seizure disorders); sensory impairments (in vision, hearing); feeding impairments including oral motor dysfunction, constipation or bowel and bladder incontinence with their associated problems (e.g., poor hygiene, skin problems), and seizure disorders.[37,49] In individuals with spastic hemiplegic, spastic quadriplegic, or diplegic CP, these comorbidities occur relatively less frequently. The rate of occurrence is significantly greater for individuals with dyskinetic, ataxic, or hypotonic CP.[60]

Microcephalus and hydrocephalus are also common findings, with the latter being the result of increased intracranial pressure. Behavioral signs of increased intracranial pressure accompanying hydrocephalus may include extreme irritability resulting from headache and vomiting. Eventually delays in reaching developmental milestones are observed, resulting from pressure-induced damage as discussed earlier.[48]

Musculoskeletal problems of altered muscle tone, muscle weakness, and joint restrictions are common and can result in functional and orthopedic impairments. For example, the abnormal pull of the spastic iliopsoas and adductor muscles are the initiating deforming force in hip dislocations (Fig. 35-5).[39]

When spasticity and contracture of the iliopsoas occur, the medial joint capsule is compressed and the femoral head is pushed laterally. As lateral drift of the femoral head occurs, the iliopsoas insertion on the lesser trochanter

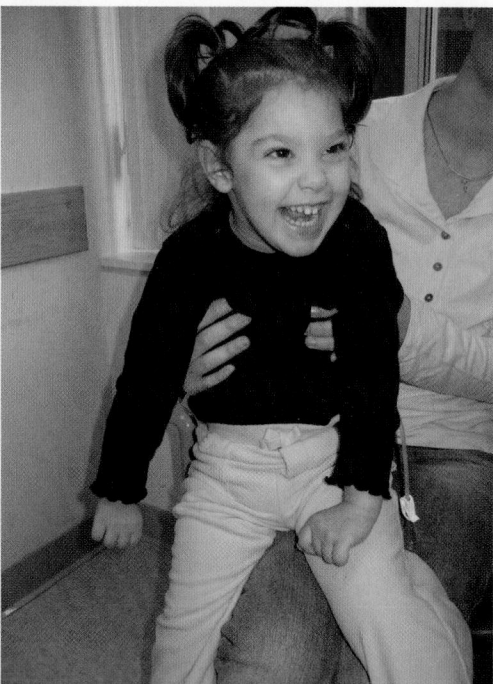

Figure 35-4

Symmetric tonic neck reflex. The same 4-year-old with quadriplegic cerebral palsy as in Figure 35-3 demonstrates another primitive reflex known as the symmetric tonic neck reflex (STNR). When the head and neck are extended, the arms extend; flexion usually predominates in the lower extremities. Flexion of the head and neck causes flexion in the upper extremities and extension in the lower extremities (not shown). In the normal infant the asymmetric tonic neck reflex and STNR are typically integrated by 6 to 8 months. Integration of the STNR allows voluntary flexion of both arms and legs needed to sit comfortably. Prior to 6 to 8 months, these reflexes can be observed in developing infants but when present are not obligatory (i.e., the person can voluntarily move out of the position). (Courtesy Allan Glanzman, Children's Seashore House of the Children's Hospital of Philadelphia, PA.)

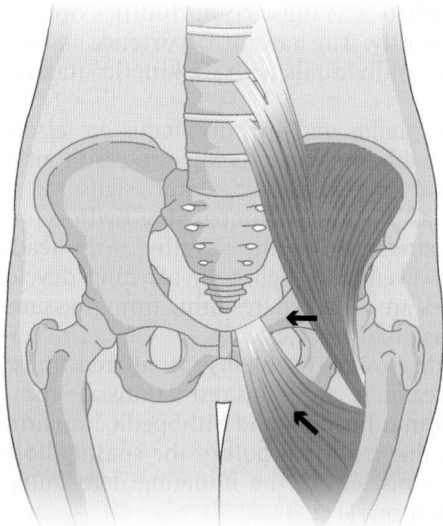

Figure 35-5

Spastic iliopsoas and adductor muscles are the initiating deforming force in acquired spastic hip dislocation.

becomes the center of rotation. Acetabular development ceases when the femoral head is completely displaced laterally, and further hip flexion pushes the head posteriorly to complete the dislocation (Fig. 35-6).[9]

Abnormalities of the muscle are also associated with CP with a decrease in the number of sarcomeres[64] per muscle fiber noted. Muscles also demonstrate an increased variation in fiber size and type[56] with both hypertrophy and atrophy present, possibly representing an ongoing dynamic process. Increases in fat and fibrous tissue and a decrease in blood flow have been identified.[55] In this process, bone grows faster than muscle, resulting in a disadvantageous length-tension relationship of the muscle and an increased risk of subsequent contracture.[63] A characteristic decrease in muscle mass also results in decreased muscle power and endurance.

Changes in muscle tone affect a person's ability to control movement, resulting in poor selective control of muscles, poor regulation of activity and muscle groups, decreased ability to learn unique movements, inappropriate sequencing of movements, and delayed anticipatory postural response. Most often, the timing and sequence of muscle activity are also affected.

A significant number of children with a diagnosis of spastic CP present with low muscle tone early in the first year of life and in the first year develop spasticity. They often have insufficient flexor skills to position themselves against gravity for activities such as lifting the head, reaching, and kicking. The child will attempt to develop alternative strategies to complete the tasks. If control is not

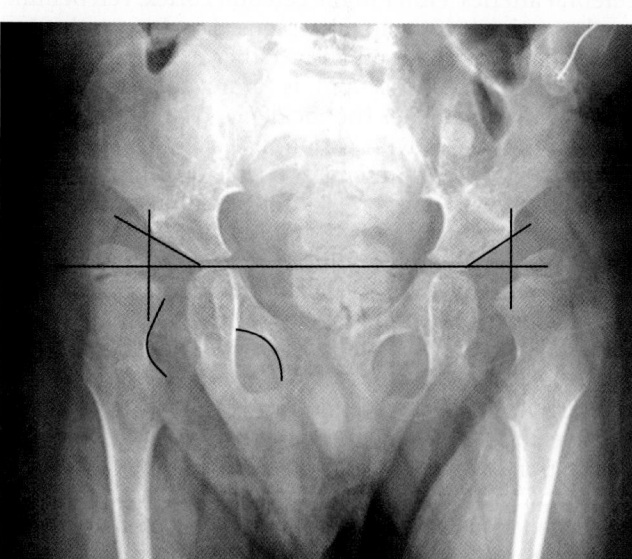

Figure 35-6

Anteroposterior radiograph of a young child with spastic quadriplegia and subsequent hip dysplasia with subluxation on the left. Note that a line drawn vertically down from the outermost edge of the acetabulum would bisect the head of the femur. Failure of the acetabulum to deepen with weight bearing resulting in hip dysplasia and subluxation occur as a result of the inability to weight bear and abnormal muscular forces pulling on the bone. The standard measurement for hip dislocation is a migration percentage. This is done by drawing Hilgenreiner's line, which provides a horizontal reference to the pelvis and then drawing Perkin's line perpendicular to Hilgenreiner's line from the outermost edge of the acetabulum. (Courtesy Allan Glanzman, Children's Seashore House of the Children's Hospital of Philadelphia, PA.)

available, these strategies result in postures that allow completion of a particular sequence but do not allow for subsequent movement and transitions.

Examples of such situations are a wide-based sitting posture that allows the child to maintain sitting but decreases the ability to turn and rotate in and out of the position. Pulling to stand with increased reliance on the arms to assist the lower extremities is another example of an alternative strategy used by children with CP.

Each type of CP is characterized by its own clinical picture based on the presence and extent of these clinical manifestations. The progression of motor development associated with each type of CP is beyond the scope of this book, but the reader should be familiar with the natural history of each as this will aid in the development of treatment goals. The reader is referred to other texts for a more detailed discussion.[17,65]

MEDICAL MANAGEMENT

DIAGNOSIS. Observation, history, and a neurologic examination will provide the physician with the information necessary to make an accurate and early diagnosis. The diagnostic studies performed depend on clinical findings. For example, electroencephalography is indicated when seizures are present or suspected; hip radiographic films are indicated to rule out hip dislocations and should be followed over time, particularly in the presence of spasticity.

Blood or urine screening tests may be used to rule out certain metabolic diseases, and a thorough workup should be undertaken if a history reveals a progressive course or positive family history. A CT or MRI scan can provide information on the location of the insult.

TREATMENT. Comprehensive and cooperative planning with an interdisciplinary team that may include physicians, therapists, nurses, special educators, psychologists, social workers, nutritionists, and family members is essential.

Some of the most common medical management strategies include pharmacologic intervention, neurosurgical intervention, and orthopedic surgery. Skeletal muscle relaxants (e.g., baclofen, diazepam, dantrolene, tizanidine, and botulinum toxin) can be used to assist in controlling increased spasticity and can be administered orally (baclofen, dantrolene, tizanidine, and diazepam), intrathecally (baclofen), or directly to muscles through injection at the motor point (botulinum toxin).[46]

Intrathecal administration of baclofen (through the sheath of the spinal cord into the subarachnoid space) uses an implantable intrathecal infusion pump to deliver medication to the spinal cord without the associated CNS sedation found with oral administration. After the pump is implanted, the dosage can be titrated to the optimal level for each person. Any attempts to control excess muscle tone (pharmaceutically or otherwise) should always be paired with functional goals to take advantage of the modulated tone.[1,3]

Motor point blocks can also be used to control spasticity and can be paired with serial casting to increase muscle length. Muscles such as the gastrocnemius, hip adductors, or hamstrings are injected with a botulinum toxin (or phenol) to create a temporary denervation and to decrease tone and increase movement.[12,33,67]

The type A botulinum toxin (Botox) is injected directly into the muscle at the motor point and is used to blockade the neuromuscular junction by acting presynaptically to reduce the release of acetylcholine, resulting in partial denervation of the muscle. Muscle weakness and decrease in muscle spasm occur in 3 to 7 days and gradually reappear in 4 to 6 months.

Successful use of botulinum toxin type A in the upper extremity has been reported,[24,25,62] as has its use to control drooling in children with CP. The effects of these injections will wear off anywhere from several weeks to several months later similar to the effect seen in lower extremity injections.[23,51]

Selective dorsal rhizotomy (surgically identifying the posterior roots of the spinal cord and selectively resecting some of them) to reduce spasticity has been used over the past decade. This is usually performed at the L2–L5 spinal levels for clients with spastic diplegia who are independent or near independent ambulators but who have spasticity that results in abnormalities of posture and gait.[73] A rhizotomy may also be used effectively for clients with severe positioning difficulties such as severe quadriplegia; however, in this population the relative benefit of rhizotomy versus intrathecal baclofen should be considered. In the population of children with quadriplegic CP, rhizotomy may reduce muscle tone enough to facilitate personal hygiene and provide improved sitting and comfort.[72]

Orthopedic surgery may include muscle lengthening or releases (e.g., adductors, iliopsoas, hamstrings) to address contracture, muscle transfers (e.g., rectus femoris or tibialis posterior) to increase control or decrease excessive muscle pull, or bone procedures (e.g., femoral derotational osteotomy [see Fig. 23-12, B]; acetabular augmentation; triple arthrodesis; spinal fusions) to correct bony deformity, hip dislocation, or scoliosis or patellar tendon advancement.[38]

Orthotic intervention may be used to maintain flexibility, support or stabilize a joint, or improve alignment. The ultimate goal is to delay the development of fixed contractures and improve function, with bracing based on both the impairment of gait deviation noted along with the anticipated gait and impairment-based natural history of the disease taken into account.

For children with a gait marked by toe walking, an articulating molded ankle-foot orthosis will aid in maintaining the flexibility of the gastrocsoleus complex and a plantar grade gait pattern, for children with lever arm dysfunction and a crouched pattern ground reaction force molded ankle-foot orthoses will restrain tibial progression through the stance phase of gait and improve the child's erect posture, and for children with spasticity of the peroneal muscles and pronation, supramalleolar orthoses (SMOs) can maintain the integrity of the midfoot and help avoid an incompetent forefoot and rocker bottom posture.

PROGNOSIS. Common causes of death in this population are related to infection, aspiration, respiratory compromise, and heart disease.[68]

Table 35-3	Predictors of Ambulation for Cerebral Palsy	
Predictors	**Ambulation Potential**	
By Diagnosis		
Monoplegia	100%	
Hemiplegia	100%*	
Ataxia	100%	
Diplegia	60%*-90%	
Spastic quadriplegia	0%-70%	
By Motor Function		
Sits independently by age 2	Good†	
Sits independently by age 3-4	50% community ambulation	
Presence of primitive reflexes beyond age 2	Poor	
Absence of postural reactions beyond age 2	Poor	
Independently crawled symmetrically or reciprocally by age 2.5	Good†	

*From Pallas Alonso CR, de La Cruz Bértolo J, Medina López MC, et al: Cerebral palsy and age of sitting and walking in very low birth weight infants. *An Esp Pediatr* 53:48-52, 2000.
†From da Paz Jr AC, Burnett SM, Braga LW: Walking prognosis in cerebral palsy: a 22-year retrospective analysis. *Dev Med Child Neurol* 36:130-134, 1994.

Most children with mild to moderate CP have a normal life span, but there is some increased mortality in the early years (before age 4) and then again with advancing age (50 and older). In those individuals with quadriplegic CP, the excess death rate declines during childhood and adulthood only to climb again after the age of 50, as is noted in the more mildly involved population.[38] In one trial, mortality was highest under 15 years and then approached twice the general population rate by 35 years of age with the nonambulatory population being at highest risk of death.

Ambulation potential may be predicted based on achievement of motor milestones (Table 35-3). Independent sitting before age 2 years is a positive indicator of future ambulation.[75] If it is going to occur, ambulation usually takes place by 8 years of age.[50]

SPECIAL IMPLICATIONS FOR THE THERAPIST 35-1

Cerebral Palsy

In addition to the treatment options discussed in the previous section, physical therapists are exploring a more focused and proactive approach of activity-based intervention through intense activity training protocols, lifestyle modifications, and mobility-enhancing devices. Increased motor activity may to lead to better physical and mental health and improve various aspects of cognitive performance.[20]

Activity-based programs for individuals with CP focus on maximizing physical function while preventing secondary musculoskeletal impairments; foster cognitive, social, and emotional development; and potentially promote or enhance neural recovery.[15a]

With new research information about the role of neural recovery in damaged nervous systems, therapists can expect to see continued changes in philosophy and intervention approaches with this unique population. Focus will continue with early intervention but include other phases through the life span. As attention is directed toward establishing, enhancing, and maintaining neural pathways, we may see changes in how CP is approached. For a more detailed discussion of traditional and emerging physical therapist practices for CP, the reader is referred to the study by Damiano.[20]

Family-Centered Care

When designing a therapy program for a child with CP, the therapist should take a broad view of the child's needs and consider the interactive effects that the child's family environment has on the goals that have been developed. To provide family-centered care, the therapist must do the following[70]:
- *Spend enough time with the family*
- *Listen carefully to the parents*
- *Make the parents feel like partners in the child's care*
- *Be sensitive to the family's values and customs*
- *Provide the specific information that the parents need*

The strengths and weaknesses of each family need to be assessed and considered when designing a given child's program, and the therapist needs to consider what the impact of carrying out the physical therapy and multidisciplinary team program will be on the family and, as a result, on the child.

If the cost (emotional, social, financial) is too great, the family may choose to abandon the intervention. As a result, the child may lose ground in terms of altered musculoskeletal alignment and decreased function, and the family must bear the emotional impact.

If the therapist is able to match the program with the family's cultural expectations, ability to participate, and emotional and financial resources, then a partnership with the family can develop that will most benefit the child in the long run. Expecting from family members only what they can succeed at and providing support and education where it is needed to help the family grow and care for the child with special needs will create the best therapeutic environment to allow the child to thrive.

There is often a fine line between balancing the natural history of the condition with the family's commitment and understanding in maximizing the child's quality of life. In addition, families make choices in terms of providing for the child with CP. Often these choices must take into consideration other family members, expectations of themselves, expectations of the child, and, as mentioned, cultural and ethnic beliefs that may or may not match up with the health care professional's defined goals and plans for intervention.

Early Intervention

A general review of intervention studies shows that children benefit from early intervention compared with those children not involved in specific programmed activities. Programming focused on cognitive outcomes has relatively stronger support[5] than programming aimed at solely motor outcomes.[31] The potential for improvement is better for children less than 9 months old but no greater than 2 years of age at a minimum frequency of intervention of two times per week.[8]

Early and accurate identification of CP provides the most likely opportunity for facilitation of optimal motor development.[37] Many motor milestone checklists are available from which a comparison with the normal can be made.[23] In fact, the gross motor function of children with CP and outcomes of intervention have often been evaluated using measures on children without motor impairment.

A more meaningful approach would be to make management decisions and evaluate intervention outcomes based on expectations for children with CP of the same age and gross motor function.[42] This type of evaluation can be made by using assessment tools specifically designed to evaluate the child with CP (e.g., Gross Motor Function Assessment[57]; Gross Motor Function Classification System[42,43]). An assessment of management practices with guidelines for the management of clients with CP is available,[16] as is a model for the acquisition of basic motor abilities and intervention implications.[6]

A significant number of children with a diagnosis of spastic CP present with low muscle tone early in the first year of life and later develop spasticity. They often have insufficient tone to sustain anti-gravity position for activities such as lifting the head, reaching, or kicking. The child will attempt to develop alternative strategies to complete the tasks. If control is not available, these strategies result in postures that allow completion of a particular sequence but do not allow for the development of the proximal strength needed for subsequent movement and transitions.

Examples of such situations are a wide-based sitting posture that allows the child to maintain sitting but decreases the ability to turn and rotate in and out of the position. Pulling to stand with the arms only (without using the lower extremities) is another example of an alternative strategy used by children with CP. If practiced and repeated over time, these abnormal movements become habitual and are difficult to change.

Postoperative Concerns

After orthopedic surgery, the therapist can assist in reducing muscle spasms that increase postoperative pain by moving and turning the child carefully and slowly; however, adequate postoperative pain management should include medication (e.g., codeine and diazepam [Valium]) prescribed by the surgeon.

In the case of postoperative casting, the therapist can instruct the family to wash and dry the skin at the edge of the cast frequently, inspecting often for signs of skin breakdown. Repositioning and ventilation under the cast with a cool-air blow dryer can also assist in preventing skin breakdown. A flashlight can be used daily to inspect beneath the cast.

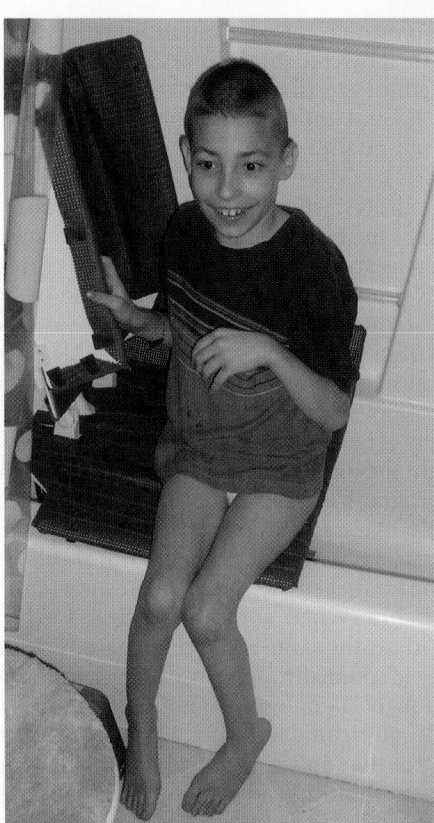

Figure 35-7

Tub lift. A battery-powered tub lift has been very successful with this child, who has spastic quadriplegic cerebral palsy. With help, he transfers from the toilet next to the tub to the tub seat. With assistance, he swings his legs into the tub, and then can independently operate the unit to lower (and later elevate) himself. (Courtesy Tamara Kittelson-Aldred, Access Therapy Services, Missoula, MT. Used with permission.)

Surgical procedures (orthopedic or neurosurgical) may expose areas of underlying muscle weakness and instability. It is critical that an intensive therapy intervention program begin after surgery to assist with strengthening and improving functional performance.

Assistive Technology

Properly prescribed assistive technology is vital in allowing the child with CP the least restrictive access to both the physical and social environment and is a critical part of the overall management of the child with CP. Assistive technology includes any device used to increase, maintain, or improve the functional ability of a person with a disability (Fig. 35-7).

This equipment can be either low tech (standers, positioning equipment, communication boards, or wheelchairs) or high tech (switch toys, power wheelchairs, or computer-based communication systems), as long as it is provided with a functional goal (Fig. 35-8).

Quality of life should be a focus in the management of all clients seeking health care services. Mobility impairment limits can negatively affect overall development, including social, cognitive, emotional, and physical development. A balanced approach to providing assistive technology as a compensation for functional limitations while focusing therapy on the impairment-based limitations that are affecting function, powered mobility is one example of assistive technology that can increase voluntary activity, function, and independence and has contributed to improved quality of life for many individuals with CP (Fig. 35-9).

For children who are dependent for mobility, power mobility can be an option and can be successful in children as young as 2 years of age with corresponding cognitive skills.[13,14,66] These systems can be controlled with a standard joystick or adapted for control with a variety of switch systems and are available both as medical equipment and as adapted play equipment.[30,47]

These power wheelchair systems allow control with a switch array or by proportional control or control through the use of a single switch through a scanning program (Fig. 35-10). Access mode needs to be carefully assessed as does switch or joystick location, hand use is obviously preferable but if this is not possible head placement is often a successful location for switches. When computer access is educationally appropriate, the same wheelchair-based control system can be adapted through an infrared link and mouse emulator to operate the computer. The mouse emulator is an electronic link that allows use of the joystick to control the mouse, usually by infrared beam.

Use of mobility and speech-generating (communication) devices is encouraged with children at all levels of motor disability, including those with severe involvement as is appropriate based on cognitive level. Differences in clinical practice and debate continue over providing an external means of mobility in favor of promoting more voluntary activity. More definitive research guidance is needed in these areas.

Proper positioning is critical to the child with CP, both from a functional perspective and to help prevent the soft tissue limitations that can develop over time. Appropriate positioning has been shown to encourage

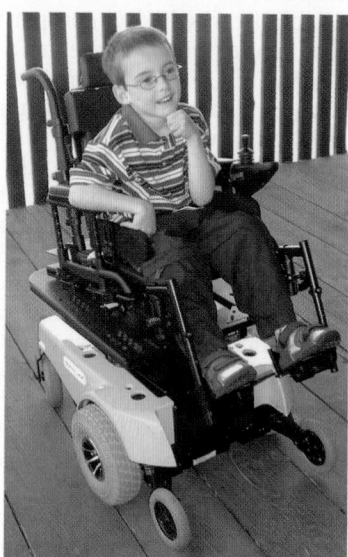

Figure 35-9

New power wheelchair. This 4-year-old child with cerebral palsy receives a new power wheelchair with a seat elevator to enable him to reach age-appropriate items on countertops and tabletops. Trunk supports and footplates help with alignment. The joystick on the left allows him to navigate independently. (Courtesy Tamara Kittelson-Aldred, Access Therapy Services, Missoula, MT. Used with permission.)

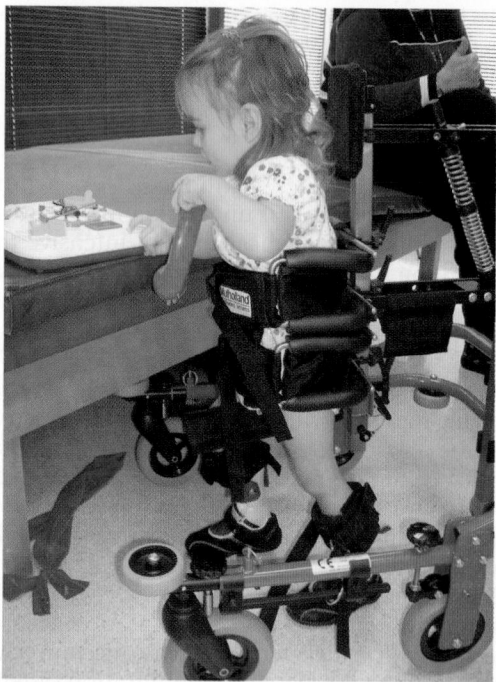

Figure 35-8

Mulholland Walkabout. This 3-year-old girl with spastic quadriplegia can propel this wheeled upright walker through space to explore her environment and play where she wants to. Although she may not become a functional ambulator, the use of this equipment is developmentally appropriate. She could be a candidate for independent wheelchair mobility, but her parents have deferred this decision for now. (Courtesy Tamara Kittelson-Aldred, Access Therapy Services, Missoula, MT. Used with permission.)

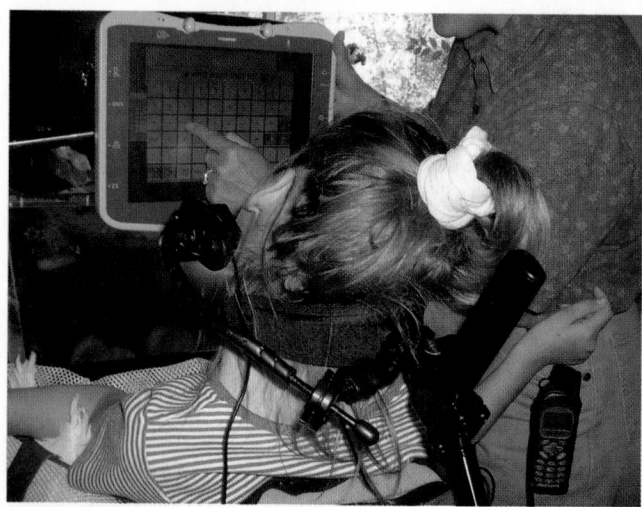

Figure 35-10

This young lady with spastic quadriplegic cerebral palsy uses a DynaVox speech-generating device with a Tash Microlite switch on the left. By moving her head, she is able to hit the switch with her cheek to stop the electronic scan where she wants it to create a message. Stealth neck rest provides suboccipital head support. (Courtesy Tamara Kittelson-Aldred, Access Therapy Services, Missoula, MT. Used with permission.)

smoother and faster reach, decrease extensor tone, increase vital capacity, and improve performance on cognitive testing.[40]

In addition to proper wheelchair position, time out of the chair to counteract the flexed posture of the body is necessary. A standing program can be initiated between 12 and 18 months of age in the child who is not pulling to stand independently to maintain flexibility and provide the normal weight-bearing forces across the hip joint.

Standing helps orient children to the upright position, assists with visual perception, and can aid in digestion and GI motility (Fig. 35-11). Standing can also be used for prolonged muscle stretching, especially in the older or larger child.

Positioning for feeding for the child with CP is often critical for his or her ultimate success and safety at this task. The child's head and neck posture is an important factor in the child's ability to protect their airway during the swallowing. Pelvic lumbar spinal postures contribute to intraabdominal volume and pressure, which can play a role in the development of gastroesophageal reflux. Inclination with respect to gravity is an important consideration when the speed of bolus progression in the mouth is considered and the child's ability to control its progression during swallowing is evaluated. A team approach using the skills of the physical and occupational therapist in conjunction with those of the speech therapist is essential in designing a program to optimize the child's oral motor skills (Fig. 35-12).

For children with expressive communication deficits, sign language, communication boards, and a variety of high-tech communication systems with voice synthesizers are available to augment spoken communication. These can also be linked with wheelchair-based control systems for the child using a power wheelchair.

When evaluating a person for assistive technology, consideration should be given both to the individual's unique abilities and challenges and to the environment in which the equipment will be used. The products should provide the person the greatest degree of functional independence in all the environmental situations encountered. The barriers in each environment may vary, and thus the solutions by necessity may be different in different environments.

Manual Passive Range-of-Motion Exercise

Splinting or positioning that offers a low-load prolonged stretch that is used throughout the day (or night if tolerated) is recommended for children with CP at risk for contracture. Splints such as lower extremity ankle-foot orthoses (AFOs) to maintain ankle ROM or supported standing to control lower extremity flexion contractures and assist with weight bearing across the hip may be implemented. Manual passive ROM exercise is not without its applications and should be applied gently and to the person's tolerance. It is best combined with a well-thought-out positioning and splinting program.

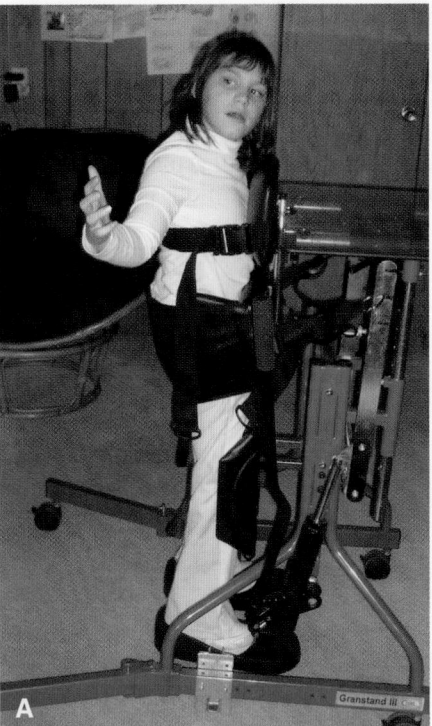

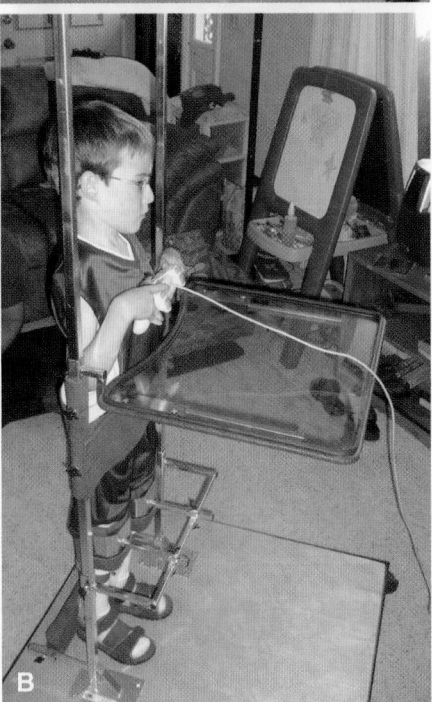

Figure 35-11

Standing frame. Many different types and styles of standers are available with a variety of adaptive features. **A,** Young girl with spastic hemiplegia from a birth injury/infection drives her power chair up to the stander. With assistance, she is able to get a seat sling under her buttocks to lift her up to standing. The sling is significant because it allows the parent to avoid lifting her into the stander. Shoe holders guide the placement of her feet. **B,** This standing frame offers an additional fun feature: the ability to operate a PlayStation. (Courtesy Tamara Kittelson-Aldred, Access Therapy Services, Missoula, MT. Used with permission.)

Other interventions used by therapists to improve ROM and facilitate motor development or improve function include relaxation techniques such as neutral warmth or pressure to acupressure points; serial or tone casts (often in conjunction with botulinum toxin A injections); therapy ball activities; aquatic programs; and manual therapy techniques.[26,45,77]

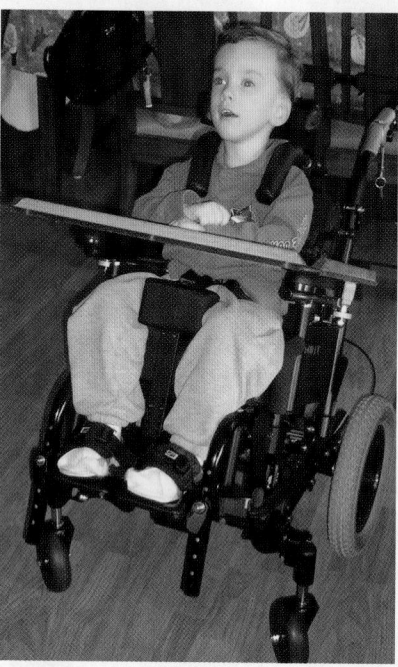

Figure 35-12

Young boy with schizencephaly and cerebral palsy with severe involvement has a planar seating system with postural components. A tilt-in-space feature and deep ischial ledge formed in the seat keep his pelvis aligned and hips back. Hip flexion is combined with the medial thigh support between his legs to keep his knees apart and allow him to relax. Shoulder pad retractors are a feature added when it was discovered that downward pressure and anterior support at the shoulders improved head control for this child. (Courtesy Tamara Kittelson-Aldred, Access Therapy Services, Missoula, MT. Used with permission.)

Orthoses

AFOs are probably the most commonly used orthoses for children with CP. A rigid polypropylene AFO is used to provide medial-lateral stability to the foot and ankle while at the same time assisting with foot clearance during gait. The AFO can be set at +3 degrees of dorsiflexion to facilitate the increased ankle dorsiflexion necessary for the swing phase of gait or to decrease genu recurvatum (hyperextension at the knee) through ground reaction forces.

Hinged AFOs may be recommended once a child is moving in the upright position, especially when the child is beginning to walk, squat, or move up and down stairs, both to allow active ankle motion and to allow normal tibial progression during the stance phase of gait. A more flexible plastic such as copolymer or a thinner polypropylene may be used in the lighter child to provide more dynamic use of the foot musculature. In this case, the term *dynamic ankle-foot orthosis* is used.

In some cases, dorsiflexion assist hinges may be used, either with a plantar flexion stop or in the more mild cases with free plantar flexion. Care must be taken to choose the correct degree of hinge strength (or an adjustable hinge) so as not to create a crouched posture.

An SMO provides medial-lateral stability for the foot and ankle while allowing free plantar flexion and dorsiflexion. It is always helpful to have whatever plantar flexion is available, since this motion helps decelerate the limb during middle and late stances and facilitates the initial progression of the limb during late stance and early swing.

The SMO can be used when decreased active ankle dorsiflexion and excessive genu recurvatum are not problems. Extending the SMO proximally to the malleoli provides important support, whereas support distal to the malleoli usually shifts the deformity in a proximal direction. General guidelines and recommendations for foot and ankle splinting can be found in Table 35-4 (Fig. 35-13).

Table 35-4	General Foot and Ankle Splinting Guidelines	
Splints	**Status**	**Application**
Adjustable dynamic response hinged AFO	Clients with some but limited, functional mobility who achieve foot flat in stance and demonstrate plantarflexion in swing	Independent standing and ambulation. Allows for both tibial progression in standing and eccentric plantarflexion loading on heel strike.
Solid AFO neutral to +3 degrees DF	Nonambulators	1. Less than 3 degrees of DF
		2. For use in stander
AFO with 90 degrees plantar flexion stop and free DF (hinged AFO)		3. Need for medial-lateral stability
		4. Nighttime/positional stretching
	Clients with some, but limited, functional mobility	Independent standing and ambulation. Allows for tibial progression for squatting, steps, ambulation and sit-to-stand
Floor reaction AFO (set dorsiflexion depending on weight line in standing)		
	Crouch gait	For clients with crouch during standing and ambulation
SMO	Full passive knee extension in standing (or set AFO to accommodate contracture)	1. Individual needs medial-lateral ankle stability
	Pronation in standing	2. Allows active plantar flexion

AFO, Ankle-foot orthosis; *DF*, dorsiflexion; *SMO*, supramalleolar orthosis.

Adolescents With Cerebral Palsy[41]

Therapists are encouraged to include older children and teens in problem solving to help them become more self-sufficient, assuming more responsibility during this developmental phase despite their limitations in physical capability. Providing adolescents the opportunity to participate in planning and decision making is important for transition planning.

This may include decisions about assistive technology, environmental modifications, health and fitness, and prevention of secondary musculoskeletal impairments. Likewise, the therapist can work closely with those individuals interested in participating in recreation and sports activities.

Client-centered assessment of strengths and needs identifying self-care, productivity, and leisure activities is possible and has been reported with this population.[41]

Adults With Cerebral Palsy

Therapists must also recognize and address the ongoing and unique needs of adults with CP (Fig. 35-14). With improved understanding of CP and its associated long-term complications and with improved health care, increased longevity has brought a new area of concern for children with CP living into adulthood: effects of the aging process. Decline of already impaired muscle strength and elasticity and bone density can lead to loss of ambulatory status.[11]

Group homes, independent living centers, and sheltered workshops are now making it possible for many nonambulatory adults with disabilities to function independently or semiindependently. Regular daily living assistance is required by adults with spastic quadriplegia, especially in the area of lifts and transfers.

Degenerative arthritis, severe joint contractures, and other orthopedic deformities present the most common and challenging problems in this population (Fig. 35-15). Moderate to intense pain is a significant problem for the majority of adults with CP, accompanied by depressive symptoms interfering with activities. Further research is needed to determine the functional impact of this problem and appropriate interventions.[22,59]

Management strategies for older children and adults are different by virtue of their ability to participate and understand the aims of therapy. Therapy to maintain functional skills through the adolescent growth spurt, when weight gain, weakness, and atrophy often result in a decline in function, is essential. Aerobic training may prevent deterioration in body composition and muscle strength.[71]

Strengthening has become an integral part of therapy programs for individuals with CP and is especially helpful in this population. Measuring isokinetic

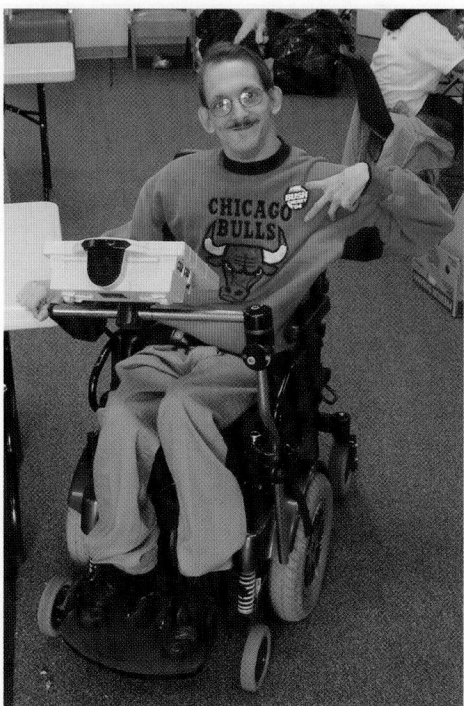

Figure 35-14

Adult with cerebral palsy. This 33-year-old man with athetoid cerebral palsy uses a speech-generating (communication) device and power chair; the joystick to operate the chair is under the client's right hand. The communication device can be folded and moved out to the side to allow for transfers. The chair has power tilt for independent position changes and pressure relief. Ankle huggers wrapped around the ankles keep his legs from flailing. A neoprene chest harness was added later to help provide external stability and increase control of his movements (not shown). This individual has clearly communicated how much he likes having the chest support, saying he feels much more in control of his body with it on. Straps and supports are fashioned with buckles, because Velcro is not strong enough to hold this client. The additional supports help reduce athetoid movements and improve function. (Courtesy Tamara Kittelson-Aldred, Access Therapy Services, Missoula, MT. Used with permission.)

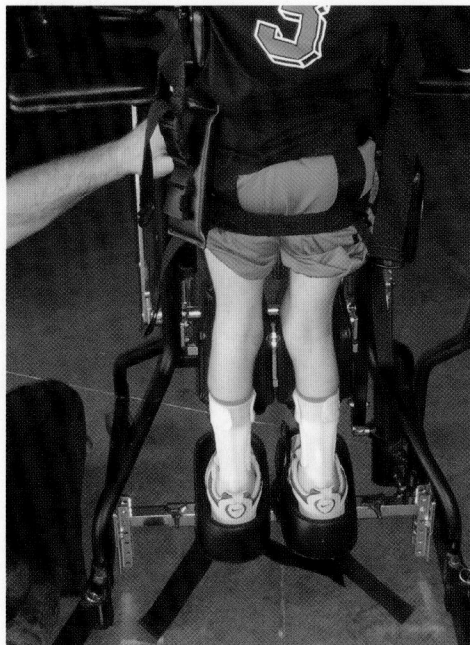

Figure 35-13

Orthoses. Ankle-foot orthoses (as seen from behind this client) in a standing frame are used for foot alignment and inhibition of tone associated with spastic quadriplegia. (Courtesy Tamara Kittelson-Aldred, Access Therapy Services, Missoula, MT. Used with permission.)

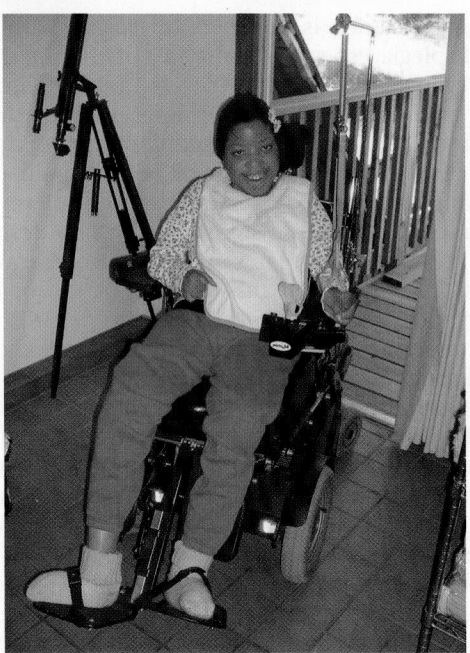

Figure 35-15

Adult with cerebral palsy. Adults with moderate to severe effects of cerebral palsy can face some difficult physical challenges. This 21-year-old woman has a power chair with seat elevator, power tilt in space, and power elevating leg rests she can operate herself. Each leg rest can be raised or lowered separately to her comfort. This client changed her lower extremity position frequently to manage pain related to spasticity and immobility. A spring upper extremity assist on the left helps keep her hand on a modified joystick to allow her to independently control her chair. (Courtesy Tamara Kittelson-Aldred, Access Therapy Services, Missoula, MT. Used with permission.)

strength is considered reliable in this population and should be used in rehabilitation protocols.[4] Isokinetic strengthening three times per week for 8 weeks can improve muscle strength and gross motor skills[36,71] and increase cadence[21] for those people who remain ambulatory into adulthood. A traditional upper extremity strengthening program of 6 to 10 repetitions three times per week for 8 weeks has been useful in improving speed and endurance in independent wheelchair propulsion.

REFERENCES

To enhance this text and add value for the reader, all references are included on the companion Evolve site that accompanies this textbook. The reader can view the reference source and access it online whenever possible.

CHAPTER 36

Seizures and Epilepsy

KENDA S. FULLER

SEIZURES AND EPILEPSY

Overview and Definition

Epilepsy comes from the Greek word meaning possession. The Greek people believed that seizures were caused by demons. Stigma and prejudice surrounding epilepsy continue, and people living with epilepsy often are reluctant to admit it or to seek treatment.[5]

A fundamental difference exists between seizure and epilepsy. A seizure is a finite event; it has a beginning and an end. Seizures are a result of paroxysmal excessive discharge of cerebral neurons resulting in transient impairment or loss of consciousness. Seizures can be induced in any normal human brain by a variety of different electrical or chemical stimuli. The cerebral cortex in particular contains within its anatomic and physiologic structure a mechanism that is inherently unstable and capable of producing a seizure. Seizures are a relatively common symptom of brain dysfunction, and they may occur in many acute medical or neurologic illnesses if brain function is temporarily disrupted. These seizures are most often self-limited and do not persist after the underlying disorder has resolved. Seizures also can occur as a reaction of the brain to physiologic stress, sleep deprivation, fever, and alcohol or sedative drug withdrawal. Isolated seizures also occur sometimes for no discernible reason as unprovoked events in presumably healthy people. None of these kinds of seizures represents epilepsy.[8]

Epilepsy is defined as a transient occurrence of signs and symptoms due to abnormal excessive or synchronous neuronal activity in the brain. Epileptic syndromes consist of clusters of clinical and electroencephalographic (EEG) features, respond to particular treatments, and may have specific prognostic implications. Epilepsy in children is usually considered constitutional, whereas in the older person, it is probably related to a provoking cause that develops over time.[35]

The International League Against Epilepsy Commission on Classification and Terminology has revised its concepts, terminology, and approaches for classifying seizures and forms of epilepsy. Organization of forms of epilepsy is first by specificity: electroclinical syndromes, non-syndromic epilepsies with structural or metabolic causes, and epilepsies of unknown cause. Recommendations of the Commission's deliberations during the 2005–2009 meetings will be used as possible in this chapter.[3]

Incidence

Acute symptomatic seizures, or provoked seizures, constitute about 40% of all episodes of seizure but are not considered epilepsy. After headache, the epilepsies are the most frequent chronic neurologic condition seen in general practice worldwide. Epilepsy affects about 45 million people worldwide. Incidence is highest among young children and the elderly, and men are affected slightly more often than women (1.5 : 1). In the United States, figures range from 31 to 57 per 100,000. The incidence of epilepsy peaks in children younger than 5 years at 60 to 70 per 100,000, decreases throughout adolescence to 30 per 100,000 in early adulthood, and rises again after the sixth decade, reaching a peak of 150 to 200 per 100,000 people older than 75 years. Epilepsy is the third most common serious neurologic disease of old age after dementia and stroke.[37] Although seizure activity in children is rare, at less than 1%, seizures are the most common symptoms requiring medical attention in the infant. It has been estimated that 75% of cases of epilepsy have their onset before 20 years of age.[31,36]

Etiologic and Risk Factors

The concept of genetic epilepsy is that epilepsy is the direct result of a known or presumed genetic defect(s) in which seizures are the core symptom of the disorder. First-degree relatives with epilepsy account for 15% of cases, and of those, about 75% have just one affected relative. However, the risk is still higher in first-degree relatives of patients with epilepsy than in the general population. Heritable factors are important in children. Common features include a variable family history, generalized spike-wave abnormality on EEG, and onset in childhood or adolescence. Because there are no consistent, demonstrable pathologic changes in the brains of individuals with idiopathic generalized epilepsy, susceptibility to these seizures most likely results from inherited biochemical, membrane, or neurotransmitter defects that result in abnormal excitability within the involved circuits.

Although mutations in single genes account for a few rare epileptic syndromes, in most cases of epilepsy, data are most consistent with complex, polygenic influences.[4,24] Complex disease genes account for about 50% of all patients with epilepsy. Multiple genes with individually small but additive effects act in combination with environmental factors will produce an increased risk for epilepsy. Neurodegenerative disorders, inherited malformations of cortical development, and inherited metabolic disorders may underlie the onset. Box 36-1 describes the current understanding of the relationship between mutations and type of epilepsy. This genetic predisposition to seizure activity may explain why one individual with brain damage develops epilepsy while another with similar damage does not develop seizure activity.[26]

Structural/metabolic causes of epilepsy are multiple, and the symptoms may be transient, resolving after treatment of the primary disorder. Box 36-2 describes some of the causes of symptomatic epilepsy. Epilepsy can be caused by virtually any major category of serious disease or human disorder. It can result from congenital malformations, infections, tumors, vascular disease, degenerative diseases, or injury. In people older than age 50 years, cerebrovascular disease is the most common cause of seizures, which often accompany or follow a stroke, and increases the risk of seizure by 17%.[18,33] It is thought that perhaps even in the absence of stroke, cerebrovascular disease may predispose an individual to seizure activity. Seizures may be the first symptom of an intracranial mass, and it is suggested that 10% to 15% of older adult-onset epilepsy is a result of neoplasm. When the seizure is because of a permanent lesion or scar, the seizure activity may persist. Head trauma is the most common preventable cause of epilepsy. More than 3000 cases of epilepsy are added every year in the U.S. population because of head injury.[32] Subdural hematoma can cause seizure activity and is common in older adults, often after a fall that may have seemed trivial.[30] Pneumonia, which carries the possibility of hypoxia, especially in the aged, can cause seizures that can become recurrent.[32] Alcohol abuse often leads to uncontrolled seizure activity.

Hormonal changes with increase in the levels of estrogen that occur during ovulation and menstruation can be a trigger for seizure in some women. Menopause tends to occur earlier in women with epilepsy, and this early menopause is associated with a history of high seizure frequency.[11] Fertility appears to be reduced by seizure activity when it is triggered by hormonal changes. Disruptions of reproductive function in women include anovulatory cycles that may increase the risk for infertility, migraine, emotional disorders, and reproductive cancers. Moreover, both epilepsy itself and use of medications have been

---

Box 36-1

MUTATION OF GENES AND SEIZURE TYPE

Benign familial neonatal seizures
  Potassium-channel *KCNQ2* and *KCNQ3*
Benign familial neonatal-infantile seizures
  Sodium-channel *SCN2A*
Generalized epilepsy with febrile seizures (+)
  Sodium-channel subunits *SCN1A*, *SCN1B*, and *SCN2A* and the *GABRG2* subunit of the GABA$_A$ receptor
Childhood absence epilepsy with febrile seizures
  GABRG2 subunit of the GABA$_A$ receptor
Autosomal dominant juvenile myoclonic epilepsy
  GABRA1 subunit of the GABA$_A$ receptor and in *EFHC1*, regulation of calcium currents
Autosomal dominant idiopathic generalized epilepsy
  Chloride-channel gene *CLCN2*
Autosomal dominant nocturnal frontal lobe epilepsy
  Nicotinic acetylcholine receptor subunits *CHRNA4* and *CHRNB2*
Autosomal dominant partial epilepsy with auditory features
  LGI1 gene, involved in development of the central nervous system (CNS)

Data from Samuel Wiebe: The epilepsies, in Goldman L, Schafer AI, eds: *Goldman's Cecil medicine*, ed 24, St. Louis, 2011, Saunders.

Box 36-2

POTENTIAL CAUSES OF ACUTE SYMPTOMATIC SEIZURES

Medical Conditions
Metabolic Derangements

- Hyponatremia (<120 mEq/L)—especially acute
- Hypernatremia (>150-155 mEq/L)—especially acute
- Hypoglycemia (<40 mg/dL)
- Hyperglycemia (>400 mg/dL)
- Hyperosmolality (>320 mOsm/L)
- Hypocalcemia (<7 mg/dl)
- Respiratory alkalosis—acute

Drug-Induced Seizures

- Isoniazid, penicillins
- Theophylline, aminophylline
- Lidocaine
- Meperidine
- Ketamine, halothane, enflurane, methohexital
- Amitriptyline, maprotiline, imipramine, doxepin, fluoxetine
- Haloperidol, trifluoperazine, chlorpromazine
- Ephedrine, phenylpropanolamine, terbutaline
- Methotrexate, BCNU (carmustine), asparaginase
- Cyclosporine
- Cocaine (crack), phencyclidine, amphetamines
- Alcohol (withdrawal)

Illnesses

- Eclampsia
- Hypertensive encephalopathy
- Liver failure
- Polyarteritis nodosa
- Porphyria
- Renal failure
- Sickle cell disease
- Syphilis
- Systemic lupus erythematosus
- Thrombotic thrombocytopenic purpura
- Whipple disease

Neurologic Conditions

- Angiitis of the nervous system
- Meningitis
- Encephalitis
- Acute head trauma (impact seizures)
- Stroke
- Brain abscess
- Brain tumor

Adapted from Pedley TA: The epilepsies. In Goldman L, ed: *Cecil textbook of medicine*, ed 22, Philadelphia, 2004, Saunders, Chap 434, Table 434-1.

implicated as causal or contributory factors that can alter reproductive hormone levels and promote the development of reproductive endocrine disorders, especially polycystic ovarian syndrome. Gestational epilepsy results from hormonal and metabolic changes that exacerbate underlying epilepsy or adversely influence serum levels of anticonvulsants. Eclampsia or toxemia is a gestational hypertensive encephalopathy manifested by seizure, hypertension, coma, proteinuria, and edema. Convulsive generalized status epilepticus in pregnancy jeopardizes both mother and fetus.

The age-dependent appearance of spontaneous seizures in the primary epilepsies appears to depend on a critical period in cerebral maturation when the genetically determined defect is expressed clinically as a manifest change in behavior. These changes include an increase in cell density, abnormal arrangements of cortical neurons, and an increase in white matter neurons.[9] Seizures may occur in the neonatal period, within the first 24 to 72 hours, and they are usually of focal cerebral origin. The seizures tend to be unilateral because of the immaturity of the forebrain and corpus callosum, limiting movement from one hemisphere to the other. Seizure activity represents the relative development of the limbic system, diencephalon, and brainstem. Hypoxic-ischemic brain insult is the most common cause of neonatal convulsions and is because of compromise of oxygen to the brain during or before delivery. The other important cause of seizures arising in the early neonatal period is hypoglycemia, most often seen in babies who are small for gestational age. The neurologic symptoms of hypoglycemia consist of irritability, drowsiness, hypotonia, and apnea. Approximately half of the babies with hypoglycemia develop neurologic symptoms, and about one fourth of these go on to develop seizures. Hypocalcemia (serum level below 7 mg/100 mL) may occur in the first 2 to 3 days of life either in low-birth-weight infants or in association with the complications of birth asphyxia. It may then contribute to seizures but is rarely the primary cause. Hypercalcemia occurring at age 6 to 8 days is usually the primary cause of the clinical features of neonatal tetany, including jitteriness and jaw, knee, and ankle clonus. Hypocalcemia is rare in infants who are breastfed or fed formula created to simulate human milk. Hypernatremia, resulting from alteration in sodium level, may also lead to neonatal seizures. Hypernatremia is associated with dehydrating illnesses. Specific syndromes are typical at particular ages, and are described at the end of this chapter.

Pathogenesis

All seizure activity is a result of chaotic electrical discharge in the central nervous system (CNS). Epileptic seizures result from the sudden, excessive electrical discharges of large aggregates of neurons. Each neuron has a stereotypic synchronized response called paroxysmal depolarization shift that consists of a sudden depolarization phase, resulting from glutamate and calcium channel activation, with a series of action potentials at its peak followed by an after-hyperpolarization phase.[20]

The original insult such as a prolonged febrile status epilepticus episode or hypoxia leads to a pathologic attempt at compensation by sprouting of the excitatory mossy fibers. Mossy fiber sprouting leads to increased excitability and to epilepsy. Other mechanisms by which neurons develop a tendency toward anomalous bursting activity include alterations in neurotransmitters and in the cholinergic, noradrenergic, serotonergic, and histaminergic afferents from the brainstem and basal forebrain structures, which modulate excitability of hemispheric motor mechanisms.

Activation of the *N*-methyl-D-aspartate type of glutamate receptors potentiates cellular excitability and leads to sustained neuronal depolarization and calcium influx. Extracellular potassium and intracellular calcium concentrations increase and contribute to the overall excitability of the epileptic neuronal aggregate. Spread of bursting activity to other neurons is normally prevented by surrounding inhibitory mechanisms, such as hyperpolarization and inhibitory interneurons. The main inhibitory neurotransmitter of the CNS is γ-aminobutyric acid (GABA). When stimulated, GABA receptors modulate chloride ion flux, inhibiting membrane depolarization. GABA antagonists or functional depletion of GABA increases membrane depolarization and may result in seizures. GABA agonists (direct or indirect) therefore play a vital role in seizure termination. Loss of GABA-mediated inhibition results in seizures.[38]

During the seizure itself, neurons are tonically depolarized and fire continuously in a sustained, high-frequency discharge (tonic phase). The seizure ends as phasic repolarizations interrupt the continuous firing pattern (clonic phase) and gradually restore membrane potentials to normal or to a temporary hyperpolarized state (postictal depression). Prolonged *N*-methyl-D-aspartate receptor activation and excessive accumulation of intracellular calcium also result in neuronal toxicity and may lead to cell death. The thalamus plays a role in generating generalized seizures and the generalized spike-wave EEG patterns that accompany them. The substantia nigra also is crucial to the expression of generalized convulsions, especially the tonic phase; GABA-ergic inhibitory transmission in the substantia nigra plays a regulatory role in the propagation of primary and secondarily generalized seizure discharges. Generalized seizures and the rhythmic spike-wave discharges are dependent on ionic conductance of the neurons in the thalamic nucleus reticularis, allowing them to function as pacemaker control cells. In the focal epilepsies, abnormal neuronal behavior originates in and may remain confined to a restricted area of the cortex.[24]

Mesial temporal sclerosis, also called hippocampal sclerosis, is characterized by neuronal loss and gliosis; whether hippocampal sclerosis is the cause or the result of seizures (or both) is not known. The scarring is characterized by variable degrees of pyramidal cell loss and gliosis in the hippocampal subfields and dentate gyrus. This condition represents the most common pathologic substrate of focal epilepsy in adolescents and adults starting between 5 and 15 years of age.[13] Hippocampal atrophy and increased hippocampal signal are best seen on T2-weighted and fluid-attenuated inversion recovery coronal MRI sequences, and widespread interictal hypometabolism is seen in the temporal lobe on positron emission tomography (PET). Figure 36-1 shows mesial sclerosis identified through coronal magnetic resonance imaging (MRI).

The hippocampus plays a critical role in both seizure activity and mood disorders. This suggests that pathology in this area of the brain might provide a link between epilepsy and depression. Remodeling of the hippocampal

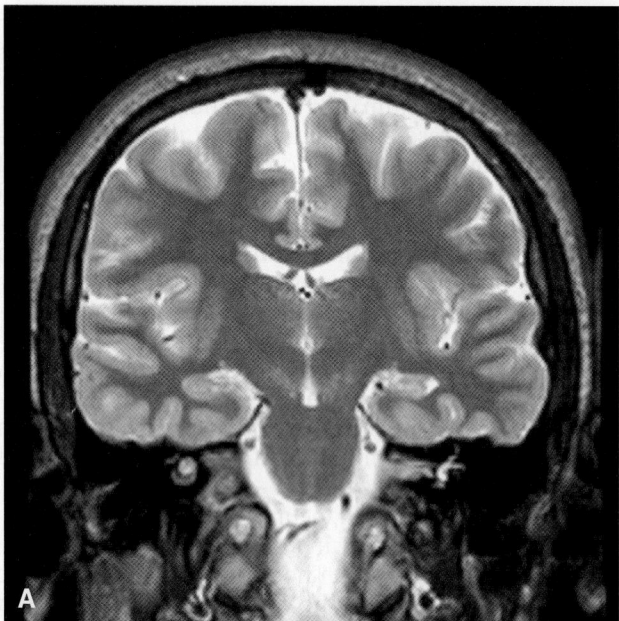

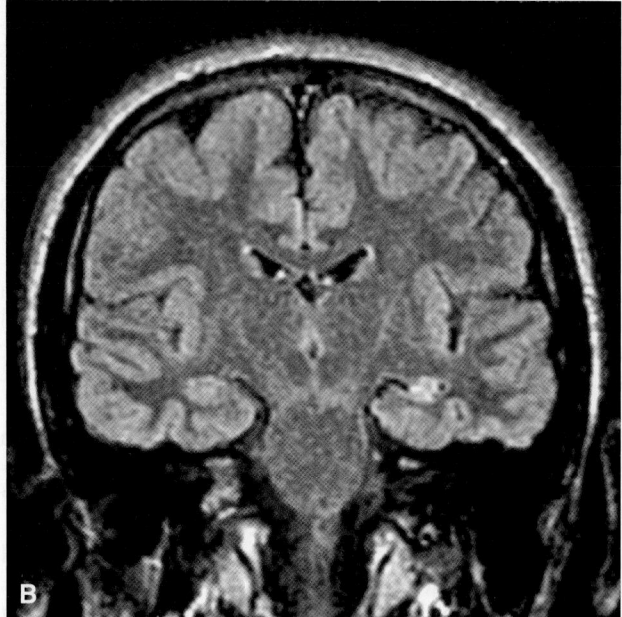

Figure 36-1

Temporal mesial sclerosis—coronal MRI. The coronal projection is essential to reveal hippocampal abnormalities. Fluid-attenuated inversion recovery MRI is superior to T2 weighting to show signal abnormalities, because the saturation nullifies the signal from the cerebrospinal fluid. **A,** A T2-weighted scan shows volume reduction of the left hippocampus. **B,** A fluid-attenuated inversion recovery sequence shows the abnormal high signal *(arrow)*, not seen on the T2 scan. (From Adam A, Dixon AK, Grainger RG, et al, eds: *Grainger and Allison's diagnostic radiology: a textbook of medical imaging*, ed 4, Philadelphia, 2001, Churchill Livingstone.)

spine synapses may play a significant role in the neurobiology of depression and the effects of antidepressant therapy. Because the effects of estrogens on hippocampus parallel those of antidepressants, loss of estrogen appears to be a critical contributor to the etiology of depressive disorders. The increased incidence of depression observed in women with epilepsy might therefore reflect a hormonal deficiency state, although it is probably not the only factor that contributes to depression.[10] Shifts in levels of brain-derived neurotrophic factor in the brain may represent another common link between the distinctive patterns of epilepsy and depression seen in women. Seizure incidence varies across the reproductive cycle, as noted above, peaking in the periovulatory period. Dramatic fluctuations in estrogen levels in women may explain their greater vulnerability to depression, even as estrogen-related surges in brain-derived neurotrophic factor expression may lead to an increased propensity for seizures.

Another potential explanation of the facilitation of seizures is *kindling.* Kindling refers to the processes that mediate long-lasting changes in brain function in response to repeated, gradually augmented stimulation of the brain resulting in epileptiform activity. Kindling also refers to sensitization of neuronal tissue by the addition of a drug or electrical stimulus that renders it susceptible to subsequent seizure activity. This may explain why exposures to localized, repetitive, low-intensity electrical stimuli induce increasingly pathologic responses. This is a possible mechanism that exists between the occurrence of a brain insult and the later onset of epilepsy. The kindling model is currently used in the study of partial epilepsy, particularly that involving the mesial temporal structures.[8] The development of seizures during the electrically induced kindling of seizures is associated with significant changes in the concentration of kynurenic acid and its precursor, tryptophan.[34] Chronic focal epileptogenic lesions can cause distant areas to become capable of generating abnormal electrical discharges and seizures. This focus continues to function independently even after ablation of the primary lesion. This has important implications for the surgical treatment of epilepsy.

The concept of epileptic encephalopathy has grown in acceptance and use. It was formally recognized in the 2006 report and is now defined within this document. Epileptic encephalopathy embodies the notion that the epileptic activity itself may contribute to severe cognitive and behavioral impairments above and beyond what might be expected from the underlying pathology alone (e.g., cortical malformation), and that these can worsen over time. These impairments may be global or more selective and they may occur along a spectrum of severity. Although certain syndromes are often referred to as epileptic encephalopathies, the encephalopathic effects of seizures and epilepsy may potentially occur in association with any form of epilepsy.[3]

Clinical Manifestations

In most individuals, seizures occur unpredictably at any time and without any relationship to posture or ongoing activities.[12,17] In some individuals, seizures are provoked by specific stimuli such as flashing lights or a flickering television. See Box 36-3 for the typical triggers to seizure. The presence of focal signs after the seizure suggests that the seizure may have a focal origin. Prodromal symptoms (premonitory symptoms that indicate an impending seizure) may include headache, mood alterations, lethargy, and myoclonic jerking. The initial events of a seizure, described either by the individual or by an observer, are usually the most reliable indication to determine whether a seizure begins focally.[7]

In the tonic phase of a tonic-clonic seizure, the body becomes rigid and the person is at risk of falling. A cry may be uttered, and the person may become cyanotic. In general, the jaw is fixed and the hands are clenched. This phase usually lasts for 30 to 60 seconds. The clonic phase begins with rhythmic, jerky contractions and relaxation of all body muscles, especially in the extremities. Figure 36-2 demonstrates the tonic and clonic phases of seizure. Biting of the tongue, lips, or inside of the mouth may occur. Saliva is blown from the mouth, with a froth appearing on the lips.

Although they do not represent a clear dichotomy, the terms of generalized and focal are still used for descriptive purposes. *Generalized epileptic seizures* are conceptualized as originating at some point in the hemisphere, activating bilaterally distributed networks. Such bilateral networks can include cortical and subcortical structures, but do not necessarily include the entire cortex. Generalized seizures can be asymmetric. *Focal seizure* describes activity either localized or more widely distributed within networks limited to one hemisphere and is characterized by the locus of onset of the attacks. These seizures are identified as temporal, frontal, parietal, or occipital. Sensory symptoms such as localized paresthesias, numbness, vertigo, auditory hallucinations, and unformed visual hallucinations occur with seizures beginning in the corresponding primary sensory areas. Focal seizures have clinical or EEG evidence of a local onset. Focal seizure originating in the cortical area that represents sensation of the hand may begin with contralateral hand tingling and then progress to involve additional cortical regions ipsilaterally, producing more extensive sensory symptoms as well as clonic motor signs. The sensation seems to march from hand to arm to leg area ipsilaterally, a process referred to as a jacksonian march. Consciousness is not depressed, and individuals can interact normally with their environment except for limitations imposed by the seizure. Minor motor seizures are reflected by myoclonus, or involuntary jerking of the major muscles, akinesia with a momentary loss of muscle movement, or atonia which causes the person to collapse. After the clonic motor activity ends, patients are often weak.[3]

In dyscognitive seizures, considered focal, alteration of cognition is major feature. Focal seizures originating from any region can become dyscognitive seizures, and unilateral focal seizures can progress to involve bilateral areas. In temporal lobe seizures, loss of consciousness results when the discharge spreads bilaterally to involve areas of the hippocampus and amygdala. The person appears dazed and confused with random walking, mumbling, head turning, or pulling at clothing. Motor tasks such as eating, drawing, and walking may continue in an awkward manner. These seizures usually last around a minute, followed by confusion and disorientation lasting several more minutes. Individuals are amnesic for details of the seizure that occurred after the aura. An olfactory relationship identifies an origin in or near the uncus of the medial temporal lobe and may have a higher association with brain tumors. Feelings of déjà vu and dreamy states, such as feelings of unreality and depersonalization; distortion of time; or depressed or fearful states are common. Visual images with illusions of multiple images or distortions regarding size can occur as well as hallucinatory phenomena. Autonomic symptoms reflect involvement of limbic structures that lie in the mesial temporal or frontal lobe and project to the hypothalamus and brainstem. Frontal lobe originations are atypical and differ dramatically from seizures originating in the temporal lobe. Although there are many variations, frontal lobe seizures tend to begin and end abruptly; have few, if any, postictal symptoms; and involve often bizarre motor manifestations, such as asynchronous thrashing or flailing of arms and legs, pelvic thrusting, pedaling leg movements, and loud vocalizations that may appear as psychiatric disorders.[24] Table 36-1 describes the symptoms and the associated area of activity in the brain.

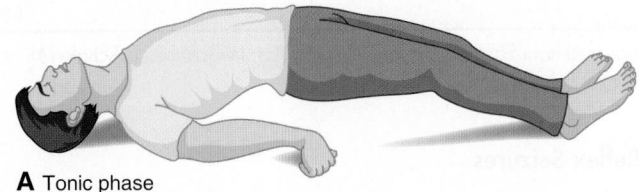

A Tonic phase

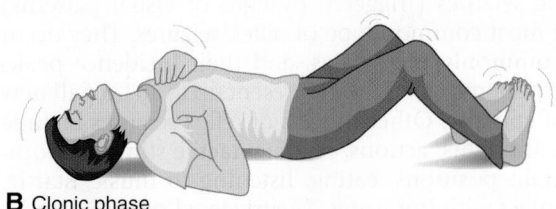

B Clonic phase

Figure 36-2

Tonic and clonic phases of seizure activity. A, Posture typical of tonic phase; **B,** movement associated with clonic phase. (From Black JM: *Medical-surgical nursing: clinical management for positive outcomes,* ed 7, Philadelphia, 2004, Saunders.)

Box 36-3

EVENTS THAT MAY TRIGGER SEIZURE

- Stress
- Poor nutrition
- Missed medication
- Skipping meals
- Flickering lights
- Illness
- Fever and allergies
- Lack of sleep
- Emotions such as anger, worry, fear
- Heat and humidity

Table 36-1	Clinical Manifestations of Focal Seizures	
Seizure Type	**Brain Activity**	**Clinical Expression**
Somatosensory	Postcentral rolandic; parietal	Contralateral tingling, numbness, hot or cold, electric. Sensation of, sense of movement or desire to move. "Marching" to other body segments.
Parietal		Contralateral agnosia of a limb, phantom limb, distortion of size or position of body part
		Ipsilateral or bilateral facial, truncal or limb tingling, numbness, or pain. Often involve lips, tongue, fingertips, feet
Motor	Precentral rolandic	Contralateral regional clonic jerking, usually rhythmic, may spread to other body segments in jacksonian motor march. Often accompanied by sensory symptoms in same area
Supplementary sensory-motor		Bilateral tonic contraction of limbs causing postural changes, may exhibit classic fencing posture, may have speech arrest or vocalization
Frontal		Contralateral head and eye version, salivation, speech arrest or vocalization; may be combined with other motor signs (as above) depending on seizure spread
Auditory	Auditory cortex in superior temporal lobe	Bilateral or contralateral buzzing, drumming, single tones, muffled sounds
Olfactory	Orbitofrontal; mesial temporal cortex	Often described as unpleasant odor
Gustatory	Parietal; rolandic operculum; insula; temporal lobe	Often unpleasant taste, acidic, metallic, salty, sweet, smoky
Vertiginous	Occipitotemporal-parietal junction; frontal lobe	Sensation of body displacement in various directions
Visual	Occipital	Contralateral static, moving, or flashing colored or uncolored lights, shapes, or spots. Contralateral or bilateral, partial or complete loss of vision.
	Temporal; occipito-temporal-parietal junction	Formed visual scenes, faces, people, objects, animals
		Autonomic: abdominal rising sensation, nausea, borborygmi, flushing, pallor, piloerection, perspiration, heart rate changes, chest pain, shortness of breath, cephalic sensation, lightheadedness, genital sensation, orgasm
Limbic	Limbic structures: amygdala, hippocampus, cingulum, olfactory cortex, hypothalamus	Psychic: déjà vu, jamais vu, depersonalization, derealization, dream-like state, forced memory or forced thinking, fear, elation, sadness, sexual pleasure, hallucinations or illusions of visual, auditory, or olfactory nature
Dyscognitive	Usually bilateral involvement of limbic structures (see above)	Previously known as "complex partial seizures," characterized by a predominant alteration of consciousness or awareness. The current definition requires involvement of at least two of five components of cognition: perception, attention, emotion, memory, and executive function.

Adapted from Samuel Wiebe: The epilepsies, in Goldman L, Schafer AI, eds: *Goldman's Cecil medicine*, ed 24, St. Louis, 2011, Saunders.

Reflex Seizures

Reflex seizures are triggered by specific simple (e.g., flashing lights) or elaborate (e.g., reading) stimuli. Visual-sensitive seizures (triggered by light or visual patterns) are the most common type of reflex seizures. They occur most commonly in females, and their incidence peaks around puberty, when they represent up to 10% of all new cases of epilepsy. Other triggers of reflex seizures include specific thoughts, actions, reading, tactile stimuli, adopting certain positions, eating, listening to music, startle, and contact with hot water. The triggered seizures can be myoclonic, convulsive, atonic, or focal, depending on the triggering stimulus. Avoiding the offending stimulus is crucial to avoid seizures, emphasizing the importance of careful questioning about seizure triggers in patients with epilepsy.[3]

Absence Seizures

Generalized absence seizures, formerly called petit mal seizures, consist of the sudden cessation of ongoing conscious activity, with only minor convulsive muscular activity or loss of postural control. Generalized seizures begin diffusely and involve both cerebral hemispheres simultaneously from the outset. The person often stares into space. Onset and termination of attacks are abrupt. Absences are not preceded by an aura and are followed by normal activity. If attacks occur during conversation, the person may miss a few words or may break off in mid-sentence for a few seconds. The person is unaware of the loss of conscious control. Often, these seizures occur in children and frequently disappear by adolescence. Atypical absence seizures are similar to absence seizures but coexist with other forms of generalized seizure.

Myoclonic Seizures

Myoclonic seizures are sudden, brief, single, or repetitive muscle contractions involving one body part or the entire body. The myoclonic jerks range from small movements of the face or hands to massive bilateral spasms that simultaneously affect the head, limbs, and trunk. Repeated myoclonic seizures may seem to crescendo and terminate in a generalized tonic-clonic convulsion. Although they can occur at any time, myoclonic seizures often cluster shortly after waking or while falling asleep.[24]

Atonic Seizures

Atonic seizures, also known as "drop attacks," are brief losses of consciousness and postural tone not associated with tonic muscular contractions. Atonic seizures occur most often in children with diffuse encephalopathies and are characterized by sudden loss of muscle tone that may result in falls with self-injury. Sometimes the loss of muscle tone is limited or fragmentary, producing only a head drop.

Seizures With Tonic and/or Clonic Manifestations

Seizures with Tonic and/or Clonic Manifestations involve brainstem, possibly prefrontal, and basal ganglia mechanisms. Ictal initiation of primarily bilateral events are predominantly disinhibitory, but other mechanisms are responsible for ictal evolution to the clonic phase, involving gradual periodic introduction of seizure-suppressing mechanisms

Formerly called grand mal seizure, tonic-clonic seizure is the archetypal seizure, which means total loss of control. The seizure begins with a sudden loss of consciousness, and falls are common. The generalized rigidity (tonic) phase is followed by very rapid generalized jerking movements (the clonic stage). In adults, incontinence of bowel and bladder occur. Generalized tonic-clonic seizures result in many striking but transient physiologic changes, including hypoxia, lactic acidosis, elevated plasma catecholamine levels, and increased concentrations of serum creatine kinase, prolactin, corticotropin, cortisol, β-endorphin, and growth hormone. In the tonic phase, respiration can cease briefly. Recovery may be swift after a short seizure, but a prolonged seizure may induce a deep sleep. Altered speech and transient paralysis or ataxia may follow, as well as headache, disorientation, or muscle soreness. Another seizure may follow without recovery of consciousness or, after recovery of consciousness, the person may experience seizure again.[26] As recovery progresses, many individuals complain of headache, muscle soreness, mental dulling, lack of energy, or mood changes lasting 24 hours. Complications include oral trauma, vertebral compression fractures, shoulder dislocation, aspiration pneumonia, and sudden death, which may be related to acute pulmonary edema, cardiac arrhythmia, or suffocation. Although this is the type of epilepsy that most people associate with the disorder, it is less common than focal seizures.

Status Epilepticus

Status epilepticus is a condition in which seizures are so prolonged or so repeated that recovery does not occur between attacks. Convulsive status epilepticus occurs when the person has generalized tonic-clonic seizures and no return to consciousness occurs between seizures. It is a medical emergency. The molecular events that cause death can occur with the first few seizures. Tonic-clonic status epilepticus is more common in people whose seizures have a known cause. Often it is the result of tumor, CNS infection, or drug abuse. Febrile seizures are a common cause of status epilepticus in children under the age of 3 years. Nonconvulsive status epilepticus is difficult to define, but it may be described as a syndrome in which the most fundamental feature is a change in the individual's behavior. A degree of clouding of mental processes occurs, ranging from drowsiness and confusion to disorientation and dysphagia. Nonconvulsive status epilepticus is seen in various neurologic diagnoses (i.e., trauma, stroke) in the acute intensive care unit setting. It also denotes a condition that can occur de novo in older adults without a precipitating cause and that is characterized by prolonged confusional episodes, which are caused by generalized slow spike-and-wave status epilepticus. There is evidence from surgically resected epileptic tissue that apoptotic pathways are activated in foci of intractable epilepsy.[3]

MEDICAL MANAGEMENT

DIAGNOSIS. Diagnosis is not the same as a classification. A syndrome is characterized with respect to many factors. Knowing a given patient's syndromic diagnosis provides key information about that patient's epilepsy, for example, likely age at onset, EEG patterns, responses to medications, and cognitive and developmental status. Focal seizures should be described according to their manifestations, for example, dyscognitive or focal motor. Genetic, structural–metabolic, and unknown represent modified concepts to replace idiopathic, symptomatic, and cryptogenic. Not all epilepsies are recognized as electroclinical syndromes. For each seizure type, ictal onset is consistent from one seizure to another, with preferential propagation patterns that can involve the contralateral hemisphere.

The history obtained from the client and the observations of bystanders are of importance in establishing a diagnosis and classifying the seizure disorder correctly. To determine seizure type, a series of questions must be answered regarding the location of the seizure activity, the level of consciousness, the level of generalized motor activity, and the preceding level of seizure activity. The state of the client after the episode, including the level of confusion, sleepiness, or headache, must be determined. These data may be gathered from the paramedic or emergency personnel in the case of an individual who has been found on the floor.

It is important to recognize events that may mimic a seizure but are not related to the diagnosis of epilepsy. Early morning confusion and headache could be related to hypoglycemia in individuals on hypoglycemic medications. If the event is a transient ischemic attack, a loss of consciousness usually does not occur, and the neurologic insult is in the form of weakness or numbness. With a seizure, however, a twitching and tingling is evident. Behavioral disturbances as seen in dementia usually have a predictable pattern, such as occurring at a certain time of day.[14] Syncope, or a transient loss of consciousness, is related to an acute change in cerebral perfusion. The related transient cerebral anoxia may itself cause seizure activity. Recurrent cardiac arrhythmia can be confused with recurrent seizures.[22]

Syncope, vasodepressive, orthostatic, or arrhythmogenic states may be confused with ictal events when episodes are recurrent. It can be a challenge to determine "fit versus faint." In general, tonic-clonic movements are much more forceful and are more prolonged than the twitches sometimes associated with fainting. Most seizures are characterized by a postictal state, not seen with syncope except for atonic drop attack. The cause of an unwitnessed, unprovoked loss of consciousness resulting in a fall may be hard to classify. Retrograde amnesia suggests an ictal diagnosis.

Epileptic seizures presenting as motor phenomena without concomitant change of consciousness may be confused with one of the paroxysmal movement disorders. Conversely, the attack of paroxysmal movement disorders may be thought to be epileptic because of a number of factors, including its sudden, unpredictable, and transient nature; its response to anticonvulsants; and the premonitory sensations preceding attacks. These two conditions frequently occur in the same families or even in the same patients. Because epilepsy and paroxysmal movement disorders may both be related to channelopathy, the pathophysiology might represent an overlap.[16] Frontal lobe seizures arise predominantly during sleep and can have dramatic motor expression. They can be confused with nonepileptic psychogenic seizures, sleep disorders, or movement disorders. Video EEG monitoring may be necessary for diagnosis.[19]

Psychogenic nonepileptic seizures, or PNES, are time-limited, paroxysmal changes in movements, sensations, behaviors, or consciousness that can resemble epileptic seizures, but they are not associated with EEG activity. Psychogenic seizures can be difficult to diagnose because they can mimic almost any type of seizure, and they often coexist with epilepsy in the same patient. When there are variable clinical manifestations across episodes, frequent and prolonged episodes, out-of-phase upper and lower body movements, pelvic thrusting, and no rigidity, PNES should be suspected. Secondary gain is usually evident, and there is often a history of sexual abuse.[19] Neuropsychological testing is not useful to differentiate PNES from epilepsy. However, psychological testing may help to determine the psychiatric diagnosis after PNES is diagnosed. Table 36-2 describes behaviors that distinguish between PENS and epilepsy.

Table 36-2	Behaviors to Distinguish Between Psychogenic Nonepileptic and Epileptic Seizures	
Observation	**PNES**	**ES**
Situational onset	Common	Rare
Gradual onset	Common	Rare
Precipitated by stimuli (noise, light)	Occasional	Rare
Purposeful movements	Occasional	Very rare
Opisthotonus (*arc de cercle*)	Occasional	Very rare
Tongue biting (tip)	Occasional	Rare
Tongue biting (side)	Very Rare	Common
Prolonged ictal atonia	Occasional	Very rare
Vocalization during tonic-clonic phase	Occasional	Very rare
Reactivity during unconsciousness	Occasional	Very rare
Rapid postictal reorientation	Common	Unusual
Undulating motor activity	Common	Very rare
Asynchronous limb movements	Common	Rare
Rhythmical pelvic movements	Occasional	Rare
Side-to-side head shaking	Common	Rare
Ictal crying	Occasional	Very rare
Ictal stuttering	Occasional	Rare
Postictal whispering	Occasional	Not present
Closed mouth in tonic phase	Occasional	Very rare
Closed eyelids during seizure onset	Very common	Rare
Convulsion >2 min	Common	Very rare
Resisted lid opening	Common	Very rare
Pupillary light reflex	Usually retained	Commonly absent
Cyanosis	Rare	Common
Ictal grasping	Rare	Occurs in FLE and TLE
Postictal nose rubbing	Not present	Can occur in TLE
Stertorous breathing postictally	Not present	Common
Self-injury	May be present (especially excoriations)	May be present (especially lacerations)
Incontinence	May be present	May be present

FLE, Frontal lobe epilepsy; TLE, temporal lobe epilepsy.
From LaFrance WC: Differentiating frontal lobe epilepsy from psychogenic nonepileptic seizures. *Neurol Clin* 29:149-162, 2011.

Epileptic encephalopathy is an electroclinical syndrome associated with a high probability that features that present will worsen after the onset of epilepsy and tends to be pharmacoresistant, Pharmacoresponsiveness relates to the prediction that the seizures will rapidly come under control with appropriate medication. Determination of an encephalopathic course requires a failure to develop as expected relative to age-matched peers or to actually regress. Epileptic encephalopathy can present along a continuum of severity and may occur at any age. The phenomenon is most common and severe in infancy and early childhood, where global and profound cognitive impairment may occur. Adults, however, can also experience cognitive losses over time from uncontrolled seizures.

Endocrine status is commonly abnormal, typically for the sex steroid hormones, presenting as sexual dysfunction in men and women resulting in lower fertility. Other signs and symptoms in women with epilepsy include menstrual irregularities, premature menopause, and polycystic ovarian syndrome. These concerns should be included in standard evaluation in individuals with epilepsy.[25]

Electroencephalography. The EEG has a central role in the diagnosis of epilepsy. The EEG records the integrated electrical activity generated by synaptic potentials in neurons in the superficial layers of a localized area of cortex. In the epileptic focus, neurons in a small area of the cortex are activated for a brief period in a synchronized pattern and then inhibited. Interictal (between-seizure) activity on the EEG provides strong presumptive evidence that the event was a seizure. The best way to diagnose the presence of seizures and to classify the seizure is to observe, simultaneously, the seizure and the associated EEG recording. A normal reading does not rule out the diagnosis, and in the older individual, it may be more difficult to distinguish normal from abnormal.[36] Prolonged EEG monitoring with simultaneous closed-circuit video recording is reserved for complicated cases of protracted and unresponsive seizures. It provides an invaluable method for recording ictal seizure events that are rarely captured during routine EEG studies. This technique is extremely helpful in the classification of seizures because it can accurately determine the location and frequency of seizure discharges while recording alterations in the level of consciousness and the presence of clinical signs.[17]

Magnetoencephalography. Magnetoencephalography measures the small magnetic fields that are generated by electrical activity in the brain and approximates their location using mathematical models. Its use is largely restricted to the evaluation of patients for epilepsy surgery, in whom it is used for mapping interictal discharges and the localization of brain function when superimposed on brain MRI.

Metabolic studies. Metabolic studies are ideally performed at the time of the seizure occurrence, when values are most likely to be abnormal. Lumbar puncture should be considered for children with repeated seizures and other evidence of neurodevelopmental disability. It may be useful for detecting low cerebrospinal fluid glucose in glucose transporter disorder; alterations in amino acids, neurotransmitters, or cofactors in metabolic disorders; or evidence of chronic infection.

Aside from glucose determination, laboratory testing such as serum electrolyte levels and toxicology screening should be based on individual clinical circumstances, such as evidence of dehydration. An EEG is not warranted after a simple febrile seizure but may be useful for evaluating individuals with an atypical feature or with other risk factors for later epilepsy. Similarly, neuroimaging is also not useful for children with simple febrile convulsions but may be considered for children with atypical features, including focal neurologic signs or preexisting neurologic deficits.[17]

Specialized neuropsychologic testing is often needed in evaluating clients with seizures. These tests not only help determine general intelligence and state of brain functioning but also often help to localize lesions.

A radiographic examination of the brain is indicated to rule out mass effect or vascular disease. MRI is the method of choice, since the lesions that cause epilepsy are often subtle.

TREATMENT. Control of seizures is paramount in the treatment of epilepsy, but it is only part of the treatment. Support and education provided by health care professionals is critical to manage the behavioral, social, and economic consequences of uncontrolled seizures. Reassurance should be given that for most individuals, epilepsy does not indicate serious brain damage. The risk-to-benefit ratio for antiepileptic treatments is one of the biggest challenges in seizure management. Because antiepileptic drugs have various adverse effects, which may interfere with normal developmental processes and affect cognitive functions, the adverse effects of more aggressive treatments compared to the benefits of complete seizure control must be considered.[6] Table 36-3 describes common side effects to typical drugs. Antiepileptic drugs carry risks of side effects that are particularly important in children. The decision as to whether or not to treat children and adolescents who have experienced a first unprovoked seizure must be based on a risk-benefit assessment that weighs the risk of having another seizure against the risks of long-term antiepileptic drug therapy. There appears to be no benefit of treatment with regard to the prognosis for long-term seizure remission.[15] Suppressing interictal discharges can improve behavior in children with epilepsy and behavioral problems, particularly focal seizures. Focal discharges may be involved in the underlying mechanisms of behavioral problems in children with epilepsy.[27]

Antiepileptic drugs are used according to the type of seizure. In most people with seizures of a single type, satisfactory control can be achieved with a single anticonvulsant drug. Monitoring of plasma drug levels has increased the ability to maintain the drug at the maximal tolerated dose. In general, drug testing should be performed during the course of treatment and again when good seizure control has been established. Continued testing may be necessary if changes in control or if side effects occur. It sometimes takes a trial of several different medications at different doses to find the best fit. In people who do not comply with the drug regimen, no drug may be better than an inconsistent dosage.[1,4] Older individuals more often have difficulty with the neurologic side effects of

Table 36-3	Side Effects of Commonly Used Antiepileptic Drugs	
Drug	**Common Side Effects**	**Serious Side Effects**
Carbamazepine	Dizziness, diplopia, blurred vision, ataxia, sedation, nausea, neutropenia, rash,* hyponatremia	Agranulocytosis, aplastic anemia, hepatic failure, Stevens-Johnson syndrome
Lacosamide	Dizziness, diplopia, blurred vision, headache, nausea	PR interval prolongation, atrial fibrillation, atrial flutter, multiorgan hypersensitivity
Lamotrigine	Dizziness, diplopia, blurred vision, insomnia, headache, rash	Stevens-Johnson syndrome, toxic epidermal necrolysis, multiorgan failure, hepatic failure
Levetiracetam	Fatigue, dizziness, somnolence, irritability, mood swings	Psychosis
Oxcarbazepine	Dizziness, diplopia, blurred vision, headache, nausea, hyponatremia	Stevens-Johnson syndrome, toxic epidermal necrolysis
Phenytoin	Fatigue, dizziness, ataxia, nausea, confusion, gingival hyperplasia, hirsutism, osteopenia, rash	Stevens-Johnson syndrome, toxic epidermal necrolysis, blood dyscrasia, pseudolymphoma, lupus-like syndrome
Pregabalin	Fatigue, dizziness, ataxia, diplopia, weight gain, edema	None reported
Rufinamide	Somnolence, headache, dizziness, diplopia, fatigue, nausea	Shortened QT interval (no known clinical risk), multiorgan hypersensitivity
Topiramate	Drowsiness, ataxia, word-finding difficulty, difficulty concentrating, anorexia, weight loss, paresthesias, metabolic acidosis, oligohidrosis, nephrolithiasis	Acute close angle glaucoma, heat stroke
Valproate	Drowsiness, ataxia, tremor, weight gain, hair loss, thrombocytopenia, hyperammonemia	Hepatic failure, pancreatitis, aplastic anemia, blood dyscrasias, lupus-like syndrome, Stevens-Johnson syndrome, toxic epidermal necrolysis
Zonisamide	Drowsiness, ataxia, difficulty concentrating, anorexia, weight loss, nausea, nephrolithiasis, oligohidrosis	Aplastic anemia, rash, Stevens-Johnson syndrome, toxic epidermal necrolysis, heat stroke

*HLA-B*1502 testing is recommended in patients of Asian descent (haplotype associated with higher risk of Stevens-Johnson syndrome).
From Asconapé JJ: The selection of antiepileptic drugs for the treatment of epilepsy in children and adults. *Neurol Clin* 28:843-852, 2010.

dizziness, imbalance, drowsiness, and tremors. Cognitive deficits may worsen with topiramate, and mood disorders may worsen with phenobarbital, topiramate, and benzodiazepines.[2]

Psychiatric comorbidities are extremely common in patients with epilepsy. Depression, anxiety disorders, panic disorder, psychosis, attention deficit disorders, and autistic disorders are overrepresented in patients with epilepsy. Antiepileptic drugs can have significant, either positive or negative, effects on mood. Some of these medications that are associated with a higher risk of depression include levetiracetam, phenobarbital, primidone, topiramate, vigabatrin, and zonisamide. Medications with a positive psychotropic effect include carbamazepine, lamotrigine, oxcarbazepine, and valproate. Almost every antiepileptic drug can cause or worsen attention deficit disorders, but the most common offenders include phenobarbital, primidone, benzodiazepines, and vigabatrin. Drugs with a favorable profile for an elderly patient include lamotrigine, pregabalin, and levetiracetam. A slow titration and conservative maintenance doses are especially important in the elderly.

The abundance of drugs makes decisions more complex, but can help manage the needs of more patients. The newer drugs have shown no better efficacy than the classic drugs, but they are easier to use, with much better pharmacokinetic profiles and fewer drug interactions. New drugs create broad-spectrum effects to control symptoms in patients with generalized epilepsies. Newer drugs are listed in Table 36-4. Comorbidities can be managed using antiepileptic drugs; positive effects or at least no negative effects can increase tolerance to the drug. Figure 36-3

Table 36-4	Antiepileptic Drugs and Year of Introduction	
Drug	**Brand Name**	**Year Introduced in USA**
felbamate[a]	Felbatol	1993
gabapentin	Neurontin	1994
lamotrigine	Lamictal	1994
lacosamide	Vimpat	2009
levetiracetam	Keppra	1999
oxcarbazepine	Trileptal	2000
pregabalin	Lyrica	2005
rufinamide	Banzel	2008
tiagabine	Gabitril	1997
topiramate	Topama	1996
vigabatrin*	Sabril	2009
zonisamide	Zonegran	2000

*Restricted use due to serious safety issues. Careful risk-benefit analysis required.
From Asconapé JJ: The selection of antiepileptic drugs for the treatment of epilepsy in children and adults. *Neurol Clin* 28:843-852, 2010.

diagrams the pharmacologic effects of some antiepileptic drugs at the GABA class A ($GABA_A$) receptor. The relationships among hormones, epilepsy, and the medications used to treat epilepsy are complex, with interactions that affect both men and women in different ways. Antiepileptic drugs and hormones have a bidirectional interaction that can impair the efficacy of contraceptive hormone treatments and the chosen epileptic drug.[25] Adrenocorticotropic hormone is the preferred drug for

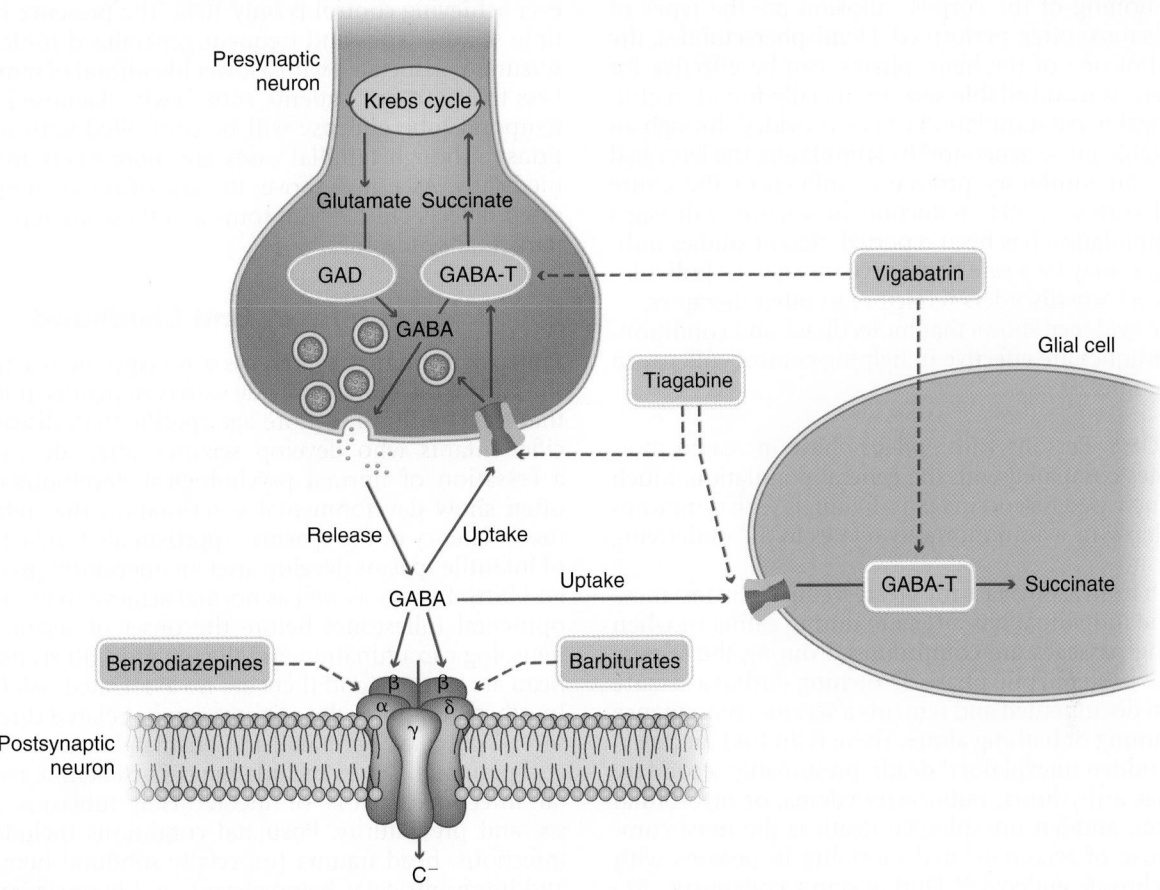

Figure 36-3

Pharmacologic effects of antiepileptic drugs at the γ-aminobutyric acid class A (GABA$_A$) receptor. Barbiturates bind to a β-subunit of the GABA$_A$ receptor to potentiate the action of the endogenous agonist GABA and prolong the opening time of the chloride ion channel. Benzodiazepines bind to an α-subunit of GABA$_A$ to potentiate the action of GABA and increase the frequency of opening of the chloride ion channel. Vigabatrin irreversibly binds to GABA transaminase (GABA-T) to inhibit degradation of the inhibitory neurotransmitter GABA. Tiagabine blocks the uptake of synaptically released GABA into both presynaptic neurons and glial cells, allowing GABA to remain at the site of action for longer periods. *GAD*, Glutamic acid decarboxylase. (From Leach JP, Brodie MJ: Tiagabine. *Lancet* 351:203, 1998.)

the management of infantile spasms, although the dose and duration of therapy are not uniform. Prednisone is also effective.

Anticonvulsive drugs are safe, but side effects do occur, especially at the start of drug therapy. Side effects of the medication may be ataxia, dysarthria, dizziness and blurring, or double vision. Fatigue is a common complaint.[5] When phenytoin is taken, osteomalacia may occur as a result of increased metabolism of vitamin D. Hyponatremia can occur at low doses of carbamazepine and should be of concern when combined with a diuretic or in individuals with cardiac failure.[28] Newer medications, such as lamotrigine, gabapentin, vigabatrin, and topiramate, are shown to be effective as add-on drugs demonstrating low interaction with other drugs.[11] These drugs are more expensive. Allergic reactions are often in the form of a rash, and in these cases a change to another medication should be made.

Ketogenic diet can be a valuable therapeutic approach for epilepsy, used mostly with children. It is a diet high in fats, with enough protein for normal growth and energy and a low threshold for carbohydrates. Although the mechanism by which the diet protects against seizures

is unknown, there is evidence that it causes effects on intermediary metabolism that influence the dynamics of the major inhibitory and excitatory neurotransmitter systems in brain. During consumption of the ketogenic diet, marked alterations in brain energy metabolism occur, with ketone bodies partly replacing glucose as fuel. Whether these metabolic changes contribute to acute seizure protection is unclear; however, the ketone body acetone has anticonvulsant activity and could play a role in the seizure protection afforded by the diet. In addition to acute seizure protection, the ketogenic diet provides protection against the development of spontaneous recurrent seizures in models of chronic epilepsy. The use of valproic acid is contraindicated in association with the ketogenic diet, because the risk of hepatotoxicity is enhanced.[12] Many people with epilepsy experience a higher frequency of seizures with large doses of caffeine. Amphetamines and other stimulants should be avoided, and some asthma drugs can increase the incidence of seizure activity.

When drug therapy does not control the seizures or drugs become toxic at effective dosages, then surgical treatment is indicated. Lobectomies, cortical resections, and sectioning of the corpus callosum are the types of surgeries most often performed. Hemispherectomies, the removal of one of the hemispheres, can be effective for the severe, uncontrollable seizures usually found in children. Vagal nerve stimulation can be provided through an implantable pulse generator. By stimulating the left vagal nucleus, an inhibitory projection influences the entire cerebral cortex. A 50% reduction in seizure with vagal nerve stimulation has been reported. Recent studies indicate that it may be a safe adjunctive therapy for individuals with seizure disorders refractory to other therapies.

Some evidence shows that biofeedback and conditioning techniques are effective in helping control epilepsy in some people.[9,29]

PROGNOSIS. Persons with epilepsy have increased mortality rates compared with the general population. Much of this increased risk occurs in individuals with symptomatic epilepsy in whom mortality relates to the underlying condition.

Death from asphyxia is the greatest concern in instances when the individual has a seizure during eating or when breathing passages are compromised during the seizure or in the postepileptic phase. Drowning during a seizure has been documented and remains a serious consequence of swimming or bathing alone. There is 20-fold increased risk of sudden unexplained death, presumably secondary to cardiac arrhythmia, pulmonary edema, or myocardial infarction. Sudden unexplained death is the most common cause of seizure-related mortality in persons with severe, chronic epilepsy.[24] During status epilepticus, 3% of children and 10% of adults die during an attack.[26] The longer an individual suffers from intractable epilepsy, the higher the possibility of exposure to factors that result in seizure-induced neuronal damage, the more prolonged the exposure to antiepilepsy drugs, and the greater the risk of seizure-related accidents, including closed head injuries.[23]

The correlation between depression and epilepsy is strong, and attempted suicide is higher than the norm in those with epilepsy. People with epilepsy are more likely to be hospitalized for depression. Young people are at particular risk for development of depression and other psychiatric disorders and are less likely to be treated. Despite evidence that two thirds of children with epilepsy have a diagnosable psychiatric disorder, only about one third receive psychiatric treatment.[11]

In people with epilepsy of no known cause and for whom a diagnosis is made before age 10, a 75% remission rate (defined as 5 seizure-free years) is seen. A child with epilepsy who has been free of seizures for more than 4 years while taking antiepileptic drugs has about a 70% chance of remaining in permanent remission when the drugs are withdrawn.

Chronic epilepsy is more likely when associated neurologic impairment is present at birth, and when the seizures begin before 2 years of age.[21] The duration of active epilepsy before achieving control is one of the most powerful predictors of remission. If seizures remain uncontrolled during the first year after diagnosis, the chance of ever achieving control is only 60%. If the period of uncontrolled seizures extends to 4 years, the chance of

ever achieving control is only 10%. The presence of multiple seizure types and frequent generalized tonic-clonic seizures is associated with a lower likelihood of remission. Less than 40% of patients with newly diagnosed mesial temporal lobe epilepsy will be controlled with medications, although familial cases are more easily managed medically. As noted above, the age of onset of epilepsy often reflects typical symptoms and these are reported as particular syndromes.

Epilepsies of Infancy and Childhood

Epilepsy in infancy represents a nonspecific reaction on the part of the brain to a wide variety of insults. It is likely that the condition is more age specific than disease specific. Infants who develop seizures often demonstrate a cessation of normal psychological development and often show developmental deterioration that relates to the frequency of the spasms. Approximately 10% to 20% of infantile spasms develop after an uneventful pregnancy and birth history as well as normal achievement of developmental milestones before the onset of seizures. The neurologic examination and the CT and MRI scans of the head are normal, and there are no associated risk factors. In other situations, the seizures can be related directly to several prenatal, perinatal, and postnatal factors. Prenatal and perinatal factors include hypoxia-ischemia, congenital infections, errors of metabolism, tuberous sclerosis, and prematurity. Postnatal conditions include CNS infections, head trauma (especially subdural hematoma and intraventricular hemorrhage), and hypoxic-ischemic encephalopathy. Dysfunction of the monoaminergic neurotransmitter system in the brainstem, derangement of neuronal structures in the brainstem, and an abnormality of the immune system may underlie the seizure activity. Stresses or injury to an infant during a critical period of neurodevelopment may cause corticotropin-releasing hormone overproduction, resulting in neuronal hyperexcitability. The number of corticotropin-releasing hormone receptors reaches a maximum in the infant brain, followed by spontaneous reduction with age, which may account for the high incidence of eventual resolution. Exogenous adrenocorticotropic hormone and glucocorticoids suppress corticotropin-releasing hormone synthesis, which may account for their effectiveness in treatment.

Febrile Convulsions

Febrile convulsions, the most common seizure disorder during childhood, generally have an excellent prognosis but may also signify a serious underlying acute infectious disease such as sepsis or bacterial meningitis. They are rare before 6 months and after age 5 and are a result of fever. The typical febrile convulsion is brief, generalized, and tonic-clonic in sequence, and the body temperature is high. The seizures occur more often when the child is asleep. The convulsion is often the first indication that the child is ill, because 90% of all seizures occur in the first 24 hours of fever. The rise in temperature, which may be a result of increased oxygen demands on cerebral oxidative mechanisms, may be the most important factor. Severe febrile seizures are most often unilateral, and a possibility exists for permanent brain damage, with the development of epilepsy, if the seizure lasts more than 30 minutes.[21]

Although most affected children have no long-term consequences, febrile seizures increase the risk of future epilepsy. This risk is low for most children, but increases when there is a family history of afebrile seizures or if there were neurologic abnormalities before the first febrile seizure. Febrile seizures are not associated with nor do they cause mental retardation, below-average IQ, poor school performance, or behavior problems. Prophylactic treatment generally is not indicated because of the benign prognosis. Routine treatment of a normal infant with simple febrile convulsions includes a careful search for the cause of the fever; active measures to control the fever, including the use of antipyretics.[17]

Severe Myoclonic Epilepsy of Infancy

Severe myoclonic epilepsy of infancy is a syndrome of early normal development followed by treatment-resistant seizures of various types and by psychomotor retardation, usually beginning at 5 to 6 months of age. These attacks are often long and may include status epilepticus. Mental retardation is noted in all cases.

Benign Myoclonic Epilepsy of Infancy

Benign myoclonus begins during infancy and consists of clusters of myoclonic movements confined to the neck, trunk, and extremities. Mutations in two potassium channel genes (*KCNQ2*, *KCNQ3*) have been associated with this syndrome. Potassium-channel regulation may be age dependent. The myoclonic activity may be confused with infantile spasms; however, the EEG is normal in individuals with benign myoclonus. The prognosis is good, with normal development and the cessation of myoclonus by 2 years of age. An anticonvulsant is not indicated.

Lennox-Gastaut Syndrome

Lennox-Gastaut syndrome usually begins between 1 and 6 years of age. The most common seizures are atonic-akinetic, resulting in loss of postural tone. Violent falls occur suddenly, followed by immediate recovery and resumption of activity, with the attack lasting less than 1 second. Injuries to the head and face are common. Tonic attacks consist of sudden flexion of the head and trunk. Clusters of attacks are common, followed by automatic behavior. Consciousness is usually clouded rather than completely lost. Neurologic abnormalities such as spasticity are common in severely affected children.[21]

Landau-Kleffner Syndrome

Landau-Kleffner syndrome is an acquired aphasia in the absence of other neurologic abnormalities. Often epileptic seizures and psychomotor disturbances develop at the same time or shortly afterward. This disorder often begins between ages 3 and 9. The age of onset is critical for the long-term loss of language. It is postulated that recently acquired skills are particularly vulnerable to any disturbance of brain function. If the formation of intracerebral connections is prevented by abnormal neuronal firings of epilepsy during optimal periods of language learning in children, then such connections may never become functional and the ability to develop language is lost.[13]

Benign Childhood Epilepsy with Centrotemporal Spikes (BECTS)

Benign childhood epilepsy with centrotemporal spikes typically occurs between the ages of 3 and 13 and is characterized by brief, simple partial hemifacial motor seizures. Childhood epilepsy with occipital paroxysms is a syndrome similar to benign childhood epilepsy with centrotemporal spikes, but it includes visual symptoms at onset, and some children have associated migraine headache. Nearly 50% of cases have a family history of epilepsy, and most have no known brain abnormality. The EEG shows spiking in the centrotemporal region. In some cases, the disorder may not require treatment because it usually remits spontaneously.

Childhood Absence Epilepsy

Childhood absence epilepsy begins between ages 4 and 10 years. The attacks may occur many times a day. Absence attacks often can be precipitated by hyperventilation. The attacks were previously described as petit mal and are characterized by a blank stare with unresponsiveness, rhythmic blinking, and, sometimes, a few small clonic jerks of arms or hands. Behavior and awareness return immediately to normal. There is no postictal period and usually no recollection that a seizure has occurred. The attacks last for between 10 and 45 seconds. Longer absence attacks accompanied by perseverative automatisms can also occur. Absence seizures commonly coexist with generalized tonic-clonic or myoclonic seizures. Untreated, absence seizures can occur hundreds of times each day, a condition referred to as pyknolepsy. Figure 36-4 shows the EEG of a child with absence epilepsy.

Lapses of awareness that have a more gradual onset, do not resolve as abruptly, and are accompanied by autonomic features or loss of muscle tone are called atypical absence seizures. These events occur most often in children with mental retardation, and they do not respond as well to antiepileptic drug treatment. Typical and atypical absence seizures also must be distinguished from dyscognitive or focal motor seizure manifested only by brief lapses of consciousness, because cause, treatment, and prognosis differ among these seizure types.[24]

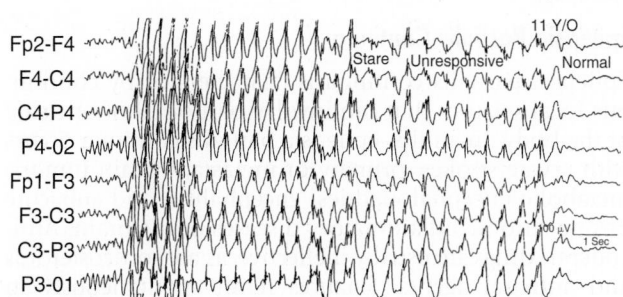

Figure 36-4

Childhood absence epilepsy. Electroencephalogram shows the typical pattern of generalized 3-Hz spike-wave complexes associated with a clinical absence seizure. (From Goldman L: *Cecil textbook of medicine,* ed 22, Philadelphia, 2004, Saunders.)

Juvenile Myoclonic Epilepsy (Janz Syndrome)

Juvenile myoclonic epilepsy (Janz syndrome) has its onset in early adolescence, between ages 8 and 20 years, in otherwise healthy individuals with normal intelligence and a family history of similar seizures. Consciousness is unimpaired, and mental retardation is not evident. It begins with early morning jerks of the head, neck, and upper limbs, making hair combing and toothbrushing difficult. As the myoclonus tends to abate later in the morning, most individuals do not seek medical advice at this stage and some deny the episodes. A few years later, early morning generalized tonic-clonic seizures develop. A gene locus has been identified on chromosome band 6p21. The seizures are especially linked to sleep deprivation and tend to appear often in college students. A proportion of these individuals have had absence seizures as well.

Epilepsy Not Related to Age

Posttraumatic Epilepsy

After penetrating wounds and other severe head injuries, about one third of individuals have seizures within 1 year. Although most individuals experience seizures within 1 to 2 years of injury, new-onset seizures still may appear 5 or more years later. Two thirds of individuals with posttraumatic epilepsy have generalized seizures. Mild head injuries (e.g., uncomplicated brief loss of consciousness, no skull fracture, absence of focal neurologic signs, no contusion or hematoma) do not increase the risk of seizures to a clinically significant degree.

Impact seizures (a generalized convulsion occurring at the time of, or immediately after, the injury) and early seizures (seizures occurring within the first 1 to 2 weeks) represent acute reactions of the brain to the trauma. Seizures beginning after 10 to 14 days reflect an increased risk of posttraumatic epilepsy development. Early seizures should be treated with phenytoin. To minimize complications from seizures occurring during acute management, phenytoin also should be given prophylactically for 1 to 2 weeks to individuals who have had severe head injuries. In the absence of overt attacks, phenytoin use should be discontinued after 2 weeks, because no data indicate that antiepileptic drugs prevent the development of later epilepsy.[24]

Epilepsia Partialis Continua

Epilepsia partialis continua is characterized by continuous focal seizures that can involve part or all of one side of the body. In adults, epilepsia partialis continua occurs with severe strokes, primary or metastatic brain tumors, metabolic encephalopathies, encephalitis, and subacute or rare chronic inflammatory diseases of the brain. Antiepileptic drugs are usually ineffective, as are corticosteroids and antiviral agents. Seizures remit spontaneously in some cases. Rasmussen encephalitis is one cause of epilepsia partialis continua. The onset is usually before age 10. Sequelae include hemiplegia, hemianopia, and aphasia. The disease is progressive and potentially lethal but more often becomes self-limited with significant neurologic deficits. The disease may be due to autoantibodies that bind to and stimulate the glutamate receptors. Studies have identified cytomegalovirus in several surgical specimens of individuals with Rasmussen encephalitis.[17]

SPECIAL IMPLICATIONS FOR THE THERAPIST 36-1

Epilepsy

Understanding the facts about epilepsy is important for therapists who may encounter an individual with epilepsy or if a seizure occurs in the work environment. Box 36-4 presents basic information regarding seizure that separates fact from myth.

The client who is experiencing a seizure normally only needs protection from injury in the environment. The therapist should make sure that no objects in the immediate area can be knocked onto the person and that the individual with seizure activity is lying on a surface that will prevent a fall. Rolling the person onto his or her side may help to keep the airway clear. Observation of physical manifestations, respiratory status, focal or general status, and duration of the seizure are important to the ongoing medical management. When the seizure appears to be generalized, observation of frothing at the mouth, deviation of the eyes, and incontinence will add information for the health practitioners attempting to control the client's seizures medically.

If the individual develops status epilepticus, emergency measures must be taken. Irreversible brain damage can result from hypoxia, and therefore an airway must be established, possibly through endotracheal intubation. Medication to suppress the CNS given at this point usually includes diazepam or lorazepam, and this is usually effective in controlling the seizure. If the seizure continues, phenobarbital may be administered, and if that is not successful, general anesthesia may be given, and the person may then require ventilatory assistance.[1,32]

The psychologic consequences are of concern. Seizure activity can often cause severe loss of confidence

---

Box 36-4

COMMON MISCONCEPTIONS ABOUT EPILEPSY

Myth: You can swallow your tongue during a seizure.
Fact: It's physically impossible to swallow your tongue.
Myth: You should restrain someone during a seizure.
Fact: Do not use restraint; the seizure will run its course and stop.
Myth: People with epilepsy should not be in jobs of responsibility and stress.
Fact: People with epilepsy hold many types of jobs; they often do not inform others of the disorder.
Myth: You can't tell what a person may do during a seizure.
Fact: The characteristic form of seizure is consistent during each episode. Behavior may be inappropriate for the time and place but will most likely not cause harm.
Myth: You can't die from epilepsy.
Fact: Status epilepticus can cause death. It should be treated as a medical emergency.

and restriction of lifestyle. For the therapist treating a client with epilepsy, it is important to have an understanding of the triggering activities associated with seizure. Knowing the type and frequency of seizures helps the therapist make recommendations regarding activities that can be engaged in safely. If compliance with the medication regimen appears to be a problem, the therapist should give the family information regarding the need to maintain consistent dosages. The therapist may be able to help the client or family understand the relationship between epilepsy and depression, and assist in the appropriate referral.

Evaluation of the home, work, and school environments should be performed so the therapist can make specific recommendations. The client sometimes needs to be encouraged to become part of the group activity. Too often, the client has been discouraged from engaging in sports or leisure activities even when the seizures are controlled. When a potential safety hazard exists, the therapist is well suited to recommend adaptations to equipment or the environment to maintain safety. Swimming can even be enjoyed as long as it is supervised directly.

Seizures often occur after activity, and so safety measures should be considered even after the activity is finished. Loss of fluids from sweating during exercise can affect the serum blood levels of medication and increase the metabolism of liver enzymes. Decisions about whether to engage in vigorous activity should be made on the basis of whether seizures are controlled by medication and only after close monitoring of blood levels of medication after exercise.

Side effects of medication can slow cognitive function or alter reaction time. Movement disorders, including nystagmus, ataxia, and dysarthria, may be related to medication. Lethargy, nausea, irritability, and skin rashes may be the result of intolerance to medication. When these symptoms are noted during intervention, the proper health care worker should be notified. The client and family should have a clear understanding of symptoms related to toxicity or nontherapeutic doses of medication.

Restriction of activity may be important in the first 2 to 3 months after the first seizure, after treatment is initiated and until it can be determined that further seizures are unlikely. When antiepileptic drugs are discontinued, activity should be limited initially. In the case of children for whom the epileptic syndrome progresses, limitations may change over time.

REFERENCES

To enhance this text and add value for the reader, all references are included on the companion Evolve site that accompanies this textbook. The reader can view the reference source and access it online whenever possible.

CHAPTER 37

Headache

KENDA S. FULLER • HEATHER CAMPBELL

OVERVIEW

Even though headache has no obvious catastrophic end point, it has the potential to erode a person's daily quality of life during what should be the most productive years. In fact, it is the rare individual who has never experienced a headache, less than 4% of the population.[136] Headache status appears on initial intakes and evaluations as it is a common primary complaint as well as a pervasive comorbidity to be managed by physical therapists. The symptoms can limit one's ability to perform daily tasks. Excess fatigue, the need to stop activity in order to limit external impact such as light and sound, and the inability to concentrate, will impact a patient's participation in therapy.

Headache can be difficult to evaluate; however, the intensity, quality, and site of pain may provide clues. Because the diagnosis of headache is essentially a clinical diagnosis, the physical therapist is often involved in the diagnosis. Awareness of the variety of manifestations can direct intervention both medically and physically. Current understanding of the pathology and physiology of the headache puts it into the realm of the neurologic evaluation. The therapist should understand the cause, precipitating factors, and typical course of both episodic and chronic headache pain. Understanding headache is a challenging task given the large number of headache syndromes and the possibility of a continuum between headache types.[48,117,124]

The International Classification of Headache Disorders 2nd Edition (ICHD 2), published in 2004 is the current standard system used for both clinical and research purposes. Box 37-1 shows the major categories and will be used as reference in this chapter. The headaches are described according to the phenomenology of the headache symptoms. Headaches are further categorized by frequency and acute or chronic states or can carry the status of probable when the symptoms lead toward a diagnosis but do not fit all criteria.

The primary headaches are those not caused by other diseases. Examples of primary headaches are migraine, tension-type, and cluster headache and other trigeminal cephalgias.

The secondary headaches are caused by associated disease or trauma, are categorized by etiology, and can have diverse causes, ranging from serious and life-threatening conditions such as brain tumors, strokes, meningitis, and subarachnoid hemorrhages to less serious but common conditions such as withdrawal from caffeine and discontinuation of analgesics. Secondary headaches can be associated with systemic illness, fever, and significantly increased blood pressure. Headache attributed to psychiatric disorder has been added as a category, and will likely expand as the understanding of the underlying physiology improves. The hallmark of secondary headaches is that they resolve when the underlying cause is successfully treated.[3] Secondary headaches will be discussed as well in the various chapters under the primary diagnosis (Stoke, Infectious Disease, Degenerative Disorders, Epilepsy and Vestibular Disorders, etc.).

Cranial Neuralgias, central and primary facial pain and other headaches, considered the third category, includes pain that projects to the face. The causes may be external or internal.

In 2006 the IHS nomenclature committee published an appendix definition for chronic migraine characterized by a pattern of headaches experienced by a patient, rather than focusing on symptoms of individual headache attacks. The potential progressive nature of migraine is addressed here, such that episodic migraine is considered a precursor to chronic migraine. The spectrum of clinical phenotypes of primary headache observed in patients with chronic migraine ranged from IHS migraine to IHS tension-type headache (TTH).[68] It has been determined that different clinical phenotypes of primary headache witnessed in a patient with migraine might share common biological mechanisms.[99] Figure 37-1 illustrates the pain patterns associated with typical complaints of headache and head pain.[29] Note that according to the ICHD 2, sinusitis would be considered Secondary Headache; categorized as 11.5 or 11.8. Trigeminal neuralgia would be classified as 13.1 and considered under part three.

PRIMARY HEADACHES

Migraine 1

Overview and Definition

Migraine is derived from the Greek word *hemicranias*. It is a neurobiologic headache disorder that is caused by increased central nervous system excitability. The definition of the World Federation of Neurology contains the

Box 37-1

IHS CLASSIFICATIONS OF HEADACHES

This classification is hierarchical and you must decide how detailed you want to make your diagnosis. This can range from the first-digit level to the fourth. First, one gets a rough idea about which group the patient belongs to. Is it, for example, 1. Migraine or 2. Tension-type headache or 3. Cluster headache and other trigeminal autonomic cephalalgias? Then one obtains information allowing a more detailed diagnosis. The desired detail depends on the purpose. In general practice, only the first- or second-digit diagnoses are usually applied, whereas in specialist practice and headache centers a diagnosis at the third- or fourth-digit levels is appropriate.

Part I: The Primary Headaches

1. Migraine
   1.1. Migraine without aura
   1.2. Migraine with aura
   1.3. Childhood periodic syndromes that are commonly precursors of migraine
   1.4. Retinal migraine
   1.5. Complications of migraine
   1.6. Probable migraine
2. Tension-type headache
   2.1. Infrequent episodic tension-type headache
   2.2. Frequent episodic tension-type headache
   2.3. Chronic tension-type headache
   2.4. Probable tension-type headache
3. Cluster headache and other trigeminal autonomic cephalalgias
   3.1. Cluster headache
   3.2. Paroxysmal hemicrania

   3.3. Short-lasting unilateral neuralgiform headache attacks with conjunctival injection and tearing (SUNCT)
   3.4. Probable trigeminal autonomic cephalalgia

Part II: The Secondary Headaches

5. Headache attributed to head and/or neck trauma
   5.1 Acute post-traumatic headache
   5.2 Chronic post-traumatic headache
   5.3 Acute headache attributed to whiplash injury [S13.4]
   5.4 Chronic headache attributed to whiplash injury [S13.4]
   5.5 Headache attributed to traumatic intracranial hematoma
   5.6 Headache attributed to other head and/or neck trauma [S06]
   5.7 Post-craniotomy headache
6. Headache attributed to cranial or cervical vascular disorder
7. Headache attributed to nonvascular intracranial disorder
8. Headache attributed to a substance or its withdrawal
9. Headache attributed to infection
10. Headache attributed to disorder of homoeostasis
11. Headache or facial pain attributed to disorder of cranium, neck, eyes, ears, nose, sinuses, teeth, mouth or other facial or cranial structures
12. Headache attributed to psychiatric disorder

Part III: Cranial Neuralgias Central and Primary Facial Pain and Other Headaches

13. Cranial neuralgias and central causes of facial pain
14. Other headache, cranial neuralgia, central or primary facial pain

From the International Headache Society Classification of Headaches.

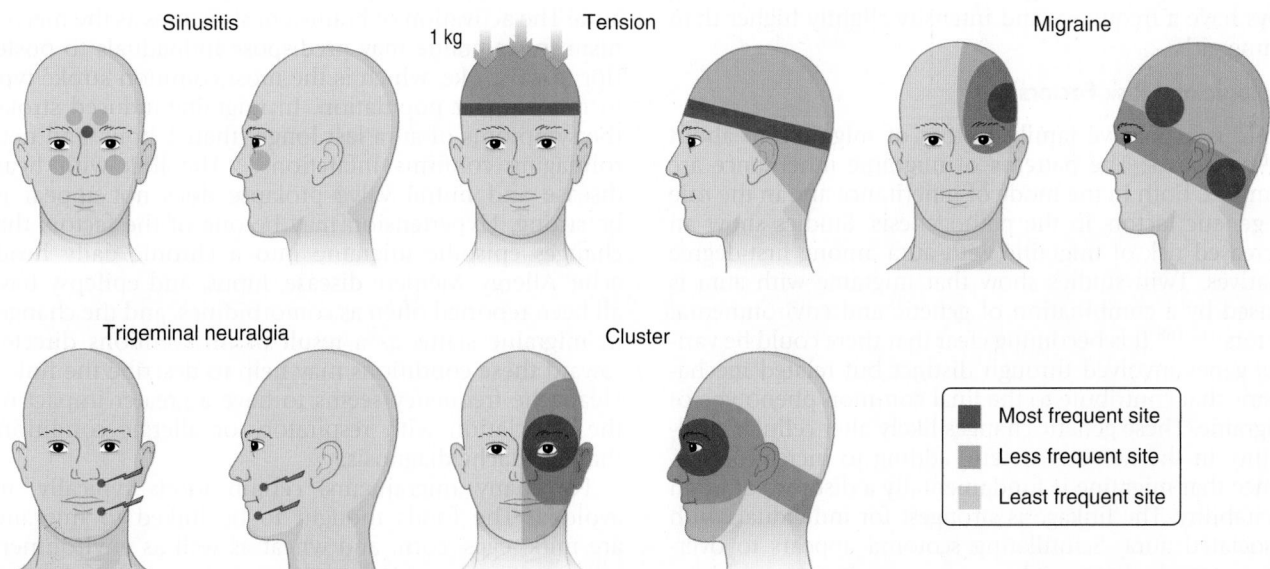

Figure 37-1

Typical headache patterns. Primary headaches include tension-type, migraine, and cluster. Sinus headache, related to infection, is a common secondary headache. Trigeminal neuralgia is an example of cranial neuralgia. (See Chapter 40.) (From Weinstein JM: Headache and facial pain. In Yanoff M, Duker JS, Augsburger JJ, et al, eds: *Ophthalmology*, ed 2, St. Louis, 2004, Mosby.)

following language regarding migraine: "a familial disorder characterized by recurrent attacks of headache widely variable in intensity, frequency and duration. Attacks are commonly unilateral and are usually associated with anorexia, nausea and vomiting. In some cases they are preceded by neurologic and mood disturbances."[180]

The World Health Organization ranks migraine among the world's most disabling medical illnesses.[181] Approximately 28 million Americans have severe, disabling migraine headaches.[100] Migraine's cost to employers is approximately $13 billion a year, and annual medical costs exceed $1 billion.[102]

Incidence

Migraine headaches are the second most common type of primary headache. An estimated 28 million people in the United States, about 12% of the population, will experience migraine headaches at some point.[136] It is now ranked by the World Health Organization as number 19 among all diseases worldwide causing disability. Migraines account for lost work days on the average of 6 days per year for an individual with significant migraine. Engaging in leisure activity is also decreased during headache periods.[27]

An estimated 6% of men and up to 18% of women have migraine headaches. In 90% of migraineurs, the first attack generally develops before the age of 40.[101] Adult women are at greater risk for the development of migraine than are adult men. In women, the frequency of headaches is highest during their reproductive years, when estrogen levels are higher, and decreases to some extent after menopause. Frequency in adult men does not appreciably change between ages 20 and 65 years.[102,137]

About 45% of cases of migraine emerge during childhood or adolescence. Migraine headaches are estimated to appear earlier in males than in females, and in both genders migraine with aura is more likely to develop at an earlier age than migraine without aura.[32,137] Young boys have a frequency and intensity slightly higher than young girls.

Etiologic and Risk Factors

There is a positive family history of migraine in about 60% of cases. The patterns of migraine inheritance are complex, both in the mode of inheritance and in the role of genetic factors in the pathogenesis. Studies show an increased risk of migraine with aura among first-degree relatives. Twin studies show that migraine with aura is caused by a combination of genetic and environmental factors.[112,168] It is becoming clear that there could be various genes involved through distinct but related mechanisms that contribute to the final common phenotype of migraine. These genetic changes likely alter cellular excitability in the nervous system, adding to increasing evidence that migraine is fundamentally a disorder of brain excitability. The linkage is strongest for individuals with associated aura. Scintillating scotoma appears to overlap a recently discovered gene for occipitotemporal lobe epilepsy. Like migraine, genetic forms of epilepsy may be related to neuronal excitability and abnormalities in ion channels, as well as the adaptive response of neurons to environmental stress.[88] These mutations may make the brain more susceptible to prolonged cortical spreading depression via excessive glutamate release or decreased removal of glutamate and potassium from the synaptic cleft.[53]

APOE epsilon2 gene appears to increase the risk of migraine, whereas APOE epsilon4 gene is protective against migraine and TTH.[66]

An allele on chromosome 8q22.1 has been found to influence the propensity for migraine by alteration of the function of astrocytes. This region is located between two genes, metadherin *MTDH* (also known as astrocyte elevated gene-1) and *PGCP* (encoding plasma glutamate carboxypeptidase). Both genes are involved in regulation of concentrations of the excitatory transmitter glutamate in the brain.[15] TRESK, which involves potassium channel currents in neuronal and non-neuronal cells, is postulated to regulate neuronal excitability and might have a particular role in pain transmission. There appears to be prominent TRESK expression in migraine-salient areas, such as the trigeminal ganglion and sensory ganglia.[93] Comorbidity, with possible association to other diseases has been studied. Some genes may predispose to both bipolar disorder and migraine.[121] Genetics have not had significant impact on The International Classification of Headache Disorders, 2nd edition. However, it is expected that within the next 10 years migraine genetics will be elucidated. It will likely change the way we classify headaches. However, the genetics of migraine may prove to be so complex that, in daily practice and research, the clinically defined diagnoses will remain as well.

Migraine is an independent risk factor for ischemic stroke, mainly in the subpopulation of women with migraine with aura who are younger than 45 years, particularly those who use estrogen-containing oral contraceptives. Migraine however should be considered a benign condition as the absolute increase of stroke risk is small.[126] There appears to be a higher incidence of stroke in between migraine attacks in individuals with aura. The activation of brainstem structures as the mechanism for migraine may predispose individuals to posterior fossa stroke, which is the most common stroke type in the younger population. In migraine-induced stroke, the symptoms of aura last longer than 1 hour, and neuroimaging confirms infarction.[115] The link with heart disease and mitral valve prolapse does not appear to be strong. Hypertension may be one of the factors that changes episodic migraine into a chronic daily headache. Allergy, Ménière disease, lupus, and epilepsy have all been reported often as comorbidities, and the changes in migraine status as a result of interventions directed toward these conditions may help to describe the link.[81] Headache frequency seems to have a greater impact on the association with respiratory or allergic conditions than headache diagnosis.[1]

For many migraineurs, certain foods typically are avoided. The foods thought to be linked to migraine are milk, eggs, corn, and wheat as well as environmental factors such as food additives, colorings, coffee, alcohol (especially red wine), and sugar.[134] It appears now that the threshold for a migraine attack probably varies according to many other factors including stress, tiredness, and hormone levels and that individuals are more vulnerable to attacks at certain times. The triggers may be confused with cravings or certain behaviors that are actually part of the start of the migraine, or a premonitory symptom. We know that migraines are often preceded by certain feelings such as tiredness, excitement, or depression or cravings for certain foods. It might be that a craving for chocolate, which is a premonitory symptom, could be misinterpreted as a migraine trigger.[76] Often the headaches are associated with hormonal changes of menstruation and use of oral contraceptives. Pure menstrual migraines appear to be more frequently migraine without aura. It appears that these migraines may be related to the abrupt decrease in estradiol that occurs immediately before menstruation after several days of exposure to high levels of estrogens. It also appears that there may be an intrinsic estrogen receptor sensitivity that differs among women.[110] There is evidence that menstrual attacks are more severe, longer, less responsive to treatment, more likely to relapse, and associated with greater disability than attacks at other times of the cycle.[107] When the headaches follow a pattern related to hormone changes, pregnancy brings periods of both exacerbation and relief. In the first trimester of pregnancy, the number and severity of migraines rise. The headaches abate during the second trimester and then increase again in the third trimester. Migraine can be triggered during delivery and may be more prevalent in the weeks and months following childbirth.[29]

It has been determined that there is not a "migraine personality" but rather that those individuals who are susceptible to migraine may also be at risk for other alterations of the nervous system. Anxiety disorders, especially panic attacks and depression, are characterized by disturbances in the same neurochemical systems, and therefore the syndromes may overlap or could even be considered one syndrome with a subset of conditions. There may also be a central serotonin demodulation that is seen within the context of psychologic disorders. Chronic pain related to migraine may also lead to changes in behavior.[40,43,114]

Pathogenesis

The components of migraine are complex; the mechanisms of dysfunction vary among individuals and among attacks in the same individual. The more that is known about migraine, the more levels of dysfunction are identified.[123] The mechanism that causes pain may be different from the mechanism that causes the neurologic symptoms. Figure 37-2 illustrates the possible mechanisms related to migraine. There appears to be factors of both central and peripheral sensitization and disinhibition resulting from hyperexcitability of cortical and brainstem neurons. The overactivation of these neurons may be the result of underlying channelopathies or ionopathies seen in the genetically predisposed individual.[52] These hyperexcitable neurons activate susceptible parts of the cortex causing aura. Meningeal vessels are sensitized and are susceptible to substances that trigger pain. The firing of these hyperexcitable neurons may be influenced by internal and external factors such as hormonal balance, foodstuffs, stress, and sleep deprivation.[140] The different symptoms observed in migraine probably reflect differential activation of cortical, brainstem, and vascular

structures. The trigger for the migraine may give the clue to the nature of the symptoms. Susceptibility to migraine during periods of recovery from prolonged stress suggests that the mechanism might involve a switch in autonomic balance from sympathetic to parasympathetic dominance.[40,62]

Central Sensitization. The central modulation of pain is related to a complex neurochemical and neurophysiologic system. The central processes of the trigeminal afferents play a major role in migraine pain. Long-lasting central sensitization, via the third-order neurons in the thalamus, may prolong the effects of a pain stimulus

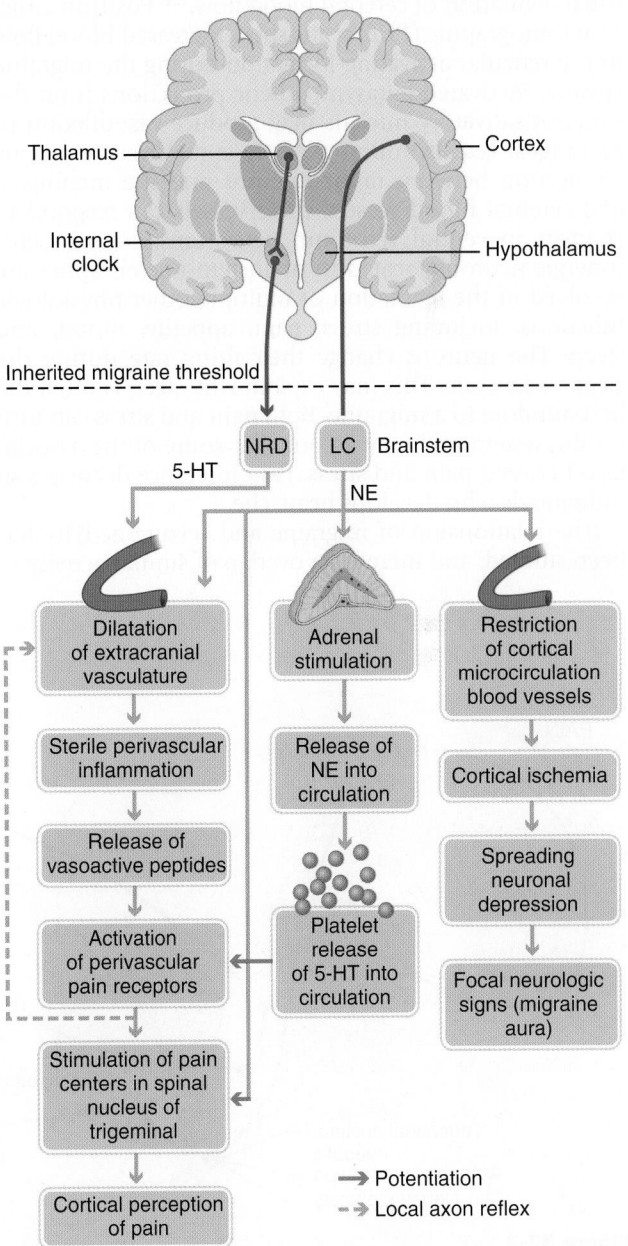

Figure 37-2

Mechanisms that are related to the pathogenesis of migraine headache based on current proposals. (From Weinstein JM: Headache and facial pain. In Yanoff M, Duker JS, Augsburger JJ, et al, eds: *Ophthalmology*, ed 2, St. Louis, 2004, Mosby.)

related to the trigeminal vascular system (Fig. 37-3). The identification of a novel retinothalamic mechanism suggests the additional existence of nontrigeminal pathways for modulation of migraine pain.[21]

Limbic structures (amygdala and insular cortices) and the rostral pons can be triggered by olfactory input and thus points to the strong physiologic relationship between the olfactory and the trigemino-nociceptive pathway in the pathophysiology of migraine disease.

Functional imaging has identified the crucial role of the brainstem in migraine with the primary dysfunction of the endogenous antinociceptive systems, including the periaqueductal gray and the dorsal raphe nucleus in the midbrain as well as the locus ceruleus involved in the neuronal regulation of cerebral blood flow.[106] Positron emission tomographic (PET) scans show increased blood flow in the reticular activating formation during the migraine episode. Activated parasympathetic projections from the superior salivatory nucleus may produce vasodilation of meningeal vessels. Although there is no direct anatomic connection between raphe neurons and the meningeal and cerebral blood vessels, these vessels can respond to changes in central serotonin neurotransmission. Serotonergic neurons located in brainstem nuclei raphes are involved in the regulation of multiple other physiologic functions, including stress, pain, appetite, mood, and sleep. The neurons change their firing rate during the sleep-wake cycle. This may explain why sleep is often the best antidote to a migraine. Both pain and stress can turn on the system and may account for some of the association between pain and stress. Pain tolerance decreases in individuals who develops headache.

The relationship of migraine and seizure activity has been studied, and there is an overlap of similar activity in the brain with cortical spreading depression and kindling (see Chapter 36). It appears that there can be evolution from visual aura to visual seizures related to the threshold of cortical hyperexcitability.[28] Cortical spreading depression may be responsible for the reflex activation of sensory pathways that induce inflammation within the meninges. Spreading depression may release a variety of substances in the cortex such as potassium, hydrogen, and nitric oxide that leak into the extracellular space and activate perivascular trigeminal nerve endings accompanied by local vascular responsiveness. Nitric oxide activates both the primary and second-order neurons of the trigeminal pain pathways. Nitric oxide is produced both immediately after cortical spreading depression and in a second prolonged wave lasting several hours. Spread of first aura symptoms and spread of cortical depression proceed at the same speed. This may explain the initial hypoperfusion that is related to the aura of headache. Cortical hyperemia may be responsible for the flashing jagged light that sometimes occurs just before the pain begins. Once the headache is underway, it appears that the vascularity changes and hyperperfusion are not related to the degree or area of the pain.[157]

Peripheral Sensitization. The trigeminal complex is a key component in the distribution of the pain within the head and neck associated with migraine primarily via the ophthalmic division of the trigeminal ganglion and the upper cervical dorsal roots. Activation of trigeminal neurons also leads to changes in adjacent glia that involve communication through gap junctions and paracrine or local signaling. It is likely that this neuronal-glial communication is involved in the development of peripheral sensitization within the trigeminal ganglion and is likely to play an important role in the initiation of migraine.[165]

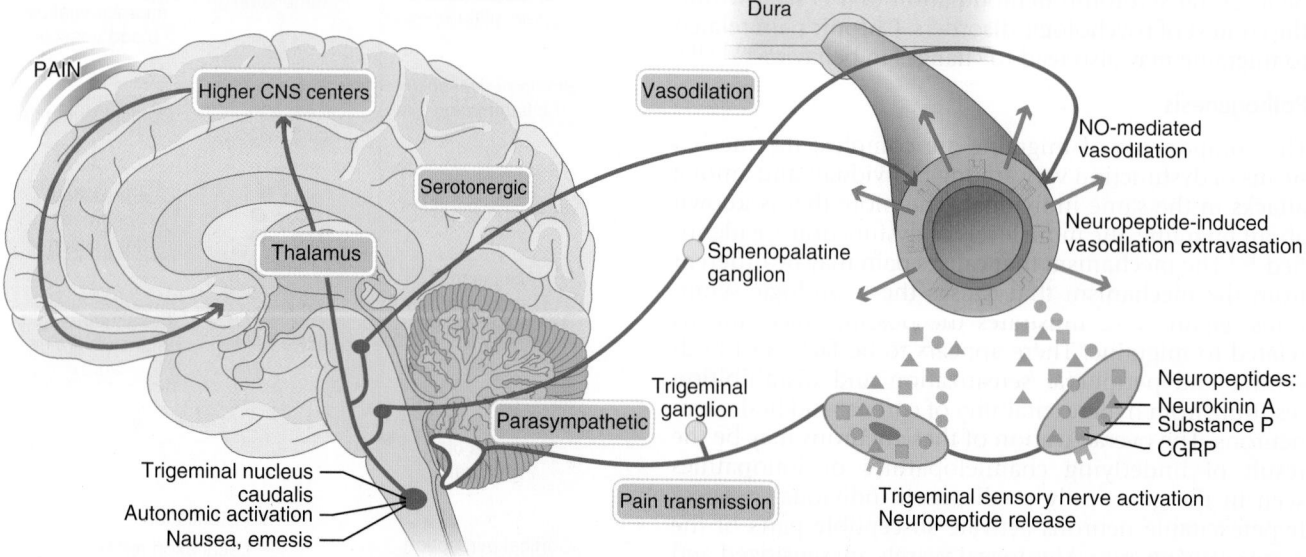

Figure 37-3

Trigeminal vascular theory of migraine headaches. Cortical hyperexcitable neurons, perhaps with an additional influence from brainstem structures, leads to activation of the trigeminovascular system. Signals reach the trigeminal nucleus caudalis in the brainstem, which in turn signals the thalamus, which innervates cortical regions, leading to the conscious sensation of headache and pain. Note that activation of the trigeminal nerve afferents leads to neuropeptide release and vasodilation of dural blood vessels, which in turn leads to release of more neuropeptides, perpetuating the cycle. (From Liu: *Neuro-ophthalmology*, ed 2, Philadelphia, 2010, Saunders.)

The meninges that cover the brain parenchyma, and the arteries of the cortex, are richly supplied by nerve fibers from the trigeminal ganglion and the upper cervical dorsal roots. The dural nerves that innervate the venous sinuses and cranial vessels consist largely of small-diameter myelinated and unmyelinated fibers that are nociceptive in function. These fibers contain substance P and calcitonin gene–related peptide that can be released when the trigeminal ganglion is stimulated, resulting in pain. Sensitization of the mechanoreceptors in these structures enhances the responses to mechanical stimuli.[116] This is thought to be responsible for the diffuse pain often noted in one area of the head and the throbbing pain that seems to be associated with the heartbeat.[29] Routine physical activities such as coughing, sneezing, bending over, or performing the Valsalva maneuver can cause pain through this mechanism. Sterile neuroinflammation is another possible result of the peptide release; however, there does not appear to be the level of tissue damage found in other inflammatory processes. As in other inflammatory disorders, inflammation in migraine is neither the original nor the leading event, but one of the mechanisms involved in its pathogenesis, helping to explain findings such as sensitization.

Visual pathways can become sensitized. A non-image-forming pathway allows maintenance of normal circadian rhythms via the suprachiasmatic nucleus and is regulated by intrinsically photosensitive retinal ganglion cells (ipRGCs). These ipRGCs are independent of the rods and cones and contain melanopsin, a photopigment. Sleep cycles are driven by light/darkness cycles. Blind persons who are able to detect light despite minimal perception of images demonstrate normal sleep patterns but had worsening migraine symptoms with light exposure, suggesting that ipRGCs, and not rods and cones, are important in photophobia. These retinal projections of non-image-forming brain areas project to the thalamus, which is dually sensitive to dural pain and light input. These neurons project widely to multiple cortical regions, including the primary somatosensory cortex, the primary and secondary motor cortices, the parietal association cortex, and the primary and secondary visual cortices.[120]

It appears that additional pain input from muscles and other cranial tissues may contribute to migraine. Modest additional input from pericranial muscles can fire the neurons and cause pain. There is often tenderness of pericranial structures during migraine. It is thought that perhaps cortical and brainstem control may enhance or diminish the pain caused by a certain pain input from these structures. It has been found that tenderness in the neck, not muscle contraction, correlates with headache development.

Neurotransmitter Substances. Neurovascular transmitters and receptors play a role in headache through their influence on the regulation of tone in cranial blood vessels. Endothelial cells found in the vessel wall synthesize and release substances that produce vasodilation and vasoconstriction of the cerebral vessels. Cerebral blood vessels are very responsive to chemical stimuli such as changes in carbon dioxide tension and oxygen level.

Bradykinin, adenosine, and histamine are released not only by neurons but also by endothelium, platelets, and mast cells. These substances have been proposed as local regulators of cerebral blood flow.[33] Study of mutations in the motor nerve terminals that contain P-type calcium channels in mice may shed some light on the mutations that would contribute to changes in acetylcholine release identified with a variety of movement disorders and may also identify part of the mechanism of the pain of migraine. Acetylcholine and vasoactive intestinal polypeptide in the cranial arteries cause relaxation of the vessels. Blood flow increases during the headache, and there appears to be some relationship to the arteries, to referred pain patterns of the veins, and to the site of pain. The middle cerebral artery and the superficial temporal artery on the pain side appear to dilate during migraine.

The neurotransmitter 5-hydroxytryptamine (5-HT), known as serotonin, is a part of the pathogenesis of migraine. Chronically low availability of serotonin is found in individuals with migraine, so a hypersensitivity to the presence of serotonin develops. Platelets contain virtually all the serotonin present in the blood and release serotonin during aggregation. Platelets play an important role in the acute inflammatory response. Aggregated platelets release catecholamines and serotonin that may cause the initial stage of vasoconstriction. Platelet aggregation is increased during the prodromal stage of migraine. This could be due to an increase in epinephrine, thrombin, or arachidonic acid in the circulation in response to anxiety. There appears to be a decrease in aggregation during the actual headache. Reported changes in plasma serotonin may be due to changes in platelet function. Serotonin also excites pain nerve endings and increases the pain response. The serotonergic neurons also have a close association with cortical astroglial cells that help to maintain homeostasis in the brain.[123]

Normally, stimulation of sensory fibers excites γ-aminobutyric acid (GABA) receptors, and the inhibition reduces the excitability of pain neurons in the dorsal horn of the spine in order to modulate pain response to stimulation. This mechanism may be aberrant in migraine sufferers, and so there is less inhibition.[123]

Endocrine Connections. In those individuals with menstrual migraine, there is a link to falling blood levels of estrogen and the migraine may be due to hormone-related pain modulation. Estrogen has a significant effect on the synaptic morphology of the neurons in the periaqueductal gray area. Afferents from the trigeminal nucleus complex and periaqueductal gray areas that project to them contain estrogen receptors. The periaqueductal gray area produces a number of behavioral and physiologic responses, including autonomic changes, sexual behavior, fear and rage reactions, and anxiety. The role of sex hormones associated with migraine may be through dysfunction of the inhibitory circuits from the locus ceruleus to the trigeminal nucleus complex. Higher levels of estrogen are correlated with activity in the locus ceruleus and inhibition of the trigeminal nucleus complex in response to painful stimulation of inflammation, so this is consistent with the typical nature of the headache, which is triggered during the time that the estrogen levels have fallen prior to the onset of menstrual bleeding.[111]

Prostaglandins could also cause the severe systemic upset and nausea and vomiting that occur. Levels of prostaglandins are elevated during migraine in the plasma, saliva, and venous blood. Prostaglandins are also implicated in the bradykinin-induced excitation of nociceptors.[48] Proinflammatory cytokines can cause sensory hypersensitivity and are expressed in the central nervous system by neurons.

Migraine associated with food with containing tyramine may occur in persons who have a deficiency of tyramine-o-sulfatase. The excess tyramine could be responsible for the release of catecholamines and could initiate the vasoconstrictive stages of migraine.

Clinical Manifestations

Migraine is a common, disabling disorder of the central nervous system. The disorder has three key features. The tendency is largely inherited, the sufferer is sensitive to exogenous and endogenous triggers that very often involve challenges to normal homeostatic biology, and the attack phenotype, when severe, is the stereotypical migraine attack. The attack itself consists of an abnormal perception of otherwise normal circumstances, such as pain without evidence of primary nociceptive activation, and light and sound sensitivity without change in ambient stimuli.[61]

Common to the complaints of migraine is the phenomenon of allodynia, or pain responses to common activities such as hair combing, shaving, or wearing earrings or a necklace. This is the result of sensitization of the neurons of the medullary dorsal horn that receive sensory input from the dura and skin. As we know from the description above, this abnormal input is sent to the thalamus and then relayed to the cortex.

Migraine without Aura 1.1. Migraine headaches may be dull or throbbing. They usually build up gradually and may last for 4 to 72 hours. Headache is aggravated by routine physical activity, and there is an association with nausea. Photophobia, or increased sensitivity to light, is common, and the migraineur will often seek a dark, quiet place. There are often various combinations of fatigue, difficulty in concentrating, neck stiffness, blurred vision, yawning, and pallor. When the headache resolves, there is commonly a feeling of heaviness and aching in the head, the scalp may be tender, and there may be considerable fatigue. At the end of the headache, there is often marked diuresis, or increased urination.[32,46]

The trigeminal brainstem nuclear complex has a somatotopic representation of the trigeminal dermatome that is continuous with the representation of the posterior head and neck region in the upper cervical dorsal horn. Pain patterns representing increased neuronal activity in the trigeminal nucleus caudalis and dorsal horn include upper cervical pain, usually on one side only.

Migraine with Aura 1.2. The headache will frequently start with a period of depression, irritability, and loss of appetite. This is often the beginning of what is known as the aura. As stated above, these symptoms are likely the result of spreading depression.

When a migraine is preceded by visual symptoms, it is known as a visual aura. The aura is usually described as changes in the visual field. Visual images change, and there can be loss of focus, spots of darkness, and zigzag flashing lights. It often begins with a hazy spot close to the center of vision; initially vision is unclear or it seems difficult to focus. The hazy spot will form into a star shape that further develops into a shape known as a fortification because it is semicircular with angles like those of fortifications. This scintillating vision consists of luminous, bright, flickering colors of the spectrum, much like a prism catching light. It can be combined with a scotoma, or an area of vision that appears to be obstructed, or missing. The visual image fades as the headache begins. The headache is intense, throbbing, and usually contralateral to the visual field changes.[32] Figure 37-4 shows the image as it would appear during a migraine.

Paresthesias can also be a part of an aura and are second in frequency to visual symptoms. Paresthesias of the hand and face are most common with tingling and numbness of the hands.[94] There is less involvement of the leg and trunk. The paresthesia often involves the tongue, something that is rarely seen in cases of stroke or transient ischemic attack (TIA). The attacks are predictable using the sensory homunculus. Speech difficulty during an aura reflects the involvement of the dominant hemisphere.[46] Vertigo and dizziness may be related to brainstem activity or changes in blood flow around the vestibular mechanism (see "Vestibular Migraine" below). For some individuals, there is a combination of aura symptoms, and the type of aura may change with each episode of headache. Neglect, spatial and geographic disorientation, anxiety, and amnesia have all been associated with the aura of migraine. Autonomic changes can also result in paresthesia of the face or extremities. The aura is fully reversible. Sometimes sensory changes are confused with motor weakness but weakness really occurs only with familial hemiplegic headache.

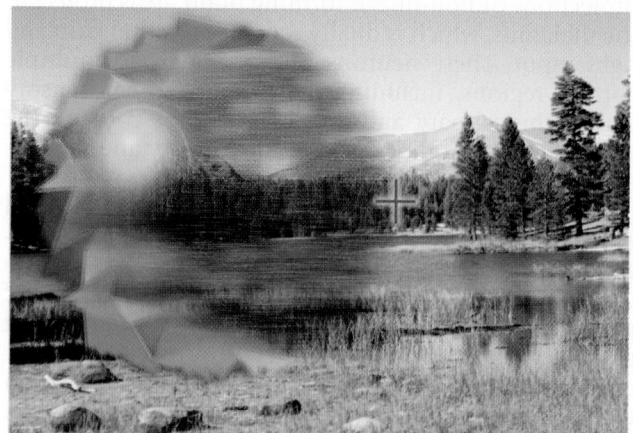

Figure 37-4

Scintillating scotoma in migraine with aura. The leading edge of the scotoma is "positive" (i.e., it consists of bright flickering imagery that obscures or replaces the normal visual field), whereas the trailing edge of the scotoma often is "negative" (i.e., it displays a relatively dark area that fully or partially obscures the visual surround). The illustration depicts a typical fortification scotoma with sharply angulated borders; many other variants of the migraine scotoma may occur. (From Weinstein JM: Headache and facial pain. In Yanoff M, Duker JS, Augsburger JJ, et al, eds: *Ophthalmology*, ed 2, St. Louis, 2004, Mosby.)

Typical Aura without Headache 1.2.3. In some cases, the aura symptoms are not followed by headache. When recurrent aura symptoms occur in the absence of headaches, the distinction from mimicking conditions becomes more important. This is especially important when the symptoms are very short or very long, or if they begin after the age of 40. Aura without headache is seen primarily in men and in advancing age.[46]

Familial Hemiplegic Migraine 1.2.4, Sporadic Familial Hemiplegic Migraine 1.2.5. Although clinicians have long recognized the genetic basis of migraine, only a few specific genes have been discovered. Most genetic advances have involved familial hemiplegic migraine (FHM). Mutations involving the *CACNA1A* gene, a P/Q-type voltage-gated calcium channel located on chromosome 19, are responsible for about half of FHM cases. In addition to hemiplegic aura, these patients with FHM may have cerebellar ataxia or severe attacks with minor head trauma. Two other FHM genes have been discovered: the *ATP1A2* gene, which produces a loss of function of the alpha-2 N^+/K^+ ATPase pump, and *SCN1A*, a neuronal voltage-gated sodium channel gene. Mutations in any of these 3 genes involved in ion transport can increase glutamate concentrations and excitatory neurotransmission, resulting in a lower threshold for cortical spreading depression and migraine.

In sporadic and familial hemiplegic migraine, the presentation is migraine with aura, including motor weakness. Paresis can be associated with impaired coordination. The person experiences symptoms of numbness and weakness preceding the onset of the headache. The numbness in the face and arm may spread to involve one side of the body. Basilar symptoms may be present with dysphasia or aphasia causing difficulty with speech. Coma and fever can occur and it can be confused with epilepsy, but does not respond to the typical seizure treatments. Attacks can be triggered by mild head injury. In 50 percent of cases with FMF1 there is a concomitant progressive cerebellar ataxia, independent of headache. This type of migraine may alternate with headaches without hemiplegic symptoms. Pain may be either contralateral or ipsilateral to symptoms, and on rare occasions there is loss of consciousness. Although the symptoms appear to resemble a TIA or mild stroke, migrainous infarction is rare. Age of onset for the hemiparetic migraine is 10 to 15 years, and there is usually a history within the family. Familial hemiplegic migraine appears to be related to genes on chromosome 19 or 1.[42] The migraine is considered sporadic if there is no first- or second-degree relative with hemiplegic migraine. There is high variability of the attacks, symptoms, and the disease course among individuals with familial hemiplegic migraine.[169]

Basilar-Type Migraine 1.2.6. Basilar migraine can occur throughout life in both sexes. Basilar migraines have a symptom profile that suggests posterior fossa involvement localizing to the vascular territory of the basilar artery—the brainstem, cerebellum, and occipital lobes. The prodromal symptoms reflect brainstem dysfunction. There are complaints of altered level of consciousness, dysarthria, tinnitus, ataxia, diplopia, symptoms in both the temporal and nasal fields of both eyes, and peripheral dysesthesias, followed by occipital headache.[5] Given how often vertigo, fluctuating hearing, and tinnitus occur together, basilar migraine may be difficult to distinguish from peripheral disorders such as hydrops (see Chapter 39) and from vertebrobasilar TIAs (see Chapter 32). The syndrome is most common in adolescent girls. The symptoms are bilateral, reflecting the bihemispheric dysfunction associated with the basilar blood flow.[12]

Childhood periodic syndromes that are commonly precursors of migraine 1.3. Childhood headaches typically include complaints of bitemporal pain and a shorter duration (less than 2 hours). Headaches appear more frequently in children than in adults. Variations of this headache type include 1.3.1 Cyclic vomiting syndrome, seen when a child vomits at least four times an hour for 1 to 5 days, and episodic vertigo are more common during an attack in a child than is headache. Cyclic vomiting syndrome appears to be a common precursor to migraine in children.

Abdominal migraine 1.3.2. Abdominal migraine 1.3.2 is named as such because the primary complaint is abdominal pain, midline periumbilical and often reported as dull or sore and autonomic responses of pallor.

Although vestibular migraine is not recognized as a headache type in the ICHD 2, it is a term that is used in reference to a particular set of symptoms. Dizziness with complaints of true vertigo is extremely common in migraine, and migraineurs often have a lifelong or childhood history of motion sensitivity, with symptoms provoked by amusement park rides, riding in the back seat of a car, or reading in the car. Most migraine sufferers will report some motion sensitivity during a severe headache and will often prefer to lie still in a dark, quiet room, although these symptoms alone are not sufficient to be considered vestibular migraine.[114]

When dizziness is the primary complaint or is the predominant component of the aura, then it may be considered as vestibular migraine. Vertigo occurring as an aura may arise from the same transient inhibition of neuronal function responsible for the visual aura. Episodic vertigo from vestibular migraine can be thought of as a subset of basilar migraine. Spells usually last approximately an hour but can last several hours or days in patients who have severe symptoms.[25] Nausea, vomiting, hypersensitivity to motion, and postural instability are cardinal signs. Some persons complain of vertigo, a swimming sensation, or imbalance without a complaint of headache. Dizziness does not always accompany the headache but may intermittently coincide with the headache. Changes are rarely seen on electronystagmography (ENG), indicating a peripheral deficit that is transient. The vestibulocochlear symptoms occur most often as a part of the headache. Auditory symptoms also occur in migraine. Phonophobia is the most common, with complaints of tinnitus more frequent than in the general population. Hearing loss alone is rarely associated with migraine.[85]

The mechanisms are still not clearly understood, but it may be that neuropeptides released during the migrainous event could increase the firing of the peripheral vestibular apparatus, or the vestibular nuclei.[128] This may result in a transient increase in the firing on one side of the system, causing the subjective sensation of moving. Changes in cerebral blood flow during the migraine may contribute to the dizziness. The inner ear is supplied by branches of the anterior inferior cerebellar artery arising from the basilar artery, and the anterior inferior cerebellar artery also supplies the anterolateral pons, middle cerebellar peduncle, and flocculus. Prolonged vasoconstriction of vertebral and basilar arteries may be responsible, or the cause could be the direct mechanical pressure of the dilated vessel during the vasodilating period of the headache. The dizziness can be associated with the position of the head, indicating an association with benign paroxysmal positional vertigo (see Chapter 39).

During perimenopause, unlike the postmenopausal period, women are under unstable fluctuations of ovarian neurosteroid levels. Such fluctuations might be an important interval-specific trigger for activating migraines. Along with migraine headache, dizziness is one of the most common complaints of perimenopause. A significant portion of this dizziness may be caused by vestibular migraine that has heterogeneous clinical features with dizziness and/or migraine headache. Because of this variation in phenomenology, the symptom of dizziness and vertigo during perimenopause is frequently misclassified as being a nonspecific climacteric symptom or having psychological origin.[127]

Ophthalmoplegic Migraine 13.17. Ophthalmoplegic migraine results in pain around the eye and paralysis in the distribution of the third, fourth, or sixth cranial nerve and can produce diplopia, or double vision. One of the features of ophthalmoplegic migraine is that the headache always precedes the oculomotor deficit by several hours or days. The paralysis can progress from being transient to lasting several days, and in some persons it becomes permanent. People with ophthalmoplegic migraine typically give a history of many years' duration of migraine without oculomotor involvement before the ophthalmoplegia develops.[12,172]

Retinal Migraine 1.4. Retinal migraine is repeated attacks of monocular visual disturbance, including scintillations, scotomata, or blindness, associated with migraine headache. Visual changes are strictly unilateral. There may be neuronal spreading depression or involvement of the posterior ciliary vasculature. TIA must be ruled out, as emboli from the carotid artery can cause similar symptoms.[9]

Status Migrainosus 1.5.1. The headache of status migrainosus (SM) lasts more than 72 hours, and a usual trigger will set it off. SM typically resembles the individual's usual severe migraine, but there may be a spread of pain to other areas as the headache persists, and the spread of allodynia occurs. The premenstrual part of the female cycle is a time of particular risk for SM, and changes in hormone status, pregnancy, miscarriage, or change in birth control pills can be factors. Upper respiratory or urinary tract infections can also be the trigger for SM. Overuse of analgesics and rebound withdrawal-type headache, the headache that comes when not taking medication, can trigger SM. Ruling out other possible causes is critical.

Prolonged vomiting to the point of dehydration is common. Severe pain and fatigue limit activity, and hospital admission may be appropriate. Ergots and antiemetics are effective to some degree. Corticosteroids may be helpful, and opioids are sometimes used. Comorbid depression is frequently seen.[20]

Persistent Aura Without Infarction 1.5.3. Migraine aura status is a rare subtype with persistent aura without infarction. One or more symptoms that the individual usually experiences as a part of his or her typical migraine aura persist for more than 1 week. Visual symptoms are most common, but it can be any symptom. Most typical treatment is ineffective, and the problem often must run its course. Acetazolamide or valproic acid has been helpful in a small number of patients.

Migraine-Triggered Seizure 1.5.5. Seizure that occurs as a result of a migraine. It is common for migraine-like symptoms to follow a seizure. Because the symptoms overlap migraine and epilepsy, it is sometimes referred to as migralepsy.

Chronic Migraine 1.6.1. Most cases of chronic migraine start as migraine without aura. The criterion for chronic migraine is headache for 15 or more days a month for more than 3 months. Medication overuse is the most common cause of chronic migraine, with rebound or withdrawal of medications as a trigger. Women predominantly report chronic migraine, and they report a change in symptoms over time, with decreasing photophobia, and nausea and a headache that resembles a mixture of TTH and migraine.[151]

MEDICAL MANAGEMENT

DIAGNOSIS. In most cases the diagnosis of migraine can be established by the history alone. The neurologic examination is normal. Diagnostic procedures can be considered unnecessary in some cases and results may lead to confusion. An EEG may show focal slowing if taken during an attack of migraine and may create the impression of a space-occupying lesion or infarction. Magnetic resonance imaging (MRI) scans show diffuse white matter changes in the frontal subcortical and deep white matter at the level of the basal ganglia. This may be due to platelet aggregation with microemboli, abnormal cerebrovascular regulation, and repeated attacks of hypoperfusion during the aura.

Migraine syndrome is difficult to define because the attacks vary widely between individuals. Within one individual, each attack may have different characteristics. The prodrome or aura, the nature of the attack, and the type of pain may represent separate pathologic processes that happen at the same time or within the cycle of the headache. The trigger that causes one type of migraine may be different from the one that causes another type. Most authors agree that stressful periods are linked to the onset of the headache, although the manifestations may be quite different.[98]

In the United States, migraine headaches often go undiagnosed or are misdiagnosed as tension-type or sinus headaches. There also seems to be two types of migraine sufferers, those who seek medical intervention and those who self-medicate without medical consultation.[30]

Severity of headache is important in determining disability, and to determine the nature of the intervention. Two common tools used to measure the impact of headache are the HIT-6 and the Migraine Disability Assessment (MIDAS) (Table 37-1).

TREATMENT. As presented above, the concept of migraine is evolving from an episodic pain disorder to a potentially

Table 37-1	Migraine Disability Assessment (MIDAS) Questionnaire

Please answer the following questions about *all* your headaches you have had over the past 3 months. Write your answer in the box next to each question. Write zero if you did not perform the activity in the past 3 months.

1. How many days in the past 3 months did you miss work or school because of your headaches?
2. How many days in the past 3 months was your productivity at work or school reduced by half or more because of your headaches? (Do not include days you counted in question 1 when you missed work or school.)
3. How many days in the past 3 months did you not do household work because of your headaches?
4. How many days in the past 3 months was your productivity in household work reduced by half or more because of your headaches? (Do not include days you counted in question 3 when you did not do household work.)
5. How many days in the past 3 months did you miss family, social, or leisure activities because of your headaches?

TOTAL days

A. How many days in the past 3 months did you have a headache (if a headache lasted more than 1 day, count each day)?
B. On a scale of 0 to 10, on average how painful were these headaches (in which 0 = no pain at all, and 10 = pain as bad as it can be)?

Once you have filled in the questionnaire, add up the total number of days from questions 1 through 5 (ignore A and B).
Grading system for the MIDAS Questionnaire:

GRADE	DEFINITION	SCORE
I	Little or no disability	0-5
II	Mild disability	6-10
III	Moderate disability	11-20
IV	Severe disability	21+

From Stewart WF, Lipton RB, Dowson AJ, et al: Development and testing of the Migraine Disability Assessment (MIDAS) Questionnaire to assess headache-related disability. *Neurology* 56:S20-S28, 2001.

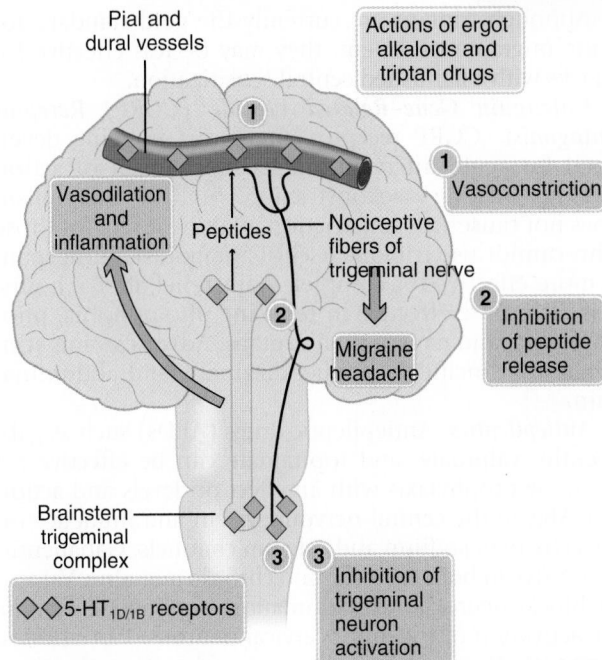

Figure 37-5

Mechanisms of ergot alkaloids and triptan drugs used in the treatment of migraine headache disorder. Ergot alkaloids and triptan drugs terminate the pain by activating serotonin 5-HT$_{1B/1D}$ receptors at several sites: (1) They activate receptors on pial and dural vessels and thereby cause vasoconstriction. (2) They activate presynaptic receptors to inhibit the release of peptides and other mediators from trigeminal neurons. (3) They activate receptors in the brainstem, which is thought to inhibit activation of trigeminal neurons responsible for migraine attacks. (From Brenner: *Pharmacology*, ed 4, Philadelphia, 2012, Saunders.)

chronic, progressive, and pervasive disease that disrupts all aspects of an individual's life. The goal is more about prevention of day-to-day attrition from disease rather than a remote catastrophic consequence.

It is clear that the causes of migraine are multifactorial, and therefore the most successful treatment is directed at the system that is most likely implicated. Avoidance of precipitating factors becomes a natural component of controlling frequency. Rest in a quiet, dark room is often necessary during the attack. Nonspecific medications control the pain of migraine or other pain disorders, whereas specific medications are effective in migraine headache attacks but are not useful for nonheadache pain disorders Pharmacologic treatment can be abortive or preventative by reducing frequency and severity. Because the migraine type may vary in one individual in different attacks, prevention is sometimes difficult. Timing of medication related to migraine type may be critical. There may be a change to the blood-brain barrier during migraine that allows inhibitory substances to pass into the brain, which changes pain perception; however, the gastric stasis that can be part of the aura can limit or slow the absorption of medication.[63] Figure 37-5 shows the mode of delivery and effects of classes of drugs used to treat migraine.

Triptans. Triptans are effective in controlling the symptoms associated with migraine. The drug action is at the level of the serotonin receptor agonist. Typically, the sensation of throbbing is diminished with use of triptans. There is evidence suggesting that triptans may also activate descending pain-modulating pathways that affect the trigeminal system. The most common triptan, sumatriptan, is a rapidly effective agent for aborting attacks when given subcutaneously by an autoinjection device. In less severe cases, sumatriptan is given orally. Other triptans now in use are zolmitriptan, rizatriptan, naratriptan, eletriptan, and frovatriptan. Headache recurrence is a problem with all triptans, and they do not appear to be effective during aura. Triptans cause constriction in the cranial arteries with an effect in the coronary arteries as well.[147] Chest tightness and pain after triptan use is common so triptans are contraindicated in patients with coronary artery disease, cerebrovascular disease, or significant risk factors due to potential vasoconstrictive effects.

Administering treatment early in the attack of migraine while the headache is mild limits attack-related disability.[38] Combination of sumatriptan and naproxen may decrease migraine recurrence and need for rescue medication in some patients.[16] Another approach is for treatment of menstrually related migraine with frovatriptan.[107,150]

Although triptans are currently the gold standard for acute migraine treatment, they may be less effective for attacks with established central sensitization.

Calcitonin Gene–Related Peptide (CGRP) Receptor Antagonist. CGRP receptor antagonist is being developed for acute intervention. Its mechanism of action does not include vasoconstriction.[122] CGRP antagonism does not cause vasoconstriction, making it safe for those who cannot use triptans. CGRP antagonist Telcagepant is more effective for complete pain relief after 2 hours. It is also more effective in reducing photophobia, phonophobia, and nausea than triptans. Adverse events seen in the trial included fatigue, dizziness, and abdominal pain.[24,71]

Antiepileptics. Antiepileptic drugs (AEDs) such as gabapentin, valproate, and topiramate can be effective for migraine prophylaxis with an effect on levels and action of GABA in the central nervous system and influence on the activity of sodium and calcium channels. Gabapentin is effective in both episodic and chronic migraine. Valproate blocks neurogenic inflammation. Topiramate inhibits the activation of trigeminocervical neurons. Paresthesias, cognitive effects, and dizziness are side effects that may limit use. Valproate should not be used during pregnancy, because of possible neural tube defects.[152,159] The mechanism by which AEDs prevent migraine is still not fully understood because other AEDs such as carisbamate, although efficacious for epilepsy, appear to be ineffective as migraine preventive medications. Divalproex and topiramate are the drugs of choice for the patient with migraine and epilepsy or migraine and bipolar illness. The pregnant migraineur who has a comorbid condition that needs treatment should be given a medication that is effective for both conditions and has the lowest potential for fetal damage.[129]

Botox. The use of Onabotulinumtoxin A (BoNTA, generally referred to as Botox) as a treatment for chronic migraine results in a significant reduction in the number of headache days. BoNTA may have other distinct properties that lead to pain relief. Central effects may be in the hippocampal neurons and astrocytes that inhibit the release of glutamate and the neuropeptides, substance P, and CGRP, from nociceptive neurons. By blocking peripheral sensitization of nociceptive fibers, it may also inhibit central sensitization and allodynia.[58] The immediate future of a preventative treatment for migraine headaches is well represented by botulinum toxin type A, glutamate NMDA receptor antagonists, gap-junction blocker tonabersat, and an angiotensin type 1 blocker candesartan.[50]

Beta Blockers. Preventive medication with documented efficacy are the beta blockers. Prophylactic treatment may be necessary if migraine occurs more than three times per month. The mode of action may involve both an effect on extracerebral vasculature and the stabilization of serotonergic neurotransmission. The beta-blocking drugs affect the central catecholaminergic system, relating to the central mechanism of the headache. In this class of drugs are propranolol, metoprolol, timolol, nadolol, and atenolol.[32] Side effects are fatigue, gastrointestinal symptoms, and dizziness. Vivid dreams, nightmares, insomnia, depression, and memory disturbances will cause termination of use.[152,164]

When migraine and hypertension or angina occur together, beta blockers or calcium channel blockers may be effective for both conditions. The athletic patient should use beta blockers with caution and beta blockers should be used with caution in the depressed migraineur unless antidepressants are used in combination. Combining a beta blocker and sodium valproate leads to an increased benefit for patients with migraine previously resistant to either alone.[130,131]

Vasoconstriction. Vasoconstricting drugs such as Cafergot, a combination of ergotamine tartrate and caffeine, are often helpful. Caffeine has several properties that may be of benefit in the treatment of migraine. Concurrent oral administration of caffeine with aspirin increases the peak plasma concentration of aspirin. It has mood-altering properties, so that the increased mental alertness, lessened fatigue, and feeling of well-being that follow caffeine ingestion counterbalance some of the symptoms of migraine. Caffeine causes cerebral vasoconstriction and may also be antiinflammatory.[152] Caffeine use is a major risk factor for development of chronic daily headache and can cause increases nervousness, sleeplessness, and anxiety.

Nonsteroidal Antiinflammatory Drugs. Nonsteroidal antiinflammatory drugs (NSAIDs) are useful analgesics for migraine-type pain. They also play a role in the inhibition of prostaglandin synthesis in brain neurons. NSAIDs are particularly effective when inflammation has caused sensitization of pain receptors to mechanical or chemical stimuli. They appear to prolong the catecholamine and serotonin turnover in brain neurons and block the release of serotonin. Antiinflammatories inhibit platelet formation that becomes abnormal during a headache phase. Aspirin and other NSAIDs are quickly absorbed. Contraindications for use are ulcers and bleeding disorders.[33] Increasing the dosage of these medications does not significantly increase their effectiveness, and there is a dose-dependent increase in the side effects, so use of aspirin and other NSAIDs at a low dose should be tried before going on to higher doses. There is no evidence that trying another type of NSAID after a failure of one type is helpful.

Ergot alkaloids provide vasoconstriction and are more active on large arteries. There is a temporary increase in blood pressure. These drugs may decrease activity in the central trigeminal neurons. Ergot alkaloid can be used to abort a headache. There is some concern about prescribing a drug that induces vasospasm in individuals with aura or those with hemiplegic migraine.[166] A short-term increase in blood pressure may limit use in some patients.

The nausea and vomiting induced by migraine can be controlled by drugs such as metoclopramide, which works as an antiemetic, counteracting gastric stasis by increasing intestinal motility and increasing the absorption of other migraine drugs.

Calcium channel antagonist drugs such as verapamil may reduce the frequency of attacks after an interval of several weeks, but the severity and duration of attacks are not influenced.[2,167] Flunarizine can be used for migraine prophylaxis if beta-blockers are ineffective or contraindicated.

The chosen drug should have the best risk-to-benefit ratio for the individual patient and take advantage of the drug's side effect profile. An underweight patient would be a candidate for one of the medications that commonly produce weight gain, such as a tricyclic antidepressant (TCA); in contrast, one would try to avoid these drugs and consider topiramate when the patient is overweight. Tertiary TCAs that have a sedating effect would be useful at bedtime for patients with insomnia. Older patients with cardiac disease or patients with significant hypotension may not be able to use TCAs or calcium channel or beta blockers, but could use divalproex or topiramate. Medication that can impair cognitive functioning should be avoided when possible.

Supplementation. Herbal therapies have also been used for many years with reported beneficial outcomes. Feverfew (*Tanacetum parthenium*) appears to decrease headache intensity and nonheadache symptoms of nausea, vomiting, photophobia, and phonophobia. Feverfew is rich in sesquiterpene lactones, which may be a nonspecific serotonin, bradykinin, prostaglandin, and acetylcholine antagonist. Other actions may include inhibition of polymorphonuclear leukocyte degranulation and phagocytosis of neutrophils, inhibit mast cell release of histamine, promote cytotoxic activity against human tumor cells, and possess both antimicrobial activity and antithrombotic potential.[69]

It appears that magnesium supplementation may specifically be effective in those individuals with low tissue or low ionized levels of magnesium. Low tissue levels of magnesium are common in patients with migraine. Magnesium also appears to have some effect on the intensity and duration of menstrual migraine, and shows promise in use in children. Taken in addition to vitamin B_6, it appears to have its best effect.[113] Riboflavin may improve oxygen metabolism at the level of the mitochondria. It has been effective in reducing attack frequency, intensity, and duration, but there are few studies to support this. Coenzyme Q10, also working at the level of the mitochondria, has been proven to decrease the frequency of migraine. Coenzyme Q10 is a critical component of the electron transport chain and functions as an important antioxidant. Evidence supports the administration of coenzyme Q10 in reducing the frequency of migraine.[15,70]

Although the mechanism of action of melatonin is not understood, melatonin is known to possess the following properties as related to migraine: antiinflammatory activity, prevention of translocation of nuclear factor kappa B to the nucleus, free radical scavenging, inhibition of CGRP-induced vasodilation, increasing inhibitory neurotransmitter activity, direct analgesic effects, inhibition of adhesion molecules, inhibition of nitric oxide synthase, and hypnotic effect from GABAergic upregulation.[133]

Beyond pharmacologic targets specific to pathophysiology in migraine is the possibility of pharmacology and supplementation that addresses the many comorbid diseases associated with migraine. Over time, many leaders in the headache field have suggested that comorbidities may in fact occur because of shared biological mechanisms, rather than as simple linear consequences. Although little has been accomplished to date, further mechanistic understanding of migraine and comorbid disease may open entirely new models and biochemical pathways of treatment. There is also the possibility that the neurobiology of headache (and pain) may cosensitize the emotional or limbic pathways, resulting in a more pervasive neurologic disease.[19]

Acupuncture has been used to control frequency and intensity of migraine. Its effect is most likely related to changes in stress levels and control of pain responses. Hypnosis has also been used, with probable similar response mechanisms. Behavioral treatment has targeted coping with pain and relaxation and examining unrealistic beliefs and their role in creating stress. It includes distraction, imagery, assertiveness training, and problem solving.[12,34,43,99]

Aerobic exercise along with progressive muscle relaxation results in reduction of self-rated migraine pain intensity. Control of symptoms with consistent exercise may be as effective as relaxation, and even topiramate.[175] Improvement in depression-related symptoms is often reported within an exercise program in migraineurs.[35,89] Distinct therapeutic targets might exist in individual patients because of their specific genetic backgrounds, suggesting that future treatments for migraine could be tailored to patient-specific mechanisms.[60] The pipeline of future compounds for the treatment of acute migraine headaches include TPRV1 antagonists, prostaglandin E receptor 4 (EP(4)) receptor antagonists, serotonin 5HT1(F) receptor agonists and nitric oxide synthase inhibitors.[18]

PROGNOSIS. Frequency and intensity of headache determine the long-term impact of migraine. Specific aspects of headache as measured by the Migraine Disability Assessment (MIDAS) and the Headache Impact Test HIT-6, can be used to help identify current status and used as an outcome measure to determine long term management, increasing communication between practitioners.[17]

Individuals with migraine typically report lower scores on the SF-36 Health Status Profile, which represents more disability than in the normal population especially in the physical and emotional areas. These low vitality scores follow the pattern of individuals with depression. Depression occurs in 30% of individuals with headache and is strongly associated with being on disability, welfare, or unemployment in individuals age under 50 years.[80]

Men have a 48% persistence rate, whereas women have a 79% rate. Menopause and the resultant decrease in estrogen usually result in a decrease in the frequency and severity of migraine. However, there have been reports of migraine attacks beginning after the onset of menopause.

There has been some question about the relationship of migraine to increased chance of stroke. Migrainous cerebral infarction is associated primarily only with an exceptionally severe migraine with changes seen on CT scan.[23]

Migraine is also associated with a high prevalence of cerebral white matter hyperintensities, occurring in the deep and periventricular white matter. Progressive gray matter volume reductions in relation to increasing headache duration and increasing headache frequency suggest that repeated migraine attacks over time result in selective structural damage to several brain regions, including the antinociceptive systems of the brainstem that results in abnormal central pain processing.[87] A long-term prospective study, assessing cognitive and memory changes in ageing individuals with and without a history of migraine showed that migraineurs do not exhibit more decline on cognitive tests over time versus controls. Migraine is certainly not a recognized risk factor for vascular dementia.[126]

SPECIAL IMPLICATIONS FOR THE THERAPIST | 37-1

Migraine

Biofeedback is the best known and most widely used nonpharmacologic procedure for the treatment of migraine. Biofeedback allows the client to make intrinsic changes in both the autonomic and somatic nervous systems. The use of biofeedback is not effective for all migraineurs, probably because of the variety of causes of migraine. The mechanism is thought to be a change in the levels of neurotransmitters produced when a person is able to control the stress response. Both thermal biofeedback (the control of temperature in the digits) and EMG feedback (the control of muscle activity) have been used by therapists in the treatment of migraine.

Because of the direct relationship between the cervical spine and the trigeminal complex causing initiation of vascular spasm, relief of some symptoms occurs when the cervical spine is treated with manipulation or other physical modalities. Although manipulation has been used for the control of migraine headache, there is an increased risk of stroke from chiropractic manipulation of the neck.

As stated above, consistent aerobic exercise may also create relief of migraine headache and should therefore be considered as a part of the intervention in a patient with a comorbidity of migraine.

Tension-Type Headache 2.1

Overview and Incidence

TTHs are the most common type of primary headache; as many as 90% of adults have had or will have tension headaches, representing 25 million people in the United States. Infrequent episodic headaches (2.1) are those that occur fewer than 12 days per year and are usually self-managed, requiring little medical attention. Prevalence appears to peak in 30- to 40-year-olds in both men and women, increasing with level of education in both genders.[148] Infrequent episodic TTH occur in 53% of 40-year-olds.[161] TTHs are more common among women than men, especially with advancing age.[11] The cost of care increases in the individual with frequent TTH, which occurs from 12 to 180 days/y. Medication cost and days of lost work increase, so the socioeconomic burden is greater. Chronic TTHs are those reported more than 180 days per year and have a different neurobiologic pathogenesis. Chronic TTHs occur most often in women older than age 50 years and have usually evolved from episodic tension headaches.[160] Distinguishing chronic TTH from migraine and from medication-induced headache is a

diagnostic challenge, and the management is different. In general, individuals with TTH seek less medical attention than migraineurs.[125]

Etiologic and Risk Factors

Frequent episodic and chronic TTH is caused by a combination of genetic and environmental factors, while infrequent episodic TTH is caused primarily by environmental factors.[146] Pain and psychological factors clearly affect one another. Individuals with TTH tend to report greater use of non-optimal coping strategies, including withdrawal, avoidance, and self-criticism when coping with negative life events. TTH sufferers appear to have a high level of fearfulness about pain and may have excess attention toward bodily function versus environmental awareness. Like migraine, central sensitization, limbic system, and reticular disinhibition play a role. Some biochemical changes are common to both migraine and TTH. Blood levels of magnesium are low in both conditions, and there is increased blood flow in anterior, middle, and posterior cerebral arteries.

Pathogenesis

Pericranial myofascial nociception represents the pathophysiology of episodic TTH. The pain input to the brain is increased because of sensitization of peripheral sensory afferent neurons, possibly by endogenous substances such as serotonin and bradykinin. Sensitization of central nociceptive pathways seems responsible for the conversion of episodic to chronic TTH.[6] This sensitization of second-order neurons and neurons at the level of the trigeminal nucleus alters nonpainful input so that it is perceived as noxious at the level of the cortex. Stimuli to skin, tendons, and muscle cause pain in the area around the head and, at the same time, in areas distant from the head. This may be consistent with referred hyperalgesia, relating to the convergence of multiple peripheral sensory afferents onto sensitized spinal cord neurons, which project to central structures that have another level of sensitization.[8,56]

Sympathetic tone is evidenced by resting heart rate, which is higher in migraine and chronic TTH than in episodic TTH.[182] Lack of normal inhibitory control in the central nervous system may also play a role in TTH. Pain that can normally be down-regulated by interneurons may lose that function, so that there is a loss of inhibitory control, or disinhibition. The neurons responsible probably belong to the bulbar reticular formation. This area receives afferents from the periphery but also from limbic structures, the orbitofrontal cortex, the nucleus raphe, and the periaqueductal gray matter.

Clinical Manifestations

Increased hardness of muscle tissue in the upper neck is found in the absence of muscle firing. Electromyographic (EMG) analysis to determine if there is increased muscle activity or increased resting tone during or between headache episodes has been inconclusive. EMG recordings do not appear to have diagnostic usefulness, and the increases that have been reported may have to do with protective adaptation rather than the cause of pain.

There is increased tenderness to palpation of the tissues around the head. Both muscles and tendon insertions have been found to be excessively tender, and pressure pain sensitivity maps appear to be different in chronic TTH.[51] The level of tenderness correlates to the intensity of the headache. The pain is usually in the whole head or in the neck and is reported as tightness or pressure. The pain is often described as dull, not throbbing. The severity of TTH increases with increasing frequency. Nausea is not typically associated with tension headache, but there are reports of anorexia, mild photophobia, and phonophobia.[82] The triggers reported most frequently for TTH are stress, both mental and physical. Irregular eating pattern and high intake of coffee or other caffeine-containing drinks causing dehydration can trigger a TTH. The relationship between sleep disturbance and headache is related to both sleep as a self-management strategy for pain and insomnia among people with TTH.[125] Abnormal responses of stretch reflex and inhibitory reflexes may occur in TTH of both chronic and episodic nature.[173] This may reflect similar sensitizations as are seen in underlying pathologies in migraine.[132]

MEDICAL MANAGEMENT

DIAGNOSIS. The diagnosis of tension headache requires the exclusion of other causative disorders. The medical history should include the evolution of the headache. A general physical and neurologic examination should be performed to rule out a disease process, including palpation of the pericranial muscles to identify tenderness and trigger points. Referred pain patterns should also be recorded. The temporal, lateral pterygoid, masseter, sternocleidomastoid, and trapezius muscles should be looked at specifically. It should be noted whether the palpation is done during the headache or nonheadache phase, as there can be up to 25% increase in pain perception during headache.

Except for their frequency and intensity, chronic TTHs are similar to frequent episodic TTHs. Chronic TTH may be linked with medication overuse (see later), and the diagnosis should be made only after there have been 15 days free of medication. It is important to recognize that individuals with confirmed migraine are prone to increased incidence of chronic TTHs between migraine attacks. The individual will usually describe a difference between the headache types.

Chronic TTHs, because they occur with greater frequency and duration and are of moderate intensity, cause a broader spectrum of fatigue and depression than a migraine might. Current studies have found that individuals with chronic TTH report a lower quality of life.

TREATMENT. The first step in treatment should be a written record of the frequency and severity of attacks by means of a headache diary for a period of 4 weeks. The diary should include triggers and medication use; often, there is more medication used than the patient had been aware of. Significant comorbidities should be identified and treated concomitantly. It should be clear to patients that frequent or chronic TTH may not be cured but improvement can be significant to lifestyle. Both pharmacologic and behavioral treatments should go hand in hand and are critical to ultimate success.

Analgesics and NSAIDs are the most typical medications used for control of TTHs, and often the individual will self-select the dosage. Most randomized placebo-controlled trials have demonstrated that aspirin (in doses of 500 and 1000 mg) and acetaminophen (1000 mg) are effective in the acute therapy for TTH. There is no consistent difference in efficacy between aspirin and acetaminophen. The NSAIDs seem to be more effective than acetaminophen and aspirin.[158] Combination therapy using analgesics can enhance the effect and allow lower dosages and lower risk of side effects. The combination of analgesics with caffeine, codeine, sedatives, or tranquilizers frequently is used and there is increased efficacy when adding caffeine to aspirin or ibuprofen.[4] Overuse of analgesics and NSAIDs may increase the frequency of TTH and estrogenic hormones, including oral contraception or hormonal replacement therapy, may worsen TTHs.

Tricyclic antidepressants such as amitriptyline are useful in chronic TTH. If depression is comorbid, tricyclics are generally regarded as more effective than selective serotonin reuptake inhibitors. As part of the differential diagnosis, Tizanidine, botulinum toxin, propranolol or valproic acid do not appear to help with TTH as they would with migraine.[7] Memantine was shown to reduce pain intensity in chronic TTH patients, albeit to a limited extent. Future NMDA antagonists with higher efficacy could be of major interest as regards the pathophysiology and future treatment of chronic TTH and other chronic pain disorders.[97]

Magnesium supplementation is effective for young patients with episodic TTH consistent with results found in young migraineurs.[65] Vitamin D and calcium supplementation provide improved control of symptoms.[135]

Physical therapy is the most used nonpharmacologic treatment of TTH and includes improvement of posture, relaxation, exercise programs, and electrical stimulation. Active treatment strategies generally are recommended.[174] Combination techniques, such as massage, relaxation, and home-based exercises and may have a modest effect. Craniocervical intervention improves outcomes in some individuals.[142] Specifically, spinal manipulation appears to have no effect on the treatment of episodic TTH.[14] However, trigger point–specific physical therapy is effective in children.[176] Active myofascial trigger points are correlated with the frequency and duration of headache.[156] Relaxation training allows patients to consciously reduce muscle tension and reduce autonomic arousal. SEMG biofeedback is used to change the amplitude of pericranial muscle tension, which is a way to establish central brain changes. Cognitive-behavioral therapy (stress management) aims to teach patients to identify thoughts and beliefs that generate stress and aggravate headaches.[74]

PROGNOSIS. Over time, there is an increased risk of the episodic TTH developing into a chronic TTH; this is likely in individuals who are unable to manage or change the internalization of negative thought. Multidisciplinary headache clinic reports the most positive results in long-term control of symptoms.[185]

Cluster Headache 3

Overview and Definition

Cluster headaches are rare but are the most painful of the primary headaches. Cluster headache is disabling to the individual as almost 20% of cluster headache patients have lost a job secondary to cluster headache, while another 8% are out of work or on disability secondary to their headaches. Suicidal ideations are substantial, occurring in 55%.[144]

There are two types of cluster headache. The episodic type is the most common, constituting 80% of all cases. **Episodic cluster headache 3.1.1** is defined by periods of susceptibility to headache, called cluster periods, alternating with periods of remission. The headache can occur daily or several times per day for a period of several weeks, known as the cluster period. The headache will go away for several months and recur as another series or cluster.[118,154] **Chronic cluster headache 3.1.2** indicates the headaches have gone on for at least 12 months and remissions last less than 14 days. Chronic cluster headache evolves from episodic cluster headache.[92]

Incidence

Cluster headaches affect approximately 1% to 4% of the population and occur predominantly in men between ages 27 and 30 years, approximately 10 years later than the typical onset of migraine. Black males appear to have a higher incidence than males of other racial backgrounds. The ratio favoring men over women is getting smaller over time.[178] Most attacks occur between early evening and early morning hours, with peak time of headache onset between midnight and 3 AM. Beer is the most common type of alcohol trigger. Migraine triggers such as weather changes and smells are also very common cluster headache triggers.

Persons with cluster headache have some similar physical characteristics, typically an average 3 inches taller than age-matched controls, hypermasculine in appearance that includes increased and asymmetric facial wrinkles and thick orange peel skin. It is common that they smoke cigarettes and drink alcohol at a rate higher than average. Cluster headache can result from secondhand cigarette smoke exposure during childhood, as greater than 60% of nonsmoking cluster headache patients had parents who smoked.[143] Personality inventories show a relationship to anxiety, compulsivity, and hypochondria.[36]

There is a correlation between cluster headache and prior head trauma with the possible relationship to venous vasculitis, because there is evidence of inflammation.[178] Studies of genetic risk are beginning to show some prevalence in certain families, with a positive history in more than 7%. The possibility of gene mutation is strong, with a high concordance found in monozygotic twin studies.[145]

Pathogenesis

Like migraine, cluster headache appears to have multifaceted components and dysfunction at many levels. There is vasodilation of the ophthalmic and internal carotid arteries, ipsilateral to the pain. The vascular changes may be a result of stimulation of the trigeminal complex, rather than a casual factor. Stimulation of the trigeminal ganglion causes a cerebral vasodilator response. There is an increase in the level of CGRP and substance P. The cerebrospinal fluid shows changes consistent with both parasympathetic and sympathetic and central involvement.

Platelet levels of histamine and serotonin increase during the episode of headache and decrease in the absence of headache. Blood pressure typically increases; heart rate decreases during attacks of cluster headache. The cluster period may be characterized by disturbances in neuroendocrine substances based on the circadian rhythm, which may explain its cyclic nature.[41,81]

The carotid body may play a major role in the pathogenesis by its receptor mechanism associated with blood pressure and heart rate. Throughout the course of the cluster period, it may be that the chemoreceptor activity is affected by central control of sympathetic and parasympathetic pathways.[64]

Hypothalamic regulation of the endocrine system may explain the cyclical nature of the headaches. There is decreased plasma testosterone during the cluster period and alterations of production of hormones and melatonin. Melatonin levels are generally low during the day and increase during the hours of darkness and sleep. The hypothalamus is involved in the fundamental processes leading to the acute attacks of cluster headache.

Brain-derived neurotrophic factor is associated with pain modulation and central sensitization. The role of brain-derived neurotrophic factor in both migraine and cluster headache pathophysiology has been suspected because of its known interaction with CGRP. Cluster headache patients showed significantly higher brain-derived neurotrophic factor concentrations both inside and outside cluster bouts.[54] Features of the microstructure of sleep and arousal mechanisms could play a role in the pathogenesis of cluster headache. Reports indicate that cluster headache and obstructive sleep apnea are associated.[5]

Clinical Manifestations

The onset is sudden, with excruciating pain. In the majority of cases, the headache remains on one side of the head in all recurrences throughout life. The headache is usually localized to one eye and the frontotemporal region (see Fig. 37-1). The pain is boring and nonthrobbing. Autonomic symptoms, which are often on the opposite side from the pain, include photophobia, tearing, and nasal congestion. Autonomic changes may be bilateral. Occasionally, Horner's syndrome (constricted pupil, droopy eyelid) or forehead sweating will appear on the uninvolved side of the face.[10] Figure 37-6 shows the interrelationship of pain and autonomic symptoms in cluster headache. Persons will occasionally complain of blurred vision on the painful side. Further, persons with cluster headache generally prefer to assume an erect rather than a reclining posture during attacks.[45]

Vasodilators such as nitroglycerin will induce cluster attacks. Often, but not always, alcohol induces an acute cluster attack while the person is in an active cluster period. Attacks are commonly induced on awakening from an afternoon nap or from sleep during the night, most commonly 90 minutes after falling asleep.

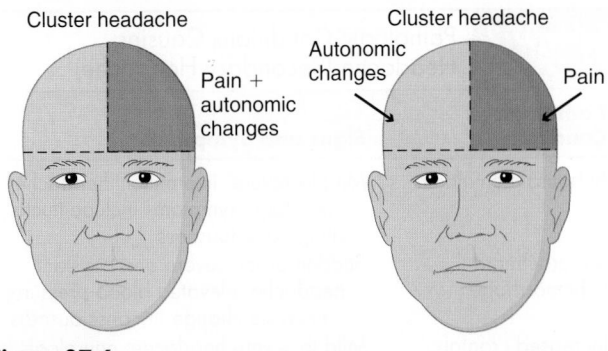

Cluster headache · Cluster headache

Pain + autonomic changes

Autonomic changes · Pain

Figure 37-6

The interrelationship of pain and autonomic symptoms and signs in cluster headache. The usual pattern is pain and autonomic changes on the same slide *(left)*. A less common pattern is pain on one side and autonomic changes on the opposite side *(right)*. (From Sjaastad O: *Cluster headache syndrome*, London, 1992, Saunders, p. 49.)

Melatonin levels are low during the day and increase during the hours of darkness and sleep; in individuals with cluster headache, the 24-hour production of melatonin is reduced, and the acrophase (the time from midnight to the moment of peak hormone level) is moved forward. Low serotonin level may be responsible for the low melatonin production.[170]

Cluster headaches follow a circadian rhythm and occur often during the same time of year. They occur most during the summer or winter solstice, appearing shortly after either the longest or shortest day of the year. Even the setting of the clock for daylight-saving time will affect the headache cycle, often bringing an end to an episode.[178]

MEDICAL MANAGEMENT

DIAGNOSIS. There remains a significant diagnostic delay for cluster headache patients, on average 5+ years, with only 21% receiving a correct diagnosis at time of initial presentation. Diagnosis is based on the symptoms and history. Paroxysmal hemicrania, trigeminal neuralgia, and temporal arteritis may have similar symptoms, but they are not episodic. Diagnostic criteria are strict unilaterality, severe intensity, orbital localization, and short duration. Differential diagnosis includes migraine, trigeminal neuralgia, chronic paroxysmal hemicrania, pericarotid syndrome, sinusitis, and glaucoma.[26]

Treatment

Management of cluster headache is divided into acute attack treatment and prophylactic treatment. Melatonin therapies can be helpful, with remission coming within 3 to 5 days.

In cluster headache, the attacks can be treated with oxygen[59] Subcutaneous sumatriptan works in cluster headache as it does in migraine. Verapamil can be used as a prophylactic drug. The dosage used in cluster headache treatment may be double the dose used in cardiology. At the start of a cluster, transitional preventive treatment such as corticosteroids or greater occipital nerve blockade can be helpful. In chronic and in long-standing clusters, lithium, methysergide, topiramate, valproic acid, and ergotamine tartrate can be used as add-on prophylactic treatment.[57] In drug-resistant chronic cluster headache, neuromodulation with either occipital nerve stimulation

or deep brain stimulation of the hypothalamus is an alternative treatment strategy.[163] Future studies are directed toward other areas of the pain matrix that may be suitable targets for neuromodulation in patients who do not respond to hypothalamic modulation.

Education should be provided regarding precipitating factors, including alcohol, abrupt changes in sleeping patterns related to travel, and work shift changes. Lack of sleep or afternoon naps may precipitate a headache. Bursts of anger or prolonged anticipatory anxiety can provoke a headache during the cluster period. Altitude hypemia can increase incidence at levels above 5000 feet, including on airplane flights. Avoiding these situations may reduce the frequency of cluster headache during a cluster period. Upright activities, including walking, appear to be of some relief. Few people choose to lie down during an attack.[36]

Surgical procedures, including radiosurgeries directed toward the sensory trigeminal nerve, have been the most successful. Hypothalamic implants have been used in individuals with an intractable chronic condition. The results are encouraging, with notable pain reduction.

Chronic cluster headache, which accounts for about 10% to 15% of patients with cluster headache, lacks the circadian pattern and is often resistant to pharmacologic management. The sphenopalatine ganglion, located in the pterygopalatine fossa, is involved in the pathophysiology of cluster headache and has been a target for blocks and other surgical approaches. Percutaneous radiofrequency ablation of the sphenopalatine ganglion was shown to have encouraging results in those patients with intractable cluster headaches.[119]

Prognosis. In the natural course of cluster headache, around 10% of those affected will transition from episodic to chronic, and that same number may change from chronic to episodic. One third will suffer for around 20 years and then experience a complete remission. In another one third, the attacks will be mild and no longer require medical intervention. The final one third of individuals continue to have attacks in the same pattern and to the same degree. Cluster headaches do not begin in old age.

SPECIAL IMPLICATIONS FOR THE THERAPIST · 37-2

Cluster Headache

It is important for the therapist to be able to recognize the symptoms of cluster headache and to differentiate it from tension headache. Tension headache often is improved when drinking alcohol. Relaxation and stress reduction may be of benefit if the client has a history of episodes triggered by stress response. Use of thermal and EMG biofeedback may be of benefit (see "Migraine" below). Aggressive exercise appears to improve symptoms in cluster headache as it does in migraine.

SECONDARY HEADACHES

A sudden onset of severe headache is usually related to an intracranial disorder such as subarachnoid hemorrhage, brain tumor, or meningitis (see Chapter 29). These headaches will most often be accompanied by other neurologic signs, such as weakness, visual disturbances, and possibly altered mental status or coma. A structural, or space-occupying, lesion is suspected in headaches that disrupt sleep, are triggered by exertion, or cause excessive drowsiness. Headaches secondary to brain tumors, endocrinopathies, and other medical problems are only a very small percentage of all headaches.[79] Even though pathologic conditions account for only a few cases of headache pain, it is critical for the therapist to understand what mechanisms may be responsible and when the client may need medical or emergent care. Table 37-2 lists some of the causes of headache that may require immediate medical attention.

Headache Attributed to Disorder of the Neck 11.2, Cervicogenic Headache 11.2.1

Overview, Definition, and Incidence

There is considerable overlap in the characteristics of migraine without aura, TTH, and cervicogenic headache due to the activation of the trigeminal complex setting into motion the cascade responsible for the particular aspects of pain. Remember that the trigeminal neurons comingle bidirectionally with the sensory distribution of C1-3 nerve roots allowing for trigeminal nociception to refer neck pain and for upper cervical spine pathology cause head pain through activation of the trigeminal complex. Neck pain is frequent with both migraine and TTH, but the pathogenesis of primary headaches does not include cervical musculoskeletal dysfunction. In order for the headache to be considered cervicogenic, the pain must be referred from a source in the neck, and perceived in one or more regions of the head and/or face.

The Cervicogenic Headache International Study Group and the Quebec Headache Study Group have expanded on the criteria from the ICHD classification as stated above and can be useful to the clinician in the differential diagnosis.

Evidence that the pain can be attributed to a neck disorder or lesion is based on at least one of the following: In cervicogenic headache, pain is localized to the neck and occipital regions and may project to the forehead, orbital region, temples, vertex, or ears. Pain is precipitated or aggravated by particular neck movements or sustained neck posture. There can be resistance or limitation of passive neck movements, with pain response to active and passive stretching or contraction. An acute onset is likely due to trauma that involves the neck, and there is a prevalence reported between 25% and 50% in patients with headache after whiplash.[103] Whiplash injuries usually affect the cervical facet joint, intervertebral disc, cervical nerve root, anterior longitudinal ligament, deep anterior flexor attachments, or a combination of these structures.

Pathogenesis

Structures innervated by C1-3 include arteries, dura, ligaments, muscles, and joints. Impairments within any of these structures have the potential to cause both head and neck pain.

Table 37-2	Pathologic Conditions Causing Headache (Secondary Headache)
Pathologic Condition	**Signs and Symptoms**
Subdural hematoma	Mild to severe, intermittent headache; neurologic symptoms include fluctuating consciousness
Subarachnoid hemorrhage	Sudden onset, severe and constant headache; elevated blood pressure; can cause change in consciousness
Increased cranial pressure	Mild to severe headache; neurologic symptoms include hemiparesis, visual changes, and brainstem symptoms, including vomiting, altered consciousness
Meningitis, viral, and bacterial	Headache severe with radiation down neck; acutely ill and febrile; positive Kernig sign
Brain abscess	Mild to severe headache; local or distant infection; may be afebrile; neurologic signs consistent with local site of infection
Central nervous system	Localized headache and focal neurologic symptoms; often see cranial nerve symptoms
Central nervous system neoplasm	Localized headache and focal neurologic symptoms; often see cranial nerve symptoms
Toxicity	Generalized headache, pulsating; may show other signs of toxicity
Sinusitis	Frontal or dull headache, usually worse in morning; increased pain in cold damp air; nasal discharge
Otitis media, mastoiditis	Feeling of fullness in ear, stabbing pains in head, vertigo, and tinnitus

Vascular disorders, primarily aneurisms, or dissection of the carotid or vertebral arteries (see chapter on stroke) cause sudden and intense neck pain with headache. There can be a sudden onset of unprovoked neck pain without headache, although this is rare. The progression to cerebrovascular events typically identifies the cause. Disorders affecting the dura of the posterior fossa can include meningitis, subdural hematoma, or subarachnoid hemorrhage, and tumor can cause concomitant neck pain and headache. (see Infectious Disorders and Neoplasm chapters.)

The remaining cervicogenic headaches are considered to be related to the ligament, muscle, and joint disorders via nociception, neuropathic pain, and central sensitization.

The transverse atlantoaxial and alar ligaments are innervated by C2 and can be damaged during injury involving acceleration–deceleration. Pain associated with their disruption may also be due to automatic cocontraction as a response to instability, surrounding tissue injury caused by excessive motion during injury, or overstretch of related structures during the movements that the ligaments are designed to limit.[13]

Suboccipital muscles are innervated by C1, and C2 innervates the prevertebrals. The accessory nerve (XI) communicates with anterior branches of C1-2 supplying the sternocleidomastoid, and with C3-4 to supply the upper trapezius. Anterior branches of the high cervical plexus also communicate with the vagus nerve (X) supplying the salivary glands, parts of the ear, pharynx, larynx, and viscera; the hypoglossal nerve (XII) supplies to the tongue and the upper cervical sympathetic ganglia.[65] The multifidus and semispinalis are part of the C3 nerve distribution and are commonly tender near their attachment sites. Spasm, sprain, or damage can be a source of pain; however, the relationship to cervicogenic headache has not been established through studies.

Alignment of the head in relationship to the cervical spine will affect the length and tension of the muscles and ligaments. When the upper back is rounded, the position of the head is adjusted to maintain the eyes in the vertical position. This often results in shortening of the suboccipital muscles and abnormal positioning of the cervical spine.[25] The C2-C3 apophyseal joint is suspected of producing cervicogenic headache related to its biomechanical vulnerability as a transitional joint between the C1 and C2 vertebra, which rotate the head, and the C3 to C7 vertebra, which flex and extend the neck. It bears both vectors of stress, and the result is a mechanical irritation of C3; this joint and the third occipital nerve appear most vulnerable to trauma from acceleration-deceleration or whiplash injuries.[2] Head and neck posture alone may not be the determining factor to cluster headache, but the posture during work tasks may contribute more to the onset.[83]

Joint dysfunction has the most closely attributable connection with the diagnosis of cervicogenic headache. The lateral atlantoaxial joint can produce referred pain to the head, and headache can be relieved with anesthetizing the joint. Traumatic damage to the capsule, including bleeding or bruising, has been found on postmortem examination. Zygapophyseal joints in the upper cervical spine appear to be the most commonly implicated as a source of cervicogenic headache. The intervertebral disc of C2-3 can reproduce headache, following nerve root distribution and connection to the trigeminal complex.

C2 neuralgia can be caused by lesions affecting the nerve via its close relationship to the lateral atlantoaxial joint, so it can be compromised in capsular changes due to inflammation or other disorders affecting the joint. Vascular system disease in the area can also lead to nociception. The neurogenic involvement explains the lancinating pain often reported in addition to the referred pattern of dull ache.

The greater occipital nerve, composed of primarily C2 and C3 dorsal root fibers, supplies sensory pathways to the occiput and parietal areas. It exits to the scalp through all extensor attachments along the nuchal ridge and lies within the occipital groove, located one-third posterior to the mastoid process and two-thirds lateral to the midpoint of the occiput. The nerve sheath may become inflamed and edematous, and easily palpated. Occiput–atlas hyperextension and chronic significant tight short extensors may compress the nerve. Pain may be aching, lancinating, or sharp, with scalp paresthesia, from occiput to temple.

Trigger point pathology of the upper cervical muscles innervated by C1 to C3 appears to be associated with headache and needs to be distinguished from upper cervical joint pain. Muscular trigger points are usually found in the suboccipital, cervical, and shoulder musculature and may refer to the head. These findings are in the absence of neurologic findings of cervical radiculopathy, although the patient might report scalp paresthesia or dysesthesia.[171,179] Trigger points may be secondary to underlying causes, or may result from chronic muscular activity without sufficient relaxation to provide normal circulation.[75] Studies show reduced efficiency of reciprocal inhibition associated with the increased motor unit excitability in trigger points.[78] Once established, trigger points may become self-perpetuating, furthering the inefficient or abnormal muscular recruitment pattern and referring pain. Pain referral maps from the cervical and scapular suspensory musculature toward and around the head as established by Travell and Simons are the currently recognized patterns.[153] For example, the forward head position assumed in response to thoracic kyphosis, as mentioned above, encourages abnormal activation and cocontraction of the sternocleidomastoid and levator scapulae, two primary appendicular muscles sharing upper cervical innervation causing both sensory and motor hyperexcitability with cephalad pain referral to head, ears, and face. Of particular interest is the sternocleidomastoid, which receives both bilateral and contralateral innervation, as well as sympathetic and vagus nerve connections, perhaps making it much more responsive, and overresponsive, to nociceptive stimuli about the head and neck.

MEDICAL MANAGEMENT

CLINICAL MANIFESTATIONS. The pain usually starts in the neck, eventually spreading to the oculofrontotemporal area. Symptoms may actually be more intense in this latter location than in the occipital or cervical region. Autonomic symptoms and signs, such as photophobia, phonophobia, nausea, vomiting, and ipsilateral periocular edema, are generally less frequent and less marked than in common migraine, but they can occur. Swallowing difficulty is reported, albeit a rarely occurring associated phenomenon. Dysphagia may occur in cervical dysfunction because of the communication of the hypoglossal and vagus nerves (cranial XII and X) with the anterior cervical plexus of C1-3. This would be a primary cervical dysfunction whether or not associated with headache.

Unilateral symptoms of occipital headaches greater than neck pain following a traumatic event are more suggestive of cervical facet joint than internal disc disruption. Examination finding of increased focal suboccipital pain with terminal cervical flexion and sequential lateral rotation suggests pain emanating from a C1-2 joint. Bilateral symptoms of neck pain with headaches would be more suggestive of cervical internal disc disruption. If reproduction of symptoms by provocative maneuvers, which facilitate closure or narrowing of the neuroforamina, are positive, then nerve root involvement rather than facet joint syndrome or internal disc disruption syndrome is of higher probability. Such compression maneuvers also provoke the uncinate joints, which begin at C2-3, and are known to be enlarged by shear forces of injury, excess mobility, and aging. In whiplash injuries, facet involvement may be more common than upper cervical nerve root injury; however, this finding may reflect paucity of epidemiologic data for whiplash-induced cervical nerve root injury.

An altered neuromuscular strategy with inhibited deep neck flexors and excessive sternocleidomastoid contraction has been noted in neck pain cases. This movement disorder may be reflected in the client with cervicogenic headache.[49]

Diagnosis

It can be difficult to readily diagnose cervicogenic headache, because there is overlap in the symptoms, including unilateral, occipital pain radiating to the upper cervical area. Criteria include the following: demonstration of clinical signs that implicate a source of pain in the neck; abolition of headache following diagnostic blockade of a cervical structure or its nerve supply; and pain that resolves within 3 months after successful treatment of the causative disorder or lesion (less than 5 on a 100-point visual analog scale).

Head movement can increase migraine pain related to allodynia but may not be the primary trigger.[39] The nature of the symptoms is not the diagnostic criteria, the manifestations are not unique and overlap with primary and other secondary headaches. It is the causal relationship to the disorder of the spine that determines the category of cervicogenic headache. Obtaining an accurate history is the initial step in formulating a differential diagnosis including neck or head trauma if there is a possible whiplash mechanism.

Biomechanical implications can be identified though reduced active range of motion (ROM) in the neck. Arm pain is common and can have either nonradicular or radicular patterns. Pain may be reproduced by external pressure over the tendinous insertions in the occipital area, along the course of the major occipital nerve, over the groove immediately behind the mastoid process, over the upper part of the sternocleidomastoid muscle on the symptomatic side, and the lateral aspect of a cervical zygapophyseal joint. Pain may be precipitated intrinsically by neck movements or sustained, awkward head positioning, especially during sleep.[67] Figure 37-7 shows the patterns of referred pain in the upper cervical area.

Radiologic examination reveals at least one of the following: movement abnormalities in flexion/extension, abnormal posture, fractures, congenital abnormalities, bone tumors, rheumatoid arthritis, or other distinct pathology (but not spondylosis or osteochondrosis, because these are conditions that are common incidental findings in asymptomatic individuals). The criteria do not insist that the lesion be located within the neural territory of C1 to C4 but that it be in the neck.[141] The mechanism, which may be related to disk disease in the lower neck, may involve compensatory increase in movement, especially in the facet joints in the upper cervical spine, thus causing pain to travel along the C1 to C4 nerve to the interface of the trigeminal complex. It is thought that nociceptive impulses and other sensory impulses can be involved in sensitization of the brainstem and thus be involved in the spread of pain into the head as described earlier. Patterns of referred pain are demonstrated in Figure 37-7.

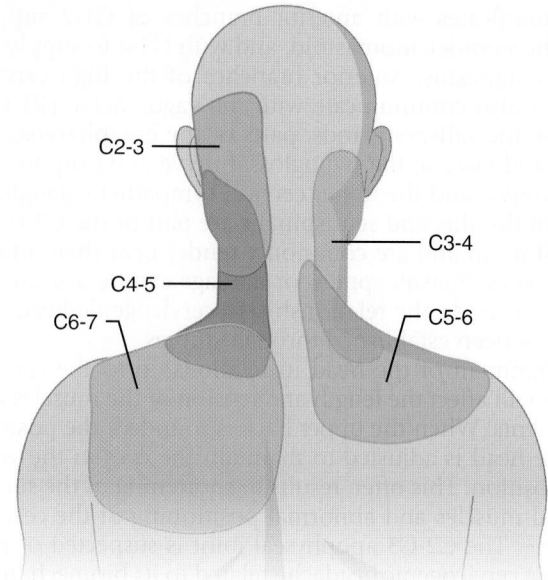

Figure 37-7

Patterns of referred pain evoked from the cervical zygapophyseal joints and intervertebral discs. (Based on Dwer et al, Schellhas et al, and Grubb and Kelly. From Bogduk N, McGuirk B: *Management of acute and chronic neck pain: An evidence-based approach.* Pain Research and Clinical Management, Philadelphia, 2006, Elsevier.)

The lack of complete response to indomethacin, sumatriptan, and ergotamine may assist in making the differential diagnosis away from primary headache. The duration of headache and pain intensity vary widely in cervical headache with a strong tendency toward chronicity. It can present as episodic in the initial phase becoming chronic in later stages. The duration of pain episodes is frequently longer than in common migraine; the pain intensity is moderate and nonexcruciating, unlike cluster headache, and it is usually of a nonthrobbing nature.

It is not acceptable to assume that a headache that follows traumatic brain injury or whiplash is necessarily cervicogenic. Neurobiologic changes may be present in the brain (see "Posttraumatic Headache" below) or TTH may develop secondary to stressors that increase after a whiplash injury.

The response to anesthesia to the upper cervical area, required in the ICHD criteria, clearly is not cost effective in the clinic to determine cause. Manual examination including valid and reliable measures need to be developed, and it is the intent of those most involved in this category of headache to come to consensus regarding appropriate measures. Physical therapists are active in this arena.[22,55,177]

There is no clear consensus on what constitutes an adequate physical examination of the neck or the techniques for performing the examination and there is question about what findings are significant.[44,186] Box 37-2 presents current testing used to lead to a diagnosis.

Treatment. Lack of response to medication is one of the considerations in making a diagnosis. However, tricyclic antidepressants have been used at a lower dosage than that required for the treatment of patients with depression with effect. Simple analgesics may be used to

Box 37-2

CLINICAL EXAMINATION AND MEASURES ASSOCIATED WITH CERVICOGENIC HEADACHE

- Neck Pain and Disability Index (NDI) (Cleland JA, Childs JD, Whitman JM: Psychometric properties of the Neck Disability Index and numeric pain rating scale in patients with mechanical neck pain. *Arch Phys Med Rehabil* 89:69-74, 2008.)
  - 0-4/50 = no disability
  - 5-14/50 = mild
  - 15-24/50 = moderate
  - 25-34/50 = severe
  - >34/50 = complete disability
- Alar and transverse ligament integrity testing
- Vertebral artery dependency test
- Headache symptoms reproduced with mechanical pressure on myofascial trigger points, myotendinous insertions, or facet capsules.
- Headache symptoms reproduced with specific head/neck motions, within available range (denotes active inflammation) or at end range.
- Symptoms reproduced with Spurling test of lateral foraminal compression (Wainner RS, Fritz JM, Irrgang JJ Boninger ML, Delitto A, Allison S: Reliability and diagnostic accuracy of the clinical examination and patient self-report measures for cervical radiculopathy. *Spine (Phila Pa 1976)* 28:52-62, 2003; Bertilson BC, Grunnesjo M, Strender LE: Reliability of clinical tests in the assessment of patients with neck/shoulder problems-impact of history, *Spine (Phila Pa 1976)* 28:2222-2231, 2003.)
- Limited C1-2 range of motion using cervical flexion rotation test (significant limitation has been identified on ipsilateral side of headache) (Hall TM: Comparative analysis and diagnostic accuracy of the cervical flexion-rotation test. *J Headache Pain* 11:391-397, 2010.)
- Limited active range of motion (Fritz JM, Brennan GP: Preliminary examination of a proposed treatment-based classification system for patients receiving physical therapy interventions for neck pain. *Phys Ther* 87:513-524, 2007.)
- Limited passive cervical and thoracic range of motion (Cleland JA, Childs JD, Fritz JM, Whitman JM: Interrater reliability of the history and physical examination in patients with mechanical neck pain. *Arch Phys Med Rehabil* 87:1388-1395, 2006; Sandmark H, Nisell R: Validity of five common manual neck pain provoking tests. *Scand J Rehab Med* 27:131-136, 1995.)
- Manual muscle test of all cervical musculature, observing substitutions and cocontractions as well as target muscle response (Jull G, et al.: Cervical musculoskeletal impairment in frequent intermittent headache. Part 1: Subjects with single headaches. *Cephalalgia* 27:793-802, 2007; Jull G, Barrett C, Magee R, et al: Further clinical clarification of the muscle dysfunction in cervical headache. *Cephalalgia* 19:179-185, 1999.)
- Craniocervical flexion test (CCFT) for assessment of deep cervical flexor strength and neuromotor pattern (Jull GA, O'Leary SP, Falla DL: Clinical assessment of the deep cervical flexor muscles: the craniocervical flexion test. *J Manipulative Physiol Therap* 7:525-533, 2008; Falla D, Jull G, Dall'Alba P, Rainoldi A, et al: An electromyographic analysis of the deep cervical flexor muscles in performance of craniocervical flexion. *Phys Ther* 83:899-906, 2003.)
- Neck Flexor Muscle Endurance Test (NFMET) results have a negative or inverse association with cervical spine dysfunction and pain (Harris KD, Heer DM, Roy TC, Santos DM, Whitman JM, Wainner RS: Reliability of a measure of neck flexor endurance. *Phys Ther* 85:1349-1355, 2005.)

---

manage pain but have long-term side effects that should considered. Muscle relaxants may be of benefit as they relate to the central nervous system.[84] Studies using botulinum toxin have been mixed, and this agent may be more effective if the "follow the pain" strategy is used, injecting the muscles that are reported as tender.[72] Cervical epidural steroid injections may be indicated for multilevel disk or spine degeneration. Nerve blocks, trigger-point injections, or radiofrequency thermal neurolysis may block the cascade of sensitization to the central mechanisms. Surgical interventions such as neurotomy, dorsal rhizotomy, and microvascular decompression of nerve roots to perform blocks or reduce pressure on a nerve often also provide only temporary relief, with the possibility of longer intensification of pain. Nerve stimulators have been used successfully in migraine and may be of some benefit in cervicogenic headache.[12]

Physical and manual therapies including exercise are the most important modalities for treatment of cervicogenic headache. Long-term prevention and control of headaches appears greatest in individuals who are involved in ongoing exercise and physical conditioning programs.[11,83,183]

SPECIAL IMPLICATIONS FOR THE THERAPIST 37-3

Cervicogenic Headaches

The chronic headache that arises from the atlantooccipital and upper cervical joints is a unique syndrome

and needs to be differentiated from disorders at other vertebral levels.[25,108]

The rich presence of sensory receptors in subcranial tissues suggests the importance of sensory feedback for head/neck function. Strong connections exist between upper cervical and oculomotor systems for gaze stability, and among the upper cervical, vestibular, and visual systems for equilibrium and spatial orientation. Rehabilitation intervention involving the upper cervical spine should therefore be based in a motor pattern and recruitment sequence approach. Task-specific activities have the most reliable and lasting effects on recovering normal movement patterns.[77] Accurate sensation recognition and motor patterns are continuously influenced by use-related experience and progressive adaptation of motor behavior.[37] If the headache is related to temporomandibular joint dysfunction, this should be addressed by the appropriate therapist. Intervention can include relaxation, body awareness, physical therapy modalities, transcutaneous electrical nerve stimulation (TENS), and soft tissue techniques.

Consider the following: (1) cervicogenic headache pain is in part a result of central sensitization, (2) abnormal neuromuscular patterns and weaknesses are identified, (3) impaired inhibition of antagonists results from myofascial trigger points, and (4) postural faults may contribute to mechanical and myofascial dysfunctions generating pain. Sensorimotor disturbances will be magnified in cases of trauma.

Addressing motor control and sensory system flexibility with differing environmental demands may better support specific treatments for joint mobility; segmental or regional stability; and length, strength, and endurance. Intentionally incorporating vestibulocolic, cervicoocular, vestibuloocular reflexes, proprioception and kinesthesia, head righting, and postural responses in varying conditions supports recovery. Neural plasticity is continuous and relies upon high repetition, sufficient intensity, variability, and feedback. Pain disturbs normal sensorimotor patterns. The presence or absence of these components in treatment programs for cervicogenic headache has not been specifically teased out of the outcome literature. However, we can make the case that neuromotor rehabilitation principles apply to the upper cervical spine.

Acute Posttraumatic Headache Syndromes 5.1, Acute Posttraumatic Headache Attributed to Mild Head Injury 5.1.2, Chronic Posttraumatic Headache 5.2

Overview, Definition, and Risk Factors

Headache is one of the most common symptoms after traumatic brain injury (TBI), and posttraumatic headache (PTH) may be part of a constellation of symptoms that is seen in the postconcussive syndrome. PTH has no defining clinical features; currently, it is classified as a secondary headache based on its close temporal relationship to the injury. Posttraumatic headache syndrome is not a single pathology but a group of traumatically induced disorders with overlapping symptoms. The headache is a manifestation of brain dysfunction and can have contribution from the musculoskeletal injuries. The headache can last longer after the trauma than the musculoskeletal problems.[109] When the headache develops within 7 days of the trauma and resolves within 3 months, it is considered acute. The headache can begin weeks or months after the trauma and can become chronic consistent with other headache types. The risk of developing chronic posttraumatic headache is greater for mild or moderate head injury than for severe head injury.[86]

The prevalence of posttraumatic headache can be as high as 60% and typically occurs within 24 hours after the trauma. The prevalence of headache can remain high over the first year.[73] A history of headache before a head injury occurs and female gender are possible risk factors for headache after TBI.[104] Preexisting episodic headaches, anxiety, and depression and a high number of other posttraumatic symptoms will increase chance of headache.[96]

Risk factors for posttraumatic headache include a blow to the head most commonly related to auto accidents, sports injury, falls, and blast injury. According to the Defense and Veterans Brain Injury Center Working Group on the Acute Management of Mild Traumatic Brain Injury in Military Operational Settings, the incidence of headache and PTSD (see Chapter 33) is greater than 90%.[90]

Pathogenesis

The pathologic mechanisms of posttraumatic headache mirror those of primary headaches. Both central and peripheral sensitization play a role in posttraumatic headache. Neurochemical changes similar to those found in migraine include excessive release of excitatory amino acids, especially glutamate; an increase in extracellular potassium, intracellular sodium, or calcium; and an abnormal accumulation of serotonin. Further, there is a decline in magnesium levels, abnormalities in nitric oxide formation, and changes in catecholamines and endogenous opioids. Chronic local inflammation can release substance P, bradykinin, and other pain-producing peptides. The nerve endings responding to these neurochemicals can trigger spasm and pain.[47]

Diffuse axonal injury resulting from the shear forces to the brain and brainstem is likely a confounding mechanism but remain difficult to image.

The connection between the cervical nerves (C1 to C3) and the cervical portion of the trigeminal nucleus forming the trigeminocervical nucleus is described above. Although there is no direct head trauma with some whiplash injury, studies show that these accidents can cause cerebral hemorrhages on the surface of the brain and upper cervical spinal cord.

Higher thermal thresholds in both the head and hand indicate central damage to the pain and temperature system. A significantly lower pressure-pain threshold in the head is related to a more severe PTSD symptomatology. This may be a form of central pain. Cranial mechanical hyperalgesia may originate from peripheral tissue damage accompanying the THI.[31]

Clinical Manifestations

Posttraumatic TTHs are generally mild to moderate with dull, aching, pressing, tightening feelings that are usually not pulsating. They are often bilateral and bandlike. These headaches do not involve nausea or vomiting and are not aggravated by bright lights. Increased stress and anxiety that may follow traumatic events may also make individuals more likely to develop TTH.

Migrainous features with unilateral pain, aggravation by physical activity, nausea, and both visual and auditory sensitivity are common. Posttraumatic migraine like headaches can become incapacitating when combined with other sequelae of brain injury. Posttraumatic cluster-like headaches appear and trauma may trigger a cluster period during what had been a remission.

Posttraumatic dysautonomic cephalalgia is rare and typically a result of anterior neck injury and is similar to migraine. The pain is unilateral and throbbing, and there are pupillary dilation and excessive sweating on the side of the headache during the headache phase. Miosis can occur between headaches.[162]

Usually there is both shear damage to the brain and musculoskeletal damage to the soft tissues in the neck, jaw, and scalp. Complaints of memory and concentration disturbances after whiplash injury are common. Dizziness and vertigo are often reported along with

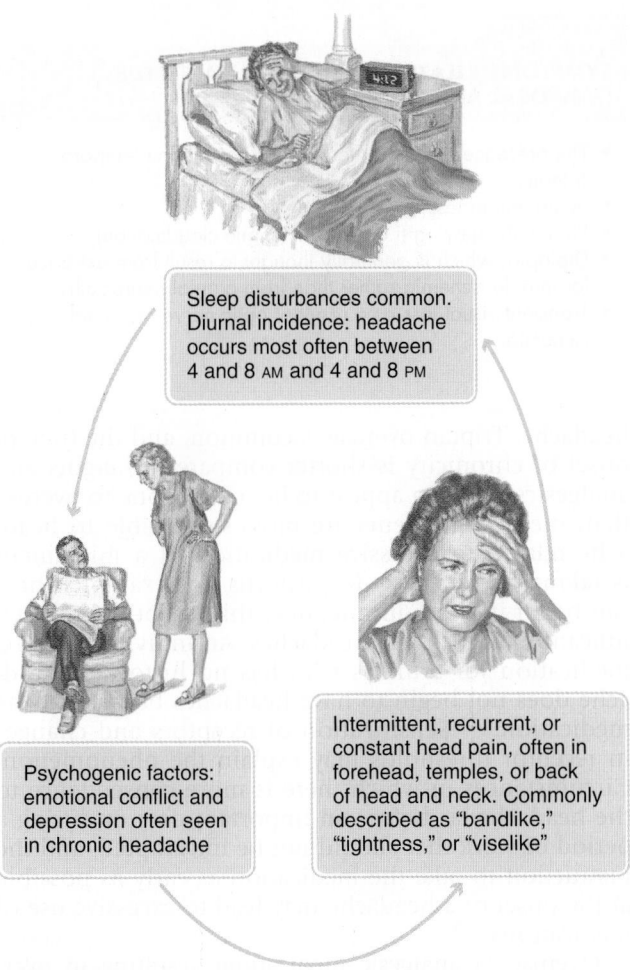

Sleep disturbances common. Diurnal incidence: headache occurs most often between 4 and 8 AM and 4 and 8 PM

Psychogenic factors: emotional conflict and depression often seen in chronic headache

Intermittent, recurrent, or constant head pain, often in forehead, temples, or back of head and neck. Commonly described as "bandlike," "tightness," or "viselike"

Figure 37-8

Tension-type headache. (From Madden: *Netter's sports medicine*, ed 1, Philadelphia, 2009, Saunders.)

headache. When the dizziness is triggered by activity, the headache can be worse. Balance deficits may be a result of sensory organization deficits typically seen with brainstem disorders. Visual dependency progressing to visual motion sensitivity, also common after vestibular disorders, cause symptoms in environments with peripheral visual movement. In an effort to control the sensation of dizziness that comes with head movement or when there is excessive visual stimulation, the individual will cocontract the muscles of the neck to limit stimulation of the vestibular system, resulting in complaints of neck soreness and stiffness and increase in headache. See Chapter 38 for further description of the mechanism of cervicogenic dizziness.[138] Common complaints in addition to head pain are irritability, lack of concentration, and memory loss. Figure 37-8 illustrates the areas of involvement and associated phenomenon. These symptoms are consistent with both chronic headache and mild or moderate head injury. Psychologic symptoms are associated with this type of headache associated with the cycle of stress, anxiety, as well as related to the neurochemical changes as stated above. Box 37-3 lists the typical complaints associated with posttraumatic headaches.

MEDICAL MANAGEMENT

DIAGNOSIS. With newer MRI techniques, PET, and single-photon emission computed tomography (SPECT), the parenchymal delayed cerebral atrophy and axonal damage related to membrane injury may be identified. The ability to detect metabolic brain changes using magnetic resonance spectroscopy will help to determine the level of brain damage sustained. Xenon inhalation techniques provide additional insight into brain perfusion abnormalities.

TREATMENT. The treatment of posttraumatic headaches proceeds in the manner described earlier for the type of headache that is manifested. Early and intensive treatment may be the main factors in stopping headache and preventing a chronic condition. Recognizing this type of headache is critical in the course of treatment of an individual with brain injury related to a blow to the head or other causes of whiplash. These headaches are often overlooked by the medical practitioners who provide the follow-up care. Individuals with persistent complaints of headache are often assigned the label of malinger or symptom magnifier. See Chapter 33 on traumatic brain injury for further discussion of treatment related to mild traumatic brain injury.

SPECIAL IMPLICATIONS FOR THE THERAPIST 37-4

Posttraumatic Headache Syndromes

Persons with posttraumatic complications are seen by therapists in many different settings. With moderate to severe head injury, the headache is a part of so many other issues that are critical to the return of function that it may be dismissed. The individual may also have difficulty in describing the headache secondary to cognitive changes. Therapists working in rehabilitation and long-term care are often confronted with vague complaints of pain and dizziness that may limit activity. With better understanding of the mechanisms of pain, and the autonomic and cognitive changes associated with these injuries, the therapist may be better able to address the specific issues.

Headache is a common complaint reported to the therapist treating soft tissue dysfunction associated with trauma. Often there are complaints of excessive fatigue, eye strain, inability to concentrate, depression, and dizziness in these same patients. The nature of the headache should be evaluated to help determine the appropriate intervention. Working with a medical practitioner to get the appropriate medication can be a part of the therapist's intervention.

Trigger-point treatment of the pericranial and cervical tissue has been used to help control the pain. As an understanding of the relationship of the pericranial structures and central modulation of pain emerges, combining treatment of soft tissue and use of CNS-mediating drugs may bring more relief from these disabling symptoms.

Headaches Attributed to Psychiatric Disorders 12

Headache that presents exclusively during and secondary to a psychiatric disturbance such as major depressive, panic, anxiety, or somatoform events may represent comorbidity and perhaps a common biological substrate. This headache category is new to the ICHD 2, and the intent is to generate more research on this topic.[155]

Medication Overuse Headaches 8.2

Frequent intake of medications used for headache can lead to chronic headache. It appears that all drugs used for the treatment of headache may lead to chronic

---

Box 37-4

SYMPTOMS RELATED TO GIANT CELL ARTERITIS (TEMPORAL ARTERITIS)

- The presence of pain or tenderness around the temporal arteries.
- Scalp tenderness.
- Pain with chewing (i.e., jaw or tongue claudication).
- Diplopia, which is generally thought to result from extraocular muscle ischemia rather than from cranial neuropathy.
- Transient visual loss as a result of optic nerve or retinal ischemia.

---

headache. Triptan overuse is common, and the time of onset of chronicity is shorter compared to ergots and analgesics. Women appear to be more prone to overuse than men. Migraineurs are most susceptible to headache related to excessive medication. If a migraineur is taking an analgesic for arthritis, for example, there can be an increase in migraine; this is not seen as significantly with cluster headaches. An individual taking medication for arthritis who has no history of headache does not begin to have headaches because of the medication.[184] Sensitization of receptors and changes in receptor thresholds may explain the phenomenon. Circumstances in which there is more consequence to the headache, as before an important date or during a period of work that should not be interrupted, and the instruction to take the medication as early as possible at the onset of a headache may lead to excessive use of medications.[139]

Overuse of analgesic medications resulting in overuse headache is common when the headache type has not been identified appropriately.[187,188] There is usually lack of response to the headache prevention medications when another medication is overused.

Headache Attributed to Giant Cell Arteritis 6.4

Headache is the most common symptom in what has been referred to in the past as temporal arteritis but is now classified as giant cell arteritis. The headache is located over a branch of the superficial temporal artery and is described as a dull ache that persists throughout the day. It may be accompanied by tenderness of the artery and overlying scalp. If severely affected, the artery may be nonpulsatile. See Chapter 12 for the description and medical management. Symptoms of vasculitis and vascular insufficiency are common relating to extracranial carotid circulation. Box 37-4 gives the typical complaints related to giant cell arteritis in the temporal region.

Sedimentation rate should be measured in individuals older than age 60 years who have headache or facial pain, unless the pain obviously results from another cause. Visual loss may result and can be avoided with early diagnosis and aggressive treatment. Findings from a temporal artery biopsy can confirm the diagnosis. Unless otherwise contraindicated, corticosteroid therapy should be instituted, pending results of the biopsy.

Headache Attributed to Rhinosinusitis 11.5

The diagnosis of pain that results from acute sinus inflammation is rarely difficult. Often a prior history of sinus inflammation or respiratory allergies is elicited. In general, the pain is of low to moderate intensity and is present on a daily basis. The pain usually is localized to the frontal or maxillary area, and there is tenderness to tapping over the affected sinus. The pain is often worsened by bending forward and may be triggered by blowing the nose or sneezing. Symptoms of nasal stuffiness are usually present, and purulent drainage from the nostrils may be seen. If the nasal passages are blocked, use of a nasal decongestant can be useful diagnostically and often results in discharge. In doubtful cases, a simple plain film of the sinuses or an opinion from an otolaryngologist should be obtained.

Postdural Puncture Headache 7.2.1

Another disabling headache can occur after lumbar puncture or with epidural anesthesia. If a myelogram is performed, it can trigger this type of headache. The headache is due to leakage of cerebrospinal fluid and changes in the pressure within the skull. The headache is usually self-limiting but can last 3 to 5 days. Symptoms include neck stiffness, tinnitus, hypacusia, photophobia, and nausea. An individual with this type of headache must lie still, because movement, including Valsalva maneuver, increases pain. Hydration helps, in combination with analgesics and antiemetics. Intravenous caffeine sodium benzoate constricts cerebral blood vessels. An epidural blood patch may be necessary. Blood taken from the peripheral vein and put into the epidural space clots and forms a patch. There is increased risk of pain, infection, and spinal cord compression. An epidural blood patch cannot be used in persons taking anticoagulants. Aspirin is not used as an analgesic because of its anticoagulant properties.[23]

Trigeminal neuralgia is a disorder of the trigeminal (fifth cranial) nerve in which there are intense and brief paroxysms of lancinating pain within the nerve's distribution. Slight pressure on a trigger zone, often in the area of the nasolabial fold, results in severe pain. Cold, intense light, taste, and sometimes a somatosensory stimulus in an extremity can cause pain most often in the cheek. Triggers that elicit this type of pain may include chewing and may lead to the erroneous diagnosis of odontogenic pain. The hallmark is no clinically evident neurologic deficit. The pain is always unilateral, and there is usually a refractory period after an episode in which the pain cannot be elicited. When there is spasm associated, it is considered tic douloureux. Trigeminal neuralgia is a rare disorder, approximately 10 cases per 100,000, affects more women than men, and is more common after the age of 50 years. Figure 37-9 shows the trigeminal distribution pattern.

Etiology

Classic trigeminal neuralgia is considered idiopathic. Symptomatic Trigeminal Neuralgia 13.1.2 is the term

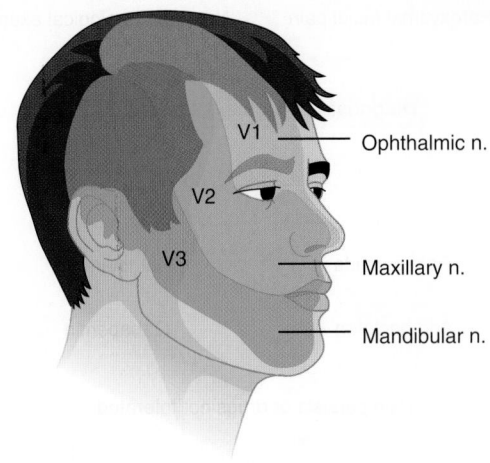

Figure 37-9

Dermatomes for trigeminal nerve. *V1*, Ophthalmic nerve; *V2*, maxillary nerve; *V3*, mandibular nerve. (From Waldman SD: Trigeminal nerve block: coronoid approach. In Waldman SD, ed: *Atlas of Interventional Pain Management*, ed 3, Philadelphia, 2009, Saunders.)

used in relation to causes such as herpes zoster, multiple sclerosis, vascular lesions, or tumors. It can be associated with inflammatory process, typically occurring in women between the ages of 50 and 70 years.

Pathogenesis

Results from experimental studies suggest that demyelinated axons are prone to ectopic impulses, which may transfer from light touch to pain fibers in proximity known as ephaptic conduction. Demyelination results from vascular compression of the nerve root by aberrant or tortuous vessels, usually the superior cerebellar artery. Demyelination has also been demonstrated in cases of trigeminal neuralgia associated with multiple sclerosis or tumors affecting the nerve root.

Clinical Manifestations

The pain associated with trigeminal neuralgia has a sudden onset and has been described as sharp, knife-like, lancinating, and "like a lightning bolt inside the head that lasts for seconds to minutes." The sensation is typically restricted to the maxillary (V2) division of the nerve, but it may involve the maxillary and mandibular divisions together. Less likely is involvement of the ophthalmic (V1) division.

The painful sensation often occurs in clusters. Any mechanical stimulation, chewing, smiling, or even a breeze, can trigger an attack. Clients avoid stimulating the trigger zone. Remissions occur between attacks, but these remission periods shorten and attacks become more frequent over the course of the disorder. In a small number of the cases, the pain occurs bilaterally, but this typically is related to probable multiple sclerosis.

MEDICAL MANAGEMENT

DIAGNOSIS. A careful neurologic examination of the head and neck is performed at initial contact. The ears, mouth, teeth, and temporomandibular joint should be examined for other problems that might cause facial

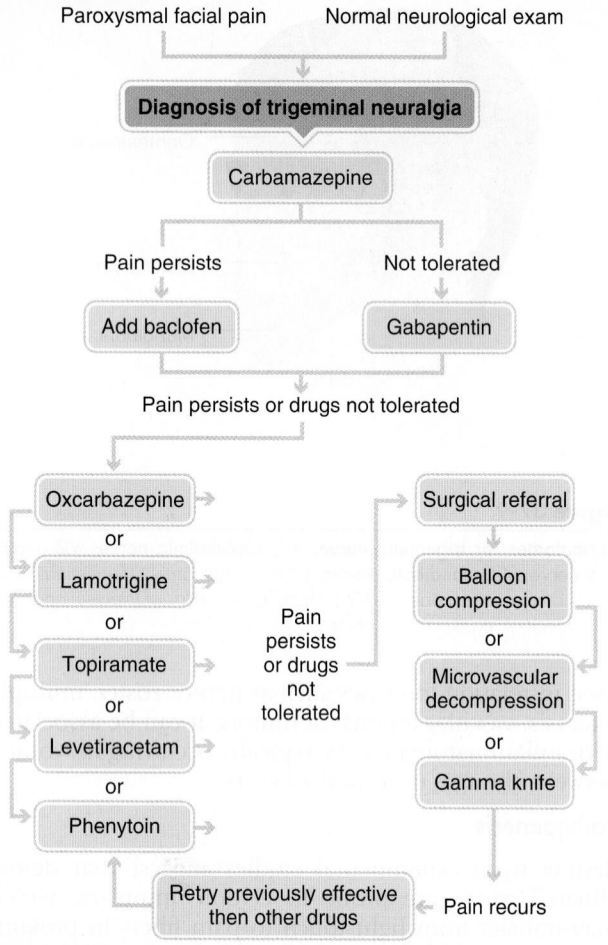

Figure 37-10

Suggested scheme for treating trigeminal neuralgia. The same pharmacologic strategy may be applied to the treatment of glossopharyngeal neuralgia. The order of choices differs for individual patients. (From: Johnson RT, Griffin JW, McArthur JC: *Current Therapy in Neurologic Disease*, ed 7, St. Louis, 2008, Mosby.)

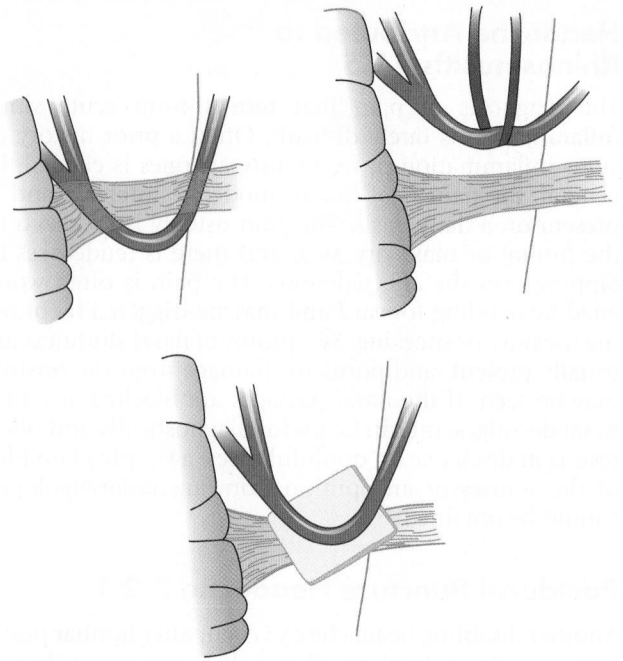

Figure 37-11

Top left, Microscopic vascular decompression to alleviate trigeminal neuralgia represents a major neurosurgical advance. The aim is to place a barrier between the vessel and trigeminal nerve. As pictured through an operating microscope, the brainstem is on the left side of the field and the trigeminal nerve lies horizontally to the right. A large, aberrant artery compresses the nerve from below. **Top right,** A surgical loop plucks the artery out from beneath the trigeminal nerve. **Bottom,** The artery is then placed over a piece of muscle or artificial material that cushions the nerve. (From Kaufman DM, Milstein MJ: *Clinical neurology for psychiatrists*, ed 6, Philadelphia, 2006, Saunders.)

pain. The finding of typical trigger zones verifies the diagnosis of trigeminal neuralgia. Sensory abnormalities in the trigeminal area, loss of corneal reflex, or evidence of any weakness in the facial muscles may indicate another cause of symptoms.[91]

Laboratory studies generally are not helpful in patients with typical symptoms of trigeminal neuralgia. Occasionally, temporomandibular joint or dental radiographs may be useful when temporomandibular joint syndrome or dental pain is in the differential diagnosis. MRI of the brain is used to look for multiple sclerosis, tumors, or other causes of secondary symptomatic trigeminal neuralgia and is typically performed early when the symptoms occur.[95]

The first line of treatment for trigeminal neuralgia is anticonvulsants; carbamazepine or Tegretol is usually tried first. Other medications are listed in Figure 37-10. Pain can be controlled about 75% of the time with oral medications. In persons whose pain is refractory to medications, neurosurgical procedures are advised and it appears that the sooner the procedure is performed the most success is obtained. Neurosurgical treatments include percutaneous procedures, stereotactic radiosurgery, and microvascular decompression.[149] Microvascular surgery is used when small blood vessels have been found to constrict the trigeminal nerve near its root. This procedure provides immediate pain relief; however, it is a major and difficult surgery. Minimal trigeminal nerve root trauma via nerve-combining technique demonstrated a beneficial impact.[105] Figure 37-11 shows the mechanism to remove pressure from the nerve from the vascular loop. Management decisions are dependent on personal preference and clinical factors such as age and overall health.

PROGNOSIS. The efficacy of evaluating treatments is complicated by the fact that the disorder may remit spontaneously. Remissions that occur soon after onset may last for years. For those who do not remit, trigeminal neuralgia can be managed medically in most cases. The Trigeminal Neuralgia Association provides information and support for persons with this diagnosis.

REFERENCES

To enhance this text and add value for the reader, all references are included on the companion Evolve site that accompanies this textbook. The reader can view the reference source and access it online whenever possible.

CHAPTER 38

Vestibular Disorders

KENDA S. FULLER

VESTIBULAR DISORDERS

Definition and Overview

Everyone is familiar with momentary feelings of dizziness related to carnival rides or great heights. Until the system fails, the activity of the vestibular system is noticed only in those particular circumstances when it is stimulated beyond normal. The dizziness that occurs when the vestibular system is overstimulated is similar to the dizziness that is perceived when the brain encounters sudden changes in the input from the vestibular system. Because the vestibular system provides information about orientation in space, disorders of the vestibular system can cause a devastating sense of abnormal movement, visual instability, and loss of balance.

The ability to maintain clear vision during head motion and to determine head position or speed and direction of movement is provided by the vestibular system. Appropriate postural reflexes are activated to maintain balance when the brain is able to interpret the forces created by gravity along with the forces generated as we move.[52] The vestibular system is critical for postural control because it uniquely identifies self-motion as different from motion in the environment. Vestibular disorders, with the exception of aggressive forms of neoplasm, are not life-threatening but can cause significant disability.[91]

The vestibular system works as part of the sensory triad for postural stability and must be integrated with somatosensory and visual input to determine appropriate postural strategies. Comorbid dysfunction can affect functional recovery, especially if it affects the visual or somatosensory inputs. Prior trauma, either physical or psychological, can cause maladaptation resulting in responses to intervention that are inconsistent with typical recovery patterns. Symptoms of dizziness and imbalance cannot always be assumed to be an actual loss of vestibular function but can reflect the inadequate use of the sensory integration appropriate for the environmental context.

At its most peripheral level, the end organ of the vestibular system is primarily a mechanical system designed to identify movement of the head. It consists of a fluid-filled labyrinth and is bordered laterally by the middle ear and medially by the petrous portion of the temporal bone. The pathologic condition at this level is related to the structures involved. Figures 38-1 and 38-2 show the mechanism of the vestibular system and the relationship of the vestibular system to the nearby structures of the brain and bony structures.

The semicircular canals are ring-shaped, fluid-filled structures oriented in three dimensions that provide sensory input about head velocity, or angular acceleration of the head. This is accomplished by movement of the endolymphatic fluid in the direction opposite to the head movement. Figure 38-3 represents the relationship of the movement of the head and the resulting effect on the direction of the endolymph movement. The ampulla is deflected away from the direction of head movement by the movement of the endolymph. Figure 38-4 shows the orientation of the labyrinths to the head and Figure 38-5 shows the relationship between the movement of the fluid within the canal, and the ampullar deflection. The speed and direction of the deflection of the hair cells of the ampulla determine the rate of firing of the vestibular nerve. The difference between the rate of firing of each vestibular nerve is interpreted by the brain as to the amount of angular acceleration of the head.[66] Disorders at this level are most often related to fluid pressures, changes in the contents of the fluid, and inflammatory or infectious agents that affect the homeostasis of the system. Blows to the head or acceleration-related injuries can cause direct damage to the labyrinthine system. Ischemia in the surrounding vasculature can cause disrupted function.

Both ends of each fluid-filled semicircular duct open into the otolith, which contains the utricle and saccule. A portion of the floor of the utricle and the saccule is thickened and contains hair cells covered with a gelatinous membrane known as the otolithic membrane. Calcium carbonate crystals, or otoconia, adhere to this membrane. Figure 38-6 shows how the otoconia sit above the hair cells. The weight of the otoconia produces a shear force on the hair cells with acceleration of the head. Information about linear acceleration, the tilt of the head, or the static position of the head with respect to gravity from the movement of the hair cells is transmitted to the vestibular nerve. There is a tonic resting firing rate of the hair cells that is carried through the vestibular nerve. The tonic firing of the vestibular system when the head is not moving is symmetrical on both sides of the system at approximately 50 spikes per second. The vestibular nerve transmits these

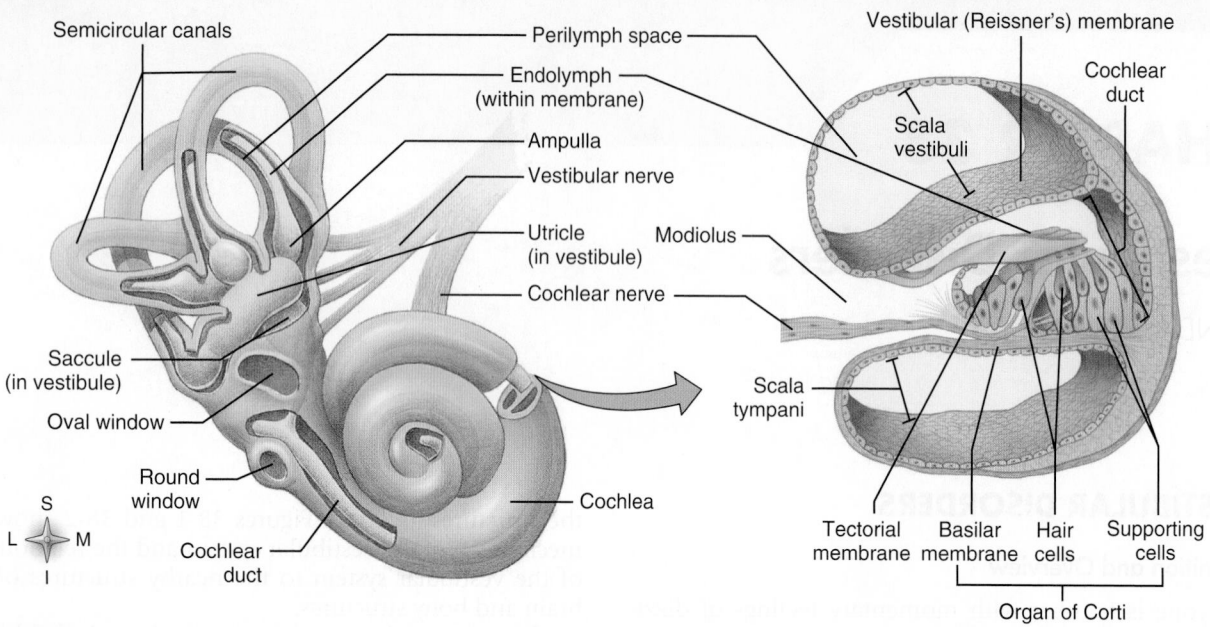

Figure 38-1

Components of the vestibular system and cochlea with distribution of neural connections. (From Thibodeau GA: *Anatomy and physiology,* ed 8, St. Louis, 2013, Mosby.)

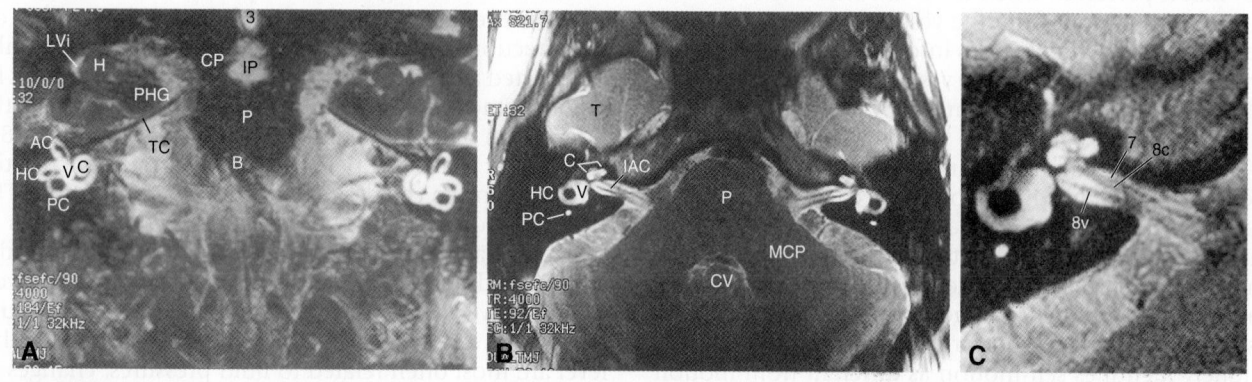

Figure 38-2

MRIs of the labyrinth. A, Coronal view. **B,** Axial view. **C,** Enlarged view. *AC,* Anterior semicircular canal; *HC,* horizontal canal; *PC,* posterior semicircular canal; *C,* cochlea; *IAC,* internal auditory canal; *P,* pons; *8v,* eighth cranial nerve (vestibulocochlear nerve). (From Nolte J: *The human brain: An introduction to its functional anatomy,* ed 5, St. Louis, 2002, Mosby.)

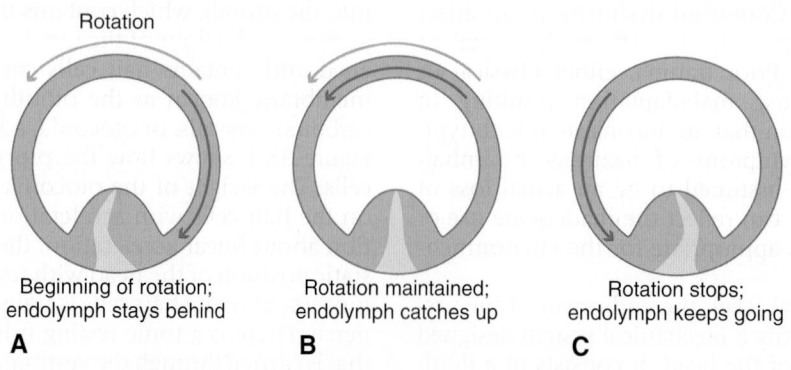

Figure 38-3

Relative movement of semicircular canals. A, Beginning of rotation. **B,** During rotation. **C,** End of rotation. (From Nolte J: *The human brain: An introduction to its functional anatomy,* ed 5, St. Louis, 2002, Mosby.)

afferent signals from the labyrinths, extending through the internal auditory canal and entering the brainstem at the pontomedullary junction. Somatosensory, visual, tactile, and auditory information is also processed in the vestibular nuclei.[19,44] The brain uses the combined input in determining orientation within the environmental context.

Changes in the position of the hair cell reflect changes in head position in relation to gravity. Figure 38-7 shows the relationship of the otolith to head positions changes. When the head is upright in the gravitational field, the acceleration due to gravity, which is 9.8 m/s^2, pulls the saccular otoconial mass toward the earth. Afferents in the inferior half of the saccule, whose hair cells are excited by this downward acceleration, have lower firing rates and lower sensitivities to linear accelerations than do those afferents in the upper half of the utricle. Excitation or inhibition of the whole utricle does not occur under normal conditions.

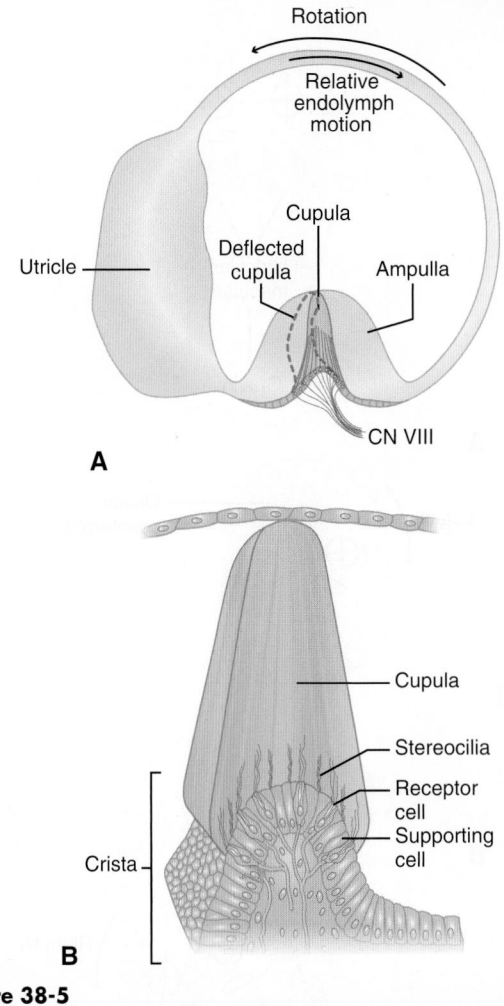

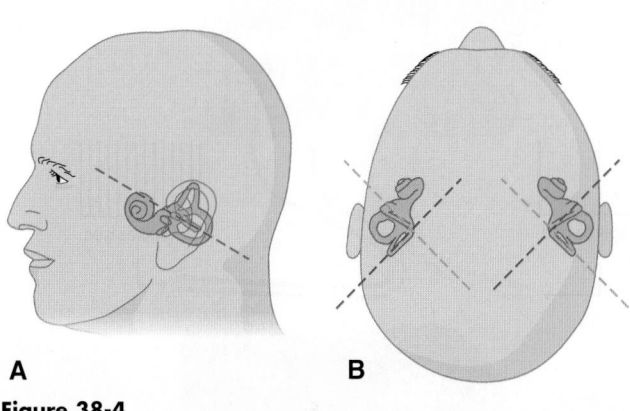

Figure 38-4

Orientation of the labyrinth. A, Side view. **B,** From the top. Labyrinth is enlarged relative to the head in this drawing for clarity. (From Nolte J: *The human brain: An introduction to its functional anatomy*, ed 5, St. Louis, 2002, Mosby.)

Figure 38-5

Two views of the ampulla. A, View of the semicircular canal and movement of the endolymph and resulting deflection of the cupula within the ampulla relative to head motion. **B,** Enlargement of the cupula showing its components. (From Nolte J: *The human brain: An introduction to its functional anatomy*, ed 5, St. Louis, 2002, Mosby.)

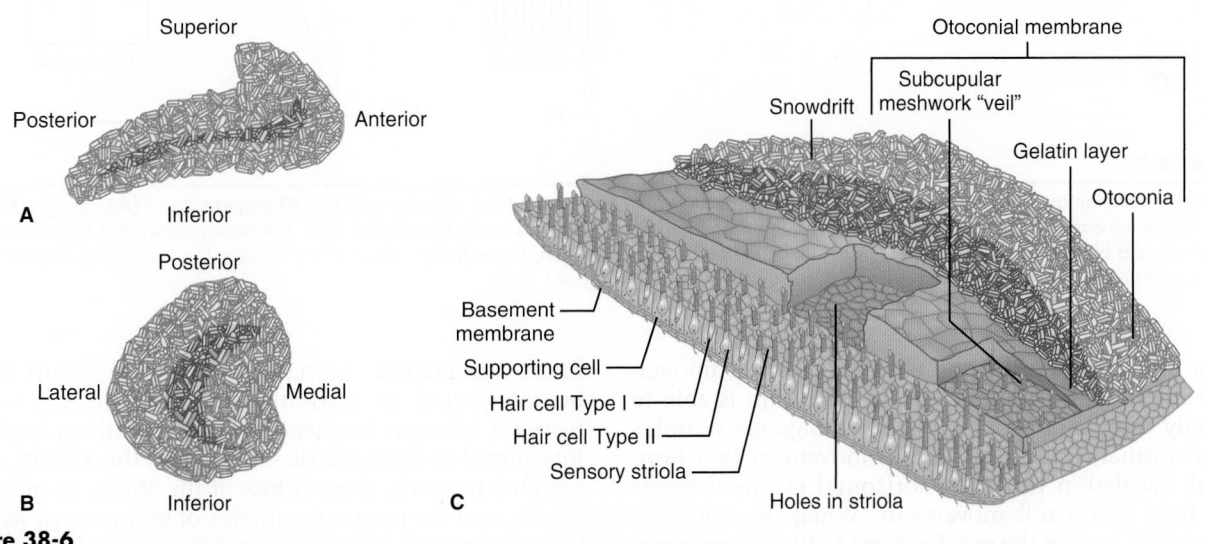

Figure 38-6

Arrangement of otoliths in the two maculae. A, Saccule. **B,** Utricle. **C,** Composition of the saccular otoconial membrane in a section taken at the level shown in **A**. (From Paparella MM, Shumrick DA, eds: *Textbook of otolaryngology, vol 1*, Philadelphia, 1980, WB Saunders.)

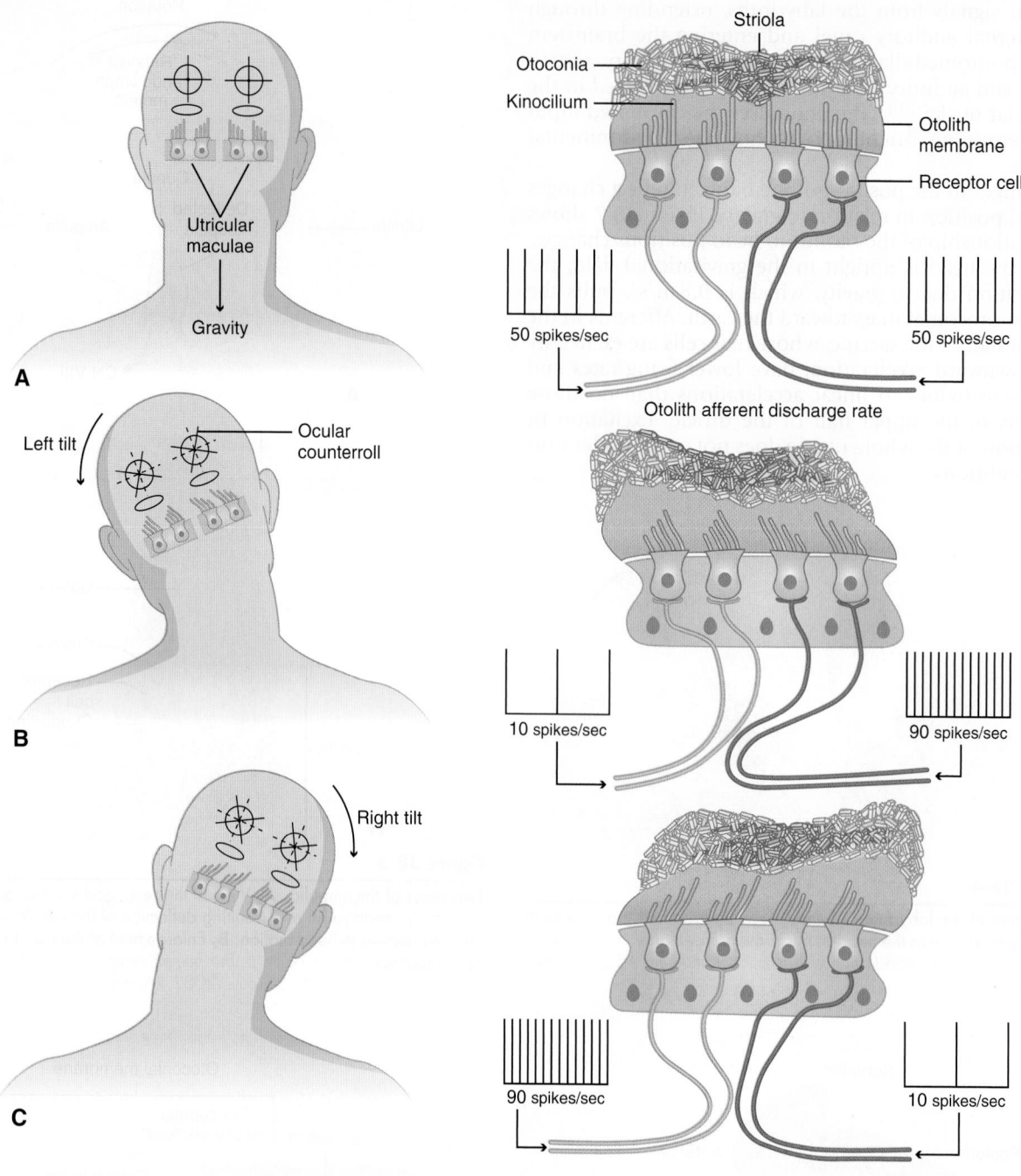

Figure 38-7

Patterns of excitation and inhibition for the left utricle and saccule when the head is tilted with the right ear 30 degrees down **(A)**, upright **(B)**, and tilted with the left ear 30 degrees down **(C)**. The utricle is seen from above and the saccule from the left side. The background color represents baseline activity and black and white represent depolarization and hyperpolarization, respectively. (Modified from Haines DE: *Fundamental neuroscience for basic and clinical applications*, ed 3, Philadelphia, 2006, Churchill Livingstone.)

The equivalence of tilt and translation causes ambiguity in the utricular afferent signals. The brain is able to correctly resolve the source of the ambiguous stimulus under normal conditions, so that movement in a horizontal translation produces horizontal eye movements with little or no roll movements. When the same net acceleration acts on the utricles during tilting movements of the head, the eyes counterroll appropriate to the tilt, but do not turn horizontally. Low-frequency or static linear accelerations acting on the otolith organs might be interpreted as gravitational accelerations resulting from tilt, whereas transient linear accelerations might be interpreted as linear translations. When this system is not working properly, there is loss of the ability to orient to gravity, and the person complains of bouncing or feels as if he or she were on a ship. It is difficult to orient to moving environments when a person is not able to orient to gravity.[11,38]

When there is disruption of the vestibular nerve on one side, causing loss of tonic firing, it results in abnormal information relayed to the brain about the position or movement of the head. The brain, as it compares the two sides, interprets the abnormal input as a perception of the head rotating toward the intact side and there will be a spontaneous nystagmus when the head is at rest. This is the true phenomenon of vertigo, or the illusion of turning or spinning. The individual will sense that the head is turning or the room is rotating. The brain quickly identifies this as an abnormal state and begins central nervous system (CNS) recalibration so that the vestibular system input from each side becomes calibrated to match the visual and somatosensory system input. There is usually adequate central adaptation to stop the spontaneous nystagmus in a lighted environment within 3 days. The spontaneous nystagmus may continue to be active in a dark room, and there may still be a sensation that the head is rotating when the eyes are closed for weeks after the onset.[11,17,29]

The vestibular system drives eye movement through its connections in the vestibular nucleus through the oculomotor nuclei to the extraocular muscles. This is known as the vestibulo-ocular reflex (VOR). The extraocular muscles are arranged in pairs and connected to the vestibular system so that a pair of canals is connected to a pair of extraocular muscles. This allows conjugate movement of the eyes as a result of head movement. Through the complex connections of the vestibular and oculomotor nuclei, information regarding direction and speed of head movement is directed to the eye muscles so that they react and move in the opposite direction at the same speed as the head is moving. This keeps the visual environment in focus during rapid head movements. Figure 38-8 shows the connection between stimulation of the semicircular canals and eye movement. Eye position signals were once thought to affect the degree of nystagmus, or to have other influence, according to Alexander's Law, but it is now apparent that they do not modulate natural vestibular responses.[6] When one side of the system is damaged or stimulated abnormally, the intricate coupling of the vestibular system and eye movements becomes disturbed.[29,53] When there is imbalance in the firing rate between the two sides of the vestibular system, the brain perceives movement of the head and the VOR mechanism causes subconscious eye movement in order to match the perception. As the eyes move, the sensation is one of the room spinning.

For head rotations at frequencies below approximately 0.1 Hz, the vestibular nerve afferent firing rate gives a poor representation of head velocity. In response to a constant velocity rotation, the cupula initially deflects but then returns back to its resting position, with a time constant of approximately 13 seconds. Neural circuits in the brainstem seem to maintain the canal signals, stretching them out in time. This effect is called *velocity storage* because it appears to "store" the head velocity information for some period of time. It appears to allow the vestibular system to function better at lower frequencies, that is, down to 0.08 Hz. There is overlap between the VOR and lower-frequency gaze-stabilizing systems of smooth pursuit and optokinetic nystagmus to allow function at all frequencies.

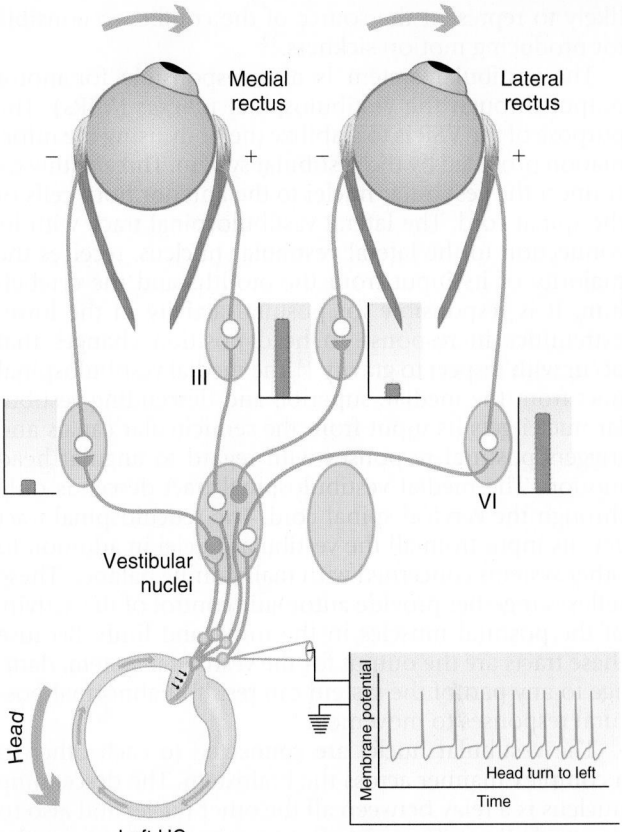

Figure 38-8

Neural connections in the direct pathway for the vestibulo-ocular reflex (VOR) from excitation of the left horizontal canal (HC). As seen from above, a leftward head rotation produces relative endolymph flow in the left HC that is clockwise and toward the utricle. The cupular deflection excites the hair cells in the left HC ampulla, and the firing rate in the afferents increases (inset). Excitatory interneurons in the vestibular nuclei connect to motor neurons for the medial rectus muscle in the ipsilateral third nucleus (III) and lateral rectus muscle in the contralateral sixth nucleus (VI). Firing rates for these motor neurons increase (mini bar graphs). The respective muscles contract and pull the eyes clockwise, opposite the head, during the slow phases of nystagmus. Inhibitory interneurons in the vestibular nuclei connect to motoneurons for the left lateral rectus and right medial rectus. Their firing rates decrease, and these antagonist muscles relax to facilitate the eye movement. (From Flint: *Cummings otolaryngology: Head & neck surgery*, ed 5, St. Louis, 2010, Mosby.)

Velocity storage creates the prolonged nystagmus that occurs after sustained constant-velocity rotation in one direction. Rotation to one side generates a positive change in afferent firing on the ipsilateral side and a negative change on the contralateral side. Because of the excitation-inhibition asymmetry inherent in the semicircular canal signals, the net result is not zero change in the afferent firing rate sensed by the brainstem, but rather a net excitation on the ipsilateral side. The excitation extends beyond the time that the cupula deflection has returned to resting state and causes the perception of rotation toward the same side. The perception and nystagmus decays with the time constant of approximately 20 seconds. The spatiotemporal properties of velocity storage, which are processed between the nodulus and uvula of the vestibulocerebellum and the vestibular nuclei, are likely to represent the source of the conflict responsible for producing motion sickness.[32]

The vestibular system is also responsible for motor output through the vestibulospinal reflexes (VSRs). The purpose of the VSR is to stabilize the body using the information provided by the vestibular system. Three pathways connect the vestibular nuclei to the anterior horn cells of the spinal cord. The lateral vestibulospinal tract, with its connection to the lateral vestibular nucleus, receives the majority of its input from the otoliths and the cerebellum. It is responsible for postural activity in the lower extremities in response to head position changes that occur with respect to gravity.[54] The medial vestibulospinal tract from the medial, superior, and descending vestibular nuclei gets its input from the semicircular canals and triggers postural responses with regard to angular head motion. The medial vestibulospinal tract descends only through the cervical spinal cord. The reticulospinal tract gets its input from all the vestibular nuclei in addition to other systems concerned with maintaining balance. These reflexes together provide automatic control of the activity of the postural muscles in the trunk and limb. Because these tracts are the output for the vestibular system, damage to any part of the system can result in abnormal postural responses to movement.[68]

The vestibular nuclei are connected to each other in a complex manner across the brainstem. The descending nucleus is a relay between all the other nuclei and also to the cerebellum. The cerebellum receives output from the vestibular nucleus. The vestibular reflexes become uncalibrated and ineffective when the cerebellum is dysfunctional (see Chapter 28).

The vertebral-basilar artery supplies blood to the components of the vestibular system. The posterior and inferior cerebellar arteries feed this area of the CNS. Because there is redundant blood supply via the circle of Willis, ischemia in this area is rare. The anterior inferior cerebellar arteries supply the peripheral mechanism via the labyrinthine, common cochlear, and anterior vestibular arteries.[19] Disorders that affect the small vessels can cause direct damage to the peripheral vestibular system, or the ischemia can cause direct damage to the vestibular nuclei. Figure 38-9 demonstrates the pathways associated with the end organ, vestibular nuclei, fibers of the cerebellum, and the extraocular muscles. This pathway involves inhibition in the process of modulating output to extraocular muscles.

Incidence and Etiologic and Risk Factors

The vestibular system can be involved in many conditions either directly or indirectly; therefore it is difficult to determine the incidence within the general population. Even the most common causes of lesions vary. Although dizziness is common in all age groups, the frequency of dizziness increases with age. Aging has a significant effect on vestibular function but may not be the primary cause of imbalance. Hair cell loss occurs with aging, particularly in the ampulla. It has been estimated that neuronal loss in the vestibular nuclei occurs at a rate of approximately 3% per decade from the age of 40 years.[83] Approximately 10% of people older than 45 years visit their physicians complaining of dizziness and it increases in those older than 75 years.[26] Changes in the vestibular system

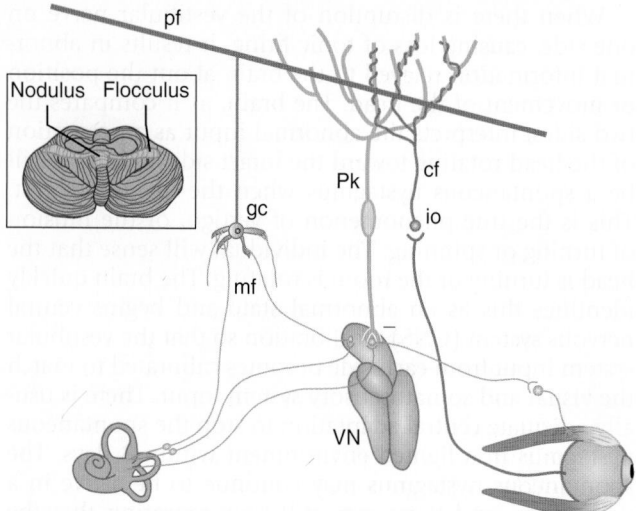

Figure 38-9

Circuitry of the cerebellum involved in modifying the vestibulo-ocular reflex (VOR). Inputs from primary vestibular afferents and secondary vestibular neurons (VN) form mossy fiber (mf) inputs to cerebellar granule cells (gc). Parallel fibers (pf) originating from these synapse weakly with Purkinje cells (Pk), causing a highly tonic inhibitory output of simple spikes from the Purkinje cells onto secondary vestibular neurons controlling the VOR. Climbing fiber (cf) input from the inferior olive (io) carries sensorimotor error information such as retinal slip. Climbing fibers make extensive and strong synapses onto Purkinje cells. Climbing fiber activity leads to complex spikes in the Purkinje cells, which can alter the efficacy of the parallel fibers' synapses onto the Purkinje cells—a form of learning. (From Flint: *Cummings otolaryngology: Head & neck surgery,* ed 5, St. Louis, 2010 Mosby.)

happen during the normal aging process, but the problems reported to physicians are most likely caused by a pathologic process. Dizziness is reported more frequently by women than by men.[36]

A dysfunction can affect the system at any level. Disorders of the labyrinth, or inner ear, can affect the sensory end organs, resulting in abnormal input into other levels of the vestibular system. Damage to the peripheral vestibular nerve can be from a neurologic pathology, mechanical deformation from a nonneurologic pathologic condition, or trauma to the structures surrounding the nerve. A central deficit can be the result of damage to the area in the brainstem or cortex that processes vestibular information. The brainstem can be affected in many ways. Pathologic processes here can also be direct, as in mechanical damage of the neurons in brain injury, bleeding disorders, and neoplasia. Hypoxic damage can occur in stroke or other conditions that cause decreased profusion of oxygen into the brainstem. Degenerative diseases such as multiple sclerosis (MS), Parkinson disease, and Alzheimer's disease can cause abnormal function in the brainstem and its connections.

Most falls in the elderly population result from an accidental slip or trip, often in association with an unsteady gait. Less than 10% of falls in the elderly population are a result of an acute attack of vertigo or dizziness. It appears that over time there is selective nonuse of vestibular cues during balance activities. Age-related increases in sway have been found for conditions that involved sway referencing of visual or somatosensory cues.

MEDICAL MANAGEMENT

DIAGNOSIS. Dizziness is the most common complaint when the vestibular system is not providing adequate information about where the head is in space. It is important to recognize that dizziness is a broad term for the sensation that results from the disruption of information from vestibular, visual, and somatosensory systems. The description of dizziness may reflect the nature of the disorder. The history of the dizziness should give an indication of the cause of the symptoms and lead toward diagnosis. The symptoms, as reported, can reflect an abnormality in the vestibular system or may indicate some other general medical cause. Often the history is complex, and much insight is gained by listening carefully and allowing the client to provide his or her own thoughts on the probable cause. Often, there is a sensation of motion when the head is stable, with the individual sitting unsupported, which can give initial cues about the system function and degree of adaptation. A sensation of rotation may represent lack of adaptation of the input, reflecting a unilateral disorder. Floating, swimming, or tilt may represent abnormal otolith response. When the report of motion is lightheaded, it is important to assess the function of the somatosensory system, and when the report is one of buzzing, disorientation, fear or panic, maladaptation of the three systems is suspected.

Because the visual system is required for adaptation, the brain will use the visual system as a substitute to determine movement of the head. The visual system can effectively determine head position in a visually stable environment. Initially, it is typical to have this visual dependency. When the CNS fails to make the appropriate adaptation back to use of the vestibular system, this dependence on vision can become chronic and cause a sense that the head is rotating when vision is occluded, or when the visual environment is not stable. Head motion–provoked disturbances reflect abnormalities in the ability of the system to identify movement accurately, related to the abnormal gain of the system. This can be tested through responses to head rotation.[63] The time it takes the brain to resettle after this motion can also reflect lack of CNS recalibration. See section on velocity storage.

When the initial description is that of feeling lightheaded, as opposed to sensation of rotation, several conditions should be considered. Presyncope is related to blood flow and may be related to orthostatic hypotension. Anxiety or panic can trigger sensation of lightheadedness, but usually there are other abnormal sensations such as paresthesia or shortness of breath. (See "Somatoform Disorders" below.) When the complaint of lightheadedness is accompanied by a lack of feeling grounded, the integration between the vestibular and somatosensory system may be disrupted. The somatosensory reference mechanism is likely the cause. (See "Special Implications for the Physical Therapist 38-1: Vestibular Dysfunction.")

Nausea is a frequent complaint associated with dizziness and reflects the stimulation of the medullary centers by abnormal sensory input. Direct damage to the medulla causes the most severe nausea, as in stroke, but it can also be reflected in traumatic brain injury. Differences in white

---

Box 38-1

THREE TYPES OF PHYSIOLOGIC NYSTAGMUS

- Vestibular induced, or spontaneous
- Visually induced, or optokinetic
- Cerebellar, or end-gaze induced

---

matter microstructure within tracts connecting visual motion and nausea-processing brain areas may contribute to nausea susceptibility. This appears to be related to an increased history of nausea episodes.[87]

Sudden-onset conditions often create a high level of nausea that decreases as the system recalibrates. Canal stimulation, especially during repositioning maneuvers, can cause nausea; horizontal canal stimulation provokes higher levels of nausea than does the posterior or anterior canal. Migraine headache and traumatic brain injury may trigger dizziness as a part of the abnormal processing of input through the brainstem. Headache pain can have a relationship to dizziness and typically reflects either a concomitant disorder of the CNS or the effort of the cervical musculature to decelerate the head. (See "Cervicogenic Headaches," Chapter 37.)

Disorientation is often described as feeling out of sync with the environment and is usually associated with other deficits, such as short-term memory loss, lack of concentration, and irritability, reflecting the intricate integration with the limbic, hippocampal, and reticular systems throughout the brainstem.[15] Disequilibrium is reported as feeling unsteady or clumsy or as if one were swaying, and a history of falls should be obtained. Fear of falling is also of importance, and the efforts made to avoid a fall can shed light on the degree of relative vestibular spinal responses. The side effects associated with use of some medications, anemia, hypoperfusion of the brain from postural hypotension, cardiac arrhythmia, endocrine disorders, and hypoglycemia may mimic a vestibular disorder. If the cause is a medical condition or the use of medications, the symptoms should decrease when the appropriate condition is treated or when the medication is stopped.[47]

The visual-ocular system is measured when looking for a disorder of the vestibular system and, when abnormal, can provide some clues as to where the damage to the system is located. If the motor component of the VOR is damaged, visual and vestibular controlled eye movements are abnormal. If the sensory component of the vestibular system is damaged, visually controlled eye movements are usually normal, but vestibular-dependent eye movements are abnormal and can cause nystagmus. Nystagmus is involuntary, rhythmic oscillation of the eye. Nystagmus can be a part of another brain dysfunction in addition to vestibular dysfunction. The nystagmus related to vestibular disorders usually has a particular direction, intensity, and shape. The characteristics can often offer clues to the pathologic condition. Pathologic nystagmus can be spontaneous, gaze evoked, or positional. Box 38-1 describes three types of physiologic nystagmus. Examination for pathologic nystagmus must include observation of the effects of fixation, eye position in the orbit, and head position.[59] Measurement of the interaction of the visual and vestibular systems can be accomplished by a variety of tests, with each test providing information that can be compared with the results of other tests to help determine the diagnosis.

Video Nystagmography or Electronystagmography. Capturing eye movements related to vestibular dysfunction can be done through use of video goggles (video nystagmography [VNG]) or by surrounding the orbit with electrodes (electronystagmography [ENG]). Most testing now is done using VNG. The angular velocity, amplitude, and frequency of nystagmus can be quantified. The ability to move the eyes quickly from one target to another intended target can be tested for accuracy and is called *saccadic eye movement.* When the target is missed on the first movement, there is a catch-up saccade used to move the eye directly to the target. Catch-up saccades are normal in some cases, such as for jumps made more than 20 degrees, because there is a consistent undershooting. Slow saccadic eye movements can be related to lesions in the central pathways that control their movement. This may be an abnormal motor response of the VOR, or it can be a part of many other degenerative or static lesions that can affect the same part of the system, such as MS or parkinsonian disorders. Saccadic eye movements can be induced by using dots or lights at different amplitudes and asking the client to move the focus quickly from target to target. Accuracy can be recorded using VNG/ENG to demonstrate the undershooting and overshooting resulting from disorders affecting control of eye movement. The direction of the nystagmus reflects possible origin. Purely vertical or torsional spontaneous nystagmus suggests a central origin. Nystagmus caused by a central lesion can be in any direction (vertical, oblique, horizontal, rotational), may change direction as gaze direction changes, and is not suppressed by fixation of gaze.[75]

The ability to follow a target through a trajectory, or smooth pursuit, is another ocular skill that reflects an intact visual-ocular system and vestibulo-ocular output. An acute vestibular lesion will cause an impairment of smooth pursuit, but accuracy should naturally return. Abnormalities of the smooth pursuit system can reflect disorders throughout the CNS. Cerebellar lesions are often a cause of abnormal smooth pursuit. Table 38-1 describes different functions of eye movements. Smooth pursuit, or tracking of the target, is observed by recording the eye movement as the client attempts to follow targets at varying velocities. Use of a pendulum or computer-generated movement of lighted targets allows a sinusoidal tracking that can be measured by electrooculographic recording. Two measures are usually applied to the recordings. Pursuit gain compares the velocity of the eye to the velocity of the target. Pursuit phase lag refers to the difference in time between waveforms of the target and the responsive eye movement. A person with normal tracking will predict the target motion and make the precise eye movements necessary to stay on target.[115]

Optokinetic nystagmus is the eye movement elicited by tracking a field instead of a target. The purpose of optokinetic nystagmus is to stabilize visually an entire moving visual field. Optokinetic nystagmus is recorded by ENG when a striped drum surrounding the client is moved at a constant velocity at a slow speed of 30 degrees and a fast speed of 60 degrees. Abnormalities of slow components parallel those of smooth pursuits and are related to disorders of the cortex, brainstem, diencephalon, or cerebellum. Abnormalities of the fast components reflect damage, as do abnormal saccades. VNG/ENG is used to measure eye movements caused by activation of the VOR and records spontaneous eye movements caused by alteration of the vestibular discharge rate. The limitations of smooth pursuit and optokinetic nystagmus illustrate the important concept that reflexive sensorimotor systems have optimal operating ranges. Smooth visual pursuit functions are best for low-frequency slow head movements. Autonomic gravity receptors function best for static and very-low-frequency conditions. These and other reflexes overlap with the vestibular system for part of its operating range, but nonvestibular systems largely break down during quick head movements. The VOR is essential for gaze stabilization during higher-frequency, velocity, and acceleration head movements.[94]

Bithermal Caloric Test. Manipulation of endolymphatic flow in the semicircular canals by creating a temperature gradient is known as *bithermal caloric stimulation.* When warm air is infused in the external auditory meatus, the skin of the horizontal canal is heated, resulting in a temperature change that is transmitted to the horizontal semicircular canal. The endolymph closest to the canal wall is heated, causing it to become relatively less dense than the surrounding endolymph. The fluid movement that results from the heating of the endolymph deflects the hair cells in the ampulla, simulating head movement; the result is a nystagmus with the fast component moving toward the canal that was stimulated. Cold air or water

Table 38-1	Different Functions of Eye Movements
Class of Eye Movement	**Main Function**
Vestibular	Holds images steady on the retina during brief head rotations
Visual fixation	Holds the image of a stationary object on the fovea
Optokinetic	Holds images steady on the retina during sustained head rotation
Smooth pursuit	Holds the image of a small moving target on the fovea or holds the image of a small near target on the retina during linear self-motion; with optokinetic responses, aids gaze stabilization during sustained head rotation
Nystagmus quick phases	Reset the eyes during prolonged rotation and direct gaze toward an oncoming visual scene
Saccades	Bring objects of interest onto the fovea
Vergence	Moves the eyes in opposite directions so that images are placed or held simultaneously on both foveas

has created movement in the opposite direction. The mnemonic COWS (*cold opposite, warm same*) describes the movement of nystagmus related to the temperature of the stimulus used. The caloric examination allows the clinician to evaluate each horizontal semicircular canal separately.[62] VNG recordings during this stimulation can indicate abnormalities in different locations of the vestibular system and brain. Paresis can indicate damage anywhere from the end organ to the entry of the nerve root in the brainstem. A central disorder that affects the nerve root, such as MS or brainstem strokes, can cause paresis recording on caloric testing. Lesions of the cerebellum evoke heightened caloric responses and a suppression fixation deficit. Abnormalities in the characteristics of the nystagmus, such as vertical or oblique responses, are associated with CNS disorders.[75] Figure 38-10 describes three ways to invoke nystagmus.

The elderly tend to show reductions in the gain of the VOR and smooth pursuit and increases in saccade latencies. Such age-related alterations might interfere with appropriate responses to fast head movements. Initially, reduction of the inhibitory system mediated through

the cerebellum can compensate for decreased sensitivity. Over time, the combination of reduced peripheral sensitivity and central inhibition decreases the range in which the system responds.[83]

Rotational Chair Testing. Rotational testing of the horizontal semicircular canal is provided by use of a motorized rotational chair. Angular acceleration can be controlled and responses to angular acceleration measured. Persons who suddenly lose vestibular function on one side have asymmetric responses to rotational stimuli. Rotational stimuli are ideally suited for testing persons with bilateral peripheral vestibular lesions because both labyrinths are stimulated simultaneously and the degree of function is accurately quantified. As with lesions of the peripheral vestibular structures, lesions of the central VOR patterns can lead to changes in the gain of rotational-induced nystagmus. Rotary chair testing may consist of either steps of constant-velocity rotation or sinusoidal harmonic oscillations, typically from 0.01 to 0.6 Hz. Velocity steps may be delivered by suddenly starting the rotation of the chair from zero velocity to a sustained constant velocity in one direction. The same stimulus may be obtained by braking the chair after a prolonged constant velocity rotation in the other direction. The horizontal canals' endolymph and cupulae tend to keep moving in the direction that the chair had been moving, so that the stimulus is equivalent to a velocity step in the direction opposite to that in which the chair had been turning.

Cerebellar dysfunction will result in abnormal amplitudes and arrhythmia. Cerebellar ataxia with bilateral vestibulopathy causes a high prevalence of subnormal function of both central and peripheral vestibular function. This is an easily missed clinical entity that is often associated with normal caloric investigations.[96] Dysfunction of the neural integrator and velocity storage can also be seen in the results of rotary chair testing.

Electrocochleography. Electrocochleography is used to record elevation of endolymphatic fluid pressure. It is the recording of acoustically evoked electrical potentials arising from the cochlea and the eighth cranial nerve. An electrode is placed on the tympanic membrane or on the wall of the external ear canal near the tympanic membrane.

Subjective Visual Vertical or Horizontal. The ability to recognize vertical and horizontal in a darkened room in relation to gravity indicates intact functioning of the utricle. This is known as *subjective visual vertical* or *subjective visual horizontal*. There is an ocular torsion that occurs after unilateral lesions of the vestibular system that is related to dysfunction of the otoliths. It is thought that this ocular rotation results in the inability, in the acute phase of vestibular damage, to accurately determine vertical or horizontal visually. This is tested in a darkened room using a light bar that is controlled by the client's relation to vertical or horizontal. Clients are asked to determine when the bar is in either a horizontal or vertical position in relationship to gravity as they sit in a chair. The offset from the true position is often up to 15 degrees. With a compensated lesion, the accuracy improves to 4 degrees but does not ever appear to return to normal. This test will not detect bilateral utricular lesions.[52,112] The "bucket test," which is a clinical simulation of visual vertical, is able to identify spatial orientation deficits in

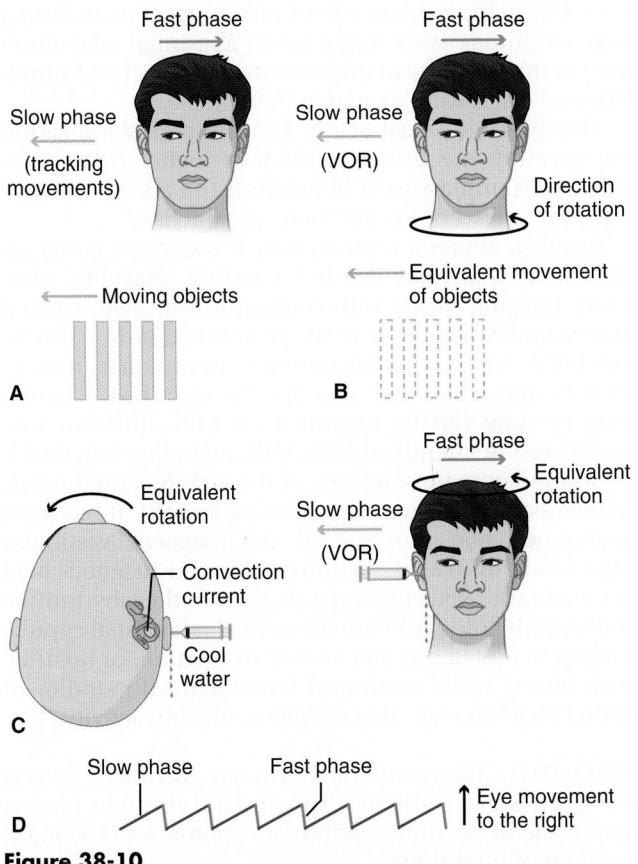

Figure 38-10

Three different ways to cause nystagmus. A, Movement of a series of objects to the individual's right causes slow tracking eye movements to the right followed by rapid movements to the left. **B,** Rotation to the left is equivalent to the movement of objects to the right as perceived by the retina. **C,** Cool water or air placed near the horizontal canal via the external ear canal causes the same movement of the endolymph as head rotation in **B. D,** Electrical recording of horizontal nystagmus with its fast phase to the left. (From Nolte J: *The human brain: An introduction to its functional anatomy,* ed 5, St. Louis, 2002, Mosby.)

clients with known vestibular disorders, but it is not useful for the diagnosis of vestibular impairment.[25]

Vestibular-Evoked Myogenic Potentials. The vestibular-evoked myogenic potential (VEMP) test can provide information in addition to the tests of the semicircular canals to isolate dysfunction in the otolith.[5] Saccular neurons have a strong projection to neck muscles and a weak projection to the oculomotor system. Utricular afferents have a strong projection to eye muscles. So measuring oculomotor responses predominantly probes utricular function, while measuring neck muscle responses to these stimuli predominantly probes saccular function.[30]

The VEMPs arise from stimulation of the saccule, and the fact that the saccule is very sensitive to sound. Click-sensitive neurons in the vestibular nerve are the same neurons that respond to tilts. VEMP testing involves generating a standard sound set and looking for inhibition of the sternocleidomastoid recorded via electromyography (EMG). When one side of the system is dysfunctional there will be a corresponding change in EMG activity in one of the sternocleidomastoid muscles. The VEMP is generated by synchronous discharges of groups of muscle cells innervated by a single motor unit, or myogenic potential; this response is found in the sternocleidomastoid as part of the vestibulocolic reflex. Recordings are made with an active electrode over the motor point.[3]

Posturography, Dynamic Visual Acuity, and Gaze Stability. Testing of vestibulospinal reflex, vision, and somatosensation influences on posture and equilibrium is performed by posturography. In the *motor control test,* the individual's postural responses are recorded during displacement of the support surface using EMG recordings that reflect the activation of the segmental, spinal, and long-loop response pathways. Prolonged motor control test latencies are evidence for abnormality in any one or a combination of components making up the long-loop automatic system and therefore are strong indications for nonvestibular, spinal cord, brainstem, and subcortical involvement.[20,89,90] The *sensory organization test,* the second component of the CDP, defines six different sensory conditions in which an individual's postural sway is measured. These six conditions vary the amount and accuracy of the sensory information (somatosensation, vision, vestibular input) available to maintain balance.[88] Vestibular dysfunction patterns are seen in virtually all persons with bilateral peripheral vestibular deficits. These persons are able to maintain balance when the vision or somatosensation is available, but they free fall repeatedly when conditions require dependence primarily on vestibular input.[12] Similar vestibular dysfunction patterns are seen in persons with peripheral vestibular lesions and CNS lesions affecting central pathways of the vestibular system. Persons who compensate after a unilateral lesion will have a normal sensory organization test result 2 to 4 weeks after the initial insult.[45] An abnormal preference for vision, either alone or in combination with vestibular dysfunction, is most frequently observed in persons with sensory dependence. In individuals with maladaptation, the balance function in the primary vestibular, or conditions 5 and 6, may be preserved on isolated testing but are not integrated during daily activity. Figure 38-11 shows sensory conditions during the sensory organization test.

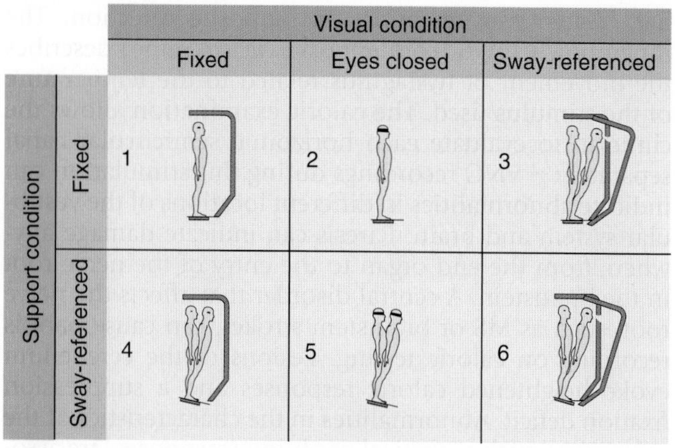

Figure 38-11

Diagram of the sensory conditions related to the sensory organization test, a component of posturography. (Courtesy NeuroCom International, Clackamas, OR.)

The addition of head movement during the SOT can increase the value of the measure.[78]

Measurement of movement strategies (ankle, hip, stepping) used to maintain balance is the third component of the CDP. Inappropriate use of ankle movements during large-amplitude sway might be an abnormal adaptation used to minimize head movements and associated stimulation of the vestibular system.[28,88]

The dynamic visual acuity and the gaze stabilization test quantify the fixation ability at higher frequencies and speeds primary to VOR function and are an objective addition to tests of the vestibulospinal reflex.[9]

Imaging. When a central cause is suspected based on clinical findings and vestibular testing, magnetic resonance imaging (MRI) with contrast is indicated. Central brainstem lesions, such as stroke, trauma, or MS, can be identified. Neoplasms, including schwannomas, meningiomas, and metastases, can also be identified. Vascular loop or sling can be identified on MRI. Inflammatory lesions can be identified with MRI, including labyrinthitis and inflammatory lesions of the eighth cranial nerve. Dizziness can be experienced during an MRI. It has been determined that during MRI the magnetic vestibular stimulation from a interaction between the magnetic field and naturally occurring ionic currents in the labyrinthine endolymph fluid pushes on the semicircular canal cupula, leading to nystagmus and a sense of rotation, or floating. Such effects could confound functional MRI studies of brain behavior, including resting-state brain activity.[98]

TREATMENT. Treatment of vestibular disorders reflects the spectrum of etiologies. The physical therapist plays a major role in the multidisciplinary approach to the management of symptoms.

When symptoms are due to a peripheral vestibular lesion, functional recovery will begin within 2 days to 4 weeks through the adaptive mechanism of the brain.[115] When the symptoms are severe, sedatives may be given, ideally for the first 24 hours only. Rehabilitation should begin within the first 3 days if possible. Treatment of recurrent dizziness depends on the nature of the underlying disorder. The goal is to eliminate the frequency and duration of the abnormal sensation of motion and the symptoms of nausea, vomiting, and anxiety.[8] If the central adaptation process is inadequate, vestibular suppression can be helpful but must be used judiciously.

Surgical intervention is considered when the symptoms are unrelenting and the underlying condition is determined but is unresponsive to other medical measures. Local application of gentamicin to selectively destroy the end organ is often used rather than ablative surgery. Surgery is indicated with neoplasia (see Chapter 30) perilymph fistula, persistent benign paroxysmal positional vertigo (BPPV), hydrops, and vascular loop. These conditions are covered later in this chapter.[72]

PROGNOSIS. When there is a unilateral lesion in the peripheral vestibular system and the CNS is intact, recovery of function is possible. The recovery related to the static imbalance, the differences in the tonic firing rate within the vestibular nuclei, is part of the adaptation process. When adaptation occurs, the spontaneous nystagmus at rest resolves, and there is no longer a sensation of movement at rest. The recovery of dynamic disturbances, reflecting the relationship of the coupling of the two sides of the system during movement, requires visual experience. The visual experience allows the brain to recognize the error of the system through the retinal slip, causing oscillopsia that occurs immediately after the lesion. It is this sensory mismatch provided by the visual system that allows the CNS to recognize the need for adaptation and drives the readjustment of motor reflexes.[69,82] The VOR should return to near normal within 2 to 6 weeks for slower movements, so that motion of the head during typical activities no longer disrupts vision or causes nausea. However, there will continue to be an abnormal reaction to rapid head turns. Recovery is minimized when the response of the individual experiencing the symptoms is to avoid the provoking motions and the CNS is never given the opportunity to adapt to the asymmetric firing patterns of the peripheral vestibular system.[74]

Complete bilateral loss is relatively rare; more often there is decreased function in both sides, often to a different degree on each side. Rehabilitation can provide adaptation to whatever degree possible and compensation for the remaining loss of function.[71] When there is complete bilateral dysfunction, substitution of the other intact sensory inputs for balance is required. The use of visual and somatosensory inputs to substitute for loss of vestibular function is possible when the environment provides adequate cues, as in well-lighted environments and firm, level surfaces. Substitution of small saccades in the direction opposite to head rotation can augment inadequate gain. Smooth pursuit accuracy can improve, and predictive strategies can improve gaze stability. More accurate use of spatial localization is reflected in the ability to imagine the location of stationary targets.[49,115]

The VSRs are slower to return, and the individual may continue to experience instability when turning quickly or walking on uneven surfaces or in the dark for weeks or months after the insult.

Recovery rate in a central vestibular system disorder causing dizziness or disequilibrium depends on the nature of the lesion and the concomitant neurologic dysfunction. If vertigo is part of a progressive disease, it should be addressed as part of the overall rehabilitation. A disease such as MS can cause episodes of symptoms and progressive dysfunction with poor adaptation and compensation because of the other damage within the CNS.[15] Vestibular rehabilitation is critical in these individuals.[57,58] In a disorder of the central as well as the peripheral vestibular system, as in head injury or multisensory disorders, the recovery is related to recognizing and treating the individual components and working on the reintegration process effectively.

Vestibular Dysfunction

Vestibular rehabilitation is used extensively for individuals with vestibular dysfunction with good evidence for effectiveness.[60,77,103] The 36-item Vestibular Rehabilitation Benefit Questionnaire (VRBQ) appears to be a concise and psychometrically robust questionnaire that addresses the main aspects of dizziness impact.[85]

The appropriate choice and progression of exercises are critical for the outcome.[89,95,107] One of the greatest challenges in working with a client with symptoms of dizziness and imbalance is making the correct determination of precipitating factors and understanding concomitant disorders of the brain and musculoskeletal system.[79] Often health care providers stop short of the success that can be achieved because they do not fully understand the very complex mechanisms related to balance and dizziness. When the system recovers, typical activity should provide adequate stimulus to maintain vestibular function.[55] Individuals will often avoid situations on the edge of their tolerance, especially if there is additional brain dysfunction. These individuals may show some decline in function over time if the system does not continue to be challenged as it is during the rehabilitation process.

Examination

Clinical evaluation by the therapist of the client with vestibular dysfunction integrates the history with the objective findings of sensory and movement disorders. The history can guide the therapist regarding the mechanism of injury and location within the system. The nature of the symptoms and the precipitating, exacerbating, and relieving factors are reviewed.[4,86,88]

The use of clinical syndromes can help make the connection between evaluation and intervention. Identification of sensation of motion at rest points to basic lack of adaptation of tonic firing rate, whereas motion-provoked dizziness occurs when the calibration between the two sides is inefficient during movement. Visual and somatosensory dependence develops early when the vestibular input is inadequate and can persist throughout the course of rehabilitation if not identified and treated. Visual motion sensitivity results from the inability to filter out movement in the peripheral fields and is related to, but not exactly the same as, visual dependency. Head-righting response should be evaluated to determine if there is ability to use the otolith mechanism without override of the somatosensory system.

Testing in the clinic includes motor control of the visual-ocular component. VOR integrity is demonstrated by the client's ability to maintain visual focus during quick head turns. Other reflexive systems can compensate for the loss of vestibular reflexes and make it appear that there is no deficit, so these factors must be recognized when performing the tests. For example, a patient with well-compensated, long-standing bilateral loss of vestibular function may appear to have no problem keeping vision fixed on the examiner as the examiner rotates the patient's head slowly from side to side. In such individuals, smooth pursuit, optokinetic nystagmus, and the cervicoocular reflex make up for the vestibular deficit. This is an example of a head movement that *can* be sensed by the vestibular system, but that is not in the range of frequencies and accelerations sensed *exclusively* by the vestibular system. However, rapid head rotation can pull the eyes off target. The vestibular deficit can thus be unmasked by very dynamic head movements.[42,110]

A careful look at the CNS, through testing of function associated with cranial nerves, cerebellum, brainstem, and cortical connections, is critical to determine if there is a central cause. Often, both central and peripheral lesions can be identified. Sensory deficits should be determined. Control of balance in altered sensory conditions that isolate vision, somatosensory, and vestibular inputs is evaluated (see earlier discussion of the sensory organization test). Musculoskeletal and neuromuscular evaluations are critical to determine compensatory movements based on deficits in these areas that may mimic vestibular dysfunction or detract from recovery. When observing upright balance, evaluation of strategy selection is helpful in identifying abnormal hip or stepping strategy, a common finding in clients with vestibular disorder.[4,56]

Seniors awaiting discharge from hospital often have impaired vestibular control of balance that is associated with impaired mobility. Evaluating vestibular function prior to discharge from hospital could improve discharge planning with respect to management of impairments that threaten balance and safe mobility.[48]

Intervention

Recovery requires both visual input and movement of the body and head. There must be an error signal produced to let the brain know that adaptation is needed. For example, when the client is unable to maintain gaze stabilization and the image moves or slips on the retina, the nervous system will identify this error and try to adapt and modify the gain of the vestibular system. This is the process of adaptation that is facilitated by vestibular rehabilitation.[42,46,51] Depending on the severity of the symptoms, these exercises may begin in a supine or sitting position in order to decrease the vestibulospinal challenge. The system is progressively challenged by adding activities incorporating movement of the eyes, head, and body, such as tracking a ball tossed from hand to hand.

Adaptation of the vestibular system is context specific. Treatment should therefore address the multitude of environments that the person will encounter. Exercises should stress the integration of all systems involved in balance, synthesizing the visual and somatosensory cues with the vestibular cues.[14] To stimulate use of somatosensory inputs, environments are designed to place less emphasis on vision while providing reliable somatosensory inputs. To stimulate the use of visual inputs, environments are designed to place less emphasis on somatosensation while providing reliable visual cues. The vestibular system is naturally stimulated when visual and somatosensory cues are distorted.[44]

Altered postural alignment is common with vestibular dysfunction. Sudden loss of vestibular function can result in both lateral flexion of the head and an abnormal shift of the center of gravity to the side of the lesion. Vestibular pathologic conditions result in an inability to accurately determine one's limits of stability, resulting in maintaining the center of gravity outside of or on the edge of the actual limits of stability, which may cause loss of balance.[54] It is often noted that the person is unable (or unwilling because of fear of falling) to move the center of gravity far enough to perform a functional task such as descending stairs.[109]

When the balance disorder results in an inability to move the center of gravity through the ranges necessary to perform mobility tasks, the client will benefit from activities directed toward increasing the limits of stability.[62] Center-of-pressure biofeedback provides input regarding control of center of gravity during weight shifts.[90] Lesions of the vestibular system can result in abnormal postural reactions to changes in head and body positions. When the individual relies on vestibular cues for the primary input for balance, the impaired system fails to provide the necessary input. Orientation to gravity or to support surface changes that include dorsiflexion or plantar flexion is inadequate to maintain upright position. This is seen in the inability to maintain balance on a compliant surface or on a surface that rotates at the ankle. It becomes difficult to walk in the dark, on soft surfaces, and up and down ramps or stairs. Postural strategies, or postural control synergies, are triggered in preparation for movement and in response to changes in the environment. An ankle strategy is used when the client is standing on a firm, flat surface. The torque for the motion is controlled at the ankle. Vestibular dysfunction does not appear to affect this strategy because the input to drive the response comes primarily from the somatosensory system. However, initially there is difficulty performing this ankle strategy without the use of vision as a second sensory system with which the brain can compare.[56]

A hip strategy is used when the client is standing on a narrow (beamlike) surface or when the surface is soft. A hip strategy is used on a flat surface when the center of gravity moves beyond the base of support. In a hip strategy, the torque is controlled at the hip. Individuals with a vestibular loss have difficulty using the hip strategy. It becomes difficult to perform activities such as single-leg stance, heel-toe walk, and standing on a beam or a compliant surface. The individual with vestibular loss can generate a hip strategy but have difficulty maintaining control with perturbations of the surface and tends to use a stepping strategy to compensate for inability to maintain balance using the hip strategy.[4,54,56] Stepping strategy is used to bring the center of gravity over the base of support when it moves too far to control with an ankle or hip strategy.

There is an abnormal perception of self-motion in relationship to movement in the environment. Therefore walking in a crowded environment, riding on an escalator, or walking in a grocery store may create increased symptoms of dizziness. Walking is easier in an empty shopping mall than in a crowded one, and walking with the crowd is less taxing than walking against the crowd.

It is important for the therapist to educate and support the individual during the natural course of the recovery. A program should be designed to facilitate the use of vestibular input for balance progressively so that the individual does not become overdependent on vision or somatosensation for balance. It appears that many individuals who have been considered compensated show less natural use of the vestibular system compared with individuals who have never had a vestibular problem. Current research is oriented toward more novel and effective ways to reestablish vestibular function. For example, use of repetitive platform perturbations at vestibular dependent velocities demonstrate improved postural stability and greater functional abilities when compared to other forms of rehabilitation.[114]

A THERAPIST'S THOUGHTS*

While this chapter demonstrates the tremendous complexity of the balance sensory and motor system, the key to successful rehabilitation of the greatest percentage of dizzy patients of all etiologies often lies in the basic understanding of the many components within the system. Simple yet critical things such as listening carefully to the patient's description of the detail in symptom onset and quality, validating the intensity of discomfort reflected in the high perception of disability, and addressing compassionately the anxiety that is often present.

The individual with BPPV or unilateral vestibular hypofunction, in the absence of comorbidities, will respond quickly and completely to the interventions of vestibular rehabilitation. However, many patients who present for help to a dizziness specialist are dealing with complex comorbidities such as atypical migraine, unidentified postconcussive syndrome, cervical somatosensory dysfunction, or disorders of the visual system either in perception or in eye position or oculomotor control. Guidance of the patient into complete adaptation and resolution of symptoms requires careful assessment and treatment of visual, oculomotor, and somatosensory system integration.

*Julie Knoll, PT, NCS

Benign Paroxysmal Positional Vertigo (BPPV)

Episodic, intense vertigo related to head position is most often a benign disorder called BPPV, also known simply as benign positional vertigo (BPV). It is considered a benign condition, because it is not the sign of a disease process but a mechanical disorder of the labyrinths.

Incidence and Risk Factors

BPPV is the most common cause of vertigo seen by otolaryngologists, representing 20% to 40% of patients with peripheral vestibular disease. The incidence is difficult to estimate given the benign, typically self-limited course of the disease. It is thought to vary from 10 to 64 cases per 100,000 persons. Affected women outnumber men by a ratio of 1.6 : 1. Involvement in more than one canal is found in 20% of cases. Spontaneous remissions are common, but the disorder can recur in up to 40% of the cases. The condition may trouble the individual intermittently for years, but in this condition a close examination of potential causes will often identify an underlying medical disorder, and recurrences decline when the disorder is managed. Increased fluid pressure within the labyrinth may dislodge otoconia (see discussion of endolymphatic hydrops below). Migraine-induced ischemia may be responsible for the release of otoconia. Head trauma or infectious or inflammatory disorders may precede the onset by months or even years. Adverse life events are reported often prior to the onset of BPPV. Aging, perhaps because of the increase of dehydration, increases incidence.[31]

Clinical Manifestations

Despite the use of the term *benign*, the symptoms related to positional vertigo are intense and can cause significant disability. There is often a strong sense of falling or spinning out of control, even when the individual is lying on a bed. Before the individual is aware of the mechanism, it seems to be something that is uncontrollable because it occurs with changes of head position. Typically, a person with BPPV will complain of brief episodes of vertigo precipitated by head movement in a specific direction. The vertigo follows getting into bed and lying down. Often the first report is that of waking up suddenly in the night with the room spinning. Bending, looking up to take an object off a shelf, tilting the head back to shave, getting a haircut, or turning the head rapidly while backing up a car can trigger symptoms. These single bouts of vertigo are frequently clustered in time and separated by remissions lasting months or more. Symptoms occur suddenly and typically last 20 seconds, but typically not more than a minute. The subjective impression of attack duration reported is frequently longer than the actual period of dizziness.[40,59] Box 38-2 gives typical complaints related to BPPV.

Pathogenesis

The otoconia in the otolith can become loose, clump together, and form densities known as canaliths. Canaliths move through the fluid and become problematic

Box 38-2

COMMON CHARACTERISTICS OF BENIGN PAROXYSMAL POSITIONAL VERTIGO

- Episodic sensation of intense vertigo with head position changes
- Sensation stops after 20 to 30 seconds in static position
- Nausea with vertigo with reports of spinning inside the head
- Autonomic changes such as sweating, feeling like passing out
- Sensation of movement of the environment and blurred vision
- Reports of disequilibrium during typical activities
- Waking up dizzy at night after rolling over in bed
- Symptoms during head movement or bending forward during typical activities

Box 38-3

CANALITHIASIS OF BENIGN PAROXYSMAL POSITIONAL VERTIGO

- The canalithiasis mechanism explains the latency of nystagmus as a result of the time needed for motion of the material within the posterior canal to be initiated by gravity.
- The nystagmus duration is correlated with the length of time required for the dense material to reach the lowest part of the canal.
- The vertical (upbeating of fast phase) and torsional (superior poles of the eyes beating toward the lower-most ear) components of the nystagmus are consistent with eye movements evoked by stimulation of the posterior canal nerve in experimental animals.
- The reversal of nystagmus when the patient returns to the sitting upright position is due to retrograde movement of material in the lumen of the posterior canal back toward the ampulla, with resulting ampullopetal deflection of the cupula.
- The fatigability of the nystagmus evoked by repeated Dix-Hallpike positional testing is explained by dispersion of material within the canal.

when they float into the semicircular canals. There is potential for them to go into any of the three canals, but most often they will move into the posterior canal because of the relationship of the posterior canal to the otolith. The posterior canal is placed in the vertical position when the body is supine and the head is extended beyond neutral and rotated 45 degrees to the same side. The canaliths drift out of the otolith through the opening to the posterior canal and begin moving through the endolymph in the semicircular canal, causing drag on the endolymph and creating cupular deflection, or movement of the ampulla. This movement of the cupula is interpreted in the brain as movement of the head. There is an intense sensation of rotation. As the canaliths reach the bottom of the semicircular canal, they slow down and stop moving, stimulation of the vestibular nerve ceases, and the sensation of movement stops. This typically takes about 15 to 60 seconds. Cana-lithiasis of the posterior semicircular is the most frequent cause of BPPV. Box 38-3 describes the phenomenon of canalithiasis.

A less common variant of BPPV is cupulolithiasis. It is thought that the otoconia can become adherent to the ampulla. In this instance, there is an inappropriate deflection of the hair cells with movement, causing vertigo and nausea. The symptoms will begin immediately with movement of the head in the provoking position and will persist as long as the head is held in the position. The symptoms may decrease slightly because of adaptation of the CNS and therefore may mimic the fatigue of canalithiasis. Cupulolithiasis, either occurring independently or in combination with canalithiasis, is more likely to be involved in the etiology of horizontal canal BPPV than is the case for posterior canal BPPV.[61]

MEDICAL MANAGEMENT

DIAGNOSIS. The diagnosis of BPPV is made based on a suggestive history and report of current clinical manifestations as described above. The classic eye movements are found when performing the Dix-Hallpike maneuver. Despite more than 20 years of information disbursed on the Epley maneuver and other provoking procedures; a patient who presents with BPPV in emergency or routine care is more likely to undergo a head CT than to be screened for BPPV.

Dix-Hallpike Maneuver. Diagnostic criteria for BPPV include spinning vertigo induced by a specific head position or movement. There is a burst of positioning nystagmus that is rotary with latency of symptoms on placing the head in a provoking position; the nystagmus is *fatigable*, that is, it diminishes with repeated positioning and lasts less than 60 seconds.

The Dix-Hallpike maneuver, or passive movement of the head from the upright position to one with the head hanging extended and rotated to 45 degrees, is the standard test performed to establish the diagnosis of BPPV. When the head is in this position, the clinician observes the eyes for evidence of nystagmus. It may take at least 20 seconds for the nystagmus to occur, and the nystagmus should fatigue within 60 seconds. The nystagmus occurs when the affected ear is placed down. Figure 38-12 shows the testing positions. The pattern of response is torsional nystagmus that is identified by rotation of the superior poles (the center, vertical component of the iris) toward the involved ear. This is accompanied by an upbeat nature to the nystagmus. There is a latency of onset of nystagmus. Duration of nystagmus is typically less than 1 minute. Vertiginous symptoms are reported as a sensation that the room is spinning, or the individual is spinning or falling out of control. Symptoms often recur, and the nystagmus beats in the opposite direction on return of the head to the upright position. BPPV can affect the anterior canal, however this is less frequent. The nystagmus expected in cases of anterior canal BPV would be torsional, such that the superior poles would beat to the right but would have a downward nature.[31] Although a positive test is pathognomonic for BPPV, a negative test indicates only that BPV is not active at that movement.

To test for BPPV in the horizontal canal (HC), the head is first brought to the supine position resting on

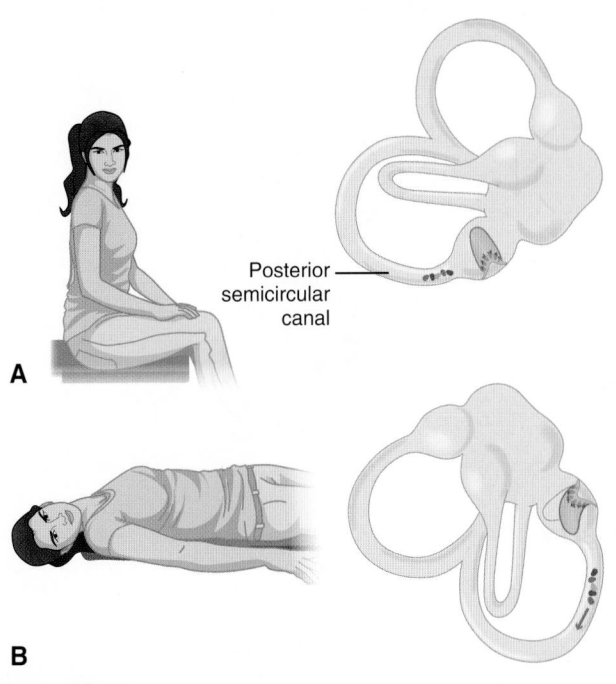

Posterior semicircular canal

A

B

Figure 38-12

The Dix-Hallpike maneuver. A, Starting position with head rotated toward the side to be tested. **B,** Lowering the patient's head backward and to the side allows debris in the posterior canal to fall to its lowest position, activating the canal and causing eye movements and vertigo. (From Lundy-Ekman L: *Neuroscience: Fundamentals for rehabilitation,* ed 4, Philadelphia, 2013, Saunders.)

the examining table or is slightly flexed. The nystagmus with horizontal canal BPV is horizontal with respect to the position of the head. HC-BPPV occurs in two forms: geotropic and apogeotropic. In geotropic HC-BPPV, the debris is in the long arm of the canal, whereas in apogeotropic it is in the short arm, close or adherent to the cupula. When a patient with right-sided geotropic HC-BPPV turns the head to the right, the debris moves toward the cupula ("ampullopetal"), which triggers right-beating nystagmus. Conversely, a right head turn in right-sided apogeotropic HC-BPPV results in debris movement away from the cupula ("ampullofugal"), which triggers left-beating nystagmus. The debris moves in opposite directions relative to the cupula in the geotropic and apogeotropic forms.[67] Figure 38-13 shows the movement of the debris in the horizontal canal.

If a brief period of dizziness is experienced during the Dix-Hallpike maneuver as the head is approaching the full supine position, and there is no evidence of posterior or anterior canal BPPV, there is a possibility of horizontal canal involvement, which should be further investigated. Horizontal canalithiasis can also occur, producing symptoms provoked by rolling in the supine position. Horizontal nystagmus may occur in either direction but will be greatest when rolling the head to the involved side.[61,93]

Another form of positional dizziness that must be ruled out in making the diagnosis of BPPV is central positional vertigo. Nystagmus that is sustained and not suppressed by visual fixation reflects a central lesion. These findings can be indicative of ischemia of the

pontomedullary brainstem or another part of the central vestibular pathway. Cerebellar involvement will cause dizziness in positions of supine, head rotated left with extension, and head rotated right with extension. Pure downbeating nystagmus in either the sitting or supine position may indicate an infratentorial disorder. This can be related to vascular insults such as Arnold-Chiari malformation, stroke, or subdural hematoma. MS lesions are common in this area and are associated with the progressive forms. Unilateral lesions, perilymphatic fistula, superior semicircular canal dehiscence, or middle ear problems can cause positional dizziness and are discussed later in this chapter. Intermittent dizziness that is made worse with position changes could also be part of the aura of migraine.

It should also be noted that it is typical to experience dizziness with the head pitched backward, as it puts the otoliths at an angle that is not a part of daily activity. Orthostatic hypotension can also create a brief episode of dizziness when going from supine to standing.

TREATMENT. Several approaches have been developed to treat persons with BPPV, including maneuvers or positions that attempt to dislodge the provoking substances and move them through the canal system back to the otolith, known as canalith repositioning procedures or the libratory maneuver. The key component is identifying the appropriate patients and then performing the correct repositioning maneuver. Canalith repositioning is a series of passive movements designed to move loose debris (otoconia) through the canal and back into the otolith. Typically 2 to 4 repeated procedures are necessary. BPPV of the posterior canal is the most common due to its position in relationship to the otolith. Figure 38-14 shows the sequence of the Epley maneuver the procedure typically used to move otoconia from the posterior canal. Even if the canalith-repositioning procedure clears the posterior canal, there is an elevated risk of reentry or canal conversion to the horizontal canal. In this case, additional maneuvers are required to clear the debris; the risk can be reduced by waiting at least 15 minutes between repetitions of canalith-repositioning procedure.[43]

When the BPV is within the horizontal canal, dizziness or vertigo is reported often associated with head turning, looking down or when rolling, especially if the head is elevated on a pillow because the canal is in a position perpendicular to gravity.

Lateral or horizontal canal BPPV responds to positional procedures that involve head rolling with the horizontal canal in the plane and allow gravity to pull the otoconia through the horizontal canal. The Gufoni and head-shaking maneuvers are effective in treating apogeotropic horizontal BPPV.[70] Oscillation to the mastoid process is effective when there is cupulolithiasis. Maneuvers should be avoided in patients who have had retinal detachment or who might be susceptible to such a detachment because of high myopia. In some cases, the canalith-repositioning procedure results in remission of symptoms and there is return of postural control under conditions of somatosensory and visual conflict and visual-vestibular interaction.[65]

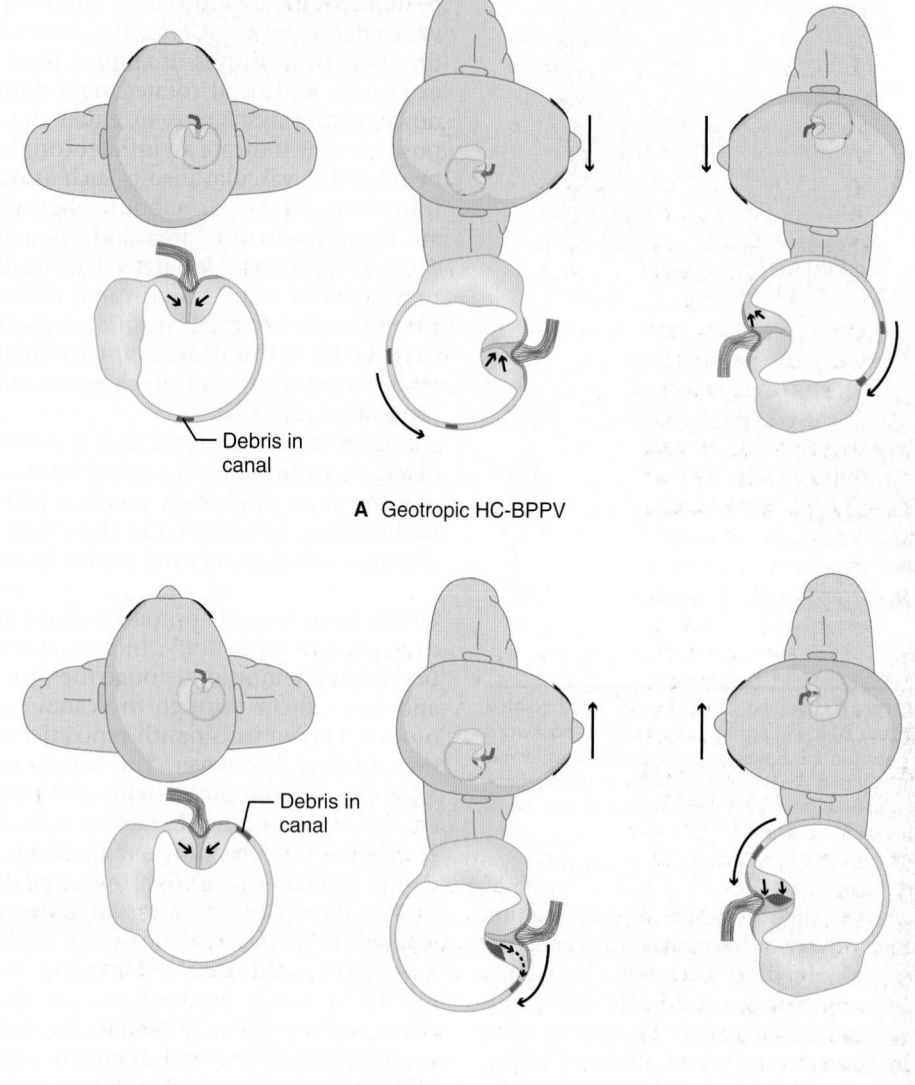

Debris in
canal

A Geotropic HC-BPPV

Debris in
canal

B Apogeotropic HC-BPPV

Figure 38-13

Relative movement of the debris in the horizontal canal during changes of head position. (From Flint: *Cummings otolaryngology: Head & neck surgery,* ed 5, St. Louis, 2010, Mosby.)

SPECIAL IMPLICATIONS FOR THE THERAPIST 38-2

BPPV

Ability to perform repositioning maneuvers is the basis for treating BPPV. It is critical to be aware of the confounding nature of multiple canal involvement. Because of the high degree of recurrence, some individuals do best with a program they can perform at home. However, because the correct canal must be identified, return to the clinic is warranted in many cases. When a client has symptoms that they are unable to control, use of anti-nausea medication prior to repositioning to control symptoms can be helpful.

When the individual has had a period of dizziness, and especially when the BPPV has recurred or has been persistent over years, there is a high incidence of maladaptation of sensory integration for balance, resulting in somatosensory and visual dependence for balance. Although the individual no longer complains of dizziness, there may be imbalance in low light or when there are compliant surface conditions. Visual motion hypersensitivity is common and responds well to intervention. Evaluation for BPPV should include the balance system, and intervention for balance disorder should follow clearing of BPPV.[61,113]

Infection

Acute unilateral vestibulopathy, or vestibular neuritis, is the second most common cause of vertigo. Viral infection is common and usually affects the vestibular nerve unilaterally. Vestibular neuritis can be a partial unilateral vestibular lesion, and this partial lesion can affect the superior division of the vestibular nerve, which includes the afferents from the horizontal and anterior semicircular canals.[39]

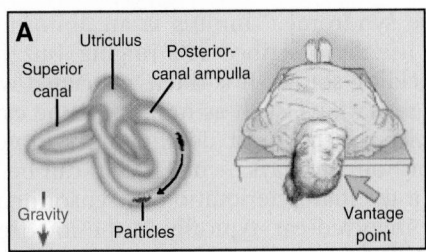

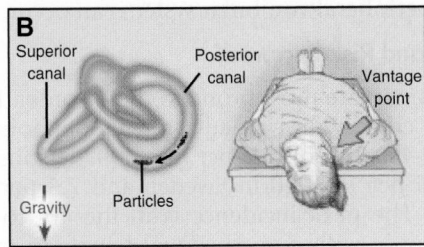

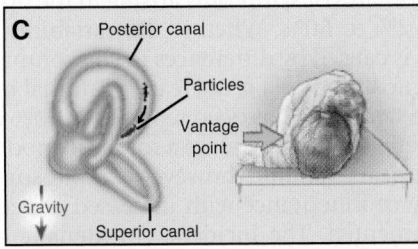

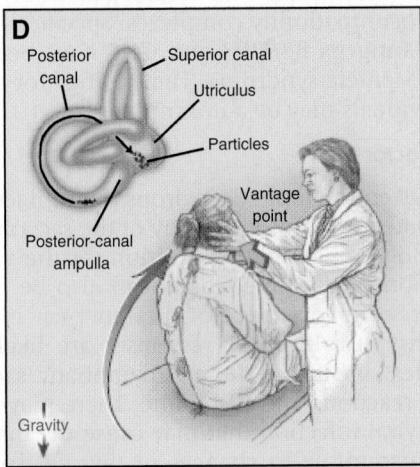

Figure 38-14

Canalith repositioning maneuver for the patient with posterior canal benign positional vertigo (BPV). Figure represents procedure for right-side BPV. Movement of particles through the canal is shown in each position.

Incidence and Etiology

Incidence is 3.5 in 100,000. Viral infections are common between the ages of 30 and 60 years, with a peak for women in the fourth decade and men in the sixth decade.[40] The apparent etiology of the disease is multifactorial. Viral pathogens include mumps, rubella, herpes simplex virus type 1, cytomegalovirus, and Epstein-Barr virus. Enteroviruses are among the other rare viral causes. Onset is often preceded by a systemic viral illness, such as an upper respiratory tract infection or gastritis. The illness may precede the vestibular dysfunction by up to 2 weeks but can happen within the course of a bout of cold or flu. When illness

such as measles, mumps, or infectious mononucleosis is the source, hearing loss may accompany the vestibular symptoms. Polyneuritis of the seventh and eighth cranial nerves, known as Ramsay Hunt syndrome, can be the result of herpes zoster, causing perivascular, perineural, and intraneural infiltration. Other viruses are suspected but have yet to be positively identified. The cortical vestibular projection fibers can be affected by herpes zoster encephalitis, which has a predilection for the temporal lobe. The use of antibiotics in general has decreased the incidence of bacterial infections affecting the vestibular system. However, infections still do arise and can be introduced into the vestibular apparatus through the various fluid systems involved or through breakdown of the bony labyrinth.

Pathogenesis

Histopathologic studies have suggested involvement of the superior vestibular nerve and vestibular ganglion, often with little or no involvement of the actual end organ. This is true of vestibular neuritis, in which there is no cochlear involvement. However, many viruses do damage throughout the labyrinth and cochlea. Typically, in vestibular neuritis, the end organ is filled with lymphocytes. Intracytoplasmic particles have been found in the vestibular ganglia. These particles are thought to be dormant forms of a virus that may produce infection, with resultant inner ear disease.[11]

Persons with bacterial meningitis develop labyrinthitis when bacteria enter the perilymphatic space from the cerebrospinal fluid by way of the cochlear aqueduct or the internal auditory canal. Some bacterial infections result in biochemical irritation of the membranes through a toxic reaction. Both congenital and acquired syphilitic infections produce labyrinthitis as a latent manifestation.

Clinical Manifestations

Unilateral vestibular neuronitis causes sudden onset of vertigo, spontaneous horizontal nystagmus, nausea, and vomiting. Immediately after the onset of unilateral vestibular hypofunction, there is intense disequilibrium. There are profound disturbances of position and motion perception. There is a false sense of angular motion (i.e., rotation). With the eyes closed, there is an illusion of spinning, or sense of motion of the body turning on its long axis toward the involved side. When the eyes are open, the illusion is of spinning of the environment in the opposite direction. There is a tonic ocular tilt reaction consisting of head tilt, conjugate eye torsion, skew deviation, and lateropulsion, seen as an abnormal weight shift toward the side of the lesion.[27] This is due to the otolithic hypofunction on the side with the lesion.[88,89]

MEDICAL MANAGEMENT

DIAGNOSIS. The VOR becomes abnormal with unilateral hypofunction. There is loss of gaze stabilization with head movement. Movement of the head then causes blurring of vision, resulting in dizziness and loss of ability to use visual cues to maintain balance. EMG testing shows a unilateral hypofunction.

A spontaneous mixed torsional and horizontal nystagmus is often present immediately after unilateral hypofunction. The slow phases are directed toward the side of the lesion, and the quick phases are to the intact side. As the eyes are observed, it is the quick phases that are apparent, and therefore the nystagmus appears to be moving away from the side with the lesion. The nystagmus is suppressed by gaze fixation, or looking at a static object.[89] Peripheral vestibular nystagmus is usually mixed torsional and horizontal in a fixed direction opposite the side of the lesion.

TREATMENT. The main groups of drugs used for symptoms of acute vertigo include antihistamines, anticholinergic agents, antidopaminergic agents, steroids, and antivirals such as acyclovir. Glucocorticoids administered within 3 days after onset of vestibular neuronitis improves long-time recovery of vestibular function and reduces length of hospital stay.[64]

Recovery of function and resolution of dizziness is accomplished through a program to facilitate the vestibular system. Recalibration, or adaptation of the system, comes by facilitating the integration of somatosensory input and recovery of normal postural responses. (See "Special Implications for the Therapist 38-1: Vestibular Dysfunction.")

PROGNOSIS. The symptoms slowly resolve over 6 weeks to 3 months, but there can be persistent complaints of imbalance, motion intolerance, and headache related to decrease in the natural motion of the head. In some cases, decreased functional use of the vestibular mechanism develops and is related to excess caution on uneven surfaces, dizziness that is more easily provoked, an overall decrease in activity level, or avoidance of activity that may cause dizziness. These individuals may continue to complain of dizziness with quick head turns, and imbalance in the dark. Often, visual motion sensitivity will develop. These conditions are justification for further rehabilitation, with a more focused approach. (See "Special Implications for the Therapist 38-1: Vestibular Dysfunction.")

Endolymphatic Hydrops and Ménière Syndrome

Definition and Overview

Endolymphatic hydrops is a disorder relating to the membranous inner ear as a consequence of the overaccumulation of endolymph compromising the perilymphatic space. Hydrops may occur in an episodic manner, as a result of sudden increases in the secretory function of the stria vascularis or of spontaneous obstruction of the endolymphatic sac. Hydropic distension may then cause a mechanical deflection of the macula and crista of the otoliths and semicircular canals, respectively, and thus vestibular hair cell depolarization, leading to the sensation of vertigo. Long-term changes to the neurosensory function of the vestibular apparatus may be the consequence of increased hydrodynamic pressure, causing increased vascular resistance, compromised blood flow, and chronic ischemic injury.[1]

Ménière syndrome is thought by many to be a form of endolymphatic hydrops but the relationship is not absolute, and it cannot be proven. The symptoms, however, lead to this hypothesis and treatments are directed toward the control of fluids. The characteristic episodic vertigo; fluctuating, sensorineural hearing loss; sensation of fullness in the ears; and tinnitus is the basis for the diagnosis

of Ménière syndrome. Tinnitus is an abnormal sound in the ear usually described as a ringing, buzzing, clicking, or crackling sound. It is often associated with other abnormal sensations, such as fullness of the ear. Vertiginous attacks are the most debilitating symptom, with intervals of hours to days. Acute attacks can be superimposed on a gradual deterioration in sensorineural hearing in the involved ear, typically in the low frequencies initially. Over time, a reduction in responsiveness of the involved peripheral vestibular system can occur.

Incidence and Risk Factors

Whites women are most prone to the disorder. However, diagnostic criteria have varied across epidemiologic studies. These vary from 157 per 100,000 persons in England to 46 per 100,000 in Sweden and 7.5 per 100,000 in France. The peak incidence is in the 40- to 60-year-old age group, with a nearly equal female to male ratio (1.3:1). Estimates of symptoms arising in the opposite ear vary from 2% to 50%. Whether the variability in prevalence rates is caused by differences in environment, genetics, or diagnostic criteria is unclear.[111] Familial occurrence of Ménière syndrome has been reported in 10% to 20% of cases. Genetic inheritance plays a role. The mode of transmission appears variable; however, an autosomal-dominant mode of inheritance with increased penetrance has been documented. The incidence of Ménière syndrome is greater in individuals with certain genetically acquired major histocompatibility complexes. Specifically, human leukocyte antigens B8/DR3 and Cw7 have been associated with Ménière syndrome. The etiology for disease in these individuals may be autoimmune.[41]

Etiologic Factors

The cause of endolymphatic hydrops is multifactorial and may be related to fibrosis, atrophy of the sac, obstruction of the endolymphatic duct, infection, or the vascularity in the region of the inner ear. It can also be caused by otosyphilis, or involvement of the inner ear in collagen vascular diseases. Immune responses are likely within the complex, including the endolymphatic sac, related to allergic reactions and histamine. There may be a predisposing viral infection that may cause the inner ear to be more susceptible to changes in thyroid, sodium, or hormone dysfunction. The deficit may also be related to overproduction of endolymph by the stria vascularis.[34] Posttraumatic endolymphatic hydrops can be observed following a blow to the head, a fall, or flexion or extension injury sustained in an automobile accident.

Pathogenesis

Despite the variety within the etiologic factors, there is a consistent disruption of homeostasis of inner ear fluid. Endolymphatic hydrops may be an epiphenomenon rather than directly responsible for the symptoms. Animal models of endolymphatic hydrops have provided a basic scientific understanding of endolymphatic hydrops, including the mechanical characteristics and the influence of hydrops on inner ear anatomy and function. These studies have shown that endolymphatic hydrops is accompanied by a cascade of subtle biochemical and morphologic alterations, each of which may contribute to the dysfunction.

Pathologic studies of the human sac in the hydrops patient have recorded ischemia and fibrosis around the endolymphatic sac. Alterations in the size of the endolymphatic duct and sac along with reductions in the lining of these structures have also been noted in both the diseased and nondiseased inner ears. This supports the theory that an abnormal endolymph drainage system may predispose individuals to the future development of Ménière syndrome. Alterations in endolymph Ca^{2+} has been shown to influence transduction in hair cells, and it is likely that endolymph Ca^{2+} changes contribute to functional losses present in the hydropic cochlea of animals, and possibly in the ears of humans with Ménière disease. These ionic disturbances may be caused by ischemia resulting from changes in local vasculature. It has been suggested that the endolymphatic sacs of patients with Ménière disease have significantly higher vasopressin receptor levels, suggesting that the ears of these patients may be more sensitive to vasopressin.[1] A common vascular mechanism for migraine headaches and Ménière disease has also been proposed. A hydropic state may leave those persons sensitive to stresses to the inner ear.[111]

Deficits are related to the volume and pressure changes within closed fluid systems. The increase in the volume of endolymph causes the membranous labyrinth to progressively dilate until the wall makes contact with the stapes footplate and the cochlear duct fills the entire scala vestibuli, causing both vestibular and cochlear dysfunction. Distension of the otoliths can put pressure on the ampulla, creating the sensation of spinning that is characteristic of acute unilateral dysfunction.

Clinical Manifestations

The typical attack of hydrops related to Ménière syndrome is experienced as an initial sensation of fullness of the ear, a reduction in hearing, and tinnitus. This is usually followed by a rotational vertigo, postural imbalance, nystagmus, and nausea. The vertigo may last from 30 minutes to 24 hours. The symptoms abate over time, and the individual regains the ability to maintain balance. However, there may still be some sense of disequilibrium. Hearing slowly returns, but over time there may be a permanent loss of hearing. Tinnitus is common in hydrops and is commonly described as a low-pitched roaring or similar to a seashell noise. Box 38-4 gives some of the characteristics consistent with the diagnosis of Ménière syndrome.

Box 38-4

SOME CHARACTERISTICS CONSISTENT FOR THE DIAGNOSIS OF MÉNIÈRE SYNDROME

The diagnosis of Ménière syndrome is primarily based on the medical history. According to established guidelines, a definite diagnosis requires the following:

- Two or more definitive episodes of spontaneous rotational vertigo lasting at least 20 minutes
- Low-frequency sensorineural hearing loss documented by audiometry
- Tinnitus or aural fullness in the affected ear
- Exclusion of other causes for the symptoms

MEDICAL MANAGEMENT

DIAGNOSIS. The complaints of vertigo, hearing loss, and tinnitus do not automatically confirm a diagnosis of endolymphatic hydrops or Ménière syndrome. The definitive vertiginous attack is sudden in onset with nausea and vomiting, lasts 20 minutes, but abates by 24 hours. Typically, any movement during an attack aggravates the vertigo. The presence of neurologic signs or symptoms such as syncope, visual aura, and motor weakness suggest another diagnosis. Disorders that can present with similar symptoms include migraine, acoustic neuroma, perilymphatic fistula, dehiscence of the superior semicircular canal, labyrinthitis, autoimmune inner ear disorder, and MS.

An audiogram, or test of hearing, typically demonstrates low-frequency hearing loss on one side. Perceived hearing loss can be difficult to verify without audiometry, especially during an exacerbation of tinnitus or aural pressure. Improvement in audiograms can reflect better control of fluid, and decreases in hearing are suggestive of progressive disease.[111]

Electrocochleography may provide objective evidence of the presence of endolymphatic hydrops in the presence of large summating potentials. However, the diagnostic utility of the test is limited by the variability of the ratio both in individuals with hydrops and in normal individuals. The results should be used in the face of other subjective history. Figure 38-15 shows typical ECoG responses. It is also important to note that elevation of SP/AP is not

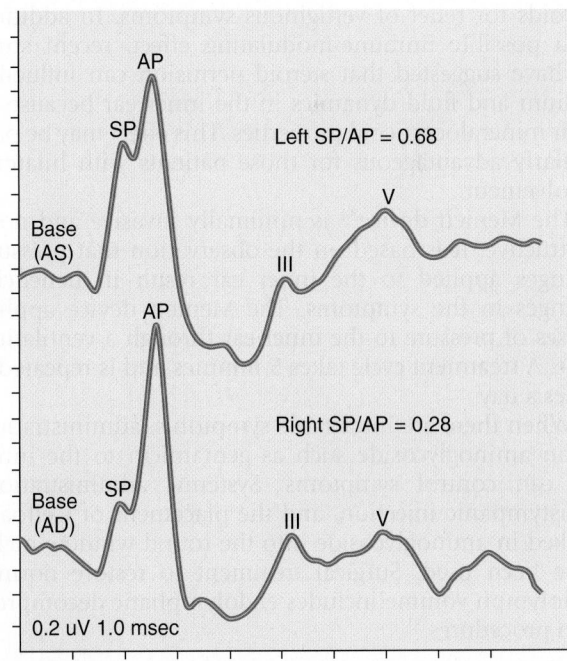

Figure 38-15

Click-evoked ECoG response recorded with a hydrogel tympanic membrane surface electrode in a patient with Ménière disease in the left ear. This response was elicited by an alternating click stimulus presented at 85 dB non-Hodgkin lymphoma. The SP and AP are measured from the prestimulus baseline. Note the increased SP in the diseased left ear. *SP,* Summating potential; *AP,* cochlear nerve action potential. (From Audiovestibular testing in patients with Meniere's disease, *Otolaryngol Clin North Am* 43(5), October 2010, Philadelphia, 2010, Saunders) specific to Ménière syndrome. Similar ECoG abnormalities have been reported in patients with perilymph fistula and superior semicircular canal dehiscence. See section below.

TREATMENT. The acute management is mainly symptomatic. Although hospitalization is rarely required, intravenous fluids may be required in the emergency department. Vestibular suppressants can be used for symptomatic control, although they can delay patients' recovery by suppressing the adaptive response if used over a longer interval. Salt restriction and lifestyle modification are typically suggested as a first course. Levels of recommended salt restriction vary; but figures often quoted range from 2 g per 24 hours down to 1 g per 24 hours with the suggestion to pay close attention to food labeling, and avoid processed foods.

Diuresis as a treatment has been advocated since at least the 1930s. Diuresis reduces the amount of endolymphatic hydrops by reducing the extracellular fluids in the body. Hydrochlorothiazide is the most widely advocated, although furosemide and spironolactone have been used as well.

Cochlear vascular insufficiency as a result of autonomic dysfunction has been proposed in hydrops. Betahistine has been used as a treatment because of its theoretic vasodilatory effects on the blood supply to the inner ear. The exact mechanism of action of betahistine in this setting is not known.

Use of transtympanic steroids to treat sudden sensorineural hearing loss have stimulated interest in the use of steroids for relief of vertiginous symptoms. In addition to a possible immune-modulating effect, recent studies have suggested that steroid perfusion can influence sodium and fluid dynamics in the inner ear because of their mineralocorticoid properties. This effect may be particularly advantageous for those patients with bilateral involvement.

The Meniett device[84] is minimally invasive and nondestructive. It is based on the observation that pressure changes applied to the inner ear result in beneficial changes in the symptoms. The Meniett device applies pulses of pressure to the inner ear through a ventilation tube. A treatment cycle takes 5 minutes and is repeated 3 times a day.

When there are intractable symptoms, administration of an aminoglycoside such as gentamicin to the inner ear can control symptoms. Systemic administration, transtympanic injection, and the placement of Gelfoam soaked in aminoglycoside into the round window niche have been used. Surgical treatment to restore normal endolymph volume includes endolymphatic decompression procedures.[31]

PROGNOSIS. The natural history of endolymphatic hydrops and Ménière syndrome is highly variable. Clusters of attacks may be separated by periods of long remission. Balance function between attacks can be normal. Over time, there is a gradual decline in the function of the vestibular system, and complaints of imbalance and mild symptoms related to a unilateral dysfunction become common. The attacks increase in frequency in the first years and then decrease. Ménière syndrome initially affects only one ear but can progress to a bilateral condition in some individuals. If bilateral involvement has not occurred within 5 years of onset of disease in the first ear, then there is less likelihood of developing bilateral involvement.

The hearing loss in Ménière syndrome is a fluctuating, low-frequency sensorineural loss early in the clinical course. Eventually, the loss becomes irreversible, often progressing in severity with involvement of higher frequencies and loss of speech discrimination.

An estimated 2% to 6% of patients with Ménière syndrome of long duration can experience "drop attacks" known as otolithic crisis of Tumarkin, characterized by being abruptly thrown to the ground without loss of consciousness and with little or no vertigo.[46]

SPECIAL IMPLICATIONS FOR THE THERAPIST 38-3

Endolymphatic Hydrops

Endolymphatic hydrops leads to great insecurity. If an acute attack occurs in social situations, it understandably can lead to social phobic reactions, even if no particular psychopathologic predisposition is present. Comorbidity with somatoform dizziness attacks may develop. Whether trigger stress that in turn leads to psychologic symptoms or stress factors are involved primarily in the pathogenesis cannot be answered at this time. The anticipation anxiety that is typical for phobic disorders arises from the unpredictable pattern of endolymphatic hydrops, the feeling of being overcome by the attacks, being completely at their mercy, and having to stop all activity until the attacks subside. The concern over not finding a place where they can stay while experiencing an acute attack, of receiving negative reactions from those around them, and of being in a situation where they are embarrassed and helpless can cause them to withdraw from social life. When invasive treatments such as gentamicin injections or sac decompression are performed, it increases the complexity of the disorder. Severe cases of Ménière syndrome ultimately can lead to reactive depressive disorders. Antidepressant medications may be helpful. The therapist role is critical to providing education, support, and the treatment of any progressive loss of vestibular function. Physical therapy is often halted during when a patient begins a course of diuretics or steroids, then resume as the system becomes more stable.

Autoimmune Ear Disease

Overview and Definition

Autoimmune ear disease (AIED) is rapidly progressive bilateral sensorineural hearing loss that responds to the administration of immunosuppressive therapy. The disease is typically characterized by symptoms of pressure and tinnitus in the ears with or without dizziness. Autoimmune disease can affect the inner ear with resultant vertigo, sensorineural hearing loss, aural fullness, and tinnitus.

Clinical Manifestations

Symptoms usually progress over weeks or months, and there is often a known systemic immune disease, such as rheumatoid arthritis. The otologic symptoms may occur as a direct assault by the immune system or as the deposition of antibody-antigen complex in the capillaries or basement membranes of inner ear structures. AIED mimics Ménière disease with fluctuating hearing loss and vestibular dysfunction. Approximately 50% of those testing positively for AIED have positive serum antibody tests. The Western blot is currently the most widely reported diagnostic tool used in the diagnosis of AIED with autoantibodies directed against the 68-kilodalton protein.[10]

Treatment

Typical patients with AIED are managed medically with corticosteroids at the lowest dose that prevents fluctuating hearing. Most patients achieve mild recovery of sensorineural hearing loss on corticosteroids. Patients with AIED present with varied symptoms, and some have only vestibular symptoms.[33] In more severe cases, there is report of medical management with methotrexate.[32]

Perilymph Fistula

Definition and Overview

Perilymph fistula, an abnormal communication of the inner and middle ear spaces, can cause vertigo. Fistulas commonly occur at the round and oval windows of the middle ear. Attempts to identify the prevalence and characterize auditory and vestibular symptoms have been inconclusive. Some studies report vestibular symptoms as the major presenting complaint, whereas others indicate hearing loss equal to or more common than balance-related symptoms. It is thought that most fistulas result from congenital malformations or prior ear surgery. Damage can also result from pressure applied via the external ear, via the eustachian tube, or by an increase in the pressure of the cerebrospinal fluid.[16]

Clinical Manifestations

Characteristics of perilymph fistula include easing of symptoms at rest and increases with activity, including the Valsalva maneuver. Barotrauma, violent exercise, heavy lifting, or even sneezing may cause a fistula. Other mechanisms include head trauma or explosive blast. Sensorineural hearing losses vary from an isolated high-frequency loss to a low-frequency or flat one. Speech discrimination test results are not characteristic. Both the pure-tone threshold and speech discrimination scores have been noted to fluctuate. Isolated mild conductive losses have been noted. Vestibular symptoms are also variable and include episodic incapacitating vertigo, equivalent to a Ménière attack, positional vertigo, motion intolerance, or occasional disequilibrium. Disequilibrium after increases in CSF pressure (e.g., nose blowing, lifting), called *Hennebert sign*, has been noted, as has

vertigo after exposure to loud noises, which is known as Tullio phenomenon.

MEDICAL MANAGEMENT

DIAGNOSIS. The inability to reliably predict the presence of a fistula before surgical exploration, as well as the lack of standard criteria for recognizing a fistula intraoperatively, have resulted in confusion and even doubt as to the existence of symptomatic fistulas. Because fistulas have been identified intraoperatively and their repair has resulted in symptomatic and objective improvement, this diagnosis must be kept in mind in the evaluation of the vertiginous patient.

Audiologic tests considered to be helpful in the diagnosis include electrocochleography. This demonstrates a larger summating potential due to endolymph/perilymph disequilibrium. However, the test is not sensitive or specific for perilymph fistula. Results of vestibular testing are nondiagnostic. The most consistent abnormality seen is a unilateral reduced caloric response in the affected ear.

A fistula test is done by introducing positive pressure into the suspected ear, either by rapid pressure on the tragus, compression of the external canal, or use of a pneumatic otoscope, while observing the eyes. A positive fistula sign consists of conjugate contralateral slow deviation of the eyes followed by three to four beats of nystagmus. Vertigo is usually elicited at the same time. Measuring body sway during pressure on the tympanic eardrum can help make the diagnosis.

TREATMENT. Recommendations with suspected inner ear fistula include the head elevation during bed rest, laxatives to reduce the risk of increased intracranial pressure, and monitoring of both hearing and vestibular function. In those instances in which hearing loss worsens or vestibular symptoms persist, surgical exploration is warranted.

Intraoperative identification of a fistula, regardless of criteria used, is reported in about 50% of individuals explored. At the time of surgery, the oval and round windows are patched with tissue, such as blood clot, fat, fascia, or absorbable gelatin sponge.[31]

PROGNOSIS. The outcome of surgical repair is variable. An appropriate surgical candidate is probably the most significant factor in outcome. Reduction in vestibular-related complaints has been reported in more than 50% of surgeries. Hearing is improved about 25% of the time.

SPECIAL IMPLICATIONS FOR THE THERAPIST 38-4

Perilymphatic Fistula

The therapist can be instrumental in helping to determine the possibility of perilymph fistula. An individual who is compliant with prescribed exercise but lacks progress over time and reports or demonstrates fluctuating symptoms and status of balance may be suspect for possible fistula. It is important to maintain close contact with the physician, as these individuals become very frustrated and may not follow through with medical attention. Vestibular therapy should be continued after surgery as good recovery is expected. Often the physician is uncertain whether the patient's complaints are because of stable vestibular disease with inadequate central compensation or by unstable labyrinthine function. In this setting, a trial of vestibular rehabilitation is appropriate and assists in the diagnosis by clarifying this important distinction. Failure to improve with vestibular rehabilitation lends further credibility to the diagnostic impression that the lesion is unstable or progressive. It is then suitable to proceed with appropriate surgical management if the symptoms are severe enough to warrant the procedure and they emanate from the end organ.

Superior Semicircular Canal Dehiscence Syndrome

Definition and Overview

Superior semicircular canal dehiscence syndrome (SCDS) is a syndrome of vertigo and oscillopsia induced by loud noises or by stimuli that change middle ear or intracranial pressure in patients with a dehiscence of bone overlying the superior semicircular canal. As seen in fistulas, Tullio phenomenon (eye movements induced by loud noises) or Hennebert sign (eye movements induced by pressure in the external auditory canal) develop and often there is chronic disequilibrium.

Pathogenesis and Clinical Manifestations

The dehiscence creates a "third mobile window" into the inner ear, thereby allowing the superior canal to respond to sound and pressure stimuli. The evoked eye movements in this syndrome typically align with the affected superior canal. Loud sounds, positive pressure in the external auditory canal, and the Valsalva maneuver can cause characteristic eye movements. A larger length of dehiscence overlying the superior canal (5 mm or greater) can lead to dysfunction in the affected canal when evaluated by responses to rapid head movements in the plane of the superior canal. Visual fixation can suppress the evoked eye movements.[35] Figure 38-16A shows the schematic representation of superior semicircular canal dehiscence; Figure 38-16B shows the condition as seen on CT scan.

Treatment

The window is repaired surgically, with good results. Bilateral superior canal (SC) dehiscence syndrome will result in some degree of oscillopsia after bilateral SCDS surgery, but provide relief from other SCDS symptoms.[2]

Ototoxicity

Overview

The aminoglycoside antibiotics can be ototoxic, with auditory toxicity estimated at 20% and vestibular toxicity affecting 15% of the individuals receiving the drug. It appears that there is a possible genetic vulnerability,

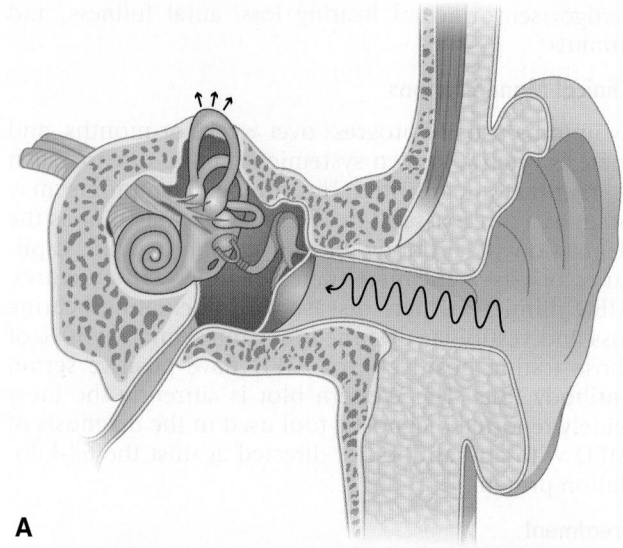

A

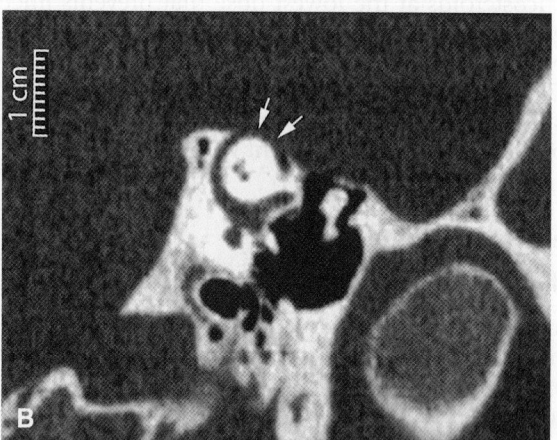

B

Figure 38-16

A, In superior semicircular canal dehiscence syndrome, sound waves can excite the superior canal because the "third mobile window" created by the dehiscence allows some sound pressure to be dissipated along a route through the superior canal in addition to the conventional route through the cochlea. **B,** CT scan demonstrating dehiscence *(arrows)* of the superior canal. (From Cummings CW, Haughey BH, Thomas R, et al: *Cummings otolaryngology: Head and neck surgery,* ed 4, St. Louis, 2004, Mosby.)

which is under study. Streptomycin and gentamicin specifically target the vestibular end organ. Other members of this group of drugs include kanamycin, tobramycin, amikacin, netilmicin, and sisomicin. Ototoxicity is usually seen in individuals who are given multiple doses over time or one large dose, usually aimed at managing a threatening infection. Damage to the hair cells in the inner ear can result in complete loss of vestibular function within 2 to 4 weeks after these drugs are given.[54]

Etiologic and Risk Factors

Approximately 3% of an orally administered aminoglycoside is absorbed from the gastrointestinal tract. They are normally injected for severe systemic infections. Penetration of the blood-brain barrier is generally poor, so that aminoglycosides are injected intrathecally to treat meningitis. Aminoglycosides are excreted primarily by the kidney by glomerular filtration, and therefore high concentrations of drug in the urine may be achieved. Impaired renal function reduces the rate of excretion. Therefore renal failure is a risk factor for ototoxicity, and dosing of aminoglycosides must be modified to compensate for delayed renal excretion. Measurement of peak and trough serum levels of aminoglycosides provides rough guidelines for therapeutic efficacy but is not an absolute guarantee for prevention of ototoxicity, particularly vestibular ototoxicity.[31]

Pathogenesis

The aminoglycoside reacts with inner ear tissues to form an active, ototoxic metabolite. The drug in its inactive form combines with iron to form an ototoxic complex. This complex reacts with oxygen to produce reactive oxygen species. These species can then react with various cell components—including the phospholipids in the cell membrane, proteins, and DNA—to disrupt the function, primarily in the outer hair cell. This process can then trigger programmed cell death, resulting in apoptosis. Histopathologic studies demonstrate that the cochlear and/or vestibular hair cells serve as primary targets for injury. Inner hair cells seem to be more resistant to injury than the outer hair cells. This could be a result of the higher concentration of the natural antioxidant glutathione in the inner hair cells. In some cases, spiral ganglion cells may be damaged directly by aminoglycosides without injury to outer hair cells. The stria vascularis may become thinner as a result of cell death. The damage is primarily bilateral, although there may be a difference in severity of loss between the two inner ear systems.

Clinical Manifestations and Treatment

One of the most debilitating early symptoms is oscillopsia. Oscillating vision is the illusion of environmental movement caused by excessive motion of images of stationary objects on the retina, known as retinal slip. Oscillopsia of vestibular origin is brought on or accentuated by head movement. It is due to insufficient VOR. When the vestibular system is unable to keep an image stationary by controlling the movement of the eyes, this slip occurs. Severe or complete bilateral loss of peripheral vestibular system function will result in inability to stabilize vision during head movement and produce oscillopsia.[47,50]

MEDICAL MANAGEMENT

PROGNOSIS. It is generally considered that the damage is permanent and that the recovery of function of the vestibular mechanism is limited. Initially there is severe disability related to sensation of dizziness, oscillopsia, and imbalance. Compensatory strategies using visual references and somatosensory input can improve mobility, taking approximately 6 weeks to become effective. There are some circumstances that will always be problematic such as walking in the dark, especially on uneven surfaces, or swimming. Night driving or driving in inclement weather should be avoided as vision is unavailable to provide stability.

Ototoxicity

When there is bilateral vestibular loss secondary to ototoxicity or by any other means that is considered permanent, the individual must be "uptrained" in the use of vision and somatosensation. They will essentially be "hanging on" with their eyes. Exercises for individuals with bilateral peripheral vestibular loss must be aimed at substitution of visual and somatosensory cues for the lost vestibular function.[60,104] The ability to maintain stable gaze is critical. Gaze stability exercise incorporates the VOR, facilitating any possible remaining vestibular function. Modifications in eye movements can be used to improve gaze stability with head movement. No mechanism to improve gaze stability will fully compensate for the loss of the VOR, and clients will continue to have difficulty seeing during rapid head movements. Some persons can learn to close their eyes during a turn and then focus quickly on a stable object to regain stability. This technique increases stability because the disruptive visual input is temporarily eliminated.[29] Strategies must be developed when the environment provides less than optimal sensory information, such as the use of an assistive device on uneven surfaces and the use of night lights to provide light at night.

Mal de Debarquement

Overview and Definition

Mal de debarquement is a syndrome that is named essentially for the symptoms related to "getting off the boat." It is usually triggered after a long time spent on a ship, such as during a cruise, or by an extended train ride. The complaints occasionally occur after international or extended air travel, especially if there is turbulence. The symptoms of dizziness and disequilibrium that usually subside within hours become persistent and can last for weeks, months, and even years. It is also reported as rocking vertigo, because the sensation is usually one of rocking back and forth and is experienced to a greater degree at rest than during movement.[18] The individual with Mal de debarquement syndrome (MdDS) would prefer to be moving in a car rather than standing still, which distinguishes it from other disorders that cause abnormal sense of movement.

Women in their third and fourth decade represent the highest percentage of people reporting symptoms; however, there has not been a clear relationship established with hormone levels. Migraine history appears to be more common in the affected group.

Pathogenesis, Clinical Manifestations, and Treatment

The basis for MdDS is uncertain but seems to be related to abnormal adaptation from one sensory context to another. An association between resting state metabolic activity and functional connectivity between the entorhinal cortex and amygdala has been found in the human disorder of abnormal motion perception.[22]

During passive motion, there may be a mismatch between the vestibular inputs that encode head motion and other sensory and motor cues. The particular movements of a boat on the water, with both a rolling (side to side) and surging (forward) cause particular referencing of the vestibular system, and the brain must decrease the use of surface reference at the ankle. Central adaptation may minimize the symptoms provoked by this mismatch, but when the movement ends, the brain must readapt to the stationary environment using an ankle strategy for balance. It has been suggested that patients with MdDS undergo a physiologic adaptive process during passive motion, but for unknown reasons they do not readily adapt back to the stable environment. This impaired return to baseline results in a perception of motion when the patient is stationary.[77] In other words, somatosensory input is no longer able to override vestibular input for stability. Providing cues outside the vestibular system is helpful, and using somatosensory weighting to providing cues about position in space appear to help the system to recalibrate. Vestibular suppressants or other medications directed at the vestibular system do not improve control of symptoms. Benzodiazepines, such as clonazepam, are of the most benefit.[21] There are some reports of MdDS following use or withdrawal from serotonergic medications. The connection here is that serotonin may inhibit glutamate, an excitatory transmitter in the vestibular nucleus.[106] Studies are underway to determine the use of transcranial magnetic stimulation for the treatment of MdDS.[23]

Prognosis

This sensation of constant motion at rest can be debilitating in that the person has difficulty managing the symptoms and tends to limit activity or overmedicate to dampen the sensation.[68] Patients with MdDS reported a poor overall quality of life especially related to role limitations due to physical problems, energy, and emotional problems. Indirect costs of lost wages during the time course add to the equation.[80]

SPECIAL IMPLICATIONS FOR THE THERAPIST 38-6

Mal de Debarquement

Traditional vestibular therapy has not proven beneficial for the treatment of MdDS in most cases. Focus on the somatosensory referencing to determine position of the head and body in space has shown clinical promise. The high degree of autonomic complaints may reflect the association of the amygdala as part of the processing deficit.

Neoplasia

Overview

Primary carcinoma can directly involve the end organ, the middle ear, or the mastoid. Glomus tumors are the most common tumor of the middle ear, arising from the chemoreceptor system of the ninth through twelfth cranial nerves and producing focal symptoms. See Chapter 30 for more information on the type of tumor presented here and information regarding treatment.

Schwann cell tumors arise from the nerve sheath of the vestibular nerve. The term *acoustic neuroma* is commonly used to describe this tumor, especially with regard to surgery. The tumor usually arises from the vestibular component of the nerve rather than the cochlea. Schwannomas are usually small, firm, encapsulated tumors that grow very slowly. They form in the internal auditory canal or cerebellopontine angle and produce symptoms by compressing the nerve. Initial symptoms are usually related to hearing loss. Eventually mild symptoms of dizziness or balance disorders can develop as the tumor increases in size and the ability to adapt to the loss of function is lost. Figure 38-17 shows the resulting findings on audiogram and imaged with MRI.

Intravestibular lipoma and intravestibular schwannoma are rare tumors occupying the intravestibular space. Patients with intravestibular lipoma or schwannoma complain of hearing impairment, tinnitus, or recurrent rotatory vertigo. Therefore, the clinical practitioner could misdiagnose them as sudden sensorineural hearing loss or Ménière disease. Because delayed diagnosis and treatment could lead to more severe and refractory symptoms, clinicians should be suspicious early.

Diagnosis

Recent advancements in imaging diagnostic tools such as computed tomography and magnetic resonance imaging have facilitated the correct diagnosis of these intravestibular tumors without surgical removal.[24] MRI with gadolinium contrast is used to diagnose these tumors. Surgical removal of schwannoma can be achieved by performing middle fossa craniotomy. The translabyrinthine approach is appropriate for tumors up to 3.0 cm. Radiosurgery (a single treatment of high-dose irradiation stereotactically administered) has been used successfully with fewer complications than surgery. There is a chance of progressive loss of hearing in the years following this procedure.

Meningiomas arise from the arachnoid layer in the area of the petrosal and sigmoid sinuses. The tumor is encapsulated and therefore does not invade the neural tissue. Displacement of the cranial nerves, brainstem, and cerebellum is common, causing complaints consistent with compressive damage.

Gliomas arising from the brainstem grow slowly and progressively disrupt the brainstem centers, invading the vestibular and auditory systems in 50% of cases.[26] Gliomas arising in the cerebellum are relatively silent until there is compression of the brainstem or obstruction of cerebrospinal fluid. Medulloblastomas, which occur primarily in children and adolescents, are rapidly growing tumors of the vermis and hemispheres of the cerebellum.

Metastatic neoplasms involve the vestibular and auditory functions primarily through involvement of the temporal bone. The internal auditory canal is a frequent site of metastatic tumor growth. Medical

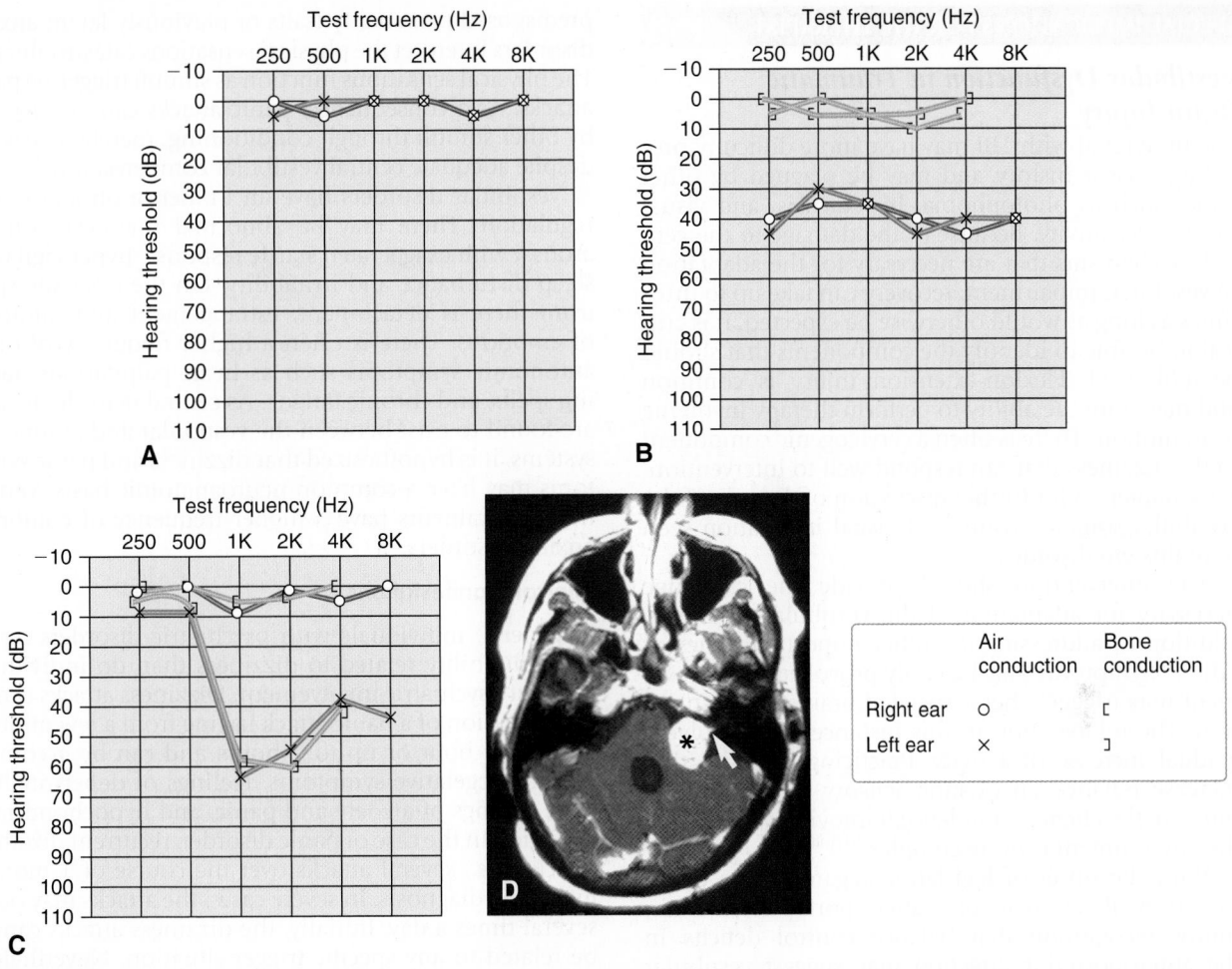

Figure 38-17

A, Normal audiogram. **B,** Abnormal audiogram in an individual with bilateral hearing loss. **C,** Abnormal audiogram in left ear with loss of both air and bone conduction. **D,** Vestibular schwannoma pressing against the left side of the brainstem and into the internal auditory canal. (**A, B,** and **C** redrawn from and **D** from Nolte J: *The human brain: an introduction to its functional anatomy,* ed 5, St Louis, 2002, Mosby.)

interventions to control growth can cause disruption of the neural tissue and trigger edema in the area of the vestibular system. This can cause acute symptoms; there is usually a good response to vestibular rehabilitation in that case.

Traumatic Brain Injury

Risk Factors

Complaints of dizziness and imbalance are common after traumatic brain injury (TBI) and may affect as many as 50% of the individuals who experience TBI. There may be direct injury to the vestibular mechanism as a result of the forces encountered during the impact. The vestibular and cochlear nerve can be damaged in the trauma, producing peripheral vestibular disorders. Labyrinthine concussion can trigger BPPV.[83] Posttraumatic endolymphatic hydrops can cause intermittent dizziness (see endolymphatic hydrops above). Perilymphatic fistula is more common after head injury and can be difficult to assess given the fluctuating nature of brain injury. Blasts or explosions are the most

common mechanisms of injury in modern warfare, and TBI is a frequent consequence of exposure to such attacks.[102] There is a greater incidence of peripheral vestibular hypofunction in dizzy service members with blast-related TBI relative to those who do not report dizziness.[10,101]

Pathogenesis

Direct damage of the vestibular nuclei or cerebellar connections can cause persistent and disabling positional dizziness.[7,73] Brainstem or midbrain damage involving the vestibular nuclei can create inability to integrate somatosensation, visual, or vestibular input. In this case, the individual will often choose to decrease the use of the vestibular system by limiting head motion and using predominantly visual or somatosensory cues for balance. The ability of the vestibular system to perform is further decreased by general lack of challenge. Then when the vestibular system is stimulated during daily activity, there is a sensation of dizziness and loss of postural stability. (See Chapter 33, "Traumatic Brain Injury," for more complete information on the pathology of brain injury.)

Vestibular Dysfunction in Traumatic Brain Injury

The individual with TBI may have more difficulty providing a clear history and may be plagued by other issues such as photophobia, hyperacusis, and visual motion sensitivity. Because of the damage to the central mechanisms that are necessary for the adaptation of vestibular impairment, recovery can take up to three times as long as would otherwise be expected. It is critical to be able to identify the components that should be addressed. Flexion-extension injury is common and may limit the ability to perform therapy involving head motion. There is often a cervicogenic component to the dizziness that can respond well to intervention. See Chapter 33 for further discussion of the role of the vestibular/somatosensory and visual integration seen in brainstem disorders.

The intervention should provide the challenge necessary for adaptation of the vestibular system in addition to addressing the other important issues of TBI.[4,83] Symptoms may be easily provoked, and movement may trigger other associated brainstem dysfunction. The intervention in this instance may involve a gradual increase of activity. Practicing activities that increase reliance on existing sensory input can also improve the client's confidence in moving about when the environment is more complex.[81,104,105]

With the onset of legislation regarding the determination of return to play after sports-related brain injury, recognition that balance control deficits in the anteroposterior direction may suggest vestibular impairment due to poor sensorimotor integration of the lateral vestibulospinal tract may lead to the sideline implementation of higher order balance tests that integrate vestibular function.[97]

Chronic Subjective Dizziness

Overview and Definition

Psychiatric processes may be the cause or the consequence of dizziness. Anxiety and phobic disorders are frequent psychiatric related disorders that include the complaint of dizziness. Terms such as *phobic vertigo* or *psychogenic dizziness* have been used in the past to describe this condition. Somatoform dizziness is also used to describe the phenomenon. A term in common use now is *chronic subjective dizziness* (CSD).[99] In some cases, the cause of the dizziness symptoms cannot be traced to any objective organic pathologic findings and in others, this appears to be sustaining of chronic symptoms following transient medical events. Secondary, reactive, or comorbid psychiatric disorders can emerge as a consequence of organic dizziness. Vestibular neuritis and BPPV are two common causes of dizziness that respond well to intervention. Sometimes these individuals are given the standard intervention and acute symptoms subside, but recovery is illusive because of the underlying psychiatric disorder. Patients who have predisposed personality traits or previously latent anxiety disorders interpret the physical sensations catastrophically. The physical sensations function as stimuli triggering panic attacks. As a consequence, panic attacks can be triggered by other stimuli through conditioning, thereby persisting despite adequate central vestibular compensation.[37]

Vestibular disorders have an influence on autonomic regulation. There may be abnormal manifestations of arousal with exaggerated startle response, hyper vigilance, sleep disturbance and irritability. On the opposite spectrum there is detachment, estrangement and numbing of emotions. There is often a higher frequency of other autonomic symptoms such as heart palpitations, fainting spells, and chronic fatigue. As central neurologic links are found to exist between the vestibular and autonomic systems, it is hypothesized that dizziness and panic symptoms may have a common neuroanatomic basis. Vertiginous migraineurs have a higher frequency of comorbid anxiety disorders.

Clinical Manifestations

In general, individuals with psychiatric disorders report more disability related to dizziness than do individuals without psychiatric involvement. Dizziness attacks can be an expression of a panic attack lasting from a few minutes to half an hour or up to 2 hours and can be accompanied by vegetative symptoms, feelings of depersonalization, feelings of anxiety and panic, and hypochondriacal anxieties. In the case of panic disorder, recurrent dizziness attacks (i.e., several attacks over the course of 1 month) justify the diagnosis. In severe cases, the attacks may occur several times a day. Initially, the dizziness attacks cannot be related to any specific trigger situation. Nevertheless, the result is that patients frequently tend to avoid those places where they experienced their first dizziness attack. Agoraphobia and social phobia are two phobic disorders underlying dizziness triggered by particular environments. However, agoraphobia when shopping in the supermarket or airports, driving a car, etc. must be distinguished from visual sensitivities related to the lack of adaptation of the vestibular mechanism.

Nighttime dizziness attacks combined with sleep disorders also can occur. The individuals subjectively believe that they have been awakened by the dizziness and afterwards often are unable to sleep for long periods. After the attacks, patients frequently feel exhausted. It is not uncommon for these patients to contact emergency medical services. Again, this must be distinguished from an attack of BPPV, which often causes symptoms during sleep when the head is turning.

Episodes of hyperventilation also may be associated with panic disorder, yet patients subjectively may not perceive them as such. The hyperventilation leads to subjective feelings and sensations, such as dizziness, emptiness, lightheadedness, fear of fainting, and paresthesias, which in turn intensify the fear in a vicious circle because patients interpret these sensations as an expression of a severe physical illness.

In generalized anxiety disorder, patients have dizziness attacks and permanent dizziness with fluctuating intensity. In addition to the symptoms, patients complain of constant inner tension and nervousness, a persistent generalized diffuse anxiety accompanied by psychomotor agitation and anxiety about the future. Anxiety disorders can be associated with depression. Often depressive disorders are not distinguished easily from each another.[37]

A depressive disorder usually takes the form of permanent diffuse dizziness. As with the anxiety disorders and phobic disorders, all further symptoms are interpreted as resulting from the dizziness. The symptoms can be manifold: depressive moods; rapid changes in mood; loss of drive and concentration; sleep disorders; or typical somatic symptoms, such as loss of appetite, loss of weight, and libidinal disorders. In severe cases, social withdrawal, fear of the future, nihilistic thoughts, and, rarely, suicidal indications may occur. Older patients often are misdiagnosed as suffering from vascular diseases or dementia. An organic lesion can act as a trigger and can make these persons feel completely unsure of themselves, leading in some instances to withdrawal from social life and isolation. Older people generally are poorly cared for in terms of psychotherapeutic and psychiatric therapy. In particular, older patients benefit most from appropriate treatment to improve their quality of life when it is hampered considerably by somatoform dizziness.

Somatoform dizziness can be an expression of a dissociative disorder, referred to as conversion disorder. In these cases, dizziness has the psychodynamic meaning of a conversion symptom. Careful clinical diagnostics commonly reveal a close temporal connection between past conflicts or stress situations and the onset of dizziness, a relationship of which patients initially are not aware. In contrast to patients who have anxiety or phobic or depressive disorders, these patients initially do not show such pronounced suffering and are less limited in their daily life and work activities. They do tend to demonstrate clear signs, however, of reaping secondary gains from the disorder, which primarily is connected with acute relief from unsolved, usually subconscious, internal conflicts. During the course of illness, however, secondary conditioning processes can start. Then the dizziness eventually occurs independently of the triggering conflict situation whenever low-level tension or mental irritation arises. In these cases, diagnosis can be difficult because the original conflict that triggered the dizziness is hidden. Therefore, it is important to identify the exact time of onset of dizziness and the associated living circumstances at that time.

Hearing disorders of a psychiatric nature are nearly always dissociative disorders, or conversion disorders. Initially, patients are not aware of the underlying conflicts and the hearing loss is attributed to an earlier illness or previously occurring event, such as loud music and noises, an upper respiratory tract infection, or an ear infection. Frequently, it is only during thorough psychiatric-psychodynamic diagnostic procedures that conflicts come to light that are connected with the hearing disorder. Depending on the underlying conflict, long-term psychotherapy may be required in some cases.

Pathogenesis

Connections between the locus coeruleus and lateral vestibular nucleus and serotonergic effects have implications for both processes. The parabrachial nucleus holds particular importance as it is tied to the central core of the amygdala and the limbic cortex through reciprocal connections and to all regions of the cerebral cortex. The amygdala is responsible for processing sensorimotor experiences when there is a threat involved. If the process is not completed efficiently, the trigger is experienced as if the threat is still going on.

A special significance is attributed to these brain structures during the development of fear and panic sensations and the conditioning of avoidance. The autonomic nervous system is unstable during this process. States of hyperventilation can alter balance of the vestibular system, induce nystagmus, and provoke dizziness sensations in patients who have subclinical vestibular disorders. Somatosensory referencing may be affected in a similar way, and there are often reports of clumsiness, bumping into doorjambs, or frequently hitting the head in these individuals. The more trauma appears to be associated, the more dissociation might be likely.[100]

MEDICAL MANAGEMENT

DIAGNOSIS. Many patients develop hypochondriac anxieties and insist on repeated diagnostic measures. Examination reveals typical symptom complexes for each of the underlying psychiatric disorders, such as anxiety, phobia, depression, or dissociation. Recognition of psychiatric factors in patients reporting dizziness creates a more accurate diagnosis, and is an important first step. Unfortunately, chronic subjective dizziness usually is included late in the differential diagnosis or not at all, which is why the diagnosis is delayed in most cases—often after several months or years of the disorder.

Individuals often consult first with an ear, nose, and throat physician, neurologist, or internist. To physicians who are less familiar with somatoform dizziness, these symptoms do not seem suspicious, and they usually are not recognized because the patients present with dizziness as the chief symptom. Initially it seems logical that, for example, a specific avoidance behavior or the reported vegetative symptoms result exclusively from organically caused dizziness. This circumstance often increases the tendency to become chronic, frequently leading to severe impairment of the quality of life, even early retirement, and high health care costs.

When complex persistent dizziness syndromes are present, careful organic diagnostics always must be performed followed by a differentiated psychiatric-psychodynamic examination performed by an experienced clinician; this practice makes possible the diagnosis of somatoform dizziness in approximately two-thirds of patients. Patients who suffer from a depersonalization or derealization syndrome often describe themselves as having diffuse dizziness or feeling dazed. Frequently, the depersonalization disorder is overlooked, but closer examination reveals that patients are not suffering from dizziness per se. The patients describe a strange feeling in their head, feeling dazed, like being wrapped in cotton, feeling unreal or foreign, as though they are outside their body. They often barely can express these symptoms in words, as they find the symptoms highly disturbing and embarrassing. Isolated depersonalization syndromes are rare; a depersonalization disorder usually is accompanied by anxiety and depressive disorders. In the presence of a depressive disorder or an anxiety disorder, the existence of a depersonalization disorder often is underestimated.

TREATMENT. Treatment is determined by clinical presentation; autonomic dysregulation should be addressed. A medical professional who is familiar with both the medical and psychiatric aspects is the best place to start. The indication is determined by the clinical findings and the underlying conflict and stress situation. Cognitive-behavioral therapy is effective for treatment of anxiety disorders. If the disorder is of short duration with mildly intrusive symptoms, focused outpatient treatment can be successful. Depending on the underlying conflict, a long-term psychodynamic therapy should be the treatment of choice. Pharmacologic interventions include selective serotonin reuptake inhibitors

PROGNOSIS. Follow-up studies of the course of complex somatoform dizziness show an urgent need for early differentiated interdisciplinary diagnostics. The follow-up period in individual studies ranges from 4 months to 2 years. Depression, anxiety, and compulsion are influenced more heavily by how the dizziness is experienced subjectively than by the objective balance disorder. Subjective experiences depend on the underlying or associated psychiatric disorder. The extent of the handicap and form of emotional distress interact with each other; depression and anxiety impede the ability to cope, thus exacerbating the dysfunction.

Attempts at symptomatic treatment such as long-term use of anti-vertiginous drugs are based on the assumption of residual signs and symptoms after a previous organic vertigo syndrome. These treatments typically lead to a short-term placebo effect, if they are successful at all, and contribute to perpetuating the dizziness symptoms by triggering the brain processes described above. When treatments are unsuccessful, this can become more depressing, and the patients may lack motivation. Clinical interactions have an important influence on the course of somatoform dizziness. When somatoform dizziness develops as a consequence of a vestibular disorder, explaining the psychosomatic connections in detail can be the first step in recovery.

Tinnitus can be a trigger for depressive disorders. Sleep disorders, concentration difficulties, irritability, and a low threshold for stress can cause depression and lead to social withdrawal. The subjectively perceived intensity of the tinnitus often depends on the level of stress. Phobic reactions may develop, particularly when the tinnitus is accompanied by hyperacusis.

SPECIAL IMPLICATIONS FOR THE THERAPIST | 38-8

Chronic Subjective Dizziness

Individuals who are predisposed to anxiety and panic reactions can interpret a physical sensation, such as dizziness, or a physical symptom of illness as catastrophic or a sign of a severe and threatening illness. This can result in an escalated anxiety or panic reaction. This anxiety reaction leads to a further increase in the level of autonomic-nervous system arousal, leading

to panic and, in some, fear of death. When this symptom complex is joined by episodes of hyperventilation with the corresponding physical consequences, such as paresthesia resulting from alkalosis, an increase in feeling of dizziness, and presyncope, this cycle can escalate further. Unexpected dizziness creates a feeling of helplessness and can trigger typical anticipation anxiety and phobic avoidance behavior. Avoidance behavior usually means avoiding body movements, thereby causing sensory integration deficits. The subjective symptoms persist, made worse by the anxious introspection, ultimately becoming chronic. Physical therapists are able to help normalize sensory references when the evaluation and examination expose this disorder. Chapter 3 provides further information on these disorders and guidelines for the appropriate strategies for intervention.

Comorbid Disorders with Vestibular Consequences

Congenital Vestibular Loss

Events before birth can cause loss of vestibular function and are related to genetics or intrauterine infection, intoxication, or anoxia. Rubella and cytomegalovirus are responsible for most cases. Thalidomide, no longer commonly used, can cause loss of vestibular function.[40]

Vascular Disease

Vertebrobasilar insufficiency is a common cause of vertigo in persons older than 50 years. This is often due to atherosclerosis of the vertebral and basilar arteries. Ischemia confined to the labyrinthine artery distribution results in infarction of the vestibular labyrinth and cochlea. Ischemia can also cause vertigo without hearing loss. A vascular loop compressing the eighth cranial nerve can cause vertigo, tinnitus, and hearing loss. Spontaneous hemorrhage into the inner ear, resulting in vertigo and hearing loss, mainly occurs in persons with underlying bleeding disorders. Leukemia is the most common disorder associated with labyrinthine hemorrhage.

Cerebellar infarction simulating vestibular neuritis is more common than previously thought. Early recognition of the pseudo-vestibular neuritis of vascular cause may allow specific management. Infarcts located dorsolateral to the fourth ventricle can cause interruption of the vestibular nuclei-archicerebellar loop seems to be responsible for central paroxysmal positional vertigo.

Vestibular dysfunction is a common component with brainstem stroke and may respond to intervention. See Chapter 32 for a more complete description of these stroke syndromes.[7]

Vestibular Migraine

A type of migraine headache that results in symptoms of dizziness is associated with vascular changes in the area of the vestibular apparatus and is common in both children and adults. (See Chapter 37 for the full description of vestibular migraine.) Approximately 30% of the population with migraine report episodic vertigo, in some cases during the headache-free period.

Diagnosis. Symptoms that qualify for a diagnosis of vestibular migraine include various types of vertigo as well as head motion-induced dizziness with nausea. Symptoms must be of moderate or severe intensity. Duration of acute episodes is limited to a window of between 5 minutes and 72 hours.[76] There seems to be more pathology in the VEMP circuitry in migraineurs than in healthy controls. We did not find support for peripheral vestibular hypersensitivity in terms of lower VEMP threshold among VM patients, but they are more sensitive for motion triggers than other migraineurs.[13] VEMP asymmetry ratios/tone bursts were significantly higher for individuals with Ménière disease than vestibular migraine.[108]

Metabolic Disorders

When vascular and nerve changes associated with diabetes mellitus occur in the area of the peripheral or central vestibular system, symptoms may develop. Loss of proprioceptive input and visual degeneration will further exacerbate the sense of disequilibrium. Metabolic disorders affecting the resorption of bone, such as *otosclerosis* and *Paget disease*, may develop to the point of causing degeneration of the labyrinths or nerves, resulting in vertigo and dizziness.

Allergies

Adverse reactions to foods and chemicals have been recognized as important etiologic agents in allergy. Otolaryngologic allergists address the clinical aspects of food sensitivity and dizziness after exposure to specific chemicals. There is clinical evidence of the relationship of dizziness with food allergies.[75,92]

Aural Cholesteatomas

Aural cholesteatomas are cysts of the middle ear or mastoid arising from squamous epithelial lining, containing keratin. Cholesteatomas erode the temporal bone and may be congenital or acquired. The cholesteatoma can cause resorption of the adjacent bone by a process of pressure erosion. This process can cause damage to the labyrinths and result in vestibular dysfunction. Annual incidence in children is 3 per 100,000 and 12.6 per 100,000 in adults. The diagnosis of aural cholesteatoma is made on otoscopic examination, including endoscopic and microscopic evaluation or surgical exploration. Special imaging procedures, such as high-resolution CT scanning and MRI, may suggest the presence of cholesteatoma within the temporal bone and may be used to complement the clinical examination. High-resolution CT scanning is useful for operative planning and is recommended for all revision mastoid operations. The symptoms of cholesteatoma vary; some cholesteatomas are asymptomatic, whereas others become infected and rapidly cause bone destruction.

Malignant External Otitis

Malignant external otitis, an infection affecting older people with diabetes or immunosuppression, begins in the external auditory canal and spreads to the temporal bone, putting pressure on the facial nerve or the surrounding nerves.

The most common intracranial complication of otitic infections is *extradural abscess*, a collection of purulent fluid between the dura mater and bone of the middle or posterior fossa. Spread of the infection across the dura from the epidural space may result in thrombophlebitis of the lateral venous sinus, subdural abscess, meningitis, and brain abscess.

In some cases, the damage is temporary, as in serous labyrinthitis, and vestibular and auditory function return to varying degrees. Permanent damage is possible when the infection causes damage to the structures of the labyrinth or the eighth cranial nerve. When the membranous labyrinth becomes permanently damaged, endolymphatic hydrops may result (see "Ménière Disease" above) and the symptoms can become episodic.

Malignant external otitis in the mastoid bone is a major clinical problem. It often occurs in persons with a chronic illness, such as diabetes, or a malignancy who are receiving broad-spectrum antibiotics. The infection enters the middle and inner ear via the nasal sinuses. The infection can spread into the intracranial cavity and create thrombosis of the cerebral arteries. The eighth cranial nerve can be affected along with surrounding cranial nerves in the presence of basilar meningitis.[11]

REFERENCES

To enhance this text and add value for the reader, all references are included on the companion Evolve site that accompanies this text book. The reader can view the reference source and access it online whenever possible.

CHAPTER 39

The Peripheral Nervous System

ROBYN GISBERT • KENDA S. FULLER

OVERVIEW

The peripheral nervous system (PNS) is composed of 31 pairs of spinal nerves that attach to the spinal cord and 10 pairs of cranial nerves that attach to the brainstem. There are 12 pairs of cranial nerves, two of which (the optic and olfactory) attach to the telencephalon and are considered part of the central nervous system (CNS).[169] The PNS serves to link the CNS to muscles for movement, and provides information back to the CNS about both internal and external conditions. Disruption of PNS function can range from a localized response that disables a single segment of an extremity to conditions that progressively degrade a person's quality of life and limit ability to work. Both the somatic and autonomic nervous systems (ANS) can be affected by PNS pathology. Although sensory loss and weakness are easily recognized hallmarks of a peripheral lesion, autonomic symptoms in the same nerve distribution may also be noted, such as lack of normal skin wrinkling and cession of sweating in the affected area. Furthermore, cardiac irregularities and circulatory problems may coexist with weakness and need to be identified properly in relationship to the PNS injury or disorder. The connections between the PNS and the CNS are complex, and in part responsible for conditions of central sensitization that result in changes to both systems that are both difficult to identify and challenging to determine appropriate interventions.

As a continuation of the description of the nervous system from Chapter 28, it is important to recall the pertinent anatomical components related to the PNS. Cell bodies of peripheral motor neurons are located within the spinal cord and brainstem, whereas those of peripheral sensory neurons reside in ganglia located outside the CNS in the periphery. Cell bodies of ANS neurons reside in the brainstem and spinal cord, and within ganglia that lie outside the CNS. Axons of PNS neurons extend from the cell bodies to form peripheral and cranial nerves (Fig. 39-1). The peripheral nerves are covered and protected by the extension of the meninges. Figure 39-2 shows the continuity of the meninges that cover the spinal cord forming the sheaths of the peripheral nerves. The *epineurium*, an extension of the dura mater, creates a substantial covering around the nerve trunks providing tensile strength through the longest part of the nerve and then becomes thinner around the smaller branches. It can continue to form encapsulated endings such as Meissner corpuscles.

The *perineurium*, extends not only the form, but the function of the arachnoid covering providing a blood–nerve barrier and continues as the capsule of some nerve endings such as Pacinian corpuscles, muscle spindles and Golgi tendon organs. In some areas, the perineurium is open ended, and can allow toxins and viruses to gain access to the nervous system. The *endoneurium* surrounds individual fibers and may contribute to directing the regrowth of nerve fibers after injury.[164]

The diameter of a nerve is associated with its function; larger fibers conduct faster than smaller fibers. The fiber type involved in the injury or dysfunction will contribute to the constellation of symptoms such as weakness or the type of sensory deficit. The surface of an axon itself is formed by a phospholipid membrane called the *axolemma*. Lying between the axolemma and the endoneurium are Schwann cells. In large-diameter axons (greater than 1 cm), the Schwann cell receives a signal to wrap its membrane around the axon, thus creating myelin (see Fig. 28-3). Myelin not only provides electrical insulation essential for rapid conduction of the axon potential but also affects axonal properties. The presence of myelin causes sodium channels to cluster at the nodes of Ranvier, thus reinforcing efficient and fast conduction.[121] As in the CNS, myelination patterns affect speed of transmission (Table 39-1). Within a peripheral nerve, only approximately 25% of the individual fibers are myelinated.[73]

Normal propagation of the action potential also requires sufficient energy, supplied by a vascular plexus interlaced between connective tissue layers. Each peripheral nerve receives an artery that penetrates the epineurium; this artery's branches extend into the perineurium as arterioles, and branches from the arterioles enter the endoneurium as capillaries. Vessels supplying peripheral nerves appear coiled when a limb is in a shortened position, but uncoiled after movement so that neural vascular supply is not impaired with a limb's normal excursion. This rich vascular supply makes peripheral nerves relatively resistant to ischemia.[191]

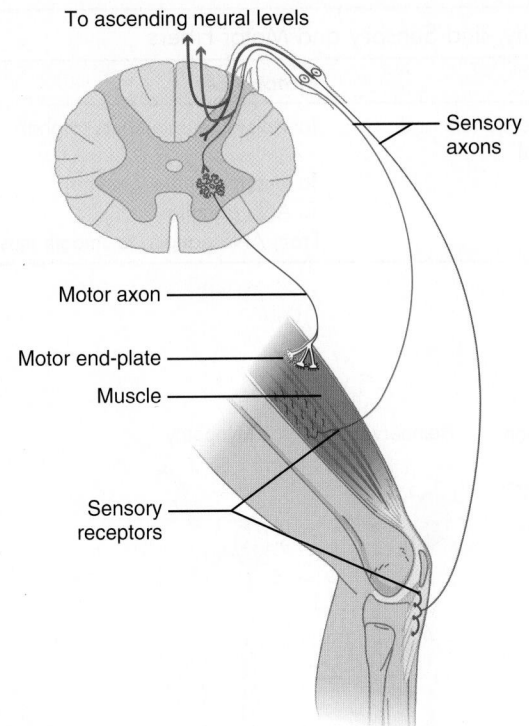

Figure 39-1

Potential sites of involvement in the peripheral nervous system. Motor: motor neuron cell body, axon, motor end plate, muscle fiber. Sensory: cell body in ganglion, axon, sensory receptor.

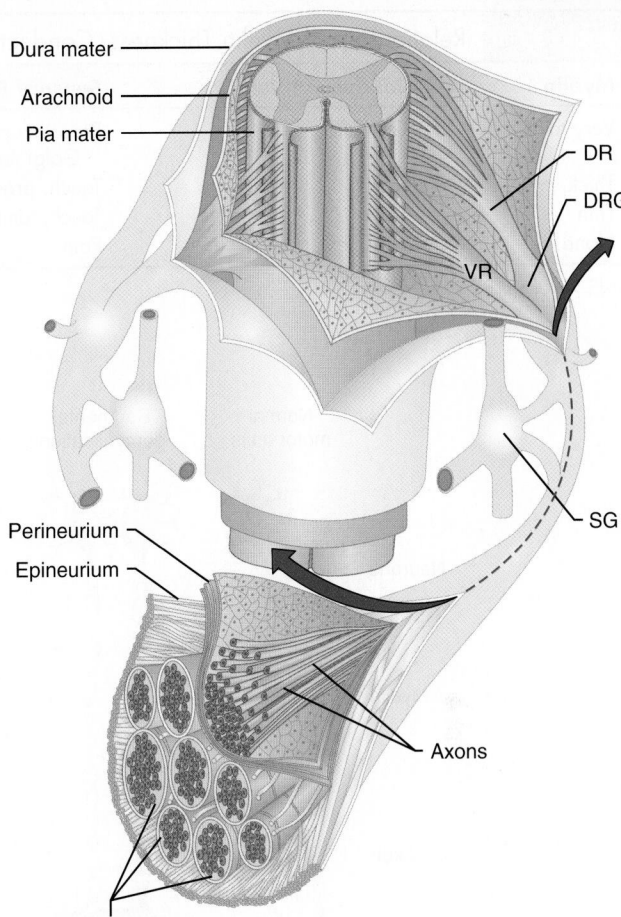

Figure 39-2

Continuity of the spinal meninges and the sheaths of peripheral nerves. The continuity between the spinal subarachnoid space and the extracellular space within nerve fascicles is indicated by the *arrow* emerging from both the cut end of the nerve and the vicinity of a dorsal root ganglion *(DRG)*. The pia mater is reflected form the exit zone of the ventral rootlets for clarity. *DR,* Dorsal root; *SG,* sympathetic ganglion; *VR,* ventral root. (Adapted from Krstic RV: *General histology of the mammal,* Berlin, 1985, Springer-Verlag. In Nolte J: *The human brain: an introduction to its functional anatomy,* ed 6, St. Louis, 2009, Mosby.)

PATHOGENESIS

Trauma, inherited disorders, environmental toxins, metabolic or nutritional disorders may affect the myelin, axon, or the adjacent motor units activated by the peripheral nerve seen in Figure 39-3. The severity of the involvement causes changes in the nerve and muscle response, so determines the amount of function lost (Table 39-2).[38] Table 39-3 describes common pathologies and level of involvement.

Lower Motor Neuron

The cell bodies of lower motor neurons (LMNs) that carry a signal to move are located in the CNS—either in the anterior horn of the spinal cord or the cranial nerve nuclei of the brainstem. Their axons travel through the ventral root to the intended target as a spinal or cranial nerve. When damage occurs to the motor portion of a peripheral nerve, paresis or paralysis will occur in muscles innervated by that nerve distal to the lesion. When spinal motor nerves are impaired, weakness occurs in all the muscles receiving axons from that spinal level (see Fig. 34-9). Deep tendon reflexes (DTRs) are diminished or absent. This is most observable in the distal regions. In the presence of axonal degeneration, rapid atrophy occurs. Prolonged paralysis gives rise to potential secondary complications such as contracture formation, deformity, and edema. In addition to the peripheral nerve, the motor end plate or muscle itself may be involved in a peripheral disorder. Involvement of muscle, termed *myopathy,* follows a different clinical pattern than nerve. When

muscle is involved, the disorder typically is reflected by proximal weakness, wasting, and hypotonia without sensory impairments (see Chapter 23).

Damage to ANS motor fibers results in alterations of involuntary motor functions such as heart rate, breathing, and gut motility. Preganglionic fibers are myelinated and can also be affected by segmental demyelination. Figure 28-17 depicts the sympathetic and parasympathetic divisions of the ANS.

Sensory Neuron

Lesions of PNS sensory fibers may occur in the dorsal root ganglion or in the nerve root proximal to the ganglia. Damage can also be to distal fibers of the peripheral nerve. Loss of sensation will follow a peripheral nerve distribution if that is the anatomic region involved, or it will follow a dermatomal pattern when the spinal nerve or dorsal root ganglia, or cell body has been affected (Fig. 39-4).

Table 39-1	Relationship of Myelin Thickness, Conduction Velocity, and Sensory and Motor Fibers		
Myelin	**Conduction Velocity**	**Sensory Fibers**	**Motor Fibers**
Very thick	Very fast	Proprioception (muscle spindle and Golgi tendon organ)	To skeletal muscle fibers (alpha)
Thick	Fast	Touch, pressure	To muscle spindle (gamma)
Thin	Slow	Touch, temperature	To ANS ganglia
None	Very slow	Pain	From ANS ganglia to smooth muscle

ANS, Autonomic nervous system.

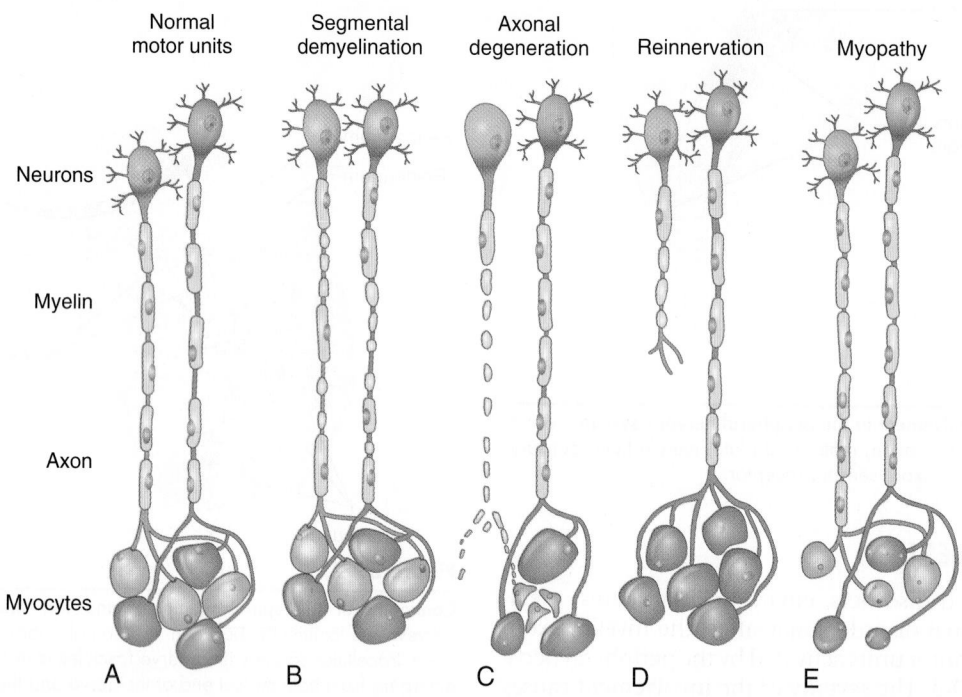

Figure 39-3

Types of nerve involvement and recovery that occur in peripheral nerves. A, Illustration of two adjacent normal myelinated nerves. **B,** Segmental demyelination. Several internodes of myelin have demyelinated, but the axons remain intact. The repair process for segmental demyelination occurs rapidly because Schwann cells divide and remyelinate the bare portion of the axon. Shorter internodal distance occurs with remyelination, thus nerve conduction velocity may not return to normal, even though muscle contracts normally. **C,** Illustration of axonal degeneration. The axon and myelin have degenerated, but the connective tissue covering remains intact in an axonotmesis. In neurotmesis, the connective tissue covering is disrupted at the lesion site. Signs of chromatolysis occur in the cell body after axonotmesis and neurotmesis. Note that muscle atrophies rapidly because it has lost the trophic influence from the nerve cell body. **D,** The repair process for axonotmesis and neurotmesis is more complex. Growth cones from the proximal axon must cross the lesion site and regrow down the connective tissue channels and reestablish a motor end plate or sensory connection before remyelination occurs. In partial nerve injuries, while the injury axon is regrowing, adjacent motor units sprout collateral fibers, leading to expansion of the size of this *(red)* motor unit. **E,** In myopathic conditions, scattered muscle fibers in adjacent motor units are small (degenerating or regenerating), while the neurons and axons are normal. (From Kumar V, Fausto N, Abbas A: *Robbins and Cotran pathologic basis of disease,* ed 7, Philadelphia, 2005, WB Saunders.)

Table 39-2	Relationship of Nerve and Muscle Responses to Disease and Trauma		
Level of Severity	**Response to Disease**	**Response to Trauma**	**Response of Muscle**
Mild	Myelinopathy (segmental demyelination)	Neurapraxia (segmental demyelination)	Paresis/paralysis, no atrophy
Severe	Axonopathy (wallerian degeneration)	Axonotmesis (wallerian degeneration)	Paresis/paralysis with atrophy
Severe	–	Neurotmesis (wallerian degeneration)	Paresis/paralysis with atrophy

Table 39-3	Causes of Peripheral Neuropathies and Myopathies and Their Effects					
	INVOLVEMENT*					
Cause	**Axonal Degeneration**	**Demyelination**	**Motor End Plate**	**Muscle**	**Motor**	**Sensory**
Charcot-Marie-Tooth disease	X	X			X	X
Mechanical compression/ entrapment						
Neurapraxia		X			X	X
Axonotmesis	X				X	X
Neurotmesis	X				X	X
Postpolio syndrome	X				X	
Diabetic mellitus	X	X			X	X
Alcohol	X	X			X	X
Guillain-Barré syndrome	X	X			X	X
Toxins						
Lead	X				X	X
Organophosphate	X	X			X	X
Myasthenia gravis			X		X	
Botulism			X		X	
Muscular dystrophy				X	X	
Inflammatory myopathy				X	X	
Steroid-induced myopathy				X	X	
Overuse myopathy				X	X	
Aging	X	X	X	X	X	X
AIDS/HIV (including associated vasculitis)	X	X			X	X
Vitamin B$_{12}$ deficiency	X	X				X
Chronic renal failure	X				X	X

AIDS, Acquired immunodeficiency syndrome; *HIV,* human immunodeficiency virus.
*The Xs indicate the most common types of involvement for each cause.

When sensory ANS fibers are affected there can be abnormal transmission of sensation into the CNS relayed from viscera, glands, or smooth muscle. Unconscious sensory functions such as baroreceptors signaling arterial pressure, receptors within organs signaling irritants, distention, or hypoxia may be affected.

PERIPHERAL NERVOUS SYSTEM CHANGES WITH AGING

Changes that occur in the PNS may be considered as one component of a continuum that relates to normal growth and development, or the changes may represent a combination of pathologic processes superimposed on the normal aging process. Because of the difficulty of studying human peripheral nerves in vivo, experimental animals have been used to assess the effects of aging.

Age does not affect the size or number of fascicles, but the perineurium and epineurium do thicken with age and the endoneurium often becomes fibrosed with increased collagen. Even with these changes, the cross-sectional area decreases slightly with age as a result of a reduced number of unmyelinated and myelinated fibers. Ventral root motor fibers are more affected than dorsal root sensory fibers. Recall that ventral roots are comprised of motor fibers, and dorsal roots are comprised of sensory fibers. Blood vessels to nerves may become atherosclerotic with aging, and occlusion may contribute to loss of nerve fibers. The prevalence of peripheral neuropathies seen in older people has been attributed to reduced microvascular caliber.[50]

Both the peripheral and central nervous systems are affected by aging. There is a reduction in β-endorphin content and γ-aminobutyric acid synthesis in the lateral thalamus and a reduced concentration of γ-aminobutyric acid and serotonin receptors. Speed of processing nociceptive stimuli and both C- and Aδ-fiber function also decrease with age, which can lead to corresponding reductions in older adults' ability to sense and respond to "first or initial pain." As a result, older adults may have greater susceptibility to burns and other injuries such as lacerations because they are not as likely to sense the initial pain.[16]

ANS dysfunction is more common in the elderly.[65] Cell bodies show chromatolysis, as well as an accumulation of lipofuscins, representing a diminished ability of the cell to rid itself of toxins. Loss of cell bodies has been observed in the sympathetic ganglia, along with a loss of unmyelinated fibers in peripheral nerves. Sympathetic control of dermal vasculature shows an age-related decline that leads to diminished wound repair efficiency. In an aging animal model, transcutaneous electrical nerve stimulation improved the vascular response. Peripheral activity of sympathetic nerves were affected by the low-frequency electrical stimulation.[100]

When the motor end plate is examined, age-related changes have occurred, but these changes are seen as early as the third decade of life and are not observed in all muscles. When sensory receptors have been evaluated, density and morphology have been found to be altered in the elderly. Altered axonal myelination creates slowing of nerve conduction velocities (NCVs). In addition,

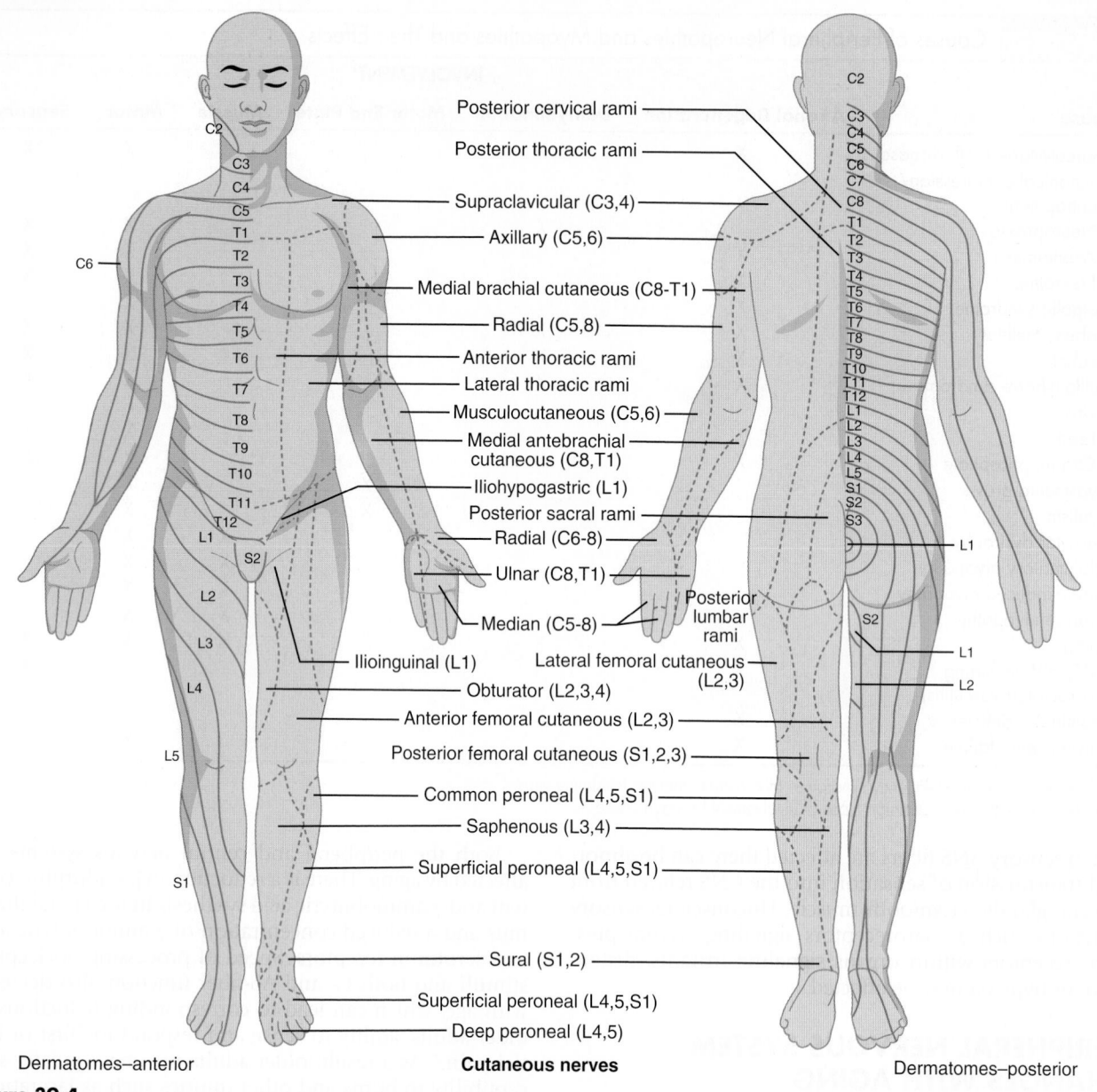

Dermatomes–anterior   **Cutaneous nerves**   Dermatomes–posterior

Figure 39-4

Dermatomal (right side of body, anterior and posterior) and peripheral sensory nerve (left side of body, anterior and posterior) patterns. (From Auerbach PS: *Wilderness medicine*, ed 5, St. Louis, Mosby, 2007.)

the loss of fibers decreases the amplitude of the potential. Decreases in protein production are hypothesized to cause myelin deterioration.[201] When individual myelinated fibers are examined, shorter internodes are seen, suggesting that a demyelinating–remyelinating process occurs with aging. This structural alteration in peripheral nerve myelination may be reflected in diminished appreciation of vibratory sense.

Simultaneous with the decreased protein production is a decrease in intraaxonal transport by cytoskeletal elements in the peripheral nerve. Electromyographic (EMG) studies of elderly people without evidence of neurologic disorders of the PNS show loss of motor units, as well as signs of reinnervation. Morphologic changes observed in people older than 60 years of age are manifested by decreased strength and sensory changes.[133] This can have consequences for movement, safety, and quality of life.

Healthy elderly, with no evidence of neurologic disease, may provide a clinical history suggestive of peripheral neuropathy. This includes numbness and tingling in the hands and feet along with mild, diffuse weakness—especially in the distal muscles of the hand. Sensory alterations may lead to poor balance and gait instability. On examination, sensory thresholds are increased.

The cause of an aging neuropathy can be attributed to a combination of factors. First, loss of both motor and sensory cell bodies; second, a dying-back condition, suggesting neurons can metabolically support a limited number of fibers or receptors, similar to that seen in other systemic neuropathies; and last, over the course of a lifetime, chronic compression of the peripheral nerves or repetitive trauma may have damaged the nerves. All these factors, combined with coexisting medical conditions, atherosclerosis, and nutritional deficiencies, may create this neuropathy of

Table 39-4	Normal Nerve Conduction Velocities and Distal Latencies*					
Nerve	Motor Conduction Velocity (m/s)	Motor Distal Latency (ms)	Motor Amplitude (mV)	Sensory Conduction Velocity (m/s)	Sensory Distal Latency (ms)	Sensory Amplitude (µV)
Median	63.5±6.2	3.49±0.34	7.0±2.7	56.2+5.8	2.84±0.34	38.5±15.6
Ulnar	61.0±5.5	2.59±0.39	5.5±1.9	54.8±5.3	2.54±0.29	35.0±14.7
Tibial	48.5±3.6	3.96±1.00	5.1±2.2			
Peroneal	52±6.2	3.77±0.86	5.1±2.3			

Normal F Wave Values

Nerve	Stimulation Site	F Wave Latency to Recording Site (ms)
Median	Elbow	22.8±1.9
Ulnar	Above Elbow	23.1±1.7
Peroneal	Above Knee	39.9±3.2
Tibial	Knee	39.6±4.4

*In general, in the upper extremities, nerve conduction velocity for motor fibers averages about 60 m/s. Investigators have reported values ranging from 45 to 75 m/s. In the lower extremity, the normal range for motor nerve conduction is in the 40 to 50 m/s range. Distal latency is a time value, reported in milliseconds, that it takes for an evoked potential to be propagated along the nerve and recorded from either the muscle (motor) or the skin (sensory). Adapted From Dyck PJ, Thomas PK, eds: *Peripheral neuropathy*, ed 3, Philadelphia, 1993, WB Saunders.

aging. In animal studies, a repetitive task performed by aging rats caused sensorimotor declines that were associated with decreased nerve conduction, and increased proinflammatory cytokines.[52] When the aging PNS is damaged, wallerian degeneration is delayed and regeneration takes longer because secretion of trophic factors is slower than in younger individuals. Density of regenerating axons is less. In a partial nerve injury, collateral sprouting is reduced, further limiting recovery of function.[201]

DIAGNOSIS OF PERIPHERAL NERVOUS SYSTEM DYSFUNCTION

Electrodiagnostic Studies

Because the nervous system is the means of signaling from the CNS to the muscle, conduction of the action potential is affected in neuropathies and myopathies. In most disorders, electrophysiologic studies are used to determine where and how the nerve or muscle may be affected. Table 39-4 lists normal values. Although the phenotype of peripheral dysfunction (i.e., physical characteristics/traits) remains unchanged, much of the current research in peripheral nerve pathophysiology is concerned with genetic and molecular changes. Findings in these areas may allow development of treatments aimed at altering cellular function and thereby preserving conduction.

Electromyography (needle EMG) involves the recording of electrical activity within muscles by way of a needle electrode similar to having an electrical microphone at the tip of the needle. Three types of information can be obtained. Healthy muscle at rest should have no spontaneous electrical activity except at the neuromuscular junction. If the muscle is denervated, there will be positive sharp waves and fibrillation potentials. Myotonia, fasciculations and cramps can also be identified in denervated muscle at rest. With slight exertion of the muscle, motor units around the needle should fire synchronously. Axon damage will result in asynchronous firing with multiphasic or complex patterns. Amplitude of the firing may also represent dysfunction. Muscle damage causes decreased

firing; in nerve injury amplitudes in a nerve may be normal above the level of damage and in the case of regeneration after injury, the axon may have spread to other muscle fibers causing the amplitude to be higher than normal. Increases in number and rate of motor unit firing reflect normal responses to maximum exertion. In muscle disease, the number of units may be increased (hyperrecruitment), whereas in nerve dysfunction, the response to maximum exertion is reduced recruitment.

Nerve conduction study involves placing two electrodes along the length of a nerve. One electrode stimulates the peripheral nerve greater than the threshold values required to cause firing. The second electrode records the characteristics of the generated action potential at a different point than the stimulation. Information is obtained about conduction velocity, wave forms, and amplitude. Nerve conduction studies will be normal even if there are just a few large fibers that can still fire. Conduction at the distal site is slowed at the site of the neuromuscular junction, and is measured as the distal latency. Because thick fibers are most vulnerable to compression injury, it can be an effective in diagnosing compression neuropathies.

Localization of injury can be confirmed, for example determining whether ulnar nerve damage is at the location of the elbow or wrist. LMN versus upper motor neuron (UMN) lesions can be identified if the cause of a motor problem is not clear. The degree of damage (neurapraxia, axonotmesis, or neurotmesis) can be identified. A clinical exam may not clearly determine the difference between myelin and axon damage, the EMG/nerve conduction study can help to clarify the state of damage. EMG/nerve conduction studies must be performed and considered in concert with the history and examination. Table 39-5 shows the relationship of findings to level of likely involvement. If a client is unable to relax properly, testing at rest may not reveal underlying fibrillations. The muscle/nerve location may be missed during the testing because of operator error, and tests may show borderline involvement despite functional loss. Conversion disorders may be identified in light of electrodiagnostic testing.

Table 39-5	Relationship of Electromyographic Findings to Innervation			
Condition	**Normal Innervation**	**Segmental Demyelination**	**Axonal/Wallerian Degeneration**	**Myopathy**
Insertion	Normal insertional noise	Normal insertional noise	Increased insertional noise	Increased insertional noise
At rest	Quiet	Quiet	Spontaneous (abnormal) potentials: fibrillation potential, positive sharp wave potential	Quiet, except end stage: fibrillation potentials
Minimal contraction	Normal motor unit potential	Affected fibers: no motor unit potential	Affected fibers: no motor unit potential	Low amplitude, polyphasic potential
Maximal contraction	Complete interference pattern	Nerve partially affected: decreased interference pattern	Nerve partially affected: decreased interference pattern; nerve completely affected: no interference pattern	Low amplitude–full interference pattern, accomplished with increased frequency of firing and with moderate effort

Table 39-6	Nerve Trauma Classifications			
		CLASSIFICATION		
Injured Tissue(s)	**Seddon**	**Sunderland**	**Modification (MacKinnon)**	
Myelin	Neurapraxia	Grade I	—	
Myelin, axon	Axonotmesis	Grade II	—	
Myelin, axon, endoneurium	Neurotmesis	Grade III	—	
Myelin, axon, endoneurium, perineurium	Neurotmesis	Grade IV	—	
Myelin, axon, endoneurium, perineurium, epineurium	Neurotmesis	Grade V	—	
Combination			Grade VI	

From Daroff: *Bradley's neurology in clinical practice*, ed 6, Philadelphia, 2012, WB Saunders.

CLASSIFICATION OF NERVE INJURY AND NEUROPATHY

Traumatic injury to peripheral nerves from mechanical involvement secondary to compression, ischemia, and stretching can be classified based on the structural and functional changes that result. Seddon[174] divided nerve injury into three categories: neurapraxia, axonotmesis, and neurotmesis. Sunderland[186] divided this classification into five categories, based on the extent of tissue injury.[187] Table 39-6 compares the classification according to Seddon and Sunderland with MacKinnon's modifications.

Demyelination: Neurapraxia

Demyelination, or loss of myelin, typically in segments, leaves the axon intact but bare where the myelin is lost. This is called *segmental demyelination*. In this scenario, the speed of transmission is decreased with effects of weakness and loss of sensory conduction. *Neurapraxia* is the temporary failure of nerve conduction in the absence of structural changes, typically the result of blunt injury, compression, or ischemia. It is caused by segmental demyelination, which slows or blocks local conduction of the action potential while conduction of the action potential remains normal above and below the point of compression. Because the axon remains intact, muscle does not atrophy. The result is paresis without degeneration and

is usually followed by slow and full recovery of function. When segmental demyelination occurs because of disease, the response may be termed a *myelinopathy*. If segmental demyelination has occurred, molecular signaling to remaining Schwann cells causes them to begin dividing mitotically. Newborn Schwann cells move to envelope the denuded segment of nerve and once these cells are in place they will begin to form myelin.

Degeneration: Axonotmesis and Neurotmesis

Degeneration occurs in any peripheral nerve disorder that directly affects the axon, including physical injury (crush, stretch, or laceration), as well as disease. *Axonotmesis* occurs when the axon has been damaged, but the connective tissue coverings that support and protect the nerve remain intact. Prolonged compression that produces an area of infarction and necrosis can cause axonotmesis. In the presence of disease, Wallerian degeneration creates an axonopathy, which is analogous to an axonotmesis. *Neurotmesis*, the most severe axonal loss, is the complete severance of the axon, as well as the disruption of its supporting connective tissue coverings (endoneurium, perineurium, and/or epineurium) at the site of injury. Neurotmesis can be caused by gunshot or stab wounds or avulsion injuries that disrupt a section of the nerve or entire nerve. When axonal continuity is lost (either axonotmesis or neurotmesis), axons degenerate distal to the lesion. Wallerian degeneration begins immediately after involvement and is completed over a period of a few weeks. The nerve cell swells and undergoes chromatolysis. The ribosomes that normally make protein for the cell disperse throughout the cytoplasm. *Chromatolysis* reflects a change in the metabolic priority of the cell as it switches from daily needs to a repair mode. Distally the axon begins to degenerate and myelin fragments within 12 hours of the lesion. This material is removed by macrophages responding to the inflammatory process. As long as the cell body remains viable, a regenerative process begins with sprouting of a growth cone as soon as new cytoplasm is synthesized and transported down the axon from the cell body As the growth cone grows, it releases proteases that dissolve material and permit the axon to enter the tissue more easily. Filopodia, which are finger-like projections extending from the growth cone, sample the environment searching for chemical and tactile cues to guide the regenerating axon; however, because the tactile cues provided by the endoneurium are absent, many times these fibers become misguided and form a neuroma. The standard used to anticipate return of function is based on a growth rate of 1 mm a day or an inch a month. In reality, this is an average reflecting the delays that occur while the growth cone crosses the repair site and makes connection with sensory end organs or motor end plate. Growth occurs faster nearer the lesion site (3 mm/day) and slower as the length of the axon increases (1 mm/day).[144]

Clinical Manifestations

Clinical presentation is correlated to the severity and location of the injury. In any case, an flaccid paralysis occurs in muscles distal to the lesion. Rapid atrophy ensues because of loss of the trophic influences of the nerve that innervated the muscle fibers. Sensory function is also lost below the level of the lesion.

MEDICAL MANAGEMENT

DIAGNOSIS. History and clinical examination are used to diagnose neurotmesis. In addition, electrophysiologic studies may be performed. EMG will demonstrate the presence of fibrillation potentials and positive sharp waves, indicating denervation of muscle fiber. EMG can be used to determine whether the lesion is complete or partial.

TREATMENT. Surgical management is needed to suture the connective tissue bundles together to guide the regenerating growth cone. Various microsurgical techniques (cable and interfascicular grafts) are used to try and direct the axon into the appropriate fascicle by restoring connective tissue continuity. After complete axonal transection, the neuron undergoes a number of degenerative processes, followed by attempts at regeneration. A distal growth cone seeks out connections with the degenerated distal fiber. The current surgical standard is epineurial repair with nylon suture. To span gaps that primary repair cannot bridge without excessive tension, nerve-cable interfascicular autografts are employed. Unfortunately, results of nerve repair to date have been no better than fair, with only 50% of patients regaining useful function. There is much ongoing research regarding pharmacologic agents, immune system modulators, enhancing factors, and entubulation chambers. Clinically applicable developments from these investigations will continue to improve the results of treatment of nerve injuries.[111] Ideally, a primary repair will be carried out; operative delays lead to shrinkage and fibrosis of the distal connective tissue support structures.[87]

Other treatments are symptomatic. For the therapist this means splinting to support structures. Use of electrical stimulation to maintain muscle bulk is controversial; recent studies have shown that the chemical signal guiding the nerve (neural cell adhesion molecule) disappears when denervated muscle receives electrical stimulation.[166] However, muscle bulk is maintained for up to 4 weeks. Because denervated skin does not wrinkle after it has been soaked in water, this has been used to evaluate denervation patterns.[151]

PROGNOSIS. Because muscle fibers innervated by the axon depend on the nerve cell body as a source of nourishment or trophic control, when axons degenerate, muscle fibers rapidly atrophy. The potential for regeneration after axonal degeneration is possible as long as the nerve cell body remains viable; new axons can sprout from the proximal end of damaged axons. However, successful functional regeneration requires that the proximal and distal ends of the connective tissue tube are aligned. This can occur in an axonotmesis because the connective tissue covering remain intact. In a neurotmesis, without surgical intervention, recovery is less likely because the proximal end of the endoneurium is not approximated to the distal endoneurium. Without surgery, axonal sprouts often enter nearby soft tissue and form a neuroma, or axonal regrowth occurs down the incorrect endoneurial tube, rendering reinnervation nonfunctional.[201] Even with surgical intervention, prognosis for recovery is poor.

Once the axon has established a distal contact either with muscle or sensory receptor, remyelination will begin. When partial axonal degeneration occurs, adjacent noninvolved axons may produce collateral sprouts that will innervate muscle fibers before the damaged axons have time to grow and reinnervate those muscle fibers. This results in an enlarged motor unit for the neuron that has collateral sprouts. Numerous reports in the literature link various molecular factors to nerve regeneration and healing following repair.[145,190]

Neuropathy

Neuropathies result from a wide variety of causes and can be classified in many ways, including the rate of onset, type and size of nerve fibers involved, distribution pattern, or pathology. For example, when a single peripheral nerve is affected the result is a *mononeuropathy*, which is commonly a result of trauma. The term *polyneuropathy* indicates involvement of several peripheral nerves. A *radiculoneuropathy* indicates involvement of the nerve root as it emerges from the spinal cord, and *polyradiculitis* indicates involvement of several nerve roots and occurs when infections create an inflammatory response. Neuropathic diseases that affect the axon or its cell body causing axonal

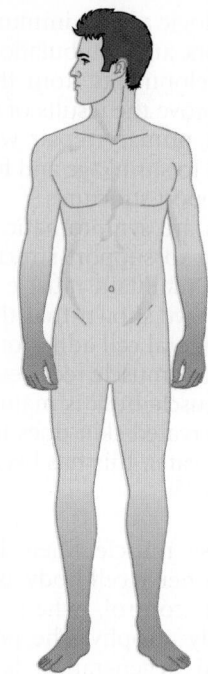

Figure 39-5

A stocking-and-glove pattern of sensory loss occurs in polyneuropathy. A gradient of greater distal loss tapering to less proximal involvement is seen.

degeneration typically affect the longest nerve fibers first with signs and symptoms beginning distally and spreading proximally as the disease progresses. Because nerves in the legs are longer, the feet and lower legs are often involved before the fingers and hands. Those conditions that affect only myelin cause segmental demyelination in both sensory and motor fibers. Thus disruption of the conduction of the action potential from proprioceptors and mechanoreceptors causes sensory changes.

The first noticeable features of neuropathies are often sensory in nature and consist of tingling, prickling, burning, or band-like *dysesthesias* and *paresthesias* in the feet. When more than one nerve is involved, the sensory loss follows a glove-and-stocking distribution that is attributed to the dying-back of the longest fibers in all nerves from distal to proximal (Fig. 39-5). The most common symptoms of motor neuropathy include distal weakness, decreases of tone (hypotonicity or flaccidity) and muscle tenderness or cramping. This can be evident when clients are asked to walk on their heels or toes, weakness of dorsiflexors or plantarflexors, respectively. It is important to recognize that the motor loss in a myopathy is opposite to that of a neuropathy. In a myopathy, the weakness tends to be proximal.

MECHANICAL INJURIES: COMPRESSION AND ENTRAPMENT SYNDROMES

Compressive neuropathies occur due to the proximity of peripheral nerves to bony, muscular, and vascular structures. Chronic nerve compression develops over time and reflects particular changes in the lining of the nerve. Mechanical injury occurs as a result of traction on a nerve, with damage occurring once tension exceeds 10% to 20% of the axon's resting length and the available slack is taken up.[13] Repetitive motion injuries affecting hands and digits can result from repeated grasping, typing, or playing a musical instrument.

Median Neuropathy (Carpal Tunnel Syndrome)

Carpal tunnel syndrome (CTS) is not a single event, but more likely a cascade of dysfunction that causes symptoms when it reaches a critical state. Described in 1854 by Paget, CTS (tardy median palsy) is the result of compression of the median nerve within the carpal tunnel in the wrist. Chronic CTS is marked by pain, paresthesia, numbness, and weakness in the distribution of the median nerve (Fig. 39-6). Although there are many causative factors, chronic CTS is most commonly associated with performance of repetitive tasks determined by position of the hand and degree of load. Physical therapists have been involved in intensive study of the causes and treatments associated with this complex disorder. Animal models exhibit the features of human CTS, including impaired sensation, motor weakness, and decreased median NCV. It is well established that a causal relationship exists between performance of a repetitive task and development of CTS.[6]

Acute CTS is less common and directly associated with fractures, dislocation, and vascular disorders of the wrist. Rheumatologic disorders and anomalous anatomy may cause sudden symptoms. The acute form of CTS may require urgent surgical intervention to avoid serious and permanent damage.[171]

Incidence

Carpal tunnel is one of the top reasons for lost workdays, with the average being between 10 and 27 days and the cost of an occurrence at more than $30,000 in medical costs. The incidence of CTS in general populations is approximately 2.8 per 1000 in studies using nerve conduction study to confirm the diagnosis. The prevalence ranges from 1% to 10% among the general population, and up to 14.5% among specific occupational groups. Nearly 70% of all CTS cases occur in women. Conventional thinking is that the tunnel is relatively smaller in females compared to males. The incidence of surgery for CTS peaks in the 45- to 55-year-old group in women and in the older-than-65-years group in men.[161]

Prevalence is increased in tasks that require gripping, holding tools which vibrate, lifting more than 12 kg, or working in an extremely cold environment.[55]

Etiology

The carpal tunnel is basically a structure with four sides, three of which are defined by the carpal bones and the fourth, the "top" of the tunnel, by the transverse carpal ligament (Fig. 39-7). Tendons passing through the tunnel with their synovial sheaths include the flexor pollicis longus, the four flexor digitorum superficialis, and the four flexor digitorum profundus tendons. Closest to the surface and most vulnerable to changes of the palm in relation to the wrist is the median nerve. The hallmark of the carpal tunnel is that it is cylindrical and inelastic. None of the sides of the tunnel yields to expansion of the

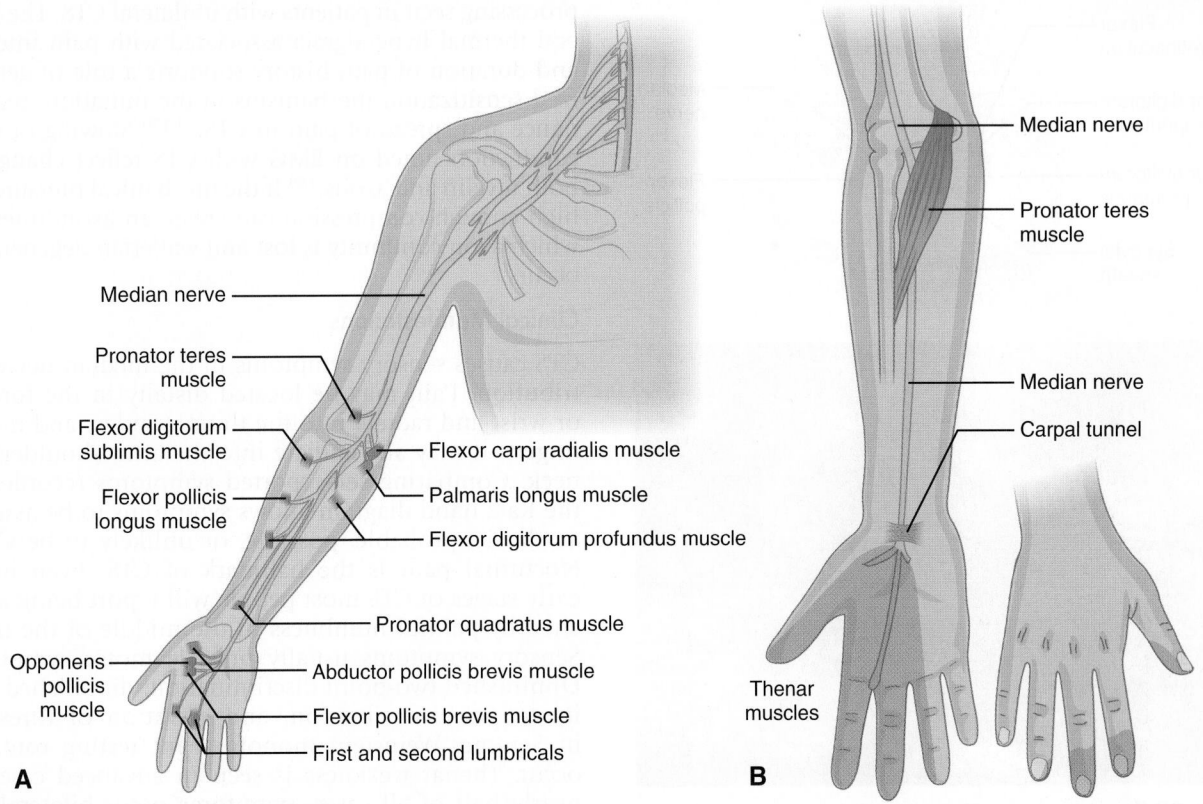

Figure 39-6

A, Median nerve course and motor innervation. **B,** The point of compression of the median nerve as it passes through the carpal tunnel. The lightly stippled area shows the sensory supply of the palmar cutaneous branch, which arises proximal to the carpal tunnel and thus is spared in the carpal tunnel syndrome. The densely stippled zone represents the cutaneous sensory area of the median nerve distal to the carpal tunnel. (A, From Canale ST: *Campbell's operative orthopaedics,* ed 10, St Louis, 2003, Mosby; B, from Noble J: *Textbook of primary care medicine,* ed 3, St Louis, 2001, Mosby.)

fluid or structures within. Change within the tunnel is the basis of study related to the etiology of carpal tunnel, but the matrix of possible causes proves to be complex and not fully understood at this time.[119] The primary problem is that pressures are increased, even at rest with the wrist held in neutral. When the individual flexes or extends the wrist, the pressure exerted on the structures can be double or triple. With sustained position of the wrist, the excessive pressure can cause neurapraxia of the median nerve.

Risk Factors

Neuropathic conditions including diabetes mellitus, alcoholism and toxic exposure can lead to carpel tunnel. Risk for developing CTS occurs in people with osteoarthritis of the carpometacarpal joint of the thumb, rheumatoid tenosynovitis, edema, pregnancy, hypothyroidism, and congestive heart failure. Physically inactive individuals are at greater risk for developing CTS over their lifetime. CTS is also 2.5 times more likely in obese individuals (body mass index >29).[57] Smoking cigarettes increases the likelihood of developing CTS, with changes in tissue common to the smoker juxtaposed to a typical extended position of the wrist while holding the cigarette. Anomalous structures within the carpal tunnel, such as variations in the branching pattern of the median nerve, range in length and width of the lumbricals, and extra tendinous slips from the long flexors within the tunnel, may

contribute to development of CTS.[14] Box 39-1 includes suggested causes of CTS.[101,147,184]

Although CTS has been reported in several occupations, the convincing link between work and CTS remains inconclusive.[57] In most cases, work acts as the "last straw" in CTS causation. Except in the case of work that involves very cold temperatures (possibly in conjunction with load and repetition) such as butchery, work is less likely than demographic and disease-related variables to cause CTS. It has been reported that computer use does not pose a severe occupational hazard for development of symptoms of CTS. The responsibility of addressing correctable lifestyle factors and treatable illnesses such as obesity, diabetes, smoking, and increased alcohol intake results in both avoidable long-term health effects and ongoing costs to the community.[57] Patients older than age 63 years have a different pattern of risk factors for CTS than do younger patients. This suggests that CTS in the elderly population may have different underlying pathogenetic mechanisms.[19] Senile systemic amyloidosis, with deposition of transthyretin in the canal may be responsible for the increase in men at that age.[175]

Pathogenesis

Schwann cell changes underlie the initial mechanism of CTS and are independent of axonal damage. Mechanical pressures induce Schwann cells to undergo apoptosis, or cell death causing demyelination at the area of the nodes

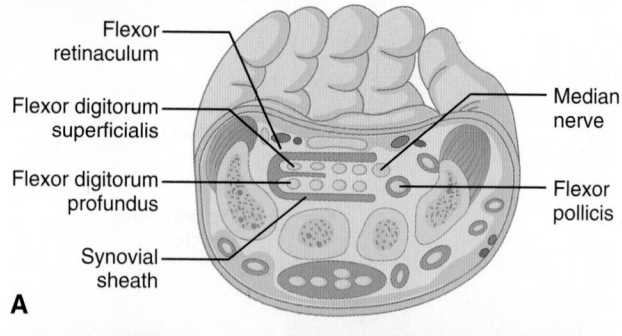

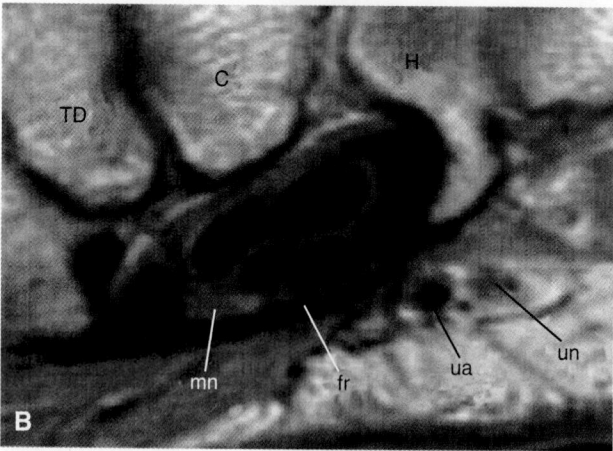

Figure 39-7

A, Cross-section of the carpal tunnel at the wrist. Contents of the tunnel include the tendon of the flexor pollicis longus *(FPL)*, the four tendons of the flexor digitorum profundus *(FDP)*, the four tendons of the flexor digitorum superficialis *(FDS)*, and the median nerve. **B,** Carpal tunnel. *C,* Capitate; *fr,* flexor retinaculum; *H,* hamate; *mn,* median nerve; *TD,* trapezoid; *ua,* ulnar artery; *un,* ulnar nerve. (**A,** From Noble J: *Textbook of primary care medicine,* ed 3, St Louis, 2001, Mosby; **B,** from Yu JS, Habib PA: Normal MR imaging anatomy of the wrist and hand, *Radiol Clin North Am* 44(4):569–581, 2006.)

of Ranvier. At the same time, proliferation of myelin is triggered. This may be caused by cell membrane proteins, known as integrins, that migrate into the area because of increased nutritive demands and appear to be involved in regulating Schwann cell activation, resulting in remyelination. However, the remyelination is not the same as the original myelin. The result is that compressed nerve segments show thinner myelin sheaths. Cytokines are most likely involved in the pathophysiology of repetitive motion injuries in peripheral nerves.[6] Interleukin-1β and tumor necrosis factor-α increase in forearm flexor muscles and tendons in study animals involving reaching and grasping involving moderate repetitive reaching with negligible force. Increases in interleukin-1β and tumor necrosis factor-α negatively correlate with grip strength. Disorganization of receptive fields and alterations of neuronal properties suggest that both peripheral inflammation and cortical neuroplasticity jointly contribute to the development of chronic repetitive motion disorders. Patterns of movement degrade over time without intervention, thus illustrating both the link between central and peripheral processing and the importance of early and appropriate intervention.[32,51] Heat and cold hyperalgesia may reflect impairments in central nociceptive

processing seen in patients with unilateral CTS. The bilateral thermal hyperalgesia associated with pain intensity and duration of pain history supports a role of generalized sensitization mechanisms in the initiation, maintenance and spread of pain in CTS.[63,170] Slowing of nerve conduction noted on EMG with CTS reflect changes in both myelin and axons.[189] If the mechanical pressures are high enough compression can create an axonotmesis in which axon continuity is lost and wallerian degeneration occurs.

Clinical Manifestations

CTS causes sensory symptoms in the median nerve distribution. Pain may be located distally in the forearm or wrist and radiate into the thumb, index, and middle fingers. It may also radiate into the arm, shoulder, and neck. Comparing self-reported symptoms recorded on the Katz hand diagram allows symptoms to be assessed as classic, probable, possible, or unlikely to be CTS.[37] Nocturnal pain is the hallmark of CTS. Even in the early stages of CTS most people will report being awakened by painful numbness in the middle of the night. Sensory symptoms usually precede motor symptoms. Diminished two-point discrimination, diminished ability to perceive vibration, and elevation of threshold in Semmes-Weinstein monofilament testing routinely occur. Thenar weakness is seen in advanced cases. In nearly half of all cases, symptoms occur bilaterally. If CTS goes untreated, symptoms escalate into persistent pain with atrophy of the thenar musculature and the person will have a loss of grip strength. The combined loss of grip strength, inability to pinch, and sensory loss causes clumsiness in the hands.[39]

MEDICAL MANAGEMENT

DIAGNOSIS. CTS appears more often as a syndrome rather than a singular finding. Diagnosis can be determined in up to 90% of instances by careful history, physical examination, and provocation tests, which are considered positive when pain, numbness, and paresthesia are produced in the median nerve distribution. The *Phalen test* involves flexing the wrist to 90 degrees for 1 minute (Fig. 39-8, *A*); the *Tinel test* is wrist percussion over the carpal tunnel (Fig. 39-8, *B*); the *Durkan carpal compression test* involves compression applied to the median nerve for 30 seconds with the thumbs or an atomizer bulb attached to a manometer. The *lumbrical incursion* test is performed by asking the patient to make a fist with the wrist in the neutral position. The test is positive if pain and paresthesia occur within 30 to 40 seconds. A full fist results in approximately 3 cm of lumbrical muscle incursion into the carpal tunnel contributing to median nerve compression.[56]

It is often suggested that the "gold standard" test of CTS is electrodiagnostic testing. Electromyography and nerve conduction studies can confirm the diagnosis, determine the severity of nerve damage, guide and measure the effect of treatment, and rule out other conditions such as radiculopathy and brachial plexus damage. Distal motor and sensory latencies and sensory NCV across the carpal tunnel are most frequently administered.[177] Changes in the sensory conduction across the wrist are reportedly the most sensitive

Box 39-1

CAUSES OF CARPAL TUNNEL SYNDROME

Neuromusculoskeletal

IDIOPATHIC
Cause unknown

Anatomic (Compression)

Small carpal canal, anomalous muscles/tendons
Basal joint (thumb) arthritis
Cervical disk lesions
Cervical spondylosis
Congenital anatomic differences or anatomic change in nerve or carpal tunnel (e.g., shape, size, volume of structures; presence of palmaris longus)
History of wrist surgery, especially previous carpal tunnel surgery
Injection: high pressure
Peripheral neuropathy
Poor posture (may also be associated with thoracic outlet syndrome)
Tendinitis
Trigger points
Tenosynovitis
Thoracic outlet syndrome

Trauma/Exertional

Swelling, hemorrhage, scar, wrist fracture, carpal dislocation
Cumulative trauma disorders*
Repetitive strain injuries*
Vibrational exposure (jackhammer or other manual labor equipment)

Systemic

Chronic kidney disease (fluid imbalance)
Congestive heart failure (fluid imbalance)
Hemochromatosis
Leukemia (tissue infiltration)
Liver disease
Medications
  • Nonsteroidal antiinflammatory drugs
  • Oral contraceptives
  • Statins
  • Alendronate (Fosamax)
  • Lithium
  • β Blocker
Obesity
Pregnancy (fluid retention)
Tumors (lipoma, hemangioma, ganglia, synovial sarcoma, fibroma, neuroma, neurofibroma)
Use of oral contraceptives
Vitamin deficiency

Endocrine

Acromegaly
Diabetes mellitus
Gout (deposits of tophi and calcium)
Hormonal imbalance (menopause; posthysterectomy)
Hyperparathyroidism
Hyperthyroidism (Graves disease)
Hypocalcemia
Hypothyroidism (myxedema)

Infectious Disease

Atypical mycobacterium
Histoplasmosis
Rubella
Sporotrichosis

Inflammatory

Amyloidosis
Arthritis (rheumatoid, gout, polymyalgia rheumatica)
Dermatomyositis
Gout/pseudogout
Scleroderma
Systemic lupus erythematosus

Neuropathic

Alcohol abuse
Chemotherapy (delayed, long-term effect)
Diabetes
Multiple myeloma (amyloidosis deposits)
Thyroid disease
Vitamin/nutritional deficiency (especially vitamin B$_6$, folic acid)
Vitamin toxicity

*The role of repetitive activities and occupational factors (e.g., hand use of any type and keyboard or computer work in particular) has been questioned as a direct cause of carpal tunnel syndrome and remains under investigation.
From Goodman CC, Snyder T: *Differential diagnosis for physical therapists: screening for referral*, ed 5, Philadelphia, 2013, WB Saunders.

indicator of CTS.[213] Ultrasound studies, which reveal an enlarged median nerve, may assist with the diagnosis.[53,99,110] The injection of corticosteroids or bupivacaine into the carpal tunnel has been used to determine involvement, therefore when the injection is accompanied by a relief of symptoms, it provides diagnostic evidence of CTS.

TREATMENT. Because the causes appear to be multifactorial, treatment approaches address several components. Early management typically involves ergonomic modification of the client's environment and lifestyle changes. A current concept in treatment of CTS involves preventing inflammation as well as minimizing cortical dedifferentiation, but there is not enough evidence yet to determine specific protocols.[32] Long-term use of antiinflammatory medications leads to gastric complications without significant change in symptoms. Steroid injection into the carpal canal shows relief up to 1 year.[36]

Surgical release of the transverse carpal ligament is indicated in when symptoms have lasted longer than 1 year and there is both motor and sensory NCV involvement, or denervation is evidenced by fibrillation potentials on EMG. Flexor tenosynovectomy with transverse carpal ligament division, endoscopic release of the ligament, and neurolysis of the median nerve are performed through limited incisions and require minimal exposure and manipulation of the nerve. Seventy-six percent of the surgical cases experience return of normal two-point discrimination and up to 70% have normal muscle strength return.[96] After surgery, nerve and tendon gliding techniques are advocated to reduce scarring, adhesions, and subsequent formation of fibrotic tissue.[198]

PROGNOSIS. Prognosis relates directly to the severity of the nerve entrapment at diagnosis, clinical cause, and mode of treatment.

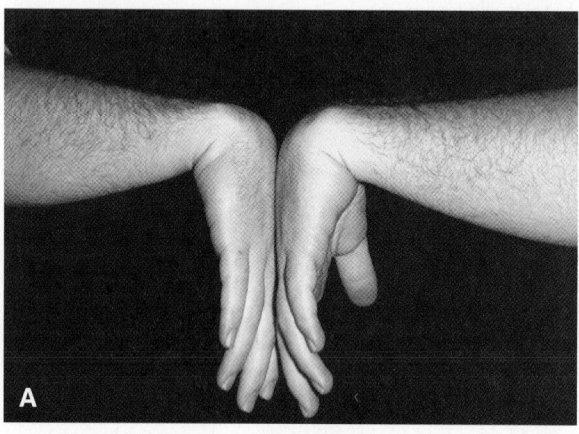

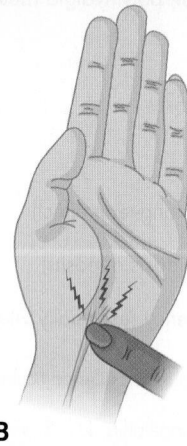

Figure 39-8

A, The Phalen test. Patients maximally flex both wrists and hold the position for 1 to 2 minutes. If symptoms of numbness or paresthesia within the median nerve distribution are reproduced, the test is positive. **B,** The Tinel sign in carpal tunnel syndrome. (A, From Frontera WR, Silver JK: *Essentials of physical medicine and rehabilitation*, Philadelphia, 2002, Hanley and Belfus; B, from Noble J: *Textbook of primary care medicine*, ed 3, St Louis, 2001, Mosby.)

Carpal Tunnel Syndrome

Overuse syndromes involve a degree of edema; consequently, icing after long periods of use is advocated to reduce the pain and swelling. Use of phonophoresis and iontophoresis can be effective to reduce local inflammation and swelling.[81] Because generalized deconditioning exacerbates the symptoms of CTS, exercise is encouraged; however, strengthening exercises in the involved wrist and hand should be avoided until symptom relief is nearly complete. Use of neutral splinting has been found to be beneficial in severe CTS when worn either at night or full time. Reductions in use of the upper extremity might be an indirect effect of daily use.[209] A combination of a cock-up splint with lumbrical intensive stretches appears to be the most effective combination for improvements in functional gains when measured at 24 weeks of intervention.[11] Therapists should not overlook the possibility that motor skill retraining may have to be included in treatment plans in order to regain function and to prevent further tissue damage when managing chronic repetitive motion injury. Proper biomechanics, frequent breaks and strategic movement patterns may prevent the persistent changes seen in these individuals.[102]

Thoracic Outlet Syndrome

Individuals with thoracic outlet syndrome (TOS) may have vague symptoms or symptoms that are difficult to interpret. Despite TOS being a common clinical disorder, conclusive evidence is lacking to support most currently used treatments.[152]

Definition

TOS is an entrapment syndrome caused by pressure from structures in the thoracic outlet on fibers of the brachial plexus at some point between the interscalene triangle and the inferior border of the axilla. In addition, vascular symptoms can occur because of compression of the subclavian artery (Fig. 39-9).

Etiology

The anatomy of the region of the thoracic outlet is extremely complex. Spinal nerve roots of the brachial plexus interact with surrounding bony ribs, muscles, and tendons (subclavius, anterior and middle scalene, and pectoralis minor) and the vascular supply (subclavian artery and vein) to the region. In addition to neurologic structures becoming entrapped, arterial and venous structures also may be affected individually or in combination. Practically, TOS can be divided into three groups: neurogenic (compression of brachial plexus), vascular (compression of subclavian artery and/or vein), and disputed (nonspecific TOS with chronic pain and symptoms of brachial plexus involvement).[21,89]

Risk Factors

Postural changes associated with growth and development, trauma to the shoulder girdle, and body composition have all been identified as contributing to the development of TOS. In human upright posture, gravity pulls on the shoulder girdle creating traction on the structures and may contribute to the development of TOS. Additionally, congenital factors that affect the bony structures, such as a cervical rib or fascial bands, also compress the neurovascular bundle. TOS is reported more commonly in women than in men, and rarely occurs in individuals younger than the age of 20 years.[64]

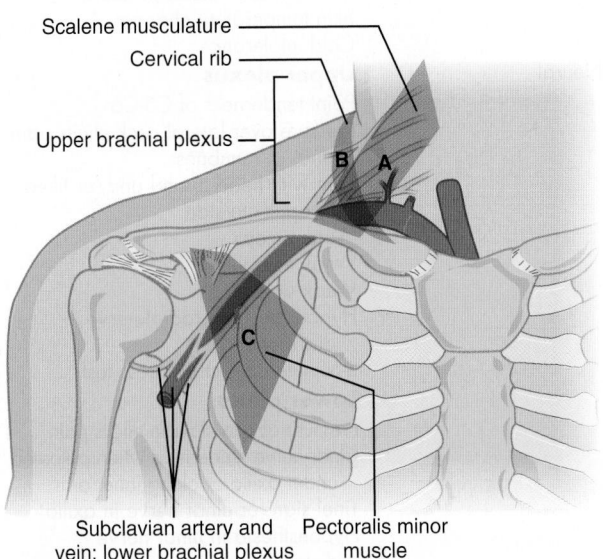

Figure 39-9

Schematic relationship of structures in development of thoracic outlet syndrome. Compression of the neurovascular bundle can occur with **(A)** hypertrophy of scalene musculature impinging on structures lying between middle and anterior scalene; **(B)** the presence of cervical rib or fibrous bands between the cervical and first rib; or **(C)** compression by pectoralis minor during hyperabduction. (From Rakel RE: *Textbook of medicine*, ed 7, Philadelphia, 2007, WB Saunders.)

Pathogenesis

Chronic compression of nerve roots or proximal plexus and arteries between the clavicle and first rib or impinging musculature results in edema and ischemia in the nerves (see Fig. 39-9). This compression initially creates a neurapraxia. After loss of myelin the axons are more vulnerable to unrelieved compression. The neurapraxia can progress to an axonotmesis in which axon continuity is lost and wallerian degeneration occurs.

Clinical Manifestations

The nerve compression in TOS results in paresthesias and pain in the arm; particularly at end of day. Other symptoms may include pain, tingling, and paresis. If the upper nerve plexus is involved (C5 to C7), pain is reported in the neck; this may radiate into the face (sometimes with ear pain) and anterior chest, as well as over the scapulae. Symptoms may also extend over the lateral aspect of the forearm into the hand. If the lower plexus is compromised (C7 to T1), pain and numbness occur in the posterior neck and shoulder, medial arm and forearm, and radiate into the ulnarly innervated digits of the hand. Weakness occurs in the muscles corresponding to nerve root innervation, and atrophy follows in severe cases. Vascular symptoms may include coldness, edema in the hand or arm, Raynaud phenomenon (cyanosis), fatigue in hand and arm, and superficial vein distention in the hand (Fig. 39-10). Overhead and lifting activities, along with movements of the head, can aggravate symptoms in the upper plexus.

MEDICAL MANAGEMENT

DIAGNOSIS. Provocative tests based on the belief that the anterior scalene can compress the neurovascular bundle are used to elicit symptoms of TOS.[199] However, these tests have a high false-positive response, and are of disputable diagnostic value.[64] Maneuvers are performed bilaterally, and the pulse is monitored to note a change in its quality.

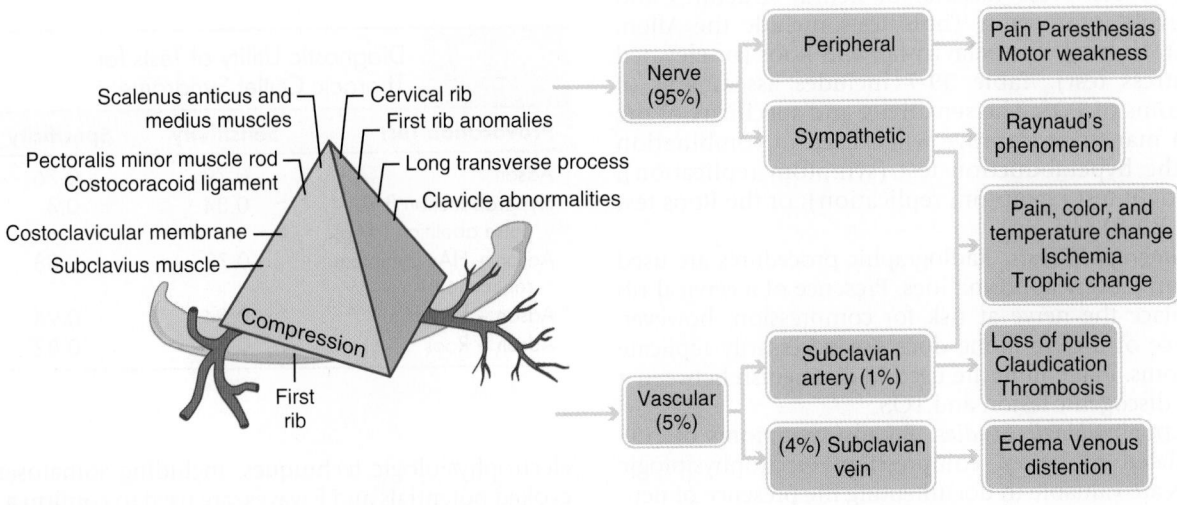

Figure 39-10

Relationship of thoracic outlet abnormalities and impairments. (From Marx RS, Hockberger RS, Walls RM: *Rosen's emergency medicine: concepts and clinical practice*, ed 6, St Louis, 2006, Mosby.)

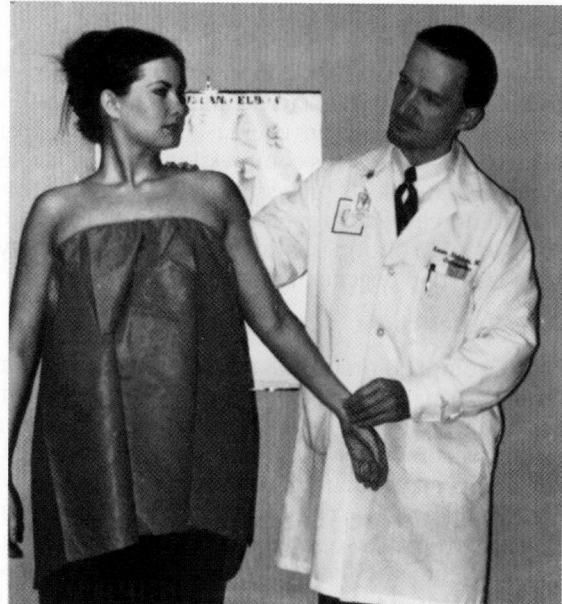

Figure 39-11

The Adson test is one of many diagnostic tests used to examine the upper extremity to determine presence of thoracic outlet syndrome: arterial or neurologic. Hold patient's arm in slight abduction while palpating the radial pulse. Ask the patient to inhale and hold the breath while extending the neck and rotating toward the affected side. The Adson test is positive if the patient reports paresthesia or if the pulse fades away. (From DeLee JC, Drez D, Miller MD: *DeLee and Drez's orthopaedic sports medicine,* ed 2, Philadelphia, 2003, WB Saunders.)

Table 39-7	Assessing Symptoms of Thoracic Outlet Syndrome*
Component	**Symptoms**
Vascular	3-Minute elevated test
	Adson test
	Swelling (arm/hand)
	Discoloration of hand
	Costoclavicular test
	Hyperabduction test
	Upper extremity claudication
	Differences in blood pressure
	Skin temperature changes
	Cold intolerance
Neural	**Upper plexus**
	Point tenderness of C5-C6
	Pressure over lateral neck elicits pain and/or numbness.
	Pain with head turned and/or tilted to opposite side
	Weak biceps
	Weak triceps
	Weak wrist
	Hypoesthesia in radial nerve distribution
	3-Minute abduction stress test
	Lower plexus
	Pressure above clavicle elicits pain
	Ulnar nerve tenderness when palpated under axilla or along inner arm
	Tinel sign for ulnar nerve in axilla
	Hypoesthesia in ulnar nerve distribution
	Serratus anterior weakness
	Weak hand grip

*Although no specific testing for thoracic outlet has proven valid in detecting upper-extremity pain of a neurogenic origin, the use of these special tests may help identify patterns of positive objective findings to help characterize thoracic outlet syndrome.
From Table 17-5 in Goodman CC, Snyder T: *Differential diagnosis for physical therapists: screening for referral,* ed 5, Philadelphia, 2013, WB Saunders.

However, mere obliteration of the peripheral pulse does not necessarily mean that TOS exists as an entrapment problem; sensory symptoms must be reproduced. For persons with a vascular component, blood pressure may differ from side to side. Although there is no universally accepted reliable diagnostic test for TOS, the *Adson maneuver* (Fig. 39-11) appears among the most effective. Several other maneuvers with a positional component of the head, shoulder, or arm have been found to compress vascular or neural structures and thus evoke symptoms. These tests include the Allen, Wright, Halsted, costoclavicular, and Roos (or elevated arm stress test). Table 39-7 includes assessment of symptoms of TOS. The sensitivity and specificity of the Adson maneuver improve when used in combination with the hyperabduction test (symptom replication), the Wright test (symptom replication), or the Roos test (Table 39-8).[72]

Radiographic Tests. Radiographic procedures are used to identify bony abnormalities. Presence of a cervical rib may place the nerve at risk for compression; however, presence of the rib alone does not necessarily replicate symptoms. Plane films are used to distinguish between a C7-T1 discogenic lesion and TOS.

Electrophysiologic Studies. Because symptoms of TOS are related to neural compression, electrophysiologic studies are valuable in documenting the presence of neuropathy. NCV allows the examiner to pinpoint the lesion, either because of a change in amplitude or a slowing in conduction velocity (Box 39-2). Other, more refined

Table 39-8	Diagnostic Utility of Tests for Thoracic Outlet Syndrome	
Provocation Test	**Sensitivity**	**Specificity**
Adson	0.79	0.76
Hyperabduction (HA)—pulse abolition (HAp)	0.84	0.4
Adson + HAs (symptom replication)	0.72	0.88
Adson + Wright's	0.54	0.94
Adson + Roos	0.72	0.82

electrophysiologic techniques, including somatosensory evoked potentials and F waves, are used to confirm a diagnosis of nerve root entrapment.

TOS should be distinguished from other disorders with similar symptoms. These include cervical

Box 39-2

TYPICAL ELECTROPHYSIOLOGIC FINDINGS IN THORACIC OUTLET SYNDROME

Upper Sensory
- Decreased amplitude

Median Sensory
- Normal

Ulnar Motor
- Normal or decreased amplitude

Median Motor
- Decreased amplitude

Electromyography
- + Positive fibrillation potentials: first dorsal interosseus

Adapted from Huang JH, Zager EL: Thoracic outlet syndrome, *Neurosurgery* 55:897–903, 2004.

Box 39-3

SURGICAL PROCEDURES AND APPROACHES FOR THORACIC OUTLET SYNDROME

Procedures
- Scalenotomy
- Scalenectomy
- Clavicle resection
- Pectoralis minor release
- First rib resection
- Cervical rib resection

Approaches
- Axillary
- Supraclavicular
- Combined axillary and supraclavicular
- Posterior
- Subclavicular
- Transclavicular

radiculopathy, reflex sympathetic dystrophy, tumors of the apex of the lung (Pancoast tumor, see Chapter 15), and ulnar nerve compression at either elbow or wrist. The sensory pattern of TOS distinguishes it from an ulnar neuropathy such as tardy ulnar palsy. Because the nerve roots are affected, the sensory changes extend above the hand and wrist into the forearm in TOS and follow a dermatomal pattern. Myofascial pain patterns may also mimic TOS symptoms.

TREATMENT. Given that TOS is a complex disorder, management is best approached by a multidisciplinary team, which may include, but is not limited to, physicians, surgeons, work-related case managers, and physical and occupational therapists.[109] Management is divided into conservative and surgical approaches. The initial treatment of the person with TOS is conservative when symptoms are mild to moderate in severity. Postural and breathing exercises and gentle stretching are the cornerstones of the initial conservative program. This is followed by strengthening exercises for shoulder girdle musculature, especially the trapezius, levator scapulae, and rhomboids. Initially, overhead exercises should be avoided because they tend to evoke symptoms. Therapists are cautioned against forceful stretching to mobilize the first rib.[78]

Surgical management of TOS is reserved for cases that are refractory to postural and exercise correction and those with vascular compromise.[31] There are at least six different surgical procedures and six different anatomic approaches for TOS (Box 39-3). In scalenotomy, the muscle is detached from the first rib; unfortunately, with this approach a high percentage of people experience recurring symptoms. Scalenectomy, removal of the scalene muscle, is advocated for people who have had recurrence of their symptoms. Clavicle resection is indicated primarily when the clavicle is damaged. When scalenectomy, with or without first rib resection, is the surgical approach used, its 5-year success rate is approximately 70%.[165]

PROGNOSIS. After surgery, 70% of cases have a good or excellent response using a supraclavicular or transaxillary resection of the first rib. Improvement in pain symptoms ranges from 70% to 80%, some patients require occasional analgesics, and 10% note no improvement. In individuals with signs and symptoms and electrophysiologic changes consistent with classic TOS, no improvement in strength is noted when atrophy was present before surgery.[31] Complications during surgery include pneumothorax, nerve compression, and transient winging of the scapula because the upper digitations of the serratus are detached.

A 4-year follow-up reported no significant difference in return to work or symptom severity when the first rib was resected compared to a conservative, nonoperative approach.[76] Factors that are associated with long-term disability include preoperative depression, single status, and less than high school education.[9]

SPECIAL IMPLICATIONS FOR THE THERAPIST   39-2

Thoracic Outlet Syndrome

Therapists need to consider using an upper-quarter screen to rule out cervical radiculopathy or shoulder dysfunction during their evaluation. If this screen is negative, range of motion and posture should be evaluated to identify soft-tissue restrictions. The client's response to provocative maneuvers should be assessed along with a sensory evaluation, preferably using Semmes-Weinstein monofilaments. Manual muscle testing or other method of evaluating strength should be performed. Treatment is aimed at pain relief along with postural correction.[210]

One reasons why TOS has been difficult to diagnose relates to the client's subjective report. Frequently, signs and symptoms do not correspond to a single lesion, but to multifocal lesions, either of vascular and/or neurogenic origin. For clients who do not respond to treatment, some believe that compression at a proximal or distal source might increase the vulnerability of nerves, making them more susceptible to compression at another site. A functional tool such as the DASH (Disabilities of the Arm, Shoulder and Hand) outcome measure should be used to track objective and functional changes. This measure has proven to be a valid, reliable, and responsive test in evaluating people with a variety of upper-extremity problems.[15]

Tardy Ulnar Palsy/Retroepicondylar Palsy

Anatomy

The ulnar nerve arises from the lower trunk of the brachial plexus and carries fibers from C8 and T1 nerve roots. At the elbow, it passes behind the medial epicondyle and then passes between the two heads of the flexor carpi ulnaris through the forearm to the wrist. The distal portion of the nerve enters the palm by crossing the flexor retinaculum and divides into a superficial and deep branch in the hand (Fig. 39-12).

Etiology

Ulnar nerve entrapment, (also called tardy ulnar palsy, cubital tunnel syndrome, and ulnar nerve neuritis) at the elbow is one of the most common entrapment neuropathies encountered in clinical practice.[208] Because of its anatomic location, ulnar nerve palsy is a common complication of fractures in the region of the elbow. A late or tardy ulnar palsy may occur years after a fracture and is associated with callus formation or a valgus deformity of the elbow. These produce a gradual stretching of the nerve in the ulnar groove of the medial epicondyle.

Risk Factors

A similar type of tardy ulnar palsy occurs with repeated trauma for relatively long periods of time in clients with a shallow ulnar groove at the elbow. Ulnar neuropathy from entrapment at the elbow is the second most frequent upper extremity neuropathy (after CTS).

Pathogenesis

The mechanism of injury compressing the ulnar nerve has been attributed to recurrent microtrauma associated with fracture and fibrous bands or recurrent cubital subluxations, as well as entrapment at the entrance or exit of the cubital tunnel.[117] Elbow flexion aggravates symptoms. Compression will initially cause a neuropraxia with demyelination of the nerve; if the pressure goes unrelieved, this will progress to an axonotmesis with denervation occurring below the level of the elbow.

Clinical Manifestations

Tardy ulnar palsy can result in a clawhand deformity with metacarpophalangeal extension and interphalangeal flexion of the ring and little fingers because of the unopposed action of the extensor muscle group and paralysis of the

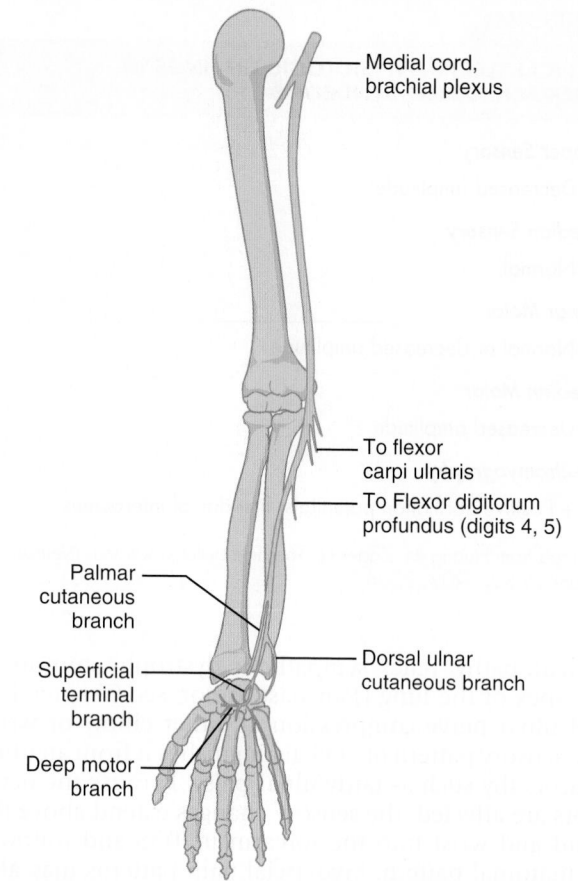

Figure 39-12

Distribution of the ulnar nerve. A tardy ulnar palsy impinges the ulnar nerve as it passes behind the medial epicondyle of the humerus. (From Steward JD: *Focal peripheral neuropathies,* ed 3, Philadelphia, 2000, Lippincott Williams & Wilkins.)

third and fourth lumbricals that normally flex the metacarpophalangeals and extend the interphalangeals (Fig. 39-13). Flattening of the hypothenar eminence along with abduction of the little finger coincides with weakness of the palmaris brevis and abductor digiti minimi. Marked atrophy of the interossei on the dorsal surface of the hand with guttering between the extensor tendons indicates the presence of denervation. Abduction and adduction movements of the fingers are impaired. Paralysis of the flexor carpi ulnaris produces a radial deviation of the hand when wrist flexion is attempted. Sensory loss is variable, but impaired sensation may be expected involving the little finger and the ulnar aspect of the ring finger and along the ulnar aspect of the palm of the hand to the wrist. Occasionally, sensory symptoms extend proximally to the wrist.

MEDICAL MANAGEMENT

DIAGNOSIS. Percussion of or bending the elbow can replicate symptoms.[117] NCV studies are helpful only when sufficient nerve damage has occurred to produce definite strength or sensory changes in the hand. NCVs are slowed through the involved region but are relatively normal above and below the epicondyle. Electromyography reports slowing of sensory or motor NCV across

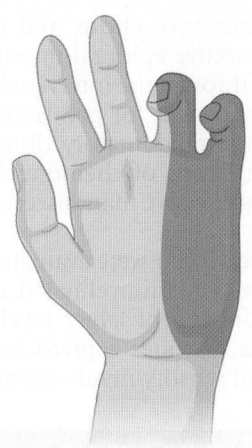

Figure 39-13

Clawing of the ring and little fingers (hyperextension of the metacarpophalangeal joint and flexion of the interphalangeal joints) from unopposed action of extensor musculature combined with paralysis of the intrinsic muscles of the hand occurs when there is involvement of the ulnar nerve. Shaded area represents ulnar nerve sensory distribution in the hand. (From Marx RS, Hockberger RS, Walls RM: *Rosen's emergency medicine: concepts and clinical practice*, ed 6, St Louis, 2006, Mosby.)

the elbow, prolonged conduction (termed a *latency*) to the flexor carpi ulnaris, along with changes in amplitude, duration, or shape of the sensory potential across the elbow. Detection of an abnormal latency requires accurate measurement of ulnar nerve segment length.[131]

TREATMENT. Mild entrapments are managed conservatively; moderate and severe compression require surgery. To relieve the compression, either decompression, the preferred method (medial epicondylectomy), or transposition of the ulnar nerve to the anterior aspect of the elbow is performed.[23,183] Symptomatically, the clawhand deformity should be treated with a splint that blocks metacarpophalangeal hyperextension (lumbrical bar) and allows the extensor digitorum to extend the interphalangeal joints.

PROGNOSIS. Results of surgery are normally good when the individual has not had a chronic tardy ulnar involvement. Decompression surgery should have complete restoration of function quickly, but recovery after transposition surgery may take up to 6 months. Surgery to treat chronic involvement (over 3 months) may have a less certain restoration of function.[183] After nerve transposition, most NCVs at follow-up are improved. However, the magnitude of change in the motor conduction velocity does not correlate well with clinical improvement. One factor that has been identified to effect outcome is body mass index; increased body weight is related slightly to patient's perception of poorer improvement.[139]

Saturday Night Palsy/Sleep Palsy

Definition and Etiology

Saturday night palsy is associated with radial nerve compression in the arm. It results from direct pressure against a firm object and typically follows deep sleep on the arm with compression of the radial nerve at the spiral groove

of the humerus in a person who is sleeping after becoming intoxicated. Sleep palsy has also been associated with lipoma compressing the radial nerve.[62] If the radial nerve is compressed in the axilla, the damage is often referred to as a crutch palsy.

Pathogenesis

Compression of the nerve causes segmental demyelination.

Clinical Manifestations

Symptoms of radial nerve paralysis depends on the level of the lesion. The more proximal the involvement, the more extensive the paralysis. When involvement occurs in the axilla, weakness occurs in elbow extension (triceps), elbow flexion (brachioradialis), and supination (supinator). If the nerve is damaged in the upper arm the triceps is spared. In addition, in both instances there will be weakness of wrist extensors and the extensors of the fingers and thumb, diminishing grip strength. Sensory loss with radial nerve involvement is variable. If present, it is typically confined to the dorsum of the hand but may extend to the dorsum of the forearm.

MEDICAL MANAGEMENT

DIAGNOSIS. Diagnosis is by history, clinical examination, and electrophysiologic examination. This type of paralysis is usually classified as a neurapraxia or conduction block, signifying demyelination. There is slowing of nerve conduction in both motor and sensory fibers across the lesion site.

TREATMENT. Medical management is aimed at asymptomatic management. A cock-up splint is used to maintain the wrist in an extended position until return of function.

PROGNOSIS. Radial nerve injuries such as Saturday night palsy have a good prognosis. Recovery rate is approximately 67% to 100% within 3 months, with the main goal being return of hand function.[211] If a neurapraxia is reported, normal conduction can be anticipated within a few months because the paralysis is related to a focal demyelination.[80]

Parsonage-Turner Syndrome

Parsonage-Turner syndrome, also known as *neuralgia amyotrophy* is a rare condition affecting the LMNs of the brachial plexus or individual nerves or nerve branches. Etiology and incidence are unknown. Clinical presentation can vary but usually involve sudden pain, muscle weakness, and eventual atrophy of affected muscles in the shoulder girdle/upper extremity. There may be a precipitating event such as a prolonged static posture or sustained or repetitive load to the arm or upper quadrant. Recovery is usually spontaneous over a period of months up to several years; some residual muscle weakness may persist. Physical therapy to assist with return of strength, motor function (including scapulohumeral rhythm), and proprioception may be needed. The therapist should assess for myofascial pain patterns, tendinitis, and other soft tissue impairments caused by compensatory movement patterns. The differential diagnosis includes cervical radiculopathy, rotator cuff disease, and TOS.[163]

Sciatica

Incidence and Etiology

Sciatica is a radiculopathy that occurs most often in individuals between the ages of 40 and 60 years in which the sciatic nerve root is affected, most typically by compression. Of those who develop lumbosacral radiculopathy, 10% to 25% develop symptoms that last more than 6 weeks. Less commonly, sciatica may occur in the presence of abscess, blood clots, or tumors. Sciatica may be mistaken for intermittent claudication or low back pain without discogenic involvement and is one of the most common conditions managed in primary care settings.

Pathogenesis

The epidural space is innervated by a meningeal branch of the spinal nerve, the recurrent sinuvertebral nerve. Arising from the dorsal root ganglion, this nerve enters through the intervertebral foramen, divides into ascending and descending branches to blood vessels, and supplies the posterior longitudinal ligament, the superficial anulus fibrosis, anterior dura mater, and dural sleeve.[89] In animal studies, the sinovertebral nerve responded to high threshold mechanical stimuli. Conduction velocity for fibers in the nerve corresponded to types III and IV, which lead researchers to correlate nerve function with nociception.[176] Herniation of the intervertebral disc can impinge on the nerve root or structures innervated by the recurrent sinuvertebral nerve to cause pain. Disc herniation, usually at the L4-5 and L5-S1 levels, is the most common cause of sciatica (i.e., pain radiating down the posterior leg from sciatic nerve root irritation).[125]

Clinical Manifestations

In addition to low back pain, when sensory fibers are affected, pain may radiate into one or both legs. The motor and sensory nerves are affected easily in a radiculopathy because compression occurs in an area where CNS connective tissue coverings meet the protective tissue coverings of the peripheral nerve, leaving that region of the nerve "at risk."[95] Coughing, sitting, and sneezing worsens the pain. For further information, see Chapter 27. Both clinical and experimental studies show that adjacent nerve roots may be affected when a lumbar disc herniates. Inflammatory chemical mediators released into the epidural space affect nearby nerve roots, without any direct compression of those roots.[142]

MEDICAL MANAGEMENT

DIAGNOSIS. Radiologic tests and electrophysiologic studies may be used in diagnosing sciatica. MRI is preferred to CT scanning for lumbar spine imaging; however, because 60% of people without back symptoms have disc bulging on MRI, protrusion and bulges may not correlate with symptoms.[12] A screening EMG examination of only four muscles in the leg identified more than 89% of surgically confirmed involvement of the nerve root.[29] Others have noted that the H-reflex has provided better predictive value of nerve root involvement than standard motor and sensory nerve conductions radiculopathies.[4] Just as radiologic studies are not sufficient alone to distinguish sciatica neither is electrophysiologic testing.

TREATMENT. Conservative efforts and rehabilitation are recommended. Selective epidural injection of steroids at target nerve roots through the intervertebral foramina has offered short-term benefit for pain relief, as has the use of nonsteroidal antiinflammatory drugs.[33] Also unclear are the long-term effects of chemonucleolysis, which is reported to be less effective than discectomy.[71]

PROGNOSIS. Subjects who were evaluated 1 year after discectomy had recovery in unmyelinated and small myelinated fibers; the function of larger myelinated fibers did not improve. This provides a physiologic rationale for residual motor and sensory involvement.[142]

SPECIAL IMPLICATIONS FOR THE THERAPIST | 39-3

Sciatica

It has been recommended that physical therapy interventions emphasize the use of joint mobilizations and exercise for improvements in health in people with sciatica.[93]

For those physical therapists using the visual analogue scale (VAS) to assess pain in sciatica, a range of minimal clinically relevant change has been reported. Using a 100-mm VAS, Todd et al[197] reported that a 13-mm change is needed to discriminate a crude change in pain, whereas Farrar et al[60] estimated a 20-mm change was needed to discriminate a crude change in pain. More recently, Giraudeau et al[74] also reported that 30 mm reflected a crude change in pain. Outcome assessments such as the Oswestry Disability Index and the Patient-Specific Functional Scale should be used to quantify meaningful functional changes with intervention.

Morton Neuroma

Morton neuroma is a common entrapment neuropathy in the forefoot, most often involving the third toe interspace. It is also called Morton metatarsalgia, interdigital neuritis, and *interdigital perineural fibroma*. The term *neuroma* is misleading, because the problem is degenerative, not proliferative as the term applies.[2]

Definition and Etiology

No incidence or prevalence for Morton neuroma has been published in any study. However, the average age of individuals diagnosed with Morton neuroma is reported to be between 45 and 60 years, with women affected more than men, in a ratio of 5:1. Bilateral involvement is uncommon.[28]

Pathogenesis

Three common digital nerves, two arising from the medial plantar nerve, and third from the lateral plantar nerve, pass between divisions of the plantar aponeurosis where each bifurcates into two interdigital nerves. The first common digital nerve supplies adjacent sides of the great and second toe, those of the second common digital nerve supply adjacent sides of the second and third toes, and the sides of the third and fourth toes are supplied by the third common digital nerve (Fig. 39-14). Mechanical irritation resulting

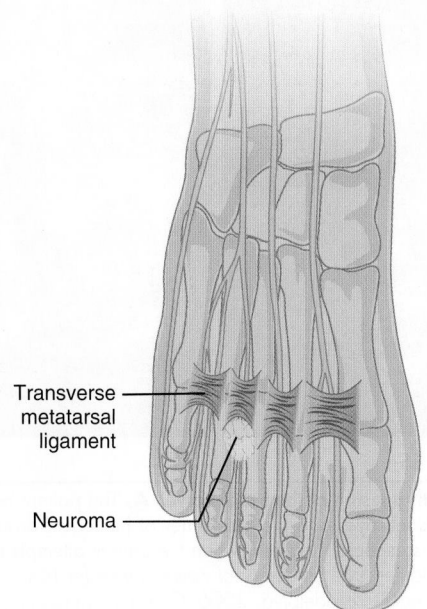

Transverse
metatarsal
ligament

Neuroma

Figure 39-14

Morton neuroma involves the common digital nerve. The most frequent location is between third and fourth metatarsals. (From Frontera WR, Silver JK: *Essentials of physical medicine and rehabilitation*, Philadelphia, 2002, Hanley and Belfus.)

from intrinsic factors, such as diminished intermetatarsal head distance[79] and poor foot mechanics (excessive pronation during gait) that pulls the nerve more medially than normal and taut as the toes extend during terminal stance, and extrinsic factors, such as high heels in which the weight is transferred onto the forefoot, maintaining the nerve in a taut condition; narrow toe box on shoe that creates a greater compression in the area; and thin-soled shoes where ground forces interact with the deep transverse metatarsal ligament, causing compression in this confined space, have been implicated as contributing to this condition. Additional inflammatory conditions, such as arthritis, and activities that involve application of repetitive forces to the plantar nerves, such as jogging on a hard surface, produce shear forces that can irritate the nerve.

Entrapment produces some or all of the following histopathology: thickening of the endoneurium, hyalization of endoneurial vessels, thickened perineurium, and demyelination of nerve fibers.[28,167]

Clinical Manifestations

Symptoms include burning, tingling, or sharp lancinating pain in one of the interspaces of the forefoot that occurs while walking. Pain may radiate into adjacent toes or proximally into the foot. Individuals may state that they must stop, remove their shoe, and massage their foot to relieve the symptoms. At its worst, the person may be apprehensive about stepping with the involved foot. Symptoms occur paroxysmally over many years and can limit participation in activities involving standing and walking.

MEDICAL MANAGEMENT

DIAGNOSIS. In 2009, a practice guideline algorithm was published that aids the clinician in management of this

common condition.[195] Typically, history and clinical examination have been used to diagnose this disorder. Two tests that provoke symptoms include plantar palpation of the involved space at the metatarsal heads as mediolateral compression is applied to the metatarsal heads (Mulder sign) and dorsiflexion of the involved toe producing symptoms and plantarflexion of the toe relieving them (Lasègue sign).[66] The reported positive predictive values of these clinical tests vary widely. Sonography and MRI have been used to assess the presence of Morton neuroma. Whereas the sensitivity for predicting the presence of Morton neuroma is reported at 0.79 and 0.86, respectively, the specificity of both sonography and MRI is 1.0[180] and has been used to diagnose Morton neuromas.[155,193]

Differential diagnoses considered would include metatarsal stress fractures, metatarsalgia, and metatarsal phalangeal derangement. Radiographs may prove helpful in differential diagnosis.

TREATMENT. Conservative, nonoperative management is directed at pressure relief and involves use of a soft orthosis (insoles) or metatarsal pad. These may provide symptom relief as long as the shoes the person is wearing have a wider toe box and a lower heel. If symptoms continue, injection of a local anesthetic or corticosteroid from the dorsal direction may be helpful. Finally, surgical treatment involves either neural decompression by releasing the intermetatarsal ligament or neurectomy, proximal to the location of the neuroma to allow retraction of the plantar nerve away from the weight-bearing surface. Individuals undergoing surgical interventions have experienced complications such as postsurgical hammertoe deformity, keloid scar formation and complex regional pain syndrome.[2]

PROGNOSIS. A systematic review of these interventions reports that for studies in which orthoses have been used, 45% to 50% of the participants reported pain relief of more than 50% up to 1 year postintervention. For various surgical approaches, pain relief of more than 50% occurred in 65% to 100% of patients up to 3 years postsurgery.[196]

Idiopathic Facial Paralysis/Bell Palsy/ Facial Nerve Compression Damage

Incidence

Bell palsy, a common clinical condition in which the facial nerve (cranial nerve [CN] VII) is unilaterally affected and is characterized by facial hemiparesis. Bell palsy affects 20 to 30 of 100,000 people each year. Although any age group can be affected, it is most common in persons between the ages of 15 and 45 years.[86]

Etiology and Pathogenesis

A direct link between Bell palsy and viral infection has been difficult to establish. Serologic studies have found a lack of signs of an acute infection immediately preceding the onset of the Bell palsy. No seasonal predilection or epidemic clustering has been documented; it is much more likely that Bell palsy is caused by reactivation of a latent virus rather than direct, communicable viral infection; most likely a latent herpes virus (herpes simplex type 1/herpes zoster). Although it is likely that the underlying disease in Bell palsy is viral polyneuropathy, an unresolved question is why such a profound effect on the facial nerve occurs, in contrast with the relatively minor and transient changes in the other cranial nerves. The major anatomic difference between the facial and other cranial nerves is in its long bony canal and because the facial nerve lies in the auditory canal, any agent that causes inflammation and swelling creates a compression that could potentially cause demyelination, ischemia and axonal degeneration.[67] In addition, centrally located structures, such as a schwannoma (acoustic neuroma) which is a slow growing tumor of the sheath of the nerve, can produce unilateral paralysis in the face by impinging on the facial nerve as it emerges from the brainstem. The weakness can appear similar; however there is slowly progressive paralysis and presence of auditory impairments. (See Chapter 26 for more information on schwannomas.)

Risk Factors

Acute facial paralysis can occur as part of many viral illnesses, including mumps, rubella, herpes simplex, and Epstein-Barr virus. People with diabetes mellitus and pregnant women[30] have an increased incidence of Bell palsy.

Clinical Manifestations

A unilateral facial paralysis develops rapidly, often overnight. Paralysis of the muscles of facial expression on one side creates an asymmetrical facial appearance (Fig. 39-15). The corner of the mouth droops, the nasolabial fold is flattened, and the palpebral fissure is widened because the eyelid does not close. In addition to the motor fibers providing innervation for facial musculature, the facial nerve also innervates the stapedius muscle of the middle ear and the sensory and autonomic fibers, which innervate for taste and lacrimation and salivation, respectively. Therefore involvement of these fibers may produce additional signs and symptoms to those of facial paralysis. If the lesion is proximal to where the fibers of the chorda tympani enter the facial nerve, the client will experience loss of taste on the affected side. In a similar fashion, if the autonomic fibers are involved, the client will experience dry eye (lack of tearing) and will produce less but thicker saliva. Some clients report that sounds are louder than normal (hyperacusis) because the stapes bone of the middle ear is less able to accommodate sound when the stapedius muscle's innervation is lost.

MEDICAL MANAGEMENT

DIAGNOSIS. Bell palsy is diagnosed in part by observation and in part by the physical examination. The individual is asked to wrinkle the forehead, close the eyes tightly, smile, and whistle while observed for facial asymmetry. In addition to the clinical presentation and history, electrodiagnostic tests can be used to demonstrate whether the lesion is one of demyelination or axonal degeneration. However, EMG as a diagnostic tool is only helpful after the nerve has degenerated; therefore testing is most

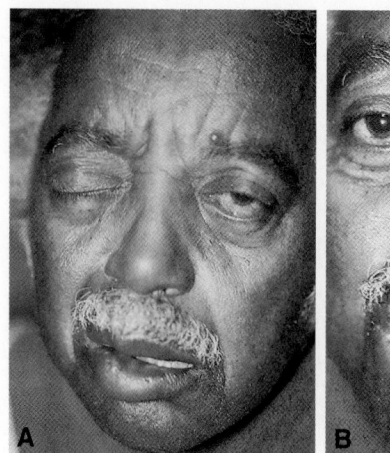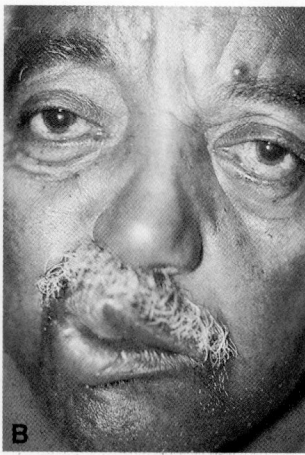

Figure 39-15

A patient with a lesion of the facial nerve. **A,** The patient has difficulty in closing his left eye, and the left corner of his mouth droops. **B,** The latter defect is especially evident when the patient attempts to purse his lips. (From Haines DE: *Fundamental neuroscience for basic and clinical applications*, ed 3, Philadelphia, 2006, Churchill Livingstone.)

accurate after 1 week. Tests of facial nerve excitability will also indicate whether the paralysis is complete.

LMN involvement of the facial nerve can be differentiated from an UMN involvement of this nerve because with UMN involvement, the client can close the eye and wrinkle the forehead but cannot smile voluntarily. With LMN involvement, the client is unable to close the eye, wrinkle the forehead, or smile voluntarily.

TREATMENT. The Quality Standards Subcommittee of the American Academy of Neurology recommends that early treatment with oral corticosteroids is probably effective in improving facial function outcomes in Bell palsy, and that the addition of acyclovir to prednisone is possibly effective; insufficient evidence exists to recommend facial nerve decompression.[94]

General medical care includes proper eye care. Reduced blinking and inability to completely close the eye increases the risk of corneal abrasion and ulceration. Artificial tears and ophthalmic ointments can prevent these complications. Patients should be instructed to use proper eye protection to prevent injuries. Facial muscle massage and facial nerve stimulation have no evidence to support their use.[134] Corticosteroids effectively reduce the risk of an unfavorable outcome. Antiviral agents, when administered concurrently with corticosteroids, may result in additional benefit.[192] However, patients offered antivirals should be counseled that a benefit from antivirals has not been established, and, if there is a benefit, it is likely that it is modest at best.[78]

PROGNOSIS. The overall prognosis of Bell palsy is favorable. In one study of untreated patients, 85% showed signs of recovery within 3 weeks. Ultimately, 71% experienced complete recovery and an additional 13% were thought to have only slight residual weakness. The degree of weakness at onset is an important prognostic indicator: 94% of patients with incomplete paralysis experienced complete recovery. At 3 to 4 months, the absence of any improvement, no matter how small, should raise concern regarding the diagnosis and lead to a search for alternative etiologies.

Motor nerve conduction studies, or electroneurography, can be used to help predict prognosis in selected patients. Patients with incomplete lesions that have an excellent prognosis do not require further evaluation. Motor nerve conduction studies involve stimulating the facial nerve electrically and recording muscle responses with surface electrodes over appropriate muscles. The amplitude of the evoked muscle response on the affected side at 10 days can be compared to the unaffected side, giving an estimate of the degree of axonal loss. A 90% drop in amplitude predicts less than complete recovery, and loss greater than 98% predicts significant residual weakness and synkinesis.

During recovery from severe nerve injury, axonal regrowth may be misdirected, resulting in synkinesis. Voluntary activation of one muscle group can cause activation of other muscles, this is known as synkinesis. Attempts at blinking can result in twitching of the mouth, or smiling can cause involuntary blinking. Misdirection of autonomic fibers can result in the syndrome of "crocodile tears," involuntary lacrimation while eating.

Recurrent attacks of facial paralysis on the ipsilateral or contralateral side occur in up to 15% of patients even after many years. Additional recurrences are quite rare, being reported at a rate between 1% and 3%.

SPECIAL IMPLICATIONS FOR THE THERAPIST   **39-4**

Bell Palsy/Facial Nerve Palsy

Because experiments using animals have indicated that electrical stimulation suppresses neuronal sprouting, electrical stimulation is no longer routinely used. Motor control of facial musculature and recovery of function using neuromuscular reeducation can be enhanced by use of surface EMG feedback. Changes in the brain map associated with individual muscles result from prolonged inactivity of the facial muscles when the course of flaccidity is prolonged. Synkinesis, or the firing of more muscle groups than necessary for the movement, occurs over time, as a result of both cortical reorganization and sprouting of recovering nerve ending to adjacent muscles. Improvement in cortical reorganization through guided facial movement with surface EMG feedback contributes to isolation and control of specific muscle groups and reduction of synkinesis.

Initially, there is profound weakness of the face with decreased firing at rest. As time passes, and neurologic recovery progresses, the resting tone tends to increase along with the synkinesis. Often, the focus of the intervention is on reducing tone at rest to improve ability to normalize facial expression and improve function during eating.[115] Bell reflex, the rolling up of the eye ball during closing of the eye, is the result of an unconscious attempt to occlude vision if the upper lid does not close far enough to meet the lower lid. The rolling of the eye is not controlled by CN VII so the movement can be extinguished by conscious downward gaze during eye closure.

HEREDITARY NEUROPATHIES

Hereditary neuropathies were once considered rare, genetically determined disorders; however, recent studies reflect, in some cases, that these represent 43% of undiagnosed neuropathies.[188] Hereditary neuropathies can be divided into two broad categories: those in which neuropathy is the primary disorder and those in which neuropathy is part of a greater multisystem disorder.[17] This section concentrates on the first group, which includes Charcot-Marie-Tooth disease and its related hereditary polyneuropathies.

Charcot-Marie-Tooth Disease

Charcot-Marie-Tooth (CMT) disease, also known as hereditary motor and sensory neuropathy, progressive muscular atrophy, or peroneal muscular atrophy, is the most common inherited disorder affecting motor and sensory nerves. It was originally described by three neurologists, Jean Martin Charcot, Pierre Marie, and Howard Henry Tooth, in the 1880s. Initially, the disorder involves the fibular (peroneal) nerve and affects muscles in the foot and lower leg. It later progresses to the muscles of the forearms and hands, making activities like buttoning or writing difficult. CMT is a genetically heterogeneous group of disorders with the same clinical phenotype, characterized by distal limb muscle wasting and weakness, usually with skeletal deformities, distal sensory loss, and abnormalities of DTRs.[148]

Incidence

Of the neuropathies, CMT is relatively common; it is estimated that 1 in 2500 persons in the United States has some form of CMT. Onset may occur in childhood or adulthood.[133]

Etiology

CMT is a genetically heterogeneous neuropathy that is most commonly inherited as autosomal dominant pattern with a genetic mutation on a chromosome other than X or Y with one normal gene and one CMT gene. Children of the affected individual will have a 50% chance of inheriting CMT. There is an autosomal recessive form of CMT in which the affected person's children have a 25% to 50% chance of inheriting the disease. It can also present as a first time occurrence in a family as a result of a spontaneous mutation.

More than 50 loci defects on chromosomes have been identified through deoxyribonucleic acid (DNA) testing.[17,141,181] These chromosomal defects create either duplication, deletion, or point mutations in the genetic code for proteins that are involved in the process of myelination. CMT1 is the most common autosomal dominant pattern and is subdivided into three forms: CMT1A, -1B, and -1C. CMT1A accounts for 70% of all CMT1 cases and is caused by a DNA duplication on chromosome 17 for peripheral myelin protein 22 (PMP22), creating segmental demyelination of the fibular (peroneal) nerve.[111] A less-common form, CMT2, has had chromosomal abnormalities mapped to chromosomes 1, 8, and X. On chromosome 1, CMT2 is associated with a mutation in human myelin protein zero (P0), which is associated with axonal dysfunction. This

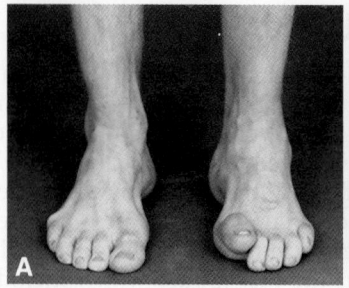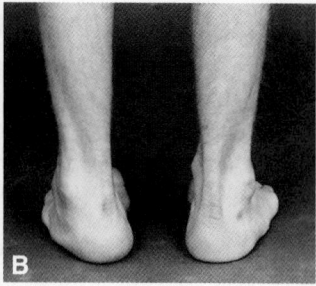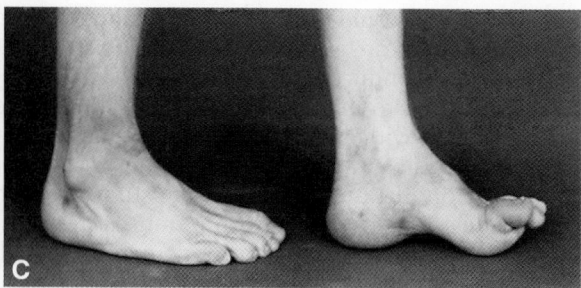

Figure 39-16

Pes cavus foot deformity in Charcot-Marie-Tooth disease. A, Clawing of left great toe. **B,** Left foot varus deformity. **C,** Cavus deformity with hammer toes. (From Canale ST: *Campbell's operative orthopaedics*, ed 10, St Louis, 2003, Mosby.)

second form of CMT is associated with axonal degeneration. CMT2 has an onset that varies between the second and seventh decades and has less involvement in the small muscles of the hands than CMT1.[36]

Pathology

Mutations in proteins (PMP, P0, and connexin) associated with Schwann cell myelination create extensive demyelination along with a hypertrophic onion bulb formation in which demyelinated axons are surrounded by Schwann cells and their processes as remyelination is attempted. The onion bulb formation creates palpable, enlarged peripheral nerves. CMT2 is associated with genetic mutations that disrupt neurofilament assembly and thus affect axonal transport, creating axonal involvement.[17]

Clinical Manifestations

Although the two major types of CMT have differing chromosomal etiologies, it is nearly impossible to tell CMT1 from CMT2 clinically. In all autosomal dominant disorders, there are degrees of genetic dominance. The presence of symptoms are not all-or-none but are graded, with differing degrees of signs and symptoms among family members who have inherited the defective gene. This is termed *variable expressivity*. In CMT1 some members of a family with the genetic mutation may have greater signs of the disorder than others who have only minor involvement.[120] In the X-linked form of CMT, men are affected and have signs of both demyelination and axonal degeneration are evident. CMT generally does not affect a person's intelligence, memory, or life span.

CMT is a slowly progressive disorder and although CMT1 begins in childhood, the actual onset may be difficult to determine. Clinical signs of CMT include distally symmetric muscle weakness, atrophy, and diminished DTRs. Because of the muscles affected, the client will have weakness of the dorsiflexors and evertors (peroneal musculature) and will ambulate with a footdrop (steppage) gait pattern. As CMT progresses, involvement will be seen distally in the upper extremities. Weakness and wasting of the intrinsic muscles of the hand occurs, followed by progressive wasting in the forearms. Because CMT1 demyelinates peripheral nerves, proprioception is lost in the feet and ankles, and cutaneous sensation is diminished in the foot and lower legs. Sensory loss is minimal in CMT2. Sensory symptoms can include tingling and burning in the feet and legs, as well as impaired proprioception.[215]

Feet have pes cavus (high arch) deformities and hammer toes (Fig. 39-16). As muscle atrophy progresses below the knee, the appearance of the client's legs takes on the shape of an inverted champagne bottle because normal muscle bulk is maintained above the knees.

MEDICAL MANAGEMENT

DIAGNOSIS. CMT is diagnosed by history and clinical examination, hereditary picture, electrophysiologic studies, and nerve biopsy. Most recently, because of the sensitivity and specificity of genetic studies, the diagnosis of CMT can be confirmed using gel electrophoresis to detect duplication, deletions, or sequence variations in genes.[17] Although CMT1 produces demyelination, electrophysiologic testing reveals underlying axonal degeneration. Slowed motor nerve conduction does not have a linear correlation with the clinical severity of the disease.[108]

Both motor and sensory NCVs will be slowed in CMT1[118] but are normal or only slightly slowed in CMT2. Abnormalities of electrophysiologic studies in CMT2 include decreased amplitude of the potential, indicating axonal loss. The nerve biopsy is abnormal and will demonstrate either a demyelinating or axonal degenerative process.

TREATMENT. CMT is an inherited disorder, and there is no specific treatment to date to alter its course. Treatment is symptomatic to ensure that function is maintained in a safe manner. Footdrop and hand deformities can be helped by orthotic devices. Because the possibility of skin ulceration exists when discriminative touch and proprioception are affected, skin care precautions should be followed when total contact orthoses are used (see Chapter 10). To prevent contractures clients should be instructed in range-of-motion exercises. Whether strengthening exercises can be used to counteract the effects of CMT has not been addressed; however, the long-term effects would be of little benefit in the presence of ongoing axonal degeneration. In a study examining the effects of weakness in CMT, results have found that individuals with CMT tend to be obese and have poor exercise tolerance. It is unknown whether exercise interventions can improve body composition and function.[27]

Studies using animal models have reported that antiprogesterone therapy combined with ascorbic acid have a positive effect on CMT1A. Although stem cell and gene therapy have been considered, the most promising treatment is pharmacologic therapies targeting the genetic mutation.[141] As specific treatments are currently lacking, and care is largely symptom based, the role of the clinician becomes increasingly important. Clinicians may contribute to accurate diagnosis based upon sensory, motor and observational findings. Individuals with CMT need lifelong support through the disease process, as well as clinicians who can modify care based on the disease progression, and develop outcome measures to monitor the disease, its progression, and the impact of interventions.[159]

PROGNOSIS. CMT is a slowly progressive disorder that is currently considered incurable. However, the CMT Association has launched a research initiative called the Strategy to Accelerate Research (STAR) to look for more effective therapies and possibly a cure for the most common forms of CMT. If unmanaged, contracture formation resulting from weakness will create further gait abnormalities, with clients reporting an increased number of falls. In the upper extremities, clients may develop problems with writing and handling objects. Individuals with CMT should be cautioned that some medications have been reported to cause an exacerbation of CMT. A database of the drugs that should be avoided is maintained by the CMT Association. Among the identified medications are several anticancer drugs, including vincristine, cisplatin, carboplatin, and taxoids.[212]

| SPECIAL IMPLICATIONS FOR THE THERAPIST | 39-5 |

Charcot-Marie-Tooth Disease

The goal in this progressive disorder is to minimize deformity and maximize function. As with other peripheral neuropathies in which muscle imbalances arise, for CMT management, the physical therapist should anticipate that deformities will arise from the imbalance between the tibialis anterior and peroneus longus and the tibialis posterior and peroneus brevis, which leads to a pes cavus and varus deformity, respectively. This weakness may be combined with diminished or lost proprioception and some degree of cutaneous involvement that can lead to an unsteady gait. These problems should be addressed with stretching, range-of-motion exercises, and bracing to improve ambulation. A recent systematic review of randomized control trials raises question about the effectiveness of stretching programs for people with CMT and other neurologic conditions that place a person at risk for deformity and contracture. In fact, this review concluded that stretching programs have little or effect when applied for less than 7 months. Effects of longer-duration stretching programs have not been elucidated.[98] An emphasis on compensation for safety with gait and function is recommended. Along with orthotic assessment and gait training, appropriate skin care should be taught to the client when total contact orthoses are used. When the individual has developed rigid deformities, a triple arthrodesis is the option to salvage remaining function.[143]

METABOLIC NEUROPATHIES

Diabetic Neuropathy

Definition

A consensus conference has agreed that a detailed definition of diabetic neuropathy (DN) is "a descriptive term meaning a demonstrable disorder, either clinically evident or subclinical, that occurs in the setting of diabetes mellitus without other causes for peripheral neuropathy."[7,112] DN is a common complication associated with diabetes mellitus (see Chapter 11) comprised of a heterogeneous group of progressive syndromes with diverse clinical manifestations. Neuropathies may be focal or diffuse and involve the autonomic or somatic PNS.[20,21,204] Typically, the involvement occurs in a distally, symmetric pattern, termed *diabetic polyneuropathy*, although single, focal nerve involvement may be seen.

Incidence

In the United States, diabetes mellitus affects more than 20 million people, and this number is expected to increase by 5% every year. The prevalence of DN is greater (54%) in type 1 diabetes (insulin-dependent diabetes mellitus) than the prevalence of DN in type 2 diabetes (noninsulin-dependent diabetes mellitus), which is 30%. The most reliable estimates from clinical studies report that DN, although present in individuals with diabetes lasting longer than 25 years, is present in 7% of people within 1 year of diagnosis with diabetes.[182]

Etiology

DN is likely caused by the chronic metabolic disturbances that affect nerve cells and Schwann cells in diabetes. For years, hyperglycemia was considered the sole cause of these secondary complications of diabetes. Although consequences of hyperglycemia include elevated levels of sorbitol and fructose, which coincides with deficiencies of sodium-potassium and adenosine triphosphate that alter the function of peripheral nerves, chronic hyperglycemia leads to abnormalities in microcirculation, creating endothelia capillary changes and local ischemia that affect the nerve. Excess sorbitol damages Schwann cells. researchers have suggested that Alterations in insulin levels appear to alter gene regulation of neurotrophic factors, adhesion molecules, and modification of proteins.[182]

Risk Factors

Although hyperglycemia is not directly attributed to damaging nerve fibers causing DN, it is a contributing factor. Conversely, some people develop neuropathies even when glycemic control is good. A clear relationship does exist between duration of diabetes and development of DN. After the onset of the neuropathy, control of hyperglycemia is known to enhance the possibility of regeneration of fibers. Although studies have confirmed a genetic predisposition to diabetes, they have not confirmed such a predisposition to development of DN nor has a familial tendency been reported. Up to 50% of all people with diabetes never develop symptoms of neuropathy.

CLASSIFICATION OF DIABETIC NEUROPATHY

Rapidly Reversible

- Hyperglycemic neuropathy

Generalized Symmetric Polyneuropathies

- Acute sensory
- Chronic sensorimotor
- Autonomic

Focal Neuropathies

- Cranial
- Focal limb

Adapted from Boulton AJ, Vinik AI, Arezzo JC, et al: Diabetic neuropathies. A statement by the American Diabetes Association, *Diabetes Care* 28:956–962, 2005.

Pathogenesis

Many hypotheses exist for the pathogenesis of this disorder. The metabolic effect of hyperglycemia exposes nerves and their associated Schwann cells to glucose. The most prominent change in DN is loss of both myelinated and unmyelinated axons. Nerves are affected distally more than proximally. Subtle changes have been reported at the nodes of Ranvier in nerves of people with DN. This is associated with slowing of the NCV.[203]

A number of studies suggest that vascular changes affect peripheral nerves in diabetes. Evidence demonstrates endoneurial microvascular thickening. In the sural nerve, this has resulted in increased numbers of closed capillaries, which are believed to cause multifocal regions of ischemia and hypoxia in the nerve, resulting in an axonal degeneration.

Another explanation for the development of DN proposes that the concentration of nerve growth factor, which has a structure that is molecularly and physiologically similar to insulin, is reduced. Because nerve growth factor acts as a trophic factor, its reduction also reduces nutrition to the nerve.

Clinical Manifestations

DN is classified in a number of ways: presumed etiology, pathologic features, anatomic location, and a mixture of these. Box 39-4 describes the disturbances that occur in DN.

Rapidly Reversible Neuropathy

Hyperglycemic Neuropathy. Hyperglycemic neuropathy occurs in individuals with poorly controlled diabetes, and in those who have been newly diagnosed, rapidly reversible nerve conduction abnormalities are reported. These abnormalities are accompanied by distally symmetric sensory changes such as burning, paresthesia, and tenderness in the feet and legs. Symptoms disappear when the individual's blood sugar is controlled, although abnormalities in nerve conduction may persist.[21]

Generalized Symmetric Polyneuropathies

Acute Sensory Neuropathy. Hallmarks of acute sensory neuropathy, are the rapid onset of severe burning pain, deep aching pain, a sudden sharp "electric shock–like" sensation, and hypersensitivity of the feet that is often worse at night. Persons with this painful condition may have mild impairments in the physical exam such as normal motor examinations in which the tendon reflexes are normal or reduced at the ankle and may have none or only mild symmetric sensory loss, with allodynia (painful sensation to nonnoxious stimuli). Testing procedures to confirm allodynia include application of a phasic stimulus (rub) to various parts of the body and asking the person whether burning occurs in a nearby region (application of a cotton ball or Semmes-Weinstein monofilament is not applied long enough for the slow summation required for allodynia). Another way of testing involves placing a towel on the body and waiting for a period of time before asking whether the cover creates pain. Nociceptive stimuli are perceived normally in acute sensory neuropathy. Electrophysiologic studies (NCV) may be normal or show minor changes. If the person can achieve and maintain stable blood glucose, recovery can occur within 1 year, even with severe symptoms.[21]

Chronic Sensorimotor Neuropathy. Chronic sensorimotor neuropathy, or diabetic polyneuropathy (DPN), is the most common type of DN and up to 50% of patients may develop this condition. Typically, its onset is insidious, but occasionally signs and symptoms appear acutely. The clinical features of DPN include sensory loss, occasionally with selective fiber-type involvement. Small fiber involvement leads to burning pain, and paresthesias, such as those described for acute sensory neuropathy, are more profound at night in the feet and lower legs (stocking pattern). Large fiber involvement results in painless paresthesia with impaired vibration, proprioception, touch, and pressure, along with loss of ankle DTRs. Clients may report that they feel as if they were walking on cotton or clouds. In DPN, motor weakness is mild but can still cause hammer toes and/or pes cavus, with wasting of small muscles in the feet and hands in more advanced cases. The presence of pronounced motor involvement implies that this is not DPN. DPN may be accompanied by clinical or subclinical autonomic involvement that can include cardiovascular and sympathetic disturbances resulting in sweating, orthostatic hypotension, and resting tachycardia with greater than 100 beats/min at rest.[21]

Autonomic Neuropathy. Sympathetic and parasympathetic involvement may occur in both type 1 and type 2 diabetes; however, in type 2 diabetes, parasympathetic functions are more affected. After 10 to 15 years, 30% of patients have subclinical manifestations of autonomic involvement. Box 39-5 shows the major manifestations associated with autonomic involvement.[158]

Focal Neuropathies

Mononeuropathies. Mononeuropathies in the limbs or cranial nerves may occur in diabetes less often than the generalized, symmetric patterns. The median, ulnar, and peroneal nerves are most commonly affected in limb focal neuropathies. The somatic division of the oculomotor nerve is most commonly involved cranial component.

MEDICAL MANAGEMENT

DIAGNOSIS. The diagnosis is based on the history, clinical examination, electrodiagnostic studies, quantitative sensory evaluation, and autonomic function testing. Diagnosis of DN should not be based on a single symptom,

MANIFESTATIONS OF AUTONOMIC DIABETIC NEUROPATHY

Cardiovascular

- Tachycardia
- Exercise intolerance
- Orthostatic hypotension
- Dizziness

Gastrointestinal

- Esophageal motility dysfunction
- Diarrhea
- Constipation

Genitourinary

- Neurogenic bladder
- Bladder urgency, incontinence
- Erectile dysfunction

Other

- Sweating, heat intolerance
- Dry skin
- Pupillary dysfunction, blurred vision

Adapted from Boulton AJ, Malik RA, Arezzo JC, et al: Diabetic somatic neuropathies, *Diabetes Care* 27:1458–1486, 2004.

sign, or test; a minimum of two abnormalities (signs and symptoms from NCV, sensory, or autonomic tests) has been recommended.[7] Tools required for the sensory examination include a 128-Hz tuning fork to assess vibration and a 1-g monofilament for touch. Autonomic functions can initially be assessed by blood pressure and heart rate response at rest, in standing and with exercise. Because diabetes is a common disorder and because neuropathies may be related to other causes, mere association of neuropathic signs and symptoms in a person with diabetes is not sufficient to diagnose DN. Other causes must be excluded.[83]

Sensory, motor, and F-responses are important to assess nerve function at baseline and intermittently at follow-up visits. The most common electrical change is a reduced amplitude in the sensory nerve action potential, which suggests axonal degeneration. A recent report found that a high percentage of newly diagnosed patients with type 2 diabetes have reduced sensory nerve action potential in upper extremity nerves.[162] Slowing of sensory and/or motor NCV suggests a demyelinating neuropathy, and pronounced slowing suggests that an alternative diagnosis should be explored.[8] Sensory fibers are generally affected first before motor fibers.

TREATMENT. Management is divided into general and specific measures. General measures include control of hyperglycemia[202] and specific measures address the symptomatic management of the disorders (see "Diabetes Mellitus" in Chapter 11). Because there is evidence that further complications can be reduced by maintaining control of the diabetes, this is one specific area addressed by health care professionals. In addition, specific drug therapies are being evaluated. Currently, studies on medications and biochemical factors, such as gangliosides and nerve growth factors, are being conducted and although

some show promise. Tricyclic antidepressants are used alone or in combination with fluphenazine to treat painful neuropathies and gabapentin or carbamazepine is an efficacious approach to the management of pain in focal neuropathies.[202] Angiotensin-converting enzyme inhibitors act on the vascular dysfunction and prevent the development and progression of DN.[124] In a systematic analysis of seven qualifying studies, researchers found vitamin B_{12} (either as B_{12} complex or as methylcobalamin, one of two coenzyme forms of B_{12}) had beneficial effects on pain and paresthesia rather than electrophysiologic changes. Methylcobalamin shows improvement in autonomic symptoms.[185]

If the person has a painful DN, an algorithm has been developed that begins with physical modalities to manage pain. This is combined with simple analgesics. Further management may include a trial of topical or benign drugs.[203] A myriad of treatments (various pharmacologic agents, topical agents, magnets, acupuncture, biofeedback, and exercise) have been suggested to manage painful DN. Of these the anticonvulsant, pregabalin, has been shown to be safe and effective and has the strongest evidence according to a 2011 guideline.[24]

A common complication of DN is the development of neuropathic foot ulcers. When great toe and ankle joint mobility is limited, greater forefoot pressures occur during gait, which may place patients with diabetes (type 1 or 2) at risk for development of metatarsal ulceration.[217] In type 2 diabetes, early detection of DN along with prophylactic foot care regimen have led to fewer foot ulcerations and amputations.[178] Institution of foot care procedures is essential (see "Special Implications for the Therapist 11-16: Diabetes Mellitus" in Chapter 11). With the development of a footdrop gait, orthotic devices should be considered for the person's safety. The type of orthosis and shoe construction prescribed should be carefully considered based on the sensory status and the person's ability to demonstrate appropriate foot care.

PROGNOSIS. DN is a slowly progressive metabolic disorder that affects many body systems. Estimates are that more than 50% of nontraumatic amputations in the United States occur in people with diabetes. The presence of autonomic involvement is associated with an increased mortality risk.

SPECIAL IMPLICATIONS FOR THE THERAPIST   39-6

Diabetic Polyneuropathy

Type 2 diabetes is established as an epidemic in developed countries such as the United States, and it is expected to increase in prevalence through the year 2050. Carrying risks and complications of many body systems, included but not limited to DN, physical therapists should focus treatments not just on the specific impairments targeting the problems of neuropathy, but also the overall health condition of the individual with diabetes. Beyond this, because there is such strong evidence that regular physical activity can prevent and delay the onset of the disease, it is suggested that the physical therapist may be ideal and uniquely trained to influence prevention programs for this population.[45] As impairments of DN can lead to problems with safety and mobility, therapists should work to maintain and improve function while preventing falls in this population. Furthermore, a 2010 randomized control trial demonstrated that gait and balance of patients with diabetes can be improved using a specific task-based exercise program.[5]

Alcoholic Neuropathy

Peripheral neuropathies, typically with distally symmetrical involvement, appear in persons with chronic alcoholism. This alcohol-related peripheral neuropathy is known to affect sensory, motor and autonomic fibers and can be a debilitating problem in people with chronic alcoholism.

Etiology and Risk Factors

Although the exact pathogenesis of alcoholic neuropathy remains unclear,[205] lesions affecting the peripheral nerves have been attributed to both the direct toxic effects of alcohol on nerve and nutritional deficiencies in thiamine and other B vitamins from poor dietary habits. However, there is more recent evidence that neither age nor nutritional status play a part in development of alcoholic neuropathies. Rather, alcohol-related neuropathies appear to be a result of the total lifetime accumulation of ethanol.[54] Patients exhibiting alcoholic neuropathy were divided into those with and without a coexisting thiamine deficiency. Researchers reported that patients without thiamine deficiency tended to have a more slowly progressive disorder in which sensory symptoms were dominant, primarily pain or a burning sensation. Along with these symptoms, the nerve biopsy demonstrated greater small fiber axonal loss. Those with alcoholic neuropathy with thiamine deficiency had large fiber involvement with segmental demyelination, and an acutely progressive motor dominant pattern along with loss of superficial and deep sensation was noted. These findings further support the view that alcohol directly and adversely affects nerve fibers.[107]

Pathogenesis

The exact pathogenesis of alcoholic neuropathy remains unclear. Segmental demyelination and axonal degeneration have been described in persons with alcoholic polyneuropathy; these differences may relate to the presence of vitamin deficiencies, as noted above. Changes occur distally at first and become more marked and proximal.[75]

Clinical Manifestations

Mild forms of alcoholic neuropathy exhibit minor loss of muscle bulk, diminished ankle reflexes, impaired sensation in the feet, and aching in the calves. Distal sensory changes include pain, paresthesia and numbness in a symmetric stocking-and-glove pattern. In addition, vibratory perception is impaired. It begins insidiously and progresses slowly; occasionally the onset may occur acutely. In the most advanced cases, symptoms involve all four extremities. Weakness and atrophy of distal musculature occurs, with lower-extremity involvement greater than upper extremity. Bilateral footdrop is observed during gait, and a wristdrop contributes to diminished grip strength because of the person's inability to extend the wrist. Both of these features are often combined with varying amounts of peripheral weakness in other muscles.

MEDICAL MANAGEMENT

DIAGNOSIS AND TREATMENT. The diagnosis is made by history, clinical examination, and electrodiagnostic testing showing loss of action potential amplitude (sensory and motor). Although diet is no longer implicated as a contributing factor in the development of alcoholic neuropathies, diet to improve nutritional status, along with vitamin supplements and abstinence from alcohol, is the treatment of choice.

It has been suggested that aerobic exercise may benefit individuals during alcohol recover by decreasing stress and improving coping mechanisms.[25] Given that alcohol-related peripheral neuropathies have a toxic cause; treatments that either block or reverse the target of the substances attack are being investigated.[129]

All other treatment is symptomatic. Orthotic devices, such as ankle–foot orthoses and cock-up splints, are used to manage weakness and improve function. Medications for sensory changes include carbamazepine, salicylates, and amitriptyline. Additional suggested therapeutic options include: benfotiamine, α-lipoic acid, acetyl-L-carnitine, vitamin E, methylcobalamin, myoinositol, N-acetylcysteine, tricyclic antidepressants, gabapentin, and topical capsaicin. Further investigations are needed to make evidence-based recommendations for the treatment and prevention of alcoholic neuropathy.[29]

PROGNOSIS. If the client totally abstains from alcohol, mild improvement can be expected, but recovery is slow (months to years) and incomplete when axonal degeneration has occurred.[146] Therefore, to anticipate the outcome, review the client's electrophysiologic studies to determine whether demyelination or degeneration is present.

Compression neuropathies, such as Saturday night palsy or peroneal nerve compression, may result from a bout of chronic alcohol intoxication where prolonged pressure compromises nerve function. Excessive alcohol intake may also produce rhabdomyolysis which produces proximal muscle weakness, swelling, and pigmented urine. Rhabdomyolysis can occur as product of renal failure after drinking.

Chronic Renal Failure

Chronic renal failure results from a gradual and progressive loss of kidney function. Electrolytes and waste products accumulate and are toxic to body systems.

Clinical Manifestations

Alteration of CNS and PNS function often occurs with chronic renal failure associated with uremia. CNS involvement (uremic encephalopathy) is manifested by recent memory loss, inability to concentrate, perceptual errors, and decreased alertness. Uremic toxins induce demyelination and atrophy, thus likewise are detrimental to both sensory and motor nerves of the PNS. The lower extremities are much more commonly affected than the upper extremities; neurologic changes are typically symmetric and can also be manifested as peripheral neuropathy or restless leg syndrome, which is more pronounced at rest. See Chapter 18 for recommendations about exercise for individuals with renal disease.

Anemia

CNS symptoms can develop in cases of severe pernicious anemia, whereas PNS symptoms of neuropathy are observed in early cases of vitamin B_{12} deficiency. The findings typically consist of a symmetric sensory neuropathy that begins in the feet and lower legs, causing moderate pain or paresthesias, although it may sometimes involve the upper extremities, especially fine motor coordination of the hands. This upper-extremity neuropathy may clinically manifest as problems with deteriorating handwriting. With a loss of proprioception, the person may interpret the neuropathy as difficulty with locomotion. The affected individual may need to hold on to the wall, countertops, or furniture at home as a result of difficulties maintaining balance. There may be an associated positive Romberg sign. Loss of motor function is a late manifestation of vitamin B_{12} deficiency. Although a symmetric neuropathy is the usual pattern, vitamin B_{12} deficiency occasionally presents as a unilateral neuropathy and/or bilateral but asymmetric neuropathy. Rarely, subacute degeneration of the spinal cord caused by vitamin B_{12} deficiency can occur in pernicious anemia, characterized by pyramidal and posterior column deficits. CNS manifestations may include headache, drowsiness, dizziness, fainting, slow thought processes, decreased attention span, apathy, depression, and irritability. See Chapter 14 for recommendations about exercise for individuals with anemia.

INFECTIONS/INFLAMMATIONS

Guillain-Barré Syndrome

Overview and Definition

Guillain-Barré syndrome (GBS) was originally described by and named for the French neurologists who published case reports describing a syndrome of flaccid paralysis, areflexia, and albuminocytologic dissociation. More recently, the syndrome has been viewed as having distinct subtypes with varying distributions worldwide. Since the virtual elimination of poliomyelitis in North America, GBS is the most common cause of rapidly evolving motor paresis and paralysis and sensory deficits. Individuals affected with GBS typically reach maximal weakness within 2 to 3 weeks, but spend weeks to months recovering. The most common form of GBS is also known as acute inflammatory demyelinating polyradiculoneuropathy.

Incidence

Annual incidence varies from 1 to 2 cases per 100,000 people. Although GBS occurs at all ages, peaks in frequency can be seen in young adults and in the fifth through the eighth decades. Occurrence is slightly greater for men than women and for whites more than blacks. Some researchers have noted a seasonal relationship associated with infections.

Etiology and Risk Factors

Evidence supports the view that GBS is an immune-mediated disorder. Bacterial (*Campylobacter jejuni*) and viral (*Haemophilus influenzae*, Epstein-Barr virus, and cytomegalovirus) infections, surgery, and vaccinations have been associated with the development of GBS. Acute infection in one study preceded onset of GBS. In one study, 90% of persons with GBS had illnesses (e.g., respiratory or gastrointestinal) during the preceding 30 days.[149]

Pathogenesis

Lesions occur throughout the PNS from the spinal nerve roots to the distal termination of both motor and sensory fibers. Originally, GBS was classified as a single entity characterized by PNS demyelination. Now, however, it is defined as several heterogeneous forms (Table 39-9). *C. jejuni* is associated more commonly with the axonal form, whereas greater sensory involvement is seen following cytomegalovirus.[90] The axonal pattern of involvement can involve motor fibers only or in the more severely involved form, motor and sensory fiber degeneration. Finally, Miller-Fisher syndrome is characterized by an acute onset of extraocular muscle paralysis with sluggish

Table 39-9	Guillain-Barré Syndrome and Its Variants	
Abbreviation	**Name**	**Clinical Characteristics**
AIDP	Acute inflammatory demyelinating polyneuropathy	Primary demyelination: progressive paralysis, areflexia
AMAN	Acute motor axonal neuropathy	Axonal variant, more severe: frequent respiratory involvement/ventilator dependence and significant residual impairments
ASAN	Acute sensory ascending neuropathy	Sensory changes more prominent than weakness
AMSAN	Acute motor and sensory axonal neuropathy	
	Acute autonomic neuropathy	Manifested by postural hypotension, impaired sweating, lacrimation, bowel and bladder function
	Fisher/Miller-Fisher syndrome	Ophthalmoplegia, ataxia, areflexia with significant weakness
CIDP	Chronic inflammatory demyelinating polyneuropathy	Slower onset, relapses and remissions or progressive course over year

pupillary light reflexes, a peripheral sensory ataxia, and loss of DTRs with relative sparing of strength in the extremities and trunk. Facial weakness and sensory loss in the limbs may also occur.

Molecular mimicry, an autoimmune theory, is the primary theory for the cause of GBS because evidence exists for antibody-mediated demyelination. Myelin of the Schwann cell is the primary target of attack. Researchers theorize that circulating antibodies to gangliosides penetrate and bind to an antigen on the surface of the myelin and activate either complement or an antibody-dependent macrophage.[91] The earliest pathologic changes in the PNS take the form of a generalized inflammatory response. Lymphocytes (T cells) and macrophages are the inflammatory cells present. Demyelination, initiated at the node of Ranvier, occurs because macrophages, responding to inflammatory signals, strip myelin from the nerves. After the initial demyelination, the body initiates a repair process. Schwann cells divide and remyelinate nerves, resulting in shorter internodal distances than were present initially.

In addition to the demyelination, there is another process that has longer-lasting effects. Although there is an axonal subtype, axonal degeneration to some degree occurs in most cases of demyelinating GBS. In the latter, many believe that the axons are damaged during the inflammatory process, according to what has been called a "bystander effect." Products that are liberated by the macrophages as they strip myelin (e.g., free oxygen radicals and proteases) also damage axons.

Axonal patterns of involvement display a diminished or absent inflammatory response seen in demyelination. Researchers have reported the presence of macrophages that invade periaxonal spaces, causing the axon to degenerate within the ventral roots. Recovery for this wallerian-like degeneration would require an extremely long period. For those individuals with acute motor axonal neuropathy, another mechanism may promote rapid recovery for what appears to be axonal involvement. Binding of antibodies to the nodes of Ranvier may cause blocking of nerve conduction by altering sodium channel conductance has been established in rabbits.

Although the autoimmune theory is the main one advanced for this disorder, it may not be the only reason for the development of GBS. Cases of GBS have been reported in immunosuppressed individuals after renal transplant.

Clinical Manifestations

Various subtypes of GBS exist; however, the classic picture is an acute form in which the time from onset to peak impairment is 4 weeks or less. A recurrent form of GBS is reported in up to 10% of cases. Acute relapses may occur in GBS and this characteristic may make it difficult to differentiate the acute from the chronic form, called *chronic inflammatory demyelinating polyradiculoneuropathy*. Most cases of chronic inflammatory demyelinating polyradiculoneuropathy progress over a period of months instead of weeks.

GBS is characterized by a rapidly ascending symmetric motor weakness and distal sensory impairments. The first neurologic symptom is often paresthesia in the toes. This is followed within hours or days by weakness distally in the legs. Weakness spreads to involve arms, trunk, and facial muscles. Flaccid paralysis is accompanied by absence of DTRs. Occasionally, sensory and motor symptoms begin in the hands and arms instead of the feet and legs. Palatal and facial muscles become involved in about half of all cases; even the muscles of mastication may be affected, but nerves to extraocular muscles typically are not involved. Up to 30% of all cases require mechanical ventilation.

Because the preganglionic fibers of the ANS are myelinated, they, too, may be subject to demyelination. If this occurs, tachycardia, abnormalities in cardiac rhythm, blood pressure changes, and vasomotor symptoms occur.

In 50% of the cases, progression of symptoms generally ceases within 2 weeks and in 90% of the cases, progression ends by 4 weeks. After the progression stops, a static phase begins, lasting 2 to 4 weeks before recovery occurs in a proximal to distal progression. This recovery may take months or even years.

MEDICAL MANAGEMENT

DIAGNOSIS. Careful clinical and neurophysiologic examinations and laboratory tests are needed to diagnosis GBS. Criteria have been developed by the National Institute of Neurologic and Communicative Disorders and Stroke (Box 39-6); however, these criteria omit the variants that have been identified.[26]

Box 39-6

CRITERIA FOR DIAGNOSIS OF GUILLAIN-BARRÉ SYNDROME

Symptoms Required for Diagnosis
- Progressive weakness in more than one extremity
- Loss of deep tendon reflexes

Symptoms Supportive of Diagnosis (in Order of Importance)
- Weakness developing rapidly that ceases to progress by 4 wk
- Symmetric weakness
- Mild sensory symptoms and signs
- Facial weakness common and symmetric; oral-bulbar
- musculature may also be involved
- Recovery usually begins 2 to 4 wk after GBS ceases to progress
- Tachycardia, cardiac arrhythmias, and labile blood pressure may occur
- Absence of fever

CSF Features
- CSF protein levels increased after 1 wk; continue to increase on serial examinations
- CSF contains 10 or fewer mononuclear leukocytes/mm^3

Electrodiagnostic Features
- Nerve conduction velocity slowed

CSF, Cerebrospinal fluid; GBS, Guillain-Barré syndrome.
Adapted from Hund EF, Borel CO, Cornblath DR, et al: Intensive management and treatment of severe Guillain-Barré syndrome, *Crit Care Med* 21:435, 1993.

To aid in diagnosis a lumbar puncture can be performed to withdraw cerebrospinal fluid. Albumin (a protein) is elevated in the cerebrospinal fluid with 10 or fewer mononuclear leukocytes present. Electrophysiologic tests will reveal slowed NCVs the entire length of the nerve when demyelination is present, as well as fibrillation potentials when axonal degeneration occurs. When both axonal involvement and demyelination occur, the amplitude of the evoked (NCV) potential will be reduced and the velocity is slowed, respectively.

These abnormalities may not be apparent during the first few weeks of the illness. In addition, to determine the extent of demyelination of the more proximal nerve roots, an F-wave electrophysiologic test may be performed; it is often prolonged or absent. As recovery occurs, slowed NCVs persist, even though the person has made a full clinical recovery. Although electrophysiologic studies are used for diagnosis, the distal compound motor action potential is a predictor of prognosis. If the compound motor action potential amplitude is less than 20% of normal limits at 3 to 5 weeks, it predicts a prolonged or poor outcome.[154]

Hysteria is the most common misdiagnosis. Because of the speed of onset, a stroke involving the brainstem will also be considered. Less-common causes of acute neuropathies must also be considered, including tick paralysis, and metabolic disorders such as porphyria. Care should be taken to rule out other potential causes of weakness including toxic exposures.

TREATMENT. Because GBS is believed to be an autoimmune disease, treatment has been aimed at controlling the response. In two major trials, plasmapheresis, a technique (also called plasma exchange) that removes plasma from circulation and filters it to remove or dilute circulating antibodies, significantly improves the impairments in GBS. Typically, the client will have four to six exchanges of 500 mL per treatment over the period of a week. Time on a respirator and time to independent ambulation (53 days) were both shorter than in the control group (85 days). Plasmapheresis is instituted when respiratory function drops precipitously (to 1.0-1.5 L), and the person is placed on a respirator.[22]

High-dose intravenous (IV) administration of immunoglobulin (Ig; a protein the immune system normally uses to attack foreign organisms) has been found safe and effective in the treatment of GBS.[200] The therapeutic dose is 0.4 g/kg/day for 5 days.[92] Practice parameter recommendations made after a review of plasma exchange and IVIg studies are that plasma exchange should be administered in nonambulatory adults seeking treatment within 4 weeks of GBS onset or ambulatory adults within 2 weeks of onset. IVIg was recommended in nonambulatory adults within 2 weeks of onset. Outcomes for either approach were equivalent. For children with severe GBS, either treatment approach is an option.[92]

PROGNOSIS. The primary methods of managing GBS have helped to improve mortality rates, which can exceed 5%. Factors that predict a poor outcome include onset at an older age, a protracted time before recovery begins, and the need for artificial respiration. An important objective evaluation finding that predicts a poor outcome is significantly reduced evoked motor potential amplitude, which correlates with the presence of axonal degeneration. A recent analysis of prognostic predictors in GBS concluded a younger age, absence of preceding diarrhea, lower levels of disability and admission, longer interval between symptoms and admission, and absence of ventilator support need all being favorable factors.[157] Although most persons recover, up to 20% can have remaining neurologic deficits. After 1 year, 67% of clients have complete recovery, but 20% remain with significant disability.[61] Even after 2 years, 8% have not recovered. Complications that can persist, even when function is recovered, include neuropathic pain, autonomic changes and distal weakness in the extremities.

SPECIAL IMPLICATIONS FOR THE THERAPIST **39-7**

Guillain-Barré Syndrome

Physical therapy is initiated at an early stage in this condition to maintain joint range of motion within the client's pain tolerance and to monitor muscle strength until active exercises can be initiated. During the ascending phase, when the person is losing function and becoming weaker, the person can become easily fatigued and overwhelmed. Focus is toward prevention of complications associated with immobilization. Physical status and gains should be monitored with outcome measures such as the functional independence measure.

Meticulous skin care is required by all staff members to prevent skin breakdown and contractures. A strict turning schedule should be established and followed by all health care providers. After each position change, skin should be inspected (especially the sacrum, heels, ankles, shoulders, and greater trochanter).

Deep muscular discomfort or pain in the proximal muscles may be reported by clients. Paresis or paralysis requires positioning and appropriate splinting, which can help alleviate muscle and joint pain. Bed cages may reduce dysesthesias that are present in the feet. Palliative modalities, such as hot packs and gentle massage, may also bring relief of musculoskeletal pain.

Care in the intensive care unit (ICU) requires observation of arterial blood gas measurements. Because the disease results in primary hypoventilation with hypoxemia and hypercapnia, watch for PO_2 below 70 mm Hg, which signals respiratory failure. Report any signs of rising PCO_2 (e.g., confusion, tachypnea). Pulse oximetry may be used to monitor peripheral oxygen saturation. Auscultate breath sounds, turn and position the person, and encourage coughing and deep breathing to maintain clear airways and prevent atelectasis. See also "Special Implications for the Therapist 15-18: Atelectasis" in Chapter 15. The therapist must also follow universal precautions to help prevent any respiratory infection for the client. Respiratory support is needed at the first sign of dyspnea (in adults, vital capacity less than 800 mL; in children, less than 12 mL/kg of body weight) or decreasing PO_2.

Ventilation is instituted when pulmonary function is compromised by loss of respiratory skeletal muscle control. Coughing and clearing of tracheal secretions becomes difficult. In addition, weakness of laryngeal and pharyngeal muscles makes swallowing difficult and increases the risk of aspiration. Early tracheostomy is indicated in people with clinical and EMG evidence of axonal involvement together with respiratory failure.

Clinical indications for weaning from the ventilator include improved forced vital capacity and improved inspiratory force concomitant with improved muscle stretch. Finally, the chest should be clear of atelectasis. Communication using a communication board or other method is needed during ventilatory support.

Exercise and Guillain-Barré Syndrome

When the person's condition stabilizes, aqua therapy can be used to initiate movement in a controlled environment. A major precaution during the early treatment phase is to provide gentle stretching and active or active-assistive exercise at a level consistent with the person's muscle strength. Overstretching and overuse of painful muscles may result in a prolonged recovery period or a lack of recovery. During the descending phase, when the paralysis slowly recedes and physical function returns, neuromuscular facilitation techniques may be integrated into the active and resistive exercises. Evidence now suggests that higher intensity rehabilitation for people with GBS produces greater functional improvements and reduces disability than does lower-intensity rehabilitation.[160]

Longer length of stay is correlated with presence of muscle belly tenderness, extreme lower-limb weakness, and low functional independence measure scores at admission. Although the presence of axonal involvement was not significantly related to length of stay, it does affect severity of involvement and the need for ventilator and orthosis, which tended to require longer stays.[69] The length of time to maximum impairment (respiratory compromise and motor involvement) has not been found to correlate with outcome. Generally, the shorter the time it takes for recovery to begin after maximum impairment has been reached, the less likely it is that long-term disability will occur.[140] When the person is discharged from therapy, recovery may not be complete. Impaired function may require the continued use of assistive devices and possibly even mobility equipment such as a wheelchair or scooter. The home may require modifications, which should be evaluated and planned for before discharge.

Postpolio Syndrome/Postpolio Muscular Atrophy

Overview

Poliomyelitis (polio) virus infection was virtually eradicated in the United States with the advent of the Salk vaccine in the 1950s and the Sabin vaccine in the 1960s. However, it remains a global health concern. It is a highly infectious and potentially deadly disease that is transmitted through person-to-person contact. Much of what is known about its course is based upon the epidemics in the United States. Clinically, the disease is characterized as one of three patterns: (1) an asymptomatic or (2) nonparalytic infection that produced gastrointestinal, flu-like symptoms and muscular pain or (3) a paralytic infection that also began with flu-like symptoms. The paralytic form generally developed within a week after the onset of the symptoms and is caused by the virus invading and anterior horn cell bodies. The extent of the asymmetric paresis and paralysis that ensued depended on the degree of anterior horn cell involvement. When cell bodies were killed, motor axons underwent wallerian degeneration and muscles rapidly atrophied. Of those persons developing acute paralysis, equal numbers (30%) recovered, had mild residual paralysis, or were left with moderate to severe paralysis. Ten percent died from respiratory involvement. Recovery was attributed to the recovery of some anterior horn cells, as well as collateral sprouting from intact peripheral nerves and to hypertrophy of spared muscle fibers.[44]

Polio is a unique neuropathy that creates only focal and asymmetric motor impairments, rather than the typical distal, symmetric motor and sensory losses associated with other neuropathies. For decades it was considered a static disease; after the initial episode there was no further progression of the disease. The last major epidemics of polio in the United States occurred in the early 1950s; thus most of the people who had paralytic polio are at least 50 years old today. Most people had significant recovery of function and went on to live very productive lives.

Definition

Postpolio syndrome (PPS), or postpolio muscular atrophy, refers to new neuromuscular symptoms that occur decades (average postpolio interval is 25 years) after recovery from the acute paralytic episode.[150] It can be difficult to diagnose as symptoms may be nonspecific.[114] PPS is generally characterized by weakness, declines in functional mobility and reports of fatigue.

Incidence and Risk Factors

It is estimated that there are 1.63 million polio survivors in the United States and that one-fourth to one-half of them will develop PPS.[82] A previous diagnosis of polio is essential for this diagnosis. As well, the degree of initial motor involvement as measured by weakness in the acute stage is a factor in the development of PPS. These combine with long-term overuse of muscle that places increased demands on joints, ligaments, and muscle.

Etiology

PPS appears to be related to the initial disorder of the motor neuron cell body affected by the poliovirus. Much of the recovery of muscle strength that occurred after the axonal degeneration can be attributed to reinnervation of denervated muscle fibers by collateral spouts from other nearby surviving axons. That is, surviving axons increased the size of their innervation ratio. For example, instead of one axon innervating 3000 muscle fibers in the quadriceps, one axon innervated 5000 fibers. Studies confirm that denervation progresses in persons with prior poliomyelitis in both clinically affected and unaffected muscles, and indicate that this progression is more rapid than that occurring in normal aging. Overall, there was a 13.4% reduction in motor-unit number and a 18.4% diminution in M-wave amplitude ($p < 0.001$). The rate of motor-unit loss was twice that occurring in healthy subjects older than age 60 years.[128]

Pathogenesis

Muscle biopsy and EMG both indicate ongoing muscle denervation. PPS seems to be an evolution of the original motor neuron dysfunction that began after the poliovirus affected the alpha motor neuron. PPS is manifested when the compensated reinnervation that occurred cannot maintain that muscle fiber innervation. The nervous system is pruning back axonal sprouts in this enlarged motor unit that it no longer has the metabolic ability to support; thus new denervation results. Symptoms are related to an attrition of oversprouting motor neurons that can no longer support these axonal spouts.[34]

Clinical Manifestations

Symptoms vary, but in general, muscle strength declines in all people, with periods of stability for 3 to 10 years in muscles that had previously been affected by polio and had fully or partially recovered. Administration of an index of postpolio sequelae has shown that pain, atrophy, and bulbar (respiratory and swallowing) problems are the three most prominent sequelae from poliomyelitis.[97] Affected persons have also reported myalgias, joint pain, increased muscle atrophy, and new weakness, as well as excessive fatigue with minimal activity, vasomotor abnormalities, and diminishing endurance. These all combine to contribute to a loss of function. Researchers report that the rate of strength deterioration is faster than would occur in normal aging. Deterioration in the lower extremity predisposes individuals to overuse of upper extremity musculature to compensate.[104]

Typically, symptoms are related to the individual's activities of daily living: crutch walking, wheelchair propulsion (Fig. 39-17). Pain is commonly located in the low back and joints of the upper extremity in women; it is worse at night and increases with physical activity and changes in climate.

MEDICAL MANAGEMENT

DIAGNOSIS. PPS is a clinical diagnosis requiring the exclusion of other medical, neurologic, orthopedic, or psychiatric disorders that could explain the new symptoms. Routine EMG can be used to confirm any new denervation, as can muscle biopsies. Single-fiber EMG and spinal fluid studies are rarely needed to establish a diagnosis.[34]

TREATMENT. Medical management is aimed at symptomatic treatment and modification of lifestyle. Surgery for residual calcaneovalgus deformities at the ankle include triple arthrodesis.[58] Perimalleolar tendon transfers have been performed to compensate for triceps surae insufficiency.[46] Small controlled studies investigating specific

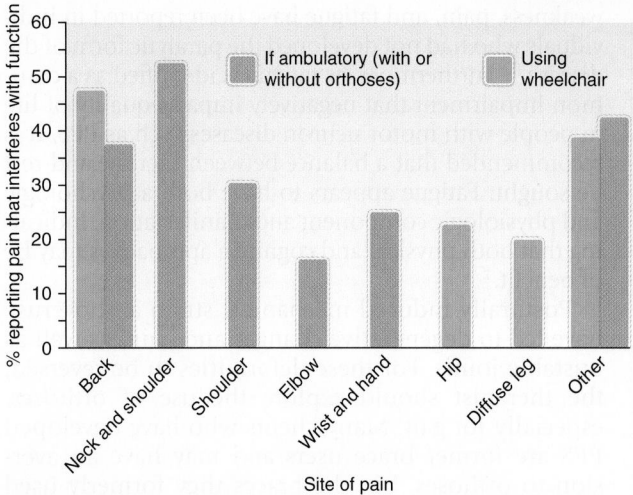

Figure 39-17

Location of pain reported in ambulatory and wheelchair-bound persons diagnosed with postpolio syndrome. (Data from Department of Physical Therapy, Institute for Rehabilitation and Research, Houston: *An instructional course on physical therapy management of post-poliomyelitis: new challenges.* Presented at the 65th American Physical Therapy Association Annual Conference, Chicago, June 1986.)

treatments with therapeutic agents such as steroids and amantadine report no definitive benefit.[59] It is recommended the care of individuals with PPS be carried out by a multidisciplinary team including specialists in rehabilitation. Treatments aimed at lifestyle intervention and activity modification are also recommended.[126]

PROGNOSIS. PPS is a slowly progressive disorder with stable periods that last 3 to 10 years. A decline in functional status is reported to correlate with a poorer quality of life in individuals affected by PPS.[105]

| SPECIAL IMPLICATIONS FOR THE THERAPIST | 39-8 |

Postpolio Syndrome

Of importance to therapists is the ongoing question of the use of exercise in the management of PPS. Partially denervated muscle does not have the physiologic capacity to respond to a conventional strengthening program. Instead, programs aimed at nonexhaustive exercise and general body conditioning are preferable.[79] The client should never exercise to the point of fatigue, and vital signs are monitored before and after exercise to assess the client's response to even mild activity. Caution the client to stop if pain persists or weakness increases. Because individuals with PPS have decreased peak workloads and decreased oxygen uptake, functional exercises of submaximal intensity are stressed with the goal of maintaining and improving endurance and functional capacity. For those with relatively good strength, a program to improve aerobic fitness is appropriate; for those with weaker leg musculature, a generalized fitness program should be aimed at endurance and improving work capacity.[214] Additionally, clients with PPS may also benefit from lifestyle modifications, including energy conservation techniques (see Box 9-8). Late-onset weakness, pain, and fatigue have been reported in individuals who had not developed the paralytic form of the disease.[82] Furthermore, as fatigue is identified as a common impairment that negatively impacts quality of life in people with motor neuron diseases such as PPS, it is recommended that a balance between exercise and rest be sought. Fatigue appears to have both a psychologic and physiologic component and manifestation, indicating that both physical and cognitive approaches may be of benefit.[1]

Posturally induced mechanical strain and overuse have led to degenerative changes and pain, as well as unstable joints. For these deformities to be reversed, the therapist should explore the use of orthoses, especially for gait. Many clients who have developed PPS are former brace users and may have an aversion to orthoses, but the braces they formerly used were not the cosmetic lightweight braces that can be constructed today. Some clients may also be resistive to the idea of using an assistive device for ambulation. Gait patterns vary among individuals with PPS as the weakness associated with the disease is variable. Individuals with PPS who report engaging in physical activity twice weekly demonstrate better gait characteristics than those who are less active. Likewise, those who use an assistive device demonstrate increased cadence.[153] The physical therapist can consider these findings in developing an overall plan of care for function and health.

Trigeminal Neuralgia/Tic Douloureux

Trigeminal neuralgia (TN), or tic douloureux, is a disorder of the trigeminal (fifth cranial) nerve in which there are intense paroxysms of lancinating pain within the nerve's distribution.

Incidence

TN is not a common disorder (5 cases per 100,000 population). It typically occurs in women between the ages of 50 and 70 years. However, TN can occur at any age, and does affect both genders.

Etiology

TN arises from many causes: herpes zoster, multiple sclerosis, vascular lesions, or tumors that can affect the nerve to produce the painful sensations. Many times it will be referred to as idiopathic because the cause remains undetermined. Physical triggers can elicit paroxysms of pain.

Pathogenesis

Researchers hypothesize that the pain is caused by ectopic activity generated at the site of involvement. Demyelinated fibers become hyperexcitable. Light mechanical stimulation recruits nearby pain fibers causing them to discharge and create the sensation of intense pain.

Clinical Manifestations

The pain associated with TN has a sudden onset and has been described as sharp, knife-like, lancinating, and "like a lightning bolt inside my head that lasts for seconds to minutes." The sensation is typically restricted to the maxillary (V2) division of the nerve, but it may involve the maxillary and mandibular divisions together. Less likely is involvement of the ophthalmic (V1) division.

The painful sensation often occurs in clusters. Any mechanical stimulation, chewing, smiling, or even a breeze can trigger an attack. Clients avoid stimulating the trigger zone. Remissions occur between attacks, but these remission periods shorten and attacks become more frequent over the course of the disorder. In approximately 10% of the cases, the pain occurs bilaterally.

MEDICAL MANAGEMENT

DIAGNOSIS. Subjective reports of pain in the typical pattern are the basis for the diagnosis. No impairment or loss of sensation or motor control is obvious on physical examination. The person can identify the trigger site. Skull radiographs, CT scans, and MRI are used to rule out tumors and vascular causes.

TREATMENT. The preferred treatment of TN is oral carbamazepine (Tegretol, an anticonvulsant). Pain can be controlled with appropriate dosage in approximately 75% of clients with TN. Side effects of this medication include blurred vision, dizziness, drowsiness, as well as hematologic changes (anemia) and altered liver function. In addition, because carbamazepine has teratogenic effects, it should not be used in the first trimester of pregnancy nor should it be used by nursing mothers.[73] Other medications, such as phenytoin (Dilantin), are less effective but should be tried in those who cannot tolerate carbamazepine. Promising new medications to manage TN include pimozide, tizanidine hydroxychloride, and topical capsaicin.[40]

In persons whose pain is refractory to medications, neurosurgical procedures are advised. Radiofrequency rhizotomy is preferred over trigeminal nerve section or alcohol ablation. Microvascular surgery has also been used when small blood vessels have been found to constrict the trigeminal nerve near its root. This procedure provides immediate pain relief; however, it is a major and difficult surgery. Individuals may also wish to consider alternative approaches to pain management. A recent review concluded that acupuncture for TN is equally effective to carbamazepine and with fewer side effects.[116]

PROGNOSIS. The efficacy of evaluating treatments for TN is complicated by the fact that the disorder may remit spontaneously. Remissions that occur soon after onset of TN may last for years. For those who do not remit, TN can be managed medically in most cases. The Trigeminal Neuralgia Association provides information and support for persons with this diagnosis.

Human Immunodeficiency Virus Advanced Disease (Acquired Immunodeficiency Syndrome)

Peripheral neuropathy, disease- or drug-induced myopathy, and musculoskeletal pain syndromes occur most often in advanced stages of human immunodeficiency virus (HIV) disease but can occur at any stage of HIV infection and may be the presenting manifestation. During the early phases of HIV when the immune system has altered responsiveness, GBS can develop. When immunoincompetence is severe, distal symmetric peripheral neuropathies occur; however, other parts of the body may be affected such as the face or trunk. The polyneuropathies are predominantly sensory. Painful dysesthesias characterized by burning, tingling, contact sensitivity and proprioceptive losses begin in the feet and ascend. Involvement of the upper extremities can occur, but this is less common and usually later in the disease progression.[32]

In severe cases, secondary motor deficits also occur. In the individual with HIV and newly acquired neuropathy with a strong major motor component, vasculitis may be the underlying etiology (see "Vasculitis" in Chapter 12). Successful treatment of HIV-related distal symmetrical peripheral neuropathies is difficult. Topical analgesics and anticonvulsants are thought to be the most effective.[172] However, pregabalin failed to prove effectiveness over a placebo in a randomized control trial. Optimizing the environment for the nerves by assuring excellent nutrition is also important in the treatment of individuals with HIV related neuropathy.[207]

Vasculitic Neuropathy

Overview, Incidence, and Risk Factors

Vasculitis can occur as a primary inflammation and necrosis of blood vessel walls (polyarteritis nodosa) or as a secondary process associated with autoimmune responses (rheumatoid vasculitis or systemic lupus erythematosus vasculitis), infections (hepatitis C with vasculitis), toxins, or drug exposure. Vasculitis can involve blood vessels of any size, type, or location and can affect any organ system, including blood vessels that supply the PNS, as well as the CNS. However, because the watershed zones between major vascular supplies exist in the PNS, peripheral nerves are likely to sustain ischemia.[135] Vasculitis may range from acute to chronic. Distribution of lesions may be irregular and segmental rather than continuous. The reported annual incidence is 40 to 54 cases per 1 million persons with variance according to age, geography, and seasonal challenges.[179]

Pathogenesis

Immune (antibody–antigen) complexes to each disorder are deposited in the blood vessels, resulting in varying symptoms, depending on the organs affected. In the case of vasculitic neuropathy, the formation of antibody–antigen complexes activates the complement cascade with generation of C3a and C5a (chemotactic agents that recruit polymorphonuclear leukocytes to the vessel walls). Phagocytosis of the immune complexes takes place, and release of free radicals and proteolytic enzymes disrupt cell membranes and damage blood vessel walls. The complement cascade generates the formation of a complement membrane attack complex that also contributes to endothelial damage (see discussion in Chapter 6 and Fig. 6-15). The resulting damage to endothelial cells results in thickening of the vessel wall, occlusion, and ischemia to the affected nerves with axonal degeneration and the resultant neuropathy. Classification is usually according to the size of the predominant vessels involved (see Chapter 12). In either case, the resulting ischemia may affect peripheral nerves.

Clinical Manifestations

Symptoms of vascular neuropathy reflect the distribution of the peripheral nerve involved. Onset is generally acute, and individuals complain of burning pain in the nerve's distribution. In addition motor weakness can be anticipated. Although a single nerve may be involved (mononeuritis), overlapping asymmetric polyneuropathies are relatively common.[77]

Peripheral neuropathy is a well-known and frequently early manifestation of many vasculitis syndromes. The pattern of neuropathic involvement depends on the extent and temporal progression of the vasculitic process that produces ischemia. A severe, burning dysesthetic pain in the involved area is present in 70% to 80% of all cases. Other symptoms may include paresthesias and sensory deficit; severe proximal muscle weakness and muscular atrophy can occur secondary to the neuropathy. In the early phase, one nerve is affected and causes focal symptoms in one extremity (mononeuritis multiplex) but can involve other nerves as the disorder progresses. The therapist should watch for anyone with neuropathy who exhibits constitutional symptoms such as fever, arthralgia, or skin involvement. This may herald a possible vasculitis syndrome and requires medical referral for accurate diagnosis. Early recognition of vasculitis can help prevent a poor outcome. Untreated or with a poor outcome to intervention, CNS involvement (e.g., encephalopathy, ischemic and hemorrhagic stroke, or cranial nerve palsy) can occur late in the course of vasculitis.

Treatment

When corticosteroids (e.g., prednisone alone or sometimes in combination with other medications) are used (such as in the case of vasculitic neuropathy), the therapist should be aware of the need for osteoporosis prevention and attend to the other potential side effects from the chronic use of these medications (see "Corticosteroids" in Chapter 5). Alternative methods of pain control may be offered in a rehabilitation setting, such as biofeedback, transcutaneous electrical nerve stimulation, and physiologic modulation (e.g., using handheld temperature sensor to control ANS function; see "Fibromyalgia" in Chapter 7).

CANCER INDUCED

Paraneoplastic Neuropathies

A little more than 50 years ago the symptoms of two individuals were reported whose autopsy revealed bronchial carcinoma. Both had developed a sensory neuropathy. Subsequent reports of similar sensory neuropathies associated with other carcinomas have been reported and it is clear that paraneoplastic syndromes can affect any portion of the nervous system (Table 39-10).

Etiology

In most individuals diagnosed with paraneoplastic neuropathy, the development of symptoms occurs subacutely

Table 39-10 Paraneoplastic Antibodies, Associated Carcinoma, and Symptoms That Develop

Antibody	Associated Carcinoma	Paraneoplastic Syndrome	Antibody Reactions with Region Involved	Signs and Symptoms
Anti-Hu	SCLC (oat cell)	Paraneoplastic sensory/sensorimotor neuropathy	Antibody affects neuronal nuclei in PNS: produces peripheral neuropathies: acute, subacute, or chronic	Sensory neuropathy Encephalomyeloneuropathy
	SCLC	Paraneoplastic encephalomyeloneuritis	Multifocal disorder Antibody affects all neuronal nuclei in PNS and CNS: produces both peripheral neuropathies and cerebellar, brainstem, cerebral and spinal signs Autonomic nervous system involvement may occur	Sensory neuropathy plus: Cerebellar ataxia, dysarthria, nystagmus Vertigo Confusion Areflexia
	SCLC lymphomas	Subacute motor neuropathy	Loss of anterior horn cells in spinal cord	Impaired motor function; sensation is spared
Anti-Yo	SCLC	LEMS	Antibodies directed against voltage-gated calcium channels that regulate ACh release in neuromuscular junction	Proximal muscle weakness
Anti-Tr	Ovarian, breast, uterine	Pancerebellar syndrome, dysarthria, and nystagmus	Purkinje cell cytoplasm and deep cerebellar neurons: subacute (weeks to months) cerebellar symptoms (limb and truncal ataxia, dysarthria, nystagmus)	Cerebellar ataxia
Anti-Ri	Hodgkin lymphoma	Slowing developing cerebellar syndrome	Purkinje cell cytoplasm	Cerebellar ataxia
Antiamphiphysin	Breast, SCLC	Opsoclonus–myoclonus	CNS nuclei: opsoclonus (involuntary conjugate multidirectional saccades)	Opsoclonus
Anti-VGC	Breast	Stiff person syndrome		
Anti-Ta	SCLC	LEMS		Proximal weakness
	Testicular	Limbic encephalitis	Limbic and brainstem neuronal nuclei	

ACh, Acetylcholine; *ANS*, autonomic nervous system; *CNS*, central nervous system; *LEMS*, Lambert-Eaton myasthenic syndrome; *PNS*, peripheral nervous system; *SCLC*, small cell lung carcinoma.
*Paraneoplastic syndromes are associated with a variety of tumors and the antibodies that are produced affect PNS, CNS, and ANS. Shaded area has PNS involvement.

or chronically over weeks to months and precedes the discovery of the tumor from months to years. The clinic features and electrophysiologic abnormalities indicate that the cell body is the primary site of involvement. Large-diameter neurons are preferentially affected.

Incidence

Numbers vary depending on how the disorder is defined, but estimates range from 10% to 50% that individuals with cancer will develop a paraneoplastic syndrome at some time during the course of their disease. Using a restrictive definition, paraneoplastic syndromes are rare.

Pathogenesis

The current theory is that an autoimmune response, initially directed against the cancer's antigen, subsequently attacks membrane receptors on or receptors within (antinuclear) neurons. See Chapter 30 for discussion of CNS neoplasms.

Clinical Manifestations

The most common symptoms are numbness and paresthesias, initially asymmetric, but progressing to involvement of all extremities. Burning and aching or lancinating pain is common. Although individuals exhibit symptoms of areflexia, weakness is not common and when it occurs, generally is related to an inability to sustain the contraction secondary to impaired proprioceptive feedback. Many individuals with paraneoplastic neuropathy develop additional symptoms demonstrating a progressive involvement of central neural structures. This includes dysarthria, cerebellar ataxia (limb and truncal), ocular nystagmus, memory loss, and ANS involvement. When these central structures are involved, the diagnosis is termed *paraneoplastic encephalomyeloneuritis*.[35]

MEDICAL MANAGEMENT

DIAGNOSIS. The differential diagnosis of paraneoplastic neuropathy is extensive and includes many disorders identified in this chapter that affect sensory nerve fibers or neurons. Recognition and diagnosis at earlier stages can expedite treatment and provides better outcomes.[106] In addition to electrophysiology findings of severely reduced amplitude or absence of sensory nerve potentials, with normal to slightly slowed sensory NCVs, nerve biopsies show nonspecific axonal degeneration and a reduction in myelinated fibers. Lumbar puncture and serum assays for antibodies may be included in the diagnostic workup. High serum titers for antibodies are suggestive of an occult tumor, but the sensitivity and specificity of these tests yields false positives and negatives. CT and MRI scanning are used to locate the tumor.[48]

TREATMENT. Typical treatments for autoimmune disorders, such as immunosuppression using prednisone, cyclophosphamide, IVIg, or plasmapheresis, generally do not work with antinuclear antibodies because receptors are located within the nucleus of the neuron.

PROGNOSIS. The course is fairly stereotypical. Individuals deteriorate over weeks or months and then stabilize at a level of severe disability; for example, sensory polyneuropathies progress proximally, then ataxias develop and become progressively greater. Neurologic improvement is rare.

SPECIAL IMPLICATIONS FOR THE THERAPIST   39-9

Polyneuropathy in Malignant Diseases

Physical therapists will want to approach the care of individual with paraneoplastic neuropathy holistically. It is important to address the symptoms of the neuropathy, the overall health condition of cancer, and the effects of immunosuppression. Recognizing and preventing problems of the integumentary system, preserving safety with mobility and gait, and prevention of falls are of great importance.

TOXINS

In addition to toxic substances in the environment, some medications prescribed to treat medical conditions can be toxic to the PNS (Table 39-11).[8]

Lead Neuropathy

Definition

Toxic substances, such as lead, affect peripheral myelin and/or axons.

Etiology and Risk Factors

Although lead has been virtually eliminated in urban environments, it may exist in third world countries or in some industries such as ceramics. The leading cause of lead neuropathy is the ingestion of lead from paint by children who live in old homes that were built before 1925. However, lead exposure may also occur after inhaling fumes from car batteries, and after drinking contaminated water or moonshine whiskey.

Table 39-11	Medications Toxic to Peripheral Nerves
Medication	**Use**
Doxorubicin (Adriamycin)	Cancer
Amiodarone	Irregular heartbeat
Chloramphenicol	Antibiotic
Cisplatin	Cancer
Dapsone	Skin diseases
Phenytoin (Dilantin)	Seizures and pain
Disulfiram (Antabuse)	Alcoholism
Ethionamide	Tuberculosis
Metronidazole (Flagyl)	*Trichomonas* infection
Gold	Rheumatoid arthritis
Isoniazid	Tuberculosis
Lithium	Manic depression and headache prevention
Nitrofurantoin (Furadantin)	Urinary tract infection
Nitrous oxide	Anesthetic
Penicillamine	Rheumatoid arthritis
Suramin	Cancer
Paclitaxel (Taxol)	Cancer
Vincristine	Cancer

Adapted from Asbury AK: Disorders of peripheral nerve. In Asbury AK, McKhann GM, McDonald WI, editors: *Disease of the nervous system: clinical neurobiology*, Philadelphia, 1986, WB Saunders, pp. 326–327.

Lead neuropathies also occur in workers in industries that use materials containing lead or who live near lead smelters. The Consumer Product Safety Commission has identified inexpensive plastic miniblinds as a source of lead exposure. As the blind is exposed to sunlight, the plastic disintegrates and sheds dust that is high in lead. Interestingly, a case report describes a woman who presented with symptoms of weakness, cognitive loss, and declines in function, and who was using heated lead as part of an unbewitching ritual. Following treatment and cessation of exposure, she recovered well.[10]

Pathogenesis

Both the CNS and PNS can be affected. In the PNS, lead exposure initially causes segmental demyelination, but with prolonged exposure damage to axon cell bodies causes axonal degeneration.[73]

Clinical Manifestations

Unlike most neuropathies, lead neuropathies primarily affect neurons innervating muscles in the upper extremity. After months of exposure, persons with a lead peripheral neuropathy will develop wrist-drop with consequences in grasping functions.

MEDICAL MANAGEMENT

DIAGNOSIS, TREATMENT, AND PROGNOSIS. Diagnosis is based on the history, clinical examination, and motor NCVs, which will be slowed. If axonal degeneration has occurred, EMG will reveal fibrillation potentials, demonstrating loss of axonal innervation. Other tests to check for concentration of lead in the body are urine evaluation and radiographs to reveal a lead line at the metaphysis in the iliac creases, long bones, and tips of the scapula.

Treatment consists of the removal of the source of the lead toxin along with the introduction of the chelating agent, edetate calcium disodium (EDTA), administered twice daily, to rid the body of lead. Symptomatic management consists of cock-up splints for the wrist-drop. Recovery depends on the length of exposure and removal of the toxin.

Pesticides and Organophosphates

Etiology

Insecticides are used extensively worldwide in industry and agriculture. Some compounds have contaminated cooking oils, and outbreaks of organophosphate poisoning have been reported after ingestion. Parathion has been responsible for more accidental poisonings and deaths than any other organophosphate.

Pathogenesis and Clinical Manifestations

All organophosphate compounds inhibit cholinesterase activity, thus creating an acute cholinergic crisis. Acutely, organophosphate toxins affect systemic functions throughout the body; they are also capable of producing a less acute, more chronic neuropathy. Nausea and vomiting, diarrhea, muscle fasciculations, weakness, and paralysis, including sudden paralysis of the respiratory musculature, can occur after overstimulation at the neuromuscular junction. Death can result from vasomotor collapse that coincides with respiratory paralysis. Symptoms of peripheral nerve involvement appear within 1 to 4 days and because they arise quickly, may resemble GBS. A chronic peripheral neuropathy may persist for months or years or a delayed neuropathy may have its onset weeks after exposure.[168]

MEDICAL MANAGEMENT

DIAGNOSIS. Overexposure to organophosphates will reduce cholinesterase activity of erythrocytes to less than 25% of normal. History and clinical evaluation may be accompanied by electrophysiologic studies to indicate the severity of the neuropathy (e.g., segmental demyelination or axonal degeneration or both).

TREATMENT. Insecticides should be washed from the skin and hair; if toxins have been ingested, emesis or lavage should be carried out. Acutely, atropine is given in doses every 10 minutes until the pupils are dilated, the skin flushed and dry, and the pulse rate rises. Neuromuscular paralysis can be reversed by injection of pralidoxime, a cholinesterase reactivator. Endotracheal intubation and ventilation may be required in the presence of respiratory paralysis. Strictly neuropathic management is aimed at symptomatic management.

PROGNOSIS. Recovery is based on removal from the toxin and the degree of involvement. If only segmental demyelination occurs, recovery will occur in weeks to months, but if axonal degeneration is present, recovery will take months to years.

MOTOR END PLATE DISORDERS

Myasthenia Gravis

Overview and Definition

Myasthenia gravis (MG) is the most common of the disorders of neuromuscular transmission. It is characterized by fluctuating weakness and fatigability of skeletal muscles.

Incidence

The incidence of MG is estimated at 1:200,000. Estimates from the National Myasthenia Gravis Foundation are that there are more than 100,000 clients with MG and an additional 25,000 undiagnosed cases. MG can affect people in any age group, but peak incidences occur in women in their twenties and thirties and in men in their fifties and sixties. Overall, the ratio of women affected compared to men is 3:2.

Etiology

MG is an autoimmune disorder whose action takes place at the site of the neuromuscular junction and motor end plate.

Risk Factors

Disorders associated with an increased incidence of MG are thymic disorders such as hyperthyroidism, thymic tumor, or thyrotoxicosis. There is an association with diabetes and immune disorders such as rheumatoid arthritis or lupus. Exacerbations may occur before the menstrual period or shortly after pregnancy. Chronic infections of any kind can exacerbate MG. Five percent to 7% appear to have a familial association.

Pathogenesis

In MG, the fundamental defect is at the neuromuscular junction. Receptors at the motor end plate normally receive acetylcholine (ACh) from the motor nerve terminal. An action potential occurs that leads to a muscle contraction. In MG, the number of ACh receptors are decreased and those that remain are flattened, which results in decreased efficiency of neuromuscular transmission. The neuromuscular junction can normally transmit at high frequencies so that the muscle does not fatigue. With fewer active ACh receptors, the nerve impulses fail to pass across the neuromuscular junction to stimulate muscle contraction. The neuromuscular abnormalities in MG are brought about by an autoimmune response mediated by specific anti-ACh receptor antibodies. The antibodies may block the site that normally binds ACh, or the antibodies may damage the postsynaptic muscle membrane. There may be endocytosis (pinching off of regions of the cell's membrane) of the receptor site.

Although the cause of the autoimmune response in MG is not well understood, the thymus appears to play a role in the disease; 75% of persons with MG have abnormalities of the thymus (e.g., thymic hyperplasia or thymoma). Cells within the thymus bear ACh receptors on their surface, and may serve as a source of autoantigen to trigger the autoimmune reaction within the thymus gland when an immunologic abnormality causes a breakdown an autoimmune attack on ACh receptors.[47]

Clinical Manifestations

Although MG can be mild to severe, its cardinal features are skeletal muscle weakness and fatigability. Repetition of activity causes fatigue, whereas rest restores activity. Other than weakness, neurologic findings are normal. A system of four major categories is used to classify MG: ocular, mild generalized, acute fulminating, or late severe.

The distribution of muscle weakness has a dichotomous pattern affecting only the ocular muscles, or a more variable, generalized pattern occurs. In approximately 85% of persons with MG, the weakness is generalized and affects the limb musculature. This fluctuating weakness is often more noticeable in proximal muscles.

Cranial muscles, particularly the eyelids and the muscles controlling eye movements, are the first to show weakness. The weakness and imbalance in the muscles controlling eye movement results in diplopia (double vision) and ptosis (drooping eyelids) as common early signs. The person will tilt the head back to accommodate (Fig. 39-18). Weak neck muscles may cause head bobbing in this position.

Chewing of meat produces fatigue, and the facial expression is one that seems to be snarling because the lips do not close. Speech tends to be nasal. Difficulty in swallowing may occur as a result of palatal, pharyngeal, and tongue weakness. Nasal regurgitation or aspiration of food is common.

MEDICAL MANAGEMENT

DIAGNOSIS. History and clinical observation of symptoms of weakness with continued use and improvement with rest are important in diagnosing MG. Several conditions that cause weakness of cranial, or somatic, muscles must also be considered. These include drug-induced myasthenia, hyperthyroidism, botulism, intracranial mass lesions, and progressive disorders of the

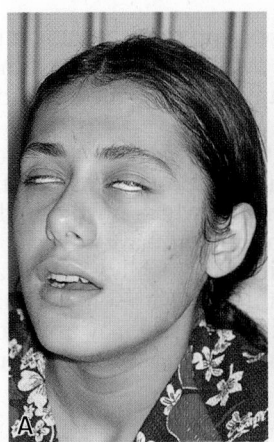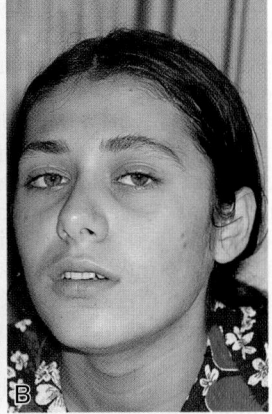

Figure 39-18

A, Facial weakness with myasthenia gravis is easily identified when the patient is asked to perform repeated facial movement. Note inability to fully open eyelids and the open jaw. **B,** Edrophonium (Tensilon) test can be used to confirm the diagnosis. Edrophonium chloride is a short-acting anticholinesterase that is injected intravenously. In myasthenia gravis, the facial weakness is rapidly relieved by this test. Similar responses occur elsewhere in the body. (From Goldman L, Ausiello D: *Cecil textbook of medicine,* ed 22, Philadelphia, 2004, WB Saunders.)

eye. Lambert-Eaton syndrome is a presynaptic disorder of the neuromuscular junction that can cause symptoms similar to those of MG. Lambert-Eaton syndrome is an autoimmune disorder associated with neoplasm, most commonly small cell (oat cell) carcinoma of the lung, which is believed to trigger the autoimmune response.

The three methods used to diagnose MG are (1) immunologic, (2) pharmacologic, and (3) electrophysiologic testing.[130] Immunologic testing detects anti-ACh receptor antibodies in the serum. The presence of anti-ACh receptor antibodies is virtually diagnostic of MG, but a negative test does not exclude diagnosis of the disease. There is no correlation between the amount of anti-ACh receptor antibodies and the severity of the disease. However, in a person with MG a treatment-induced fall in the antibody level often correlates with clinical improvement.

The drug edrophonium (Tensilon) is used to demonstrate improvement in the myasthenic muscles by inhibiting acetylcholinesterase (AChE), an enzyme required for ACh uptake. Muscle strength and endurance are measured before and after administration of the drug. This test confirms that ACh uptake is part of the pathologic status; however, a control test of saline should also be used for comparison.

Electrophysiologic testing of myasthenic disorders demonstrates a normal EMG at rest. Specialized testing must be employed using repetitive stimulation to demonstrate a rapid decrement in the motor action potential's amplitude. Absence of sensory deficits and retention of tendon reflexes throughout the course of the disease also tend to confirm the diagnosis of MG. Because respiratory impairment is a serious complication of MG, measurements of ventilatory function should be performed.[194]

TREATMENT. AChE inhibitor medication provides for improvement of weakness but does not treat the underlying disease. Administration of this medication is tailored to the individual's requirements throughout the day. For example, a person with difficulty chewing and swallowing would take the medication before meals. Side effects of AChE inhibitors include gastrointestinal effects such as nausea and vomiting, abdominal cramping, and increased bronchial and oral secretions.

Surgical removal of the thymus is successful in 85% of persons with MG. Up to 35% of those undergoing thymectomy achieve a drug-free remission, although this may take years.

Immunosuppression using drugs, such as corticosteroids (prednisone) and azathioprine, are effective in nearly all persons with MG. Initially, high daily doses are begun and then followed by alternate-day high doses that are tapered slowly over a period of months. Unfortunately, adverse side effects are associated with high-dose steroids. These include cushingoid appearance, weight gain, hypertension, and osteoporosis (see Chapter 7).

Plasmapheresis is performed to remove substances that affect ACh receptors. However, plasmapheresis produces only short-term reduction in anti-AChE antibodies and is not effective for long-term symptom control.

PROGNOSIS. The course of MG is variable, typified by remissions and exacerbations, especially within the first year after onset. Symptoms often fluctuate in intensity during the day. This daily variability is superimposed on longer-term spontaneous relapses that may last for weeks. Remissions are rarely complete or permanent. This disorder follows a slowly progressive course. Onset of other systemic disorders and infections may precipitate an exacerbation of the disease and are the most common cause of a crisis. A myasthenic crisis is a medical emergency requiring attention to life-endangering weakening of the respiratory muscles and requires ventilatory assistance. Treatment of a crisis occurs in the ICU because the client requires careful, immediate control of medications for survival.[216]

When MG begins in children, it is important to establish the form it takes. Because AChE antibodies cross the placenta, 10% of newborns of mothers with MG develop a myasthenic reaction. Newborns with neonatal MG have a weak suck and cry and are hypotonic. Fortunately, this resolves in a few weeks.

SPECIAL IMPLICATIONS FOR THE THERAPIST | 39-10

Myasthenia Gravis

Physical and occupational therapy may be indicated as supportive care to assist the client with MG. In the acute care setting, the therapist must establish an accurate neurologic and respiratory baseline. Tidal volume, vital capacity, and inspiratory force should be monitored regularly during treatment. Deep breathing and coughing should be encouraged. When eating, the person should be instructed to sit upright and to swallow when the chin is tipped slightly downward toward the chest and never with the neck extended because of the risk of aspiration. Finally, the client should never speak with food in the mouth.

The therapist must also be alert to signs of an impending myasthenic crisis (increasing muscle weakness; respiratory distress; or difficulty while talking, chewing, or swallowing). Make sure the client recognizes the side effects and signs of toxicity of AChE inhibitor medications. For those receiving a prolonged course of corticosteroids, report adverse side effects to the physician.

Plan therapy and teach the client to plan activities to coincide with periods of maximum energy (see Box 9-8 for energy conservation tips). The home should be arranged to help prevent unnecessary energy expenditure. Frequent rest periods help conserve energy and give muscles a chance to regain strength. The person with MG should avoid strenuous exercise, stress, and excessive exposure to the sun or cold weather. All of these can exacerbate signs and symptoms.

Researchers report that a strength training program eliciting maximal isometric contractions could be instituted in clients with mild-to-moderate MG. As long as participants were monitored for fatigue during periods of exercise, improvements were noted in all muscles.[82] After 3 months, participants' knee extensor muscles showed the most significant strength gains without adverse reactions. The use of a cooling vest to decrease core body temperature to determine whether

pulmonary function and subjective perceptions of strength and fatigue would improve in persons with MG has been investigated. All measures were improved in the majority of participants.[132]

Because individuals diagnosed as having MG are placed on long-term corticosteroid medication, the treatment may induce a secondary condition: osteoporosis. These individuals should be encouraged to undergo dual energy x-ray absorptiometry (previously DEXA, now DXA) scan and to receive calcium supplements to counteract osteoporosis.[113]

Importantly, clinicians should monitor signs and symptoms and the impact on participation and quality of life. A preliminary version of a MG specific, patient reported disability assessment instrument has been developed called the MG_DIS. It is based on the International Classification of Functioning, Disability, and Health (ICF) and is designed to monitor changes of functioning in people with MG as well as serve as an outcome measure in clinical trials.[156]

BOTULISM

Definition and Incidence

Botulism is a rare, often fatal condition (20% mortality) caused by ingestion of a potent neurotoxin produced by *Clostridium botulinum*, which is found in improperly preserved or canned foods, as well as in contaminated wounds. The Centers for Disease Control and Prevention recognizes four categories of botulism: (1) foodborne, (2) wound, (3) infant, and (4) unclassified.[43] Approximately 10 adult cases and 100 cases of infant botulism are reported each year in the United States.

Etiology and Pathogenesis

The anaerobic bacillus releases a protein neurotoxin that is heat labile; it is destroyed by boiling food for 10 minutes; inadequate food preparation allows the neurotoxin to be ingested.

Infant botulism affects babies ages 3 weeks to 9 months; the most common source of infant botulism arises from the ingestion of honey, which is why children younger than 1 year are not allowed to have honey.

Botulism is not always ingested orally. Some cases occur after wounds are contaminated with soil, in chronic drug abusers, after cesarean delivery, and may even occur when antibiotics are administered to prevent wound infection.

When the neurotoxin is ingested, digestive acids and proteolytic enzymes cannot destroy the molecules of the toxin and it is absorbed into the blood from the small intestine. Minute amounts of circulating toxin reach the cholinergic nerve endings at the motor end plate and bind to gangliosides of the presynaptic nerve terminals. Flaccid paralysis is caused by inhibition of ACh released from cholinergic terminals at the motor end plate. Inhibition of ACh release causes a symmetric paralysis with normal sensory and mental status.

Clinical Manifestations

Onset of symptoms develops 12 to 36 hours after ingestion of food containing the toxin. Signs and symptoms include malaise, weakness, blurred and double vision (diplopia), dry mouth, and nausea and vomiting. Progression is variable, but respiratory failure can occur in 6 to 8 hours. People may also report difficulty swallowing (dysphagia), dysarthria (slurred speech), and photophobia. Because the motor end plate is involved, there are no direct sensory changes. Motor weakness of the face and neck muscles progresses to involve the diaphragm, accessory muscles of respiration, and muscles controlling the extremities. Secondary effects from the flaccid paralysis, such as severe muscle wasting, pressure sores, and aspiration pneumonia, may occur.

MEDICAL MANAGEMENT

DIAGNOSIS, TREATMENT, AND PROGNOSIS. A history suggesting a food source, and toxin identification made by serum or stool analysis are used in the diagnosis. EMG testing demonstrates a decreasing amplitude and facilitation of muscle action potential after tetanic stimulation. Differential diagnosis includes disorders that also display a rapidly evolving flaccid paralysis, such as GBS, MG, and tick paralysis.

Immediate treatment is directed toward neutralizing the toxin using injectable trivalent ABE (botulism equine trivalent antitoxin) serum, an antitoxin. Antitoxin prevents further binding of free botulism toxin to the presynaptic endings. If paralysis occurs because of wound botulism, care should include debridement and antibiotics.

Removal of unabsorbed toxin from the gastrointestinal tract is accomplished by gastric lavage and induced emesis. Finally, supportive measures should be instituted in the hospital; intubation and mechanical ventilation are needed when the individual's vital capacity is compromised.

If untreated, this disorder can be fatal within 24 hours of ingestion. Respiratory failure leads to death. In mild-to-moderate cases, a gradual recovery of muscle strength can take as long as 12 months after onset. After hospitalization, graded rehabilitation is instituted to treat muscle wasting, deconditioning, and orthostatic hypotension.

ABNORMAL RESPONSE IN PERIPHERAL NERVES

Complex Regional Pain Syndrome/Reflex Sympathetic Dystrophy/Causalgia

Complex regional pain syndrome (CRPS), first described in 1864, is characterized by sensory, autonomic, motor, and dystrophic signs and symptoms. CRPS includes disorders of the sympathetic nervous system with or without known trauma. New insights into nervous system function and pain mechanisms have led to reclassification of the syndrome.

CRPS I (formerly reflex sympathetic dystrophy) is the label used to describe this syndrome when there is an absence of known traumatic nerve injury; however, there is usually an initiating noxious event. CRPS II (formerly causalgia) refers to a similar condition associated with known traumatic nerve injury. A third type (CRPS-NOS) (not otherwise specified) only partially meets CRPS criteria and cannot be explained by any other condition.

Incidence

CRPS I may occur after 5% of all injuries with a reported number of new cases each year of approximately 50,000 in the United States. Because the diagnosis is often missed or delayed, estimates on incidence may be underreported. Some very mild cases may resolve and others may progress to become a chronic, debilitating disorder. Although the average age of an individual with CRPS is in the mid-30s, it has been reported in all age groups, including children as young as 3 years. Women are three times more likely to develop CRPS than men.[42]

Etiology

CRPS has its origin in a variety of conditions: it can follow medical procedures, including surgery, such as arthroscopy; it can occur after an UMN lesion arising from traumatic brain injury, cerebrovascular accidents (often in the presence of flaccidity), or destructive lesions of the CNS; or it can occur after LMN disorders from peripheral nerve injuries, neuropathies, and entrapments. CRPS has been reported following motor vehicle accidents, fractures, bites (human, animal), falls, assault, after shoulder subluxation or dislocation and even what seem like minor strains or sprains. Any event that causes traction of the brachial plexus and nerve roots resulting in constant nerve irritation may result in CRPS.

Pathogenesis

CRPS is now regarded as a systemic condition that involves both central and peripheral components of the neuraxis and interactions between the immune and nervous systems. No one knows for sure what causes the cascade of neurogenic responses that leads to CRPS. Laboratory studies of blood and tissue samples appear normal; although there is some evidence of elevated systemic levels of inflammatory markers and catecholamines (mediators in sympathetic hyperactivity).[41] There is no apparent inflammation of the affected soft tissues (e.g., skin, muscles). There is some evidence that the cellular changes are occurring within the nerve fibers to the affected tissues.

An injury at one somatic level initiates sympathetic efferent activity that affects many segmental levels. CRPS is thought to represent a reflex neurogenic inflammation. Facilitation of the sympathetic nervous system (SNS) and its neurotransmitters and catecholamines activates primary afferent nociceptors to create the sensation of pain. Deterioration of the SNS function is common. Excess release of substance P from terminal sensory nerves is part of the overreaction of the neurogenic inflammatory process.

Migraine headaches appear to overlap with CRPS. The signaling neuropeptide CGRP (calcitonin gene-related peptide) appears to be linked to the hyperresponsiveness in both migraine headaches and CRPS. Loss of inhibition in the complex cascade of nerve-related inflammatory chemicals that can occur after major or minor trauma suggests it's not the trauma itself that exaggerates the process, but rather, the nervous system's response to injury.[18] It has been suggested that people with CRPS who lose their automatic nervous system reflex responses might have a faulty nervous system to begin with, which could explain why they develop CRPS when others with similar injuries recover normally.[206]

Thermal dysfunctions are related to either the inhibition of SNS vasoconstriction or facilitation of the SNS causing excessive vasoconstriction (Fig. 39-19). Clinical studies have shown abnormal SNS reflexes that indicate CNS dysfunction exists as well.[213]

Clinical Manifestations

The natural history of CRPS is one of change over time. CRPS has overlapping but identifiable clinical stages (Table 39-12). The primary clinical features of CRPS fall into 4 distinct subgroups: (1) abnormalities in pain processing, (2) skin color and temperature changes, (3) edema, vasomotor, and sudomotor abnormalities, and (4) motor dysfunction and trophic changes. Intense, burning pain in a specific area, most often an extremity, is the most commonly reported symptom. Other clinical manifestations vary widely and can include, headache, difficulty sleeping, fatigue, difficulty concentrating, memory loss, edema, inability to initiate movement, weakness, tremor, muscle spasms, dystrophy, and atrophy.

The pain that occurs is disproportionate to what would be expected. The overall pain intensity increases with disease duration. Even tactile stimulation may be perceived as pain (allodynia).[70] The pain spreads from localized to

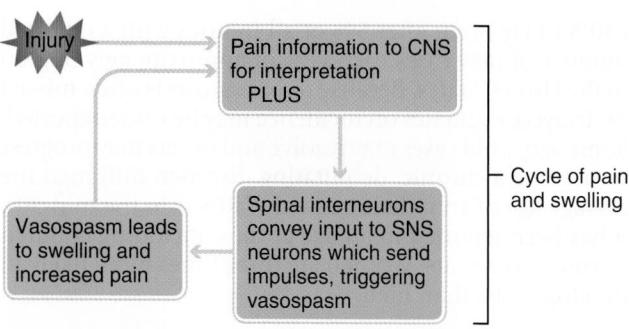

Figure 39-19

The exaggerated pain associated with sympathetic over activity occurs after minor trauma. Normally, the response of the sympathetic nervous system after injury causes cutaneous blood vessels to contract. This response shuts down appropriately within minutes to hours. In complex regional pain syndrome, the sympathetic nervous system functions abnormally and causes vasospasm, which creates cycles of swelling and pain. Initially, vasodilation occurs that increases skin temperature. Later in the course of the disorder, symptoms consist of cyanosis and coldness in the involved extremity.

Table 39-12	Complex Regional Pain Syndrome: Progressive Clinical Stages	
Stage		**Classic Signs and Symptoms**
Stage I: Acute inflammation: denervation and sympathetic hypoactivity	Begins up to 10 days following injury; lasts 3-6 months	**Pain**—more severe than expected; burning or aching character; increased by dependent position, physical contact or emotional disturbances **Hyperalgesia** (lower pain threshold, increased sensitivity), **allodynia** (all stimuli are perceived as pain), and **hyperpathia** (threshold to pain is increased, once exceeded, sensation intensity increased more rapidly and greater than expected) **Edema**—soft and localized **Vasomotor/thermal changes**—affected limb is warmer **Skin—Hyperthermia** and **dry** Increased hair and nail growth
Stage II: Dystrophic: paradoxic sympathetic hyperactivity	Occurs 3-6 months after onset of pain, lasts about 6 months	**Pain**—worsens: constant, burning and aching **Allodynia, hyperalgesia,** and **hyperpathia** almost always present **Edema**—becomes thicker and more fibrotic causing joint stiffness **Vasomotor/thermal changes**—neither warm, nor cold **Skin**—thin, glossy, cool (vasoconstriction) and sweaty Thin, ridged nails X-rays reveal disuse **osteoporosis**, cystic and subchondral bone erosion
Stage III: Atrophic	Begins about 6-12 months after onset; may last for years, or may resolve and reoccur	**Pain**—spreads proximally, occasionally to entire skin surface or plateaus; joint stiffness progresses **Edema**—continues to harden **Vasomotor/thermal changes**—sympathetic nervous system regulation is decreased on affected extremity, affected limb is cooler **Skin**—thin, shiny, cyanotic, and dry Fingertips and toes on involved extremity are atrophic Fascia is thickened; contractures may occur X-ray demonstrates bony **demineralization and ankylosis**

a regional distribution, including to the same extremity on the contralateral side of the body in a mirror pattern (e.g., right arm to left arm), to the other extremity on the ipsilateral side (e.g., right arm to right leg), and to the other extremity on the opposite side (e.g., right arm to left leg).

Although sensory impairments are most often the hallmark of CRPS, movement disorders also occur. Motor symptoms may precede the appearance of other impairments by weeks or months or may appear on the contralateral extremity in a mirror fashion but most often they occur concomitantly with autonomic changes and pain. All manifestations contribute to impairments of function and alter quality of life.

Despite the fact that three stages of CRPS were originally identified and are still referred to, the course of this disorder is more unpredictable than the stages imply.[103] Individuals typically remain in a specific stage for 6 to 8 months; however, some may progress rapidly to and through the next stage. As the condition progresses, symptoms may spread proximally and even spread to affect other extremities. In a few cases, the entire body may become involved.[123]

Three abnormal vasomotor patterns have been identified; these relate to the temperature and color (warmth or heat with redness, cool with bluish tint) of the extremity and the acuity of CRPS. Hypersensitivity and abnormal sweating may be followed by dry skin. Other vasomotor changes include changes in the nails in which they become thick, brittle, and ridged.

MEDICAL MANAGEMENT

DIAGNOSIS. In the absence of a specific biomarker, the diagnosis of CRPS is based primarily on the clinical examination and history. Proposed diagnostic criteria for CRPS requires at least one symptom in each of the four subgroups, and one sign in at least two of the four subgroups. A combination of diagnostic tests aimed at assessing secondary changes (radiographic examinations, thermographic studies, sudomotor function tests, NCV or somatosensory evoked potentials, and laser Doppler flowmetry) may aid in establishing a diagnosis. Because of the evolutionary nature of CRPS, a correct diagnosis may be delayed, especially in children.[49,84]

TREATMENT. Treatment for CRPS tends to be multifactorial and prolonged. Successful treatment depends on early diagnosis, treatment of the underlying cause, and aggressive and sustained physical therapy.[88] Although stellate ganglion blocks or sympathectomy are used to alleviate pain and early symptoms, this approach is based on weak evidence.[122] All of the following treatments have limited evidence for their effectiveness.[68] Medications such as corticosteroids, nonsteroidal antiinflammatory drugs, antidepressants, antianxiety agents, and anticonvulsants may offer pain relief by normalizing overactive pain pathways but do not vary the duration of the disease. Amitriptyline has been used to facilitate sleep and relieve depression. Calcium channel blockers help to improve peripheral circulation through their effect on the SNS. Newer, more selective drugs (e.g., immunomodulators) are showing promising results.[173]

IV ketamine infusion has been used in severe cases unresponsive to other therapies. This drug works by shutting off the N-methyl-D-aspartate receptors in the brain but must be supported by a wide range of other management tools (e.g., good nutrition, physical and occupational therapy, exercise, cognitive behavioral counseling).[70]

Sympathetic, somatic, and trigger point blocks, spinal cord stimulators, and intrathecal pumps for the delivery of baclofen or morphine decrease pain intensity and perception of pain, but do not alter the disease progression. A less-expensive alternative may be the use of hyperbaric oxygenation therapy used to restore circulation, reduce inflammation, and eliminate swelling in affected limbs while also changing pain processing in the brain. This is not yet approved by the FDA and results reported so far are based on case studies.[127]

Integrative medicine has a role in the treatment of chronic conditions like CRPS. Some people find relief from their symptoms (or at least an ability to cope better and improve function) when traditional allopathic medicine is augmented by acupuncture, craniosacral therapy, BodyTalk, Reiki, tai chi, yoga, or other forms of complementary care. Cognitive behavioral therapy, although not a cure for CRPS, can help improve pain, mood, and function.[84,85]

PROGNOSIS. CRPS is a complex syndrome with varying severity and disability. In many cases, the pain continues for years or, less frequently, it may remit, then recur after another injury. Spontaneous remission is unusual; only modest improvements have been reported with most current therapies.[173]

In some cases, malingering for secondary gain has been documented.[218] Outcome measures for CRPS I typically concentrate on impairments, leaving measurement of disability, which is the most relevant to function, with few assessments.[168] Physical therapy is indicated, particularly as part of a program of pain control. Although the goal is to maintain function so that the individual can perform normal activities, a vigorous approach is not indicated. Current research is aimed at understanding physiologic processes and finding the most effective interventions.

SPECIAL IMPLICATIONS FOR THE THERAPIST   39-11

Complex Regional Pain Syndrome

Goals for physical therapy include educating the client and encouraging normal positioning and use of the involved extremity while minimizing pain and normalizing sensation. Stress loading (loading and scrubbing) is a key part of the rehabilitation program. Weight bearing and compression through the affected extremity is followed by a distraction force (e.g., carrying weights or a bucket with weights inside. Scrubbing is performed on hands and knees or for just lower-extremity involvement in the standing position. A scrub brush held in the hand or attached to the foot is held with constant pressure against the contact surface and a scrubbing motion applied in various directions.

All scrubbing and loading activities are done daily with gradual progression to tolerance.

At first, there is often an increase in pain and swelling with this type of program, but these symptoms decrease after a few days. Desensitization techniques may also assist in normalizing sensation to the affected area. This consists of progressive stimulation with very soft material to more textured fabrics or materials. Sensory input is graded from light touch to deep pressure and from consistent to intermittent duration with each material.

There is evidence that graded motor imagery reduces pain and swelling in some people with CRPS. This approach involves recognizing pictured hands (or whatever body part is affected) as being right or left, imagining movements, and mirroring movements. The affected individual must practice hourly for several weeks to have an effect.[136-138]

Although modalities are used to provide pain relief, the greatest success occurs when they are administered during earlier stages of CRPS. External transcutaneous electrical nerve stimulator units are reported to be minimally effective.[31] When the lower extremity is involved, aquatic therapy is helpful for improving mobility when weight bearing on land is problematic.

The therapist should be aware of the potential for significant psychologic, emotional, social, and spiritual issues associated with any chronic condition, but especially one as painful and debilitating as CRPS can become. Furthermore, because the pain is often disproportionate to the incident, people with CRPS may be misunderstood by their loved ones and by clinicians. Attentive listening; acknowledging and validating feelings of anger, worthlessness, anxiety/depression, and hopelessness; referral to support groups; and communication with the physician about the individual's needs are essential during the long process of recovery.

A report of increased spontaneous falls throughout the course of the illness has been documented for more than a quarter of individuals with CRPS. It would be advisable to conduct a falls assessment and institute client safety education and falls prevention.[173]

REFERENCES

To enhance this text and add value for the reader, all references are included on the companion Evolve site that accompanies this textbook. The reader can view the reference source and access it online whenever possible.

CHAPTER 40

Laboratory Tests and Values

GLENN L. IRION

INTRODUCTION

Laboratory tests may be used by the physician for screening (searching for an occult disease process in an otherwise healthy person), diagnosis (identifying or ruling out potential causes of symptoms), or to monitor a patient's condition following the diagnosis of a disease.[53] Specific tests may be used for any of these purposes, depending on what information is needed. For example, a glucose test may be used for screening a population, for diagnosis of diabetes mellitus, or to monitor the effectiveness of an individual's therapy for diabetes mellitus.

Screening tests may be used on populations in an effort to identify individuals who are at risk for certain diseases, for example, those with high cholesterol who could benefit from treatment before disease manifestations become evident. Screening is also done for genetic or metabolic diseases to find individuals before disease occurs. State laws generally require routine screening in newborns for a number of disorders, notably phenylketonuria, sickle cell disease, and hypothyroidism.

Certain lab tests are very sensitive and specific for certain pathologic conditions, whereas others may only provide one piece of evidence suggesting a health problem without actually providing a certain diagnosis. For the therapist, laboratory values assist in deciding whether therapy should be provided at that time, should be scaled back, or should be more aggressive.[16]

Some lab values are clear contraindications for receiving therapy, whereas others are suggestive that therapy provided should be less physiologically demanding. In almost all cases, therapists should not rely solely upon a lab value that is printed in a chart or on a computer screen for a number of reasons. The therapist must communicate with other members of the health care team to determine what aspects of therapy should be held until physiologic improvement, what should be modified, and what should be done in place of the prescribed treatment plan.[30]

For example, an individual who is short of breath with blood gas values that indicate no physiologic reserve for increasing metabolic demand should not undergo therapy that involves activity; other aspects may be addressed such as positioning, pressure relief, and educating caregivers. Note also that different physicians or facilities may adopt criteria for holding therapy that vary from those suggested in the text. In addition, lab values may not always reflect an individual's current physiologic status. Other members of the health care team may be aware of the person's situation and give advice on that individual's current physiologic status. Other reasons for not relying solely on reading numbers are discussed below under limitations of lab testing.

Limitations of Lab Testing

The range of values for a given test in a healthy person is known as the *reference range* or *expected value*, formerly known as the normal range. The reference range depends on the methods used for the test and must be compared against the reference range specific to that laboratory. How well that reference range depicts homeostasis may vary with sex, age, weight, physiologic changes (such as pregnancy), and fluid status.

Each laboratory will include a means of assessing the results—sometimes by placing *L* for low or *H* for high after a test result or by providing the range of reference lab values for the tests performed. Although lab tests are generally reliable, a test may fail to produce a result that should indicate an abnormal condition that truly exists (false negative) or the results may falsely indicate that an abnormal condition exists (false positive). Laboratory tests are frequently "rechecked" so as to ensure a higher degree of diagnostic accuracy.

Some tests may have less predictive value regarding the individual's physiology than we would expect. The positive predictive value of a test depends on the prevalence of the disease in a population. The less prevalent the disease, the less accurate laboratory results may be. Statistically, as the number of tests performed on a single individual increase, the possibility of an incorrect conclusion also increases, regardless of whether the person is sick.[41] This phenomenon is purely related to chance because a significant margin of error arises from the arbitrary setting of limits for normal or reference values.

Results may be inaccurate, outdated, or the abnormality indicated by the test may not have the expected impact on the person. Inaccurate values may be obtained if samples used for lab analysis are contaminated, mishandled, or mislabeled, or testing materials and techniques are flawed. Results may not accurately portray a person's physiologic status as a result of other substances present in the sample, such as medications that the person is taking.

In some cases, the condition of the individual may have changed between obtaining the sample and when receiving physical therapy. Therefore the values recorded in the medical record may not reflect the person's current condition, resulting in a false-positive or false-negative result. Alternately, the person may have recovered spontaneously or received treatment that has restored normal physiology. For example, a lab report may indicate that the person is anemic, but the individual may have received a blood transfusion since the lab report was generated. For these reasons communication with other members of the health care team is essential as interventions to correct the person's condition may not have been noted in the medical record.

People may have vastly different tolerances for the alterations in homeostasis implied by abnormal lab test results. In particular, the chronicity of the condition may affect an individual's tolerance. For example, a person with chronic anemia may be able to ambulate freely, and another person with similar lab values, but with acute anemia may not be able to sit upright. Often a discussion with the patient and the nurse in addition to monitoring vital signs help guide the intensity and duration of activity that will be tolerated by that individual.

In summary, reference values or "normal" ranges provided in this chapter are not meant to be memorized and applied as a standard to every case. Instead, the reference ranges provided in this chapter give the therapist a general idea of the values expected for each test, but interpretation of specific individual values must be done using the laboratory reference values (usually provided on most laboratory reports) not these figures.

In addition to the material in this chapter, the reader may wish to refer to a website provided by the American Association for Clinical Chemistry (www.labtestsonline.org).[1] This website will cover any additional lab tests the therapist might encounter, including the opportunity to enter a condition and determine which lab tests might be employed.

Abbreviations

Box 40-1 provides recommended units for clinical laboratory data. Table 40-1 lists The Joint Commission's official "do not use" list of abbreviations. The list was originally created in 2004 by The Joint Commission as part of the requirements for meeting National Patient Safety Goal requirement 2B, which required a standardized list of abbreviations, acronyms, and symbols that are not to be used throughout the organization.

APACHE

The Acute Physiology and Chronic Health Evaluation (APACHE), a system for prognosis development for critically ill patients, has been developed using a number of lab and other values. Based on data entered regarding admission diagnosis, age, health history, and the physiologic measurements taken during the first 24 hours, a

---

Box 40-1

UNITS FOR CLINICAL LABORATORY DATA*

g	gram
ng	nanogram
mg	milligram
mL	milliliter
L	liter
dL	deciliter (100 mL)
pg	picogram
mm³	cubic millimeter
mmol	millimole
U	unit
IU	international unit
mU	milliunit
μg	microgram
μU	microunit
μm	micron
mEq	milliequivalent

*Note: Some of the items in this box are on the official Do Not Use List (see Table 40-1) but are still commonly used and thus listed.

---

predicted death rate is calculated. Length of stay in the intensive care unit (ICU) can also be predicted.

Measurements include body temperature, mean arterial pressure, heart rate, respiratory rate, partial pressure of arterial pressure, hematocrit, white blood cell (WBC) count, arterial pH, Glasgow coma scale, and serum bicarbonate, potassium, and creatinine.[63,80] A particularly important calculation is the ratio of the partial pressure of arterial oxygen (PaO_2) to the fraction of inspired oxygen (FIO_2). Room air has a FIO_2 of approximately 21%. If PaO_2 remains low despite increasing the concentration of oxygen in the inspired air, the individual has a poor prognosis for recovery. Newer variables (use of mechanical ventilation and thrombolytic therapy) and adjustment to the equations used for predictions have been used to generate the latest version (APACHE IV).[44,81]

BASIC METABOLIC PANEL

The most common lab tests constitute what are now known as the *basic metabolic panel* (BMP),[30] *comprehensive metabolic panel*, and *hepatic function panel*. These three terms are based on current procedural terminology (CPT) codes.[9] These replace a variety of other names, such as SMA-6, SMA-7, SMA-12, SMA-20, Chemistry Panel, Chem Screen, Chem-6, Chem-7, Chem-12, Chem-20, SMAC-6, SMAC-7, SMAC-12, and SMAC-20.

The BMP is a group of eight specific tests for electrolyte level, acid–base balance, blood sugar, and kidney status. The tests consist of serum concentrations of sodium, potassium, chloride, calcium, blood urea nitrogen (BUN), creatinine, glucose, and carbon dioxide. The BMP may be done as part of a routine physical examination as an outpatient, routine testing of inpatients, or when a physician suspects an abnormality that may be detected by one or more components of the BMP.

Normal values for BMP are given in Table 40-2, along with possible causes and consequences of abnormal

Table 40-1	Official "Do Not Use" List*	
Do Not Use	**Potential Problem**	**Use Instead**
U (unit)	Mistaken for "0" (zero), the number "4" (four) or "cc"	Write "unit"
IU (International Unit)	Mistaken for IV (intravenous) or the number 10 (ten)	Write "International Unit"
Q.D., QD, q.d., qd (daily)	Mistaken for each other	Write "daily"
Q.O.D., QOD, q.o.d., qod (every other day)	Period after the Q mistaken for "1" and the "O" mistaken for "I"	Write "every other day"
Trailing zero (X.0 mg)†	Decimal point is missed	Write X mg
Lack of leading zero (.X mg)		Write 0.X mg
MS	Can mean morphine sulfate or magnesium sulfate	Write "morphine sulfate"
MSO_4 and $MgSO_4$	Confused for one another	Write "magnesium sulfate"

*Applies to all orders and all medication-related documentation that is handwritten (including free-text computer entry) or on preprinted forms.
†**Exception:** A "trailing zero" may be used where required to demonstrate the level of precision of the value being reported, such as for laboratory results, imaging studies that report size of lesions, or catheter/tube sizes. It may not be used in medication orders or other medication-related documentation.

Additional Abbreviations, Acronyms and Symbols (for *possible* future inclusion in the Official "Do Not Use" List)

Do Not Use	**Potential Problem**	**Use Instead**
> (greater than)	Misinterpreted as the number "7" (seven) or the letter "L";	Write "greater than"
< (less than)	confused for one another	Write "less than"
Abbreviations for drug names	Misinterpreted because of similar abbreviations for multiple drugs	Write drug names in full
Apothecary units	Unfamiliar to many practitioners; confused with metric units	Use metric units
@	Mistaken for the number "2" (two)	Write "at"
cc	Mistaken for U (units) when poorly written	Write "mL" or "milliliters"
μ	Mistaken for mg (milligrams) resulting in 1000-fold overdose	Write "mcg" or "micrograms"

Data from The Joint Commission: Official "Do Not Use" List. Available at http://www.jointcommission.org/facts_about_the_official_/. Accessed August 11, 2014.

values. BMP may be used as a screening tool, especially for diabetes and kidney disease. The sample is obtained by venipuncture, preferably after 10 to 12 hours of fasting.[1]

As an indicator of current status of electrolytes, acid–base balance, renal function, and blood sugar, significant changes in BMP values may indicate a number of acute problems, such as kidney failure, insulin shock, diabetic coma, and respiratory distress.[1] Changes in sodium, potassium, and calcium, in particular, alter the excitability of neurons, cardiac, and skeletal muscle and can produce weakness, spasms, altered sensation, cardiac arrhythmias, and, potentially, death.[3] Each component of the BMP is described below. For companion information regarding fluid and electrolyte balance–imbalance, the reader is directed to Chapter 5; see also Tables 5-9 through 5-12.

Sodium

Sodium is a critical determinant of fluid volume in the body. Under normal circumstances, increases in the amount of sodium in the body lead to retention of water and a loss of sodium leads to loss of water in the body. Normally, small increases in sodium concentration increase thirst, which corrects sodium concentration. Derangement of homeostatic mechanisms may impair the linkage between thirst and sodium concentration. Sodium concentration may be decreased (hyponatremia) by excessive infusion or ingestion of water, excessive production of antidiuretic hormone, or by diseases that cause retention of water, such as heart failure, cirrhosis, nephrotic syndrome, and syndrome of inappropriate

antidiuretic hormone release (SIADH). Increased fluid volume increases blood pressure and may increase cell volume. Neurons are especially vulnerable to cell swelling, leading to neurologic dysfunction, possibly progressing to coma or death.

Sodium concentration may increase (hypernatremia) when excessive water is lost from the body, such as in profuse sweating or decreased antidiuretic hormone (ADH) production (diabetes insipidus). Changes in sodium concentration may lead to visible changes in body fluid volume manifested as dehydration or edema.

Potassium

Potassium is particularly important for function of excitable cells—nerves, muscles, and heart. Therefore, the normal range for potassium is very narrow. Excitable cells remove the vast majority of potassium from surrounding fluids to maintain their resting potentials. Small alterations in extracellular potassium have profound effects on these cells. The heart muscle is very susceptible to potassium disturbances; arrhythmias and cardiac arrest can result from hypokalemia or hyperkalemia. Abnormal values in either direction can also lead to muscle weakness or irritability. Potassium measurements provide useful information about renal and adrenal disorders and about water and acid–base imbalances.

Use of loop diuretics in particular can lead to compensatory reabsorption of sodium at the expense of losing potassium in the urine. In addition to cardiac arrhythmia, signs of hypokalemia include mental

Table 40-2	Reference Values for Basic Metabolic Profile and Magnesium	
Test	**Reference Value**	**Critical Value**
Sodium	Infant: 134-150 mEq/L Child: 135-145 mEq/L Adult, older: 135-145 mEq/L	Adult: ≤110
Potassium	Infant: 3.6-5.8 mEq/L Child: 3.5-5.5 mEq/L Adult, older: 3.5-5.0 mEq/L	Newborn: <2.5 or >8.1 mEq/L Adult: <2.5 or >6.6 mEq/L For the physical therapist: <3.2 or >5.1 (some facilities use a slightly higher reference range (5.1 up to 5.3)
Chloride	Infant: 95-110 mEq/L Child: 98-105 mEq/L Adult, older: 95-105 mEq/L	Adult: <80 or >115 mEq/L
Calcium	Infant: 10-12 mg/dL Child: 9-11.5 mg/dL Adult, older: 9-11 mg/dL	<7 mg/dL (tetany), >12 mg/dL (coma)
Blood urea nitrogen (BUN)	Newborn: 3-12 mg/dL Infant: 5-18 Child: 5-18 Adolescent: — Adult female: 10-20 Adult male: 10-20	
Creatinine	Newborn: 0.3-1.2 mg/dL Infant: 0.2-0.4 mg/dL Child: 0.3-0.7 mg/dL Adolescent: 0.5-1.0 mg/dL Adult female: 0.5-1.1 mg/dL Adult male: 0.6-1.2 mg/dL	
Magnesium	Infant: 1.4-2.9 mEq/L Child: 1.6-2.6 mEq/L Adult, older: 1.5-2.5 mEq/L	<0.5 or >3.0 mEq/L

Creatinine for older adult decreases with decreased muscle mass. BUN may be slightly higher than adult level. A normal BUN-to-creatinine ratio is 10:1 to 20:1 for all ages.

status changes, dizziness, weakness, myalgia, muscle twitches, nausea, vomiting, clammy skin, and potentially respiratory failure caused by weakness of muscles of inspiration.

Hyperkalemia may result from excessive potassium replacement, consumption of foods such as many fruits with high potassium content, and several drugs such as angiotensin-converting enzyme inhibitors. Hyperkalemia can also produce numbness, tingling, flaccid paralysis, nausea, vomiting, diarrhea, and anorexia. Any abnormal value should lead to consultation before treatment due to the potential for severe consequences.

Chloride

Chloride levels tend to change along with changes in sodium and water. It may also change in response to alterations in cellular pH. Carbon dioxide that diffuses into cells, especially red blood cells, generates carbonic acid that must be managed by exchanging bicarbonate ions for chloride ions. As carbon dioxide is added to the blood, chloride moves into red cells and bicarbonate moves out. In the lungs, the process is reversed. Hyperchloremia is usually found with hypernatremia because they usually have the same causes, but hyperchloremia can occur as a result of hyperventilation. Conversely, hypochloremia

can occur with hypoventilation, which is usually caused by chronic respiratory disease resulting from the chloride shift in response to changes in pH.

Calcium

Calcium is tested most commonly to rule in or rule out kidney or bone disease and to rule out changes in ionized calcium as a cause of neuromuscular dysfunction. It is commonly tested along with phosphorus and vitamin D because of kidney disease and osteoporosis and with parathyroid hormone as serum calcium concentration can be altered by various forms of parathyroid disorders.

Hypercalcemia may also be present with kidney stones and certain forms of cancer, especially multiple myeloma. Arrhythmias may result from the role of calcium in some specific forms of electrical potentials of the heart. Calcium is also responsible for neuronal excitability. Hypercalcemia decreases the firing of neurons, resulting in muscle weakness, fatigability, and decreased muscle tone and reflexes. Decreased ionized calcium can cause numbness around the mouth and in the fingers and toes, and muscle spasms, often secondary to respiratory alkalosis that may result from hyperventilation.

Table 40-3	Blood Glucose Tests

Fasting Plasma (Blood) Glucose (mg/dL)

Adults	70-100 mg/dL
Adults older than 60 yr	80-110 mg/dL
Children	60-100 mg/dL
Neonates	40-80 mg/dL

World Health Organization* Diabetes Criteria: Interpretation of Oral Glucose Tolerance Test

Glucose Levels	Normal		IFG		IGT		Diabetes Mellitus	
	Fasting	2 hr	Fasting	2 hr	Fasting	2 hr	Fasting	2 hr
Venous plasma (mmol/L)	<6.1	<7.8	≥6.1 & <7.0	<7.8	<7.0	≥7.8	≥7.0	≥11.1
(mg/dL)	<110	<140	≥110 & <126	<140	<126	≥140	≥126	≥200

Hemoglobin A$_{1c}$

Adult:	Normal reference range: 4.0%-6.0%[†]
Good glucose control:	2.5%-5.9%
Fair glucose control:	6.0%-7.0%
Poor glucose control:	less than 7.0%

*Available at: http://www.who.org. Accessed August 11, 2014.

[†]An HbA$_{1c}$ of 6.5% is recommended by the World Health Organization (WHO) as the cutpoint for diagnosing diabetes. A value of less than 6.5% does not exclude diabetes diagnosed using glucose tests.

From World Health Organization (2011). *Use of glycated haemoglobin (HbA1c) in the diagnosis of diabetes mellitus. Report of a WHO Consultation.* Available online at http://www.who.int/diabetes/publications/diagnosis_diabetes2011/en/. Accessed August 11, 2014.

Magnesium

Magnesium, like calcium, is involved in regulation of excitable cells but is not part of the BMP and must be ordered separately. Low magnesium also results in arrhythmias, weakness, muscle spasms, and numbness. Magnesium (see Table 40-2) may be reduced in diabetes, with the use of diuretics, as a result of chronic vomiting or diarrhea, and may be increased by renal failure, hyperparathyroidism, or hypothyroidism.

Blood Urea Nitrogen and Creatinine

BUN and creatinine (see Table 40-2) are used to evaluate kidney function in individuals with kidney failure, for differential diagnosis if kidney disease is suspected, to monitor treatment of kidney disease, and to monitor kidney function while clients are using certain drugs.[1] Creatinine is a normal waste product related to creatine phosphate, a mechanism of regenerating adenosine triphosphate in skeletal muscle. Normally, the amount of creatinine in the blood is kept at a normal level by clearance in the kidneys. Because release of creatinine into the blood from muscle remains constant, a rise in serum creatinine usually represents a decline in the kidney's capacity for excreting wastes.

The rise in creatinine levels is directly correlated with the amount of loss of nephron function. With aging, a decrease in lean body mass (muscle tissue), may result in decreasing creatinine values. However, serum creatinine may remain normal in an older person even with significant declines in creatinine clearance and renal function because of the decline in lean body mass.

Causes for elevated creatinine may include glomerulonephritis, pyelonephritis, acute tubular necrosis, obstruction by prostate disease or kidney stones, or decreased renal blood flow. Creatinine may also be elevated as a result of excessive release of creatine caused by muscle injury.

BUN also rises with decreased renal function, caused in particular by decreased renal blood flow, as opposed to decreased glomerular filtration (creatinine). Because BUN reflects a balance of nitrogen added to the blood and excreted by the kidney, BUN may be elevated by increased protein catabolism or dietary intake of protein.

Gastrointestinal bleeding will increase BUN because of the breakdown of protein from the blood within the gastrointestinal tract. The synthesis of urea also depends on the liver. People with severe primary liver disease will have a decreased BUN. With combined liver and renal disease (as occurs in hepatorenal syndrome), the BUN can be normal, not because renal excretory function is good, but because poor hepatic functioning resulted in decreased formation of urea. Failure of the liver to convert nitrogen from amino acids to urea results in accumulation of ammonia, which is discussed in "Comprehensive Metabolic Panel: Blood Ammonia" section.

Blood Glucose

In addition to being part of the BMP, blood glucose may be measured under particular conditions to diagnose a suspected alteration in glucose homeostasis. Table 40-3 lists reference values for glucose testing. BMP glucose testing only reflects the blood glucose at the time the sample is obtained. Understanding how well a person manages glucose requires testing the body's ability to clear glucose from the blood over time, whereas a blood draw for BMP may be done at random times with respect to eating.

Individuals may be allowed to have a blood glucose concentration above normal for exercise (up to 240 mg/dL), but blood glucose below 100 is considered unsafe because of the risk of driving blood glucose even farther below normal. A value below 60 may cause diabetic shock and a value above 300 may lead to ketoacidosis with strenuous exercise. Release of glucose from the liver during exercise in the presence of already elevated blood glucose (above 240 mg/dL) is feared to lead to further increase and therefore, exercise with a value above 240 is considered risky.

Signs of hypoglycemia are related to activation of the sympathetic nervous system as a compensation for low blood sugar and to signs of decreased neural function. These signs include diaphoresis, tachycardia, increased respiratory rate, hypotension, inability to follow commands, tingling, visual changes, seizures, and unresponsiveness. Signs of hyperglycemia are related to dehydration and acidosis. They include lethargy, acetone breath, dehydration, polyuria, thirst, lethargy, confusion, nausea and vomiting, weak rapid pulse, and Kussmaul breathing, which is a deep, rapid, labored breathing pattern unique to ketoacidosis.

Fasting blood sugar, as the name implies, is done after fasting (at least 8 hours). Not eating overnight should allow blood sugar to fall to normal, whereas a random measurement as part of the BMP may be elevated from eating close to the time of the test. Another test is the *2-hour postprandial blood sugar*; 2 hours should be sufficient time for blood glucose to return to normal following eating. A more rigorous test of the ability to clear glucose from the blood is the *oral glucose tolerance test*. This test involves consumption of a fixed amount of glucose and measurement of blood glucose at fixed intervals afterward to determine how quickly blood sugar can be brought back to normal. A person with a normal response will have a modest elevation in blood glucose after 1 hour and a return to normal by 2 hours. Blood glucose in an individual with either a lack of insulin or lack of insulin response will remain elevated after more than 2 hours.

A test for long-term glycemic control (ability to maintain a steady blood sugar concentration over a period of many days) is glycosylated hemoglobin (HbA1c). The amount of HbA1c measured in the red blood cells (RBCs) depends on the amount of glucose available in the bloodstream over the 120-day life span of the RBC, thereby reflecting the average blood sugar level for the 100- to 120-day period before the test.

The A1c test determines the fraction of hemoglobin containing bound glucose and reflects the average blood glucose concentration over a number of weeks to months, as opposed to the snapshot view provided by blood glucose monitoring. The more glucose the RBC was exposed to, the greater the HbA1c percentage. An important advantage of this test is that the sample is not affected by short-term variations such as food intake, exercise, stress, hypoglycemic agents, or compliance. The HbA1c measurement is now used more frequently than the 2-hour postprandial blood sugar in monitoring people with diabetes.

Oral hypoglycemic agents are usually recommended when A1c levels are greater than 7.0%. Lowering hemoglobin A(1c) to less than 7% reduces the risk of microvascular complications of diabetes, but the importance of maintaining this target in the presence of kidney failure is still under investigation.[54] Although the high analytical quality of the HbA1c test is recognized and accepted, the clinical relevance of this marker regarding risk reduction of cardiovascular morbidity and mortality is still being debated.[26] Fructosamine is an alternative to using HbA1c to identify persons at risk for diabetes[31] and/or monitor long-term control of diabetes mellitus.[31] Fructosamine is formed by the glycosylation of proteins by excessive serum glucose. Whereas HbA1c reflects average blood glucose of 2 to 3 months, fructosamine indicates the average over a 2- to 3-week period because of the shorter life span of individual protein molecules as opposed to RBC life span. Measurement of fructosamine may be preferred in circumstances in which A1c measurement is unavailable or unreliable (such as in the case of disorders of RBCs, hemolytic anemia or chronic blood loss).[32]

Diabetes-related antibodies can be measured to distinguish type 1 from 2 upon diagnosis of diabetes mellitus. Several different antibodies may be responsible for type 1 diabetes mellitus. The ability to determine whether a person has type 1 or 2 diabetes can aid in the treatment protocol and prognosis of the disease, particularly because of the greater risk of ketoacidosis in type 1. See Chapter 11 for further details.

Carbon Dioxide

Carbon dioxide is a byproduct of aerobic metabolism and is intimately involved in the regulation of acid–base balance. Bicarbonate ion is produced in a reaction between carbon dioxide and water, producing bicarbonate and hydrogen ions. Therefore, each bicarbonate ion available to fluids negates the effect of a single hydrogen ion on a fluid's pH. As such, bicarbonate ion acts as a buffer, preventing changes in plasma pH. Low HCO_3^- occurs in conditions that produce metabolic acidosis such as diabetic ketoacidosis and compensation for hypoventilation (respiratory acidosis) in chronic respiratory disease.

Respiratory compensation for metabolic acidosis results in the loss of carbon dioxide from the plasma, which in return, reduces the amount of HCO_3^- in the plasma. The renal system also contributes to pH regulation by altering the amount of H+ that passes in the urine and by synthesizing HCO_3^-. Renal compensation is slower to correct pH, requiring several days, as opposed to the more rapid respiratory response. The ability to regulate pH can be compromised by either respiratory or renal disease. Hypoventilation allows carbon dioxide, and thereby acid, to accumulate. Renal disease decreases the ability of the kidney to selectively alter fluid concentration, usually resulting in acidosis. Table 40-4 provides lab values that indicate whether acidosis or alkalosis is metabolic or respiratory and whether it is compensated or uncompensated. Further discussion of acid–base balance in disease is found in Chapter 5.

Blood lactate is a result of metabolism exceeding what can be supplied by aerobic metabolism. Although this

Table 40-4 Laboratory Values in Acid–Base Disorders*

	ARTERIAL BLOOD			
	pH (7.35-7.45)	PCO₂ (35-45 mm Hg)	HCO₃⁻ (22-26 mEq/L)	Signs
Metabolic Acidosis				
Uncompensated	<7.35	Normal	<22	Headache, fatigue; nausea, vomiting, diarrhea, muscular twitching; convulsions; coma, hyperventilation
Compensated	Normal	<35	<22	Increased respiratory rate
Metabolic Alkalosis				
Uncompensated	>7.45	Normal	>26	Nausea, vomiting, diarrhea, confusion, irritability agitation; muscle twitching, muscle cramping, muscle weakness, paresthesias, convulsions, slow breathing
Compensated	Normal	>45	>26	Decreased respiratory rate
Respiratory Acidosis				
Uncompensated	<7.35	>45	Normal	Headache, diaphoresis, tachycardia, disorientation, agitation, cyanosis, lethargy, ↓ deep tendon reflex
Compensated	Normal	>45	>26	–
Respiratory Alkalosis				
Uncompensated	>7.45	<35	Normal	Rapid, deep respirations, light headedness, muscle twitching, anxiety and fears; paresthesias, cardiac arrhythmia
Compensated	Normal	<35	<22	–

PCO_2, Partial pressure of carbon dioxide.
*See also Table 5-13.
Modified from Goodman CC, Snyder TE: *Differential diagnosis for physical therapists: screening for referral*, ed 4, Philadelphia, 2007, WB Saunders, p. 498.

is usually associated with athletes performing anaerobic exercise, blood lactate can increase significantly in critically ill patients. Lack of cardiac output, anemia, and low hemoglobin saturation may lead to inadequate oxygen transport and promote anaerobic metabolism and lactate accumulation in a resting critically ill patient. Elevated lactate is associated with poor outcomes.

COMPREHENSIVE METABOLIC PANEL

The comprehensive metabolic panel is composed of the BMP with the addition of tests related to liver and other functions. These additional tests may be conducted separately as the liver panel. Decreased liver function is associated with increased risk of infection because of the role of the liver in producing globulins, edema as a result of the requirement for the liver's production of albumin, and excessive coagulation because of the liver's role in producing molecules involved in regulating coagulation.

The liver panel consists of bilirubin, total protein, albumin, and serum enzymes that are altered when liver function is compromised. These tests are aspartate aminotransferase (AST, formerly called serum glutamic-oxaloacetic transaminase), alanine aminotransferase (ALT, formerly called serum glutamic-pyruvic transaminase), lactate dehydrogenase (LDH), γ-glutamyl transferase (GGT), and alkaline phosphatase (ALP).

> **Note to Reader:** Please note that even though these tests are collectively known as the liver panel, diseases of other tissues or organs may cause deviations from the reference values.

Hepatic Function Panel

These tests consist of enzymes that are abundant in hepatocytes (AST, ALT, LDH, GGT, ALP), a substance that indicates the effectiveness of the liver in clearing a product from the blood (bilirubin), and products of the liver (total protein and albumin). Therefore, injury to cells of the liver (hepatocytes) may cause AST, ALT, LDH, GGT, and ALP concentrations in the blood to increase. However, these enzymes are not unique to the liver and individual abnormal values are usually not sufficient to diagnose a particular liver dysfunction. Consequently, physicians rely on various tests and measures in conjunction with clinical observations and other diagnostic tests (Table 40-5).

Measuring transaminases (enzymes) released into the blood from liver cells when they are damaged provides information about liver function and, in particular, the amount of inflammation in the liver. ALT, AST, GGT, and LDH are elevated with injury to hepatocytes. For example, ALT is an enzyme that serves as a sensitive indicator of hepatocellular damage; it is the primary test for detecting hepatitis.

Table 40-5 Laboratory Tests for Liver and Biliary Tract Disease

	Normal Range	Comment
Serum bilirubin		
Direct (conjugated)	0.1-0.3mg/dL	Increased with obstruction
Indirect (unconjugated)	0.2-0.8 mg/dL	Increased with other problems
Total	0.1-1.0 mg/dL	Increased with cirrhosis; hepatitis, hemolytic anemia, jaundice, transfusion reaction
Urine bilirubin	0	—
Serum proteins		
Albumin (A)	3.5-5.0 g/dL	Decreased in liver damage, burns, Crohn disease, SLE, malnutrition (e.g., anorexia nervosa) digoxin (digitalis) toxicity
Globulin (G)	2.5-3.5 g/dL	Increased in hepatitis
Total	6-8.5 g/dL	Decreased in liver damage (synthesis is impaired)
A/G ratio	1.5:1 to 2.5:1	Ratio reverses with chronic hepatitis or other chronic liver disease
Transferrin (iron levels)	250-300 g/dL	Decreased in liver damage, increased in iron deficiency
α-Fetoprotein	6-20 ng/mL	Cancer associated antigen; made by fetus but not by healthy adults value >1000 ng/mg indicates likely hepatocellular carcinoma
Serum enzymes		
AST	8-20 U/L	Increased in liver damage, released by liver when damage occurs to liver cells; increased with primary muscle diseases (e.g., myopathy)
ALT	5-35 U/L	Same as above
LDH	45-90 U/L	Same as above; increased with metastatic disease osteosarcoma
GGT	5-38 U/L	Age- and gender-dependent elevated with significant liver disorder
Alkaline phosphatase	30-85 U/L	Increased with liver tumor, biliary obstruction, rheumatoid arthritis, hyperparathyroidism, Paget disease of bone
Blood ammonia	<75 ng/dL	Great variation in reported values because of methods used; increased in severe liver damage
Coagulation functions		
Prothrombin time	12-15 sec	Prolonged in liver damage; salicylate intoxication, intake of anticoagulants (warfarin), DIC
INR	0.9-1.1 (ratio)	Prolonged in clotting factor, deficiencies (e.g., hemophilia), leukemia, DIC, with administration of heparin
Activated partial thromboplastin time	30-40 sec; therapeutic level 2-25 times normal	
Platelets	150,000-400,000/mm³	May drop when spleen is enlarged from portal hypertension, decreased in DIC and burns; increased with inflammation (see Tables 40-6, 40-12)

AST, Aspartate aminotransferase; *ALT*, alanine aminotransferase; *DIC*, disseminated intravascular coagulation; *LDH*, lactate dehydrogenase; *GGT*, γ-glutamyl transferase; *INR*, international normalized ratio; *SLE*, systemic lupus erythematosus.
Modified from Goodman CC, Snyder TE: *Differential diagnosis for therapists*, ed 5, Philadelphia, 2013.

ALP is related to the bile ducts and is increased when they are blocked and may indicate gallbladder, liver, and bile duct disease,[1] but may also be elevated from increased bone turnover in chronic renal failure.[42] Increased levels of this enzyme may be caused by hyperparathyroidism, Paget disease of bone, or rheumatoid arthritis. It is also elevated in biliary obstruction or with hepatocytic carcinoma.

AST is also abundant in kidney cells. It is used in conjunction with ALT to determine the possible cause of liver injury. LDH is also found in the heart and skeletal muscles and historically had been used for differential diagnosis of chest pain. LDH may be elevated by injury to cancer cells. Therefore, elevated LDH may raise the suspicion of metastatic disease, particularly osteosarcoma.

Elevated bilirubin indicates the inability to clear sufficient bilirubin from the blood, similar to the way BUN and creatinine are instrumental in clearing the kidneys. Bilirubin is measured as either total bilirubin, or direct and indirect bilirubin separately, to determine the cause of elevated bilirubin. Total bilirubin can be elevated by liver disease or other causes such as bile duct occlusion and hemolytic anemia in which the amount of bilirubin to be cleared is elevated by excessive destruction of RBCs. Levels of albumin and total protein reflect the ability of the liver to synthesize proteins.[1]

Total protein and albumin may be decreased because of their excretion in the urine as a result of kidney disease. Therefore, the results of multiple tests must be combined with other clinical data to determine the causes of changes in total protein and albumin. Decreased albumin results in edema, including ascites and pulmonary edema. It also alters the serum concentration of drugs that would normally bind to albumin. Lack of albumin also impairs wound healing and leads to muscle atrophy. Because albumin has a half-life of 18 to 20 days, production of proteins by the liver may be impaired for several days before showing up in a comprehensive metabolic panel. If malnutrition is suspected, prealbumin with a half-life of 24 to 48 hours may be measured to give an indication of the direction that albumin concentration is heading.

The albumin-to-globulin ratio (A/G) may provide additional information to the comprehensive metabolic panel. The ratio of albumin to globulin is normally slightly greater than 1.0. The ratio may change either from an increase or decrease in albumin or globulin,

Table 40-6	Complete Blood Count	
Abbreviation	**Measure of**	**Significance**
Leukocytes (WBCs)	Total number of WBCs; fight infection and react against foreign bodies or tissues	*Decreased:* infection, bone marrow suppression or failure (e.g., following neoplastic chemotherapy/radiotherapy, bone marrow infiltrative diseases), AIDS, alcoholism, diabetes, autoimmune diseases; lowest in morning *Increased:* indicates infection, inflammation, tissue necrosis, leukemia, tissue trauma or stress (physical or emotional), burns, thyroid storm, dehydration
Red blood cells (RBCs)	Erythrocyte (red cell count)	*Decreased:* anemia, blood loss, dietary insufficiency of iron and vitamins essential in RBC production, chemotherapy, various disorders/disease (e.g., Hodgkin disease, multiple myeloma, leukemia, SLE, rheumatic fever, endocarditis) *Increased:* polycythemia vera, dehydration, severe diarrhea, poisoning, pulmonary fibroses, high altitude, chronic heart disease
	Hematocrit (Hct) is percentage of whole blood occupied by RBCs	*Decreased:* anemia caused by blood loss (e.g., gastrointestinal bleeding trauma), nutritional deficiency (e.g., folate, iron, vitamin B_{12}), leukemia, hyperthyroidism cirrhosis, hemolytic reaction (e.g., blood transfusion, chemicals or drugs, severe burns, prosthetic heart valve) *Increased:* erythrocytosis, polycythemia, severe dehydration, shock caused by severe dehydration or burns, cor pulmonale
	Hemoglobin (Hb) measures O_2-carrying capacity of RBCs	*Decreased:* hemoglobinopathy (e.g., sickle cell disease), pregnancy, hyperthyroidism, some medications (e.g., antibiotics, antineoplastic drugs, aspirin, rifampin, sulfonamides), cirrhosis, severe hemorrhage, severe burns, systemic disease (e.g., Hodgkin disease, leukemia, lymphoma, SLE, sarcoidosis) *Increased:* living in high altitudes, some medications (e.g., gentamicin, methyldopa [Aldomet]), COPD, congestive heart failure, dehydration, polycythemia vera
Platelets (thrombocytes)	Clotting potential	*Decreased:* anemia, use of antibiotics, toxic effect of many drugs (e.g., antiinflammatories, steroids), pneumonia and other infections, HIV infection, cancer chemotherapy, bone marrow involvement *Increased:* inflammation, infection, cancer, splenectomy, trauma, rheumatoid arthritis, heart disease, cirrhosis, recovery from bone marrow suppression

AIDS, Acquired immunodeficiency syndrome; *COPD,* chronic obstructive pulmonary disease; *HIV,* human immunodeficiency virus; *SLE,* systemic lupus erythematosus.

suggesting a number of potential problems. A/G may be decreased by underproduction of albumin as a result of liver disease, loss of albumin as a result of nephrotic syndrome, or excessive production of globulins in multiple myeloma and autoimmune disorders. The ratio can be increased by diminished immunoglobulin production caused by either genetic disorders or some forms of leukemia. Abnormal A/G requires further investigation into the cause.[37]

Blood Ammonia

Ammonia is an intermediate product of breaking down amino acids. Severe liver injury results in the inability to convert ammonia into urea to be excreted by the kidneys and leads to accumulation of ammonia. Ammonia accumulation because of hepatic disease may result in hepatic encephalopathy, including confusion, lethargy, dementia, daytime sleepiness, tremors, deterioration of fine motor skills, and speech impairment. Ammonia may be tested if hepatic encephalopathy or Reye syndrome is suspected as a cause of unexplained mental status or coma. A combination of elevated ammonia and decreased glucose in a child is indicative of Reye syndrome.

Other causes of elevated ammonia may include gastrointestinal bleeding and genetic defects in the enzymes of the urea cycle.[1] Table 40-5 lists reference values and interpretations for the hepatic function panel and ammonia. When liver dysfunction results in increased serum ammonia and urea levels, peripheral nerve function can also be impaired. Asterixis and numbness or tingling (misinterpreted as carpal or tarsal tunnel syndrome) can occur as a result of this ammonia abnormality causing intrinsic nerve pathologic findings (see further discussion in Chapter 17).

COMPLETE BLOOD COUNT

The complete blood count (CBC) is a common laboratory test performed routinely in many clinical settings. Although the term *complete* is commonly used, different degrees of detail are available. The term *CBC* implies that RBCs (erythrocytes), WBCs (leukocytes), and platelets are counted from a sample of blood. CBC is an automated test that provides results regarding the concentration of RBCs, WBCs, and platelets.

Table 40-6 lists normal and abnormal values related to blood testing with a number of potential causes and

Table 40-7	Complete Blood Count Reference Values				
Age	**WBCs (cells/mm³)**	**RBCs (10⁶/mm³)**	**Erythrocyte Sedimentation Rate (ESR; mm/hr)**	**Hematocrit (Hct; %)**	**Hemoglobin (Hb; g/dL)**
Newborn	18,000-40,000 (drops to adult levels in 2-3 wk)	5.5-6.0	–	Up to 60	17-19
Children	4500-14,500 (varies with age)	4.6-4.8 (varies with age)	1-13	30-49 (varies with age)	14-17
Adult men	4500-11,000	4.5-5.3	0-17*	37-39	13-18
Adult women	4500-11,000	4.1-5.1	1-25†	36-46	12-16
Pregnant women	4500-16,000	Slightly lower	44-114 (increases because of increase serum globulins and fibrinogen)	Decreases in third trimester because of hemodilution	11-12

*Upper limit for men after age 50 years is 20.
†Upper limit for women after age 50 years is 30.
Data from Corbett J: *Laboratory tests and diagnostic procedures with nursing diagnoses,* ed 8, Upper Saddle River, NJ, 2012, Prentice Hall Health.

the consequences of abnormal values. A simple count of RBCs, WBCs, and platelets may be sufficient for determining the appropriate level of mobilization and exercise. Table 40-7 lists reference values for the CBC.

Red Blood Cells

RBC count, and simpler forms of assessing the capacity of the blood to carry oxygen such as hemoglobin concentration (Hb) or hematocrit (Hct) correlate with a person's endurance and orthostatic tolerance. A relative decrease in the capacity of blood to carry oxygen is termed *anemia*. Several additional tests may be required to determine the cause of anemia, including intrinsic factor, and vitamin B_{12} and folic acid, which are necessary for erythropoiesis. Mean cell volume, mean cell Hb, red cell distribution width (variation in RBC size), presence of immature cells (reticulocytes), and ferritin may be necessary to diagnose the cause of anemia.

Ferritin is an intracellular store of iron. Its value declines in anemia caused by chronic iron deficiency and severe protein depletion that may occur in conditions such as burns or malnutrition. Elevation of ferritin is also used as an indicator of states of chronic iron excess such as hemochromatosis.[1]

Men with essential hypertension may have a syndrome known as insulin-resistance–associated hepatic iron overload syndrome, which is characterized by increased iron stores and metabolic abnormalities.[52] In general, individuals with elevated ferritin are at increased risk for insulin-resistance syndrome.[19,77] Ferritin can also be elevated in conditions that do not reflect iron stores, such as acute inflammatory diseases, infections, and metastatic malignancies.

White Blood Cells

WBC count can be provided as a total, a count of individual types of leukocytes, or subtypes of leukocytes. WBCs may either increase or decrease in disease. In general, an increase suggests infection or other inflammatory response. WBC count may decrease as a result of bone marrow disease or chemotherapy for either cancer or to prevent transplant rejection.

The primary therapy implications are related to the presence of infection with elevated leukocyte count (leukocytosis) or risk of patients/clients becoming infected with a low WBC count (leukopenia). In particular, neutropenia is a risk factor for nosocomial infection. Facility policy may require supply of individual equipment, air filtration systems, gowning, gloving, and facemasks.[75]

Platelets

Indications for platelet count include unexplained bruising and long coagulation time. Increased platelet count is termed *thrombocytosis*. Although uncommon, it may be caused by splenectomy, some forms of leukemia, other forms of cancer, and iron-deficiency anemia. Decreases in platelet count (thrombocytopenia) are much more likely to be found in clinical situations.

Platelet count is decreased by excessive bleeding, coagulation disorders, autoimmune disorders, or histocompatibility problems caused by transfusion of incompatible platelets, bone marrow diseases such as aplastic anemia, some forms of leukemia, multiple myeloma, and other cancer involving the bone marrow. In addition, chronic bleeding, autoimmune disease, and drugs that suppress cell production by the bone marrow such as cancer or other chemotherapies may be causes of thrombocytopenia.[33,69]

Thrombocytopenia increases the risk of bleeding into muscles and joints with activity. Caution should be taken with manual therapy, wound debridement, physical therapy modalities and equipment that may cause minor trauma such as blood pressure cuffs, pneumatic therapies, compression hose, elastic or resistive bands, cuff weights, and heavy lifting in general. The person's cognition, safety awareness, strength, balance, and coordination become more important considerations with low platelet counts.

Table 40-8	Complete Blood Count: Exercise Guidelines (Adult)*	
White blood cell (WBC) count	<1000/mm³	No exercise*; wear protective mask
	<5000/mm³ or 10,000 with fever	No exercise permitted*
	4,800-10,800 mm³	Normal reference range; no activity restriction in healthy adults but some modifications may be needed in clients who are ill or during recovery after chemotherapy
Hematocrit (Hct)	>5000/mm³	Light exercise: progress to resistive exercise as tolerated
	<25%	No exercise permitted
	>25%	Light exercise permitted
	30%-32%	Add resistive exercise as tolerated
Hemoglobin (Hb)	<8 g/dL	No exercise permitted
	8-10 g/dL	Light exercise permitted
	>10 g/dL	Resistive exercise permitted
Platelets	<20,000/mm³	No exercise†
Prothrombin time (PT)	Values ≥2.5 times the reference range	Physical and occupational therapy contraindicated
Clients receiving anticoagulant therapy (PT)	INR ≥2.5-3.0	Consult with physician (treat this value as a precaution or red flag for consultation rather than a strict "do not treat" guideline); INR between 4 and 5: individual may be allowed to participate in familiar exercise routine; INR greater than 6 requires bed rest until corrected (Tuzson 2009). For an excellent review of this topic see Tuzson (2009).

INR, International normalized ratio.

The definition of exercise is not standard when applying these lab values. The therapist must keep in mind that what constitutes "aerobic exercise" for one individual (e.g., getting on and off the toilet) may not raise the heart rate of someone else who is in good condition. The recommendation for "no exercise" must be interpreted carefully as well, and does not necessarily mean "no physical therapy." Practicing safe bed-to-commode transfers, gait in room or hallway, and activities of daily living may be appropriate and indicated when lab values fall into the "no exercise" category.

*Any of these exercise guidelines are only meant as a general recommendation, especially those that indicate "no exercise." The therapist must make individual determinations depending on the total picture taking into consideration the consequences of treatment versus no treatment, client's age, general health status, and disease or condition present. For example, someone with an acute episode of urinary tract infection with altered WBC count and fever would be treated differently from someone with a chronic condition, such as diabetes mellitus. An important question to ask yourself is: Will the person fare better or worse with physical therapy intervention? Consult with the physician and other members of the team for guidance and restrictions when needed.

†See Table 40-9.

Data from Garritan S, Jones P, Kornberg T, Parkin C: Laboratory values in the intensive care unit, *Acute Care Perspectives, Newsletter of the Acute Care/Hospital Clinical Practice Section,* APTA, Winter 1995; and Tuzson A: How high is too high? *Acute Care Perspectives* 18(1):8–11, 2009.

Table 40-8 provides guidelines for exercise related to CBC values and Table 40-9 provides more specific guideline for anyone with thrombocytopenia. As noted in the introduction, these guidelines should be used in conjunction with clinical judgment and in consultation with other responsible health care providers.

BLOOD TESTS

Tests may be conducted on characteristics and subpopulations of different cells to determine the causes of altered blood counts. Bone marrow disease may be suspected for a number of reasons, particularly a global decrease of blood cells (pancytopenia).

Aspiration of bone marrow may also be required when cancer involving the bone marrow is suspected.[62] Bone marrow aspiration or biopsy allows evaluation of blood formation (hematopoiesis) by quantifying blood elements and precursor blood cells, as well as any abnormal or malignant cells.

Tests of Red Blood Cells

Symptoms of anemia may be present in spite of normal RBC count, or the cause of anemia may need to be identified. Therefore more specific testing of RBCs may be needed. These include tests of RBC size, shape, maturity, and the type and concentration of Hb inside them.

Hematocrit

Hct is a simple test involving a small quantity of blood that can be obtained with a simple skin prick. The blood is drawn into a small pipette and placed into a centrifuge to determine the relative volume of RBCs expressed as the percentage of total volume of the blood sample occupied by RBCs. This test is a quick screen for anemia. A low Hct is indicative of anemia, but anemia could still exist in the presence of a normal *relative* volume of RBCs. A condition of excessive numbers of RBCs is termed *polycythemia*. It may be present with dehydration (relative loss of water from the blood) or as a response to hypoxemia caused by chronic pulmonary disease or living at a high altitude. Polycythemia vera is a disease in which Hct is elevated and is discussed in Chapter 14. Hct values that are even slightly out of the normal range put older adults at increased risk for heart problems and even death when undergoing major surgery.[78] Note that the Wu 2007 study[78] demonstrated increased mortality with both anemia and polycythemia.

Hemoglobin

Because Hb is packaged in RBCs, the relative volume of red cells (Hct) and the concentration of molecules carrying oxygen in the blood are usually highly correlated. However, certain disease states may allow normal numbers of RBCs, but result in reduced concentration of Hb

Table 40-9	Exercise Guidelines for Thrombocytopenia*
Platelet Count (cells/mm³)	**Exercise**
>150,000 (normal range: 150,000-450,000)	Normal activity (unrestricted)
50,000-150,000	Progressive resistive exercise (as tolerated); manual muscle testing without restrictions Swimming Sexual intercourse Low bench stepping Bicycling (no grade; flat only)
20,000-50,000	Active range of motion (AROM) exercise Moderate exercise; light weights Stationary bicycling Walking as tolerated; no prolonged stretching Aquatic therapy
10,000-20,000	Light exercise; no resistive training or exercise; avoid Valsalva AROM exercise only Walking as tolerated; guard carefully, especially on stairs Aquatic therapy with physician approval
Less than 10,000	Some advocate no exercise, others permit AROM exercise Restricted to activities of daily living; walking with physician approval; dependent upon individual risk factors and characteristics

*These guidelines vary from institution to institution; the therapist should check with each facility for its specific guidelines. Some therapists working in oncology settings report a more liberal exercise guideline. For example, in some centers, restriction to active range of motion and activities of daily living is indicated only when platelet counts drop below 5000/mm³. See also comments regarding exercise and decision making at the bottom of Table 40-8.

within individual cells. Therefore a person with normal Hct may have reduced Hb concentration. Hct and Hb concentration are frequently tested simultaneously. When done this way, the term *H&H* is generally used.

Mean corpuscular Hb concentration is used to determine whether RBCs have reduced Hb concentration within them. This test would not be necessary if Hct and Hb concentration show the same changes from normal or both were normal.

Mean corpuscular volume is also used in the differential diagnosis of anemia. Different disease states may increase mean corpuscular volume, such as vitamin B_{12} or folic acid deficiency (macrocytic anemia), or mean corpuscular volume may be decreased as in iron-deficiency anemia (hypochromic anemia) or other causes of decreased cell volume (microcytic anemia).

Hb levels of 12 to 16 g/dL are considered normal, but studies show that older adults with a low-normal value of 12 g/dL are more likely to have difficulty performing daily tasks. Mild anemia may cause significant functional problems. Difficulty walking, climbing stairs, or doing house or yard work may be an early sign of low-normal Hb levels.[10]

In individuals with anemia, we expect to find decreased tolerance of activity and upright positioning, dyspnea, tachycardia, and subjective complaints of fatigue/feeling weak. Severe anemia may also produce angina in some individuals. H&H alone may not be sufficient predictors of a person's tolerance of activity. In particular, individuals with chronic anemia may have much better tolerance than those with more acute anemia.

In most people with anemia, exercise and upright positioning will need to be progressed more gradually with close monitoring of vital signs. In some cases of anemia, Borg's Rating of Perceived Exertion may be a better predictor of exercise tolerance than heart rate alone.

In hospitalized patients, a decrease in Hb to 8 or below should trigger discussion with the patient's nurse and physician concerning activity level and need for transfusion or other interventions to improve Hb. However, note that the number of transfusions received by a patient is an independent predictor of patient outcome. As the number of transfusions received by a patient increases, patients have longer ICU stays, longer hospital stays, increased mortality, and more complications.[11] Anemia is common in patients in ICUs. Although trauma and bleeding may produce anemia in many patients seen in an ICU, most cases of anemia in ICUs are not a result of bleeding, but are the effects of inflammatory cytokines associated with poor health suppressing RBC production.

Red Blood Cell Shape

The normal biconcave disc of RBCs may be altered in a number of diseases. The crescent shape of RBCs may be seen microscopically to confirm the diagnosis of sickle cell disease. A number of rare genetic diseases may also alter the shape of RBCs. For example, hereditary spherocytosis, as the name implies, allows red cells to take on a spherical shape.

Reticulocyte Count

Immature RBCs are termed *reticulocytes*. Increased numbers of reticulocytes in the blood indicate compensation by the bone marrow for RBC loss, typically as a result of bleeding. This condition is termed *reticulocytosis*.

Iron

Iron is required for the synthesis of Hb. Lack of iron results in small, hypochromic (pale) RBCs that cannot carry as much oxygen as normal. Iron status is determined by serum transferrin receptor assay[51] and serum ferritin.[12] Iron-deficiency anemia is discussed further in Chapter 14.

Vitamin B_{12} and Folic Acid

Both of these vitamins are critical to the production of RBCs. Deficiency results in release of large immature RBCs from the bone marrow. Vitamin B_{12} is obtained from ingesting animal protein and requires intrinsic factor, which is produced by the gastric mucosa for absorption in the distal part of the ileum. When absorption of vitamin B_{12} is inadequate because of a malabsorption syndrome or from lack of intrinsic factor, pernicious anemia may develop.

Vitamin B_{12} shots may be recommended when serum levels are too low. Folic acid (folate), one of the B vitamins, is also necessary for normal function of RBCs and WBCs and for the adequate synthesis of certain purines and pyrimidines, which are precursors to deoxyribonucleic acid (DNA). As with vitamin B_{12}, folate depends on normal absorption in the intestinal mucosa.

Haptoglobin may be used in the work up for anemia. Haptoglobin is a protein produced by the liver that binds free Hb in the blood. As it binds Hb it is cleared by the liver. Haptoglobin will decrease in the presence of hemolytic anemia as more haptoglobin binds Hb and is removed from the blood by the liver. Haptoglobin will also decrease if liver disease results in decreased production of haptoglobin and diminished uptake haptoglobin bound to Hb by the liver.

Erythrocyte Sedimentation Rate

Although not related to anemia, erythrocyte sedimentation rate (ESR) is clustered with other tests of RBCs and is presented in Table 40-7. ESR is a nonspecific test for inflammatory disorders, which is associated with a number of potential disorders including cancer, autoimmune diseases, and infection. As the name implies, the test is based on how quickly RBCs sink to the bottom of a test solution containing anticoagulated (unclotted) blood. ESR is increased in the sense that sedimentation is more rapid (more cells sink to the bottom per time) when they clump together.

Clumping is caused by a change in blood proteins brought on by inflammation, specifically the presence of globulins or fibrinogen in the blood. The more severe the inflammation, the faster the sedimentation rate or settling of cells and the higher the ESR; a significant increase in the ESR warrants closer investigation.

By itself, this test is nonspecific and therefore not diagnostic for any particular organ disease or injury, but the ESR may be used as a screening test to rule out certain diseases or to monitor treatment in specific diseases such as juvenile rheumatoid arthritis, Kawasaki disease, temporal arteritis, gout, and polymyalgia rheumatica. It can be used as an index of musculoskeletal dysfunction such as tissue injury or inflammation or bone infections.

ESR is a fairly reliable indicator of the course of many diseases and, therefore, may be used to monitor the course of such diseases or responses to treatment of these diseases. In general, as the disease worsens, the ESR increases and as the disease improves, the ESR decreases. ESR also increases with age.[5,67]

White Blood Cell Tests

Various disease states are characterized by their effects on specific types of WBCs. The elevation or depression of one type may be useful in diagnosis. A CBC can demonstrate a normal level, a decreased level (leukopenia), or an elevated level (leukocytosis). Leukopenia can result from cancer, cancer chemotherapy, aplastic anemia and other causes. Leukocytosis is produced primarily by infection and in some forms of leukemia. Both the absolute numbers and the numbers of white cells relative to each other can be useful in diagnosis. An analysis of the relative numbers of different types of white cells is known as a white cell differential or *diff*.

Neutrophils

Neutrophils normally represent the majority of WBCs present in the blood. A decreased number is termed *neutropenia* and an increased number is termed *neutrophilia*. Neutropenia is clinically significant as a risk factor for infection and may result from a large number of causes. In general, neutrophilia suggests the presence of infection.

Because of their appearance, neutrophils are also called polymorphonuclear (PMN) cells. Mature cells are segmented (called segs), whereas immature cells appear to be banded (bands). Bands make up approximately 3% to 5% of WBCs and circulate for about 6 hours before they mature into segmented neutrophils. During counting, PMNs are divided into bands and segs. The presence of relatively high numbers of immature PMNs (bands) indicates rapid production of neutrophils in response to events such as acute infection, necrosis, or autoimmune disease. This may be referred to as a left shift because of the historic method of hand counting the white cell differential.

Absolute neutrophil count (ANC) is determined by multiplying the WBC count by the percentage of cells that are neutrophils. ANC is an indication of a person's ability to prevent infection. This measurement is particularly important for individuals receiving cancer chemotherapy and those who have received bone marrow transplants. Individuals with low ANC may be placed on neutropenic precautions. These precautions include protective isolation and either not allowing the individual to leave the individual's room or a requirement to wear a mask. Neutropenic precautions may be put into effect with a WBC count less than 1000 or an ANC less than 500/μL.[38]

Basophils, Eosinophils, and Monocytes

Basophils are implicated in immune responses, particularly allergies. Eosinophils are elevated (*eosinophilia*) in the presence of certain disease states, worm infestation, or allergies. Monocytes are blood cells that migrate into tissues as needed during injury or infection. After migration they are referred to as macrophages. Chapter 7 describes the role of macrophages in immunity.

Lymphocytes

(See complete description and discussion in Chapter 7.)

Lymphocytes are divided into B cells (capable of producing antibodies) and T cells that either produce toxic granules containing powerful enzymes to destroy pathogen-infected or otherwise damaged cells (cytotoxic or killer T cells), produce direct injury to cells carrying foreign markers (helper T cells), or assist in modulating B- and T-cell function (regulator T cells). A third type of lymphocyte (natural killer [NK] cells) is part of the innate immune system; NK cells respond to common patterns on antigens rather than (like B and T cells) requiring an antigen-presenting cell to initiate action.

Interest in lymphocyte subtypes is primarily a result of the effect of acquired immunodeficiency syndrome (AIDS) on particular subtypes of WBCs. In particular, helper T cells are vulnerable to human immunodeficiency virus (HIV) destruction, resulting in immunosuppression. The relative populations of each is determined by the presence of cell markers denoted CD2, CD4, CD8, and CD19. Cytotoxic (killer) T cells have CD2; helper T cells have CD4; regulatory T cells have CD8; and B cells are detected by CD19. Table 40-10 lists the relative numbers of these cells. Table 40-11 lists the potential indications of varying proportions in the WBC differential.

HEMOSTASIS

The process of hemostasis is described in Chapter 14. Both excessive and deficient hemostasis can lead to problems. Tests relevant to hemostasis involve platelets; enzymes required to initiate, promote, or inhibit hemostasis; binding of coagulation factors; and calcium. Platelets are discussed in the previous section on CBC. Lab values related to tests of coagulation listed in Table 40-12 are referred to as the coagulation profile. Coagulation tests are important to determine whether the person clots too easily or does not clot sufficiently to prevent excessive bleeding.

In addition to thrombocytopenia, disorders such as hemophilia, von Willebrand disease, and bone marrow suppression may lead to excessive bleeding. Therefore, coagulation status should be known before therapy that might cause bleeding is performed. This might include resistance exercise, activities with risk of falling, or sharp debridement.

Patients/clients may be anticoagulated for a number of reasons. When individuals are treated for venous thrombosis, atrial fibrillation, or coronary artery disease, they may become overly anticoagulated and bleed excessively. Tests for coagulation involve the function of the terminal products of the coagulation cascade. As discussed in Chapter 6, coagulation factors interact and result in the production of thrombin, which activates the reaction to convert fibrinogen to fibrin. The tests in the next section evaluate bleeding time, but because of how the test is performed, the tests indicate the effectiveness of different mechanisms within the coagulation cascade.

Tests of Coagulation

Several tests are related to coagulability. Historically, prothrombin time (PT) and activated partial thromboplastin time (aPTT) have been used to determine coagulability either diagnostically or to monitor anticoagulant therapy with heparin and warfarin. These medications are used for many conditions, including atrial fibrillation; prevention of acute myocardial infarction (MI) in people with peripheral arterial disease; prevention of stroke, recurrent MI, or death in people who have had an MI; valvular heart disease (native and prosthetic); and venous thromboembolism (prevention or treatment).[13,27]

The international normalized ratio (INR) was developed to provide PT results that would not vary between laboratories. Individuals receiving anticoagulation therapy because of coronary artery disease, cerebrovascular disease, atrial fibrillation, history of deep venous thrombosis, and other reasons are anticoagulated to an INR of 2 to 3.[22]

As INR increases, however, the risk of bleeding with minor trauma increases and excessive bleeding may occur during surgery, as well as spontaneous bleeding. Note, however, that INR and other tests of coagulation are tests of how quickly a person will coagulate with a standardized stimulus; they are not tests of whether a person will bleed with trauma. Therefore, some people may experience excessive bleeding with minor trauma at a therapeutic INR and others with supratherapeutic INR may not experience significant bleeding episodes with trauma.

Within the past few years, low-molecular-weight heparins (LMWHs) have been developed. In spite of the greater cost, use of LMWHs has increased because of the more rapid onset of anticoagulation, lower risk of platelet-dependent thrombus formation,[25] and less prolongation of bleeding time indices.[20,46]

Although INR has been an effective test for anticoagulation produced by unfractionated heparin (an historically

Table 40-10	T- and B-Cell Lymphocyte Surface Markers	
Surface Markers	**Reference Value**	
T cells (CD2)	95%	
Helper T cells (CD4)	24%-62%	
Suppressor T cells (CD8)	19%-65%	
B cells (CD19)	4%-25%	
T helper–to–suppressor cell ratio	0.5-2.0	

Data from Corbett JV: *Laboratory tests and diagnostic proceedings*, ed 8, Upper Saddle River, NJ, 2012, Prentice Hall Health.

Table 40-11	Differential White Blood Cell Count Reference Values		
Cell	**Function**	**Absolute Count (cells/mm³)**	**Differential Count (%)**
Neutrophils (PMNs, polyps, segs, bands)	Segmented or mature neutrophils are WBCs that constitute a defense against foreign substances (usually bacterial infection); band cells are immature neutrophils that may be called up from bone marrow to help fight severe (usually bacterial) infections	1800-7000*	50-60
Lymphocytes	Produce antibodies, fight tumor cells, and respond to viral infection	1500-4000	30-40
Monocytes	Clean up debris after neutrophils have done their job	0-800	1-9
Eosinophils	Attack parasites and play a role in asthma and allergy	0-450	0-3
Basophils	Release histamines during allergic reactions	0-200	0-1

*Level less than 500 is referred to as *nadir;* individuals undergoing chemotherapy may exhibit an ANC nadir because of bone marrow suppression.

Table 40-12	Coagulation Profile (Platelets)			
		COAGULATION STUDY		
Age	**Platelet Count (cells/mm³)**	**International Normalized Ratio (INR)**	**Prothrombin Time (PT)**	**Activated Partial Thromboplastin Time (aPTT)**
Premature infant	100,000-300,000			
Newborn	150,000-300,000			
Infant	200,000-475,000			
Child	150,000-400,000			
Adult, older	150,000-400,000	0.9-1.1 (ratio)*	12-15 sec	30-40 sec

*Minimal interlaboratory variability.

manufactured heparin consists of a wide range of sizes of individual heparin molecules as opposed to LMWH) and warfarin, aPTT is used to monitor the effectiveness of LMWH. Therapeutic INR takes days to reach with unfractionated heparin or warfarin and is related more to extrinsic coagulation pathway, whereas LMWH can reduce coagulability much more rapidly as measured by aPTT, which is a better measure of intrinsic coagulation pathway.

Heparin anti-Xa is an alternative test that can be used to assess the effectiveness of both unfractionated and LMWH. Heparin impairs the coagulation sequence primarily through inhibiting coagulation factors Xa and thrombin. Whereas unfractionated heparin exerts its effect through both factors Xa and thrombin and has more variable effects on coagulation, LMWH acts primarily on factor Xa and produces a more predictable anticoagulant effect. Although routine monitoring of LMWH is not needed to the extent that it is needed for unfractionated heparin, heparin anti-Xa is preferred for special circumstances such as during pregnancy, in the presence of kidney disease, or other populations.

Heparin anti-Xa may also be used for some individuals who do not respond as expected to heparin because of an underlying disorder such as lupus, which affects partial thromboplastin time.[23]

Side effects of heparin in addition to excessive bleeding include hypersensitivity reaction, osteopenia in elderly or bed-bound patients and heparin-induced thrombocytopenia. Heparin-induced thrombocytopenia is caused by heparin-dependent platelet activating antibodies that cause a paradoxical thrombosis as a result of release of microparticles from platelet surfaces and is potentially fatal. It is more common with unfractionated heparin than with LMWH. Thrombosis occurs prior to the decrease in platelet count. Consequences of heparin-induced thrombocytopenia include deep venous thrombosis, pulmonary embolism, gangrene, MI, cardiovascular accident, skin lesions at injection sites, and disseminate intravascular coagulation. Nonheparin anticoagulants are needed to reduce the risk of thrombosis.

Platelet function tests are separate tests run on specialized devices to determine how well platelets aggregate and initiate the coagulation sequence.[14] These tests may be run either because of increased risk of excessive coagulation or because of deficient coagulation. The tests consist of the time to form a clot (closure time assay), the strength of the clot (viscoelastometry), and the rate of platelet aggregation (end point platelet aggregation assay). Different disorders of coagulation can be determined by the combination of results from these assays.

Components of Coagulation

Specific components of coagulation may be tested on suspicion of their involvement in bleeding disorders. These include specific coagulation factors that produce hemophilia and von Willebrand factor.

Coagulation Factors

Individual factor testing may also be performed as a follow-up to abnormal PT, aPTT, or because of suspected coagulation factor deficiencies. Deficiencies may be genetic, for example, hemophilias A and B, or acquired in conditions such as disseminated intravascular coagulation, liver disease, or vitamin K deficiency.[1,8]

Of particular interest are factors VIII and IX. Genetic defects in the production of these factors produce hemophilia A and B, respectively. Hemophilia B is also known as Christmas disease. Genetic defects may also occur in coagulation factors other than VIII and IX, but are very rare. Abnormal aPTT (intrinsic pathway) with normal PT indicates involvement of factors VIII, IX, XI, or XII, whereas normal aPTT with prolonged PT (extrinsic pathway) suggests factor I, II, V, VII, or X.[1]

von Willebrand disease, a genetic disease like hemophilia, impairs coagulation because of a lack of effective von Willebrand factor, which along with factor VIII, is necessary for binding of platelets to collagen.

Antiphospholipid antibodies are associated with inappropriate coagulation and autoimmune diseases, especially systemic lupus erythematosus. Cardiolipin antibodies are the most common, along with lupus anticoagulant and anti-β_2 glycoprotein I. Cardiolipins are a class of phospholipid molecules found on the membranes of a number of cells, notably platelets.

Antibodies to cardiolipin increase the risk of inappropriate coagulation and are associated with thrombocytopenia, premature labor and preeclampsia. Antiphospholipid syndrome is the term used for the clinical syndrome associated with elevated antiphospholipid antibodies and morbidity resulting from inappropriate clotting and recurrent spontaneous abortion. Secondary antiphospholipid syndrome is secondary to an autoimmune disease such as systemic lupus erythematosus (SLE), whereas primary disease is not.[55]

Regulation of Coagulation

Either excessive or deficient clotting may occur as a consequence of deficiencies or defective components of the system to regulate coagulation. Antithrombin is naturally produced as a means of counterbalancing the coagulation sequence. The balance of thrombin produced by the coagulation cascade and antithrombin produced by the liver determines the likelihood of coagulation/thrombosis.

Antithrombin inhibits both thrombin itself and several of the factors involved in the coagulation cascade that culminates in thrombin production. Antithrombin deficiency can be inherited or acquired. Heterozygous individuals experience episodes of excessive coagulation in early adulthood, whereas homozygous individuals develop excessive coagulation early in life. Antithrombin deficiency can result in either normally functional, but insufficient quantities of antithrombin or in sufficient quantities, but dysfunctional antithrombin. Testing can determine which is the case. Acquired antithrombin deficiency can result from liver disease, disseminated intravascular coagulation, cancer, and nephrotic syndrome.

Proteins C and S are measured in the routine work up for unexplained excessive coagulation. Deficiencies of proteins C and S are both associated with excessive coagulation. These proteins, along with thrombin, are responsible for preventing dysfunction of the coagulation cascade. As the coagulation cascade is activated, the mechanism for halting it is also activated. Thrombin is activated by the coagulation cascade resulting in clotting, but it also combines with thrombomodulin to activate protein C. Activated protein C combines with protein S to degrade factors VIIIa and Va, the factors that are responsible for the production of thrombin itself. When functioning normally, the production of thrombin with an appropriate stimulus leads to coagulation sufficient to stop bleeding and then halting of the coagulation process.

Genetic defects may result in insufficient quantities of either protein C or S, abnormal function of either protein C or S, or increased clearance of protein S with the result that these proteins are not capable of halting thrombin production in a timely manner and either excessive or inappropriate coagulation/thrombosis may occur. The excessive clotting usually occurs in veins, increasing the risk of pulmonary embolism, but can also occur in arteries.[34]

Factor V Leiden mutation and Prothrombin 20210A are genetic mutations associated with increased risk of venous thromboembolism.[71] Tests for these genetic mutations may be performed in the presence of unexplained excessive coagulation or a family history of thrombotic disease. Factor V Leiden is a mutation that results in a form of factor V that degrades more slowly following coagulation and therefore promotes extended coagulation. Factor V Leiden is fairly common (5% of white population). The risk of thromboembolic events is increased three to eight times in heterozygous individuals and 50 to 80 times in those who are homozygous for this gene.

Those who are heterozygous for the Prothrombin 20210A gene produce excess thrombin and have approximately three times the risk of thromboembolic events of those without the gene. This gene is less prevalent and being homozygous for this gene is extremely rare.[17]

D-Dimer

D-dimer is a specific type of fragment produced by lysis of products of coagulation by plasmin. These fragments of crosslinked fibrin are not detectible under normal circumstances, but in the presence of clotting or coagulation, these fibrin degradation products will be released in proportion to the quantities of fibrin and plasmin in the circulation. A negative test for D-dimer suggests a low likelihood of a large thrombus or clot. Elevated D-dimer suggests that possibility of a number of unfavorable coagulation conditions including pulmonary embolism, intravascular coagulation in addition to thromboembolism associated with surgery, immobilization, and atherosclerosis. Further testing is required to determine the cause of elevated D-dimer.[36]

Warfarin Sensitivity Testing

Two genotypes, CYP2C9 and VKORC1, are associated with abnormal sensitivity to warfarin (Coumadin). These genetic variations alter the doses necessary to produce optimum anticoagulation with warfarin. Warfarin prevents the recycling of vitamin K, which, in turn, reduces the production of a number of factors in the coagulation cascade, and thereby decreases the risk of coagulation.

Vitamin K epoxide reductase (VKOR) is the protein responsible for the production of clotting factors II, VII, IX, and X. Variations in the gene VKORC1 alter the sensitivity of VKOR to warfarin requiring either an increase or decrease in the normal dose of warfarin to produce the desired anticoagulation response.

Another protein, cytochrome P450 2C9 (CYP2C9) is important because of its role in degrading warfarin. Genetic variations in this gene lead to slower breakdown and greater accumulation of warfarin, which then leads to excessive anticoagulation. Individuals with this gene mutation require a lower dose of warfarin or risk excessive bleeding.[68]

CARDIOVASCULAR LAB TESTS

Tests in this section are related to the diagnosis of heart failure, MI, and assessing the risk of coronary artery disease.

Congestive Heart Failure

Atrial natriuretic peptide was discovered many years ago and found to provide a minor contribution to regulation of body fluid composition. As blood volume increases, stretching the atria, the amount of atrial natriuretic peptide released increases, causing the loss of sodium and water in the urine to correct excessive volume.

A similar peptide, brain natriuretic peptide (BNP), was discovered in the brain. Subsequent research showed that BNP was also found in the ventricles of the heart, but the name was retained. Testing for BNP has gained in popularity. Like atrial natriuretic peptide, BNP is related to excessive blood volume. It is used for differential diagnosis of shortness of breath as BNP is elevated in congestive heart failure.[17,22] A value of greater than 100 pg/mL is considered positive for congestive heart failure. Levels of BNP rise with disease severity, so levels from 100 to 300 pg/mL generally indicate mild heart failure; 300 to 700 pg/mL indicates moderate heart failure; and levels above 700 pg/mL indicate severe heart failure.[65] Even smaller elevations of BNP above normal are indicative of impaired cardiac pump function[25] and future mortality.[73,74] The BNP test can also be used to monitor disease progression in individuals with left-sided heart failure.

Cardiac Enzymes and Markers

As described with the liver panel, injured cells release some of their intracellular enzymes. The greater the damage, the higher the concentration of these enzymes becomes in the blood. The release and clearance of different enzymes after cell injury varies widely. In some cases, enzymes rise rapidly, but also are cleared rapidly. For this reason, more than one enzyme is generally measured for diagnostic purposes, and evaluated in conjunction with clinical signs and symptoms. Table 40-13 lists some of the enzymes released into plasma with injury and which cells (and therefore which organs) are damaged.

Creatine Kinase

Creatine kinase (CK) is a major cytoplasmic enzyme of muscle present in three major isoenzymatic forms—skeletal muscle (MM), brain (BB), and cardiac muscle (MB). CK-MM constitutes more than 90% of serum total CK. Trauma to skeletal muscle can cause CK release, and elevation of total serum CK levels is associated with muscle soreness. Increase in serum CK occurs within 6 to 24 hours of direct muscle injury.[66] Although CK-MB is very specific to myocardial muscle, CK-MB may not reach the threshold required to diagnose MI for several hours.[1] Other tests that provide results more rapidly include troponin and myoglobin.

Myoglobin

Myoglobin is a small protein involved in the transport and storage of oxygen in muscle cells. This molecule leaks out of cells soon after injury. It starts to rise within 2 to 3 hours of a MI and reaches its peak in 8 to 12 hours.[1] However, it falls rapidly back to normal within 1 to 2 days after the MI and thus could be missed as a serum marker of MI if medical attention is delayed. Myoglobin may also be elevated by trauma to muscle, including the use of defibrillators and drugs used in the field to degrade the clots or thrombi responsible for chest pain.

Troponin

Three types of troponin have been described in heart and skeletal muscle—troponin C, T, and I (TnC, TnT, TnI). Enzymes more specific to cardiac muscle are called cTnI and cTnT. The isozymes of troponin used are quite specific for myocardial injury.[57] Normally, these troponin isozymes are found at very low to undetectable levels in the blood. Elevations suggestive of cardiac muscle injury are detectible within 3 to 4 hours and can remain sufficiently elevated for diagnosis up to 14 days, depending on the extent of the cardiac muscle injury.

Slight elevations are indicative of unstable angina or MI[20] and predict whether a person is at risk of having a future coronary event and/or can benefit from early revascularization compared with conservative medical treatment.[47] Those individuals with elevated troponin are also at increased risk for mortality for the next few months.[29,35]

Table 40-13	Serum Isoenzymes and Markers	
Isoenzyme	**Where Found**	**Increased in**
CK-BB	Brain	Central nervous system surgery, cardiac arrest, Reye syndrome, cerebral contusion, cerebrovascular accident, malignant hyperthermia, bowel infarction, renal failure
CK-MB	Myocardium	MI, cardiac contusion, cardiac trauma, congestive heart failure without MI, tachyarrhythmias with underlying coronary artery disease, cardiac surgery, myocarditis
CK-MM	Skeletal muscle	Intramuscular injections, skeletal muscle trauma, extreme muscle exertion, tonic clonic seizures, surgery, excess alcohol (toxic effect on muscle), alcohol withdrawal syndrome, seizures, electric countershock, muscular dystrophy, severe hypokalemia, hypothyroidism, extreme hypothermia or hyperthermia
LDH-1	Heart, kidney, red blood cells	MI, cardiac contusion or trauma, myocarditis, cardiac surgery; also, renal disease and infarction, hemolysis, hemolytic anemia, hemolysis with prosthetic heart valves, leukemia, pernicious or megaloblastic anemia
LDH-2	Almost all tissues except skeletal muscle	Injury to any tissue except skeletal muscle
Troponins (I, T, C)	Contractile proteins found in heart and skeletal muscle	MI (specific isoforms or troponin I and T)
Myoglobin	Skeletal and cardiac muscle	Immediate rise when cardiac or skeletal muscle is damaged

CK-BB, -MB, -MM, Creatinine kinase subunits; *LDH*, lactate dehydrogenase.

Although cardiac troponins are more specific than CK-MB and myoglobin, cardiac troponins may be elevated for reasons other than MI. They may be slightly elevated with vigorous exercise (e.g., marathon), traumatic injury (including defibrillation, ablation, cardiac surgery), inflammatory disease involving the heart, high-dose chemotherapy, sepsis, or accumulation in the blood secondary to kidney disease. This may not be significant for an evolving MI, but an elevated troponin level is still an indication of compromised cardiac status and must be evaluated in context of the whole picture (i.e., patient's medical status and physiology, trend or pattern of serial troponin values). Table 40-14 lists reference values for the cardiac isozymes.

Risk Factors for Atherosclerotic Disease

Although lipids are important molecules involved in the storage of energy, production of steroids and bile acids, and maintenance of cell membranes, inappropriate serum levels of certain lipids are associated with atherosclerotic vascular disease. Those of particular interest include triglycerides, cholesterol, and lipoproteins. Several blood lipids are used for screening in certain populations based on age or presence of risk factors.

Lipids

The liver metabolizes cholesterol to its free form, which is then transported in the bloodstream by lipoproteins. Lipid measurements are important in detecting genetically determined disorders of lipid metabolism and in assessing the risk of coronary artery disease and other diseases caused by atherosclerosis. In particular, elevation of low-density lipoprotein (LDL) is a strong predictor of cardiovascular disease. Lower-than-normal levels of high-density lipoprotein (HDL) also increase the risk. In addition to genetic defects associated with elevated LDL, other factors, such as smoking, diet, certain drugs (oral contraceptives, sulfonamides, aspirin, and steroids), hypothyroidism, exercise, and alcohol, alter one or both. A full lipid profile includes total cholesterol, LDL, HDL, and triglycerides (Table 40-15). The tests may also be used to assess the need for and the efficacy of treatment.

For screening purposes, total cholesterol may be used. Unlike HDL, LDL, and triglycerides, total cholesterol does not need to be measured after fasting. Approximately 75% of cholesterol is bound to LDL and 25% to HDL.

LDL can accumulate in the blood as a result of genetic defects in its metabolism by the liver and become incorporated into atherosclerotic plaques, thereby increasing the risk of coronary artery disease, stroke, and other vascular disease. The predictive accuracy of lipoprotein testing is improved by measuring specific subtypes of LDL, especially the very-low-density forms. HDL is associated with removing excess cholesterol from the blood and the risk of coronary artery disease is decreased as HDL concentration increases. Therefore, the combination of high LDL and low HDL indicates a greater risk of coronary artery disease.

Triglycerides are a component of fat and are converted between glycerol, free fatty acids, and monoglycerides within the liver and adipose tissue as the need to either store or release energy arises. The liver can convert glycerol, fatty acids, and monoglycerides back to triglycerides in adipose tissue when the body requires an additional source of energy.

Elevated serum triglyceride will usually occur in conjunction with elevated cholesterol and is a risk factor for atherosclerotic disease. Because cholesterol and triglycerides can vary independently, measurement of both values is more meaningful than the measurement of either substance alone. Elevated levels of triglyceride may require treatment with lipid-lowering medications. Poor glycemic control can also elevate triglycerides. A very high level of triglycerides (1000 mg/dL) is also a risk factor for pancreatitis.[1]

Direct LDL cholesterol (direct LDL-C) as the name implies, measures LDL directly rather than calculating it from measures of total cholesterol, HDL, and cholesterol. In standard serum cholesterol testing, LDL cannot be computed accurately in the presence of high triglyceride concentration either because of a recent meal or a metabolic disorder. Measurement of lipoprotein-associated phospholipase A_2 may also be used to determine risk of heart disease. This substance is produced by macrophages. Lipoprotein-associated phospholipase A_2 in the blood is largely bound to LDL and is speculated to promote the inflammation of blood vessels responsible for atherosclerosis. Table 40-15 lists reference values for the lipid profile.[15]

Homocysteine

Other cardiac markers include homocysteine and C-reactive protein (CRP), which are both risk factors and

Table 40-14	Cardiac Enzymes and Markers (Serum)				
Enzyme	**Normal Range (%)**	**Appears (hr)**	**Peaks (hr)**	**Normalizes (days)**	
CK-MB	<3	3-6	18-24	2-3	
LDH-1	17-27	12-24	48-72	6-12	
LDH-2	23-28	12-24	48-78	6-12	
LDH-1>LDH-2 (flipped ratio)	*	12-24	48-72	6-12	
Myoglobin	50-120 µg/mL	0-2	3+	—	
Troponin I	<0.6 ng/mL	3-6	14-48	7-14	
Troponin T	<0.1 ng/mL	3-6	14-48	7-14	

CK-MB, Creatine kinase submit; *LDH*, lactate dehydrogenase.
*No actual value is reported, only that LDH-1 becomes higher than LDH-2 for a short period.
Data from Corbett J: *Laboratory tests and diagnosis procedures*, ed 8, Upper Saddle River, NJ, 2012, Prentice Hall Health.

cardiac markers. Homocysteine is a naturally occurring amino acid in the blood produced by the breakdown of various proteins in the body. It is related to free radicals, which may be involved in the oxidation of LDL and plaque formation in arteries. Homocysteine levels increase with age; high levels have a significant effect in accelerating the aging process of the arteries caused by atherosclerosis.

Homocysteine is also linked to the development of early arterial changes characteristic of development of Alzheimer disease,[6,7] hypertension,[79] and the risk of stroke.[40,49] An elevated homocysteine level is also an independent risk factor for osteoporotic fractures in older adults.[2] The magnitude of the effect of homocysteine level on fracture risk is similar to its observed effect on the risk of cardiovascular disease and dementia.[18,72]

Because of its role in homocysteine metabolism, methylenetetrahydrofolate reductase mutations C677T and A1298C (MTHFR mutation) are additional genetic risk factors for development of thrombosis or premature cardiovascular disease. These two mutations result in elevated homocysteine. The effect of these mutations depends on which mutation(s) are present and whether the person is heterozygous or homozygous for one or both mutations.

C-Reactive Protein

CRP is produced by the liver in response to the presence of inflammation anywhere in the body. Systemic inflammation has been implicated in the pathogenesis of atherosclerosis and in particular an association with high-sensitivity CRP (hs-CRP). CRP is an indicator of systemic inflammation[61] and may be directly involved in the atherothrombotic process itself.[59]

Clinically, levels of hs-CRP above 3 mg/L indicate elevated risk for MI and stroke, even among apparently healthy individuals with low-to-normal lipid levels.[32] Elevated CRP is an independent predictor of future cardiovascular events that also predicts the risk of hypertension, diabetes, and restenosis after angioplasty.[28,58] Table 40-16 lists the values for these tests.

Half of all heart attacks and strokes in the United States occur in people with normal cholesterol levels, and 20% of all cardiac-related events occur in people with no major risk factors. People with low LDL and high CRP have more cardiovascular events than people with high LDL and low CRP. Using hs-CRP along with traditional methods of measuring risk may help prevent morbidity and mortality associated with vascular disease.[59]

CRP is associated with elevated blood sugar and triglycerides, poor diet, and sedentary lifestyle. Genetic factors may also play a significant role in CRP levels. Although the 2007 American Heart Association Guidelines for Cardiovascular Disease Prevention advise physicians to consider family history of heart attack before age 60 years but not CRP values, some independent researchers are including CRP in the development of risk scores (e.g., Reynolds Risk score).[60]

CRP levels are also measured in secondary prevention (individuals already diagnosed at high risk for coronary events) toward dual-goal therapy of LDL reduction and reduction of CRP levels, because CRP levels correlate with progression of atherosclerosis and clinical outcomes in individuals with coronary artery disease who are treated with statins. This reflects a change from previous policies in which it was assumed CRP levels did not provide additional information for at-risk individuals.[48,56]

Elevated levels of CRP have been identified as a predictive factor in HIV disease progression, independent of CD4 T-cell count and HIV ribonucleic acid (RNA) level.

Table 40-15	Full Lipid Profile	
Lipids, Lipoprotein	**(Expected)**	**Comments Values (mg/dL)**
LDL	<70	Recommended target value if at very high risk for heart disease
	<100	Recommended if heart disease or diabetes is present
	<130	Recommended if two or more risk factors are present
	<160	Recommended if one or no risk factors present
	160-189	High
	>189	Very high
HDL	<40	Desirable
	>60	Represents a negative risk factor; the higher the number, the better
Total cholesterol	<200	Desirable; recommended
	200-239	Borderline high; moderate risk
	≥240	Higher risk
Triglycerides	<150	Recommended
	<100	Desirable
	150-199	Moderate risk
	200-499	High risk
	>499	Very high risk
	>1000	At risk for pancreatitis

Risk factors include cigarette smoking, male older than age 45 years, female older than age 55 years, low HDL (less than 40 mg/dL), hypertension, and family history of premature heart disease.[15]

Data from Executive Summary of the Third Report of The National Cholesterol Education Program (NCEP) Expert Panel on Detection, Evaluation, and Treatment of High Blood Cholesterol in Adults (Adult Treatment Panel III), *JAMA* 285(19):2486–2497, 2001.

Table 40-16	Homocysteine and High-Sensitivity C-Reactive Protein	
Homocysteine	5-15 µmol/L	Normal
	16-100	Mild hyperhomocysteinemia
	>100	Severe hyperhomocysteinemia
hs-CRP	<1.0 mg/L	Low risk
	1-3 mg/L	Average risk
	>3 mg/L	High risk

hs-CRP, High-sensitivity C-reactive protein.

Data from Bortolotto LA, Safar ME, Billaud E, et al: Plasma homocysteine, aortic stiffness, and renal function in hypertensive patients. *Hypertension* 34(4 Pt 2):837–842, 1999; and American Association for Clinical Chemistry (AACC): Lab Tests Online. http://www.labtestsonline.org/. Accessed August 11, 2014.

Levels of CRP above 2.3 mg/L may signal faster progression of HIV to AIDS and may provide additional prognostic information.[39]

Cardiovascular Pressures

A number of physiologic measurements are made in the ICU or coronary care unit to monitor cardiovascular health and response to treatment. These include central venous pressure (CVP), pulmonary artery wedge pressure (PAWP), and pulmonary artery pressure. CVP is measured from a catheter introduced from a peripheral vein such as the subclavian or jugular into the right atrium. CVP indicates the working pressure of the right ventricle, which can either indicate the effectiveness of the right ventricle as a pump or the fluid status of the individual. Increased CVP indicates either poor pumping function of the right ventricle or fluid overload. Dehydration, on the other hand, causes CVP to decrease.

PAWP is an indicator of the effectiveness of the left ventricle as a pump. A balloon-tipped catheter is inserted from a central vein, through the right side of the heart, through the pulmonary artery, and advanced into progressively smaller branches of pulmonary arterial vessels. The balloon tip is then forced or wedged into a small arterial vessel, and the balloon is inflated. With the balloon inflated, the catheter is exposed only to the pressure present in the fluid between the catheter tip and the left atrium. Poor pumping function of the left ventricle leads to increased pressure as determined by PAWP. PAWP is falling out of favor because of the risk and cost of the instrumentation and the availability of other means of assessing the pumping function of the left ventricle.

Pulmonary artery pressure is also determined by a catheter inserted through a central vein, through the right side of the heart, and into the pulmonary arterial circulation. However, no balloon is inflated. The catheter is exposed to the fluctuations in pressure that occur with the cardiac cycle as blood fills and is emptied from the pulmonary arterial vessels. Generally, one is interested in whether pulmonary hypertension exists. Pulmonary artery pressure can be measured by the same catheter used for PAWP by deflating the balloon and withdrawing the tip so it is no longer wedged. Manipulating this catheter is not considered part of physical therapy practice. Table 40-17 lists reference values for vascular pressures.

PULMONARY FUNCTION TESTS

Tests may be performed for screening purposes or for diagnosis of specific pulmonary diseases. Pulmonary function studies may reveal abnormalities in the airways, alveoli, and pulmonary vascular bed early in the course of disease when physical examinations and x-ray studies are still normal. In addition, the location of an airway abnormality can be determined (i.e., upper airway, large airway, or small airway).

Tests include static lung volumes, dynamic breathing tests, and physiologic tests. Imaging may also be used to augment these tests. These tests can provide additional information for the physical examination of the person with compromised respiratory function such as

Table 40-17	Vascular Pressures	
Pressure		**Reference Range (mm Hg)**
Pulmonary artery systolic		20-30
Pulmonary artery diastolic		8-15
Pulmonary artery wedge pressure		4-12
Central venous pressure		0-5

distinguishing obstructive from restrictive disease, separating airway disease from issues with elasticity, and determining central from peripheral causes of breathing disorders.

A spirometer can be used to measure the movement of air in and out of the lungs during various breathing maneuvers. Lung volumes are measured from a reference point of the muscles of inspiration being relaxed. Table 40-18 lists the names given to these lung volumes. Norms based on height, age, and sex are available for comparison of the individual's results. These values include tidal volume (TV), inspiratory reserve volume (IRV), expiratory reserve volume (ERV), and vital capacity (VC).

TV is the amount that is inspired with a normal breath. The amount that can be inspired beyond normal inspiration with a maximal inspiratory effort is the IRV. The name implies that it is a reserve for increasing the volume of air inspired if needed during exercise or other stress. The amount of air that can be expired beyond the normal expiration using maximal expiratory effort is the ERV. VC represents the maximal volume that can be moved. Mathematically, it is the sum of the IRV, TV, and ERV and represents tapping the total reserves of both inspiration and expiration.

However, the volumes measured with a spirometer are only the changes that occur with breathing and not the actual volume contained in the lungs. Additional volumes are determined by dilution techniques that can be used to compute the volume of air present in the lungs. Residual volume (RV) is the volume of air present in the lungs at the end of maximal expiration as a result of anatomical and physiologic properties of the lungs and airways. RV is increased in obstructive diseases and decreased in restrictive diseases. It is determined by use of helium or nitrogen dilution techniques in pulmonary function labs. An amount of helium or nitrogen is added from a known volume after maximal expiration occurs. The subject breathes in and out of the closed system until the helium or nitrogen concentration equilibrates. Then the unknown volume of the lungs (RV) is computed. When this volume is determined, both functional residual capacity (FRC) and total lung capacity can be determined. FRC represents the actual volume of the lungs when the muscles of inspiration are relaxed. It is the volume of the lungs before normal tidal inspiration and after normal tidal expiration. FRC, like RV is increased in obstructive disease and decreased in restrictive diseases. FRC is computed by adding RV to ERV. Total lung capacity is computed as RV plus ERV, TV, and IRV (see Table 40-18).

A number of time-based tests are also used to assess pulmonary function. In addition to the changes in volumes characteristic of obstructive and restrictive

| Table 40-18 | Pulmonary Function Test Components |

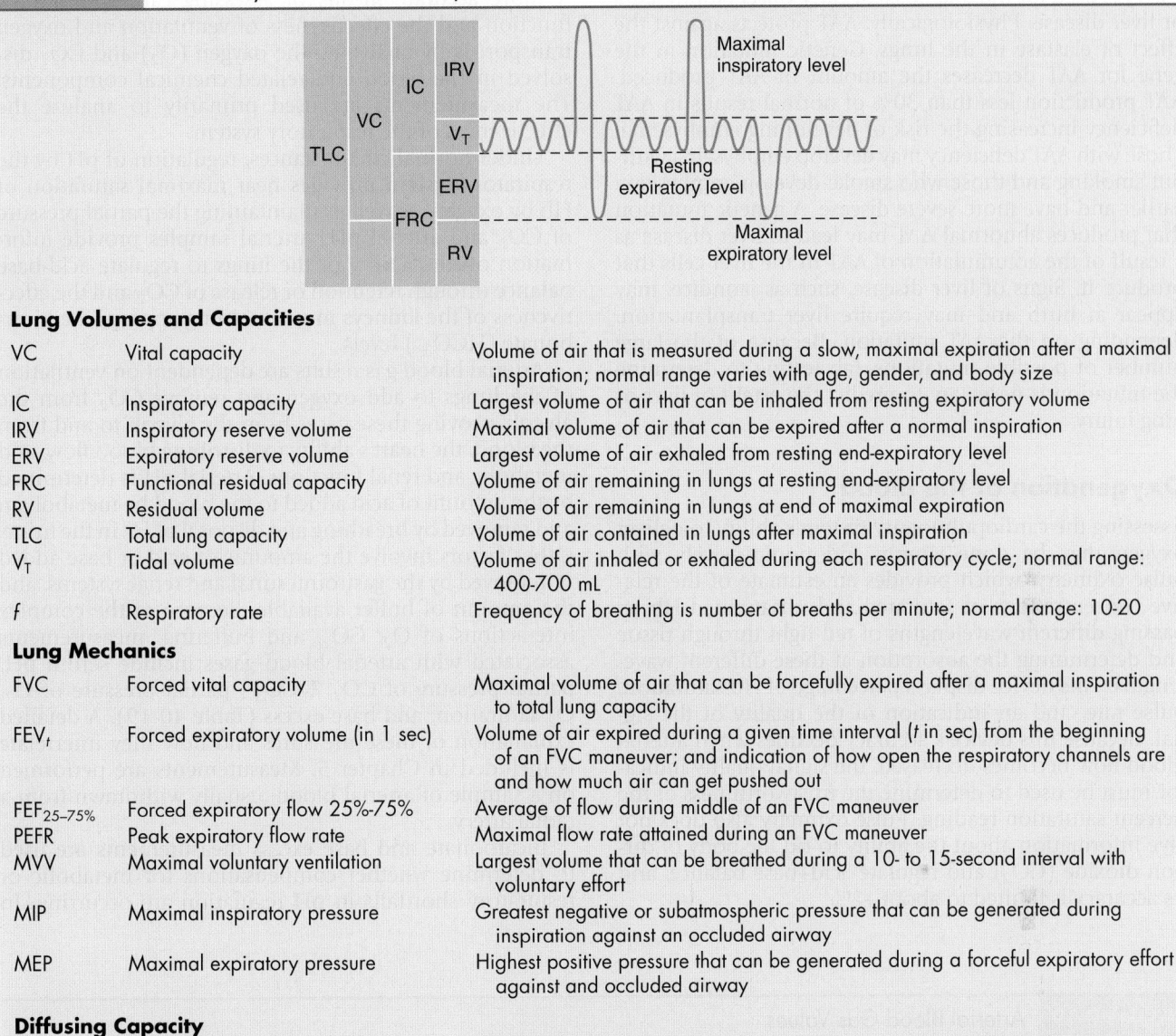

Lung Volumes and Capacities

VC	Vital capacity	Volume of air that is measured during a slow, maximal expiration after a maximal inspiration; normal range varies with age, gender, and body size
IC	Inspiratory capacity	Largest volume of air that can be inhaled from resting expiratory volume
IRV	Inspiratory reserve volume	Maximal volume of air that can be expired after a normal inspiration
ERV	Expiratory reserve volume	Largest volume of air exhaled from resting end-expiratory level
FRC	Functional residual capacity	Volume of air remaining in lungs at resting end-expiratory level
RV	Residual volume	Volume of air remaining in lungs at end of maximal expiration
TLC	Total lung capacity	Volume of air contained in lungs after maximal inspiration
V_T	Tidal volume	Volume of air inhaled or exhaled during each respiratory cycle; normal range: 400-700 mL
f	Respiratory rate	Frequency of breathing is number of breaths per minute; normal range: 10-20

Lung Mechanics

FVC	Forced vital capacity	Maximal volume of air that can be forcefully expired after a maximal inspiration to total lung capacity
FEV_t	Forced expiratory volume (in 1 sec)	Volume of air expired during a given time interval (t in sec) from the beginning of an FVC maneuver; and indication of how open the respiratory channels are and how much air can get pushed out
$FEF_{25-75\%}$	Forced expiratory flow 25%-75%	Average of flow during middle of an FVC maneuver
PEFR	Peak expiratory flow rate	Maximal flow rate attained during an FVC maneuver
MVV	Maximal voluntary ventilation	Largest volume that can be breathed during a 10- to 15-second interval with voluntary effort
MIP	Maximal inspiratory pressure	Greatest negative or subatmospheric pressure that can be generated during inspiration against an occluded airway
MEP	Maximal expiratory pressure	Highest positive pressure that can be generated during a forceful expiratory effort against and occluded airway

Diffusing Capacity

D_LCO	Diffusing capacity for carbon monoxide	Reflects ability of lung to transfer gas across the alveolar/capillary interface (assists in diagnosis of diffuse infiltrative lung disease and emphysema)

From Black JM, Hawks J, editors: *Medical-surgical nursing: clinical management for positive outcomes*, ed 7, Philadelphia, 2005, WB Saunders.

diseases, more detailed information about the disease processes and which structures are involved can be obtained with time-based tests. A simple, but powerful diagnostic test is the computation of the ratio of forced expiratory volume in 1 second (FEV_1) to forced vital capacity (FVC). With normal lung function, a person will have expired 80% of FVC in 1 second with maximal effort. This is expressed as $FEV_1/FVC = 0.8$. With obstructive disease, a person will be unable to expire 80% within 1 second and the FEV_1/FVC declines to 0.6 and lower as severity of obstructive disease increases. Restrictive disease is characterized by diminished volumes of all types and difficulty taking a deep breath, although FEV_1/FVC may be normal or greater than normal because of excessive stiffness of the lungs. Further information can be obtained by computing the slope of the middle 50% of the maximum VC as an index of small airway resistance.

Physiologic testing may also include maximum inspiratory pressure, which is measured with a manometer attached to a mouthpiece. Maximum inspiratory pressure is an index of the strength of the muscles of inspiration. Other functional testing includes the maximum voluntary ventilation, which tests physiologic components of strength and endurance of breathing.

A simple device frequently used for monitoring airway resistance in persons with asthma is the peak flow meter. The person expires as forcefully as possible for one breath. The device is individualized for a given person with areas of the scale marked with colors to indicate whether function is adequate (green), some intervention is needed (yellow), or emergency care should be sought (red).

Measurement of the quantity of serum α1-antitrypsin (AAT) is used for the diagnosis of early-onset emphysema or liver disease. Physiologically, AAT protects against the effect of elastase in the lungs. Genetic mutation in the gene for AAT decreases the amount of AAT produced. AAT production less than 30% of normal results in AAT deficiency increasing the risk of developing emphysema. Those with AAT deficiency may develop emphysema without smoking and those who smoke develop emphysema earlier and have more severe disease. A genetic mutation that produces abnormal AAT may lead to liver disease as a result of the accumulation of AAT in the liver cells that produce it. Signs of liver disease, such as jaundice, may appear at birth and may require liver transplantation, depending on the AAT mutation. Because of the large number of possible mutations, lab testing to determine the mutation is necessary to predict the extent of liver or lung injury.

Oxygenation of the Blood

Assessing the cardiopulmonary system's ability to deliver oxygen may be done simply and noninvasively with pulse oximetry, which provides an estimate of the relative concentrations of saturated and unsaturated Hb by passing different wavelengths of red light through tissue and determining the absorption at these different wavelengths. This device displays percentage of Hb saturation, pulse rate, and an indication of the quality of the signal. Because this device's accuracy declines when arterial blood flow becomes decreased, the signal quality indicator must be used to determine the trustworthiness of the percent saturation reading. Pulse oximetry also does not give information about the ability to rid the body of carbon dioxide (CO_2) and regulate acid–base balance, and its accuracy is limited to about ±2%.

Arterial Blood Gases

A more accurate means of assessing cardiopulmonary function and the effectiveness of ventilation and oxygen transport is by analyzing the oxygen (O_2) and CO_2 dissolved in the blood and related chemical components. The measurements are used primarily to analyze the effectiveness of the respiratory system.

Under normal circumstances, regulation of pH by the respiratory system provides near maximal saturation of Hb by oxygen, as well as maintaining the partial pressure of CO_2 and arterial pH. Arterial samples provide information on the ability of the lungs to regulate acid-base balance through retention or release of CO_2 and the effectiveness of the kidneys in maintaining appropriate bicarbonate (HCO_3^-) levels.

Arterial blood gas results are dependent on ventilation of the lungs to add oxygen and remove CO_2 from the alveoli, moving these gases from the alveoli to and from the blood, the heart's ability to distribute blood flow, and metabolic and renal functions. Arterial pH is determined by the amount of acid added to the blood by metabolism and removed by breathing and disposal of H^+ in the urine. Other factors involve the amounts of acid or base added or removed by the gastrointestinal and renal systems, and the amount of buffer available. Because of the complex interactions of O_2, CO_2, and buffering, measurements associated with arterial blood gases include serum pH, partial pressure of CO_2, HCO_3^-, partial pressure of O_2, O_2 saturation, and base excess (Table 40-19). A detailed explanation of these measures and how they interrelate is included in Chapter 5. Measurements are performed on a sample of arterial blood, usually withdrawn from a radial artery.

Bicarbonate and base excess measurements are used to determine whether compensations for metabolic or respiratory shortfalls in pH regulation are occurring. In

Table 40-19	Arterial Blood Gas Values	
Term	**Definition**	**Reference Value**
pH	Measure of blood acidity; ratio of acids to bases	7.35-7.45
$PaCO_2$	Pressure or tension exerted by CO_2 dissolved in arterial blood; measures effectiveness of alveolar ventilation (i.e., how well air is exchanging with blood in the lungs)	35-45 mm Hg
HCO_3^-	Amount of bicarbonate or alkaline substance dissolved in blood; influenced mainly by metabolic changes	22-26 mEq/L
PaO_2	Pressure exerted by O_2 dissolved in arterial blood in attempting to diffuse through pulmonary membrane	75-100 mm Hg
O_2 saturation	Oxyhemoglobin saturation: percentage of O_2 carried by hemoglobin	96-100%
Critical Values		
pH	≤7.20 or >7.60	
PCO_2	≤20 or >70 mm Hg	
HCO_3^-	≤10 or >40 mEq/L	
PO_2	≤40 mm Hg	
O_2 saturation	<95%*	

CO_2, Carbon dioxide; HCO_3^-, bicarbonate ion; O_2, oxygen; $PaCO_2$, partial pressure of arterial carbon dioxide; PaO_2, partial pressure of arterial oxygen; PO_2, partial pressure of oxygen; PCO_2, partial pressure of carbon dioxide.
*This value varies depending on the clinical situation. For example, a healthy adult with O_2 saturation levels less than 95% would bear further investigation, whereas in someone who smokes 95% saturation level would not be suspect; resting PO_2 declines with aging after age 70 years.
Modified from Goodman CC, Snyder TE: *Differential diagnosis for physical therapists: screening for referral*, ed 5, Philadelphia, 2013, WB Saunders.

addition to the typical radial artery sample site, samples from other vessels can be taken to determine the performance of the cardiac and ventilatory pumps in their roles of gas exchange. For example, a person with poor cardiac pump performance but normal gas exchange in the lungs may initially demonstrate good arterial blood gases, but low venous O_2 and high venous CO_2.

SERUM HORMONES

Several hormones are frequently affected in populations seen in physical therapy and may impact systems relevant to the provision of therapy. Most common is hypothyroidism. Alterations in parathyroid hormone, cortisol, and adrenocorticotropic hormone may also occur.

Thyroid hormone is necessary initially for normal growth and development. It is routinely tested in newborns in all states to detect hypothyroidism, a potential cause of cognitive delays or developmental disability when left untreated or when treatment is delayed.

In adults, a slowing of metabolism with hypothyroidism may cause sensitivity to cold; brittle, coarse skin and nails; bradycardia; constipation; and slower cognitive processing. Hypothyroidism has also been linked to musculoskeletal injuries and affective changes, including depression and anxiety.

Severe chronic hypothyroidism may progress to a condition known as myxedemic coma. Hypothyroidism may be caused by either pituitary dysfunction or thyroid dysfunction. Thyroid testing includes both thyroid-stimulating hormone (TSH) and thyroxine (T_4). TSH (produced in the pituitary) stimulates the thyroid to produce thyroid hormones (T_3 and T_4). Elevated TSH with decreased T_4 indicates thyroid disease, whereas depressed TSH indicates pituitary disease. Hyperthyroidism, most notably from Graves disease, may produce atrial fibrillation and exophthalmos, which is a protrusion of the eyes.

Parathyroid hormone regulates calcium metabolism. In the face of hypocalcemia, release of parathyroid hormone causes bones to release calcium into the blood. Cortisol and adrenocorticotropic hormone are related to adrenal cortex function. Adrenocorticotropic hormone is released by the anterior pituitary to stimulate release of cortisol by cells of the adrenal cortex. Cortisol, a glucocorticoid, is released in response to stress and provides glucose to circulate in the blood. In particular, protein reservoirs are made available for conversion of amino acids into fuel sources, which can damage musculoskeletal structures. Cortisol also inhibits the immune system.

Fluid volume and composition may be altered by changes in the release of several hormones. ADH may be either elevated or depressed as a result of injury to or disease of the posterior pituitary. ADH is increased in what is termed SIADH, causing fluid retention and hyponatremia.

The potentially life-threatening disease, diabetes insipidus, results in decreased ADH with extreme loss of water in the urine and hypernatremia. Tests may also be performed for renin, angiotensin, and aldosterone as part of a workup for low potassium (hypokalemia), muscle weakness, hypertension, or hypotension. Table 40-20 lists reference values for serum thyroid hormones.

IMMUNOLOGIC

Diagnostic immunology or serodiagnostic testing uses blood tests to aid in the diagnosis of infectious disease, immune disorders, allergic reactions, neoplastic disease (e.g., genetic changes and tumor-related antigens), and in blood grouping and typing (not discussed further here). Blood tests can be used to determine whether particular antigens are present (bacteria, viruses, parasites, fungi, or enzymes).

Immunoglobulins, the general term for antibodies that are produced in response to antigens, are divided into five subclasses (IgA, IgD, IgE, IgG, and IgM). These classes of immunoglobulins can be differentiated by morphology and by their roles in the immune system. During lab testing, the globulins are separated by electrophoresis into different fractions. Different fractions are indicative of different diseases. For example, α-globulin is elevated in rheumatoid arthritis and β- and γ-globulins are elevated in multiple myeloma.

Ideally, serum is collected at the beginning of the illness during the acute phase and again 3 to 4 weeks later during the convalescent phase. An increase in the quantity (titer) of a specific antibody between these two phases is diagnostically significant. The specific antibody tests for individual antigens are beyond the scope of this chapter. The reader is referred to more comprehensive laboratory and diagnostic manuals.

Tumor-Associated Antigens

Knowledge of the interactions between tumor cells and the immune system has made identification of tumor-associated antigens possible. Tumor-associated antigens discovered by these methods are being used to develop passive (humoral), as well as active immunotherapy strategies to stimulate the immune system. Development of biomarkers is ongoing in hopes of developing better screening techniques for early detection,[24,43] along with identifying strategies for personalized cancer

Table 40-20	Thyroid Function Reference Values				
Age	Thyroxine (T_4) (µg/dL)	Triiodothyronine (T_3) (ng/dL)	Free T_4 Index (ng/dL)	Thyroid-Stimulating Hormone (TSH) (µIU/L)
Adolescent, adult, older adult	4.5-11.5	80-200	4.6-11.2	0.35-5.5 (newer recommendations are for 0.3-3.0)

Data from Corbett JV: *Laboratory tests and diagnostic procedures with nursing diagnoses*, ed 8, Upper Saddle River, NJ, 2012, Prentice Hall.

immunotherapy (targeted therapies),[21] and even better—prevention with antitumor vaccines.[70,76]

Investigations and identification of gene expression profiles and prognostic markers for different types of cancer (e.g., breast, prostate, ovarian, or lung) are ongoing. Efforts to find molecular methods to detect disease recurrence and micrometastases using biomarkers are also underway. Although not completely reliable, tumor-antigen markers such as prostate-specific antigen and CA-125 for ovarian cancer are already in use.

Rheumatoid Factor

Rheumatoid factor (RF), an anti–γ-globulin antibody, is elevated in rheumatoid arthritis and Sjögren syndrome. However, a negative test does not rule out either disease. Approximately 20% of those diagnosed with these diseases are negative for RF. A positive RF test may also occur with chronic diseases such as SLE, endocarditis, syphilis, tuberculosis, sarcoidosis, cancer, and viral infections, as well as other diseases.[1]

Cyclic citrullinated peptide antibody is also used to assist in the diagnosis of rheumatoid arthritis. Excessive conversion of the amino acid arginine to citrulline leads to the production of abnormal structures called cyclic citrullinated peptides. Cyclic citrullinated peptide antibodies are produced against these abnormal protein products that are associated with the disease process of rheumatoid arthritis. Both RF and cyclic citrullinated peptide antibody testing are requirements of the American College of Rheumatology Rheumatoid Arthritis Classification Criteria.[4]

Human Leukocyte Antigen

Human leukocyte antigen (HLA) refers to inherited components of the immune system. Inheritance of certain HLA proteins increases the risk of specific diseases, especially spondyloarthropathies such as ankylosing spondylitis, reactive arthropathy, Reiter syndrome, and psoriatic arthropathy (arthritis). Not all persons with a certain HLA pattern will develop the disease, but those who do have that HLA pattern have a greater probability for its development than the general population. Table 40-21 lists other diseases and related HLA proteins.

Antinuclear Antibodies

Measurement of serum antinuclear antibodies is used in the diagnosis of autoimmune diseases, such as polymyositis, scleroderma, mixed connective tissue disease, Sjögren syndrome and SLE. Exacerbations of SLE are related to elevations in antinuclear antibody (ANA), which may occur with events such as exposure to sunlight.

Individuals with signs suggestive of these diseases may have a blood sample examined for the presence of a number of ANAs for diagnosis and prognosis of these diseases. Different patterns of ANA assist in the diagnosis of different diseases and subtypes of them. Other indicators of systemic inflammation, such as CRP and ESR, are likely to be ordered at the same time. A generalized test of ANA may be followed up by tests of subsets of ANA for diagnosis and prognosis. The pattern of ANA is used

Table 40-21	Diseases Associated with HLA Antigens*
Disease	**HLA Antigen**
Ankylosing spondylitis	HLA-B27 (present in 90% of cases)
Multiple sclerosis	HLA-B27, HLA-Dw2, HLA-A3, HLA-B18
Myasthenia gravis	HLA-B8
Psoriasis	HLA-B13, HLA-B17
Reiter syndrome; reactive arthritis	HLA-B27
Juvenile insulin-dependent diabetes	HLA-Bw15, HLA-B8
Graves disease	HLA-B27
Juvenile rheumatoid arthritis	HLA-B27, HLA-DR4
Autoimmune chronic active hepatitis	HLA-B8
Polymyalgia rheumatica	HLA-DR4

HLA, Human leukocyte antigen.
*HLA testing is used to confirm the diagnosis and is not usually regarded as diagnostic by itself.
Data from Pagana KD, Pagana JJ: *Mosby's diagnostic and laboratory test reference*, ed 11, St Louis, 2012, Mosby.

along with clinical signs and symptoms for diagnosis and prognosis.[45]

URINALYSIS

Urine is composed of 95% water and 5% solids, although its composition may vary from almost 100% water. It is the end product of metabolic processes carried out in the body. Although urine contains thousands of dissolved substances, the three main components are water, urea, and sodium chloride.

Urine is created through the processes available to the kidney. With a large number of nephrons and long, coiled tubules, healthy kidneys have the opportunity to maintain the composition of body fluids by the filtration of blood and both passive and active mechanisms that result in its final composition. Many substances dissolved in the blood are reabsorbed, including glucose. However, the ability of the kidneys to reabsorb some of them is limited. If the concentration of glucose in the blood becomes great enough, it will exceed the kidney's ability to reabsorb what was filtered and it will begin to appear in the urine.

The kidney has a remarkable ability to rid the body of a number of substances, especially urea. Urea, for example, is present in the blood but at a much lower concentration than in the excreted urine. Testing of urine is centuries old. Simple yet important screening tests are done easily with small patches placed on urine dipsticks. Important components of urinalysis include color, specific gravity, glucose, ketone, WBCs, RBCs (occult blood), electrolytes, and drug screens.

Color and Appearance

The color of urine is related to a number of factors and the most important is its concentration. A pale yellow color is considered normal. Dilution of solute by increased volume of water in the urine decreases its color, whereas reduced volume caused by dehydration increases its yellow appearance. The presence of blood with intact RBCs produces a more purple-to-red color and hemolyzed blood produces a smoky appearance.

Color may also be altered by medications, including antibiotics, some laxatives, chlorzoxazone (a muscle relaxant), and Pyridium. Pyridium is an anesthetic used for treating the burning pain of urinary tract infection that colors the urine orange. The ingestion of certain foods, such as rhubarb, carrots, and beets, and some vitamins and supplements can cause a change in the color of urine.

Dark brown urine may occur with liver disease or with disseminated intravascular coagulation. Highly concentrated urine (e.g., decreased hydration or renal dysfunction) is also colored differently depending on the individual and may appear dark yellow, gold, or orange, often accompanied by a strong odor. Asparagus can also bring about a characteristic odor to the urine, and certain vitamin and herbal supplements can change the color (e.g., vitamin C can cause the urine to turn a bright yellow or orange).

Bleeding from the upper urinary tract (kidney and ureters) may produce dark red urine, whereas bleeding in the lower urinary tract (bladder and urethra) produces bright red urine. Occult blood, meaning hidden blood, represents a more subtle change in urine color than the red, purple, or smoky-appearing urine and is tested as part of urinalysis. Bleeding can indicate a number of disorders such as kidney stones, infection, or cancer. Frank purulence (visible pus in the urine) or a cloudy appearance is indicative of infection of the urinary tract.

When urine gives a positive result for occult blood but no RBCs are seen on a microscopic examination, myoglobinuria is suspected. Myoglobinuria is the excretion of myoglobin, a muscle protein, into the urine as a result of traumatic muscle injury (e.g., automobile accident, football injury, or electric shock), muscle disorder (e.g., muscular dystrophy, arterial occlusion to a muscle), certain kinds of poisoning (e.g., carbon monoxide) or heat stroke.

Specific Gravity

Specific gravity is a test performed to assess the kidney's ability to vary the concentration of solute in the urine appropriately. The specific gravity measured is determined by the amount of solute present. Urine with no solute has a specific gravity of 1.0; specific gravity increases with the concentration of solute present in urine. A high specific gravity indicates concentrated urine, whereas a low specific gravity indicates dilute urine. Renal dysfunction is suspected when the kidney is unable to concentrate or dilute the urine as needed for homeostasis. Dilute urine has a specific gravity approaching 1.0, whereas the specific gravity caused by dehydration may reach 1.2 or greater. Specific gravity correlates with color. Urine with a specific gravity close to 1.0 will be clear, whereas specific gravity closer to 1.2 produces dark yellow urine.

Glucose and Ketones

Glucose and ketones present in the urine represent alterations in glucose metabolism. Glucose present in the urine indicates saturation of the active transport mechanism for glucose from the filtered urine. Under normal circumstances, virtually all glucose that filters from the blood can be reabsorbed from the urine.

When the blood glucose level exceeds the reabsorption capacity of the renal tubules, glucose will be spilled into the urine. Failure to absorb all of the glucose indicates a very high plasma glucose concentration and most likely diabetes mellitus. Metabolism of triglycerides by the Krebs cycle requires glucose. When intracellular glucose becomes low from starvation or insufficient insulin, excess fatty acids that cannot be metabolized by the Krebs cycle are converted to ketones.

In healthy individuals, the quantity of ketone bodies formed in the liver is completely metabolized so that only negligible amounts (if any) appear in the urine. However, excessive production of ketones caused by either diabetes mellitus or starvation (including eating disorders) results in detectible concentrations of ketones in the urine. Table 40-22 lists reference values for urinalysis.

DRUG SCREENING

Employees of health care institutions may be subjected to preemployment screening, random tests, and testing after significant incidents at work. Policies vary between facilities and may include screening of students on clinical affiliations. Patients may also be tested as part of the diagnostic process. Tests may be performed for a number of substances, including alcohol, amphetamines,

Table 40-22	Routine Urinalysis and Related Tests		
General Characteristics and Measurements	**Chemical Determinations**		**Microscopic Examination of Sediment**
Color: pale yellow to amber Turbidity: clear to slightly hazy Specific gravity (with a normal fluid intake): 1.015-1.025 pH: 4.5-8.0 (average pH: 5-6)	Glucose: negative Ketones: negative Blood: negative Bilirubin: negative Urobilinogen: 0.1-1.0 Nitrate for bacteria: negative Leukocyte esterase: negative		Casts: negative, occasional hyaline casts Red blood cells: negative or rare Crystals: negative White blood cells: negative or rare Epithelial cells: few

Data from Pagana KD, Pagana TJ: *Mosby's diagnostic and laboratory test reference*, ed 11, St. Louis, 2012, Mosby.

methamphetamines, barbiturates, cocaine, LSD, marijuana, opiates, phencyclidine, and other drugs that might impair employee performance or confound patient diagnosis including analgesics, tranquilizers, sedatives, and stimulants.

MICROBIOLOGIC STUDIES

A large number of microbiologic studies are available to identify potential causes of infection. Identification of the pathogen aids in the prognosis and treatment of infectious disease. In particular, patients may be placed in isolation, requiring special attention to their therapy and the most effective antimicrobial agents for the person's condition may be prescribed. Gram stains and cultures are the most commonly encountered microbiologic studies in the therapy practice.

Tests for Rapid Identification

Gram stain is used to distinguish organisms that take up this stain (gram positive) from those that do not (gram negative). A number of common pathogens are gram positive, including *Staphylococcus* and *Streptococcus* species. Gram-negative organisms frequently require different antimicrobial drugs.

Acid-fast testing is generally for determining tuberculosis infection. Acid-fast bacillus is a term generally applied to *Mycobacterium tuberculosis*. Testing is done on sputum samples, but may also be done with samples obtained from bronchoscopy or other tissue or fluid samples.

Potassium hydroxide is used for identifying fungal infection.

Cultures

Cultures are obtained to detect the presence of bacteria in the blood (e.g., bacteremia), sputum (e.g., pneumonia or tuberculosis), pleural fluid (e.g., empyema), throat (e.g., streptococci, meningococci, or gonococci), urine (e.g., urinary tract infection), skin (e.g., staphylococci, streptococci, or *Pseudomonas*), and wounds (e.g., staphylococci, streptococci, or *Pseudomonas*).

Other cultures may include stool and anal, cerebrospinal fluid (CSF), cervical, and urethral cultures. Cultures are usually performed when clinical presentation is suggestive of infection (e.g., chills, fever, or pus). Cultures should be performed before antibiotic therapy is initiated (often the culture is taken and the antibiotic dispensed before results are known); otherwise, the antibiotic may interrupt the organism's growth in the laboratory.

Samples of tissue or body fluids are used to determine the species or quantity of microbes present. A quantitative culture by tissue biopsy or fluid obtained by needle aspiration is best to determine the number of organisms present. Infection, delayed wound healing, and failure of skin grafts are associated with cultures numbering 100,000 or more organisms per gram. β-Hemolytic *Streptococcus* causes infection at a lower number per gram of tissue.[64]

Blood cultures are taken when systemic infection is suspected. These may be done when individuals have indwelling catheters, localized infection, and other risk factors in the presence of fever, malaise, or anorexia. Skin, even in healthy individuals, is expected to have a number of organisms on its surface. In particular, species of *Streptococcus*, *Staphylococcus*, and various fungi are commonly present. In some cases, virulent strains may become present and lead to infection. Infection may take the form of a crusty, honey-colored area (impetigo), spread through follicles (folliculitis), cause abscess formation (furuncles), spread through fascial planes (carbuncles), or appear as fungal manifestations such as ringworm or athlete's foot.

Wounds are frequently cultured for a number of reasons. Both quantitative and qualitative cultures may be taken to determine the appropriate medical treatment. Swab cultures with culturettes are still used frequently, but only represent surface bacteria, which may not be the source of the infection. Biopsy of the wound or removal of fluid deep in the wound is more likely to identify the problematic microbes than a swab.

FLUID ANALYSIS

Samples of fluid may be drawn from a number of body compartments. Tests are performed for a variety of reasons including determining the cause of fluid accumulation in these spaces, determining whether these compartments are infected, or whether cancer or other cells or substances are present. Compartments may include the area around the brain and spinal cord, joints, the spaces around the lungs or heart, and in the abdomen.

Cerebrospinal Fluid

This fluid surrounds the brain and spinal cord and also exists in cavities within the brain called ventricles and within the central canal of the spinal cord. CSF is typically collected by a *lumbar puncture*. At this site distal to the end of the spinal cord, a needle can be introduced without risk of injuring the spinal cord.

Both the composition and pressure of CSF may be analyzed. Infections (meningitis) may be determined by both presence of bacteria and by alterations in the normal composition of CSF. Pressure within the CSF space may be altered through blockage of the normal flow and reabsorption mechanisms of the brain, which may alter cerebral function or even cause death.

The presence of immunoglobulins may be indicative of other disorders, especially the presence of IgG with multiple sclerosis. Box 40-2 includes other indications for lumbar puncture.

Appearance

Testing of CSF involves measurement of a variety of substances and states. Box 40-3 lists standard pathologic levels of substances found in the CSF. Appearance is normally clear; cloudiness indicates a disease state, graded from 0 to 4 (indicating progressive levels of cloudiness)—0 denotes a clear fluid, and 4 indicates inability to see newsprint through the fluid. Bilirubin accumulating in the body (jaundice) can give the CSF a yellow tinge, and blood in the fluid will cause it to turn pink.

DIAGNOSTIC LUMBAR PUNCTURE IN ADULTS

Diseases detected with high sensitivity and high specificity
  Bacterial meningitis
  Tuberculous meningitis
  Fungal meningitis
Diseases detected with high sensitivity and moderate specificity
  Viral meningitis
  Subarachnoid hemorrhage
  Multiple sclerosis
  Neurosyphilis
  Infectious polyneuritis
  Paraspinal abscess
Disease detected with moderate sensitivity and high specificity
  Meningeal malignancy
Diseases detected with moderate sensitivity and moderate specificity
  Intracranial hemorrhage
  Viral encephalitis
Other recognized indications for lumbar puncture
  Toxoplasmosis
  Amebic infections
  Aseptic meningitis
  Inflammatory neuropathies
  Metastatic brain tumors
  Normal-pressure hydrocephalus
  Hepatic encephalopathy
  Systemic lupus erythematosus

Modified from McConnell H: Current and future clinical utility of cerebrospinal fluid in neurology and psychiatry. In McConnell H, Bianchine J, editors: *Cerebrospinal fluid in neurology and psychiatry*, London, 1998, Chapman & Hall; and Irani DN. *Cerebrospinal fluid in clinical practice*, Philadelphia, WB Saunders, 2008.

FACTORS EVALUATED IN CEREBROSPINAL FLUID

Appearance
Cells
Inorganic compounds
Acid–base status

Organic compounds
  Lactate
  Glucose
  Proteins
  Immunoglobulins
  Enzymes
  Amino acids
  Peptides, neuropeptides

Cells found in the CSF usually indicate an abnormality in the central nervous system, as the CSF is normally virtually free of cells. Cell types found in disease or trauma include WBCs, macrophages, cartilage cells, glial cells, bone marrow, and various tumor cells.

Levels of inorganic compounds in the CSF can reflect disorders of the nervous system. Calcium can alter the activation of various neurotransmitters, and low levels are implicated in seizure disorders. Low levels of calcium are also associated with tetany and tumors of the diencephalon. Increased levels of calcium are seen in meningitis.

Magnesium levels will drop in the person with meningitis and ischemic brain disorders. Increased levels of magnesium are seen after intracranial hemorrhage. CSF sodium levels normally change as the plasma levels change. Sodium levels can be out of proportion in the CSF in encephalomalacia and tuberculous meningitis. Elevated potassium levels are seen in neonatal hemorrhage, aspiration pneumonia, seizure disorders, and cardiac arrest.

Glucose concentrations in CSF usually parallel plasma levels but have a 4-hour lag period. Decreased levels are seen as a result of subarachnoid hemorrhage, hypoglycemia, neoplastic or inflammatory infiltration of the meninges, and many forms of meningitis. LDH is increased in meningitis. Amino acids acting as neurotransmitters in CSF represent an important regulatory mechanism. Levels are increased in meningitis and in CSF blocks and are decreased in multiple sclerosis. Abnormalities are found in Parkinson disease and depression.

The CSF plays an important role in the transport of peptides to target areas of the brain. Neuropeptides (e.g., endorphins) are related to higher brain functions, such as learning, memory, posture, and movement, as well as to emotions[50] and pain mechanisms. Persons with phantom and neurogenic pain have been found to have low CSF endorphin levels.

Synovial Fluid Analysis

Arthrocentesis, the surgical puncture of a joint cavity for aspiration (withdrawal) of fluid, is performed by inserting a sterile needle into the joint space. Although the knee is the most commonly aspirated joint, arthrocentesis can be done on any major joint (e.g., shoulder, hip, elbow, wrist, ankle). This test is performed for many different reasons, such as to establish the presence of infection, crystal-induced arthritis, synovitis, or neoplasms.

Fluid may be aspirated from joints to determine the cause of joint effusion, or simply to relieve pressure caused by effusion due to acute trauma. Joint aspiration also offers the potential benefit of removing WBCs, a source of destructive enzymes, from the joint. Joint effusions may increase intraarticular pressure impairing synovial capillary perfusion. Removing synovial fluid via arthrocentesis could potentially improve the delivery of nutrients to cartilage and surrounding tissues.

Once the fluid sample is obtained, it is examined microscopically and chemically. Table 40-23 describes the classification of synovial fluid. Normal joint fluid is clear, colorless or straw-colored, and viscous because of hyaluronic acid in the absence of inflammation. A small amount of blood may be caused by needle trauma; true hemarthrosis gives the fluid a homogeneous pink or red appearance. Viscosity is reduced in people with inflammatory arthritis, and the synovial fluid tends to drip like water; fluid of high viscosity forms a string several inches long.

The mucin clot test correlates with the viscosity and is performed by adding acetic acid to joint fluid. Cell counts are also performed, including a WBC count (normal joint fluid contains fewer than 200/mm³) and neutrophils (PMNs). The concentration of WBCs determines cloudiness.

Although a low WBC count usually indicates a noninflammatory condition, a higher count does not exclude

Table 40-23	Classification of Synovial Fluid			
	Normal	**Noninflammatory**	**Inflammatory**	**Infectious/Septic**
Color	Clear to yellow	Straw-colored, yellow	Yellow to white	Yellow to white, cloudy to opaque
Clarity	Transparent	Transparent	Translucent to cloudy	Opaque
WBCs/mm³	<200	200-2000	2000-100,000	>75,000
PMNs	<25%	<25%	>50%	>75% (tuberculosis: 20%-80%)
Crystals	0	0	May be +	0
Examples		Osteoarthritis, trauma, aseptic necrosis, SLE	RA, gout, pseudogout, SLE, seronegative spondyloarthropathies	Bacterial infection, tuberculosis, fungal disease

PMNs, Neutrophils; *RA,* rheumatoid arthritis; *SLE,* systemic lupus erythematosus; *WBCs,* white blood cells.

traumatic effusion. Synovial fluid WBC counts may approach 100,000/μL immediately after joint surgery. Normal synovial fluid contains 25% or fewer neutrophils. A very high percentage of PMNs (>75%) is found in most people with acute bacterial infectious arthritis (see Table 40-23).

Fluid containing 70% or more of PMNs may indicate an inflammatory process, even if the total WBC count is low. The presence of crystals, which is usually associated with an inflammatory process, can be determined by examining the synovial fluid under polarized light. This test is used to differentiate between gout and pseudogout and other crystal-induced arthropathies. Finding characteristic crystals does not rule out concomitant infection.

Pleural and Pericardial Fluid Analysis

Accumulations of fluid around the lungs and heart may result from inflammatory diseases, neoplastic disease, infection, or altered lymphatic drainage. Either of these compartments may be affected in isolation or both may be affected, particularly in systemic inflammatory diseases such as amyloidosis, sarcoidosis, rheumatoid arthritis, or SLE. Accumulation of fluid in the pleural space may impair inspiration, increase the work of breathing, and in severe cases, cause respiratory failure.

The pericardial space may be filled with inflammatory fluid or blood. Pericarditis may produce audible changes (friction rub) and electrocardiographic changes and other symptoms. Filling of the pericardium with blood, however, is a potentially life-threatening condition called *hemopericardium.*

When the right side of the heart cannot fill sufficiently to maintain cardiac output, the condition is known as *cardiac tamponade* resulting in acute heart failure. Fluid can be drawn from either the pleural (pleurocentesis) or pericardial spaces (pericardiocentesis) with a needle for either analysis or to relieve pressure within these spaces.

Peritoneal fluid may accumulate for a large number of reasons, including hepatic failure and cancer metastasizing to the peritoneum. Fluid drawn from the peritoneum will be analyzed for infectious agents, cancer cells, electrolytes, and other fluid components to investigate the reason for ascites, the term used to describe peritoneal fluid accumulation. Withdrawal of fluid from the peritoneum is paracentesis.

REFERENCES

To enhance this text and add value for the reader, all references are included on the companion Evolve site that accompanies this textbook. The reader can view the reference source and access it online whenever possible.

APPENDIX A

Summary of Standard Precautions[11]

KIMBERLY LEVENHAGEN

HISTORICAL PERSPECTIVE

The Centers for Disease Control and Prevention (CDC) and the Healthcare Infection Control Practices Advisory Committee have developed (and continue to revise) the CDC Guideline for Isolation Precautions in Hospitals.[12] These guidelines were developed to assist hospitals in maintaining up-to-date isolation practices governing infection control and strategies for surveillance, prevention, and control of nosocomial/health care associated infections in U.S. hospitals.

Nosocomial infection is a term used to refer only to infections acquired in hospitals. A new term, *health care–associated infection* (HAI), is used now to refer to infections associated with health care delivery in any setting, such as hospitals, long-term care facilities, ambulatory settings, and home care.

Both terms are still in use but HAI is the preferred nomenclature. This updated term (HAI) reflects the inability to determine with certainty where the pathogen is acquired, since people can be colonized with or exposed to potential pathogens outside of the health care setting, before receiving health care, or while moving among the various settings within the health care system.[12]

The guideline recommendations are based on the latest epidemiologic information on transmission of infection in hospitals. The recommendations are intended primarily for use in the care of patients in acute care hospitals, although many of the recommendations are applicable for individuals receiving care in subacute care, extended care facilities, or other outpatient settings, including home health.

The recommendations are not intended for use in day care, well care, or domiciliary care programs. Because there have been few studies to test the efficacy of isolation precautions and gaps still exist in the knowledge of the epidemiology and modes of transmission of some diseases; disagreement with some of the recommendations is expected.

The Healthcare Infection Control Practices Advisory Committee recognizes that the goal of preventing transmission of infections in hospitals can be accomplished by multiple means and that hospitals will modify the recommendations according to their needs and circumstances and as directed by federal, state, or local regulations.

No guideline can address all the needs of the more than 6000 U.S. hospitals, which range in size from 5 beds to more than 1500 and serve very different client populations. Modification of the recommendations is encouraged if (1) the principles of epidemiology and disease transmission are maintained, and (2) precautions are included to interrupt spread of infection by all routes likely to be encountered in the hospital.

UNIVERSAL PRECAUTIONS (Formerly Used Terminology)

In 1985, largely because of the human immunodeficiency virus (HIV) epidemic, isolation practices in the United States were altered dramatically by the introduction of a new strategy for isolation precautions, which became known as universal precautions. Following the initial reports of hospital personnel becoming infected with HIV through needlesticks and skin contamination with blood, a widespread outcry created the urgent need for new isolation strategies to protect hospital personnel from bloodborne infections.

The subsequent modification of isolation precautions in some hospitals produced several major strategic changes and sacrificed some measures of protection against client-to-client transmission in the process of adding protection against client-to-personnel transmission.

In acknowledgment of the fact that many clients with bloodborne infections are not recognized, the universal precautions approach at that time placed emphasis on applying blood and body fluid precautions universally to all people regardless of their presumed infection status. Until this time, most clients placed on isolation precautions were those with a diagnosis or a suspicion of an infectious disease. This provision led to the term *universal precautions*.

In addition to emphasizing prevention of needlestick injuries and the use of traditional barriers such as gloves and gowns, universal precautions expanded blood and body fluid precautions to include the use of masks and eye coverings to prevent mucous membrane exposure during certain procedures and the use of individual ventilation devices when the need for resuscitation was predictable. This approach, and particularly the techniques

1731

for preventing mucous membrane exposures, was reemphasized in subsequent CDC reports that contained recommendations for prevention of HIV transmission in health care settings.

STANDARD PRECAUTIONS (Currently Accepted Nomenclature)

Universal precautions were further revised to be replaced by *standard precautions*. The revised guideline contains two tiers of precautions to update universal precautions: standard precautions and transmission-based precautions. Components of all standard precautions are listed in Table A-1.

Standard Precautions

Most important, standard precautions assume any person may be contagious and addresses the care of all patients in hospitals regardless of their diagnosis or presumed infection status. Implementation of these standard precautions is the primary strategy for successful HAI control.

Standard precautions synthesize the major features of universal (blood and body fluid) precautions (designed to reduce the risk of transmission of bloodborne pathogens) and body substance isolation (designed to reduce the risk of transmission of pathogens from moist body substances). Standard precautions apply to (1) blood; (2) all body fluids, secretions, and excretions, except sweat, regardless of whether or not they contain visible blood; (3) nonintact skin; and (4) mucous membranes.

Standard precautions are designed to reduce the risk of transmission of microorganisms from both recognized and unrecognized sources of infection in hospitals.

Preventive Environment

A set of preventive measures termed *protective environment* has been added to the standard precautions used to prevent HAI. These measures consist of engineering and design interventions that decrease the risk of exposure to environmental fungi for severely immunocompromised recipients of allogeneic hematopoietic stem cell transplant during their highest-risk phase, usually the first 100 days after transplantation, or longer in the presence of graft-versus-host disease.[11]

Protective Environment

A protective environment is a specialized patient care area, usually in a hospital, with a positive airflow relative to the corridor (i.e., air flows from the room to the outside adjacent space). The combination of high-efficiency particulate air filtration, high numbers of air changes per hour (ACH; 12 or more), and minimal leakage of air into the room creates an environment that can safely accommodate anyone who has undergone hematopoietic stem cell transplant.[29]

Table A-1	Recommendations for Application of Standard Precautions for the Care of All Individuals in All Health Care Settings
Component	**Recommendations**
Hand hygiene	After touching blood, body fluids, secretions, excretions, contaminated items; immediately after removing gloves; between patient contacts
Personal protective equipment (PPE)	See Appendix text
Gloves	For touching blood, body fluids, secretions, excretions, contaminated items; for touching mucous membranes and nonintact skin
Mask, eye protection, face shield	During procedures and patient care activities likely to generate splashes or sprays of blood, body fluids, secretions
Gown	During procedures and patient care activities when contact of clothing/exposed skin with blood/body fluids, secretions, and excretions is anticipated
Soiled patient care equipment	Handle in a manner that prevents transfer of microorganisms to others and to the environment; wear gloves if visibly contaminated; perform hand hygiene
Environmental control	Develop procedures for routine care, cleaning, and disinfection of environmental surfaces, especially frequently touched surfaces in patient care areas
Textiles (linen and laundry)	Handle in a manner that prevents transfer of microorganisms to others and to the environment
Needles and other sharps	Do not recap, bend, break, or hand-manipulate used needles; use safety features when available; place used sharps in puncture-resistant container
Patient resuscitation	Use mouthpiece, resuscitation bag, other ventilation devices to prevent mouth contact
Patient placement	Prioritize for single-patient room if patient is at increased risk of transmission, is likely to contaminate the environment or does not maintain appropriate hygiene, or is at increased risk of acquiring infection or developing adverse outcome following infection
Respiratory hygiene/cough etiquette (source containment of infectious respiratory secretions in symptomatic patients, beginning at initial point of encounter)	Instruct symptomatic persons to cover mouth/nose when sneezing/coughing; use tissues and dispose in no-touch receptacle; observe hand hygiene after soiling of hands with respiratory secretions; wear surgical mask if tolerated or maintain spatial separation, more than 3 feet if possible

From Department of Health and Human Services, Centers for Disease Control and Prevention: *Supplement I: Infection control in healthcare, home, and community settings,* Atlanta, 2005, Centers for Disease Control and Prevention.

Transmission-Based Precautions

Transmission-based precautions are designed only for the care of specified individuals known or suspected to be infected or colonized by epidemiologically important pathogens that can be transmitted by airborne or droplet transmission or by contact with dry skin or contaminated surfaces.

Transmission-based precautions are designed for individuals documented or suspected to be infected or colonized by highly transmissible or epidemiologically important pathogens for which additional precautions beyond standard precautions are needed to interrupt transmission in hospitals.

There are three types of transmission-based precautions (see Table 8-3):

- Airborne precautions/airborne infection isolation room
- Droplet precautions
- Contact precautions

Precautions may be combined for diseases that have multiple routes of transmission. When used either singly or in combination, they are to be used in addition to standard precautions.

Specific recommendations have been published according to the type of infection and condition and can be found at www.cdc.gov/hicpac/2007IP/2007ip_appendA.html. Guidelines are also given for colonization or infections with multidrug resistant organisms at www.cdc.gov/hicpac/mdro/mdro_toc.html.

Airborne Infection Isolation (see Table 8-3)

Airborne infection isolation refers to the isolation of individuals infected with organisms spread via airborne droplet nuclei less than 5 μm in diameter. The isolation area receives numerous ACH (12 or more ACH for new construction as of 2001; 6 or more ACH for construction before 2001) and is under negative pressure, such that the direction of the airflow is from the outside adjacent space (e.g., the corridor) into the room.[29]

The air in an airborne infection isolation room is preferably exhausted to the outside but may be recirculated provided that the return air is filtered through a high-efficiency particulate air filter. The use of personal respiratory protection is also indicated for persons entering these rooms when caring for tuberculosis or smallpox patients and for staff who lack immunity to airborne viral diseases (e.g., measles or varicella zoster virus infection).[29]

Questions arise when it comes to carrying out isolation procedures in the acute care setting. Can training take place outside of the room? If gait training is done in the hallway, what infection control measures are necessary? Although we do not yet have evidence-based clinical practice guidelines to follow in this area, the consensus has been that the therapist should wash hands and use gown/glove/mask as appropriate for the patient's precautions.

Isolation procedures can prevent taking patients out of the room in order to practice gait, stair climbing, or other important functional activities. Leaving the room or unit is not usually possible when there are documented multidrug resistant organisms. If procedures established by the epidemiology/infection control department prevent the therapist from delivering adequate care, the therapist will need to consult with members of that department to find ways to remove or minimize these barriers.

Ambulation is done in the individual's room as much as possible. If the patient is taken into the hallway, the patient sits on the edge of the bed or in a chair close to the door and given a clean hospital gown to don. The patient washes his or her hands before leaving the room. The therapist removes any personal protective equipment (PPE) defined as specialized clothing or equipment worn by an employee for protection against infectious materials.[10] Gloves can be kept on if needed and proceeds to ambulate the individual in the hallway.

Once the therapist (or staff) reenters the room, it is necessary to re-gown/glove as indicated. If the patient touches anything in the hallway other than the assistive device (i.e., handrails, etc.) the area must be cleaned with sani-wipes. This protocol has been developed by experts in infection control and will likely change as new information about transmission protection is published.

Each therapist should check with the individual facility's infection control department regarding specific in-house recommendations/requirements. The 2007 CDC guidelines[12] for isolation precaution (contact or droplet precautions) recommend caregivers don PPE upon entry into the patient's room; previous guidelines were for PPE when working within 3 feet of the individual.

Droplet Precautions (see Table 8-3)

Pathogens can be acquired from contact with infected airborne droplets (from coughing or sneezing) into the respiratory tract or by direct contact with vesicular fluid to mucous membranes or eye. Droplet transmission can be controlled through airborne infection isolation just discussed and respiratory hygiene (see further discussion of respiratory hygiene below).

Contact Precautions (see Table 8-3)

When contact precautions are in place, patients may be ambulated in the hallways provided they do not touch any objects in the hall, including the wall, railings, doorways, etc. Anything they do touch must be cleaned with an approved cleaner. Isolation procedures for patient and therapist (hand washing, glove and gown donning, and removal in and out of the room) may vary from institution to institution. The therapist is advised to always read the instructions and follow them unless alternate practices have been requested and approved.

SOURCES OF POTENTIAL EXPOSURE FOR THE THERAPIST

Standard precautions are intended to prevent occupational transmission of infectious diseases such as tuberculosis, HIV infection, hepatitis B, and hepatitis C. All body secretions and moist membranes and tissues (excluding perspiration) are considered to be potentially infectious and require the use of barriers and/or isolation techniques to prevent transmission of organisms.[11,19]

Therapists at greatest risk include those who perform electromyographic studies, therapists in direct contact with clients with tuberculosis (see also Box 15-4), therapists who provide wound management, and those who assess or treat temporomandibular joint disorder or perform manual lymphatic drainage inside the mouth.

Any therapist who assists in toileting or changing diapers (in adults or children) is at increased risk. Other risk factors include human bites and contact with sputum and pleural fluid tinged with blood (bloodborne pathogens). Health care workers are at increased risk of bacterial colonization from damaged skin on the hands after frequent handwashing.

Mode of Transmission

Blood is the single most important source of HIV, HBV, and HCV in the workplace.

The potential for hepatitis B virus (HBV) and hepatitis C virus (HCV) transmission in the workplace is 20 times greater than that for HIV, but the modes of transmission for these viruses are similar. All have been transmitted in occupational settings *only* by percutaneous inoculation or contact with an open wound, nonintact skin (e.g., cutaneous scratches; chapped, abraded, weeping, burned, or dermatitic skin), or bloody mucous membranes, blood-contaminated body fluids, or concentrated virus.

In the hospital and other health care settings, standard precautions should be followed when workers are exposed to blood, certain other body fluids (amniotic fluid, pericardial fluid, peritoneal fluid, pleural fluid, synovial fluid, cerebrospinal fluid, semen, and vaginal secretions), or any body fluid visibly contaminated with blood.

HBV can be transmitted through infected saliva, but saliva has not been implicated in HIV transmission except in the dental setting, in which saliva may be contaminated with blood. HBV and HIV transmission have not been documented from exposure to other body fluids, such as nasal secretions, sweat, tears, urine, or vomitus. However, standard precautions still apply whenever handling any body secretions. People who are sexually active should be aware that HIV is intermittently shed in semen.[5]

These fluids are most likely to transmit bloodborne pathogens. The hepatitis B vaccine substantially reduces the risk of infection and is available at no charge to all employees who have occupational exposure to the virus. It is considered so important that an employee must sign a letter of declination if declining the vaccine. Currently there are no vaccines available for HCV or HIV.

Guidelines for Infected Health Care Workers

Any health care worker with HIV or the most virulent form of hepatitis B or C should not perform exposure-prone procedures in which blood contact might occur. Permission and guidance from special review committees are required before an infected health care worker can perform such procedures.

For the therapist, this would primarily exclude wound care, including debridement and dressing changes. According to guidelines drafted by the CDC, at a minimum, the potential client must be informed of the worker's HIV, hepatitis B, or hepatitis C status if the health care worker will be performing specific exposure-prone procedures.

Control of Transmission

Hand Hygiene

Hand hygiene is a general term that applies to either hand washing, antiseptic hand wash, antiseptic hand rub, or surgical hand antisepsis. *Handwashing* refers to washing hands with plain (i.e., non-antimicrobial) soap and water. Hand hygiene is the term used when discussing reducing transmission.

Guidelines for hand hygiene in health care settings have been published by the CDC and are available online at http://www.cdc.gov/mmwr/PDF/rr/rr5116.pdf. For visual orientation to handwashing and hand rubbing, see the World Health Organization's posters available online at http://www.cdc.gov/handhygiene/Basics. html. Video presentations are also available at http://www. who.int/gpsc/5may/ and http://www.nejm.org/doi/full/ 10.1056/NEJMvcm0903599?query=TOC.[23]

Second to immunization, hand hygiene is the most effective disease-preventing measure anyone can practice. Hand hygiene is important in any and all settings and at all times. Despite compelling evidence that proper hand hygiene can reduce the transmission of pathogens to others and decrease the occurrence of antimicrobial resistance (e.g., methicillin-resistant *Staphylococcus aureus*), the adherence of health care workers (HCWs) to recommended hand hygiene practices remains unacceptably low.[1,14,17,30] According to the World Health Organization, hand-hygiene initiatives are ignored in up to 50% of all cases.[2,3]

To quote two prominent voices (Doron and Allegranzi 2011) in regards to the importance of hand-hygiene:[16]

> *Hand-hygiene campaigns can help address the problem, but can also suffer from their own success as a sense of urgency wanes. "Commonly, once success is achieved in hand hygiene, resources within the hospital are redirected to other important programs. As a result, hand-hygiene observations may be less frequent and less abundant, compliance rates may not be fed back to personnel as regularly as they had been, and incentive programs may be discontinued. The biggest challenge for institutions is, therefore, not how to improve hand-hygiene compliance, but how to maintain it in the face of the many other important patient safety goals that hospitals are focusing on these days.*

And there is evidence to suggest glove use lowers appropriate hand hygiene. Wearing gloves is not a substitute for proper hand hygiene; infection control requires following well-established standards for both.[18]

Hand hygiene is an integral part of reducing transmission of harmful microbes in a health care setting. Streptococci and coagulase-negative staphylococci are the most common bacteria residing on the skin. HCWs can transiently obtain other pathogens after patient care or from the areas immediately surrounding a client, which can then be transmitted to others. Transient organisms are more likely to be transmitted to others than are resident flora of the skin. Hand hygiene significantly reduces transient bacteria on HCWs' hands and the risk of transmitting infection.

Proper hand hygiene consists of using soap (antimicrobial or non-antimicrobial) and water when hands are visibly soiled with blood or other body fluid, before and after eating, and after using the restroom (see Box 8-4). If hands are not visibly soiled, decontamination may be accomplished by using an alcohol-based rub for the following instances: before and after direct contact with a client, before putting on gloves and after removing gloves for a nonsurgical procedure or client contact, after contact with inanimate objects (including medical equipment) in the client's vicinity, and before moving to a clean part of the same person.

Alcohol Rub. Hands may also be decontaminated with an alcohol-based rub after contact with body fluids or excretions, mucous membranes, nonintact skin, and wound dressings if hands are not visibly soiled. In the case of *Clostridium difficile*, spores are resistant to alcohol so alcohol-based hand rubs are not considered adequate when the disease is in a spore state; most *C. difficile* organisms released during disease outbreaks are in the vegetative form and can be killed by alcohol.[31] Without knowing the exact state of the condition, it is difficult to know when alcohol-based products will be effective. Currently, washing hands with an antimicrobial soap and water after removing gloves (see Box 8-5) is recommended by the CDC during outbreaks or if a client is suspected of having *C. difficile*.

Jewelry and Artificial Nails. Other pertinent recommendations have been made by the CDC in regard to wearing jewelry and artificial nails (acrylics) (available on-line at http://www.cdc.gov/mmwr/PDF/rr/rr5116.pdf). Although rings have been shown to harbor organisms, more studies are needed to determine if this leads to an increase in transmission of these microbes; the CDC has not made specific recommendations in this area.

Available studies suggest that the areas under the fingernails contain significant amounts of bacteria, especially coagulase-negative staphylococci and gram-negative rods. Artificial nails harbor even larger concentrations than natural nails. It is unknown if long or artificial nails contribute to transmission of these organisms, although a few reports have linked outbreaks of *Pseudomonas* and *Serratia* to artificial nails worn by nurses.[20]

More studies are needed to determine the significance of artificial nails, but the CDC recommends that artificial nails should not be worn if the HCW is in contact with clients at high risk for infection and adverse outcome.[8]

Respiratory Hygiene

Respiratory hygiene/cough etiquette addresses the education of HCWs and clients on the importance of controlling respiratory secretions to prevent the spread of respiratory pathogens, particularly during seasonal outbreaks of viral pathogens such as influenza and respiratory syncytial virus infections.

Signs should be posted in strategic locations such as reception and waiting areas in emergency departments and outpatient clinics that remind all persons to cover their mouths/noses when coughing or sneezing, using and disposing of tissues, and perform hand hygiene after contact with respiratory sections. During seasonal outbreaks, masks may be offered to clients who are coughing or otherwise symptomatic. They should also be encouraged to remain at least 3 feet from others in waiting areas or other similar locations.

Barrier Precautions (Personal Protective Equipment)

All health care workers should routinely use appropriate barrier precautions to prevent skin and mucous membrane exposure when contact with blood or other body fluids of any person is anticipated. Exposure to blood and body fluids can be minimized through the proper use of PPE. Personal protective equipment (gloves, gowns, and masks) provides a barrier to the transmission of infections to HCWs and other clients. However, *PPE is not a substitute for good engineering, work practice, and administrative controls, but should be used in conjunction with these controls to provide for a safe and healthy workplace.*

Gloves. The Occupational Safety and Health Administration has mandated that gloves be worn by HCWs when caring for clients when they may be exposed to blood or body fluids that can be contaminated with blood. Gloves have been shown to reduce contamination of hands as well as reduce the transmission of pathogens by HCWs. However, gloves do not completely protect against hand contamination; therefore decontamination of the hands before and after use is essential. Keep in mind that gloves can fail with clinical activity, allowing transmission of microbes. Pathogens can penetrate to the health care worker's hand, resulting in transference to others.

The CDC has provided the following important guidelines to protect yourself as well as the patient/client. You can find the complete guidelines available online at Centers for Disease Control and Prevention: Healthcare Associated Infections. Available on-line at http://www.cdc.gov/HAI/prevent/ppe_train.html.[13]

- Gloves should be worn for touching blood and body fluids, mucous membranes, blisters, lesions, and nonintact skin of all persons; gloves should be pulled up over the cuffs of the gown.
- Keep your gloved hands away from your face. Remove and replace the gloves if they become torn, heavily soiled, or contaminated. Perform hand hygiene before putting on new gloves.
- Gloves should be changed and hands washed after contact with each client.
- Wearing gloves is not a substitute for hand hygiene; well-established standards and guidelines as discussed in this Appendix must be followed with and without glove use.[18]
- A thin layer of water-based skin care product (e.g., Aquafor, Eucerin, O'Keeffe's Working Hands Creme) should be applied after glove removal to prevent skin chapping, which is a potential risk factor for employees. Petroleum-based hand creams or lotions, which can damage latex gloves, should not be used.

Face Protection

- Masks and protective eyewear or face shields should be worn during procedures that are likely to generate splashes, sprays, or droplets of blood or other body fluids to prevent exposure of mucous membranes of the mouth, nose, and eyes. Goggles or face shields should come equipped with a foam brow band, which prevents blood and body fluids from dripping from the forehead into the eyes. See also Box 15-4 for additional information regarding specific protective masks (called respirators) to wear when treating clients with active tuberculosis.
- Pocket masks or mechanical ventilation devices should be available in areas in which cardiopulmonary resuscitation procedures are likely.
- A mask or particulate respirator should be worn over the nose, mouth, and chin; the flexible nosepiece should be fit over the bridge of the nose and secured with fasteners or elastic. Particulate respirators must fit properly; to check the fit, inhale then exhale: the respirator should collapse during inhalation and there should be no air leaking out during exhalation.

Gowns

- Gowns should be of a material that prevents penetration by microorganisms and subsequent contamination of the skin or clothing.
- Gowns should be worn for direct patient contact if the patient has uncontained secretions or excretions. Fluid-proof gowns or aprons should be worn during procedures that are likely to generate splashes of blood or other body fluids.
- The opening is worn in the back and the gown should be secured. If the gown does not close, a second gown with the opening in the front should be worn.
- Gowns should not be reused, even for the same patient.
- Therapists treating clients with whirlpool or pulsatile lavage with suction should wear hair cover; mask; face shield; fluid-proof, long-sleeved gown; knee-high, fluid-resistant boots; and gloves covering the gown cuffs. Shoulder-length gloves should be available for those working with whirlpools. See Box A-1.
- Hands should be washed before and after client contact, after removing PPE, before and after gloving, and immediately if hands are grossly contaminated with blood.
- Hands and other skin surfaces should be washed immediately and thoroughly if contaminated with blood or other body fluids. Hands should be washed immediately after gloves are removed. Antiseptic hand cleaner should be used when handwashing facilities are unavailable.

Other

- Remember to clean noncritical items between patients (e.g., pens, pencils, walkers, or other assistive devices).
- Eating, drinking, applying lip balm or lipstick, and handling contact lenses are prohibited in any area where clients or their body fluids are present.
- Sharp instruments, such as scissors or scalpels, should be handled with great care and disposed of in puncture-resistant containers. Needles should never be manipulated, bent, broken, or recapped.

Box A-1

STANDARD PRECAUTIONS IN THE USE OF PULSATILE LAVAGE WITH SUCTION (PLWS)

PLWS Use and Maintenance

- Read all device instructions for use and recommended techniques to minimize environmental contamination.
- Use continuous suction (60–100 mm Hg).
- Position the splash shield to remain in contact with the wound/periwound area at all times.
- Dispose of the suction waste canister after each use.
- Dispose of all single-use pulsatile lavage components immediately after use.
- Disinfect any reusable item(s). (Only a suction diverter handpiece can be reused—nothing can be sterilized to be reused.)

Environmental Controls

- Always perform PLWS in an appropriately ventilated private room enclosed with walls and doors that shut.
- Minimize potential contamination of equipment and supplies; do not leave shelves or cabinets open.
- Cover surfaces at risk for aerosol contamination.
- After each treatment, clean and disinfect environmental surfaces that can be touched by hand.

Personal Protective Equipment

- Wear a fluid-proof gown; gloves; mask, goggles, or face shield; and hair and shoe covers.
- Provide patient/client with a droplet barrier (e.g., surgical mask) when appropriate during PLWS treatment.
- Cover all entrance sites of lines and ports, and wounds that are not being treated.

Data from Loehne HB: Pulsatile lavage with concurrent suction. In Sussman C, Bates-Jensen B, eds: *Wound care: A collaborative practice manual for health professionals*, ed 4, Philadelphia, 2011, Lippincott Williams & Wilkins.

- Health care workers who have exudative lesions or weeping dermatitis should refrain from all direct client care and from handling equipment belonging to the client until the condition resolves.

Once the PPE is in use properly, the therapist should avoid touching or adjusting the PPE.

When the procedure or client visit is completed, remove all PPE except respirators at the doorway before leaving the room.

Respirators can be removed outside the client's door, after closing the door. Continue to practice standard precautions by removing remaining pieces of PPE carefully and correctly.[11] Mask/respirator is only to be removed by the ties/elastics not the front since it is considered contaminated. Avoid contact with the potentially contaminated exterior surfaces of gloves, face shield, gowns, and so on. Turn gloves and gown inside out as you remove them and discard appropriately. Perform hand hygiene when all pieces of equipment are removed and discarded.[27]

Hydrotherapy and Therapeutic Pool Protocol[9]

In the past, routine cultures of hydrotherapy and pool equipment were performed to identify and supposedly eliminate colonization of infectious bacteria. In this way, the spread of infection was prevented from equipment to client and from client to client, especially in the acute care setting.

Now, under the outcomes-based management philosophy, infection control is cost driven so that the outcome is managed, as long as the outcome is what was predicted and intended or improving. For example, in the case of preventing the spread of infection through hydrotherapy or therapeutic pool equipment, good disinfection and cleaning procedures are practiced and monitored closely. This plan is both cost effective and accompanied by a high degree of safety. The CDC offers guidelines for preferred methods for cleaning, disinfection, and sterilization of patient-care medical devices and environment. They are available online at http://www.cdc.gov/hicpac/pdf/guidelines/Disinfection_Nov_2008.pdf.

Routine environmental cultures are not cost effective and therefore are not performed. Many organisms are present normally, and if present and no one is infected, these pathogens are not considered a functional problem. Under outcomes-based management, when an infectious problem develops, the cause is traced back to the source and eliminated at that point.

Pulsatile Lavage With Suction

Pulsatile lavage with suction (PLWS), a high-pressure irrigation treatment used by physical therapists as a wound debridement system, can aerosolize infectious agents at least 8 feet. Infection control precautions must be used routinely during the procedure (see Box A-1) and all surfaces wiped down after the procedure. Failure to do so has been linked with an outbreak of multidrug-resistant *Acinetobacter baumannii* from environmental contamination.[25]

When using pulsatile lavage with suction for wound care, clients should be treated in a private treatment room with all walls and doors closed.[22] Proper personal protective equipment, such as masks, gloves, and eyewear, must be worn by the therapist when treating the individual and cleaning hydrotherapy equipment. Tip or suction diverter cannot be reused from treatment to treatment.

Outpatient and Home Health Care

Preventing spread of an infectious disease to the family, the home health therapist, and perhaps the community is a primary concern when preparing the client to return home. The therapist should work closely with outpatient staff or the home health nurse and seek guidance if unsure how to handle a specific situation.

Individuals leaving the hospital and then following up with the outpatient facility may still be colonized. If a person was recently hospitalized, it should be standard practice to ask if that individual was in a room in which people taking care of him/her had to wear special outfits.

A list of helpful hints for outpatient and home health care includes the following:

- Hand hygiene is the best protection against transmission of infectious diseases, and it is essential after providing direct care and before touching anything when gloves are removed.
- Staff should leave extraneous clothing and equipment outside the client's area and take in only items that are needed.

- Equipment needed on a regular basis, such as the blood pressure cuff and stethoscope, should be in the room at the beginning of home health care. Single-use equipment is often available. Stethoscopes can be contaminated with staphylococci and are therefore a potential vector of infection.[24,33] Such contamination poses a risk to people with open wounds such as burns. This contamination is greatly reduced by frequent cleaning with alcohol or nonionic detergent; cleaning with antiseptic soap is only 75% effective in reducing the bacterial count.[4]
- When it is no longer needed, equipment should be bagged or covered and taken to the appropriate area for decontamination and reprocessing. Disposable equipment should be contained, labeled, and discarded.
- The therapist should be adequately supplied with gloves, masks, gowns, and disposable plastic aprons. Some plastic bags of different sizes should be carried for the therapist's own use and to demonstrate to the client's family how to handle soiled linens and trash.
- Paper towels are useful when working in the client's area. Use them as a clean surface during care and to wipe your hands.
- Before going into the client's area, plan what to do and gather the items needed.
- It is important to remember that isolation or precautions can have a negative effect on the family. Help the family feel comfortable with the techniques needed for isolation. Encourage them to visit with the client and not just be with him or her during care.
- Should the client have a feces-borne infectious disease such as hepatitis A or *salmonellosis*, it is important to show the family how to bag and launder soiled linens. It is equally important to demonstrate how to bag and dispose of soiled paper products such as linen savers, which cannot be flushed down the toilet. Remind the family to wash their hands afterward, and the therapist should do so as well.
- If the client has hepatitis A or *salmonellosis*, the family and the client should be reminded not to handle raw food served to others, such as lettuce or tomatoes, until the physician determines the client is past the infectious stage.
- In treating clients with bloodborne illnesses, if the client accidentally sustains a cut, any spilled blood on inanimate objects or surfaces should be cleaned off with household bleach and water. Razors and toothbrushes should not be shared.
- The therapist should practice self-protection at all times. Use good hand hygiene and, when in doubt, ask for assistance from other, more knowledgeable health care staff.

Environmental Surfaces, Medical and Other Equipment

Medical equipment and other articles in a health care facility may be contaminated and precautions must be taken to avoid transmitting pathogens after touching items in a room. Studies have shown that methicillin-resistant *Staphylococcus* aureus and vancomycin-resistant *Enterococcus* can live for days to weeks on medical equipment,[6] and environmental contamination with these organisms is a major risk factor in transmission.

Norovirus, *C. difficile*, and *Acinetobacter* are all able to survive for extended periods of time in the environment, and infections caused by these organisms can be traced to environment or health-care worker hands.[34] Numerous studies report noncompliance of health care staff with routine cleaning practices of hands, hospital surfaces, and inanimate objects such as stethoscopes.[26,28,35]

Studies[34] have detected Norovirus on toilet lids, door handles, and phones. *C. difficile* was isolated on rectal thermometers and commodes, among other equipment, and *Acinetobacter* was found extensively during outbreaks in the intensive care setting (bed rails, bedside tables, surfaces of ventilators, sinks, suction equipment, mattresses, resuscitation equipment, curtains, slings for patient lifting, mops, buckets, door handles, stethoscopes, incubators, and computer keyboards). Paper has also been implicated as a possible source of bacteria, with organisms shown to remain stable for 72 hours.[21] These organisms are easily picked up on hands or gloves and transmitted to other clients.

Cell Phones. Although these guidelines do not address the issue of contaminated cell phones, several studies have demonstrated the presence of microbes on cell phones. There is some evidence that cell phones carried by patients and visitors are twice as likely as the mobile phones of health workers to carry pathogens.[32] Patient phones also tested for higher rates of multidrug-resistant bacteria, including methicillin-resistant *Staphylococcus aureus*.

More studies are needed to determine if this leads to an increase in the transmission of microbes and the most appropriate method of decontamination.[7]

A THERAPIST'S THOUGHTS

Infectious Control Practices

There is growing evidence that disinfecting a client's environment can reduce the risk for heath care–associated infections.[15,34] Please refer to CDC guidelines for preferred cleaning, disinfection, and sterilization methods. Available online at http://www.cdc.gov/hicpac/pdf/guidelines/Disinfection_Nov_2008.pdf. See also Guide to Elimination of *Clostridium difficile* in health care settings, Washington, DC, Association for Professionals in Infection Control and Epidemiology, 2008 [http://www.apic.org/Resource_/EliminationGuideForm/5de5d1c1-316a-4b5e-b9b4-c3fbeac1b53e/File/APIC-Cdiff-Elimination-Guide.pdf].

Interpretation on how to handle individuals on infection precautions is per the compliance officer at your facility, accrediting bodies, and state practice acts. It is my experience that guidelines change often due to current evidence, staffing changes, and increased prevalence/incidence of infectious diseases in a facility. Other physical therapists have observed this phenomenon in their facilities as well. It is imperative the physical therapist remain current with infection control practices and policies to ensure patient safety.

Kimberly Levenhagen, PT, DPT, WCC

SUMMARY

Evidence suggests that up to 30% of health care associated infections are preventable through adherence to good infection control procedures. Adherence to infection control practices is a Joint Commission National Patient Safety Goal. Here is a link to this area: http://www.jointcommission.org/standards_information/npsgs.aspx.

Environmental surfaces are an issue and physical therapists can play an important role in improving patient care outcomes by implementing these guidelines into their daily practice. Because of the increase of microorganisms on fomites, the therapist should wash hands even after touching environmental surfaces. Environmental surfaces need to be cleaned with U.S. Environmental Protection Agency–approved products (e.g., bleach for *C. difficile*) when there is a risk of infection and cross contamination in all settings.

Physical therapists in hospital, home health, and skilled nursing facilities are aware of the risk of transfer of infectious diseases via fomites and now there is increasing concern in the outpatient and school-based systems due to community-associated methicillin-resistant *Staphylococcus aureus*.

In all situations, the physical therapist has a responsibility to select appropriate equipment (e.g., vinyl or wipeable gait belts) that can be cleaned appropriately with Environmental Protection Agency–approved products between uses. For example, with approved disposable wipes, the amount of wait-time after cleaning is dependent on the type of germicidal wipes in use. The time necessary to disinfect is indicated on the product (e.g., "Treated surface must remain visibly wet for a full 3 minutes"). With the rising number of patients requiring contact isolation precautions and the average size of patients rising, patient gowns can be rolled up as a gait belt and as a sheet for the larger patients. It is single use and goes to the laundry. [Thanks to Alisa Curry, PT, DPT, for this tip!]

Cleaning equipment used between different individuals needs to be stressed (i.e., mats, walkers, chairs, portable stairs, blood pressure cuffs, stethoscopes, therapist's ID badge, and writing utensil). Any visible soiling must be removed first and then the item wiped a second time, leaving the surface wet for 3 minutes after the initial cleaning. Equipment that cannot be cleaned should be issued to the individual (cloth gait belts, blood pressure cuffs, etc.).

In any setting, if you are a manager or administrator of your facility, it is important to ensure appropriate compliance with guidelines and cleaning recommendations. Watch for future publications on the role of allied health professionals in this area (e.g., publication by Kimberly Levenhagen, in process).

REFERENCES

To enhance this text and add value for the reader, all references are included on the companion Evolve site that accompanies this textbook. The reader can view the reference source and access it online whenever possible.

APPENDIX B

Guidelines for Activity and Exercise

Frequently, older adults with orthopedic dysfunction are inactive, hypertensive, and have multiple risk factors for comorbidities. These factors often are not documented, and the client is treated as an orthopedic case without regard for the past medical history or current cardiopulmonary (or other) condition.

For these reasons, the health care provider must view the effect of other systems on the client's orthopedic condition and rehabilitation outcome. A thorough evaluation may be necessary, and monitoring cardiopulmonary responses to exercise may be required. Postoperative considerations for various conditions are important when planning a rehabilitation program; these guidelines are listed in each section throughout this text whenever possible.

Exercise should be specific to the functional and medical needs of each individual. Whenever possible, physical activity and exercise should be at a level that causes minimal to no symptoms, and progression should be built into the program. For the aging adult, physiologic homeostasis may be altered by stress, medications, illness, and exercise. To assist in balancing and maintaining homeostasis, 1 day of rest between each day of exercise may be recommended for some individuals.

Interval training, consisting of short-term periods of ambulation followed by rest, is now recommended. Such a program activates the oxygen transport to skeletal and circulatory systems for completion of an activity of daily living to develop endurance. Progress slowly by increasing duration to 30 minutes before increasing intensity. Encourage the client to keep an exercise diary that includes any symptoms that may occur during or after exercise. Review the diary and compare this report to the client's verbal report, because the person may forget or deny important information.

MEDICATIONS AND EXERCISE

Some clients may be taking medications that can have considerable side effects and interactions when combined with other medications, including effects on exercise parameters such as heart rate, blood pressure, or respiratory rate. Medications can also affect balance, posture, motor control, sleep, and mood, which may affect the individual's performance in rehabilitation. Common drugs with side effects that may affect an exercise program are listed in Table B-1.

People who are taking drugs that can cause volume depletion or orthostatic hypotension should have their blood pressure and pulse checked in both reclining and standing positions. Avoiding sudden postural changes or activities, limiting activities that promote vasodilation, and providing an adequate warm-up and cool-down period are essential. See also "Special Implications for the Therapist 12-8: Orthostatic Hypotension" in Chapter 12. Therapeutic intervention, especially exercise, should be scheduled according to medication peak blood levels to minimize effects on participation and to enhance rehabilitation performance.

GUIDELINES FOR MONITORING VITAL SIGNS

It is important to know normal responses to movement and activity (including exercise) to be able to identify abnormal responses in the client with a medical diagnosis. Safe and effective exercise can be measured in part by monitoring vital sign responses (temperature, heart rate, respiratory rate, blood pressure, oxygen saturation, pain levels). Such data can be used as specific outcome measures to substantiate decision making. For example, how quickly the heart rate returns to normal is an outcome measurement of fitness and conditioning.

The use of walking velocity has been proposed as the "sixth vital sign." Walking speed is a general indicator of function[27] and, as such, a reflection of many variables such as health status, motor control, muscle strength, and endurance. It is a reliable, valid, and sensitive measure of functional ability with additional predictive value in assessing future health status, functional decline, potential for hospitalization, and even mortality.[15]

The test is conducted using a timed 10-meter walk test on a 20-meter-long straight path. Complete descriptions of the test and expected results are available.[5,6,15,27] As specialists in human movement and function, the therapist can use walking speed as a practical and predictive "vital sign" of general health that can be used to monitor change (improvement or decline) in health and function.

Table B-1	Common Drugs That May Affect an Exercise Program
Drugs	**Effects**
Anticoagulants	Bleeding into tissues; see Table 40-9
Antidepressants, antipsychotics	Sedation, lethargy, muscle weakness; orthostasis and falls, arrhythmias
	Antipsychotics only: extrapyramidal motor effects (change in posture, balance, and involuntary movements)
Antihypertensive agents	Hypotension; orthostasis and falls
	Reduced exercise capacity (β-blockers)
β-Adrenergic blockers	Decreased heart rate (resting and exercise), fatigue, masking of hypoglycemic symptoms
Corticosteroids	See Table 5-4
Immunosuppressants	See Table 5-3
Nonsteroidal antiinflammatory drugs (NSAIDs)	See Table 5-2
Diuretics	Hypokalemia—arrhythmias, muscle cramps (see Chapter 5)
	Dehydration—orthostasis and falls, thermoregulatory disturbance
	Elevated heart rate with all activity
Insulin, oral hypoglycemics	Hypoglycemia
Pain medication, narcotics, opioids	Blunted respiratory response, sedation, lethargy, muscle weakness, incoordination
Thyroid medication	Altered metabolic state (see Chapter 5)
	Impaired cardiopulmonary function
	Myalgias, stiffness, trigger points
	See further discussion in Chapter 11
Tranquilizers, sedatives	Relaxation, reduced coordination; orthostasis and falls

See also Table 12-5 and Box 5-2.

Table B-2	Body Temperature Conversions	
Celsius (° C)		**Fahrenheit (° F)**
34.0		93.2
35.0		95.0
35.6		96.1
35.8		96.4
36.0		96.8
36.2		97.2
36.4		97.5
36.6		97.9
36.8		98.2
37.0		**98.6**
37.2		99.0
37.4		99.3
37.6		99.7
37.8		100.0
38.0		100.4
38.2		100.8
38.4		101.1
38.6		101.5
38.8		101.8
39.0		102.2
39.2		102.6
39.4		102.9
39.6		103.3
39.8		103.6
40.0		104.0
40.2		104.4
40.4		104.7
40.6		105.2
40.8		105.4
41.0		105.9
41.2		106.1
41.4		106.5
42.0		107.6
42.4		108.3
43.0		109.4

Anyone with a significant past medical history of cardiovascular or pulmonary disease requires monitoring of vital signs and perceived exertion during exercise. The more coronary risk factors present (see Table 12-3), the greater the need for monitoring. For any client with known coronary artery disease and/or previous history of myocardial infarction, exercise testing should be performed before an exercise program is undertaken.

If this testing has not been accomplished and baseline measurements are unavailable for use in planning exercise, the therapist must monitor the client's heart rate and blood pressure and note any accompanying symptoms during exercise. Too rapid a rise in heart rate, respiratory rate, or blood pressure for the workload is a general indication for modifying the activity or exercise program (see "Abnormal Heart Rate Response" and "Abnormal Respiratory Rate Response" below).

Type of exercise may make a difference in the changes observed in vital signs in older adults. Measurement of heart rate and blood pressure responses to typical isometric, isokinetic, and eccentric resistance-training protocols in older adults showed that changes in blood pressure, arterial pressure, and rate-pressure product were significantly greater during isometric exercise than during eccentric exercise. Clinically, an isokinetic eccentric exercise program enables older adults to work at the same torque output with less cardiovascular stress than isometric exercise.[24]

Temperature

Normal body temperature is not a specific number but a range of values that depends on factors such as the time of day, age, medical status, and presence or absence of infection. Oral body temperature ranges from 96.8° to 99.5° F (36° to 37.5° C) with an average of 98.6° F (37° C) (Table B-2).

The clinical implications of fever and approach to fever vary considerably from person to person, institution to institution, and physician to physician. For example, there is a tendency among the aging population to develop an increase in temperature on hospital admission or in response to any change in homeostasis. Alternatively, fever in older adults residing in extended care facilities may suggest an infectious process, whereas postoperative fever can indicates a surgical complication, such as intraabdominal abscess, leaking anastomosis with peritonitis, or an infected surgical site or prosthesis (e.g., valve, joint, graft). Fever response in adults older than 75 years is often blunted and sometimes even absent.

Others who may remain afebrile in the presence of significant infectious pathology include those who are immunocompromised (e.g., transplant recipients, corticosteroid users, individuals with cancer undergoing treatment), alcoholics, individuals with chronic renal insufficiency, and anyone taking excessive antipyretic medications. Establishing a basal body temperature and monitoring for changes in temperature (of more than 2.4° F [1.3° C]) can assist in early detection of infection (see Box 8-1 for other manifestations of infection).[10,37]

Single temperature spikes (sudden elevation that returns to normal without intervention) is usually of no diagnostic significance unless it occurs in an immunocompromised individual.[13] Common causes of sustained fever are listed in Box 8-2 and Table 8-1. Unexplained fever in adolescents may be a manifestation of drug abuse or endocarditis.

The therapist should use discretionary caution with anyone who has a fever. Exercise with a fever stresses the cardiopulmonary and immune systems, which may be further complicated by dehydration.

Heart Rate (Pulse Rate)

Measuring the heart rate by taking the pulse is really a measurement of the pulse rate. A true measure of the heart rate requires measurement of the electrical impulses of the heart. Resting heart rate is age dependent, with minimal variation for each individual within the normal ranges.

The normal range for the resting pulse rate is 60–100 beats/min (or bpm). A rate above 100 beats/min indicates tachycardia; below 60 beats/min indicates bradycardia. Some variations occur with age and training (Table B-3). For example, a well-trained athlete whose heart muscle develops along with the skeletal muscle may have a resting heart rate of less than 60 beats/min.

The force of the pulse represents the strength of the heart's stroke volume. A weak, thready pulse reflects a decreased stroke volume, such as occurs with hemorrhagic shock. A full, bounding pulse indicates an increased stroke volume, possibly associated with anxiety, exercise, or some pathologic condition. The pulse force (pulse amplitude) is recorded using the following three-point scale (some physicians/nurses use a four-point scale):

3+	Full, bounding
2+	Normal
1+	Weak, thready
0	Absent

The pulse should be measured before and during the activity using the same position both times. Count for 6 seconds and add a 0 to that number for a beats-per-minute

Table B-3	Normal Resting Pulse Rates Across Age Groups	
Age	**Average Beats/Min**	**Normal Limits (Beats/Min)**
Newborn	125	70–190
1 y	120	80–160
2 y	110	80–130
4 y	100	80–120
6 y	100	70–110
8–10 y	90	70–110
12 y		
Female	90	70–110
Male	85	65–105
14 y		
Female	85	65–105
Male	80	60–100
16 y		
Female	80	60–100
Male	75	55–95
18 y		
Female	75	55–95
Male	70	50–90
Well-conditioned athlete	May be 50–60	50–100
Adult	—	60–80
Aging	—	60–100

From Behrman RE, Kliegman RM, Jenson HB: *Nelson textbook of pediatrics,* ed 17, Philadelphia, 2004, Saunders.

count or count for 10 seconds and multiply by 6. Heart rate response should increase gradually with an increase in the workload of the heart. Once a steady state has been achieved, little change should occur in heart rate during sustained endurance activities (e.g., water aerobics, riding a stationary bicycle). Factors affecting heart rate responses are listed in Box B-1.

Effect of Deconditioning

Heart rate responses are different in the deconditioned person because the resting heart rate is higher to begin with. The heart rate increases more rapidly for the same workload compared to the change in a healthy individual. A rapid heart rate may occur during activity in response to dehydration, because the decreased plasma volume results in decreased blood volume and subsequent decreased blood to the heart.

A decreased stroke volume (volume ejected per heartbeat) is compensated for by a higher heart rate to match the demands for oxygen caused by the activity. *Cardiac muscle dysfunction* is the term used when a decreased stroke volume occurs as a result of diseased cardiac muscle that can no longer contract and pump blood out of the heart normally. Decreased stroke volume results in a more rapid rise in heart rate unless the person is taking beta-blocking medication.

Effect of Age

Aging is accompanied by a decreasing maximum heart rate. The age-predicted method for calculating the predicted maximal (target) heart rate (PMHR) is 220 – age.

FACTORS AFFECTING HEART RATE

- Age
- Anemia
- Anxiety, panic
- Autonomic dysfunction (e.g., diabetes, spinal cord injury)
- Caffeine
- Cardiac muscle dysfunction
- Deconditioned state
- Dehydration (decreased blood volume causes increased heart rate)
- Drugs (e.g., blood pressure medication; asthma inhalants; antihistamines, such as over-the-counter cold medications; narcotics)
- Emotional or psychologic stress
- Exercise
- Fear
- Fever
- Hyperthyroidism
- Infection
- Pain
- Potassium level
- Sleep disturbances/sleep deprivation
- Stress

For example, for a 70-year-old the PMHR = 220 − 70, or 150 beats/min. This principle is based on the fact that the heart's maximal rate is 220 beats/min and that this maximal rate declines by one beat each year (probably as a result of the heart's stiffening and becoming less compliant).[26] Target heart rate is the first number calculated in determining the *training zone*—that is, keeping the heart rate during exercise between 65% and 85% of the estimated peak heart rate. The lower end of the range is for strengthening the heart, lungs, and circulatory system; the upper end builds endurance. Lower targets are used for those who are just beginning an exercise program, those who are deconditioned, and individuals with known heart disease.

Some concern about the use of this formula has been raised; some consider it inaccurate because it was based on early research that only examined sedentary men under the age of 60. The formula does not take into account female gender, older age, diagnosis, fitness level, or the presence of comorbidities. It has been suggested that the standard formula overestimates maximum heart rate in older adults. This would have the effect of underestimating the true level of physical stress imposed during exercise testing and the appropriate intensity of prescribed exercise programs.[36]

This method should not be applied to individuals with peripheral neuropathies, those with chronotropic incompetence (irregular contraction of the heart), or clients taking β-blockers for hypertension and angina. The β-blockers are medications that block the sympathetic nervous system's input to the β_1-receptors in the heart, thus affecting heart rate and contractility. The net effect is a decrease in the resting and exercise heart rate (drug-induced bradycardia).

The most accurate way to determine maximum heart rate is a stress test in consultation with a cardiologist.

Since this is not practical or cost effective, the therapist can teach the client how to use rating of perceived exertion (RPE) as a more user-friendly method. For most clients, it is best to wait until the person has exercised for at least 5 minutes before applying the formula. When using the 6–20 scale (very, very light effort to very, very hard effort), multiply the RPE number that matches the client's effort and multiply by 10 (or simply add a zero after the number). This figure gives a close estimate of the expected heart rate in a healthy individual; cardiovascular (aerobic) exercise should be in the 11–14 RPE range.[7]

There is a revised age-adjusted formula to calculate target heart rate *training zone* that may be more accurate: 208 − (age × 0.70).[28] For a 70-year-old, using this formula would suggest a maximum heart rate of 159 beats/min. This method does require accurate measurement of the pulse and a calculator and may still be off by up to 8 beats/min. For the active, healthy older adult, another formula has been proposed: PMHR = 205 minus − ½ age.[27] For example, evaluating the same 70-year-old under these conditions would be 205 − ½(70), or 205 − 35 (PMHR = 170).

Preliminary work has also been done to modify the heart rate equation for women undergoing treatment for cancer using the equation: 207 − 0.86 × age.[19] A subsequent article will come out for men and women during cancer treatment. The equation has not been tested for cancer survivors. But there are plans to do that in a future study.[31]

There is a revised gender-adjusted formula for women based on the St. James Women Take Heart Project launched in 1992 with published recommendations in 2010.[18] The new formula for estimating peak heart rate in women is 206 − (age × 0.88). Under the old formula (220 − age), the estimated peak heart rate for women was higher, so it could lead to overdiagnosis of heart disease and less conclusive results of stress tests. The 220 − age formula sets a higher-than-necessary heart rate target that may discourage some women from exercising at an appropriately vigorous rate. This is an especially important point knowing the many pieces of exercise equipment (in home and at gyms) use the 220 − age formula, thus misleading women in exercising at an uncomfortable level to achieve an artificially determined goal for peak heart rate.

Keep in mind that anyone taking cardiac medications may not be able to achieve a target heart rate above 90 beats/min. For example, β-blockers slow the heart at rest and limit how fast it can beat during exercise. Therefore, symptoms of shortness of breath, the use of RPE, or the "talk test" may be much better ways to determine exercise intensity. According to the talk test, an individual is exercising at a moderate intensity if able to talk (or sing) out loud while exercising. Anyone having trouble finishing a sentence should slow down. Many individuals who are compromised need more time to work up to the exercise load and to cool down. Using RPE still requires close monitoring of heart rate and blood pressure.

Other methods for prescribing exercise intensity by target heart rate include the Heart Rate Reserve (Karvonen) Method, which takes into account the person's resting heart rate; the rate-pressure product method (valid indicator of myocardial oxygen uptake); maximal oxygen consumption (VO_{2max} or maximal functional capacity); and the systolic blood pressure method. Information on each of these methods and their recommended applications and known limitations is available.[26]

Most methods for determining exercise intensity are based on target heart rates that are 40–85% of VO_{2max}. However, there are some people for whom exercise intensity should not be prescribed by a target heart rate method, such as those who are deconditioned. In such cases, exercise should be prescribed at the lower end of the intensity continuum.

A safe rate of exercise will allow the heart rate to return to the resting level within 5 minutes after stopping exercise (blood pressure returns to resting levels after heart rate). Avoid increases of more than 20 beats/min over resting heart rate. (See "Exercise and Antihypertensive Medications," Chapter 12.) Do not remove telemetry immediately after exercise (wait 5–10 minutes); in the case of cardiac transplantation, cool down may take up to 1 hour (warm-up should last 30–45 minutes).

Abnormal Heart Rate Response

Heart rate should increase commensurately with exercise; as the intensity of exercise increases, the heart rate increases (e.g., like blood pressure, heart rate also increases according to metabolic equivalent [MET]; only a minimal increase in heart rate would be expected with a low-MET activity). The MET system provides one way of measuring the amount of oxygen needed to perform an activity: 1 MET = 3.5 mL of oxygen uptake, which a person requires when resting.

If the pulse is irregular, count the pulse for a full minute and document the number of beats per minute as well as the number of irregular beats (see next section). Abnormal heart rate responses include a rapid rate of rise in heart rate (judging from the activity, age, and training history) or a decreased heart rate with activity (e.g., arrhythmias or pauses in pulse). For example, a doubling of the heart rate with walking on a flat surface (no incline) would be considered outside normal parameters.

A decreased heart rate with activity may occur as a normal response when the person is sympathetically overloaded before treatment. For example, a person who takes inhalants for asthma just before therapy or who drinks more than three cups of coffee within 2 hours of the therapy appointment may have an artificially elevated baseline heart rate. Over the course of therapy, without further stimulation, this person's heart rate may decrease, especially if the therapy session has no exercise component. Factors such as these require individual evaluation of abnormal responses for each person.

Pulse amplitude (weak or bounding quality of the pulse) that fades with inspiration and strengthens with expiration is paradoxic (paradoxical pulse) and should be reported to the physician. When there is compression or constriction around the heart (e.g., pericardial effusion, tension pneumothorax, pericarditis with fluid, pericardial tamponade) and the person breathes in, the increased mechanical pressure of inspiration added to the physiologic compression from the underlying disease prevents the heart from contracting fully and results in reduced pulse. When the individual expires, the pressure from chest expansion is reduced and the pulse increases.

Table B-4	Normal Resting Respiratory Rates
Age	**Breaths/Min**
Premature	40–70
Birth–3 mo	35–55
3–6 mo	30–45
6–12 mo	25–40
1–3 y	20–30
3–6 y	20–25
6–10 y	15–25
10–16 y	12–30
18 y	12–20
Adult	10–12*

*Typical for average, healthy adult; low for older adult.
From Behrman RE, Kliegman RM, Jenson HB: *Nelson textbook of pediatrics*, ed 17, Philadelphia, 2004, Saunders.

A pulse increase of more than 20 beats/min lasting for more than 3 minutes after rest or changing position should also be reported.

If ischemia occurs as evidenced by angina or (on visual readout) depression of ST segment on electrocardiogram, the person should rest and then return to an activity level below ischemic level. For example, if the ST segment drops below baseline with activity or the client experiences angina when the heart rate is at 140 beats/min, the activity level should be reduced so that the heart rate remains below 140 beats/min.

Heart Rhythm

For the person with an abnormal heart rhythm, the pulse should be palpated throughout the activity if no electrocardiogram or Holter monitor reading is available during exercise. If any abnormal pulse beats are noted (e.g., absent, irregular), the number of pauses per minute should be counted at rest and during activity. There should be no more than six abnormal or absent beats per minute. The normal heart rhythm should not change, and individuals with arrhythmias at rest should not show an increase in number of irregular heartbeats with increased activity.

Respiratory Rate

Normal resting respiratory rates are presented in Table B-4. The ratio of pulse rate to respiratory rate is fairly constant (4:1). The respirations can be counted at the same time that the pulse is counted. If an abnormality is suspected, these measurements should be taken for a full minute. A normal pulmonary response to exercise is an increase in breathing rate and depth based on body type and disease present. Factors that can affect respiratory rate include the following:
- Altered lung compliance (chronic obstructive pulmonary disease [COPD], hyaline membrane disease) or any other restrictive condition
- Airway resistance (asthma)
- Alterations in lung volumes/lung capacity (smokers, persons with emphysema or occupational lung disease)

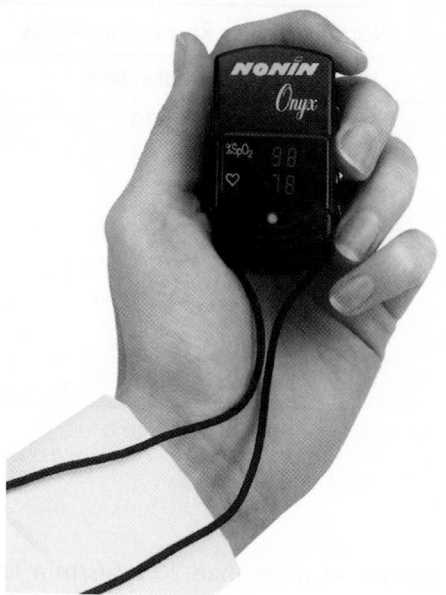

Figure B-1

Noninvasive monitoring of oxygen saturation (Sao_2), sometimes referred to as the fifth vital sign, can be done with a pulse oximeter. A finger probe is used most frequently during stationary activities. This compact unit (Onyx) is small enough to carry and ideal for spot checks anytime. The person slips this digital pulse oximeter onto a finger for an immediate pulse rate and oxygen saturation percentage. An ear probe (not shown) can be used to measure oxygen saturation continuously during exercise. (Courtesy Nonin, Inc., Plymouth, MN.)

- Body position (diaphragm cannot drop down enough to expand the lungs in the fully supine position in the pregnant, obese, or spinal cord–injured client)

Abnormal Respiratory Rate Response

An abnormal respiratory rate response is usually characterized by too rapid a rise in respiratory rate for the activity and medical condition of the client. Increases in respiratory rate greater than 10 respirations/min must be monitored carefully. Measuring the respiratory rate may be difficult. The client must be observed for how much work is required to breathe, and whenever possible, a pulse oximeter should be used to measure arterial oxygen saturation noninvasively (Fig. B-1).

Pulse Oximetry

The saturation of hemoglobin with oxygen can be measured via pulse oximetry (Spo_2) or arterial blood gas (ABG) analysis (Sao_2). A normal Spo_2 or Sao_2 value is 95% or higher. An Sao_2 or Sao_2 value below 90% means the Pao_2 is below 60 mm Hg, indicating the person is not adequately oxygenated (Pao_2 is a measure of the pressure of oxygen dissolved in plasma as measured by ABG analysis).

The Pao_2 at rest may decline with age because of a loss of surface respiratory space for ventilatory exchange, especially in adults aged 70 years or older. The Pao_2 increases with activity in older adults as blood volume and respiratory volume increase.[11]

Using a pulse oximeter with the pulmonary population can provide an outcome measure with exercise for

documentation. Oxygen saturation values must be interpreted within the context of the person's medical status as well as respiratory and metabolic status (as determined by ABG measurements). Respiratory and metabolic status are taken into consideration, because shifts in the oxyhemoglobin curve caused by factors such as temperature fluctuations or acidosis will change the affinity of oxygen to the hemoglobin.

Normal oxygen saturation is 98%, with no change in this measurement during activity or exercise. Clients with chronic respiratory disease may experience a drop in oxygen saturation that is considered normal for them, but this represents a normal response to pathology and is not truly normal.

There has been some question as to whether nail polish can affect the accuracy of pulse oximetry readings. Studies to date have not shown a statistically or clinically significant difference in readings with nail polish of any color (including colorless) in healthy or critically ill and mechanically ventilated individuals.[8,12,23,34]

Activity should be terminated if oxygen saturation drops to 90% or less in the acutely ill individual or 86% in the person with chronic lung disease. Individuals with decreased oxygen saturation may require more time to accomplish tasks and often experience fatigue and/or shortness of breath. Panic values may vary according to institution and physician. Increased oxygen during activity may prevent such drops but should be discussed with the physician before it is instituted.

At all times, other vital signs should be monitored (heart rate, respiratory rate, and blood pressure) to assess how well the person is tolerating the activity and oxygen desaturation. In the event of large changes in oxygen saturation as determined by pulse oximetry with no changes in vital signs, the pulse oximetry may not be accurate, thus requiring a mechanical check.

Caution is advised when using a finger probe on an individual with cold, discolored hands (blue or white), which is an indication that blood has already been shunted from the fingers. Pulse oximetry as a measure of oxygen saturation would not be accurate in such a situation.[21] Peripheral arterial vasoconstriction during the early phases of treadmill exercise has been documented in individuals with vascular pathology secondary to atherosclerosis.[35]

Supplemental Oxygen

Supplemental oxygen is given if an individual has documented or suspected hypoxemia or deficient oxygenation of the blood, defined as a Pao_2 below 60 mm Hg, an Sao_2 or Spo_2 below 90%, or either value below the desirable range for the clinical situation.[32]

Other times, supplemental oxygen may be needed include severe trauma, acute myocardial infarction, during or after labor and delivery, and as part of procedural sedation or general anesthesia. The therapist should be alert for any signs of increasing hypoxia (reduced tissue oxygenation despite adequate perfusion) indicating a possible need for supplemental oxygen. These include increasing tachypnea and dyspnea, skin color changes (pale, cyanotic), increasing tachycardia, hypertension, restlessness, and/or disorientation.[32]

Table B-5	Normal Blood Pressures for Children*
Age	**Blood Pressure Systolic Range/Diastolic Range (mm Hg)**
Premature	55–75/35–45
0–3 mo	65–85/45–55
3–6 mo	70–90/50–65
6–12 mo	80–100/55–65
1–3 y	90–105/55–70
3–6 y	95–110/60–75
6–12 y	100–120/60–75
12 y	110–135/65–85

*Normal blood pressure values for children and adolescents of various ethnic groups are under investigation.
From Behrman RE, Kliegman RM, Jenson HB: *Nelson textbook of pediatrics*, ed 17, Philadelphia, 2004, Saunders.

Oxygen supplementation in anyone with COPD must be prescribed and monitored very carefully to avoid oxygen toxicity and absorption atelectasis. The therapist should watch for blunting of the respiratory drive. Too much oxygen can depress the respiratory drive of a person with COPD. For example, in the person with emphysema, low arterial oxygen levels are the respiratory drive triggers. For this reason, too much oxygen delivered as an intervention can depress the respiratory drive, which is now reliant on lower levels of arterial oxygen.

The drive to breathe in a normal person results from an increase in the arterial carbon dioxide level (PCO_2). Since the individual with COPD chronically retains excessive amounts of carbon dioxide, an increased arterial PCO_2 is no longer an effective respiratory drive mechanism.[30]

If oxygen flow rate must be increased during exercise for individuals with chronic lung disease, oxygen flow rate must be returned promptly to its set value at the end of exercise. Failure to return flow rate to the value determined by the physician may result in hypoventilation, retention of carbon dioxide, and respiratory acidosis.

Blood Pressure

To monitor blood pressure effectively, the therapist must be familiar with normal (see Table 12-8; Table B-5) and abnormal blood pressure responses to exercise and must keep in mind that arterial blood pressure is a general indicator of the function of the heart as a pump and a measure of the peripheral arterial resistance. Systolic pressure measures the force exerted against the arteries during the ejection cycle, and diastolic pressure measures the force exerted against the arteries during rest or against peripheral resistance.

Systolic blood pressure normally rises with increased exertion in proportion to the workload (approximately 7–10 mm Hg/MET) with little or no change in diastolic blood pressure,[2] and it rises more quickly in males than in females. For example, during endurance activities, the systolic blood pressure gradually increases, but with sustained activity no further change should occur. Exercise involving a small total muscle mass, such as a single extremity, typically elicits minimal incremental changes in systolic blood pressure and greater increases in diastolic blood pressure.[4]

Diastolic blood pressure may increase or decrease a maximum of 10 mm Hg due to adaptive dilatation of peripheral vasculature. A highly trained athlete may exhibit more than a 10 mm Hg drop in diastolic blood pressure as a result of increased vasodilation, but this would be considered an abnormal response in an older or untrained adult. A sustained elevation of the diastolic blood pressure during the recovery phase of activity is also considered abnormal. More specific abnormal responses to activity are discussed in detail elsewhere.[22]

If the resting blood pressure is excessively high (systolic blood pressure 200 mm Hg or diastolic blood pressure 105–110 mm Hg), physician clearance should be obtained before continuing with evaluation or treatment. Exercise should be terminated if blood pressure becomes excessively high (systolic blood pressure higher than 250 mm Hg or diastolic blood pressure higher than 110 mm Hg). Systolic blood pressure rise during exercise (19.7 mm Hg/min of exercise duration) and a relatively slow recovery in systolic pressure after exercise are associated with the risk of any stroke and of ischemic stroke.[25]

Blood pressure should always be measured in the same position, because it can drop quickly with cessation of activity (e.g., do not measure blood pressure while the client is sitting, then ambulate, and recheck blood pressure in the standing position; measure in the standing position, ambulate, and remeasure while standing). In fact, because blood pressure changes can occur within 10 seconds, a truly accurate postexercise blood pressure may be difficult to obtain. Always observe for associated symptoms, such as shortness of breath, dizziness, palpitations, or increase in heart rate.

Blood Pressure Poststroke

Patients in the acute care setting poststroke may have orders for permissive hypertension (e.g., up to 220 mm Hg systolic and up to 120 mm Hg diastolic). This is important to facilitate brain tissue perfusion with ischemic strokes. The therapist may find that even basic bed mobility (e.g., moving from supine to sitting) can increase blood pressure beyond acceptable limits. Concern for complications such as hemorrhagic conversion may dictate the need to return the individual to a resting position and notify nursing/physician before proceeding further.

Some therapists do not immediately return the patient to a supine resting position but rather try to obtain blood pressure measurements in sitting, standing, and return to supine. This gives the physician a better idea of what is needed to control blood pressure with daily activities. For example, if the diastolic blood pressure is 180 mm Hg when sitting but increases to 200 mm Hg when standing, then medicating for a diastolic measurement of 160 mm Hg while resting in supine is not likely going to provide adequate (functional) control needed for daily activities.

Pediatrics

A child's blood pressure is usually much lower than an adult's. Children are at risk for developing high blood pressure if they exceed the guidelines listed in Table B-5. About 1% of children (including very young babies) have blood pressure that is too high. The cause is often unknown. When a child's high blood pressure is severe, it is often because of another serious condition, such as kidney disease or heart disease.

Children can inherit high blood pressure from their parents. Overweight children are also at higher risk. Children who both have a family history of hypertension and are overweight should be screened for aberrant blood pressure. The American Heart Association recommends that all children 3 years of age and older have their blood pressure checked once a year.

A child's sex, age, and height are used to determine age-, sex-, and height-specific systolic and diastolic blood pressure percentiles (see Table 12-8). This approach provides information that lets researchers consider different levels of growth in evaluating blood pressure. It also demonstrates the blood pressure standards that are based on sex, age, and height and allows a more precise classification of blood pressure according to body size. More importantly, the approach avoids misclassifying children at the extremes of normal growth.[1]

The therapist can provide an important service by including this type of assessment. In children, even a mild elevation of blood pressure can lead to serious medical conditions such as cardiomyopathy and kidney or visual impairments. Medical evaluation and monitoring for signs of early organ damage are needed for any child or adolescent with high blood pressure.

Current guidelines for children may not be very accurate. "Normal" blood pressure values may be different for children and adolescents of various ethnic groups. Heretofore, values have been established without consideration of ethnicity and/or culture and were based mostly on normal values for Anglo children. Investigation to establish more accurate norms and to verify standards for current blood pressure guidelines set by national committees are under way.[29]

Abnormal Blood Pressure Response

An abnormal blood pressure response may result in hypotension or hypertension as reflected by any of the following responses:

- Too rapid a rise in systolic blood pressure for the workload; in the healthy adult, the systolic blood pressure should go up by 20 mm Hg with minimal to moderate exercise and 40–50 mm Hg with intensive exercise. These values are less likely with cardiac clients.
- Very little change in systolic blood pressure with excessive workload in an unfit or deconditioned person.
- Progressive rise of diastolic blood pressure.
- Diastolic blood pressure should remain the same or change slightly (less than 5 mm Hg increase/decrease should be noted); a drop of more than 10 mm Hg in diastolic blood pressure is considered abnormal.
- Drop in systolic pressure (or both systolic and diastolic pressure) of 10–20 mm Hg or more associated with an increase in pulse rate of more than 15 beats/min (depleted intravascular volume).
- Narrowing of pulse pressure (systolic blood pressure – diastolic blood pressure).

An increase in diastolic blood pressure of 20 mm Hg or more may be a sign that the person has exceeded cardiac reserve capacity and that blood flow to the liver,

Box B-2
FACTORS AFFECTING BLOOD PRESSURE

- Age
- Blood vessel size
- Blood viscosity
- Force of heart contraction
- Medications
  - Angiotensin-converting enzyme inhibitors
  - Adrenergic inhibitors
  - β-Blockers
  - Diuretics
  - Narcotic analgesics
- Diet and exercise
- Obesity
- Time of recent meal (eating increases systolic pressure)
- Caffeine
- Nicotine
- Alcohol and other drugs
- Cocaine
- Anxiety, panic
- Presence or perceived degree of pain
- Living at higher altitudes
- Distended urinary bladder
- Sleep apnea
- Pregnancy
- Pain

kidneys, and digestive tract has been critically reduced. A decrease in diastolic blood pressure may occur as a result of rapid vasodilation, an effect of training in the athletic individual.

A drop in diastolic blood pressure may also indicate normalization in a hypertensive individual as a result of vasodilation and decreased peripheral resistance. For example, this may occur if the hypertensive person experiences a calming effect as a result of participating in a regular routine of exercise after driving in heavy traffic to get to the clinic on time. Other factors that affect blood pressure are listed in Box B-2.

GUIDELINES FOR AQUATIC PHYSICAL THERAPY

Paula Richley Geigle and Charlotte O. Norton

The decision to include aquatic physical therapy in a treatment regime is made for each client based on the *Guide to Physical Therapist Practice*.[16] For each individual, a risk-benefit analysis is completed at each intervention point, wellness through tertiary care.[28] Sound clinical decision making is required to determine if the positive impact of hydrostatic principles offsets any potential risks created by the aquatic environment.[17]

The clinician must consider the static properties of water, including density and specific gravity, hydrostatic pressure, and the effects of buoyancy on each client. For example, aquatic therapy is very useful to initiate gait training as the amount of weightbearing force is reduced to approximately 25% of body weight when the person is in the water to the level of the axilla and to 50% body weight when in the water to the level of the waist.[20]

Table B-6	Precautions and Contraindications for Aquatic Physical Therapy	
Precautions	**Contraindications**

Precautions	Contraindications
Cardiac conditions	Uncontrolled seizure activity
Unstable vital signs	Unstable medical condition
Incontinence	Client behavior that compromises patient or staff safety
Severe/chronic ear infections	Phobia of water
Chronic obstructive pulmonary disease (COPD)	Fragile medical condition that places client at risk in an aquatic environment may be a contraindication; decided on a case-by-case basis
Pregnancy (complex or involved)	
Any land exercise precaution	
Inability to perceive overworking	
Anxiety regarding water	
Open skin areas	
Low body fat with decreased ability to generate heat with movement	

Courtesy Paula Richley Geigle, PT, PhD, and Charlotte Norton, DPT, ATC, CSCS. Used with permission.

The effects of time-dependent properties such as viscosity, laminar flow, turbulent flow, and their effects on the amount of resistance encountered with water activity are additional critical elements considered in the thought process determining whether to include or not include aquatic therapy and, if included, under what conditions the therapist develops the program.[3] Additionally, thermodynamics and its respective interaction with varied client presentations plays a key role in directing the appropriate use of aquatic physical therapy.

In each practice environment, therapists must assess the precautions and contraindications for each respective clientele category. Precautions for aquatic physical therapy participation include but are not limited to the conditions listed in Table B-6.[17]

An overview of examination components, organized by *Guide* categories and systems review, is provided in Table B-7. The therapist can use this tool to guide the examination performed prior to aquatic intervention. Categories of test and measurement tools are also included from which clinicians can choose to complete these additional assessment components.

Studies on the comparative value of aquatic therapy over other forms of treatment are limited. One study has reported on the benefit of aquatic therapy in the early days after hip or knee joint replacement. When all other variables were compared among the various treatment groups, the aquatic group had the best short-term improvements. At the end of 6 months, there was no difference in outcomes from one group to the next. There were overall trends that seemed to support the idea that aquatic therapy was slightly more beneficial than either land-based or nonspecific water-based exercises.[33]

Despite the lack of evidence to support the application of aquatic exercise, therapists do have an excellent resource for applying aquatic exercise to a wide range of settings (rehabilitation, wellness, and fitness).[9] This text provides the therapist with an approach to applying aquatic exercise following the ICF model. Prescribing optimal, safe, and effective exercise programming to address deficits in function, activity, and participation is demonstrated in this text.

One example of the clinical decision-making process used in determining if and how the aquatic medium should be used in rehabilitation is the case of Viola, an 80-year-old woman living independently with her husband in a full-spectrum retirement community. She was referred to aquatic physical therapy for severe back pain, after having undergone several spinal fusions. The back pain was interfering with her activity level.

Viola participated in an initial land-based physical therapy examination and a course of therapeutic exercise and manual therapy. After a 3- to 4-week land-based physical therapy intervention, an aquatic physical therapy referral was recommended with the goals of reducing lumbar spasm and pain that interfered with her functional activities. Viola reported several comorbidities, including a 15-year history of Parkinson disease.

For Viola's program, the clinician must consider the client's body type and structure, and whether she demonstrates any changes in muscle tone as a result of Parkinson disease. Changes in tone must be considered in relation to density and specific gravity, as both affect the amount of buoyancy support the person may need while participating in aquatic physical therapy.

The use of hydrostatic pressure and the effects of buoyancy in deeper water to minimize the effects of gravity may help decrease the amount of muscle spasm and pain (*Guide* Musculoskeletal category) Viola experiences from both her spinal involvement and tone changes from a longstanding neuromuscular pathology. The increased movement that buoyancy offers allows Viola to increase her cardiovascular reserve (*Guide* Cardiovascular/Pulmonary category) without increasing her back pain.

Scaling of speed and amplitude[14] is enabled by the buoyancy principle, both from ease of movement and decreased fear of balance loss (*Guide* Neuromuscular and Musculoskeletal categories). In other words, the aquatic environment facilitates larger, full range-of-motion movement as a result of a decreased falling anxiety and the increased proprioceptive input from hydrostatic pressure.

Examination of her postural control in a variety of positions with particular attention to safety issues (*Guide* Neuromuscular category) associated with Parkinson disease–related muscle tone fluctuations during positioning transitions will allow the clinician to determine the most appropriate application of viscosity and resistance for her exercise program. For example, Viola demonstrates the "typical" Parkinson rigidity when in a full supine position. Any horizontal aquatic techniques should place Viola in about 25–30 degrees of trunk flexion via flotation supports.

Finally, the clinician must consider the water temperature (*Guide* Neuromuscular category). Warmer temperatures, approximating 90° F (32.2° C), will facilitate relaxation of the muscles and help to reduce the rigidity associated with Parkinson disease and may increase the ease of spinal muscle activation.

Using the *Guide to Physical Therapist Practice* and hydrodynamic principles as a conceptual framework for clinical decision making, optimal aquatic care can be initiated.

Table B-7	Aquatic Practice for the Physical Therapist

Systems Review	Evaluation/Examination	Tests and Measures	Date/Results/Initials
Cardiovascular/pulmonary	Dyspnea on exertion Decreased endurance	Vital signs, EEG, exertion scales Physiologic response to position changes • Vital signs (HR, BP) • Observations • Laboratory values	
	Increased pulmonary response to low-level activity loads	Increased cardiopulmonary responses to low load: • Breath/voice sounds • Cyanosis • Respiratory pattern/rate/rhythm • Ventilatory flow/force/volume (spirometry, oximetry)	
	Increased cardiovascular response to low-level activity loads	Increased cardiovascular responses to low load: • BP • HR/rhythm/sounds • Angina/claudication/dyspnea • ECG	
	Impaired ventilatory forces and flow	Impaired ventilation: • Gas analyses from chart • Observations • Oximetry • Airway clearance tests • Pulmonary function tests	
	Impaired ventilatory volumes	Impaired ventilation: • Gas analyses from chart • Observations • Oximetry • Airway clearance tests • Pulmonary function tests	
	Integrity of tracheotomy	Observation, blood gas analysis, oximetry	
Integumentary	Impaired sensation: abrasion injury from bottom/sides/underwater lights Discontinuity of skin integrity: vascular disease—arterial/diabetic/venous Long-term medication use Lymphedema: skin integrity/drainage/hydrostatic pressure effect Skin lesions: trauma—burns/frostbite, cellulitis, postradiation, postsurgical status surgery	Observation: • Light touch, hot/cold • Sensory integration • Inspection of integument • Augmented photography • Thermography	
Musculoskeletal	Strength/power/endurance: ability to control center of balance, equipment use Recent surgical episodes: passive/active/active assist Fatigue issues: changing presession/postsession; access in/out of pool; during/after aquatic session	• Manual muscle test • Dynamometry • Performance tests • Technology-assisted analysis (PEAK Biodex platform, etc) • Activities of daily living scales • Postural analysis grids • Videography	
Neuromuscular	Seizure activity (within last 3–6 mo)	Client/caregiver/medical record/review of current medications	
	Alteration in auditory/sensory/somatosensory/position sense	Stereognosis Tactile discrimination Kinesthesiometry Observations Vibration Hot/cold	
	Vestibular dysfunction: moderate to severe	Vestibuloocular reflex, nystagmus	

Table B-7	Aquatic Practice for the Physical Therapist—cont'd		
Systems Review	**Evaluation/Examination**	**Tests and Measures**	**Date/Results/ Initials**
	Decreased strength	Dynamometry	
		Manual muscle testing	
		Timed activities	
		Physical capacity scales	
		Electromyography	
	Dysfunction: recruitment/timing/ sequencing	Coordination	
		Motor proficiency	
		Motor planning	
		Postural challenge tests	
	General deconditioning	Vital signs	
		Perceived exertion scales	
		Spirometer	
		Aerobic capacity measurement	
	Postural control issues in varied positions	Observations	
		Technology-assisted analyses	
		Grid measurement	
		Functional assessment in pool: can client reposition head out of water independently?	
	Oral motor control	Coordinated breath control	
		Mouth closure	
		Controlled exhalation/inhalation on request (blowing bubbles)	
	Peripheral nerve integrity	Motor and sensory integrity tests	
Psychologic	Fear of water	Quality-of-life scales	
	Impulsivity	Orientation assessment	
	Aggression	Communication assessment	
	Confusion	Ability to follow directions: safety of client/ staff/other clients and caregivers	
	Short-term memory issues		
	Attention to task difficulties		
Endocrine/ metabolic	Immune system compromise: waterborne/ airborne infections		
	Systemic issues: diabetes mellitus, kidney function		
	Dialysis/chemotherapy ports		
Gastrointestinal/ genitourinary	Bowel incontinence		
	Bladder incontinence		
	Unpredictable vomiting		
	PEG tube/stoma		
	Catheter care		
Obstetric	Pregnancy (before/after): water temperature, infection risk, discharge into pool		
	Incontinence		
	Pelvic floor surgery: risk of infection, discharge into pool		

ECG, Electrocardiogram; *HR,* heart rate; *BP,* blood pressure; *PEG,* percutaneous endoluminal gastrostomy.
Courtesy Paula Richley Geigle, PT, PhD, and Charlotte O. Norton, DPT, MS, ATC, CSCS. Used with permission.

The Aquatic Physical Therapy Section of the American Physical Therapy Association provides current clinical information on its website and produces both a how-to manual on aquatic programming and a bibliography updated every 2 years (www.aquaticpt.org).

REFERENCES
To enhance this text and add value for the reader, all references are included on the companion Evolve site that accompanies this textbook. The reader can view the reference source and access it online whenever possible.

INDEX

Page numbers followed by f indicated figure(s); t, table(s); b, box(es).

1750